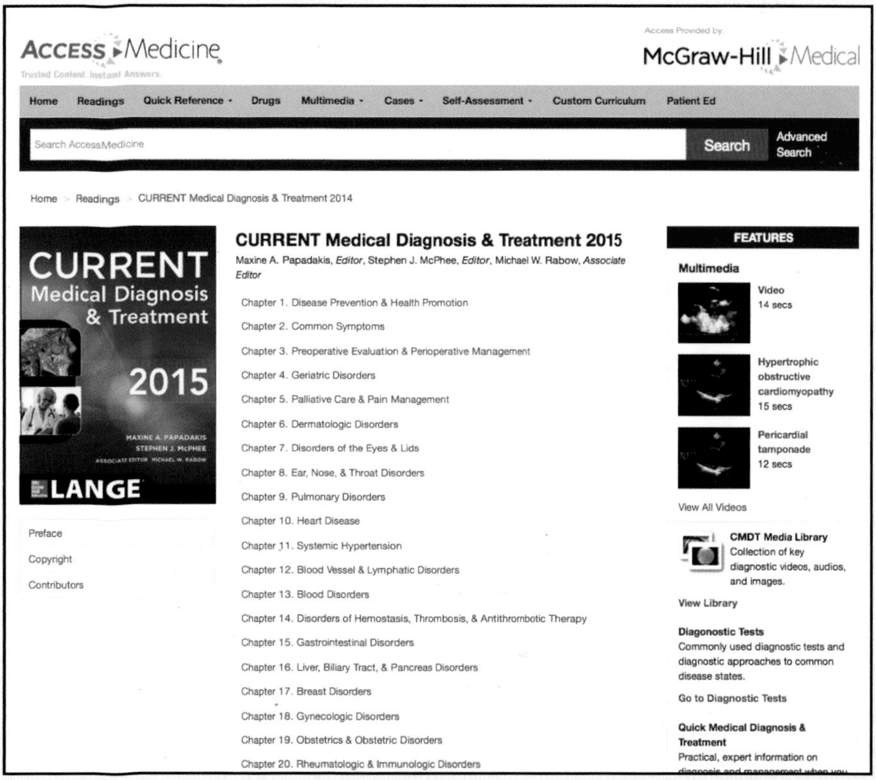

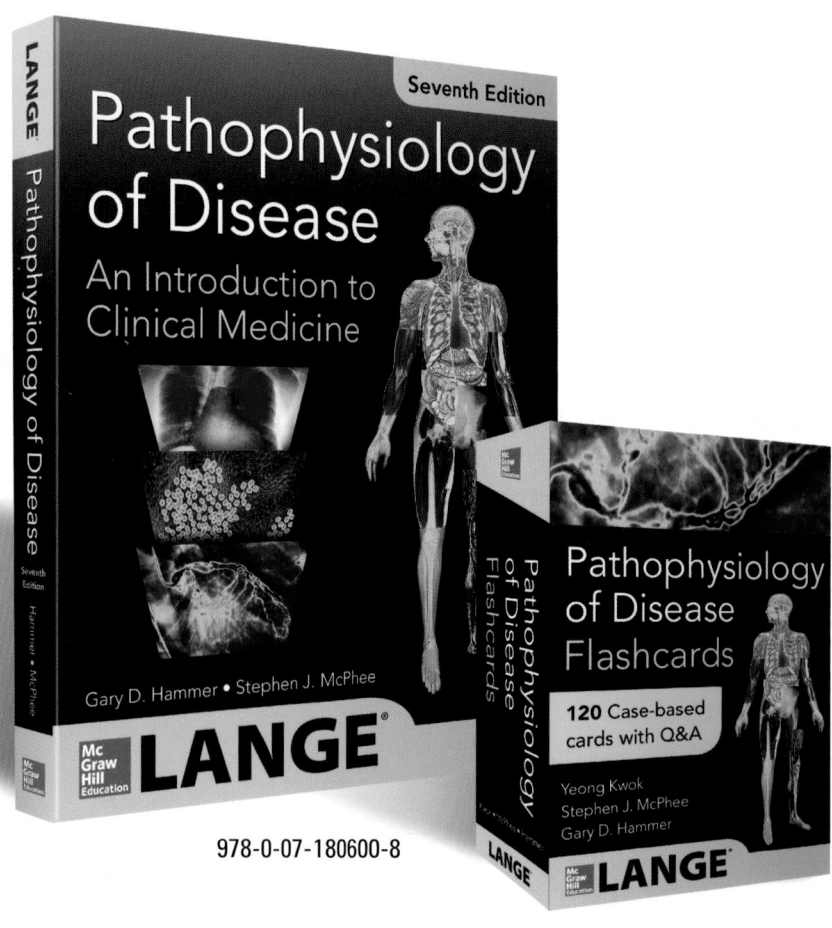

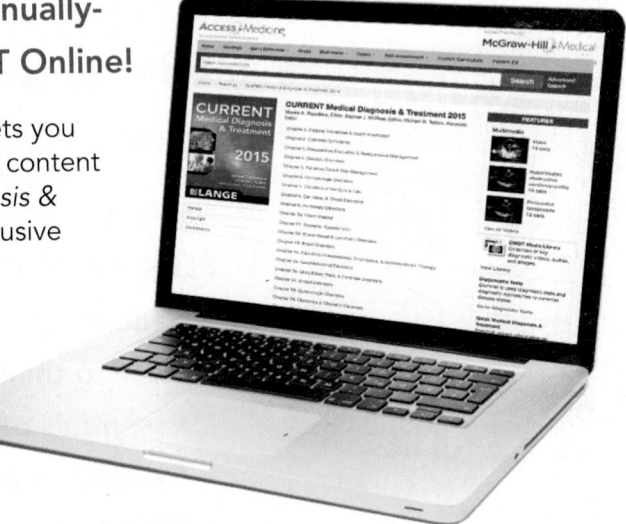
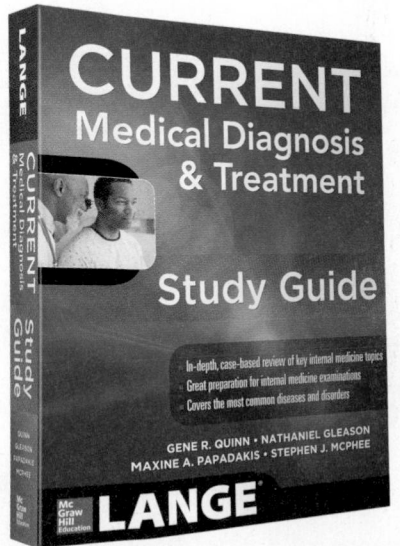

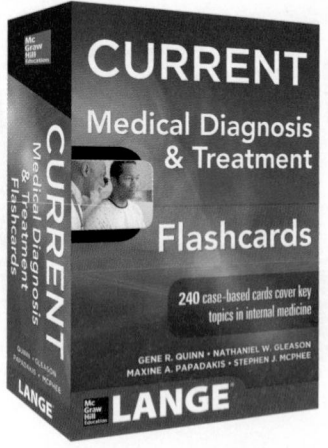
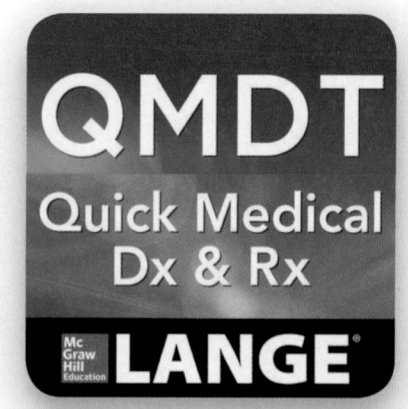

a LANGE medical book

2015
CURRENT
Medical Diagnosis
& Treatment

FIFTY-FOURTH EDITION

Edited by

Maxine A. Papadakis, MD
Professor of Medicine
Associate Dean of Students
School of Medicine
University of California, San Francisco

Stephen J. McPhee, MD
Professor of Medicine, Emeritus
Division of General Internal Medicine
Department of Medicine
University of California, San Francisco

Associate Editor

Michael W. Rabow, MD
Professor of Medicine
Division of General Internal Medicine
Department of Medicine
University of California, San Francisco

With Associate Authors

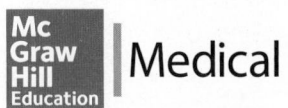

New York   Chicago   San Francisco   Athens   London   Madrid   Mexico City
Milan   New Delhi   Singapore   Sydney   Toronto

Current Medical Diagnosis & Treatment 2015, Fifty-Fourth Edition

Previous editions copyright 2000 through 2014 by McGraw-Hill Education; copyright © 1987 through 1999 by Appleton & Lange; copyright 1962 through 1986 by Lange Medical Publications.

1 2 3 4 5 6 7 8 9 0   DOW/DOW   19 18 17 16 15 14

ISBN 978-0-07-182486-6
MHID 0-07-182486-3
ISSN 0092-8682

Notice

Medicine is an ever-changing science. As new research and clinical experience broaden our knowledge, changes in treatment and drug therapy are required. The authors and the publisher of this work have checked with sources believed to be reliable in their efforts to provide information that is complete and generally in accord with the standards accepted at the time of publication. However, in view of the possibility of human error or changes in medical sciences, neither the authors nor the publisher nor any other party who has been involved in the preparation or publication of this work warrants that the information contained herein is in every respect accurate or complete, and they disclaim all responsibility for any errors or omissions or for the results obtained from use of the information contained in this work. Readers are encouraged to confirm the information contained herein with other sources. For example and in particular, readers are advised to check the product information sheet included in the package of each medication they plan to administer to be certain that the information contained in this work is accurate and that changes have not been made in the recommended dose or in the contraindications for administration. This recommendation is of particular importance in connection with new or infrequently used medications.

This book was set by Cenveo Publisher® Services.
The editors were Harriet Lebowitz, Barbara Holton, and Sarah Henry.
The production supervisor was Jeffrey Herzich.
Project management was provided by Yashmita Hota at Cenveo Publisher Services.
The copyeditor was Jennifer Bernstein.
Design modified from original by Alan Barnett; the cover designer was Thomas DePierro.
The index was prepared by Katherine Pitcoff.
RR Donnelley was printer and binder.

This book is printed on acid-free paper.

McGraw-Hill Education books are available at special quantity discounts to use as premiums and sales promotions, or for use in corporate training programs. To contact a representative please visit the Contact Us pages at www.mhprofessional.com.

Contents

---

*Free access to online chapters at www.accessmedicine.com/cmdt

Authors

Michael J. Aminoff, MD, DSc, FRCP
Distinguished Professor and Executive Vice Chair,
Department of Neurology, University of California,
San Francisco; Attending Physician, University of
California Medical Center, San Francisco
aminoffm@neurology.ucsf.edu
Nervous System Disorders

Charalambos Babis Andreadis, MD, MSCE
Assistant Professor of Medicine, Division of Hematology/
Oncology, University of California, San Francisco
candreadis@medicine.ucsf.edu
Blood Disorders

Alicia Y. Armstrong, MD, MHSCR
Medical Monitor, Contraceptive and Reproductive Health
Branch, Eunice Kennedy Shriver National Institute for
Child Health and Human Development, National
Institutes for Health, Rockville, Maryland
ayba55@aol.com
Gynecologic Disorders

David M. Barbour, PharmD, BCPS
Pharmacist, Denver, Colorado
dbarbour99@gmail.com
Drug References

Robert B. Baron, MD, MS
Professor of Medicine; Associate Dean for Graduate and
Continuing Medical Education; Vice Chief, Division of
General Internal Medicine, University of California,
San Francisco
baron@medicine.ucsf.edu
Lipid Disorders; Nutritional Disorders

Kevin Barrows, MD
Associate Clinical Professor of Family and Community
Medicine, Medical Director, Osher Center for
Integrative Medicine; Department of Family and
Community Medicine, University of California,
San Francisco
barrowsk@ocim.ucsf.edu
CMDT Online—Integrative Medicine

Thomas M. Bashore, MD
Professor of Medicine; Clinical Chief, Division of
Cardiology, Duke University Medical Center, Durham,
North Carolina
thomas.bashore@duke.edu
Heart Disease

Timothy G. Berger, MD
Professor of Clinical Dermatology, Department of
Dermatology, University of California, San Francisco
bergert@derm.ucsf.edu
Dermatologic Disorders

Brook Calton, MD, MHS
Assistant Clinical Professor, Division of Geriatrics,
Department of Medicine, University of California,
San Francisco
References

Matt Cascino, MD
Chief Medical Resident, Department of Medicine,
University of California, San Francisco
References

Hugo Q. Cheng, MD
Clinical Professor of Medicine, University of California,
San Francisco
quinny@medicine.ucsf.edu
Preoperative Evaluation & Perioperative Management

Mark S. Chesnutt, MD
Clinical Professor, Pulmonary & Critical Care Medicine,
Dotter Interventional Institute, Oregon Health &
Science University, Portland, Oregon; Director, Critical
Care, Portland Veterans Affairs Medical Center
chesnutm@ohsu.edu
Pulmonary Disorders

Thomas D. Chi, MD
Assistant Professor, Department of Urology, University of
California, San Francisco
TChi@urology.ucsf.edu
Urologic Disorders

Peter V. Chin-Hong, MD
Associate Professor, Division of Infectious Diseases,
Department of Medicine, University of California,
San Francisco
peter.chin-hong@ucsf.edu
*Common Problems in Infectious Diseases & Antimicrobial
Therapy*

Kerry C. Cho, MD
Assistant Clinical Professor of Medicine, Division of
Nephrology, University of California, San Francisco
kerry.cho@ucsf.edu
Electrolyte & Acid-Base Disorders

Patricia A. Cornett, MD
Professor of Medicine, University of California, San
Francisco; Chief, Hematology/Oncology, San Francisco
Veterans Affairs Medical Center, San Francisco, California
patricia.cornett@va.gov
Cancer

Marisa L. Cruz, MD
Fellow, Division of Endocrinology and Metabolism,
University of California, San Francisco
References

Russ Cucina, MD, MS
Associate Professor of Hospital Medicine; Medical
Director, Information Technology, UCSF Medical
Center; University of California, San Francisco
rcucina@medicine.ucsf.edu
CMDT Online—Information Technology in Patient Care

Lloyd E. Damon, MD
Professor of Clinical Medicine, Department of Medicine,
Division of Hematology/Oncology; Director of Adult
Hematologic Malignancies and Blood and Marrow
Transplantation, University of California, San Francisco
damonl@medicine.ucsf.edu
Blood Disorders

Tiffany O. Dea, PharmD, BCOP
Oncology Pharmacist, Veterans Affairs Medical Center,
San Francisco, California; Adjunct Professor, Thomas J.
Long School of Pharmacy and Health Sciences,
Stockton, California
tiffany.dea@va.gov
Cancer

Charles DeBattista, DMH, MD
Professor of Psychiatry and Behavioral Sciences Director:
Depression Clinic and Research Program Director of
Medical Student Education in Psychiatry, Stanford
University School of Medicine, Stanford, California
debattista@stanford.edu
Psychiatric Disorders

Tonja Dirkx, MD
Assistant Professor of Medicine, Division of Nephrology,
Department of Medicine, Oregon Health & Science
University, Portland, Oregon; Renal Clinic Director,
Portland Veterans Affairs Medical Center
dirkxt@ohsu.edu
Kidney Disease

Stuart J. Eisendrath, MD
Professor of Psychiatry; Director of The UCSF Depression
Center, Langley Porter Psychiatric Hospital and Clinics,
University of California, San Francisco
stuart.eisendrath@ucsf.edu
Psychiatric Disorders

Paul A. Fitzgerald, MD
Clinical Professor of Medicine, Department of Medicine,
Division of Endocrinology, University of California,
San Francisco
paul.fitzgerald@ucsf.edu
Endocrine Disorders

Patrick F. Fogarty, MD
Assistant Professor of Medicine, Department of Medicine;
Director, Penn Comprehensive Hemophilia and
Thrombosis Program, Hospital of the University of
Pennsylvania, Philadelphia, Pennsylvania
patrick.fogarty@uphs.upenn.edu
*Disorders of Hemostasis, Thrombosis, & Antithrombotic
Therapy*

Lawrence S. Friedman, MD
Professor of Medicine, Harvard Medical School;
Professor of Medicine, Tufts University School of
Medicine, Boston, Massachusetts; Chair, Department
of Medicine, Newton-Wellesley Hospital, Newton,
Massachusetts; Assistant Chief of Medicine,
Massachusetts General Hospital, Boston,
Massachusetts
lfriedman@partners.org
*Liver, Biliary Tract, & Pancreas Disorders; Hepatobiliary
Cancers (in Chapter 39)*

Warren J. Gasper, MD
Clinical Instructor of Surgery, Division of Vascular and
Endovascular Surgery, Department of Surgery,
University of California, San Francisco
warren.gasper@ucsf.edu
Blood Vessel & Lymphatic Disorders

Armando E. Giuliano, MD, FACS, FRCSEd
Executive Vice Chair of Surgery, Associate Director of
Surgical Oncology, Cedars-Sinai Medical Center, Los
Angeles, California
armando.giuliano@cshs.org
Breast Disorders

Ralph Gonzales, MD, MSPH
Professor of Medicine; Professor of Epidemiology &
Biostatistics, Division of General Internal Medicine,
Department of Medicine, University of California,
San Francisco
ralphg@medicine.ucsf.edu
Common Symptoms

Christopher B. Granger, MD
Professor of Medicine; Director, Cardiac Care
Unit, Duke University Medical Center,
Duke Clinical Research Institute, Durham,
North Carolina
christopher.granger@dm.duke.edu
Heart Disease

Blake Gregory, MD
Chief Resident, Department of Medicine, University of
California, San Francisco
References; Illustrations

B. Joseph Guglielmo, PharmD
Professor and Dean, School of Pharmacy, University of
California, San Francisco
guglielmoj@pharmacy.ucsf.edu
*Common Problems in Infectious Diseases & Antimicrobial
Therapy; CMDT Online—Anti-infective
Chemotherapeutic & Antibiotic Agents*

David L. Hamel, Jr., MD
Chief Medical Resident, Department of Medicine,
University of California, San Francisco
References

Richard J. Hamill, MD
Professor, Division of Infectious Diseases, Departments of
    Medicine and Molecular Virology & Microbiology,
    Baylor College of Medicine, Houston, Texas
rhamill@bcm.edu
Mycotic Infections

G. Michael Harper, MD
Associate Professor, Department of Medicine, University
    of California San Francisco School of Medicine;
    Associate Chief of Staff for Geriatrics, Palliative and
    Extended Care, San Francisco Veterans Affairs Medical
    Center, San Francisco, California
michael.harper3@med.va.gov
Geriatric Disorders

David B. Hellmann, MD, MACP
Aliki Perroti Professor of Medicine; Vice Dean for
    Johns Hopkins Bayview; Chairman, Department of
    Medicine, Johns Hopkins Bayview Medical Center,
    Johns Hopkins University School of Medicine,
    Baltimore, Maryland
hellmann@jhmi.edu
Rheumatologic & Immunologic Disorders

Carolyn Hendrickson, MD
Fellow, Division of Pulmonary & Critical Care Medicine,
    University of California, San Francisco
References

Sara A. Hurvitz, MD
Assistant Professor; Director, Breast Oncology Program,
    Division of Hematology/Oncology, Department of
    Internal Medicine, University of California, Los
    Angeles
shurvitz@mednet.ucla.edu
Breast Disorders

John B. Imboden, Jr., MD
Alice Betts Endowed Chair for Arthritis Research;
    Professor of Medicine, University of California,
    San Francisco; Chief, Division of Rheumatology,
    San Francisco General Hospital
John.Imboden@ucsf.edu
Rheumatologic & Immunologic Disorders

Kevin Jackson, MD
Assistant Professor of Medicine, Director of
    Electrophysiology, Duke Raleigh Hospital,
    Duke University Medical Center, Durham,
    North Carolina
k.j@duke.edu
Heart Disease

Jane Jih, MD, MPH
Primary Care Research Fellow, Division of General
    Internal Medicine, Department of Medicine, University
    of California, San Francisco
References

Meshell D. Johnson, MD
Assistant Professor, Division of Pulmonary and Critical
    Care Medicine, Department of Medicine, University of
    California, San Francisco
meshell.johnson@ucsf.edu
Blood Vessel & Lymphatic Disorders

C. Bree Johnston, MD, MPH
Director of Palliative and Supportive Care,
    PeaceHealth St. Joseph Medical Center, Bellingham,
    Washington; Clinical Professor of Medicine,
    Division of Geriatrics, University of California,
    San Francisco
bjohnston@peacehealth.org
Geriatric Disorders

Mitchell H. Katz, MD
Clinical Professor of Medicine, Epidemiology &
    Biostatistics, University of California, San Francisco;
    Director of Health Services, Los Angeles County
mkatz@dhs.lacounty.gov
HIV Infection & AIDS

Robin K. Kelley, MD
Assistant Professor of Medicine, Division of
    Hematology/Oncology, University of California,
    San Francisco
katie.kelley@ucsf.edu
Alimentary Tract Cancers (in Chapter 39)

J. Daniel Kelly, MD
Fellow, Division of Infectious Diseases, Center for AIDS
    Prevention Studies, Department of Medicine,
    University of California, San Francisco
Dan.Kelly@ucsf.edu
Viral & Rickettsial Infections

Geoffrey A. Kerchner, MD, PhD
Assistant Professor of Neurology and Neurological
    Sciences, Stanford Center for Memory Disorders,
    Stanford University School of Medicine, Stanford,
    California
kerchner@stanford.edu
Nervous System Disorders

C. Seth Landefeld, MD
Professor; Chief, Division of Geriatrics; Associate
    Chair for Strategic Planning and Implementation,
    Department of Medicine, University of California,
    San Francisco; Staff Physician, San Francisco Veterans
    Affairs Medical Center
sethl@medicine.ucsf.edu
Geriatric Disorders

David Lange, MD
Fellow, Division of Cardiology, Department of Medicine,
    Cedars-Sinai Medical Center, Los Angeles, California
References

Sarah Lee, MD
Pediatric Neurology Resident, Department of Neurology & Neurological Sciences, Stanford Hospital and Clinics, Stanford, California
References

Jonathan E. Lichtmacher, MD
Health Sciences Clinical Professor of Psychiatry; Director, Adult Psychiatry Clinic, Langley Porter Hospitals and Clinics, University of California, San Francisco
jonathanl@lppi.ucsf.edu
Psychiatric Disorders

Chuanyi Mark Lu, MD, PhD
Associate Professor, Department of Laboratory Medicine, University of California, San Francisco; Chief, Hematology and Hematopathology, Laboratory Medicine Service, Veterans Affairs Medical Center, San Francisco, California
mark.lu@va.gov
Appendix: Therapeutic Drug Monitoring & Laboratory Reference Intervals (includes Pharmacogenetic Testing online); CMDT Online—Diagnostic Testing & Medical Decision Making

Anthony Luke, MD, MPH
Professor of Clinical Orthopaedics, Department of Orthopaedics; Director, UCSF Primary Care Sports Medicine; Director, Human Performance Center at the Orthopaedic Institute, University of California, San Francisco
LukeA@orthosurg.ucsf.edu
Sports Medicine & Outpatient Orthopedics

Lawrence R. Lustig, MD
Francis A. Sooy, MD Professor of Otolaryngology—Head & Neck Surgery; Division Chief of Otology & Neurotology, Department of Otolaryngology—Head & Neck Surgery, University of California, San Francisco
llustig@ohns.ucsf.edu
Ear, Nose, & Throat Disorders

C. Benjamin Ma, MD
Associate Professor, Department of Orthopaedic Surgery; Chief, Sports Medicine and Shoulder Service, University of California, San Francisco
MaBen@orthosurg.ucsf.edu
Sports Medicine & Outpatient Orthopedics

H. Trent MacKay, MD, MPH
Professor of Obstetrics and Gynecology, Uniformed Services University of the Health Sciences, Bethesda, Maryland; Staff Physician, Department of Obstetrics and Gynecology, Walter Reed National Military Medical Center, Bethesda, Maryland
mackayt@mail.nih.gov
Gynecologic Disorders

Umesh Masharani, MB, BS, MRCP(UK)
Professor of Medicine, Division of Endocrinology and Metabolism, Department of Medicine, University of California, San Francisco
umesh.masharani@ucsf.edu
Diabetes Mellitus & Hypoglycemia

Megan McNamara, MD, MSc
Assistant Professor of Medicine, Department of Medicine, Case Western Reserve University, Cleveland, Ohio; Director of the Center for the Advancement of Medical Learning, Case Western Reserve School of Medicine, Cleveland, Ohio
Megan.Mcnamara@va.gov
Women's Health Issues

Kenneth R. McQuaid, MD
Professor of Clinical Medicine, University of California, San Francisco; Chief, Gastroenterology Section, San Francisco Veterans Affairs Medical Center
kenneth.mcquaid@med.va.gov
Gastrointestinal Disorders; Alimentary Tract Cancers (in Chapter 39)

Maxwell V. Meng, MD, FACS
Associate Professor, Department of Urology, University of California, San Francisco
mmeng@urology.ucsf.edu
Urologic Disorders; Cancers of the Genitourinary Tract (in Chapter 39)

Tracy Minichiello, MD
Associate Professor of Medicine, University of California, San Francisco; Chief, Anticoagulation and Thrombosis Services, San Francisco Veterans Affairs Medical Center
minichie@medicine.ucsf.edu
Disorders of Hemostasis, Thrombosis, & Antithrombotic Therapy

Paul L. Nadler, MD
Clinical Professor of Medicine; Director, Screening and Acute Care Clinic, Division of General Internal Medicine, Department of Medicine, University of California, San Francisco
nadler@medicine.ucsf.edu
Common Symptoms

Jacqueline A. Nemer, MD, FACEP
Associate Professor of Emergency Medicine, Department of Emergency Medicine, University of California, San Francisco
jacqueline.nemer@ucsf.edu
Disorders Related to Environmental Emergencies

Anna Neumeier, MD
Chief Medical Resident, Department of Medicine, University of California, San Francisco
References

C. Diana Nicoll, MD, PhD, MPA

Clinical Professor and Vice Chair, Department of Laboratory Medicine; Associate Dean, University of California, San Francisco; Chief of Staff and Chief, Laboratory Medicine Service, San Francisco Veterans Affairs Medical Center

diana.nicoll@va.gov

Appendix: Therapeutic Drug Monitoring & Laboratory Reference Intervals (includes Pharmacogenetic Testing online); CMDT Online—Diagnostic Testing & Medical Decision Making

Kent R. Olson, MD

Clinical Professor of Medicine, Pediatrics, and Pharmacy, University of California, San Francisco; Medical Director, San Francisco Division, California Poison Control System

kent.olson@ucsf.edu

Poisoning

Christopher D. Owens, MD, MSc

Associate Professor of Surgery, Division of Vascular and Endovascular Surgery, Department of Surgery, University of California, San Francisco

christopher.owens@ucsfmedctr.org

Blood Vessel & Lymphatic Disorders

Steven Z. Pantilat, MD

Professor of Clinical Medicine, Department of Medicine; Alan M. Kates and John M. Burnard Endowed Chair in Palliative Care; Director, Palliative Care Program, University of California, San Francisco

stevep@medicine.ucsf.edu

Palliative Care & Pain Management

Manesh R. Patel, MD

Assistant Professor of Medicine, Division of Cardiology, Department of Medicine, Duke University Medical Center, Durham, North Carolina

patel017@notes.duke.edu

Heart Disease

Susan S. Philip, MD, MPH

Assistant Clinical Professor, Division of Infectious Diseases, Department of Medicine, University of California, San Francisco; Director, STD Prevention and Control Section, San Francisco Department of Public Health, San Francisco, California

susan.philip@sfdph.org

Spirochetal Infections

Michael Pignone, MD, MPH

Professor of Medicine, Division of General Internal Medicine, Department of Medicine, University of North Carolina, Chapel Hill

pignone@med.unc.edu

Disease Prevention & Health Promotion; CMDT Online— Diagnostic Testing & Medical Decision Making

Thomas J. Prendergast, MD

Associate Professor of Medicine, Oregon Health & Science University; Pulmonary Critical Care Section Chief, Portland Veterans Affairs Medical Center, Portland, Oregon

thomas.prendergast@va.gov

Pulmonary Disorders

Reed E. Pyeritz, MD, PhD

Professor of Medicine and Genetics; Vice-Chair for Academic Affairs, Department of Medicine, Raymond and Ruth Perelman School of Medicine of the University of Pennsylvania, Philadelphia

reed.pyeritz@uphs.upenn.edu

Clinical Genetic Disorders; CMDT Online—Fundamentals of Human Genetics

Michael W. Rabow, MD, FAAHPM

Professor of Clinical Medicine, Division of General Internal Medicine, Department of Medicine; Director, Symptom Management Service, Helen Diller Family Comprehensive Cancer Center, University of California, San Francisco

mrabow@medicine.ucsf.edu

Palliative Care & Pain Management

Joseph H. Rapp, MD

Professor of Surgery in Residence, University of California, San Francisco; Chief, Vascular Surgery Service, Veterans Affairs Medical Center, San Francisco, California

rappj@surgery.ucsf.edu

Blood Vessel & Lymphatic Disorders

Paul Riordan-Eva, FRCOphth

Consultant Ophthalmologist, King's College Hospital, London, United Kingdom

paul.riordan-eva@nhs.net

Disorders of the Eyes & Lids

Vanessa L. Rogers, MD

Associate Professor, Obstetrics and Gynecology, University of Texas Southwestern Medical Center, Dallas, Texas

vanessa.rogers@utsouthwestern.edu

Obstetrics & Obstetric Disorders

Philip J. Rosenthal, MD

Professor, Division of Infectious Diseases, Department of Medicine, University of California, San Francisco; San Francisco General Hospital

prosenthal@medsfgh.ucsf.edu

Protozoal & Helminthic Infections

René Salazar, MD

Associate Professor of Clinical Medicine, Division of General Internal Medicine, Department of Medicine, University of California, San Francisco

salazarr@medicine.ucsf.edu

Disease Prevention & Health Promotion

Joshua S. Schindler, MD
Assistant Professor, Department of Otolaryngology, Oregon Health & Science University, Portland, Oregon; Medical Director, OHSU-Northwest Clinic for Voice and Swallowing
schindlj@ohsu.edu
Ear, Nose, & Throat Disorders

Brian S. Schwartz, MD
Assistant Clinical Professor, Division of Infectious Diseases, Department of Medicine, University of California, San Francisco
brian.schwartz@ucsf.edu
Bacterial & Chlamydial Infections

Wayne X. Shandera, MD
Assistant Professor, Department of Internal Medicine, Baylor College of Medicine, Houston, Texas
shandera@bcm.tmc.edu
Viral & Rickettsial Infections

Samuel A. Shelburne, MD, PhD
Assistant Professor, Department of Infectious Diseases, MD Anderson Cancer Center, Houston, Texas
sshelburne@mdanderson.org
Mycotic Infections

Scott Steiger, MD
Assistant Clinical Professor, Division of General Internal Medicine, University of California, San Francisco
Opiods for Chronic, Noncancer Pain (in Chapter 5)

Michael Sutters, MD, MRCP(UK)
Attending Nephrologist, Virginia Mason Medical Center, Seattle, Washington; Affiliate Assistant Professor of Medicine, Division of Nephrology, University of Washington School of Medicine, Seattle, Washington
michael.sutters@vmmc.org
Systemic Hypertension

Philip Tiso
Principal Editor, Division of General Internal Medicine, University of California, San Francisco
References

Shivani V. Tripathi, MD
Fellow, Department of Dermatology, University of California, San Francisco
References

Julian Villar, MD, MPH
Chief Resident, Department of Emergency Medicine, San Francisco General Hospital, University of California, San Francisco
References

Judith Walsh, MD, MPH
Professor of Clinical Medicine, Division of General Internal Medicine, Women's Health Center of Excellence, University of California, San Francisco
Judith.Walsh@ucsf.edu
Women's Health Issues

Thomas J. Walsh, MD, MS
Assistant Professor, Department of Urology, University of Washington School of Medicine, Seattle, Washington
walsht@u.washington.edu
Urologic Disorders

Sunny Wang, MD
Assistant Clinical Professor of Medicine, Division of Hematology and Oncology, University of California, San Francisco; San Francisco Veterans Affairs Medical Center
sunny.wang@ucsf.edu
Lung Cancer (in Chapter 39)

Suzanne Watnick, MD
Associate Professor of Medicine, Division of Nephrology and Hypertension, Oregon Health & Science University, Portland; Portland Veterans Affairs Medical Center, Portland, Oregon
watnicks@ohsu.edu
Kidney Disease

CAPT Jason Woo, MD, MPH, FACOG
Medical Monitor, Contraceptive and Reproductive Health Branch, Eunice Kennedy Shriver National Institute for Child Health and Human Development, National Institutes for Health, Rockville, Maryland
jasonwoo@pol.net
Gynecologic Disorders

Kevin C. Worley, MD
Assistant Professor of Obstetrics and Gynecology, Department of Obstetrics and Gynecology, Division of Maternal-Fetal Medicine, University of Texas Southwestern Medical Center, Dallas, Texas Kevin.Worley@UTSouthwestern.edu
Obstetrics & Obstetric Disorders

Andrew R. Zolopa, MD
Professor of Medicine, Division of Infectious Diseases and Geographic Medicine, Stanford University, Stanford, California
azolopa@stanford.edu
HIV Infection & AIDS

Preface

Current Medical Diagnosis & Treatment 2015 (CMDT 2015) is the 54th edition of this single-source reference for practitioners in both hospital and ambulatory settings. The book emphasizes the practical features of clinical diagnosis and patient management in all fields of internal medicine and in specialties of interest to primary care practitioners and to subspecialists who provide general care.

INTENDED AUDIENCE FOR *CMDT*

House officers, medical students, and all other health professions students will find the descriptions of diagnostic and therapeutic modalities, with citations to the current literature, of everyday usefulness in patient care.

Internists, family physicians, hospitalists, nurse practitioners, physicians' assistants, and all primary care providers will appreciate *CMDT* as a ready reference and refresher text. Physicians in other specialties, pharmacists, and dentists will find the book a useful basic medical reference text. Nurses, nurse-practitioners, and physicians' assistants will welcome the format and scope of the book as a means of referencing medical diagnosis and treatment.

Patients and their family members who seek information about the nature of specific diseases and their diagnosis and treatment may also find this book to be a valuable resource.

NEW IN THIS EDITION OF *CMDT*

- The latest 2014 American Heart Association/American College of Cardiology/Heart Rhythm Society (AHA/ACC/HRS) guidelines for anticoagulation recommendations for atrial fibrillation
- New table comparing the features of dabigatran, rivaroxaban, and apixaban for stroke prevention in nonvalvular atrial fibrillation
- Updated information and algorithms incorporating the guidelines for treatment of valvular heart disease and indications for interventions based on the 2014 AHA/ACC guidelines
- Discussion about the four groups of patients who benefit from statin medications based on the 2014 AHA/ACC guidelines
- Indications for high intensity and moderate intensity statins based on the 2014 AHA/ACC guidelines
- New evidence suggesting a cardiovascular cause for palpitations
- Updates on target specific oral anticoagulants
- Inclusion of Juvenile Nephronophthisis-Medullary Cystic Disease
- Revised psychiatric diagnoses in accordance with the *Diagnostic Statistical Manual,* 5th edition (DSM-5), including the identification of obsessive-compulsive disorder (OCD) spectrum disorders as a separate category from the anxiety disorders and updating of terms such as the subtypes of schizophrenia, somatization disorder, hypochondriasis, and substance abuse and dependence
- Positive and negative likelihood ratios for history, physical examination, and laboratory findings in the diagnosis of pneumonia
- Information about contact dermatitis from cellphone covers
- Use of omalizumab for refractory chronic urticaria
- New discussion about electronic cigarettes and tobacco cigarette cessation
- The new US Preventive Services Task Force (USPSTF) recommendation for universal HIV screening
- Update on HIV/TB coinfection
- New section on Middle East Respiratory Syndrome
- Extensive update on Arbovirus Encephalitides, Dengue, and Influenza
- Update on chronic pelvic pain
- New information about breast cancer risk for women with a family history of *BRCA* mutation
- An update on mammography screening for breast cancer
- Current recommendations for Papanicolaou smear screening
- Updated guidelines for management of abnormal cervical cytology
- Update on management of women at risk for preterm delivery
- Recommendations for low-dose CT screening of the lung in high-risk patients in relatively good health who meet National Lung Screening Trial criteria
- Risk prediction tools identifying variables that predicted postoperative myocardial infarction and cardiac arrest as well as postoperative respiratory failure
- New section on opioids for chronic, noncancer pain
- Update on the epidemic of opioid-based prescription drug abuse, misuse, and overdose

- Alternatives for treatment of diabetic retinopathy, anterior ischemic optic neuropathy, and optic neuritis
- Guidelines regarding use of ambulatory and home blood pressure measurements
- Guidelines for initiating antihypertensive therapy based on the UK's 2013 National Institute of Health and Care Excellence (NICE) and for blood pressure targets from the 2013 US Joint National Committee Report (JNC8) and Kidney Disease Improving Global Outcomes (KDIGO)
- Updated classification of glucose-6-phosphate dehydrogenase (G6PD) isoenzyme activity
- Updated treatment options for *Helicobacter pylori*
- Clarification of the best tests for celiac disease
- Clarification of the best test for *Clostridium difficile* infection, and an update on when to consider "fecal microbiota transplantation" for its treatment
- Update on use of immunomodulators, anti-TNF agents, and anti-integrins in Crohn disease
- New antivirals for treatment of hepatitis C
- Scoring tools for assessing the severity of acute pancreatitis
- New information on the antiphospholipid syndrome
- Update on surgical treatment of spinal stenosis
- New sections on IgG4-related disease and Takayasu arteritis
- Update on HLA-B alleles and risk of serious drug-induced hypersensitivity reactions
- New information on functional hypopituitarism, isolated hypogonadotropic hypogonadism, diagnosis of growth hormone deficiency in adults, treatment of diabetes insipidus, classification of amiodarone-induced thyrotoxicosis, preoperative parathyroid imaging, adrenal incidentaloma
- Latest recommendations for vaccinations

OUTSTANDING FEATURES OF *CMDT*

- Medical advances up to time of annual publication
- Detailed presentation of all primary care topics, including gynecology, obstetrics, dermatology, ophthalmology, otolaryngology, psychiatry, neurology, toxicology, urology, geriatrics, orthopedics, women's health, preventive medicine, and palliative care
- Concise format, facilitating efficient use in any practice setting
- More than 1000 diseases and disorders
- Annual update on HIV infection and AIDS
- Specific disease prevention information
- Easy access to medication dosages, with trade names indexed and costs updated in each edition
- Recent references, with unique identifiers (PubMed, PMID numbers) for rapid downloading of article abstracts and, in some instances, full-text reference articles

CMDT Online (www.AccessMedicine.com) provides full electronic access to *CMDT 2015* plus expanded basic science information and five additional chapters. The five online-only chapters (Anti-infective Chemotherapeutic & Antibiotic Agents, Fundamentals of Human Genetics, Diagnostic Testing & Medical Decision Making, Information Technology in Patient Care, and Integrative Medicine) are available at www.AccessMedicine.com/CMDT. CMDT Online is updated throughout the year and includes an expanded, dedicated Media Gallery as well as links to related Web sites. Subscribers also receive access to Diagnosaurus with 1000+ differential diagnoses, *Pocket Guide to Diagnostic Tests, Quick Medical Diagnosis & Treatment*, and *CURRENT Practice Guidelines in Primary Care.*

ACKNOWLEDGMENTS

We wish to thank our associate authors for participating once again in the annual updating of this important book. We are especially grateful to Patrick Hranitzky, MD, Ingrid L. Roig, MD, Marshall L. Stoller, MD, and Emmanuel T. Tavan, MD who are leaving *CMDT* this year. We have all benefited from their clinical wisdom and commitment. We gratefully acknowledge and thank Phil Tiso for his years of collegial work on CMDT, and the expertise and enthusiasm that he brings to the team.

Many students and physicians also have contributed useful suggestions to this and previous editions, and we are grateful. We continue to welcome comments and recommendations for future editions in writing or via electronic mail. The editors' and authors' institutional and e-mail addresses are given in the Authors section.

Maxine A. Papadakis, MD
papadakM@medsch.ucsf.edu
Stephen J. McPhee, MD
smcphee@medicine.ucsf.edu
Michael W. Rabow, MD
mrabow@medicine.ucsf.edu
San Francisco, California

From inability to let alone; from too much zeal for the new and contempt for what is old; from putting knowledge before wisdom, and science before art and cleverness before common sense; from treating patients as cases; and from making the cure of the disease more grievous than the endurance of the same, Good Lord, deliver us.

—Sir Robert Hutchison

Disease Prevention & Health Promotion

Michael Pignone, MD, MPH
René Salazar, MD

GENERAL APPROACH TO THE PATIENT

The medical interview serves several functions. It is used to collect information to assist in diagnosis (the "history" of the present illness), to understand patient values, to assess and communicate prognosis, to establish a therapeutic relationship, and to reach agreement with the patient about further diagnostic procedures and therapeutic options. It also serves as an opportunity to influence patient behavior, such as in motivational discussions about smoking cessation or medication adherence. Interviewing techniques that avoid domination by the clinician increase patient involvement in care and patient satisfaction. Effective clinician-patient communication and increased patient involvement can improve health outcomes.

Patient Adherence

For many illnesses, treatment depends on difficult fundamental behavioral changes, including alterations in diet, taking up exercise, giving up smoking, cutting down drinking, and adhering to medication regimens that are often complex. Adherence is a problem in every practice; up to 50% of patients fail to achieve full adherence, and one-third never take their medicines. Many patients with medical problems, even those with access to care, do not seek appropriate care or may drop out of care prematurely. Adherence rates for short-term, self-administered therapies are higher than for long-term therapies and are inversely correlated with the number of interventions, their complexity and cost, and the patient's perception of overmedication.

As an example, in HIV-infected patients, adherence to antiretroviral therapy is a crucial determinant of treatment success. Studies have unequivocally demonstrated a close relationship between patient adherence and plasma HIV RNA levels, CD4 cell counts, and mortality. Adherence levels of > 95% are needed to maintain virologic suppression. However, studies show that over 60% of patients are < 90% adherent and that adherence tends to decrease over time.

Patient reasons for nonadherence include simple forgetfulness, being away from home, being busy, and changes in daily routine. Other reasons include psychiatric disorders (depression or substance abuse), uncertainty about the effectiveness of treatment, lack of knowledge about the consequences of poor adherence, regimen complexity, and treatment side effects.

Patients seem better able to take prescribed medications than to adhere to recommendations to change their diet, exercise habits, or alcohol intake or to perform various self-care activities (such as monitoring blood glucose levels at home). For short-term regimens, adherence to medications can be improved by giving clear instructions. Writing out advice to patients, including changes in medication, may be helpful. Because low functional health literacy is common (almost half of English-speaking US patients are unable to read and understand standard health education materials), other forms of communication—such as illustrated simple text, videotapes, or oral instructions—may be more effective. For non–English-speaking patients, clinicians and health care delivery systems can work to provide culturally and linguistically appropriate health services.

To help improve adherence to long-term regimens, clinicians can work with patients to reach agreement on the goals for therapy, provide information about the regimen, ensure understanding by using the "teach-back" method, counsel about the importance of adherence and how to organize medication-taking, reinforce self-monitoring, provide more convenient care, prescribe a simple dosage regimen for all medications (preferably one or two doses daily), suggest ways to help in remembering to take doses (time of day, mealtime, alarms) and to keep appointments, and provide ways to simplify dosing (medication boxes). Single-unit doses supplied in foil wrappers can increase adherence but should be avoided for patients who have difficulty opening them. Medication boxes with compartments (eg, Medisets) that are filled weekly are useful. Microelectronic devices can provide feedback to show patients whether they have taken doses as scheduled or to notify patients within a day if doses are skipped. Reminders, including cell phone text messages, are another effective means of encouraging adherence. The clinician can also enlist social support from family and friends, recruit an adherence monitor, provide a more convenient care environment, and provide rewards and recognition for the patient's efforts to follow the regimen. Collaborative programs that utilize pharmacists to help ensure adherence are also effective.

Adherence is also improved when a trusting doctor-patient relationship has been established and when patients actively participate in their care. Clinicians can improve patient adherence by inquiring specifically about the behaviors in question. When asked, many patients admit to incomplete adherence with medication regimens, with advice about giving up cigarettes, or with engaging only in "safer sex" practices. Although difficult, sufficient time must be made available for communication of health messages.

Medication adherence can be assessed generally with a single question: "In the past month, how often did you take your medications as the doctor prescribed?" Other ways of assessing medication adherence include pill counts and refill records; monitoring serum, urine, or saliva levels of drugs or metabolites; watching for appointment nonattendance and treatment nonresponse; and assessing predictable drug effects such as weight changes with diuretics or bradycardia from beta-blockers. In some conditions, even partial adherence, as with drug treatment of hypertension and diabetes mellitus, improves outcomes compared with nonadherence; in other cases, such as HIV antiretroviral therapy or treatment of tuberculosis, partial adherence may be worse than complete nonadherence.

Guiding Principles of Care

Ethical decisions are often called for in medical practice, at both the "micro" level of the individual patient-clinician relationship and at the "macro" level of the allocation of resources. Ethical principles that guide the successful approach to diagnosis and treatment are honesty, beneficence, justice, avoidance of conflict of interest, and the pledge to do no harm. Increasingly, Western medicine involves patients in important decisions about medical care, eg, which colorectal screening test to obtain or modality of therapy for breast cancer or how far to proceed with treatment of patients who have terminal illnesses (see Chapter 5).

The clinician's role does not end with diagnosis and treatment. The importance of the empathic clinician in helping patients and their families bear the burden of serious illness and death cannot be overemphasized. "To cure sometimes, to relieve often, and to comfort always" is a French saying as apt today as it was five centuries ago—as is Francis Peabody's admonition: "The secret of the care of the patient is in caring for the patient." Training to improve mindfulness and enhance patient-centered communication increases patient satisfaction and may also improve clinician satisfaction.

Coleman CI et al. Dosing frequency and medication adherence in chronic disease. J Manag Care Pharm. 2012 Sep;18(7):527–39. [PMID: 22971206]

Desroches S et al. Interventions to enhance adherence to dietary advice for preventing and managing chronic diseases in adults. Cochrane Database Syst Rev. 2013 Feb 28;2:CD008722. [PMID: 23450587]

Inadomi JM et al. Adherence to colorectal cancer screening: a randomized clinical trial of competing strategies. Arch Intern Med. 2012 Apr 9;172(7):575–82. [PMID: 22493463]

Viswanathan M et al. Interventions to improve adherence to self-administered medications for chronic diseases in the United States: a systematic review. Ann Intern Med. 2012 Dec 4;157(11):785–95. [PMID: 22964778]

HEALTH MAINTENANCE & DISEASE PREVENTION

Preventive medicine can be categorized as primary, secondary, or tertiary. Primary prevention aims to remove or reduce disease risk factors (eg, immunization, giving up or not starting smoking). Secondary prevention techniques promote early detection of disease or precursor states (eg, routine cervical Papanicolaou screening to detect carcinoma or dysplasia of the cervix). Tertiary prevention measures are aimed at limiting the impact of established disease (eg, partial mastectomy and radiation therapy to remove and control localized breast cancer). Tables 1–1 and 1–2 give leading causes of death in the United States and estimates of deaths from preventable causes.

Many effective preventive services are underutilized, and few adults receive all of the most strongly recommended services. The three highest-ranking services in terms of potential health benefits and cost-effectiveness include discussing aspirin use with high-risk adults, tobacco-use screening and brief interventions, and immunizing children. Other high-ranking services with data indicating substantial room for improvement in utilization are screening adults aged 50 and older for colorectal cancer, immunizing adults aged 65 and older against pneumococcal disease, and screening young women for *Chlamydia*.

Several methods, including the use of provider or patient reminder systems (including interactive patient health records), reorganization of care environments, and possibly provision of financial incentives (though this remains controversial), can increase utilization of preventive services, but such methods have not been widely adopted.

Table 1–1. Leading causes of death in the United States, 2011.

Category	Estimate
All causes	**2,437,163**
1. Diseases of the heart	596,339
2. Malignant neoplasms	575,313
3. Chronic lower respiratory diseases	143,382
4. Cerebrovascular diseases	128,931
5. Accidents (unintentional injuries)	122,777
6. Alzheimer disease	84,691
7. Diabetes mellitus	73,282
8. Influenza and pneumonia	53,667
9. Nephritis, nephrotic syndrome, and nephrosis	45,731
10. Intentional self-harm (suicide)	38,285

Source: National Center for Health Statistics 2012.

Table 1–2. Deaths from all causes attributable to common preventable risk factors. (Numbers given in the thousands.)

Risk Factor	Male (95% CI)	Female (95% CI)	Both Sexes (95% CI)
Tobacco smoking	248 (226–269)	219 (196–244)	467 (436–500)
High blood pressure	164 (153–175)	231 (213–249)	395 (372–414)
Overweight–obesity (high BMI)	114 (95–128)	102 (80–119)	216 (188–237)
Physical inactivity	88 (72–105)	103 (80–128)	191 (164–222)
High blood glucose	102 (80–122)	89 (69–108)	190 (163–217)
High LDL cholesterol	60 (42–70)	53 (44–59)	113 (94–124)
High dietary salt (sodium)	49 (46–51)	54 (50–57)	102 (97–107)
Low dietary omega-3 fatty acids (seafood)	45 (37–52)	39 (31–47)	84 (72–96)
High dietary trans fatty acids	46 (33–58)	35 (23–46)	82 (63–97)
Alcohol use	45 (32–49)	20 (17–22)	64 (51–69)
Low intake of fruits and vegetables	33 (23–45)	24 (15–36)	58 (44–74)
Low dietary polyunsaturated fatty acids (in replacement of saturated fatty acids)	9 (6–12)	6 (3–9)	15 (11–20)

BMI, body mass index; CI, confidence interval; LDL, low-density lipoprotein.
Note: Numbers of deaths cannot be summed across categories.
Used, with permission, from Danaei G et al. The preventable causes of death in the United States: comparative risk assessment of dietary, lifestyle, and metabolic risk factors. PLoS Med. 2009 Apr 28;6(4):e1000058.

Cruz M et al. Predicting 10-year mortality for older adults. JAMA. 2013 Mar 6;309(9):874–6. [PMID: 23462780]

Danaei G et al. The preventable causes of death in the United States: comparative risk assessment of dietary, lifestyle, and metabolic risk factors. PLoS Med. 2009 Apr 28;6(4):e1000058. [PMID: 19399161]

Krogsbøll LT et al. General health checks in adults for reducing morbidity and mortality from disease: Cochrane systematic review and meta-analysis. BMJ. 2012 Nov 20;345:e7191. [PMID: 23169868]

Maciosek MV et al. Greater use of preventive services in U.S. health care could save lives at little or no cost. Health Aff (Millwood). 2010 Sep;29(9):1656–60. [PMID: 20820022]

Scott A et al. The effect of financial incentives on the quality of health care provided by primary care physicians. Cochrane Database Syst Rev. 2011 Sep 7;(9):CD008451. [PMID: 21901722]

US Burden of Disease Collaborators. The state of US health, 1990–2010: burden of diseases, injuries, and risk factors. JAMA. 2013 Aug 14;310(6):591–608. [PMID: 23842577]

PREVENTION OF INFECTIOUS DISEASES

Much of the decline in the incidence and fatality rates of infectious diseases is attributable to public health measures—especially immunization, improved sanitation, and better nutrition.

Immunization remains the best means of preventing many infectious diseases. Recommended immunization schedules for children and adolescents can be found online at http://www.cdc.gov/vaccines/schedules/hcp/child-adolescent.html and the schedule for adults is outlined in Table 30–7. Substantial vaccine-preventable morbidity and mortality continue to occur among adults from vaccine-preventable diseases, such as hepatitis A, hepatitis B, influenza, and pneumococcal infections. Strategies to improve vaccination rates include increasing community demand for vaccinations; enhancing access to vaccination services; provider- or system-based interventions, such as reminder systems; assigning vaccination responsibilities to non-physician personnel and interventions that activate patients through personal contact.

Evidence suggests annual **influenza vaccination** is safe and effective with potential benefit in all age groups, and the Advisory Committee on Immunization Practices (ACIP) recommends routine influenza vaccination for all persons aged 6 months and older, including all adults. When vaccine supply is limited, certain groups should be given priority, such as adults 50 years and older, individuals with chronic illness or immunosuppression, and pregnant women. An alternative high-dose inactivated vaccine is available for adults 65 years and older. Adults 65 years and older can receive either the standard dose or high-dose vaccine, whereas those younger than 65 years should receive a standard-dose preparation.

Increasing reports of **pertussis** among US adolescents, adults, and their infant contacts have stimulated vaccine development for older age groups. The ACIP recommends routine use of a single dose of tetanus, diphtheria, and 5-component acellular pertussis vaccine (Tdap) for adults aged 19–64 years to replace the next booster dose of tetanus and diphtheria toxoids vaccine (Td). Due to increasing reports of pertussis in the United States, clinicians may choose to give Tdap to persons aged 65 years and older (particularly to those who might risk transmission to at-risk infants who are most susceptible to complications, including death), despite limited published data on the safety and efficacy of the vaccine in this age group.

Both **hepatitis A vaccine** and immune globulin provide protection against hepatitis A; however, administration of immune globulin may provide a modest benefit over vaccination in some settings. A recombinant protein **hepatitis E vaccine** has been developed that has proven safe and efficacious in preventing hepatitis E among high-risk populations. Hepatitis B vaccine administered as a three-dose series is recommended for all children aged 0–18 years and high-risk individuals (ie, health care workers, injection drug users, people with end-stage renal disease). Adults with diabetes are also at increased risk for hepatitis B infection, and in October 2011, the ACIP recommended **vaccination for hepatitis B** in diabetic patients aged 19–59 years. In diabetic persons aged 60 and older, hepatitis B vaccination should be considered.

Human papillomavirus (HPV) virus-like particle (VLP) vaccines have demonstrated effectiveness in preventing persistent HPV infections, and thus may impact the rate of cervical intraepithelial neoplasia (CIN) II–III. The American Academy of Pediatrics (AAP) recommends routine HPV vaccination for girls aged 11–12 years. The AAP also recommends that all unvaccinated girls and women aged 13–26 years receive the HPV vaccine. In October 2011, the ACIP approved recommendations for routine vaccination of males 11 or 12 years of age with three doses of HPV4 (quadrivalent vaccine). Vaccination of males with HPV may lead to indirect protection of women by reducing transmission of HPV and may prevent anal intraepithelial neoplasia and squamous cell carcinoma in men who have sex with men. Despite the effectiveness of the vaccine, rates of immunization are low. Interventions addressing personal beliefs and system barriers to vaccinations may help address the slow adoption of this vaccine.

Persons traveling to countries where infections are endemic should take precautions described in Chapter 30 and at http://wwwnc.cdc.gov/travel/destinations/list.htm. Immunization registries—confidential, population-based, computerized information systems that collect vaccination data about all residents of a geographic area—can be used to increase and sustain high vaccination coverage.

The rate of tuberculosis in the United States has been declining since 1992. In 2011, the US tuberculosis rate was 3.4 cases per 100,000 population, a decrease of 6.4% from the 2010 rate. This represents the lowest recorded rate since national tuberculosis surveillance began in 1953. Skin testing for **tuberculosis** (see Table 9–13) and treating selected patients reduce the risk of reactivation tuberculosis. Two blood tests, which are not confounded by prior BCG (bacillus Calmette-Guérin) vaccination, have been developed to detect tuberculosis infection by measuring in vitro T-cell interferon-gamma release in response to two antigens (one, the enzyme-linked immunospot [ELISpot], [T-SPOT.TB] and the other, a quantitative ELISA [QuantiFERON-TBGold] test). These T-cell–based assays have an excellent specificity that is higher than tuberculin skin testing in BCG-vaccinated populations.

The Advisory Council for the Elimination of Tuberculosis has called for a renewed commitment to eliminating tuberculosis in the United States, and the Institute of Medicine has published a detailed plan for achieving that goal. Patients with HIV infection are at an especially high risk for tuberculosis. In 2010, there were an estimated 1.1 million incident cases of tuberculosis among the 34 million people living with HIV. Early initiation of antiretroviral therapy may help control the HIV-associated tuberculosis syndemic.

Treatment of tuberculosis poses a risk of hepatotoxicity and thus requires close monitoring of liver transaminases. Alanine aminotransferase (ALT) monitoring during the treatment of latent tuberculosis infection is recommended for certain individuals (preexisting liver disease, pregnancy, chronic alcohol consumption). ALT should be monitored in HIV-infected patients during treatment of tuberculosis disease and should be considered in patients over the age of 35. Symptomatic patients with an ALT elevation three times the upper limit of normal or asymptomatic patients with an elevation five times the ULN should be treated with a modified or alternative regimen.

In 2010, the Centers for Disease Control and Prevention (CDC) updated guidelines for the prevention and treatment of **sexually transmitted diseases**. Highlights of these guidelines include updated treatments for bacterial vaginosis and genital warts as well as antibiotic-resistant *Neisseria gonorrhoeae*, the prevalence of which has risen (see Chapter 30).

HIV infection is a major infectious disease problem in the world. Since sexual contact is a common mode of transmission, primary prevention relies on eliminating unsafe sexual behavior by promoting abstinence, later onset of first sexual activity, decreased number of partners, and use of latex condoms. Unfortunately, as many as one-third of HIV-positive persons continue unprotected sexual practices after learning that they are HIV-infected. Preexposure prophylaxis with antiretroviral drugs in men who have sex with men could have a major impact on preventing HIV infection, and studies evaluating the impact in other groups are underway. Postexposure prophylaxis is widely used after occupational and nonoccupational contact, and it has been estimated to reduce the risk of transmission by approximately 80%.

The CDC recommends universal HIV screening of all patients age 13–64, and the US Preventive Services Task Force (USPSTF) recommends that clinicians screen adolescents and adults age 15 to 65 years. In addition to reducing sexual transmission of HIV, initiation of antiretroviral therapy reduces the risk for AIDS-defining events and death among patients with less immunologically advanced disease.

In immunocompromised patients, live vaccines are contraindicated but many killed or component vaccines are safe and recommended. *Asymptomatic* HIV-infected patients have not shown adverse consequences when given live MMR and influenza vaccinations as well as tetanus, hepatitis B, *H influenza* type b and pneumococcal vaccinations—all should be given. However, if poliomyelitis immunization is required, the inactivated poliomyelitis vaccine is indicated. In *symptomatic* HIV-infected patients, live virus vaccines such as MMR should generally be avoided, but annual influenza vaccination is safe.

Herpes zoster, caused by reactivation from previous varicella zoster virus infection, affects many older adults and people with immune system dysfunction. Whites are at higher risk than other ethnic groups and the incidence in adults aged 65 and older may be higher than previously described. It can cause postherpetic neuralgia, a potentially debilitating chronic pain syndrome. A varicella vaccine is available for the prevention of herpes zoster. The ACIP recommends routine zoster vaccination, administered as a one-time subcutaneous dose (0.65 mL), of all persons aged 60 years or older. Persons who report a previous episode of zoster can be vaccinated; however, the vaccine is contraindicated in immunocompromised (primary or acquired) individuals. The durability of vaccine response and whether any booster vaccination is needed are still uncertain. The cost-effectiveness of the vaccine varies substantially, and the patient's age should be considered in vaccine recommendations. One study reported a cost-effectiveness exceeding $100,000 per quality-adjusted life year saved. Despite its availability, uptake of the vaccine remains low at 2–7% nationally. Financial barriers (cost, limited knowledge of reimbursement) have had a significant impact on its underutilization.

Methicillin-resistant *Staphylococcus aureus* **(MRSA)**, previously recognized as a nosocomial pathogen, has emerged as a common cause of staphylococcal infection in the outpatient setting; it accounts for more than 50% of outpatient staphylococcal infections. Strategies to prevent MRSA infection include screening asymptomatic carriers; however, universal screening of large populations is not cost-effective. Screening high-risk populations needs additional study. Diligent hand hygiene, rigorous infection control policies, and appropriate use of antibiotics remain key to preventing MRSA infections.

Cataldo MA et al. Methicillin-resistant *Staphylococcus aureus*: a community health threat. Postgrad Med. 2010 Nov;122(6): 16–23. [PMID: 21084777]

Centers for Disease Control and Prevention (CDC). ACIP recommends all 11–12 year-old males get vaccinated against HPV. http://www.cdc.gov/media/releases/2011/a1025_ACIP_HPV_Vote.html

Centers for Disease Control and Prevention (CDC). Child, Adolescent & "Catch-up" Immunization Schedules, United States, 2014. http://www.cdc.gov/vaccines/schedules/hcp/child-adolescent.html

Centers for Disease Control and Prevention (CDC). HIV/AIDS, 2014. https://www.cdc.gov/hiv/basics/index.html.

Centers for Disease Control and Prevention (CDC). Pertussis (whooping cough) outbreaks, 2013. http://www.cdc.gov/pertussis/outbreaks.html

Centers for Disease Control and Prevention (CDC). Adult Immunization Schedules, United States, 2014. http://www.cdc.gov/vaccines/schedules/hcp/adult.html.

Centers for Disease Control and Prevention (CDC). Trends in tuberculosis—United States, 2011. MMWR Morb Mortal Wkly Rep. 2012 Mar 23;61(11):181–5. [PMID: 22437911]

Centers for Disease Control and Prevention (CDC). Use of hepatitis B vaccination for adults with diabetes mellitus: recommendations of the Advisory Committee on Immunization Practices (ACIP). MMWR Morb Mortal Wkly Rep. 2011 Dec 23;60(5):1709–11. [PMID: 22189894]

Chou R et al. Screening for HIV: systematic review to update the 2005 U.S. Preventive Services Task Force recommendation. Ann Intern Med. 2012 Nov 20;157(10):706–18. [PMID: 23165662]

Gagliardi AM et al. Vaccines for preventing herpes zoster in older adults. Cochrane Database Syst Rev. 2012 Oct 17;10: CD008858. [PMID: 23076951]

Hurley LP et al. Barriers to the use of herpes zoster vaccine. Ann Intern Med. 2010 May 4;152(9):555–60. [PMID: 20439573]

Kelesidis T et al. Preexposure prophylaxis for HIV prevention. Curr HIV/AIDS Rep. 2011 Jun;8(2):94–103. [PMID: 21465112]

Lau D et al. Interventions to improve influenza and pneumococcal vaccination rates among community-dwelling adults: a systematic review and meta-analysis. Ann Fam Med. 2012 Nov–Dec;10(6):538–46. [PMID: 23149531]

Mazurek GH et al. Updated guidelines for using interferon gamma release assays to detect *Mycobacterium tuberculosis* infection—United States, 2010. MMWR Recomm Rep. 2010 Jun 25;59(RR-5):1–25. [PMID: 20577159]

Paisley RD et al. Whooping cough in adults: an update on a reemerging infection. Am J Med. 2012 Feb;125(2):141–3. [PMID: 22269615]

Parks NA et al. Routine screening for methicillin-resistant *Staphylococcus aureus*. Surg Infect (Larchmt). 2012 Aug;13(4): 223–7. [PMID: 22913747]

Rey D. Post-exposure prophylaxis for HIV infection. Expert Rev Anti Infect Ther. 2011 Apr;9(4):431–42. [PMID: 21504400]

Ridda I et al. The importance of pertussis in older adults: a growing case for reviewing vaccination strategy in the elderly. Vaccine. 2012 Nov 6;30(48):6745–52. [PMID: 22981762]

Sanford M et al. Zoster vaccine (Zostavax): a review of its use in preventing herpes zoster and postherpetic neuralgia in older adults. Drugs Aging. 2010 Feb 1;27(2):159–76. [PMID: 20104941]

Suthar AB et al. Antiretroviral therapy for prevention of tuberculosis in adults with HIV: a systematic review and meta-analysis. PLoS Med. 2012;9(7):e1001270. [PMID: 22911011]

Williams WW et al; Centers for Disease Control and Prevention (CDC). Influenza vaccination coverage among adults—National Health Interview Survey, United States, 2008–09 influenza season. MMWR Morb Mortal Wkly Rep. 2012 Jun 15;61(Suppl):65–72. [PMID: 22695466]

Wolfe RM. Update on adult immunizations. J Am Board Fam Med. 2012 Jul–Aug;25(4):496–510. [PMID: 22773718]

Workowski KA et al; Centers for Disease Control and Prevention (CDC). Sexually transmitted diseases treatment guidelines, 2010. MMWR Recomm Rep. 2010 Dec 17;59(RR-12):1–110. Erratum in MMWR Recomm Rep. 2011 Jan 14;60(1):18. [PMID: 21160459]

Zhu FC et al. Efficacy and safety of a recombinant hepatitis E vaccine in healthy adults: a large-scale, randomized, double-blind placebo-controlled, phase 3 trial. Lancet. 2010 Sep 11;376(9744):895–902. [PMID: 20728932]

PREVENTION OF CARDIOVASCULAR DISEASE

Cardiovascular diseases, including coronary heart disease (CHD) and stroke, represent two of the most important causes of morbidity and mortality in developed countries. Several risk factors increase the risk for coronary disease and stroke. These risk factors can be divided into those that are modifiable (eg, lipid disorders, hypertension, cigarette smoking) and those that are not (eg, age, sex, family history of early coronary disease). Impressive declines in age-specific mortality rates from heart disease and stroke have been achieved in all age groups in North America during the past two decades, in large part through improvement of modifiable risk factors: reductions in cigarette smoking, improvements in lipid levels, and more aggressive detection and treatment of hypertension. This section considers the role of screening for cardiovascular risk and the use of effective therapies to reduce such risk. Key recommendations for cardiovascular prevention are shown in Table 1–3. New guidelines issued in 2013 encourage regular assessment of global cardiovascular risk in adults 40–79 years of age without known cardiovascular disease.

Goff DC Jr et al. 2013 ACC/AHA Guideline on the assessment of cardiovascular risk: a report of the American College of Cardiology/American Heart Association Task Force on Practice Guidelines. Circulation. 2013 Nov 12. [Epub ahead of print] [PMID: 24222018]

Sugerman DT et al. JAMA patient page. Statins. JAMA. 2013 Apr 3;309(13):1419. [PMID: 23549589]

Taylor F et al. Statins for the primary prevention of cardiovascular disease. Cochrane Database Syst Rev. 2013 Jan 31;1: CD004816. [PMID: 23440795]

Table 1–3. Expert recommendations for cardiovascular prevention methods: US Preventive Services Task Force (USPSTF).[1]

Prevention Method	Recommendation
Screening for abdominal aortic aneurysm	Recommends one-time screening for abdominal aortic aneurysm (AAA) by ultrasonography in men aged 65–75 years who have ever smoked. (B) No recommendation for or against screening for AAA in men aged 65–75 years who have never smoked. (C) Recommends against routine screening for AAA in women. (D)
Aspirin use	Recommends the use of aspirin for men aged 45–79 years when the potential benefit due to a reduction in myocardial infarctions outweighs the potential harm due to an increase in gastrointestinal hemorrhage. (A) Recommends the use of aspirin for women aged 55–79 years when the potential benefit of a reduction in ischemic strokes outweighs the potential harm of an increase in gastrointestinal hemorrhage. (A) Current evidence is insufficient to assess the balance of benefits and harms of aspirin for cardiovascular disease prevention in men and women 80 years or older. (I) Recommends against the use of aspirin for stroke prevention in women younger than 55 years and for myocardial infarction prevention in men younger than 45. (D)
Blood pressure screening	Recommends screening for high blood pressure in adults aged 18 and older. (A)
Serum lipid screening	Strongly recommends screening men aged 35 and older for lipid disorders. (A) Recommends screening men aged 20–35 for lipid disorders if they are at increased risk for coronary heart disease. (B) Strongly recommends screening women aged 45 and older for lipid disorders if they are at increased risk for coronary heart disease. (A) Recommends screening women aged 20–45 for lipid disorders if they are at increased risk for coronary heart disease. (B) No recommendation for or against routine screening for lipid disorders in men aged 20–35, or in women aged 20 and older who are not at increased risk for coronary heart disease. (C)
Counseling about healthy diet and physical activity	Although the correlation among healthful diet, physical activity, and the incidence of cardiovascular disease is strong, existing evidence indicates that the health benefit of initiating behavioral counseling in the primary care setting to promote a healthful diet and physical activity is small. Clinicians may choose to selectively counsel patients rather than incorporate counseling into the care of all adults in the general population. (C)
Screening for diabetes mellitus	Recommends screening for type 2 diabetes mellitus in asymptomatic adults with sustained blood pressure (either treated or untreated) > 135/80 mm Hg. (B) Current evidence is insufficient to assess the balance of benefits and harms of screening for type 2 diabetes mellitus in asymptomatic adults with blood pressure of 135/80 mm Hg or lower. (I)
Screening for smoking and counseling to promote cessation	Recommends that clinicians ask all adults about tobacco use and provide tobacco cessation interventions for those who use tobacco products. (A)

[1]**Recommendation A:** The USPSTF strongly recommends that clinicians routinely provide the service to eligible patients. (The USPSTF found good evidence that the service improves important health outcomes and concludes that benefits substantially outweigh harms.)
Recommendation B: The USPSTF recommends that clinicians routinely provide the service to eligible patients. (The USPSTF found at least fair evidence that the service improves important health outcomes and concludes that benefits substantially outweigh harms.)
Recommendation C: The USPSTF makes no recommendation for or against routine provision of the service.
Recommendation D: The USPSTF recommends against routinely providing the service to asymptomatic patients. (The USPSTF found at least fair evidence that the service is ineffective or that harms outweigh benefits.)
Recommendation I: The USPSTF concludes that the evidence is insufficient to recommend for or against routinely providing the service.
http://www.uspreventiveservicestaskforce.org/adultrec.htm

Abdominal Aortic Aneurysm

One-time screening for abdominal aortic aneurysm (AAA) by ultrasonography in men aged 65–75 years is associated with a significant reduction in AAA-related mortality (odds ratio, 0.55 [95% CI, 0.36 to 0.86]) and possibly a reduction in all-cause mortality (OR = 0.98, 95% CI, 0.95, 1.00). Women do not appear to benefit from screening, and most of the benefit in men appears to accrue among current or former smokers. Recent analyses suggest that screening men aged 65 years and older is highly cost-effective.

Søgaard R et al. Cost effectiveness of abdominal aortic aneurysm screening and rescreening in men in a modern context: evaluation of a hypothetical cohort using a decision analytical model. BMJ. 2012 Jul 5;345:e4276. [PMID: 22767630]

Cigarette Smoking

Cigarette smoking remains the most important cause of preventable morbidity and early mortality. In 2000, there were an estimated 4.8 million premature deaths in the world attributable to smoking, 2.4 million in developing countries and 2 million in industrialized countries. More than three-quarters (3.8 million) of these deaths were in men. The leading causes of death from smoking were cardiovascular diseases (1.7 million deaths), chronic obstructive pulmonary disease (COPD) (1 million deaths), and lung cancer (0.9 million deaths). Cigarettes are responsible for one in every four deaths in the United States: in 2005, over 250,000 deaths in men and over 225,000 deaths in women were attributable to smoking. Annual costs of smoking-related health care is approximately $96 billion per year in the United States, with another $97 billion in productivity losses. Fortunately, US smoking rates are declining; in 2012, 18% of US adults were smokers.

Nicotine is highly addictive, raises brain levels of dopamine, and produces withdrawal symptoms on discontinuation. Smokers die 5–8 years earlier than never-smokers. They have twice the risk of fatal heart disease, 10 times the risk of lung cancer, and several times the risk of cancers of the mouth, throat, esophagus, pancreas, kidney, bladder, and cervix; a twofold to threefold higher incidence of stroke and peptic ulcers (which heal less well than in non-smokers); a twofold to fourfold greater risk of fractures of the hip, wrist, and vertebrae; four times the risk of invasive pneumococcal disease; and a twofold increase in cataracts.

In the United States, over 90% of cases of COPD occur among current or former smokers. Both active smoking and passive smoking are associated with deterioration of the elastic properties of the aorta (increasing the risk of aortic aneurysm) and with progression of carotid artery atherosclerosis. Smoking has also been associated with increased risks of leukemia, of colon and prostate cancers, of breast cancer among postmenopausal women who are slow acetylators of N-acetyltransferase-2 enzymes, of osteoporosis, and of Alzheimer disease. In cancers of the head and neck, lung, esophagus, and bladder, smoking is linked to mutations of the $P53$ gene, the most common genetic change in human cancer. Patients with head and neck cancer who continue to smoke during radiation therapy have lower rates of response than those who do not smoke. Olfaction and taste are impaired in smokers, and facial wrinkles are increased. Heavy smokers have a 2.5 greater risk of age-related macular degeneration.

The children of smokers have lower birth weights, are more likely to be mentally retarded, have more frequent respiratory infections and less efficient pulmonary function, have a higher incidence of chronic ear infections than children of nonsmokers, and are more likely to become smokers themselves.

In addition, exposure to environmental tobacco smoke has been shown to increase the risk of cervical cancer, lung cancer, invasive pneumococcal disease, and heart disease; to promote endothelial damage and platelet aggregation; and to increase urinary excretion of tobacco-specific lung carcinogens. The incidence of breast cancer may be increased as well. Of approximately 450,000 smoking-related deaths in the United States annually, as many as 53,000 are attributable to environmental tobacco smoke.

Smoking cessation reduces the risks of death and of myocardial infarction in people with coronary artery disease; reduces the rate of death and acute myocardial infarction in patients who have undergone percutaneous coronary revascularization; lessens the risk of stroke; slows the rate of progression of carotid atherosclerosis; and is associated with improvement of COPD symptoms. On average, women smokers who quit smoking by age 35 add about 3 years to their life expectancy, and men add more than 2 years to theirs. Smoking cessation can increase life expectancy even for those who stop after the age of 65.

Although tobacco use constitutes the most serious common medical problem, it is undertreated. Almost 40% of smokers attempt to quit each year, but only 4% are successful. Persons whose clinicians advise them to quit are 1.6 times as likely to attempt quitting. Over 70% of smokers see a physician each year, but only 20% of them receive any medical quitting advice or assistance.

Factors associated with successful cessation include having a rule against smoking in the home, being older, and having greater education. Several effective interventions are available to promote smoking cessation, including counseling, pharmacotherapy, and combinations of the two. The five steps for helping smokers quit are summarized in Table 1–4.

Common elements of supportive smoking cessation treatments are reviewed in Table 1–5. A system should be implemented to identify smokers, and advice to quit should be tailored to the patient's level of readiness to change. Pharmacotherapy to reduce cigarette consumption is ineffective in smokers who are unwilling or not ready to quit. Conversely, all patients trying to quit should be offered pharmacotherapy except those with medical contraindications, women who are pregnant or breast-feeding, and adolescents. Weight gain occurs in most patients (80%) following smoking cessation. Average weight gain is 2 kg, but for some (10–15%), major weight gain—over 13 kg—may occur. Planning for the possibility of weight gain, and means of mitigating it, may help with maintenance of cessation.

Table 1–4. Actions and strategies for the primary care clinician to help patients quit smoking.

Action	Strategies for Implementation
Step 1. Ask—Systematically Identify All Tobacco Users at Every Visit	
Implement an officewide system that ensures that for *every* patient at *every* clinic visit, tobacco-use status is queried and documented[1]	Expand the vital signs to include tobacco use. Data should be collected by the health care team. The action should be implemented using preprinted progress note paper that includes the expanded vital signs, a vital signs stamp or, for computerized records, an item assessing tobacco-use status. Alternatives to the vital signs stamp are to place tobacco-use status stickers on all patients' charts or to indicate smoking status using computerized reminder systems.
Step 2. Advise—Strongly Urge All Smokers to Quit	
In a clear, strong, and personalized manner, urge every smoker to quit	Advice should be **Clear** : "I think it is important for you to quit smoking now, and I will help you. Cutting down while you are ill is not enough." **Strong:** "As your clinician, I need you to know that quitting smoking is the most important thing you can do to protect your current and future health." **Personalized:** Tie smoking to current health or illness and/or the social and economic costs of tobacco use, motivational level/readiness to quit, and the impact of smoking on children and others in the household. Encourage clinic staff to reinforce the cessation message and support the patient's quit attempt.
Step 3. Attempt—Identify Smokers Willing to Make a Quit Attempt	
Ask every smoker if he or she is willing to make a quit attempt at this time	If the patient is willing to make a quit attempt at this time, provide assistance (see step 4). If the patient prefers a more intensive treatment or the clinician believes more intensive treatment is appropriate, refer the patient to interventions administered by a smoking cessation specialist and follow up with him or her regarding quitting (see step 5). If the patient clearly states he or she is not willing to make a quit attempt at this time, provide a motivational intervention.
Step 4. Assist—Aid the Patient in Quitting	
A. Help the patient with a quit plan	**Set a quit date.** Ideally, the quit date should be within 2 weeks, taking patient preference into account. **Help the patient prepare for quitting.** The patient must: **Inform** family, friends, and coworkers of quitting and request understanding and support. **Prepare the environment** by removing cigarettes from it. Prior to quitting, the patient should avoid smoking in places where he or she spends a lot of time (eg, home, car). **Review** previous quit attempts. What helped? What led to relapse? **Anticipate** challenges to the planned quit attempt, particularly during the critical first few weeks.
B. Encourage nicotine replacement therapy except in special circumstances	Encourage the use of the nicotine patch or nicotine gum therapy for smoking cessation.
C. Give key advice on successful quitting	**Abstinence:** Total abstinence is essential. Not even a single puff after the quit date. **Alcohol:** Drinking alcohol is highly associated with relapse. Those who stop smoking should review their alcohol use and consider limiting or abstaining from alcohol use during the quit process. **Other smokers in the household:** The presence of other smokers in the household, particularly a spouse, is associated with lower success rates. Patients should consider quitting with their significant others and/or developing specific plans to maintain abstinence in a household where others still smoke.
D. Provide supplementary materials	**Source:** Federal agencies, including the National Cancer Institute and the Agency for Health Care Policy and Research; nonprofit agencies (American Cancer Society, American Lung Association, American Heart Association); or local or state health departments. **Selection concerns:** The material must be culturally, racially, educationally, and age appropriate for the patient. **Location:** Readily available in every clinic office.

(continued)

Table 1–4. Actions and strategies for the primary care clinician to help patients quit smoking. (continued)

Action	Strategies for Implementation
	Step 5. Arrange—Schedule Follow-Up Contact
Schedule follow-up contact, either in person or via telephone	**Timing:** Follow-up contact should occur soon after the quit date, preferably during the first week. A second follow-up contact is recommended within the first month. Schedule further follow-up contacts as indicated. **Actions** during follow-up: Congratulate success. If smoking occurred, review the circumstances and elicit recommitment to total abstinence. Remind the patient that a lapse can be used as a learning experience and is not a sign of failure. Identify the problems already encountered and anticipate challenges in the immediate future. Assess nicotine replacement therapy use and problems. Consider referral to a more intense or specialized program.

[1]Repeated assessment is not necessary in the case of the adult who has never smoked or not smoked for many years and for whom the information is clearly documented in the medical record.

Several pharmacologic therapies have been shown to be effective in promoting cessation. Nicotine replacement therapy doubles the chance of successful quitting. The nicotine patch, gum, and lozenges are available over-the-counter, and nicotine nasal spray and inhalers by prescription. The sustained-release antidepressant drug bupropion (150–300 mg/d orally) is an effective smoking cessation agent and is associated with minimal weight gain, although seizures are a contraindication. It acts by boosting brain levels of dopamine and norepinephrine, mimicking the effect of nicotine. More recently, varenicline, a partial nicotinic acetylcholine-receptor agonist, has been shown to improve cessation rates; however, its adverse effects, particularly its effects on mood, are not completely understood and warrant careful consideration. No single pharmacotherapy is clearly more effective than others, so patient preferences and data on adverse effects should be taken into account in selecting a treatment. Recently, e-cigarettes have become popular; some serve as a nicotine-delivery device, but others deliver water vapor. Their efficacy in smoking cessation, however, has not been well evaluated, and some users may find them addictive.

Clinicians should not show disapproval of patients who failed to stop smoking or who are not ready to make a quit attempt. Thoughtful advice that emphasizes the benefits of cessation and recognizes common barriers to success can increase motivation to quit and quit rates. An intercurrent illness such as acute bronchitis or acute myocardial infarction may motivate even the most addicted smoker to quit.

Individualized or group counseling is very cost-effective, even more so than in treating hypertension. Smoking cessation counseling by telephone ("quitlines") and text messaging-based intervention have both proved effective. An additional strategy is to recommend that any smoking take place out of doors to limit the effects of passive smoke on housemates and coworkers. This can lead to smoking reduction and quitting.

The clinician's role in smoking cessation is summarized in Table 1–4. Public policies, including higher cigarette taxes and more restrictive public smoking laws, have also been shown to encourage cessation, as have financial incentives directed to patients.

Table 1–5. Common elements of supportive smoking treatments.

Component	Examples
Encouragement of the patient in the quit attempt	Note that effective cessation treatments are now available. Note that half the people who have *ever* smoked have now quit. Communicate belief in the patient's ability to quit.
Communication of caring and concern	Ask how the patient feels about quitting. Directly express concern and a willingness to help. Be open to the patient's expression of fears of quitting, difficulties experienced, and ambivalent feelings.
Encouragement of the patient to talk about the quitting process	Ask about: Reasons that the patient wants to quit. Difficulties encountered while quitting. Success the patient has achieved. Concerns or worries about quitting.
Provision of basic information about smoking and successful quitting	Inform the patient about: The nature and time course of withdrawal. The addictive nature of smoking. The fact that any smoking (even a single puff) increases the likelihood of full relapse.

Cahill K et al. Pharmacological interventions for smoking cessation: an overview and network meta-analysis. Cochrane Database Syst Rev. 2013 May 31;5:CD009329. [PMID: 23728690]

Carson KV et al. Training health professionals in smoking cessation. Cochrane Database Syst Rev. 2012 May 16;5:CD000214. [PMID: 22592671]

Centers for Disease Control and Prevention (CDC). Current cigarette smoking among adults—United States, 2011. MMWR Morb Mortal Wkly Rep. 2012 Nov 9;61(44):889–94. [PMID: 23134971]

Free C et al. Smoking cessation support delivered via mobile phone text messaging (txt2stop): a single-blind, randomised trial. Lancet. 2011 Jul 2;378(9785):49–55. [PMID: 21722952]

Lindson-Hawley N et al. Reduction versus abrupt cessation in smokers who want to quit. Cochrane Database Syst Rev. 2012 Nov 14;11:CD008033. [PMID: 23152252]

Moore D et al. Effectiveness and safety of nicotine replacement therapy assisted reduction to stop smoking: systematic review and meta-analysis. BMJ. 2009 Apr 2;338:b1024. [PMID: 19342408]

Mottillo S et al. Behavioural interventions for smoking cessation: a meta-analysis of randomized controlled trials. Eur Heart J. 2009 Mar;30(6):718–30. [PMID: 19109354]

Oza S et al. How many deaths are attributable to smoking in the United States? Comparison of methods for estimating smoking-attributable mortality when smoking prevalence changes. Prev Med. 2011 Jun;52(6):428–33. [PMID: 21530575]

Pierce JP et al. What public health strategies are needed to reduce smoking initiation? Tob Control. 2012 Mar;21(2):258–64. [PMID: 22345263]

Rigotti NA et al. Interventions for smoking cessation in hospitalised patients. Cochrane Database Syst Rev. 2012 May 16;5:CD001837. [PMID: 22592676]

Stead LF et al. Combined pharmacotherapy and behavioural interventions for smoking cessation. Cochrane Database Syst Rev. 2012 Oct 17;10:CD008286. [PMID: 23076944]

Tahiri M et al. Alternative smoking cessation aids: a meta-analysis of randomized controlled trials. Am J Med. 2012 Jun;125(6):576–84. [PMID: 22502956]

Whittaker R et al. Mobile phone-based interventions for smoking cessation. Cochrane Database Syst Rev. 2012 Nov 14;11:CD006611. [PMID: 23152238]

► Lipid Disorders (see Chapter 28)

Higher low-density lipoprotein (LDL) cholesterol concentrations and lower high-density lipoprotein (HDL) levels are associated with an increased risk of CHD. Cholesterol lowering therapy reduces the relative risk of CHD events, with the degree of reduction proportional to the reduction in LDL cholesterol achieved. The absolute benefits of screening for—and treating—abnormal lipid levels depend on the presence and number of other cardiovascular risk factors, including hypertension, diabetes mellitus, smoking, age, and gender. If other risk factors are present, cardiovascular risk is higher and the benefits of therapy are greater. Patients with known cardiovascular disease are at higher risk and have larger benefits from reduction in LDL cholesterol.

Evidence for the effectiveness of statin-type drugs is better than for the other classes of lipid-lowering agents or dietary changes specifically for improving lipid levels. Multiple large randomized, placebo-controlled trials have demonstrated important reductions in total mortality, major coronary events, and strokes with lowering levels of LDL cholesterol by statin therapy for patients with known cardiovascular disease. Statins also reduce cardiovascular events for patients with diabetes mellitus. For patients with no previous history of cardiovascular events or diabetes, meta-analyses have shown important reductions of cardiovascular events.

Guidelines for therapy are discussed in Chapter 28.

Cholesterol Treatment Trialists' (CTT) Collaborators. The effects of lowering LDL cholesterol with statin therapy in people at low risk of vascular disease: meta-analysis of individual data from 27 randomised trials. Lancet. 2012 Aug 11;380(9841):581–90. [PMID: 22607822]

Mitchell AP et al. Statin cost effectiveness in primary prevention: a systematic review of the recent cost-effectiveness literature in the United States. BMC Res Notes. 2012 Jul 24;5:373. [PMID: 22828389]

Taylor F et al. Statins for the primary prevention of cardiovascular disease. Cochrane Database Syst Rev. 2013 Jan 31;1:CD004816. [PMID: 23440795]

► Hypertension (see Chapter 11)

Over 66 million adults in the United States have hypertension. In over half of these adults (35.8 million), hypertension is not controlled. Among the 35.8 million whose hypertension is not well-controlled, nearly 40% are unaware of their elevated blood pressure; almost 16% are aware but not being treated, and 45% are being treated but the hypertension is not controlled. In every adult age group, higher values of systolic and diastolic blood pressure carry greater risks of stroke and heart failure. Systolic blood pressure is a better predictor of morbid events than diastolic blood pressure. Home monitoring is better correlated with target organ damage than clinic-based values. Clinicians can apply specific blood pressure criteria, such as those of the Joint National Committee, along with consideration of the patient's cardiovascular risk and personal values, to decide at what levels treatment should be considered in individual cases.

Primary prevention of hypertension can be accomplished by strategies aimed at both the general population and special high-risk populations. The latter include persons with high-normal blood pressure or a family history of hypertension, blacks, and individuals with various behavioral risk factors such as physical inactivity; excessive consumption of salt, alcohol, or calories; and deficient intake of potassium. Effective interventions for primary prevention of hypertension include reduced sodium and alcohol consumption, weight loss, and regular exercise. Potassium supplementation lowers blood pressure modestly, and a diet high in fresh fruits and vegetables and low in fat, red meats, and sugar-containing beverages also reduces blood pressure. Interventions of unproven efficacy include pill supplementation of potassium, calcium, magnesium, fish oil, or fiber; macronutrient alteration; and stress management.

Improved identification and treatment of hypertension is a major cause of the recent decline in stroke deaths as well as the reduction in incidence of heart failure–related hospitalizations. Because hypertension is usually asymptomatic, screening is strongly recommended to identify patients for treatment. Despite strong recommendations in favor of screening and treatment, hypertension control remains suboptimal. An intervention that included patient education and provider education was more effective than provider education alone in achieving control of hypertension, suggesting the benefits of patient participation; another trial found that home monitoring combined with telephone-based nurse support was more effective than home monitoring alone for blood pressure control. Pharmacologic management of hypertension is discussed in Chapter 11.

Centers for Disease Control and Prevention (CDC). Vital signs: awareness and treatment of uncontrolled hypertension among adults—United States, 2003–2010. MMWR Morb Mortal Wkly Rep. 2012 Sep 7;61:703–9. [PMID: 22951452]

Glynn LG et al. Interventions used to improve control of blood pressure in patients with hypertension. Cochrane Database Syst Rev. 2010 Mar 17;(3):CD005182. [PMID: 20238338]

▶ **Chemoprevention**

Regular use of low-dose aspirin (81–325 mg) can reduce the incidence of myocardial infarction in men (see Chapter 10). Low-dose aspirin reduces stroke but not myocardial infarction in middle-aged women (see Chapter 24). Based on its ability to prevent cardiovascular events, aspirin use appears cost-effective for men and women who are at increased cardiovascular risk, which can be defined as 10-year risk over 10%. Results from a meta-analysis suggest that aspirin may also reduce the risk of death from several common types of cancer (colorectal, esophageal, gastric, breast, prostate, and possibly lung).

Nonsteroidal anti-inflammatory drugs may reduce the incidence of colorectal adenomas and polyps but may also increase heart disease and gastrointestinal bleeding, and thus are not recommended for colon cancer prevention in average risk patients.

Antioxidant vitamin (vitamin E, vitamin C, and beta-carotene) supplementation produced no significant reductions in the 5-year incidence of—or mortality from—vascular disease, cancer, or other major outcomes in high-risk individuals with coronary artery disease, other occlusive arterial disease, or diabetes mellitus.

Antithrombotic Trialists' (ATT) Collaboration; Baigent C et al. Aspirin in the primary and secondary prevention of vascular disease: collaborative meta-analysis of individual participant data from randomised trials. Lancet. 2009 May 30;373(9678):1849–60. [PMID: 19482214]

Gaziano JM et al. Multivitamins in the prevention of cancer in men: the Physicians' Health Study II randomized controlled trial. JAMA. 2012 Nov 14;308(18):1871–80. [PMID: 23162860]

Macpherson H et al. Multivitamin-multimineral supplementation and mortality: a meta-analysis of randomized controlled trials. Am J Clin Nutr. 2013 Feb;97(2):437–44. [PMID: 23255568]

Rothwell P et al. Effect of daily aspirin on long-term risk of death due to cancer: analysis of individual patient data from randomised trials. Lancet. 2011 Jan 1;377(9759):31–41. [PMID: 21144578]

Sesso HD et al. Multivitamins in the prevention of cardiovascular disease in men: the Physicians' Health Study II randomized controlled trial. JAMA. 2012 Nov 7;308(17):1751–60. [PMID: 23117775]

PREVENTION OF OSTEOPOROSIS

See Chapters 26 and 42.

Osteoporosis, characterized by low bone mineral density, is common and associated with an increased risk of fracture. The lifetime risk of an osteoporotic fracture is approximately 50% for women and 30% for men. Osteoporotic fractures can cause significant pain and disability. As such, research has focused on means of preventing osteoporosis and related fractures. Primary prevention strategies include calcium supplementation, vitamin D supplementation, and exercise programs. Calcium supplementation can decrease fracture risk but may also increase risk of cardiovascular events. Vitamin D supplements alone do not appear to reduce fracture risk, although higher dosages (800 international units/d orally) may be effective.

Screening for osteoporosis on the basis of low bone mineral density is also recommended for women over age 60, based on indirect evidence that screening can identify women with low bone mineral density and that treatment of women with low bone density with bisphosphonates is effective in reducing fractures. However, real-world adherence to pharmacologic therapy for osteoporosis is low: one-third to one-half of patients do not take their medication as directed. The effectiveness of screening for osteoporosis in younger women and in men has not been established. Concern has been raised that bisphosphonates may increase the risk of certain types of fractures and osteonecrosis of the jaw, making consideration of the benefits and risks of therapy important when considering screening.

Bischoff-Ferrari HA et al. A pooled analysis of vitamin D dose requirements for fracture prevention. N Engl J Med. 2012 Jul 5;367(1):40–9. [PMID: 22762317]

Bolland MJ et al. Calcium supplements with or without vitamin D and risk of cardiovascular events: reanalysis of the Women's Health Initiative limited access dataset and meta-analysis. BMJ. 2011 Apr 19;342:d2040. [PMID: 21505219]

Chung M et al. Vitamin D with or without calcium supplementation for prevention of cancer and fractures: an updated meta-analysis for the U.S. Preventive Services Task Force. Ann Intern Med. 2011 Dec 20;155(12):827–38. [PMID: 22184690]

Giusti A et al. Atypical fractures of the femur and bisphosphonate therapy: a systematic review of case/case series studies. Bone. 2010 Aug;47(2):169–80. [PMID: 20493982]

Hiligsmann M et al. Cost-effectiveness of osteoporosis screening followed by treatment: the impact of medication adherence. Value Health. 2010 Jun–Jul;13(4):394–401. [PMID: 20102558]

Marjoribanks J et al. Long term hormone therapy for perimenopausal and postmenopausal women. Cochrane Database Syst Rev. 2012 Jul 11;7:CD004143. [PMID: 22786488]

Nelson HD et al. Screening for osteoporosis: an update for the U.S. Preventive Services Task Force. Ann Intern Med. 2010 Jul 20;153(2):99–111. [PMID: 20621892]

PREVENTION OF PHYSICAL INACTIVITY

Lack of sufficient physical activity is the second most important contributor to preventable deaths, trailing only tobacco use. A sedentary lifestyle has been linked to 28% of deaths from leading chronic diseases. Worldwide, approximately 30% of adults are physically inactive. Inactivity rates are higher in women, those from high-income countries (such as the Americas), and increase with age. Among teens age 13–15, 80% report doing fewer than 60 minutes of moderate to vigorous intensity per day and boys are more active than girls.

The US Department of Health and Human Services and the CDC recommends that adults and older adults engage in 150 minutes of moderate-intensity (such as brisk walking) or 75 minutes of vigorous-intensity aerobic activity (such as jogging or running) or an equivalent mix of moderate- and vigorous-intensity aerobic activity each week. In addition to the activity recommendations, the CDC recommends activities to strengthen all major muscle groups (abdomen, arms, back, chest, hips, legs, and shoulders) at least twice a week.

Patients who engage in regular moderate to vigorous exercise have a lower risk of myocardial infarction, stroke, hypertension, hyperlipidemia, type 2 diabetes mellitus, diverticular disease, and osteoporosis. Evidence supports the recommended guidelines of 30 minutes of moderate physical activity on most days of the week in both the primary and secondary prevention of CHD.

In longitudinal cohort studies, individuals who report higher levels of leisure time physical activity are less likely to gain weight. Conversely, individuals who are overweight are less likely to stay active. However, at least 60 minutes of daily moderate-intensity physical activity may be necessary to maximize weight loss and prevent significant weight regain. Moreover, adequate levels of physical activity appear to be important for the prevention of weight gain and the development of obesity. Physical activity also appears to have an independent effect on health-related outcomes such as development of type 2 diabetes mellitus in patients with impaired glucose tolerance when compared with body weight, suggesting that adequate levels of activity may counteract the negative influence of body weight on health outcomes.

Physical activity can be incorporated into any person's daily routine. For example, the clinician can advise a patient to take the stairs instead of the elevator, to walk or bike instead of driving, to do housework or yard work, to get off the bus one or two stops earlier and walk the rest of the way, to park at the far end of the parking lot, or to walk during the lunch hour. The basic message should be the more the better and anything is better than nothing.

To be more effective in counseling about exercise, clinicians can also incorporate motivational interviewing techniques, adopt a whole practice approach (eg, use practice nurses to assist), and establish linkages with community agencies. Clinicians can incorporate the "5 As" approach:

1. Ask (identify those who can benefit).
2. Assess (current activity level).
3. Advise (individualize plan).
4. Assist (provide a written exercise prescription and support material).
5. Arrange (appropriate referral and follow-up).

Such interventions have a moderate effect on self-reported physical activity and cardiorespiratory fitness, even if they do not always help patients achieve a predetermined level of physical activity. In their counseling, clinicians should advise patients about both the benefits and risks of exercise, prescribe an exercise program appropriate for each patient, and provide advice to help prevent injuries or cardiovascular complications.

Behavioral change interventions have been proven effective in increasing physical activity in sedentary older women, although evidence is lacking to support the use of pedometers to increase physical activity in this population. Although primary care providers regularly ask patients about physical activity and advise them with verbal counseling, few providers provide written prescriptions or perform fitness assessments. Tailored interventions may potentially help increase physical activity in individuals. Exercise counseling with a prescription, eg, for walking at either a hard intensity or a moderate intensity-high frequency, can produce significant long-term improvements in cardiorespiratory fitness. To be effective, exercise prescriptions must include recommendations on type, frequency, intensity, time, and progression of exercise and must follow disease-specific guidelines.

Several factors influence physical activity behavior, including personal, social (eg, family and work factors), and environmental (eg, access to exercise facilities and well-lit parks). Broad-based interventions targeting various factors are often the most successful, and interventions to promote physical activity are more effective when health agencies work with community partners. such as schools, businesses, and health-care organizations. Enhanced community awareness through mass media campaigns, school-based strategies, and policy approaches are proven strategies to increase physical activity.

Center for Disease Control and Prevention (CDC). How much physical activity do adults need? http://www.cdc.gov/physicalactivity/everyone/guidelines/adults.html

Hallal PC et al; Lancet Physical Activity Series Working Group. Global physical activity levels: surveillance progress, pitfalls, and prospects. Lancet. 2012 Jul 21;380(9838):247–57. [PMID: 22818937]

Hunter GR et al. Combined aerobic and strength training and energy expenditure in older women. Med Sci Sports Exerc. 2013 Jul;45(7):1386–93. [PMID: 23774582]

McMurdo ME et al. Do pedometers increase physical activity in sedentary older women? A randomized controlled trial. J Am Geriatr Soc. 2010 Nov;58(11):2099–106. [PMID: 21054290]

Orrow G et al. Effectiveness of physical activity promotion based in primary care: systematic review and meta-analysis of randomised controlled trials. BMJ. 2012 Mar 26;344:e1389. [PMID: 22451477]

Thomas GN et al. A systematic review of lifestyle modification and glucose intolerance in the prevention of type 2 diabetes. Curr Diabetes Rev. 2010 Nov;6(6):378–87. [PMID: 20879973]

PREVENTION OF OVERWEIGHT & OBESITY

Obesity is now a true epidemic and public health crisis that both clinicians and patients must face. Normal body weight is defined as a body mass index (BMI), calculated as the weight in kilograms divided by the height in meters squared, of < 25 kg/m^2; overweight is defined as a BMI = $25.0–29.9$ kg/m^2, and obesity as a BMI > 30 kg/m^2. Over the last several years, the prevalence of obesity in the US population has increased dramatically. The most recent national data reveal that one-third of adults in the United States are obese, and prevalence rates are higher in blacks and Hispanics compared to non-Hispanic whites.

Risk assessment of the overweight and obese patient begins with determination of BMI, waist circumference for those with a BMI of 35 or less, presence of comorbid conditions, and a fasting blood glucose and lipid panel. Obesity is clearly associated with type 2 diabetes mellitus, hypertension, hyperlipidemia, cancer, osteoarthritis, cardiovascular disease, obstructive sleep apnea, and asthma.

Obesity is associated with a higher all-cause mortality rate. Data suggest an increase among those with grades 2 and 3 obesity (BMI > 35); however, the impact on all-cause mortality among overweight (BMI 25–30) and grade 1 obesity (BMI 30–35) is questionable. Nonetheless, there is a strong relationship between overweight and obesity and many chronic diseases. One of the most important sequelae of the rapid surge in prevalence of obesity has been a dramatic increase in the prevalence of diabetes. In addition, almost one-quarter of the US population currently has the metabolic syndrome. Both of these factors put affected obese individuals at high risk for the development of CHD.

Metabolic syndrome is defined as the presence of any three of the following: waist measurement of 40 inches or more for men and 35 inches or more for women, triglyceride levels of 150 mg/dL (1.70 mmol/L) or above, HDL cholesterol level < 40 mg/dL (< 1.44 mmol/L) for men and < 50 mg/dL (< 1.80 mmol/L) for women, blood pressure of 130/85 mm Hg or above, and fasting blood glucose levels of 100 mg/dL (5.55 mmol/L) or above. The relationship between overweight and obesity and diabetes, hypertension, and coronary artery disease is thought to be due to insulin resistance and compensatory hyperinsulinemia. Persons with a BMI ≥ 40 have death rates from cancers that are 52% higher for men and 62% higher for women than the rates in men and women of normal weight. Significant trends of increasing risk of death with higher BMIs are observed for cancers of the stomach and prostate in men and for cancers of the breast, uterus, cervix, and ovary in women, and for cancers of the esophagus, colon and rectum, liver, gallbladder, pancreas, and kidney, non-Hodgkin lymphoma, and multiple myeloma in both men and women.

Clinicians must work to identify and provide the best prevention and treatment strategies for patients who are overweight and obese.

Prevention of overweight and obesity involves both increasing physical activity and dietary modification to reduce caloric intake. Adequate levels of physical activity appear to be important for the prevention of weight gain and the development of obesity. Despite this, only 49% of Americans are physically active at a moderate level and 20% at a more vigorous level. In addition, only 3% of Americans meet four of the five USDA recommendations for the intake of grains, fruits, vegetables, dairy products, and meat. Only one of four Americans eats the recommended five or more fruits and vegetables per day.

Clinicians can help guide patients to develop personalized eating plans to reduce energy intake, particularly by recognizing the contributions of fat, concentrated carbohydrates, and large portion sizes (see Chapter 29). Patients typically underestimate caloric content, especially when consuming food away from home. Providing patients with caloric and nutritional information may help address the current obesity epidemic. To prevent the long-term chronic disease sequelae of overweight or obesity, clinicians must work with patients to modify other risk factors, eg, by smoking cessation—see above) and strict blood pressure and glycemic control (see Chapters 11 and 27).

Lifestyle modification, including diet, physical activity, and behavior therapy has been shown to induce clinically significant weight loss. Other treatment options for obesity include pharmacotherapy and surgery (see Chapter 29). In overweight and obese persons, at least 60 minutes of moderate-high intensity physical activity may be necessary to maximize weight loss and prevent significant weight regain. Counseling interventions or pharmacotherapy can produce modest (3–5 kg) sustained weight loss over 6–12 months. Counseling appears to be most effective when intensive and combined with behavioral therapy. Pharmacotherapy appears safe in the short term; long-term safety is still not established. Lorcaserin, a selective 5-hydroxytryptamine (5-HT) (2C) agonist, has been shown to reduce body weight through a reduction of energy intake without influencing energy expenditure. It was approved by the US Food and Drug Administration (FDA) in June 2012 for adults with a BMI ≥ 30 or adults with a BMI ≥ 27 who have at least one obesity-related condition, such as hypertension, type 2 diabetes mellitus, or hypercholesterolemia.

Finally, clinicians seem to share a general perception that almost no one succeeds in long-term maintenance of weight loss. However, research demonstrates that approximately 20% of overweight individuals are successful at long-term weight loss (defined as losing ≥ 10% of initial body weight and maintaining the loss for ≥ 1 year). National Weight Control Registry members who lost an average of 33 kg and maintained the loss for more than 5 years have provided useful information about how to maintain weight loss. Members report engaging in high levels of physical activity (approximately 60 min/d), eating a low-calorie, low-fat diet, eating breakfast regularly, self-monitoring weight, and maintaining a consistent eating pattern from weekdays to weekends.

Flegal KM et al. Association of all-cause mortality with overweight and obesity using standard body mass index categories: a systematic review and meta-analysis. JAMA. 2013 Jan 2;309(1):71–82. [PMID: 23280227]

Ogden CL et al. Prevalence of obesity in the United States, 2009–2010. NCHS Data Brief. 2012 Jan;(82):1–8. [PMID: 22617494]

Rock CL et al. Effect of a free prepared meal and incentivized weight loss program on weight loss maintenance in obese and overweight women: a randomized controlled trial. JAMA. 2010 Oct 27;304(16):1803–10. [PMID: 20935388]

CANCER PREVENTION

▶ Primary Prevention

Cancer mortality rates continue to decrease in the United States; part of this decrease results from reductions in tobacco use, since cigarette smoking is the most important preventable cause of cancer. Primary prevention of skin cancer consists of restricting exposure to ultraviolet light by wearing appropriate clothing and use of sunscreens. In the past two decades, there has been a threefold increase in the incidence of squamous cell carcinoma and a fourfold increase in melanoma in the United States. Persons who engage in regular physical exercise and avoid obesity have lower rates of breast and colon cancer. Prevention of occupationally induced cancers involves minimizing exposure to carcinogenic substances such as asbestos, ionizing radiation, and benzene compounds. Chemoprevention has been widely studied for primary cancer prevention (see above Chemoprevention section and Chapter 39). Use of tamoxifen, raloxifene, and aromatase inhibitors for breast cancer prevention is discussed in Chapters 17 and 39. Hepatitis B vaccination can prevent hepatocellular carcinoma (HCC), and screening and vaccination programs may be cost-effective and useful in preventing HCC in high-risk groups such as Asians and Pacific Islanders. The use of HPV vaccine to prevent cervical and possibly anal cancer is discussed above. In addition to preventing anogenital cancers,

HPV vaccines may have a role in the prevention of HPV-related head and neck cancers. Studies evaluating the long-term efficacy of the vaccine against non-anogenital cancers are ongoing.

Centers for Disease Control and Prevention (CDC). Cancer screening—United States, 2010. MMWR Morb Mortal Wkly Rep. 2012 Jan 27;61(3):41–5. [PMID: 22278157]

D'Souza G et al. The role of HPV in head and neck cancer and review of the HPV vaccine. Prev Med. 2011 Oct;53(Suppl 1):S5–S11. [PMID: 21962471]

Smith RA et al. Cancer screening in the United States, 2012: a review of current American Cancer Society guidelines and current issues in cancer screening. CA Cancer J Clin. 2012;62: 129–42. [PMID: 22261986]

▶ Screening & Early Detection

Screening prevents death from cancers of the breast, colon, and cervix. Current cancer screening recommendations from the USPSTF are shown in Table 1–6. Despite an

Table 1–6. Cancer screening recommendations for average-risk adults: US Preventive Services Task Force (USPSTF).[1]

Test	USPSTF Recommendations
Breast self-examination	Recommends against teaching breast self-examination (D).
Clinical breast examination	Insufficient evidence to recommend for or against.
Mammography	Recommends biennial screening mammography for women aged 50–74 years (B). Decision to start biennial screening before the age of 50 should be an individual one and take patient context into account, including the patient's values regarding specific benefits and harms (C).
Cervical cancer screening	Recommends screening for cervical cancer in women aged 21–65 years with cytology (Pap smear) every 3 years or, for women aged 30–65 years who want to lengthen the screening interval, screening with a combination of cytology and human papillomavirus (HPV) testing every 5 years (A). Recommends against screening for cervical cancer in women younger than 21 years (D). Recommends against screening for cervical cancer in women older than 65 years who have had adequate prior screening and are not otherwise at high risk for cervical cancer (D). Recommends against screening for cervical cancer in women who have had a hysterectomy with removal of the cervix and who do not have a history of a high-grade precancerous lesion (ie, cervical intraepithelial neoplasia [CIN] grade 2 or 3) or cervical cancer (D). Recommends against screening for cervical cancer with HPV testing, alone or in combination with cytology, in women younger than 30 years (D).
Colorectal cancer (CRC) screening	Recommends CRC screening using fecal occult blood testing,[2] sigmoidoscopy, or colonoscopy, in adults, beginning at age 50 years and continuing until age 75 years (A). Recommends against routine screening in adults aged 76–85 years (C). Recommends against screening in adults older than aged 85 years (D).
Prostate cancer screening	Recommends against PSA-based screening for prostate cancer (D).
Testicular cancer screening	Recommends against screening for testicular cancer in adolescent or adult males.

[1]United States Preventive Services Task Force recommendations available at http://www.ahrq.gov/clinic/pocketgd1011/gcp10s2.htm.
[2]Home test with three samples.

Recommendation A: The USPSTF strongly recommends that clinicians routinely provide the service to eligible patients. (The USPSTF found good evidence that the service improves important health outcomes and concludes that benefits substantially outweigh harms.)

Recommendation B: The USPSTF recommends that clinicians routinely provide the service to eligible patients. (The USPSTF found at least fair evidence that the service improves important health outcomes and concludes that benefits substantially outweigh harms.)

Recommendation C: The USPSTF recommends against routinely providing the service. There may be considerations that support providing the service in an individual patient. There is at least moderate certainty that the net benefit is small.

Recommendation D: The USPSTF recommends against routinely providing the service to asymptomatic patients. (The USPSTF found at least fair evidence that the service is ineffective or that harms outweigh benefits.)

increase in rates of screening for breast, cervical, and colon cancer over the last decade, overall screening for these cancers is suboptimal. Interventions including group education, one-on-one education, patient reminders, reduction of structural barriers, reduction of out-of-pocket costs, and provider assessment and feedback are effective in promoting recommended cancer screening.

Evidence from randomized trials suggests that screening mammography has both benefits and downsides. A 2011 Cochrane review estimated that screening with mammography led to a reduction in breast cancer mortality of 15% but resulted in 30% overdiagnosis and overtreatment. Currently, the appropriate form and frequency of screening for breast cancer remains controversial and screening guidelines vary. Clinicians should discuss the risks and benefits with each patient and consider individual patient preferences when deciding when to begin screening (see Chapters 17 and 42).

Digital mammography is more sensitive in women with dense breasts and younger women; however, studies exploring outcomes are lacking. MRI is not currently recommended for general screening, and its impact on breast cancer mortality is uncertain; however, the American Cancer Society recommends it for women at high risk ($\geq$ 20–25%), including those with a strong family history of breast or ovarian cancer. Screening with both MRI and mammography might be superior to mammography alone in ruling out cancerous lesions in women with an inherited predisposition to breast cancer.

All current recommendations call for cervical and colorectal cancer screening. Screening for testicular cancers among asymptomatic adolescent or adult males is not recommended by the USPSTF. Prostate cancer screening remains controversial, since no completed studies have answered the question whether early detection and treatment after screen detection produce sufficient benefits to outweigh harms of treatment. A 2013 Cochrane systematic review revealed that prostate cancer screening with PSA testing did not decrease all-cause mortality and may not decrease prostate cancer-specific mortality. Any benefits in terms of reduction in prostate cancer-related mortality would take more than 10 years to become evident. Men with less than 10–15 years life expectancy should be informed that screening for prostate cancer is unlikely to be beneficial. In May 2012, the USPSTF recommended against PSA-based screening for prostate cancer (Grade: D Recommendation).

Annual or biennial fecal occult blood testing reduces mortality from colorectal cancer by 16–33%. Fecal immunochemical tests (FIT) are superior to guaiac-based fecal occult blood tests (gFOBT) in detecting advanced adenomatous polyps and colorectal cancer, and patients are more likely to favor FIT over gFOBTs. The risk of death from colon cancer among patients undergoing at least one sigmoidoscopic examination is reduced by 60–80% compared with that among those not having sigmoidoscopy. Colonoscopy has also been advocated as a screening examination. It is more accurate than flexible sigmoidoscopy for detecting cancer and polyps, but its value in reducing colon cancer mortality has not been studied directly. CT colonography (virtual colonoscopy) is a noninvasive option in screening for colorectal cancer. It has been shown to have a high safety profile and performance similar to colonoscopy.

The USPSTF recommends screening for cervical cancer in women aged 21–65 years with a Papanicolaou smear (cytology) every 3 years or, for women aged 30–65 years who desire longer intervals, screening with cytology and HPV testing every 5 years. The USPSTF recommends against screening in women younger than 21 years of age and average-risk women over 65 with adequate prior screening. Receipt of HPV vaccination has no impact on screening intervals.

In 2012, the American Cancer Society, the American Society for Colposcopy and Cervical Pathology, and the American Society for Clinical Pathology published updated guidelines for management of abnormal results. Women whose cervical specimen HPV tests are positive but cytology results are otherwise negative should repeat co-testing in 12 months (option 1) or undergo HPV-genotype-specific testing for types 16 or 16/18 (option 2). Colposcopy is recommended in women who test positive for types 16 or 16/18. Women with ASCUS (atypical squamous cells of undetermined significance) on cytology and a negative HPV test result should continue routine screening as per age-specific guidelines.

Evidence suggests that chest CT is significantly more sensitive that chest radiography in identifying small asymptomatic lung cancers; however, controversy exists regarding the efficacy and cost-effectiveness of low-dose CT screening in high-risk individuals. The National Lung Screening Trial (NLST), a randomized clinical trial of over 53,000 individuals at high risk for lung cancer, revealed a 20% relative reduction and 6.7% absolute reduction in lung cancer mortality in those who were screened with annual low-dose CTs for 3 years compared with those who had chest radiographs. There were a greater number of false-positive results in the low-dose CT group compared with those in the radiography group (23.3% vs 6.5%) (see Chapter 39). The Multicentric Italian Lung Detection (MILD) study, a randomized trial of over 4000 participants comparing annual or biennial low-dose CT with observation revealed no evidence of a protective effect with annual or biennial low-dose CT screening.

The American Cancer Society recommends that clinicians with access to high quality lung cancer screening and treatment centers utilize an informed and shared decision making process to discuss low-dose CT screening in high-risk patients in relatively good health who meet NLST criteria (age 55–74 with a $\geq$ 30 pack-year smoking history, current smokers, or $\leq$ 15 years since quitting). Screening should not be viewed as an alternative to smoking cessation.

Buys SS et al; PLCO Project Team. Effect of screening on ovarian cancer mortality: the Prostate, Lung, Colorectal and Ovarian (PLCO) Cancer Screening Randomized Controlled Trial. JAMA. 2011 Jun 8;305(22):2295–303. [PMID: 21642681]

Deutekom M et al. Comparison of guaiac and immunological fecal occult blood tests in colorectal cancer screening: the patient perspective. Scand J Gastroenterol. 2010 Nov;45(11): 1345–9. [PMID: 20560814]

Goodman DM et al. JAMA patient page: Screening tests. JAMA. 2013 Mar 20;309(11):1185. [PMID: 23512066]

Gotzsche PC et al. Screening for breast cancer with mammography. Cochrane Database Syst Rev. 2011 Jan 19;(1):CD001877. [PMID: 21249649]

Ilic D et al. Screening for prostate cancer. Cochrane Database Syst Rev. 2013 Jan 31;1:CD004720. [PMID: 23440794]

Levi Z et al. A higher detection rate for colorectal cancer and advanced adenomatous polyp for screening with immuno-chemical fecal occult blood test than guaiac fecal occult blood test, despite lower compliance rate. A prospective, controlled, feasibility study. Int J Cancer. 2011 May 15;128(10):2415–24. [PMID: 20658527]

Moyer VA; U.S. Preventive Services Task Force. Screening for cervical cancer: U.S. Preventive Services Task Force recommendation statement. Ann Intern Med. 2012 Jun 19;156(12):880–91. [PMID: 22711081]

Moyer VA; U.S. Preventive Services Task Force. Screening for prostate cancer: U.S. Preventive Services Task Force recommendation statement. Ann Intern Med. 2012 Jul 17;157(2):120–34. [PMID: 22801674]

National Lung Screening Trial Research Team; Aberle DR et al. Reduced lung-cancer mortality with low-dose computed tomographic screening. N Engl J Med. 2011. Aug 4;365(5):395–409. [PMID: 21714641]

Oken MM et al; PLCO Project Team. Screening by chest radiograph and lung cancer mortality: the Prostate, Lung, Colorectal, and Ovarian (PLCO) randomized trial. JAMA. 2011 Nov 2;306(17):1865–73. [PMID: 22031728]

Pastorino U et al. Annual or biennial CT screening versus observation in heavy smokers: 5-year results of the MILD trial. Eur J Cancer Prev. 2012 May;21(3):308–15. [PMID: 22465911]

Saslow D et al. American Cancer Society, American Society for Colposcopy and Cervical Pathology, and American Society for Clinical Pathology screening guidelines for the prevention and early detection of cervical cancer. J Low Genit Tract Dis. 2012 Jul;16(3):175–204. [PMID: 22418039]

Tria Tirona M. Breast cancer screening update. Am Fam Physician. 2013 Feb 15;87(4):274–8. [PMID: 23418799]

U.S. Preventive Services Task Force. Screening for testicular cancer: U.S. Preventive Services Task Force reaffirmation recommendation statement. Ann Intern Med. 2011 Apr 5;154(7):483–6. [PMID: 21464350]

Wender R et al. American Cancer Society lung cancer screening guidelines. CA Cancer J Clin. 2013 Mar–Apr;63(2):107–17. [PMID: 23315954]

PREVENTION OF INJURIES & VIOLENCE

Injuries remain the most important cause of loss of potential years of life before age 65. Homicide and motor vehicle accidents are a major cause of injury-related deaths among young adults, and accidental falls are the most common cause of injury-related death in the elderly. Approximately one-third of all injury deaths include a diagnosis of traumatic brain injury. Other causes of injury-related deaths include suicide and accidental exposure to smoke, fire, and flames.

Motor vehicle accident deaths per miles driven continue to decline in the United States. Each year in the United States, more than 500,000 people are nonfatally injured while riding bicycles. The rate of helmet use by bicyclists and motorcyclists is significantly increased in states with helmet laws. Young men appear most likely to resist wearing helmets. Clinicians should try to educate their patients about seat belts, safety helmets, the risks of using cellular telephones while driving, drinking and driving—or using other intoxicants or long-acting benzodiazepines and then driving—and the risks of having guns in the home.

Long-term alcohol abuse adversely affects outcome from trauma and increases the risk of readmission for new trauma. Alcohol and illicit drug use are associated with an increased risk of violent death.

Males aged 16–35 are at especially high risk for serious injury and death from accidents and violence, with blacks and Latinos at greatest risk. For 16- and 17-year-old drivers, the risk of fatal crashes increases with the number of passengers. Deaths from firearms have reached epidemic levels in the United States and will soon surpass the number of deaths from motor vehicle accidents. Having a gun in the home increases the likelihood of homicide nearly threefold and of suicide fivefold. Educating clinicians to recognize and treat depression as well as restricting access to lethal methods have been found to reduce suicide rates.

Clinicians have a critical role in detection, prevention, and management of intimate partner violence (see Chapter 42). Inclusion of a single question in the medical history—"At any time, has a partner ever hit you, kicked you, or otherwise physically hurt you?"—can increase identification of this common problem. Another screen consists of three questions: (1) "Have you ever been hit, kicked, punched, or otherwise hurt by someone within the past year? If so, by whom?" (2) "Do you feel safe in your current relationship?" (3) "Is there a partner from a previous relationship who is making you feel unsafe now?" Assessment for abuse and offering of referrals to community resources creates potential to interrupt and prevent recurrence of domestic violence and associated trauma. Screening patients in emergency departments for intimate partner violence appears to have no adverse effects related to screening and may lead to increased patient contact with community resources. Clinicians should take an active role in following up with patients whenever possible, since intimate partner violence screening with passive referrals to services may not be adequate. A randomized control trial to assess the impact of intimate partner violence screening on violence reduction and health outcomes in women revealed no difference in violence occurrence between screened and nonscreened women. Evaluation of services for patients *after* identification of intimate partner violence should be a priority.

Physical and psychological abuse, exploitation, and neglect of older adults are serious underrecognized problems. Risk factors for elder abuse include a culture of violence in the family; a demented, debilitated, or depressed and socially isolated victim; and a perpetrator profile of mental illness, alcohol or drug abuse, or emotional and/or financial dependence on the victim. Clues to elder mistreatment include the patient's appearance, recurrent urgent-care visits, missed appointments, suspicious physical findings, and implausible explanations for injuries.

Amstadter AB et al. Prevalence and correlates of poor self-rated health in the United States: the national elder mistreatment study. Am J Geriatr Psychiatry. 2010 Jul;18(7):615–23. [PMID: 20220579]

Centers for Disease Control and Prevention (CDC). CDC Grand Rounds: reducing severe traumatic brain injury in the United States. MMWR Morb Mortal Wkly Rep. 2013 Jul 12;62(27):549–52. [PMID: 23842444]

Centers for Disease Control and Prevention (CDC). Vital signs: nonfatal, motor vehicle-occupant injuries (2009) and seat belt use (2008) among adults—United States. MMWR Morb Mortal Wkly Rep. 2011 Jan 7;59(51):1681–6. [PMID: 21209609]

Murphy K et al. A literature review of findings in physical elder abuse. Can Assoc Radiol J. 2013 Feb;64(1):10–4. [PMID: 23351969]

National Highway Traffic Safety Administration (NHTSA). Fatality Analysis Reporting System: national statistics summary, 2010. http://www-fars.nhtsa.dot.gov/Main/index.aspx

Turner S et al. Modification of the home environment for the reduction of injuries. Cochrane Database Syst Rev. 2011 Feb 16;(2):CD003600. [PMID: 21328262]

PREVENTION OF SUBSTANCE ABUSE: ALCOHOL & ILLICIT DRUGS

Substance abuse is a major public health problem in the United States. In the United States, approximately 51% of adults 18 years and older are current regular drinkers (at least 12 drinks in the past year). Maximum recommended consumption for adult women and those older than 65 years is three or fewer drinks per day (seven per week), and for adult men, four or fewer drinks per day (14 per week). The spectrum of **alcohol misuse** includes **risky drinking** (alcohol consumption above the recommended daily, weekly, or per occasion amounts), harmful use (a pattern causing damage to health), **alcohol abuse** (a pattern leading to clinically significant impairment or distress), and **alcohol dependence** (includes three or more of the following: tolerance, withdrawal, increased consumption, desire to cut down use, giving up social activities, increased time using alcohol or recovering from use, continued use despite known adverse effects). Estimating the prevalence of alcohol misuse is challenging; however, it has been suggested that 30% of the US population is affected. Underdiagnosis and treatment of alcohol misuse is substantial, both because of patient denial and lack of detection of clinical clues. Treatment rates for alcohol dependence have slightly declined over the last several years. Only a quarter of alcohol-dependent patients have ever been treated.

As with cigarette use, clinician identification and counseling about alcohol misuse is essential. An estimated 15–30% of hospitalized patients have problems with alcohol abuse or dependence, but the connection between patients' presenting complaints and their alcohol use is often missed.

The Alcohol Use Disorder Identification Test (AUDIT) consists of questions on the quantity and frequency of alcohol consumption, on alcohol dependence symptoms, and on alcohol-related problems (Table 1–7). The AUDIT questionnaire is a cost-effective and efficient diagnostic tool for routine screening of alcohol use disorders in primary care settings. Choice of therapy remains controversial. However, use of screening procedures and brief intervention methods (see Chapter 25) can produce a 10–30% reduction in long-term alcohol use and alcohol-related problems. Brief advice and counseling without regular follow-up and reinforcement cannot sustain significant long-term reductions in unhealthy drinking behaviors.

Time restraints may prevent clinicians from screening patients and single-question screening tests for unhealthy alcohol use may help increase the frequency of screening in primary care settings. Clinical trials support the use of screening and brief intervention for unhealthy alcohol use in adults. The National Institute on Alcohol Abuse and Alcoholism recommends the following single-question screening test: "How many times in the past year have you had X or more drinks in a day?" (X is 5 for men and 4 for women, and a response of > 1 is considered positive.) The single-item screening test has been validated in primary care settings.

Several pharmacologic agents are effective in reducing alcohol consumption. In acute alcohol detoxification, standard treatment regimens use long-acting benzodiazepines, the preferred medications for alcohol detoxification, because they can be given on a fixed schedule or through "front-loading" or "symptom-triggered" regimens. Adjuvant sympatholytic medications can be used to treat hyper-adrenergic symptoms that persist despite adequate sedation. Three drugs are FDA approved for treatment of alcohol dependence—disulfiram, naltrexone, and acamprosate. Disulfiram, an aversive agent, has significant adverse effects and consequently, compliance difficulties have resulted in no clear evidence that it increases abstinence rates, decreases relapse rates, or reduces cravings. Persons who receive short-term treatment with naltrexone have a lower chance of alcoholism relapse. Compared with placebo, naltrexone can lower the risk of treatment withdrawal in alcohol-dependent patients, and long-acting intramuscular formulation of naltrexone has been found to be well-tolerated and to reduce drinking significantly among treatment-seeking alcoholics over a 6-month period. In a randomized, controlled trial, patients receiving medical management with naltrexone, a combined behavioral intervention, or both, fared better on drinking outcomes, whereas acamprosate showed no evidence of efficacy with or without combined behavioral intervention. A depot formulation of naltrexone is available with good evidence for clinical efficacy. Topiramate is a promising treatment for alcohol dependence. A 6-month randomized trial of topiramate versus naltrexone revealed a greater reduction of alcohol intake and cravings in participants receiving topiramate. Topiramate's side effect profile is favorable, and the benefits appear to increase over time. Clinicians should be aware that although topiramate appears to be an effective treatment for alcohol dependence, the manufacturer has not pursued FDA approval for this indication.

Over the last decade, the rate of **prescription drug abuse** has increased dramatically, particularly at both ends of the age spectrum. The most commonly abused classes of medications are pain relievers, tranquilizers, stimulants, and sedatives. Opioid-based prescription drug abuse, misuse, and overdose has reached epidemic proportions in the

Table 1–7. Screening for alcohol abuse using the Alcohol Use Disorder Identification Test (AUDIT).[1]

(Scores for response categories are given in parentheses. Scores range from 0 to 40, with a cutoff score of ≥ 5 indicating hazardous drinking, harmful drinking, or alcohol dependence.)

1. How often do you have a drink containing alcohol?

| (0) Never | (1) Monthly or less | (2) Two to four times a month | (3) Two or three times a week | (4) Four or more times a week |

2. How many drinks containing alcohol do you have on a typical day when you are drinking?

| (0) 1 or 2 | (1) 3 or 4 | (2) 5 or 6 | (3) 7 to 9 | (4) 10 or more |

3. How often do you have six or more drinks on one occasion?

| (0) Never | (1) Less than monthly | (2) Monthly | (3) Weekly | (4) Daily or almost daily |

4. How often during the past year have you found that you were not able to stop drinking once you had started?

| (0) Never | (1) Less than monthly | (2) Monthly | (3) Weekly | (4) Daily or almost daily |

5. How often during the past year have you failed to do what was normally expected of you because of drinking?

| (0) Never | (1) Less than monthly | (2) Monthly | (3) Weekly | (4) Daily or almost daily |

6. How often during the past year have you needed a first drink in the morning to get yourself going after a heavy drinking session?

| (0) Never | (1) Less than monthly | (2) Monthly | (3) Weekly | (4) Daily or almost daily |

7. How often during the past year have you had a feeling of guilt or remorse after drinking?

| (0) Never | (1) Less than monthly | (2) Monthly | (3) Weekly | (4) Daily or almost daily |

8. How often during the past year have you been unable to remember what happened the night before because you had been drinking?

| (0) Never | (1) Less than monthly | (2) Monthly | (3) Weekly | (4) Daily or almost daily |

9. Have you or has someone else been injured as a result of your drinking?

| (0) No | (2) Yes, but not in the past year | (4) Yes, during the past year |

10. Has a relative or friend or a doctor or other health worker been concerned about your drinking or suggested you cut down?

| (0) No | (2) Yes, but not in the past year | (4) Yes, during the past year |

[1]Adapted, with permission, from BMJ Publishing Group Ltd. and Piccinelli M et al. Efficacy of the alcohol use disorders identification test as a screening tool for hazardous alcohol intake and related disorders in primary care: a validity study. BMJ. 1997 Feb 8;314 (7078):420–4.

United States. Strategies to address this epidemic include establishing and strengthening prescription drug monitoring programs, regulating pain management facilities and establishing dosage thresholds requiring consultation with pain specialists; however, further evaluation is necessary to determine the impact of these strategies on opioid abuse and misuse. (See Chapter 5.)

Use of illegal drugs—including cocaine, methamphetamine, and so-called "designer drugs"—either sporadically or episodically remains an important problem. Lifetime prevalence of drug abuse is approximately 8% and is generally greater among men, young and unmarried individuals, Native Americans, and those of lower socioeconomic status. As with alcohol, drug abuse disorders often coexist with personality, anxiety, and other substance abuse disorders. Abuse of anabolic-androgenic steroids has been associated with use of other illicit drugs, alcohol, and cigarettes and with violence and criminal behavior.

As with alcohol abuse, the lifetime treatment rate for drug abuse is low (8%). The recognition of drug abuse presents special problems and requires that the clinician actively consider the diagnosis. Clinical aspects of substance abuse are discussed in Chapter 25.

Buprenorphine has potential as a medication to ameliorate the symptoms and signs of withdrawal from opioids and has been shown to be effective in reducing concomitant cocaine and opioid abuse. The risk of overdose is lower with buprenorphine than methadone and is preferred for patients at high risk for methadone toxicity. Evidence does not support the use of naltrexone in maintenance treatment of opioid addiction. Rapid opioid detoxification with opioid antagonist induction using general anesthesia has emerged as an approach to treat opioid dependence. However, a randomized comparison of buprenorphine-assisted rapid opioid detoxification with naltrexone induction and clonidine-assisted opioid detoxification with delayed naltrexone induction found no significant differences in rates of completion of inpatient detoxification, treatment retention, or proportions of opioid-positive urine specimens, and the anesthesia procedure was associated with more potentially life-threatening adverse events. Finally, cognitive behavior therapy, contingency management, couples and family therapy, and other types of behavioral treatment have been shown to be effective interventions for drug addiction.

Flórez G et al. Topiramate for the treatment of alcohol dependence: comparison with naltrexone. Eur Addict Res. 2011; 17(1):29–36. [PMID: 20975274]

Garcia AM. State laws regulating prescribing of controlled substances: balancing the public health problems of chronic pain and prescription painkiller abuse and overdose. J Law Med Ethics. 2013 Mar;41(Suppl 1):42–5. [PMID: 23590739]

Jonas DE et al. Behavioral counseling after screening for alcohol misuse in primary care: a systematic review and meta-analysis for the U.S. Preventive Services Task Force. Ann Intern Med. 2012 Nov 6;157(9):645–54 [PMID: 23007881]

Kahan M et al. Buprenorphine: new treatment of opioid addiction in primary care. Can Fam Physician. 2011 Mar;57(3): 281–9. [PMID: 21402963]

Manubay JM et al. Prescription drug abuse: epidemiology, regulatory issues, chronic pain management with narcotic analgesics. Prim Care. 2011 Mar;38(1):71–90. [PMID: 21356422]

National Institute on Drug Abuse. Topics in brief: prescription drug abuse—December 2011. http://www.drugabuse.gov/publications/topics-in-brief/prescription-drug-abuse

Schiller JS et al. Summary health statistics for U.S. adults: National Health Interview Survey, 2010, Table 27. Vital Health Stat 10. 2012 Jan;(252):94–96. [PMID: 22834228]

Soyka M et al. Emerging drugs to treat alcoholism. Expert Opin Emerg Drugs. 2010 Dec;15(4):695–711. [PMID: 20560783]

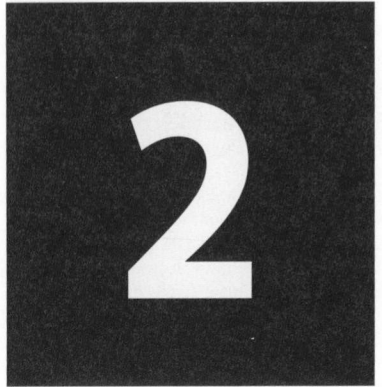

Common Symptoms

Ralph Gonzales, MD, MSPH
Paul L. Nadler, MD

COUGH

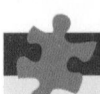

▶ General Considerations

Cough adversely affects personal and work-related interactions, disrupts sleep, and often causes discomfort of the throat and chest wall. Most people seeking medical attention for acute cough desire symptom relief; few are worried about serious illness. Cough results from stimulation of mechanical or chemical afferent nerve receptors in the bronchial tree. Effective cough depends on an intact afferent–efferent reflex arc, adequate expiratory and chest wall muscle strength, and normal mucociliary production and clearance.

▶ Clinical Findings

A. Symptoms

Distinguishing **acute** (< 3 weeks), **persistent** (3–8 weeks), and **chronic** (> 8 weeks) cough illness syndromes is a useful first step in evaluation. Postinfectious cough lasting 3–8 weeks has also been referred to as **subacute** cough to distinguish this common, distinct clinical entity from acute and chronic cough.

1. Acute cough—In healthy adults, most acute cough syndromes are due to viral respiratory tract infections. Additional features of infection such as fever, nasal congestion, and sore throat help confirm the diagnosis. Dyspnea (at rest or with exertion) may reflect a more serious condition, and further evaluation should include assessment of oxygenation (pulse oximetry or arterial blood gas measurement), airflow (peak flow or spirometry), and pulmonary parenchymal disease (chest radiography). The timing and character of the cough have not been found to be very useful in establishing the cause of acute cough syndromes, although cough-variant asthma should be considered in adults with prominent nocturnal cough, and persistent cough with phlegm increases the patient's likelihood of chronic obstructive pulmonary disease (COPD). The presence of post-tussive emesis or inspiratory whoop modestly increases the likelihood of pertussis, and the absence of paroxysmal cough decreases the likelihood of pertussis in adolescents and adults with cough lasting more than 1 week. Uncommon causes of acute cough should be suspected in those with heart disease (heart failure [HF]) or hay fever (allergic rhinitis) and those with environmental risk factors (such as farm workers).

2. Persistent and chronic cough—Cough due to acute respiratory tract infection resolves within 3 weeks in the vast majority of patients (over 90%). Pertussis infection should be considered in adolescents and adults with persistent or severe cough lasting more than 3 weeks. In selected geographic areas, the prevalence of pertussis approaches 20% when cough has persisted beyond 3 weeks, although the exact prevalence of pertussis is difficult to ascertain due to the limited sensitivity of diagnostic tests.

When angiotensin-converting enzyme (ACE) inhibitor therapy, acute respiratory tract infection, and chest radiograph abnormalities are absent, most cases of persistent and chronic cough are due to or exacerbated by postnasal drip, asthma, or gastroesophageal reflux disease (GERD), or some combination of these three entities. A history of nasal or sinus congestion, wheezing, or heartburn should direct subsequent evaluation and treatment, though these conditions frequently cause persistent cough in the absence of typical symptoms. Dyspnea at rest or with exertion is not commonly reported among patients with persistent cough; dyspnea requires assessment for chronic lung disease, HF, or anemia.

Bronchogenic carcinoma is suspected when cough is accompanied by unexplained weight loss and fevers with night sweats, particularly in persons with significant tobacco or occupational exposures (asbestos, radon, diesel exhaust, and metals). Persistent and chronic cough accompanied by excessive mucus secretions increases the likelihood of COPD, particularly among smokers, or bronchiectasis in a patient with a history of recurrent or complicated pneumonia; chest radiographs are helpful in diagnosis.

B. Physical Examination

Examination can direct subsequent diagnostic testing for acute cough. Pneumonia is suspected when acute cough is accompanied by vital sign abnormalities (tachycardia, tachypnea, fever). Findings suggestive of airspace consolidation (rales, decreased breath sounds, fremitus, egophony) are significant predictors of community-acquired pneumonia but are present in the minority of cases. Purulent sputum is associated with bacterial infections in patients with structural lung disease (eg, COPD, cystic fibrosis), but it is a poor predictor of pneumonia in the otherwise healthy adult. Wheezing and rhonchi are frequent findings in adults with acute bronchitis and do not represent consolidation or adult-onset asthma in most cases.

Examination of patients with persistent cough should look for evidence of chronic sinusitis, contributing to postnasal drip syndrome or asthma. Chest and cardiac signs may help distinguish COPD from HF. In patients with cough and dyspnea, a normal match test (ability to blow out a match from 25 cm away) and maximum laryngeal height > 4 cm (measured from the sternal notch to the cricoid cartilage at end expiration) substantially decrease the likelihood of COPD. Similarly, normal jugular venous pressure and no hepatojugular reflux decrease the likelihood of biventricular HF.

C. Diagnostic Studies

1. Acute cough—Chest radiography should be considered for any adult with acute cough whose vital signs are abnormal or whose chest examination suggests pneumonia. The relationship between specific clinical findings and the probability of pneumonia is shown in Table 2–1. A large, multicenter randomized clinical trial found that an elevated serum C-reactive protein (levels > 30 mg/dL) improves diagnostic accuracy of clinical prediction rules for pneumonia in adults with acute cough illness. In patients with dyspnea, pulse oximetry and peak flow help exclude hypoxemia or obstructive airway disease. However, a normal pulse oximetry value (eg, > 93%) does not rule out a significant alveolar–arterial (A–a) gradient when patients have effective respiratory compensation. During documented outbreaks, clinical diagnosis of influenza has a positive predictive value of ~70%; it usually obviates the usefulness of rapid diagnostic tests.

2. Persistent and chronic cough—Chest radiography is indicated when ACE inhibitor therapy–related and postinfectious cough are excluded by history or further diagnostic testing. If pertussis infection is suspected, polymerase chain reaction testing should be performed on a nasopharyngeal swab or nasal wash specimen—although the ability to detect pertussis decreases as the duration of cough increases. When the chest film is normal, postnasal drip, asthma, and GERD are the most likely causes. The presence

of typical symptoms of these conditions directs further evaluation or empiric therapy, though typical symptoms are often absent. Definitive tests for determining the presence of each are available (Table 2–2). However, empiric treatment with a maximum-strength regimen for postnasal drip, asthma, or GERD for 2–4 weeks is one recommended approach since documenting the presence of postnasal drip, asthma, and GERD does not mean they are the cause of the cough. Alternative approaches to identifying patients

Table 2–1. Positive and negative likelihood ratios for history, physical examination, and laboratory findings in the diagnosis of pneumonia.

Finding	Positive Likelihood Ratio	Negative Likelihood Ratio
Medical history		
Fever	1.7–2.1	0.6–0.7
Chills	1.3–1.7	0.7–0.9
Physical examination		
Tachypnea (RR > 25 breaths/min)	1.5–3.4	0.8
Tachycardia (> 100 beats/min in two studies or > 120 beats/min in one study)	1.6–2.3	0.5–0.7
Hyperthermia (> 37.8°C)	1.4–4.4	0.6–0.8
Chest examination		
Dullness to percussion	2.2–4.3	0.8–0.9
Decreased breath sounds	2.3–2.5	0.6–0.8
Crackles	1.6–2.7	0.6–0.9
Rhonchi	1.4–1.5	0.8–0.9
Egophony	2.0–8.6	0.8–1.0
Laboratory findings		
Leukocytosis (> 11 × 10⁹/L in one study or ≥ 10.4 × 10⁹/L in another study)	1.9–3.7	0.3–0.6

RR, respiratory rate.

Table 2–2. Empiric treatments or tests for persistent cough.

Suspected Condition	Step 1 (Empiric Therapy)	Step 2 (Diagnostic Testing)
Postnasal drip	Therapy for allergy or chronic sinusitis	ENT referral; sinus CT scan
Asthma	Beta-2-agonist	Spirometry; consider methacholine challenge if normal
GERD	Proton pump inhibitors	Esophageal pH monitoring

ENT, ear, nose, and throat; GERD, gastroesophageal reflux disease.

who have asthma with its corticosteroid-responsive cough include examining induced sputum for increased eosinophil counts (> 3%); measuring increased exhaled nitric oxide levels; or providing an empiric trial of prednisone, 30 mg daily orally for 2 weeks. Spirometry may help identify large airway obstruction in patients who have persistent cough and wheezing and who are not responding to asthma treatment. When empiric treatment trials are not successful, additional evaluation with pH manometry, endoscopy, barium swallow, sinus CT or high-resolution chest CT may identify the cause.

▶ Differential Diagnosis

A. Acute Cough

Acute cough may be a symptom of acute respiratory tract infection, asthma, allergic rhinitis, and HF, as well as many less common causes.

B. Persistent and Chronic Cough

Causes of persistent cough include environmental exposures (cigarette smoke, air pollution), pertussis infection, postnasal drip (upper airway cough syndrome), asthma (including cough-variant asthma), GERD, COPD, bronchiectasis, eosinophilic bronchitis, tuberculosis or other chronic infection, interstitial lung disease, and bronchogenic carcinoma. COPD is a common cause of persistent cough among patients > 50 years of age. Persistent cough may also be psychogenic.

▶ Treatment

A. Acute Cough

Treatment of acute cough should target the underlying etiology of the illness, the cough reflex itself, and any additional factors that exacerbate the cough. There is substantial evidence showing that antibiotics do not improve cough severity or duration in patients with uncomplicated acute bronchitis. Cough duration is typically 1–3 weeks; yet patients frequently expect cough to last less than 10 days. When influenza is diagnosed (including H1N1 influenza), treatment with oseltamivir or zanamivir is equally effective (1 less day of illness) when initiated within 30–48 hours of illness onset, although treatment is recommended regardless of illness duration when patients present with severe illness requiring hospitalization. In the setting of *Chlamydophila* or *Mycoplasma*-documented infection or outbreaks, first-line antibiotics include erythromycin, 250 mg orally four times daily for 7 days, or doxycycline, 100 mg orally twice daily for 7 days. In patients diagnosed with acute bronchitis, inhaled beta-2-agonist therapy reduces severity and duration of cough in some patients. Evidence supports a modest benefit of dextromethorphan, but not codeine, on cough severity in adults with cough due to acute respiratory tract infections. Treatment of postnasal drip (with antihistamines, decongestants, or nasal corticosteroids) or GERD (with H_2-blockers or proton-pump inhibitors), when accompanying acute cough illness, can also be helpful. There is good evidence that vitamin C and echinacea are not effective in reducing the severity of acute cough after it develops; however, evidence does support vitamin C (at least 1 g daily) for prevention of colds among persons with major physical stressors (eg, post-marathon) or malnutrition. Treatment with zinc lozenges, when initiated within 24 hours of symptom onset, reduces the duration and severity of cold symptoms.

B. Persistent and Chronic Cough

Evaluation and management of persistent cough often requires multiple visits and therapeutic trials, which frequently lead to frustration, anger, and anxiety. When pertussis infection is suspected early in its course, treatment with a macrolide antibiotic (azithromycin 500 mg on day 1, then 250 mg once daily for days 2–5; clarithromycin 500 mg twice daily for 7 days; erythromycin 250 mg four times daily for 14 days) is appropriate to reduce shedding and transmission of the organism. When pertussis infection has lasted more than 7–10 days, antibiotic treatment does not affect the duration of cough, which can last up to 6 months. Early identification, revaccination with Tdap, and treatment of adult patients who work or live with persons at high-risk for complications from pertussis is encouraged (pregnant women, infants [particularly younger than 1 year], and immunosuppressed individuals). Table 2–2 outlines empiric treatments for persistent cough. There is no evidence to guide how long treatment for persistent cough due to postnasal drip, asthma, or GERD should be continued. Studies have not found a consistent benefit of inhaled corticosteroid therapy in adults with persistent cough.

When empiric treatment trials fail, consider other causes of chronic cough such as obstructive sleep apnea, tonsillar enlargement, and environmental fungi. The small percentage of patients with idiopathic chronic cough should be managed in consultation with an otolaryngologist or a pulmonologist; consider high-resolution CT scan of the lungs. Treatment options include nebulized lidocaine therapy and morphine sulfate, 5–10 mg orally twice daily.

▶ When to Refer

- Failure to control persistent or chronic cough following empiric treatment trials.
- Patients with recurrent symptoms should be referred to an otolaryngologist or a pulmonologist.
- Adults needing Tdap vaccination to enable "cocooning" of at-risk individuals (eg, infants age < 1 year).

▶ When to Admit

- Patient at high risk for tuberculosis for whom compliance with respiratory precautions is uncertain.
- Need for urgent bronchoscopy, such as suspected foreign body.
- Smoke or toxic fume inhalational injury.
- Intractable cough despite treatment, when cough impairs gas exchange, or in patients at high risk for barotrauma (eg, recent pneumothorax).

Benich JJ 3rd et al. Evaluation of the patient with chronic cough. Am Fam Physician. 2011 Oct 15;84(8):887–92. [PMID: 22010767]

Birring SS. Controversies in the evaluation and management of chronic cough. Am J Respir Crit Care Med. 2011 Mar 15;183(6):t708–15. [PMID: 21148722]

Broekhuizen BD et al. Undetected chronic obstructive pulmonary disease and asthma in people over 50 years with persistent cough. Br J Gen Pract. 2010 Jul;60(576):489–94. [PMID: 20594438]

Centers for Disease Control and Prevention (CDC). Updated recommendations for use of tetanus toxoid, reduced diphtheria toxoid and acellular pertussis vaccine (Tdap) in pregnant women and persons who have or anticipate having close contact with an infant aged <12 months—Advisory Committee on Immunization Practices (ACIP), 2011. MMWR Morb Mortal Wkly Rep. 2011 Oct 21;60(41):1424–6. [PMID: 22012116]

Centers for Disease Control and Prevention (CDC). Updated recommendations for use of tetanus toxoid, reduced diphtheria toxoid, and acellular pertussis (Tdap) vaccine in adults aged 65 years and older—Advisory Committee on Immunization Practices (ACIP), 2012. MMWR Morb Mortal Wkly Rep. 2012 Jun 29;61(25):468–70. Erratum in: MMWR Morb Mortal Wkly Rep. 2012 Jul 13;61(27):515. [PMID: 22739778]

Cornia PB et al. Does this coughing adolescent or adult patient have pertussis? JAMA. 2010 Aug 25;304(8):890–6. [PMID: 20736473]

Held U et al. Diagnostic aid to rule out pneumonia in adults with cough and feeling of fever. A validation study in the primary care setting. BMC Infect Dis. 2012 Dec 17;12:355. [PMID: 23245504]

Johnstone KJ et al. Inhaled corticosteroids for subacute and chronic cough in adults. Cochrane Database Syst Rev. 2013 Mar 28;3:CD009305. [PMID: 23543575]

Lim KG et al. Long-term safety of nebulized lidocaine for adults with difficult-to-control chronic cough: a case series. Chest. 2013 Apr;143(4):1060–5. [PMID: 23238692]

van Vugt SF et al. Use of serum C reactive protein and procalcitonin concentrations in addition to symptoms and signs to predict pneumonia in patients presenting to primary care with acute cough: diagnostic study. BMJ. 2013 Apr 30;346: f2450. [PMID: 23633005]

DYSPNEA

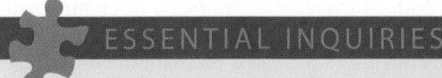

▶ Fever, cough, and chest pain.

▶ Vital sign measurements; pulse oximetry.

▶ Cardiac and chest examination.

▶ Chest radiography and arterial blood gas measurement in selected patients.

▶ General Considerations

Dyspnea is a subjective experience or perception of uncomfortable breathing. However, the relationship between level of dyspnea and the severity of underlying disease varies widely across individuals. Dyspnea can result from conditions that increase the mechanical effort of breathing (eg, COPD, restrictive lung disease, respiratory muscle weakness), conditions that produce compensatory tachypnea (eg, hypoxemia or acidosis), or psychogenic conditions. The following factors play a role in how and when dyspnea presents in patients: rate of onset, previous dyspnea, medications, comorbidities, psychological profile, and severity of underlying disorder. In patients with established COPD, the patient-reported severity of dyspnea is superior to forced expiratory volume in 1 second (FEV_1) in predicting quality of life and 5-year mortality.

▶ Clinical Findings

A. Symptoms

The duration, severity, and periodicity of dyspnea influence the tempo of the clinical evaluation. Rapid onset, severe dyspnea in the absence of other clinical features should raise concern for pneumothorax, pulmonary embolism, or increased left ventricular end-diastolic pressure (LVEDP). Spontaneous pneumothorax is usually accompanied by chest pain and occurs most often in thin, young males, or in those with underlying lung disease. Pulmonary embolism should always be suspected when a patient with new dyspnea reports a recent history (previous 4 weeks) of prolonged immobilization or hospitalization, estrogen therapy, or other risk factors for deep venous thrombosis (DVT) (eg, previous history of thromboembolism, cancer, obesity, lower extremity trauma) and when the cause of dyspnea is not apparent. Silent myocardial infarction, which occurs more frequently in diabetic persons and women, can result in acute heart failure and dyspnea.

Accompanying symptoms provide important clues to causes of dyspnea. When cough and fever are present, pulmonary disease (particularly infections) is the primary concern; myocarditis, pericarditis, and septic emboli can present in this manner. Chest pain should be further characterized as acute or chronic, pleuritic or exertional. Although acute pleuritic chest pain is the rule in acute pericarditis and pneumothorax, most patients with pleuritic chest pain in the outpatient clinic have pleurisy due to acute viral respiratory tract infection. Periodic chest pain that precedes the onset of dyspnea suggests myocardial ischemia or pulmonary embolism. When associated with wheezing, most cases of dyspnea are due to acute bronchitis; however, other causes include new-onset asthma, foreign body, and vocal cord dysfunction.

When a patient reports prominent dyspnea with mild or no accompanying features, consider noncardiopulmonary causes of impaired oxygen delivery (anemia, methemoglobinemia, cyanide ingestion, carbon monoxide), metabolic acidosis due to a variety of conditions, panic disorder, neuromuscular disorders, and chronic pulmonary embolism.

B. Physical Examination

A focused physical examination should include evaluation of the head and neck, chest, heart, and lower extremities. Visual inspection of the patient can suggest obstructive airway disease (pursed-lip breathing, use of accessory respiratory muscles, barrel-shaped chest), pneumothorax

Table 2–3. Clinical findings suggesting obstructive airway disease.

	Adjusted Likelihood Ratios	
	Factor Present	Factor Present
> 40 pack-years smoking	11.6	0.9
Age ≥ 45 years	1.4	0.5
Maximum laryngeal height ≤ 4 cm	3.6	0.7
All three factors	58.5	0.3

Reproduced, with permission, from Straus SE et al. The accuracy of patient history, wheezing, and laryngeal measurements in diagnosing obstructive airway disease. CARE-COAD1 Group. Clinical Assessment of the Reliability of the Examination—Chronic Obstructive Airways Disease. JAMA. 2000 Apr 12;283(14):1853–7.

(asymmetric excursion), or metabolic acidosis (Kussmaul respirations). Patients with impending upper airway obstruction (eg, epiglottitis, foreign body), or severe asthma exacerbation, sometimes assume a tripod position. Focal wheezing raises the suspicion for a foreign body or other bronchial obstruction. Maximum laryngeal height (the distance between the top of the thyroid cartilage and the suprasternal notch at end expiration) is a measure of hyperinflation. Obstructive airway disease is virtually nonexistent when a nonsmoking patient younger than 45 years has a maximum laryngeal height > 4 cm (Table 2–3). Absent breath sounds suggests a pneumothorax. An accentuated pulmonic component of the second heart sound (loud P2) is a sign of pulmonary hypertension and pulmonary embolism.

Table 2–4 shows clinical predictors of increased LVEDP in dyspneic patients with no prior history of HF. When none is present, there is a very low probability (< 10%) of

Table 2–4. Clinical findings suggesting increased left ventricular end-diastolic pressure.

Tachycardia
Systolic hypotension
Jugular venous distention (> 5–7 cm H$_2$O)[1]
Hepatojugular reflux (> 1 cm)[2]
Crackles, especially bibasilar
Third heart sound[3]
Lower extremity edema
Radiographic pulmonary vascular redistribution or cardiomegaly[1]

[1]These findings are particularly helpful.
[2]Proper abdominal compression for evaluating hepatojugular reflux requires > 30 seconds of sustained right upper quadrant abdominal compression.
[3]Cardiac auscultation of the patient at 45-degree angle in left lateral decubitus position doubles the detection rate of third heart sounds.
Source: Badgett RG et al. Can the clinical examination diagnose left-sided heart failure in adults? JAMA. 1997 Jun 4;277(21):1712–9.

increased LVEDP, and when two or more are present, there is a very high probability (> 90%) of increased LVEDP.

C. Diagnostic Studies

Causes of dyspnea that can be managed without chest radiography are few: ingestions causing lactic acidosis, anemia, methemoglobinemia, and carbon monoxide poisoning. The diagnosis of pneumonia should be confirmed by chest radiography in most patients. When COPD exacerbation is severe enough to require hospitalization, results of chest radiography can influence management decisions in up to 20% of patients. Chest radiography is fairly sensitive and specific for new-onset HF (represented by redistribution of pulmonary venous circulation) and can help guide treatment of patients with other cardiac disease. End-expiratory chest radiography enhances detection of a small pneumothorax.

A normal chest radiograph has substantial diagnostic value. When there is no physical examination evidence of COPD or HF and the chest radiograph is normal, the major remaining causes of dyspnea include pulmonary embolism, *Pneumocystis jirovecii* infection (initial radiograph may be normal in up to 25%), upper airway obstruction, foreign body, anemia, and metabolic acidosis. If a patient has tachycardia and hypoxemia but a normal chest radiograph and electrocardiogram (ECG), then tests to exclude pulmonary emboli (see Chapter 9), anemia, or metabolic acidosis are warranted. High-resolution chest CT is particularly useful in the evaluation of pulmonary embolism and interstitial and alveolar lung disease.

Table 2–4 shows clinical findings suggesting increased LVEDP. Elevated serum or B-type natriuretic peptide (BNP or NT-proBNP) levels are both sensitive and specific for increased LVEDP in symptomatic persons. However, the systematic use of BNP in the evaluation of dyspnea in the emergency department does not appear to have clinically significant impact on patient or system outcomes and it does not conclusively affect hospital mortality rates.

Arterial blood gas measurement may be considered if clinical examination and routine diagnostic testing are equivocal. With two notable exceptions (carbon monoxide poisoning and cyanide toxicity), arterial blood gas measurement distinguishes increased mechanical effort causes of dyspnea (respiratory acidosis with or without hypoxemia) from compensatory tachypnea (respiratory alkalosis with or without hypoxemia or metabolic acidosis) from psychogenic dyspnea (respiratory alkalosis). An observational study, however, found that arterial blood gas measurement had little value in determining the cause of dyspnea in patients presenting to the emergency department. Carbon monoxide and cyanide impair oxygen delivery with minimal alterations in PO$_2$; percent carboxyhemoglobin identifies carbon monoxide toxicity. Cyanide poisoning should be considered in a patient with profound lactic acidosis following exposure to burning vinyl (such as a theater fire or industrial accident). Suspected carbon monoxide poisoning or methemoglobinemia can also be confirmed with venous carboxyhemoglobin or methemoglobin levels.

Because arterial blood gas testing is impractical in most outpatient settings, **pulse oximetry** has assumed a central role in the office evaluation of dyspnea. Oxygen saturation values above 96% almost always correspond with a $Po_2 > 70$ mm Hg, and values < 94% almost always represent clinically significant hypoxemia. Important exceptions to this rule include carbon monoxide toxicity, which leads to a normal oxygen saturation (due to the similar wavelengths of oxyhemoglobin and carboxyhemoglobin), and methemoglobinemia, which results in an oxygen saturation of about 85% that fails to increase with supplemental oxygen. A delirious or obtunded patient with obstructive lung disease warrants immediate measurement of arterial blood gases to exclude hypercapnia and the need for intubation, regardless of the oxygen saturation. If a patient reports dyspnea with exertion, but resting oximetry is normal, assessment of desaturation with ambulation (eg, a brisk walk around the clinic) can be useful for confirming impaired gas exchange.

Episodic dyspnea can be challenging if an evaluation cannot be performed during symptoms. Life-threatening causes include recurrent pulmonary embolism, myocardial ischemia, and reactive airway disease. When associated with audible wheezing, vocal cord dysfunction should be considered, particularly in a young woman who does not respond to asthma therapy. Spirometry is very helpful in further classifying patients with obstructive airway disease but is rarely needed in the initial or emergent evaluation of patients with acute dyspnea.

Differential Diagnosis

Urgent and emergent conditions causing acute dyspnea include pneumonia, COPD, asthma, pneumothorax, pulmonary embolism, cardiac disease (eg, HF, acute myocardial infarction, valvular dysfunction, arrhythmia, cardiac shunt), metabolic acidosis, cyanide toxicity, methemoglobinemia, and carbon monoxide poisoning.

Treatment

The treatment of urgent or emergent causes of dyspnea should aim to relieve the underlying cause. Pending diagnosis, patients with hypoxemia should be immediately provided supplemental oxygen unless significant hypercapnia is present or strongly suspected pending arterial blood gas measurement. Dyspnea frequently occurs in patients nearing the end of life. Opioid therapy, anxiolytics, and corticosteroids can provide substantial relief independent of the severity of hypoxemia. Oxygen therapy is most beneficial to patients with significant hypoxemia ($Pao_2 < 55$ mm Hg) (see Chapter 5). In patients with severe COPD and hypoxemia, oxygen therapy improves mortality and exercise performance. It may relieve dyspnea in mildly and non-hypoxemic patients with COPD. Pulmonary rehabilitation programs are another therapeutic option for patients with moderate to severe COPD or interstitial pulmonary fibrosis. Noninvasive ventilation may be considered for patients with dyspnea caused by an acute COPD exacerbation, but the efficacy of this treatment is still uncertain.

▶ When to Refer

- Following acute stabilization, patients with advanced COPD should be referred to a pulmonologist, and patients with HF or valvular heart disease should be referred to a cardiologist.
- Cyanide toxicity or carbon monoxide poisoning should be managed in conjunction with a toxicologist.

▶ When to Admit

- Impaired gas exchange from any cause or high risk of pulmonary embolism pending definitive diagnosis.
- Suspected cyanide toxicity or carbon monoxide poisoning.

Amimoto Y et al. Lung sound analysis in a patient with vocal cord dysfunction and bronchial asthma. J Asthma. 2012 Apr;49(3):227–9. [PMID: 22335255]

Burri E et al. Value of arterial blood gas analysis in patients with acute dyspnea: an observational study. Crit Care. 2011;15(3):R145. [PMID: 21663600]

Cranston JM et al. Oxygen therapy for dyspnoea in adults. Cochrane Database Syst Rev. 2008 Jul 16;(3):CD004769. [PMID: 18646110]

Gallagher R. The use of opioids for dyspnea in advanced disease. CMAJ. 2011 Jul 12;183(10):1170. [PMID: 21746829]

Jang TB et al. The predictive value of physical examination findings in patients with suspected acute heart failure syndrome. Intern Emerg Med. 2012 Jun;7(3):271–4. [PMID: 22094407]

Junker C et al. Are arterial blood gases necessary in the evaluation of acutely dyspneic patients? Crit Care. 2011 Aug 2;15(4):176. [PMID: 21892979]

Kamal AH et al. Dyspnea review for the palliative care professional: assessment, burdens, and etiologies. J Palliat Med. 2011 Oct;14(10):1167–72. [PMID: 21895451]

Lin RJ et al. Dyspnea in palliative care: expanding the role of corticosteroids. J Palliat Med. 2012 Jul;15(7):834–7. [PMID: 22385025]

Parshall MB et al; American Thoracic Society Committee on Dyspnea. An official American Thoracic Society statement: update on the mechanisms, assessment, and management of dyspnea. Am J Respir Crit Care Med. 2012 Feb 15;185(4):435–52. [PMID: 22336677]

Shreves A et al. Emergency management of dyspnea in dying patients. Emerg Med Pract. 2013 May;15(5):1–20. [PMID: 23967787]

Smith TA et al. The use of non-invasive ventilation for the relief of dyspnoea in exacerbations of chronic obstructive pulmonary disease; a systematic review. Respirology. 2012 Feb;17(2):300–7. [PMID: 22008176]

Trinquart L et al. Natriuretic peptide testing in EDs for managing acute dyspnea: a meta-analysis. Am J Emerg Med. 2011 Sep;29(7):757–67. [PMID: 20825895]

Troughton RW et al. B-type natriuretic peptides: looking to the future. Ann Med. 2011 May;43(3):188–97. [PMID: 20961274]

Uronis H et al. Symptomatic oxygen for non-hypoxaemic chronic obstructive pulmonary disease. Cochrane Database Syst Rev. 2011 Jun 15;(6):CD006429. [PMID: 21678356]

Weintraub NL et al. Acute heart failure syndromes: emergency department presentation, treatment, and disposition: current approaches and future aims: a scientific statement from the American Heart Association. Circulation. 2010 Nov 9;122(19):1975–96. [PMID: 20937981]

HEMOPTYSIS

General Considerations

Hemoptysis is the expectoration of blood that originates below the vocal cords. It is commonly classified as trivial, mild, or massive—the latter defined as more than 200–600 mL (about 1–2 cups) in 24 hours. Massive hemoptysis can be usefully defined as any amount that is hemodynamically significant or threatens ventilation. Its in-hospital mortality was 6.5% in a recent study. The initial goal of management of massive hemoptysis is therapeutic, not diagnostic.

The lungs are supplied with a dual circulation. The pulmonary arteries arise from the right ventricle to supply the pulmonary parenchyma in a low-pressure circuit. The bronchial arteries arise from the aorta or intercostal arteries and carry blood under systemic pressure to the airways, blood vessels, hila, and visceral pleura. Although the bronchial circulation represents only 1–2% of total pulmonary blood flow, it can increase dramatically under conditions of chronic inflammation—eg, chronic bronchiectasis—and is frequently the source of hemoptysis.

The causes of hemoptysis can be classified anatomically. Blood may arise from the airways in COPD, bronchiectasis, and bronchogenic carcinoma; from the pulmonary vasculature in left ventricular failure, mitral stenosis, pulmonary embolism, pulmonary arterial hypertension, and arteriovenous malformations; or from the pulmonary parenchyma in pneumonia, inhalation of crack cocaine, or granulomatosis with polyangiitis (formerly Wegener granulomatosis). Diffuse alveolar hemorrhage is due to small vessel bleeding usually caused by autoimmune or hematologic disorders and results in alveolar infiltrates on chest radiography. Most cases of hemoptysis presenting in the outpatient setting are due to infection (eg, acute or chronic bronchitis, pneumonia, tuberculosis). Hemoptysis due to lung cancer increases with age, accounting for up to 20% of cases among the elderly. Less commonly (< 10% of cases), pulmonary venous hypertension (eg, mitral stenosis, pulmonary embolism) causes hemoptysis. Most cases of hemoptysis that have no visible cause on CT scan or bronchoscopy will resolve within 6 months without treatment, with the notable exception of patients at high risk for lung cancer (smokers older than 40 years). Iatrogenic hemorrhage may follow transbronchial lung biopsies, anticoagulation, or pulmonary artery rupture due to distal placement

of a balloon-tipped catheter. No cause is identified in up to 15–30% of cases.

▶ Clinical Findings

A. Symptoms

Blood-tinged sputum in the setting of an upper respiratory tract infection in an otherwise healthy, young (age < 40 years) nonsmoker does not warrant an extensive diagnostic evaluation if the hemoptysis subsides with resolution of the infection. However, hemoptysis is frequently a sign of serious disease, especially in patients with a high prior probability of underlying pulmonary pathology. One should not distinguish between blood-streaked sputum and cough productive of blood alone with regard to the evaluation plan. The goal of the history is to identify patients at risk for one of the disorders listed above. Pertinent features include duration of symptoms, presence of respiratory infection, and past or current tobacco use. Nonpulmonary sources of hemorrhage—from the sinuses or the gastrointestinal tract—must be excluded.

B. Physical Examination

Elevated pulse, hypotension, and decreased oxygen saturation suggest large volume hemorrhage that warrants emergent evaluation and stabilization. The nares and oropharynx should be carefully inspected to identify a potential upper airway source of bleeding. Chest and cardiac examination may reveal evidence of HF or mitral stenosis.

C. Diagnostic Studies

Diagnostic evaluation should include a chest radiograph and complete blood count. Kidney function tests, urinalysis, and coagulation studies are appropriate in specific circumstances. Hematuria that accompanies hemoptysis may be a clue to Goodpasture syndrome or vasculitis. Flexible bronchoscopy reveals endobronchial cancer in 3–6% of patients with hemoptysis who have a normal (non-lateralizing) chest radiograph. Nearly all of these patients are smokers over the age of 40, and most will have had symptoms for more than 1 week. Bronchoscopy is indicated in such patients. High-resolution chest CT scan complements bronchoscopy and should be strongly considered in patients with normal chest radiograph and low risk for malignancy. It can visualize unsuspected bronchiectasis and arteriovenous malformations and will show central endobronchial lesions in many cases. High-resolution chest CT scanning is the test of choice for suspected small peripheral malignancies. Helical CT pulmonary angiography has become the initial test of choice for evaluating patients with suspected pulmonary embolism, although caution should be taken to avoid large contrast loads in patients with even mild chronic kidney disease (serum creatinine > 2.0 g/dL or rapidly rising creatinine in normal range). Helical CT scanning can be avoided in patients who are at "unlikely" risk for pulmonary embolism using the Wells score for pulmonary embolism and the sensitive D-dimer test. Echocardiography may reveal evidence of HF or mitral stenosis.

Treatment

Management of mild hemoptysis consists of identifying and treating the specific cause. Massive hemoptysis is life-threatening. The airway should be protected with endotracheal intubation, ventilation ensured, and effective circulation maintained. If the location of the bleeding site is known, the patient should be placed in the decubitus position with the involved lung dependent. Uncontrollable hemorrhage warrants rigid bronchoscopy and surgical consultation. In stable patients, flexible bronchoscopy may localize the site of bleeding, and angiography can embolize the involved bronchial arteries. Embolization is effective initially in 85% of cases, although rebleeding may occur in up to 20% of patients during the following year. The anterior spinal artery arises from the bronchial artery in up to 5% of people, and paraplegia may result if it is inadvertently cannulated and embolized. There is limited evidence that antifibrinolytics may reduce the duration of bleeding.

When to Refer

- Patients should be referred to a pulmonologist when bronchoscopic evaluation of lower respiratory tract is required.
- Patients should be referred to an otolaryngologist when an upper respiratory tract bleeding source is identified.
- Patients with severe coagulopathy complicating management should be referred to a hematologist.

When to Admit

- To stabilize bleeding process in patients at risk for or experiencing massive hemoptysis.
- To correct disordered coagulation (using clotting factors or platelets, or both).
- To stabilize gas exchange.

Conway AJ et al. Is investigation of patients with haemoptysis and normal chest radiograph justified? Thorax. 2011 Apr; 66(4):352. [PMID: 20805153]

Fartoukh M et al. Early prediction of in-hospital mortality of patients with hemoptysis: an approach to defining severe hemoptysis. Respiration. 2012;83(2):106–14. [PMID: 22025193]

Hurt K et al. Haemoptysis: diagnosis and treatment. Acute Med. 2012;11(1):39–45. [PMID: 22423349]

Jeudy J et al; Expert Panel on Thoracic Imaging. ACR Appropriateness Criteria hemoptysis. J Thorac Imaging. 2010 Aug;25(3):W67–9. [PMID: 20711032]

Pasha SM et al. Safety of excluding acute pulmonary embolism based on an unlikely clinical probability by the Wells rule and normal D-dimer concentration: a meta-analysis. Thromb Res. 2010 Apr;125(4):e123–7. [PMID: 19942258]

Shigemura N et al. Multidisciplinary management of life-threatening massive hemoptysis: a 10-year experience. Ann Thorac Surg. 2009 Mar;87(3):849–53. [PMID: 19231404]

CHEST PAIN

ESSENTIAL INQUIRIES

- ▶ Chest pain onset, character, location/size, duration, periodicity, and exacerbators; and shortness of breath.
- ▶ Vital signs; chest and cardiac examination.
- ▶ Electrocardiography and biomarkers of myocardial necrosis in selected patients.

General Considerations

Chest pain (or chest discomfort) is a common symptom that can occur as a result of cardiovascular, pulmonary, pleural, or musculoskeletal disease, esophageal or other gastrointestinal disorders, or anxiety states. The frequency and distribution of life-threatening causes of chest pain, such as acute coronary syndrome (ACS), pericarditis, aortic dissection, pulmonary embolism, pneumonia, and esophageal perforation, vary substantially between clinical settings. Systemic lupus erythematosus, rheumatoid arthritis, and HIV are conditions that confer a strong risk for coronary artery disease. Because pulmonary embolism can present with a wide variety of symptoms, consideration of the diagnosis and rigorous risk factor assessment for venous thromboembolism (VTE) is critical. Classic VTE risk factors include cancer, trauma, recent surgery, prolonged immobilization, pregnancy, oral contraceptives, and family history and prior history of VTE. Other conditions associated with increased risk of pulmonary embolism include HF and COPD. Sickle cell anemia can cause acute chest syndrome. Patients with this syndrome often have chest pain, fever, and cough.

Clinical Findings

A. Symptoms

Myocardial ischemia is usually described as dull, aching sensation of "pressure," "tightness," "squeezing," or "gas," rather than as sharp or spasmodic. Ischemic symptoms usually subside within 5–20 minutes but may last longer. Progressive symptoms or symptoms at rest may represent unstable angina. Prolonged chest pain episodes might represent myocardial infarction, although up to one-third of patients with acute myocardial infarction do not report chest pain. When present, pain due to myocardial ischemia is commonly accompanied by a sense of anxiety or uneasiness. The location is usually retrosternal or left precordial. Because the heart lacks somatic innervation, precise localization of pain due to cardiac ischemia is difficult; the pain is commonly referred to the throat, lower jaw, shoulders, inner arms, upper abdomen, or back. Ischemic pain may be precipitated or exacerbated by exertion, cold temperature, meals, stress, or combinations of these factors and is usually relieved by rest. However, many episodes do not conform to these patterns; and atypical presentations of ACS are more common in the elderly, women, and persons with diabetes mellitus. Other symptoms that are associated with ACS include shortness of breath; dizziness; a feeling of impending doom; and vagal symptoms, such as nausea and diaphoresis. In the elderly, fatigue is a common presenting complaint of ACS. Likelihood ratios for cardinal symptoms considered in the evaluation of acute myocardial infarction are summarized in Table 2–5.

Hypertrophy of either ventricle or aortic stenosis may also give rise to chest pain with less typical features. Pericarditis may produce pain that is greater when supine than upright and may increase with respiration, coughing, or swallowing. Pleuritic chest pain is usually not ischemic, and pain on palpation may indicate a musculoskeletal cause. Aortic dissection classically produces an abrupt onset of tearing pain of great intensity that often radiates to the back; however, this classic presentation occurs in a

small proportion of cases. Anterior aortic dissection can also lead to myocardial or cerebrovascular ischemia.

Pulmonary embolism has a wide range of clinical presentations, with chest pain present in about 75% of cases. The chief objective in evaluating patients with suspected pulmonary embolism is to assess the patient's clinical risk for VTE based on medical history and associated signs and symptoms (see above and Chapter 9). Rupture of the thoracic esophagus iatrogenically or secondary to vomiting is another cause of chest pain.

B. Physical Examination

Findings on physical examination can occasionally yield important clues to the underlying cause of chest pain; however, a normal physical examination should never be used as the sole basis for ruling-out most diagnoses, particularly ACS and aortic dissection. Vital signs (including pulse oximetry) and cardiopulmonary examination are always the first steps for assessing the urgency and tempo of the subsequent examination and diagnostic work-up.

Findings that increase the likelihood of ACS include diaphoresis, hypotension, S_3 or S_4 gallop, pulmonary crackles, or elevated jugular venous pressure (see Table 2–5). Although chest pain that is reproducible or worsened with palpation strongly suggests a musculoskeletal cause, up to 15% of patients with ACS will have reproducible chest wall tenderness. Pointing to the location of the pain with one finger has been shown to be highly correlated with nonischemic chest pain. Aortic dissection can result in differential blood pressures (> 20 mm Hg), pulse amplitude deficits, and new diastolic murmurs. Although hypertension is considered the rule in patients with aortic dissection, systolic blood pressure < 100 mm Hg is present in up to 25% of patients.

A cardiac friction rub represents pericarditis until proven otherwise. It can best be heard with the patient sitting forward at end-expiration. Tamponade should be excluded in all patients with a clinical diagnosis of pericarditis by assessing pulsus paradoxus (a decrease in systolic blood pressure during inspiration > 10 mm Hg) and inspection of jugular venous pulsations. Subcutaneous emphysema is common following cervical esophageal perforation but present in only about one-third of thoracic perforations (ie, those most commonly presenting with chest pain).

The absence of abnormal physical examination findings in patients with suspected pulmonary embolism usually serves to *increase* the likelihood of pulmonary embolism, although a normal physical examination is also compatible with the much more common conditions of panic/anxiety disorder and musculoskeletal disease.

C. Diagnostic Studies

Unless a competing diagnosis can be confirmed, an ECG is warranted in the initial evaluation of most patients with acute chest pain to help exclude ACS. ST segment elevation is the ECG finding that is the strongest predictor of acute myocardial infarction (see Table 2–5); however, up to 20% of patients with ACS can have a normal ECG. In the emergency department, patients with suspected ACS can be safely removed from cardiac monitoring if they are pain-free at initial

Table 2–5. Likelihood ratios (LRs) for clinical features associated with acute myocardial infarction.

Clinical Feature	LR+ (95% CI)
History	
Chest pain that radiates to the left arm	2.3 (1.7–3.1)
Chest pain that radiates to the right shoulder	2.9 (1.4–3.0)
Chest pain that radiates to both arms	7.1 (3.6–14.2)
Pleuritic chest pain	0.2 (0.2–0.3)
Sharp or stabbing chest pain	0.3 (0.2–0.5)
Positional chest pain	0.3 (0.2–0.4)
Chest pain reproduced by palpation	0.2–0.41
Nausea or vomiting	1.9 (1.7–2.3)
Diaphoresis	2.0 (1.9–2.2)
Physical examination	
Systolic blood pressure ≤ 80 mm Hg	3.1 (1.8–5.2)
Pulmonary crackles	2.1 (1.4–3.1)
Third heart sound	3.2 (1.6–6.5)
Electrocardiogram	
Any ST segment elevation (≥ 1 mm)	11.2 (7.1–17.8)
Any ST segment depression	3.2 (2.5–4.1)
Any Q wave	3.9 (2.7–7.7)
Any conduction defect	2.7 (1.4–5.4)
New ST segment elevation (≥ 1 mm)	5.7–53.91
New ST segment depression	3.0–5.21
New Q wave	5.3–24.81
New conduction defect	6.3 (2.5–15.7)

[1]Heterogenous studies do not allow for calculation of a point estimate.

Adapted, with permission, from Panju AA et al. The rational clinical examination. Is this patient having a myocardial infarction? JAMA. 1998 Oct 14;280(14):1256–63.

physician assessment and have a normal or nonspecific ECG. This decision rule had 100% sensitivity for serious arrhythmia (95% confidence interval, 80–100%), but deserves further validation. Clinically stable patients with cardiovascular disease risk factors, normal ECG, normal cardiac biomarkers, and no alternative diagnoses (such as typical GERD or costochondritis) should be followed-up with a timely exercise stress test that includes perfusion imaging. The ECG can also provide evidence for alternative diagnoses, such as pericarditis and pulmonary embolism. Chest radiography is often useful in the evaluation of chest pain, and is always indicated when cough or shortness of breath accompanies chest pain. Findings of pneumomediastinum or new pleural effusion are consistent with esophageal perforation.

The ADAPT trial found that an accelerated diagnostic protocol that included a TIMI score, electrocardiography, and 0 + 2 hour values of troponin I could identify patients at low short-term risk for a major adverse cardiac event within 30 days.

The TIMI score was shown in a study to be useful for risk stratification of significant cardiac events in patients selected for an emergency department observation unit, with intermediate risk scores (3–5) requiring admission (15.4% vs 9.8%, $P = 0.048$).

The MIDAS study found that patients in whom ACS was suspected who sought medical attention within 8 hours of symptom onset could undergo 3 hours of serial testing with the point-of-care troponin I assay with similar diagnostic accuracy.

Patients presenting to the emergency department with chest pain of intermediate or high probability for ACS without electrocardiographic or biomarker evidence of a myocardial infarction can be safely discharged from an observation unit after stress cardiac magnetic resonance imaging. An alternative to stress testing in the emergency department, sixty-four–slice CT coronary angiography (CTA) has been studied for diagnosing ACS among patients with normal or nonspecific ECG and normal biomarkers. A meta-analysis of nine studies found ACS in 10% of patients, and an estimated sensitivity of CTA for ACS of 95%, specificity of 87%, yielding a negative likelihood ratio (LR) of 0.06 and positive LR of 7.4. A study that examined the prognostic implications of nonobstructing coronary artery disease determined by CTA during acute chest pain found a low incidence of major adverse cardiac events (0.6% vs 1.3%, for the normal and nonobstructive groups, respectively, $P = 0.2$). Multidetector CTA enables diagnosis (or exclusion) of coronary artery disease, ACS, and pulmonary emboli (so-called "triple rule-out") but involves both radiation and contrast exposure. Helical CT is the study of choice at most centers for the diagnosis of aortic dissection as well as for esophageal perforation.

In the evaluation of pulmonary embolism, diagnostic test decisions and results must be interpreted in the context of the clinical likelihood of VTE. A negative D-dimer test is helpful for excluding pulmonary embolism in patients with low clinical probability of VTE (3-month incidence = 0.5%); however, the 3-month risk of VTE among patients with intermediate and high risk of VTE is sufficiently high in the setting of a negative D-dimer test (3.5% and 21.4%, respectively) to warrant further imaging given the life-threatening nature of this condition if left untreated. CT angiography (with helical or multidetector CT imaging) has replaced ventilation-perfusion scanning as the preferred initial diagnostic test, having approximately 90–95% sensitivity and 95% specificity for detecting pulmonary embolism (compared with pulmonary angiography). However, for patients with high clinical probability of VTE, lower extremity ultrasound or pulmonary angiogram may be indicated even with a normal helical CT.

Panic disorder is a common cause of chest pain, accounting for up to 25% of cases that present to emergency departments and a higher proportion of cases presenting in primary care office practices. Features that correlate with an increased likelihood of panic disorder include absence of coronary artery disease, atypical quality of chest pain, female sex, younger age, and a high level of self-reported anxiety.

▶ Treatment

Treatment of chest pain should be guided by the underlying etiology. The term "noncardiac chest pain" is used to describe patients who evade diagnosis after receiving extensive work-up. Almost half reported symptom improvement with high-dose proton-pump inhibitor therapy. A systematic review found modest benefit of antidepressants in reducing noncardiac chest pain and a meta-analysis of 15 trials suggested modest to moderate benefit for psychological (especially cognitive-behavioral) interventions. Hypnotherapy may have some benefit.

▶ When to Refer

- Refer patients with poorly controlled, noncardiac chest pain to a pain specialist.
- Refer patients with sickle cell anemia to a hematologist.

▶ When to Admit

- Failure to adequately exclude (to a sufficient degree) life-threatening causes of chest pain, particularly myocardial infarction, dissecting aortic aneurysm, pulmonary embolism, and esophageal rupture.
- Pain control for rib fracture that impairs gas exchange.

Beigel R et al. Prognostic implications of nonobstructive coronary artery disease in patients undergoing coronary computed tomographic angiography for acute chest pain. Am J Cardiol. 2013 Apr 1;111(7):941–5. [PMID: 23332596]

Diercks DB et al. Diagnostic accuracy of a point-of-care troponin I assay for acute myocardial infarction within 3 hours after presentation in early presenters to the emergency department with chest pain. Am Heart J. 2012 Jan;163(1):74–80.e4. [PMID: 22172439]

Geersing GJ et al. Excluding venous thromboembolism using point of care D-dimer tests in outpatients: a diagnostic meta-analysis. BMJ. 2009 Aug 14;339:b2990. [PMID: 19684102]

Goldstein JA et al; CT-STAT Investigators. The CT-STAT (Coronary Computed Tomographic Angiography for Systematic Triage of Acute Chest Pain Patients to Treatment) trial. J Am Coll Cardiol. 2011 Sep 27;58(14):1414–22. [PMID: 21939822]

Hoffmann U et al; ROMICAT-II Investigators. Coronary CT angiography versus standard evaluation in acute chest pain. N Engl J Med. 2012 Jul 26;367(4):299–308. [PMID: 22830462]

Holly J et al. Prospective evaluation of the use of the thrombolysis in myocardial infarction score as a risk stratification tool for chest pain patients admitted to an ED observation unit. Am J Emerg Med. 2013 Jan;31(1):185–9. [PMID: 22944539]

Kisely SR et al. Psychological interventions for symptomatic management of non-specific chest pain in patients with normal coronary anatomy. Cochrane Database Syst Rev. 2012 Jun 13;6:CD004101. [PMID: 22696339]

Kosowsky JM. Approach to the ED patient with "low risk" chest pain. Emerg Med Clin North Am. 2011 Nov;29(4):721–7. [PMID: 22040703]

McConaghy JR et al. Outpatient diagnosis of acute chest pain in adults. Am Fam Physician. 2013 Feb 1;87(3):177–82. [PMID: 23418761]

Mills NL et al. Implementation of a sensitive troponin I assay and risk of recurrent myocardial infarction and death in patients with suspected acute coronary syndrome. JAMA. 2011 Mar 23;305(12):1210–6. [PMID: 21427373]

Nguyen TM et al. Systematic review: the treatment of noncardiac chest pain with antidepressants. Aliment Pharmacol Ther. 2012 Mar;35(5):493–500. [PMID: 22239853]

Ranasinghe AM et al. Acute aortic dissection. BMJ. 2011 Jul 29;343:d4487. [PMID: 21803810]

Rogers IS et al. Usefulness of comprehensive cardiothoracic computed tomography in the evaluation of acute undifferentiated chest discomfort in the emergency department (CAPTURE). Am J Cardiol. 2011 Mar 1;107(5):643–50. [PMID: 21247533]

Scheuermeyer FX et al. Safety and efficiency of a chest pain diagnostic algorithm with selective outpatient stress testing for emergency department patients with potential ischemic chest pain. Ann Emerg Med. 2012 Apr;59(4):256–64. [PMID: 22221842]

Than M et al. 2-Hour accelerated diagnostic protocol to assess patients with chest pain symptoms using contemporary troponins as the only biomarker: the ADAPT trial. J Am Coll Cardiol. 2012 Jun 5;59(23):2091–8. [PMID: 22578923]

Yoon YE et al. Evaluation of acute chest pain in the emergency department: "triple rule-out" computed tomography angiography. Cardiol Rev. 2011 May–Jun;19(3):115–21. [PMID: 21464639]

PALPITATIONS

ESSENTIAL INQUIRIES

- ▶ Forceful, rapid, or irregular beating of the heart.
- ▶ Rate, duration, and degree of regularity of heart beat; age at first episode.
- ▶ Factors that precipitate or terminate episodes.
- ▶ Light-headedness or syncope; neck pounding.
- ▶ Chest pain.

▶ General Considerations

Palpitations are defined as an unpleasant awareness of the forceful, rapid, or irregular beating of the heart. They are the primary symptom for approximately 16% of patients presenting to an outpatient clinic with a cardiac complaint. While palpitations are usually benign, they are occasionally the symptom of a life-threatening arrhythmia. To avoid

Table 2–6. Palpitations: Patients at high risk for a cardiovascular cause.

Historical risk factors
Family history of significant arrhythmias
Personal or family history of syncope or resuscitated sudden death
History of myocardial infarction (and likely scarred myocardium)
Physical examination findings
Structural heart disease such as dilated or hypertrophic cardiomyopathies
Valvular disease (stenotic or regurgitant)
ECG findings
Long QT syndrome
Bradycardia
Second- or third-degree heart block
Sustained ventricular arrhythmias

missing a dangerous cause of the patient's symptom, clinicians sometimes pursue expensive and invasive testing when a conservative diagnostic evaluation is sufficient. The converse is also true; in one study, 54% of patients with supraventricular tachycardia were initially wrongly diagnosed with panic, stress, or anxiety disorder. A disproportionate number of these misdiagnosed patients are women. Table 2–6 lists history, physical examination, and ECG findings suggesting a cardiovascular cause for the palpitations.

▶ Clinical Findings

A. Symptoms

Although described by patients in a myriad of ways, guiding the patient through a careful description of their palpitations may indicate a mechanism and narrow the differential diagnosis. Pertinent questions include the age at first episode; precipitants; and the rate, duration, and degree of regularity of the heart beat during the subjective palpitations. Palpitations lasting less than 5 minutes, and a family history of panic disorder reduce the likelihood of an arrhythmic cause (LR = 0.38 and LR = 0.26, respectively). To better understand the symptom, the examiner can ask the patient to "tap out" the rhythm with their fingers. The circumstances associated with onset and termination can also be helpful in determining the cause. Palpitations that start and stop abruptly suggest supraventricular or ventricular tachycardias. Termination of palpitations using vagal maneuvers (eg, Valsalva maneuver) suggests supraventricular tachycardia.

Three common descriptions of palpitations are (1) "flip-flopping" (or "stop and start"), often caused by premature contraction of the atrium or ventricle, with the perceived "stop" from the pause following the contraction, and the "start" from the subsequent forceful contraction; (2) rapid "fluttering in the chest," with regular "fluttering" suggesting supraventricular or ventricular arrhythmias (including sinus tachycardia) and irregular "fluttering" suggesting atrial fibrillation, atrial flutter, or tachycardia with variable block; and (3) "pounding in the neck" or neck pulsations, often due to "cannon" A waves in the jugular venous pulsations that occur when the right atrium contracts against a closed tricuspid valve.

Palpitations associated with chest pain suggests ischemic heart disease, or if the chest pain is relieved by leaning forward, pericardial disease is suspected. Palpitations associated with light-headedness, presyncope, or syncope suggest hypotension and may signify a life-threatening cardiac arrhythmia. Palpitations that occur regularly with exertion suggests a rate-dependent bypass tract or hypertrophic cardiomyopathy. If a benign etiology for these concerning symptoms cannot be ascertained at the initial visit, then ambulatory monitoring or prolonged cardiac monitoring in the hospital might be warranted.

Noncardiac symptoms should also be elicited since the palpitations may be caused by a normal heart responding to a metabolic or inflammatory condition. Weight loss suggests hyperthyroidism. Palpitations can be precipitated by vomiting or diarrhea that leads to electrolyte disorders and hypovolemia. Hyperventilation, hand tingling, and nervousness are common when anxiety or panic disorder is the cause of the palpitations.

B. Physical Examination

Rarely does the clinician have the opportunity to examine a patient during an episode of palpitations. However, careful cardiovascular examination can find abnormalities that can increase the likelihood of specific cardiac arrhythmias. The midsystolic click of mitral valve prolapse can suggest the diagnosis of a supraventricular arrhythmia. The harsh holosystolic murmur of hypertrophic cardiomyopathy, which occurs along the left sternal border and increases with the Valsalva maneuver, suggests atrial fibrillation or ventricular tachycardia. The presence of dilated cardiomyopathy, suggested on examination by a displaced and enlarged cardiac point-of-maximal impulse, increases the likelihood of ventricular tachycardia and atrial fibrillation. In patients with chronic atrial fibrillation, in-office exercise (eg, a brisk walk in the hallway) may reveal an intermittent accelerated ventricular response as the cause of the palpitations. The clinician should also look for signs of hyperthyroidism (eg, tremulousness, brisk deep tendon reflexes, or fine hand tremor), or signs of stimulant drug use (eg, dilated pupils or skin or nasal septal lesions). Visible neck pulsations (LR, 2.68; 95% CI, 1.25–5.78) in association with palpitations increases the likelihood of atrioventricular nodal reentry tachycardia.

C. Diagnostic Studies

Commonly used studies in the initial evaluation of a patient with palpitations are the 12-lead ECG and ambulatory ECG monitoring devices (eg, the Holter monitor or the event recorder).

A 12-lead ECG should be performed on all patients reporting palpitations because it can provide evidence for a wide variety of causes. Although in most instances a specific arrhythmia will not be detected on the tracing, a careful evaluation of the ECG can help the clinician deduce a likely etiology in certain circumstances.

For instance, bradyarrhythmias and heart block can be associated with ventricular ectopy or escape beats that may

be experienced as palpitations by the patient. Evidence of prior myocardial infarction by history or on ECG (eg, Q waves) increases the patient's risk for nonsustained or sustained ventricular tachycardia. Ventricular preexcitation (Wolff-Parkinson-White syndrome) is suggested by a short PR interval (< 0.20 ms) and delta waves (upsloping PR segments). Left ventricular hypertrophy with deep septal Q waves in I, AVL, and V4 through V6 is seen in patients with hypertrophic obstructive cardiomyopathy. The presence of left atrial enlargement as suggested by a terminal P-wave force in V1 more negative than 0.04 msec and notched in lead II reflects a patient at increased risk for atrial fibrillation. A prolonged QT interval and abnormal T-wave morphology suggests the long-QT syndrome, which puts patients at increased risk for ventricular tachycardia.

For high-risk patients (Table 2–6), further diagnostic studies are warranted. A step-wise approach has been suggested—starting with ambulatory monitoring devices (Holter monitoring if the palpitations are expected to occur within the subsequent 72-hour period, event monitoring if less frequent), followed by invasive electrophysiologic testing if the ambulatory monitor records a worrisome arrhythmia or if serious arrhythmias are strongly suspected despite normal findings on the appropriate ambulatory monitor.

In patients with a prior myocardial infarction, ambulatory cardiac monitoring or signal-averaged-ECG are appropriate next steps to assess ventricular tachycardia. ECG exercise testing is appropriate in patients who have palpitations with physical exertion and patients with suspected coronary artery disease. Echocardiography is useful when physical examination or ECG suggests structural abnormalities or decreased ventricular function.

▶ Differential Diagnosis

When assessing a patient with palpitations in an urgent care setting, the clinician must ascertain whether the symptoms represent (1) an arrhythmia that is minor and transient, (2) significant cardiovascular disease, (3) a cardiac manifestation of a systemic disease such as thyrotoxicosis, or (4) a benign somatic symptom that is amplified by underlying psychosocial characteristics of the patient.

Palpitations in patients with a known history of cardiac disease or palpitations that occur during sleep increase the likelihood of a cardiac arrhythmia. A history of panic disorder or palpitations that last less than 5 minutes make a cardiac arrhythmia slightly less likely. Patients who seek medical attention in the emergency department instead of a medical clinic are more likely to have a cardiac etiology (47% versus 21%), whereas psychiatric causes are more common among patients with palpitations who seek medical attention in office practices (45% versus 27%). In a study of patients who went to a university medical clinic with the chief complaint of palpitations, etiologies were cardiac in 43%, psychiatric in 31%, and miscellaneous in 10% (including illicit drugs, medications, anemia, thyrotoxicosis, and mastocytosis).

Cardiac arrhythmias that can result in symptoms of palpitations include sinus bradycardia; sinus, supraventricular, and ventricular tachycardia; premature ventricular and atrial contractions; sick sinus syndrome; and advanced atrioventricular block.

Nonarrhythmic cardiac causes of palpitations include valvular heart diseases, such as aortic insufficiency or stenosis, atrial or ventricular septal defect, cardiomyopathy, congenital heart disease, and pericarditis.

Noncardiac causes of palpitations include fever, dehydration, hypoglycemia, anemia, thyrotoxicosis, and pheochromocytoma. Drugs such as cocaine, alcohol, caffeine, and pseudoephedrine can precipitate palpitations, as can prescription medications, including digoxin, phenothiazines, theophylline, and beta-agonists.

The most common psychiatric causes of palpitations are anxiety and panic disorder. The release of catecholamines during a panic attack or significant stress can trigger an arrhythmia. Asking a single question, "Have you experienced brief periods, for seconds or minutes, of an overwhelming panic or terror that was accompanied by racing heartbeats, shortness of breath, or dizziness?" can help identify patients with panic disorder.

▶ Treatment

After ambulatory monitoring, most patients with palpitations are found to have benign atrial or ventricular ectopy and nonsustained ventricular tachycardia. In patients with structurally normal hearts, these arrhythmias are not associated with adverse outcomes. Abstention from caffeine and tobacco may help. Often, reassurance suffices. If not, or in very symptomatic patients, a trial of a beta-blocker may be prescribed. A three-session course of cognitive behavioral therapy that includes some physical activity has proven effective for patients with benign palpitations with or without chest pain. For treatment of specific atrial or ventricular arrhythmias, see Chapter 10.

▶ When to Refer

• For electrophysiologic studies.
• For advice regarding treatment of atrial or ventricular arrhythmias.

▶ When to Admit

• Palpitations associated with syncope or near-syncope, particularly when the patient is aged 75 years or older and has an abnormal ECG, hematocrit < 30%, shortness of breath, respiratory rate > 24/min, or a history of HF.
• Patients with risk factors for a serious arrhythmia.

Indik JH. When palpitations worsen. Am J Med. 2010 Jun;123(6):517–9. [PMID: 20569756]
Jamshed N et al. Emergency management of palpitations in the elderly: epidemiology, diagnostic approaches, and therapeutic options. Clin Geriatr Med. 2013 Feb;29(1):205–30. [PMID: 23177608]
Jellins J et al. Brugada syndrome. Hong Kong Med J. 2013 Apr;19(2):159–67. [PMID: 23535677]
Jonsbu E et al. Short-term cognitive behavioral therapy for non-cardiac chest pain and benign palpitations: a randomized controlled trial. J Psychosom Res. 2011 Feb;70(2):117–23. [PMID: 21262413]

Misiri J et al. Evaluation of syncope and palpitations in women. J Womens Health (Larchmt). 2011 Oct;20(10):1505–15. [PMID: 21819232]
Thavendiranathan P et al. Does this patient with palpitations have a cardiac arrhythmia? JAMA. 2009 Nov 18;302(19):2135–43. [PMID: 19920238]
Vallès E et al. Diagnostic and prognostic value of electrophysiologic study in patients with nondocumented palpitations. Am J Cardiol. 2011 May 1;107(9):1333–7. [PMID: 21371684]
Wexler RK et al. Outpatient approach to palpitations. Am Fam Physician. 2011 Jul 1;84(1):63–9. [PMID: 21766757]

LOWER EXTREMITY EDEMA

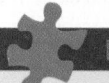

ESSENTIAL INQUIRIES

▶ History of venous thromboembolism.
▶ Symmetry of swelling.
▶ Pain.
▶ Change with dependence.
▶ Skin findings: hyperpigmentation, stasis dermatitis, lipodermatosclerosis, atrophie blanche, ulceration.

▶ General Considerations

Acute and chronic lower extremity edema present important diagnostic and treatment challenges. Lower extremities can swell in response to increased venous or lymphatic pressures, decreased intravascular oncotic pressure, increased capillary leak, and local injury or infection. **Chronic venous insufficiency** is by far the most common cause, affecting up to 2% of the population, and the incidence of venous insufficiency has not changed during the past 25 years. Venous insufficiency is a common complication of DVT; however, only a small number of patients with chronic venous insufficiency report a history of this disorder. Venous ulceration commonly affects patients with chronic venous insufficiency, and its management is labor-intensive and expensive. Other causes of lower extremity edema include cellulitis, musculoskeletal disorders (Baker cyst rupture, gastrocnemius tear or rupture), lymphedema, HF, cirrhosis, nephrotic syndrome, and medication side effects (eg, calcium channel blockers, minoxidil, or pioglitazone).

▶ Clinical Findings

A. Symptoms and Signs

Normal lower extremity venous pressure (in the erect position: 80 mm Hg in deep veins, 20–30 mm Hg in superficial veins) and cephalad venous blood flow require competent bicuspid venous valves, effective muscle contractions, and normal respirations. When one or more of these components fail, venous hypertension may result. Chronic exposure to elevated venous pressure by the postcapillary venules in the legs leads to leakage of fibrinogen and growth factors into the interstitial space, leukocyte aggregation and activation, and obliteration of the cutaneous lymphatic network. These changes account for the brawny, fibrotic skin changes observed in patients with chronic venous insufficiency, and the predisposition toward skin ulceration, particularly in the medial malleolar area.

Among common causes of lower extremity swelling, DVT is the most life-threatening. Clues suggesting DVT include a history of cancer, recent limb immobilization, or confinement to bed for at least 3 days following major surgery within the past month (Table 2–7). A search for alternative explanations is equally important in excluding DVT. Bilateral involvement and significant improvement upon awakening favor systemic causes (eg, venous insufficiency, HF, and cirrhosis). The sensation of "heavy legs" is the most frequent symptom of chronic venous insufficiency, followed by itching. Pain, particularly if severe, is uncommon in uncomplicated venous insufficiency. Lower extremity swelling and inflammation in a limb recently affected by DVT could represent anticoagulation failure and thrombus recurrence but more often are caused by **postphlebitic syndrome** with valvular incompetence. Other causes of a painful, swollen calf include ruptured popliteal cyst ("pseudothrombophlebitis"), calf strain or trauma, and cellulitis.

Lower extremity swelling is a familiar complication of therapy with calcium channel blockers (particularly felodipine and amlodipine), pioglitazone, and minoxidil. Bilateral lower extremity edema can be a presenting symptom of nephrotic syndrome or volume overload caused by renal failure or cirrhosis. Prolonged airline flights (> 10 hours)

are associated with edema. In addition, among those with low to medium risk of thromboembolism (eg, women taking oral contraceptives), long flights are associated with a 2% incidence of asymptomatic popliteal DVT.

B. Physical Examination

Physical examination should include assessment of the heart, lungs, and abdomen for evidence of pulmonary hypertension (primary, or secondary to chronic lung disease), HF, or cirrhosis. Some patients with cirrhosis have pulmonary hypertension without lung disease. There is a spectrum of skin findings related to chronic venous insufficiency that depends on the severity and chronicity of the disease, ranging from hyperpigmentation and stasis dermatitis to abnormalities highly specific for chronic venous insufficiency: lipodermatosclerosis (thick brawny skin; in advanced cases, the lower leg resembles an inverted champagne bottle) and atrophie blanche (small depigmented macules within areas of heavy pigmentation). The size of both calves should be measured 10 cm below the tibial tuberosity and elicitation of pitting and tenderness performed. Swelling of the entire leg or swelling of one leg 3 cm more than the other suggests deep venous obstruction. It is normal for the left calf to be slightly larger than the right as a result of the left common iliac vein coursing under the aorta.

An ulcer located over the medial malleolus is a hallmark of chronic venous insufficiency but can be due to other causes. Shallow, large, modestly painful ulcers are characteristic of venous insufficiency, whereas small, deep, and more painful ulcers are more apt to be due to arterial insufficiency, vasculitis, or infection (including cutaneous diphtheria). Diabetic vascular ulcers, however, may be painless. When an ulcer is on the foot or above the mid calf, causes other than venous insufficiency should be considered.

C. Diagnostic Studies

Most causes of lower extremity swelling can be demonstrated with color duplex ultrasonography. Patients without an obvious cause of acute lower extremity swelling (eg, calf strain) should have an ultrasound performed, since DVT is difficult to exclude on clinical grounds. A predictive rule allows a clinician to exclude a lower extremity DVT in patients without an ultrasound if the patient has low pretest probability for DVT and has a negative sensitive D-dimer test (the "Wells prediction rule"). Assessment of the ankle-brachial pressure index (ABPI) is important in the management of chronic venous insufficiency, since peripheral arterial disease may be exacerbated by compression therapy. This can be performed at the same time as ultrasound. Caution is required in interpreting the results of ABPI in older patients and diabetics due to decreased compressibility of their arteries. A dipstick urine test that is strongly positive for protein can suggest nephrotic syndrome, and a serum creatinine can help estimate kidney function.

▶ Treatment

Treatment of lower extremity edema should be guided by the underlying etiology. See relevant chapters for treatment of edema in patients with HF (see Chapter 10), nephrosis

Table 2–7. Risk stratification of adults referred for ultrasound to rule out DVT.

Step 1: Calculate risk factor score
Score 1 point for each
Untreated malignancy
Paralysis, paresis, or recent plaster immobilization
Recently bedridden for > 3 days due to major surgery within 4 weeks
Localized tenderness along distribution of deep venous system
Entire leg swelling
Swelling of one calf > 3 cm more than the other (measured 10 cm below tibial tuberosity)
Ipsilateral pitting edema
Collateral superficial (nonvaricose) veins
Previously documented DVT
Alternative diagnosis as likely as or more likely than DVT: subtract 2 points

Step 2: Obtain ultrasound		
Score	Ultrasound Positive	Ultrasound Negative
≤ 0	Confirm with venogram	DVT ruled out
1–2	Treat for DVT	Repeat ultrasound in 3–7 days
≥ 3	Treat for DVT	Confirm with venogram

DVT, deep venous thrombosis.

(see Chapter 22), cirrhosis (see Chapter 16), and lymphedema (see Chapter 12). Edema resulting from calcium channel blocker therapy responds to concomitant therapy with ACE inhibitors or angiotensin receptor blockers.

In patients with chronic venous insufficiency without a comorbid volume overload state (eg, HF), it is best to avoid diuretic therapy. These patients have relatively decreased intravascular volume, and administration of diuretics may first enhance sodium retention through increased secretion of renin and angiotensin and then result in acute kidney injury and oliguria. Instead, the most effective treatment involves (1) leg elevation, above the level of the heart, for 30 minutes three to four times daily, and during sleep; (2) compression therapy; and (3) ambulatory exercise to increase venous return through calf muscle contractions. A wide variety of stockings and devices are effective in decreasing swelling and preventing ulcer formation. They should be put on with awakening, before hydrostatic forces result in edema. To control simple edema, 20–30 mm Hg is usually sufficient; whereas, 30–40 mm Hg is usually required to control moderate to severe edema associated with ulcer formation. Patients with decreased ABPI should be managed in concert with a vascular surgeon. Compression stockings (12–18 mm Hg at the ankle) are effective in preventing edema and asymptomatic thrombosis associated with long airline flights in low- to medium-risk persons. For lymphedema, new bandaging systems applied twice weekly can be effective. See Chapter 12 for treatment of venous stasis ulcers.

▶ When to Refer

- Chronic lower extremity ulcerations requiring specialist wound care.
- Refer patients with nephrotic syndrome to a nephrologist.
- Refer patients with coexisting severe arterial insufficiency (claudication) that would complicate treatment with compression stockings to a vascular surgeon.

▶ When to Admit

- Pending definitive diagnosis in patients at high risk for DVT despite normal lower extremity ultrasound.
- Severe, acute swelling raising concern for an impending compartment syndrome.
- Severe edema that impairs ability to ambulate or perform activities of daily living.

Hamdan A. Management of varicose veins and venous insufficiency. JAMA. 2012 Dec 26;308(24):2612–21. [PMID: 23268520]

Moffatt CJ et al. A preliminary randomized controlled study to determine the application frequency of a new lymphoedema bandaging system. Br J Dermatol. 2012 Mar;166(3):624–32. [PMID: 22059933]

Partsch H et al. Dose finding for an optimal compression pressure to reduce chronic edema of the extremities. Int Angiol. 2011 Dec;30(6):527–33. [PMID: 22233613]

Word R. Medical and surgical therapy for advanced chronic venous insufficiency. Surg Clin North Am. 2010 Dec;90(6):1195–214. [PMID: 21074036]

FEVER & HYPERTHERMIA

ESSENTIAL INQUIRIES

- ▶ Age; injection substance use.
- ▶ Localizing symptoms; weight loss; joint pain.
- ▶ Immunosuppression or neutropenia; history of cancer.
- ▶ Medications.
- ▶ Travel.

▶ General Considerations

The average normal oral body temperature taken in midmorning is 36.7°C (range 36–37.4°C). This range includes a mean and 2 standard deviations, thus encompassing 95% of a normal population (normal diurnal temperature variation is 0.5–1°C). The normal rectal or vaginal temperature is 0.5°C higher than the oral temperature, and the axillary temperature is 0.5°C lower. Rectal temperature is more reliable than oral temperature, particularly in patients who breathe through their mouth or in tachypneic states.

Fever is a regulated rise to a new "set point" of body temperature. When stimuli act on monocyte-macrophages, these cells elaborate pyrogenic cytokines, causing elevation of the set point through effects in the hypothalamus. These cytokines include interleukin-1 (IL-1), tumor necrosis factor (TNF), interferon-gamma, and interleukin-6 (IL-6). The elevation in temperature results from either increased heat production (eg, shivering) or decreased heat loss (eg, peripheral vasoconstriction). Body temperature in cytokine-induced fever seldom exceeds 41.1°C unless there is structural damage to hypothalamic regulatory centers.

▶ Clinical Findings

A. Fever

Fever as a symptom provides important information about the presence of illness—particularly infections—and about changes in the clinical status of the patient. The fever pattern, however, is of marginal value for most specific diagnoses except for the relapsing fever of malaria, borreliosis, and occasional cases of lymphoma, especially Hodgkin disease. Furthermore, the degree of temperature elevation does not necessarily correspond to the severity of the illness. In general, the febrile response tends to be greater in children than in adults. In older persons, neonates, and in persons receiving certain medications (eg, NSAIDs or corticosteroids), a normal temperature or even hypothermia may be observed. Markedly elevated body temperature may result in profound metabolic disturbances. High temperature during the first trimester of pregnancy may cause birth defects, such as anencephaly. Fever increases insulin requirements and alters the metabolism and disposition of drugs used for the treatment of the diverse diseases associated with fever.

B. Hyperthermia

Hyperthermia—not mediated by cytokines—occurs when body metabolic heat production or environmental heat load exceeds normal heat loss capacity or when there is impaired heat loss; heat stroke is an example. Body temperature may rise to levels (> 41.1°C) capable of producing irreversible protein denaturation and resultant brain damage; no diurnal variation is observed.

Neuroleptic malignant syndrome is a rare and potentially lethal idiosyncratic reaction to neuroleptic medications, particularly haloperidol and fluphenazine; however, it has also been reported with the atypical neuroleptics (such as olanzapine or risperidone) (see Chapter 25). Serotonin syndrome resembles neuroleptics malignant syndrome but occurs within hours of ingestion of agents that increase levels of serotonin in the central nervous system, including serotonin reuptake inhibitors, monoamine oxidase inhibitors, tricyclic antidepressants, meperidine, dextromethorphan, bromocriptine, tramadol, lithium, and psychostimulants (such as cocaine, methamphetamine, and MDMA) (see Chapter 38). Clonus and hyperreflexia are more common in serotonin syndrome, whereas "lead pipe" rigidity is more common in neuroleptic malignant syndrome. Neuroleptic malignant and serotonin syndromes share common clinical and pathophysiologic features to malignant hyperthermia of anesthesia (see Chapter 38).

C. Fever of Undetermined Origin

See Fever of Unknown Origin, Chapter 30.

▶ Treatment

Most fever is well tolerated. When the temperature is > 40°C, symptomatic treatment may be required. A temperature > 41°C is likely to be hyperthermia and thus not cytokine mediated, and emergent management is indicated. (See Heat Stroke, Chapter 37.)

A. General Measures for Removal of Heat

Regardless of the cause of the fever, alcohol sponges, cold sponges, ice bags, ice-water enemas, and ice baths will lower body temperature (see Chapter 37). They are more useful in hyperthermia, since patients with cytokine-related fever will attempt to override these therapies.

B. Pharmacologic Treatment of Fever

1. Antipyretic drugs—Antipyretic therapy is not needed except for patients with marginal hemodynamic status. Aspirin or acetaminophen, 325–650 mg every 4 hours, is effective in reducing fever. These drugs are best administered around-the-clock rather than as needed, since "as needed" dosing results in periodic chills and sweats due to fluctuations in temperature caused by varying levels of drug.

2. Antimicrobial therapy—Antibacterial and antifungal prophylactic regimens are only recommended for patients expected to have < 100 neutrophils/mcL for more than 7 days, unless other factors increase risks for complications or mortality. In most febrile patients, empiric antibiotic therapy should be deferred pending further evaluation. However, empiric antibiotic therapy is sometimes warranted. Prompt broad-spectrum antimicrobials are indicated for febrile patients who are clinically unstable, even before infection can be documented. These include patients with hemodynamic instability, those with neutropenia (neutrophils < 500/mcL), others who are asplenic (surgically or secondary to sickle cell disease) or immunosuppressed (including individuals taking systemic corticosteroids, azathioprine, cyclosporine, or other immunosuppressive medications) (Tables 30–4 and 30–5), and those who are HIV infected (see Chapter 31).

Inpatient treatment is standard to manage febrile neutropenic episodes, although carefully selected patients may be managed as outpatients after systematic assessment beginning with a validated risk index (eg, Multinational Association for Supportive Care in Cancer [MASCC] score or Talcott rules). Patients with MASCC scores ≥ 21 or in Talcott group 4, and without other risk factors, can be managed safely as outpatients. Febrile neutropenic patients should receive initial doses of empiric antibacterial therapy within an hour of triage and should either be monitored for at least 4 hours to determine suitability for outpatient management or be admitted to the hospital.

The carefully selected outpatients determined to be at low risk by the MASCC score or Talcott rules can be managed with an oral fluoroquinolone plus amoxicillin/clavulanate (or clindamycin, if penicillin allergic), unless fluoroquinolone prophylaxis was used before fever developed. For treatment of fever during neutropenia following chemotherapy, outpatient parenteral antimicrobial therapy can be provided effectively and safely (in low-risk patients) with a single agent such as cefepime, piperacillin/tazobactam, imipenem, meropenem or doripenem; or (in high-risk patients) with a combination of agents such as an aminoglycoside *plus* one of the following agents: piperacillin/tazobactam, cefepime (or ceftazidime), imipenem, meropenem (or doripenem); *or* vancomycin *plus* one of the following: piperacillin/tazobactam, cefepime (or ceftazidime), imipenem, meropenem, aztreonam *and* an aminoglycoside, or ciprofloxacin *and* an aminoglycoside. If a fungal infection is suspected in patients with prolonged fever and neutropenia, fluconazole is an equally effective but less toxic alternative to amphotericin B.

C. Treatment of Hyperthermia

Discontinuation of the offending agent is mandatory. Treatment of neuroleptic malignant syndrome includes dantrolene in combination with bromocriptine or levodopa (see Chapter 25). Treatment of serotonin syndrome includes administration of a central serotonin receptor antagonist—cyproheptadine or chlorpromazine—alone or in combination with a benzodiazepine (see Chapter 38). In patients for whom it is difficult to distinguish which syndrome is present, treatment with a benzodiazepine may be the safest therapeutic option.

▶ When to Admit

- Neuroleptic malignant syndrome; serotonin syndrome; malignant hyperthermia of anesthesia.
- Heat stroke.
- For measures to control temperature when it is > 41°C or when associated with seizure or other mental status changes.

Affronti M et al. Low-grade fever: how to distinguish organic from non-organic forms. Int J Clin Pract. 2010 Feb;64(3): 316–21. [PMID: 20456171]

Coburn B et al. Does this adult patient with suspected bacteremia require blood cultures? JAMA. 2012 Aug 1;308(5): 502–11. [PMID: 22851117]

Flowers CR et al. Antimicrobial prophylaxis and outpatient management of fever and neutropenia in adults treated for malignancy: American Society of Clinical Oncology clinical practice guideline. J Clin Oncol. 2013 Feb 20;31(6):794–810. [PMID: 23319691]

Kim YJ et al. Diagnostic value of 18F-FDG PET/CT in patients with fever of unknown origin. Intern Med J. 2012 Jul;42(7):834–7. [PMID: 22805689]

Worth LJ et al; Australian Consensus Guidelines 2011 Steering Committee. Use of risk stratification to guide ambulatory management of neutropenic fever. Intern Med J. 2011 Jan;41(1b):82–9. [PMID: 21272172]

INVOLUNTARY WEIGHT LOSS

ESSENTIAL INQUIRIES

- ▶ Age; caloric intake; secondary confirmation (eg, changes in clothing size).
- ▶ Fever; change in bowel habits.
- ▶ Substance use.
- ▶ Age-appropriate cancer screening history.

▶ General Considerations

Body weight is determined by a person's caloric intake, absorptive capacity, metabolic rate, and energy losses. Body weight normally peaks by the fifth or sixth decade and then gradually declines at a rate of 1–2 kg per decade. In NHANES II, a national survey of community-dwelling elders (age 50–80 years), recent involuntary weight loss (> 5% usual body weight) was reported by 7% of respondents, and this was associated with a 24% higher mortality.

▶ Etiology

Involuntary weight loss is regarded as clinically significant when it exceeds 5% or more of usual body weight over a 6- to 12-month period. It often indicates serious physical or psychological illness. Physical causes are usually evident during the initial evaluation. The most common causes are cancer (about 30%), gastrointestinal disorders (about 15%), and dementia or depression (about 15%). When an adequately nourished-appearing patient complains of weight loss, inquiry should be made about exact weight changes (with approximate dates) and about changes in clothing size. Family members can provide confirmation of weight loss, as can old documents such as driver's licenses. A mild, gradual weight loss occurs in some older individuals. However, rapid involuntary weight loss is predictive of morbidity and mortality. In addition to various disease states, causes in older individuals include loss of teeth and consequent difficulty with chewing, alcoholism, and social isolation.

▶ Clinical Findings

Once the weight loss is established, the history, medication profile, physical examination, and conventional laboratory and radiologic investigations (such as complete blood count, serologic tests including HIV, thyroid-stimulating hormone [TSH] level, urinalysis, fecal occult blood test, chest radiography, and upper gastrointestinal series) usually reveal the cause. When these tests are normal, the second phase of evaluation should focus on more definitive gastrointestinal investigation (eg, tests for malabsorption; endoscopy) and cancer screening (eg, Papanicolaou smear, mammography, prostate specific antigen [PSA]). A prospective case study in patients with unintentional weight loss showed that colonoscopy did not find colorectal cancer if weight loss was the sole indication for the test.

If the initial evaluation is unrevealing, follow-up is preferable to further diagnostic testing. Death at 2-year follow-up was not nearly as common in patients with unexplained involuntary weight loss (8%) as in those with weight loss due to malignant (79%) and established nonmalignant diseases (19%). Psychiatric consultation should be considered when there is evidence of depression, dementia, anorexia nervosa, or other emotional problems. Ultimately, in approximately 15–25% of cases, no cause for the weight loss can be found.

▶ Differential Diagnosis

Malignancy, gastrointestinal disorders (poorly fitting dentures, cavities, swallowing or malabsorption disorders, pancreatic insufficiency), psychological problems (dementia, depression, paranoia), endocrine disorders (hyperthyroidism, hypothyroidism, hyperparathyroidism, hypoadrenalism), eating problems (dietary restrictions, lack of money for food), social problems (alcoholism, and social isolation), and medication side effects are all established causes.

▶ Treatment

Weight stabilization occurs in most surviving patients with both established and unknown causes of weight loss through treatment of the underlying disorder and caloric supplementation. Nutrient intake goals are established in relation to the severity of weight loss, in general ranging from 30 to 40 kcal/kg/d. In order of preference, route of administration options include oral, temporary nasojejunal tube, or percutaneous gastric or jejunal tube. Parenteral nutrition is reserved for patients with serious associated problems. A variety of pharmacologic agents have been proposed for the treatment of weight loss. These can be categorized into appetite stimulants (corticosteroids, progestational agents, dronabinol, and serotonin antagonists); anabolic agents (growth hormone and testosterone derivatives); and anticatabolic agents (omega-3 fatty acids, pentoxifylline, hydrazine sulfate, and thalidomide).

▶ When to Refer

- Weight loss caused by malabsorption.
- Persistent nutritional deficiencies despite adequate supplementation.
- Weight loss as a result of anorexia or bulimia.

When to Admit

- Severe protein-energy malnutrition, including the syndromes of kwashiorkor and marasmus.
- Vitamin deficiency syndromes.
- Cachexia with anticipated progressive weight loss secondary to unmanageable psychiatric disease.
- To carefully manage electrolyte and fluid replacement in protein-energy malnutrition and avoid "re-feeding syndrome."

Chapman IM. Weight loss in older persons. Med Clin North Am. 2011 May;95(3):579–93. [PMID: 21549879]

Davis IJ et al. Unintentional weight loss as the sole indication for colonoscopy is rarely associated with colorectal cancer. J Am Board Fam Med. 2011 Mar–Apr;24(2):218–9. [PMID: 21383224]

Morley JE. Undernutrition in older adults. Fam Pract. 2012 Apr;29(Suppl 1):i89–i93. [PMID: 22399563]

Murphy RA et al. Nutritional intervention with fish oil provides a benefit over standard of care for weight and skeletal muscle mass in patients with nonsmall cell lung cancer receiving chemotherapy. Cancer. 2011 Apr 15;117(8):1775–82. [PMID: 21360698]

Schilp J et al. Early determinants for the development of undernutrition in an older general population: Longitudinal Aging Study Amsterdam. Br J Nutr. 2011 Sep;106(5):708–17. [PMID: 21450117]

Visvanathan R et al. Undernutrition and anorexia in the older person. Gastroenterol Clin North Am. 2009 Sep;38(3):393–409. [PMID: 19699404]

FATIGUE & CHRONIC FATIGUE SYNDROME

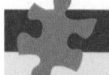

ESSENTIAL INQUIRIES

- ► Weight loss; fever.
- ► Sleep-disordered breathing.
- ► Medications; substance use.

General Considerations

Fatigue, as an isolated symptom, accounts for 1–3% of visits to generalists. The symptom of fatigue is often poorly described and less well defined by patients than symptoms associated with specific dysfunction of organ systems. Fatigue or lassitude and the closely related complaints of weakness, tiredness, and lethargy are often attributed to overexertion, poor physical conditioning, sleep disturbance, obesity, undernutrition, and emotional problems. A history of the patient's daily living and working habits may obviate the need for extensive and unproductive diagnostic studies.

Investigated causes of chronic fatigue syndrome include an occult retrovirus infection or an immune dysregulation mechanism, or both. Recent studies, however, have failed to show any differences in levels of xenotropic murine leukemia-virus-related virus in US patients with and without chronic fatigue syndrome. The diagnosis of chronic fatigue syndrome remains hotly debated because of the lack of a gold standard. Persons with chronic fatigue syndrome meeting specific criteria (such as those from the CDC) report a greater frequency of childhood trauma and psychopathology and demonstrate higher levels of emotional instability and self-reported stress than persons who do not have chronic fatigue. Neuropsychological and neuroendocrine studies reveal neurobiologic abnormalities in most patients, but none with a consistent pattern. A longitudinal MRI study showed that no abnormal patterns in rate and extent of brain atrophy, ventricle volume, white matter lesions, cerebral blood flow, or aqueductal cerebrospinal fluid flow were detected in the chronic fatigue syndrome population. Sleep disorders have been reported in 40–80% of patients with chronic fatigue syndrome, but their treatment has provided only modest benefit, suggesting that it is an effect rather than a cause of the fatigue. Veterans of the Gulf War show a tenfold greater incidence of chronic fatigue syndrome compared with nondeployed military personnel.

Clinical Findings

A. Fatigue

Clinically relevant fatigue is composed of three major components: generalized weakness (difficulty in initiating activities); easy fatigability (difficulty in completing activities); and mental fatigue (difficulty with concentration and memory). Important diseases that can cause fatigue include hyperthyroidism and hypothyroidism, HF, infections (endocarditis, hepatitis), COPD, sleep apnea, anemia, autoimmune disorders, irritable bowel syndrome, and cancer. Alcoholism, side effects from such drugs as sedatives, and beta-blockers may be the cause. Psychological conditions, such as insomnia, depression, anxiety, panic attacks, dysthmia, and somatization disorder, may cause fatigue. Common outpatient infectious causes include mononucleosis and sinusitis. These conditions are usually associated with other characteristic signs, but patients may emphasize fatigue and not reveal their other symptoms unless directly asked. The lifetime prevalence of significant fatigue (present for at least 2 weeks) is about 25%. Fatigue of unknown cause or related to psychiatric illness exceeds that due to physical illness, injury, medications, drugs, or alcohol.

B. Chronic Fatigue Syndrome

A working case definition of chronic fatigue syndrome indicates that it is not a homogeneous abnormality, and there is no single pathogenic mechanism (Figure 2–1). No physical finding or laboratory test can be used to confirm the diagnosis of this disorder.

The evaluation of chronic fatigue syndrome includes a history and physical examination as well as complete blood count, erythrocyte sedimentation rate, serum chemistries—blood urea nitrogen (BUN), electrolytes, glucose, creatinine, and calcium; liver and thyroid function tests—antinuclear antibody, urinalysis, and tuberculin skin test; and screening questionnaires for psychiatric disorders. Other tests to be performed as clinically indicated are serum cortisol, rheumatoid factor, immunoglobulin levels, Lyme serology in endemic areas, and HIV antibody. More extensive testing is usually unhelpful, including antibody to Epstein-Barr virus. There may be an abnormally high rate

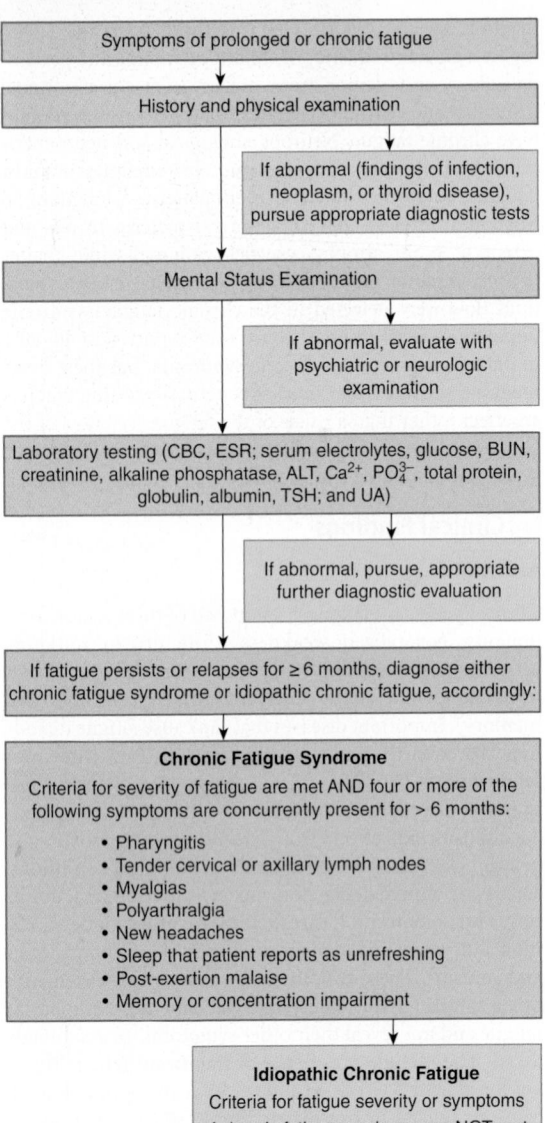

Symptoms of prolonged or chronic fatigue

↓

History and physical examination

↓

If abnormal (findings of infection, neoplasm, or thyroid disease), pursue appropriate diagnostic tests

↓

Mental Status Examination

↓

If abnormal, evaluate with psychiatric or neurologic examination

↓

Laboratory testing (CBC, ESR; serum electrolytes, glucose, BUN, creatinine, alkaline phosphatase, ALT, Ca^{2+}, PO_4^{3-}, total protein, globulin, albumin, TSH; and UA)

↓

If abnormal, pursue, appropriate further diagnostic evaluation

↓

If fatigue persists or relapses for ≥ 6 months, diagnose either chronic fatigue syndrome or idiopathic chronic fatigue, accordingly:

Chronic Fatigue Syndrome

Criteria for severity of fatigue are met AND four or more of the following symptoms are concurrently present for > 6 months:

- Pharyngitis
- Tender cervical or axillary lymph nodes
- Myalgias
- Polyarthralgia
- New headaches
- Sleep that patient reports as unrefreshing
- Post-exertion malaise
- Memory or concentration impairment

↓

Idiopathic Chronic Fatigue

Criteria for fatigue severity or symptoms of chronic fatigue syndrome are NOT met

▲ **Figure 2–1.** Classification of chronic fatigue patients. ALT, alanine aminotransferase; BUN, blood urea nitrogen; Ca^{2+}, calcium; CBC, complete blood count; ESR, erythrocyte sedimentation rate; PO_4^{3-}, phosphate; TSH, thyroid-stimulating hormone; UA, urinalysis.

of postural hypotension. MRI scans may show brain abnormalities on T_2-weighted images—chiefly small, punctate, subcortical white matter hyperintensities, predominantly in the frontal lobes, although a 2010 study found no such abnormalities. Brain MRI is not recommended in the routine evaluation of chronic fatigue syndrome.

▶ Treatment

A. Fatigue

Management of fatigue involves identification and treatment of conditions that contribute to fatigue, such as

cancer, pain, depression, disordered sleep, weight loss, and anemia. Resistance training and aerobic exercise lessens fatigue and improves performance for a number of chronic conditions associated with a high prevalence of fatigue, including HF, COPD, arthritis, and cancer. Continuous positive airway pressure is an effective treatment for obstructive sleep apnea. Psychostimulants such as methylphenidate have shown inconsistent results in randomized trials of treatment of cancer-related fatigue. Modafinil and armodafinil appear to be effective and well-tolerated in HIV-positive patients with fatigue and with depression.

B. Chronic Fatigue Syndrome

A variety of agents and modalities have been tried for the treatment of chronic fatigue syndrome. Acyclovir, intravenous immunoglobulin, nystatin, and low-dose hydrocortisone do not improve symptoms. Some patients with postural hypotension report response to increases in dietary sodium as well as fludrocortisone, 0.1 mg orally daily. In a phase III double-blind placebo-controlled randomized trial evaluating the experimental toll-like receptor 3-agonist rintatolimod, administered twice weekly intravenously to 243 cases of severe chronic fatigue syndrome, the patients receiving the rintatolimod were shown to improve exercise tolerance and reduce use of other medications; confirmation of these results is needed. There is a greater prevalence of past and current psychiatric diagnoses in patients with this syndrome. Affective disorders are especially common. Patients with chronic fatigue syndrome have benefited from a comprehensive multidisciplinary intervention, including optimal medical management, treating any ongoing affective or anxiety disorder pharmacologically, and implementing a comprehensive cognitive-behavioral treatment program. At present, cognitive-behavioral therapy and graded exercise are the treatments of choice for patients with chronic fatigue syndrome. **Cognitive-behavioral therapy,** a form of nonpharmacologic treatment emphasizing self-help and aiming to change perceptions and behaviors that may perpetuate symptoms and disability, is helpful. Although few patients are cured, the treatment effect is substantial. Response to cognitive-behavioral therapy is not predictable on the basis of severity or duration of chronic fatigue syndrome, although patients with low interest in psychotherapy rarely benefit. **Graded exercise** has also been shown to improve functional work capacity and physical function. A 2011 randomized trial (PACE trial) has confirmed the independent benefits of cognitive behavioral therapy and graded exercise, and found no benefit of adaptive pacing therapy.

In addition, the clinician's sympathetic listening and explanatory responses can help overcome the patient's frustrations and debilitation by this still mysterious illness. All patients should be encouraged to engage in normal activities to the extent possible and should be reassured that full recovery is eventually possible in most cases.

▶ When to Refer

- Infections not responsive to standard treatment.
- Difficult to control hyperthyroidism or hypothyroidism.
- Severe psychological disease.
- Malignancy.

When to Admit

- Failure to thrive.
- Fatigue severe enough to impair activities of daily living.

Kerr CW et al. Effects of methylphenidate on fatigue and depression: a randomized, double-blind, placebo-controlled trial. J Pain Symptom Manage. 2012 Jan;43(1):68–77. [PMID: 22208450]

Kitai E et al. Fatigue as a first-time presenting symptom: management by family doctors and one year follow-up. Isr Med Assoc J. 2012 Sep;14(9):555–9. [PMID: 23101419]

McMillan EM et al. Exercise is an effective treatment modality for reducing cancer-related fatigue and improving physical capacity in cancer patients and survivors: a meta-analysis. Appl Physiol Nutr Metab. 2011 Dec;36(6):892–903. [PMID: 22067010]

Perrin R et al. Longitudinal MRI shows no cerebral abnormality in chronic fatigue syndrome. Br J Radiol. 2010 May;83(989): 419–23. [PMID: 20223910]

Rabkin JG et al. Treatment of HIV-related fatigue with armodafinil: a placebo-controlled randomized trial. Psychosomatics. 2011 Jul–Aug;52(4):328–36. [PMID: 21777715]

Strayer DR et al; Chronic Fatigue Syndrome AMP-516 Study Group. A double-blind, placebo-controlled, randomized, clinical trial of the TLR-3 agonist rintatolimod in severe cases of chronic fatigue syndrome. PLoS One. 2012; 7(3):e31334. [PMID: 22431963]

White PD et al; PACE Trial Management Group. Comparison of adaptive pacing therapy, cognitive behaviour therapy, graded exercise therapy, and specialist medical care for chronic fatigue syndrome (PACE): a randomized trial. Lancet. 2011 Mar 5;377(9768):823–36. [PMID: 21334061]

Wiborg JF et al. Towards an evidence-based treatment model for cognitive behavioral interventions focusing on chronic fatigue syndrome. J Psychosom Res. 2012 May;72(5): 399–404. [PMID: 22469284]

ACUTE HEADACHE

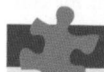

ESSENTIAL INQUIRIES

- Age > 50 years.
- Rapid onset and severe intensity (ie, "thunderclap" headache); trauma.
- Fever; vision changes.
- HIV infection.
- Current or past history of hypertension.
- Neurologic findings (mental status changes, motor or sensory deficits).

General Considerations

Headache is a common reason that adults seek medical care, accounting for approximately 13 million visits each year in the United States to physicians' offices, urgent care clinics, and emergency departments. A broad range of disorders can cause headache (see Chapter 24). This section deals only with acute nontraumatic headache in adolescents and adults. The challenge in the initial evaluation of acute headache is to identify which patients are presenting with an uncommon but life-threatening condition, approximately 1% of patients seeking care in emergency department settings and considerably less in office practice settings.

Diminution of headache in response to typical migraine therapies (such as serotonin receptor antagonists or ketorolac) does not rule out critical conditions such as subarachnoid hemorrhage or meningitis as the underlying cause.

Clinical Findings

A. Symptoms

A careful history and physical examination should aim to identify causes of acute headache that require immediate treatment. These causes can be broadly classified as imminent or completed **vascular events** (intracranial hemorrhage, thrombosis, vasculitis, malignant hypertension, arterial dissection, or aneurysm), **infections** (abscess, encephalitis, meningitis), **intracranial masses** causing intracranial hypertension, **preeclampsia,** and **carbon monoxide poisoning.** Having the patient carefully describe the onset of headache can be helpful in diagnosing a serious cause. Report of a sudden-onset headache that reaches maximal and severe intensity within seconds or a few minutes is the classic description of a "thunderclap" headache and should precipitate work-up for subarachnoid hemorrhage, since the estimated prevalence of subarachnoid hemorrhage in patients with "thunderclap" headache is 43%. Other historical features that raise the need for diagnostic testing include headache brought on by the Valsalva maneuver, cough, exertion, or sexual activity.

The general medical history can also guide the need for additional work-up. A new headache in a patient over the age of 50 or with a history of HIV disease under most circumstances (including a normal neurologic examination) warrants immediate neuroimaging (Table 2–8). When the patient has a medical history of hypertension—particularly uncontrolled hypertension—a complete

Table 2–8. Clinical features associated with acute headache that warrant urgent or emergent neuroimaging.

Prior to lumbar puncture
Abnormal neurologic examination
Abnormal mental status
Abnormal funduscopic examination (papilledema; loss of venous pulsations)
Meningeal signs
Emergent (conduct prior to leaving office or emergency department)
Abnormal neurologic examination
Abnormal mental status
"Thunderclap" headache
Urgent (scheduled prior to leaving office or emergency department)
HIV-positive patient[1]
Age > 50 years (normal neurologic examination)

[1]Use CT with or without contrast or MRI if HIV positive.
Source: American College of Emergency Physicians. Clinical Policy: critical issues in the evaluation and management of patients presenting to the emergency department with acute headache. Ann Emerg Med. 2002 Jan;39(1):108–22.

Table 2–9. Summary likelihood ratios (LRs) for individual clinical features associated with migraine diagnosis.

Clinical Feature	LR+ (95% CI)	LR– (95% CI)
Nausea	19 (15–25)	0.19 (0.18–0.20)
Photophobia	5.8 (5.1–6.6)	0.24 (0.23–0.26)
Phonophobia	5.2 (4.5–5.9)	0.38 (0.36–0.40)
Exacerbation by physical activity	3.7 (3.4–4.0)	0.24 (0.23–0.26)

search for criteria satisfying a diagnosis of "malignant hypertension" is appropriate to determine the correct urgency level of hypertension management (see Chapter 11). Headache and hypertension associated with pregnancy may be due to preeclampsia. Episodic headache associated with the triad of hypertension, heart palpitations, and sweats is suggestive of pheochromocytoma. In the absence of "thunderclap" headache, advanced age, and HIV disease, a careful physical examination and detailed neurologic examination will usually determine acuity of the work-up and need for further diagnostic testing.

Patient symptoms can also be useful for diagnosing migraine headache in the absence of the "classic" migraine pattern involving scintillating scotoma followed by unilateral headache, photophobia, and nausea and vomiting (Table 2–9). The presence of three or more of these features can establish the diagnosis of migraine (in the absence of other clinical features that warrant neuroimaging studies), and the presence of none or one of these features (provided it is not nausea) can help to rule out migraine.

B. Physical Examination

Critical components of the physical examination of the patient with acute headache include vital signs, neurologic examination, and vision testing with funduscopic examination. The finding of fever with acute headache warrants additional maneuvers to elicit evidence of meningeal inflammation, such as Kernig and Brudzinski signs. Besides malignant hypertension, significant hypertension can also be a sign of intracranial hemorrhage, preeclampsia, and pheochromocytoma. Patients over 60 years of age should be examined for scalp or temporal artery tenderness.

Careful assessment of visual acuity, ocular gaze, visual fields, pupillary defects, optic disks, and retinal vein pulsations is crucial. Diminished visual acuity is suggestive of glaucoma, temporal arteritis, or optic neuritis. Ophthalmoplegia or visual field defects may be signs of venous sinus thrombosis, tumor, or aneurysm. Afferent pupillary defects can be due to intracranial masses or optic neuritis. Ipsilateral ptosis and miosis suggest Horner syndrome and in conjunction with acute headache may signify carotid artery dissection. Finally, papilledema or absent retinal venous pulsations are signs of elevated intracranial pressure—findings that should be followed by neuroimaging prior to performing lumbar puncture (Table 2–8). Nonmydriatic fundoscopy reveals up to 8.5% of patients who arrive at the emergency department complaining of headache show abnormalities, of which few had other significant physical examination findings and 41% had normal neuroimaging studies.

Mental status and complete neurologic evaluations are also critical and should include assessment of motor and sensory systems, reflexes, gait, cerebellar function, and pronator drift. Any abnormality on mental status or neurologic evaluation warrants emergent neuroimaging (Table 2–8).

C. Diagnostic Studies

Neuroimaging is summarized in Table 2–8. Under most circumstances, a noncontrast head CT is sufficient to exclude intracranial hypertension with impending herniation, intracranial hemorrhage, and many types of intracranial masses (notable exceptions include lymphoma and toxoplasmosis in HIV-positive patients, herpes simplex encephalitis, and brain abscess). When needed, a contrast study can be ordered to follow a normal noncontrast study. A normal neuroimaging study does not sufficiently exclude subarachnoid hemorrhage and should be followed by lumbar puncture. In patients for whom there is a high level of suspicion for subarachnoid hemorrhage or aneurysm, a normal CT and lumbar puncture should be followed by angiography within the next few days (provided the patient is medically stable). Lumbar puncture is also indicated to exclude infectious causes of acute headache, particularly in patients with fever or meningeal signs. Cerebrospinal fluid tests should routinely include Gram stain, white blood cell count with differential, red blood cell count, glucose, total protein, and bacterial culture. In appropriate patients, also consider testing cerebrospinal fluid for VDRL (syphilis), cryptococcal antigen (HIV-positive patients), acid-fast bacillus stain and culture, and complement fixation and culture for coccidioidomycosis. Storage of an extra tube with 5 mL of cerebrospinal fluid is also prudent for conducting unanticipated tests in the immediate future. Polymerase chain reaction tests for specific infectious pathogens (eg, herpes simplex 2) should also be considered in patients with evidence of central nervous system infection but no identifiable pathogen.

In addition to neuroimaging and lumbar puncture, additional diagnostic tests for exclusion of life-threatening causes of acute headache include erythrocyte sedimentation rate (temporal arteritis; endocarditis), urinalysis (malignant hypertension; preeclampsia), and sinus CT or radiograph (bacterial sinusitis, independently or as a cause of venous sinus thrombosis).

▶ Treatment

Treatment should be directed at the cause of acute headache. In patients in whom migraine or migraine-like headache has been diagnosed, early treatment with NSAIDs or triptans can often abort or provide significant relief of symptoms (see Chapter 24). High-flow oxygen therapy may also provide effective treatment for all headache types in emergency department setting. Other causes of acute headache, such as subarachnoid hemorrhage, intracranial mass, or meningitis, usually require emergent treatment in the hospital.

When to Refer

- Frequent migraines not responsive to standard therapy.
- Migraines with atypical features.
- Chronic daily headaches due to medication overuse.

When to Admit

- Need for repeated doses of parenteral pain medication.
- To facilitate an expedited work-up requiring a sequence of neuroimaging and procedures.
- Monitoring for progression of symptoms and neurologic consultation when the initial emergency department work-up is inconclusive.
- Pain severe enough to impair activities of daily living or limit participation in follow-up appointments or consultation.

De Luca GC et al. When and how to investigate the patient with headache. Semin Neurol. 2010 Apr;30(2):131–44. [PMID: 20352583]

Derry CJ et al. Sumatriptan (oral route of administration) for acute migraine attacks in adults. Cochrane Database Syst Rev. 2012 Feb 15;2:CD008615. [PMID: 22336849]

Edlow JA et al. Clinical policy: critical issues in the evaluation and management of adult patients presenting to the emergency department with acute headache. Ann Emerg Med. 2008 Oct;52(4):407–36. [PMID: 18809105]

Friedman BW et al. Headache in the emergency department. Curr Pain Headache Rep. 2011 Aug;15(4):302–7. [PMID: 21400252]

Friedman BW et al. Metoclopramide for acute migraine: a dose-finding randomized clinical trial. Ann Emerg Med. 2011 May;57(5):475–82.e1. [PMID: 21227540]

Jamshidi S et al. Clinical predictors of significant findings on head computed tomographic angiography. J Emerg Med. 2011 Apr;40(4):469–75. [PMID: 19854018]

Loder E. Triptan therapy in migraine. N Engl J Med. 2010 Jul 1;363(1):63–70. [PMID: 20592298]

Ozkurt B et al. Efficacy of high-flow oxygen therapy in all types of headache: a prospective, randomized, placebo-controlled trial. Am J Emerg Med. 2012 Nov;30(9):1760–4. [PMID: 22560101]

Thulasi P et al. Nonmydriatic ocular fundus photography among headache patients in an emergency department. Neurology. 2013 Jan 29;80(5):432–7. [PMID: 23284060]

DYSURIA

ESSENTIAL INQUIRIES

- ► Fever; new back or flank pain; nausea or vomiting.
- ► Vaginal discharge.
- ► Pregnancy risk.
- ► Structural abnormalities.
- ► Instrumentation of urethra or bladder.

General Considerations

Dysuria (painful urination) is a common reason for adolescents and adults to seek urgent medical attention. An inflammatory process (eg, infection; autoimmune disorder) underlies most causes of dysuria. In women, cystitis will be diagnosed in up to 50–60% of cases and has an incidence of 0.5–0.7% per year in sexually active young women. The key objective in evaluating women with dysuria is to exclude serious upper urinary tract disease, such as acute pyelonephritis, and sexually transmitted diseases. In elderly men, dysuria may be a symptom of prostatitis. In contrast, in younger men, urethritis accounts for the vast majority of cases of dysuria.

Clinical Findings

A. Symptoms

Well-designed cohort studies have shown that some women can be reliably diagnosed with uncomplicated cystitis without a physical examination or urinalysis, and randomized controlled trials show that telephone management of uncomplicated cystitis is safe and effective. An increased likelihood of cystitis is present when women report multiple irritative voiding symptoms (dysuria, urgency, frequency), fever, or back pain (LRs = 1.6–2.0). Inquiring about symptoms of vulvovaginitis is imperative. When women report dysuria and urinary frequency, and deny vaginal discharge and irritation, the likelihood ratio for culture-confirmed cystitis is 24.5. In contrast, when vaginal discharge or irritation is present, as well as dysuria or urinary frequency, the LR is 0.7. Gross hematuria in women with voiding symptoms usually represents hemorrhagic cystitis but can also be a sign of bladder cancer (particularly in older patients) or upper tract disease. Failure of hematuria to resolve with antibiotic treatment should prompt further evaluation of the bladder and kidneys. Chlamydial infection should be strongly considered among women age 25 years or younger who are sexually active and seeking medical attention for a suspected urinary tract infection for the first time or have a new partner.

Because fever and back pain, as well as nausea and vomiting, are considered harbingers of (or clinical criteria for) acute pyelonephritis, women with these symptoms should usually be examined by a clinician prior to treatment in order to exclude coexistent urosepsis, hydronephrosis, or nephrolithiasis. Other major risk factors for acute pyelonephritis (among women 18–49 years of age) relate to sexual behaviors (frequency of sexual intercourse three or more times per week, new sexual partner in previous year, recent spermicide use), as well as diabetes mellitus and recent urinary tract infection or incontinence. Finally, pregnancy, underlying structural factors (polycystic kidney disease, nephrolithiasis, neurogenic bladder), immunosuppression, diabetes mellitus, and a history of recent bladder or urethral instrumentation usually alter the treatment regimen (antibiotic choice or duration of treatment, or both) of uncomplicated cystitis.

B. Physical Examination

Fever, tachycardia, or hypotension suggest the possibility of urosepsis and potential need for hospitalization. A focused examination in women, in uncomplicated circumstances, could be limited to ascertainment of costovertebral angle tenderness and to a lower abdominal and pelvic examination, if the history suggests vulvovaginitis or cervicitis.

▶ C. Diagnostic Studies

1. Urinalysis—Urinalysis is probably overutilized in the evaluation of dysuria. The probability of culture-confirmed urinary tract infection among women with a history and physical examination compatible with uncomplicated cystitis is about 70–90%. Urinalysis is most helpful in

atypical presentations of cystitis. Dipstick detection (> trace) of leukocytes, nitrites, or blood supports a diagnosis of cystitis. When both leukocyte and nitrite tests are positive, the LR is 4.2, and when both are negative, the LR is 0.3. The negative predictive value of urinalysis is not sufficient to exclude culture-confirmed urinary tract infection in women with multiple and typical symptoms; and randomized trial evidence shows that antibiotic treatment is beneficial to women with typical symptoms and negative urinalysis dipstick tests. Microscopy of unspun urine may also be helpful in diagnosis and reduce unnecessary use of

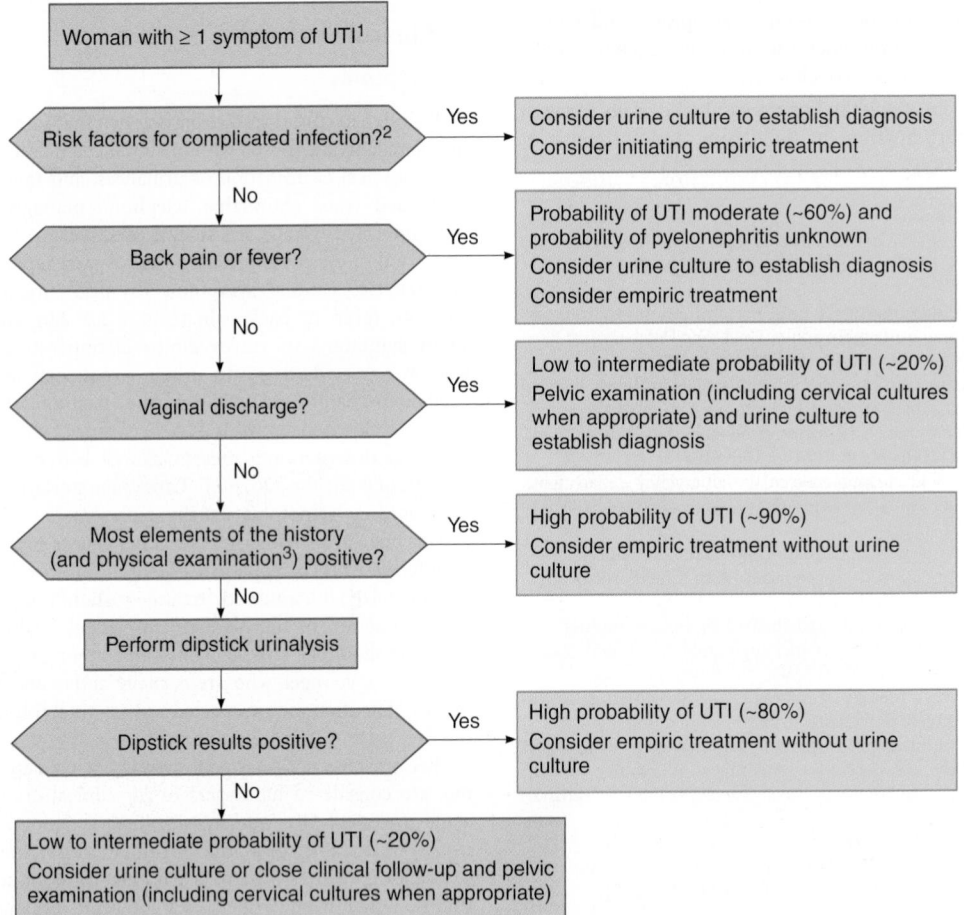

[1]In women who have risk factors for sexually transmitted diseases, consider testing for *Chlamydia*. The US Preventive Services Task Force recommends screening for *Chlamydia* for all women 25 years or younger and women of any age with more than one sexual partner, a history of sexually transmitted disease, or inconsistent use of condoms.

[2]A complicated UTI is one in an individual with a functional or anatomic abnormality of the urinary tract, including a history of polycystic renal disease, nephrolithiasis, neurogenic bladder, diabetes mellitus, immunosuppression, pregnancy, indwelling urinary catheter, or recent urinary tract instrumentation.

[3]The only physical examination finding that increases the likelihood of UTI is costovertebral angle tenderness, and clinicians may consider not performing this test in patients with typical symptoms of acute uncomplicated UTI (as in telephone management).

▲ **Figure 2–2.** Proposed algorithm for evaluating women with symptoms of acute urinary tract infection (UTI). (Modified and reproduced, with permission, from Bent S et al. Does this woman have an acute uncomplicated urinary tract infection? JAMA. 2002 May 22–29;287(20):2701–10.)

antibiotics. The combination of urgency, dysuria, and pyuria (assessed with the high power objective (40 ×) for pus cells (> 1 pus cell/7 high power fields) had a positive predictive value of 71.71 and LR of 2.97.

2. Urine culture—Urine culture should be considered for all women with upper tract symptoms (prior to initiating antibiotic therapy), as well as those with dysuria and a negative urine dipstick test. In symptomatic women, a clean-catch urine culture is considered positive when 10^2–10^3 colony-forming units/mL of a uropathogenic organism is detected.

3. Renal imaging—When severe flank or back pain is present, the possibility of complicated kidney infection (perinephric abscess, nephrolithiasis) or of hydronephrosis should be considered. Renal ultrasound or CT scanning should be done to rule out abscess or hydronephrosis. To exclude nephrolithiasis, noncontrast helical CT scanning is more accurate than intravenous urography and is rapidly becoming the diagnostic test of choice. In a meta-analysis, the positive and negative likelihood ratios of helical CT scanning for diagnosis of nephrolithiasis were 23.2 and 0.05, respectively.

Differential Diagnosis

The differential diagnosis of dysuria in women includes acute cystitis, acute pyelonephritis, vaginitis (*Candida*, bacterial vaginosis, *Trichomonas*, herpes simplex), urethritis/cervicitis (*Chlamydia*, gonorrhea), and interstitial cystitis/painful bladder syndrome. Nucleic acid amplification tests from first-void urine or vaginal swab specimens are highly sensitive for detecting chlamydial infection. Other infectious pathogens associated with dysuria and urethritis in men include *Mycoplasma genitalium* and Enterobacteriacea.

Treatment

Definitive treatment is directed to the underlying cause of the dysuria. An evidence-informed algorithm for managing suspected urinary tract infection in women is shown in Figure 2–2. This algorithm supports antibiotic treatment of most women with multiple and typical symptoms of urinary tract infection without performing urinalysis or urine culture. Antibiotic selection should be guided by local resistance patterns; major options for uncomplicated cystitis include nitrofurantoin, cephalosporins, ciprofloxacin, and trimethoprim-sulfamethoxazole. Prolonged treatment of urinary tract infections (> 7 days) in men does not appear to reduce early or late recurrences. Symptomatic relief can be provided with phenazopyridine, a urinary analgesic that is available over-the-counter; it is used in combination with antibiotic therapy (when a urinary tract infection has been confirmed) but for no more than 2 days. Patients should be informed that phenazopyridine will

cause orange/red discoloration of their urine and other bodily fluids (eg, some contact lens wearers have reported discoloration of their lenses). Rare cases of methemoglobinemia and hemolytic anemia have been reported, usually with overdoses or underlying renal dysfunction.

In cases of interstitial cystitis/painful bladder syndrome (see Chapter 23), patients will often respond to a multimodal approach that may include urethral/vesicular dilation, biofeedback, cognitive behavioral therapy, antidepressants, dietary changes, vaginal emollients, and other supportive measures.

▶ When to Refer

- Anatomic abnormalities leading to repeated urinary infections.
- Infections associated with nephrolithiasis.
- Persistent interstitial cystitis/painful bladder syndrome.

▶ When to Admit

- Severe pain requiring parenteral medication or impairing ambulation or urination (such as severe primary herpes simplex genitalis).
- Dysuria associated with urinary retention or obstruction.
- Pyelonephritis with ureteral obstruction.

Abrams P et al. Evaluation and treatment of lower urinary tract symptoms in older men. J Urol. 2009 Apr;181(4):1779–87. [PMID: 19233402]

Blozik E et al. UTI in women. Consider telemedical management. BMJ. 2010 Mar 16;340:c1464. [PMID: 20233765]

Drekonja DM et al. Urinary tract infection in male veterans: treatment patterns and outcomes. JAMA Intern Med. 2013 Jan 14;173(1):62–8. [PMID: 23212273]

Hanno PM et al; Interstitial Cystitis Guidelines Panel of the American Urological Association Education and Research, Inc. AUA guideline for the diagnosis and treatment of interstitial cystitis/bladder pain syndrome. J Urol. 2011 Jun;185(6):2162–70. [PMID: 21497847]

Heytens S et al. Cystitis: symptomatology in women with suspected uncomplicated urinary tract infection. J Womens Health (Larchmt). 2011 Jul;20(7):1117–21. [PMID: 21671766]

Hooton TM et al. Cefpodoxime vs ciprofloxacin for short-course treatment of acute uncomplicated cystitis: a randomized trial. JAMA. 2012 Feb 8;307(6):583–9. [PMID: 22318279]

Little P et al. Validating the prediction of lower urinary tract infection in primary care: sensitivity and specificity of urinary dipsticks and clinical scores in women. Br J Gen Pract. 2010 Jul;60(576):495–500. [PMID: 20594439]

Mishra B et al. Symptom-based diagnosis of urinary tract infection in women: are we over-prescribing antibiotics? Int J Clin Pract. 2012 May;66(5):493–8. [PMID: 22512608]

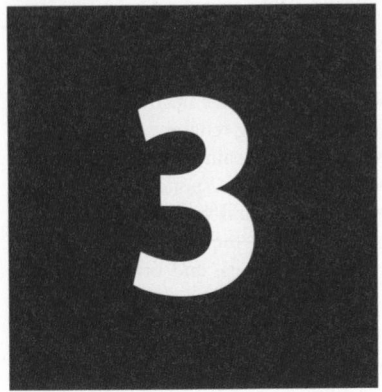

Preoperative Evaluation & Perioperative Management

Hugo Q. Cheng, MD

EVALUATION OF THE ASYMPTOMATIC PATIENT

Patients without significant medical problems—especially those under age 50—are at very low risk for perioperative complications. Their preoperative evaluation should include a history and physical examination. Special emphasis is placed on obtaining a careful pharmacologic history and assessment of functional status, exercise tolerance, and cardiopulmonary symptoms and signs in an effort to reveal previously unrecognized disease that may require further evaluation prior to surgery. In addition, a directed bleeding history (Table 3–1) should be taken to uncover coagulopathy that could contribute to excessive surgical blood loss. Routine preoperative laboratory tests in asymptomatic healthy patients under age 50 have not been found to help predict or prevent complications. Even elderly patients undergoing minor or minimally invasive procedures (such as cataract surgery) are unlikely to benefit from preoperative screening tests.

Chopra V et al. Perioperative practice: time to throttle back. Ann Intern Med. 2010 Jan 5;152(1):47–51. [PMID: 19949135]

Gupta A. Preoperative screening and risk assessment in the ambulatory surgery patient. Curr Opin Anaesthesiol. 2009 Dec;22(6):705–11. [PMID: 19633545]

Laine C et al. In the clinic. Preoperative evaluation. Ann Intern Med. 2009 Jul 7;151(1):ITC1–15. [PMID: 19581642]

CARDIAC RISK ASSESSMENT & REDUCTION IN NONCARDIAC SURGERY

Cardiac complications of noncardiac surgery are a major cause of perioperative morbidity and mortality. The most important perioperative cardiac complications are myocardial infarction (MI) and cardiac death. Other complications include heart failure (HF), arrhythmias, and unstable angina. The principal patient-specific risk factor is the presence of end-organ cardiovascular disease. This includes not only coronary artery disease and HF, but also cerebrovascular disease and chronic kidney disease if due to atherosclerosis. Diabetes mellitus, especially if treated with insulin, is considered a cardiovascular disease equivalent and has also been shown to increase the risk of cardiac complications. Major abdominal, thoracic, and vascular

surgical procedures (especially abdominal aortic aneurysm repair) carry a higher risk of postoperative cardiac complications, likely due to their associated major fluid shifts, hemorrhage, and hypoxemia. These risk factors were identified in a validated multifactorial risk prediction tool: the Revised Cardiac Risk Index (RCRI) (Table 3–2). The RCRI is widely used for assessing and communicating cardiac risk and has been incorporated into perioperative management guidelines. Limited exercise capacity (eg, the inability to walk for two blocks at a normal pace or climb a flight of stairs without resting) also predicts higher cardiac risk. Emergency operations are also associated with greater cardiac risk. However, emergency operations should not be delayed by extensive cardiac evaluation. Instead, patients facing emergency surgery should be medically optimized for surgery as quickly as possible and closely monitored for cardiac complications during the perioperative period.

Another risk prediction tool, derived from the American College of Surgeons' National Surgical Quality Improvement Program (NSQIP) patient database, identified five variables that predicted postoperative MI and cardiac arrest. These include patient age, the location or type of operation, serum creatinine > 1.5 g/dL (132.6 mcmol/L), dependency in activities of daily living, and the patient's American Society of Anesthesiologists physical status classification. An online risk calculator using the NSQIP tool can be found at http://www.qxmd.com/calculate-online/cardiology/gupta-perioperative-cardiac-risk.

▶ Role of Preoperative Noninvasive Ischemia Testing

Most patients can be accurately risk-stratified by history and physical examination. A resting electrocardiogram (ECG) should also be obtained in patients with at least one RCRI predictor prior to major surgery. Additional noninvasive stress testing rarely improves risk stratification or management, especially in patients without RCRI predictors, in those who are undergoing minor operations, or those who have at least fair functional capacity. Patients with poor functional capacity or a high RCRI score are much more likely to suffer cardiac complications. Stress testing prior to vascular surgery in these patients can stratify them into

Table 3–1. Findings suggestive of a bleeding disorder.

Unprovoked bruising on the trunk of > 5 cm in diameter
Frequent unprovoked epistaxis or gingival bleeding
Menorrhagia with iron deficiency
Hemarthrosis with mild trauma
Prior excessive surgical blood loss or reoperation for bleeding
Family history of abnormal bleeding
Presence of severe kidney or liver disease
Use of medications that impair coagulation, including nutritional
    supplements and herbal remedies

low-risk and high-risk subgroups. The absence of ischemia on dipyridamole scintigraphy or dobutamine stress echocardiography is reassuring. In contrast, extensive inducible ischemia in this population predicts a very high risk of cardiac complications, which may not be modifiable by either medical management or coronary revascularization. The predictive value of an abnormal stress test result for nonvascular surgery patients is less well established. An approach to perioperative cardiac risk assessment and management in patients with known or suspected stable coronary artery disease is shown in Figure 3–1.

> **Perioperative Management of Patients with Coronary Artery Disease**

Patients with acute coronary syndromes require immediate management of their cardiac disease prior to any preoperative evaluation (see Chapter 10). In a large cohort study, postoperative MI typically occurred within 3 days of surgery, and was associated with a 30-day mortality rate of 11.6%. Postoperative MI is usually silent or may present without

Table 3–2. Revised Cardiac Risk Index.

Independent Predictors of Postoperative Cardiac Complications	
1. Intrathoracic, intraperitoneal, or suprainguinal vascular surgery	
2. History of ischemic heart disease	
3. History of heart failure	
4. Insulin treatment for diabetes mellitus	
5. Serum creatinine level > 2 mg/dL [> 176.8 mcmol/L]	
6. History of cerebrovascular disease	
Scoring (Number of Predictors Present)	Risk of Major Cardiac Complications[1]
None	0.4%
One	1%
Two	2.4%
More than two	5.4%

[1]Cardiac death, myocardial infarction or nonfatal cardiac arrest. Data from Devereaux PJ et al. Perioperative cardiac events in patients undergoing noncardiac surgery: a review of the magnitude of the problem, the pathophysiology of the events and methods to estimate and communicate risk. CMAJ. 2005 Sept 13;173(6):627–34.

chest pain. Symptoms and signs that should prompt consideration of postoperative MI include unexplained hypotension, hypoxemia, or delirium. Screening asymptomatic patients for postoperative MI through the use of ECG or cardiac enzyme monitoring remains controversial, since it has not yet been demonstrated to improve outcomes.

A. Medications

Preoperative antianginal medications, including beta-blockers, calcium channel blockers, and nitrates, should be continued throughout the perioperative period. Beta-adrenergic blocking drugs exert a cardioprotective effect in surgical patients. A small, randomized trial in vascular surgery patients with ischemia on dobutamine stress echocardiography found that bisoprolol reduced the 30-day risk of cardiac mortality or nonfatal MI from 34% to 3% in these high-risk patients. In contrast, subsequent larger trials found less benefit and potential harm in lower risk patients. In the largest of these studies, a high, fixed dose of metoprolol succinate given to patients with at least one RCRI predictor reduced the absolute risk of cardiac complications by 1.1%. However, this benefit was offset by a 0.8% absolute increase in total mortality, driven by greater incidence of stroke and death from sepsis. Because of the uncertain benefit-to-risk ratio of perioperative beta-blockade, it should be reserved for patients with a relatively high risk of cardiac complications. Suggested indications and starting doses for prophylactic beta-blockade are presented in Table 3–3. Ideally, beta-blockers should be started well in advance of surgery, to allow time to gradually titrate up the dose without causing excessive bradycardia or hypotension. The dose should be adjusted to maintain a heart rate between 50 and 70 beats per minute while keeping systolic blood pressure above 100 mm Hg. Beta-blockers should be continued for at least 3–7 days after surgery.

A meta-analysis of randomized trials found that the use of HMG-CoA reductase inhibitors (statins) prevents MI in patients undergoing noncardiac surgery. Safety concerns, such as liver failure or rhabdomyolysis, have not materialized in these studies. Statins should be considered in all patients undergoing vascular surgery and other patients deemed to be at high risk for cardiac complications, regardless of lipid levels. Patients already taking statins should continue these agents during the perioperative period.

B. Coronary Revascularization

Retrospective studies suggest that patients who had previously undergone coronary artery bypass grafting (CABG) surgery or percutaneous coronary interventions (PCI) have a relatively low risk of cardiac complications when undergoing subsequent noncardiac surgery. However, one trial randomized over 500 patients with angiographically proven coronary artery disease to either coronary revascularization (with either CABG or PCI) or medical management alone before vascular surgery. Postoperative nonfatal MI, 30-day mortality, and long-term mortality did not differ, suggesting that prophylactic revascularization before noncardiac surgery does not prevent cardiac complications. Thus, preoperative CABG or PCI should only be

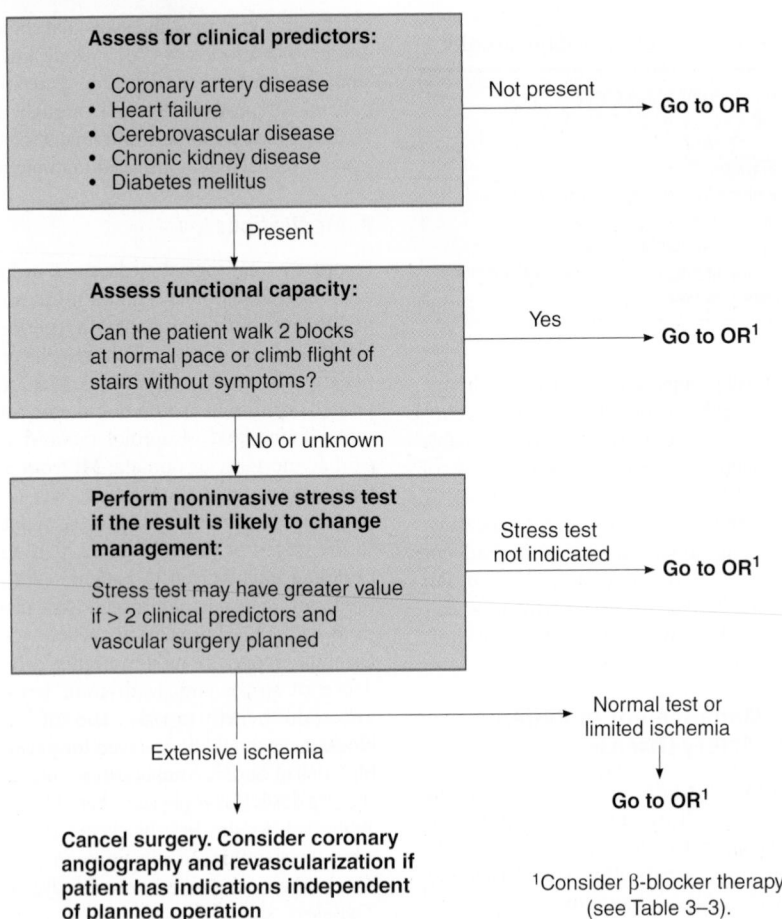

▲ **Figure 3–1.** Assessment and management of patients with known or suspected stable coronary artery disease (CAD) undergoing elective major noncardiac surgery. (OR, operating room.)

performed on patients who have indications for the procedure independent of the planned noncardiac operation. In addition, the perioperative cardiac mortality rate may be very high in patients who have undergone recent intracoronary stenting, if antiplatelet therapy is stopped prematurely. The presumed mechanism of this increased mortality is acute stent thrombosis. Therefore, elective surgery should be deferred for at least 4–6 weeks after placement of a bare-metal stent and for a full year after placement of a drug-eluting stent if antiplatelet therapy must be stopped perioperatively.

▶ Heart Failure & Left Ventricular Dysfunction

Decompensated HF, manifested by an elevated jugular venous pressure, an audible third heart sound, or evidence of pulmonary edema on physical examination or chest radiography, significantly increases the risk of perioperative cardiac complications. Elective surgery should be postponed in patients with decompensated HF until it can be evaluated and brought under control.

Patients with compensated left ventricular dysfunction are at increased risk for cardiac complications. In vascular surgery patients who had preoperative echocardiography, asymptomatic left ventricular dysfunction (either systolic or diastolic) was associated with a twofold increase in cardiac complications. In contrast, a history of symptomatic HF was associated with a sevenfold increase in risk. Current guidelines recommend preoperative echocardiography in patients without known HF with unexplained dyspnea and in patients with known HF with clinical deterioration.

Table 3–3. Indications for prophylactic perioperative beta-blockade.[1]

Strong indications	Patient already taking beta-blocker to treat ischemia, arrhythmia, or hypertension
Possible indications	Patients with coronary artery disease undergoing vascular or other major surgery Patient with multiple Revised Cardiac Risk Index predictors (see Table 3–2) undergoing vascular or other major surgery

[1]Initial dose recommendations: atenolol 25 mg orally daily, bisoprolol 2.5 mg orally daily, or metoprolol 25 mg orally twice daily. The dose of beta-blocker should be carefully titrated to keep heart rate < 70 beats per minute and systolic blood pressure > 100 mm Hg.

A small observational study found that routine echocardiography in patients with suspected heart disease or age ≥ 65 years old prior to emergency noncardiac surgery frequently led to a change in diagnosis or management plan. While this is not an established practice, preoperative echocardiography should be considered when there is uncertainty about the patient's cardiac status.

Patients receiving diuretics and digoxin should have serum electrolyte and digoxin levels measured prior to surgery because abnormalities in these levels may increase the risk of perioperative arrhythmias. Clinicians must be cautious not to give too much diuretic, since the volume-depleted patient will be much more susceptible to intraoperative hypotension. The surgeon and anesthesiologist should be made aware of the presence and severity of left ventricular dysfunction so that appropriate decisions can be made regarding perioperative fluid management and intraoperative monitoring.

Valvular Heart Disease

If the severity of valvular lesions is unknown, echocardiography should be performed prior to noncardiac surgery. Candidates for valve replacement surgery or valvuloplasty independent of the planned noncardiac surgery should have the valve correction procedure performed first. Patients with uncorrected severe or symptomatic aortic stenosis are at particular risk for cardiac complications. They should only undergo surgery after consultation with a cardiologist and anesthesiologist. In a series of patients with aortic stenosis who underwent noncardiac surgery, death or nonfatal MI occurred in 31% in patients with severe aortic stenosis (aortic valve area < 0.7 cm²), in 11% in those with moderate aortic stenosis (aortic valve area 0.7–1.0 cm²), and in 2% in those without aortic stenosis. Patients with asymptomatic aortic stenosis appeared to be at lower risk than patients with symptomatic aortic stenosis. Patients with mitral stenosis require heart rate control to prolong diastolic filling time. Regurgitant lesions are generally less problematic during surgery because the vasodilatory effect of anesthetics promotes forward flow. Patients with aortic regurgitation or aortic insufficiency likely benefit from afterload reduction and careful attention to volume status.

Arrhythmias

The finding of a rhythm disturbance on preoperative evaluation should prompt consideration of further cardiac evaluation, particularly when the finding of structural heart disease would alter perioperative management. Patients with a rhythm disturbance without evidence of underlying heart disease are at low risk for perioperative cardiac complications. There is no evidence that the use of antiarrhythmic medications to suppress an asymptomatic arrhythmia alters perioperative risk.

Patients with symptomatic arrhythmias should not undergo elective surgery until their cardiac condition has been addressed. Thus, in patients with atrial fibrillation or other supraventricular arrhythmias, adequate rate control should be established prior to surgery. Symptomatic ventricular tachycardia must be thoroughly evaluated and controlled prior to surgery. Patients who have independent indications for a permanent pacemaker or implanted defibrillator should have it placed prior to noncardiac surgery. The anesthesiologist must be notified that a patient has an implanted pacemaker or defibrillator so that steps may be taken to prevent device malfunction caused by electromagnetic interference from the intraoperative use of electrocautery.

▶ Hypertension

Mild to moderate hypertension (systolic blood pressure below 180 mm Hg and diastolic blood pressure below 110 mm Hg) is associated with intraoperative blood pressure lability and asymptomatic myocardial ischemia but does not appear to be an independent risk factor for more serious cardiac complications. No evidence supports delaying surgery in order to better control mild to moderate hypertension. Most medications for chronic hypertension should generally be continued up to and including the day of surgery. Consideration should be given to holding angiotensin-converting enzyme inhibitors and angiotensin receptor blockers on the day of surgery in the absence of HF, since these agents may increase the risk of intraoperative hypotension. Diuretic agents, if not needed to control HF, are also frequently held on the day of surgery to prevent hypovolemia and electrolyte disorders.

Severe hypertension, defined as a systolic pressure > 180 mm Hg or diastolic pressure > 110 mm Hg, appears to be an independent predictor of perioperative cardiac complications, including MI and HF. It is reasonable to consider delaying surgery in patients with severe hypertension until blood pressure can be controlled, although it is not known whether the risk of cardiac complications is reduced with this approach.

Chopra V et al. Effect of perioperative statins on death, myocardial infarction, atrial fibrillation, and length of stay: a systematic review and meta-analysis. Arch Surg. 2012 Feb;147(2):181–9. [PMID: 22351917]

Devereaux PJ et al. Characteristics and short-term prognosis of perioperative myocardial infarction in patients undergoing noncardiac surgery: a cohort study. Ann Intern Med. 2011 Apr 19;154(8):523–8. [PMID: 21502650]

Gupta PK et al. Development and validation of a risk calculator for prediction of cardiac risk after surgery. Circulation. 2011 Jul 26;124(4):381–7. [PMID: 21730309]

Task Force for Preoperative Cardiac Risk Assessment and Perioperative Cardiac Management in Non-cardiac Surgery; European Society of Cardiology (ESC) et al. Guidelines for pre-operative cardiac risk assessment and perioperative cardiac management in non-cardiac surgery. Eur Heart J. 2009 Nov;30(22):2769–812. [PMID: 19713421]

PULMONARY EVALUATION IN NON–LUNG RESECTION SURGERY

Pneumonia and respiratory failure requiring prolonged mechanical ventilation are the most important postoperative pulmonary complications. The occurrence of these complications has been associated with a significant increase in mortality and hospital length of stay.

Pulmonary thromboembolism is another serious complication; prophylaxis against venous thromboembolic disease is described in Chapter 14.

Risk Factors for the Development of Postoperative Pulmonary Complications

The risk of developing a pulmonary complication is highest in patients undergoing cardiac, thoracic, and upper abdominal surgery, with reported complication rates ranging from 9% to 19%. The risk in patients undergoing lower abdominal or pelvic procedures ranges from 2% to 5%, and for extremity procedures the range is < 1–3%. The pulmonary complication rate for laparoscopic procedures appears to be much lower than that for open procedures. In one series of over 1500 patients who underwent laparoscopic cholecystectomy, the pulmonary complication rate was < 1%. Other procedure-related risk factors include prolonged anesthesia time, need for general anesthesia, and emergency operations.

Among the many patient-specific risk factors for postoperative pulmonary complications, the strongest predictor appears to be advanced age. Surgical patients in their seventh decade had a fourfold higher risk of pulmonary complications compared with patients under age 50. The presence and severity of systemic disease of any type is associated with pulmonary complications. In particular, patients with chronic obstructive pulmonary disease (COPD) or HF have at least twice the risk compared with patients without these conditions. A risk calculator for assessing the risk of postoperative respiratory failure was derived from the NSQIP patient database (http://www.qxmd.com/calculate-online/respirology/postoperative-respiratory-failure-risk-calculator). Predictors in this model include the type of surgery, emergency surgery, preoperative sepsis, dependency in activities of daily living, and the patient's American Society of Anesthesiologists physical status classification.

Patients with well-controlled asthma at the time of surgery are not at increased risk for pulmonary complications. Obesity causes restrictive pulmonary physiology, which may increase pulmonary risk in surgical patients. However, it is unclear if obesity is an independent risk predictor. Obstructive sleep apnea has been associated with a variety of postoperative complications, particularly in patients undergoing bariatric surgery. The STOP screening questionnaire asks whether a patient has snoring, tiredness during the day, observed apnea, and high blood pressure. The presence of two or more of these findings had a 78% positive predictive value for obstructive sleep apnea and was associated with a doubled risk for postoperative pulmonary complications. A summary of risk factors for pulmonary complications is presented in Table 3–4.

Pulmonary Function Testing & Laboratory Studies

Few data support the use of preoperative testing to assess pulmonary risk. The main role for preoperative pulmonary function testing (PFT) is to help identify and characterize

Table 3–4. Clinical risk factors for postoperative pulmonary complications.

Upper abdominal or cardiothoracic surgery
Prolonged anesthesia time (> 4 hours)
Emergency surgery
Age > 60 years
Chronic obstructive pulmonary disease
Heart failure
Severe systemic disease
Tobacco use (> 20 pack-years)
Impaired cognition or sensorium
Functional dependency or prior stroke
Preoperative sepsis
Low serum albumin level
Obstructive sleep apnea

pulmonary disease in patients with unexplained symptoms prior to major abdominal or cardiothoracic surgery. In patients with diagnosed lung disease, PFT often adds little information above clinical assessment. Furthermore, there is no clear degree of PFT abnormality that can be used as an absolute contraindication to non–lung resection surgery. Chest radiographs in unselected patients also rarely add clinically useful information. In one study, only 0.1% of routine preoperative chest radiographs changed clinical management. They may be more useful in patients who are undergoing abdominal or thoracic surgery who are over age 50 or have known cardiopulmonary disease. Some experts have also advocated polysomnography to diagnose obstructive sleep apnea prior to bariatric surgery, but the benefits of this approach are unproven. Abnormally low or high blood urea nitrogen levels (indicating malnutrition or kidney disease, respectively) and hypoalbuminemia predict higher risk of pulmonary complications and mortality, although the added value of laboratory testing over clinical assessment is uncertain. Arterial blood gas measurement is not routinely recommended except in patients with known lung disease and suspected hypoxemia or hypercapnia.

Perioperative Management

Retrospective studies have shown that smoking cessation reduced the incidence of pulmonary complications, but only if it was initiated at least 1–2 months before surgery. A meta-analysis of randomized trials found that preoperative smoking cessation programs reduced both pulmonary and surgical wound complications, especially if smoking cessation was initiated at least 4 weeks prior to surgery. The preoperative period may be an optimal time to initiate smoking cessation efforts. A systematic review found that smoking cessation programs started in a preoperative evaluation clinic increased the odds of abstinence at 3–6 months by nearly 60%.

The incidence of postoperative pulmonary complications in patients with COPD or asthma may be reduced by preoperative optimization of pulmonary function. Patients who are wheezing should receive preoperative therapy with bronchodilators and, in certain cases, corticosteroids.

Antibiotics may be beneficial for patients with COPD who cough with purulent sputum. Patients receiving oral theophylline should continue taking the drug perioperatively. A serum theophylline level should be measured to rule out toxicity.

Postoperative risk reduction strategies have centered on promoting lung expansion through the use of incentive spirometry, continuous positive airway pressure (CPAP), intermittent positive-pressure breathing (IPPB), and deep breathing exercises. Although trial results have been mixed, all these techniques have been shown to reduce the incidence of postoperative atelectasis and, in a few studies, to reduce the incidence of postoperative pulmonary complications. In most comparative trials, these methods were equally effective. Given the higher cost of CPAP and IPPB, incentive spirometry and deep breathing exercises are the preferred methods for most patients. Incentive spirometry must be performed for 15 minutes every 2 hours. Deep breathing exercises must be performed hourly and consist of 3-second breath-holding, pursed lip breathing, and coughing. These measures should be started preoperatively and be continued for 1–2 days postoperatively.

Johnson DC et al. Perioperative pulmonary complications. Curr Opin Crit Care. 2011 Aug;17(4):362–9. [PMID: 21734490]
Mills E et al. Smoking cessation reduces postoperative complications: a systematic review and meta-analysis. Am J Med. 2011 Feb;124(2):144–54. [PMID: 21295194]
Qaseem A et al; Clinical Efficacy Assessment Subcommittee of the American College of Physicians. Risk assessment for and strategies to reduce perioperative pulmonary complications for patients undergoing noncardiothoracic surgery: a guideline from the American College of Physicians. Ann Intern Med. 2006 Apr 18;144(8):575–80. [PMID: 16618955]

EVALUATION OF THE PATIENT WITH LIVER DISEASE

Patients with serious liver disease are at increased risk for perioperative morbidity and demise. Appropriate preoperative evaluation requires consideration of the effects of anesthesia and surgery on postoperative liver function and of the complications associated with anesthesia and surgery in patients with preexisting liver disease.

▶ The Effects of Anesthesia & Surgery on Liver Function

Postoperative elevation of serum aminotransferase levels is a relatively common finding after major surgery. Most of these elevations are transient and not associated with hepatic dysfunction. While direct hepatotoxicity is rare with modern anesthetics agents, these drugs may cause deterioration of hepatic function via intraoperative reduction in hepatic blood flow leading to ischemic injury. Medications used for regional anesthesia produce similar reductions in hepatic blood flow and thus may be equally likely to lead to ischemic liver injury. Intraoperative hypotension, hemorrhage, and hypoxemia may also contribute to liver injury.

▶ Risk Assessment in Surgical Patients with Liver Disease

Screening unselected patients with liver function tests has a low yield and is not recommended. Patients with suspected or known liver disease based on history or physical examination, however, should have measurement of liver enzyme levels as well as tests of hepatic synthetic function performed prior to surgery.

Acute hepatitis increases surgical mortality risk. In three small series of patients with acute viral hepatitis who underwent abdominal surgery, the mortality rate was roughly 10%. Similarly, patients with undiagnosed alcoholic hepatitis had high mortality rates when undergoing abdominal surgery. Thus, elective surgery in patients with acute viral or alcoholic hepatitis should be delayed until the acute episode has resolved. In the absence of cirrhosis or synthetic dysfunction, chronic viral hepatitis is unlikely to increase risk significantly. A large cohort study of hepatitis C seropositive patients who underwent surgery found a mortality rate of less than 1%. Similarly, nonalcoholic fatty liver disease by itself probably does not pose a serious risk in surgical patients.

In patients with cirrhosis, postoperative complication rates correlate with the severity of liver dysfunction. Traditionally, severity of dysfunction has been assessed with the Child-Turcotte-Pugh score (see Chapter 16). Patients with Child-Turcotte-Pugh class C cirrhosis who underwent portosystemic shunt surgery, biliary surgery, or trauma surgery during the 1970s and 1980s had a 50–85% mortality rate. Patients with Child-Turcotte-Pugh class A or B cirrhosis who underwent abdominal surgery during the 1990s, however, had relatively low mortality rates (hepatectomy 0–8%, open cholecystectomy 0–1%, laparoscopic cholecystectomy 0–1%). A conservative approach would be to avoid elective surgery in patients with Child-Turcotte-Pugh class C cirrhosis and pursue it with great caution in class B patients. The Model for End-stage Liver Disease (MELD) score, based on bilirubin and creatinine levels, and the prothrombin time expressed as the International Normalized Ratio, also predicted surgical mortality and outperformed the Child-Turcotte-Pugh classification in some studies. A web-based risk assessment calculator incorporating age and MELD score can predict both perioperative and long-term mortality (mayoclinic.org/meld/mayomodel9.html).

In addition, when surgery is elective, it is prudent to attempt to reduce the severity of ascites, encephalopathy, and coagulopathy preoperatively. Ascites is a particular problem in abdominal operations, where it can lead to wound dehiscence or hernias. Great care should be taken when using analgesics and sedatives, as this can worsen hepatic encephalopathy. In general, short-acting agents and lower doses should be used. Patients with coagulopathy should receive vitamin K (if there is concern for concomitant malnutrition) and may need fresh frozen plasma transfusion at the time of surgery.

O'Leary JG et al. Surgery in the patient with liver disease. Clin Liver Dis. 2009 May;13(2):211–31. [PMID: 19442915]

PREOPERATIVE HEMATOLOGIC EVALUATION

Three of the more common clinical situations faced by the medical consultant are the patient with anemia, the assessment of bleeding risk, and the perioperative management of oral anticoagulation.

Preoperative anemia is common, with·a prevalence of 43% in a large cohort of elderly veterans undergoing surgery. The main goals of the preoperative evaluation of the anemic patient are to determine the need for preoperative diagnostic evaluation and the need for transfusion. When feasible, the diagnostic evaluation of the patient with previously unrecognized anemia should be done prior to surgery because certain types of anemia (particularly that due to sickle cell disease, hemolysis, and acute blood loss) have implications for perioperative management. These types of anemia are typically associated with an elevated reticulocyte count. While preoperative anemia is associated with higher perioperative morbidity and mortality, it is not known whether correction of preoperative anemia with transfusions or erythropoiesis stimulating agents will improve postoperative outcomes. Determination of the need for preoperative transfusion in an individual patient must consider factors other than the absolute hemoglobin level, including the presence of cardiopulmonary disease, the type of surgery, and the likely severity of surgical blood loss. The few studies that have compared different postoperative transfusion thresholds failed to demonstrate improved outcomes with a more aggressive transfusion strategy. One trial randomized hip fracture patients, most of whom with cardiovascular disease, to either transfusion to maintain a hemoglobin level > 10 g/dL (100 g/L) or transfusion for symptomatic anemia. Patients receiving symptom-triggered transfusion received far few units of packed red blood cells without increased mortality or complication rates.

The most important component of the bleeding risk assessment is a directed bleeding history (see Table 3–1). Patients who are reliable historians and who reveal no suggestion of abnormal bleeding on directed bleeding history and physical examination are at very low risk for having an occult bleeding disorder. Laboratory tests of hemostatic parameters in these patients are generally not needed. When the directed bleeding history is unreliable or incomplete or when abnormal bleeding is suggested, a formal evaluation of hemostasis should be done prior to surgery and should include measurement of the prothrombin time, activated partial thromboplastin time, and platelet count (see Chapter 13).

Patients receiving long-term oral anticoagulation are at risk for thromboembolic complications when an operation requires interruption of this therapy. A recent meta-analysis of cohort studies found that approximately 1% of patients who had interruption of anticoagulation for a procedure suffered a thrombotic complication. "Bridging" anticoagulation, where unfractionated or low-molecular-weight heparin is administered parenterally while oral anticoagulants are held, is commonly practiced but its benefits are uncertain. In the same meta-analysis, there was no reduction in thrombotic risk with bridging anticoagulation. In addition, the patients who received bridging anticoagulation had a 3.7% incidence of serious bleeding, compared with 0.9% for patients who did not receive bridging anticoagulation. Most experts recommend bridging therapy only in patients at high risk for thromboembolism. An approach to perioperative anticoagulation management is shown in Table 3–5, but the recommendations must be considered in the context of patient preference and hemorrhagic risk. Oral direct thrombin inhibitors should be withheld several days prior to surgery, based on the patient's renal function (Table 3–6). There is no antidote to reverse the anticoagulant effect of

Table 3–5. Recommendations for perioperative anticoagulation management.

Thromboembolic Risk without Anticoagulation	Recommendation
Low (eg, atrial fibrillation with no more than two other stroke risk factors,[1] mechanical bileaflet aortic valve prosthesis with no other stroke risk factors, or single venous thromboembolism > 3 months ago without hypercoagulable condition[2])	1. Stop warfarin 5 days before surgery 2. Measure INR the day before surgery to confirm that it is < 1.6 3. If hemostasis permits, resume warfarin 12–24 hours after surgery 4. No bridging with parenteral anticoagulants before or after surgery
High (eg, atrial fibrillation or mechanical heart valve with stroke < 3 months prior, mechanical mitral valve prosthesis, caged-ball or tilting disk valve prosthesis, or venous thrombosis < 3 months ago or associated with hypercoagulable condition[2])	1. Stop warfarin 5 days before surgery 2. Begin bridging with therapeutic dose UFH infusion or LMWH 2 days after stopping oral anticoagulation 3. Administer last dose of LMWH 24 hours before surgery; discontinue UFH 4–6 hours before surgery 4. Measure INR the day before surgery to confirm that it is < 1.6 5. If hemostasis permits, resume warfarin 12–24 hours after surgery 6. If hemostasis permits, resume bridging with therapeutic dose UFH infusion or LMWH beginning 48 hours after surgery and continuing until the INR is therapeutic

[1]Heart failure, hypertension, diabetes mellitus, age > 75 years.
[2]Patients should receive venous thromboembolism prophylaxis after surgery (see Chapter 14).
INR, international normalized ratio; LMWH, low-molecular-weight heparin; UFH, unfractionated heparin.

Table 3–6. Recommendations for preoperative management of oral direct thrombin inhibitors.[1]

Creatinine Clearance	Dabigatran	Rivaroxaban
> 50 mL/min/1.73m² (0.83 mL/s/m²)	Hold 2–3 days prior	Hold 3–4 days prior
30–50 mL/min/1.73m² (0.5–0.83 mL/s/m²)	Hold 4 days prior	No data available
< 30 mL/min/1.73m² (< 0.5 mL/s/m²)	Hold at least 5 days prior	Contraindicated

[1]Recommended times are for complete reversal of anticoagulant effect. If mild to moderate anticoagulant effect at time of procedure is desired, the holding times should be reduced by 50%.

Table 3–7. Risk factors for the development of postoperative delirium.

Preoperative factors
  Age > 70 years
  Alcohol abuse
  Cognitive impairment
  Poor physical function status
  Markedly abnormal serum sodium, potassium, or glucose level
  Aortic, thoracic, hip fracture surgery, or emergency surgery
Postoperative factors
  Use of meperidine or benzodiazepines, anticholinergics, antihistamines
  Postoperative hematocrit < 30%
  Use of urinary catheters

these medications, so they should only be restarted after surgery when adequate hemostasis is assured.

Douketis JD et al. Perioperative management of antithrombotic therapy: Antithrombotic Therapy and Prevention of Thrombosis, 9th ed: American College of Chest Physicians Evidence-Based Clinical Practice Guidelines. Chest. 2012 Feb;141 (2 Suppl):e326S–50S. Erratum in: Chest. 2012 Apr;141(4):1129 [PMID: 22315266]

Mussallam KM et al. Preoperative anaemia and postoperative outcomes in non-cardiac surgery: a retrospective cohort study. Lancet. 2011 Oct 15;378(9800):1396–407. [PMID: 21982521]

Siegal D et al. Periprocedural heparin bridging in patients receiving vitamin K antagonists: systematic review and meta-analysis of bleeding and thromboembolic rates. Circulation. 2012 Sept 25;126(13):1630–9. [PMID: 22912386]

NEUROLOGIC EVALUATION

Delirium can occur after any major operation but is particularly common after hip fracture repair and cardiovascular surgery, where the incidence is 30–60%. Postoperative delirium has been associated with higher rates of major postoperative cardiac and pulmonary complications, poor functional recovery, an increased length of hospital stay, an increased risk of subsequent dementia and functional decline, and increased mortality. Several preoperative and postoperative factors have been associated with the development of postoperative delirium, most notably age, preoperative functional or cognitive impairment, preoperative psychotropic drug use, and derangements of serum chemistry. Patients with multiple risk factors are at especially high risk. Delirium occurred in half of the patients with at least three of the risk factors listed in Table 3–7.

Two types of interventions to prevent delirium have been evaluated: focused geriatric care and psychotropic medications. In a randomized, controlled trial of hip fracture surgery patients, those who received daily visits and targeted recommendations from a geriatrician had a lower risk of postoperative delirium (32%) than the control patients (50%). Common interventions to prevent delirium were maintenance of the hematocrit > 30%; minimizing the use of benzodiazepines and anticholinergic medications; maintenance of regular bowel function; and early discontinuation of urinary catheters. Other studies comparing postoperative care in specialized geriatrics units with standard wards have shown similar reductions in the incidence of delirium. Limited data support the effectiveness of using low doses of neuroleptics to prevent postoperative delirium, but this practice is uncommon. While clinically apparent delirium usually resolves over several days, some patients will suffer from subtler postoperative cognitive dysfunction that can last for weeks or months after surgery. Patients who experienced postoperative delirium are more likely to have subsequent postoperative cognitive dysfunction.

Stroke complicates < 1% of all surgical procedures but may occur in 1–6% of patients undergoing cardiac or carotid artery surgery. Most of the strokes in cardiac surgery patients are embolic in origin, and about half occur within the first postoperative day. Stroke after cardiac surgery is associated with significantly increased mortality, up to 22% in some studies. A prediction model for stroke after CABG surgery includes the following risk factors: age > 60 years, female sex, urgent or emergency surgery, diabetes mellitus, chronic kidney disease, peripheral vascular disease, and systolic dysfunction.

Symptomatic carotid artery stenosis is associated with a high risk of stroke in patients undergoing cardiac surgery. In general, symptomatic carotid lesions should be treated prior to elective cardiac surgery. In contrast, most studies suggest that asymptomatic carotid bruits and asymptomatic carotid stenosis are associated with little or no increased risk of stroke in surgical patients. Prophylactic carotid endarterectomy or stenting in patients with asymptomatic carotid artery disease is unlikely to be beneficial in most patients, as the stroke risk of the carotid procedure likely outweighs any risk reduction it provides in a subsequent operation. On the other hand, patients with independent indications for such procedures (see Chapter 12) should probably have the carotid operation prior to the elective surgery. A meta-analysis of trials comparing carotid endarterectomy to carotid stenting found that endarterectomy led to fewer periprocedural strokes.

Bateman BT et al. Perioperative acute ischemic stroke in noncardiac and nonvascular surgery: incidence, risk factors, and outcomes. Anesthesiology. 2009 Feb;110(2):231–8. [PMID: 19194149]

Robinson TN et al. Preoperative cognitive dysfunction is related to adverse postoperative outcomes in the elderly. J Am Coll Surg. 2012 Jul;215(1):12–8. [PMID: 22626912]
Saczynski JS et al. Cognitive trajectories after postoperative delirium. N Engl J Med. 2012 Jul 5;367(1):30–9. [PMID: 22762316]

MANAGEMENT OF ENDOCRINE DISEASES

▶ Diabetes Mellitus

Patients with diabetes mellitus are at increased risk for postoperative infections, particularly those involving the surgical site. Patients with a preoperative hemoglobin A_{1c} < 7% have roughly half the risk for developing a postoperative infection compared with those with a hemoglobin A_{1c} > 7%. Even in patients without diabetes, hyperglycemia is associated with surgical site infection although proof of a causal relationship is lacking. The most challenging issue in diabetic patients, however, is the maintenance of glucose control during the perioperative period. The increased secretion of cortisol, epinephrine, glucagon, and growth hormone during surgery is associated with insulin resistance and hyperglycemia in diabetic patients. The goal of management is the prevention of severe hyperglycemia or hypoglycemia in the perioperative period.

The ideal postoperative blood glucose level is not known. Trials have demonstrated that tighter perioperative glycemic control leads to better clinical outcomes in cardiac surgery patients in a critical care unit. This finding is not generally applicable to other surgical patients, however, as a subsequent trial demonstrated **increased** mortality with tight control in surgical patients in an intensive care unit. Data are lacking on risks and benefits of tight control in patients outside of intensive care units. The American College of Physicians recommends maintaining serum glucose between 140 mg/dL and 200 mg/dL (7.8–11.1 mmol/L), whereas the British National Health Service guidelines recommend a range of 108–180 mg/dL (6–10 mmol/L).

The specific pharmacologic management of diabetes during the perioperative period depends on the type of diabetes (insulin-dependent or not), the level of glycemic control, and the type and length of surgery. In general, all patients with type 1 diabetes and some with type 2 diabetes will need an intravenous insulin infusion perioperatively. Perioperative management of all diabetic patients requires frequent blood glucose monitoring to prevent hypoglycemia and to ensure prompt treatment of hyperglycemia. Recommendations for glycemic control in patients who generally do not need intraoperative insulin are shown in Table 3–8. Perioperative use of corticosteroids, common in neurosurgical and organ transplant procedures, increases glucose intolerance. Patients receiving corticosteroids often require additional regular insulin with meals, while their fasting glucose levels may remain relatively unchanged.

▶ Corticosteroid Replacement

Perioperative complications (predominantly hypotension) resulting from primary or secondary adrenocortical insufficiency are rare. The common practice of administering

Table 3–8. Perioperative management of diabetic patients who do not need insulin.

Patient	Recommended Management
Diabetes well controlled on diet alone	Measure glucose every 4 hours while fasting or NPO and give subcutaneous regular insulin as needed to maintain blood glucose at 140–200 mg/dL (7.8–11.1 mmol/L)[1] Avoid glucose-containing solutions during surgery
Diabetes well controlled on an oral medication	The last dose of medication should be taken on the evening before surgery Measure glucose every 4 hours while fasting or NPO and give subcutaneous regular insulin as needed to maintain blood glucose at 140–200 mg/dL (7.8–11.1 mmol/L)[1] Measure blood glucose level every 4 hours (or more frequently as indicated) during surgery Resume oral hypoglycemic therapy when the patient returns to baseline diet

[1]Glycemic target should be individualized, but tight glycemic control is generally not indicated (see text).
NPO, nothing by mouth.

high-dose corticosteroids during the perioperative period in patients at risk for adrenocortical insufficiency has not been rigorously studied. While definitive recommendations regarding perioperative corticosteroid therapy cannot be made, a conservative approach would be to consider any patient who has received the equivalent of at least 7.5 mg of prednisone daily for 3 weeks within the past year to be at risk for having adrenocortical insufficiency. Patients who have been taking less than 5 mg of prednisone daily and those receiving alternate day corticosteroid dosing are unlikely to require supplemental coverage. A commonly used regimen is 100 mg of hydrocortisone given intravenously daily, divided every 8 hours, beginning before induction of anesthesia and continuing for 24–48 hours. Tapering the dose is not necessary. Patients receiving long-term maintenance corticosteroid therapy should also continue their usual dose throughout the perioperative period.

▶ Thyroid Disease

Severe symptomatic hypothyroidism has been associated with perioperative complications, including intraoperative hypotension, HF, cardiac arrest, and death. Elective surgery should be delayed in patients with severe hypothyroidism until adequate thyroid hormone replacement can be achieved. Similarly, patients with symptomatic hyperthyroidism are at risk for perioperative thyroid storm and should not undergo elective surgery until their thyrotoxicosis is controlled. An endocrinologist should be consulted if emergency surgery is needed in such patients. Conversely, patients with asymptomatic or mild hypothyroidism generally tolerate surgery well, with only a slight increase in the incidence of intraoperative hypotension; surgery need not be delayed for the month or more required to ensure adequate thyroid hormone replacement.

Dhatariya K et al; Joint British Diabetes Societies. NHS Diabetes guideline for the perioperative management of the adult patient with diabetes. Diabet Med. 2012 Apr;29(4):420–33. [PMID: 22288687]

Qaseem A et al. Use of intensive insulin therapy for the management of glycemic control in hospitalized patients: a clinical practice guideline from the American College of Physicians. Ann Intern Med. 2011 Feb 15;154(4):260–7. [PMID: 21320941]

Richards JE et al. Relationship of hyperglycemia and surgical-site infection in orthopaedic surgery. J Bone Joint Surg Am. 2012 Jul 3;94(13):1181–6. [PMID: 22760385]

KIDNEY DISEASE

Approximately 1% of patients suffer a significant reduction in kidney function after major surgery. The risk is much higher, however, in patients undergoing cardiac operations, where 10–30% of patients develop acute kidney injury. The development of acute kidney injury is an independent predictor of mortality, even if renal dysfunction resolves. The mortality associated with the development of perioperative acute kidney injury that requires dialysis exceeds 50%. Risk factors associated with postoperative deterioration in kidney function are shown in Table 3–9. Several medications, including "renal dose" dopamine, mannitol, N-acetylcysteine, and furosemide, have been evaluated in an attempt to preserve kidney function during the perioperative period. None of these have proved effective in clinical trials and generally should not be used for this indication. Maintenance of adequate intravascular volume is likely to be the most effective method to reduce the risk of perioperative deterioration in kidney function. Exposure to renal toxic agents such as nonsteroidal anti-inflammatory drugs and intravenous contrast should be minimized or avoided. Angiotensin-converting enzyme inhibitors and angiotensin receptor blockers reduce renal perfusion and may increase the risk of perioperative acute kidney injury. Although firm evidence is lacking, it may be useful to temporarily discontinue these medications in patients at risk for perioperative acute kidney injury.

Although the mortality rate for elective major surgery is low (1–4%) in patients with dialysis-dependent chronic kidney disease, the risk for perioperative complications, including postoperative hyperkalemia, pneumonia, fluid overload, and bleeding, is substantially increased. Postoperative hyperkalemia requiring emergent hemodialysis has been reported to occur in 20–30% of patients. Patients should undergo dialysis preoperatively within 24 hours before surgery, and their serum electrolyte levels should be measured just prior to surgery and monitored closely during the postoperative period.

Borthwick E et al. Perioperative acute kidney injury: risk factors, recognition, management, and outcomes. BMJ. 2010 Jul 5;341: c3365. [PMID: 20603317]

ANTIBIOTIC PROPHYLAXIS OF SURGICAL SITE INFECTIONS

There are an estimated 0.5–1 million surgical site infections annually in the United States. Surgical site infection is estimated to occur in roughly 4% of general or vascular operations. For most major procedures, the use of prophylactic antibiotics has been demonstrated to reduce the incidence of surgical site infections significantly. For example, antibiotic prophylaxis in colorectal surgery reduces the incidence of surgical site infection from 25–50% to below 20%. In addition, in a case-control study of Medicare beneficiaries, the use of preoperative antibiotics within 2 hours of surgery was associated with a twofold reduction in 60-day mortality.

Multiple studies have evaluated the effectiveness of different antibiotic regimens for various surgical procedures. In most cases, no single antibiotic regimen has been shown to be superior. Several general conclusions can be drawn from these data. First, substantial evidence suggests that a single dose of an appropriate intravenous antibiotic—or combination of antibiotics—is as effective as multiple-dose regimens that extend into the postoperative period. For longer procedures, the dose should be repeated every 3–4 hours to ensure maintenance of a therapeutic serum level. In colorectal surgery, however, three doses of an intravenous cephalosporin have been shown to reduce surgical site infection incidence compared with a single dose. Similarly, at least 24 hours of postoperative antibiotic therapy is recommended after cardiac surgery. Second, for most procedures, a first-generation cephalosporin is as effective as later-generation agents. However, in a large randomized trial of colorectal surgery patients, the use of prophylactic ertapenem significantly reduced the surgical site infection rate compared to that for cefotetan. Third, prophylactic antibiotics should be given intravenously at induction of anesthesia or roughly 30–60 minutes prior to the skin incision. Although the type of procedure is the main factor determining the risk of developing a surgical site infection, certain patient factors have been associated with increased risk, including diabetes mellitus, older age, obesity, heavy alcohol consumption, admission from a long-term care facility, and multiple medical comorbidities.

Other strategies to prevent surgical site infections have proven to be controversial. Evidence suggests that nasal carriage with *Staphylococcus aureus* is associated with a twofold to ninefold increased risk of surgical site and catheter-related infections in surgical patients. Treatment of nasal carriers of *S aureus* with 2% mupirocin ointment (twice daily intranasally for 3 days) prior to cardiac surgery decreases the risk of surgical site infections. However, in a 2008 cohort study, universal screening for methicillin-resistant *S aureus* in surgical patients failed to reduce

Table 3–9. Risk factors for the development of postoperative acute kidney failure.

Preoperative chronic kidney disease
Aortic and major peripheral vascular surgery
Cardiac surgery
Severe heart failure
Preoperative jaundice
Age > 70 years
Diabetes mellitus
COPD requiring daily bronchodilator therapy

COPD, chronic obstructive pulmonary disease.

infection rates from this pathogen. High concentration oxygen delivered in the immediate postoperative period may reduce surgical site infections in patients undergoing colorectal surgery or operations requiring general anesthesia. Preoperative bathing with antiseptic agents and preoperative hair removal are common practices but have not demonstrated a reduction in surgical site infections in randomized trials. The use of razors for hair removal actually seems to increase the risk of surgical site infections and is therefore specifically not recommended. If preoperative hair removal is indicated, the use of clippers is preferred.

Guidelines for antibiotic prophylaxis against infective endocarditis in patients undergoing invasive procedures are presented in Chapter 33. The American Association of Orthopaedic Surgeons recommends consideration of prophylactic antibiotics in patients with prosthetic joints on a case-by-case basis. More definitive or evidence-based guidelines for antibiotic prophylaxis against prosthetic joint infection are lacking.

Enzler MJ et al. Antimicrobial prophylaxis in adults. Mayo Clin Proc. 2011 Jul;86(7):686–701. [PMID: 21719623]

Suzuki T et al. Optimal duration of prophylactic antibiotic administration for elective colon cancer surgery: a randomized, clinical trial. Surgery. 2011 Feb;149(2):171–8. [PMID: 20655559]

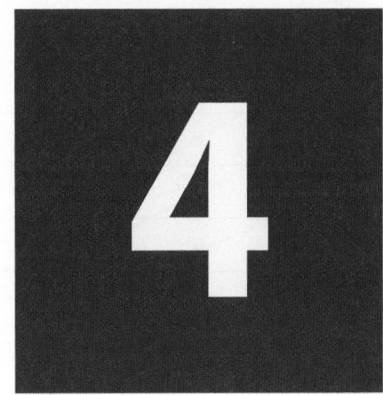

Geriatric Disorders

G. Michael Harper, MD
C. Bree Johnston, MD, MPH
C. Seth Landefeld, MD

GENERAL PRINCIPLES OF GERIATRIC CARE

The following principles help in caring for older adults:

1. Many disorders are multifactorial in origin and are best managed by multifactorial interventions.
2. Diseases often present atypically.
3. Not all abnormalities require evaluation and treatment.
4. Complex medication regimens, adherence problems, and polypharmacy are common challenges.

ASSESSMENT OF THE OLDER ADULT

Comprehensive assessment addresses three topics in addition to conventional assessment of symptoms and diseases: prognosis, values and preferences, and ability to function independently. Comprehensive assessment is warranted before major clinical decisions are made.

▶ Assessment of Prognosis

When an older person's life expectancy is > 10 years (ie, 50% of similar persons live longer than 10 years), it is reasonable to consider effective tests and treatments much as they are considered in younger persons. When life expectancy is < 10 years (and especially when it is much less), choices of tests and treatments should be made on the basis of their ability to improve that particular patient's prognosis and quality of life in the shorter term of that patient's life expectancy. The relative benefits and harms of tests and treatments often change as prognosis worsens.

When an older patient's clinical situation is dominated by a single disease process (eg, lung cancer metastatic to brain), prognosis can be estimated well with a disease-specific instrument. Even in this situation, however, prognosis generally worsens with age (especially age > 90 years) and with the presence of serious age-related conditions, such as dementia, malnutrition, or impaired ability to walk.

When an older patient's clinical situation is not dominated by a single disease process, prognosis can be estimated initially by considering the patient's age, sex, and general health (Figure 4–1). For example, < 25% of men age 95 years will live 5 years, whereas nearly 75% of women age 70 years will live 10 years.

The prognosis of older persons living at home can be estimated by considering age, sex, comorbid conditions, and function (Table 4–1). The prognosis of older persons discharged from the hospital is worse than that of those living at home and can be estimated by considering gender, comorbid conditions, and function at discharge (Table 4–2).

▶ Assessment of Values & Preferences

Although patients vary in their values and preferences, most frail older patients prioritize maintaining their independence over prolonging survival. Values and preferences are determined by speaking directly with a patient or, when the patient cannot express preferences reliably, with the patient's surrogate. The clinician might ask a patient considering a hip replacement, "How would you like your hip pain and function to be different? Tell me about the risk and discomfort you are willing to go through to achieve that improvement."

In assessing values and preferences, it is important to keep in mind the following:

1. Patients are experts about their preferences for outcomes and experiences; however, they often do not have adequate information to express informed preferences for specific tests or treatments.
2. Patients' preferences often change over time. For example, some patients find living with a disability more acceptable than they thought before experiencing it.

▶ Assessment of Function

People often lose function in multiple domains as they age, with the results that they may not be able to do some activities as quickly or capably and may need assistance with other activities. Assessment of function improves prognostic estimates (see above). Assessment of function is essential to determining an individual's needs in the context of their values and preferences, and the possible effects of prescribed treatment.

Women

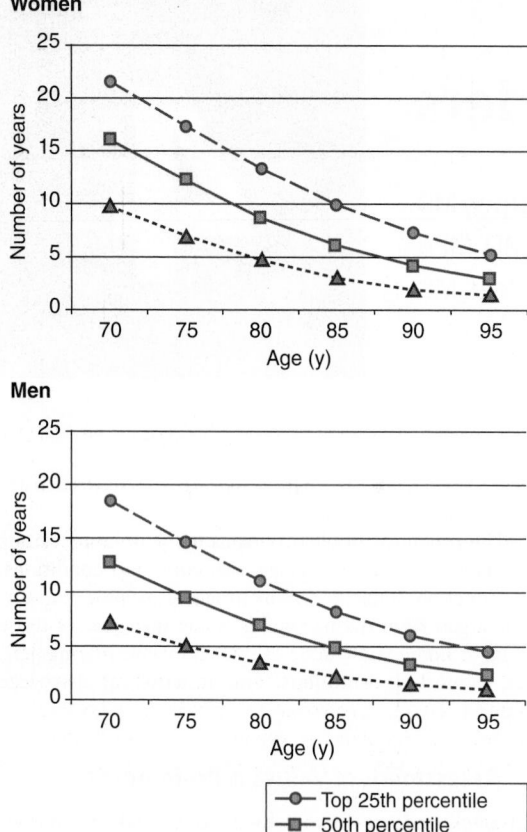

Men

Legend:
- —○— Top 25th percentile
- —■— 50th percentile
- --▲-- Lowest 25th percentile

▲ **Figure 4–1.** Median life expectancy of older women and men. (Adapted, with permission, from Walter LC et al. Screening for colorectal, breast, and cervical cancer in the elderly: a review of the evidence. Am J Med. 2005 Oct;118(10):1078–86.) Copyright © Elsevier.

Table 4–1. Prognostic factors, "risk points," and 4-year mortality rates for older persons living at home.

Prognostic Factor	Risk Points
Age	
60–64 years	1
64–69 years	2
70–74 years	3
74–79 years	4
80–84 years	5
85 years and older	7
Male sex	2
Comorbid conditions reported by patients	
Diabetes mellitus	1
Cancer	2
Lung disease	2
Heart failure	2
Body mass index < 25	1
Current smoker	2
Function	
Bathing difficulty	2
Difficulty handling finances	2
Difficulty walking several blocks	2
Sum of Risk Points	**4-year Mortality Rate**
1–2	2%
3–6	7%
7–10	19%
> 10	53%

Reprinted, with permission, from Lee SJ et al. Development and validation of a prognostic index for 4-year mortality in older adults. JAMA. 2006 Feb 15;295(7):801–8. Copyright © 2006 American Medical Association. All rights reserved.

About one-fourth of patients over 65 have impairments in their IADLs (instrumental activities of daily living: transportation, shopping, cooking, using the telephone, managing money, taking medications, housecleaning, laundry) or ADLs (basic activities of daily living: bathing, dressing eating, transferring from bed to chair, continence, toileting). Half of those persons older than 85 years have these latter impairments.

▶ **Functional Screening Instrument**

Functional screening should include assessment of ADL and IADL and questions to detect weight loss, falls, incontinence, depressed mood, self neglect, fear for personal safety, and common serious impairments (eg, hearing, vision, cognition, and mobility). Standard functional screening measures may not be useful in capturing subtle impairments in highly functional independent elders. One technique for these patients is to identify and regularly ask about a target activity, such as bowling or gardening. If the

patient begins to have trouble with or discontinues an "advanced activity of daily living," it may indicate early impairment, such as onset of cognitive impairment, incontinence, or worsening hearing loss, which additional gentle questioning or assessment may uncover.

▶ **Frailty**

"Frailty" is a term that describes older adults who experience decreased functional reserve. Frailty is characterized by multisystem dysregulation that usually includes chronic inflammation, sarcopenia, and alterations in neuroendocrine function. Persons with frailty are at increased risk for functional decline and death. There is no standard

Table 4–2. Prognostic factors, "risk points," and 1-year mortality rates for older patients discharged from the hospital after an acute medical illness.

Prognostic Factor	Risk Points
Male sex	1
Comorbid conditions reported by patients	
Cancer, metastatic	8
Cancer, not metastatic	3
Serum creatinine > 3 mg/dL	2
Albumin < 3 mg/dL	2
Albumin 3.0–3.4 mg/dL	1
Function	
Dependent in 1–4 ADL[1]	2
Dependent in 5 ADL[1]	5
Sum of Risk Points	**1-year Mortality Rate**
0–1	4%
2–3	19%
4–6	34%
> 6	64%

[1]ADL refers to five activities of daily living: bathing, dressing, transferring, using the toilet, and eating.
Reprinted, with permission, from Walter LC et al. Development and validation of a prognostic index for 1-year mortality in older adults after hospitalization. JAMA. 2001 Jun 20;285(23):2987–94. Copyright © 2006 American Medical Association. All rights reserved.

assessment tool for frailty. Elements of the frailty syndrome include slow gait speed, low hand grip strength, weight loss, low energy expenditure, and in some models, cognitive decline. The ideal strategies for preventing and treating the frailty syndrome are unknown. At present, treatment is largely supportive, multifactorial, and individualized based on patient goals, life expectancy, and comorbidities. Exercise, particularly strength and resistance training, is the intervention with the strongest evidence for benefit. Sometimes, transitioning a patient to a palliative approach or a hospice program is the most appropriate clinical intervention when efforts to prevent functional decline fail.

Clegg A et al. Frailty in elderly people. Lancet. 2013 Mar 2; 381(9868):752–62. Erratum in: Lancet.2013 Oct 19; 382(9901): 1328 [PMID: 23395245]
Fried TR et al. Health outcome prioritization to elicit preferences of older persons with multiple health conditions. Patient Educ Couns. 2011 May;83(2):278–82. [PMID: 20570078]
Sudore RL et al. Redefining the "planning" in advance care planning: preparing for end-of-life decision making. Ann Intern Med. 2010 Aug 17;153(4):256–261. [PMID: 20713793]

MANAGEMENT OF COMMON GERIATRIC PROBLEMS

1. Dementia

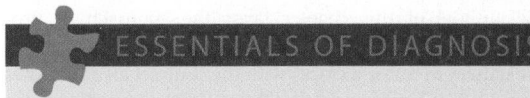

ESSENTIALS OF DIAGNOSIS

▶ Progressive decline of intellectual function.
▶ Loss of short-term memory and at least one other cognitive deficit.
▶ Deficit severe enough to cause impairment of function.
▶ Not delirious.

▶ General Considerations

Dementia is an acquired persistent and progressive impairment in intellectual function, with compromise of memory and at least one other cognitive domain, most commonly aphasia (typically, word finding difficulty), apraxia (inability to perform motor tasks, such as cutting a loaf of bread, despite intact motor function), agnosia (inability to recognize objects), and impaired executive function (poor abstraction, mental flexibility, planning, and judgment). The diagnosis of dementia requires a significant decline in function that is severe enough to interfere with work or social life.

Dementia has a prevalence that doubles every 5 years in the older population, reaching 30–50% at age 85. Alzheimer disease accounts for roughly two-thirds of dementia cases in the United States, with vascular dementia (either alone or combined with Alzheimer disease) and dementia with Lewy bodies accounting for much of the rest.

Depression and delirium are also common in elders, may coexist with dementia, and may also present with cognitive impairment. Depression is a common concomitant of early dementia. A patient with depression and cognitive impairment whose intellectual function improves with treatment of the mood disorder has an almost fivefold greater risk of suffering irreversible dementia later in life. Delirium, characterized by acute confusion, occurs much more commonly in patients with underlying dementia.

▶ Clinical Findings

A. Screening

1. Cognitive impairment—The Medicare Annual Wellness Visit mandates that clinicians assess patients for cognitive impairment. However, according to the US Preventive Services Task Force, there is insufficient evidence to recommend for or against screening all older adults for cognitive impairment. While there is logic in the argument that early detection may improve future planning and patient outcomes, empiric evidence that demonstrates a clear benefit for either patients or caregivers remains lacking.

When there is suspicion of cognitive impairment, the combination of a three-item word recall with a clock drawing task (also known as the "mini-cog") is a **simple screening test** that is fairly quick to administer. Ask the patient to repeat three items followed by instructions to draw the face of a clock. While different methods for administering and scoring the clock draw test have been described, the authors of this chapter favor the approach of predrawing a four inch circle on a sheet of paper and instructing the patient to "draw a clock" with the time set at 10 minutes after 11. If the patient recalls all three items after 3 minutes the test is considered normal, and there is no need to score the clock. Conversely, if the patient recalls zero items, the test is considered abnormal, and similarly there is no need to score the clock. When the patient recalls one or two items, the test is normal when the clock is drawn correctly (numbers in the proper position and the time accurately portrayed). When a patient fails this simple screen, further cognitive evaluation with a standardized instrument is warranted. The Montreal Cognitive Assessment (MoCA ©) is a 30-point test that takes about 10 minutes to administer and examines several areas of cognitive function. A score below 26 is considered abnormal. Free downloadable versions in multiple languages are available at http://www.mocatest.org.

2. Decision-making capacity—Cognitively impaired elders commonly face serious medical decisions, and the clinicians involved in their care must ascertain whether the capacity exists to make the choice. The following five elements should be considered in a thorough assessment: (1) ability to express a choice; (2) understanding relevant information about the risks and benefits of planned therapy and the alternatives, in the context of one's values, including no treatment; (3) comprehension of the problem and its consequences; (4) ability to reason; and (5) consistency. A patient's choice should follow from an understanding of the consequences.

Sensitivity must be used in applying these five components to people of various cultural backgrounds. Decision-making capacity varies over time. Furthermore, the capacity to make a decision is a function of the decision in question. A woman with mild dementia may lack the capacity to consent to coronary artery bypass grafting yet retain the capacity to designate a surrogate decision-maker.

B. Symptoms and Signs

The clinician can gather important information about the type of dementia that may be present by asking about: (1) the rate of progression of the deficits as well as their nature (including any personality or behavioral change); (2) the presence of other neurologic symptoms, particularly motor problems; (3) risk factors for HIV; (4) family history of dementia; and (5) medications, with particular attention to recent changes.

Work-up is directed at identifying any potentially reversible causes of dementia. However, such cases are indeed rare. For a detailed description of the symptoms and signs of different forms of dementia, see Chapter 24.

C. Physical Examination

The neurologic examination emphasizes assessment of mental status but should also include evaluation for sensory deficits, possible previous strokes, parkinsonism, or peripheral neuropathy. The remainder of the physical examination should focus on identifying comorbid conditions that may aggravate the individual's disability. For a detailed description of the neuropsychological assessment, see Chapter 24.

D. Laboratory Findings

Laboratory studies should include a complete blood count, electrolytes, calcium, creatinine, glucose, thyroid-stimulating hormone (TSH), and vitamin B_{12} levels. While hypothyroidism or vitamin B_{12} deficiency may contribute to the cognitive impairment, treating these conditions typically does not completely reverse the dementia. HIV testing, RPR (rapid plasma reagin) test, heavy metal screen, and liver biochemical tests may be informative in selected patients but should not be considered part of routine testing. For a detailed description of laboratory findings, see Chapter 24.

E. Imaging

Most patients should receive neuroimaging as part of the diagnostic work-up to rule out subdural hematoma, tumor, previous stroke, and hydrocephalus (usually normal pressure). Those who are younger and those who have focal neurologic symptoms or signs, seizures, gait abnormalities, and an acute or subacute onset are most likely to yield positive findings and most likely to benefit from MRI scanning. In older patients with a more classic picture of Alzheimer disease in whom neuroimaging is desired, a noncontrast CT scan is sufficient. For a detailed description of imaging, see Chapter 24.

▶ Differential Diagnosis

Older individuals experience occasional difficulty retrieving items from memory (usually manifested as word-finding complaints) and experience a slowing in their rate of information processing. In **mild cognitive impairment,** a patient complains of memory problems, demonstrates mild deficits (most commonly in short-term memory) on formal testing, but does not meet criteria for dementia. Dementia will develop in more than half of people with mild cognitive impairment within 5 years. Acetylcholinesterase inhibitors have not consistently demonstrated a delay in the progression of mild cognitive impairment to Alzheimer disease. An elderly patient with intact cognition but with severe impairments in vision or hearing commonly becomes confused in an unfamiliar medical setting and consequently may be falsely labeled as demented.

Delirium can be distinguished from dementia by its acute onset, fluctuating course, and deficits in attention rather than memory. Because delirium and dementia often coexist, it may not be possible to determine how much impairment is attributable to each condition until the patient is fully recovered and back in their usual setting. Many medications have been associated with delirium and other types of cognitive impairment in older patients. Anticholinergic agents, hypnotics, neuroleptics, opioids, nonsteroidal anti-inflammatory drugs (NSAIDs), antihistamines (including H$_1$ and H$_2$-antagonists), and corticosteroids are just some of the medications that have been associated with cognitive impairment in elders.

▶ Treatment

Patients and families should be made aware of the Alzheimer's Association (http://www.alz.org) as well as the wealth of helpful community and online resources and publications available. Caregiver support, education, and counseling may prevent or delay nursing home placement. Education should include the manifestations and natural history of dementia as well as the availability of local support services such as respite care. Even under the best of circumstances, caregiver stress can be substantial. Collaborative care models and disease management programs appear to improve the quality of care for patients with dementia.

A. Cognitive Impairment

1. Acetylcholinesterase inhibitors—Many experts recommend considering a trial of acetylcholinesterase inhibitors (eg, donepezil, galantamine, rivastigmine) in most patients with mild to moderate Alzheimer disease. These medications produce a modest improvement in cognitive function that is not likely to be detected in routine clinical encounters. Acetylcholinesterase inhibitors may also have similarly modest cognitive benefits in patients with vascular dementia or dementia with Lewy bodies. However, acetylcholinesterase inhibitors have not convincingly been shown to delay institutionalization or functional decline. There is insufficient evidence to recommend their use in mild cognitive impairment to slow the progression toward dementia or to improve cognitive test scores.

Starting doses, respectively, of donepezil, galantamine, and rivastigmine, are 5 mg orally once daily (maximum 10 mg once daily), 4 mg orally twice daily (maximum 12 mg twice daily), and 1.5 mg orally twice daily (maximum 6 mg twice daily). The doses are increased gradually as tolerated. The most bothersome side effects include diarrhea, nausea, anorexia, weight loss, and syncope. Some patients with moderate to severe cognitive impairment continue to experience benefits from acetylcholinesterase inhibitors. In those patients who have had no apparent benefit, experience side effects, or for whom the financial outlay is a burden, the drug should be discontinued.

2. Memantine—In clinical trials, patients with more advanced disease have been shown to have statistical benefit from the use of memantine, an N-methyl-D-aspartate (NMDA) antagonist, with or without concomitant use of an acetylcholinesterase inhibitor. Long-term and meaningful functional outcomes have yet to be demonstrated.

B. Behavioral Problems

1. Nonpharmacologic approaches—Behavioral problems in demented patients are often best managed with a nonpharmacologic approach. Initially, it should be established that the problem is not unrecognized delirium, pain, urinary obstruction, or fecal impaction. It also helps to inquire whether the caregiver or institutional staff can tolerate the behavior, as it is often easier to find ways to accommodate to the behavior than to modify it. If not, the caregiver should keep a brief log in which the behavior is described along with antecedent events and consequences. Recurring precipitants of the behavior are often found to be present or it may be that the behavior is rewarded. Caregivers are taught to use simple language when communicating with the patient, to break down activities into simple component tasks, and to use a "distract, not confront" approach when the patient seems disturbed by a troublesome issue. Additional steps to address behavioral problems include providing structure and routine, discontinuing all medications except those considered absolutely necessary, and correcting, if possible, sensory deficits.

2. Pharmacologic approaches—There is no clear consensus about pharmacologic approaches to treatment of behavioral problems in patients who have not benefited from nonpharmacologic therapies. The target symptoms—depression, anxiety, psychosis, mood lability, or pain—may suggest which class of medications might be most helpful in a given patient. Patients with depressive symptoms may show improvement with antidepressant therapy. Patients with dementia with Lewy bodies have shown clinically significant improvement in behavioral symptoms when treated with rivastigmine (3–6 mg orally twice daily).

Despite the lack of strong evidence, antipsychotic medications have remained a mainstay for the treatment of behavioral disturbances, particularly agitation and aggression, largely because of the lack of alternatives. The atypical antipsychotic agents (risperidone, olanzapine, quetiapine, aripiprazole, clozapine, ziprasidone) are reported to be better tolerated than older agents but should be avoided in patients with vascular risk factors due to an increased risk of stroke; they can cause weight gain and are also associated with hyperglycemia in diabetic patients and are considerably more expensive. Both typical and atypical antipsychotics in several short-term trials and one long-term trial increased mortality compared with placebo when used to treat elderly demented patients with behavioral disturbances. Starting and target dosages should be much lower than those used in schizophrenia (eg, haloperidol, 0.5–2 mg orally; risperidone, 0.25–2 mg orally).

C. Driving

Although drivers with dementia are at an increased risk for motor vehicle accidents, many patients continue to drive safely well beyond the time of diagnosis, making the timing of when to recommend that a patient stop driving particularly challenging.

There is no clear-cut evidence to suggest a single best approach to determining an individual patient's risk, and there is no accepted "gold standard" test. The result is that clinicians must consider several factors upon which to base their judgment. For example, determining the severity of dementia can be useful. Patients with very mild or mild dementia according to the Clinical Dementia Rating Scale were able to pass formal road tests at rates of 88% and 69%, respectively. Experts agree that patients with moderately severe or more advanced dementia should be counseled to stop driving. Although not well studied, clinicians should also consider the effects of comorbid conditions and medications and the role each may play in contributing to the risk of driving by a patient with dementia. Assessment of the ability to carry out IADLs may also add to the determination of risk. Finally, in some cases of mild dementia, referral may be needed to a driver rehabilitation specialist for evaluation. Although not standardized, this evaluation often consists of both off- and on-road testing. The cost for this assessment can be substantial, and it is typically not covered by health insurance. Experts recommend such an evaluation for patients with mild dementia, for those with dementia for whom new impairment in driving skills is observed, and for those with significant deficits in cognitive domains such as attention, executive function, and visuospatial skills.

Clinicians must also be aware of the reporting requirements in their individual jurisdictions. Some states have mandatory reporting laws for clinicians, but in other states, the decision to report an unsafe driver with dementia is voluntary. When a clinician has made the decision to report an unsafe driver to the Department of Motor Vehicles, he or she must consider the impact as a potential breach in confidentiality and must weigh and address, in advance when possible, the consequences from the loss of driving independence.

D. Advance Financial Planning

Difficulty in managing financial affairs often develops early in the course of dementia. The patient's caregiver may seek advice from the patient's primary care clinician. Although expertise is not expected, clinicians should have some proficiency to address financial concerns. Just as clinicians counsel patients and families about advance care planning, the same should be done to educate about the need for advance financial planning and to recommend that patients complete a durable power of attorney for finance matters (DPOAF) when the capacity to do so still exists. In most states the DPOAF can be executed with or without the aid of an attorney. Other options to assist in managing and monitoring finances include online banking, automatic bill payments, direct deposits and joint bank accounts. A potential risk of the joint account is that the joint account holder has no obligation to act in the best interest of the patient.

No gold standard test is available to identify when a patient with dementia no longer has financial capacity. However, the clinician should be on the lookout for signs that a patient is either at risk for or actually experiencing financial incapacity. Because financial impairment can occur when dementia is mild, making that diagnosis should alone be enough to warrant further investigation. Questioning patients and caregivers about late, missed or repeated bill payments, unusual or uncharacteristic purchases or gifts, overdrawn bank accounts and reports of missing funds can provide evidence of suspected financial impairment. Patients with dementia are also at increased risk for becoming victims of financial abuse and some

answers to these same questions might also be signs of potential financial abuse. When financial abuse is suspected, clinicians should be aware of the reporting requirements in their local jurisdictions. Social workers can aid with this reporting.

▶ Prognosis

Life expectancy after a diagnosis of Alzheimer disease is typically 3–15 years; it may be shorter than previously reported. Other neurodegenerative dementias, such as dementia with Lewy bodies, show more rapid decline. Hospice is often appropriate for patients with end-stage dementia.

▶ When to Refer

Referral for neuropsychological testing may be helpful in the following circumstances: to distinguish dementia from depression, to diagnose dementia in persons of very poor education or very high premorbid intellect, and to aid diagnosis when impairment is mild.

Devanand DP et al. Relapse risk after discontinuation of risperidone in Alzheimer's disease. N Engl J Med. 2012 Oct 18; 367(16):1497–507. [PMID: 23075176]

Howard R et al. Donepezil and memantine for moderate-to-severe Alzheimer's disease. N Engl J Med. 2012 Mar 8; 366(10):893–903. [PMID: 22397651]

Lin JS et al. Screening for cognitive impairment in older adults: a systematic review for the U.S. Preventive Services Task Force Ann Intern Med. 2013 November 5;159(9):601–12. [PMID: 24145578]

Russ TC et al. Cholinesterase inhibitors for mild cognitive impairment. Cochrane Database Syst Rev. 2012 Sep 12;9: CD009132. [PMID: 22972133]

Widera E et al. Finances in the older patient with cognitive impairment: "He didn't want me to take over". JAMA. 2011 Feb 16; 305(7):698–706. [PMID: 21325186]

2. Depression

ESSENTIALS OF DIAGNOSIS

▶ Depressed elders may not admit to depressed mood.

▶ Depression screening in elders should include a question about anhedonia.

▶ General Considerations

Depressive symptoms—often related to loss, disease, and life changes—may be present in more than 25% of elders; however, the prevalence of major depression is similar in younger and older populations. Depression is particularly common in hospitalized and institutionalized elders. Older single men have the highest suicide rate of any demographic group. Older patients with depression are more likely to have somatic complaints, less likely to report depressed mood, and more likely to experience delusions than younger patients. In addition, depression may be an early symptom of a neurodegenerative condition such as dementia. Depressed patients who have comorbid conditions (such as heart failure) are at higher risk for hospitalization, tend to have longer hospital stays, and have worse outcomes than their nondepressed counterparts.

Clinical Findings

A simple two-question screen—which consists of asking "During the past 2 weeks, have you felt down, depressed, or hopeless?" and "During the past 2 weeks, have you felt little interest or pleasure in doing things?"—is highly sensitive for detecting major depression in persons over age 65. Positive responses can be followed up with more comprehensive, structured interviews, such as the Geriatric Depression Scale (http://www.stanford.edu/~yesavage/GDS.html) or the PHQ-9.

Elderly patients with depressive symptoms should be questioned about medication use, since drugs (eg, benzodiazepines, corticosteroids) may contribute to the clinical picture. Similarly, several medical problems can cause fatigue, lethargy, or hypoactive delirium, all of which may be mistaken for depression. Particularly when delirium is the differential diagnosis, laboratory testing should include a complete blood count; liver, thyroid, and kidney function tests; serum calcium; urinalysis; and electrocardiogram.

Treatment

Choice of antidepressant agent in elders is usually based on side effect profile, cost, and patient specific factors such as presenting symptoms and comorbidities. Selective serotonin reuptake inhibitors (SSRIs) are often used as first-line agents because of their relatively benign side-effect profiles (see Table 25–7). In general, fluoxetine is avoided because of its long duration of action and tricyclic antidepressants are avoided because of their high anticholinergic side effects. Mirtazapine is often used for patients with weight loss, anorexia, or insomnia. Venlafaxine or duloxetine may be useful in patients who also have neuropathic pain. Regardless of the drug chosen, many experts recommend starting elders at a relatively low dose, titrating to full dose slowly, and continuing for a longer trial (at least 8 weeks) before trying a different medication. For patients experiencing their first episode of depression, drug treatment should continue for at least 6 months after remission of the depression. Recurrence of major depression is common enough among elders that long-term maintenance medication therapy should be considered.

Problem-solving therapy and cognitive behavioral therapy can be effective alone or in combination with medication therapy. Depressed elders may do better with a collaborative or multidisciplinary care model that includes socialization and other support elements than with usual care.

When to Refer

Referral should be considered for patients who have not responded to an initial antidepressant drug trial and for patients with have symptoms of mania, suicidality, or psychosis.

When to Admit

Patients who are suicidal, homicidal, psychotic, or a danger to self or others should be considered for acute psychiatric hospitalization.

Kok RM et al. Continuing treatment of depression in the elderly: a systematic review and meta-analysis of double-blinded randomized controlled trials with antidepressants. Am J Geriatr Psychiatry. 2011 March;19(3):249–55. [PMID: 21425505]
Leontjevas R et al. A structural multidisciplinary approach to depression management in nursing-home residents: a multi-centre, stepped-wedge cluster-randomised trial. Lancet. 2013 Jun 29;381(9885):2255–64. [PMID: 23643110]
Prina AM et al. Association between depression and hospital outcomes among older men. CMAJ. 2013 Feb 5;185(2):117–23. [PMID: 23228999]

3. Delirium

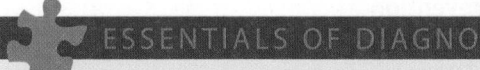

ESSENTIALS OF DIAGNOSIS

▶ Rapid onset and fluctuating course.
▶ Primary deficit in attention rather than memory.
▶ May be hypoactive or hyperactive.
▶ Dementia frequently coexists.

General Considerations

Delirium is an acute, fluctuating disturbance of consciousness, associated with a change in cognition or the development of perceptual disturbances (see also Chapter 25). It is the pathophysiologic consequence of an underlying general medical condition such as infection, coronary ischemia, hypoxemia, or metabolic derangement. Delirium persists in up to 25% of patients and is associated with worse clinical outcomes (higher in-hospital and postdischarge mortality, longer lengths of stay, greater probability of placement in a nursing facility).

Although the acutely agitated elderly patient often comes to mind when considering delirium, many episodes are more subtle. Such quiet, or hypoactive, delirium may only be suspected if one notices new cognitive slowing or inattention.

Cognitive impairment is an important risk factor for delirium. Approximately 25% of delirious patients are demented, and 40% of demented hospitalized patients are delirious. Other risk factors are male sex, severe illness, hip fracture, fever or hypothermia, hypotension, malnutrition, polypharmacy and use of psychoactive medications, sensory impairment, use of restraints, use of intravenous lines or urinary catheters, metabolic disorders, depression, and alcoholism.

Clinical Findings

A number of bedside instruments for the assessment of delirium are available. The confusion assessment method (CAM), which requires (1) acute onset and fluctuating course and (2) inattention and *either* (3) disorganized thinking *or* (4) altered level of consciousness, is easy to administer and performs well.

A key component of a delirium work-up is review of medications because a large number of drugs, the addition of a new drug, or the discontinuation of a drug known to cause withdrawal symptoms are all associated with the development of delirium. Medications that are particularly likely to increase the risk of delirium include opioids, benzodiazepines, as well as H_1- and H_2-antihistamines.

Laboratory evaluation of most patients should include a complete blood count, electrolytes, blood urea nitrogen (BUN) and serum creatinine, glucose, calcium, albumin, liver function studies, urinalysis, and electrocardiography. In selected cases, serum magnesium, serum drug levels, arterial blood gas measurements, blood cultures, chest radiography, urinary toxin screen, head CT scan, and lumbar puncture may be helpful.

Prevention

Prevention is the best approach in the management of delirium. Measures include improving cognition (frequent reorientation, activities, socialization with family and friends, when possible), sleep (massage, noise reduction, minimizing interruptions at night), mobility, vision (visual aids and adaptive equipment), hearing (portable amplifiers, cerumen disimpaction), and hydration status (volume repletion). No medications have been consistently shown to prevent delirium or reduce its duration or severity.

Treatment

Management of established episodes of delirium is largely supportive and includes reassurance and reorientation, treatment of underlying causes, eliminating unnecessary medications, and avoidance of indwelling catheters and restraints. Antipsychotic agents (such as haloperidol, 0.5–1 mg orally, or quetiapine, 25 mg orally, at bedtime or twice daily) are considered the medication of choice when drug treatment of delirium is necessary. As with dementia, caution should be used when prescribing antipsychotic medications, including checking the QTc interval, eliminating other QTc prolonging medications, and correcting any deficiencies of electrolytes. Benzodiazepines should be avoided except in the circumstance of alcohol or benzodiazepine withdrawal. In ventilated patients in the intensive care unit setting, dexmedetomidine or propofol (or both) may also be useful alternatives or adjuncts to antipsychotic therapy in patients with delirium.

Most episodes of delirium clear in a matter of days after correction of the precipitant, but some patients suffer episodes of much longer duration, and a significant percentage never return to their former baseline level of functioning.

When to Refer

If an initial evaluation does not reveal the cause of delirium or if entities other than delirium are in the differential diagnosis, referral to a neuropsychologist, neurologist, or geropsychiatrist should be considered.

When to Admit

Patients with delirium of unknown cause should be admitted for an expedited work-up if consistent with the patient's goals of care.

Clegg A et al. Which medications to avoid in people at risk of delirium: a systematic review. Age Aging. 2011 Jan;40(1):23–9. [PMID: 21068014]

Vidal EI et al. Delirium in older adults. BMJ. 2013 Apr 9;346: f2031. [PMID: 23571740]

4. Immobility

Although common in older people, reduced mobility is never normal and is often treatable if its causes are identified. Bed rest is an important cause of hospital-induced functional decline. Among hospitalized medical patients over 70, about 10% experience a decline in function, much of which results from preventable reductions in mobility.

The hazards of bed rest in older adults are multiple, serious, quick to develop, and slow to reverse. Deconditioning of the cardiovascular system occurs within days and involves fluid shifts, decreased cardiac output, decreased peak oxygen uptake, and increased resting heart rate. More striking changes occur in skeletal muscle, with loss of contractile velocity and strength. Pressure ulcers, deep venous thrombosis, and pulmonary embolism are additional serious risks. Within days after being confined to bed, the risk of postural hypotension, falls, and skin breakdown rises rapidly in the older patient. Moreover, recovery from these changes usually takes weeks to months.

Prevention & Treatment

When immobilization cannot be avoided, several measures can be used to minimize its consequences. Skin should be inspected at least daily. If the patient is unable to shift position, staff should do so every 2 hours. To minimize cardiovascular deconditioning, patients should be positioned as close to the upright position as possible, several times daily. To reduce the risks of contracture and weakness, range of motion and strengthening exercises should be started immediately and continued as long as the patient is in bed. Whenever possible, patients should assist with their own positioning, transferring, and self-care. For patients at high risk for venous thromboembolism, antithrombotic measures should be used if that is consistent with the patient's goals of care (see Chapter 14).

Avoiding restraints and discontinuing intravenous lines and urinary catheters will increase opportunities for early mobility. Graduated ambulation should begin as soon as it is feasible. Advice from a physical therapist is often helpful both before and after discharge. Prior to discharge, physical therapists can recommend appropriate exercises and assistive devices; after discharge, they can recommend safety modifications and maintenance exercises.

Brown CJ et al. Mobility limitation in the older patient: a clinical review. JAMA. 2013 Sep 18;310(11):1168–77. [PMID: 24045741]

Covinsky KE et al. Hospitalization-associated disability: "She was probably able to ambulate, but I 'm not sure". JAMA. 2011 Oct 26;306(16):1782–93. [PMID: 22028354]

5. Falls & Gait Disorders

About one-third of people over age 65 fall each year, and the frequency of falls increases markedly with advancing age. About 10% of falls result in serious injuries such as fractures, soft tissue injuries, and traumatic brain injuries. Complications from falls are the leading cause of death from injury in persons over age 65. Hip fractures are common precursors to functional impairment, nursing home placement, and death.

Every older person should be asked about falls. Assessment of patients who fall should include postural blood pressure and pulse, thorough cardiac examination, evaluations of strength, range of motion, cognition, and proprioception, and examination of feet and footwear. A thorough gait assessment should be performed in all older people. Gait and balance can be readily assessed by the "Up and Go Test," in which the patient is asked to stand up from a sitting position without use of hands, walk 10 feet, turn around, walk back, and sit down. Patients who take < 10 seconds are usually normal, patients who take longer than 30 seconds tend to need assistance with many mobility tasks, and those in between tend to vary widely with respect to gait, balance, and function. The ability to recognize common patterns of gait disorders is an extremely useful clinical skill to develop. Examples of gait abnormalities and their causes are listed in Table 4–3.

▶ Causes of Falls

Balance and ambulation require a complex interplay of cognitive, neuromuscular, and cardiovascular function. With age, balance mechanisms can become compromised and postural sway increases. These changes predispose the older person to a fall when challenged by an additional insult to any of these systems.

A fall may be the clinical manifestation of an occult problem, such as pneumonia or myocardial infarction, but much more commonly falls are due to the interaction between an impaired patient and an environmental risk factor. Falls in older people are rarely due to a single cause, and effective intervention entails a comprehensive assessment of the patient's intrinsic deficits (usually diseases and medications), the activity engaged in at the time of the fall, and environmental obstacles.

Intrinsic deficits are those that impair sensory input, judgment, blood pressure regulation, reaction time, and balance and gait. Dizziness may be closely related to the deficits associated with falls and gait abnormalities. While it may be impossible to isolate a sole "cause" or a "cure" for falls, gait abnormalities, or dizziness, it is often possible to identify and ameliorate some of the underlying contributory conditions and improve the patient's overall function.

Medication use is one of the most common, significant, and reversible causes of falling. A meta-analysis found that sedative/hypnotics, antidepressants, and benzodiazepines were the classes of drugs most likely to be associated with falling. The use of multiple medications simultaneously has also been associated with an increased fall risk. Other often overlooked but treatable contributors include postural hypotension (including postprandial, which peaks 30–60 minutes after a meal), insomnia, use of multifocal lenses, and urinary urgency.

Since most falls occur in or around the home, a visit by a visiting nurse, physical therapist, or health care provider for a home safety evaluation reaps substantial benefits in identifying environmental obstacles and is generally reimbursed by third-party payers, including Medicare.

▶ Complications of Falls

The most common fractures resulting from falls are of the wrist, hip, and vertebrae. There is a high mortality rate (approximately 20% in 1 year) in elderly women with hip fractures, particularly if they were debilitated prior to the time of the fracture.

Table 4–3. Evaluation of gait abnormalities.

Gait Abnormality	Possible Cause
Inability to stand without use of hands	Deconditioning Myopathy (hyperthyroidism, alcohol, statin-induced) Hip or knee pain
Unsteadiness upon standing	Orthostatic hypotension Balance problem (peripheral neuropathy, vision problem, vestibular, other central nervous system causes) Generalized weakness
Stagger with eyes closed	Often indicates that vision is compensating for another deficit
Short steps	Weakness Parkinson disease or related condition
Asymmetry	Cerebrovascular accident Focal pain or arthritis
Wide-based gait	Fear, balance problems
Flexed knees	Contractures, quadriceps weakness
Slow gait	Fear of falling, weakness, deconditioning, peripheral vascular disease, chronic obstructive pulmonary disease, heart failure, angina pectoris

Fear of falling again is a common, serious, but treatable factor in the elderly person's loss of confidence and independence. Referral to a physical therapist for gait training with special devices is often all that is required.

Chronic subdural hematoma is an easily overlooked complication of falls that must be considered in any elderly patient presenting with new neurologic symptoms or signs. Headache or known history of trauma may both be absent.

Patients who are unable to get up from a fall are at risk for dehydration, electrolyte imbalance, pressure sores, rhabdomyolysis, and hypothermia.

▶ Prevention & Management

The risk of falling and consequent injury, disability, and potential institutionalization can be reduced by modifying those factors outlined in Table 4–4. Emphasis is placed on treating all contributory medical conditions (eg, cataracts), minimizing environmental hazards, and eliminating medications where the harms may outweigh the benefits—particularly those that induce orthostasis and parkinsonism (eg, alpha-blockers, nitrates, antipsychotics). Also important are strength, balance, and gait training as well as screening and treatment for osteoporosis, if present. Falls and fractures may be prevented by prescribing vitamin D at a dose of 800 international units daily or higher.

Assistive devices, such as canes and walkers, are useful for many older adults but are often used incorrectly. Canes should be used on the "good" side. The height of walkers and canes should generally be about the level of the wrist. Physical therapists are invaluable in assessing the need for an assistive device, selecting the best device, and training a patient in its correct use.

Early surgery for patients with cataracts may reduce falls, but eyeglasses, particularly bifocal or graduated lenses, may actually increase the risk of falls, particularly in the early weeks of use. Patients should be counseled about the need to take extra care when new eyeglasses are being used.

Patients with repeated falls are often reassured by the availability of phones at floor level, a portable phone, or a lightweight radio call system. Their therapy should also include training in techniques for arising after a fall. The clinical utility of anatomically designed external hip protectors in reducing fractures is currently uncertain.

▶ When to Refer

Patients with a recent history of falls should be referred for physical therapy, eye examination, and home safety evaluation.

▶ When to Admit

If the patient has new falls that are unexplained, particularly in combination with a change in the physical examination, hospitalization should be considered.

Chang HJ et al. JAMA patient page. Falls and older adults. JAMA. 2010 Jan 20;303(3):288. [PMID: 20085959]

Moyer VA. Prevention of falls in community-dwelling older adults: U.S. Preventive Health Services Task Force recommendation statement. Ann Intern Med. 2012 Aug 7;157(3):197–204. [PMID: 22868837]

Tinetti ME et al. The patient who falls: "It's always a trade-off". JAMA. 2010 Jan 20;303(3):258–66. [PMID: 20085954]

Table 4–4. Fall risk factors and targeted interventions and best evidence for fall prevention.

Risk Factor	Targeted Intervention
Postural hypotension (> 20 mm Hg drop in systolic blood pressure, or systolic blood pressure < 90 mm Hg)	Behavioral recommendations, such as hand clenching, elevation of head of bed; discontinuation or substitution of high-risk medications
Use of benzodiazepine or sedative-hypnotic agent	Education about sleep hygiene; discontinuation or substitution of medications
Use of multiple prescription medications	Review of medications
Environmental hazards	Appropriate changes; installation of safety equipment (eg, grab bars)
Gait impairment	Gait training, assistive devices, balance or strengthening exercises
Impairment in transfer or balance	Balance exercises, training in transfers, environmental alterations (eg, grab bars)
Impairment in leg or arm muscle strength or limb range of motion	Exercise with resistance bands or putty, with graduated increases in resistance
Best Evidence for Fall Prevention[1]	**Number of Trials and Risk Ratios**
Exercise or physical therapy	16 randomized controlled trials Risk ratio for falls 0.87 (confidence interval 0.81–0.94)
Vitamin D supplementation	9 randomized controlled trials Risk ratio for falls 0.83 (confidence interval 0.77–0.89)
Multifactorial intervention	19 randomized controlled trials Risk ratio for falls 0.94 (confidence interval 0.87–1.02)

[1]Adapted, with permission, from Michael YL et al. Primary care-relevant interventions to prevent falling in older adults: a systematic evidence review for the U.S. Preventive Services Task Force. Ann Intern Med. 2010 Dec 21;153(12):815–25. [PMID: 21173416]

6. Urinary Incontinence

> ### ESSENTIALS OF DIAGNOSIS
>
> ▶ Involuntary loss of urine.
> ▶ *Stress* incontinence: leakage of urine upon coughing, sneezing, or standing.
> ▶ *Urge* incontinence: urgency and inability to delay urination.
> ▶ *Overflow* incontinence: may have variable presentation.

▶ General Considerations

Incontinence in older adults is common, and interventions can improve most patients. Many patients fail to tell their providers about it. A simple question about involuntary leakage of urine is a reasonable screen: "Do you have a problem with urine leaks or accidents?"

▶ Classification

Because continence requires adequate mobility, mentation, motivation, and manual dexterity, problems outside the bladder often result in incontinence. In general, the authors of this chapter find it useful to differentiate between "transient" or "potentially reversible" causes of incontinence and more "established" causes.

A. Transient Causes

Use of the mnemonic "DIAPPERS" may be helpful in remembering the categories of transient incontinence.

1. Delirium—A clouded sensorium impedes recognition of both the need to void and the location of the nearest toilet. Delirium is the most common cause of incontinence in hospitalized patients; once it clears, incontinence usually resolves.

2. Infection—Symptomatic urinary tract infection commonly causes or contributes to urgency and incontinence. Asymptomatic bacteriuria does not.

3. Atrophic urethritis or vaginitis—Atrophic urethritis can usually be diagnosed presumptively by the presence of vaginal mucosal telangiectasia, petechiae, erosions, erythema, or friability. Urethral inflammation, if symptomatic, may contribute to incontinence in some women. Some experts suggest a trial of topical estrogen in these cases.

4. Pharmaceuticals—Drugs are one of the most common causes of transient incontinence. Typical offending agents include potent diuretics, anticholinergics, psychotropics, opioid analgesics, alpha-blockers (in women), alpha-agonists (in men), and calcium channel blockers.

5. Psychological factors—Severe depression with psychomotor retardation may impede the ability or motivation to reach a toilet.

6. Excess urinary output—Excess urinary output may overwhelm the ability of an older person to reach a toilet in time. In addition to diuretics, common causes include excess fluid intake; metabolic abnormalities (eg, hyperglycemia, hypercalcemia, diabetes insipidus); and disorders associated with peripheral edema, with its associated heavy nocturia when previously dependent legs assume a horizontal position in bed.

7. Restricted mobility—(See Immobility section, above.) If mobility cannot be improved, access to a urinal or commode (eg, at the bedside) may improve continence.

8. Stool impaction—This is a common cause of urinary incontinence in hospitalized or immobile patients. Although the mechanism is still unknown, a clinical clue to its presence is the onset of both urinary and fecal incontinence. Disimpaction usually restores urinary continence.

B. Established Causes

Causes of established incontinence should be addressed after the transient causes have been uncovered and managed appropriately.

1. Detrusor overactivity (urge incontinence)—Detrusor overactivity refers to uninhibited bladder contractions that cause leakage. It is the most common cause of established geriatric incontinence, accounting for two-thirds of cases, and is usually idiopathic. Women will complain of urinary leakage after the onset of an intense urge to urinate that cannot be forestalled. In men, the symptoms are similar, but detrusor overactivity commonly coexists with urethral obstruction from benign prostatic hyperplasia. Because detrusor overactivity also may be due to bladder stones or tumor, the abrupt onset of otherwise unexplained urge incontinence—especially if accompanied by perineal or suprapubic discomfort or sterile hematuria—should be investigated by cystoscopy and cytologic examination of a urine specimen.

2. Urethral incompetence (stress incontinence)—Urethral incompetence is the second most common cause of established urinary incontinence in older women. Stress incontinence is most commonly seen in men after radical prostatectomy. Stress incontinence is characterized by instantaneous leakage of urine in response to a stress maneuver. It commonly coexists with detrusor overactivity. Typically, urinary loss occurs with laughing, coughing, or lifting heavy objects. Leakage is worse or occurs only during the day, unless another abnormality (eg, detrusor overactivity) is also present. To test for stress incontinence, have the patient relax her perineum and cough vigorously (a single cough) while standing with a full bladder. Instantaneous leakage indicates stress incontinence if urinary retention has been excluded by postvoiding residual determination using ultrasound. A delay of several seconds or persistent leakage suggests that the problem is instead caused by an uninhibited bladder contraction induced by coughing.

3. Urethral obstruction—Urethral obstruction (due to prostatic enlargement, urethral stricture, bladder neck contracture, or prostatic cancer) is a common cause of established incontinence in older men but is rare in older women. It can present as dribbling incontinence after voiding, urge incontinence due to detrusor overactivity (which coexists in two-thirds of cases), or overflow incontinence due to urinary retention. Renal ultrasound is required to exclude hydronephrosis in men whose postvoiding residual urine exceeds 150 mL.

4. Detrusor underactivity (overflow incontinence)— Detrusor underactivity is the least common cause of incontinence. It may be idiopathic or due to sacral lower motor nerve dysfunction. When it causes incontinence, detrusor underactivity is associated with urinary frequency, nocturia, and frequent leakage of small amounts. The elevated postvoiding residual urine (generally over 450 mL) distinguishes it from detrusor overactivity and stress incontinence, but only urodynamic testing differentiates it from urethral obstruction in men. Such testing usually is not required in women, in whom obstruction is rarely present.

▶ **Treatment**

A. Transient Causes

Each identified transient cause should be treated regardless of whether an established cause coexists. For patients with urinary retention induced by an anticholinergic agent, discontinuation of the drug should first be considered. If this is not feasible, substituting a less anticholinergic agent may be useful.

B. Established Causes

1. Detrusor overactivity—The cornerstone of treatment is bladder training. Patients start by voiding on a schedule based on the shortest interval recorded on a bladder record. They then gradually lengthen the interval between voids by 30 minutes each week using relaxation techniques to postpone the urge to void. Lifestyle modifications, including weight loss and caffeine reduction, may also improve incontinence symptoms. For cognitively impaired patients and nursing home residents who are unable to manage on their own, timed and prompted voiding initiated by caregivers is effective.

Pelvic floor muscle ("Kegel") exercises can reduce the frequency of incontinence episodes when performed correctly and sustained. If behavioral approaches prove insufficient, drug therapy with antimuscarinic agents may provide additional benefit. The two oral drugs for which there is the most experience are tolterodine and oxybutynin. Available regimens of these drugs follow: short-acting tolterodine, 1–2 mg twice a day; long-acting tolterodine, 2–4 mg daily; short-acting oxybutynin, 2.5–5 mg twice or three times a day; long-acting oxybutynin, 5–15 mg daily; and oxybutynin transdermal patch, 3.9 mg per day applied twice weekly. All of these agents can produce delirium, dry mouth, or urinary retention; long-acting preparations may be better tolerated. Agents such as fesoterodine (4–8 mg orally once daily), trospium chloride (20 mg orally once or twice daily), long-acting trospium chloride (60 mg orally

daily), darifenacin (7.5–15 mg orally daily), and solifenacin (5–10 mg orally daily) appear to have similar efficacy and have not been clearly demonstrated to be better tolerated than the older agents in long-acting form.

The beta-3-agonist, mirabegron, 25–50 mg orally daily, is the first of a novel class of drugs approved for overactive bladder symptoms, which includes urge urinary incontinence. In trials comparing mirabegron with antimuscarinic drugs, the efficacy and safety profiles have been comparable, with less dry mouth reported in persons who received mirabegron. However, because of its potential cardiac effects and the relatively small number of adults over the age of 70 who have been studied in trials, mirabegron's role in the treatment of urge urinary incontinence in frail older adults or those with hypertension or cardiac conditions remains to be determined.

An alternative to oral agents is an injection of onabotulinumtoxinA into the detrusor muscle. In a head-to-head comparison of onabotulinumtoxinA with antimuscarinic drugs, patients had similar rates of reduction of incontinence episodes. Persons who received onabotulinumtoxinA had higher rates of complete resolution of incontinence and lower rates of dry mouth but were more likely to experience urinary retention and urinary tract infections than those who did not receive onabotulinumtoxinA.

The combination of behavioral therapy and antimuscarinics appears to be more effective than either alone although one study in a group of younger women showed that adding behavioral therapy to individually titrated doses of extended-release oxybutynin was no better than drug treatment alone.

In men with both benign prostatic hyperplasia and detrusor overactivity and who have postvoid residual volumes of ≤ 150 mL, an antimuscarinic agent added to an alpha-blocker may provide additional relief of lower urinary tract symptoms.

2. Urethral incompetence (stress incontinence)—Lifestyle modifications, including limiting caffeine intake and timed voiding, may be helpful for some women, particularly women with mixed stress/urge incontinence. Pelvic floor muscle exercises are effective for women with mild to moderate stress incontinence; the exercises can be combined, if necessary, with biofeedback, electrical stimulation, or vaginal cones. Instruct the patient to pull in the pelvic floor muscles and hold for 6–10 seconds and to perform three sets of 8–12 contractions daily. Benefits may not be seen for 6 weeks. Pessaries or vaginal cones may be helpful in some women but should be prescribed by providers who are experienced with using these modalities.

Although a last resort, surgery is the most effective treatment for stress incontinence; cure rates as high as 96% can result, even in older women. Drug therapy is limited. Clinical trials have shown that duloxetine, a serotonin and norepinephrine reuptake inhibitor, reduces stress incontinence episodes in women but efficacy in older women remains unknown. It is approved for use for this indication in some countries but not the United States. Side effects, including nausea, are common.

3. Urethral obstruction—Surgical decompression is the most effective treatment for obstruction, especially in the setting of urinary retention due to benign prostatic hyperplasia. A variety of nonsurgical techniques make decompression feasible even for frail men. For the nonoperative candidate with urinary retention, intermittent or indwelling catheterization is used. For a man with prostatic obstruction who does not require or desire immediate surgery, treatment with alpha-blocking agents (eg, terazosin, 1–10 mg daily; prazosin, 1–5 mg orally twice daily; tamsulosin, 0.4–0.8 mg daily) can improve symptoms and delay obstruction. Finasteride, 5 mg daily, can provide additional benefit to an alpha-blocking agent in men with an enlarged prostate.

4. Detrusor underactivity—For the patient with a poorly contractile bladder, augmented voiding techniques (eg, double voiding, suprapubic pressure) often prove effective. If further emptying is needed, intermittent or indwelling catheterization is the only option. Antibiotics should be used only for symptomatic upper urinary tract infection or as prophylaxis against recurrent symptomatic infections in a patient using intermittent catheterization; they should not be used as prophylaxis with an indwelling catheter.

When to Refer

- Men with urinary obstruction who do not respond to medical therapy should be referred to a urologist.
- Women who do not respond to medical and behavioral therapy should be referred to a urogynecologist or urologist.

Chapple CR et al. Randomized double-blind, active-controlled phase 3 study to assess 12-month safety and efficacy of mirabegron, a β_3-adrenoreceptor agonist, in overactive bladder. Eur Urol. 2013 Feb;63(2):296–305. [PMID: 23195283]
Goode PS et al. Incontinence in older women. JAMA. 2010 Jun 2; 303(21):2172–81. [PMID: 20516418]
Visco AG et al. Anticholinergic therapy vs. onabotulinumtoxinA for urgency urinary incontinence. N Engl J Med. 2012 Nov 8; 367(19):1803–13. [PMID: 23036134]

7. Weight Loss

General Considerations

Weight loss affects substantial numbers of elderly. The degree of unintended weight loss that deserves evaluation is not agreed upon, although a reasonable threshold is loss of 5% of body weight in 1 month or 10% of body weight in 6 months.

Clinical Findings

Useful laboratory and radiologic studies for the patient with weight loss include complete blood count, serum chemistries (including glucose, TSH, creatinine, calcium, and in men, testosterone), urinalysis, and chest radiograph. These studies are intended to uncover an occult metabolic or neoplastic cause but are not exhaustive. Exploring the patient's social situation, cognition, mood, and dental health are at least as important as looking for a purely medical cause of weight loss.

Treatment

Oral nutritional supplements of 200–1000 kcal/d can increase weight and improve outcomes in malnourished hospitalized elders. Megestrol acetate as an appetite stimulant has not been shown to increase body mass or lengthen life in among elders and has significant side effects. For those who have lost the ability to feed themselves, assiduous hand feeding may allow maintenance of weight. Although artificial nutrition and hydration ("tube feeding") may seem a more convenient alternative, it deprives the patient of the enjoyment associated with eating as well as the social milieu typically associated with mealtime; before this option is chosen, the patient or his or her surrogate should be offered the opportunity to review the benefits and burdens of the treatment in light of overall goals of care. If tube feeding is initiated and the patient makes repeated attempts to pull out the tube, the utility of tube feeding should be reconsidered. Tube feeding is not recommended for patients with end-stage dementia.

Abellan van Kan G et al. The assessment of frailty in older adults. Clin Geriatr Med. 2010 May;26(2):275–86. [PMID: 20497846]
Boockvar KS et al. Chapter 8: Palliative care for frail older adults: "There are things I can't do anymore that I wish I could…". In: McPhee SJ et al (editors): *Care at the Close of Life: Evidence and Experience.* McGraw-Hill, 2010
Srinivas-Shankar U et al. Effects of testosterone on muscle strength, physical function, body composition, and quality of life in intermediate-frail and frail elderly men: a randomized, double-blind, placebo controlled study. J Clin Endocrinol Metab. 2010 Feb;95(2):639–50. [PMID: 20061435]

8. Pressure Ulcers

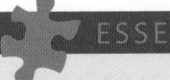

ESSENTIALS OF DIAGNOSIS

► Examine at-risk patients on admission to the hospital and daily thereafter.

► Pressure ulcers should be described by one of six stages:

- Non-blanchable hyperemia (stage I).
- Extension through epidermis (stage II).
- Full thickness skin loss (stage III).
- Full thickness wounds with extension into muscle, bone, or supporting structures (stage IV).
- If eschar or slough overlies the wound, the wound is unstageable.
- Suspected deep tissue injury is an area of discolored or blistered skin.

General Considerations

The majority of pressure ulcers develop during a hospital stay for an acute illness. Incident rates range from 3% to 30% and vary according to patient characteristics. The primary risk factor for pressure ulcers is immobility. Other contributing risk factors include reduced sensory perception, moisture (urinary and fecal incontinence), poor nutritional status, and friction and shear forces.

Suspected deep tissue injury and unstageable are included in the six pressure ulcer stages. Ulcers in which the base is covered by slough (yellow, tan, gray, green, or brown) or eschar (tan, brown, or black) are considered unstageable. Suspected deep tissue injury is an area of purple or maroon discolored intact skin or blood-filled blister. The area may be preceded by tissue that is painful, firm, mushy, boggy, warmer, or cooler compared with adjacent tissue.

A number of risk assessment instruments including the Braden Scale and the Norton score can be used to assess the risk of developing pressure ulcers; both have reasonable performance characteristics. These instruments can be used to identify the highest risk patients who might benefit most from scarce resources such as mattresses that reduce or relieve pressure.

While Medicare does not reimburse for hospital-acquired pressure ulcers, there is a higher reimbursement for pressure ulcers present on admission. Therefore, clinicians should include a full skin assessment on every admission evaluation.

Prevention

Using specialized support surfaces (including mattresses, beds, and cushions), patient repositioning, optimizing nutritional status, and moisturizing sacral skin are strategies that have been shown to reduce pressure ulcers. For moderate- to high-risk patients, mattresses or overlays that reduce tissue pressure below a standard mattress appear to be superior to standard mattresses. The literature comparing specific products is sparse and inconclusive.

Evaluation

Evaluation of pressure ulcers should include patient's risk factors and goals of care, wound stage, size, depth, presence or absence of exudate, type of exudate present, appearance of the wound bed, and whether there appears to be surrounding infection, sinus tracking, or cellulitis. In poorly healing or atypical pressure ulcers, biopsy should be performed to rule out malignancy or other less common lesions such as pyoderma gangrenosum.

Treatment

Treatment is aimed toward removing necrotic debris and maintaining a moist wound bed that will promote healing and formation of granulation tissue. The type of dressing that is recommended depends on the location and depth of the wound, whether necrotic tissue or dead space is present, and the amount of exudate (Table 4–5). Pressure-reducing devices (eg, air-fluid beds and low air loss beds) are associated with improved healing rates. Although poor

Table 4–5. Treatment of pressure ulcers.

Ulcer Type	Dressing Type and Considerations
Stage I and suspected deep tissue injury	Polyurethane film Hydrocolloid wafer Semipermeable foam dressing
Stage II	Hydrocolloid wafers Semipermeable foam dressing Polyurethane film
Stage III/IV	**For highly exudative wounds,** use highly absorptive dressing or packing, such as calcium alginate Wounds with necrotic debris must be debrided Debridement can be autolytic, mechanical (wet to moist), or surgical **Shallow, clean wounds** can be dressed with hydrocolloid wafers, semipermeable foam, or polyurethane film **Deep wounds** can be packed with gauze; if the wound is deep and highly exudative, an absorptive packing should be used
Heel ulcer	Do not remove eschar on heel ulcers because it can help promote healing (eschar in other locations should be debrided)
Unstageable	Debride before deciding on further therapy

nutritional status is a risk factor for the development of pressure ulcers, the results of trials of nutritional supplementation in the treatment of pressure ulcers have been disappointing.

Providers can become easily overwhelmed by the array of products available for treatment of established pressure ulcers. Most institutions should designate a wound care expert or wound care team to select a streamlined wound care product line that has simple guidelines. In a patient with end-stage disease who is receiving palliative care, appropriate treatment might be directed toward comfort (including minimizing dressing changes and odors) rather than efforts directed at healing.

Complications

Pressure ulcers are associated with increased mortality rates, although a causal link has not been proven. Complications include pain, cellulitis, osteomyelitis, systemic sepsis, and prolongation of lengths of stay in the inpatient or nursing home setting.

When to Refer

Ulcers that are large or nonhealing should be referred to a plastic or general surgeon or dermatologist for biopsy, debridement, and possible skin grafting.

When to Admit

Patients with pressure ulcers should be admitted if the primary residence is unable to provide adequate wound care or pressure reduction, if the wound is infected, or for complex or surgical wound care.

Langemo DK et al; National Pressure Ulcer Advisory Panel. Pressure ulcers in individuals receiving palliative care: a National Pressure Ulcer Advisory Panel white paper. Adv Skin Wound Care. 2010 Feb;23(2):59–72. [PMID: 20087072]
Lohi J et al. Local dressings for pressure ulcers: what is the best tool to apply in primary and secondary care? Wound Care. 2010 Mar;19(3):123–7. [PMID: 20559190]
National Pressure Ulcer Advisory Panel Website: http://www.npuap.org/pr2.htm

9. Pharmacotherapy & Polypharmacy

There are several reasons for the greater incidence of iatrogenic drug reactions in the elderly population, the most important of which is the high number of medications that elders take. Drug metabolism is often impaired in this group due to a decrease in glomerular filtration rate as well as reduced hepatic clearance. Older individuals often have varying responses to a given serum drug level. Thus, they are more sensitive to some drugs (eg, opioids) and less sensitive to others (eg, beta-blocking agents). Most emergency hospitalizations for recognized adverse drug events among older persons result from only a few medications used alone or in combination; examples include warfarin, antiplatelet agents, insulins, oral hypoglycemic agents, and to a lesser extent, opioid analgesics and digoxin.

▶ Precautions in Administering Drugs

Nonpharmacologic interventions can often be a first-line alternative to drugs (eg, diet for mild hypertension or type 2 diabetes mellitus). Therapy is begun with less than the usual adult dosage and the dosage increased slowly, consistent with its pharmacokinetics in older patients. However, age-related changes in drug distribution and clearance are variable among individuals, and some require full doses. After determining acceptable measures of success and toxicity, the dose is increased until one or the other is reached.

Despite the importance of beginning new drugs in a slow, measured fashion, all too often an inadequate trial is attempted (in terms of duration or dose) before discontinuation. Antidepressants, in particular, are frequently stopped before therapeutic dosages are reached.

A number of simple interventions can help improve adherence to the prescribed medical regimen. When possible, the clinician should keep the dosing schedule simple, the number of pills low, the medication changes as infrequent as possible, and encourage the patient to use a single pharmacy. Pillboxes or "medi-sets" help some patients with adherence.

Having the patient or caregiver bring in all medications at each visit can help the clinician perform medication reconciliation and reinforce reasons for drug use, dosage, frequency of administration, and possible adverse effects. Medication reconciliation is particularly important if the patient sees multiple providers.

The risk of toxicity goes up with the number of medications prescribed. Certain combinations of medications (eg, warfarin and many types of antibiotics, digoxin and clarithromycin, angiotensin-converting enzyme inhibitors and NSAIDs) are particularly likely to cause drug-drug interactions and should be watched carefully.

Trials of individual drug discontinuation should be considered (including sedative-hypnotics, antipsychotic medications, digoxin, proton pump inhibitors, NSAIDs) when the original indication is unclear, the goals of care have changed, or the patient might be experiencing side effects.

▶ When to Refer

Patients with poor or uncertain adherence may benefit from referral to a pharmacist or a home health nurse.

Budnitz DS et al. Emergency hospitalizations for adverse drug events in older Americans. N Engl J Med. 2011 Nov 24; 365(21):2002–12. [PMID: 22111719]
Gallagher PF et al. Prevention of potentially inappropriate prescribing for elderly patients: a randomized controlled trial using STOPP/START criteria. Clin Pharmacol Ther. 2011 Jun; 89(6):845–54. [PMID: 21508941]
Steinman MA et al. Managing medications in clinically complex elders: "There's got to be a happy medium". JAMA. 2010 Oct 13; 304(14):1592–601. [PMID: 20940385]

10. Vision Impairment

Visual impairment due to age-related refractive error ("presbyopia"), macular degeneration, cataracts, glaucoma, and diabetic retinopathy contributes to impaired quality of life for many older adults. The prevalence of serious and correctable visual disorders in elders is sufficient to warrant a complete eye examination by an ophthalmologist or optometrist annually or biannually for most elders. Many patients with visual loss benefit from a referral to a low vision program, and primary care providers should not assume that an ophthalmologist or optometrist will automatically make this referral.

Rosenberg EA et al. The visually impaired patient. Am Fam Physician. 2008 May 15;77(10):1431–6. [PMID: 18533377]

11. Hearing Impairment

Over one-third of persons over age 65 and half of those over age 85 have some hearing loss. Hearing loss is associated with social isolation, depression, and an increased risk of cognitive impairment. A reasonable screen is to ask patients if they have hearing impairment. Those who answer "yes" should be referred for audiometry. Those who answer "no" may still have hearing impairment and can be screened by a handheld audioscope or the whispered voice test. The whispered voice test is administered by standing 2 feet behind the subject, whispering three random numbers, and simultaneously rubbing the external auditory canal of the non-tested ear to mask the sound. If the patient is unable to identify all three numbers, the test should be repeated with different numbers, and if still abnormal, a referral should be made to audiometry. To determine the degree to which hearing impairment interferes with functioning, the provider may ask if the patient becomes frustrated when conversing with family members, is embarrassed when meeting new people, has difficulty watching TV, or has problems understanding conversations. Caregivers or family members often have important information on the impact of hearing loss on the patient's social interactions.

Hearing amplification can improve hearing-related quality of life in patients with hearing loss. However, compliance with hearing amplification can be a challenge because of dissatisfaction with performance; stigma associated with hearing aid use; and cost, since hearing amplification is not paid for under most Medicare plans. Newer digital devices may perform better but are considerably more expensive. Special telephones, amplifiers for the television, and other devices are helpful to many patients. Portable amplifiers are pager-sized units with earphones attached; they can be purchased inexpensively at many electronics stores and can be useful in health care settings for improving communication with hearing impaired patients. In general, facing the patient and speaking slowly in a low tone is a more effective communication strategy than shouting.

Chou R et al. Screening adults aged 50 years or older for hearing loss: a review of the evidence for the U.S. Preventive Service Task Force. Ann Intern Med. 2011 March 1;154(5):347–55. [PMID: 21357912]
Lin FR et al; Health ABC Study Group. Hearing loss and cognitive decline in older adults. JAMA Intern Med. 2013 Feb 25;173(4):293–9. [PMID: 23337978]
Pacala JT et al. Hearing deficits in the older patient: "I didn't notice anything". JAMA. 2012 Mar 21;307(11):1185–94. [PMID: 22436959]

12. Elder Mistreatment & Self Neglect

Elder mistreatment is defined as "actions that cause harm or create a serious risk of harm to an older adult by a caregiver or other person who stands in a trust relationship to the older adult, or failure by a caregiver to satisfy the elder's basic needs or to protect the elder from harm." Self neglect is the most common form of elder mistreatment and occurs among all demographic strata of the aging population. According to the best available estimates, the prevalence of potential neglect and psychological and financial abuse is about 5% each, with other forms of abuse being less common.

Clues to the possibility of elder abuse include behavioral changes in the presence of the caregiver, delays between occurrences of injuries and when treatment was sought, inconsistencies between an observed injury and associated explanation, lack of appropriate clothing or hygiene, and not filling prescriptions. Many elders with cognitive impairment become targets of financial abuse. Both elder abuse and self neglect are associated with an increased risk of mortality.

It is helpful to observe and talk with every older person alone for at least part of a visit in order to ask questions directly about possible abuse and neglect (Table 4–6). When self neglect is suspected, it is critical to establish whether a patient has decision-making capacity in order to determine what course of action needs to be taken. A patient who has full decision-making capacity should be

Table 4–6. Phrases and actions that may be helpful in situations of suspected abuse or neglect.

Questions for the Elder
1. Has anyone hurt you?
2. Are you afraid of anybody?
3. Is anyone taking or using your money without your permission?

Questions for the Caregiver
1. Are your dad's needs more than you can handle?
2. Are you worried that you might hit your dad?
3. Have you hit your dad?

If abuse is suspected
Tell the patient that you are concerned, want to help, and will call Adult Protective Services to see if there is anything that they can do to help
Document any injuries
Document the patient's words
Document whether or not the patient has decision-making capacity using a tool such as "Aid to Capacity Evaluation"

provided with help and support but can choose to live in conditions of self neglect, providing that the public is not endangered by the actions of the person. In contrast, a patient who lacks decision-making capacity who lives in conditions of self neglect will require more aggressive intervention, which may include guardianship, in-home help, or placement in a supervised setting. Mental state scores, such as the MoCA, may provide some insight into the patient's cognitive status but are not designed to assess decision-making capacity. A standardized tool, such as the "Aid to Capacity Evaluation," is easy to administer, has good performance characteristics for determining decision-making capacity, and is available free online at www.jointcentreforbioethics.ca/tools/ace_download.shtml.

▶ **When to Refer**

The laws in most states require health care providers to report suspected abuse or neglect to Adult Protective Services; agencies are available in all 50 states to assist in cases of suspected elder abuse. The Web site for the National Center for Elder Abuse is http://www.ncea.aoa.gov. When it is unclear whether a patient has decision-making capacity after an initial assessment, or whether an untreated mental health disorder is contributing to the problem, a referral to a mental health professional is appropriate.

▶ **When to Admit**

Hospital admission is appropriate when a patient is unsafe in the community and an alternate plan cannot be put into place in a timely manner.

Mosqueda L et al. Elder abuse and self-neglect: "I don't care anything about going to the doctor, to be honest…". JAMA. 2011 Aug 3;306(5):532–40. [PMID: 21813431]
Sessums LL et al. Does this patient have medical decision-making capacity? JAMA. 2011 July 27;306(4):420–7. [PMID: 21791691]

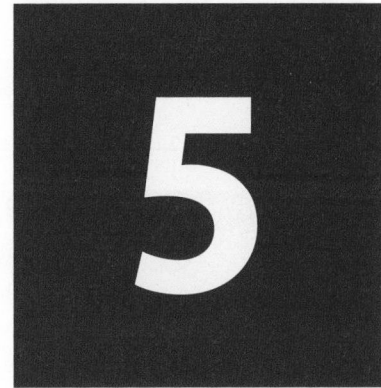

Palliative Care & Pain Management

Michael W. Rabow, MD
Steven Z. Pantilat, MD

DEFINITION & SCOPE OF PALLIATIVE CARE

The focus of palliative care is to improve symptoms and quality of life at any stage of any serious illness, to support patients' family and loved ones, and to help align patients' care with their preferences and goals. At the end of life, palliative care often becomes the sole focus of care, but palliative care alongside cure-focused treatment is beneficial throughout the course of a serious illness, regardless of prognosis, whether the goal is to cure disease or manage it.

Palliative care includes management of pain, dyspnea, nausea and vomiting, constipation, and agitation; emotional distress, such as depression, anxiety, and interpersonal strain; and existential distress, such as spiritual crisis. While palliative care is a medical subspecialty recognized by the American Board of Medical Specialties, all clinicians should possess the basic skills to be able to manage pain; treat dyspnea; identify possible depression; communicate about important issues, such as prognosis and patient preferences for care; and help address spiritual distress. Advanced certification in palliative care is offered by the Joint Commission to hospitals providing high quality palliative services.

During any stage of illness, symptoms that cause significant suffering are a medical emergency that should be managed aggressively with frequent elicitation, continuous reassessment, and individualized treatment. While patients at the end of life may experience a host of distressing symptoms, pain, dyspnea, and delirium are among the most feared and burdensome. Management of these common symptoms is described later in this chapter. The principles of palliative care dictate that properly informed patients or their surrogates may decide to pursue aggressive symptom relief at the end of life even if, as a known but unintended consequence, the treatments preclude further unwanted curative interventions or even hasten death, although increasingly palliative care has been shown to prolong life.

Quill TE et al. Generalist plus specialist palliative care—creating a more sustainable model. N Engl J Med. 2013 Mar 28;368(13):1173–5. [PMID: 23465068]
Rabow M et al. Moving upstream: a review of the evidence of the impact of outpatient palliative care. J Palliat Med. 2013 Dec;16(12):1540–9. [PMID: 24225013]

Smith TJ et al. American Society of Clinical Oncology provisional clinical opinion: the integration of palliative care into standard oncology care. J Clin Oncol. 2012 Mar 10;30(8):880–7. [PMID: 22312101]
Temel JS et al. Early palliative care for patients with metastatic non-small-cell lung cancer. N Engl J Med. 2010 Aug 19;363(8):733–42. [PMID: 20818875]

PAIN MANAGEMENT

PRINCIPLES OF PAIN MANAGEMENT

The experience of pain includes the patient's emotional reaction to it and is influenced by many factors, including the patient's prior experiences with pain, meaning given to the pain, emotional stresses, and family and cultural influences. Pain is a subjective phenomenon, and clinicians cannot reliably detect its existence or quantify its severity without asking the patient directly. A useful means of assessing pain and evaluating the effectiveness of analgesia is to ask the patient to rate the degree of pain along a numeric or visual pain scale (Table 5–1).

General guidelines for management of pain are recommended for the treatment of all patients with pain. Clinicians should ask about the nature, severity, timing, location, quality, and aggravating and relieving factors of the pain. Distinguishing between neuropathic and nociceptive (somatic or visceral) pain is essential to proper tailoring of pain treatments. The goal of pain management is properly decided by the patient. Some patients may wish to be completely free of pain even at the cost of significant sedation, while others will wish to control pain to a level that still allows maximal functioning.

Chronic severe pain should be treated continuously. For ongoing pain, a long-acting analgesic can be given around the clock with a short-acting medication as needed for "breakthrough" pain. Whenever possible, the oral route of administration is preferred because it is easier to administer at home, is not painful, and imposes no risk from needle exposure. Patient-controlled analgesia (PCA) of intravenous medications can achieve better analgesia faster with less medication use and its principles have been adapted for use with oral administration.

Table 5–1. Pain assessment scales.

A. Numeric Rating Scale

No pain   Worst pain

0   1   2   3   4   5   6   7   8   9   10

B. Numeric Rating Scale Translated into Word and Behavior Scales

Pain intensity	Word scale	Nonverbal behaviors
0	No pain	Relaxed, calm expression
1–2	Least pain	Stressed, tense expression
3–4	Mild pain	Guarded movement, grimacing
5–6	Moderate pain	Moaning, restless
7–8	Severe pain	Crying out
9–10	Excruciating pain	Increased intensity of above

C. Wong Baker FACES Pain Rating Scale[1]

0 No hurt	1 Hurts Little Bit	2 Hurts Little More	3 Hurts Even More	4 Hurts Whole Lot	5 Hurts Worst

0 No hurt	1 Hurts Little Bit	2 Hurts Little More	3 Hurts Even More	4 Hurts Whole Lot	5 Hurts Worst

[1]Especially useful for patients who cannot read English and for pediatric patients.
Reprinted, with permission, from Hockenberry M, Wilson D, Winkelstein ML. *Wong's Essentials of Pediatric Nursing*, ed. 8. Copyright © 2009, Mosby, St. Louis.

The underlying cause of pain should be diagnosed and treated, balancing the burden of diagnostic tests or therapeutic interventions with the patient's suffering. For example, radiation therapy for painful bone metastases or nerve blocks for neuropathic pain may obviate the need for ongoing treatment with analgesics and their side effects. Regardless of decisions about seeking and treating the underlying cause of pain, every patient should be offered prompt relief.

PAIN MANAGEMENT FOR PATIENTS WITH SERIOUS ILLNESS

▶ Definition & Prevalence

Pain is a common problem for patients with serious illness. Up to 75% of patients dying of cancer, heart failure, COPD, or other diseases experience pain. Pain is what many people say they fear most about dying and is routinely undertreated. Joint Commission reviews of healthcare organizations now include pain management standards.

▶ Barriers to Good Care

Deficiencies in pain management in the seriously ill have been documented in many settings. Many clinicians have limited training and clinical experience with pain management and thus are understandably reluctant to attempt to manage severe pain. Lack of knowledge about the proper selection and dosing of analgesic medications carries with it attendant and typically exaggerated fears about the side effects of pain medications, including the possibility of respiratory depression from opioids. Most clinicians, however, can develop good pain management skills, and nearly all pain, even at the end of life, can be managed without hastening death through respiratory depression. In rare instances, palliative sedation may be necessary to control intractable suffering as an intervention of last resort.

A misunderstanding of the physiologic effects of opioids can lead to unfounded concerns on the part of clinicians, patients, or family members that patients will become addicted to opioids. While physiologic **tolerance** (requiring increasing dosage to achieve the same analgesic effect) and **dependence** (requiring continued dosing to prevent symptoms of medication withdrawal) are expected with regular opioid use, the use of opioids at the end of life for relief of pain and dyspnea is not generally associated with a risk of psychological **addiction** (misuse of a substance for purposes other than one for which it was prescribed and despite negative consequences in health, employment, or legal and social spheres). The risk for problematic use of pain medications is higher, however, in patients with a history of addiction or substance abuse. Yet even patients with such a history need pain relief, albeit with closer monitoring. Some patients who demonstrate behaviors associated with addiction (demand for specific medications and doses, anger and irritability, poor cooperation or disturbed interpersonal reactions) may have **pseudo-addiction,** defined as exhibiting behaviors associated with addiction but only because their pain is inadequately treated. Once pain is relieved, these behaviors cease. In all cases, clinicians must be prepared to use appropriate doses of opioids in order to relieve distressing symptoms for patients at the end of life.

Harms from the use of opioid analgesics, including medication diversion or death from accidental or intentional overdose, are known and significant risks. Some clinicians fear legal repercussions from prescribing the high doses of opioids sometimes necessary to control pain at the end of life. The US Food and Drug Administration (FDA) released a Risk Evaluation and Management Strategy for long-acting and extended-release opioids to help inform physicians about appropriate prescribing and reduce abuse [http://www.fda.gov/Drugs/DrugSafety/Informationby-DrugClass/ucm163647.htm]. Some states have special training, licensing and documentation requirements for opioid prescribing. However, governmental and professional medical groups, regulators (including the FDA), and the US Supreme Court have made it clear that appropriate treatment of pain is the right of the patient and a fundamental responsibility of the clinician. Although clinicians may feel trapped between consequences of over- or underprescribing opioids, there remains a wide range of practice in which clinicians can appropriately treat pain. Referral to pain management or palliative care experts is appropriate whenever pain cannot be controlled expeditiously or safely by the primary clinician. In the field of chronic, nonmalignant pain management, many clinicians are using pain medication contracts and urine drug testing to help decrease the chance of abuse and diversion (see Box, Opioids for Chronic, Noncancer Pain). Clinicians who are caring for patients earlier in the course of life-threatening illness and are concerned that their patient may be misusing opioids (with serious negative consequences) can conduct periodic urine toxicology screening to confirm that the patient is taking the medication as prescribed and not using other medications.

PHARMACOLOGIC PAIN MANAGEMENT STRATEGIES

In general, pain can be well controlled with opioid and nonopioid analgesic medications. For mild to moderate pain, acetaminophen, aspirin, and nonsteroidal anti-inflammatory drugs (NSAIDs) may be sufficient. For moderate to severe pain, opioids often are necessary. In all cases, the choice of analgesics must be guided by a careful consideration of the physiology of the pain and the benefits and risks of the particular analgesic being considered.

▶ Acetaminophen & NSAIDs

Appropriate doses of acetaminophen may be just as effective an analgesic and antipyretic as NSAIDs but without the risk of gastrointestinal bleeding or ulceration. Acetaminophen can be given at a dosage of 500–1000 mg orally every 6 hours, although it can be taken every 4 hours as long as the risk of hepatotoxicity is kept in mind. Hepatotoxicity is of particular concern because of how commonly acetaminophen is also an ingredient in various over-the-counter medications and because of failure to account for the acetaminophen dose included in combination acetaminophen-opioid medications such as Vicodin or Norco. With a recognition that total acetaminophen doses should not exceed 3000 mg/d long-term or 2000 mg/d for older patients and for those with liver disease, the FDA is now limiting the amount of acetaminophen available in combination analgesics.

Commonly used NSAIDs and their dosages are listed in Table 5–2. The NSAIDs are antipyretic, analgesic, and anti-inflammatory. NSAIDs increase the risk of gastrointestinal bleeding by 1.5 times normal. The risks of bleeding and nephrotoxicity from NSAIDs are both increased in elders. Gastrointestinal bleeding and ulceration may be prevented with the concurrent use of proton pump inhibitors (eg, omeprazole, 20–40 mg orally daily) or with the class of NSAIDs that inhibit only cyclooxygenase (COX)-2. Celecoxib (100 mg/d to 200 mg orally twice daily) is the only COX-2 inhibitor available and should be used with caution in patients with cardiac disease. The NSAIDs, including COX-2 inhibitors, can lead to fluid retention and exacerbations of heart failure and should be used with caution in patients with that condition. Unlike all other NSAIDs, naproxen has not been shown to increase the risk of major cardiovascular events and thus may be preferred in patients with coronary artery disease or at risk for cardiac disease. Topical formulations of NSAIDs (such as diclofenac 1.3% patch or 1% gel), placed over the painful body part for treatment of musculoskeletal pain, are associated with fewer side effects than oral administration.

▶ Opioid Medications

A. Formulations and Regimens

For many patients, opioids are the mainstay of pain management. Opioids are appropriate for severe pain due to any cause, including neuropathic pain. Opioid medications are listed in Table 5–3. Full opioid agonists such as morphine, hydromorphone, oxycodone, methadone, fentanyl, hydrocodone, and codeine are used most commonly. Hydrocodone and codeine are typically combined with acetaminophen or an NSAID, although acetaminophen in these combinations is restricted to 325 mg per unit dose due to the risk for toxicity. Extended-release hydrocodone without acetaminophen is FDA approved. **Short-acting formulations** of oral morphine sulfate (starting dosage 4–8 mg orally every 3–4 hours), hydromorphone (1–2 mg orally every 3–4 hours), or oxycodone (5 mg orally every 3–4 hours) are useful for acute pain not controlled with other analgesics. These same oral medications, or oral transmucosal fentanyl (200 mcg oralet dissolved in mouth) or buccal fentanyl (100 mcg dissolved in the mouth), can be used for "rescue" or "breakthrough" treatment for patients experiencing pain that breaks through long-acting medications.

OPIOIDS FOR CHRONIC, NONCANCER PAIN

Scott Steiger, MD

The potential harms and benefits of taking opioids daily to manage chronic, noncancer pain (CNCP) may be different than receiving opioids to manage the pain associated with a life-limiting illness in the setting of palliative and end-of-life care, as discussed elsewhere in this chapter.

CNCP is common in the United States. The Institute of Medicine estimates that CNCP afflicts 100 million adults and costs $635 billion annually in treatment and lost productivity. Efforts by medical societies, patient advocacy groups, and pharmaceutical companies led to an increased awareness of the magnitude of this problem and more aggressive treatment over the last two decades. Consequently, the prescription of opioids has undergone a dramatic increase. Hydrocodone has been the most commonly prescribed medication in the United States since at least 2008, and prescriptions for methadone for pain increased 1300% between 1997 and 2006. The total amount of opioid prescriptions filled in 2007 would have been enough for each adult in the United States to receive 700 mg of morphine.

The increased attention to treating CNCP has undoubtedly improved the lives of many patients, but the increase in prescribing opioids has had a deleterious effect on the health of the population as a whole. From 1991 to 2008, the number of deaths from opioid overdose quadrupled, and the number of patients admitted to treatment for addiction to opioids has quintupled. The Centers for Disease Control and Prevention has named prescription drug abuse an epidemic in the United States.

ASSESSING BENEFITS OF OPIOIDS

Research demonstrates that the beneficial effect of opioids for CNCP is modest at best and no measures have been identified to predict a good response. The improvements are generally measured in terms of a reduction in the analog pain score of 2–3 points on a 10-point scale or in improvements in the less precise outcome of *function*. Before considering a trial of prolonged opioid therapy, clinicians should discuss these modest possible benefits with patients in order to help set realistic goals of treatment (eg, moving from an average pain of 7 to a 4). Clinicians should also consider a deadline for reaching the patient's goals. Since the published trials have generally lasted less than 16 weeks, it is reasonable to set a deadline before that, with some experts advocating a 90-day trial period. Limiting the time of a trial also helps prevent dose escalation to levels associated with increased risk of adverse effects, including overdose.

Many experts recommend developing a specific goal of improved function, and tracking the patient's progress toward achieving this goal over time. But for the many patients who do not have specific, measurable goals—or who come to the clinician already taking daily opioid medication—monitoring response to treatment over time can be difficult. A useful tracking measure is the PEG, which directly patients to quantify on a scale of 0–10 the following three outcomes: **Pain** intensity on average over the last week; how the pain has affected their **Energy** level; and how much pain has impacted their **General activity.** Patients who do not progress toward their goal or whose PEG scores remain high over time may have pain that is unresponsive to opioids, and clinicians should reconsider the original diagnosis and use other modalities (both pharmacologic and nonpharmacologic) to provide analgesia. Without a clear analgesic benefit from opioids for CNCP, the risks may predominate, and the ineffective therapy should be discontinued.

RISKS OF PROLONGED OPIOID THERAPY

The risks of opioids are different than most other medications. One of the most attractive features of opioids as a class is the absence specific organ toxicity attendant to most other kinds of medications. However, not every CNCP patient is a good candidate for prolonged opioid therapy. In addition to the grave risks of addiction and death to patients and the common side effects of sedation and constipation, prolonged opioid use leads to increased risk of many problems, including hypogonadism, fracture, hyperalgesia, psychosocial problems, and fraught interactions with the health care team. When considering whether to initiate or continue opioids for CNCP, clinicians should delineate these specific risks for patients to inform decision-making.

In addition to overdose, the biggest concern of many patients and clinicians is addiction. The level of risk to the individual CNCP patient is uncertain. While physical opioid dependence has been demonstrated with daily use in virtually all patients, the published risk of addiction in patients prescribed opioids for CNCP varies between less than 1% to more than 20%, with the lowest frequencies observed in studies that excluded patients with a history of substance abuse or addiction. Recent survey data found that nearly 80% of people in the United States who tried heroin for the first time in the prior year had already abused opioid medications.

Importantly, diversion of medication from patients to whom they are prescribed into other hands is another risk that must be considered when prescribing prolonged opioid therapy for CNCP. Diversion can represent opportunism, as when a patient sells medication in order to make money. Family members, acquaintances, or strangers may steal or extort medication for their own use or gain.

LIMITING RISKS

In an effort to limit the risks of opioids for patients with CNCP, nearly all medical society consensus panels and experts guidelines recommend using a risk assessment tool, patient-provider agreements, urine drug testing, dose limitations, and limits on the use of some medications. However, data demonstrating the effectiveness of such measures are limited.

Risk Assessment Tool

Although there are no highly predictive models for who will benefit from prolonged opioid therapy for CNCP, some models can identify patients most likely to exhibit aberrant or addictive behaviors. Most published guidelines recommend using one of these tools to determine how closely to monitor patients who are taking opioids daily, or whether to offer prolonged opioid therapy at all.

Patient-Provider Agreements

Also known as "pain contracts," these agreements have a modest effect with 7–23% reduction in aberrant behaviors reported. They do represent an opportunity for the clinician to discuss explicitly the risks and benefits of opioids for CNCP, protocols and procedures for refills and monitoring, and consequences of worrisome behaviors.

Urine Drug Testing

Toxicology testing is a tool borrowed from addiction treatment with goals of limiting diversion and identifying risky secondary drug use. Guidelines recommend increasing frequency of testing with increased risk as determined by dose, risk assessment tool, or recent behavior. It is imperative that clinicians choose their tests appropriately and understand the limitations of toxicology testing when using this tool. **Universal testing is recommended** due to the inability of most clinicians to judge misuse of medication as well as documented racial differences in monitoring.

Dose Limitations

No published data support the use of daily doses of opioids above approximately 200 mg of morphine for CNCP, while risk of overdose increases approximately linearly with dose in observational studies. This has led some guideline authors—and one state, Washington—to impose limits on the amount of opioid a prescriber can offer.

Special Medication Limitations

The US Food and Drug Administration requires companies making extended-release opioid formulations to provide trainings for prescribers. Many guidelines recommend that the prescription of methadone and fentanyl be limited to specialists, and some recommend against concurrent prescription of opioids and benzodiazepines.

A SHARED DECISION-MAKING APPROACH

Prescribing opioids for patients with CNCP is fraught with challenges for clinicians, but taking the approach of carefully evaluating risks and benefits allows the opportunity for shared decision-making in individual cases. Clinical trials do not suggest that the majority of people with CNCP will benefit significantly from daily opioids, and the dramatic increase in morbidity and mortality witnessed with the increased availability of these medications warrants very careful patient selection. It is incumbent upon the clinician to provide frank advice to patients prescribed ongoing opioid therapy for CNCP and offer safer alternatives when the benefit is insufficient or the risks too high.

Bohnert AS et al. Association between opioid prescribing patterns and opioid overdose-related deaths. JAMA. 2011 Apr 6;305(13):1315–21. [PMID: 21467284]

Noble M et al. Long-term opioid management for chronic noncancer pain. Cochrane Database Syst Rev. 2010 Jan 20;(1):CD006605. [PMID: 20091598]

Nuckols TK et al. Opioid prescribing: a systematic review and critical appraisal of guidelines for chronic pain. Ann Intern Med. 2014 Jan 7;160(1):38–47. [PMID: 24217469]

Starrels JL et al. Systematic review: treatment agreements and urine drug testing to reduce opioid misuse in patients with chronic pain. Ann Intern Med. 2010 Jun 1;152(11):712–20. [PMID: 20513829]

Warner M et al. Drug poisoning deaths in the U.S., 1980–2008. NCHS Data Brief. 2011 Dec;(81):1–8. [PMID: 22617462] http://www.cdc.gov/nchs/data/databriefs/db81.pdf

Table 5–2. Acetaminophen, COX-2 inhibitors, and useful nonsteroidal anti-inflammatory drugs.

Drug	Usual Dose for Adults ≥ 50 kg	Usual Dose for Adults < 50 kg[1]	Cost per Unit	Cost for 30 Days[2]	Comments[3]
Acetaminophen[4] (Tylenol, Datril, etc)	325–500 mg every 4 hours or 750 mg every 6 hours, up to 2000–3000 mg/d	10–15 mg/kg every 4 hours (oral); 15–20 mg/kg every 4 hour (rectal), up to 2000–3000 mg/d	$0.02/500 mg (oral) OTC; $0.71/650 mg (rectal) OTC	$3.60 (oral); $127.80 (rectal)	Not an NSAID because it lacks peripheral anti-inflammatory effects. Equivalent to aspirin as analgesic and antipyretic agent. Limit dose to 3000 mg/d and to 2000 mg/d in older patients and those with liver disease. Be mindful of multiple sources of acetaminophen as in combination analgesics, cold remedies, and sleep aids.
Aspirin[5]	650 mg every 4 hours or 975 mg every 6 hours	10–15 mg/kg every 4 hours (oral); 15–20 mg/kg every 4 hours (rectal)	$0.02/325 mg OTC; $1.51/600 mg (rectal) OTC	$7.20 (oral); $271.80 (rectal)	Available also in enteric-coated form that is more slowly absorbed but better tolerated.
Celecoxib[4] (Celebrex)	200 mg once daily (osteoarthritis); 100–200 mg twice daily (RA)	100 mg once or twice daily	$4.95/100 mg; $7.52/200 mg	$225.60 OA; $451.20 RA	Cyclooxygenase-2 inhibitor. No antiplatelet effects. Lower doses for elderly who weigh < 50 kg. Lower incidence of endoscopic gastrointestinal ulceration. Not known if true lower incidence of gastrointestinal bleeding. Possible link to cardiovascular toxicity. Celecoxib is contraindicated in sulfonamide allergy.
Choline magnesium salicylate[6] (Trilasate, others)	1000–1500 mg three times daily	25 mg/kg three times daily	$0.46/500 mg	$124.20	Salicylates cause less gastrointestinal distress and kidney impairment than NSAIDs but are probably less effective in pain management than NSAIDs.
Diclofenac (Voltaren, Cataflam, others)	50–75 mg orally two or three times daily; 1% gel 2–4 g four times daily; 1.3% patch two times daily		$1.47/50 mg; $1.77/75 mg	$132.30; $159.30	May impose higher risk of hepatotoxicity. Enteric-coated product; slow onset. Topical formulations may result in fewer side effects than oral formulations.
Diclofenac sustained release (Voltaren-XR, others)	100–200 mg once daily		$2.81/100 mg	$168.60	
Diflunisal[7] (Dolobid, others)	500 mg every 12 hours		$1.70/500 mg	$102.00	Fluorinated acetylsalicylic acid derivative.
Etodolac (Lodine, others)	200–400 mg every 6–8 hours		$1.32/400 mg	$158.40	
Fenoprofen calcium (Nalfon, others)	300–600 mg every 6 hours		$2.19/600 mg	$262.80	Perhaps more side effects than others, including tubulointerstitial nephritis.
Flurbiprofen (Ansaid)	50–100 mg three or four times daily		$0.79/50 mg; $1.18/100 mg	$94.80; $141.60	Adverse gastrointestinal effects may be more common among elderly.
Ibuprofen (Motrin, Advil, Rufen, others)	400–800 mg every 6 hours	10 mg/kg every 6–8 hours	$0.28/600 mg Rx; $0.05/200 mg OTC	$33.60; $9.00	Relatively well tolerated and inexpensive.
Indomethacin (Indocin, Indometh, others)	25–50 mg two to four times daily		$0.38/25 mg; $0.64/50 mg	$45.60; $76.80	Higher incidence of dose-related toxic effects, especially gastrointestinal and bone marrow effects.
Ketoprofen (Orudis, Oruvail, others)	25–75 mg every 6–8 hours (max 300 mg/d)		$1.12/50 mg Rx; $1.241.07/75 mg Rx; $0.50/12.5 mg OTC	$126.00; $148.80; $90.00	Lower doses for elderly.

(continued)

Table 5–2. Acetaminophen, COX-2 inhibitors, and useful nonsteroidal anti-inflammatory drugs. (continued)

Drug	Usual Dose for Adults ≥ 50 kg	Usual Dose for Adults < 50 kg[1]	Cost per Unit	Cost for 30 Days[2]	Comments[3]
Ketorolac tromethamine (Toradol)	10 mg every 4–6 hours to a maximum of 40 mg/d orally		$1.14/10 mg	Not recommended	Short-term use (< 5 days) only; otherwise, increased risk of gastrointestinal side effects.
Ketorolac tromethamine[8] (Toradol	60 mg intramuscularly or 30 mg intravenously initially, then 30 mg every 6 hours intramuscularly or intravenously		$2.52/30 mg	Not recommended	Intramuscular or intravenous NSAID as alternative to opioid. Lower doses for elderly. Short-term use (< 5 days) only.
Magnesium salicylate (various)	467–934 mg every 6 hours		$0.23/467 mg OTC	$55.20	
Meclofenamate sodium[9] (Meclomen)	50–100 mg every 6 hours		$5.37/100 mg	$644.40	Diarrhea more common.
Mefenamic acid (Ponstel)	250 mg every 6 hours		$17.41/250 mg	$2089.20	
Nabumetone (Relafen)	500–1000 mg once daily (max dose 2000 mg/d)		$1.38/500 mg; $1.62/750 mg	$97.20	May be less ulcerogenic than ibuprofen, but overall side effects may not be less.
Naproxen (Naprosyn, Anaprox, Aleve [OTC], others)	250–500 mg every 6–8 hours	5 mg/kg every 8 hours	$1.29/500 mg Rx; $0.08/220 mg OTC	$154.80; $7.20 OTC	Generally well tolerated. Lower doses for elderly.
Oxaprozin (Daypro, others)	600–1200 mg once daily		$1.50/600 mg	$90.00	Similar to ibuprofen. May cause rash, pruritus, photosensitivity.
Piroxicam (Feldene, others)	20 mg daily		$2.64/20 mg	$79.20	Not recommended in the elderly due to high adverse drug reaction rate. Single daily dose convenient. Long half-life. May cause higher rate of gastrointestinal bleeding and dermatologic side effects.
Sodium salicylate	325–650 mg every 3–4 hours				No longer available in the United States
Sulindac (Clinoril, others)	150–200 mg twice daily		$0.98/150 mg; $1.21/200 mg	$58.80; $72.60	May cause higher rate of gastrointestinal bleeding. May have less nephrotoxic potential.
Tolmetin (Tolectin)	200–600 mg four times daily		$0.75/200 mg; $3.98/600 mg	$90.00; $477.60	Perhaps more side effects than others, including anaphylactic reactions.

[1]Acetaminophen and NSAID dosages for adults weighing < 50 kg should be adjusted for weight.
[2]Average wholesale price (AWP, for AB-rated generic when available) for quantity listed. Source: *Red Book Online, 2014, Truven Health Analytics, Inc.* AWP may not accurately represent the actual pharmacy cost because wide contractual variations exist among institutions.
[3]The adverse effects of headache, tinnitus, dizziness, confusion, rashes, anorexia, nausea, vomiting, gastrointestinal bleeding, diarrhea, nephrotoxicity, visual disturbances, etc, can occur with any of these drugs. Tolerance and efficacy are subject to great individual variations among patients. Note: All NSAIDs can increase serum lithium levels.
[4]Acetaminophen and celecoxib lack antiplatelet effects.
[5]May inhibit platelet aggregation for 1 week or more and may cause bleeding.
[6]May have minimal antiplatelet activity.
[7]Administration with antacids may decrease absorption.
[8]Has the same gastrointestinal toxicities as oral NSAIDs.
[9]Coombs-positive autoimmune hemolytic anemia has been associated with prolonged use.
COX-2, cyclooxygenase-2; OA, osteoarthritis; RA, rheumatoid arthritis; OTC, over-the-counter; Rx, prescription.
Data from Jacox AK et al. *Management of Cancer Pain: Quick Reference Guide for Clinicians No. 9.* AHCPR Publication No. 94–0593. Rockville, MD: Agency for Health Care Policy and Research, Public Health Service, U.S. Department of Health and Human Services. March 1994.

Table 5–3. Useful opioid agonist analgesics.

Drug	Approximate Equianalgesic Dose (compared to morphine 30 mg orally or 10 mg IV/SC)[1]		Usual Starting Dose				Potential Advantages	Potential Disadvantages
			Adults ≥ 50 kg Body Weight		Adults < 50 kg Body Weight			
	Oral	Parenteral	Oral	Parenteral	Oral	Parenteral		
Opioid agonists[2]								
Buprenorphine transdermal	Not available	Not available	Not available orally. Transdermal doses available: 5, 10, and 20 mcg/h Initiate 5 mcg/h patch for opioid-naïve patients (may currently be using nonopioid analgesics) $72.39/10 mcg/h	Not available	Not available	Not available	7-day analgesia, may be initiated in opioid-naïve patients. Can titrate up dose after 72 hours.	QT prolongation
Fentanyl	Not available	100 mcg every hour	Not available	50–100 mcg IV/IM every hour or 0.5–1.5 mcg/kg/h IV infusion $0.37/100 mcg	Not available	0.5–1 mcg/kg IV every 1–4 hours or 1–2 mcg/kg IV × 1, then 0.5–1 mcg/kg/h infusion	Possibly less neuroexcitatory effects, including in kidney failure.	
Fentanyl oral transmucosal (Actiq); buccal (Fentora)	Not available	Not available	200 mcg transmucosal; 100 mcg buccal; $18.80/200 mcg transmucosal; $47.96/200 mcg buccal	Not available	Not available	Not available	For pain breaking through long-acting opioid medication.	Transmucosal and buccal formulations are not bioequivalent; there is higher bioavailability of buccal formulation.

Drug								
Fentanyl transdermal	Conversion to fentanyl patch is based on total daily dose of oral morphine[2]: morphine 60–134 mg/d orally = fentanyl 25 mcg/h patch; morphine 135–224 mg/d orally = fentanyl 50 mcg/h patch; morphine 225–314 mg/d orally = fentanyl 75 mcg/h patch; and morphine 315–404 mg/d orally = fentanyl 100 mcg/h patch	Not available	Not available orally 12.5–25 mcg/h patch every 72 hours; $16.65/25 mcg/h	Not available	12.5–25 mcg/h patch every 72 hours	Not available	Stable medication blood levels.	Not for use in opioid-naive patients. Minimum starting dose is 25 mcg/h patch in patients who have been taking stable dose of opioids for at least 1 week at the equivalent of at least 60 mg/d of oral morphine.
Hydrocodone, extended release (Zohydro ER)	20 mg[1]	Not available	10 mg every 12 hours Cost not yet published)	Not available	Not available	Not available	Available as an extended release formulation without acetaminophen	
Hydromorphone[3] (Dilaudid)	7.5 mg every 3–4 hours	1.5 mg every 3–4 hours	1–2 mg every 3–4 hours; $0.45/2 mg	1.5 mg every 3–4 hours; $1.02/2 mg	0.06 mg/ every 3–4 hours	0.015 mg/kg every 3–4 hours	Similar to morphine. Available in injectable high-potency preparation, rectal suppository.	Short duration.
Hydromorphone extended release (Exalgo)	45–60 mg every 24 hours	Not available	8 mg every 24 hours; 13.58/8 mg	Not available	Not available	Not available	Similar to morphine	
Levorphanol (Levo-Dromoran)	4 mg every 6–8 hours	2 mg every 6–8 hours	4 mg every 6–8 hours; $1.07/2 mg	Not available	0.04 mg/kg every 6–8 hours	Not available	Longer-acting than morphine sulfate.	
Meperidine[4] (Demerol)	300 mg every 2–3 hours; normal dose 50–150 mg every 3–4 hours	100 mg every 3 hours	Not recommended	100 mg every 3 hours; $3.29/100 mg	Not recomended	0.75 mg/kg every 2–3 hours	Use only when single dose, short duration analgesia is needed as for outpatient procedures like colonoscopy. Not recommended for chronic pain or for repeated dosing.	Short duration. Normeperidine metabolite accumulates in kidney failure and other situations, and in high concentrations may cause irritability and seizures.

(continued)

Table 5–3. Useful opioid agonist analgesics. (continued)

| Drug | Approximate Equianalgesic Dose (compared to morphine 30 mg orally or 10 mg IV/SC)[1] | | Usual Starting Dose | | | | Potential Advantages | Potential Disadvantages |
| | | | Adults ≥ 50 kg Body Weight | | Adults < 50 kg Body Weight | | | |
	Oral	Parenteral	Oral	Parenteral	Oral	Parenteral		
Methadone (Dolophine, others)	10–20 mg every 6–8 hours (when converting from < 100 mg long-term daily oral morphine[5])	5–10 mg every 6–8 hours	5–20 mg every 6–8 hours; $0.14/10 mg	2.5–10 mg every 6–8 hours; $9.33/10 mg	0.2 mg/kg every 6–8 hours	0.1 mg/kg every 6–8 hours	Somewhat longer-acting than morphine. Useful in cases of intolerance to morphine. May be particularly useful for neuropathic pain. Available in liquid formulation.	Analgesic duration shorter than plasma duration. May accumulate, requiring close monitoring during first weeks of treatment. Equianalgesic ratios vary with opioid dose.
Morphine[3] immediate release (Morphine sulfate tablets, Roxanol liquid)	30 mg every 3–4 hours (repeat around-the-clock dosing); 60 mg every 3–4 hours (single or intermittent dosing)	10 mg every 3–4 hours	4–8 mg every 3–4 hours; Used for breakthrough pain in patients already taking controlled-release preparations $0.32/15 mg tab; 0.80/20 mg liquid	10 mg every 3–4 hours; $1.96/10 mg	0.3 mg/kg every 3–4 hours	0.1 mg/kg every 3–4 hours	Standard of comparison; multiple dosage forms available.	No unique problems when compared with other opioids.
Morphine controlled-release[3] (MS Contin Oramorph)	90–120 mg every 12 hours	Not available	15–60 mg every 12 hours; $1.70/30 mg	Not available	Not available	Not available		
Morphine extended release (Kadian, Avinza)	180–240 mg every 24 hours	Not available	20–30 mg every 24 hours; $5.69/30 mg	Not available	Not available	Not available	Once-daily dosing possible.	
Oxycodone (Roxicodone, OxyIR)	20–30 mg every 3–4 hours	Not available	5–10 mg every 3–4 hours; $0.48/5 mg	Not available	0.2 mg/kg every 3–4 hours	Not available		
Oxycodone controlled release (Oxycontin)	40 mg every 12 hours	Not available	20–40 mg every 12 hours; $5.24/20 mg				Similar to morphine.	
Oxymorphone[6] oral, immediate release (Opana)	10 mg every 6 hours	Not available	5–10 mg every 6 hours; $2.95/5 mg	Not available				Taking with food can increase serum levels by 50%. Equianalgesic dosing conversion range is wide.

Drug							Comments
Oxymorphone[6] extended release (Opana ER)	30–40 mg every 12 hours	Not available	15–30 mg every 12 hours; $3.34/10 mg	Not available				Taking with food can increase serum levels by 50%. Equianalgesic dosing conversion range is wide.
Combination Opioid-Nonopioid Preparations							
Codeine[7,8] (with aspirin or acetaminophen)[9]	180–200 mg every 3–4 hours; commonly available dose in combination with acetaminophen, 15–60 mg of codeine every 4–6 hours	130 mg every 3–4 hours	60 mg every 4–6 hours; $0.54/60 mg	60 mg every 2 hours (IM/SC); price not available in the United States	0.5–1 mg/kg every 3–4 hours	Not recommended	Similar to morphine.	Closely monitor for efficacy as patients vary in their ability to convert the prodrug codeine to morphine.
Hydrocodone[6] (in Lorcet, Lortab, Vicodin, others)[9]	30 mg every 3–4 hours	Not available	10 mg every 3–4 hours; $0.54/5 mg	Not available	0.2 mg/kg every 3–4 hours	Not available		Combination with acetaminophen limits dosage titration.
Oxycodone[7] (in Percocet, Percodan, Tylox, others)[9]	30 mg every 3–4 hours	Not available	10 mg every 3–4 hours; $0.43/5 mg	Not available	0.2 mg/kg every 3–4 hours	Not available	Similar to morphine.	Combination with acetaminophen and aspirin limits dosage titration.

[1] Published tables vary in the suggested doses that are equianalgesic to morphine. Clinical response is the criterion that must be applied for each patient; titration to clinical efficacy is necessary. Because there is not complete cross-tolerance among these drugs, it is usually necessary to use a lower than equianalgesic dose initially when changing drugs and to retitrate to response.

[2] Conversion is conservative; therefore, do not use these equianalgesic doses for converting back from fentanyl patch to other opioids because they may lead to inadvertent overdose. Patients may require breakthrough doses of short-acting opioids during conversion to transdermal fentanyl.

[3] Caution: For morphine, hydromorphone, and oxymorphone, rectal administration is an alternative route for patients unable to take oral medications. Equianalgesic doses may differ from oral and parenteral doses. A short-acting opioid should normally be used for initial therapy.

[4] Not recommended for chronic pain. Doses listed are for brief therapy of acute pain only. Switch to another opioid for long-term therapy.

[5] Methadone conversion varies depending on the equivalent total daily dose of morphine. Consult with a pain management or palliative care expert for conversion.

[6] Caution: Recommended doses do not apply for adult patients with kidney or hepatic insufficiency or other conditions affecting drug metabolism.

[7] Caution: Doses of aspirin and acetaminophen in combination products must also be adjusted to the patient's body weight.

[8] Caution: Doses of codeine above 60 mg often are not appropriate because of diminishing incremental analgesia with increasing doses but continually increasing nausea, constipation, and other side effects.

[9] Caution: Monitor total acetaminophen dose carefully, including any OTC use. Total acetaminophen dose maximum 3 g/d. If liver impairment or heavy alcohol use, maximum is 2 g/d. Available dosing formulations of these combination medications are being adjusted to reflect increased caution about acetaminophen toxicity. Acetaminophen doses in a single combination tablet or capsule will be limited to no more than 325 mg.

Note: Average wholesale price (AWP, generic when available) for quantity listed. Source: *Red Book Online, 2014, Truven Health Analytics, Inc.* AWP may not accurately represent the actual pharmacy cost because wide contractual variations exist among institutions.

Data from Jacox AK et al. *Management of Cancer Pain: Quick Reference Guide for Clinicians No. 9.* AHCPR Publication No. 94–0593. Rockville, MD. Agency for Health Care Policy and Research, Public Health Service, U.S. Department of Health and Human Services. March 1994, and from Erstad BL. A rational approach to the management of acute pain states. Hosp Formul 1994;29 (8 Part 2):586.

For chronic stable pain, **long-acting medications** are preferred, such as oral sustained-release morphine (one to three times a day), oxycodone (two or three times a day), hydrocodone (two times a day), or methadone (three or four times a day) (Table 5–3). A useful technique for opioid management of chronic pain is equianalgesic dosing (Table 5–3). The dosages of any full opioid agonists used to control pain can be converted into an equivalent dose of any other opioid. This approach is helpful in estimating the appropriate dose of a long-acting opioid based on the amount of short-acting opioid required over the preceding days. For example, 24-hour opioid requirements established using short-acting opioid medications can be converted into equivalent dosages of long-acting medications or formulations. Cross-tolerance is often incomplete, however, so generally only two-thirds to three-quarters of the full, calculated equianalgesic dosage is administered initially when switching between opioid formulations.

Methadone deserves special consideration among the long-acting opioids because it is inexpensive, available in a liquid formulation, and may have added efficacy for neuropathic pain. However, equianalgesic dosing is complex because it varies with the patient's opioid dose and caution must be used at higher methadone doses (generally > 100–150 mg/d) because of the risk of QT prolongation. Baseline ECG is recommended before starting methadone except at the very end of life where comfort is the only goal. Given the complexities of management and the increasing prevalence of methadone overdose in the United States, consultation with a palliative medicine or pain specialist may be appropriate.

Transdermal fentanyl is appropriate for patients already tolerant to other opioids for at least 1 week at a dose equivalent to at least 60 mg/d of oral morphine (equivalent to transdermal fentanyl 25 mcg/h every 72 hours) and therefore should not be used in the postoperative setting or be the first opioid used. Medications that inhibit cytochrome P450 3A4, such as ritonavir, ketoconazole, itraconazole, troleandomycin, clarithromycin, nelfinavir, nefazodone, amiodarone, amprenavir, aprepitant, diltiazem, erythromycin, fluconazole, fosamprenavir, and verapamil, and grapefruit juice can cause increased levels and duration of transdermal fentanyl. Since transdermal fentanyl can require 24–48 hours to achieve pharmacologic "steady state," patients should be given short-acting opioids while awaiting the full analgesic effect of transdermal fentanyl, and changes in dose of transdermal fentanyl should be made no more frequently than every 6 days.

While some clinicians and patients inexperienced with the management of severe chronic pain may feel more comfortable with combined nonopioid-opioid agents, full agonist opioids are typically a better choice in patients with severe pain because the dose of opioid is not limited by the toxicities of the acetaminophen, aspirin, or NSAID component of combination preparations. There is no maximal allowable or effective dose for full opioid agonists. The dose should be increased to whatever is necessary to relieve pain, remembering that certain types of pain, such as neuropathic pain, may respond better to agents other than opioids, or to combinations of opioids with co-analgesics (see below).

While physiologic tolerance is possible with opioids, failure of a previously effective opioid dose to adequately relieve pain is usually due to worsening of the underlying condition causing pain, such as tumor growth or new metastasis in a patient with cancer. In this case, for moderate unrelieved pain, the dose of opioid can be increased by 25–50%. For severe unrelieved pain, a dose increase of 50–100% may be appropriate. The frequency of dosing should be adjusted so that pain control is continuous. Long-term dosing may then be adjusted by adding the average daily amount of short-acting opioid necessary for breakthrough pain over the preceding 72–96 hours to the long-acting medication dose. In establishing or reestablishing adequate dosing, frequent reassessment of the patient's pain and medication side effects is necessary.

B. Opioid Adverse Effects

As opioids are titrated upward, increasing difficulty with the side effects can be expected. Constipation is common at any dose of opioid, and tolerance to this side effect does not develop over time. Opioid-induced constipation should be anticipated and prevented in all patients (see below).

Sedation can be expected with opioids, although tolerance to this effect and to other nonconstipation side effects typically develops within 24–72 hours at a stable dose. Sedation typically appears well before significant respiratory depression. If treatment for sedation is desired, dextroamphetamine (2.5–7.5 mg orally at 8 AM and noon) or methylphenidate (2.5–10 mg orally at 8 AM and noon) may be helpful. Caffeinated beverages can also ameliorate minor opioid sedation.

Opioid-induced neurotoxicity—including myoclonus, hyperalgesia, delirium with hallucinosis, and seizures—may develop in patients who take high doses of opioids for a prolonged period. These symptoms may resolve after lowering the dose or switching opioids, especially to ones like fentanyl or methadone that do not have active metabolites. While waiting for the level of the offending opioid to fall, low doses of lorazepam, baclofen, or gabapentin may be helpful for treating myoclonus; haloperidol may be useful for treating delirium. Avoiding or correcting dehydration may be helpful for prevention and treatment of opioid-induced neurotoxicity.

Nausea due to opioids may occur with initiation of therapy and resolve after a few days. Notably, unrelieved constipation may be a more common cause of nausea in the setting of opioid use than opioid-induced nausea. Severe or persistent nausea despite treatment of constipation can be managed by switching opioids or by giving haloperidol, 0.5–4 mg orally, subcutaneously, or intravenously every 6 hours; prochlorperazine, 10 mg orally or intravenously or 25 mg rectally every 6 hours; or metoclopramide, 5–20 mg orally, subcutaneously, or intravenously before meals and bed. Ondansetron, 4–8 mg orally or intravenously every 6 hours, also relieves nausea but can contribute to constipation. Most antiemetic treatments can contribute to sedation.

Although clinicians may worry about respiratory depression with opioids, this side effect is uncommon when a low dose is given initially and titrated upward slowly.

Patients at particular risk for respiratory depression include those with chronic obstructive pulmonary disease, obstructive sleep apnea, and baseline CO_2 retention, those with liver or kidney or combined liver-kidney failure, and those with adrenal insufficiency or frank myxedema. Yet, even patients with severe pulmonary disease and obstructive sleep apnea can tolerate low-dose opioids, but they should be monitored carefully. Hospitalized patients with these conditions who require increased doses of opioids should be monitored with continuous pulse oximetry. Clinicians should not allow unfounded concerns about respiratory depression to prevent them from treating pain adequately.

▶ Medications for Neuropathic Pain

It is essential when taking a patient's history to listen for descriptions such as burning, shooting, pins and needles, or electricity, and for pain associated with numbness. Such a history suggests neuropathic pain, which is treated with some medications not typically used for other types of pain. While opioids are effective for neuropathic pain, a number of nonopioid medications also have been found to be effective in randomized trials (Table 5–4). Successful management of neuropathic pain often requires the use of more than one effective medication.

The tricyclic antidepressants (TCAs) are good first-line therapy. Nortriptyline and desipramine are preferred because they cause less orthostatic hypotension and have fewer anticholinergic effects than amitriptyline. Start with a low dosage (10–25 mg orally daily) and titrate upward in 10 mg increments every 4 or 5 days to 50 mg. It may take several weeks for a TCA to have its full effect as a neuropathic pain analgesic.

The calcium channel alpha2-delta ligands gabapentin and pregabalin are also first-line therapies for neuropathic pain. Both medications can cause sedation, dizziness, ataxia, and gastrointestinal side effects but have no significant drug interactions. Both drugs require dose adjustments in patients with kidney dysfunction. Gabapentin should be started at low dosages of 100–300 mg orally three times a day and titrated upward by 300 mg/d every 4 or 5 days with a typical effective dose of 1800–3600 mg/d. Pregabalin should be started at 150 mg/d in two or three divided doses. If necessary, the dose of pregabalin can be titrated upward to 300–600 mg/d in two or three divided doses. Both drugs are relatively safe in accidental overdose and may be preferred over TCAs for a patient with a history of heart failure or arrhythmia or if there is a risk of suicide. Prescribing both gabapentin and morphine for neuropathic pain may provide better analgesia at lower doses than if each is used as a single agent.

The selective serotonin norepinephrine reuptake inhibitors (SSNRIs), duloxetine and venlafaxine, are also first-line treatments for neuropathic pain. Patients should be advised to take duloxetine on a full stomach because nausea is a common side effect. Duloxetine generally should not be combined with other serotonin or norepinephrine uptake inhibitors, but it can be combined with gabapentin or pregabalin. Because venlafaxine can cause hypertension and

Table 5–4. Pharmacologic management of neuropathic pain.

Drug[1]	Starting Dose	Typical Dose
Antidepressants[2]		
Nortriptyline	10 mg orally at bedtime	10–50 mg orally at bedtime
Desipramine	10 mg orally at bedtime	10–50 mg orally at bedtime
Calcium-channel alpha2-delta ligands		
Gabapentin[3]	100–300 mg orally once to three times daily	300–1200 mg orally three times daily
Pregabalin[4]	50 mg orally three times daily	100 mg orally three times daily
Selective serotonin norepinephrine reuptake inhibitors		
Duloxetine	60 mg orally daily or 20 mg orally twice daily in elders	60–120 mg orally daily
Venlafaxine[5]	75 mg orally daily divided into two or three doses	150–225 mg orally daily divided into two or three doses
Opioids	**(see Table 5–3)**	**(see Table 5–3)**
Other medications		
Lidocaine transdermal	5% patch applied daily, for a maximum of 12 hours	1–3 patches applied daily for a maximum of 12 hours
Tramadol hydrochloride	50 mg orally four times daily	100 mg orally two to four times daily

[1]Begin at the starting dose and titrate up every 4 or 5 days. Within each category, drugs listed in order or prescribing preference.
[2]Begin with a low dose. Pain relief may be achieved at doses below antidepressant doses, thereby minimizing adverse side effects.
[3]Common side effects include nausea, somnolence, and dizziness. Take medication on a full stomach. Do not combine with serotonin or norepinephrine uptake inhibitors, or with tricyclic antidepressants.
[4]Common side effects include dizziness, somnolence, peripheral edema, and weight gain. Must adjust dose for kidney impairment.
[5]*Caution:* Can cause hypertension and ECG changes. Obtain baseline ECG and monitor.

induce ECG changes, patients with cardiovascular risk factors should be carefully monitored when starting this drug.

Other medications effective for neuropathic pain include tramadol and the 5% lidocaine patch. The 5% lidocaine patch is effective in postherpetic neuralgia and may be effective in other types of localized neuropathic pain.

▶ Adjuvant Pain Medications & Treatments

If pain cannot be controlled without uncomfortable medication side effects, clinicians should consider using lower doses of multiple medications, as is done commonly for neuropathic pain, rather than larger doses of one or two medications. For metastatic bone pain, the anti-inflammatory effect of NSAIDs can be particularly helpful. Radiation therapy (including single-fraction treatments) and bisphosphonates may also relieve bone pain. For some patients, a nerve block can provide substantial relief, such as a celiac plexus block for pain from pancreatic cancer. Intrathecal pumps may be useful for patients with severe pain responsive to opioids but who require such large doses that systemic side effects (eg, sedation and constipation) become limiting. There is some evidence for the use of cannabinoids as analgesics.

Corticosteroids such as dexamethasone or prednisone can be helpful for patients with headache due to increased intracranial pressure, pain from spinal cord compression, metastatic bone pain, and neuropathic pain due to invasion or infiltration of nerves by tumor. Because of the side effects of long-term corticosteroid administration, they are most appropriate for short-term use and in patients with end-stage disease. Low-dose intravenous or oral ketamine has been used successfully for neuropathic and other pain syndromes refractory to opioids.

NONPHARMACOLOGIC TREATMENTS

Nonpharmacologic therapies are valuable in treating pain. Hot or cold packs, massage, and physical therapy can be helpful for musculoskeletal pain. Similarly, biofeedback, acupuncture, chiropractic, meditation, music therapy, cognitive behavioral therapy, guided imagery, cognitive distraction, and framing may be of help in treating pain. Because mood and psychological issues play an important role in the patient's perception of and response to pain, psychotherapy, support groups, prayer, and pastoral counseling can also help in the management of pain. Major depression, which may be instigated by chronic pain or may alter the response to pain, should be treated aggressively.

▶ When to Refer

- Pain not responding to opioids at typical doses.
- Neuropathic pain not responding to first-line treatments.
- Complex methadone management issues.
- Intolerable side effects from oral opioids.
- Severe pain from bone metastases.
- For a surgical or anesthesia-based procedure, intrathecal pump, or nerve block.

▶ When to Admit

- Severe exacerbation of pain that is not responsive to previous stable oral opioid around-the-clock plus breakthrough doses.
- Patients whose pain is so severe that they cannot be cared for at home.
- Uncontrollable side effects from opioids, including nausea, vomiting, and altered mental status.

Bengoechea I et al. Opioid use at the end of life and survival in a Hospital at Home unit. J Palliat Med. 2010 Sep;13(9):1079–83. [PMID: 20799903]

Dworkin RH et al. Recommendations for the pharmacological management of neuropathic pain: an overview and literature update. Mayo Clin Proc. 2010 Mar;85(3 Suppl):S3–14. [PMID: 20194146]

Salpeter SR et al. The use of very-low-dose methadone for palliative pain control and the prevention of opioid hyperalgesia. J Palliat Med. 2013 Jun;16(6):616–22. [PMID: 23556990]

Smith EM et al; Alliance for Clinical Trials in Oncology. Effect of duloxetine on pain, function, and quality of life among patients with chemotherapy-induced painful peripheral neuropathy: a randomized clinical trial. JAMA. 2013 Apr 3;309(13):1359–67. [PMID: 23549581]

PALLIATION OF OTHER COMMON SYMPTOMS

DYSPNEA

Dyspnea is the subjective experience of difficulty breathing and may be characterized by patients as tightness in the chest, shortness of breath, or a feeling of suffocation. Up to 50% of terminally ill patients may experience severe dyspnea.

Treatment of dyspnea is usually first directed at the cause (see Chapter 9). At the end of life, dyspnea is often treated nonspecifically with opioids. **Immediate-release morphine** given orally (2–4 mg every 4 hours) or intravenously (1–2 mg every 4 hours) treats dyspnea effectively. Doses are typically lower than would be necessary for the relief of moderate pain. **Sustained-release morphine** given orally at 10 mg daily appears to be safe and effective for most patients with dyspnea. Supplemental oxygen may be useful for the dyspneic patient *who is hypoxic*. However, a nasal cannula and face mask are sometimes not well tolerated, and fresh air from a window or fan may provide relief. Judicious use of noninvasive ventilation as well as nonpharmacologic relaxation techniques such as meditation and guided imagery may be beneficial for some patients. Benzodiazepines may be useful adjuncts for treatment of dyspnea-related agitation. Nonpharmacologic treatments, including acupuncture, may be quite effective.

NAUSEA & VOMITING

Nausea and vomiting are common and distressing symptoms. As with pain, the management of nausea may be maximized by regular dosing and often requires multiple medications. An understanding of the four major inputs to the vomiting center may help direct treatment (see Chapter 15).

Vomiting associated with opioids is discussed above. When vomiting is due to stimulation of peripheral afferent nerves from the gut, offering patients small amounts of food only when they are hungry may be helpful. Nasogastric suction may provide rapid, short-term relief for vomiting associated with constipation (in addition to laxatives), gastroparesis, or gastric outlet or bowel obstruction. Prokinetic agents, such as metoclopramide (5–20 mg orally or intravenously four times a day), can be helpful in the setting of partial bowel obstruction. Transdermal scopolamine (1.5-mg patch every 3 days) can reduce peristalsis and reduce cramping pain, and ranitidine (50 mg intravenously every 6 hours) and octreotide (starting at 50–100 mcg subcutaneously every 8 hours) or as continuous intravenous or subcutaneous infusion, beginning at 10–20 mcg/h) can reduce gut secretions improving nausea and vomiting. High-dose corticosteroids (eg, dexamethasone, 20 mg orally or intravenously daily in divided doses) can be used in refractory cases of nausea or vomiting or when it is due to bowel obstruction or increased intracranial pressure.

Vomiting due to disturbance of the vestibular apparatus may be treated with anticholinergic and antihistaminic agents (including diphenhydramine, 25 mg orally or intravenously every 8 hours, or scopolamine, 1.5-mg patch every 3 days).

Benzodiazepines can be effective in preventing the anticipatory nausea associated with chemotherapy. Finally, many patients find medical cannabis (in particular strains with high cannabidiol [CBD] content) or dronabinol (2.5–20 mg orally every 4–6 hours) helpful in the management of nausea and vomiting.

CONSTIPATION

Given the frequent use of opioids, poor dietary intake, and physical inactivity, constipation is a common problem in the seriously ill or dying. Clinicians must inquire about any difficulty with hard or infrequent stools. Constipation is an easily preventable and treatable cause of discomfort, distress, and nausea and vomiting (see above and Chapter 15).

Constipation may be prevented or relieved if patients can increase their activity and their intake of fluids. Simple considerations such as privacy, undisturbed toilet time, and a bedside commode rather than a bedpan may be important for some patients.

For patients taking opioids, anticipating and preventing constipation is key. A prophylactic bowel regimen with a stimulant laxative (senna or bisacodyl) should be started when opioid treatment is begun. Table 15–4 lists other agents (including polyethylene glycol) that can be added as needed. Docusate, a stool softener, adds little to senna in hospitalized patients and is not recommended. Methylnaltrexone, a subcutaneous medication, is a peripherally acting mu-receptor antagonist and is available for severe, unrelieved, opioid-induced constipation.

FATIGUE

Fatigue is a distressing symptom and is the most common complaint among cancer patients. Specific abnormalities that can contribute to fatigue, including anemia, hypothyroidism, hypogonadism, cognitive and functional impairment, and malnutrition, should be corrected. Because pain, depression, and fatigue often coexist in patients with cancer, pain and depression should be managed adequately in the setting of patients with fatigue. Fatigue from medication adverse effects and polypharmacy is common and should be addressed. For nonspecific fatigue, exercise and physical rehabilitation may be most effective. Low doses of psychostimulants, such as methylphenidate 5–10 mg orally in the morning and afternoon or modafinil 200 mg orally in the morning, can be effective. Corticosteroids may have a short-term benefit. American Ginseng has been shown to be effective for cancer-related fatigue.

DELIRIUM & AGITATION

Many patients die in a state of delirium—a disturbance of consciousness and a change in cognition that develops over a short time and is manifested by misinterpretations, illusions, hallucinations, disturbances in the sleep-wake cycle, psychomotor disturbances (eg, lethargy, restlessness), and mood disturbance (eg, fear, anxiety). Delirium may be hyperactive, hypoactive, or mixed. Agitated delirium at the end of life has been called **terminal restlessness.**

Careful attention to patient safety and nonpharmacologic strategies to help the patient remain oriented (clocks, calendars, a familiar environment, reassurance and redirection from caregivers) may be sufficient to prevent or manage mild delirium. Some delirious patients may be "pleasantly confused," and a decision by the patient's family and the clinician not to treat delirium may be considered.

More commonly, however, delirium at the end of life is distressing to patients and family and requires treatment. Delirium may interfere with the family's ability to feel comforting to the patient and may prevent a patient from being able to recognize and report important symptoms. While there are many reversible causes of delirium (see Chapter 25), identifying and correcting the underlying cause at the end of life is often complex because a patient may have many possible causes. When the cause of delirium cannot be identified, treated, or corrected rapidly enough, delirium may be treated symptomatically with neuroleptic agents, such as haloperidol (1–10 mg orally, subcutaneously, intramuscularly, or intravenously twice or three times a day) or risperidone (1–3 mg orally twice a day). The benefits of neuroleptic agents in the treatment of agitation must be weighed carefully against potential harms, based on evidence showing an association between antipsychotic medications and increased mortality for older adults with dementia. The role of hydration as a treatment of delirium at the end of life is unclear but intravenous fluids do not appear to attenuate most instances of delirium. When delirium is refractory to treatment and remains intolerable, sedation may be required to provide relief and may be achieved rapidly with midazolam (0.5–5 mg/h subcutaneously or intravenously) or barbiturates (especially useful in the outpatient setting).

Candy B et al. Laxatives or methylnaltrexone for the management of constipation in palliative care patients. Cochrane Database Syst Rev. 2011 Jan 19;(1):CD003448. [PMID: 21249653]

Currow DC et al. Once-daily opioids for chronic dyspnea: a dose increment and pharmacovigilance study. J Pain Symptom Manage. 2011 Sep;42(3):388–99. [PMID: 21458217]

Davidson PM et al. Update on the role of palliative oxygen. Curr Opin Support Palliat Care. 2011 Jun;5(2):87–91. [PMID: 21532348]

Kerr CW et al. Effects of methylphenidate on fatigue and depression: a randomized, double-blind, placebo-controlled trial. J Pain Symptom Manage. 2012 Jan;43(1):68–77. [PMID: 22208450]

Peuckmann V et al. Pharmacological treatments for fatigue associated with palliative care. Cochrane Database Syst Rev. 2010 Nov 10;(11):CD006788. [PMID: 21069692]

Suzuki M et al. A randomized, placebo-controlled trial of acupuncture in patients with chronic obstructive pulmonary disease (COPD): the COPD-acupuncture trial (CAT). Arch Intern Med. 2012 Jun 11;172(11):878–86. [PMID: 22905352]

Tarumi Y et al. Randomized, double-blind, placebo-controlled trial of oral docusate in the management of constipation in hospice patients. J Pain Symptom Manage. 2013 Jan;45(1):2–13. [PMID: 22889861]

CARE OF PATIENTS AT THE END OF LIFE

In the United States, nearly 2.5 million people die each year. Caring for patients at the end of life is an important responsibility and a rewarding opportunity for clinicians. From the medical perspective, the end of life may be defined as that time when death—whether due to terminal illness or acute or chronic illness—is expected within weeks to months and can no longer be reasonably forestalled by medical intervention. Palliative care at the end of life focuses on relieving distressing symptoms and promoting quality of life (as with all other stages of illness). For patients at the end of life, palliative care may become the sole focus of care.

▶ Prognosis at the End of Life

Clinicians must help patients understand when they are approaching the end of life. Most patients want prognostic information. This information influences patients' treatment decisions and may change how they spend their remaining time, but does not negatively impact patient survival. One-half or more of patients do not understand that many treatments they might be offered are palliative and not curative. Patients require support for distress that may accompany discussions of prognostic information.

While certain diseases such as cancer are more amenable to prognostic estimates regarding the time course to death, the other common causes of mortality in the United States—including heart disease, stroke, chronic lung disease, and dementia—have more variable trajectories and difficult to predict prognoses. Even for patients with cancer, clinician estimates of prognosis are often inaccurate and generally overly optimistic. Nonetheless, clinical experience, epidemiologic data, guidelines from professional organizations (eg, the National Hospice and Palliative Care Organization), and computer modeling and prediction tools (eg, the Palliative Performance Scale or www.eprognosis.org) may be used to help patients identify the end period of their lives. Clinicians can also ask themselves

"Would I be surprised if this patient died in the next year?" to determine whether a discussion of prognosis would be appropriate. If the answer is "no," then the clinician should initiate a discussion. Recognizing that patients may have different levels of comfort with prognostic information, clinicians can introduce the topic by simply saying, "I have information about the likely time course of your illness. Would you like to talk about it?"

▶ Expectations About the End of Life

Patients' experiences at the end of life are influenced by their expectations about how they will die and the meaning of death. Many people fear how they will die more than death itself. Patients report fears of dying in pain or of suffocation, of loss of control, indignity, isolation, and of being a burden to their families. All of these anxieties may be ameliorated with good supportive care provided by an attentive group of caretakers.

Death is often regarded by clinicians, patients, and families as a failure of medical science. This attitude can create or heighten a sense of guilt about the failure to prevent dying. Both the general public and clinicians often are complicit in denying death, treating dying persons merely as patients and death as an enemy to be battled furiously in hospitals rather than as an inevitable outcome to be experienced as a part of life at home. As a result, approximately 75–80% of people in the United States die in hospitals or long-term care facilities.

Even when the clinician continues to pursue cure of potentially reversible disease, relieving suffering, providing support, and helping the patient prepare for death are foremost considerations. Patients at the end of life and their families identify a number of elements as important to quality end-of-life care: managing pain and other symptoms adequately, avoiding inappropriate prolongation of dying, preserving dignity, preparing for death, achieving a sense of control, relieving the burden on others, and strengthening relationships with loved ones.

▶ Communication & Care of the Patient

Caring for patients at the end of life requires the same skills clinicians use in other tasks of medical care: diagnosing treatable conditions, providing patient education, facilitating decision-making, and expressing understanding and caring. Higher-quality communication is associated with greater satisfaction and awareness of patient wishes. Clinicians must become proficient at delivering bad news and then dealing with its consequences (Table 5–5). When needed, the use of a professional interpreter can facilitate clear communication and help broker cultural issues.

Three further obligations are central to the clinician's role at this time. First, he or she must work to identify, understand, and relieve physical, psychological, social, and spiritual distress or suffering. Second, clinicians can serve as facilitators or catalysts for hope. While hope for a particular outcome may fade (such as cure of advanced cancer following exhaustive conventional and experimental treatments), it can be redefined by the patient's belief of what is *still* possible. Although expecting a "miraculous cure" may

Table 5–5. Suggestions for the delivery of bad news.

Prepare an appropriate place and time.
Address basic information needs.
Be direct; avoid jargon and euphemisms.
Allow for silence and emotional ventilation.
Assess and validate patient reactions.
Respond to immediate discomforts and risks.
Listen actively and express empathy.
Achieve a common perception of the problem.
Reassure about pain relief.
Ensure basic follow-up and make specific plans for the future.

Table 5–6. Clinician interventions helpful to families of dying patients.

Excellent communication, including clinician willingness to talk about death, timely and clear information, proactive guidance, listening, and empathic responses.
Advance care planning and clear decision-making, including culturally sensitive communication, achieving consensus among family members and an understanding that surrogate decision-makers are trying to determine what the *patient* would have wanted, not what the surrogate would want.
Support for home care, including orienting family members to the scope and details of family caregiving, providing clear direction about how to contact professional caregivers, and informing patients and families of the benefits of hospice care.
Empathy for family emotions and relationships, including recognizing and validating common positive and negative feelings.
Attention to grief and bereavement, including support for anticipatory grief and follow-up with the family after the patient's death.

Data from Rabow MW et al. Supporting family caregivers at the end of life: "they don't know what they don't know." JAMA. 2004 Jan 28;291(4):483–91.

be simplistic, hope for relief of pain, for reconciliation with loved ones, for discovery of meaning, and for spiritual transformation is realistic at the end of life. With such questions as "What is still possible now for you?" "When you look to the future, what do you hope for?" "What good might come of this?" clinicians can help patients uncover hope, explore meaningful and realistic goals, and develop strategies to realize them.

Finally, dying patients' feelings of isolation and fear demand that clinicians assert that they will care for the patient throughout the final stage of life. The promise of nonabandonment is perhaps the central principle of end-of-life care and is a clinician's pledge to an individual patient to serve as a caring partner, a resource for creative problem-solving and relief of suffering, a guide during uncertain times, and a witness to the patient's experiences—no matter what happens. Clinicians can say to a patient, "I will care for you whatever happens." Dying patients need their clinicians to offer their presence—not necessarily the ability to solve all problems but rather a commitment to recognize and receive the patients' difficulties and experiences with respect and empathy. At its best, the patient-clinician relationship can be a covenant of compassion and a recognition of common humanity.

▶ Caring for the Family

In caring for patients at the end of life, clinicians must appreciate the central role played by family, friends, and partners and often must deal with strong emotions of fear, anger, shame, sadness, and guilt experienced by those individuals. While significant others may support and comfort a patient at the end of life, the threatened loss of a loved one may also create or reveal dysfunctional or painful family dynamics. Furthermore, clinicians must be attuned to the potential impact of illness on the patient's family: substantial physical caregiving responsibilities and financial burdens as well as increased rates of anxiety, depression, chronic illness, and even mortality. Family caregivers, typically women, commonly provide the bulk of care for patients at the end of life, yet their work is often not acknowledged or compensated.

Clinicians can help families confront the imminent loss of a loved one (Table 5–6) and often must negotiate amid complex and changing family needs. Identifying a spokesperson for the family, conducting family meetings, allowing all to be heard, and providing time for consensus may

help the clinician work effectively with the family. Providing good palliative care to the patient can reduce the risk of depression and complicated grief in loved ones after the patient's death.

▶ Clinician Self-Care

Many clinicians find caring for patients at the end of life to be one of the most rewarding aspects of practice. However, working with the dying requires tolerance of uncertainty, ambiguity, and existential challenges. Clinicians must recognize and respect their own limitations and attend to their own needs in order to avoid being overburdened, overly distressed, or emotionally depleted.

Candy B et al. Interventions for supporting informal caregivers of patients in the terminal phase of a disease. Cochrane Database Syst Rev. 2011 Jun 15;(6):CD007617. [PMID: 21678368]

El-Jawahri A et al. Associations among prognostic understanding, quality of life, and mood in patients with advanced cancer. Cancer. 2014 Jan 15;120(2):278–85. [PMID: 24122784]

Hudson PL et al. A systematic review of psychosocial interventions for family carers of palliative care patients. BMC Palliat Care. 2010 Aug 5;9:17. [PMID: 20687960]

Kearney MK et al. Self-care of physicians caring for patients at the end of life: "Being connected. . . a key to my survival". JAMA. 2009 Mar 18;301(11):1155–64. [PMID: 19293416]

Lennes IT et al. Predictors of newly diagnosed cancer patients' understanding of the goals of their care at initiation of chemotherapy. Cancer. 2013 Feb 1;119(3):691–9. [PMID: 23011902]

Moon JR et al. Short- and long-term associations between widowhood and mortality in the United States: longitudinal analyses. J Public Health (Oxf). 2013 Oct 28. [Epub ahead of print.] [PMID: 24167198]

Pantilat SZ. Communicating with seriously ill patients: better words to say. JAMA. 2009 Mar 25;301(12):1279–81. [PMID: 19318656]

Sinclair S. Impact of death and dying on the personal lives and practices of palliative and hospice care professionals. CMAJ. 2011 Feb 8;183(2):180–7. [PMID: 21135081]

Weeks JC et al. Patients' expectations about effects of chemotherapy for advanced cancer. N Engl J Med. 2012 Oct 25;367(17):1616–25. [PMID: 23094723]

▶ Decision-Making, Advance Care Planning, & Advance Directives

Patients deserve to have their health care be consistent with their preferences and goals of care. Well-informed, competent adults have a right to refuse medical intervention even if this is likely to result in death. Many are willing to sacrifice some quantity of life to protect a certain quality of life. In order to promote patient autonomy, clinicians are obligated to inform patients about the risks, benefits, alternatives, and expected outcomes of medical interventions such as cardiopulmonary resuscitation (CPR), mechanical ventilation, hospitalization and ICU care, and artificial nutrition and hydration. **Advance directives** are oral or written statements made by patients when they are competent that are intended to guide care should they become incompetent. Advance directives allow patients to project their autonomy into the future and are an important part of **advance care planning**—a process whereby clinicians help patients match treatments and care to their goals and values. Advance directives take effect when the patient can no longer communicate his or her preferences directly. While oral statements about these matters are ethically binding, they are not legally binding in all states. State-specific advance directive forms are available from a number of sources, including http://www.caringinfo.org.

Clinicians should facilitate the process for all patients—ideally, well before the end of life—to consider their preferences, to appoint a surrogate and talk to that person about their preferences, and to formulate an advance directive. Most patients with a serious illness have already thought about end-of-life issues, want to discuss them with their clinician, want the clinician to bring up the subject, and feel better for having had the discussion. Patients who have such discussions with their clinicians are perceived by their family as having a better quality of life at the end of life, are less likely to die in the hospital, and more likely to utilize hospice care. With advance care planning discussions, patients' loved ones are less likely to suffer from depression during bereavement.

One type of advance directive is the **Durable Power of Attorney for Health Care (DPOA-HC)** that, in addition to documenting patient preferences for care, allows the patient to designate a surrogate decision-maker. The DPOA-HC is particularly useful because it is often difficult to anticipate what decisions will need to be made. The responsibility of the surrogate is to provide "substituted judgment"—to decide as the *patient* would, not as the *surrogate* wants. Clinicians should encourage patients to talk with their surrogates about their preferences generally and about scenarios that are likely to arise, such as the need for mechanical ventilation in a patient with end-stage emphysema. Clear clinician communication is important to correct misunderstandings and address biases. In the absence of a designated surrogate, clinicians usually turn to family members or next of kin. Despite regulations requiring health care institutions to inform patients of their rights to formulate an advance directive, only a minority of people in the United States (including clinicians themselves as well as patients with advanced illness) have completed them. **POLST (Physician Orders for Life-Sustaining Treatment)** forms are physician orders that accompany patients wherever they are cared for—home, hospital, or nursing home—and are an increasingly widely used complement to advance directives for patients at the end of life.

▶ Do Not Attempt Resuscitation Orders

As part of advance care planning, clinicians can elicit patient preferences about CPR. Most patients and many clinicians overestimate the chances of success of CPR. Only about 15% of all patients who undergo CPR in the hospital survive to hospital discharge. Moreover, among certain populations—especially those with multisystem organ failure, metastatic cancer, and sepsis—the likelihood of survival to hospital discharge following CPR is virtually nil. Patients may ask their clinician to write an order that CPR not be attempted on them.

For some patients at the end of life, decisions about CPR may not be about *whether* they will live but about *how* they will die. Clinicians should correct the misconception that withholding CPR in appropriate circumstances is tantamount to "not doing everything" or "just letting someone die." While respecting the patient's right ultimately to make the decision—and keeping in mind their own biases and prejudices—clinicians should offer explicit recommendations about DNAR orders and protect dying patients and their families from feelings of guilt and from the sorrow associated with vain hopes. Clinicians should discuss what interventions will be continued and started to promote quality of life rather than focusing only on what is not to be done. For patients with implantable cardioverter defibrillators (ICDs), clinicians must also address issues of turning off these devices as death approaches to prevent them from discharging during the dying process.

▶ Hospice & Other Palliative Care Institutions

In the United States, hospice is a specific type of palliative care service focused on comprehensively addressing the needs of the dying. In the United States, 45% of people who die use hospice with about 66% of hospice patients die at home where they can be cared for by their family and visiting hospice staff. Hospice care can also be provided in hospitals and institutional residences. As is true of all types of palliative care, hospice emphasizes individualized attention, human contact, and an interdisciplinary team approach. Hospice care can include arranging for respite for family caregivers and assisting with referrals for legal, financial, and other services. Patients in hospice require a physician who is responsible for their care. Primary care clinicians are strongly encouraged to fulfill this role.

Hospice care is highly rated by families and has been shown to increase patient satisfaction, to reduce costs (depending on when patients are referred to hospice care), and to decrease family caregiver mortality. Despite evidence that suggests that hospice care does not increase mortality and may even extend life, hospice care tends to be used very near the end of life. The average length of stay in hospices in the United States is 69 days, with 36% of patients dying within 7 of beginning hospice care.

In the United States, most hospice organizations require clinicians to estimate the patient's probability of survival to be < 6 months, since this is a criterion for eligibility to receive Medicare or other insurance coverage. Regrettably, the hospice benefit can be difficult to provide to people who are homeless or isolated or who have terminal prognoses that are difficult to quantify.

► Cultural Issues

The individual patient's experience of dying occurs in the context of a complex interaction of personal, philosophic, and cultural influences. Various religious, ethnic, gender, class, and cultural traditions help determine patients' styles of communication, comfort in discussing particular topics, expectations about dying and medical interventions, and attitudes about the appropriate disposition of dead bodies. While each patient is an individual, being sensitive to a person's cultural beliefs and respecting ethnic traditions are important responsibilities of the clinician caring for a patient at the end of life, especially when the cultures of origin of the clinician and patient differ. A clinician may ask a patient, "What do I need to know about you and your beliefs that will help me take care of you?"

Bischoff KE et al. Advance care planning and the quality of end-of-life care in older adults. J Am Geriatr Soc. 2013 Feb;61(2):209–14. [PMID: 23350921]
Wendler D et al. Systematic review: the effect on surrogates of making treatment decisions for others. Ann Intern Med. 2011 Mar 1;154(5):336–46. [PMID: 21357911]
Zier LS et al. Surrogate decision makers' interpretation of prognostic information: a mixed-methods study. Ann Intern Med. 2012 Mar 6;156(5):360–6. [PMID: 22393131]

► Nutrition & Hydration

People approaching the end of life often lose their appetite and most ultimately stop eating and drinking. The anorexia-cachexia syndrome frequently occurs in patients with advanced cancer, and cachexia is a common and poor prognostic sign in patients with heart failure. Ill people often have no hunger with total caloric deprivation, and the associated ketonemia produces a sense of well-being, analgesia, and mild euphoria. Although it is unclear to what extent withholding hydration at the end of life creates an uncomfortable sensation of thirst, any such sensation is usually relieved by simply moistening the dry mouth. Ice chips, hard candy, swabs, popsicles, or minted mouthwash may be effective. Although this normal process of diminishing oral intake and accompanying weight loss is very common, it can be distressing to patients and families who may associate the offering of food with compassion and love and lack of eating with distressing images of

starvation. In response, patients and families often ask about supplemental enteral or parenteral nutrition.

Unfortunately supplemental, artificial nutrition and hydration offers little benefit to those at the end of life and rarely achieves patient and family goals. For example, although tube feedings are often considered in patients with advanced dementia who aspirate, they do not prevent aspiration pneumonia and there is debate about whether artificial nutrition prolongs life in the terminally ill. Furthermore, force feeding may cause nausea and vomiting in ill patients, and eating can lead to diarrhea in the setting of malabsorption. Artificial nutrition and hydration may increase oral and airway secretions as well as increase the risk of choking, aspiration, and dyspnea; ascites, edema, and effusions may be worsened. Nasogastric and gastrostomy tube feeding and parenteral nutrition impose risks of infection, epistaxis, pneumothorax, electrolyte imbalance, and aspiration—as well as the need to physically restrain the delirious patient to prevent dislodgment of catheters and tubes.

Individuals at the end of life have a right to refuse all nutrition and hydration. Because they may have deep social and cultural significance for patients, families, and clinicians themselves, decisions about artificial nutrition and hydration are not simply medical. Eliciting perceived goals of artificial nutrition and hydration and correcting misperceptions can help patients and families make clear decisions. Family and friends can be encouraged to express their love and caring in ways other than intrusive attempts at force feeding or hydration.

► Withdrawal of Curative Efforts

Requests from appropriately informed and competent patients or their surrogates for withdrawal of life-sustaining interventions must be respected. Limitation of life sustaining interventions prior to death is an increasingly common practice in intensive care units. The withdrawal of life-sustaining interventions such as mechanical ventilation must be approached carefully to avoid needless patient suffering and distress for those in attendance. Clinicians should educate the patient and family about the expected course of events and the difficulty of determining the precise timing of death after withdrawal of interventions. Sedative and analgesic agents should be administered to ensure patient comfort even at the risk of respiratory depression or hypotension. Scopolamine (10 mcg/h subcutaneously or intravenously, or a 1.5-mg patch every 3 days), glycopyrrolate (1 mg orally every 4 hours), or atropine (1% ophthalmic solution, 1 or 2 drops sublingually as often as every hour) can be used for controlling airway secretions and the resultant "death rattle." A guideline for withdrawal of mechanical ventilation is provided in Table 5–7.

► Psychological, Social, & Spiritual Issues

Dying is not exclusively or even primarily a biomedical event. It is an intimate personal experience with profound psychological, interpersonal, and existential meanings. For many people at the end of life, the prospect of impending death stimulates a deep and urgent assessment of their

Table 5–7. Guidelines for withdrawal of mechanical ventilation.

1. Stop neuromuscular blocking agents.
2. Administer opioids or sedatives to eliminate distress. If not already sedated, begin with fentanyl 100 mcg (or morphine sulfate 10 mg). Provide repeated boluses as needed during the process of withdrawing mechanical ventilation. Patients who require repeated boluses may benefit from a continuous infusion of fentanyl 100 mcg/h intravenously (or morphine sulfate 10 mg/h intravenously). Distress is indicated by RR > 24, nasal flaring, use of accessory muscles of respiration, HR increase > 20%, MAP increase > 20%, grimacing, clutching.
3. Discontinue vasoactive agents and other agents unrelated to patient comfort, such as antibiotics, intravenous fluids, and diagnostic procedures.
4. Decrease Flo_2 to room air and PEEP to 0 cm H_2O.
5. Observe patient for distress. If patient is distressed, increase opioids by repeating bolus dose and increasing hourly infusion rate by 50 mcg fentanyl (or 5 mg morphine sulfate),[1] then return to observation. If patient is not distressed, place on T piece and observe. If patient continues without distress, extubate patient and continue to observe for distress.

[1]Ventilatory support may be increased until additional opioids have effect.
RR, respiratory rate; HR, heart rate; MAP, mean airway pressure; Flo_2, fraction of inspired oxygen; PEEP, positive end-expiratory pressure.
Adapted, with permission, from San Francisco General Hospital Guidelines for Withdrawal of Mechanical Ventilation/Life Support.

identity, the quality of their relationships, and the meaning and purpose of their existence.

A. Psychological Challenges

In 1969, Elisabeth Kübler-Ross identified five psychological stages or patterns of emotions that patients at the end of life may experience: denial and isolation, anger, bargaining, depression, and acceptance. Not every patient will experience all these emotions, and typically not in an orderly progression. In addition to these five stages are the perpetual challenges of anxiety and fear of the unknown. Simple information, listening, assurance, and support may help patients with these psychological challenges. In fact, patients and families rank emotional support as one of the most important aspects of good end-of-life care. Psychotherapy and group support may be beneficial as well.

Despite the significant emotional stress of facing death, clinical depression is not normal at the end of life and should be treated. Cognitive and affective signs of depression (such as hopelessness or helplessness) may help distinguish depression from the low energy and other vegetative signs common with end-stage illness. Although traditional antidepressant treatments such as selective serotonin reuptake inhibitors are effective, more rapidly acting medications such as dextroamphetamine or methylphenidate (in doses used for sedation described earlier in this chapter) may be particularly useful when the end of life is near or while waiting for other antidepressant medication to take effect. Oral ketamine is emerging as a promising, rapid-onset treatment for anxiety and depression at the end of

Table 5–8. Five statements often necessary for the completion of important interpersonal relationships.

(1) "Forgive me."	(An expression of regret)
(2) "I forgive you."	(An expression of acceptance)
(3) "Thank you."	(An expression of gratitude)
(4) "I love you."	(An expression of affection)
(5) "Goodbye."	(Leave-taking)

Reprinted, with permission, from Byock I. *Dying Well: Peace and Possibilities at the End of Life.* New York: Riverhead Books, 1997.

life. Some research suggests a mortality benefit from treating depression in the setting of serious illness.

B. Social Challenges

At the end of life, patients should be encouraged to discharge personal, professional, and business obligations. This might include completing important work or personal projects, distributing possessions, writing a will, and making funeral and burial arrangements. The prospect of death often prompts patients to examine the quality of their interpersonal relationships and to begin the process of saying goodbye (Table 5–8). Dying may intensify a patient's need to feel cared for by the clinician and the need for clinician empathy and compassion. Concern about estranged relationships or "unfinished business" with significant others and interest in reconciliation may become paramount at this time.

C. Spiritual Challenges

Spirituality is the attempt to understand or accept the underlying meaning of life, one's relationships to oneself and other people, one's place in the universe, one's legacy, and the possibility of a "higher power" in the universe. Spirituality is distinguished from particular religious practices or beliefs and is generally considered a universal human concern.

Unlike physical ailments such as infections and fractures, which usually require a clinician's intervention to be treated, the patient's spiritual concerns often require only a clinician's attention, listening, and witness. Clinicians might choose to inquire about the patient's spiritual concerns and ask whether the patient wishes to discuss them. For example, asking, "How are you within yourself?" or "Are you at peace?" communicates that the clinician is interested in the patient's whole experience and provides an opportunity for the patient to share perceptions about his or her inner life. Questions that might constitute an existential "review of systems" are presented in Table 5–9. Formal legacy work and dignity therapy have been shown to be effective in improving quality of life and spiritual well-being. Patients should be supported by clinicians, but engagement with religious communities and professional chaplains as part of comprehensive care are key.

While dying may be a period of inevitable loss of physical functioning, the end of life also offers an opportunity for psychological, interpersonal, and spiritual development. Individuals may grow—even achieve a heightened

Table 5–9. An existential review of systems.

Intrapersonal
What does your illness/dying mean to you?
What do you think caused your illness?
How have you been healed in the past?
What do you think is needed for you to be healed now?
What is right with you now?
What do you hope for?
Are you at peace?
Interpersonal
Who is important to you?
To whom does your illness/dying matter?
Do you have any unfinished business with significant others?
Transpersonal
What is your source of strength, help, or hope?
Do you have spiritual concerns or a spiritual practice?
If so, how does your spirituality relate to your illness/dying, and how can I help integrate your spirituality into your health care?
What do you think happens after we die?
What purpose might your illness/dying serve?
What do you think is trying to happen here?

sense of well-being or transcendence—in the process of dying. Through listening, support, and presence, clinicians may help foster this learning and be a catalyst for this transformation. Rather than thinking of dying simply as the termination of life, clinicians and patients may be guided by a developmental model of dying that recognizes a series of lifelong developmental tasks and landmarks and allows for growth at the end of life.

Balboni TA et al. Provision of spiritual support to patients with advanced cancer by religious communities and associations with medical care at the end of life. JAMA Intern Med. 2013 Jun 24;173(12):1109–17. [PMID: 23649656]

Chochinov HM et al. Effect of dignity therapy on distress and end-of-life experience in terminally ill patients: a randomised controlled trial. Lancet Oncol. 2011 Aug;12(8):753–62. [PMID: 21741309]

Rayner L et al. Antidepressants for the treatment of depression in palliative care: systematic review and meta-analysis. Palliat Med. 2011 Jan;25(1):36–51. [PMID: 20935027]

TASKS AFTER DEATH

After the death of a hospitalized patient, the clinician is called upon to perform a number of tasks, both required and recommended. The clinician must plainly and directly inform the family of the death, complete a death certificate, contact an organ procurement organization, and request an autopsy. Providing words of sympathy and reassurance, time for questions and initial grief, and a quiet private room for the family is appropriate and much appreciated.

▶ The Pronouncement & Death Certificate

In the United States, state policies direct clinicians to confirm the death of a patient in a formal process called "pronouncement." The diagnosis of death is typically easy to make and the clinician need only verify the absence of spontaneous respirations and cardiac activity. Attempting to elicit pain in a patient who has died is unnecessary and disrespectful and should be avoided. A note describing these findings and the time of death is entered in the patient's medical record. In many states, when a patient whose death is expected dies outside of the hospital (at home or in prisons, for example) nurses may be authorized to report the death over the telephone to a physician who assumes responsibility for signing the death certificate within 24 hours. For traumatic deaths, some states allow emergency medical technicians to pronounce a patient dead at the scene based on clearly defined criteria and with physician telephonic or radio supervision.

While the pronouncement may often seem like an awkward and unnecessary formality, clinicians may use this time to reassure the patient's loved ones at the bedside that the patient died peacefully and that all appropriate care had been given. Both clinicians and families may use the ritual of the pronouncement as an opportunity to begin to process emotionally the death of the patient.

Physicians are legally required to accurately report the underlying cause of death on the death certificate. This reporting is important both for patients' families (for insurance purposes and the need for an accurate family medical history) and for the epidemiologic study of disease and public health. The physician should be specific about the major cause of death being the condition without which the patient would not have died (eg, "decompensated cirrhosis") and its contributory cause (eg, "hepatitis B and hepatitis C infections and chronic alcoholic hepatitis") as well as any associated conditions (eg, "acute kidney injury")—and not simply put down "cardiac arrest" as the cause of death.

▶ Autopsy & Organ Donation

Discussing the options and obtaining consent for autopsy and organ donation with patients prior to death is usually the best practice. This approach advances the principle of patient autonomy and lessens the responsibilities of distressed family members during the period immediately following the death. However, after a patient dies, or in the case of brain death, designated organ transplant personnel are more successful than the treating clinicians at obtaining consent for organ donation from surviving family members. Federal regulations require that a designated representative of an organ procurement organization approach the family about organ donation if the organs are appropriate for transplantation. Most people in the United States support the donation of organs for transplants. Currently, however, organ transplantation is severely limited by the availability of donor organs. Many potential donors and the families of actual donors experience a sense of reward in contributing, even through death, to the lives of others.

Clinicians must be sensitive to ethnic and cultural differences in attitudes about autopsy and organ donation. Patients or their families should be reminded of their right to limit autopsy or organ donation in any way they choose, although such restriction may limit the utility of autopsy. Pathologists can perform autopsies without interfering with funeral plans or the appearance of the deceased.

The results of an autopsy may help surviving family members and clinicians understand the exact cause of a patient's death and foster a sense of closure. A clinician-family conference to review the results of the autopsy provides a good opportunity for clinicians to assess how well families are grieving and to answer questions. Despite the advantages of conducting postmortem examinations, autopsy rates are approximately 5%. Families report refusing autopsies out of fear of disfigurement of the body or delay of the funeral or say they were simply not asked. They allow autopsies in order to advance medical knowledge, to identify the exact cause of their loved one's death, and to be reassured that appropriate care was given. Routinely addressing these issues when discussing autopsy may help increase the autopsy rate; the most important mistake is the failure to ask for permission to perform it.

Follow-up & Grieving

Proper care of patients at the end of life includes following up with surviving family members after the patient has died. Following up by telephone enables the clinician to assuage any guilt about decisions the family may have made, assess how families are grieving, reassure them about the nature of normal grieving, and identify complicated grief or depression. Clinicians can recommend support groups and counseling as needed. A card or telephone call from the clinician to the family days to weeks after the patient's death (and perhaps on the anniversary of the death) allows the clinician to express concern for the family and the deceased.

After a patient dies, the clinician too may need to grieve. Although clinicians may be relatively unaffected by the deaths of some patients, other deaths may cause feelings of sadness, loss, and guilt. These emotions should be recognized as the first step toward processing and healing them. Each clinician may find personal or communal resources that help with the process of grieving. Shedding tears, the support of colleagues, time for reflection, and traditional or personal mourning rituals all may be effective. Attending the funeral of a patient who has died can be a satisfying personal experience that is almost universally appreciated by families and that may be the final element in caring well for people at the end of life.

Chau NG et al. Bereavement practices of physicians in oncology and palliative care. Arch Intern Med. 2009 May 25;169(10):963–71. [PMID: 19468090]

Simon NM. Treating complicated grief. JAMA. 2013 Jul 24;310(4):416–23. [PMID: 23917292]

Thornton JD et al. Effect of an iPod video intervention on consent to donate organs: a randomized trial. Ann Intern Med. 2012 Apr 3;156(7):483–90. [PMID: 22473435]

Dermatologic Disorders

Timothy G. Berger, MD

Dermatologic diseases are diagnosed by the types of lesions they cause. To make a diagnosis: (1) identify the type of lesion(s) the patient exhibits by morphology establishing a differential diagnosis (Table 6–1); and (2) obtain the elements of the history, physical examination, and appropriate laboratory tests to confirm the diagnosis. Unique clinical situations, such as the ill ICU patient, lead to different diagnostic considerations.

PRINCIPLES OF DERMATOLOGIC THERAPY

▶ Frequently Used Treatment Measures

A. Bathing

Soap should be used only in the axillae and groin and on the feet by persons with dry or inflamed skin. Soaking in water for 10–15 minutes before applying topical corticosteroids enhances their efficacy (Soak and Smear). Bath oils can be used, but add little above the use of moisturizers, and may make the tub slippery, increasing the risk of falling.

B. Topical Therapy

Nondermatologists should become familiar with a representative agent in each category for each indication (eg, topical corticosteroid, topical retinoid, etc).

1. Corticosteroids—Topical corticosteroid creams, lotions, ointments, gels, foams, and sprays are presented in Table 6–2 Topical corticosteroids are divided into classes based on potency. There is little (except price) to recommend one agent over another within the same class. For a given agent, an ointment is more potent than a cream. The potency of a topical corticosteroid may be dramatically increased by occlusion (covering with a water impermeable barrier) for at least 4 hours. Depending on the location of the skin condition, gloves, plastic wrap, moist pajamas covered by dry pajamas (wet wraps) or plastic occlusive suits for patients can be used. Caution should be used in applying topical corticosteroids to areas of thin skin (face, scrotum, vulva, skin folds). Topical corticosteroid use on the eyelids may result in glaucoma or cataracts. One may estimate the amount of topical corticosteroid needed by using the "rule of

nines" (as in burn evaluation; see Figure 37–2). In general, it takes an average of 20–30 g to cover the body surface of an adult once. Systemic absorption does occur, but adrenal suppression, diabetes mellitus, hypertension, osteoporosis, and other complications of systemic corticosteroids are very rare with topical corticosteroid therapy.

2. Emollients for dry skin ("moisturizers")—Dry skin is not related to water intake but to abnormal function of the epidermis. Many types of emollients are available. Petrolatum, mineral oil, Aquaphor, Vanicream, and Eucerin cream are the heaviest and best. Emollients are most effective when applied to wet skin. If the skin is too greasy after application, pat dry with a damp towel. Vanicream is relatively allergen-free and can be used if allergic contact dermatitis to topical products is suspected.

The scaly appearance of dry skin may be improved by urea, lactic acid, or glycolic acid-containing products provided no inflammation (erythema or pruritus) is present.

3. Drying agents for weepy dermatoses—If the skin is weepy from infection or inflammation, drying agents may be beneficial. The best drying agent is water, applied as repeated compresses for 15–30 minutes, alone or with aluminum salts (Burow solution, Domeboro tablets).

4. Topical antipruritics—Lotions that contain 0.5% each of camphor and menthol (Sarna) or pramoxine hydrochloride 1% (with or without 0.5% menthol, eg, Prax, PrameGel, Aveeno Anti-Itch lotion) are effective antipruritic agents. Hydrocortisone, 1% or 2.5%, may be incorporated for its anti-inflammatory effect (Pramosone cream, lotion, or ointment). Doxepin cream 5% may reduce pruritus but may cause drowsiness. Pramoxine and doxepin are most effective when applied with topical corticosteroids. Topical capsaicin can be effective in some forms of neuropathic itch. Ice in a plastic bag covered by a thin cloth applied to itchy spots can be effective.

C. Systemic Antipruritic Drugs

1. Antihistamines—H_1-blockers are the agents of choice for pruritus when due to histamine, such as in urticaria. Otherwise, they appear to benefit itchy patients only by their sedating effects. Hydroxyzine 25–50 mg nightly is a

Table 6–1. Morphologic categorization of skin lesions and diseases.

Pigmented	Freckle, lentigo, seborrheic keratosis, nevus, blue nevus, halo nevus, atypical nevus, melanoma
Scaly	Psoriasis, dermatitis (atopic, stasis, seborrheic, chronic allergic contact or irritant contact), xerosis (dry skin), lichen simplex chronicus, tinea, tinea versicolor, secondary syphilis, pityriasis rosea, discoid lupus erythematosus, exfoliative dermatitis, actinic keratoses, Bowen disease, Paget disease, intertrigo
Vesicular	Herpes simplex, varicella, herpes zoster, pompholyx (vesicular dermatitis of palms and soles), vesicular tinea, dermatophytid, dermatitis herpetiformis, miliaria crystallina, scabies, photosensitivity
Weepy or encrusted	Impetigo, acute contact allergic dermatitis, any vesicular dermatitis
Pustular	Acne vulgaris, acne rosacea, folliculitis, candidiasis, miliaria pustulosa, any vesicular dermatitis
Figurate ("shaped") erythema	Urticaria, erythema multiforme, erythema migrans, cellulitis, erysipelas, erysipeloid, arthropod bites
Bullous	Impetigo, blistering dactylitis, pemphigus, pemphigoid, porphyria cutanea tarda, drug eruptions, erythema multiforme, toxic epidermal necrolysis
Papular	Hyperkeratotic: warts, corns, seborrheic keratoses Purple-violet: lichen planus, drug eruptions, Kaposi sarcoma Flesh-colored, umbilicated: molluscum contagiosum Pearly: basal cell carcinoma, intradermal nevi Small, red, inflammatory: acne, miliaria rubra, candidiasis, scabies, folliculitis
Pruritus[1]	Xerosis, scabies, pediculosis, bites, systemic causes, anogenital pruritus
Nodular, cystic	Erythema nodosum, furuncle, cystic acne, follicular (epidermal) inclusion cyst
Photodermatitis (photodistributed rashes)	Drug, polymorphic light eruption, lupus erythematosus
Morbilliform	Drug, viral infection, secondary syphilis
Erosive	Any vesicular dermatitis, impetigo, aphthae, lichen planus, erythema multiforme
Ulcerated	Decubiti, herpes simplex, skin cancers, parasitic infections, syphilis (chancre), chancroid, vasculitis, stasis, arterial disease

[1]Not a morphologic class but included because it is one of the most common dermatologic presentations.

Table 6–2. Useful topical dermatologic therapeutic agents.

Agent	Formulations, Strengths, and Prices[1]	Apply	Potency Class	Common Indications	Comments
Corticosteroids					
Hydrocortisone acetate	Cream 1%: $3.00/30 g Ointment 1%: $3.00/30 g Lotion 1%: $7.20/120 mL	Twice daily	Low	Seborrheic dermatitis Pruritus ani Intertrigo	Not the same as hydrocortisone butyrate or valerate Not for poison oak OTC lotion (Aquinil HC) OTC solution (Scalpicin, T Scalp)
	Cream 2.5%: $11.00/30 g	Twice daily	Low	As for 1% hydrocortisone	Perhaps better for pruritus ani Not clearly better than 1% More expensive Not OTC
Alclometasone dipropionate (Aclovate)	Cream 0.05%: $48.08/15 g Ointment 0.05%: $20.00/15 g	Twice daily	Low	As for hydrocortisone	More efficacious than hydrocortisone Perhaps causes less atrophy
Desonide	Cream 0.05%: $77.08/15 g Ointment 0.05%: $240.40/60 g Lotion 0.05%: $284.26/60 mL	Twice daily	Low	As for hydrocortisone For lesions on face or body folds resistant to hydrocortisone	More efficacious than hydrocortisone Can cause rosacea or atrophy Not fluorinated
Clocortolone (Cloderm)	Cream 0.1%: $238.87/30 g	Three times daily	Medium	Contact dermatitis Atopic dermatitis	Does not cross-react with other corticosteroids chemically and can be used in patients allergic to other corticosteroids

(continued)

Table 6–2. Useful topical dermatologic therapeutic agents. (continued)

Agent	Formulations, Strengths, and Prices[1]	Apply	Potency Class	Common Indications	Comments
Prednicarbate (Dermatop)	Emollient cream 0.1%: $126.19/60 g Ointment 0.1%: $30.00/15 g	Twice daily	Medium	As for triamcinolone	May cause less atrophy No generic formulations Preservative-free
Triamcinolone acetonide	Cream 0.1%: $5.58/15 g Ointment 0.1%: $5.58/15 g Lotion 0.1%: $42.44/60 mL	Twice daily	Medium	Eczema on extensor areas Used for psoriasis with tar Seborrheic dermatitis and psoriasis on scalp	Caution in body folds, face Economical in 0.5-lb and 1-lb sizes for treatment of large body surfaces Economical as solution for scalp
	Cream 0.025%: $6.12/15 g Ointment 0.025%: $10.11/80 g	Twice daily	Medium	As for 0.1% strength	Possibly less efficacy and few advantages over 0.1% formulation
Fluocinolone acetonide	Cream 0.025%: $33.77/15 g Ointment 0.025%: $33.77/15 g	Twice daily	Medium	As for triamcinolone	
	Solution 0.01%: $180.00/60 mL	Twice daily	Medium	As for triamcinolone solution	
Mometasone furoate (Elocon)	Cream 0.1%: $26.75/15 g Ointment 0.1%: $24.30/15 g Lotion 0.1%: $55.71/60 mL	Once daily	Medium	As for triamcinolone	Often used inappropriately on the face or on children Not fluorinated
Diflorasone diacetate	Cream 0.05%: $84.61/15 g Ointment 0.05%: $179.54/30 g	Twice daily	High	Nummular dermatitis Allergic contact dermatitis Lichen simplex chronicus	
Amcinonide (Cyclocort)	Cream 0.1%: $151.20/15 g Ointment 0.1%: $388.80/60 g	Twice daily	High	As for betamethasone	
Fluocinonide (Lidex)	Cream 0.05%: $15.95/15 g Gel 0.05%: $18.83/15 g Ointment 0.05%: $6.54/15 g Solution 0.05%: $97.19/60 mL	Twice daily	High	As for betamethasone Gel useful for poison oak	Economical generics Lidex cream can cause stinging on eczema Lidex emollient cream preferred
Betamethasone dipropionate (Diprolene)	Cream 0.05%: $41.60/15 g Ointment 0.05%: $43.22/15 g Lotion 0.05%: $45.00/60 mL	Twice daily	Ultra-high	For lesions resistant to high-potency corticosteroids Lichen planus Insect bites	Economical generics available
Clobetasol propionate (Temovate)	Cream 0.05%: $24.71/15 g Ointment 0.05%: $24.71/15 g Lotion 0.05%: $277.20/60 mL	Twice daily	Ultra-high	As for betamethasone dipropionate	Somewhat more potent than diflorasone Limited to 2 continuous weeks of use Limited to 50 g or less per week Cream may cause stinging; use "emollient cream" formulation Generic available
Halobetasol propionate (Ultravate)	Cream 0.05%: $31.49/15 g Ointment 0.05%: $31.49/15 g	Twice daily	Ultra-high	As for clobetasol	Same restrictions as clobetasol Cream does not cause stinging Compatible with calcipotriene (Dovonex)
Flurandrenolide (Cordran)	Tape: $459.47/80" × 3" roll Lotion 0.05%: $394.68/60 mL	Every 12 hours	Ultra-high	Lichen simplex chronicus	Protects the skin and prevents scratching

(continued)

Table 6–2. Useful topical dermatologic therapeutic agents. (continued)

Agent	Formulations, Strengths, and Prices[1]	Apply	Potency Class	Common Indications	Comments
Nonsteroidal anti-inflammatory agents					
Tacrolimus[2] (Protopic)	Ointment 0.1%: $254.87/30 g Ointment 0.03%: $254.87/30 g	Twice daily	N/A	Atopic dermatitis	Steroid substitute not causing atrophy or striae Burns in ≥ 40% of patients with eczema
Pimecrolimus[2] (Elidel)	Cream 1%: $214.46/30 g	Twice daily	N/A	Atopic dermatitis	Steroid substitute not causing atrophy or striae
Antibiotics (for acne)					
Clindamycin phosphate	Solution 1%: $39.18/30 mL Gel 1%: $68.99/30 mL Lotion 1%: $95.98/60 mL Pledget 1%: $46.40/60	Twice daily	N/A	Mild papular acne	Lotion is less drying for patients with sensitive skin
Erythromycin	Solution 2%: $47.63/60 mL Gel 2%: $31.35/30 g Pledget 2%: $94.55/60	Twice daily	N/A	As for clindamycin	Many different manufacturers Economical
Erythromycin/ Benzoyl peroxide (Benzamycin)	Gel: $58.35/23.3 g Gel: $111.64/46.6 g	Twice daily	N/A	As for clindamycin Can help treat comedonal acne	No generics More expensive More effective than other topical antibiotic Main jar requires refrigeration
Clindamycin/ Benzoyl peroxide (BenzaClin)	Gel: $134.52/25 g Gel: $269.03/50 g	Twice daily		As for benzamycin	No generic More effective than either agent alone
Antibiotics (for impetigo)					
Mupirocin (Bactroban)	Ointment 2%: $42.50/22 g Cream 2%: $75.82/15 g	Three times daily	N/A	Impetigo, folliculitis	Because of cost, use limited to tiny areas of impetigo Used in the nose twice daily for 5 days to reduce staphylococcal carriage
Antifungals: *Imidazoles*					
Clotrimazole	Cream 1%: $5.12/15 g OTC Solution 1%: $9.23/10 mL	Twice daily	N/A	Dermatophyte and Candida infections	Available OTC Inexpensive generic cream available
Econazole (Spectazole)	Cream 1%: $17.50/15 g	Once daily	N/A	As for clotrimazole	No generic Somewhat more effective than clotrimazole and miconazole
Ketoconazole	Cream 2%: $16.43/15 g	Once daily	N/A	As for clotrimazole	No generic Somewhat more effective than clotrimazole and miconazole
Miconazole	Cream 2%: $3.30/30 g OTC	Twice daily	N/A	As for clotrimazole	As for clotrimazole
Oxiconazole (Oxistat)	Cream 1%: $280.82/30 g Lotion 1%: $280.82/30 mL	Twice daily	N/A		
Sertaconazole (Ertaczo)	Cream 2%: $439.61/60 g	Twice daily	N/A	Refractory tinea pedis	By prescription More expensive
Sulconazole (Exelderm)	Cream 1%: $62.05/15 g Solution 1%: $163.76/30 mL	Twice daily	N/A	As for clotrimazole	No generic Somewhat more effective than clotrimazole and miconazole

(continued)

Table 6–2. Useful topical dermatologic therapeutic agents. (continued)

Agent	Formulations, Strengths, and Prices[1]	Apply	Potency Class	Common Indications	Comments
Other antifungals					
Butenafine (Mentax)	Cream 1%: $100.59/15 g	Once daily	N/A	Dermatophytes	Fast response; high cure rate; expensive Available OTC
Ciclopirox (Loprox) (Penlac)	Cream 0.77%: $51.10/30 g Lotion 0.77%: $96.15/60 mL Solution 8%: $25.00/6.6 mL	Twice daily	N/A	As for clotrimazole	No generic Somewhat more effective than clotrimazole and miconazole
Naftifine (Naftin)	Cream 1%: $331.37/60 g Gel 1%: $331.37/60 mL	Once daily	N/A	Dermatophytes	No generic Somewhat more effective than clotrimazole and miconazole
Terbinafine (Lamisil)	Cream 1%: $8.72/12 g OTC	Once daily	N/A	Dermatophytes	Fast clinical response OTC
Antipruritics					
Camphor/ menthol (Sarna)	Lotion 0.5%/0.5%: $7.80/222 mL	Two to three times daily	N/A	Mild eczema, xerosis, mild contact dermatitis	
Pramoxine hydrochloride (Prax)	Lotion 1%: $17.86/120 mL OTC	Four times daily	N/A	Dry skin, varicella, mild eczema, pruritus ani	OTC formulations (Prax, Aveeno Anti-Itch Cream or Lotion; Itch-X Gel) By prescription mixed with 1% or 2% hydrocortisone
Doxepin (Zonalon)	Cream 5%: $262.00/30 g	Four times daily	N/A	Topical antipruritic, best used in combination with appropriate topical corticosteroid to enhance efficacy	Can cause sedation
Emollients					
Aveeno	Cream, lotion, others	Once to three times daily	N/A	Xerosis, eczema	Choice is most often based on personal preference by patient
Aqua glycolic	Cream, lotion, shampoo, others	Once to three times daily	N/A	Xerosis, ichthyosis, keratosis pilaris Mild facial wrinkles Mild acne or seborrheic dermatitis	Contains 8% glycolic acid Available from other makers, eg, Alpha Hydrox, or generic 8% glycolic acid lotion May cause stinging on eczematous skin
Aquaphor	Ointment: $13.99/396 g	Once to three times daily	N/A	Xerosis, eczema For protection of area in pruritus ani	Not as greasy as petrolatum
Urea (various)	Cream 20%: $14.00/90 g Lotion 10%: $1400/240 mL	Twice daily	N/A	Xerosis	Contains urea as humectant Nongreasy hydrating agent (10%); debrides keratin (20%)
Complex 15	Lotion: $6.48/240 mL Cream: $4.82/75 g	Once to three times daily	N/A	Xerosis Lotion or cream recommended for split or dry nails	Active ingredient is a phospholipid
DML	Cream, lotion, facial moisturizer: $5.95/240 mL	Once to three times daily	N/A	As for Complex 15	Face cream has sunscreen
Eucerin	Cream: $7.37/240 g Lotion: $5.10/240 mL	Once to three times daily	N/A	Xerosis, eczema	Many formulations made Eucerin Plus contains alphahydroxy acid and may cause stinging on eczematous skin Facial moisturizer has SPF 25 sunscreen

(continued)

Table 6–2. Useful topical dermatologic therapeutic agents. (continued)

Agent	Formulations, Strengths, and Prices[1]	Apply	Potency Class	Common Indications	Comments
Lac-Hydrin-Five	Lotion: $11.37/226 g OTC	Twice daily	N/A	Xerosis, ichthyosis, keratosis pilaris	Prescription strength is 12%
Lubriderm	Lotion: $7.37/473 mL	Once to three times daily	N/A	Xerosis, eczema	Unscented usually preferred
Neutrogena	Cream, lotion, facial moisturizer: $7.15/240 mL	Once to three times daily	N/A	Xerosis, eczema	Face cream has titanium-based sunscreen
Ceratopic Cream	Cream: $60.00/6 oz	Twice daily	N/A	Xerosis, eczema	Contains ceramide; anti-inflammatory and nongreasy moisturizer
U-Lactin	Lotion: $12.00/240 mL OTC	Once daily	N/A	Hyperkeratotic heels	Moisturizes and removes keratin

[1]Average wholesale price (AWP, for AB-rated generic when available) for quantity listed. AWP may not accurately represent the actual pharmacy cost because wide contractual variations exist among institutions. Source: *Red Book Online, 2014, Truven Health Analytics, Inc.* Thomson Reuters (Healthcare) Inc.

[2]Topical tacrolimus and pimecrolimus should only be used when other topical treatments are ineffective. Treatment should be limited to an area and duration to be as brief as possible. Treatment with these agents should be avoided in persons with known immunosuppression, HIV infection, bone marrow and organ transplantation, lymphoma, at high risk for lymphoma, and those with a prior history of lymphoma. N/A, not applicable; OTC, over-the-counter.

typical dose. Sedating and nonsedating antihistamines are of limited value for the treatment of pruritus associated with inflammatory skin disease. Agents that may treat pruritus better include antidepressants (such as doxepin, mirtazapine, and paroxetine) as well as agents that may act either centrally or peripherally directly on the neurons that perceive or modulate pruritus (such as gabapentin, pregabalin, and duloxetine). Aprepitant and opioid antagonists such as naltrexone and butorphanol can be very effective in select patients, but their exact role in the management of the pruritic patient is not yet defined.

2. Systemic corticosteroids—(See Chapter 26.)

American Academy of Dermatology. Medical student core curriculum. http://www.aad.org/education-and-quality-care/medical-student-core-curriculum

Apfelbacher CJ et al. Oral H1 antihistamines as monotherapy for eczema. Cochrane Database Syst Rev. 2013 Feb28;2: CD00770. [PMID: 23450580]

Berger TG et al. Pruritus in the older patient: a clinical review. JAMA. 2013 Dec11;310(22): 2443–50. [PMID: 24327039]

Elmariah SB et al. Topical therapies for pruritus. Semin Cutan Med Surg. 2011 Jun;30(2):118–26. [PMID: 21767774]

Ständer S et al. Medical treatment of pruritus. Expert Opin Emerg Drugs. 2012 Sep;17(3):335–45. [PMID: 22870909]

Steinhoff M et al. Pruritus: management algorithms and experimental therapies. Semin Cutan Med Surg. 2011 Jun;30(2): 127–37. [PMID: 21767775]

▶ **Sunscreens**

Protection from ultraviolet light should begin at birth and will reduce the incidence of actinic keratoses, melanoma, and some nonmelanoma skin cancers when initiated at any age. The best protection is shade, but protective clothing,

avoidance of direct sun exposure during the peak hours of the day, and daily use of chemical sunscreens are important.

Fair-complexioned persons should use a sunscreen with an SPF (sun protective factor) of at least 15 and preferably 30–40 every day. Sunscreens with high SPF values (> 30) usually afford some protection against UVA as well as UVB and are helpful in managing photosensitivity disorders. The actual SPF achieved is about one-quarter or less than that listed on the product, since patients apply only one-quarter as much sunscreen per unit area when compared with the amount used in tests to determine the listed SPF. Repeated daily applications enhance sunscreen efficacy. Aggressive sunscreen use should be accompanied by vitamin D supplementation in persons at risk for osteopenia (eg, organ transplant recipients).

Bodekær M et al. Accumulation of sunscreen in human skin after daily applications: a study of sunscreens with different ultraviolet radiation filters. Photodermatol Photoimmunol Photomed. 2012 Jun;28(3):127–32. [PMID: 22548393]

Jou PC et al. UV protection and sunscreens: what to tell patients. Cleve Clin J Med. 2012 Jun;79(6):427–36. [PMID: 22660875]

Liu W et al. Sunburn protection as a function of sunscreen application thickness differs between high and low SPFs. Photodermatol Photoimmunol Photomed. 2012 Jun;28(3):120–6. [PMID: 22548392]

Mar V et al. Nodular melanoma: a distinct clinical entity and the largest contributor to melanoma deaths in Victoria, Australia. J Am Acad Dermatol. 2013 Apr;68(4):568–75. [PMID: 23182058]

Ou-Yang H et al. High-SPF sunscreens (SPF≥70) may provide ultraviolet protection above minimal recommended levels by adequately compensating for lower sunscreen user application amounts. J Am Acad Dermatol. 2012 Dec;67(6):1220–7. [PMID: 22463921]

Petersen B et al. Sunscreen use and failures—on site observations on a sun-holiday. Photochem Photobiol Sci. 2012 Dec13;12(1):190–6. [PMID: 23023728]

Robinson JK et al. Prevention of melanoma with regular sunscreen use. JAMA. 2011 Jul20;306(3):302–3. [PMID: 21712528]

Complications of Topical Dermatologic Therapy

Complications of topical therapy can be largely avoided. They fall into several categories: allergy, irritation, and overuse.

A. Allergy

Of the topical antibiotics, neomycin and bacitracin have the greatest potential for sensitization. Diphenhydramine, benzocaine, vitamin E, aromatic essential oils, bee pollen, preservatives, fragrances, and even the topical corticosteroids themselves can cause allergic contact dermatitis.

B. Irritation

Preparations of tretinoin, benzoyl peroxide, and other acne medications should be applied sparingly to the skin.

C. Overuse

Topical corticosteroids may induce acne-like lesions on the face (steroid rosacea) and atrophic striae in body folds.

▼ COMMON DERMATOSES

PIGMENTED LESIONS

MELANOCYTIC NEVI (NORMAL MOLES)

In general, a **benign mole** is a small (< 6 mm) lesion with a well-defined border and a single shade of pigment from beige or pink to dark brown. The physical examination must take precedence over the history.

Moles have a normal natural history. In the patient's first decade of life, moles often appear as flat, small, brown lesions. They are called junctional nevi because the nevus cells are at the junction of the epidermis and dermis. Over the next two decades, these moles grow in size and often become raised, reflecting the appearance of a dermal component, giving rise to compound nevi (Figure 6–1). Moles may darken and grow during pregnancy. As white patients enter their seventh and eighth decades, most moles have lost their junctional component and dark pigmentation. At every stage of life, normal moles should be well-demarcated, symmetric, and uniform in contour and color.

Boulos S et al. Free skin cancer screening provides access to care. J Am Acad Dermatol. 2012 Oct;67(4):787–8. [PMID: 22980248]

McWhirter JE et al. Visual images for patient skin self-examination and melanoma detection: a systematic review of published studies. J Am Acad Dermatol. 2013 Jul;69(1):47–55. [PMID: 23474227]

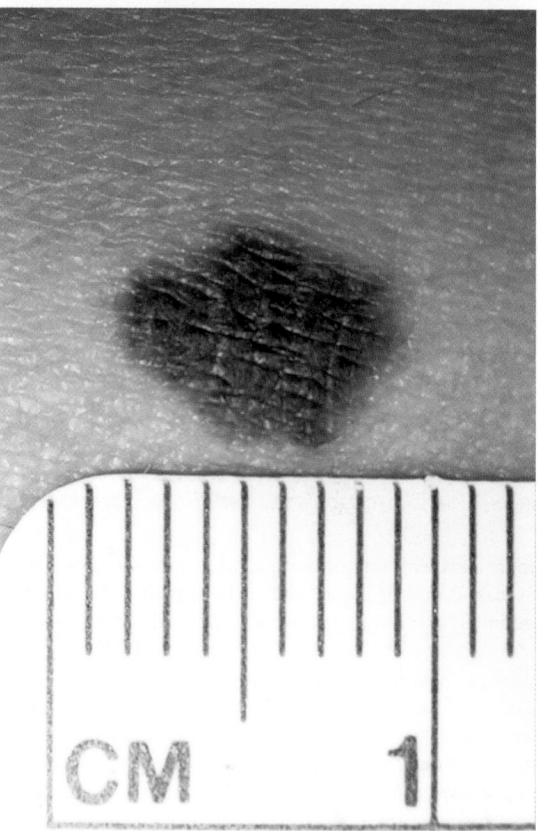

▲ **Figure 6–1.** Benign, flat and macular compound nevus on the arm. (Courtesy of Richard P. Usatine, MD; used, with permission, from Usatine RP, Smith MA, Mayeaux EJ Jr, Chumley H, Tysinger J. *The Color Atlas of Family Medicine*. McGraw-Hill, 2009.)

U.S. Preventive Services Task Force. Screening for skin cancer: U.S. Preventive Services Task Force recommendation statement. Ann Intern Med. 2009 Feb3;150(3):188–93. [PMID: 19189908]

Walter FM et al. Effect of adding a diagnostic aid to best practice to manage suspicious pigmented lesions in primary care: randomised controlled trial. BMJ. 2012 Jul4; 345:e4110. [PMID: 22763392]

ATYPICAL NEVI

The term "atypical nevus" or "atypical mole" has supplanted "dysplastic nevus." The diagnosis of atypical moles is made clinically and not histologically, and moles should be removed only if they are suspected to be melanomas. Clinically, these moles are large (≥ 6 mm in diameter), with an ill-defined, irregular border and irregularly distributed pigmentation (Figure 6–2). It is estimated that 5–10% of the white population in the United States has one or more atypical nevi, and recreational sun exposure is a primary risk for the development of atypical nevi in nonfamilial settings. Studies have defined an increased risk of melanoma in the following populations: patients with 50 or

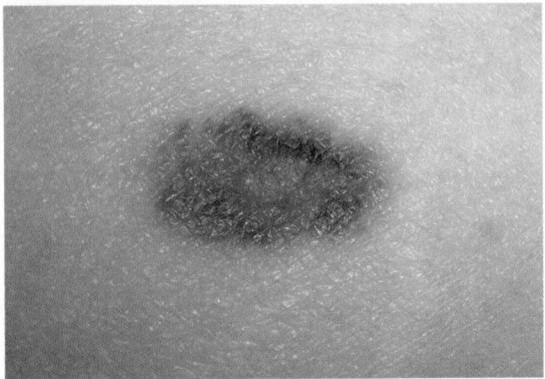

▲ **Figure 6–2.** Atypical (dysplastic) nevus on the chest. (Courtesy of Richard P. Usatine, MD; used, with permission, from Usatine RP, Smith MA, Mayeaux EJ Jr, Chumley H, Tysinger J. *The Color Atlas of Family Medicine.* McGraw-Hill, 2009.)

more nevi with one or more atypical moles and one mole at least 8 mm or larger, and patients with a few to many definitely atypical moles. These patients deserve education and regular (usually every 6–12 months) follow-up. Kindreds with familial melanoma (numerous atypical nevi and a family history of two first-degree relatives with melanoma) deserve even closer attention, as the risk of developing single or even multiple melanomas in these individuals approaches 50% by age 50.

Duffy K et al. The dysplastic nevus: from historical perspective to management in the modern era: part I. Historical, histologic, and clinical aspects. J Am Acad Dermatol. 2012 Jul;67(1): 1.e1–16. [PMID: 22703915]

Duffy K et al. The dysplastic nevus: from historical perspective to management in the modern era: part II. Molecular aspects and clinical management. J Am Acad Dermatol. 2012 Jul;67(1):19.e1–12. [PMID: 22703916]

BLUE NEVI

Blue nevi are small, slightly elevated, blue-black lesions (Figure 6–3) that favor the dorsal hands. They are common in persons of Asian descent, and an individual patient may have several of them. If present without change for many years, they may be considered benign, since malignant blue nevi are rare. However, blue-black papules and nodules that are new or growing must be evaluated to rule out nodular melanoma.

Barros JA et al. Comparative dermatology: blue nevus. An Bras Dermatol. 2012 Jul–Aug;87(4):661–2. [PMID: 22892793]

Longo C et al. Blue lesions. Dermatol Clin. 2013 Oct;31(4): 637–47. [PMID: 24075551]

Phadke PA et al. Blue nevi and related tumors. Clin Lab Med. 2011 Jun;31(2):345–58. [PMID: 21549247]

FRECKLES & LENTIGINES

Freckles (ephelides) and lentigines are flat brown spots. Freckles first appear in young children, darken with ultraviolet exposure, and fade with cessation of sun exposure.

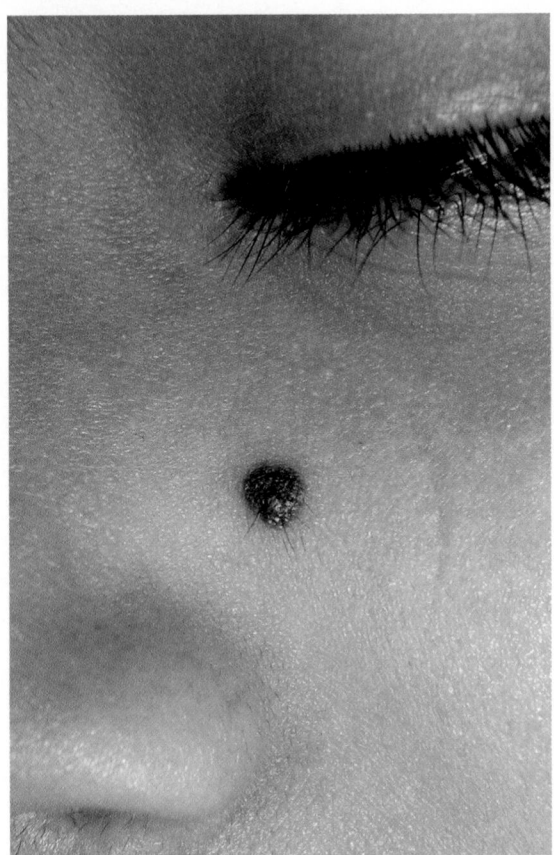

▲ **Figure 6–3.** Blue nevus on the left cheek, with some resemblance to a melanoma. (Courtesy of Richard P. Usatine, MD; used, with permission, from Usatine RP, Smith MA, Mayeaux EJ Jr, Chumley H, Tysinger J. *The Color Atlas of Family Medicine.* McGraw-Hill, 2009.)

They are determined by genetic factors. In adults lentigines gradually appear in sun-exposed areas, particularly the dorsa of the hands, upper back, and upper chest, starting in the fourth to fifth decade of life, and are associated with photoaging and estrogen and progesterone use. They are macular, usually 3–5 mm in diameter. On the upper back, they may have a very irregular border (inkspot lentigines). They do not fade with cessation of sun exposure. They should be evaluated like all pigmented lesions: If the pigmentation is homogeneous and they are symmetric and flat, they are most likely benign. They can be treated with topical 0.1% tretinoin, 0.1% tazarotene, 2% 4-hydroxyanisole with 0.01% tretinoin, laser therapy, or cryotherapy.

Ezzedine K et al. Freckles and solar lentigines have different risk factors in Caucasian women. J Eur Acad Dermatol Venereol. 2013 Mar;27(3):e345–56. [PMID: 22924836]

SEBORRHEIC KERATOSES

Seborrheic keratoses are benign plaques, beige to brown or even black, 3–20 mm in diameter, with a velvety or warty surface (Figure 6–4). They appear to be stuck or pasted

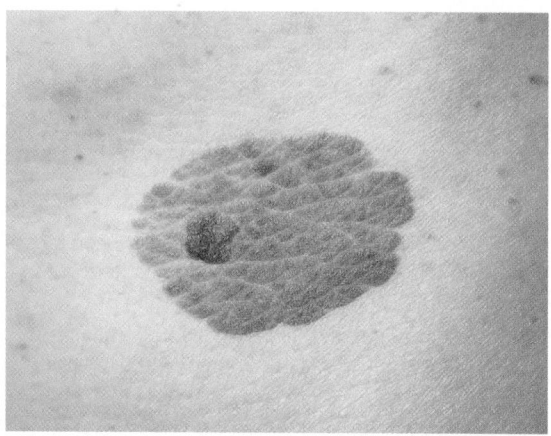

▲ **Figure 6–4.** Seborrheic keratosis with "stuck on appearance" but irregular borders and color variation suspicious for possible melanoma. (Courtesy of Richard P. Usatine, MD; used, with permission, from Usatine RP, Smith MA, Mayeaux EJ Jr, Chumley H, Tysinger J. *The Color Atlas of Family Medicine.* McGraw-Hill, 2009.)

onto the skin. They are extremely common—especially in the elderly—and may be mistaken for melanomas or other types of cutaneous neoplasms. Although they may be frozen with liquid nitrogen or curetted if they itch or are inflamed, no treatment is needed.

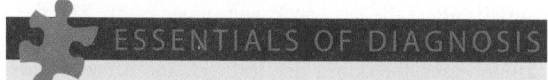

Choi JW et al. Differentiation of benign pigmented skin lesions with the aid of computer image analysis: a novel approach. Ann Dermatol. 2013 Aug;25(3):340–7. [PMID: 24003278]

MALIGNANT MELANOMA

ESSENTIALS OF DIAGNOSIS

► May be flat or raised.

► Should be suspected in any pigmented skin lesion with recent change in appearance.

► Examination with good light may show varying colors, including red, white, black, and bluish.

► Borders typically irregular.

General Considerations

Malignant melanoma is the leading cause of death due to skin disease. In 2013, approximately 76,690 new melanomas were diagnosed in the United States, with 45,060 cases in men and 31,630 in women. Melanoma will cause an estimated 9480 deaths (two-thirds in men). One in four cases of melanoma occurs before the age of 40. Increased detection of early melanomas has led to increased survival, but melanoma fatalities continue to increase, especially in elderly men.

Tumor thickness is the single most important prognostic factor. Ten-year survival rates—related to thickness in millimeters—are as follows: < 1 mm, 95%; 1–2 mm, 80%; 2–4 mm, 55%; and > 4 mm, 30%. With lymph node involvement, the 5-year survival rate is 30%; with distant metastases, it is < 10%.

► Clinical Findings

Primary malignant melanomas may be classified into various clinicohistologic types, including lentigo maligna melanoma (arising on chronically sun-exposed skin of older individuals); superficial spreading malignant melanoma (two-thirds of all melanomas arising on intermittently sun-exposed skin); nodular malignant melanoma; acral-lentiginous melanomas (arising on palms, soles, and nail beds); ocular melanoma; and malignant melanomas on mucous membranes. These different clinical types of melanoma appear to have different oncogenic mutations, which may be important in the treatment of patients with advanced disease. Clinical features of pigmented lesions suspicious for melanoma are an irregular notched border where the pigment appears to be leaking into the normal surrounding skin; a topography that may be irregular, ie, partly raised and partly flat (Figure 6–5). Color variegation is present, and colors such as pink, blue, gray, white, and black are indications for referral. A useful mnemonic is the ABCD rule: "ABCD = Asymmetry, Border irregularity, Color variegation, and Diameter > 6 mm." "E" for Evolution can be added. The history of a changing mole (evolution) is the single most important historical reason for close evaluation and possible referral. Bleeding and ulceration are ominous signs. A mole that stands out from the patient's other moles deserves special scrutiny—the "ugly duckling sign." A patient with a large number of moles is statistically at increased risk for melanoma and deserves careful and periodic examination, particularly if the lesions are atypical. Referral of suspicious pigmented lesions is always appropriate.

While superficial spreading melanoma is largely a disease of whites, persons of other races are still at risk for this

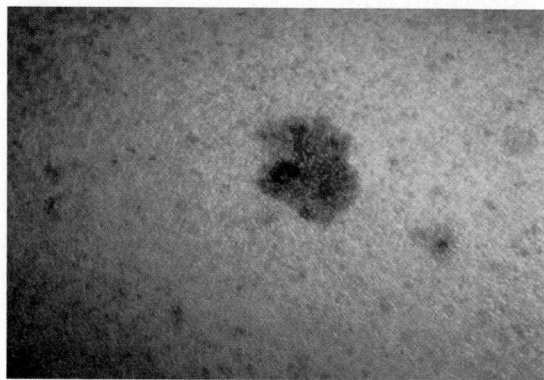

▲ **Figure 6–5.** Malignant melanoma, with multiple colors and classic "ABCDE" features. (Used, with permission, from Berger TG, Dept Dermatology, UCSF.)

and other types of melanoma, particularly acral lentiginous melanoma. These occur as dark, sometimes irregularly shaped lesions on the palms and soles and as new, often broad and solitary, darkly pigmented longitudinal streaks in the nails. Acral lentiginous melanoma may be a difficult diagnosis because benign pigmented lesions of the hands, feet, and nails occur commonly in more darkly pigmented persons and clinicians may hesitate to biopsy the palms, soles, and nail beds. As a result, the diagnosis is often delayed until the tumor has become clinically obvious and histologically thick. Clinicians should give special attention to new or changing lesions in these areas.

▶ Treatment

Treatment of melanoma consists of excision. After histologic diagnosis, the area is usually reexcised with margins dictated by the thickness of the tumor. Thin low-risk and intermediate-risk tumors require only conservative margins of 1–3 cm. Surgical margins of 0.5–1 cm for melanoma in situ and 1 cm for lesions < 1 mm in thickness are recommended.

Sentinel lymph node biopsy (selective lymphadenectomy) using preoperative lymphoscintigraphy and intraoperative lymphatic mapping is effective for staging melanoma patients with intermediate risk without clinical adenopathy and is recommended for all patients with lesions over 1 mm in thickness or with high-risk histologic features. Referral of intermediate-risk and high-risk patients to centers with expertise in melanoma is strongly recommended. Identifying the oncogenic mutations in patients with advanced melanoma may be important in their treatment. The long-term use of beta-blockers may reduce the risk of progression of high-risk melanoma.

Bichakjian CK et al; American Academy of Dermatology. Guidelines of care for the management of primary cutaneous melanoma. J Am Acad Dermatol. 2011 Nov;65(5):1032–47. [PMID: 21868127]

Coit DG et al. Melanoma, versions 2.2013: featured updates to the NCCN guidelines. J Natl Compr Canc Netw. 2013 Apr1;11(4):395–407. [PMID: 23584343]

Council ML. Common skin cancers in older adults: approach to diagnosis and management. Clin Geriatr Med. 2013 May;29(2):361–72. [PMID: 23571033]

De G iorgi V et al. Treatment with beta-blockers and reduced disease progression in patients with thick melanoma. Arch Intern Med. 2011 Apr25;171(8):779–81. [PMID: 21518948]

Fox MC et al. Management options for metastatic melanoma in the era of novel therapies: a primer for the practicing dermatologist: PartI: management of stage III disease. J Am Acad Dermatol. 2013 Jan;68(1):1.e1–9. [PMID: 23244383]

Fox MC et al. Management options for metastatic melanoma in the era of novel therapies: a primer for the practicing dermatologist: Part II: management of stage IV disease. J Am Acad Dermatol. 2013 Jan;68(1):13.e1–13. [PMID: 23244384]

Menzies AM et al. New combinations and immunotherapies for melanoma: latest evidence and clinical utility. Ther Adv Med Oncol. 2013 Sep;5(5):278–85. [PMID: 23997828]

Scolyer RA. Evolving concepts in melanoma classification and their relevance to multidisciplinary melanoma patient care. Mol Oncol. 2011 Apr;5(2):124–36. [PMID: 21482206]

Tuong W et al. Melanoma: epidemiology, diagnosis, treatment, and outcomes. Dermatol Clin. 2012 Jan;30(1):113–24. [PMID: 22117873]

SCALING DISORDERS

ATOPIC DERMATITIS

 ESSENTIALS OF DIAGNOSIS

▶ Pruritic, exudative, or lichenified eruption on face, neck, upper trunk, wrists, and hands and in the antecubital and popliteal folds.

▶ Personal or family history of allergic manifestations (eg, asthma, allergic rhinitis, atopic dermatitis).

▶ Tendency to recur.

▶ Onset in childhood in most patients. Onset after age 30 is very uncommon.

▶ General Considerations

Atopic dermatitis looks different at different ages and in people of different races. Diagnostic criteria for atopic dermatitis must include pruritus, typical morphology and distribution (flexural lichenification, hand eczema, nipple eczema, and eyelid eczema in adults), onset in childhood, and chronicity. Also helpful are: (1) a personal or family history of atopic disease (asthma, allergic rhinitis, atopic dermatitis), (2) xerosis-ichthyosis, (3) facial pallor with infraorbital darkening, (4) elevated serum IgE, and (5) repeated skin infections.

▶ Clinical Findings

A. Symptoms and Signs

Itching may be severe and prolonged. Rough, red plaques usually without the thick scale and discrete demarcation of psoriasis affect the face, neck, and upper trunk. The flexural surfaces of elbows and knees are often involved. In chronic cases, the skin is dry, leathery, and lichenified. In black patients with severe disease, pigmentation may be lost in lichenified areas. During acute flares, widespread redness with weeping, either diffusely or in discrete plaques, is common.

B. Laboratory Findings

Food allergy is an uncommon cause of flares of atopic dermatitis in adults. Eosinophilia and increased serum IgE levels may be present.

▶ Differential Diagnosis

Atopic dermatitis must be distinguished from seborrheic dermatitis (less pruritic, frequent scalp and face involvement, greasy and scaly lesions, and quick response to therapy). Secondary staphylococcal infections may exacerbate atopic dermatitis, and should be considered during hyperacute, weepy flares of atopic dermatitis. Fissuring where the earlobe connects to the neck is a cardinal sign of secondary infection. Since virtually all patients with atopic dermatitis have skin disease before age 5, a new diagnosis of atopic dermatitis in an adult over age 30 should be made cautiously and only after consultation.

Treatment

Patient education regarding gentle skin care and exactly how to use medications is critical in the successful management of atopic dermatitis.

A. General Measures

Atopic patients have hyperirritable skin. Anything that dries or irritates the skin will potentially trigger dermatitis. Atopic individuals are sensitive to low humidity and often get worse in the winter. Adults with atopic disorders should not bathe more than once daily. Soap should be confined to the armpits, groin, scalp, and feet. Washcloths and brushes should not be used. After rinsing, the skin should be patted dry (not rubbed) and then immediately—within three minutes—covered with a thin film of an emollient such as Aquaphor, Eucerin, petrolatum, Vanicream, or a corticosteroid as needed. Vanicream can be used if contact dermatitis resulting from additives in medication is suspected. Atopic patients may be irritated by scratchy fabrics, including wools and acrylics. Cottons are preferable, but synthetic blends also are tolerated. Other triggers of eczema in some patients include sweating, ointments, hot baths, and animal danders.

B. Local Treatment

Corticosteroids should be applied sparingly to the dermatitis once or twice daily and rubbed in well. Their potency should be appropriate to the severity of the dermatitis. In general, one should begin with triamcinolone 0.1% or a stronger corticosteroid then taper to hydrocortisone or another slightly stronger mild corticosteroid (alclometasone, desonide). It is vital that patients taper off corticosteroids and substitute emollients as the dermatitis clears to avoid the side effects of corticosteroids. Tapering is also important to avoid rebound flares of the dermatitis that may follow their abrupt cessation. Tacrolimus ointment (Protopic 0.03% or 0.1%) and pimecrolimus cream (Elidel 1%) can be effective in managing atopic dermatitis when applied twice daily. Burning on application occurs in about 50% of patients using Protopic and in 10–25% of Elidel users, but it may resolve with continued treatment. These medications do not cause skin atrophy or striae, avoiding the complications of long-term topical corticosteroid use. They are safe for application on the face and even the eyelids.

The US Food and Drug Administration (FDA) has issued a black box warning for both topical tacrolimus and pimecrolimus due to concerns about the development of T-cell lymphoma. The agents should be used sparingly and only in locations where less expensive corticosteroids cannot be used. Tacrolimus and pimecrolimus should be avoided in patients at high risk for lymphoma (ie, those with HIV, iatrogenic immunosuppression, prior lymphoma).

The treatment of atopic dermatitis is dictated by the pattern and stage of the dermatitis—acute/weepy, subacute/scaly, or chronic/lichenified.

1. Acute weeping lesions—Use water or aluminum subacetate solution (Domeboro tablets, one in a pint of cool water) or colloidal oatmeal (Aveeno; dispense one box, and use as directed on box) as soothing or astringent soaks, baths, or wet dressings for 10–30 minutes two to four times daily. Lesions on extremities particularly may be bandaged for protection at night. Use high-potency corticosteroids after soaking but spare the face and body folds. Tacrolimus is usually not tolerated at this stage. Systemic corticosteroids may be required (see below).

2. Subacute or scaly lesions—At this stage, the lesions are dry but still red and pruritic. Mid- to high-potency corticosteroids in ointment form should be continued until scaling and elevated skin lesions are cleared and itching is decreased substantially. At that point, patients should begin a 2- to 4-week taper from twice-daily to daily to alternate-day dosing with topical corticosteroids to reliance on emollients, with occasional use of corticosteroids on specific itchy areas. Instead of tapering the frequency of usage of a more potent corticosteroid, it may be preferable to switch to a low-potency corticosteroid. Tacrolimus and pimecrolimus are more expensive alternatives and may be added if corticosteroids cannot be stopped.

3. Chronic, dry, lichenified lesions—Thickened and usually well-demarcated, they are best treated with high-potency to ultra-high-potency corticosteroid ointments. Nightly occlusion for 2–6 weeks may enhance the initial response. Occasionally, adding tar preparations such as LCD (liquor carbonis detergens) 10% in Aquaphor or 2% crude coal tar may be beneficial.

4. Maintenance treatment—Once symptoms have improved, constant application of effective moisturizers is recommended to prevent flares. In patients with moderate disease, use of topical anti-inflammatories only on weekends or three times weekly can prevent flares.

C. Systemic and Adjuvant Therapy

Systemic corticosteroids are indicated only for severe acute exacerbations. Oral prednisone dosages should be high enough to suppress the dermatitis quickly, usually starting with 40–60 mg daily for adults. The dosage is then tapered to nil over a period of 2–4 weeks. Owing to the chronic nature of atopic dermatitis and the side effects of chronic systemic corticosteroids, long-term use of these agents is not recommended for maintenance therapy. Bedtime doses of hydroxyzine, diphenhydramine, or doxepin may be helpful via their sedative properties in reducing perceived pruritus. Fissures, crusts, erosions, or pustules indicate staphylococcal infection clinically. Antistaphylococcal antibiotics given systemically—such as a first-generation cephalosporin or doxycycline if methicillin-resistant *Staphylococcus aureus* is suspected—may be helpful. Cultures to exclude methicillin-resistant *S aureus* are recommended. However, in this setting, continuing and augmenting the topical anti-inflammatory treatment often improves the dermatitis, despite the presence of infection. Phototherapy can be an important adjunct for severely affected patients, and the properly selected patient with recalcitrant disease may benefit greatly from therapy with UVB with or without coal tar or PUVA (psoralen plus ultraviolet A). Oral cyclosporine, mycophenolate mofetil, methotrexate, or azathioprine may be used for the most severe and recalcitrant cases.

► Complications of Treatment

The clinician should monitor for skin atrophy. **Eczema herpeticum,** a generalized herpes simplex infection manifested by monomorphic vesicles, crusts, or scalloped erosions superimposed on atopic dermatitis or other extensive eczematous processes, is treated successfully with oral acyclovir, 200 mg five times daily, or intravenous acyclovir in a dose of 10 mg/kg intravenously every 8 hours (500 mg/m^2 every 8 hours). Smallpox vaccination is absolutely contraindicated in patients with atopic dermatitis or a history thereof because of the risk of eczema vaccinatum (widespread vaccinia infection, preferentially in areas of dermatitis).

► Prognosis

Atopic dermatitis runs a chronic or intermittent course. Affected adults may have only hand dermatitis. Poor prognostic factors for persistence into adulthood in atopic dermatitis include onset early in childhood, early generalized disease, and asthma. Only 40–60% of these patients have lasting remissions.

Eichenfield LF et al. Guidelines of care for the management of atopic dermatitis: section 1. Diagnosis and assessment of atopic dermatitis. J Am Acad Dermatol. 2014 Feb;70(2): 338–51. [PMID: 24290431]

Eichenfield LF et al. Guidelines of care for the management of atopic dermatitis: section 2. Guidelines of care for the management and treatment of atopic dermatitis with topical therapies. J Am Acad Dermatol. In press.

Kwatra SG et al. The infra-auricular fissure: a bedside marker of disease severity in patients with atopic dermatitis. J Am Acad Dermatol. 2012 Jun;66(6):1009–10. [PMID: 22583715]

Ring J et al. Guidelines for treatment of atopic eczema (atopic dermatitis) part I. J Eur Acad Dermatol Venereol. 2012 Aug;26(8):1045–60. [PMID: 22805051]

Ring J et al. Guidelines for treatment of atopic eczema (atopic dermatitis) part II. J Eur Acad Dermatol Venereol. 2012 Sep;26(9):1175–93. [PMID: 22813359]

Schmitt J et al. Efficacy and tolerability of proactive treatment with topical corticosteroids and calcineurin inhibitors for atopic eczema: systematic review and meta-analysis of randomized controlled trials. Br J Dermatol. 2011 Feb;164(2): 415–28. [PMID: 20819086]

Sidbury R et al. Guidelines of care for the management of atopic dermatitis: section 3. Management and treatment with phototherapy and systemic agents. J Am Acad Dermatol. In press.

Sidbury R et al. Guidelines of care for the management of atopic dermatitis: section 4. Prevention of disease flares and use of adjunctive therapies and approaches. J Am Acad Dermatol. In press.

Torrelo A et al. Atopic dermatitis: impact on quality of life and patients' attitudes toward its management. Eur J Dermatol. 2012 Jan–Feb;22(1):97–105. [PMID: 22237114]

Van Onselen J. Skin care in the older person: identifying and managing eczema. Br J Community Nurs. 2011 Dec;16(12): 576, 578–80, 582. [PMID: 22413402]

Van Velsen SG et al. Two-year assessment of effect of topical corticosteroids on bone mineral density in adults with moderate to severe atopic dermatitis. J Am Acad Dermatol. 2012 Apr;66(4):691–3. [PMID: 22421118]

LICHEN SIMPLEX CHRONICUS (Circumscribed Neurodermatitis)

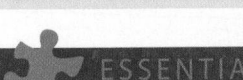

ESSENTIALS OF DIAGNOSIS

► Chronic itching and scratching.

► Lichenified lesions with exaggerated skin lines overlying a thickened, well-circumscribed scaly plaque.

► Predilection for nape of neck, wrists, external surfaces of forearms, lower legs, scrotum, and vulva.

► General Considerations

Lichen simplex chronicus represents a self-perpetuating scratch-itch cycle—a learned behavior that is hard to disrupt.

► Clinical Findings

Intermittent itching incites the patient to scratch the lesions. Itching may be so intense as to interfere with sleep. Dry, leathery, hypertrophic, lichenified plaques appear on the neck, ankles, or perineum (Figure 6–6). The patches are rectangular, thickened, and hyperpigmented. The skin lines are exaggerated.

► Differential Diagnosis

This disorder can be differentiated from plaque-like lesions such as psoriasis (redder lesions having whiter scales on the elbows, knees, and scalp and nail findings), lichen planus (violaceous, usually smaller polygonal papules), and nummular (coin-shaped) dermatitis. Lichen simplex chronicus may complicate chronic atopic dermatitis.

► Treatment

For lesions in extra-genital regions, superpotent topical corticosteroids are effective, with or without occlusion, when used twice daily for several weeks. In some patients, flurandrenolide (Cordran) tape may be effective, since it prevents scratching and rubbing of the lesion. The injection of triamcinolone acetonide suspension (5–10 mg/mL) into the lesions may occasionally be curative. Continuous occlusion with a flexible hydrocolloid dressing for 7 days at a time for 1–2 months may also be helpful. For genital lesions, see the section Pruritus Ani.

► Prognosis

The disease tends to remit during treatment but may recur or develop at another site.

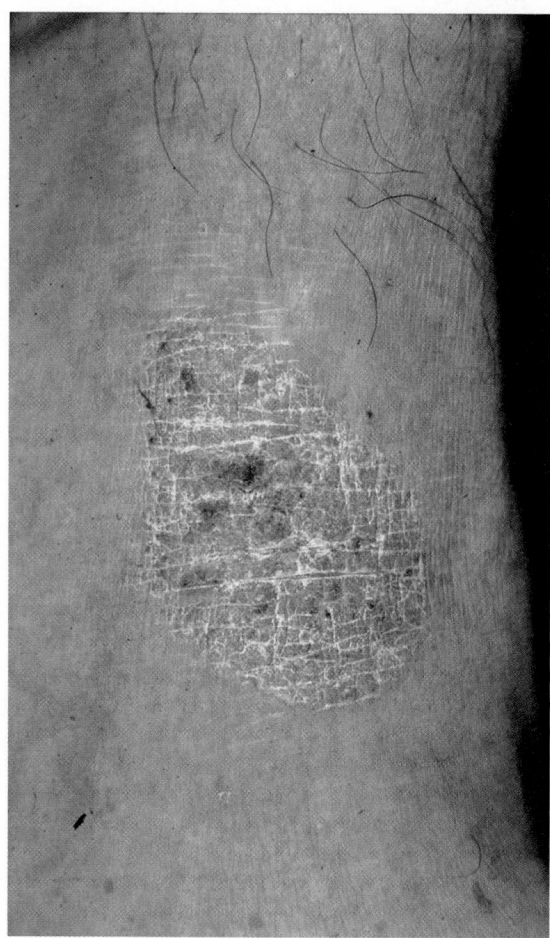

▲ **Figure 6–6.** Lichen simplex chronicus. (Used, with permission, from Berger TG, Dept Dermatology, UCSF.)

Szegedi K et al. Increased frequencies of IL-31-producing T cells are found in chronic atopic dermatitis skin. Exp Dermatol. 2012 Jun;21(6):431–6. [PMID: 22621183]

PSORIASIS

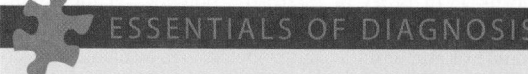

ESSENTIALS OF DIAGNOSIS

▶ Silvery scales on bright red, well-demarcated plaques, usually on the knees, elbows, and scalp.

▶ Nail findings including pitting and onycholysis (separation of the nail plate from the bed).

▶ Mild itching (usually).

▶ May be associated with psoriatic arthritis.

▶ Psoriasis patients are at increased risk for metabolic syndrome and lymphoma.

▶ Histopathology is not often useful and can be confusing.

▶ General Considerations

Psoriasis is a common benign, chronic inflammatory skin disease with both a genetic basis and known environmental triggers. Injury or irritation of normal skin tends to induce lesions of psoriasis at the site (Koebner phenomenon). Obesity worsens psoriasis, and significant weight loss in obese persons may lead to substantial improvement of their psoriasis. Psoriasis has several variants—the most common is the plaque type. Eruptive (guttate) psoriasis consisting of myriad lesions 3–10 mm in diameter occurs occasionally after streptococcal pharyngitis. Rarely, grave, occasionally life-threatening forms (generalized pustular and erythrodermic psoriasis) may occur. Plaque type or extensive erythrodermic psoriasis with abrupt onset may accompany HIV infection.

▶ Clinical Findings

There are often no symptoms, but itching may occur and be severe. Favored sites include the scalp, elbows, knees, palms and soles, and nails. The lesions are red, sharply defined plaques covered with silvery scales (Figure 6–7). The glans penis and vulva may be affected. Occasionally, only the flexures (axillae, inguinal areas) are involved. Fine stippling ("pitting") in the nails is highly suggestive of

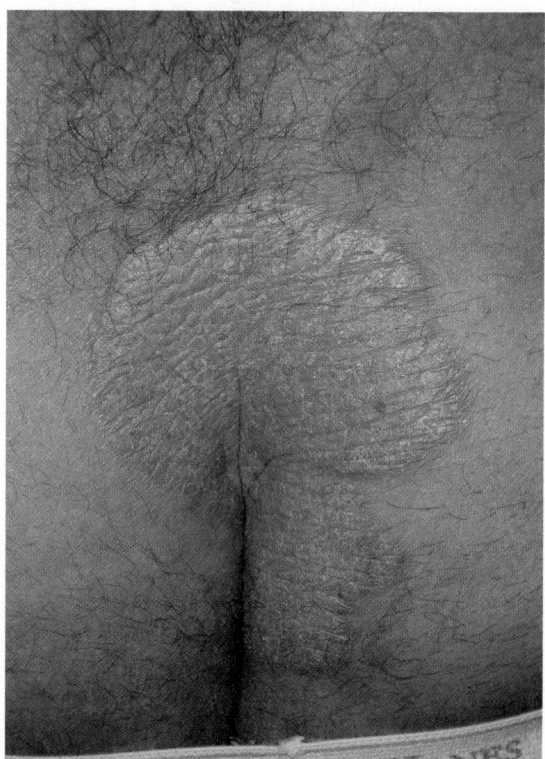

▲ **Figure 6–7.** Plaque psoriasis in the sacral region and intergluteal fold. (Courtesy of Richard P. Usatine, MD; used, with permission, from Usatine RP, Smith MA, Mayeaux EJ Jr, Chumley H, Tysinger J. *The Color Atlas of Family Medicine.* McGraw-Hill, 2009.)

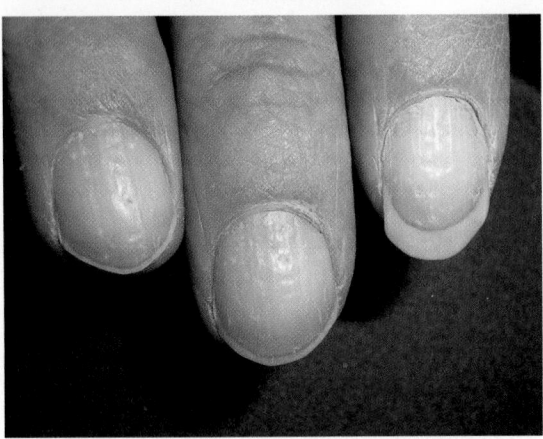

▲ **Figure 6–8.** Nail pitting due to psoriasis. (Courtesy of Richard P. Usatine, MD; used, with permission, from Usatine RP, Smith MA, Mayeaux EJ Jr, Chumley H, Tysinger J. *The Color Atlas of Family Medicine.* McGraw-Hill, 2009.)

psoriasis (Figure 6–8). Patients with psoriasis often have a pink or red intergluteal fold. Not all patients have findings in all locations, but the occurrence of a few may help make the diagnosis when other lesions are not typical. Some patients have mainly hand or foot dermatitis and only minimal findings elsewhere. There may be associated arthritis that is most commonly distal and oligoarticular, although the rheumatoid variety with a negative rheumatoid factor may occur. The psychosocial impact of psoriasis is a major factor in determining the treatment of the patient.

▶ **Differential Diagnosis**

The combination of red plaques with silvery scales on elbows and knees, with scaliness in the scalp or nail findings, is diagnostic. Psoriasis lesions are well demarcated and affect extensor surfaces—in contrast to atopic dermatitis, with poorly demarcated plaques in flexural distribution. In body folds, scraping and culture for *Candida* and examination of scalp and nails will distinguish psoriasis from intertrigo and candidiasis. Dystrophic changes in nails may simulate onychomycosis, but again, the general examination combined with a potassium hydroxide (KOH) preparation or fungal culture will be valuable in diagnosis. The cutaneous features of reactive arthritis (Reiter syndrome) mimic psoriasis.

▶ **Treatment**

There are many therapeutic options in psoriasis to be chosen according to the extent (body surface area [BSA] affected) and the presence of other findings (for example, arthritis). Certain drugs, such as beta-blockers, antimalarials, statins, and lithium, may flare or worsen psoriasis. Even tiny doses of systemic corticosteroids given to patients with psoriasis may lead to severe rebound flares of their disease when they are tapered. **Never use systemic corticosteroids to treat flares of psoriasis.** In general, patients with moderate to severe psoriasis should be managed by or in conjunction with a dermatologist.

A. Limited Disease

For patients with numerous small plaques, phototherapy is the best therapy (see below). For patients with large plaques and < 10% of the BSA involved, the easiest regimen is to use a high-potency to ultra-high-potency topical corticosteroid cream or ointment. It is best to restrict the ultra-high-potency corticosteroids to 2–3 weeks of twice-daily use and then use them in a pulse fashion three or four times on weekends or switch to a midpotency corticosteroid. Topical corticosteroids rarely induce a lasting remission. Additional measures are therefore commonly added to topical corticosteroid therapy. Calcipotriene ointment 0.005% or calcitriol ointment 0.003%, both vitamin D analogs, are used twice daily for plaque psoriasis. Initially, patients are treated with twice-daily corticosteroids plus a vitamin D analog twice daily. This rapidly clears the lesions. The vitamin D analog is then used alone once daily and with the corticosteroid once daily for several weeks. Eventually, the topical corticosteroids are stopped, and once- or twice-daily application of the vitamin D analog is continued long-term. Calcipotriene usually cannot be applied to the groin or on the face because of irritation. Treatment of extensive psoriasis with vitamin D analogs may result in hypercalcemia, so that the maximum dose for calcipotriene is 100 g/week and for calcitriol is 200 g/week. Calcipotriene is incompatible with many topical corticosteroids (but not halobetasol), so if used concurrently it must be applied at a different time. Tar preparations such as Fototar cream, LCD (liquor carbonis detergens) 10% in Nutraderm lotion, alone or mixed directly with triamcinolone 0.1%, are useful adjuncts when applied twice daily. Occlusion alone has been shown to clear isolated plaques in 30–40% of patients. Thin, occlusive hydrocolloid dressings are placed on the lesions and left undisturbed for as long as possible (a minimum of 5 days, up to 7 days) and then replaced. Responses may be seen within several weeks.

For the scalp, start with a tar shampoo, used daily if possible. For thick scales, use 6% salicylic acid gel (eg, Keralyt), P & S solution (phenol, mineral oil, and glycerin), or fluocinolone acetonide 0.01% in oil (Derma-Smoothe/FS) under a shower cap at night, and shampoo in the morning. In order of increasing potency, triamcinolone 0.1%, or fluocinolone, betamethasone dipropionate, fluocinonide or amcinonide, and clobetasol are available in solution form for use on the scalp twice daily. For psoriasis in the body folds, treatment is difficult, since potent corticosteroids cannot be used and other agents are poorly tolerated. Tacrolimus ointment 0.1% or 0.03% or pimecrolimus cream 1% may be effective in penile, groin, and facial psoriasis.

B. Moderate Disease

Psoriasis affecting 10–30% of the patient's BSA is frequently treated with UV phototherapy, either in a medical office or via a home light unit. Systemic agents listed below may also be used.

C. Generalized Disease

If psoriasis involves > 30% of the body surface, it is difficult to treat with topical agents. The treatment of choice is outpatient narrowband UVB (NB-UVB) three times weekly. Clearing occurs in an average of 7 weeks, but maintenance may be required. Severe psoriasis unresponsive to outpatient ultraviolet light may be treated in a psoriasis day care center with the Goeckerman regimen, which involves use of crude coal tar for many hours and exposure to UVB light. Such treatment may offer the best chance for prolonged remissions.

Psoralen plus UVA (PUVA) photochemotherapy may be effective even in patients who have not responded to standard NB-UVB treatment. Long-term use of PUVA is associated with an increased risk of skin cancer (especially squamous cell carcinoma and perhaps melanoma), particularly in persons with fair complexions. Thus, periodic examination of the skin is imperative. Atypical lentigines are a common complication. There can be rapid aging of the skin in fair individuals. Cataracts have not been reported with proper use of protective glasses. PUVA may be used in combination with other therapy, such as acitretin or methotrexate.

Methotrexate is very effective for severe psoriasis in doses up to 25 mg once weekly. It should be used according to published protocols. Long-term methotrexate use may be associated with cirrhosis. After receiving a 3.5–4 g cumulative dose, the patient should be referred to a hepatologist for consideration of a liver biopsy. Administration of folic acid, 1–2 mg daily, can eliminate nausea caused by methotrexate without compromising efficacy.

Acitretin, a synthetic retinoid, is most effective for pustular psoriasis in dosages of 0.5–0.75 mg/kg/d. Liver enzymes and serum lipids must be checked periodically. Because acitretin is a teratogen and persists for long periods in fat, women of childbearing age must wait at least 3 years after completing acitretin treatment before considering pregnancy. When used as single agents, retinoids will flatten psoriatic plaques, but will rarely result in complete clearing. Retinoids find their greatest use when combined with phototherapy—either UVB or PUVA, with which they are synergistic.

Cyclosporine dramatically improves psoriasis and may be used to control severe cases. Rapid relapse (rebound) is the rule after cessation of therapy, so another agent must be added if cyclosporine is stopped. The tumor necrosis factor (TNF) inhibitors etanercept (Enbrel), infliximab (Remicade), and adalimumab (Humira) are effective in pustular and chronic plaque psoriasis and are also effective for the associated arthritis. Infliximab provides the most rapid response and can be used for severe pustular or erythrodermic flares. Etanercept is used more frequently for long-term treatment at a dose of 50 mg twice weekly for 3 months, then 50 mg once weekly. All three TNF inhibitors can also induce or worsen psoriasis. IL-12/23 monoclonal antibodies (ustekinumab [Stelara]) are also effective and may be considered instead of using a TNF inhibitor. Given the large number of immunosuppressive and biologic agents available, consultation with a dermatologist is recommended when considering institution of treatment with a systemic agent for moderate to severe psoriasis.

► Prognosis

The course tends to be chronic and unpredictable, and the disease may be refractory to treatment. Patients (especially those older than 40 years) should be monitored for metabolic syndrome, which correlates with the severity of their skin disease.

Arias-Santiago S et al. Atheroma plaque, metabolic syndrome and inflammation in patients with psoriasis. Eur J Dermatol. 2012 May– Jun;22(3):337–44. [PMID: 22503884]

Armstrong AW et al. Psoriasis and the risk of diabetes mellitus: a systematic review and meta-analysis. JAMA Dermatol. 2013 Jan;149(1):84–91. [PMID: 23407990]

Bailey EE et al. Combination treatments for psoriasis: a systematic review and meta-analysis. Arch Dermatol. 2012 Apr;148(4):511–22. [PMID: 22184718]

Gelfand JM et al. Comparative effectiveness of commonly used systemic treatments of phototherapy for moderate to severe plaque psoriasis in the clinical practice setting. Arch Dermatol. 2012 Apr;148(4):487–94. [PMID: 22508874]

Hendriks AG et al. Combinations of classical time-honoured topicals in plaque psoriasis: a systematic review. J Eur Acad Dermatol Venereol. 2013 Apr;27(4):399–410. [PMID: 22779910]

Hsu S et al. Consensus guidelines for the management of plaque psoriasis. Arch Dermatol. 2012 Jan;148(1):95–102. [PMID: 22250239]

Kim IH et al. Comparative efficacy of biologics in psoriasis: a review. Am J Clin Dermatol. 2012 Dec1;13(6):365–74. [PMID: 22967166]

Lebwohl MG et al. A randomized study to evaluate the efficacy and safety of adding topical therapy to etanercept in patients with moderate to severe plaque psoriasis. J Am Acad Dermatol. 2013 Sep;69(3):385–92. [PMID: 23643256]

Mason A et al. Topical treatments for chronic plaque psoriasis: an abridged Cochrane Systematic Review. J Am Acad Dermatol. 2013 Nov;69(5):799–807. [PMID: 24124809]

Reich K et al. Efficacy of biologics in the treatment of moderate to severe psoriasis: a network meta-analysis of randomized controlled trials. Br J Dermatol. 2012 Jan;166(1):179–88. [PMID: 21910698]

Ryan C et al. Association between biologic therapies for chronic plaque psoriasis and cardiovascular events: a meta-analysis of randomized controlled trials. JAMA. 2011 Aug24;306(8): 864–71. [PMID: 21862748]

Samarasekere EJ et al. Topical therapies for the treatment of plaque psoriasis: systematic review and network meta-analyses. Br J Dermatol. 2013 May;168(5):954–67. [PMID: 23413913]

PITYRIASIS ROSEA

ESSENTIALS OF DIAGNOSIS

- ► Oval, fawn-colored, scaly eruption following cleavage lines of trunk.
- ► Herald patch precedes eruption by 1–2 weeks.
- ► Occasional pruritus.

► General Considerations

This is a common mild, acute inflammatory disease that is 50% more common in females. Young adults are

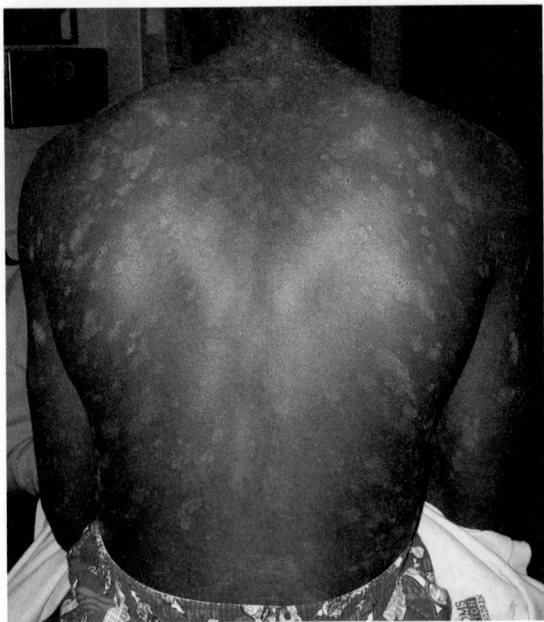

▲ **Figure 6–9.** Pityriasis rosea with scaling lesions following skin lines and resembling a Christmas tree. (Courtesy of EJ Mayeaux, MD; used, with permission, from Usatine RP, Smith MA, Mayeaux EJ Jr, Chumley H, Tysinger J. *The Color Atlas of Family Medicine.* McGraw-Hill, 2009.)

principally affected, mostly in the spring or fall. Concurrent household cases have been reported.

Clinical Findings

Itching is common but is usually mild. The diagnosis is made by finding one or more classic lesions. The lesions consist of oval, fawn-colored plaques up to 2 cm in diameter. The centers of the lesions have a crinkled or "cigarette paper" appearance and a collarette scale, ie, a thin bit of scale that is bound at the periphery and free in the center. Only a few lesions in the eruption may have this characteristic appearance, however. Lesions follow cleavage lines on the trunk (so-called Christmas tree pattern, Figure 6–9), and the proximal portions of the extremities are often involved. A variant that affects the flexures (axillae and groin), so called inverse pityriasis rosea, and a papular variant, especially in black patients, also occur. An initial lesion ("herald patch") that is often larger than the later lesions often precedes the general eruption by 1–2 weeks. The eruption usually lasts 6–8 weeks and heals without scarring.

Differential Diagnosis

A serologic test for syphilis should be performed if at least a few perfectly typical lesions are not present and especially if there are palmar and plantar or mucous membrane lesions or adenopathy, features that are suggestive of secondary syphilis. For the nonexpert, an RPR (rapid plasma reagin) test in all cases is not unreasonable. Tinea corporis may present with red, slightly scaly plaques, but rarely are there more than a few lesions of tinea corporis compared to the many lesions of pityriasis rosea. Seborrheic dermatitis on occasion

presents on the body with poorly demarcated patches over the sternum, in the pubic area, and in the axillae. Tinea versicolor lacks the typical collarette rimmed lesions. Certain drugs (eg, angiotensin-converting enzyme [ACE] inhibitors and metronidazole) and influenza immunization rarely may induce a skin eruption mimicking pityriasis rosea.

Treatment

Pityriasis rosea often requires no treatment. In Asians, Hispanics, or blacks, in whom lesions may remain hyperpigmented for some time, more aggressive management may be indicated. Treatment is, otherwise, only indicated if the patient is symptomatic. While adequately controlled and reproduced trials have not demonstrated widely effective treatments, most dermatologists recommend UVB treatments, or prednisone as used for contact dermatitis for severe or severely symptomatic cases. For mild to moderate cases, topical corticosteroids of medium strength (triamcinolone 0.1%) and oral antihistamines may also be used if pruritus is bothersome.

Prognosis

Pityriasis rosea is usually an acute self-limiting illness that disappears in about 6 weeks.

Polate M et al. Palmar herald patch in pityriasis rosea. Australas J Dermatol. 2012 Aug;53(3):e64–5. [PMID: 22881477]
Sinha S et al. Coexistence of two atypical variants of pityriasis rosea: a case report and review of literature. Pediatr Dermatol. 2012 Jul–Aug;29(4):538–40. [PMID: 21906158]

SEBORRHEIC DERMATITIS & DANDRUFF

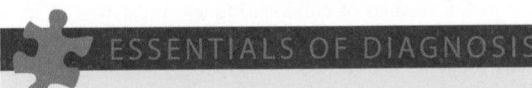

> ESSENTIALS OF DIAGNOSIS

> ▶ Dry scales and underlying erythema.
> ▶ Scalp, central face, presternal, interscapular areas, umbilicus, and body folds.

General Considerations

Seborrheic dermatitis is an acute or chronic papulosquamous dermatitis that often coexists with psoriasis.

Clinical Findings

Pruritus is an inconstant finding. The scalp, face, chest, back, umbilicus, eyelid margins, and body folds have dry scales or oily yellowish scurf (Figure 6–10). Patients with Parkinson disease, HIV infection, and patients who become acutely ill and are hospitalized often have seborrheic dermatitis.

Differential Diagnosis

There is a spectrum from seborrheic dermatitis to scalp psoriasis. Extensive seborrheic dermatitis may simulate intertrigo in flexural areas, but scalp, face, and sternal involvement suggests seborrheic dermatitis.

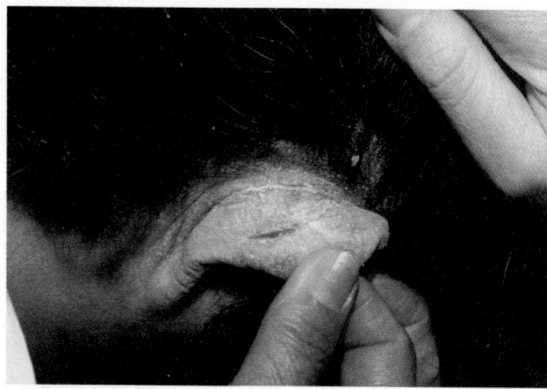

▲ **Figure 6–10.** Seborrheic dermatitis. (Used, with permission, from Berger TG, Dept Dermatology, UCSF.)

► **Treatment**

A. Seborrhea of the Scalp

Shampoos that contain zinc pyrithione or selenium are used daily if possible. These may be alternated with ketoconazole shampoo (1% or 2%) used twice weekly. A combination of shampoos is used in refractory cases. Tar shampoos are also effective for milder cases and for scalp psoriasis. Topical corticosteroid solutions or lotions are then added if necessary and are used twice daily. (See treatment for scalp psoriasis, above.)

B. Facial Seborrheic Dermatitis

The mainstay of therapy is a mild corticosteroid (hydrocortisone 1%, alclometasone, desonide) used intermittently and not near the eyes. If the disorder cannot be controlled with intermittent use of a mild topical corticosteroid alone, ketoconazole (Nizoral) 2% cream is added twice daily. Topical tacrolimus (Protopic) and pimecrolimus (Elidel) are steroid-sparing alternatives.

C. Seborrheic Dermatitis of Nonhairy Areas

Low-potency corticosteroid creams—ie, 1% or 2.5% hydrocortisone, desonide, or alclometasone dipropionate—are highly effective.

D. Seborrhea of Intertriginous Areas

Apply low-potency corticosteroid lotions or creams twice daily for 5–7 days and then once or twice weekly for maintenance as necessary. Ketoconazole or clotrimazole cream may be a useful adjunct. Tacrolimus or pimecrolimus topically may avoid corticosteroid atrophy in chronic cases.

E. Involvement of Eyelid Margins

"Marginal blepharitis" usually responds to gentle cleaning of the lid margins nightly as needed, with undiluted Johnson & Johnson Baby Shampoo using a cotton swab.

► **Prognosis**

The tendency is for lifelong recurrences. Individual outbreaks may last weeks, months, or years.

Hay RJ. Malassezia, dandruff and seborrhoeic dermatitis: an overview. Br J Dermatol. 2011 Oct;165(Suppl 2):2–8. [PMID: 21919896]

FUNGAL INFECTIONS OF THE SKIN

Mycotic infections are traditionally divided into two principal groups—superficial and deep. In this chapter, we will discuss only the superficial infections: tinea corporis and tinea cruris; dermatophytosis of the feet and dermatophytid of the hands; tinea unguium (onychomycosis); and tinea versicolor. See Chapter 36 for discussion of deep mycoses.

The diagnosis of fungal infections of the skin is usually based on the location and characteristics of the lesions and on the following laboratory examinations: (1) Direct demonstration of fungi in 10% KOH of scrapings from suspected lesions. "If it's scaly, scrape it" is a time-honored maxim (Figure 6–11). (2) Cultures of organisms from skin scrapings. (3) Histologic sections of biopsies stained with periodic acid-Schiff (Hotchkiss-McManus) technique may be diagnostic if scrapings and cultures are falsely negative.

► **Principles of Treatment**

A diagnosis should always be confirmed by KOH preparation, culture, or biopsy. Many other diseases cause scaling, and use of an antifungal agent without a firm diagnosis

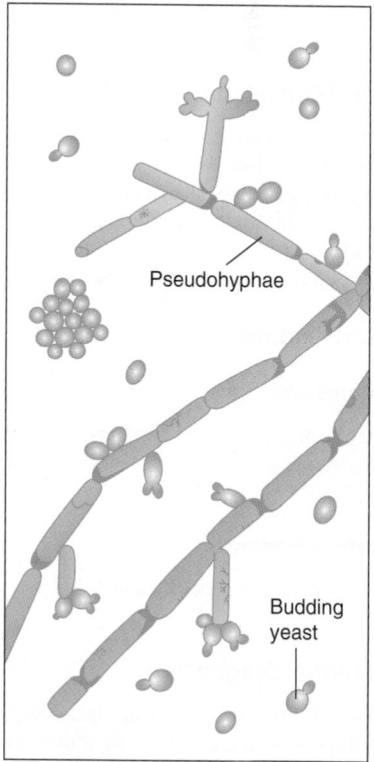

▲ **Figure 6–11.** KOH preparation of fungus demonstrating pseudohyphae and budding yeast forms. (Reproduced, with permission, from Nicoll D et al. *Pocket Guide to Diagnostic Tests,* 6th ed. McGraw-Hill, 2012.)

makes subsequent diagnosis more difficult. In general, fungal infections are treated topically except for those involving the nails, those that are very extensive, or those that involve the hair follicles. In these situations, oral agents may be useful, with special attention to their side effects and complications, including hepatic toxicity.

General Measures & Prevention

Since moist skin favors the growth of fungi, dry the skin carefully after bathing or after perspiring heavily. Talc or other drying powders may be useful. The use of topical corticosteroids for other diseases may be complicated by intercurrent tinea or candidal infection, and topical antifungals are often used in intertriginous areas with corticosteroids to prevent this.

1. Tinea Corporis or Tinea Circinata (Body Ringworm)

> ### ESSENTIALS OF DIAGNOSIS
>
> ▶ Ring-shaped lesions with an advancing scaly border and central clearing or scaly patches with a distinct border.
>
> ▶ On exposed skin surfaces or the trunk.
>
> ▶ Microscopic examination of scrapings or culture confirms the diagnosis.

General Considerations

The lesions are often on exposed areas of the body such as the face and arms. A history of exposure to an infected cat may occasionally be obtained, usually indicating *Microsporum* infection. *Trichophyton rubrum* is the most common pathogen, usually representing extension onto the trunk or extremities of tinea cruris, pedis, or manuum.

Clinical Findings

A. Symptoms and Signs

Itching may be present. In classic lesions, rings of erythema have an advancing scaly border and central clearing (Figure 6–12).

B. Laboratory Findings

The diagnosis should be confirmed by KOH preparation or culture.

Differential Diagnosis

Positive fungal studies distinguish tinea corporis from other skin lesions with annular configuration, such as the annular lesions of psoriasis, lupus erythematosus, syphilis, granuloma annulare, and pityriasis rosea. Psoriasis has typical lesions on elbows, knees, scalp, and nails. Secondary syphilis is often manifested by characteristic palmar,

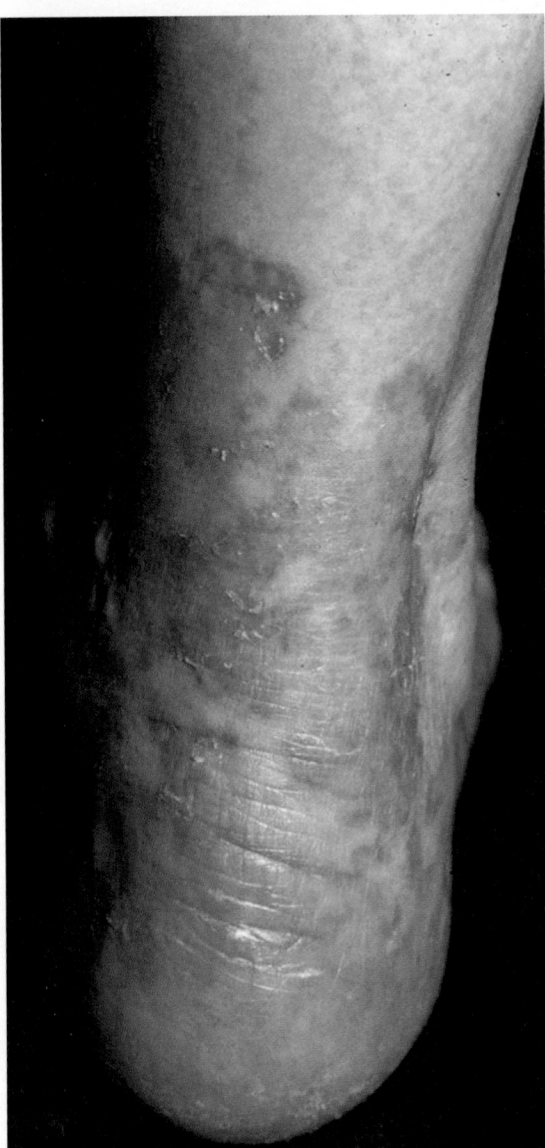

▲ **Figure 6–12.** Tinea pedis and corporis. (Used, with permission, from Berger TG, Dept Dermatology, UCSF.)

plantar, and mucous membrane lesions. Tinea corporis rarely has the large number of symmetric lesions seen in pityriasis rosea. Granuloma annulare lacks scales.

Complications

Complications include extension of the disease down the hair follicles (in which case it becomes much more difficult to cure) and pyoderma.

Prevention

Treat infected household pets (*Microsporum* infections). To prevent recurrences, the use of foot powder and keeping feet dry by wearing sandals, or changing socks can be useful.

Treatment

A. Local Measures

Tinea corporis responds to most topical antifungals, including miconazole, clotrimazole, butenafine, and terbinafine, which are available over the counter (see Table 6–2). Terbinafine and butenafine require shorter courses and lead to the most rapid response. Treatment should be continued for 1–2 weeks after clinical clearing. Betamethasone dipropionate with clotrimazole (Lotrisone) is not recommended. Long-term improper use may result in side effects from the high-potency corticosteroid component, especially in body folds. Cases of tinea that are clinically resistant to this combination but respond to topical antifungals without the topical corticosteroid can occur.

B. Systemic Measures

Griseofulvin (ultramicrosize), 250–500 mg twice daily, is used. Typically, 4–6 weeks of therapy are required. Itraconazole as a single week-long pulse of 200 mg daily is also effective in tinea corporis. Terbinafine, 250 mg daily for 1 month, is an alternative.

Prognosis

Body ringworm usually responds promptly to conservative topical therapy or to an oral agent within 4 weeks.

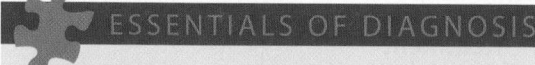

Rotta I et al. Efficacy of topical antifungals in the treatment of dermatophytosis: a mixed-treatment comparison meta-analysis involving 14 treatments. JAMA Dermatol. 2013 Mar;149(3):341–9. [PMID: 23553036]

2. Tinea Cruris (Jock Itch)

ESSENTIALS OF DIAGNOSIS

▸ Marked itching in intertriginous areas, usually sparing the scrotum.

▸ Peripherally spreading, sharply demarcated, centrally clearing erythematous lesions.

▸ May have associated tinea infection of feet or toenails.

▸ Laboratory examination with microscope or culture confirms diagnosis.

General Considerations

Tinea cruris lesions are confined to the groin and gluteal cleft. Intractable pruritus ani may occasionally be caused by a tinea infection.

Clinical Findings

A. Symptoms and Signs

Itching may be severe, or the rash may be asymptomatic. The lesions have sharp margins, cleared centers, and active, spreading scaly peripheries. Follicular pustules are sometimes encountered. The area may be hyperpigmented on resolution.

B. Laboratory Findings

Hyphae can be demonstrated microscopically in KOH preparations. The organism may be cultured.

Differential Diagnosis

Tinea cruris must be distinguished from other lesions involving the intertriginous areas, such as candidiasis, seborrheic dermatitis, intertrigo, psoriasis of body folds ("inverse psoriasis"), and erythrasma. Candidiasis is generally bright red and marked by satellite papules and pustules outside of the main border of the lesion. *Candida* typically involves the scrotum. Seborrheic dermatitis also often involves the face, sternum, and axillae. Intertrigo tends to be more red, less scaly, and present in obese individuals in moist body folds with less extension onto the thigh. Inverse psoriasis is characterized by distinct plaques. Other areas of typical psoriatic involvement should be checked, and the KOH examination will be negative. Erythrasma is best diagnosed with Wood (ultraviolet) light—a brilliant coral-red fluorescence is seen.

Treatment

A. General Measures

Drying powder (eg, miconazole nitrate [Zeasorb-AF]) can be dusted into the involved area in patients with excessive perspiration or occlusion of skin due to obesity.

B. Local Measures

Any of the topical antifungal preparations listed in Table 6–2 may be used. Terbinafine cream is curative in over 80% of cases after once-daily use for 7 days.

C. Systemic Measures

Griseofulvin ultramicrosize is reserved for severe cases. Give 250–500 mg orally twice daily for 1–2 weeks. One week of either itraconazole, 200 mg daily, or terbinafine, 250 mg daily, can be effective.

Prognosis

Tinea cruris usually responds promptly to topical or systemic treatment but often recurs.

3. Tinea Manuum & Tinea Pedis (Dermatophytosis, Tinea of Palms & Soles, "Athlete's Foot")

ESSENTIALS OF DIAGNOSIS

▸ Most often presenting with asymptomatic scaling.

▸ May progress to fissuring or maceration in toe web spaces.

► Common cofactor in lower leg cellulitis.

► Itching, burning, and stinging of interdigital web; scaling palms, and soles; vesicles of soles in inflammatory cases.

► The fungus is shown in skin scrapings examined microscopically or by culture of scrapings.

General Considerations

Tinea of the feet is an extremely common acute or chronic dermatosis. Most infections are caused by Trichophyton species.

Clinical Findings

A. Symptoms and Signs

The presenting symptom may be itching, burning, or stinging. Pain may indicate secondary infection with complicating cellulitis. **Interdigital tinea pedis is the most common predisposing cause of lower leg cellulitis in healthy individuals.** Regular examination of the feet of diabetic patients for evidence of scaling and fissuring and treatment of any identified tinea pedis may prevent complications. Tinea pedis has several presentations that vary with the location. On the sole and heel, tinea may appear as chronic noninflammatory scaling, occasionally with thickening and fissuring. This may extend over the sides of the feet in a "moccasin" distribution. The KOH preparation is usually positive. Tinea pedis often appears as a scaling or fissuring of the toe webs, perhaps with sodden maceration (Figure 6–13). As the web spaces become more macerated, the KOH preparation and fungal culture are less often positive because bacterial species begin to dominate. Finally, there may also be grouped vesicles distributed anywhere on the soles, generalized exfoliation of the skin of the soles, or nail

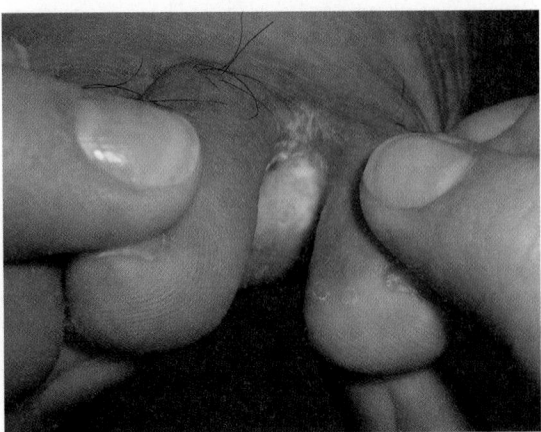

▲ **Figure 6–13.** Tinea pedis in the interdigital space between fourth and fifth digits. (Courtesy of Richard P. Usatine, MD; used, with permission, from Usatine RP, Smith MA, Mayeaux EJ Jr, Chumley H, Tysinger J. *The Color Atlas of Family Medicine*. McGraw-Hill, 2009.)

involvement in the form of discoloration and thickening and crumbling of the nail plate.

B. Laboratory Findings

KOH and culture does not always demonstrate pathogenic fungi from macerated areas.

Differential Diagnosis

Differentiate from other skin conditions involving the same areas, such as interdigital erythrasma (use Wood light). Psoriasis may be a cause of chronic scaling on the palms or soles and may cause nail changes. Repeated fungal cultures should be negative, and the condition will not respond to antifungal therapy. Contact dermatitis will often involve the dorsal surfaces and will respond to topical or systemic corticosteroids. Vesicular lesions should be differentiated from pompholyx (dyshidrosis) and scabies by proper scraping of the roofs of individual vesicles. Rarely, gram-negative organisms may cause toe web infections, manifested as an acute erosive flare of interdigital disease. This entity is treated with aluminum salts (see below) and imidazole antifungal agents or ciclopirox.

Prevention

The essential factor in prevention is personal hygiene. Wear open-toed sandals if possible. Use of sandals in community showers and bathing places is often recommended, though the effectiveness of this practice has not been studied. Careful drying between the toes after showering is essential. A hair dryer used on low setting may be used. Socks should be changed frequently, and absorbent nonsynthetic socks are preferred. Apply dusting and drying powders as necessary. The use of powders containing antifungal agents (eg, Zeasorb-AF) or chronic use of antifungal creams may prevent recurrences of tinea pedis.

Treatment

A. Local Measures

1. Macerated stage—Treat with aluminum subacetate solution soaks for 20 minutes twice daily. Broad-spectrum antifungal creams and solutions (containing imidazoles or ciclopirox instead of tolnaftate and haloprogin) will help combat diphtheroids and other gram-positive organisms present at this stage and alone may be adequate therapy. If topical imidazoles fail, 1 week of once-daily topical allylamine treatment (terbinafine or butenafine) will often result in clearing.

2. Dry and scaly stage—Use any of the antifungal agents listed in Table 6–2. The addition of urea 10–20% lotion or cream may increase the efficacy of topical treatments in thick ("moccasin") tinea of the soles.

B. Systemic Measures

Griseofulvin may be used for severe cases or those recalcitrant to topical therapy. If the infection is cleared by systemic therapy, the patient should be encouraged to begin maintenance with topical therapy, since recurrence is common. Itraconazole, 200 mg daily for 2 weeks or 400 mg daily for 1 week, or terbinafine, 250 mg daily for 2–4 weeks, may be used in refractory cases.

Prognosis

For many individuals, tinea pedis is a chronic affliction, temporarily cleared by therapy only to recur.

Bell-Syer SE et al. Oral treatments for fungal infections of the skin of the foot. Cochrane Database Syst Rev. 2012 Oct17;10: CD003584. [PMID: 23076898]

Matricciani L et al. Safety and efficacy of tinea pedis and onycho-mycosis treatment in people with diabetes: a systematic review. J Foot Ankle Res. 2011 Dec4;4:26. [PMID: 22136082]

Parish LC et al. A randomized, double-blind, vehicle-controlled efficacy and safety study of naftifine 2% cream in the treatment of tinea pedis. J Drugs Dermatol. 2011 Nov1;10(11): 1282–8. [PMID: 22052309]

Vanhooteghem O et al. Chronic interdigital dermatophytic infection: a common lesion associated with potentially severe consequences. Diabetes Res Clin Pract. 2011 Jan;91(1):23–5. [PMID: 21035887]

4. Tinea Versicolor (Pityriasis Versicolor)

ESSENTIALS OF DIAGNOSIS

- ▶ Velvety, tan, or pink macules or white macules that do not tan.
- ▶ Fine scales that are not visible but are seen by scraping the lesion.
- ▶ Central upper trunk the most frequent site.
- ▶ Yeast and short hyphae observed on microscopic examination of scales.

General Considerations

Tinea versicolor is a mild, superficial *Malassezia* infection of the skin (usually of the upper trunk). This yeast is a colonizer of all humans, which accounts for the high recurrence rate after treatment. The eruption is often called to patients' attention by the fact that the involved areas will not tan, and the resulting hypopigmentation may be mistaken for vitiligo. A hyperpigmented form is not uncommon.

Clinical Findings

A. Symptoms and Signs

Lesions are asymptomatic, but a few patients note itching. The lesions are velvety, tan, pink, or white macules that vary from 4–5 mm in diameter to large confluent areas. The lesions initially do not look scaly, but scales may be readily obtained by scraping the area. Lesions may appear on the trunk, upper arms, neck, and groin.

B. Laboratory Findings

Large, blunt hyphae and thick-walled budding spores ("spaghetti and meatballs") are seen on KOH. Fungal culture is not useful.

Differential Diagnosis

Vitiligo usually presents with larger periorificial lesions. Vitiligo (and not tinea versicolor) is characterized by total depigmentation, not just a lessening of pigmentation. Vitiligo does not scale. Pink and red-brown lesions on the chest are differentiated from seborrheic dermatitis of the same areas by the KOH preparation.

Treatment & Prognosis

Topical treatments include selenium sulfide lotion, which may be applied from neck to waist daily and left on for 5–15 minutes for 7 days; this treatment is repeated weekly for a month and then monthly for maintenance. Ketoconazole shampoo, 1% or 2%, lathered on the chest and back and left on for 5 minutes may also be used weekly for treatment and to prevent recurrence. Clinicians must stress to the patient that the raised and scaly aspects of the rash are being treated; the alterations in pigmentation may take months to fade or fill in.

Ketoconazole, 200 mg daily orally for 1 week or 400 mg as a single oral dose, with exercise to the point of sweating after ingestion, results in short-term cure of 90% of cases. Patients should be instructed not to shower for 8–12 hours after taking ketoconazole, because it is delivered in sweat to the skin. The single dose may not work in more hot and humid areas, and more protracted therapy carries a small risk of drug-induced hepatitis. Two doses of oral fluconazole, 300 mg, 14 days apart has similar efficacy. Without maintenance therapy, recurrences will occur in over 80% of "cured" cases over the subsequent 2 years. Imidazole creams, solutions, and lotions are quite effective for localized areas but are too expensive for use over large areas such as the chest and back.

Framil VM et al. New aspects in the clinical course of pityriasis versicolor. An Bras Dermatol. 2011 Nov–Dec;86(6):1135–40. [PMID: 22281901]

DISCOID & SUBACUTE LUPUS ERYTHEMATOSUS
(Chronic Cutaneous Lupus Erythematosus)

ESSENTIALS OF DIAGNOSIS

- ▶ Localized red plaques, usually on the face.
- ▶ Scaling, follicular plugging, atrophy, dyspigmentation, and telangiectasia of involved areas.
- ▶ Histology distinctive.
- ▶ Photosensitive.

General Considerations

The two most common forms of chronic cutaneous lupus erythematosus (CCLE) are chronic scarring (discoid) lesions (DLE) and erythematous non-scarring red plaques (subacute cutaneous LE) (SCLE). Both occur most frequently in areas exposed to solar irradiation. Permanent hair loss and loss of pigmentation are common sequelae of discoid lesions. Systemic lupus erythematosus (SLE) is discussed in Chapter 20. Patients with SLE may have DLE or SCLE lesions.

▶ Clinical Findings

A. Symptoms and Signs

Symptoms are usually mild. The lesions consist of dusky red, well-localized, single or multiple plaques, 5–20 mm in diameter, usually on the head in DLE and the trunk in SCLE. In DLE, the scalp, face, and external ears may be involved. In discoid lesions, there is atrophy, telangiectasia, depigmentation, and follicular plugging. On the scalp, significant permanent hair loss may occur in lesions of DLE. In SCLE, the lesions are erythematous annular or psoriasiform plaques up to several centimeters in diameter and favor the upper chest and back.

B. Laboratory Findings

In patients with DLE, the possibility of SLE should be considered if the following findings are present: positive antinuclear antibody (ANA), other positive serologic studies (eg, anti-double stranded DNA or anti-Smith antibody), high erythrocyte sedimentation rate, arthralgias/arthritis, presence of hypocomplementemia, widespread lesions (not localized to the head), or nail changes. Patients with marked photosensitivity and a picture otherwise suggestive of lupus may have negative ANA tests but are positive for antibodies against Ro/SSA or La/SSB (SCLE).

▶ Differential Diagnosis

The diagnosis is based on the clinical appearance confirmed by skin biopsy in all cases. In DLE, the scales are dry and "thumbtack-like" and can thus be distinguished from those of seborrheic dermatitis and psoriasis. Older lesions that have left depigmented scarring (classically in the concha of the ear) or areas of hair loss will also differentiate lupus from these diseases. Ten percent of patients with SLE have discoid skin lesions, and 5% of patients with discoid lesions have SLE. Medications (most commonly, hydrochlorothiazide, calcium channel blockers, H_2-blockers and proton pump inhibitors, ACE inhibitors, TNF inhibitors, and terbinafine) may induce SCLE with a positive Ro/SSA.

▶ Treatment

A. General Measures

Protect from sunlight. Use high-SPF (> 50) sunblock with UVB and UVA coverage daily. **Caution:** Do not use any form of radiation therapy. Avoid using drugs that are potentially photosensitizing when possible.

B. Local Treatment

For limited lesions, the following should be tried before systemic therapy: high-potency corticosteroid creams applied each night and covered with airtight, thin, pliable plastic film (eg, Saran Wrap); or Cordran tape; or ultra-high-potency corticosteroid cream or ointment applied twice daily without occlusion.

C. Local Infiltration

Triamcinolone acetonide suspension, 2.5–10 mg/mL, may be injected into the lesions of DLE once a month.

D. Systemic Treatment

1. Antimalarials—Caution: These drugs should be used only when the diagnosis is secure because they have been associated with flares of psoriasis, which may be in the differential diagnosis.

A. Hydroxychloroquine sulfate—0.2–0.4 g orally daily for several months may be effective and is often used prior to chloroquine. A minimum 3-month trial is recommended.

B. Chloroquine sulfate—250 mg daily may be effective in some cases where hydroxychloroquine is not.

C. Quinacrine (atabrine)—100 mg daily may be the safest of the antimalarials, since eye damage has not been reported. It colors the skin yellow and is therefore not acceptable to some patients. It may be added to the other antimalarials for incomplete responses.

2. Isotretinoin—Isotretinoin, 1 mg/kg/d, is effective in hypertrophic DLE lesions.

3. Thalidomide—Thalidomide is effective in refractory cases in doses of up to 300 mg daily. Monitor for neuropathy.

Both isotretinoin and thalidomide are teratogens and should be used with appropriate contraception and monitoring in women of childbearing age.

▶ Prognosis

The disease is persistent but not life-endangering unless systemic lupus is present. Treatment with one or more antimalarials is effective in more than half of cases. Although the only morbidity may be cosmetic, this can be of overwhelming significance in more darkly pigmented patients with widespread disease. Scarring alopecia can be prevented or lessened with close attention and aggressive therapy. Over years, DLE tends to become inactive. Drug-induced SCLE usually resolves over months when the inciting medication is stopped.

Cheeley J et al. Acitretin for the treatment of cutaneous T-cell lymphoma. J Am Acad Dermatol. 2013 Feb;68(2):247–54. [PMID: 22917895]

Chong BF et al. Determining risk factors for developing systemic lupus erythematosus in patients with discoid lupus erythematosus. Br J Dermatol. 2012 Jan;166(1):29–35. [PMID: 21910708]

Duarte-García A et al. Seasonal variation in the activity of systemic lupus erythematosus. J Rheumatol. 2012 Jul;39(7):1392–8. [PMID: 22660806]

Francès C et al. Low blood concentration of hydroxychloroquine in patients with refractory cutaneous lupus erythematosus: a French multicenter prospective study. Arch Dermatol. 2012 Apr;148(4):479–84. [PMID: 22508872]

Grönhagen CM et al. Subacute cutaneous lupus erythematosus and its association with drugs: a population-based matched case-control study of 234 patients in Sweden. Br J Dermatol. 2012 Aug;167(2):296–305. [PMID: 22458771]

Kuhn A et al. Photoprotective effects of a broad-spectrum sunscreen in ultraviolet-induced cutaneous lupus erythematosus: a randomized, vehicle-controlled, double-blind study. J Am Acad Dermatol. 2011 Jan;64(1):37–48. [PMID: 21167404]

Lowe G et al. A systematic review of drug-induced subacute cutaneous lupus erythematosus. Br J Dermatol. 2011 Mar;164(3):465–72. [PMID: 21039412]

Merola JF et al. Association of discoid lupus erythematosus with other clinical manifestations among patients with systemic lupus erythematosus. J Am Acad Dermatol. 2013 Jul;69(1):19–24. [PMID: 23541758]

Wahie S et al. Long-term response to hydroxychloroquine in patients with discoid lupus erythematosus. Br J Dermatol. 2013 Sep;169(3):653–9. [PMID: 23581274]

CUTANEOUS T-CELL LYMPHOMA
(Mycosis Fungoides)

ESSENTIALS OF DIAGNOSIS

► Localized or generalized erythematous scaling patches and plaques.

► Pruritus.

► Lymphadenopathy.

► Distinctive histology.

General Considerations

Mycosis fungoides is a cutaneous T-cell lymphoma that begins on the skin and may involve only the skin for years or decades. Certain medications (including selective serotonin reuptake inhibitors) and photoallergy may produce eruptions clinically and histologically identical to those of mycosis fungoides.

Clinical Findings

A. Symptoms and Signs

Localized or generalized erythematous patches or plaques are present usually on the trunk. Plaques are almost always over 5 cm in diameter. Pruritus is a frequent complaint and can be severe. IL-31 may mediate the pruritus of Sézary syndrome. The lesions often begin as nondescript or nondiagnostic patches, and it is not unusual for the patient to have skin lesions for more than a decade before the diagnosis can be confirmed. Follicular involvement with hair loss is characteristic of mycosis fungoides, and its presence should raise the suspicion of mycosis fungoides for any pruritic eruption. In more advanced cases, tumors appear. Lymphadenopathy may occur locally or widely. Lymph node enlargement may be due to benign expansion of the node (dermatopathic lymphadenopathy) or by specific involvement with mycosis fungoides.

B. Laboratory Findings

The skin biopsy remains the basis of diagnosis, though at times numerous biopsies are required before the diagnosis can be confirmed. In more advanced disease, circulating malignant T cells (Sézary cells) can be detected in the blood (T-cell gene rearrangement test). Eosinophilia may be present.

Differential Diagnosis

Mycosis fungoides may be confused with psoriasis, a drug eruption, an eczematous dermatitis, or tinea corporis. Histologic examination can distinguish these conditions.

Treatment

The treatment of mycosis fungoides is complex. Early and aggressive treatment has not proved to cure or prevent progression of the disease. Skin-directed therapies, including topical corticosteroids, topical mechlorethamine, bexarotene gel, and UV phototherapy, are used initially. If the disease progresses, PUVA plus retinoids, PUVA plus interferon, extracorporeal photophoresis, bexarotene, alpha-interferon with or without retinoids, interleukin 12, denileukin, and total skin electron beam treatment are used.

Prognosis

Mycosis fungoides is usually slowly progressive (over decades). Prognosis is better in patients with patch or plaque stage disease and worse in patients with erythroderma, tumors, and lymphadenopathy. Survival is not reduced in patients with limited patch disease. Elderly patients with limited patch and plaque stage disease commonly die of other causes. Overly aggressive treatment may lead to complications and premature demise.

Cheeley J et al. Acitretin for the treatment of cutaneous T-cell lymphoma. J Am Acad Dermatol. 2013 Feb;68(2):247–54. [PMID: 22917895]

Deonizio JM et al. The role of molecular analysis in cutaneous lymphomas. Semin Cutan Med Surg. 2012 Dec;31(4):234–40. [PMID: 23174493]

Ohmatsu H et al. Serum IL-31 levels are increased in patients with cutaneous T-cell lymphoma. Acta Derm Venereol. 2012 May;92(3):282–3. [PMID: 22456907]

Olsen EA et al. Clinical end points and response criteria in mycosis fungoides and Sézary syndrome: a consensus statement of the International Society for Cutaneous Lymphomas, the United States Cutaneous Lymphoma Consortium, and the Cutaneous Lymphoma Task Force of the European Organisation for the Research and Treatment of Cancer. J Clin Oncol. 2011 Jun20;29(18):2598–607. [PMID: 21576639]

Weberschock T et al. Interventions for mycosis fungoides. Cochrane Database Syst Rev. 2012 Sep12;9: CD008946. [PMID: 22972128]

EXFOLIATIVE DERMATITIS
(Exfoliative Erythroderma)

ESSENTIALS OF DIAGNOSIS

► Scaling and erythema over most of the body.

► Itching, malaise, fever, chills, weight loss.

General Considerations

Erythroderma describes generalized redness and scaling of the skin of > 30% BSA. A preexisting dermatosis is the cause of exfoliative dermatitis in two-thirds of cases, including psoriasis, atopic dermatitis, contact dermatitis, pityriasis rubra pilaris, and seborrheic dermatitis. Reactions to topical or systemic drugs account for about 15% of cases, cancer (underlying lymphoma, solid tumors and, most commonly, cutaneous T-cell lymphoma) for about 10%, and 10% are idiopathic. Causation of the remainder is indeterminable. At the time of acute presentation, without a clear-cut prior history of skin disease or drug exposure, it may be impossible to make a specific diagnosis of the underlying condition, and diagnosis may require continued observation.

Clinical Findings

A. Symptoms and Signs

Symptoms may include itching, weakness, malaise, fever, and weight loss. Chills are prominent. Redness and scaling is widespread. Loss of hair and nails can occur. Generalized lymphadenopathy may be due to lymphoma or leukemia or may be reactive. The mucosae are spared.

B. Laboratory Findings

A skin biopsy is required and may show changes of a specific inflammatory dermatitis or cutaneous T-cell lymphoma. Peripheral leukocytes may show clonal rearrangements of the T-cell receptor in Sézary syndrome.

Differential Diagnosis

It may be impossible to identify the cause of exfoliative erythroderma early in the course of the disease, so careful follow-up is necessary.

Complications

Debility (protein loss) and dehydration may develop in patients with generalized inflammatory exfoliative erythroderma; or sepsis may occur.

Treatment

A. Topical Therapy

Home treatment is with cool to tepid baths and application of mid-potency corticosteroids under wet dressings or with the use of an occlusive plastic suit. If the exfoliative erythroderma becomes chronic and is not manageable in an outpatient setting, the patient should be hospitalized. Keep the room at a constant warm temperature and provide the same topical treatment as for an outpatient.

B. Specific Measures

Stop all medications, if possible. Systemic corticosteroids may provide spectacular improvement in severe or fulminant exfoliative dermatitis, but long-term therapy should be avoided (see Chapter 26). In addition, systemic corticosteroids must be used with caution because some patients with erythroderma have psoriasis and could develop pustular psoriasis. For cases of psoriatic erythroderma and pityriasis rubra pilaris, acitretin, methotrexate, cyclosporine, or a TNF inhibitor may be indicated. Erythroderma secondary to lymphoma or leukemia requires specific topical or systemic chemotherapy. Suitable antibiotic drugs with coverage for *Staphylococcus* should be given when there is evidence of bacterial infection.

Prognosis

Most patients recover completely or improve greatly over time but may require long-term therapy. Deaths are rare in the absence of cutaneous T-cell lymphoma. A minority of patients will suffer from undiminished erythroderma for indefinite periods.

Bhandarkar AP et al. Nevirapine induced exfoliative dermatitis in an HIV-infected patient. Indian J Pharmacol. 2011 Nov;43(6):738–9. [PMID: 22144790]

Li J et al. Erythroderma: a clinical and prognostic study. Dermatology. 2012;225(2):154–62. [PMID: 23037884]

Mumoli N et al. Severe exfoliative dermatitis caused by esomeprazole. J Am Geriatr Soc. 2011 Dec;59(12):2377–8. [PMID: 22188084]

Zattra E et al. Erythroderma in the era of biological therapies. Eur J Dermatol. 2012 Mar–Apr;22(2):167–71. [PMID: 22321651]

MISCELLANEOUS SCALING DERMATOSES

Isolated scaly patches may represent actinic (solar) keratoses, nonpigmented seborrheic keratoses, or Bowen or Paget disease.

1. Actinic Keratoses

Actinic keratoses are small (0.2–0.6 cm) macules or papules—flesh-colored, pink, or slightly hyperpigmented—that feel like sandpaper and are tender when the finger is drawn over them. They occur on sun-exposed parts of the body in persons of fair complexion. Actinic keratoses are considered premalignant, but only 1:1000 lesions per year progress to become squamous cell carcinomas.

Application of liquid nitrogen is a rapid method of eradication. The lesions crust and disappear in 10–14 days. "Field treatment" with a topical agent to the anatomic area where the actinic keratoses are most prevalent (eg, forehead, dorsal hands, etc) can be considered in patients with multiple lesions in one region. The topical agents used for field treatment include fluorouracil, imiquimod, and ingenol mebutate. Photodynamic therapy can be effective in cases refractory to topical treatment. Any lesions that persist should be evaluated for possible biopsy.

Berman B et al. What is the role of field-directed therapy in the treatment of actinic keratosis? Part 2: commonly used field-directed and lesion-directed therapies. Cutis. 2012 Jun;89(6):294–301. [PMID: 22838095]

Gupta AK et al. Interventions for actinic keratoses. Cochrane Database Syst Rev. 2012 Dec12;12: CD004415. [PMID: 23235610]

Lebwohl M et al. Ingenol mebutate gel for actinic keratosis. N Engl J Med. 2012 Mar15;366(11):1010–9. [PMID: 22417254]

Morton CA et al. European guidelines for topical photodynamic therapy part 1: treatment delivery and current indications—actinic keratoses, Bowen's disease, basal cell carcinoma. J Eur Acad Dermatol Venereol. 2013 May;27(5):536–44. [PMID: 23181594]

Werner RN et al. The natural history of actinic keratosis: a systematic review. Br J Dermatol. 2013 Sep;169(3):502–18. [PMID: 23647091]

2. Bowen Disease & Paget Disease

Bowen disease (intraepidermal squamous cell carcinoma) can develop on both sun-exposed and non–sun-exposed skin. The lesion is usually a small (0.5–3 cm), well-demarcated, slightly raised, pink to red, scaly plaque and may resemble psoriasis or a large actinic keratosis. These lesions may progress to invasive squamous cell carcinoma. Excision or other definitive treatment is indicated.

Extramammary Paget disease, a manifestation of intraepidermal carcinoma or underlying genitourinary or gastrointestinal cancer, resembles chronic eczema and usually involves apocrine areas such as the genitalia. Mammary Paget disease of the nipple, a unilateral or rarely bilateral red scaling plaque that may ooze, is associated with an underlying intraductal mammary carcinoma (Figure 6–14). While these lesions appear as red patches and plaques in fair-skinned persons, in Asians, Hispanics, and other persons of color, hyperpigmentation may be prominent.

Bath-Hextall FJ et al. Interventions for cutaneous Bowen's disease. Cochrane Database Syst Rev. 2013 Jun24;6: CD007281. [PMID: 23794286]

Hida T et al. Pigmented mammary Paget's disease mimicking melanoma: report of three cases. Eur J Dermatol. 2012 Jan–Feb;22(1):121–4. [PMID: 22064040]

Sandoval-Leon AC et al. Paget's disease of the nipple. Breast Cancer Res Treat. 2013 Aug;141(1):1–12. [PMID: 23929251]

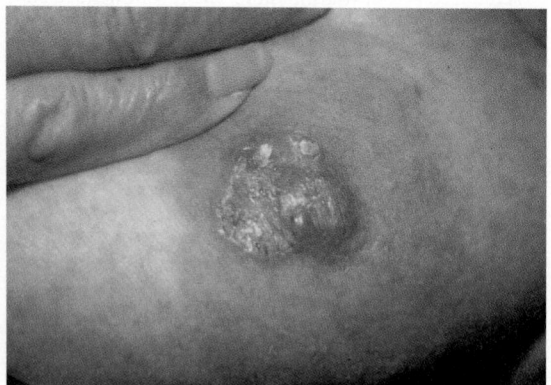

▲ **Figure 6–14.** Paget disease of the breast surrounding the nipple. (Courtesy of the University of Texas Health Sciences Center, Division of Dermatology; used, with permission, from Usatine RP, Smith MA, Mayeaux EJ Jr, Chumley H, Tysinger J. *The Color Atlas of Family Medicine.* McGraw-Hill, 2009.)

INTERTRIGO

Intertrigo is caused by the macerating effect of heat, moisture, and friction. It is especially likely to occur in obese persons and in humid climates. The symptoms are itching, stinging, and burning. The body folds develop fissures, erythema, and sodden epidermis, with superficial denudation. Candidiasis may complicate intertrigo. "Inverse psoriasis," seborrheic dermatitis, tinea cruris, erythrasma, and candidiasis must be ruled out.

Maintain hygiene in the area, and keep it dry. Compresses may be useful acutely. Hydrocortisone 1% cream plus an imidazole or nystatin cream is effective. Recurrences are common.

VESICULAR DERMATOSES

HERPES SIMPLEX
(Cold or Fever Sore; Genital Herpes)

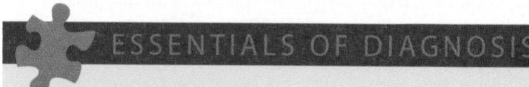

ESSENTIALS OF DIAGNOSIS

► Recurrent small grouped vesicles on an erythematous base, especially in the orolabial and genital areas.

► May follow minor infections, trauma, stress, or sun exposure; regional lymph nodes may be swollen and tender.

► Viral cultures and direct fluorescent antibody tests are positive.

► General Considerations

Over 85% of adults have serologic evidence of herpes simplex type 1 (HSV-1) infections, most often acquired asymptomatically in childhood. Occasionally, primary infections may be manifested as severe gingivostomatitis. Thereafter, the patient may have recurrent self-limited attacks, provoked by sun exposure, orofacial surgery, fever, or a viral infection.

About 25% of the United States population has serologic evidence of infection with herpes simplex type 2 (HSV-2). HSV-2 causes lesions whose morphology and natural history are similar to those caused by HSV-1 but are typically located on the genitalia of both sexes. The infection is acquired by sexual contact. In monogamous heterosexual couples where one partner has HSV-2 infection, seroconversion of the noninfected partner occurs in 10% over a 1-year period. Up to 70% of such infections appeared to be transmitted during periods of asymptomatic shedding. Genital herpes may also be due to HSV-1.

► Clinical Findings

A. Symptoms and Signs

The principal symptoms are burning and stinging. Neuralgia may precede or accompany attacks. The lesions consist

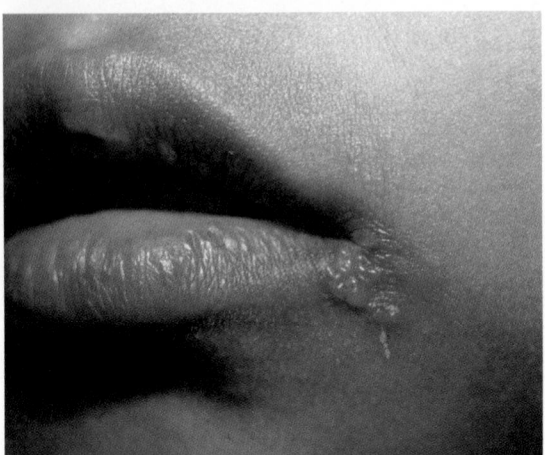

▲ **Figure 6–15.** Herpes simplex type 1 vesicles at the vermillion border of the lip. (Courtesy of Richard P. Usatine, MD; used, with permission, from Usatine RP, Smith MA, Mayeaux EJ Jr, Chumley H, Tysinger J. *The Color Atlas of Family Medicine.* McGraw-Hill, 2009.)

of small, grouped vesicles that can occur anywhere but which most often occur on the vermilion border of the lips (Figure 6–15), the penile shaft, the labia, the perianal skin, and the buttocks. Any erosion in the anogenital region can be due to herpes simplex. Regional lymph nodes may be swollen and tender. The lesions usually crust and heal in 1 week.

B. Laboratory Findings

Lesions of herpes simplex must be distinguished from chancroid, syphilis, pyoderma, or trauma. Direct fluorescent antibody slide tests offer rapid, sensitive diagnosis. Viral culture may also be helpful. Herpes serology is not used in the diagnosis of an acute genital ulcer. However, specific HSV-2 serology by Western blot assay or enzyme-linked immunosorbent assay (ELISA) can determine who is HSV-infected and potentially infectious. Such testing is very useful in couples in which only one partner reports a history of genital herpes.

► Complications

Complications include pyoderma, eczema herpeticum, herpetic whitlow, herpes gladiatorum (epidemic herpes in wrestlers transmitted by contact), proctitis, esophagitis, neonatal infection, keratitis, and encephalitis.

► Prevention

The use of latex condoms and patient education have proved effective in reducing genital herpes transmission in some studies but have not proved beneficial in others. No single or combination intervention absolutely prevents transmission. Sunscreens are useful adjuncts in preventing sun-induced HSV-1 recurrences. Prophylactic use of oral acyclovir (200 mg four times daily) may prevent herpes recurrences. Comparable doses are 500 mg twice daily for

valacyclovir and 250 mg twice daily for famciclovir. A preventive antiviral medication should be started beginning 24 hours prior to ultraviolet light exposure, dental surgery, or orolabial cosmetic surgery.

► Treatment

A. Systemic Therapy

Three systemic agents are available for the treatment of herpes infections: acyclovir, its valine analog valacyclovir, and famciclovir. All three agents are very effective and, when used properly, virtually nontoxic. Only acyclovir is available for intravenous administration. In the immunocompetent, with the exception of severe orolabial herpes, only genital disease is treated. For first clinical episodes of herpes simplex, the dosage of acyclovir is 400 mg orally five times daily (or 800 mg three times daily); of valacyclovir, 1000 mg twice daily; and of famciclovir, 250 mg three times daily. The duration of treatment is from 7 to 10 days depending on the severity of the outbreak.

Most cases of recurrent herpes are mild and do not require therapy. In addition, pharmacotherapy of recurrent HSV is of limited benefit, with studies finding a reduction in the average outbreak by only 12–24 hours. To be effective, the treatment must be initiated by the patient at the first sign of recurrence. If treatment is desired, recurrent genital herpes outbreaks may be treated with 3 days of valacyclovir, 500 mg twice daily, 5 days of acyclovir, 200 mg five times a day, or 5 days of famciclovir, 125 mg twice daily. Valacyclovir, 2 g twice daily for 1 day, or famciclovir, 1 g once or twice in 1 day, are equally effective short-course alternatives, and can abort impending recurrences of both orolabial and genital herpes. The addition of a potent topical corticosteroid three times daily reduces the duration, size, and pain of orolabial herpes treated with an oral antiviral agent.

In patients with frequent or severe recurrences, suppressive therapy is most effective in controlling disease. Suppressive treatment will reduce outbreaks by 85% and reduces viral shedding by > 90%. This results in about a 50% reduced risk of transmission. The recommended suppressive doses, taken continuously, are acyclovir, 400 mg twice daily; valacyclovir, 500 mg once daily; or famciclovir, 125–250 mg twice daily. Long-term suppression appears very safe, and after 5–7 years a substantial proportion of patients can discontinue treatment.

B. Local Measures

In general, topical therapy has only limited efficacy. It is strongly urged that 5% acyclovir ointment, if used at all, be limited to the restricted indications for which it has been approved, ie, initial herpes genitalis and mucocutaneous herpes simplex infections in immunocompromised patients. Penciclovir cream, to be applied at the first symptom every 2 hours while awake for 4 days for recurrent orolabial herpes, reduces the average attack duration from 5 days to 4.5 days.

► Prognosis

Aside from the complications described above, recurrent attacks last several days, and patients recover without sequelae.

Antonelli G et al. Antiviral therapy: old and current issues. Int J Antimicrob Agents. 2012 Aug;40(2):95–102. [PMID: 22727532]

Kinchington PR et al. Herpes simplex virus and varicella zoster virus, the house guests who never leave. Herpesviridae. 2012 Jun12;3(1): 5. [PMID: 22691604]

HERPES ZOSTER (Shingles)

ESSENTIALS OF DIAGNOSIS

▶ Pain along the course of a nerve followed by grouped vesicular lesions.

▶ Involvement is unilateral; some lesions (< 20) may occur outside the affected dermatome.

▶ Lesions are usually on face or trunk.

▶ Direct fluorescent antibody positive, especially in vesicular lesions.

General Considerations

Herpes zoster is an acute vesicular eruption due to the varicella-zoster virus. It usually occurs in adults. With rare exceptions, patients suffer only one attack. Dermatomal herpes zoster does not imply the presence of a visceral malignancy. Generalized disease, however, raises the suspicion of an associated immunosuppressive disorder such as HIV infection. HIV-infected patients are 20 times more likely to develop zoster, often before other clinical findings of HIV disease are present. A history of HIV risk factors and HIV testing when appropriate should be considered, especially in patients with zoster who are younger than 55 years.

Clinical Findings

Pain usually precedes the eruption by 48 hours or more and may persist and actually increase in intensity after the lesions have disappeared. The lesions consist of grouped, tense, deep-seated vesicles distributed unilaterally along a dermatome (Figure 6–16). The most common distributions are on the trunk or face. Up to 20 lesions may be found outside the affected dermatomes, even in immune-competent persons. Regional lymph glands may be tender and swollen.

Differential Diagnosis

Since poison oak and poison ivy dermatitis can occur unilaterally, they must be differentiated at times from herpes zoster. Allergic contact dermatitis is pruritic; zoster is painful. One must differentiate herpes zoster from lesions of herpes simplex, which occasionally occurs in a dermatomal distribution. Doses of antivirals appropriate for zoster should be used in the absence of a clear diagnosis. Facial zoster may simulate erysipelas initially, but zoster is unilateral and shows vesicles after 24–48 hours. Depending on the dermatome involved, the pain of preeruptive herpes

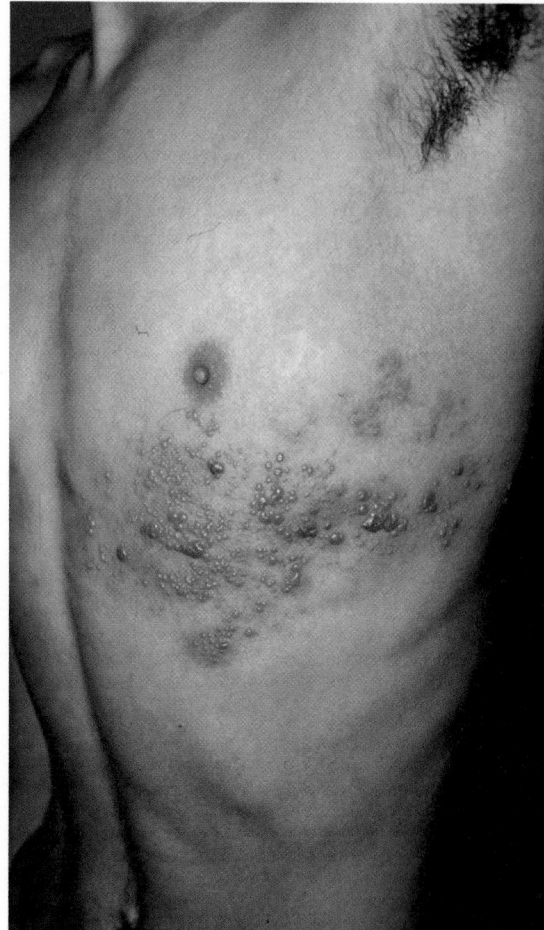

▲ **Figure 6–16.** Herpes zoster. (Used, with permission, from Berger TG, Dept Dermatology, UCSF.)

zoster may lead the clinician to diagnose migraine, myocardial infarction, acute abdomen, herniated disk, etc.

Complications

Sacral zoster may be associated with bladder and bowel dysfunction. Persistent neuralgia, anesthesia or scarring of the affected area, facial or other nerve paralysis, and encephalitis may occur. Postherpetic neuralgia is most common after involvement of the trigeminal region, and in patients over the age of 55. Early (within 72 hours after onset) and aggressive antiviral treatment of herpes zoster reduces the severity and duration of postherpetic neuralgia. Zoster ophthalmicus (V_1) can result in visual impairment.

Prevention

An effective live herpes zoster vaccine (Zostavax) is available and recommended to prevent both herpes zoster and postherpetic neuralgia. It is approved for persons over the age of 50 and recommended in persons aged 60 and older, even in those who have had zoster.

Treatment

A. General Measures

1. Immunocompetent host—Antiviral treatment within 72 hours of rash decreases the duration and severity of acute herpes zoster. Since such treatment also reduces postherpetic neuralgia, those with a risk of developing this complication should be treated (ie, those over age 50 and those with nontruncal eruption). In addition, younger patients with acute moderate to severe pain or rash may benefit from effective antiviral therapy. Treatment can be given with oral acyclovir, 800 mg five times daily; famciclovir, 500 mg three times daily; or valacyclovir, 1 g three times daily—all for 7 days (see Chapter 32). For reasons of increased bioavailability and ease of dosing schedule, the preferred agents are those given three times daily. Patients should maintain good hydration. The dose of antiviral should be adjusted for kidney function as recommended. Nerve blocks may be used in the management of initial severe pain. Ophthalmologic consultation is vital for involvement of the first branch of the trigeminal nerve, even if the patient has no ocular symptoms.

Systemic corticosteroids are effective in reducing acute pain, improving quality of life, and returning patients to normal activities much more quickly. They do not increase the risk of dissemination in immunocompetent hosts. If not contraindicated, a tapering 3-week course of prednisone, starting at 60 mg/d, should be considered for its adjunctive benefit in immunocompetent patients. Oral corticosteroids do not reduce the prevalence, severity, or duration of postherpetic neuralgia beyond that achieved by effective antiviral therapy. Adequate analgesia, including the use of opioids, tricyclic antidepressants, and gabapentin as necessary, should be given from the onset of zoster-associated pain.

2. Immunocompromised host—Given the safety and efficacy of currently available antivirals, most immunocompromised patients with herpes zoster are candidates for antiviral therapy. The dosage schedule is as listed above, but treatment should be continued until the lesions have completely crusted and are healed or almost healed (up to 2 weeks). Because corticosteroids increase the risk of dissemination in immunosuppressed patients, they should not be used in these patients. Progression of disease may necessitate intravenous therapy with acyclovir, 10 mg/kg intravenously, three times daily. After 3–4 days, oral therapy may be substituted if there has been a good response to intravenous therapy. Adverse effects include decreased kidney function from crystallization, nausea and vomiting, and abdominal pain.

Foscarnet, administered in a dosage of 40 mg/kg two or three times daily intravenously, is indicated for treatment of acyclovir-resistant varicella-zoster virus infections.

B. Local Measures

Calamine or starch shake lotions may be of some help.

C. Postherpetic Neuralgia Therapy

The most effective treatment is prevention with vaccination of those at risk for developing zoster and early and aggressive antiviral therapy once zoster has occurred. Once established, postherpetic neuralgia may be treated with capsaicin ointment, 0.025–0.075%, or lidocaine (Lidoderm) topical patches. Chronic postherpetic neuralgia may be relieved by regional blocks (stellate ganglion, epidural, local infiltration, or peripheral nerve), with or without corticosteroids added to the injections. Tricyclic antidepressants, such as amitriptyline, 25–75 mg orally as a single nightly dose, are the first-line therapy beyond simple analgesics. Gabapentin, up to 3600 mg orally daily (starting at 300 mg orally three times daily), or duloxetine, up to 60–120 mg orally daily (starting at 30–60 mg orally daily) may be added for additional pain relief. Long-acting opioids may be appropriate. Referral to a pain management clinic should be considered in moderate to severe cases and in those failing the above treatments.

Prognosis

The eruption persists 2–3 weeks and usually does not recur. Motor involvement in 2–3% of patients may lead to temporary palsy.

Bruxelle J et al. Effectiveness of antiviral treatment on acute phase of herpes zoster and development of post herpetic neuralgia: review of international publications. Med Mal Infect. 2012 Feb;42(2):53–8. [PMID: 22169279]

Eilers R et al. Assessment of vaccine candidates for persons aged 50 and older: a review. BMC Geriatr. 2013 Apr15;13:32. [PMID: 23586926]

Gagliardi AM et al. Vaccines for preventing herpes zoster in older adults. Cochrane Database Syst Rev. 2012 Oct17;10: CD008858. [PMID: 23076951]

O'Connor KM et al. Herpes zoster. Med Clin North Am. 2013 Jul;97(4):503–22. [PMID: 23809711]

Thyssen JP et al. Coin exposure may cause allergic nickel dermatitis: a review. Contact Dermatitis. 2013 Jan;68(1):3–14. [PMID: 22762130]

POMPHOLYX; VESICULOBULLOUS HAND ECZEMA (Formerly Known as Dyshidrosis, Dyshidrotic Eczema)

ESSENTIALS OF DIAGNOSIS

► Pruritic "tapioca" vesicles of 1–2 mm on the palms, soles, and sides of fingers.

► Vesicles may coalesce to form multiloculated blisters.

► Scaling and fissuring may follow drying of the blisters.

► Appearance in the third decade, with lifelong recurrences.

General Considerations

This is an extremely common form of hand dermatitis, preferably called pompholyx (Gr "bubble") or vesiculobullous dermatitis of the palms and soles. About half of patients have an atopic background and many patients report flares with stress. Patients with widespread dermatitis due to any cause may develop pompholyx-like eruptions as a part of an autoeczematization response. A bullous hand dermatitis that is followed by a widespread dermatitis may develop in patients taking intravenous immunoglobin (IVIG), particularly those being treated for neurologic conditions; the dermatitis resolves over weeks to months.

Clinical Findings

Small clear vesicles stud the skin at the sides of the fingers and on the palms (Figure 6–17) or soles. They look like the grains in tapioca. They may be associated with intense itching. Later, the vesicles dry and the area becomes scaly and fissured.

Differential Diagnosis

Unroofing the vesicles and examining the blister roof with a KOH preparation will reveal hyphae in cases of bullous tinea. Always examine the feet of a patient with a hand eruption because patients with inflammatory tinea pedis may have a vesicular dermatophytid of the palms. Nonsteroidal anti-inflammatory drugs (NSAIDs) may produce

an eruption very similar to that of dyshidrosis on the hands.

▶ Prevention

There is no known way to prevent attacks if the condition is idiopathic. About one-third to one-half of patients with vesiculobullous hand dermatitis have a relevant contact allergen, especially nickel. Patch testing and avoidance of identified allergens can lead to improvement.

▶ Treatment

Topical and systemic corticosteroids help some patients dramatically. Since this is a chronic problem, systemic corticosteroids are generally not appropriate therapy. A high-potency topical corticosteroid used early in the attack may help abort the flare and ameliorate pruritus. Topical corticosteroids are also important in treating the scaling and fissuring that are seen after the vesicular phase. It is essential that patients avoid anything that irritates the skin; they should wear cotton gloves inside vinyl gloves when doing dishes or other wet chores, use long-handled brushes instead of sponges, and use a hand cream after washing the hands. Patients respond to PUVA therapy and injection of botulinum toxin into the palms as for hyperhidrosis.

▶ Prognosis

For most patients, the disease is an inconvenience. For some, vesiculobullous hand eczema can be incapacitating.

Apfelbacher C et al. Characteristics and provision of care in patients with chronic hand eczema: updated data from the CARPE Registry. Acta Derm Venereol. 2014 Feb 26;94(2): 163–7. [PMID: 23995048]
Coenraads PJ. eczema. N Engl J Med. 2012 Nov8;367(19): 1829–37. [PMID: 23134383]

PORPHYRIA CUTANEA TARDA

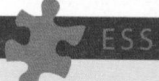

ESSENTIALS OF DIAGNOSIS

▶ Noninflammatory blisters on sun-exposed sites, especially the dorsal surfaces of the hands.

▶ Hypertrichosis, skin fragility.

▶ Associated liver disease.

▶ Elevated urine porphyrins.

▶ General Considerations

Porphyria cutanea tarda is the most common type of porphyria. Cases are sporadic or hereditary. The disease is associated with ingestion of certain medications (eg, estrogens), and liver disease from alcoholism or hepatitis C. In patients with liver disease, hemosiderosis is often present.

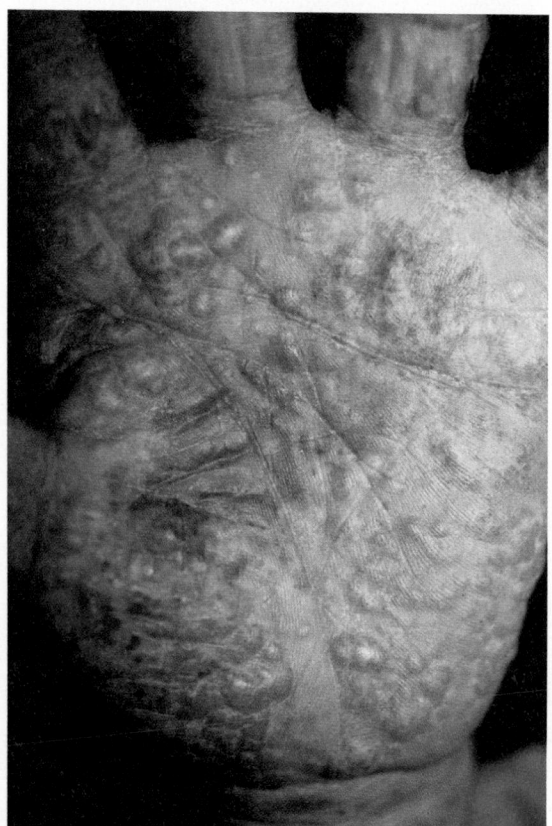

▲ **Figure 6–17.** Pompholyx (acute vesiculobullous hand eczema). (Used, with permission, from Berger TG, Dept Dermatology, UCSF.)

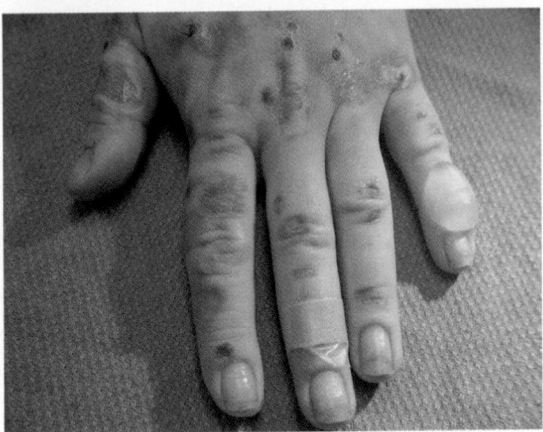

▲ **Figure 6–18.** Porphyria cutanea tarda. (Courtesy of Lewis Rose, MD; used, with permission, from Usatine RP, Smith MA, Mayeaux EJ Jr, Chumley H, Tysinger J. *The Color Atlas of Family Medicine.* McGraw-Hill, 2009.)

▶ Clinical Findings

A. Symptoms and Signs

Patients complain of painless blistering and fragility of the skin of the dorsal surfaces of the hands (Figure 6–18). Facial hypertrichosis and hyperpigmentation are common.

B. Laboratory Findings

Urinary uroporphyrins are elevated twofold to fivefold above coproporphyrins. Patients may also have abnormal liver function tests, evidence of hepatitis C infection, increased liver iron stores, and hemochromatosis gene mutations.

▶ Differential Diagnosis

Skin lesions identical to those of porphyria cutanea tarda may be seen in patients who receive maintenance dialysis and in those who take certain medications (tetracyclines and NSAIDs, especially naproxen, and voriconazole). In this so-called pseudoporphyria, the biopsy results are identical to those associated with porphyria cutanea tarda, but urine porphyrins are normal.

▶ Prevention

Barrier sun protection with clothing is required. Although the lesions are triggered by sun exposure, the wavelength of light triggering the lesions is beyond that absorbed by sunscreens.

▶ Treatment

Stopping all triggering medications and substantially reducing or stopping alcohol consumption may alone lead to improvement. Phlebotomy without oral iron supplementation at a rate of 1 unit every 2–4 weeks will gradually lead to improvement. Very low dose antimalarials (as low as 200 mg of hydroxychloroquine twice weekly), alone or in combination with phlebotomy, will increase the excretion of porphyrins, improving the skin disease. Deferasirox, an iron chelator can also improve porphyria cutanea tarda. Treatment is continued until the patient is asymptomatic. Urine porphyrins may be monitored.

▶ Prognosis

Most patients improve with treatment. Sclerodermoid skin lesions may develop on the trunk, scalp, and face.

Balwani M et al. The porphyrias: advances in diagnosis and treatment. Hematology Am Soc Hematol Educ Program. 2012;2012:19–27. [PMID: 23233556]

Borghi A et al. Prolonged cyclosporine treatment of severe or recalcitrant psoriasis: descriptive study in a series of 20 patients. Int J Dermatol. 2012 Dec;51(12):1512–6. [PMID: 23171021]

Gerstenblith MR et al. Pompholyx and eczematous reactions associated with intravenous immunoglobulin therapy. J Am Acad Dermatol. 2012 Feb;66(2):312–6. [PMID: 21601310]

Pandya AG et al. Deferasirox for porphyria cutanea tarda: a pilot study. Arch Dermatol. 2012 Aug;148(8):898–901. [PMID: 22911183]

Poh-Fitzpatrick MB. Porphyria cutanea tarda: treatment options revisited. Clin Gastroenterol Hepatol. 2012 Dec;10(12):1410–1. [PMID: 22982098]

Singal AK et al. Low-dose hydroxychloroquine is as effective as phlebotomy in treatment of patients with porphyria cutanea tarda. Clin Gastroenterol Hepatol. 2012 Dec;10(12):1402–9. [PMID: 22985607]

Van Meter JR et al. Iron, genes, and viruses: the porphyria cutanea tarda triple threat. Cutis. 2011 Aug;88(2):73–6. [PMID: 21916273]

DERMATITIS HERPETIFORMIS

Dermatitis herpetiformis is an uncommon disease manifested by pruritic papules, vesicles, and papulovesicles mainly on the elbows, knees, buttocks, posterior neck, and scalp. It appears to have its highest prevalence in Scandinavia and is associated with HLA antigens -B8, -DR3, and -DQ2. The diagnosis is made by light microscopy. Circulating antibodies to tissue transglutaminase are present in 90% of cases. NSAIDs may cause flares. Patients have gluten-sensitive enteropathy, but for the great majority it is subclinical. However, ingestion of gluten is the cause of the disease, and strict long-term avoidance of dietary gluten has been shown to decrease the dose of dapsone (usually 100–200 mg daily) required to control the disease and may even eliminate the need for treatment. Patients with dermatitis herpetiformis are at increased risk for development of gastrointestinal lymphoma, and this risk is reduced by a gluten-free diet.

Bolotin D et al. Dermatitis herpetiformis. Part I. Epidemiology, pathogenesis, and clinical presentation. J Am Acad Dermatol. 2011 Jun;64(6):1017–24. [PMID: 21571167]

Bolotin D et al. Dermatitis herpetiformis. Part II. Diagnosis, management, and prognosis. J Am Acad Dermatol. 2011 Jun;64(6):1027–33. [PMID: 21571168]

Cardones AR et al. Management of dermatitis herpetiformis. Immunol Allergy Clin North Am. 2012 May;32(2):275–81. [PMID: 22560140]

Kárpáti S et al. Dermatitis herpetiformis. Clin Dermatol. 2012 Jan–Feb;30(1):56–9. [PMID: 22137227]

WEEPING OR CRUSTED LESIONS

IMPETIGO

ESSENTIALS OF DIAGNOSIS

▸ Superficial blisters filled with purulent material that rupture easily.

▸ Crusted superficial erosions.

▸ Positive Gram stain and bacterial culture.

▸ General Considerations

Impetigo is a contagious and autoinoculable infection of the skin caused by staphylococci or streptococci.

▸ Clinical Findings

A. Symptoms and Signs

The lesions consist of macules, vesicles, bullae, pustules, and honey-colored gummy crusts that when removed leave denuded red areas (Figure 6–19). The face and other exposed parts are most often involved. **Ecthyma** is a deeper form of impetigo caused by staphylococci or streptococci, with ulceration and scarring. It occurs frequently on the extremities.

B. Laboratory Findings

Gram stain and culture confirm the diagnosis. In temperate climates, most cases are associated with *S aureus* infection. *Streptococcus* species are more common in tropical infections.

▸ Differential Diagnosis

The main differential diagnoses are acute allergic contact dermatitis and herpes simplex. Contact dermatitis may be suggested by the history or by linear distribution of the lesions, and culture should be negative for staphylococci and streptococci. Herpes simplex infection usually presents with grouped vesicles or discrete erosions and may be associated with a history of recurrences. Viral cultures are positive.

▸ Treatment

Soaks and scrubbing can be beneficial, especially in unroofing lakes of pus under thick crusts. Topical agents such as bacitracin, mupirocin, or retapamulin can be attempted for infections limited to small areas. Mupirocin and retapamulin are more expensive than systemic treatments. In most cases, systemic antibiotics are indicated. Cephalexin, 250 mg four times daily, is usually effective. Doxycycline, 100 mg twice daily, is a reasonable alternative. Community-associated methicillin-resistant *S aureus* (CA-MRSA) may cause impetigo, and initial coverage for MRSA could include doxycycline, clindamycin, or trimethoprim-sulfamethoxazole (TMP-SMZ). About 50% of CA-MRSA cases are quinolone resistant. Recurrent impetigo is associated with nasal carriage of *S aureus* and is treated with rifampin, 600 mg daily for 5 days. Intranasal mupirocin ointment twice daily for 5 days clears the carriage of 40% of MRSA strains. Bleach baths (¼ to ½ cup per 20 liters of bathwater for 15 minutes 3–5 times weekly) for all family members, and the use of dilute household bleach to clean showers and other bath surfaces may help reduce the spread. Individuals should not share towels if there is a case of impetigo in the household.

Koning S et al. Interventions for impetigo. Cochrane Database Syst Rev. 2012 Jan18;1: CD003261. [PMID: 22258953]

CONTACT DERMATITIS

ESSENTIALS OF DIAGNOSIS

▸ Erythema and edema, with pruritus, often followed by vesicles and bullae (in allergic contact dermatitis) in an area of contact with a suspected agent.

▸ Later, weeping, crusting, or secondary infection.

▸ A history of previous reaction to suspected contactant.

▸ Positive patch test (in allergic contact dermatitis).

▸ General Considerations

Contact dermatitis (irritant or allergic) is an acute or chronic dermatitis that results from direct skin contact with chemicals or allergens. Eighty percent of cases are due to excessive exposure to or additive effects of primary or universal irritants (eg, soaps, detergents, organic solvents) and are called irritant contact dermatitis. This appears red

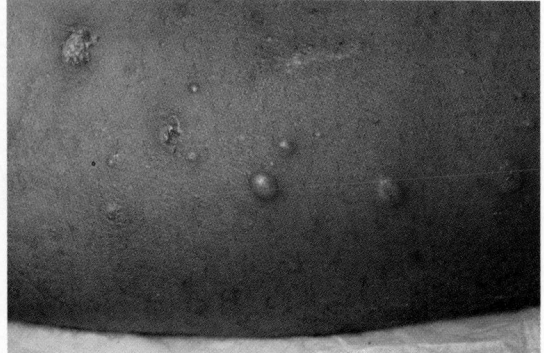

▲ **Figure 6–19.** Bullous impetigo. (Used, with permission, from Berger TG, Dept Dermatology, UCSF.)

and scaly but not vesicular. The most common causes of allergic contact dermatitis are poison ivy or poison oak, topically applied antimicrobials (especially bacitracin and neomycin), anesthetics (benzocaine), hair-care products, preservatives, jewelry (nickel), rubber, essential oils, propolis (from bees), and adhesive tape. Occupational exposure is an important cause of allergic contact dermatitis. Weeping and crusting are typically due to allergic and not irritant dermatitis.

▶ Clinical Findings

A. Symptoms and Signs

In allergic contact dermatitis, the acute phase is characterized by tiny vesicles and weepy and crusted lesions, whereas resolving or chronic contact dermatitis presents with scaling, erythema, and possibly thickened skin. Itching, burning, and stinging may be severe. The lesions, distributed on exposed parts or in bizarre asymmetric patterns, consist of erythematous macules, papules, and vesicles. The affected area is often hot and swollen, with exudation and crusting, simulating—and at times complicated by—infection. The pattern of the eruption may be diagnostic (eg, typical linear streaked vesicles on the extremities in poison oak or ivy dermatitis [Figure 6–20]) The location will often suggest the cause: Scalp involvement suggests hair dyes or shampoos; face involvement, creams, cosmetics, soaps, shaving materials, nail polish; and neck involvement, jewelry, hair dyes. Unilateral facial involvement suggests nickel contact dermatitis from cellphone cover (about 25% of which have free nickel on their surface).

B. Laboratory Findings

Gram stain and culture will rule out impetigo or secondary infection (impetiginization). If itching is generalized, then scabies should be considered. After the episode of allergic contact dermatitis has cleared, patch testing may be useful if the triggering allergen is not known.

▶ Differential Diagnosis

Asymmetric distribution, blotchy erythema around the face, linear lesions, and a history of exposure help distinguish acute contact dermatitis from other skin lesions. The most commonly mistaken diagnosis is impetigo. Chronic allergic contact dermatitis must be differentiated from scabies, atopic dermatitis, pompholyx, and other eczemas.

▶ Prevention

Prompt and thorough removal of the causative oil by washing with liquid dishwashing soap (eg, Dial Ultra) may be effective if done within 30 minutes after exposure to poison oak or ivy. Goop and Tecnu are also effective but much more costly without increased efficacy. The three most effective over-the-counter barrier creams that are applied prior to exposure and prevent/reduce the severity of the dermatitis are Stokogard, Hollister Moisture Barrier, and Hydropel.

The mainstay of prevention is identification of the agent causing the dermatitis and avoidance of exposure or use of

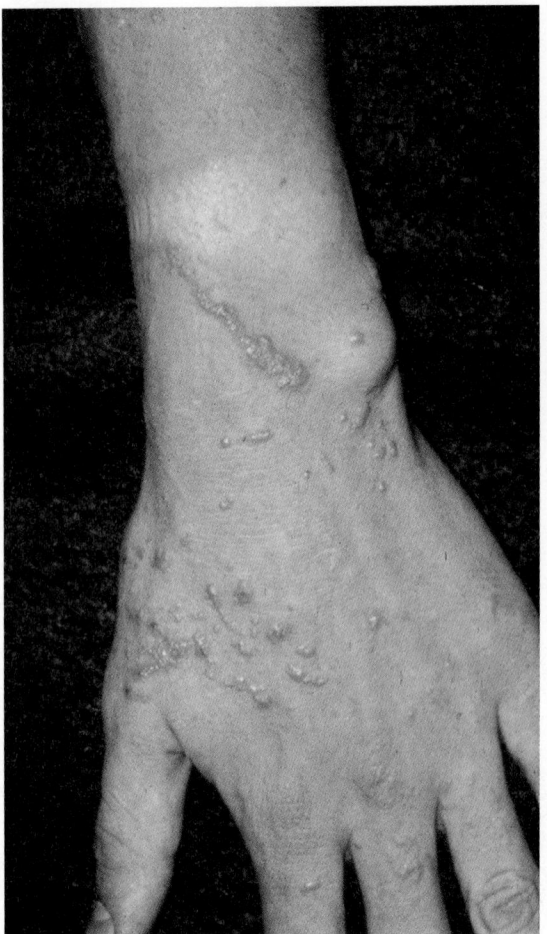

▲ **Figure 6–20.** Contact dermatitis with linear pattern due to poison ivy. (Used, with permission, from Berger TG, Dept Dermatology, UCSF.)

protective clothing and gloves. In industry-related cases, prevention may be accomplished by moving or retraining the worker.

▶ Treatment

A. Overview

While local measures are important, severe or widespread involvement is difficult to manage without systemic corticosteroids because even the highest-potency topical corticosteroids seem not to work well on vesicular and weepy lesions. Localized involvement (except on the face) can often be managed solely with topical agents. Irritant contact dermatitis is treated by protection from the irritant and use of topical corticosteroids as for atopic dermatitis (described above). The treatment of allergic contact dermatitis is detailed below.

B. Local Measures

1. Acute weeping dermatitis—Compresses are most often used. It is unwise to scrub lesions with soap and water. Calamine lotion may be used between wet dressings, especially for involvement of intertriginous areas or when oozing is not marked. Lesions on the extremities may be bandaged with wet dressings for 30–60 minutes several times a day. High potency topical corticosteroids in gel or cream form (eg, fluocinonide, clobetasol, or halobetasol) may help suppress acute contact dermatitis and relieve itching. This treatment should be followed by tapering of the number of applications per day or use of a mid-potency corticosteroid such as triamcinolone 0.1% cream to prevent rebound of the dermatitis. A soothing formulation is 2 oz of 0.1% triamcinolone acetonide cream in 7.5 oz Sarna lotion (0.5% camphor, 0.5% menthol, 0.5% phenol) mixed by the patient.

2. Subacute dermatitis (subsiding)—Mid-potency (triamcinolone 0.1%) to high-potency corticosteroids (clobetasol, amcinonide, fluocinonide, desoximetasone) are the mainstays of therapy.

3. Chronic dermatitis (dry and lichenified)—High-potency to superpotency corticosteroids are used in ointment form.

C. Systemic Therapy

For acute severe cases, prednisone may be given orally for 12–21 days. Prednisone, 60 mg for 4–7 days, 40 mg for 4–7 days, and 20 mg for 4–7 days without a further taper is one useful regimen. Another is to dispense seventy-eight 5-mg pills to be taken 12 the first day, 11 the second day, and so on. The key is to use enough corticosteroid (and as early as possible) to achieve a clinical effect and to taper slowly enough to avoid rebound. A Medrol Dosepak (methylprednisolone) with 5 days of medication is inappropriate on both counts. (See Chapter 26.)

▶ Prognosis

Allergic contact dermatitis is self-limited if reexposure is prevented but often takes 2–3 weeks for full resolution.

Jensen P et al. Excessive nickel release from mobile phones—a persistent cause of nickel allergy and dermatitis. Contact Dermatitis. 2011 Dec;65(6):354–8. [PMID: 22077435]
Thyssen JP et al. Coin exposure may cause allergic nickel dermatitis: a review. Contact Dermatitis. 2013 Jan;68(1):3–14. [PMID: 22762130]

PUSTULAR DISORDERS

ACNE VULGARIS

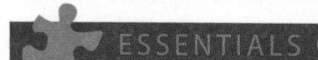

ESSENTIALS OF DIAGNOSIS

▶ Occurs at puberty, though onset may be delayed into the third or fourth decade.

▶ Open and closed comedones are the hallmark of acne vulgaris.

▶ The most common of all skin conditions.

▶ Severity varies from purely comedonal to papular or pustular inflammatory acne to cysts or nodules.

▶ Face and upper trunk may be affected.

▶ Scarring may be a sequela of the disease or picking and manipulating by the patient.

▶ General Considerations

Acne vulgaris is polymorphic. Open and closed comedones, papules, pustules, and cysts are found. The disease is activated by androgens in those who are genetically predisposed.

In younger persons, acne vulgaris is more common and more severe in males. It does not always clear spontaneously when maturity is reached. Twelve percent of women and 3% of men over age 25 have acne vulgaris. This rate does not decrease until after age 44. The skin lesions parallel sebaceous activity. Pathogenic events include plugging of the infundibulum of the follicles, retention of sebum, overgrowth of the acne bacillus (*Propionibacterium acnes*) with resultant release of and irritation by accumulated fatty acids, and foreign body reaction to extrafollicular sebum. The mechanism of antibiotics in controlling acne is not clearly understood, but they may work because of their antibacterial or anti-inflammatory properties.

When a resistant case of acne is encountered in a woman, hyperandrogenism may be suspected. This may or may not be accompanied by hirsutism, irregular menses, or other signs of virilism. Polycystic ovary syndrome (PCOS) is the most common identifiable cause.

▶ Clinical Findings

There may be mild soreness, pain, or itching. The lesions occur mainly over the face, neck, upper chest, back, and shoulders. Comedones are the hallmark of acne vulgaris. Closed comedones are tiny, flesh-colored, noninflamed bumps that give the skin a rough texture or appearance. Open comedones typically are a bit larger and have black material in them. Inflammatory papules, pustules, ectatic pores, acne cysts, and scarring are also seen (Figure 6–21)

Acne may have different presentations at different ages. Preteens often present with comedones as their first lesions. Inflammatory lesions in young teenagers are often found in the middle of the face, extending outward as the patient becomes older. Women in their third and fourth decades (often with no prior history of acne) commonly present with papular lesions on the chin and around the mouth.

▶ Differential Diagnosis

In adults, acne rosacea presents with papules and pustules in the middle third of the face, but telangiectasia, flushing, and the absence of comedones distinguish this disease from acne vulgaris. A pustular eruption on the face in patients receiving antibiotics or with otitis externa should be investigated with culture to rule out an uncommon gram-negative folliculitis. Acne may develop in patients

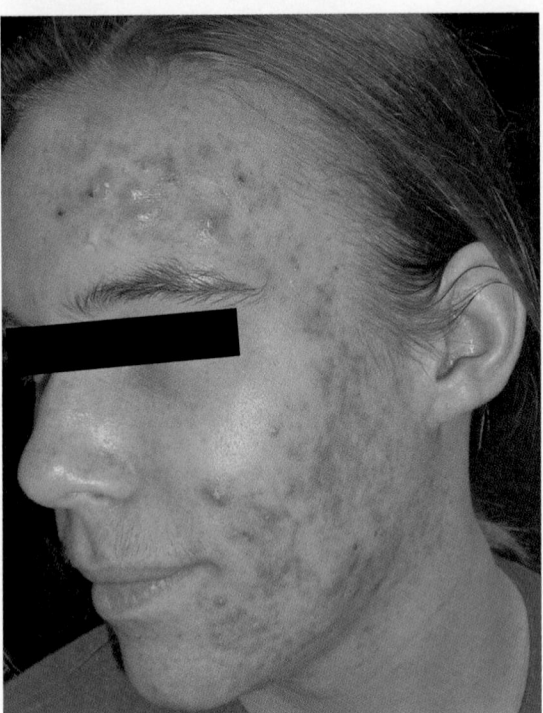

▲ **Figure 6–21.** Acne vulgaris, severe nodular cystic form with scarring. (Courtesy of Richard P. Usatine, MD; used, with permission, from Usatine RP, Smith MA, Mayeaux EJ Jr, Chumley H, Tysinger J. *The Color Atlas of Family Medicine.* McGraw-Hill, 2009.)

who use systemic corticosteroids or topical fluorinated corticosteroids on the face. Acne may be exacerbated or caused by irritating creams or oils. Pustules on the face can also be caused by tinea infections. Lesions on the back are more problematic. When they occur alone, staphylococcal folliculitis, miliaria ("heat rash") or, uncommonly, *Malassezia* folliculitis should be suspected. Bacterial culture, trial of an antistaphylococcal antibiotic, and observing the response to therapy will help in the differential diagnosis. In patients with HIV infection, folliculitis is common and may be either staphylococcal folliculitis or eosinophilic folliculitis.

▶ **Complications**

Cyst formation, pigmentary changes in pigmented patients, severe scarring, and psychological problems may result.

▶ **Treatment**

A. General Measures

1. Education of the patient—When scarring seems out of proportion to the severity of the lesions, clinicians must suspect that the patient is manipulating the lesions. It is essential that the patient be educated in a supportive way about this complication. Anxiety and depression are often the underlying cause of young women excoriating minor acne. It is wise to let the patient know that at least 4–6

weeks will be required to see improvement and that old lesions may take months to fade. Therefore, improvement will be judged according to the number of new lesions forming after 6–8 weeks of therapy. Additional time will be required to see improvement on the back and chest, as these areas are slowest to respond. If hair pomades are used, they should contain glycerin and not oil. Avoid topical exposure to oils, cocoa butter (theobroma oil), and greases.

2. Diet—A low glycemic diet that results in weight loss has been reported to improve acne in males aged 18–25. This improvement was associated with a reduction in insulin resistance. Hyperinsulinemia has also been associated with acne in eumenorrheic women. The metabolic syndrome with insulin resistance can also be a feature of PCOS in women. This finding suggests a possible common pathogenic mechanism for acne in both adult women and men.

B. Comedonal Acne

Treatment of acne is based on the type and severity of lesions. Comedones require treatment different from that of pustules and cystic lesions. In assessing severity, take the sequelae of the lesions into account. An individual who gets only a few new lesions per month that scar or leave postinflammatory hyperpigmentation must be treated much more aggressively than a comparable patient whose lesions clear without sequelae. Soaps play little role in acne treatment, and unless the patient's skin is exceptionally oily, a mild soap should be used to avoid irritation that will limit the usefulness of other topicals, all of which are themselves somewhat irritating. The agents effective in comedonal acne are listed below in the order in which they should be tried.

1. Topical retinoids—Tretinoin is very effective for comedonal acne or for treatment of the comedonal component of more severe acne, but its usefulness is limited by irritation. Start with 0.025% cream (not gel) and have the patient use it at first twice weekly at night, then build up to as often as nightly. A few patients cannot use even this low-strength preparation more than three times weekly but even that may cause improvement. A lentil-sized amount is sufficient to cover the entire face. To avoid irritation, have the patient wait 20 minutes after washing to apply. Adapalene gel 0.1% and reformulated tretinoin (Renova, Retin A Micro, Avita) are other options for patients irritated by standard tretinoin preparations. Some patients—especially teenagers—do best on 0.01% gel. Although the absorption of tretinoin is minimal, its use during pregnancy is contraindicated. Patients should be warned that their acne may flare in the first 4 weeks of treatment. Tazarotene gel (0.05% or 0.1%) (Tazorac) is another topical retinoid approved for treatment of psoriasis and acne, and may be used in patients intolerant of the other retinoids.

2. Benzoyl peroxide—Benzoyl peroxide products are available in concentrations of 2.5%, 4%, 5%, 8%, and 10%, but it appears that 2.5% is as effective as 10% and less irritating. In general, water-based and not alcohol-based gels should be used to decrease irritation. Benzoyl peroxide in combination with adapalene is available as a single formulation.

3. Antibiotics—Use of topical antibiotics (see below) has been demonstrated to decrease pustular and comedonal lesions.

C. Papular or Cystic Inflammatory Acne

Topical or oral antibiotics are the mainstay for treatment of inflammatory acne. The oral antibiotics of choice are tetracycline and doxycycline. Minocycline is often effective in acne unresponsive or resistant to treatment with these antibiotics but it is more expensive. Rarely, other antibiotics such as TMP-SMZ (one double-strength tablet twice daily), clindamycin (150 mg twice daily), or a cephalosporin (cefadroxil or cephalexin) may be used. Topical clindamycin phosphate and erythromycin are also used (see below). Topicals are probably the equivalent of about 500 mg/d of tetracycline given orally, which is half the usual starting dose. Topical antibiotics are used in three situations: for mild papular acne that can be controlled by topicals alone, for patients who refuse or cannot tolerate oral antibiotics, or to wean patients under good control from oral to topical preparations. To decrease resistance, benzoyl peroxide should be used in combination with the topical antibiotic.

1. Mild acne—The first choice of topical antibiotics in terms of efficacy and relative lack of induction of resistant *P acnes* is the combination of erythromycin or clindamycin with benzoyl peroxide topical gel. Clindamycin (Cleocin T) lotion (least irritating), gel, or solution, or one of the many brands of topical erythromycin gel or solution, may be used twice daily and the benzoyl peroxide in the morning. (A combination of erythromycin or clindamycin with benzoyl peroxide is available.) The addition of tretinoin 0.025% cream or 0.01% gel at night may increase improvement, since it works via a different mechanism. Combination preparations of an antibiotic and benzoyl peroxide and antibiotic plus tretinoin are available, but there is no evidence that they are superior to the individual agents used separately.

2. Moderate acne—Tetracycline, 500 mg twice daily, doxycycline, 100 mg twice daily, and minocycline, 50–100 mg twice daily, are all effective. When initiating minocycline therapy, start at 100 mg in the evening for 4–7 days, then 100 mg twice daily, to decrease the incidence of vertigo. Plan a return visit in 6 weeks and at 3–4 months after that. If the patient's skin is quite clear, instructions should be given for tapering the dose by 250 mg for tetracycline, by 100 mg for doxycycline, or by 50 mg for minocycline every 6–8 weeks—while treating with topicals—to arrive at the lowest systemic dose needed to maintain clearing. In general, immediately lowering the dose to zero without other therapy results in prompt recurrence.

Tetracycline, minocycline, and doxycycline are contraindicated in pregnancy, but oral erythromycin may be used. It is important to discuss the issue of contraceptive failure when prescribing antibiotics for women taking oral contraceptives. Women may need to consider using barrier methods as well, and should report breakthrough bleeding.

Oral contraceptives or spironolactone (50–200 mg daily) may be added as an antiandrogen in women with antibiotic-resistant acne or in women in whom relapse occurs after isotretinoin therapy.

3. Severe acne—

A. ISOTRETINOIN—A vitamin A analog, isotretinoin is used for the treatment of severe cystic acne that has not responded to conventional therapy. A dosage of 0.5–1 mg/kg/d for 20 weeks for a cumulative dose of at least 120 mg/kg is usually adequate for severe cystic acne. Patients should be offered isotretinoin therapy before they experience significant scarring if they are not promptly and adequately controlled by antibiotics. The drug is *absolutely contraindicated during pregnancy* because of its teratogenicity; two serum pregnancy tests should be obtained before starting the drug in women and every month thereafter. Sufficient medication for only 1 month should be dispensed. Two forms of effective contraception must be used. Informed consent must be obtained before its use and patients must be enrolled in a monitoring program (iPledge). Side effects occur in most patients, usually related to dry skin and mucous membranes (dry lips, nosebleed, and dry eyes). If headache occurs, pseudotumor cerebri must be considered. Depression has been reported. Hypertriglyceridemia will develop in about 25% of patients, hypercholesterolemia in 15%, and a lowering of high-density lipoproteins in 5%. Minor elevations in liver function tests may develop in some patients. Fasting blood sugar may be elevated. Miscellaneous adverse reactions include decreased night vision, musculoskeletal symptoms, dry skin, thinning of hair, exuberant granulation tissue in lesions, and bony hyperostoses (seen only with very high doses or with long duration of therapy). Moderate to severe myalgias rarely necessitate decreasing the dosage or stopping the drug. Inflammatory bowel disease has first appeared after acne treatment with both tetracyclines and isotretinoin at a rate of 1:1000 cases treated or less. Causality of this association has not been established. Young adults with severe acne who are potential candidates for isotretinoin should be asked about any bowel symptoms prior to starting isotretinoin. Laboratory tests to be performed in all patients before treatment and after 4 weeks on therapy include complete blood cell count (CBC), cholesterol, triglycerides, and liver function studies.

Elevations of liver enzymes and triglycerides return to normal upon conclusion of therapy. The drug may induce long-term remissions in 40–60%, or acne may recur that is more easily controlled with conventional therapy. Occasionally, acne does not respond or promptly recurs after therapy, but it may clear after a second course.

B. INTRALESIONAL INJECTION—In otherwise moderate acne, intralesional injection of dilute suspensions of triamcinolone acetonide (2.5 mg/mL, 0.05 mL per lesion) will often hasten the resolution of deeper papules and occasional cysts.

C. LASER DERMABRASION—Cosmetic improvement may be achieved by excision and punch-grafting of deep scars and by abrasion of inactive acne lesions, particularly flat, superficial scars. The technique is not without untoward effects, since hyperpigmentation, hypopigmentation, grooving, and scarring have been known to occur. Dark-skinned individuals do poorly. Corrective surgery within 12 months after isotretinoin therapy may not be advisable. Active acne of all types can be treated with certain laser and photodynamic therapies. This can be considered when standard treatments are contraindicated or fail.

▶ Prognosis

Acne vulgaris eventually remits spontaneously, but when this will occur cannot be predicted. The condition may persist throughout adulthood and may lead to severe scarring if left untreated. Patients treated with antibiotics continue to improve for the first 3–6 months of therapy. Relapse during treatment may suggest the emergence of resistant *P acnes*. The disease is chronic and tends to flare intermittently in spite of treatment. Remissions following systemic treatment with isotretinoin may be lasting in up to 60% of cases. Relapses after isotretinoin usually occur within 3 years and require a second course in up to 20% of patients.

Arowojolu AO et al. Combined oral contraceptive pills for treatment of acne. Cochrane Database Syst Rev. 2012 Jul11;7: CD004425. [PMID: 22786490]

Garner SE et al. Minocycline for acne vulgaris: efficacy and safety. Cochrane Database Syst Rev. 2012 Aug15;8: CD002086. [PMID: 22895927]

Purdy S et al. Acne vulgaris. Clin Evid (Online). 2011 Jan5; 2011. [PMID: 21477388]

Rademaker M. Isotretinoin: dose, duration and relapse. What does 30 years of usage tell us? Australas J Dermatol. 2013 Aug;54(3):157–62. [PMID: 23013115]

Torrelo A et al. Atopic dermatitis: impact on quality of life and patients' attitudes toward its management. Eur J Dermatol. 2012 Jan–Feb;22(1):97–105. [PMID: 22237114]

Williams HC et al. Acne vulgaris. Lancet. 2012 Jan 28;379(9813):361–72. [PMID: 21880356]

ROSACEA

ESSENTIALS OF DIAGNOSIS

▶ A chronic facial disorder.

▶ A neurovascular component (erythema and telangiectasis and a tendency to flush easily).

▶ An acneiform component (papules and pustules) may also be present.

▶ A glandular component accompanied by hyperplasia of the soft tissue of the nose (rhinophyma).

▶ General Considerations

The pathogenesis of this disorder is not known. Topical corticosteroids applied to the face can induce rosacea-like conditions.

▶ Clinical Findings

Patients frequently report flushing or exacerbation of their rosacea due to heat, hot drinks, spicy food, sunlight, exercise, alcohol, emotions, or menopausal flushing. The cheeks, nose, and chin—at times the entire face—may have a rosy hue. No comedones are seen. In its mildest form, erythema and dilated vessels are seen on the cheeks. Inflammatory papules may be superimposed on this background and may evolve to pustules (Figure 6–22). Associated seborrhea may be found. The patient often complains of burning or stinging with episodes of flushing. Patients may have associated ophthalmic disease, including blepharitis and keratitis, that often requires systemic antibiotic therapy.

▶ Differential Diagnosis

Rosacea is distinguished from acne by the presence of the neurovascular component and the absence of comedones. The rosy hue of rosacea and telangiectasis will pinpoint the diagnosis. Lupus is often misdiagnosed, but the presence of pustules excludes that diagnosis.

▶ Treatment

Educating patients to avoid the factors they know to produce exacerbations is important. Patients should wear a broad-spectrum sunscreen with UVA coverage; however, exquisite sensitivity to topical preparations may limit patient options. Zinc- or titanium-based sunscreens are

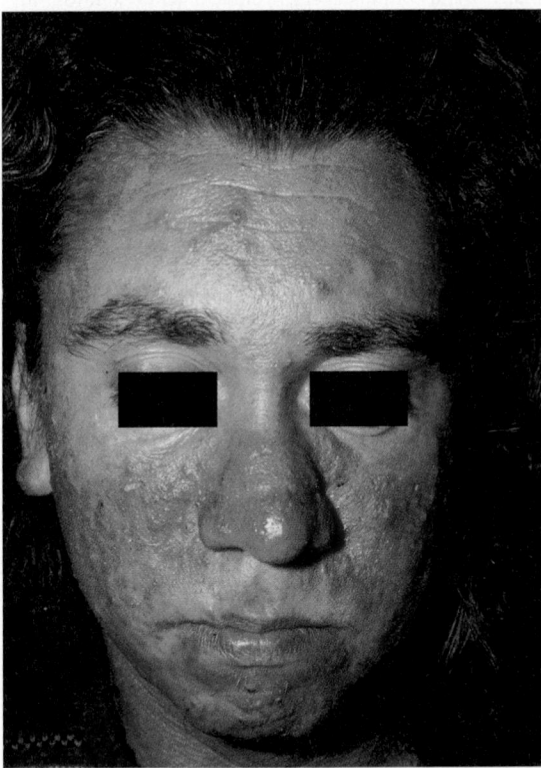

▲ **Figure 6–22.** Rosacea. (Used, with permission, from Berger TG, Dept Dermatology, UCSF.)

better tolerated, and barrier protective silicones in the sunblock may enhance tolerance. Medical management is most effective for the inflammatory papules and pustules and the erythema that surrounds them. Rosacea is usually a lifelong condition, so maintenance therapy is required.

A. Local Therapy

Avoidance of triggers (especially alcohol) and sucking on an ice cube may be effective in reducing facial erythema and flushing. Metronidazole (available as creams, gels, or lotions), 0.75% applied twice daily or 1% applied once daily, is the topical treatment of choice. If metronidazole is not tolerated, topical clindamycin (solution, gel, or lotion) 1% applied twice daily is effective. Response is noted in 4–8 weeks. Sulfur-sodium sulfacetamide-containing topicals are helpful in patients only partially responsive to topical antibiotics. Benzoyl peroxide, as in acne vulgaris, may be helpful in reducing the pustular component. Topical retinoids can be carefully added for maintenance. Topical brimonidine tartrate gel 0.5% can temporarily reduce the flush/redness of rosacea patients. Prolonged use did not lead to tachyphylaxis in short trials.

B. Systemic Therapy

Tetracycline, 250 or 500 mg orally twice daily on an empty stomach, should be used when topical therapy is inadequate. Minocycline or doxycycline, 50–100 mg orally daily to twice daily, is also effective. Metronidazole or amoxicillin, 250–500 mg orally twice daily, or rifaximin, 550 mg orally twice daily, may be used in refractory cases. Side effects are few, although metronidazole may produce a disulfiram-like effect when the patient ingests alcohol and it may cause neuropathy with long-term use. Isotretinoin may succeed where other measures fail. A dosage of 0.5 mg/kg/d orally for 12–28 weeks is recommended. See precautions above. Telangiectases are benefitted by laser therapy, and phymatous overgrowth of the nose can be treated by surgical reduction.

▶ Prognosis

Rosacea tends to be a persistent process. With the regimens described above, it can usually be controlled adequately.

Baldwin HE. Diagnosis and treatment of rosacea: state of the art. J Drugs Dermatol. 2012 Jun;11(6):725–30. [PMID: 22648219]

Moore A et al. Long-term safety and efficacy of once-daily topical brimonidine tartrate gel 0.5% for the treatment of moderate to severe facial erythema of rosacea: results of a 1-year open-label study. J Drugs Dermatol. 2014 Jan1;13(1):56–61. [PMID: 24385120]

Rice SA et al. Repeatedly red faced. Lancet. 2012 Apr21;379(9825): 1560. [PMID: 22521073]

Torpy JM et al. JAMA patient page. Rosacea. JAMA. 2012 Jun6;307(21): 2333. [PMID: 22706840]

van Zuuren EJ et al. Effective and evidence-based management strategies for rosacea: summary of a Cochrane systematic review. Br J Dermatol. 2011 Oct;165(4):760–81. [PMID: 21692773]

van Zuuren EJ et al. Interventions for rosacea. Cochrane Database Syst Rev. 2011 Mar16;(3): CD003262. [PMID: 21412882]

FOLLICULITIS (Including Sycosis)

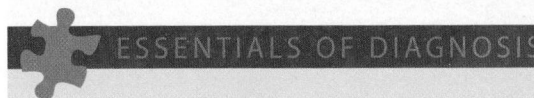

ESSENTIALS OF DIAGNOSIS

▶ Itching and burning in hairy areas.

▶ Pustules in the hair follicles.

▶ General Considerations

Folliculitis has multiple causes. It is frequently caused by staphylococcal infection and may be more common in the diabetic patient. When the lesion is deep-seated, chronic, and recalcitrant on the head and neck, it is called sycosis.

Gram-negative folliculitis, which may develop during antibiotic treatment of acne, may present as a flare of acne pustules or nodules. *Klebsiella, Enterobacter, Escherichia coli,* and *Proteus* have been isolated from these lesions.

"Hot tub folliculitis," caused by *Pseudomonas aeruginosa,* is characterized by pruritic or tender follicular, pustular lesions occurring within 1–4 days after bathing in a contaminated hot tub, whirlpool, or swimming pool. Rarely, systemic infections may result. Neutropenic patients should avoid these exposures.

Nonbacterial folliculitis may also be caused by friction and oils. Occlusion, perspiration, and rubbing, such as that resulting from tight jeans and other heavy fabrics on the upper legs can worsen this type of folliculitis.

Steroid acne may be seen during topical or systemic corticosteroid therapy.

A form of sterile folliculitis called eosinophilic folliculitis consisting of urticarial papules with prominent eosinophilic infiltration is common in patients with AIDS. It may appear first with institution of highly active antiretroviral therapy (HAART) and be mistaken for a drug eruption.

Pseudofolliculitis is caused by ingrowing hairs in the beard area. It occurs in men and women with tightly curled beard hair. In this entity, the papules and pustules are located at the side of and not in follicles. It may be treated by growing a beard, by using chemical depilatories, or by shaving with a foil-guard razor. Laser hair removal is dramatically beneficial in patients with pseudofolliculitis, requires limited maintenance, and can be done on patients of any skin color. Pseudofolliculitis is a true medical indication for such a procedure and should not be considered cosmetic.

▶ Clinical Findings

The symptoms range from slight burning and tenderness to intense itching. The lesions consist of pustules of hair follicles (Figure 6–23).

▶ Differential Diagnosis

It is important to differentiate bacterial from nonbacterial folliculitis. The history is important for pinpointing the causes of nonbacterial folliculitis, and a Gram stain and

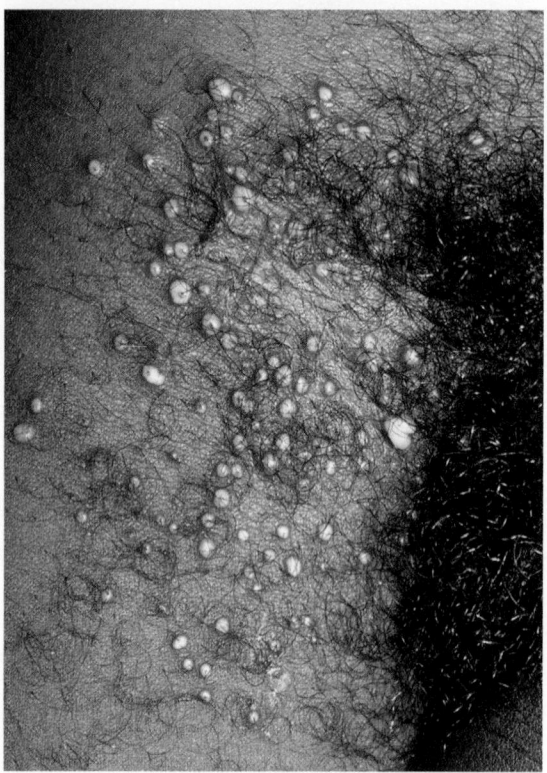

▲ **Figure 6–23.** Bacterial folliculitis. (Used, with permission, from Berger TG, Dept Dermatology, UCSF.)

culture are indispensable. One must differentiate folliculitis from acne vulgaris or pustular miliaria (heat rash) and from infections of the skin such as impetigo or fungal infections. Pseudomonas folliculitis is often suggested by the history of hot tub use. Eosinophilic folliculitis in AIDS often requires biopsy for diagnosis.

► Complications

Abscess formation is the major complication of bacterial folliculitis.

► Prevention

Correct any predisposing local causes such as oils or friction. Be sure that the water in hot tubs and spas is treated properly. If staphylococcal folliculitis is persistent, treatment of nasal or perineal carriage with rifampin, 600 mg daily for 5 days, or with topical mupirocin ointment 2% twice daily for 5 days, may help. Prolonged oral clindamycin, 150–300 mg/d for 4–6 weeks, or oral TMP-SMZ given 1 week per month for 6 months can be effective in preventing recurrent staphylococcal folliculitis and furunculosis. Bleach baths (¼ to ½ cup per 20 liters of bathwater for 15 minutes 3–5 times weekly) may reduce cutaneous staphylococcal carriage and not contribute to antibiotic resistance. Control of blood glucose in diabetes may reduce the number of these infections.

► Treatment

A. Local Measures

Anhydrous ethyl alcohol containing 6.25% aluminum chloride (Xerac AC), applied three to seven times weekly to lesions and environs, may be helpful, especially for chronic frictional folliculitis of the buttocks. Topical antibiotics are generally ineffective if bacteria have invaded the hair follicle, but may be prophylactic if used as an aftershave in patients with recurrent folliculitis after shaving.

B. Specific Measures

Pseudomonas folliculitis will clear spontaneously in non-neutropenic patients if the lesions are superficial. It may be treated with ciprofloxacin, 500 mg twice daily for 5 days.

Systemic antibiotics are recommended for bacterial folliculitis due to other organisms. Extended periods of treatment (4–8 weeks or more) with antistaphylococcal antibiotics are required if infection has involved the scalp or densely hairy areas such as the axilla, beard, or groin.

Gram-negative folliculitis in acne patients may be treated with isotretinoin in compliance with all precautions discussed above (see Acne Vulgaris).

Eosinophilic folliculitis may be treated initially by the combination of potent topical corticosteroids and oral antihistamines. In more severe cases, treatment is with one of the following: topical permethrin (application for 12 hours every other night for 6 weeks); itraconazole, 200–400 mg daily; UVB or PUVA phototherapy; or isotretinoin, 0.5 mg/kg/d for up to 5 months. A remission may be induced by some of these therapies, but long-term treatment may be required.

► Prognosis

Bacterial folliculitis is occasionally stubborn and persistent, requiring prolonged or intermittent courses of antibiotics.

Lutz JK et al. Prevalence and antimicrobial-resistance of *Pseudomonas aeruginosa* in swimming pools and hot tubs. Int J Environ Res Public Health. 2011 Feb;8(2):554–64. [PMID: 21556203]
Weingartner JS et al. What is your diagnosis? Demodex folliculitis. Cutis. 2012 Aug;90(2): 62, 65–6, 69. [PMID: 22988646]

MILIARIA (Heat Rash)

 ESSENTIALS OF DIAGNOSIS

► Burning, itching, superficial aggregated small vesicles, papules, or pustules on covered areas of the skin, usually the trunk.

► More common in hot, moist climates.

► Rare forms associated with fever and even heat prostration.

General Considerations

Miliaria occurs most commonly on the trunk and intertriginous areas. A hot, moist environment is the most frequent cause. Occlusive clothing required for certain occupations may increase the risk. Bedridden febrile patients are susceptible. Plugging of the ostia of sweat ducts occurs, with ultimate rupture of the sweat duct, producing an irritating, stinging reaction. Increase in numbers of resident aerobes, notably cocci, plays a role. Medications that enhance sweat gland function (eg, clonidine, beta-blockers, opioids) may contribute.

Clinical Findings

The usual symptoms are burning and itching. The lesions consist of small, superficial, red, thin-walled, discrete vesicles (miliaria crystallina), papules (miliaria rubra), or vesicopustules or pustules (miliaria pustulosa). The reaction virtually always affects the back in a hospitalized patient.

Differential Diagnosis

Miliaria is to be distinguished from drug eruption and folliculitis.

Prevention

Use of an antibacterial preparation such as chlorhexidine prior to exposure to heat and humidity may help prevent the condition. Frequent turning or sitting of the hospitalized patient may reduce miliaria on the back.

Treatment

The patient should keep cool and wear light clothing. Triamcinolone acetonide, 0.1% in Sarna lotion, or a mid-potency corticosteroid in a lotion or cream should be applied two to four times daily. Secondary infections (superficial pyoderma) are treated with appropriate antistaphylococcal antibiotics. Anticholinergic drugs given by mouth may be helpful in severe cases, eg, glycopyrrolate, 1 mg twice daily.

Prognosis

Miliaria is usually a mild disorder, but severe forms (tropical anhidrosis and asthenia) result from interference with the heat-regulating mechanism.

Carter R 3rd et al. Patients presenting with miliaria while wearing flame resistant clothing in high ambient temperatures: a case series. J Med Case Rep. 2011 Sep22;5:474. [PMID: 21939537]

Carvalho R et al. sQUIZ your knowledge! "Water-drop" lesions in a febrile patient. Miliaria crystalline (MC). Eur J Dermatol. 2012 Jan–Feb;22(1):160–1. [PMID: 22370171]

MUCOCUTANEOUS CANDIDIASIS

ESSENTIALS OF DIAGNOSIS

▶ Severe pruritus of vulva, anus, or body folds.

▶ Superficial denuded, beefy-red areas with or without satellite vesicopustules.

▶ Whitish curd-like concretions on the oral and vaginal mucous membranes.

▶ Yeast and pseudohyphae on microscopic examination of scales or curd.

General Considerations

Mucocutaneous candidiasis is a superficial fungal infection that may involve almost any cutaneous or mucous surface of the body. It is particularly likely to occur in diabetics, during pregnancy, and in obese persons. Systemic antibiotics, oral corticosteroids, and oral contraceptive agents may be contributory. Oral candidiasis may be the first sign of HIV infection (see Chapter 31).

Clinical Findings

A. Symptoms and Signs

Itching may be intense. Burning is reported, particularly around the vulva and anus. The lesions consist of superficially denuded, beefy-red areas in the depths of the body folds such as in the groin and the intergluteal cleft, beneath the breasts, at the angles of the mouth, and in the umbilicus. The peripheries of these denuded lesions are superficially undermined, and there may be satellite vesicopustules. Whitish, curd-like concretions may be present on mucosal lesions (Figure 6–24). Paronychia may occur (Figure 6–25).

B. Laboratory Findings

Clusters of budding yeast and pseudohyphae can be seen under high power (400×) when skin scales or curd-like

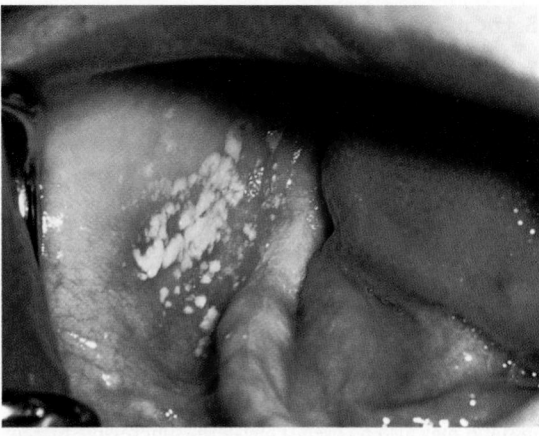

▲ **Figure 6–24.** Oral mucosal candidiasis. (Courtesy of Sol Silverman, Jr., DDS, Public Health Image Library, CDC.)

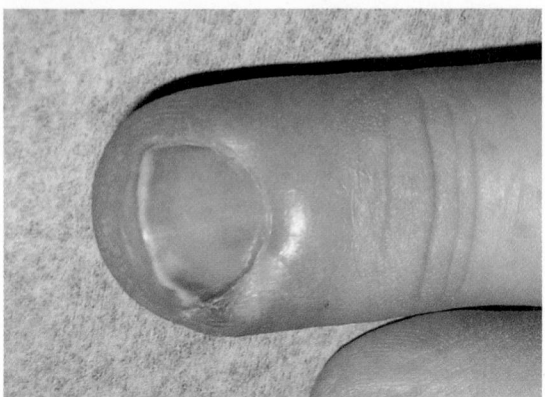

▲ **Figure 6–25.** Acute paronychia. (Courtesy of EJ Mayeaux, MD; used, with permission, from Usatine RP, Smith MA, Mayeaux EJ Jr, Chumley H, Tysinger J. *The Color Atlas of Family Medicine.* McGraw-Hill, 2009.)

lesions have been cleared in 10% KOH. Culture can confirm the diagnosis.

▶ Differential Diagnosis

Intertrigo, seborrheic dermatitis, tinea cruris, "inverse psoriasis," and erythrasma involving the same areas may mimic mucocutaneous candidiasis.

▶ Complications

Systemic invasive candidiasis with candidemia may be seen with immunosuppression and in patients receiving broad-spectrum antibiotic and hypertonic glucose solutions, as in hyperalimentation. There may or may not be clinically evident mucocutaneous candidiasis.

▶ Treatment

A. General Measures

Affected parts should be kept dry and exposed to air as much as possible. If possible, discontinue systemic antibiotics. For treatment of systemic invasive candidiasis, see Chapter 36.

B. Local Measures

1. Nails and paronychia—Apply clotrimazole solution 1% twice daily. Thymol 4% in ethanol applied once daily is an alternative.

2. Skin—Apply nystatin ointment or clotrimazole cream 1%, either with hydrocortisone cream 1%, twice daily. Gentian violet 0.5% solution is economical and highly effective in treating cutaneous candidiasis (and also mucosal disease), but the purple discoloration represents a cosmetic issue for some patients.

3. Vulvar and anal mucous membranes—For vaginal candidiasis, single-dose fluconazole (150 mg orally) is effective. Intravaginal clotrimazole, miconazole, terconazole, or nystatin may also be used. Long-term suppressive therapy may be required for recurrent or "intractable" cases. Non-*albicans* candidal species may be identified by culture in

some refractory cases and may respond to oral itraconazole, 200 mg twice daily for 2–4 weeks.

4. Balanitis—This is most frequent in uncircumcised men, and *Candida* usually plays a role. Topical nystatin ointment is the initial treatment if the lesions are mildly erythematous or superficially erosive. Soaking with dilute aluminum acetate for 15 minutes twice daily may quickly relieve burning or itching. Chronicity and relapses, especially after sexual contact, suggest reinfection from a sexual partner who should be treated. Severe purulent balanitis is usually due to bacteria. If it is so severe that phimosis occurs, oral antibiotics—some with activity against anaerobes—are required; if rapid improvement does not occur, urologic consultation is indicated.

5. Mastitis—Lancinating breast pain and nipple dermatitis in breast-feeding women may be a manifestation of *Candida* colonization/infection of the breast ducts. Treatment with oral fluconazole, 200 mg daily can be dramatically effective. Topical gentian violet 0.5% is also useful in these cases.

▶ Prognosis

Cases of cutaneous candidiasis range from the easily cured to the intractable and prolonged.

Amir LH et al. The role of micro-organisms (*Staphylococcus aureus* and *Candida albicans*) in the pathogenesis of breast pain and infection in lactating women: study protocol. BMC Pregnancy Childbirth. 2011 Jul22;11:54. [PMID: 21777483]

Pienaar ED et al. Interventions for the prevention and management of oropharyngeal candidiasis associated with HIV infection in adults and children. Cochrane Database Syst Rev. 2010 Nov10;(11): CD003940. [PMID: 21069679]

Ray A et al. Interventions for prevention and treatment of vulvovaginal candidiasis in women with HIV infection. Cochrane Database Syst Rev. 2011 Aug10;(8): CD008739. [PMID: 21833970]

ERYTHEMAS

REACTIVE ERYTHEMAS

1. Urticaria & Angioedema

> ### ESSENTIALS OF DIAGNOSIS
>
> ▶ Eruptions of evanescent wheals or hives.
>
> ▶ Itching is usually intense but may on rare occasions be absent.
>
> ▶ Special forms of urticaria have special features (dermatographism, cholinergic urticaria, solar urticaria, or cold urticaria).
>
> ▶ Most incidents are acute and self-limited over a period of 1–2 weeks.
>
> ▶ Chronic urticaria (episodes lasting > 6 weeks) may have an autoimmune basis.

General Considerations

Urticaria can result from many different stimuli on an immunologic or nonimmunologic basis. The most common immunologic mechanism is mediated by IgE, as seen in the majority of patients with acute urticaria; another involves activation of the complement cascade. Some patients with chronic urticaria demonstrate autoantibodies directed against mast cell IgE receptors. ACE inhibitor and angiotensin receptor blocker therapy may be complicated by urticaria or angioedema. In general, extensive costly workups are not indicated in patients who have urticaria. A careful history and physical examination are more helpful.

Clinical Findings

A. Symptoms and Signs

Lesions are itchy red swellings of a few millimeters to many centimeters (Figure 6–26). The morphology of the lesions may vary over a period of minutes to hours, resulting in geographic or bizarre patterns. Individual lesions in true urticaria last < 24 hours, and often only 2–4 hours. Angioedema is involvement of deeper subcutaneous tissue with swelling of the lips, eyelids, palms, soles, and genitalia. **Angioedema is no more likely than urticaria to be associated with systemic complications such as laryngeal edema or hypotension.** In cholinergic urticaria, triggered by a rise in core body temperature (hot showers, exercise), wheals are 2–3 mm in diameter with a large surrounding red flare. Cold urticaria is acquired or inherited and triggered by exposure to cold and wind (see Chapter 37).

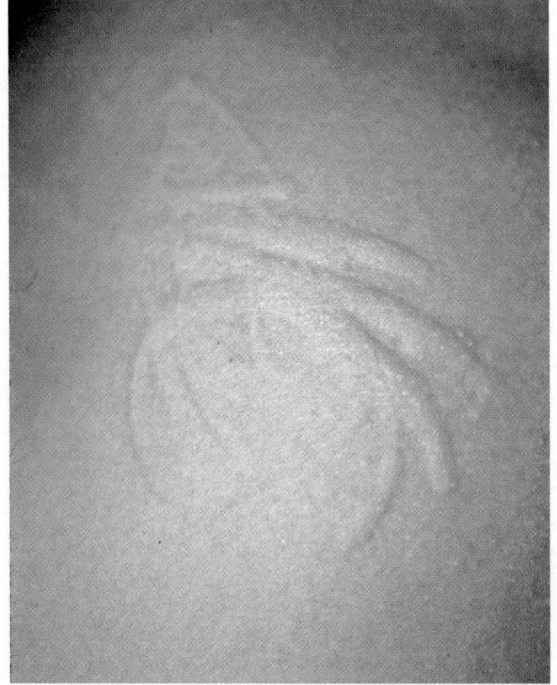

▲ **Figure 6–26.** Urticaria. (Used, with permission, from Berger TG, Dept Dermatology, UCSF.)

B. Laboratory Findings

Laboratory studies are not likely to be helpful in the evaluation of acute or chronic urticaria. The most common causes of acute urticaria are foods, infections, and medications. The cause of chronic urticaria is often not found. In patients with individual lesions that persist past 24 hours, skin biopsy may confirm neutrophilic urticaria or urticarial vasculitis. A functional ELISA test can detect patients with an autoimmune basis for their chronic urticaria.

Differential Diagnosis

Papular urticaria resulting from insect bites persists for days. A central punctum can usually be seen. Streaked urticarial lesions may be seen in the 24–48 hours before blisters appear in acute allergic plant dermatitis, eg, poison ivy, oak, or sumac. Urticarial response to heat, sun, water, and pressure are quite rare. Urticarial vasculitis may be seen as part of serum sickness, associated with fever and arthralgia. In this setting, a low serum complement level may be associated with severe systemic disease.

In hereditary angioedema, there is generally a positive family history and gastrointestinal or respiratory symptoms. Urticaria is not part of the syndrome, and lesions are not pruritic.

Treatment

A. General Measures

A detailed search by history for a cause of acute urticaria should be undertaken, and treatment may then be tailored to include the provocative condition. The chief causes are medications—eg, aspirin, NSAIDs, morphine, and codeine; arthropod bites—eg, insect bites and bee stings (though the latter may cause anaphylaxis as well as angioedema); physical factors such as heat, cold, sunlight, and pressure; and, presumably, neurogenic factors, as in cholinergic urticaria induced by exercise, excitement, hot showers, etc. Other causes may include penicillins and other medications; inhalants such as feathers and animal danders; ingestion of shellfish, tomatoes, or strawberries; infections such as viral hepatitis (causing urticarial vasculitis); and in selected patients salicylates and tartrazine dyes.

B. Systemic Treatment

The mainstay of treatment initially includes H_1-antihistamines (see above). Initial therapy is hydroxyzine, 10 mg twice daily to 25 mg three times daily, or as a single nightly dose of 50–75 mg to reduce daytime sedation. Cyproheptadine, 4 mg four times daily, may be especially useful for cold urticaria. "Nonsedating" or less sedating antihistamines are added if the generic sedating antihistamines are not effective. Options include fexofenadine, 60 mg twice daily (or 180 mg once daily); or cetirizine or loratadine, 10 mg daily. Higher doses of these second-generation antihistamines may be required to suppress urticaria (up to four times the standard recommended dose) than are required for allergic rhinitis. These high doses are safe and can be used in refractory cases.

Doxepin (a tricyclic antidepressant), 10–75 mg at bedtime, can be very effective in chronic urticaria. It has anticholinergic side effects.

H_2-antihistamines in combination with H_1-blockers may be helpful in patients with symptomatic dermatographism and to a lesser degree in chronic urticaria. UVB phototherapy can suppress some cases of chronic urticaria. If neutrophils are a significant component of the inflammatory infiltrate in chronic urticaria, dapsone or colchicine (or both) may be useful.

A few patients with chronic urticaria may respond to elimination of salicylates and tartrazine (coloring agent). Asymptomatic foci of infection—sinusitis, vaginal candidiasis, cholecystitis, and intestinal parasites—may rarely cause chronic urticaria. Systemic corticosteroids in a dose of about 40 mg daily will usually suppress acute and chronic urticaria. However, the use of corticosteroids is rarely indicated, since properly selected combinations of antihistamines with less toxicity are usually effective. Once corticosteroids are withdrawn, the urticaria virtually always returns if it had been chronic. Instead of instituting systemic corticosteroids, consultation should be sought from a dermatologist or allergist with experience in managing severe urticaria. Cyclosporine (3–5 mg/kg/d) and other immunosuppressives may be effective in severe cases of chronic urticaria. Omalizumab can be highly effective in patients with refractory chronic urticaria and should be considered when severe chronic urticaria fails to respond to high-dose antihistamines.

C. Local Treatment

Local treatment is rarely rewarding.

▶ Prognosis

Acute urticaria usually lasts only a few days to weeks. Half of patients whose urticaria persists for > 6 weeks will have it for years. Patients in whom angioedema develops with an ACE inhibitor may be switched to an angiotensin receptor blocker with caution (estimated cross reaction about 10%).

Ben-Shoshan M et al. Psychosocial factors and chronic spontaneous urticaria: a systematic review. Allergy. 2013 Feb;68(2):131–41. [PMID: 23157275]

Carr TF et al. Chapter 21: Urticaria and angioedema. Allergy Asthma Proc. 2012 May–Jun;33(Suppl 1):S70–2. [PMID: 22794694]

Church MK et al. H(1)-antihistamines and urticaria: how can we predict the best drug for our patient? Clin Exp Allergy. 2012 Oct;42(10):1423–9. [PMID: 22994340]

Maurer M et al. Omalizumab for the treatment of chronic idiopathic or spontaneous urticaria. N Engl J Med. 2013 Mar7;368(10):924–35.Erratum in: N Engl J Med. 2013 Jun13;368(24):2340–1. [PMID: 23432142]

2. Erythema Multiforme

▶ Sudden onset of symmetric erythematous skin lesions with history of recurrence.

▶ May be macular, papular, urticarial, bullous, or purpuric.

▶ "Target" lesions with clear centers and concentric erythematous rings or "iris" lesions may be noted in erythema multiforme minor. These are rare in drug-associated erythema multiforme major.

▶ Erythema multiforme minor on extensor surfaces, palms, soles, or mucous membranes. Erythema multiforme major favors the trunk.

▶ Herpes simplex is the most common cause of erythema multiforme minor.

▶ Drugs are the most common cause of erythema multiforme major in adults.

▶ General Considerations

Erythema multiforme is an acute inflammatory skin disease that is divided clinically into minor and major types based on the clinical findings. Approximately 90% of cases of erythema multiforme minor follow outbreaks of herpes simplex, and so is now preferably termed "herpes-associated erythema multiforme." The term "erythema multiforme major" has been replaced by three terms: Stevens-Johnson syndrome (SJS), with < 10% BSA skin loss; toxic epidermal necrolysis (TEN) when there is > 30% BSA skin loss; and SJS/TEN overlap for cases with between 10% and 30% BSA denudation. The abbreviation SJS/TEN is often used to refer to these three variants of what is considered one syndrome. All these clinical scenarios are characterized by toxicity and involvement of two or more mucosal surfaces (often oral and conjunctival). They are most often caused by medications, especially sulfonamides, NSAIDs, allopurinol, and anticonvulsants. *Mycoplasma pneumoniae* may trigger a skin eruption closely resembling SJS and may be the cause of SJS in up to 50% of children in some series. Erythema multiforme may also present as chronic or recurring ulceration localized to the oral mucosa, with skin lesions present in only half of the cases. The exposure to drugs associated with SJS/TEN may be systemic or topical (eg, eyedrops).

▶ Clinical Findings

A. Symptoms and Signs

A classic target lesion, found most commonly in herpes-associated erythema multiforme, consists of three concentric zones of color change, most often found acrally on the hands and feet. Not all lesions will have this appearance (Figure 6–27). Drug-associated bullous eruptions in the SJS/TEN spectrum present with raised purpuric target-like

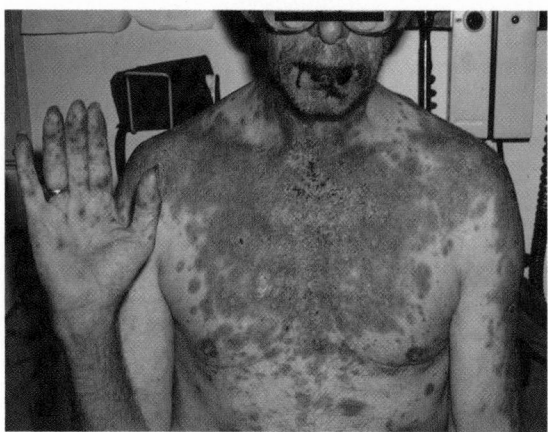

▲ **Figure 6–27.** Erythema multiforme. (Used, with permission, from Berger TG, Dept Dermatology, UCSF.)

lesions, with only two zones of color change and a central blister, or nondescript reddish or purpuric macules. Pain on eating, swallowing, and urination can occur if the appropriate mucosae are involved.

B. Laboratory Findings

Blood tests are not useful for diagnosis. Skin biopsy is diagnostic. Direct immunofluorescence studies are negative.

▶ Differential Diagnosis

Urticaria and drug eruptions are the chief entities that must be differentiated from erythema multiforme minor. Individual lesions of true urticaria should come and go within 24 hours and are usually responsive to antihistamines. In erythema multiforme major, the differential diagnosis includes autoimmune bullous diseases (including pemphigus and pemphigoid), acute generalized exanthematous pustulosis, and, rarely, pustular psoriasis. The presence of a blistering eruption requires biopsy and consultation for appropriate diagnosis and treatment.

▶ Complications

The tracheobronchial mucosa and conjunctiva may be involved in severe cases with resultant scarring. Ophthalmologic consultation is required if ocular involvement is present because vision loss is the major consequence of SJS/TEN.

▶ Treatment

A. General Measures

TEN is best treated in a burn unit, or hospital setting with similar support. Otherwise, patients need not be admitted unless mucosal involvement interferes with hydration and nutrition. Patients who begin to blister should be seen daily. Open lesions should be managed like second-degree burns. Immediate discontinuation of the inciting medication (before blistering occurs) is a significant predictor of

outcome. Delay in establishing the diagnosis and inadvertently continuing the offending medication results in higher morbidity and mortality.

B. Specific Measures

The most important aspect of treatment is to stop the offending medication and to move patients with > 25–30% BSA involvement to an appropriate acute care environment. Nutritional and fluid support and high vigilance for infection are the most important aspects of care. Recent reviews of systemic treatments for SJS and TEN have been conflicting, but the largest series have failed to show statistically significant benefit with treatment. Some data support the use of high-dose corticosteroids. If corticosteroids are to be tried in more severe cases, they should be used early, before blistering occurs, and in moderate to high doses (prednisone, 100–250 mg) and stopped within days if there is no dramatic response. IVIG (1 g/kg/d for 4 days) has become standard of care at some centers for TEN cases. It has not been proven to reduce mortality. Oral and topical corticosteroids are useful in the oral variant of erythema multiforme. Oral acyclovir prophylaxis of herpes simplex infections may be effective in preventing recurrent herpes-associated erythema multiforme minor.

C. Local Measures

Topical therapy is not very effective in this disease. For oral lesions, 1% diphenhydramine elixir mixed with Kaopectate or with 1% dyclonine may be used as a mouth rinse several times daily.

▶ Prognosis

Erythema multiforme minor usually lasts 2–6 weeks and may recur. SJS/TEN may be serious with a mortality of about 30% in cases with > 30% BSA involvement.

Huang YC et al. The efficacy of intravenous immunoglobulin for the treatment of toxic epidermal necrolysis: a systematic review and meta-analysis. Br J Dermatol. 2012 Aug;167(2):424–32. [PMID: 22458671]

Sokumbi O et al. Clinical features, diagnosis, and treatment of erythema multiforme: a review for the practicing dermatologist. Int J Dermatol. 2012 Aug;51(8):889–902. [PMID: 22788803]

Vern-Gross TZ et al. Erythema multiforme, Stevens Johnson syndrome, and toxic epidermal necrolysis syndrome in patients undergoing radiation therapy: a literature review. Am J Clin Oncol. 2012 Aug13. [Epub ahead of print] [PMID: 22892429]

Zhu QY et al. Toxic epidermal necrolysis: performance of SCORTEN and the score-based comparison of the efficacy of corticosteroid therapy and intravenous immunoglobulin combined therapy in China. J Burn Care Res. 2012 Nov;33(6):e295–308. [PMID: 22955159]

Ziemer M et al. Stevens-Johnson syndrome and toxic epidermal necrolysis in patients with lupus erythematosus: a descriptive study of 17 cases from a national registry and review of the literature. Br J Dermatol. 2012 Mar;166(3):575–600. [PMID: 22014091]

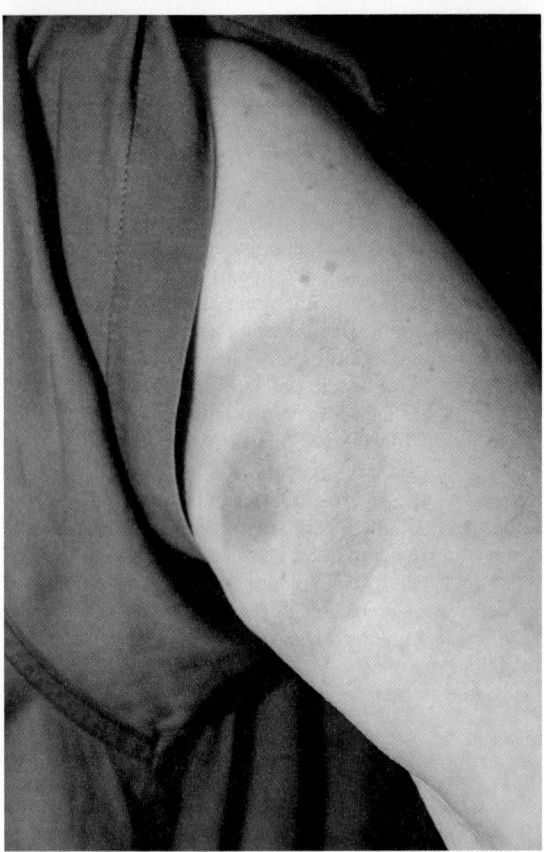

▲ **Figure 6–28.** Erythema migrans due to *Borrelia burgdorferi* (Lyme disease). (Courtesy of James Gathany, Public Health Image Library, CDC.)

3. Erythema Migrans (See also Chapter 34)

Erythema migrans is a unique cutaneous eruption that characterizes the localized or generalized early stage of Lyme disease (borreliosis) (Figure 6–28).

INFECTIOUS ERYTHEMAS

1. Erysipelas

ESSENTIALS OF DIAGNOSIS

▸ Edematous, spreading, circumscribed, hot, erythematous area, with or without vesicles or bullae.

▸ Central face frequently involved.

▸ Pain, chills, fever, and systemic toxicity may be striking.

General Considerations

Erysipelas is a superficial form of cellulitis that occurs classically on the cheek, caused by beta-hemolytic streptococci.

▸ Clinical Findings

A. Symptoms and Signs

The symptoms are pain, malaise, chills, and moderate fever. A bright red spot appears first, very often near a fissure at the angle of the nose. This spreads to form a tense, sharply demarcated, glistening, smooth, hot plaque. The margin characteristically makes noticeable advances in days or even hours. The lesion is somewhat edematous and may pit slightly with the finger. Vesicles or bullae occasionally develop on the surface. The lesion does not usually become pustular or gangrenous and heals without scar formation. The disease may complicate any break in the skin that provides a portal of entry for the organism.

B. Laboratory Findings

Leukocytosis is almost invariably present; blood cultures may be positive.

▸ Differential Diagnosis

Erysipeloid is a benign bacillary infection producing cellulitis of the skin of the fingers or the backs of the hands in fishermen and meat handlers.

▸ Complications

Unless erysipelas is promptly treated, death may result from extension of the process and systemic toxicity, particularly in the elderly.

▸ Treatment

Place the patient at bed rest with the head of the bed elevated. Intravenous antibiotics effective against group A beta-hemolytic streptococci and staphylococci should be considered, but outpatient treatment with oral antibiotics have demonstrated equal efficacy. A 7-day course with penicillin VK, 250 mg, dicloxacillin, 250 mg, or a first-generation cephalosporin, 250 mg, orally four times a day. Alternatives in penicillin-allergic patients are clindamycin (250 mg twice daily orally for 7–14 days) or erythromycin (250 mg four times daily orally for 7–14 days), the latter only if the infection is known to be due to streptococci.

▸ Prognosis

With appropriate treatment, rapid improvement is expected. Recurrence is uncommon.

Mortazavi M et al. Incidence of deep vein thrombosis in erysipelas or cellulitis of the lower extremities. Int J Dermatol. 2013 Mar;52(3):279–85. [PMID: 22913433]

Perelló-Alzamora MR et al. Clinical and epidemiological characteristics of adult patients hospitalized for erysipelas and cellulitis. Eur J Clin Microbiol Infect Dis. 2012 Sep;31(9):2147–52. [PMID: 22298240]

Picard D et al. Risk factors for abscess formation in patients with superficial cellulitis (erysipelas) of the leg. Br J Dermatol. 2013 Apr;168(4):859–63. [PMID: 23210619]

2. Cellulitis

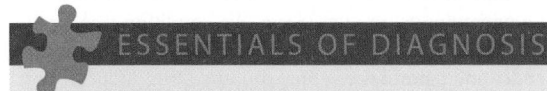

▶ Edematous, expanding, erythematous, warm plaque with or without vesicles or bullae.

▶ Lower leg is frequently involved.

▶ Pain, chills, and fever are commonly present.

▶ Septicemia may develop.

General Considerations

Cellulitis, a diffuse spreading infection of the dermis and subcutaneous tissue, is usually on the lower leg (Figure 6–29) and most commonly due to gram-positive cocci, especially group A beta-hemolytic streptococci and *S aureus*. Rarely, gram-negative rods or even fungi can produce a similar picture. In otherwise healthy persons, the most common portal of entry for lower leg cellulitis is toe web intertrigo with fissuring, usually a complication of interdigital tinea pedis. Venous insufficiency can also predispose to lower leg cellulitis. Injection drug use and open ulcerations may also be complicated by cellulitis. Cellulitis in the diabetic foot may be a major problem and is often associated with neuropathy and hyperkeratotic nodules from ill-fitting shoes and abnormal weight bearing.

Clinical Findings

A. Symptoms and Signs

Cellulitis begins as a small patch, which from its onset is tender. Swelling, erythema, and pain are often present. The lesion expands over hours, so that from onset to presentation is usually 6 to 36 hours. As the lesion grows, the patient becomes more ill with progressive chills, fever, and malaise. If septicemia develops, hypotension may develop, followed by shock.

B. Laboratory Findings

Leukocytosis or at least a neutrophilia (left shift) is present from early in the course. Blood cultures may be positive. If a central ulceration, pustule, or abscess is present, culture may be of value. Aspiration of the advancing edge has a low yield (20%) and is usually not performed. Instead, if an unusual organism is suspected and there is no loculated site to culture, a full thickness skin biopsy taken before antibiotics are given can be useful. Part is cultured and part processed for histologic evaluation with Gram stain. This technique is particularly useful in the immunocompromised patient. If a primary source for the infection is identified (wound, leg ulcer, toe web intertrigo), cultures from these sites isolate the causative pathogen in half of cases and can be used to guide antibiotic therapy.

Differential Diagnosis

Two potentially life-threatening entities that can mimic cellulitis (ie, present with a painful, red, swollen lower extremity) include deep venous thrombosis and necrotizing fasciitis. The diagnosis of necrotizing fasciitis should be suspected in a patient who has a very toxic appearance, bullae, crepitus or anesthesia of the involved skin, overlying skin necrosis, and laboratory evidence of rhabdomyolysis (elevated creatine kinase [CK]) or disseminated intravascular coagulation. While these findings may be present with severe cellulitis and bacteremia, it is essential to rule out necrotizing fasciitis because rapid surgical debridement is essential. Other skin lesions that may resemble cellulitis include sclerosing panniculitis, an acute, exquisitely tender red plaque on the medial lower legs above the malleolus in patients with venous stasis or varicosities, and acute severe contact dermatitis on a limb, which produces erythema, vesiculation, and edema as seen in cellulitis, but with itching instead of pain. Bilateral lower leg cellulitis is rare and other diagnoses, especially severe stasis dermatitis, should be considered in this setting. Severe lower extremity stasis dermatitis usually develops over days to

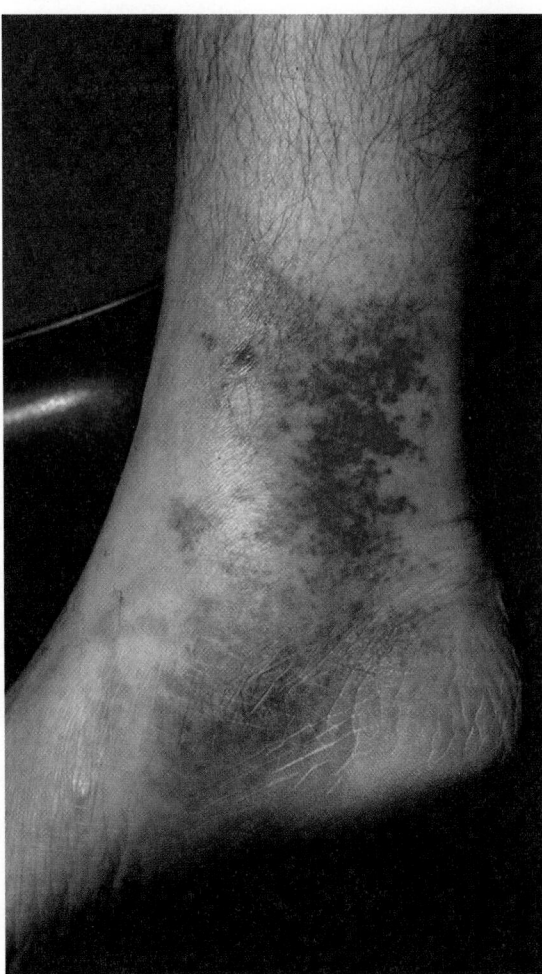

▲ **Figure 6–29.** Cellulitis. (Used, with permission, from Berger TG, Dept Dermatology, UCSF.)

weeks rather than the hours of cellulitis. It is also not as tender to palpation as cellulitis.

▶ Treatment

Intravenous or parenteral antibiotics may be required for the first 2–5 days, with adequate coverage for *Streptococcus* and *Staphylococcus*. Hospitalization is required in cases with severe local symptoms and signs, hypotension, elevated serum creatinine, low serum bicarbonate, elevated creatine kinase, elevated white blood cell count with marked left shift, or elevated C-reactive protein. If CA-MRSA is suspected, therapy is vancomycin, clindamycin, or TMP-SMZ plus a beta-lactam. In mild cases or following the initial parenteral therapy, dicloxacillin or cephalexin, 250–500 mg four times daily for 5–10 days, is usually adequate. If MRSA is suspected, use of TMP-SMZ, clindamycin, or the combination of doxycycline plus rifampin should be considered. In patients in whom intravenous treatment is not instituted, the first dose of oral antibiotic can be doubled to achieve rapid high blood levels. In patients with recurrent lower leg cellulitis, oral penicillin 250 mg twice daily can delay the appearance of the next episode.

Hirschmann JV et al. Lower limb cellulitis and its mimics: part I. Lower limb cellulitis. J Am Acad Dermatol. 2012 Aug;67(2):163.e1–12. [PMID: 22794815]

Hirschmann JV et al. Lower limb cellulitis and its mimics: part II. Conditions that simulate lower limb cellulitis. J Am Acad Dermatol. 2012 Aug;67(2):177.e1–9. [PMID: 227948156]

Lazzarini L et al. Erysipelas-cellulitis of the leg: impact of the application of a guideline in an infectious diseases unit. J Chemother. 2011 Dec;23(6): 378. [PMID: 22233827]

Picard D et al. Risk factors for abscess formation in patients with superficial cellulitis (erysipelas) of the leg. Br J Dermatol. 2013 Apr;168(4):859–63. [PMID: 23210619]

BLISTERING DISEASES

PEMPHIGUS

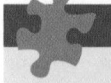

ESSENTIALS OF DIAGNOSIS

▶ Relapsing crops of bullae.

▶ Often preceded by mucous membrane bullae, erosions, and ulcerations.

▶ Superficial detachment of the skin after pressure or trauma variably present (Nikolsky sign).

▶ Acantholysis on biopsy.

▶ Immunofluorescence studies and serum ELISA for pathogenic antibodies are confirmatory.

▶ General Considerations

Pemphigus is an uncommon intraepidermal blistering disease occurring on skin and mucous membranes. It is caused

by autoantibodies to adhesion molecules expressed in the skin and mucous membranes. The cause is unknown, and in the preantibiotic, presteroid era, the condition was usually fatal within 5 years. The bullae appear spontaneously and are tender and painful when they rupture. Drug-induced pemphigus from penicillamine, captopril, and others has been reported. There are several forms of pemphigus: **pemphigus vulgaris** and its variant, **pemphigus vegetans**; and the more superficially blistering **pemphigus foliaceus** and its variant, **pemphigus erythematosus**. All forms may occur at any age but most commonly in middle age. The vulgaris form begins in the mouth in over 50% of cases. The foliaceus form is especially apt to be associated with other autoimmune diseases, or it may be drug-induced. Paraneoplastic pemphigus, a unique form of the disorder, is associated with numerous types of benign and malignant neoplasms but most frequently non-Hodgkin lymphoma.

▶ Clinical Findings

A. Symptoms and Signs

Pemphigus is characterized by an insidious onset of *flaccid* bullae, crusts, and erosions in crops or waves (Figure 6–30). In pemphigus vulgaris, lesions often appear first on the oral mucous membranes. These rapidly become erosive. The scalp is another site of early involvement. Rubbing a cotton swab or finger laterally on the surface of uninvolved skin may cause easy separation of the epidermis (**Nikolsky sign**).

B. Laboratory Findings

The diagnosis is made by light microscopy and by direct and indirect immunofluorescence (IIF) microscopy. Autoantibodies to intercellular adhesion molecules can be detected with ELISA assays and have replaced the use of IIF in some centers.

▶ Differential Diagnosis

Blistering diseases include erythema multiforme, drug eruptions, bullous impetigo, contact dermatitis, dermatitis

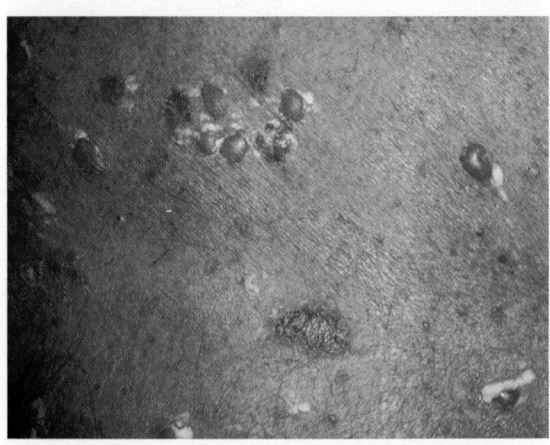

▲ **Figure 6–30.** Pemphigus. (Used, with permission, from Berger TG, Dept Dermatology, UCSF.)

herpetiformis, and bullous pemphigoid, but flaccid blisters are not typical of these diseases, and acantholysis is not seen on biopsy. All of these diseases have clinical characteristics and different immunofluorescence test results that distinguish them from pemphigus.

Paraneoplastic pemphigus is clinically, histologically, and immunologically distinct from other forms of the disease. Oral erosions and erythematous plaques resembling erythema multiforme are seen. Survival rates are low because of the underlying malignancy.

▶ **Complications**

Secondary infection commonly occurs; this is a major cause of morbidity and mortality. Disturbances of fluid, electrolyte, and nutritional intake can occur as a result of painful oral ulcers.

▶ **Treatment**

A. General Measures

When the disease is severe, hospitalize the patient at bed rest and provide antibiotics and intravenous feedings as indicated. Anesthetic troches used before eating ease painful oral lesions.

B. Systemic Measures

Pemphigus requires systemic therapy as early in its course as possible. However, the main morbidity in this disease is due to the side effects of such therapy. Initial therapy is with systemic corticosteroids: prednisone, 60–80 mg daily. In all but the most mild cases, a steroid-sparing agent is added from the beginning, since the course of the disease is long and the steroid-sparing agents take several weeks to exert their activity. Azathioprine (100–200 mg daily) or mycophenolate mofetil (1–1.5 g twice daily) are used most frequently. Rituximab treatment, especially early in the course, appears to be associated with therapeutic induction of a complete remission. Monthly IVIG at 2 g/kg intravenously over 3–4 days frequently is beneficial. In refractory cases, cyclophosphamide, pulse intravenous corticosteroids, and plasmapheresis can be used. Increased risk of thromboembolism is associated with IVIG therapy in these doses.

C. Local Measures

In patients with limited disease, skin and mucous membrane lesions should be treated with topical corticosteroids. Complicating infection requires appropriate systemic and local antibiotic therapy.

▶ **Prognosis**

The course tends to be chronic in most patients, though about one-third appear to experience remission. Infection is the most frequent cause of death, usually from *S aureus* septicemia.

Cianchini G et al. Therapy with rituximab for autoimmune pemphigus: results from a single-center observational study on 42 cases with long-term follow-up. J Am Acad Dermatol. 2012 Oct;67(4):617–22. [PMID: 22243765]

Leshem YA et al. Successful treatment of pemphigus with biweekly 1-g infusions of rituximab: A retrospective study of 47 patients. J Am Acad Dermatol. 2013 Mar;68(3);404–11. [PMID: 23044076]

Martin LK et al. A systematic review of randomized controlled trials for pemphigus vulgaris and pemphigus foliaceus. J Am Acad Dermatol. 2011 May;64(5):903–8. [PMID: 21353333]

Tsuruta D et al. Diagnosis and treatment of pemphigus. Immunotherapy. 2012 Jul;4(7):735–45. [PMID: 22853759]

Venugopal SS et al. Diagnosis and clinical features of pemphigus vulgaris. Immunol Allergy Clin North Am. 2012 May;32(2):233–43. [PMID: 22560136]

BULLOUS PEMPHIGOID

Many other autoimmune skin disorders are characterized by formation of bullae, or blisters. These include bullous pemphigoid, cicatricial pemphigoid, dermatitis herpetiformis, and pemphigoid gestationis.

Bullous pemphigoid is a relatively benign pruritic disease characterized by *tense* blisters in flexural areas, usually remitting in 5 or 6 years, with a course characterized by exacerbations and remissions. Most affected persons are over the age of 60 (often in their 70s or 80s), and men are affected twice as frequently as women. The appearance of blisters may be preceded by urticarial or edematous lesions for months. Oral lesions are present in about one-third of affected persons. The disease may occur in various forms, including localized, vesicular, vegetating, erythematous, erythrodermic, and nodular.

The diagnosis is made by biopsy and direct immunofluorescence examination. Light microscopy shows a subepidermal blister. With direct immunofluorescence, IgG and C3 are found at the dermal-epidermal junction. If the patient has mild disease, ultrapotent corticosteroids may be adequate. Prednisone at a dosage of 0.75 mg/kg daily is often used to achieve rapid control of more widespread disease. Although slower in onset of action, tetracycline or erythromycin, 500 mg three times daily, alone or combined with nicotinamide—*not nicotinic acid or niacin*—(up to 1.5 g/d), if tolerated, may control the disease in patients who cannot use corticosteroids or may allow decreasing or eliminating corticosteroids after control is achieved. Dapsone is particularly effective in mucous membrane pemphigoid. If these drugs are not effective, methotrexate, 5–25 mg weekly, or azathioprine, 50 mg one to three times daily, or mycophenolate mofetil (1 g twice daily) may be used as steroid-sparing agents.

Gaitanis G et al. High-dose intravenous immunoglobulin in the treatment of adult patients with bullous pemphigoid. Eur J Dermatol. 2012 May–Jun;22(3):363–9. [PMID: 22548754]

Schmidt E et al. Pemphigoid diseases. Lancet. 2013 Jan26;381(9863):320–32. [PMID: 23237497]

Tampoia M et al. Diagnostic accuracy of enzyme-linked immunosorbent assays (ELISA) to detect anti-skin autoantibodies in autoimmune blistering skin diseases: A systematic review and meta-analysis. Autoimmun Rev. 2012 Dec;12(2):121–6. [PMID: 22781589]

PAPULES

WARTS

ESSENTIALS OF DIAGNOSIS

- ▶ Verrucous papules anywhere on the skin or mucous membranes, usually no larger than 1 cm in diameter.
- ▶ Prolonged incubation period (average 2–18 months).
- ▶ Spontaneous "cures" are frequent in common warts (50% at 2 years).
- ▶ "Recurrences" (new lesions) are frequent.

▶ General Considerations

Warts (common, plantar, and genital) are caused by human papillomaviruses (HPVs). Typing of HPV lesions is NOT a part of standard medical evaluation except in the case of genital dysplasia.

▶ Clinical Findings

There are usually no symptoms. Tenderness on pressure occurs with plantar warts; itching occurs with anogenital warts (Figure 6–31). Flat warts are most evident under oblique illumination. Periungual warts may be dry, fissured, and hyperkeratotic and may resemble hangnails or other nonspecific changes. Plantar warts resemble plantar corns or calluses.

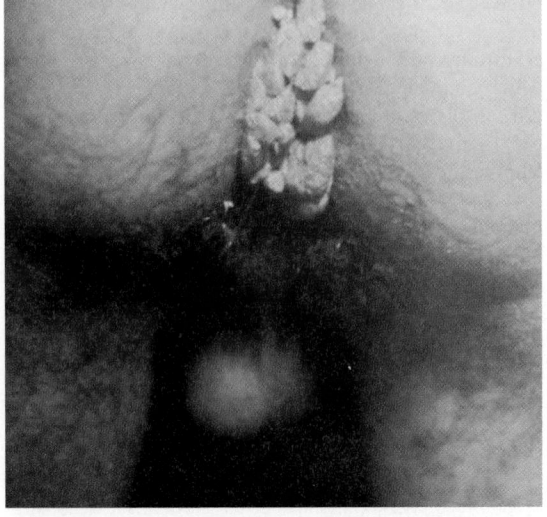

▲ **Figure 6–31.** Condylomata acuminata, or genital warts, of the anal region due to human papillomavirus. (Public Health Image Library, CDC.)

▶ Differential Diagnosis

Some warty-looking lesions are actually hypertrophic actinic keratoses or squamous cell carcinomas. Some genital warty lesions may be due to secondary syphilis (condylomata lata). The lesions of molluscum contagiosum are pearly with a central dell. In AIDS, wart-like lesions may be caused by varicella zoster virus.

▶ Prevention

Administration of a vaccine against certain genital HPV types can prevent infection with these wart types and reduce cervical dysplasia. It is recommended for teenagers and young adults (see Chapters 1 and 18).

▶ Treatment

Treatment is aimed at inducing "wart-free" intervals for as long as possible without scarring, since no treatment can guarantee a remission or prevent recurrences. In immunocompromised patients, the goal is even more modest, ie, to control the size and number of lesions present.

A. Removal

For common warts of the hands, patients are usually offered liquid nitrogen or keratolytic agents. The former may work in fewer treatments but requires office visits and is painful.

1. Liquid nitrogen—Liquid nitrogen is applied to achieve a thaw time of 30–45 seconds. Two freeze-thaw cycles are given every 2–4 weeks for several visits. Scarring will occur if it is used incorrectly. Liquid nitrogen may cause permanent depigmentation in pigmented individuals. Cryotherapy is first-line physician applied surgical treatment for genital warts (condyloma acuminata).

2. Keratolytic agents and occlusion—Salicylic acid products may be used against common warts or plantar warts. They are applied then occluded. Plantar warts may be treated by applying a 40% salicylic acid plaster after paring. The plaster may be left on for 5–6 days, then removed, the lesion pared down, and another plaster applied. Although it may take weeks or months to eradicate the wart, the method is safe and effective with almost no side effects. Chronic occlusion alone with water-impermeable tape (duct tape, adhesive tape) is less effective than cryotherapy.

3. Podophyllum resin—For genital warts, the purified active component of the podophyllum resin, podofilox, is applied by the patient twice daily 3 consecutive days a week for cycles of 4–6 weeks. It is less irritating and more effective than "physician-applied" podophyllum resin. After a single 4-week cycle, 45% of patients were wart-free; but of these, 60% relapsed at 6 weeks. Thus, multiple cycles of treatment are often necessary. Patients unable to obtain the take home podofilox may be treated in the clinician's office by painting each wart carefully (protecting normal skin) every 2–3 weeks with 25% podophyllum resin (podophyllin) in compound tincture of benzoin. Pregnant patients should not be so treated. Podophyllin is ineffective for common warts and plantar warts.

4. Imiquimod—A 5% cream of this local interferon inducer has moderate activity in clearing external genital warts (EGWs). Treatment is once daily on 3 alternate days per week. Response may be slow, with patients who eventually cleared having responses at 8 weeks (44%) or 12 weeks (69%). There is a marked gender difference with respect to response, with 77% of women and 40% of men having complete clearing of their lesions. Once cleared, about 13% have recurrences in the short term.

In accidental exposure during pregnancy, there is less risk with imiquimod than with podophyllum resin (category B versus category X). Imiquimod is considerably more expensive than podophyllotoxin, but given the high rate of response in women and its safety, it appears to be the "patient-administered" treatment of choice for EGWs in women. In men, the more rapid response, lower cost, and similar efficacy make podophyllotoxin the initial treatment of choice, with imiquimod used for recurrences or refractory cases. Imiquimod has no demonstrated efficacy for—and should not be used to treat—plantar or common warts.

5. Operative removal—Plantar warts may be removed by blunt dissection. For genital warts, snip biopsy (scissors) removal followed by light electrocautery is more effective than cryotherapy, especially for patients with pedunculated or large lesions.

6. Laser therapy—The CO_2 laser can be effective for treating recurrent warts, periungual warts, plantar warts, and condylomata acuminata. It leaves open wounds that must fill in with granulation tissue over 4–6 weeks and is best reserved for warts resistant to all other modalities. Lasers with emissions of 585, 595, or 532 nm may also be used every 3–4 weeks to gradually ablate common or plantar warts. This is no more effective than cryotherapy in controlled trials. For genital warts, it has not been shown that laser therapy is more effective than electrosurgical removal. Photodynamic therapy can be considered in refractory widespread flat and genital warts.

7. Other agents—Bleomycin diluted to 1 unit/mL may be injected into common and plantar warts. It has been shown to have a high cure rate. It should be used with caution on digital warts because of the potential complications of Raynaud phenomenon, nail loss, and terminal digital necrosis.

B. Immunotherapy

Squaric acid dibutylester may be effective. It is applied in a concentration of 0.2–2% directly to the warts from once weekly to five times weekly to induce a mild contact dermatitis. Between 60% and 80% of warts clear over 10–20 weeks. Injection of *Candida* antigen starting at 1:50 dilution and repeated every 3–4 weeks may be similarly effective in stimulating immunologic regression of common and plantar warts.

C. Physical Modalities

Soaking warts in hot (42.2°C) water for 10–30 minutes daily for 6 weeks has resulted in involution in some cases.

▶ Prognosis

There is a striking tendency to the development of new lesions. Warts may disappear spontaneously or may be unresponsive to treatment.

Chelimo C et al. Risk factors for and prevention of human papillomaviruses (HPV), genital warts and cervical cancer. J Infect. 2013 Mar;66(3):207–17. [PMID: 23103285]

Chesson HW et al. Estimates of the annual direct medical costs of the prevention and treatment of disease associated with human papillomavirus in the United States. Vaccine. 2012 Sep14;30(42):6016–9. [PMID: 22867718]

Giuliano AR et al. Efficacy of quadrivalent HPV vaccine against HPV Infection and disease in males. N Engl J Med. 2011 Feb3;364(5):401–11. [PMID: 21288094]

Hathaway JK. HPV: diagnosis, prevention, and treatment. Clin Obstet Gynecol. 2012 Sep;55(3):671–80. [PMID: 22828099]

Jemal A et al. Annual Report to the Nation on the Status of Cancer, 1975–2009, featuring the burden and trends in human papillomavirus (HPV)-associated cancers and HPV vaccination coverage levels. J Natl Cancer Inst. 2013 Feb6;105(3): 175–201. [PMID: 23297039]

Komericki P et al. Efficacy and safety of imiquimod versus podophyllotoxin in the treatment of anogenital warts. Sex Transm Dis. 2011 Mar;38(3):216–8. [PMID: 20938374]

Kwok CS et al. Topical treatments for cutaneous warts. Cochrane Database Syst Rev. 2012 Sep12;9: CD001781. [PMID: 22972052]

Patel H et al. Systematic review of the incidence and prevalence of genital warts. BMC Infect Dis. 2013 Jan25;13:39. [PMID: 23347441]

MOLLUSCUM CONTAGIOSUM

Molluscum contagiosum, caused by a poxvirus, presents as single or multiple dome-shaped, waxy papules 2–5 mm in diameter that are umbilicated (Figure 6–32). Lesions at first are firm, solid, and flesh-colored but upon reaching

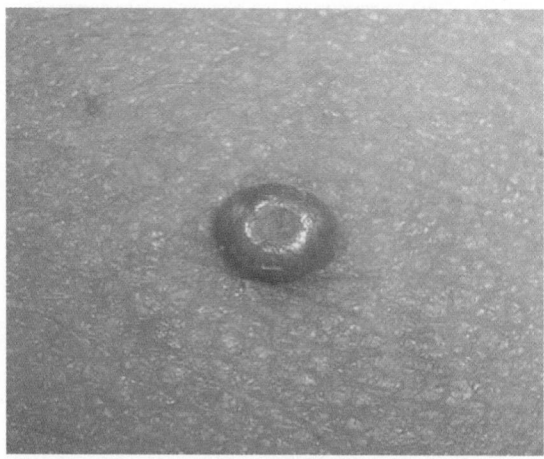

▲ **Figure 6–32.** Molluscum contagiosum lesion on the back. (Courtesy of Richard P. Usatine, MD; used, with permission, from Usatine RP, Smith MA, Mayeaux EJ Jr, Chumley H, Tysinger J. *The Color Atlas of Family Medicine.* McGraw-Hill, 2009.)

maturity become soft, whitish, or pearly gray and may suppurate. The principal sites of involvement are the face, lower abdomen, and genitals.

The lesions are autoinoculable and spread by wet skin-to-skin contact. In sexually active individuals, they may be confined to the penis, pubis, and inner thighs and are considered a sexually transmitted infection.

Molluscum contagiosum is common in patients with AIDS, usually with a helper T-cell count < 100/mcL. Extensive lesions tend to develop over the face and neck as well as in the genital area.

The diagnosis is easily established in most instances because of the distinctive central umbilication of the dome-shaped lesion. The best treatment is by curettage or applications of liquid nitrogen as for warts—but more briefly. When lesions are frozen, the central umbilication often becomes more apparent. Light electrosurgery with a fine needle is also effective. It has been estimated that individual lesions persist for about 2 months. They are difficult to eradicate in patients with AIDS unless immunity improves. However, in AIDS, with highly effective antiretroviral treatment, molluscum do not need to be treated because they usually spontaneously clear.

Chen X et al. Molluscum contagiosum virus infection. Lancet Infect Dis. 2013 Oct;13(10):877–88. [PMID: 23972567]

BASAL CELL CARCINOMA

ESSENTIALS OF DIAGNOSIS

▶ Pearly papule, erythematous patch > 6 mm, or nonhealing ulcer, in sun exposed areas (face, trunk, lower legs).

▶ History of bleeding.

▶ Fair-skinned person with a history of sun exposure (often intense, intermittent).

▶ General Considerations

Basal cell carcinomas are the most common form of cancer. They occur on sun-exposed skin in otherwise normal, fair-skinned individuals; ultraviolet light is the cause. The most common presentation is a papule or nodule that may have a central scab or erosion (Figure 6–33). Occasionally the nodules have stippled pigment (pigmented basal cell carcinoma). Intradermal nevi without pigment on the face of older white individuals may resemble basal cell carcinomas. Basal cell carcinomas grow slowly, attaining a size of 1–2 cm or more in diameter, usually only after years of growth. There is a waxy, "pearly" appearance, with telangiectatic vessels easily visible. It is the pearly or translucent quality of these lesions that is most diagnostic, a feature best appreciated if the skin is stretched. On the back and chest, basal cell carcinomas appear as reddish, somewhat shiny, scaly patches.

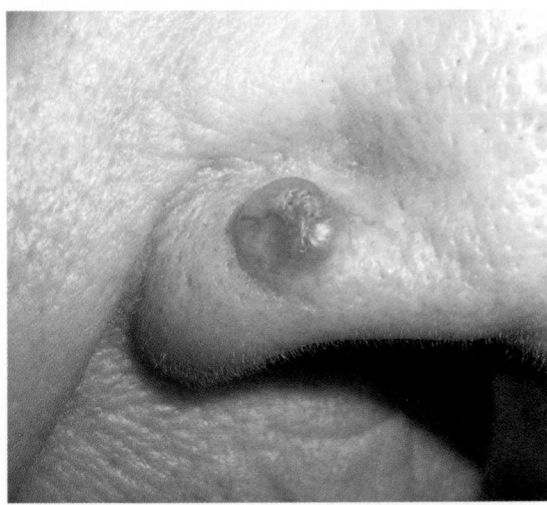

▲ **Figure 6–33.** Nodular basal cell carcinoma of the nose. (Courtesy of Richard P. Usatine, MD; used, with permission, from Usatine RP, Smith MA, Mayeaux EJ Jr, Chumley H, Tysinger J. *The Color Atlas of Family Medicine.* McGraw-Hill, 2009.)

Clinicians should examine the whole skin routinely, looking for bumps, patches, and scabbed lesions. When examining the face, look at the eyelid margins and medial canthi, the nose and alar folds, the lips, and then around and behind the ears.

▶ Treatment

Lesions suspected to be basal cell carcinomas should be biopsied, by shave or punch biopsy. Therapy is then aimed at eradication with minimal cosmetic deformity, often by excision and suturing with recurrence rates of 5% or less. The technique of three cycles of curettage and electrodesiccation depends on the skill of the operator and is not recommended for head and neck lesions. After 4–6 weeks of healing, it leaves a broad, hypopigmented, at times hypertrophic scar. Radiotherapy is effective and sometimes appropriate for older individuals (over age 65), but recurrent tumors after radiation therapy are more difficult to treat and may be more aggressive. Radiation therapy is the most expensive method to treat basal cell carcinoma and should only be used if other treatment options are not appropriate. Mohs surgery—removal of the tumor followed by immediate frozen section histopathologic examination of margins with subsequent reexcision of tumor-positive areas and final closure of the defect—gives the highest cure rates (98%) and results in least tissue loss. It is appropriate therapy for tumors of the eyelids, nasolabial folds, canthi, external ear, and temple; for recurrent lesions; or where tissue sparing is needed for cosmesis. Since up to half of patients with a basal cell carcinoma will develop a second lesion, patients with basal cell carcinomas must be monitored at least yearly to detect new or recurrent lesions.

Ad Hoc Task Force; Connolly SM et al. AAD/ACMS/ASDSA/ASMS 2012 appropriate use criteria for Mohs micrographic surgery: a report of the American Academy of Dermatology, American College of Mohs Surgery, American Society for Dermatologic Surgery Association, and the American Society for Mohs Surgery. J Am Acad Dermatol. 2012 Oct;67(4): 531–50. [PMID: 22959232]

Flohil SC et al. Trends in basal cell carcinoma incidence rates: a 37-Year Dutch observational study. J Invest Dermatol. 2013 Apr;133(4):913–8. [PMID: 23190883]

SQUAMOUS CELL CARCINOMA

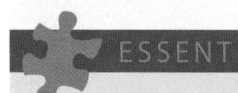

ESSENTIALS OF DIAGNOSIS

▸ Nonhealing ulcer or warty nodule.

▸ Skin damage due to long-term sun exposure.

▸ Common in fair-skinned organ transplant recipients.

Squamous cell carcinoma usually occurs subsequent to prolonged sun exposure on exposed parts in fair-skinned individuals who sunburn easily and tan poorly. It may arise from an actinic keratosis. The lesions appear as small red, conical, hard nodules that occasionally ulcerate (Figure 6–34). In actinically induced squamous cell cancers, rates of metastasis are estimated from retrospective studies to be 3–7%. Squamous cell carcinomas of the ear, temple, lip, oral cavity, tongue, and genitalia have much higher rates of recurrence or metastasis and require special management.

Examination of the skin and therapy are essentially the same as for basal cell carcinoma. The preferred treatment of squamous cell carcinoma is excision. Electrodesiccation and curettage and x-ray radiation may be used for some lesions, and fresh tissue microscopically controlled excision (Mohs) is recommended for high-risk lesions (lips, temples, ears, nose) and for recurrent tumors. Follow-up for squamous cell carcinoma must be more frequent and thorough than for basal cell carcinoma, starting at every 3 months, with careful examination of lymph nodes for 1 year, then twice yearly thereafter. In addition, palpation of the lips is essential to detect hard or indurated areas that represent early squamous cell carcinoma. All such cases must be biopsied. Multiple squamous cell carcinomas are very common on the sun-exposed skin of organ transplant patients. The intensity of immunosuppression, not the use of any particular immunosuppressive agent, is the primary risk factor in determining the development of skin cancer after transplant. The tumors begin to appear after 5 years of immunosuppression. Voriconazole treatment appears to increase the risk of development of squamous cell carcinoma, especially in lung transplant patients. Regular dermatologic evaluation in at-risk organ transplant recipients is recommended. Biologic behavior of skin

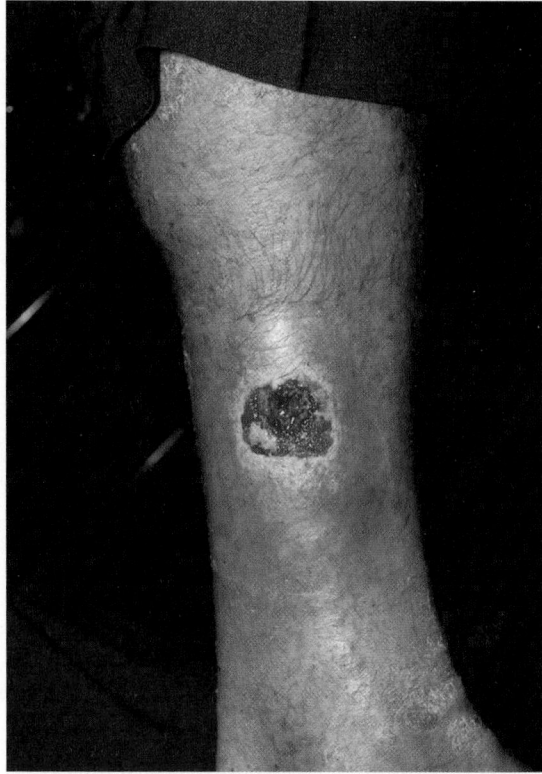

▲ **Figure 6–34.** Squamous cell carcinoma. (Used, with permission, from Berger TG, Dept Dermatology, UCSF.)

cancer in organ transplant recipients may be aggressive, and careful management is required. Other forms of immunosuppression such as chronic lymphocytic leukemia, HIV/AIDS, and chronic iatrogenic immunosuppression may also increase skin cancer risk and be associated with more aggressive skin cancer behavior.

Behshad R et al. Systemic treatment of locally advanced non-metastatic cutaneous squamous cell carcinoma: a review of the literature. Br J Dermatol. 2011 Dec;165(6):1169–77. [PMID: 21777215]

Carroll RP et al. Conversion to sirolimus in kidney transplant recipients with squamous cell cancer and changes in immune phenotype. Nephrol Dial Transplant. 2013 Feb; 28(2):462–5. [PMID: 23223314]

Roozeboom MH et al. Clinical and histological prognostic factors for local recurrence and metastasis of cutaneous squamous cell carcinoma: analysis of a defined population. Acta Derm Venereol. 2013 Jul6;93(4):417–21. [PMID: 23138613]

Schmults CD et al. Factors predictive of recurrence and death from cutaneous squamous cell carcinoma: a 10-year, single-institution cohort study. JAMA Dermatol. 2013 May;149(5):541–7. [PMID: 23677079]

Zwald FO et al. Skin cancer in solid organ transplant recipients: advances in therapy and management: part I. Epidemiology of skin cancer in solid organ transplant recipients. J Am Acad Dermatol. 2011 Aug;65(2):253–61. [PMID: 21763561]

VIOLACEOUS TO PURPLE PAPULES & NODULES

LICHEN PLANUS

► Pruritic, violaceous, flat-topped papules with fine white streaks and symmetric distribution.

► Lacy or erosive lesions of the buccal and vaginal mucosa; nail dystrophy.

► Commonly seen along linear scratch marks (Koebner phenomenon) on anterior wrists, penis, legs.

► Histopathologic examination is diagnostic.

► General Considerations

Lichen planus is an inflammatory pruritic disease of the skin and mucous membranes characterized by distinctive papules with a predilection for the flexor surfaces and trunk. The three cardinal findings are typical skin lesions, mucosal lesions, and histopathologic features of band-like infiltration of lymphocytes in the upper dermis. The most common drugs causing lichen planus-like reactions include sulfonamides, tetracyclines, quinidine, NSAIDs, beta-blockers, and hydrochlorothiazide. Lichenoid drug eruptions can resemble lichen planus clinically and histologically. Hepatitis C infection is found with greater frequency in lichen planus patients than in controls. Allergy to mercury and other metal containing amalgams can trigger oral lesions identical to lichen planus. Lichenoid drug eruptions can resemble lichen planus clinically and histologically.

► Clinical Findings

Itching is mild to severe. The lesions are violaceous, flat-topped, angulated papules, up to 1 cm in diameter, discrete or in clusters, with very fine white streaks (Wickham striae) on the flexor surfaces of the wrists and on the penis, lips, tongue as well as buccal, vaginal, esophageal, and anorectal mucous membranes. The papules may become bullous or eroded. The disease may be generalized (Figure 6–35). Mucous membrane lesions have a lacy white network overlying them that may be confused with leukoplakia. The presence of oral and vaginal lichen planus in the same patient is common. Patients with both these mucous membranes involved are at much higher risk for esophageal lichen planus. The Koebner phenomenon (appearance of lesions in areas of trauma) may be seen.

A special form of lichen planus is the erosive or ulcerative variety, a major problem in the mouth or genitalia. Squamous cell carcinoma develops in 5% of patients with erosive oral or genital lichen planus and may occur in esophageal lichen planus.

► Differential Diagnosis

Lichen planus must be distinguished from similar lesions produced by medications (see above) and other papular

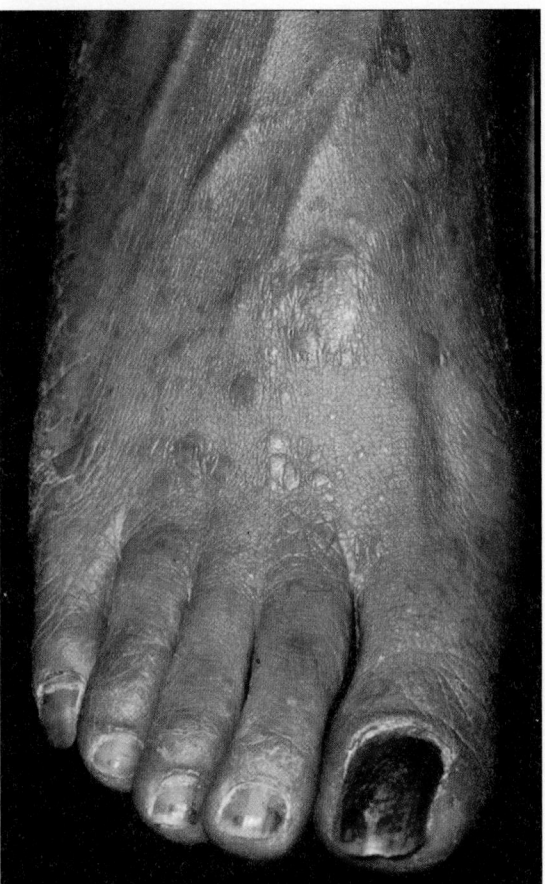

⏶ **Figure 6–35.** Lichen planus. (Used, with permission, from Berger TG, Dept Dermatology, UCSF.)

lesions such as psoriasis, lichen simplex chronicus, graft-versus-host disease, and syphilis. Lichen planus on the mucous membranes must be differentiated from leukoplakia. Erosive oral lesions require biopsy and often direct immunofluorescence for diagnosis since lichen planus may simulate other erosive diseases.

► Treatment

A. Topical Therapy

Superpotent topical corticosteroids applied twice daily are most helpful for localized disease in nonflexural areas. Alternatively, high-potency corticosteroid cream or ointment may be used nightly under thin pliable plastic film.

Topical tacrolimus appears effective in oral and vaginal erosive lichen planus, but long-term therapy is required to prevent relapse. If tacrolimus is used, lesions must be observed carefully for development of cancer. Since absorption can occur through mucous membranes, serum tacrolimus levels should be checked at least once if widespread mucosal application (> 5–10 cm²) is used. If the erosive oral lichen planus lesions are adjacent to a metal containing amalgam, removal of the amalgam may result in clearing of the erosions.

B. Systemic Therapy

Corticosteroids (see Chapter 26) may be required in severe cases or in circumstances where the most rapid response to treatment is desired. Unfortunately, relapse almost always occurs as the corticosteroids are tapered, making systemic corticosteroid therapy an impractical option for the management of chronic lichen planus. NB-UVB, bath PUVA, oral PUVA, and the combination of an oral retinoid plus PUVA (re-PUVA) are all forms of phototherapy that can improve lichen planus. Hydroxychloroquine, 200 mg orally twice daily, can also be effective in mucosal and cutaneous lichen planus.

Prognosis

Lichen planus is a benign disease, but it may persist for months or years and may be recurrent. Hypertrophic lichen planus and oral lesions tend to be especially persistent, and neoplastic degeneration has been described in chronically eroded lesions.

Cheng S et al. Interventions for erosive lichen planus affecting mucosal sites. Cochrane Database Syst Rev. 2012 Feb15;2: CD008092. [PMID: 22336835]

García-García V et al. New perspectives on the dynamic behaviour of oral lichen planus. Eur J Dermatol. 2012 Mar-Apr;22(2):172–7. [PMID: 22381396]

Le Cleach L et al. Clinical practice. Lichen planus. N Engl J Med. 2012 Feb23;366(8):723–32. [PMID: 22356325]

Sharma A et al. Lichen planus: an update and review. Cutis. 2012 Jul;90(1):17–23. [PMID: 22908728]

Throngprasom K et al. Interventions for treating oral lichen planus. Cochrane Database Syst Rev. 2011 Jul6;(7): CD001168. [PMID: 21735381]

KAPOSI SARCOMA

General Considerations

Before 1980 in the United States, this rare malignant skin lesion was seen mostly in elderly men, had a chronic clinical course, and was rarely fatal. Kaposi sarcoma occurs endemically in an often aggressive form in young black men of equatorial Africa, but it is rare in American blacks. Kaposi sarcoma continues to occur largely in homosexual men with HIV infection as an AIDS-defining illness. Kaposi sarcoma may complicate immunosuppressive therapy, and stopping the immunosuppression may result in improvement. Human herpes virus 8 (HHV-8), or Kaposi sarcoma-associated herpes virus (KSHV), is universally present in all forms of Kaposi sarcoma.

Red or purple plaques or nodules on cutaneous or mucosal surfaces are characteristic. Marked edema may occur with few or no skin lesions. Kaposi sarcoma commonly involves the gastrointestinal tract and can be screened for by fecal occult blood testing. In asymptomatic patients, these lesions are not sought or treated. Pulmonary Kaposi sarcoma can present with shortness of breath, cough, hemoptysis, or chest pain; it may be asymptomatic, appearing only on chest radiograph. Bronchoscopy may be indicated. The incidence of AIDS-associated Kaposi sarcoma is diminishing; however, chronic Kaposi sarcoma can develop in patients with HIV infection, high CD4 counts, and low viral loads. In this setting, the Kaposi sarcoma usually resembles the endemic form, being indolent and localized. At times, however, it can be clinically aggressive.

Treatment

For Kaposi sarcoma in the elderly, palliative local therapy with intralesional chemotherapy or radiation is usually all that is required. In the setting of iatrogenic immunosuppression, the treatment of Kaposi sarcoma is primarily reduction of doses of immunosuppressive medications. In AIDS-associated Kaposi sarcoma, the patient should first be given effective anti-HIV antiretrovirals because in most cases this treatment alone is associated with improvement. Other therapeutic options include cryotherapy or intralesional vinblastine (0.1–0.5 mg/mL) for cosmetically objectionable lesions; radiation therapy for accessible and space-occupying lesions; and laser surgery for certain intraoral and pharyngeal lesions. Systemic therapy is indicated in patients with rapidly progressive skin disease (more than ten new lesions per month), with edema or pain, and with symptomatic visceral disease or pulmonary disease. Liposomal doxorubicin is highly effective in controlling these cases and has considerably less toxicity—and greater efficacy—than anthracycline monotherapy or combination chemotherapeutic regimens. Alpha-interferon may also be used. Paclitaxel and other taxanes can be effective even in patients who do not respond to anthracycline treatment.

La Ferla L et al. Kaposi's sarcoma in HIV-positive patients: the state of art in the HAART-era. Eur Rev Med Pharmacol Sci. 2013 Sep;17(17):2354–65. [PMID: 24065230]

Lu CL et al. Immune reconstitution inflammatory syndrome of Kaposi's sarcoma in an HIV-infected patient. J Microbiol Immunol Infect. 2013 Aug;46(4):309–12. [PMID: 22503798]

Régnier-Rosencher E et al. Treatments for classic Kaposi sarcoma: a systematic review of the literature. J Am Acad Dermatol. 2013 Feb;68(2):313–31. [PMID: 22695100]

PRURITUS (ITCHING)

Pruritus is a disagreeable sensation that provokes a desire to scratch. It is modulated by multiple factors, including anxiety, depression, and amphetamine and cocaine use. Calcium channel blockers can cause pruritus with or without eczema, even years after they have been started, and it may take up to 1 year for the pruritus to resolve after the calcium channel blocker has been stopped. Pruritus as a medical complaint is 40% as common as low back pain. Elderly Asian men are most significantly affected with 20% of all healthcare visits in Asian men over the age of 65 involving the complaint of itch. The quality of life of a patient with chronic pruritus is the same as a patient on hemodialysis. **Most cases of pruritus are not mediated by histamine,** hence the poor response of many pruritic patients to antihistamines. Neuropathic disease, especially in diabetics, is associated with pruritus, making neurally acting agents attractive new approaches to the management of pruritus.

Dry skin is the first cause of itch that should be sought, since it is common and easily treated. Other causes include scabies, atopic dermatitis, insect bites, pediculosis, contact dermatitis, drug reactions, urticaria, psoriasis, lichen planus, lichen simplex chronicus, and fiberglass dermatitis.

Persistent pruritus not explained by cutaneous disease or association with a primary skin eruption should prompt a staged workup for systemic causes. Perhaps the most common cause of pruritus associated with systemic disease is uremia in conjunction with hemodialysis. This condition and to a lesser degree the pruritus of liver disease may be helped by phototherapy with ultraviolet B or PUVA. Naltrexone and nalmefene have been shown to relieve the pruritus of liver disease. Naltrexone is not effective in pruritus associated with advanced chronic kidney disease, but gabapentin may be effective. Endocrine disorders such as hypothyroidism, hyperthyroidism, or hyperparathyroidism, psychiatric disturbances, lymphoma, leukemia, and other internal malignant disorders, iron deficiency anemia, and certain neurologic disorders may also cause pruritus. The treatment of chronic pruritus can be frustrating. Combinations of antihistamines, sinequan, gabapentin, mirtazapine, and opioid antagonists can be attempted in refractory cases. In cancer-associated and other forms of pruritus, aprepitant (Emend) 80 mg daily for several days can be dramatically effective.

▶ Prognosis

Elimination of external factors and irritating agents may give complete relief. Pruritus accompanying a specific skin disease will subside when the skin disease is controlled. Pruritus accompanying serious internal disease may not respond to any type of therapy.

Bergasa NV. The itch of liver disease. Semin Cutan Med Surg. 2011 Jun;30(2):93–8. [PMID: 21767769]

Berger TG et al. Pruritus and renal failure. Semin Cutan Med Surg. 2011 Jun;30(2):99–100. [PMID: 21767770]

Berger TG et al. Pruritus in the older patient: a clinical review. JAMA. 2013 Dec11;310(22):2443–50. [PMID: 24327039]

Chiang HC et al. Cancer and itch. Semin Cutan Med Surg. 2011 Jun;30(2):107–12. [PMID: 21767772]

Serling SL et al. Approach to pruritus in the adult HIV-positive patient. Semin Cutan Med Surg. 2011 Jun;30(2):101–6. [PMID: 21767771]

Shive M et al. Itch as a patient-reported symptom in ambulatory care visits in the United States. J Am Acad Dermatol. 2013 Oct;69(4):550–6. [PMID: 23870201]

Summers EM et al. Chronic eczematous eruptions in the aging: further support for an association with exposure to calcium channel blockers. JAMA Dermatol. 2013 Jul;149(7):814–8. [PMID: 23636109]

ANOGENITAL PRURITUS

ESSENTIALS OF DIAGNOSIS

▶ Itching, chiefly nocturnal, of the anogenital area.

▶ Examination is highly variable, ranging from no skin findings to excoriations and inflammation of any degree, including lichenification.

▶ General Considerations

Anogenital pruritus may be due to intertrigo, psoriasis, lichen simplex chronicus, or seborrheic or contact dermatitis (from soaps, colognes, douches, and various topical treatments) or it may be due to irritating secretions, as in diarrhea, leukorrhea, or trichomoniasis, or to local disease (candidiasis, dermatophytosis, erythrasma), and at times oxyuriasis (pinworms). Lichen sclerosus may at times be the cause. Erythrasma at any anatomic location (Figure 6–36) is easily diagnosed by demonstration of coral-red fluorescence with Wood light; it is easily cured with erythromycin orally or topically.

In pruritus ani, hemorrhoids are often found, and leakage of mucus and bacteria from the distal rectum onto the perianal skin may be important in cases in which no other skin abnormality is found.

Many women experience pruritus vulvae. Pruritus vulvae does not usually involve the anal area, though anal itching may spread to the vulva. In men, pruritus of the scrotum is most commonly seen in the absence of pruritus ani. Up to one-third of causes of anogenital pruritus may be due to nerve impingements of the lumbosacral spine, so referral for evaluation of lumbosacral spine disease is appropriate if no skin disorder is identified, and topical therapy is ineffective.

Squamous cell carcinoma of the anus and extramammary Paget disease are rare causes of genital pruritus.

▶ Clinical Findings

A. Symptoms and Signs

The only symptom is itching. Physical findings are usually not present, but there may be erythema, fissuring, maceration, lichenification, excoriations, or changes suggestive of candidiasis or tinea.

B. Laboratory Findings

Urinalysis and blood glucose testing may lead to a diagnosis of diabetes mellitus. Microscopic examination or

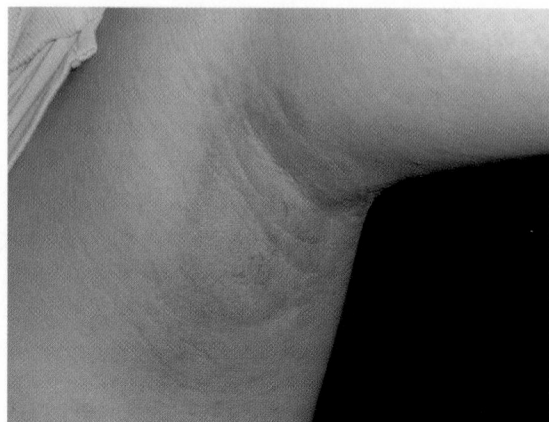

▲ **Figure 6–36.** Erythrasma of the axilla. (Courtesy of Richard P. Usatine, MD; used, with permission, from Usatine RP, Smith MA, Mayeaux EJ Jr, Chumley H, Tysinger J. *The Color Atlas of Family Medicine*. McGraw-Hill, 2009.)

culture of tissue scrapings may reveal yeasts or fungi. Stool examination may show pinworms. Radiologic studies may demonstrate spinal disease.

▶ Differential Diagnosis

The etiologic differential diagnosis consists of *Candida* infection, parasitosis, local irritation from contactants or irritants, nerve impingement and other primary skin disorders of the genital area such as psoriasis, seborrhea, intertrigo, or lichen sclerosus.

▶ Prevention

Instruct the patient in proper anogenital hygiene after treating systemic or local conditions. If appropriate, physical therapy and exercises to support the lower spine are recommended.

▶ Treatment

A. General Measures

Treating constipation, preferably with high-fiber management (psyllium), may help. Instruct the patient to use very soft or moistened tissue or cotton after bowel movements and to clean the perianal area thoroughly with cool water if possible. Women should use similar precautions after urinating. Avoid "baby wipes" as they frequently contain preservatives that cause allergic contact dermatitis.

B. Local Measures

Pramoxine cream or lotion or hydrocortisone-pramoxine (Pramosone), 1% or 2.5% cream, lotion, or ointment, is helpful in managing pruritus in the anogenital area. The ointment or cream should be applied after a bowel movement. Topical doxepin cream 5% is similarly effective, but it may be sedating. The use of strong corticosteroids on the scrotum may lead to persistent severe burning upon withdrawal of the drug. Underclothing should be changed daily, and in men, the seam of their "boxers" should not rub against or contact the scrotum. Balneol Perianal Cleansing Lotion or Tucks premoistened pads, ointment, or cream may be very useful for pruritus ani. About one-third of patients with scrotal or anal pruritus will respond to capsaicin cream 0.006%. Treatment for underlying spinal neurologic disease may be required.

▶ Prognosis

Although benign, anogenital pruritus is often persistent and recurrent.

Serling SL et al. Approach to pruritus in the adult HIV-positive patient. Semin Cutan Med Surg. 2011 Jun;30(2):101–6. [PMID: 21767771]

Thorstensen KA et al. Recognition and management of vulvar dermatologic conditions: sclerosus, lichen planus, and lichen simplex chronicus. J Midwifery Womens Health. 2012 May–Jun;57(3):260–75. [PMID: 22594865]

SCABIES

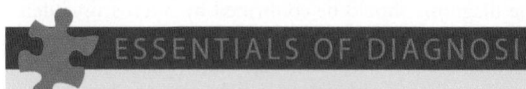

ESSENTIALS OF DIAGNOSIS

- ▶ Generalized very severe itching.
- ▶ Burrows, vesicles and pustules, especially on finger webs and in wrist creases.
- ▶ Mites, ova, and brown dots of feces visible microscopically.
- ▶ Red papules or nodules on the scrotum and on the penile glans and shaft are pathognomonic.

▶ General Considerations

Scabies is caused by infestation with *Sarcoptes scabiei*. The infestation usually spares the head and neck (though even these areas may be involved in infants, in the elderly, and in patients with AIDS). Scabies is usually acquired by sleeping with or in the bedding of an infested individual or by other close contact. The entire household may be affected. Facility-associated scabies is increasingly common, primarily in long-term care facilities. Index patients are usually elderly and immunosuppressed. When these patients are hospitalized, hospital-based epidemics can occur. These epidemics are difficult to eradicate since many health care workers become infected and spread the infestation to other patients.

▶ Clinical Findings

A. Symptoms and Signs

Itching is almost always present and can be quite severe. The lesions consist of more or less generalized excoriations with small pruritic vesicles, pustules, and "burrows" in the web spaces and on the heels of the palms, wrists (Figure 6–37), elbows, around the axillae, and on the breasts of women. The feet are a good place to identify burrows, since they may have been scratched off in other locations. The burrow appears as a short irregular mark, 2–3 mm long and the width of a hair. Characteristic nodular lesions may occur on the scrotum or penis and along the posterior axillary line.

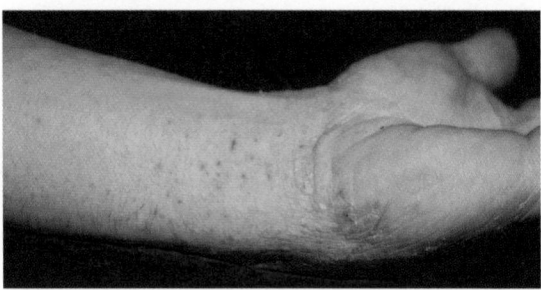

▲ **Figure 6–37.** Scabies. (Used, with permission, from Berger TG, Dept Dermatology, UCSF.)

B. Laboratory Findings

The diagnosis should be confirmed by microscopic demonstration of the organism, ova, or feces in a mounted specimen, examined with tap water. Best results are obtained when multiple lesions are scraped, choosing the best unexcoriated lesions from interdigital webs, wrists, elbows, or feet. A No. 15 blade is used to scrape each lesion until it is flat. Pinpoint bleeding may result from the scraping. Patients with crusted/hyperkeratotic scabies must be evaluated for immunosuppression (especially HIV and HTLV-1 infections) if no iatrogenic cause of immunosuppression is present.

► Differential Diagnosis

Scabies must be distinguished from the various forms of pediculosis, from bedbug and flea bites, and from other causes of pruritus.

► Treatment & Prognosis

Treatment is aimed at killing scabies mites and controlling the dermatitis, which can persist for months after effective eradication of the mites. Bedding and clothing should be laundered or cleaned or set aside for 14 days in plastic bags. High heat (60°C) is required to kill the mites and ova. Unless treatment is aimed at all infected persons in a family or institutionalized group, reinfestations will probably occur.

Permethrin 5% cream is highly effective and safe in the management of scabies. Treatment consists of a single application for 8–12 hours, repeated in 1 week.

Pregnant patients should be treated only if they have documented scabies themselves. Permethrin 5% cream once for 12 hours—or 5% or 6% sulfur in petrolatum applied nightly for 3 nights from the collarbones down—may be used.

Patients will continue to itch for several weeks after treatment. Use of triamcinolone 0.1% cream will help resolve the dermatitis. Scabies in nursing home patients, institutionalized or mentally impaired (especially Down syndrome) patients, and AIDS patients may be much more difficult to treat.

Most failures in normal persons are related to incorrect use or incomplete treatment of the housing unit. In these cases, repeat treatment with permethrin once weekly for 2 weeks, with reeducation regarding the method and extent of application, is suggested. In immunocompetent individuals, ivermectin in a dose of 200 mcg/kg is effective in about 75% of cases with a single dose and 95% of cases with two doses 2 weeks apart. In immunosuppressed hosts and those with crusted (hyperkeratotic) scabies, multiple doses of ivermectin (every 2 weeks for two or three doses) plus topical therapy with permethrin once weekly may be effective when topical treatment and oral therapy alone fail. Oral ivermectin can be very beneficial in mass treatment to eradicate infections in institutions or villages.

If secondary pyoderma is present, it is treated with systemic antibiotics. In areas where nephritogenic streptococcal strains are prevalent, infestation with scabies or exposure to scabies-infested dogs may be followed by acute post-streptococcal glomerulonephritis.

Persistent pruritic postscabietic papules may be treated with mid- to high-potency corticosteroids or with intralesional triamcinolone acetonide (2.5–5 mg/mL).

Currier RW et al. Scabies in animals and humans: history, evolutionary perspectives, and modern clinical management. Ann N Y Acad Sci. 2011 Aug; 1230:E50–60. [PMID: 22417107]

Gunning K et al. Pediculosis and scabies: treatment update. Am Fam Physician. 2012 Sep15;86(6):535–41. [PMID: 23062045]

Monsel G et al. Management of scabies. Skin Therapy Lett. 2012 Mar;17(3):1–4. [PMID: 22446818]

Shimose L et al. Diagnosis, prevention, and treatment of scabies. Curr Infect Dis Rep. 2013 Oct;15(5):426–31. [PMID: 23904181]

PEDICULOSIS

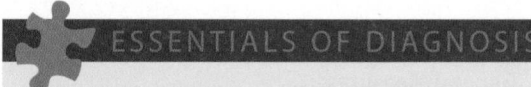

ESSENTIALS OF DIAGNOSIS

- ► Pruritus with excoriation.
- ► Nits on hair shafts; lice on skin or clothes.
- ► Occasionally, sky-blue macules (maculae ceruleae) on the inner thighs or lower abdomen in pubic louse infestation.

► General Considerations

Pediculosis is a parasitic infestation of the skin of the scalp, trunk, or pubic areas. Body lice usually occur among people who live in overcrowded dwellings with inadequate hygiene facilities. Pubic lice may be sexually transmitted. Head lice may be transmitted by shared use of hats or combs. Adults contacting children with head lice frequently acquire the infestation.

There are three different varieties: (1) pediculosis pubis, caused by *Phthirus pubis* (pubic louse, "crabs"); (2) pediculosis corporis, caused by *Pediculus humanus* var *corporis* (body louse); and (3) pediculosis capitis, caused by *Pediculus humanus* var *capitis* (head louse).

Head and body lice are similar in appearance and are 3–4 mm long. The body louse can seldom be found on the body, because the insect comes onto the skin only to feed and must be looked for in the seams of the clothing. Trench fever, relapsing fever, and typhus are transmitted by the body louse in countries where those diseases are endemic.

► Clinical Findings

Itching may be very intense in body louse infestations, and scratching may result in deep excoriations, especially over the upper shoulders, posterior flanks, and neck. In some cases, only itching is present, with few excoriations seen. Pyoderma may be the presenting sign. Head lice can be found on the scalp or may be manifested as small nits resembling pussy willow buds on the scalp hairs close to the skin. They are easiest to see above the ears and at the nape of the neck. Pubic louse infestations are occasionally generalized, particularly in hairy individuals; the lice may even be found on the eyelashes and in the scalp.

Differential Diagnosis

Head louse infestation must be distinguished from seborrheic dermatitis, body louse infestation from scabies and bedbug bites, and pubic louse infestation from anogenital pruritus and eczema.

Treatment

Body lice are treated by disposing of the infested clothing and addressing the patient's social situation. For pubic lice, permethrin rinse 1% for 10 minutes and permethrin cream 5% applied for 8 hours are effective. Sexual contacts should be treated. Clothes and bedclothes should be washed and dried at high temperature.

Permethrin 1% cream rinse (Nix) is a topical over-the-counter pediculicide and ovicide and is the treatment of choice for head lice. It is applied to the scalp and hair and left on for 8 hours before being rinsed off. Permethrin resistance of head lice is common. Malathion lotion 1% (Ovide) is very effective, but it is highly volatile and flammable, so application must be done in a well-ventilated room or out of doors. Topical ivermectin and spinosad 0.9% suspension are new agents that appear superior to previous treatments. For involvement of eyelashes, petrolatum is applied thickly twice daily for 8 days, and remaining nits are then plucked off.

Gunning K et al. Pediculosis and scabies: treatment update. Am Fam Physician. 2012 Sep15;86(6):535–41. [PMID: 23062045]
Ivermectin (Sklice) topical lotion for head lice. Med Lett Drugs Ther. 2012 Aug6;54(1396):61–3. [PMID: 22869290]

SKIN LESIONS DUE TO OTHER ARTHROPODS

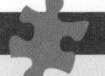 ESSENTIALS OF DIAGNOSIS

▶ Localized rash with pruritus.

▶ Furuncle-like lesions containing live arthropods.

▶ Tender erythematous patches that migrate ("larva migrans").

▶ Generalized urticaria or erythema multiforme in some patients.

General Considerations

Some arthropods (eg, mosquitoes and biting flies) are readily detected as they bite. Many others are not because they are too small, because there is no immediate reaction, or because they bite during sleep. Reactions are allergic and may be delayed for hours to days. Patients are most apt to consult a clinician when the lesions are multiple and pruritus is intense.

Many persons will react severely only to their earliest contacts with an arthropod, thus presenting pruritic lesions when traveling, moving into new quarters, etc. Body lice, fleas, bedbugs, and mosquitoes should be considered. Bedbug exposure typically occurs in hotels and in housing with inadequate hygiene but also may occur in stable domiciles. Spiders are often incorrectly believed to be the source of bites; they rarely attack humans, though the brown recluse spider (Loxosceles laeta, L reclusa) may cause severe necrotic reactions and death due to intravascular hemolysis, and the black widow spider (Latrodectus mactans) may cause severe systemic symptoms and death. (See also Chapter 38.) The majority of patient-diagnosed, physician-diagnosed, and even published cases of brown recluse spider bites (or loxoscelism) are incorrect, especially if made in areas where these spiders are not endemic. Many of these lesions are actually due to CA-MRSA.

In addition to arthropod bites, the most common lesions are venomous stings (wasps, hornets, bees, ants, scorpions) or bites (centipedes), furuncle-like lesions due to fly maggots or sand fleas in the skin, and a linear creeping eruption due to a migrating larva.

Clinical Findings

The diagnosis may be difficult when the patient has not noticed the initial attack but suffers a delayed reaction. Individual bites are often in clusters and tend to occur either on exposed parts (eg, midges and gnats) or under clothing, especially around the waist or at flexures (eg, small mites or insects in bedding or clothing). The reaction is often delayed for 1–24 hours or more. Pruritus is almost always present and may be all but intolerable once the patient starts to scratch. Secondary infection may follow scratching. Urticarial wheals are common. Papules may become vesicular. The diagnosis is aided by searching for exposure to arthropods and by considering the patient's occupation and recent activities.

The principal arthropods are as follows:

1. **Fleas:** Fleas are bloodsucking ectoparasites that feed on dogs, cats, humans, and other species. Flea saliva produces papular urticaria in sensitized individuals. To break the life cycle of the flea, one must treat the home and pets, using quick-kill insecticides, residual insecticides, and a growth regulator.

2. **Bedbugs:** In crevices of beds or furniture; bites tend to occur in lines or clusters. Papular urticaria is a characteristic lesion of bedbug (Cimex lectularius) bites. Bedbugs are not restricted to any socioeconomic group and are a major health problem in some major metropolitan areas, especially in commercial and residential hotels.

3. **Ticks:** Usually picked up by brushing against low vegetation.

4. **Chiggers or red bugs:** These are larvae of trombiculid mites. A few species confined to particular regions and locally recognized habitats (eg, berry patches, woodland edges, lawns, brush turkey mounds in Australia, poultry farms) attack humans, often around the waist, on the ankles, or in flexures, raising intensely itching erythematous papules after a delay of many hours.

The red chiggers may sometimes be seen in the center of papules that have not yet been scratched.

5. **Bird and rodent mites:** Larger than chiggers, bird mites infest birds and their nests. Bites are multiple anywhere on the body. Room air conditioning units may suck in bird mites and infest the inhabitants of the room. Rodent mites from mice or rats may cause similar effects. If the domicile has evidence of rodent activity, then rodent mite dermatitis should be suspected, as the mites are rarely found. Pet rodents or birds may be infested with mites, maintaining the infestation.

6. **Mites in stored products:** These are white and almost invisible and infest products such as copra, vanilla pods, sugar, straw, cottonseeds, and cereals. Persons who handle these products may be attacked, especially on the hands and forearms and sometimes on the feet.

7. **Caterpillars of moths with urticating hairs:** The hairs are blown from cocoons or carried by emergent moths, causing severe and often seasonally recurrent outbreaks after mass emergence. The gypsy moth is a cause in the eastern United States.

8. **Tungiasis:** Tungiasis is due to the burrowing flea known as *Tunga penetrans* and is found in Africa, the West Indies, and South and Central America. The female burrows under the skin, sucks blood, swells to 0.5 cm, and then ejects her eggs onto the ground. Ulceration, lymphangitis, gangrene, and septicemia may result, in some cases with lethal effect. Simple surgical removal is usually performed.

▶ Prevention

Arthropod infestations are best prevented by avoidance of contaminated areas, personal cleanliness, and disinfection of clothing, bedclothes, and furniture as indicated. Chiggers and mites can be repelled by permethrin applied to the head and clothing. (It is not necessary to remove clothing.) Bedbugs are no longer repelled by permethrin. Aggressive cleaning, usually requiring removal of the affected occupant from the domicile, may be necessary to eradicate bedbug infestation in a residence.

▶ Treatment

Living arthropods should be removed carefully with tweezers after application of alcohol and preserved in alcohol for identification. In endemic Rocky Mountain spotted fever areas, ticks should not be removed with the bare fingers.

Corticosteroid lotions or creams are helpful. Topical antibiotics may be applied if secondary infection is suspected. Localized persistent lesions may be treated with intralesional corticosteroids.

Stings produced by many arthropods may be alleviated by applying papain powder (Adolph's Meat Tenderizer) mixed with water, or aluminum chloride hexahydrate (Xerac AC).

Extracts from venom sacs of bees, wasps, yellow jackets, and hornets are available for immunotherapy of patients at risk for anaphylaxis.

Doggett SL et al. Bed bugs: clinical relevance and control options. Clin Microbiol Rev. 2012 Jan;25(1):164–92. [PMID: 22232375]

Haddad V Jr et al. Tropical dermatology: venomous arthropods and human skin: Part I. Insecta. J Am Acad Dermatol. 2012 Sep;67(3):331.e1–14. [PMID: 22890734]

Haddad V Jr et al. Tropical dermatology: venomous arthropods and human skin: Part II. Diplopoda, Chilopoda, and Arachnida. J Am Acad Dermatol. 2012 Sep;67(3):347.e1–9. [PMID: 22890735]

INFLAMMATORY NODULES

ERYTHEMA NODOSUM

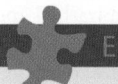

ESSENTIALS OF DIAGNOSIS

▶ Painful red nodules without ulceration on anterior aspects of legs.

▶ Slow regression over several weeks to resemble contusions.

▶ Women are predominantly affected by a ratio of 10:1 compared to men.

▶ Some cases associated with infection, inflammatory bowel disease, or drug exposure.

▶ General Considerations

Erythema nodosum is a symptom complex characterized by tender, erythematous nodules that appear most commonly on the extensor surfaces of the lower legs. It usually lasts about 6 weeks and may recur. The disease may be associated with various infections—streptococcosis, primary coccidioidomycosis, other deep fungal infections, tuberculosis, *Yersinia pseudotuberculosis* and *Y enterocolitica* infection, diverticulitis, or syphilis. It may accompany sarcoidosis, Behçet disease, and inflammatory bowel disease. Erythema nodosum may be associated with pregnancy or with use of oral contraceptives.

▶ Clinical Findings

A. Symptoms and Signs

The subcutaneous swellings are exquisitely tender and may be preceded by fever, malaise, and arthralgia. They are most often located on the anterior surfaces of the legs below the knees but may occur on the arms, trunk, and face. The lesions, 1–10 cm in diameter, are at first pink to red; with regression, all the various hues seen in a contusion can be observed (Figure 6–38).

B. Laboratory Findings

Evaluation of patients presenting with acute erythema nodosum should include a careful history (including drug exposures) and physical examination for prior upper respiratory infection or diarrheal illness, symptoms of any deep fungal infection endemic to the area, a chest radiograph, a

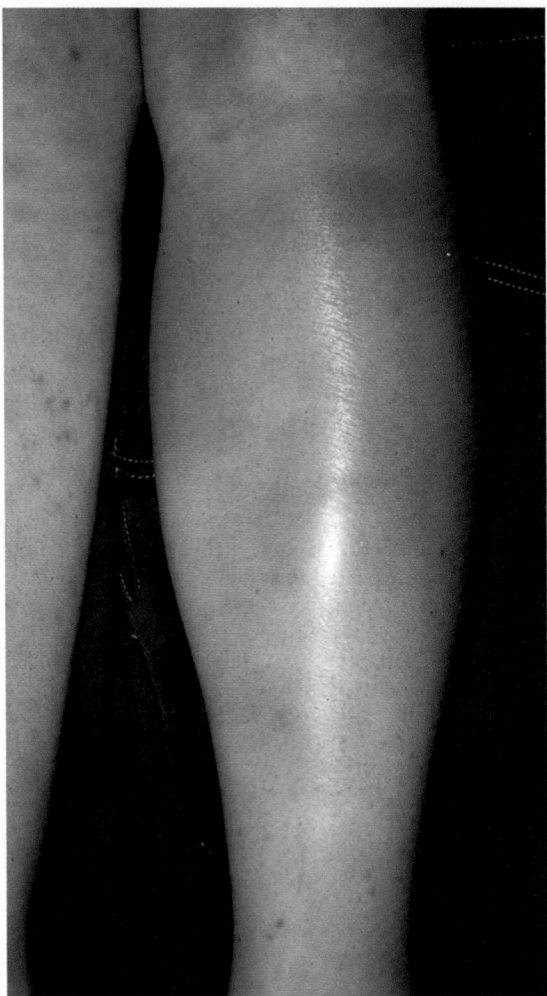

▲ **Figure 6–38.** Erythema nodosum. (Used, with permission, from Berger TG, Dept Dermatology, UCSF.)

PPD, and two consecutive ASO/DNAse B titers at 2- to 4-week intervals. If no underlying cause is found, only a small percentage of patients will go on to develop a significant underlying illness (usually sarcoidosis) over the next year.

▶ **Differential Diagnosis**

Erythema induratum from tuberculosis is seen on the posterior surfaces of the legs and may ulcerate. Lupus panniculitis presents as tender nodules on the buttocks and posterior arms that heal with depressed scars. In polyarteritis nodosa, the subcutaneous nodules are often associated with a fixed livedo. In the late stages, erythema nodosum must be distinguished from simple bruises and contusions.

▶ **Treatment**

First, the underlying cause should be identified and treated. Primary therapy is with NSAIDs in usual doses. Saturated solution of potassium iodide, 5–15 drops three times daily, results in prompt involution in many cases. Complete bed rest may be advisable if the lesions are painful. Systemic therapy directed against the lesions themselves may include corticosteroid therapy (see Chapter 26) unless contraindicated by associated infection.

▶ **Prognosis**

The lesions usually disappear after about 6 weeks, but they may recur.

Chen S et al. *Mycobacterium tuberculosis* infection is associated with the development of erythema nodosum and nodular vasculitis. PLoS One. 2013 May1;8(5):e62653. [PMID: 23650522]

Chong TA et al. Diverticulitis: an inciting factor in erythema nodosum. J Am Acad Dermatol. 2012 Jul;67(1):e60–2. [PMID: 22703921]

Eimpunth S et al. Tender cutaneous nodules of the legs: diagnosis and clinical clues to diagnosis. Int J Dermatol. 2013 May;52(5):560–6. [PMID: 22928517]

Passarini B et al. Erythema nodosum. G Ital Dermatol Venereol. 2013 Aug;148(4):413–7. [PMID: 23900162]

FURUNCULOSIS (Boils) & CARBUNCLES

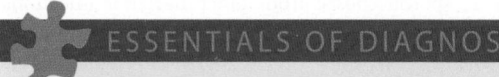

ESSENTIALS OF DIAGNOSIS

▶ Extremely painful inflammatory swelling based on a hair follicle that forms an abscess.

▶ Predisposing condition (diabetes mellitus, HIV disease, injection drug use) sometimes present.

▶ Coagulase-positive *S aureus* is the causative organism.

▶ **General Considerations**

A furuncle (boil) is a deep-seated infection (abscess) caused by *S aureus* and involving the entire hair follicle and adjacent subcutaneous tissue. The most common sites of occurrence are the hairy parts exposed to irritation and friction, pressure, or moisture. Because the lesions are autoinoculable, they are often multiple. Diabetes mellitus (especially if using insulin injections), injection drug use, allergy injections, and HIV disease all increase the risk of staphylococcal infections by increasing the rate of carriage. Certain other exposures including hospitalization, athletic teams, prisons, military service, and homelessness may also increase the risk of infection.

A carbuncle consists of several furuncles developing in adjoining hair follicles and coalescing to form a conglomerate, deeply situated mass with multiple drainage points.

▶ **Clinical Findings**

A. Symptoms and Signs

Pain and tenderness may be prominent. The abscess is either rounded or conical. It gradually enlarges, becomes fluctuant, and then softens and opens spontaneously after a few days to 1–2 weeks to discharge a core of necrotic tissue and pus. The inflammation occasionally subsides before necrosis occurs. Infection of the soft tissue around the nails (paronychia) may be due to staphylococci when it is acute or *Candida* when chronic.

B. Laboratory Findings

There may be slight leukocytosis, but a white blood cell count is rarely required. Pus can be cultured to rule out MRSA or other bacteria. Culture of the anterior nares may identify chronic staphylococcal carriage in cases of recurrent cutaneous infection.

▶ Differential Diagnosis

The most common entity in the differential is an inflamed epidermal inclusion cyst that suddenly becomes red, tender, and expands greatly in size over one to a few days. The history of a prior cyst in the same location, the presence of a clearly visible cyst orifice, and the extrusion of malodorous cheesy rather than purulent material helps in the diagnosis. Tinea profunda (deep dermatophyte infection of the hair follicle) may simulate recurrent furunculosis. Furuncle is also to be distinguished from deep mycotic infections, such as sporotrichosis; from other bacterial infections, such as anthrax and tularemia (rare); from atypical mycobacterial infections; and from acne cysts. Hidradenitis suppurativa (acne inversa) presents with recurrent tender sterile abscesses in the axillae and groin, on the buttocks, or below the breasts. The presence of old scars or sinus tracts plus negative cultures suggests this diagnosis.

▶ Complications

Serious and sometimes fatal complications of staphylococcal infection such as septicemia can occur.

▶ Prevention

Identifying and eliminating the source of infection is critical to prevent recurrences after treatment. The source individual may have chronic dermatitis or be an asymptomatic carrier. Local measures such as meticulous handwashing; no sharing of towels and clothing; aggressive scrubbing of showers, bathrooms and surfaces with bleach; bleach baths (¼–½ cup per 20 liters of bathwater for 15 minutes 3–5 times weekly) and isolation of infected patients who reside in institutions to prevent spread are all effective measures.

▶ Treatment

A. Specific Measures

Incision and drainage is recommended for all loculated suppurations and is the mainstay of therapy. Systemic antibiotics are usually given, although they offer little beyond adequate incision and drainage. Sodium dicloxacillin or cephalexin, 1 g daily in divided doses by mouth for 10 days, is usually effective. Doxycycline 100 mg twice daily, trimethoprim-sulfamethoxazole double-strength one tablet

twice daily, and clindamycin 150–300 mg twice daily are effective in treating MRSA. Recurrent furunculosis may be effectively treated with a combination of cephalexin (250–500 mg four times daily) **or** doxycycline (100 mg twice daily) for 2–4 weeks **plus** either rifampin (300 mg twice daily for 5 days for 2–4 weeks) **or** long-term clindamycin (150–300 mg daily for 1–2 months). Shorter courses of antibiotics (7–14 days) plus longer-term daily chlorhexidine whole body washing and intranasal, axilla, and anogenital mupirocin may also cure recurrent furunculosis. Family members, pets, and intimate contacts may need evaluation for staphylococcal carrier state and perhaps concomitant treatment. Stopping high-risk behavior such as injection drug use can also prevent recurrence of furunculosis.

B. Local Measures

Immobilize the part and avoid overmanipulation of inflamed areas. Use moist heat to help larger lesions "localize." Use surgical incision and drainage *after* the lesions are "mature." To incise and drain an acute staphylococcal paronychia, insert a flat metal spatula or sharpened hardwood stick into the nail fold where it adjoins the nail. This will release pus from a mature lesion.

▶ Prognosis

Recurrent crops may harass the patient for months or years.

Daly JM et al. Management of skin and soft tissue infections in community practice before and after implementing a "best practice" approach: an Iowa Research Network (IRENE) intervention study. J Am Board Fam Med. 2011 Sep–Oct;24(5):524–33. [PMID: 21900435]

Davido B et al. Recurrent furunculosis: Efficacy of the CMC regimen—skin disinfection (chlorhexidine), local nasal antibiotic (mupirocin), and systemic antibiotic (clindamycin). Scand J Infect Dis. 2013 Nov;45(11):837–41. [PMID: 23848409]

Demos M et al. Recurrent furunculosis: a review of the literature. Br J Dermatol. 2012 Oct;167(4):725–32. [PMID: 22803835]

Parnes B et al. Improving the management of skin and soft tissue infections in primary care: a report from State Networks of Colorado Ambulatory Practices and Partners (SNOCAP-USA) and the Distributed Ambulatory Research in Therapeutics Network (DARTNet). J Am Board Fam Med. 2011 Sep–Oct;24(5):534–42. [PMID: 21900436]

EPIDERMAL INCLUSION CYST

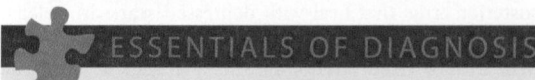

ESSENTIALS OF DIAGNOSIS

- ▶ Firm dermal papule or nodule.
- ▶ Overlying black comedone or "punctum."
- ▶ Expressible foul-smelling cheesy material.
- ▶ May become red and drain, mimicking an abscess.

General Considerations

Epidermal inclusion cysts (EICs) are common, benign growths of the upper portion of the hair follicle. They are common in Gardner syndrome and may be the first stigmata of the condition.

EICs favor the face and trunk and may complicate nodulocystic acne vulgaris. Individual lesions range in size from 0.3 cm to several centimeters. An overlying pore or punctum is characteristic. Lateral pressure may lead to extrusion of a foul-smelling, cheesy material.

Differential Diagnosis

EICs are distinguished from lipomas by being more superficial (in the dermis not the subcutaneous fat) and by their overlying punctum. Many other benign and malignant tumors may superficially resemble EICs, but all lack the punctum.

Complications

EICs may rupture, creating an acute inflammatory nodule very similar to an abscess. Cultures of the expressed material will be sterile.

Treatment

Treatment is not required if asymptomatic. Inflamed lesions may be treated with incision and drainage or intralesional triamcinolone acetomide 5–10 mg/mL. For large or symptomatic cysts, surgical excision is curative.

Baek SO et al. Giant epidermal inclusion facial cyst. J Craniofac Surg. 2011 May;22(3):1149–51. [PMID: 21586975]

PHOTODERMATITIS

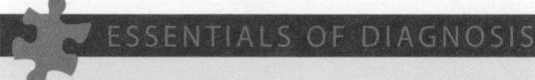

ESSENTIALS OF DIAGNOSIS

► Painful or pruritic erythema, edema, or vesiculation on sun-exposed surfaces: the face, neck, hands, and "V" of the chest.

► Inner upper eyelids spared, as is the area under the chin.

General Considerations

In most cases, photosensitivity is an acute or chronic skin reaction due to hypersensitivity to ultraviolet radiation. It is caused by certain medications, by lupus erythematosus, and some inherited disorders including the porphyrias. Contact photosensitivity may occur with plants, perfumes, and sunscreens. Three percent of persons with atopic dermatitis, especially middle-aged women, are photosensitive.

Photodermatitis is manifested as phototoxicity—a tendency for the individual to sunburn more easily than expected—or, as photoallergy, a true immunologic reaction that often presents with dermatitis.

Clinical Findings

A. Symptoms and Signs

The acute inflammatory phase of phototoxicity, if severe enough, is accompanied by pain, fever, gastrointestinal symptoms, malaise, and even prostration. Signs include erythema, edema, and possibly vesiculation and oozing on exposed surfaces. Peeling of the epidermis and pigmentary changes often result. The key to diagnosis is localization of the rash to photoexposed areas, though these eruptions may become generalized with time to involve even photoprotected areas. The lower lip may be affected.

B. Laboratory Findings

Blood and urine tests are generally not helpful unless porphyria cutanea tarda is suggested by the presence of blistering, scarring, milia (white cysts 1–2 mm in diameter) and skin fragility of the dorsal hands, and facial hypertrichosis. Eosinophilia may be present in chronic photoallergic responses.

Differential Diagnosis

The differential diagnosis is long. If a clear history of the use of a topical or systemic photosensitizer is not available and if the eruption is persistent, then a workup including biopsy and light testing may be required. Photodermatitis must be differentiated from contact dermatitis that may develop from one of the many substances in suntan lotions and oils, as these may often have a similar distribution. Sensitivity to actinic rays may also be part of a more serious condition such as porphyria cutanea tarda or lupus erythematosus. These disorders are diagnosed by appropriate blood or urine tests. Phenothiazines, quinine or quinidine, griseofulvin, sulfonamides (especially hydrochlorothiazide), NSAIDs, and antibiotics (eg, some tetracyclines, quinolones, TMP-SMZ) may photosensitize the skin. Polymorphous light eruption (PMLE) is a very common idiopathic photodermatitis and often has its onset in the third to fourth decades except in Native Americans and Latinos, in whom it may present in childhood. PMLE is chronic in nature. Transitory periods of spontaneous remission do occur. The action spectrum of PMLE may also extend into the long ultraviolet wavelengths (UVA; 320–400 nm). Drug-induced photosensitivity is triggered by UVA.

Complications

Some individuals continue to be chronic light reactors even when they apparently are no longer exposed to photosensitizing drugs.

Prevention

While sunscreens are useful agents in general and should be used by persons with photosensitivity, patients may react to such low amounts of energy that sunscreens alone may not be sufficient. Sunscreens with an SPF of 30–60 and broad UVA coverage, containing dicamphor sulfonic acid (Mexoryl SX), avobenzone (Parasol 1789), titanium dioxide, and micronized zinc oxide, are especially useful in patients with photoallergic dermatitis. Photosensitivity due to porphyria is not prevented by sunscreens and requires barrier protection (clothing) to prevent outbreaks.

▶ Treatment

A. Specific Measures

Medications should be suspected in cases of photosensitivity even if the particular medication (such as hydrochlorothiazide) has been used for months.

B. Local Measures

When the eruption is vesicular or weepy, treatment is similar to that of any acute dermatitis, using cooling and soothing wet dressing.

Sunscreens should be used as described above. Mid-potency to high-potency topical corticosteroids are of limited benefit in sunburn reactions but may help in PMLE and photoallergic reactions. Since the face is often involved, close monitoring for corticosteroid side effects is recommended.

C. Systemic Measures

Aspirin may have some value for fever and pain of acute sunburn. Systemic corticosteroids in doses as described for acute contact dermatitis may be required for severe photosensitivity reactions. Otherwise, different photodermatoses are treated in specific ways.

Patients with severe photoallergy may require immunosuppressives, such as azathioprine, in the range of 50–300 mg/d, or cyclosporine, 3–5 mg/kg/d.

▶ Prognosis

The most common phototoxic sunburn reactions are usually benign and self-limited. PMLE and some cases of photoallergy can persist for years.

Kiss F et al. A review of UVB-mediated photosensitivity disorders. Photochem Photobiol Sci. 2012 Dec13;12(1):37–46. [PMID: 23023766]
Sharma VK et al. Photodermatoses in pigmented skin. Photochem Photobiol Sci. 2013 Jan;12(1):65–77. [PMID: 23123922]

ULCERS

LEG ULCERS SECONDARY TO VENOUS INSUFFICIENCY

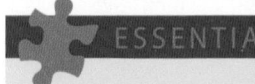

ESSENTIALS OF DIAGNOSIS

▶ Past history of varicosities, thrombophlebitis, or postphlebitic syndrome.

▶ Irregular ulceration, often on the medial aspect of the lower legs above the malleolus.

▶ Edema of the legs, varicosities, hyperpigmentation, and red and scaly areas (stasis dermatitis) and scars from old ulcers support the diagnosis.

▶ General Considerations

Patients at risk may have a history of venous insufficiency, either with obvious varicosities or with a past history of thrombophlebitis, or with immobility of the calf muscle group (paraplegics, etc). Red, pruritic patches of stasis dermatitis often precede ulceration. Because venous insufficiency plays a role in between 75% and 90% of lower leg ulcerations, testing of venous competence is a required part of a leg ulcer evaluation even when no changes of venous insufficiency are present. The left leg is usually more severely affected than the right.

▶ Clinical Findings

A. Symptoms and Signs

Classically, chronic edema is followed by a dermatitis, which is often pruritic. These changes are followed by hyperpigmentation, skin breakdown, and eventually sclerosis of the skin of the lower leg (Figure 6–39). The ulcer base may be clean, but it often has a yellow fibrin eschar that may require surgical removal . Ulcers that appear on the feet, toes, or above the knees should be approached with other diagnoses in mind.

B. Laboratory Findings

Thorough evaluation of the patient's vascular system (including measurement of the ankle/brachial index [ABI]) is essential. If the ABI is < 0.7, the patient should be referred to a vascular surgeon for surgical evaluation. Doppler and light rheography examinations as office procedures are usually sufficient (except in the diabetic) to elucidate the cause of most vascular cases of lower leg ulceration.

▶ Differential Diagnosis

The differential includes vasculitis, pyoderma gangrenosum, arterial ulcerations, infection, trauma, skin cancer,

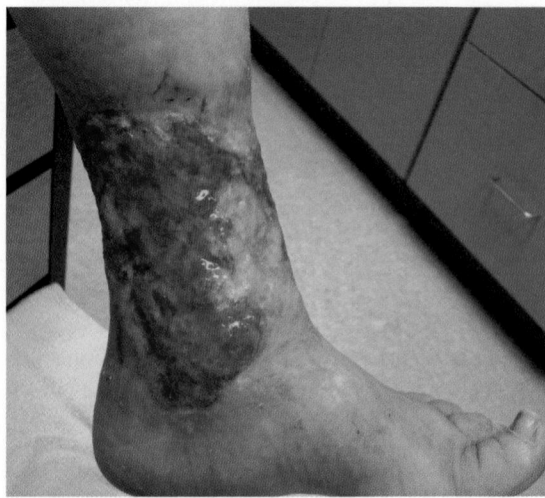

▲ **Figure 6–39.** Venous stasis ulcer near the medial malleolus. (Courtesy of Maureen Sheehan, MD; used, with permission, from Usatine RP, Smith MA, Mayeaux EJ Jr, Chumley H, Tysinger J. *The Color Atlas of Family Medicine.* McGraw-Hill, 2009.)

arachnid bites, and sickle cell anemia. When the diagnosis is in doubt, a punch biopsy from the border (not base) of the lesion may be helpful.

► Prevention

Compression stockings to reduce edema are the most important means of prevention. Compression should achieve a pressure of 30 mm Hg below the knee and 40 mm Hg at the ankle. The stockings should not be used in patients with arterial insufficiency with an ABI < 0.7. Pneumatic sequential compression devices may be of great benefit when edema is refractory to standard compression dressings.

► Treatment

A. Local Measures

Clean the base of the ulcer with saline or cleansers such as Saf-Clens. A curette or small scissors can be used to remove the yellow fibrin eschar; local anesthesia may be used if the areas are very tender.

The ulcer is treated with metronidazole gel to reduce bacterial growth and odor. Any red dermatitic skin is treated with a medium- to high-potency corticosteroid ointment. The ulcer is then covered with an occlusive hydroactive dressing (DuoDerm, Hydrasorb or Cutinova) or a polyurethane foam (Allevyn) followed by an Unna zinc paste boot. This is changed weekly. The ulcer should begin to heal within weeks, and healing should be complete within 4–6 months. If the patient is diabetic, becaplermin (Regranex) may be applied to those ulcers that are not becoming smaller or developing a granulating base. Some ulcerations require grafting. Full- or split-thickness grafts often do not take, and pinch grafts (small shaves of skin laid onto the bed) may be effective. Cultured epidermal cell grafts may accelerate wound healing, but they are very expensive. They should be considered in refractory ulcers, especially those that have not healed after a year or more of conservative therapy. Manuka honey has been purported to accelerate wound healing, but comparative controlled trials of efficacy are lacking.

No topical intervention has evidence to suggest that it will improve healing of arterial leg ulcers.

B. Systemic Therapy

Pentoxifylline, 400 mg three times daily administered with compression dressings, is beneficial in accelerating healing of venous insufficiency leg ulcers. Zinc supplementation is occasionally beneficial in patients with low serum zinc levels. The diagnosis of cellulitis in the setting of a venous insufficiency ulcer can be very difficult. Surface cultures are of limited value. The diagnosis of cellulitis should be considered in the following settings: 1) expanding warmth and erythema surrounding the ulceration with or without 2) increasing pain of the ulceration. The patient may also report increased exudate from the ulceration, but this without the other cardinal findings of cellulitis does not confirm the diagnosis of cellulitis. If cellulitis accompanies the ulcer, systemic antibiotics are recommended: dicloxacillin, 250 mg orally four times a day, or levofloxacin, 500 mg once daily for 1–2 weeks is usually adequate. Routine use of antibiotics and treating bacteria isolated from a chronic ulcer without clinical evidence of infection is discouraged. If the ulcer fails to heal or there is a persistent draining tract in the ulcer, an underlying osteomyelitis should be sought.

► Prognosis

The combination of limited debridement, compression dressings or stockings, and newer moist dressings will heal the majority of venous stasis ulcers within months (average 18 months). These need to be applied at least 80% of the time to optimize ulcer healing. Topical growth factors, antibiotics, debriding agents, and xenografts and autografts can be considered in recalcitrant cases, but they are usually not required in most patients. The failure of venous insufficiency ulcerations to heal is most often related to not using the basic treatment methods consistently, rather than failure to use these specific modalities. **Ongoing control of edema is essential to prevent recurrent ulceration.** The use of compression stockings following ulcer healing is critical to prevent recurrence, with recurrence rates 2–20 times higher if patients do not comply with compression stocking use. If the ABI is < 0.5, the prognosis for healing is poor. Patients with an ABI below 0.5 or refractory ulcerations (or both) should be considered for surgical procedure (artery-opening procedures or ablation of the incompetent superficial vein).

Bryan LJ et al. Higher soluble P-selectin is associated with chronic venous insufficiency: the San Diego Population Study. Thromb Res. 2012 Nov;130(5):716–9. [PMID: 22892384]

Chaby G et al; Angio-Dermatology Group of the French Society of Dermatology. Prognostic factors associated with healing of venous leg ulcers: a multicentre, prospective, cohort study. Br J Dermatol. 2013 Nov;169(5):1106–13. [PMID: 23909381]

Mosti G et al. High compression pressure over the calf is more effective than graduated compression in enhancing venous pump function. Eur J Vasc Endovasc Surg. 2012 Sep;44(3): 332–6. [PMID: 22819741]

Mowatt-Larssen E et al. Treatment of primary varicose veins has changed with the introduction of new techniques. Semin Vasc Surg. 2012 Mar;25(1):18–24. [PMID: 22595477]

Uhl JF et al. Anatomy of the foot venous pump: physiology and influence on chronic venous disease. Phlebology. 2012 Aug;27(5):219–30. [PMID: 22847928]

MISCELLANEOUS DERMATOLOGIC DISORDERS[1]

PIGMENTARY DISORDERS

Although the color of skin may be altered by many diseases and agents, the vast majority of patients have either an increase or decrease in pigment secondary to some inflammatory disease such as acne or atopic dermatitis.

---

[1]Hirsutism is discussed in Chapter 26.

Other pigmentary disorders include those resulting from exposure to exogenous pigments such as carotenemia, argyria, and tattooing. Other endogenous pigmentary disorders are attributable to metabolic substances—including hemosiderin (iron)—in purpuric processes; or to homogentisic acid in ochronosis; and bile pigments.

Classification

First, determine whether the disorder is hyperpigmentation or hypopigmentation, ie, an increase or decrease in normal skin colors. Each may be considered to be primary or to be secondary to other disorders.

A. Primary Pigmentary Disorders

1. Hyperpigmentation—The disorders in this category are nevoid, congenital or acquired, and include pigmented nevi, ephelides (juvenile freckles), and lentigines (senile freckles). Hyperpigmentation occurs also in arsenical melanosis or in association with Addison disease. **Melasma (chloasma)** occurs as patterned hyperpigmentation of the face, usually as a direct effect of estrogens. It occurs not only during pregnancy but also in 30–50% of women taking oral contraceptives, and rarely in men. One report suggests that such men have low testosterone and elevated luteinizing hormone levels.

2. Hypopigmentation and depigmentation—The disorders in this category are vitiligo, albinism, and piebaldism. In vitiligo, pigment cells (melanocytes) are destroyed (Figure 6–40). Vitiligo, present in approximately 1% of the population, may be associated with other autoimmune disorders such as autoimmune thyroid disease, pernicious anemia, diabetes mellitus, and Addison disease.

B. Secondary Pigmentary Disorders

Any damage to the skin (irritation, allergy, infection, excoriation, burns, or dermatologic therapy such as chemical peels and freezing with liquid nitrogen) may result in hyperpigmentation or hypopigmentation. Several disorders of clinical importance are described below.

1. Hyperpigmentation—The most common type of secondary hyperpigmentation occurs after another dermatologic condition, such as acne, and is most commonly seen in moderately complexioned persons (Asians, Hispanics, and light-skinned African Americans). It is called postinflammatory hyperpigmentation.

Pigmentation may be produced by certain drugs, eg, chloroquine, chlorpromazine, minocycline, and amiodarone. Fixed drug eruptions to phenolphthalein in laxatives, to TMP-SMZ, to NSAIDs, and to tetracyclines, for example, are further causes.

2. Hypopigmentation—**Leukoderma** may complicate atopic dermatitis, lichen planus, psoriasis, DLE, and lichen simplex chronicus. Practitioners must exercise special care in using liquid nitrogen on any patient with olive or darker complexions, since doing so may result in hypopigmentation or depigmentation, at times permanent. Intralesional or intra-articular injections of high concentrations of corticosteroids may also cause localized temporary hypopigmentation.

Differential Diagnosis

The evaluation of pigmentary disorders is helped by Wood's light, which accentuates epidermal pigmentation and highlights hypopigmentation. Depigmentation, as seen in vitiligo, enhances with Wood's light examination, whereas postinflammatory hypopigmentation does not.

Complications

Actinic keratoses and skin cancers are more likely to develop in persons with vitiligo. Severe emotional trauma may occur in extensive vitiligo and other types of hypopigmentation and hyperpigmentation, particularly in naturally dark-skinned persons.

Treatment & Prognosis

A. Hyperpigmentation

Therapeutic bleaching preparations generally contain hydroquinone. Hydroquinone has occasionally caused unexpected hypopigmentation, hyperpigmentation, or even secondary ochronosis and pigmented milia, particularly with prolonged use.

The role of exposure to ultraviolet light cannot be overstressed as a factor promoting or contributing to most disorders of hyperpigmentation, and such exposure should be minimized. Melasma, ephelides, and postinflammatory hyperpigmentation may be treated with varying success with 3–4% hydroquinone cream, gel, or solution and a sunscreen containing UVA photoprotectants (Avobenzone, Mexoryl, zinc oxide, titanium dioxide). Tretinoin cream, 0.025–0.05%, may be added. Superficial melasma responds well, but if there is predominantly dermal deposition of pigment (does *not* enhance with Wood's light), the prognosis is poor. Response to therapy may take months and requires avoidance of sunlight. Hyperpigmentation often recurs after treatment if the skin is exposed to ultraviolet

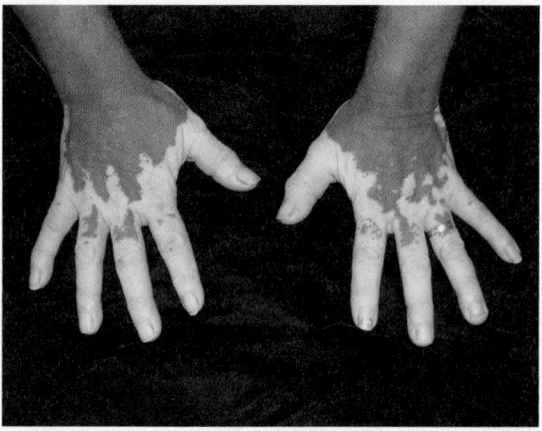

▲ **Figure 6–40.** Vitiligo of the hands. (Courtesy of Richard P. Usatine, MD; used, with permission, from Usatine RP, Smith MA, Mayeaux EJ Jr, Chumley H, Tysinger J. *The Color Atlas of Family Medicine.* McGraw-Hill, 2009.)

light. Solar lentigines respond to liquid nitrogen application. Tretinoin, 0.1% cream and tazarotene 0.1% used over 10 months, will fade solar lentigines (liver spots), hyperpigmented facial macules in Asians, and postinflammatory hyperpigmentation in blacks. New laser systems for the removal of epidermal and dermal pigments are available, and referral should be considered for patients whose responses to medical treatment are inadequate.

B. Hypopigmentation

In secondary hypopigmentation, repigmentation may occur spontaneously. Cosmetics such as Covermark and Dermablend are highly effective for concealing disfiguring patches. Therapy of vitiligo is long and tedious, and the patient must be strongly motivated. If < 20% of the skin is involved (most cases), topical tacrolimus 0.1% twice daily is the first-line therapy. A superpotent corticosteroid may also be used, but local skin atrophy from prolonged use may ensue. With 20–25% involvement, narrowband UVB or oral PUVA is best. Severe phototoxic response (sunburn) may occur with PUVA. The face and upper chest respond best, and the fingertips and the genital areas do not respond as well to treatment. Years of treatment may be required.

Korobko IV. Review of current clinical studies of vitiligo treatments. Dermatol Ther. 2012 Nov;25(Suppl 1):S17–27. [PMID: 23237034]

Passeron T. Melasma pathogenesis and influencing factors—an overview of the latest research. J Eur Acad Dermatol Venereol. 2013 Jan;27(Suppl 1):5–6. [PMID: 23205539]

Rivas S et al. Treatment of melasma with topical agents, peels and lasers: an evidence-based review. Am J Clin Dermatol. 2013 Oct;14(5):359–76. [PMID: 23881551]

Sheth VM et al. Comorbidities associated with vitiligo: a ten-year retrospective study. Dermatology. 2013;227(4):311–5. [PMID: 24107643]

Vrijman C et al. The prevalence of thyroid disease in patients with vitiligo: a systematic review. Br J Dermatol. 2012 Dec;167(6):1224–35. [PMID: 22860695]

BALDNESS (Alopecia)

▶ Baldness Due to Scarring (Cicatricial Alopecia)

Cicatricial baldness may occur following chemical or physical trauma, lichen planopilaris, bacterial or fungal infections, severe herpes zoster, chronic DLE, scleroderma, and excessive ionizing radiation. The specific cause is often suggested by the history, the distribution of hair loss, and the appearance of the skin, as in lupus erythematosus. Biopsy is useful in the diagnosis of scarring alopecia, but specimens must be taken from the active border and not from the scarred central zone.

Scarring alopecias are irreversible and permanent. It is important to diagnose and treat the scarring process as early in its course as possible.

▶ Baldness Not Associated with Scarring

Nonscarring alopecia may occur in association with various systemic diseases such as SLE, secondary syphilis,

hyperthyroidism or hypothyroidism, iron deficiency anemia, and pituitary insufficiency. The only treatment necessary is prompt and adequate control of the underlying disorder and usually leads to regrowth of the hair.

Androgenetic (male pattern) baldness, the most common form of alopecia, is of genetic predetermination. The earliest changes occur at the anterior portions of the calvarium on either side of the "widow's peak" and on the crown (vertex). The extent of hair loss is variable and unpredictable. Minoxidil 5% is available over the counter and can be specifically recommended for persons with recent onset (< 5 years) and smaller areas of alopecia. Approximately 40% of patients treated twice daily for a year will have moderate to dense growth. Finasteride (Propecia), 1 mg orally daily, has similar efficacy and may be additive to minoxidil. As opposed to minoxidil, finasteride is used only in males.

Hair loss or thinning of the hair in women results from the same cause as common baldness in men (androgenetic alopecia) and may be treated with topical minoxidil. A workup consisting of determination of serum testosterone, DHEAS, iron, total iron-binding capacity, thyroid function tests, and a complete blood count will identify most other causes of hair thinning in premenopausal women. Women who complain of thin hair but show little evidence of alopecia need follow-up, because > 50% of the scalp hair can be lost before the clinician can perceive it.

Telogen effluvium is transitory increase in the number of hairs in the telogen (resting) phase of the hair growth cycle. This may occur spontaneously, may appear at the termination of pregnancy, may be precipitated by "crash dieting," high fever, stress from surgery or shock, malnutrition, or may be provoked by hormonal contraceptives. Whatever the cause, telogen effluvium usually has a latent period of 2–4 months. The prognosis is generally good. The condition is diagnosed by the presence of large numbers of hairs with white bulbs coming out upon gentle tugging of the hair. Counts of hairs lost by the patient on combing or shampooing often exceed 150 per day, compared to an average of 70–100. In one study, a major cause of telogen effluvium was found to be iron deficiency, and the hair counts bore a clear relationship to serum iron levels. If iron deficiency is suspected, a serum ferritin should be obtained, and the value followed with supplementation.

Alopecia areata is of unknown cause but is believed to be an immunologic process. Typically, there are patches that are perfectly smooth and without scarring. Tiny hairs 2–3 mm in length, called "exclamation hairs," may be seen. Telogen hairs are easily dislodged from the periphery of active lesions. The beard, brows, and lashes may be involved. Involvement may extend to all of the scalp hair (alopecia totalis) or to all scalp and body hair (alopecia universalis). Severe forms may be treated by systemic corticosteroid therapy, although recurrences follow discontinuation of therapy. Alopecia areata is occasionally associated with Hashimoto thyroiditis, pernicious anemia, Addison disease, and vitiligo.

Intralesional corticosteroids are frequently effective for alopecia areata. Triamcinolone acetonide in a concentration of 2.5–10 mg/mL is injected in aliquots of 0.1 mL at approximately 1- to 2-cm intervals, not exceeding a total dose of 30 mg per month for adults. Alopecia areata is usually self-limiting, with complete regrowth of hair in 80% of patients with focal disease. Some mild cases are resistant to treatment, as are the extensive totalis and universalis types. Support groups for patients with extensive alopecia areata are very beneficial.

In trichotillomania (the pulling out of one's own hair), the patches of hair loss are irregular and short growing hairs are always present, since they cannot be pulled out until they are long enough. The patches are often unilateral, occurring on the same side as the patient's dominant hand. The patient may be unaware of the habit.

Alkhalifah A. Alopecia areata update. Dermatol Clin. 2013 Jan;31(1):93–108. [PMID: 23159179]

Mirmirani P. Managing hair loss in midlife women. Maturitas. 2013 Feb;74(2):119–22. [PMID: 23182767]

Ucak H et al. Prognostic factors that affect the response to topical treatment in patchy alopecia areata. J Eur Acad Dermatol Venereol. 2014 Jan;28(1):34–40. [PMID: 23181708]

NAIL DISORDERS

1. Morphologic Abnormalities of the Nails

▶ Classification

Acquired nail disorders may be classified as local or those associated with systemic or generalized skin diseases.

A. Local Nail Disorders

Onycholysis (distal separation of the nail plate from the nail bed, usually of the fingers) is caused by excessive exposure to water, soaps, detergents, alkalies, and industrial cleaning agents. Candidal infection of the nail folds and subungual area, nail hardeners, and drug-induced photosensitivity may cause onycholysis, as may hyperthyroidism, hypothyroidism, and psoriasis.

1. Distortion of the nail occurs as a result of chronic inflammation of the nail matrix underlying the eponychial fold. Such changes may also be caused by warts, tumors, or cysts, impinging on the nail matrix.

2. Discoloration and crumbly thickened nails are noted in dermatophyte infection and psoriasis.

3. Allergic reactions (to resins in undercoats and polishes or to nail glues) are characterized by onycholysis or by grossly distorted, hypertrophic, and misshapen nails.

B. Nail Changes Associated with Systemic or Generalized Skin Diseases

Beau lines (transverse furrows) may follow any serious systemic illness.

1. Atrophy of the nails may be related to trauma or to vascular or neurologic disease.

2. Clubbed fingers may be due to the prolonged hypoxemia associated with cardiopulmonary disorders (Figure 6–41) (See Chapter 9).

3. Spoon nails may be seen in anemic patients.

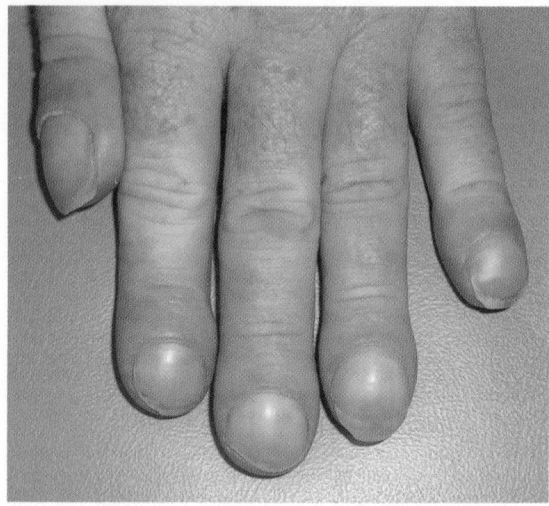

▲ **Figure 6–41.** Clubbing of the fingers in congenital heart disease. (Courtesy of Richard P. Usatine, MD; used, with permission, from Usatine RP, Smith MA, Mayeaux EJ Jr, Chumley H, Tysinger J. *The Color Atlas of Family Medicine.* McGraw-Hill, 2009.)

4. Stippling or pitting of the nails is seen in psoriasis, alopecia areata, and hand eczema.

5. Nail hyperpigmentation may be caused by many chemotherapeutic agents, but especially the taxanes.

▶ Differential Diagnosis

Onychomycosis may cause nail changes identical to those seen in psoriasis. Careful examination for more characteristic lesions elsewhere on the body is essential to the diagnosis of the nail disorders. Cancer should be suspected (eg, Bowen disease or squamous cell carcinoma) as the cause of any persistent solitary subungual or periungual lesion.

▶ Complications

Toenail changes may lead to an ingrown nail—in turn often complicated by bacterial infection and occasionally by exuberant granulation tissue. Poor manicuring and poorly fitting shoes may contribute to this complication. Cellulitis may result.

▶ Treatment & Prognosis

Treatment consists usually of careful debridement and manicuring and, above all, reduction of exposure to irritants (soaps, detergents, alkali, bleaches, solvents, etc). Longitudinal grooving due to temporary lesions of the matrix, such as warts, synovial cysts, and other impingements, may be cured by removal of the offending lesion.

2. Tinea Unguium (Onychomycosis)

Tinea unguium is a trichophyton infection of one or more (but rarely all) fingernails or toenails. The species most commonly found is *T rubrum*. "Saprophytic" fungi may rarely (< 5%) cause onychomycosis.

The nails are lusterless, brittle, and hypertrophic, and the substance of the nail is friable. Laboratory diagnosis is mandatory since only 50% of dystrophic nails are due to dermatophytosis. Portions of the nail should be cleared with 10% KOH and examined under the microscope for hyphae. Fungi may also be cultured. Periodic acid-Schiff stain of a histologic section of the nail plate will also demonstrate the fungus readily. Each technique is positive in only 50% of cases so several different tests may need to be performed.

Onychomycosis is difficult to treat because of the long duration of therapy required and the frequency of recurrences. Fingernails respond more readily than toenails. For toenails, treatment is limited to patients with discomfort, inability to exercise, and immune compromise.

In general, systemic therapy is required to effectively treat nail onychomycosis. Topical therapy has limited value and the adjunctive value of surgical procedures is unproven. Efficacy of laser treatments is lacking, especially with regard to long-term cures. Fingernails can virtually always be cured and toenails are cured 35–50% of the time and are clinically improved about 75% of the time. In all cases, before treatment, the diagnosis should be confirmed. The costs of the various treatment options should be known and the most cost-effective treatment chosen. Drug interactions must be avoided. Ketoconazole, due to its higher risk for hepatotoxicity, is not recommended to treat any form of onychomycosis. For fingernails, ultramicronized griseofulvin 250 mg orally three times daily for 6 months can be effective. Alternative treatments are (in order of preference) oral terbinafine 250 mg daily for 6 weeks, oral itraconazole 400 mg daily for 7 days each month for 2 months, and oral itraconazole 200 mg daily for 2 months. Off-label use of fluconazole, 400 mg once weekly for 6 months, can also be effective, but there is limited evidence for this option. Once clear, fingernails usually remain free of disease for some years.

Onychomycosis of the toenails does not respond to griseofulvin therapy or topical treatments. The best treatment, which is also FDA approved, is oral terbinafine 250 mg daily for 12 weeks. Liver function tests and a complete blood count with platelets are performed monthly during treatment. Pulse oral itraconazole 200 mg twice daily for 1 week per month for 3 months is inferior to standard terbinafine treatments, but it is an acceptable alternative for those unable to take terbinafine. The courses of terbinafine or itraconazole may need to be repeated 6 months after the first treatment cycle if fungal cultures of the nail are still positive.

Bergstrom KG. Onychomycosis: is there a role for lasers? J Drugs Dermatol. 2011 Sep1;10(9):1074–75. [PMID: 22052283]
Dehesa L et al. Treatment of inflammatory nail disorders. Dermatol Ther. 2012 Nov–Dec;25(6):525–34. [PMID: 23210751]
Gupta AK et al. New therapeutic options for onychomycosis. Expert Opin Pharmacother. 2012 Jun;13(8):1131–42. Erratum in: Expert Opin Pharmacother.2013 Jan;14(1):149. [PMID: 22533461]
Shemer A. Update: medical treatment of onychomycosis. Dermatol Ther. 2012 Nov;25(6):582–93. [PMID: 23210757]

DERMATITIS MEDICAMENTOSA (Drug Eruption)

ESSENTIALS OF DIAGNOSIS

▶ Usually, abrupt onset of widespread, symmetric erythematous eruption.

▶ May mimic any inflammatory skin condition.

▶ Constitutional symptoms (malaise, arthralgia, headache, and fever) may be present.

▶ General Considerations

As is well recognized, only a minority of cutaneous drug reactions result from allergy. True allergic drug reactions involve prior exposure, an "incubation" period, reactions to doses far below the therapeutic range, manifestations different from the usual pharmacologic effects of the drug, involvement of only a small portion of the population at risk, restriction to a limited number of syndromes (anaphylactic and anaphylactoid, urticarial, vasculitic, etc), and reproducibility.

Rashes are among the most common adverse reactions to drugs and occur in 2–3% of hospitalized patients. Amoxicillin, TMP-SMZ, and ampicillin or penicillin are the most common causes of urticarial and maculopapular reactions. Toxic epidermal necrolysis and Stevens-Johnson syndrome are most commonly produced by sulfonamides and anticonvulsants. Phenolphthalein, pyrazolone derivatives, tetracyclines, NSAIDs, TMP-SMZ, and barbiturates are the major causes of fixed drug eruptions. Calcium channel blockers are a common cause of pruritus and eczemas in the elderly.

▶ Clinical Findings

A. Symptoms and Signs

Drug eruptions are generally classified as "simple" or "complex." Simple drug eruptions involve an exanthem, usually appear in the second week of drug therapy, and have no associated constitutional or laboratory findings. Antibiotics, including the penicillins and quinolones are the most common causes. Complex drug eruptions (also called drug-induced hypersensitivity syndromes [DIHS]) occur during the third week of treatment on average and have constitutional and laboratory findings. These may include fevers, chills, hematologic abnormalities (especially eosinophilia), and abnormal liver or kidney function. A mnemonic for complex eruptions is "DRESS" (DRug Eruption with Eosinophilia and Systemic Symptoms). The most common causes are the long-acting sulfonamides, allopurinol, and anticonvulsants. The use of anticonvulsants to treat bipolar disorder and chronic pain has led to an apparent increase in these reactions. In patients of certain races, polymorphisms of antigen presenting major histocompatibility (MHC) loci increases risk for the development of severe drug eruptions. In Han Chinese, HLA typing is indicated before institution of carbamazepine treatment,

Table 6–3. Skin reactions due to systemic drugs.

Reaction	Appearance	Distribution and Comments	Common Offenders
Toxic erythema	Morbilliform, maculopapular, exanthematous reactions.	The most common skin reaction to drugs. Often more pronounced on the trunk than on the extremities. In previously exposed patients, the rash may start in 2–3 days. In the first course of treatment, the eruption often appears about the seventh to ninth days. Fever may be present.	Antibiotics (especially ampicillin and TMP-SMZ), sulfonamides and related compounds (including thiazide diuretics, furosemide, and sulfonylurea hypoglycemic agents), and barbiturates.
SJS/TEN	Target-like lesions. Bullae may occur. Mucosal involvement.	Usually trunk and proximal extremities.	Sulfonamides, anticonvulsants, allopurinol, and NSAIDs.
Erythema nodosum	Inflammatory cutaneous nodules.	Usually limited to the extensor aspects of the legs. May be accompanied by fever, arthralgias, and pain.	Oral contraceptives.
Allergic vasculitis	Inflammatory changes may present as urticaria that lasts over 24 hours, hemorrhagic papules ("palpable purpura"), vesicles, bullae, or necrotic ulcers.	Most severe on the legs.	Sulfonamides, phenytoin, propylthiouracil.
Exfoliative dermatitis and erythroderma	Red and scaly.	Entire skin surface.	Allopurinol, sulfonamides, isoniazid, anticonvulsants, or carbamazepine.
Photosensitivity: increased sensitivity to light, often of ultraviolet A wavelengths, but may be due to UVB or visible light as well	Sunburn, vesicles, papules in photodistributed pattern.	Exposed skin of the face, the neck, and the backs of the hands and, in women, the lower legs. Exaggerated response to ultraviolet light.	Sulfonamides and sulfonamide-related compounds (thiazide diuretics, furosemide, sulfonylureas), tetracyclines, phenothiazines, sulindac, amiodarone, voriconazole, and NSAIDs.
Drug-related lupus erythematosus	May present with a photosensitive rash, annular lesions, or psoriasis on upper trunk.	Less severe than systemic lupus erythematosus, sparing the kidneys and central nervous system. Recovery often follows drug withdrawal.	Diltiazem, etanercept, hydrochlorothiazide, infliximab, lisinopril, terbinafine.
Lichenoid and lichen planus–like eruptions	Pruritic, erythematous to violaceous polygonal papules that coalesce or expand to form plaques.	May be in photo- or nonphoto-distributed pattern.	Carbamazepine, furosemide, hydroxychloroquine, phenothiazines, beta-blockers, quinidine, quinine, sulfonylureas, tetracyclines, thiazides, and triprolidine.
Fixed drug eruptions	Single or multiple demarcated, round, erythematous plaques that often become hyperpigmented.	Recur at the same site when the drug is repeated. Hyperpigmentation, if present, remains after healing.	Numerous drugs, including antimicrobials, analgesics, barbiturates, cardiovascular drugs, heavy metals, antiparasitic agents, antihistamines, phenolphthalein, ibuprofen, and naproxen.
Urticaria	Red, itchy wheals that vary in size from < 1 cm to many centimeters. May be accompanied by angioedema.	Chronic urticaria is rarely caused by drugs.	Acute urticaria: penicillins, NSAIDs, sulfonamides, opioids, and salicylates. Angioedema is common in patients receiving ACE inhibitors and angiotensin receptor blockers.

(continued)

Table 6–3. Skin reactions due to systemic drugs. (continued)

Reaction	Appearance	Distribution and Comments	Common Offenders
Pigmentary changes	Flat hyperpigmented areas.	Forehead and cheeks (chloasma, melasma). The most common pigmentary disorder associated with drug ingestion. Improvement is slow despite stopping the drug.	Oral contraceptives are the usual cause.
	Blue-gray discoloration.	Light-exposed areas.	Chlorpromazine and related phenothiazines.
	Brown or blue-gray pigmentation.	Generalized.	Heavy metals (silver, gold, bismuth, and arsenic).
	Yellow color.	Generalized.	Quinacrine.
	Blue-black patches on the shins.		Minocycline, chloroquine.
	Blue-black pigmentation of the nails and palate and depigmentation of the hair.		Chloroquine.
	Slate-gray color.	Primarily in photoexposed areas.	Amiodarone.
	Brown discoloration of the nails.	Especially in more darkly pigmented patients.	Hydroxyurea.
Psoriasiform eruptions	Scaly red plaques.	May be located on trunk and extremities. Palms and soles may be hyperkeratotic. May cause psoriasiform eruption or worsen psoriasis.	Antimalarials, lithium, beta-blockers, and TNF inhibitors.
Pityriasis rosea–like eruptions	Oval, red, slightly raised patches with central scale.	Mainly on the trunk.	Barbiturates, bismuth, captopril, clonidine, methopromazine, metoprolol, metronidazole, and tripelennamine.

ACE, angiotensin-converting enzyme; NSAIDs, nonsteroidal anti-inflammatory drugs; SJS/TEN, Stevens-Johnson syndrome/toxic epidermal necrolysis; TMP-SMZ, trimethoprim-sulfamethoxazole; TNF, tumor necrosis factor.

for example. Coexistent reactivation of Epstein-Barr virus, HHV-6, or cytomegalovirus is often present and may be important in the pathogenesis of these complex drug eruptions. Table 6–3 summarizes the types of skin reactions, their appearance and distribution, and the common offenders in each case.

B. Laboratory Findings

Routinely ordered blood work is of no value in the diagnosis of simple drug eruptions. In complex drug eruptions, the CBC, liver biochemical tests, and renal function tests should be monitored. Skin biopsies may be helpful in making the diagnosis.

▶ Differential Diagnosis

Observation after discontinuation, which may be a slow process, helps establish the diagnosis. Rechallenge, though of theoretical value, may pose a danger to the patient and is best avoided.

▶ Complications

Some cutaneous drug reactions may be associated with visceral involvement. The organ systems involved depend on the individual medication or drug class. Most common is an infectious mononucleosis-like illness and hepatitis associated with administration of anticonvulsants. Myocarditis may be a serious complication of drug-induced hypersensitivity syndrome. Months after recovering from DRESS, patients may suffer hypothyroidism.

▶ Treatment

A. General Measures

Systemic manifestations are treated as they arise (eg, anemia, icterus, purpura). Antihistamines may be of value in urticarial and angioneurotic reactions. Epinephrine 1:1000, 0.5–1 mL intravenously or subcutaneously, should be used as an emergency measure. In DIHS, systemic corticosteroids may be required, starting at about 1 mg/kg/d and tapering very slowly.

B. Local Measures

SJS/TEN with extensive blistering eruptions resulting in erosions and superficial ulcerations, which demand hospitalization and nursing care as for burn patients, develops in some DIHS patients.

▶ Prognosis

Drug rash usually disappears upon withdrawal of the drug and proper treatment. DIHS may be associated with auto-immune phenomena, including abnormal thyroid function. This can occur months after the hypersensitivity syndrome has resolved.

Bourgeois GP et al. A review of DRESS-associated myocarditis. J Am Acad Dermatol. 2012 Jun;66(6):e229–36. [PMID: 21658796]

Hausmann O et al. Etiology and pathogenesis of adverse drug reactions. Chem Immunol Allergy. 2012;97:32–46. [PMID: 22613852]

Summers EM et al. Chronic eczematous eruptions in the aging: further support for an association with exposure to calcium channel blockers. JAMA Dermatol. 2013 Jul;149(7):814–8. [PMID: 23636109]

Walsh S et al. Drug Reaction with Eosinophilia and Systemic Symptoms (DRESS): is cutaneous phenotype a prognostic marker for outcome? A review of clinicopathological features of 27 cases. Br J Dermatol. 2013 Feb;168(2):391–401. [PMID: 23034060]

Wei CY et al. A recent update of pharmacogenomics in drug-induced severe skin reactions. Drug Metab Pharmacokinet. 2012;27(1):132–41. [PMID: 22041139]

Winnicki M et al. A systematic approach to systemic contact dermatitis and symmetric drug-related intertriginous and flexural exanthema (SDRIFE): a closer look at these conditions and an approach to intertriginous eruptions. Am J Clin Dermatol. 2011 Jun1;12(3):171–80. [PMID: 21469762]

Yin ZQ et al. Meta-analysis on the comparison between two topical calcineurin inhibitors in atopic dermatitis. J Dermatol. 2012 Jun;39(6):520–6. [PMID: 22409418]

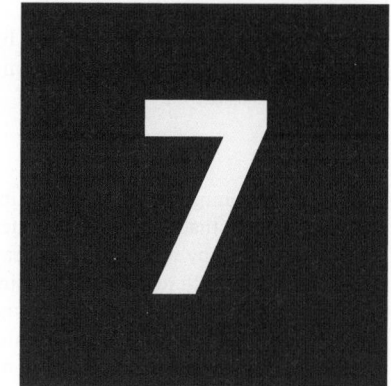

Disorders of the Eyes & Lids

7

Paul Riordan-Eva, FRCOphth

REFRACTIVE ERRORS

Refractive errors are the most common cause of reduced clarity of vision (visual acuity) and may be a readily treatable component of poor vision in patients with other diagnoses.

Use of a pinhole will overcome most refractive errors and thus allows their identification as a cause of reduced visual acuity.

1. Contact Lenses

Contact lenses are used mostly for correction of refractive errors, for which they provide better optical correction than glasses, as well as for management of diseases of the cornea, conjunctiva, or lids. Colored contact lenses are being used increasingly for cosmesis.

The major risk from contact lens wear is bacterial, amebic, or fungal corneal infection, potentially a blinding condition. Such infections occur more commonly with soft lenses, particularly extended wear, for which there is at least a five-fold increase in risk of corneal ulceration compared with daily wear. Contact lens wearers including those using lenses for cosmesis should be made aware of the risks they face and ways to minimize them, such as avoiding overnight wear or use of lenses past their replacement date and maintaining meticulous lens hygiene, including not using tap water or saliva for lens cleaning. Contact lenses should be removed whenever there is ocular discomfort or redness. Ophthalmologic care should be sought if symptoms persist.

▶ When to Refer

Any contact lens wearer with an acute painful red eye must be referred emergently to an ophthalmologist.

American Academy of Ophthalmology Refractive Management/ Intervention Panel. Preferred Practice Pattern® Guidelines – Summary Benchmark. Refractive errors & refractive surgery. San Francisco, CA: American Academy of Ophthalmology; 2013. Available at: http://one.aao.org/summary-benchmark-detail/refractive-errors--surgery-summary-benchmark-octob

Lee SY et al. Contact lens complications in an urgent-care population: the University of California, Los Angeles, Contact Lens Study. Eye Contact Lens. 2012 Jan;38(1):49–52. [PMID: 22157395]

Singh S et al. Colored cosmetic contact lenses: an unsafe trend in the younger generation. Cornea. 2012 Jul;31(7):777–9. [PMID: 22378117]

2. Surgical Correction

Various surgical techniques are available for the correction of refractive errors, particularly nearsightedness. Laser corneal refractive surgery reshapes the middle layer (stroma) of the cornea with an excimer laser. Other refractive surgery techniques are extraction of the clear crystalline lens with insertion of a single vision, multifocal or accommodative intraocular lens; insertion of an intraocular lens without removal of the crystalline lens (phakic intraocular lens); intrastromal corneal ring segments (INTACS); collagen cross-linking; laser thermal keratoplasty; and conductive keratoplasty (CK). Topical atropine and pirenzepine, a selective muscarinic antagonist, and rigid contact lens wear during sleep (orthokeratology) are also being investigated for nearsightedness.

American Academy of Ophthalmology Refractive Management/ Intervention Panel. Preferred Practice Pattern® Guidelines. Refractive errors & refractive surgery. San Francisco, CA: American Academy of Ophthalmology; 2013. Available at: http://one.aao.org/preferred-practice-pattern/refractive-errors--surgery-ppp-2013

Bastawrous A et al. Laser refractive eye surgery. BMJ. 2011 Apr 20; 342:d2345. [PMID: 21508060]

DISORDERS OF THE LIDS & LACRIMAL APPARATUS

1. Hordeolum

Hordeolum is a common staphylococcal abscess that is characterized by a localized red, swollen, acutely tender area on the upper or lower lid. Internal hordeolum is a meibomian gland abscess that usually points onto the conjunctival surface of the lid; external hordeolum or sty usually is smaller and on the margin.

Warm compresses are helpful. Incision may be indicated if resolution does not begin within 48 hours.

An antibiotic ointment (bacitracin or erythromycin) applied to the eyelid every 3 hours may be beneficial during the acute stage. Internal hordeolum may lead to generalized cellulitis of the lid.

2. Chalazion

Chalazion is a common granulomatous inflammation of a meibomian gland that may follow an internal hordeolum. It is characterized by a hard, nontender swelling on the upper or lower lid with redness and swelling of the adjacent conjunctiva. If the chalazion is large enough to impress the cornea, vision will be distorted. Treatment is usually by incision and curettage but corticosteroid injection may also be effective.

Arbabi EM et al. Chalazion. BMJ. 2010 Aug 10;341:c4044. [PMID: 21155069]

3. Blepharitis

Blepharitis is a common chronic bilateral inflammatory condition of the lid margins. **Anterior blepharitis** involves the eyelid skin, eyelashes, and associated glands. It may be ulcerative, because of infection by staphylococci, or seborrheic in association with seborrhea of the scalp, brows, and ears. **Posterior blepharitis** results from inflammation of the meibomian glands. There may be bacterial infection, particularly with staphylococci, or primary glandular dysfunction, in which there is a strong association with acne rosacea.

▶ Clinical Findings

Symptoms are irritation, burning, and itching. In **anterior blepharitis**, the eyes are "red-rimmed" and scales or granulations can be seen clinging to the lashes. In **posterior blepharitis**, the lid margins are hyperemic with telangiectasias, and the meibomian glands and their orifices are inflamed. The lid margin is frequently rolled inward to produce a mild entropion, and the tears may be frothy or abnormally greasy.

Blepharitis is a common cause of recurrent conjunctivitis. Both anterior and, more particularly, posterior blepharitis may be complicated by hordeola or chalazia; abnormal lid or lash positions, producing trichiasis; epithelial keratitis of the lower third of the cornea; marginal corneal infiltrates; and inferior corneal vascularization and thinning.

▶ Treatment

Anterior blepharitis is usually controlled by cleanliness of the lid margins, eyebrows, and scalp. Scales should be removed from the lids daily with a hot wash cloth or a damp cotton applicator and baby shampoo. In acute exacerbations, an antistaphylococcal antibiotic eye ointment such as bacitracin or erythromycin is applied daily to the lid margins. Antibiotic sensitivity studies may be helpful in severe cases.

In **mild posterior blepharitis**, regular meibomian gland expression may be sufficient to control symptoms. Inflammation of the conjunctiva and cornea indicates a need for more active treatment, including long-term low-dose oral antibiotic therapy, usually with tetracycline (250 mg twice daily), doxycycline (100 mg daily), minocycline (50–100 mg daily) or erythromycin (250 mg three times daily), and possibly short-term topical corticosteroids, eg, prednisolone, 0.125% twice daily. Topical therapy with antibiotics such as ciprofloxacin 0.3% ophthalmic solution twice daily may be helpful but should be restricted to short courses.

American Academy of Ophthalmology Cornea/External Disease Panel. Preferred Practice Pattern® Guidelines. Blepharitis. San Francisco, CA: American Academy of Ophthalmology; 2013. Available at: http://one.aao.org/preferred-practice-pattern/blepharitis-ppp--2013
American Academy of Ophthalmology Cornea/External Disease Panel. Preferred Practice Pattern® Guidelines – Summary Benchmark. Blepharitis. San Francisco, CA: American Academy of Ophthalmology; 2013. Available at: http://one.aao.org/summary-benchmark-detail/blepharitis-summary-benchmark--october-2012

4. Entropion & Ectropion

Entropion (inward turning of usually the lower lid) occurs occasionally in older people as a result of degeneration of the lid fascia, or may follow extensive scarring of the conjunctiva and tarsus. Surgery is indicated if the lashes rub on the cornea. Botulinum toxin injections may also be used for temporary correction of the involutional lower eyelid entropion of older people.

Ectropion (outward turning of the lower lid) is common with advanced age (Figure 7–1). Surgery is indicated if there is excessive tearing, exposure keratitis, or a cosmetic problem.

Bedran EG et al. Ectropion. Semin Ophthalmol. 2010 May; 25(3):59–65. [PMID: 20590414]
Ferreira IS et al. Trichiasis. Semin Ophthalmol. 2010 May; 25(3):66–71. [PMID: 20590415]
Pereira MG et al. Eyelid entropion. Semin Ophthalmol. 2010 May;25(3):52–8. [PMID: 20590413]

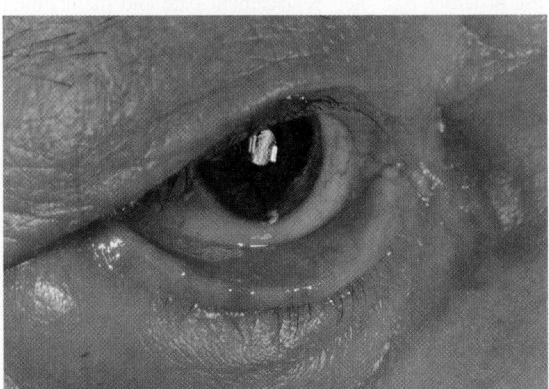

▲ **Figure 7–1.** Involutional ectropion of right lower eyelid. (From M. Reza Vagefi and John H Sullivan. Reproduced, with permission, from Riordan-Eva P, Cunningham ET Jr. *Vaughan & Asbury's General Ophthalmology*, 18th edition. McGraw-Hill, 2011.)

5. Tumors

Eyelid tumors are usually benign. Basal cell carcinoma is the most common malignant tumor. Squamous cell carcinoma, meibomian gland carcinoma, and malignant melanoma also occur. Surgery for any lesion involving the lid margin should be performed by an ophthalmologist or suitably trained plastic surgeon to avoid deformity of the lid. Otherwise, small lesions can often be excised by the nonophthalmologist. Histopathologic examination of eyelid tumors should be routine, since 2% of lesions thought to be benign clinically are found to be malignant. The Mohs technique of intraoperative examination of excised tissue is particularly valuable in ensuring complete excision so that the risk of recurrence is reduced. The role of vismodegib in the treatment of eyelid basal cell carcinoma is being investigated.

Dekmezian MS et al. Malignancies of the eyelid: a review of primary and metastatic cancers. Int J Dermatol. 2013 Aug;52(8):903–26. [PMID: 23869923]
Gill HS et al. Vismodegib for periocular and orbital basal cell carcinoma. JAMA Ophthalmol. 2013 Dec 1;131(12):1591–4. [PMID: 24136169]
Wang CJ et al. Clinicopathologic features and prognostic factors of malignant eyelid tumors. Int J Ophthalmol. 2013 Aug 18;6(4):442–7. [PMID: 23991375]

6. Dacryocystitis

Dacryocystitis is infection of the lacrimal sac usually due to congenital or acquired obstruction of the nasolacrimal system. It may be acute or chronic and occurs most often in infants and in persons over 40 years. It is usually unilateral. The usual infectious organisms are *Staphylococcus aureus* and beta-hemolytic streptococci in acute dacryocystitis and *S epidermidis*, anaerobic streptococci, or *Candida albicans* in chronic dacryocystitis.

Acute dacryocystitis is characterized by pain, swelling, tenderness, and redness in the tear sac area; purulent material may be expressed. In chronic dacryocystitis, tearing and discharge are the principal signs, and mucus or pus may also be expressed.

Acute dacryocystitis responds well to systemic antibiotic therapy. Surgical relief of the underlying obstruction is usually done electively but may be performed urgently in acute cases. The chronic form may be kept latent with antibiotics, but relief of the obstruction is the only cure. In adults, the standard procedure for obstruction of the lacrimal drainage system is dacryocystorhinostomy, which involves surgical exploration of the lacrimal sac and formation of a fistula into the nasal cavity; if necessary, the procedure can be supplemented by nasolacrimal intubation. Congenital nasolacrimal duct obstruction is common and often resolves spontaneously. It can be treated by probing of the nasolacrimal system and supplemented by nasolacrimal intubation or balloon catheter dilation, if necessary. Dacryocystorhinostomy is rarely required.

Ali MJ et al. Clinical profile and management outcome of acute dacryocystitis: two decades of experience in a tertiary eye care center. Semin Ophthalmol. 2013 Oct 30. [Epub ahead of print] [PMID: 24171807]

American Academy of Ophthalmology Preferred Practice Pattern® Clinical Question. Nasolacrimal duct obstruction. San Francisco, CA: American Academy of Ophthalmology;2013.http://one.aao.org/clinical-questions/nasolacrimal-duct-obstruction-3
Pinar-Sueiro S et al. Dacryocystitis: systematic approach to diagnosis and therapy. Curr Infect Dis Rep. 2012 Jan 29. [Epub ahead of print] [PMID: 22286338]

CONJUNCTIVITIS

Conjunctivitis is the most common eye disease. It may be acute or chronic. Most cases are due to viral or bacterial (including gonococcal and chlamydial) infection. Other causes include keratoconjunctivitis sicca, allergy, chemical irritants, and deliberate self-harm. The mode of transmission of infectious conjunctivitis is usually direct contact via fingers, towels, handkerchiefs, etc, to the fellow eye or to other persons. It may be through contaminated eye drops.

Conjunctivitis must be differentiated from acute uveitis, acute glaucoma, and corneal disorders (Table 7–1).

American Academy of Ophthalmology Cornea/External Disease Panel. Preferred Practice Pattern® Guidelines. Conjunctivitis. San Francisco, CA: American Academy of Ophthalmology; 2013.http://one.aao.org/preferred-practice-pattern/conjunctivitis-ppp--2013
American Academy of Ophthalmology Cornea/External Disease Panel. Preferred Practice Pattern® Guidelines – Summary Benchmark. Conjunctivitis. San Francisco, CA: American Academy of Ophthalmology; 2013. http://one.aao.org/summary-benchmark-detail/conjunctivitis-summary-benchmark--october-2012
Azari AA et al. Conjunctivitis: a systematic review of diagnosis and treatment. JAMA. 2013 Oct 23;310(16):1721–9. [PMID: 24150468]
Goodman DM et al. JAMA patient page. Conjunctivitis. JAMA. 2013 May 22;309(20):2176. [PMID: 23695487]

1. Viral Conjunctivitis

Adenovirus is the most common cause of viral conjunctivitis. There is usually bilateral disease with copious watery discharge, often with marked foreign body sensation, and a follicular conjunctivitis. Infection spreads easily. Eye clinics and contaminated swimming pools are sometimes the source of infection. Epidemic keratoconjunctivitis, which may result in visual loss due to corneal subepithelial infiltrates, is usually caused by adenovirus types 8, 19, and 37. The disease lasts at least 2 weeks. Infection with adenovirus types 3, 4, 7, and 11 is typically associated with pharyngitis, fever, malaise, and preauricular adenopathy (pharyngoconjunctival fever). The disease usually lasts 10 days. Viral conjunctivitis may also be due to herpes simplex virus (HSV), when it is usually unilateral and may be associated with lid vesicles, and enterovirus 70 or coxsackievirus A24 that characteristically cause acute hemorrhagic conjunctivitis (see Chapter 32).

Except for HSV infection for which treatment with topical (eg, ganciclovir 0.15% gel) and/or systemic (eg, oral acyclovir) antivirals is recommended, there is no specific treatment. Cold compresses reduce discomfort and topical

Table 7–1. The inflamed eye: Differential diagnosis of common causes.

	Acute Conjunctivitis	Acute Anterior Uveitis (Iritis)	Acute Angle-Closure Glaucoma	Corneal Trauma or Infection
Incidence	Extremely common	Common	Uncommon	Common
Discharge	Moderate to copious	None	None	Watery or purulent
Vision	No effect on vision	Often blurred	Markedly blurred	Usually blurred
Pain	Mild	Moderate	Severe	Moderate to severe
Conjunctival injection	Diffuse; more toward fornices	Mainly circumcorneal	Mainly circumcorneal	Mainly circumcorneal
Cornea	Clear	Usually clear	Cloudy	Clarity change related to cause
Pupil size	Normal	Small	Moderately dilated	Normal or small
Pupillary light response	Normal	Poor	None	Normal
Intraocular pressure	Normal	Usually normal but may be low or elevated	Markedly elevated	Normal
Smear	Causative organisms	No organisms	No organisms	Organisms found only in corneal infection

sulfonamides (or oral antibiotics) can be prescribed to prevent secondary bacterial infection. The value of weak topical corticosteroids or topical cyclosporine for corneal infiltrates due to adenoviral infection is uncertain.

Kaufman HE. Adenovirus advances: new diagnostic and therapeutic options. Curr Opin Ophthalmol. 2011 Jul;22(4):290–3. [PMID: 21537185]
Skevaki CL et al. Treatment of viral conjunctivitis with antiviral drugs. Drugs. 2011 Feb 12;71(3):331–47. [PMID: 21319870]

2. Bacterial Conjunctivitis

The organisms isolated most commonly in bacterial conjunctivitis are staphylococci, including methicillin-resistant *S aureus* (MRSA); streptococci, particularly *S pneumoniae*; *Haemophilus* species; *Pseudomonas*; and *Moraxella*. All may produce a copious purulent discharge. There is no blurring of vision and only mild discomfort. In severe (hyperpurulent) cases, examination of stained conjunctival scrapings and cultures is recommended, particularly to identify gonococcal infection.

The disease is usually self-limited, lasting about 10–14 days if untreated. A topical sulfonamide or oral antibiotic will usually clear the infection in 2–3 days. Except in special circumstances, the use of topical fluoroquinolones is rarely justified for treatment of a generally self-limiting, benign infection.

Epling J. Bacterial conjunctivitis. Clin Evid (Online). 2012 Feb 20; 2012. [PMID: 22348418]
Sheikh A et al. Antibiotics versus placebo for acute bacterial conjunctivitis. Cochrane Database Syst Rev. 2012 Sep 12; (9):CD001211. [PMID: 22972049]

A. Gonococcal Conjunctivitis

Gonococcal conjunctivitis, usually acquired through contact with infected genital secretions, typically causes copious purulent discharge. It is an ophthalmologic emergency because corneal involvement may rapidly lead to perforation. The diagnosis should be confirmed by stained smear and culture of the discharge. A single 1-g dose of intramuscular ceftriaxone is usually adequate. (Fluoroquinolone resistance is common.) Topical antibiotics such as erythromycin and bacitracin may be added. Other sexually transmitted diseases, including chlamydiosis, syphilis, and HIV infection, should be considered. Routine treatment for chlamydial infection is recommended.

Mayor MT et al. Diagnosis and management of gonococcal infections. Am Fam Physician. 2012 Nov 15;86(10):931–8. [PMID: 23157146]

B. Chlamydial Keratoconjunctivitis

1. Trachoma—Trachoma is the most common infectious cause of blindness worldwide, with approximately 40 million people affected and 1.3 million with profound vision loss. Recurrent episodes of infection in childhood manifest as bilateral follicular conjunctivitis, epithelial keratitis, and corneal vascularization (pannus). Cicatrization of the tarsal conjunctiva leads to entropion and trichiasis in adulthood, with secondary central corneal scarring.

Immunologic tests or polymerase chain reaction on conjunctival samples will confirm the diagnosis but treatment should be started on the basis of clinical findings. A single 1-g dose of oral azithromycin is the preferred drug treatment, but improvements in hygiene and living conditions probably have contributed more to the marked reduction in the prevalence of trachoma during the past 25 years. Local treatment is not necessary. Surgical treatment includes correction of eyelid deformities and corneal transplantation.

Bhosai SJ et al. Trachoma: an update on prevention, diagnosis, and treatment. Curr Opin Ophthalmol. 2012 Jul;23(4):288–95. [PMID: 22569465]

Taylor HR et al. Trachoma in Australia: an update. Clin Experiment Ophthalmol. 2013 Jul;41(5):508–12. [PMID: 23078264]

2. Inclusion conjunctivitis—The agent of inclusion conjunctivitis is a common cause of genital tract disease in adults. The eye is usually involved following contact with genital secretions. The disease starts with acute redness, discharge, and irritation. The eye findings consist of follicular conjunctivitis with mild keratitis. A nontender preauricular lymph node can often be palpated. Healing usually leaves no sequelae. Diagnosis can be rapidly confirmed by immunologic tests or polymerase chain reaction on conjunctival samples. Treatment is with a single-dose of azithromycin, 1 g orally. Before treatment, all cases should be assessed for genital tract infection so that management can be adjusted accordingly, and other venereal diseases sought.

Malamos P et al. Evaluation of single-dose azithromycin versus standard azithromycin/doxycycline treatment and clinical assessment of regression course in patients with adult inclusion conjunctivitis. Curr Eye Res. 2013 Dec;38(12):1198–206. [PMID: 24047438]

Mishori R et al. *Chlamydia trachomatis* infections: screening, diagnosis, and management. Am Fam Physician. 2012 Dec 15; 86(12):1127–32. [PMID: 23316985]

3. Dry Eyes (Keratoconjunctivitis Sicca)

This is a common disorder, particularly in older women. Hypofunction of the lacrimal glands, causing loss of the aqueous component of tears, may be due to aging, hereditary disorders, systemic disease (eg, Sjögren syndrome), or systemic drugs. Excessive evaporation of tears may be due to environmental factors (eg, a hot, dry, or windy climate) or abnormalities of the lipid component of the tear film, as in blepharitis. Mucin deficiency may be due to vitamin A deficiency, or conjunctival scarring from trachoma, Stevens-Johnson syndrome and related conditions, mucous membrane pemphigoid, burns, or topical drugs or their preservatives.

▶ Clinical Findings

The patient complains of dryness, redness, or foreign body sensation. In severe cases, there is persistent marked discomfort, with photophobia, difficulty in moving the eyelids, and often excessive mucus secretion. In many cases, inspection reveals no abnormality, but on slit-lamp examination there are subtle abnormalities of tear film stability and reduced volume of the tear film meniscus along the lower lid. In more severe cases, damaged corneal and conjunctival cells stain with 1% rose Bengal. In the most severe cases, there is marked conjunctival injection, loss of the normal conjunctival and corneal luster, epithelial keratitis that may progress to frank ulceration, and mucous strands. The Schirmer test, which measures the rate of production of the aqueous component of tears, may be helpful.

▶ Treatment

Aqueous deficiency can be treated with various types of artificial tears. The simplest preparations are physiologic (0.9%) or hypo-osmotic (0.45%) solutions of sodium chloride, which can be used as frequently as every half-hour, but in most cases are needed only three or four times a day. More prolonged duration of action can be achieved with drop preparations containing methylcellulose, polyvinyl alcohol, or polyacrylic acid (carbomers) or by using petrolatum ointment or a hydroxypropyl cellulose (Lacrisert) insert. Such mucomimetics are particularly indicated when there is mucin deficiency. If there is tenacious mucus, mucolytic agents (eg, acetylcysteine, 20% one drop six times daily) may be helpful. Autologous serum eye drops are used for severe dry eyes. Presumably due to its effects on ocular surface and lacrimal gland inflammation, cyclosporine (0.05% ophthalmic emulsion [Restasis] twice a day) has been shown to be beneficial in moderate and severe dry eyes with few adverse effects even in individuals treated for up to 4 years. Increased dietary intake of omega-3 fatty acids has been reported to be beneficial.

Lacrimal punctal occlusion by canalicular plugs or cautery is useful in severe cases. Blepharitis is treated as described above. Associated blepharospasm may benefit from botulinum toxin injections.

Artificial tear preparations are generally very safe and without side effects. Preservatives included in some preparations to maintain sterility are potentially toxic and allergenic and may cause keratitis and cicatrizing conjunctivitis in frequent users. The development of such reactions may be misinterpreted as a worsening of the dry eye state requiring more frequent use of the artificial tears and leading in turn to further deterioration, rather than being recognized as a need to change to a preservative-free preparation.

American Academy of Ophthalmology Cornea/External Disease Panel. Preferred Practice Pattern® Guidelines. Dry eye syndrome. San Francisco, CA: American Academy of Ophthalmology;2013. http://one.aao.org/preferred-practice-pattern/dry-eye-syndrome-ppp--2013

American Academy of Ophthalmology Cornea/External Disease Panel. Preferred Practice Pattern® Guidelines – Summary Benchmark. Dry eye syndrome. San Francisco, CA: American Academy of Ophthalmology;2013. http://one.aao.org/summary-benchmark-detail/dry-eye-syndrome-summary-benchmark--october-2012

Fraunfelder FT et al. The role of medications in causing dry eye. J Ophthalmol. 2012;2012:285851. [PMID: 23050121]

Tong L et al. Choice of artificial tear formulation for patients with dry eye: where do we start? Cornea. 2012 Nov;31(Suppl 1): S32–6. [PMID: 23038032]

Torpy JM et al. JAMA patient page. Dry eye. JAMA. 2012 Aug 8; 308(6):632. [PMID: 22871877]

4. Allergic Eye Disease

Allergic eye disease is common and takes a number of different forms but all are expressions of atopy, which may also manifest as atopic asthma, atopic dermatitis, or allergic rhinitis.

▶ Clinical Findings

Symptoms include itching, tearing, redness, stringy discharge and, occasionally, photophobia and visual loss.

Allergic conjunctivitis is a benign disease, occurring usually in late childhood and early adulthood. It may be seasonal (hay fever), developing usually during the spring or summer, or perennial. Clinical signs are limited to conjunctival hyperemia and edema (chemosis), the latter at times being marked and sudden in onset. **Vernal keratoconjunctivitis** also tends to occur in late childhood and early adulthood. It is usually seasonal, with a predilection for the spring. Large "cobblestone" papillae are noted on the upper tarsal conjunctiva. There may be lymphoid follicles at the limbus. **Atopic keratoconjunctivitis** is a more chronic disorder of adulthood. Both the upper and the lower tarsal conjunctivas exhibit a fine papillary conjunctivitis with fibrosis, resulting in forniceal shortening and entropion with trichiasis. Staphylococcal blepharitis is a complicating factor. Corneal involvement, including refractory ulceration, is frequent during exacerbations of both vernal and atopic keratoconjunctivitis. The latter may be complicated by herpes simplex keratitis.

▶ Treatment

A. Mild and Moderately Severe Allergic Eye Disease

Topical treatments include emedastine, epinastine, alcaftadine, ketotifen, or bepotastine (which have histamine H_1-receptor antagonist, mast cell stabilizer, and eosinophil inhibitor activity) or ketorolac (a nonsteroidal anti-inflammatory drug) (Table 7–2). Olopatadine and azelastine reduce symptoms by similar mechanisms. Topical mast cell stabilizers, such as cromolyn, lodoxamide, nedocromil, and pemirolast produce longer-term prophylaxis but the therapeutic response may be delayed. Topical vasoconstrictors and antihistamines are of limited efficacy in allergic eye disease and may produce rebound hyperemia and follicular conjunctivitis. Systemic antihistamines (eg, loratadine 10 mg orally daily) may be useful in prolonged atopic keratoconjunctivitis. In allergic conjunctivitis, specific allergens may be avoidable. In vernal keratoconjunctivitis, a cooler climate often provides significant benefit.

B. Acute Exacerbations and Severe Allergic Eye Disease

Topical corticosteroids (Table 7–2) are essential to the control of acute exacerbations of both vernal and atopic keratoconjunctivitis. Corticosteroid-induced side effects, including cataracts, glaucoma, and exacerbation of herpes simplex keratitis, are major problems but may be attenuated by the ester corticosteroid, loteprednol. Topical cyclosporine or tacrolimus is also effective. Systemic corticosteroid or other immunosuppressant therapy and even plasmapheresis may be required in severe atopic keratoconjunctivitis.

Kari O et al. Diagnostics and new developments in the treatment of ocular allergies. Curr Allergy Asthma Rep. 2012 Jun;12(3):232–9. [PMID: 22382607]

O'Brien TP. Allergic conjunctivitis: an update on diagnosis and management. Curr Opin Allergy Clin Immunol. 2013 Oct;13(5):543–9. [PMID: 23974684]

Sy H et al. Atopic keratoconjunctivitis. Allergy Asthma Proc. 2013 Jan–Feb;34(1):33–41. [PMID: 23406935]

PINGUECULA & PTERYGIUM

Pinguecula is a yellow elevated conjunctival nodule, more commonly on the nasal side, in the area of the palpebral fissure. It is common in persons over age 35 years. Pterygium is a fleshy, triangular encroachment of the conjunctiva onto the nasal side of the cornea and is usually associated with prolonged exposure to wind, sun, sand, and dust. Pinguecula and pterygium are often bilateral.

Pingueculae rarely grow but may become inflamed (pingueculitis). Pterygia become inflamed and may grow. No treatment is usually required for inflammation of pinguecula or pterygium, but artificial tears are often beneficial, and short courses of topical nonsteroidal anti-inflammatory agents or weak corticosteroids (loteprednol or fluorometholone four times a day) may be necessary.

The indications for excision of pterygium are growth that threatens vision by encroaching on the visual axis, marked induced astigmatism, or severe ocular irritation. Recurrence is common and often more aggressive than the primary lesion.

Liu T et al. Progress in the pathogenesis of pterygium. Curr Eye Res. 2013 Dec;38(12):1191–7. [PMID: 24047084]

CORNEAL ULCER

Corneal ulcers are most commonly due to infection by bacteria, viruses, fungi, or amebas. Noninfectious causes—all of which may be complicated by infection—include neurotrophic keratitis (resulting from loss of corneal sensation), exposure keratitis (due to inadequate eyelid closure), severe dry eye, severe allergic eye disease, and various inflammatory disorders that may be purely ocular or part of a systemic vasculitis. Delayed or ineffective treatment of corneal ulceration may lead to devastating consequences with corneal scarring or intraocular infection. Prompt referral is essential.

Patients complain of pain, photophobia, tearing, and reduced vision. The eye is red, with predominantly circumcorneal injection, and there may be purulent or watery discharge. The corneal appearance varies according to the underlying cause.

▶ When to Refer

Any patient with an acute painful red eye and corneal abnormality should be referred emergently to an ophthalmologist.

Table 7–2. Topical ophthalmic agents.

Agent	Cost/Size[1]	Recommended Regimen	Indications
Antibacterial Agents[2]			
Azithromycin (AzaSite)	$116.58/2.5 mL	1 drop two times daily for 2 days, then once daily for 5 days	Bacterial conjunctivitis.
Bacitracin 500 units/g ointment (various)[3]	$69.34/3.5 g	Refer to package insert (instructions vary)	
Bacitracin/Polymyxin ointment (Polysporin, AK-Poly)	$25.70/3.5 g	Refer to package insert (instructions vary)	
Besifloxacin ophthalmic suspension, 0.6% (Besivance)	$139.72/5 mL	1 drop three times daily for 7 days	Bacterial conjunctivitis.
Cefazolin 10% (fortified) solution	Compounding pharmacy		
Chloramphenicol 1% ointment[4]	Compounding pharmacy		
Chloramphenicol 0.5% solution[4]	Compounding pharmacy		
Ciprofloxacin HCl 0.3% solution (Ciloxan)	$40.44/5 mL	1–2 drops every 2 hours while awake for 2 days, then every 4 hours for 5 days	Bacterial conjunctivitis.
Ciprofloxacin HCl 0.3% ointment	$144.90/3.5 g	Apply small amount (0.5 inch) into lower conjunctival sac three times daily for 2 days, then two times daily for 5 days	Bacterial conjunctivitis.
Erythromycin 0.5% ointment (various)[5]	$19.00/3.5 g	1 cm ribbon up to six times daily (depending on severity of infection)	Bacterial infection of the eye.
Fusidic acid 1% in gel (Fucithalmic)	Not available in United States		
Gatifloxacin 0.5% solution (Zymaxid)	$118.16/2.5 mL	1 drop every 2 hours while awake, up to eight times on day 1, then two to four times daily while awake, days 2–7	
Gentamicin sulfate 0.3% solution (various)	$17.93/5 mL	1–2 drops every 4 hours up to 2 drops every hour for severe infections	Ocular surface infection.
Gentamicin sulfate 0.3% ointment (various)	$18.03/3.5 g	Apply small amount (0.5 inch) into lower conjunctival sac two to three times daily	Ocular surface infection.
Levofloxacin 0.5% solution (various),	$74.76/5 mL	1–2 drops every 2 hours while awake for 2 days (maximum eight times per day), then every 4 hours for 5 days (maximum four times per day)	Bacterial conjunctivitis.
Moxifloxacin 0.5% solution (Vigamox)	$126.48/3 mL	1 drop three times daily for 7 days	Bacterial conjunctivitis.
Neomycin/Polymyxin B/Gramicidin (Neosporin)	$55.74/10 mL	1–2 drops every 4 hours for 7–10 days or more frequently, as required	Ocular surface infection.
Norfloxacin 0.3% solution	Compounding pharmacy		Ocular surface infection.
Ofloxacin 0.3% solution (Ocuflox)	$13.75/5 mL	1–2 drops every 2–4 hours for 2 days, then four times daily for 5 days	Bacterial conjunctivitis.
Polymyxin B/Trimethoprim sulfate 10,000 U/mL/1 mg/mL (Polytrim)[6]	$17.42/10 mL	1 drop every 3 hours for 7–10 days (maximum of 6 doses per day)	Ocular surface infection.
Propamidine isetionate 0.1% solution	Not available in the United States	1–2 drops every 2–4 hours for 2 days, then four times daily for 5 days	Ocular surface infection (including *Ancanthamoeba* keratitis).
Propamidine isetionate 0.1% ointment	Not available in the United States	Apply small amount (0.5 inch) into lower conjunctival sac up to four times daily	Ocular surface infection (including *Ancanthamoeba* keratitis).
Sulfacetamide sodium 10% solution (various)	$58.50/15 mL	1 or 2 drops every 2–3 hours initially; taper by increasing time intervals as condition responds; usual duration 7–10 days	Bacterial infection of the eye.

(continued)

Table 7–2. Topical ophthalmic agents. (continued)

Agent	Cost/Size[1]	Recommended Regimen	Indications
Sulfacetamide sodium 10% ointment (various)	$65.86/3.5 g	Apply small amount (0.5 inch) into lower conjunctival sac once every 3–4 hours and at bedtime; taper by increasing time intervals as condition responds; usual duration 7–10 days	Bacterial infection of the eye.
Tobramycin 0.3% solution (various)	$14.10/5 mL	1–2 drops every 4 hours for a mild to moderate infection or hourly until improvement (then reduce prior to discontinuation) for a severe infection	Eye infection.
Tobramycin 1.5% (fortified) solution	Compounding pharmacy		
Tobramycin 0.3% ointment (Tobrex)	$118.80/3.5 g	Apply small amount (0.5 inch) into lower conjunctival sac two to three times daily for a mild to moderate infection or every 3–4 hours until improvement (then reduce prior to discontinuation) for a severe infection	Eye infection.
Antifungal Agents			
Amphotericin 0.1–0.5% solution	Compounding pharmacy		
Natamycin 5% suspension (Natacyn)	$315.84/15 mL	1 drop every 1–2 hours initially; see prescribing information for further recommendations	Fungal blepharitis, conjunctivitis, keratitis.
Voriconazole 1% solution	Compounding pharmacy		
Antiviral Agents			
Acyclovir 3% ointment (Zovirax)	Not available in United States	Five times daily	Herpes simplex virus keratitis.
Ganciclovir 0.15% gel (Zirgan)	$283.04/5 g	Five times daily	
Trifluridine 1% solution (Viroptic)	$178.28/7.5 mL	1 drop onto cornea every 2 hours while awake for a maximum daily dose of 9 drops until resolution occurs; then an additional 7 days of 1 drop every 4 hours while awake (minimum five times daily)	
Anti-Inflammatory Agents			
Antihistamines[7]			
Alcaftadine 0.25% ophthalmic solution (Lastacaft)	$155.39/3 mL	1 drop once daily	Allergic eye disease.
Azelastine HCl 0.05% ophthalmic solution (Optivar)	$104.06/6 mL	1 drop two to four times daily (up to 6 weeks)	
Bepotastine besilate 1.5% solution (Bepreve)	$342.52/10 mL	1 drop twice daily	
Emedastine difumarate 0.05% solution (Emadine)	$115.80/5 mL	1 drop four times daily	
Epinastine hydrochloride 0.05% ophthalmic solution (Elestat)	$106.99/5 mL	1 drop twice daily (up to 8 weeks)	
Mast cell stabilizers			
Cromolyn sodium 4% solution (Crolom)	$37.20/10 mL	1 drop four to six times daily	Allergic eye disease.
Ketotifen fumarate 0.025% solution (Zaditor)	$64.86/5 mL	1 drop two to four times daily	
Lodoxamide tromethamine 0.1% solution (Alomide)	$149.40/10 mL	1 or 2 drops four times daily (up to 3 months)	

(continued)

Table 7–2. Topical ophthalmic agents. (continued)

Agent	Cost/Size[1]	Recommended Regimen	Indications
Nedocromil sodium 2% solution (Alocril)	$161.66/5 mL	1 drop twice daily	
Olopatadine hydrochloride 0.1% solution (Patanol)	$174.60/5 mL	1 drop twice daily	
Pemirolast potassium 0.1% solution (Alamast)	Not available in the United States	1 drop four times daily	
Nonsteroidal anti-inflammatory agents[8]			
Bromfenac 0.09% solution (Xibrom)	$144.54/2.5 mL	1 drop to operated eye twice daily beginning 24 hours after cataract surgery and continuing through first 2 postoperative weeks	Treatment of postoperative inflammation following cataract extraction.
Diclofenac sodium 0.1% solution (Voltaren)	$73.03/5 mL	1 drop to operated eye four times daily beginning 24 hours after surgery and continuing through first 2 postoperative weeks.	Treatment of postoperative inflammation following cataract extraction and laser corneal surgery.
Flurbiprofen sodium 0.03% solution (various)	$8.73/2.5 mL	1 drop every half hour beginning 2 hours before surgery; 1 drop to operated eye four times daily beginning 24 hours after cataract surgery	Inhibition of intraoperative miosis. Treatment of cystoid macular edema and inflammation after cataract surgery.
Ketorolac tromethamine 0.5% solution (Acular)	$106.87/5 mL	1 drop four times daily	Treatment of allergic eye disease, postoperative inflammation following cataract extraction and laser corneal surgery.
Nepafenac 0.1% suspension (Nevanac)	$189.00/3 mL	1 drop to operated eye three times daily beginning 24 hours after cataract surgery and continuing through first 2 postoperative weeks	Treatment of postoperative inflammation following cataract extraction.
Corticosteroids[9]			
Dexamethasone sodium phosphate 0.1% solution (various)	$20.34/5 mL	1 or 2 drops as often as indicated by severity; use every hour during the day and every 2 hours during the night in severe inflammation; taper off as inflammation decreases	Treatment of steroid-responsive inflammatory conditions of anterior segment.
Dexamethasone sodium phosphate 0.05% ointment	Compounding pharmacy	Apply thin coating on lower conjunctival sac three or four times daily	
Fluorometholone 0.1% suspension (various)[10]	$105.60/10 mL	1 or 2 drops as often as indicated by severity; use every hour during the day and every 2 hours during the night in severe inflammation; taper off as inflammation decreases	
Fluorometholone 0.25% suspension (FML Forte)[10]	$213.60/10 mL	1 drop two to four times daily	
Fluorometholone 0.1% ointment (FML S.O.P.)	$106.80/3.5 g	Apply thin coating on lower conjunctival sac three or four times daily	
Loteprednol etabopate 0.5% (Lotemax)	$343.16/10 mL	1 or 2 drops four times daily	
Prednisolone acetate 0.12% suspension (Pred Mild)	$42.62/10 mL	1 or 2 drops as often as indicated by severity of inflammation; use every hour during the day and every 2 hours during the night in severe inflammation; taper off as inflammation decreases	

(continued)

Table 7–2. Topical ophthalmic agents. (continued)

Agent	Cost/Size[1]	Recommended Regimen	Indications
Prednisolone sodium phosphate 0.125% solution	Compounding pharmacy		
Prednisolone acetate 1% suspension (various)	$105.60/10 mL	2 drops four times daily	
Prednisolone sodium phosphate 1% solution (various)	$57.55/10 mL	1–2 drops two to four times daily	
Rimexolone 1% suspension (Vexol)	$107.76/10 mL	1–2 drops four times daily for 2 weeks	Treatment of postoperative inflammation.
Immunomodulator			
Cyclosporine 0.05% emulsion (Restasis) 0.4 mL/container	$191.27/30 containers	1 drop twice daily	Dry eyes and severe allergic eye disease.
Tacrolimus 0.1% ointment	$231.91/30 g tube	Not yet established (no label to support)	Severe allergic eye disease; no indication in United States.
Agents for Glaucoma and Ocular Hypertension			
Sympathomimetics			
Apraclonidine HCl 0.5% solution (Iopidine)	$86.77/5 mL	1 drop three times daily	Reduction of intraocular pressure. Expensive. Reserve for treatment of resistant cases.
Apraclonidine HCl 1% solution (Iopidine)	$24.21/unit dose	1 drop 1 hour before and immediately after anterior segment laser surgery	To control or prevent elevations of intraocular pressure after laser trabeculoplasty or iridotomy.
Brimonidine tartrate 0.2% solution (Alphagan)	$18.13/5 mL	1 drop two or three times daily	Reduction of intraocular pressure.
Beta-adrenergic blocking agents			
Betaxolol HCl 0.5% solution (Betoptic) and 0.25% suspension (Betoptic S)[11]	0.5%: $123.28/10 mL 0.25%: $206.58/10 mL	1 drop twice daily	Reduction of intraocular pressure.
Carteolol HCl 1% and 2% solution (Various, Teoptic)[12]	1%: $37.07/10 mL	1 drop twice daily	
Levobunolol HCl 0.25% and 0.5% solution (Betagan)[13]	0.5%: $32.25/10 mL	1 drop once or twice daily	
Metipranolol HCl 0.3% solution (OptiPranolol)[13]	$50.17/10 mL	1 drop twice daily	
Timolol 0.25% and 0.5% solution (Betimol)[13]	0.5%: $155.40/10 mL	1 drop once or twice daily	
Timolol maleate 0.25% and 0.5% solution (Timoptic) and 0.25% and 0.5% gel (Timoptic-XE, Timoptic GFS)[13]	0.5% solution: $32.35/10 mL 0.5% gel: $174.24/5 mL	1 drop once or twice daily	
Miotics			
Pilocarpine HCl (various)[14] 1–4%, 6%, 8%, and 10%	2%: $95.13/15 mL	1 drop three or four times daily	Reduction of intraocular pressure, treatment of acute or chronic angle-closure glaucoma, and pupillary constriction.
Pilocarpine HCl 4% gel (Pilopine HS)	$109.50/4 g	Apply 0.5-inch ribbon in lower conjunctival sac at bedtime	

(continued)

Table 7–2. Topical ophthalmic agents. (continued)

Agent	Cost/Size[1]	Recommended Regimen	Indications
Carbonic anhydrase inhibitors			
Brinzolamide 1% suspension (Azopt)	$171.00/10 mL	1 drop three times daily	Reduction of intraocular pressure.
Dorzolamide HCl 2% solution (Trusopt)	$66.75/10 mL	1 drop three times daily	
Prostaglandin analogs			
Bimatoprost 0.03% solution (Lumigan, Latisse)	$132.28/3 mL	1 drop once daily at night	Reduction of intraocular pressure.
Latanoprost 0.005% solution (Xalatan)	$21.60/2.5 mL	1 drop once or twice daily at night	
Tafluprost 0.0015% solution (Zioptan, Saflutan)	$124.55/30 Units	1 drop once daily at night	
Travoprost 0.004% solution (Travatan)	$104.05/2.5 mL	1 drop once daily at night	
Unoprostone isopropyl 0.15% solution (Rescula)	$129.49/5 mL	1 drop twice daily	
Combined preparations			
Brinzolamide 1% and timolol 0.5% (Azarga)	Not available in United States	1 drop twice daily	Reduction of intraocular pressure.
Brimonidine 0.2% and timolol 0.5% (Combigan)	$240.79/10 mL	1 drop twice daily	
Dorzolamide 2% and timolol 0.5% (Cosopt)	$122.60/10 mL	1 drop twice daily	
Travoprost 0.004% and timolol 0.5% (DuoTrav)	Not available in United States	1 drop daily	
Bimatoprost 0.03% and timolol 0.5% (Ganfort)	Not available in United States	1 drop daily in the morning	
Latanoprost 0.005% and timolol 0.5% (Xalacom)	Not available in United States	1 drop daily in the morning	

[1]Average wholesale price (AWP, for AB-rated generic when available) for quantity listed. Source: *Red Book Online, 2014, Truven Health Analytics, Inc.* AWP may not accurately represent the actual pharmacy cost because wide contractual variations exist among institutions.
[2]Many combination products containing antibacterials or antibacterials and corticosteroids are available.
[3]Little efficacy against gram-negative organisms (except *Neisseria*).
[4]Aplastic anemia has been reported with prolonged ophthalmic use.
[5]Also indicated for prophylaxis of neonatal conjunctivitis due to *Neisseria gonorrhoeae* or *Chlamydia trachomatis*.
[6]No gram-positive coverage.
[7]May produce rebound hyperemia and local reactions.
[8]Cross-sensitivity to aspirin and other nonsteroidal anti-inflammatory drugs.
[9]Long-term use increases intraocular pressure, causes cataracts and predisposes to bacterial, herpes simplex virus, and fungal keratitis.
[10]Less likely to elevate intraocular pressure.
[11]Cardioselective (beta-1) beta-blocker.
[12]Teoptic is not available in the United States.
[13]Nonselective (beta-1 and beta-2) beta-blocker. Monitor all patients for systemic side effects, particularly exacerbation of asthma.
[14]Decreased night vision, headaches possible.

INFECTIOUS KERATITIS

1. Bacterial Keratitis

Bacterial keratitis usually pursues an aggressive course. Precipitating factors include contact lens wear—especially overnight wear—and corneal trauma, including refractive surgery. The pathogens most commonly isolated are *Pseudomonas aeruginosa, Moraxella* species, and other gram-negative bacilli; staphylococci, including MRSA; and streptococci. The cornea is hazy, with a central ulcer and adjacent stromal abscess. Hypopyon is often present. The ulcer is scraped to recover material for Gram stain and culture prior to starting treatment with high concentration topical antibiotic drops applied hourly day and night for at least the first 48 hours. Fluoroquinolones such as levofloxacin

0.5%, ofloxacin 0.3%, norfloxacin 0.3%, or ciprofloxacin 0.3% are commonly used as first-line agents as long as local prevalence of resistant organisms is low (Table 7–2). The fourth-generation fluoroquinolones (moxifloxacin 0.5% and gatifloxacin 0.3%) may be preferable because they are also active against mycobacteria. Gram-positive cocci can also be treated with a cephalosporin such as fortified cefazolin 10%, but vancomycin may be required for MRSA; and gram-negative bacilli can be treated with an aminoglycoside such as fortified tobramycin 1.5%. If no organisms are seen on Gram stain, these two agents can be used together in areas where resistance to fluoroquinolones is common. Adjunctive topical corticosteroid therapy should only be prescribed by an ophthalmologist.

▶ When to Refer

American Academy of Ophthalmology Cornea/External Disease Panel. Preferred Practice Pattern® Guidelines. Bacterial keratitis. San Francisco, CA: American Academy of Ophthalmology; 2013. http://one.aao.org/preferred-practice-pattern/bacterial-keratitis-ppp--2013

American Academy of Ophthalmology Cornea/External Disease Panel. Preferred Practice Pattern® Guidelines – Summary Benchmark. Bacterial keratitis. San Francisco, CA: American Academy of Ophthalmology; 2013. http://one.aao.org/summary-benchmark-detail/bacterial-keratitis-summary-benchmark--october-201

Ray KJ et al. Fluoroquinolone treatment and susceptibility of isolates from bacterial keratitis. JAMA Ophthalmol. 2013 Mar;131(3):310–3. [PMID: 23307105]

Sharma N et al. Steroid associated infective keratitis—case studies for caution. Aust Fam Physician. 2011 Nov;40(11):888–90. [PMID: 22059219]

2. Herpes Simplex Keratitis

Herpes simplex keratitis is an important cause of ocular morbidity. The ability of the virus to colonize the trigeminal ganglion leads to recurrences that may be precipitated by fever, excessive exposure to sunlight, or immunodeficiency.

The dendritic (branching) ulcer is the most characteristic manifestation. More extensive ("geographic") ulcers also occur, particularly if topical corticosteroids have been used. These ulcers are most easily seen after instillation of fluorescein and examination with a blue light. Such epithelial disease in itself does not lead to corneal scarring. It responds well to simple debridement and patching. More rapid healing can be achieved by the addition of topical antivirals, such as trifluridine drops, ganciclovir gel, or acyclovir ointment (Table 7–2), or oral antivirals, such as acyclovir, 400 mg five times daily. Long-term oral acyclovir, 400 mg twice daily, or valacyclovir, 500 mg once daily, reduces the rate of recurrent epithelial disease, particularly in atopic individuals.

Stromal herpes simplex keratitis produces increasingly severe corneal opacity with each recurrence. Topical antivirals alone are insufficient to control stromal disease, so topical corticosteroids are used as well but they may enhance viral replication, exacerbating epithelial disease; steroid dependence is common. Oral acyclovir, 200–400 mg five times a day, is often helpful in the treatment of severe herpetic keratitis. The role of topical cyclosporine is being determined. Severe stromal scarring may require corneal

grafting, but the overall outcome is relatively poor. **Caution:** For patients with known or possible herpetic disease, topical corticosteroids should be prescribed only with ophthalmologic supervision.

▶ When to Refer

Any patient with a history of herpes simplex keratitis and an acute red eye should be referred urgently to an ophthalmologist.

American Academy of Ophthalmology Preferred Practice Pattern® Clinical Question. Herpes simplex virus epithelial keratitis. San Francisco, CA: American Academy of Ophthalmology; 2013. http://one.aao.org/clinical-questions/herpes-simplex-virus-epithelial-keratitis

Rowe AM et al. Herpes keratitis. Prog Retin Eye Res. 2013 Jan;32:88–101. [PMID: 22944008]

Sharma N et al. Steroid associated infective keratitis—case studies for caution. Aust Fam Physician. 2011 Nov;40(11):888–90. [PMID: 22059219]

3. Herpes Zoster Ophthalmicus

Herpes zoster frequently involves the ophthalmic division of the trigeminal nerve. It presents with malaise, fever, headache, and periorbital burning and itching. These symptoms may precede the eruption by a day or more. The rash is initially vesicular, quickly becoming pustular and then crusting. Involvement of the tip of the nose or the lid margins predicts involvement of the eye. Ocular signs include conjunctivitis, keratitis, episcleritis, and anterior uveitis, often with elevated intraocular pressure. Recurrent anterior segment inflammation, neurotrophic keratitis, and posterior subcapsular cataract are long-term complications. Optic neuropathy, cranial nerve palsies, acute retinal necrosis, and cerebral angiitis occur infrequently. HIV infection is an important risk factor for herpes zoster ophthalmicus and increases the likelihood of complications.

High-dose oral acyclovir (800 mg five times a day), valacyclovir (1 g three times a day), or famciclovir (250–500 mg three times a day) started within 72 hours after the appearance of the rash reduces the incidence of ocular complications but not of postherpetic neuralgia. Anterior uveitis requires treatment with topical corticosteroids and cycloplegics. Neurotrophic keratitis is an important cause of long-term morbidity.

▶ When to Refer

Any patient with herpes zoster ophthalmicus and ocular symptoms or signs should be referred urgently to an ophthalmologist.

Borkar DS et al. Incidence of herpes zoster ophthalmicus: results from the Pacific Ocular Inflammation Study. Ophthalmology. 2013 Mar;120(3):451–6. [PMID: 23207173]

Yawn BP et al. Herpes zoster eye complications: rates and trends. Mayo Clin Proc. 2013 Jun;88(6):562–70. [PMID: 23664666]

4. Fungal Keratitis

Fungal keratitis tends to occur after corneal injury involving plant material or in an agricultural setting, in eyes with chronic ocular surface disease, and increasingly in contact lens wearers. It is usually an indolent process, with the cornea characteristically having multiple stromal abscesses and relatively little epithelial loss. Intraocular infection is common. Corneal scrapings should be cultured on media suitable for fungi whenever the history or corneal appearance is suggestive of fungal disease. Diagnosis is often delayed and treatment is difficult. Natamycin 5%, amphotericin 0.1-0.5%, and voriconazole 1% are the most commonly used topical agents. Systemic imidazoles may be helpful. Corneal grafting is often required.

Prajna NV et al. The mycotic ulcer treatment trial: a randomized trial comparing natamycin vs voriconazole. JAMA Ophthalmol. 2013 Apr;131(4):422–9. [PMID: 23710492]

Sharma S. Diagnosis of fungal keratitis: current options. Expert Opin Med Diagn. 2012 Sep;6(5):449–55. [PMID: 23480809]

Thomas PA et al. Mycotic keratitis: epidemiology, diagnosis and management. Clin Microbiol Infect. 2013 Mar;19(3):210–20. [PMID: 23398543]

5. Acanthamoeba Keratitis

Acanthamoeba infection is an important cause of keratitis in contact lens wearers. Although severe pain with perineural and ring infiltrates in the corneal stroma is characteristic, it is not specific and earlier forms with changes confined to the corneal epithelium are identifiable. Diagnosis is facilitated by confocal microscopy. Culture requires specialized media. Long-term treatment is required because of the organism's ability to encyst within the corneal stroma. Topical biguanides are probably the only effective primary treatment. Corneal grafting may be required after resolution of infection to restore vision. Systemic anti-inflammatory therapy is helpful if there is scleral involvement.

Clarke B et al. Advances in the diagnosis and treatment of *Acanthamoeba* keratitis. J Ophthalmol. 2012;2012:484892. [PMID: 23304449]

Kaiserman I et al. Prognostic factors in *Acanthamoeba* keratitis. Can J Ophthalmol. 2012 Jun;47(3):312–7. [PMID: 22687314]

Pacella E et al. Results of case-control studies support the association between contact lens use and *Acanthamoeba* keratitis. Clin Ophthalmol. 2013;7:991–4. [PMID: 23761962]

Page MA et al. *Acanthamoeba* keratitis: a 12-year experience covering a wide spectrum of presentations, diagnoses, and outcomes. J Ophthalmol. 2013;2013:670242. [PMID: 23840938]

ACUTE ANGLE-CLOSURE GLAUCOMA

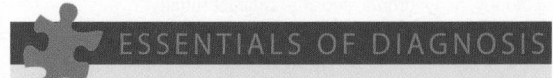

ESSENTIALS OF DIAGNOSIS

► Older age group, particularly farsighted individuals.

► Rapid onset of severe pain and profound visual loss with "halos around lights."

► Red eye, cloudy cornea, dilated pupil.

► Hard eye on palpation.

► General Considerations

Primary acute angle-closure glaucoma (acute angle-closure crisis) occurs only with closure of a preexisting narrow anterior chamber angle, for which the predisposing factors are shallow anterior chamber, which may be associated with farsightedness or short stature (or both); enlargement of the crystalline lens with age causing further shallowing; and inheritance, being particularly prevalent among Inuits and Asians. It may be precipitated by pupillary dilation and thus can occur from sitting in a darkened theater, during times of stress, following nonocular administration of anticholinergic or sympathomimetic agents (eg, nebulized bronchodilators, atropine for preoperative medication, antidepressants, bowel or bladder antispasmodics, nasal decongestants, or tocolytics) or, rarely, from pharmacologic mydriasis (see Precautions in Management of Ocular Disorders, below). Secondary acute angle-closure glaucoma may occur in anterior uveitis or dislocation of the lens or due to various drugs paradoxically including acetazolamide (see Table 7–3). Symptoms are the same as in primary acute angle-closure glaucoma, but differentiation is important because of differences in management. Acute glaucoma, for which the mechanism may not be the same in all cases, can occur in association with hemodialysis. (Chronic angle-closure glaucoma presents in the same way as chronic open-angle glaucoma [see below]).

► Clinical Findings

Patients with acute glaucoma usually seek treatment immediately because of extreme pain and blurred vision, though there are subacute cases. The blurred vision is associated with halos around lights. Nausea and abdominal pain may occur. The eye is red, the cornea cloudy, and the pupil moderately dilated and nonreactive to light. Intraocular pressure is usually over 50 mm Hg, producing a hard eye on palpation.

► Differential Diagnosis

Acute glaucoma must be differentiated from conjunctivitis, acute uveitis, and corneal disorders (Table 7–1).

► Treatment

Initial treatment in acute glaucoma is reduction of intraocular pressure. A single 500-mg intravenous dose of acetazolamide, followed by 250 mg orally four times a day, together with topical medications is usually sufficient. Osmotic diuretics such as oral glycerin and intravenous urea or mannitol—the dosage of all three being 1–2 g/kg—may be necessary if there is no response to acetazolamide.

A. Primary

In primary acute angle-closure glaucoma, once the intraocular pressure has started to fall, topical 4% pilocarpine, 1 drop every 15 minutes for 1 hour and then four times a day, is used to reverse the underlying angle closure. The definitive treatment is laser peripheral iridotomy or surgical peripheral iridectomy. Cataract extraction is a possible alternative. If it is

Table 7–3. Adverse ophthalmic effects of systemic drugs.

Drug	Possible Side Effects
Ophthalmic drugs	
Carbonic anhydrase inhibitors (eg, acetazolamide, methazolamide)	Stevens-Johnson syndrome, nearsightedness, angle-closure glaucoma due to ciliary body swelling.
Respiratory drugs	
Anticholinergic bronchodilators (eg, ipratropium)	Angle-closure glaucoma due to mydriasis, blurring of vision due to cycloplegia, dry eyes.
Oxygen	Retinopathy of prematurity.
Sympathomimetic bronchodilators (eg, salbutamol) and decongestants (eg, ephedrine)	Angle-closure glaucoma due to mydriasis.
Cardiovascular system drugs	
Alpha-2-antagonists (eg, terazosin, doxazosin)	Complications during (floppy-iris syndrome) and after cataract surgery.
Amiodarone	Corneal deposits (vortex keratopathy), optic neuropathy, thyroid ophthalmopathy.
Digitalis	Disturbance of color vision, photopsia.
Phosphodiesterase type 5 inhibitors (eg, sildenafil, udenafil)	Disturbance of color vision, ischemic optic neuropathy.
Statins	Extraocular muscle paralysis (myasthenic syndrome).
Thiazides (eg, indapamide)	Angle-closure glaucoma due to ciliary body swelling, nearsightedness, xanthopsia (yellow vision).
Gastrointestinal drugs	
Anticholinergic agents	Angle-closure glaucoma due to mydriasis, blurring of vision due to cycloplegia, dry eyes.
Urinary tract drugs	
Alpha-2-antagonists (eg, tamsulosin, alfuzosin, terazosin, doxazosin)	Complications during (floppy-iris syndrome) and after cataract surgery.
Anticholinergic agents	Angle-closure glaucoma due to mydriasis, blurring of vision due to cycloplegia, dry eyes.
Central nervous system drugs	
Amphetamines	Widening of palpebral fissure, blurring of vision due to mydriasis, elevated intraocular pressure.
Anticholinergic agents including preoperative medications	Angle-closure glaucoma due to mydriasis, blurring of vision due to cycloplegia, dry eyes.
Diazepam	Nystagmus.
Haloperidol	Capsular cataract.
Lithium carbonate	Proptosis, oculogyric crisis, nystagmus.
Monoamine oxidase inhibitors	Nystagmus.
Morphine	Miosis.
Neostigmine	Nystagmus, miosis.
Phenothiazines	Pigmentary deposits in conjunctiva, cornea, lens, and retina, oculogyric crisis.
Phenytoin	Nystagmus.
Retigabine	Ocular pigmentation and retinopathy.
Risperidone, paliperidone	Complications during (floppy-iris syndrome) and after cataract surgery.
Selective serotonin reuptake inhibitors (SSRI) (eg, paroxetine, sertraline)	Angle-closure glaucoma.
Serotonin and noradrenaline reuptake inhibitors (eg, venlafaxine)	Angle-closure glaucoma.
Thioridazine	Corneal and lens deposits, retinopathy, oculogyric crisis.
Topiramate	Angle-closure glaucoma due to ciliary body swelling, nearsightedness, macular folds, anterior uveitis.

(continued)

Table 7–3. Adverse ophthalmic effects of systemic drugs. (continued)

Drug	Possible Side Effects
Tricyclic agents (eg, imipramine)	Angle-closure glaucoma due to mydriasis, blurring of vision due to cycloplegia.
Vigabatrin	Visual field constriction.
Obstetric drugs	
Sympathomimetic tocolytics	Angle-closure glaucoma due to mydriasis.
Hormonal agents	
Aromatase inhibitors (eg, anastrozole)	Dry eye, vitreo-retinal traction, retinal hemorrhages.
Cabergoline	Angle-closure glaucoma.
Female sex hormones	Retinal artery occlusion, retinal vein occlusion, papilledema, cranial nerve palsies, ischemic optic neuropathy.
Tamoxifen	Crystalline retinal and corneal deposits, altered color perception, cataract, optic neuropathy.
Immunomodulators	
Alpha-interferon	Retinopathy, keratoconjunctivitis, dry eyes, optic neuropathy.
Corticosteroids	Cataract (posterior subcapsular); susceptibility to viral (herpes simplex), bacterial, and fungal infections; steroid-induced glaucoma.
Cyclosporine	Posterior reversible leukoencephalopathy.
Tacrolimus	Optic neuropathy, posterior reversible leukoencephalopathy.
Antibacterials	
Chloramphenicol	Optic neuropathy.
Ethambutol	Optic neuropathy.
Fluoroquinolones	Diplopia, retinal detachment.
Isoniazid	Optic neuropathy.
Linezolid	Optic neuropathy.
Streptomycin	Optic neuropathy, Stevens-Johnson syndrome.
Sulfonamides	Stevens-Johnson syndrome, nearsightedness, angle-closure glaucoma due to ciliary body swelling.
Tetracycline, doxycycline, minocycline	Papilledema.
Antimalarial agents	
Chloroquine, hydroxychloroquine	Retinal degeneration principally involving the macula, keratopathy.
Quinine	Retinal toxicity, pupillary abnormalities.
Amebicides	
Iodochlorhydroxyquin	Optic neuropathy.
Chemotherapeutic agents	
Chlorambucil	Optic neuropathy.
Cisplatin	Optic neuropathy.
Docetaxel	Lacrimal (canalicular) obstruction.
Fluorouracil	Lacrimal (canalicular) obstruction.
Vincristine	Optic neuropathy.
Chelating agents	
Deferoxamine, deferasirox	Retinopathy, optic neuropathy, lens opacity.
Penicillamine	Ocular pemphigoid, optic neuropathy, extraocular muscle paralysis (myasthenic syndrome).
Oral hypoglycemic agents	
Chlorpropamide	Refractive error, Stevens-Johnson syndrome, optic neuropathy.

(continued)

Table 7–3. Adverse ophthalmic effects of systemic drugs. (continued)

Drug	Possible Side Effects
Vitamins	
Vitamin A	Papilledema.
Vitamin D	Band-shaped keratopathy.
Antirheumatic agents	
Chloroquine, hydroxychloroquine	Retinal degeneration principally involving the macula, keratopathy.
Gold salts	Deposits in the cornea, conjunctiva, and lens.
Indomethacin	Corneal deposits.
Penicillamine	Ocular pemphigoid, optic neuropathy, extraocular muscle paralysis (myasthenic syndrome).
Phenylbutazone	Retinal hemorrhages.
Salicylates	Subconjunctival and retinal hemorrhages, nystagmus.
Dermatologic agents	
Retinoids (eg, isotretinoin, tretinoin, acitretin, and etretinate)	Papilledema, blepharoconjunctivitis, corneal opacities, decreased contact lens tolerance, decreased dark adaptation, teratogenic ocular abnormalities.
Bisphosphonates	
Alendronate, pamidronate	Scleritis, episcleritis, uveitis.

not possible to control the intraocular pressure medically, the angle closure may be overcome by corneal indentation, laser treatment (argon laser peripheral iridoplasty), cyclodiode laser treatment, or paracentesis; or by glaucoma drainage surgery as for uncontrolled open-angle glaucoma (see below).

All patients with primary acute angle-closure should undergo prophylactic laser peripheral iridotomy to the unaffected eye, unless that eye has already undergone cataract or glaucoma surgery. Whether prophylactic laser peripheral iridotomy should be undertaken in asymptomatic patients with narrow anterior chamber angles is uncertain and mainly influenced by the risk of the more common chronic angle-closure (see below).

B. Secondary

In secondary acute angle-closure glaucoma, additional treatment is determined by the cause.

▶ Prognosis

Untreated acute angle-closure glaucoma results in severe and permanent visual loss within 2–5 days after onset of symptoms. Affected patients need to be monitored for development of chronic glaucoma.

▶ When to Refer

Any patient with suspected acute angle-closure glaucoma must be referred emergently to an ophthalmologist.

American Academy of Ophthalmology Glaucoma Panel. Preferred Practice Pattern® Guidelines. Primary open-angle closure glaucoma suspect. San Francisco, CA: American Academy of Ophthalmology; 2010. http://one.aao.org/preferred-practice-pattern/primary-openangle-glaucoma-suspect-ppp--october-20

American Academy of Ophthalmology Glaucoma Panel. Preferred Practice Pattern® Guidelines – Summary Benchmark. Primary angle closure. San Francisco, CA: American Academy of Ophthalmology; 2013. http://one.aao.org/summary-benchmark-detail/primary-angle-closure-summary-benchmark--october-2

Gracitelli CP et al. Ability of non-ophthalmologist doctors to detect eyes with occludable angles using the flashlight test. Int Ophthalmol. 2013 Oct 1. [Epub ahead of print] [PMID: 24081914]

Thomas R et al. Management algorithms for primary angle closure disease. Clin Experiment Ophthalmol. 2013 Apr;41(3):282–92. [PMID: 23009061]

White J. Diagnosis and management of acute angle-closure glaucoma. Emerg Nurse. 2011 Jun;19(3):27. [PMID: 21823566]

CHRONIC GLAUCOMA

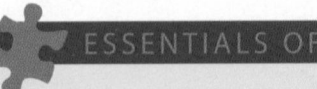

ESSENTIALS OF DIAGNOSIS

▶ No symptoms in early stages.

▶ Insidious progressive bilateral loss of peripheral vision, resulting in tunnel vision but preserved visual acuities until advanced disease.

▶ Pathologic cupping of the optic disks.

▶ Intraocular pressure is usually elevated.

▶ General Considerations

Chronic glaucoma is characterized by gradually progressive excavation ("cupping") and corresponding pallor of the optic disk with loss of vision progressing from slight visual field loss to complete blindness. In chronic open-angle glaucoma, primary or secondary, the intraocular pressure is elevated due to reduced drainage of aqueous fluid through the trabecular meshwork. In chronic angle-closure glaucoma, which is particularly common in Inuits and eastern Asians, flow of aqueous fluid into the anterior chamber angle is obstructed. In normal-tension glaucoma, intraocular pressure is not elevated but the same pattern of optic nerve damage occurs, probably due to vascular insufficiency.

Primary open-angle glaucoma is usually bilateral. There is an increased prevalence in first-degree relatives of affected individuals and in diabetic patients. In Afro-Caribbeans and Africans, and probably in Hispanics, it is more frequent, occurs at an earlier age, and results in more severe optic nerve damage. Secondary open-angle glaucoma may result from ocular disease, eg, pigment dispersion, pseudoexfoliation, uveitis, or trauma; or corticosteroid therapy, whether it is intraocular, topical, systemic, inhaled, or administered by nasal spray.

In the United States, it is estimated that 2% of people over 40 years of age have glaucoma, affecting over 2.5 million individuals. At least 25% of cases are undetected. Over 90% of cases are of the open-angle type. Worldwide, about 45 million people have open-angle-glaucoma, of whom about 4.5 million are bilaterally blind. About 4 million people, of whom approximately 50% live in China, are bilaterally blind from chronic angle-closure glaucoma.

Clinical Findings

Because initially there are no symptoms, chronic glaucoma is often suspected at a routine eye test. Diagnosis requires consistent and reproducible abnormalities in at least two of three parameters—optic disk or retinal nerve fiber layer (or both), visual field, and intraocular pressure. Optic disk cupping is identified as an absolute increase or an asymmetry between the two eyes of the ratio of the diameter of the optic cup to the diameter of the whole optic disk (cup-disk ratio). (Cup-disk ratio greater than 0.5 or 0.2 or more asymmetry between eyes is suggestive.) Detection of optic disk cupping and associated abnormalities of the retinal nerve fiber layer is facilitated by optical coherence tomography scans. Visual field abnormalities initially develop in the paracentral region, followed by constriction of the peripheral visual field. Central vision remains good until late in the disease. The normal range of intraocular pressure is 10–21 mm Hg. Its measurement is more complicated after corneal refractive surgery.

In many individuals (about 4.5 million in the United States), elevated intraocular pressure is not associated with optic disk or visual field abnormalities (**ocular hypertension**). Treatment to reduce intraocular pressure is justified if there is a moderate to high risk of progression to glaucoma, determined by several factors, including age, optic disk appearance, level of intraocular pressure, and corneal thickness, but monitoring for development of glaucoma is required in all cases. A significant proportion of eyes with primary open-angle glaucoma have normal intraocular pressure when it is first measured, and only repeated measurements identify the abnormally high pressure. In normal-tension glaucoma, intraocular pressure is always within the normal range.

Prevention

There are many causes of optic disk abnormalities or visual field changes that mimic glaucoma and visual field testing may prove unreliable in some patients, particularly in the older age group. The diagnosis of glaucoma is not always straightforward and screening programs need to involve ophthalmologists.

Although all persons over age 50 years may benefit from intraocular pressure measurement and optic disk examination every 3–5 years, population-based screening for glaucoma is not cost-effective. Screening for chronic open-angle glaucoma should be targeted at individuals with an affected first-degree relative, at persons who have diabetes mellitus, and at older individuals with African or Hispanic ancestry. Screening may also be warranted in patients taking long-term oral or combined intranasal and inhaled corticosteroid therapy. Screening for chronic angle-closure glaucoma should be targeted at Inuits and Asians.

Treatment

A. Medications

The prostaglandin analogs (bimatoprost 0.03%, latanoprost 0.005%, tafluprost 0.0015%, and travoprost 0.004% each used once daily at night, and unoprostone 0.15%, twice daily) are commonly used as first-line therapy because of their efficacy, their lack of systemic side effects, and the convenience of once-daily dosing (except unoprostone) (Table 7–2). All may produce conjunctival hyperemia, permanent darkening of the iris and eyebrow color, and increased eyelash growth. Latanoprost has been associated with reactivation of uveitis and macular edema.

Topical beta-adrenergic blocking agents (such as timolol 0.25% or 0.5%, carteolol 1% or 2%, levobunolol 0.5%, and metipranolol 0.3% solutions twice daily *or* timolol 0.1%, 0.25%, or 0.5% gel once daily) may be used alone or in combination with a prostaglandin analog. They are contraindicated in patients with reactive airway disease or heart failure. Betaxolol, 0.25% or 0.5%, a beta-receptor selective blocking agent, is theoretically safer in reactive airway disease but less effective at reducing intraocular pressure. Brimonidine 0.2%, a selective alpha-2-agonist, and dorzolamide 2% or brinzolamide 1%, topical carbonic anhydrase inhibitors, also can be used in addition to a prostaglandin analog or a beta-blocker (twice daily) or as initial therapy when prostaglandin analogs and beta-blockers are contraindicated (brimonidine twice daily, dorzolamide and brinzolamide three times daily). All three are associated with allergic reactions. Combination drops latanoprost 0.005% and timolol 0.5% (Xalacom), bimatoprost 0.03% and timolol 0.5% (Ganfort), and travoprost 0.004% and timolol 0.5% (DuoTrav), each used once daily, and dorzolamide 2% and timolol 0.5% (Cosopt), brinzolamide 1% and timolol 0.5% (Azarga), and brimonidine 0.2% and timolol 0.5% (Combigan), each used twice daily improve compliance when multiple medications are required.

Apraclonidine, 0.5–1%, another alpha-2-agonist, can be used three times a day to postpone the need for surgery in patients receiving maximal medical therapy, but long-term use is limited by drug reactions. It is more commonly used to control acute rises in intraocular pressure such as after laser therapy. Pilocarpine 1–4%, epinephrine, 0.5–1%, and the prodrug dipivefrin, 0.1%, are rarely used because of adverse effects. Oral carbonic anhydrase inhibitors (eg, acetazolamide) may still be used on a long-term basis if topical therapy is inadequate and surgical or laser therapy is inappropriate.

Formulations of topical agents without preservative or not including benzalkonium chloride as the preservative are available.

B. Laser Therapy and Surgery

Laser trabeculoplasty is used as an adjunct to topical therapy to defer surgery and is also advocated as primary treatment. Surgery is generally undertaken when intraocular pressure is inadequately controlled by medical and laser therapy, but it may also be used as primary treatment. Trabeculectomy remains the standard procedure. Adjunctive treatment with subconjunctival mitomycin or fluorouracil is used perioperatively or postoperatively in difficult cases. Viscocanalostomy, deep sclerectomy with collagen implant and Trabectome—two alternative procedures that avoid a full-thickness incision into the eye—are associated with fewer complications but are less effective than trabeculectomy and more difficult to perform.

In chronic angle-closure glaucoma, laser peripheral iridotomy or surgical peripheral iridectomy may be helpful. In patients with asymptomatic narrow anterior chamber angles, which includes about 10% of Chinese adults, prophylactic laser peripheral iridotomy can be performed to reduce the risk of acute and chronic angle-closure glaucoma. However, there are concerns about the efficacy of such treatment and the risk of cataract progression and corneal decompensation. In the United States, about 1% of people over age 35 years have narrow anterior chamber angles, but acute and chronic angle-closure are sufficiently uncommon that prophylactic therapy is not generally advised.

▶ Prognosis

Untreated chronic glaucoma that begins at age 40–45 years will probably cause complete blindness by age 60–65. Early diagnosis and treatment can preserve useful vision throughout life. In primary open-angle glaucoma—and if treatment is required in ocular hypertension—the aim is to reduce intraocular pressure to a level that will adequately reduce progression of visual field loss. In eyes with marked visual field or optic disk changes, intraocular pressure must be reduced to less than 16 mm Hg. In normal-tension glaucoma with progressive visual field loss, it is necessary to achieve even lower intraocular pressure such that surgery is often required.

▶ When to Refer

All patients with suspected chronic glaucoma should be referred to an ophthalmologist.

American Academy of Ophthalmology Glaucoma Panel. Preferred Practice Pattern® Guidelines - Summary Benchmark. Primary open-angle glaucoma. San Francisco, CA: American Academy of Ophthalmology;2013. http://one.aao.org/summary-benchmark-detail/primary-openangle-glaucoma-summary-benchmark--octo

American Academy of Ophthalmology Glaucoma Panel. Preferred Practice Pattern® Guidelines - Summary Benchmark. Primary open-angle glaucoma suspect. San Francisco, CA: American Academy of Ophthalmology;2010. http://one.aao.org/summary-benchmark-detail/primary-openangle-glaucoma-suspect-summary-benchma

Burr J et al. Medical versus surgical interventions for open angle glaucoma. Cochrane Database Syst Rev. 2012 Sep 12;9:CD004399. [PMID: 22972069]

Peters D et al. Lifetime risk of blindness in open-angle glaucoma. Am J Ophthalmol. 2013 Oct;156(4):724–30. [PMID: 23932216]

Quigley HA. Glaucoma. Lancet. 2011 Apr 16;377(9774):1367–77. [PMID: 21453963]

UVEITIS

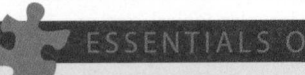

ESSENTIALS OF DIAGNOSIS

▶ Usually immunologic but possibly infective or neoplastic.

▶ Acute nongranulomatous anterior uveitis: pain, redness, photophobia, and visual loss.

▶ Granulomatous anterior uveitis: blurred vision in a mildly inflamed eye.

▶ Posterior uveitis: gradual loss of vision in a quiet eye.

▶ General Considerations

Intraocular inflammation (uveitis) is classified into acute or chronic, into nongranulomatous or granulomatous according to the clinical signs, and into anterior or posterior by its distribution—involving the anterior or posterior segments of the eye—or into panuveitis in which both segments are affected. The common types are acute nongranulomatous anterior uveitis, granulomatous anterior uveitis, and posterior uveitis.

In most cases, the pathogenesis of uveitis is primarily immunologic but infection may be the cause, particularly in immunodeficiency states. The systemic disorders associated with acute nongranulomatous anterior uveitis are the HLA-B27-related conditions (ankylosing spondylitis, reactive arthritis, psoriasis, ulcerative colitis, and Crohn disease). Chronic nongranulomatous anterior uveitis occurs in juvenile idiopathic arthritis. Behçet syndrome produces both anterior uveitis, with recurrent hypopyon but little discomfort, and posterior uveitis, characteristically with branch retinal vein occlusions. Both herpes simplex and herpes zoster infections may cause nongranulomatous anterior uveitis as well as retinitis (acute retinal necrosis), which has a very poor prognosis.

Diseases producing granulomatous anterior uveitis also tend to be causes of posterior uveitis. These include sarcoidosis, toxoplasmosis, tuberculosis, syphilis, Vogt-Koyanagi-Harada syndrome (bilateral uveitis associated with alopecia, poliosis [depigmented eyelashes, eyebrows, or hair], vitiligo, and hearing loss), and sympathetic ophthalmia that occurs after penetrating ocular trauma.

In toxoplasmosis there may be evidence of previous episodes of retinochoroiditis. Syphilis characteristically produces a "salt and pepper" fundus but may present with a wide variety of clinical manifestations. The other principal pathogens responsible for ocular inflammation in HIV infection (see below) are cytomegalovirus (CMV), herpes simplex and herpes zoster viruses, mycobacteria, *Cryptococcus*, *Toxoplasma*, and *Candida*.

Autoimmune retinal vasculitis and pars planitis (intermediate uveitis) are idiopathic conditions that cause posterior uveitis.

Clinical Findings

Anterior uveitis is characterized by inflammatory cells and flare within the aqueous. In severe cases there may be hypopyon (layered collection of white cells) and fibrin within the anterior chamber. Cells may also be seen on the corneal endothelium as keratic precipitates (KPs). In granulomatous uveitis there are large "mutton-fat" KPs (Figure 7–2), and iris nodules may be seen. In nongranulomatous uveitis the KPs are smaller and iris nodules are not seen. The pupil is usually small, and with the development of posterior synechiae (adhesions between the iris and anterior lens capsule) it also becomes irregular.

Nongranulomatous anterior uveitis tends to present acutely with unilateral pain, redness, photophobia, and visual loss. In juvenile idiopathic arthritis there tends to be an indolent often initially asymptomatic process with a high risk of sight-threatening complications. Granulomatous anterior uveitis is usually indolent, causing blurred vision in a mildly inflamed eye.

In **posterior uveitis** there are cells in the vitreous. Inflammatory lesions may be present in the retina or choroid. Fresh lesions are yellow with indistinct margins and there may be retinal hemorrhages, whereas older lesions have more definite margins and are commonly pigmented. Retinal vessel sheathing may occur adjacent to such lesions

or more diffusely. In severe cases, vitreous opacity precludes visualization of retinal details.

Posterior uveitis tends to present with gradual visual loss in a relatively quiet eye. Bilateral involvement is common. Visual loss may be due to vitreous haze and opacities, inflammatory lesions involving the macula, macular edema, retinal vein occlusion, or rarely associated optic neuropathy.

Differential Diagnosis

Retinal detachment, intraocular tumors, and central nervous system lymphoma may all masquerade as uveitis.

Treatment

Anterior uveitis usually responds to topical corticosteroids. Occasionally periocular corticosteroid injections or even systemic corticosteroids may be required. Dilation of the pupil is important to relieve discomfort and prevent posterior synechiae. **Posterior uveitis** more commonly requires systemic, periocular or intravitreal corticosteroid therapy and occasionally systemic immunosuppression with agents such as azathioprine, tacrolimus, cyclosporine, mycophenolate, or methotrexate, of which the last also can be administered by intraocular injection. The use of biologic therapies is increasing. Pupillary dilation is not usually necessary.

If an infectious cause is identified, specific antimicrobial therapy may be indicated. In general, the prognosis for anterior uveitis, particularly the nongranulomatous type, is better than for posterior uveitis.

When to Refer

- Any patient with suspected acute uveitis should be referred urgently to an ophthalmologist or emergently if visual loss or pain is severe.
- Any patient with suspected chronic uveitis should be referred to an ophthalmologist, urgently if there is more than mild visual loss.

When to Admit

Patients with severe uveitis, particularly those requiring intravenous therapy, may require hospital admission.

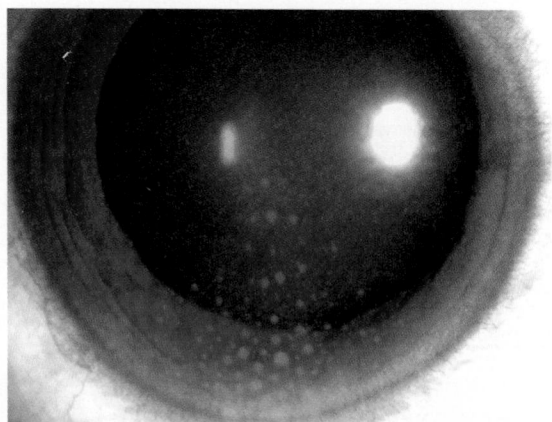

▲ **Figure 7–2.** Granulomatous keratic precipitates located on the inferior corneal endothelium. (From Emmett T Cunningham, Jr. Reproduced, with permission, from Riordan-Eva P, Cunningham ET Jr. *Vaughan & Asbury's General Ophthalmology*, 18th ed. McGraw-Hill, 2011.)

Deibel JP et al. Ocular inflammation and infection. Emerg Med Clin North Am. 2013 May;31(2):387–97. [PMID: 23601478]

Denniston AK et al. Systemic therapies for inflammatory eye disease: past, present and future. BMC Ophthalmol. 2013 Apr 24; 13:18. [PMID: 23617902]

Jabs DA et al. Approach to the diagnosis of the uveitides. Am J Ophthalmol. 2013 Aug;156(2):228–36. [PMID: 23668682]

Kruh J et al. Corticosteroid-sparing agents: conventional systemic immunosuppressants. Dev Ophthalmol. 2012;51:29–46. [PMID: 22517202]

Lin P et al. The future of uveitis treatment. Ophthalmology. 2014 Jan;121(1):365–76. [PMID: 24169255]

CATARACT

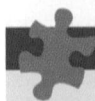

ESSENTIALS OF DIAGNOSIS

▶ Gradually progressive blurred vision.

▶ No pain or redness.

▶ Lens opacities (may be grossly visible).

General Considerations

Cataract is opacity of the crystalline lens. It is the leading cause of blindness worldwide, but access to treatment and quality of outcome are still limited in many areas. Cataracts are usually bilateral. They may be congenital (owing to intrauterine infections such as rubella and CMV, or inborn errors of metabolism such as galactosemia); traumatic; secondary to systemic disease (diabetes, myotonic dystrophy, atopic dermatitis), systemic or inhaled corticosteroid treatment, uveitis, or radiation exposure; or associated with other drugs, including statins; but age-related cataract is by far the most common type. Most persons over age 60 have some degree of lens opacity. Cigarette smoking increases the risk of cataract formation. No dietary modification has been shown to prevent age-related cataract or slow its progression.

Clinical Findings

The predominant symptom is progressive blurring of vision. Glare, especially in bright light or when driving at night; change of focusing, particularly development of near-sightedness; and monocular double vision may also occur.

Even in its early stages, a cataract can be seen through a dilated pupil with an ophthalmoscope or slit lamp. As the cataract matures, the retina will become increasingly more difficult to visualize, until finally the fundus reflection is absent and the pupil is white.

Treatment

In adults functional visual impairment is the prime criterion for surgery. The cataract is usually removed by one of the techniques in which the posterior lens capsule remains (extracapsular), thus providing support for a prosthetic intraocular lens. Laser treatment may be used during surgery and may be required subsequently if the posterior capsule opacifies. Ultrasonic fragmentation (phacoemulsification) of the lens nucleus and foldable intraocular lenses allow cataract surgery to be performed through a small incision without the need for sutures, thus reducing the postoperative complication rate and accelerating visual rehabilitation. Multifocal and accommodative intraocular lenses reduce the need for both distance and near vision correction. In the developing world, manual small incision surgery in which the lens nucleus is removed intact, is increasingly popular.

Management of congenital cataract is complicated by additional technical difficulties during surgery, changes in the optics of the eye with growth influencing choice of intraocular lens power, and treatment of associated amblyopia.

Prognosis

Cataract surgery is cost-effective in improving survival and quality of life. In the developed world, it improves visual acuity in 95% of cases. In the other 5%, there is preexisting retinal damage or operative or postoperative complications. In less developed areas overall, the outcome is less good, in part due to uncorrected refractive error postoperatively. Treatment with an alpha-1-antagonist, such as tamsulosin or alfuzosin for benign prostatic hyperplasia or risperidone or paliperidone for psychiatric disease, increases the risk of complications during surgery (floppy iris syndrome) and in the early postoperative period. Nasolacrimal duct obstruction increases the risk of intraocular infection (endophthalmitis).

When to Refer

Patients with cataracts should be referred to an ophthalmologist when their visual impairment adversely affects their everyday activities.

American Academy of Ophthalmology Cataract and Anterior Segment Panel. Preferred Practice Panel® Guidelines. Cataract in the adult eye. San Francisco, CA: American Academy of Ophthalmology; 2011. http://one.aao.org/preferred-practice-pattern/cataract-in-adult-eye-ppp--october-2011

American Academy of Ophthalmology Cataract and Anterior Segment Panel. Preferred Practice Panel® Guidelines – Summary Benchmark. Cataract in the adult eye. San Francisco, CA: American Academy of Ophthalmology;2013. http://one.aao.org/summary-benchmark-detail/cataract-in-adult-eye-summary-benchmark--october-2

Eichenbaum JW. Geriatric vision loss due to cataracts, macular degeneration, and glaucoma. Mt Sinai J Med. 2012 Mar–Apr;79(2): 276–94. [PMID: 22499498]

Kam JK et al. Nasolacrimal duct screening to minimise post-cataract surgery endophthalmitis. Clin Experiment Ophthalmol. 2013 Oct 3. [Epub ahead of print] [PMID: 24118663]

RETINAL DETACHMENT

ESSENTIALS OF DIAGNOSIS

▶ Rapid loss of vision in one eye possibly with "curtain" spreading across field of vision.

▶ No pain or redness.

▶ Detachment seen by ophthalmoscopy.

General Considerations

Most cases of retinal detachment are due to development of one or more peripheral retinal tears or holes or both (rhegmatogenous retinal detachment). This is usually spontaneous, related to degenerative changes in the vitreous, and generally occurs in persons over 50 years of age. Nearsightedness and cataract extraction are the two most common predisposing causes. Peripheral retinal defects may also be caused by penetrating or blunt ocular trauma.

Tractional retinal detachment occurs when there is preretinal fibrosis, such as in association with proliferative retinopathy secondary to diabetic retinopathy or retinal vein occlusion. Serous retinal detachment results from accumulation of subretinal fluid, such as in neovascular age-related macular degeneration or secondary to choroidal tumor.

▶ Clinical Findings

Rhegmatogenous retinal detachment usually starts in the superior temporal area and spreads rapidly, causing visual field loss that starts inferiorly and expands upwards. Central vision remains intact until the macula becomes detached. On ophthalmoscopic examination, the retina is seen hanging in the vitreous like a gray cloud (Figure 7–3). One or more retinal tears or holes (or both) will usually be found on further examination.

In traction retinal detachment, there is irregular retinal elevation with fibrosis. With serous retinal detachment, the retina is dome-shaped and the subretinal fluid may shift position with changes in posture.

▶ Treatment

Treatment of rhegmatogenous retinal detachments is directed at closing all of the retinal tears. A permanent adhesion between the neurosensory retina, the retinal pigment epithelium, and the choroid is produced in the region of the defects by laser photocoagulation to the retina or cryotherapy to the sclera. Indentation of the sclera with a silicone sponge or buckle; subretinal fluid drainage via an incision in the sclera; or injection of an expansile gas into the vitreous cavity, possibly following intraocular surgery to remove the vitreous (pars plana vitrectomy), may be required to achieve apposition of the neurosensory retina to the retinal pigment epithelium while the adhesion is developing. Certain types of uncomplicated retinal detachment may be treated by pneumatic retinopexy, in which an expansile gas is injected into the vitreous cavity followed by positioning of the patient's head to facilitate reattachment of the retina. Once the retina is repositioned, the defects are sealed by laser photocoagulation or cryotherapy; these two methods are also used to seal retinal defects without associated detachment. Intravitreal injection of ocriplasmin (Jetrea), a serine protease, may release vitreo-macular traction to avoid the need for vitrectomy.

In complicated retinal detachments—particularly those in which fibroproliferative tissue has developed on the surface of the retina or within the vitreous cavity, ie, traction retinal detachments—retinal reattachment can be accomplished only by pars plana vitrectomy, direct manipulation of the retina, and internal tamponade of the retina with air, expansile gas, or silicone oil. (The presence of an expansile gas within the eye is a contraindication to air travel, mountaineering at high altitude, and nitrous oxide anesthesia. Such gases persist in the globe for weeks after surgery.) Treatment of serous retinal detachments is determined by the underlying cause.

▶ Prognosis

About 90% of uncomplicated rhegmatogenous retinal detachments can be cured with one operation. The visual prognosis is worse if the macula is detached or if the detachment is of long duration.

▶ When to Refer

All cases of retinal detachment must be referred urgently to an ophthalmologist, emergently if central vision is good because this indicates that the macula has not detached. During transportation the patient's head is positioned so that the detached portion of the retina will fall back with the aid of gravity.

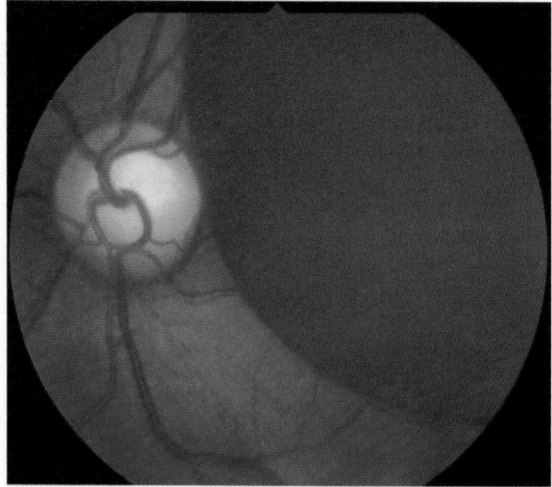

▲ **Figure 7–3.** Large preretinal hemorrhage. (Reproduced, with permission, from Riordan-Eva P, Cunningham ET Jr. *Vaughan & Asbury's General Ophthalmology*, 18th ed. McGraw-Hill, 2011.)

American Academy of Ophthalmology Retina Panel. Preferred Practice Panel® Guidelines. Posterior vitreous detachment, retinal breaks and lattice degeneration. San Francisco, CA: American Academy of Ophthalmology; 2013. http://one.aao.org/preferred-practice-pattern/posterior-vitreous-detachment-retinal-breaks-latti-5

American Academy of Ophthalmology Retina Panel. Preferred Practice Panel® Guidelines – Summary Benchmark. Idiopathic macular hole. San Francisco, CA: American Academy of Ophthalmology; 2013. http://one.aao.org/summary-benchmark-detail/idiopathic-macular-hole-summary-benchmark--october

Chang HJ et al. JAMA patient page. Retinal detachment. JAMA. 2012 Apr 4;307(13):1447. [PMID: 22474209]

Dorrepaal SJ et al. Using patient positioning to promote resorption of subretinal fluid in rhegmatogenous retinal detachment before pneumatic retinopexy. Retina. 2014 Mar;34(3): 477–82. [PMID: 23903793]

Hatten B et al. Retinal detachment. Emerg Med J. 2011 Jan;28(1):83. [PMID: 20378746]
Olsen T et al. The incidence of retinal detachment after cataract surgery. Open Ophthalmol J. 2012;6:79–82. [PMID: 23002414]
Schwartz SG et al. Update on retinal detachment surgery. Curr Opin Ophthalmol. 2013 May;24(3):255–61. [PMID: 23429600]

VITREOUS HEMORRHAGE

Patients with vitreous hemorrhage complain of sudden visual loss, abrupt onset of floaters that may progressively increase in severity, or occasionally, "bleeding within the eye." Visual acuity ranges from 20/20 (6/6) to light perception only. The eye is not inflamed, and clues to diagnosis are inability to see fundal details clearly despite the presence of a clear lens or localized collection of blood in front of the retina (Figure 7–3). Causes of vitreous hemorrhage include retinal tear (with or without detachment), diabetic or sickle cell retinopathy, retinal vein occlusion, retinal vasculitis, neovascular age-related macular degeneration, blood dyscrasia, trauma, subarachnoid hemorrhage, and severe straining.

When to Refer

All patients with suspected vitreous hemorrhage must be referred urgently to an ophthalmologist.

Schweitzer KD et al. Predicting retinal tears in posterior vitreous detachment. Can J Ophthalmol. 2011 Dec;46(6):481–5. [PMID: 22153633]
Takkar A et al. Teaching NeuroImages: Terson syndrome in cortical venous sinus thrombosis. Neurology. 2013 Aug 6;81(6):e40–1. [PMID: 23918868]

AGE-RELATED MACULAR DEGENERATION

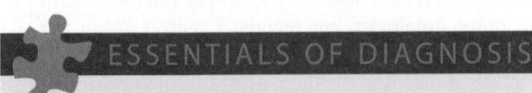

ESSENTIALS OF DIAGNOSIS

- ▶ Older age group.
- ▶ Acute or chronic deterioration of central vision in one or both eyes.
- ▶ Distortion or abnormal size of images.
- ▶ No pain or redness.
- ▶ Macular abnormalities seen by ophthalmoscopy.

General Considerations

In developed countries, age-related macular degeneration is the leading cause of permanent visual loss in the older population. Its prevalence increases with each decade over age 50 years (to almost 30% by age 75). Its occurrence and response to treatment are influenced by genetically determined variations in the complement pathway and in lipoprotein metabolism. Other associated factors are race (usually white), sex (slight female predominance), family history, cigarette smoking, and possibly regular aspirin use.

Age-related macular degeneration is classified into atrophic ("dry," "geographic") and neovascular ("wet," "exudative"). Although both are progressive and usually bilateral, they differ in manifestations, prognosis, and management.

Clinical Findings

The precursor to age-related macular degeneration is age-related maculopathy, characterized by retinal drusen. Hard drusen appear ophthalmoscopically as discrete yellow deposits. Soft drusen are larger, paler, and less distinct. Large, confluent soft drusen are particularly associated with neovascular age-related macular degeneration.

Atrophic degeneration is characterized by gradually progressive bilateral visual loss of moderate severity due to atrophy and degeneration of the outer retina and retinal pigment epithelium. In **neovascular degeneration** choroidal new vessels grow between the retinal pigment epithelium and Bruch membrane, leading to accumulation of serous fluid, hemorrhage, and fibrosis. The onset of visual loss is more rapid and more severe than in atrophic degeneration. The two eyes are frequently affected sequentially over a period of a few years. Neovascular disease accounts for about 90% of all cases of legal blindness due to age-related macular degeneration. Macular degeneration results in loss of central vision only. Peripheral fields and hence navigational vision are maintained, though these may become impaired by cataract formation for which surgery may be helpful.

Treatment

No dietary modification has been shown to prevent the development of age-related maculopathy. In patients with age-related maculopathy, oral treatment with antioxidants (vitamins C and E), zinc, copper and carotenoids (lutein and zeaxanthin, rather than vitamin A [beta-carotene]) is recommended to reduce the risk of progression to advanced disease. Oral omega-3 fatty acids do not provide additional benefit. Laser retinal photocoagulation results in regression of drusen but does not reduce the risk of disease progression.

Inhibitors of vascular endothelial growth factors (VEGF), such as ranibizumab (Lucentis), pegaptanib (Macugen), bevacizumab (Avastin), and aflibercept (VEGF Trap-Eye, Eylea), reverse choroidal neovascularization, resulting in stabilization and less frequently improvement in vision in neovascular degeneration. They have to be administered directly into the vitreous, although topical and oral administration are being investigated. Initial trials involved monthly injections for 2 years but less frequent treatment may be sufficient when there is evidence of reactivation of disease. Treatment is well tolerated with minimal adverse effects, although there is a risk of intraocular complications. There is some concern about nonocular adverse effects of bevacizumab but it is more cost-effective than other VEGF inhibitors. Long-term outcome studies show that about one-third of eyes have a poor outcome even with prolonged treatment.

There is no specific treatment for atrophic degeneration, but—as with the neovascular form—patients may benefit from low vision aids.

When to Refer

Older patients developing sudden visual loss due to macular disease—particularly paracentral distortion or scotoma with preservation of central acuity—should be referred urgently to an ophthalmologist.

Age-Related Eye Disease Study 2 Research Group. Lutein + zea-xanthin and omega-3 fatty acids for age-related macular degeneration: the Age-Related Eye Disease Study 2 (AREDS2) randomized clinical trial. JAMA. 2013 May 15;309(19):2005–15. [PMID: 23644932]

American Academy of Ophthalmology Retina Panel. Preferred Practice Panel° Guidelines – Summary Benchmark. Age-related macular degeneration. San Francisco, CA: American Academy of Ophthalmology; 2013. http://one.aao.org/summary-benchmark-detail/agerelated-macular-degeneration-summary-benchmark-

American Academy of Ophthalmology Vision Rehabilitation Committee. Preferred Practice Panel° Guidelines. Vision rehabilitation. San Francisco, CA: American Academy of Ophthalmology; 2013. http://one.aao.org/preferred-practice-pattern/vision-rehabilitation-ppp--2013

Cheung CM et al. Treatment of age-related macular degeneration. Lancet. 2013 Oct 12;382(9900):1230–2. [PMID: 23870812]

Goodman DM et al. JAMA patient page. Age-related macular degeneration. JAMA. 2012 Oct 24;308(16):1702. [PMID: 23093172]

Kolber MR et al. Vitamins for age-related macular degeneration demonstrate minimal differences. Can Fam Physician. 2013 May;59(5):503. [PMID: 23673586]

CENTRAL & BRANCH RETINAL VEIN OCCLUSIONS

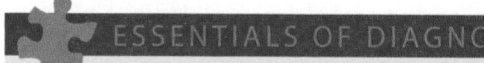
ESSENTIALS OF DIAGNOSIS

- ► Sudden monocular loss of vision.
- ► No pain or redness.
- ► Widespread or sectoral retinal hemorrhages.

General Considerations

All patients with retinal vein occlusion should be screened for diabetes, systemic hypertension, hyperlipidemia, and glaucoma. Estrogen therapy (including combined oral contraceptives), antiphospholipid syndromes, inherited thrombophilia, and hyperhomocysteinemia should be considered particularly in younger patients. Rarely, hyperviscosity syndromes, including myeloproliferative disorders, are associated with retinal vein occlusions and especially should be considered in simultaneous bilateral disease.

Clinical Findings

A. Symptoms and Signs

The visual impairment in **central retinal vein occlusion** is commonly first noticed upon waking. Ophthalmoscopic signs include widespread retinal hemorrhages, retinal venous dilation and tortuosity, retinal cotton-wool spots, and optic disk swelling.

Branch retinal vein occlusion may present in a variety of ways. Sudden loss of vision may occur at the time of occlusion if the fovea is involved or some time afterward from vitreous hemorrhage due to retinal new vessels. More gradual visual loss may occur with development of macular edema. In acute branch retinal vein occlusion, the retinal abnormalities (hemorrhages, venous dilation and tortuosity, and cotton-wool spots) are confined to the area drained by the obstructed vein.

Check blood pressure in all patients.

B. Laboratory Findings

Obtain screening studies for diabetes mellitus, hyperlipidemia, and hyperviscosity, including a serum protein electrophoresis especially to identify IgM paraproteinemia. Particularly in younger patients, consider obtaining antiphospholipid antibodies, lupus anticoagulant, tests for inherited thrombophilia, and plasma homocysteine levels.

Complications

If central retinal vein occlusion is associated with widespread retinal ischemia, manifesting as poor visual acuity (20/200 (6/60) or worse), florid retinal abnormalities, and extensive areas of capillary closure on fluorescein angiography, there is a high risk of development of neovascular (rubeotic) glaucoma, typically within the first 3 months.

Branch retinal vein occlusion may be complicated by peripheral retinal neovascularization or chronic macular edema.

Treatment

Eyes at risk for neovascular glaucoma following ischemic central retinal vein occlusion can be treated by panretinal laser photocoagulation prophylactically or as soon as there is evidence of neovascularization, the latter approach necessitating frequent monitoring. Regression of iris neovascularization has been achieved with intravitreal injections of bevacizumab, an inhibitor of VEGF. In branch retinal vein occlusion complicated by retinal neovascularization, the ischemic retina should be laser photocoagulated.

Intravitreal injection of a VEGF inhibitor, such as ranibizumab (Lucentis), pegaptanib (Macugen), bevacizumab (Avastin), or aflibercept (VEGF Trap-Eye, Eylea), is beneficial in chronic macular edema due to either branch or nonischemic central retinal vein occlusion. Intravitreal triamcinolone improves vision in chronic macular edema due to nonischemic central retinal vein occlusion, whereas an intravitreal implant containing dexamethasone is beneficial in both central and branch retinal vein occlusion. Retinal laser photocoagulation may be indicated in chronic macular edema due to branch but not central retinal vein occlusion.

Prognosis

In central retinal vein occlusion, severity of visual loss initially is a good guide to visual outcome. Initial visual acuity of 20/60 (6/18) or better indicates a good prognosis. Visual prognosis is poor for eyes with neovascular glaucoma.

Visual outcome in branch retinal vein occlusion is determined by the severity of macular damage from hemorrhage, ischemia, or edema.

When to Refer

All patients with retinal vein occlusion should be referred urgently to an ophthalmologist.

Kiire CA et al. Managing retinal vein occlusion. BMJ. 2012 Feb 22; 344:e499. [PMID: 22362114]

Macdonald D. The ABCs of RVO: A review of retinal venous occlusion. Clin Exp Optom. 2013 Nov 20. [Epub ahead of print] [PMID: 24256639]

Scott IU. Management of macular edema associated with retinal vein occlusion. Arch Ophthalmol. 2012 Oct 1;130(10):1314–6. [PMID: 23044946]

Shirodkhar AL et al. Management of branch retinal vein occlusion. Br J Hosp Med (Lond). 2012 Jan;73(1):20–3. [PMID: 22241405]

CENTRAL & BRANCH RETINAL ARTERY OCCLUSIONS

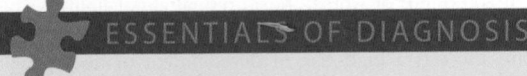

ESSENTIALS OF DIAGNOSIS

- ► Sudden monocular loss of vision.
- ► No pain or redness.
- ► Widespread or sectoral retinal pallid swelling.

General Considerations

In patients 50 years of age or older with central retinal artery occlusion, giant cell arteritis must be considered (see Ischemic Optic Neuropathy and Chapter 20). Otherwise, even if no retinal emboli are identified on ophthalmoscopy, urgent investigation for carotid and cardiac sources of emboli must be undertaken in central and particularly in branch retinal artery occlusion, so that timely treatment can be given to reduce the risk of stroke (see Chapters 12, 14, and 24). Diabetes mellitus, hyperlipidemia, and systemic hypertension should be considered as etiologic factors in patients with retinal artery occlusion. Migraine, oral contraceptives, systemic vasculitis, congenital or acquired thrombophilia, and hyperhomocysteinemia should be considered, particularly in young patients. Internal carotid artery dissection should be considered when there is neck pain or a recent history of neck trauma. Multiple branch retinal artery occlusions, which may be asymptomatic, along with encephalopathy and hearing loss are the characteristic features of Susac syndrome.

Clinical Findings

A. Symptoms and Signs

Central retinal artery occlusion presents as sudden profound monocular visual loss. Visual acuity is usually reduced to counting fingers or worse, and visual field is

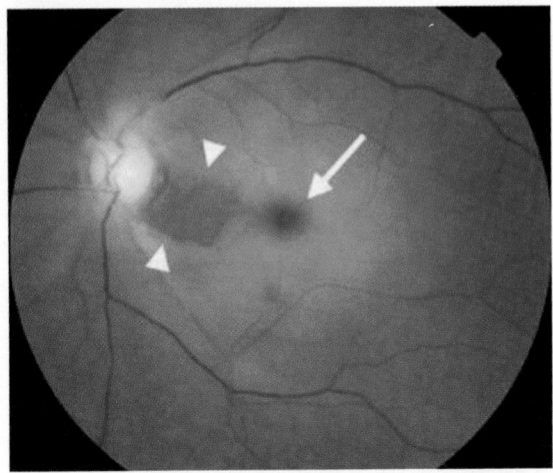

▲ **Figure 7–4.** Acute central retinal artery occlusion with cherry-red spot and preserved retina adjacent to the optic disk due to cilioretinal artery supply. (From Esther Posner. Reproduced, with permission, from Riordan-Eva P, Cunningham ET Jr. *Vaughan & Asbury's General Ophthalmology*, 18th ed. McGraw-Hill, 2011.)

restricted to an island of vision in the temporal field. Ophthalmoscopy reveals pallid swelling of the retina with a cherry-red spot at the fovea (Figure 7–4). The retinal arteries are attenuated, and "box-car" segmentation of blood in the veins may be seen. Occasionally, emboli are seen in the central retinal artery or its branches. The retinal swelling subsides over a period of 4–6 weeks, leaving a pale optic disk and attenuated arterioles.

Branch retinal artery occlusion may also present with sudden loss of vision if the fovea is involved, but more commonly sudden loss of visual field is the presenting complaint. Fundal signs of retinal swelling and adjacent cotton-wool spots are limited to the area of retina supplied by the occluded artery.

Identify risk factors for cardiac source of emboli including arrhythmia, particularly atrial fibrillation, and cardiac valvular disease, and check the blood pressure. Clinical features of giant cell arteritis include age 50 years or older, jaw claudication (which is very specific), headache, scalp tenderness, general malaise, weight loss, symptoms of polymyalgia rheumatica, and tenderness, thickening, or absence of pulse of the superficial temporal arteries. Table 20–12 lists the clinical manifestations of vasculitis.

B. Laboratory Findings

Erythrocyte sedimentation rate and C-reactive protein are usually markedly elevated in giant cell arteritis but one or both may be normal. Consider screening for other types of vasculitis (see Table 20–13). Screen for diabetes mellitus and hyperlipidemia in all patients. Particularly in younger patients, consider testing for antiphospholipid antibodies, lupus anticoagulant, inherited thrombophilia, and elevated plasma homocysteine.

C. Imaging

To identify carotid and cardiac sources of emboli, obtain duplex ultrasonography of the carotid arteries, ECG, and echocardiography, with transesophageal studies (if necessary). When indicated, obtain CT or MR studies for internal carotid artery dissection.

▶ Treatment

If the patient is seen within a few hours after onset, emergency treatment—including laying the patient flat, ocular massage, high concentrations of inhaled oxygen, intravenous acetazolamide, and anterior chamber paracentesis—may influence the visual outcome. Studies of early thrombolysis, particularly by local intra-arterial injection but also intravenously, have shown good results in central retinal artery occlusion not due to giant cell arteritis but the former method has a high incidence of adverse effects and may be difficult to accomplish within the required time.

In giant cell arteritis there is risk—highest in the first few days—of involvement of the other eye. When the diagnosis is suspected, high-dose corticosteroids (oral prednisolone 1–1.5 mg/kg/d, if necessary preceded by intravenous hydrocortisone 250–500 mg immediately or, especially in patients with bilateral visual loss, methylprednisolone 0.5–1 g/d for 1–3 days) must be instituted immediately, possibly together with low-dose aspirin (~81 mg/d orally). The patient must be monitored closely to ensure that treatment is adequate. A temporal artery biopsy should be performed promptly, and if necessary, assistance should be sought from a rheumatologist.

Patients with embolic retinal artery occlusion and 70–99% ipsilateral carotid artery stenosis and possibly those with 50–69% stenosis should be considered for carotid endarterectomy or possibly angioplasty with stenting to be performed within 2 weeks (see Chapters 12 and 24). Retinal embolization due to cardiac disease such as atrial fibrillation or a hypercoagulable state usually requires anticoagulation.

▶ When to Refer

- Patients with central retinal artery occlusion should be referred emergently to an ophthalmologist.
- Patients with branch retinal artery occlusion should be referred urgently.

▶ When to Admit

Patients with visual loss due to giant cell arteritis may require emergency admission for high-dose corticosteroid therapy and close monitoring to ensure that treatment is adequate.

Cugati S et al. Treatment options for central retinal artery occlusion. Curr Treat Options Neurol. 2013 Feb;15(1):63–77. [PMID: 23070637]

Kennedy S. Polymyalgia rheumatica and giant cell arteritis: an in-depth look at diagnosis and treatment. J Am Acad Nurse Pract. 2012 May;24(5):277–85. [PMID: 22551331]

Salvarani C et al. Clinical features of polymyalgia rheumatica and giant cell arteritis. Nat Rev Rheumatol. 2012 Sep;8(9):509–21. [PMID: 22825731]

Varma DD et al. A review of central retinal artery occlusion: clinical presentation and management. Eye (Lond). 2013 Jun;27(6): 688–97. [PMID: 23470793]

TRANSIENT MONOCULAR VISUAL LOSS

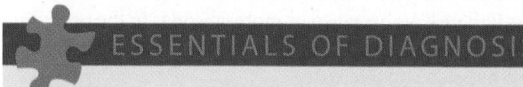

ESSENTIALS OF DIAGNOSIS

▶ Monocular loss of vision usually lasting a few minutes with complete recovery.

Transient monocular visual loss ("ocular transient ischemic attack [TIA]") is usually caused by a retinal embolus from ipsilateral carotid disease or the heart. The visual loss is characteristically described as a curtain passing vertically across the visual field with complete monocular visual loss lasting a few minutes and a similar curtain effect as the episode passes (amaurosis fugax; also called "fleeting blindness"). An embolus is rarely seen on ophthalmoscopy. Other causes of transient, often recurrent, visual loss due to ocular ischemia are giant cell arteritis, hypercoagulable state (such as antiphospholipid syndrome), hyperviscosity, and severe occlusive carotid disease; in the last case, the visual loss characteristically occurs on exposure to bright light. More transient visual loss, lasting only a few seconds to 1 minute, usually recurrent, and affecting one or both eyes, occurs in patients with optic disk swelling, for example in those with raised intracranial pressure. In young patients, there is a benign form of transient recurrent visual loss that has been ascribed to choroidal or retinal vascular spasm.

▶ Diagnostic Studies

In most cases, clinical assessment and investigations are much the same as for retinal artery occlusion (see above) with greater emphasis on identifying a source of emboli. Optic disk swelling requires different investigations (see below).

▶ Treatment

All patients with possible embolic transient visual loss should be treated immediately with oral aspirin (at least 81 mg daily), or another antiplatelet drug, until the cause has been determined. Affected patients with 70–99% (and possibly those with 50–69%) ipsilateral carotid artery stenosis should be considered for urgent carotid endarterectomy or possibly angioplasty with stenting (see Chapters 12 and 24). In all patients, vascular risk factors (eg, hypertension) need to be controlled. Retinal embolization due to a cardiac disease, such as atrial fibrillation, or a hypercoagulable state usually requires anticoagulation. In younger patients with the benign variant of transient monocular blindness, calcium channel blockers, such as slow-release nifedipine, 60 mg/d, may be effective.

▶ When to Refer

In all cases of episodic visual loss, early ophthalmologic consultation is advisable.

▶ When to Admit

Hospital admission is advisable in embolic transient visual loss if there have been two or more episodes in the preceding week ("crescendo TIA") or the underlying cause is cardiac or a hypercoagulable state.

Barbetta I et al. Outcomes of urgent carotid endarterectomy for stable and unstable acute neurologic deficits. J Vasc Surg. 2014 Feb;59(2):440–6. [PMID: 24246539]

Carmo GA et al. Carotid stenosis management: a review for the internist. Intern Emerg Med. 2014 Mar;9(2):133–42. [PMID: 24057347]

Petzold A et al. Patterns of non-embolic transient monocular visual field loss. J Neurol. 2013 Jul;260(7):1889–900. [PMID: 23564298]

Ritter JC et al. Carotid endarterectomy: where do we stand at present? Curr Opin Cardiol. 2013 Nov;28(6):619–24. [PMID: 24100648]

Ritter JC et al. The current management of carotid atherosclerotic disease: who, when and how? Interact Cardiovasc Thorac Surg. 2013 Mar;16(3):339–46. [PMID: 23197661]

Simmons BB et al. Transient ischemic attack: part I. Diagnosis and evaluation. Am Fam Physician. 2012 Sep 15;86(6):521–6. [PMID: 23062043]

RETINAL DISORDERS ASSOCIATED WITH SYSTEMIC DISEASES

1. Diabetic Retinopathy

ESSENTIALS OF DIAGNOSIS

- ▶ Present in about 35% of all diagnosed diabetic patients.
- ▶ Present in about 20% of type 2 diabetic patients at diagnosis.
- ▶ Background retinopathy: mild retinal abnormalities without visual loss.
- ▶ Maculopathy: macular edema, exudates, or ischemia.
- ▶ Proliferative retinopathy: new retinal vessels.

▶ General Considerations

Diabetic retinopathy is broadly classified as **nonproliferative**, which is subclassified as mild, moderate, or severe, or **proliferative**, which is less common but causes more severe visual loss. Diabetic retinopathy is present in about 35% of diagnosed diabetic patients. In the United States, it affects about 4 million people; it is the leading cause of new

blindness among adults aged 20–65 years; and the number of affected individuals aged 65 years or older is increasing. Worldwide, there are approximately 93 million people with diabetic retinopathy, including 28 million with vision-threatening disease. Retinopathy increases in prevalence and severity with increasing duration and poorer control of diabetes. In type 1 diabetes, retinopathy is not detectable for at least 3 years after diagnosis. In type 2 diabetes, retinopathy is present in about 20% of patients at diagnosis and may be the presenting feature.

▶ Clinical Findings

Clinical assessment uses stereoscopic examination of the retina, retinal imaging with optical coherence tomography, and sometimes fluorescein angiography.

Nonproliferative retinopathy manifests as microaneurysms, retinal hemorrhages, venous beading, retinal edema, and hard exudates (Figure 7–5). Reduction of vision is most commonly due to **diabetic macular edema**, which may be focal or diffuse, but it can also be due to macular ischemia. Macular involvement is the most common cause of legal blindness in type 2 diabetes. Macular edema is associated with treatment with thiazolidinediones (glitazones).

Proliferative retinopathy is characterized by neovascularization, arising from either the optic disk or the major vascular arcades. Vitreous hemorrhage is a common sequel. Proliferation into the vitreous of blood vessels, with their associated fibrous component, may lead to tractional retinal detachment.

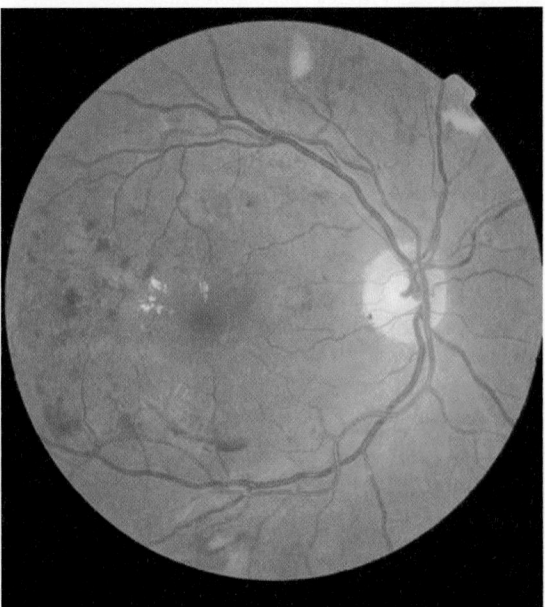

▲ **Figure 7–5.** Moderate nonproliferative diabetic retinopathy with multiple microaneurysms and hemorrhages, mild macular hard exudates, and two cotton-wool spots in the superior retina. (Reproduced, with permission, from Riordan-Eva P, Cunningham ET Jr. *Vaughan & Asbury's General Ophthalmology,* 18th ed. McGraw-Hill, 2011.)

Screening

Visual symptoms and visual acuity are poor guides to the presence of diabetic retinopathy. Adult and adolescent patients with diabetes mellitus should undergo at least yearly screening by fundal photography, commonly with centralized screening that may involve computer detection software programs, or slit-lamp examination. (Failure to identify diabetic retinopathy by direct ophthalmoscopy is common, particularly if the pupils are not dilated.) More frequent monitoring is required in women during pregnancy and in those planning pregnancy. Patients with type 2 diabetes mellitus should be screened shortly after diagnosis.

Treatment

Treatment includes optimizing blood glucose, blood pressure, renal function, and serum lipids, although such measures are probably more important in preventing the development of retinopathy than in influencing its subsequent course. Fenofibrate seems to have beneficial effects beyond reduction of serum lipids.

Macular edema and exudates, but not ischemia, may respond to laser photocoagulation; to intravitreal administration of a VEGF inhibitor (ranibizumab [Lucentis], pegaptanib [Macugen], bevacizumab [Avastin] or aflibercept [VEGF Trap-Eye, Eylea]) or corticosteroid (triamcinolone, dexamethasone implant [Ozurdex], or fluocinolone implant [Retisert, Iluvien]); to vitrectomy; or to intravitreal injection of a serine protease (ocriplasmin [Jetrea]) to release vitreo-retinal traction.

Proliferative retinopathy is usually treated by panretinal laser photocoagulation, preferably before vitreous hemorrhage or tractional detachment has occurred. Regression of neovascularization can also be achieved by intravitreal injection of a VEGF inhibitor. In patients with severe **nonproliferative retinopathy,** fluorescein angiography can help determine whether panretinal laser photocoagulation should be undertaken prophylactically by visualizing the extent of retinal ischemia. Vitrectomy is necessary for removal of persistent vitreous hemorrhage, to improve vision and allow panretinal laser photocoagulation for the underlying retinal neovascularization, for treatment of tractional retinal detachment involving the macula, and for management of rapidly progressive proliferative disease.

Proliferative diabetic retinopathy, especially after successful laser treatment, is not a contraindication to treatment with thrombolytic agents, aspirin, or warfarin unless there has been recent vitreous or pre-retinal hemorrhage.

When to Refer

- All diabetic patients with sudden loss of vision or retinal detachment should be referred emergently to an ophthalmologist.
- Proliferative retinopathy or macular involvement requires urgent referral to an ophthalmologist.
- Severe nonproliferative retinopathy or unexplained reduction of visual acuity requires early referral to an ophthalmologist.

American Academy of Ophthalmology Retina Panel. Preferred Practice Panel* Guidelines – Summary Benchmark. Diabetic retinopathy. San Francisco, CA: American Academy of Ophthalmology; 2013. http://one.aao.org/summary-benchmark-detail/diabetic-retinopathy-summary-benchmark--october-20

Antonetti DA et al. Diabetic retinopathy. N Engl J Med. 2012 Mar 29;366(13):1227–39. [PMID: 22455417]

Bressler NM et al. Panretinal photocoagulation for proliferative diabetic retinopathy. N Engl J Med. 2011 Oct 20;365(16):1520–6. [PMID: 22010918]

Errera MH et al. Pregnancy-associated retinal diseases and their management. Surv Ophthalmol. 2013 Mar–Apr;58(2):127–42. [PMID: 23410822]

Guigui S et al. Screening for diabetic retinopathy: review of current methods. Hosp Pract (Minneap). 2012 Apr;40(2):64–72. [PMID: 22615080]

Kiire CA et al. Medical management for the prevention and treatment of diabetic macular edema. Surv Ophthalmol. 2013 Sep–Oct;58(5):459–65. [PMID: 23969020]

2. Hypertensive Retinochoroidopathy

Systemic hypertension affects both the retinal and choroidal circulations. The clinical manifestations vary according to the degree and rapidity of rise in blood pressure and the underlying state of the ocular circulation. The most florid ocular changes occur in young patients with abrupt elevations of blood pressure, such as may occur in pheochromocytoma, malignant hypertension, or preeclampsia-eclampsia. Hypertensive retinopathy can be a surrogate marker for current and future nonocular end-organ damage.

Chronic hypertension accelerates the development of atherosclerosis. The retinal arterioles become more tortuous and narrow and develop abnormal light reflexes ("silver-wiring" and "copper-wiring"). There is increased venous compression at the retinal arteriovenous crossings ("arteriovenous nicking"), an important factor predisposing to branch retinal vein occlusions. Flame-shaped hemorrhages occur in the nerve fiber layer of the retina.

Acute elevations of blood pressure result in loss of autoregulation in the retinal circulation, leading to the breakdown of endothelial integrity and occlusion of precapillary arterioles and capillaries. These pathologic changes are manifested as cotton-wool spots, retinal hemorrhages, retinal edema, and retinal exudates, often in a stellate appearance at the macula (Figure 7–6). In the choroid, vasoconstriction and ischemia result in serous retinal detachments and retinal pigment epithelial infarcts that later develop into pigmented lesions that may be focal, linear, or wedge-shaped. The abnormalities in the choroidal circulation may also affect the optic nerve head, producing ischemic optic neuropathy with optic disk swelling. Fundal abnormalities are the hallmark of hypertensive crisis with retinopathy (previously known as malignant hypertension) that requires emergency treatment. Marked fundal abnormalities are likely to be associated with permanent retinal, choroidal, or optic nerve damage. Precipitous reduction of blood pressure may exacerbate such damage.

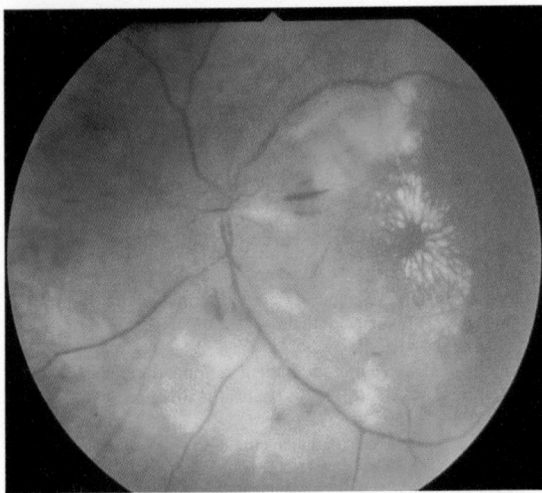

▲ **Figure 7–6.** Accelerated hypertension in a young woman manifesting as marked optic disk edema, macular star of hard exudates, serous retinal detachment, and retinal hemorrhages and cotton-wool spots. (Reproduced, with permission, from Riordan-Eva P, Cunningham ET Jr. *Vaughan & Asbury's General Ophthalmology,* 18th ed. McGraw-Hill, 2011.)

Bhargava M et al. How does hypertension affect your eyes? J Hum Hypertens. 2012 Feb;26(2):71–83. [PMID: 21509040]

Chatziralli IP et al. The value of fundoscopy in general practice. Open Ophthalmol J. 2012;6:4–5. [PMID: 22435081]

Errera MH et al. Pregnancy-associated retinal diseases and their management. Surv Ophthalmol. 2013 Mar–Apr;58(2):127–42. [PMID: 23410822]

3. Blood Dyscrasias

Severe **thrombocytopenia** or **anemia** may result in various types of retinal or choroidal hemorrhages, including white centered retinal hemorrhages (Roth spots) that occur in leukemia and many other situations besides bacterial endocarditis. Involvement of the macula may result in permanent visual loss.

Sickle cell retinopathy is particularly common in hemoglobin SC disease but may also occur with other hemoglobin S variants. Manifestations include "salmon-patch" preretinal/intraretinal hemorrhages, "black sunbursts" resulting from intraretinal hemorrhage, and new vessels. Severe visual loss is rare. Retinal laser photocoagulation reduces the frequency of vitreous hemorrhage from new vessels. Surgery is occasionally needed for persistent vitreous hemorrhage or tractional retinal detachment.

Charles KS et al. Ophthalmic manifestations of haematological disorders. West Indian Med J. 2013 Jan;62(1):99–103. [PMID: 24171339]

4. HIV Infection/AIDS

HIV retinopathy, the most common ophthalmic abnormality in HIV infection, manifests clinically as cotton-wool spots, retinal hemorrhages, and microaneurysms but may also cause reduced contrast sensitivity, and retinal nerve fiber layer and outer retinal damage.

CMV retinitis has become less common with the availability of highly active antiretroviral therapy (HAART) but continues to be prevalent where resources are limited. It usually occurs when CD4 counts are below 50/mcL (or 0.05×10^9/L) and is characterized by progressively enlarging yellowish-white patches of retinal opacification, accompanied by retinal hemorrhages and usually beginning adjacent to the major retinal vascular arcades. Patients are often asymptomatic until there is involvement of the fovea or optic nerve, or until retinal detachment develops.

Choices for initial therapy are (1) valganciclovir 900 mg orally twice daily for 3 weeks; (2) ganciclovir 5 mg/kg intravenously twice a day, foscarnet 60 mg/kg intravenously three times a day, or cidofovir 5 mg/kg intravenously once weekly, for 2–3 weeks; or (3) local administration, using either intravitreal injection of ganciclovir or foscarnet, or the sustained-release ganciclovir intravitreal implant. All available agents are virostatic. Maintenance therapy can be achieved with lower-dose therapy (oral valganciclovir 900 mg once daily, intravenous ganciclovir 5 mg/kg/d, intravenous foscarnet 90 mg/kg/d, or intravenous cidofovir 5 mg/kg once every 2 weeks) or with intravitreal therapy. Systemic therapy has a greater risk of nonocular adverse effects but reduces mortality, incidence of nonocular CMV disease, and incidence of retinitis in the fellow eye and avoids intraocular complications of intravitreal administration. Pharmacologic prophylaxis against CMV retinitis in patients with low CD4 counts or high CMV burdens has not been found to be worthwhile.

In all patients with CMV retinitis, HAART needs to be instituted or adjusted. This may lead to the immune reconstitution inflammatory syndrome (IRIS), of which the immune recovery uveitis may lead to visual loss, predominantly due to cystoid macular edema. If the CD4 count is maintained above 100/mcL (0.1×10^9/L), it may be possible to discontinue maintenance anti-CMV therapy.

Other ophthalmic manifestations of opportunistic infections occurring in AIDS patients include herpes simplex retinitis, which usually manifests as acute retinal necrosis; toxoplasmic and candidal chorioretinitis possibly progressing to endophthalmitis; herpes zoster ophthalmicus and herpes zoster retinitis, which can manifest as acute retinal necrosis or progressive outer retinal necrosis; and various entities due to syphilis, tuberculosis, or cryptococcosis. Kaposi sarcoma of the conjunctiva (see Chapter 31) and orbital lymphoma may also be seen on rare occasions.

Carmichael A. Cytomegalovirus and the eye. Eye (Lond). 2012 Feb;26(2):237–40. [PMID: 22173076]

Gangaputra S et al. Non-cytomegalovirus ocular opportunistic infections in patients with AIDS. Am J Ophthalmol. 2013 Feb;155(2):206–12. [PMID: 23068916]

Jabs DA et al. Comparison of treatment regimens for cytomegalovirus retinitis in patients with AIDS in the era of highly active antiretroviral therapy. Ophthalmology. 2013 Jun;120(6):1262–70. [PMID: 23419804]

Sugar EA et al. Incidence of cytomegalovirus retinitis in the era of highly active antiretroviral therapy. Am J Ophthalmol. 2012 Jun;153(6):1016–24.e5. [PMID: 22310076]

Wong RW et al. Emerging concepts in the management of acute retinal necrosis. Br J Ophthalmol. 2013 May;97(5):545–52. [PMID: 23235944]

ISCHEMIC OPTIC NEUROPATHY

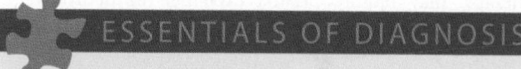

ESSENTIALS OF DIAGNOSIS

► Sudden painless visual loss with signs of optic nerve dysfunction.

► Optic disk swelling in anterior ischemic optic neuropathy.

Anterior ischemic optic neuropathy—due to inadequate perfusion of the posterior ciliary arteries that supply the anterior portion of the optic nerve—produces sudden visual loss, usually with an altitudinal field defect, and optic disk swelling. In older patients it may be caused by giant cell arteritis (arteritic anterior ischemic optic neuropathy). The predominant factor predisposing to nonarteritic anterior ischemic optic neuropathy, which subsequently affects the fellow eye in up to 25% of cases, is a congenitally crowded optic disk. Other causative factors include systemic hypertension, diabetes mellitus, hyperlipidemia, systemic vasculitis, inherited or acquired thrombophilia, and possibly ingestion of phosphodiesterase type 5 inhibitors, interferon-alpha therapy, and obstructive sleep apnea. Diabetic papillopathy is a cause of chronic (possibly ischemic) optic disk swelling that generally has a better visual outcome. Rarely, an optic neuropathy that can be difficult to differentiate from nonarteritic anterior optic neuropathy, but typically affecting both eyes simultaneously and having a more chronic course, develops in patients taking amiodarone.

Ischemic optic neuropathy, usually involving the retrobulbar optic nerve and thus not causing any optic disk swelling (**posterior ischemic optic neuropathy**), may occur after severe blood loss or nonocular surgery, particularly prolonged lumbar spine surgery in the prone position, or in association with dialysis. In both situations there may be several contributory factors.

▶ Treatment

Arteritic anterior ischemic optic neuropathy necessitates emergency high-dose systemic corticosteroid treatment to prevent visual loss in the other eye. (See Central & Branch Retinal Artery Occlusions, above and Polymyalgia Rheumatica & Giant Cell Arteritis, Chapter 20.) Similar treatment is required in anterior ischemic optic neuropathy due to systemic vaculitis, which may also be classified as arteritic anterior ischemic optic neuropathy. It is uncertain whether systemic or intravitreal corticosteroid therapy influences the outcome in nonarteritic anterior ischemic optic neuropathy or whether oral low-dose (~81 mg daily) aspirin reduces the risk of fellow eye involvement. In ischemic optic neuropathy after nonocular surgery, marked anemia should be treated by blood transfusion.

▶ When to Refer

Patients with ischemic optic neuropathy should be referred urgently to an ophthalmologist.

▶ When to Admit

Patients with ischemic optic neuropathy due to giant cell arteritis may require emergency admission for high-dose corticosteroid therapy and close monitoring to ensure that treatment is adequate.

Hayreh SS. Ischemic optic neuropathies—where are we now? Graefes Arch Clin Exp Ophthalmol. 2013 Aug;251(8):1873–84. [PMID: 23821118]
Kitaba A et al. Perioperative visual loss after nonocular surgery. J Anesth. 2013 Dec;27(6):919–26. [PMID: 23775280]
Passman RS et al. Amiodarone-associated optic neuropathy: a critical review. Am J Med. 2012 May;125(5):447–53. [PMID: 22385784]
Postoperative Visual Loss Study Group. Risk factors associated with ischemic optic neuropathy after spinal fusion surgery. Anesthesiology. 2012 Jan;116(1):15–24. [PMID: 22185873]
Warner MA. Cracking open the door on perioperative visual loss. Anesthesiology. 2012 Jan;116(1):1–2. [PMID: 22185869]

OPTIC NEURITIS

ESSENTIALS OF DIAGNOSIS

► Subacute unilateral visual loss with signs of optic nerve dysfunction.

► Pain exacerbated by eye movements.

► Optic disk usually normal in acute stage but subsequently develops pallor.

▶ General Considerations

Inflammatory optic neuropathy (optic neuritis) is strongly associated with demyelinating disease, particularly multiple sclerosis but also acute disseminated encephalomyelitis. It also occurs in sarcoidosis; as a component of neuromyelitis optica (Devic syndrome), which is associated with serum antibodies to aquaporin-4; particularly in children following viral infection; related to infection with varicella zoster virus; with various autoimmune disorders, particularly systemic lupus erythematosus; related to treatment with biologics; and by spread of inflammation from the meninges, orbital tissues, or paranasal sinuses.

▶ Clinical Findings

Optic neuritis in demyelinating disease is characterized by unilateral loss of vision that usually develops over a few days. Vision ranges from 20/30 (6/9) to no perception of light. Commonly there is pain behind the eye, particularly on eye movements. Field loss is usually central. There is particular loss of color vision and a relative afferent pupillary defect. In about two-thirds of cases, the optic nerve is normal during the acute stage (retrobulbar optic neuritis). In the remainder, the optic disk is swollen (papillitis) with occasional flame-shaped peripapillary hemorrhages. Visual acuity usually improves within 2–3 weeks and returns to 20/40 (6/12) or better in 95% of previously unaffected eyes. Optic atrophy subsequently develops if there has been destruction of sufficient optic nerve fibers. Any patient with presumed demyelinating optic neuritis in which visual recovery does not occur or there are other atypical features, including continuing deterioration of vision or persisting pain after 2 weeks, should undergo further investigation, including CT or MRI of the head and orbits to exclude a lesion compressing the optic nerve.

▶ **Treatment**

In acute demyelinating optic neuritis, intravenous methyl-prednisolone (1 g daily for 3 days followed by a tapering course of oral prednisolone) has been shown to accelerate visual recovery, although in clinical practice, the oral taper is not often prescribed and oral methylprednisolone may be used. Use in an individual patient is determined by the degree of visual loss, the state of the fellow eye, and the patient's visual requirements.

Optic neuritis due to sarcoidosis, neuromyelitis optica, herpes zoster, or systemic lupus erythematosus generally has a poorer prognosis, requires more prolonged corticosteroid therapy, may require plasma exchange in neuromyelitis optica, and may necessitate long-term immunosuppression.

▶ **Prognosis**

Among patients with a first episode of clinically isolated optic neuritis, multiple sclerosis will develop in 50% within 15 years but the visual and neurologic prognosis is good. The major risk factors are female sex and multiple white matter lesions on brain MRI. Various disease-modifying drugs including interferon (Avonex, Rebif, Betaseron, Extavia), glatiramer acetate (Copaxone), mitoxantrone (Novantrone), natazilumab (Tysabri), and fingolimod (Gilenya) are available, and others such as teriflunomide, BG-12 (dimethyl fumarate), laquinimod, and alemtuzumab are available, to reduce the risk of further neurologic episodes and potentially the accumulation of disability but each has its own range of adverse effects that in some instances are life-threatening. Fingolimod is associated with macular edema.

▶ **When to Refer**

All patients with optic neuritis should be referred urgently for ophthalmologic or neurologic assessment.

American Academy of Ophthalmology Preferred Practice Pattern® Clinical Question. Corticosteroids for optic neuritis treatment. San Francisco, CA: American Academy of Ophthalmology 2013. http://one.aao.org/clinical-questions/corticosteroids-optic-neuritis-treatment--2013
Hoorbakht H et al. Optic neuritis, its differential diagnosis and management. Open Ophthalmol J. 2012;6:65–72. [PMID: 22888383]
Jeffery DR. Recent advances in treating multiple sclerosis: efficacy, risks and place in therapy. Ther Adv Chronic Dis. 2013 Jan;4(1):45–51. [PMID: 23342246]

Morrow MJ et al. Neuromyelitis optica. J Neuroophthalmol. 2012 Jun;32(2):154–66. [PMID: 22617743]
Perumal J et al. Emerging disease-modifying therapies in multiple sclerosis. Curr Treat Options Neurol. 2012 Jun;14(3):256–63. [PMID: 22426573]
Trebst C et al. Update on the diagnosis and treatment of neuromyelitis optica: recommendations of the Neuromyelitis Optica Study Group (NEMOS). J Neurol. 2014 Jan;26(1):1–16. [PMID: 24272588]

OPTIC DISK SWELLING

Optic disk swelling may result from intraocular disease, orbital and optic nerve lesions, severe hypertensive retino-choroidopathy, or raised intracranial pressure, the last necessitating urgent imaging to exclude an intracranial mass or cerebral venous sinus occlusion but potentially being caused by numerous conditions. Intraocular causes include central retinal vein occlusion, posterior uveitis, and posterior scleritis. Optic nerve lesions causing disk swelling include anterior ischemic optic neuropathy; optic neuritis; optic disk drusen; optic nerve sheath meningioma; and infiltration by sarcoidosis, leukemia, or lymphoma. Any orbital lesion causing nerve compression may produce disk swelling.

Papilledema (optic disk swelling due to raised intracranial pressure) is usually bilateral and most commonly produces enlargement of the blind spot without loss of acuity. Chronic papilledema, as in idiopathic intracranial hypertension and cerebral venous sinus occlusion, or severe acute papilledema may be associated with visual field loss and occasionally with profound loss of acuity. All patients with chronic papilledema must be monitored carefully—especially their visual fields—and cerebrospinal fluid shunt or optic nerve sheath fenestration should be considered in those with progressive visual failure not controlled by medical therapy (weight loss where appropriate and acetazolamide).

Optic disk drusen and congenitally crowded optic disks, which are associated with farsightedness, cause optic disk elevation that may be mistaken for swelling (pseudo-papilledema). Exposed optic disk drusen may be obvious clinically or can be demonstrated by their autofluorescence. Buried drusen are best detected by orbital ultrasound or CT scanning. Other family members may be similarly affected.

Biousse V. Idiopathic intracranial hypertension: diagnosis, monitoring and treatment. Rev Neurol (Paris). 2012 Oct;168(10):673–83. [PMID: 22981270]
Biousse V et al. Update on the pathophysiology and management of idiopathic intracranial hypertension. J Neurol Neurosurg Psychiatry. 2012 May;83(5):488–94. [PMID: 22423118]
Sergott RC. Headaches associated with papilledema. Curr Pain Headache Rep. 2012 Aug;16(4):354–8. [PMID: 22669513]

OCULAR MOTOR PALSIES

In complete **third nerve paralysis**, there is ptosis with a divergent and slightly depressed eye. Extraocular movements are restricted in all directions except laterally (preserved lateral rectus function). Intact fourth nerve (superior oblique) function is detected by the presence of inward rotation on attempted depression of the eye. Pupillary involvement (relatively dilated pupil that does not constrict normally to light) is an important sign differentiating "surgical," including traumatic, from "medical" causes of isolated third nerve palsy. Compressive lesions of the third nerve—eg, aneurysm of the posterior communicating artery and uncal herniation due to a supratentorial mass lesion—characteristically have pupillary involvement. Patients with painful acute isolated third nerve palsy and pupillary involvement should be assumed to have a posterior communicating artery aneurysm until this has been excluded. Pituitary apoplexy is a rarer cause. Medical causes of isolated third nerve palsy include diabetes mellitus, hypertension, giant cell arteritis, and herpes zoster.

Fourth nerve paralysis causes upward deviation of the eye with failure of depression on adduction. In acquired cases, there is vertical and torsional diplopia that are most apparent on looking down. Trauma is a major cause of acquired—particularly bilateral—fourth nerve palsy, but posterior fossa tumor and medical causes such as in third nerve palsies should also be considered. Similar clinical features are seen in congenital cases due to developmental anomaly of the nerve, muscle or tendon.

Sixth nerve paralysis causes convergent squint in the primary position with failure of abduction of the affected eye, producing horizontal diplopia that increases on gaze to the affected side and on looking into the distance. It is an important sign of raised intracranial pressure. Sixth nerve palsy may also be due to trauma, neoplasms, brainstem lesions, or medical causes such as in third nerve palsy.

An intracranial or intraorbital mass lesion should be considered in any patient with an isolated ocular motor palsy. In patients with isolated ocular motor nerve palsies presumed to be due to medical causes, brain MRI is generally only necessary if recovery has not begun within 3 months, although some authors suggest that it should be undertaken in all cases.

Ocular motor nerve palsies occurring in association with other neurologic signs may be due to lesions in the brainstem, cavernous sinus, or orbit. Lesions around the cavernous sinus involve the upper divisions of the trigeminal nerve, the ocular motor nerves, and occasionally the optic chiasm. Orbital apex lesions involve the optic nerve and the ocular motor nerves.

Myasthenia gravis and Graves ophthalmopathy (thyroid eye disease) should also be considered in the differential diagnosis of disordered extraocular movements.

When to Refer

- Any patient with recent onset isolated third nerve palsy, particularly if there is pupillary involvement or pain, must be referred emergently for neurologic assessment and CT, MR, or catheter angiography for intracranial aneurysm.

- All patients with recent onset double vision should be referred urgently to an ophthalmologist or neurologist, particularly if there is multiple cranial nerve dysfunction or other neurologic abnormalities.

When to Admit

Patients with double vision due to giant cell arteritis may require emergency admission for high-dose corticosteroid therapy and close monitoring to ensure that treatment is adequate. (See Central & Branch Retinal Artery Occlusions and Chapter 20.)

Cordonnier M et al. Neuro-ophthalmological emergencies: which ocular signs or symptoms for which diseases? Acta Neurol Belg. 2013 Sep;113(3):215–24. [PMID: 23475430]

Gräf M et al. How to deal with diplopia. Rev Neurol (Paris). 2012 Oct;168(10):720–8. [PMID: 22986079]

Lo CP et al. Neuroimaging of isolated and non-isolated third nerve palsies. Br J Radiol. 2012 Apr;85(1012):460–7. [PMID: 22253341]

Lueck CJ. Infranuclear ocular motor disorders. Handb Clin Neurol. 2011;102:281–318. [PMID: 21601071]

Pierrot-Deseilligny C. Nuclear, internuclear, and supranuclear ocular motor disorders. Handb Clin Neurol. 2011;102:319–31. [PMID: 21601072]

Sadagopan KA et al. Managing the patient with oculomotor nerve palsy. Curr Opin Ophthalmol. 2013 Sep;24(5):438–47. [PMID: 23872817]

Tamhankar MA et al. Isolated third, fourth, and sixth cranial nerve palsies from presumed microvascular versus other causes: a prospective study. Ophthalmology. 2013 Nov;120(11): 2264–9. [PMID: 23747163]

THYROID EYE DISEASE (Graves Ophthalmopathy)

Thyroid eye disease is a syndrome of clinical and orbital imaging abnormalities caused by deposition of mucopolysaccharides and infiltration with chronic inflammatory cells of the orbital tissues, particularly the extraocular muscles. It usually occurs in association with autoimmune hyperthyroidism. Clinical or laboratory evidence of thyroid dysfunction and thyroid antibodies may not be detectable at presentation or even on long-term follow-up, but their absence requires consideration of other disease entities. Radioiodine therapy, possibly indirectly due to induction of hypothyroidism, and cigarette smoking increase the severity of thyroid eye disease and ethanol injection of thyroid nodules has been reported to be followed by severe disease. Ocular myasthenia and thyroid eye disease are associated and may coexist, the presence of ptosis rather than eyelid retraction being a characteristic feature.

Clinical Findings

The primary clinical features are proptosis, lid retraction and lid lag, conjunctival chemosis and episcleral inflammation, and extraocular muscle dysfunction. Resulting symptoms are cosmetic abnormalities, surface irritation, which usually responds to artificial tears, and diplopia, which should be treated conservatively (eg, with prisms) in the active stages of the disease and only by surgery when the disease has been static for at least 6 months. The important complications are corneal exposure and optic nerve compression, both of which may lead to marked visual loss. The primary imaging features are enlargement of the extraocular muscles, usually affecting both orbits. The clinical and imaging abnormalities of thyroid eye disease may be mimicked by dural carotico-cavernous fistula.

▶ Treatment

Treatment options for optic nerve compression or severe corneal exposure are intravenous pulse methylprednisolone therapy (eg, 1 g daily for 3 days, repeated weekly for 3 weeks), oral prednisolone 80–100 mg/d, radiotherapy, or surgery (usually consisting of extensive removal of bone from the medial, inferior, and lateral walls of the orbit), either singly or in combination. The role of systemic or orbital rituximab is uncertain.

The optimal management of moderately severe thyroid eye disease without visual loss is controversial. Systemic corticosteroids and radiotherapy may be beneficial. Peribulbar corticosteroid injections have been advocated. Surgical decompression may be justified in patients with marked proptosis. Lateral tarsorrhaphy may be used for moderately severe corneal exposure. Other procedures are particularly useful for correcting lid retraction but should not be undertaken until the orbital disease is quiescent and orbital decompression or extraocular muscle surgery has been undertaken. Oral selenium seems to be beneficial in mild disease. Establishing and maintaining euthyroidism are important in all cases.

▶ When to Refer

All patients with thyroid eye disease should be referred to an ophthalmologist, urgently if there is reduced vision.

Alhambra Expósito MR et al. Clinical efficacy of intravenous glucocorticoid treatment in Graves' ophthalmopathy. Endocrinol Nutr. 2013 Jan;60(1):10–4. [PMID: 23177093]

Bartalena L. Diagnosis and management of Graves disease: a global overview. Nat Rev Endocrinol. 2013 Dec;9(12):724–34. [PMID: 24126481]

Dolman PJ. Evaluating Graves' orbitopathy. Best Pract Res Clin Endocrinol Metab. 2012 Jun;26(3):229–48. [PMID: 22632361]

Hegedüs L et al. Treating the thyroid in the presence of Graves' ophthalmopathy. Best Pract Res Clin Endocrinol Metab. 2012 Jun;26(3):313–24. [PMID: 22632368]

Menconi F et al. Spontaneous improvement of untreated mild Graves' ophthalmopathy: the Rundle curve revisited. Thyroid. 2014 Jan;24(1):60–6. [PMID: 23980907]

ORBITAL CELLULITIS

Orbital cellulitis is characterized by fever, proptosis, restriction of extraocular movements, and swelling with redness of the lids. Immediate treatment with intravenous antibiotics is necessary to prevent optic nerve damage and spread of infection to the cavernous sinuses, meninges, and brain. Infection of the paranasal sinuses is the usual underlying cause; examples of infecting organisms include

S pneumoniae, the incidence of which has been reduced by the administration of pneumococcal vaccine, other streptococci such as the anginosus group, *H influenzae* and, less commonly, *S aureus*. Penicillinase-resistant penicillin, such as nafcillin, is recommended, possibly together with metronidazole or clindamycin to treat anaerobic infections (Table 30–5). If trauma is the underlying cause, a cephalosporin, such as cefazolin or ceftriaxone, should be added to ensure coverage for *S aureus* and group A beta-hemolytic streptococci. Vancomycin or clindamycin may be required if there is concern about MRSA, which is infrequently associated with paranasal sinus infection. MRSA may cause multiple orbital abscesses and delay in the institution of vancomycin or clindamycin frequently necessitates surgery with a poor visual outcome. For patients with penicillin hypersensitivity, vancomycin, levofloxacin, and metronidazole are recommended. The response to antibiotics is usually excellent, but surgery may be required to drain the paranasal sinuses or orbital abscess. In immunocompromised patients, zygomycosis must be considered.

▶ When to Refer

All patients with suspected orbital cellulitis must be referred emergently to an ophthalmologist.

Mathias MT et al. Atypical presentations of orbital cellulitis caused by methicillin-resistant *Staphylococcus aureus*. Ophthalmology. 2012 Jun;119(6):1238–43. [PMID: 22406032]

OCULAR TRAUMA

Ocular trauma, which occurs in many different circumstances and by a variety of mechanisms, is an important cause of severe visual impairment at all ages but particularly in young adult males and is the leading cause of monocular blindness in the United States. Thorough but safe clinical assessment, supplemented when necessary by imaging, is crucial to effective management.

Huang YH et al. Ocular trauma. JAMA. 2012 Aug 15;308(7):710–1. [PMID: 22893168]

Powell J et al. Surgical ophthalmologic examination. Oral Maxillofac Surg Clin North Am. 2012 Nov;24(4):557–72. [PMID: 22995153]

Scruggs D et al. Ocular injuries in trauma patients: an analysis of 28,340 trauma admissions in the 2003–2007 National Trauma Data Bank National Sample Program. J Trauma Acute Care Surg. 2012 Nov;73(5):1308–12. [PMID: 22914085]

1. Conjunctival & Corneal Foreign Bodies

If a patient complains of "something in my eye" and gives a consistent history, a foreign body is usually present on the cornea or under the upper lid even though it may not be visible. Visual acuity should be tested before treatment is instituted, to assess the severity of the injury and as a basis for comparison in the event of complications.

After a local anesthetic (eg, proparacaine, 0.5%) is instilled, the eye is examined with a hand flashlight, using

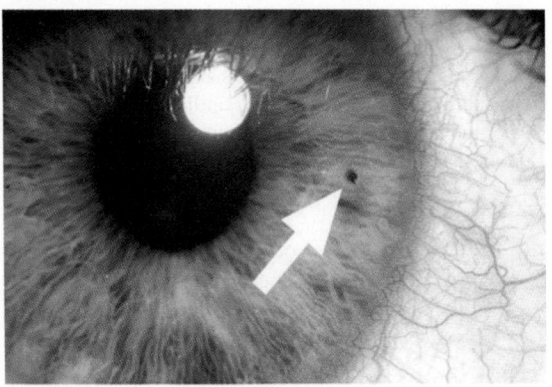

▲ **Figure 7–7.** Corneal rust stain from metallic foreign body (arrow). (From James J Augsburger and Zélia M Corrêa. Reproduced, with permission, from Riordan-Eva P, Cunningham ET Jr. *Vaughan & Asbury's General Ophthalmology*, 18th ed. McGraw-Hill, 2011.)

oblique illumination, and loupe. Corneal foreign bodies may be made more apparent by the instillation of sterile fluorescein. They are then removed with a sterile wet cotton-tipped applicator or hypodermic needle. Bacitracin-polymyxin ophthalmic ointment should be instilled. It is not necessary to patch the eye.

Steel foreign bodies usually leave a diffuse rust ring (Figure 7–7). This requires excision of the affected tissue and is best done under local anesthesia using a slit lamp. **Caution:** Anesthetic drops should not be given to the patient for self-administration.

If there is no infection, a layer of corneal epithelial cells will line the crater within 24 hours. The intact corneal epithelium forms an effective barrier to infection, but once it is disturbed the cornea becomes extremely susceptible to infection. Early infection is manifested by a white necrotic area around the crater and a small amount of gray exudate.

In the case of a foreign body under the upper lid, a local anesthetic is instilled and the lid is everted by grasping the lashes gently and exerting pressure on the mid portion of the outer surface of the upper lid with an applicator. If a foreign body is present, it can easily be removed by passing a wet sterile cotton-tipped applicator across the conjunctival surface.

► When to Refer

Urgent referral to an ophthalmologist should be arranged if a corneal foreign body cannot be removed or if there is suspicion of corneal infection.

2. Intraocular Foreign Body

Intraocular foreign body requires emergency treatment by an ophthalmologist. Patients giving a history of "something hitting the eye"—particularly while hammering on metal or using grinding equipment—must be assessed for this possibility, especially when no corneal foreign body is seen, a corneal or scleral wound is apparent, or there is marked visual loss or media opacity. Such patients must be treated as for corneal laceration (see below) and referred without delay. Intraocular foreign bodies significantly increase the risk of intraocular infection.

► When to Refer

Patients with suspected intraocular foreign body must be referred emergently to an ophthalmologist.

Faghihi H et al. Posttraumatic endophthalmitis: report No. 2. Retina. 2012 Jan;32(1):146–51. [PMID: 21775927]

3. Corneal Abrasions

A patient with a corneal abrasion complains of severe pain and photophobia. There is often a history of trauma to the eye, commonly involving a fingernail, piece of paper, or contact lens. Visual acuity is recorded, and the cornea and conjunctiva are examined with a light and loupe to rule out a foreign body. If an abrasion is suspected but cannot be seen, sterile fluorescein is instilled into the conjunctival sac: the area of corneal abrasion will stain a deeper green than the surrounding cornea.

Treatment includes bacitracin-polymyxin ophthalmic ointment, mydriatic (cyclopentolate 1%), and analgesics either topical or oral nonsteroidal anti-inflammatory agents. Padding the eye is probably not helpful for small abrasions. Recurrent corneal erosion may follow corneal abrasions.

Riordan-Eva P. Ophthalmic emergencies. In: *Vaughan & Asbury's General Ophthalmology*, 18th ed. Riordan-Eva P et al (editors). McGraw-Hill, 2011.
Wipperman JL et al. Evaluation and management of corneal abrasions. Am Fam Physician. 2013 Jan 15;87(2):114–20. [PMID: 23317075]

4. Contusions

Contusion injuries of the eye and surrounding structures may cause ecchymosis ("black eye"), subconjunctival hemorrhage, edema or rupture of the cornea, hemorrhage into the anterior chamber (hyphema), rupture of the root of the iris (iridodialysis), paralysis of the pupillary sphincter, paralysis of the muscles of accommodation, cataract, dislocation of the lens, vitreous hemorrhage, retinal hemorrhage and edema (most common in the macular area), detachment of the retina, rupture of the choroid, fracture of the orbital floor ("blowout fracture"), or optic nerve injury. Many of these injuries are immediately obvious; others may not become apparent for days or weeks. The possibility of globe injury must always be considered in patients with facial injury, particularly if there is an orbital fracture. Patients with moderate to severe contusions should be seen by an ophthalmologist.

Any injury causing hyphema involves the danger of secondary hemorrhage, which may cause intractable glaucoma with permanent visual loss. The patient should be advised to rest until complete resolution has occurred. Daily ophthalmologic assessment is essential. Aspirin and any drugs inhibiting coagulation increase the risk of secondary hemorrhage and are to be avoided. Sickle cell anemia or trait adversely affects outcome.

▶ When to Refer

Patients with moderate or severe ocular contusion should be referred to an ophthalmologist, emergently if there is hyphema.

Blice JP. Ocular injuries, triage, and management in maxillofacial trauma. Atlas Oral Maxillofac Surg Clin North Am. 2013 Mar;21(1):97–103. [PMID: 23498334]

5. Lacerations

A. Lids

If the lid margin is lacerated, the patient should be referred for specialized care, since permanent notching may result. Lacerations of the lower eyelid near the inner canthus often sever the lower canaliculus, for which canalicular intubation is likely to be required. Lid lacerations not involving the margin may be sutured like any skin laceration.

B. Conjunctiva

In lacerations of the conjunctiva, sutures are not necessary. To prevent infection, topical sulfonamide or antibiotic is used until the laceration is healed.

C. Cornea or Sclera

Patients with suspected corneal or scleral lacerations must be seen promptly by an ophthalmologist (Figure 7–8). Manipulation is kept to a minimum, since pressure may result in extrusion of the intraocular contents. The eye is bandaged lightly and covered with a metal shield that rests on the orbital bones above and below. The patient should be

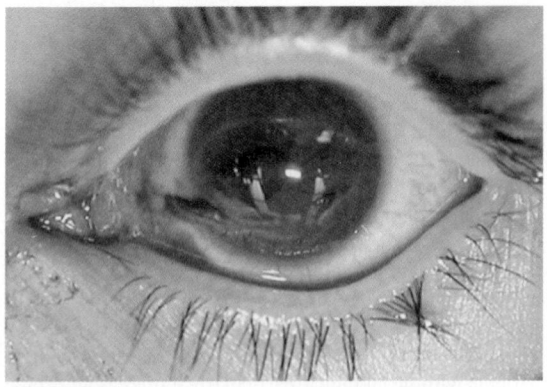

▲ **Figure 7–8.** Corneoscleral laceration inferonasally with pupil displaced toward the laceration and iris incarcerated in wound. (From James J Augsburger and Zélia M Corrêa. Reproduced, with permission, from Riordan-Eva P, Cunningham ET Jr. *Vaughan & Asbury's General Ophthalmology*, 18th ed. McGraw-Hill, 2011.)

instructed not to squeeze the eye shut and to remain still. The eye is routinely imaged by radiography, and CT scanning if necessary, to identify and localize any metallic intraocular foreign body. MRI is contraindicated because of the risk of movement of the foreign body in the magnetic field. Endophthalmitis occurs in over 5% of open globe injuries.

▶ When to Refer

Patients with suspected globe laceration must be referred emergently to an ophthalmologist.

Agrawal R et al. Pre-operative variables affecting final vision outcome with a critical review of ocular trauma classification for posterior open globe (zone III) injury. Indian J Ophthalmol. 2013 Oct;61(10):541–5. [PMID: 24212303]

Agrawal R et al. Prognostic factors for open globe injuries and correlation of ocular trauma score at a tertiary referral eye care centre in Singapore. Indian J Ophthalmol. 2013 Sep;61(9):502–6. [PMID: 24104709]

Bunting H et al. Prediction of visual outcomes after open globe injury in children: a 17-year Canadian experience. J AAPOS. 2013 Feb;17(1):43–8. [PMID: 23363881]

Nishide T et al. Preoperative factors associated with improvement in visual acuity after globe rupture treatment. Eur J Ophthalmol. 2013 Sep–Oct;23(5):718–22. [PMID: 23483506]

Patel SN et al. Diagnostic value of clinical examination and radiographic imaging in identification of intraocular foreign bodies in open globe injury. Eur J Ophthalmol. 2012 Mar–Apr;22(2):259–68. [PMID: 21607931]

ULTRAVIOLET KERATITIS (Actinic Keratitis)

Ultraviolet burns of the cornea are usually caused by use of a sunlamp without eye protection, exposure to a welding arc, or exposure to the sun when skiing ("snow blindness"). There are no immediate symptoms, but about 6–12 hours later the patient complains of agonizing pain and severe photophobia. Slit-lamp examination after instillation of sterile fluorescein shows diffuse punctate staining of both corneas.

Treatment consists of binocular patching and instillation of 1–2 drops of 1% cyclopentolate (to relieve the discomfort of ciliary spasm). All patients recover within 24–48 hours without complications. Local anesthetics should not be prescribed because they delay corneal epithelial healing.

CHEMICAL CONJUNCTIVITIS & KERATITIS

Chemical burns are treated by copious irrigation of the eyes with tap water, saline solution, or buffering solution if available as soon as possible after exposure. Neutralization of an acid with an alkali or vice versa generates heat and may cause further damage. Alkali injuries are more serious and require prolonged irrigation, since alkalies are not precipitated by the proteins of the eye as are acids. It is important to remove any retained particulate matter such as is typically present in injuries involving cement and building plaster. This may require double eversion of the upper lid. The pupil should be dilated with 1% cyclopentolate, 1 drop twice a day, to relieve discomfort and prophylactic topical antibiotics should be started. In moderate to severe injuries, intensive topical corticosteroids and topical and systemic vitamin C are also necessary. Complications include mucus deficiency, scarring of the cornea and conjunctiva, symblepharon (adhesions between the tarsal and bulbar conjunctiva), tear duct obstruction, and secondary infection. It can be difficult to assess severity of chemical burns without slit-lamp examination.

Chau JP et al. A systematic review of methods of eye irrigation for adults and children with ocular chemical burns. Worldviews Evid Based Nurs. 2012 Aug;9(3):129–38. [PMID: 21649853]
Singh P et al. Ocular chemical injuries and their management. Oman J Ophthalmol. 2013 May;6(2):83–86. [PMID: 24082664]

TREATMENT OF OCULAR DISORDERS

Table 7–2 lists commonly used ophthalmic drugs and their indications and costs.

PRECAUTIONS IN MANAGEMENT OF OCULAR DISORDERS

1. Use of Local Anesthetics

Unsupervised self-administration of local anesthetics is dangerous because the patient may further injure an anesthetized eye without knowing it. The drug may also interfere with the normal healing process.

2. Pupillary Dilation

Dilating the pupil can very occasionally precipitate acute glaucoma if the patient has a narrow anterior chamber angle and should be undertaken with caution if the anterior chamber is obviously shallow (readily determined by oblique illumination of the anterior segment of the eye). A short-acting mydriatic such as tropicamide should be used and the patient warned to report immediately if ocular discomfort or redness develops. Angle closure is more likely to occur if pilocarpine is used to overcome pupillary dilation than if the pupil is allowed to constrict naturally.

Gracitelli CP et al. Ability of non-ophthalmologist doctors to detect eyes with occludable angles using the flashlight test. Int Ophthalmol. 2013 Oct 1. [Epub ahead of print] [PMID: 24081914]
Lavanya R et al. Risk of acute angle closure and changes in intraocular pressure after pupillary dilation in Asian subjects with narrow angles. Ophthalmology. 2012 Mar;119(3):474–80. [PMID: 22118999]

3. Corticosteroid Therapy

Repeated use of local corticosteroids presents several hazards: herpes simplex (dendritic) keratitis, fungal infection, open-angle glaucoma, and cataract formation. Furthermore, perforation of the cornea may occur when corticosteroids are used for herpes simplex keratitis. Topical nonsteroidal anti-inflammatory agents are being used increasingly. The potential for causing or exacerbating systemic hypertension, diabetes mellitus, gastritis, osteoporosis, or glaucoma must always be borne in mind when systemic corticosteroids are prescribed, such as for uveitis or giant cell arteritis.

4. Contaminated Eye Medications

Ophthalmic solutions are prepared with the same degree of care as fluids intended for intravenous administration, but once bottles are opened there is always a risk of contamination, particularly with solutions of tetracaine, proparacaine, fluorescein, and any preservative-free preparations. The most dangerous is fluorescein, as this solution is frequently contaminated with *P aeruginosa*, which can rapidly destroy the eye. Sterile fluorescein filter paper strips are recommended for use in place of fluorescein solutions.

Whether in plastic or glass containers, eye solutions should not remain in use for long periods after the bottle is opened. Four weeks after opening is an absolute maximal time to use a solution containing preservatives before discarding. Preservative-free preparations should be kept refrigerated and discarded within 1 week after opening. Single-use vials should not be reused.

If the eye has been injured accidentally or by surgical trauma, it is of the greatest importance to use freshly opened bottles of sterile medications or single-use eyedropper units.

5. Toxic & Hypersensitivity Reactions to Topical Therapy

In patients receiving long-term topical therapy, local toxic or hypersensitivity reactions to the active agent or preservatives may develop, especially if there is inadequate tear secretion. Preservatives in contact lens cleaning solutions may produce similar problems. Burning and soreness are exacerbated by drop instillation or contact lens insertion; occasionally, fibrosis and scarring of the conjunctiva and cornea may occur. Preservative-free topical medication and contact lens solutions are available.

An antibiotic instilled into the eye can sensitize the patient to that drug and cause an allergic reaction upon subsequent systemic administration. Potentially fatal anaphylaxis is known to occur in up to 0.3% of patients after intravenous fluorescein for fluorescein angiography. Anaphylaxis also has been reported after topical fluorescein.

6. Systemic Effects of Ocular Drugs

The systemic absorption of certain topical drugs (through the conjunctival vessels and lacrimal drainage system) must be considered when there is a systemic medical contraindication to the use of the drug. Ophthalmic solutions of the nonselective beta-blockers, eg, timolol, may worsen bradycardia, heart failure, or asthma. Phenylephrine eye drops may precipitate hypertensive crises and angina. Also to be considered are adverse interactions between systemically administered and ocular drugs. Using only 1 or 2 drops at a time and a few minutes of nasolacrimal occlusion or eyelid closure ensure maximum efficacy and decrease systemic side effects of topical agents.

ADVERSE OCULAR EFFECTS OF SYSTEMIC DRUGS

Systemically administered drugs produce a wide variety of adverse effects on the visual system. Table 7–3 lists the major examples. Routine periodic screening is recommended to exclude retinopathy in patients treated with hydroxychloroquine.

Blomquist PH. Ocular complications of systemic medications. Am J Med Sci. 2011 Jul;342(1):62–9. [PMID: 21139494]

Fraunfelder FW. Ocular & systemic side effects of drugs. In: *Vaughan & Asbury's General Ophthalmology*, 18th ed. Riordan-Eva P et al (editors). McGraw-Hill, 2011.

González-Martín-Moro J et al. Impact of tamsulosin exposure on late complications following cataract surgery: retrospective cohort study. Int Ophthalmol. 2013 Oct 25. [Epub ahead of print] [PMID: 24158613]

Marmor MF. Comparison of screening procedures in hydroxychloroquine toxicity. Arch Ophthalmol. 2012 Apr;130(4): 461–9. [PMID: 22159170]

Marmor MF et al. Revised recommendations on screening for chloroquine and hydroxychloroquine retinopathy. Ophthalmology. 2011 Feb;118(2):415–22. [PMID: 21292109]

Stelton CR et al. Hydrochloroquine retinopathy: characteristic presentation with review of screening. Clin Rheumatol. 2013 Jun;32(6):895–8. [PMID: 23515601]

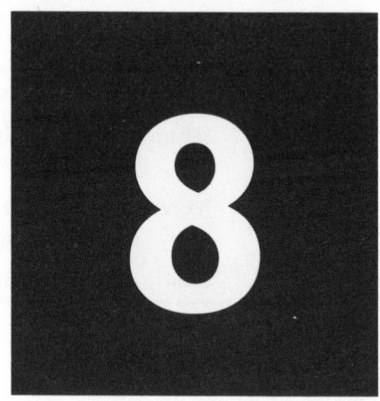

Ear, Nose, & Throat Disorders

8

Lawrence R. Lustig, MD

Joshua S. Schindler, MD

DISEASES OF THE EAR

HEARING LOSS

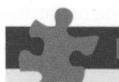

ESSENTIALS OF DIAGNOSIS

▶ Three main types of hearing loss: conductive, sensory, and neural.

▶ Most commonly due to cerumen impaction, transient eustachian tube dysfunction associated with upper respiratory tract infection, or age-related hearing loss.

▶ Classification & Epidemiology

Table 8–1 categorizes hearing loss as normal, mild, moderate, severe, and profound and outlines the vocal equivalent as well as the decibel range.

A. Conductive Hearing Loss

Conductive hearing loss results from dysfunction of the external or middle ear. There are four mechanisms, each resulting in impairment of the passage of sound vibrations to the inner ear: (1) obstruction (eg, cerumen impaction), (2) mass loading (eg, middle ear effusion), (3) stiffness effect (eg, otosclerosis), and (4) discontinuity (eg, ossicular disruption). Conductive losses in adults are most commonly due to cerumen impaction or transient eustachian tube dysfunction associated with upper respiratory tract infection. Persistent conductive losses usually result from chronic ear infection, trauma, or otosclerosis. Conductive hearing loss is often correctable with medical or surgical therapy—or in some cases both.

B. Sensory Hearing Loss

Sensory and neural causes of hearing loss are difficult to differentiate due to testing methodology, thus often referred to as "sensorineural." Sensory hearing loss results from deterioration of the cochlea, usually due to loss of hair cells from the organ of Corti. Sensorineural losses in adults are common. The most common form is a gradually progressive, predominantly high-frequency loss with advancing age (presbyacusis). Additional common causes include excessive noise exposure, head trauma, and systemic diseases. An individual's genetic make-up influences all of these causes of hearing loss. Sensory hearing loss is usually not correctable with medical or surgical therapy but often may be prevented or stabilized. An exception is a sudden sensory hearing loss, which may respond to corticosteroids if delivered within several weeks of onset.

C. Neural Hearing Loss

Neural hearing loss occurs with lesions involving the eighth nerve, auditory nuclei, ascending tracts, or auditory cortex. It is the least common clinically recognized cause of hearing loss. Causes include acoustic neuroma, multiple sclerosis, and auditory neuropathy.

▶ Evaluation of Hearing (Audiology)

In a quiet room, the hearing level may be estimated by having the patient repeat aloud words presented in a soft whisper, a normal spoken voice, or a shout. A 512-Hz tuning fork is useful in differentiating conductive from sensorineural losses. In the **Weber test,** the tuning fork is placed on the forehead or front teeth. In conductive losses, the sound appears louder in the poorer-hearing ear, whereas in sensorineural losses it radiates to the better side. In the **Rinne test,** the tuning fork is placed alternately on the mastoid bone and in front of the ear canal. In conductive losses > 25 dB, bone conduction exceeds air conduction; in sensorineural losses, the opposite is true.

Formal audiometric studies are performed in a sound-proofed room. Pure-tone thresholds in decibels (dB) are obtained over the range of 250–8000 Hz for both air and bone conduction. Conductive losses create a gap between the air and bone thresholds, whereas in sensorineural losses both air and bone thresholds are equally diminished. Speech discrimination measures the clarity of hearing, reported as percentage correct (90–100% is normal). The site of the lesion responsible for sensorineural loss (cochlea versus central auditory system) may be determined with auditory brainstem-evoked responses; however, an MRI

Table 8–1. Hearing loss classification.

Classification	Vocal Equivalent	Decibel (dB) Range
Normal	Soft whisper	0–20 dB
Mild	Soft spoken voice	20–40 dB
Moderate	Normal spoken	40–60 dB
Severe	Loud spoken voice	60–80 dB
Profound	Shout	>80 dB

scan is preferred for its better sensitivity and specificity in the evaluation of central lesions.

Every patient who complains of a hearing loss should be referred for audiologic evaluation unless the cause is easily remediable (eg, cerumen impaction, otitis media). Because idiopathic sudden sensorineural hearing loss requires treatment (corticosteroids) within a limited several week time period, any new-onset hearing loss without obvious ear pathology needs an immediate audiometric referral. Routine audiologic screening is recommended for adults who have been exposed to potentially injurious levels of noise or in those who have reached the age of 65, after which screening evaluations may be done every few years.

Isaacson B. Hearing loss. Med Clin North Am. 2010 Sep;94(5):973–88. [PMID: 20736107]

Walker JJ et al. Audiometry screening and interpretation. Am Fam Physician. 2013 Jan 1;87(1):41–7. [PMID: 23317024]

▶ **Hearing Amplification**

Patients with hearing loss not correctable by medical therapy may benefit from hearing amplification. Contemporary hearing aids are comparatively free of distortion and have been miniaturized to the point where they often may be contained entirely within the ear canal or lie inconspicuously behind the ear. To optimize the benefit, a hearing aid must be carefully selected to conform to the nature of the hearing loss.

For patients with conductive loss or unilateral profound sensorineural loss, bone-conducting hearing aids directly stimulate the ipsilateral cochlea (for conductive losses) or contralateral ear (profound unilateral sensorineural loss).

For patients with severe to profound sensory hearing loss, the cochlear implant—an electronic device that is surgically implanted into the cochlea to stimulate the auditory nerve—offers socially beneficial auditory rehabilitation to most adults with acquired deafness and children with congenital or genetic deafness. New trends in cochlear implantation include its use for patients with only partial deafness, preserving residual hearing and allowing both acoustic and electrical hearing in the same ear, as well as bilateral cochlear implantation.

Gaylor JM et al. Cochlear implantation in adults: a systematic review and meta-analysis. JAMA Otolaryngol Head Neck Surg. 2013 Mar;139(3):265–72. [PMID: 23429927]

Pai I et al. Outcome of bone-anchored hearing aids for single-sided deafness: a prospective study. Acta Otolaryngol. 2012 Jul;132(7):751–5. [PMID: 22497318]

Woodson EA et al. The hybrid cochlear implant: a review. Adv Otorhinolaryngol. 2010;67:125–34. [PMID: 19955729]

DISEASES OF THE AURICLE

Disorders of the auricle are for the most part dermatologic. Skin cancers due to sun exposure are common and may be treated with standard techniques. Traumatic auricular hematoma must be recognized and drained to prevent significant cosmetic deformity (cauliflower ear) or canal blockage resulting from dissolution of supporting cartilage. Similarly, cellulitis of the auricle must be treated promptly to prevent development of perichondritis and its resultant deformity. Relapsing polychondritis is a rheumatologic disorder often associated with recurrent, frequently bilateral, painful episodes of auricular erythema and edema. Treatment with corticosteroids may help forestall cartilage dissolution. Respiratory compromise may occur as a result of progressive involvement of the cartilaginous tracheobronchial tree. Chondritis and perichondritis may be differentiated from auricular cellulitis by sparing of involvement of the lobule, which does not contain cartilage.

Lambru G et al. The red ear syndrome. J Headache Pain. 2013 Oct 4;14(1):83. [PMID: 24093332]

Summers A. Managing auricular haematoma to prevent 'cauliflower ear'. Emerg Nurse. 2012 Sep;20(5):28–30. [PMID: 23256352]

DISEASES OF THE EAR CANAL

1. Cerumen Impaction

Cerumen is a protective secretion produced by the outer portion of the ear canal. In most persons, the ear canal is self-cleansing. Recommended hygiene consists of cleaning the external opening with a washcloth over the index finger without entering the canal itself. In most cases, cerumen impaction is self-induced through ill-advised attempts at cleaning the ear. It may be relieved with detergent ear drops (eg, 3% hydrogen peroxide; 6.5% carbamide peroxide), mechanical removal, suction, or irrigation. Irrigation is performed with water at body temperature to avoid a vestibular caloric response. The stream should be directed at the posterior ear canal wall adjacent to the cerumen plug. Irrigation should be performed only when the tympanic membrane is known to be intact.

Use of jet irrigators designed for cleaning teeth (eg, WaterPik) for wax removal should be avoided since they may result in tympanic membrane perforations. Following professional irrigation, the ear canal should be thoroughly dried (eg, by instilling isopropyl alcohol or using a hair blow-dryer on low-power setting) to reduce the likelihood of inducing external otitis. Specialty referral for cleaning under microscopic guidance is indicated when the impaction is frequently recurrent, has not responded to routine measures, or if the patient has a history of chronic otitis media or tympanic membrane perforation.

Roland PS et al. Clinical practice guideline: cerumen impaction. Otolaryngol Head Neck Surg. 2008 Sep;139(3 Suppl 2): S1–S21. [PMID: 18707628]

2. Foreign Bodies

Foreign bodies in the ear canal are more frequent in children than in adults. Firm materials may be removed with a loop or a hook, taking care not to displace the object medially toward the tympanic membrane; microscopic guidance is helpful. Aqueous irrigation should not be performed for organic foreign bodies (eg, beans, insects), because water may cause them to swell. Living insects are best immobilized before removal by filling the ear canal with lidocaine.

Williams J et al. Removal of foreign bodies from children's ears: a nurse-led clinic. Nurs Stand. 2013 Aug 21–27;27(51):43–6. [PMID: 23965098]

3. External Otitis

ESSENTIALS OF DIAGNOSIS

▶ Painful erythema and edema of the ear canal skin.

▶ Often with purulent exudate.

▶ May evolve into osteomyelitis of the skull base, often called malignant external otitis, particularly in the diabetic or immunocompromised patient.

▶ General Considerations

External otitis presents with otalgia, frequently accompanied by pruritus and purulent discharge. There is often a history of recent water exposure (ie, swimmer's ear) or mechanical trauma (eg, scratching, cotton applicators). External otitis is usually caused by gram-negative rods (eg, *Pseudomonas*, *Proteus*) or fungi (eg, *Aspergillus*), which grow in the presence of excessive moisture. Persistent external otitis in the diabetic or immunocompromised patient may evolve into osteomyelitis of the skull base, often called **malignant external otitis.** Usually caused by *Pseudomonas aeruginosa*, osteomyelitis begins in the floor of the ear canal and may extend into the middle fossa floor, the clivus, and even the contralateral skull base.

▶ Clinical Findings

Examination reveals erythema and edema of the ear canal skin, often with a purulent exudate. Manipulation of the auricle often elicits pain. Because the lateral surface of the tympanic membrane is ear canal skin, it is often erythematous. However, in contrast to acute otitis media, it moves normally with pneumatic otoscopy. When the canal skin is very edematous, it may be impossible to visualize the tympanic membrane. **Malignant external otitis** usually presents with persistent foul aural discharge, granulations in the ear canal, deep otalgia, and in advanced cases,

progressive cranial nerve palsies involving nerves VI, VII, IX, X, XI, or XII. Diagnosis is confirmed by the demonstration of osseous erosion on CT and radionuclide scanning.

▶ Treatment

Fundamental to the treatment of external otitis is protection of the ear from additional moisture and avoidance of further mechanical injury by scratching. In cases of swimmer's ear, acidification with a drying agent (ie, a 50/50 mixture of isopropyl alcohol/white vinegar) after getting moisture into the ear is often helpful. When infected, acidic otic antibiotic drops that contain either an aminoglycoside or fluoroquinolone antibiotic, with or without corticosteroids, are usually effective (eg, neomycin sulfate, polymyxin B sulfate, and hydrocortisone). Purulent debris filling the ear canal should be gently removed to permit entry of the topical medication. Drops should be used abundantly (five or more drops three or four times a day) to penetrate the depths of the canal. When substantial edema of the canal wall prevents entry of drops into the ear canal, a wick is placed to facilitate entry of the medication. In recalcitrant cases—particularly when cellulitis of the periauricular tissue has developed—oral fluoroquinolones (eg, ciprofloxacin, 500 mg twice daily for 1 week) are the drugs of choice because of their effectiveness against *Pseudomonas* species. Any case of persistent otitis externa in an immunocompromised or diabetic individual must be referred for specialty evaluation.

Treatment of **malignant external otitis** is medical, requiring prolonged antipseudomonal antibiotic administration, often for several months. Although intravenous therapy is often required (eg, ciprofloxacin 200–400 mg every 12 hours), selected patients may be treated with oral ciprofloxacin (500–1000 mg twice daily), which has proved effective against many of the causative *Pseudomonas* strains. To avoid relapse, antibiotic therapy should be continued, even in the asymptomatic patient, until gallium scanning indicates a marked reduction in the inflammatory process.

Kaushik V et al. Interventions for acute otitis externa. Cochrane Database Syst Rev. 2010 Jan 20;(1): CD004740. [PMID: 20091565]

Mahdyoun P et al. Necrotizing otitis externa: a systematic review. Otol Neurotol. 2013 Jun;34(4):620–9. [PMID: 23598690]

4. Pruritus

Pruritus of the external auditory canal, particularly at the meatus, is a common problem. While it may be associated with external otitis or with dermatologic conditions such as seborrheic dermatitis and psoriasis, most cases are self-induced either from excoriation or by overly zealous ear cleaning. To permit regeneration of the protective cerumen blanket, patients should be instructed to avoid use of soap and water or cotton swabs in the ear canal and avoid any scratching. Patients with excessively dry canal skin may benefit from application of mineral oil, which helps counteract dryness and repel moisture. When an inflammatory component is present, topical application of a corticosteroid (eg, 0.1% triamcinolone) may be beneficial.

Acar B et al. New treatment strategy and assessment question-naire for external auditory canal pruritus: topical pimecroli-mus therapy and Modified Itch Severity Scale. J Laryngol Otol. 2010 Feb;124(2):147–51. [PMID: 19922703]

5. Exostoses & Osteomas

Bony overgrowths of the ear canal are a frequent incidental finding and occasionally have clinical significance. Clini-cally, they present as skin-covered bony mounds in the medial ear canal obscuring the tympanic membrane to a variable degree. Solitary osteomas are of no significance as long as they do not cause obstruction or infection. Multiple exostoses, which are generally acquired from repeated exposure to cold water (eg, "surfer's ear") may progress and require surgical removal.

Spielmann PM et al. Surgical management of external auditory canal lesions. J Laryngol Otol. 2013 Mar;127(3):246–51. [PMID: 23351401]

6. Neoplasia

The most common neoplasm of the ear canal is squamous cell carcinoma. When an apparent otitis externa does not resolve on therapy, a malignancy should be suspected and biopsy performed. This disease carries a very high 5-year mortality rate because the tumor tends to invade the lym-phatics of the cranial base and must be treated with wide surgical resection and radiation therapy. Adenomatous tumors, originating from the ceruminous glands, generally follow a more indolent course.

Bacciu A et al. Guidelines for treating temporal bone carcinoma based on long-term outcomes. Otol Neurotol. 2013 Jul;34(5):898–907. [PMID: 23507994]
Lassig AA et al. Squamous cell carcinoma involving the temporal bone: lateral temporal bone resection as primary interven-tion. Otol Neurotol. 2013 Jan;34(1):141–50. [PMID: 23202152]

DISEASES OF THE EUSTACHIAN TUBE

1. Eustachian Tube Dysfunction

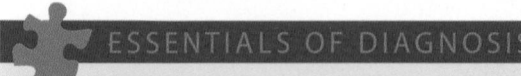

ESSENTIALS OF DIAGNOSIS

► Aural fullness.
► Fluctuating hearing.
► Discomfort with barometric pressure change.
► At risk for serous otitis media.

The tube that connects the middle ear to the nasophar-ynx—the eustachian tube—provides ventilation and drain-age for the middle ear cleft. It is normally closed, opening only during swallowing or yawning. When eustachian tube function is compromised, air trapped within the middle ear becomes absorbed and negative pressure results. The most common causes of eustachian tube dysfunction are diseases associated with edema of the tubal lining, such as viral upper respiratory tract infections and allergy. The patient usually reports a sense of fullness in the ear and mild to moderate impairment of hearing. When the tube is only partially blocked, swallowing or yawning may elicit a popping or crackling sound. Examination may reveal retraction of the tympanic membrane and decreased mobility on pneumatic otoscopy. Following a viral illness, this disorder is usually transient, lasting days to weeks. Treatment with systemic and intranasal decongestants (eg, pseudoephedrine, 60 mg orally every 4 hours; oxymetazo-line, 0.05% spray every 8–12 hours) combined with autoin-flation by forced exhalation against closed nostrils may hasten relief. Autoinflation should not be recommended to patients with active intranasal infection, since this maneu-ver may precipitate middle ear infection. Allergic patients may also benefit from desensitization or intranasal cortico-steroids (eg, beclomethasone dipropionate, two sprays in each nostril twice daily for 2–6 weeks). Air travel, rapid altitudinal change, and underwater diving should be avoided during an active phase of the disease.

Conversely, an overly patent eustachian tube, termed "patulous eustachian tube," is a relatively uncommon prob-lem, though may be quite distressing. Typical complaints include fullness in the ear and autophony, an exaggerated ability to hear oneself breathe and speak. A patulous eusta-chian tube may develop during rapid weight loss, or it may be idiopathic. In contrast to a hypofunctioning eustachian tube, the aural pressure is often made worse by exertion and may diminish during an upper respiratory tract infec-tion. Although physical examination is usually normal, respiratory excursions of the tympanic membrane may occasionally be detected during vigorous breathing. Treat-ment includes avoidance of decongestant products, inser-tion of a ventilating tube to reduce the outward stretch of the eardrum during phonation, and, rarely, surgical nar-rowing of the eustachian tube.

Caffier PP et al. Impact of laser eustachian tuboplasty on middle ear ventilation, hearing, and tinnitus in chronic tube dysfunc-tion. Ear Hear. 2011 Feb;32(1):132–9. [PMID: 20585250]
Park MS et al. Clinical manifestations of aural fullness. Yonsei Med J. 2012 Sep;53(5):985–91. [PMID: 22869482]

2. Serous Otitis Media

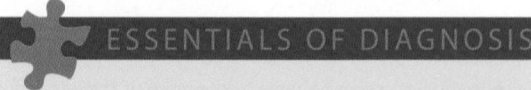

ESSENTIALS OF DIAGNOSIS

► Blocked eustachian tube remains for a prolonged period.
► Resultant negative pressure will result in transuda-tion of fluid.

Prolonged eustachian tube dysfunction with resultant negative middle ear pressure may cause a transudation of fluid. This condition, known as serous otitis media, is especially common in children because their eustachian tubes are narrower and more horizontal in orientation than those in adults. Serous otitis media is less common in adults, in whom it usually occurs after an upper respiratory tract infection, with barotrauma, or with chronic allergic rhinitis. In any adult with persistent unilateral serous otitis media, nasopharyngeal carcinoma must be excluded. The tympanic membrane in serous otitis media is dull and hypomobile, occasionally accompanied by air bubbles in the middle ear and conductive hearing loss. The treatment of serous otitis media is similar to that for eustachian tube dysfunction. A short course of oral corticosteroids (eg, prednisone, 40 mg/d for 7 days) has been advocated by some clinicians, as have oral antibiotics (eg, amoxicillin, 250 mg three times daily for 7 days)—or even a combination of the two. The role of these regimens remains controversial, but they are probably of little lasting benefit.

When medication fails to bring relief after several months, a ventilating tube placed through the tympanic membrane may restore hearing and alleviate the sense of aural fullness. Endoscopically guided laser expansion of the nasopharyngeal orifice of the eustachian tube may improve function in recalcitrant cases.

Harmes KM et al. Otitis media: diagnosis and treatment. Am Fam Physician. 2013 Oct 1;88(7):435–40. [PMID: 24134083]
Khodaverdi M et al. Hearing 25 years after surgical treatment of otitis media with effusion in early childhood. Int J Pediatr Otorhinolaryngol. 2013 Feb;77(2):241–7. [PMID: 23218983]

3. Barotrauma

Persons with poor eustachian tube function (eg, congenital narrowness or acquired mucosal edema) may be unable to equalize the barometric stress exerted on the middle ear by air travel, rapid altitudinal change, or underwater diving. The problem is generally most acute during airplane descent, since the negative middle ear pressure tends to collapse and block the eustachian tube. Several measures are useful to enhance eustachian tube function and avoid otic barotrauma. The patient should be advised to swallow, yawn, and autoinflate frequently during descent, which may be painful if the eustachian tube collapses. Oral decongestants (eg, pseudoephedrine, 60–120 mg) should be taken several hours before anticipated arrival time so that they will be maximally effective during descent. Topical decongestants such as 1% phenylephrine nasal spray should be administered 1 hour before arrival.

For acute negative middle ear pressure that persists on the ground, treatment includes decongestants and attempts at autoinflation. Myringotomy (creation of a small eardrum perforation) provides immediate relief and is appropriate in the setting of severe otalgia and hearing loss. Repeated episodes of barotrauma in persons who must fly frequently may be alleviated by insertion of ventilating tubes.

Underwater diving may represent an even a greater barometric stress to the ear than flying. The problem occurs most commonly during the descent phase, when pain develops within the first 15 feet if inflation of the middle ear via the eustachian tube has not occurred. Divers must descend slowly and equilibrate in stages to avoid the development of severely negative pressures in the tympanum that may result in hemorrhage (hemotympanum) or perilymphatic fistula. In the latter, the oval or round window ruptures, resulting in sensory hearing loss and acute vertigo. Sensory hearing loss or vertigo, which develops during the ascent phase of a saturation dive, may be the first (or only) symptom of decompression sickness. Immediate recompression will return intravascular gas bubbles to solution and restore the inner ear microcirculation. Patients should be warned to avoid diving when they have upper respiratory infections or episodes of nasal allergy. Tympanic membrane perforation is an absolute contraindication to diving, as the patient will experience an unbalanced thermal stimulus to the semicircular canals and may experience vertigo, disorientation, and even emesis.

Klingmann C. Inner ear decompression sickness in compressed-air diving. Undersea Hyperb Med. 2012 Jan–Feb;39(1): 589–94. [PMID: 22400449]
Magliulo G et al. Pneumolabyrinth following eustachian tube insufflation. Otolaryngol Head Neck Surg. 2012 Nov;147(5): 980–1. [PMID: 22927699]

DISEASES OF THE MIDDLE EAR

1. Acute Otitis Media

ESSENTIALS OF DIAGNOSIS

► Otalgia, often with an upper respiratory tract infection.

► Erythema and hypomobility of tympanic membrane.

► General Considerations

Acute otitis media is a bacterial infection of the mucosally lined air-containing spaces of the temporal bone. Purulent material forms not only within the middle ear cleft but also within the pneumatized mastoid air cells and petrous apex. Acute otitis media is usually precipitated by a viral upper respiratory tract infection that causes eustachian tube obstruction. This results in accumulation of fluid and mucus, which becomes secondarily infected by bacteria. The most common pathogens are *Streptococcus pneumoniae*, *Haemophilus influenzae*, and *Streptococcus pyogenes*.

► Clinical Findings

Acute otitis media is most common in infants and children, although it may occur at any age. Presenting symptoms and signs include otalgia, aural pressure, decreased hearing, and often fever. The typical physical findings are erythema and decreased mobility of the tympanic membrane. Occasionally, bullae will be seen on the tympanic membrane.

Rarely, when middle ear empyema is severe, the tympanic membrane can bulge outward. In such cases, tympanic membrane rupture is imminent. Rupture is accompanied by a sudden decrease in pain, followed by the onset of otorrhea. With appropriate therapy, spontaneous healing of the tympanic membrane occurs in most cases. When perforation persists, chronic otitis media may evolve. Mastoid tenderness often accompanies acute otitis media and is due to the presence of pus within the mastoid air cells. This alone does not indicate suppurative (surgical) mastoiditis. Frank swelling over the mastoid bone or the association of cranial neuropathies or central findings indicates severe disease requiring urgent care.

▶ Treatment

The treatment of acute otitis media is specific antibiotic therapy, often combined with nasal decongestants. The first-choice oral antibiotic treatment is amoxicillin (80–90 mg/kg/d divided twice daily) (*or* erythromycin [50 mg/kg/d]) plus sulfonamide (150 mg/kg/d) for 10 days. Alternatives useful in resistant cases are cefaclor (20–40 mg/kg/d) or amoxicillin-clavulanate (20–40 mg/kg/d) combinations.

Tympanocentesis for bacterial (aerobic and anaerobic) and fungal culture may be performed by any experienced physician. A 20-gauge spinal needle bent 90 degrees to the hub attached to a 3-mL syringe is inserted through the inferior portion of the tympanic membrane. Interposition of a pliable connecting tube between the needle and syringe permits an assistant to aspirate without inducing movement of the needle. Tympanocentesis is useful for otitis media in immunocompromised patients and when infection persists or recurs despite multiple courses of antibiotics.

Surgical drainage of the middle ear (myringotomy) is reserved for patients with severe otalgia or when complications of otitis (eg, mastoiditis, meningitis) have occurred.

Recurrent acute otitis media may be managed with long-term antibiotic prophylaxis. Single daily oral doses of sulfamethoxazole (500 mg) or amoxicillin (250 or 500 mg) are given over a period of 1–3 months. Failure of this regimen to control infection is an indication for insertion of ventilating tubes.

Harmes KM et al. Otitis media: diagnosis and treatment. Am Fam Physician. 2013 Oct 1;88(7):435–40. [PMID: 24134083]

2. Chronic Otitis Media

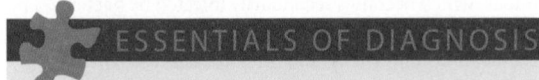

ESSENTIALS OF DIAGNOSIS

▶ Chronic otorrhea with or without otalgia.

▶ Tympanic membrane perforation with conductive hearing loss.

▶ Often amenable to surgical correction.

▶ General Considerations

Chronic infection of the middle ear and mastoid generally develops as a consequence of recurrent acute otitis media, although it may follow other diseases and trauma.

Perforation of the tympanic membrane is usually present. The bacteriology of chronic otitis media differs from that of acute otitis media. Common organisms include *P aeruginosa, Proteus* species, *Staphylococcus aureus,* and mixed anaerobic infections.

▶ Clinical Findings

The clinical hallmark of chronic otitis media is purulent aural discharge. Drainage may be continuous or intermittent, with increased severity during upper respiratory tract infection or following water exposure. Pain is uncommon except during acute exacerbations. Conductive hearing loss results from destruction of the tympanic membrane or ossicular chain, or both.

▶ Treatment

The medical treatment of chronic otitis media includes regular removal of infected debris, use of earplugs to protect against water exposure, and topical antibiotic drops (ofoxacin 0.3% or ciprofloxacin with dexamethasone) for exacerbations. The activity of ciprofloxacin against *Pseudomonas* may help dry a chronically discharging ear when given in a dosage of 500 mg orally twice a day for 1–6 weeks.

Definitive management is surgical in most cases. Tympanic membrane repair may be accomplished with temporalis muscle fascia. Successful reconstruction of the tympanic membrane may be achieved in about 90% of cases, often with elimination of infection and significant improvement in hearing. When the mastoid air cells are involved by irreversible infection, they should be exenterated at the same time through a mastoidectomy.

Shinnabe A et al. Clinical characteristics and surgical benefits and problems of chronic otitis media and middle ear cholesteatoma in elderly patients older than 70 years. Otol Neurotol. 2012 Sep;33(7):1213–7. [PMID: 22801042]

▶ Complications of Otitis Media

A. Cholesteatoma

Cholesteatoma is a special variety of chronic otitis media (Figure 8–1). The most common cause is prolonged eustachian tube dysfunction, with resultant chronic negative middle ear pressure that draws inward the upper flaccid portion of the tympanic membrane. This creates a squamous epithelium-lined sac, which—when its neck becomes obstructed—may fill with desquamated keratin and become chronically infected. Cholesteatomas typically erode bone, with early penetration of the mastoid and destruction of the ossicular chain. Over time they may erode into the inner ear, involve the facial nerve, and on rare occasions spread intracranially. Otoscopic examination may reveal an epitympanic retraction pocket or a marginal tympanic membrane perforation that exudes keratin debris, or granulation tissue. The treatment of cholesteatoma is surgical marsupialization of the sac or its complete removal. This may require the creation of a "mastoid bowl" in which the ear canal and mastoid are joined into a large common cavity that must be periodically cleaned.

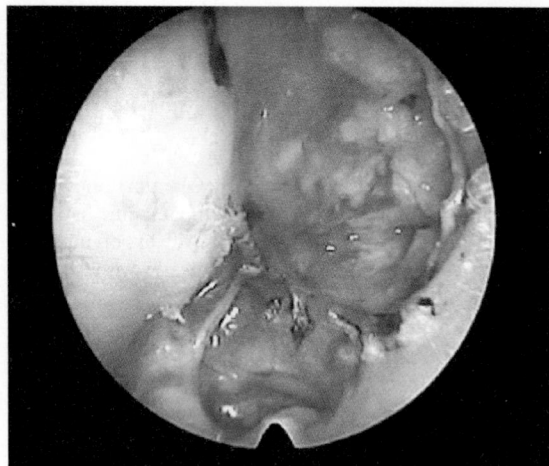

▲ **Figure 8–1. Cholesteatoma.** (From Vladimir Zlinksy, MD in Roy F. Sullivan, PhD: Audiology Forum: Video Otoscopy, www.RCSullivan.com; reproduced with permissions from Usatine RP, Smith MA, Mayeaux EJ Jr, Chumley H, Tysinger J. *The Color Atlas of Family Medicine*. McGraw-Hill, 2009.)

Nankivell PC et al. Surgery for tympanic membrane retraction pockets. Cochrane Database Syst Rev. 2010 Jul 7;(7): CD007943. [PMID: 20614467]

Prasad SC et al. Current trends in the management of the complications of chronic otitis media with cholesteatoma. Curr Opin Otolaryngol Head Neck Surg. 2013 Oct;21(5):446–54. [PMID: 23892792]

B. Mastoiditis

Acute suppurative mastoiditis usually evolves following several weeks of inadequately treated acute otitis media. It is characterized by postauricular pain and erythema accompanied by a spiking fever. CT scan reveals coalescence of the mastoid air cells due to destruction of their bony septa. Initial treatment consists of intravenous antibiotics (eg, cefazolin 0.5–1.5 g every 6–8 hours) directed against the most common offending organisms (*S pneumoniae, H influenzae*, and *S pyogenes)*, and myringotomy for culture and drainage. Failure of medical therapy indicates the need for surgical drainage (mastoidectomy).

C. Petrous Apicitis

The medial portion of the petrous bone between the inner ear and clivus may become a site of persistent infection when the drainage of its pneumatic cell tracts becomes blocked. This may cause foul discharge, deep ear and retro-orbital pain, and sixth nerve palsy (Gradenigo syndrome); meningitis may be a complication. Treatment is with prolonged antibiotic therapy (based on culture results) and surgical drainage via petrous apicectomy.

Yorgancilar E et al. Complications of chronic suppurative otitis media: a retrospective review. Eur Arch Otorhinolaryngol. 2013 Jan;270(1):69–76. [PMID: 22249835]

D. Facial Paralysis

Facial palsy may be associated with either acute or chronic otitis media. In the acute setting, it results from inflammation of the seventh nerve in its middle ear segment, perhaps mediated through bacterially secreted neurotoxins. Treatment consists of myringotomy for drainage and culture, followed by intravenous antibiotics (based on culture results). The use of corticosteroids is controversial. The prognosis is excellent, with complete recovery in most cases.

Facial palsy associated with chronic otitis media usually evolves slowly due to chronic pressure on the seventh nerve in the middle ear or mastoid by cholesteatoma. Treatment requires surgical correction of the underlying disease. The prognosis is less favorable than for facial palsy associated with acute otitis media.

Kim J et al. Facial nerve paralysis due to chronic otitis media: prognosis in restoration of facial function after surgical intervention. Yonsei Med J. 2012 May;53(3):642–8. [PMID: 22477011]

E. Sigmoid Sinus Thrombosis

Trapped infection within the mastoid air cells adjacent to the sigmoid sinus may cause septic thrombophlebitis. This is heralded by signs of systemic sepsis (spiking fevers, chills), at times accompanied by signs of increased intracranial pressure (headache, lethargy, nausea and vomiting, papilledema). Diagnosis can be made noninvasively by magnetic resonance venography. Primary treatment is with intravenous antibiotics (based on culture results). Surgical drainage with ligation of the internal jugular vein may be indicated when embolization is suspected.

Ropposch T et al. Management of otogenic sigmoid sinus thrombosis. Otol Neurotol. 2011 Sep;32(7):1120–3. [PMID: 21817936]

F. Central Nervous System Infection

Otogenic meningitis is by far the most common intracranial complication of ear infection. In the setting of acute suppurative otitis media, it arises from hematogenous spread of bacteria, most commonly *H influenzae* and *S pneumoniae*. In chronic otitis media, it results either from passage of infections along preformed pathways such as the petrosquamous suture line or from direct extension of disease through the dural plates of the petrous pyramid.

Epidural abscesses arise from direct extension of disease in the setting of chronic infection. They are usually asymptomatic but may present with deep local pain, headache, and low-grade fever. They are often discovered as an incidental finding at surgery. Brain abscess may arise in the temporal lobe or cerebellum as a result of septic thrombophlebitis adjacent to an epidural abscess. The predominant causative organisms are *S aureus, S pyogenes*, and *S pneumoniae*. Rupture into the subarachnoid space results in meningitis and often death. (See Chapter 30.)

Yorgancilar E et al. Complications of chronic suppurative otitis media: a retrospective review. Eur Arch Otorhinolaryngol. 2013 Jan;270(1):69–76. [PMID: 22249835]

3. Otosclerosis

Otosclerosis is a progressive disease with a marked familial tendency that affects the bony otic capsule. Lesions involving the footplate of the stapes result in increased impedance to the passage of sound through the ossicular chain, producing conductive hearing loss. This may be treated either through the use of a hearing aid or surgical replacement of the stapes with a prosthesis (stapedectomy). When otosclerotic lesions impinge on the cochlea ('cochlear otosclerosis'), permanent sensory hearing loss occurs.

Bloch SL. On the biology of the bony otic capsule and the pathogenesis of otosclerosis. Dan Med J. 2012 Oct;59(10):B4524. [PMID: 23158898]

4. Trauma to the Middle Ear

Tympanic membrane perforation may result from impact injury or explosive acoustic trauma (Figure 8–2). Spontaneous healing occurs in most cases. Persistent perforation may result from secondary infection brought on by exposure to water. Patients should be advised to wear earplugs while swimming or bathing during the healing period. Hemorrhage behind an intact tympanic membrane (hemotympanum) may follow blunt trauma or extreme barotrauma. Spontaneous resolution over several weeks is the usual course. When a conductive hearing loss > 30 dB persists for more than 3 months following trauma, disruption of the ossicular chain should be suspected. Middle ear exploration with reconstruction of the ossicular chain, combined with repair of the tympanic membrane when required, will usually restore hearing.

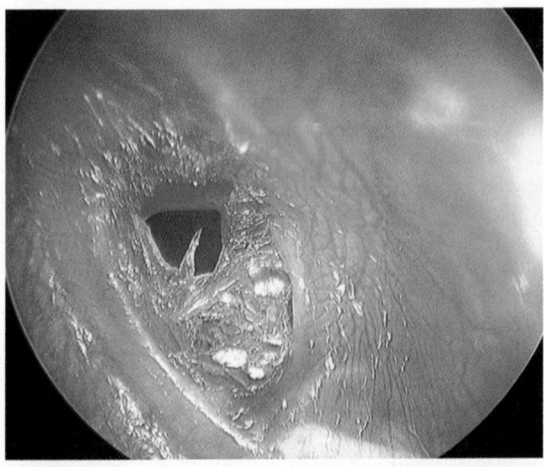

▲ **Figure 8–2.** Traumatic perforation of the left tympanic membrane. (From William Clark, MD; reproduced with permission, from Usatine RP, Smith MA, Mayeaux EJ Jr, Chumley H, Tysinger J. *The Color Atlas of Family Medicine.* McGraw-Hill, 2009.)

Darley DS et al. Otologic considerations of blast injury. Disaster Med Public Health Prep. 2010 Jun;4(2):145–52. [PMID: 20526137]

5. Middle Ear Neoplasia

Primary middle ear tumors are rare. Glomus tumors arise either in the middle ear (glomus tympanicum) or in the jugular bulb with upward erosion into the hypotympanum (glomus jugulare). They present clinically with pulsatile tinnitus and hearing loss. A vascular mass may be visible behind an intact tympanic membrane. Large glomus jugulare tumors are often associated with multiple cranial neuropathies, especially involving nerves VII, IX, X, XI, and XII. Treatment usually requires surgery, radiotherapy, or both. Pulsatile tinnitus thus warrants magnetic resonance angiography and venography to rule out a vascular mass.

EARACHE

Earache can be caused by a variety of otologic problems, but external otitis and acute otitis media are the most common. Differentiation of the two should be apparent by pneumatic otoscopy (see above relevant sections on otitis externa and otitis media). Pain out of proportion to the physical findings may be due to herpes zoster oticus, especially when vesicles appear in the ear canal or concha. Persistent pain and discharge from the ear suggest osteomyelitis of the skull base or cancer, and patients with these complaints should be referred for specialty evaluation.

Nonotologic causes of otalgia are numerous. The sensory innervation of the ear is derived from the trigeminal, facial, glossopharyngeal, vagal, and upper cervical nerves. Because of this rich innervation, referred otalgia is quite frequent. Temporomandibular joint dysfunction is a common cause of referred ear pain. Pain is exacerbated by chewing or psychogenic grinding of the teeth (bruxism) and may be associated with dental malocclusion. Repeated episodes of severe lancinating otalgia may occur in glossopharyngeal neuralgia. Infections and neoplasia that involve the oropharynx, hypopharynx, and larynx frequently cause otalgia. Persistent earache demands specialty referral to exclude cancer of the upper aerodigestive tract.

Conover K. Earache. Emerg Med Clin North Am. 2013 May;31(2):413–42. [PMID: 23601480]

DISEASES OF THE INNER EAR

1. Sensory Hearing Loss

Diseases of the cochlea result in sensory hearing loss, a condition that is usually irreversible. Most cochlear diseases result in bilateral symmetric hearing loss. The presence of unilateral or asymmetric sensorineural hearing loss suggests a lesion proximal to the cochlea. Lesions affecting the eighth cranial nerve and central auditory system are discussed in the section on neural hearing loss. The primary goals in the management of sensory hearing loss are prevention of further losses and functional improvement with amplification and auditory rehabilitation.

A. Presbyacusis

Presbyacusis, or age-related hearing loss, is the most frequent cause of sensory hearing loss and is progressive, predominantly high-frequency, and symmetrical. It is difficult to separate the various etiologic factors (eg, noise trauma, drug exposure) that may contribute to presbyacusis, but genetic predisposition and prior noise exposure appear to play an important role. Most patients notice a loss of speech discrimination that is especially pronounced in noisy environments. About 25% of people between the ages of 65 and 75 years and almost 50% of those over 75 experience hearing difficulties.

Humes LE et al. Central presbycusis: a review and evaluation of the evidence. J Am Acad Audiol. 2012 Sep;23(8):635–66. [PMID: 22967738]

Kidd Iii AR et al. Recent advances in the study of age-related hearing loss: a mini-review. Gerontology. 2012;58(6):490–6. [PMID: 22710288]

B. Noise Trauma

Noise trauma is the second most common cause of sensory hearing loss. Sounds exceeding 85 dB are potentially injurious to the cochlea, especially with prolonged exposures. The loss typically begins in the high frequencies (especially 4000 Hz) and progresses to involve the speech frequencies with continuing exposure. Among the more common sources of injurious noise are industrial machinery, weapons, and excessively loud music. Personal music devices (eg, MP3 and CD players) used at excessive loudness levels may also be potentially injurious. Monitoring noise levels in the workplace by regulatory agencies has led to preventive programs that have reduced the frequency of occupational losses. Individuals of all ages, especially those with existing hearing losses, should wear earplugs when exposed to moderately loud noises and specially designed earmuffs when exposed to explosive noises.

Henderson E et al. Prevalence of noise-induced hearing-threshold shifts and hearing loss among US youths. Pediatrics. 2011 Jan;127(1):e39–46. [PMID: 21187306]

Thurston FE. The worker's ear: A history of noise-induced hearing loss. Am J Ind Med. 2013 Mar;56(3):367–77. [PMID: 22821731]

C. Physical Trauma

Head trauma has effects on the inner ear similar to those of severe acoustic trauma. Some degree of sensory hearing loss may occur following simple concussion and is frequent after skull fracture. Deployment of air bags during an automobile accident has also been associated with hearing loss.

Ohki M et al. Sensorineural hearing loss due to air bag deployment. Case Report Otolaryngol. 2012;2012:203714. [PMID: 22953102]

D. Ototoxicity

Ototoxic substances may affect both the auditory and vestibular systems. The most commonly used ototoxic medications are aminoglycosides; loop diuretics; and several antineoplastic agents, notably cisplatin. These medications may cause irreversible hearing loss even when administered in therapeutic doses. When using these medications, it is important to identify high-risk patients such as those with preexisting hearing losses or kidney disease. Patients simultaneously receiving multiple ototoxic agents are at particular risk owing to ototoxic synergy. Useful measures to reduce the risk of ototoxic injury include serial audiometry and monitoring of serum peak and trough levels and substitution of equivalent nonototoxic drugs whenever possible.

It is possible for topical agents that enter the middle ear to be absorbed into the inner ear via the round window. When the tympanic membrane is perforated, use of potentially ototoxic ear drops (eg, neomycin, gentamicin) is best avoided.

Schacht J et al. Cisplatin and aminoglycoside antibiotics: hearing loss and its prevention. Anat Rec (Hoboken). 2012 Nov;295(11):1837–50. [PMID: 23045231]

E. Sudden Sensory Hearing Loss

Idiopathic sudden loss of hearing in one ear may occur at any age, but typically, it occurs in persons over age 20 years. The cause is unknown; however, one hypothesis is that it results from a viral infection or a sudden vascular occlusion of the internal auditory artery. Prognosis is mixed, with many patients suffering permanent deafness in the involved ear while others have complete recovery. Prompt treatment with corticosteroids has been shown to improve the odds of recovery. A common regimen is oral prednisone, 1 mg/kg/d, followed by a tapering dose over a 10-day period. Intratympanic administration of corticosteroids alone or in association with oral corticosteroids has been associated with an equal or more favorable prognosis in some reports. Because treatment appears to be most effective as close to the onset of the loss as possible, and appears not to be effective after 6 weeks, a prompt audiogram should be obtained in all patients who present with sudden hearing loss without obvious middle ear pathology.

Labus J et al. Meta-analysis for the effect of medical therapy vs. placebo on recovery of idiopathic sudden hearing loss. Laryngoscope. 2010 Sep;120(9):1863–71. [PMID: 20803741]

Rauch SD et al. Oral vs intratympanic corticosteroid therapy for idiopathic sudden sensorineural hearing loss: a randomized trial. JAMA. 2011 May 25;305(20):2071–9. [PMID: 21610239]

Wei BP et al. Steroids for idiopathic sudden sensorineural hearing loss. Cochrane Database Syst Rev. 2013 Jul 2;7: CD003998. [PMID: 23818120]

F. Hereditary Hearing Loss

Sensory hearing loss with onset during adult life often runs in families. The mode of inheritance may be either autosomal dominant or recessive. The age at onset, the rate of progression of hearing loss, and the audiometric pattern (high-frequency, low-frequency, or flat) can often be predicted by studying family members. Great strides have been made in identifying the molecular genetic errors associated with hereditary hearing loss. The connexin-26 mutation, the most common cause of genetic deafness, may be tested clinically. Hearing loss is also frequently found in hereditary mitochondrial disorders.

Angeli S et al. Genetics of hearing and deafness. Anat Rec (Hoboken). 2012 Nov;295(11):1812–29. [PMID: 23044516]
Shearer AE et al. Deafness in the genomics era. Hear Res. 2011 Dec;282(1–2):1–9. [PMID: 22016077]

G. Autoimmune Hearing Loss

Sensory hearing loss may be associated with a wide array of systemic autoimmune disorders such as systemic lupus erythematosus, granulomatosis with polyangiitis (formerly Wegener granulomatosis), and Cogan syndrome (hearing loss, keratitis, aortitis). The loss is most often bilateral and progressive. The hearing level often fluctuates, with periods of deterioration alternating with partial or even complete remission. The tendency is for the gradual evolution of permanent hearing loss, which usually stabilizes with some remaining auditory function but occasionally proceeds to complete deafness. Vestibular dysfunction, particularly dysequilibrium and postural instability, may accompany the auditory symptoms. A syndrome resembling Ménière disease may also occur with intermittent attacks of severe vertigo.

In many cases, the autoimmune pattern of audiovestibular dysfunction presents in the absence of recognized systemic autoimmune disease. Use of laboratory tests to screen for autoimmune disease (eg, antinuclear antibody, rheumatoid factor, erythrocyte sedimentation rate) may be informative. Specific tests of immune reactivity against inner ear antigens (anticochlear antibodies, lymphocyte transformation tests) are current research tools and have limited clinical value to date. Responsiveness to oral corticosteroid treatment is helpful in making the diagnosis and constitutes first-line therapy. If stabilization of hearing becomes dependent on long-term corticosteroid use, steroid-sparing immunosuppressive regimens may become necessary.

Greco A et al. Cogan's syndrome: an autoimmune inner ear disease. Autoimmun Rev. 2013 Jan;12(3):396–400. [PMID: 22846458]
Malik MU et al. Spectrum of immune-mediated inner ear disease and cochlear implant results. Laryngoscope. 2012 Nov;122(11):2557–62. [PMID: 22991211]

2. Tinnitus

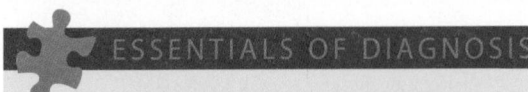

ESSENTIALS OF DIAGNOSIS

► Perception of abnormal ear or head noises.

► Persistent tinnitus often, though not always, indicates the presence of sensory hearing loss.

► Intermittent periods of mild, high-pitched tinnitus lasting seconds to minutes are common in normal-hearing persons.

► General Considerations

Tinnitus is defined as the sensation of sound in the absence of an exogenous sound source. Tinnitus can accompany any form of hearing loss, and its presence provides no diagnostic value in determining the cause of a hearing loss. Approximately 15% of the general population experience some type of tinnitus, with prevalence beyond 20% in aging populations.

► Clinical Findings

A. Symptoms and Signs

Though tinnitus is commonly associated with hearing loss, tinnitus severity correlates poorly with the degree of hearing loss. About one in seven tinnitus sufferers experience severe annoyance and 4% are severely disabled. When severe and persistent, tinnitus may interfere with sleep and the ability to concentrate, resulting in considerable psychological distress.

Pulsatile tinnitus—often described by the patient as listening to one's own heartbeat—should be distinguished from tonal tinnitus. Although often ascribed to conductive hearing loss, this symptom may be far more serious and may indicate a vascular abnormality such as glomus tumor, venous sinus stenosis, carotid vaso-occlusive disease, arteriovenous malformation, or aneurysm. In contrast, a staccato "clicking" tinnitus may result from middle ear muscle spasm, sometimes associated with palatal myoclonus. The patient typically perceives a rapid series of popping noises, lasting seconds to a few minutes, accompanied by a fluttering feeling in the ear.

B. Diagnostic Testing

For routine, nonpulsatile tinnitus, audiometry should be ordered to rule out an associated hearing loss. For unilateral tinnitus, particularly associated with hearing loss in the absence of an obvious causative factor (ie, noise trauma), an MRI should be obtained to rule out a retrocochlear lesion, such as vestibular schwannoma. Magnetic resonance angiography and venography should be considered for patients who have pulsatile tinnitus to rule out a vascular lesion as causative.

► Treatment

The most important treatment of tinnitus is avoidance of exposure to excessive noise, ototoxic agents, and other factors that may cause cochlear damage. Masking the tinnitus with music or through amplification of normal sounds with a hearing aid may also bring some relief. Among the numerous drugs that have been tried, oral antidepressants (eg, nortriptyline at an initial dosage of 50 mg orally at bedtime) have proved to be the most effective. Habituation techniques, such as tinnitus retraining therapy, and masking techniques may prove beneficial in those with refractory symptoms. Transcranial magnetic stimulation of the central auditory system has been shown to improve symptoms in some patients. Progress is also being made toward implantable brain stimulators to treat tinnitus.

Hoare DJ et al. Systematic review and meta-analyses of randomized controlled trials examining tinnitus management. Laryngoscope. 2011 Jul;121(7):1555–64. [PMID: 21671234]

Langguth B et al. Tinnitus: causes and clinical management. Lancet Neurol. 2013 Sep;12(9):920–30. [PMID: 23948178]

Meng Z et al. Repetitive transcranial magnetic stimulation for tinnitus. Cochrane Database Syst Rev. 2011 Oct 5;(10): CD007946. [PMID: 21975776]

3. Hyperacusis

Excessive sensitivity to sound may occur in normal-hearing individuals either in association with ear disease, following noise trauma, in patients susceptible to migraines, or for psychological reasons. Patients with cochlear dysfunction commonly experience "recruitment," an abnormal sensitivity to loud sounds despite a reduced sensitivity to softer ones. Fitting hearing aids and other amplification devices to patients with recruitment requires use of compression circuitry to avoid uncomfortable overamplification. For normal-hearing individuals with hyperacusis, use of an earplug in noisy environments may be beneficial, though attempts should be made at habituation.

Knipper M et al. Advances in the neurobiology of hearing disorders: recent developments regarding the basis of tinnitus and hyperacusis. Prog Neurobiol. 2013 Dec;111:17–33. [PMID: 24012803]

Levine RA. Tinnitus: diagnostic approach leading to treatment. Semin Neurol. 2013 Jul;33(3):256–69. [PMID: 24057829]

4. Vertigo

ESSENTIALS OF DIAGNOSIS

▶ Either a sensation of motion when there is no motion or an exaggerated sense of motion in response to movement.

▶ Duration of vertigo episodes and association with hearing loss is the key to diagnosis.

▶ Must differentiate peripheral from central etiologies of vestibular dysfunction.

▶ **Peripheral:** Onset is sudden; often associated with tinnitus and hearing loss; horizontal nystagmus may be present.

▶ **Central:** Onset is gradual; no associated auditory symptoms.

▶ Evaluation includes audiogram and electronystagmography (ENG) or videonystagmography (VNG) and MRI.

▶ General Considerations

Vertigo can be caused by either a peripheral and central etiology, or both (Table 8–2).

▶ Clinical Findings

A. Symptoms and Signs

Vertigo is the cardinal symptom of vestibular disease. While vertigo is typically experienced as a distinct

Table 8–2. Causes of vertigo.

Peripheral causes
Vestibular neuritis/labyrinthitis
Ménière disease
Benign positional vertigo
Ethanol intoxication
Inner ear barotrauma
Semicircular canal dehiscence
Central causes
Seizure
Multiple sclerosis
Wernicke encephalopathy
Chiari malformation
Cerebellar ataxia syndromes
Mixed central and peripheral causes
Migraine
Stroke and vascular insufficiency
Posterior inferior cerebellar artery stroke
Anterior inferior cerebellar artery stroke
Vertebral artery insufficiency
Vasculitides
Cogan syndrome
Susac syndrome
Granulomatosis with polyangiitis (formerly Wegener granulomatosis)
Behçet disease
Cerebellopontine angle tumors
Vestibular schwannoma
Meningioma
Infections
Lyme disease
Syphilis
Vascular compression
Hyperviscosity syndromes
Waldenström macroglobulinemia
Endocrinopathies
Hypothyroidism
Pendred syndrome

"spinning" sensation, it may also present as a sense of tumbling or of falling forward or backward. It should be distinguished from imbalance, light-headedness, and syncope, all of which are nonvestibular in origin (Table 8–3).

1. Peripheral vestibular disease—Peripheral vestibulopathy usually causes vertigo of sudden onset, may be so severe that the patient is unable to walk or stand, and is frequently accompanied by nausea and vomiting. Tinnitus

Table 8–3. Common vestibular disorders: differential diagnosis based on classic presentations.

Duration of Typical Vertiginous Episodes	Auditory Symptoms Present	Auditory Symptoms Absent
Seconds	Perilymphatic fistula	Positioning vertigo (cupulolithiasis), vertebrobasilar insufficiency, migraine-associated vertigo
Hours	Endolymphatic hydrops (Ménière syndrome, syphilis)	Migraine-associated vertigo
Days	Labyrinthitis, labyrinthine concussion, autoimmune inner ear disease	Vestibular neuronitis, migraine-associated vertigo
Months	Acoustic neuroma, ototoxicity	Multiple sclerosis, cerebellar degeneration

and hearing loss may be associated and provide strong support for a peripheral (ie, otologic) origin.

A thorough history will often narrow down, if not confirm the diagnosis. Critical elements of the history include the duration of the discrete vertiginous episodes (seconds, minutes to hours, or days), and associated symptoms. Triggers should also be sought, including diet (eg, high salt in the case of Ménière disease), stress, fatigue, and bright lights (eg, migraine-associated dizziness).

The physical examination of the patient with vertigo includes evaluation of the ears, eye motion in response to head turning and observation for nystagmus, cranial nerve examination, and Romberg testing. In acute peripheral lesions, nystagmus is usually horizontal with a rotatory component; the fast phase usually beats away from the diseased side. Visual fixation tends to inhibit nystagmus except in very acute peripheral lesions or with central nervous system disease. Dix-Hallpike testing (quickly lowering the patient to the supine position with the head extending over the edge and placed 30 degrees lower than the body, turned either to the left or right) will elicit a delayed onset (~10 sec) fatiguable nystagmus in cases of benign positional vertigo. Nonfatigable nystagmus in this position indicates a central etiology for the dizziness.

Since visual fixation often suppresses observed nystagmus, many of these maneuvers are performed with Frenzel goggles, which prevent visual fixation, and often bring out subtle forms of nystagmus. The Fukuda test can demonstrate vestibular asymmetry when the patient steps in place with eyes closed and consistently rotates.

2. Central disease—In contrast to peripheral forms of vertigo, dizziness arising from central etiologies (Table 8–2) tends to develop gradually and then become progressively more severe and debilitating. Nystagmus is not always present but can occur in any direction and may be dissociated in the two eyes. The associated nystagmus is often nonfatigable, vertical rather than horizontal in orientation, without latency, and unsuppressed by visual fixation. ENG is useful in documenting these characteristics. The evaluation of central audiovestibular dysfunction requires imaging of the brain with MRI.

Episodic vertigo can occur in patients with diplopia from external ophthalmoplegia and is maximal when the patient looks in the direction where the separation of images is greatest. Cerebral lesions involving the temporal cortex may also produce vertigo, which is sometimes the initial symptom of a seizure. Finally, vertigo may be a feature of a number of systemic disorders and can occur as a side effect of certain anticonvulsant, antibiotic, hypnotic, analgesic, and tranquilizing drugs or of alcohol.

B. Laboratory Findings

Laboratory investigations such as audiologic evaluation, caloric stimulation, ENG, VNG, vestibular-evoked myogenic potentials (VEMPs), and MRI are indicated in patients with persistent vertigo or when central nervous system disease is suspected. These studies will help distinguish between central and peripheral lesions and to identify causes requiring specific therapy. ENG consists of objective recording of the nystagmus induced by head and body movements, gaze, and caloric stimulation. It is helpful in quantifying the degree of vestibular hypofunction. Computer-driven rotatory chairs and posturography platforms offer additional diagnostic modalities from specialized centers.

Kantner C et al. Characteristics and clinical applications of ocular vestibular evoked myogenic potentials. Hear Res. 2012 Dec;294(1–2):55–63. [PMID: 23123220]

Kaylie D et al. Evaluation of the patient with recurrent vertigo. Arch Otolaryngol Head Neck Surg. 2012 Jun;138(6):584–7. [PMID: 22710511]

► Vertigo Syndromes Due to Peripheral Lesions

A. Endolymphatic Hydrops (Ménière Syndrome)

The cause of Ménière syndrome is unknown. Distention of the endolymphatic compartment of the inner ear is a pathologic finding and thought to be part of the pathogenesis of the disorder. Although a precise cause of hydrops cannot be established in most cases, two known causes are syphilis and head trauma. The classic syndrome consists of episodic vertigo, with discrete vertigo spells lasting 20 minutes to several hours in association with fluctuating low-frequency sensorineural hearing loss, tinnitus (usually low-tone and "blowing" in quality), and a sensation of unilateral aural pressure (Table 8–3). These symptoms in the absence of hearing fluctuations suggests migraine-associated dizziness. Symptoms wax and wane as the endolymphatic pressure rises and falls. Caloric testing commonly reveals loss or impairment of thermally induced nystagmus on the involved side. Primary treatment involves a low salt diet and diuretics (eg, acetazolamide). In refractory cases, patients may undergo intratympanic corticosteroid injections, endolymphatic sac decompression or vestibular ablation either through transtympanic gentamicin, vestibular nerve section, or surgical labyrinthectomy.

Herraiz C et al. Transtympanic steroids for Ménière's disease. Otol Neurotol. 2010 Jan;31(1):162–7. [PMID: 19924013]
Le CH et al. Novel techniques for the diagnosis of Ménière's disease. Curr Opin Otolaryngol Head Neck Surg. 2013 Oct;21(5):492–6. [PMID: 23995329]

B. Labyrinthitis

Patients with labyrinthitis suffer from acute onset of continuous, usually severe vertigo lasting several days to a week, accompanied by hearing loss and tinnitus. During a recovery period that lasts for several weeks, the vertigo gradually improves. Hearing may return to normal or remain permanently impaired in the involved ear. The cause of labyrinthitis is unknown. Treatment consists of antibiotics if the patient is febrile or has symptoms of a bacterial infection, and supportive care. Vestibular suppressants are useful during the acute phase of the attack (eg, diazepam or meclizine) but should be discontinued as soon as feasible to avoid long-term dysequilibrium from inadequate compensation.

Beyea JA et al. Recent advances in viral inner ear disorders. Curr Opin Otolaryngol Head Neck Surg. 2012 Oct;20(5):404–8. [PMID: 22902415]
Post RE. Dizziness: a diagnostic approach. Am Fam Physician. 2010 Aug 15;82(4):361–8. [PMID: 20704166]

C. Benign Paroxysmal Positioning Vertigo

Patients suffering from recurrent spells of vertigo, lasting a few minutes per spell, associated with changes in head position (often provoked by rolling over in bed), usually have benign paroxysmal positioning vertigo. The term "positioning vertigo" is more accurate than "positional vertigo" because it is provoked by changes in head position rather than by the maintenance of a particular posture.

The typical symptoms of positioning vertigo occur in clusters that persist for several days. There is a brief (10–15 sec) latency period following a head movement before symptoms develop, and the acute vertigo subsides within 10–60 seconds, though the patient may remain imbalanced for several hours. Constant repetition of the positional change leads to habituation. Since some central nervous system disorders can mimic BPPV (eg, vertebrobasilar insufficiency), recurrent cases warrant MRI scanning of the head. In central lesions, there is no latent period, fatigability, or habituation of the symptoms and signs. Treatment of BPPV involves physical therapy protocols (eg, the Epley maneuver or Brandt-Daroff exercises), based on the theory that peripheral positioning vertigo results from free-floating otoconia within a semicircular canal.

Kollén L et al. Benign paroxysmal positional vertigo is a common cause of dizziness and unsteadiness in a large population of 75-year-olds. Aging Clin Exp Res. 2012 Aug;24(4):317–23. [PMID: 23238307]
Prokopakis E et al. Canalith repositioning procedures among 965 patients with benign paroxysmal positional vertigo. Audiol Neurootol. 2012 Nov 6;18(2):83–8. [PMID: 23147839]

D. Vestibular Neuronitis

In vestibular neuronitis, a paroxysmal, usually single attack of vertigo occurs without accompanying impairment of auditory function and will persist for several days to a week before gradually clearing. During the acute phase, examination reveals nystagmus and absent responses to caloric stimulation on one or both sides. The cause of the disorder is unclear though presumed to be viral. Treatment consists of supportive care, including diazepam or meclizine during the acute phases of the vertigo only, followed by vestibular therapy if the patient does not completely compensate.

Jeong SH et al. Vestibular neuritis. Semin Neurol. 2013 Jul;33(3):185–94. [PMID: 24057821]
Koors PD et al. Investigation of seasonal variability of vestibular neuronitis. J Laryngol Otol. 2013 Oct;127(10):968–71. [PMID: 24063368]

E. Traumatic Vertigo

The most common cause of vertigo following head injury is labyrinthine concussion. Symptoms generally diminish within several days but may linger for a month or more. Basilar skull fractures that traverse the inner ear usually result in severe vertigo lasting several days to a week and deafness in the involved ear. Chronic posttraumatic vertigo may result from cupulolithiasis. This occurs when traumatically detached statoconia (otoconia) settle on the ampulla of the posterior semicircular canal and cause an excessive degree of cupular deflection in response to head motion. Clinically, this presents as episodic positioning vertigo. Treatment consists of supportive care and vestibular suppressant medication (diazepam or meclizine) during the acute phase of the attack, and vestibular therapy.

Liu H. Presentation and outcome of post-traumatic benign paroxysmal positional vertigo. Acta Otolaryngol. 2012 Aug;132(8):803–6. [PMID: 22404210]

F. Perilymphatic Fistula

Leakage of perilymphatic fluid from the inner ear into the tympanic cavity via the round or oval window is a rare cause of vertigo and sensory hearing loss. Most cases result from either physical injury (eg, blunt head trauma, hand slap to ear); extreme barotrauma during airflight, scuba diving, etc; or vigorous Valsalva maneuvers (eg, during weight lifting). Treatment may require middle ear exploration and window sealing with a tissue graft; however, this is seldom indicated without a clear-cut history of a precipitating traumatic event.

Fife TD et al. Posttraumatic vertigo and dizziness. Semin Neurol. 2013 Jul;33(3):238–43. [PMID: 24057827]

G. Cervical Vertigo

Position receptors located in the facets of the cervical spine are important physiologically in the coordination of head and eye movements. Cervical proprioceptive dysfunction is a common cause of vertigo triggered by neck movements. This disturbance often commences after neck injury, particularly hyperextension. An association also exists with degenerative cervical spine disease. Although symptoms vary, vertigo may be triggered by assuming a particular head position as opposed to moving to a new head position (the latter typical of labyrinthine dysfunction). Diagnosis may often be confused with migraine-associated vertigo, which is also associated with head movement. Management consists of neck movement exercises to the extent permitted by orthopedic considerations.

Ogawa Y et al. Intermittent positional downbeat nystagmus of cervical origin. Auris Nasus Larynx. 2013 Oct 24. [Epub ahead of print] [PMID: 24206826]

H. Migrainous Vertigo

Episodic vertigo is frequently associated with a migraine type of headache. Head trauma may also be a precipitating feature. The vertigo may be temporally related to the headache and last up to several hours, although the vertigo may also occur in the absence of any headache. It may appear identical to Ménière disease but without associated hearing loss or tinnitus. Accompanying symptoms may include head pressure, visual and motion sensitivity, auditory sensitivity, and photosensitivity. Symptoms typically worsen with lack of sleep and anxiety or stress. There is often a history of motion intolerance (easily carsick as a child) and there may be a familial tendency. Food triggers may also be common, including caffeine, chocolate, and alcohol among others. Treatment includes dietary and lifestyle changes (improved sleep pattern, avoidance of stress) and antimigraine prophylactic medication.

Furman JM et al. Vestibular migraine: clinical aspects and pathophysiology. Lancet Neurol. 2013 Jul;12(7):706–15. [PMID: 23769597]
Lempert T. Vestibular migraine. Semin Neurol. 2013 Jul;33(3):212–8. [PMID: 24057824]

I. Superior Semicircular Canal Dehiscence

Deficiency in the bony covering of the superior semicircular canal may be associated with vertigo triggered by loud noise exposure, straining, and an apparent conductive hearing loss. Diagnosis is with coronal high-resolution CT scan and VEMPs. Surgically sealing the dehiscent canal can improve symptoms.

Shaia WT et al. Evolution in surgical management of superior canal dehiscence syndrome. Curr Opin Otolaryngol Head Neck Surg. 2013 Oct;21(5):497–502. [PMID: 23989599]

Zuniga MG et al. Ocular versus cervical VEMPs in the diagnosis of superior semicircular canal dehiscence syndrome. Otol Neurotol. 2013 Jan;34(1):121–6. [PMID: 23183641]

▶ Vertigo Syndromes Due to Central Lesions

Central nervous system causes of vertigo include brainstem vascular disease, arteriovenous malformations, tumor of the brainstem and cerebellum, multiple sclerosis, and vertebrobasilar migraine (Table 8–2). Vertigo of central origin often becomes unremitting and disabling. The associated nystagmus is often nonfatigable, vertical rather than horizontal in orientation, without latency, and unsuppressed by visual fixation. ENG is useful in documenting these characteristics. There are commonly other signs of brainstem dysfunction (eg, cranial nerve palsies; motor, sensory, or cerebellar deficits in the limbs) or of increased intracranial pressure. Auditory function is generally spared. The underlying cause should be treated.

Kutz JW Jr. The dizzy patient. Med Clin North Am. 2010 Sep;94(5):989–1002. [PMID: 20736108]
Lempert T et al. Management of common central vestibular disorders. Curr Opin Otolaryngol Head Neck Surg. 2010 Oct;18(5):436–40. [PMID: 20639762]

DISEASES OF THE CENTRAL AUDITORY & VESTIBULAR SYSTEMS (Table 8–3)

Lesions of the eighth cranial nerve and central audiovestibular pathways produce neural hearing loss and vertigo. One characteristic of neural hearing loss is deterioration of speech discrimination out of proportion to the decrease in pure tone thresholds. Another is auditory adaptation, wherein a steady tone appears to the listener to decay and eventually disappear. Auditory evoked responses are useful in distinguishing cochlear from neural losses and may give insight into the site of lesion within the central pathways.

The evaluation of central audiovestibular disorders usually requires imaging of the internal auditory canal, cerebellopontine angle, and brain with enhanced MRI.

1. Vestibular Schwannoma (Acoustic Neuroma)

Eighth cranial nerve schwannomas are among the most common intracranial tumors. Most are unilateral, but about 5% are associated with the hereditary syndrome, neurofibromatosis type 2, in which bilateral eighth nerve tumors may be accompanied by meningiomas and other intracranial and spinal tumors. These benign lesions arise within the internal auditory canal and gradually grow to involve the cerebellopontine angle, eventually compressing the pons and resulting in hydrocephalus. Their typical auditory symptoms are unilateral hearing loss with a deterioration of speech discrimination exceeding that predicted by the degree of pure tone loss. Nonclassic presentations, such as sudden unilateral hearing loss, are fairly common. Any individual with a unilateral or asymmetric sensorineural hearing loss should be evaluated for an intracranial mass lesion. Vestibular dysfunction more often takes the form of continuous dysequilibrium than episodic vertigo. Diagnosis is made by enhanced MRI. Treatment consists of observation, microsurgical excision, or stereotactic radiotherapy, depending on such factors as patient age, underlying health, and size of the tumor at presentation. Bevacizumab (vascular endothelial growth factor blocker) has shown promise for treatment of tumors in patients with neurofibromatosis type 2.

Patel J et al. The changing face of acoustic neuroma management in the USA: Analysis of the 1998 and 2008 patient surveys from the acoustic neuroma association. Br J Neurosurg. 2013 Jul 19. [Epub ahead of print] [PMID: 23869572]
Plotkin SR et al. Bevacizumab for progressive vestibular schwannoma in neurofibromatosis type 2: a retrospective review of 31 patients. Otol Neurotol. 2012 Aug;33(6):1046–52. [PMID: 22805104]
Quesnel AM et al. Current strategies in management of intracanalicular vestibular schwannoma. Curr Opin Otolaryngol Head Neck Surg. 2011 Oct;19(5):335–40. [PMID: 22552696]

2. Vascular Compromise

Vertebrobasilar insufficiency is a common cause of vertigo in the elderly. It is often triggered by changes in posture or extension of the neck. Reduced flow in the vertebrobasilar system may be demonstrated noninvasively through magnetic resonance angiography. Empiric treatment is with vasodilators and aspirin.

Karatas M. Vascular vertigo: epidemiology and clinical syndromes. Neurologist. 2011 Jan;17(1):1–10. [PMID: 21192184]
Schneider JI et al. Vertigo, vertebrobasilar disease, and posterior circulation ischemic stroke. Emerg Med Clin North Am. 2012 Aug;30(3):681–93. [PMID: 22974644]

3. Multiple Sclerosis

Patients with multiple sclerosis may suffer from episodic vertigo and chronic imbalance. Hearing loss in this disease is most commonly unilateral and of rapid onset. Spontaneous recovery may occur.

Pula JH et al. Multiple sclerosis as a cause of the acute vestibular syndrome. J Neurol. 2013 Jun;260(6):1649–54. [PMID: 23392781]

OTOLOGIC MANIFESTATIONS OF AIDS

The otologic manifestations of AIDS are protean. The pinna and external auditory canal may be affected by Kaposi sarcoma as well as persistent and potentially invasive fungal infections, particularly due to *Aspergillus fumigatus*. The most common middle ear manifestation of AIDS is serous otitis media due to eustachian tube dysfunction arising from adenoidal hypertrophy (HIV lymphadenopathy), recurrent mucosal viral infections, or an obstructing nasopharyngeal tumor (eg, lymphoma). For middle ear effusions, ventilating tubes are seldom helpful and may trigger profuse watery otorrhea. Acute otitis media is usually caused by the typical bacterial organisms that occur in nonimmunocompromised patients, although *Pneumocystis jirovecii* otitis has been reported. Sensorineural hearing loss is common and in some cases appears to result from viral central nervous system infection. In cases of progressive hearing loss, it is important to evaluate for cryptococcal meningitis and syphilis. Acute facial paralysis due to herpes zoster infection (Ramsay Hunt syndrome) is quite common and follows a clinical course similar to that in nonimmunocompromised patients. Treatment is primarily with high-dose acyclovir (see Chapters 6 and 32). Corticosteroids may also be effective.

DISEASES OF THE NOSE & PARANASAL SINUSES

INFECTIONS OF THE NOSE & PARANASAL SINUSES

1. Acute Viral Rhinosinusitis (Common Cold)

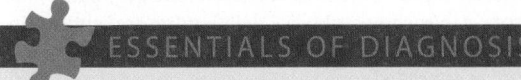

ESSENTIALS OF DIAGNOSIS

- ▶ Clear rhinorrhea, hyposmia, and nasal congestion.
- ▶ Associated symptoms, including malaise, headache, and cough.
- ▶ Erythematous, engorged nasal mucosa on examination without intranasal purulence.
- ▶ Symptoms last < 4 weeks and typically < 10 days.
- ▶ Symptoms are self-limited.

▶ Clinical Findings

The nonspecific symptoms of the ubiquitous common cold are present in the early phases of many diseases that affect the upper aerodigestive tract. Because there are numerous serologic types of rhinoviruses, adenoviruses, and other viruses, patients remain susceptible throughout life. These infections, while generally quite benign and self-limited, have been implicated in the development or exacerbation of more serious conditions, such as acute bacterial sinusitis, acute otitis media, asthma and cystic fibrosis exacerbation, and bronchitis. Nasal congestion, decreased sense of smell, watery rhinorrhea, and sneezing accompanied by general malaise, throat discomfort and, occasionally, headache are typical in viral infections. Nasal examination usually shows erythematous, edematous mucosa and a watery discharge. The presence of purulent nasal discharge suggests bacterial rhinosinusitis.

▶ Treatment

Even though there are no effective antiviral therapies for either the prevention or treatment of viral rhinitis, there is a common misperception among patients that antibiotics are helpful. Zinc for the treatment of viral rhinitis has been controversial. A 2011 meta-analysis of randomized controlled trials demonstrated no benefit in five studies that used < 75 mg of zinc acetate daily, but significant reduction in duration of cold symptoms was noted in all three studies that used zinc acetate in daily doses of over 75 mg. The effect with zinc salts other than acetate was also significant at doses > 75 mg/d, but not as high as the zinc acetate lozenge studies (20% vs 42% reduction in cold duration). Buffered hypertonic saline (3–5%) nasal irrigation has been shown to improve symptoms and reduce the need for nonsteroidal anti-inflammatory drugs. Other supportive measures, such as oral decongestants (pseudoephedrine, 30–60 mg every 4–6 hours or 120 mg twice daily), may provide some relief of rhinorrhea and nasal obstruction. Nasal sprays, such as oxymetazoline or phenylephrine, are rapidly effective but should not be used for more than a few days to prevent rebound congestion. Withdrawal of the drug after prolonged use leads to **rhinitis medicamentosa,** an almost addictive need for continuous usage. Treatment of rhinitis medicamentosa requires mandatory cessation of the sprays, and this is often extremely frustrating for patients. Topical intranasal corticosteroids (eg, flunisolide, 2 sprays in each nostril twice daily), intranasal anticholinergic (ipratropium 0.06% nasal spray, 2–3 sprays every 8 hours as needed) or a short tapering course of oral prednisone may help during the process of withdrawal.

► Complications

Other than mild eustachian tube dysfunction or transient middle ear effusion, complications of viral rhinitis are unusual. Secondary acute bacterial rhinosinusitis may occur and is suggested by persistence of symptoms beyond 10 days, accompanied both by purulent green or yellow nasal secretions and unilateral facial or tooth pain. (See Acute Bacterial Rhinosinusitis below.)

While the symptoms of influenza A/H1N1 (swine flu) are much the same as other respiratory viruses, certain persons (including children younger than 5 years, adults older than 65 years, pregnant women, patients with underlying respiratory or immune disorders, and adolescents younger than 19 years receiving aspirin therapy) are at particular risk for the development of hypoxia and acute respiratory distress syndrome (ARDS). Mortality in those in whom ARDS developed was > 17%. Diagnosis of influenza A/H1N1 is confirmed by nasopharyngeal, oropharyngeal, or endobronchial swab or aspirate and identification of the virus by reverse transcriptase-polymerase chain reaction (RT-PCR). Treatment with oseltamivir or zanamivir has been effective, but up to date diagnosis, treatment, and containment guidelines should be sought from the Centers for Disease Control and Prevention at http://www.cdc.gov/flu/ if the diagnosis is suspected.

Hemilä H. Zinc lozenges may shorten the duration of colds: a systematic review. Open Respir Med J. 2011;5:51–8. [PMID: 21769305]
Sullivan SJ et al. 2009 H1N1 Influenza. Mayo Clin Proc. 2010 Jan;85(1):64–76. [PMID: 20007905]

2. Acute Bacterial Rhinosinusitis (Sinusitis)

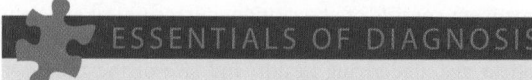

ESSENTIALS OF DIAGNOSIS

► Purulent yellow-green nasal discharge or expectoration.

► Facial pain or pressure over the affected sinus or sinuses.

► Nasal obstruction.

► Acute onset of symptoms (between 1 and 4 weeks duration).

► Associated symptoms, including cough, malaise, fever, and headache.

► General Considerations

Acute sinus infections are uncommon compared with viral rhinitis, but they still affect nearly 20 million Americans annually, accounting for over 2 billion dollars in health care expenditures for sinusitis annually. Such infections are often associated with inflammation of the nasal cavity mucosa near the drainage pores of the sinuses. To acknowledge this inflammation as a major component of the disease and to differentiate it from such processes as allergic or acute viral rhinitis, otolaryngologists prefer the term "bacterial rhinosinusitis."

Acute bacterial rhinosinusitis usually is a result of impaired mucociliary clearance and obstruction of the osteomeatal complex, or sinus "pore." Edematous mucosa causes obstruction of the complex, resulting in the accumulation of mucous secretion in the sinus cavity that becomes secondarily infected by bacteria. The largest of these osteomeatal complexes is deep to the middle turbinate in the middle meatus. This complex is actually a confluence of complexes draining the maxillary, ethmoid, and frontal sinuses. The sphenoid drains from a separate complex between the septum and superior turbinate.

The typical pathogens of bacterial sinusitis are the same as those that cause acute otitis media: *S pneumoniae*, other streptococci, *H influenzae* and, less commonly, *S aureus* and *Moraxella catarrhalis*. Pathogens vary regionally in both prevalence and drug resistance; about 25% of healthy asymptomatic individuals may, if sinus aspirates are cultured, harbor such bacteria as well. Understanding of the anatomy, pathogenesis and microbiology of acute bacterial rhinosinusitis can help the clinician make the most expeditious and cost-effective diagnosis and treatment while avoiding serious complications.

► Clinical Findings

A. Symptoms and Signs

There are no agreed upon criteria for the diagnosis of acute bacterial rhinosinusitis in adults. All study groups note a number of major symptoms, including purulent nasal drainage, nasal obstruction or congestion, facial pain/pressure, altered smell, cough, and fever. Minor symptoms include headache, otalgia, halitosis, dental pain, and fatigue. Many of the more specific signs and symptoms may be related to the affected sinuses. It is important to note that studies have demonstrated no correlation between patient reports of "sinus headache" and presence of sinusitis on CT scan. Bacterial rhinosinusitis can be distinguished from viral rhinitis by persistence of symptoms more than 10 days after onset or worsening of symptoms within 10 days after initial improvement. Acute infections are defined as those lasting less than 4 weeks, with subacute infections lasting between 4 weeks and 12 weeks.

Acute maxillary sinusitis is the most common form of acute bacterial rhinosinusitis because the maxillary is the largest sinus with a single drainage pathway that is easily obstructed. Unilateral facial fullness, pressure and tenderness over the cheek are common symptoms, but may not be present in many cases. Pain may refer to the upper incisor and canine teeth via branches of the trigeminal nerve, which traverse the floor of the sinus. Purulent nasal drainage should be noted with nasal airway obstruction or facial pain (pressure). Maxillary sinusitis may result from dental infection, and teeth that are tender should be carefully examined for signs of abscess. Removal of the diseased tooth or drainage of the periapical abscess typically resolves the sinus infection.

Acute ethmoiditis in adults is often accompanied by maxillary sinusitis and symptoms are similar to those described above. Localized ethmoid sinusitis may present with pain and pressure over the high lateral wall of the nose between the eyes that may radiate to the orbit.

Sphenoid sinusitis is usually seen in the setting of pansinusitis, or infection of all the paranasal sinuses on at least one side. The patient may complain of a headache "in the middle of the head" and often points to the vertex.

Acute frontal sinusitis may cause pain and tenderness of the forehead. This is most easily elicited by palpation of the orbital roof just below the medial end of the eyebrow.

Hospital-associated sinusitis is a form of acute bacterial rhinosinusitis that may present without any symptoms in the head and neck. It is a common source of fever in critically ill patients and is often associated with prolonged presence of a nasogastric or, rarely, nasotracheal tube causing inflammation of the nasal mucosa and osteomeatal complex obstruction. Pansinusitis on the side of the tube is common on imaging studies.

B. Imaging

It is usually possible to make the diagnosis of acute bacterial rhinosinusitis on clinical grounds alone. Although more sensitive than clinical examination, routine radiographs are not cost-effective and are not recommended by the Agency for Health Care Policy and Research or American Association of Otolaryngology Guidelines in the routine diagnosis of acute bacterial rhinosinusitis. Consensus guidelines report that imaging may be helpful when clinically based criteria are difficult to evaluate, when the patient does not respond to appropriate therapy, when patients have been treated repeatedly with antibiotics for presumed sinusitis, when intracranial involvement or cerebrospinal fluid rhinorrhea is suspected, when complicated dental infection is suspected, or when symptoms of more serious infection are noted.

When necessary, noncontrast, screening coronal CT scans are more cost-effective and provide more information than conventional sinus films. CT provides a rapid and effective means to assess all of the paranasal sinuses, identify areas of greater concern (such as bony dehiscence, periosteal elevation or maxillary tooth root exposure within the sinus), and speed appropriate therapy.

CT scans are reasonably sensitive but are not specific. Swollen soft tissue and fluid may be difficult to distinguish when opacification of the sinus is present from other conditions, such as chronic rhinosinusitis, nasal polyposis, or mucus retention cysts. Sinus abnormalities can be seen in most patients with an upper respiratory infection, while bacterial rhinosinusitis develops in only 2%.

▶ Treatment

All patients with acute bacterial rhinosinusitis should have careful evaluation of pain. Nonsteroidal anti-inflammatory drugs are generally recommended. Sinus symptoms may be improved with oral or nasal decongestants (or both)—eg, oral pseudoephedrine, 30–120 mg per dose, up to 240 mg/d; nasal oxymetazoline, 0.05%, or xylometazoline, 0.05–0.1%, one or two sprays in each nostril every 6–8 hours for up to 3 days. All clinical practice guidelines recommend using intranasal corticosteroids in the first 5 days of symptoms that could be acute bacterial rhinosinusitis or acute viral rhinitis since meta-analysis demonstrates a small, but significant reduction in facial pain and congestion scores with use. Recommendations exist for high-dose mometasone furoate (200 mcg each nostril twice daily) for 21 days. However, this indication is not approved by the US Food and Drug Administration.

Eighty percent of patients with acute bacterial rhinosinusitis improve symptomatically within 2 weeks without antibiotic therapy. Antibiotic treatment is controversial in uncomplicated cases of clinically diagnosed acute bacterial rhinosinusitis because only 5% of patients will note a shorter duration of illness with treatment, and antibiotic treatment is associated with nearly twice the number of adverse events compared with placebo. Antibiotics may be considered when symptoms last more than 10–14 days or when symptoms (including fever, facial pain, and swelling of the face) are severe or when cases are complicated (such as immunodeficiency). In these patients, administration of antibiotics does reduce the incidence of clinical failure by 50% and represents the most cost-effective treatment strategy. Double-blinded studies exist to support numerous antibiotic choices. A summary of national guidelines for the treatment of acute sinusitis can be found in Table 8–4. Selection of antibiotics is usually empiric and based on a number of factors including regional patterns of antibiotic resistance, antibiotic allergy, cost, and patient tolerance. Unless the patient is allergic to penicillin, amoxicillin should be used as the first-line agent. Treatment is usually for 7–10 days, although longer courses are sometimes required to prevent relapses. Macrolide therapy has been recommended as first-line therapy in patients with penicillin allergy, and tetracyclines have also been used.

Table 8–4. Oral antibiotic regimens for acute sinusitis.

Drug	Dose	Duration	Notes
First-line therapy			
Amoxicillin	1000 mg three times daily	7–10 days	
Trimethoprim-sulfamethoxazole	160 mg–800 mg twice daily	7–10 days	Suitable in penicillin allergy
Doxycycline	200 mg once daily × 1 day, 100 mg twice daily thereafter	7–10 days	Suitable in penicillin allergy
Amoxicillin-clavulanate[1]	1000/62.5 mg ER 2 tablets twice daily	10 days	If no improvement after 3 days on first-line therapy
First-line therapy after recent antibiotic use (within 4–6 weeks)			
Levofloxacin	500 mg once daily	10 days	
Amoxicillin-clavulanate	875/125 mg twice daily	10 days	
Second-line therapy			
Amoxicillin-clavulanate	1000/62.5 mg ER 2 tablets twice daily	10 days	If no improvement after 3 days on first-line therapy
Moxifloxacin	400 mg once daily	10 days	If no improvement after 3 days on first-line therapy

[1]In communities where there is multidrug-resistant *S pneumoniae* and beta-lactamase beta-lactam inhibitor–producing strains of *H influenza* and *M catarrhalis*.

Adapted, with permission, from Marple BF et al. Acute bacterial rhinosinusitis: a review of US treatment guidelines. Otolaryngol Head Neck Surg. 2006 Sep;135(3):341–8. Copyright © 2006 Sage Publications. Reprinted by permission of Sage Publications.

Multidrug resistant *S pneumoniae* prevalence is growing in many urban areas of the United States as are beta-lactamase beta-lactam inhibitor producing strains of *H influenza* and *M catarrhalis*. In such regions, guidelines call for empiric use of amoxicillin-clavulanate or second- or third-generation cephalosporins. Fluoroquinolones are reserved for treatment failures or for patients with a recent history of antibiotic therapy for another infection. Recurrent sinusitis or sinusitis that does not appear to respond clinically warrants CT imaging and evaluation by a specialist.

Hospital-associated infections in critically ill patients are treated differently from community-acquired infections. Broad-spectrum antibiotic coverage for bacteria including *P aeruginosa*, *S aureus* (including methicillin-resistant strains), and anaerobes must be considered. Removal of the nasogastric tube and improved nasal hygiene (nasal saline sprays, humidification of supplemental nasal oxygen, and nasal decongestants) are critical interventions and often curative in mild cases without aggressive antibiotic use. Endoscopic or transantral cultures may help direct medical therapy in complicated cases.

▶ Complications

Local complications of acute bacterial rhinosinusitis include orbital cellulitis and abscess, osteomyelitis, intracranial extension and cavernous sinus thrombosis.

Any change in the ocular examination in a patient with acute bacterial rhinosinusitis necessitates immediate CT imaging. Orbital complications typically occur by extension of ethmoid sinusitis through the lamina papyracea, a thin layer of bone that comprises the medial orbital wall. Extension in this area may cause orbital cellulitis leading to proptosis, gaze restriction, and orbital pain. Select cases are responsive to intravenous antibiotics with or without corticosteroids and should be managed in close conjunction with an ophthalmologist or otolaryngologist, or both. Extension through the lamina papyracea can also lead to subperiosteal abscess formation (orbital abscess). Such abscesses cause marked proptosis, ophthalmoplegia, and pain with medial gaze. While some of these abscesses will respond to antibiotics, such findings should prompt an immediate referral to a specialist for consideration of decompression and evacuation. Failure to intervene quickly may lead to permanent visual impairment and a "frozen globe."

Osteomyelitis requires prolonged antibiotics as well as removal of necrotic bone. The frontal sinus is most commonly affected, with bone involvement suggested by a tender puffy swelling of the forehead (Pott puffy tumor). Following treatment, secondary cosmetic reconstructive procedures may be necessary.

Intracranial complications of sinusitis can occur either through hematogenous spread, as in cavernous sinus thrombosis and meningitis, or by direct extension, as in epidural and intraparenchymal brain abscesses. Fortunately, they are rare today. Cavernous sinus thrombosis is heralded by ophthalmoplegia, chemosis, and visual loss. The diagnosis is most commonly confirmed by MRI and, when identified early, it typically responds to intravenous antibiotics. Frontal epidural and intracranial abscesses are often clinically silent, but may present with altered metal status, persistent fever, or severe headache.

When to Refer

Failure of acute bacterial rhinosinusitis to resolve after an adequate course of oral antibiotics may necessitate referral to an otolaryngologist for evaluation. Endoscopic cultures may direct further treatment choices. Nasal endoscopy and CT scan are indicated when symptoms persist longer than 4–12 weeks. Any patients with suspected extension of disease outside the sinuses should be evaluated urgently by an otolaryngologist and imaging should be obtained.

When to Admit

- Facial swelling and erythema indicative of facial cellulitis.
- Proptosis.
- Vision change or gaze abnormality indicative of orbital cellulitis.
- Abscess or cavernous sinus involvement.
- Mental status changes suggestive of intracranial extension.
- Immunocompromised status.
- Failure to respond to appropriate first-line treatment for acute bacterial rhinosinusitis or symptoms persisting longer than 4 weeks.

Bhattacharyya N et al. Patterns of care before and after the adult sinusitis clinical practice guideline. Laryngoscope. 2013 Jul;123(7):1588–91. [PMID: 23417327]

Hayward G et al. Intranasal corticosteroids in management of acute sinusitis: a systematic review and meta-analysis. Ann Fam Med. 2012 May–Jun;10(3):241–9. [PMID: 22585889]

Lemiengre MB et al. Antibiotics for clinically diagnosed acute rhinosinusitis in adults. Cochrane Database Syst Rev. 2012 Oct 17;10: CD006089. [PMID: 23076918]

Meltzer EO et al. Rhinosinusitis diagnosis and management for the clinician: a synopsis of recent consensus guidelines. Mayo Clin Proc. 2011 May86(5):427–43. [PMID: 21490181]

3. Nasal Vestibulitis & *S aureus* Nasal Colonization

Inflammation of the nasal vestibule may result from folliculitis of the hairs that line this orifice and is usually the result of nasal manipulation or hair trimming. Systemic antibiotics effective against *S aureus* (such as dicloxacillin, 250 mg orally four times daily for 7–10 days) are indicated. Topical mupirocin or bacitracin (applied two or three times daily) may be a helpful addition and may prevent future occurrences. If recurrent, the addition of rifampin (10 mg/kg orally twice daily for the last 4 days of treatment) may eliminate the *S aureus* carrier state. If a furuncle exists, it should be incised and drained, preferably intranasally. Adequate treatment of these infections is important to prevent retrograde spread of infection through valveless veins into the cavernous sinus and intracranial structures.

S aureus is the leading nosocomial pathogen in the world, and nasal carriage is a well-defined risk factor in the development and spread of nosocomial infections. While the vast majority of patients have no vestibulitis symptoms, screening methods (including nasal swabs and PCR-based assays) have demonstrated rates of *S aureus* nasal colonization at around 30% and methicillin-resistant *S aureus* colonization in patients in the intensive care unit to be as high as 11%. Elimination of the carrier state is challenging, but studies of mupirocin (2% topical nasal application twice daily) have demonstrated efficacy in reducing surgical and catheter/hardware infections. Consensus screening and treatment recommendations are not yet available.

Mehta MS et al. Dose-ranging study to assess the application of intranasal 2% mupirocin calcium ointment to eradicate Staphylococcus aureus nasal colonization. Surg Infect (Larchmt). 2013 Feb;14(1):69–72. [PMID: 23448592]

4. Invasive Fungal Sinusitis

Invasive fungal sinusitis is rare and includes both rhinocerebral mucormycosis (*Mucor, Absidia,* and *Rhizopus sp.*) and other invasive fungal infections, such as *Aspergillus.* The fungus spreads rapidly through vascular channels and may be lethal if not detected early. Patients with mucormycosis almost invariably have a contributing factor that results in some degree of immunocompromise, such as diabetes mellitus, long-term corticosteroid therapy, or end-stage renal disease. Mucormycosis is more common, however, in patients who are profoundly immunocompromised for the treatment of hematologic malignancies. Occasional cases have been reported in patients with AIDS though *Aspergillus sp.* is more common in this setting. The initial symptoms may be similar to those of acute bacterial rhinosinusitis, although facial pain is often more severe. Nasal drainage is typically clear or straw-colored, rather than purulent, and visual symptoms may be noted at presentation in the absence of significant nasal findings. On examination, the classic finding of mucormycosis is a black eschar on the middle turbinate. This finding is not universal and may be inapparent if the infection is deep or high within the nasal bones. Often the mucosa appears normal or simply pale and dry. Early diagnosis requires suspicion of the disease and nasal biopsy with silver stains, revealing broad nonseptate hyphae within tissues and necrosis with vascular occlusion. Because CT or MRI may initially show only soft tissue changes, biopsy and ultimate debridement should be based on the clinical setting rather than radiographic demonstration of bony destruction or intracranial changes.

Invasive fungal sinusitis represents a medical and surgical emergency. Once recognized, prompt wide surgical debridement and amphotericin B by intravenous infusion are indicated for patients with reversible immune deficiency. Lipid-based amphotericin B (Ambisome) may be used in patients who have kidney disease or in those in whom it develops secondary to nephrotoxic doses of nonlipid amphotericin. Other antifungals, including voriconazole and caspofungin, may be appropriate therapy depending on the speciation of the organism. There is evidence that suggests that iron chelator therapy may also be a useful adjunct. While necessary for any possibility of cure, surgical management often results in tremendous disfigurement and functional deficits. Even with early diagnosis and immediate appropriate intervention, the prognosis is guarded and often results in the loss of at least one eye. In persons with diabetes, the mortality rate is about 20%. If kidney disease is present or develops, mortality is over 50%; in the setting of AIDS or hematologic malignancy with neutropenia, mortality approaches 100%. Aggressive management with surgery should be considered carefully, since the disease-specific survival is only about 57% and because many patients are gravely ill at the time of diagnosis, the overall survival is about 18%.

Monroe MM et al. Invasive fungal rhinosinusitis: a 15-year experience with 29 patients. Laryngoscope. 2013 Jul;123(7): 1583–7. [PMID: 23417294]

ALLERGIC RHINITIS

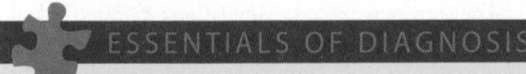

ESSENTIALS OF DIAGNOSIS

- ▶ Clear rhinorrhea, sneezing, tearing, eye irritation, and pruritus.
- ▶ Associated symptoms, including cough, bronchospasm, eczematous dermatitis.
- ▶ Environmental allergen exposure with presence of allergen specific IgE.

▶ General Considerations

Allergic rhinitis is very common in the United States. Population studies have reported the prevalence as between 14% and 40% among Americans, with most consensus panels agreeing on 20%. Allergic rhinitis adversely affects school and work performance, costing about $6 billion annually in the United States. These costs may be underestimated as epidemiology studies consistently show an association with asthma. Seasonal allergic rhinitis is most commonly caused by pollens and spores. Flowering shrub and tree pollens are most common in the spring, flowering plants and grasses in the summer, and ragweed and molds in the fall. Dust, household mites, air pollution, and pet dander may produce year-round symptoms, termed "perennial rhinitis."

Allergic rhinitis is caused by exposure to an airborne allergen in a predisposed individual. Activation of both humoral (B-cell) and cytotoxic (T-cell) immune responses with subsequent allergen-specific IgE responses causes release of inflammatory mediators. The response is increased as antigen is passed to regional lymph nodes for greater T-cell activation. Interleukin and cytokine release causes specific activation of mast cells, eosinophils, plasma cells, basophils, and other T-cells. Many of these circulating cells then migrate into the nasal and ocular epithelium where they contribute directly to symptoms through proinflammatory mediators, including histamine, prostaglandins, and kinins.

▶ Clinical Findings

The symptoms of "hay fever" are similar to those of viral rhinitis but are usually persistent and may show seasonal variation. Nasal symptoms are often accompanied by eye irritation, pruritus, conjunctival erythema, and excessive tearing. Many patients will note a strong family history of atopy or allergy.

The clinician should be careful to distinguish allergic rhinitis from nonallergic or vasomotor rhinitis. **Vasomotor rhinitis** is caused by increased sensitivity of the vidian nerve and is a common cause of clear rhinorrhea in the elderly. Often patients will report that they have troubling rhinorrhea in response to numerous nasal stimuli, including warm or cold air, odors or scents, light, or particulate matter.

On physical examination, the mucosa of the turbinates is usually pale or violaceous because of venous engorgement. This is in contrast to the erythema of viral rhinitis. Nasal polyps, which are yellowish boggy masses of hypertrophic mucosa, are associated with long-standing allergic rhinitis.

▶ Treatment

A. Intranasal Corticosteroids

Intranasal corticosteroid sprays have revolutionized the treatment of allergic rhinitis. Evidence-based literature reviews show that these are more effective—and frequently less expensive—than nonsedating antihistamines. Patients should be reminded that there may be a delay in onset of relief of 2 or more weeks. Corticosteroid sprays may also shrink hypertrophic nasal mucosa and nasal polyps, thereby providing an improved nasal airway and osteomeatal complex drainage. Because of this effect, intranasal corticosteroids are critical in treating allergy in patients prone to recurrent acute bacterial rhinosinusitis or chronic rhinosinusitis. There are many available preparations, including beclomethasone (42 mcg/spray twice daily per nostril), flunisolide (25 mcg/spray twice daily per nostril), mometasone furoate (200 mcg once daily per nostril), budesonide (100 mcg twice daily per nostril), and fluticasone propionate (200 mcg once daily per nostril). All intranasal corticosteroids are considered equally effective. Probably the most critical factor is compliance with regular use and proper introduction into the nasal cavity. In order to deliver medication to the region of the middle meatus, proper application involves holding the bottle straight up with the head tilted forward and pointing the bottle toward the ipsilateral ear when spraying. Side effects are limited and the most annoying is epistaxis. Some experts believe that this is related to incorrect delivery of the drug to the nasal septum.

B. Antihistamines

Treatment of allergic and perennial rhinitis has improved in recent years. Antihistamines offer temporary, but immediate, control of many of the most troubling symptoms of allergic rhinitis. Effective antihistamines include nonsedating loratadine (10 mg orally once daily), desloratadine (5 mg once daily), and fexofenadine (60 mg twice daily or 120 mg once daily) and minimally sedating cetirizine (10 mg orally once daily). Brompheniramine or chlorpheniramine (4 mg orally every 6–8 hours, or 8–12 mg orally every 8–12 hours as a sustained-release tablet) and clemastine (1.34–2.68 mg orally twice daily) may be less expensive, although usually associated with some drowsiness. The H_1-receptor antagonist nasal spray azelastine (1–2 sprays per nostril daily) has also been shown to be effective in a randomized trial, although many patients object to its bitter taste. Topical nasal sprays are particularly useful in patients who experience side effects, mostly xerostomia and sedation, of oral antihistamines. Many patients who find initial benefit from an antihistamine complain that allergy symptoms eventually return after several months of use. In such patients, typically with perennial allergy problems, antihistamine tolerance seems to develop and alternating effective antihistamines periodically can control symptoms over the long term.

C. Adjunctive Treatment Measures

In addition to intranasal corticosteroid sprays and antihistamines, including H_1-receptor antagonists, the literature supports the use of antileukotriene medications such as montelukast (10 mg/d orally) alone or with cetirizine (10 mg/d orally) or loratadine (10 mg/d orally). There are proinflammatory effects of cysteinyl leukotrienes in upper airway disease, including allergic rhinitis, and hyperplastic polyposis, and sinusitis. Improved nasal rhinorrhea, sneezing, and congestion are seen with the use of leukotriene receptor antagonists, often in conjunction with antihistamines. Cromolyn sodium and sodium nedocromil are also useful adjunct agents for allergic rhinitis. They work by stabilizing mast cells and preventing proinflammatory mediator release. They are not absorbed by the gastrointestinal tract but do function topically and have very few side effects. The most useful form of cromolyn is probably the ophthalmologic preparation; the nasal preparation is not nearly as effective as inhaled corticosteroids. Intranasal cromolyn is cleared rapidly and must be administered four times daily for continued relief of symptoms.

Intranasal anticholinergic agents, such as ipratropium bromide 0.03% or 0.06% sprays (42–84 mcg per nostril three times daily), may be helpful adjuncts when rhinorrhea is a major symptom. Ipratropium nasal sprays are not as effective as intranasal corticosteroids for treating allergic rhinitis but are particularly useful for treating **vasomotor rhinitis**.

Avoiding or reducing exposure to airborne allergens is the most effective means of alleviating symptoms of allergic rhinitis. Depending on the allergen, this can be extremely difficult. Maintaining an allergen-free environment by covering pillows and mattresses with plastic covers, substituting synthetic materials (foam mattress, acrylics) for animal products (wool, horsehair), and removing dust-collecting household fixtures (carpets, drapes, bedspreads, wicker) is worth the attempt to help more troubled patients. Air purifiers and dust filters may also aid in maintaining an allergen-free environment. Nasal saline irrigations are a useful adjunct in the treatment of allergic rhinitis to mechanically flush the allergens from the nasal cavity. Though debated, there is no clear benefit to hypertonic saline over commercially available normal saline preparations (eg, Ayr or Ocean Spray). When symptoms are extremely bothersome, a search for offending allergens may prove helpful. This can either be done by serum radioallergosorbent test (RAST) testing or skin testing by an allergist.

In some cases, allergic rhinitis symptoms are inadequately relieved by medication and avoidance measures. Often, such patients have a strong family history of atopy and may also have lower respiratory manifestations such as allergic asthma. Referral to an allergist may be appropriate for consideration of immunotherapy. This treatment course is quite involved, with proper identification of offending allergens, progressively increasing doses of allergen(s) and eventual maintenance dose administration over a period of 3–5 years. Immunotherapy has been proven to reduce circulating IgE levels in patients with allergic rhinitis and reduce the need for allergy medications. Both subcutaneous and sublingual immunotherapy have been shown to be effective in the long-term treatment of refractory allergic rhinitis. Treatments are given at a suitable medical facility with monitoring following treatment because of the risk of anaphylaxis during dose escalation. Local reactions from injections are common and usually self-limited.

Bernstein DI et al. Current standards and future directions in immunotherapy: perspectives on challenges and opportunities for the allergist. Ann Allergy Asthma Immunol. 2011 Nov;107(5):422–5. [PMID: 22018613]

Uzzaman A et al. Chapter 5: Allergic rhinitis. Allergy Asthma Proc. 2012 May–Jun;33(Suppl 1):S15–8. [PMID: 22794678]

OLFACTORY DYSFUNCTION

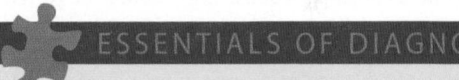

ESSENTIALS OF DIAGNOSIS

▶ Subjective diminished smell or taste sensation.

▶ Lack of objective nasal obstruction.

▶ Objective decrease in olfaction demonstrated by testing.

▶ General Considerations

Anatomic blockage of the nasal cavity with subsequent airflow disruption is the most common cause of olfactory dysfunction (hyposmia or anosmia). Polyps, septal deformities, and nasal tumors may be the cause. Transient olfactory dysfunction often accompanies the common cold, nasal allergies, and perennial rhinitis through changes in the nasal and olfactory epithelium. About 20% of olfactory dysfunction is idiopathic, although it often follows a viral illness. Central nervous system neoplasms, especially those that involve the olfactory groove or temporal lobe, may affect olfaction and must be considered in patients with no other explanation for their hyposmia or other neurologic signs. Head trauma accounts for < 5% of cases of hyposmia but is more commonly associated with anosmia. Absent, diminished, or distorted smell or taste has been reported in a wide variety of endocrine, nutritional, and nervous disorders. In particular, olfactory dysfunction in Parkinson disease and Alzheimer disease has been the subject of research. A great many medications have also been implicated in altering olfaction.

Clinical Findings

Evaluation of olfactory dysfunction should include a thorough history of systemic illnesses and medication use as well as a physical examination focusing on the nose and nervous system. Nasal obstruction (from polyps, trauma, foreign bodies, or nasal masses) can cause functional hyposmia and should be excluded before concluding that the disruption of olfaction is primary. Most clinical offices are not set up to test olfaction, but such tests may at times be worthwhile if only to assess whether a patient possesses any sense of smell at all. The University of Pennsylvania Smell Identification Test (UPSIT) is available commercially and is a simple, self-administered "scratch-and-sniff" test that is useful in differentiating hyposmia, anosmia, and malingering. Odor threshold can be tested at regional specialty centers using increasing concentrations of various odorants.

Treatment

Hyposmia secondary to nasal polyposis, obstruction, and chronic rhinosinusitis may respond to endoscopic sinus surgery. Unfortunately, there is no specific treatment for primary disruption of olfaction. While some disturbances spontaneously resolve, little evidence supports the use of large doses of vitamin A and zinc to patients with transient olfactory dysfunction. The degree of hyposmia is the greatest predictor of recovery, with less severe hyposmia recovering at a much higher rate. In permanent hyposmia, counseling should be offered about seasoning foods with spices (eg, pepper) that stimulate the trigeminal as well as olfactory chemoreceptors, abuse of table salt as a seasoning, and safety issues such as the use of smoke alarms and electric rather than gas home appliances.

Hong SC et al. Distorted olfactory perception: a systematic review. Acta Otolaryngol. 2012 Jun;132(Suppl 1):S27–31. [PMID: 22582778]
Rudmik L et al. Olfactory improvement after endoscopic sinus surgery. Curr Opin Otolaryngol Head Neck Surg. 2012 Feb;20(1):29–32. [PMID: 22143338]

EPISTAXIS

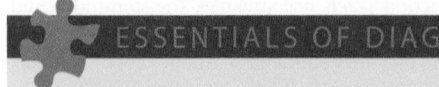

ESSENTIALS OF DIAGNOSIS

▶ Bleeding from the unilateral anterior nasal cavity most commonly.

▶ Most cases may be successfully treated by direct pressure on the bleeding site for 15 minutes. When this is inadequate, topical sympathomimetics and various nasal tamponade methods are usually effective.

▶ Posterior, bilateral, or large volume epistaxis should be triaged immediately to a specialist in a critical care setting.

General Considerations

Epistaxis is an extremely common problem in the primary care setting. Predisposing factors include nasal trauma (nose picking, foreign bodies, forceful nose blowing), rhinitis, drying of the nasal mucosa from low humidity or supplemental nasal oxygen, deviation of the nasal septum, hypertension, atherosclerotic disease, hereditary hemorrhagic telangiectasia (Osler-Weber-Rendu syndrome), inhaled nasal cocaine or other drug use, and alcohol use. Anticoagulation or antiplatelet medications may be associated with a higher incidence of epistaxis, more frequent recurrence of epistaxis, and greater difficulty controlling bleeding, but they do not cause epistaxis. Bleeding is most common in the anterior septum where a confluence of veins creates a superficial venous plexus (Kiesselbach plexus).

Clinical Findings

It is important in all patients with epistaxis to consider underlying causes of the bleeding. Laboratory assessment of bleeding parameters may be indicated, especially in recurrent cases. Once the acute episode has passed, careful examination of the nose and paranasal sinuses to rule out neoplasia and hereditary hemorrhagic telangiectasia is wise.

Patients presenting with epistaxis often have higher blood pressures than control patients, but in many cases, blood pressure returns to normal following treatment of acute bleeding. Repeat evaluation for clinically significant hypertension and treatment should be performed following control of epistaxis and removal of any packing.

Treatment

Most cases of anterior epistaxis may be successfully treated by direct pressure on the site by compression of the nares continuously for 15 min. Venous pressure is reduced in the sitting position, and slight leaning forward lessens the swallowing of blood. Short-acting topical nasal decongestants (eg, phenylephrine, 0.125–1% solution, one or two sprays), which act as vasoconstrictors, may also be helpful. When the bleeding does not readily subside, the nose should be examined, using good illumination and suction, in an attempt to locate the bleeding site. Topical 4% cocaine applied either as a spray or on a cotton strip serves both as an anesthetic and a vasoconstrictor. If cocaine is unavailable, a topical decongestant (eg, oxymetazoline) and a topical anesthetic (eg, tetracaine or lidocaine) provide similar results. When visible, the bleeding site may be cauterized with silver nitrate, diathermy, or electrocautery. A supplemental patch of Surgicel or Gelfoam may be helpful with a moisture barrier, such as petroleum-based ointment, to prevent drying and crusting.

Occasionally, a site of bleeding may be inaccessible to direct control, or attempts at direct control may be unsuccessful. In such cases there are a number of alternatives. When the site of bleeding is anterior, a hemostatic sealant, pneumatic nasal tamponade, or anterior packing may suffice. There are a number of ways to do this, such as with several feet of lubricated iodoform packing systematically placed in the floor of the nose and then the vault of the nose, or with various manufactured products designed for nasal tamponade.

About 5% of nasal bleeding originates in the **posterior nasal cavity.** Such bleeds are more commonly associated with atherosclerotic disease and hypertension. If an anteriorly placed pneumatic nasal tamponade is unsuccessful, it may be necessary to consult an otolaryngologist for a pack to occlude the choana before placing a pack anteriorly. In emergency settings, double balloon packs (Epistat) may facilitate rapid control of bleeding with little or no mucosal trauma. Because such packing is uncomfortable, bleeding may persist, and vasovagal syncope is quite possible, hospitalization for monitoring and stabilization is indicated. Opioid analgesics are needed to reduce the considerable discomfort and elevated blood pressure caused by a posterior pack.

Surgical management of epistaxis, through ligation of the nasal arterial supply (internal maxillary artery and ethmoid arteries) is an alternative to posterior nasal packing. Endovascular embolization of the internal maxillary artery or facial artery is also quite effective and can allow very specific control of hemorrhage. Such alternatives are necessary when packing fails to control life-threatening hemorrhage. On very rare occasions, ligation of the external carotid artery may be necessary.

After control of epistaxis, the patient is advised to avoid straining and vigorous exercise for several days. Nasal saline should be applied to the packing frequently to keep the packing moist. Avoidance of hot or spicy foods and tobacco is also advisable, since these may cause nasal vasodilation. Avoiding nasal trauma, including nose picking, is an obvious necessity. Lubrication with petroleum jelly or bacitracin ointment and increased home humidity may also be useful ancillary measures. Finally, antistaphylococcal antibiotics (eg, cephalexin, 500 mg orally four times daily, or clindamycin, 150 mg orally four times daily) are indicated to reduce the risk of toxic shock syndrome developing while the packing remains in place (at least 5 days).

▶ When to Refer

- Patients with recurrent epistaxis, large volume epistaxis, and episodic epistaxis with associated nasal obstruction should be referred to an otolaryngologist for endoscopic evaluation and possible imaging.
- Those with ongoing bleeding beyond 15 minutes should be taken to a local emergency department if the clinician is not prepared to manage acute epistaxis.

Manes RP. Evaluating and managing the patient with nosebleeds. Med Clin North Am. 2010 Sep;94(5):903–12. [PMID: 20736102]
Schlosser RJ. Clinical practice. Epistaxis. N Engl J Med. 2009 Feb 19;360(8):784–9. [PMID: 19228621]

NASAL TRAUMA

The nasal pyramid is the most frequently fractured bone in the body. Fracture is suggested by crepitance or palpably mobile bony segments. Epistaxis and pain are common, as are soft tissue hematomas ("black eye"). It is important to make certain that there is no palpable step-off of the infraorbital rim, which would indicate the presence of a zygomatic complex fracture. Radiologic confirmation may at times be helpful but is not necessary in uncomplicated nasal fractures. It is also important to assess for possible concomitant additional facial, pulmonary, or intracranial injuries when the circumstances of injury are suggestive, as in the case of automobile and motorcycle accidents.

Treatment is aimed at maintaining long-term nasal airway patency and cosmesis. Closed reduction, using topical 4% cocaine and locally injected 1% lidocaine, should be attempted within 1 week of injury. In the presence of marked nasal swelling, it is best to wait several days for the edema to subside before undertaking reduction. Persistent functional or cosmetic defects may be repaired by delayed reconstructive nasal surgery.

Intranasal examination should be performed in all cases to rule out septal hematoma, which appears as a widening of the anterior septum, visible just posterior to the columella. The septal cartilage receives its only nutrition from its closely adherent mucoperichondrium. An untreated subperichondrial hematoma will result in loss of the nasal cartilage with resultant saddle nose deformity. Septal hematomas may become infected, with *S aureus* most commonly, and should be drained with an incision in the inferior mucoperichondrium on both sides.

Packing for 2–5 days is often helpful to help prevent reformation of the hematoma. Antibiotics with antistaphylococcal efficacy (eg, cephalexin, 500 mg four times daily, or clindamycin, 150 mg four times daily) should be given for 3–5 days or the duration of the packing to reduce the risk of toxic shock syndrome and the drained fluid sent for culture.

Ziccardi VB et al. Management of nasal fractures. Oral Maxillofac Surg Clin North Am. 2009 May;21(2):203–8. [PMID: 19348986]

TUMORS & GRANULOMATOUS DISEASE

1. Benign Nasal Tumors

A. Nasal Polyps

Nasal polyps are pale, edematous, mucosally covered masses commonly seen in patients with allergic rhinitis, but compelling evidence argues against a purely allergic pathogenesis. They may result in chronic nasal obstruction and a diminished sense of smell. In patients with nasal polyps and a history of asthma, aspirin should be avoided as it may precipitate a severe episode of bronchospasm, known as **triad asthma** (Samter triad). Such patients may have an immunologic salicylate sensitivity. The presence of polyps in children should suggest the possibility of cystic fibrosis.

Use of topical intranasal corticosteroids improves the quality of life in patients with nasal polyposis and chronic rhinosinusitis. Initial treatment with topical nasal corticosteroids (see Allergic Rhinitis section for specific drugs) for 1–3 months is usually successful for small polyps and may reduce the need for operation. A short course of oral corticosteroids (eg, prednisone, 6-day course using 21 5-mg tablets: 30 mg on day 1 and tapering by 5 mg each day) may also be of benefit.

When polyps are massive or medical management is unsuccessful, polyps may be removed surgically. In healthy persons, this is a minor outpatient procedure. In recurrent cases or when surgery itself is associated with increased risk (such as in patients with asthma), a more complete procedure, such as ethmoidectomy, may be advisable. In recurrent polyposis, it may be necessary to remove polyps from the ethmoid, sphenoid, and maxillary sinuses to provide longer-lasting relief. Intranasal corticosteroid should be continued following polyp removal to prevent recurrence, and the clinician should consider allergen testing to determine the offending allergen and avoidance measures.

Martinez-Devesa P et al. Oral steroids for nasal polyps. Cochrane Database Syst Rev. 2011 Jul 6;(7): CD005232. [PMID: 21735400]
Rudmik L et al. Impact of topical nasal steroid therapy on symptoms of nasal polyposis: a meta-analysis. Laryngoscope. 2012 Jul;122(7):1431–7. [PMID: 22410935]

B. Inverted Papilloma

Inverted papillomas are benign tumors caused by human papillomavirus (HPV) that usually arise on the lateral nasal wall. They present with unilateral nasal obstruction and occasionally hemorrhage. They are often easily seen on anterior rhinoscopy as cauliflower-like growths in or around the middle meatus. Because squamous cell carcinoma is seen in about 10% of inverted or schneiderian papillomas, complete excision is strongly recommended. This usually requires a medial maxillectomy, but in selected cases an endoscopic approach may be possible. Because recurrence rates for inverted papilloma are reported to be as high as 20%, subsequent clinical and radiologic follow-up is imperative. All excised tissue (not just a portion) should be carefully reviewed by the pathologist to be sure no carcinoma is present.

Carta F et al. Role of endoscopic approach in the management of inverted papilloma. Curr Opin Otolaryngol Head Neck Surg. 2011 Feb;19(1):21–4. [PMID: 21191294]
Syrjänen K et al. Detection of human papillomavirus in sinonasal papillomas: systematic review and meta-analysis. Laryngoscope. 2013 Jan;123(1):181–92. [PMID: 23161522]

2. Malignant Nasopharyngeal & Paranasal Sinus Tumors

Though rare, malignant tumors of the nose, nasopharynx, and paranasal sinuses are quite problematic because they tend to remain asymptomatic until late in their course. Squamous cell carcinoma is the most common cancer found in the sinuses and nasopharynx. It is especially common in the nasopharynx, where it obstructs the eustachian tube and results in serous otitis media. Nasopharyngeal carcinoma (nonkeratinizing squamous cell carcinoma or lymphoepithelioma) is usually associated with elevated IgA antibody to the viral capsid antigen of the Epstein-Barr virus (EBV). It is particularly common in patients of southern Chinese descent and has a weaker association with tobacco exposure than other head and neck squamous cell carcinomas. Adenocarcinomas, mucosal melanomas, sarcomas, and non-Hodgkin lymphomas are less commonly encountered neoplasms of this area.

Early symptoms are nonspecific, mimicking those of rhinitis or sinusitis. Unilateral nasal obstruction, otitis media, and discharge are common, with pain and recurrent hemorrhage often clues to the diagnosis of cancer. Any adult with persistent unilateral nasal symptoms or new otitis media should be thoroughly evaluated with nasal endoscopy and nasopharyngoscopy. A high index of suspicion remains a key to early diagnosis of these tumors. Patients often present with advanced symptoms such as proptosis, expansion of a cheek, or ill-fitting maxillary dentures. Malar hypesthesia, due to involvement of the infraorbital nerve, is common in maxillary sinus tumors. Biopsy is necessary for definitive diagnosis, and MRI is the best imaging study to delineate the extent of disease and plan appropriate surgery and radiation.

Treatment depends on the tumor type and the extent of disease. Very early stage disease may be treated with megavoltage radiation therapy alone, but advanced nasopharyngeal carcinoma is best treated with concurrent radiation and cisplatin followed by adjuvant chemotherapy with cisplatin and fluorouracil. This chemoradiation therapy protocol significantly decreases local, nodal, and distant failures and increases progression-free and overall survival in advanced stage disease. Locally recurrent nasopharyngeal carcinoma may in selected cases be treated with repeat irradiation protocols or surgery with moderate success and a high degree of concern about local wound healing. Other squamous cell carcinomas are best treated—when resectable—with a combination of surgery and irradiation. Cranial base surgery, which can be done endoscopically using image navigation, appears to be an effective modality in improving the overall prognosis in paranasal sinus malignancies eroding the ethmoid roof. Although the prognosis is poor for advanced tumors, the results of treating resectable tumors of paranasal sinus origin have improved with the wider use of skull base resections and intensity-modulated radiation therapy. Cure rates are often 45–60%.

Lee AW et al. Current management of nasopharyngeal cancer. Semin Radiat Oncol. 2012 Jul;22(3):233–44. [PMID: 22687948]
Xue WQ et al. Quantitative association of tobacco smoking with the risk of nasopharyngeal carcinoma: a comprehensive meta-analysis of studies conducted between 1979 and 2011. Am J Epidemiol. 2013 Aug 1;178(3):325–38. [PMID: 23785114]

3. Sinonasal Inflammatory Disease (Granulomatosis with Polyangiitis & Sarcoidosis)

The nose and paranasal sinuses are involved in over 90% of cases of **granulomatosis with polyangiitis**. It is often not realized that involvement at these sites is more common than involvement of lungs or kidneys. Examination shows bloodstained crusts and friable mucosa. Biopsy, when positive, shows necrotizing granulomas and vasculitis. Other recognized sites of granulomatosis with polyangiitis in the head and neck include the subglottis and the middle ear.

Sarcoidosis commonly involves the paranasal sinuses and is clinically similar to other chronic sinonasal inflammatory processes. Sinonasal symptoms, including rhinorrhea, nasal obstruction, and hyposmia or anosmia may precede diagnosis of sarcoidosis in other organ systems. Clinically, the turbinates appear engorged with small white granulomas. Biopsy shows classic noncaseating granulomas. Notably, patients with sinonasal involvement generally have more trouble managing sarcoidosis in other organ systems.

Polymorphic reticulosis (midline malignant reticulosis, idiopathic midline destructive disease, lethal midline granuloma)—as the multitude of apt descriptive terms suggest—is not well understood but appears to be a nasal T-cell or NK cell lymphoma. In contrast to granulomatosis with polyangiitis, involvement is limited to the mid face, and there may be extensive bone destruction. Many destructive lesions of the mucosa and nasal structures labeled as polymorphic reticulosis are in fact non-Hodgkin lymphoma of either NK cell or T cell origin. Immunophenotyping, especially for CD56 expression, is essential in the histologic evaluation. Even when apparently localized, these lymphomas have a poor prognosis, with progression and death within a year the rule.

For treatment of granulomatosis with polyangiitis, see Chapter 20.

Gulati S et al. Sinonasal involvement in sarcoidosis: a report of seven cases and review of literature. Eur Arch Otorhinolaryngol. 2012 Mar;269(3):891–6. [PMID: 21947433]
Taylor SC et al. Progression and management of Wegener's granulomatosis in the head and neck. Laryngoscope. 2012 Aug;122(8):1695–700. [PMID: 22674560]

DISEASES OF THE ORAL CAVITY & PHARYNX

LEUKOPLAKIA, ERYTHROPLAKIA, ORAL LICHEN PLANUS, & ORAL CANCER

 ESSENTIALS OF DIAGNOSIS

- ► **Leukoplakia**—A white lesion that cannot be removed by rubbing the mucosal surface.
- ► **Erythroplakia**—Similar to leukoplakia except that it has a definite erythematous component.
- ► **Oral Lichen Planus**—Most commonly presents as lacy leukoplakia but may be erosive; definitive diagnosis requires biopsy.
- ► **Oral Cancer**—Early lesions appear as leukoplakia or erythroplakia; more advanced lesions will be larger, with invasion into tongue such that a mass lesion is palpable. Ulceration may be present.

Leukoplakic regions range from small to several centimeters in diameter (Figure 8–3). Histologically, they are often hyperkeratoses occurring in response to chronic irritation

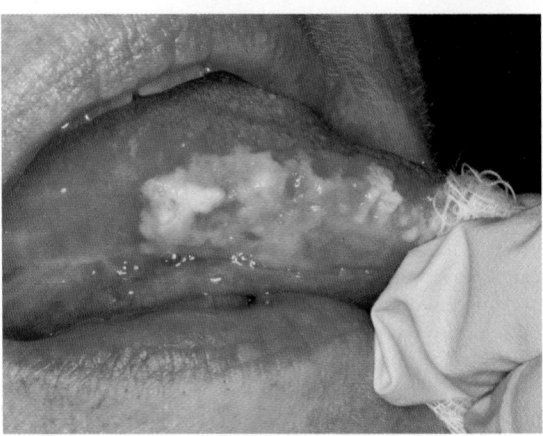

▲ **Figure 8–3.** Leukoplakia with moderate dysplasia on the lateral border of the tongue. (From Ellen Eisenberg, DMD; reproduced with permission, from Usatine RP, Smith MA, Mayeaux EJ Jr, Chumley H, Tysinger J. *The Color Atlas of Family Medicine.* McGraw-Hill, 2009.)

(eg, from dentures, tobacco, lichen planus); about 2–6%, however, represent either dysplasia or early invasive squamous cell carcinoma. Distinguishing between **erythroplakia** and **leukoplakia** is important because about 90% of cases of erythroplakia are either dysplasia or carcinoma. **Squamous cell carcinoma** accounts for 90% of oral cancer. Alcohol and tobacco use are the major epidemiologic risk factors.

The differential diagnosis may include oral candidiasis, necrotizing sialometaplasia, pseudoepitheliomatous hyperplasia, median rhomboid glossitis, and vesiculoerosive inflammatory disease such as erosive lichen planus. This should not be confused with the brown-black gingival melanin pigmentation—diffuse or speckled—common in nonwhites, blue-black embedded fragments of dental amalgam, or other systemic disorders associated with general pigmentation (neurofibromatosis, familial polyposis, Addison disease). Intraoral melanoma is extremely rare and carries a dismal prognosis.

Any area of **erythroplakia**, enlarging area of **leukoplakia**, or a lesion that has submucosal depth on palpation should have an incisional biopsy or an exfoliative cytologic examination. Ulcerative lesions are particularly suspicious and worrisome. Specialty referral should be sought early both for diagnosis and treatment. A systematic intraoral examination—including the lateral tongue, floor of the mouth, gingiva, buccal area, palate, and tonsillar fossae—and palpation of the neck for enlarged lymph nodes should be part of any general physical examination, especially in patients over the age of 45 who smoke tobacco or drink immoderately. Indirect or fiberoptic examination of the nasopharynx, oropharynx, hypopharynx, and larynx by an otolaryngologist, head and neck surgeon, or radiation oncologist should also be considered for such patients when there is unexplained or persistent throat or ear pain, oral or nasal bleeding, or oral erythroplakia. Fine-needle aspiration (FNA) biopsy may expedite the diagnosis if an enlarged lymph node is found. To date, there are no approved therapies for reversing or stabilizing leukoplakia or erythroplakia.

Oral lichen planus is a relatively common (0.5–2% of the population) chronic inflammatory autoimmune disease that may be difficult to diagnose clinically because of its numerous distinct phenotypic subtypes. For example, the reticular pattern may mimic candidiasis or hyperkeratosis, while the erosive pattern may mimic squamous cell carcinoma. Management begins with distinguishing it from other oral lesions. Exfoliative cytology or a small incisional or excisional biopsy is indicated, especially if squamous cell carcinoma is suspected. Therapy is aimed at managing pain and discomfort. Corticosteroids have been used widely both locally and systemically. Cyclosporines and retinoids have also been used. Many think there is a low rate (1%) of squamous cell carcinoma arising within lichen planus (in addition to the possibility of clinical misdiagnosis).

Hairy leukoplakia occurs on the lateral border of the tongue and is a common early finding in HIV infection (see Chapter 31). It often develops quickly and appears as slightly raised leukoplakic areas with a corrugated or "hairy" surface (Figure 8–4). Clinical response following administration of zidovudine or acyclovir has been reported, and treatment is under active investigation.

Early detection of **squamous cell carcinoma** is the key to successful management (Figure 8–5). Lesions < 4 mm in depth have a low propensity to metastasize. Most patients in whom the tumor is detected before it is 2 cm in diameter are cured by local resection. Radiation is an alternative but not generally used as first-line therapy for small lesions. Large tumors are usually treated with a combination of resection, neck dissection, and external beam radiation. Reconstruction, if required, is done at the time of resection and can involve the use of myocutaneous flaps or vascularized free flaps with or without bone.

Clinical trials have suggested a role for beta-carotene, cyclooxygenase (COX)-2 inhibitors, vitamin E, and retinoids in producing regression of leukoplakia and reducing the incidence of recurrent squamous cell carcinomas. Retinoids suppress head and neck and lung carcinogenesis in animal models and inhibit carcinogenesis in individuals with premalignant lesions. They also seem to reduce the

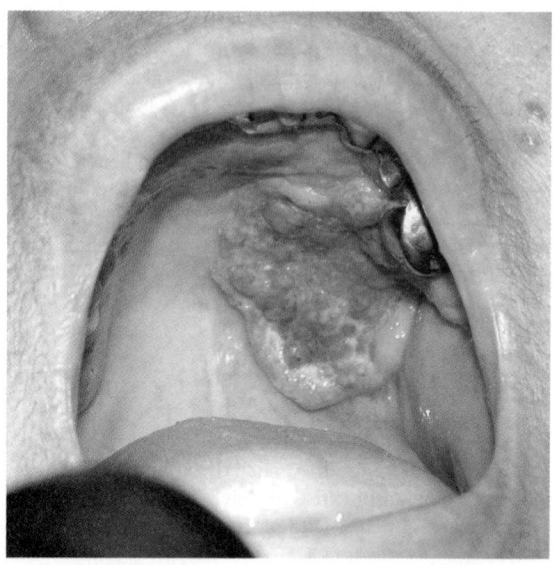

▲ **Figure 8–5.** Squamous cell carcinoma of the palate. (From Frank Miller, MD; reproduced with permission, from Usatine RP, Smith MA, Mayeaux EJ Jr, Chumley H, Tysinger J. *The Color Atlas of Family Medicine.* McGraw-Hill, 2009.)

incidence of second primary cancers in head and neck and lung cancer patients previously treated for a primary.

Amagasa T et al. Oral premalignant lesions: from a clinical perspective. Int J Clin Oncol. 2011 Feb;16(1):5–14. [PMID: 21225307]
García-García V et al. New perspectives on the dynamic behaviour of oral lichen planus. Eur J Dermatol. 2012 Mar–Apr;22(2):172–7. [PMID: 22381396]
Liu W et al. Malignant transformation of oral leukoplakia: a retrospective cohort study of 218 Chinese patients. BMC Cancer. 2010 Dec 16;10:685. [PMID: 21159209]

ORAL CANDIDIASIS

ESSENTIALS OF DIAGNOSIS

▶ Fluctuating throat or mouth discomfort.
▶ Systemic or local immunosuppression, such as recent corticosteroid, chemotherapy, or antibiotic use.
▶ Erythema of the oral cavity or oropharynx with fluffy, white patches.
▶ Rapid resolution of symptoms with appropriate treatment.

► Clinical Findings

A. Symptoms and Signs

Oral candidiasis (thrush) is usually painful and looks like creamy-white curd-like patches overlying erythematous mucosa (see Figure 6–24). Because these white areas are

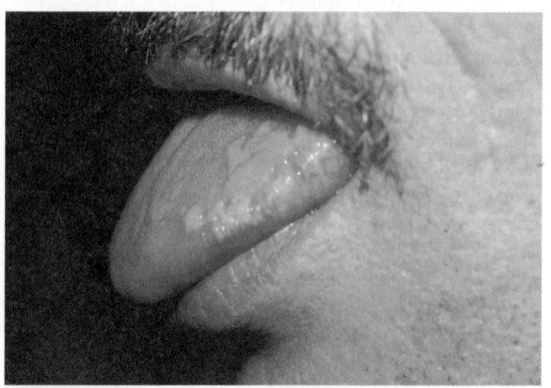

▲ **Figure 8–4.** Oral hairy leukoplakia on the side of the tongue in AIDS. (From Richard P. Usatine, MD; reproduced with permission, from Usatine RP, Smith MA, Mayeaux EJ Jr, Chumley H, Tysinger J. *The Color Atlas of Family Medicine.* McGraw-Hill, 2009.)

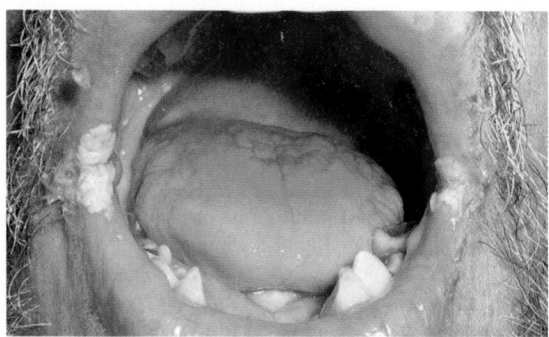

▲ **Figure 8–6.** Severe angular cheilitis in HIV-positive man with oral thrush. (From Richard P. Usatine, MD; reproduced with permission, from Usatine RP, Smith MA, Mayeaux EJ Jr, Chumley H, Tysinger J. *The Color Atlas of Family Medicine.* McGraw-Hill, 2009.)

easily rubbed off (eg, by a tongue depressor)—unlike leu-koplakia or lichen planus—only the underlying irregular erythema may be seen. Oral candidiasis is commonly encountered among the following adult patients: (1) those who wear dentures, (2) those who are debilitated and have poor oral hygiene, (3) those with diabetes, (4) those with anemia, (5) those undergoing chemotherapy or local irra-diation, and (6) those receiving corticosteroids (oral or systemic) or broad-spectrum antibiotics. Angular cheilitis is another manifestation of candidiasis, although it is also seen in nutritional deficiencies (Figure 8–6).

B. Diagnostic Studies

The diagnosis is made clinically. A wet preparation using potassium hydroxide will reveal spores and may show non-septate mycelia. Biopsy will show intraepithelial pseudo-mycelia of *Candida albicans.*

Candidiasis is often the first manifestation of HIV infec-tion, and HIV testing should be considered in patients with no known predisposing cause for *Candida* overgrowth (see also Chapter 31). The US Department of Health Services Clinical Practice Guideline for Evaluation and Management of Early HIV Infection recommends examination of the oral mucosa with each clinician visit as well as at a dental exami-nation every 6 months for individuals infected with HIV.

▶ Treatment

Effective antifungal therapy may be achieved with any of the following: fluconazole (100 mg orally daily for 7 days), ketoconazole (200–400 mg orally with breakfast [requires acidic gastric environment for absorption] for 7–14 days), clotrimazole troches (10 mg dissolved orally five times daily), or nystatin mouth rinses (500,000 units [5 mL of 100,000 units/mL] held in the mouth before swallowing three times daily). In patients with HIV infection, however, longer courses of therapy with fluconazole may be needed, and oral itraconazole (200 mg/d) may be indicated in flu-conazole-refractory cases. Many of the *Candida* species in these patients are resistant to first-line azoles and may require newer drugs, such as voriconazole. In addition,

0.12% chlorhexidine or half-strength hydrogen peroxide mouth rinses may provide local relief. Nystatin powder (100,000 units/g) applied to dentures three or four times daily for several weeks may help denture wearers.

Giannini PJ et al. Diagnosis and management of oral candidiasis. Otolaryngol Clin North Am. 2011 Feb;44(1):231–40. [PMID: 21093632]

Pienaar ED et al. Interventions for the prevention and manage-ment of oropharyngeal candidiasis associated with HIV infec-tion in adults and children. Cochrane Database Syst Rev. 2010 Nov 10;11: CD003940. [PMID: 21069679]

GLOSSITIS, GLOSSODYNIA, DYSGEUSIA, & BURNING MOUTH SYNDROME

Inflammation of the tongue with loss of filiform papillae leads to a red, smooth-surfaced tongue (glossitis). Rarely painful, it may be secondary to nutritional deficiencies (eg, niacin, riboflavin, iron, or vitamin E), drug reactions, dehydration, irritants, foods and liquids, and possibly auto-immune reactions or psoriasis. If the primary cause cannot be identified and corrected, empiric nutritional replace-ment therapy may be of value.

Glossodynia is burning and pain of the tongue, which may occur with or without glossitis. In the absence of any clinical findings, it has been termed "burning mouth syn-drome." Glossodynia with glossitis has been associated with diabetes mellitus, drugs (eg, diuretics), tobacco, xerosto-mia, and candidiasis as well as the listed causes of glossitis. Periodontal disease is not apt to be a factor. The burning mouth syndrome typically has no identifiable associated risk factors and seems to be most common in postmeno-pausal women. Treating possible underlying causes, chang-ing long-term medications to alternative ones, and smoking cessation may resolve symptoms of glossitis. Both gloss-odynia and the burning mouth syndrome are benign, and reassurance that there is no infection or tumor is likely to be appreciated. Effective treatments for the burning mouth syndrome include alpha-lipoic acid and clonazepam. Clon-azepam is most effective as a rapid dissolving tablet placed on the tongue in doses from 0.25 mg to 0.5 mg every 8–12 hours. Behavioral therapy has also been shown to be effec-tive. Unilateral symptoms, symptoms that cannot be related to a specific medication, and symptoms and signs involving regions supplied by other cranial nerves all may suggest neuropathology, and imaging of the brain, brainstem, and skull base with MRI should be considered.

Minor JS et al. Burning mouth syndrome and secondary oral burning. Otolaryngol Clin North Am. 2011 Feb;44(1): 205–19. [PMID: 21093630]

INTRAORAL ULCERATIVE LESIONS

1. Necrotizing Ulcerative Gingivitis (Trench Mouth, Vincent Angina)

Necrotizing ulcerative gingivitis, often caused by an infec-tion of both spirochetes and fusiform bacilli, is common in young adults under stress (classically at examination time).

Underlying systemic diseases may also predispose to this disorder. Clinically, there is painful acute gingival inflammation and necrosis, often with bleeding, halitosis, fever, and cervical lymphadenopathy. Warm half-strength peroxide rinses and oral penicillin (250 mg three times daily for 10 days) may help. Dental gingival curettage may prove necessary.

Feller L et al. Necrotizing periodontal diseases in HIV-seropositive subjects: pathogenic mechanisms. J Int Acad Periodontol. 2008 Jan;10(1):10–5. [PMID: 18333595]

2. Aphthous Ulcer (Canker Sore, Ulcerative Stomatitis)

Aphthous ulcers are very common and easy to recognize. Their cause remains uncertain, although an association with human herpesvirus 6 has been suggested. Found on freely moving, nonkeratinized mucosa (eg, buccal and labial mucosa and not attached gingiva or palate), they may be single or multiple, are usually recurrent, and appear as painful small round ulcerations with yellow-gray fibrinoid centers surrounded by red halos (Figure 8–7). Minor aphthous ulcers are < 1 cm and generally heal in 10–14 days. Major aphthous ulcers are > 1 cm and can be disabling due to the degree of associated oral pain.

Treatment is challenging because no single systemic treatment has proven effective. Topical corticosteroids (triamcinolone acetonide, 0.1%, or fluocinonide ointment, 0.05%) in an adhesive base (Orabase Plain) do appear to provide symptomatic relief in many patients. Other topical therapies shown to be effective in controlled studies include diclofenac 3% in hyaluronan 2.5%, doxymycine-cyanoacrylate, mouthwashes containing the enzymes amyloglucosidase and glucose oxidase, and amlexanox 5% oral paste. A 1-week tapering course of prednisone (40–60 mg/d) has also been used successfully. Cimetidine maintenance therapy may be useful in patients with recurrent aphthous ulcers. Thalidomide has been used selectively in recurrent aphthous ulcerations in HIV-positive patients.

Large or persistent areas of ulcerative stomatitis may be secondary to erythema multiforme or drug allergies, acute herpes simplex, pemphigus, pemphigoid, epidermolysis bullosa acquisita, bullous lichen planus, Behçet disease, or inflammatory bowel disease. Squamous cell carcinoma may occasionally present in this fashion. When the diagnosis is not clear, incisional biopsy is indicated.

Brocklehurst P et al. Systemic interventions for recurrent aphthous stomatitis (mouth ulcers). Cochrane Database Syst Rev. 2012 Sep 12;9: CD005411. [PMID: 22972085]
Chattopadhyay A et al. Recurrent aphthous stomatitis. Otolaryngol Clin North Am. 2011 Feb;44(1):79–88. [PMID: 21093624]

3. Herpes Stomatitis

Herpes gingivostomatitis is common, mild, and short-lived and requires no intervention in most adults. In immunocompromised persons, however, reactivation of herpes simplex virus infection is frequent and may be severe. Clinically, there is initial burning, followed by typical small vesicles that rupture and form scabs. Lesions are most commonly found on the attached gingiva and mucocutaneous junction of the lip, but lesions can also form on the tongue, buccal mucosa, and soft palate. Acyclovir (200–800 mg orally five times daily for 7–14 days) may shorten the course and reduce postherpetic pain. Differential diagnosis includes aphthous stomatitis (see above), erythema multiforme, syphilitic chancre, and carcinoma. Coxsackievirus-caused lesions (grayish white tonsillar plaques and palatal ulcers of herpangina or buccal and lip ulcers in hand-foot-and-mouth disease) are seen more commonly in children under age 6.

Nasser M et al. Acyclovir for treating primary herpetic gingivostomatitis. Cochrane Database Syst Rev. 2008 Oct 8;(4): CD006700. [PMID: 18843726]
Westley S et al. Recurrent intra-oral herpes simplex 1 infection. Dent Update. 2011 Jul–Aug;38(6):368–70,372–4. [PMID: 21905349]

PHARYNGITIS & TONSILLITIS

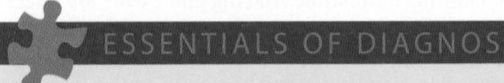

ESSENTIALS OF DIAGNOSIS

► Sore throat.

► Fever.

► Anterior cervical adenopathy.

► Tonsillar exudate.

► Focus is to treat group A beta-hemolytic streptococcus infection to prevent rheumatic sequelae.

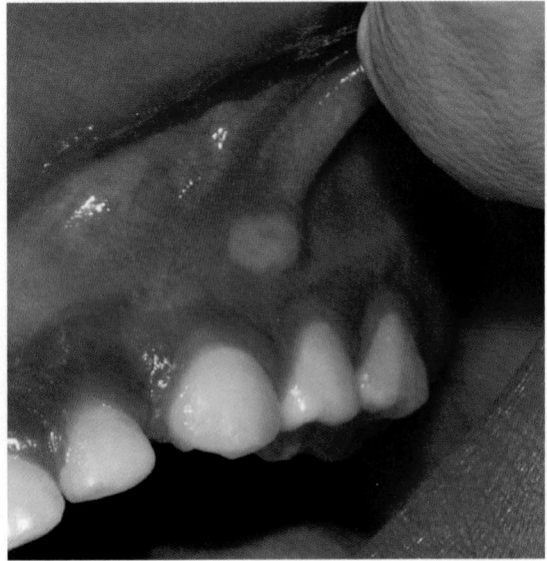

▲ **Figure 8–7.** Aphthous stomatitis. (From Ellen Eisenberg, MD and Dr. Joanna Douglas; reproduced with permission, from Usatine RP, Smith MA, Mayeaux EJ Jr, Chumley H, Tysinger J. *The Color Atlas of Family Medicine.* McGraw-Hill, 2009.)

General Considerations

Pharyngitis and tonsillitis account for over 10% of all office visits to primary care clinicians and 50% of outpatient antibiotic use. The most appropriate management continues to be debated because some of the issues are deceptively complex, but consensus has increased in recent years. The main concern is determining who is likely to have a group A beta-hemolytic streptococcal infection (GABHS), as this can lead to subsequent complications such as rheumatic fever and glomerulonephritis. A second public health policy concern is reducing the extraordinary cost (both in dollars and in the development of antibiotic-resistant *S pneumoniae*) in the United States associated with unnecessary antibiotic use. Questions now being asked: Is there still a role for culturing a sore throat, or have the rapid antigen tests supplanted this procedure under most circumstances? Are clinical criteria alone a sufficient basis for decisions about which patients should be given antibiotics? Should any patient receive any antibiotic other than penicillin (or erythromycin if penicillin-allergic)? For how long should treatment be continued? Numerous well-done studies in the past few years as well as increasing experience with rapid laboratory tests for detection of streptococci (eliminating the delay caused by culturing) appear to make a consensus approach more possible.

Clinical Findings

A. Symptoms and Signs

The clinical features most suggestive of GABHS pharyngitis include fever over 38°C, tender anterior cervical adenopathy, lack of a cough, and a pharyngotonsillar exudate (Figures 8–8 and 8–9). These four features (the Centor criteria), when present, strongly suggest GABHS, and some would treat regardless of laboratory results. When three of the four are present, laboratory sensitivity of rapid antigen testing for GABHS exceeds 90%. When only one criterion is present,

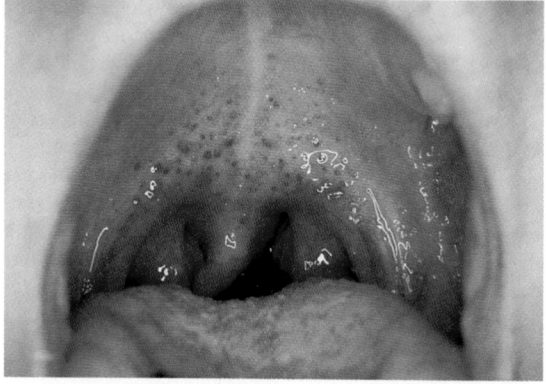

▲ **Figure 8–9.** Pharyngeal inflammation and petechiae of the soft palate caused by group A streptococcus. (From Dr. Heinz F. Eichenwald, Public Health Image Library, CDC.)

GABHS is unlikely. Sore throat may be severe, with odynophagia, tender adenopathy, and a scarlatiniform rash. An elevated white count and left shift are also possible. Hoarseness, cough, and coryza are not suggestive of this disease.

Marked lymphadenopathy and a shaggy white-purple tonsillar exudate, often extending into the nasopharynx, suggest mononucleosis, especially if present in a young adult. With about 90% sensitivity, lymphocyte to white blood cell ratios of > 35% suggest EBV infection and not tonsillitis. Hepatosplenomegaly and a positive heterophil agglutination test or elevated anti-EBV titer are corroborative. However, about one-third of patients with infectious mononucleosis have secondary streptococcal tonsillitis, requiring treatment. Ampicillin should routinely be avoided if mononucleosis is suspected because it induces a rash that might be misinterpreted by the patient as a penicillin allergy. Diphtheria (extremely rare but described in the alcoholic population) presents with low-grade fever and an ill patient with a gray tonsillar pseudomembrane.

The most common pathogens other than GABHS in the differential diagnosis of "sore throat" are viruses, *Neisseria gonorrhoeae*, *Mycoplasma*, and *Chlamydia trachomatis*. Rhinorrhea and lack of exudate would suggest a virus, but in practice it is not possible to confidently distinguish viral upper respiratory infection from GABHS on clinical grounds alone. Infections with *Corynebacterium diphtheria*, anaerobic streptococci, and *Corynebacterium haemolyticum* (which responds better to erythromycin than penicillin) may also mimic pharyngitis due to GABHS.

B. Laboratory Findings

A single-swab throat culture is 90–95% sensitive and the rapid antigen detection testing (RADT) is 90–99% sensitive for GABHS. Results from the RADT are available in about 15 minutes, much sooner than from the throat culture.

Treatment

Given the availability of many well-documented studies in recent years, one would think that a consensus might

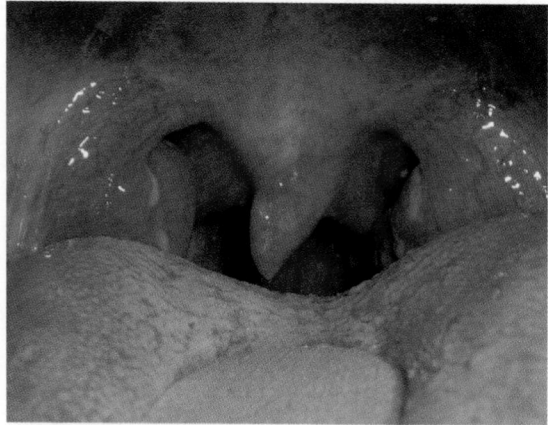

▲ **Figure 8–8.** Streptococcal pharyngitis showing tonsillar exudate and erythema. (From Michael Nguyen, MD; reproduced with permission, from Usatine RP, Smith MA, Mayeaux EJ Jr, Chumley H, Tysinger J. *The Color Atlas of Family Medicine.* McGraw-Hill, 2009.)

develop as to the most appropriate way to treat a sore throat. The Infectious Diseases Society of America recommends laboratory confirmation of the clinical diagnosis by means of either throat culture or RADT of the throat swab. The American College of Physicians–American Society of Internal Medicine (ACP-ASIM), in collaboration with the Centers for Disease Control and Prevention, advocates use of a clinical algorithm alone—in lieu of microbiologic testing—for confirmation of the diagnosis in adults for whom the suspicion of streptococcal infection is high. Others examine the assumptions of the ACP-ASIM guideline for using a clinical algorithm alone and question whether those recommendations will achieve the stated objective of dramatically decreasing excess antibiotic use. A reasonable strategy to follow is that patients with zero or one Centor criteria are at very low risk for GABHS and therefore, do not need throat cultures or RADT of the throat swap and should not receive antibiotics. Patients with two or three Centor criteria need throat cultures or RADT of the throat swap, since positive results would warrant antibiotic treatment. Patients who have four Centor criteria are likely to have GABHS and can receive empiric therapy without throat culture or RADT.

Forty years ago, a single intramuscular injection of benzathine penicillin or procaine penicillin, 1.2 million units once, was the standard antibiotic treatment. This remains effective, but the injection is painful. It is now used for patients if compliance with an oral regimen is an issue. Currently, oral treatment is effective and preferred. Antibiotic choice aims to reduce the already low (10–20%) incidence of treatment failures (positive culture after treatment despite symptomatic resolution) and recurrences. Penicillin V potassium (250 mg orally three times daily or 500 mg twice daily for 10 days) or cefuroxime axetil (250 mg orally twice daily for 5–10 days) are both effective. The efficacy of a 5-day regimen of penicillin V potassium appears to be similar to that of a 10-day course, with a 94% clinical response rate and an 84% streptococcal eradication rate. Erythromycin (also active against *Mycoplasma* and *Chlamydia*) is a reasonable alternative to penicillin in allergic patients. Cephalosporins are somewhat more effective than penicillin in producing bacteriologic cures; 5-day administration has been successful for cefpodoxime and cefuroxime. The macrolide antibiotics have also been reported to be successful in shorter-duration regimens. Azithromycin (500 mg once daily), because of its long half-life, need be taken for only 3 days.

Adequate antibiotic treatment usually avoids the streptococcal complications of scarlet fever, glomerulonephritis, rheumatic myocarditis, and local abscess formation.

Antibiotics for treatment failures are also somewhat controversial. Surprisingly, penicillin-tolerant strains are not isolated more frequently in those who fail treatment than in those treated successfully with penicillin. The reasons for failure appear to be complex, and a second course of treatment with the same drug is reasonable. Alternatives to penicillin include cefuroxime and other cephalosporins, dicloxacillin (which is beta-lactamase–resistant), and amoxicillin with clavulanate. When there is a history of penicillin allergy, alternatives should be used, such as erythromycin. Erythromycin resistance—with failure rates

of about 25%—is an increasing problem in many areas. In cases of severe penicillin allergy, cephalosporins should be avoided as the cross-reaction is common (8% or more).

Ancillary treatment of pharyngitis includes analgesics and anti-inflammatory agents, such as aspirin, acetaminophen, and corticosteroids. In meta-analysis, corticosteroids increased the likelihood of complete pain resolution at 24 hours by threefold without an increase in recurrence or adverse events. Some patients find that salt water gargling is soothing. In severe cases, anesthetic gargles and lozenges (eg, benzocaine) may provide additional symptomatic relief. Occasionally, odynophagia is so intense that hospitalization for intravenous hydration and antibiotics is necessary. (See Chapter 33.)

Patients who have had rheumatic fever should be treated with a continuous course of antimicrobial prophylaxis (erythromycin, 250 mg twice daily orally, or penicillin G, 500 mg once daily orally) for at least 5 years.

Hayward G et al. Corticosteroids as standalone or add-on treatment for sore throat. Cochrane Database Syst Rev. 2012 Oct 17;10: CD008268. [PMID: 23076943]

Kociolek LK et al. In the clinic. Pharyngitis. Ann Intern Med. 2012 Sep 4;157(5):ITC3-1–16. [PMID: 22944886]

van Driel ML et al. Different antibiotic treatments for group A streptococcal pharyngitis. Cochrane Database Syst Rev. 2010 Oct 6;(10): CD004406. [PMID: 20927734]

PERITONSILLAR ABSCESS & CELLULITIS

When infection penetrates the tonsillar capsule and involves the surrounding tissues, peritonsillar cellulitis results. Peritonsillar abscess (**quinsy**) and cellulitis present with severe sore throat, odynophagia, trismus, medial deviation of the soft palate and peritonsillar fold, and an abnormal muffled ("hot potato") voice. Following therapy, peritonsillar cellulitis usually either resolves over several days or evolves into peritonsillar abscess. The existence of an abscess may be confirmed by aspirating pus from the peritonsillar fold just superior and medial to the upper pole of the tonsil. A 19-gauge or 21-gauge needle should be passed medial to the molar and no deeper than 1 cm, because the internal carotid artery may lie more medially than its usual location and pass posterior and deep to the tonsillar fossa. Most commonly, patients with peritonsillar abscess present to the emergency department and receive a dose of parenteral amoxicillin (1 g), amoxicillin-sulbactam (3 g), or clindamycin (600–900 mg). Less severe cases and patients who are able to tolerate oral intake may be treated for 7–10 days with oral antibiotics, including amoxicillin, 500 mg three times a day; amoxicillin-clavulanate, 875 mg twice a day; or clindamycin, 300 mg four times daily. Although antibiotic treatment is generally undisputed, there is controversy regarding the surgical management of peritonsillar abscess. Methods include needle aspiration, incision and drainage, and tonsillectomy. Some clinicians incise and drain the area and continue with parenteral antibiotics, whereas others aspirate only and monitor as an outpatient. To drain the abscess and avoid recurrence, it may be appropriate to consider immediate tonsillectomy (quinsy tonsillectomy). About 10% of patients with peritonsillar abscess exhibit relative indications for tonsillectomy. All three approaches are effective and have support in the literature. Regardless of the method used, one must be sure the abscess is adequately treated, since complications such as extension to the retropharyngeal, deep neck, and posterior mediastinal spaces are possible. Bacteria may also be aspirated into the lungs, resulting in pneumonia. There is controversy about whether a single abscess is a sufficient indication for tonsillectomy; about 30% of patients aged 17–30 who do not undergo early planned tonsillectomy following peritonsillar abscess ultimately undergo surgery and only about 13% of those over 30 have their tonsils removed.

Tagliareni JM et al. Tonsillitis, peritonsillar and lateral pharyngeal abscesses. Oral Maxillofac Surg Clin North Am. 2012 May;24(2):197–204. [PMID: 22503067]
Wikstén J et al. Who ends up having tonsillectomy after peritonsillar infection? Eur Arch Otorhinolaryngol. 2012 Apr;269(4):1281–4. [PMID: 22037720]

DEEP NECK INFECTIONS

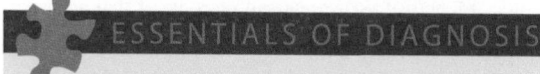

ESSENTIALS OF DIAGNOSIS

▸ Marked acute neck pain and swelling.

▸ Abscesses are emergencies because rapid airway compromise may occur.

▸ May spread to the mediastinum or cause sepsis.

▸ General Considerations

Ludwig angina is the most commonly encountered neck space infection. It is a cellulitis of the sublingual and submaxillary spaces, often arising from infection of the mandibular dentition. **Deep neck abscesses** most commonly originate from odontogenic infections. Other causes include suppurative lymphadenitis, direct spread of pharyngeal infection, penetrating trauma, pharyngoesophageal foreign bodies, cervical osteomyelitis, and intravenous injection of the internal jugular vein, especially in drug abusers. Recurrent deep neck infection may suggest an underlying congenital lesion such as a branchial cleft cyst. Suppurative lymphadenopathy in middle-age persons who smoke and drink alcohol regularly should be considered a manifestation of malignancy (typically metastatic squamous cell carcinoma) until proven otherwise.

▸ Clinical Findings

Patients with **Ludwig angina** have edema and erythema of the upper neck under the chin and often of the floor of the mouth. The tongue may be displaced upward and backward by the posterior spread of cellulitis and coalescence of pus is often present in the floor of mouth. This may lead to occlusion of the airway. Microbiologic isolates include streptococci, staphylococci, *Bacteroides*, and *Fusobacterium*.

Patients with **deep neck abscesses** usually present with marked neck pain and swelling. Fever is common but not always present. *Deep neck abscesses are emergencies because they may rapidly compromise the airway.* Untreated or inadequately treated, they may spread to the mediastinum or cause sepsis.

Contrast-enhanced CT usually augments the clinical examination in defining the extent of the infection. It often will distinguish inflammation and phlegmon (requiring antibiotics) from abscess (requiring drainage), and define for the surgeon the extent of an abscess. CT with MRI may also identify thrombophlebitis of the internal jugular vein secondary to oropharyngeal inflammation. This condition, known as **Lemierre syndrome**, is rare and usually associated with severe headache. The presence of pulmonary infiltrates consistent with septic emboli in the setting of a neck abscess should lead one to suspect Lemierre syndrome.

▸ Treatment

Usual doses of penicillin plus metronidazole, ampicillin-sulbactam, clindamycin, or selective cephalosporins are good initial choices for treatment of **Ludwig angina**. Culture and sensitivity data are then used to refine the choice. Dental consultation is advisable to address the offending tooth or teeth. External drainage via bilateral submental incisions is required if the airway is threatened or when medical therapy has not reversed the process.

Treatment of **deep neck abscesses** includes securing the airway, intravenous antibiotics, and incision and drainage. When the infection involves the floor of mouth, base of tongue, supraglottic or paraglottic space, the airway may be secured either by intubation or tracheotomy. Tracheotomy is preferable in the patients with substantial pharyngeal edema, since attempts at intubation may precipitate acute airway obstruction. Bleeding in association with a deep neck abscess is very rare but suggests carotid artery or internal jugular vein involvement and requires prompt neck exploration both for drainage of pus and for vascular control.

Patients with **Lemierre syndrome** require prompt institution of antibiotics appropriate for *Fusobacterium necrophorum* as well as the more usual upper airway pathogens. The use of anticoagulation in treatment is debated and of no proven benefit.

Dahlén G et al. Necrobacillosis in humans. Expert Rev Anti Infect Ther. 2011 Feb;9(2):227–36. [PMID: 21342070]
Vieira F et al. Deep neck infection. Otolaryngol Clin North Am. 2008 Jun;41(3):459–83. [PMID: 18435993]

SNORING

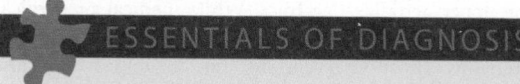

ESSENTIALS OF DIAGNOSIS

▸ Noise produced on inspiration during sleep.

▸ Snoring is associated with obstructive sleep apnea (OSA) but has no disruption of sleep by clinical sleep evaluation.

▶ General Considerations

Ventilation disorders during sleep are extremely common. While OSA occurs in 5–10% of Americans, clinically relevant snoring may occur in as many as 59%. In general, sleep-disordered breathing problems are attributed to narrowing of the upper aerodigestive tract during sleep due to changes in position, muscle tone, and soft tissue hypertrophy or laxity. The most common sites of obstruction are the oropharynx and the base of the tongue. The spectrum of the problem ranges from simple snoring without cessation of airflow to OSA with long periods of apnea and life-threatening physiologic sequelae. OSA is discussed in Chapter 9. In contrast to OSA, snoring is almost exclusively a social problem, and despite its prevalence and association with OSA, there is comparatively little known about the management of this problem.

▶ Clinical Findings

A. Symptoms and Signs

All patients who complain of snoring should be evaluated for OSA as discussed in Chapter 9. Symptoms of OSA (including snoring, excessive daytime somnolence, daytime headaches, and weight gain) may be present in as many as 30% of patients without demonstrable apnea or hypopnea on formal testing. Clinical examination should include examination of the nasal cavity, nasopharynx, oropharynx, and larynx to help exclude other causes of dynamic airway obstruction. In many cases of isolated snoring, the palate and uvula appear enlarged and elongated with excessive mucosa hanging below the muscular portion of the soft palate.

B. Imaging and Diagnostic Testing

Sleep examination with polysomnography is strongly advised in the evaluation of a patient with complaints of snoring. Radiographic imaging of the head or neck is generally not necessary for management of primary snoring.

▶ Treatment

Expeditious and inexpensive management solutions of snoring are sought, often with little or no benefit. Diet modification and a regimen of physical exercise can lead to improvement in snoring through weight loss and improvement in pharyngeal tone that accompanies overall physical conditioning. Position change during sleep can be effective, and time-honored treatments such as taping or sewing a tennis ball to the back of a shirt worn during sleep may satisfactorily eliminate symptoms by ensuring recumbency on one side.

Anatomic management of snoring can be challenging. As with OSA, snoring can come from a number of sites in the upper aerodigestive tract. While medical or surgical correction of nasal obstruction may help alleviate snoring problems, most interventions aim to improve airflow through the nasopharynx and oropharynx. Nonsurgical options include mandibular advancement appliances designed to pull the base of tongue forward and continuous positive airway pressure via face or nasal mask. Compliance with both of these treatment options is problematic

because snorers without OSA do not notice the physiologic benefits of these devices noted by patients with sleep apnea.

Surgical correction of snoring is most commonly directed at the soft palate. Historical approaches involved resection of redundant mucosa and the uvula similar to uvulopalatopharyngoplasty that is used for OSA. Regardless of how limited the procedure or what technique was used, postoperative pain, expense of general anesthesia and high recurrence rates limit the utility of these procedures. Office-based approaches are more widely used because of these limitations. Most of these procedures aim to stiffen the palate to prevent vibration rather than remove it. A series of procedures, including injection snoreplasty, radiofrequency thermal fibrosis, and implantable palatal device have been used with variable success and patient tolerance. The techniques can be technically challenging. Persistent symptoms may occur following initial treatment necessitating costly (and sometimes painful) repeat procedures. The durability of these procedures in alleviating symptoms is also poorly understood and late failures can lead to patient and clinician frustration.

Bäck LJ et al. Radiofrequency ablation treatment of soft palate for patients with snoring: a systematic review of effectiveness and adverse effects. Laryngoscope. 2009 Jun;119(6):1241–50. [PMID: 19365852]

Pliska BT et al. Effectiveness and outcome of oral appliance therapy. Dent Clin North Am. 2012 Apr;56(2):433–44. [PMID: 22480812]

Ulualp SO. Snoring and obstructive sleep apnea. Med Clin North Am. 2010 Sep;94(5):1047–55. [PMID: 20736112]

▼ DISEASES OF THE SALIVARY GLAND

ACUTE INFLAMMATORY SALIVARY GLAND DISORDERS

1. Sialadenitis

Acute bacterial sialadenitis most commonly affects either the parotid or submandibular gland. It typically presents with acute swelling of the gland, increased pain and swelling with meals, and tenderness and erythema of the duct opening. Pus often can be massaged from the duct. Sialadenitis often occurs in the setting of dehydration or in association with chronic illness. Underlying Sjögren syndrome may contribute. Ductal obstruction, often by an inspissated mucous plug, is followed by salivary stasis and secondary infection. The most common organism recovered from purulent draining saliva is *S aureus*. Treatment consists of intravenous antibiotics such as nafcillin (1 g intravenously every 4–6 hours) and measures to increase salivary flow, including hydration, warm compresses, sialagogues (eg, lemon drops), and massage of the gland. Treatment can usually then be switched to an oral agent based on clinical and microbiologic improvement to complete a 10-day treatment course. Less severe cases can often be treated with oral antibiotics with similar spectrum. Complete resolution of parotid swelling and pain can take 2–3 weeks. Failure of the process to improve and ultimately resolve on this regimen suggests abscess formation, ductal stricture, stone, or tumor causing obstruction. Ultrasound or CT scan may be helpful in establishing the diagnosis. In the setting of acute illness, a severe and potentially life-threatening form of sialadenitis, sometimes called **suppurative sialadenitis**, may develop. The causative organism is usually *S aureus*, but often no pus will drain from Stensen papilla. These patients often do not respond to rehydration and intravenous antibiotics and thus may require operative incision and drainage to resolve the infection.

2. Sialolithiasis

Calculus formation is more common in Wharton duct (draining the submandibular glands) than in Stensen duct (draining the parotid glands). Clinically, a patient may note postprandial pain and local swelling, often with a history of recurrent acute sialadenitis. Stones in Wharton duct are usually large and radiopaque, whereas those in Stensen duct are usually radiolucent and smaller. Those very close to the orifice of Wharton duct may be palpated manually in the anterior floor of the mouth and removed intraorally by dilating or incising the distal duct. The duct proximal to the stone must be temporarily clamped (using, for instance, a single throw of a suture) to keep manipulation of the stone from pushing it back toward the submandibular gland. Those more than 1.5–2 cm from the duct are too close to the lingual nerve to be removed safely in this manner. Similarly, dilation of Stensen duct, located on the buccal surface opposite the second maxillary molar, may relieve distal stricture or allow a small stone to pass. Extracorporeal shock-wave lithotripsy and fluoroscopically guided basket retrieval have been used successfully, but are being replaced by sialoendoscopy for the management of chronic sialolithiasis. Repeated episodes of sialadenitis are usually associated with stricture and chronic infection. If the obstruction cannot be safely removed or dilated, excision of the gland may be necessary to relieve recurrent symptoms.

Harrison JD. Causes, natural history, and incidence of salivary stones and obstructions. Otolaryngol Clin North Am. 2009 Dec;42(6):927–47. [PMID: 19962002]

Wallace E et al. Management of giant sialoliths: review of the literature and preliminary experience with interventional sialendoscopy. Laryngoscope. 2010 Oct;120(10):1974–8. [PMID: 20824782]

CHRONIC INFLAMMATORY & INFILTRATIVE DISORDERS OF THE SALIVARY GLANDS

Numerous infiltrative disorders may cause unilateral or bilateral parotid gland enlargement. Sjögren syndrome and sarcoidosis are examples of lymphoepithelial and granulomatous diseases that may affect the salivary glands. Metabolic disorders, including alcoholism, diabetes mellitus, and vitamin deficiencies, may also cause diffuse enlargement. Several drugs have been associated with parotid enlargement, including thioureas, iodine, and drugs with cholinergic effects (eg, phenothiazines), which stimulate salivary flow and cause more viscous saliva.

Salomonsson S et al. Minor salivary gland immunohistology in the diagnosis of primary Sjögren's syndrome. J Oral Pathol Med. 2009 Mar;38(2):282–8. [PMID: 18793250]

SALIVARY GLAND TUMORS

Approximately 80% of salivary gland tumors occur in the parotid gland. In adults, about 80% of these are benign. In the submandibular triangle, it is sometimes difficult to distinguish a primary submandibular gland tumor from a metastatic submandibular space node. Only 50–60% of primary submandibular tumors are benign. Tumors of the minor salivary glands are most likely to be malignant, with adenoid cystic carcinoma predominating, and may be found throughout the oral cavity or oropharynx.

Most parotid tumors present as an asymptomatic mass in the superficial part of the gland. Their presence may have been noted by the patient for months or years. Facial nerve involvement correlates strongly with malignancy. Tumors may extend deep to the plane of the facial nerve or may originate in the parapharyngeal space. In such cases, medial deviation of the soft palate is visible on intraoral examination. MRI and CT scans have largely replaced sialography in defining the extent of tumor.

When the clinician encounters a patient with an otherwise asymptomatic salivary gland mass where tumor is the most likely diagnosis, the choice is whether to simply excise the mass via a parotidectomy with facial nerve dissection or submandibular gland excision or to first obtain an FNA biopsy. Although the accuracy of FNA biopsy for malignancy has been reported to be quite high, results vary among institutions. If a negative FNA biopsy would lead to a decision not to proceed to surgery, then it should be considered. Poor overall health of the patient and the possibility of inflammatory disease as the cause of the mass are situations where FNA biopsy might be helpful. In otherwise straightforward nonrecurrent cases, excision is indicated. In benign and small low-grade malignant tumors, no additional treatment is needed. Postoperative irradiation is indicated for larger and high-grade cancers.

Adelstein DJ et al. Biology and management of salivary gland cancers. Semin Radiat Oncol. 2012 Jul;22(3):245–53. [PMID: 22687949]

Carrillo JF et al. Diagnostic accuracy of fine needle aspiration biopsy in preoperative diagnosis of patients with parotid gland masses. J Surg Oncol. 2009 Aug 1;100(2):133–8. [PMID: 19507187]

► DISEASES OF THE LARYNX

DYSPHONIA, HOARSENESS, & STRIDOR

The primary symptoms of laryngeal disease are hoarseness and stridor. Hoarseness is caused by an abnormal vibration of the vocal folds. The voice is breathy when too much air passes incompletely apposed vocal folds, as in unilateral vocal fold paralysis or vocal fold mass. The voice is harsh when the vocal folds are stiff and vibrate irregularly, as is the case in laryngitis or malignancy. Heavy, edematous vocal folds produce a rough, low-pitched vocal quality. Stridor (a high-pitched, typically inspiratory, sound) is the result of turbulent airflow from a narrowed upper airway. Airway narrowing at or above the vocal folds produces inspiratory stridor. Airway narrowing below the vocal fold level produces either expiratory or biphasic stridor. The timing and rapidity of onset of stridor are critically important in determining the seriousness of the airway problem. *All cases of stridor should be evaluated by a specialist and rapid-onset stridor should be evaluated emergently.*

Evaluation of an abnormal voice begins with obtaining a history of the circumstances preceding its onset and an examination of the airway.

Any patient with hoarseness that has persisted beyond 2 weeks should be evaluated by an otolaryngologist with laryngoscopy. Especially when the patient has a history of tobacco use, laryngeal cancer or lung cancer (leading to paralysis of a recurrent laryngeal nerve) must be strongly considered. In addition to structural causes of dysphonia, laryngoscopy can help identify functional problems with the voice including vocal fold paralysis, muscle tension dysphonia, and spasmodic dysphonia.

Johns MM 3rd et al. Shortfalls of the American Academy of Otolaryngology-Head and Neck Surgery's Clinical practice guideline: Hoarseness (Dysphonia). Otolaryngol Head Neck Surg. 2010 Aug;143(2):175–7. [PMID: 20647114]

Schwartz SR et al. Clinical practice guideline: hoarseness (dysphonia). Otolaryngol Head Neck Surg. 2009 Sep;141(3 Suppl 2):S1–S31. [PMID: 19729111]

COMMON LARYNGEAL DISORDERS

1. Acute Laryngitis

Acute laryngitis is probably the most common cause of hoarseness, which may persist for a week or so after other symptoms of an upper respiratory infection have cleared. The patient should be warned to avoid vigorous use of the voice (singing, shouting) until their voice returns to normal, since persistent use may lead to the formation of traumatic vocal fold hemorrhage, polyps, and cysts. Although thought to be usually viral in origin, both *M catarrhalis* and *H influenzae* may be isolated from the nasopharynx at higher than expected frequencies. Despite this finding, a meta-analysis has failed to demonstrate any convincing evidence that antibiotics significantly alter the natural resolution of acute laryngitis. Erythromycin may speed subjective perception of hoarseness and cough. Oral or intramuscular corticosteroids may be used in highly selected cases of professional vocalists to speed recovery and allow scheduled performances. Examination of the vocal folds and assessment of vocal technique are mandatory prior to corticosteroid initiation, since inflamed vocal folds are at greater risk for hemorrhage and the subsequent development of traumatic vocal fold pathology.

Reveiz L et al. Antibiotics for acute laryngitis in adults. Cochrane Database Syst Rev. 2013 Mar 28;3: CD004783. [PMID: 23543536]

Schomacker H et al. Pathogenesis of acute respiratory illness caused by human parainfluenza viruses. Curr Opin Virol. 2012 Jun;2(3):294–9. [PMID: 22709516]

2. Laryngopharyngeal Reflux

ESSENTIALS OF DIAGNOSIS

▶ Commonly associated with hoarseness, throat irritation, and chronic cough.

▶ Symptoms typically occur when upright and half of patients do not experience heartburn.

▶ Laryngoscopy is critical to exclude other causes of hoarseness.

▶ Diagnosis is made based on response to proton pump inhibitor therapy, as no gold standard for the condition exists.

▶ Treatment failure with proton pump inhibitors is common and may suggest other etiologies.

Gastroesophageal reflux into the larynx (laryngopharyngeal reflux) is considered a cause of chronic hoarseness when other causes of abnormal vocal fold vibration (such as tumor or nodules) have been excluded by laryngoscopy. Gastroesophageal reflux disease (GERD) has also been suggested as a contributing factor to other symptoms such as throat clearing, throat discomfort, chronic cough, a sensation of postnasal drip, esophageal spasm, and some cases of asthma. Since less than half of patients with laryngeal acid exposure have typical symptoms of heartburn and regurgitation, the lack of such symptoms should not be construed as eliminating this cause. Indeed, most patients with symptomatic laryngopharyngeal reflux, as it is now called, do not meet criteria for GERD by pH probe testing and these entities must be considered separately. The prevalence of this condition is hotly debated in the literature and laryngopharyngeal reflux may not be as common as once thought.

Evaluation should initially exclude other causes of dysphonia through laryngoscopy; consultation with an otolaryngologist is advisable. Many clinicians opt for an empiric trial of a proton pump inhibitor. Such an empiric trial should not precede visualization of the vocal folds to exclude other causes of hoarseness. When used, the American Academy of Otolaryngology Head and Neck Surgery recommends twice daily therapy with full strength proton pump inhibitor (eg, omeprazole 40 mg orally twice daily, or equivalent) for a minimum of 3 months. Patients may note improvement in symptoms after 3 months, but the changes in the larynx often take 6 months to resolve. If symptoms improve and cessation of therapy leads to symptoms again, then a proton pump inhibitor is resumed at the lowest dose effective for remission, usually daily but at times on a demand basis. Although H_2-receptor antagonists are an alternative to proton pump inhibitors, they are generally both less clinically effective and less cost-effective. Nonresponders should undergo pH testing and manometry. Twenty-four-hour pH monitoring of the pharynx should best document laryngopharyngeal reflux and is advocated by some as the initial management step but it is costly, more difficult, and less available than lower esophageal monitoring alone. Double pH probe (proximal and distal esophageal probes) testing is the best option for evaluation, since lower esophageal pH monitoring alone does not correlate well with laryngopharyngeal reflux symptoms. Oropharyngeal pH probe testing is available, but its ability to predict response to reflux treatment in patients with laryngopharyngeal reflux is not known.

Altman KW et al. The challenge of protocols for reflux disease: a review and development of a critical pathway. Otolaryngol Head Neck Surg. 2011 Jul;145(1):7–14. [PMID: 21493264]

Ford CN. GERD-related chronic laryngitis: pro. Arch Otolaryngol Head Neck Surg. 2010 Sep;136(9):910–3. [PMID: 20855685]

Vaezi MF. Gastroesophageal reflux-related chronic laryngitis: con. Arch Otolaryngol Head Neck Surg. 2010 Sep;136(9):908–9. [PMID: 20855684]

3. Recurrent Respiratory Papillomatosis

Papillomas are common lesions of the larynx and other sites where ciliated and squamous epithelia meet. Unlike oral papillomas, recurrent respiratory papillomatosis typically becomes symptomatic, with hoarseness that occasionally progresses over weeks to months. These papillomas are almost always due to HPV types 6 and 11. The disease is more common in children where it causes hoarseness and stridor. Repeated laser vaporizations or cold knife resections via operative laryngoscopy are the mainstay of treatment. Severe cases can cause airway compromise even in adults and require treatment as often as every 6 weeks to maintain airway patency. Extension can occur into the trachea and lungs. Tracheotomy should be avoided, if possible, since it introduces an additional squamociliary junction for which papillomas appear to have an affinity. Interferon treatment has been under investigation for many years but is only indicated in severe cases with pulmonary involvement. Rarely, cases of malignant transformation have been reported (often in smokers), but recurrent respiratory papillomatosis should generally be thought of as a benign condition. Cidofovir (a cytosine nucleotide analog in use to treat cytomegalovirus retinitis) has been used with success as intralesional therapy for recurrent respiratory papillomatosis. Because cidofovir causes adenocarcinomas in laboratory animals, its potential for carcinogenesis is being monitored. The quadrivalent recombinant human HPV vaccine (Gardasil) offers hope for the eventual eradication of this benign, but terribly morbid, disease.

Blumin JH et al. Dysplasia in adults with recurrent respiratory papillomatosis: incidence and risk factors. Ann Otol Rhinol Laryngol. 2009 Jul;118(7):481–5. [PMID: 19708485]

Bonagura VR et al. Recurrent respiratory papillomatosis: a complex defect in immune responsiveness to human papillomavirus-6 and -11. APMIS. 2010 Jun;118(6–7):455–70. [PMID: 20553528]

Carvalho CM et al. Prognostic factors of recurrent respiratory papillomatosis from a registry of 72 patients. Acta Otolaryngol. 2009 Apr;129(4):462–70. [PMID: 19235575]

4. Epiglottitis

Epiglottitis (or, more correctly, supraglottitis) should be suspected when a patient presents with a rapidly developing sore throat or when odynophagia (pain on swallowing) is out of proportion to apparently minimal oropharyngeal findings on examination. It is more common in diabetic patients and may be viral or bacterial in origin. Rarely in the era of *H influenzae* type b vaccine is this bacterium isolated in adults. Unlike in children, indirect laryngoscopy is generally safe and may demonstrate a swollen, erythematous epiglottis. Lateral plain radiographs may demonstrate an enlarged epiglottis (the epiglottis "thumb sign"). Initial treatment is hospitalization for intravenous antibiotics—eg, ceftizoxime, 1–2 g intravenously every 8–12 hours; or cefuroxime, 750–1500 mg intravenously every 8 hours; and dexamethasone, usually 4–10 mg as initial bolus, then 4 mg intravenously every 6 hours—and observation of the airway. Corticosteroids may be tapered as symptoms and signs resolve. Similarly, substitution of oral antibiotics may be appropriate to complete a 10-day course. Less than 10% of adults require intubation. Indications for intubation are dyspnea, rapid pace of sore throat (where progression to airway compromise may occur before the effects of corticosteroids and antibiotics), and endolaryngeal abscess noted on CT imaging. If the patient is not intubated, prudence suggests monitoring oxygen saturation with continuous pulse oximetry and initial admission to a monitored unit.

Verbruggen K et al. Epiglottitis and related complications in adults. Case reports and review of the literature. B-ENT. 2012;8(2):143–8. [PMID: 22896936]

MASSES OF THE LARYNX

1. Traumatic Lesions of the Vocal Folds

Vocal fold nodules are smooth, paired lesions that form at the junction of the anterior one-third and posterior two-thirds of the vocal folds. They are a common cause of hoarseness resulting from vocal abuse. In adults, they are referred to as "singer's nodules" and in children, as "screamer's nodules." Treatment requires modification of voice habits, and referral to a speech therapist is indicated. While nearly all true nodules will resolve with behavior modification, recalcitrant nodules may require surgical excision. Often, additional pathology, such as a polyp or cyst, may be encountered.

Vocal fold polyps are unilateral masses that form within the superficial lamina propria of the vocal fold. They are related to vocal trauma and seem to follow resolution of vocal fold hemorrhage. Small, sessile polyps may resolve with conservative measures, such as voice rest and corticosteroids, but larger polyps are often irreversible and require operative removal to restore normal voice.

Vocal fold cysts are also considered traumatic lesions of the vocal folds and are either true cysts with an epithelial lining or pseudocysts. They typically form from mucus-secreting glands on the inferior aspect of the vocal folds. Cysts may fluctuate in size from week to week and cause a variable degree of hoarseness. They rarely, if ever, resolve completely and may leave behind a sulcus, or vocal fold scar, if they decompress or are marsupialized. Such scarring can be a frustrating cause of permanent dysphonia.

Polypoid corditis is different from vocal fold polyps and may form from loss of elastin fibers and loosening of the intracellular junctions within the lamina propria. This loss allows swelling of the gelatinous matrix of the superficial lamina propria (called **Reinke edema**). These changes in the vocal folds are strongly associated with smoking, but also with vocal abuse, chemical industrial irritants, and hypothyroidism. While this problem is common in both male and female smokers, women seem more troubled by the characteristic decline in modal pitch caused by the increased mass of the vocal folds. If the patient stops smoking or the lesions cause stridor and airway obstruction, surgical resection of the hyperplastic vocal fold mucosa may be indicated to improve the voice or airway, or both.

A common but often unrecognized cause of hoarseness and odynophonia are **contact ulcers** or their close relatives, **granulomas**. Both lesions form on the vocal processes of the arytenoid cartilages, and patients often can correctly inform the clinician which side is affected. The cause of these ulcers and granulomas is disputed, but they are clearly related to trauma and may be related to exposure of the underlying perichondrium. They are common following intubation and generally resolve quite quickly. Chronic ulceration or granuloma formation has been associated with gastroesophageal reflux but is also common in patients with muscle tension dysphonia. Treatment is often multimodal and an inhaled corticosteroid (eg, fluticasone 440 mcg twice daily) may be the most effective pharmacologic therapy. Adjunct treatment measures include proton pump inhibitor therapy (omeprazole 40 mg orally twice daily, or equivalent) and voice therapy with special attention to vocal hygiene. Rare cases can be quite stubborn and persistent without adequate therapy. Surgical removal is rarely, if ever, required for nonobstructive lesions.

Gökcan KM et al. Vascular lesions of the vocal fold. Eur Arch Otorhinolaryngol. 2009 Apr;266(4):527–33. [PMID: 18704472]

2. Laryngeal Leukoplakia

Leukoplakia of the vocal folds is commonly found in association with hoarseness in smokers. Direct laryngoscopy with biopsy is advised in almost all cases. Histologic examination usually demonstrates mild, moderate, or severe dysplasia. In some cases, invasive squamous cell carcinoma is present in the initial biopsy specimen. Cessation of smoking may reverse or stabilize mild or moderate dysplasia. Some patients—estimated to be < 5% of those with mild dysplasia and about 35–60% of those with severe dysplasia—will subsequently develop squamous cell carcinoma. Treatment options include close follow-up with laryngovideostroboscopy, serial resection, and external beam radiation therapy. Despite their cost and the lack of any evidence for their use in the treatment of leukoplakia, proton pump inhibitors have become the mainstay of treatment for these lesions.

Isenberg JS et al. Institutional and comprehensive review of laryngeal leukoplakia. Ann Otol Rhinol Laryngol. 2008 Jan;117(1):74–9. [PMID: 18254375]

3. Squamous Cell Carcinoma of the Larynx

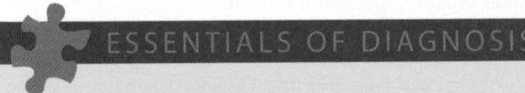
ESSENTIALS OF DIAGNOSIS

► New and persistent (more than 2 weeks duration) hoarseness in a smoker.

► Persistent throat or ear pain, especially with swallowing.

► Neck mass.

► Hemoptysis.

► Stridor or other symptoms of a compromised airway.

► General Considerations

Squamous cell carcinoma of the larynx, the most common malignancy of the larynx, occurs almost exclusively in patients with a history of significant tobacco use. Squamous cell carcinoma is usually seen in men age 50–70 years; about 13,000 new cases are seen in United States each year. There may be an association between laryngeal cancer and HPV type 16 or 18 infection, but this association is much less strong than that between HPV 16 or 18 and oropharyngeal cancer. In both cancer types, the association with HPV seems to be strongest in nonsmokers. Laryngeal cancer is very treatable and early detection is the key to maximizing posttreatment voice, swallowing, and breathing function.

► Clinical Findings

A. Symptoms and Signs

A change in voice quality is most often the presenting complaint, although throat or ear pain, hemoptysis, dysphagia, weight loss, and airway compromise may occur. Because of their early impact on vocal quality, glottic cancers are among the smallest detectable human malignancies and treatment success is very high with early lesions. Neck metastases are not common in early glottic (true vocal fold) cancer in which the vocal folds are mobile, but a third of patients in whom there is impaired fold mobility will also have involved lymph nodes at neck dissection. Supraglottic carcinoma (false vocal folds, aryepiglottic folds, epiglottis), on the other hand, often metastasizes to both sides of the neck early in the disease. Complete head and neck examination, including laryngoscopy, by an experienced clinician is mandated for any person with the concerning symptoms listed under Essentials of Diagnosis.

B. Imaging and Laboratory Studies

Radiologic evaluation by CT or MRI is helpful in assessing tumor extent. Imaging evaluates neck nodes, tumor volume, and cartilage sclerosis or destruction. A chest CT scan is indicated if there are level VI enlarged nodes (around the trachea and the thyroid gland) or IV enlarged nodes (inferior to the cricoid cartilage along the internal jugular vein) or if a chest film is concerning for a second primary lesion or metastases. Laboratory evaluation includes complete blood count and liver function tests. Formal cardiopulmonary evaluation may be indicated, especially if partial laryngeal surgery is being considered. All partial laryngectomy candidates should have good to excellent lung function and exercise tolerance because chronic microaspiration may be expected following the procedure. A positron emission tomography (PET) scan or CT-PET scan may be indicated to assess for distant metastases when there appears to be advanced local or regional disease.

C. Biopsy

Diagnosis is made by biopsy at the time of laryngoscopy when true fold mobility and arytenoid fixation, as well as surface tumor extent, can be evaluated. Most otolaryngologists recommend esophagoscopy and bronchoscopy at the same time to exclude synchronous primary tumor. Although an FNA biopsy of an enlarged neck node may have already been done, it is generally acceptable to assume radiographically enlarged neck nodes (> 1–1.5 cm) or nodes with necrotic centers are neck metastases. Open biopsies of nodal metastases should be discouraged because they may lead to higher rates of tumor treatment failure.

D. Tumor Staging

The American Joint Committee on Cancer (AJCC) staging of laryngeal cancers uses the TNM system to describe tumor extent and can be used for prognosis. Early laryngeal cancers, T1 and T2 (stage I and II) lesions, involve 1–2 laryngeal subsites locally and have no nodal metastases or profound functional abnormalities. T3 and T4 lesions may involve multiple laryngeal subsites with limitation of laryngeal mobility. These locally advanced lesions are stage III or IV cancers and any size tumor with regional nodal metastases is at least a stage III tumor. Stage I and II lesions are generally treated with single modality therapy (surgery or radiation) while multimodality therapy, usually including chemotherapy with radiation therapy, is reserved for more advanced stage III and IV lesions.

▶ Treatment

Treatment of laryngeal carcinoma has four goals: cure, preservation of safe effective swallowing, preservation of useful voice, and avoidance of a permanent tracheostoma. For early glottic and supraglottic cancers, radiation therapy is the standard of care since cure rates are > 95% and 80%, respectively. That said, radiation therapy carries substantial morbidity and many early tumors (T1 and T2 lesions, without involved nodes) and selected advanced tumors (T3 and T4) may be treated with partial laryngectomy if at least one cricoarytenoid unit can be preserved. Five-year locoregional cure rates exceed 80–90% with surgery, and

patient-reported satisfaction is excellent. In supraglottic tumors, even when clinically N0, elective limited neck dissection is indicated following surgical resection because of the high risk of neck node involvement.

Advanced stage III and IV tumors represent a challenging and ever changing treatment dilemma. Twenty-five years ago, total laryngectomy was often recommended for such patients. However, the 1994 VA study (with induction cisplatin and 5-fluorouracil followed by irradiation alone in responders) demonstrated that two-thirds of patients could preserve their larynx. Subsequent studies have further defined multimodal therapy. Cisplatin-based chemotherapy concomitant with radiation therapy has been shown to be superior to either irradiation alone or induction chemotherapy followed by radiation. The same benefits have been demonstrated with the epidermal growth factor receptor blocker cetuximab with lower overall systemic toxicity and better patient tolerance. However, chemoradiation using either cetuximab or cisplatin is associated with prolonged gastrostomy-dependent dysphagia.

The high rate of dysphagia and morbidity associated with severe laryngeal stenosis following chemoradiation has prompted a reevaluation of the role of extended, but less-than-total, laryngeal resection for selected advanced laryngeal carcinoma in which at least one cricoarytenoid unit is intact (organ preservation surgery). In addition to the late complications, clinicians have noted that the overall success in the treatment of larynx cancer has declined in parallel with the increase in organ preservation chemoradiation therapy over the past 20 years. Some experts have proposed that this decline is the direct result of the shift in management of advanced laryngeal cancer away from surgery. Organ preservation surgery should be considered and discussed as an alternative to chemoradiation but may require referral to an appropriate regional center where such techniques are offered. After thorough evaluation of candidacy and discussion of the treatment options, patient choice plays a critical role in the ultimate decision to pursue surgery or chemoradiation as a definitive treatment modality. The patient and treating clinicians must carefully consider *different* early and late side effects and complications associated with different treatment modalities.

The presence of malignant adenopathy in the neck affects the prognosis greatly. Supraglottic tumors metastasize early and bilaterally to the neck, and this must be included in the treatment plans even when the neck is apparently uninvolved. Glottic tumors in which the true vocal folds are mobile (T1 or T2) have less than a 5% rate of nodal involvement; when a fold is immobile, the rate of ipsilateral nodal involvement climbs to about 30%. An involved neck is treated by surgery or chemoradiation, or both. This decision will depend on the treatment chosen for the larynx and the extent of neck involvement.

Total laryngectomy is largely reserved for patients with advanced resectable tumors with extralaryngeal spread or cartilage involvement, for those with persistent tumor following chemoradiation, and for patients with recurrent or second primary tumor following previous radiation therapy. Voice rehabilitation via a primary (or at times secondary) tracheoesophageal puncture produces intelligible and serviceable speech in about 75–85% of patients. Indwelling prostheses that are changed every 3–6 months are a common alternative to patient-inserted prostheses, which need changing more frequently.

Long-term follow-up is critical in head and neck cancer patients. In addition to the 3–4% annual rate of second tumors and monitoring for recurrence, psychosocial aspects of treatment are common. Dysphagia, impaired communication, and altered appearance, may result in patient difficulties adapting to the workplace and to social interactions. In addition, smoking cessation and alcohol abatement are common challenges. Nevertheless, about 65% of patients with larynx cancer are cured, most have useful speech, and many resume their prior livelihoods with adaptations.

Bonner JA et al. Radiotherapy plus cetuximab for locoregionally advanced head and neck cancer: 5-year survival data from a phase 3 randomised trial, and relation between cetuximab-induced rash and survival. Lancet Oncol. 2010 Jan;11(1):21–8. [PMID: 19897418]

Suárez C et al. Transoral microsurgery for treatment of laryngeal and pharyngeal cancers. Curr Oncol Rep. 2013 Apr;15(2):134–41. [PMID: 23275183]

Wang CJ et al. Current concepts of organ preservation in head and neck cancer. Eur Arch Otorhinolaryngol. 2011 Apr;268(4):481–7. [PMID: 21107854]

VOCAL FOLD PARALYSIS

Vocal fold paralysis can result from a lesion or damage to either the vagus or recurrent laryngeal nerve and usually results in breathy dysphonia and effortful voicing. Common causes of **unilateral recurrent laryngeal nerve** involvement include thyroid surgery (and occasionally thyroid cancer), other neck surgery (anterior discectomy and carotid endarterectomy), and mediastinal or apical involvement by lung cancer. Skull base tumors often involve or abut upon lower cranial nerves and may affect the vagus nerve directly, or the vagus nerve may be damaged during surgical management of the lesion. While iatrogenic injury is the most common cause of unilateral vocal fold paralysis, the second most common cause is idiopathic. However, before deciding whether the paralysis is due to iatrogenic injury or is idiopathic, the clinician must exclude other causes, such as malignancy. In the absence of other cranial neuropathies, a CT scan with contrast from the skull base to the aorto-pulmonary window (the span of the recurrent laryngeal nerve) should be performed. If other cranial nerve deficits or high vagal weakness with palate paralysis is noted, a MRI scan of the brain and brainstem is warranted.

Unlike unilateral fold paralysis, **bilateral fold paralysis** usually causes inspiratory stridor with deep inspiration. If the onset of bilateral fold paralysis is insidious, it may be asymptomatic at rest and the patient may have a normal voice. However, the acute onset of bilateral vocal fold paralysis with inspiratory stridor at rest should be managed by a specialist immediately in a critical care environment. Causes of bilateral fold paralysis include thyroid surgery, esophageal cancer, and ventricular shunt malfunction.

Unilateral or bilateral fold immobility may also be seen in cricoarytenoid arthritis secondary to advanced rheumatoid arthritis, intubation injuries, glottic and subglottic stenosis and, of course, laryngeal cancer. The goal of intervention is the creation of a safe airway with minimal reduction in voice quality and airway protection from aspiration. A number of fold lateralization procedures for bilateral paralysis have been advocated as a means of removing the tracheotomy tube.

Unilateral vocal fold paralysis is occasionally temporary and may take over a year to resolve spontaneously. Surgical management of persistent or irrecoverable symptomatic unilateral vocal fold paralysis has evolved over the last several decades. The primary goal is medialization of the paralyzed fold in order to create a stable platform for vocal fold vibration. Additional goals include improving pulmonary toilet by facilitating of cough and advancing diet. Success has been reported for years with injection laryngoplasty using Teflon, Gelfoam, fat, and collagen. Teflon is the only permanent injectable material, but its use is discouraged because of granuloma formation within the vocal folds of some patients. Temporary injectable materials, such as collagen or fat, provide excellent temporary restoration of voice and can be placed under local or general anesthesia. Once the paralysis is determined to be permanent, formal medialization thyroplasty may be performed by creating a small window in the thyroid cartilage and placing an implant between the thyroarytenoid muscle and inner table of the thyroid cartilage. This procedure moves the vocal fold medially and creates a stable platform for bilateral, symmetric mucosal vibration.

Gardner GM et al. The cost of vocal fold paralysis after thyroidectomy. Laryngoscope. 2013 Jun;123(6):1455–63. [PMID: 23703383]

Misono S et al. Evidence-based practice: evaluation and management of unilateral vocal fold paralysis. Otolaryngol Clin North Am. 2012 Oct;45(5):1083–108. [PMID: 22980687]

TRACHEOSTOMY & CRICOTHYROTOMY

There are two primary indications for tracheotomy: airway obstruction at or above the level of the larynx and respiratory failure requiring prolonged mechanical ventilation. In an acute emergency, cricothyrotomy secures an airway more rapidly than tracheotomy, with fewer potential immediate complications such as pneumothorax and hemorrhage. Percutaneous dilatational tracheotomy as an elective bedside (or intensive care unit) procedure has undergone scrutiny in recent years as an alternative to tracheotomy. In experienced hands, the various methods of percutaneous tracheotomy have been documented to be safe in carefully selected patients. Simultaneous videobronchoscopy can reduce the incidence of major complications. The major cost reduction comes from avoiding the operating room. Bedside tracheotomy (in the intensive care unit) achieves similar cost reduction and is advocated by some experts as slightly less costly than the percutaneous procedures.

The most common indication for elective tracheotomy is the need for prolonged mechanical ventilation. There is no firm rule about how many days a patient must be intubated before conversion to tracheotomy should be advised. The incidence of serious complications such as subglottic stenosis increases with extended endotracheal intubation. As soon as it is apparent that the patient will require protracted ventilatory support, tracheotomy should replace the endotracheal tube. Less frequent indications for tracheostomy are life-threatening aspiration pneumonia, the need to improve pulmonary toilet to correct problems related to insufficient clearing of tracheobronchial secretions, and sleep apnea.

Posttracheotomy care requires humidified air to prevent secretions from crusting and occluding the inner cannula of the tracheotomy tube. The tracheotomy tube should be cleaned several times daily. The most frequent early complication of tracheotomy is dislodgment of the tracheotomy tube. Surgical creation of an inferiorly based tracheal flap sutured to the inferior neck skin may make reinsertion of a dislodged tube easier. It should be recalled that the act of swallowing requires elevation of the larynx, which is limited by tracheotomy. Therefore, frequent tracheal and bronchial suctioning is often required to clear the aspirated saliva as well as the increased tracheobronchial secretions. Care of the skin around the stoma is important to prevent maceration and secondary infection.

Down J et al. Early vs late tracheostomy in critical care. Br J Hosp Med (Lond). 2009 Sep 9;70(9):510–13. [PMID: 19749640]

Halum SL et al. A multi-institutional analysis of tracheotomy complications. Laryngoscope. 2012 Jan;122(1):38–45. [PMID: 22183627]

FOREIGN BODIES IN THE UPPER AERODIGESTIVE TRACT

FOREIGN BODIES OF THE TRACHEA & BRONCHI

Aspiration of foreign bodies occurs much less frequently in adults than in children. The elderly and denture wearers appear to be at greatest risk. Wider familiarity with the Heimlich maneuver has reduced deaths. If the maneuver is unsuccessful, cricothyrotomy may be necessary. Plain chest radiographs may reveal a radiopaque foreign body. Detection of radiolucent foreign bodies may be aided by inspiration-expiration films that demonstrate air trapping distal to the obstructed segment. Atelectasis and pneumonia may occur later.

Tracheal and bronchial foreign bodies should be removed under general anesthesia with rigid bronchoscopy by a skilled endoscopist working with an experienced anesthesiologist.

Digoy GP. Diagnosis and management of upper aerodigestive tract foreign bodies. Otolaryngol Clin North Am. 2008 Jun;41(3):485–96. [PMID: 18435994]

ESOPHAGEAL FOREIGN BODIES

Foreign bodies in the esophagus create urgent but not life-threatening situations as long as the airway is not compromised. There is probably time to consult an experienced clinician for management. It is a useful diagnostic sign of complete obstruction if the patient is drooling or cannot handle secretions. Patients may often point to the exact level of the obstruction. Indirect laryngoscopy often shows pooling of saliva at the esophageal inlet. Plain films may detect radiopaque foreign bodies such as chicken bones. Coins tend to align in the coronal plane in the esophagus and sagittally in the trachea. If a foreign body is suspected, a barium swallow may help make the diagnosis.

The treatment of an esophageal foreign body depends very much on identification of its nature. In children, swallowed nonfood objects are common. In adults, however, food foreign bodies are more common, and there is the greater possibility of underlying esophageal pathology. Endoscopic removal and examination is usually best via flexible esophagoscopy or rigid laryngoscopy and esophagoscopy. If there is nothing sharp such as a bone, some clinicians advocate a hospitalized 24-hour observation period prior to esophagoscopy, noting that spontaneous passage of the foreign body will occur in 50% of adult patients. In the management of meat obstruction, the use of papain (meat tenderizer) should be discouraged because it can damage the esophageal mucosa and lead to stenosis or perforation.

Weissberg D et al. Foreign bodies in the esophagus. Ann Thorac Surg. 2007 Dec;84(6):1854–7. [PMID: 18036898]

DISEASES PRESENTING AS NECK MASSES

The differential diagnosis of neck masses is heavily dependent on the location in the neck, the age of the patient, and the presence of associated disease processes. Rapid growth and tenderness suggest an inflammatory process, while firm, painless, and slowly enlarging masses are often neoplastic. In young adults, most neck masses are benign (branchial cleft cyst, thyroglossal duct cyst, reactive lymphadenitis), although malignancy should always be considered (lymphoma, metastatic thyroid carcinoma). Lymphadenopathy is common in HIV-positive persons, but a growing or dominant mass may well represent lymphoma. In adults over age 40, cancer is the most common cause of persistent neck mass. A metastasis from squamous cell carcinoma arising within the mouth, pharynx, larynx, or upper esophagus should be suspected, especially if there is a history of tobacco or significant alcohol use. Especially among patients younger than 30 or older than 70, lymphoma should be considered. In any case, a comprehensive otolaryngologic examination is needed. Cytologic evaluation of the neck mass via FNA biopsy is likely to be the next step if an obvious primary tumor is not obvious on physical examination.

CONGENITAL LESIONS PRESENTING AS NECK MASSES IN ADULTS

1. Branchial Cleft Cysts

Branchial cleft cysts usually present as a soft cystic mass along the anterior border of the sternocleidomastoid muscle. These lesions are usually recognized in the second or third decades of life, often when they suddenly swell or become infected. To prevent recurrent infection and possible carcinoma, they should be completely excised, along with their fistulous tracts.

First branchial cleft cysts present high in the neck, sometimes just below the ear. A fistulous connection with the floor of the external auditory canal may be present. Second branchial cleft cysts, which are far more common, may communicate with the tonsillar fossa. Third branchial cleft cysts, which may communicate with the piriform sinus, are rare and present low in the neck.

Magdy EA et al. First branchial cleft anomalies: presentation, variability and safe surgical management. Eur Arch Otorhinolaryngol. 2013 May;270(6):1917–25. [PMID: 23192665]

2. Thyroglossal Duct Cysts

Thyroglossal duct cysts occur along the embryologic course of the thyroid's descent from the tuberculum impar of the tongue base to its usual position in the low neck. Although they may occur at any age, they are most common before age 20. They present as a midline neck mass, often just below the hyoid bone, which moves with swallowing. Surgical excision is recommended to prevent recurrent infection. This requires removal of the entire fistulous tract along with the middle portion of the hyoid bone through which many of the fistulas pass. Preoperative evaluation should include a thyroid ultrasound to confirm anatomic position of the thyroid.

Lin ST et al. Thyroglossal duct cyst: a comparison between children and adults. Am J Otolaryngol. 2008 Mar–Apr;29(2):83–7. [PMID: 18314017]

INFECTIOUS & INFLAMMATORY NECK MASSES

1. Reactive Cervical Lymphadenopathy

Normal lymph nodes in the neck are usually < 1 cm in length. Infections involving the pharynx, salivary glands, and scalp often cause tender enlargement of neck nodes. Enlarged nodes are common in HIV-infected persons. Except for the occasional node that suppurates and requires incision and drainage, treatment is directed against the underlying infection. An enlarged node (> 1.5 cm) or node with a necrotic center that is not associated with an obvious infection should be further evaluated, especially if the patient has a history of smoking, alcohol use, or prior cancer. Other common indications for FNA biopsy of a node include its persistence or continued enlargement. Common causes of cervical adenopathy include tumor (squamous cell carcinoma, lymphoma, occasional metastases from non-head and neck sites) and infection (eg, reactive nodes, mycobacteria [discussed below], and cat scratch disease). Rare causes of adenopathy include Kikuchi disease (histiocytic necrotizing lymphadenopathy) and autoimmune adenopathy.

Leung AK et al. Cervical lymphadenitis: etiology, diagnosis, and management. Curr Infect Dis Rep. 2009 May;11(3):183–9. [PMID: 19366560]

2. Tuberculous & Nontuberculous Mycobacterial Lymphadenitis

Granulomatous neck masses are not uncommon. The differential diagnosis includes mycobacterial adenitis, sarcoidosis, and cat-scratch disease due to *Bartonella henselae*. Mycobacterial lymphadenitis is on the rise both in immunocompromised and immunocompetent individuals. The usual presentation of granulomatous disease in the neck is simply single or matted nodes. Although mycobacterial adenitis can extend to the skin and drain externally (as described for atypical mycobacteria and referred to as scrofula), this late presentation is no longer common.

FNA biopsy is usually the best initial diagnostic approach: cytology, smear for acid-fast bacilli, culture, and sensitivity test can all be done. Excisional biopsy of a node may be needed.

PCR from FNA (or from excised tissue) is the single most sensitive test and is particularly useful when conventional methods have not been diagnostic but clinical impression remains consistent for tuberculous infection.

See Table 9–15 for current recommended treatment of tuberculous lymphadenopathy. For atypical (nontuberculous) lymphadenopathy, treatment depends on sensitivity results of culture, but antibiotics likely to be useful include 6 months of isoniazid and rifampin and, for at least the first 2 months, ethambutol—all in standard dosages. Some would totally excise the involved nodes prior to chemotherapy, depending on location and other factors, but this can lead to chronic draining fistulas.

Fontanilla JM et al. Current diagnosis and management of peripheral tuberculous lymphadenitis. Clin Infect Dis. 2011 Sep;53(6):555–62. [PMID: 21865192]
Polesky A et al. Peripheral tuberculous lymphadenitis: epidemiology, diagnosis, treatment, and outcome. Medicine (Baltimore). 2005 Nov;84(6):350–62. [PMID: 16267410]

3. Lyme Disease

Lyme disease, caused by the spirochete *Borrelia burgdorferi* and transmitted by ticks of the *Ixodes* genus, may have protean manifestation, but over 75% of patients have symptoms involving the head and neck. Facial paralysis, dysesthesias, dysgeusia, or other cranial neuropathies are most common. Headache, pain, and cervical lymphadenopathy may occur. See Chapter 34 for a more detailed discussion.

Ljøstad U et al. Chronic Lyme; diagnostic and therapeutic challenges. Acta Neurol Scand Suppl. 2013;(196):38–47. [PMID: 23190290]

TUMOR METASTASES

In older adults, 80% of firm, persistent, and enlarging neck masses are metastatic in origin. The great majority of these arise from squamous cell carcinoma of the upper aerodigestive tract. A complete head and neck examination may reveal the tumor of origin, but examination under anesthesia with direct laryngoscopy, esophagoscopy, and bronchoscopy is usually required to fully evaluate the tumor and exclude second primaries.

It is often helpful to obtain a cytologic diagnosis if initial head and neck examination fails to reveal the primary tumor. An open biopsy should be done only when neither physical examination by an experienced clinician specializing in head and neck cancer nor FNA biopsy performed by an experienced cytopathologist yields a diagnosis. In such a setting, one should strongly consider obtaining an MRI or PET scan prior to open biopsy, as these methods may yield valuable information about a possible presumed primary site or another site for FNA.

With the exception of papillary thyroid carcinoma, non–squamous cell metastases to the neck are infrequent. While tumors that are not primary in the head or neck seldom metastasize to the cervical lymph nodes, the supraclavicular lymph nodes are quite often involved by lung, gastroesophageal, and breast tumors. Infradiaphragmatic tumors, with the exception of renal cell carcinoma and testicular cancer, rarely metastasize to the neck.

Barzilai G et al. Pattern of regional metastases from cutaneous squamous cell carcinoma of the head and neck. Otolaryngol Head Neck Surg. 2005 Jun;132(6):852–6. [PMID: 15944554]

LYMPHOMA

About 10% of lymphomas present in the head and neck. Multiple rubbery nodes, especially in the young adult or in patients who have AIDS, are suggestive of this disease. A thorough physical examination may demonstrate other sites of nodal or organ involvement. FNA biopsy may be diagnostic, but open biopsy is often required to determine architecture and an appropriate treatment course.

Bryson TC et al. Cervical lymph node evaluation and diagnosis. Otolaryngol Clin North Am. 2012 Dec;45(6):1363–83. [PMID: 23153753]

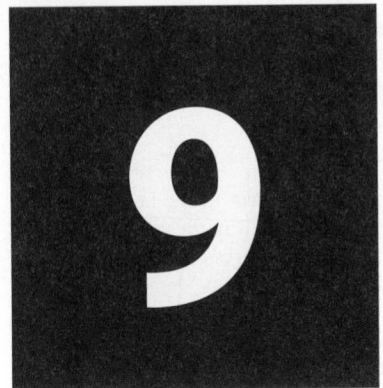

Pulmonary Disorders

Mark S. Chesnutt, MD
Thomas J. Prendergast, MD

DISORDERS OF THE AIRWAYS

Airway disorders have diverse causes but share certain common pathophysiologic and clinical features. Airflow limitation is characteristic and frequently causes dyspnea and cough. Other symptoms are common and typically disease-specific. Disorders of the airways can be classified as those that involve the upper airways—loosely defined as those above and including the vocal folds—and those that involve the lower airways.

DISORDERS OF THE UPPER AIRWAYS

Acute upper airway obstruction can be immediately life-threatening and must be relieved promptly to avoid asphyxia. Causes of acute upper airway obstruction include trauma to the larynx or pharynx, foreign body aspiration, laryngospasm, laryngeal edema from thermal injury or angioedema, infections (acute epiglottitis, Ludwig angina, pharyngeal or retropharyngeal abscess), and acute allergic laryngitis.

Chronic obstruction of the upper airway may be caused by carcinoma of the pharynx or larynx, laryngeal or subglottic stenosis, laryngeal granulomas or webs, or bilateral vocal fold paralysis. Laryngeal or subglottic stenosis may become evident weeks or months after translaryngeal endotracheal intubation. Inspiratory stridor, intercostal retractions on inspiration, a palpable inspiratory thrill over the larynx, and wheezing localized to the neck or trachea on auscultation are characteristic findings. Flow-volume loops may show flow limitations characteristic of obstruction. Soft-tissue radiographs of the neck may show supraglottic or infraglottic narrowing. CT and MRI scans can reveal exact sites of obstruction. Flexible endoscopy may be diagnostic, but caution is necessary to avoid exacerbating upper airway edema and precipitating critical airway narrowing.

Vocal fold dysfunction syndrome is characterized by paradoxical vocal fold adduction, resulting in both acute and chronic upper airway obstruction. It can cause dyspnea and wheezing that may be distinguished from asthma or exercise-induced asthma by the lack of response to bronchodilator therapy, normal spirometry immediately after an attack, spirometric evidence of upper airway obstruction, a negative bronchial provocation test, or direct visualization of adduction of the vocal folds on both inspiration and expiration. The condition appears to be psychogenic in nature. Bronchodilators are of no therapeutic benefit. Treatment consists of speech therapy, which uses breathing, voice, and neck relaxation exercises to abort the symptoms.

Gimenez LM et al. Vocal cord dysfunction: an update. Ann Allergy Asthma Immunol. 2011 Apr;106(4):267–75. [PMID: 21457874]

DISORDERS OF THE LOWER AIRWAYS

Tracheal obstruction may be intrathoracic (below the suprasternal notch) or extrathoracic. Fixed tracheal obstruction may be caused by acquired or congenital tracheal stenosis, primary or secondary tracheal neoplasms, extrinsic compression (tumors of the lung, thymus, or thyroid; lymphadenopathy; congenital vascular rings; aneurysms, etc), foreign body aspiration, tracheal granulomas and papillomas, and tracheal trauma. Tracheomalacia, foreign body aspiration, and retained secretions may cause variable tracheal obstruction.

Acquired **tracheal stenosis** is usually secondary to previous tracheotomy or endotracheal intubation. Dyspnea, cough, and inability to clear pulmonary secretions occur weeks to months after tracheal decannulation or extubation. Physical findings may be absent until tracheal diameter is reduced 50% or more, when wheezing, a palpable tracheal thrill, and harsh breath sounds may be detected. The diagnosis is usually confirmed by plain films or CT of the trachea. Complications include recurring pulmonary infection and life-threatening respiratory failure. Management is directed toward ensuring adequate ventilation and oxygenation and avoiding manipulative procedures that may increase edema of the tracheal mucosa. Surgical reconstruction, endotracheal stent placement, or laser photoresection may be required.

Bronchial obstruction may be caused by retained pulmonary secretions, aspiration, foreign bodies, bronchomalacia, bronchogenic carcinoma, compression by extrinsic masses, and tumors metastatic to the airway. Clinical and radiographic findings vary depending on the location of the obstruction and the degree of airway narrowing. Symptoms include dyspnea, cough, wheezing, and, if infection is present, fever and chills. A history of recurrent pneumonia in the same lobe or segment or slow resolution (> 3 months) of pneumonia on successive radiographs suggests the possibility of bronchial obstruction and the need for bronchoscopy.

Roentgenographic findings include **atelectasis** (local parenchymal collapse), postobstructive infiltrates, and air trapping caused by unidirectional expiratory obstruction. CT scanning may demonstrate the nature and exact location of obstruction of the central bronchi. MRI may be superior to CT for delineating the extent of underlying disease in the hilum, but it is usually reserved for cases in which CT findings are equivocal. Bronchoscopy is the definitive diagnostic study, particularly if tumor or foreign body aspiration is suspected. The finding of bronchial breath sounds on physical examination or an air bronchogram on chest radiograph in an area of atelectasis rules out complete airway obstruction. Bronchoscopy is unlikely to be of therapeutic benefit in this situation.

Brigger MT et al. Management of tracheal stenosis. Curr Opin Otolaryngol Head Neck Surg. 2012 Dec;20(6):491–6. [PMID: 22929114]

ASTHMA

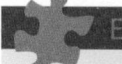

ESSENTIALS OF DIAGNOSIS

▸ Episodic or chronic symptoms of airflow obstruction.

▸ Reversibility of airflow obstruction, either spontaneously or following bronchodilator therapy.

▸ Symptoms frequently worse at night or in the early morning.

▸ Prolonged expiration and diffuse wheezes on physical examination.

▸ Limitation of airflow on pulmonary function testing or positive bronchoprovocation challenge.

General Considerations

Asthma is a common disease, affecting approximately 7–10% of the population. It is slightly more common in male children (< 14 years old) and in female adults. There is a genetic predisposition to asthma. Prevalence, hospitalizations, and fatal asthma have all increased in the United States over the past 20 years. Each year, approximately 500,000 hospital admissions and 4500 deaths in the United States are attributed to asthma. Hospitalization rates have been highest among blacks and children, and death rates are consistently highest among blacks aged 15–24 years.

Definition & Pathogenesis

Asthma is a chronic inflammatory disorder of the airways. No single histopathologic feature is pathognomonic but common findings include inflammatory cell infiltration with eosinophils, neutrophils, and lymphocytes (especially T lymphocytes); goblet cell hyperplasia, sometimes with plugging of small airways with thick mucus; collagen deposition beneath the basement membrane; hypertrophy of bronchial smooth muscle; airway edema; mast cell activation; and denudation of airway epithelium. This airway inflammation underlies disease chronicity and contributes to airway hyper-responsiveness and airflow limitation.

The strongest identifiable predisposing factor for the development of asthma is atopy, but obesity is increasingly recognized as a risk factor. Exposure of sensitive patients to inhaled allergens increases airway inflammation, airway hyper-responsiveness, and symptoms. Symptoms may develop immediately (immediate asthmatic response) or 4–6 hours after allergen exposure (late asthmatic response). Common allergens include house dust mites (often found in pillows, mattresses, upholstered furniture, carpets, and drapes), cockroaches, cat dander, and seasonal pollens. Substantially reducing exposure reduces pathologic findings and clinical symptoms.

Nonspecific precipitants of asthma include exercise, upper respiratory tract infections, rhinosinusitis, postnasal drip, aspiration, gastroesophageal reflux, changes in the weather, and stress. Exposure to **products of combustion** (eg, tobacco smoke, crack cocaine, methamphetamines, and other agents) increases asthma symptoms and the need for medications and reduces lung function. **Air pollution** (increased air levels of respirable particles, ozone, SO_2, and NO_2) precipitate asthma symptoms and increase emergency department visits and hospitalizations. Selected individuals may experience asthma symptoms after exposure to aspirin, nonsteroidal anti-inflammatory drugs, or tartrazine dyes. Other **medications** may precipitate asthma symptoms (see Table 9–23). **Occupational asthma** is triggered by various agents in the workplace and may occur weeks to years after initial exposure and sensitization. Women may experience catamenial asthma at predictable times during the menstrual cycle. **Exercise-induced bronchoconstriction** begins during exercise or within 3 minutes after its end, peaks within 10–15 minutes, and then resolves by 60 minutes. This phenomenon is thought to be a consequence of the airways' attempt to warm and humidify an increased volume of expired air during exercise. "Cardiac asthma" is wheezing precipitated by decompensated heart failure.

Clinical Findings

Symptoms and signs vary widely between patients as well as individually over time. General clinical findings in stable asthma patients are listed in Figure 9–1 and Table 9–1; Table 9–2 lists findings seen during asthma exacerbations.

Components of Severity		Classification of Asthma Severity ≥12 years of age			
			Persistent		
		Intermittent	Mild	Moderate	Severe
Impairment Normal FEV₁/FVC: 8–19 yr 85% 20–39 yr 80% 40–59 yr 75% 60–80 yr 70%	Symptoms	≤ 2 days/week	> 2 days/week but not daily	Daily	Throughout the day
	Nighttime awakenings	≤ 2x/month	3–4x/month	> 1x/week but not nightly	Often 7x/week
	Short-acting β₂-agonist use for symptom control (not prevention of EIB)	≤ 2 days/week	> 2 days/week but not daily, and not more than 1x on any day	Daily	Several times per day
	Interference with normal activity	None	Minor limitation	Some limitation	Extremely limited
	Lung function	• Normal FEV₁ between exacerbations • FEV₁ > 80% predicted • FEV₁/FVC normal	• FEV₁ > 80% predicted • FEV₁/FVC normal	• FEV₁ > 60% but < 80% predicted • FEV₁/FVC reduced 5%	• FEV₁ < 60% predicted • FEV₁/FVC reduced > 5%
Risk	Exacerbations requiring oral systemic corticosteroids	0–1/year (see note)	≥ 2/year (see note) ⟶ ⟵ Consider severity and interval since last exacerbation. ⟶ Frequency and severity may fluctuate over time for patients in any severity category. Relative annual risk of exacerbations may be related to FEV₁.		
Recommended Step for Initiating Treatment (See Figure 9–2 for treatment steps.)		Step 1	Step 2	Step 3 and consider short course of oral systemic corticosteroids	Step 4 or 5
		In 2–6 weeks, evaluate level of asthma control that is achieved and adjust therapy accordingly.			

EIB, exercise-induced bronchospasm; FEV₁, forced expiratory volume in 1 second; FVC, forced vital capacity; ICU, intensive care unit.

Notes:

- The stepwise approach is meant to assist, not replace, the clinical decision-making required to meet individual patient needs.

- Level of severity is determined by assessment of both impairment and risk. Assess impairment domain by patient's/caregiver's recall of previous 2–4 weeks and spirometry. Assign severity to the most severe category in which any feature occurs.

- At present, there are inadequate data to correspond frequencies of exacerbations with different levels of asthma severity. In general, more frequent and intense exacerbations (eg, requiring urgent, unscheduled care, hospitalization, or ICU admission) indicate greater underlying disease severity. For treatment purposes, patients who had ≥ 2 exacerbations requiring oral systemic corticosteroids in the past year may be considered the same as patients who have persistent asthma, even in the absence of impairment levels consistent with persistent asthma.

▲ **Figure 9–1.** Classifying asthma severity and initiating treatment. (Adapted from National Asthma Education and Prevention Program. Expert Panel Report 3: Guidelines for the Diagnosis and Management of Asthma. National Institutes of Health Pub. No. 08-4051. Bethesda, MD, 2007. http://www.nhlbi.nih.gov/guidelines/asthma/asthgdln.htm.)

Table 9–1. Assessing asthma control.

Components of Control		Classification of Asthma Control (≥12 years of age)		
		Well Controlled	Not Well Controlled	Very Poorly Controlled
Impairment	Symptoms	≤ 2 days/week	> 2 days/week	Throughout the day
	Nighttime awakenings	≤ 2×/month	1–3×/week	≥ 4×/week
	Interference with normal activity	None	Some limitation	Extremely limited
	Short-acting beta-2-agonist use for symptom control (not prevention of EIB)	≤ 2 days/week	> 2 days/week	Several times/day
	FEV_1 or peak flow Validated questionnaires	> 80% predicted/personal best	60–80% predicted/personal best	< 60% predicted/personal best
	ATAQ	0	1–2	3–4
	ACQ	≤ 0.75[1]	≥ 1.5	N/A
	ACT	≥ 20	16–19	≤ 15
Risk	**Exacerbations requiring oral system corticosteroids**	0–1/year	≥ 2/year (see note)	
		Consider severity and interval since last exacerbation		
	Progressive loss of lung function	Evaluation requires long-term follow-up care		
	Treatment-related adverse effects	Medication side effects can vary in intensity from none to very troublesome and worrisome. The level of intensity does not correlate to specific levels of control but should be considered in the overall assessment of risk.		
Recommended Action for Treatment (see Figure 9–2 for steps)		• Maintain current step. • Regular follow-ups every 1–6 months to maintain control. • Consider step down if well controlled for at least 3 months.	• Step up 1 step and • Reevaluate in 2–6 weeks. • For side effects, consider alternative treatment options.	• Consider short course of oral systemic corticosteroids, • Step up 1–2 steps, and • Reevaluate in 2 weeks. • For side effects, consider alternative treatment options.

[1]ACQ values of 0.76–1.4 are indeterminate regarding well-controlled asthma.
EIB, exercise-induced bronchospasm; ICU, intensive care unit.
Notes:
• The stepwise approach is meant to assist, not replace, the clinical decision-making required to meet individual patient needs.
• The level of control is based on the most severe impairment or risk category. Assess impairment domain by patient's recall of previous 2–4 weeks and by spirometry or peak flow measures. Symptom assessment for longer periods should reflect a global assessment, such as inquiring whether the patient's asthma is better or worse since the last visit.
• At present, there are inadequate data to correspond frequencies of exacerbations with different levels of asthma control. In general, more frequent and intense exacerbations (eg, requiring urgent, unscheduled care, hospitalization, or ICU admission) indicate poorer disease control. For treatment purposes, patients who had ≥ 2 exacerbations requiring oral systemic corticosteroids in the past year may be considered the same as patients who have not-well-controlled asthma, even in the absence of impairment levels consistent with not-well-controlled asthma.
• Validated Questionnaires for the impairment domain (the questionnaire did not assess lung function or the risk domain).
  ATAQ = Asthma Therapy Assessment Questionnaire©
  ACQ = Asthma Control Questionnaire© (user package may be obtained at www.qoltech.co.uk or juniper@qoltech.co.uk)
  ACT = Asthma Control Test™
  Minimal Importance Difference: 1.0 for the ATAQ; 0.5 for the ACQ; not determined for the ACT.
• Before step up in therapy:
  —Review adherence to medication, inhaler.
  —If an alternative treatment option was used in a step, discontinue and use the preferred treatment for that step.
Adapted from National Asthma Education and Prevention Program. Expert Panel Report 3: Guidelines for the Diagnosis and Management of Asthma. National Institutes of Health Pub. No. 08-4051. Bethesda, MD, 2007. http://www.nhlbi.nih.gov/guidelines/asthma/asthgdln.htm

Table 9–2. Evaluation and classification of severity of asthma exacerbations.

	Mild	Moderate	Severe	Respiratory Arrest Imminent
Symptoms				
Breathlessness	While walking	At rest, limits activity	At rest, interferes with conversation	While at rest, mute
Talks in	Sentences	Phrases	Words	Silent
Alertness	May be agitated	Usually agitated	Usually agitated	Drowsy or confused
Signs				
Respiratory rate	Increased	Increased	Often > 30/minute	> 30/minute
Body position	Can lie down	Prefers sitting	Sits upright	Unable to recline
Use of accessory muscles; suprasternal retractions	Usually not	Commonly	Usually	Paradoxical thoracoabdominal movement
Wheeze	Moderate, often only end expiratory	Loud; throughout exhalation	Usually loud; throughout inhalation and exhalation	Absent
Pulse/minute	< 100	100–120	> 120	Bradycardia
Pulsus paradoxus	Absent < 10 mm Hg	May be present 10–25 mm Hg	Often present > 25 mm Hg	Absence suggests respiratory muscle fatigue
Functional Assessment				
PEF or FEV$_1$ % predicted or % personal best	≥ 70%	40–69%	< 40%	< 25%
PaO$_2$ (on air, mm Hg)	Normal[1]	≥ 60[1]	< 60: possible cyanosis	< 60: possible cyanosis
PCO$_2$ (mm Hg)	< 42 mm Hg[1]	< 42 mm Hg[1]	≥ 42[1]	≥ 42[1]
SaO$_2$ (on air, %)	> 95%[1]	90–95%[1]	< 90%[1]	< 90%[1]

[1]Test not usually necessary.
PEF, peak expiratory flow; SaO$_2$, oxygen saturation.
Adapted from National Asthma Education and Prevention Program. Expert Panel Report 3: Guidelines for the Diagnosis and Management of Asthma. National Institutes of Health Pub. No. 08-4051. Bethesda, MD, 2007. http://www.nhlbi.nih.gov/guidelines/asthma/asthgdln.htm

A. Symptoms and Signs

Asthma is characterized by episodic wheezing, difficulty in breathing, chest tightness, and cough. Excess sputum production is common. The frequency of asthma symptoms is highly variable. Some patients have infrequent, brief attacks of asthma while others may suffer nearly continuous symptoms. Asthma symptoms may occur spontaneously or be precipitated or exacerbated by many different triggers as discussed above. Asthma symptoms are frequently worse at night; circadian variations in bronchomotor tone and bronchial reactivity reach their nadir between 3 AM and 4 AM, increasing symptoms of bronchoconstriction.

Some physical examination findings increase the probability of asthma. Nasal mucosal swelling, secretion increases, and polyps are often seen in patients with allergic asthma. Eczema, atopic dermatitis, or other allergic skin disorders may also be present. Wheezing or a prolonged expiratory phase during normal breathing correlates well with the presence of airflow obstruction. (Wheezing during forced expiration does not.) Chest examination may be normal between exacerbations in patients with mild asthma. During severe asthma exacerbations, airflow may be too limited to produce wheezing,

and the only diagnostic clue on auscultation may be globally reduced breath sounds with prolonged expiration. Hunched shoulders and use of accessory muscles of respiration suggest an increased work of breathing.

B. Laboratory Findings

Arterial blood gas measurements may be normal during a mild asthma exacerbation, but respiratory alkalosis and an increase in the alveolar-arterial oxygen difference (A–a–Do$_2$) are common. During severe exacerbations, hypoxemia develops and the Paco$_2$ returns to normal. The combination of an increased Paco$_2$ and respiratory acidosis may indicate impending respiratory failure and the need for mechanical ventilation.

C. Pulmonary Function Testing

Clinicians are able to identify airflow obstruction on examination, but they have limited ability to assess its severity or to predict whether it is reversible. The evaluation for asthma should therefore include **spirometry** (forced expiratory volume in 1 second [FEV$_1$], forced vital capacity [FVC], FEV$_1$/FVC) before and after the administration of a short-acting bronchodilator. These measurements help determine the presence and extent of airflow obstruction and whether it is immediately reversible. Airflow obstruction is indicated by a reduced FEV_1/FVC ratio. Significant reversibility of airflow obstruction is defined by an increase of $\geq$ 12% and 200 mL in FEV_1 or $\geq$ 15% and 200 mL in FVC after inhaling a short-acting bronchodilator. **A positive bronchodilator response strongly confirms the diagnosis of asthma but a lack of responsiveness in the pulmonary function laboratory does not preclude success in a clinical trial of bronchodilator therapy.** Severe airflow obstruction results in significant air trapping, with an increase in residual volume and consequent reduction in FVC, resulting in a pattern that may mimic a restrictive ventilatory defect.

Bronchial provocation testing with inhaled histamine or methacholine may be useful when asthma is suspected but spirometry is nondiagnostic. Bronchial provocation is not recommended if the FEV_1 is less than 65% of predicted. A positive methacholine test is defined as a $\geq$ 20% fall in the FEV_1 at exposure to a concentration of 8 mg/mL or less. A negative test has a negative predictive value for asthma of 95%. Exercise challenge testing may be useful in patients with symptoms of exercise-induced bronchospasm.

Peak expiratory flow (PEF) meters are handheld devices designed as personal monitoring tools. PEF monitoring can establish peak flow variability, quantify asthma severity, and provide both patient and clinician with objective measurements on which to base treatment decisions. There are conflicting data about whether measuring PEF improves asthma outcomes, but doing so is recommended to help confirm the diagnosis of asthma, to improve asthma control in patients with poor perception of airflow obstruction, and to identify environmental and occupational causes of symptoms. Predicted values for PEF vary with age, height, and gender but are poorly standardized. Comparison with reference values is less helpful than comparison with the patient's own baseline. PEF shows diurnal variation. It is generally lowest on first awakening and highest several hours before the midpoint of the waking day. PEF should be measured in the morning before the administration of a bronchodilator and in the afternoon after taking a bronchodilator. A 20% change in PEF values from morning to afternoon or from day to day suggests inadequately controlled asthma. PEF values less than 200 L/min indicate severe airflow obstruction.

D. Additional Testing

Routine chest radiographs in patients with asthma are usually normal or show only hyperinflation. Other findings may include bronchial wall thickening and diminished peripheral lung vascular shadows. Chest imaging is indicated when pneumonia, another disorder mimicking asthma, or a complication of asthma such as pneumothorax is suspected.

Skin testing or in vitro testing to assess sensitivity to environmental allergens can identify atopy in patients with persistent asthma who may benefit from therapies directed at their allergic diathesis. Evaluations for paranasal sinus

disease or gastroesophageal reflux should be considered in patients with pertinent, severe or refractory asthma symptoms.

▶ Complications

Complications of asthma include exhaustion, dehydration, airway infection, and tussive syncope. Pneumothorax occurs but is rare. Acute hypercapnic and hypoxemic respiratory failure occurs in severe disease.

▶ Differential Diagnosis

Patients who have atypical symptoms or poor response to therapy may have a condition that mimics asthma. These disorders typically fall into one of four categories: upper airway disorders, lower airway disorders, systemic vasculitides, and psychiatric disorders. **Upper airway disorders** that mimic asthma include vocal fold paralysis, vocal fold dysfunction syndrome, foreign body aspiration, laryngotracheal masses, tracheal narrowing, tracheomalacia, and airway edema (eg, angioedema or inhalation injury). **Lower airway disorders** include nonasthmatic chronic obstructive pulmonary disease (COPD) (chronic bronchitis or emphysema), bronchiectasis, allergic bronchopulmonary mycosis, cystic fibrosis, eosinophilic pneumonia, and bronchiolitis obliterans. **Systemic vasculitides** with pulmonary involvement may have an asthmatic component, such as Churg-Strauss syndrome. **Psychiatric causes** include conversion disorders ("functional" asthma), emotional laryngeal wheezing, vocal fold dysfunction, or episodic laryngeal dyskinesis. Rarely, Münchausen syndrome or malingering may explain a patient's complaints.

▶ NAEPP 3 Diagnosis & Management Guidelines

The third Expert Panel Report of the National Asthma Education and Prevention Program (NAEPP), in conjunction with the Global Initiative for Asthma (GINA), a collaboration between the National Institutes of Health (NIH)/National Heart, Lung, and Blood Institute (NHLBI) and the World Health Organization (WHO), provides guidelines for diagnosis and management of asthma (NAEPP 3) (Figure 9–2). This report identifies four components of chronic asthma diagnosis and management: (1) assessing and monitoring asthma severity and asthma control, (2) patient education designed to foster a partnership for care, (3) control of environmental factors and comorbid conditions that affect asthma, and (4) pharmacologic agents for asthma.

1. Assessing and monitoring asthma severity and asthma control—**Severity** is the intrinsic intensity of the disease process. **Control** is the degree to which symptoms and limitations on activity are minimized by therapy. **Responsiveness** is the ease with which control is achieved with therapy. NAEPP 3 guidelines emphasize control over classifications of severity, since the latter is variable over time and in response to therapy. A measure of severity on initial presentation (see Figure 9–1) is helpful, however, in

Intermittent Asthma	Persistent Asthma: Daily Medication
	Consult with asthma specialist if step 4 care or higher is required. Consider consultation at step 3.

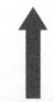

Step 1

Preferred:

SABA PRN

Step 2

Preferred:

Low-dose ICS

Alternative:

Cromolyn, LTRA, nedocromil, or theophylline

Step 3

Preferred:

Low-dose ICS + LABA
OR
Medium-dose ICS

Alternative:

Low-dose ICS + either LTRA, theophylline, or zileuton

Step 4

Preferred:

Medium-dose ICS + LABA

Alternative:

Low-dose ICS + either LTRA, theophylline, or zileuton

Step 5

Preferred:

High-dose ICS + LABA

AND

Consider omalizumab for patients who have allergies

Step 6

Preferred:

High-dose ICS + LABA + oral corticosteroid

AND

Consider omalizumab for patients who have allergies

Step up if needed

(first, check adherence, environmental control, and comorbid conditions)

Assess control

Step down if possible

(and asthma is well controlled at least 3 months)

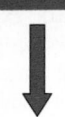

Each step: Patient education, environmental control, and management of comorbidities.

Steps 2–4: Consider subcutaneous allergen immunotherapy for patients who have allergic asthma (see notes).

Quick-Relief Medication for All Patients

- SABA as needed for symptoms. Intensity of treatment depends on severity of symptoms: up to three treatments at 20-minute intervals as needed. Short course of oral systemic corticosteroids may be needed.
- Use of SABA > 2 days a week for symptom relief (not prevention of EIB) generally indicates inadequate control and the need to step up treatment.

Key: *Alphabetical order is used when more than one treatment option is listed within either preferred or alternative therapy.* EIB, exercise-induced bronchospasm; ICS, inhaled corticosteroid; LABA, inhaled long-acting beta-2-agonist; LTRA, leukotriene receptor antagonist; SABA, inhaled short-acting beta-2-agonist

Notes:

- The stepwise approach is meant to assist, not replace, the clinical decision-making required to meet individual patient needs.
- If alternative treatment is used and response is inadequate, discontinue it and use the preferred treatment before stepping up.
- Zileuton is a less desirable alternative as adjunctive therapy due to limited studies and the need to monitor liver function. Theophylline requires monitoring of serum concentration levels.
- In step 6, before oral systemic corticosteroids are introduced, a trial of high-dose ICS + LABA + either LTRA, theophylline, or zileuton may be considered, although this approach has not been studied in clinical trials.
- Step 1, 2, and 3 preferred therapies are based on Evidence A; step 3 alternative therapy is based on Evidence A for LTRA, Evidence B for theophylline, and Evidence D for zileuton. Step 4 preferred therapy is based on Evidence B, and alternative therapy is based on Evidence B for LTRA and theophylline and Evidence D for zileuton. Step 5 preferred therapy is based on Evidence B. Step 6 preferred therapy is based on (EPR 2 1997) and Evidence B for omalizumab.
- Immunotherapy for steps 2–4 is based on Evidence B for house-dust mites, animal danders, and pollens; evidence is weak or lacking for molds and cockroaches. Evidence is strongest for immunotherapy with single allergens. The role of allergy in asthma is greater in children than in adults.
- Clinicians who administer immunotherapy or omalizumab should be prepared and equipped to identify and treat anaphylaxis that may occur.

▲ **Figure 9–2.** Stepwise approach to managing asthma. (Adapted from National Asthma Education and Prevention Program. Expert Panel Report 3: Guidelines for the Diagnosis and Management of Asthma. National Institutes of Health Pub. No. 08-4051. Bethesda, MD, 2007. http://www.nhlbi.nih.gov/guidelines/asthma/asthgdln.htm.)

guiding the initiation of therapy. Control of asthma is assessed in terms of **impairment** (frequency and intensity of symptoms and functional limitations) and **risk** (the likelihood of acute exacerbations or chronic decline in lung function). A key insight is that these two domains of control may respond differently to treatment: some patients may have minimal impairment yet remain at risk for severe exacerbations, for example, in the setting of an upper respiratory tract infection. Table 9–1 is used to assess the adequacy of asthma control and is used in conjunction with Figure 9–2 to guide adjustments in therapy based on the level of control.

2. Patient education designed to foster a partnership for care—Active self-management reduces urgent care visits and hospitalizations and improves perceived control of asthma. Therefore, an outpatient preventive approach that includes self-management education is an integral part of effective asthma care.

All patients, but particularly those with poorly controlled symptoms or history of severe exacerbations, should have a written **asthma action plan** that includes instructions for daily management and measures to take in response to specific changes in status. Patients should be taught to recognize symptoms—especially patterns indicating inadequate asthma control or predicting the need for additional therapy.

3. Control of environmental factors and comorbid conditions that affect asthma—Significant reduction in exposure to nonspecific airway irritants or to inhaled allergens in atopic patients may reduce symptoms and medication needs. Comorbid conditions that impair asthma management, such as rhinosinusitis, gastroesophageal reflux, obesity, and obstructive sleep apnea, should be identified and treated. This search for complicating conditions is particularly crucial in the initial evaluation of new asthma, and in patients who have difficult to control symptoms or frequent exacerbations.

4. Pharmacologic agents for asthma—Asthma medications can be divided into two categories: quick-relief (**reliever**) medications that act principally by direct relaxation of bronchial smooth muscle, thereby promoting prompt reversal of acute airflow obstruction to relieve accompanying symptoms, and long-term control (**controller**) medications that act primarily to attenuate airway inflammation and that are taken daily independent of symptoms to achieve and maintain control of persistent asthma.

Most asthma medications are administered orally or by inhalation. Inhalation of an appropriate agent results in a more rapid onset of pulmonary effects as well as fewer systemic effects compared with oral administration of the same dose. Proper inhaler technique and the use of an inhalation chamber with metered-dose inhalers (MDIs) decrease oropharyngeal deposition and improve drug delivery to the lung. Nebulizer therapy is reserved for acutely ill patients and those who cannot use inhalers because of difficulties with coordination, understanding, or cooperation.

▶ Treatment

The goals of asthma therapy are to minimize chronic symptoms that interfere with normal activity (including exercise), to prevent recurrent exacerbations, to reduce or eliminate the need for emergency department visits or hospitalizations, and to maintain normal or near-normal pulmonary function. These goals should be met while providing pharmacotherapy with the fewest adverse effects and while satisfying patients' and families' expectations of asthma care. **NAEPP 3 recommendations emphasize daily anti-inflammatory therapy with inhaled corticosteroids as the cornerstone of treatment of persistent asthma.**

A. Long-Term Control Medications

Anti-inflammatory agents, long-acting bronchodilators, and leukotriene modifiers comprise the important long-term control medications (Tables 9–3 and 9–4). Other classes of agents are mentioned briefly below as well.

1. Anti-inflammatory agents—Corticosteroids are the most potent and consistently effective anti-inflammatory agents currently available. They reduce both acute and chronic inflammation, resulting in fewer asthma symptoms, improved airflow, decreased airway hyper-responsiveness, and fewer asthma exacerbations. These agents may also potentiate the action of beta-adrenergic agonists.

Inhaled corticosteroids are preferred, first-line agents for all patients with persistent asthma. Patients with persistent symptoms or asthma exacerbations who are not taking an inhaled corticosteroid should be started on one. The most important determinants of agent selection and appropriate dosing are the patient's status and response to treatment. Dosages for inhaled corticosteroids vary depending on the specific agent and delivery device. For most patients, twice-daily dosing provides adequate control of asthma. Once-daily dosing may be sufficient in selected patients. Maximum responses from inhaled corticosteroids may not be observed for months. The use of an inhalation chamber ("spacer") coupled with mouth washing after inhaled corticosteroid use decreases local side effects (cough, dysphonia, oropharyngeal candidiasis) and systemic absorption. Dry powder inhalers (DPIs) are not used with an inhalation chamber. Systemic effects (adrenal suppression, osteoporosis, skin thinning, easy bruising, and cataracts) may occur with high-dose inhaled corticosteroid therapy.

Systemic corticosteroids (oral or parenteral) are most effective in achieving prompt control of asthma during exacerbations or when initiating long-term asthma therapy in patients with severe symptoms. In patients with refractory, poorly controlled asthma, systemic corticosteroids may be required for the long-term suppression of symptoms. Repeated efforts should be made to reduce the dose to the minimum needed to control symptoms. Alternate-day treatment is preferred to daily treatment. Concurrent treatment with calcium supplements and vitamin D should be initiated to prevent corticosteroid-induced bone mineral loss in long-term administration. Bone mineral density testing after 3 or more months of systemic corticosteroid lifetime use can guide the use of

Table 9–3. Long-term control medications for asthma.

Medication	Dosage Form	Adult Dose	Comments
Inhaled Corticosteroids			**(See Table 9–4)**
Systemic Corticosteroids			**(Applies to all three corticosteroids)**
Methylprednisolone	2-, 4-, 6-, 8-, 16-, 32-mg tablets	7.5–60 mg	• Administer single dose in AM either daily or on alternate days (alternate-day therapy may produce less adrenal suppression) as needed for control.
Prednisolone	5-mg tablets, 5 mg/5 mL, 15 mg/5 mL	40–60 mg	• Short courses or "bursts" as single or two divided doses for 3–10 days are effective for establishing control when initiating therapy or during a period of gradual
Prednisone	1, 2.5, 5, 10, 20, 50 mg tablets; 5 mg/mL		deterioration. • There is no evidence that tapering the dose following improvement in symptom control and pulmonary function prevents relapse.
Inhaled Long-Acting Beta-2-Agonists			**Should not be used for symptom relief or exacerbations. Use with inhaled corticosteroids.**
Salmeterol	DPI 50 mcg/actuation	1 blister every 12 hours	• Decreased duration of protection against EIB may occur with regular use.
Formoterol	DPI 12 mcg/single-use capsule	1 capsule every 12 hours	• Additional doses should not be administered for at least 12 hours. • Agents should be used only with their specific inhaler and should not be taken orally.
Combined Medication			
Fluticasone/Salmeterol	DPI 100 mcg/50 mcg 250 mcg/50 mcg 500 mcg/50 mcg HFA 45 mcg/21 mcg 115 mcg/21 mcg 230 mcg/21 mcg	1 inhalation twice daily; dose depends on severity of asthma	• 100/50 DPI or 45/21 HFA for patient not controlled on low- to medium-dose inhaled corticosteroids. • 250/50 DPI or 115/21 HFA for patients not controlled on medium- to high-dose inhaled corticosteroids.
Budesonide/Formoterol	HFA MDI 80 mcg/4.5 mcg 160 mcg/4.5 mcg	2 inhalations twice daily; dose depends on severity of asthma	• 80/4.5 for asthma not controlled on low- to medium-dose inhaled corticosteroids. • 160/4.5 for asthma not controlled on medium- to high-dose inhaled corticosteroids.
Cromolyn and Nedocromil			
Cromolyn	MDI 0.8 mg/puff	2 puffs four times daily	• 4 to 6-week trial may be needed to determine maximum benefit.
	Nebulizer 20 mg/ampule	1 ampule four times daily	• Dose by MDI may be inadequate to affect hyperresponsiveness.
Nedocromil	MDI 1.75 mg/puff	2 puffs four times daily	• One dose before exercise or allergen exposure provides effective prophylaxis for 1–2 hours. Not as effective for EIB as SABA. • Once control is achieved, the frequency of dosing may be reduced.
Inhaled Long-Acting Anticholinergic			**Should not be used for symptom relief or exacerbations. Use with inhaled corticosteroids.**
Tiotropium	DPI 18 mcg/blister	1 blister daily	
Leukotriene Modifiers			
Leukotriene Receptor Antagonists			
Montelukast	4-mg or 5-mg chewable tablet 10-mg tablet	10 mg daily at bedtime	• Exhibits a flat dose-response curve. Doses > 10 mg will not produce a greater response in adults.

(Continued)

Table 9–3. Long-term control medications for asthma. (Continued)

Medication	Dosage Form	Adult Dose	Comments
Zafirlukast	10- or 20-mg tablet	20-mg tablet twice daily	• Administration with meals decreases bioavailability; take at least 1 hour before or 2 hours after meals. • Monitor for symptoms and signs of hepatic dysfunction.
5-Lipoxygenase Inhibitor			
Zileuton	600-mg tablet	600 mg four times daily	• Monitor hepatic enzyme (ALT).
Methylxanthines			
Theophylline	Liquids, sustained-release tablets, and capsules	Starting dose 10 mg/kg/d up to 300 mg maximum; usual maximum dose 800 mg/d	• Adjust dose to achieve serum concentration of 5–15 mcg/mL after at least 48 hours on same dose. • Due to wide interpatient variability in theophylline metabolic clearance, routine serum theophylline level monitoring is important.
Immunomodulators			
Omalizumab	Subcutaneous injection, 150 mg/1.2 mL following reconstitution with 1.4 mL sterile water for injection	150–375 mg subcutaneously every 2–4 weeks, depending on body weight and pretreatment serum IgE level	• Do not administer more than 150 mg per injection site. • Monitor for anaphylaxis for 2 hours following at least the first three injections.

Table 9–4. Estimated comparative daily dosages for inhaled corticosteroids for asthma.

Drug	Low Daily Dose Adult	Medium Daily Dose Adult	High Daily Dose Adult
Beclomethasone HFA 40 or 80 mcg/puff	80–240 mcg	> 240–480 mcg	> 480 mcg
Budesonide DPI 90, 180, or 200 mcg/inhalation	180–600 mcg	> 600–1200 mcg	> 1200 mcg
Flunisolide 250 mcg/puff	500–1000 mcg	> 1000–2000 mcg	> 2000 mcg
Flunisolide HFA 80 mcg/puff	320 mcg	> 320–640 mcg	> 640 mcg
Fluticasone **HFA/MDI:** 44, 110, or 220 mcg/puff	88–264 mcg	> 264–440 mcg	> 440 mcg
DPI: 50, 100, or 250 mcg/inhalation	100–300 mcg	> 300–500 mcg	> 500 mcg
Mometasone DPI 200 mcg/puff	200 mcg	400 mcg	> 400 mcg
Triamcinolone acetonide 75 mcg/puff	300–750 mcg	> 750–1500 mcg	> 1500 mcg

DPI, dry power inhaler; HFA, hydrofluoroalkaline; MDI, metered-dose inhaler.

Notes:

• The most important determinant of appropriate dosing is the clinician's judgment of the patient's response to therapy.

• Potential drug interactions:
A number of the inhaled corticosteroids, including fluticasone, budesonide, and mometasone, are metabolized in the gastrointestinal tract and liver by CYP 3A4 isoenzymes. Potent inhibitors of CYP 3A4, such as ritonavir and ketoconazole, have the potential for increasing systemic concentrations of these inhaled corticosteroids by increasing oral availability and decreasing systemic clearance. Some cases of clinically significant Cushing syndrome and secondary adrenal insufficiency have been reported.

Adapted from National Asthma Education and Prevention Program. Expert Panel Report 3: Guidelines for the Diagnosis and Management of Asthma. National Institutes of Health Pub. No. 08-4051. Bethesda, MD, 2007. http://www.nhlbi.nih.gov/guidelines/asthma/asthgdln.htm

bisphosphonates for treatment of steroid-induced osteoporosis. Rapid discontinuation of systemic corticosteroids after long-term use may precipitate adrenal insufficiency.

2. Long-acting bronchodilators

A. Mediator inhibitors—Cromolyn sodium and nedocromil are long-term control medications that prevent asthma symptoms and improve airway function in patients with mild persistent or exercise-induced asthma. These agents modulate mast cell mediator release and eosinophil recruitment and inhibit both early and late asthmatic responses to allergen challenge and exercise-induced bronchospasm. They can be effective when taken before an exposure or exercise but do not relieve asthmatic symptoms once present. The clinical response to these agents is less predictable than to inhaled corticosteroids. Nedocromil may help reduce the dose requirements for inhaled corticosteroids. Both agents have excellent safety profiles.

B. Beta-adrenergic agonists—Long-acting beta-2-agonists provide bronchodilation for up to 12 hours after a single dose. Salmeterol and formoterol are the two long-acting beta-2-agonists available for asthma in the United States. They are administered via dry powder delivery devices. They are indicated for long-term prevention of asthma symptoms, nocturnal symptoms, and for prevention of exercise-induced bronchospasm. When added to low and medium daily doses of inhaled corticosteroids (Table 9–4), long-acting beta-2-agonists provide control equivalent to what is achieved by doubling the inhaled corticosteroid dose. Side effects are minimal at standard doses. **Long-acting beta-2-agonists should not be used as monotherapy** since they have no anti-inflammatory effect and since monotherapy with long-acting beta-2-agonists has been associated in two large studies with a small but statistically significant increased risk of severe or fatal asthma attacks. This increased risk has not been fully explained but may relate to genetic variation in the beta-adrenergic receptor, and remains an area of controversy. The efficacy of combined inhaled corticosteroid and long-acting beta-2-agonist therapy has led to marketing of combination medications that deliver both agents simultaneously (see Table 9–3). Combination inhalers containing formoterol and budesonide have shown efficacy in both maintenance and rescue, given formoterol's short time to onset.

C. Anticholinergics—The long-acting anticholinergic tiotropium has been studied as add-on therapy for patients who have either a bronchodilator response or a positive methacholine challenge that is not adequately controlled with low-dose inhaled corticosteroid. After 14 weeks of treatment, the addition of tiotropium resulted in improvements in PEF, FEV_1, and symptom control; the improvements were greater than those achieved by doubling the dose of the inhaled corticosteroid for the same period of time. The addition of tiotropium was not inferior to the addition of salmeterol. In patients with asthma receiving inhaled corticosteroids and long-acting beta-2-agonists who suffered at least one exacerbation in the preceding year, the addition of tiotropium resulted in a small improvement in peak FEV_1 as well as a modest increase in time to next exacerbation.

D. Phosphodiesterase inhibitors—Theophylline provides mild bronchodilation in asthmatic patients. Theophylline also has anti-inflammatory and immunomodulatory properties, enhances mucociliary clearance, and strengthens diaphragmatic contractility. Sustained-release theophylline preparations are effective in controlling nocturnal symptoms and as added therapy in patients with moderate or severe persistent asthma whose symptoms are inadequately controlled by inhaled corticosteroids. When added to inhaled corticosteroids, theophylline may allow equivalent control at lower corticosteroid doses.

Theophylline serum concentrations need to be monitored closely owing to the drug's narrow toxic-therapeutic range, individual differences in metabolism, and the effects of many factors on drug absorption and metabolism. At therapeutic doses, potential adverse effects include insomnia, aggravation of dyspepsia and gastroesophageal reflux, and urination difficulties in men with prostatic hyperplasia. Dose-related toxicities include nausea, vomiting, tachyarrhythmias, headache, seizures, hyperglycemia, and hypokalemia.

3. Leukotriene modifiers

—Leukotrienes are potent biochemical mediators that contribute to airway obstruction and asthma symptoms by contracting airway smooth muscle, increasing vascular permeability and mucus secretion, and attracting and activating airway inflammatory cells. Zileuton is a 5-lipoxygenase inhibitor that decreases leukotriene production, and zafirlukast and montelukast are cysteinyl leukotriene receptor antagonists. In randomized controlled trials (RCTs), these agents cause modest improvements in lung function and reductions in asthma symptoms and lessen the need for beta-2-agonist rescue therapy. These agents are alternatives to low-dose inhaled corticosteroids in patients with mild persistent asthma, although, as monotherapy, their effect is generally less than inhaled corticosteroids. In real-life community trials, leukotriene receptor antagonists were equivalent in efficacy to an inhaled corticosteroid as first-line long-term controller medication or to a long-acting beta-2-agonist as add-on therapy. Zileuton can cause reversible elevations in plasma aminotransferase levels. Churg-Strauss syndrome has been diagnosed in a small number of patients who have taken montelukast or zafirlukast, perhaps due to corticosteroid withdrawal rather than a direct drug effect.

4. Desensitization

—Immunotherapy for specific allergens may be considered in selected asthma patients who have exacerbations when exposed to allergens to which they are sensitive and when unresponsive to environmental control measures or other therapies. Studies show a reduction in asthma symptoms in patients treated with single-allergen immunotherapy. Because of the risk of immunotherapy-induced bronchoconstriction, it should be administered only in a setting where such complications can be immediately treated.

5. Omalizumab

—Omalizumab is a recombinant antibody that binds IgE without activating mast cells. In clinical trials in patients with moderate to severe asthma and elevated IgE levels, omalizumab reduced the need for corticosteroids.

6. Vaccination—Patients with asthma should receive pneumococcal vaccination (Pneumovax) and annual influenza (both seasonal and epidemic influenza A [H1N1]) vaccinations. Inactive vaccines (Pneumovax) are associated with few side effects but use of the live attenuated influenza vaccine intranasally may be associated with asthma exacerbations in young children.

7. Oral sustained-release beta-2-agonists—These agents are reserved for patients with bothersome nocturnal asthma symptoms or moderate to severe persistent asthma who do not respond to other therapies.

B. Quick-Relief Medications

Short-acting bronchodilators and systemic corticosteroids are the important quick-relief medications (Table 9–5).

1. Beta-adrenergic agonists—Short-acting inhaled beta-2-agonists, including albuterol, levalbuterol, bitolterol, pirbuterol, and terbutaline, are the most effective bronchodilators during exacerbations. All patients with acute symptoms should be prescribed one of these agents. There is no convincing evidence to support the use of one agent over another. Beta-2-agonists relax airway smooth muscle and cause a prompt increase in airflow and decrease in symptoms. Administration before exercise effectively prevents exercise-induced bronchoconstriction. Beta-2-selective agents may produce less cardiac stimulation than those with mixed beta-1 and beta-2 activities, although clinical trials have not consistently demonstrated this finding.

Inhaled beta-adrenergic therapy is as effective as oral or parenteral therapy in relaxing airway smooth muscle and improving acute asthma and offers the advantages of rapid onset of action (< 5 minutes) with fewer systemic side effects. Repetitive administration produces incremental bronchodilation. One or two inhalations of a short-acting inhaled beta-2-agonist from an MDI are usually sufficient for mild to moderate symptoms. Severe exacerbations frequently require higher doses: 6–12 puffs every 30–60 minutes of albuterol by MDI with an inhalation chamber or 2.5 mg by nebulizer provide equivalent bronchodilation. Administration by nebulization does not offer more effective delivery than MDIs used correctly but does provide higher doses. With most beta-2-agonists, the recommended dose by nebulizer for acute asthma (albuterol, 2.5 mg) is 25–30 times that delivered by a single activation of the MDI (albuterol, 0.09 mg). This difference suggests that **standard dosing of inhalations from an MDI will often be insufficient in the setting of an acute exacerbation.** Independent of dose, nebulizer therapy may be more effective in patients who are unable to coordinate inhalation of medication from an MDI because of age, agitation, or severity of the exacerbation.

Scheduled daily use of short-acting beta-2-agonists is not recommended. Increased use (more than one canister a month) or lack of expected effect indicates diminished asthma control and indicates the need for additional long-term control therapy.

2. Anticholinergics—Anticholinergic agents reverse vagally mediated bronchospasm but not allergen- or exercise-induced bronchospasm. They may decrease mucus gland hypersecretion. Ipratropium bromide, a quaternary derivative of atropine free of atropine's side effects, is less effective than beta-2-agonists for relief of acute bronchospasm, but it is the inhaled drug of choice for patients with intolerance to beta-2-agonists or with bronchospasm due to beta-blocker medications. Ipratropium bromide reduces the rate of hospital admissions when added to inhaled short-acting beta-2-agonists in patients with moderate to severe asthma exacerbations.

3. Corticosteroids—Systemic corticosteroids are effective primary treatment for patients with moderate to severe asthma exacerbations and for patients with exacerbations who do not respond promptly and completely to inhaled beta-2-agonist therapy. These medications speed the resolution of airflow obstruction and reduce the rate of relapse. Delays in administering corticosteroids may result in delayed benefits from these important agents. Therefore, oral corticosteroids should generally be **prescribed for early administration at home** in patients with moderate to severe asthma. The minimal effective dose of systemic corticosteroids for asthma patients has not been identified. Outpatient prednisone "burst" therapy is 0.5–1 mg/kg/d (typically 40–60 mg) in 1–2 doses for 3–10 days. Severe exacerbations requiring hospitalization typically require 1 mg/kg of prednisone or methylprednisolone every 6–12 hours for 48 hours or until the FEV_1 (or PEF rate) returns to 50% of predicted (or 50% of baseline). The dose is then decreased to 60–80 mg/d until the PEF reaches 70% of predicted or personal best. No clear advantage has been found for higher doses of corticosteroids. It may be prudent to administer corticosteroids intravenously to critically ill patients to avoid concerns about altered gastrointestinal absorption.

4. Antimicrobials—Multiple studies suggest that infections with viruses (rhinovirus) and bacteria (*Mycoplasma pneumoniae, Chlamydophila pneumoniae*) predispose to acute exacerbations of asthma and may underlie chronic, severe asthma. **The use of empiric antibiotics is, however, not recommended in routine asthma exacerbations because there is no consistent evidence to support improved clinical outcomes.** Antibiotics should be considered when there is a high likelihood of acute bacterial respiratory tract infection, such as for patients with fever or purulent sputum and evidence of pneumonia or bacterial sinusitis.

5. Phosphodiesterase inhibitors—Methylxanthines are not recommended for therapy of asthma exacerbations. Aminophylline has clearly been shown to be less effective than beta-2-agonists when used as single-drug therapy for acute asthma; it adds little except toxicity to the acute bronchodilator effects achieved by nebulized metaproterenol alone. Patients with exacerbations who are currently taking theophylline should have its serum concentration measured to exclude theophylline toxicity.

Table 9–5. Quick-relief medications for asthma.

Medication	Dosage Form	Adult Dose	Comments
Inhaled Short-Acting Beta-2-Agonists			
	MDI		
Albuterol CFC	90 mcg/puff, 200 puffs/ canister	2 puffs 5 minutes before exercise	• An increasing use or lack of expected effect indicates diminished control of asthma.
Albuterol HFA	90 mcg/puff, 200 puffs/ canister	2 puffs every 4–6 hours as needed	• Not recommended for long-term daily treatment. Regular use exceeding 2 days/week for symptom control (not prevention of EIB) indicates the need to step up therapy.
Pirbuterol CFC	200 mcg/puff, 400 puffs/ canister		• Differences in potency exist, but all products are essentially comparable on a per puff basis.
Levalbuterol HFA	45 mcg/puff, 200 puffs/ canister		• May double usual dose for mild exacerbations. • Prime the inhaler by releasing four actuations prior to use. • Periodically clean HFA activator, as drug may block/ plug orifice.
	Nebulizer solution		
Albuterol	0.63 mg/3 mL 1.25 mg/3 mL 2.5 mg/3 mL 5 mg/mL (0.5%)	1.25–5 mg in 3 mL of saline every 4–8 hours as needed	• May mix with budesonide inhalant suspension, cromolyn or ipratropium nebulizer solutions. • May double dose for severe exacerbations.
Levalbuterol (R-albuterol)	0.31 mg/3 mL 0.63 mg/3 mL 1.25 mg/0.5 mL 1.25 mg/3 mL	0.63 mg–1.25 mg every 8 hours as needed	• Compatible with budesonide inhalant suspension. The product is a sterile-filled, preservative-free, unit dose vial.
Anticholinergics			
	MDI		
Ipratropium HFA	17 mcg/puff, 200 puffs/ canister	2–3 puffs every 6 hours	• Evidence is lacking for anticholinergics producing added benefit to beta-2-agonists in long-term control asthma therapy.
	Nebulizer solution		
	0.25 mg/mL (0.025%)	0.25 mg every 6 hours	
	MDI		
Ipratropium with albuterol	18 mcg/puff of ipratropium bromide and 90 mcg/ puff of albuterol, 200 puffs/ canister	2–3 puffs every 6 hours	
	Nebulizer solution		
	0.5 mg/3 mL ipratropium bromide and 2.5 mg/ 3 mL albuterol	3 mL every 4–6 hours	• Contains EDTA to prevent discolorations of the solution. This additive does not induce bronchospasm.
Systemic Corticosteroids			
Methylprednisolone	2, 4, 6, 8, 16, 32 mg tablets	40–60 mg/d as single or 2 divided doses	• Short courses or "bursts" are effective for establishing control when initiating therapy or during a period of gradual deterioration. • The burst should be continued until symptoms resolve and the PEF is at least 80% of personal best. This usually requires 3–10 days but may require longer. There is no evidence that tapering the dose following improvements prevents relapse.
Prednisolone	5 mg tablets, 5 mg/5 mL, 15 mg/5 mL		
Prednisone	1, 2.5, 5, 10, 20, 50 mg tablets; 5 mg/mL		

(continued)

Table 9–5. Quick-relief medications for asthma. (continued)

Medication	Dosage Form	Adult Dose	Comments
	Repository injection		
Methylprednisolone acetate	40 mg/mL 80 mg/mL	240 mg intramuscularly once	May be used in place of a short burst of oral corticosteroids in patients who are vomiting or if adherence is a problem.

CFC, chlorofluorocarbon; EIB, exercise-induced bronchospasm; HFA, hydrofluoroalkane; MDI, metered-dose inhaler; PEF, peak expiratory flow. Adapted from National Asthma Education and Prevention Program. Expert Panel Report 3: Guidelines for the Diagnosis and Management of Asthma. National Institutes of Health Pub. No. 08-4051. Bethesda, MD, 2007. http://www.nhlbi.gov/guidelines/asthma/asthgdln.htm

► Treatment of Asthma Exacerbations

NAEPP 3 asthma treatment algorithms begin with an assessment of the severity of a patient's baseline asthma. Adjustments to that algorithm follow a stepwise approach based on a careful assessment of asthma control. Most instances of uncontrolled asthma are mild and can be managed successfully by patients at home with the telephone assistance of a clinician (Figure 9–3). More severe exacerbations require evaluation and management in an urgent care or emergency department setting (Figure 9–4).

A. Mild Exacerbations

Mild asthma exacerbations are characterized by only minor changes in airway function (PEF > 80%) and minimal symptoms and signs of airway dysfunction (see Table 9–2). Many such patients respond quickly and fully to an inhaled short-acting beta-2-agonist alone. However, an inhaled short-acting beta-2-agonist may need to be continued at increased doses, eg, every 3–4 hours for 24–48 hours. In patients not taking an inhaled corticosteroid, initiating one should be considered during the mild exacerbation. In patients already taking an inhaled corticosteroid, a 7-day course of oral corticosteroids (0.5–1.0 mg/kg/d) may be necessary. Doubling the dose of inhaled corticosteroid is not effective and is not recommended in the NAEPP 3 guidelines.

B. Moderate Exacerbations

The principal goals of treatment of moderate asthma exacerbations are correction of hypoxemia, reversal of airflow obstruction, and reduction of the likelihood of recurrence of obstruction. Early intervention may lessen the severity and shorten the duration of an exacerbation. Of paramount importance is correction of hypoxemia through the use of supplemental oxygen. Airflow obstruction is treated with continuous administration of an inhaled short-acting beta-2-agonist and the early administration of systemic corticosteroids. Serial measurements of lung function to quantify the severity of airflow obstruction and its response to treatment are useful. The improvement in FEV_1 after 30 minutes of treatment correlates significantly with the severity of the asthma exacerbation. Serial measurement of airflow in the emergency department may reduce the rate of hospital admissions for asthma exacerbations. The post-exacerbation care plan is important. **Regardless of the severity, all patients should be provided with necessary medications and education in how to use them, instruction in self-assessment, a follow-up appointment, and an action plan for managing recurrence.**

C. Severe Exacerbations

Severe exacerbations of asthma can be life-threatening, so treatment should be started immediately. All patients with a severe exacerbation should immediately receive oxygen, high doses of an inhaled short-acting beta-2-agonist, and systemic corticosteroids. A brief history pertinent to the exacerbation can be completed while such treatment is being initiated. More detailed assessments, including laboratory studies, usually add little early on and so should be postponed until after therapy is instituted.

Oxygen therapy is very important because asphyxia is a common cause of asthma deaths. Supplemental oxygen should be given to maintain an Sao_2 > 90% or a Pao_2 > 60 mm Hg. Oxygen-induced hypoventilation is extremely rare, and concern for hypercapnia should never delay correction of hypoxemia.

Frequent high-dose delivery of an **inhaled short-acting beta-2-agonist** is indicated and usually well tolerated in severe airway obstruction. Some studies suggest that continuous therapy is more effective than intermittent administration of these agents, but there is no clear consensus as long as similar doses are administered. At least three MDI or nebulizer treatments should be given in the first hour of therapy. Thereafter, the frequency of administration varies according to the improvement in airflow and symptoms and the occurrence of side effects. Ipratropium bromide reduces the rate of hospital admissions when added to inhaled short-acting beta-2-agonists in patients with moderate to severe asthma exacerbations.

Systemic corticosteroids are administered as detailed above. **Intravenous magnesium** sulfate (2 g intravenously over 20 minutes) produces a detectable improvement in airflow and may reduce hospitalization rates in acute severe asthma (FEV_1 < 25% of predicted on presentation, or failure to respond to initial treatment).

Mucolytic agents (eg, acetylcysteine, potassium iodide) may worsen cough or airflow obstruction. Anxiolytic and hypnotic drugs are generally contraindicated in severe asthma exacerbations because of their respiratory depressant effects.

Assess Severity

- **Patients at high risk for a fatal attack require immediate medical attention after initial treatment.**

- Symptoms and signs suggestive of a more serious exacerbation such as marked breathlessness, inability to speak more than short phrases, use of accessory muscles, or drowsiness (see Table 9–3) should result in initial treatment while immediately consulting with a clinician.

- Less severe symptoms and signs can be treated initially with assessment of response to therapy and further steps as listed below.

- If available, measure PEF—values of 50–79% predicted or personal best indicate the need for quick-relief medication. Depending on the response to treatment, contact with a clinician may also be indicated. Values below 50% indicate the need for immediate medical care.

Initial Treatment

- Inhaled SABA: up to two treatments 20 minutes apart of 2–6 puffs by MDI or nebulizer treatments.

- Note: Medication delivery is highly variable. Children and individuals who have exacerbations of lesser severity may need fewer puffs than suggested above.

Good Response

No wheezing or dyspnea (assess tachypnea in young children).

PEF ≥ 80% predicted or personal best.

- Contact clinician for follow-up instructions and further management.

- May continue inhaled SABA every 3–4 hours for 24–48 hours.

- Consider short course of oral systemic corticosteroids.

Incomplete Response

Persistent wheezing and dyspnea (tachypnea).

PEF 50–79% predicted or personal best.

- Add oral systemic corticosteroid.

- Continue inhaled SABA.

- Contact clinician urgently (this day) for further instruction.

Poor Response

Marked wheezing and dyspnea.

PEF < 50% predicted or personal best.

- Add oral systemic corticosteroid.

- Repeat inhaled SABA immediately.

- If distress is severe and nonresponsive to initial treatment:

  —Call your doctor AND
  —**PROCEED TO ED;**
  —Consider calling 9-1-1 (ambulance transport).

- To ED.

ED, emergency department; MDI, metered-dose inhaler; PEF, peak expiratory flow; SABA short-acting beta-2-agonist (quick-relief inhaler).

▲ **Figure 9–3.** Management of asthma exacerbations: home treatment. (Adapted from National Asthma Education and Prevention Program. Expert Panel Report 3: Guidelines for the Diagnosis and Management of Asthma. National Institutes of Health Pub. No. 08-4051. Bethesda, MD, 2007. http://www.nhlbi.nih.gov/guidelines/asthma/asthgdln.htm.)

In the **emergency department setting, repeat assessment** of patients with severe exacerbations should be done after the initial dose of inhaled bronchodilator and again after three doses of inhaled bronchodilators (60–90 minutes after initiating treatment). The response to initial treatment is a better predictor of the need for hospitalization than is the severity of an exacerbation on presentation. The decision to hospitalize a patient should be based on the duration and severity of symptoms, severity of airflow obstruction, arterial blood gas results (if available), course and severity of prior exacerbations, medication use at the time of the exacerbation, access to

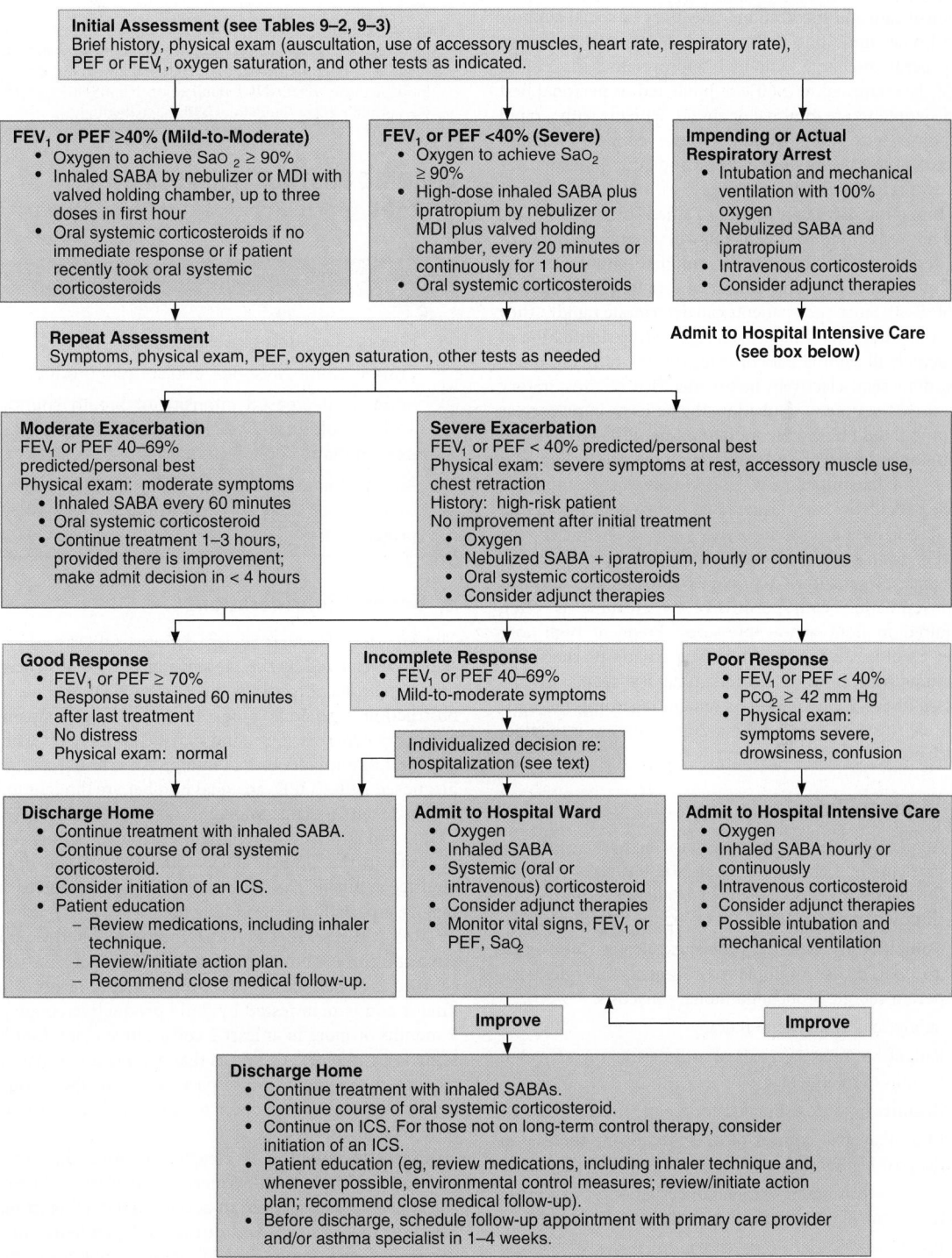

FEV$_1$, forced expiratory volume in 1 second; ICS, inhaled corticosteroid; MDI, metered-dose inhaler; PEF, peak expiratory flow; SABA, short-acting β_2-agonist; SaO$_2$, oxygen saturation.

▲ **Figure 9–4.** Management of asthma exacerbations: emergency department and hospital-based treatment. (Adapted from National Asthma Education and Prevention Program. Expert Panel Report 3: Guidelines for the Diagnosis and Management of Asthma. National Institutes of Health Pub. No. 08-4051. Bethesda, MD, 2007. http://www.nhlbi.nih.gov/guidelines/asthma/asthgdln.htm.)

medical care and medications, adequacy of social support and home conditions, and presence of psychiatric illness. In general, discharge to home is appropriate if the PEF or FEV_1 has returned to $\geq 60\%$ of predicted or personal best and symptoms are minimal or absent. Patients with a rapid response to treatment should be observed for 30 minutes after the most recent dose of bronchodilator to ensure stability of response before discharge.

In the **intensive care setting,** a small subset of patients will not respond to treatment and will progress to impending respiratory failure due to a combination of worsening airflow obstruction and respiratory muscle fatigue (see Table 9–2). Since such patients can deteriorate rapidly, they must be monitored in a critical care setting. Intubation of an acutely ill asthma patient is technically difficult and is best done semi-electively, before the crisis of a respiratory arrest. At the time of intubation, the patient's intravascular volume should be closely monitored because hypotension commonly follows the administration of sedative medications and the initiation of positive-pressure ventilation; these patients are often dehydrated due to poor recent oral intake and high insensible losses.

The main goals of mechanical ventilation are to ensure adequate oxygenation and to avoid barotrauma. Controlled hypoventilation with permissive hypercapnia is often required to limit airway pressures. Frequent high-dose delivery of inhaled short-acting beta-2-agonists should be continued along with anti-inflammatory agents as discussed above. Many questions remain regarding the optimal delivery of inhaled beta-2-agonists to intubated, mechanically ventilated patients.

▶ When to Refer

- Atypical presentation or uncertain diagnosis of asthma, particularly if additional diagnostic testing is required (bronchoprovocation challenge, allergy skin testing, rhinoscopy, consideration of occupational exposure).

- Complicating comorbid problems, such as rhinosinusitis, tobacco use, multiple environmental allergies, suspected allergic bronchopulmonary mycosis.

- Suboptimal response to therapy.

- Patient not meeting goals of asthma therapy after 3–6 months of treatment.

- Requires high-dose inhaled corticosteroids for control.

- More than two courses of oral prednisone therapy in the past 12 months.

- Any life-threatening asthma exacerbation or exacerbation requiring hospitalization in the past 12 months.

- Presence of social or psychological issues interfering with asthma management.

Barnes PJ. Severe asthma: advances in current management and future therapy. J Allergy Clin Immunol. 2012 Jan;129(1): 48–59. [PMID: 22196524]

Hopkin JM. The diagnosis of asthma, a clinical syndrome. Thorax. 2012 Jul;67(7):660–2. [PMID: 22561527]

Lazarus SC. Clinical practice. Emergency treatment of asthma. N Engl J Med. 2010 Aug19;363(8):755–64. [PMID: 20818877]

National Asthma Education and Prevention Program: Expert panel report III: Guidelines for the diagnosis and management of asthma. Bethesda, MD: National Heart, Lung, and Blood Institute, 2007. (NIH publication No. 08-4051). http://www.nhlbi.nih.gov/guidelines/asthma/asthgdln.htm

CHRONIC OBSTRUCTIVE PULMONARY DISEASE

ESSENTIALS OF DIAGNOSIS

- ▶ History of cigarette smoking
- ▶ Chronic cough, dyspnea, and sputum production.
- ▶ Rhonchi, decreased intensity of breath sounds, and prolonged expiration on physical examination.
- ▶ Airflow limitation on pulmonary function testing that is not fully reversible and most often progressive.

▶ General Considerations

The American Thoracic Society defines COPD as a disease state characterized by the presence of airflow obstruction due to chronic bronchitis or emphysema; the airflow obstruction is generally progressive, may be accompanied by airway hyperreactivity, and may be partially reversible. The NHLBI estimates that 14 million Americans have been diagnosed with COPD; an equal number are thought to be afflicted but remain undiagnosed. Grouped together, COPD and asthma now represent the fourth leading cause of death in the United States, with over 130,000 deaths reported annually. The death rate from COPD is increasing rapidly, especially among elderly men.

Most patients with COPD have features of both emphysema and chronic bronchitis. **Chronic bronchitis** is a clinical diagnosis defined by excessive secretion of bronchial mucus and is manifested by daily productive cough for 3 months or more in at least 2 consecutive years. **Emphysema** is a pathologic diagnosis that denotes abnormal permanent enlargement of air spaces distal to the terminal bronchiole, with destruction of their walls and without obvious fibrosis.

Cigarette smoking is clearly the most important cause of COPD in North America and Western Europe. Nearly all smokers suffer an accelerated decline in lung function that is dose- and duration-dependent. Fifteen percent develop progressively disabling symptoms in their 40s and 50s. Approximately 80% of patients seen for COPD have significant exposure to tobacco smoke. The remaining 20% frequently have a combination of exposures to environmental tobacco smoke, occupational dusts and chemicals, and indoor air pollution from biomass fuel used for cooking and heating in poorly ventilated buildings. Outdoor air pollution, airway infection, familial factors, and allergy have also been implicated in chronic bronchitis, and hereditary factors (deficiency of alpha-1-antiprotease [alpha-1-antitrypsin]) have been implicated. Atopy and the tendency for bronchoconstriction to develop in response to nonspecific airway stimuli may be important risks.

► Clinical Findings

A. Symptoms and Signs

Patients with COPD characteristically present in the fifth or sixth decade of life complaining of excessive cough, sputum production, and shortness of breath. Symptoms have often been present for 10 years or more. Dyspnea is noted initially only on heavy exertion, but as the condition progresses it occurs with mild activity. In severe disease, dyspnea occurs at rest. As the disease progresses, two symptom patterns tend to emerge, historically referred to as "pink puffers" and "blue bloaters" (Table 9–6). Most COPD patients have pathologic evidence of both disorders, and their clinical course may involve other factors such as central control of ventilation and concomitant sleep-disordered breathing.

Pneumonia, pulmonary hypertension, cor pulmonale, and chronic respiratory failure characterize the late stage of COPD. A hallmark of COPD is the periodic exacerbation of symptoms beyond normal day-to-day variation, often including increased dyspnea, an increased frequency or severity of cough, increased sputum volume or change in sputum character. These exacerbations are commonly precipitated by infection (more often viral than bacterial) or environmental factors. Exacerbations of COPD vary widely in severity but typically require a change in regular therapy.

B. Laboratory Findings

Spirometry provides objective information about pulmonary function and assesses the response to therapy. Pulmonary function tests early in the course of COPD reveal only evidence of abnormal closing volume and reduced midexpiratory flow rate. Reductions in FEV_1 and in the ratio of forced expiratory volume to vital capacity ($FEV_1\%$ or FEV_1/FVC ratio) (Table 9–6) occur later. In severe disease, the FVC is markedly reduced. Lung volume measurements reveal a marked increase in residual volume (RV), an increase in total lung capacity (TLC), and an elevation of the RV/TLC ratio, indicative of air trapping, particularly in emphysema.

Arterial blood gas measurements characteristically show no abnormalities early in COPD other than an

Table 9–6. Patterns of disease in advanced COPD.

	Type A: Pink Puffer (Emphysema Predominant)	Type B: Blue Bloater (Bronchitis Predominant)
History and physical examination	Major complaint is dyspnea, often severe, usually presenting after age 50. Cough is rare, with scant clear, mucoid sputum. Patients are thin, with recent weight loss common. They appear uncomfortable, with evident use of accessory muscles of respiration. Chest is very quiet without adventitious sounds. No peripheral edema.	Major complaint is chronic cough, productive of mucopurulent sputum, with frequent exacerbations due to chest infections. Often presents in late 30s and 40s. Dyspnea usually mild, though patients may note limitations to exercise. Patients frequently overweight and cyanotic but seem comfortable at rest. Peripheral edema is common. Chest is noisy, with rhonchi invariably present; wheezes are common.
Laboratory studies	Hemoglobin usually normal (12–15 g/dL). PaO_2 normal to slightly reduced (65–75 mm Hg) but SaO_2 normal at rest. $PaCO_2$ normal to slightly reduced (35–40 mm Hg). Chest radiograph shows hyperinflation with flattened diaphragms. Vascular markings are diminished, particularly at the apices.	Hemoglobin usually elevated (15–18 g/dL). PaO_2 reduced (45–60 mm Hg) and $PaCO_2$ slightly to markedly elevated (50–60 mm Hg). Chest radiograph shows increased interstitial markings ("dirty lungs"), especially at bases. Diaphragms are not flattened.
Pulmonary function tests	Airflow obstruction ubiquitous. Total lung capacity increased, sometimes markedly so. DL_{CO} reduced. Static lung compliance increased.	Airflow obstruction ubiquitous. Total lung capacity generally normal but may be slightly increased. DL_{CO} normal. Static lung compliance normal.
Special evaluations		
(V̇/Q̇) matching	Increased ventilation to high (V̇/Q̇) areas, ie, high dead space ventilation.	Increased perfusion to low (V̇/Q̇) areas.
Hemodynamics	Cardiac output normal to slightly low. Pulmonary artery pressures mildly elevated and increase with exercise.	Cardiac output normal. Pulmonary artery pressures elevated, sometimes markedly so, and worsen with exercise.
Nocturnal ventilation	Mild to moderate degree of oxygen desaturation not usually associated with obstructive sleep apnea.	Severe oxygen desaturation, frequently associated with obstructive sleep apnea.
Exercise ventilation	Increased minute ventilation for level of oxygen consumption. PaO_2 tends to fall, $PaCO_2$ rises slightly.	Decreased minute ventilation for level of oxygen consumption. PaO_2 may rise; $PaCO_2$ may rise significantly.

DL_{CO}, single-breath diffusing capacity for carbon monoxide; (V̇/Q̇), ventilation-perfusion.

increased A–a–Do$_2$. Indeed, measurement is unnecessary unless (1) hypoxemia or hypercapnia is suspected, (2) the FEV$_1$ is < 40% of predicted, or (3) there are clinical signs of right heart failure. Hypoxemia occurs in advanced disease, particularly when chronic bronchitis predominates. Compensated respiratory acidosis occurs in patients with chronic respiratory failure, particularly in chronic bronchitis, with worsening of acidemia during acute exacerbations.

Examination of the sputum may reveal *Streptococcus pneumoniae, H influenzae,* or *Moraxella catarrhalis.* Positive sputum cultures are poorly correlated with acute exacerbations, and research techniques demonstrate evidence of preceding viral infection in a majority of patients with exacerbations. The ECG may show sinus tachycardia and, in advanced disease, chronic pulmonary hypertension may produce electrocardiographic abnormalities typical of cor pulmonale. Supraventricular arrhythmias (multifocal atrial tachycardia, atrial flutter, and atrial fibrillation) and ventricular irritability also occur.

C. Imaging

Radiographs of patients with chronic bronchitis typically show only nonspecific peribronchial and perivascular markings. Plain radiographs are insensitive for the diagnosis of emphysema; they show hyperinflation with flattening of the diaphragm or peripheral arterial deficiency in about half of cases. CT of the chest, particularly using high-resolution CT, is more sensitive and specific than plain radiographs for its diagnosis. In advanced disease, pulmonary hypertension may be suggested by enlargement of central pulmonary arteries on radiographs and Doppler echocardiography provides an estimate of pulmonary artery pressure.

▶ Differential Diagnosis

Clinical, imaging, and laboratory findings should enable the clinician to distinguish COPD from other obstructive pulmonary disorders such as asthma, bronchiectasis, cystic fibrosis, bronchopulmonary mycosis, and central airflow obstruction. Asthma is characterized by complete or near-complete reversibility of airflow obstruction. Bronchiectasis is distinguished from COPD by recurrent pneumonia and hemoptysis, digital clubbing, and characteristic imaging abnormalities. Patients with severe alpha-1-antitrypsin deficiency have a family history of the disorder and the finding of panacinar bibasilar emphysema early in life, usually in the third or fourth decade; hepatic cirrhosis and hepatocellular carcinoma may develop. Cystic fibrosis occurs in children, adolescents and young adults. Mechanical obstruction of the central airways can be distinguished from COPD by flow-volume loops.

▶ Complications

Acute bronchitis, pneumonia, pulmonary thromboembolism, atrial dysrhythmias (such as atrial fibrillation, atrial flutter, and multifocal atrial tachycardia), and concomitant left ventricular failure may worsen otherwise stable COPD. Pulmonary hypertension, cor pulmonale, and chronic respiratory failure are common in advanced COPD. Spontaneous pneumothorax occurs in a small fraction of patients with emphysema. Hemoptysis may result from chronic bronchitis or may signal bronchogenic carcinoma.

▶ Prevention

COPD is largely preventable through elimination of long-term exposure to tobacco smoke or other inhaled toxins. Smokers with early evidence of airflow limitation can significantly alter their disease by smoking cessation. Smoking cessation slows the decline in FEV$_1$ in middle-aged smokers with mild airways obstruction. Vaccination against seasonal and epidemic influenza A (H1N1) and pneumococcal infection may also be of benefit.

▶ Treatment

The treatment of COPD is guided by the severity of symptoms or the presence of an exacerbation of stable symptoms. Standards for the management of patients with stable COPD and COPD exacerbations from the American Thoracic Society and the Global Initiative for Obstructive Lung Disease (GOLD), a joint expert committee of the NHLBI and the WHO, are incorporated in the recommendations below. See Chapter 37 for a discussion of air travel in patients with lung disease.

A. Ambulatory Patients

1. Smoking cessation—The single most important intervention in smokers with COPD is to encourage smoking cessation (discussed further in Chapter 1).

2. Oxygen therapy—**Supplemental oxygen for patients with resting hypoxemia is the only therapy with evidence of improvement in the natural history of COPD.** Proved benefits of home oxygen therapy in hypoxemic patients include longer survival, reduced hospitalizations, and better quality of life. Survival in hypoxemic patients with COPD treated with supplemental oxygen therapy is directly proportionate to the number of hours per day oxygen is administered: in COPD hypoxemic patients treated with continuous oxygen for 24 hours daily, the survival after 36 months is about 65%—significantly better than the survival rate of about 45% in those treated with only nocturnal oxygen. Oxygen by nasal prongs must be given for at least 15 hours a day unless therapy is specifically intended only for exercise or sleep. In COPD patients with borderline low-normal resting oxygen levels (Pao$_2$ between 56 mm Hg and 69 mm Hg), however, several studies of supplemental oxygen therapy showed no survival benefit. COPD patients with normal or low-normal resting oxygen levels who desaturate with exertion improve their exercise tolerance and shorten recovery from dyspnea when supplemental oxygen therapy is used during activity, but there is no evidence of a mortality benefit. Requirements for US Medicare coverage for a patient's home use of oxygen and oxygen equipment are listed in Table 9–7. Arterial blood gas analysis is preferred over oximetry to guide initial oxygen therapy. Hypoxemic patients with pulmonary hypertension, chronic cor pulmonale, erythrocytosis, impaired cognitive

Table 9–7. Home oxygen therapy: Requirements for Medicare coverage.[1]

Group I (any of the following):

1. $PaO_2 \leq 55$ mm Hg or $SaO_2 \leq 88\%$ taken while awake, at rest, breathing room air.
2. During sleep (prescription for nocturnal oxygen use only):
   a. $PaO_2 \leq 55$ mm Hg or $SaO_2 \leq 88\%$ for a patient whose awake, resting, room air PaO_2 is ≥ 56 mm Hg or $SaO_2 \geq 89\%$,
      or
   b. Decrease in $PaO_2 > 10$ mm Hg or decrease in $SaO_2 > 5\%$ associated with symptoms or signs reasonably attributed to hypoxemia (eg, impaired cognitive processes, nocturnal restlessness, insomnia).
3. During exercise (prescription for oxygen use only during exercise):
   a. $PaO_2 \leq 55$ mg Hg or $SaO_2 \leq 88\%$ taken during exercise for a patient whose awake, resting, room air PaO_2 is ≥ 56 mm Hg or $SaO_2 \geq 89\%$, *and*
   b. There is evidence that the use of supplemental oxygen during exercise improves the hypoxemia that was demonstrated during exercise while breathing room air.

Group II[2]:

$PaO_2 = 56–59$ mm Hg or $SaO_2 = 89\%$ if there is evidence of any of the following:

1. Dependent edema suggesting heart failure.
2. P pulmonale on ECG (P wave > 3 mm in standard leads II, III, or aVF).
3. Hematocrit > 56%.

[1]Centers for Medicare & Medicaid Services, US, 2003.
[2]Patients in this group must have a second oxygen test 3 months after the initial oxygen set-up.

function, exercise intolerance, nocturnal restlessness, or morning headache are particularly likely to benefit from home oxygen therapy.

Home oxygen may be supplied by liquid oxygen systems, compressed gas cylinders, or oxygen concentrators. Most patients benefit from having both stationary and portable systems. For most patients, a flow rate of 1–3 L/min achieves a PaO_2 greater than 55 mm Hg. The monthly cost of home oxygen therapy ranges from $300 to $500 or more, higher for liquid oxygen systems. Medicare covers approximately 80% of home oxygen expenses. **Transtracheal oxygen** is an alternative method of delivery and may be useful for patients who require higher flows of oxygen than can be delivered via the nose or who are experiencing troublesome side effects from nasal delivery such as nasal drying or epistaxis. Reservoir nasal cannulas or "pendants" and demand (pulse) oxygen delivery systems are also available to conserve oxygen.

3. Inhaled bronchodilators—Bronchodilators do not alter the inexorable decline in lung function that is a hallmark of COPD, but they improve symptoms, exercise tolerance, and overall health status. Aggressiveness of bronchodilator therapy should be matched to the severity of the patient's disease. In patients who experience no symptomatic improvement, bronchodilators should be discontinued.

The most commonly prescribed short-acting bronchodilators are the anticholinergic ipratropium bromide and beta-2-agonists (eg, albuterol, metaproterenol), delivered by MDI or as an inhalation solution by nebulizer. **Ipratropium bromide is generally preferred to the short-acting beta-2-agonists as a first-line agent because of its longer duration of action and absence of sympathomimetic side effects.** Some studies have suggested that ipratropium achieves superior bronchodilation in COPD patients. Typical doses are two to four puffs (36–72 mcg) every 6 hours. Short-acting beta-2-agonists are less expensive and have a more rapid onset of action, commonly leading to greater patient satisfaction. At maximal doses, beta-2-agonists have bronchodilator action equivalent to that of ipratropium but may cause tachycardia, tremor, or hypokalemia. There does not appear to be any advantage of scheduled use of short-acting beta-2-agonists compared with as-needed administration. Use of both short-acting beta-2-agonists and anticholinergics at submaximal doses leads to improved bronchodilation compared with either agent alone but does not improve dyspnea.

Long-acting beta-2-agonists (eg, formoterol, salmeterol, indacaterol, arformoterol) and anticholinergics (tiotropium) appear to achieve bronchodilation that is equivalent or superior to what is experienced with ipratropium, in addition to similar improvements in health status. Although more expensive than short-acting agents, long-acting bronchodilators may have superior clinical efficacy in persons with advanced disease. One RCT of long-term administration of tiotropium added to standard therapy reported fewer exacerbations or hospitalizations, and improved dyspnea scores, in the tiotropium group. Tiotropium had no effect on long-term decline in lung function, however. Another RCT comparing the effects of tiotropium with those of salmeterol-fluticasone over 2 years reported no difference in the risk of COPD exacerbation. The incidence of pneumonia was higher in the salmeterol-fluticasone group, yet dyspnea scores were lower and there was a mortality benefit compared with tiotropium. This last finding awaits confirmation in further studies.

The symptomatic benefits of long-acting bronchodilators are firmly established. Increased exacerbations and mortality in patients treated with salmeterol have not been observed in COPD patients, and several studies report a trend toward lower mortality in patients treated with salmeterol alone, compared with placebo. In addition, a 4-year tiotropium trial reported fewer cardiovascular events in the intervention group. Subsequent meta-analyses that include the 4-year tiotropium trial did not find an increase in cardiovascular events in treated patients and most practitioners believe that the documented benefits of anticholinergic therapy outweigh any potential risks.

4. Corticosteroids—Multiple large clinical trials have reported a reduction in the frequency of COPD exacerbations and an increase in self-reported functional status in COPD patients treated with inhaled corticosteroids. These same trials demonstrate no effect of inhaled corticosteroids on mortality or the characteristic decline in lung function experienced by COPD patients. Thus, inhaled corticosteroids alone should not be considered first-line therapy in stable COPD patients.

However, combination therapy with an inhaled corticosteroid and a long-acting beta-2-agonist reduces the frequency of exacerbations and improves self-reported functional status in COPD patients, compared with placebo or with sole use of inhaled corticosteroids, long-acting beta-2-agonists, or anticholinergics. In one RCT, addition of an inhaled corticosteroid/long-acting beta-2-agonist to tiotropium therapy in COPD patients did not reduce the frequency of exacerbations but did improve hospitalization rates and functional status.

Apart from acute exacerbations, COPD is not generally responsive to oral corticosteroid therapy. Compared with patients receiving placebo, only 10–20% of stable outpatients with COPD given oral corticosteroids will have a > 20% increase in FEV_1. There may be a subset of steroid-responsive COPD patients more likely to benefit from long-term oral or inhaled corticosteroids. Since there are no clinical predictors to identify such responders, empiric trials of oral corticosteroids are common. If an empiric trial of oral corticosteroid is conducted, a baseline FEV_1 should be documented when the patient is stable (ie, not measured during an exacerbation), on maximal long-term bronchodilator therapy, and obtained immediately after a bronchodilator administration. After a 3- to 4-week trial of 0.25–0.5 mg/kg oral prednisone, the corticosteroid should only be continued if there is a 20% or greater increase in FEV_1 over this baseline value. Responders to oral corticosteroids are usually switched to inhaled agents, but there are few data to guide this practice. Oral corticosteroids have well-recognized adverse effects, so it is prudent to minimize cumulative exposure. It is rare for a patient to be truly "corticosteroid-dependent" when all other available therapies are optimized.

5. Theophylline—Oral theophylline is a fourth-line agent for treating COPD patients who do not achieve adequate symptom control with inhaled anticholinergic, beta-2-agonist, and corticosteroid therapies. Sustained-release theophylline improves hemoglobin saturation during sleep in COPD patients and is a first-line agent for those with sleep-related breathing disorders. Theophylline improves dyspnea ratings, exercise performance, and pulmonary function in many patients with stable COPD. Its benefits result from bronchodilation; anti-inflammatory properties; and extrapulmonary effects on diaphragm strength, myocardial contractility, and kidney function. Theophylline toxicity is a significant concern due to the drug's narrow therapeutic window, and long-term administration requires careful monitoring of serum levels. Despite potential for adverse effects, theophylline continues to have a beneficial role in carefully selected patients.

6. Antibiotics—Antibiotics are commonly prescribed to outpatients with COPD for the following indications: (1) to treat an acute exacerbation, (2) to treat acute bronchitis, and (3) to prevent acute exacerbations of chronic bronchitis (prophylactic antibiotics). In patients with COPD, antibiotics appear to improve outcomes slightly in the first two situations, but not the third. **Patients with a COPD exacerbation associated with increased sputum purulence accompanied by dyspnea or an increase in the quantity of sputum are thought to benefit the most from antibiotic therapy.** The choice of antibiotic depends on local bacterial resistance patterns and individual risk of *Pseudomonas aeruginosa* infection (history of *Pseudomonas* isolation, FEV_1 < 50% of predicted, recent hospitalization [2 or more days in the past 3 months], more than three courses of antibiotics within the past year, use of systemic corticosteroids). Oral antibiotic options include doxycycline (100 mg every 12 hours), trimethoprim-sulfamethoxazole (160/800 mg every 12 hours), a cephalosporin (eg, cefpodoxime 200 mg every 12 hours or cefprozil 500 mg every 12 hours), a macrolide (eg, azithromycin 500 mg followed by 250 mg daily for 5 days), a fluoroquinolone (eg, ciprofloxacin 500 mg every 12 hours), and amoxicillin-clavulanate (875/125 mg every 12 hours). Suggested duration of therapy is 3–7 days and depends on response to therapy; some studies suggest that 5 days is as effective as 7 days but with fewer adverse effects. There are few controlled trials of antibiotics in severe COPD exacerbations, but prompt administration is appropriate, particularly in persons with risk factors for poor outcomes (age > 65 years, FEV_1 < 50% predicted, three or more exacerbations in the past year, antibiotic therapy within the past 3 months, comorbid conditions such as cardiac disease).

7. Pulmonary rehabilitation—Graded aerobic physical exercise programs (eg, walking 20 minutes three times weekly or bicycling) are helpful to prevent deterioration of physical condition and to improve patients' ability to carry out daily activities. Training of inspiratory muscles by inspiring against progressively larger resistive loads reduces dyspnea and improves exercise tolerance, health status, and respiratory muscle strength in some but not all patients. Pursed-lip breathing to slow the rate of breathing and abdominal breathing exercises to relieve fatigue of accessory muscles of respiration may reduce dyspnea in some patients. Many patients undergo these exercise and educational interventions in a structured rehabilitation program. In a number of studies, pulmonary rehabilitation has been shown to improve exercise capacity, decrease hospitalizations, and enhance quality of life. Referral to a comprehensive rehabilitation program is recommended in patients who have severe dyspnea, reduced quality of life, or frequent hospitalizations despite optimal medical therapy.

8. Other measures—In patients with chronic bronchitis, increased mobilization of secretions may be accomplished through the use of adequate systemic hydration, effective cough training methods, or use of a hand-held flutter device and postural drainage, sometimes with chest percussion or vibration. Postural drainage and chest percussion should be used only in selected patients with excessive amounts of retained secretions that cannot be cleared by coughing and other methods; these measures are of no benefit in pure emphysema. Expectorant-mucolytic therapy has generally been regarded as unhelpful in patients with chronic bronchitis. Cough suppressants and sedatives should be avoided.

Human alpha-1-antitrypsin is available for replacement therapy in emphysema due to congenital deficiency (PiZZ or null genotype) of alpha-1-antiprotease (alpha-1-antitrypsin). Patients over 18 years of age with airflow obstruction by spirometry and serum levels less than 11 mcmol/L (~50 mg/dL) are potential candidates for replacement therapy. Alpha-1-antitrypsin is administered intravenously in a dose of 60 mg/kg body weight once weekly. There is no evidence that replacement therapy is beneficial to heterozygotes (eg, PiMZ) with low-normal serum levels, although such patients may be at slightly increased risk for emphysema, especially in the setting of tobacco smoke exposure. Severe dyspnea in spite of optimal medical management may warrant a clinical trial of an opioid (eg, morphine 5–10 mg orally every 3–4 hours, oxycodone 5–10 mg orally every 4–6 hours, sustained-release morphine 10 mg orally once daily). Sedative-hypnotic drugs (eg, diazepam, 5 mg three times daily) marginally improve intractable dyspnea but cause significant drowsiness; they may benefit very anxious patients. Transnasal positive-pressure ventilation at home to rest the respiratory muscles is an approach to improve respiratory muscle function and reduce dyspnea in patients with severe COPD. A bilevel transnasal ventilation system has been reported to reduce dyspnea in ambulatory patients with severe COPD, but the long-term benefits of this approach and compliance with it have not been defined.

B. Hospitalized Patients

Management of the hospitalized patient with an acute exacerbation of COPD includes (1) supplemental oxygen (titrated to maintain Sao$_2$ between 90% and 94% or Pao$_2$ between 60 mm Hg and 70 mm Hg), (2) inhaled ipratropium bromide (500 mcg by nebulizer, or 36 mcg by MDI with spacer, every 4 hours as needed) plus beta-2-agonists (eg, albuterol 2.5 mg diluted with saline to a total of 3 mL by nebulizer, or MDI, 90 mcg per puff, four to eight puffs via spacer, every 1–4 hours as needed), (3) corticosteroids (prednisone 30–40 mg orally per day for 7–10 days is usually sufficient, even 5 days may be adequate), (4) broad-spectrum antibiotics and, (5) in selected cases, chest physiotherapy.

For patients without risk factors for *Pseudomonas*, management options include a fluoroquinolone (eg, levofloxacin 750 mg orally or intravenously per day, or moxifloxacin 400 mg orally or intravenously every 24 hours) or a third-generation cephalosporin (eg, ceftriaxone 1 g intravenously per day, or cefotaxime 1 g intravenously every 8 hours).

For patients with risk factors for *Pseudomonas,* therapeutic options include piperacillin-tazobactam (4.5 g intravenously every 6 hours), ceftazidime (1 g intravenously every 8 hours), cefepime (1 g intravenously every 12 hours), or levofloxacin (750 mg orally or intravenously per day for 3–7 days).

Theophylline should not be initiated in the acute setting, but patients taking theophylline prior to acute hospitalization should have their theophylline serum levels measured and maintained in the therapeutic range. Oxygen therapy should not be withheld for fear of worsening respiratory acidemia; hypoxemia is more detrimental than hypercapnia. Cor pulmonale usually responds to measures that reduce pulmonary artery pressure, such as

supplemental oxygen and correction of acidemia; bed rest, salt restriction, and diuretics may add some benefit. Cardiac dysrhythmias, particularly multifocal atrial tachycardia, usually respond to aggressive treatment of COPD itself. Atrial flutter may require DC cardioversion after initiation of the above therapy. If progressive respiratory failure ensues, tracheal intubation and mechanical ventilation are necessary. In clinical trials of COPD patients with hypercapnic acute respiratory failure, noninvasive positive-pressure ventilation (NPPV) delivered via face mask reduced the need for intubation and shortened lengths of stay in the intensive care unit (ICU). Other studies have suggested a lower risk of nosocomial infections and less use of antibiotics in COPD patients treated with NPPV. These benefits do not appear to extend to hypoxemic respiratory failure or to patients with acute lung injury or acute respiratory distress syndrome (ARDS).

C. Surgery for COPD

1. Lung transplantation—Experience with both single and bilateral sequential lung transplantation for severe COPD is extensive. Requirements for lung transplantation are severe lung disease, limited activities of daily living, exhaustion of medical therapy, ambulatory status, potential for pulmonary rehabilitation, limited life expectancy without transplantation, adequate function of other organ systems, and a good social support system. Average total charges for lung transplantation through the end of the first postoperative year exceed $250,000. The 2-year survival rate after lung transplantation for COPD is 75%. Complications include acute rejection, opportunistic infection, and obliterative bronchiolitis. Substantial improvements in pulmonary function and exercise performance have been noted after transplantation.

2. Lung volume reduction surgery—Lung volume reduction surgery (LVRS), or reduction pneumoplasty, is a surgical approach to relieve dyspnea and improve exercise tolerance in patients with advanced diffuse emphysema and lung hyperinflation. Bilateral resection of 20–30% of lung volume in selected patients results in modest improvements in pulmonary function, exercise performance, and dyspnea. The duration of any improvement as well as any mortality benefit remains uncertain. Prolonged air leaks occur in up to 50% of patients postoperatively. Mortality rates in centers with the largest experience with LVRS range from 4% to 10%.

The National Emphysema Treatment Trial compared LVRS with medical treatment in a randomized, multicenter clinical trial of 1218 patients with severe emphysema. Overall, surgery improved exercise capacity but not mortality when compared with medical therapy. The persistence of this benefit remains to be defined. Subgroup analysis suggested that patients with upper lobe predominant emphysema and low exercise capacity might have improved survival, while other groups suffered excess mortality when randomized to surgery.

3. Bullectomy—Bullectomy is an older surgical procedure for palliation of dyspnea in patients with severe bullous emphysema. Bullectomy is most commonly pursued when a single bulla occupies at least 30–50% of the hemithorax. In this procedure, the surgeon removes a large emphysematous bulla that demonstrates no ventilation or perfusion on lung scanning and compresses adjacent lung with preserved function. Bullectomy can be performed with a CO_2 laser via thoracoscopy.

Prognosis

The outlook for patients with clinically significant COPD is poor. The degree of pulmonary dysfunction at the time the patient is first seen is an important predictor of survival: median survival of patients with $FEV_1 \leq 1$ L is about 4 years. A multidimensional index (the BODE index), which includes body mass index (BMI), airway obstruction (FEV_1), dyspnea (Medical Research Council dyspnea score), and exercise capacity is a tool that predicts death and hospitalization better than FEV_1 alone. Comprehensive care programs, cessation of smoking, and supplemental oxygen may reduce the rate of decline of pulmonary function, but therapy with bronchodilators and other approaches probably has little, if any, impact on the natural course of COPD.

Dyspnea at the end of life can be extremely uncomfortable and distressing to the patient and family. As patients near the end of life, meticulous attention to palliative care is essential to effectively manage dyspnea (see Chapter 5).

When to Refer

- COPD onset occurs before the age of 40.
- Frequent exacerbations (two or more a year) despite optimal treatment.
- Severe or rapidly progressive COPD.
- Symptoms disproportionate to the severity of airflow obstruction.
- Need for long-term oxygen therapy.
- Onset of comorbid illnesses (such as bronchiectasis, heart failure, or lung cancer).

When to Admit

- Severe symptoms or acute worsening that fails to respond to outpatient management.
- Acute or worsening hypoxemia, hypercapnia, peripheral edema, or change in mental status.
- Inadequate home care, or inability to sleep or maintain nutrition/hydration due to symptoms.
- The presence of high-risk comorbid conditions.

Leuppi JD et al. Short-term vs conventional glucocorticoid therapy in acute exacerbations of chronic obstructive pulmonary disease: the REDUCE randomized clinical trial. JAMA. 2013 Jun 5;309(21):2223–31. [PMID: 23695200]

Littner MR. In the clinic. Chronic obstructive pulmonary disease. Ann Intern Med. 2011 Apr 5;154(7):ITC4–15. [PMID: 21464346]

Miles MC et al. Optimum bronchodilator combinations in chronic obstructive pulmonary disease: what is the current evidence? Drugs. 2012 Feb 12;72(3):301–8. [PMID: 22316346]

Qaseem A et al. Diagnosis and management of stable chronic obstructive pulmonary disease: a clinical practice guideline update from the American College of Physicians, American College of Chest Physicians, American Thoracic Society, and European Respiratory Society. Ann Intern Med. 2011 Aug 2;155(3):179–91. [PMID: 21810710]

Rabe KF et al; Global Initiative for Chronic Obstructive Lung Disease. Global strategy for the diagnosis, management, and prevention of chronic obstructive pulmonary disease: GOLD executive summary. Am J Respir Crit Care Med. 2007 Sep 15;176(6):532–55. [PMID: 17507545]

Torpy JM et al. JAMA patient page. Chronic obstructive pulmonary disease. JAMA. 2012 Sep 26;308 (12):1281. [PMID: 23011720]

BRONCHIECTASIS

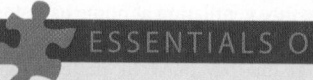

ESSENTIALS OF DIAGNOSIS

- ▶ Chronic productive cough with dyspnea and wheezing.
- ▶ Radiographic findings of dilated, thickened airways and scattered, irregular opacities.

General Considerations

Bronchiectasis is a congenital or acquired disorder of the large bronchi characterized by permanent, abnormal dilation and destruction of bronchial walls. It may be caused by recurrent inflammation or infection of the airways and may be localized or diffuse. Cystic fibrosis causes about half of all cases of bronchiectasis. Other causes include lung infection (tuberculosis, fungal infections, lung abscess, pneumonia), abnormal lung defense mechanisms (humoral immunodeficiency, alpha-1-antiprotease [alpha-1-antitrypsin] deficiency with cigarette smoking, mucociliary clearance disorders, rheumatic diseases), and localized airway obstruction (foreign body, tumor, mucoid impaction). Immunodeficiency states that may lead to bronchiectasis include congenital or acquired panhypogammaglobulinemia; common variable immunodeficiency; selective IgA, IgM, and IgG subclass deficiencies; and acquired immunodeficiency from cytotoxic therapy, AIDS, lymphoma, multiple myeloma, leukemia, and chronic kidney and liver diseases. Most patients with bronchiectasis have panhypergammaglobulinemia, however, presumably reflecting an immune system response to chronic airway infection. Acquired primary bronchiectasis is now uncommon in the United States because of improved control of bronchopulmonary infections.

Clinical Findings

A. Symptoms and Signs

Symptoms of bronchiectasis include chronic cough with production of copious amounts of purulent sputum, hemoptysis, and pleuritic chest pain. Dyspnea and wheezing occur in 75% of patients. Weight loss, anemia, and other systemic manifestations are common. Physical findings are nonspecific, but persistent crackles at the lung bases are common. Clubbing is infrequent in mild cases but is common in severe disease (see Figure 6–41). Copious, foul-smelling, purulent sputum is characteristic. Obstructive pulmonary dysfunction with hypoxemia is seen in moderate or severe disease.

B. Imaging

Radiographic abnormalities include dilated and thickened bronchi that may appear as "tram-tracks" or as ring-like markings. Scattered irregular opacities, atelectasis, and focal consolidation may be present. High-resolution CT is the diagnostic study of choice.

C. Microbiology

Haemophilus influenzae is the most common organism recovered from non–cystic fibrosis patients with bronchiectasis. *P aeruginosa, S pneumoniae,* and *Staphylococcus aureus* are commonly identified. Nontuberculous mycobacteria are seen less commonly. Patients with *Pseudomonas* infection experience an accelerated course, with more frequent exacerbations and more rapid decline in lung function.

▶ Treatment

Treatment of acute exacerbations consists of antibiotics, daily chest physiotherapy with postural drainage and chest percussion, and inhaled bronchodilators. Hand-held flutter valve devices may be as effective as chest physiotherapy in clearing secretions. Antibiotic therapy should be guided by sputum smears and cultures. If a specific bacterial pathogen cannot be isolated, then empiric oral antibiotic therapy for 10–14 days is appropriate. Common regimens include amoxicillin or amoxicillin-clavulanate (500 mg every 8 hours), ampicillin or tetracycline (250–500 mg four times daily), trimethoprim-sulfamethoxazole (160/800 mg every 12 hours), or ciprofloxacin (500–750 mg twice daily). It is important to screen patients for infection with nontuberculous mycobacteria because these organisms may underlie a lack of treatment response. Preventive or suppressive treatment is sometimes given to stable outpatients with bronchiectasis who have copious purulent sputum. Prolonged macrolide therapy (azithromycin 500 mg three times a week for 6 months or 250 mg daily for 12 months) has been found to decrease the frequency of exacerbations compared to placebo. High-dose amoxicillin (3 g/d) or alternating cycles of the antibiotics listed above given orally for 2–4 weeks are also used, although this practice is not supported by clinical trial data. In patients with underlying cystic fibrosis, inhaled aerosolized aminoglycosides reduce colonization by *Pseudomonas* species, improve FEV_1 and reduce hospitalizations; in non–cystic fibrosis bronchiectasis, adding inhaled tobramycin to oral ciprofloxacin for acute exacerbations due to *Pseudomonas* decreases microbial sputum burden but without apparent clinical benefit. Complications of bronchiectasis include hemoptysis, cor

pulmonale, amyloidosis, and secondary visceral abscesses at distant sites (eg, brain). Bronchoscopy is sometimes necessary to evaluate hemoptysis, remove retained secretions, and rule out obstructing airway lesions. Massive hemoptysis may require embolization of bronchial arteries or surgical resection. Surgical resection is otherwise reserved for the few patients with localized bronchiectasis and adequate pulmonary function in whom conservative management fails.

Altenburg J et al. Effect of azithromycin maintenance treatment on infectious exacerbations among patients with non–cystic fibrosis bronchiectasis: the BAT randomized controlled trial. JAMA. 2013 Mar27;309(12):1251–9. [PMID: 23532241]

Feldman C. Bronchiectasis: new approaches to diagnosis and management. Clin Chest Med. 2011 Sep;32(3):535–46. [PMID: 21867821]

Wong C et al. Azithromycin for prevention of exacerbations in non–cystic fibrosis bronchiectasis (EMBRACE): a randomised, double-blind, placebo-controlled trial. Lancet. 2012 Aug18;380(9842):660–7. [PMID: 22901887]

ALLERGIC BRONCHOPULMONARY MYCOSIS

Allergic bronchopulmonary mycosis is a pulmonary hypersensitivity disorder caused by allergy to fungal antigens that colonize the tracheobronchial tree. It usually occurs in atopic asthmatic individuals who are 20–40 years of age, in response to antigens of *Aspergillus* species. For this reason, the disorder is commonly referred to as allergic bronchopulmonary aspergillosis (ABPA). Primary criteria for the diagnosis of ABPA include (1) a clinical history of asthma, (2) peripheral eosinophilia, (3) immediate skin reactivity to *Aspergillus* antigen, (4) precipitating antibodies to *Aspergillus* antigen, (5) elevated serum IgE levels, (6) pulmonary infiltrates (transient or fixed), and (7) central bronchiectasis. If the first six of these seven primary criteria are present, the diagnosis is almost certain. Secondary diagnostic criteria include identification of *Aspergillus* in sputum, a history of brown-flecked sputum, and late skin reactivity to *Aspergillus* antigen. High-dose prednisone (0.5–1 mg/kg orally per day) for at least 2 months is the treatment of choice, and the response in early disease is usually excellent. Depending on the overall clinical situation, prednisone can then be cautiously tapered. Relapses are frequent, and protracted or repeated treatment with corticosteroids is not uncommon. Patients with corticosteroid-dependent disease may benefit from itraconazole (200 mg orally three times a day with food for 3 days followed by twice daily for at least 16 weeks) without added toxicity. Bronchodilators (Table 9–5) are also helpful. Complications include hemoptysis, severe bronchiectasis, and pulmonary fibrosis.

Bains SN et al. Allergic bronchopulmonary aspergillosis. Clin Chest Med. 2012 Jun;33(2):265–81. [PMID: 22640845]

Mahdavinia M et al. Management of allergic bronchopulmonary aspergillosis: a review and update. Ther Adv Respir Dis. 2012 Jun;6(3):173–87. [PMID: 22547692]

CYSTIC FIBROSIS

► Chronic or recurrent productive cough, dyspnea, and wheezing.

► Recurrent airway infections or chronic colonization of the airways with *H influenzae, P aeruginosa, S aureus,* or *Burkholderia cepacia*. Bronchiectasis and scarring on chest radiographs.

► Airflow obstruction on spirometry.

► Pancreatic insufficiency, recurrent pancreatitis, distal intestinal obstruction syndrome, chronic hepatic disease, nutritional deficiencies, or male urogenital abnormalities.

► Sweat chloride concentration > 60 mEq/L on two occasions or gene mutation known to cause cystic fibrosis.

► General Considerations

Cystic fibrosis is the most common cause of severe chronic lung disease in young adults and the most common fatal hereditary disorder of whites in the United States. It is an autosomal recessive disorder affecting about 1 in 3200 whites; 1 in 25 is a carrier. Cystic fibrosis is caused by abnormalities in a membrane chloride channel (the cystic fibrosis transmembrane conductance regulator [CFTR] protein) that results in altered chloride transport and water flux across the apical surface of epithelial cells. Almost all exocrine glands produce an abnormal mucus that obstructs glands and ducts and leads to tissue damage. In the respiratory tract, inadequate hydration of the tracheobronchial epithelium impairs mucociliary function. High concentration of extracellular DNA in airway secretions (due to chronic airway inflammation and autolysis of neutrophils) increases sputum viscosity.

Over one-third of the nearly 30,000 cystic fibrosis patients in the United States are adults. Because of the wide range of alterations seen in the CFTR protein structure and function, cystic fibrosis in adults may present with a variety of pulmonary and nonpulmonary manifestations. Patients with cystic fibrosis have an increased risk of malignancies of the gastrointestinal tract, osteopenia, and arthropathies.

► Clinical Findings

A. Symptoms and Signs

Cystic fibrosis should be suspected in a young adult with a history of chronic lung disease (especially bronchiectasis), pancreatitis, or infertility. Cough, sputum production, decreased exercise tolerance, and recurrent hemoptysis are typical complaints. Patients also often complain of chronic rhinosinusitis symptoms, steatorrhea, diarrhea, and abdominal pain. Patients with cystic fibrosis are often malnourished with low body mass index. Digital clubbing, increased anteroposterior chest diameter, hyperresonance

to percussion, and apical crackles are noted on physical examination. Sinus tenderness, purulent nasal secretions, and nasal polyps may also be seen. Nearly all men with cystic fibrosis have congenital bilateral absence of the vas deferens with azoospermia. Biliary cirrhosis and gallstones may occur.

B. Laboratory Findings

Arterial blood gas studies often reveal hypoxemia and, in advanced disease, a chronic, compensated respiratory acidosis. Pulmonary function studies show a mixed obstructive and restrictive pattern. There is a reduction in FVC, airflow rates, and TLC. Air trapping (high ratio of RV to TLC) and reduction in pulmonary diffusing capacity are common.

C. Imaging

Hyperinflation is seen early in the disease process. Peribronchial cuffing, mucus plugging, bronchiectasis (ring shadows and cysts), increased interstitial markings, small rounded peripheral opacities, and focal atelectasis are common findings. Pneumothorax can also be seen. Thin-section CT scanning often confirms the presence of bronchiectasis.

D. Diagnosis

The quantitative pilocarpine iontophoresis sweat test reveals elevated sodium and chloride levels (> 60 mEq/L) in the sweat of patients with cystic fibrosis. Two tests on different days performed in experienced laboratories are required for accurate diagnosis. A normal sweat chloride test does not exclude the diagnosis in which case genotyping or other alternative diagnostic studies (such as measurement of nasal membrane potential difference, semen analysis, or assessment of pancreatic function) should be pursued, especially if there is a high clinical suspicion of cystic fibrosis. Standard genotyping is a limited diagnostic tool because it screens for only a fraction of the known cystic fibrosis mutations, although complete genetic testing is available.

► Treatment

Early recognition and comprehensive multidisciplinary therapy improve symptom control and the chances of survival. Referral to a regional cystic fibrosis center is strongly recommended. Conventional treatment programs focus on the following areas: clearance and reduction of lower airway secretions, reversal of bronchoconstriction, treatment of respiratory tract infections and airway bacterial burden, pancreatic enzyme replacement, and nutritional and psychosocial support (including genetic and occupational counseling). The Pulmonary Therapies Committee, established by the Cystic Fibrosis Foundation, has issued evidenced-based recommendations regarding long-term use of medications for maintenance of lung function and reduction of exacerbations in patients with cystic fibrosis.

Clearance of lower airway secretions can be promoted by postural drainage, chest percussion or vibration techniques, positive expiratory pressure (PEP) or flutter valve breathing devices, directed cough, and other breathing techniques; these approaches require detailed patient instruction by experienced personnel. Inhaled recombinant human deoxyribonuclease (rhDNase, dornase alpha) cleaves extracellular DNA in sputum, decreasing sputum viscosity; when administered long-term at a daily nebulized dose of 2.5 mg, this therapy leads to improved FEV_1 and reduces the risk of cystic fibrosis–related respiratory exacerbations and the need for intravenous antibiotics. Inhalation of hypertonic saline twice daily has been associated with small improvements in pulmonary function and fewer pulmonary exacerbations. The beneficial effects of hypertonic saline may derive from improved airway mucous clearance.

Short-term antibiotics are used to treat active airway infections based on results of culture and susceptibility testing of sputum. *S aureus* (including methicillin-resistant strains) and a mucoid variant of *P aeruginosa* are commonly present. *H influenzae*, *Stenotrophomonas maltophilia*, and *B cepacia* (a highly drug-resistant organism) are occasionally isolated. **Long-term antibiotic therapy** is helpful in slowing disease progression and reducing exacerbations in patients with sputum cultures positive for *P aeruginosa*. These antibiotics include azithromycin 500 mg orally three times a week, which has immunomodulatory properties, and various inhaled antibiotics (eg, tobramycin, aztreonam, colistin, and levofloxacin) taken two to three times a day. The length of therapy depends on the persistent presence of *P aeruginosa* in the sputum. The incidence of atypical mycobacterial colonization is higher in cystic fibrosis patients and directed antibiotic treatment is recommended for frequent exacerbations, progressive decline in lung function, or failure to thrive. Yearly screening with sputum acid-fast bacilli cultures is advised.

Inhaled bronchodilators (eg, albuterol, two puffs every 4 hours as needed) should be considered in patients who demonstrate an increase of at least 12% in FEV_1 after an inhaled bronchodilator. An inhaled corticosteroid should be added to the treatment regimen for patients who have cystic fibrosis with persistent asthma or allergic bronchopulmonary mycosis.

Ivacaftor is an oral drug, available for the 5% of cystic fibrosis patients with a G551D mutation. Ivacaftor is a potentiator of the CFTR channel that works by increasing the time the channel remains open after being activated; it has been found to improve lung function by 10% within 2 weeks of treatment, decrease pulmonary exacerbations by 55%, and decrease sweat chloride into the indeterminate range. CFTR corrector therapy for the most common mutation (DeltaF508) is currently under trial.

Lung transplantation is currently the only definitive treatment for advanced cystic fibrosis. Double-lung or heart-lung transplantation is required. A few transplant centers offer living lobar lung transplantation to selected patients. The 3-year survival rate following transplantation for cystic fibrosis is about 55%.

Vaccination against pneumococcal infection and annual influenza vaccination are advised. **Screening** of family members and genetic counseling are suggested.

Prognosis

The longevity of patients with cystic fibrosis is increasing, and the median survival age is over 35 years. Death occurs from pulmonary complications (eg, pneumonia, pneumothorax, or hemoptysis) or as a result of terminal chronic respiratory failure and cor pulmonale.

Braun AT et al. Cystic fibrosis lung transplantation. Curr Opin Pulm Med. 2011 Nov;17(6):467–72. [PMID: 21897255]

Cohen-Cymberknoh M et al. Managing cystic fibrosis: strategies that increase life expectancy and improve quality of life. Am J Respir Crit Care Med. 2011 Jun1;183(11):1463–71. [PMID: 21330455]

Flume PA et al; Cystic Fibrosis Foundation Pulmonary Therapies Committee. Cystic fibrosis pulmonary guidelines: treatment of pulmonary exacerbations. Am J Respir Crit Care Med. 2009 Nov1;180(9):802–8. [PMID: 19729669]

Flume PA et al; Cystic Fibrosis Foundation Pulmonary Therapies Committee. Cystic fibrosis pulmonary guidelines: pulmonary complications: hemoptysis and pneumothorax. Am J Respir Crit Care Med. 2010 Aug1;182(3):298–306. [PMID: 20675678]

BRONCHIOLITIS

ESSENTIALS OF DIAGNOSIS

▶ Insidious onset of cough and dyspnea.

▶ Irreversible airflow obstruction on pulmonary function testing.

▶ Minimal findings on chest radiograph.

▶ Relevant exposure or risk factor: toxic fumes, viral infections, organ transplantation, connective tissue disease.

General Considerations

Bronchiolitis is a generic term applied to varied inflammatory processes that affect the bronchioles, which are small conducting airways < 2 mm in diameter. In infants and children, bronchiolitis is common and usually caused by respiratory syncytial virus or adenovirus infection. In adults, bronchiolitis is less common but is encountered in multiple clinical settings. Disorders associated with bronchiolitis include organ transplantation, connective tissue diseases, and hypersensitivity pneumonitis. Inhalational injuries as well as postinfectious and drug-induced causes are identified by association with a known exposure or illness prior to the onset of symptoms. Idiopathic cases are characterized by the insidious onset of dyspnea or cough and include cryptogenic organizing pneumonitis (COP).

The clinical approach to bronchiolitis divides patients into groups based on etiology, but different clinical syndromes may have identical histopathological findings. As a result, no single classification scheme has been widely accepted, and there is an overlapping array of terms to describe these disorders from the viewpoints of the clinician, the pathologist, and the radiologist.

Clinical Findings

Acute bronchiolitis is most commonly seen following viral infection in children.

Constrictive bronchiolitis (also referred to as obliterative bronchiolitis, or bronchiolitis obliterans) is relatively infrequent although it is the most common finding following inhalation injury. It may also be seen in rheumatoid arthritis; drug reactions; and chronic rejection following heart-lung, lung, or bone marrow transplant. Patients with constrictive bronchiolitis have airflow obstruction on spirometry; minimal radiographic abnormalities; and a progressive, deteriorating clinical course.

Proliferative bronchiolitis is associated with diverse pulmonary disorders including infection, aspiration, ARDS, hypersensitivity pneumonitis, connective tissue diseases, and organ transplantation. Compared with constrictive bronchiolitis, proliferative bronchiolitis is more likely to have an abnormal chest radiograph.

Cryptogenic organizing pneumonitis (COP) formally referred to as **bronchiolitis obliterans with organizing pneumonia** (BOOP) (see Table 9–17) affects men and women between the ages of 50 and 70 years, typically with a dry cough, dyspnea, and constitutional symptoms that may be present for weeks to months prior to seeking medical attention. A history of a preceding viral illness is present in half of cases. Pulmonary function testing typically reveals a restrictive ventilatory defect and impaired oxygenation. The chest radiograph frequently shows bilateral patchy, ground-glass or alveolar infiltrates, although other patterns have been described (see Table 9–17).

Follicular bronchiolitis is most commonly associated with connective tissue disease, especially rheumatoid arthritis, and with immunodeficiency states.

Respiratory bronchiolitis usually occurs without symptoms or physiologic evidence of lung impairment.

Diffuse panbronchiolitis is most frequently diagnosed in Japan. Men are affected about twice as often as women, two-thirds are nonsmokers, and most patients have a history of chronic pansinusitis. Patients complain of dyspnea, cough, and sputum production, and chest examination shows crackles and rhonchi. Pulmonary function tests reveal obstructive abnormalities, and the chest radiograph shows a distinct pattern of diffuse, small, nodular shadows with hyperinflation.

Treatment

Constrictive bronchiolitis is relatively unresponsive to corticosteroids and is frequently progressive. Corticosteroids are effective in two-thirds of patients with **proliferative bronchiolitis,** and improvement can be prompt. Therapy is initiated with prednisone at 1 mg/kg/d orally for 1–3 months. The dose is then tapered slowly to 20–40 mg/d, depending on the response, and weaned over the subsequent 3–6 months as tolerated. Relapses are common if corticosteroids are stopped prematurely or tapered too quickly. Most patients with COP recover following corticosteroid treatment.

Drakopanagiotakis F et al. Cryptogenic and secondary organizing pneumonia: clinical presentation, radiographic findings, treatment response, and prognosis. Chest. 2011 Apr;139(4):893–900. [PMID: 20724743]

Nakaseko C et al. Incidence, risk factors and outcomes of bronchiolitis obliterans after allogeneic stem cell transplantation. Int J Hematol. 2011 Mar;93(3):375–82. [PMID: 21424350]

PULMONARY INFECTIONS

PNEUMONIA

This section sets forth the evaluation and management of pulmonary infiltrates in immunocompetent persons separately from the approach to immunocompromised persons—defined as those with HIV disease, absolute neutrophil counts < 1000/mcL (1.0×10^9/L), current or recent exposure to myelosuppressive or immunosuppressive drugs, or those currently taking prednisone in a dosage > 5 mg/d.

1. Community-Acquired Pneumonia

 ESSENTIALS OF DIAGNOSIS

▶ Fever or hypothermia, tachypnea, cough with or without sputum, dyspnea, chest discomfort, sweats or rigors (or both).

▶ Bronchial breath sounds or inspiratory crackles on chest auscultation.

▶ Parenchymal opacity on chest radiograph.

▶ Occurs outside of the hospital or within 48 hours of hospital admission in a patient not residing in a long-term care facility.

General Considerations

Community-acquired pneumonia (CAP) is a common disorder, with approximately 4–5 million cases diagnosed each year in the United States, 25% of which require hospitalization. It is the most deadly infectious disease in the United States and the eighth leading cause of death. Mortality in milder cases treated as outpatients is < 1%. Among patients hospitalized for CAP, in-hospital mortality is approximately 10–12% and 1-year mortality (in those over age 65) is > 40%. Risk factors for the development of CAP include advanced age; alcoholism; tobacco use; comorbid medical conditions, especially asthma or COPD; and immunosuppression.

The patient's history, physical examination, and imaging studies are essential to establishing a diagnosis of CAP. None of these efforts identifies a specific microbiologic cause, however. Sputum examination may be helpful in selected patients but 40% of patients cannot produce an evaluable sputum sample and Gram stain and culture lack sensitivity for the most common causes of pneumonia. Since patient outcomes improve when the

Table 9–8. Recommended empiric antibiotics for community-acquired pneumonia.

Outpatient management

1. For previously healthy patients who have not taken antibiotics within the past 3 months:
   a. A macrolide (clarithromycin, 500 mg orally twice a day; or azithromycin, 500 mg orally as a first dose and then 250 mg orally daily for 4 days, or 500 mg orally daily for 3 days), or
   b. Doxycycline, 100 mg orally twice a day.
2. For patients with such comorbid medical conditions as chronic heart, lung, liver, or renal disease; diabetes mellitus; alcoholism; malignancy; asplenia; immunosuppressant conditions or use of immunosuppressive drugs; or use of antibiotics within the previous 3 months (in which case, an alternative from a different antibiotic class should be selected):
   a. A respiratory fluoroquinolone (moxifloxacin, 400 mg orally daily; gemifloxacin, 320 mg orally daily; levofloxacin, 750 mg orally daily) or
   b. A macrolide (as above) plus a beta-lactam (amoxicillin, 1 g orally three times a day; amoxicillin-clavulanate, 2 g orally twice a day are preferred to cefpodoxime, 200 mg orally twice a day; cefuroxime, 500 mg orally twice a day).
3. In regions with a high rate (> 25%) of infection with high level (MIC ≥ 16 mcg/mL) macrolide-resistant *Streptococcus pneumoniae*, consider use of alternative agents listed above in (2) for patients with comorbidities.

Inpatient management not requiring intensive care

1. A respiratory fluoroquinolone
   a. See above for oral therapy.
   b. For intravenous therapy, moxifloxacin, 400 mg daily; levofloxacin, 750 mg daily; ciprofloxacin, 400 mg every 8–12 hours or
2. A macrolide *plus* a beta-lactam
   a. See above for oral therapy.
   b. For intravenous therapy, ampicillin, 1–2 g every 4–6 hours; cefotaxime, 1–2 g every 4–12 hours; ceftriaxone, 1–2 g every 12–24 hours.

Inpatient intravenous management requiring intensive care

1. Azithromycin (500 mg orally as a first dose and then 250 mg orally daily for 4 days, or 500 mg orally daily for 3 days) or a respiratory fluoroquinolone plus an antipneumococcal beta-lactam (cefotaxime, ceftriaxone, or ampicillin-sulbactam, 1.5–3 g every 6 hours).
2. For patients allergic to beta-lactam antibiotics, a fluoroquinolone *plus* aztreonam (1–2 g every 6–12 hours).
3. For patients at risk for *Pseudomonas* infection
   a. An antipneumococcal, antipseudomonal beta-lactam (piperacillin-tazobactam, 3.375–4.5 g every 6 hours; cefepime, 1–2 g twice a day; imipenem, 0.5–1 g every 6–8 hours; meropenem, 1 g every 8 hours) *plus* ciprofloxacin (400 mg every 8–12 hours) or levofloxacin, *or*
   b. The above beta-lactam *plus* an aminoglycoside (gentamicin, tobramycin, amikacin, all weight-based dosing administered daily adjusted to appropriate trough levels) *plus* azithromycin or a respiratory fluoroquinolone.
4. For patients at risk for methicillin-resistant *Staphylococcus* aureus infection, add vancomycin (interval dosing based on renal function to achieve serum trough concentration 15–20 mcg/mL) *or* linezolid (600 mg twice a day).

MIC, minimum inhibitory concentration.
Recommendations assembled from Mandell LA et al. Infectious Diseases Society of America/American Thoracic Society consensus guidelines on the management of community-acquired pneumonia in adults. Clin Infect Dis. 2007;44:S27–72. [PMID: 17278083]

initial antibiotic choice is appropriate for the infecting organism, the American Thoracic Society and Infectious Disease Society of America recommend empiric treatment based on epidemiologic data (see Table 9–8). Such treatment improves initial antibiotic coverage, reduces unnecessary hospitalization, and appears to improve 30-day survival.

Decisions regarding hospitalization and ICU care should be based on prognostic criteria (see below).

▶ **Definition & Pathogenesis**

CAP is diagnosed outside of the hospital in ambulatory patients who are not residents of nursing homes or other long-term care facilities. It may also be diagnosed in a previously ambulatory patient within 48 hours after admission to the hospital.

Pulmonary defense mechanisms (cough reflex, mucociliary clearance system, immune responses) normally prevent the development of lower respiratory tract infections following aspiration of oropharyngeal secretions containing bacteria or inhalation of infected aerosols. CAP

occurs when there is a defect in one or more of these normal defense mechanisms or when a large infectious inoculum or a virulent pathogen overwhelms the immune response.

Prospective studies fail to identify the cause of CAP in 40–60% of cases; two or more causes are identified in up to 5% of cases. Bacteria are more commonly identified than viruses. The most common bacterial pathogen identified in most studies of CAP is *S pneumoniae*, accounting for approximately two-thirds of bacterial isolates. Other common bacterial pathogens include *H influenzae*, *M pneumoniae*, *C pneumoniae*, *S aureus*, *Neisseria meningitidis*, *M catarrhalis*, *Klebsiella pneumoniae*, other gram-negative rods, and *Legionella* species. Common viral causes of CAP include influenza virus, respiratory syncytial virus, adenovirus, and parainfluenza virus. A detailed assessment of epidemiologic risk factors may aid in diagnosing pneumonias due to the following uncommon causes: *Chlamydophila psittaci* (psittacosis), *Coxiella burnetii* (Q fever), *Francisella tularensis* (tularemia), endemic fungi (*Blastomyces*, *Coccidioides*, *Histoplasma*), and sin nombre virus (hantavirus pulmonary syndrome).

▶ Clinical Findings

A. Symptoms and Signs

Most patients with CAP experience an acute or subacute onset of fever, cough with or without sputum production, and dyspnea. Other common symptoms include sweats, chills, rigors, chest discomfort, pleurisy, hemoptysis, fatigue, myalgias, anorexia, headache, and abdominal pain.

Common physical findings include fever or hypothermia, tachypnea, tachycardia, and arterial oxygen desaturation. Many patients appear acutely ill. Chest examination often reveals inspiratory crackles and bronchial breath sounds. Dullness to percussion may be observed if lobar consolidation or a parapneumonic pleural effusion is present. **The clinical evaluation is < 50% sensitive compared to chest imaging for the diagnosis of CAP** (see Imaging section below). In most patients, therefore, a chest radiograph is essential to the evaluation of suspected CAP.

B. Diagnostic Testing

Diagnostic testing for a specific infectious cause of CAP is not generally indicated in ambulatory patients treated as outpatients because empiric antibiotic therapy is almost always effective in this population. In ambulatory outpatients whose presentation (travel history, exposure) suggests an etiology not covered by standard therapy (eg, *Coccidioides*) or public health concerns (eg, *Mycobacterium tuberculosis*, influenza), diagnostic testing is appropriate. Diagnostic testing is recommended in hospitalized CAP patients for multiple reasons: the likelihood of an infectious cause unresponsive to standard therapy is higher in more severe illness, the inpatient setting allows narrowing of antibiotic coverage as specific diagnostic information is available, and the yield of testing is improved in more acutely ill patients.

Diagnostic testing results are used to guide initial antibiotic therapy, permit adjustment of empirically chosen therapy to a specific infectious cause or resistance pattern, and facilitate epidemiologic analysis. There are three widely available, rapid point-of-care diagnostic tests that may guide initial therapy: the sputum Gram stain, urinary antigen tests for *S pneumonia* and *Legionella* species, and rapid antigen detection tests for influenza. Sputum Gram stain is neither sensitive nor specific for *S pneumonia*, the most common cause of CAP. The usefulness of a sputum Gram stain lies in broadening initial coverage in patients to be hospitalized for CAP, most commonly to cover *S aureus* (including community-acquired methicillin-resistant strains, CA-MRSA) or gram-negative rods. Urinary antigen assays for *Legionella pneumophilia* and *S pneumoniae* are at least as sensitive and specific as sputum Gram stain and culture. Results are available immediately and are not affected by early initiation of antibiotic therapy. Positive tests may allow narrowing of initial antibiotic coverage. Urinary antigen assay for *S pneumoniae* should be ordered for patients with leukopenia, asplenia, active alcohol use, chronic severe liver disease, pleural effusion, and those requiring ICU admission. Urinary antigen assay for *L pneumophilia* should be ordered for patients with active alcohol use, travel within 2 weeks, pleural effusion and those requiring ICU admission. Rapid influenza testing has intermediate sensitivity but high specificity. Positive tests may reduce unnecessary antibacterial use and direct isolation of hospitalized patients.

Additional microbiologic testing including pre-antibiotic sputum and blood cultures (at least two sets with needle sticks at separate sites) has been standard practice for patients with CAP who require hospitalization. The yield of blood and sputum cultures is low. However, false-positive results are common, and the impact of culture results on patient outcomes is small. As a result, targeted testing based on specific indications is recommended. Culture results are not available prior to initiation of antibiotic therapy. Their role is to allow narrowing of initial empiric antibiotic coverage, adjustment of coverage based on specific antibiotic resistance patterns, to identify unsuspected pathogens not covered by initial therapy, and to provide information for epidemiologic analysis.

Apart from microbiologic testing, hospitalized patients should undergo complete blood count with differential and a chemistry panel (including serum glucose, electrolytes, urea nitrogen, creatinine, bilirubin, and liver enzymes). Hypoxemic patients should have arterial blood gases sampled. Test results help assess severity of illness and guide evaluation and management. HIV testing should be considered in all adult patients, and performed in those with risk factors.

C. Imaging

A pulmonary opacity on chest radiography or CT scan is required to establish a diagnosis of CAP. Radiographic findings range from patchy airspace opacities to lobar consolidation with air bronchograms to diffuse alveolar or interstitial opacities. Additional findings can include pleural effusions and cavitation. Chest imaging cannot identify a specific microbiologic cause of CAP, however. There is no pattern of radiographic abnormalities pathognomonic of any infectious cause.

Chest imaging may help assess severity and response to therapy over time. Progression of pulmonary opacities during antibiotic therapy or lack of radiographic improvement over time are poor prognostic signs and also raise concerns about secondary or alternative pulmonary processes. **Clearing of pulmonary opacities in patients with CAP can take 6 weeks or longer.** Clearance is usually quickest in younger patients, nonsmokers, and those with only single lobe involvement.

D. Special Examinations

Patients with CAP who have significant pleural fluid collections may require diagnostic thoracentesis (glucose, lactate dehydrogenase [LD], and total protein levels; leukocyte count with differential; pH determination) with pleural fluid Gram stain and culture. Positive pleural cultures indicate the need for tube thoracostomy drainage.

Patients with cavitary opacities should have sputum fungal and mycobacterial cultures.

Sputum induction and fiberoptic bronchoscopy to obtain samples of lower respiratory secretions are indicated in patients who cannot provide expectorated sputum samples or who may have *Pneumocystis jirovecii* or *M tuberculosis* pneumonia.

Serologic assays, polymerase chain reaction tests, specialized culture tests, and other diagnostic tests for organisms such as viruses, *Legionella*, *M pneumoniae*, and *C pneumoniae* may be performed when these diagnoses are suspected.

▶ Differential Diagnosis

The differential diagnosis of lower respiratory tract infection is extensive and includes upper respiratory tract infections, reactive airway diseases, heart failure, cryptogenic organizing pneumonitis, lung cancer, pulmonary vasculitis, pulmonary thromboembolic disease, and atelectasis.

▶ Treatment

Two general principles guide antibiotic therapy once the diagnosis of CAP is established: **prompt** initiation of a drug to which the etiologic pathogen is **susceptible.**

In patients who require specific diagnostic evaluation, sputum and culture specimens should be obtained prior to initiation of antibiotics. Since early administration of antibiotics to acutely ill patients is associated with improved outcomes, obtaining diagnostic specimens or test results should not delay the initial dose of antibiotics by more than 6 hours from presentation.

Optimal antibiotic therapy would be pathogen directed, but a definitive microbiologic diagnosis is rarely available on or within 6 hours of presentation. A syndromic approach to therapy, based on clinical presentation and chest imaging, does not reliably predict the microbiology of CAP. Therefore, initial antibiotic choices are typically empiric, based on acuity (treatment as an outpatient, inpatient, or in the ICU), patient risk factors for specific pathogens, and local antibiotic resistance patterns (Table 9–8).

Since *S pneumoniae* remains a common cause of CAP in all patient groups, local prevalence of drug-resistant *S pneumoniae* significantly affects initial antibiotic choice. Prior treatment with one antibiotic in a pharmacologic class (eg, beta-lactam, macrolide, fluoroquinolone) predisposes the emergence of drug-resistant *S pneumoniae,* with resistance developing against that class of antibiotics to which the pathogen was previously exposed. Definitions of resistance have shifted based on observations of continued clinical efficacy at achievable serum levels. In CAP, for parenteral penicillin G or oral amoxicillin, susceptible strains have a minimum inhibitory concentration (MIC) ≤ 2 mcg/mL; intermediate resistance is defined as an MIC between 2 mcg/mL and 4 mcg/mL because treatment failures are uncommon with MIC ≤ 4 mcg/mL. Macrolide resistance has increased; approximately one-third of *S pneumoniae* isolates now show in vitro resistance to macrolides. Treatment failures have been reported but remain rare compared to the number of patients treated; current in vivo efficacy appears to justify maintaining

macrolides as first-line therapy except in areas where there is a high prevalence of resistant strains. *S pneumoniae* resistant to fluoroquinolones is rare in the United States (1% to levofloxacin, 2% to ciprofloxacin) but is increasing.

Community-acquired methicillin-resistant *S aureus* (CA-MRSA) is genetically and phenotypically different from hospital-acquired MRSA strains. CA-MRSA is a rare cause of necrotizing pneumonia, empyema, respiratory failure, and shock; it appears to be associated with prior influenza infection. Linezolid may be preferred to vancomycin in treatment of CA-MRSA pulmonary infection. For expanded discussions of specific antibiotics, see Chapter 30.

A. Treatment of Outpatients

See Table 9–8 for specific drug dosages. The most common etiologies of CAP in outpatients who do not require hospitalization are *S pneumoniae*; *M pneumoniae*; *C pneumoniae*; and respiratory viruses, including influenza. For previously healthy patients with no recent (90 days) use of antibiotics, the recommended treatment is a macrolide (clarithromycin or azithromycin) or doxycycline.

In patients at risk for drug resistance (antibiotic therapy within the past 90 days, age > 65 years, comorbid illness, immunosuppression, exposure to a child in daycare), the recommended treatment is a respiratory fluoroquinolone (moxifloxacin, gemifloxacin, or levofloxacin) or a macrolide plus a beta-lactam (high-dose amoxicillin and amoxicillin-clavulanate are preferred to cefpodoxime and cefuroxime).

In regions where there is a high incidence of macrolide-resistant *S pneumoniae*, initial therapy in patients with no comorbidities may include a respiratory fluoroquinolone or the combination of a beta-lactam added to a macrolide.

There are limited data to guide recommendations for duration of treatment. The decision should be influenced by the severity of illness, etiologic pathogen, response to therapy, other medical problems, and complications. Most experts recommend administering a minimum of 5 days of therapy and continuing antibiotics until the patient is afebrile for 48–72 hours. There appears to be no advantage to routinely extending antibiotic therapy beyond 3 days following clinical improvement with defervescence.

B. Treatment of Hospitalized and ICU Patients

The most common etiologies of CAP in patients who require hospitalization but not intensive care are *S pneumoniae, M pneumoniae, C pneumoniae, H influenza, Legionella* species, and respiratory viruses. Some patients have aspiration as an immediate precipitant to the CAP without a specific bacterial etiology. First-line therapy in hospitalized patients is a respiratory fluoroquinolone (eg, moxifloxacin, gemifloxacin, or levofloxacin) or the combination of a macrolide (clarithromycin or azithromycin) plus a beta-lactam (cefotaxime, ceftriaxone, or ampicillin) (see Table 9–8).

Almost all patients admitted to a hospital for treatment of CAP receive intravenous antibiotics. However, no studies in hospitalized patients demonstrated superior outcomes with intravenous antibiotics compared with oral antibiotics, as long as patients were able to tolerate the oral therapy and the drug was well absorbed. Duration of inpatient antibiotic treatment is the same as for outpatients.

The most common etiologies of CAP in patients who require admission to intensive care are *S pneumoniae*, Legionella species, *H influenza, Enterobacteriaceae* species, *S aureus,* and *Pseudomonas species.* First-line therapy in ICU patients with CAP is either azithromycin or a respiratory fluoroquinolone (moxifloxacin, gemifloxacin, or levofloxacin) combined with an antipneumococcal beta-lactam (cefotaxime, ceftriaxone, or ampicillin-sulbactam). In patients at risk for *Pseudomonas* infection, one of two following regimens can be used: an antipneumococcal, antipseudomonal beta-lactam (piperacillin-tazobactam, cefepime, imipenem, meropenem) plus ciprofloxacin or levofloxacin **or** the above antipneumococcal beta-lactam plus an aminoglycoside (gentamicin, tobramycin, amikacin) plus either azithromycin or a respiratory fluoroquinolone (moxifloxacin, gemifloxacin, or levofloxacin).

▶ **Prevention**

Polyvalent pneumococcal vaccine (containing capsular polysaccharide antigens of 23 common strains of *S pneumoniae*) has the potential to prevent or lessen the severity of the majority of pneumococcal infections in immunocompetent patients. Indications for pneumococcal vaccination include age ≥ 65 years or any chronic illness that increases the risk of CAP (see Chapter 30). Immunocompromised patients and those at highest risk for fatal pneumococcal infections should receive a single revaccination 6 years after the first vaccination. Immunocompetent persons 65 years of age or older should receive a second dose of vaccine if the patient first received the vaccine 6 or more years previously and was under 65 years old at the time of vaccination.

The seasonal influenza vaccine is effective in preventing severe disease due to influenza virus with a resulting positive impact on both primary influenza pneumonia and secondary bacterial pneumonias. The seasonal influenza vaccine is administered annually to persons at risk for complications of influenza infection (age ≥ 65 years, residents of long-term care facilities, patients with pulmonary or cardiovascular disorders, patients recently hospitalized with chronic metabolic disorders) as well as health care workers and others who are able to transmit influenza to high-risk patients.

Hospitalized patients who would benefit from pneumococcal and influenza vaccines should be vaccinated during hospitalization. The vaccines can be given simultaneously, and may be administered as soon as the patient has stabilized.

▶ **When to Admit**

Once a diagnosis of CAP is made, the first management decision is to determine the site of care: Is it safe to treat the patient at home or does he or she require hospital or intensive care admission? There are two widely used clinical

prediction rules available to guide admission and triage decisions, the Pneumonia Severity Index (PSI) and the CURB-65.

A. Hospital Admission Decision

The PSI is a validated prediction model that uses 20 items from demographics, medical history, physical examination, laboratory and imaging to stratify patients into five risk groups. The PSI is weighted toward discrimination at low predicted mortality. In conjunction with clinical judgment, it facilitates safe decisions to treat CAP in the outpatient setting. An on-line PSI risk calculator is available at http://pda. ahrq.gov/clinic/psi/psicalc.asp. The CURB-65 assesses five simple, independent predictors of increased mortality (**c**onfusion, **u**remia, **r**espiratory rate, **b**lood pressure, and age > 65) to calculate a 30-day predicted mortality (http://www. mdcalc.com/curb-65-severity-score-community-acquired-pneumonia/). Compared with the PSI, the simpler CURB-65 is less discriminating at low mortality but excellent at identifying patients with high mortality who may benefit from ICU level care. A modified version (CRB-65) dispenses with serum blood urea nitrogen and eliminates the need for laboratory testing. Both have the advantage of simplicity: Patients with zero CRB-65 predictors have a low predicted mortality (< 1%) and usually do not need hospitalization; hospitalization should be considered for those with one or two predictors, since they have an increased risk of death; and urgent hospitalization (with consideration of ICU admission) is required for those with three or four predictors.

B. Intensive Care Unit Admission Decision

Expert opinion has defined major and minor criteria to identify patients at high risk for death. Major criteria are septic shock with need for vasopressor support and respiratory failure with need for mechanical ventilation. Minor criteria are respiratory rate ≥ 30 breaths per minute, hypoxemia (defined as $Pao_2/Fio_2 \leq 250$), hypothermia (core temperature < 36.0°C), hypotension requiring aggressive fluid resuscitation, confusion/disorientation, multilobar pulmonary opacities, leukopenia due to infection with WBC < 4000/mcL (< 4.0 × 10⁹/L), thrombocytopenia with platelet count < 100,000/mcL (< 100 × 10⁹/L), uremia with blood urea nitrogen ≥ 20 mg/dL (> 7.1 mmol/L), metabolic acidosis, or elevated lactate level. Either one major criterion or three or more minor criteria of illness severity generally require ICU level care.

In addition to pneumonia-specific issues, good clinical practice always makes an admission decision in light of the whole patient. Additional factors suggesting need for inpatient hospitalization include the following:

- Exacerbations of underlying disease (eg, heart failure) that would benefit from hospitalization.

- Other medical or psychosocial needs (such as cognitive dysfunction, psychiatric disease, homelessness, drug abuse, lack of outpatient resources, or poor overall functional status).

- Failure of outpatient therapy, including inability to maintain oral intake and medications.

Mandell LA et al. Infectious Diseases Society of America/ American Thoracic Society consensus guidelines on the management of community-acquired pneumonia in adults. Clin Infect Dis. 2007 Mar1;44(Suppl 2):S27–72. [PMID: 17278083]

Richards G et al. CURB-65, PSI, and APACHE II to assess mortality risk in patients with severe sepsis and community acquired pneumonia in PROWESS. J Intensive Care Med. 2011 Jan–Feb;26(1):34–40. [PMID: 21341394]

Waterer GW et al. Management of community-acquired pneumonia in adults. Am J Respir Crit Care Med. 2011 Jan15;183(2):157–64. [PMID: 20693379]

Watkins RR et al. Diagnosis and management of community-acquired pneumonia in adults. Am Fam Physician. 2011 Jun1;83(11):1299–306. [PMID: 21661712]

2. Nosocomial Pneumonia (Hospital-Acquired, Ventilator-Associated, and Health Care–Associated)

ESSENTIALS OF DIAGNOSIS

▶ **Hospital-acquired pneumonia (HAP)** occurs > 48 hours after admission to the hospital or other health care facility and excludes any infection present at the time of admission.

▶ **Health care–associated pneumonia (HCAP)** occurs in community members whose extensive contact with healthcare has changed their risk for virulent and drug resistant organisms.

▶ **Ventilator-associated pneumonia (VAP)** develops following endotracheal intubation and mechanical ventilation.

▶ At least two of the following: fever, leukocytosis, purulent sputum.

▶ New or progressive parenchymal opacity on chest radiograph.

▶ Especially common in patients requiring intensive care or mechanical ventilation.

General Considerations

Hospitalized patients carry different flora with different resistance patterns than healthy patients in the community, and their health status may place them at higher risk for more severe infection. The diagnostic approach and antibiotic treatment of patients with hospital-acquired pneumonia (HAP) is, therefore, different from patients with CAP. Similarly, management of patients in whom pneumonia develops following endotracheal intubation and mechanical ventilation (ventilator-associated pneumonia or VAP) should address issues specific to this group of patients. Some community members have extensive contact with the healthcare system and carry flora that more closely resemble hospitalized patients than healthy community residents. When pneumonia develops in these persons, the infection is referred to as health care–associated pneumonia (HCAP). Initial management and antibiotic therapy should be targeted to the common flora and specific risk factors for severe disease.

Considered together, these nosocomial pneumonias (HAP/VAP/HCAP) represent an important cause of morbidity and mortality despite widespread use of preventive measures, advances in diagnostic testing, and potent new antimicrobial agents. HAP is the second most common cause of infection among hospital inpatients and is the leading cause of death due to infection with mortality rates ranging from 20% to 50%. While a minority of cases occurs in ICU patients, the highest-risk patients are those in ICUs or who are being mechanically ventilated; these patients also experience higher morbidity and mortality from HAP. As management of more chronic illnesses shifts to the outpatient setting, more cases of HCAP are caused by unusual organisms, and there is a high frequency of drug resistance. Definitive identification of the infectious cause of a lower respiratory infection is rarely available on presentation, thus, rather than pathogen-directed antibiotic treatment, the choice of empiric therapy is informed by epidemiologic and patient data.

▶ Definition & Pathogenesis

HAP develops more than 48 hours after admission to the hospital and VAP develops in a mechanically ventilated patient more than 48 hours after endotracheal intubation. HCAP is defined as pneumonia that occurs in a nonhospitalized patient with extensive healthcare contact (see Table 9–9).

Three factors distinguish nosocomial pneumonia from CAP: (1) different infectious causes; (2) different antibiotic susceptibility patterns, specifically, a higher incidence of drug resistance; and (3) poorer underlying health status of patients putting them at risk for more severe infections. Since access to the lower respiratory tract occurs primarily through microaspiration, nosocomial pneumonia starts with a change in upper respiratory tract flora. Colonization of the pharynx and possibly the stomach with bacteria is the most important step in the pathogenesis of nosocomial

Table 9–9. Risk factors for health care–associated pneumonia.

- Antibiotic therapy in the preceding 90 days.
- Acute care hospitalization for at least 2 days in the preceding 90 days.
- Residence in a nursing home or extended care facility.
- Home infusion therapy, including chemotherapy, within the past 30 days.
- Long-term dialysis within the past 30 days.
- Home wound care.
- Family member with an infection involving a multiple drug-resistant pathogen.
- Immunosuppressive disease or immunosuppressive therapy.

Adapted with permission of the American Thoracic Society. Copyright © American Thoracic Society. American Thoracic Society, Infectious Diseases Society of America. Guidelines for the management of adults with hospital-acquired, ventilator-associated and healthcare-associated pneumonia. Am J Respir Crit Care Med. 2005; 171(4):388-416. [PMID: 15699079] pneumonia. Pharyngeal colonization is promoted by exogenous factors (eg, instrumentation of the upper airway with nasogastric and endotracheal tubes; contamination by dirty hands, equipment, and contaminated aerosols; and treatment with broad-spectrum antibiotics that promote the emergence of drug-resistant organisms) and patient factors (eg, malnutrition, advanced age, altered consciousness, swallowing disorders, and underlying pulmonary and systemic diseases). Within 48 hours of admission, 75% of seriously ill hospitalized patients have their upper airway colonized with organisms from the hospital environment.

Impaired cellular and mechanical defense mechanisms in the lungs of hospitalized patients raise the risk of infection after aspiration has occurred.

Gastric acid may play a role in protection against nosocomial pneumonias. Observational studies have suggested that elevation of gastric pH due to antacids, H_2-receptor antagonists, proton pump inhibitors (PPIs), or enteral feeding is associated with gastric microbial overgrowth, tracheobronchial colonization, and HAP/VAP. Sucralfate, a cytoprotective agent that does not alter gastric pH, is associated with a trend toward a lower incidence of VAP. The Infectious Disease Society of America and other professional organizations recommend that acid suppressive medications (H_2-receptor antagonists and PPIs) only be given to patients at high risk for stress gastritis.

The microbiology of the nosocomial pneumonias differs from CAP but is substantially the same among HAP, VAP, and HCAP (Table 9–10). The most common organisms responsible for HAP include *S aureus* (both methicillin-sensitive *S aureus* and MRSA), *P aeruginosa*, gram-negative rods including non-extended spectrum beta-lactamase (non-ESBL)–producing and ESBL-producing (*Enterobacter* species, *K pneumoniae*, and *Escherichia coli*) organisms. VAP patients may be infected with *Acinetobacter* species and *Stenotrophomonas maltophilia*. HCAP patients may have common organisms (*S pneumoniae, H influenzae*) that are more likely to be drug-resistant, or flora that resembles HAP. Anaerobic organisms (bacteroides, anaerobic streptococci, fusobacterium) may also cause pneumonia in the hospitalized patient; when isolated, they are commonly part of a polymicrobial flora. Mycobacteria, fungi, chlamydiae, viruses, rickettsiae, and protozoal organisms are uncommon causes of nosocomial pneumonias.

▶ Clinical Findings

A. Symptoms and Signs

The symptoms and signs associated with nosocomial pneumonias are nonspecific; however, two or more clinical findings (fever, leukocytosis, purulent sputum) in the setting of a new or progressive pulmonary opacity on chest radiograph were approximately 70% sensitive and 75% specific for the diagnosis of VAP in one study. Other findings include those listed above for CAP.

The differential diagnosis of new lower respiratory tract symptoms and signs in hospitalized patients includes heart failure, atelectasis, aspiration, ARDS, pulmonary thromboembolism, pulmonary hemorrhage, and drug reactions.

B. Laboratory Findings

Diagnostic evaluation for suspected nosocomial pneumonia includes blood cultures from two different sites. Blood cultures can identify the pathogen in up to 20% of all patients with nosocomial pneumonias; positivity is associated with increased risk of complications and other sites of infection. Blood counts and clinical chemistry tests do not establish a specific diagnosis of HCAP; however, they help define the severity of illness and identify complications. The assessment of oxygenation by an arterial blood gas or pulse oximetry determination helps define the severity of illness and determines the need for assisted ventilation. Thoracentesis for pleural fluid analysis should be considered in patients with pleural effusions.

Examination of sputum is attended by the same disadvantages as in CAP. Gram stains and cultures of sputum are neither sensitive nor specific in the diagnosis of nosocomial pneumonias. The identification of a bacterial organism by culture of sputum does not prove that the organism is a lower respiratory tract pathogen. However, it can be used to help identify bacterial antibiotic sensitivity patterns and as a guide to adjusting empiric therapy.

C. Imaging

Radiographic findings in HAP/VAP are nonspecific and often confounded by other processes that led initially to hospitalization or ICU admission. (See CAP above.)

D. Special Examinations

Endotracheal aspiration using a sterile suction catheter and fiberoptic bronchoscopy with bronchoalveolar lavage or a protected specimen brush can be used to obtain lower respiratory tract secretions for analysis, most commonly in patients with VAP. Endotracheal aspiration cultures have significant negative predictive value but limited positive predictive value in the diagnosis of specific infectious causes of HAP/VAP. An invasive diagnostic approach using quantitative culture of bronchoalveolar lavage samples or protected specimen brush samples in patients in whom VAP is suspected leads to significantly less antibiotic use, earlier attenuation of organ dysfunction, and fewer deaths at 14 days.

Table 9–10. Organisms prevalent in nosocomial pneumonias.[1]

- *Streptococcus pneumonia,* often drug-resistant, in HCAP
- *Staphylococcus aureus,* methicillin-sensitive (MSSA)
- *S aureus,* methicillin-resistant (MRSA)
- Gram-negative rods, non-ESBL
- ESBL-producing gram-negative rods including *Klebsiella pneumonia, Escherichia coli* and *Enterobacter* species
- *Pseudomonas aeruginosa*
- Acinetobacter species

ESBL, extended spectrum beta-lactamase.
[1]Nosocomial pneumonias include hospital-associated pneumonia (HAP), ventilator-associated pneumonia (VAP), and health care–associated pneumonia (HCAP).

Table 9–11. Recommended empirical antibiotics for nosocomial pneumonias.[1]

When there is low risk for multiple drug–resistant pathogens, use **one** of the following:
    Ceftriaxone, 1–2 g intravenously every 12–24 hours
    Gemifloxacin, 320 mg orally daily
    Moxifloxacin, 400 mg orally or intravenously daily
    Levofloxacin, 750 mg orally or intravenously daily
    Ciprofloxacin, 400 mg intravenously every 8–12 hours
    Ampicillin-sulbactam, 1.5–3 g intravenously every 6 hours
    Piperacillin-tazobactam 3.375–4.5 g intravenously every 6 hours
    Ertapenem, 1 g intravenously daily

When there is higher risk for multiple drug-resistant pathogens, use **one** agent from **each** of the following categories:
  1. Antipseudomonal coverage
    a. Cefipime, 1–2 g intravenously twice a day *or* ceftazidime, 1–2 g intravenously every 8 hours
    b. Imipenem, 0.5–1 g intravenously every 6–8 hours *or* meropenem, 1 g intravenously every 8 hours
    c. Piperacillin-tazobactam, 3.375–4.5 g intravenously every 6 hours
    d For penicillin-allergic patients, aztreonam, 1–2 g intravenously every 6–12 hours
  2. A second antipseudomonal agent
    a. Levofloxacin, 750 mg intravenously daily or ciprofloxacin, 400 mg intravenously every 8–12 hours
    b. Intravenous gentamicin, tobramycin, amikacin, all weight-based dosing administered daily adjusted to appropriate trough levels
  3. Coverage for MRSA if appropriate with either
    a. Intravenous vancomycin (interval dosing based on renal function to achieve serum trough concentration 15–20 mcg/mL) *or*
    b. Linezolid, 600 mg intravenously twice a day

[1]Nosocomial pneumonias includes hospital-acquired pneumonia (HAP), ventilator-associated pneumonia (VAP), and health care–associated pneumonia (HCAP).
MRSA, methicillin-resistant *Staphylococcus aureus.*
Adapted with permission of the American Thoracic Society. Copyright © American Thoracic Society. American Thoracic Society, Infectious Diseases Society of America. Guidelines for the management of adults with hospital-acquired, ventilator-associated and healthcare-associated pneumonia. Am J Respir Crit Care Med. 2005;171(4):388-416. [PMID:15699079]

▶ Treatment

Treatment of the nosocomial pneumonias, like treatment of CAP, is usually empiric (Table 9–11). Because of the high mortality rate, therapy should be started as soon as pneumonia is suspected. There is no consensus on the best regimens because this patient population is heterogeneous and local flora and resistance patterns must be taken into account.

After results of sputum, blood, and pleural fluid cultures are available, it may be possible to de-escalate initially broad therapy. Duration of antibiotic therapy should be individualized based on the pathogen, severity of illness, response to therapy, and comorbid conditions. Data from one large trial assessing treatment outcomes in VAP suggested that 8 days of antibiotics is as effective as 15 days, except in cases caused by *P aeruginosa.*

For expanded discussions of specific antibiotics, see Chapter 30.

Falcone M et al. Healthcare-associated pneumonia: diagnostic criteria and distinction from community-acquired pneumonia. Int J Infect Dis. 2011 Aug;15(8):e545–50. [PMID: 21616695]

Labelle A et al. Healthcare-associated pneumonia: approach to management. Clin Chest Med. 2011 Sep;32(3):507–15. [PMID: 21867819]

Zilberberg MD et al. Healthcare-associated pneumonia: the state of evidence to date. Curr Opin Pulm Med. 2011 May;17(3):142–7. [PMID: 21252678]

3. Anaerobic Pneumonia & Lung Abscess

ESSENTIALS OF DIAGNOSIS

- ▶ History of or predisposition to aspiration.
- ▶ Indolent symptoms, including fever, weight loss, malaise.
- ▶ Poor dentition.
- ▶ Foul-smelling purulent sputum (in many patients).
- ▶ Infiltrate in dependent lung zone, with single or multiple areas of cavitation or pleural effusion.

▶ General Considerations

Aspiration of small amounts of oropharyngeal secretions occurs during sleep in normal individuals but rarely causes disease. Sequelae of aspiration of larger amounts of material include nocturnal asthma, chemical pneumonitis, mechanical obstruction of airways by particulate matter, bronchiectasis, and pleuropulmonary infection. Individuals predisposed to disease induced by aspiration include those with depressed levels of consciousness due to drug or alcohol use, seizures, general anesthesia, or central nervous system disease; those with impaired deglutition due to esophageal disease or neurologic disorders; and those with tracheal or nasogastric tubes, which disrupt the mechanical defenses of the airways.

Periodontal disease and poor dental hygiene, which increase the number of anaerobic bacteria in aspirated material, are associated with a greater likelihood of anaerobic pleuropulmonary infection. Aspiration of infected oropharyngeal contents initially leads to pneumonia in dependent lung zones, such as the posterior segments of the upper lobes and superior and basilar segments of the lower lobes. Body position at the time of aspiration determines which lung zones are dependent. The onset of symptoms is insidious. By the time the patient seeks medical attention, necrotizing pneumonia, lung abscess, or empyema may be apparent.

In most cases of aspiration and necrotizing pneumonia, lung abscess, and empyema, multiple species of anaerobic bacteria are causing the infection. Most of the remaining cases are caused by infection with both anaerobic and aerobic bacteria. *Prevotella melaninogenica*, *Peptostreptococcus*, *Fusobacterium nucleatum*, and *Bacteroides* species are commonly isolated anaerobic bacteria.

▶ Clinical Findings

A. Symptoms and Signs

Patients with anaerobic pleuropulmonary infection usually present with constitutional symptoms such as fever, weight loss, and malaise. Cough with expectoration of foul-smelling purulent sputum suggests anaerobic infection, though the absence of productive cough does not rule out such an infection. Dentition is often poor. Patients are rarely edentulous; if so, an obstructing bronchial lesion is usually present.

B. Laboratory Findings

Expectorated sputum is inappropriate for culture of anaerobic organisms because of contaminating mouth flora. Representative material for culture can be obtained only by transthoracic aspiration, thoracentesis, or bronchoscopy with a protected brush. Transthoracic aspiration is rarely indicated, because drainage occurs via the bronchus and anaerobic pleuropulmonary infections usually respond well to empiric therapy.

C. Imaging

The different types of anaerobic pleuropulmonary infection are distinguished on the basis of their radiographic appearance. **Lung abscess** appears as a thick-walled solitary cavity surrounded by consolidation. An air-fluid level is usually present. Other causes of cavitary lung disease (tuberculosis, mycosis, cancer, infarction, granulomatosis with polyangiitis [formerly Wegener granulomatosis]) should be excluded. **Necrotizing pneumonia** is distinguished by multiple areas of cavitation within an area of consolidation. **Empyema** is characterized by the presence of purulent pleural fluid and may accompany either of the other two radiographic findings. Ultrasonography is of value in locating fluid and may also reveal pleural loculations.

▶ Treatment

Drugs of choice are clindamycin (600 mg intravenously every 8 hours until improvement, then 300 mg orally every 6 hours) or amoxicillin-clavulanate (875 mg/125 mg orally every 12 hours). Penicillin (amoxicillin, 500 mg every 8 hours, or penicillin G, 1–2 million units intravenously every 4–6 hours) plus metronidazole (500 mg orally or intravenously every 8–12 hours) is another option. Penicillin alone is inadequate treatment for anaerobic pleuropulmonary infections because an increasing number of anaerobic organisms produce beta-lactamases, and up to 20% of patients do not respond to penicillins. Antibiotic therapy for anaerobic pneumonia should be continued until the chest radiograph improves, a process that may take a month or more; patients with lung abscesses should be treated until radiographic resolution of the abscess cavity is demonstrated. Anaerobic pleuropulmonary disease requires adequate drainage with tube thoracostomy for the treatment of empyema. Open pleural drainage is sometimes necessary because of the propensity of these infections to produce loculations in the pleural space.

Bartlett JG. Anaerobic bacterial infection of the lung. Anaerobe. 2012 Apr;18(2):235–9. [PMID: 22209937]

Desai H et al. Pulmonary emergencies: pneumonia, acute respiratory distress syndrome, lung abscess, and empyema. Med Clin North Am. 2012 Nov;96(6):1127–48. [PMID: 23102481]

Kwong JC et al. New aspirations: the debate on aspiration pneumonia treatment guidelines. Med J Aust. 2011 Oct 3;195(7):380–1. [PMID: 21978335]

PULMONARY INFILTRATES IN THE IMMUNOCOMPROMISED HOST

Pulmonary infiltrates in immunocompromised patients (patients with HIV disease, absolute neutrophil counts < 1000/mcL (< 1.0×10^9/L), current or recent exposure to myelosuppressive or immunosuppressive drugs, or those currently taking > 5 mg/d of prednisone) may arise from infectious or noninfectious causes. Infection may be due to bacterial, mycobacterial, fungal, protozoal, helminthic, or viral pathogens. Noninfectious processes such as pulmonary edema, alveolar hemorrhage, drug reactions, pulmonary thromboembolic disease, malignancy, and radiation pneumonitis may mimic infection.

Although almost any pathogen can cause pneumonia in an immunocompromised host, two clinical tools help the clinician narrow the differential diagnosis. The first is knowledge of the underlying immunologic defect. Specific immunologic defects are associated with particular infections. Defects in humoral immunity predispose to bacterial infections; defects in cellular immunity lead to infections with viruses, fungi, mycobacteria, and protozoa. Neutropenia and impaired granulocyte function predispose to infections from *S aureus*, *Aspergillus*, gram-negative bacilli, and *Candida*. Second, the time course of infection also provides clues to the etiology of pneumonia in immunocompromised patients. A fulminant pneumonia is often caused by bacterial infection, whereas an insidious pneumonia is more apt to be caused by viral, fungal, protozoal, or mycobacterial infection. Pneumonia occurring within 2–4 weeks after organ transplantation is usually bacterial, whereas several months or more after transplantation *P jirovecii*, viruses (eg, cytomegalovirus), and fungi (eg, *Aspergillus*) are encountered more often.

Clinical Findings

Chest radiography is rarely helpful in narrowing the differential diagnosis. Examination of expectorated sputum for bacteria, fungi, mycobacteria, *Legionella*, and *P jirovecii* is important and may preclude the need for expensive, invasive diagnostic procedures. Sputum induction is often necessary for diagnosis. The sensitivity of induced sputum for detection of *P jirovecii* depends on institutional expertise, number of specimens analyzed, and detection methods.

Routine evaluation frequently fails to identify a causative organism. The clinician may begin empiric antimicrobial therapy before proceeding to invasive procedures such as bronchoscopy, transthoracic needle aspiration, or open lung biopsy. The approach to management must be based on the severity of the pulmonary infection, the underlying disease, the risks of empiric therapy, and local expertise and experience with diagnostic procedures. Bronchoalveolar lavage using the flexible bronchoscope is a safe and effective method for obtaining representative pulmonary secretions for microbiologic studies. It involves less risk of bleeding and other complications than bronchial brushing and transbronchial biopsy. Bronchoalveolar lavage is especially suitable for the diagnosis of *P jirovecii* pneumonia in patients with AIDS when induced sputum analysis is negative. Surgical lung biopsy, now often performed by video-assisted thoracoscopy, provides the definitive option for diagnosis of pulmonary infiltrates in the immunocompromised host. However, a specific diagnosis is obtained in only about two-thirds of cases, and the information obtained rarely affects the outcome.

Corti M et al. Respiratory infections in immunocompromised patients. Curr Opin Pulm Med. 2009 May;15(3):209–17. [PMID: 19276812]

Crothers K et al. HIV infection and risk for incident pulmonary diseases in the combination antiretroviral therapy era. Am J Respir Crit Care Med. 2011 Feb1;183(3):388–95. [PMID: 20851926]

Limper AH et al. An official American Thoracic Society statement: treatment of fungal infections in adult pulmonary and critical care patients. Am J Respir Crit Care Med. 2011 Jan1;183(1):96–128. [PMID: 21193785]

Marom EM et al. Imaging studies for diagnosing invasive fungal pneumonia in immunocompromised patients. Curr Opin Infect Dis. 2011 Aug;24(4):309–14. [PMID: 21673574]

PULMONARY TUBERCULOSIS

ESSENTIALS OF DIAGNOSIS

► Fatigue, weight loss, fever, night sweats, and productive cough.

► Risk factors for acquisition of infection: household exposure, incarceration, drug use, travel to an endemic area.

► Chest radiograph: pulmonary opacities, most often apical.

► Acid-fast bacilli on smear of sputum or sputum culture positive for *M tuberculosis*.

General Considerations

Tuberculosis is one of the world's most widespread and deadly illnesses. *M tuberculosis*, the organism that causes tuberculosis infection and disease, infects one-third of the world's population. In 2012, there were 8.6 million new cases of tuberculosis worldwide with 1.3 million people dying of the disease. In the United States, an estimated 11 million people are infected with *M tuberculosis*. Tuberculosis occurs disproportionately among disadvantaged populations such as the malnourished, homeless, and those living in overcrowded and substandard housing. There is an increased occurrence of tuberculosis among HIV-positive individuals.

Infection with *M tuberculosis* begins when a susceptible person inhales airborne droplet nuclei containing viable organisms. Tubercle bacilli that reach the alveoli are ingested by alveolar macrophages. Infection follows if the inoculum escapes alveolar macrophage microbicidal activity. Once infection is established, lymphatic and hematogenous dissemination of tuberculosis typically occurs before the development of an effective immune response. This stage of infection, **primary tuberculosis**, is usually clinically and radiographically silent. In most persons with intact cell-mediated immunity, T-cells and macrophages surround the organisms in granulomas that limit their multiplication and spread. The infection is contained but not eradicated, since viable organisms may lie dormant within granulomas for years to decades.

Individuals with **latent tuberculosis infection** do not have active disease and cannot transmit the organism to others. However, reactivation of disease may occur if the host's immune defenses are impaired. **Active tuberculosis will develop in approximately 6% of individuals with latent tuberculosis infection who are not given preventive therapy;** half of these cases occur in the 2 years following primary infection. Diverse conditions such as gastrectomy, silicosis, diabetes mellitus, and an impaired immune response (eg, HIV infection; therapy with corticosteroids, tumor necrosis factor inhibitors or other immunosuppressive drugs) are associated with an increased risk of reactivation.

In approximately 5% of cases, the immune response is inadequate to contain the primary infection and **progressive primary tuberculosis** develops, accompanied by both pulmonary and constitutional symptoms as described below. The clinical presentation does not definitively distinguish primary disease from reactivation of latent tuberculosis infection. Standard teaching has held that 90% of tuberculosis in adults represents activation of latent disease. However, DNA fingerprinting of the bacillus suggests that as many as one-third of new cases of tuberculosis in urban populations are primary infections resulting from person-to-person transmission.

The prevalence of drug-resistant strains is increasing worldwide; however, in the United States, the rate of drug-resistant isolates has fallen to < 1%. Risk factors for drug resistance include immigration from countries with a high prevalence of drug-resistant tuberculosis, close and prolonged contact with individuals with drug-resistant tuberculosis, unsuccessful previous therapy, and nonadherence to treatment. Drug resistance may be single or multiple. **Drug-resistant tuberculosis** is resistant to one first-line antituberculous drug, either isoniazid or rifampin. **Multidrug-resistant tuberculosis** is resistant to isoniazid and rifampin, and possibly additional agents. **Extensively drug-resistant tuberculosis** is resistant to isoniazid, rifampin, fluoroquinolones, and either aminoglycosides or capreomycin or both. Outcomes of drug-resistant tuberculosis treatment are worse than when the isolate is drug-sensitive, but outcomes appear to vary with HIV status. In a review of extensively drug-resistant tuberculosis cases in the United States, mortality was 10% and 68% in HIV-negative and HIV-positive patients, respectively.

▶ **Clinical Findings**

A. Symptoms and Signs

The patient with pulmonary tuberculosis typically presents with slowly progressive constitutional symptoms of malaise, anorexia, weight loss, fever, and night sweats. Chronic cough is the most common pulmonary symptom. It may be dry at first but typically becomes productive of purulent sputum as the disease progresses. Blood-streaked sputum is common, but significant hemoptysis is rarely a presenting symptom; life-threatening hemoptysis may occur in advanced disease. Dyspnea is unusual unless there is extensive disease. Rarely, the patient is asymptomatic. On physical examination, the patient appears chronically ill and malnourished. On chest examination, there are no physical findings specific for tuberculosis infection. The examination may be normal or may reveal classic findings such as posttussive apical rales.

B. Laboratory Findings

Definitive diagnosis depends on recovery of *M tuberculosis* from cultures or identification of the organism by DNA or RNA amplification techniques. Three consecutive morning sputum specimens are advised. Fluorochrome staining with rhodamine-auramine of concentrated, digested sputum specimens is performed initially as a screening method, with confirmation by the Kinyoun or Ziehl-Neelsen stains. Demonstration of acid-fast bacilli on sputum smear does not establish a diagnosis of *M tuberculosis,* since nontuberculous mycobacteria may colonize the airways and are increasingly recognized to cause clinical illness in patients with underlying structural lung disease.

In patients thought to have tuberculosis who cannot produce satisfactory specimens or when the smear of the spontaneously expectorated sputum is negative for acid-fast bacilli, sputum induction with 3% hypertonic saline should be performed. Flexible bronchoscopy with bronchial washings has similar diagnostic yield to induced sputum; transbronchial lung biopsies do not significantly increase the diagnostic yield but may lead to earlier diagnosis by identifying tissue granulomas. Post-bronchoscopy expectorated sputum specimens should be collected. Early morning aspiration of gastric contents after an overnight fast is suitable only for culture and not for stained smear because nontuberculous mycobacteria may be present in the stomach in the absence of tuberculous infection. Positive blood cultures for *M tuberculosis* are uncommon in patients with normal CD4 cell counts but the organism may be cultured from blood in up to 50% of HIV-seropositive patients with tuberculosis whose CD4 cell counts are < 100/mcL (< 0.1×10^9/L).

Traditional light-microscopic examination of stained sputum for acid-fast bacilli and culture of sputum specimens remain the mainstay of tuberculosis diagnosis. The slow rate of mycobacterial growth, the urgency to provide early, appropriate treatment to patients to improve their outcomes and limit community spread, and concerns about potential drug toxicities in patients treated empirically who do not have tuberculosis infection, have fostered interest in rapid diagnostic techniques (see Table 9–12). Molecular diagnostics offer multiple options and many advantages at significantly increased expense. Nucleic acid amplification testing not only detects *M tuberculosis* (NAAT-TB) but it also identifies resistance markers (NAAT-R). NAAT-TB can identify *M tuberculosis* within hours of sputum processing, allowing early isolation and treatment, but the negative predictive value is low in smear-negative patients. NAAT-R allows rapid identification of primary drug resistance and is indicated in the following patients: (1) those treated previously for tuberculosis, (2) those born (or who lived for > 1 year) in a country with moderate tuberculosis incidence or a high incidence of multiple drug-resistant isolates, (3) contacts of patients with multidrug-resistant tuberculosis, or (4) those who are HIV seropositive. Clinical suspicion remains the critical factor in interpreting all these studies. Standard drug susceptibility testing of culture isolates is considered routine for the first isolate of *M tuberculosis*, when a treatment regimen is failing, and when sputum cultures remain positive after 2 months of therapy.

Needle biopsy of the pleura reveals granulomatous inflammation in approximately 60% of patients with pleural effusions caused by *M tuberculosis.* Pleural fluid cultures are positive for *M tuberculosis* in less than 23–58% of cases of pleural tuberculosis. Culture of three pleural biopsy specimens combined with microscopic examination

Table 9–12. Essential laboratory tests for the detection of *Mycobacterium tuberculosis*.[1]

Test	Time to Result	Test Characteristics
Acid-fast bacilli light microscopy	1 day	Three morning specimens recommended. Combined sensitivity of 70% (54% for the first specimen, 11% for the second specimen, and 5% for the third specimen). First morning specimen increased yield by 12% compared to spot specimen.
Nucleic acid amplification test, detection (NAAT-TB)	1 day	Sensitivity/specificity high for smear-positive specimens, 85–97% for both, but sensitivity falls in smear-negative specimens to ~66%. Therefore, a positive NAAT in smear-negative patients with intermediate to high (> 30%) pretest probability of *M tuberculosis* infection is helpful while a negative NAAT is not. Should not be ordered in patients with low pretest probability of *M tuberculosis* infection.
Nucleic acid amplification test, resistance markers (NAAT-R)	1–2 days	Multiple assays for rifampin and isoniazid are available. Specificity uniformly high, > 98%. Sensitivity varies from about 84% to 96% increases with multiple specimens. See text for indications for testing.
Mycobacterial growth detection Liquid (broth based) medium Solid (agar or egg based) medium	Up to 6–8 weeks Avg 10–14 days Avg 3–4 weeks	Liquid culture methods are more sensitive (~90% and 76%, respectively) with shorter time to detection but higher contamination with bacterial growth than solid culture methods. Specificity exceeds 99% for all methods.
Identification of *M tuberculosis* complex by DNA probe or high performance liquid chromatography	1 day[1]	May be useful in areas of low *M tuberculosis* incidence where nontuberculous mycobacteria are commonly isolated.
First-line drug susceptibility testing (liquid medium)	1–2 weeks[1]	Gold standard. Should be performed routinely on the initial isolate.
Second-line and novel compound drug susceptibility testing Liquid (broth based) medium Solid (agar or egg based) medium	1–2 weeks[1] 3–4 weeks[1]	

[1]Following detection of mycobacterial growth.
Adapted, with permission, from Diagnostic Standards and Classification of Tuberculosis in Adults and Children. This official statement of the American Thoracic Society and the Centers for Disease Control and Prevention was adopted by the ATS Board of Directors, July 1999. This statement was endorsed by the Council of the Infectious Disease Society of America, September 1999. Am J Respir Crit Care Med. 2000 Apr;161(4 Pt 1):1376-95.

of a pleural biopsy yields a diagnosis in up to 90% of patients with pleural tuberculosis. Tests for pleural fluid adenosine deaminase (approximately 90% sensitivity and specificity for pleural tuberculosis at levels > 70 units/L) and interferon-gamma (89% sensitivity, 97% specificity in a recent meta-analysis) can be extremely helpful diagnostic aids, particularly in making decisions to pursue invasive testing in complex cases.

C. Imaging

Contrary to traditional teaching, molecular analysis demonstrates that radiographic abnormalities in pulmonary tuberculosis do not distinguish primary disease from reactivation of latent tuberculosis (Figure 9–5). The only independent predictor of an atypical pattern on chest radiograph—that is, not associated with upper lobe or cavitary disease—is an impaired host immune response. In elderly patients, lower lobe infiltrates with or without pleural effusion are frequently encountered. Lower lung tuberculosis may masquerade as pneumonia or lung cancer. A "miliary" pattern (diffuse small nodular densities) can be seen with hematologic or lymphatic dissemination of the organism. Immunocompromised patients—particularly those with late-stage HIV infection—often display lower

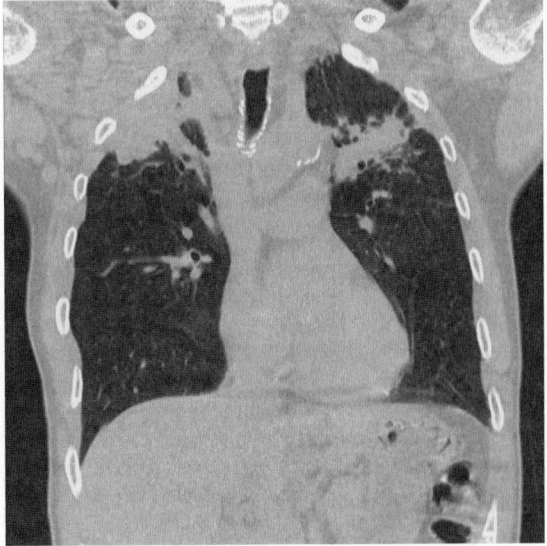

▲ **Figure 9–5. Pulmonary tuberculosis.** Chest CT scan showing biapical noncavitary consolidation consistent with pulmonary tuberculosis and associated right axillary lymphadenopathy.

lung zone, diffuse, or miliary infiltrates; pleural effusions; and involvement of hilar and, in particular, mediastinal lymph nodes.

Resolution of active tuberculosis leaves characteristic radiographic findings. Dense nodules in the pulmonary hila, with or without obvious calcification, upper lobe fibronodular scarring, and bronchiectasis with volume loss are common findings. Ghon (calcified primary focus) and Ranke (calcified primary focus and calcified hilar lymph node) complexes are seen in a minority of patients.

D. Special Examinations

Testing for latent tuberculosis infection is used to evaluate an asymptomatic person in whom M tuberculosis infection is suspected (eg, following contact exposure) or to establish the prevalence of tuberculosis infection in a population. Testing may be used in a person with symptoms of active tuberculosis, but a positive test does not distinguish between active and latent infection. Routine testing of individuals at low risk for tuberculosis is not recommended.

The traditional approach to latent tuberculosis infection is the **tuberculin skin test**. The Mantoux test is the preferred method: 0.1 mL of purified protein derivative (PPD) containing 5 tuberculin units is injected intradermally on the volar surface of the forearm using a 27-gauge needle on a tuberculin syringe. The **transverse width in millimeters of induration** at the skin test site is measured after 48–72 hours. To optimize test performance, criteria for determining a positive reaction vary depending on the likelihood of infection. Table 9–13 summarizes the criteria

established by the Centers for Disease Control and Prevention (CDC) for interpretation of the Mantoux tuberculin skin test. Sensitivity and specificity of the tuberculin skin test are high: 77% and 97%, respectively. Specificity falls to 59% in populations previously vaccinated with bacillus Calmette-Guérin (BCG, an extract of *Mycobacterium bovis*). False-negative tuberculin skin test reactions may result from improper testing technique; concurrent infections, including fulminant tuberculosis; malnutrition; advanced age; immunologic disorders; malignancy; corticosteroid therapy; chronic kidney disease; and HIV infection. Some individuals with latent tuberculosis infection may have a negative tuberculin skin test when tested many years after exposure. **Anergy testing is not recommended for routine use to distinguish a true-negative result from anergy.** Poor anergy test standardization and lack of outcome data limit the evaluation of its effectiveness. Interpretation of the tuberculin skin test in persons who have previously received BCG vaccination is the same as in those who have not had BCG.

Interferon gamma release assays are in vitro assays of CD4+ T-cell–mediated interferon gamma release in response to stimulation by specific *M tuberculosis* antigens. The antigens are absent from all BCG strains and most nontuberculous mycobacteria; therefore, in whole blood, the specificity of interferon gamma release assays is superior to the tuberculin skin test in BGC-vaccinated individuals. Sensitivity is comparable to the tuberculin skin test: 60–90% depending on the specific assay and study population. Sensitivity is reduced by HIV infection, particularly in patients with low CD4 counts. Specificity is high, > 95%.

Table 9–13. Classification of positive tuberculin skin test reactions.[1]

Induration Size	Group
≥ 5 mm	1. HIV-positive persons. 2. Recent contacts of individuals with active tuberculosis. 3. Persons with fibrotic changes on chest films suggestive of prior tuberculosis. 4. Patients with organ transplants and other immunosuppressed patients (receiving the equivalent of > 15 mg/d of prednisone for 1 month or more).
≥ 10 mm	1. Recent immigrants (< 5 years) from countries with a high prevalence of tuberculosis (eg, Asia, Africa, Latin America). 2. HIV-negative injection drug users. 3. Mycobacteriology laboratory personnel. 4. Residents of and employees[2] in the following high-risk congregate settings: correctional institutions; nursing homes and other long-term facilities for the elderly; hospitals and other health care facilities; residential facilities for AIDS patients; and homeless shelters. 5. Persons with the following medical conditions that increase the risk of tuberculosis: gastrectomy, ≥ 10% below ideal body weight, jejunoileal bypass, diabetes mellitus, silicosis, advanced chronic kidney disease, some hematologic disorders, (eg, leukemias, lymphomas), and other specific malignancies (eg, carcinoma of the head or neck and lung). 6. Children < 4 years of age or infants, children, and adolescents exposed to adults at high risk.
≥ 15 mm	1. Persons with no risk factors for tuberculosis.

[1]A tuberculin skin test reaction is considered positive if the transverse diameter of the *indurated* area reaches the size required for the specific group. All other reactions are considered negative.
[2]For persons who are otherwise at low risk and are tested at entry into employment, a reaction of > 15 mm induration is considered positive. Data from Screening for tuberculosis and tuberculosis infection in high-risk populations: recommendations of the Advisory Council for the Elimination of Tuberculosis. MMWR Morb Mortal Wkly Rep 1995 Sep 8;44(RR-11):19–34. [PMID: 7565540]

Potential advantages of interferon gamma release assay testing include fewer false-positive results from prior BCG vaccination, better discrimination of positive responses due to nontuberculous mycobacteria, and the requirement for only one patient contact (ie, no need for the patient to return to have the tuberculin skin test read 48–72 hours later). Disadvantages include the need for specialized laboratory equipment and personnel, and the substantially increased cost compared to the tuberculin skin test.

In endemic areas, interferon gamma release assays are no more sensitive than the tuberculin skin test in active tuberculosis (20–40% false-negative rate) and cannot distinguish active from latent disease. Interferon gamma release assays should not be used to exclude active tuberculosis.

Guidelines established by the CDC allow interferon gamma release assays to be used interchangeably with the tuberculin skin testing in the diagnosis of latent tuberculosis infection. Interferon gamma release assays are preferred in patients with prior BCG vaccination; the tuberculin skin test is preferred in children under 5 years old. Routine use of both tests is not recommended. In individuals with a positive tuberculin skin test but a low prior probability of latent tuberculosis infection and low risk for progression to active disease, the interferon gamma release assay may be helpful as a confirmatory test to exclude a false-positive tuberculin skin test.

▶ **Treatment**

A. General Measures

The goals of therapy are to eliminate all tubercle bacilli from an infected individual while avoiding the emergence of clinically significant drug resistance. The basic principles of antituberculous treatment are (1) to administer multiple drugs to which the organisms are susceptible; (2) to add at least two new antituberculous agents to a regimen when treatment failure is suspected; (3) to provide the safest, most effective therapy in the shortest period of time; and (4) to ensure adherence to therapy.

All suspected and confirmed cases of tuberculosis should be reported promptly to local and state public health authorities. Public health departments will perform case investigations on sources and patient contacts to determine if other individuals with untreated, infectious tuberculosis are present in the community. They can identify infected contacts eligible for treatment of latent tuberculous infection, and ensure that a plan for monitoring adherence to therapy is established for each patient with tuberculosis. Patients with tuberculosis should be treated by clinicians who are skilled in the management of this infection. Clinical expertise is especially important in cases of drug-resistant tuberculosis.

Nonadherence to antituberculous treatment is a major cause of treatment failure, continued transmission of tuberculosis, and the development of drug resistance. Adherence to treatment can be improved by providing detailed patient education about tuberculosis and its treatment in addition to a case manager who oversees all aspects of an individual patient's care. **Directly observed therapy (DOT)**, which requires that a health care worker physically observe the patient ingest antituberculous medications in the home, clinic, hospital, or elsewhere, also improves adherence to treatment. The importance of direct observation of therapy cannot be overemphasized. The CDC recommends DOT for all patients with drug-resistant tuberculosis and for those receiving intermittent (twice- or thrice-weekly) therapy.

Hospitalization for initial therapy of tuberculosis is not necessary for most patients. It should be considered if a patient is incapable of self-care or is likely to expose new, susceptible individuals to tuberculosis. Hospitalized patients with active disease require a private room with negative-pressure ventilation until tubercle bacilli are no longer found in their sputum ("smear-negative") on three consecutive smears taken on separate days.

Characteristics of antituberculous drugs are provided in Table 9–14. Additional treatment considerations can be found in Chapter 33. More complete information can be obtained from the CDC's Division of Tuberculosis Elimination Web site at http://www.cdc.gov/tb/.

B. Treatment of Tuberculosis in HIV-Negative Persons

Most patients with previously untreated pulmonary tuberculosis can be effectively treated with either a 6-month or a 9-month regimen, though the 6-month regimen is preferred. The initial phase of a 6-month regimen consists of 2 months of daily isoniazid, rifampin, pyrazinamide, and ethambutol. Once the isolate is determined to be isoniazid-sensitive, ethambutol may be discontinued. If the M tuberculosis isolate is susceptible to isoniazid and rifampin, the second phase of therapy consists of isoniazid and rifampin for a minimum of 4 additional months, with treatment to extend at least 3 months beyond documentation of conversion of sputum cultures to negative for M tuberculosis. If DOT is used, medications may be given intermittently using one of three regimens: (1) Daily isoniazid, rifampin, pyrazinamide, and ethambutol for 2 months, followed by isoniazid and rifampin two or three times each week for 4 months if susceptibility to isoniazid and rifampin is demonstrated. (2) Daily isoniazid, rifampin, pyrazinamide, and ethambutol for 2 weeks, then administration of the same agents twice a week for 6 weeks followed by administration of isoniazid and rifampin twice each week for 4 months if susceptibility to isoniazid and rifampin is demonstrated. (3) Isoniazid, rifampin, pyrazinamide, and ethambutol three times a week for 6 months.

Patients who cannot or should not (eg, pregnant women) take pyrazinamide should receive daily isoniazid and rifampin along with ethambutol for 4–8 weeks. If susceptibility to isoniazid and rifampin is demonstrated or drug resistance is unlikely, ethambutol can be discontinued and isoniazid and rifampin may be given twice a week for a total of 9 months of therapy. If drug resistance is a concern, patients should receive isoniazid, rifampin, and ethambutol for 9 months. Patients with smear- and culture-negative disease (eg, pulmonary tuberculosis diagnosed on clinical grounds) and patients for whom drug susceptibility testing is not available can be treated with

Table 9–14. Characteristics of antituberculous drugs.

Drug	Most Common Side Effects	Tests for Side Effects	Drug Interactions	Remarks
Isoniazid	Peripheral neuropathy, hepatitis, rash, mild CNS effects.	AST and ALT; neurologic examination.	Phenytoin (synergistic); disulfiram.	Bactericidal to both extracellular and intracellular organisms. Pyridoxine, 10 mg orally daily as prophylaxis for neuritis; 50–100 mg orally daily as treatment.
Rifampin	Hepatitis, fever, rash, flu-like illness, gastrointestinal upset, bleeding problems, kidney failure.	CBC, platelets, AST and ALT.	Rifampin inhibits the effect of oral contraceptives, quinidine, corticosteroids, warfarin, methadone, digoxin, oral hypoglycemics; aminosalicylic acid may interfere with absorption of rifampin. Significant interactions with protease inhibitors and non-nucleoside reverse transcriptase inhibitors.	Bactericidal to all populations of organisms. Colors urine and other body secretions orange. Discoloring of contact lenses.
Pyrazinamide	Hyperuricemia, hepatotoxicity, rash, gastrointestinal upset, joint aches.	Uric acid, AST, ALT.	Rare.	Bactericidal to intracellular organisms.
Ethambutol	Optic neuritis (reversible with discontinuance of drug; rare at 15 mg/kg); rash.	Red-green color discrimination and visual acuity.	Rare.	Bacteriostatic to both intracellular and extracellular organisms. Mainly used to inhibit development of resistant mutants. Use with caution in kidney disease or when ophthalmologic testing is not feasible.
Streptomycin	Eighth nerve damage, nephrotoxicity.	Vestibular function (audiograms); BUN and creatinine.	Neuromuscular blocking agents may be potentiated and cause prolonged paralysis.	Bactericidal to extracellular organisms. Use with caution in older patients or those with kidney disease.

ALT, alanine aminotransferase; AST, aspartate aminotransferase; BUN, blood urea nitrogen; CBC, complete blood count.

6 months of isoniazid and rifampin combined with pyrazinamide for the first 2 months. This regimen assumes low prevalence of drug resistance. Previous guidelines have used streptomycin interchangeably with ethambutol. Increasing worldwide streptomycin resistance has made this drug less useful as empiric therapy.

When a twice-weekly or thrice-weekly regimen is used instead of a daily regimen, the dosages of isoniazid, pyrazinamide, and ethambutol or streptomycin must be increased. Recommended dosages for the initial treatment of tuberculosis are listed in Table 9–15. Fixed-dose combinations of isoniazid and rifampin (Rifamate) and of isoniazid, rifampin, and pyrazinamide (Rifater) are available to simplify treatment. Single tablets improve compliance but are more expensive than the individual drugs purchased separately.

C. Treatment of Tuberculosis in HIV-Positive Persons

Management of tuberculosis is complex in patients with concomitant HIV disease. Experts in the management of both tuberculosis and HIV disease should be involved in the care of such patients. The CDC has published detailed recommendations for the treatment of tuberculosis in HIV-positive patients (http://www.cdc.gov/tb/).

The basic approach to HIV-positive patients with tuberculosis is similar to that detailed above for patients without HIV disease. Additional considerations in HIV-positive patients include: (1) longer duration of therapy and (2) drug interactions between rifamycin derivatives such as rifampin and rifabutin used to treat tuberculosis and some of the protease inhibitors and nonnucleoside reverse transcriptase inhibitors (NNRTIs), used to treat HIV (see http://www.cdc.gov/tb/). DOT should be used for all HIV-positive tuberculosis patients. Pyridoxine (vitamin B_6), 25–50 mg orally each day, should be administered to all HIV-positive patients being treated with isoniazid to reduce central and peripheral nervous system side effects.

D. Treatment of Drug-Resistant Tuberculosis

Patients with drug-resistant *M tuberculosis* infection require careful supervision and management. Clinicians

Table 9–15. Recommended dosages for the initial treatment of tuberculosis.

Drugs	Daily	Cost[1]	Twice a Week[2]	Cost[1]/wk	Three Times a Week[2]	Cost[1]/wk
Isoniazid	5 mg/kg Max: 300 mg/dose	$0.16/300 mg	15 mg/kg Max: 900 mg/dose	$0.96	15 mg/kg Max: 900 mg/dose	$1.44
Rifampin	10 mg/kg Max: 600 mg/dose	$6.08/600 mg	10 mg/kg Max: 600 mg/dose	$12.16	10 mg/kg Max: 600 mg/dose	$18.24
Pyrazinamide	15–30 mg/kg Max: 2 g/dose	$4.80/2 g	50–70 mg/kg Max: 4 g/dose	$19.20	50–70 mg/kg Max: 3 g/dose	$21.60
Ethambutol	5–25 mg/kg Max: 2.5 g/dose	$11.33/2.5 g	50 mg/kg Max: 2.5 g/dose	$22.66	25–30 mg/kg Max: 2.5 g/dose	$33.99
Streptomycin	15 mg/kg Max: 1 g/dose	$22.50/1 g	25–30 mg/kg Max: 1.5 g/dose	$90.00	25–30 mg/kg Max: 1.5 g/dose	$135.00

[1]Average wholesale price (AWP, for AB-rated generic when available) for quantity listed. Source: *Red Book Online, 2014 Truven Health Analytics, Inc.* AWP may not accurately represent the actual pharmacy cost because wide contractual variations exist among institutions.
[2]All intermittent dosing regimens should be used with directly observed therapy.

who are unfamiliar with the treatment of drug-resistant tuberculosis should seek expert advice. Tuberculosis resistant only to isoniazid can be successfully treated with a 6-month regimen of rifampin, pyrazinamide, and ethambutol or streptomycin or a 12-month regimen of rifampin and ethambutol. When isoniazid resistance is documented during a 9-month regimen without pyrazinamide, isoniazid should be discontinued. If ethambutol was part of the initial regimen, rifampin and ethambutol should be continued for a minimum of 12 months. If ethambutol was not part of the initial regimen, susceptibility tests should be repeated and two other drugs to which the organism is susceptible should be added. Treatment of *M tuberculosis* isolates resistant to agents other than isoniazid and treatment of drug resistance in HIV-infected patients require expert consultation.

Multidrug-resistant tuberculosis and extensively drug-resistant tuberculosis call for an individualized daily DOT plan under the supervision of an experienced clinician. Treatment regimens are based on the patient's overall status and the results of susceptibility studies. Most drug-resistant isolates are resistant to at least isoniazid and rifampin and require a minimum of three drugs to which the organism is susceptible. These regimens are continued until culture conversion is documented, and then a two-drug regimen is continued for at least another 12 months. Some experts recommend at least 18–24 months of a three-drug regimen.

E. Treatment of Extrapulmonary Tuberculosis

In most cases, regimens that are effective for treating pulmonary tuberculosis are also effective for treating extrapulmonary disease. However, many experts recommend 9 months of therapy when miliary, meningeal, or bone and joint disease is present. Treatment of skeletal tuberculosis is enhanced by early surgical drainage and debridement of necrotic bone. Corticosteroid therapy has been shown to help prevent constrictive pericarditis from tuberculous pericarditis and to reduce neurologic complications from tuberculous meningitis (see Chapter 33).

F. Treatment of Pregnant or Lactating Women

Tuberculosis in pregnancy is usually treated with isoniazid, rifampin, and ethambutol for 2 months, followed by isoniazid and rifampin for an additional 7 months. Ethambutol can be stopped after the first month if isoniazid and rifampin susceptibility is confirmed. Since the risk of teratogenicity with pyrazinamide has not been clearly defined, pyrazinamide should be used only if resistance to other drugs is documented and susceptibility to pyrazinamide is likely. Streptomycin is contraindicated in pregnancy because it may cause congenital deafness. Pregnant women taking isoniazid should receive pyridoxine (vitamin B_6), 10–25 mg orally once a day, to prevent peripheral neuropathy.

Small concentrations of antituberculous drugs are present in breast milk. First-line therapy is not known to be harmful to nursing newborns at these concentrations. Therefore, breastfeeding is not contraindicated while receiving first-line antituberculous therapy. Lactating women receiving other agents should consult a tuberculosis expert.

G. Treatment Monitoring

Adults should have measurements of a complete blood count (including platelets) and serum bilirubin, hepatic enzymes, urea nitrogen, and creatinine before starting therapy for tuberculosis. Visual acuity and red-green color vision tests are recommended before initiation of ethambutol and serum uric acid, before starting pyrazinamide. Audiometry should be performed if streptomycin therapy is initiated.

Routine monitoring of laboratory tests for evidence of drug toxicity during therapy is not recommended, unless baseline results are abnormal or liver disease is suspected. Monthly questioning for symptoms of drug toxicity is advised. Patients should be educated about common side effects of antituberculous medications and instructed to seek medical attention should these symptoms occur.

Monthly follow-up of outpatients is recommended, including sputum smear and culture for *M tuberculosis*, until cultures convert to negative. Patients with negative sputum cultures after 2 months of treatment should have at least one additional sputum smear and culture performed at the end of therapy. Patients with drug-resistant isolates should have sputum cultures performed monthly during the entire course of treatment. A chest radiograph at the end of therapy provides a useful baseline for any future films.

Patients whose cultures do not become negative or whose symptoms do not resolve despite 3 months of therapy should be evaluated for nonadherence to the regimen and for drug-resistant organisms. DOT is required for the remainder of the treatment regimen, and the addition of at least two drugs not previously given should be considered pending repeat drug susceptibility testing. The clinician should seek expert assistance if drug resistance is newly found, if the patient remains symptomatic, or if smears or cultures remain positive.

Patients with only a clinical diagnosis of pulmonary tuberculosis (smears and cultures negative for *M tuberculosis*) whose symptoms and radiographic abnormalities are unchanged after 3 months of treatment usually either have another process or have had tuberculosis in the past.

H. Treatment of Latent Tuberculosis

Treatment of latent tuberculous infection is essential to controlling and eliminating tuberculosis. Treatment of latent tuberculous infection substantially reduces the risk that infection will progress to active disease. Targeted testing with the tuberculin skin test or interferon gamma release assays is used to identify persons who are at high risk for tuberculosis and who stand to benefit from treatment of latent infection. Table 9–13 gives the tuberculin skin test criteria for treatment of latent tuberculous infection. In general, patients with a positive tuberculin skin test or interferon gamma release assay who are at increased risk for exposure or disease are treated. It is essential that each person who meets the criteria for treatment of latent tuberculous infection undergo a careful assessment to exclude active disease. A history of past treatment for tuberculosis and contraindications to treatment should be sought. All patients at risk for HIV infection should be tested for HIV. Patients suspected of having tuberculosis should receive one of the recommended multidrug regimens for active disease until the diagnosis is confirmed or excluded.

Some close contacts of persons with active tuberculosis should be evaluated for treatment of latent tuberculous infection despite a negative tuberculin skin test reaction (< 5 mm induration). These include immunosuppressed persons and those who may develop disease quickly after tuberculous infection. Close contacts who have a negative tuberculin skin test reaction on initial testing should be retested 10–12 weeks later.

Several treatment regimens for both HIV-negative and HIV-positive persons are available for the treatment of latent tuberculous infection: (1) **Isoniazid:** A 9-month oral regimen (minimum of 270 doses administered within 12 months) is considered optimal. Dosing options include a daily dose of 300 mg or twice-weekly doses of 15 mg/kg. Persons at risk for developing isoniazid-associated peripheral neuropathy (diabetes mellitus, uremia, malnutrition, alcoholism, HIV infection, pregnancy, seizure disorder) may be given supplemental pyridoxine (vitamin B_6), 10–50 mg/d. (2) **Rifampin and pyrazinamide:** A 2-month oral regimen (60 doses administered within 3 months) of daily rifampin (10 mg/kg up to a maximum dose of 600 mg) and pyrazinamide (15–20 mg/kg up to a maximum dose of 2 g) is recommended. This regimen has been associated with significant hepatotoxicity, so careful laboratory monitoring is required. (3) **Rifampin:** Patients who cannot tolerate isoniazid or pyrazinamide can be considered for a 4-month regimen (minimum of 120 doses administered within 6 months) of rifampin. HIV-positive patients receiving protease inhibitors or NNRTIs who are given rifampin require management by experts in both tuberculosis and HIV disease (see Treatment of Tuberculosis in HIV-Positive Persons, above).

Contacts of persons with isoniazid-resistant, rifampin-sensitive tuberculosis should receive a 2-month regimen of rifampin and pyrazinamide or a 4-month regimen of daily rifampin alone. Contacts of persons with drug-resistant tuberculosis should receive two drugs to which the infecting organism has demonstrated susceptibility. Contacts in whom the tuberculin skin test or interferon gamma release assay is negative and contacts who are HIV seronegative may be observed without treatment or treated for 6 months. HIV-positive contacts should be treated for 12 months. All contacts of persons with multidrug-resistant tuberculosis or extensively drug-resistant tuberculosis should have 2 years of follow-up regardless of treatment.

Persons with a positive tuberculin skin test (≥ 5 mm of induration) and fibrotic lesions suggestive of old tuberculosis on chest radiographs who have no evidence of active disease and no history of treatment for tuberculosis should receive 9 months of isoniazid, or 2 months of rifampin and pyrazinamide, or 4 months of rifampin (with or without isoniazid). Pregnant or breastfeeding women with latent tuberculosis should receive either daily or twice-weekly isoniazid with pyridoxine (vitamin B_6).

Baseline laboratory testing is indicated for patients at risk for liver disease, patients with HIV infection, women who are pregnant or within 3 months of delivery, and persons who use alcohol regularly. Patients receiving treatment for latent tuberculous infection should be evaluated once a month to assess for symptoms and signs of active tuberculosis and hepatitis and for adherence to their treatment regimen. Routine laboratory testing during treatment is indicated for those with abnormal baseline laboratory tests and for those at risk for developing liver disease.

Vaccine BCG is an antimycobacterial vaccine developed from an attenuated strain of *M bovis*. Millions of individuals worldwide have been vaccinated with BCG. However, it is not generally recommended in the United States because of the low prevalence of tuberculous infection, the vaccine's interference with the ability to determine latent tuberculous infection using tuberculin skin test reactivity, and its variable effectiveness in prophylaxis of pulmonary tuberculosis. BCG vaccination in the United States should only be undertaken after consultation with local health officials and tuberculosis experts. Vaccination of health care workers should be considered on an individual basis in settings in which a high percentage of tuberculosis patients are infected with strains resistant to both isoniazid and rifampin, in which transmission of such drug-resistant *M tuberculosis* and subsequent infection are likely, and in which comprehensive tuberculous infection-control precautions have been implemented but have not been successful. The BCG vaccine is contraindicated in persons with impaired immune responses due to disease or medications.

▶ Prognosis

Almost all properly treated immunocompetent patients with tuberculosis can be cured. Relapse rates are less than 5% with current regimens. The main cause of treatment failure is nonadherence to therapy.

American Thoracic Society; Centers for Disease Control and Prevention. Diagnostic Standards and Classification of Tuberculosis in Adults and Children. Am J Respir Crit Care Med. 2000 Apr;161(4 Part 1):1376–95. [PMID: 10764337]

American Thoracic Society; Centers for Disease Control and Prevention; Infectious Diseases Society of America. Controlling tuberculosis in the United States. Am J Respir Crit Care Med. 2005 Nov1;172(9):1169–227. [PMID: 16249321]

Blumberg HM et al; American Thoracic Society/Centers for Disease Control and Prevention/Infectious Diseases Society of America. Treatment of tuberculosis. Am J Respir Crit Care Med. 2003 Feb15;167(4):603–62. [PMID: 12588714]

Horsburgh CR Jret al. Clinical practice. Latent tuberculosis infection in the United States. N Engl J Med. 2011 Apr14;364(15):1441–8. [PMID: 21488766]

Punnoose AR et al. JAMA patient page. Tuberculosis. JAMA. 2013 Mar6;309(9):938. [PMID: 23462792]

Sia IG et al. Current concepts in the management of tuberculosis. Mayo Clin Proc. 2011 Apr;86(4):348–61. [PMID: 21454737]

PULMONARY DISEASE CAUSED BY NONTUBERCULOUS MYCOBACTERIA

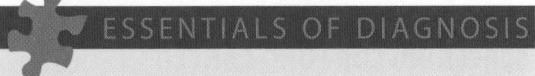

ESSENTIALS OF DIAGNOSIS

▶ Chronic cough, sputum production, and fatigue; less commonly: malaise, dyspnea, fever, hemoptysis, and weight loss.

▶ Parenchymal opacities on chest radiograph, often with thin-walled cavities, that spread contiguously and often involve overlying pleura.

▶ Isolation of nontuberculous mycobacteria in a sputum culture.

▶ General Considerations

Mycobacteria other than *M tuberculosis*—nontuberculous mycobacteria (NTM), sometimes referred to as "atypical" mycobacteria—are ubiquitous in water and soil and have

been isolated from tap water. There appears to be a continuing increase in the number and prevalence of NTM species. Marked geographic variability exists, both in the NTM species responsible for disease and in the prevalence of disease. These organisms are not considered communicable from person to person, have distinct laboratory characteristics, and are often resistant to most antituberculous drugs. (See Chapter 33.)

▶ Definition & Pathogenesis

The diagnosis of lung disease caused by NTM is based on a combination of clinical, radiographic, and bacteriologic criteria and the exclusion of other diseases that can resemble the condition. Specific diagnostic criteria are discussed below. Complementary data are important for diagnosis because NTM organisms can reside in or colonize the airways without causing clinical disease.

Mycobacterium avium complex (MAC) is the most frequent cause of NTM pulmonary disease in humans in the United States. *Mycobacterium kansasii* is the next most frequent pulmonary pathogen. Other NTM causes of pulmonary disease include *Mycobacterium abscessus*, *Mycobacterium xenopi*, and *Mycobacterium malmoense*; the list of more unusual etiologic NTM species is long. Most NTM cause a chronic pulmonary infection that resembles tuberculosis but tends to progress more slowly. Disseminated disease is rare in immunocompetent hosts; however, disseminated MAC disease is common in patients with AIDS.

▶ Clinical Findings

A. Symptoms and Signs

NTM infection among immunocompetent hosts frequently presents in one of three prototypical patterns: cavitary, upper lobe lesions in older male smokers that may mimic *M tuberculosis*; nodular bronchiectasis affecting the mid lung zones in middle-aged women with chronic cough; and hypersensitivity pneumonitis following environmental exposure. Most patients with NTM infection experience a chronic cough, sputum production, and fatigue. Less common symptoms include malaise, dyspnea, fever, hemoptysis, and weight loss. Symptoms from coexisting lung disease (COPD, bronchiectasis, previous mycobacterial disease, cystic fibrosis, and pneumoconiosis) may confound the evaluation. In patients with bronchiectasis, coinfection with NTM and *Aspergillus* is a negative prognostic factor. New or worsening infiltrates as well as adenopathy or pleural effusion (or both) are described in HIV-positive patients with NTM infection as part of the immune reconstitution inflammatory syndrome following institution of highly active antiretroviral therapy.

B. Laboratory Findings

The diagnosis of NTM infection rests on recovery of the pathogen from cultures. Sputum cultures positive for atypical mycobacteria do not prove infection because NTM may exist as saprophytes colonizing the airways or may be environmental contaminants. Bronchial washings are considered to be more sensitive than expectorated sputum samples; however, their specificity for clinical disease is not known.

Bacteriologic criteria have been proposed based on studies of patients with cavitary disease with MAC or *M kansasii*. Diagnostic criteria in immunocompetent persons include the following: positive culture results from at least two separate expectorated sputum samples; or positive culture from at least one bronchial wash; or a positive culture from pleural fluid or any other normally sterile site. The diagnosis can also be established by demonstrating NTM cultured from a lung biopsy, bronchial wash, or sputum plus histopathologic changes such as granulomatous inflammation in a lung biopsy. Rapid species identification of some NTM is possible using DNA probes or high-pressure liquid chromatography.

Diagnostic criteria are less stringent for patients with severe immunosuppression. HIV-infected patients may show significant MAC growth on culture of bronchial washings without clinical infection; therefore, HIV patients being evaluated for MAC infection must be considered individually.

Drug susceptibility testing on cultures of NTM is recommended for the following NTM: (1) *Mycobacterium avium intracellulare* to macrolides only (clarithromycin and azithromycin); (2) *M kansasii* to rifampin; and (3) rapid growers (such as *Mycobacterium fortuitum*, *Mycobacterium chelonae*, *M abscessus*) to amikacin, doxycycline, imipenem, fluoroquinolones, clarithromycin, cefoxitin, and sulfonamides.

C. Imaging

Chest radiographic findings include infiltrates that are progressive or persist for at least 2 months, cavitary lesions, and multiple nodular densities. The cavities are often thin-walled and have less surrounding parenchymal infiltrate than is commonly seen with MTB infections. Evidence of contiguous spread and pleural involvement is often present. High-resolution CT of the chest may show multiple small nodules with or without multifocal bronchiectasis. Progression of pulmonary infiltrates during therapy or lack of radiographic improvement over time are poor prognostic signs and also raise concerns about secondary or alternative pulmonary processes. Clearing of pulmonary infiltrates due to NTM is slow.

▶ Treatment

Establishing NTM infection does not mandate treatment in all cases, for two reasons. First, clinical disease may never develop in some patients, particularly asymptomatic patients with few organisms isolated from single specimens. Second, the spectrum of clinical disease severity is very wide; in patients with mild or slowly progressive symptoms, traditional chemotherapeutic regimens using a combination of agents may lead to drug-induced side effects worse than the disease itself.

Specific treatment regimens and responses to therapy vary with the species of NTM. HIV-seronegative patients with MAC pulmonary disease usually receive a combination of daily clarithromycin or azithromycin, rifampin or rifabutin, and ethambutol (Table 9–15). For patients with severe fibrocavitary disease, streptomycin or amikacin is added for the first 2 months. The optimal duration of treatment is unknown, but therapy should be continued for 12 months after sputum conversion. Medical treatment is initially successful in about two-thirds of cases, but relapses after treatment are common; long-term benefit is demonstrated in about half of all patients. Those who do not respond favorably generally have active but stable disease. Surgical resection is an alternative for the patient with progressive disease that responds poorly to chemotherapy; the success rate with surgical therapy is good. Disease caused by *M kansasii* responds well to drug therapy. A daily regimen of rifampin, isoniazid, and ethambutol for at least 18 months with a minimum of 12 months of negative cultures is usually successful. Rapidly growing mycobacteria (*M abscessus*, *M fortuitum*, *M chelonae*) are generally resistant to standard antituberculous therapy.

▶ When to Refer

Patients with rapidly growing mycobacteria infection should be referred for expert management.

Adjemian J et al. Prevalence of nontuberculous mycobacterial lung disease in U.S. Medicare beneficiaries. Am J Respir Crit Care Med. 2012 Apr15;185(8):881–6. [PMID: 22312016]

Esteban J et al. Current treatment of nontuberculous mycobacteriosis: an update. Expert Opin Pharmacother. 2012 May;13(7):967–86. [PMID: 22519767]

Griffith DE et al. An official ATS/IDSA statement: diagnosis, treatment, and prevention of nontuberculous mycobacterial diseases. Am J Respir Crit Care Med. 2007 Feb15;175(4): 367–416. [PMID: 17277290]

Iseman MD. Mycobacterial infections in the era of modern biologic agents. Am J Med Sci. 2011 Apr;341(4):278–80. [PMID: 21378550]

▼ PULMONARY NEOPLASMS

See Chapter 39 for discussions of Lung Cancer, Secondary Lung Cancer, and Mesothelioma.

SCREENING FOR LUNG CANCER

Two large RCTs reported findings in 2011 that clarify the utility of lung cancer screening. The Prostate, Lung, Colorectal and Ovarian Randomized Trial (PLCO) randomized 154,901 adults (52% current or former smokers) between the ages of 55 and 74 years to receive either no screening or annual posterior-anterior chest radiographs for 4 consecutive years. The investigators monitored the participants after screening for an average of 12 years. Results showed no mortality benefit from four annual chest radiographs either in the whole cohort or in a subset of heavy smokers who met the entry criteria for the other major trial, the National Lung Screening Trial (NLST). The NLST enrolled 53,454 current or former smokers (minimum 30-pack year exposure history) between the ages of 55 and 74 years who were randomly assigned to one of two screening modalities: three annual posterior-anterior chest radiographs or three annual low-dose chest CT scans. They were monitored for an additional 6.5 years after screening. Compared with chest radiography, low-dose chest CT detected more early-stage lung cancers and fewer advanced-stage lung cancers, indicating that CT screening systematically shifted the time of diagnosis to earlier stages, thereby providing more persons the opportunity for effective treatment. Furthermore, compared with chest radiographs, the cohort that received three annual CT scans had a statistically significant mortality benefit, with reductions in both lung cancer deaths (20.0%) and all-cause mortality (6.7%). This is the first time that evidence from a RCT demonstrated that lung cancer screening reduces all-cause mortality.

Additional information from PLCO, the NLST, and multiple other ongoing randomized trials is available. Salient issues that temper enthusiasm for widespread screening at this time include the following: **(1) Generalizability to community practice:** NLST-participating institutions demonstrated a high level of expertise in imaging interpretation and diagnostic evaluation. Ninety-six percent of findings on CT were false positives but the vast majority of patients were monitored with serial imaging. Invasive diagnostic evaluations were uncommon and were associated with a low complication rate (1.4%). **(2) Duration of screening:** The rate of detection of new lung cancers did not fall with each subsequent annual screening over 3 years. Since each year lung cancers first become detectable during that screening interval, the optimal number of annual CT scans is unknown as is the optimal screening interval. **(3) Overdiagnosis:** After 6.4 years of post-screening observation, there were more lung cancers in the NLST CT cohort than the chest radiography cohort (1089 and 969, respectively). Since the groups were randomized and well matched, lung cancer incidence should have been identical. Therefore, 18.5% of the lung cancers detected by CT remained clinically silent and invisible on chest radiograph for 6.4 years. Many, perhaps most, of these lung cancers will never cause clinical disease and represent overdiagnosis. **(4) Cost effectiveness:** The number needed to screen with three annual chest CT scans to prevent one death from lung cancer was 320.

Clear evidence exists showing the benefit of screening with low-dose chest CT in high-risk individuals and, since late 2013, screening has been recommended by the US Preventive Services Task Force. There is no evidence of benefit in a mixed population screened with chest radiography.

Aberle DR et al; National Lung Screening Trial Research Team. Results of the two incidence screenings in the National Lung Screening Trial. N Engl J Med. 2013 Sep5;369(10):920–31. [PMID: 24004119]

Field JK et al. Prospects for population screening and diagnosis of lung cancer. Lancet. 2013 Aug24;382(9893):732–41. [PMID: 23972816]

Humphrey LL et al. Screening for lung cancer with low-dose computed tomography: a systematic review to update the US Preventive services task force recommendation. Ann Intern Med. 2013 Sep17;159(6):411–20. [PMID: 23897166]

Kovalchik SA et al. Targeting of low-dose CT screening according to the risk of lung-cancer death. N Engl J Med. 2013 Jul18;369(3):245–54. [PMID: 23863051]

Moyer VA. Screening for Lung Cancer: U.S. Preventive Services Task Force Recommendation Statement. Ann Intern Med. 2013 Dec31. [Epub ahead of print] [PMID: 24378917]

National Lung Screening Trial Research Team. Reduced lung-cancer mortality with low-dose computed tomographic screening. N Engl J Med. 2011 Aug4;365(5):395–409. [PMID: 21714641]

Oken MM et al. Screening by chest radiograph and lung cancer mortality: the Prostate, Lung, Colorectal, and O varian (PLCO) randomized trial. JAMA. 2011 Nov2;306(17):1865–73. [PMID: 22031728]

Patz EF Jret al. Overdiagnosis in low-dose computed tomography screening for lung cancer. JAMA Intern Med. 2013 Dec9. [Epub ahead of print] [PMID: 24322569]

SOLITARY PULMONARY NODULE

A solitary pulmonary nodule, sometimes referred to as a "coin lesion," is a < 3 cm isolated, rounded opacity on chest imaging outlined by normal lung and not associated with infiltrate, atelectasis, or adenopathy. Most are asymptomatic and represent an unexpected finding on chest radiography or CT scanning. The finding is important because it carries a significant risk of malignancy. The frequency of malignancy in surgical series ranges from 10% to 68% depending on patient population. Most benign nodules are infectious granulomas. **Benign neoplasms** such as hamartomas account for less than 5% of solitary nodules.

The goals of evaluation are to identify and resect malignant tumors in patients who will benefit from resection while avoiding invasive procedures in benign disease. The task is to identify nodules with a sufficiently high probability of malignancy to warrant biopsy or resection or a sufficiently low probability of malignancy to justify observation.

Symptoms alone rarely establish the cause, but clinical and imaging data can be used to assess the probability of malignancy. Malignant nodules are rare in persons under age 30. Above age 30, the likelihood of malignancy increases with age. Smokers are at increased risk, and the likelihood of malignancy increases with the number of cigarettes smoked daily. Patients with a prior malignancy have a higher likelihood of having a malignant solitary nodule.

The first and most important step in the imaging evaluation is to review old imaging studies. Comparison with prior studies allows estimation of doubling time, which is an important marker for malignancy. Rapid progression (doubling time less than 30 days) suggests infection while long-term stability (doubling time greater than 465 days) suggests benignity. Certain radiographic features help in estimating the probability of malignancy. Size is correlated with malignancy. A study of solitary nodules identified by CT scan showed a 1% malignancy rate in those measuring 2–5 mm, 24% in 6–10 mm, 33% in 11–20 mm, and 80% in 21–45 mm. The appearance of a smooth, well-defined edge is characteristic of a benign process. Ill-defined margins or a lobular appearance suggest malignancy. A high-resolution CT finding of spiculated margins and a peripheral halo are both highly associated with malignancy. Calcification and its pattern are also helpful clues. Benign lesions tend to have dense calcification in a central or laminated pattern. Malignant lesions are associated with sparser calcification that is typically stippled or eccentric. Cavitary lesions with thick (> 16 mm) walls are much more likely to be malignant. High-resolution CT offers better resolution of these characteristics than chest radiography and is more likely to detect lymphadenopathy or the presence of multiple lesions. Chest CT is indicated in any suspicious solitary pulmonary nodule.

▶ Treatment

Based on clinical and radiologic data, the clinician should assign a specific probability of malignancy to the lesion. The decision whether to recommend a biopsy or surgical excision depends on the interpretation of this probability in light of the patient's unique clinical situation. The probabilities in parentheses below represent guidelines only and should not be interpreted as prescriptive.

In the case of solitary pulmonary nodules, a continuous probability function may be grouped into three categories. In patients with a **low probability** (< 5%) **of malignancy** (eg, age under 30, lesions stable for more than 2 years, characteristic pattern of benign calcification), watchful waiting is appropriate. Management consists of serial imaging studies (CT scans or chest radiographs) at intervals that identify growth suggestive of malignancy. Three-dimensional reconstruction of high-resolution CT images provides a more sensitive test for growth.

Patients with a **high probability** (> 60%) **of malignancy** should proceed directly to resection following staging, provided the surgical risk is acceptable. Biopsies rarely yield a specific benign diagnosis and are not indicated.

Optimal management of patients with an **intermediate probability of malignancy** (5–60%) remains controversial. The traditional approach is to obtain a diagnostic biopsy either through transthoracic needle aspiration (TTNA) or bronchoscopy. Bronchoscopy yields a diagnosis in 10–80% of procedures depending on the size of the nodule and its location. In general, the bronchoscopic yield for nodules that are < 2 cm and peripheral is low, although complications are generally rare. Newer bronchoscopic modalities such as electromagnetic navigation and ultrathin bronchoscopy are being studied, although their impact upon diagnostic yield remains uncertain. TTNA has a higher diagnostic yield, reported to be between 50% and 97%. The yield is strongly operator-dependent, however, and is affected by the location and size of the lesion. Complications are higher than bronchoscopy, with pneumothorax occurring in up to 30% of patients, with up to one-third of these patients requiring placement of a chest tube.

Disappointing diagnostic yields and a high false-negative rate (up to 20–30% in TTNA) have prompted alternative approaches. **Positron emission tomography** (PET) detects increased glucose metabolism within malignant lesions with high sensitivity (85–97%) and specificity (70–85%). Many diagnostic algorithms have incorporated PET into the assessment of patients with inconclusive high-resolution CT findings. A positive PET increases the likelihood of malignancy, and a negative PET correctly excludes cancer in most cases. False-negative PET scans can occur with tumors with low metabolic activity (well-differentiated adenocarcinomas, carcinoids, and bronchioloalveolar tumors), and follow-up CT imaging is typically performed at discrete intervals to ensure absence of growth. PET has several drawbacks, however: resolution below 1 cm is poor, the test is expensive, and availability remains limited.

Sputum cytology is highly specific but lacks sensitivity. It is used in central lesions and in patients who are poor candidates for invasive diagnostic procedures.

Some centers recommend **video-assisted thoracoscopic surgery** (VATS) resection of all solitary pulmonary nodules with intermediate probability of malignancy. In some cases, the surgeon will remove the nodule and evaluate it in the operating room with frozen section. If the nodule is malignant, he or she will proceed to lobectomy and lymph node sampling, either thoracoscopically or through conversion to standard thoracotomy. This approach is less common when PET scanning is available.

All patients should be provided with an estimate of the likelihood of malignancy, and their preferences should be used to help guide diagnostic and therapeutic decisions. A strategy that recommends observation may not be preferred by a patient who desires a definitive diagnosis. Similarly, a surgical approach may not be agreeable to all patients unless the presence of cancer is definitive. Patient preferences should be elicited, and patients should be well informed regarding the specific risks and benefits associated with the recommended approach as well as the alternative strategies.

Ost DE et al. Decision making in patients with pulmonary nodules. Am J Respir Crit Care Med. 2012 Feb15;185(4):363–72. [PMID: 21980032]

Wang Memoli JS et al. Meta-analysis of guided bronchoscopy for the evaluation of the pulmonary nodule. Chest. 2012 Aug;142(2):385–93. [PMID: 21980059]

RIGHT MIDDLE LOBE SYNDROME

Right middle lobe syndrome is recurrent or persistent atelectasis of the right middle lobe. This collapse is related to the relatively long length and narrow diameter of the right middle lobe bronchus and the oval ("fish mouth") opening to the lobe, in the setting of impaired collateral ventilation. Fiberoptic bronchoscopy or CT scan is often necessary to rule out obstructing tumor. Foreign body or other benign causes are common.

Gudbjartsson T et al. Middle lobe syndrome: a review of clinicopathological features, diagnosis and treatment. Respiration. 2012;84(1):80–6. [PMID: 22377566]

BRONCHIAL CARCINOID TUMORS

Carcinoid and bronchial gland tumors are sometimes termed "bronchial adenomas." This term should be avoided because it implies that the lesions are benign when, in fact, carcinoid tumors and bronchial gland carcinomas are low-grade malignant neoplasms.

Carcinoid tumors are about six times more common than bronchial gland carcinomas, and most of them occur as pedunculated or sessile growths in central bronchi. Men and women are equally affected. Most patients are under 60 years of age. Common symptoms of bronchial carcinoid tumors are hemoptysis, cough, focal wheezing, and recurrent pneumonia. Peripherally located bronchial carcinoid tumors are rare and present as asymptomatic solitary pulmonary nodules. **Carcinoid syndrome** (flushing, diarrhea, wheezing, hypotension) is rare. Fiberoptic bronchoscopy may reveal a pink or purple tumor in a central airway. These lesions have a well-vascularized stroma, and biopsy may be complicated by significant bleeding. CT scanning is helpful to localize the lesion and to follow its growth over time. Octreotide scintigraphy is also available for localization of these tumors.

Bronchial carcinoid tumors grow slowly and rarely metastasize. Complications involve bleeding and airway obstruction rather than invasion by tumor and metastases. Surgical excision of clinically symptomatic lesions is often necessary, and the prognosis is generally favorable. Most bronchial carcinoid tumors are resistant to radiation and chemotherapy (see Chapter 39).

Aydin E et al. Long-term outcomes and prognostic factors of patients with surgically treated pulmonary carcinoid: our institutional experience with 104 patients. Eur J Cardiothorac Surg. 2011 Apr;39(4):549–54. [PMID: 21282063]

Cakir M et al. The molecular pathogenesis and management of bronchial carcinoids. Expert Opin Ther Targets. 2011 Apr;15(4):457–91. [PMID: 21275849]

MEDIASTINAL MASSES

Various developmental, neoplastic, infectious, traumatic, and cardiovascular disorders may cause masses that appear in the mediastinum on chest radiograph. A useful convention arbitrarily divides the mediastinum into three compartments—anterior, middle, and posterior—in order to classify mediastinal masses and assist in differential diagnosis. Specific mediastinal masses have a predilection for one or more of these compartments; most are located in the anterior or middle compartment. The differential diagnosis of an **anterior mediastinal mass** includes thymoma, teratoma, thyroid lesions, lymphoma, and mesenchymal tumors (lipoma, fibroma). The differential diagnosis of a **middle mediastinal mass** includes lymphadenopathy, pulmonary artery enlargement, aneurysm of the aorta or innominate artery, developmental cyst (bronchogenic, enteric, pleuropericardial), dilated azygous or hemiazygous vein, and foramen of Morgagni hernia. The differential diagnosis of a **posterior mediastinal mass** includes hiatal hernia, neurogenic tumor, meningocele, esophageal tumor, foramen of Bochdalek hernia, thoracic spine disease, and extramedullary hematopoiesis. The neurogenic tumor group includes neurilemmoma, neurofibroma, neurosarcoma, ganglioneuroma, and pheochromocytoma.

Symptoms and signs of mediastinal masses are nonspecific and are usually caused by the effects of the mass on surrounding structures. Insidious onset of retrosternal chest pain, dysphagia, or dyspnea is often an important clue to the presence of a mediastinal mass. In about half of cases, symptoms are absent, and the mass is detected on routine chest radiograph. Physical findings vary depending on the nature and location of the mass.

CT scanning is helpful in management; additional radiographic studies of benefit include barium swallow if esophageal disease is suspected, Doppler sonography or venography of brachiocephalic veins and the superior vena cava, and angiography. MRI is useful; its advantages include better delineation of hilar structures and distinction between vessels and masses. MRI also allows imaging in multiple planes, whereas CT permits only axial imaging. Tissue diagnosis is necessary if a neoplastic disorder is suspected. Treatment and prognosis depend on the underlying cause of the mediastinal mass.

Fujii Y. Published guidelines for management of thymoma. Thorac Surg Clin. 2011 Feb;21(1):125–9. [PMID: 21070994]

Gubens MA. Treatment updates in advanced thymoma and thymic carcinoma. Curr Treat Options Oncol. 2012 Dec;13 (4):527–34. [PMID: 22961051]

Mikhail M et al. Thymic neoplasms: a clinical update. Curr Oncol Rep. 2012 Aug;14(4):350–8. [PMID: 22639107]

Nakazono T et al. MRI findings of mediastinal neurogenic tumors. AJR Am J Roentgenol. 2011 Oct;197(4):W643–52. [PMID: 21940535]

INTERSTITIAL LUNG DISEASE (DIFFUSE PARENCHYMAL LUNG DISEASE)

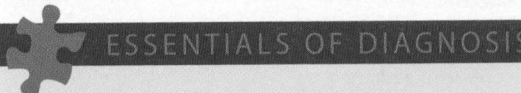

ESSENTIALS OF DIAGNOSIS

► Insidious onset of progressive dyspnea and nonproductive chronic cough; extrapulmonary findings may accompany specific diagnoses.

► Tachypnea, small lung volumes, bibasilar dry rales; digital clubbing and right heart failure with advanced disease.

► Chest radiographs with low lung volumes and patchy distribution of ground glass, reticular, nodular, reticulonodular, or cystic opacities.

► Reduced lung volumes, pulmonary diffusing capacity and 6-minute walk distance; hypoxemia with exercise.

Interstitial lung disease, or diffuse parenchymal lung disease, comprises a heterogeneous group of disorders that share common presentations (dyspnea), physical findings (late inspiratory crackles), and chest radiographs (septal thickening and reticulonodular changes).

The term "interstitial" is misleading since the pathologic process usually begins with injury to the alveolar epithelial or capillary endothelial cells (alveolitis). Persistent alveolitis may lead to obliteration of alveolar capillaries and reorganization of the lung parenchyma, accompanied by irreversible fibrosis. The process does not affect the airways proximal to the respiratory bronchioles. At least 180 disease entities may present as interstitial lung disease. Table 9–16 outlines a selected list of differential diagnoses of interstitial lung disease. In most patients, no specific cause can be identified. In the remainder, medications and a variety of organic and inorganic dusts are the principal causes. The history—particularly the occupational and medication history—may provide evidence of a specific cause.

Table 9–16. Differential diagnosis of interstitial lung disease.

Medication-related
Antiarrhythmic agents (amiodarone)
Antibacterial agents (nitrofurantoin, sulfonamides)
Antineoplastic agents (bleomycin, cyclophosphamide, methotrexate, nitrosoureas)
Antirheumatic agents (gold salts, penicillamine)
Phenytoin

Environmental and occupational (inhalation exposures)
Dust, inorganic (asbestos, silica, hard metals, beryllium)
Dust, organic (thermophilic actinomycetes, avian antigens, *Aspergillus* species)
Gases, fumes, and vapors (chlorine, isocyanates, paraquat, sulfur dioxide)
Ionizing radiation
Talc (injection drug users)

Infections
Fungus, disseminated (*Coccidioides immitis, Blastomyces dermatitidis, Histoplasma capsulatum*) Mycobacteria, disseminated
Pneumocystis jirovecii
Viruses

Primary pulmonary disorders
Cryptogenic organizing pneumonia (COP)
Idiopathic interstitial pneumonia: Acute interstitial pneumonia, desquamative interstitial pneumonia, nonspecific interstitial pneumonia, usual interstitial pneumonia, respiratory bronchiolitis-associated interstitial lung disease
Pulmonary alveolar proteinosis

Systemic disorders
Acute respiratory distress syndrome
Amyloidosis
Ankylosing spondylitis
Autoimmune disease: Dermatomyositis, polymyositis, rheumatoid arthritis, systemic sclerosis (scleroderma), systemic lupus erythematosus
Chronic eosinophilic pneumonia
Goodpasture syndrome
Idiopathic pulmonary hemosiderosis
Inflammatory bowel disease
Langerhans cell histiocytosis (eosinophilic granuloma)
Lymphangitic spread of cancer (lymphangitic carcinomatosis)
Lymphangioleiomyomatosis
Pulmonary edema
Pulmonary venous hypertension, chronic
Sarcoidosis
Granulomatosis polyangiitis (formerly Wegener granulomatosis)

The connective tissue diseases are a group of immunologically mediated inflammatory disorders including rheumatoid arthritis, systemic lupus erythematosus, scleroderma, polymyositis-dermatomyositis, Sjögren syndrome, and other overlap conditions. The presence of diffuse parenchymal lung disease in the setting of an established connective tissue disease is suggestive of the etiology. In some cases, lung disease precedes the more typical manifestations of the underlying connective tissue disease by months or years.

Known causes of interstitial lung disease are dealt with in their specific sections. The important idiopathic forms are discussed below.

IDIOPATHIC INTERSTITIAL PNEUMONIAS

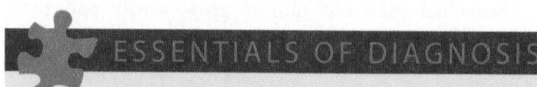
ESSENTIALS OF DIAGNOSIS

► Important to identify specific fibrosing disorders.
► Idiopathic disease may require biopsy for diagnosis.
► Accurate diagnosis identifies patients most likely to benefit from therapy.

► General Considerations

The most common diagnosis among patients with interstitial lung disease is idiopathic interstitial pneumonia. Historically, this diagnosis was based on clinical and radiographic criteria with only a small number of patients undergoing surgical lung biopsy. When biopsies were obtained, the common element of fibrosis led to the grouping together of several histologic patterns under the category of idiopathic interstitial pneumonia. These distinct histopathologic features are now recognized as being associated with different natural histories and responses to therapy (see Table 9–17). Therefore, in the evaluation of patients with interstitial lung disease, clinicians should attempt to identify specific disorders.

Patients with idiopathic interstitial pneumonia may have any of the histologic patterns described in Table 9–17. The first step in evaluation is to identify patients whose disease is truly idiopathic. As indicated in Table 9–16, most identifiable causes of interstitial lung disease are infectious, medication-related, or environmental or occupational agents. Interstitial lung diseases associated with other medical conditions (pulmonary-renal syndromes, collagen-vascular disease) may be identified through a careful medical history. Apart from acute interstitial pneumonia, the clinical presentations of the idiopathic interstitial pneumonias are sufficiently similar to preclude a specific diagnosis. Chest radiographs and high-resolution CT scans are occasionally diagnostic. Ultimately, many patients with apparently idiopathic disease require surgical lung biopsy to make a definitive diagnosis. The importance of accurate diagnosis is twofold. First, it allows the clinician to provide accurate information about the cause and natural history of

Table 9–17. Idiopathic interstitial pneumonias.

Name and Clinical Presentation	Histopathology	Radiographic Pattern	Response to Therapy and Prognosis
Usual interstitial pneumonia (UIP) Age 55–60, slight male predominance. Insidious dry cough and dyspnea lasting months to years. Clubbing present at diagnosis in 25–50%. Diffuse fine late inspiratory crackles on lung auscultation. Restrictive ventilatory defect and reduced diffusing capacity on pulmonary function tests. ANA and RF positive in ~25% in the absence of documented collagen-vascular disease.	Patchy, temporally and geographically nonuniform distribution of fibrosis, honeycomb change, and normal lung. Type I pneumocytes are lost, and there is proliferation of alveolar type II cells. "Fibroblast foci" of actively proliferating fibroblasts and myofibroblasts. Inflammation is generally mild and consists of small lymphocytes. Intra-alveolar macrophage accumulation is present but is not a prominent feature.	Diminished lung volume. Increased linear or reticular bibasilar and subpleural opacities. Unilateral disease is rare. High-resolution CT scanning shows minimal ground-glass and variable honeycomb change. Areas of normal lung may be adjacent to areas of advanced fibrosis. Between 2% and 10% have normal chest radiographs and high-resolution CT scans on diagnosis.	No randomized study has demonstrated improved survival compared with untreated patients. Inexorably progressive. Response to corticosteroids and cytotoxic agents at best 15%, and these probably represent misclassification of histopathology. Median survival approximately 3 years, depending on stage at presentation. Current interest in antifibrotic agents.
Respiratory bronchiolitis–associated interstitial lung disease (RB-ILD)[1] Age 40–45. Presentation similar to that of UIP though in younger patients. Similar results on pulmonary function tests, but less severe abnormalities. Patients with respiratory bronchiolitis are invariably heavy smokers.	Increased numbers of macrophages evenly dispersed within the alveolar spaces. Rare fibroblast foci, little fibrosis, minimal honeycomb change. In RB-ILD the accumulation of macrophages is localized within the peribronchiolar air spaces; in DIP,[1] it is diffuse. Alveolar architecture is preserved.	May be indistinguishable from UIP. More often presents with a nodular or reticulonodular pattern. Honeycombing rare. High-resolution CT more likely to reveal diffuse ground-glass opacities and upper lobe emphysema.	Spontaneous remission occurs in up to 20% of patients, so natural history unclear. Smoking cessation is essential. Prognosis clearly better than that of UIP: median survival greater than 10 years. Corticosteroids thought to be effective, but there are no randomized clinical trials to support this view.
Acute interstitial pneumonia (AIP) Clinically known as Hamman-Rich syndrome. Wide age range, many young patients. Acute onset of dyspnea followed by rapid development of respiratory failure. Half of patients report a viral syndrome preceding lung disease. Clinical course indistinguishable from that of idiopathic ARDS.	Pathologic changes reflect acute response to injury within days to weeks. Resembles organizing phase of diffuse alveolar damage. Fibrosis and minimal collagen deposition. May appear similar to UIP but more homogeneous and there is no honeycomb change—though this may appear if the process persists for more than a month in a patient on mechanical ventilation.	Diffuse bilateral airspace consolidation with areas of ground-glass attenuation on high-resolution CT scan.	Supportive care (mechanical ventilation) critical but effect of specific therapies unclear. High initial mortality: Fifty to 90 percent die within 2 months after diagnosis. Not progressive if patient survives. Lung function may return to normal or may be permanently impaired.
Nonspecific interstitial pneumonia (NSIP) Age 45–55. Slight female predominance. Similar to UIP but onset of cough and dyspnea over months, not years.	Nonspecific in that histopathology does not fit into better-established categories. Varying degrees of inflammation and fibrosis, patchy in distribution but uniform in time, suggesting response to single injury. Most have lymphocytic and plasma cell inflammation without fibrosis. Honeycombing present but scant. Some have advocated division into cellular and fibrotic subtypes.	May be indistinguishable from UIP. Most typical picture is bilateral areas of ground-glass attenuation and fibrosis on high-resolution CT. Honeycombing is rare.	Treatment thought to be effective, but no prospective clinical studies have been published. Prognosis overall good but depends on the extent of fibrosis at diagnosis. Median survival greater than 10 years.
Cryptogenic organizing pneumonia (COP, formerly bronchiolitis obliterans organizing pneumonia [BOOP]) Typically age 50–60 but wide variation. Abrupt onset, frequently weeks to a few months following a flu-like illness. Dyspnea and dry cough prominent, but constitutional symptoms are common: fatigue, fever, and weight loss. Pulmonary function tests usually show restriction, but up to 25% show concomitant obstruction.	Included in the idiopathic interstitial pneumonias on clinical grounds. Buds of loose connective tissue (Masson bodies) and inflammatory cells fill alveoli and distal bronchioles.	Lung volumes normal. Chest radiograph typically shows interstitial and parenchymal disease with discrete, peripheral alveolar and ground-glass infiltrates. Nodular opacities common. High-resolution CT shows subpleural consolidation and bronchial wall thickening and dilation.	Rapid response to corticosteroids in two-thirds of patients. Long-term prognosis generally good for those who respond. Relapses are common.

[1]Includes desquamative interstitial pneumonia (DIP).

ANA, antinuclear antibody; ARDS, acute respiratory distress syndrome; RF, rheumatoid factor; UIP, usual interstitial pneumonia.

the illness. Second, accurate diagnosis helps distinguish patients most likely to benefit from therapy.

▶ Clinical Findings

A. Symptoms, Signs, and Imaging

The diagnosis of usual interstitial pneumonia (UIP) can be made on clinical grounds alone in selected patients (Table 9–17). A diagnosis of UIP can be made with 90% confidence in patients over 65 years of age who have (1) idiopathic disease by history and who demonstrate inspiratory crackles on physical examination; (2) restrictive physiology on pulmonary function testing; (3) characteristic radiographic evidence of progressive fibrosis over several years; and (4) diffuse, patchy fibrosis with pleural-based honeycombing on high-resolution CT scan (Figure 9–6). Such patients do not need surgical lung biopsy.

B. Special Studies

Three diagnostic techniques are in common use: bronchoalveolar lavage, transbronchial biopsy, and surgical lung biopsy, either through an open procedure or using VATS.

Bronchoalveolar lavage may provide a specific diagnosis in cases of infection, particularly with *P jirovecii* or mycobacteria, or when cytologic examination reveals the presence of malignant cells. The findings may be suggestive and sometimes diagnostic of eosinophilic pneumonia, Langerhans cell histiocytosis, or alveolar proteinosis. Analysis of the cellular constituents of lavage fluid may suggest a specific disease, but these findings are not diagnostic.

Transbronchial biopsy through the flexible bronchoscope is easily performed in most patients. The risks of pneumothorax (5%) and hemorrhage (1–10%) are low.

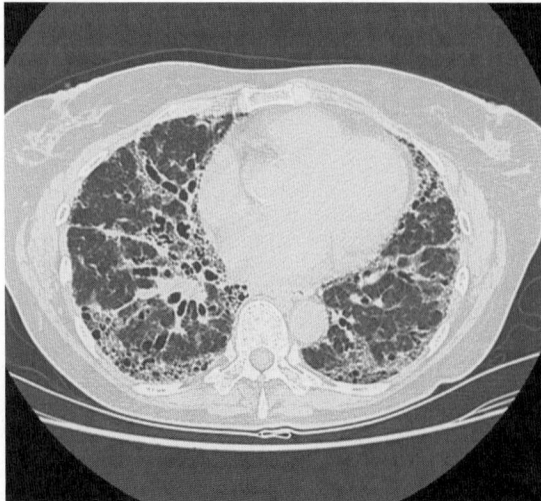

▲ **Figure 9–6. Idiopathic pulmonary fibrosis.** CT scan of the lungs showing the typical radiographic pattern of idiopathic pulmonary fibrosis, with a predominantly basilar, peripheral pattern of traction bronchiectasis, reticulation, and early honeycombing.

However, the tissue specimens recovered are small, sampling error is common, and crush artifact may complicate diagnosis. Transbronchial biopsy can make a definitive diagnosis of sarcoidosis, lymphangitic spread of carcinoma, pulmonary alveolar proteinosis, miliary tuberculosis, and Langerhans cell histiocytosis. Note that the diagnosis of UIP cannot be confirmed on transbronchial lung biopsy since the histologic diagnosis requires a pattern of changes rather than a single pathognomonic finding. Transbronchial biopsy may exclude UIP by confirming a specific alternative diagnosis. Transbronchial biopsy also cannot establish a specific diagnosis of idiopathic interstitial pneumonia. These patients generally require surgical lung biopsy.

Surgical lung biopsy is the standard for diagnosis of interstitial lung disease. Two or three biopsies taken from multiple sites in the same lung, including apparently normal tissue, may yield a specific diagnosis as well as prognostic information regarding the extent of fibrosis versus active inflammation. Patients under age 60 without a specific diagnosis generally should undergo surgical lung biopsy. In older and sicker patients, the risks and benefits must be weighed carefully for three reasons: (1) the morbidity of the procedure can be significant; (2) a definitive diagnosis may not be possible even with surgical lung biopsy; and (3) when a specific diagnosis is made, there may be no effective treatment. Empiric therapy or no treatment may be preferable to surgical lung biopsy in some patients.

▶ Treatment

Treatment of idiopathic interstitial pneumonia is controversial. No randomized study has demonstrated that any treatment improves survival or quality of life compared with no treatment. Clinical experience suggests that patients with RB-ILD, nonspecific interstitial pneumonia (NSIP), or COP (see Table 9–17) frequently respond to corticosteroids and should be given a trial of therapy—typically prednisone, 1–2 mg/kg/d for a minimum of 2 months. The same therapy is almost uniformly ineffective in patients with UIP. Since this therapy carries significant morbidity, experts do not recommend routine use of corticosteroids in patients with UIP. A number of antifibrotic (pirfenidone, interferon gamma 1b) and immunomodulator/immunosuppressant (cyclosporine A, azathioprine, etanercept) agents have been investigated and none of them are recommended for the treatment of UIP, either in monotherapy or combination therapy. The only definitive treatment for UIP is lung transplantation, with a 5-year survival rate estimated at 50%.

Ferguson EC et al. Lung CT: part 2, the interstitial pneumonias—clinical, histologic, and CT manifestations. AJR Am J Roentgenol. 2012 Oct;199(4):W464–76. [PMID: 22997396]

Poletti V et al. Current status of idiopathic nonspecific interstitial pneumonia. Semin Respir Crit Care Med. 2012 Oct;33(5):440–9. [PMID: 23001799]

Raghu G et al. An official ATS/ERS/JRS/ALAT statement: idiopathic pulmonary fibrosis: evidence-based guidelines for diagnosis and management. Am J Respir Crit Care Med. 2011 Mar15;183(6):788–824. [PMID: 21471066]

SARCOIDOSIS

► General Considerations

Sarcoidosis is a systemic disease of unknown etiology characterized in about 90% of patients by granulomatous inflammation of the lung. The incidence is highest in North American blacks and northern European whites; among blacks, women are more frequently affected than men. Onset of disease is usually in the third or fourth decade.

► Clinical Findings

A. Symptoms and Signs

Patients may have malaise, fever, and dyspnea of insidious onset. Symptoms from skin involvement (erythema, lupus pernio [Figure 9–7]), iritis, peripheral neuropathy, arthritis (see Chapter 20), or cardiomyopathy may also cause the patient to seek care. Some individuals are asymptomatic and come to medical attention after abnormal findings (typically bilateral hilar and right paratracheal

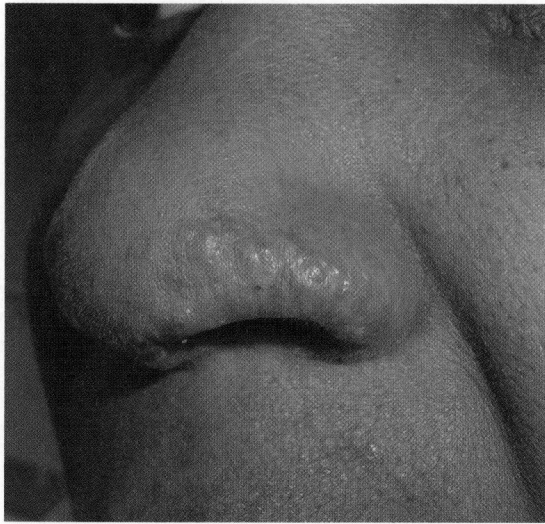

▲ **Figure 9–7.** Skin involvement in sarcoidosis (lupus pernio), here involving the nasal rim. (From Richard P. Usatine, MD; reproduced with permission, from Usatine RP, Smith MA, Mayeaux EJ Jr, Chumley H, Tysinger J. *The Color Atlas of Family Medicine.* McGraw-Hill, 2009.)

lymphadenopathy) on chest radiographs. Physical findings are atypical of interstitial lung disease in that crackles are uncommon on chest examination. Other symptoms and findings may include parotid gland enlargement, hepatosplenomegaly, and lymphadenopathy.

B. Laboratory Findings

Laboratory tests may show leukopenia, an elevated erythrocyte sedimentation rate, and hypercalcemia (about 5% of patients) or hypercalciuria (20%). Angiotensin-converting enzyme (ACE) levels are elevated in 40–80% of patients with active disease. This finding is neither sensitive nor specific enough to have diagnostic significance. Physiologic testing may reveal evidence of airflow obstruction, but restrictive changes with decreased lung volumes and diffusing capacity are more common. Skin test anergy is present in 70%. ECG may show conduction disturbances and dysrhythmias.

C. Imaging

Radiographic findings are variable and include bilateral hilar adenopathy alone (radiographic stage I), hilar adenopathy and parenchymal involvement (radiographic stage II), or parenchymal involvement alone (radiographic stage III). Parenchymal involvement is usually manifested radiographically by diffuse reticular infiltrates, but focal infiltrates, acinar shadows, nodules and, rarely, cavitation may be seen. Pleural effusion is noted in less than 10% of patients.

D. Special Examinations

The diagnosis of sarcoidosis generally requires histologic demonstration of noncaseating granulomas in biopsies from a patient with other typical associated manifestations. Other granulomatous diseases (eg, berylliosis, tuberculosis, fungal infections) and lymphoma must be excluded. Biopsy of easily accessible sites (eg, palpable lymph nodes, skin lesions, or salivary glands) is likely to be positive. Transbronchial lung biopsy has a high yield (75–90%) as well, especially in patients with radiographic evidence of parenchymal involvement. Some clinicians believe that tissue biopsy is not necessary when stage I radiographic findings are detected in a clinical situation that strongly favors the diagnosis of sarcoidosis (eg, a young black woman with erythema nodosum). Biopsy is essential whenever clinical and radiographic findings suggest the possibility of an alternative diagnosis such as lymphoma. Bronchoalveolar lavage fluid in sarcoidosis is usually characterized by an increase in lymphocytes and a high CD4/CD8 cell ratio. Bronchoalveolar lavage does not establish a diagnosis but may be useful in following the activity of sarcoidosis in selected patients. All patients require a complete ophthalmologic evaluation.

► Treatment

Indications for treatment with oral corticosteroids (prednisone, 0.5–1.0 mg/kg/d) include disabling constitutional symptoms, hypercalcemia, iritis, uveitis, arthritis, central nervous system involvement, cardiac involvement, granulomatous hepatitis, cutaneous lesions other than erythema nodosum, and progressive pulmonary lesions. Long-term therapy is usually required over months to years. Serum ACE levels usually fall with clinical improvement. Immunosuppressive drugs and cyclosporine have been tried, primarily when corticosteroid therapy has been exhausted, but experience with these drugs is limited.

▶ **Prognosis**

The outlook is best for patients with hilar adenopathy alone; radiographic involvement of the lung parenchyma is associated with a worse prognosis. Erythema nodosum portends a good outcome. About 20% of patients with lung involvement suffer irreversible lung impairment, characterized by progressive fibrosis, bronchiectasis, and cavitation. Pneumothorax, hemoptysis, mycetoma formation in lung cavities, and respiratory failure often complicate this advanced stage. Myocardial sarcoidosis occurs in about 5% of patients, sometimes leading to restrictive cardiomyopathy, cardiac dysrhythmias, and conduction disturbances. Death from respiratory insufficiency occurs in about 5% of patients.

Patients require long-term follow-up: at a minimum, yearly physical examination, pulmonary function tests, chemistry panel, ophthalmologic evaluation, chest radiograph, and ECG.

Baughman RP et al. A concise review of pulmonary sarcoidosis. Am J Respir Crit Care Med. 2011 Mar1;183(5):573–81. [PMID: 21037016]
Iannuzzi MC et al. Sarcoidosis: clinical presentation, immunopathogenesis, and therapeutics. JAMA. 2011 Jan26;305(4):391–9. [PMID: 21266686]
Morgenthau AS et al. Recent advances in sarcoidosis. Chest. 2011 Jan;139(1):174–82. [PMID: 21208877]

PULMONARY ALVEOLAR PROTEINOSIS

Pulmonary alveolar proteinosis is a rare disease in which phospholipids accumulate within alveolar spaces. The condition may be primary (idiopathic) or secondary (occurring in immunodeficiency; hematologic malignancies; inhalation of mineral dusts; or following lung infections, including tuberculosis and viral infections). Progressive dyspnea is the usual presenting symptom, and chest radiograph shows bilateral alveolar infiltrates suggestive of pulmonary edema. The diagnosis is based on demonstration of characteristic findings on bronchoalveolar lavage (milky appearance and PAS-positive lipoproteinaceous material) in association with typical clinical and radiographic features. In some cases, transbronchial or surgical lung biopsy (revealing amorphous intra-alveolar phospholipid) is necessary.

The course of the disease varies. Some patients experience spontaneous remission; others develop progressive respiratory insufficiency. Pulmonary infection with *Nocardia* or fungi may occur. Therapy for alveolar proteinosis consists of periodic whole lung lavage.

Borie R et al. Pulmonary alveolar proteinosis. Eur Respir Rev. 2011 Jun;20(120):98–107. [PMID: 21632797]
Patel SM et al. Pulmonary alveolar proteinosis. Can Respir J. 2012 Jul–Aug;19(4):243–5. [PMID: 22891182]

EOSINOPHILIC PULMONARY SYNDROMES

Eosinophilic pulmonary syndromes are a diverse group of disorders typically characterized by eosinophilic pulmonary infiltrates, dyspnea, and cough. Many patients have constitutional symptoms, including fever. Common causes include exposure to medications (nitrofurantoin, phenytoin, ampicillin, acetaminophen, ranitidine) or infection with helminths (eg, *Ascaris,* hookworms, *Strongyloides*) or filariae (eg, *Wuchereria bancrofti, Brugia malayi,* tropical pulmonary eosinophilia). **Löffler syndrome** refers to acute eosinophilic pulmonary infiltrates in response to transpulmonary passage of helminth larvae. Pulmonary eosinophilia can also be a feature of other illnesses, including allergic bronchopulmonary mycosis, Churg-Strauss syndrome, systemic hypereosinophilic syndromes, eosinophilic granuloma of the lung (properly referred to as pulmonary Langerhans cell histiocytosis), neoplasms, and numerous interstitial lung diseases. If an extrinsic cause is identified, therapy consists of removal of the offending drug or treatment of the underlying parasitic infection.

One-third of cases are idiopathic, and there are two common syndromes. **Chronic eosinophilic pneumonia** is seen predominantly in women and is characterized by fever, night sweats, weight loss, and dyspnea. Asthma is present in half of cases. Chest radiographs often show peripheral infiltrates, the "photographic negative" of pulmonary edema. Bronchoalveolar lavage typically has a marked eosinophilia; peripheral blood eosinophilia is present in greater than 80%. Therapy with oral prednisone (1 mg/kg/d for 1–2 weeks followed by a gradual taper over many months) usually results in dramatic improvement; however, most patients require at least 10–15 mg of prednisone every other day for a year or more (sometimes indefinitely) to prevent relapses. **Acute eosinophilic pneumonia** is an acute, febrile illness characterized by cough and dyspnea, sometimes rapidly progressing to respiratory failure. The chest radiograph is abnormal but nonspecific. Bronchoalveolar lavage frequently shows eosinophilia but peripheral blood eosinophilia is rare at the onset of symptoms. The response to corticosteroids is usually dramatic.

Cottin V et al. Eosinophilic lung diseases. Immunol Allergy Clin North Am. 2012 Nov;32(4):557–86. [PMID: 23102066]
Rose DM et al. Primary eosinophilic lung diseases. Allergy Asthma Proc. 2013 Jan–Feb;34(1):19–25. [PMID: 23406932]

DISORDERS OF THE PULMONARY CIRCULATION

PULMONARY VENOUS THROMBOEMBOLISM

ESSENTIALS OF DIAGNOSIS

▸ Predisposition to venous thrombosis, usually of the lower extremities.

▸ One or more of the following: dyspnea, chest pain, hemoptysis, syncope.

▸ Tachypnea and a widened alveolar-arterial PO_2 difference.

▸ Elevated rapid D-dimer and characteristic defects on CT arteriogram of the chest, ventilation-perfusion lung scan, or pulmonary angiogram.

▶ General Considerations

Pulmonary venous thromboembolism, often referred to as pulmonary embolism (PE), is a common, serious, and potentially fatal complication of thrombus formation within the deep venous circulation. PE is the third leading cause of death among hospitalized patients. Despite this prevalence, most cases are not recognized antemortem, and less than 10% of patients with fatal emboli have received specific treatment for the condition. Management demands a vigilant systematic approach to diagnosis and an understanding of risk factors so that appropriate preventive therapy can be given.

Many substances can embolize to the pulmonary circulation, including air (during neurosurgery, from central venous catheters), amniotic fluid (during active labor), fat (long bone fractures), foreign bodies (talc in injection drug users), parasite eggs (schistosomiasis), septic emboli (acute infectious endocarditis), and tumor cells (renal cell carcinoma). The most common embolus is thrombus, which may arise anywhere in the venous circulation or heart but most often originates in the deep veins of the lower extremities. Thrombi confined to the calf rarely embolize to the pulmonary circulation. However, about 20% of calf vein thrombi propagate proximally to the popliteal and ileofemoral veins, at which point they may break off and embolize to the pulmonary circulation. Pulmonary emboli will develop in 50–60% of patients with proximal deep venous thrombosis (DVT); half of these embolic events will be asymptomatic. **Approximately 50–70% of patients who have symptomatic pulmonary emboli will have lower extremity DVT when evaluated.**

PE and DVT are two manifestations of the same disease. The risk factors for PE are the risk factors for thrombus formation within the venous circulation: venous stasis, injury to the vessel wall, and hypercoagulability (Virchow triad). Venous stasis increases with immobility (bed rest—especially postoperative—obesity, stroke), hyperviscosity (polycythemia), and increased central venous pressures (low cardiac output states, pregnancy). Vessels may be damaged by prior episodes of thrombosis, orthopedic surgery, or trauma. Hypercoagulability can be caused by medications (oral contraceptives, hormonal replacement therapy) or disease (malignancy, surgery) or may be the result of inherited gene defects. The most common inherited cause in white populations is resistance to activated protein C, also known as factor V Leiden. The trait is present in approximately 3% of healthy American men and in 20–40% of patients with idiopathic venous thrombosis. Other major risks for hypercoagulability include the following: deficiencies or dysfunction of protein C, protein S, and antithrombin; prothrombin gene mutation; hyperhomocysteinemia and the presence of antiphospholipid antibodies (lupus anticoagulant and anticardiolipin antibody).

PE has multiple physiologic effects. Physical obstruction of the vascular bed and vasoconstriction from neurohumoral reflexes both increase pulmonary vascular resistance. Massive thrombus may cause right ventricular failure. Vascular obstruction increases physiologic dead space (wasted ventilation) and leads to hypoxemia through right-to-left shunting, decreased cardiac output, and surfactant depletion causing atelectasis. Reflex bronchoconstriction promotes wheezing and increased work of breathing.

▶ Clinical Findings

A. Symptoms and Signs

The clinical diagnosis of PE is notoriously difficult for two reasons. First, the clinical findings depend on both the size of the embolus and the patient's preexisting cardiopulmonary status. Second, common symptoms and signs of pulmonary emboli are not specific to this disorder (Table 9–18).

Indeed, no single symptom or sign or combination of clinical findings is specific to PE. Some findings are fairly sensitive: dyspnea and pain on inspiration occur in 75–85% and 65–75% of patients, respectively. Tachypnea is the only sign reliably found in more than half of patients. A common clinical strategy is to use combinations of clinical findings to identify patients' risk for PE. For example, 97% of patients in the original Prospective Investigation of Pulmonary Embolism Diagnosis (PIOPED I) study with angiographically proved pulmonary emboli had one or more of three findings: dyspnea, chest pain with breathing, or tachypnea. Wells and colleagues have published and validated a simple clinical decision rule that quantifies and dichotomizes this clinical risk assessment, allowing diversion of patients deemed unlikely to have PE to a simpler diagnostic algorithm (see Integrated Approach to Diagnosis of Pulmonary Embolism).

B. Laboratory Findings

The **ECG** is abnormal in 70% of patients with PE. However, the most common abnormalities are sinus tachycardia and nonspecific ST and T wave changes, each seen in approximately 40% of patients. Five percent or less of patients in

Table 9–18. Frequency of specific symptoms and signs in patients at risk for pulmonary thromboembolism.

	UPET[1] PE + (n = 327)	PIOPEDI[2] PE + (n = 117)	PIOPEDI[2] PE − (n = 248)
Symptoms			
Dyspnea	84%	73%	72%
Respirophasic chest pain	74%	66%	59%
Cough	53%	37%	36%
Leg pain	NR	26%	24%
Hemoptysis	30%	13%	8%
Palpitations	NR	10%	18%
Wheezing	NR	9%	11%
Anginal pain	14%	4%	6%
Signs			
Respiratory rate ≥ 16 UPET, ≥ 20 PIOPED I	92%	70%	68%
Crackles (rales)	58%	51%	40%[3]
Heart rate ≥ 100/min	44%	30%	24%
Fourth heart sound (S_4)	NR	24%	13%[3]
Accentuated pulmonary component of second heart sound (S_2P)	53%	23%	13%[3]
T ≥ 37.5°C UPET, ≥ 38.5°C PIOPED	43%	7%	12%
Homans sign	NR	4%	2%
Pleural friction rub	NR	3%	2%
Third heart sound (S_3)	NR	3%	4%
Cyanosis	19%	1%	2%

[1]Data from the Urokinase-Streptokinase Pulmonary Embolism Trial (UPET), as reported in Bell WR et al. The clinical features of submassive and massive pulmonary emboli. Am J Med. 1977 Mar;62(3):355–60. [PMID: 842555]
[2]Data from patients enrolled in the PIOPED I study, as reported in Stein PD et al. Clinical, laboratory, roentgenographic, and electrocardiographic findings in patients with acute pulmonary embolism and no preexisting cardiac or pulmonary disease. Chest. 1991 Sep; 100(3):598–603. [PMID: 1909617]
[3]$P < 0.05$ comparing patients in the PIOPED I study.
PE+, confirmed diagnosis of pulmonary embolism; PE-, diagnosis of pulmonary embolism ruled out; NR, not reported.

the PIOPED I study had P pulmonale, right ventricular hypertrophy, right axis deviation, and right bundle branch block.

Arterial blood gases usually reveal acute respiratory alkalosis due to hyperventilation. The arterial Po_2 and the alveolar-arterial oxygen difference ($A-a-Do_2$) are usually abnormal in patients with PE compared with healthy, age-matched controls. However, arterial blood gases are not diagnostic: among patients who were evaluated in the PIOPED I study, neither the Po_2 nor the $A-a-Do_2$ differentiated between those with and those without pulmonary emboli. Profound hypoxia with a normal chest radiograph in the absence of preexisting lung disease is highly suspicious for PE.

Plasma levels of **D-dimer**, a degradation product of cross-linked fibrin, are elevated in the presence of thrombus. Using a D-dimer threshold between 300 and 500 ng/mL (300 and 500 mcg/L), a rapid quantitative enzyme-linked immunosorbent assay (ELISA) has shown a sensitivity for venous thromboembolism of 95–97% and a

specificity of 45%. Therefore, a D-dimer < 500 ng/mL (< 500 mcg/L) using a rapid quantitative ELISA provides strong evidence against venous thromboembolism, with a likelihood ratio of 0.11–0.13. Appropriate diagnostic thresholds have not been established for patients in whom D-dimer is elevated.

Serum troponin I, troponin T, and plasma B-type natriuretic peptide (BNP) levels are typically higher in patients with PE compared with those without embolism; the presence and magnitude of the elevation are not useful in diagnosis, but correlate with adverse outcomes, including mechanical ventilation, prolonged hospitalization, and death.

C. Imaging and Special Examinations

1. Chest radiography—The chest radiograph is necessary to exclude other common lung diseases and to permit interpretation of the ventilation-perfusion ($\dot{V}/\dot{Q}$) scan, but it does not establish the diagnosis by itself. The chest

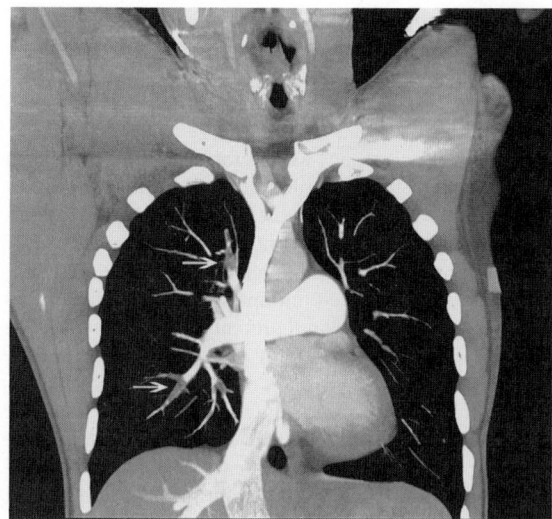

▲ **Figure 9–8. Pulmonary emboli.** Pulmonary CT angiogram demonstrating multiple segmental and subsegmental pulmonary emboli (arrows) in the right lung in a patient with a spontaneous upper extremity deep venous thrombosis.

radiograph was normal in only 12% of patients with confirmed PE in the PIOPED I study. The most frequent findings were atelectasis, parenchymal infiltrates, and pleural effusions. However, the prevalence of these findings was the same in hospitalized patients without PE. A prominent central pulmonary artery with local oligemia (Westermark sign) or pleural-based areas of increased opacity that represent intraparenchymal hemorrhage (Hampton hump) are uncommon. Paradoxically, the chest radiograph may be most suggestive of PE when normal in the setting of hypoxemia.

2. CT—Helical CT pulmonary angiography is used as the initial diagnostic study in North America for suspected PE (Figure 9–8). Helical CT pulmonary angiography requires administration of intravenous radiocontrast dye but is otherwise noninvasive. A high quality study is very sensitive for the detection of thrombus in the proximal pulmonary arteries but less so in more distal arteries where it may miss as many as 75% of subsegmental defects, compared with pulmonary angiography. Comparing helical CT pulmonary angiography to the (V̇/Q̇) scan as the initial test for PE, detection of thrombi is roughly comparable, although more alternative pulmonary diagnoses are made with CT scanning.

Test characteristics of helical CT pulmonary angiography vary widely by study and facility. Factors influencing results include patient size and cooperation, the type and quality of the scanner, the imaging protocol, and the experience of the interpreting radiologist. The 2006 PIOPED II study, using multidetector (four-row) helical CT and excluding the 6% of patients whose studies were "inconclusive," reported sensitivity of 83% and specificity of 96%.

A 15–20% false-negative rate is high for a screening test, and raises the practical question whether it is safe to withhold anticoagulation in patients with a negative helical CT. Research data provide two complementary answers. The insight of PIOPED I, that the clinical assessment of pretest probability improves the performance of the (V̇/Q̇) scan, was confirmed with helical CT pulmonary angiography in PIOPED II, where positive and negative predictive values were highest in patients with concordant clinical assessments but poor with conflicting assessments. The negative predictive value of a normal helical CT in patients with a high pretest probability was only 60%. Therefore, a normal helical CT alone does not exclude PE in high-risk patients, and either empiric therapy or further testing is indicated.

A large, prospective trial, the Christopher Study, incorporated objective, validated pretest clinical assessment into diagnostic algorithms using D-dimer measurement. In this study, patients with a high pretest probability and a negative helical CT pulmonary angiogram who were not receiving anticoagulation had a low (< 2%) 3-month incidence of subsequent PE. This low rate of complications supports the contention that many false-negative studies represent clinically insignificant, small distal thrombi and provides support for monitoring most patients with a high-quality negative helical CT pulmonary angiogram off therapy (see Integrated Approach to Diagnosis of Pulmonary Embolism below). The rate of false-positive helical CT pulmonary angiograms and overtreatment of PE has not been as well studied to date.

3. Ventilation-perfusion lung scanning—A perfusion scan is performed by injecting radiolabeled microaggregated albumin into the venous system, allowing the particles to embolize to the pulmonary capillary bed. To perform a ventilation scan, the patient breathes a radioactive gas or aerosol while the distribution of radioactivity in the lungs is recorded. A defect on perfusion scanning represents diminished blood flow to that region of the lung. This finding is not specific for PE. Defects in the perfusion scan are interpreted in conjunction with the ventilation scan to give a high, low, or intermediate (indeterminate) probability that PE is the cause of the abnormalities. Criteria for the combined interpretation of ventilation and perfusion scans (commonly referred to as a single test, the (V̇/Q̇) scan) are complex, confusing, and not completely standardized. A normal perfusion scan excludes the diagnosis of clinically significant PE (negative predictive value of 91% in the PIOPED I study). A high-probability (V̇/Q̇) scan is most often defined as having two or more segmental perfusion defects in the presence of normal ventilation and is sufficient to make the diagnosis of PE in most instances (positive predictive value of 88% among PIOPED I patients). (V̇/Q̇) scans are most helpful when they are either normal or indicate a high probability of PE. Such readings are reliable—interobserver agreement is best for normal and high-probability scans—and they carry predictive power. The likelihood ratios associated with normal and high-probability scans are 0.10 and 18, respectively, indicating significant and frequently conclusive changes from pretest to posttest probability.

However, 75% of PIOPED I ($\dot{V}/\dot{Q}$) scans were nondiagnostic, ie, of low or intermediate probability. At angiography, these patients had an overall incidence of PE of 14% and 30%, respectively.

One of the most important findings of PIOPED I was that the clinical assessment of pretest probability could be used to aid the interpretation of the ($\dot{V}/Q$) scan. For patients with low-probability ($\dot{V}/Q$) scans and a low (20% or less) clinical pretest probability of PE, the diagnosis was confirmed in only 4%. Such patients may reasonably be observed off therapy without angiography. All other patients with nondiagnostic ($\dot{V}/Q$) scans require further testing to determine the presence of venous thromboembolism.

4. Venous thrombosis studies—Seventy percent of patients with PE will have DVT on evaluation, and approximately half of patients with DVT will have PE on angiography. Since the history and physical examination are neither sensitive nor specific for PE and since the results of ($\dot{V}/Q$) scanning are frequently equivocal, documentation of DVT in a patient with suspected PE establishes the need for treatment and may preclude further testing.

Commonly available diagnostic techniques include venous ultrasonography, impedance plethysmography, and contrast venography. In most centers, **venous ultrasonography** is the test of choice to detect proximal DVT. Inability to compress the common femoral or popliteal veins in symptomatic patients is diagnostic of first-episode DVT (positive predictive value of 97%); full compressibility of both sites excludes proximal DVT (negative predictive value of 98%). The test is less accurate in distal thrombi, recurrent thrombi, or in asymptomatic patients. Impedance plethysmography relies on changes in electrical impedance between patent and obstructed veins to determine the presence of thrombus. Accuracy is comparable though not quite as high as ultrasonography. Both ultrasonography and impedance plethysmography are useful in the serial examination of patients with high clinical suspicion of venous thromboembolism but negative leg studies. In patients with suspected first-episode DVT and a negative ultrasound or impedance plethysmography examination, multiple studies have confirmed the safety of withholding anticoagulation while conducting two sequential studies on days 1–3 and 7–10. Similarly, patients with nondiagnostic ($\dot{V}/Q$) scans and an initial negative venous ultrasound or impedance plethysmography examination may be monitored off therapy with serial leg studies over 2 weeks. When serial examinations are negative for proximal DVT, the risk of subsequent venous thromboembolism over the following 6 months is less than 2%.

Contrast venography remains the reference standard for the diagnosis of DVT. An intraluminal filling defect is diagnostic of venous thrombosis. However, venography has significant shortcomings and has been replaced by venous ultrasound as the diagnostic procedure of choice. Venography may be useful in complex situations where there is discrepancy between clinical suspicion and noninvasive testing.

5. Pulmonary angiography—Pulmonary angiography remains the reference standard for the diagnosis of PE.

An intraluminal filling defect in more than one projection establishes a definitive diagnosis. Secondary findings highly suggestive of PE include abrupt arterial cutoff, asymmetry of blood flow—especially segmental oligemia—or a prolonged arterial phase with slow filling. Pulmonary angiography was performed in 755 patients in the PIOPED I study. A definitive diagnosis was established in 97%; in 3% the studies were nondiagnostic. Four patients (0.8%) with negative angiograms subsequently had pulmonary thromboemboli at autopsy. Serial angiography has demonstrated minimal resolution of thrombus prior to day 7 following presentation. Thus, negative angiography within 7 days of presentation excludes the diagnosis.

Pulmonary angiography is a safe but invasive procedure with well-defined morbidity and mortality data. Minor complications occur in approximately 5% of patients. Most are allergic contrast reactions, transient kidney injury, or percutaneous catheter–related injuries; cardiac perforation and arrhythmias are reported but rare. Among the PIOPED I patients who underwent angiography, there were five deaths (0.7%) directly related to the procedure.

The appropriate role of pulmonary angiography in the diagnosis of PE remains a subject of ongoing debate. There is wide agreement that angiography is indicated in any patient in whom the diagnosis is in doubt when there is a high clinical pretest probability of PE or when the diagnosis of PE must be established with certainty, as when anticoagulation is contraindicated or placement of an inferior vena cava filter is contemplated.

▶ **Integrated Approach to Diagnosis of Pulmonary Embolism**

An integrated approach to diagnosis of PE uses the clinical likelihood of venous thromboembolism derived from a clinical prediction rule (Table 9–19) along with the results of diagnostic tests to come to one of three decision points: to establish venous thromboembolism (PE or DVT) as the diagnosis, to exclude venous thromboembolism with sufficient confidence to follow the patient off anticoagulation, or to refer the patient for additional testing. An ideal diagnostic algorithm would proceed in a cost-effective, stepwise fashion to come to these decision points at minimal risk to the patient. Most North American centers use a rapid D-dimer and helical CT pulmonary angiography based diagnostic algorithm (Figure 9–9). The standard ($\dot{V}/Q$) scan based algorithm (Table 9–20) remains useful in many patients, especially those who are not able to undergo CT pulmonary angiography (eg, those with advanced chronic kidney disease). In the rigorously conducted Christopher Study, the incidence of venous thromboembolism was only 1.3% and fatal PE occurred in just 0.5% of persons monitored for 3 months off anticoagulation therapy after objective, validated tools for clinical assessment, quantitative rapid D-dimer assays and a negative helical CT pulmonary angiography. The incidence of PE following a negative evaluation by these three means is comparable to that seen following negative pulmonary angiography.

Table 9–19. Clinical prediction rule for pulmonary embolism (PE).

Variable	Points
Clinical symptoms and signs of deep venous thrombosis (DVT) (leg swelling and pain with palpation of deep veins)	3.0
Alternative diagnosis less likely than PE	3.0
Heart rate > 100 beats/min	1.5
Immobilization for more than 3 days or surgery in previous 4 weeks	1.5
Previous PE or DVT	1.5
Hemoptysis	1.0
Cancer (with treatment within past 6 months or palliative care)	1.0
Three-tiered clinical probability assessment	**Score**
High	> 6.0
Moderate	2.0 to 6.0
Low	< 2.0
Dichotomous clinical probability assessment	**Score**
PE likely	> 4.0
PE unlikely	< or = 4.0

Data from Wells PS et al. Derivation of a simple clinical model to categorize patients' probability of pulmonary embolism: increasing the models' utility with the SimpliRED D-dimer. Thromb Haemost. 2000 Mar;83(3):416–20. [PMID: 10744147]

Prevention

Venous thromboembolism is often clinically silent until it presents with significant morbidity or mortality. It is a prevalent disease, clearly associated with identifiable risk factors. For example, the incidence of proximal DVT, PE, and fatal PE in untreated patients undergoing hip fracture surgery is reported to be 10–20%, 4–10%, and 0.2–5%, respectively. There is unambiguous evidence of the efficacy of prophylactic therapy in this and other clinical situations, yet it remains underused. Only about 50% of surgical deaths from PE had received any form of preventive therapy. Discussion of strategies for the prevention of venous thromboembolism can be found in Chapter 14.

Treatment

A. Anticoagulation

Anticoagulation is not definitive therapy but a form of secondary prevention. Heparin binds to and accelerates the ability of antithrombin to inactivate thrombin, factor Xa, and factor IXa. It thus retards additional thrombus formation, allowing endogenous fibrinolytic mechanisms to lyse existing clot. The standard regimen of heparin followed by 6 months of oral warfarin results in an 80–90% reduction in the risk of both recurrent venous thrombosis and death from PE. LMWHs are as effective as unfractionated heparin in the treatment of venous thromboembolism (see Tables 14–15, 14–18, 14–19).

The optimal duration of anticoagulation therapy for venous thromboembolism is unknown. There appears to be a protective benefit to continued anticoagulation in first-episode venous thromboembolism (twice the rate of recurrence in 6 weeks compared with 6 months of therapy) and recurrent disease (eightfold risk of recurrence in 6 months compared with 4 years of therapy). These studies do not distinguish patients with reversible risk factors, such as surgery or transient immobility, from patients who have a nonreversible hypercoagulable state such as factor V Leiden, inhibitor deficiency, antiphospholipid syndrome, or malignancy. An RCT of low-dose warfarin (INR 1.5–2.0) versus no therapy following 6 months of standard therapy in patients with idiopathic DVT was stopped early. The protective benefits of continued

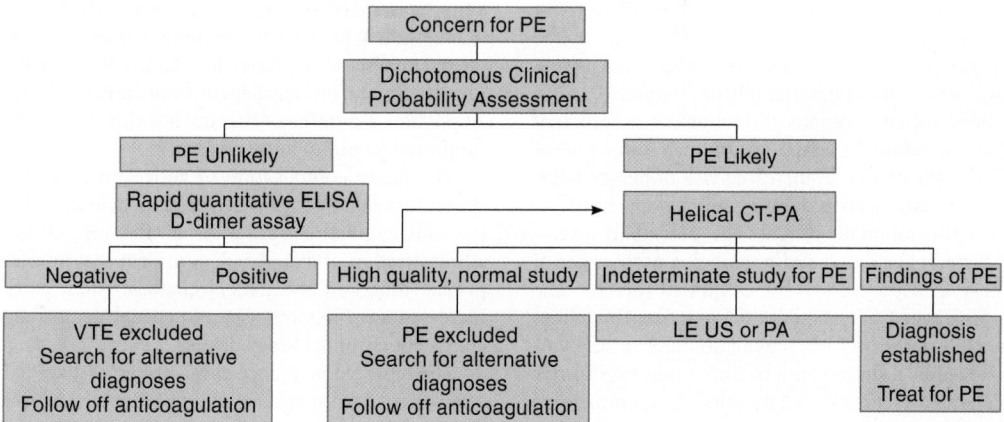

▲ **Figure 9–9.** D-dimer and helical CT-PA based diagnostic algorithm for PE. CT-PA, CT pulmonary angiogram; PE, pulmonary embolism; ELISA, enzyme-linked immunosorbent assay; VTE, venous thromboembolic disease; LE US, lower extremity venous ultrasound for deep venous thrombosis; PA, pulmonary angiogram. (Reproduced, with permission, from van Belle A et al. Effectiveness of managing suspected pulmonary embolism using an algorithm combining clinical probability, D-dimer testing, and computed tomography. JAMA. 2006 Jan 11;295(2):172–9.)

Table 9–20. Pulmonary ventilation-perfusion scan based diagnostic algorithm for PE.

Clinical concern for PE:
1. Analyze by three-tiered clinical probability assessment (Table 9–19)
2. Obtain (V̇/Q̇) scan
3. Match results in the following table

	Clinical suspicion for PE by clinical probability assessment		
	HIGH	**MODERATE**	**LOW**
High probability	STOP. Diagnosis established. Treat for PE.	STOP. Diagnosis established. Treat for PE.	Diagnosis likely (56% in PIOPED I, but small number of patients). Treat for PE or evaluate further with LE US or CT-PA.
Indeterminate	Diagnosis highly likely (66% in PIOPED I). Treat for PE or evaluate further with LE US or CT-PA.	Uncertain diagnosis. Evaluate further with LE US or CT-PA.	Uncertain diagnosis. Evaluate further with LE US or CT-PA.
Low probability	Uncertain diagnosis. Evaluate further with LE US or CT-PA.	Uncertain diagnosis. Evaluate further with LE US or CT-PA.	STOP. Diagnosis excluded; monitor off anticoagulation. Consider alternative diagnoses.
Normal	STOP. Diagnosis excluded; monitor off anticoagulation. Consider alternative diagnoses.	STOP. Diagnosis excluded; monitor off anticoagulation. Consider alternative diagnoses.	STOP. Diagnosis excluded; monitor off anticoagulation. Consider alternative diagnoses.

Data from The PIOPED Investigators. Value of the ventilation/perfusion scan in acute pulmonary embolism: results of the Prospective Investigation of Pulmonary Embolism Diagnosis (PIOPED). JAMA. 1990 May 23–30;263(20):2753–9. [PMID: 2332918]

CT-PA, helical CT pulmonary angiography; LE US, lower extremity venous ultrasound for DVT; PE, pulmonary embolism.

anticoagulation include fewer DVTs in addition to a trend toward lower mortality despite more hemorrhage in the warfarin group. Risk reductions were consistent across groups with and without inherited thrombophilia.

For many patients, venous thrombosis is a recurrent disease, and continued therapy results in a lower rate of recurrence at the cost of an increased risk of hemorrhage. Therefore, the appropriate duration of therapy needs to take into consideration the patient's age, potentially reversible risk factors, likelihood and potential consequences of hemorrhage, and preferences for continued therapy. The current American College of Chest Physician Guidelines recommend 3 months of anticoagulation after a first episode provoked by a surgery or a transient nonsurgical risk factor. Extended therapy (6–12 months) is recommended for unprovoked or recurrrent episode with a low to moderate risk of bleeding. For patients with cancer, extended therapy is recommended regardless of bleeding risk and LMWH is preferred over vitamin K antagonists. It is reasonable to continue therapy for 6 months after a first episode when there is a reversible risk factor, 12 months after

a first-episode of idiopathic thrombosis, and 6–12 months to indefinitely in patients with nonreversible risk factors or recurrent disease. D-dimer testing has been suggested to identify those who may benefit from continued anticoagulation after 3 months of therapy but clinical data have not supported its utility in this regard.

The major complication of anticoagulation is hemorrhage. Risk factors for hemorrhage include the intensity of the anticoagulation; duration of therapy; concomitant administration of drugs such as aspirin that interfere with platelet function; and patient characteristics, particularly increased age, previous gastrointestinal hemorrhage, and coexistent chronic kidney disease.

The reported incidence of major hemorrhage following intravenous administration of unfractionated heparin is nil to 7%; that of fatal hemorrhage is nil to 2%. The incidence with LMWHs is not statistically different. There is no information comparing hemorrhage rates at different doses of heparin. The risk of death from another pulmonary embolism during subtherapeutic heparin administration in the first 24–48 hours after diagnosis is significant; it appears to outweigh the risk of short-term supratherapeutic heparin levels. The incidence of hemorrhage during therapy with warfarin is reported to be between 3% and 4% per patient year. The frequency varies with the target INR and is consistently higher when the INR exceeds 4.0. There is no apparent additional antithrombotic benefit in venous thromboembolism with a target INR above 2.0–3.0 (see Chapter 14).

B. Thrombolytic Therapy

Streptokinase, urokinase, and recombinant tissue plasminogen activator (rt-PA; alteplase) increase plasmin levels and thereby directly lyse intravascular thrombi. In patients with established PE, thrombolytic therapy accelerates resolution of emboli within the first 24 hours compared with standard heparin therapy. This is a consistent finding using angiography, ($\dot{V}/\dot{Q}$) scanning, echocardiography, and direct measurement of pulmonary artery pressures. However, at 1 week and 1 month after diagnosis, these agents show no difference in outcome compared with heparin and warfarin. There is no evidence that thrombolytic therapy improves mortality. Subtle improvements in pulmonary function, including improved single-breath diffusing capacity and a lower incidence of exercise-induced pulmonary hypertension, have been observed. The reliability and clinical importance of these findings is unclear. The major disadvantages of thrombolytic therapy compared with heparin are its greater cost and significant increase in major hemorrhagic complications. The incidence of intracranial hemorrhage in patients with PE treated with alteplase is 2.1% compared with 0.2% in patients treated with heparin.

Current evidence supports thrombolytic therapy for PE in patients at high risk for death in whom the more rapid resolution of thrombus may be lifesaving. Such patients are usually hemodynamically unstable despite heparin therapy. Absolute contraindications to thrombolytic therapy include active internal bleeding and stroke within the past 2 months. Major contraindications include uncontrolled hypertension and surgery or trauma within the past 6 weeks. The role of thrombolysis in patients who are hemodynamically stable but with echocardiographic evidence of right heart strain from acute pulmonary embolism is unclear and is subject to considerable practice variation.

C. Additional Measures

Interruption of the inferior vena cava may be indicated in patients with a major contraindication to anticoagulation who have or are at high risk for development of proximal DVT or PE. Placement of an inferior vena cava filter is also recommended for recurrent thromboembolism despite adequate anticoagulation, for chronic recurrent embolism with a compromised pulmonary vascular bed (eg, in pulmonary hypertension), and with the concurrent performance of surgical pulmonary embolectomy or pulmonary thromboendarterectomy. Percutaneous transjugular placement of a mechanical filter is the preferred mode of inferior vena cava interruption. These devices reduce the short-term incidence of PE in patients presenting with proximal lower extremity DVT. However, they are associated with a twofold increased risk of recurrent DVT in the first 2 years following placement so plans must be usually made for their subsequent removal.

In rare critically ill patients for whom thrombolytic therapy is contraindicated or unsuccessful, mechanical or surgical extraction of thrombus may be indicated. Pulmonary embolectomy is an emergency procedure of last resort with a very high mortality rate. It is performed only in a few specialized centers. Several catheter devices to fragment and extract thrombus through a transvenous approach have been reported in small numbers of patients. Comparative outcomes with surgery, thrombolytic therapy, or heparin have not been studied.

▶ Prognosis

PE is estimated to cause more than 50,000 deaths annually. **In the majority of deaths, PE is not recognized antemortem or death occurs before specific treatment can be initiated.** These statistics highlight the importance of preventive therapy in high-risk patients (see Chapter 14). The outlook for patients with diagnosed and appropriately treated PE is generally good. Overall prognosis depends on the underlying disease rather than the PE itself. Death from recurrent thromboemboli is uncommon, occurring in less than 3% of cases. Perfusion defects resolve in most survivors. Chronic thromboembolic pulmonary hypertension develops in approximately 1% of patients. Selected patients may benefit from pulmonary endarterectomy.

American College of Emergency Physicians Clinical Policies Subcommittee on Critical Issues in the Evaluation and Management of Adult Patients Presenting to the Emergency Department With Suspected Pulmonary Embolism, Fesmire FM et al. Critical issues in the evaluation and management of adult patients presenting to the emergency department with suspected pulmonary embolism. Ann Emerg Med. 2011 Jun;57(6):628–652.e75. [PMID: 21621092]

Burns SK et al. Diagnostic imaging and risk stratification of patients with acute pulmonary embolism. Cardiol Rev. 2012 Jan–Feb;20(1):15–24. [PMID: 22143281]

Goldhaber SZ et al. Pulmonary embolism and deep vein thrombosis. Lancet. 2012 May12;379(9828):1835–46. [PMID: 22494827]

Jaff MR et al; American Heart Association Council on Cardiopulmonary, Critical Care, Perioperative and Resuscitation; American Heart Association Council on Peripheral Vascular Disease; American Heart Association Council on Arteriosclerosis, Thrombosis and Vascular Biology. Management of massive and submassive pulmonary embolism, iliofemoral deep vein thrombosis, and chronic thromboembolic pulmonary hypertension: a scientific statement from the American Heart Association. Circulation. 2011 Apr26;123(16):1788–830. [PMID: 21422387]

Kearon C et al. Antithrombotic therapy for VTE disease: Antithrombotic Therapy and Prevention of Thrombosis, 9th ed: American College of Chest Physicians Evidence-Based Clinical Practice Guideline. Chest. 2012 Feb;141(2 Suppl): e419S–94S. [PMID: 22315268]

Merrigan JM et al. JAMA patient page. Pulmonary embolism. JAMA. 2013 Feb6;309(5):504. [PMID: 23385279]

PULMONARY HYPERTENSION

▶ Dyspnea, fatigue, chest pain, and syncope on exertion.

▶ Narrow splitting of second heart sound with loud pulmonary component; findings of right ventricular hypertrophy and heart failure in advanced disease.

▶ Electrocardiographic evidence of right ventricular strain or hypertrophy and right atrial enlargement.

▶ Enlarged central pulmonary arteries on chest radiograph.

▶ Elevated right ventricular systolic pressure on two-dimensional echocardiography with Doppler flow studies.

▶ General Considerations

Pulmonary hypertension is a complex problem characterized by pathologic elevation in pulmonary arterial pressure. Normal pulmonary artery systolic pressure at rest is 15–30 mm Hg, with a mean pressure between 10 mm Hg and 18 mm Hg. The pulmonary circulation is a low pressure, low resistance system due to its large cross-sectional area and it can accommodate significant increase in blood flow during exercise. The primary pathologic mechanism in pulmonary hypertension is an increase in pulmonary vascular resistance that leads to an increase in the pulmonary systolic pressure > 30 mm Hg or the mean pressure > 20 mm Hg.

The World Health Organization currently classifies pulmonary hypertension based on similarities in pathologic mechanisms and includes the following five groups.

Group 1 (pulmonary arterial hypertension secondary to various disorders): This group gathers diseases that localize directly to the pulmonary arteries leading to structural changes, smooth muscle hypertrophy, and endothelial dysfunction. This group includes idiopathic (formerly primary) pulmonary arterial hypertension, heritable pulmonary arterial hypertension, HIV infection, portal hypertension, drugs and toxins, connective tissue disorders, congenital heart disease, schistosomiasis, chronic hemolytic anemia, primary veno-occlusive disease, and pulmonary capillary hemangiomatosis.

Group 2 (pulmonary venous hypertension secondary to left heart disease): Often referred to as pulmonary venous hypertension or "post-capillary" pulmonary hypertension, this group includes left ventricular systolic or diastolic dysfunction and valvular heart disease.

Group 3 (pulmonary hypertension secondary to lung disease or hypoxemia): This group is caused by advanced obstructive and restrictive lung disease including COPD, interstitial lung disease, pulmonary fibrosis, bronchiectasis, as well as other causes of chronic hypoxemia such as sleep-disordered breathing, alveolar hypoventilation syndromes, and high altitude exposure.

Group 4 (pulmonary hypertension secondary to chronic thromboembolism): This group consists of patients with pulmonary hypertension due to thromboembolic occlusion of the proximal and distal pulmonary arteries. (The current classification no longer includes patients with non-thrombotic occlusion such as tumors or foreign objects.)

Group 5 (pulmonary arterial hypertension secondary to hematologic, systemic, metabolic, or miscellaneous causes): These patients have pulmonary hypertension secondary to hematologic disorders (eg, myeloproliferative disorders, splenectomy), systemic disorders (eg, sarcoidosis, vasculitis, pulmonary Langerhans cell histiocytosis, neurofibromatosis type 1), metabolic disorders (eg, glycogen storage disease, Gaucher disease, thyroid disease), and miscellaneous causes (tumor embolization, external compression of the pulmonary vasculature, end-stage renal disease on dialysis).

The clinical severity of pulmonary hypertension is classified according to the New York Heart Association (NYHA) classification system, which was originally developed for heart failure but subsequently modified by the World Health Organization; it is based primarily on symptoms and functional status.

Class I: Pulmonary hypertension without limitation of physical activity. No dyspnea, fatigue, chest pain or near syncope with exertion.

Class II: Pulmonary hypertension resulting in slight limitation of physical activity. No symptoms at rest but ordinary physical activity causes dyspnea, fatigue, chest pain, or near syncope.

Class III: Pulmonary hypertension resulting in marked limitation of physical activity. No symptoms at rest but less than ordinary activity causes dyspnea, fatigue, chest pain, or near syncope.

Class IV: Pulmonary hypertension with inability to perform any physical activity without symptoms. Evidence of right heart failure. Dyspnea and fatigue at rest and worsening of symptoms with any activity.

▶ Clinical Findings

A. Symptoms and Signs

There are no specific symptoms or signs but patients with pulmonary hypertension typically experience dyspnea with exertion and even, with advanced disease, at rest. Anginal pain, nonproductive cough, malaise, and fatigue may be present. Syncope occurs with exertion when there is insufficient cardiac output or if there is an arrhythmia. Hemoptysis is a rare but life-threatening event in pulmonary hypertension usually caused by the rupture of a pulmonary artery.

Findings on physical examination can include jugular venous distention, accentuated pulmonary valve component of the second heart sound, right-sided third heart sound, tricuspid regurgitation murmur, hepatomegaly, and lower extremity edema. Cyanosis can occur in patients with an open patent foramen ovale and right-to-left shunt due to increased right atrial pressure.

B. Laboratory Findings

Routine blood work is often normal; any abnormalities noted are usually related to the underlying disease in secondary pulmonary hypertension. On arterial blood gas analysis, patients with idiopathic pulmonary arterial hypertension often have normal Pao_2 at rest but show evidence of hyperventilation with a decrease in $Paco_2$. All patients should be screened for HIV and collagen vascular disease.

The ECG is typically normal except in advanced disease where right ventricular hypertrophy (right axis deviation, incomplete right bundle branch block) and right atrial enlargement (peaked P wave in the inferior and right-sided leads) can be noted.

C. Imaging and Special Examinations

Radiographs and CT scans of the chest are useful in diagnosis. Enlargement of the right and left main pulmonary arteries is common; right ventricular and right atrial enlargement is seen in advanced disease. Chest imaging and pulmonary function testing are also useful in determining the cause of pulmonary hypertension for patients in Group 3 (pulmonary hypertension due to lung disease). On pulmonary function testing, the combination of decreased single-breath diffusing capacity, normal FVC on spirometry, normal TLC on lung volume measurement, and increased wasted ventilation on cardiopulmonary exercise testing is suggestive of pathologically increased pulmonary arterial pressures.

Patients in whom pulmonary hypertension is suspected should undergo echocardiography with Doppler flow. The echocardiogram is useful in the assessment of underlying cardiac disease while Doppler flow can estimate the right ventricular systolic pressure. Right ventricular systolic pressure can be estimated based on tricuspid jet velocity and right atrial pressure. The severity of pulmonary hypertension can also be assessed based on the right ventricular size and function. Right-sided cardiac catheterization remains the gold standard for the diagnosis and quantification of pulmonary hypertension and should be performed prior to initiation of advanced therapies. Estimated pressures on echocardiogram correlate with right heart catheterization measurement but can vary by at least 10 mm Hg in > 50% of cases so should not be used to direct therapy. Cardiac catheterization is particularly helpful in differentiating pulmonary arterial hypertension from pulmonary venous hypertension by assessment of the drop in pressure across the pulmonary circulation, also known as the transpulmonary gradient. Vasodilator challenge is often performed during right heart catheterization and for a significant acute vasodilator response consists of a drop in mean pulmonary pressure of > 10 mm Hg (or 20%) to < 40 mm Hg.

In patients with unexplained pulmonary hypertension who have a history of PE or risk factors for thromboembolic disease, chronic thromboembolic disease (Group 4 pulmonary hypertension) should be excluded prior to diagnosing idiopathic pulmonary hypertension. (V̇/Q̇) lung scanning is a very sensitive test that can differentiate chronic thromboembolic pulmonary hypertension from idiopathic pulmonary arterial hypertension. Currently, pulmonary angiography is considered the most definitive diagnostic procedure for defining the distribution and extent of disease in chronic thromboembolic pulmonary hypertension.

▶ Treatment

Primary therapy refers to treatment directed at the underlying cause of pulmonary hypertension. Currently, there are no primary therapies available targeting the underlying lesion for patients in Group 1 (pulmonary arterial hypertension) but advanced therapies are available directly targeting the pulmonary hypertension itself. The advanced therapy chosen is typically based on patient symptoms and functional status according to the NYHA/WHO classification. Based on observational studies showing improved functional status and possible decreased mortality, first-line therapy consists of oral calcium channel blockers. However, these drugs should only be given to patients with positive acute vasodilator response when tested in the cardiac catheterization laboratory because they may be harmful to nonresponders. Preferred treatments for Group 1 patients in functional class II include oral endothelin receptor antagonists (ambrisentan, bosentan), and phosphodiesterase inhibitors (sildenafil, tadalafil). RCTs using either endothelin receptor antagonists or phosphodiesterase inhibitors have shown improvement in symptoms, 6-minute walk distance, WHO functional status, and hemodynamic measurements. For Group 1 patients in functional classes III and IV or Group 1 patients who are not responsive to previous therapies, prostanoid agents are available. Continuous long-term intravenous epoprostenol infusion improved mortality in a prospective RCT. Limitations to intravenous prostacyclins (epoprostenol, treprostinil) include short medication half-life requiring a reliable continuous infusion, difficulty in titration, and high cost of therapy. Inhaled prostanoids (iloprost, treprostinil) and subcutaneous prostanoids (treprostinil) are available for patients unable to tolerate continuous intravenous infusion. Oral formulation of prostacyclin analogs are in clinical trials.

Treatment of patients with Group 2 pulmonary hypertension (secondary to left heart failure) is discussed in Chapter 10.

Patients with Group 3 pulmonary hypertension (due to lung disease) and hypoxemia at rest or with physical activity should receive supplemental oxygen. In patients with COPD and hypoxemia, administration of supplemental oxygen for ≥ 15 hours per day has been shown to slow the progression of pulmonary hypertension. The main goal is to decrease pulmonary venous pressure by treating heart failure and volume overload.

For patients with Group 1 pulmonary hypertension and Group 4 pulmonary hypertension (due to thromboembolic disease), long-term anticoagulation is recommended and generally accepted, based solely on observational studies suggesting improvement in survival. For Group 4 patients in functional class IV and no response to other advanced therapies, thromboendarterectomy is recommended.

Only patients with surgically accessible lesions and acceptable perioperative risk should undergo this procedure.

Lung transplantation is a treatment option for selected patients with pulmonary hypertension when medical therapy is no longer effective. Double-lung transplant is the preferred method although single lung transplant is routinely done as well. In some cases, transplantation of the heart and both lungs is needed.

► Prognosis

The prognosis of idiopathic (some Group 1) pulmonary hypertension is poor and is not affected by therapies primarily used to treat symptoms. Conversely, the prognosis for patients with secondary pulmonary hypertension (some Group 1 and Groups 2–5) depends on the underlying disease and its response to treatment. In all cases, right ventricular function is one of the most important prognostic factors. The presence of cor pulmonale carries a poor survival outcome regardless of the underlying cause.

► When to Refer

Patients with pulmonary arterial hypertension and symptoms of dyspnea, fatigue, chest pain, or near syncope should be referred to a pulmonologist or cardiologist at a specialized center for expert management.

► When to Admit

- Patients with pulmonary hypertension, severe symptoms, and evidence of decompensated right heart failure with volume overload should be admitted to the hospital for aggressive diuresis.
- Patients with Group 1 pulmonary hypertension and functional class IV symptoms should be admitted to a specialized center for initiation of advanced therapies such as intravenous prostacyclins.

Hassoun PM et al. Update in pulmonary vascular diseases 2011. Am J Respir Crit Care Med. 2012 Jun;185(11):1177–82. [PMID: 22661524]
Lourenço AP et al. Current pathophysiological concepts and management of pulmonary hypertension. Int J Cardiol. 2012 Mar22;155(3):350–61. [PMID: 21641060]

PULMONARY VASCULITIS

Granulomatosis with polyangiitis is an idiopathic disease manifested by a combination of glomerulonephritis, necrotizing granulomatous vasculitis of the upper and lower respiratory tracts, and varying degrees of small vessel vasculitis. Chronic sinusitis, arthralgias, fever, skin rash, and weight loss are frequent presenting symptoms. Specific pulmonary complaints occur less often. The most common sign of lung disease is nodular pulmonary infiltrates, often with cavitation, seen on chest radiography. Tracheal stenosis and endobronchial disease are sometimes seen. The diagnosis is most often based on serologic testing and biopsy of lung, sinus tissue, or kidney with demonstration of necrotizing granulomatous vasculitis (see Chapter 20).

Allergic angiitis and granulomatosis (Churg-Strauss syndrome) is an idiopathic multisystem vasculitis of small and medium-sized arteries that occurs in patients with asthma. The skin and lungs are most often involved, but other organs, including the paranasal sinuses, the heart, gastrointestinal tract, liver, and peripheral nerves, may also be affected. Peripheral eosinophilia > 1500 cells/mcL (> 1.5 × 10^9/L) or > 10% of peripheral WBCs is the rule. Abnormalities on chest radiographs range from transient opacities to multiple nodules. This illness may be part of a spectrum that includes polyarteritis nodosa. The diagnosis requires demonstration of histologic features including fibrinoid necrotizing epithelioid and eosinophilic granulomas.

► Treatment

Treatment of pulmonary vasculitis usually requires corticosteroids and cyclophosphamide. Oral prednisone (1 mg/kg ideal body weight per day initially, tapering slowly to alternate-day therapy over 3–6 months) is the corticosteroid of choice; in granulomatosis with polyangiitis, some clinicians may use cyclophosphamide alone. For fulminant vasculitis, therapy may be initiated with intravenous methylprednisolone (up to 1 g intravenously per day) for several days. Cyclophosphamide (1–2 mg/kg ideal body weight orally per day initially, with dosage adjustments to avoid neutropenia) is given until complete remission is obtained and then is slowly tapered, and often replaced with methotrexate or azathioprine for maintenance therapy.

► Prognosis

Five-year survival rates in patients with these vasculitis syndromes have been improved by the combination therapy. Complete remissions can be achieved in over 90% of patients with granulomatosis with polyangiitis. The addition of trimethoprim-sulfamethoxazole (one double-strength tablet by mouth twice daily) to standard therapy may help prevent relapses.

Gibelin A et al. Epidemiology and etiology of wegener granulomatosis, microscopic polyangiitis, churg-strauss syndrome and goodpasture syndrome: vasculitides with frequent lung involvement. Semin Respir Crit Care Med. 2011 Jun;32(3): 264–73. [PMID: 21674413]

ALVEOLAR HEMORRHAGE SYNDROMES

Diffuse alveolar hemorrhage may occur in a variety of immune and nonimmune disorders. Hemoptysis, alveolar infiltrates on chest radiograph, anemia, dyspnea, and occasionally fever are characteristic. Rapid clearing of diffuse lung infiltrates within 2 days is a clue to the diagnosis of diffuse alveolar hemorrhage. Pulmonary hemorrhage can be associated with an increased single-breath diffusing capacity for carbon monoxide ($D_{L_{CO}}$).

Causes of **immune alveolar hemorrhage** have been classified as anti-basement membrane antibody disease (Goodpasture syndrome), vasculitis and collagen vascular disease (systemic lupus erythematosus, granulomatosis with polyangiitis, systemic necrotizing vasculitis, and others), and pulmonary capillaritis associated with idiopathic rapidly progressive glomerulonephritis. **Nonimmune causes** of diffuse hemorrhage include coagulopathy, mitral stenosis, necrotizing pulmonary infection, drugs (penicillamine), toxins (trimellitic anhydride), and idiopathic pulmonary hemosiderosis.

Goodpasture syndrome is idiopathic recurrent alveolar hemorrhage and rapidly progressive glomerulonephritis. The disease is mediated by anti-glomerular basement membrane antibodies. Goodpasture syndrome occurs mainly in men who are in their 30s and 40s. Hemoptysis is the usual presenting symptom, but pulmonary hemorrhage may be occult. Dyspnea, cough, hypoxemia, and diffuse bilateral alveolar infiltrates are typical features. Iron deficiency anemia and microscopic hematuria are usually present. The diagnosis is based on characteristic linear IgG deposits detected by immunofluorescence in glomeruli or alveoli and on the presence of anti-glomerular basement membrane antibody in serum. Combinations of immunosuppressive drugs (initially methylprednisolone, 30 mg/kg intravenously over 20 minutes every other day for three doses, followed by daily oral prednisone, 1 mg/kg/d; with cyclophosphamide, 2 mg/kg orally per day) and plasmapheresis have yielded excellent results.

Idiopathic pulmonary hemosiderosis is a disease of children or young adults characterized by recurrent pulmonary hemorrhage; in contrast to Goodpasture syndrome, renal involvement and anti-glomerular basement membrane antibodies are absent, but iron deficiency is typical. Treatment of acute episodes of hemorrhage with corticosteroids may be useful. Recurrent episodes of pulmonary hemorrhage may result in interstitial fibrosis and pulmonary failure.

de Prost N et al. Diffuse alveolar hemorrhage in immunocompetent patients: etiologies and prognosis revisited. Respir Med. 2012 Jul;106(7):1021–32. [PMID: 22541718]
Newsome BR et al. Diffuse alveolar hemorrhage. South Med J. 2011 Apr;104(4):269–74. [PMID: 21606695]

ENVIRONMENTAL & OCCUPATIONAL LUNG DISORDERS

SMOKE INHALATION

The inhalation of products of combustion may cause serious respiratory complications. As many as one-third of patients admitted to burn treatment units have pulmonary injury from smoke inhalation. **Morbidity and mortality due to smoke inhalation may exceed those attributed to the burns themselves.** The death rate of patients with both severe burns and smoke inhalation exceeds 50%.

All patients in whom significant smoke inhalation is suspected must be assessed for three consequences of smoke inhalation: impaired tissue oxygenation, thermal injury to the upper airway, and injury to the lower airways and lung parenchyma. Impaired tissue oxygenation may result from inhalation of a hypoxemia gas mixture, carbon monoxide or cyanide, or from alterations in $\dot{V}/\dot{Q}$ matching, and is an immediate threat to life. Immediate treatment with 100% oxygen is essential. The management of patients with carbon monoxide and cyanide poisoning is discussed in Chapter 38. The clinician must recognize that patients with carbon monoxide poisoning display a normal partial pressure of oxygen in arterial blood (Pao_2) but have a low *measured* (ie, not oximetric) hemoglobin saturation (Sao_2). Treatment with 100% oxygen should be continued until the measured carboxyhemoglobin level falls to less than 10% and concomitant metabolic acidosis has resolved.

Thermal injury to the mucosal surfaces of the upper airway occurs from inhalation of super-heated gases. Complications including mucosal edema, upper airway obstruction, and impaired ability to clear oral secretions usually become evident by 18–24 hours and produce inspiratory stridor. Respiratory failure occurs in severe cases. Early management (see Chapter 37) includes the use of a high-humidity face mask with supplemental oxygen, gentle suctioning to evacuate oral secretions, elevation of the head 30 degrees to promote clearing of secretions, and topical epinephrine to reduce edema of the oropharyngeal mucous membrane. Helium-oxygen gas mixtures (Heliox) may reduce labored breathing due to critical upper airway narrowing. Close monitoring with arterial blood gases and later with oximetry is important. Examination of the upper airway with a fiberoptic laryngoscope or bronchoscope is superior to routine physical examination. Endotracheal intubation is often necessary to establish airway patency and is likely to be necessary in patients with deep facial burns or oropharyngeal or laryngeal edema. Tracheotomy should be avoided if possible because of an increased risk of pneumonia and death from sepsis.

Injury to the lower airways and lung parenchyma results from inhalation of toxic gases and products of combustion, including aldehydes and organic acids. The site of lung injury depends on the solubility of the gases inhaled, the duration of exposure, and the size of inhaled particles that transport noxious gases to distal lung units. Bronchorrhea and bronchospasm are seen early after exposure along with dyspnea, tachypnea, and tachycardia. Labored breathing and cyanosis may follow. Physical examination at this stage reveals diffuse wheezing and rhonchi. Bronchiolar and alveolar edema (eg, ARDS) may develop within 1–2 days after exposure. Sloughing of the bronchiolar mucosa may occur within 2–3 days, leading to airway obstruction, atelectasis, and worsening hypoxemia. Bacterial colonization and pneumonia are common by 5–7 days after the exposure.

Treatment of smoke inhalation consists of supplemental oxygen, bronchodilators, suctioning of mucosal debris and mucopurulent secretions via an indwelling endotracheal tube, chest physical therapy to aid clearance of secretions, and adequate humidification of inspired gases. Positive end-expiratory pressure (PEEP) has been advocated to treat bronchiolar edema. Judicious fluid management and close monitoring for secondary bacterial infection with daily sputum Gram stains round out the management protocol.

The routine use of corticosteroids for lung injury from smoke inhalation has been shown to be ineffective and may even be harmful. Routine or prophylactic use of antibiotics is not recommended.

Patients who survive should be watched for the late development of bronchiolitis obliterans.

Albright JM et al. The acute pulmonary inflammatory response to the graded severity of smoke inhalation injury. Crit Care Med. 2012 Apr;40(4):1113–21. [PMID: 22067627]

PULMONARY ASPIRATION SYNDROMES

Aspiration of material into the tracheobronchial tree results from various disorders that impair normal deglutition, especially disturbances of consciousness and esophageal dysfunction.

1. Acute Aspiration of Gastric Contents (Mendelson Syndrome)

Acute aspiration of gastric contents may be catastrophic. The pulmonary response depends on the characteristics and amount of gastric contents aspirated. The more acidic the material, the greater the degree of chemical pneumonitis. Aspiration of pure gastric acid (pH < 2.5) causes extensive desquamation of the bronchial epithelium, bronchiolitis, hemorrhage, and pulmonary edema. Acute gastric aspiration is one of the most common causes of ARDS. The clinical picture is one of abrupt onset of respiratory distress, with cough, wheezing, fever, and tachypnea. Crackles may be audible at the bases of the lungs. Hypoxemia may be noted immediately after aspiration occurs. Radiographic abnormalities, consisting of patchy alveolar opacities in dependent lung zones, appear within a few hours. If particulate food matter has been aspirated along with gastric acid, radiographic features of bronchial obstruction may be observed. Fever and leukocytosis are common even in the absence of infection.

Treatment of acute aspiration of gastric contents consists of supplemental oxygen, measures to maintain the airway, and the usual measures for treatment of acute respiratory failure. There is no evidence to support the routine use of prophylactic antibiotics or corticosteroids after gastric aspiration. Secondary pulmonary infection, which occurs in about one-fourth of patients, typically appears 2–3 days after aspiration. Management of infection depends on the observed flora of the tracheobronchial tree. Hypotension secondary to alveolar capillary membrane injury and intravascular volume depletion is common and is managed with the judicious administration of intravenous fluids.

2. Chronic Aspiration of Gastric Contents

Chronic aspiration of gastric contents may result from primary disorders of the larynx or the esophagus, such as achalasia, esophageal stricture, systemic sclerosis (scleroderma), esophageal carcinoma, esophagitis, and gastroesophageal reflux. In the last condition, relaxation of the tone of the lower esophageal sphincter allows reflux of gastric contents into the esophagus and predisposes to chronic pulmonary aspiration, especially at night. Cigarette smoking, consumption of alcohol or caffeine, and use of theophylline are known to relax the lower esophageal sphincter. Pulmonary disorders linked to gastroesophageal reflux and chronic aspiration include asthma, chronic cough, bronchiectasis, and pulmonary fibrosis. Even in the absence of aspiration, acid in the esophagus may trigger bronchospasm or bronchial hyperreactivity through reflex mechanisms.

The diagnosis and management of gastroesophageal reflux and chronic aspiration is challenging. A discussion of strategies for the evaluation, prevention, and management of extraesophageal reflux manifestations can be found in Chapter 15.

3. "Café Coronary"

Acute obstruction of the upper airway by food is associated with difficulty swallowing, old age, dental problems that impair chewing, and use of alcohol and sedative drugs. The Heimlich procedure is lifesaving in many cases.

4. Retention of an Aspirated Foreign Body

Retention of an aspirated foreign body in the tracheobronchial tree may produce both acute and chronic conditions, including atelectasis, postobstructive hyperinflation, both acute and recurrent pneumonia, bronchiectasis, and lung abscess. Occasionally, a misdiagnosis of asthma, COPD, or lung cancer is made in adult patients who have aspirated a foreign body. The plain chest radiograph usually suggests the site of the foreign body. In some cases, an expiratory film, demonstrating regional hyperinflation due to a check-valve effect, is helpful. Bronchoscopy is usually necessary to establish the diagnosis and attempt removal of the foreign body.

5. Aspiration of Inert Material

Most patients suffer no serious sequelae from aspiration of inert material. However, it may cause asphyxia if the amount aspirated is massive and if cough is impaired, in which case immediate tracheobronchial suctioning is necessary.

6. Aspiration of Toxic Material

Aspiration of toxic material into the lung usually results in clinically evident pneumonia. **Hydrocarbon pneumonitis** is caused by aspiration of ingested petroleum distillates, eg, gasoline, kerosene, furniture polish, and other household petroleum products. Lung injury results mainly from vomiting of ingested products and secondary aspiration. Therapy is supportive. The lung should be protected from repeated aspiration with a cuffed endotracheal tube if necessary. **Lipoid pneumonia** is a chronic syndrome related to the repeated aspiration of oily materials, eg, mineral oil, cod liver oil, and oily nose drops; it usually occurs in elderly patients with impaired swallowing. Patchy opacities in dependent lung zones and lipid-laden macrophages in expectorated sputum are characteristic findings.

Kwong JC et al. New aspirations: the debate on aspiration pneumonia treatment guidelines. Med J Aust. 2011 Oct3; 195(7): 380–1. [PMID: 21978335]

Raghavendran K et al. Aspiration-induced lung injury. Crit Care Med. 2011 Apr;39(4):818–26. [PMID: 21263315]

OCCUPATIONAL PULMONARY DISEASES

Many acute and chronic pulmonary diseases are directly related to inhalation of noxious substances encountered in the workplace. Disorders that are linked to occupational exposures may be classified as follows: (1) pneumoconioses, (2) hypersensitivity pneumonitis, (3) obstructive airway disorders, (4) pulmonary edema, (5) lung cancer, (6) pleural diseases, and (7) miscellaneous disorders.

1. Pneumoconioses

Pneumoconioses are chronic fibrotic lung diseases caused by the inhalation of inorganic dusts. Pneumoconioses due to inhalation of inert dusts may be asymptomatic disorders with diffuse nodular opacities on chest radiograph or may be severe, symptomatic, life-shortening disorders. Clinically important pneumoconioses include coal worker's pneumoconiosis, silicosis, and asbestosis (Table 9–21). Treatment for each is supportive.

Table 9–21. Selected pneumoconioses.

Disease	Agent	Occupations
Metal dusts		
Siderosis	Metallic iron or iron oxide	Mining, welding, foundry work
Stannosis	Tin, tin oxide	Mining, tin-working, smelting
Baritosis	Barium salts	Glass and insecticide manufacturing
Coal dust		
Coal worker's pneumoconiosis	Coal dust	Coal mining
Inorganic dusts		
Silicosis	Free silica (silicon dioxide)	Rock mining, quarrying, stone cutting, tunneling, sandblasting, pottery, diatomaceous earth
Silicate dusts		
Asbestosis	Asbestos	Mining, insulation, construction, shipbuilding
Talcosis	Magnesium silicate	Mining, insulation, construction, shipbuilding
Kaolin pneumoconiosis	Sand, mica, aluminum silicate	Mining of china clay; pottery and cement work
Shaver disease	Aluminum powder	Manufacture of corundum

A. Coal Worker's Pneumoconiosis

In coal worker's pneumoconiosis, ingestion of inhaled coal dust by alveolar macrophages leads to the formation of coal macules, usually 2–5 mm in diameter, that appear on chest radiograph as diffuse small opacities that are especially prominent in the upper lung. Simple coal worker's pneumoconiosis is usually asymptomatic; pulmonary function abnormalities are unimpressive. Cigarette smoking does not increase the prevalence of coal worker's pneumoconiosis but may have an additive detrimental effect on ventilatory function. In complicated coal worker's pneumoconiosis (**"progressive massive fibrosis"**), conglomeration and contraction in the upper lung zones occur, with radiographic features resembling complicated silicosis. **Caplan syndrome** is a rare condition characterized by the presence of necrobiotic rheumatoid nodules (1–5 cm in diameter) in the periphery of the lung in coal workers with rheumatoid arthritis.

B. Silicosis

In silicosis, extensive or prolonged inhalation of free silica (silicon dioxide) particles in the respirable range (0.3–5 mcm) causes the formation of small rounded opacities (silicotic nodules) throughout the lung. Calcification of the periphery of hilar lymph nodes ("eggshell" calcification) is an unusual radiographic finding that strongly suggests silicosis. Simple silicosis is usually asymptomatic and has no effect on routine pulmonary function tests; in complicated silicosis, large conglomerate densities appear in the upper lung and are accompanied by dyspnea and obstructive and restrictive pulmonary dysfunction. The incidence of pulmonary tuberculosis is increased in patients with silicosis. All patients with silicosis should have a tuberculin skin test and a current chest radiograph. If old, healed pulmonary tuberculosis is suspected, multidrug treatment for tuberculosis (not single-agent preventive therapy) should be instituted.

C. Asbestosis

Asbestosis is a nodular interstitial fibrosis occurring in workers exposed to asbestos fibers (shipyard and construction workers, pipe fitters, insulators) over many years (typically 10–20 years). Patients with asbestosis usually first seek medical attention at least 15 years after exposure with the following symptoms and signs: progressive dyspnea, inspiratory crackles, and in some cases, clubbing and cyanosis. The radiographic features of asbestosis include linear streaking at the lung bases, opacities of various shapes and sizes, and honeycomb changes in advanced cases. The presence of pleural calcifications may be a clue to diagnosis. High-resolution CT scanning is the best imaging method for asbestosis because of its ability to detect parenchymal fibrosis and define the presence of coexisting pleural plaques. Cigarette smoking in asbestos workers increases the prevalence of radiographic pleural and parenchymal changes and markedly increases the incidence of lung carcinoma. It may also interfere with the clearance of short asbestos fibers from the lung. Pulmonary function studies show restrictive dysfunction and reduced diffusing capacity. The presence of a ferruginous body in tissue suggests significant asbestos exposure; however, other histologic features must be present for diagnosis. There is no specific treatment.

Centers for Disease Control and Prevention (CDC). Pneumoconiosis and advanced occupational lung disease among surface coal miners—16 states, 2010–2011. MMWR Morb Mortal Wkly Rep. 2012 Jun15;61(23):431–4. [PMID: 22695382]
Lazarus A et al. Asbestos-related pleuropulmonary diseases: benign and malignant. Postgrad Med. 2012 May;124(3):116–30. [PMID: 22691906]
Leung CC et al. Silicosis. Lancet. 2012 May26;379(9830):2008–18. [PMID: 22534002]

2. Hypersensitivity Pneumonitis

Hypersensitivity pneumonitis (also called extrinsic allergic alveolitis) is a nonatopic, nonasthmatic inflammatory pulmonary disease. It is manifested mainly as an occupational disease (Table 9–22), in which exposure to inhaled organic antigens leads to an acute illness. Prompt diagnosis is essential since symptoms are usually reversible if the offending antigen is removed from the patient's environment early in the course of illness. Continued exposure may lead to progressive disease. The histopathology of acute hypersensitivity pneumonitis is characterized by interstitial infiltrates of lymphocytes and plasma cells, with noncaseating granulomas in the interstitium and air spaces.

► **Clinical Findings**

A. Acute Illness

The symptoms are characterized by sudden onset of malaise, chills, fever, cough, dyspnea, and nausea 4–8 hours after exposure to the offending antigen. This may occur after the patient has left work or even at night and thus may mimic paroxysmal nocturnal dyspnea. Bibasilar crackles, tachypnea, tachycardia, and (occasionally) cyanosis are noted. Small nodular densities sparing the apices and bases of the lungs are noted on chest radiograph. Laboratory studies reveal an increase in the white blood cell count with a shift to the left, hypoxemia, and the presence of precipitating antibodies to the offending agent in serum. Hypersensitivity pneumonitis antibody panels against common offending antigens are available; positive results, while supportive, do not establish a definitive diagnosis. Pulmonary function studies reveal restrictive dysfunction and reduced diffusing capacity.

B. Subacute Illness

A subacute hypersensitivity pneumonitis syndrome (15% of cases) is characterized by the insidious onset of chronic cough and slowly progressive dyspnea, anorexia, and weight loss. Chronic exposure leads to progressive respiratory insufficiency and the appearance of pulmonary fibrosis on chest imaging. Surgical lung biopsy may be necessary for the diagnosis of subacute and chronic hypersensitivity pneumonitis. Even with surgical lung biopsy, however, chronic hypersensitivity pneumonitis may be difficult to diagnose because histopathologic patterns overlap with several idiopathic interstitial pneumonias.

► **Treatment**

Treatment of acute hypersensitivity pneumonitis consists of identification of the offending agent and avoidance of further exposure. In severe acute or protracted cases, oral corticosteroids (prednisone, 0.5 mg/kg daily as a single morning dose for 2 weeks, tapered to nil over 4–6 weeks) may be given. Change in occupation is often unavoidable.

Lacasse Y et al. Recent advances in hypersensitivity pneumonitis. Chest. 2012 Jul;142(1):208–17. [PMID: 22796841]

3. Obstructive Airway Disorders

Occupational pulmonary diseases manifested as obstructive airway disorders include occupational asthma, industrial bronchitis, and byssinosis.

A. Occupational Asthma

It has been estimated that from 2% to 5% of all cases of asthma are related to occupation. Offending agents in the workplace are numerous; they include grain dust, wood dust, tobacco, pollens, enzymes, gum arabic, synthetic dyes, isocyanates (particularly toluene diisocyanate), rosin

Table 9–22. Selected causes of hypersensitivity pneumonitis.

Disease	Antigen	Source
Farmer's lung	*Micropolyspora faeni, Thermoactinomyces vulgaris*	Moldy hay
"Humidifier" lung	Thermophilic actinomycetes	Contaminated humidifiers, heating systems, or air conditioners
Bird fancier's lung ("pigeon-breeder's disease")	Avian proteins	Bird serum and excreta
Bagassosis	*Thermoactinomyces sacchari* and *T vulgaris*	Moldy sugar cane fiber (bagasse)
Sequoiosis	Graphium, Aureobasidium, and other fungi	Moldy redwood sawdust
Maple bark stripper's disease	*Cryptostroma (Coniosporium) corticale*	Rotting maple tree logs or bark
Mushroom picker's disease	Same as farmer's lung	Moldy compost
Suberosis	*Penicillium frequentans*	Moldy cork dust
Detergent worker's lung	*Bacillus subtilis* enzyme	Enzyme additives

(soldering flux), inorganic chemicals (salts of nickel, platinum, and chromium), trimellitic anhydride, phthalic anhydride, formaldehyde, and various pharmaceutical agents. Diagnosis of occupational asthma depends on a high index of suspicion, an appropriate history, spirometric studies before and after exposure to the offending substance, and peak flow rate measurements in the workplace. Bronchial provocation testing may be helpful in some cases. Treatment consists of avoidance of further exposure to the offending agent and bronchodilators, but symptoms may persist for years after workplace exposure has been terminated.

B. Industrial Bronchitis

Industrial bronchitis is chronic bronchitis found in coal miners and others exposed to cotton, flax, or hemp dust. Chronic disability from industrial bronchitis is infrequent.

C. Byssinosis

Byssinosis is an asthma-like disorder in textile workers caused by inhalation of cotton dust. The pathogenesis is obscure. Chest tightness, cough, and dyspnea are characteristically worse on Mondays or the first day back at work, with symptoms subsiding later in the week. Repeated exposure leads to chronic bronchitis.

4. Toxic Lung Injury

Toxic lung injury from inhalation of irritant gases is discussed in the section on smoke inhalation. **Silo-filler's disease** is acute toxic high-permeability pulmonary edema caused by inhalation of nitrogen dioxide encountered in recently filled silos. Bronchiolitis obliterans is a common late complication, which may be prevented by early treatment of the acute reaction with corticosteroids. Extensive exposure to silage gas may be fatal. Inhalation of the compound diacetyl, a constituent of butter-flavoring, has been linked to the development of bronchiolitis obliterans among microwave popcorn production workers.

5. Lung Cancer

Many industrial pulmonary carcinogens have been identified, including asbestos, radon gas, arsenic, iron, chromium, nickel, coal tar fumes, petroleum oil mists, isopropyl oil, mustard gas, and printing ink. Cigarette smoking acts as a cocarcinogen with asbestos and radon gas to cause bronchogenic carcinoma. Asbestos alone causes malignant mesothelioma. Almost all histologic types of lung cancer have been associated with these carcinogens. Chloromethyl methyl ether specifically causes small cell carcinoma of the lung.

6. Pleural Diseases

Occupational diseases of the pleura may result from exposure to asbestos (see above) or talc. Inhalation of talc causes pleural plaques that are similar to those caused by asbestos. Benign asbestos pleural effusion occurs in some asbestos workers and may cause chronic blunting of the costophrenic angle on chest radiograph.

7. Other Occupational Pulmonary Diseases

Occupational agents are also responsible for other pulmonary disorders. These include exposure to beryllium, which now occurs in machining and handling of beryllium products and alloys. Beryllium miners are not at risk for berylliosis and beryllium is no longer used in fluorescent lamp production, which was a source of exposure before 1950. **Berylliosis**, an acute or chronic pulmonary disorder, occurs from absorption of beryllium through the lungs or skin and wide dissemination throughout the body. Acute berylliosis is a toxic, ulcerative tracheobronchitis and chemical pneumonitis following intense and severe exposure to beryllium. Chronic berylliosis, a systemic disease closely resembling sarcoidosis, is more common. Chronic pulmonary beryllium disease is thought to be an alveolitis mediated by the proliferation of beryllium-specific helper-inducer T cells in the lung.

Cartier A et al. Clinical assessment of occupational asthma and its differential diagnosis. Immunol Allergy Clin North Am. 2011 Nov;31(4):717–28. [PMID: 21978853]

Henneberger PK et al; ATS Ad Hoc Committee on Work-Exacerbated Asthma. An official American Thoracic Society statement: work-exacerbated asthma. Am J Respir Crit Care Med. 2011 Aug1;184(3):368–78. [PMID: 21804122]

Malo JL et al. Definitions and classification of work-related asthma. Immunol Allergy Clin North Am. 2011 Nov;31(4):645–62. [PMID: 21978849]

Myers R. Asbestos-related pleural disease. Curr Opin Pulm Med. 2012 Jul;18(4):377–81. [PMID: 22617814]

Smith AM. The epidemiology of work-related asthma. Immunol Allergy Clin North Am. 2011 Nov;31(4):663–75. [PMID: 21978850]

MEDICATION-INDUCED LUNG DISEASE

Typical patterns of pulmonary response to medications implicated in medication-induced respiratory disease are summarized in Table 9–23. Pulmonary injury due to medications occurs as a result of allergic reactions, idiosyncratic reactions, overdose, or undesirable side effects. In most patients, the mechanism of pulmonary injury is unknown.

Precise diagnosis of medication-induced pulmonary disease is often difficult because results of routine laboratory studies are not helpful and radiographic findings are not specific. A high index of suspicion and a thorough history of medication usage are critical to establishing the diagnosis of medication-induced lung disease. The clinical response to cessation of the suspected offending agent is also helpful. Acute episodes of medication-induced pulmonary disease usually disappear 24–48 hours after the medication has been discontinued, but chronic syndromes may take longer to resolve. Challenge tests to confirm the diagnosis are risky and rarely performed.

Treatment of medication-induced lung disease consists of discontinuing the offending agent immediately and managing the pulmonary symptoms appropriately.

Inhalation of crack cocaine may cause a spectrum of acute pulmonary syndromes, including pulmonary infiltration with eosinophilia, pneumothorax and pneumomediastinum, bronchiolitis obliterans, and acute respiratory

Table 9–23. Pulmonary manifestations of selected medication toxicities.

Asthma	Pulmonary edema
Beta-blockers	Noncardiogenic
Aspirin	Aspirin
Nonsteroidal anti-inflammatory drugs	Chlordiazepoxide
	Cocaine
Histamine	Ethchlorvynol
Methacholine	Heroin
Acetylcysteine	Cardiogenic
Aerosolized pentamidine	Beta-blockers
Any nebulized medication	**Pleural effusion**
Chronic cough	Bromocriptine
Angiotensin-converting enzyme inhibitors	Nitrofurantoin
	Any drug inducing systemic lupus erythematosus
Pulmonary infiltration	Methysergide
Without eosinophilia	Chemotherapeutic agents (eg, carmustine, cyclophosphamide, dasatinib, docetaxel, GM-CSF, methotrexate)
Amitriptyline	
Azathioprine	
Amiodarone	
With eosinophilia	
Sulfonamides	**Mediastinal widening**
L-Tryptophan	Phenytoin
Nitrofurantoin	Corticosteroids
Penicillin	Methotrexate
Methotrexate	**Respiratory failure**
Crack cocaine	Neuromuscular blockade
Drug-induced systemic lupus erythematosus	Aminoglycosides
Hydralazine	Succinylcholine
Procainamide	Gallamine
Isoniazid	Dimethyltubocurarine (metocurine)
Chlorpromazine	Central nervous system depression
Phenytoin	Sedatives
Interstitial pneumonitis/fibrosis	Hypnotics
Nitrofurantoin	Opioids
Bleomycin	Alcohol
Busulfan	Tricyclic antidepressants
Cyclophosphamide	Oxygen
Methysergide	
Phenytoin	

GM-CSF, granulocyte-macrophage colony-stimulating factor.

failure associated with diffuse alveolar damage and alveolar hemorrhage. Corticosteroids have been used with variable success to treat alveolar hemorrhage.

Piciucchi S et al. Prospective evaluation of drug-induced lung toxicity with high-resolution CT and transbronchial biopsy. Radiol Med. 2011 Mar;116(2):246–63. [PMID: 21311994]

Schwaiblmair M et al. Cytochrome P450 polymorphisms and drug-induced interstitial lung disease. Expert Opin Drug Metab Toxicol. 2011 Dec;7(12):1547–60. [PMID: 22070131]

RADIATION LUNG INJURY

The lung is an exquisitely radiosensitive organ that can be damaged by external beam radiation therapy. The degree of pulmonary injury is determined by the volume of lung irradiated, the dose and rate of exposure, and potentiating factors (eg, concurrent chemotherapy, previous radiation therapy in the same area, and simultaneous withdrawal of corticosteroid therapy). Symptomatic radiation lung injury occurs in about 10% of patients treated for carcinoma of the breast, 5–15% of patients treated for carcinoma of the lung, and 5–35% of patients treated for lymphoma. Two phases of the pulmonary response to radiation are apparent: an acute phase (radiation pneumonitis) and a chronic phase (radiation fibrosis).

1. Radiation Pneumonitis

Acute radiation pneumonitis usually occurs 2–3 months (range 1–6 months) after completion of radiotherapy and is characterized by insidious onset of dyspnea, intractable dry cough, chest fullness or pain, weakness, and fever. Late radiation pneumonitis may develop 6–12 months after completion of radiation. The pathogenesis of acute radiation pneumonitis is unknown, but there is speculation that hypersensitivity mechanisms are involved. The dominant histopathologic findings are a lymphocytic interstitial pneumonitis progressing to an exudative alveolitis. Inspiratory crackles may be heard in the involved area. In severe disease, respiratory distress and cyanosis occur that are characteristic of ARDS. An increased white blood cell count and elevated sedimentation rate are common. Pulmonary function studies reveal reduced lung volumes, reduced lung compliance, hypoxemia, reduced diffusing capacity, and reduced maximum voluntary ventilation. Chest radiography, which correlates poorly with the presence of symptoms, usually demonstrates alveolar or nodular opacities limited to the irradiated area. Air bronchograms are often observed. Sharp borders of an opacity may help distinguish radiation pneumonitis from other conditions such as infectious pneumonia, lymphangitic spread of carcinoma, and recurrent tumor; however, the opacity may extend beyond the radiation field. No specific therapy is proved to be effective in radiation pneumonitis, but prednisone (1 mg/kg/d orally) is commonly given immediately for about 1 week. The dose is then reduced and maintained at 20–40 mg/d for several weeks, then slowly tapered. Radiation pneumonitis may improve in 2–3 weeks following onset of symptoms as the exudative phase resolves. Acute respiratory failure, if present, is treated supportively. Death from ARDS is unusual in radiation pneumonitis.

2. Pulmonary Radiation Fibrosis

Radiation fibrosis may occur with or without antecedent radiation pneumonitis. Cor pulmonale and chronic respiratory failure are rare. Radiographic findings include obliteration of normal lung markings, dense interstitial and pleural fibrosis, reduced lung volumes, tenting of the diaphragm, and sharp delineation of the irradiated area. No specific therapy is proven effective, and corticosteroids have no value. Pulmonary fibrosis may develop after an intervening period (6–12 months) of well-being in patients who experience radiation pneumonitis. Pulmonary radiation fibrosis occurs in most patients who receive a full course of radiation therapy for cancer of the lung or breast. Most patients are asymptomatic, although slowly progressive dyspnea may occur.

3. Other Complications of Radiation Therapy

Other complications of radiation therapy directed to the thorax include pericardial effusion, constrictive pericarditis, tracheoesophageal fistula, esophageal candidiasis, radiation dermatitis, and rib fractures. Small pleural effusions, radiation pneumonitis outside the irradiated area, spontaneous pneumothorax, and complete obstruction of central airways are unusual occurrences.

PLEURAL DISEASES

PLEURITIS

Pain due to acute pleural inflammation is caused by irritation of the parietal pleura. Such pain is localized, sharp, and fleeting; it is made worse by coughing, sneezing, deep breathing, or movement. When the central portion of the diaphragmatic parietal pleura is irritated, pain may be referred to the ipsilateral shoulder. There are numerous causes of pleuritis. The setting in which pleuritic pain develops helps narrow the differential diagnosis. In young, otherwise healthy individuals, pleuritis is usually caused by viral respiratory infections or pneumonia. The presence of pleural effusion, pleural thickening, or air in the pleural space requires further diagnostic and therapeutic measures. Simple rib fracture may cause severe pleurisy.

Treatment of pleuritis consists of treating the underlying disease. Analgesics and anti-inflammatory drugs (eg, indomethacin, 25 mg orally two or three times daily) are often helpful for pain relief. Codeine (30–60 mg orally every 8 hours) or other opioids may be used to control cough associated with pleuritic chest pain if retention of airway secretions is not a likely complication. Intercostal nerve blocks are sometimes helpful but the benefit is usually transient.

PLEURAL EFFUSION

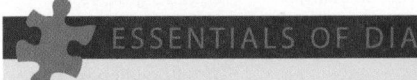
ESSENTIALS OF DIAGNOSIS

► May be asymptomatic; chest pain frequently seen in the setting of pleuritis, trauma, or infection; dyspnea is common with large effusions.

► Dullness to percussion and decreased breath sounds over the effusion.

► Radiographic evidence of pleural effusion.

► Diagnostic findings on thoracentesis.

► General Considerations

There is constant movement of fluid from parietal pleural capillaries into the pleural space at a rate of 0.01 mL/kg body weight/h. Absorption of pleural fluid occurs through parietal pleural lymphatics. The resultant homeostasis leaves 5–15 mL of fluid in the normal pleural space. A pleural effusion is an abnormal accumulation of fluid in

Table 9–24. Causes of pleural fluid transudates and exudates.

Transudates	Exudates
Heart failure (> 90% of cases)	Pneumonia (parapneumonic effusion)
Cirrhosis with ascites	Cancer
Nephrotic syndrome	Pulmonary embolism
Peritoneal dialysis	Bacterial infection
Myxedema	Tuberculosis
Atelectasis (acute)	Connective tissue disease
Constrictive pericarditis	Viral infection
Superior vena cava obstruction	Fungal infection
Pulmonary embolism	Rickettsial infection
	Parasitic infection
	Asbestos
	Meigs syndrome
	Pancreatic disease
	Uremia
	Chronic atelectasis
	Trapped lung
	Chylothorax
	Sarcoidosis
	Drug reaction
	Post-myocardial injury syndrome

the pleural space. Pleural effusions may be classified by differential diagnosis (Table 9–24) or by underlying pathophysiology. Five pathophysiologic processes account for most pleural effusions: increased production of fluid in the setting of normal capillaries due to increased hydrostatic or decreased oncotic pressures (**transudates**); increased production of fluid due to abnormal capillary permeability (**exudates**); decreased lymphatic clearance of fluid from the pleural space (**exudates**); infection in the pleural space (**empyema**); and bleeding into the pleural space (**hemothorax**). **Parapneumonic** pleural effusions are exudates that accompany bacterial pneumonias.

Diagnostic thoracentesis should be performed whenever there is a new pleural effusion and no clinically apparent cause. Observation is appropriate in some situations (eg, symmetric bilateral pleural effusions in the setting of heart failure), but an atypical presentation or failure of an effusion to resolve as expected warrants thoracentesis. Sampling allows visualization of the fluid in addition to chemical and microbiologic analyses to identify the underlying pathophysiologic process.

► Clinical Findings

A. Symptoms and Signs

Patients with pleural effusions most often report dyspnea, cough, or respirophasic chest pain. Symptoms are more common in patients with existing cardiopulmonary disease. Small pleural effusions are less likely to be symptomatic than larger effusions. Physical findings are usually absent in small effusions. Larger effusions may present with dullness to percussion and diminished or absent breath sounds over the effusion. Compressive atelectasis may cause bronchial breath sounds and egophony just above the effusion. A massive effusion with increased intrapleural pressure may cause contralateral shift of the trachea and bulging of the intercostal spaces. A pleural friction rub indicates infarction or pleuritis.

B. Laboratory Findings

The gross appearance of pleural fluid helps identify several types of pleural effusion. Grossly purulent fluid signifies empyema. Milky white pleural fluid should be centrifuged. A clear supernatant above a pellet of white cells indicates empyema, whereas a persistently turbid supernatant suggests a **chylous effusion**; analysis of this supernatant reveals chylomicrons and a high triglyceride level (> 100 mg/dL [1 mmol/L]), often from disruption of the thoracic duct. **Hemorrhagic pleural effusion** is a mixture of blood and pleural fluid. Ten thousand red cells per milliliter create blood-tinged pleural fluid; 100,000 red cells/mL create grossly bloody pleural fluid. **Hemothorax** is the presence of gross blood in the pleural space, usually following chest trauma or instrumentation. It is defined as a ratio of pleural fluid hematocrit to peripheral blood hematocrit > 0.5.

Pleural fluid samples should be sent for measurement of protein, glucose, and LD in addition to total and differential white blood cell counts. Chemistry determinations are used to classify effusions as transudates or exudates. This classification is important because the differential diagnosis and subsequent evaluation for each entity is vastly different (Table 9–24). A **pleural exudate** is an effusion that has one or more of the following laboratory features: (1) ratio of pleural fluid protein to serum protein > 0.5; (2) ratio of pleural fluid LD to serum LD > 0.6; (3) pleural fluid LD greater than two-thirds the upper limit of normal serum LD. **Pleural transudates** occur in the setting of normal capillary integrity and demonstrate none of the laboratory features of exudates. A transudate suggests the absence of local pleural disease; characteristic laboratory findings include a glucose equal to serum glucose, pH between 7.40 and 7.55, and fewer than 1.0×10^3 white blood cells/mcL (1.0×10^9/L) with a predominance of mononuclear cells.

Heart failure accounts for 90% of transudates. Bacterial pneumonia and cancer are the most common causes of exudative effusion. Other causes of exudates with characteristic laboratory findings are summarized in Table 9–25.

Table 9–25. Characteristics of important exudative pleural effusions.

Etiology or Type of Effusion	Gross Appearance	White Blood Cell Count (cells/mcL)	Red Blood Cell Count (cells/mcL)	Glucose	Comments
Malignancy	Turbid to bloody; occasionally serous	1000 to < 100,000 M	100 to several hundred thousand	Equal to serum levels; < 60 mg/dL in 15% of cases	Eosinophilia uncommon; positive results on cytologic examination
Uncomplicated parapneumonic	Clear to turbid	5000–25,000 P	< 5000	Equal to serum levels	Tube thoracostomy unnecessary
Empyema	Turbid to purulent	25,000–100,000 P	< 5000	Less than serum levels; often very low	Drainage necessary; putrid odor suggests anaerobic infection
Tuberculosis	Serous to serosanguineous	5000–10,000 M	< 10,000	Equal to serum levels; occasionally < 60 mg/dL	Protein > 4.0 g/dL and may exceed 5 g/dL; eosinophils (> 10%) or mesothelial cells (> 5%) make diagnosis unlikely; see text for discussion of additional diagnostic tests
Rheumatoid	Turbid; greenish yellow	1000–20,000 M or P	< 1000	< 40 mg/dL	Secondary empyema common; high LD, low complement, high rheumatoid factor, cholesterol crystals are characteristic
Pulmonary infarction	Serous to grossly bloody	1000–50,000 M or P	100 to > 100,000	Equal to serum levels	Variable findings; no pathognomonic features
Esophageal rupture	Turbid to purulent; red-brown	< 5000 to > 50,000 P	1000–10,000	Usually low	High amylase level (salivary origin); pneumothorax in 25% of cases; effusion usually on left side; pH < 6.0 strongly suggests diagnosis
Pancreatitis	Turbid to sero-sanguineous	1000–50,000 P	1000–10,000	Equal to serum levels	Usually left-sided; high amylase level

LD, lactate dehydrogenase; M, mononuclear cell predominance; P, polymorphonuclear leukocyte predominance.

Pleural fluid pH is useful in the assessment of parapneumonic effusions. A pH below 7.30 suggests the need for drainage of the pleural space. An elevated amylase level in pleural fluid suggests pancreatitis, pancreatic pseudocyst, adenocarcinoma of the lung or pancreas, or esophageal rupture.

Suspected tuberculous pleural effusion should be evaluated by thoracentesis with culture along with pleural biopsy, since pleural fluid culture positivity for *M tuberculosis* is low (< 23–58% of cases). Closed pleural biopsy reveals granulomatous inflammation in approximately 60% of patients, and culture of three pleural biopsy specimens combined with histologic examination of a pleural biopsy for granulomas yields a diagnosis in up to 90% of patients. Tests for pleural fluid adenosine deaminase (approximately 90% sensitivity and specificity for pleural tuberculosis at levels >70 units/L) and interferon-gamma (89% sensitivity, 97% specificity in a meta-analysis) can be extremely helpful diagnostic aids, particularly in making decisions to pursue invasive testing in complex patients.

Between 40% and 80% of exudative pleural effusions are malignant, while over 90% of malignant pleural effusions are exudative. Almost any form of cancer may cause effusions, but the most common causes are lung cancer (one-third of cases) and breast cancer. In 5–10% of malignant pleural effusions, no primary tumor is identified. The term "**paramalignant**" pleural effusion refers to an effusion in a patient with cancer when repeated attempts to identify tumor cells in the pleura or pleural fluid are nondiagnostic but when there is a presumptive relation to the underlying malignancy. For example, superior vena cava syndrome with elevated systemic venous pressures causing a transudative effusion would be "paramalignant."

Pleural fluid specimens should be sent for cytologic examination in all cases of exudative effusions in patients suspected of harboring an underlying malignancy. The diagnostic yield depends on the nature and extent of the underlying malignancy. Sensitivity is between 50% and 65%. A negative cytologic examination in a patient with a high prior probability of malignancy should be followed by one repeat thoracentesis. If that examination is negative, thoracoscopy is preferred to closed pleural biopsy. The sensitivity of thoracoscopy is 92–96%.

C. Imaging

The lung is less dense than water and floats on pleural fluid that accumulates in dependent regions. Subpulmonary fluid may appear as lateral displacement of the apex of the diaphragm with an abrupt slope to the costophrenic sulcus or a greater than 2 cm separation between the gastric air bubble and the lung. On a standard upright chest radiograph, approximately 75–100 mL of pleural fluid must accumulate in the posterior costophrenic sulcus to be visible on the lateral view, and 175–200 mL must be present in the lateral costophrenic sulcus to be visible on the frontal view. Chest CT scans may identify as little as 10 mL of fluid. At least 1 cm of fluid on the decubitus view is necessary to permit blind thoracentesis. Ultrasonography is useful to guide thoracentesis in the setting of smaller effusions.

Pleural fluid may become trapped (loculated) by pleural adhesions, thereby forming unusual collections along the lateral chest wall or within lung fissures. Round or oval fluid collections in fissures that resemble intraparenchymal masses are called pseudotumors. Massive pleural effusion causing opacification of an entire hemithorax is most commonly caused by cancer but may be seen in tuberculosis and other diseases.

▶ Treatment

A. Transudative Pleural Effusion

Transudative pleural effusions characteristically occur in the absence of pleural disease. Therefore, treatment is directed at the underlying condition. Therapeutic thoracentesis for severe dyspnea typically offers only transient benefit. Pleurodesis and tube thoracostomy are rarely indicated.

B. Malignant Pleural Effusion

Chemotherapy or radiation therapy or both offer temporary control in some malignant effusions but are generally ineffective in lung cancer in the pleural space except for small cell lung cancer. Asymptomatic malignant effusions usually do not require specific treatment. Symptomatic patients should have a therapeutic thoracentesis. If symptoms are relieved but the effusion returns, the options are serial thoracenteses, attempted pleurodesis, or placement of an indwelling drainage catheter that the patient can access at home. Choice among these options depends on the rate of reaccumulation in addition to the functional status, tolerance for discomfort, and life expectancy of the patient. Consultation with a thoracic specialist is advised. (See Chapter 39.)

C. Parapneumonic Pleural Effusion

Parapneumonic pleural effusions are divided into three categories: simple or uncomplicated, complicated, and empyema. **Uncomplicated parapneumonic effusions** are free-flowing sterile exudates of modest size that resolve quickly with antibiotic treatment of pneumonia. They do not need drainage. **Empyema** is gross infection of the pleural space indicated by positive Gram stain or culture. Empyema should always be drained by tube thoracostomy to facilitate clearance of infection and to reduce the probability of fibrous encasement of the lung, causing permanent pulmonary impairment.

Complicated parapneumonic effusions present the most difficult management decisions. They tend to be larger than simple parapneumonic effusions and to show more evidence of inflammatory stimuli such as low glucose level, low pH, or evidence of loculation. Inflammation probably reflects ongoing bacterial invasion of the pleural space despite rare positive bacterial cultures. The morbidity associated with complicated effusions is due to their tendency to form a fibropurulent pleural "peel," trapping otherwise functional lung and leading to permanent impairment. Tube thoracostomy is indicated when pleural fluid glucose is < 60 mg/dL (< 3.3 mmol/L) or the pH is

< 7.2. These thresholds have not been prospectively validated and should not be interpreted strictly. The clinician should consider drainage of a complicated effusion if the pleural fluid pH is between 7.2 and 7.3 or the LD is > 1000 units/L (> 20 mckat/L). Pleural fluid cell count and protein have little diagnostic value in this setting.

Tube thoracostomy drainage of empyema or complicated parapneumonic effusions is frequently complicated by loculation that prevents adequate drainage. Intrapleural instillation of fibrinolytic agents has not been shown in controlled trials to improve drainage. The combination of intrapleural tissue plasminogen activator and deoxyribonuclease (DNase), an enzyme that catalyses extracellular DNA and degrades biofilm formation within the pleural cavity, has been found to improve clinical outcome (increased drainage, decrease length of stay and surgical referral) compared with placebo or either agent alone.

D. Hemothorax

A small-volume hemothorax that is stable or improving on chest radiographs may be managed by close observation. In all other cases, hemothorax is treated by immediate insertion of a large-bore thoracostomy tube to: (1) drain existing blood and clot, (2) quantify the amount of bleeding, (3) reduce the risk of fibrothorax, and (4) permit apposition of the pleural surfaces in an attempt to reduce hemorrhage. Thoracotomy may be indicated to control hemorrhage, remove clot, and treat complications such as bronchopleural fistula formation.

Light RW. Pleural effusions. Med Clin North Am. 2011 Nov;95(6):1055–70. [PMID: 22032427]

Rahman NM et al. Intrapleural use of tissue plasminogen activator and DNase in pleural infection. N Engl J Med. 2011 Aug11;365(6):518–26. [PMID: 21830966]

Rodriguez-Panadero F et al. Management of malignant pleural effusions. Curr Opin Pulm Med. 2011 Jul;17(4):269–73. [PMID: 21519264]

Ryu JH et al. Update on uncommon pleural effusions. Respirology. 2011 Feb;16(2):238–43. [PMID: 21073678]

SPONTANEOUS PNEUMOTHORAX

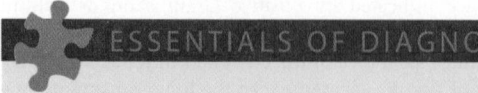

ESSENTIALS OF DIAGNOSIS

► Acute onset of unilateral chest pain and dyspnea.

► Minimal physical findings in mild cases; unilateral chest expansion, decreased tactile fremitus, hyperresonance, diminished breath sounds, mediastinal shift, cyanosis and hypotension in tension pneumothorax.

► Presence of pleural air on chest radiograph.

► General Considerations

Pneumothorax, or accumulation of air in the pleural space, is classified as spontaneous (primary or secondary) or traumatic. Primary spontaneous pneumothorax occurs in the absence of an underlying lung disease, whereas secondary spontaneous pneumothorax is a complication of preexisting pulmonary disease. Traumatic pneumothorax results from penetrating or blunt trauma. Iatrogenic pneumothorax may follow procedures such as thoracentesis, pleural biopsy, subclavian or internal jugular vein catheter placement, percutaneous lung biopsy, bronchoscopy with transbronchial biopsy, and positive-pressure mechanical ventilation. Tension pneumothorax usually occurs in the setting of penetrating trauma, lung infection, cardiopulmonary resuscitation, or positive-pressure mechanical ventilation. In tension pneumothorax, the pressure of air in the pleural space exceeds ambient pressure throughout the respiratory cycle. A check-valve mechanism allows air to enter the pleural space on inspiration and prevents egress of air on expiration.

Primary pneumothorax affects mainly tall, thin boys and men between the ages of 10 and 30 years. It is thought to occur from rupture of subpleural apical blebs in response to high negative intrapleural pressures. Family history and cigarette smoking may also be important factors.

Secondary pneumothorax occurs as a complication of COPD, asthma, cystic fibrosis, tuberculosis, *Pneumocystis* pneumonia, menstruation (catamenial pneumothorax), and a wide variety of interstitial lung diseases including sarcoidosis, lymphangioleiomyomatosis, Langerhans cell histiocytosis, and tuberous sclerosis. Aerosolized pentamidine and a prior history of *Pneumocystis* pneumonia are considered risk factors for the development of pneumothorax. One-half of patients with pneumothorax in the setting of recurrent (but not primary) *Pneumocystis* pneumonia will develop pneumothorax on the contralateral side. The mortality rate of pneumothorax in *Pneumocystis* pneumonia is high.

► Clinical Findings

A. Symptoms and Signs

Chest pain ranging from minimal to severe on the affected side and dyspnea occur in nearly all patients. Symptoms usually begin during rest and usually resolve within 24 hours even if the pneumothorax persists. Alternatively, pneumothorax may present with life-threatening respiratory failure if underlying COPD or asthma is present.

If pneumothorax is small (< 15% of a hemithorax), physical findings, other than mild tachycardia, are normal. If pneumothorax is large, diminished breath sounds, decreased tactile fremitus, and decreased movement of the chest are often noted. Tension pneumothorax should be suspected in the presence of marked tachycardia, hypotension, and mediastinal or tracheal shift.

B. Laboratory Findings

Arterial blood gas analysis is often unnecessary but reveals hypoxemia and acute respiratory alkalosis in most patients. Left-sided primary pneumothorax may produce QRS axis and precordial T wave changes on the ECG that may be misinterpreted as acute myocardial infarction.

C. Imaging

Demonstration of a visceral pleural line on chest radiograph is diagnostic and may only be seen on an expiratory film. A few patients have secondary pleural effusion that demonstrates a characteristic air-fluid level on chest radiography. In supine patients, pneumothorax on a conventional chest radiograph may appear as an abnormally radiolucent costophrenic sulcus (the "deep sulcus" sign). In patients with tension pneumothorax, chest radiographs show a large amount of air in the affected hemithorax and contralateral shift of the mediastinum.

▶ Differential Diagnosis

If the patient is a young, tall, thin, cigarette-smoking man, the diagnosis of primary spontaneous pneumothorax is usually obvious and can be confirmed by chest radiograph. In secondary pneumothorax, it is sometimes difficult to distinguish loculated pneumothorax from an emphysematous bleb. Occasionally, pneumothorax may mimic myocardial infarction, pulmonary embolism, or pneumonia.

▶ Complications

Tension pneumothorax may be life-threatening. Pneumomediastinum and subcutaneous emphysema may occur as complications of spontaneous pneumothorax. If pneumomediastinum is detected, rupture of the esophagus or a bronchus should be considered.

▶ Treatment

Treatment depends on the severity of pneumothorax and the nature of the underlying disease. In a reliable patient with a small (< 15% of a hemithorax), stable spontaneous primary pneumothorax, observation alone may be appropriate. Many small pneumothoraces resolve spontaneously as air is absorbed from the pleural space; supplemental oxygen therapy may increase the rate of reabsorption. Simple aspiration drainage of pleural air with a small-bore catheter (eg, 16 gauge angiocatheter or larger drainage catheter) can be performed for spontaneous primary pneumothoraces that are large or progressive. Placement of a small-bore chest tube (7F to 14F) attached to a one-way Heimlich valve provides protection against development of tension pneumothorax and may permit observation from home. The patient should be treated symptomatically for cough and chest pain, and followed with serial chest radiographs every 24 hours.

Patients with secondary pneumothorax, large pneumothorax, tension pneumothorax, or severe symptoms or those who have a pneumothorax on mechanical ventilation should undergo chest tube placement (tube thoracostomy). The chest tube is placed under water-seal drainage, and suction is applied until the lung expands. The chest tube can be removed after the air leak subsides.

All patients who smoke should be advised to discontinue smoking and warned that the risk of recurrence is 50% if cigarette smoking is continued. Future exposure to high altitudes, flying in unpressurized aircraft, and scuba diving should be avoided.

Indications for thoracoscopy or open thoracotomy include recurrences of spontaneous pneumothorax, any occurrence of bilateral pneumothorax, and failure of tube thoracostomy for the first episode (failure of lung to reexpand or persistent air leak). Surgery permits resection of blebs responsible for the pneumothorax and pleurodesis by mechanical abrasion and insufflation of talc.

Management of pneumothorax in patients with *Pneumocystis* pneumonia is challenging because of a tendency toward recurrence, and there is no consensus on the best approach. Use of a small chest tube attached to a Heimlich valve has been proposed to allow the patient to leave the hospital. Some clinicians favor its insertion early in the course.

▶ Prognosis

An average of 30% of patients with spontaneous pneumothorax experience recurrence of the disorder after either observation or tube thoracostomy for the first episode. Recurrence after surgical therapy is less frequent. Following successful therapy, there are no long-term complications.

Grundy S et al. Primary spontaneous pneumothorax: a diffuse disease of the pleura. Respiration. 2012;83(3):185–9. [PMID: 22343477]

▼ DISORDERS OF CONTROL OF VENTILATION

The principal influences on ventilatory control are arterial P_{CO_2}, pH, P_{O_2}, and brainstem tissue pH. These variables are monitored by peripheral and central chemoreceptors. Under normal conditions, the ventilatory control system maintains arterial pH and P_{CO_2} within narrow limits; arterial P_{O_2} is more loosely controlled.

Abnormal control of ventilation can be seen with a variety of conditions ranging from rare disorders such as Ondine curse, neuromuscular disorders, myxedema, starvation, and carotid body resection to more common disorders such as asthma, COPD, obesity, heart failure, and sleep-related breathing disorders. A few of these disorders will be discussed in this section.

Silvestrelli G et al. Ventilatory disorders. Front Neurol Neurosci. 2012;30:90–3. [PMID: 22377872]

OBESITY-HYPOVENTILATION SYNDROME (Pickwickian Syndrome)

In obesity-hypoventilation syndrome, alveolar hypoventilation appears to result from a combination of blunted ventilatory drive and increased mechanical load imposed upon the chest by obesity. Voluntary hyperventilation returns the P_{CO_2} and the P_{O_2} toward normal values, a correction not seen in lung diseases causing chronic respiratory failure such as COPD. Most patients with obesity-hypoventilation syndrome also suffer from obstructive sleep apnea (see below), which must be treated aggressively if identified as a comorbid disorder. Therapy of obesity-hypoventilation syndrome consists mainly of weight loss, which improves hypercapnia and hypoxemia as well as the ventilatory responses to hypoxia and hypercapnia. NPPV is helpful in some patients. Respiratory stimulants may be helpful and include theophylline, acetazolamide, and medroxyprogesterone acetate, 10–20 mg every 8 hours orally. Improvement in hypoxemia, hypercapnia, erythrocytosis, and cor pulmonale are goals of therapy.

Piper AJ et al. Obesity hypoventilation syndrome: mechanisms and management. Am J Respir Crit Care Med. 2011 Feb1;183(3):292–8. [PMID: 21037018]

HYPERVENTILATION SYNDROMES

Hyperventilation is an increase in alveolar ventilation that leads to hypocapnia. It may be caused by a variety of conditions, such as pregnancy, hypoxemia, obstructive and infiltrative lung diseases, sepsis, hepatic dysfunction, fever, and pain. The term "central neurogenic hyperventilation" denotes a monotonous, sustained pattern of rapid and deep breathing seen in comatose patients with brainstem injury of multiple causes. Functional hyperventilation may be acute or chronic. **Acute hyperventilation** presents with hyperpnea, paresthesias, carpopedal spasm, tetany, and anxiety. **Chronic hyperventilation** may present with various nonspecific symptoms, including fatigue, dyspnea, anxiety, palpitations, and dizziness. The diagnosis of chronic hyperventilation syndrome is established if symptoms are reproduced during voluntary hyperventilation. Once organic causes of hyperventilation have been excluded, treatment of acute hyperventilation consists of breathing through pursed lips or through the nose with one nostril pinched, or rebreathing expired gas from a paper bag held over the face in order to decrease respiratory alkalemia and its associated symptoms. Anxiolytic drugs may also be useful.

SLEEP-RELATED BREATHING DISORDERS

Abnormal ventilation during sleep is manifested by apnea (breath cessation for at least 10 seconds) or hypopnea (decrement in airflow with drop in hemoglobin saturation of at least 4%). Episodes of apnea are **central** if ventilatory effort is absent for the duration of the apneic episode, **obstructive** if ventilatory effort persists throughout the apneic episode but no airflow occurs because of transient obstruction of the upper airway, and **mixed** if absent ventilatory effort precedes upper airway obstruction during the apneic episode. Pure central sleep apnea is uncommon; it may be an isolated finding or may occur in patients with primary alveolar hypoventilation or with lesions of the brainstem. Obstructive and mixed sleep apneas are more common and may be associated with life-threatening cardiac arrhythmias, severe hypoxemia during sleep, daytime somnolence, pulmonary hypertension, cor pulmonale, systemic hypertension, and secondary erythrocytosis.

OBSTRUCTIVE SLEEP APNEA

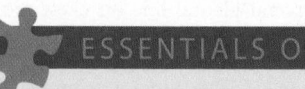 ESSENTIALS OF DIAGNOSIS

► Daytime somnolence or fatigue.
► A history of loud snoring with witnessed apneic events.
► Overnight polysomnography demonstrating apneic episodes with hypoxemia.

► General Considerations

Upper airway obstruction during sleep occurs when loss of normal pharyngeal muscle tone allows the pharynx to collapse passively during inspiration. Patients with anatomically narrowed upper airways (eg, micrognathia, macroglossia, obesity, tonsillar hypertrophy) are predisposed to the development of obstructive sleep apnea. Ingestion of alcohol or sedatives before sleeping or nasal obstruction of any type, including the common cold, may precipitate or worsen the condition. Hypothyroidism and cigarette smoking are additional risk factors for obstructive sleep apnea. Before making the diagnosis of obstructive sleep apnea, a drug history should be obtained and a seizure disorder, narcolepsy, and depression should be excluded.

► Clinical Findings

A. Symptoms and Signs

Most patients with obstructive or mixed sleep apnea are obese, middle-aged men. Systemic hypertension is common. Patients may complain of excessive daytime somnolence, morning sluggishness and headaches, daytime fatigue, cognitive impairment, recent weight gain, and impotence. Bed partners usually report loud cyclical snoring, breath cessation, witnessed apneas, restlessness, and thrashing movements of the extremities during sleep. Personality changes, poor judgment, work-related problems, depression, and intellectual deterioration (memory impairment, inability to concentrate) may also be observed.

Physical examination may be normal or may reveal systemic and pulmonary hypertension with cor pulmonale. The patient may appear sleepy or even fall asleep during the evaluation. The oropharynx is frequently found to be narrowed by excessive soft tissue folds, large tonsils, pendulous uvula, or prominent tongue. Nasal obstruction by a deviated nasal septum, poor nasal airflow, and a nasal twang to the speech may be observed. A "bull neck" appearance is common.

B. Laboratory Findings

Erythrocytosis is common. Thyroid function tests (serum, TSH, FT_4) should be obtained to exclude hypothyroidism.

C. Other Studies

Observation of the sleeping patient may reveal loud snoring interrupted by episodes of increasingly strong ventilatory effort that fail to produce airflow. A loud snort often accompanies the first breath following an apneic episode. Definitive diagnostic evaluation for suspected sleep apnea includes otorhinolaryngologic examination and overnight polysomnography (the monitoring of multiple physiologic factors during sleep). Screening may be performed using home nocturnal pulse oximetry, which when normal has a high negative predictive value in ruling out significant sleep apnea. A complete **polysomnography** examination includes electroencephalography, electro-oculography, electromyography, ECG, pulse oximetry, and measurement of respiratory effort and airflow. Polysomnography reveals apneic episodes lasting as long as 60 seconds. Oxygen saturation falls, often to very low levels. Bradydysrhythmias, such as sinus bradycardia, sinus arrest, or atrioventricular block, may occur. Tachydysrhythmias, including paroxysmal supraventricular tachycardia, atrial fibrillation, and ventricular tachycardia, may be seen once airflow is reestablished.

▶ Treatment

Weight loss and strict avoidance of alcohol and hypnotic medications are the first steps in management. Weight loss may be curative, but most patients are unable to lose the 10–20% of body weight required. **Nasal continuous positive airway pressure (nasal CPAP)** at night is curative in many patients. Polysomnography is frequently necessary to determine the level of CPAP (usually 5–15 cm H_2O) necessary to abolish obstructive apneas. Unfortunately, only about 75% of patients continue to use nasal CPAP after 1 year. Pharmacologic therapy for obstructive sleep apnea is disappointing. Supplemental oxygen may lessen the severity of nocturnal desaturation but may also lengthen apneas; it should not be routinely prescribed. Polysomnography is necessary to assess the effects of oxygen therapy. Mechanical devices inserted into the mouth at bedtime to hold the jaw forward and prevent pharyngeal occlusion have modest effectiveness in relieving apnea; however, patient compliance is not optimal.

Uvulopalatopharyngoplasty (UPPP), a procedure consisting of resection of pharyngeal soft tissue and amputation of approximately 15 mm of the free edge of the soft palate and uvula, is helpful in approximately 50% of selected patients. It is more effective in eliminating snoring than apneic episodes. UPPP may be performed on an outpatient basis with a laser. **Nasal septoplasty** is performed if gross anatomic nasal septal deformity is present. **Tracheostomy** relieves upper airway obstruction and its physiologic consequences and represents the definitive treatment for obstructive sleep apnea. However, it has numerous adverse effects, including granuloma formation, difficulty with speech, and stoma and airway infection. Furthermore, the long-term care of the tracheostomy, especially in obese patients, can be difficult. Tracheostomy and other maxillofacial surgery approaches are reserved for patients with life-threatening arrhythmias or severe disability who have not responded to conservative therapy.

Aurora RN et al. The treatment of central sleep apnea syndromes in adults: practice parameters with an evidence-based literature review and meta-analyses. Sleep. 2012 Jan1;35(1):17–40. [PMID: 22215916]
Park JG et al. Updates on definition, consequences, and management of obstructive sleep apnea. Mayo Clin Proc. 2011 Jun;86(6):549–54. [PMID: 21628617]
Piper AJ et al. Obesity hypoventilation syndrome: mechanisms and management. Am J Respir Crit Care Med. 2011 Feb1;183(3):292–8. [PMID: 21037018]

ACUTE RESPIRATORY FAILURE

Respiratory failure is defined as respiratory dysfunction resulting in abnormalities of oxygenation or ventilation (CO_2 elimination) severe enough to threaten the function of vital organs. Arterial blood gas criteria for respiratory failure are not absolute but may be arbitrarily established as a Po_2 under 60 mm Hg (7.8 kPa) or a Pco_2 over 50 mm Hg (6.5 kPa). Acute respiratory failure may occur in a variety of pulmonary and nonpulmonary disorders (Table 9–26). Only a few selected general principles of management will be reviewed here.

▶ Clinical Findings

Symptoms and signs of acute respiratory failure are those of the underlying disease combined with those of hypoxemia or hypercapnia. The chief symptom of hypoxemia is dyspnea, though profound hypoxemia may exist in the absence of complaints. Signs of hypoxemia include cyanosis, restlessness, confusion, anxiety, delirium, tachypnea, bradycardia or tachycardia, hypertension, cardiac dysrhythmias, and tremor. Dyspnea and headache are the cardinal symptoms of hypercapnia. Signs of hypercapnia include peripheral and conjunctival hyperemia, hypertension, tachycardia, tachypnea, impaired consciousness, papilledema, and asterixis. The symptoms and signs of acute respiratory failure are both insensitive and nonspecific; therefore, the clinician must maintain a high index of suspicion and obtain arterial blood gas analysis if respiratory failure is suspected.

▶ Treatment

Treatment of the patient with acute respiratory failure consists of: (1) specific therapy directed toward the underlying disease; (2) respiratory supportive care directed toward the maintenance of adequate gas exchange; and (3) general supportive care. Only the last two aspects are discussed below.

A. Respiratory Support

Respiratory support has both nonventilatory and ventilatory aspects.

1. Nonventilatory aspects—The main therapeutic goal in acute hypoxemic respiratory failure is to ensure adequate

Table 9–26. Selected causes of acute respiratory failure in adults.

Airway disorders	Neuromuscular and related disorders
Asthma	Primary neuromuscular diseases
Acute exacerbation of chronic bronchitis or emphysema	Guillain-Barré syndrome
Obstruction of pharynx, larynx, trachea, main stem bronchus, or lobar bronchus by edema, mucus, mass, or foreign body	Myasthenia gravis
	Poliomyelitis
	Polymyositis
Pulmonary edema	Drug- or toxin-induced
Increased hydrostatic pressure	Botulism
Left ventricular dysfunction (eg, myocardial ischemia, heart failure)	Organophosphates
	Neuromuscular blocking agents
Mitral regurgitation	Aminoglycosides
Left atrial outflow obstruction (eg, mitral stenosis)	Spinal cord injury
	Phrenic nerve injury or dysfunction
Volume overload states	Electrolyte disturbances: hypokalemia, hypophosphatemia
Increased pulmonary capillary permeability	
Acute respiratory distress syndrome	Myxedema
Acute lung injury	**Central nervous system disorders**
Unclear etiology	
Neurogenic	Drugs: sedative, hypnotic, opioid, anesthetics
Negative pressure (inspiratory airway obstruction)	Brainstem respiratory center disorders: trauma, tumor, vascular disorders, hypothyroidism
Reexpansion	
Tocolytic-associated	
Parenchymal lung disorders	Intracranial hypertension
Pneumonia	Central nervous system infections
Interstitial lung diseases	
Diffuse alveolar hemorrhage syndromes	**Increased CO_2 production**
Aspiration	Fever
Lung contusion	Infection
Pulmonary vascular disorders	Hyperalimentation with excess caloric and carbohydrate intake
Thromboembolism	
Air embolism	Hyperthyroidism
Amniotic fluid embolism	Seizures
Chest wall, diaphragm, and pleural disorders	Rigors
Rib fracture	Drugs
Flail chest	
Pneumothorax	
Pleural effusion	
Massive ascites	
Abdominal distention and abdominal compartment syndrome	

oxygenation of vital organs. Inspired oxygen concentration should be the lowest value that results in an arterial hemoglobin saturation of $\geq 90\%$ ($PO_2 \geq 60$ mm Hg [≥ 7.8 kPa]). Higher arterial oxygen tensions are of no proven benefit. Restoration of normoxia may rarely cause hypoventilation in patients with chronic hypercapnia; however, **oxygen therapy should not be withheld for fear of causing progressive respiratory acidemia.** Hypoxemia in patients with obstructive airway disease is usually easily corrected by administering low-flow oxygen by nasal cannula (1–3 L/min) or

Venturi mask (24–40%). Higher concentrations of oxygen are necessary to correct hypoxemia in patients with ARDS, pneumonia, and other parenchymal lung diseases.

2. Ventilatory aspects—Ventilatory support consists of maintaining patency of the airway and ensuring adequate alveolar ventilation. Mechanical ventilation may be provided via face mask (noninvasive) or through tracheal intubation.

A. Noninvasive positive-pressure ventilation— NPPV delivered via a full face mask or nasal mask is first-line therapy in COPD patients with hypercapnic respiratory failure who can protect and maintain the patency of their airway, handle their own secretions, and tolerate the mask apparatus. Several studies have demonstrated the effectiveness of this therapy in reducing intubation rates and ICU stays in patients with ventilatory failure. A bilevel positive-pressure ventilation mode (BiPAP) is preferred for most patients. Patients with acute lung injury or ARDS or those who suffer from severely impaired oxygenation do not benefit and should be intubated if they require mechanical ventilation.

B. Tracheal intubation—Indications for tracheal intubation include: (1) hypoxemia despite supplemental oxygen, (2) upper airway obstruction, (3) impaired airway protection, (4) inability to clear secretions, (5) respiratory acidosis, (6) progressive general fatigue, tachypnea, use of accessory respiratory muscles, or mental status deterioration, and (7) apnea. In general, orotracheal intubation is preferred to nasotracheal intubation in urgent or emergency situations because it is easier, faster, and less traumatic. The position of the tip of the endotracheal tube at the level of the aortic arch should be verified by chest radiograph immediately following intubation, and auscultation should be performed to verify that both lungs are being inflated. Only tracheal tubes with high-volume, low-pressure air-filled cuffs should be used. Cuff inflation pressure should be kept below 20 mm Hg if possible to minimize tracheal mucosal injury.

C. Mechanical ventilation—Indications for mechanical ventilation include: (1) apnea, (2) acute hypercapnia that is not quickly reversed by appropriate specific therapy, (3) severe hypoxemia, and (4) progressive patient fatigue despite appropriate treatment.

Several modes of positive-pressure ventilation are available. Controlled mechanical ventilation (CMV; also known as assist-control or A-C) and synchronized intermittent mandatory ventilation (SIMV) are ventilatory modes in which the ventilator delivers a minimum number of breaths of a specified tidal volume each minute. In both CMV and SIMV, the patient may trigger the ventilator to deliver additional breaths. In CMV, the ventilator responds to breaths initiated by the patient above the set rate by delivering additional full tidal volume breaths. In SIMV, additional breaths are not supported by the ventilator unless the pressure support mode is added. Numerous alternative modes of mechanical ventilation now exist, the most popular being pressure support ventilation (PSV), pressure control ventilation (PCV), and CPAP.

PEEP is useful in improving oxygenation in patients with diffuse parenchymal lung disease such as ARDS. It should be used cautiously in patients with localized parenchymal disease, hyperinflation, or very high airway pressure requirements during mechanical ventilation.

D. Complications of mechanical ventilation— Potential complications of mechanical ventilation are numerous. Migration of the tip of the endotracheal tube into a main bronchus can cause atelectasis of the contralateral lung and overdistention of the intubated lung. Barotrauma (alternatively referred to as "volutrauma"), manifested by subcutaneous emphysema, pneumomediastinum, subpleural air cysts, pneumothorax, or systemic gas embolism, may occur in patients whose lungs are overdistended by excessive tidal volumes, especially those with hyperinflation caused by airflow obstruction. Subtle parenchymal lung injury due to overdistention of alveoli is another potential hazard. Strategies to avoid barotrauma include deliberate hypoventilation through the use of low mechanical tidal volumes and respiratory rates, resulting in "permissive hypercapnia."

Acute respiratory alkalosis caused by overventilation is common. Hypotension induced by elevated intrathoracic pressure that results in decreased return of systemic venous blood to the heart may occur in patients treated with PEEP, those with severe airflow obstruction, and those with intravascular volume depletion. Ventilator-associated pneumonia is another serious complication of mechanical ventilation.

B. General Supportive Care

Maintenance of adequate nutrition is vital; parenteral nutrition should be used only when conventional enteral feeding methods are not possible. Overfeeding, especially with carbohydrate-rich formulas, should be avoided, because it can increase CO_2 production and may potentially worsen or induce hypercapnia in patients with limited ventilatory reserve. However, failure to provide adequate nutrition is more common. Hypokalemia and hypophosphatemia may worsen hypoventilation due to respiratory muscle weakness. Sedative-hypnotics and opioid analgesics are frequently used. They should be titrated carefully to avoid oversedation, leading to prolongation of intubation. Temporary paralysis with a nondepolarizing neuromuscular blocking agent is occasionally used to facilitate mechanical ventilation and to lower oxygen consumption. Prolonged muscle weakness due to an acute myopathy is a potential complication of these agents. Myopathy is more common in patients with kidney injury and in those given concomitant corticosteroids.

Psychological and emotional support of the patient and family, skin care to avoid pressure ulcers, and meticulous avoidance of health care–associated infection and complications of tracheal tubes are vital aspects of comprehensive care for patients with acute respiratory failure.

Attention must also be paid to preventing complications associated with serious illness. Stress gastritis and ulcers may be avoided by administering sucralfate (1 g orally twice a day), histamine H_2-receptor antagonists, or PPIs. There is some concern that the latter two agents, which raise the gastric pH, may permit increased growth of gram-negative bacteria in the stomach, predisposing to pharyngeal colonization and ultimately HCAP; many clinicians therefore prefer sucralfate. The risk of DVT and PE may be reduced by subcutaneous administration of heparin (5000 units every 12 hours), the use of LMWH (see Table 14–15), or placement of sequential compression devices on the lower extremities.

▶ Course & Prognosis

The course and prognosis of acute respiratory failure vary and depend on the underlying disease. The prognosis of acute respiratory failure caused by uncomplicated sedative or opioid overdose is excellent. Acute respiratory failure in patients with COPD who do not require intubation and mechanical ventilation has a good immediate prognosis. On the other hand, ARDS associated with sepsis has an extremely poor prognosis, with mortality rates of about 90%. Overall, adults requiring mechanical ventilation for all causes of acute respiratory failure have survival rates of 62% to weaning, 43% to hospital discharge, and 30% to 1 year after hospital discharge.

Carrillo A et al. Non-invasive ventilation in community-acquired pneumonia and severe acute respiratory failure. Intensive Care Med. 2012 Mar;38(3):458–66. [PMID: 22318634]

Nee PA et al. Critical care in the emergency department: acute respiratory failure. Emerg Med J. 2011 Feb;28(2):94–7. [PMID: 21112972]

Soeiro A de M et al. Demographic, etiological, and histological pulmonary analysis of patients with acute respiratory failure: a study of 19 years of autopsies. Clinics (Sao Paulo). 2011;66(7):1193–7. [PMID: 21876973]

ACUTE RESPIRATORY DISTRESS SYNDROME

 ESSENTIALS OF DIAGNOSIS

▶ Acute onset of respiratory failure.

▶ Bilateral radiographic pulmonary opacities.

▶ Respiratory failure not fully explained by heart failure or volume overload.

▶ Ratio of partial pressure of oxygen in arterial blood (PaO_2) to fractional concentration of inspired oxygen (FIO_2) < 300 mm Hg, with PEEP ≥ 5 cm H_2O.

▶ General Considerations

ARDS denotes acute hypoxemic respiratory failure following a systemic or pulmonary insult without evidence of heart failure. ARDS is the most severe form of acute lung injury and is characterized by an acute onset within 1 week of a known clinical insult, bilateral radiographic pulmonary infiltrates, respiratory failure not fully explained by heart failure or volume overload, and a PaO_2/FIO_2

Table 9–27. Selected disorders associated with ARDS.

Systemic Insults	Pulmonary Insults
Trauma	Aspiration of gastric contents
Sepsis	Embolism of thrombus, fat, air,
Pancreatitis	or amniotic fluid
Shock	Miliary tuberculosis
Multiple transfusions	Diffuse pneumonia (eg, SARS)
Disseminated intravascular	Acute eosinophilic pneumonia
coagulation	Cryptogenic organizing
Burns	pneumonitis
Drugs and drug overdose	Upper airway obstruction
Opioids	Free-base cocaine smoking
Aspirin	Near-drowning
Phenothiazines	Toxic gas inhalation
Tricyclic antidepressants	Nitrogen dioxide
Amiodarone	Chlorine
Chemotherapeutic agents	Sulfur dioxide
Nitrofurantoin	Ammonia
Protamine	Smoke
Thrombotic thrombocytopenic	Oxygen toxicity
purpura	Lung contusion
Cardiopulmonary bypass	Radiation exposure
Head injury	High-altitude exposure
Paraquat	Lung reexpansion or reperfusion

ARDS, acute respiratory distress syndrome; SARS, severe acute respiratory syndrome.

ratio < 300 mm Hg (according to the Berlin Definition). The severity of ARDS is based on the level of oxygenation impairment. Mild ARDS is defined by a Pao_2/Fio_2 ratio of between 200 and 300 mm Hg, moderate ARDS is defined by a Pao_2/Fio_2 ratio between 100 and 200 mm Hg, and severe ARDS is defined by a Pao_2/Fio_2 ratio less than 100 mm Hg. ARDS may follow a wide variety of clinical events (Table 9–27). Common risk factors for ARDS include sepsis, aspiration of gastric contents, shock, infection, lung contusion, nonthoracic trauma, toxic inhalation, near-drowning, and multiple blood transfusions. About one-third of ARDS patients initially have sepsis syndrome. Although the mechanism of lung injury varies with the cause, damage to capillary endothelial cells and alveolar epithelial cells is common to ARDS regardless of cause. Damage to these cells causes increased vascular permeability and decreased production and activity of surfactant; these abnormalities lead to interstitial and alveolar pulmonary edema, alveolar collapse, and hypoxemia.

▶ **Clinical Findings**

ARDS is marked by the rapid onset of profound dyspnea that usually occurs 12–48 hours after the initiating event. Labored breathing, tachypnea, intercostal retractions, and crackles are noted on physical examination. Chest radiography shows diffuse or patchy bilateral infiltrates that rapidly become confluent; these characteristically spare the costophrenic angles. Air bronchograms occur in about 80% of cases. Upper lung zone venous engorgement is distinctly uncommon. Heart size is normal, and pleural effusions are small or nonexistent. Marked hypoxemia occurs

that is refractory to treatment with supplemental oxygen. Many patients with ARDS demonstrate multiple organ failure, particularly involving the kidneys, liver, gut, central nervous system, and cardiovascular system.

▶ **Differential Diagnosis**

Since ARDS is a physiologic and radiographic syndrome rather than a specific disease, the concept of differential diagnosis does not strictly apply. Normal-permeability ("cardiogenic" or hydrostatic) pulmonary edema must be excluded, however, because specific therapy is available for that disorder. Measurement of pulmonary capillary wedge pressure by means of a flow-directed pulmonary artery catheter may be required in selected patients with suspected cardiac dysfunction. Routine use of the Swan-Ganz catheter in ARDS is discouraged.

▶ **Prevention**

No measures that effectively prevent ARDS have been identified; specifically, prophylactic use of PEEP in patients at risk for ARDS has not been shown to be effective. Intravenous methylprednisolone does not prevent ARDS when given early to patients with sepsis syndrome or septic shock.

▶ **Treatment**

Treatment of ARDS must include identification and specific treatment of the underlying precipitating and secondary conditions (eg, sepsis). Meticulous supportive care must then be provided to compensate for the severe dysfunction of the respiratory system associated with ARDS and to prevent complications (see above).

Treatment of the hypoxemia seen in ARDS usually requires tracheal intubation and positive-pressure mechanical ventilation. The lowest levels of PEEP (used to recruit atelectatic alveoli) and supplemental oxygen required to maintain the Pao_2 above 55 mm Hg (7.13 kPa) or the Sao_2 above 88% should be used. Efforts should be made to decrease Fio_2 to less than 60% as soon as possible in order to avoid oxygen toxicity. PEEP can be increased as needed as long as cardiac output and oxygen delivery do not decrease and airway pressures do not increase excessively. Prone positioning may transiently improve oxygenation in selected patients by helping recruit atelectatic alveoli; however, great care must be taken during the maneuver to avoid dislodging catheters and tubes.

A variety of mechanical ventilation strategies are available. A multicenter study of 800 patients demonstrated that a protocol using volume-control ventilation with low tidal volumes (6 mL/kg of ideal body weight) resulted in a 10% absolute mortality reduction over therapy with standard tidal volumes (defined as 12 mL/kg of ideal body weight); this trial reported the lowest mortality (31%) of any intervention to date for ARDS.

Approaches to hemodynamic monitoring and fluid management in patients with acute lung injury have been carefully studied. A prospective RCT comparing hemodynamic management guided either by a pulmonary artery catheter or a central venous catheter using an explicit management protocol demonstrated that a pulmonary artery catheter should not be routinely used for the management of acute lung injury. A subsequent randomized, prospective clinical study of restrictive fluid intake and diuresis as needed to maintain central venous pressure < 4 mm Hg or pulmonary artery occlusion pressure < 8 mm Hg (conservative strategy group) versus a fluid management protocol to target a central venous pressure of 10–14 mm Hg or a pulmonary artery occlusion pressure 14–18 mm Hg (liberal strategy group), showed that patients in the conservative strategy group experienced faster improvement in lung function and spent significantly fewer days on mechanical ventilation and in the ICU without an improvement in death by 60 days or worsening nonpulmonary organ failure at 28 days. Oxygen delivery can be increased in anemic patients by ensuring that hemoglobin concentrations are at least 7 g/dL (70 g/L); patients are not likely to benefit from higher levels. Increasing oxygen delivery to supranormal levels through the use of inotropes and high hemoglobin concentrations is not clinically useful and may be harmful. Strategies to decrease oxygen consumption include the appropriate use of sedatives, analgesics, and antipyretics.

A large number of innovative therapeutic interventions to improve outcomes in ARDS patients have been or are being investigated. Unfortunately, to date, none have consistently shown benefit in clinical trials. Systemic corticosteroids have been studied extensively with variable and inconsistent results. While a few small studies suggest some specific improved outcomes when given within the first 2 weeks after the onset of ARDS, the routine use of corticosteroids is not recommended.

▶ Course & Prognosis

The mortality rate associated with ARDS is 30–40%. If ARDS is accompanied by sepsis, the mortality rate may reach 90%. The major causes of death are the primary illness and secondary complications such as multiple organ system failure or sepsis. Median survival is about 2 weeks. Many patients who succumb to ARDS and its complications die after withdrawal of ventilator support (see Chapter 5). Most survivors of ARDS are left with some pulmonary symptoms (cough, dyspnea, sputum production), which tend to improve over time. Mild abnormalities of oxygenation, diffusing capacity, and lung mechanics persist in some individuals.

Saguil A et al. Acute respiratory distress syndrome: diagnosis and management. Am Fam Physician. 2012 Feb15;85(4):352–8. [PMID: 22335314]

The ARDS Definition Task Force; Ranieri VM et al. Acute respiratory distress syndrome: the Berlin Definition. JAMA. 2012 Jun20;307(23):2526–33. [PMID: 22797452]

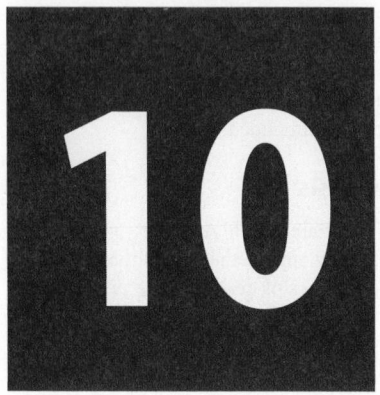

Heart Disease

Thomas M. Bashore, MD

Christopher B. Granger, MD

Kevin Jackson, MD

Manesh R. Patel, MD

CONGENITAL HEART DISEASE

In the United States, there are more adults with congenital heart disease than children, with over 1.5 million adults in the United States surviving with congenital heart disease.

Baumgartner H et al; Task Force on the Management of Grown-up Congenital Heart Disease of the European Society of Cardiology (ESC); Association for European Paediatric Cardiology (AEPC); ESC Committee for Practice Guidelines (CPG). ESC Guidelines for the management of grown-up congenital heart disease (new version 2010). Eur Heart J. 2010 Dec;31(23):2915–57. [PMID: 20801927]

Warnes CA et al. ACC/AHA 2008 Guidelines for the Management of Adults With Congenital Heart Disease. A Report of the American College of Cardiology/American Heart Association Task Force on Practice Guidelines. Circulation. 2008 Dec 2;118(23):e714–833. [PMID: 18997169]

PULMONARY VALVE STENOSIS

 ESSENTIALS OF DIAGNOSIS

- Severe cases may present with right-sided heart failure.
- P_2 delayed and soft or absent.
- Ejection click often present and decreases with inspiration—the only right heart auscultatory event that decreases with inspiration, all others increase.
- Echocardiography/Doppler is diagnostic.
- Patients with peak pulmonic valve gradients > 60 mm Hg or mean of 40 mm Hg by echocardiography/Doppler should undergo intervention regardless of symptoms.

General Considerations

Stenosis of the pulmonary valve or right ventricular (RV) infundibulum increases the resistance to RV outflow, raises the RV pressure, and limits pulmonary blood flow.

Pulmonic stenosis is often congenital, associated with other cardiac lesions. Pulmonary blood flow preferentially goes to the left lung in valvular pulmonic stenosis. In the absence of associated shunts, arterial saturation is normal. Infundibular stenosis may be so severe that the RV is divided into a low-pressure and high-pressure chamber (double-chambered RV). Peripheral pulmonic stenosis can accompany valvular pulmonic stenosis and may be part of a variety of clinical syndromes, including the congenital rubella syndrome. Patients who have had the Ross procedure for aortic valve disease (transfer of the pulmonary valve to the aortic position with a homograft pulmonary valve placed in the pulmonary position) may experience postoperative (noncongenital) pulmonic stenosis due to an immune response in the homograft. RV outflow obstructions can also occur when there is a conduit from the RV to the pulmonary artery (PA) that becomes stenotic.

▶ Clinical Findings

A. Symptoms and Signs

Mild cases of pulmonic stenosis are asymptomatic; moderate to severe pulmonic stenosis may cause symptoms of dyspnea on exertion, syncope, chest pain, and eventually RV failure.

On examination, there is often a palpable parasternal lift due to right ventricular hypertrophy (RVH) and the pulmonary outflow tract may be palpable if it is enlarged. A loud, harsh systolic murmur and occasionally a prominent thrill are present in the left second and third interspaces parasternally. The murmur radiates toward the left shoulder due to the flow pattern and increases with inspiration. In mild to moderate pulmonic stenosis, a loud ejection click can be heard to precede the murmur; this sound decreases with inspiration as the increased RV filling from inspiration prematurely opens the valve during atrial systole. This is the only right-sided auscultatory event that decreases with inspiration. The reason for this is that the valve excursion in systole is less with inspiration than with expiration. This relates to premature opening of the pulmonary valve with the atrial kick into the RV. The click therefore diminishes in intensity when more volume is ejected into the RV with inspiration, raising the RV diastolic pressure. The second sound is obscured by the murmur in severe cases; the pulmonary component may be diminished, delayed, or absent. A right-sided S_4 and a prominent *a* wave in the venous pulse are present when there is RV diastolic dysfunction or a *c-v* wave if there is tricuspid regurgitation present. Pulmonary valve regurgitation is relatively uncommon in primary pulmonic stenosis and may be very difficult to hear, as the gradient between the reduced PA diastolic pressure and the elevated RV diastolic pressure may be quite small (low-pressure pulmonary valve regurgitation).

B. ECG and Chest Radiography

Right axis deviation or RVH is noted; peaked P waves provide evidence of right atrial (RA) overload. Heart size may be normal on radiographs, or there may be a prominent RV and RA or gross cardiac enlargement, depending on the severity. There is often poststenotic dilation of the main and left pulmonary arteries. Pulmonary vascularity is usually normal.

C. Diagnostic Studies

Echocardiography/Doppler is the diagnostic tool of choice, can provide evidence for a doming valve versus a dysplastic valve, can determine the gradient across the valve, and can provide information regarding subvalvular obstruction and the presence or absence of tricuspid or pulmonic valvular regurgitation. Mild pulmonic stenosis is present if the peak gradient by echocardiography/Doppler is < 30 mm Hg, moderate pulmonic stenosis is present if the peak gradient is between 30 mm Hg and 60 mm Hg, and severe pulmonic stenosis is present if the peak gradient is > 60 mm Hg or the mean gradient is > 40 mm Hg. Catheterization is usually unnecessary for the diagnosis; it should be used only if the data are unclear or in preparation for either a percutaneous intervention or surgery.

► Prognosis & Treatment

Patients with mild pulmonic stenosis have a normal life span with no intervention. Moderate stenosis may be asymptomatic in childhood and adolescence, but symptoms often appear as patients grow older. The degree of stenosis does worsen with time in many patients, so serial follow-up is important. Severe stenosis is rarely associated with sudden death but can cause right heart failure in patients as early as in their 20s and 30s. Pregnancy and exercise tends to be well tolerated except in severe stenosis.

Class I indications for intervention include all symptomatic patients and all those with a resting peak gradient > 60 mm Hg or mean > 40 mm Hg, regardless of symptoms. Percutaneous balloon valvuloplasty is highly successful in domed valve patients and is the treatment of choice. Surgical commissurotomy can also be done, or pulmonary valve replacement (with either a bioprosthetic valve or homograft) when pulmonary valve regurgitation is too severe or the valve is dysplastic. Pulmonary outflow tract obstruction due to RV to PA conduit obstruction or to homograft pulmonary valve stenosis can be relieved with a percutaneously implanted pulmonary valve. The applicability of this approach to primary pulmonic valve stenosis remains under investigation.

Endocarditis prophylaxis is unnecessary for native valves even after valvuloplasty unless there has been prior pulmonary valve endocarditis (a very rare entity) (see Table 33–4).

► When to Refer

All symptomatic patients, and all asymptomatic patients whose peak pulmonary valve gradient is > 60 mm Hg or mean gradient > 40 mm Hg, should be referred to a cardiologist with expertise in adult congenital heart disease.

Bashore TM. Adult congenital heart disease: right ventricular outflow tract lesions. Circulation. 2007 Apr 10;115(14):1933–47. [PMID: 17420363]
Odenwald T et al. Pulmonary valve interventions. Expert Rev Cardiovasc Ther. 2011 Nov;9(11):1445–57. [PMID: 22059793]
Warnes CA et al. ACC/AHA 2008 Guidelines for the Management of Adults With Congenital Heart Disease. A Report of the American College of Cardiology/American Heart Association Task Force on Practice Guidelines. Circulation. 2008 Dec 2;118(23):e714–833. [PMID: 18997169]

COARCTATION OF THE AORTA

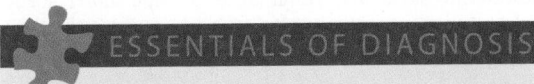

ESSENTIALS OF DIAGNOSIS

- ► Usual presentation is systemic hypertension.
- ► Echocardiography/Doppler is diagnostic; a gradient of > 20 mm Hg may be significant due to collaterals around the coarctation, reducing gradient despite severe obstruction.
- ► Associated bicuspid aortic valve (in 50–80% of patients).
- ► Systolic pressure is higher in upper extremities than in lower extremities; diastolic pressures are similar.

► General Considerations

Coarctation of the aorta consists of localized narrowing of the aortic arch just distal to the origin of the left subclavian artery. Collateral circulation develops around the coarctation through the intercostal arteries and the branches of the subclavian arteries and can result in a lower transcoarctation gradient by enabling blood flow to bypass the obstruction. Coarctation is a cause of secondary hypertension and should be considered in young patients with elevated blood pressure (BP). The renin–angiotensin system is reset, however, and contributes to the hypertension occasionally seen even after coarctation repair. A bicuspid valve is seen in over 50–80% of the cases, and there is an increased incidence of cerebral berry aneurysms.

► Clinical Findings

A. Symptoms and Signs

If cardiac failure does not occur in infancy, there are usually no symptoms until the hypertension produces left ventricular (LV) failure or cerebral hemorrhage occurs.

Strong arterial pulsations are seen in the neck and supra-sternal notch. Hypertension is present in the arms, but the pressure is normal or low in the legs. This difference is exaggerated by exercise. Femoral pulsations are weak and are delayed in comparison with the brachial or radial pulse. Patients may have severe coarctation, but with large collateral blood vessels may have relatively small gradients across the coarctation because of high flow through the collaterals to the aorta distal to the coarctation. A continuous murmur heard superiorly and midline in the back or over the left anterior chest may be present when large collaterals are present. The coarctation itself may result in systolic ejection murmurs at the base, often heard posteriorly. There may be an associated aortic regurgitation or stenosis murmur due to the bicuspid aortic valve.

B. ECG and Chest Radiography

The ECG usually shows LV hypertrophy (LVH). Radiography shows scalloping of the ribs due to enlarged collateral intercostal arteries, dilation of the left subclavian artery and poststenotic aortic dilation, and LV enlargement. The coarctation region and the poststenotic dilation of the descending aorta may result in a "3" sign along aortic shadow on the PA chest radiograph (the notch in the "3" representing the area of coarctation).

C. Diagnostic Studies

Echocardiography/Doppler is usually diagnostic and may provide additional evidence for a bicuspid aortic valve. Both MRI and CT can also provide excellent images of the coarctation local anatomy and one or the other should be done in all patients to define the coarctation structure. MRI and echocardiography/Doppler can also provide estimates of the gradient across the lesion. A significant peak-to-peak gradient is > 20 mm Hg. Cardiac catheterization provides definitive gradient information and is necessary if percutaneous stenting is to be considered.

▶ Prognosis & Treatment

Cardiac failure is common in infancy and in older untreated patients; it is uncommon in late childhood and young adulthood. Patients with a demonstrated peak gradient of > 20 mm Hg should be considered for intervention, especially if there is evidence of collateral blood vessels. Most untreated patients with severe coarctation die of hypertension, rupture of the aorta, infective endarteritis, or cerebral hemorrhage before the age of 50. Aortic dissection also occurs with increased frequency. Coarctation of any significance may be poorly tolerated in pregnancy because of the inability to support the placental flow.

Resection of the coarctation site has a surgical mortality rate of 1–4% and includes risk of spinal cord injury. The percutaneous interventional procedure of choice is endovascular stenting when anatomically feasible; self-expanding and balloon-expandable covered stents have been shown to be advantageous over bare metal stents. Otherwise, surgical resection (usually with end-to-end anastomosis) should be performed. About 25% of surgically corrected patients

continue to be hypertensive years after surgery because of permanent changes in the renin–angiotensin system, endothelial dysfunction, aortic stiffness, altered arch morphology, and increased ventricular stiffness. Recurrence of the coarctation stenosis following intervention requires long-term follow-up.

▶ When to Refer

All patients with coarctation and a detectable gradient should be referred to a cardiologist with expertise in adult congenital heart disease.

Brown ML et al. Coarctation of the aorta: lifelong surveillance is mandatory following surgical repair. J Am Coll Cardiol. 2013 Sep 10;62(11):1020–5. [PMID: 23850909]

Vergales JE et al. Coarctation of the aorta—the current state of surgical and transcatheter therapies. Curr Cardiol Rev. 2013 Aug;9(3):211–9. [PMID: 23909637]

Warnes CA et al. ACC/AHA 2008 Guidelines for the Management of Adults With Congenital Heart Disease. A Report of the American College of Cardiology/American Heart Association Task Force on Practice Guidelines. Circulation. 2008 Dec 2;118(23):e714–833. [PMID: 18997169]

ATRIAL SEPTAL DEFECT & PATENT FORAMEN OVALE

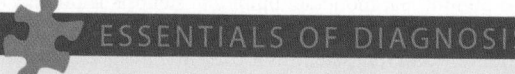

ESSENTIALS OF DIAGNOSIS

- ▶ Often asymptomatic and discovered on routine physical examination.

- ▶ Echocardiography/Doppler is diagnostic.

- ▶ All atrial septal defects (ASD) should be closed either by a percutaneous device or by surgery if there is any evidence of an RV volume overload regardless of symptoms.

- ▶ A patent foramen ovale (PFO), present in 25% of the population, rarely can lead to paradoxic emboli. Suspicion should be highest in patients who have cryptogenic stroke before age 55 years.

▶ General Considerations

The most common form of ASD (80% of cases) is persistence of the ostium secundum in the mid septum. A less common abnormality is persistence of the ostium primum (low in the septum). In many patients with an ostium primum defect, there are mitral or tricuspid valve "clefts" as well as a ventricular septal defect (VSD) as part of the atrioventricular (AV) septal defect. A third form of ASD is the **sinus venosus defect,** a hole usually at of the upper or (rarely) the lower part of the atrial septum due to failure of the embryonic superior vena cava or the inferior vena cava to merge with the atria properly. The inferior vena cava sinus venosus defect is uncommon. The superior vena cava sinus venosus defect is usually associated with an anomalous connection of the right upper pulmonary vein into the superior vena cava. The **coronary sinus ASD** is also rare and basically an unroofed coronary sinus. In all cases, normally oxygenated blood from the higher-pressure LA passes into the RA, increasing RV output and pulmonary blood flow. In children, the degree of shunting across these defects may be quite large (pulmonary to systemic blood flow ratios of 3:1 or so). As the RV diastolic pressure rises from the chronic volume overload, the RA pressure may rise and the degree of left-to-right shunting may decrease. Eventually, if the RA pressure exceeds the LA, the shunt may reverse and be primarily right-to-left and systemic cyanosis appears. The major factor in the direction of shunt flow is thus the compliance of the respective atrial chambers.

The pulmonary pressures are modestly elevated in most patients with an ASD due to the high pulmonary blood flow, but severe pulmonary hypertension with cyanosis (Eisenmenger physiology) is actually unusual, occurring in only about 15% of the patients with an ASD alone. Eventual RV failure may occur though, and most shunts should be corrected unless they are quite small (< 1.5:1 left-to-right shunt). In adults, a large left-to-right shunt may have begun to reverse, so the absolute left-to-right shunt measurement (Qp/Qs, where Qp = pulmonary flow and Qs = systemic flow) at the time the patient is studied may underestimate the original shunt size. In addition, in most patients the LV and LA compliance normally declines more over time than the RV and RA, and the natural history of small atrial septal shunts is to increase the left-to-right shunt as the patient ages.

ASDs predispose to atrial fibrillation due to RA enlargement, and paradoxic right-to-left emboli do occur. Interestingly, paradoxic emboli may be more common in patients with a PFO than a true ASD. An **aneurysm of the atrial septum** is not a true aneurysm but rather simply redundancy of the atrial septum. When present with a PFO, the back and forth swinging of the redundant atrial septum ("jump rope septum") tends to pull open the PFO. This helps explain why more right-to-left shunting occurs in patients with an atrial septal aneurysm and PFO than in those with a PFO alone and creates the anatomic substrate for the occurrence of paradoxical emboli. Other factors may distort the atrial septum (such as an enlarged aorta) and increase shunting in patients with a PFO. Right to left PFO shunting may be more prominent upright, creating orthostatic hypoxemia (platypnea orthodeoxia).

▶ Clinical Findings

A. Symptoms and Signs

Patients with a small or moderate ASD or with a PFO are asymptomatic unless a complication occurs. There is only trivial shunting in a PFO unless the RA pressure increases for some other reason or the atrial septum is distorted. Shunting in a PFO is more common if an atrial septal aneurysm is present. With larger ASD shunts, exertional dyspnea or heart failure may develop, most commonly in the fourth decade of life or later. Prominent RV and PA pulsations are then readily visible and palpable. A moderately loud systolic ejection murmur can be heard in the second and third interspaces parasternally as a result of increased flow through the pulmonary valve. S_2 is widely split and does not vary with breathing due to the fact that the left-to-right shunt decreases as the RA pressure increases with inspiration and the RV stroke volume is held relatively constant in inspiration and expiration ("fixed" splitting of the second sound results). In very large left-to-right shunts, a tricuspid rumble may be heard due to the high flow across the tricuspid valve.

B. ECG and Chest Radiography

Right axis deviation or RVH may be present depending on the size of the RV volume overload. Incomplete or complete right bundle branch block is present in nearly all cases of ASD, and superior axis deviation is noted in the complete AV septal defect, where complete heart block is often seen as well. With sinus venosus defects, the P axis is leftward of +15° due to abnormal atrial activation with loss of the upper RA tissue from around the sinus node. In some patients with a secundum defect, there is notching in the inferior QRS leads (sometimes referred to as crochetage since the negative spike within the QRS resembles a crochet needle). The chest radiograph shows large pulmonary arteries, increased pulmonary vascularity, an enlarged RA and RV, and a small aortic knob as with all pre-tricuspid valve cardiac left-to-right shunts.

C. Diagnostic Studies

Echocardiography demonstrates evidence of RA and RV volume overload. The atrial defect is usually observed, although sinus venosus defects may be elusive. Many patients with a PFO also have an atrial septal aneurysm (defined as > 10 mm excursion of the septum from the static position). Echocardiography with agitated saline bubble contrast can demonstrate a right-to-left shunt, and both pulsed and color flow Doppler flow studies can demonstrate shunting in either direction. In platypnea orthodeoxia, the shunt may primarily result from inferior vena cava blood, and a femoral vein saline injection may be required to demonstrate the shunt. Transesophageal echocardiography (TEE) is helpful when transthoracic echocardiography quality is not optimal because it improves the sensitivity for detection of small shunts and provides a better assessment of PFO anatomy. Both CT and MRI can elucidate the atrial septal anatomy and demonstrate associated lesions, such as anomalous pulmonary venous connections. Atrial septal anatomy can be complex, and MRI can both define multiple fenestrations and reveal whether there is an adequate rim around the defect to allow for safe positioning of an atrial septal device. Cardiac catheterization can define the size and location of the shunt and determine the pulmonary pressure and pulmonary vascular resistance (PVR).

▶ Prognosis & Treatment

Patients with small atrial shunts live a normal life span with no intervention. Large shunts usually cause disability by age 40 years. Because left-to-right shunts tend to increase with age-related changes in LV (and subsequently LA) compliance, guidelines suggest that closure of all left-to-right shunts over 1.5:1 should be accomplished. This situation always results in RV volume overload. Increased PVR and pulmonary hypertension secondary to pulmonary vascular disease rarely occur in childhood or young adult life in secundum defects but are more common in primum defects. If the pulmonary systolic pressure is > two-thirds the systemic pressure, the pulmonary hypertension may preclude ASD closure. After age 40 years, cardiac arrhythmias (especially atrial fibrillation) and heart failure occur with increased frequency due to the chronic right heart volume overload. Paradoxical systemic arterial embolization also becomes more of a concern as RV compliance is lost and the left-to-right shunt begins to reverse.

PFOs are usually not associated with significant shunting, and therefore the patients are asymptomatic and the heart size is normal. However, PFOs are responsible for most paradoxical emboli and are one of the most frequent causes of cryptogenic strokes in patients under age 55 years. An associated atrial septal aneurysm increases the risk of right-to-left shunting.

Occasionally, a PFO may be responsible for cyanosis, especially if the RA pressure is elevated from pulmonary or RV hypertension or from severe tricuspid regurgitation.

Surgery involves anything from simple stitching of the foramen closed to patching of the hole with Dacron or a pericardial patch. For ostium secundum ASDs, percutaneous closure by use of a variety of devices is preferred over surgery when the anatomy is appropriate.

Patients with a PFO who have symptoms related to stroke or transient ischemic attack (especially if the age is under 55) or who have hypoxemia (especially upon standing) should have the PFO closed if no other cause for symptoms is evident. For patients with cryptogenic stroke or transient ischemic attack, it remains uncertain whether closure of the PFO, either by open surgical or percutaneous techniques, has any advantage over anticoagulation with either warfarin or aspirin. RESPECT (Randomized Evaluation of recurrent Stroke comparing PFO Closure to current standard Treatment) randomized 980 patients, and PCTRIAL (Percutaneous Closure of patent foramen ovale versus medical treatment in patients with cryptogenic stroke TRIAL) randomized 414 patients. Neither trial met the superiority composite end point (death, nonfatal stroke, transient ischemic attack, or peripheral embolism), but both trials had much fewer events in the medical arms than prior studies had suggested. Practically, young patients (< 55 years of age) with cryptogenic stroke and no other identifiable cause except for the presence of a PFO may still be considered for PFO closure in many centers, but the data suggest medical therapy remains an equally viable option.

When cyanosis might be improved by PFO closure, it is appropriate to consider it. PFO closure is also occasionally recommended for deep sea divers to help prevent the "bends" due to nitrous oxide shunting. A case-control study did not confirm the relationship between migraine plus aura and a PFO.

▶ When to Refer

- All patients with an ASD should be evaluated by a cardiologist with expertise in adult congenital disease to ensure no other structural disease is present and to investigate whether the RV is enlarged.

- If the RA and RV sizes remain normal, serial echocardiography should be performed.

- If the RA and RV volumes increase, then referral to a cardiologist who performs percutaneous closure is warranted.

- Patients < 55 years of age with an apparent paradoxical embolus and a PFO should be referred for possible closure of the defect, although studies have yet to prove the effectiveness of percutaneous closure and medical therapy appears equally effective.

- Patients with cyanosis and a PFO with evidence for a right-to-left shunt by agitated saline bubble contrast on echocardiography.

Carroll JD et al; RESPECT Investigators. Closure of patent foramen ovale versus medical therapy after cryptogenic stroke. N Engl J Med. 2013 Mar 21;368(12):1092–100. [PMID: 23514286]

Di Tullio MR et al. Patent foramen ovale, subclinical cerebrovascular disease, and ischemic stroke in a population-based cohort. J Am Coll Cardiol. 2013 Jul 2;62(1):35–41. [PMID: 23644084]

Garg P et al. Lack of association between migraine headache and patent foramen ovale: results of a case-control study. Circulation. 2010 Mar 30;121(12):1406–12. [PMID: 20231534]

Hoffmann A et al. Cerebrovascular accidents in adult patients with congenital heart disease. Heart. 2010 Aug;96(15):1223–6. [PMID: 20639238]

Landzberg MJ et al. Patent foramen ovale: when is intervention warranted? Can J Cardiol. 2013 Jul;29(7):890–2. [PMID: 23790552]

Tobis J et al. Percutaneous treatment of patent foramen ovale and atrial septal defects. J Am Coll Cardiol. 2012 Oct 30;60 (18): 1722–32. [PMID: 23040567]

Warnes CA et al. ACC/AHA 2008 Guidelines for the Management of Adults With Congenital Heart Disease. A Report of the American College of Cardiology/American Heart Association Task Force on Practice Guidelines. Circulation. 2008 Dec 2;118(23):e714–833. [PMID: 18997169]

VENTRICULAR SEPTAL DEFECT

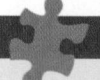

ESSENTIALS OF DIAGNOSIS

▶ A restrictive VSD is small and makes a louder murmur than an unrestricted one. The higher the gradient across the septum, the smaller the left-to-right shunt.

▶ Small defects may be asymptomatic.

▶ Larger defects may result in pulmonary hypertension (Eisenmenger physiology) if not repaired.

▶ Echocardiography/Doppler is diagnostic.

General Considerations

De novo VSDs are uncommon in adults. Congenital VSDs occur in various parts of the ventricular septum. Four types are often described: in **type A,** the VSD lies underneath the semilunar valves; in **type B,** the VSD is membranous with three variations; in **type C,** the inlet VSD is present below the tricuspid valve and often part of the AV canal defect; and **type D** is the muscular VSD. Membranous and muscular septal defects may spontaneously close in childhood as the septum grows and hypertrophies. A left-to-right shunt is present unless there is associated RV hypertension. The smaller the defect, the greater the gradient from the LV to the RV and the louder the murmur. The presentation in adults depends on the size of the shunt and whether there is associated pulmonic or subpulmonic stenosis that has protected the lung from the systemic pressure and volume. Unprotected lungs with large shunts invariably lead to pulmonary vascular disease and severe pulmonary hypertension (Eisenmenger physiology).

Clinical Findings

A. Symptoms and Signs

The clinical features depend on the size of the defect and the presence or absence of RV outflow obstruction or increased PVR. Small shunts are associated with loud, harsh holosystolic murmurs in the left third and fourth interspaces along the sternum. A systolic thrill is common. Larger shunts may create RV volume and pressure overload. If pulmonary hypertension occurs, high-pressure pulmonary valve regurgitation may result. Right heart failure may gradually become evident late in the course, and the shunt will begin to balance or reverse as RV and LV systolic pressures equalize with the advent of pulmonary hypertension. Cyanosis from right-to-left shunting may then occur.

B. ECG and Chest Radiography

The ECG may be normal or may show right, left, or biventricular hypertrophy, depending on the size of the defect and the PVR. With large shunts, the RV, the LV, the LA, and the pulmonary arteries are enlarged and pulmonary vascularity is increased on chest radiographs. The RV is often normal until late in the process. If an increased PVR (pulmonary hypertension) evolves, an enlarged PA with pruning of the distal pulmonary vascular bed is seen. In rare cases of a VSD high in the ventricular septum, an aortic cusp may prolapse into the VSD and reduce the VSD shunt but result in acute aortic regurgitation.

C. Diagnostic Studies

Echocardiography can demonstrate the size of the overloaded chambers and can usually define the defect anatomy. Doppler can qualitatively assess the magnitude of shunting by noting the gradient from LV to RV and, if some tricuspid regurgitation is present, the RV systolic pressure can be estimated. The septal leaflet of the tricuspid valve may be part of the VSD anatomy and the complex

appears as a ventricular septal "aneurysm." These membranous septal aneurysms may fenestrate and result in a VSD shunt or may remain intact. Color flow Doppler helps delineate the shunt severity and the presence of valvular regurgitation. MRI and cardiac CT can often visualize the defect and describe any other anatomic abnormalities. MRI can provide quantitative shunt data as well. Cardiac catheterization is usually reserved for those with at least moderate shunting to determine the PVR and the degree of pulmonary hypertension. A PVR of > 7.0 absolute units or a PVR/systemic vascular resistance ratio of > 0.67 (two-thirds systemic) usually implies inoperability. The vasoreactivity of the pulmonary circuit may be tested at catheterization using agents such as inhaled nitric oxide.

Prognosis & Treatment

Patients with a small VSD as the only abnormality have a normal life expectancy except for the small threat of infective endocarditis. Antibiotic prophylaxis after dental work is only recommended when the VSD is residual from a prior patch closure or when there is associated pulmonary hypertension and cyanosis (see Tables 33–4, 33–5, and 33–6). With large shunts, heart failure may develop early in life, and survival beyond age 40 years is unusual without intervention.

The 2008 ACC/AHA guidelines for the management of patients with VSD include the following:

1. Medical management (class 2b recommendation): Pulmonary vasodilatory therapy is appropriate for adults with a VSD and severe pulmonary hypertension. The response to inhaled nitric oxide is used to guide which agent would be the best option.

2. Surgical management (class 1 recommendation): Closure is indicated when the left-to-right shunt ratio is > 2.0 or there is clinical LV volume overload. In addition, closure is recommended if there has been a history of infective endocarditis.

3. Surgical management (class 2b recommendation): Closure is reasonable if the left-to-right shunt is > 1.5 and pulmonary pressure and PVR are less than two-thirds systemic pressure and systemic vascular resistance. Closure is also reasonable if the shunt ratio is > 1.5 and there is evidence of heart failure.

Small shunts (pulmonary-to-systemic flow ratio < 1.5) in asymptomatic patients do not require surgery or other intervention. The presence of RV infundibular stenosis or pulmonary valve stenosis may protect the pulmonary circuit such that some patients even with a large VSD may still be operable as adults.

Surgical repair of a VSD is generally a low-risk procedure unless there is significant Eisenmenger physiology. Devices for nonsurgical closure of muscular VSDs are approved and those for membranous VSDs are being implanted with promising results; however, conduction disturbance is a major complication. The percutaneous devices are also approved for closure of a VSD related to acute myocardial infarction, although the results in this very high-risk patient population have not been encouraging. The drugs used to treat pulmonary hypertension secondary to VSD are similar to those used to treat idiopathic ("primary") pulmonary hypertension (see below).

▶ When to Refer

All patients with a VSD should be referred to a cardiologist with expertise in adult congenital disease to decide if long-term follow-up is warranted.

Anderson BR et al. Contemporary outcomes of surgical ventricular septal defect closure. J Thorac Cardiovasc Surg. 2013 Mar;145(3):641–7. [PMID: 23414985]

Penny DJ et al. Ventricular septal defect. Lancet. 2011 Mar 26;377(9771):1103–12. [PMID: 21349577]

Warnes CA et al. ACC/AHA 2008 Guidelines for the Management of Adults With Congenital Heart Disease. A Report of the American College of Cardiology/American Heart Association Task Force on Practice Guidelines. Circulation. 2008 Dec 2;118(23):e714–833. [PMID: 18997169]

TETRALOGY OF FALLOT

ESSENTIALS OF DIAGNOSIS

▶ Five features are characteristic:
- VSD.
- RVH.
- RV outflow obstruction from infundibular stenosis.
- Overriding aorta in half (< 50% of the aorta over the septum).
- A right-sided aortic arch is seen in 25%.

▶ Echocardiography/Doppler and the examination may underestimate significant pulmonary valve regurgitation. Be wary if the RV is enlarged.

▶ Arrhythmias are common; periodic Holter monitoring is recommended.

▶ Serious arrhythmias and sudden death may occur if the QRS width is > 180 msec.

▶ General Considerations

Patients with tetralogy of Fallot have a VSD, RV infundibular stenosis, RVH, and a dilated aorta (in about 50% of patients it overrides the septum). If there is an associated ASD, the complex is referred to as pentalogy of Fallot. There may or may not be pulmonary valve stenosis as well, usually due to a bicuspid pulmonary valve. The aorta can be quite enlarged and aortic regurgitation may occur. If more than 50% of the aorta overrides into the RV outflow tract, the anatomy is considered as double outlet RV. Two vascular abnormalities are common: a right-sided aortic arch (in 25%) and anomalous left anterior descending coronary artery from the right cusp (7–9%). The latter is important in that surgical correction must avoid injuring the coronary artery when repairing the RV outflow obstruction.

Most adult patients have undergone prior surgery. If significant RV outflow obstruction is present in infancy, a systemic arterial to pulmonary artery shunt is often the initial surgical procedure to improve pulmonary blood flow. This procedure enables blood to reach the underperfused lung either by directly attaching one of the subclavian arteries to the PA (**classic Blalock shunt**) or by creating a conduit between the two (**modified Blalock shunt**). Other types of systemic to pulmonary shunts no longer in use include a window between the right PA and the aorta (**Waterston-Cooley shunt**) or a window between the left PA and the descending aorta (**Potts shunt**). In the adult, there may be a reduced upper extremity pulse on the side used for the classic Blalock procedure. **Total repair** of the tetralogy of Fallot generally includes a VSD patch and usually an enlarging RV outflow tract patch, as well as a takedown of the arterial-pulmonary artery shunt. Often the RV outflow tract patch extends through the pulmonary valve into the PA (trans-annular patch), and the patient is left with varying degrees of pulmonary valve regurgitation. Over the years, the volume overload from severe pulmonary valve regurgitation becomes the major hemodynamic problem seen in adults. Ventricular arrhythmias can also originate from the edge of the patch, and tend to increase with the size of the RV.

▶ Clinical Findings

Most adult patients in whom tetralogy of Fallot has been repaired are relatively asymptomatic unless right heart failure occurs or arrhythmias become an issue. Patients can be active and generally require no specific therapy except endocarditis prophylaxis.

A. Symptoms and Signs

Physical examination should include checking both arms for any loss of pulse from a prior shunt procedure in infancy. The jugular venous pulsations (JVP) may reveal an increased *a* wave from poor RV compliance or rarely a *c-v* wave due to tricuspid regurgitation. The right-sided arch has no consequence. The precordium may be active, often with a persistent pulmonary outflow murmur. P_2 may or may not be audible. A right-sided gallop may be heard. A residual VSD or aortic regurgitation murmur may be present. At times, the insertion site of a prior Blalock or other shunt may create a stenotic area in the branch PA and a continuous murmur occurs as a result.

B. ECG and Chest Radiography

The ECG reveals RVH and right axis deviation; in repaired tetralogy, there is often a right bundle branch block pattern. The chest radiograph shows a classic boot-shaped heart with prominence of the RV and a concavity in the RV outflow tract. This may be less impressive following repair. The aorta may be enlarged and right-sided. Importantly, the width of the QRS should be examined yearly. There are data that persons at greatest risk for sudden death are those with a QRS width of > 180 msec. Most experts recommend Holter monitoring as well, especially if patients experience palpitations. The width of the QRS corresponds to the RV size, and in some patients, the QRS width actually decreases following relief of the pulmonary valve regurgitation with use of a prosthetic pulmonary valve.

C. Diagnostic Studies

Echocardiography/Doppler usually establishes the diagnosis by noting the unrestricted (large) VSD, the RV infundibular stenosis, and the enlarged aorta. In patients who have had tetralogy of Fallot repaired, echocardiography/Doppler also provides data regarding the amount of pulmonary valve regurgitation, RV and LV function, and the presence of aortic regurgitation.

Cardiac MRI and CT can quantitate both the pulmonary insufficiency and the RV volumes. In addition, cardiac MRI and CT can identify whether there is either a native pulmonary arterial branch stenosis or a stenosis at the distal site of a prior arterial-to-PA shunt or other anomalies such as an ASD. Cardiac catheterization is occasionally required to document the degree of pulmonary valve regurgitation because noninvasive studies depend on velocity gradients. Pulmonary angiography demonstrates the degree of pulmonary valve regurgitation, and RV angiography helps assess any postoperative outflow tract aneurysm.

▶ Prognosis & Treatment

A few patients with "just the right amount" of subpulmonic stenosis enter adulthood without having had surgery. However, most adult patients have had surgical repair of tetralogy of Fallot, including VSD closure, resection of infundibular muscle, and insertion of an outflow tract patch to relieve the subpulmonic obstruction. Many have a transannular patch resulting in pulmonary valve regurgitation. Patients should be monitored to ensure the RV volume does not increase. Low-pressure pulmonary valve regurgitation is difficult to diagnose due to the fact that the RV diastolic pressures tend to be high and the pulmonary arterial diastolic pressure is low. This means there is little gradient between the PA and the RV in diastole, so that there may be little murmur or evidence for turbulence on color flow Doppler. If the RV begins to enlarge, it must be assumed that this is due to pulmonary valve regurgitation until proven otherwise. Early surgical pulmonary valve replacement is increasingly being favored. A percutaneous approach is not approved at this point.

If an anomalous coronary artery is present, then an extracardiac conduit around it from the RV to the PA may be necessary. By 20-year follow-up, reoperation is needed in about 10–15%, not only for severe pulmonary valve regurgitation but also for residual infundibular stenosis. Usually the pulmonary valve is replaced with a pulmonary homograft, although a porcine bioprosthetic valve is also suitable. Cryoablation of tissue giving rise to arrhythmias is sometimes performed at the time of reoperation. Branch pulmonary stenosis may be percutaneously opened by stenting. If a conduit has been used already for repair of the RV outflow obstruction, a percutaneous approach with a stented pulmonary valve may be possible. All patients require endocarditis prophylaxis (see Tables 33–4, 33–5, and 33–6). Most adults with stable hemodynamics can be quite active, and most women can carry a pregnancy adequately.

Arrhythmias are not uncommon with both atrial fibrillation and ventricular ectopy noted especially after the age of 45. Left heart disease appears to cause these arrhythmias more often than right heart disease. Biventricular dysfunction is not an uncommon consequence as the patient ages. The cause of associated LV dysfunction is often multifactorial and frequently unclear.

▶ When to Refer

All patients with tetralogy of Fallot should be referred to a cardiologist with expertise in adult congenital heart disease.

Aboulhosn JA et al; Alliance for Adult Research in Congenital Cardiology (AARCC). Left and right ventricular diastolic function in adults with surgically repaired tetralogy of Fallot: a multi-institutional study. Can J Cardiol. 2013 Jul;29(7): 866–72. [PMID: 23369488]

Apitz C et al. Tetralogy of Fallot. Lancet. 2009 Oct 24;374(9699): 1462–71. [PMID: 19683809]

Bashore TM. Adult congenital heart disease: right ventricular outflow tract lesions. Circulation. 2007 Apr 10;115(14):1933–47. [PMID: 17420363]

Khairy P et al; Alliance for Adult Research in Congenital Cardiology (AARCC). Arrhythmia burden in adults with surgically repaired tetralogy of Fallot: a multi-institutional study. Circulation. 2010 Aug 31;122(9):868–75. [PMID: 20713900]

Scherptong RW et al. Follow-up after pulmonary valve replacement in adults with tetralogy of Fallot: association between QRS duration and outcome. J Am Coll Cardiol. 2010 Oct 26;56:1486–92. [PMID: 20951325]

PATENT DUCTUS ARTERIOSUS

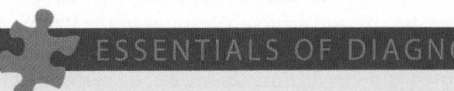

ESSENTIALS OF DIAGNOSIS

▶ Rare in adults.

▶ Adults with a small or moderate size patent ductus arteriosus are usually asymptomatic, at least until middle age.

▶ The lesion is best visualized by MRI, CT, or contrast angiography.

▶ General Considerations

The embryonic ductus arteriosus allows shunting of blood from the PA to the aorta in utero. The ductus arteriosus normally closes immediately after birth so that right heart blood flows only to the pulmonary arteries. Failure to close results in a persistent shunt connecting the left PA and aorta, usually near the origin of the left subclavian artery. Prior to birth, the ductus is kept patent by the effect of circulating prostaglandins; in the neonate, a patent ductus can often be closed by administration of a prostaglandin inhibitor such as indomethacin. The effect of the persistent left-to-right shunt on the pulmonary circuit is dependent on the size of the ductus. If large enough, pulmonary hypertension (Eisenmenger physiology) may occur. A small ductus may be well tolerated until adulthood.

▶ **Clinical Findings**

A. Symptoms and Signs

There are no symptoms unless LV failure or pulmonary hypertension develops. The heart is of normal size or slightly enlarged, with a hyperdynamic apical impulse. The pulse pressure is wide, and diastolic pressure is low. A continuous rough "machinery" murmur, accentuated in late systole at the time of S_2, is heard best in the left first and second interspaces at the left sternal border. Thrills are common. If pulmonary hypertension is present (Eisenmenger physiology), the shunt may reverse and the lower body receives desaturated blood, while the upper body receives saturated blood. Thus, the hands appear normal while the toes are cyanotic and clubbed (differential cyanosis).

B. ECG and Chest Radiography

A normal ECG tracing or LVH is found, depending on the magnitude of shunting. On chest radiographs, the heart is normal in size and contour, or there may be LV and LA enlargement. The PA, aorta, and LA are prominent because they all are in the shunt pathway.

C. Diagnostic Studies

Echocardiography/Doppler can determine LV, RV, and atrial dimensions. Color flow Doppler allows visualization of the high velocity shunt jet into the proximal left PA. Cardiac MRI and CT, however, are the best noninvasive modalities to demonstrate the abnormality and its shape and to assess the size of the pulmonary arteries. Cardiac catheterization can establish the shunt size and direction, and define the size and anatomic features of the ductus. It can also help determine whether pulmonary hypertension has occurred and vasodilatory testing can be performed to see if some of the pulmonary hypertension is reactive.

▶ **Prognosis & Treatment**

Large shunts cause a high mortality rate from cardiac failure early in life. Smaller shunts are compatible with long survival, heart failure being the most common late complication. Infective endocarditis or endarteritis may rarely occur, and antibiotic prophylaxis for dental procedures continues to be recommended by some clinicians (see Tables 33–4, 33–5, and 33–6).

Surgical ligation of the patent ductus can be accomplished with excellent results. If the ductus has a "neck" and is of small enough size, percutaneous approaches using either coils or occluder devices are the preferred therapy. Newer duct occluder devices have a high success rate at a very low risk and are preferred. Patients with Eisenmenger physiology who have not undergone surgical ligation may benefit from pulmonary vasodilator therapy. To monitor these latter patients, serial assessment of toe oxygen saturation as a marker of improvement in the right-to-left shunt is important because of the reversal in flow in the ductus. On rare occasions the ductus may become aneurysmal and require repair.

Table 10–1. Recommendations for interventions in patients with patent ductus arteriosus.[1]

Class I
A. Closure of a patent ductus arteriosus either percutaneously or surgically is indicated for the following:
1. Presence of left atrial or left ventricular enlargement, pulmonary artery hypertension, or net left-to-right shunting (level of evidence: C).
2. Prior endarteritis (level of evidence: C).
B. Consultation with adult congenital heart disease interventional cardiologists is recommended before surgical closure is selected as the method of repair for patients with a calcified patent ductus arteriosus (level of evidence: C).
C. Surgical repair by a surgeon experienced in coronary heart disease surgery is recommended when:
1. The patent ductus arteriosus is too large for device closure (level of evidence: C).
2. Distorted ductal anatomy precludes device closure (eg, aneurysm or endarteritis) (level of evidence: B).
Class IIa
A. It is reasonable to close an asymptomatic small patent ductus arteriosus by catheter device (level of evidence: C).
B. Patent ductus arteriosus closure is reasonable for patients with pulmonary artery hypertension with a net left-to-right shunt (level of evidence: C).
Class III
Patent ductus arteriosus closure is not indicated for patients with pulmonary artery hypertension and net right-to-left shunt (level of evidence: C).

[1]Class I indicates treatment is useful and effective, class IIa indicates weight of evidence is in favor of usefulness/efficacy, class IIb indicates weight of evidence is less well established, and class III indicates intervention is not useful/effective and may be harmful. Type A recommendations are based on data derived from multiple randomized clinical trials or meta-analyses. Type B recommendations are based on data derived from a single randomized clinical trials or large nonrandomized studies. Type C recommendations are based on consensus of opinion of the experts or on data derived from small studies, retrospective studies, or registries. ACC/AHA, American College of Cardiology/American Heart Association.

Table 10–1 outlines the current recommendations for intervention in adult patients with a patent ductus arteriosus. Note it is the only lesion that depends on auscultation; if the murmur is audible, it should be repaired.

▶ **When to Refer**

All patients with patent ductus arteriosus should be referred to a cardiologist with expertise in adult congenital disease.

Laughon M et al. Patent ductus arteriosus management: what are the next steps? J Pediatr. 2010 Sep;157(3):355–7. [PMID: 20580017]

Song S et al. Hybrid approach for aneurysm of patent ductus arteriosus in an adult. Ann Thorac Surg. 2013 Jan;95(1):e15–7. [PMID: 23272885]

Warnes CA et al. ACC/AHA 2008 Guidelines for the Management of Adults With Congenital Heart Disease. A Report of the American College of Cardiology/American Heart Association Task Force on Practice Guidelines. Circulation. 2008 Dec 2;118(23):e714–833. [PMID: 18997169]

VALVULAR HEART DISEASE

A 2014 update of the ACCF/AHA valvular guidelines suggests all lesions may be best classified clinically into one of six categories:

Stage A: Patients at risk for valvular heart disease (VHD).

Stage B: Patients with progressive VHD (mild to moderate severity) and asymptomatic.

Stage C: Asymptomatic patients who have reached criteria for severe VHD.

　C1: Normal LV function.

　C2: Abnormal LV function.

Stage D: Symptomatic patients as a result of VHD.

Nishimura RA et al. 2014 AHA/ACC Guideline for the Management of Patients With Valvular Heart Disease: A Report of the American College of Cardiology/American Heart Association Task Force on Practice Guidelines. Circulation. 2014 Mar 3. [Epub ahead of print] [PMID: 24589853]

MITRAL STENOSIS

 ESSENTIALS OF DIAGNOSIS

▶ Fatigue, exertional dyspnea, orthopnea, and paroxysmal nocturnal dyspnea when the stenosis becomes severe.

▶ Symptoms often precipitated by onset of atrial fibrillation or pregnancy.

▶ Two syndromes occur; one with moderate mitral stenosis and dyspnea and one with severe mitral stenosis, pulmonary hypertension, and low cardiac output.

▶ Echocardiography/Doppler is diagnostic.

▶ Intervention indicated for symptoms or evidence of pulmonary hypertension. Most symptomatic patients have a valve area < 1.5 cm^2.

▶ General Considerations

Most patients with mitral stenosis are usually presumed to have underlying rheumatic heart disease, though a history of rheumatic fever is usually noted in only about one-third. Rheumatic mitral stenosis results in thickening of the leaflets, fusion of the mitral commissures, retraction, thickening and fusion of the chordae, and calcium deposition in the valve. Mitral stenosis can also occur due to congenital disease with chordal fusion or papillary muscle malposition. The papillary muscles may be abnormally close together, sometimes so close they merge into a single papillary muscle (the parachute mitral valve). In these patients, the chordae or valvular tissue (or both) may also be fused. In other patients, mitral annular calcification may stiffen the mitral valve and reduce its motion to the point where a mitral gradient is present, most often in the elderly or patients with end-stage renal disease. Calcium in the mitral annulus virtually invades the mitral leaflet from the annulus inward as opposed to the calcium buildup from rheumatic heart disease, where it is commonly in the commissures and leaflet edges. Mitral valve obstruction may also develop in patients who have had mitral valve repair with a mitral annular ring that is too small, or in patients who have had a surgical valve replacement (prosthetic valve-patient mismatch).

▶ Clinical Findings

A. Symptoms and Signs

Two clinical syndromes occur with mitral stenosis. In **mild** to **moderate mitral stenosis,** LA pressure and cardiac output may be essentially normal, and the patient is either asymptomatic or symptomatic only with extreme exertion. The measured valve area is usually between 1.5 cm^2 and 1.0 cm^2. In **severe mitral stenosis** (valve area < 1.0 cm^2), severe pulmonary hypertension develops due to a "secondary stenosis" of the pulmonary vasculature. In this condition, pulmonary edema is uncommon, but symptoms of low cardiac output and right heart failure predominate.

A characteristic finding of rheumatic mitral stenosis is an opening snap following A$_2$ due to the stiff mitral valve. The interval between the opening snap and aortic closure sound is long when the LA pressure is low but shortens as the LA pressure rises and approaches the aortic diastolic pressure. As mitral stenosis worsens, there is a localized diastolic murmur low in pitch whose duration increases with the severity of the stenosis. The heart murmur is best heard at the apex with the patient in the left lateral position (Table 10–2).

Paroxysmal or chronic atrial fibrillation eventually develops in 50–80% of patients. Any increase in the heart rate reduces diastolic filling time and increases the mitral gradient. A sudden increase in heart rate may precipitate pulmonary edema. Therefore, heart rate control is important to maintain, with slow heart rates allowing for more diastolic filling of the LV.

B. Diagnostic Studies

Echocardiography is the most valuable technique for assessing mitral stenosis (Table 10–2). A scoring system is helpful in defining which patients are eligible for percutaneous valvuloplasty. One to four points are assigned to each of four observed parameters, with one being the least involvement and four the greatest: mitral leaflet thickening, mitral leaflet mobility, submitral scarring, and commissural calcium. Patients with a total valve score of 8 or less respond best to balloon valvuloplasty. LA size can also be determined by echocardiography: increased size denotes an increased likelihood of atrial fibrillation and thrombus formation. The effective mitral valve area can be determined by planimetering the smallest mitral orifice or by using the continuous-wave Doppler gradient. Some determination of the pulmonary pressure can also be quantitated by measuring the peak RV pressure from the tricuspid velocity jet signal.

Because echocardiography and careful symptom evaluation provide most of the needed information, cardiac catheterization is used primarily to detect associated coronary or myocardial disease—usually after the decision to intervene has been made.

Table 10–2. Differential diagnosis of valvular heart disease.

	Mitral Stenosis	Mitral Regurgitation	Aortic Stenosis	Aortic Regurgitation	Tricuspid Stenosis	Tricuspid Regurgitation
Inspection	Malar flush, precordial bulge, and diffuse pulsation in young patients.	Usually prominent and hyperdynamic apical impulse to left of MCL.	Sustained PMI, prominent atrial filling wave.	Hyperdynamic PMI to left of MCL and downward. Visible carotid pulsations. Pulsating nailbeds (Quincke), head bob (deMusset).	Giant *a* wave in jugular pulse with sinus rhythm. Peripheral edema or ascites, or both.	Large *v* wave in jugular pulse; time with carotid pulsation. Peripheral edema or ascites, or both.
Palpation	"Tapping" sensation over area of expected PMI. Right ventricular pulsation left third to fifth ICS parasternally when pulmonary hypertension is present. P_2 may be palpable.	Forceful, brisk PMI; systolic thrill over PMI. Pulse normal, small, or slightly collapsing.	Powerful, heaving PMI to left and slightly below MCL. Systolic thrill over aortic area, sternal notch, or carotid arteries in severe disease. Small and slowly rising carotid pulse. If bicuspid AS, check for delay at femoral artery to exclude coarctation.	Apical impulse forceful and displaced significantly to left and downward. Prominent carotid pulses. Rapidly rising and collapsing pulses (Corrigan pulse).	Pulsating, enlarged liver in ventricular systole.	Right ventricular pulsation. Systolic pulsation of liver.
Heart sounds, rhythm, and blood pressure	S_1 loud if valve mobile. Opening snap following S_2. The worse the disease, the closer the S_2-opening snap interval.	S_1 normal or buried in early part of murmur (exception in mitral prolapse where murmur may be late). Prominent third heart sound when severe MR. Atrial fibrillation common. Blood pressure normal. Midsystolic clicks may be present and may be multiple.	A_2 normal, soft, or absent. Prominent S_4. Blood pressure normal, or systolic pressure normal with high diastolic pressure.	S_1 normal or reduced, A_2 loud. Wide pulse pressure with diastolic pressure < 60 mm Hg. When severe, gentle compression of femoral artery with diaphragm of stethoscope may reveal diastolic flow (Duroziez) and pressure in leg on palpation > 40 mm Hg than arm (Hill).	S_1 often loud.	Atrial fibrillation may be present.
Murmurs						
Location and transmission	Localized at or near apex. Diastolic rumble best heard in left lateral position; may be accentuated by having patient do sit-ups. Rarely, short diastolic murmur along lower left sternal border (Graham Steell) in severe pulmonary hypertension.	Loudest over PMI; posteriorly directed jets (ie, anterior mitral prolapse) transmitted to left axilla, left infrascapular area; anteriorly directed jets (ie, posterior mitral prolapse) heard over anterior precordium. Murmur unchanged after premature beat.	Right second ICS parasternally or at apex, heard in carotid arteries and occasionally in upper interscapular area. May sound like MR at apex (Gallaverdin phenomenon), but murmur occurs after S_1 and stops before S_2.	Diastolic: louder along left sternal border in third to fourth interspace. Heard over aortic area and apex. May be associated with low-pitched middiastolic murmur at apex (Austin Flint) due to functional mitral stenosis. If due to an enlarged aorta, murmur may radiate to right sternal border.	Third to fifth ICS along left sternal border to apex. Murmur increases with inspiration.	Third to fifth ICS along left sternal border. Murmur hard to hear but increases with inspiration. Sit-ups can increase cardiac output and accentuate murmur.

Timing	Relation of opening snap to A₂ important. The higher the LA pressure, the earlier the opening snap. Presystolic accentuation before S₁ if in sinus rhythm. Graham Steell begins with P₂ (early diastole) if associated pulmonary hypertension.	Pansystolic: begins with S₁ and ends at or after A₂. May be late systolic in mitral valve prolapse.	Begins after S₁ ends before A₂. The more severe the stenosis, the later the murmur peaks.	Begins immediately after aortic second sound and ends before first sound (blurring both); helps distinguish from MR.	Rumble often follows audible opening snap.	At times, hard to hear. Begins with S1 and fills systole. Increases with inspiration.
Character	Low-pitched, rumbling; presystolic murmur merges with loud S₁.	Blowing, high-pitched; occasionally harsh or musical.	Harsh, rough.	Blowing, often faint.	As for mitral stenosis.	Blowing, coarse, or musical.
Optimum auscultatory conditions	After exercise, left lateral recumbency. Bell chest piece lightly applied.	After exercise; use diaphragm chest piece. In prolapse, findings may be more evident whilestanding.	Use stethoscope diaphragm. Patient resting, leaning forward, breath held in full expiration.	Use stethoscope diaphragm. Patient leaning forward, breath held in expiration.	Use stethoscope bell. Murmur usually louder and at peak during inspiration. Patient recumbent.	Use stethoscope diaphragm. Murmur usually becomes louder during inspiration.
Radiography	Straight left heart border from enlarged LA appendage. Elevation of left mainstem bronchus. Large right ventricle and pulmonary artery if pulmonary hypertension is present. Calcification in mitral valve in rheumatic mitral stenosis or in annulus in calcific mitral stenosis.	Enlarged left ventricle and LA.	Concentric left ventricular hypertrophy. Prominent ascending aorta. Calcified aortic valve common.	Moderate to severe left ventricular enlargement. Aortic root often dilated.	Enlarged right atrium with prominent SVC and azygous shadow.	Enlarged right atrium and right ventricle.

(continued)

Table 10–2. Differential diagnosis of valvular heart disease. (continued)

	Mitral Stenosis	Mitral Regurgitation	Aortic Stenosis	Aortic Regurgitation	Tricuspid Stenosis	Tricuspid Regurgitation
ECG	Broad P waves in standard leads; broad negative phase of diphasic P in V_1. If pulmonary hypertension is present, tall peaked P waves, right axis deviation, or right ventricular hypertrophy appears.	Left axis deviation or frank left ventricular hypertrophy. P waves broad, tall, or notched in standard leads. Broad negative phase of diphasic P in V_1.	Left ventricular hypertrophy.	Left ventricular hypertrophy.	Tall, peaked P waves. Possible right ventricular hypertrophy.	Right axis usual.
Echocardiography						
Two-dimensional echocardiography	Thickened, immobile mitral valve with anterior and posterior leaflets moving together. "Hockey stick" shape to opened anterior leaflet in rheumatic mitral stenosis. Annular calcium with thin leaflets in calcific mitral stenosis. LA enlargement, normal to small left ventricle. Orifice can be traced to approximate mitral valve orifice area.	Thickened mitral valve in rheumatic disease; mitral valve prolapse; flail leaflet or vegetations may be seen. Dilated left ventricle in volume overload. Operate for left ventricular end-systolic dimension > 4.5 cm.	Dense persistent echoes from the aortic valve with poor leaflet excursion. Left ventricular hypertrophy late in the disease. Bicuspid valve in younger patients.	Abnormal aortic valve or dilated aortic root. Diastolic vibrations of the anterior leaflet of the mitral valve and septum. In acute aortic regurgitation, premature closure of the mitral valve before the QRS. When severe, dilated left ventricle with normal or decreased contractility. Operate when left ventricular end-systolic dimension > 5.0 cm.	In rheumatic disease, tricuspid valve thickening, decreased early diastolic filling slope of the tricuspid valve. In carcinoid, leaflets fixed, but no significant thickening.	Enlarged right ventricle with paradoxical septal motion. Tricuspid valve often pulled open by displaced chordae.
Continuous and color flow Doppler and TEE	Prolonged pressure half-time across mitral valve allows estimation of gradient. MVA estimated from pressure half-time. Indirect evidence of pulmonary hypertension by noting elevated right ventricular systolic pressure measured from the tricuspid regurgitation jet.	Regurgitant flow mapped into LA. Use of PISA helps assess MR severity. TEE important in prosthetic mitral valve regurgitation.	Increased transvalvular flow velocity; severe AS when peak jet > 4 m/sec (64 mm Hg). Valve area estimate using continuity equation is poorly reproducible.	Demonstrates regurgitation and qualitatively estimates severity based on percentage of left ventricular outflow filled with jet and distance jet penetrates into left ventricle. TEE important in aortic valve endocarditis to exclude abscess. Mitral inflow pattern describes diastolic dysfunction.	Prolonged pressure half-time across tricuspid valve can be used to estimate mean gradient. Severe tricuspid stenosis present when mean gradient > 5 mm Hg.	Regurgitant flow mapped into right atrium and venae cavae. Right ventricular systolic pressure estimated by tricuspid regurgitation jet velocity.

A_2, aortic second sound; AS, aortic stenosis; ICS, intercostal space; LA, left atrial; MCL, midclavicular line; MR, mitral regurgitation; MVA, measured valve area; P_2, pulmonary second sound; PISA, proximal isovelocity surface area; PMI, point of maximal impulse; S_1, first heart sound; S_2, second heart sound; S_4, fourth heart sound; SVC, superior vena cava; TEE, transesophageal echocardiography; V_1, chest ECG lead 1.

Treatment & Prognosis

In most cases, there is a long asymptomatic phase after the initial rheumatic infection, followed by subtle limitation of activity. Pregnancy and its associated increase in cardiac output, which results in an increased transmitral pressure gradient, often precipitate symptoms. Toward the end of pregnancy, the cardiac output is also maintained by an increase in heart rate, further increasing the mitral gradient by shortening diastolic time. Patients with moderate to severe mitral stenosis should have the condition corrected prior to becoming pregnant if possible. Pregnant patients who become symptomatic can undergo successful surgery, preferably in the third trimester, although balloon valvuloplasty is the treatment of choice if the echo score is low enough.

The onset of atrial fibrillation often precipitates symptoms, which usually initially improve with control of the ventricular rate or restoration of sinus rhythm. Conversion to and subsequent maintenance of sinus rhythm are most commonly successful when the duration of atrial fibrillation is brief (< 6–12 months) and the LA is not severely dilated (diameter < 4.5 cm). Once atrial fibrillation occurs, the patient should receive warfarin anticoagulation therapy even if sinus rhythm is restored, since atrial fibrillation often recurs even with antiarrhythmic therapy and 20–30% of these patients will have systemic embolization if untreated. Systemic embolization in the presence of only mild to moderate disease is not an indication for surgery but should be treated with warfarin anticoagulation. Newer target specific anticoagulants (dabigatran, apixaban, and rivaroxaban) have not been studied for the prevention of stroke and non–central nervous system embolism in patients with moderate or severe mitral stenosis and atrial fibrillation, and they are not approved for these patients.

Indications for intervention focus on symptoms such as an episode of pulmonary edema, a decline in exercise capacity, or any evidence for pulmonary hypertension (peak systolic pulmonary pressure > 50 mm Hg). Some experts believe that the presence of atrial fibrillation should be a consideration for an intervention. Most interventions are not pursued until the patient is symptomatic (stage D) (Figure 10–1). In some patients, symptoms develop with calculated mitral valve areas between 1.5 cm² and 1.0 cm². Symptoms should drive the decision to intervene in these patients, not the estimated valve area.

Open mitral commissurotomy is now rarely performed and has given way to percutaneous balloon valvuloplasty.

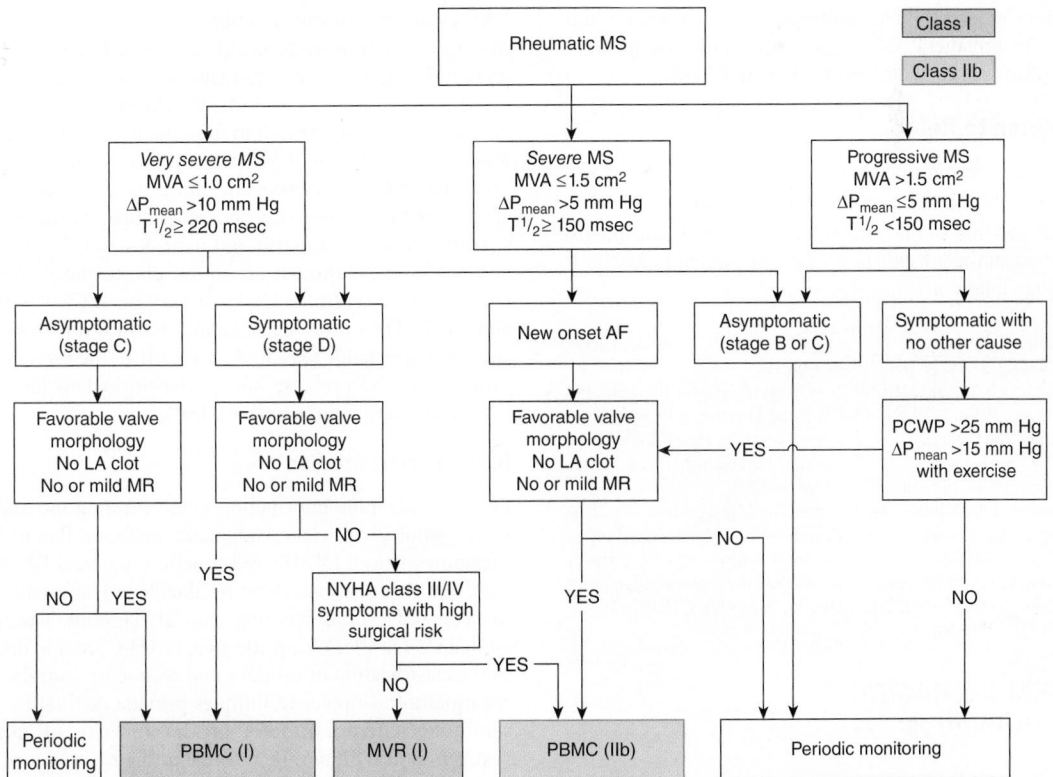

▲ Figure 10–1. The 2014 AHA/ACC guidelines for intervention in mitral stenosis. (Reproduced with permission from Nishimura RA et al. 2014 AHA/ACC Guideline for the Management of Patients With Valvular Heart Disease: A Report of the American College of Cardiology/American Heart Association Task Force on Practice Guidelines. Circulation. 2014 Mar 3. [Epub ahead of print] [PMID: 24589853])

Ten-year follow-up data comparing surgery to balloon valvuloplasty suggest no real difference in outcome between the two modalities. Replacement of the valve is indicated when combined stenosis and regurgitation are present or when the mitral valve echo score is > 8–10. Percutaneous mitral valvuloplasty has a very low mortality rate (< 0.5%) and low morbidity rate (3–5%). Operative mortality rates are also low: 1–3% in most institutions. Repeat balloon valvuloplasty can be done if the morphology of the valve is suitable. At surgery, a Maze procedure may be done at the same time to reduce recurrent atrial arrhythmias. It involves a number of endocardial incisions across the right and left atria to disrupt the electrical activity that sustains atrial arrhythmias.

Mechanical mitral prosthetic valves are more prone to thrombosis than aortic prosthetic valves. Bioprosthetic valves degenerate after about 10–15 years and percutaneous balloon valvuloplasty procedures are not effective on bioprosthetic valves when stenosis occurs, although the emergence of improved percutaneous stented valve technology suggests this may be used to relieve bioprosthetic mitral stenosis in high-risk patients. Younger patients and those with end-stage renal disease are generally felt to do least well with bioprosthetic heart valves, although recent data have questioned the role of chronic kidney disease as a major risk factor. Endocarditis prophylaxis is always indicated for prosthetic valves but is not indicated in native valve disease (see Tables 33–4, 33–5, and 33–6).

When to Refer

- Patients with mitral stenosis should be monitored with yearly examinations and echocardiograms.
- All patients should initially be seen by a cardiologist, who can then decide how often the patient needs cardiology follow-up.

Chandrashekhar Y et al. Mitral stenosis. Lancet. 2009 Oct 10;374 (9697):271–83. [PMID: 19747723]

Nishimura RA et al. 2014 AHA/ACC Guideline for the Management of Patients With Valvular Heart Disease: A Report of the American College of Cardiology/American Heart Association Task Force on Practice Guidelines. Circulation. 2014 Mar 3. [Epub ahead of print] [PMID: 24589853]

Vahanian A et al; Joint Task Force on the Management of Valvular Heart Disease of the European Society of Cardiology (ESC); European Association for Cardio-Thoracic Surgery (EACTS). Guidelines on the management of valvular heart disease (version 2012). Eur Heart J. 2012 Oct;33(19):2451–96. [PMID: 22922415]

MITRAL REGURGITATION
(Mitral Insufficiency)

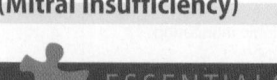

ESSENTIALS OF DIAGNOSIS

- ▶ May be asymptomatic for years (or for life) or may cause left-sided heart failure.
- ▶ Echocardiographic findings can help decide when to operate.

- ▶ For chronic primary mitral regurgitation, surgery is indicated for symptoms or when the LV ejection fraction (LVEF) is < 60% or the echocardiographic LV end-systolic dimension is > 4.0 cm.
- ▶ In patients with mitral prolapse and severe mitral regurgitation, earlier surgery is indicated if mitral repair can be performed.

General Considerations

Mitral regurgitation places a volume load on the heart (increases preload) but reduces afterload. The result is an enlarged LV with an increased EF. Over time, the stress of the volume overload reduces myocardial contractile function; when this occurs, there is a drop in EF and a rise in end-systolic volume.

Clinical Findings

A. Symptoms and Signs

In acute mitral regurgitation, the LA size is not large, and LA pressure rises abruptly, leading to pulmonary edema if severe. When chronic, the LA enlarges progressively and the increased volume can be handled without a major rise in the LA pressure; the pressure in pulmonary veins and capillaries may rise only transiently during exertion. Exertional dyspnea and fatigue progress gradually over many years.

Mitral regurgitation leads to chronic LA and LV enlargement and may result in subsequent atrial fibrillation and LV dysfunction. Clinically, mitral regurgitation is characterized by a pansystolic murmur maximal at the apex, radiating to the axilla and occasionally to the base; a hyperdynamic LV impulse and a brisk carotid upstroke; and a prominent third heart sound due to the increased volume returning to the LV in early diastole (Tables 10–2 and 10–3). The mitral regurgitation murmur due to mitral valve prolapse tends to radiate anteriorly in the presence of posterior leaflet prolapse and posteriorly when the prolapse is primarily of the anterior leaflet.

B. Diagnostic Studies

Echocardiographic information demonstrating the underlying pathologic process (rheumatic, prolapse, flail leaflet, cardiomyopathy), LV size and function, LA size, PA pressure, and RV function can be invaluable in planning treatment as well as in recognizing associated lesions. The 2014 guidelines for VHD from the ACCF/AHA provide details of the classification of primary and secondary mitral valve regurgitation. Doppler techniques provide qualitative and semiquantitative estimates of the severity of mitral regurgitation. TEE may help reveal the cause of regurgitation and is especially useful in patients who have had mitral valve replacement, in suspected endocarditis, and in identifying candidates for valvular repair. Echocardiographic dimensions and measures of systolic function are critical in deciding the timing of surgery. In patients with severe mitral regurgitation (stage C1) but preserved LV dimensions should undergo at least yearly echocardiography. Exercise hemodynamics with

Table 10–3. Effect of various interventions on systolic murmurs.

Intervention	Hypertrophic Obstructive Cardiomyopathy	Aortic Stenosis	Mitral Regurgitation	Mitral Prolapse
Valsalva	↑	↓	↓ or ×	↑ or ↓
Standing	↑	↑ or ×	↓ or ×	↑
Handgrip or squatting	↓	↓ or ×	↑	↓
Supine position with legs elevated	↓	↑ or ×	×	↓
Exercise	↑	↑ or ×	↓	↑

↑, increased; ↓, decreased; ×, unchanged.
Modified, with permission, from Paraskos JA. Combined valvular disease. In: *Valvular Heart Disease*. Dalen JE, Alpert JS (editors). Little, Brown, LWW, 2000.

either Doppler echocardiography or cardiac catheterization may be useful when the symptoms do not fit the anatomic severity of mitral regurgitation. B-type natriuretic peptide (BNP) is useful in the early identification of LV dysfunction in the presence of mitral regurgitation, and asymptomatic patients with BNP values > 105 pg/mL are at higher risk for developing heart failure. Conversely, low values of BNP appear to have a negative predictive value.

Cardiac MRI is occasionally useful, if specific myocardial causes are being sought (such as amyloid or myocarditis) or if myocardial viability assessment is needed prior to deciding whether to add coronary artery bypass grafting to mitral repair in patients with chronic ischemic mitral regurgitation.

Cardiac catheterization provides a further assessment of regurgitation and its hemodynamic impact along with LV function, resting cardiac output, and PA pressure. The 2014 ACCF/AHA guidelines recommend coronary angiography to determine the presence of CAD prior to valve surgery in all men over age 40 years and in menopausal women with coronary risk factors. In younger patients (< 50 years of age), cardiac multidetector CT may be adequate to screen patients with VHD for asymptomatic CAD. A normal CT angiogram identifies normal or insignificant disease in a very high percentage of patients.

▶ **Treatment & Prognosis**

A. Primary Mitral Regurgitation

The degree of LV enlargement usually reflects the severity and chronicity of regurgitation. LV volume overload may ultimately lead to LV failure and reduced cardiac output. LA enlargement may be considerable in **chronic mitral regurgitation** and considerable mitral regurgitation regurgitant volume may be tolerated. Patients with chronic lesions may remain asymptomatic for many years. Surgery is necessary when symptoms develop. However, because progressive and irreversible deterioration of LV function may occur prior to the onset of symptoms, early surgery is indicated even in asymptomatic patients with a reduced EF (< 60%) or marked LV dilation (end-systolic dimension > 4.0 cm on echocardiography) (Figure 10–2). Pulmonary hypertension development suggests the mitral regurgitation is severe as well and should prompt intervention.

Nonrheumatic mitral regurgitation may develop abruptly, such as with papillary muscle dysfunction following myocardial infarction, valve perforation in infective endocarditis, in patients with hypertrophic cardiomyopathy, or when there are ruptured chordae tendineae in mitral valve prolapse. Emergency surgery may be required for acute nonrheumatic mitral regurgitation.

Some patients may become hemodynamically unstable and can be initially treated with vasodilators or intra-aortic balloon counterpulsation, which reduce the amount of retrograde regurgitant flow by lowering systemic vascular resistance. There is controversy regarding the role of afterload reduction in chronic mitral regurgitation, since the lesion inherently results in a reduction in afterload, and there are no data that chronic afterload reduction is effective. A heightened sympathetic state has led some experts to suggest that beta-blockade be considered routinely. Cardiomyopathy and mitral regurgitation due to persistent tachycardia may also improve with normalization of the heart rate.

B. Myocardial Disease and Mitral Regurgitation

When mitral regurgitation is due to papillary dysfunction, it may subside as the infarction heals or LV dilation diminishes. The cause of the regurgitation in most situations is displacement of the papillary muscles and an enlarged mitral annulus rather than true papillary muscle ischemia. The fundamental problem is the lack of leaflet coaptation during systole. In acute infarction, rupture of the papillary muscle may occur with catastrophic results. Transient—but sometimes severe—mitral regurgitation may occur during episodes of myocardial ischemia and contribute to flash pulmonary edema. Patients with dilated cardiomyopathies of any origin may have **secondary mitral regurgitation** due to papillary muscle displacement or dilation of the mitral annulus. In patients with ischemic cardiomyopathy, ventricular reconstructive surgery to restore the mitral apparatus anatomy and reshape the ventricle (Dor procedure) has had limited success and is now rarely performed. If mitral valve replacement is performed, preservation of the chordae to the native valve helps prevent further ventricular dilation following surgery. Several groups have reported good results with mitral valve repair in patients with LVEF < 30% and secondary mitral regurgitation. The 2014 ACCF/AHA guidelines (Figure 10–2) advise that mitral valve repair/replacement can be attempted in

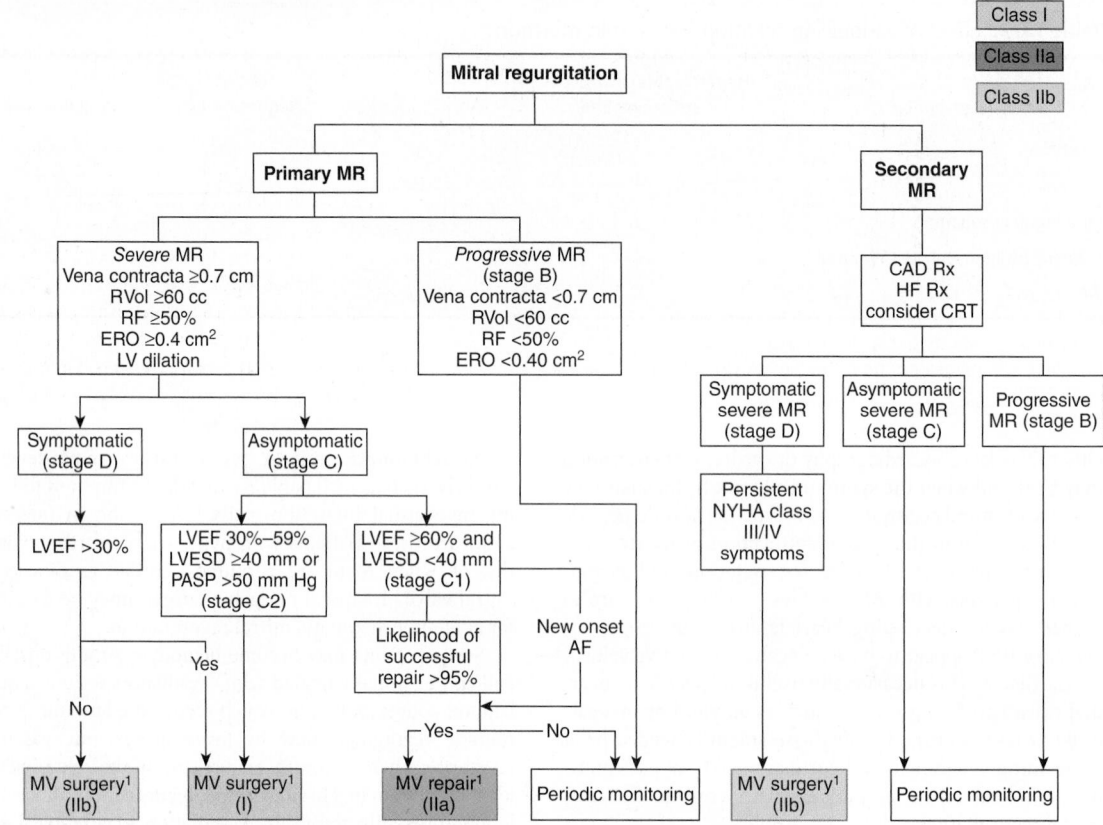

Class I
Class IIa
Class IIb

Mitral regurgitation

Primary MR

Secondary MR

Severe MR
Vena contracta ≥0.7 cm
RVol ≥60 cc
RF ≥50%
ERO ≥0.4 cm²
LV dilation

Progressive MR
(stage B)
Vena contracta <0.7 cm
RVol <60 cc
RF <50%
ERO <0.40 cm²

CAD Rx
HF Rx
consider CRT

Symptomatic
severe MR
(stage D)

Asymptomatic
severe MR
(stage C)

Progressive
MR (stage B)

Symptomatic
(stage D)

Asymptomatic
(stage C)

Persistent
NYHA class
III/IV
symptoms

LVEF >30%

LVEF 30%–59%
LVESD ≥40 mm or
PASP >50 mm Hg
(stage C2)

LVEF ≥60% and
LVESD <40 mm
(stage C1)

New onset
AF

Likelihood of
successful
repair >95%

Yes

No

Yes — No

MV surgery[1]
(IIb)

MV surgery[1]
(I)

MV repair[1]
(IIa)

Periodic monitoring

MV surgery[1]
(IIb)

Periodic monitoring

[1]Mitral valve repair preferred over MVR when possible.
AF, atrial fibrillation; CAD, coronary artery disease; CRT, cardiac resynchronization therapy; ERO, effective regurgitant orifice; HF, heart failure; LV, left ventricular; LVEF, left ventricular ejection fraction; LVESD, left ventricular end-systolic dimension; MR, mitral regurgitation, MV, mitral valve; MVR, mitral valve replacement; NYHA, New York Heart association; PASP, pulmonary artery systolic pressure; RF, regurgitant fraction; R Vol, regurgitant volume; Rx, prescription.

▲ **Figure 10–2.** The 2014 AHA/ACC guidelines for intervention in mitral regurgitation. (Reproduced with permission from Nishimura RA et al. 2014 AHA/ACC Guideline for the Management of Patients With Valvular Heart Disease: A Report of the American College of Cardiology/American Heart Association Task Force on Practice Guidelines. Circulation. 2014 Mar 3. [Epub ahead of print] [PMID: 24589853])

patients with an EF < 30% or an LV end-systolic dimension > 5.5 cm, or both, as long as repair and preservation of the chordae are possible. Recent data suggest that mitral valve replacement with chordal preservation may be as effective as mitral valve repair. There may also be a role for cardiac resynchronization therapy with biventricular pacemaker insertion, which has been found to reduce mitral regurgitation due to cardiomyopathy in many patients.

Currently, there are several ongoing trials of percutaneous approaches to reducing mitral regurgitation. These approaches include the use of a mitral clip device to create a double orifice mitral valve, various coronary catheter devices to reduce the mitral annular area, and devices to reduce the septal-lateral ventricular size and consequent mitral orifice size. Some success has been noted with the mitral clip device. A complete understanding about when this may be useful is still under investigation. The device is reserved for patients in whom surgical risk is considered excessive. In addition, vascular plugging and occluder devices are being used in selected patients to occlude perivalvular leaks around prosthetic mitral valves.

▶ When to Refer

All patients with more than mild mitral regurgitation should be referred to a cardiologist for an evaluation. Serial examinations and echocardiograms (usually yearly) should be obtained, and referral made if there is any increase in the LV end-systolic dimensions, a fall in the EF to < 60%, or symptoms.

Ahmed MI et al. A randomized controlled phase IIb trial of beta(1)-receptor blockade for chronic degenerative mitral regurgitation. J Am Coll Cardiol. 2012 Aug 28;60(9):833–8. [PMID: 22818065]

Mauri L et al; EVEREST II Investigators. 4-year results of a randomized controlled trial of percutaneous repair versus surgery for mitral regurgitation. J Am Coll Cardiol. 2013 Jul 23;62(4):317–28. [PMID: 23665364]

Nishimura RA et al. 2014 AHA/ACC Guideline for the Management of Patients With Valvular Heart Disease: A Report of the American College of Cardiology/American Heart Association Task Force on Practice Guidelines. Circulation. 2014 Mar 3. [Epub ahead of print] [PMID: 24589853]

Suri RM et al. Association between early surgical intervention vs watchful waiting and outcomes for mitral regurgitation due to flail mitral valve leaflets. JAMA. 2013 Aug 14;310(6):609–16. [PMID: 23942679]

Vahanian A et al; Joint Task Force on the Management of Valvular Heart Disease of the European Society of Cardiology (ESC); European Association for Cardio-Thoracic Surgery (EACTS). Guidelines on the management of valvular heart disease (version 2012). Eur Heart J. 2012 Oct;33(19):2451–96. [PMID: 22922415]

Whitlow PL et al; EVEREST II Investigators. Acute and 12-month results with catheter-based mitral valve leaflet repair: The EVEREST II (Endovascular Valve Edge-to-Edge Repair) High Risk Study. J Am Coll Cardiol. 2012 Jan 10;59(2):130–9. [PMID: 22222076]

MITRAL VALVE PROLAPSE SYNDROME

 ESSENTIALS OF DIAGNOSIS

► Single or multiple mid-systolic clicks often heard on auscultation.

► Murmur may be pansystolic or only late in systole.

► Often associated with skeletal changes (straight back, pectus excavatum, and scoliosis) or hyper-flexibility of joints.

► Echocardiography is confirmatory with prolapse of mitral leaflets in systole into the LA.

► Chest pain and palpitations common symptoms in the young adult.

General Considerations

The significance of mild mitral valve prolapse ("floppy" or myxomatous mitral valve), also commonly referred to as "degenerative" mitral valve disease, has been in dispute because of the frequency with which it is diagnosed by echocardiography even in healthy young women (up to 10%). A controversial hyperadrenergic syndrome has also been described (especially in young females) that may be responsible for some of the noncardiac symptoms observed. Fortunately, this hyperadrenergic component attenuates with age. Some patients with mitral prolapse have findings of a systemic collagen abnormality (Marfan or Ehlers-Danlos syndrome). In these conditions, a dilated aortic root and aortic regurgitation may coexist. In many persons, the "degenerative" myxomatous mitral valve clearly leads to long-term sequelae and is the most common cause of mitral regurgitation in developing countries.

Patients who have only a mid-systolic click usually have no immediate clinical issues, but significant mitral regurgitation may develop, occasionally suddenly due to rupture of chordae tendineae (flail leaflet) or gradually due to progressive annular dilation. The need for valve repair or replacement increases with age, so that approximately 2% per year of patients with clinically significant regurgitation over age 60 years will eventually require surgery.

Clinical Findings

A. Symptoms and Signs

Mitral valve prolapse is usually asymptomatic but may be associated with nonspecific chest pain, dyspnea, fatigue, or palpitations. Most patients are female, many are thin, and some have skeletal deformities such as pectus excavatum or scoliosis. On auscultation, there are characteristic mid-systolic clicks that may be multiple and emanate from the chordae or redundant valve tissue. If leaflets fail to come together properly, the clicks will be followed by a late systolic murmur. As the mitral regurgitation worsens, the murmur is heard more and more throughout systole. The smaller the LV chamber, the greater the degree of prolapse, and thus auscultatory findings are often accentuated in the standing position or during the Valsalva maneuver.

B. Diagnostic Studies

The diagnosis is primarily clinical and confirmed echocardiographically. Mitral prolapse is often associated with aortic root disease, and any evidence for a dilated aorta by chest radiography should prompt either CT or MRI angiography. If palpitations are an issue, an ambulatory monitor is often helpful to distinguish atrial from ventricular tachyarrhythmias.

Treatment

Beta-blockers in low doses are used to treat the hyperadrenergic state when present and are usually satisfactory for treatment of arrhythmias (see Table 11–6). Selective serotonin reuptake inhibitors have also been used, especially if orthostatic hypotension or anxiety is associated with mitral valve prolapse; results have been mixed. Afterload reduction has not been shown to be effective when mitral regurgitation is present.

Mitral valve repair is strongly favored over valve replacement, and its efficacy has led many to recommend intervention earlier and earlier in the course of the disease process. Mitral repair may include shortening of chordae, chordae transfers, wedge resection of redundant valve tissue, or the insertion of a mitral annular ring to reduce the annular size, or some combination of these techniques. Stitching of the leaflets together to create a double orifice mitral valve is also used at times (Alfieri procedure) and can be performed percutaneously. Mitral repair or replacement can be achieved through a right minithoracotomy with or without the use of a robotic device. Endocarditis prophylaxis is no longer recommended for most patients with mitral valve prolapse regardless of the degree of mitral regurgitation. A variety of percutaneous techniques and devices have been tried with some success (notably in the mitral clip trials), although results suggest that surgical repair may be more durable.

When to Refer

• All patients with mitral valve prolapse and audible mitral regurgitation should be seen at least once by a cardiologist.

- Periodic echocardiography is warranted to assess LV size (especially end-systolic dimensions) and EF when mitral regurgitation is present. If only mitral clicks are audible, then serial echocardiography is not warranted.

Filho AS et al. Mitral valve prolapse and anxiety disorders. Br J Psychiatry. 2011 Sep;199(3):247–8. [PMID: 21881100]

Mauri L et al; EVEREST II Investigators. 4-year results of a randomized controlled trial of percutaneous repair versus surgery for mitral regurgitation. J Am Coll Cardiol. 2013 Jul 23;62(4):317–28. [PMID: 23665364]

Whitlow PL et al; EVEREST II Investigators. Acute and 12-month results with catheter-based mitral valve leaflet repair: The EVEREST II (Endovascular Valve Edge-to-Edge Repair) High Risk Study. J Am Coll Cardiol. 2012 Jan 10;59(2):130–9. [PMID: 22222076]

AORTIC STENOSIS

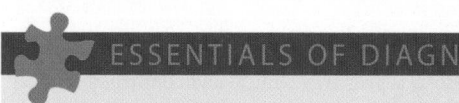

ESSENTIALS OF DIAGNOSIS

► Congenital bicuspid aortic valve, usually asymptomatic until middle or old age.

► "Degenerative" or calcific aortic stenosis; same risk factors as atherosclerosis.

► Symptoms likely once the mean gradient is > 40 mm Hg.

► Echocardiography/Doppler is diagnostic.

► Surgery indicated for symptoms.

► Surgery considered for asymptomatic patients with severe aortic stenosis (mean gradient > 50 mm Hg).

► Emerging role for BNP as marker of early LV myocardial failure.

► General Considerations

There are two common clinical scenarios in which aortic stenosis is prevalent. The first is due to a congenitally abnormal **unicuspid** or **bicuspid valve,** rather than tricuspid. Symptoms occur in young or adolescent individuals if the stenosis is severe, but more often emerge at age 50–65 years when calcification and degeneration of the valve becomes manifest. A dilated ascending aorta, primarily due to an intrinsic defect in the aortic root media, may accompany the bicuspid valve in about half of these patients. Coarctation of the aorta is also seen in a number of patients with congenital aortic stenosis. Offspring of patients with a bicuspid valve have a much higher incidence of the disease as well (up to 30% in some series).

A second group develops what has traditionally been called **degenerative** or **calcific aortic stenosis**, which is thought to be related to calcium deposition due to processes similar to what occurs in atherosclerotic vascular disease. Approximately 25% of patients over age 65 years and 35% of those over age 70 years have echocardiographic evidence of

aortic valve thickening (sclerosis). About 10–20% of these will progress to hemodynamically significant aortic stenosis over a period of 10–15 years. Certain genetic markers are now being discovered that are associated with aortic stenosis (most notably Notch 1), so a genetic component appears a likely contributor, at least in some patients. Other associated genetic markers have also been described.

Aortic stenosis has become the most common surgical valve lesion in developed countries, and many patients are elderly. The risk factors include hypertension, hypercholesterolemia, and smoking. Hypertrophic obstructive cardiomyopathy (HOCM) may also coexist with valvular aortic stenosis.

► Clinical Findings

A. Symptoms and Signs

Slightly narrowed, thickened, or roughened valves (aortic sclerosis) or aortic dilation may produce the typical ejection murmur of aortic stenosis. In mild or moderate cases where the valve is still pliable, an ejection click may precede the murmur. The characteristic systolic ejection murmur is heard at the aortic area and is usually transmitted to the neck and apex. In some cases, only the high-pitched components of the murmur are heard at the apex, and the murmur may sound like mitral regurgitation (so-called Gallaverdin phenomenon). In severe aortic stenosis, a palpable LV heave or thrill, a weak to absent aortic second sound, or reversed splitting of the second sound is present (see Table 10–2). When the valve area is < 0.8–1.0 cm² (normal, 3–4 cm²), ventricular systole becomes prolonged and the typical carotid pulse pattern of delayed upstroke and low amplitude is present. This may be an unreliable finding in older patients with extensive arteriosclerotic vascular disease and a stiff aorta. LVH increases progressively due to the pressure overload, eventually resulting in elevation in ventricular end-diastolic pressure. Cardiac output is maintained until the stenosis is severe (with a valve area < 0.8 cm²). LV failure, angina pectoris, or syncope may be presenting symptoms and signs of significant aortic stenosis; importantly, all symptoms tend to occur with exertion.

In a few patients, there appears to be a mismatch among the typical aortic stenosis assessments: the aortic valve gradient severity (low), the aortic valve area (severe), the degree of the LVH (severe), and the EF (normal). These "paradoxical" low flow aortic stenosis patients may have significant LV afterload due to increased aortic vascular impedance as well as the valvular stenosis resistance. The 2014 ACCF/AHA and the European valvular guidelines acknowledge the possible inclusion of these patients in the treatment algorithms for aortic stenosis (Table 10–4).

Symptoms of LV failure may be sudden in onset or may progress gradually. Angina pectoris frequently occurs in aortic stenosis due to underperfusion of the endocardium. Of patients with calcific aortic stenosis and angina, 50% have significant associated CAD. Syncope, a late finding, occurs with exertion as the LV pressures rises, stimulating the LV baroreceptors to cause peripheral vasodilation. This vasodilation results in the need for an increase in stroke volume, which increases the LV systolic pressure

Table 10–4. 2014 ACCF/ACC guidelines for surgical indications in aortic stenosis.

Recommendations	COR	LOE
AVR is recommended in symptomatic patients with severe AS (stage D)	I	B
AVR is recommended for asymptomatic patients with severe AS (stage C2 or D) and LVEF < 50%	I	B
AVR is indicated for patients with severe AS (stage C or D) when undergoing other cardiac surgery	I	B
AVR is reasonable for asymptomatic patients with very severe AS (aortic velocity ≥ 5 m/s) (stage C2) and low surgical risk	IIa	B
AVR is reasonable in asymptomatic patients (stage C1) with severe AS and an abnormal exercise test	IIa	B
AVR is reasonable in symptomatic patients with low-flow/low-gradient severe AS with reduced LVEF (stage S1) with a low-dose dobutamine stress study that shows an aortic velocity ≥4 m/s (or mean gradient ≥ 40 mm Hg) with a valve area ≤ 1.0 cm^2 at any dobutamine dose	IIa	B
AVR is reasonable for patients with moderate AS (stage B) (velocity 3.0–3.9 m/s) who are undergoing other cardiac surgery	IIa	C
AVR may be considered for asymptomatic patients with severe AS (stage C1) and rapid disease progression and low surgical risk	IIb	C
AVR may be considered in symptomatic patients who have low-flow/low-gradient severe AS (stage S2) who are normotensive and have an LVEF ≥50% if clinical, hemodynamic, and anatomic data support valve obstruction as the most likely cause of symptoms	IIb	C

AS, aortic stenosis, AVR, aortic valve replacement; COR, class of recommendation; LOE, level of evidence; LVEF, left ventricular ejection fraction; N/A, not applicable.
Reproduced, with permission, from Nishimura RA et al. 2014 AHA/ACC Guideline for the Management of Patients With Valvular Heart Disease: A Report of the American College of Cardiology/American Heart Association Task Force on Practice Guidelines. Circulation. 2014 Mar 3. [Epub ahead of print] [PMID: 24589853].

again, creating a cycle of vasodilation and stimulation of the baroreceptors that eventually results in a drop in BP, as the stenotic valve prevents further increase in stroke volume. Less commonly, syncope may be due to arrhythmias (usually ventricular tachycardia but sometimes AV block as calcific invasion of the conduction system from the aortic valve may occur).

B. Diagnostic Studies

The ECG reveals LVH or secondary repolarization changes in most patients but can be normal in up to 10%. The chest radiograph may show a normal or enlarged cardiac silhouette, calcification of the aortic valve, and dilation and calcification of the ascending aorta. The echocardiogram provides useful data about aortic valve calcification and opening and the severity of LV wall thickness and overall ventricular function, while Doppler can provide an excellent estimate of the aortic valve gradient. The 2014 ACCF/AHA guidelines provide echo/Doppler criteria for identifying aortic stenosis severity. Valve area estimation by echocardiography is less reliable but a critical component to the diagnosis of paradoxical low flow aortic stenosis (low gradient, low flow, normal LVEF patients). Cardiac catheterization mostly provides an assessment of the hemodynamic consequence of the aortic stenosis, and the anatomy of the coronary arteries. In younger patients, and in patients with high aortic gradients the aortic valve need not be crossed at catheterization. If the valve is crossed, the valve gradient can be measured at catheterization and an estimated valve area calculated; a valve area < 1.0 cm^2 indicates significant stenosis. Aortic regurgitation can be semiquantified by aortic root angiography.

In patients with a low LVEF and both low output and a low valve gradient (< 40 mm Hg), it may be unclear if an increased afterload is responsible for the low EF or if there is an associated cardiomyopathy. To sort this out, the patient should be studied at baseline and then during an intervention that increases cardiac output (eg, dobutamine or nitroprusside infusion). If the valve area increases, then the flow-limiting problem is not the valve, but rather a cardiomyopathy with low cardiac output, and surgery is generally not warranted. If the valve area remains unchanged at the higher induced outputs and there remains contractile reserve (an increase in the stroke volume > 20%), then the valve is generally considered flow limiting and surgery is indicated. Recent data have suggested the use of BNP may provide prognostic data in the setting of poor LV function and aortic stenosis. A BNP > 550 pg/mL has been associated with a poor outcome in these patients regardless of the results of dobutamine testing.

▶ Prognosis & Treatment

Valve replacement is usually not indicated in asymptomatic individuals, though a class II indication is to operate once the peak valve gradient by Doppler exceeds 64 mm Hg or the mean gradient exceeds 60 mm Hg. Stress testing and perhaps the use of BNP may help identify patients who deny symptoms but have compromised ventricular

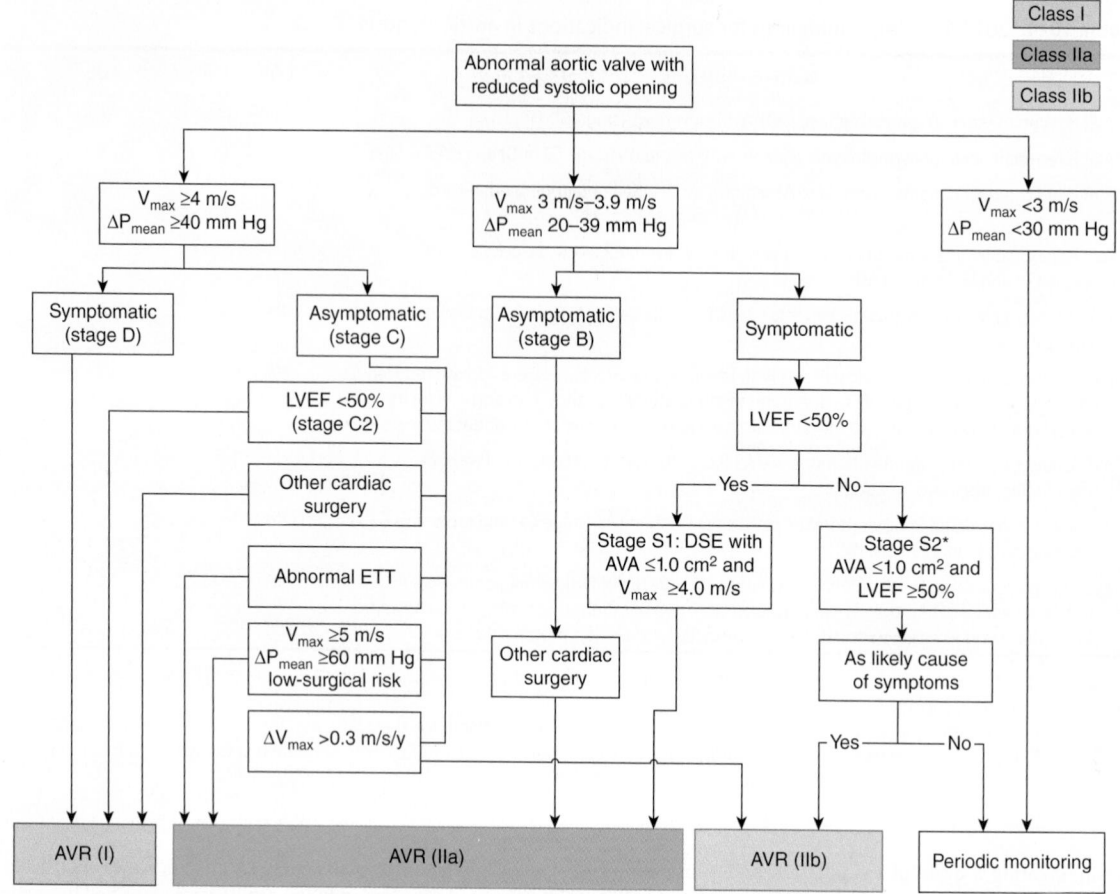

Class I
Class IIa
Class IIb

*AVR should be considered with stage S2 AS only if valve obstruction is the most likely cause of symptoms, stroke volume index is <35 mL/m², indexed AVA is ≤0.6 cm²/m² and data are recorded when the patient is normotensive (systolic BP <140 mm Hg).

As indicates aortic stenosis; AVA, aortic valve area; AVR, aortic valve replacement; BP, blood pressure; DSE, dobutamine stress echocardiography; ETT, exercise treadmill test; LVEF, left ventricular ejection fraction; ΔP_{mean}, mean pressure gradient; and V_{max}, maximum velocity.

▲ **Figure 10–3.** Algorithm for the management of aortic valve stenosis. (Reproduced, with permission from Nishimura RA et al. 2014 AHA/ACC Guideline for the Management of Patients With Valvular Heart Disease: A Report of the American College of Cardiology/American Heart Association Task Force on Practice Guidelines. Circulation. 2014 Mar 3. [Epub ahead of print] [PMID: 24589853])

function. Following the onset of heart failure, angina, or syncope, the prognosis without surgery is poor (50% 3-year mortality rate). Medical treatment may stabilize patients in heart failure, but surgery is indicated for all symptomatic patients with evidence of significant aortic stenosis.

The surgical mortality rate for valve replacement is low, even in the elderly, and ranges from 2% to 5%. This low risk is due to the dramatic hemodynamic improvement that occurs with relief of the increased afterload. Mortality rates are substantially higher when there is an associated ischemic cardiomyopathy. Severe coronary lesions are usually bypassed at the same time, although there are little data to suggest this practice affects outcome. Around one-third to one-half of all patients with aortic stenosis has significant CAD.

Statins have not been shown to be beneficial in preventing the progression of aortic stenosis but longer-term studies in patients with early disease are still pending. If patients with aortic stenosis have concomitant CAD, the guidelines for use of statins should be followed. Control of systemic hypertension is also an important adjunct, and inadequate systemic BP control is common due to unreasonable concerns about providing too much afterload reduction in patients with aortic stenosis.

The interventional options in patients with aortic stenosis are variable and dependent on the patient's lifestyle and age. The algorithm to decide when an intervention is appropriate in various situations is outlined in Figure 10–3.

In the young and adolescent patient, percutaneous balloon valvuloplasty still has a role but is associated with early restenosis in the elderly, and thus is rarely used except as a temporizing measure in calcific aortic stenosis. Data suggest aortic balloon valvuloplasty in the elderly has an advantage only in those with preserved LV function, and such patients are usually excellent candidates for surgical aortic valve replacement (AVR). Middle-aged adults generally can tolerate the anticoagulation therapy necessary for the use of mechanical AVR, so most undergo AVR with a bileaflet mechanical valve. If the aortic root is severely dilated as well (> 4.5 cm), then the valve may be housed in a Dacron sheath (Bentall procedure) and the root replaced. Alternatively, a human homograft root and valve replacement can be used. In the elderly, bioprosthetic (either porcine or bovine pericardial) valves with a life expectancy of about 10–15 years are routinely used instead of mechanical valves to avoid need for anticoagulation. Data favor the bovine pericardial valve over the porcine aortic valve. If the aortic annulus is small, a bioprosthetic valve with a short sheath can be sewn to the aortic wall (the stentless AVR) rather than sewing the prosthetic annulus to the aortic annulus. (Annulus is a relative term when speaking of the aortic valve, since there is no true annulus.) Another popular surgical option is the Wheat procedure; it involves aortic root replacement above the coronary arteries and AVR. The coronary arteries thus remain attached to the native aorta between the new graft and prosthetic valve rather than being reimplanted onto an artificial sheath or homograft.

In patients with a bicuspid aortic valve, there is often an associated ascending aortic aneurysm. If the maximal dimension of the aortic root exceeds 5.5 cm, it is recommended to proceed with root replacement regardless of the severity of the aortic valve disease. The aortic valve may be replaced at the same time or may be left alone (valve sparing operation).

Anticoagulation is required with the use of mechanical valves, and the international normalized ratio (INR) should be maintained between 2.0 and 3.0 or between 2.5 and 3.5, depending on type and position of valve and patient risk factors. In general, mechanical aortic valves are less subject to thrombosis than mechanical mitral valves. Some newer bileaflet mechanical valves (On-X) that require either no or a reduced dose of warfarin therapy are being evaluated, although the final data regarding the safety of this particular design are not available. The Prospective Randomized On-X valve AntiCoagulation Trial (PROACT) was begun in 2006 and is ongoing. Preliminary results have been reported and are very promising.

The use of transcutaneous aortic valve replacement (TAVR) has grown dramatically, with over 60,000 implants reported. In the United States, the Food and Drug Administration (FDA) has granted limited approval for one device (Edwards SAPIEN™), and trials of a second device (CoreValve™) have been reported in high-risk patients. The devices use either a stent with a trileaflet bovine pericardial valve constructed in it or a stent with a large valve from a cow's jugular vein mounted inside. There are a variety of approaches, though most valves are placed via a femoral artery approach. Other options include an antegrade approach via transseptal across the atrial septum, via the LV apex with a small surgical incision, via the subclavian arteries, or via a minithoracotomy. The Edwards SAPIEN valve is a balloon-expandable valvular stent, while the CoreValve is a valvular stent that self-expands when pushed out of the catheter sheath. Multiple other devices are in trials; these allow for repositioning and may result in less paravalvular regurgitation.

Table 10–5 outlines the suggested indications for TAVR. TAVR has also been used in "valve-in-valve" procedures to reduce the gradient in patients with prosthetic valve stenosis. A high incidence of heart block has been noted after CoreValve and many require permanent pacing. After placement of the SAPIEN device, residual aortic regurgitation remains a concern and has impact on its long-term success. TAVR has been remarkably successful in very high-risk and very elderly patients, and ongoing studies are addressing its usefulness in lower-risk patients compared to surgical AVR.

Table 10–5. Recommendations for use of TAVR.

Recommendations	COR	LOE
Surgical AVR is recommended in patients who meet indication for AVR with low or intermediate surgical risk	I	A
TAVR is recommended in patients who meet an indication for AVR for AS who have a prohibitive surgical risk and a predicted post-TAVR surival > 12 mo	I	B
For patient in whom TAVR or high-risk surgical AVR is being considered, members of a Heart Valve Team should collaborate closely to provide optimal patient care	I	C
TAVR is a reasonable alternative to surgical AVR for AS in patients who meet indication for AVR and who have high surgical risk	IIa	B
Percutaneous aortic balloon dilation may be considered as a bridge to surgical or transcatheter AVR in severely symptomatic patients (NYHA class III-IV) with severe AS	IIb	C
TAVR is not recommended in patients in whom the existing comorbidities would preclude the expected benefit from correction of AS	III: No Benefit	B

AS, aortic stenosis; AVR, aortic valve replacement; COR, class of recommendation; LOE, level of evidence; N/A, not applicable; NYHA, New York Heart Association; TVAR, transcatheter aortic valve replacement.

Reproduced, with permission, from Nishimura RA et al. 2014 AHA/ACC Guideline for the Management of Patients With Valvular Heart Disease: A Report of the American College of Cardiology/American Heart Association Task Force on Practice Guidelines. Circulation. 2014 Mar 3. [Epub ahead of print] [PMID: 24589853]

When to Refer

- All patients with echocardiographic evidence for mild-to-moderate aortic stenosis (estimated peak valve gradient > 30 mm Hg by echocardiography/Doppler) should be referred to a cardiologist for evaluation and to determine the frequency of follow-up.

- Any patients with symptoms suggestive of aortic stenosis should be seen by a cardiologist.

Chan KL et al; ASTRONOMER Investigators. Effect of lipid lowering with rosuvastatin on progression of aortic stenosis: results of the aortic stenosis progression observation: measuring effects of rosuvastatin (ASTRONOMER) trial. Circulation. 2010 Jan 19;121(2):306–14. [PMID: 20048204]

Goel SS et al. Severe aortic stenosis and coronary artery disease—implications for management in the transcatheter aortic valve replacement era: a comprehensive review. J Am Coll Cardiol. 2013 Jul 2;62(1):1–10. [PMID: 23644089]

Herrmann HC et al. Predictors of mortality and outcomes of therapy in low-flow severe aortic stenosis: a Placement of Aortic Transcatheter Valves (PARTNER) trial analysis. Circulation. 2013 Jun 11;127(23):2316–26. [PMID: 23661722]

Holmes DR Jr et al. 2012 ACCF/AATS/SCAI/STS expert consensus document on transcatheter aortic valve replacement. J Am Coll Cardiol. 2012 Mar 27;59(13):1200–54. [PMID: 22300974]

Jander N et al. Outcome of patients with low-gradient "severe" aortic stenosis and preserved ejection fraction. Circulation. 2011 Mar 1;123(8):887–95. [PMID: 21321152]

Leon MB et al; PARTNER Trial Investigators. Transcatheter aortic-valve implantation for aortic stenosis in patients who cannot undergo surgery. N Engl J Med. 2010 Oct 21;363(17):1597–607. [PMID: 20961243]

Lindman BR et al. Current management of calcific aortic stenosis. Circ Res. 2013 Jul 5;113(2):223–37. [PMID: 23833296]

Nishimura RA et al. 2014 AHA/ACC Guideline for the Management of Patients With Valvular Heart Disease: A Report of the American College of Cardiology/American Heart Association Task Force on Practice Guidelines. Circulation. 2014 Mar 3. [Epub ahead of print] [PMID: 24589853]

Vahanian A et al; Joint Task Force on the Management of Valvular Heart Disease of the European Society of Cardiology (ESC); European Association for Cardio-Thoracic Surgery (EACTS). Guidelines on the management of valvular heart disease (version 2012). Eur Heart J. 2012 Oct;33(19):2451–96. [PMID: 22922415]

AORTIC REGURGITATION

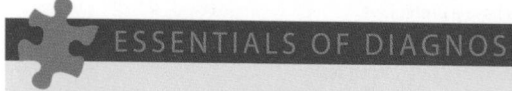

ESSENTIALS OF DIAGNOSIS

- ▶ Usually asymptomatic until middle age; presents with left-sided failure or chest pain.

- ▶ Echocardiography/Doppler is diagnostic.

- ▶ Surgery indicated for symptoms, EF < 55%, or LV end-systolic dimension > 5.0–5.5 cm.

General Considerations

Rheumatic aortic regurgitation has become much less common than in the preantibiotic era, and nonrheumatic causes now predominate. These include congenitally bicuspid valves, infective endocarditis, and hypertension. Many patients have aortic regurgitation secondary to aortic root diseases such as that associated with Marfan syndrome or to aortic dissection. Rarely, inflammatory diseases, such as ankylosing spondylitis or reactive arthritis, may be causative.

Clinical Findings

A. Symptoms and Signs

The clinical presentation is determined by the rapidity with which regurgitation develops. In chronic aortic regurgitation, the only sign for many years may be a soft aortic diastolic murmur. As the severity of the aortic regurgitation increases, diastolic BP falls, and the LV progressively enlarges. Most patients remain asymptomatic even at this point. LV failure is a late event and may be sudden in onset. Exertional dyspnea and fatigue are the most frequent symptoms, but paroxysmal nocturnal dyspnea and pulmonary edema may also occur. Angina pectoris or atypical chest pain may occasionally be present. Associated CAD and presyncope or syncope are less common than in aortic stenosis.

Hemodynamically, because of compensatory LV dilation, patients eject a large stroke volume, which is adequate to maintain forward cardiac output until late in the course of the disease. LV diastolic pressure may rise when heart failure occurs. Abnormal LV systolic function, as manifested by reduced EF < 55%) and increasing end-systolic LV volume (>5.0 cm), is a sign that surgical intervention is warranted.

The major physical findings in **chronic aortic regurgitation** relate to the high stroke volume being ejected into the systemic vascular system with rapid runoff as the regurgitation takes place (see Table 10–2). This results in a wide arterial pulse pressure. The pulse has a rapid rise and fall (water-hammer pulse or Corrigan pulse), with an elevated systolic and low diastolic pressure. The large stroke volume is also responsible for characteristic findings such as Quincke pulses (nailbed capillary pulsations), Duroziez sign (to and fro murmur over a partially compressed peripheral artery, commonly the femoral), and Musset sign (head bob with each pulse). In younger patients, the increased stroke volume may summate with the pressure wave reflected from the periphery and create a higher than expected systolic pressure in the lower extremities compared with the central aorta. Since the peripheral bed is much larger in the leg than the arm, the BP in the leg may be over 40 mm Hg higher than in the arm (Hill sign) in severe aortic regurgitation. The apical impulse is prominent, laterally displaced, usually hyperdynamic, and may be sustained. A systolic murmur is usually present and may be quite soft and localized; the aortic diastolic murmur is usually high-pitched and decrescendo. A mid or late diastolic low-pitched mitral murmur (Austin Flint murmur) may be heard in advanced aortic regurgitation, owing to relative obstruction of mitral inflow produced by partial closure of the mitral valve by the rapidly rising LV diastolic pressure due to the aortic regurgitation.

In **acute aortic regurgitation** (usually from aortic dissection or infective endocarditis), LV failure is manifested primarily as pulmonary edema and may develop rapidly; surgery is urgently required in such cases. Patients with acute aortic regurgitation do not have the dilated LV of chronic aortic regurgitation and the extra LV volume is handled poorly. For the same reason, the diastolic murmur is shorter, may be minimal in intensity, and the pulse pressure may not be widened—making clinical diagnosis difficult. The mitral valve may close prematurely even before LV systole has been initiated (pre-closure) due to the rapid rise in the LV diastolic pressure, and the first heart sound is thus diminished or inaudible. Pre-closure of the mitral valve can be readily detected on echocardiography and is considered an indication for surgical intervention.

B. Diagnostic Studies

The ECG usually shows moderate to severe LVH. Radiographs show cardiomegaly with LV prominence and sometimes a dilated aorta.

Echocardiography demonstrates the major diagnostic features, including whether the lesion involves the proximal aortic root and what valvular pathology is present. Annual assessments of LV size and function are critical in determining the timing for valve replacement. The 2014 ACCF/ACC valvular guidelines provides criteria for assessing the severity of aortic regurgitation. Cardiac MRI and CT can estimate aortic root size, particularly when there is concern for an ascending aneurysm. MRI can provide a regurgitant fraction to help confirm severity. Cardiac catheterization may be unnecessary in younger patients, particularly those with acute aortic regurgitation, but can help define hemodynamics, aortic root abnormalities, and associated CAD preoperatively in older patients. Increasing data are emerging that serum BNP or pro-NT BNP may be an early sign of LV dysfunction, and it is possible that these data will be added to recommendations for surgical intervention in the future.

▶ Treatment & Prognosis

Aortic regurgitation that appears or worsens during or after an episode of infective endocarditis or aortic dissection may lead to acute severe LV failure or subacute progression over weeks or months. The former usually presents as pulmonary edema; surgical replacement of the valve is indicated even during active infection. These patients may be transiently improved or stabilized by vasodilators.

Chronic aortic regurgitation may be tolerated for many years, but the prognosis without surgery becomes poor when symptoms occur. Since aortic regurgitation places both a preload (volume) and afterload increase on the LV, medications that decrease afterload can reduce regurgitation severity. Current recommendations advocate afterload reduction in aortic regurgitation when there is associated systolic hypertension (systolic BP > 140 mm Hg). Afterload reduction in normotensive patients remains controversial. Angiotensin receptor blockers (ARBs), rather than beta-blockers, are the preferred additions to the medical therapy in patients with **Marfan disease** because of the ARBs ability to reduce aortic stiffness (by blocking TGF-beta) and to slow the rate of aortic dilation. The role of beta-blockers continues to be explored in aortic regurgitation in an attempt to reduce adverse neuroendocrine activation.

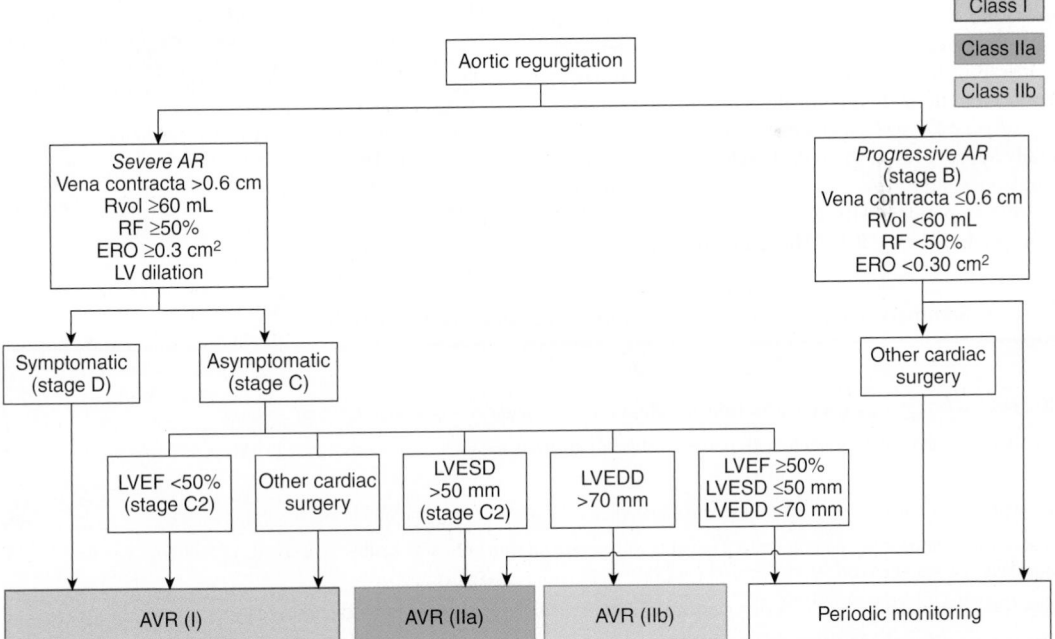

▲ **Figure 10–4.** Algorithm for the management of chronic aortic regurgitation. (Reproduced with permission from Nishimura RA et al. 2014 AHA/ACC Guideline for the Management of Patients With Valvular Heart Disease: A Report of the American College of Cardiology/American Heart Association Task Force on Practice Guidelines. Circulation. 2014 Mar 3. [Epub ahead of print] [PMID: 24589853]

Surgery is indicated once symptoms emerge or for any evidence of LV dysfunction. Figure 10–4 outlines the recommendations for intervention in chronic aortic regurgitation.

LV dysfunction in this situation can be defined by echocardiography if the EF is < 55% or if the LV end-systolic dimension is > 5.0 cm (class 2b indication), even in the asymptomatic patient. In addition, aortic root diameters of > 4.5 cm in Marfan or > 5.0 cm in non-Marfan patients are indications for surgery to avoid the rapid expansion that occurs when the root diameter exceeds 6.0 cm. Although the operative mortality rate is higher when LV function is severely impaired, valve replacement or repair is still likely indicated, since LV function often improves and the long-term prognosis is thereby enhanced even in this situation. The issues with AVR covered in the above section concerning aortic stenosis pertain here. Currently, however, there are no percutaneous approaches to aortic regurgitation. Aortic regurgitation due to a paravalvular prosthetic valve defect can occasionally be occluded with percutaneous occluder devices. The choice of prosthetic valve for AVR depends on the patient's age and compatibility with warfarin anticoagulation. Table 10–6 summarizes the recommendations for aortic regurgitation intervention.

The operative mortality for AVR is usually in the 3–5% range. Aortic regurgitation due to aortic root disease requires repair or replacement of the root. Though valve-sparing operations have improved recently, most patients with root replacement undergo valve replacement at the same time. Root replacement in association with valve replacement may require reanastomosis of the coronary arteries, and thus the procedure is more complex than valve replacement alone. The Wheat procedure replaces the aortic root but spares the area where the coronaries attach to avoid the necessity for their reimplantation. Following surgery, LV size usually decreases and LV function generally improves even when the baseline EF is depressed.

Guidelines vary regarding when intervention on the aortic root in patients with bicuspid aortic valve disease is appropriate. The ACCF/AHA guidelines suggest the "cutoff" diameter value for repair should be 5.5 cm, while the ESC recommendation is still 5.0 cm. There are data that the root expands more rapidly or dissection is much more prevalent when the aortic root diameter exceeds 6.0 cm, and the general sense is not to let it approach that diameter. The following classifications outline when to operate on the aortic root in patients with a bicuspid aortic valve based on the former and more recent guidelines:

Class 1 indication (LOE C): aortic root diameter of sinuses or ascending aorta > 5.5 cm.

Class 2a indication (LOE C): aortic root diameter of sinuses or ascending aorta > 5.0 cn with associated risk factors (family history of dissection or increase in size .0.5 cm per year).

Class 2a indication (LOE C): aortic root diameter > 4.5 cm if patient undergoing AVR for clinical reasons.

▶ When to Refer

- Patients with audible aortic regurgitation should be seen, at least initially, by a cardiologist who can determine whether the patient needs follow-up.

- Patients with a dilated aortic root should be monitored by a cardiologist, since imaging studies other than the chest radiograph or echocardiogram may be required to decide surgical timing.

Bonow RO. Chronic mitral regurgitation and aortic regurgitation: have indications for surgery changed? J Am Coll Cardiol. 2013 Feb 19;61(7):693–701. [PMID: 23265342]

Elder DH et al. The impact of renin-angiotensin-aldosterone system blockade on heart failure outcomes and mortality in patients identified to have aortic regurgitation: a large population study. J Am Coll Cardiol. 2011 Nov 8;58(20):2084–91. [PMID: 22051330]

Nishimura RA et al. 2014 AHA/ACC Guideline for the Management of Patients With Valvular Heart Disease: A Report of the American College of Cardiology/American Heart Association Task Force on Practice Guidelines. Circulation. 2014 Mar 3. [Epub ahead of print] [PMID: 24589853]

Table 10–6. Summary of recommendations for aortic regurgitation: intervention.

Recommendations	COR	LOE
AVR or repair is indicated for symptomatic patients with severe AR regardless of LV systolic function (stage D)	I	B
AVR or repair is indicated for asymptomatic patients with chronic severe AR and LV systolic dysfunction (LVEF < 50%) (stage C2)	I	B
AVR or repair is indicated for patients with severe AR (stage C or D) while undergoing other cardiac surgery	I	C
AVR or repair is reasonable for asymptomatic patients with severe AR with normal LV systolic function (LVEF ≥ 50%), but severe LV dilatation (LVESD >50 mm) (stage C2)	IIa	B
AVR or repair is reasonable in patients with moderate AR (stage B) while undergoing other cardiac surgery	IIa	C
AVR or repair may be considered for asymptomatic patients with severe AR and normal LV systolic function (LVEF ≥50%) when there is evidence of progressive increases in LV dimension (LVEDD >65 mm)	IIb	C

AR, aortic regurgitation; AVR, aortic valve replacement; COR, class of recommendation; LOE, level of evidence; LV, left ventricular; LVEDD, left ventricular end-diastolic dimension; LVEF, left ventricular ejection fraction; LVESD, left ventricular end-systolic dimension; N/A, not applicable. Reproduced, with permission, from Nishimura RA et al. 2014 AHA/ACC Guideline for the Management of Patients With Valvular Heart Disease: A Report of the American College of Cardiology/American Heart Association Task Force on Practice Guidelines. Circulation. 2014 Mar 3. [Epub ahead of print] [PMID: 24589853]

Vahanian A et al; Joint Task Force on the Management of Valvular Heart Disease of the European Society of Cardiology (ESC); European Association for Cardio-Thoracic Surgery (EACTS). Guidelines on the management of valvular heart disease (version 2012). Eur Heart J. 2012 Oct;33(19):2451–96. [PMID: 22922415]

TRICUSPID STENOSIS

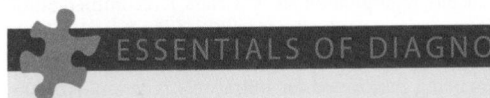

ESSENTIALS OF DIAGNOSIS

- ▶ Female predominance.
- ▶ History of rheumatic heart disease. Carcinoid disease or prosthetic valve degeneration are the most common etiologies in the United States.
- ▶ Echocardiography/Doppler is diagnostic; mean valve gradient > 5 mm Hg indicates severe tricuspid stenosis.

▶ General Considerations

Tricuspid valve stenosis is usually rheumatic in origin, although in the United States, tricuspid stenosis is more commonly due to tricuspid valve repair or replacement or to the carcinoid syndrome. Tricuspid regurgitation frequently accompanies the lesion. It should be suspected when "right heart failure" appears in the course of mitral valve disease or in the postoperative period after tricuspid valve repair or replacement. Congenital forms of tricuspid stenosis may also be rarely observed, as have case reports of multiple pacemaker leads creating RV inflow obstruction at the tricuspid valve.

▶ Clinical Findings

A. Symptoms and Signs

Tricuspid stenosis is characterized by right heart failure with hepatomegaly, ascites, and dependent edema. In sinus rhythm, giant **a** wave is seen in the JVP, which is elevated (see Table 10–2). The typical diastolic rumble along the lower left sternal border mimics mitral stenosis, though in tricuspid stenosis the rumble increases with inspiration. In sinus rhythm, a presystolic liver pulsation may be found.

B. Diagnostic Studies

In the absence of atrial fibrillation, the ECG reveals RA enlargement. The chest radiograph may show marked cardiomegaly with a normal PA size. A dilated superior vena cava and azygous vein may be evident.

The normal valve area of the tricuspid valve is 10 cm², so significant stenosis must be present to produce a gradient. Hemodynamically, a mean diastolic pressure gradient of > 5 mm Hg is considered significant, although even a 2 mm Hg gradient can be considered abnormal. This can be demonstrated by echocardiography or cardiac catheterization.

▶ Treatment & Prognosis

Tricuspid stenosis may be progressive, eventually causing severe right-sided heart failure. Initialtherapy is directed at reducing the fluid congestion, with diuretics the mainstay (see Treatment, Heart Failure, below). When there is considerable bowel edema, torsemide may have an advantage over other loop diuretics, such as furosemide, because it is better absorbed from the gut. Aldosterone inhibitors also help, particularly if there is liver engorgement or ascites. Neither surgical nor percutaneous valvuloplasty is particularly effective for relief of tricuspid stenosis, as residual tricuspid regurgitation is common. Tricuspid valve replacement is clearly the preferred surgical approach. Mechanical tricuspid valve replacement is rarely done because the low flow predisposes to thrombosis and because the mechanical valve cannot be crossed should the need arise for right heart catheterization or pacemaker implantation. Therefore, bioprosthetic valves are almost always preferred. Often tricuspid valve replacement is done in conjunction with mitral valve replacement for mitral stenosis. The indications for valve replacement in severe tricuspid stenosis are straightforward:

Class 1 indication (LOE C); at time of operation for left-sided valve disease.

Class 1 indication (LOE C); if symptomatic.

Class 2b indication (LOE C): rarely percutaneous balloon commissurotomy for isolated tricuspid stenosis in high-risk patients with no significant tricuspid regurgitation.

Hong SN. Carcinoid heart disease. J Am Coll Cardiol. 2010 May 4;55(18):1996. [PMID: 20430272]
Nishimura RA et al. 2014 AHA/ACC Guideline for the Management of Patients With Valvular Heart Disease: A Report of the American College of Cardiology/American Heart Association Task Force on Practice Guidelines. Circulation. 2014 Mar 3. [Epub ahead of print] [PMID: 24589853]
Yeter E et al. Tricuspid balloon valvuloplasty to treat tricuspid stenosis. J Heart Valve Dis. 2010 Jan;19(1):159–60. [PMID: 20329507]

TRICUSPID REGURGITATION

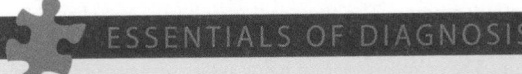

ESSENTIALS OF DIAGNOSIS

- ▶ Frequently occurs in patients with pulmonary or cardiac disease with pressure or volume overload on the right ventricle.
- ▶ Tricuspid valve regurgitation from pacemaker lead placement is becoming more common.
- ▶ Echocardiography useful in determining cause (low- or high-pressure tricuspid regurgitation).

▶ General Considerations

Tricuspid valvular regurgitation often occurs whenever there is RV dilation from any cause. As tricuspid regurgitation increases, the RV size increases further, and this in turn worsens the severity of the tricuspid regurgitation. The causes of tricuspid regurgitation thus relate to anatomic issues with either the valve itself or to the RV geometry. In most cases, the cause is the RV geometry and not primary tricuspid valve disease. An enlarged, dilated RV may be present if there is pulmonary hypertension for any reason, in severe pulmonary valve regurgitation, or in cardiomyopathy. The RV may be injured from myocardial infarction or may be inherently dilated due to infiltrative diseases (RV dysplasia or sarcoidosis). RV dilation is often secondary to left heart failure. Inherent abnormalities of the tricuspid valve include Ebstein anomaly (displacement of the septal and posterior, but not the anterior, leaflets into the RV), tricuspid valve prolapse, carcinoid plaque formation, collagen disease inflammation, valvular tumors, or tricuspid endocarditis. In addition, pacemaker lead valvular injury is becoming an increasingly recognized iatrogenic cause.

► Clinical Findings

A. Symptoms and Signs

The symptoms and signs of tricuspid regurgitation are identical to those resulting from RV failure due to any cause. As a generality, the diagnosis can be made by careful inspection of the JVP (see Table 10–2). The JVP waveform should decline during ventricular systole (the x descent). The timing of this decline can be observed by palpating the opposite carotid artery. As tricuspid regurgitation worsens, more and more of this x descent valley in the JVP is filled with the regurgitant wave until all of the x descent is obliterated and a positive systolic waveform will be noted in the JVP. An associated tricuspid regurgitation murmur may or may not be audible and can be distinguished from mitral regurgitation by the left parasternal location and increase with inspiration. An S_3 may accompany the murmur and is related to the high flow returning from the RA. Cyanosis may be present if the increased RA pressure stretches the atrial septum and opens a PFO or there is a true ASD (eg, in about 50% of patients with Ebstein anomaly). Severe tricuspid regurgitation results in hepatomegaly, edema, and ascites.

B. Diagnostic Studies

The ECG is usually nonspecific, though atrial fibrillation is not uncommon. The chest radiograph may reveal evidence of an enlarged RA or dilated azygous vein and pleural effusion. The echocardiogram helps assess severity of tricuspid regurgitation, RV systolic pressure, and RV size and function. A paradoxically moving interventricular septum may be present due to the volume overload on the RV. Catheterization confirms the presence of the regurgitant wave in the RA and elevated RA pressures. If the PA or RV systolic pressure is < 40 mm Hg, primary valvular tricuspid regurgitation should be suspected.

► Treatment & Prognosis

Mild tricuspid regurgitation is common and generally can be well managed with diuretics. When present, bowel edema may reduce the effectiveness of diuretics such as furosemide, and intravenous diuretics should initially be used. Torsemide is better absorbed in this situation when oral diuretics are added. Aldosterone antagonists have a role as well, particularly if ascites is present. At times, the efficacy of loop diuretics can be enhanced by adding a thiazide diuretic (see Treatment, Heart Failure, below).

Aquapheresis has also been proven helpful to reduce the edema in marked right heart failure.

Definitive treatment usually requires elimination of the cause of the tricuspid regurgitation. If the problem is left heart disease, then treatment of the left heart issues may lower pulmonary pressures, reduce RV size, and resolve the tricuspid regurgitation. Treatment for primary and secondary causes of pulmonary hypertension will generally reduce the tricuspid regurgitation. It is a class I recommendation that tricuspid annuloplasty be performed when tricuspid regurgitation is present and mitral valve replacement or repair is being performed for mitral regurgitation. Annuloplasty without insertion of a prosthetic ring (DeVega annuloplasty) may also be effective in reducing the tricuspid annular dilation. The valve leaflet itself can occasionally be repaired in tricuspid valve endocarditis. In years past, tricuspid regurgitation due to endocarditis in substance abuse patients was treated temporarily with removal of the valve, although it had to be replaced eventually (usually by 3–6 months); this practice is rarely done now. If there is an inherent defect in the tricuspid valve apparatus that cannot be repaired, then replacement of the tricuspid valve is warranted. Almost always, a bioprosthetic valve, and not a mechanical valve, is used. Anticoagulation is not required for bioprosthetic valves unless there is associated atrial fibrillation. The indications for surgical intervention are summarized in Figure 10–5.

► When to Refer

- Anyone with moderate or severe tricuspid regurgitation should be seen at least once by a cardiologist to determine whether studies and intervention are needed.
- Severe tricuspid regurgitation requires regular follow-up by a cardiologist.

Kim JB et al. Surgical outcomes of severe tricuspid regurgitation: predictors of adverse clinical outcomes. Heart. 2013 Feb;99(3):181–7. [PMID: 23038792]

Nishimura RA et al. 2014 AHA/ACC Guideline for the Management of Patients With Valvular Heart Disease: A Report of the American College of Cardiology/American Heart Association Task Force on Practice Guidelines. Circulation. 2014 Mar 3. [Epub ahead of print] [PMID: 24589853]

Vahanian A et al; Joint Task Force on the Management of Valvular Heart Disease of the European Society of Cardiology (ESC); European Association for Cardio-Thoracic Surgery (EACTS). Guidelines on the management of valvular heart disease (version 2012). Eur Heart J. 2012 Oct;33(19):2451–96. [PMID: 22922415]

PULMONARY VALVE REGURGITATION

ESSENTIALS OF DIAGNOSIS

- ► Most cases are due to pulmonary hypertension.
- ► Echocardiogram is definitive in high-pressure, but may be less definitive in low-pressure, pulmonary valve regurgitation.
- ► Low-pressure pulmonary valve regurgitation is well tolerated.

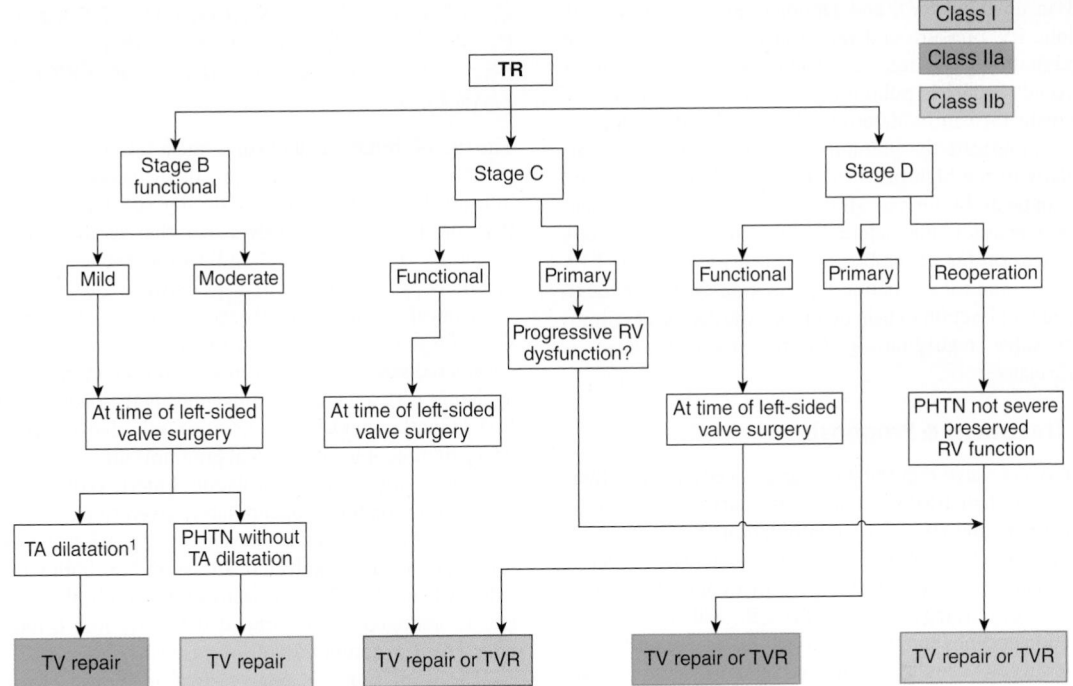

Class I
Class IIa
Class IIb

Figure 10–5. The 2014 AHA/ACC guidelines on the indications for surgical intervention in tricuspid regurgitation. (Reproduced with permission from Nishimura RA et al. 2014 AHA/ACC Guideline for the Management of Patients With Valvular Heart Disease: A Report of the American College of Cardiology/ American Heart Association Task Force on Practice Guidelines. Circulation. 2014 Mar 3. [Epub ahead of print] [PMID: 24589853])

General Considerations

Pulmonary valve regurgitation can be divided into **high-pressure causes** (due to pulmonary hypertension) and **low-pressure causes** (usually due to a dilated pulmonary annulus, to a congenitally abnormal [bicuspid or dysplastic] pulmonary valve, or to plaque from carcinoid disease). It may also follow surgical repair, eg, frequently occurring after repair of tetralogy of Fallot with a transannular patch. Because the RV tolerates a volume load better than a pressure load, it tends to tolerate low pressure pulmonary valve regurgitation for long periods of time without dysfunction.

Clinical Findings

Most patients are asymptomatic. Others show symptoms of right heart volume overload. On examination, a hyperdynamic RV can usually be palpated (RV lift). If the PA is enlarged, it may be palpated along the left sternal border. P_2 will be palpable in pulmonary hypertension and both systolic and diastolic thrills are occasionally noted. On auscultation, the second heart sound may be widely split due to prolonged RV systole. A pulmonary valve systolic click may be noted as well as a

right-sided gallop. If pulmonic stenosis is also present, the ejection click may decline with inspiration while any associated systolic murmur will increase. In high-pressure pulmonary valve regurgitation, the pulmonary diastolic (Graham Steell) murmur is readily audible. It is often due to a dilated pulmonary annulus. The murmur increases with inspiration and diminishes with the Valsalva maneuver. In low-pressure pulmonary valve regurgitation, the PA diastolic pressure may be only a few mm Hg higher than the RV diastolic pressure, and there is little diastolic gradient to produce a murmur or characteristic echocardiography/Doppler findings. At times, only contrast angiography or MRI of the main PA will show the free flowing pulmonary valve regurgitation in low-pressure pulmonary valve regurgitation. This situation is common in following patients with repair of tetralogy of Fallot where, despite little murmur, there may be free flowing pulmonary valve regurgitation. This can be suspected by noting an enlarging right ventricle.

The ECG is generally of little value, although right bundle branch block is common, and there may be ECG criteria for RVH. The chest radiograph may show only the enlarged RV and PA. Echocardiography may demonstrate evidence of RV volume overload (paradoxic septal motion and an enlarged RV), and Doppler can determine peak systolic RV pressure and reveal any associated tricuspid regurgitation. The interventricular septum may appear flattened if there is pulmonary hypertension. The size of the main PA can be determined and color flow Doppler can demonstrate the pulmonary valve regurgitation, particularly in the high-pressure situation. Cardiac MRI and CT can be useful for assessing the size of the PA, for imaging the jet lesion, for excluding other causes of pulmonary hypertension (eg, thromboembolic disease, peripheral PA stenosis), and for evaluating RV function. MRI provides a regurgitant fraction to help quantitate the degree of pulmonary valve regurgitation. Cardiac catheterization is confirmatory.

▶ **Treatment & Prognosis**

Pulmonary valve regurgitation rarely needs specific therapy other than treatment of the primary cause. In low-pressure pulmonary valve regurgitation due to surgical patch repair of tetralogy of Fallot, pulmonary valve replacement may be indicated if RV enlargement or dysfunction is present. In tetralogy of Fallot, the QRS will widen as RV function declines and the ECG is helpful here (a QRS > 180 msec suggests a higher risk for sudden death) and increasing RV volumes should trigger an evaluation for potential pulmonary valve regurgitation. In carcinoid heart disease, pulmonary valve replacement with a porcine bioprosthesis may be undertaken, though the plaque from this disorder eventually covers the prosthetic pulmonary valve, and this tends to limit the lifespan of these valves. In high-pressure pulmonary valve regurgitation, treatment to control the cause of the pulmonary hypertension is key. Low-pressure pulmonary valve regurgitation is well tolerated over many years; exercise and pregnancy are well tolerated. High-pressure pulmonary valve regurgitation is poorly tolerated and is a serious condition that needs a thorough evaluation for cause and therapy. High pulmonary pressures require a thorough evaluation to distinguish a primary pulmonary cause versus one due to left-sided heart disease. Pulmonary valve replacement requires a bioprosthetic valve in most cases. Pulmonary regurgitation due to an RV to PA conduit or due to a pulmonary autograft replacement as part of the Ross procedure can be repaired with a percutaneous pulmonary valve (Melody valve).

▶ **When to Refer**

- Patients with pulmonary valve regurgitation that results in RV enlargement should be referred to a cardiologist regardless of the estimated pulmonary pressures.

McElhinney DB et al. Short- and medium-term outcomes after transcatheter pulmonary valve replacement in the expanded multicenter US Melody valve trial. Circulation. 2010 Aug 3;122(5):507–16. [PMID: 20644013]

Warnes CA et al. ACC/AHA 2008 Guidelines for the Management of Adults With Congenital Heart Disease. A Report of the American College of Cardiology/American Heart Association Task Force on Practice Guidelines. Circulation. 2008 Dec 2;118(23):e714–833. [PMID: 18997169]

MANAGEMENT OF ANTICOAGULATION FOR PROSTHETIC HEART VALVES DURING PREGNANCY & NONCARDIAC SURGERY OR PROCEDURES

The risk of thromboembolism is much lower with bioprosthetic valves than mechanical prosthetic valves. Mechanical mitral valve prostheses pose a greater risk for thrombosis than mechanical aortic valves. For that reason, the INR should be kept between 2.5 and 3.5 for mechanical mitral prosthetic valves but can be kept between 2.0 and 2.5 for mechanical aortic prosthetic valves. Recent data suggest that with some bileaflet AVRs, an INR as low as 1.5 may be considered safely. Most guidelines recommend that anticoagulation with a vitamin K antagonist is reasonable for the first 3 months after a bioprosthetic mitral valve replacement or repair, though many surgical programs do not feel that is necessary without atrial fibrillation. Enteric-coated aspirin (81 mg once daily) is concomitantly given to patients with both types of mechanical valves but appears to be more important for mitral valve prostheses and for both types of valves when other high-risk factors for thrombosis are present. Clopidogrel is recommended for the first 6 months after TAVR in addition to lifelong aspirin.

The use of vitamin K antagonists, unfractionated heparin, low-molecular-weight heparin and antifibrinolytics in various clinical situations in patients with VHD is summarized in Table 10–7 and the issues are covered in depth in both the 2102 ESC and the 2014 ACCF/AHA VHD guidelines.

Warfarin causes fetal skeletal abnormalities in up to 2% of women who become pregnant while taking it, so every effort is made to defer valve replacement in women until after childbearing age. However, if a woman with a mechanical valve becomes pregnant while taking warfarin, the risk of stopping warfarin may be higher for the mother than the risk of continuing warfarin for the fetus. The risk of warfarin to the fetal skeleton is greatest during the first trimester. Current guidelines suggest warfarin and low-dose aspirin are safe during the second and third trimester and should be stopped at time of delivery. At time of vaginal delivery, unfractionated heparin with activated partial thromboplastin time (aPTT) at least two times control is desirable. The risk of warfarin embryopathy has been related to the dose, and guidelines suggest it is reasonable to continue warfarin for the first trimester if the dose is ≤ 5 mg/d. If the dose is > 5 mg/d, it is appropriate to consider either low-molecular-weight heparin as long as the anti-Xa is being monitored (range 0.8 units/mL to 1.2 units/mL) or unfractionated heparin if the aPTT can be monitored and is at least two times control. Target specific oral anticoagulants (antithrombin or Xa inhibitors) should not be used in place of warfarin for mechanical prosthetic valves. This is based on the RE-ALIGN trial that showed that carefully-dosed dabigatran had both more thrombotic complications and more bleeding than warfarin.

Eikelboom JW et al; RE-ALIGN Investigators. Dabigatran versus warfarin in patients with mechanical heart valves. N Engl J Med. 2013 Sep 26;369(13):1206–14. [PMID: 23991661]

Holbrook A et al. Evidence-based management of anticoagulant therapy: Antithrombotic Therapy and Prevention of Thrombosis, 9th ed: American College of Chest Physicians

Table 10–7. Recommendations for administering vitamin K antagonist (VKA) therapy in patients undergoing procedures or patients with certain clinical conditions.

Procedures	Recommendations
General	Stop VKA 5 days prior and resume 12–24 hours after procedure
Bridging for mechanical heart valves	Required only for those at high risk for thromboembolism Bridge with UFH or LMWH and stop UFH 4–6 hours before procedure or stop LMWH 24 hours before procedure Resume 48–72 hours after the procedure

Clinical Situations	Recommendations
Atrial fibrillation and moderate or severe mitral stenosis	VKA (target INR 2.0–3.0) If patient refuses, aspirin (50–100 mg) plus clopidogrel (75 mg)
Sinus rhythm and mitral stenosis	If left atrial size > 5.5 cm, then consider VKA (target 2.0–3.0)
Intermittent atrial fibrillation or history of systemic embolus and mitral stenosis	VKA (target INR 2.0–3.0)

Endocarditis
   Native valve or bioprosthetic valve endocarditis
   Mechanical valve endocarditis
	No anticoagulation recommended
	Hold VKA until "safe to resume" (generally when mycotic aneurysm is ruled out or there is no need for urgent surgery)

First 3 months following valve replacement
   Bioprosthetic aortic valve replacement
   Transcatheter valve replacement
   Mitral or aortic repair
   Bioprosthetic mitral valve
	
	Aspirin (50–100 mg)
	Aspirin (50–100 mg) plus clopidogrel (75 mg)
	Aspirin (50–100 mg)
	VKA (target INR 2.0–3.0)

Long-term anticoagulation after valve replacement
   Bioprosthetic valve in normal sinus rhythm
   Mechanical valve replacement
	
	Aspirin (50–100 mg)
	VKA (target INR 2.0–3.0 for aortic, target INR 2.5–3.5 for mitral) plus aspirin (50–100 mg)

Prosthetic valve thrombosis
   Right sided valve
   Left sided valve
	
	Fibrinolytic therapy
	Early surgery if thrombus large (> 0.8 cm² area), otherwise either fibrinolytic therapy or UFH

Pregnancy and a mechanical heart valve	Add aspirin (50–100 mg) for high risk Adjusted dose LMWH twice daily throughout pregnancy (follow anti-Xa 4 hours after dose) *or* Adjusted dose UFH every 12 hours throughout pregnancy (aPTT > 2 times control or anti-Xa between 0.35 and 0.70) *or* Adjusted dose UFH or LMWH until 13th week of pregnancy then VKA until close to deliver then resume UFH or LMWH

aPTT, activated partial thromboplastin time; INR, international normalized ratio; LMWH, low-molecular-weight heparin; UFH, unfractionated heparin.
Modified, with permission, from Holbrook A et al. Evidence-based management of anticoagulant therapy: Antithrombotic Therapy and Prevention of Thrombosis, 9th ed: American College of Chest Physicians Evidence-Based Clinical Practice Guidelines. Chest 2012;141: (Suppl 2:e152S–e184S).

Evidence-Based Clinical Practice Guidelines. Chest. 2012 Feb;141(2 Suppl):e152S–84S. [PMID: 22315259]
Nishimura RA et al. 2014 AHA/ACC Guideline for the Management of Patients With Valvular Heart Disease: A Report of the American College of Cardiology/American Heart Association Task Force on Practice Guidelines. Circulation. 2014 Mar 3. [Epub ahead of print] [PMID: 24589853]
Vahanian A et al; Joint Task Force on the Management of Valvular Heart Disease of the European Society of Cardiology (ESC); European Association for Cardio-Thoracic Surgery (EACTS). Guidelines on the management of valvular heart disease (version 2012). Eur Heart J. 2012 Oct;33(19):2451–96. [PMID: 22922415]

CORONARY HEART DISEASE (ATHEROSCLEROTIC CAD, ISCHEMIC HEART DISEASE)

Coronary heart disease, or atherosclerotic CAD, is the number one killer in the United States and worldwide. Every minute, an American dies of coronary heart disease. About 37% of people who experience an acute coronary event, either angina or myocardial infarction, will die of it in the same year. Death rates of coronary heart disease have declined every year since 1968, with about half of the decline from 1980 to 2000 due to treatments and half due to improved risk factors. Coronary heart disease is still responsible for approximately one of five deaths and over 600,000 deaths per year in the United States. Coronary heart disease afflicts nearly 16 million Americans and the prevalence rises steadily with age; thus, the aging of the US population promises to increase the overall burden of coronary heart disease.

Risk Factors for CAD

Most patients with coronary heart disease have some identifiable risk factor. These include a positive family history (the younger the onset in a first-degree relative, the greater the risk), male sex, blood lipid abnormalities, diabetes mellitus, hypertension, physical inactivity, abdominal obesity, and cigarette smoking, psychosocial factors, consumption of too few fruits and vegetables, and too much alcohol. Smoking remains the number one preventable cause of death and illness in the United States. Although smoking rates have declined in the United States in recent decades, 18% of women and 21% of men still smoke. According to the World Health Organization, 1 year after quitting, the risk of coronary heart disease decreases by 50%. Various interventions have been shown to increase the likelihood of successful smoking cessation (see Chapter 1).

Hypercholesterolemia provides an important modifiable risk factor for coronary heart disease. Risk increases progressively with higher levels of low-density lipoprotein (LDL) cholesterol and declines with higher levels of high-density lipoprotein (HDL) cholesterol. Composite risk scores, such as the Framingham score (see Table 28–2) and the 10-year atherosclerotic cardiovascular disease risk calculator (http://my.americanheart.org/cvriskcalculator), provide estimates of 10-year probability of development of coronary heart disease that can guide primary prevention strategies. The 2013 ACC/AHA Guideline on the Treatment of Blood Cholesterol to Reduce Atherosclerotic Cardiovascular Risk in Adults suggests statin therapy in four populations: patients with (1) clinical atherosclerotic disease, (2) LDL cholesterol ≥ 190 mg/dL, (3) diabetes who are aged 40–75 years, and (4) an estimated 10-year atherosclotic risk of ≥ 7.5% aged 40–75 years (Figure 10–6). Importantly, the updated guidelines no longer recommend treating to a target LDL cholesterol, an approach that has never been shown to be effective in randomized trials. Patients in these categories should be treated with moderate or high intensity statin, with high intensity statin for the higher risk populations (Table 10–8).

Myocardial Hibernation & Stunning

Areas of myocardium that are persistently underperfused but still viable may develop sustained contractile dysfunction. This phenomenon, which is termed "myocardial hibernation," appears to represent an adaptive response that maybe associated with depressed LV function. It is important to recognize this phenomenon, since this form of dysfunction is reversible following coronary revascularization. Hibernating myocardium can be identified by radionuclide testing, positron emission tomography (PET), contrast-enhanced MRI, or its retained response

to inotropic stimulation with dobutamine. A related phenomenon, termed "myocardial stunning," is the occurrence of persistent contractile dysfunction following prolonged or repetitive episodes of myocardial ischemia. Clinically, myocardial stunning is often seen after reperfusion of acute myocardial infarction and is defined with improvement following revascularization.

Stone NJ et al. 2013 ACC/AHA Guideline on the Treatment of Blood Cholesterol to Reduce Atherosclerotic Cardiovascular Risk in Adults: a report of the American College of Cardiology/American Heart Association Task Force on Practice Guidelines. Circulation. 2013 Nov 12. [Epub ahead of print] [PMID: 24222016]

CHRONIC STABLE ANGINA PECTORIS

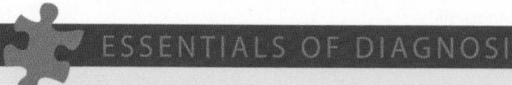
ESSENTIALS OF DIAGNOSIS

► Precordial chest pain, usually precipitated by stress or exertion, relieved rapidly by rest or nitrates.

► ECG or scintigraphic evidence of ischemia during pain or stress testing.

► Angiographic demonstration of significant obstruction of major coronary vessels.

General Considerations

Angina pectoris is usually due to atherosclerotic heart disease. Coronary vasospasm may occur at the site of a lesion or, less frequently, in apparently normal vessels. Other unusual causes of coronary artery obstruction such as congenital anomalies, emboli, arteritis, or dissection may cause ischemia or infarction. Angina may also occur in the absence of coronary artery obstruction as a result of severe myocardial hypertrophy, severe aortic stenosis or regurgitation, or in response to increased metabolic demands, as in hyperthyroidism, marked anemia, or paroxysmal tachycardias with rapid ventricular rates. Rarely, angina occurs with angiographically normal coronary arteries and without other identifiable causes. This presentation has been labeled **syndrome X** and is most likely due to inadequate flow reserve in the resistance vessels (microvasculature). Syndrome X remains difficult to diagnose. Although treatment is often not very successful in relieving symptoms, the prognosis of syndrome X is good.

Clinical Findings

A. Symptoms

The diagnosis of angina pectoris depends principally upon the history, which should specifically include the following information: circumstances that precipitate and relieve angina, characteristics of the discomfort, location and radiation, duration of attacks, and effect of nitroglycerin.

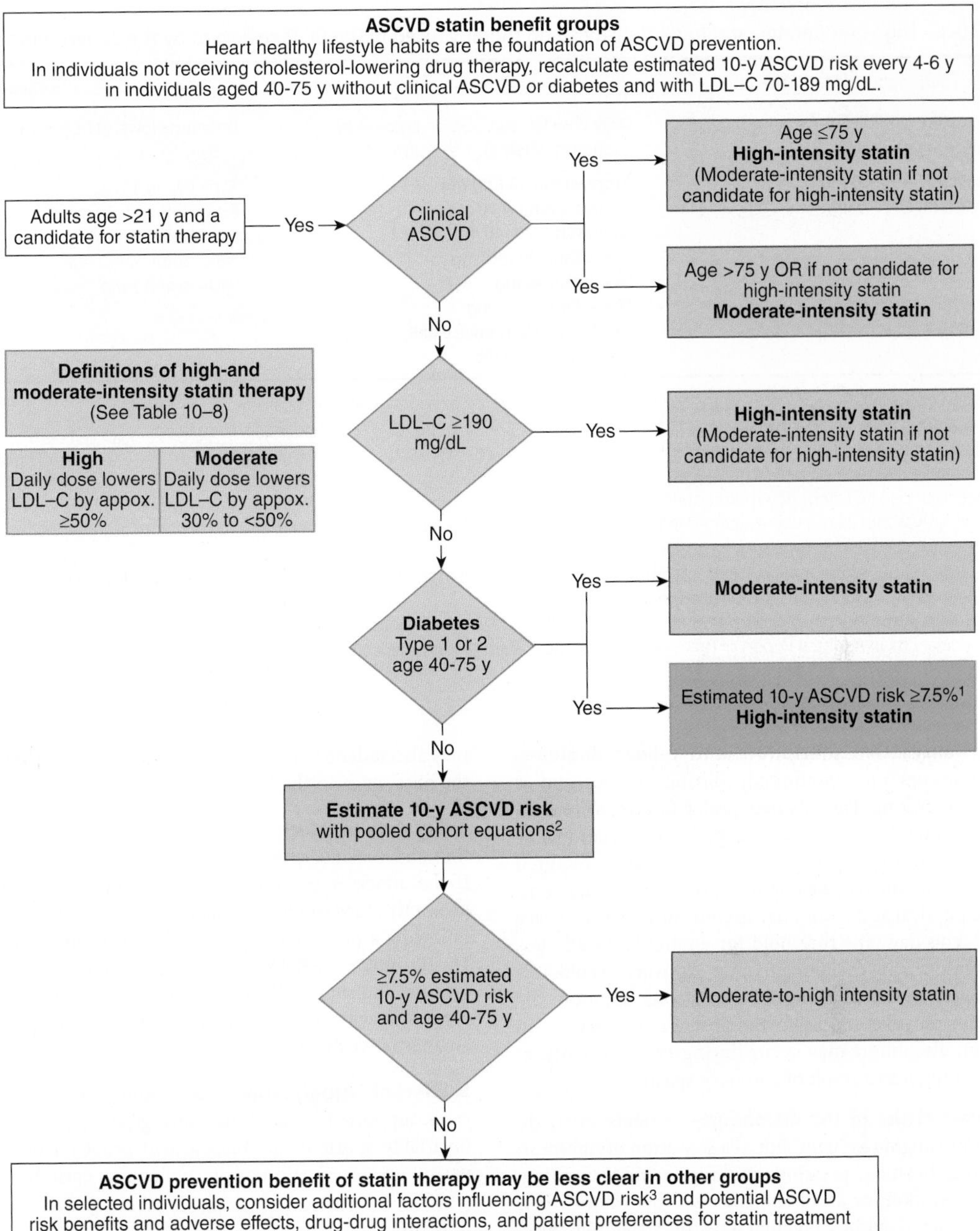

ASCVD statin benefit groups
Heart healthy lifestyle habits are the foundation of ASCVD prevention.
In individuals not receiving cholesterol-lowering drug therapy, recalculate estimated 10-y ASCVD risk every 4-6 y in individuals aged 40-75 y without clinical ASCVD or diabetes and with LDL–C 70-189 mg/dL.

Adults age >21 y and a candidate for statin therapy

Clinical ASCVD

Age ≤75 y
High-intensity statin
(Moderate-intensity statin if not candidate for high-intensity statin)

Age >75 y OR if not candidate for high-intensity statin
Moderate-intensity statin

Definitions of high- and moderate-intensity statin therapy
(See Table 10–8)

High	Moderate
Daily dose lowers LDL–C by appox. ≥50%	Daily dose lowers LDL–C by appox. 30% to <50%

LDL–C ≥190 mg/dL

High-intensity statin
(Moderate-intensity statin if not candidate for high-intensity statin)

Diabetes
Type 1 or 2
age 40-75 y

Moderate-intensity statin

Estimated 10-y ASCVD risk ≥7.5%[1]
High-intensity statin

Estimate 10-y ASCVD risk
with pooled cohort equations[2]

≥7.5% estimated 10-y ASCVD risk and age 40-75 y

Moderate-to-high intensity statin

ASCVD prevention benefit of statin therapy may be less clear in other groups
In selected individuals, consider additional factors influencing ASCVD risk[3] and potential ASCVD risk benefits and adverse effects, drug-drug interactions, and patient preferences for statin treatment

[1]Percent reduction in LDL–C can be used as an indication of response and adherence to therapy, but is not in itself a treatment goal.

[2]The Pooled Cohort Equations can be used to estimate 10-year ASCVD risk in individuals with and without diabetes. A downloadable spreadsheet enabling estimation of 10-year and lifetime risk for ASCVD and a web-based calculator are available at http://my.americanheart.org/cvriskcalculator and http://www.cardiosource.org/science-and-quality/practice-guidelines-and-quality-standards/2013-prevention-guideline-tools.aspx.

[3]Primary LDL–C ≥160 mg/dL or other evidence of genetic hyperlipidemias, family history of premature ASCVD with onset <55 years of age in a first degree male relative or <65 years of age in a first degree female relative, high-sensitivity C-reactive protein >2 mg/L, CAC score ≥300 Agatston units or ≥75 percentile for age, sex, and ethnicity, ankle-brachial index <0.9, or elevated lifetime risk of ASCVD.

ASCVD, atherosclerotic cardiovascular disease; CAC, coronary artery calcium; LDL–C, low-density lipoprotein cholesterol.

▲ **Figure 10–6.** Major recommendation for statin therapy for ASCVD prevention. (Reproduced, with permission, from Stone NJ et al. 2013 ACC/AHA Guideline on the Treatment of Blood Cholesterol to Reduce Atherosclerotic Cardiovascular Risk in Adults: A Report of the American College of Cardiology/American Heart Association Task Force on Practice Guidelines. Circulation. 2013 Nov 12. [Epub ahead of print])

Table 10–8. High-, moderate-, and low-intensity statin therapy (used in the RCTs reviewed by the expert panel).[1,2]

High-Intensity Statin Therapy	Moderate-Intensity Statin Therapy	Low-Intensity Statin Therapy
Daily dose lowers LDL-C on average by approximately ≥ 50%	Daily dose lowers LDL-C on average by approximately 30% to < 50%	Daily dose lowers LDL-C on average by < 30%
Atorvastatin (40[3])–80 mg Rosuvastatin 20 *(40)* mg	Atorvastatin 10 *(20)* mg Rosuvastatin *(5)* 10 mg Simvastatin 20–40 mg[4] Pravastatin 40 *(80)* mg Lovastatin 40 mg *Fluvastatin XL 80 mg* **Fluvastatin 40 mg twice daily** **Pitavastatin 2–4 mg**	*Simvastatin 10 mg* *Pravastatin 10–20 mg* *Lovastatin 20 mg* *Fluvastatin 20–40 mg* *Pitavastatin 1 mg*

[1]Statins and doses in boldface were evaluated in RCTs; all demonstrated a reduction in major cardiovascular events. Statins and doses that are approved by the US FDA but were not tested in the RCTs reviewed are listed in italics.

[2]Individual responses to statin therapy varied in the RCTs and should be expected to vary in clinical practice. There might be a biologic basis for a less-than-average response.

[3]Evidence from one RCT only: down-titration if unable to tolerate atorvastatin 80 mg in IDEAL.

[4]Although simvastatin 80 mg was evaluated in RCTs, initiation of simvastatin 80 mg or titration to 80 mg is not recommended by the FDA due to the increased risk of myopathy, including rhabdomyolysis.

FDA, Food and Drug Administration; IDEAL, Incremental Decrease through Aggressive Lipid Lowering study; LDL–C, low-density lipoprotein cholesterol; and RCTs, randomized controlled trials.

Modified, with permission, from Stone NJ et al. 2013 ACC/AHA Guideline on the Treatment of Blood Cholesterol to Reduce Atherosclerotic Cardiovascular Risk in Adults: A Report of the American College of Cardiology/American Heart Association Task Force on Practice Guidelines. Circulation. 2013 Nov 12. [Epub ahead of print]

Circumstances that precipitate and relieve angina— Angina occurs most commonly during activity and is relieved by resting. Patients may prefer to remain upright rather than lie down, as increased preload in recumbency increases myocardial work. The amount of activity required to produce angina may be relatively consistent under comparable physical and emotional circumstances or may vary from day to day. The threshold for angina is usually less after meals, during excitement, or on exposure to cold. It is often lower in the morning or after strong emotion; the latter can provoke attacks in the absence of exertion. In addition, discomfort may occur during sexual activity, at rest, or at night as a result of coronary spasm.

2. Characteristics of the discomfort—Patients often do not refer to angina as "pain" but as a sensation of tightness, squeezing, burning, pressing, choking, aching, bursting, "gas," indigestion, or an ill-characterized discomfort. It is often characterized by clenching a fist over the mid chest. The distress of angina is rarely sharply localized and is not spasmodic.

3. Location and radiation—The distribution of the distress may vary widely in different patients but is usually the same for each patient unless unstable angina or myocardial infarction supervenes. In most cases, the discomfort is felt behind or slightly to the left of the mid sternum. When it begins farther to the left or, uncommonly, on the right, it characteristically moves centrally substernally. Although angina may radiate to any dermatome from C8 to T4, it radiates most often to the left shoulder and upper arm, frequently moving down the inner volar aspect of the arm to the elbow, forearm, wrist, or fourth and fifth fingers. It

may also radiate to the right shoulder or arm, the lower jaw, the neck, or even the back.

4. Duration of attacks—Angina is generally of short duration and subsides completely without residual discomfort. If the attack is precipitated by exertion and the patient promptly stops to rest, it usually lasts < 3 minutes. Attacks following a heavy meal or brought on by anger often last 15–20 minutes. Attacks lasting more than 30 minutes are unusual and suggest the development of an acute coronary syndrome with unstable angina, myocardial infarction, or an alternative diagnosis.

5. Effect of nitroglycerin—The diagnosis of angina pectoris is supported if sublingual nitroglycerin promptly and invariably shortens an attack and if prophylactic nitrates permit greater exertion or prevent angina entirely.

B. Signs

Examination during angina frequently reveals a significant elevation in systolic and diastolic BP, although hypotension may also occur, and may reflect more severe ischemia or inferior ischemia (especially with bradycardia) due to a Bezold–Jarisch reflex. Occasionally, a gallop rhythm and an apical systolic murmur due to transient mitral regurgitation from papillary muscle dysfunction are present during pain only. Supraventricular or ventricular arrhythmias may be present, either as the precipitating factor or as a result of ischemia.

It is important to detect signs of diseases that may contribute to or accompany atherosclerotic heart disease, eg, diabetes mellitus (retinopathy or neuropathy), xanthelasma tendinous xanthomas,, hypertension, thyrotoxicosis, myxedema, or peripheral artery disease. Aortic stenosis or regurgitation, hypertrophic cardiomyopathy, and mitral valve prolapse should be sought, since they may produce angina or other forms of chest pain.

C. Laboratory Findings

Other than standard laboratory tests to evaluate for acute coronary syndrome (troponin and CK-MB), factors contributing to ischemia (such as anemia), and to screen for risk factors that may increase the probability of true coronary heart disease (such as hyperlipidemia and diabetes mellitus), blood tests are not helpful to diagnose chronic angina.

D. ECG

The resting ECG is often normal in patients with angina. In the remainder, abnormalities include old myocardial infarction, nonspecific ST–T changes, and changes of LVH. During anginal episodes, as well as during asymptomatic ischemia, the characteristic ECG change is horizontal or downsloping ST-segment depression that reverses after the ischemia disappears. T wave flattening or inversion may also occur. Less frequently, transient ST-segment elevation is observed; this finding suggests severe (transmural) ischemia from coronary occlusion, and it can occur with coronary spasm.

E. Pretest Probability

The history as detailed above, the physical examination findings, and laboratory and ECG findings are used to develop a pretest probability of CAD as the cause of the clinical symptoms. Other important factors to include in calculating the pretest probability of CAD are patient age, sex, and clinical symptoms. Patients with low to intermediate pretest probability for CAD should undergo noninvasive stress testing whereas patients with high pretest probability are generally referred for cardiac catheterization.

F. Exercise ECG

Exercise testing is the most commonly used noninvasive procedure for evaluating for inducible ischemia in the patient with angina. Exercise testing is often combined with imaging studies (nuclear, echocardiography, or MRI [see below]), but in low-risk patients without baseline ST segment abnormalities or in whom anatomic localization is not necessary, the exercise ECG remains the recommended initial procedure because of considerations of cost and convenience.

Exercise testing can be done on a motorized treadmill or with a bicycle ergometer. A variety of exercise protocols are utilized, the most common being the Bruce protocol, which increases the treadmill speed and elevation every 3 minutes until limited by symptoms. At least two ECG leads should be monitored continuously.

1. Precautions and risks—The risk of exercise testing is about one infarction or death per 1000 tests, but individuals who have pain at rest or minimal activity are at higher risk and should not be tested. Many of the traditional exclusions, such as recent myocardial infarction or heart failure, are no longer used *if the patient is stable and ambulatory*, but symptomatic aortic stenosis remains a contraindication.

2. Indications—Exercise testing is used (1) to confirm the diagnosis of angina; (2) to determine the severity of limitation of activity due to angina; (3) to assess prognosis in patients with known coronary disease, including those recovering from myocardial infarction, by detecting groups at high or low risk; and (4) to evaluate responses to therapy. Because false-positive tests often exceed true positives, leading to much patient anxiety and self-imposed or mandated disability, exercise testing of asymptomatic individuals should be done only for those whose occupations place them or others at special risk (eg, airline pilots), and older individuals commencing strenuous activity.

3. Interpretation—The usual ECG criterion for a positive test is 1 mm (0.1 mV) horizontal or downsloping ST-segment depression (beyond baseline) measured 80 milliseconds after the J point. By this criterion, 60–80% of patients with anatomically significant coronary disease will have a positive test, but 10–30% of those without significant disease will also be positive. False positives are uncommon when a 2-mm depression is present. Additional information is inferred from the time of onset and duration of the ECG changes, their magnitude and configuration, BP and heart rate changes, the duration of exercise, and the presence of associated symptoms. In general, patients exhibiting more severe ST-segment depression (> 2 mm) at low workloads (< 6 minutes on the Bruce protocol) or heart rates (< 70% of age-predicted maximum)—especially when the duration of exercise and rise in BP are limited or when hypotension occurs during the test—have more severe disease and a poorer prognosis. Depending on symptom status, age, and other factors, such patients should be referred for coronary arteriography and possible revascularization. On the other hand, less impressive positive tests in asymptomatic patients are often "false positives." Therefore, exercise testing results that do not conform to the clinical picture should be confirmed by stress imaging.

G. Myocardial Stress Imaging

Myocardial stress imaging (scintigraphy, echocardiography, or MRI) is indicated (1) when the resting ECG makes an exercise ECG difficult to interpret (eg, left bundle branch block, baseline ST–T changes, low voltage); (2) for confirmation of the results of the exercise ECG when they are contrary to the clinical impression (eg, a positive test in an asymptomatic patient); (3) to localize the region of ischemia; (4) to distinguish ischemic from infarcted myocardium; (5) to assess the completeness of revascularization following bypass surgery or coronary angioplasty; or (6) as a prognostic indicator in patients with known coronary disease. Published criteria summarize these indications for stress testing.

1. Myocardial perfusion scintigraphy—This test, also known as radionuclide imaging, provides images in which radionuclide uptake is proportionate to blood flow at the time of injection.

Stress imaging is positive in about 75–90% of patients with anatomically significant coronary disease and in 20–30% of those without it. Occasionally, other conditions, including infiltrative diseases (sarcoidosis, amyloidosis), left bundle branch block, and dilated cardiomyopathy, may produce resting or persistent perfusion defects. False-positive radionuclide tests may occur as a result of diaphragmatic attenuation or, in women, attenuation through breast tissue. Tomographic imaging (single-photon emission computed tomography, SPECT) can reduce the severity of artifacts.

2. Radionuclide angiography—This procedure, also known as Multi Gated Acquisition Scan, or MUGA scan, uses radionuclide tracers to image the LV and measures its EF and wall motion. In coronary disease, resting abnormalities usually represent infarction, and those that occur only with exercise usually indicate stress-induced ischemia. Exercise radionuclide angiography has approximately the same sensitivity as myocardial perfusion scintigraphy, but it is less specific in older individuals and those with other forms of heart disease. In addition, because of the precision around LVEF, the test is also used for monitoring patients exposed to cardiotoxic therapies (such as chemotherapeutic agents).

3. Stress echocardiography—Echocardiograms performed during supine exercise or immediately following upright exercise may demonstrate exercise-induced segmental wall motion abnormalities as an indicator of ischemia. In experienced laboratories, the test accuracy is comparable to that obtained with scintigraphy—though a higher proportion of tests is technically inadequate. While exercise is the preferred stress because of other information derived, pharmacologic stress with high-dose dobutamine (20–40 mcg/kg/min) can be used as an alternative to exercise.

H. Other Imaging

1. Positron emission tomography—PET and SPECT scanning can accurately distinguish transiently dysfunctional ("stunned") myocardium from scar tissue.

2. CT and MRI scanning—CT scanning can image the heart and, with contrast medium and multislice technology, the coronary arteries. Multislice CT angiography may be useful in evaluating patients with low likelihood of significant CAD to rule out disease. CT angiography may also be useful for evaluating chest pain and suspected acute coronary syndrome. However, the role of CT angiography in routine practice is yet to be established, since it currently requires both radiation exposure and contrast load. Radionuclide SPECT imaging also has similar radiation exposure. CT angiography with noninvasive functional assessment of coronary stenosis (Fractional flow reserve) termed "CT-FFR" is also being evaluated in patients with low-intermediate likelihood of CAD.

Electron beam CT (EBCT) can quantify coronary artery calcification, which is highly correlated with atheromatous plaque and has high sensitivity, but low specificity, for obstructive coronary disease. Thus, although this test can stratify patients into lower and higher risk groups, the appropriate management of individual patients with asymptomatic coronary artery calcification—beyond aggressive risk factors modification—is unclear. This test has not traditionally been used in symptomatic patients. According to the American Heart Association, persons who are at low risk (< 10% 10-year risk) or at high risk (>20% 10-year risk) do not benefit from coronary calcium assessment (class III, level of evidence: B) (see Tables 28–1 and 28–2). However, in clinically selected, intermediate-risk patients, it may be reasonable to determine the atherosclerosis burden using EBCT in order to refine clinical risk prediction and to select patients for more aggressive target values for lipid-lowering therapies (class IIb, level of evidence: B).

Cardiac MRI using gadolinium provides high-resolution images of the heart and great vessels without radiation exposure or use of iodinated contrast media. Gadolinium has been associated with a rare but fatal complication in patients with severe kidney disease, called necrotizing systemic fibrosis. Gadolinium can demonstrate perfusion using dobutamine or adenosine to produce pharmacologic stress. Advances have been made in imaging the proximal coronary arteries, but this application remains investigational.

I. Ambulatory ECG Monitoring

Ambulatory ECG recorders can monitor for ischemic ST-segment depression but this modality is rarely used for ischemia detection.

J. Coronary Angiography

Selective coronary arteriography is the definitive diagnostic procedure for CAD. It can be performed with low mortality (about 0.1%) and morbidity (1–5%), but due to the invasive nature and cost, it is currently only recommended in patients with a high pretest probability of CAD.

Coronary arteriography should be performed in the following circumstances if percutaneous transluminal coronary angioplasty or bypass surgery is a consideration:

1. Limiting stable angina despite an adequate medical regimen.

2. Clinical presentation (unstable angina, postinfarction angina, etc) or noninvasive testing suggests high-risk disease (see Indications for Revascularization).

3. Concomitant aortic valve disease and angina pectoris, to determine whether the angina is due to accompanying coronary disease.

4. Asymptomatic older patients undergoing valve surgery so that concomitant bypass may be done if the anatomy is propitious.

5. Recurrence of symptoms after coronary revascularization to determine whether bypass grafts or native vessels are occluded.

6. Cardiac failure where a surgically correctable lesion, such as LV aneurysm, mitral regurgitation, or reversible ischemic dysfunction, is suspected.

7. Survivors of sudden death or symptomatic or life-threatening arrhythmias when CAD may be a correctable cause.

8. Chest pain of uncertain cause or cardiomyopathy of unknown cause.

9. Emergently performed cardiac catheterization with intention to perform primary PCI in patients with suspected acute myocardial infarction.

Appropriate use criteria for the use of diagnostic heart catheterization and coronary angiography were developed by the ACC/AHA in 2012.

A narrowing > 50% of the luminal diameter is considered hemodynamically (and clinically) significant, although most lesions producing ischemia are associated with narrowing in excess of 70%. In those with strongly positive exercise ECGs or scintigraphic studies, three-vessel or left main disease may be present in 75–95% depending on the criteria used. **Intravascular ultrasound** (IVUS) is useful when the angiogram is equivocal as well as for assessing the results of angioplasty or stenting. In addition, IVUS is the invasive diagnostic method of choice for ostial left main lesions and coronary dissections. In fractional flow reserve (FFR), a pressure wire is used to measure the relative change in pressure across a coronary lesion after the administration of adenosine. Revascularization based on abnormal FFR improves clinical outcomes compared to revascularization of all angiographically stenotic lesions. FFR is an important invasive tool to aid with ischemia driven revascularization and has become the standard tool to evaluate borderline lesions in cases in which the clinical team is evaluating the clinical and hemodynamic significance of a coronary stenosis.

LV angiography is usually performed at the same time as coronary arteriography. Global and regional LV function are visualized, as well as mitral regurgitation if present. LV function is a major determinant of prognosis in coronary heart disease.

▶ Differential Diagnosis

When atypical features are present—such as prolonged duration (hours or days) or darting, knifelike pains at the apex or over the precordium—ischemia is less likely.

Anterior chest wall syndrome is characterized by sharply localized tenderness of intercostal muscles. Inflammation of the chondrocostal junctions may result in diffuse chest pain that is also reproduced by local pressure (Tietze syndrome). Intercostal neuritis (due to herpes zoster, diabetes mellitus, for example) also mimics angina.

Cervical or thoracic spine disease involving the dorsal roots produces sudden sharp, severe chest pain suggesting angina in location and "radiation" but related to specific movements of the neck or spine, recumbency, and straining or lifting. Pain due to cervical or thoracic disk disease involves the outer or dorsal aspect of the arm and the thumb and index fingers rather than the ring and little fingers.

Reflux esophagitis, peptic ulcer, chronic cholecystitis, esophageal spasm, and functional gastrointestinal disease may produce pain suggestive of angina pectoris. The picture may be especially confusing because ischemic pain may also be associated with upper gastrointestinal symptoms, and esophageal motility disorders may be improved by nitrates and calcium channel blockers. Assessment of esophageal motility may be helpful.

Degenerative and inflammatory lesions of the left shoulder and thoracic outlet syndromes may cause chest pain due to nerve irritation or muscular compression; the symptoms are usually precipitated by movement of the arm and shoulder and are associated with paresthesias.

Pneumonia, pulmonary embolism, and spontaneous pneumothorax may cause chest pain as well as dyspnea. Dissection of the thoracic aorta can cause severe chest pain that is commonly felt in the back; it is sudden in onset, reaches maximum intensity immediately, and may be associated with changes in pulses. Other cardiac disorders such as mitral valve prolapse, hypertrophic cardiomyopathy, myocarditis, pericarditis, aortic valve disease, or RVH may cause atypical chest pain or even myocardial ischemia.

▶ Treatment

Sublingual nitroglycerin is the drug of choice for acute management; it acts in about 1–2 minutes. As soon as the attack begins, one fresh tablet is placed under the tongue. This may be repeated at 3- to 5-minute intervals, but current recommendations are that if pain is not relieved or improving after 5 minutes, that the patient call 9-1-1; pain not responding to three tablets or lasting more than 20 minutes may represent evolving infarction. The dosage (0.3, 0.4, or 0.6 mg) and the number of tablets to be used before seeking further medical attention must be individualized. Nitroglycerin buccal spray is also available as a metered (0.4 mg) delivery system. It has the advantage of being more convenient for patients who have difficulty handling the pills and of being more stable.

▶ Prevention of Further Attacks

A. Aggravating Factors

Angina may be aggravated by hypertension, LV failure, arrhythmia (usually tachycardias), strenuous activity, cold temperatures, and emotional states. These factors should be identified and treated when possible.

B. Nitroglycerin

Nitroglycerin, 0.3–0.6 mg sublingually or 0.4–0.8 mg translingually by spray, should be taken 5 minutes before any activity likely to precipitate angina. Sublingual isosorbide dinitrate (2.5–10 mg) is only slightly longer-acting than sublingual nitroglycerin.

C. Long-Acting Nitrates

Longer-acting nitrate preparations include isosorbide dinitrate, 10–40 mg orally three times daily; isosorbide mononitrate, 10–40 mg orally twice daily or 60–120 mg once daily in a sustained-release preparation; oral sustained-release nitroglycerin preparations, 6.25–12.5 mg two to four times daily; nitroglycerin ointment, 6.25–25 mg applied two to four times daily; and transdermal nitroglycerin patches that deliver nitroglycerin at a predetermined rate (usually 5–20 mg/24 h). The main limitation to long-term nitrate therapy is tolerance, which can be limited by using a regimen that includes a minimum 8- to 10-hour period per day without nitrates. Isosorbide dinitrate can be given three times daily, with the last dose after dinner, or longer-acting isosorbide mononitrate once daily. Transdermal nitrate preparations should be removed overnight in most patients.

Nitrate therapy is often limited by headache. Other side effects include nausea, light-headedness, and hypotension.

D. Beta-Blockers

Beta-blockers are the only antianginal agents that have been demonstrated to prolong life in patients with coronary disease (post-myocardial infarction). Beta-blockers should be considered for first-line therapy in most patients with chronic angina and are recommened as such by the Stable Ischemic Heart disease guidelines (Figure 10–7).

Beta-blockers with intrinsic sympathomimetic activity, such as pindolol, are less desirable because they may exacerbate angina in some individuals and have not been effective in secondary prevention trials. The pharmacology and side effects of the beta-blockers are discussed in Chapter 11 (see Table 11–6). The dosages of all these drugs when given for angina are similar. The major contraindications are severe bronchospastic disease, bradyarrhythmias, and decompensated heart failure.

E. Ranolazine

Ranolazine is indicated as first-line use for chronic angina. Ranolazine has no effect on heart rate and BP, and it has been shown in clinical trials to prolong exercise duration and time to angina, both as monotherapy and when administered with conventional antianginal therapy. It is safe to use with erectile dysfunction drugs. The usual dose is 500 mg orally twice a day. Because it can cause QT prolongation, it is contraindicated in patients with existing QT prolongation; in patients taking QT prolonging drugs, such as class I or III antiarrhythmics (eg, quinidine, dofetilide, sotalol); and in those taking potent and moderate CYP450 3A inhibitors (eg, clarithromycin and rifampin). Of interest, in spite of the QT prolongation, there is a significantly lower rate of ventricular arrhythmias with its use following acute coronary syndromes, as shown in the MERLIN trial. It also decreases occurrence of atrial fibrillation and results in a small decrease in HbA_{1c}. It is contraindicated in patients with significant liver and kidney disease. Ranolazine is not to be used for treatment of acute anginal episodes.

F. Calcium Channel Blocking Agents

Unlike the beta-blockers, calcium channel blockers have not been shown to reduce mortality postinfarction and in some cases have increased ischemia and mortality rates. This appears to be the case with some dihydropyridines (eg, nifedipine) and with diltiazem and verapamil in patients with clinical heart failure or moderate to severe LV dysfunction. Meta-analyses have suggested that short-acting nifedipine in moderate to high doses causes an increase in mortality. It is uncertain whether these findings are relevant to longer-acting dihydropyridines. Nevertheless, considering the uncertainties and the lack of demonstrated favorable effect on outcomes, calcium channel blockers should be considered third-line anti-ischemic drugs in the postinfarction patient. Similarly, these agents, with the exception of amlodipine (which proved safe in patients with heart failure in the PRAISE-2 trial), should be avoided in patients with heart failure or low EFs.

The pharmacologic effects and side effects of the calcium channel blockers are discussed in Chapter 11 and summarized in Table 11–8. Diltiazem, amlodipine, and verapamil are preferable because they produce less reflex tachycardia and because the former, at least, may cause fewer side effects. Nifedipine, nicardipine, and amlodipine are also approved agents for angina. Isradipine, felodipine, and nisoldipine are not approved for angina but probably are as effective as the other dihydropyridines.

G. Alternative and Combination Therapies

Patients who do not respond to one class of antianginal medication often respond to another. It may, therefore, be worthwhile to use an alternative agent before progressing to combinations. The stable ischemic heart disease guidelines recommend starting with a beta-blocker as initial therapy, followed by calcium channel blockers, long-acting nitrates, or ranolazine. A few patients will have further response to a regimen including all four agents.

H. Platelet-Inhibiting Agents

Several studies have demonstrated the benefit of antiplatelet drugs for patients with stable and unstable vascular disease. Therefore, unless contraindicated, aspirin (81–325 mg orally daily) should be prescribed for all patients with angina. Clopidogrel, 75 mg orally daily, reduces vascular events in patients with stable vascular disease (as an alternative to aspirin) and in patients with acute coronary syndromes (in addition to aspirin). Thus, it is also a good alternative in aspirin-intolerant patients. Clopidogrel did not reduce myocardial infarction, stroke, or cardiovascular death in the CHARISMA trial of patients with cardiovascular disease or multiple risk factors, with about a 50% increase in bleeding. However, it might be reasonable to use combination clopidogrel and aspirin for certain high-risk patients with established coronary disease.

I. Risk Reduction

Patients with coronary disease should undergo aggressive risk factor modification. This approach, with a particular focus on statin treatment, treating hypertension, stopping smoking, and exercise and weight control (especially for patients with metabolic syndrome or at risk for diabetes), may markedly improve outcome. For patients with diabetes and cardiovascular disease, there is uncertainty about the optimal target blood sugar control. The ADVANCE trial suggested some benefit for tight blood sugar control with

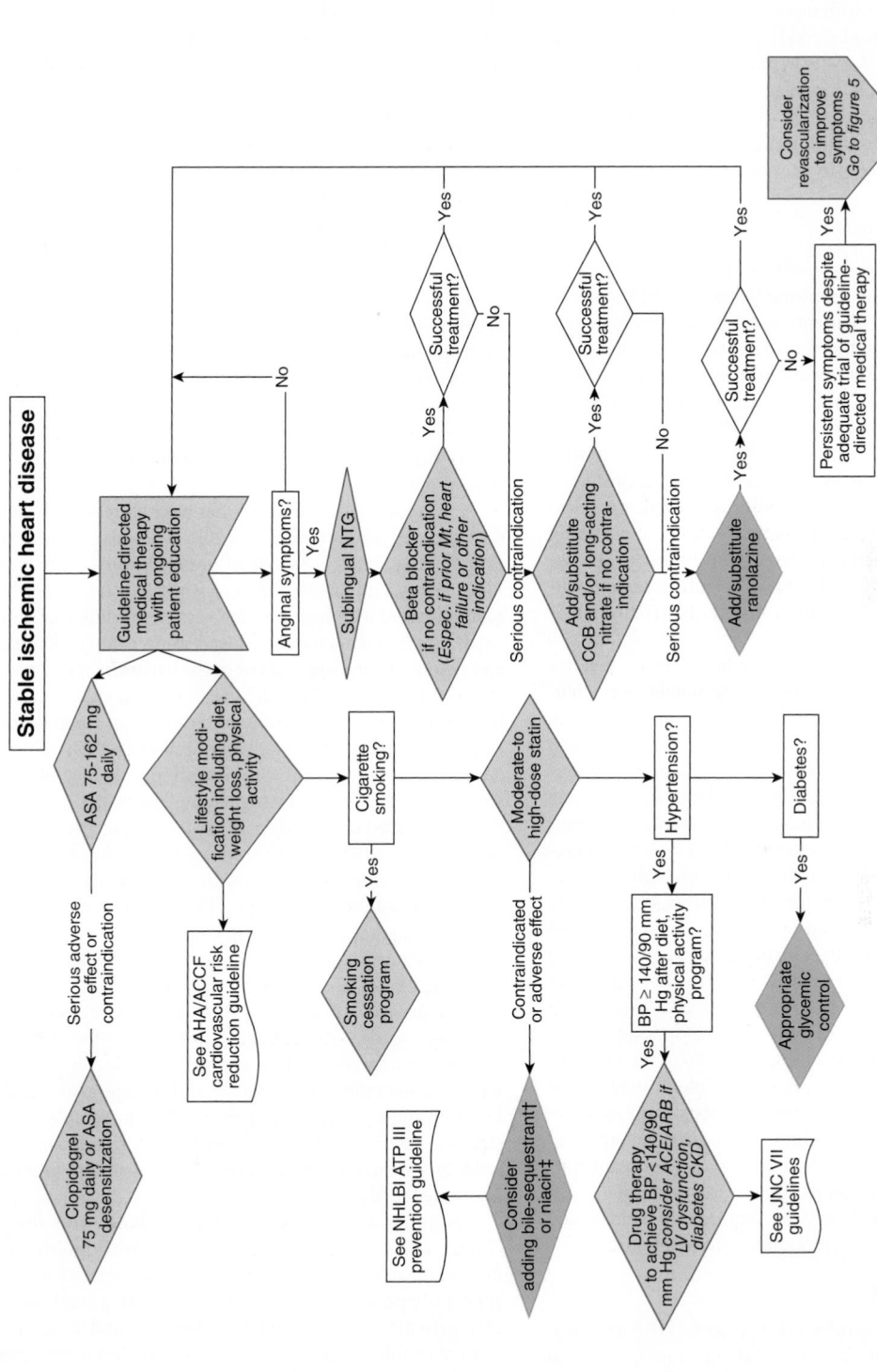

▲ **Figure 10–7.** Algorithm for guideline-directed medical therapy for patients with stable ischemic heart disease. The use of bile acid sequestrant is relatively contraindicated when triglycerides are ≥ 200 mg/dL and contraindicated when triglycerides are ≥ 500 mg/dL. Dietary supplement niacin must not be used as a substitute for prescription niacin. (Reproduced, with permission, from Fihn SD et al; American College of Cardiology Foundation/American Heart Association Task Force. 2012 ACCF/AHA/ACP/AATS/PCNA/SCAI/STS guideline for the diagnosis and management of patients with stable ischemic heart disease. Circulation. 2012 Dec 18;126(25):e354-471.)

target $HbA_{1C} \leq 6.5\%$ but the ACCORD trial found that routine aggressive targeting for blood sugar control to HbA_{1C} to < 6.0% in patients with diabetes and coronary disease was associated with increased mortality. Therefore, tight blood sugar control should be avoided particularly in patients with history of severe hypoglycemia, long-standing diabetes, and advanced vascular disease. Aggressive BP control (target systolic BP < 120 mm Hg) in the ACCORD trial was not associated with reduction in coronary heart disease events, although stroke was reduced.

J. Revascularization

1. Indications—There is general agreement that otherwise healthy patients in the following groups should undergo revascularization: (1) Patients with unacceptable symptoms despite medical therapy to its tolerable limits. (2) Patients with left main coronary artery stenosis > 50% with or without symptoms. (3) Patients with three-vessel disease with LV dysfunction (EF < 50% or previous transmural infarction). (4) Patients with unstable angina who after symptom control by medical therapy continue to exhibit ischemia on exercise testing or monitoring. (5) Post-myocardial infarction patients with continuing angina or severe ischemia on noninvasive testing. The use of revascularization for patients with acute coronary syndromes and acute ST elevation myocardial infarction is discussed below.

Data from the COURAGE trial have shown that for patients with chronic angina and disease suitable for percutaneous coronary intervention (PCI), PCI in addition to stringent guideline-directed medical therapy aimed at both risk reduction and anti-anginal care offers no mortality benefit beyond excellent medical therapy alone, and relatively moderate long-term symptomatic improvement. Also, drug-eluting stents, widely used because of their benefits in preventing restenosis, have been associated with higher rates of late stent thrombosis. Therefore, for patients with mild to moderate CAD and limited symptoms, revascularization may not provide significant functional status quality of life benefit. For patients with moderate to significant coronary stenosis, such as those who have two-vessel disease associated with underlying LV dysfunction, anatomically critical lesions (> 90% proximal stenoses, especially of the proximal left anterior descending artery), or physiologic evidence of severe ischemia (early positive exercise tests, large exercise-induced thallium scintigraphic defects, or frequent episodes of ischemia on ambulatory monitoring), a heart team consisting of revascularization physicians (interventional cardiologists and surgeons) may be required to review and provide patients with best revascularization options.

2. Type of procedure

A. Percutaneous coronary intervention including stenting—PCI, including balloon angioplasty and coronary stenting, can effectively open stenotic coronary arteries. Coronary stenting, with either bare metal stents or drug-eluting stents, has substantially reduced restenosis. Stenting can also be used selectively for left main coronary stenosis, particularly when coronary artery bypass grafting (CABG) is contraindicated.

PCI is possible but often less successful in bypass graft stenoses. Experienced operators are able to successfully dilate > 90% of lesions attempted. The major early complication is intimal dissection with vessel occlusion, although this is rare with coronary stenting. The use of intravenous platelet glycoprotein IIb/IIIa inhibitors (abciximab, eptifibatide, tirofiban) substantially reduce the rate of periprocedural myocardial infarction, and placement of intracoronary stents markedly improve initial and long-term angiographic results, especially with complex and long lesions. After percutaneous coronary intervention, all patients should have CK-MB and troponin measured. The definition of a periprocedural infarction is still under debate with many experts advocating for a clinical definition that incorporates enzymes, angiographic findings, and electrocardiographic evidence. Acute thrombosis after stent placement can largely be prevented by aggressive antithrombotic therapy (long-term aspirin, 81–325 mg, plus clopidogrel, 300–600 mg loading dose followed by 75 mg daily, for between 30 days and 1 year, and with acute use of platelet glycoprotein IIb/IIIa inhibitors).

A major limitation with PCI has been **restenosis,** which occurs in the first 6 months in < 10% of vessels treated with drug-eluting stents, 15–30% of vessels treated with bare metal stents, and 30–40% of vessels without stenting. Factors associated with higher restenosis rates include diabetes, small luminal diameter, longer and more complex lesions, and lesions at coronary ostia or in the left anterior descending coronary artery. Drug-eluting stents that elute antiproliferative agents such as sirolimus, everolimus, zotarolimus, or paclitaxel have substantially reduced restenosis. In-stent restenosis is often treated with restenting with drug-eluting stents, and rarely with brachytherapy. The nearly 2 million PCIs performed worldwide per year far exceeds the number of CABG operations, but the rationale for many of the procedures performed in patients with stable angina should be for angina symptom reduction. The COURAGE trial has confirmed earlier studies in showing that even for patients with moderate anginal symptoms and positive stress tests PCI provides no benefit over medical therapy with respect to death or myocardial infarction. PCI was more effective at relieving angina, although most patients in the medical group had improvement in symptoms. Thus, in patients with mild or moderate stable symptoms, aggressive lipid-lowering and antianginal therapy may be a preferable initial strategy, reserving PCI for patients with significant and refractory symptoms or for those who are unable to take the prescribed medicines.

Several studies of PCI, including those with drug-eluting stents, versus CABG in patients with multivessel disease have been reported. The SYNTAX trial as well as previously performed trials with drug-eluting stent use in PCI patients show comparable mortality and infarction rates over follow-up periods of 1–3 years but a high rate (approximately 40%) of repeat procedures following PCI. Stroke rates are higher with CABG. As a result, the choice of revascularization procedure may depend on details of coronary anatomy and is often a matter of patient preference. However, it should be noted that < 20% of patients with multivessel disease meet the entry criteria for the clinical trials, so these results cannot be generalized to all multivessel disease patients. Outcomes with percutaneous revascularization in diabetics have generally been inferior to those with CABG. The FREEDOM trial demonstrated that CABG surgery was superior to PCI with regards to death, myocardial infarction, and stroke for patients with diabetes and multivessel coronary disease at 5 years across all subgroups of SYNTAX score anatomy.

B. CORONARY ARTERY BYPASS GRAFTING—CABG can be accomplished with a very low mortality rate (1–3%) in otherwise healthy patients with preserved cardiac function. However, the mortality rate of this procedure rises to 4–8% in older individuals and in patients who have had a prior CABG.

Grafts using one or both internal mammary arteries (usually to the left anterior descending artery or its branches) provide the best long-term results in terms of patency and flow. Segments of the saphenous vein (or, less optimally, other veins) or the radial artery interposed between the aorta and the coronary arteries distal to the obstructions are also used. One to five distal anastomoses are commonly performed.

Minimally invasive surgical techniques may involve a limited sternotomy, lateral thoracotomy (MIDCAB), or thoracoscopy (port-access). They are more technically demanding, usually not suitable for more than two grafts, and do not have established durability. Bypass surgery can be performed both on circulatory support (on pump) and without direct circulatory support (off-pump). Randomized trial data have not shown a benefit with off-pump bypass surgery but minimally invasive surgical techniques allow earlier postoperative mobilization and discharge.

The operative mortality rate is increased in patients with poor LV function (LVEF < 35%) or those requiring additional procedures (valve replacement or ventricular aneurysmectomy). Patients over 70 years of age, patients undergoing repeat procedures, or those with important noncardiac disease (especially chronic kidney disease and diabetes) or poor general health also have higher operative mortality and morbidity rates, and full recovery is slow. Thus, CABG should be reserved for more severely symptomatic patients in this group. Early (1–6 months) graft patency rates average 85–90% (higher for internal mammary grafts), and subsequent graft closure rates are about 4% annually. Early graft failure is common in vessels with poor distal flow, while late closure is more frequent in patients who continue smoking and those with untreated hyperlipidemia. Antiplatelet therapy with aspirin improves graft patency rates. Smoking cessation and vigorous treatment of blood lipid abnormalities (particularly with statins) are necessary. Repeat revascularization (see below) may be necessitated because of recurrent symptoms due to progressive native vessel disease and graft occlusions. Reoperation is technically demanding and less often fully successful than the initial operation.

K. Mechanical Extracorporeal Counterpulsation

Extracorporeal counterpulsation entails repetitive inflation of a high-pressure chamber surrounding the lower half of the body during the diastolic phase of the cardiac cycle for daily 1-hour sessions over a period of 7 weeks. Randomized trials have shown that extracorporeal counterpulsation reduces angina thus it may be considered for relief of refractory angina in patients with stable coronary disease.

L. Neuromodulation

Spinal cord stimulation can be used to relieve chronic refractory angina. Spinal cord stimulators are subcutaneously implantable via a minimally invasive procedure under local anesthesia.

▶ Prognosis

The prognosis of angina pectoris has improved with development of therapies aimed at secondary prevention. Mortality rates vary depending on the number of vessels diseased, the severity of obstruction, the status of LV function, and the presence of complex arrhythmias. Mortality rates are progressively higher in patients with one-, two-, and three-vessel disease and those with left main coronary artery obstruction (ranging from 1% per year to 25% per year). The outlook in individual patients is unpredictable, and nearly half of the deaths are sudden. Therefore, risk stratification is attempted. Patients with accelerating symptoms have a poorer outlook. Among stable patients, those whose exercise tolerance is severely limited by ischemia (< 6 minutes on the Bruce treadmill protocol) and those with extensive ischemia by exercise ECG or scintigraphy have more severe anatomic disease and a poorer prognosis. The Duke Treadmill Score, based on a standard Bruce protocol exercise treadmill test, provides an estimate of risk of death at 1 year. The score uses time on the treadmill, amount of ST-segment depression, and presence of angina (Table 10–9).

▶ When to Refer

All patients with new or worsening symptoms believed to represent progressive angina or a positive stress test for myocardial ischemia with continued angina despite medical therapy (or both) should be referred to a cardiologist.

Table 10–9. Duke treadmill score: Calculation and interpretation.

Time in minutes on Bruce protocol	= _____
−5 × amount of depression (in mm)	= _____

−4 × angina index
    0 = no angina on test
    1 = angina, not limiting
    2 = limiting angina
	= _____

Total Score	Risk Group	Annual Mortality
≥ 5	Low	0.25%
−10 to +4	Intermediate	1.25%
≤ −11	High	5.25%

When to Admit

- Patients with elevated cardiac biomarkers, ischemic ECG findings, or hemodynamic instability.

- Patients with new or worsened symptoms possibly thought to be ischemic but who lack high-risk features can be observed with serial ECGs and biomarkers, and discharged if stress testing shows low-risk findings.

Boden WE et al; COURAGE Trial Research Group. Optimal medical therapy with or without PCI for stable coronary disease. N Engl J Med. 2007 Apr 12;356(15):1503–16. [PMID: 17387127]

Cassar A et al. Chronic coronary artery disease: diagnosis and management. Mayo Clin Proc. 2009 Dec;84(12):1130–46. [PMID: 19955250]

Fihn SD et al. 2012 ACCF/AHA/ACP/AATS/PCNA/SCAI/STS Guideline for the Diagnosis and Management of Patients With Stable Ischemic Heart Disease: a report of the American College of Cardiology Foundation/American Heart Association task force on practice guidelines, and the American College of Physicians, American Association for Thoracic Surgery, Preventive Cardiovascular Nurses Association, Society for Cardiovascular Angiography and Interventions, and Society of Thoracic Surgeons. Circulation. 2012 Dec 18;126(25):e354–471. [PMID: 23166211]

Grines CL et al. Prevention of premature discontinuation of dual antiplatelet therapy in patients with coronary artery stents: a science advisory from the American Heart Association, American College of Cardiology, Society for Cardiovascular Angiography and Interventions, American College of Surgeons, and American Dental Association, with representation from the American College of Physicians. Circulation. 2007 Feb 13;115(6):813–8. [PMID: 17224480]

Levine GN et al. 2011 ACCF/AHA/SCAI Guideline for Percutaneous Coronary Intervention: a report of the American College of Cardiology Foundation/American Heart Association Task Force on Practice Guidelines and the Society for Cardiovascular Angiography and Interventions. Circulation. 2011 Dec 6;124(23):e574–651. [PMID: 22064601]

Min JK et al. Diagnostic accuracy of fractional flow reserve from anatomic CT angiography. JAMA. 2012 Sep 26;308(12):1237–45. [PMID: 22922562]

Moussa ID et al. Consideration of a new definition of clinically relevant myocardial infarction after coronary revascularization: an expert consensus document from the Society for Cardiovascular Angiography and Interventions (SCAI). J Am Coll Cardiol. 2013 Oct 22;62(17):1563–70. [PMID: 24135581]

Patel MR et al. ACCF/SCAI/STS/AATS/AHA/ASNC 2009 Appropriateness Criteria for Coronary Revascularization: a report by the American College of Cardiology Foundation Appropriateness Criteria Task Force, Society for Cardiovascular Angiography and Interventions, Society of Thoracic Surgeons, American Association for Thoracic Surgery, American Heart Association, and the American Society of Nuclear Cardiology Endorsed by the American Society of Echocardiography, the Heart Failure Society of America, and the Society of Cardiovascular Computed Tomography. J Am Coll Cardiol. 2009 Feb 10;53(6):530–53. [PMID: 19195618]

Patel MR et al. ACCF/SCAI/AATS/AHA/ASE/ASNC/HFSA/HRS/SCCM/SCCT/SCMR/STS 2012 appropriate use criteria for diagnostic catheterization: a report of the American College of Cardiology Foundation Appropriate Use Criteria Task Force, Society for Cardiovascular Angiography and Interventions, American Association for Thoracic Surgery, American Heart Association, American Society of Echocardiography, American Society of Nuclear Cardiology, Heart Failure Society of America, Heart Rhythm Society, Society of Critical Care Medicine, Society of Cardiovascular Computed Tomography, Society for Cardiovascular Magnetic Resonance, and Society of Thoracic Surgeons. J Am Coll Cardiol. 2012 May 29;59(22):1995–2027. [PMID: 22578925]

Patel MR et al. Low diagnostic yield of elective coronary angiography. N Engl J Med. 2010 Mar 11;362(10):886–95. [PMID: 20220183]

Skyler JS et al. Intensive glycemic control and the prevention of cardiovascular events: implications of the ACCORD, ADVANCE, and VA Diabetes Trials: a position statement of the American Diabetes Association and a Scientific Statement of the American College of Cardiology Foundation and the American Heart Association. J Am Coll Cardiol. 2009 Jan 20;53(3):298–304. [PMID: 19147051]

Torpy JM et al. JAMA patient page. Cardiac stress testing. JAMA. 2008 Oct 15;300(15):1836. [PMID: 18854548]

CORONARY VASOSPASM & ANGINA WITH NORMAL CORONARY ARTERIOGRAMS

 ESSENTIALS OF DIAGNOSIS

▶ Precordial chest pain, often occurring at rest during stress or without known precipitant, relieved rapidly by nitrates.

▶ ECG evidence of ischemia during pain, sometime with ST-segment elevation.

▶ Angiographic demonstration of:

– No significant obstruction of major coronary vessels.

– Coronary spasm that responds to intra-coronary nitroglycerin or calcium channel blockers.

General Considerations

Although most symptoms of myocardial ischemia result from fixed stenosis of the coronary arteries or intraplaque hemorrhage or thrombosis at the site of lesions, some ischemic events may be precipitated or exacerbated by coronary vasoconstriction.

Spasm of the large coronary arteries with resulting decreased coronary blood flow may occur spontaneously or may be induced by exposure to cold, emotional stress, or vasoconstricting medications, such as ergot derivative drugs. Spasm may occur both in normal and in stenosed coronary arteries. Even myocardial infarction may occur as a result of spasm in the absence of visible obstructive coronary heart disease, although most instances of such coronary spasm occur in the presence of coronary stenosis.

Cocaine can induce myocardial ischemia and infarction by causing coronary artery vasoconstriction or by increasing myocardial energy requirements. It also may contribute to accelerated atherosclerosis and thrombosis. The ischemia in **Prinzmetal (variant) angina** usually results from coronary vasoconstriction. It tends to involve the right coronary artery and there may be no fixed stenoses. Myocardial ischemia may also occur in patients with normal coronary arteries as a result of disease of the coronary microcirculation or abnormal vascular reactivity. This has been termed "syndrome X."

Clinical Findings

Ischemia may be silent or result in angina pectoris.

Prinzmetal (variant) angina is a clinical syndrome in which chest pain occurs without the usual precipitating factors and is associated with ST-segment elevation rather than depression. It often affects women under 50 years of age. It characteristically occurs in the early morning, awakening patients from sleep, and is apt to be associated with arrhythmias or conduction defects. It may be diagnosed by challenge with ergonovine (a vasoconstrictor), although the results of such provocation are not specific and it entails risk.

Treatment

Patients with chest pain associated with ST-segment elevation should undergo coronary arteriography to determine whether fixed stenotic lesions are present. If they are, aggressive medical therapy or revascularization is indicated, since this may represent an unstable phase of the disease. If significant lesions are not seen and spasm is suspected, avoidance of precipitants such as cigarette smoking and cocaine is the top priority. Episodes of coronary spasm generally respond well to nitrates, and both nitrates and calcium channel blockers (including long-acting nifedipine, diltiazem, or amlodipine, [see Table 11–8]) are effective prophylactically. By allowing unopposed alpha-1-mediated vasoconstriction, beta-blockers have exacerbated coronary vasospasm, but they may have a role in management of patients in whom spasm is associated with fixed stenoses.

When to Refer

All patients with persistent symptoms of chest pain that may represent spasm should be referred to a cardiologist.

Agarwal M et al. Nonacute coronary syndrome anginal chest pain. Med Clin North Am. 2010 Mar;94(2):201–16. [PMID: 20380951]

ACUTE CORONARY SYNDROMES WITHOUT ST-SEGMENT ELEVATION

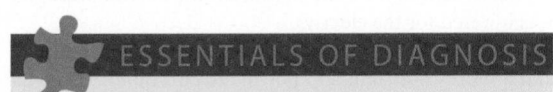

ESSENTIALS OF DIAGNOSIS

► Distinction in acute coronary syndrome between patients with and without ST-segment elevation at presentation is essential to determine need for reperfusion therapy.

► Fibrinolytic therapy is harmful in acute coronary syndrome without ST-segment elevation, unlike with ST-segment elevation where acute reperfusion saves lives.

► Antiplatelet and anticoagulation therapies and coronary intervention are mainstays of treatment.

General Considerations

Acute coronary syndromes comprise the spectrum of unstable cardiac ischemia from unstable angina to acute myocardial infarction. Acute coronary syndromes are classified based on the presenting ECG as either "ST-segment elevation" (STEMI) or "non–ST-segment elevation" (NSTEMI). This allows for immediate classification and guides determination of whether patients should be considered for acute reperfusion therapy. The evolution of cardiac biomarkers then allows determination of whether myocardial infarction has occurred.

Acute coronary syndromes represent a dynamic state in which patients frequently shift from one category to another, as new ST elevation can develop after presentation and cardiac biomarkers can become abnormal with recurrent ischemic episodes.

Clinical Findings

A. Symptoms and Signs

Patients with acute coronary syndromes generally have symptoms and signs of myocardial ischemia either at rest or with minimal exertion. These symptoms and signs are similar to chronic angina symptoms described above, consisting of substernal chest pain or discomfort that may radiate to the jaw, left shoulder or arm. Dyspnea, nausea, diaphoresis, or syncope may either accompany the chest discomfort or may be the only symptom of acute coronary syndrome. About one-third of patients with myocardial infarction have no chest pain per se—these patients tend to be older, female, have diabetes, and be at higher risk for subsequent mortality. Patients with acute coronary syndromes have signs of heart failure in about 10% of cases, and this is also associated with higher risk of death.

Many hospitals have developed **chest pain observation units** to provide a systematic approach toward serial risk stratification to improve the triage process. In many cases, those who have not experienced new chest pain and have insignificant ECG changes and no cardiac biomarker elevation undergo treadmill exercise tests or imaging procedures to exclude ischemia at the end of an 8- to 24-hour period and are discharged directly from the emergency department if these tests are negative.

B. Laboratory Findings

Depending on the time from symptom onset to presentation, initial laboratory findings may be normal. The markers of cardiac myocyte necrosis, myoglobin, CK-MB, and troponin I and T may all be used to identify acute myocardial infarction. These markers have a well-described pattern of release over time in patients with myocardial infarction (see Laboratory Findings, Acute Myocardial Infarction with ST-Segment Elevation, below). In patients with STEMI, these initial markers are often within normal limits as the patient is being rushed to immediate reperfusion. In patients without ST-segment elevation, it is the presence of abnormal CK-MB or troponin values that are associated with myocyte necrosis and the diagnosis of myocardial infarction. **The universal definition of myocardial infarction** is a rise of cardiac biomarkers with at least one value above the 99th percentile of the upper reference limit together with evidence of myocardial ischemia with at least one of the following: symptoms of ischemia, ECG changes of new ischemia, new Q waves, or imaging evidence of new loss of viable myocardium or new wall motion abnormality.

Serum creatinine is an important determinant of risk, and estimated creatinine clearance is important to guide dosing of certain antithrombotics, including eptifibatide and enoxaparin.

C. ECG

Many patients with acute coronary syndromes will exhibit ECG changes during pain—either ST-segment elevation, ST-segment depression, or T wave flattening or inversion. Dynamic ST segment shift is the most specific for acute coronary syndrome. ST segment elevation in lead aVR suggests left main or three vessel disease.

► Treatment

A. General Measures

Treatment of acute coronary syndromes without ST elevation should be multifaceted. Patients who are at medium or high risk should be hospitalized, maintained at bed rest or at very limited activity for the first 24 hours, monitored, and given supplemental oxygen. Sedation with a benzodiazepine agent may help if anxiety is present.

B. Specific Measures

Figure 10–8 provides an algorithm for initial management of non-ST segment myocardial infarction.

C. Antiplatelet and Anticoagulation Therapy

Patients should receive a combination of antiplatelet and anticoagulant agents on presentation. *Fibrinolytic therapy should be avoided in patients without ST-segment elevation since they generally do not have an acute coronary occlusion, and the risk of such therapy appears to outweigh the benefit.*

1. Antiplatelet therapy

A. ASPIRIN—Aspirin, 81–325 mg daily, should be commenced immediately and continued for the first month. The 2012 ACC/AHA guidelines for longer-term aspirin treatment recommend aspirin 75–162 mg/d as preferable to higher doses with or without coronary stenting.

B. P_2Y_{12} INHIBITORS—ACC/AHA guidelines call for either a P_2Y_{12} inhibitor (clopidogrel, prasugrel [at the time

of PCI], or ticagrelor) or a glycoprotein IIb/IIIa inhibitor "up-front" (prior to coronary angiography) as a class I recommendation. The European Society of Cardiology guidelines provide a stronger recommendation for a P_2Y_{12} inhibitor up-front, as a class IA recommendation for all patients. Both sets of guidelines recommend postponing elective CABG surgery for at least 5 days after the last dose of clopidogrel or ticagrelor and at least 7 days after the last dose of prasugrel due to risk of bleeding.

The **Clopidogrel** in Unstable Angina to Prevent Recurrent Events (CURE) trial demonstrated a 20% reduction in the composite end point of cardiovascular death, myocardial infarction, and stroke with the addition of clopidogrel (300 mg loading dose, 75 mg/d for 9–12 months) to aspirin in patients with non–ST-segment elevation acute coronary syndromes. The large CURRENT trial showed that "double-dose" clopidogrel (600 mg initial oral loading dose, followed by 150 mg orally daily) for 7 days reduced stent thrombosis with a modest increase in major (but not fatal) bleeding and, therefore, it is an option for patients with acute coronary syndrome undergoing PCI.

The European Society of Cardiology guidelines recommend ticagrelor for all patients at moderate to high risk for acute coronary syndrome (class 1 recommendation). Prasugrel is recommended for patients who have not yet received another P_2Y_{12} inhibitor, for whom a PCI is planned, and who are not at high risk for life-threatening bleeding. Clopidogrel is reserved for patients who cannot receive either ticagrelor or prasugrel. Some studies have shown an association between assays of residual platelet function and thrombotic risk during P_2Y_{12} inhibitor therapy, and both the European and the US guidelines recommend only selective use of platelet function testing to guide therapy (class IIb recommendation).

Prasugrel is both more potent and has a faster onset of action than clopidogrel. The TRITON trial compared prasugrel with clopidogrel in patients with STEMI or NSTEMI in whom PCI was planned; prasugrel resulted in a 19% relative reduction in death from cardiovascular causes, myocardial infarction, or stroke, at the expense of an increase in serious bleeding (including fatal bleeding). Stent thrombosis was reduced by half. Because patients with prior stroke or transient ischemic attack had higher risk of intracranial hemorrhage, prasugrel is contraindicated in such patients. Bleeding was also higher in patients with low body weight (< 60 kg) and older age (≥ 75 years), and caution should be used in these populations. For patients with STEMI treated with PCI, prasugrel appears to be especially effective without a substantial increase in bleeding. For patients who will not receive revascularization, prasugrel, when compared to clopidogrel, had no overall benefit in the TRILOGY trial (the dose of prasugrel was lowered for the elderly).

Ticagrelor has a faster onset of action than clopidogrel and a more consistent and potent effect. The PLATO trial showed that when ticagrelor was started at the time of presentation in acute coronary syndrome patients (UA/NSTEMI and STEMI), it reduced cardiovascular death, myocardial infarction, and stroke by 16% when compared with clopidogrel. In addition, there was a 22% relative risk

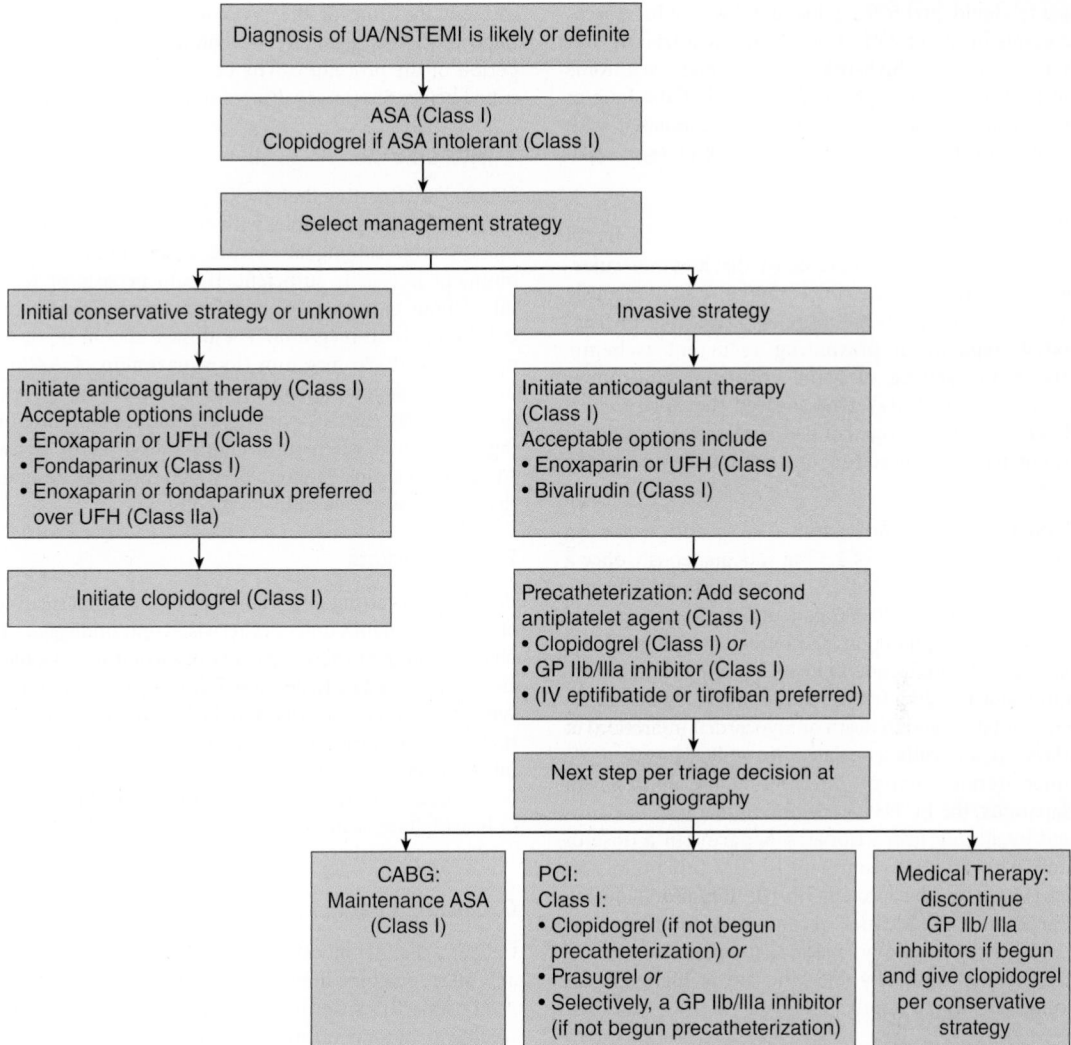

▲ **Figure 10–8.** Flowchart for class 1 and class II a recommendations for initial management of unstable angina/ non– ST-segment elevation myocardial infarction (UA/NS TEMI). ASA, aspirin; CABG, coronary artery bypass grafting; GP IIb/IIIa, glycoprotein IIb/IIIa; LOE, level of evidence; UFH, unfractionated heparin. (Reproduced, with permission, from Wright RS et al. 2011 ACCF/AHA Focused Update of the Guidelines for the Management of Patients With Unstable Angina/ Non-ST-Elevation Myocardial Infarction (Updating the 2007 Guideline): a report of the American College of Cardiology Foundation/American Heart Association Task Force on Practice Guidelines. Circulation. 2011 May 10;123(18):2022–60. Erratum in: Circulation. 2011 Sep 20;124(12):e337–40; Circulation. 2011 Jun 7;123(22):e625–6. [PMID: 21444889])

reduction in mortality with ticagrelor. The overall rates of bleeding were similar between ticagrelor and clopidogrel, although non-CABG related bleeding was modestly higher. The finding of a lesser treatment effect in the United States may have been related to use of higher-dose aspirin, and thus when using ticagrelor, low-dose aspirin (81 mg/d) is recommended.

C. GLYCOPROTEIN IIB/IIIA INHIBITORS—Small molecule inhibitors of the platelet glycoprotein IIb/IIIa receptor are useful adjuncts in high-risk patients (usually defined by fluctuating ST-segment depression or positive biomarkers)

with acute coronary syndromes, particularly when they are undergoing PCI. **Tirofiban,** 0.4 mcg/kg/min for 30 minutes followed by 0.1 mcg/kg/min, and **eptifibatide,** 180 mcg/kg bolus followed by a continuous infusion of 2 mcg/kg/min, have both been shown to be effective. Downward dose adjustments (1 mcg/kg/min) are required in patients with reduced kidney function. For example, if the estimated creatinine clearance is below 50 mL/min, the eptifibatide infusion should be cut in half to 1 mcg/kg/min. The ISAR-REACT 2 trial showed that for patients undergoing PCI with high-risk acute coronary syndrome, especially with elevated troponin, intravenous **abciximab** (added to clopidogrel 600 mg loading dose) reduces ischemic events by about 25%. The EARLY-ACS trial in over 10,000 patients with high-risk acute coronary syndrome found no benefit from eptifibatide started at the time of admission and higher rates of bleeding compared with eptifibatide treatment started at the time of invasive coronary angiography.

2. Anticoagulant therapy

A. Heparin—Several trials have shown that **low-molecular-weight heparin** (enoxaparin 1 mg/kg subcutaneously every 12 hours) is somewhat more effective than **unfractionated heparin** in preventing recurrent ischemic events in the setting of acute coronary syndromes. However, the SYNERGY trial showed that unfractionated heparin and enoxaparin had similar rates of death or (re)infarction in the setting of frequent early coronary intervention.

B. Fondaparinux—Fondaparinux, a specific factor Xa inhibitor given in a dose of 2.5 mg subcutaneously once a day, was found in the OASIS-5 trial to be equally effective as enoxaparin among 20,000 patients at preventing early death, myocardial infarction, and refractory ischemia, and resulted in a 50% reduction in major bleeding. This reduction in major bleeding translated into a significant reduction in mortality (and in death or myocardial infarction) at 30 days. While catheter-related thrombosis was more common during coronary intervention procedures with fondaparinux, the FUTURA trial found that it can be controlled by adding unfractionated heparin (in a dose of 85 units/kg without glycoprotein IIb/IIIa inhibitors, and 60 units/kg with glycoprotein IIb/IIIa inhibitors) during the procedure. Guidelines recommend fondaparinux, describing it as especially favorable for patients who are initially treated medically and who are at high risk for bleeding, such as the elderly.

C. Direct thrombin inhibitors—The ACUITY trial showed that **bivalirudin** appears to be a reasonable alternative to heparin (unfractionated heparin or enoxaparin) plus a glycoprotein IIb/IIIa antagonist for many patients with acute coronary syndromes who are undergoing early coronary intervention. Bivalirudin (without routine glycoprotein IIb/IIIa inhibitor) is associated with substantially less bleeding than heparin plus glycoprotein IIb/IIIa inhibitor. The ISAR REACT-4 trial showed that bivalirudin has similar efficacy compared to abciximab but better bleeding outcomes in NSTEMI patients.

D. Temporary Discontinuation of Antiplatelet Therapy for Procedures

Patients who have had recent coronary stents are at risk for thrombotic events, including **stent thrombosis,** if $P2Y_{12}$ inhibitors are discontinued for procedures (eg, dental procedures or colonoscopy). If possible, these procedures should be delayed until the end of the necessary treatment period with $P2Y_{12}$ inhibitors, which generally is at least 1 month with bare metal stents and 3–6 months with drug-eluting stents. Before that time, if a procedure is necessary, risk and benefit of continuing the antiplatelet therapy

through the time of the procedure should be assessed. Aspirin should generally be continued throughout the period of the procedure. The cardiologist should be consulted before temporary discontinuation of these agents.

E. Nitroglycerin

Nitrates are first-line therapy for patients with acute coronary syndromes presenting with chest pain. Nonparenteral therapy with sublingual or oral agents or nitroglycerin ointment is usually sufficient. If pain persists or recurs, intravenous nitroglycerin should be started. The usual initial dosage is 10 mcg/min. The dosage should be titrated upward by 10–20 mcg/min (to a maximum of 200 mcg/min) until angina disappears or mean arterial pressure drops by 10%. Careful—usually continuous—BP monitoring is required when intravenous nitroglycerin is used. Avoid hypotension (systolic BP < 100 mm Hg). Tolerance to continuous nitrate infusion is common.

F. Beta-Blockers

Beta-blockers are an important part of the initial treatment of unstable angina unless otherwise contraindicated. The pharmacology of these agents is discussed in Chapter 11 and summarized in Table 11–6. Use of agents with intrinsic sympathomimetic activity should be avoided in this setting. Oral medication is adequate in most patients, but intravenous treatment with metoprolol, given as three 5-mg doses 5 minutes apart as tolerated and in the absence of heart failure, achieves a more rapid effect. Oral therapy should be titrated upward as BP permits.

G. Calcium Channel Blockers

Calcium channel blockers have not been shown to favorably affect outcome in unstable angina, and they should be used primarily as third-line therapy in patients with continuing symptoms on nitrates and beta-blockers or those who are not candidates for these drugs. In the presence of nitrates and without accompanying beta-blockers, diltiazem or verapamil is preferred, since nifedipine and the other dihydropyridines are more likely to cause reflex tachycardia or hypotension. The initial dosage should be low, but upward titration should proceed steadily (see Table 11–8).

H. Statins

The PROVE-IT trial provides evidence for starting a statin in the days immediately following an acute coronary syndrome. In this trial, more intensive therapy with atorvastatin 80 mg/d, regardless of total or LDL cholesterol level, improved outcome compared to pravastatin 40 mg/d, with the curves of death or major cardiovascular event separating as early as 3 months after starting therapy. High-dose statins are recommended for all patients with acute coronary syndromes (Table 10–8).

▶ **Indications for Coronary Angiography**

For patients with acute coronary syndrome, including non–ST-segment elevation myocardial infarction, risk stratification is important for determining intensity of care. Several therapies, including glycoprotein IIb/IIIa inhibitors, low-molecular-weight heparin, and early invasive catheterization, have been shown to have the greatest benefit in higher-risk patients with acute coronary syndrome. As outlined in the ACC/AHA guidelines, patients with any high-risk feature (Table 10–10) generally warrant an early invasive strategy with catheterization and revascularization. For patients without these high-risk features, either an invasive or noninvasive approach, using exercise (or pharmacologic stress for patients unable to exercise) stress testing to identify patients who have residual ischemia and/or high risk, can be used. Moreover, based on the ICTUS trial, a strategy based on selective coronary angiography and revascularization for instability or inducible ischemia, or both, even for patients with positive troponin, is acceptable (ACC/AHA class IIb recommendation).

Two risk-stratification tools are available that can be used at the bedside, the GRACE Risk Score (http://www.out-comes-umassmed.org/grace) and the TIMI Risk Score (available for PDA download at http://www.timi.org). The GRACE risk score, which applies to patients with or without ST elevation, was developed in a more generalizable registry population and includes Killip class, BP, ST-segment deviation, cardiac arrest at presentation, serum creatinine, elevated creatine kinase (CK)-MB or troponin, and heart rate. The TIMI Risk Score includes seven variables: age $\geq$ 65, three or more cardiac risk factors, prior coronary stenosis $\geq$ 50%, ST-segment deviation, two anginal events in prior 24 hours, aspirin in prior 7 days, and elevated cardiac markers.

▶ **When to Refer**

- All patients with acute myocardial infarction should be referred to a cardiologist.
- Patients who are taking a $P2Y_{12}$ inhibitor following coronary stenting should consult a cardiologist before discontinuing treatment for nonemergency procedures.

Gurbel PA et al. Platelet function during extended prasugrel and clopidogrel therapy for patients with ACS treated without revascularization: the TRILOGY ACS Platelet Function Substudy. JAMA. 2012 Nov 7;308(17):1785–94. [PMID: 23124119]

Hamm CW et al. ESC Guidelines for the management of acute coronary syndromes in patients presenting without persistent ST-segment elevation: The Task Force for the management of acute coronary syndromes (ACS) in patients presenting without persistent ST-segment elevation of the European Society of Cardiology (ESC). Eur Heart J. 2011 Dec;32(23):2999–3054. [PMID: 21873419]

Jneid H et al. 2012 ACCF/AHA focused update of the guideline for the management of patients with unstable angina/non–ST-elevation myocardial infarction (updating the 2007 guideline and replacing the 2011 focused update): a report of the American College of Cardiology Foundation/American Heart Association Task Force on Practice Guidelines. Circulation. 2012 Aug 14;126(7):875–910. [PMID: 22800849]

Levine GN et al. 2011 ACCF/AHA/SCAI Guideline for Percutaneous Coronary Intervention: a report of the American College of Cardiology Foundation/American Heart Association Task Force on Practice Guidelines and the Society for Cardiovascular Angiography and Interventions. Circulation. 2011 Dec 6;124(23):e574–651. [PMID: 22064601]

Table 10–10. Indications for catheterization and percutaneous coronary intervention.[1]

Acute coronary syndromes (unstable angina and non-ST elevation MI)	
Class I	Early invasive strategy for any of the following high-risk indicators:
	Recurrent angina/ischemia at rest or with low-level activity
	Elevated troponin
	ST-segment depression
	Recurrent ischemia with evidence of HF
	High-risk stress test result
	EF < 40%
	Hemodynamic instability
	Sustained ventricular tachycardia
	PCI within 6 months
	Prior CABG
	In the absence of these findings, either an early conservative or early invasive strategy
Class IIa	Early invasive strategy for patients with repeated presentations for ACS despite therapy
Class III	Extensive comorbidities in patients in whom benefits of revascularization are not likely to outweigh the risks
	Acute chest pain with low likelihood of ACS
Acute MI after fibrinolytic therapy (2013 ACCF/AHA guidelines)	
Class I	Cardiogenic shock or acute severe heart failure that develops after initial presentation
	Intermediate or high-risk findings on predischarge noninvasive ischemia testing
	Spontaneous or easily provoked myocardial ischemia
Class IIa	Failed reperfusion or reocclusion after fibrinolytic therapy
Class IIa	Stable[2] patients after successful fibrinolysis, before discharge and ideally between 3 and 24 hours

[1]Class I indicates treatment is useful and effective, IIa indicates weight of evidence is in favor of usefulness/efficacy, class IIb indicates weight of evidence is less well established, and class III indicates intervention is not useful/effective and may be harmful. Level of evidence A recommendations are derived from large-scale randomized trials, and B recommendations are derived from smaller randomized trials or carefully conducted observational analyses.

[2]Although individual circumstances will vary, clinical stability is defined by the absence of low output, hypotension, persistent tachycardia, apparent shock, high-grade ventricular or symptomatic supraventricular tachyarrhythmias, and spontaneous recurrent ischemia.

ACCF/AHA, American College of Cardiology Foundation/American Heart Association; ACS, acute coronary syndrome; AMI, acute myocardial infarction; CABG, coronary artery bypass grafting; HF, heart failure; EF, ejection fraction; LVEF, left ventricular ejection fraction; MI, myocardial infarction; PCI, percutaneous coronary intervention.

Source: O'Gara PT et al. 2013 ACCF/AHA guideline for the management of ST-elevation myocardial infarction: a report of the American College of Cardiology Foundation/American Heart Association Task Force on Practice Guidelines. Circulation. 2013;127.

Thygesen K et al. Third universal definition of myocardial infarction. Circulation. 2012 Oct 16;126(16):2020–35. [PMID: 22923432]

Wallentin L et al; PLATO Investigators. Ticagrelor versus clopidogrel in patients with acute coronary syndromes. N Engl J Med. 2009 Sep 10;361(11):1045–57. [PMID: 19717846]

ACUTE MYOCARDIAL INFARCTION WITH ST-SEGMENT ELEVATION

ESSENTIALS OF DIAGNOSIS

► Sudden but not instantaneous development of prolonged (> 30 minutes) anterior chest discomfort (sometimes felt as "gas" or pressure).

► Sometimes painless, masquerading as acute heart failure, syncope, stroke, or shock.

► ECG: ST-segment elevation or left bundle branch block.

► Immediate reperfusion treatment is warranted.

► Primary PCI within 90 minutes of first medical contact is the goal and is superior to fibrinolytic therapy.

► Fibrinolytic therapy within 30 minutes of hospital presentation is the goal, and if given within 12 hours of onset of symptoms reduces mortality.

► General Considerations

STEMI results, in most cases, from an occlusive coronary thrombus at the site of a preexisting (though not necessarily severe) atherosclerotic plaque. More rarely, infarction may result from prolonged vasospasm, inadequate myocardial blood flow (eg, hypotension), or excessive metabolic demand. Very rarely, myocardial infarction may be caused by embolic occlusion, vasculitis, aortic root or coronary artery dissection, or aortitis. Cocaine is a cause of infarction, which should be considered in young individuals without risk factors. A condition that may mimic STEMI is stress cardiomyopathy (also referred to as Tako-Tsubo or apical ballooning syndrome) (see below).

ST elevation connotes an acute coronary occlusion and thus warrants immediate reperfusion therapy.

► Clinical Findings

A. Symptoms

1. Premonitory pain—There is usually a worsening in the pattern of angina preceding the onset of symptoms of myocardial infarction; classically the onset of angina occurs with minimal exertion or at rest.

2. Pain of infarction—Unlike anginal episodes, most infarctions occur at rest, and more commonly in the early morning. The pain is similar to angina in location and radiation but it may be more severe, and it builds up rapidly or in waves to maximum intensity over a few minutes or longer. Nitroglycerin has little effect; even opioids may not relieve the pain.

3. Associated symptoms—Patients may break out in a cold sweat, feel weak and apprehensive, and move about, seeking a position of comfort. They prefer not to lie quietly. Light-headedness, syncope, dyspnea, orthopnea, cough, wheezing, nausea and vomiting, or abdominal bloating may be present singly or in any combination.

4. Painless infarction—One-third of patients with acute myocardial infarction present without chest pain, and these patients tend to be undertreated and have poor outcomes. Older patients, women, and patients with diabetes mellitus are more likely to present without classic chest pain. As many as 25% of infarctions are detected on routine ECG without any recallable acute episode.

5. Sudden death and early arrhythmias—Of all deaths from myocardial infarction, about 50% occur before the patients arrive at the hospital, with death presumably caused by ventricular fibrillation.

B. Signs

1. General—Patients may appear anxious and sometimes are sweating profusely. The heart rate may range from marked bradycardia (most commonly in inferior infarction) to tachycardia, low cardiac output, or arrhythmia. The BP may be high, especially in former hypertensive patients, or low in patients with shock. Respiratory distress usually indicates heart failure. Fever, usually low grade, may appear after 12 hours and persist for several days.

2. Chest—The **Killip classification** is the standard way to classify heart failure in patients with acute myocardial infarction and has powerful prognostic value. Killip class I is absence of rales and S_3, class II is rales that do not clear with coughing over one-third or less of the lung fields or presence of an S_3, class III is rales that do not clear with coughing over more than one-third of the lung fields, and class IV is cardiogenic shock (rales, hypotension, and signs of hypoperfusion).

3. Heart—The cardiac examination may be unimpressive or very abnormal. Jugular venous distention reflects RA hypertension, and a Kussmaul sign (failure of decrease of jugular venous pressure with inspiration) is suggestive of RV infarction. Soft heart sounds may indicate LV dysfunction. Atrial gallops (S_4) are the rule, whereas ventricular gallops (S_3) are less common and indicate significant LV dysfunction. Mitral regurgitation murmurs are not uncommon and may indicate papillary muscle dysfunction or, rarely, rupture. Pericardial friction rubs are uncommon in the first 24 hours but may appear later.

4. Extremities—Edema is usually not present. Cyanosis and cold temperature indicate low output. The peripheral pulses should be noted, since later shock or emboli may alter the examination.

C. Laboratory Findings

Cardiac-specific markers of myocardial damage include quantitative determinations of CK-MB, highly sensitive and conventional troponin I, and troponin T. Each of these tests may become positive as early as 4–6 hours after the onset of a myocardial infarction and should be abnormal by 8–12 hours. Troponins are more sensitive and specific than CK-MB. "Highly sensitive" or "fourth-generation" troponin assays, which are not yet approved in the United States but are the standard assays in most of Europe, have a 10- to 100-fold lower limit of detection with high analytic precision, enabling quantification of levels even in most normal individuals and allowing myocardial infarction to be detected earlier, using the change in value over 3 hours.

Circulating levels of troponins may remain elevated for 5–7 days or longer and therefore are generally not useful for evaluating suspected early reinfarction. Elevated CK-MB generally normalizes within 24 hours, thus being more helpful for evaluation of reinfarction. Low level elevations of troponin in patients with severe chronic kidney disease may not be related to acute coronary disease but rather a function of the physiologic washout of the marker. While many conditions including chronic heart failure are associated with elevated levels of the high-sensitivity troponin assays, these assays may be especially useful when negative to exclude myocardial infarction in patients complaining of chest pain.

D. ECG

The extent of the ECG abnormalities, especially the sum of the total amount of ST-segment deviation, is a good indicator of extent of acute infarction and risk of subsequent adverse events. The classic evolution of changes is from peaked ("hyperacute") T waves, to ST-segment elevation, to Q wave development, to T-wave inversion. This may occur over a few hours to several days. The evolution of new Q waves (> 30 milliseconds in duration and 25% of the R wave amplitude) is diagnostic, but Q waves do not occur in 30–50% of acute infarctions (non-Q wave infarctions). Left bundle branch block, especially when new (or not known to be old), in a patient with symptoms of an acute myocardial infarction, is considered to be a "STEMI equivalent"; reperfusion therapy is indicated for the affected patient. Concordant ST elevation (ie, ST elevation in leads with an overall positive QRS complex) with left bundle branch block is a specific finding indicating STEMI.

E. Chest Radiography

The chest radiograph may demonstrate signs of heart failure, but these changes often lag behind the clinical findings. Signs of aortic dissection, including mediastinal widening, should be sought as a possible alternative diagnosis.

F. Echocardiography

Echocardiography provides convenient bedside assessment of LV global and regional function. This can help with the diagnosis and management of infarction; echocardiography has been used successfully to make judgments about admission and management of patients with suspected infarction, including in patients with ST-segment elevation or left bundle branch block of uncertain significance, since normal wall motion makes an infarction unlikely. Doppler echocardiography is generally the most convenient procedure for diagnosing postinfarction mitral regurgitation or VSD.

G. Other Noninvasive Studies

Diagnosis of myocardial infarction and extent of myocardial infarction can be assessed by various imaging studies in addition to echocardiography. **MRI** with gadolinium contrast enhancement is the most sensitive test to detect and quantitate extent of infarction, with the ability to detect as little as 2 g of myocardial infarction. **Technetium-99m pyrophosphate scintigraphy,** when injected at least 18 hours postinfarction, complexes with calcium in necrotic myocardium to provide a "hot spot" image of the infarction. This test is insensitive to small infarctions, and false-positive studies occur, so its use is limited to patients in whom the diagnosis by ECG and enzymes is not possible—principally those who present several days after the event or have intraoperative infarctions. **Scintigraphy with thallium-201** or technetium-based perfusion tracers will demonstrate "cold spots" in regions of diminished perfusion, which usually represent infarction when the radiotracer is administered at rest, but abnormalities do not distinguish recent from old damage. All of these tests may be considered after the patient has had revascularization.

H. Hemodynamic Measurements

These can be helpful in managing the patient with suspected cardiogenic shock. Use of PA catheters, however, has generally not been associated with better outcomes and should be limited to patients with severe hemodynamic compromise for whom the information would be anticipated to change management.

▶ Treatment

A. Aspirin, P2Y$_{12}$ Inhibitors (Prasugrel, Ticagrelor, and Clopidogrel)

All patients with definite or suspected myocardial infarction should receive aspirin at a dose of 162 mg or 325 mg at once regardless of whether fibrinolytic therapy is being considered or the patient has been taking aspirin. Chewable aspirin provides more rapid blood levels. Patients with a definite aspirin allergy should be treated with a P2Y$_{12}$ inhibitor (clopidogrel, prasugrel, or ticagrelor). Clopidogrel at a loading dose of 600 mg orally (or 300 mg) will result in faster onset of action than the standard 75 mg maintenance dose.

P2Y$_{12}$ inhibitors, *in combination with aspirin,* have also been shown to provide important benefits in patients with acute STEMI. Thus, guidelines call for a P2Y$_{12}$ inhibitor to be added to aspirin to all patients with STEMI, regardless of whether or not reperfusion is given, and continued for at least 14 days, and generally for 1 year. The preferred P2Y$_{12}$ inhibitors are prasugrel (60 mg orally on day 1, then 10 mg daily) or ticagrelor (150 mg orally on day 1, then 90 mg twice daily). Both of these drugs demonstrated superior outcomes to clopidogrel in clinical studies of primary PCI. With fibrinolytic therapy, there are no randomized trial data regarding when the early use of prasugrel or ticagrelor and clopidogrel is indicated (at the dose of 300-mg loading dose for patients < 75 years of age and no loading dose for patients > 75 years of age). Prasugrel is contraindicated in patients with history of stroke or who are older than 75 years.

B. Reperfusion Therapy

The current recommendation is to treat patients with STEMI who seek medical attention within 12 hours of the onset of symptoms with reperfusion therapy, either primary PCI or fibrinolytic therapy. Patients without ST-segment elevation (previously labeled "non-Q wave" infarctions) do not benefit, and may derive harm, from thrombolysis.

1. Primary percutaneous coronary intervention—Immediate coronary angiography and primary PCI (including stenting) of the infarct-related artery have been shown to be superior to thrombolysis when done by experienced operators in high-volume centers with rapid time from first medical contact to intervention ("door-to-balloon"). US and European guidelines call for first medical contact or "door-to-balloon" times of ≤ 90 minutes. Several trials have shown that if efficient transfer systems are in place, transfer of patients with acute myocardial infarction from hospitals without primary PCI capability to hospitals with primary PCI capability with first door-to-device times of ≤ 120 minutes can improve outcome compared with fibrinolytic therapy at the presenting hospital, although this requires sophisticated systems to ensure rapid identification, transfer, and expertise in PCI. Because PCI also carries a lower risk of hemorrhagic complications including intracranial hemorrhage, it may be the preferred strategy in many older patients and others with contraindications to fibrinolytic therapy (see Table 10–10 for factors to consider in choosing fibrinolytic therapy or primary PCI).

In general, **stenting** is standard for patients with acute myocardial infarction. Primary PCI stenting is done with bivalirudin or unfractionated heparin with glycoprotein IIb/IIIa inhibitors. Although randomized trials have shown a benefit with regards to fewer repeat interventions for restenosis with use of drug-eluting stents in STEMI patients, bare metal stents are used more commonly since the patient's ability to obtain and comply with P2Y$_{12}$ inhibitor therapy is often not known at the time of PCI. In the subgroup of patients with cardiogenic shock, early catheterization and percutaneous or surgical revascularization are the preferred management and have been shown to reduce mortality.

There was a signal of early (< 24 hours) increased stent thrombosis with bivalirudin in HORIZONS that was also seen in the EUROMAX trial despite prolongation of the bivalirudin infusion.

"Facilitated" PCI, whereby a combination of medications (full- or reduced-dose fibrinolytic agents with or without glycoprotein IIb/IIIa inhibitors) is given followed

by immediate PCI is not recommended. Patients should be treated either with primary PCI or with fibrinolytic agents (and immediate rescue PCI for reperfusion failure), if it can be done promptly as outlined in the ACC/AHA and European guidelines. Timely access to most appropriate reperfusion, including primary PCI, can be expanded with development of regional systems of care, including emergency medical systems and networks of hospitals. Patients treated with fibrinolytic therapy appear to have improved outcomes if transferred for routine coronary angiography and PCI within 24 hours. The American Heart Association has a program called Mission: Lifeline to support development of regional systems of care (see http://www.heart.org/missionlifeline).

2. Fibrinolytic therapy

A. Benefit—Fibrinolytic therapy reduces mortality and limits infarct size in patients with acute myocardial infarction associated with ST-segment elevation (defined as ≥ 0.1 mV in two inferior or lateral leads or two contiguous precordial leads), or with left bundle branch block (not known to be old). The greatest benefit occurs if treatment is initiated within the first 3 hours, when up to a 50% reduction in mortality rate can be achieved. The magnitude of benefit declines rapidly thereafter, but a 10% relative mortality reduction can be achieved up to 12 hours after the onset of chest pain. The survival benefit is greatest in patients with large—usually anterior—infarctions. Primary PCI (including stenting) of the infarct-related artery, however, is superior to thrombolysis when done by experienced operators with rapid time from first medical contact to intervention ("door-to-balloon") (see above).

B. Contraindications—Major bleeding complications occur in 0.5–5% of patients, the most serious of which is intracranial hemorrhage. The major risk factors for intracranial bleeding are older age (≥ 75 years), hypertension at presentation (especially over 180/110 mm Hg), low body weight (< 70 kg), and the use of fibrin-specific fibrinolytic agents (alteplase, reteplase, tenecteplase). Although patients over age 75 years have a much higher mortality rate with acute myocardial infarction and therefore may derive greater benefit, the risk of severe bleeding is also higher, particularly among patients with risk factors for intracranial hemorrhage, such as severe hypertension or recent stroke. Patients presenting more than 12 hours after the onset of chest pain may also derive a small benefit, particularly if pain and ST-segment elevation persist, but rarely does this benefit outweigh the attendant risk.

Contraindications to fibrinolytic therapy include previous hemorrhagic stroke, other strokes or cerebrovascular events within 1 year, known intracranial neoplasm, recent head trauma (including minor trauma), active internal bleeding (excluding menstruation), or suspected aortic dissection. Relative contraindications are BP > 180/110 mm Hg at presentation, other intracerebral pathology not listed above as a contraindication, known bleeding diathesis, trauma (including minor head trauma) within 2–4 weeks, major surgery within 3 weeks, prolonged > 10 minutes) or traumatic cardiopulmonary resuscitation, recent (within 2–4 weeks) internal bleeding, noncompressible vascular punctures, active diabetic retinopathy, pregnancy, active peptic ulcer disease, a history of severe hypertension, current use of anticoagulants (INR > 2.0–3.0), and (for streptokinase) prior allergic reaction or exposure to streptokinase or anistreplase within 2 years.

C. Fibrinolytic agents—The following fibrinolytic agents are available for acute myocardial infarction and are characterized in Table 10–11.

Alteplase (recombinant tissue plasminogen activator; t-PA) results in about a 50% reduction in circulating fibrinogen. In the first GUSTO trial, which compared a 90-minute dosing of t-PA (with unfractionated heparin) with streptokinase, the 30-day mortality rate with t-PA was one absolute percentage point lower (one additional life saved per 100 patients treated), though there was also a small *increase* in the rate of intracranial hemorrhage. An angiographic substudy confirmed a higher 90-minute patency rate and a higher rate of normal (TIMI grade 3) flow in patients.

Reteplase is a recombinant deletion mutant of t-PA that is slightly less fibrin specific. In comparative trials, it appears to have efficacy similar to that of alteplase, but it has a longer duration of action and can be administered as two boluses 30 minutes apart.

Tenecteplase (TNK-t-PA) is a genetically engineered substitution mutant of native t-PA that has reduced plasma clearance, increased fibrin sensitivity, and increased resistance to plasminogen activator inhibitor-1. It can be given as a single weight-adjusted bolus. In a large comparative trial, this agent was equivalent to t-PA with regard to efficacy and resulted in significantly less noncerebral bleeding. In the STREAM trial, as part of pharmacoinvasive therapy with use of clopidogrel, aspirin, and enoxaparin and routine catheterization within 24 hours, the tenecteplase dose was reduced in half for patients ≥ age 75 with an apparent reduction in intracranial hemorrhage. **Streptokinase**, commonly used outside of the United States, is somewhat less effective at opening occluded arteries and less effective at reducing mortality. It is non–fibrin-specific, causes depletion of circulating fibrinogen, and has a tendency to induce hypotension, particularly if infused rapidly. This can be managed by slowing or interrupting the infusion and administering fluids. There is controversy as to whether adjunctive heparin is beneficial in patients given streptokinase, unlike its administration with the more clot-specific agents. Allergic reactions, including anaphylaxis, occur in 1–2% of patients, and this agent should generally not be administered to patients with prior exposure.

(1) Selection of a fibrinolytic agent—In the United States, most patients are treated with alteplase, reteplase, or tenecteplase. The differences in efficacy between them are small compared with the potential benefit of treating a greater proportion of appropriate candidates in a more

Table 10–11. Fibrinolytic therapy for acute myocardial infarction.

	Alteplase; Tissue Plasminogen Activator (t-PA)	Reteplase	Tenecteplase (TNK-t-PA)	Streptokinase
Source	Recombinant DNA	Recombinant DNA	Recombinant DNA	Group C streptococcus
Half-life	5 minutes	15 minutes	20 minutes	20 minutes
Usual dose	100 mg	20 units	40 mg	1.5 million units
Administration	Initial bolus of 15 mg, followed by 50 mg infused over the next 30 minutes and 35 mg over the following 60 minutes	10 units as a bolus over 2 minutes, repeated after 30 minutes	Single weight-adjusted bolus, 0.5 mg/kg	750,000 units over 20 minutes followed by 750,000 units over 40 minutes
Anticoagulation after infusion	Aspirin, 325 mg daily; heparin, 5000 units as bolus, followed by 1000 units per hour infusion, subsequently adjusted to maintain PTT 1.5–2 times control	Aspirin, 325 mg; heparin as with t-PA	Aspirin, 325 mg daily	Aspirin, 325 mg daily; there is no evidence that adjunctive heparin improves outcome following streptokinase
Clot selectivity	High	High	High	Low
Fibrinogenolysis	+	+	+	+++
Bleeding	+	+	+	+
Hypotension	+	+	+	+++
Allergic reactions	0	0	+	++
Reocclusion	10–30%	—	5–20%	5–20%
Approximate cost[1]	$6712.54	$5211.86	$4194.30	Not available in the United States

[1]Average wholesale price (AWP, for AB-rated generic when available) for quantity listed.
Source: *Red Book Online, 2013, Truven Health Analytics, Inc.* AWP may not accurately represent the actual pharmacy cost because wide contractual variations exist among institutions.
PTT, partial thromboplastin time.

prompt manner. The principal objective should be to administer a thrombolytic agent within 30 minutes of presentation—or even during transport. The ability to administer tenecteplase as a single bolus is an attractive feature that may facilitate earlier treatment. The combination of a reduced-dose thrombolytic given with a platelet glycoprotein IIb/IIIa inhibitor does not reduce mortality but does cause a modest increase in bleeding complications.

(2) Postfibrinolytic management—After completion of the fibrinolytic infusion, aspirin (81–325 mg/d) and anticoagulation should be continued until revascularization or for the duration of the hospital stay (or up to 8 days) with some anticoagulant, with advantages favoring either enoxaparin or fondaparinux.

(A) LOW-MOLECULAR-WEIGHT HEPARIN—In the EXTRACT trial, enoxaparin significantly reduced death and myocardial infarction at day 30 (compared with unfractionated heparin), at the expense of a modest increase in bleeding. In patients younger than age 75, enoxaparin was given as a 30-mg intravenous bolus and 1 mg/kg every 12 hours; in patients age 75 years and older, it was given with no bolus and 0.75 mg/kg intravenously every 12 hours. This appeared to attenuate the risk of intracranial hemorrhage in the elderly that had been seen with full-dose enoxaparin. Another antithrombotic option is fondaparinux, given at a dose of 2.5 mg subcutaneously once a day. There is no benefit of fondaparinux among patients undergoing primary PCI, and fondaparinux is not recommended as a sole anticoagulant during PCI due to risk of catheter thrombosis.

(B) UNFRACTIONATED HEPARIN—Anticoagulation with intravenous heparin (initial dose of 60 units/kg bolus to a maximum of 4000 units, followed by an infusion of 12 units/kg/min to a maximum of 1000 units, then adjusted to maintain an aPTT of 50–75 seconds beginning with an aPTT drawn 3 hours after thrombolytic) is continued for at least 48 hours after alteplase, reteplase, or tenecteplase, and with continuation of an anticoagulant until revascularization (if performed) or until hospital discharge (or day 8).

For all patients with acute myocardial infarction treated with intensive antithrombotic therapy, prophylactic treatment with proton pump inhibitors or antacids and an H_2-blocker is advisable, although certain proton pump inhibitors, such as omeprazole and esomeprazole, decrease the effect of clopidogrel.

3. Assessment of myocardial reperfusion, recurrent ischemic pain, reinfarction—Myocardial reperfusion can be recognized clinically by the early cessation of pain and the resolution of ST-segment elevation. Although at least 50% resolution of ST-segment elevation by 90 minutes may occur without coronary reperfusion, ST resolution is a strong predictor of better outcome. Even with anticoagulation, 10–20% of reperfused vessels will reocclude during hospitalization, although reocclusion and reinfarction appear to be reduced following intervention. Reinfarction, indicated by recurrence of pain and ST-segment elevation, can be treated by readministration of a thrombolytic agent or immediate angiography and PCI.

C. General Measures

Cardiac care unit monitoring should be instituted as soon as possible. Patients without complications can be transferred to a telemetry unit after 24 hours. Activity should initially be limited to bed rest but can be advanced within 24 hours. Progressive ambulation should be started after 24–72 hours if tolerated. For patients without complications, discharge by day 4 appears to be appropriate. Low-flow oxygen therapy (2–4 L/min) should be given if oxygen saturation is reduced.

D. Analgesia

An initial attempt should be made to relieve pain with sublingual nitroglycerin. However, if no response occurs after two or three tablets, intravenous opioids provide the most rapid and effective analgesia and may also reduce pulmonary congestion. Morphine sulfate, 4–8 mg, or meperidine, 50–75 mg, should be given. Subsequent small doses can be given every 15 minutes until pain abates.

Nonsteroidal anti-inflammatory agents, other than aspirin, should be avoided during hospitalization for STEMI due to increased risk of mortality, myocardial rupture, hypertension, heart failure, and kidney injury with their use.

E. Beta-Adrenergic Blocking Agents

Trials have shown modest short-term benefit from beta-blockers started during the first 24 hours after acute myocardial infarction if there are no contraindications (metoprolol 25–50 mg orally twice daily). Aggressive beta-blockade can increase shock, with overall harm in patients with heart failure. Thus, early beta-blockade should be avoided in patients with any degree of heart failure, evidence of low output state, increased risk of cardiogenic shock, or other relative contraindications to beta-blockade. Carvedilol (beginning at 6.25 mg twice a day, titrated to 25 mg twice a day) was shown to be beneficial in the CAPRICORN trial following the acute phase of large myocardial infarction.

F. Nitrates

Nitroglycerin is the agent of choice for continued or recurrent ischemic pain and is useful in lowering BP or relieving pulmonary congestion. However, routine nitrate administration is not recommended, since no improvement in outcome has been observed in the ISIS-4 or GISSI-3 trials. Nitrates should be avoided in patients who received phosphodiesterase inhibitors (sildenafil, vardenafil, and tadalafil) in the prior 24 hours.

G. Angiotensin-Converting Enzyme (ACE) Inhibitors

A series of trials (SAVE, AIRE, SMILE, TRACE, GISSI-III, and ISIS-4) have shown both short- and long-term improvement in survival with ACE inhibitor therapy. The benefits are greatest in patients with EF ≤ 40%, large infarctions, or clinical evidence of heart failure. Because substantial amounts of the survival benefit occur on the first day, ACE inhibitor treatment should be commenced early in patients without hypotension, especially patients with large or anterior myocardial infarction. Given the benefits of ACE inhibitors for patients with vascular disease, it is reasonable to use ACE inhibitors for all patients following STEMI who do not have contraindications (see Table 11–4).

H. Angiotensin Receptor Blockers

Although there has been inconsistency in the effects of different ARBs on mortality for patients post-myocardial infarction with heart failure and/or LV dysfunction, the VALIANT trial showed that valsartan 160 mg orally twice a day is equivalent to captopril in reducing mortality. Thus, valsartan should be used for all patients with ACE inhibitor intolerance, and is a reasonable, albeit more expensive, alternative to captopril. The combination of captopril and valsartan (at reduced dose) was no better than either agent alone and resulted in more side effects.

I. Aldosterone Antagonists

The RALES trial showed that 25 mg spironolactone can reduce the mortality rate of patients with advanced heart failure, and the EPHESUS trial showed a 15% relative risk reduction in mortality with eplerenone 25 mg daily for patients post-myocardial infarction with LV dysfunction and either clinical heart failure or diabetes. Kidney dysfunction or hyperkalemia are contraindications, and patients must be monitored carefully for development of hyperkalemia.

J. Calcium Channel Blockers

There are no studies to support the routine use of calcium channel blockers in most patients with acute myocardial infarction—and indeed, they have the potential to exacerbate ischemia and cause death from reflex tachycardia or myocardial depression. Long-acting calcium channel blockers should generally be reserved for management of hypertension or ischemia as second- or third-line drugs after beta-blockers and nitrates.

K. Long-Term Antithrombotic Therapy

Discharge on aspirin, 81–325 mg/d, since it is highly effective, inexpensive, and well tolerated, is a key quality indicator of myocardial infarction care. In the CURE trial, clopidogrel, 75 mg/d, (in addition to aspirin) for 3–12 months for non-ST elevation acute coronary syndromes resulted in a similar 20% relative risk reduction in cardiovascular death, myocardial infarction, and stroke, and continuing clopidogrel for 1 year for patients with STEMI is reasonable, regardless of whether they underwent reperfusion therapy. The TRITON trial showed that prasugrel was more beneficial than clopidogrel in reducing ischemic events in patients undergoing PCI, but it resulted in more bleeding. The PLATO trial showed that long-term therapy with ticagrelor and low-dose aspirin was superior to clopidogrel and aspirin. In the WARIS-II trial, long-term anticoagulation with warfarin post-myocardial infarction was associated with a reduction in the composite of death, reinfarction, and stroke, with substantially higher rates of bleeding.

Patients who have received a coronary stent and who require warfarin anticoagulation present a particular challenge, since "triple therapy" with aspirin, clopidogrel, and warfarin has a high risk of bleeding. Triple therapy should be (1) limited to patients with a clear indication for warfarin (such as $CHADS_2$ score of 2 or more or a mechanical prosthetic valve), (2) used for the shortest period of time (such as 1 month after placement of bare metal stent; drug-eluting stents that would require longer clopidogrel duration should be avoided if possible), (3) used with low-dose aspirin and with strategies to reduce risk of bleeding (eg, proton pump inhibitors for patients with history of gastrointestinal bleeding), and (4) used with consideration of a lower target anticoagulation intensity (INR 2.0 to 2.5, at least for the indication of atrial fibrillation) during the period of concomitant treatment with aspirin and $P2Y_{12}$ therapy. Several ongoing studies will evaluate the target specific oral anticoagulants in this area.

L. Coronary Angiography

For patients who do not reperfuse based on lack of at least 50% resolution of ST elevation, rescue angioplasty should be performed and has been shown to reduce the composite of death, reinfarction, stroke, or severe heart failure. According to the evidence in the 2012 European and ACC/AHA guidelines, patients treated with coronary angiography and PCI 3–24 hours after fibrinolytic therapy showed improved outcomes. Patients with recurrent ischemic pain prior to discharge should undergo catheterization and, if indicated, revascularization. PCI of a totally occluded infarct-related artery > 24 hours after STEMI should generally not be performed in asymptomatic patients with one or two vessel disease without evidence of severe ischemia.

▶ When to Refer

All patients with acute myocardial infarction should be referred to a cardiologist.

Armstrong PW et al; STREAM Investigative Team. Fibrinolysis or primary PCI in ST-segment elevation myocardial infarction. N Engl J Med. 2013 Apr 11;368(15):1379–87. [PMID: 23473396]

Fox KA et al; FIR Collaboration. Long-term outcome of a routine versus selective invasive strategy in patients with non-ST-segment elevation acute coronary syndrome a meta-analysis of individual patient data. J Am Coll Cardiol. 2010 Jun 1;55(22):2435–45. [PMID: 20359842]

Kushner FG et al. 2009 Focused Updates: ACC/AHA Guidelines for the Management of Patients With ST-Elevation Myocardial Infarction (updating the 2004 Guideline and 2007 Focused Update) and ACC/AHA/SCAI Guidelines on Percutaneous Coronary Intervention (updating the 2005 Guideline and 2007 Focused Update): a report of the American College of Cardiology Foundation/American Heart Association Task Force on Practice Guidelines. Circulation. 2009 Dec 1;120(22):2271–306. Erratum in: Circulation. 2010 Mar 30;121(12):e257. Dosage error in article text. [PMID: 19923169]

Levine GN et al. 2011 ACCF/AHA/SCAI Guideline for Percutaneous Coronary Intervention: a report of the American College of Cardiology Foundation/American Heart Association Task Force on Practice Guidelines and the Society for Cardiovascular Angiography and Interventions. Circulation. 2011 Dec 6;124(23):e574–651. [PMID: 22064601]

Mehta S et al. Adjunct therapy in STEMI intervention. Cardiol Clin. 2010 Feb;28(1):107–25. [PMID: 19962053]

Steg PG et al. ESC Guidelines for the management of acute myocardial infarction in patients presenting with ST-segment elevation: The Task Force on the management of ST-segment elevation acute myocardial infarction of the European Society of Cardiology (ESC). Eur Heart J. 2012 Oct;33(20):2569–619. [PMID: 22922416]

Torpy JM et al. JAMA patient page. Myocardial infarction. JAMA. 2008 Jan 30;299(4):476. [PMID: 18230786]

Wijns W et al. Guidelines on myocardial revascularization: The Task Force on Myocardial Revascularization of the European Society of Cardiology (ESC) and the European Association for Cardio-Thoracic Surgery (EACTS). Eur Heart J. 2010 Oct;31(20):2501–55. [PMID: 20802248]

▶ Complications

A variety of complications can occur after myocardial infarction even when treatment is initiated promptly.

A. Postinfarction Ischemia

In clinical trials of thrombolysis, recurrent ischemia occurred in about one-third of patients, was more common following non–ST elevation myocardial infarction than after STEMI, and had important short- and long-term prognostic implications. Vigorous medical therapy should be instituted, including nitrates and beta-blockers as well as aspirin 81–325 mg/d, anticoagulant therapy (unfractionated heparin, enoxaparin, or fondaparinux) and clopidogrel. Most patients with postinfarction angina—and all who are refractory to medical therapy—should undergo early catheterization and revascularization by PCI or CABG.

B. Arrhythmias

Abnormalities of rhythm and conduction are common.

1. Sinus bradycardia—This is most common in inferior infarctions or may be precipitated by medications. Observation or withdrawal of the offending agent is usually sufficient. If accompanied by signs of low cardiac output, atropine, 0.5–1 mg intravenously, is usually effective. Temporary pacing is rarely required.

2. Supraventricular tachyarrhythmias—Sinus tachycardia is common and may reflect either increased adrenergic stimulation or hemodynamic compromise due to hypovolemia or pump failure. In the latter, beta-blockade is contraindicated. Supraventricular premature beats are common and may be premonitory for atrial fibrillation. Electrolyte abnormalities and hypoxia should be corrected and causative agents (especially aminophylline) stopped. Atrial fibrillation should be rapidly controlled or converted to sinus rhythm. Intravenous beta-blockers such as metoprolol (2.5–5 mg/h) or short-acting esmolol (50–200 mcg/kg/min)

are the agents of choice if cardiac function is adequate. Intravenous diltiazem (5–15 mg/h) may be used if beta-blockers are contraindicated or ineffective. Digoxin (0.5 mg as initial dose, then 0.25 mg every 90–120 minutes [up to 1–1.25 mg] for a loading dose, followed by 0.25 mg daily if kidney function is normal) is preferable if heart failure is present with atrial fibrillation, but the onset of action is delayed. Electrical cardioversion (commencing with 100 J) may be necessary if atrial fibrillation is complicated by hypotension, heart failure, or ischemia, but the arrhythmia often recurs. Amiodarone (150 mg intravenous bolus and then 15–30 mg/h intravenously, or rapid oral loading with 400 mg three times daily) may be helpful to restore or maintain sinus rhythm.

3. Ventricular arrhythmias—Ventricular arrhythmias are most common in the first few hours after infarction and are a marker of high risk. Ventricular premature beats may be premonitory for ventricular tachycardia or fibrillation but generally should not be treated in the absence of frequent or sustained ventricular tachycardia. Lidocaine is *not* recommended as a prophylactic measure.

Sustained ventricular tachycardia should be treated with a 1 mg/kg bolus of lidocaine if the patient is stable or by electrical cardioversion (100–200 J) if not. If the arrhythmia cannot be suppressed with lidocaine, procainamide (100 mg boluses over 1–2 minutes every 5 minutes to a cumulative dose of 750–1000 mg) or intravenous amiodarone (150 mg over 10 minutes, which may be repeated as needed, followed by 360 mg over 6 hours and then 540 mg over 18 hours) should be initiated, followed by an infusion of 0.5 mg/min (720 mg/ 24 hours). Ventricular fibrillation is treated electrically (300–400 J). Unresponsive ventricular fibrillation should be treated with additional amiodarone and repeat cardioversion while cardiopulmonary resuscitation (CPR) is administered.

Accelerated idioventricular rhythm is a regular, wide-complex rhythm at a rate of 70–100/min. It may occur with or without reperfusion and should not be treated with antiarrhythmics, which could cause asystole.

4. Conduction disturbances—All degrees of AV block may occur in the course of acute myocardial infarction. Block at the level of the AV node is more common than infranodal block and occurs in approximately 20% of inferior myocardial infarctions. First-degree block is the most common and requires no treatment. Second-degree block is usually of the Mobitz type I form (Wenckebach), is often transient, and requires treatment only if associated with a heart rate slow enough to cause symptoms. Complete AV block occurs in up to 5% of acute inferior infarctions, usually is preceded by Mobitz I second-degree block, and generally resolves spontaneously, though it may persist for hours to several weeks. The escape rhythm originates in the distal AV node or AV junction and hence has a narrow QRS complex and is reliable, albeit often slow (30–50 beats/min). Treatment is often necessary because of resulting hypotension and low cardiac output. Intravenous atropine (1 mg) usually restores AV conduction temporarily, but if the escape complex is wide or if repeated atropine treatments are needed, temporary ventricular pacing is indicated. The prognosis for these patients is only slightly worse than for patients in whom AV block did not develop.

In anterior infarctions, the site of block is distal, below the AV node, and usually a result of extensive damage of the His-Purkinje system and bundle branches. New first-degree block (prolongation of the PR interval) is unusual in anterior infarction; Mobitz type II AV block or complete heart block may be preceded by intraventricular conduction defects or may occur abruptly. The escape rhythm, if present, is an unreliable wide-complex idioventricular rhythm. *Urgent ventricular pacing is mandatory*, but even with successful pacing, morbidity and mortality are high because of the extensive myocardial damage. New conduction abnormalities such as right or left bundle branch block or fascicular blocks may presage progression, often sudden, to second- or third-degree AV block. Temporary ventricular pacing is recommended for new-onset alternating bilateral bundle branch block, bifascicular block, or bundle branch block with worsening first-degree AV block. Patients with anterior infarction who progress to second- or third-degree block even transiently should be considered for insertion of a prophylactic permanent ventricular pacemaker before discharge.

C. Myocardial Dysfunction

Persons with hypotension not responsive to fluid resuscitation or refractory heart failure or cardiogenic shock should be considered for urgent echocardiography to assess left and right ventricular function and for mechanical complications, right heart catheterization, and continuous measurements of arterial pressure. These measurements permit the accurate assessment of volume status and may facilitate decisions about volume resuscitation, selective use of pressors and inotropes, and mechanical support.

1. Acute LV failure—Dyspnea, diffuse rales, and arterial hypoxemia usually indicate LV failure. General measures include supplemental oxygen to increase arterial saturation to above 95% and elevation of the trunk. Diuretics are usually the initial therapy unless RV infarction is present. Intravenous furosemide (10–40 mg) or bumetanide (0.5–1 mg) is preferred because of the reliably rapid onset and short duration of action of these drugs. Higher dosages can be given if an inadequate response occurs. Morphine sulfate (4 mg intravenously followed by increments of 2 mg) is valuable in acute pulmonary edema.

Diuretics are usually effective; however, because most patients with acute infarction are not volume overloaded, the hemodynamic response may be limited and may be associated with hypotension. In mild heart failure, sublingual isosorbide dinitrate (2.5–10 mg every 2 hours) or nitroglycerin ointment (6.25–25 mg every 4 hours) may be adequate to lower PCWP. In more severe failure, especially if cardiac output is reduced and BP is normal or high, sodium nitroprusside may be the preferred agent. It should be initiated only with arterial pressure monitoring; the initial dosage should be low (0.25 mcg/kg/min) to avoid excessive hypotension, but the dosage can be increased by increments of 0.5 mcg/kg/min every 5–10 minutes up to 5–10 mcg/kg/min until the desired hemodynamic response

is obtained. Excessive hypotension (mean BP < 65–75 mm Hg) or tachycardia (> 10/min increase) should be avoided.

Intravenous nitroglycerin (starting at 10 mcg/min) also may be effective but may lower PCWP with less hypotension. Oral or transdermal vasodilator therapy with nitrates or ACE inhibitors is often necessary after the initial 24–48 hours (see below).

Inotropic agents should be avoided if possible, because they often increase heart rate and myocardial oxygen requirements and worsen clinical outcomes. Dobutamine has the best hemodynamic profile, increasing cardiac output and modestly lowering PCWP, usually without excessive tachycardia, hypotension, or arrhythmias. The initial dosage is 2.5 mcg/kg/min, and it may be increased by similar increments up to 15–20 mcg/kg/min at intervals of 5–10 minutes. Dopamine is more useful in the presence of hypotension (see below), since it produces peripheral vasoconstriction, but it has a less beneficial effect on PCWP. Digoxin has not been helpful in acute infarction except to control the ventricular response in atrial fibrillation, but it may be beneficial if chronic heart failure persists.

2. Hypotension and shock—Patients with hypotension (systolic BP < 90 mm Hg, individualized depending on prior BP) and signs of diminished perfusion (low urinary output, confusion, cold extremities) that does not respond to fluid resuscitation should be presumed to have cardiogenic shock and should be considered for urgent catheterization and revascularization as well as selective use of intra-aortic balloon pump (IABP) support and hemodynamic monitoring with a PA catheter, although these later measures have not been shown to improve outcome. Up to 20% will have findings indicative of intravascular hypovolemia (due to diaphoresis, vomiting, decreased venous tone, medications—such as diuretics, nitrates, morphine, beta-blockers, calcium channel blockers, and thrombolytic agents—and lack of oral intake). These should be treated with successive boluses of 100 mL of normal saline until PCWP reaches 15–18 mm Hg to determine whether cardiac output and BP respond. **Pericardial tamponade** due to hemorrhagic pericarditis (especially after thrombolytic therapy or cardiopulmonary resuscitation) or ventricular rupture should be considered and excluded by echocardiography if clinically indicated. RV infarction, characterized by a normal PCWP but elevated RA pressure, can produce hypotension. This is discussed below.

Most patients with cardiogenic shock will have moderate to severe LV systolic dysfunction, with a mean EF of 30% in the SHOCK trial. If hypotension is only modest (systolic pressure > 90 mm Hg) and the PCWP is elevated, diuretics should be administered. If the BP falls, inotropic support will need to be added. A large randomized trial showed no benefit of IABP support in cardiogenic shock.

Dopamine is generally considered to be the most appropriate pressor for cardiogenic hypotension. It should be initiated at a rate of 2–4 mcg/kg/min and increased at 5-minute intervals to the appropriate hemodynamic end point. At low dosages (< 5 mcg/kg/min), it improves renal blood flow; at intermediate dosages (2.5–10 mcg/kg/min), it stimulates myocardial contractility; at higher dosages (> 8 mcg/kg/min), it is a potent alpha-1-adrenergic agonist. In general, BP and cardiac index rise, but PCWP does not fall. Dopamine may be combined with nitroprusside or dobutamine (see above for dosing), or the latter may be used in its place if hypotension is not severe. Norepinephrine (0.1–0.5 mcg/kg/min) is generally reserved for failure of other vasopressors, since epinephrine produces less vasoconstriction and does not increase coronary perfusion pressure (aortic diastolic pressure), but it does tend to worsen the balance between myocardial oxygen delivery and utilization.

Patients with cardiogenic shock not due to hypovolemia have a poor prognosis, with 30-day mortality rates of 40–80%. If they do not respond rapidly, IABP may be considered to both reduce myocardial energy requirements (systolic unloading) and improve diastolic coronary blood flow. However, the SHOCK II trial did not find a difference in all-cause mortality at 30-days between patients randomized to IABP versus routine care with rapid revascularization. Longer term outcomes from this trial failed to identify any situation in which IABP use was helpful. Surgically implanted (or percutaneous) ventricular assist devices may be used in refractory cases. Emergent cardiac catheterization and coronary angiography followed by percutaneous or surgical revascularization offer the best chance of survival.

D. RV Infarction

RV infarction is present in one-third of patients with inferior wall infarction but is clinically significant in < 50% of these. It presents as hypotension with relatively preserved LV function and should be considered whenever patients with inferior infarction exhibit low BP, raised venous pressure, and clear lungs. Hypotension is often exacerbated by medications that decrease intravascular volume or produce venodilation, such as diuretics, nitrates, and opioids. RA pressure and JVP are high, while PCWP is normal or low and the lungs are clear. The diagnosis is suggested by ST-segment elevation in right-sided anterior chest leads, particularly RV_4. The diagnosis can be confirmed by echocardiography or hemodynamic measurements. Treatment consists of fluid loading beginning with 500 mL of 0.9% saline over 2 hours to improve LV filling, and inotropic agents only if necessary.

E. Mechanical Defects

Partial or complete rupture of a papillary muscle or of the interventricular septum occurs in < 1% of acute myocardial infarctions and carries a poor prognosis. These complications occur in both anterior and inferior infarctions, usually 3–7 days after the acute event. They are detected by the appearance of a new systolic murmur and clinical deterioration, often with pulmonary edema. The two lesions are distinguished by the location of the murmur (apical versus parasternal) and by Doppler echocardiography. Hemodynamic monitoring is essential for appropriate management and demonstrates an increase in oxygen saturation between the RA and PA in VSD and, often, a large v wave with mitral regurgitation. Treatment by nitroprusside and, preferably, intra-aortic balloon

counterpulsation (IABC) reduces the regurgitation or shunt, but surgical correction is mandatory. In patients remaining hemodynamically unstable or requiring continuous parenteral pharmacologic treatment or counterpulsation, early surgery is recommended, though mortality rates are high (15% to nearly 100%, depending on residual ventricular function and clinical status). Patients who are stabilized medically can have delayed surgery with lower risks (10–25%), although this may be due to the death of sicker patients, some of whom may have been saved by earlier surgery.

F. Myocardial Rupture

Complete rupture of the LV free wall occurs in < 1% of patients and usually results in immediate death. It occurs 2–7 days postinfarction, usually involves the anterior wall, and is more frequent in older women. Incomplete or gradual rupture may be sealed off by the pericardium, creating a **pseudoaneurysm**. This may be recognized by echocardiography, radionuclide angiography, or LV angiography, often as an incidental finding. It demonstrates a narrow-neck connection to the LV. Early surgical repair is indicated, since delayed rupture is common.

G. LV Aneurysm

An LV aneurysm, a sharply delineated area of scar that bulges paradoxically during systole, develops in 10–20% of patients surviving an acute infarction. This usually follows anterior Q wave infarctions. Aneurysms are recognized by persistent ST-segment elevation (beyond 4–8 weeks), and a wide neck from the LV can be demonstrated by echocardiography, scintigraphy, or contrast angiography. They rarely rupture but may be associated with arterial emboli, ventricular arrhythmias, and heart failure. Surgical resection may be performed for these indications if other measures fail. The best results (mortality rates of 10–20%) are obtained when the residual myocardium contracts well and when significant coronary lesions supplying adjacent regions are bypassed.

H. Pericarditis

The pericardium is involved in approximately 50% of infarctions, but pericarditis is often not clinically significant. Twenty percent of patients with Q wave infarctions will have an audible friction rub if examined repetitively. Pericardial pain occurs in approximately the same proportion after 2–7 days and is recognized by its variation with respiration and position (improved by sitting). Often, no treatment is required, but aspirin (650 mg every 4–6 hours) will usually relieve the pain. Indomethacin and corticosteroids can cause impaired infarct healing and predispose to myocardial rupture, and therefore should generally be avoided in the early post-myocardial infarction period. Likewise, anticoagulation should be used cautiously, since hemorrhagic pericarditis may result.

One week to 12 weeks after infarction, Dressler syndrome (post-myocardial infarction syndrome) occurs in < 5% of patients. This is an autoimmune phenomenon and presents as pericarditis with associated fever, leukocytosis and, occasionally, pericardial or pleural effusion. It may recur over months. Treatment is the same as for other forms of pericarditis. A short course of nonsteroidal agents or corticosteroids may help relieve symptoms.

I. Mural Thrombus

Mural thrombi are common in large anterior infarctions but not in infarctions at other locations. Arterial emboli occur in approximately 2% of patients with known infarction, usually within 6 weeks. Anticoagulation with heparin followed by short-term (3-month) warfarin therapy prevents most emboli and should be considered in all patients with large anterior infarctions. Mural thrombi can be detected by echocardiography or cardiac MRI, but these procedures should not be relied upon for determining the need for anticoagulation.

Thiele H et al; IABP-SHOCK II Trial Investigators. Intraaortic balloon support for myocardial infarction with cardiogenic shock. N Engl J Med. 2012 Oct 4;367(14):1287-96. [PMID: 22920912]

► Postinfarction Management

After the first 24 hours, the focus of patient management is to prevent recurrent ischemia, improve infarct healing and prevent remodeling, and prevent recurrent vascular events. Patients with hemodynamic compromise, who are at high risk for death, need careful monitoring and management of volume status.

A. Risk Stratification

Risk stratification is important for management of STEMI. GRACE and TIMI risk scores can be helpful tools. The GRACE risk score is available for web access and/or PDA download at http://www.outcomes-umassmed.org/grace, and the TIMI Risk Score is available at http://www.timi. org. Patients with recurrent ischemia (spontaneous or provoked), hemodynamic instability, impaired LV function, heart failure, or serious ventricular arrhythmias should undergo cardiac catheterization (Table 10–10). ACE inhibitor (or ARB) therapy is indicated in patients with clinical heart failure or LVEF ≤ 40%. Aldosterone blockade is indicated for patients with an LVEF ≤ 40% and either heart failure or diabetes mellitus.

For patients not undergoing cardiac catheterization, submaximal exercise (or pharmacologic stress testing for patients unable to exercise) before discharge or a maximal test after 3–6 weeks (the latter being more sensitive for ischemia) helps patients and clinicians plan the return to normal activity. Imaging in conjunction with stress testing adds additional sensitivity for ischemia and provides localizing information. Both exercise and pharmacologic stress imaging have successfully predicted subsequent outcome. One of these tests should be used prior to discharge in patients who have received thrombolytic therapy as a means of selecting appropriate candidates for coronary angiography.

B. Secondary Prevention

Postinfarction management should begin with identification and modification of risk factors. Treatment of hyperlipidemia and smoking cessation both prevent recurrent infarction and death. Statin therapy should be started before the patient is discharged from the hospital to reduce recurrent atherothrombotic events. BP control and cardiac rehabilitation or exercise are also recommended.

Beta-blockers improve survival rates, primarily by reducing the incidence of sudden death in high-risk subsets of patients, though their value may be less in patients without complications with small infarctions and normal exercise tests. While a variety of beta-blockers have been shown to be beneficial, for patients with LV dysfunction managed with contemporary treatment, carvedilol titrated to 25 mg orally twice a day has been shown to reduce mortality. Beta-blockers with intrinsic sympathomimetic activity have not proved beneficial in postinfarction patients.

Antiplatelet agents are beneficial; aspirin (81–325 mg daily, with 81 mg daily the preferred long-term dose) is recommended, and adding clopidogrel (75 mg daily) has been shown to provide additional benefit short term after STEMI. Prasugrel provides further reduction in thrombotic outcomes compared with clopidogrel, at the cost of more bleeding. Likewise, ticagrelor provides benefit over clopidogrel but should be used with low-dose aspirin (81 mg/d). Warfarin anticoagulation for 3 months reduces the incidence of arterial emboli after large anterior infarctions, and according to the results of at least one study it improves long-term prognosis, but these studies were before routine use of aspirin and clopidogrel. An advantage to combining low-dose aspirin and warfarin has not been demonstrated, except perhaps in patients with atrial fibrillation.

Calcium channel blockers have not been shown to improve prognoses overall and should not be prescribed purely for secondary prevention. Antiarrhythmic therapy other than with beta-blockers has not been shown to be effective except in patients with symptomatic arrhythmias. Amiodarone has been studied in several trials of postinfarct patients with either LV dysfunction or frequent ventricular ectopy. Although survival was not improved, amiodarone was not harmful—unlike other agents in this setting. Therefore, it is the agent of choice for individuals with symptomatic postinfarction supraventricular arrhythmias. While implantable defibrillators improve survival for patients with postinfarction LV dysfunction and heart failure, the DINAMIT trial found no benefit to implantable defibrillators implanted in the 40 days following acute myocardial infarction.

Cardiac rehabilitation programs and exercise training can be of considerable psychological benefit and appear to improve prognosis.

C. ACE Inhibitors and ARBs in Patients with LV Dysfunction

Patients who sustain substantial myocardial damage often experience subsequent progressive LV dilation and dysfunction, leading to clinical heart failure and reduced long-term survival. In patients with EFs < 40%, long-term ACE inhibitor (or ARB) therapy prevents LV dilation and the onset of heart failure and prolongs survival. The HOPE trial, as well as an overview of trials of ACE inhibitors for secondary prevention, also demonstrated a reduction of approximately 20% in mortality rates and the occurrence of nonfatal myocardial infarction and stroke with ramipril treatment of patients with coronary or peripheral vascular disease and without confirmed LV systolic dysfunction. Therefore, ACE inhibitor therapy should be strongly considered in this broader group of patients—and especially in patients with diabetes and those with even mild systolic hypertension, in whom the greatest benefit was observed (see Table 11–7).

D. Revascularization

Postinfarction patients not treated with primary PCI who appear likely to benefit from early revascularization if the anatomy is appropriate are (1) those who have undergone fibrinolytic therapy, especially if they have high-risk features (including systolic BP of < 100 mm Hg, heart rate of > 100 bpm, Killip class II or III, ST-segment depression of 2 mm or more in the anterior leads); (2) patients with LV dysfunction (EF < 30–40%); (3) patients with non–ST elevation MI and high-risk features; and (4) patients with markedly positive exercise tests and multi-vessel disease. The value of revascularization in patients not treated with acute reperfusion therapy with preserved LV function who have mild ischemia and are not symptom limited is less clear. In general, patients without high-risk features who survive infarctions without complications, have preserved LV function (EF > 50%), and have no exercise-induced ischemia have an excellent prognosis and do not require invasive evaluation.

O'Gara PT et al. 2013 ACCF/AHA guideline for the management of ST-elevation myocardial infarction: a report of the American College of Cardiology Foundation/American Heart Association Task Force on Practice Guidelines. Circulation. 2013 Jan 29;127(4):e362–425. Erratum in: Circulation. 2013 Dec 24;128(25):e481. [PMID: 23247304]

▼ DISORDERS OF RATE & RHYTHM

Abnormalities of cardiac rhythm and conduction can be symptomatic (syncope, near syncope, dizziness, fatigue, or palpitations), or asymptomatic. In addition, they can be lethal (sudden cardiac death) or dangerous to the extent that they reduce cardiac output, so that perfusion of the brain and myocardium is impaired. Stable supraventricular tachycardia is generally well tolerated in patients without underlying heart disease but may lead to myocardial ischemia or heart failure in patients with coronary disease, valvular abnormalities, and systolic or diastolic myocardial dysfunction. Ventricular tachycardia, if prolonged (lasting more than 10–30 seconds), often results in hemodynamic compromise and may deteriorate into ventricular fibrillation if left untreated.

Whether slow heart rates produce symptoms at rest or with exertion depends on whether cerebral and peripheral

perfusion can be maintained, which is generally a function of whether the patient is upright or supine and whether LV function is adequate to maintain stroke volume. If the heart rate abruptly slows, as with the onset of complete heart block or sinus arrest, syncope or convulsions (or both) may result.

Arrhythmias are detected either because they produce symptoms or because they are detected during the course of monitoring. Arrhythmias causing sudden death, syncope, or near syncope require further evaluation and treatment unless they are related to conditions that are reversible or immediately treatable (eg, electrolyte abnormalities or acute myocardial infarction). In contrast, there is controversy over when and how to evaluate and treat rhythm disturbances that are not symptomatic but are possible markers for more serious abnormalities (eg, nonsustained ventricular tachycardia [NSVT]). This uncertainty reflects two issues: (1) the difficulty of reliably stratifying patients into high-risk and low-risk groups; and (2) the lack of treatments that are both effective and safe. Thus, screening patients for these so-called "premonitory" abnormalities is often not productive.

A number of procedures are used to evaluate patients with symptoms who are believed to be at risk for life-threatening arrhythmias, including in-hospital and ambulatory ECG monitoring, event recorders (instruments that can be used for prolonged periods to record or transmit rhythm tracings when infrequent episodes occur), exercise testing, catheter-based electrophysiologic studies (to assess sinus node function, AV conduction, and inducibility of arrhythmias), and tests of autonomic nervous system function (tilt-table testing).

Treatment of arrhythmias varies and can include modalities such as antiarrhythmic drugs (see Table 10–12) and more invasive techniques such as catheter ablation.

▶ Antiarrhythmic Drugs (Table 10–12)

Antiarrhythmic drugs are frequently used to treat arrhythmias, but have variable efficacy and produce frequent side effects. They are often divided into classes based on their electropharmacologic actions and many of these drugs have multiple actions. The most frequently used classification scheme is the Vaughan-Williams, which consists of four classes.

Class I agents block membrane sodium channels. Three subclasses are further defined by the effect of the agents on the Purkinje fiber action potential. Class Ia drugs (ie, quinidine, procainamide, disopyramide) slow the rate of rise of the action potential (V_{max}) and prolong its duration, thus slowing conduction and increasing refractoriness (moderate depression of phase 0 upstroke of the action potential). Class Ib agents (ie, lidocaine, mexiletine) shorten action potential duration; they do not affect conduction or refractoriness (minimal depression of phase 0 upstroke of the action potential). Class Ic agents (ie, flecainide, propafenone) prolong V_{max} and slow repolarization, thus slowing conduction and prolonging refractoriness, but more so than class Ia drugs (maximal depression of phase 0 upstroke of the action potential).

Table 10–12. Antiarrhythmic drugs.

Agent	Intravenous Dosage	Oral Dosage	Therapeutic Plasma Level	Route of Elimination	Side Effects
Class Ia: Action: Sodium channel blockers: Depress phase 0 depolarization; slow conduction; prolong repolarization.					
Indications: Supraventricular tachycardia, ventricular tachycardia, prevention of ventricular fibrillation, symptomatic ventricular premature beats.					
Quinidine	6–10 mg/kg (intramuscularly or intravenously) over 20 min (rarely used parenterally)	200–400 mg every 4–6 h or every 8 h (long-acting)	2–5 mg/mL	Hepatic	GI, ↓ LVF, ↑ Dig
Procainamide	100 mg/1–3 min to 500–1000 mg; maintain at 2–6 mg/min	50 mg/kg/d in divided doses every 3–4 h or every 6 h (long-acting)	4–10 mg/mL; NAPA (active metabolite), 10–20 mcg/mL	Renal	SLE, hypersensitivity, ↓ LVF
Disopyramide		100–200 mg every 6–8 h	2–8 mg/mL	Renal	Urinary retention, dry mouth, markedly ↓ LVF
Class Ib: Action: Shorten repolarization.					
Indications: Ventricular tachycardia, prevention of ventricular fibrillation, symptomatic ventricular beats.					
Lidocaine	1–2 mg/kg at 50 mg/min; maintain at 1–4 mg/min		1–5 mg/mL	Hepatic	CNS, GI
Mexiletine		100–300 mg every 6–12 h; maximum: 1200 mg/d	0.5–2 mg/mL	Hepatic	CNS, GI, leukopenia
Class Ic: Action: Depress phase 0 repolarization; slow conduction. Propafenone is a weak calcium channel blocker and beta-blocker and prolongs action potential and refractoriness.					
Indications: Life-threatening ventricular tachycardia or fibrillation, refractory supraventricular tachycardia.					
Flecainide		50–150 mg twice daily	0.2–1 mg/mL	Hepatic	CNS, GI, ↓ ↓ LVF, incessant VT, sudden death
Propafenone		150–300 mg every 8–12 h	**Note:** Active metabolites	Hepatic	CNS, GI, ↓ ↓ LVF, ↑ Dig
Class II: Action: Beta-blocker, slows AV conduction. Note: Other beta-blockers may also have antiarrhythmic effects but are not yet approved for this indication in the United States.					
Indications: Supraventricular tachycardia; may prevent ventricular fibrillation.					
Esmolol	500 mcg/kg over 1–2 min; maintain at 25–200 mcg/kg/min	Other beta-blockers may be used concomitantly	Not established	Hepatic	↓ LVF, bronchospasm
Propranolol	1–5 mg at 1 mg/min	40–320 mg in 1–4 doses daily (depending on preparation)	Not established	Hepatic	↓ LVF, bradycardia, AV block, bronchospasm
Metoprolol	2.5–5 mg	50–200 mg daily	Not established	Hepatic	↓ LVF, bradycardia, AV block
Class III: Action: Prolong action potential.					
Indications: *Amiodarone:* refractory ventricular tachycardia, supraventricular tachycardia, prevention of ventricular tachycardia, atrial fibrillation, ventricular fibrillation; *dofetilide:* atrial fibrillation and flutter; *sotalol:* ventricular tachycardia, atrial fibrillation; *ibutilide:* conversion of atrial fibrillation and flutter.					
Amiodarone	150–300 mg infused rapidly, followed by 1-mg/min infusion for 6 h (360 mg) and then 0.5 mg/min	800–1600 mg/d for 7–21 days; maintain at 100–400 mg/d (higher doses may be needed)	1–5 mg/mL	Hepatic	Pulmonary fibrosis, hypothyroidism, hyperthyroidism, photosensitivity corneal and skin deposits, hepatitis, ↑ Dig, neurotoxicity, GI

(continued)

Table 10–12. Antiarrhythmic drugs. (continued)

Agent	Intravenous Dosage	Oral Dosage	Therapeutic Plasma Level	Route of Elimination	Side Effects
Dronedarone		400 mg twice daily		Hepatic (contraindicated in severe impairment)	QTc prolongation, HF. Contraindicated in HF (NYHA class IV and class II and III if recent decompensation)
Sotalol		80–160 mg every 12 h (higher doses may be used for life-threatening arrhythmias)		Renal (dosing interval should be extended if creatinineclearance is < 60 mL/min)	Early incidence of torsades de pointes, LVF, bradycardia, fatigue (and otherside effects associated with beta-blockers)
Dofetilide		125–500 mcg every 12 h		Renal (dose must be reduced with kidney dysfunction)	Torsades de pointes in 3%; interaction with cytochrome P-450 inhibitors
Ibutilide	1 mg over 10 min, followed by a second infusion of 0.5–1 mg over 10 min			Hepatic and renal	Torsades de pointes in up to 5% of patients within 3 h after administration; patients must be monitored with defibrillator nearby
Class IV: Action: Slow calcium channel blockers.					
Indications: Supraventricular tachycardia.					
Verapamil	2.5 mg bolus followed by additional boluses of 2.5–5 mg every 1–3 min; total 20 mg over 20 min; maintain at 5 mg/kg/min	80–120 mg every 6–8 h; 240–360 mg once daily with sustained-release preparation	0.1–0.15 mg/mL	Hepatic	↓ LVF, constipation, ↑ Dig, hypotension
Diltiazem	0.25 mg/kg over 2 min; second 0.35-mg/kg bolus after 15 min if response is inadequate; infusion rate, 5–15 mg/h	180–360 mg daily in 1–3 doses depending on preparation (oral forms not approved for arrhythmias)		Hepatic metabolism, renal excretion	Hypotension, ↓ LVF
Miscellaneous: Indications: Supraventricular tachycardia.					
Adenosine	6 mg rapidly followed by 12 mg after 1–2 min if needed; use half these doses if administered via central line			Adenosine receptor stimulation, metabolized in blood	Transient flushing, dyspnea, chest pain, AV block, sinus bradycardia; effect ↓ by theophylline, by dipyridamole
Digoxin	0.5 mg over 20 min followed by increment of 0.25 or 0.125 mg to 1–1.5 mg over 24 h	1–1.5 mg over 24–36 h in 3 or 4 doses; maintenance, 0.125–0.5 mg/d	0.7–2 mg/mL	Renal	AV block, arrhythmias, GI, visual changes

AV, atrioventricular; HF, heart failure; CNS, central nervous system; Dig, elevation of serum digoxin level; GI, gastrointestinal (nausea, vomiting, diarrhea); ↓LVF, reduced left ventricular function; NAPA, N-acetylprocainamide; NYHA, New York Heart Association; SLE, systemic lupus erythematosus; VT, ventricular tachycardia.

Class II agents are the beta-blockers, which decrease automaticity, prolong AV conduction, and prolong refractoriness.

Class III agents (ie, amiodarone, dronedarone, sotalol, dofetilide, ibutilide) block potassium channels and prolong repolarization, widening the QRS and prolonging the QT interval. They decrease automaticity and conduction and prolong refractoriness. Dronedarone has been shown to reduce cardiovascular hospitalizations when used in patients with paroxysmal atrial fibrillation in the absence of heart failure; however, the PALLAS trial found an *increase* in cardiovascular events when dronedarone was used in patients with permanent atrial fibrillation.

Class IV agents are the calcium channel blockers, which decrease automaticity and AV conduction.

There are some antiarrhythmic agents that do not fall into one of these categories. The most frequently used are digoxin and adenosine. Digoxin inhibits the Na+, K+-ATPase pump. Digoxin prolongs AV nodal conduction and the AV nodal refractory period, but it shortens the action potential and decreases the refractoriness of the ventricular myocardium and Purkinje fibers. Adenosine can block AV nodal conduction and shortens atrial refractoriness.

Although the in vitro electrophysiologic effects of most of these agents have been defined, their use remains largely empiric. All can exacerbate arrhythmias (proarrhythmic effect), and many depress LV function.

The risk of antiarrhythmic agents has been highlighted by many studies, most notably the Coronary Arrhythmia Suppression Trial (CAST), in which two class Ic agents (flecainide, encainide) and a class Ia agent (moricizine) increased mortality rates in patients with asymptomatic ventricular ectopy after myocardial infarction. A similar result has been reported in the Mortality in the Survival With Oral D-sotalol (SWORD) study with d-sotalol, a class III agent without the beta-blocking activity of the currently marketed formulation d,l-sotalol. Class 1c antiarrhythmic agents should therefore not be used in patients with prior myocardial infarction or structural heart disease.

The use of antiarrhythmic agents for specific arrhythmias is discussed below.

Connolly SJ et al; PALLAS Investigators. Dronedarone in high-risk permanent atrial fibrillation. N Engl J Med. 2011 Dec 15;365(24):2268–76. [PMID: 22082198]

Ganjehei L et al. Pharmacologic management of arrhythmias. Tex Heart Inst J. 2011;38(4):344–9. [PMID: 21841856]

Li EC et al. Drug-induced QT-interval prolongation: considerations for clinicians. Pharmacotherapy. 2010 Jul;30(7):684–701. [PMID: 20575633]

Shu J et al. Pharmacotherapy of cardiac arrhythmias—basic science for clinicians. Pacing Clin Electrophysiol. 2009 Nov;32(11):1454–65. [PMID: 19744278]

Thireau J et al. New drugs vs. old concepts: a fresh look at antiarrhythmics. Pharmacol Ther. 2011 Nov;132(2):125–45. [PMID: 21420430]

Torp-Pedersen C et al. Antiarrhythmic drugs: safety first. J Am Coll Cardiol. 2010 April 13;55(15):1569–76. [PMID: 20378074]

▶ Catheter Ablation for Cardiac Arrhythmias

Catheter ablation has become the primary modality of therapy for many symptomatic supraventricular arrhythmias, including AV nodal reentrant tachycardia, tachycardias involving accessory pathways, paroxysmal atrial tachycardia, and atrial flutter. Catheter ablation of atrial fibrillation is more complex and usually involves complete electrical isolation of the pulmonary veins (which are often the sites of initiation of atrial fibrillation) or placing linear lesions within the atria to prevent propagation throughout the atrial chamber. This technique is currently considered a reasonable second-line therapy (after pharmacologic treatment) for certain patients with symptomatic drug-refractory atrial fibrillation. Catheter ablation of ventricular arrhythmias has proved more difficult, but experienced centers have demonstrated reasonable success with all types of ventricular tachycardias including bundle-branch reentry, tachycardia originating in the ventricular outflow tract or papillary muscles, tachycardias originating in the left side of the interventricular septum (fascicular ventricular tachycardia), and ventricular tachycardias occurring in patients with ischemic or dilated cardiomyopathy. Ablation of many of these arrhythmias can be performed from the epicardial surface of the heart via a percutaneous subxiphoid approach.

Catheter ablation has also been successfully performed for the treatment of ventricular fibrillation when a uniform premature ventricular contraction (PVC) can be identified. In addition, patients with symptomatic PVCs or PVCs occurring at a high enough burden to result in a cardiomyopathy (usually > 10,000/day) are often referred for catheter ablation as well.

Catheter ablation procedures are generally safe, with an overall major complication rate ranging from 2% to 8%. Major vascular damage during catheter insertion occurs in < 2% of patients. There is a low incidence of perforation of the myocardial wall resulting in pericardial tamponade. Sufficient damage to the AV node to require permanent cardiac pacing occurs in < 1% of patients. When transseptal access through the interatrial septum or retrograde LV catheterization is required, additional potential complications include damage to the heart valves, damage to a coronary artery, or systemic emboli. A rare but potentially fatal complication after catheter ablation of atrial fibrillation is the development of an atrio-esophageal fistula resulting from ablation on the posterior wall of the LA just overlying the esophagus.

Aliot EM et al. EHRA/HRS Expert Consensus on Catheter Ablation of Ventricular Arrhythmias: developed in a partnership with the European Heart Rhythm Association (EHRA), a Registered Branch of the European Society of Cardiology (ESC), and the Heart Rhythm Society (HRS); in collaboration with the American College of Cardiology (ACC) and the American Heart Association (AHA). Heart Rhythm. 2009 Jun;6(6):886–933. [PMID: 19467519]

Bohnen M et al. Incidence and predictors of major complications from contemporary catheter ablation to treat cardiac arrhythmias. Heart Rhythm. 2011 Nov;8(11):1661–6. [PMID: 21699857]

Calkins H et al. HRS/HERA/ECAS Expert Consensus Statement on Catheter and Surgical Ablation of Atrial Fibrillation: recommendations for patient selection, procedural techniques, patient management and follow-up, definitions, end-points and research trial design: a report of the Heart Rhythm Society (HRS) Task Force on Catheter and Surgical Ablation of Atrial Fibrillation. Developed in partnership with the European Heart Rhythm Association (EHRA), a registered branch of the European Society of Cardiology (ESC) and the European Cardiac Arrhythmia Society (ECAS); and in collaboration with the American College of Cardiology (ACC), American Heart Association (AHA), the Asia Pacific Heart Rhythm Society (APHRS), and the Society of Thoracic Surgeons (STS). Heart Rhythm. 2012 Apr;9(4):632–96.e21. [PMID: 22386883]

Wazni O et al. Catheter ablation for atrial fibrillation. N Engl J Med. 2011 Dec 15;365(24):2296–304. [PMID: 22168644]

SINUS ARRHYTHMIA, BRADYCARDIA, & TACHYCARDIA

Sinus arrhythmia is a cyclic increase in normal heart rate with inspiration and decrease with expiration. It results from reflex changes in vagal influence on the normal pacemaker and disappears with breath holding or increase of heart rate. It is common in both the young and the elderly and is not a pathologic arrhythmia.

Sinus bradycardia is a heart rate slower than 60 beats/min due to increased vagal influence on the normal pacemaker or organic disease of the sinus node. The rate usually increases during exercise or administration of atropine. In healthy individuals, and especially in patients who are in excellent physical condition, sinus bradycardia to rates of 50 beats/min or even lower is a normal finding. However, severe sinus bradycardia (< 45 beats/min) may be an indication of sinus node pathology (see below), especially in elderly patients and individuals with heart disease. It may cause weakness, confusion, or syncope if cerebral perfusion is impaired. Atrial, junctional and ventricular ectopic rhythms are more apt to occur with slow sinus rates. Pacing may be required if symptoms correlate with the bradycardia.

Sinus tachycardia is defined as a heart rate faster than 100 beats/min that is caused by rapid impulse formation from the sinoatrial node; it occurs with fever, exercise, emotion, pain, anemia, heart failure, shock, thyrotoxicosis, or in response to many drugs. Alcohol and alcohol withdrawal are common causes of sinus tachycardia and other supraventricular arrhythmias. The onset and termination are usually gradual, in contrast to paroxysmal supraventricular tachycardia due to reentry. The rate infrequently exceeds 160 beats/min but may reach 180 beats/min in young persons. The rhythm is generally regular, but serial 1-minute counts of the heart rate indicate that it varies five or more beats per minute with changes in position, with breath holding, or with sedation. In rare instances, otherwise healthy individuals may present with "inappropriate" sinus tachycardia where persistently elevated basal heart rates are not in-line with physiologic demands. Long-term consequences of this disorder are few. While the exact mechanism underlying "inappropriate" sinus tachycardia are unclear, pharmacologic agents, such as beta-blockers or ivabradine (which selectively blocks the I_f current within the sinus node), have been shown to have varying success in improving symptoms. Catheter ablation aimed at modifying the sinus node to lower mean heart rate has been reported, however recurrence rates are high.

▶ When to Refer

Patients with symptoms related to bradycardia or tachycardia when reversible etiologies have been excluded.

▶ When to Admit

Patients with bradycardia and recent or recurrent syncope.

ATRIAL PREMATURE BEATS (Atrial Extrasystoles)

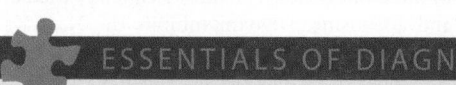

ESSENTIALS OF DIAGNOSIS

▶ Usually asymptomatic.

▶ Isolated interruption in regular rhythm.

▶ P-wave morphology on ECG usually differs from sinus P-wave morphology.

▶ Can be harbinger of future development of atrial fibrillation.

Atrial premature beats occur when an ectopic focus in the atria fires before the next sinus node impulse. The contour of the P wave usually differs from the patient's normal complex, unless the ectopic focus is near the sinus node. Such premature beats occur frequently in normal hearts. Acceleration of the heart rate by any means usually abolishes most premature beats. Early atrial premature beats may cause aberrant QRS complexes (left or right bundle branch block) or may not be conducted to the ventricles because the AV node or ventricles are still refractory.

Differentiation of Aberrantly Conducted Supraventricular Beats from Ventricular Beats

This distinction can be very difficult in patients with a wide QRS complex; it is important because of the differing prognostic and therapeutic implications of each type. Findings favoring a ventricular origin include (1) AV dissociation; (2) a QRS duration exceeding 0.14 second; (3) capture or fusion beats (infrequent); (4) left axis deviation with right bundle branch block morphology; (5) monophasic (R) or biphasic (qR, QR, or RS) complexes in V_1; and (6) a qR or QS complex in V_6. Supraventricular origin is favored by (1) a triphasic QRS complex, especially with initial negativity in leads I and V_6; (2) ventricular rates exceeding 170 beats/min; (3) QRS duration longer than 0.12 second but not longer than 0.14 second; and (4) the presence of preexcitation syndrome.

The relationship of the P waves to the tachycardia complex is helpful. A 1:1 relationship usually means a supraventricular origin, except in the case of ventricular tachycardia with retrograde atrial activation.

Treatment of this arrhythmia is rarely indicated.

PAROXYSMAL SUPRAVENTRICULAR TACHYCARDIA

- ► Frequently associated with palpitations.
- ► Abrupt onset/offset.
- ► Rapid, regular rhythm.
- ► Most commonly seen in young adults.
- ► Rarely causes syncope.
- ► Usually have a narrow QRS complex on ECG.
- ► Often responsive to vagal maneuvers, AV nodal blockers, or adenosine.

► General Considerations

This is a common paroxysmal tachycardia and often occurs in patients without structural heart disease. The most common mechanism for paroxysmal supraventricular tachycardia is reentry, which may be initiated or terminated by a fortuitously timed atrial or ventricular premature beat. The reentrant circuit most commonly involves dual pathways (a slow and a fast pathway) within the AV node. This is referred to as AV nodal reentrant tachycardia (AVNRT). Less commonly, reentry is due to an accessory pathway between the atria and ventricles, referred to as atrioventricular reciprocating tachycardia (AVRT). Approximately one-third of patients with supraventricular tachycardia have accessory pathways to the ventricles. The pathophysiology and management of arrhythmias due to accessory pathways differ in important ways and are discussed separately below.

► Clinical Findings

A. Symptoms and Signs

Patients may be asymptomatic except for awareness of rapid heart action, but some experience mild chest pain or shortness of breath, especially when episodes are prolonged, even in the absence of associated cardiac abnormalities. Episodes begin and end abruptly and may last a few seconds to several hours or longer.

B. ECG

The heart rate may be 140–240 beats/min (usually 160–220 beats/min) and is regular (despite exercise or change in position). The P wave usually differs in contour from sinus beats and is often buried in the QRS complex.

► Treatment

In the absence of structural heart disease, serious effects are rare, and most episodes resolve spontaneously. Particular effort should be made to terminate the episode quickly if cardiac failure, syncope, or anginal pain develops or if there is underlying cardiac or (particularly) coronary disease. Because reentry is the most common mechanism for paroxysmal supraventricular tachycardia, effective therapy requires that conduction be interrupted at some point in the reentry circuit and the vast majority of these circuits involve the AV node.

A. Mechanical Measures

A variety of maneuvers have been used to interrupt episodes, and patients may learn to perform these themselves. These maneuvers result in an acute increase in vagal tone and include the Valsalva maneuver, stretching the arms and body, lowering the head between the knees, coughing, splashing cold water on the face, and breath holding. Carotid sinus massage is often performed by physicians but should be avoided if the patient has carotid bruits or a history of transient cerebral ischemic attacks. Firm but gentle pressure and massage are applied first over the right carotid sinus for 10–20 seconds and, if unsuccessful, then over the left carotid sinus. Pressure should not be exerted on both sides at the same time. Continuous ECG or auscultatory monitoring of the heart rate is essential so that pressure can be relieved as soon as the rhythm is broken or if excessive bradycardia occurs. Carotid sinus pressure will interrupt up to half of the attacks, especially if the patient has received a digitalis glycoside or other agent (such as a calcium channel blocker) that delays AV conduction. These maneuvers stimulate a vagal outpouring, delay AV conduction, and block the reentry mechanism at the level of the AV node, terminating the arrhythmia.

B. Drug Therapy

If mechanical measures fail, two rapidly acting intravenous agents will terminate more than 90% of episodes. Intravenous **adenosine** has a very brief duration of action and minimal negative inotropic activity (Table 10–12). Because the half-life of adenosine is < 10 seconds, the drug must be given rapidly (in 1–2 seconds from a peripheral intravenous line); use half the dose if given through a central line. Adenosine causes block of electrical conduction through the AV node. Adenosine is very well tolerated, but nearly 20% of patients will experience transient flushing, and some patients experience severe chest discomfort. Caution must be taken when adenosine is given to elderly patients because the resulting pause can be prolonged. Adenosine must also be used with caution in patients with reactive airways disease because it can promote bronchospasm.

Calcium channel blockers also rapidly induce AV block and break many episodes of reentrant supraventricular tachycardia (Table 10–12). These agents should be used with caution in patients with heart failure due to their negative inotropic effects. These agents include verapamil and diltiazem. Diltiazem may cause less hypotension and myocardial depression than verapamil.

Intravenous beta-blockers include **esmolol** (a very short-acting beta-blocker), propranolol, and metoprolol. All may be effective for virtually any type of supraventricular tachycardia and cause less myocardial depression than the calcium channel blockers. If the tachycardia is believed to be mediated by an accessory pathway, intravenous **procainamide** may terminate the tachycardia by prolonging refractoriness in the accessory pathway; however, because it facilitates AV conduction and an initial increase in rate may occur, it is usually not given until after a calcium channel blocker or a beta-blocker has been administered. Although intravenous amiodarone is safe, it is usually not required and often ineffective for treatment of these arrhythmias.

C. Cardioversion

If the patient is hemodynamically unstable or if adenosine, beta-blockers, and calcium channel blockers are contraindicated or ineffective, synchronized electrical cardioversion (beginning at 100 J) is almost universally successful. If digitalis toxicity is present or strongly suspected, as in the case of paroxysmal tachycardia with block, electrical cardioversion should be avoided.

▶ Prevention

A. Catheter Ablation

Because of concerns about the safety and the intolerability of antiarrhythmic medications, radiofrequency ablation is the preferred approach to patients with recurrent symptomatic reentrant supraventricular tachycardia, whether it is due to dual pathways within the AV node or to accessory pathways.

B. Drugs

AV nodal blocking agents are the drugs of choice as first-line medical therapy (Table 10–12). Beta-blockers or non-dihydropyridine calcium channel blockers, such as diltiazem and verapamil, are typically used first. Patients who do not respond to agents that increase refractoriness of the AV node may be treated with antiarrhythmics. The class Ic agents (flecainide, propafenone) can be used in patients without underlying structural heart disease. In patients with evidence of structural heart disease, class III agents, such as sotalol or amiodarone, are probably a better choice because of the lower incidence of ventricular proarrhythmia during long-term therapy.

Colucci RA et al. Common types of supraventricular tachycardia: diagnosis and management. Am Fam Physician. 2010 Oct 15;82(8):942–52. [PMID: 20949888]

Link MS. Clinical practice. Evaluation and initial treatment of supraventricular tachycardia. N Engl J Med. 2012 Oct 11;367(15):1438–48. [PMID: 23050527]

Linton NW et al. Narrow complex (supraventricular) tachycardias. Postgrad Med J. 2009 Oct;85(1008):546–51. [PMID: 19789194]

Marill KA et al. Adenosine for wide-complex tachycardia: efficacy and safety. Crit Care Med. 2009 Sep;37(9):2512–8. [PMID: 19623049]

Rosso R et al. Focal atrial tachycardia. Heart. 2010 Feb;96(3):181–5. [PMID: 19443472]

Tabatabaei N et al. Supravalvular arrhythmia: identifying and ablating the substrate. Circ Arrhythm Electrophysiol. 2009 Jun;2(3):316–26. [PMID: 19808482]

SUPRAVENTRICULAR TACHYCARDIAS DUE TO ACCESSORY AV PATHWAYS (Preexcitation Syndromes)

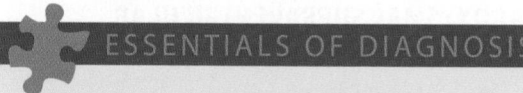

▶ Frequently associated with palpitations.

▶ Can be associated with syncope.

▶ Rapid, regular rhythm.

▶ May have narrow or wide QRS complex on ECG.

▶ Often have preexcitation (delta wave) on baseline ECG.

▶ General Considerations

Accessory pathways or bypass tracts between the atrium and the ventricle bypass the compact AV node and can predispose to reentrant arrhythmias, such as AV reciprocating tachycardia (AVRT) and atrial fibrillation. These may be wholly or partly within the node (eg, Mahaim fibers), yielding a short PR interval and normal QRS morphology. More commonly, they make direct connections between the atrium and ventricle through Kent bundles **(Wolff-Parkinson-White syndrome)**. This often produces a short PR interval with a delta wave (preexcitation) at the onset of the wide, slurred QRS complex owing to early ventricular depolarization of the region adjacent to the pathway. Although the morphology and polarity of the delta wave can suggest the location of the pathway, mapping by intracardiac recordings is required for precise anatomic localization.

Accessory pathways occur in 0.1–0.3% of the population and facilitate reentrant arrhythmias owing to the disparity in refractory periods of the AV node and accessory pathway. Whether the tachycardia is associated with a narrow or wide QRS complex is frequently determined by whether antegrade conduction is through the node (narrow) or the bypass tract (wide). Some bypass tracts only conduct in a retrograde direction. In these cases, the bypass tract is termed "concealed" because it is not readily apparent on a baseline (sinus) ECG. Orthodromic reentrant tachycardia is a reentrant rhythm that conducts antegrade down the AV node and retrograde up the accessory pathway, resulting in a narrow QRS complex unless an underlying bundle branch block or interventricular conduction delay is present. Antidromic reentrant tachycardia conducts antegrade down the accessory pathway and retrograde through the AV node, resulting in a wide and often bizarre appearing QRS complex. Accessory pathways are often less refractory than specialized conduction tissue and thus tachycardias involving accessory pathways have the potential to be more rapid. Up to 30% of patients with Wolff-Parkinson-White syndrome will develop atrial fibrillation or flutter with antegrade conduction down the accessory pathway and a rapid ventricular response. If this conduction is very rapid, it can potentially degenerate to ventricular fibrillation.

▶ Clinical Findings & Treatment

Some patients have a delta wave found incidentally on ECG (Wolff-Parkinson-White pattern). Even in the absence of palpitations, light-headedness, or syncope, these patients are at higher risk for sudden cardiac death than the general population. Risk factors include younger age (< 30), male sex, history of atrial fibrillation and associated congenital heart disease. Multiple risk stratification strategies have been proposed to identify asymptomatic patients with Wolff-Parkinson-White pattern ECG who may be at higher risk for lethal cardiac arrhythmias. A sudden loss of preexcitation during exercise testing likely indicates an accessory pathway with poor conduction properties and therefore low risk for rapid anterograde conduction. In the absence of this finding or other signs of weak anterograde properties (intermittent preexcitation on resting ECG or Holter monitoring), patients may be referred for invasive electrophysiology testing. During the study, patients found to have the shortest preexcited R-R interval (SPERRI) during atrial fibrillation of ≤ 250 msec or inducible supraventricular tachycardia are at increased risk for sudden cardiac death and should undergo catheter ablation.

A. Catheter Ablation

As with AVNRT, radiofrequency catheter ablation has become the procedure of choice in patients with accessory pathways and recurrent symptoms or asymptomatic patients with Wolff-Parkinson-White pattern ECG and high risk features at baseline or during electrophysiology study. Success rates for ablation of accessory pathways with radiofrequency catheters exceed 95% in appropriate patients. Major complications from catheter ablation are rare but include AV block, cardiac tamponade, and thromboembolic events. Minor complications, including hematoma at the catheter access site, occurs in 1–2% of procedures.

B. Pharmacologic Therapy

Narrow-complex reentrant rhythms involving a bypass tract can be managed as discussed for AVNRT. Atrial fibrillation and flutter with a concomitant antegrade conducting bypass tract must be managed differently, since agents such as digoxin, calcium channel blockers, and even beta-blockers may increase the refractoriness of the AV node with minimal or no effect on the accessory pathway, often leading to faster ventricular rates. Therefore, these agents should be avoided. The class Ia, class Ic, and class III antiarrhythmic agents will increase the refractoriness of the bypass tract and are the drugs of choice for wide-complex tachycardias involving accessory pathways. If hemodynamic compromise is present, electrical cardioversion is warranted.

Long-term therapy often involves a combination of agents that increase refractoriness in the bypass tract (class Ia or Ic agents) and in the AV node (calcium channel blockers and beta-blockers), provided that atrial fibrillation or flutter with short RR cycle lengths is not present (see above). The class III agent, amiodarone, can be effective in refractory cases. Patients who are difficult to manage should undergo electrophysiologic evaluation.

▶ When to Refer

- Patients with an incidental finding of Wolff-Parkinson-White pattern on ECG without evidence of loss of preexcitation spontaneously or during exercise testing.
- Patients with recurrent symptoms or episodes despite treatment with AV nodal blocking agents.
- Patients with preexcitation and a history of atrial fibrillation.

▶ When to Admit

- Patients with paroxysmal supraventricular tachycardia and syncope.
- Patients with a history of syncope and preexcitation identified on an ECG.

Cohen MI et al. PACES/HRS expert consensus statement on the management of the asymptomatic young patient with a Wolff-Parkinson-White (WPW, ventricular preexcitation) electrocardiographic pattern: developed in partnership between the Pediatric and Congenital Electrophysiology Society (PACES) and the Heart Rhythm Society (HRS). Endorsed by the governing bodies of PACES, HRS, the American College of Cardiology Foundation (ACCF), the American Heart Association (AHA), the American Academy of Pediatrics (AAP), and the Canadian Heart Rhythm Society (CHRS). Heart Rhythm. 2012 Jun;9(6):1006–24. [PMID: 22579340]

Czosek RJ et al. Cost-effectiveness of various risk stratification methods for asymptomatic ventricular pre-excitation. Am J Cardiol. 2013 Jul 15;112(2):245–50. [PMID: 23587276]

Mark DG et al. Preexcitation syndromes: diagnostic consideration in the ED. Am J Emerg Med. 2009 Sep;27(7):878–88. [PMID: 19683122]

Obeyesekere MN et al. Risk of arrhythmia and sudden death in patients with asymptomatic preexcitation: a meta-analysis. Circulation. 2012 May 15;125(19):2308–15. [PMID: 22532593]

ATRIAL FIBRILLATION

 ESSENTIALS OF DIAGNOSIS

- ▶ Irregularly irregular heart rhythm.
- ▶ Usually tachycardic.
- ▶ Often associated with palpitations (acute onset) or fatigue (chronic).
- ▶ ECG shows erratic atrial activity with irregular ventricular response.
- ▶ High risk for thromboembolism: common cause of stroke.
- ▶ High incidence and prevalence in the elderly population.

▶ General Considerations

Atrial fibrillation is the most common chronic arrhythmia, with an incidence and prevalence that rise with age, so that it affects approximately 9% of individuals over age

80 years. It occurs in rheumatic and other forms of VHD, dilated cardiomyopathy, ASD, hypertension, and coronary heart disease as well as in patients with no apparent cardiac disease; it may be the initial presenting sign in thyrotoxicosis, and this condition should be excluded with the initial episode. The atrial activity may be very fine and difficult to detect on the ECG, or quite coarse and often mistaken for atrial flutter. Atrial fibrillation often appears in a paroxysmal fashion before becoming the established rhythm. Pericarditis, chest trauma, thoracic or cardiac surgery, thyroid disorders, obstructive sleep apnea, or pulmonary disease (as well as medications such as theophylline and beta-adrenergic agonists) may cause attacks in patients with normal hearts. Acute alcohol excess and alcohol withdrawal—and, in predisposed individuals, even consumption of small amounts of alcohol—may precipitate atrial fibrillation. This latter presentation, which is often termed "holiday heart," is usually transient and self-limited. Short-term rate control usually suffices as treatment. Perhaps the most serious consequence of atrial fibrillation is the propensity for thrombus formation due to stasis in the atria (particularly the left atrial appendage) and consequent embolization, most devastatingly to the cerebral circulation. Overall, the rate of stroke is approximately 5% per year. However, patients with significant obstructive valvular disease, chronic heart failure or LV dysfunction, diabetes mellitus, hypertension, or age over 75 years and those with a history of prior stroke or other embolic events are at substantially higher risk (up to nearly 20% per year in patients with multiple risk factors) (Table 10–13). A substantial portion of the aging population with hypertension has asymptomatic or "subclinical" atrial fibrillation that is also associated with increased risk of stroke.

▶ Clinical Findings

A. Symptoms and Signs

Atrial fibrillation itself is rarely life-threatening; however, it can have serious consequences if the ventricular rate is sufficiently rapid to precipitate hypotension, myocardial ischemia, or tachycardia-induced myocardial dysfunction. Moreover, particularly in patients with risk factors, atrial fibrillation is a major preventable cause of stroke. Although many patients—particularly older or inactive individuals—have relatively few symptoms if the rate is controlled, some patients are aware of the irregular rhythm and may find it very uncomfortable. Most patients will complain of fatigue whether they experience other symptoms or not. The heart rate may range from quite slow to extremely rapid, but is uniformly irregular unless underlying complete heart block with junctional escape rhythm or a permanent ventricular pacemaker is in place. Atrial fibrillation is the only common arrhythmia in which the ventricular rate is rapid and the rhythm very irregular. Because of the varying stroke volumes resulting from fluctuating periods of diastolic filling, not all ventricular beats produce a palpable peripheral pulse. The difference between the apical rate and the pulse rate is the "pulse deficit"; this deficit is greater when the ventricular rate is high.

Table 10–13. CHADS$_2$ Risk Score for assessing risk of stroke and for selecting antithrombotic therapy for patients with atrial fibrillation.

	Condition	Points
C	Congestive heart failure	1
H	Hypertension (current or treated)	1
A	Age ≥ 75 years	1
D	Diabetes mellitus	1
S$_2$	Stroke or transient ischemic attack	2
CHADS$_2$ Score	**Adjusted Stroke Rate,%/year (95% Confidence Interval)**	**Patients[1] (n = 1733)**
0	1.9 (1.2 to 3.0)	120
1	2.8 (2.0 to 3.8)	463
2	4.0 (3.1 to 5.1)	523
3	5.9 (4.6 to 7.3)	337
4	8.5 (6.3 to 11)	220
5	12.5 (8.2 to 17.5)	65

[1]Validation performed in a population of Medicare beneficiaries age 65 to 95 years who were not prescribed warfarin at hospital discharge.

Reproduced, with permission, from Gage BF et al. Validation of clinical classification schemes for predicting stroke: results from the National Registry of Atrial Fibrillation. JAMA. 2001;285(22): 2864–70.

B. ECG

The surface ECG typically demonstrates erratic, disorganized atrial activity between discrete QRS complexes occurring in an irregular pattern. The atrial activity may be very fine and difficult to detect on the ECG, or quite coarse and often mistaken for atrial flutter.

▶ Treatment

A. Newly Diagnosed Atrial Fibrillation

1. Initial management

A. HEMODYANMICALIY UNSTABLE PATIENT—If the patient is hemodynamically unstable—usually as a result of a rapid ventricular rate or associated cardiac or noncardiac conditions—hospitalization and immediate treatment of atrial fibrillation are required. Urgent cardioversion is usually indicated in patients with shock or severe hypotension, pulmonary edema, or ongoing myocardial infarction or ischemia. There is a potential risk of thromboembolism in patients undergoing cardioversion who have not received anticoagulation therapy if atrial fibrillation has been present for >48 hours; however, in hemodynamically unstable patients the need for immediate rate control outweighs that risk. Electrical cardioversion is usually preferred in unstable patients. An initial shock with 100–200 J is administered in synchrony with the R wave. If sinus rhythm is not restored, an additional attempt with 360 J is indicated. If this fails, cardioversion may be successful after loading with intravenous **ibutilide** (1 mg over 10 minutes, repeated in 10 minutes if necessary).

B. HEMODYNAMICALIY STABLE PATIENT—If, as is often the case—particularly in older individuals—the patient has no symptoms, hemodynamic instability, or evidence of important precipitating conditions (such as silent myocardial infarction or ischemia, decompensated heart failure, pulmonary embolism, or hemodynamically significant valvular disease), hospitalization is usually not necessary. In most of these cases, atrial fibrillation is an unrecognized chronic or paroxysmal condition and should be managed accordingly (see Subsequent Management, below). For new onset atrial fibrillation, thyroid function tests and assessment for occult valvular or myocardial disease should be performed.

In more stable patients or those at particularly high risk for embolism (ie, underlying mitral stenosis, a history of prior embolism, or severe heart failure), a strategy of rate control and anticoagulation is appropriate. This is also true when the conditions that precipitated atrial fibrillation are likely to persist (such as following cardiac or noncardiac surgery, with respiratory failure, or with pericarditis). Rate control and anticoagulation is also appropriate even when the conditions causing the atrial fibrillation might resolve spontaneously over a period of hours to days (such as atrial fibrillation due to excessive alcohol intake, electrolyte imbalance or atrial fibrillation due to exposure to excessive theophylline or sympathomimetic agents). The choice of agent is guided by the hemodynamic status of the patient, associated conditions, and the urgency of achieving rate control. Although both hypotension and heart failure may improve when the ventricular rate is slowed, calcium channel blockers and beta-blockers may themselves precipitate hemodynamic deterioration. Digoxin is less risky, but even when used aggressively (0.5 mg intravenously over 30 minutes, followed by increments of 0.25 mg every 1–2 hours to a total dose of 1–1.5 mg over 24 hours in patients not previously receiving this agent), rate control is rather slow and may be inadequate, particularly in patients with sympathetic activation.

In the setting of myocardial infarction or ischemia, beta-blockers are the preferred agent. The most frequently used agents are either metoprolol (administered as a 5 mg intravenous bolus, repeated twice at intervals of 5 minutes and then given as needed by repeat boluses or orally at total daily doses of 50–400 mg) or, in very unstable patients, esmolol (0.5 mg/kg intravenously, repeated once if necessary, followed by a titrated infusion of 0.05–0.2 mg/kg/min). If beta-blockers are contraindicated, calcium channel blockers are immediately effective. Diltiazem (20 mg bolus, repeated after 15 minutes if necessary, followed by a maintenance infusion of 5–15 mg/h) is the preferred calcium blocker if hypotension or LV dysfunction is present. Otherwise, verapamil (5–10 mg intravenously over 2–3 minutes, repeated after 30 minutes if necessary) may be used. Amiodarone, even when administered intravenously, has a relatively slow onset but is often a useful adjunct when rate control with the previously cited agents is incomplete or contraindicated or when cardioversion is planned in the near future. However, amiodarone should not be used in this setting if long-term therapy is planned with other antiarrhythmic agents.

If the onset of atrial fibrillation was > 48 hours prior to presentation (or unknown) and early cardioversion is considered necessary due to inability to adequately rate control, a transesophageal echocardiogram should be performed prior to cardioversion to exclude left atrial thrombus. If thrombus is present, the cardioversion is delayed until after a 4-week period of therapeutic anticoagulation. In any case, because atrial contractile activity may not recover for several weeks after restoration of sinus rhythm in patients who have been in atrial fibrillation for more than several days, cardioversion should be followed by anticoagulation for at least 1 month unless there is a strong contraindication.

2. Subsequent management—Up to two-thirds of patients experiencing a first episode of atrial fibrillation will spontaneously revert to sinus rhythm within 24 hours. In the absence of VHD, diabetes, hypertension or other risk factors for stroke, these patients may not require long-term anticoagulation beyond aspirin. If atrial fibrillation persists or has been present for more than a week, spontaneous conversion is unlikely. In most cases immediate cardioversion is not required and management consists of rate control and anticoagulation whether or not the patient has been admitted to the hospital. Rate control is usually relatively easy to achieve with beta-blockers, rate-slowing calcium blockers and, occasionally, digoxin, used as single agents or more often in combination. In older patients, who often have diminished AV nodal function and relatively limited activity, modest rate control can often be achieved with a single agent. Many younger or more active individuals require a combination of two agents. Choice of the initial medication is best based on the presence of accompanying conditions: Hypertensive patients should be given beta-blockers or calcium blockers (see Tables 11–6 and 11–8); coronary patients should usually receive a beta-blocker; and patients with heart failure should be given a beta-blocker with consideration of adding digoxin. Adequacy of rate control should be evaluated by recording the apical pulse rate both at rest and with an appropriate level of activity (such as after brisk walking around the corridor or climbing stairs).

A. ANTICOAGULATION—For patients with atrial fibrillation, even when it is paroxysmal or occurs rarely, the need for oral anticoagulation should be evaluated and treatment initiated for those without strong contraindication. Patients with "**lone atrial fibrillation**" (eg, no evidence of associated heart disease, hypertension, atherosclerotic vascular disease, diabetes mellitus, or history of stroke or TIA) under age 65 years need no antithrombotic treatment. Patients with **transient atrial fibrillation**, such as in the setting of acute myocardial infarction or pneumonia, but no prior history of arrhythmia, are at high risk for future development of atrial fibrillation and appropriate anticoagulation should be initiated based on risk factors (see Table 10–13). If the cause is **reversible**, such as after coronary artery bypass surgery or associated with hyperthyroidism, then long term anticoagulation is not necessary.

In addition to the traditional five risk factors that comprise the CHADS$_2$ score (heart failure, hypertension, age ≥ 75 years, diabetes mellitus, and [2 points for] history of

Table 10–14. CHA$_2$DS$_2$-VASc Risk Score for assessing risk of stroke and for selecting antithrombotic therapy for patients with atrial fibrillation.

CHA$_2$DS$_2$-VASc Risk Score	
Heart failure or LVEF ≤ 40% 1	1
Hypertension	1
Age ≥ 75 years	2
Diabetes mellitus	1
Stroke, transient ischemic attack, or thromboembolism	2
Vascular disease (previous myocardial infarction, peripheral artery disease, or aortic plaque)	1
Age 65–74 years	1
Sex category (ie, female sex)	1
Maximum score	9

Adjusted stroke rate according to CHA$_2$DS$_2$-VASc score

CHA$_2$DS$_2$-VASc Score	Patients (n=7329)	Adjusted stroke rate (%/year)
0	1	0%
1	422	1.3%
2	1230	2.2%
3	1730	3.2%
4	1718	4.0%
5	1159	6.7%
6	679	9.8%
7	294	9.6%
8	82	6.7 %
9	14	15.2%

CHA$_2$DS$_2$-VASc score = 0: recommend no antithrombotic therapy

CHA$_2$DS$_2$-VASc score = 1: recommend antithrombotic therapy with oral anticoagulation or antiplatelet therapy but preferably oral anticoagulation.

CHA$_2$DS$_2$-VASc score = 2: recommend oral anticoagulation

Modified, with permission, from Camm AJ et al. 2012 focused update of the ESC Guidelines for the management of atrial fibrillation: an update of the 2010 ESC Guidelines for the management of atrial fibrillation. Developed with the special contribution of the European Heart Rhythm Association. Eur Heart J. 2012 Nov;33(21) 2719–47. [PMID: 22922413]

CHA$_2$DS$_2$-VASc, Cardiac failure, Hypertension, Age ≥ 75 years (Doubled), Diabetes, Stroke (Doubled), Vascular disease, Age 65–74, and Sex category (Female); LVEF, left ventricular ejection fraction.

stroke or transient ischemic attack), the European and American guidelines recommend that three additional factors included in the CHA$_2$DS$_2$-VASc score be considered: age 65–74 years, female gender, and presence of vascular disease (Table 10–14). The CHA$_2$DSv-VASc score is especially relevant for patients who have a CHADS$_2$ score of 0 or 1; if the CHA$_2$DS$_2$-VASc score is ≥ 2, oral anticoagulation is recommended, and if CHA$_2$DS$_2$-VASc score is 1, oral anticoagulation, aspirin, or no anticoagulation can be used, with a preference for oral anticoagulation, taking into account risk, benefit, and patient preferences. The use of warfarin is discussed in the section on Selecting Appropriate Anticoagulant Therapy in Chapter 14. Unfortunately, studies show that only about half of patients with atrial fibrillation and an indication for oral anticoagulation are receiving it, and even when treated with warfarin, they are out of the target INR range nearly half the time. Cardioversion, if planned, should be performed after at least 3–4 weeks of anticoagulation at a therapeutic level (or after exclusion of left atrial appendage thrombus by transesophageal echocardiogram as discussed above). Anticoagulation clinics with systematic management of warfarin dosing and adjustment have been shown to result in better maintenance of target anticoagulation.

Three target specific (or direct acting) oral anticoagulants—dabigatran, rivaroxaban, and apixaban—have been shown to be at least as effective as warfarin for stroke prevention in patients with nonvalvular atrial fibrillation (Table 10–15).

Dabigatran was compared with warfarin (in the RELY trial) for prevention of stroke and systemic embolism for patients with atrial fibrillation and at least one additional risk factor for stroke. The lower dabigatran dose (110 mg orally twice daily) was noninferior to warfarin in stroke prevention and caused significantly less bleeding, and a second higher (150 mg orally twice daily) dose, which has been approved by the FDA, resulted in significantly fewer strokes with similar bleeding rates. Both doses of dabigatran caused substantially less intracerebral hemorrhage than warfarin. There is higher incidence of gastrointestinal bleeding with dabigatran, and there is no readily available direct reversal agent. In spite of this, when oral anticoagulation with either dabigatran or warfarin was stopped for elective or emergency procedures or surgery in the RELY trial, the risk of bleeding was numerically lower with dabigatran than with warfarin. Dabigatran is 80% renally metabolized. In the United States, the 110 mg dose is not approved, and creatinine clearance should be calculated before initiating therapy. The lower dose of 75 mg twice a day is recommended for patients with creatinine clearances 15–30 mL/min, although clinical practice guidelines recommend avoiding any of the target specific oral anticoagulants in patients with an estimated creatine clearance < 30 mL/min since these patients were excluded from the clinical trials. There is no widely available test to accurately measure the effect of dabigatran, although the aPTT is affected by dabigatran and a normal aPTT suggests little if any dabigatran effect. Patients may be converted from warfarin to dabigatran by stopping the warfarin and beginning dabigatran once the INR is ≤ 2.0, and this is a reasonable approach for transition from warfarin to any of the target specific oral anticoagulants. Neither dabigatran nor any of the target specific oral anticoagulants should be used in patients with mechanical prosthetic heart valves.

Rivaroxaban is approved by the FDA for stroke prevention in nonvalvular atrial fibrillation. In the ROCKET-AF trial, rivaroxaban proved noninferior to warfarin for stroke prevention for patients with high-risk features of thromboembolism, with half of the patients in the ROCKET-AF trial having a history of stroke. Rivaroxaban is dosed at 20 mg once daily, with a reduced dose (15 mg/d) for patients with creatinine clearances < 50 mL/min. Similar to dabigatran,

Table 10–15. Target specific oral anticoagulants for stroke prevention in patients with nonvalvular atrial fibrillation.

	Dabigatran	Rivaroxaban	Apixaban
Class	Antithrombin	Factor Xa inhibitor	Factor Xa inhibitor
Bleeding risk compared to warfarin	Less intracranial bleeding Higher incidence of gastrointestinal bleeding	Less intracranial bleeding Higher incidence of gastro-intestinal bleeding	Substantially lower risk of major bleeding Less intracranial bleeding
Dosage	110 mg twice daily 150 mg twice daily	20 mg once daily	5 mg twice daily
Dosage adjustments	75 mg twice daily for GFR 15-30 mL/min (approved but not tested in clinical trials)	15 mg once daily for GFR <50 mL/min	2.5 mg twice daily for patients with at least two of three risk factors: 1. Age ≥ 80 years 2. Body weight ≤ 60 kg 3. Serum creatinine ≥ 1.5 mg/dL

(Reproduced, with permission, from Nishimura RA et al. 2014 AHA/ACC Guideline for the Management of Patients With Valvular Heart Disease: A Report of the American College of Cardiology/American Heart Association Task Force on Practice Guidelines. Circulation. 2014 Mar 3. [Epub ahead of print] [PMID: 24589853]

there was substantially less intracranial hemorrhage with rivaroxaban than warfarin.

Apixaban is more effective than warfarin at stroke prevention while having a substantially lower risk of major bleeding (in the ARISOTLE trial) and a lower risk of all-cause mortality. Apixaban is approved by the FDA and its dosage is 5 mg twice daily or 2.5 mg twice daily for patients with two of three high-risk criteria (age ≥ 80 years, body weight ≤ 60 kg, and serum creatinine ≥ 1.5 mg/dL). Apixaban is associated with less intracranial hemorrhage and is well tolerated. Apixaban was also shown to be superior to aspirin (and better tolerated) in the AVER-ROES trial of patients deemed not suitable for warfarin. These target specific oral anticoagulants have important advantages over warfarin, and therefore they are recommended preferentially over vitamin K antagonists in the European Guidelines (Figure 10–9).

There are some patients with atrial fibrillation, however, who should be treated with vitamin K antagonists. These patients include those who have mechanical prosthetic valves, advanced kidney disease (creatinine clearance < 30 mL/min), moderate or severe mitral stenosis, and those who cannot afford the newer drugs. Patients who have been stable on warfarin for a long period of time, with a high time in target INR range, and who are at lower risk for intracranial hemorrhage will have relatively less benefit to switch to a newer drug.

There are some important practical issues with using the newer drugs. It is important to monitor kidney function at baseline and at least once a year, or more often for those with impaired kidney function. Each of the drugs interacts with other drugs affecting the P-glycoprotein pathway, like oral ketoconazole, verapamil, and dronederone. To transition patients from warfarin to a direct-acting drug, wait until the INR decreases to about 2.0. Each of the drugs has a half-life of about 10 hours for patients with normal kidney function. For elective procedures, stop the drugs two to three half-lives before procedures with low to moderate bleeding risk (ie, colonoscopy, dental extraction, cardiac catheterization), and five half-lives before procedures like major surgery. There are no practical tests to

immediately measure the effect of the drugs, although a normal aPTT suggests little effect with dabigatran, and a normal prothrombin suggests little effect with rivaroxaban. For rivaroxaban and apixaban, chromogenic Xa assays will measure the effect, but may not be readily available. For bleeding, standard measures (eg, diagnosing and controlling the source, stopping antithrombotic agents, and replacing blood products) should be taken. If the direct-acting drug was taken in the prior 2–4 hours, use activated oral charcoal to reduce absorption. If the patient is taking aspirin, consider platelet transfusion. For life-threatening bleeding, prothrombin complex concentrate may have an effect, but this should generally be used in consultation with hematology. For cardioversion, the target specific drugs appear to have similar rates of subsequent stroke as warfarin, as long as patients have been taking the drugs and adherent for at least several weeks. Like with warfarin, there appears to be a 1.5- to 2-fold increased rate of bleeding associated with the use of aspirin, which therefore should not be used with the oral anticoagulants unless there is a clear indication, like acute coronary syndrome within the prior year.

The management of serious bleeding events for patients on target specific oral anticoagulants is under investigation, however preliminary data suggest that administration of coagulation factors (activated or four-factor prothrombin complex concentrate) may quickly reverse the effects of these agents. Due to the short half-life of the target specific oral anticoagulants (9–12 hours with normal kidney function), supportive measures (packed red blood cells, FFP, platelets) may suffice until the drug has cleared.

The safety of electrical cardioversion has not been specifically studied for any of the three target specific agents, although there is experience with several hundred patients in each of the clinical trials comparing the new agents to warfarin. While the experience is limited, stroke risk following cardioversion was reported to be low and similar to the risk in patients treated with warfarin. Most patients had been taking anticoagulants for at least several weeks prior to cardioversion and therefore the strategy of 3–4 weeks of stable anticoagulation or transesophageal echocardiogram to exclude left atrial thrombus prior to cardioversion applies.

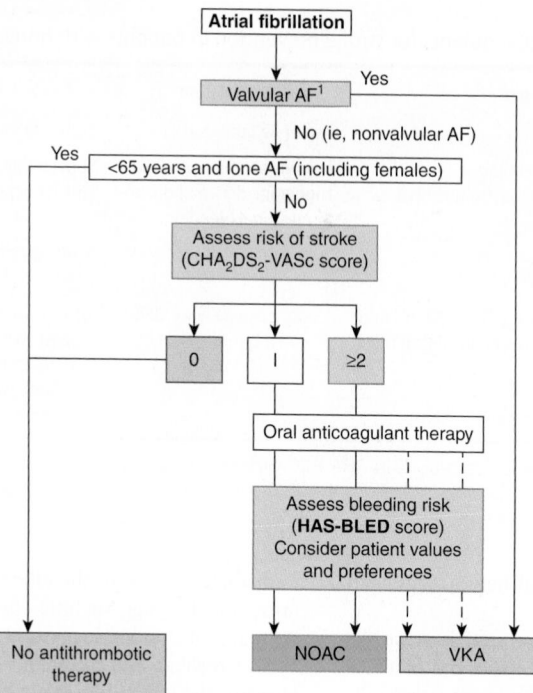

Antiplatelet therapy with aspirin plus clopidogrel, or–less effectively–aspirin only, should be considered in patients who refuse any OAC, or cannot tolerate anticoagulants for reasons unrelated to bleeding. If there are contraindications to OAC or antiplatelet therapy, left atrial appendage occlusion, closure or excision may be considered.
Colour: CHA_2DS_2-VASc; green = 0, blue = I, red ≥2.
Line: solid = best option; dashed = alternative option.
AF = atrial fibrillation; CHA_2DS_2-VASc = see text; HAS-BLED = see text; NOAC = novel oral anticoagulant; OAC = oral anticoagulant; VKA = vitamin K antagonist.
[1]Includes rheumatic valvular disease and prosthetic valves.

▲ **Figure 10–9.** Choice of anticoagulant. (Reproduced, with permission, from Camm AJ et al. 2012 focused update of the ESC Guidelines for the management of atrial fibrillation: an update of the 2010 ESC Guidelines for the management of atrial fibrillation. Developed with the special contribution of the European Heart Rhythm Association. Eur Heart J. 2012 Nov;33(21):2719-47.)

B. Rate control or elective cardioversion—Two large randomized controlled trials (the 4060-patient Atrial Fibrillation Follow-up Investigation of Rhythm Management, or AFFIRM trial; and the Rate Control Versus Electrical Cardioversion for Persistent Atrial Fibrillation, or RACE trial) compared strategies of rate control and rhythm control. In both, a strategy of rate control and long-term anticoagulation was associated with no higher rates of death or stroke—both, if anything, favored rate control—and only a modestly increased risk of hemorrhagic events than a strategy of restoring sinus rhythm and maintaining it with antiarrhythmic drug therapy. Of note is that exercise tolerance and quality of life were not significantly better in the rhythm control group. Nonetheless, the decision of whether to attempt to restore sinus rhythm following the initial episode remains controversial. Elective cardioversion following an appropriate period of anticoagulation is generally recommended for the initial episode in patients in whom atrial fibrillation is thought to be of recent onset and when there is an identifiable precipitating factor. Similarly, cardioversion is appropriate in patients who remain symptomatic from the rhythm despite aggressive efforts to achieve rate control.

In cases in which elective cardioversion is required, it may be accomplished electrically or pharmacologically. **Intravenous ibutilide** may be used as described above in a setting in which the patient can undergo continuous ECG monitoring for at least 4–6 hours following administration. In patients in whom a decision has been made to continue antiarrhythmic therapy to maintain sinus rhythm (see next paragraph), cardioversion can be attempted with an agent that is being considered for long-term use. For instance, after therapeutic anticoagulation has been established, amiodarone can be initiated on an outpatient basis (400 mg twice daily for 2 weeks, followed by 200 mg twice daily for at least 2–4 weeks and then a maintenance dose of 200 mg daily). Because amiodarone increases the prothrombin time in patients taking warfarin and increases digoxin levels, careful monitoring of anticoagulation and drug levels is required.

Other agents that may be used for both cardioversion and maintenance therapy include dofetilide, propafenone, flecainide, and sotalol. **Dofetilide** (125–500 mcg twice daily orally) must be initiated in hospital due to the potential risk of torsades de pointes and the downward dose adjustment that is required for patients with renal impairment. Propafenone (150–300 mg orally every 8 hours) should be avoided in patients with structural heart disease (CAD, systolic dysfunction, or significant LVH). **Flecainide** (50–150 mg twice daily orally) should be used in conjunction with an AV nodal blocking drug if there is a history of atrial flutter and should be avoided in patients with structural heart disease. **Sotalol** (80–160 mg orally twice daily) should be initiated in the hospital in patients with structural heart disease due to a risk of torsades de pointes; it is not very effective for converting atrial fibrillation but can be used to maintain sinus rhythm following cardioversion.

In patients treated long-term with an antiarrhythmic agent, sinus rhythm will persist in approximately 50%. The most commonly used medications are amiodarone, dronedarone, sotalol, propafenone, flecainide, and dofetilide, but the latter four agents are associated with a clear risk of proarrhythmia in certain populations; dronedarone has less efficacy than amiodarone, and amiodarone frequently causes other adverse effects. Therefore, after an initial presentation of atrial fibrillation, it may be prudent to determine whether atrial fibrillation recurs during a period of 6 months without antiarrhythmic drugs (during which anticoagulation is maintained). If it does recur, the decision to restore sinus rhythm and initiate long-term antiarrhythmic therapy can be based on how well the patient tolerates atrial fibrillation. The decision to maintain long-term anticoagulation should be based on risk factors (CHADS$_2$ or CHA$_2$DSv-VASc score) and not on the perceived presence or absence of atrial fibrillation as future episodes may be asymptomatic.

B. Paroxysmal and Refractory Atrial Fibrillation

1. Recurrent paroxysmal atrial fibrillation—Patients with recurrent paroxysmal atrial fibrillation are at similar stroke risk as those who are in atrial fibrillation chronically. Although these episodes may be apparent to the patient, many are not recognized and may be totally asymptomatic. Thus, ambulatory ECG monitoring or event recorders are indicated in those in whom paroxysmal atrial fibrillation is suspected. Antiarrhythmic agents are usually not successful in preventing all paroxysmal atrial fibrillation episodes. However, dofetilide has been shown to be as effective as amiodarone in maintaining sinus rhythm in certain patients and does not have as many untoward long-term effects. Long-term anticoagulation should be considered for all patients except in those who are under 65 years of age and have no additional stroke risk factors (see above).

2. Refractory atrial fibrillation—Because of trial results indicating that important adverse clinical outcomes (death, stroke, hemorrhage, heart failure) are no more common with rate control than rhythm control, atrial fibrillation should generally be considered refractory if it causes persistent symptoms or limits activity. This is much more likely in younger individuals and those who are active or engage in strenuous exercise. Even in such individuals, two-drug or three-drug combinations of a beta-blocker, rate-slowing calcium blocker, and digoxin usually can

prevent excessive ventricular rates, though in some cases they are associated with excessive bradycardia during sedentary periods.

If antiarrhythmic or rate-control medications fail to improve the symptoms of atrial fibrillation, catheter ablation of foci in and around the pulmonary veins that initiate atrial fibrillation may be considered. Pulmonary vein isolation is a reasonable second-line therapy for individuals with symptomatic atrial fibrillation that is refractory to pharmacologic therapy. Ablation is successful about 70% of the time but more than one procedure may be required. The procedure is routinely performed in the electrophysiology laboratory using a catheter-based approach and can also be performed via a subxiphoid approach thorascopically, via thoracotomy, or via median sternotomy in the operating room by experienced surgeons. In patients deemed inappropriate for pulmonary vein isolation, radiofrequency ablation of the AV node and permanent pacing ensure rate control and may facilitate a more physiologic rate response to activity, but this is used only as a last resort.

▶ When to Refer

- Symptomatic atrial fibrillation with or without rate control.
- Asymptomatic atrial fibrillation with poor rate control despite AV nodal blockers.

▶ When to Admit

- Atrial fibrillation with rapid ventricular response resulting in hemodynamic compromise.
- Atrial fibrillation resulting in acute heart failure.

Bishara R et al. Transient atrial fibrillation and risk of stroke after acute myocardial infarction. Thromb Haemost. 2011 Nov; 106(5): 877–84. [PMID: 21866303]

Calkins H et al. HRS/HERA/ECAS Expert Consensus Statement on Catheter and Surgical Ablation of Atrial Fibrillation: recommendations for patient selection, procedural techniques, patient management and follow-up, definitions, end-points and research trial design: a report of the Heart Rhythm Society (HRS) Task Force on Catheter and Surgical Ablation of Atrial Fibrillation. Developed in partnership with the European Heart Rhythm Association (EHRA), a registered branch of the European Society of Cardiology (ESC) and the European Cardiac Arrhythmia Society (ECAS); and in collaboration with the American College of Cardiology (ACC), American Heart Association (AHA), the Asia Pacific Heart Rhythm Society (APHRS), and the Society of Thoracic Surgeons (STS). Heart Rhythm. 2012 Apr;9(4):632–96, e21 [PMID: 22386883]

Connolly SJ et al; RELY Steering Committee and Investigators. Dabigatran versus warfarin in patients with atrial fibrillation. N Engl J Med. 2009 Sep 17;361(12):1139–51. Erratum in: N Engl J Med. 2010 Nov 4;363(19):1877. [PMID: 19717844]

Durrant J et al. Stroke risk stratification scores in atrial fibrillation: current recommendations for clinical practice and future perspectives. Expert Rev Cardiovasc Ther. 2013 Jan;11(1): 77–90. [PMID: 23259448]

Granger CB et al; ARISTOTLE Committees and Investigators. Apixaban versus warfarin in patients with atrial fibrillation. N Engl J Med. 2011 Sep 15;365(11):981–92. [PMID: 21870978]

Healey JS et al; ASSERT Investigators. Subclinical atrial fibrillation and the risk of stroke. N Engl J Med. 2012 Jan 12;366(2): 120–9. [PMID: 22236222]

January CT et al. 2014 AHA/ACC/HRS Guideline for the Management of Patients With Atrial Fibrillation: A Report of the American College of Cardiology/American Heart Association Task Force on Practice Guidelines and the Heart Rhythm Society. Circulation. 2014 Apr 10. [Epub ahead of print] No abstract available. [PMD: 24682347]

Nagarakanti R et al. Dabigatran versus warfarin in patients with atrial fibrillation: an analysis of patients undergoing cardioversion. Circulation. 2011 Jan 18;123(2):131–6. [PMID: 21200007]

Patel MR et al; ROCKET AF Investigators. Rivaroxaban versus warfarin in nonvalvular atrial fibrillation. N Engl J Med. 2011 Sep 8;365(10):883–91. [PMID: 21830957]

Van Gelder IC et al; RACE II Investigators. Lenient versus strict rate control in patients with atrial fibrillation. N Engl J Med. 2010 Apr 15;362(15):1363–73. [PMID: 20231232]

ATRIAL FLUTTER

ESSENTIALS OF DIAGNOSIS

▶ Usually regular heart rhythm.

▶ Often tachycardic (100–150 beats/min).

▶ Often associated with palpitations (acute onset) or fatigue (chronic).

▶ ECG shows "sawtooth" pattern of atrial activity in leads II, III, and AVF.

▶ Often seen in conjunction with structural heart disease or chronic obstructive pulmonary disease (COPD).

Atrial flutter is less common than fibrillation. It occurs most often in patients with COPD but may be seen also in those with rheumatic or coronary heart disease, heart failure, ASD, or surgically repaired congenital heart disease. The reentrant circuit generates atrial rates of 250–350 beats/min, usually with transmission of every second, third, or fourth impulse through the AV node to the ventricles. The ECG typically demonstrates a "sawtooth" pattern of atrial activity in the inferior leads (II, III, and AVF).

▶ Treatment

Ventricular rate control is accomplished using the same agents used in atrial fibrillation, but it is much more difficult with atrial flutter than with atrial fibrillation. Conversion of atrial flutter to sinus rhythm with class I antiarrhythmic agents is also difficult to achieve, and administration of these drugs has been associated with slowing of the atrial flutter rate to the point at which 1:1 AV conduction can occur at rates in excess of 200 beats/min, with subsequent hemodynamic collapse. The intravenous class III antiarrhythmic agent ibutilide has been significantly more successful in converting atrial flutter (Table 10–12). About 50–70% of patients return to sinus rhythm within 60–90 minutes following the infusion of 1–2 mg of this agent. Electrical cardioversion is also very effective for atrial flutter, with approximately 90% of patients converting following synchronized shocks of as little as 25–50 J.

The persistence of atrial contractile function in this arrhythmia provides some protection against thrombus formation, though the risk of systemic embolization remains increased. Precardioversion anticoagulation is not necessary for atrial flutter of < 48 hours duration except in the setting of mitral valve disease. However, **anticoagulation** with warfarin or the newer anticoagulants (dabigatran, rivaroxaban, or apixaban) is necessary in chronic atrial flutter, given that the stroke risk is the same as with chronic atrial fibrillation, perhaps because transient periods of atrial fibrillation are common in these patients.

Chronic atrial flutter is often a difficult management problem, as rate control is difficult. If pharmacologic therapy is chosen, amiodarone and dofetilide are the antiarrhythmics of choice (Table 10–12). Dofetilide is often given in conjunction with an AV nodal blocker (other than verapamil). Atrial flutter can follow a typical or atypical reentry circuit around the atrium. The anatomy of the typical circuit has been well defined and allows for catheter ablation within the atrium to interrupt the circuit and eliminate atrial flutter. Catheter ablation is a highly successful treatment that has become the preferred approach for recurrent typical atrial flutter.

▶ When to Refer

• Symptomatic atrial flutter with or without rate control.

• Asymptomatic atrial flutter with poor rate control despite AV nodal blockers.

▶ When to Admit

• Atrial flutter with 1:1 conduction resulting in hemodynamic compromise.

• Atrial flutter resulting in acute heart failure.

Parikh MG et al. Usefulness of transesophageal echocardiography to confirm clinical utility of CHA2DS2-VASc and CHADS2 scores in atrial flutter. Am J Cardiol. 2012 Feb 15;109(4):550–5. [PMID: 22133753]

Scheuermeyer FX et al. Emergency department management and 1-year outcomes of patients with atrial flutter. Ann Emerg Med. 2011 Jun;57(6):564–71. [PMID: 21257230]

Spector P et al. Meta-analysis of ablation of atrial flutter and supraventricular tachycardia. Am J Cardiol. 2009 Sep 1;104(5):671–7. [PMID: 19699343]

MULTIFOCAL ATRIAL TACHYCARDIA

ESSENTIALS OF DIAGNOSIS

▶ ECG reveals three or more distinct P-wave morphologies.

▶ Often associated with palpitations.

▶ Associated with severe COPD.

▶ Treatment of the underlying lung disease is the most effective therapy.

This is a rhythm characterized by varying P wave morphology (by definition, three or more foci) and markedly irregular PP intervals. The rate is usually between 100 and 140 beats/min, and AV block is unusual. Most patients have concomitant severe COPD. Treatment of the underlying condition is the most effective approach; verapamil, 240–480 mg orally daily in divided doses, is also of value in some patients, but this particular arrhythmia is very difficult to manage.

Spodick DH. Multifocal atrial arrhythmia. Am J Geriatr Cardiol. 2005 May–Jun;14(3):162. [PMID: 15886545]

AV JUNCTIONAL RHYTHM

ESSENTIALS OF DIAGNOSIS

► Regular heart rhythm.
► Can have wide or narrow QRS complex.
► Often seen in digitalis toxicity.

The atrial-nodal junction or the nodal-His bundle junction may assume pacemaker activity for the heart, usually at a rate of 35–60 beats/min. This may occur in patients with myocarditis, CAD, and digitalis toxicity as well as in individuals with normal hearts. The rate responds normally to exercise, and the diagnosis is often an incidental finding on ECG monitoring, but it can be suspected if the jugular venous pulse shows cannon *a* waves. Junctional rhythm is often an escape rhythm because of depressed sinus node function with sinoatrial block or delayed conduction in the AV node. **Nonparoxysmal junctional tachycardia** results from increased automaticity of the junctional tissues in digitalis toxicity or ischemia and is associated with a narrow QRS complex and a rate usually < 120–130 beats/min. It is usually considered benign when it occurs in acute myocardial infarction, but the ischemia that induces it may also cause ventricular tachycardia and ventricular fibrillation.

VENTRICULAR PREMATURE BEATS (Ventricular Extrasystoles)

Ventricular premature beats, also called PVCs, are typically isolated beats originating from ventricular tissue. Sudden death occurs more frequently (presumably as a result of ventricular fibrillation) when ventricular premature beats occur in the presence of organic heart disease but not in individuals with no known cardiac disease.

▶ Clinical Findings

The patient may or may not sense the irregular beat, usually as a skipped beat. Exercise generally abolishes premature beats in normal hearts, and the rhythm becomes regular. Ventricular premature beats are characterized by wide QRS complexes that differ in morphology from the patient's normal beats. They are usually not preceded by a P wave, although retrograde ventriculoatrial conduction

may occur. Unless the latter is present, there is a fully compensatory pause (ie, without change in the PP interval). Bigeminy and trigeminy are arrhythmias in which every second or third beat is premature; these patterns confirm a reentry mechanism for the ectopic beat. Ambulatory ECG monitoring or monitoring during graded exercise may reveal more frequent and complex ventricular premature beats than occur in a single routine ECG. An increased frequency of ventricular premature beats during exercise is associated with a higher risk of cardiovascular mortality, though there is no evidence that specific therapy has a role.

▶ Treatment

If no associated cardiac disease is present and if the ectopic beats are asymptomatic, no therapy is indicated. If they are frequent, electrolyte abnormalities (especially hypokalemia or hyperkalemia and hypomagnesemia), hyperthyroidism, and occult heart disease should be excluded. Pharmacologic treatment is indicated only for patients who are symptomatic. If the underlying condition is mitral prolapse, hypertrophic cardiomyopathy, LVH, or coronary disease—or if the QT interval is prolonged—beta-blocker therapy is appropriate. The class I and III agents (see Table 10–12) are all effective in reducing ventricular premature beats but may exacerbate serious arrhythmias in 5–20% of patients; sudden death may occur. Therefore, every attempt should be made to avoid using class I or III antiarrhythmic agents in patients without symptoms. Catheter ablation is a well-established therapy for symptomatic individuals who do not respond to antiarrhythmic drugs or for those patients whose burden of ectopic beats has resulted in a tachycardia-induced cardiomyopathy.

Chen T et al. Ventricular ectopy in patients with left ventricular dysfunction: should it be treated? J Card Fail. 2013 Jan;19(1):40–9. [PMID: 23273593]
Yokokawa M et al. Recovery from left ventricular dysfunction after ablation of frequent premature ventricular complexes. Heart Rhythm. 2013 Feb;10(2):172–5. [PMID: 23099051]

VENTRICULAR TACHYCARDIA

ESSENTIALS OF DIAGNOSIS

► Fast, wide QRS complex on ECG.
► Often associated with structural heart disease.
► Frequently associated with syncope.
► In the absence of reversible cause, implantable cardioverter defibrillator (ICD) is recommended.

▶ General Considerations

Ventricular tachycardia is defined as three or more consecutive ventricular premature beats. The usual rate is 160–240 beats/min and is moderately regular but less so than atrial tachycardia. The usual mechanism is reentry, but abnormally triggered rhythms occur.

Ventricular tachycardia is a frequent complication of acute myocardial infarction and dilated cardiomyopathy but may occur in chronic coronary disease, hypertrophic cardiomyopathy, mitral valve prolapse, myocarditis, and in most other forms of myocardial disease. It can also be a consequence of atypical forms of cardiomyopathies, such as arrhythmogenic right ventricular cardiomyopathy. However, ventricular tachycardia can also occur in patients with structurally normal hearts. **Torsades de pointes**, a form of ventricular tachycardia in which QRS morphology twists around the baseline, may occur in the setting of severe hypokalemia, hypomagnesemia, or after administration of a drug that prolongs the QT interval. In nonacute settings, most patients with ventricular tachycardia have known or easily detectable cardiac disease, and the finding of ventricular tachycardia is an unfavorable prognostic sign.

▶ Clinical Findings

A. Symptoms and Signs

Patients may be asymptomatic or experience syncope or milder symptoms of impaired cerebral perfusion.

B. Laboratory Findings

Ventricular tachycardia can occur in the setting of hypokalemia and hypomagnesemia. Cardiac markers may be elevated when ventricular tachycardia presents in the setting of acute myocardial infarction or as a consequence of underlying coronary disease and demand ischemia.

C. Differentiation of Aberrantly Conducted Supraventricular Beats from Ventricular Beats

Ventricular tachycardia is either nonsustained (three or more consecutive beats lasting < 30 seconds and terminating spontaneously) or sustained. The distinction from aberrant conduction of supraventricular tachycardia may be difficult in patients with a wide QRS complex; it is important because of the differing prognostic and therapeutic implications of each type. Findings favoring a ventricular origin include (1) AV dissociation; (2) a QRS duration exceeding 0.14 second; (3) capture or fusion beats (infrequent); (4) left axis deviation with right bundle branch block morphology; (5) monophasic (R) or biphasic (qR, QR, or RS) complexes in V_1; and (6) a qR or QS complex in V_6. Supraventricular origin is favored by (1) a triphasic QRS complex, especially if there was initial negativity in leads I and V_6; (2) ventricular rates exceeding 170 beats/min; (3) QRS duration longer than 0.12 second but not longer than 0.14 second; and (4) the presence of preexcitation syndrome.

The relationship of the P waves to the tachycardia complex is helpful. A 1:1 relationship usually means a supraventricular origin, except in the case of ventricular tachycardia with retrograde P waves.

▶ Treatment

A. Acute Ventricular Tachycardia

The treatment of acute ventricular tachycardia is determined by the degree of hemodynamic compromise and the duration of the arrhythmia. The management of ventricular tachycardia in acute myocardial infarction is discussed in the Complications section of Acute Myocardial Infarction with ST-Segment Elevation, above. In other patients, if ventricular tachycardia causes hypotension, heart failure, or myocardial ischemia, synchronized DC cardioversion with 100–360 J should be performed immediately. If the patient is tolerating the rhythm, amiodarone 150 mg as a slow intravenous bolus over 10 minutes, followed by an infusion of 1 mg/min for 6 hours and then a maintenance infusion of 0.5 mg/min for an additional 18–42 hours can be used. Lidocaine, 1 mg/kg as an intravenous bolus injection, can also be used. If the ventricular tachycardia recurs, supplemental amiodarone infusions of 150 mg over 10 minutes can be given. If the patient is stable, intravenous procainamide, 20 mg/min intravenously (up to 1000 mg), followed by an infusion of 20–80 mcg/kg/min could also be tried. Empiric magnesium replacement (1–2 g intravenously) may help. Ventricular tachycardia can also be terminated by ventricular overdrive pacing (through a pacemaker or ICD), and this approach is useful when the rhythm is recurrent.

B. Chronic Recurrent Ventricular Tachycardia

1. Sustained ventricular tachycardia—Patients with symptomatic or sustained ventricular tachycardia in the absence of a reversible precipitating cause (acute myocardial infarction or ischemia, electrolyte imbalance, drug toxicity, etc) are at high risk for recurrence. In those with significant LV dysfunction, subsequent sudden death is common. Several trials, including the Antiarrhythmics Versus Implantable Defibrillator (AVID) and the Canadian Implantable Defibrillator trials, strongly suggest that these patients should be managed with ICDs. In those with preserved LV function, the mortality rate is lower and the etiology is often different than in those with depressed ventricular function. Treatment with amiodarone, optimally in combination with a beta-blocker, may be adequate. Sotalol may be an alternative, though there is less supporting evidence. However, many times if ventricular tachycardia occurs in a patient with preserved ventricular function, it is either an outflow tract tachycardia or a fascicular ventricular tachycardia, and these arrhythmias will often respond to AV nodal blockers or can be effectively treated with catheter ablation. The role of electrophysiologic study in this group may help identify patients who are candidates for radiofrequency ablation of a ventricular tachycardia focus. This is particularly the case for arrhythmias that originate in the ventricular outflow tract (often appearing as left bundle branch block with inferior axis on the surface ECG), the left posterior fascicle (right bundle branch block, superior axis morphology), or sustained bundle branch reentry. Catheter ablation can be used as a palliative therapy for those patients with recurrent tachycardia who receive ICD shocks despite antiarrhythmic therapy.

2. Nonsustained ventricular tachycardia (NSVT)—NSVT is defined as runs of three or more ventricular beats lasting < 30 seconds and terminating spontaneously. These may be symptomatic (usually experienced as light-headedness) or asymptomatic. In individuals without heart disease, NSVT is not clearly associated with a poor prognosis. However, in patients with structural heart disease, particularly when they have reduced LVEF, there is an increased risk of subsequent symptomatic ventricular tachycardia or sudden death. Beta-blockers reduce these risks in patients who have coronary disease with significant LV systolic dysfunction (EF < 40%), but if sustained ventricular tachycardia has been induced during electrophysiologic testing, an implantable defibrillator may be indicated. In patients with chronic heart failure and reduced EF—whether due to coronary disease or primary cardiomyopathy and regardless of the presence of asymptomatic ventricular arrhythmias—beta-blockers reduce the incidence of sudden death by 40–50% and should be routine therapy (see section on Heart Failure).

Although there are no definitive data with amiodarone in this group, trends from a number of studies suggest that it may be beneficial. Other antiarrhythmic agents should generally be avoided because their proarrhythmic risk appears to outweigh any benefit, even in patients with inducible arrhythmias that are successfully suppressed in the electrophysiology laboratory.

▶ When to Admit

Any sustained ventricular tachycardia.

Chen J et al. Rapid-rate nonsustained ventricular tachycardia found on implantable cardioverter-defibrillator interrogation: relationship to outcomes in the SCD-HeFT (Sudden Cardiac Death in Heart Failure Trial). J Am Coll Cardiol. 2013 May 28;61(21):2161–8. [PMID: 23541974]

Kuck KH et al; VTACH study group. Catheter ablation of stable ventricular tachycardia before defibrillator implantation in patients with coronary heart disease (VTACH): a multicentre randomised controlled trial. Lancet. 2010 Jan 2;375(9708): 31–40. [PMID: 20109864]

VENTRICULAR FIBRILLATION & DEATH

Sudden cardiac death is defined as unexpected nontraumatic death in clinically well or stable patients who die within 1 hour after onset of symptoms. The causative rhythm in most cases is ventricular fibrillation, which is usually preceded by ventricular tachycardia except in the setting of acute ischemia or infarction. Complete heart block and sinus node arrest may also cause sudden death. A disproportionate number of sudden deaths occur in the early morning hours and this suggests that there is a strong interplay with the autonomic nervous system. Over 75% of victims of sudden cardiac death have severe CAD. Many have old myocardial infarctions. Sudden death may be the initial manifestation of coronary disease in up to 20% of patients and accounts for approximately 50% of deaths from coronary disease. Other conditions that predispose to sudden death include severe LVH, hypertrophic cardiomyopathy, congestive cardiomyopathy, aortic stenosis, pulmonic stenosis, primary pulmonary hypertension, cyanotic congenital heart disease, atrial myxoma, mitral valve prolapse, hypoxia, electrolyte abnormalities, prolonged QT interval syndrome, the Brugada syndrome, arrhythmogenic right ventricular cardiomyopathy, catecholaminergic polymorphic ventricular tachycardia, and conduction system disease.

▶ Treatment

Unless ventricular fibrillation occurs shortly after myocardial infarction, is associated with ischemia, or is seen with an unusual correctable process (such as an electrolyte abnormality, drug toxicity, or aortic stenosis), surviving patients require evaluation and intervention since recurrences are frequent. Coronary arteriography should be performed to exclude coronary disease as the underlying cause, since revascularization may prevent recurrence. When ventricular fibrillation occurs in the initial 24 hours after infarction, long-term management is no different from that of other patients with acute infarction. Conduction disturbances should be managed as described in the next section. Survivors of ventricular fibrillation or cardiac arrest have improved long-term outcomes if a hypothermia protocol is rapidly initiated and continued for 24–36 hours after cardiac arrest.

The current consensus is that if myocardial infarction or ischemia, bradyarrhythmias and conduction disturbances or other identifiable and correctable precipitating causes of ventricular fibrillation are not found to be the cause of the sudden death episode, an ICD is the treatment of choice. In addition, evidence from the MADIT II study and Sudden Cardiac Death in Heart Failure Trial (SCD-HeFT) suggest that patients with severe LV dysfunction—whether due to an ischemic cause such as a remote myocardial infarction or a nonischemic cause of advanced heart failure—have a reduced risk of death with the prophylactic implantation of an ICD. However, the DINAMIT study demonstrated that implanting prophylactic ICDs in patients early after myocardial infarction is associated with a trend toward worse outcomes. These patients may be managed with a wearable defibrillator vest until recovery of ventricular function can be assessed at a later date.

Brodine WN et al; MADIT-II Research Group. Effects of beta-blockers on implantable cardioverter defibrillator therapy and survival in the patients with ischemic cardiomyopathy (from the Multicenter Automatic Defibrillator Implantation Trial-II). Am J Cardiol. 2005 Sep 1;96(5):691–5. [PMID: 16125497]

Hohnloser SH et al; DINAMIT Investigators. Prophylactic use of an implantable cardioverter-defibrillator after acute myocardial infarction. N Engl J Med. 2004 Dec 9;351(24):2481–8. [PMID: 15590950]

Kadish A et al; Defibrillators in Non-Ischemic Cardiomyopathy Treatment Evaluation (DEFINITE) Investigators. Prophylactic defibrillator implantation in patients with nonischemic dilated cardiomyopathy. N Engl J Med. 2004 May 20;350(21): 2151–8. [PMID: 15152060]

Nielsen N et al; TTM Trial Investigators. Targeted temperature management at 33 degrees C versus 36 degrees C after cardiac arrest. N Engl J Med. 2013 Dec 5;369(23):2197–206. [PMID: 24237006]

Olasveengen TM et al. Intravenous drug administration during out-of-hospital cardiac arrest: a randomized trial. JAMA. 2009 Nov 25;302(20):2222–9. [PMID: 19934423]

Sasson C et al. Predictors of survival from out-of-hospital cardiac arrest: a systematic review and meta-analysis. Circulation. 2010 Jan 1;3(1):63–81. [PMID: 20123673]

ACCELERATED IDIOVENTRICULAR RHYTHM

Accelerated idioventricular rhythm is a regular wide complex rhythm with a rate of 60–120 beats/min, usually with a gradual onset. Because the rate is often similar to the sinus rate, fusion beats and alternating rhythms are common. Two mechanisms have been invoked: (1) an escape rhythm due to suppression of higher pacemakers resulting from sinoatrial and AV block or from depressed sinus node function; and (2) slow ventricular tachycardia due to increased automaticity or, less frequently, reentry. It occurs commonly in acute infarction and following reperfusion with thrombolytic drugs. The incidence of associated ventricular fibrillation is much less than that of ventricular tachycardia with a rapid rate, and treatment is not indicated unless there is hemodynamic compromise or more serious arrhythmias. This rhythm also is common in digitalis toxicity.

Accelerated idioventricular rhythm must be distinguished from the idioventricular or junctional rhythm with rates < 40–45 beats/min that occurs in the presence of complete AV block. AV dissociation—where ventricular rate exceeds sinus—but not AV block occurs in most cases of accelerated idioventricular rhythm.

LONG QT SYNDROME

Congenital long QT syndrome is an uncommon disease that is characterized by recurrent syncope, a long QT interval (usually 0.5–0.7 second), documented ventricular arrhythmias, and sudden death. It may occur in the presence (Jervell-Lange-Nielsen syndrome) or absence (Romano-Ward syndrome) of congenital deafness. Inheritance may be autosomal recessive or autosomal dominant (Romano-Ward). Specific genetic mutations affecting membrane potassium and sodium channels have been identified and help delineate the mechanisms and susceptibility to arrhythmia.

Because this is a primary electrical disorder usually with no evidence of structural heart disease or LV dysfunction, the long-term prognosis is excellent if arrhythmia is controlled. Long-term treatment with beta-blockers or permanent pacing has been shown to be effective. ICD implantation is recommended for patients in whom recurrent syncope, sustained ventricular arrhythmias, or sudden cardiac death occurs despite drug therapy. An ICD should be considered as primary therapy in certain patients, such as those in whom aborted sudden cardiac death is the initial presentation of the long-QT syndrome, when there is a strong family history of sudden cardiac death, or when compliance or intolerance to drugs is a concern.

Acquired long QT interval secondary to use of antiarrhythmic agents, methadone, antidepressant drugs, or certain antibiotics; electrolyte abnormalities; myocardial ischemia; or significant bradycardia may result in ventricular tachycardia (particularly torsades de pointes). Notably, many antiarrhythmic drugs that are effective for the treatment of atrial and ventricular arrhythmias may significantly prolong the QT interval (sotalol, dofetilide). If a drug therapy is found to prolong the QT interval beyond 500 ms or 15% longer than the baseline QT, it should be discontinued.

The management of torsades de pointes differs from that of other forms of ventricular tachycardia. Class Ia, Ic, or III antiarrhythmics, which prolong the QT interval, should be avoided—or withdrawn immediately if being used. Intravenous beta-blockers may be effective, especially in congenital forms of long-QT syndrome; intravenous magnesium should be given acutely. Increasing the heart rate, whether by infusion of beta-agonist (dopamine or isoproterenol) or temporary atrial or ventricular pacing, is an effective approach that can both break and prevent the rhythm.

Moskovitz JB et al. Electrocardiographic implications of the prolonged QT interval. Am J Emerg Med. 2013 May;31(5):866–71. [PMID: 23602761]

Roden DM. Clinical practice. Long-QT syndrome. N Engl J Med. 2008 Jan 10;358(2):169–76. [PMID: 18184962]

Schwartz P et al. Who are the long-QT syndrome patients who receive an implantable cardioverter-defibrillator and what happens to them?: data from the European Long-QT Syndrome Implantable Cardioverter-Defibrillator (LQTS ICD) Registry. Circulation. 2010 Sep 28;122(13):1272–82. [PMID: 20837891]

BRADYCARDIAS & CONDUCTION DISTURBANCES

SICK SINUS SYNDROME

ESSENTIALS OF DIAGNOSIS

► Most patients are asymptomatic.

► More common in elderly population.

► May have recurrent supraventricular arrhythmia and bradyarrhythmia.

► Frequently seen in patients with concomitant atrial fibrillation.

► Often chronotropically incompetent.

► May be caused by drug therapy.

► General Considerations

This imprecise diagnosis is applied to patients with sinus arrest, sinoatrial exit block (recognized by a pause equal to a multiple of the underlying PP interval or progressive shortening of the PP interval prior to a pause), or persistent sinus bradycardia. These rhythms are often caused or exacerbated by drug therapy (digitalis, calcium channel blockers, beta-blockers, sympatholytic agents, antiarrhythmics), and agents that may be responsible should be withdrawn prior to making the diagnosis. Another presentation is of recurrent supraventricular tachycardias (paroxysmal reentry tachycardias, atrial flutter, and atrial fibrillation), associated with bradyarrhythmias ("tachy-brady syndrome"). The long pauses that often follow the termination of tachycardia cause the associated symptoms.

Sick sinus syndrome occurs most commonly in elderly patients and is frequently seen in patients with concomitant atrial fibrillation. The pathologic changes are usually nonspecific, characterized by patchy fibrosis of the sinus node and cardiac conduction system. Sick sinus syndrome may be caused by other conditions, including sarcoidosis, amyloidosis, Chagas disease, and various cardiomyopathies. Coronary disease is an uncommon cause.

▶ Clinical Findings

Most patients with ECG evidence of sick sinus syndrome are asymptomatic, but rare individuals may experience syncope, dizziness, confusion, palpitations, heart failure, or angina. Because these symptoms are either nonspecific or are due to other causes, it is essential that they be demonstrated to coincide temporally with arrhythmias. This may require prolonged ambulatory monitoring or the use of an event recorder.

▶ Treatment

Most symptomatic patients will require permanent pacing (see AV block, below). Dual-chamber pacing is preferred because ventricular pacing is associated with a higher incidence of subsequent atrial fibrillation, and subsequent AV block occurs at a rate of 2% per year. In addition, resultant "pacemaker syndrome" can result from loss of AV synchrony. Treatment of associated tachyarrhythmias is often difficult without first instituting pacing, since beta-blockers, calcium-channel blockers, digoxin, and other antiarrhythmic agents may exacerbate the bradycardia. Unfortunately, symptomatic relief following pacing has not been consistent, largely because of inadequate documentation of the etiologic role of bradyarrhythmias in producing the symptom. Furthermore, many of these patients may have associated ventricular arrhythmias that may require treatment. Permanent pacing may alleviate symptoms in carefully selected patients.

Alboni P et al. Treatment of persistent sinus bradycardia with intermittent symptoms: are guidelines clear? Europace. 2009 May;11(5):562–4. [PMID: 19213798]
Riahi S et al; DANPACE Investigators. Heart failure in patients with sick sinus syndrome treated with single lead atrial or dual-chamber pacing: no association with pacing mode or right ventricular pacing site. Europace. 2012 Oct;14(10):1475–82. [PMID: 22447958]

AV BLOCK

AV block is categorized as first-degree (PR interval > 0.21 second with all atrial impulses conducted), second-degree (intermittent blocked beats), or third-degree (complete heart block, in which no supraventricular impulses are conducted to the ventricles).

Second-degree block is further subclassified. In **Mobitz type I (Wenckebach)** AV block, the AV conduction time (PR interval) progressively lengthens, with the RR interval shortening before the blocked beat; this phenomenon is almost always due to abnormal conduction within the AV node. In **Mobitz type II** AV block, there are intermittently nonconducted atrial beats not preceded by lengthening AV conduction. It is usually due to block within the His bundle system. The classification as Mobitz type I or Mobitz type II is only partially reliable because patients may appear to have both types on the surface ECG, and the site of origin of 2:1 AV block cannot be predicted from the ECG. The width of the QRS complexes assists in determining whether the block is nodal or infranodal. When they are narrow, the block is usually nodal; when they are wide, the block is usually infranodal. Electrophysiologic studies may be necessary for accurate localization. Management of AV block in acute myocardial infarction has already been discussed.

First-degree and **Mobitz type I block** may occur in normal individuals with heightened vagal tone . They may also occur as a drug effect (especially digitalis, calcium channel blockers, beta-blockers, or other sympatholytic agents), often superimposed on organic disease. These disturbances also occur transiently or chronically due to ischemia, infarction, inflammatory processes (including Lyme disease), fibrosis, calcification, or infiltration. The prognosis is usually good, since reliable alternative pacemakers arise from the AV junction below the level of block if higher degrees of block occur.

Mobitz type II block is almost always due to organic disease involving the infranodal conduction system. In the event of progression to complete heart block, alternative pacemakers are not reliable. Thus, prophylactic ventricular pacing is required.

Complete (third-degree) heart block is a more advanced form of block often due to a lesion distal to the His bundle and associated with bilateral bundle branch block. The QRS is wide and the ventricular rate is slower, usually < 50 beats/min. Transmission of atrial impulses through the AV node is completely blocked, and a ventricular pacemaker maintains a slow, regular ventricular rate, usually < 45 beats/min. Exercise does not increase the rate. The first heart sound varies in intensity; wide pulse pressure, a changing systolic BP level, and cannon venous pulsations in the neck are also present. Patients may be asymptomatic or may complain of weakness or dyspnea if the rate is < 35 beats/min; symptoms may occur at higher rates if the left ventricle cannot increase its stroke output. During periods of transition from partial to complete heart block, some patients have ventricular asystole that lasts several seconds to minutes. Syncope occurs abruptly.

Patients with episodic or chronic infranodal complete heart block require permanent pacing, and temporary pacing is indicated if implantation of a permanent pacemaker is delayed.

▶ Treatment

The indications for **permanent pacing** have been discussed: symptomatic bradyarrhythmias, asymptomatic

Mobitz II AV block, or complete heart block. A standardized nomenclature for pacemaker generators is used, usually consisting of four letters. The first letter refers to the chamber that is stimulated (A = atrium, V = ventricle, D = dual, for both). The second letter refers to the chamber in which sensing occurs (also A, V, or D). The third letter refers to the sensory mode (I = inhibition by a sensed impulse, T = triggering by a sensed impulse, D = dual modes of response). The fourth letter refers to the programmability or rate modulation capacity (usually P for programming for two functions, M for programming more than two, and R for rate modulation).

A dual-chamber multiple programmable pacemaker that senses and paces in both chambers is the most physiologic approach to pacing patients who remain in sinus rhythm. AV synchrony is particularly important in patients in whom atrial contraction produces a substantial increment in stroke volume and in those in whom sensing the atrial rate to provide rate-responsive ventricular pacing is useful. Dual-chamber pacing is most useful for individuals with LV systolic or—perhaps more importantly—diastolic dysfunction and for physically active individuals. In patients with single-chamber ventricular pacemakers, the lack of an atrial kick may lead to the so-called pacemaker syndrome, in which the patient experiences signs of low cardiac output while upright.

Pulse generators are also available that can increase their rate in response to motion or respiratory rate when the intrinsic atrial rate is inappropriately low. These are most useful in active individuals. Follow-up after pacemaker implantation, usually by telephonic monitoring, is essential. All pulse generators and lead systems have an early failure rate that is now below 1% and an expected battery life varying from 4 years to 10 years.

Epstein AE et al. 2012 ACCF/AHA/HRS focused update incorporated into the ACCF/AHA/HRS 2008 guidelines for device-based therapy of cardiac rhythm abnormalities: a report of the American College of Cardiology Foundation/American Heart Association Task Force on Practice Guidelines and the Heart Rhythm Society. Circulation. 2013 Jan 22;127(3):e283–352. [PMID: 23255456]

AV DISSOCIATION

When a ventricular pacemaker is firing at a rate faster than or close to the sinus rate (accelerated idioventricular rhythm, ventricular premature beats, or ventricular tachycardia), atrial impulses arriving at the AV node when it is refractory may not be conducted. This phenomenon is AV dissociation but does not necessarily indicate AV block. No treatment is required aside from management of the causative arrhythmia.

INTRAVENTRICULAR CONDUCTION DEFECTS

Intraventricular conduction defects, including bundle branch block, are common in individuals with otherwise normal hearts and in many disease processes, including ischemic heart disease, inflammatory disease, infiltrative disease, cardiomyopathy, and postcardiotomy. Bifascicular

block is present when two of these—right bundle, left anterior, and left posterior fascicle—are involved. Trifascicular block is defined as right bundle branch block with alternating left hemiblock, alternating right and left bundle branch block, or bifascicular block with documented prolonged infranodal conduction (long His-ventricular interval).

The prognosis of intraventricular block is generally related to the underlying myocardial process. Patients with no apparent heart disease have an overall survival rate similar to that of matched controls. However, left bundle branch block—but not right—is associated with a higher risk of development of overt cardiac disease and cardiac mortality. With bifascicular block, the incidence of occult complete heart block or progression to it is low, and pacing is not usually warranted in asymptomatic patients. However, in patients with bifascicular block that presents with syncope where no other readily identifiable cause is found, early pacemaker implantation has been shown to reduce further episodes.

Garcia D et al. Intraventricular conduction abnormality—an electrocardiographic algorithm for rapid detection and diagnosis. Am J Emerg Med. 2009 May;27(4):492–502. [PMID: 19555622]
Santini M et al. Prevention of syncope through permanent cardiac pacing in patients with bifascicular block and syncope of unexplained origin: the PRESS study. Circ Arrhythm Electrophysiol. 2013 Feb;6(1):101–7. [PMID: 23390123]

SYNCOPE

ESSENTIALS OF DIAGNOSIS

▶ Transient loss of consciousness and postural tone from vasodepressor or cardiogenic causes.

▶ Prompt recovery without resuscitative measures.

▶ Common clinical problem.

▶ General Considerations

Syncope is a symptom defined as a transient, self-limited loss of consciousness, usually leading to a fall. Thirty percent of the adult population will experience at least one episode of syncope. It accounts for approximately 3% of emergency department visits. A specific cause of syncope is identified in about 50% of cases during the initial evaluation. The prognosis is relatively favorable except when accompanying cardiac disease is present. In many patients with recurrent syncope or near syncope, arrhythmias are not the cause. This is particularly true when the patient has no evidence of associated heart disease by history, examination, standard ECG, or noninvasive testing. The history is the most important of the evaluation to identify the cause of syncope.

Vasodepressor syncope may be due to excessive vagal tone or impaired reflex control of the peripheral circulation. The most frequent type of vasodepressor syncope is vasovagal hypotension or the "common faint," which is often initiated by a stressful, painful, or claustrophobic experience, especially in young women. Enhanced vagal tone with resulting hypotension is the cause of syncope in carotid sinus hypersensitivity and postmicturition syncope; vagal-induced sinus bradycardia, sinus arrest, and AV block are common accompaniments and may themselves be the cause of syncope.

Orthostatic (postural) hypotension is another common cause of vasodepressor syncope, especially in the elderly; in diabetic patients or others with autonomic neuropathy; in patients with blood loss or hypovolemia; and in patients taking vasodilators, diuretics, and adrenergic-blocking drugs. In addition, a syndrome of chronic idiopathic orthostatic hypotension exists primarily in older men. In most of these conditions, the normal vasoconstrictive response to assuming upright posture, which compensates for the abrupt decrease in venous return, is impaired.

Cardiogenic syncope can occur on a mechanical or arrhythmic basis. There is usually no prodrome; thus, injury secondary to falling is common. Mechanical problems that can cause syncope include aortic stenosis (where syncope may occur from autonomic reflex abnormalities or ventricular tachycardia), pulmonary stenosis, HOCM, congenital lesions associated with pulmonary hypertension or right-to-left shunting, and LA myxoma obstructing the mitral valve. Episodes are commonly exertional or postexertional. More commonly, cardiac syncope is due to disorders of automaticity (sick sinus syndrome), conduction disorders (AV block), or tachyarrhythmias (especially ventricular tachycardia and supraventricular tachycardia with rapid ventricular rate).

► Clinical Findings

A. Symptoms and Signs

Syncope is characteristically abrupt in onset, often resulting in injury, transient (lasting for seconds to a few minutes), and followed by prompt recovery of full consciousness.

Vasodepressor premonitory symptoms, such as nausea, diaphoresis, tachycardia, and pallor, are usual in the "common faint." Episodes can be aborted by lying down or removing the inciting stimulus. In **orthostatic (postural) hypotension,** a greater than normal decline (20 mm Hg) in BP immediately upon arising from the supine to the standing position is observed, with or without tachycardia depending on the status of autonomic (baroreceptor) function.

B. Diagnostic Tests

The evaluation for syncope depends on findings from the history and physical examination (especially orthostatic BP evaluation, examination of carotid and other arteries, and cardiac examination).

1. ECG—The resting ECG may reveal arrhythmias, evidence of accessory pathways, prolonged QT interval, and other signs of heart disease (such as infarction or hypertrophy). If the history is consistent with syncope, ambulatory ECG monitoring is essential. This may need to be repeated several times, since yields increase with longer periods of monitoring, at least up to 3 days. Event recorder and transtelephone ECG monitoring may be helpful in patients with intermittent presyncopal episodes. Caution is required before attributing a patient's symptom to rhythm or conduction abnormalities observed during monitoring without concomitant symptoms. In many cases, the symptoms are due to a different arrhythmia or to noncardiac causes. For instance, dizziness or syncope in older patients may be unrelated to concomitantly observed bradycardia, sinus node abnormalities, and ventricular ectopy.

2. Autonomic testing—Orthostatic hypotension from autonomic function can be diagnosed with more certainty by observing BP and heart rate responses to Valsalva maneuver and by tilt testing.

Carotid sinus massage in patients who do not have carotid bruits or a history of cerebral vascular disease can precipitate sinus node arrest or AV block in patients with carotid sinus hypersensitivity. **Head-up tilt-table testing** can identify patients whose syncope may be on a vasovagal basis. In older patients, vasoconstrictor abnormalities and autonomic insufficiency are perhaps the most common causes of syncope. Thus, tilt testing should be done before proceeding to invasive studies unless clinical and ambulatory ECG evaluation suggests a cardiac abnormality. Although different testing protocols are used, passive tilting to at least 70 degrees for 10–40 minutes—in conjunction with isoproterenol infusion or sublingual nitroglycerin, if necessary—is typical. Syncope due to bradycardia, hypotension, or both will occur in approximately one-third of patients with recurrent syncope. Some studies have suggested that, at least with some of the more extreme protocols, false-positive responses may occur.

3. Electrophysiologic studies—Electrophysiologic studies to assess sinus node function and AV conduction and to induce supraventricular or ventricular tachycardia are indicated in patients with recurrent episodes, nondiagnostic ambulatory ECGs, and negative autonomic testing if vasomotor syncope is a consideration. Electrophysiologic studies reveal an arrhythmic cause in 20–50% of patients, depending on the study criteria, and are most often diagnostic when the patient has had multiple episodes and has identifiable cardiac abnormalities.

4. Exercise testing—When the symptoms are associated with exertion or stress, exercise testing may be helpful.

► Treatment

Treatment consists largely of counseling patients to avoid predisposing situations. Paradoxically, beta-blockers have been used in patients with altered autonomic function uncovered by head-up tilt testing but they have provided only minimal benefit. If symptomatic bradyarrhythmias or supraventricular tachyarrhythmias are detected, therapy can usually be initiated without additional diagnostic studies. Permanent pacing has little benefit except in patients with documented severe pauses and bradycardiac responses.

Volume expanders, such as fludrocortisone, or vasoconstrictors, such as midodrine, have also been tried but with minimal benefit. Selective serotonin reuptake inhibitors have shown some benefit in select patients.

See Recommendations for Resumption of Driving, below.

▶ When to Admit

- Patients with syncope and concomitant structural heart disease or when a primary cardiac etiology is suspected.
- Patients with recent or recurrent syncope are often monitored in the hospital.
- Those with less ominous symptoms may be monitored as outpatients.

Benditt DG. Syncope risk assessment in the emergency department and clinic. Prog Cardiovasc Dis. 2013 Jan–Feb;55(4): 376–81. [PMID: 23472774]

Kessler C et al. The emergency department approach to syncope: evidence-based guidelines and prediction rules. Emerg Med Clin North Am. 2010 Aug;28(3):487–500. [PMID: 20709240]

Krahn AD et al. Selecting appropriate diagnostic tools for evaluating the patient with syncope/collapse. Prog Cardiovasc Dis. 2013 Jan–Feb;55(4):402–9. [PMID: 23472778]

RECOMMENDATIONS FOR RESUMPTION OF DRIVING

An important management problem in patients who have experienced syncope, symptomatic ventricular tachycardia, or aborted sudden death is to provide recommendations concerning automobile driving. Patients with syncope or aborted sudden death thought to have been due to temporary factors (acute myocardial infarction, bradyarrhythmias subsequently treated with permanent pacing, drug effect, electrolyte imbalance) should be strongly advised after recovery not to drive for at least 1 month. Other patients with symptomatic ventricular tachycardia or aborted sudden death, whether treated pharmacologically, with antitachycardia devices, or with ablation therapy, should not drive for at least 6 months. Longer restrictions are warranted in these patients if spontaneous arrhythmias persist. The clinician should comply with local reporting and driving restriction regulations and consult local authorities concerning individual cases where required.

Sakaguchi S et al. Syncope and driving, flying and vocational concerns. Prog Cardiovasc Dis. 2013 Jan–Feb;55(4):454–63. [PMID: 23472784]

HEART FAILURE

ESSENTIALS OF DIAGNOSIS

- ▶ **LV failure:** Either due to systolic or diastolic dysfunction. Predominant symptoms are those of low cardiac output and congestion, including dyspnea.
- ▶ **RV failure:** Symptoms of fluid overload predominate; usually RV failure is secondary to LV failure.
- ▶ Assessment of LV function is a crucial part of diagnosis and management.
- ▶ Optimal management of chronic heart failure includes combination medical therapies, such as ACE inhibitors, aldosterone antagonists, and beta-blockers.

▶ General Considerations

Heart failure is a common syndrome that is increasing in incidence and prevalence. Approximately 5 million patients in the United States have heart failure, and there are nearly 500,000 new cases each year. Each year in the United States, over 1 million patients are discharged from the hospital with a diagnosis of heart failure. It is primarily a disease of aging, with over 75% of existing and new cases occurring in individuals over 65 years of age. The prevalence of heart failure rises from < 1% in individuals below 60 years to nearly 10% in those over 80 years of age.

Heart failure may be right sided or left sided (or both). Patients with **left heart failure** may have symptoms of low cardiac output and elevated pulmonary venous pressure; dyspnea is the predominant feature. Signs of fluid retention predominate in **right heart failure**. Most patients exhibit symptoms or signs of both right- and left-sided failure, and LV dysfunction is the primary cause of RV failure. Approximately half of patients with heart failure have **preserved LV systolic function** and usually have some degree of diastolic dysfunction. Patients with reduced or preserved systolic function may have similar symptoms and it may be difficult to distinguish clinically between the two based on signs and symptoms. In developed countries, CAD with resulting myocardial infarction and loss of functioning myocardium (ischemic cardiomyopathy) is the most common cause of **systolic heart failure**. Systemic hypertension remains an important cause of heart failure and, even more commonly in the United States, an exacerbating factor in patients with cardiac dysfunction due to other causes such as CAD. Several processes may present with dilated or congestive cardiomyopathy, which is characterized by LV or biventricular dilation and generalized systolic dysfunction. These are discussed elsewhere in this chapter, but the most common are alcoholic cardiomyopathy, viral myocarditis (including infections by HIV), and dilated cardiomyopathies with no obvious underlying cause (idiopathic cardiomyopathy). Rare causes of dilated cardiomyopathy include infiltrative diseases (hemochromatosis, sarcoidosis, amyloidosis, etc), other infectious agents, metabolic disorders, cardiotoxins, and drug toxicity. VHDs—particularly degenerative aortic stenosis and chronic aortic or mitral regurgitation—are not infrequent causes of heart failure. The most frequent cause of **diastolic cardiac dysfunction** is LVH, commonly resulting from hypertension, but conditions such as hypertrophic or restrictive cardiomyopathy, diabetes, and pericardial disease can produce the same clinical picture. Atrial fibrillation with or without rapid ventricular response may contribute to impaired left ventricular filling, and aging itself contributes to impaired left ventricular relaxation.

Heart failure is often preventable by early detection of patients at risk and by early intervention. The importance of these approaches is emphasized by US guidelines that have incorporated a classification of heart failure that includes four stages. Stage A includes patients at risk for developing heart failure (such as patients with hypertension or CAD without current or previous symptoms or identifiable structural abnormalities of the myocardium). In the majority of these patients, development of heart failure can be prevented with interventions such as the aggressive treatment of hypertension, modification of coronary risk factors, and reduction of excessive alcohol intake. Stage B includes patients who have structural heart disease but no current or previously recognized symptoms of heart failure. Examples include patients with previous myocardial infarction, other causes of reduced systolic function, LVH, or asymptomatic valvular disease. Both ACE inhibitors and beta-blockers prevent heart failure in the first two of these conditions, and more aggressive treatment of hypertension and early surgical intervention are effective in the latter two. Stages C and D include patients with clinical heart failure and the relatively small group of patients that has become refractory to the usual therapies, respectively. These are discussed below.

▶ Clinical Findings

A. Symptoms

The most common symptom of patients with **left heart failure** is shortness of breath, chiefly exertional dyspnea at first and then progressing to orthopnea, paroxysmal nocturnal dyspnea, and rest dyspnea. Chronic nonproductive cough, which is often worse in the recumbent position, may occur. Nocturia due to excretion of fluid retained during the day and increased renal perfusion in the recumbent position is a common nonspecific symptom of heart failure, as is fatigue and exercise intolerance. These symptoms correlate poorly with the degree of cardiac dysfunction. Patients with **right heart failure** have predominate signs of fluid retention, with the patient exhibiting edema, hepatic congestion and, on occasion, loss of appetite and nausea due to edema of the gut or impaired gastrointestinal perfusion and ascites. Surprisingly, some individuals with severe LV dysfunction will display few signs of left heart failure and appear to have isolated right heart failure. Indeed, they may be clinically indistinguishable from patients with cor pulmonale, who have right heart failure secondary to pulmonary disease.

Patients with acute heart failure from myocardial infarction, myocarditis, and acute valvular regurgitation due to endocarditis or other conditions usually present with pulmonary edema. Patients with episodic symptoms may be having LV dysfunction due to intermittent ischemia. Patients may also present with acute exacerbations of chronic, stable heart failure. Exacerbations are usually caused by alterations in therapy (or patient noncompliance), excessive salt and fluid intake, arrhythmias, excessive activity, pulmonary emboli, intercurrent infection, or progression of the underlying disease.

Patients with heart failure are often categorized by the NYHA classification as class I (asymptomatic), class II (symptomatic with moderate activity), class III (symptomatic with mild activity), or class IV (symptomatic at rest). This classification is important since some of the treatments are indicated based on NYHA classification.

B. Signs

Many patients with heart failure, including some with severe symptoms, appear comfortable at rest. Others will be dyspneic during conversation or minor activity, and those with long-standing severe heart failure may appear cachectic or cyanotic. The vital signs may be normal, but tachycardia, hypotension, and reduced pulse pressure may be present. Patients often show signs of increased sympathetic nervous system activity, including cold extremities and diaphoresis. Important peripheral signs of heart failure can be detected by examination of the neck, the lungs, the abdomen, and the extremities. RA pressure may be estimated through the height of the pulsations in the jugular venous system. In addition to the height of the venous pressure, abnormal pulsations such as regurgitant v waves should be sought. Examination of the carotid pulse may allow estimation of pulse pressure as well as detection of aortic stenosis. Thyroid examination may reveal occult hyperthyroidism or hypothyroidism, which are readily treatable causes of heart failure. Crackles at the lung bases reflect transudation of fluid into the alveoli. Pleural effusions may cause bibasilar dullness to percussion. Expiratory wheezing and rhonchi may be signs of heart failure. Patients with severe right heart failure may have hepatic enlargement—tender or nontender—due to passive congestion. Systolic pulsations may be felt in tricuspid regurgitation. Sustained moderate pressure on the liver may increase jugular venous pressure (a positive hepatojugular reflux is an increase of > 1 cm). Ascites may also be present. Peripheral pitting edema is a common sign in patients with right heart failure and may extend into the thighs and abdominal wall.

Cardinal cardiac examination signs are a parasternal lift, indicating pulmonary hypertension; an enlarged and sustained LV impulse, indicating LV dilation and hypertrophy; a diminished first heart sound, suggesting impaired contractility; and an S_3 gallop originating in the LV and sometimes the RV. An S_4 is usually present in diastolic heart failure. Murmurs should be sought to exclude primary valvular disease; secondary mitral regurgitation and tricuspid regurgitation murmurs are common in patients with dilated ventricles. In chronic heart failure, many of the expected signs of heart failure may be absent despite markedly abnormal cardiac function and hemodynamic measurements.

C. Laboratory Findings

A blood count may reveal anemia and a high red-cell distribution width (RDW), both of which are associated with poor prognosis in chronic heart failure through poorly understood mechanisms. Renal function tests can determine whether cardiac failure is associated with impaired renal function that may reflect poor renal perfusion. Chronic kidney disease is another poor prognostic factor in heart failure and may limit certain treatment options. Serum electrolytes may disclose hypokalemia, which increases the risk of arrhythmias; hyperkalemia, which may limit the use of inhibitors of the renin–angiotensin system; or hyponatremia, an indicator of marked activation of the renin–angiotensin system and a poor prognostic sign. Thyroid function should be assessed to detect occult thyrotoxicosis or myxedema and iron studies test should be checked to test for hemochromatosis. In unexplained cases, appropriate biopsies may lead to a diagnosis of amyloidosis. Myocardial biopsy may exclude specific causes of dilated cardiomyopathy but rarely reveals specific reversible diagnoses.

Serum BNP is a powerful prognostic marker that adds to clinical assessment in differentiating dyspnea due to heart failure from noncardiac causes. Two markers—BNP and N-terminal pro-BNP—provide similar diagnostic and prognostic information. BNP is expressed primarily in the ventricles and is elevated when ventricular filling pressures are high. It is quite sensitive in patients with symptomatic heart failure—whether due to systolic or to diastolic dysfunction—but less specific in older patients, women, and patients with COPD. Studies have shown that BNP can help in emergency department triage in diagnosis of acute decompensated heart failure, such that a NT-proBNP < 300 pg/mL or BNP < 100 pg/mL, combined with a normal ECG, makes heart failure unlikely. BNP is less sensitive and specific to diagnose heart failure in the chronic setting. BNP may be helpful in guiding intensity of diuretic and other therapies for monitoring and management of chronic heart failure. Worsening breathlessness or weight associated with a rising BNP (or both) might prompt increasing the dose of diuretics. However, to date, the routine use of BNP to guide therapy has not been shown to be beneficial in randomized trials. Elevation of serum troponin, and especially of high-sensitivity troponin, is common in both chronic and acute heart failure, and it is associated with higher risk of adverse outcomes.

D. ECG and Chest Radiography

ECG may indicate an underlying or secondary arrhythmia, myocardial infarction, or nonspecific changes that often include low voltage, intraventricular conduction defects, LVH, and nonspecific repolarization changes. Chest radiographs provide information about the size and shape of the cardiac silhouette. Cardiomegaly is an important finding and is a poor prognostic sign. Evidence of pulmonary venous hypertension includes relative dilation of the upper lobe veins, perivascular edema (haziness of vessel outlines), interstitial edema, and alveolar fluid. In acute heart failure, these findings correlate moderately well with pulmonary venous pressure. However, patients with chronic heart failure may show relatively normal pulmonary vasculature despite markedly elevated pressures. Pleural effusions are common and tend to be bilateral or right-sided.

E. Additional Studies

Many studies have indicated that the clinical diagnosis of systolic myocardial dysfunction is often inaccurate. The primary confounding conditions are diastolic dysfunction of the heart with decreased relaxation and filling of the LV (particularly in hypertension and in hypertrophic states) and pulmonary disease. Because patients with heart failure usually have significant resting ECG abnormalities, stress imaging procedures such as perfusion scintigraphy or dobutamine echocardiography are often indicated.

The most useful test is the echocardiogram because it can differentiate heart failure with and without preserved LV systolic function. The echocardiogram can define the size and function of both ventricles and of the atria. It will also allow detection of pericardial effusion, valvular abnormalities, intracardiac shunts, and segmental wall motion abnormalities suggestive of old myocardial infarction as opposed to more generalized forms of dilated cardiomyopathy.

Radionuclide angiography as well as cardiac MRI also measure LVEF and permit analysis of regional wall motion. These tests are especially useful when echocardiography is technically suboptimal, such as in patients with severe pulmonary disease. When myocardial ischemia is suspected as a cause of LV dysfunction, stress testing should be performed.

F. Cardiac Catheterization

In most patients with heart failure, clinical examination and noninvasive tests can determine LV size and function and valve function to confirm the diagnosis. Left heart catheterization may be helpful to define the presence and extent of CAD, although CT angiography may also be appropriate, especially when the likelihood of coronary disease is low. Evaluation for coronary disease is particularly important when LV dysfunction may be partially reversible by revascularization. The combination of angina or noninvasive evidence of significant myocardial ischemia with symptomatic heart failure is often an indication for coronary angiography if the patient is a potential candidate for revascularization. Right heart catheterization may be useful to select and monitor therapy in patients refractory to standard therapy.

▶ Treatment

The treatment of heart failure is aimed at relieving symptoms, improving functional status, and preventing death and hospitalizations. Figure 10–10 outlines the role of the major pharmacologic and device therapies for chronic heart failure. The evidence of clinical benefit, including reducing death and hospitalization, of most therapies is limited to patients with heart failure with reduced LVEF. Treatment of heart failure with preserved LV ejection is aimed at improving symptoms and treating comorbidities.

A. Correction of Reversible Causes

The major reversible causes of chronic heart failure include valvular lesions, myocardial ischemia, uncontrolled hypertension, arrhythmias (especially persistent tachycardias), alcohol- or drug-induced myocardial depression, intracardiac shunts, and high-output states. Calcium

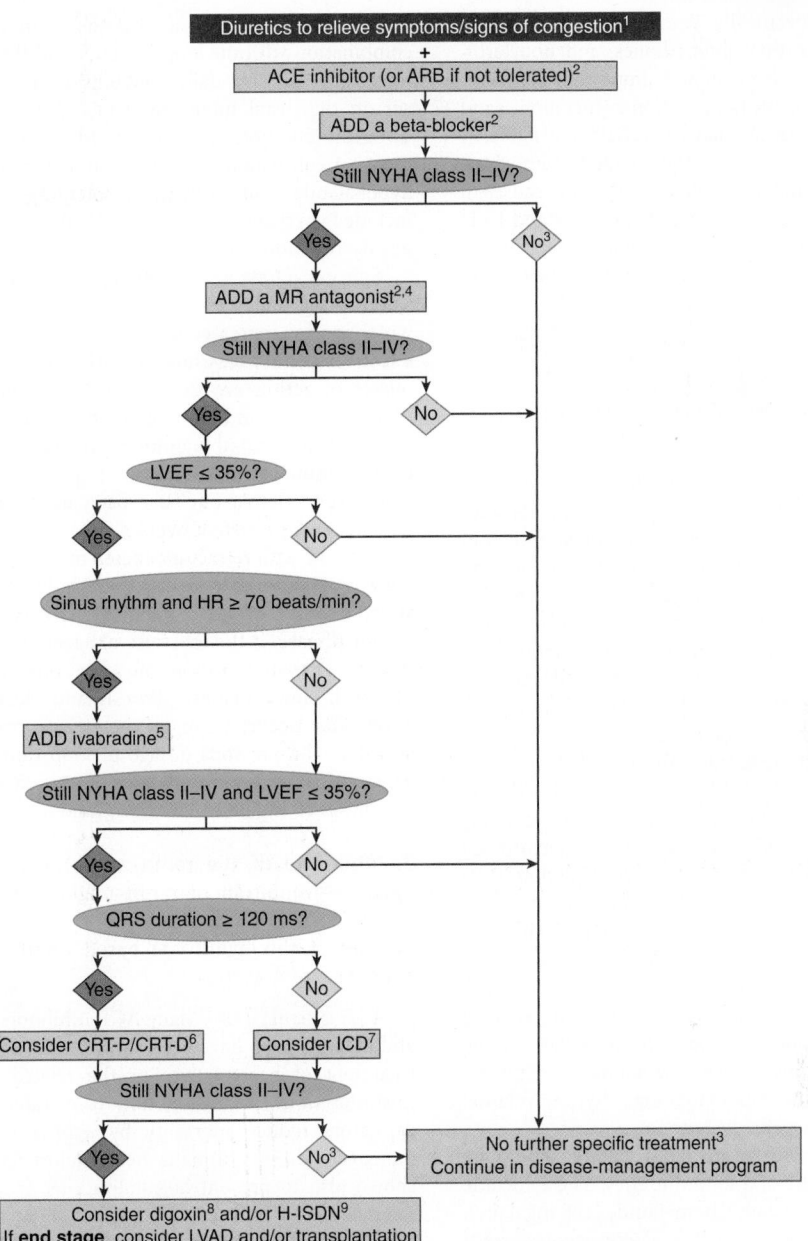

Diuretics to relieve symptoms/signs of congestion[1]
+
ACE inhibitor (or ARB if not tolerated)[2]

ADD a beta-blocker[2]

Still NYHA class II–IV?

Yes → ADD a MR antagonist[2,4]

No[3]

Still NYHA class II–IV?

Yes → LVEF ≤ 35%?

No

LVEF ≤ 35%?

Yes → Sinus rhythm and HR ≥ 70 beats/min?

No

Sinus rhythm and HR ≥ 70 beats/min?

Yes → ADD ivabradine[5]

No

Still NYHA class II–IV and LVEF ≤ 35%?

Yes → QRS duration ≥ 120 ms?

No

QRS duration ≥ 120 ms?

Yes → Consider CRT-P/CRT-D[6]

No → Consider ICD[7]

Still NYHA class II–IV?

Yes

No[3] → No further specific treatment[3]
Continue in disease-management program

Consider digoxin[8] and/or H-ISDN[9]
If **end stage**, consider LVAD and/or transplantation

[1]Diuretics may be used as needed to relieve the signs and symptoms of congestion (see Section 7.5) but they have not been shown to reduce hospitalization of death.
[2]Should be titrated to evidence-based dose or maximum tolerated dose below the evidence-based dose.
[3]Asymptomatic patients with an LVEF ≤ 35% and a history of myocardial infarction should be considered for an ICD.
[4]If mineralocorticoid receptor antagonist not tolerated, an ARB may be added to an ACE inhibitor as an alternative.
[5]European Medicines Agency has approved ivabradine for use in patients with a heart rate ≥ 75 b.p.m. May also be considered in patients with a contraindication to a beta-blocker or beta-blocker intolerance.
[6]See Section 9.2 for details—indication differs according to heart rhythm, NYHA class, QRS duration, QRS morphology, and LVEF.
[7]Not indicated in NYHA class IV.
[8]Digoxin may be used earlier to control the ventricular rate in patients with atrial fibrillation—usually in conjunction with a beta-blocker.
[9]The combination of hydralazine and isosorbide dinitrate may also be considered earlier in patients unable to tolerate an ACE inhibitor or an ARB.

▲ **Figure 10–10.** Treatment options for patients with chronic symptomatic systolic heart failure. ACE, angiotensin-converting enzyme; ARB, angiotensin receptor blocker; CRT-D, cardiac resynchronization therapy defibrillator; CRT-P, cardiac resynchronization therapy pacemaker; H-ISDN, hydralazine and isosorbide dinitrate; HR, heart rate; ICD, implantable cardioverter defibrillator; LBBB, left bundle branch block; LVAD, left ventricular assist device; LVEF, left ventricular ejection fraction; MR antagonist, mineralocorticoid receptor antagonist; NYHA, New York Heart Association. (Modified, with permission, from McMurray JJ et al. ESC guidelines for the diagnosis and treatment of acute and chronic heart failure 2012: the Task Force for the Diagnosis and Treatment of Acute and Chronic Heart Failure 2012 of the European Society of Cardiology. Eur J Heart Fail. 2012 Aug;14(8):803–69. [PMID: 22828712]) channel blockers (specifically verapamil or diltiazem), antiarrhythmic drugs, thiazolidinediones, and nonsteroidal anti-inflammatory agents may be important contributors to worsening heart failure. Some metabolic and infiltrative cardiomyopathies may be partially reversible, or their progression may be slowed; these include hemochromatosis, sarcoidosis, and amyloidosis. Reversible causes of diastolic dysfunction include pericardial disease and LVH due to hypertension. Once possible reversible components are being addressed, the measures outlined below are appropriate.

B. Pharmacologic

See also the following section on Acute Heart Failure & Pulmonary Edema.

1. Diuretic therapy—Diuretics are the most effective means of providing symptomatic relief to patients with moderate to severe heart failure with dyspnea and fluid overload. Few patients with symptoms or signs of fluid retention can be optimally managed without a diuretic. However, excessive diuresis can lead to electrolyte imbalance and neurohormonal activation. *A combination of a diuretic and an ACE inhibitor should be the initial treatment in most symptomatic patients with heart failure and reduced LVEF, with the early addition of a beta-blocker.*

When fluid retention is mild, thiazide diuretics or a similar type of agent (hydrochlorothiazide, 25–100 mg; metolazone, 2.5–5 mg; chlorthalidone, 25–50 mg; etc) may be sufficient. Thiazide or related diuretics often provide better control of hypertension than short-acting loop agents. The thiazides are generally ineffective when the glomerular filtration rate falls below 30–40 mL/min, a not infrequent occurrence in patients with severe heart failure. Metolazone maintains its efficacy down to a glomerular filtration rate of approximately 20–30 mL/min. Adverse reactions include hypokalemia and intravascular volume depletion with resulting prerenal azotemia, skin rashes, neutropenia and thrombocytopenia, hyperglycemia, hyperuricemia, and hepatic dysfunction.

Patients with more severe heart failure should be treated with one of the oral loop diuretics. These include furosemide (20–320 mg daily), bumetanide (1–8 mg daily), and torsemide (20–200 mg daily). These agents have a rapid onset and a relatively short duration of action. In patients with preserved kidney function, two or more daily doses are preferable to a single larger dose. In acute situations or when gastrointestinal absorption is in doubt, they should be given intravenously. Torsemide may be effective when furosemide is not, including related to better absorption and a longer half life. Larger doses (up to 500 mg of furosemide or equivalent) may be required with severe renal impairment. The major adverse reactions include intravascular volume depletion, prerenal azotemia, and hypotension. Hypokalemia, particularly with accompanying digitalis therapy, is a major problem. Less common side effects include skin rashes, gastrointestinal distress, and ototoxicity (the latter more common with ethacrynic acid and possibly less common with bumetanide).

The oral potassium-sparing agents are often useful in combination with the loop diuretics and thiazides. Triamterene (37.5–75 mg daily) and amiloride (5–10 mg daily) act on the distal tubule to reduce potassium secretion. Their diuretic potency is only mild and not adequate for most patients with heart failure, but they may minimize the hypokalemia induced by more potent agents. Side effects include hyperkalemia, gastrointestinal symptoms, and kidney dysfunction.

Spironolactone (12.5–100 mg daily) and eplerenone (25–100 mg daily) are specific inhibitors of aldosterone, which is often increased in heart failure and has important effects beyond potassium retention (see below). Their onsets of action are slower than the other potassium-sparing agents, and spironolactone's side effects include gynecomastia. Combinations of potassium supplements or ACE inhibitors and potassium-sparing drugs can produce hyperkalemia but have been used with success in patients with persistent hypokalemia.

Patients with refractory edema may respond to combinations of a loop diuretic and thiazide-like agents. Metolazone, because of its maintained activity with chronic kidney disease, is the most useful agent for such a combination. Extreme caution must be observed with this approach, since massive diuresis and electrolyte imbalances often occur; 2.5 mg of metolazone orally should be added to the previous dosage of loop diuretic. In many cases this is necessary only once or twice a week, but dosages up to 10 mg daily have been used in some patients.

2. Inhibitors of the renin–angiotensin–aldosterone system—Inhibition of renin–angiotensin–aldosterone system with ACE inhibitors should be part of the initial therapy of this syndrome based on their life-saving benefits.

A. ACE INHIBITORS—Many ACE inhibitors are available, and at least seven have been shown to be effective for the treatment of heart failure or the related indication of postinfarction LV dysfunction (see Table 11–7). ACE inhibitors reduce mortality by approximately 20% in patients with symptomatic heart failure and have been shown also to prevent hospitalizations, increase exercise tolerance, and reduce symptoms in these patients. As a result, ACE inhibitors should be part of first-line treatment of patients with symptomatic LV systolic dysfunction (EF < 40%), usually in combination with a diuretic. They are also indicated for the management of patients with reduced EFs without symptoms because they prevent the progression to clinical heart failure.

Because ACE inhibitors may induce significant hypotension, particularly following the initial doses, they must be started with caution. Hypotension is most prominent in patients with already low BPs (systolic pressure < 100 mm Hg), hypovolemia, prerenal azotemia (especially if it is diuretic induced), and hyponatremia (an indicator of activation of the renin–angiotensin system). These patients should generally be started at low dosages (captopril 6.25 mg orally three times daily, enalapril 2.5 mg orally daily, or the equivalent), but other patients may be started at twice these dosages. Within several days (for those with the markers of higher risk) or at most 2 weeks, patients should be questioned about symptoms of hypotension, and both kidney function and K^+ levels should be monitored.

ACE inhibitors should be titrated to the dosages proved effective in clinical trials (captopril 50 mg three times daily, enalapril 10 mg twice daily, ramipril 10 mg daily, lisinopril 20 mg daily, or the equivalent) over a period of 1–3 months. Most patients will tolerate these doses. Asymptomatic hypotension is not a contraindication to up-titrating or continuing ACE inhibitors. Some patients exhibit increases in serum creatinine or K^+, but they do not require discontinuation if the levels stabilize—even at values as high as 3 mg/dL and 5.5 mEq/L, respectively. Kidney dysfunction is more frequent in diabetic patients, older patients, and those with low systolic pressures, and these groups should be monitored more closely. The most common side effects of ACE inhibitors in heart failure patients are dizziness (often not related to the level of BP) and cough, though the latter is often due as much to heart failure or intercurrent pulmonary conditions as to the ACE inhibitor.

B. Angiotensin II receptor blockers—Another approach to inhibiting the renin–angiotensin–aldosterone system is the use of specific ARBs (see Table 11–7), which will decrease adverse effects of angiotensin II by blocking the AT_1 receptor. In addition, because there are alternative pathways of angiotensin II production in many tissues, the receptor blockers may provide more complete blockade of the AT_1 receptor.

However, these agents do not share the effects of ACE inhibitors on other potentially important pathways that produce increases in bradykinin, prostaglandins, and nitric oxide in the heart, blood vessels, and other tissues. The Valsartan in Heart Failure Trial (Val-HeFT) examined the efficacy of adding valsartan (titrated to a dose of 160 mg orally twice a day) to ACE inhibitor therapy. While the addition of valsartan did not reduce mortality, the composite of death or hospitalization for heart failure was significantly reduced. The CHARM trial randomized 7601 patients with chronic heart failure with or without LV systolic dysfunction and with or without background ACE inhibitor therapy to candesartan (titrated to 32 mg orally daily) or placebo. Among patients with an LVEF of < 40%, there was an 18% reduction in cardiovascular death or heart failure hospitalization and a statistically significant 12% reduction in all-cause mortality. The benefits were similar among patients on ACE inhibitors, including among patients on full-dose ACE inhibitors. Thus, ARBs, specifically candesartan or valsartan, provide important benefits as an alternative to, and in addition to, ACE inhibitors in chronic heart failure with reduced LVEF. A large trial of patients with chronic heart failure and preserved LVEF found no benefit from the ARB irbesartan.

C. Spironolactione and eplerenone—Inhibiting aldosterone has become a mainstay of management of symptomatic heart failure with reduced LVEF. The RALES trial compared spironolactone 25 mg daily with placebo in patients with advanced heart failure (current or recent class IV) already receiving ACE inhibitors and diuretics and showed a 29% reduction in mortality as well as similar decreases in other clinical end points. Hyperkalemia was uncommon in this severe heart failure clinical trial population, which was maintained on high doses of diuretic, but hyperkalemia with spironolactone appears to be common in general practice. Potassium levels should be monitored closely during initiation of spironolactone (after 1 and 4 weeks of therapy), particularly for patients with even mild degrees of kidney injury, and in patients receiving ACE inhibitors. Based on the EMPHASIS-HF trial, the efficacy and safety of aldosterone antagonism—in the form of eplerenone, 25–50 mg orally daily—is established for patients with mild or moderate heart failure. This trial showed a significant reduction in cardiovascular death as well as in hospitalization for heart failure among patients with NYHA class II heart failure and LVEF< 30%. Most experts believe that spironolactone is likely to provide similar benefit. *Careful monitoring of serum potassium levels, in particular for patients with any degree of kidney insufficiency, is important to avoid life-threatening hyperkalemia. Serum potassium should be checked within 1 week of initiating an aldosterone blocker and periodically thereafter.*

While the TOPCAT trial failed to show that spironolactone improved cardiovascular mortality and morbidity in a population of patients with heart failure and preserved LVEF (≥ 45%), there appeared to be a reduction in heart failure hospitalization, but at the cost of increased hyperkalemia and renal dysfunction.

3. Beta-blockers—Beta-blockers are part of the foundation of care of chronic heart failure based on their life-saving benefits. The mechanism of this benefit remains unclear, but it is likely that chronic elevations of catecholamines and sympathetic nervous system activity cause progressive myocardial damage, leading to worsening LV function and dilation. The primary evidence for this hypothesis is that over a period of 3–6 months, beta-blockers produce consistent substantial rises in EF (averaging 10% absolute increase) and reductions in LV size and mass.

Three drugs have strong evidence of reducing mortality: carvedilol (a nonselective beta-1- and beta-2-receptor blocker), the beta-1-selective extended-release agent metoprolol succinate, (but not short-acting metoprolol tartrate), and bisoprolol (beta-1-selective agent).

This has led to a strong recommendation that *stable* patients (defined as having no recent deterioration or evidence of volume overload) with mild, moderate, and even severe heart failure should be treated with a beta-blocker unless there is a noncardiac contraindication. In the COPERNICUS trial, carvedilol was both well tolerated and highly effective in reducing both mortality and heart failure hospitalizations in a group of patients with severe (NYHA class III or IV) symptoms, but care was taken to ensure that they were free of fluid retention at the time of initiation. In this study, one death was prevented for every 13 patients treated for 1 year—as dramatic an effect as has been seen with a pharmacologic therapy in the history of cardiovascular medicine. One trial comparing carvedilol and (short-acting) metoprolol tartrate (COMET) found significant reductions in all-cause mortality and cardiovascular mortality with carvedilol. Thus, patients with chronic heart failure should be treated with extended-release metoprolol succinate, bisoprolol, or carvedilol, but not short-acting metoprolol tartrate.

Because even apparently stable patients may deteriorate when beta-blockers are initiated, initiation must be done gradually and with great care. Carvedilol is initiated at a dosage of 3.125 mg orally twice daily and may be increased to 6.25, 12.5, and 25 mg twice daily at intervals of approximately 2 weeks. The protocols for sustained-release metoprolol use were started at 12.5 or 25 mg orally daily and doubled at intervals of 2 weeks to a target dose of 200 mg daily (using the Toprol XL sustained-release preparation). Bisoprolol was administered at a dosage of 1.25, 2.5, 3.75, 5, 7.5, and 10 mg orally daily, with increments at 1- to 4-week intervals. More gradual up-titration is often more convenient and may be better tolerated. The SENIORS trial of 2135 patients found that nebivolol was effective in elderly patients (70 years and older) with chronic heart failure, although the evidence of degree of benefit was not as strong as with the three proven beta-blockers carvedilol, metoprolol succinate, or bisoprolol.

Patients should be instructed to monitor their weights at home as an indicator of fluid retention and to report any increase or change in symptoms immediately. Before each dose increase, the patient should be seen and examined to ensure that there has not been fluid retention or worsening of symptoms. If heart failure worsens, this can usually be managed by increasing diuretic doses and delaying further increases in beta-blocker doses, though downward adjustments or discontinuation is sometimes required. Carvedilol, because of its beta-blocking activity, may cause dizziness or hypotension. This can usually be managed by reducing the doses of other vasodilators and by slowing the pace of dose increases.

4. Digitalis glycosides—The efficacy of digitalis glycosides in reducing the symptoms of heart failure has been established in at least four multicenter trials that have demonstrated that digoxin withdrawal is associated with worsening symptoms and signs of heart failure, more frequent hospitalizations for decompensation, and reduced exercise tolerance. This was also seen in the 6800-patient Digitalis Investigators Group (DIG) trial, though that study found no benefit (or harm) with regard to survival. A reduction in deaths due to progressive heart failure was balanced by an increase in deaths due to ischemic and arrhythmic events. Based on these results, digoxin should be used for patients who remain symptomatic when taking diuretics and ACE inhibitors as well as for patients with heart failure who are in atrial fibrillation and require rate control.

Digoxin has a half-life of 24–36 hours and is eliminated almost entirely by the kidneys. The oral maintenance dose may range from 0.125 mg three times weekly to 0.5 mg daily. It is lower in patients with kidney dysfunction, in older patients, and in those with smaller lean body mass. Although an oral loading dose of 0.75–1.25 mg (depending primarily on lean body size) over 24–48 hours may be

given if an early effect is desired, in most patients with chronic heart failure it is sufficient to begin with the expected maintenance dose (usually 0.125–0.25 mg daily). Amiodarone, quinidine, propafenone, and verapamil are among the drugs that may increase digoxin levels up to 100%. It is prudent to measure a blood level after 7–14 days (and at least 6 hours after the last dose was administered). Optimum serum digoxin levels are 0.7–1.2 ng/mL, though clinically evident toxicity is rare with levels < 1.8 ng/mL. Digoxin may induce ventricular arrhythmias, especially when hypokalemia or myocardial ischemia is present. Once an appropriate maintenance dose is established, subsequent levels are usually not indicated unless there is a change in kidney function or medications that affects digoxin levels or a significant deterioration in cardiac status that may be associated with reduced clearance. Digoxin toxicity is discussed in Chapter 38.

5. Vasodilators—Although ACE inhibitors, which have vasodilating properties, improve prognosis, such a benefit is not established with the direct-acting vasodilators. The combination of hydralazine and isosorbide dinitrate has been shown to improve outcome in African Americans, but the effect is less clear than the well-established benefits of ACE inhibitors. The 2012 European guidelines give hydralazine and isosorbide dinitrate a modest class IIb recommendation for patients with reduced LVEF who are unable to tolerate ACE inhibitor and ARB therapy, or who have persistent symptoms despite treatment with a beta-blocker, ACE inhibitor, and aldosterone antagonist.

See section on Acute Myocardial Infarction earlier in this chapter for a discussion on the intravenous vasodilating drugs and their dosages.

A. Nitrates—Intravenous vasodilators (sodium nitroprusside or nitroglycerin) are used primarily for acute or severely decompensated chronic heart failure, especially when accompanied by hypertension or myocardial ischemia. If neither of the latter is present, therapy is best initiated and adjusted based on hemodynamic measurements. The starting dosage for nitroglycerin is generally about 10 mcg/min, which is titrated upward by 10–20 mcg/min (to a maximum of 200 mcg/min) until mean arterial pressure drops by 10%. Hypotension (BP < 100 mm Hg systolic) should be avoided. For sodium nitroprusside, the starting dosage is 0.3–0.5 mcg/kg/min with upward titration to a maximum dose of 10 mcg/kg/min.

Isosorbide dinitrate, 20–80 mg orally three times daily, and nitroglycerin ointment, 12.5–50 mg (1–4 inches) every 6–8 hours, appears to be equally effective although the ointment is somewhat inconvenient for long-term therapy. The nitrates are moderately effective in relieving shortness of breath, especially in patients with mild to moderate symptoms, but less successful—probably because they have little effect on cardiac output—in advanced heart failure. Nitrate therapy is generally well tolerated, but headaches and hypotension may limit the dose of all agents. The development of tolerance to long-term nitrate therapy occurs. This is minimized by intermittent therapy, especially if a daily 8- to 12-hour nitrate-free interval is used, but probably develops to some extent in most patients receiving these agents. Transdermal nitroglycerin patches have no sustained effect in patients with heart failure and should not be used for this indication.

B. Hydralazine—Oral hydralazine is a potent arteriolar dilator; when used as a single agent, it has not been shown to improve symptoms or exercise tolerance during long-term treatment. The combination of nitrates and oral hydralazine produces greater hemodynamic effects.

Hydralazine therapy is frequently limited by side effects. Approximately 30% of patients are unable to tolerate the relatively high doses required to produce hemodynamic improvement in heart failure (200–400 mg daily in divided doses). The major side effect is gastrointestinal distress, but headaches, tachycardia, and hypotension are relatively common. ARBs have largely supplanted the use of the hydralazine–isosorbide dinitrate combination in ACE-intolerant patients.

6. Ivabradine—Ivabradine inhibits the If channel in the sinus node and has the specific effect of slowing sinus rate. The SHIFT trial enrolled 6588 patients with symptomatic heart failure, LVEF ≤ 35%, and sinus rhythm with rate ≥ 70 beats per minute. Most patients were receiving an ACE inhibitor, a beta-blocker, and an aldosterone antagonist, although a minority were on full-dose beta-blocker. Cardiovascular death and hospitalizaiton for heart failure were reduced by 18%, with an absolute reduction of 4.2% over 23 months, mainly driven by less heart failure hospitalization. Ivabradine is not approved for use in the United States; it is approved by the European Medicines Agency for use in patients with a heart rate ≥ 75 beats per minute. The European guidelines give it a class IIa recommendation for patients in sinus rhythm with heart rate ≥ 70 beats per minute with an EF ≤ 35%, and persisting symptoms despite treatment with an evidence-based dose of beta-blocker (or maximum tolerated dose below that), ACE inhibitor (or ARB), and an aldosterone antagonist (or ARB).

7. Combination of medical therapies—Optimal management of chronic heart failure involves using combinations of proven life-saving therapies. In addition to ACE inhibitors and beta-blockers, patients who remain symptomatic should be considered for additional therapy, in the form of ARBs (best proven in class II–III heart failure), mineralocorticoid (aldosterone) receptor antagonists, or hydralazine and isosorbide dinitrate (with some evidence of benefit in African Americans).

8. Treatments that may cause harm in heart failure with reduced LVEF—Several therapies should be avoided, when possible, in patients with systolic heart failure, and therefore are listed as class III recommendations in the European guidelines. These include thiazoladinediones (glitazones) that cause worsening heart failure, most calcium channel blockers (with the exception of amlodipine and felodipine), nonsteroidal anti-inflammatory drugs, and cyclooxygenase-2 inhibitors that cause sodium and water retention and renal impairment, and the combination of an ACE inhibitor, ARB, and aldosterone blocker that increases the risk of hyperkalemia.

9. Anticoagulation—Patients with LV failure and reduced EF are at somewhat increased risk for developing intracardiac thrombi and systemic arterial emboli. However, this risk appears to be primarily in patients who are in atrial fibrillation, who have had thromboemboli, or who have large recent anterior myocardial infarction. In general, these patients should receive warfarin for 3 months following the myocardial infarction. Other patients with heart failure have embolic rates of approximately two per 100 patient-years of follow-up, which approximates the rate of major bleeding, and routine anticoagulation does not appear warranted except in patients with prior embolic events or mobile LV thrombi.

10. Antiarrhythmic therapy—Patients with moderate to severe heart failure have a high incidence of both symptomatic and asymptomatic arrhythmias. Although < 10% of patients have syncope or presyncope resulting from ventricular tachycardia, ambulatory monitoring reveals that up to 70% of patients have asymptomatic episodes of NSVT. These arrhythmias indicate a poor prognosis independent of the severity of LV dysfunction, but many of the deaths are probably not arrhythmia related. Beta-blockers, because of their marked favorable effect on prognosis in general and on the incidence of sudden death specifically, should be initiated in these as well as all other patients with heart failure (see Beta-Blockers, above). Empiric antiarrhythmic therapy with amiodarone did not improve outcome in the SCD-HeFT trial, and most other agents are contraindicated because of their proarrhythmic effects in this population and their adverse effect on cardiac function. For patients with systolic heart failure and atrial fibrillation, a rhythm control strategy has not been shown to improve outcome compared to a rate control strategy and thus should be reserved for patients with a reversible cause of atrial fibrillation or refractory symptoms. Then, amiodarone is the drug of choice.

11. Statin therapy—Even though vascular disease is present in many patients with chronic heart failure, the role of statins has not been well defined in the heart failure population. Two trials—the CORONA and the GISSI-HF trials—have failed to show benefits of statins in the chronic heart failure population.

C. Nonpharmacologic Treatment

1. Implantable cardioverter defibrillators—Randomized clinical trials have extended the indications for ICDs beyond patients with symptomatic or asymptomatic arrhythmias to the broad population of patients with chronic heart failure and LV systolic dysfunction who are receiving contemporary heart failure treatments, including beta-blockers. In the second Multicenter Automatic Defibrillator Implantation Trial (MADIT II), 1232 patients with prior myocardial infarction and an EF < 30% were randomized to an ICD or a control group. Mortality was 31% lower in the ICD group, which translated into nine lives saved for each 100 patients who received a device and were monitored for 3 years. The United States Centers for Medicare and Medicaid Services provides reimbursement coverage to include patients with chronic heart failure and ischemic or nonischemic cardiomyopathy with an EF ≤ 35%.

2. Biventricular pacing (resynchronization)—Many patients with heart failure due to systolic dysfunction have abnormal intraventricular conduction that results in dyssynchronous and hence inefficient contractions. Several studies have evaluated the efficacy of "multisite" pacing, using leads that stimulate the RV from the apex and the LV from the lateral wall via the coronary sinus. Patients with wide QRS complexes (generally ≥ 120 milliseconds), reduced EFs, and moderate to severe symptoms have been evaluated. Results from trials with up to 2 years of follow-up have shown an increase in EF, improvement in symptoms and exercise tolerance, and reduction in death and hospitalization. The best responders to cardiac resynchronization therapy are patients with wider QRS, left bundle branch block, and nonischemic cardiomyopathy, and the lowest responders are those with narrow QRS and non–left bundle branch block pattern. Thus, as recommended in the 2013 European guidelines, resynchronization therapy is indicated for patients with class II, III, and ambulatory class IV heart failure, EF ≤ 35%, and left bundle branch blockpattern with QRS duration of ≥ 120 msec. Patients with non–left bundle branch block pattern and prolonged QRS duration may be considered for treatment.

3. Case management, diet, and exercise training—Thirty to 50 percent of heart failure patients who are hospitalized will be readmitted within 3–6 months. Strategies to prevent clinical deterioration, such as case management, home monitoring of weight and clinical status, and patient adjustment of diuretics, can prevent rehospitalizations and should be part of the treatment regimen of advanced heart failure. Involvement of a multidisciplinary team (rather than a single physician) and in-person (rather than telephonic) communication appear to be important features of successful programs.

Patients should routinely practice moderate salt restriction (2–2.5 g sodium or 5–6 g salt per day). More severe sodium restriction is usually difficult to achieve and unnecessary because of the availability of potent diuretic agents.

Exercise training improves activity tolerance in significant part by reversing the peripheral abnormalities associated with heart failure and deconditioning. In severe heart failure, restriction of activity may facilitate temporary recompensation. A large trial (HF ACTION, 2331 patients) showed no significant benefit (nor harm) from a structured exercise training program on death or hospitalization, although functional status and symptoms were improved. Thus, in stable patients, a prudent increase in activity or a regular exercise regimen can be encouraged. Indeed, a gradual exercise program is associated with diminished symptoms and substantial increases in exercise capacity.

4. Coronary revascularization—Since underlying CAD is the cause of heart failure in the majority of patients, coronary revascularization has been thought to be able to both improve symptoms and prevent progression. However, the STITCH trial failed to show an overall survival benefit from CABG among patients with multivessel coronary disease who were candidates for CABG but who had heart failure and a LVEF of ≤ 35%. Revascularization does appear warranted for some patients with heart failure, including those with more severe angina or left main coronary disease (excluded from the STITCH trial), or selected patients with less severe symptoms.

5. Cardiac transplantation—Because of the poor prognosis of patients with advanced heart failure, cardiac transplantation is widely used. Many centers have 1-year survival rates exceeding 80–90%, and 5-year survival rates above 70%. Infections, hypertension and kidney dysfunction caused by cyclosporine, rapidly progressive coronary atherosclerosis, and immunosuppressant-related cancers have been the major complications. The high cost and limited number of donor organs require careful patient selection early in the course.

6. Other surgical treatment options—Externally powered and implantable ventricular assist devices can be used in patients who require ventricular support either to allow the heart to recover or as a bridge to transplantation. The latest generation devices are small enough to allow patients unrestricted mobility and even discharge from the hospital. Continuous flow devices appear to be more effective than pulsatile flow devices. However, complications are frequent, including bleeding, thromboembolism, and infection, and the cost is very high, exceeding $200,000 in the initial 1–3 months.

Although 1-year survival was improved in the REMATCH randomized trial, all 129 patients died by 26 months.

7. Palliative care—Despite the technologic advances of recent years, it should be remembered that many patients with chronic heart failure are elderly and have multiple comorbidities. Many of them will not experience meaningful improvements in survival with aggressive therapy, and the goal of management should be symptomatic improvement and palliation (see Chapter 5).

► **Prognosis**

Once manifest, heart failure carries a poor prognosis. Even with modern treatment, the 5-year mortality is approximately 50%. Mortality rates vary from < 5% per year in those with no or few symptoms to > 30% per year in those with severe and refractory symptoms. These figures emphasize the critical importance of early detection and intervention. Higher mortality is related to older age, lower LVEF, more severe symptoms, chronic kidney disease, and diabetes. The prognosis of heart failure has improved in the past two decades, probably at least in part because of the more widespread use of ACE inhibitors and beta-blockers, which markedly improve survival.

► **When to Refer**

Patients with new symptoms of heart failure not explained by an obvious cause should be referred to a cardiologist.

Patients with continued symptoms of heart failure and reduced LVEF (≤ 35%) should be referred to a cardiologist for consideration of placement of an ICD or cardiac resynchronization therapy (if QRS duration is ≥ 120 msec especially with left bundle branch block pattern).

When to Admit

- Patients with unexplained new or worsened symptoms, or positive cardiac biomarkers concerning for acute myocardial necrosis.

- Patients with hypoxia, fluid overload, or pulmonary edema not readily resolved in outpatient setting.

Brignole M et al. 2013 ESC Guidelines on cardiac pacing and cardiac resynchronization therapy: the Task Force on cardiac pacing and resynchronization therapy of the European Society of Cardiology (ESC). Developed in collaboration with the European Heart Rhythm Association (EHRA). Eur Heart J. 2013 Aug;34(29):2281–329. [PMID: 23801822]

Davies EJ et al. Exercise based rehabilitation for heart failure. Cochrane Database Syst Rev. 2010 Apr 14;4: CD003331. [PMID: 20393935]

Ezekowitz JA et al. Standardizing care for acute decompensated heart failure in a large megatrial: the approach for the Acute Studies of Clinical Effectiveness of Nesiritide in Subjects with Decompensated Heart Failure (ASCEND-HF). Am Heart J. 2009 Feb;157(2):219–28. [PMID: 19185628]

Hunt SA et al. 2009 focused update incorporated into the ACC/AHA 2005 Guidelines for the Diagnosis and Management of Heart Failure in Adults: a report of the American College of Cardiology Foundation/American Heart Association Task Force on Practice Guidelines: developed in collaboration with the International Society for Heart and Lung Transplantation. Circulation. 2009 Apr 14;119(14):e391–479. [PMID: 19324966]

McMurray JJ et al. ESC guidelines for the diagnosis and treatment of acute and chronic heart failure 2012: the Task Force for the Diagnosis and Treatment of Acute and Chronic Heart Failure 2012 of the European Society of Cardiology. Eur J Heart Fail. 2012 Aug;14(8):803–69. [PMID: 22828712]

Moss AJ et al. Cardiac-resynchronization therapy for the prevention of heart-failure events. N Engl J Med. 2009 Oct 1;361(14): 1329–38. [PMID: 19723701]

Shah AM et al; TOPCAT Investigators. Cardiac structure and function in heart failure with preserved ejection fraction: baseline findings from the echocardiographic study of the treatment of preserved cardiac function heart failure with an aldosterone antagonist trial. Circ Heart Fail. 2014 Jan 1;7(1): 104–15. [PMID: 24249049]

Swedberg K et al. Ivabradine and outcomes in chronic heart failure (SHIFT): a randomised placebo-controlled study. Lancet. 2010 Sep 11;376(9744):875–85. [PMID: 20801500]

Tang AS et al; Resynchronization-Defibrillation for Ambulatory Heart Failure Trial Investigators. Cardiac-resynchronization therapy for mild-to-moderate heart failure. N Engl J Med. 2010 Dec 16;363(25):2385–95. [PMID: 21073365]

Torpy JM et al. JAMA patient page. Heart failure. JAMA. 2009 May 13;301(18):1950. [PMID: 19436025]

Velazquez EJ et al; STICH Investigators. Coronary-artery bypass surgery in patients with left ventricular dysfunction. N Engl J Med. 2011 Apr 28;364(17):1607–16. [PMID: 21463150]

Zannad F et al; EMPHASIS-HF Study Group. Eplerenone in patients with systolic heart failure and mild symptoms. N Engl J Med. 2011 Jan 6;364(1):11–21. [PMID: 21073363]

ACUTE HEART FAILURE & PULMONARY EDEMA

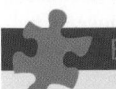 ESSENTIALS OF DIAGNOSIS

- ▶ Acute onset or worsening of dyspnea at rest.
- ▶ Tachycardia, diaphoresis, cyanosis.
- ▶ Pulmonary rales, rhonchi; expiratory wheezing.
- ▶ Radiograph shows interstitial and alveolar edema with or without cardiomegaly.
- ▶ Arterial hypoxemia.

General Considerations

Typical causes of acute cardiogenic pulmonary edema include acute myocardial infarction or severe ischemia, exacerbation of chronic heart failure, acute severe hypertension, acute kidney injury, acute volume overload of the LV (valvular regurgitation), and mitral stenosis. By far the most common presentation in developed countries is one of acute or subacute deterioration of chronic heart failure, precipitated by discontinuation of medications, excessive salt intake, myocardial ischemia, tachyarrhythmias (especially rapid atrial fibrillation), or intercurrent infection. Often in the latter group, there is preceding volume overload with worsening edema and progressive shortness of breath for which earlier intervention can usually avoid the need for hospital admission.

Clinical Findings

Acute pulmonary edema presents with a characteristic clinical picture of severe dyspnea, the production of pink, frothy sputum, and diaphoresis and cyanosis. Rales are present in all lung fields, as are generalized wheezing and rhonchi. Pulmonary edema may appear acutely or subacutely in the setting of chronic heart failure or may be the first manifestation of cardiac disease, usually acute myocardial infarction, which may be painful or silent. Less severe decompensations usually present with dyspnea at rest and rales and other evidence of fluid retention but without severe hypoxia.

Noncardiac causes of pulmonary edema include intravenous opioids, increased intracerebral pressure, high altitude, sepsis, several medications, inhaled toxins, transfusion reactions, shock, and disseminated intravascular coagulation. These are distinguished from cardiogenic pulmonary edema by the clinical setting, the history, and the physical examination. Conversely, in most patients with cardiogenic pulmonary edema, an underlying cardiac abnormality can usually be detected clinically or by the ECG, chest radiograph, or echocardiogram.

The chest radiograph reveals signs of pulmonary vascular redistribution, blurriness of vascular outlines, increased interstitial markings, and, characteristically, the butterfly pattern of distribution of alveolar edema. The heart may be enlarged or normal in size depending on whether heart failure was previously present. Assessment of cardiac function by echocardiography is important, since a substantial proportion of patients has normal EFs with elevated atrial pressures due to diastolic dysfunction. In cardiogenic pulmonary edema, BNP is elevated, and the PCWP is invariably elevated, usually over 25 mm Hg. In noncardiogenic pulmonary edema, the wedge pressure may be normal or even low.

▶ Treatment

In full-blown pulmonary edema, the patient should be placed in a sitting position with legs dangling over the side of the bed; this facilitates respiration and reduces venous return. Oxygen is delivered by mask to obtain an arterial $Po_2 > 60$ mm Hg. Noninvasive pressure support ventilation may improve oxygenation and prevent severe CO_2 retention while pharmacologic interventions take effect. However, if respiratory distress remains severe, endotracheal intubation and mechanical ventilation may be necessary.

Morphine is highly effective in pulmonary edema and may be helpful in less severe decompensations when the patient is uncomfortable. The initial dosage is 2–8 mg intravenously (subcutaneous administration is effective in milder cases) and may be repeated after 2–4 hours. Morphine increases venous capacitance, lowering LA pressure, and relieves anxiety, which can reduce the efficiency of ventilation. However, morphine may lead to CO_2 retention by reducing the ventilatory drive. It should be avoided in patients with opioid-induced pulmonary edema, who may improve with opioid-antagonists, and in those with neurogenic pulmonary edema.

Intravenous diuretic therapy (furosemide, 40 mg, or bumetanide, 1 mg—or higher doses if the patient has been receiving long-term diuretic therapy) is usually indicated even if the patient has not exhibited prior fluid retention. These agents produce venodilation prior to the onset of diuresis. The DOSE trial has shown that, for acute decompensated heart failure, bolus doses of furosemide are of similar efficacy as continuous intravenous infusion, and that higher dose furosemide (2.5 times the prior daily dose) resulted in more rapid fluid removal without a substantially higher risk of kidney impairment.

Nitrate therapy accelerates clinical improvement by reducing both BP and LV filling pressures. Sublingual nitroglycerin or isosorbide dinitrate, topical nitroglycerin, or intravenous nitrates will ameliorate dyspnea rapidly prior to the onset of diuresis, and these agents are particularly valuable in patients with accompanying hypertension.

Intravenous nesiritide, a recombinant form of human BNP, is a potent vasodilator that reduces ventricular filling pressures and improves cardiac output. Its hemodynamic effects resemble those of intravenous nitroglycerin with a more predictable dose–response curve and a longer duration of action. In clinical studies, nesiritide (administered as 2 mcg/kg by intravenous bolus injection followed by an infusion of 0.01 mcg/kg/min, which may be up-titrated if needed) produced a rapid improvement in both dyspnea and hemodynamics. The primary adverse effect is hypotension, which may be symptomatic and sustained. The ASCEND trial randomized nearly 7000 patients with acute decompensated heart failure to receive either nesiritide or placebo; results showed a reduction in dyspnea, worsening in kidney function, and no effect on death or heart failure rehospitalization. Because most patients with acute heart failure respond well to conventional therapy, the role of nesiritide may be primarily in patients who continue to be symptomatic after initial treatment with diuretics and nitrates.

A randomized placebo-controlled trial of 950 patients evaluating intravenous milrinone in patients admitted for decompensated heart failure who had no definite indications for inotropic therapy showed no benefit in increasing survival, decreasing length of admission, or preventing readmission. In addition, rates of sustained hypotension and atrial fibrillation were significantly increased. Thus, the role of positive inotropic agents appears to be limited in patients with refractory symptoms and signs of low cardiac output, particularly if life-threatening vital organ hypoperfusion (such as deteriorating kidney function) is present. In some cases, dobutamine or milrinone may help maintain patients who are awaiting cardiac transplantation.

Bronchospasm may occur in response to pulmonary edema and may itself exacerbate hypoxemia and dyspnea. Treatment with inhaled beta-adrenergic agonists or intravenous aminophylline may be helpful, but both may also provoke tachycardia and supraventricular arrhythmias.

In most cases, pulmonary edema responds rapidly to therapy. When the patient has improved, the cause or precipitating factor should be ascertained. In patients without prior heart failure, evaluation should include echocardiography and in many cases cardiac catheterization and coronary angiography. Patients with acute decompensation of chronic heart failure should be treated to achieve a euvolemic state and have their medical regimen optimized. Generally, an oral diuretic and an ACE inhibitor should be initiated, with efficacy and tolerability confirmed prior to discharge. In selected patients, early but careful initiation of beta-blockers in low doses should be considered.

Felker GM et al; NHLBI Heart Failure Clinical Research Network. Diuretic strategies in patients with acute decompensated heart failure. N Engl J Med. 2011 Mar 3;364(9):797–805. [PMID: 21366472]

Gray AJ et al; 3CPO Study Investigators. A multicentre randomised controlled trial of the use of continuous positive airway pressure and non-invasive positive pressure ventilation in the early treatment of patients presenting to the emergency department with severe acute cardiogenic pulmonary oedema: the 3CPO trial. Health Technol Assess. 2009 Jul;13(33):1–106. [PMID: 19615296]

Weng CL et al. Meta-analysis: noninvasive ventilation in acute cardiogenic pulmonary edema. Ann Intern Med. 2010 May 4;152(9):590–600. [PMID: 20439577]

West RL et al. A review of dyspnea in acute heart failure syndromes. Am Heart J. 2010 Aug;160(2):209–14. [PMID: 20691823]

MYOCARDITIS & THE CARDIOMYOPATHIES

INFECTIOUS MYOCARDITIS

ESSENTIALS OF DIAGNOSIS

► Often follows an upper respiratory infection.

► May present with chest pain (pleuritic or nonspecific) or signs of heart failure.

► Echocardiogram documents cardiomegaly and contractile dysfunction.

► Myocardial biopsy, though not sensitive, may reveal a characteristic inflammatory pattern. MRI may now have a role in diagnosis.

► General Considerations

Cardiac dysfunction due to primary myocarditis is presumed generally to be caused by either an acute viral infection or a postviral immune response. Secondary myocarditis is the result of inflammation caused by nonviral pathogens, drugs, chemicals, physical agents, or inflammatory diseases such as systemic lupus erythematosus. The list of both infectious and noninfectious causes of myocarditis is extensive (Table 10–16).

Early phase myocarditis is initiated by infection of cardiac tissue. Both cellular and humoral inflammatory processes contribute to the progression to chronic injury, and there are subgroups that might benefit from immunosuppression.

Genetic predisposition is a likely factor in some cases. Autoimmune myocarditis (eg, giant cell myocarditis) may occur with no identifiable viral infection.

► Clinical Findings

A. Symptoms and Signs

Patients may present several days to a few weeks after the onset of an acute febrile illness or a respiratory infection or with heart failure without antecedent symptoms. The onset of heart failure may be gradual or may be abrupt and fulminant. Emboli may occur. Pleural-pericardial chest pain is common. Examination reveals tachycardia, a gallop rhythm, and other evidence of heart failure or conduction defect. Many acute infections are subclinical, though they may present later as idiopathic cardiomyopathy or with ventricular arrhythmias. At times, the presentation may mimic an acute myocardial infarction with ST changes, positive cardiac markers, and regional wall motion abnormalities despite normal coronaries. Microaneurysms may also occur and may be associated with serious ventricular arrhythmias. Patients may present in a variety of ways with fulminant, subacute, or chronic myocarditis. In the European Study of Epidemiology and Treatment of Inflammatory Heart Disease, 72% had dyspnea, 32% had chest pain, and 18% had arrhythmias.

Table 10–16. Causes of myocarditis.

1. INFECTIOUS CAUSES

RNA viruses: Picornaviruses (coxsackie A and B, echovirus, poliovirus, hepatitis virus), orthomyxovirus (Iinfluenza), paramyxoviruses (respiratory syncytial virus, mumps), togaviruses (rubella), flaviviruses (dengue fever, yellow fever)

DNA viruses: Adenovirus (A1, 2, 3 and 5), erythrovirus (Bi9V and 2), herpesviruses (human herpes virus 6 A and B, cytomegalovirus, Epstein-Barr virus, varicella-zoster), retrovirus (HIV)

Bacteria: Chlamydia (*Chlamydophila pneumoniae, C psittaci*), *Haemophilus influenzae, Legionella, Pneumophilia, Brucella, Clostridium, Francisella tularensis, Neisseria meningitis, Mycobacterium* (tuberculosis), *Salmonella, Staphylococcus,* streptococcus A, *Streptococcus, pneumoniae,* tularemia, tetanus, syphilis, *Vibrio cholera*

Spirocheta: *Borrelia recurrentis,* leptospira, *Treponema pallidum*

Rickettsia: *Coxiella burnetti, R rickettsii, R prowazekii*

Fungi: *Actinomyces, Aspergillus, Candida, Cryptococcus, Histoplasma, Nocardia*

Protozoa: *Entamoeba histolytica, Plasmodium falciparum, Trypanosoma cruzi, T burcei, T gondii, Leishmania.*

Helminthic: *Ascaris, Echinococcus granulosus, Schistosoma, Trichenella spiralis, Wuchereria bancrofti*

2. NONINFECTIOUS CAUSES

Autoimmune diseases: Dermatomyositis, inflammatory bowel disease, rheumatoid arthritis, Sjögren syndrome, systemic lupus erythematosus, granulomatosis with polyangiitis (formerly Wegener granulomatosis), giant cell myocarditis

Drugs: Aminophyllin, amphetamine, anthracyclin, catecholamines, chloramphenicol, cocaine, cyclophosphamide, doxorubicin, 5-FU, mesylate, methysergide, phenytoin, trastuzumab, zidovudine

Hypersensitivity reactions due to drugs: Azithromycin, benzodiazepines, clozapine, cephalosporins, dapsone, dobutamine, lithium, diuretics, thiazide, methyldopa, mexiletine, streptomycin, sulfonamides, nonsteroidal anti-inflammatory drugs, tetanus toxoid, tetracycline, tricyclic antidepressants

Hypersensitivity reactions due to venoms: Bee, wasp, black widow spider, scorpion, snakes

Systemic diseases: Churg-Strauss syndrome, collagen diseases, sarcoidosis, Kawasaki disease, scleroderma

Other: Heat stroke, hypothermia, transplant rejection, radiation injury

Modified, with permission, from Schultheiss HP et al. The management of myocarditis. Eur Heart J. 2011;32:2616–25.

B. ECG and Chest Radiography

ECG may show sinus tachycardia, other arrhythmias, nonspecific repolarization changes, and intraventricular conduction abnormalities. The presence of Q waves or left bundle branch block portends a higher rate of death or cardiac transplantation. Ventricular ectopy may be the initial and only clinical finding. Chest radiograph is nonspecific, but cardiomegaly is frequent, though not universal. Evidence for pulmonary venous hypertension is common and frank pulmonary edema may be present.

C. Diagnostic Studies

There is no specific laboratory study that is consistently present, though the white blood cell count is usually elevated and the sedimentation rate and CRP may be increased. Troponin I levels are elevated in about one-third of patients, but CK-MB is elevated in only 10%. Echocardiography provides the most convenient way of evaluating cardiac function and can exclude many other processes. MRI with gadolinium enhancement reveals spotty areas of injury throughout the myocardium, but both T2 and T1-weighted images are needed to achieve optimal results; correlation with endomyocardial biopsy results has been poor.

D. Endomyocardial Biopsy

Confirmation of myocarditis still requires histologic evidence. An AHA/ACCF/ESC joint statement in 2007 made a class 1 recommendation for biopsy under the following situations: (1) in patients with heart failure, a normal-sized or dilated LV < 2 weeks after onset of symptoms, and hemodynamic compromise; or (2) in patients with a dilated LV 2 weeks to 3 months after onset of symptoms, new ventricular arrhythmias or AV nodal block (Mobitz II or complete heart block) or who do not respond to usual care after 1–2 weeks. In some cases, the identification of inflammation without viral genomes by PCR suggests that immunosuppression might be useful.

▶ Treatment & Prognosis

Patients with fulminant myocarditis may present with acute cardiogenic shock. The ventricles are usually not dilated, but thickened (possibly due to myoedema). There is a high death rate, but if the patients recover, they are often left with no residual cardiomyopathy. Patients with subacute disease have a dilated cardiomyopathy and generally make an incomplete recovery. Those who present with chronic disease tend to have only mild dilation of the LV and eventually present with a more restrictive cardiomyopathy. Treatment is directed toward the clinical scenario with ACE inhibitors and beta-blockers if LVEF is < 40%. Nonsteroidal anti-inflammatory drugs should be used if myopericarditis-related chest pain occurs. Colchicine has been suggested if pericarditis predominates. Arrhythmias should be suppressed.

Specific antimicrobial therapy is indicated when an infecting agent is identified. Exercise should be limited during the recovery phase. Some experts believe digoxin should be avoided, and it likely has little value in this setting. Immunosuppressive therapy with corticosteroids and intravenous immunoglobulin (IVIG) has been used in the hopes of improving the outcome when the process is acute (< 6 months) and if the biopsy suggests ongoing inflammation. However, controlled trials have not suggested a benefit. Uncontrolled trials suggest that interferon might have a role. Studies are lacking as to when to discontinue the chosen therapy if the patient improves. Patients with fulminant myocarditis require aggressive short-term support including an IABP or an LV assist device. If severe pulmonary infiltrates accompany the fulminant myocarditis, extracorporeal membrane oxygenation (ECMO) support may be temporarily required and has had notable success. Ongoing studies are addressing whether patients with giant

cell myocarditis may be responsive to immunosuppressive agents, as a special case. Overall, if improvement does not occur, many patients may be eventual candidates for cardiac transplantation or long-term use of the newer LV assist devices.

▶ When to Refer

Patients in whom myocarditis is suspected should be seen by a cardiologist at a tertiary care center where facilities are available for diagnosis and therapies available should a fulminant course ensue. The facility should have ventricular support devices and transplantation options available.

Cooper LT et al. The role of endomyocardial biopsy in the management of cardiovascular disease: a scientific statement from the American Heart Association, the American College of Cardiology, and the European Society of Cardiology. J Am Coll Cardiol. 2007 Nov 6;50(19):1914–31. [PMID: 17980265]
Schultheiss HP et al. The management of myocarditis. Eur Heart J. 2011 Nov;32(21):2616–25. [PMID: 21705357]

DRUG-INDUCED & TOXIC MYOCARDITIS

A variety of medications, illicit drugs, and toxic substances can produce acute or chronic myocardial injury; the clinical presentation varies widely. The phenothiazines, lithium, chloroquine, disopyramide, antimony-containing compounds, and arsenicals can also cause ECG changes, arrhythmias, or heart failure. Hypersensitivity reactions to sulfonamides, penicillins, and aminosalicylic acid as well as other drugs can result in cardiac dysfunction. Radiation can cause an acute inflammatory reaction as well as a chronic fibrosis of heart muscle, usually in conjunction with pericarditis.

The incidence of cocaine cardiotoxicity has increased markedly. Cocaine can result in coronary artery spasm, myocardial infarction, arrhythmias, and myocarditis. Because many of these processes are believed to be mediated by cocaine's inhibitory effect on norepinephrine reuptake by sympathetic nerves, beta-blockers have been used in patients with fixed stenosis. In documented coronary spasm, calcium channel blockers and nitrates may be effective. Usual therapy for heart failure or conduction system disease is warranted when symptoms occur. Other illicit drug use has been associated with myocarditis in various case reports.

The problem of cardiovascular side effects from cancer chemotherapy agents is a growing one. Anthracyclines remain the cornerstone of treatment of many malignancies. Heart failure can be expected in 5% of patients treated with a cumulative dose of 400–450 mg/m^2, and this rate is doubled if the patient is over age 65. The major mechanism of cardiotoxicity is thought to be due to oxidative stress inducing both apoptosis and necrosis of myocytes. There is also disruption of the sarcomere. This is the rationale behind the superoxide dismutase mimetic and iron-chelating agent, dexrazoxane, to protect from the injury. The use of trastuzumab in combination with anthracyclines increases the risk of cardiac dysfunction to up to 28%; this has been an issue since combined use of these agents is particularly effective in *HER*2-positive breast cancer.

In patients receiving chemotherapy, it is important to look for subtle signs of cardiovascular compromise. Echocardiography, cardiac MRI, and serial multigated acquisition (MUGA) studies can provide concrete data regarding LV function. Serum troponin and BNP levels as markers of cardiac injury, and the neutrophil glucosamine-associated lipocalcin as a marker of renal injury, are often elevated in patients with significant cardiotoxicity.

▶ When to Refer

Many patients with myocardial injury from toxic agents can be monitored safely if ventricular function remains relatively preserved (EF > 40%) and no heart failure symptoms occur. Diastolic dysfunction may be subtle.

Once heart failure becomes evident or significant conduction system disease becomes manifest, the patient should be evaluated and monitored by a cardiologist in case myocardial dysfunction worsens and further intervention becomes warranted.

Eschenhagen T et al. Cardiovascular side effects of cancer therapies: a position statement from the Heart Failure Association of the European Society of Cardiology. Eur J Heart Fail. 2011 Jan;13(1):1–10. [PMID: 21169385]

Riezzo I et al. Side effects of cocaine abuse: multiorgan toxicity and pathological consequences. Curr Med Chem. 2012;19 (33):5624–46. [PMID: 22934772]

DILATED CARDIOMYOPATHY

ESSENTIALS OF DIAGNOSIS

▶ Symptoms and signs of heart failure.

▶ Echocardiogram confirms LV dilation, thinning, and global dysfunction.

▶ Severity of RV dysfunction critical in long-term prognosis.

▶ General Considerations

The cardiomyopathies are a heterogeneous group of entities primarily affecting the myocardium and not associated with other major causes of cardiac disease, such as ischemic heart disease, hypertension, pericardial disease, valvular disease, or congenital defects. Although some have specific causes, many cases are idiopathic. The classification of cardiomyopathies is based on features of presentation and pathophysiology (Table 10–17).

Dilated cardiomyopathies cause about 25% of all cases of heart failure. They usually present with symptoms and signs of heart failure (most commonly dyspnea). Occasionally, symptomatic ventricular arrhythmias are the presenting event. LV dilation and systolic dysfunction (EF < 50%)

Table 10–17. Classification of the cardiomyopathies.

	Dilated	Hypertrophic	Restrictive
Frequent causes	Idiopathic, alcoholic, major catecholamine discharge, myocarditis, postpartum, doxorubicin, endocrinopathies, genetic diseases	Hereditary syndrome, possibly chronic hypertension in the elderly	Amyloidosis, post-radiation, post-open heart surgery, diabetes, endomyocardial fibrosis
Symptoms	Left or biventricular heart failure	Dyspnea, chest pain, syncope	Dyspnea, fatigue, right-sided heart failure > left heart failure
Physical examination	Cardiomegaly, S_3, elevated jugular venous pressure, rales	Sustained point of maximal impulse, S_4, variable systolic murmur, bisferiens carotid pulse	Elevated jugular venous pressure, Kussmaul sign
Electrocardiogram	ST–T changes, conduction abnormalities, ventricular ectopy	Left ventricular hypertrophy, exaggerated septal Q waves	ST–T changes, conduction abnormalities, low voltage
Chest radiograph	Enlarged heart, pulmonary congestion	Mild cardiomegaly	Mild to moderate cardiomegaly
Echocardiogram, nuclear studies, MRI	Left ventricular dilation and dysfunction	Left ventricular hypertrophy, asymmetric septal hypertrophy, small left ventricular size, normal or supranormal function, systolic anterior mitral motion, diastolic dysfunction	Small or normal left ventricular size, normal or mildly reduced left ventricular function. Gadolinium-hyperenhancement on MRI.
Cardiac catheterization	Left ventricular dilation and dysfunction, high diastolic pressures, low cardiac output. Coronary angiography important to exclude ischemic cause.	Small, hypercontractile left ventricle, dynamic outflow gradient, diastolic dysfunction	High diastolic pressure, "square root" sign, normal or mildly reduced left ventricular function

are essential for diagnosis. Dilated cardiomyopathy occurs more often in blacks than whites and in men more than women. A growing number of cardiomyopathies due to genetic abnormalities are being recognized, and it is estimated these may represent up to 30–48% of cases. Often no cause can be identified, but chronic alcohol abuse and unrecognized myocarditis are probably frequent causes. Chronic tachycardia may also precipitate a dilated cardiomyopathy that may improve over time if rate control can be achieved. Amyloidosis, sarcoidosis, hemochromatosis, and diabetes may rarely present as dilated cardiomyopathies, as well as the more classic restrictive picture. The RV may be primarily involved in arrhythmogenic RV dysplasia, an unusual cardiomyopathy with displacement of myocardial cells by adipose tissue, or in Uhl disease, in which there is extreme thinning of the RV walls. The function of the RV often determines how well patients do over the long term since RV dysfunction may or may not be present in patients with severe LV dysfunction. An embryologic defect can result in massive trabeculation in the LV (ventricular noncompaction). Intraventricular thrombus is not uncommon in dilated cardiomyopathy.

Clinical Findings

A. Symptoms and Signs

In most patients, symptoms of heart failure develop gradually. The physical examination reveals rales, an elevated JVP, cardiomegaly, S_3 gallop rhythm, often the murmurs of functional mitral or tricuspid regurgitation, peripheral edema, or ascites. In severe heart failure, Cheyne-Stokes breathing, pulsus alternans, pallor, and cyanosis may be present.

B. ECG and Chest Radiography

The major findings are listed in Table 10–17. Sinus tachycardia is common. Other common abnormalities include left bundle branch block and ventricular or atrial arrhythmias. The chest radiograph reveals cardiomegaly, evidence for left and/or right heart failure, and pleural effusions (right > left).

C. Diagnostic Studies

An echocardiogram is indicated to exclude unsuspected valvular or other lesions and confirm the presence of dilated cardiomyopathy and the reduced systolic function (as opposed to pure diastolic heart failure). Mitral Doppler inflow patterns also help in the diagnosis of associated diastolic dysfunction. Color flow Doppler can reveal tricuspid or mitral regurgitation, and continuous Doppler can help define PA pressures. Exercise or pharmacologic stress myocardial perfusion imaging may suggest the possibility of underlying coronary disease. Radionuclide ventriculography provides a noninvasive measure of the EF and both RV and LV wall motion, though its use is now being supplanted by cardiac MRI in many institutions. Cardiac MRI is particularly helpful in inflammatory or infiltrative processes, such as sarcoidosis or hemochromatosis, and is the diagnostic study of choice for RV dysplasia

where there is fatty infiltration. MRI can also help define an ischemic etiology by noting gadolinium hyperenhancement consistent with myocardial scar. Cardiac catheterization is seldom of specific value unless myocardial ischemia or LV aneurysm is suspected. The serum ferritin is an adequate screening study for hemochromatosis. The erythrocyte sedimentation rate may be low due to liver congestion if right heart failure is present. The serum level of BNP or pro-BNP can be used to help quantitate the severity of heart failure. Intracavitary thrombosis is not uncommon. Myocardial biopsy is rarely useful in establishing the diagnosis, though occasionally the underlying cause (eg, sarcoidosis, hemochromatosis) can be discerned. Biopsy is most useful in transplant rejection.

Treatment

Standard therapy for heart failure should include ACE inhibitors or ARBs, beta-blockers, diuretics, and an aldosterone antagonist. Systemic BP control is important. Digoxin is a second-line drug but remains favored as an adjunct by some clinicians. Calcium channel blockers should generally be avoided unless absolutely necessary for rate control in atrial fibrillation. Sodium restriction is helpful, especially in acute heart failure. When atrial fibrillation is present, heart rate control is vital if sinus rhythm cannot be established or maintained. There are little data to suggest an advantage of sinus rhythm over atrial fibrillation on long-term outcomes. Many patients may be candidates for cardiac synchronization therapy with biventricular pacing and an implantable defibrillator. Few cases of cardiomyopathy are amenable to specific therapy for the underlying cause. Alcohol use should be discontinued, since there is often marked recovery of cardiac function following a period of abstinence in alcoholic cardiomyopathy. Endocrine causes (hyperthyroidism or hypothyroidism, acromegaly, and pheochromocytoma) should be treated. Immunosuppressive therapy is not indicated in chronic dilated cardiomyopathy. The management of heart failure is outlined in the section on heart failure. There are some patients who may benefit from implantable LV assist devices either as a bridge to transplantation or to temporize while cardiac function returns. LV assist devices are also being considered as destination therapy in patients who are not candidates for cardiac transplantation. Arterial and pulmonary emboli are more common in dilated cardiomyopathy than in ischemic cardiomyopathy. Suitable candidates may benefit from long-term anticoagulation, and all patients with atrial fibrillation should be so treated. Some clinicians use warfarin to prevent or treat an LV thrombus when discovered on an echocardiogram.

Prognosis

The prognosis of dilated cardiomyopathy without clinical heart failure is variable, with some patients remaining stable, some deteriorating gradually, and others declining rapidly. Once heart failure is manifest, the natural history is similar to that of other causes of heart failure, with an annual mortality around 11–13%.

When to Refer

Patients with new or worsened symptoms of heart failure with dilated cardiomyopathy should be referred to a cardiologist. Patients with continued symptoms of heart failure and reduced LVEF (≤ 35%) should be referred to a cardiologist for consideration of placement of an ICD or cardiac resynchronization therapy (if QRS duration is ≥ 120 msec especially with left bundle branch block pattern). Patients with advanced refractory symptoms should be referred for consideration of heart transplant or LV assist device therapy.

When to Admit

Patients with hypoxia, fluid overload, or pulmonary edema not readily resolved in outpatient setting should be admitted.

Anderson L et al. The role of endomyocardial biopsy in the management of cardiovascular disease: a scientific statement from the American Heart Association, the American College of Cardiology, and the European Society of Cardiology. Eur Heart J. 2008 Dec;29(13):1696–97. [PMID: 18456711]
Jefferies JL et al. Dilated cardiomyopathy. Lancet. 2010 Feb 27;375(9716):752–62. [PMID: 20189027]
McNally EM et al. Genetic mutations and mechanisms in dilated cardiomyopathy. J Clin Invest. 2013 Jan 2;123(1): 19–26. [PMID: 23281406]

TAKO-TSUBO CARDIOMYOPATHY

ESSENTIALS OF DIAGNOSIS

- ▶ Occurs after a major catecholamine discharge.
- ▶ Acute chest pain or shortness of breath.
- ▶ Predominately affects postmenopausal women.
- ▶ Presents as an acute anterior myocardial infarction, but coronaries normal at cardiac catheterization.
- ▶ Imaging reveals apical left ventricular ballooning due to anteroapical stunning of the myocardium.
- ▶ Most patients recover completely.

General Considerations

LV apical ballooning (Tako-Tsubo syndrome) follows a high catecholamine surge. The resulting shape of the LV suggests a rounded ampulla form similar to a Japanese octopus pot (tako-tsubo pot). Mid-ventricular ballooning has also been described. The key feature is that the myocardial stunning that occurs does not follow the pattern suggestive of coronary ischemia. The acute myocardial injury is more common in postmenopausal women. It has been described following some stressful event, such as hypoglycemia, lightning strikes, earthquakes, postventricular tachycardia, during alcohol withdrawal, following surgery, during hyperthyroidism, after stroke, and following emotional stress ("broken-heart syndrome"). Virtually any event that triggers excess catecholamines may be implicated.

Pericarditis and even tamponade has been described in isolated cases.

Clinical Findings

A. Symptoms and Signs

The symptoms are similar to any acute coronary syndrome. Typical angina and dyspnea are usually present. Syncope is rare, although arrhythmias are not uncommon.

B. ECG and Chest Radiography

The ECG reveals ST-segment elevation as well as deep anterior T wave inversion. The chest radiograph is either normal or reveals pulmonary congestion. The dramatic T wave inversions gradually resolve over time.

C. Diagnostic Studies

The echocardiogram reveals LV apical dyskinesia usually not consistent with any particular coronary distribution. The urgent cardiac catheterization reveals the LV apical ballooning in association with normal coronaries. Initial cardiac enzymes are positive but often taper quickly. In almost all cases, MRI hyperenhancement studies reveal no long-term scarring.

Treatment

Immediate therapy is similar to any acute myocardial infarction. Initiation of long-term therapy depends on whether LV dysfunction persists. Most patients receive aspirin, beta-blockers, and ACE inhibitors until the LV fully recovers. See Treatment of Heart Failure, above.

Prognosis

Prognosis is good unless there is a serious complication (such as mitral regurgitation, ventricular rupture, ventricular tachycardia). Recovery is expected in most cases after a period of weeks to months. At times, the LV function recovers in days. Rarely, repeat episodes have been reported.

Eitel I et al. Clinical characteristics and cardiovascular magnetic resonance findings in stress (takotsubo) cardiomyopathy. JAMA. 2011 Jul 20;306(3):277–86. [PMID: 21771988]
Milinis K et al. Takotsubo cardiomyopathy: pathophysiology and treatment. Postgrad Med J. 2012 Sep;88(1043):530–8. [PMID: 22647668]

HYPERTROPHIC CARDIOMYOPATHY

ESSENTIALS OF DIAGNOSIS

- ▶ May present with dyspnea, chest pain, syncope.
- ▶ Though LV outflow gradient is classic, symptoms are primarily related to diastolic dysfunction.
- ▶ Echocardiogram is diagnostic.
- ▶ Increased risk of sudden death.

General Considerations

Hypertrophic cardiomyopathy is noted when there is LV hypertrophy unrelated to any pressure or volume overload. The increased wall thickness reduces LV systolic stress, increases the EF, and can result in an "empty ventricle" at end-systole. The interventricular septum may be disproportionately involved (asymmetric septal hypertrophy), but in some cases the hypertrophy is localized to the mid ventricle or to the apex. The LV outflow tract is narrowed during systole due to the hypertrophied septum and systolic anterior motion of the mitral valve. The obstruction is worsened by factors that increase myocardial contractility (sympathetic stimulation, digoxin, and postextrasystolic beat) or that decrease LV filling (Valsalva maneuver, peripheral vasodilators). The amount of obstruction is preload and afterload dependent and can vary from day to day. The consequence of the hypertrophy is elevated LV diastolic pressures rather than systolic dysfunction. Rarely, systolic dysfunction develops late in the disease. The LV is usually more involved than the RV and the atria are frequently significantly enlarged.

HOCM is inherited as an autosomal dominant trait with variable penetrance and is caused by mutations of one of a large number of genes, most of which code for myosin heavy chains or proteins regulating calcium handling. The prognosis is related to the specific gene mutation. Patients usually present in early adulthood. Elite athletes may demonstrate considerable hypertrophy that can be confused with HOCM, but generally diastolic dysfunction is not present in the athlete. The apical variety is particularly common in those of Asian descent. A mid-ventricular obstructive form is also known where there is contact between the septum and papillary muscles. A hypertrophic cardiomyopathy in the elderly (usually in association with hypertension) has also been defined as a distinct entity. Mitral annular calcification is often present. Mitral regurgitation is variable and often dynamic, depending on the degree of outflow tract obstruction.

Clinical Findings

A. Symptoms and Signs

The most frequent symptoms are dyspnea and chest pain (Table 10–17). Syncope is also common and is typically postexertional, when diastolic filling diminishes and outflow obstruction increases due to residual circulating catecholamines. Arrhythmias are an important problem. Atrial fibrillation is a long-term consequence of chronically elevated LA pressures and is a poor prognostic sign. Ventricular arrhythmias are also common, and sudden death may occur, often in athletes after extraordinary exertion.

Features on physical examination include a bisferiens carotid pulse, triple apical impulse (due to the prominent atrial filling wave and early and late systolic impulses), and a loud S_4. The JVP may reveal a prominent a wave due to reduced RV compliance. In cases with outflow obstruction, a loud systolic murmur is present along the left sternal border that increases with upright posture or Valsalva maneuver and decreases with squatting. These maneuvers help differentiate the murmur of HOCM from that of aortic stenosis, since in HOCM, reducing the LV volume increases obstruction and the murmur intensity; whereas in valvular aortic stenosis, reducing the stroke volume across the valve decreases the murmur. Mitral regurgitation is frequently present as well.

B. ECG and Chest Radiography

LVH is nearly universal in symptomatic patients, though entirely normal ECGs are present in up to 25%, usually in those with localized hypertrophy. Exaggerated septal Q waves inferolaterally may mimic myocardial infarction. The chest radiograph is often unimpressive. Unlike aortic stenosis, the ascending aorta is not dilated.

C. Diagnostic Studies

The echocardiogram is diagnostic, revealing asymmetric LVH, systolic anterior motion of the mitral valve, early closing followed by reopening of the aortic valve, a small and hypercontractile LV, and delayed relaxation and filling of the LV during diastole. The septum is usually 1.3–1.5 times the thickness of the posterior wall. Septal motion tends to be reduced. Doppler ultrasound reveals turbulent flow and a dynamic gradient in the LV outflow tract and, commonly, mitral regurgitation. Abnormalities in the diastolic filling pattern are present in 80% of patients. Echocardiography can usually differentiate the disease from ventricular noncompaction. Myocardial perfusion imaging may suggest septal ischemia in the presence of normal coronary arteries. Cardiac MRI confirms the hypertrophy and contrast enhancement frequently reveals evidence for scar at the junction of the RV attachment to the septum. Cardiac catheterization confirms the diagnosis and defines the presence or absence of CAD. Frequently, coronary arterial bridging (squeezing in systole) occurs, especially of the septal arteries. Exercise studies are recommended to assess for ventricular arrhythmias and to document the BP response. Holter monitoring is recommended for determination of ventricular ectopy.

Treatment

Beta-blockers should be the initial drug in symptomatic individuals, especially when dynamic outflow obstruction is noted on the echocardiogram. The resulting slower heart rates assist with diastolic filling of the stiff LV. Dyspnea, angina, and arrhythmias respond in about 50% of patients. Calcium channel blockers, especially verapamil, have also been effective in symptomatic patients. Their effect is due primarily to improved diastolic function; however, their vasodilating actions can also increase outflow obstruction and cause hypotension. Disopyramide is also used because of its negative inotropic effects; it is usually used in addition to the medical regimen rather than as primary therapy or to help control atrial arrhythmias. Diuretics are frequently necessary due to the high diastolic pressure and PCWP. Patients do best in sinus rhythm, and atrial fibrillation should be aggressively treated with antiarrhythmics or radiofrequency ablation. Dual-chamber pacing may prevent the progression of hypertrophy and obstruction. There appears to be an advantage to the use of short-AV delay biventricular pacing. Nonsurgical septal ablation has been performed by injection of alcohol into septal branches of the left coronary artery with good results in small series of patients. Patients with malignant ventricular arrhythmias and unexplained syncope in the presence of a positive family history for sudden death with or without an abnormal BP response to exercise are probably best managed with an implantable defibrillator. Excision of part of the outflow myocardial septum (myotomy–myomectomy) by experienced surgeons has been successful in patients with severe symptoms unresponsive to medical therapy. A few surgeons advocate mitral valve replacement, as this results in resolution of the gradient as well, and prevents associated mitral regurgitation. In some cases, myomectomy has been combined with an Alfieri stitch on the mitral valve with success. Rare cases with progression to dilation or with intractable symptoms can be considered for cardiac transplantation. Figure 10–11 provides an algorithm for the treatment of HOCM.

Pregnancy results in an increased risk in patients with symptoms or outflow tract gradients of > 50 mm Hg. Genetic counseling is indicated before planned conception. In pregnant patients with HOCM, continuation of beta-blocker therapy is recommended.

Prognosis

The natural history of HOCM is highly variable. Several specific mutations are associated with a higher incidence of early malignant arrhythmias and sudden death, and definition of the genetic abnormality provides the best estimate of prognosis. Some patients remain asymptomatic for many years or for life. Sudden death, especially during exercise, may be the initial event. The highest risk patients are those with (1) a personal history of serious ventricular arrhythmias or survival of a sudden death episode; (2) a family history of sudden death; (3) unexplained syncope; (4) documented NSVT, defined as three or more beats of ventricular tachycardia at ≥ 120 beats per minute on ambulatory Holter monitoring; and (5) maximal LV wall thickness ≥ 30 mm. In addition, patients whose BP does not increase during treadmill stress testing are also at risk, as are those with double and compound genetic mutations and those with marked LV outflow tract obstruction. MRI data suggest that the extent of scarring on hyperenhancement may also be predictive of adverse events. HOCM is the pathologic feature most frequently associated with sudden death in athletes. Pregnancy is generally well tolerated. Endocarditis prophylaxis is no longer indicated. A final stage may be a transition into dilated cardiomyopathy in 5–10% of patients due to the long-term effects of LV remodeling; treatment at that stage is similar to that for dilated cardiomyopathy.

When to Refer

Patients should be referred to a cardiologist when symptoms are difficult to control, syncope has occurred, or there are any of the high-risk features present as noted above.

Gersh BJ et al. 2011 ACCF/AHA guideline for the treatment of hypertrophic cardiomyopathy. J Am Coll Cardiol. 2011 Dec 13;58(25):e212–60. [PMID: 22075469]
Maron BJ et al. Hypertrophic cardiomyopathy. Lancet. 2013 Jan 19;381(9862):242–55. [PMID: 22874472]

RESTRICTIVE CARDIOMYOPATHY

 ESSENTIALS OF DIAGNOSIS

► Right heart failure tends to dominate over left heart failure.
► Pulmonary hypertension is present.
► Amyloidosis is the most common cause.
► Echocardiography is key to diagnosis.
► Myocardial biopsy or cardiac MRI can confirm amyloid.

General Considerations

Restrictive cardiomyopathy is characterized by impaired diastolic filling with reasonably preserved contractile function. The condition is relatively uncommon, with the most frequent cause being amyloidosis. Cardiac amyloidosis is more common in men than in women and rarely manifests before the age of 40. The AL type is the most common. In the elderly, secondary amyloidosis can occur (AA type). It may manifest secondarily to multiple myeloma. A familiar type (most often seen in elderly blacks) occurs due to a build-up of transthyretin.

In Africa, endomyocardial fibrosis, a specific entity in which there is severe fibrosis of the endocardium, often with eosinophilia (Löffler syndrome), is seen. Other causes of restrictive cardiomyopathy are infiltrative cardiomyopathies (eg, hemochromatosis, sarcoidosis) and connective tissue diseases (eg, scleroderma).

Clinical Findings

A. Symptoms and Signs

Restrictive cardiomyopathy must be distinguished from constrictive pericarditis (Table 10–17). The key feature is that ventricular interaction is accentuated with respiration in constrictive pericarditis and that interaction is absent in restrictive cardiomyopathy. In addition, the pulmonary arterial pressure is invariably elevated in restrictive cardiomyopathy due to the high pulmonary capillary wedge pressure (PCWP) and is normal in uncomplicated constrictive pericarditis.

B. Diagnostic Studies

Conduction disturbances are frequently present. Low voltage on the ECG combined with ventricular hypertrophy on the echocardiogram is suggestive of disease. Cardiac MRI presents a distinctive pattern of diffuse hyperenhancement of the gadolinium image in amyloidosis

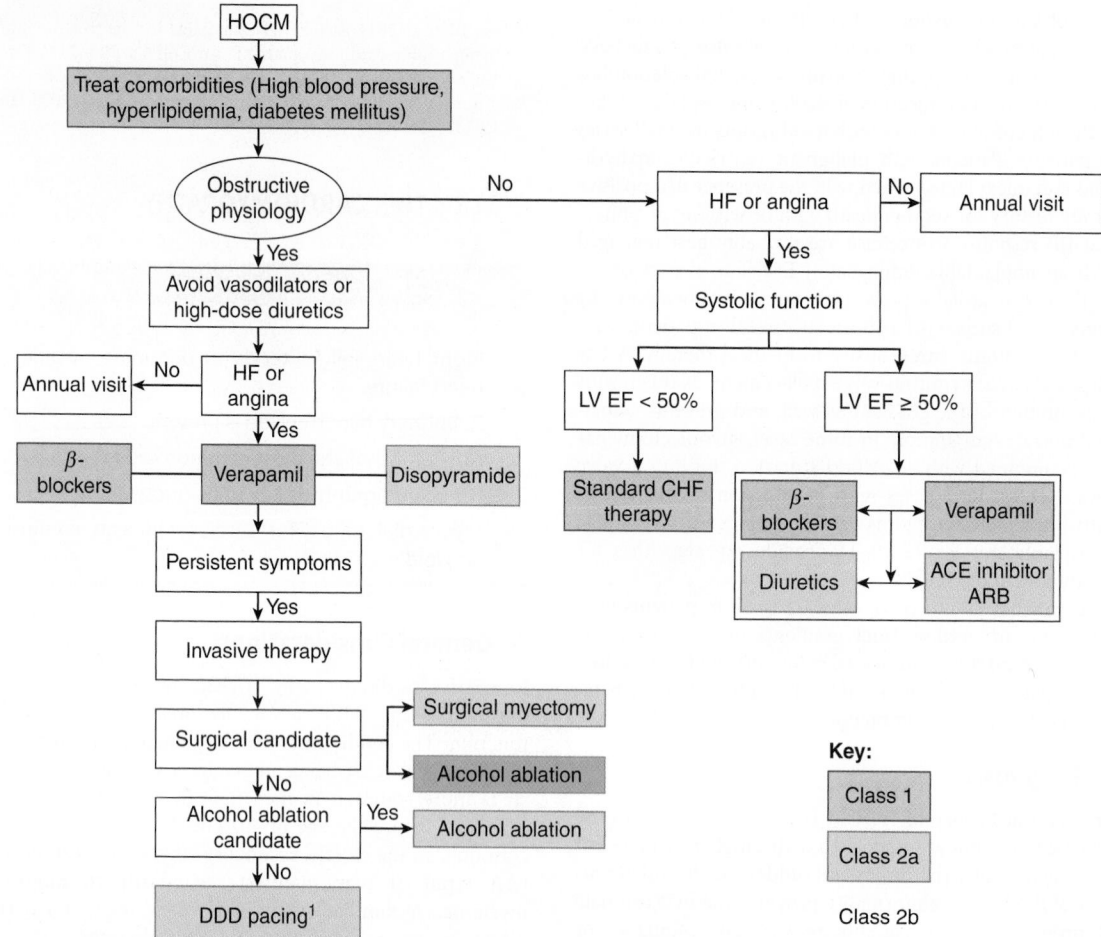

¹See section on AV Block in the text.

▲ **Figure 10–11.** Recommended therapeutic approach to the patient with hypertrophic obstructive cardiomyopathy (HOCM). ACE, angiotensin-converting enzyme; ARB, angiotensin receptor blockers; HF, heart failure; LVEF, left ventricular ejection fraction. (Reproduced, with permission, from Gersh BJ et al. 2011 ACCF/AHA Guideline for the Diagnosis and Treatment of Hypertrophic Cardiomyopathy A Report of the American College of Cardiology Foundation/ American Heart Association Task Force on Practice Guidelines Developed in Collaboration With the American Association for Thoracic Surgery, American Society of Echocardiography, American Society of Nuclear Cardiology, Heart Failure Society of America, Heart Rhythm Society, Society for Cardiovascular Angiography and Interventions, and Society of Thoracic Surgeons. J Am Coll Cardiol. 2011 Dec 13;58(25):e212–60.)

and is a useful screening test. The echocardiogram reveals a small thickened LV with bright myocardium (speckled), rapid early diastolic filling revealed by the mitral inflow Doppler, and biatrial enlargement. The LV chamber size is usually normal with a reduced LVEF. Atrial septal thickening may be evident. Rectal, abdominal fat, or gingival biopsies can confirm systemic involvement, but myocardial involvement may still be present if these are negative, and requires endomyocardial biopsy for the confirmation of cardiac amyloid. Demonstration of tissue infiltration on biopsy specimens using special stains followed by immunohistochemical studies and genetic testing is essential to define which specific protein is involved.

▶ Treatment

Unfortunately, little useful therapy is available for either the causative conditions or the restrictive cardiomyopathy itself. Diuretics can help, but excessive diuresis can produce worsening kidney dysfunction. As with most patients with severe right heart failure, loop diuretics, thiazides, and aldosterone antagonists are all useful. Recently, the use of ultrafiltration devices have allowed for improved diuresis, although it is not clear if prognosis is improved. Digoxin may precipitate arrhythmias and generally should not be used. Beta-blockers help slow heart rates and improve filling. Corticosteroids may be helpful in sarcoidosis but they are more effective for the conduction abnormalities than heart failure. In amyloidosis, the therapeutic strategy depends on the characterization of the type of amyloid protein and extent of disease and may include chemotherapy or bone marrow transplantation. In familial amyloidosis, liver transplantation may be an option. Cardiac transplantation has also been used in patients with primary cardiac amyloidosis and no evidence of systemic involvement.

▶ **When to Refer**

All patients with the diagnosis of a restrictive cardiomyopathy should be referred to a cardiologist to decide etiology and plan appropriate treatment. This is especially true if amyloidosis is suspected because the prognosis is poor.

Kapoor P et al. Cardiac amyloidosis: a practical approach to diagnosis and management. Am J Med. 2011 Nov;124(11): 1006–15. [PMID: 22017778]
Quarta CC et al. Amyloidosis. Circulation. 2012 Sep18;126(12): e178–82. [PMID: 22988049]
Sharma N et al. Current state of cardiac amyloidosis. Curr Opin Cardiol. 2013 Mar;28(2):242–8. [PMID: 23324855]

RHEUMATIC FEVER

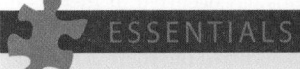
ESSENTIALS OF DIAGNOSIS

▶ More common in developing countries (100 cases/100,000 population) than in the United States (~2 cases/100,000 population).

▶ Peak incidence ages 5–15 years.

▶ Diagnosis based on Jones criteria and confirmation of streptococcal infection.

▶ May involve mitral and other valves acutely, rarely leading to heart failure.

▶ **General Considerations**

Rheumatic fever is a systemic immune process that is a sequela of a beta-hemolytic streptococcal infection of the pharynx. It is a major scourge in developing countries and responsible for 250,000 deaths in young people worldwide each year. Signs of rheumatic fever usually commence 2–3 weeks after infection but may appear as early as 1 week or as late as 5 weeks. The disease has become quite uncommon in the United States, except in immigrants; however, there have been reports of new outbreaks in several regions of the United States. The peak incidence is between ages 5 and 15 years; rheumatic fever is rare before age 4 years or after age 40 years. Rheumatic carditis and valvulitis may be self-limited or may lead to slowly progressive valvular deformity. The characteristic lesion is a perivascular granulomatous reaction with vasculitis. The mitral valve is acutely attacked in 75–80% of cases, the aortic valve in 30%

(but rarely as the sole valve involved), and the tricuspid and pulmonary valves in under 5% of. Overall, carditis is thought to occur in about 30–45% of cases of acute rheumatic fever.

Chronic rheumatic heart disease results from single or repeated attacks of rheumatic fever that produce rigidity and deformity of valve cusps, fusion of the commissures, or shortening and fusion of the chordae tendineae. Valvular stenosis or regurgitation results, and the two often coexist. In chronic rheumatic heart disease, the mitral valve alone is affected in 50–60% of cases; combined lesions of the aortic and mitral valves occur in 20%; pure aortic lesions are less common. Tricuspid involvement occurs in about 10% of cases but only in association with mitral or aortic disease and is thought to be more common when recurrent infections have occurred. The pulmonary valve is rarely affected long term. A history of rheumatic fever is obtainable in only 60% of patients with rheumatic heart disease.

▶ **Clinical Findings**

The presence of two major criteria—or one major and two minor criteria—establishes the diagnosis. Echocardiographic studies revealing valvular abnormalities have suggested that subclinical cardiac involvement may be missed using the strict Jones criteria. India, New Zealand, and Australia have all published revised guidelines.

A. Major Criteria

1. Carditis—Carditis is most likely to be evident in children and adolescents. Any of the following suggests the presence of carditis: (1) pericarditis; (2) cardiomegaly, detected by physical signs, radiography, or echocardiography; (3) heart failure, right- or left-sided—the former perhaps more prominent in children, with painful liver engorgement due to tricuspid regurgitation; and (4) mitral or aortic regurgitation murmurs, indicative of dilation of a valve ring with or without associated valvulitis The Carey–Coombs short mid-diastolic mitral murmur may be present due to inflammation of the mitral valve.

In the absence of any of the above definitive signs, the diagnosis of carditis depends on the following less specific abnormalities: (1) ECG changes, including changing contour of P waves or inversion of T waves; (2) changing quality of heart sounds; and (3) sinus tachycardia, arrhythmia, or ectopic beats.

2. Erythema marginatum and subcutaneous nodules—Erythema marginatum begins as rapidly enlarging macules that assume the shape of rings or crescents with clear centers. They may be raised, confluent, and either transient or persistent.

Subcutaneous nodules are uncommon except in children. They are small (≤ 2 cm in diameter), firm, and nontender and are attached to fascia or tendon sheaths over bony prominences. They persist for days or weeks, are recurrent, and are indistinguishable from rheumatoid nodules.

3. Sydenham chorea—This is the least common (3% of cases) but most diagnostic manifestation of acute rheumatic fever. Defined as involuntary choreoathetoid movements primarily of the face, tongue, and upper extremities, sydenham chorea may be the sole manifestation of rheumatic fever; only 50% of cases have other overt signs. Girls are more frequently affected, and occurrence in adults is rare.

4. Polyarthritis—This is a migratory polyarthritis that involves the large joints sequentially. In adults, only a single joint may be affected. The arthritis lasts 1–5 weeks and subsides without residual deformity. Prompt response of arthritis to therapeutic doses of salicylates or nonsteroidal agents is characteristic.

B. Minor Criteria

These include fever, polyarthralgias, reversible prolongation of the PR interval, and an elevated erythrocyte sedimentation rate or CRP. Supporting evidence includes positive throat culture or rapid streptococcal antigen test and elevated or rising streptococcal antibody titer.

C. Laboratory Findings

There is nonspecific evidence of inflammatory disease, as shown by a rapid sedimentation rate. High or increasing titers of antistreptococcal antibodies (antistreptolysin O and anti-DNase B) are used to confirm recent infection; 10% of cases lack this serologic evidence.

▶ Treatment

A. General Measures

The patient should be kept at strict bed rest until the temperature returns to normal (without the use of antipyretic medications) and the sedimentation rate, plus the resting pulse rate, and the ECG have all returned to baseline.

B. Medical Measures

1. Salicylates—The salicylates markedly reduce fever and relieve joint pain and swelling. They have no effect on the natural course of the disease. Adults may require large doses of aspirin, 0.6–0.9 g every 4 hours; children are treated with lower doses.

2. Penicillin—Penicillin (benzathine penicillin, 1.2 million units intramuscularly once, or procaine penicillin, 600,000 units intramuscularly daily for 10 days) is used to eradicate streptococcal infection if present. Erythromycin may be substituted (40 mg/kg/d).

3. Corticosteroids—There is no proof that cardiac damage is prevented or minimized by corticosteroids. A short course of corticosteroids (prednisone, 40–60 mg orally daily, with tapering over 2 weeks) usually causes rapid improvement of the joint symptoms and is indicated when response to salicylates has been inadequate.

▶ Prevention of Recurrent Rheumatic Fever

Improvement in socioeconomic conditions and public health are critical to reducing bouts of rheumatic fever. The initial episode of rheumatic fever can usually be prevented by early treatment of streptococcal pharyngitis. (See Chapter 33.) Prevention of recurrent episodes of rheumatic fever is critical. Recurrences of rheumatic fever are most common in patients who have had carditis during their initial episode and in children, 20% of whom will have a second episode within 5 years. The preferred method of prophylaxis is with benzathine penicillin G, 1.2 million units intramuscularly every 4 weeks. Oral penicillin (200,000–250,000 units twice daily) is less reliable.

If the patient is allergic to penicillin, sulfadiazine (or sulfisoxazole), 1 g daily, or erythromycin, 250 mg orally twice daily, may be substituted. The macrolide azithromycin is similarly effective against group A streptococcal infection. If the patient has not had an immediate hypersensitivity (anaphylactic-type) reaction to penicillin, then cephalosporin may also be used.

Recurrences are uncommon after 5 years following the first episode and in patients over 25 years of age. Prophylaxis is usually discontinued after these times except in groups with a high risk of streptococcal infection—parents or teachers of young children, nurses, military recruits, etc. Secondary prevention of rheumatic fever depends on whether carditis has occurred. If there is no evidence for carditis, preventive therapy can be stopped at age 21 years. If carditis has occurred but there is no residual valvular disease, it can be stopped at 10 years after the episode. If carditis has occurred with residual valvular involvement, it should be continued for 10 years after the last episode or until age 40 years if the patient is in a situation in which reexposure would be expected.

▶ Prognosis

Initial episodes of rheumatic fever may last months in children and weeks in adults. The immediate mortality rate is 1–2%. Persistent rheumatic carditis with cardiomegaly, heart failure, and pericarditis implies a poor prognosis; 30% of children thus affected die within 10 years after the initial attack. After 10 years, two-thirds of patients will have detectable valvular abnormalities (usually thickened valves with limited mobility), but significant symptomatic VHD or persistent cardiomyopathy occurs in < 10% of patients with a single episode. In developing countries, acute rheumatic fever occurs earlier in life, recurs more frequently, and the evolution to chronic valvular disease is both accelerated and more severe.

Lee JL et al. Acute rheumatic fever and its consequences: a persistent threat to developing nations in the 21st century. Autoimmun Rev. 2009 Dec;9(2):117–23. [PMID: 19386288]

Marijon E et al. Rheumatic heart disease. Lancet. 2012 Mar 10;379(9819):953–64. [PMID: 22405798]

Roberts K et al. Screening for rheumatic heart disease: current approaches and controversies. Nat Rev Cardiol. 2013 Jan; 10(1): 49–58. [PMID: 23149830]

DISEASES OF THE PERICARDIUM

ACUTE INFLAMMATORY PERICARDITIS

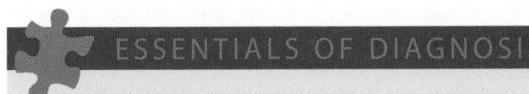

ESSENTIALS OF DIAGNOSIS

- ▶ Anterior pleuritic chest pain that is worse supine than upright.
- ▶ Pericardial rub.
- ▶ Fever common.
- ▶ Erythrocyte sedimentation rate usually elevated.
- ▶ ECG reveals diffuse ST-segment elevation with associated PR depression.

► General Considerations

Acute (< 2 weeks) inflammation of the pericardium may be infectious in origin or may be due to systemic diseases (autoimmune syndromes, uremia), neoplasm, radiation, drug toxicity, hemopericardium, postcardiac surgery, or contiguous inflammatory processes in the myocardium or lung. In many of these conditions, the pathologic process involves both the pericardium and the myocardium.

Viral infections (especially infections with coxsackieviruses and echoviruses but also influenza, Epstein–Barr, varicella, hepatitis, mumps, and HIV viruses) are the most common cause of acute pericarditis and probably are responsible for many cases classified as idiopathic. Males—usually under age 50 years—are most commonly affected. The differential diagnosis primarily requires exclusion of acute myocardial infarction. **Tuberculous pericarditis** has become rare in developed countries but remains common in certain areas of the world. It results from direct lymphatic or hematogenous spread; clinical pulmonary involvement may be absent or minor, although associated pleural effusions are common. **Bacterial pericarditis** is rare and usually results from direct extension from pulmonary infections. Pneumococci can cause a primary pericardial infection. *Borrelia burgdorferi,* the organism responsible for Lyme disease, can also cause myopericarditis. **Uremic pericarditis** is a common complication of chronic kidney disease. The pathogenesis is uncertain; it occurs both with untreated uremia and in otherwise stable dialysis patients. Spread of adjacent lung cancer as well as invasion by breast cancer, renal cell carcinoma, Hodgkin disease, and lymphomas are the most common **neoplastic processes** involving the pericardium and have become the most frequent causes of pericardial tamponade in many countries. Pericarditis may occur 2–5 days after infarction due to an inflammatory reaction to transmural myocardial necrosis [**postmyocardial infarction or postcardiotomy pericarditis (Dressler syndrome)**]. **Radiation** can initiate a fibrinous and fibrotic process in the pericardium, presenting as subacute pericarditis or constriction. Radiation pericarditis usually follows treatments of more than 4000 cGy delivered to ports including more than 30% of the heart.

Other causes of pericarditis include connective tissue diseases, such as lupus erythematosus and rheumatoid arthritis, drug-induced pericarditis (minoxidil, penicillins, clozapine), and myxedema.

► Clinical Findings

A. Symptoms and Signs

The presentation and course of inflammatory pericarditis depend on its cause, but most syndromes have associated chest pain, which is usually pleuritic and postural (relieved by sitting). The pain is substernal but may radiate to the neck, shoulders, back, or epigastrium. Dyspnea may also be present and the patient is often febrile. A pericardial friction rub is characteristic, with or without evidence of fluid accumulation or constriction (see below). The presentation of **tuberculous pericarditis** tends to be subacute, but nonspecific symptoms (fever, night sweats, fatigue) may be present for days to months. Pericardial involvement develops in 1–8% of patients with pulmonary tuberculosis. Symptoms and signs of **bacterial pericarditis** are similar to those of other types of inflammatory pericarditides, but patients appear toxic and are often critically ill. **Uremic pericarditis** can present with or without symptoms; fever is absent. Often **neoplastic pericarditis** is painless, and the presenting symptoms relate to hemodynamic compromise or the primary disease. At times the pericardial effusion is very large, consistent with its chronic nature. **Postmyocardial infarction or postcardiotomy pericarditis (Dressler syndrome)** usually presents as a recurrence of pain with pleural-pericardial features. A rub is often audible, and repolarization changes on the ECG may be confused with ischemia. Large effusions are uncommon, and spontaneous resolution usually occurs in a few days. Dressler syndrome occurs days to weeks to several months after myocardial infarction or open heart surgery, may be recurrent, and probably represents an autoimmune syndrome. Patients present with typical pain, fever, malaise, and leukocytosis. Rarely, other symptoms of an autoimmune disorder, such as joint pain and fever, may occur. Tamponade is rare with Dressler syndrome after myocardial infarction but not when it occurs postoperatively. The clinical onset of **radiation pericarditis** is usually within the first year but may be delayed for many years; often a full decade or more may pass before constriction becomes evident.

B. Laboratory Findings and Diagnostic Studies

The diagnosis of **viral pericarditis** is usually clinical, and leukocytosis is often present. Rising viral titers in paired sera may be obtained for confirmation but are rarely done. Cardiac enzymes may be slightly elevated, reflecting an epicardial myocarditis component. The echocardiogram is often normal or reveals only a trivial amount of extra fluid during the acute inflammatory process. The diagnosis of **tuberculous pericarditis** can be inferred if acid-fast bacilli are found elsewhere. The tuberculous pericardial effusions are usually small or moderate but may be large when chronic. The yield of organisms by pericardiocentesis is low; pericardial biopsy has a higher yield but may also be negative, and pericardiectomy may be required. If bacterial pericarditis is suspected on clinical grounds, diagnostic pericardiocentesis can be confirmatory. In **uremic patients** not on dialysis, the incidence of pericarditis correlates roughly with the level of blood urea nitrogen (BUN) and creatinine. The pericardium is characteristically "shaggy" in uremic pericarditis, and the effusion is hemorrhagic and exudative. The diagnosis of **neoplastic pericarditis** can occasionally be made by cytologic examination of the effusion or by pericardial biopsy, but it may be difficult to establish clinically if the patient has received mediastinal radiation within the previous year. Neoplastic pericardial effusions develop over a long period of time and may become quite huge (> 2 L). The sedimentation rate is high in **postmyocardial infarction or postcardiotomy pericarditis** and can help confirm the diagnosis. Large pericardial effusions and accompanying pleural effusions are frequent. Myxedema pericardial effusions due to hypothyroidism usually are characterized by the presence of cholesterol crystals within the fluid.

C. Other Studies

The ECG usually shows generalized ST and T wave changes and may manifest a characteristic progression beginning with diffuse ST elevation, followed by a return to baseline and then to T wave inversion. Atrial injury is often present and manifested by PR depression especially in the limb leads. The chest radiograph is frequently normal, but may show cardiac enlargement if pericardial fluid is present, as well as signs of related pulmonary disease. Mass lesions and enlarged lymph nodes may suggest a neoplastic process. MRI and CT scan can visualize neighboring tumor in neoplastic pericarditis. A screening chest CT or MRI is often recommended to ensure there are no extracardiac diseases contiguous to the pericardium.

▶ Treatment

Most experts suggest a restriction in activity until symptom resolution. Nonsteroidal anti-inflammatory drugs are generally effective. Studies also suggest that the initial treatment of the acute episode with colchicine helps prevent recurrences. Current recommendations include ibuprofen 600–800 mg three times daily for 1–2 weeks or indomethacin 50 mg three times daily for 1–2 weeks. Doses can be decreased once symptoms resolve. Colchicine should be added to the nonsteroidal anti-inflammatory drug at 0.5–0.6 mg twice daily and continued for 3 months. Colchicine should also be the initial therapy in all refractory cases and in recurrent pericarditis. Its use should be for 6 months in such cases. Aspirin and colchicine should be used instead of nonsteroidal anti-inflammatory drugs in postmyocardial infarction pericarditis (Dressler syndrome) since nonsteriodal anti-inflammatory drugs may have an adverse effect on myocardial healing. Aspirin in doses of 650–1000 mg three times daily for 1–2 weeks plus 3 months of colchicine is the recommended treatment. Systemic corticosteroids can be used in patients with severe symptoms, in refractory cases, or in patients with immune-mediated etiologies, but such therapy may entail a higher risk of recurrence and colchicine is recommended in addition, again for 3 months, to help prevent recurrences. Prednisone in doses of 0.25–0.5 mg/kg/d is suggested. In general, symptoms subside in several days to weeks. The major early complication is tamponade, which occurs in < 5% of patients. There may be recurrences in the first few weeks or months. Rarely, when colchicine therapy alone fails, recurrent pericarditis may require more significant immunosuppression, such as cyclophosphamide or methotrexate. If colchicine plus more significant immunosuppression fails, surgical pericardial stripping may be required in recurrent cases even without clinical evidence for constrictive pericarditis.

Standard antituberculous drug therapy is usually successful for **tuberculous pericarditis** (see Chapter 9), but constrictive pericarditis can occur. **Uremic pericarditis** usually resolves with the institution of—or with more aggressive—dialysis. Tamponade is fairly common, and partial pericardiectomy (pericardial window) may be necessary. Whereas anti-inflammatory agents may relieve the pain and fever associated with uremic pericarditis, indomethacin and systemic corticosteroids do not affect its natural history. The prognosis with **neoplastic effusion** is poor, with only a small minority surviving 1 year. If it is compromising the clinical comfort of the patient, the effusion is initially drained percutaneously. A pericardial window, either by a subxiphoid approach or via video-assisted thoracic surgery, allows for partial pericardiectomy. Instillation of chemotherapeutic agents or tetracycline may be used to reduce the recurrence rate. Symptomatic therapy is the initial approach to **radiation pericarditis,** but recurrent effusions and constriction often require surgery.

▶ When to Refer

Patients who do not respond initially to conservative management, who have recurrences, or who appear to be developing constrictive pericarditis should be referred to a cardiologist for further assessment.

Lotrionte M et al. International collaborative systematic review of controlled clinical trials on the pharmacologic treatment of acute pericarditis and its recurrences. Am Heart J. 2010 Oct;160(4):662–70. [PMID: 20934560]

Markel G et al. Prevention of recurrent pericarditis with colchicine in 2012. Clin Cardiol. 2013 Mar;36(3):125–8. [PMID: 23404655]

Sparano DM et al. Pericarditis and pericardial effusion: management update. Curr Treat Options Cardiovasc Med. 2011 Dec; 13(6):543–55. [PMID: 21989746]

Spodick DH. Colchicine effectively and safely treats acute pericarditis and prevents and treats recurrent pericarditides. Heart. 2012 Jul;98(14):1035–6. [PMID: 22634168]

PERICARDIAL EFFUSION & TAMPONADE

Pericardial effusion can develop during any of the pericarditis processes. The speed of accumulation determines the physiologic importance of the effusion. Because the pericardium stretches, large effusions (> 1000 mL) that develop slowly may produce no hemodynamic effects. Conversely, smaller effusions that appear rapidly can cause tamponade due to the curvilinear relationship between the volume of fluid and the intrapericardial pressure. Tamponade is characterized by elevated intrapericardial pressure (> 15 mm Hg), which restricts venous return and ventricular filling. As a result, the stroke volume and arterial pulse pressure fall, and the heart rate and venous pressure rise. Shock and death may result.

▶ **Clinical Findings**

A. Symptoms and Signs

Pericardial effusions may be associated with pain if they occur as part of an acute inflammatory process or may be painless, as is often the case with neoplastic or uremic effusion. Dyspnea and cough are common, especially with tamponade. Other symptoms may result from the primary disease.

A pericardial friction rub may be present even with large effusions. In cardiac tamponade, tachycardia, tachypnea, a narrow pulse pressure, and a relatively preserved systolic pressure are characteristic. Pulsus paradoxus is defined as a > 10 mm Hg decline in systolic pressure during inspiration. Since the RV and LV share the same pericardium, when there is significant pericardial effusion, as the RV enlarges with inspiratory filling, septal motion toward the LV reduces LV filling and results in an accentuated drop in the stroke volume and BP with inspiration. Central venous pressure is elevated and since the intrapericardial, and thus intracardiac, pressures are high even at the initiation of diastole, there is no evident *y* descent in the RA, RV, or LV hemodynamic tracings. This differs from constriction where most of the initial filling of the RV and LV occurs during early diastole (the Y descent), and it is only in mid to late diastole that the ventricles can no longer fill. Edema or ascites are rarely present in tamponade; these signs favor a more chronic process.

B. Laboratory Findings

Laboratory tests tend to reflect the underlying processes (see causes of pericarditis above).

C. Diagnostic Studies

Chest radiograph can suggest chronic effusion by an enlarged cardiac silhouette with a globular configuration but may appear normal in acute situations. The ECG often reveals nonspecific T wave changes and reduced QRS voltage. Electrical alternans is present occasionally but is pathognomonic due to the heart swinging within the large effusion. Echocardiography is the primary method for demonstrating pericardial effusion and is quite sensitive. If tamponade is present, the high intrapericardial pressure may collapse lower pressure cardiac structures, such as the RA and RV. In tamponade, the normal inspiratory reduction in LV filling is accentuated due to RV/LV interaction and there is a > 25% reduction in maximal mitral inflow velocities. RV collapse is particularly evident in diastole as the enlarging diastolic LV crowds out the RV within the fixed space provided by the ventricles and pericardium. The apparent RV diastolic "collapse" is due to the thinner

RV being unable to fill appropriately during diastole at the same time that the thicker and more powerful LV enters diastole. Cardiac CT and MRI also demonstrate pericardial fluid, pericardial thickening, and any associated contiguous lesions. Diagnostic pericardiocentesis or biopsy is often indicated for microbiologic and cytologic studies; a pericardial biopsy may be performed relatively simply through a small subxiphoid incision or by use of a video-assisted thoracoscopic surgical procedure. Unfortunately, the quality of the pericardial fluid itself rarely leads to a diagnosis, and any type of fluid (serous, serosanguinous, bloody, etc) can be seen in most diseases. Pericardial fluid analysis is most useful in excluding a bacterial cause. Effusions due to hypothyroidism or lymphatic obstruction may contain cholesterol or be chylous in nature, respectively.

▶ **Treatment**

Small effusions can be followed clinically by careful observations of the JVP and by testing for a change in the paradoxical pulse. Serial echocardiograms are indicated if no intervention is immediately contemplated. When tamponade is present, urgent pericardiocentesis is required. Because the pressure–volume relationship in the pericardial fluid is curvilinear and upsloping, removal of a small amount of fluid often produces a dramatic fall in the intrapericardial pressure and immediate hemodynamic benefit; but complete drainage with a catheter is preferable. Continued or repeat drainage may be indicated, especially in malignant effusions. Pericardial windows via video-assisted thorascopy have been particularly effective in preventing recurrences. Effusions related to recurrent inflammatory pericarditis can be treated as noted above (see Acute Inflammatory Pericarditis).

Additional therapy is determined by the nature of the primary process. Recurrent effusion in neoplastic disease and uremia, in particular, may require partial pericardiectomy.

▶ **When to Refer**

- Any unexplained pericardial effusion should be referred to a cardiologist.

- Trivial pericardial effusions are common, especially in heart failure, and need not be referred unless symptoms of pericarditis are evident.

- Hypotension or a paradoxical pulse suggesting the pericardial effusion is hemodynamically compromising the patient should prompt an immediate referral.

- Echocardiographic signs of tamponade should always trigger referral.

Bodson L et al. Cardiac tamponade. Curr Opin Crit Care. 2011 Oct;17(5):416–24. [PMID: 21716107]

Imazio M et al. Medical therapy of pericardial diseases: part II: noninfectious pericarditis, pericardial effusions and constrictive pericarditis. J Cardiovasc Med (Hagerstown). 2010 Nov;11(11): 785–94. [PMID: 20925146]

Refaat MM et al. Neoplastic pericardial effusion. Clin Cardiol. 2011 Oct;34(10):593–8. [PMID: 21928406]

CONSTRICTIVE PERICARDITIS

ESSENTIALS OF DIAGNOSIS

► Evidence of right heart failure.

► No fall or an elevation of the JVP with inspiration (Kussmaul sign).

► Echocardiographic evidence for septal bounce and reduced mitral inflow velocities with inspiration.

► May be difficult to differentiate from restrictive cardiomyopathy.

► Cardiac catheterization may be necessary.

► General Considerations

Inflammation can lead to a thickened, fibrotic, adherent pericardium that restricts diastolic filling and produces chronically elevated venous pressures. In the past, tuberculosis was the most common cause of constrictive pericarditis, but the process now more often occurs after radiation therapy, cardiac surgery, or viral pericarditis; histoplasmosis is another uncommon cause, occurring mainly in individuals who live in the Ohio River Valley.

At times, both pericardial tamponade and constrictive pericarditis may coexist, a condition referred to as effusive-constrictive pericarditis. The only definitive way to diagnose this condition is to reveal the underlying constrictive physiology once the pericardial fluid is drained.

► Clinical Findings

A. Symptoms and Signs

The principal symptoms are slowly progressive dyspnea, fatigue, and weakness. Chronic edema, hepatic congestion, and ascites are usually present. Ascites often seems out of proportion to the degree of peripheral edema. The examination reveals these signs and a characteristically elevated jugular venous pressure with a rapid y descent. This can be detected at bedside by careful observation of the jugular pulse and noting an apparent increased pulse wave at the end of ventricular systole (due to an apparent accentuation of the v wave by the rapid y descent). Kussmaul sign—a failure of the JVP to fall with inspiration—is also a frequent finding. The apex may actually retract with systole and a pericardial "knock" may be heard in early diastole. Pulsus paradoxus is unusual. Atrial fibrillation is common.

B. Diagnostic Studies

At times constrictive pericarditis is extremely difficult to differentiate from restrictive cardiomyopathy. When unclear, the use of both noninvasive testing and cardiac catheterization is required to sort out the difference.

1. Radiographic findings—The chest radiograph may show normal heart size or cardiomegaly. Pericardial calcification is best seen on the lateral view and is uncommon. It rarely involves the LV apex, and finding of calcification at the LV apex is more consistent with LV aneurysm.

2. Echocardiography—Echocardiography rarely demonstrates a thickened pericardium. A septal "bounce" reflecting the rapid early filling is common, though. RV/LV interaction may be demonstrated by a reduction in the mitral inflow Doppler pattern of > 25%, much as in tamponade. The Doppler mitral inflow pattern should demonstrate at least a 25% fall with inspiration. Usually the initial inflow into the LV is very rapid and this can be demonstrated as well by the Doppler inflow (E wave) pattern.

3. Cardiac CT and MRI—These imaging tests are only occasionally helpful. Pericardial thickening of > 4 mm must be present to establish the diagnosis, and no pericardial thickening is demonstrable in 20–25% of patients with constrictive pericarditis. Some MRI techniques demonstrate the septal bounce and can provide evidence for ventricular interaction.

4. Cardiac catheterization—This procedure is often confirmatory or can be diagnostic in difficult cases where the echocardiographic features are unclear or mixed. As a generality, the pulmonary pressure is low in constriction (as opposed to restrictive cardiomyopathy). In constrictive pericarditis, because of the need to demonstrate RV/LV interaction, cardiac catheterization should include simultaneous measurement of both the LV and RV pressure tracings with inspiration and expiration. Hemodynamically, patients with constriction have equalization of end-diastolic pressures throughout their cardiac chambers, there is rapid early filling then an abrupt increase in diastolic pressure ("square-root" sign), the RV end-diastolic pressure is more than one-third the systolic pressure, simultaneous measurements of RV and LV systolic pressure reveal a discordance with inspiration (the RV rises as the LV falls), and there is usually a Kussmaul sign (failure of the RA pressure to fall with inspiration). The area of the RV pressure tracing may also be less in expiration and greater during inspiration, reflecting the variability in filling of the RV with respiration. The ratio of the RV tracing area to the LV tracing area should increase with inspiration if constriction is present; this is due to the increased RV filling and higher RV systolic pressure with inspiration while the LV systolic pressure falls and the LV tracing area becomes less. These findings differ from restrictive cardiomyopathy in which the LV diastolic pressure is usually greater than the RV diastolic pressure by 5 mm Hg, there is pulmonary hypertension, and simultaneous measurements of the RV and LV systolic pressure reveal a concordant drop in the peak systolic ventricular pressures during inspiration with no change in the RV/LV tracing area ratio with inspiration.

► Treatment

Initial treatment consists of diuresis. As in other disorders of right heart failure, the diuresis should be aggressive, using loop diuretics (torsemide if bowel edema is suspected), thiazides, and aldosterone antagonists (especially if ascites is present). At times, aquaphoresis may be of value. Surgical pericardiectomy should be done when diuretics are unable to control symptoms. Pericardiectomy removes only the pericardium between the phrenic nerve pathways, however, and most patients still require diuretics after the procedure, though symptoms are usually dramatically improved. Morbidity and mortality after pericardiectomy are high (up to 15%) and are greatest in those with the most disability prior to the procedure.

► When to Refer

If the diagnosis of constrictive pericarditis is unclear or the symptoms resist medical therapy, then referral to a cardiologist is warranted to both establish the diagnosis and recommend therapy.

Imazio M. Contemporary management of pericardial diseases. Curr Opin Cardiol. 2012 May;27(3):308–17. [PMID: 22450720]

Talreja DR et al. Constrictive pericarditis in the modern era: novel criteria for diagnosis in the cardiac catheterization laboratory. J Am Coll Cardiol. 2008 Jan22;51(3):315–9. [PMID: 18206742]

PULMONARY HYPERTENSION & PULMONARY HEART DISEASE

PULMONARY HYPERTENSION

ESSENTIALS OF DIAGNOSIS

► Mean PA pressure ≥ 25 mm Hg with normal PCWP.

► Dyspnea, and often cyanosis, with no evidence of left heart disease.

► Enlarged pulmonary arteries on chest radiograph.

► Elevated JVP and RV heave.

► Echocardiography is often diagnostic.

► General Considerations

The normal pulmonary bed offers about one-tenth as much resistance to blood flow as the systemic arterial system. Experts recommend that a diagnosis of idiopathic pulmonary hypertension should be firmly based on a mean PA pressure of ≥ 25 mm Hg in association with a PCWP of < 16 mm Hg at rest.

The clinical classification of pulmonary hypertension by the Fourth World Symposium on Pulmonary Hypertension is outlined in Table 10–18.

Group 1 includes pulmonary arterial hypertension related to an underlying pulmonary vasculopathy. It includes the former "primary" pulmonary hypertension under the term "idiopathic pulmonary hypertension" and is defined as pulmonary hypertension and elevated PVR in the absence of other disease of the lungs or heart. Its cause is unknown. Drug and toxic pulmonary hypertension has

Table 10–18. Clinical classification of pulmonary hypertension.

I. Pulmonary arterial hypertension from pulmonary vasculopathy
Idiopathic pulmonary arterial hypertension
Heritable gene mutations
BMPR2 (bone morphogenic protein receptor type 2)
ALK1 (activin A receptor type II-like kinase-1), *endoglin* (with or without hereditary hemorrhagic telangiectasia)
Unknown
Drug and toxin-induced
Associated with
Connective tissue diseases
HIV infection
Portal hypertension
Congenital heart disease
Schistosomiasis
Chronic hemolytic anemia
Persistent pulmonary hypertension of the newborn
Pulmonary veno-occlusive disease and/or pulmonary capillary hemangiomatosis
II. Pulmonary hypertension due to left heart disease
Systolic dysfunction
Diastolic dysfunction
III. Pulmonary hypertension due to lung disease and/or hypoxia
Chronic obstructive pulmonary disease
Interstitial lung disease
Other pulmonary disease with mixed restrictive and obstructive pattern
IV. Chronic thromboembolic pulmonary hypertension
V. Pulmonary hypertension with unclear multifactorial mechanisms
Hematologic disorders: myeloproliferative disorders, lenectomy
Systemic disorders: sarcoidosis, pulmonary Langerhans cell histiocytosis: lymphangioleimyomatosis, neurofibromatosis, vasculitis
Metabolic disorders: glycogen storage disease, Gaucher disease, thyroid disorders
Others: tumoral obstruction, fibrosing mediastinitis, chronic renal failure on dialysis

Modified, with permission, from Simonneau G et al. Updated clinical classification of pulmonary hypertension. J Am Coll Cardiol. 2009; 54:S43–54.

been described associated with the use of anorexigenic agents that increase serotonin release and block its uptake. These include aminorex fumarate, fenfluramine, and dexfenfluramine. In some cases, there is epidemiologic linkage to ingestion of rapeseed oil or L-tryptophan and use of illicit drugs, such as amphetamines. Pulmonary hypertension associated with connective tissue disease includes cases associated with scleroderma—up to 8–12% of patients with scleroderma may be affected.

Group 2 includes all cases related to left heart disease. **Group 3** includes cases due to parenchymal lung disease, impaired control of breathing, or living at high altitude.

This group encompasses those with idiopathic pulmonary fibrosis and COPD. **Group 4** represents patients with chronic thromboemboli. **Group 5** includes multifactorial cases.

► **Clinical Findings**

A. Symptoms and Signs

The clinical picture is similar to that of pulmonary hypertension from other causes. Dyspnea, chest pain, fatigue, and lightheadedness are early symptoms; later symptoms include syncope, abdominal distention, ascites, and peripheral edema. Chronic lung disease, especially sleep apnea, often is overlooked as a cause for pulmonary hypertension as is chronic thromboembolic disease. Patients with idiopathic pulmonary hypertension are characteristically young women who have evidence of right heart failure that is usually progressive, leading to death in 2–8 years without therapy. This is a decidedly different prognosis than patients with Eisenmenger physiology due to a left-to-right shunt; 40% of patients with Eisenmenger physiology are alive 25 years after the diagnosis has been made. Patients have manifestations of low cardiac output, with weakness and fatigue, as well as edema and ascites as right heart failure advances. Peripheral cyanosis is present, and syncope on effort may occur.

B. Diagnostic Studies

The laboratory evaluation of idiopathic pulmonary hypertension must exclude a secondary cause. A hypercoagulable state should be sought by measuring proteins C and S levels, the presence of a lupus anticoagulant, the level of factor V Leiden, prothrombin gene mutations, and D-dimer. Chronic pulmonary emboli must be excluded (usually by ventilation-perfusion lung scan or contrast spiral CT); the ventilation-perfusion scan is the more sensitive test. The chest radiograph helps exclude a primary pulmonary etiology—evidence for patchy pulmonary edema may raise the suspicion of pulmonary veno-occlusive disease due to obstruction in pulmonary venous drainage. A sleep study may be warranted if sleep apnea is suspected. The ECG is generally consistent with RVH and RA enlargement. Echocardiography with Doppler helps exclude an intracardiac shunt and usually demonstrates an enlarged RV and RA—at times they may be huge and hypocontractile. Severe pulmonic or tricuspid regurgitation may be present. Septal flattening is consistent with pulmonary hypertension. Doppler interrogation of the tricuspid regurgitation jet helps provide an estimate of RV systolic pressure. Pulmonary function tests help exclude other disorders, though primary pulmonary hypertension may present with a reduced carbon monoxide diffusing capacity of the lung ($D_{L_{CO}}$) and severe desaturation (particularly if a PFO has been stretched open and a right-to-left shunt is present). A declining $D_{L_{CO}}$ in a scleroderma patient may precede the development of pulmonary hypertension. Chest CT demonstrates enlarged pulmonary arteries and excludes other causes (such as emphysema or interstitial lung disease). Pulmonary angiography (or MR

angiography or CT angiography) reveals loss of the smaller acinar pulmonary vessels and tapering of the larger ones. Catheterization allows measurement of pulmonary pressures and testing for vasoreactivity using a variety of agents, including 100% oxygen, adenosine, epoprostenol, and nitric oxide. Nitric oxide is preferred due to its ease of use and short half-life. A positive response is defined as one that decreases the pulmonary mean pressure by 10 mm Hg with the final mean PA pressure < 40 mm Hg.

► **Treatment & Prognosis**

General measures include the use of warfarin in all patients with idiopathic pulmonary hypertension who have no contraindication to its use, diuretics in patients with right-sided heart failure, oxygen (especially during sleep) with a goal of maintaining an oxygen saturation of> 90%, and occasionally, digoxin. Patients are advised against heavy physical exertion. A sodium restricted diet (< 2400 mg/d) is advised. The therapeutic algorithm is based on the response to an intravenous vasodilator trial and the clinical risk assessment (Figure 10–12). Patients with a positive response to the intravenous vasodilator should first be tried on oral calcium channel blockers or sildenafil, or both. Patients who do not have a positive response are then divided into those of **lower risk** (no RV failure, > 400 meters on a 6-minute walk test, peak VO_2 max > 10.4 mL/kg/min, minimal RV dysfunction, normal right heart hemodynamics and minimally elevated BNP) and those of **highest risk** (RV failure, rapidly progressive symptoms, < 300 meters on a 6-minute walk, peak VO_2 max < 10.4 mL/kg/min, abnormal echocardiographic findings (pericardial effusion, severe RV enlargement and dysfunction, RA pressure > 20 mm Hg, cardiac index < 2.0 L/min/m2, or significantly elevated BNP). A negative response to vasodilators in a low-risk patient suggests the next line of therapy be endothelin receptor blockers or phosphodiesterase-5 inhibitors as initial oral treatment. If the patient does not respond, then the use of epoprostenol (intravenously) or treprostinil (intravenously), iloprost (inhaled), or treprostinil (subcutaneously) may be tried. For those high-risk patients who do not respond, then therapy consists of use of an intravenous prostacyclin (epoprostenol or treprostinil). Failure of all of these therapies suggests that lung transplantation should be considered. Palliation of patients who are not too cyanotic can be achieved by atrial septostomy to increase forward cardiac output.

In a few patients with acute or chronic pulmonary emboli or both, pulmonary thrombectomy may be effective. In chronic thromboembolic disease, a new soluble guanylate cyclase stimulator, riociguat, has also been found to be of value in patients who cannot undergo thrombectomy or who have undergone the procedure but still experience symptoms.

Most patients die of RV failure; a severely dilated RV with poor contractile function (cor pulmonale) has been shown to predict early mortality. Pregnancy is potentially life-threatening and must be avoided or terminated early to save the mother's life if the pulmonary hypertension is severe. Survival has improved with idiopathic pulmonary

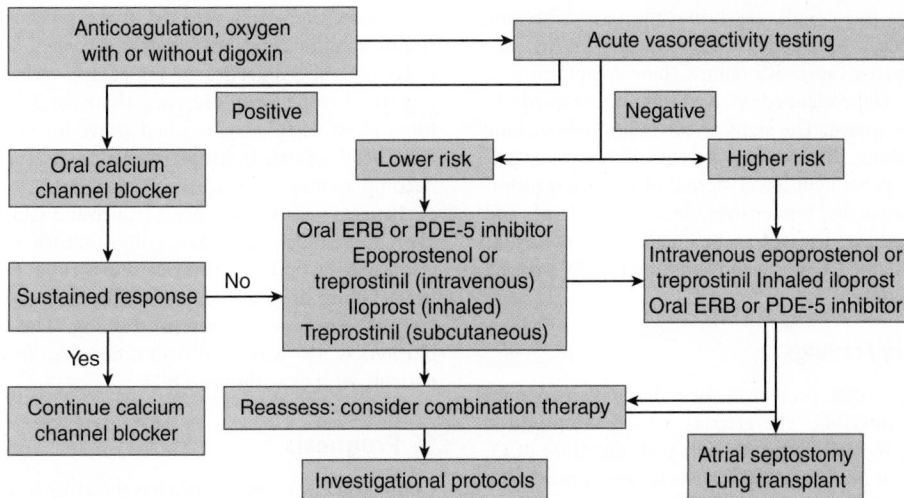

▲ **Figure 10–12.** Pulmonary hypertension treatment algorithm. ERB, endothelin receptor blockers; PDE-5, phospho-diesterase- 5. (Modified, with permission, from McLaughlin VV et al; American College of Cardiology Foundation Task Force on Expert Consensus Documents; American Heart Association; American College of Chest Physicians; American Thoracic Society, Inc; Pulmonary Hypertension Association. ACCF/AHA 2009 expert consensus document on pulmonary hypertension a report of the American College of Cardiology Foundation Task Force on Expert Consensus Documents and the American Heart Association developed in collaboration with the American College of Chest Physicians; American Thoracic Society, Inc.; and the Pulmonary Hypertension Association. J Am Coll Cardiol. 2009 Apr 28;53(17):1573–619.)

hypertension, though it still remains a dread disease. One, 2- and 3-year survival rates of 85.7%, 69.5%, and 54.9% are still reported. Men fare worse than women, and etiology, functional class, exercise tolerance, and RV hemodynamics all adversely affect outcome.

▶ When to Refer

All patients with suspected pulmonary hypertension should be referred to either a cardiologist or pulmonologist who specializes in the evaluation and treatment of patients with unexplained pulmonary hypertension.

Benza RL et al. Predicting survival in pulmonary arterial hypertension: insights from the Registry to Evaluate Early and Long-term Pulmonary Arterial Hypertension Disease Management (REVEAL). Circulation. 2010 Jul 13;122(2):164–72. [PMID: 20585012]

Ghofrani HA et al; PATENT-1 Study Group. Riociguat for the treatment of pulmonary arterial hypertension. N Engl J Med. 2013 Jul 25;369(4):330–40. [PMID: 23883378]

Hoeper MM et al. Diagnosis, assessment and treatment of non-pulmonary arterial pulmonary hypertension. J Am Coll Cardiol. 2009 Jun 30;54(1 Suppl):S85–96. [PMID: 19555862]

McLaughlin VV et al. ACCF/AHA 2009 expert consensus document on pulmonary hypertension: a report of the American College of Cardiology Foundation Task Force on Expert Consensus Documents and the American Heart Association developed in collaboration with the American College of Chest Physicians; American Thoracic Society, Inc.; and the Pulmonary Hypertension Association. J Am Coll Cardiol. 2009 Apr 28;53(17):1573–619. [PMID: 19389575]

Pulido T et al; SERAPHIN Investigators. Macitentan and morbidity and mortality in pulmonary arterial hypertension. N Engl J Med. 2013 Aug 29;369(9):809–18. [PMID: 23984728]

PULMONARY HEART DISEASE (Cor Pulmonale)

ESSENTIALS OF DIAGNOSIS

▶ Associated with chronic bronchitis or emphysema or pulmonary hypertension.

▶ Elevated jugular venous pressure, parasternal lift, edema, hepatomegaly, ascites.

▶ ECG shows tall, peaked P waves (P pulmonale), right axis deviation, and RVH.

▶ Echocardiogram excludes primary LV dysfunction.

▶ General Considerations

The term "cor pulmonale" denotes RV systolic and diastolic failure resulting from pulmonary disease and the attendant hypoxia or from pulmonary vascular disease (pulmonary hypertension). Its clinical features depend on both the primary underlying disease and its effects on the heart.

Cor pulmonale is most commonly caused by pulmonary hypertension from any cause (see above), COPD or idiopathic pulmonary fibrosis. Less frequent causes include pneumoconiosis and kyphoscoliosis.

▶ Clinical Findings

A. Symptoms and Signs

The predominant symptoms of compensated cor pulmonale are related to the pulmonary disorder and include chronic productive cough, exertional dyspnea, wheezing respirations, easy fatigability, and weakness. When the pulmonary disease causes RV failure, these symptoms may be intensified. Dependent edema and right upper quadrant pain may also appear. The signs of cor pulmonale include cyanosis, clubbing, distended neck veins, RV heave or gallop (or both), prominent lower sternal or epigastric pulsations, an enlarged and tender liver, dependent edema, and ascites. Severe lung disease can be a cause of low cardiac output by reducing LV filling and subsequently LV preload and stroke volume.

B. Laboratory Findings

Polycythemia is often present in cor pulmonale secondary to chronic hypoxemia. The arterial oxygen saturation is often below 85% and frequently falls with exertion; PCO_2 may or may not be elevated. Cyanosis is more prevalent if there is right to left shunting via a PFO.

C. ECG and Chest Radiography

The ECG may show right axis deviation and peaked P waves. Deep S waves are present in lead V_6. Right axis deviation and low voltage may be noted in patients with pulmonary emphysema. Frank RVH is uncommon except in pulmonary hypertension. The ECG often mimics myocardial infarction; Q waves may be present in leads II, III, and aVF because of the vertically placed heart, but they are rarely deep or wide, as in inferior myocardial infarction. Supraventricular arrhythmias are frequent and nonspecific.

The chest radiograph discloses the presence or absence of parenchymal disease and a prominent or enlarged RV and PA.

D. Diagnostic Studies

Pulmonary function tests usually confirm the underlying lung disease. The echocardiogram should show normal LV size and function but RV and RA dilation and RV dysfunction. Perfusion lung scans are rarely of value, but, if negative, they help exclude chronic pulmonary emboli. Multislice CT has replaced pulmonary angiography as the most specific method of diagnosis for the pulmonary emboli. The serum BNP level may be elevated from RV dysfunction.

▶ Differential Diagnosis

In its early stages, cor pulmonale can be diagnosed on the basis of the clinical examination and radiologic, echocardiographic or ECG evidence. Catheterization of the right heart will establish a definitive diagnosis but is more often performed to exclude left-sided heart failure or pulmonary venous disease, which can be an unrecognized cause of right-sided failure in some patients. Differential diagnostic considerations relate primarily to the specific pulmonary disease that has produced RV failure (see above).

▶ Treatment

The details of the treatment of chronic pulmonary disease (chronic respiratory failure) are discussed in Chapter 9.

Otherwise, therapy is directed at the pulmonary process responsible for right heart failure. Oxygen, salt and fluid restriction, and diuretics are mainstays, with combination diuretic therapy (loop diuretics, thiazides and spironolactone) often useful, as described above for other causes of right heart failure. Inotropic agents are useful when acute decompensation occurs.

Patients with systolic heart failure and COPD are more likely to be older, have more comorbidities, reduced exercise capacity, and increased cardiovascular mortality and heart failure hospitalization, but they do not have a differential response to exercise training. The use of beta-blockers is not associated with differences in outcome for patients with or without COPD.

▶ Prognosis

Compensated cor pulmonale has the same prognosis as the underlying pulmonary disease. Once signs of heart failure appear, the average life expectancy is 2–5 years, but survival is significantly longer when uncomplicated emphysema is the cause.

▶ When to Refer

Patients with unexplained or difficult to manage right heart failure should be referred to a cardiologist or a pulmonologist in an effort to uncover correctable causes and to address therapeutic options.

Barr RG et al. Percent emphysema, airflow obstruction and impaired left ventricular filling. N Engl J Med. 2010 Jan 21; 362(3):217–27. [PMID: 20089972]

Hoeper MM et al. Diagnosis, assessment and treatment of non-pulmonary arterial pulmonary hypertension. J Am Coll Cardiol. 2009 Jun 30;54(1 Suppl):S85–96. [PMID: 19555862]

Mentz RJ et al. Clinical characteristics, response to exercise training, and outcomes in patients with heart failure and chronic obstructive pulmonary disease: findings from Heart Failure and A Controlled Trial Investigating Outcomes of Exercise TraiNing (HF-ACTION). Am Heart J. 2013 Feb;165(2):193–9. [PMID: 23351822]

Stone IS et al. Chronic obstructive pulmonary disease: a modifiable risk factor for cardiovascular disease? Heart. 2012 Jul;98(14):1055–62. [PMID: 22739636]

NEOPLASTIC DISEASES OF THE HEART

Primary cardiac tumors are rare and constitute only a small fraction of all tumors that involve the heart or pericardium. The most common primary tumor is atrial myxoma; it comprises about 50% of all tumors in adult case series. It is generally attached to the atrial septum and is more likely to affect the LA than the RA. Patients with myxoma can present with the characteristics of a systemic illness, with obstruction of blood flow through the heart, or with signs of peripheral embolization. The characteristics include fever, malaise, weight loss, leukocytosis, elevated sedimentation rate, and emboli (peripheral or pulmonary, depending on the location of the tumor). This is often confused with infective endocarditis, lymphoma, other cancers, or autoimmune diseases. In other cases, the tumor may grow to considerable size and produce symptoms by obstructing mitral inflow. Episodic pulmonary edema (classically occurring when an upright posture is assumed) and signs of low output may result. Physical examination may reveal a diastolic sound related to motion of the tumor ("tumor plop") or a diastolic murmur similar to that of mitral stenosis. Right-sided myxomas may cause symptoms of right-sided failure. Familial myxomas occur as part of the **Carney complex**—that consists of myxomas, pigmented skin lesions, and endocrine neoplasia.

The diagnosis is established by echocardiography or by pathologic study of embolic material. Cardiac MRI is useful as an adjunct. Contrast angiography is frequently unnecessary. Surgical excision is usually curative, though recurrences do occur and serial echocardiographic follow-up, on at least a yearly basis, is recommended.

The second most common primary cardiac tumors are valvular papillary fibroelastomas and atrial septal lipomas. These tend to be benign and usually require no therapy, although large ones may embolize or cause valvular dysfunction. Other primary cardiac tumors include rhabdomyomas (that often appear multiple in both the RV and LV), fibrous histiocytomas, hemangiomas, and a variety of unusual sarcomas. The diagnosis may be supported by an abnormal cardiac contour on radiograph. Echocardiography is usually helpful but may miss tumors infiltrating the ventricular wall. Cardiac MRI is emerging as the diagnostic procedure of choice.

Metastases from malignant tumors can also affect the heart. Most often this occurs in malignant melanoma, but other tumors involving the heart include bronchogenic carcinoma, carcinoma of the breast, the lymphomas, renal cell carcinoma, and, in patients with AIDS, Kaposi sarcoma. These are often clinically silent but may lead to pericardial tamponade, arrhythmias and conduction disturbances, heart failure, and peripheral emboli. ECG may reveal regional Q waves. The diagnosis is often made by echocardiography, but cardiac MRI and CT scanning can often better delineate the extent of involvement. The prognosis is poor for secondary cardiac tumors; effective treatment is not available. On rare occasions, surgical resection for debulking or removal and chemotherapy is warranted. Primary pericardial tumors, such as mesotheliomas related to asbestos exposure, may also occur.

Many primary tumors may be resectable. Atrial myxomas should be removed surgically due to the high incidence of embolization from these friable tumors. Papillary fibroelastomas are usually benign but may embolize and large ones should be considered for surgical excision. Large pericardial effusions from metastatic tumors may be drained for comfort, but the fluid invariably recurs. Rhabdomyomas may be surgically cured if the tumor is accessible and can be removed while still leaving enough functioning myocardium intact.

▶ When to Refer

All patients with suspected cardiac tumors should be referred to a cardiologist or cardiac surgeon for evaluation and possible therapy.

Burnside N et al. Malignant primary cardiac tumours. Interact Cardiovasc Thorac Surg. 2012 Dec;15(6):1004–6. [PMID: 22922450]

Michael RJ. Cardiac tumor issue overview. Methodist DeBakey Cardiovasc J. 2010 Jul–Sep;6(3):2–3. [PMID: 20834204]

Motwani M et al. MR imaging of cardiac tumors and masses: a review of methods and clinical applications. Radiology. 2013 Jul;268(1):26–43. [PMID: 23793590]

▼ TRAUMATIC HEART DISEASE

Trauma is the leading cause of death in patients aged 1–44 years of age; cardiac and vascular trauma is second only to neurologic injury as the reason for these deaths. Penetrating wounds to the heart are usually lethal unless surgically repaired. Stab wounds to the RV occasionally lead to hemopericardium without progressing to tamponade.

Blunt trauma is a more frequent cause of cardiac injuries, particularly outside of the emergency department setting. This type of injury is quite frequent in motor vehicle accidents and may occur with any form of chest trauma, including CPR efforts. The most common injuries are myocardial contusions or hematomas. Other forms of nonischemic cardiac injury include metabolic injury due to burns, electrical current, or sepsis. These may be asymptomatic (particularly in the setting of more severe injuries) or may present with chest pain of a nonspecific nature or, not uncommonly, with a pericardial component. Elevations of cardiac enzymes are frequent but the levels do not correlate with prognosis. Echocardiography may reveal an akinetic segment or pericardial effusion. Pericardiocentesis is warranted if tamponade is evident. Heart failure is uncommon if there are no associated cardiac or pericardial injuries, and conservative management is usually sufficient.

Severe trauma may also cause myocardial or valvular rupture. Cardiac rupture may involve any chamber, but survival is most likely if injury is to one of the atria or the RV. Hemopericardium or pericardial tamponade is the usual clinical presentation, and surgery is almost always necessary. Mitral and aortic valve rupture may occur during severe blunt trauma—the former presumably if the impact occurs during systole and the latter if during diastole. Patients reach the hospital in shock or severe heart failure. Immediate surgical repair is essential. The same types of injuries may result in transection of the aorta, either at the level of the arch or distal to the takeoff of the left subclavian artery. Transthoracic echocardiography and TEE are the most helpful and immediately available diagnostic techniques.

Blunt trauma may also result in damage to the coronary arteries. Acute or subacute coronary thrombosis is the most common presentation. The clinical syndrome is one of acute myocardial infarction with attendant ECG, enzymatic, and contractile abnormalities. Emergent revascularization is sometimes feasible, either by the percutaneous route or by coronary artery bypass surgery. LV aneurysms are common outcomes of traumatic coronary occlusions, likely due to sudden occlusion with no collateral vascular support. Coronary artery dissection or rupture may also occur in the setting of blunt cardiac trauma.

As expected, patients with severe preexisting conditions fare the least well after cardiac trauma. Data from ReCONECT, a trauma consortium, reveals that mortality is linked to volume of cases seen at various centers, preexisting coronary disease or heart failure, intubation, age, and a severity scoring index.

Bock JS et al. Blunt cardiac injury. Cardiol Clin. 2012 Nov; 30(4):545–55. [PMID: 23102031]

Clancy K et al. Screening for blunt cardiac injury: an Eastern Association for the Surgery of Trauma practice management guideline. J Trauma Acute Care Surg. 2012 Nov;73(5 Suppl 4): S301–6. [PMID: 23114485]

Harrington DL et al; Research Consortium of New England Centers for Trauma (ReCONECT). Factors associated with survival following blunt chest trauma in older patients: results from a large regional trauma cooperative. Arch Surg. 2010 May;145(5):432–7. [PMID: 20479340]

Restrepo CS et al. Imaging patients with cardiac trauma. Radiographics. 2012 May–Jun;32(3):633–49. [PMID: 22582351]

RISK OF SURGERY IN THE CARDIAC PATIENT

See Chapter 3.

HEART DISEASE & PREGNANCY

The management of cardiac disease in pregnancy is discussed in the references listed below, including the available scoring systems to assess risk. Only a few major points can be covered in this brief section. Fundamentally, the highest risk patients are those with pulmonary hypertension, severe valvular stenosis, cyanosis, and heart failure. Regurgitant valve disease patients tolerate pregnancy better than stenotic valve disease patients due to the afterload reducing effect of pregnancy.

A comprehensive review of the safety of drugs in pregnancy and during breast-feeding can be found at www. perinatology.com/exposures/druglist.htm.

CARDIOVASCULAR COMPLICATIONS OF PREGNANCY

Pregnancy-related hypertension (eclampsia and preeclampsia) is discussed in Chapter 19.

1. Cardiomyopathy of Pregnancy (Peripartum Cardiomyopathy)

In approximately 1 in 3000 to 4000 live births, dilated cardiomyopathy develops in the mother in the final month of pregnancy or within 6 months after delivery. The disease may be related to a cathepsin-D cleavage product of the hormone prolactin, suggesting blockage of prolactin may be a potential therapeutic strategy if proven in clinical trials using bromocriptine. Immune and viral causes have also been postulated. Small studies have suggested some improvement with the use of intravenous immunoglobulin and pentoxifylline. The disease occurs more frequently in women over age 30 years, is usually related to the first or second pregnancy, and there has been some association with gestational hypertension and drugs used to stop uterine contractions. Risk factors include obesity, a history of cardiac disorders such as myocarditis, use of certain medications, smoking, alcoholism, multiple pregnancies, being African American, and being malnourished.

The course of the disease is variable; most cases improve or resolve completely over several months, but others progress to refractory heart failure. About 60% of patients make a complete recovery. Serum BNP levels are routinely elevated in pregnancy, but serial values may be useful in predicting who may be at increased risk for a worse outcome. Beta-blockers have been administered judiciously to these patients, with at least anecdotal success. Diuretics, hydralazine, and nitrates help treat the heart failure with minimal risk to the fetus. Some experts advocate anticoagulation because of an increased risk of thrombotic events, and both warfarin and heparin have their proponents. In severe cases, transient use of extracorporeal oxygenation (ECMO) has been lifesaving. Recurrence in subsequent pregnancies is common, particularly if cardiac function has not completely recovered, and subsequent pregnancies are to be discouraged if the EF remains < 55%. The risk of recurrent heart failure in a subsequent pregnancy has been estimated to be about 1 in 5 (21%).

Biteker M et al. Role of bromocriptine in peripartum cardiomyopathy. Am J Obstet Gynecol. 2009 Aug;201(2):e13. [PMID: 19306960]

Elkayam U et al. Peripartum cardiomyopathy. Cardiol Clin. 2012 Aug;30(3):435–40. [PMID: 22813368]

Johnson-Coyle L et al; American College of Cardiology Foundation; American Heart Association. Peripartum cardiomyopathy: review and practice guidelines. Am J Crit Care. 2012 Mar;21(2):89–98. Erratum in: Am J Crit Care. 2012 May;21 (3):155. Dosage error in article text. [PMID: 22381985]

Rutherford JD. Heart failure in pregnancy. Curr Heart Fail Rep. 2012 Dec;9(4):277–81. [PMID: 22821089]

Shah T et al. Peripartum cardiomyopathy: a contemporary review. Methodist Debakey Cardiovasc J. 2013 Jan–Mar;9(1): 38–43. [PMID: 23519269]

2. Coronary Artery & Other Vascular Abnormalities During Pregnancy

There have been a number of reports of myocardial infarction during pregnancy. It is known that pregnancy predisposes to dissection of the aorta and other arteries, perhaps because of the accompanying connective tissue changes. The risk may be particularly high in patients with Marfan, Ehlers-Danlos, or Loeys-Dietz syndromes. However, coronary artery dissection is responsible for only a minority of the infarctions; most are caused by atherosclerotic CAD or coronary emboli. The majority of the events occur near term or shortly following delivery, and paradoxical emboli through a PFO has been implicated in a few instances. Clinical management is essentially similar to that of other patients with acute infarction, unless there is a connective tissue disorder. If nonatherosclerotic dissection is present, coronary intervention may be risky as further dissection can be aggravated. In most instances, conservative management is warranted. At times, extensive aortic dissection requires surgical intervention. Recent studies suggest Marfan patients are particularly susceptible to further aortic expansion during pregnancy when the aortic diameter is > 4.5 cm and guidelines suggest pregnancy be discouraged in these situations.

Donnelly RT et al. The immediate and long-term impact of pregnancy on aortic growth rate and mortality in women with Marfan syndrome. J Am Coll Cardiol. 2012 Jul 17;60(3):224–9. [PMID: 22789886]

El-Deeb M et al. Acute coronary syndrome in pregnant women. Expert Rev Cardiovasc Ther. 2011 Apr;9(4):505–15. [PMID: 21517733]

Goland S et al. Pregnancy in Marfan syndrome: maternal and fetal risks and recommendations for patient assessment and management. Cardiol Rev. 2009 Nov–Dec;17(6):253–62. [PMID: 19829173]

Kealey A. Coronary artery disease and myocardial infarction in pregnancy: a review of epidemiology, diagnosis, medical and surgical management. Can J Cardiol. 2010 Jun;26(6):185–9. [PMID: 20548979]

3. Prophylaxis for Infective Endocarditis During Pregnancy & Delivery

The 2007 ACC/AHA Task Force addressing adults with congenital heart disease has formulated guidelines outlining recommendations for pregnant women during labor and delivery. Pregnancy itself is not considered a risk for endocarditis. Since vaginal delivery might include bacteremia, the guidelines advocated endocarditis prophylaxis to cover the same high-risk groups as in the traditional endocarditis recommendations from the ACC/AHA, acknowledging the data are lacking to support this approach. It is reasonable (Class 2a, LOE C) to consider antibiotic prophylaxis against infective endocarditis before vaginal delivery at the time of membrane rupture in select patients with the highest risk of adverse outcomes, which include those with the following indications: (1) prosthetic cardiac valve or prosthetic material used for cardiac valve repair, and (2) unrepaired and palliated cyanotic congenital heart disease, including surgically constructed palliative shunts conduits.

Duval X et al; AEPEI Study Group. Temporal trends in infective endocarditis in the context of prophylaxis guideline modifications: three successive population-based surveys. J Am Coll Cardiol. 2012 May 29;59(22):1968–76. [PMID: 22624837]

Warnes CA et al. ACC/AHA 2008 Guidelines for the Management of Adults With Congenital Heart Disease. A Report of the American College of Cardiology/American Heart Association Task Force on Practice Guidelines. Circulation. 2008 Dec 2;118(23):e714–833. [PMID: 18997169]

▶ Management of Labor

Although vaginal delivery is usually well tolerated, unstable patients (including patients with severe hypertension and worsening heart failure) should have planned cesarean section. An increased risk of aortic rupture has been noted during delivery in patients with coarctation of the aorta and severe aortic root dilation with Marfan syndrome, and vaginal delivery should be avoided in these conditions. For most patients, even those with congenital heart disease, vaginal delivery is preferred.

▼ CARDIOVASCULAR SCREENING OF ATHLETES

The sudden death of a competitive athlete inevitably becomes an occasion for local if not national publicity. On each occasion, the public and the medical community ask whether such events could be prevented by more careful or complete screening. Although each event is tragic, it must be appreciated that there are approximately 5 million competitive athletes at the high school level or above in any given year in the United States. The number of cardiac deaths occurring during athletic participation is unknown, but estimates at the high school level range from one in 300,000 to one in 100,000 participants. Death rates among more mature athletes increase as the prevalence of CAD rises. These numbers highlight the problem of how to screen individual participants. Even an inexpensive test such as an ECG would generate an enormous cost if required of all athletes, and it is likely that few at-risk individuals would be detected. Echocardiography, either as a routine test or as a follow-up examination for abnormal ECGs, would be prohibitively expensive except for the elite professional athlete. Thus, the most feasible approach is that of a careful medical history and cardiac examination performed by personnel aware of the conditions responsible for most sudden deaths in competitive athletes. In a series of 158 athletic deaths in the United States between 1985 and 1995, hypertrophic cardiomyopathy (36%) and coronary anomalies (19%) were by far the most frequent underlying conditions. LV hypertrophy was present in another 10%, ruptured aorta (presumably due to Marfan syndrome or cystic medial necrosis) in 6%, myocarditis or dilated cardiomyopathy in 6%, aortic stenosis in 4%, and arrhythmogenic RV dysplasia in 3%. In addition, commotio cordis, or sudden death due to direct myocardial injury, may occur. More common in children, ventricular tachycardia or ventricular fibrillation may occur even after a minor direct blow to the heart; it is thought to be due to the precipitation of a PVC just prior to the peak of the T wave on ECG.

It is likely that a careful family and medical history and cardiovascular examination will identify some individuals at risk. A family history of premature sudden death or cardiovascular disease or of any of these predisposing conditions should mandate further workup, including an ECG and echocardiogram. Symptoms of unexplained fatigue or dyspnea, exertional chest pain, syncope, or near-syncope also warrant further evaluation. A Marfan-like appearance, significant elevation of BP or abnormalities of heart rate or rhythm, and pathologic heart murmurs or heart sounds should also be investigated before clearance for athletic participation is given. Such an evaluation is recommended before participation at the high school and college levels and every 2 years during athletic competition.

Stress-induced syncope or chest pressure may be the first clue to an anomalous origin of a coronary artery. Anatomically, this lesion occurs most often when the left

Table 10–19. Recommendations for competitive sports participation among athletes with potential causes of SCD.

Condition	36th Bethesda Conference	European Society of Cardiology
Structural cardiac abnormilities		
HCM	Exclude athletes with a probable or definitive clinical diagnosis from all competitive sports. Genotype-positive/phenotype-negative athletes may still compete.	Exclude athletes with a probable or definitive clinical diagnosis from all competitive sports. Exclude genotype-positive/phenotype-negative individuals from competitive sports.
ARVC	Exclude athletes with a probable or definitive diagnosis from competitive sports.	Exclude athletes with a probable or definitive diagnosis from competitive sports.
CCAA	Exclude from competitive sports. Participation in all sports 3 months after successful surgery would be permitted for an athlete with ischemia, ventricular arrhythmia or tachyarrhythmia, or LV dysfunction during maximal exercise testing.	Not applicable.
Electrical cardiac abnormalities		
WPW	Athletes without structural heart disease, without a history of palpitations, or without tachycardia can participate in all competitive sports. In athletes with symptoms, electrophysiological study and ablation are recommended. Return to competitive sports is allowed after corrective ablation, provided that the ECG has normalized.	Athletes without structural heart disease, without a history of palpitations, or without tachycardia can participate in all competitive sports. In athletes with symptoms, electrophysiological study and ablation are recommended. Return to competitive sport is allowed after corrective ablation, provided that the ECG has normalized.
LQTS	Exclude any athlete with a previous cardiac arrest or syncopal episode from competitive sports. Asymptomatic patients restricted to competitive low-intensity sports. Genotype-positive/phenotype-negative athletes may still compete.	Exclude any athlete with a clinical or genotype diagnosis from competitive sports.
BrS	Exclude from all competitive sports except those of low intensity.	Exclude from all competitive sports.
CPVT	Exclude all patients with a clinical diagnosis from competitive sports. Genotype-positive/phenotype-negative patients may still compete in low-intensity sports.	Exclude all patients with a clinical diagnosis from competitive sports. Genotype-positive/phenotype-negative patients are also excluded.
Acquired cardiac abnormalities		
Commotio cordis	Eligibility for returning to competitive sport in survivors is a matter of individual clinical judgment. Survivors must undergo a thorough cardiovascular workup including 12-lead electrocardiography, ambulatory Holter monitoring, and echocardiography	Not applicable.
Mycordidits	Exclude from all competitive sports. Convalescent period of 6 months. Athletes may return to competitive when test results normalize.	Exclude from all competitive sports. Convalescent period of 6 months. Athletes may return to competition when test results normalize.

ARVC, arrhythmogenic right ventricular cardiomyopathy; BrS, Brugada syndrome: CCAA, congenital coronary artery anomalies; CPVT, cathecholaminergic polymorphic ventricular tachycardia; ECG, electrocardiogram; HCM, hypertrophic cardiomyopathy; LQTS, long QT syndrome; LV, left ventricular: WPW, Wolff-Parkinson-White syndrome.
Reproduced, with permission, from Chandra N et al. Sudden Cardiac Death in Young Athletes: Practical Challenges and Diagnostic Dilemmas. J Am Coll Cardiol. 2013;61:1027-40.

anterior descending artery or left main coronary arises from the right coronary cusp and traverses between the aorta and pulmonary trunks. The "slit-like" orifice that results from the angulation at the vessel origin is thought to cause ischemia when the aorta and pulmonary arteries enlarge during rigorous exercise.

The toughest distinction may be in sorting out the healthy athlete with LVH from the athlete with hypertrophic cardiomyopathy. In general, the healthy athlete's heart is *less* likely to have an unusual pattern of LVH, or to have LA enlargement, an abnormal ECG, an LV cavity < 45 mm in diameter at end-diastole, an abnormal diastolic filling pattern, or a family history of hypertrophic cardiomyopathy. In addition, the athlete is more likely to be male than the individual with hypertrophic cardiomyopathy. Increased risk is also evident in patients with the Wolff-Parkinson-White syndrome, a prolonged QTc interval, or the Brugada syndrome on their ECG.

Selective use of routine ECG and stress testing is recommended in men above age 40 years and women above age 50 years who continue to participate in vigorous exercise and at earlier ages when there is a positive family history for premature CAD, hypertrophic cardiomyopathy, or multiple risk factors. Because at least some of the risk features (long QT, LVH, Brugada syndrome, Wolff-Parkinson-White syndrome) may be evident on routine ECG screening, several cost-effectiveness studies have been done. Most suggest that pre-participation ECGs are of potential value, though what to do when the QTc is mildly increased is unclear. Many experts feel the high incidence of false-positive ECG studies make it very ineffective as a screening tool. With the low prevalence of cardiac anomalies in the general public, it has been estimated that 200,000 individual athletes would need to be screened to identify the single individual who would die suddenly. The issue of routine screening, therefore, remains controversial.

Once a high-risk individual has been identified, guidelines from the Bethesda conference and the ESC have been provided to help determine whether the athlete may continue to participate in sporting events. Table 10–19 summarizes these recommendations.

Chandra N et al. Sudden cardiac death in young athletes: practical challenges and diagnostic dilemmas. J Am Coll Cardiol. 2013 Mar 12;61(10):1027–40. [PMID: 23473408]

Higgins JP et al. Sudden cardiac death in young athletes: preparticipation screening for underlying cardiovascular abnormalities and approaches to prevention. Phys Sportsmed. 2013 Feb;41(1):81–93. [PMID: 23445863]

Paterick TE et al. March Madness 2011: for whom the bell tolls? Am J Med. 2012 Mar;125(3):231–5. [PMID: 22340916]

Schoenbaum M et al. Economic evaluation of strategies to reduce sudden cardiac death in young athletes. Pediatrics. 2012 Aug;130(2):e380–9. [PMID: 22753553]

Systemic Hypertension

Michael Sutters, MD, MRCP (UK)

An estimated 77.9 million Americans have elevated blood pressure (systolic blood pressure ≥140 mm Hg or diastolic blood pressure ≥ 90 mm Hg); of these, 78% are aware of their diagnosis, but only 68% are receiving treatment and only 64% of those treated are under control (using the threshold criterion of 140/90 mm Hg). By convention, hypertension is categorized based on office measurements as stage 1 (140–159/90–99 mm Hg) and stage 2 (> 160/100 mm Hg). Cardiovascular morbidity and mortality increase as both systolic and diastolic blood pressures rise, but in individuals over age 50 years, the systolic pressure and pulse pressure are better predictors of complications than diastolic pressure. The prevalence of hypertension increases with age, and it is more common in blacks than in whites. The mortality rates for stroke and coronary heart disease, two of the major complications of hypertension, have declined by 50–60% over the past three decades but have recently leveled off. The number of patients with end-stage kidney disease and heart failure—two other conditions in which hypertension plays a major causative role—continues to rise.

HOW IS BLOOD PRESSURE MEASURED & HYPERTENSION DIAGNOSED?

Blood pressure should be measured with a well-calibrated sphygmomanometer. The bladder width within the cuff should encircle at least 80% of the arm circumference. Readings should be taken after the patient has been resting comfortably, back supported in the sitting or supine position, for at least 5 minutes and at least 30 minutes after smoking or coffee ingestion. A video demonstrating the correct technique can be found at http://www.abdn.ac.uk/medical/bhs/tutorial/tutorial.htm. Office-based devices that permit multiple automated measurements after a pre-programmed rest period produce blood pressure readings that are independent of the white coat effect and digit preference. Blood pressure measurements taken outside the office environment, either by intermittent self monitoring (home blood pressure) or with an automated device programmed to take measurements at regular intervals (ambulatory blood pressure) are more powerful predictors of outcomes and are increasingly advocated in clinical

guidelines. Home measurements are also helpful in differentiating "white coat" hypertension (where blood pressure is elevated in the clinic but normal at home) from hypertension that is resistant to treatment and in diagnosis of "masked hypertension" (where blood pressure is normal in the clinic but elevated at home). The cardiovascular risk associated with masked hypertension is similar to that observed in sustained hypertension.

A single elevated blood pressure reading is not sufficient to establish the diagnosis of hypertension. The major exceptions to this rule are hypertensive presentations with unequivocal evidence of life-threatening end-organ damage, as seen in hypertensive emergency, or in hypertensive urgency where blood pressure is > 220/125 mm Hg but life-threatening end-organ damage is absent. In less severe cases, the diagnosis of hypertension depends on a series of measurements of blood pressure, since readings can vary and tend to regress toward the mean with time. Patients whose initial blood pressure is in the hypertensive range exhibit the greatest fall toward the normal range between the first and second encounters. However, the concern for diagnostic precision needs to be balanced by an appreciation of the importance of establishing the diagnosis of hypertension as quickly as possible, since a 3-month delay in treatment of hypertension in high-risk patients is associated with a twofold increase in cardiovascular morbidity and mortality. The Canadian Hypertension Education Program provides an algorithm designed to expedite the diagnosis of hypertension (Figure 11–1). To this end, these guidelines recommend short intervals between initial office visits and stress the importance of early identification of target organ damage or diabetes mellitus, which, if present, justifies pharmacologic intervention if blood pressure remains above 140/90 mm Hg after just two visits. The Canadian guidelines suggest the use of ambulatory and home blood pressure measurements as complements to office-based evaluations. Guidelines from the United Kingdom go further in suggesting that ambulatory or home BP measurements should be used in preference to office-based measurements in the diagnosis of hypertension. When measured by automated office devices, manual home cuffs, or daytime ambulatory equipment,

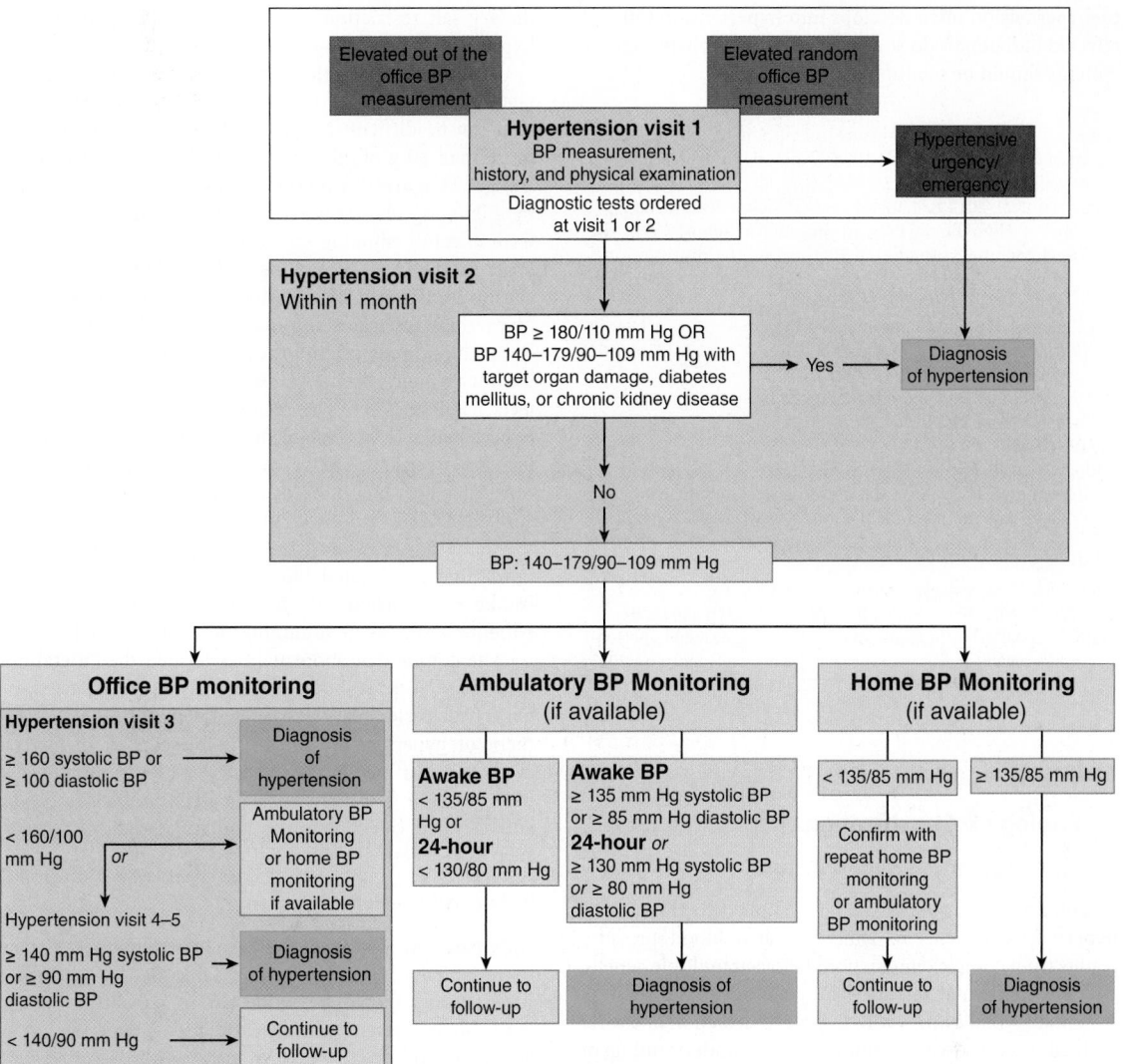

△ Figure 11–1. The Canadian Hypertension Education Program expedited assessment and diagnosis of patients with hypertension: Focus on validated technologies for blood pressure (BP) assessment. (Reprinted, with permission, from the Canadian Hypertension Education Program. The 2012 Canadian Hypertension Education Program recommendations for the management of hypertension: blood pressure management, diagnosis, assessment of risk, and therapy. http://www.hypertension.ca)

stage 1 hypertension is diagnosed at an average blood pressure > 135/85 mm Hg; for 24-hour ambulatory measurement, the diagnostic threshold for stage 1 hypertension is still lower at 130/80 mm Hg.

Ambulatory blood pressure readings are normally lowest at night and the loss of this nocturnal dip is a dominant predictor of cardiovascular risk, particularly risk of thrombotic stroke. An accentuation of the normal morning increase in blood pressure is associated with increased likelihood of cerebral hemorrhage. Furthermore, variability of systolic blood pressure predicts cardiovascular events independently of mean systolic blood pressure. It is becoming increasingly clear that in diagnosing and monitoring hypertension, there should be a move away from isolated office

readings and toward a more integrated view based on repeated measurements in a more "real world" environment. The diagnosis of hypertension does not automatically entail drug treatment; this decision depends on the clinical setting, as discussed below.

PREHYPERTENSION

Data from the Framingham cohort indicate that blood pressure bears a linear relationship with cardiovascular risk down to a systolic blood pressure of 115 mm Hg; based on these data, it has been suggested that individuals with blood pressures in the gray area of 120–139/80–89 mm Hg be categorized as having "prehypertension." Because prehypertension often develops into hypertension (50% of affected individuals do so within 4 years), prehypertensive patients should be monitored annually.

Drawz PE et al. Blood pressure measurement: clinic, home, ambulatory, and beyond. Am J Kidney Dis. 2012 Sep;60(3): 449–62. [PMID: 22521624]

James PA et al. 2014 Evidence-Based Guideline for the Management of High Blood Pressure in Adults: Report From the Panel Members Appointed to the Eighth Joint National Committee (JNC 8). JAMA. 2013 Dec18. 2014 Feb 5;311(5):507–20. [PMID: 24352797]

McCormack T et al. Management of hypertension in adults in primary care: NICE guideline. Br J Gen Pract. 2012 Mar;62 (596):163–4. [PMID: 22429432]

Pimenta E et al. Prehypertension: epidemiology, consequences and treatment. Nat Rev Nephrol. 2010 Jan;6(1):21–30. [PMID: 19918256]

Sidney S et al; National Forum for Heart Disease and Stroke Prevention. The "heart disease and stroke statistics—2013 update" and the need for a national cardiovascular surveillance system. Circulation. 2013 Jan 1;127(1):21–3. [PMID: 23239838]

Stern HR. The new hypertension guidelines. J Clin Hypertens (Greenwich). 2013 Oct;15(10):748–51. [PMID: 24088284]

Yano Y et al. Recognition and management of masked hypertension: a review and novel approach. J Am Soc Hypertens. 2013 May–Jun;7(3):244–52. [PMID: 23523411]

APPROACH TO HYPERTENSION

▶ Etiology & Classification

A. Primary Essential Hypertension

Essential hypertension is the term applied to the 95% of hypertensive patients in which elevated blood pressure results from complex interactions between multiple genetic and environmental factors. The proportion regarded as "essential" will diminish with improved detection of clearly defined secondary causes and with better understanding of pathophysiology. Essential hypertension occurs in 10–15% of white adults and 20–30% of black adults in the United States. The onset is usually between ages 25 and 50 years; it is uncommon before age 20 years. The best understood endogenous and environmental determinants of blood pressure include overactivation of the sympathetic nervous and renin-angiotensin-aldosterone systems, blunting of the pressure-natriuresis relationship, variation in cardiovascular and renal development, and elevated intracellular sodium and calcium levels.

Exacerbating factors include obesity, sleep apnea, increased salt intake, excessive alcohol use, cigarette smoking, polycythemia, nonsteroidal anti-inflammatory (NSAID) therapy, and low potassium intake. **Obesity** is associated with an increase in intravascular volume, elevated cardiac output, activation of the renin-angiotensin system and, probably, increased sympathetic outflow. Weight reduction lowers blood pressure modestly. In patients with **sleep apnea,** treatment with continuous positive airway pressure (CPAP) has been associated with improvements in blood pressure. **Increased salt intake** probably elevates blood pressure in some individuals so

dietary salt restriction is recommended in patients with hypertension (see below).

Excessive use of **alcohol** also raises blood pressure, perhaps by increasing plasma catecholamines. Hypertension can be difficult to control in patients who consume more than 40 g of ethanol (two drinks) daily or drink in "binges." **Cigarette smoking** raises blood pressure, again by increasing plasma norepinephrine. Although the long-term effect of smoking on blood pressure is less clear, the synergistic effects of smoking and high blood pressure on cardiovascular risk are well documented. The relationship of **exercise** to hypertension is variable. Aerobic exercise lowers blood pressure in previously sedentary individuals, but increasingly strenuous exercise in already active subjects has less effect. The relationship between stress and hypertension is not established. **Polycythemia,** whether primary, drug-induced, or due to diminished plasma volume, increases blood viscosity and may raise blood pressure. **NSAIDs** produce increases in blood pressure averaging 5 mm Hg and are best avoided in patients with borderline or elevated blood pressures. Low **potassium intake** is associated with higher blood pressure in some patients; an intake of 90 mmol/d is recommended.

The complex of abnormalities termed the **"metabolic syndrome"** (upper body obesity, insulin resistance, and hypertriglyceridemia) is associated with both the development of hypertension and an increased risk of adverse cardiovascular outcomes. Affected patients usually also have low high-density lipoprotein (HDL) cholesterol levels and elevated catecholamines and inflammatory markers such as C-reactive protein.

B. Secondary Hypertension

Approximately 5% of patients have hypertension secondary to identifiable specific causes (Table 11–1). Secondary hypertension should be suspected in patients in whom hypertension develops at an early age or after the age of 50 years, and in those previously well controlled who become refractory to treatment. Hypertension resistant to three medications is another clue although multiple medications are usually required to control hypertension in persons with diabetes. Secondary causes include genetic syndromes, kidney disease, renal vascular hypertension, primary hyperaldosteronism, Cushing syndrome, pheochromocytoma,

Table 11–1. Identifiable causes of hypertension.

Sleep apnea
Drug-induced or drug-related
Chronic kidney disease
Primary aldosteronism
Renovascular disease
Long-term corticosteroid therapy and Cushing syndrome
Pheochromocytoma
Coarctation of the aorta
Thyroid or parathyroid disease

Data from Chobanian AV et al. The Seventh Report of the Joint National Committee on Prevention, Detection, Evaluation, and Treatment of High Blood Pressure: the JNC 7 report. JAMA. 2003 May 21;289(19):2560–72.

coarctation of the aorta, and hypertension associated with pregnancy, estrogen use, hypercalcemia and medications.

1. Genetic causes—Hypertension can be caused by mutations in single genes, inherited on a Mendelian basis. Although rare, these conditions provide important insight into blood pressure regulation and possibly the genetic basis of essential hypertension. **Glucocorticoid remediable aldosteronism** is an autosomal dominant cause of early-onset hypertension with normal or high aldosterone and low renin levels. It is caused by the formation of a chimeric gene encoding both the enzyme responsible for the synthesis of aldosterone (transcriptionally regulated by angiotensin II) and an enzyme responsible for synthesis of cortisol (transcriptionally regulated by ACTH). As a consequence, aldosterone synthesis becomes driven by ACTH, which can be suppressed by exogenous cortisol. In the **syndrome of apparent mineralocorticoid excess,** early-onset hypertension with hypokalemic metabolic alkalosis is inherited on an autosomal recessive basis. Although plasma renin is low and plasma aldosterone level is very low in these patients, aldosterone antagonists are effective in controlling hypertension. This disease is caused by loss of the enzyme, 11beta-hydroxysteroid dehydrogenase, which normally metabolizes cortisol and thus protects the otherwise "promiscuous" mineralocorticoid receptor in the distal nephron from inappropriate glucocorticoid activation. Similarly, glycyrrhetinic acid, found in licorice, causes increased blood pressure through inhibition of 11beta-hydroxysteroid dehydrogenase. The syndrome of **hypertension exacerbated in pregnancy** is inherited as an autosomal dominant trait. In these patients, a mutation in the mineralocorticoid receptor makes it abnormally responsive to progesterone and, paradoxically, to spironolactone. **Liddle syndrome** is an autosomal dominant condition characterized by early-onset hypertension, hypokalemic alkalosis, low renin, and low aldosterone levels. This is caused by a mutation that results in constitutive activation of the epithelial sodium channel of the distal nephron, with resultant unregulated sodium reabsorption and volume expansion.

2. Renal disease—Renal parenchymal disease is the most common cause of secondary hypertension and is related to increased intravascular volume or increased activity of the renin–angiotensin–aldosterone system.

3. Renal vascular hypertension—Renal artery stenosis is present in 1–2% of hypertensive patients. Its cause in most younger individuals is fibromuscular dysplasia, particularly in women under 50 years of age. The remainder is due to atherosclerotic stenoses of the renal arteries. The mechanisms of hypertension relate to excessive renin release due to reduction in renal perfusion pressure and attenuation of pressure natriuresis with stenosis affecting a single kidney or with bilateral renal artery stenosis. Activation of the renal sympathetic nerves may also be important.

Renal vascular hypertension should be suspected in the following circumstances: (1) if the documented onset is before age 20 or after age 50 years, (2) hypertension is resistant to three or more drugs, (3) if there are epigastric or renal artery bruits, (4) if there is atherosclerotic disease of the aorta or peripheral arteries (15–25% of patients with symptomatic lower limb atherosclerotic vascular disease have renal artery stenosis), (5) if there is an abrupt increase (> 25%) in the level of serum creatinine after administration of angiotensin-converting enzyme (ACE) inhibitors, or (6) if episodes of pulmonary edema are associated with abrupt surges in blood pressure. There is no ideal screening test for renal vascular hypertension. If suspicion is sufficiently high and endovascular intervention is a viable option, renal arteriography, the definitive diagnostic test, is the best approach. Renal arteriography is not recommended as a routine adjunct to coronary studies. Where suspicion is moderate to low, noninvasive angiography using magnetic resonance (MR) or CT are reasonable approaches. With improvements in technology and operator expertise, Doppler sonography may play an increasing role in detection of renal artery stenosis, providing physiologic indices of stenosis severity and ease of repeated examination to detect progression. Gadolinium, a contrast agent used in MR angiography, is contraindicated in patients with an estimated glomerular filtration rate (GFR) of < 30 mL/min because it might precipitate nephrogenic systemic fibrosis in patients with advanced kidney disease. In young patients with fibromuscular disease, angioplasty is very effective, but there is controversy regarding the best approach to the treatment of atheromatous renal artery stenosis. Correction of the stenosis in selected patients might reduce the number of medications required to control blood pressure and could protect kidney function, but the extent of preexisting parenchymal damage to the affected and contralateral kidney has a significant influence on both blood pressure and kidney function outcomes following revascularization. The real challenge is identifying those patients likely to benefit from intervention: in this regard, a hyperemic (papaverine-induced) systolic gradient > 21 mm Hg appears to predict a good response to renal artery angioplasty or stenting. A reasonable approach advocates medical therapy as long as hypertension can be well controlled and there is no progression of kidney disease. The addition of a statin should be considered. Endovascular intervention might be considered in patients with uncontrollable hypertension, progressive kidney disease, or episodic pulmonary edema attributable to the lesion. Angioplasty might also be warranted when progression of stenosis is either demonstrated or is predicted by a constellation of risk factors, including systolic blood pressure > 160 mm Hg, advanced age, diabetes mellitus or high-grade stenosis (> 60%) at the time of diagnosis. However, multiple studies have failed to identify an overall advantage of stenting over medical management in patients with atherosclerotic renal artery stenosis. The CORAL study utilized a distal capture device to prevent embolization into the kidney, but the conclusion was once again that stenting is not superior to medical therapy (incorporating a statin) in the management of atherosclerotic renal artery stenosis. Although drugs modulating the renin-angiotensin system have improved the success rate of medical therapy of hypertension due to renal artery stenosis, they may trigger hypotension and (usually reversible) kidney dysfunction in individuals with bilateral disease. Thus, kidney function and blood pressure should be closely monitored during the first weeks of therapy in patients in whom this is a consideration.

4. Primary hyperaldosteronism—Hyperaldosteronism is suggested when the plasma aldosterone concentration is elevated (normal: 1–16 ng/dL) in association with suppression of plasma renin activity (normal: 1–2.5 ng/mL/h). However, the plasma aldosterone/renin ratio (normal < 30) is not highly specific as a screening test. This is because "bottoming out" of renin assays leads to exponential increases in the plasma aldosterone/renin ratio even when aldosterone levels are normal. Hence, an elevated plasma aldosterone/renin ratio should probably not be taken as evidence of hyperaldosteronism unless the aldosterone level is actually supranormal. The lesion responsible for hyperaldosteronism is an adrenal adenoma or bilateral adrenal hyperplasia. At least some aldosterone-secreting adenomas arise as a consequence of somatic mutations in a potassium channel gene in glomerulosa cells. Screening is appropriate in patients with resistant hypertension, (needing more than three drugs for control) and those with spontaneous or thiazide-induced hypokalemia, incidentaloma, or family history of primary hyperaldosteronism.

During the workup for hyperaldosteronism, medications that alter renin and aldosterone levels, including ACE inhibitors, angiotensin receptor blockers (ARBs), diuretics, beta-blockers, and clonidine, should be discontinued for 2 weeks before sampling; spironolactone and eplerenone should be held for 4 weeks. Calcium channel and alpha-receptor blockers can be used to control blood pressure during this drug washout period. Patients with a plasma aldosterone level > 16 ng/dL and an aldosterone/renin ratio of ≥ 30 might require further evaluation for primary hyperaldosteronism.

5. Cushing syndrome—Hypertension occurs in about 80% of patients with spontaneous Cushing syndrome. Excess glucocorticoid may act through salt and water retention (via mineralocorticoid effects), increased angiotensinogen levels, or permissive effects in the regulation of vascular tone.

Diagnosis and treatment of Cushing syndrome are discussed in Chapter 26.

6. Pheochromocytoma—Pheochromocytomas are uncommon; they are probably found in < 0.1% of all patients with hypertension and in approximately two individuals per million population. However, autopsy studies indicate that pheochromocytomas are very often undiagnosed in life. The blood pressure elevation caused by the catecholamine excess results mainly from alpha-receptor–mediated vasoconstriction of arterioles, with a contribution from beta-1-receptor-mediated increases in cardiac output and renin release. Chronic vasoconstriction of the arterial and venous beds leads to a reduction in plasma volume and predisposes to postural hypotension. Glucose intolerance develops in some patients. Hypertensive crisis in pheochromocytoma may be precipitated by a variety of drugs, including tricyclic antidepressants, antidopaminergic agents, metoclopramide, and naloxone. The diagnosis and treatment of pheochromocytoma are discussed in Chapter 26.

7. Coarctation of the aorta—This uncommon cause of hypertension is discussed in Chapter 10. Evidence of radial-femoral delay should be sought in all younger patients with hypertension.

8. Hypertension associated with pregnancy—Hypertension occurring de novo or worsening during pregnancy, including preeclampsia and eclampsia, is one of the most common causes of maternal and fetal morbidity and mortality (see Chapter 19). Autoantibodies with the potential to activate the angiotensin II type 1 receptor have been causally implicated in preeclampsia, in resistant hypertension, and in progressive systemic sclerosis.

9. Estrogen use—A small increase in blood pressure occurs in most women taking oral contraceptives. However, a more significant increase above 140/90 mm Hg is noted in about 5% of women, mostly in obese individuals older than age 35 who have been treated for more than 5 years. This is caused by increased hepatic synthesis of angiotensinogen. Postmenopausal estrogen does not generally cause hypertension but rather maintains endothelium-mediated vasodilation.

10. Other causes of secondary hypertension—Hypertension has also been associated with hypercalcemia, acromegaly, hyperthyroidism, hypothyroidism, baroreceptor denervation, compression of the rostral ventrolateral medulla, and increased intracranial pressure. A number of medications may cause or exacerbate hypertension—most importantly cyclosporine, tacrolimus, angiogenesis inhibitors, and erythrocyte-stimulating agents (such as erythropoietin, decongestants, and NSAIDs); cocaine and alcohol should also be considered.

▶ When to Refer

Referral to a hypertension specialist should be considered in cases of severe, resistant or early-/late-onset hypertension or when secondary hypertension is suggested by screening.

Chrysant SG. The current status of angioplasty of atherosclerotic renal artery stenosis for the treatment of hypertension. J Clin Hypertens (Greenwich). 2013 Sep;15(9):694–8. [PMID: 24034664]

Cooper CJ et al; the CORAL Investigators. Stenting and medical therapy for atherosclerotic renal-artery stenosis. N Engl J Med. 2013 Nov18. 2014 Jan 2;370(1):13–22. [PMID: 24245566]

Manger WM. The protean manifestations of pheochromocytoma. Horm Metab Res. 2009 Sep;41(9):658–63. [PMID: 19242899]

Messerli FH et al. Essential hypertension. Lancet. 2007 Aug 18;370(9587):591–603. [PMID: 17707755]

Xia Y et al. Angiotensin receptor agonistic autoantibodies and hypertension: preeclampsia and beyond. Circ Res. 2013 Jun 21;113(1):78–87. [PMID: 23788505]

▶ Complications of Untreated Hypertension

Elevated blood pressure results in structural and functional changes in the vasculature and heart. Most of the adverse outcomes in hypertension are associated with thrombosis rather than bleeding, possibly because increased vascular shear stress converts the normally anticoagulant endothelium to a prothrombotic state. The excess morbidity and mortality related to hypertension approximately doubles for each 6 mm Hg increase in diastolic blood pressure. However, target-organ damage varies markedly between individuals with similar levels of office hypertension; home and ambulatory pressures are superior to office readings in the prediction of end-organ damage and variability in blood pressure from visit to visit predicts cardiovascular endpoints independently of mean office-based systolic blood pressure.

A. Hypertensive Cardiovascular Disease

Cardiac complications are the major causes of morbidity and mortality in primary (essential) hypertension. For any level of blood pressure, left ventricular hypertrophy is associated with incremental cardiovascular risk in association with heart failure (through systolic or diastolic dysfunction), ventricular arrhythmias, myocardial ischemia, and sudden death.

The occurrence of heart failure is reduced by 50% with antihypertensive therapy. Hypertensive left ventricular hypertrophy regresses with therapy and is most closely related to the degree of systolic blood pressure reduction. Diuretics have produced equal or greater reductions of left ventricular mass when compared with other drug classes. Conventional beta-blockers are less effective in reducing left ventricular hypertrophy but play a specific role in patients with established coronary artery disease or impaired left ventricular function.

B. Hypertensive Cerebrovascular Disease and Dementia

Hypertension is the major predisposing cause of hemorrhagic and ischemic stroke. Cerebrovascular complications are more closely correlated with systolic than diastolic blood pressure. The incidence of these complications is markedly reduced by antihypertensive therapy. Preceding hypertension is associated with a higher incidence of subsequent dementia of both vascular and Alzheimer types. Home and ambulatory blood pressure may be a better predictor of cognitive decline than office readings in older people. Effective blood pressure control may reduce the risk of development of cognitive dysfunction later in life, but once cerebral small vessel disease is established, low blood pressure might exacerbate this problem.

C. Hypertensive Kidney Disease

Chronic hypertension leads to nephrosclerosis, a common cause of kidney disease that is particularly prevalent in blacks, in whom susceptibility is linked to *APOL1* mutations. These mutations became prevalent in people of African descent because they also conferred resistance to trypanosomal infection. Aggressive blood pressure control, to 130/80 mm Hg or lower, slows the progression of all forms of chronic kidney disease, especially when proteinuria is present.

D. Aortic Dissection

Hypertension is a contributing factor in many patients with dissection of the aorta. Its diagnosis and treatment are discussed in Chapter 12.

E. Atherosclerotic Complications

Most Americans with hypertension die of complications of atherosclerosis, but antihypertensive therapy seems to have a lesser impact on atherosclerotic complications compared with the other effects of treatment outlined above. Prevention of cardiovascular outcomes related to atherosclerosis probably requires control of multiple risk factors, of which hypertension is only one.

Duron E et al. Antihypertensive treatments, cognitive decline, and dementia. J Alzheimers Dis. 2010;20(3):903–14. [PMID: 20182022]

White WB et al. Average daily blood pressure, not office blood pressure, is associated with progression of cerebrovascular disease and cognitive decline in older people. Circulation. 2011 Nov 22;124(21):2312–9. [PMID: 22105196]

▶ Clinical Findings

The clinical and laboratory findings are mainly referable to involvement of the target organs: heart, brain, kidneys, eyes, and peripheral arteries.

A. Symptoms

Mild to moderate primary (essential) hypertension is largely asymptomatic for many years. The most frequent symptom, headache, is also very nonspecific. Accelerated hypertension is associated with somnolence, confusion, visual disturbances, and nausea and vomiting (hypertensive encephalopathy).

Hypertension in patients with **pheochromocytomas** that secrete predominantly norepinephrine is usually sustained but may be episodic. The typical attack lasts from minutes to hours and is associated with headache, anxiety, palpitation, profuse perspiration, pallor, tremor, and nausea and vomiting. Blood pressure is markedly elevated, and angina or acute pulmonary edema may occur. In **primary aldosteronism,** patients may have muscular weakness, polyuria, and nocturia due to hypokalemia; malignant hypertension is rare. **Chronic hypertension** often leads to left ventricular hypertrophy and diastolic dysfunction, which can present with exertional and paroxysmal nocturnal dyspnea. Cerebral involvement causes stroke due to thrombosis or hemorrhage from microaneurysms of small penetrating intracranial arteries. **Hypertensive encephalopathy** is probably caused by acute capillary congestion and exudation with cerebral edema, which is reversible.

B. Signs

Like symptoms, physical findings depend on the cause of hypertension, its duration and severity, and the degree of effect on target organs.

1. Blood pressure—Blood pressure is taken in both arms and, if lower extremity pulses are diminished or delayed, in the legs to exclude coarctation of the aorta. An orthostatic drop of at least 20/10 mm Hg is often present in pheochromocytoma. Older patients may have falsely elevated readings by sphygmomanometry because of noncompressible vessels.

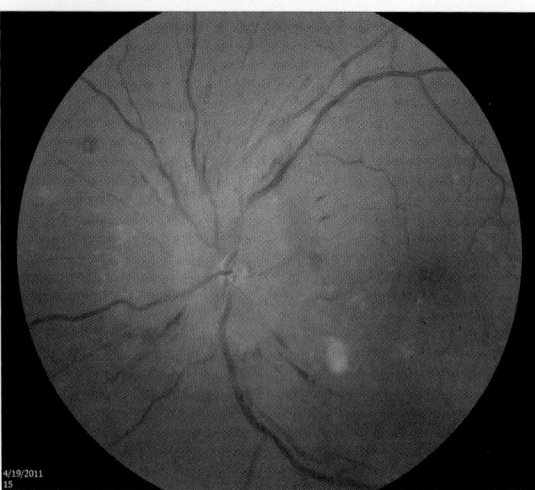

4/19/2011
15

▲ **Figure 11–2.** This image shows severe acute hypertensive retinopathy with hypertensive retinopathy, intraretinal hemorrhages, nerve fiber layer infarcts (cotton-wool spots) and arteriovenous nicking. Retinal arteries show irregular thinning. (Used, with permission, from Dr. Richard S. Munsen, Department of Ophthalmology, University of Washington School of Medicine.)

This may be suspected in the presence of Osler sign—a palpable brachial or radial artery when the cuff is inflated above systolic pressure. Occasionally, it may be necessary to make direct measurements of intra-arterial pressure, especially in patients with apparent severe hypertension who do not tolerate therapy.

2. Retinas—Narrowing of arterial diameter to < 50% of venous diameter, copper or silver wire appearance, exudates, hemorrhages, or hypertensive retinopathy are associated with a worse prognosis. The typical changes of hypertensive retinopathy are shown in Figure 11–2.

3. Heart—A left ventricular heave indicates severe or long-standing hypertrophy. Aortic insufficiency may be auscultated in up to 5% of patients, and hemodynamically insignificant aortic insufficiency can be detected by Doppler echocardiography in 10–20%. A presystolic (S_4) gallop due to decreased compliance of the left ventricle is quite common in patients in sinus rhythm .

4. Pulses—Radial-femoral delay suggests coarctation of the aorta; loss of peripheral pulses occurs due to atherosclerosis, less commonly aortic dissection, and rarely Takayasu arteritis, all of which can involve the renal arteries.

C. Laboratory Findings

Recommended testing includes the following: hemoglobin; urinalysis and serum creatinine; fasting blood sugar level (hypertension is a risk factor for the development of diabetes, and hyperglycemia can be a presenting feature of pheochromocytoma); plasma lipids (necessary to calculate cardiovascular risk and as a modifiable risk factor); serum uric acid (hyperuricemia is a relative contraindication to diuretic therapy); and serum electrolytes.

D. Electrocardiography and Chest Radiographs

Electrocardiographic criteria are highly specific but not very sensitive for left ventricular hypertrophy . The "strain" pattern of ST–T wave changes is a sign of more advanced disease and is associated with a poor prognosis. A chest radiograph is not necessary in the workup for uncomplicated hypertension.

E. Echocardiography

The primary role of echocardiography should be to evaluate patients with clinical symptoms or signs of cardiac disease.

F. Diagnostic Studies

Additional diagnostic studies are indicated only if the clinical presentation or routine tests suggest secondary or complicated hypertension. These may include 24-hour urine free cortisol, urine or plasma metanephrines and plasma aldosterone and renin concentrations to screen for endocrine causes of hypertension. Renal ultrasound will detect structural changes (such as polycystic kidneys, asymmetry and hydronephrosis) as well as echogenicity and reduced cortical volume, which are reliable indicators of advanced chronic kidney disease. Evaluation for renal artery stenosis should be undertaken in concert with subspecialist consultation.

G. Summary

Since most hypertension is essential or primary, few studies are necessary beyond those listed above. If conventional therapy is unsuccessful or if secondary hypertension is suspected, further studies and perhaps referral to a hypertension specialist are indicated.

DellaCroce JT. Hypertension and the eye. Curr Opin Ophthalmol. 2008 Nov;19(6):493–8. [PMID: 18854694]

▶ Nonpharmacologic Therapy

Lifestyle modification may have an impact on morbidity and mortality. A diet rich in fruits, vegetables, and low-fat dairy foods and low in saturated and total fats (DASH diet) has been shown to lower blood pressure. Additional measures, listed in Table 11–2, can prevent or mitigate hypertension or its cardiovascular consequences.

All patients with high-normal or elevated blood pressures, those who have a family history of cardiovascular complications of hypertension, and those who have multiple coronary risk factors should be counseled about nonpharmacologic approaches to lowering blood pressure. Approaches of proved but modest value include weight reduction, reduced alcohol consumption and, in some patients, reduced salt intake. Gradually increasing activity levels should be encouraged in previously sedentary patients, but strenuous exercise training programs in already active individuals may have less benefit. Alternative approaches that may be modestly effective include relaxation techniques and biofeedback. Calcium and potassium supplements have been advocated, but their ability to lower

Table 11–2. Lifestyle modifications to manage hypertension.[1]

Modification	Recommendation	Approximate Systolic BP Reduction, Range
Weight reduction	Maintain normal body weight (BMI, 18.5–24.9)	5–20 mm Hg/10 kg weight loss
Adopt DASH eating plan	Consume a diet rich in fruits, vegetables, and low-fat dairy products with a reduced content of saturated fat and total fat	8–14 mm Hg
Dietary sodium reduction	Reduce dietary sodium intake to no more than 100 mEq/d (2.4 g sodium or 6 g sodium chloride)	2–8 mm Hg
Physical activity	Engage in regular aerobic physical activity such as brisk walking (at least 30 minutes per day, most days of the week)	4–9 mm Hg
Moderation of alcohol consumption	Limit consumption to no more than two drinks per day (1 oz or 30 mL ethanol [eg, 24 oz beer, 10 oz wine, or 3 oz 80-proof whiskey]) in most men and no more than one drink per day in women and lighter-weight persons	2–4 mm Hg

[1]For overall cardiovascular risk reduction, stop smoking. The effects of implementing these modifications are dose- and time-dependent and could be higher for some individuals.
BMI, body mass index calculated as weight in kilograms divided by the square of height in meters; BP, blood pressure; DASH, Dietary Approaches to Stop Hypertension.
Data from Chobanian AV et al. The Seventh Report of the Joint National Committee on Prevention, Detection, Evaluation, and Treatment of High Blood Pressure: the JNC 7 report. JAMA. 2003 May 21;289(19):2560–72.

blood pressure is limited. Smoking cessation will reduce cardiovascular risk. Overall, the effects of lifestyle modification on blood pressure are modest.

Aburto NJ et al. Effect of lower sodium intake on health: systematic review and meta-analyses. BMJ. 2013 Apr 3;346:f1326. [PMID: 23558163]
Blumenthal JA et al. Effects of the DASH diet alone and in combination with exercise and weight loss on blood pressure and cardiovascular biomarkers in men and women with high blood pressure: the ENCORE study. Arch Intern Med. 2010 Jan 25;170(2):126–35. [PMID: 20101007]
Brook RD et al; American Heart Association Professional Education Committee of the Council for High Blood Pressure Research, Council on Cardiovascular and Stroke Nursing, Council on Epidemiology and Prevention, and Council on Nutrition, Physical Activity. Beyond medications and diet: alternative approaches to lowering blood pressure: a scientific statement from the American Heart Association. Hypertension. 2013 Jun;61(6):1360–83. [PMID: 23608661]
Sacks FM et al. Dietary therapy in hypertension. N Engl J Med. 2010 Jun 3;362(22):2102–12. [PMID: 20519681]

▶ Who Should Be Treated with Medications?

Treatment should ideally be offered to all persons in whom blood pressure reduction, irrespective of initial blood pressure levels, will appreciably reduce overall cardiovascular risk with an acceptably low rate of medication-associated adverse effects. Outcomes data indicate that patients with office-based blood pressure measurements that consistently exceed 160/100 mm Hg (stage 2 hypertension) will benefit from antihypertensive therapy irrespective of cardiovascular risk. Several international guidelines suggest that treatment thresholds evaluated by home-based measurements should be lower, perhaps 150/95 mm Hg using

home blood pressure or daytime ambulatory measurements. However, prospective outcomes data for treatment based on measurements taken outside the clinic are lacking. As outlined in Figure 11–3, treatment should be offered at lower thresholds in those with elevated cardiovascular risk or in the presence of existing end-organ damage. The corollary of this is that treatment thresholds might reasonably be set higher for young people with extremely low cardiovascular risk; the Canadian guidelines suggest a threshold of > 160/100 mm Hg.

Since evaluation of total cardiovascular risk (Table 11–3) is important in deciding who to treat with antihypertensive medications, risk calculators are becoming essential clinical tools. A reliable and regularly updated calculator is available at Qrisk.org. Free smart phone (eg, iPhone) applications are also available to estimate coronary heart disease risk. In general, a 20% total cardiovascular risk (which includes stroke) is equivalent to a 15% coronary heart disease risk.

▶ Goals of Treatment

Most experts believe that blood pressure targets for hypertensive patients at the greatest risk for cardiovascular events, particularly patients with diabetes, should be lower (< 130/80 mm Hg) than for individuals at lower total cardiovascular risk (< 140/90 mm Hg). Observational studies suggest that there does not seem to be a blood pressure level below which decrements in risk taper off. However, this may not be true with respect to pharmacologically modulated blood pressure. In fact, over-enthusiastic treatment may have adverse consequences in certain settings. There is an association between lower blood pressure and cognitive decline in elderly patients subjected to intensification of antihypertensive treatment later in life. Excessive lowering of diastolic pressure, perhaps below 70 mm Hg,

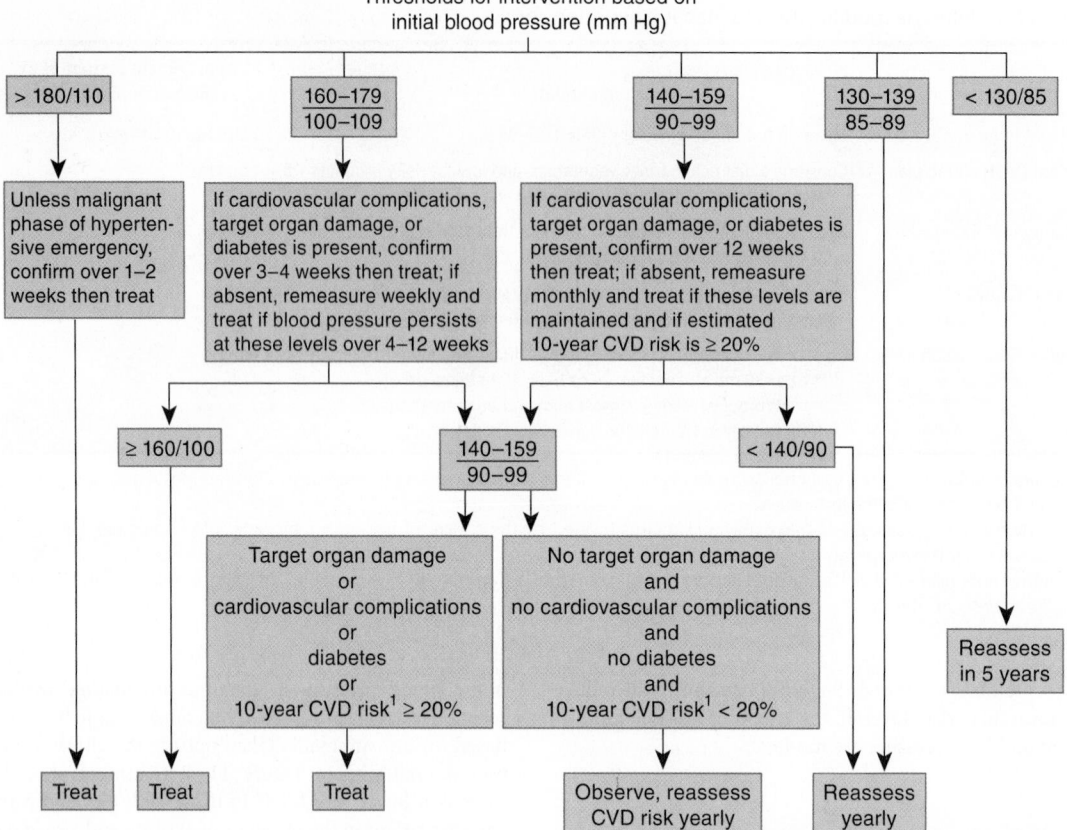

Thresholds for intervention based on initial blood pressure (mm Hg)

- **> 180/110** → Unless malignant phase of hypertensive emergency, confirm over 1–2 weeks then treat → **Treat**

- **160–179 / 100–109** → If cardiovascular complications, target organ damage, or diabetes is present, confirm over 3–4 weeks then treat; if absent, remeasure weekly and treat if blood pressure persists at these levels over 4–12 weeks

- **140–159 / 90–99** → If cardiovascular complications, target organ damage, or diabetes is present, confirm over 12 weeks then treat; if absent, remeasure monthly and treat if these levels are maintained and if estimated 10-year CVD risk is ≥ 20%

- **130–139 / 85–89**

- **< 130/85**

≥ 160/100 → **Treat**

140–159 / 90–99

< 140/90

Target organ damage or cardiovascular complications or diabetes or 10-year CVD risk[1] ≥ 20% → **Treat**

No target organ damage and no cardiovascular complications and no diabetes and 10-year CVD risk[1] < 20% → **Observe, reassess CVD risk yearly**

Reassess yearly

Reassess in 5 years

[1]Assessed with CVD risk chart.

▲ **Figure 11–3.** British Hypertension Society algorithm for diagnosis and treatment of hypertension, incorporating total cardiovascular risk in deciding which "prehypertensive" patients to treat. (CVD, cardiovascular disease.) CVD risk chart available at qrisk.org. (Reproduced, with permission, from Guidelines for management of hypertension: report of the Fourth Working Party of the British Hypertension Society, 2004-BHS IV. J Hum Hypertens. 2004 Mar;18(3):139–85.)

should be avoided in patients with coronary artery disease. In diabetic patients, treatment of systolic pressures to below 130–135 mm Hg significantly increases the risk of serious adverse effects with no additional gain in terms of cardiac, renal, or retinal disease. On the other hand, reducing systolic pressure below 130 mm Hg does seem to further lower the risk of stroke, so lower targets might be justified in patients at high risk for cerebrovascular events.

The SPS3 trial in patients recovering from a lacunar stroke indicated that treating the systolic blood pressure to < 130 mm Hg (mean systolic blood pressure of 127 mm Hg among treated vs mean systolic blood pressure 138 mm Hg among untreated patients) probably reduced the risk of recurrent stroke (and with an acceptably low rate of adverse effects from treatment).

Large-scale trials in hypertension have focused on discrete end points occurring over relatively short intervals, thereby placing the emphasis on the prevention of catastrophic events in advanced disease. There is an ongoing shift in emphasis in viewing hypertension in the context of overall cardiovascular risk. Accordingly, treatment of persons with hypertension should focus on comprehensive

risk reduction with more careful consideration of the possible long-term adverse effects of antihypertensive medications, which include the metabolic derangements linked to conventional beta-blockers and thiazide diuretics and possible modest elevations in the risk of malignancy associated with several antihypertensive drugs.

Statins should be more widely used. In this respect, there is evidence from the Anglo-Scandinavian Cardiac Outcomes Trial (ASCOT) that statins can significantly improve outcomes in persons with hypertension (with modest background cardiovascular risk) whose total cholesterol is < 250 mg/dL (6.5 mmol/L). Notably, the effect of statins appeared to be synergistic with calcium channel blocker/ACE inhibitor regimens but not beta-blocker/diuretic regimens. The British Hypertension Society guidelines recommend that statins be offered as secondary prevention to patients whose total cholesterol exceeds 135 mg/dL (3.5 mmol/L) if they have documented coronary artery disease or a history of ischemic stroke. In addition, statins should be considered as primary prevention in patients with long-standing type 2 diabetes or in those with type 2 diabetes who are older than age 50 years, and perhaps in all

Table 11–3. Cardiovascular risk factors.

Major risk factors
Hypertension[1]
Cigarette smoking
Obesity (BMI ≥ 30)[1]
Physical inactivity
Dyslipidemia[1]
Diabetes mellitus[1]
Microalbuminuria or estimated GFR < 60 mL/min
Age (> 55 years for men, > 65 years for women)
Family history of premature cardiovascular disease (men < 55 years or women < 65 years)
Target-organ damage
Heart
Left ventricular hypertrophy
Angina or prior myocardial infarction
Prior coronary revascularization
Heart failure
Brain
Stroke or transient ischemic attack
Chronic kidney disease
Peripheral arterial disease
Retinopathy

[1]Components of the metabolic syndrome.
BMI indicates body mass index calculated as weight in kilograms divided by the square of height in meters; GFR, glomerular filtration rate.
Data from Chobanian AV et al. The Seventh Report of the Joint National Committee on Prevention, Detection, Evaluation, and Treatment of High Blood Pressure: the JNC 7 report. JAMA. 2003 May 21; 289(19):2560–72.

persons with type 2 diabetes. Ideally, total and low-density lipoprotein (LDL) cholesterol should be reduced by 30% and 40% respectively, or to approximately < 155 mg/dL (4 mmol/L) and < 77 mg/dL (2 mmol/L), whichever is the greatest reduction. However, total and LDL cholesterol levels of < 194 mg/dL (5 mmol/L) and < 116 mg/dL (3 mmol/L) respectively, or reductions of 25% and 30% are regarded as clinically acceptable objectives. Low-dose aspirin (81 mg/d) is likely to be beneficial in patients older than age 50 with either target organ damage or elevated total cardiovascular risk (> 20–30%). Care should be taken to ensure that blood pressure is controlled to the recommended levels before starting aspirin to minimize the risk of intracranial hemorrhage.

Bangalore S et al. Blood pressure targets in subjects with type 2 diabetes mellitus/impaired fasting glucose:observations from traditional and bayesian random-effects meta-analyses of randomized trials. Circulation. 2011 Jun 21;123(24):2776–8. [PMID: 21632497]

McInnes G. Pre-hypertension: how low to go and do drugs have a role? Br J Clin Pharmacol. 2012 Feb;73(2):187–93. [PMID: 21883385]

Sever PS et al; ASCOT Investigators. Prevention of coronary and stroke events with atorvastatin in hypertensive patients who have average or lower-than-average cholesterol concentrations, in the Anglo-Scandinavian Cardiac Outcomes Trial—Lipid Lowering Arm (ASCOT-LLA): a multicentre randomised controlled trial. Lancet. 2003 Apr 5;361(9364):1149–58. [PMID: 12686036]

Sever P et al; ASCOT Steering Committee Members. Potential synergy between lipid-lowering and blood-pressure-lowering in the Anglo-Scandinavian Cardiac Outcomes Trial. Eur Heart J. 2006 Dec;27(24):2982–8. [PMID: 17145722]

SPS3 Study Group; Benavente OR et al. Blood-pressure targets in patients with recent lacunar stroke: the SPS3 randomised trial. Lancet. 2013 Aug 10;382(9891):507–15.Erratum in: Lancet. 2013 Aug 10;382(9891):506. [PMID: 23726159]

Turnbull F et al; Blood Pressure Lowering Treatment Trialists' Collaboration. Effects of different blood pressure-lowering regimens on major cardiovascular events in individuals with and without diabetes mellitus: results of prospectively designed overviews of randomized trials. Arch Intern Med. 2005 Jun 27;165(12):1410–9. [PMID: 15983291]

DRUG THERAPY: CURRENT ANTIHYPERTENSIVE AGENTS

There are now many classes of antihypertensive drugs of which six (diuretics, beta-blockers, renin inhibitors, ACE inhibitors, calcium channel blockers, and ARBs) are suitable for initial therapy based on efficacy and tolerability (Table 11–4). A number of considerations enter into the selection of the initial regimen for a given patient. These include the weight of evidence for beneficial effects on clinical outcomes, the safety and tolerability of the drug, its cost, demographic differences in response, concomitant medical conditions, and lifestyle issues. The specific classes of antihypertensive medications are discussed below, and guidelines for the choice of initial medications are offered.

A. Diuretics

Thiazide diuretics (Table 11–5) are the antihypertensives that have been most extensively studied and most consistently effective in clinical trials. They lower blood pressure initially by decreasing plasma volume, but during long-term therapy, their major hemodynamic effect is reduction of peripheral vascular resistance. Most of the antihypertensive effect of these agents is achieved at lower dosages than used previously (typically, 12.5 mg of hydrochlorothiazide or equivalent), but their biochemical and metabolic effects are dose related. Chlorthalidone has the advantage of better 24-hour blood pressure control than hydrochlorothiazide. The loop diuretics (such as furosemide) may lead to electrolyte and volume depletion more readily than the thiazides and have short durations of action. Because of these adverse effects, loop diuretics should be reserved for use in patients with kidney dysfunction (serum creatinine > 2.5 mg/dL [208.3 mcmol/L]) in which case they are more effective than thiazides. Relative to beta-blockers and ACE inhibitors, diuretics are more potent in blacks, older individuals, the obese, and other subgroups with increased plasma volume or low plasma renin activity (or both). They are relatively more effective in smokers than in nonsmokers. Long-term thiazide administration also mitigates the loss of bone mineral content in older women at risk for osteoporosis.

Overall, diuretics administered alone control blood pressure in 50% of patients with mild to moderate hypertension and can be used effectively in combination with all other agents. They are also useful for lowering isolated or predominantly systolic hypertension. The adverse effects of

Table 11–4. Clinical trial and guideline basis for compelling indications for individual drug classes.[1]

High-Risk Conditions with Compelling Indication[2]	Recommended Drugs						Clinical Trial Basis
	Diuretic	Beta-Blockers	ACE Inhibitors	ARB	CCB	Aldosterone Antagonist	
Heart failure	•	•	•	•		•	ACC/AHA Heart Failure Guideline, MERIT-HF, COPERNICUS, CIBIS, SOLVD, AIRE, TRACE, ValHEFT, RALES
Post-myocardial infarction		•	•			•	ACC/AHA Post-MI Guideline, BHAT, SAVE, Capricorn, EPHESUS
High coronary disease risk	•	•	•		•		ALLHAT, HOPE, ANBP2, LIFE, CONVINCE
Diabetes mellitus	•	•	•	•	•		NKF-ADA Guideline, UKPDS, ALLHAT
Chronic kidney disease			•	•			NKF Guideline, Captopril Trial, RENAAL, IDNT, REIN, AASK
Recurrent stroke prevention	•		•				PROGRESS

[1]Compelling indications for antihypertensive drugs are based on benefits from outcome studies or existing clinical guidelines; the compelling indication is managed in parallel with the blood pressure.
[2]Conditions for which clinical trials demonstrate benefit of specific classes of antihypertensive drugs.
AASK, African American Study of Kidney Disease and Hypertension; ACC/AHA, American College of Cardiology/American Heart Association; ACE, angiotensin converting enzyme; AIRE, Acute Infarction Ramipril Efficacy; ALLHAT, Antihypertensive and Lipid-Lowering Treatment to Prevent Heart Attack Trial; ANBP2, Second Australian National Blood Pressure Study; ARB, angiotensin receptor blocker; BHAT, Beta-Blocker Heart Attack Trial; CCB, calcium channel blocker; CIBIS, Cardiac Insufficiency Bisoprolol Study; CONVINCE, Controlled Onset Verapamil Investigation of Cardiovascular End Points; COPERNICUS, Carvedilol Prospective Randomized Cumulative Survival Study; EPHESUS, Eplerenone Post-Acute Myocardial Infarction Heart Failure Efficacy and Survival Study; HOPE, Heart Outcomes Prevention Evaluation Study; IDNT, Irbesartan Diabetic Nephropathy Trial; LIFE, Losartan Intervention For Endpoint Reduction in Hypertension Study; MERIT-HF, Metoprolol CR/XL Randomized Intervention Trial in Congestive Heart Failure; NKF-ADA, National Kidney Foundation–American Diabetes Association; PROGRESS, Perindopril Protection Against Recurrent Stroke Study; RALES, Randomized Aldactone Evaluation Study; REIN, Ramipril Efficacy in Nephropathy Study; RENAAL, Reduction of Endpoints in Non-Insulin-Dependent Diabetes Mellitus with the Angiotensin II Antagonist Losartan Study; SAVE, Survival and Ventricular Enlargement Study; SOLVD, Studies of Left Ventricular Dysfunction; TRACE, Trandolapril Cardiac Evaluation Study; UKPDS, United Kingdom Prospective Diabetes Study; ValHEFT, Valsartan Heart Failure Trial.
Data from Chobanian AV et al. The Seventh Report of the Joint National Committee on Prevention, Detection, Evaluation, and Treatment of High Blood Pressure: the JNC 7 report. JAMA. 2003 May 21;289(19): 2560–72.

diuretics relate primarily to the metabolic changes listed in Table 11–5. Erectile dysfunction, skin rashes, and photosensitivity are less frequent. Hypokalemia has been a concern but is uncommon at the recommended dosages. The risk can be minimized by limiting dietary salt or increasing dietary potassium; potassium replacement is not usually required to maintain serum K$^+$ at > 3.5 mmol/L. Higher serum K levels are prudent in patients at special risk from intracellular potassium depletion, such as those taking digoxin or with a history of ventricular arrhythmias in which case a potassium-sparing agent could be used. Compared with ACE inhibitors and ARBs, diuretic therapy is associated with a slightly higher incidence of mild new-onset diabetes. Diuretics also increase serum uric acid and may precipitate gout. Increases in blood glucose, triglycerides, and LDL cholesterol may occur but are relatively minor during long-term low-dose therapy.

B. Beta-Adrenergic Blocking Agents

These drugs are effective in hypertension because they decrease the heart rate and cardiac output. Even after continued use of beta-blockers, cardiac output remains lower and systemic vascular resistance higher with agents that do not have intrinsic sympathomimetic or alpha-blocking activity. The beta-blockers also decrease renin release and are more efficacious in populations with elevated plasma renin activity, such as younger white patients. They neutralize the reflex tachycardia caused by vasodilators and are especially useful in patients with associated conditions that benefit from the cardioprotective effects of these agents. These include individuals with angina pectoris, previous myocardial infarction, and stable heart failure as well as those with migraine headaches and somatic manifestations of anxiety.

Although all beta-blockers appear to be similar in antihypertensive potency, they differ in a number of pharmacologic properties (these differences are summarized in Table 11–6), including specificity to the cardiac beta-1-receptors (cardioselectivity) and whether they also block the beta-2-receptors in the bronchi and vasculature; at higher dosages, however, all agents are nonselective. The beta-blockers also differ in their pharmacokinetics, lipid solubility—which determines whether they cross the blood–brain

Table 11–5. Antihypertensive drugs: Diuretics. (In descending order of preference.)

Drugs	Proprietary Names	Initial Oral Doses	Dosage Range	Cost per Unit	Cost of 30 Days Treatment[1] (Average Dosage)	Adverse Effects	Comments
Thiazides and related diuretics							
Hydrochloro-thiazide	Esidrix, Microzide	12.5 or 25 mg once daily	12.5–50 mg once daily	$0.08/25 mg	$2.40	$\downarrow$ K$^+$, $\downarrow$ Mg^{2+}, $\uparrow$ Ca^{2+}, $\downarrow$ Na, $\uparrow$ uric acid, $\uparrow$ glucose, $\uparrow$ LDL cholesterol, $\uparrow$ triglycerides; rash, erectile dysfunction.	Low dosages effective in many patients without associated metabolic abnormalities; metolazone more effective with concurrent kidney disease; indapamide does not alter serum lipid levels.
Chlorthalidone	Thalitone	12.5 or 25 mg once daily	12.5–50 mg once daily	$0.55/25 mg	$16.50		
Metolazone	Zaroxolyn	1.25 or 2.5 mg once daily	1.25–5 mg once daily	$1.48/5 mg	$44.40		
Indapamide	Lozol	2.5 mg once daily	2.5–5 mg once daily	$0.83/2.5 mg	$24.90		
Loop diuretics							
Furosemide	Lasix	20 mg twice daily	40–320 mg in 2 or 3 doses	$0.14/40 mg	$8.40	Same as thiazides, but higher risk of excessive diuresis and electrolyte imbalance. Increases calcium excretion.	Furosemide: Short duration of action a disadvantage; should be reserved for patients with kidney disease or fluid retention. Poor antihypertensive.
Ethacrynic acid	Edecrin	50 mg once daily	50–100 mg once or twice daily	$8.29/25 mg	$497.40		
Bumetanide	Bumex	0.25 mg twice daily	0.5–10 mg in 2 or 3 doses	$0.45/1 mg	$27.00		Torsemide: Effective blood pressure medication at low dosage.
Torsemide	Demadex	2.5 mg once daily	5–10 mg once daily	$0.70/10 mg	$21.00		
Aldosterone receptor blockers							
Spironolac-tone	Aldactone	12.5 or 25 mg once daily	12.5–100 mg once daily	$0.46/25 mg	$13.80	Hyperkalemia, metabolic acidosis, gynecomastia.	Can be useful add-on therapy in patients with refractory hypertension.
Amiloride	Midamor	5 mg once daily	5–10 mg once daily	$1.28/5 mg	$38.40		
Eplerenone	Inspra	25 mg once daily	25–100 mg once daily	$4.10/25 mg	$123.00		
Combination products							
Hydrochloro-thiazide and triamterene	Dyazide (25/50 mg); Maxzide (25/37.5 mg; 50/75 mg)	1 tab once daily	1 or 2 tabs once daily	$0.39	$11.70	Same as thiazides plus GI disturbances, hyperkalemia rather than hypokalemia, headache; triamterene can cause kidney stones and kidney dysfunction; spironolactone causes gynecomastia. Hyperkalemia can occur if this combination is used in patients with advanced kidney disease or those taking ACE inhibitors.	Use should be limited to patients with demonstrable need for a potassium-sparing agent.
Hydrochloro-thiazide and amiloride	Moduretic (50/5 mg)	½ tab once daily	1 or 2 tabs once daily	$0.33	$9.90		
Hydrochloro-thiazide and spironol-actone	Aldactazide (25/25 mg; 50/50 mg)	1 tab (25/25 mg) once daily	1 or 2 tabs once daily	$1.28	$38.40		

[1]Average wholesale price (AWP, for AB-rated generic when available) for quantity listed.
Source: *Red Book* Online, 2014, Truven Health Analytics, Inc. AWP may not accurately represent the actual pharmacy cost because wide contractual variations exist among institutions.
ACE, angiotensin-converting enzyme; GI, gastrointestinal; LDL, low-density lipoprotein.

Table 11–6. Antihypertensive drugs: Beta-adrenergic blocking agents.

Drug	Proprietary Name	Initial Oral Dosage	Dosage Range	Cost per Unit	Cost of 30 Days Treatment (Based on Average Dosage)[1]	Special Properties					Comments[5]
						Beta-1 Selectivity[2]	ISA[3]	MSA[4]	Lipid Solubility	Renal vs Hepatic Elimination	
Acebutolol	Sectral	400 mg once daily	200–1200 mg in 1 or 2 doses	$1.34/400 mg	$40.20	+	+	+	+	H > R	Positive ANA; rare LE syndrome; also indicated for arrhythmias. Doses > 800 mg have beta-1 and beta-2 effects.
Atenolol	Tenormin	25 mg once daily	25–100 mg once daily	$0.85/50 mg	$25.50	+	0	0	0	R	Also indicated for angina pectoris and post-MI. Doses > 100 mg have beta-1 and beta-2 effects.
Betaxolol	Kerlone	10 mg once daily	10–40 mg once daily	$0.78/10 mg	$23.40	+	0	0	+	H > R	
Bisoprolol and hydrochlorothiazide	Ziac	2.5 mg/6.25 mg once daily	2.5 mg/6.25 mg–10 mg/6.25 mg once daily	$1.14/2.5/6.25 mg	$34.20	+	0	0	0	R = H	Low-dose combination approved for initial therapy. Bisoprolol also effective for heart failure.
Carvedilol	Coreg	6.25 mg twice daily	12.5–50 mg in 2 doses	$2.13/25 mg	$127.80 (25 mg twice a day)	0	0	0	+++	H > R	Alpha:beta blocking activity 1:9; may cause orthostatic symptoms; effective for heart failure. Nitric oxide potentiating vasodilatory activity.
Labetalol	Normodyne, Trandate	100 mg twice daily	200–2400 mg in 2 doses	$0.73/200 mg	$43.80	0	0/+	0	++	H	Alpha:beta blocking activity 1:3; more orthostatic hypotension, fever, hepatotoxicity.
Metoprolol	Lopressor	50 mg twice daily	50–200 mg twice daily	$0.56/50 mg	$33.60	+	0	+	+++	H	Also indicated for angina pectoris and post-MI. Approved for heart failure. Doses > 100 mg have beta-1 and beta-2 effects.
	Toprol XL (SR preparation)	25 mg once daily	25–400 mg once daily	$1.58/100 mg	$47.40						

Drug	Brand name	Proprietary Dose	Dosage Range	Cost per Unit	Cost[1]	β₁ Selectivity[2]	ISA[3]	MSA[4]	Lipid Solubility	Renal vs Hepatic Elimination	Comments[5]
Metoprolol and hydrochlorothiazide	Lopressor HCT	50 mg/25 mg once daily	50 mg/25 mg–200 mg/50 mg	$1.13/50 mg/25 mg	$33.90	+	0	+	0	+++	H	
Nadolol	Corgard	20 mg once daily	20–320 mg once daily	$3.97/40 mg	$119.10	0	0	0	0	0	R	
Nebivolol	Bystolic	5 mg once daily	40 mg once daily	$3.15/5 mg	$94.50	+	0	0	0	++	H	Nitric oxide potentiating vasodilatory activity.
Penbutolol	Levatol	20 mg once daily	20–80 mg once daily	$4.07/20 mg	$122.10	0	+	0	+	++	R > H	
Pindolol	Visken	5 mg twice daily	10–60 mg in 2 doses	$1.10/5 mg	$66.60	0	++	+	++	+	H > R	In adults, 35% renal clearance.
Propranolol	Inderal	20 mg twice daily	40–640 mg in 2 doses	$0.51/40 mg	$30.60	0	0	++	0	+++	H	Once-daily SR preparation also available. Also indicated for angina pectoris and post-MI.
Timolol	Blocadren	5 mg twice daily	10–60 mg in 2 doses	$0.83/10 mg	$49.80	0	0	0	0	++	H > R	Also indicated for post-MI. 80% hepatic clearance.

[1] Average wholesale price (AWP, for AB-rated generic when available) for quantity listed. Source: Red Book Online 2014, Truven Health Analytics, Inc. AWP may not accurately represent the actual pharmacy cost because wide contractual variations exist among institutions.

[2] Agents with beta-1 selectivity are less likely to precipitate bronchospasm and decreased peripheral blood flow in low doses, but selectivity is only relative.

[3] Agents with ISA cause less resting bradycardia and lipid changes.

[4] MSA generally occurs at concentrations greater than those necessary for beta-adrenergic blockade. The clinical importance of MSA by beta-blockers has not been defined.

[5] Adverse effects of all beta-blockers: bronchospasm, fatigue, sleep disturbance and nightmares, bradycardia and atrioventricular block, worsening of heart failure, cold extremities, gastrointestinal disturbances, erectile dysfunction, ↑ triglycerides, ↓HDL cholesterol, rare blood dyscrasias.

ANA, antinuclear antibody; ISA, intrinsic sympathomimetic activity; LE, lupus erythematosus; MI, myocardial infarction; MSA, membrane-stabilizing activity; SR, sustained release; 0, no effect;+, some effect;++, moderate effect;+++, most effect.

barrier and affect the incidence of central nervous system side effects—and route of metabolism. Unlike the traditional beta-blockers, carvedilol and nebivolol also diminish peripheral vascular resistance through concomitant alpha-blockade and increased nitric oxide release, respectively. The implications of this distinction are discussed below.

The side effects of beta-blockers include inducing or exacerbating bronchospasm in predisposed patients; sinus node dysfunction and atrioventricular (AV) conduction depression (resulting in bradycardia or AV block); nasal congestion; Raynaud phenomenon; and central nervous system symptoms with nightmares, excitement, depression, and confusion. Fatigue, lethargy, and erectile dysfunction may occur. The traditional beta-blockers (but not the vasodilator beta-blockers carvedilol and nebivolol) have an adverse effect on lipids and glucose metabolism. Metoprolol reduces mortality and morbidity in patients with chronic stable heart failure and systolic left ventricular dysfunction (see Chapter 10). Carvedilol and nebivolol, which maintain cardiac output, are also beneficial in patients with systolic left ventricular dysfunction. Beta-blockers are used cautiously in patients with type 1 diabetes, since they can mask the symptoms of hypoglycemia and prolong these episodes by inhibiting gluconeogenesis. These drugs should also be used with caution in patients with advanced peripheral vascular disease associated with rest pain or nonhealing ulcers, but they are generally well tolerated in patients with mild claudication. Nebivolol can be safely used in patients with stage II claudication (claudication at 200 m).

In treatment of pheochromocytoma, beta-blockers should not be administered until alpha-blockade has been established. Otherwise, blockade of vasodilatory beta-2-adrenergic receptors will allow unopposed vasoconstrictor alpha-adrenergic receptor activation with worsening of hypertension. *For the same reason, beta-blockers should not be used to treat hypertension arising from cocaine use.*

In addition to adverse metabolic changes associated with their use, some experts have suggested that the therapeutic shortcomings of traditional beta-blockers are the consequence of the particular hemodynamic profile associated with these drugs. Pressure peaks in the aorta are augmented by reflection of pressure waves from the peripheral circulation. These reflected waves are delayed in patients taking ACE inhibitors and thiazide diuretics, resulting in decreased central systolic and pulse pressures. By contrast, traditional beta-blockers appear to potentiate reflection of pressure waves, possibly because peripheral resistance vessels are a reflection point and peripheral resistance is increased by these drugs. This might explain why the traditional beta-blockers are less effective at controlling systolic and pulse pressure.

Because of the lack of efficacy in primary prevention of myocardial infarction and inferiority compared with other drugs in prevention of stroke and left ventricular hypertrophy, traditional beta-blockers should not be regarded as ideal first-line agents in the treatment of hypertension without specific compelling indications (such as active coronary artery disease). It might be that vasodilating beta-blockers will emerge as alternative first-line antihypertensives,

but this possibility has yet to be rigorously tested in outcomes studies.

Great care should be exercised if the decision is made, in the absence of compelling indications, to remove beta-blockers from the treatment regimen because abrupt withdrawal can precipitate acute coronary events and severe increases in blood pressure.

C. Renin Inhibitors

Since renin cleavage of angiotensinogen is the rate-limiting step in the renin-angiotensin cascade, the most efficient inactivation of this system would be expected with renin inhibition. Conventional ACE inhibitors and ARBs probably offer incomplete blockade, even in combination. Aliskiren, a renin inhibitor, binds the proteolytic site of renin, thereby preventing cleavage of angiotensinogen. As a consequence, levels of angiotensins I and II are reduced and renin concentration is increased. Aliskiren effectively lowers blood pressure, reduces albuminuria, and limits left ventricular hypertrophy but it has yet to be established as a first-line drug based on outcomes data. The combination of aliskiren with ACE inhibitors or ARBs in persons with type 2 diabetes mellitus certainly offers no advantage and might even increase the risk of adverse cardiac or renal consequences.

D. Angiotensin-Converting Enzyme Inhibitors

ACE inhibitors are being increasingly used as the initial medication in mild to moderate hypertension (Table 11–7). Their primary mode of action is inhibition of the renin–angiotensin–aldosterone system, but they also inhibit bradykinin degradation, stimulate the synthesis of vasodilating prostaglandins, and can reduce sympathetic nervous system activity. These latter actions may explain why they exhibit some effect even in patients with low plasma renin activity. ACE inhibitors appear to be more effective in younger white patients. They are relatively less effective in blacks and older persons and in predominantly systolic hypertension. Although as single therapy they achieve adequate antihypertensive control in only about 40–50% of patients, the combination of an ACE inhibitor and a diuretic or calcium channel blocker is potent.

ACE inhibitors are the agents of choice in persons with type 1 diabetes with frank proteinuria or evidence of kidney dysfunction because they delay the progression to end-stage kidney disease. Many authorities have expanded this indication to include persons with type 1 and type 2 diabetics with microalbuminuria who do not meet the usual criteria for antihypertensive therapy. ACE inhibitors may also delay the progression of nondiabetic kidney disease. The Heart Outcomes Prevention Evaluation (HOPE) trial demonstrated that the ACE inhibitor ramipril reduced the number of cardiovascular deaths, nonfatal myocardial infarctions, and nonfatal strokes and also reduced the incidence of new-onset heart failure, kidney dysfunction, and new-onset diabetes in a population of patients at high risk for vascular events. Although this was not specifically a

Table 11–7. Antihypertensive drugs: Renin and ACE inhibitors and angiotensin II receptor blockers.

Drug	Proprietary Name	Initial Oral Dosage	Dosage Range	Cost per Unit	Cost of 30 Days Treatment (Average Dosage)[1]	Adverse Effects	Comments
Renin inhibitors							
Aliskiren	Tekturna	150 mg once daily	150–300 mg once daily	$4.16/150 mg	$124.80	Angioedema, hypotension, hyperkalemia Contraindicated in pregnancy.	Probably metabolized by CYP3A4. Absorption is inhibited by high fat meal.
Aliskiren and HCTZ	Tekturna HCT	150 mg/12.5 mg once daily	150 mg/12.5 mg–300 mg/25 mg once daily	$4.16/150 mg/12.5 mg	$124.80		
ACE inhibitors							
Benazepril	Lotensin	10 mg once daily	5–40 mg in 1 or 2 doses	$1.05/20 mg	$31.50	Cough, hypotension, dizziness, kidney dysfunction, hyperkalemia, angioedema; taste alteration and rash (may be more frequent with captopril); rarely, proteinuria, blood dyscrasia. Contraindicated in pregnancy.	More fosinopril is excreted by the liver in patients with renal dysfunction (dose reduction may or may not be necessary). Captopril and lisinopril are active without metabolism. Captopril, enalapril, lisinopril, and quinapril are approved for heart failure.
Benazepril and HCTZ	Lotensin HCT	5 mg/6.25 mg once daily	5 mg/6.25 mg–20 mg/25 mg	$2.07/any dose	$62.10		
Benazepril and amlodipine	Lotrel	10 mg/2.5 mg once daily	10 mg/2.5 mg–40 mg/10 mg	$3.32/20 mg/10 mg	$99.60		
Captopril	Capoten	25 mg twice daily	50–450 mg in 2 or 3 doses	$1.20/25 mg	$72.00		
Captopril and HCTZ	Capozide	25 mg/15 mg twice daily	25 mg/15 mg–50 mg/25 mg	$0.72/25 mg/15 mg	$43.20		
Enalapril	Vasotec	5 mg once daily	5–40 mg in 1 or 2 doses	$1.68/20 mg	$50.40		
Enalapril and HCTZ	Vaseretic	5 mg/12.5 mg once daily	5 mg/12.5 mg–10 mg/25 mg	$1.19/10 mg/25 mg	$35.70		
Fosinopril	Monopril	10 mg once daily	10–80 mg in 1 or 2 doses	$1.19/20 mg	$35.70		
Fosinopril and HCTZ	Monopril HCT	10 mg/12.5 mg once daily	10 mg/12.5 mg–20 mg/12.5 mg	$1.26/any dose	$37.80		
Lisinopril	Prinivil, Zestril	5–10 mg once daily	5–40 mg once daily	$1.06/20 mg	$31.80		
Lisinopril and HCTZ	Prinzide or Zestoretic	10 mg/12.5 mg once daily	10 mg/12.5 mg–20 mg/12.5 mg	$1.20/20 mg/12.5 mg	$36.00		
Moexipril	Univasc	7.5 mg once daily	7.5–30 mg in 1 or 2 doses	$1.39/7.5 mg	$41.70		
Moexipril and HCTZ	Uniretic	7.5 mg/12.5 mg once daily	7.5 mg/12.5 mg–15 mg/25 mg	$1.34/7.5 mg/12.5 mg	$40.20		
Perindopril	Aceon	4 mg once daily	4–16 mg in 1 or 2 doses	$3.57/8 mg	$107.10		
Quinapril	Accupril	10 mg once daily	10–80 mg in 1 or 2 doses	$1.22/20 mg	$36.60		
Quinapril and HCTZ	Accuretic	10 mg/12.5 mg once daily	10 mg/12.5 mg–20 mg/25 mg	$1.22/20 mg/12.5 mg	$36.60		
Ramipril	Altace	2.5 mg once daily	2.5–20 mg in 1 or 2 doses	$1.89/5 mg	$56.70		

(continued)

Table 11–7. Antihypertensive drugs: Renin and ACE inhibitors and angiotensin II receptor blockers. (continued)

Drug	Proprietary Name	Initial Oral Dosage	Dosage Range	Cost per Unit	Cost of 30 Days Treatment (Average Dosage)[1]	Adverse Effects	Comments
Trandolapril	Mavik	1 mg once daily	1–8 mg once daily	$1.24/4 mg	$37.20		
Trandolapril and verapamil	Tarka	2 mg/180 mg ER once daily	2 mg/180 mg ER–8 mg/480 mg ER	$3.12/any dose	$93.60		
Angiotensin II receptor blockers							
Candesartan cilexitil	Atacand	16 mg once daily	8–32 mg once daily	$3.31/16 mg	$99.30	Hyperkalemia, kidney dysfunction, rare angioedema. Combinations have additional side effects. Contraindicated in pregnancy.	Losartan has a very flat dose-response curve. Valsartan and irbesartan have wider dose-response ranges and longer durations of action. Addition of low-dose diuretic (separately or as combination pills) increases the response.
Candesartan cilexitil/ HCTZ	Atacand HCT	16 mg/12.5 mg once daily	32 mg/12.5 mg once daily	$4.09/16 mg/12.5 mg	$122.70		
Eprosartan	Teveten	600 mg once daily	400–800 mg in 1–2 doses	$5.06/600 mg	$151.80		
Eprosartan/HCTZ	Teveten HCT	600 mg/12.5 mg once daily	600 mg/12.5 mg–600 mg/25 mg once daily	$5.36/600 mg/12.5 mg	$160.80		
Irbesartan	Avapro	150 mg once daily	150–300 mg once daily	$3.07/150 mg	$92.10		
Irbesartan and HCTZ	Avalide	150 mg/12.5 mg once daily	150–300 mg irbesartan once daily	$3.71/150 mg	$111.30		
Losartan	Cozaar	50 mg once daily	25–100 mg in 1 or 2 doses	$2.42/50 mg	$72.60		
Losartan and HCTZ	Hyzaar	50 mg/12.5 mg once daily	50 mg/12.5 mg–100 mg/25 mg tablets once daily	$2.67/50 mg/12.5 mg/ tablet	$80.10		
Olmesartan	Benicar	20 mg once daily	20–40 mg once daily	$4.27/20 mg	$128.10		
Olmesartan and HCTZ	Benicar HCT	20 mg/12.5 mg once daily	20 mg/12.5 mg–40 mg/25 mg once daily	$4.27/20 mg/12.5 mg	$128.10		
Olmesartan and amlodipine	Azor	20 mg/5 mg once daily	20 mg/5 mg–40 mg/10 mg	$5.83/20 mg/5 mg	$159.90		
Olmesartan and amlodipine and HCTZ	Tribenzor	20 mg/5 mg/12.5 mg once daily	20 mg/5 mg/12.5 mg–40 mg/10 mg/25 mg once daily	$5.33/20 mg/5 mg/ 12.5 mg	$159.90		
Telmisartan	Micardis	40 mg once daily	20–80 mg once daily	$4.63/40 mg	$138.90		
Telmisartan and HCTZ	Micardis HCT	40 mg/12.5 mg once daily	40 mg/12.5 mg–80 mg/25 mg once daily	$5.89/40 mg/12.5 mg	$176.70		

Drug	Proprietary Name	Initial Dose	Dosage Range	Cost per Unit	Cost for 30 Days' Treatment	Adverse Effects	Comments
Telmisartan and amlodipine	Twynsta	40 mg/5 mg once daily	40 mg/5 mg–80 mg/10 mg once daily	$5.71/any dose	$171.30	Hyperkalemia, kidney dysfunction, rare angioedema. Combinations have additional side effects. Contraindicated in pregnancy.	Losartan has a very flat dose-response curve. Valsartan and irbesartan have wider dose-response ranges and longer durations of action. Addition of low-dose diuretic (separately or as combination pills) increases the response.
Valsartan	Diovan	80 mg once daily	80–320 mg once daily	$5.56/160 mg	$166.80		
Valsartan and HCTZ	Diovan HCT	80 mg/12.5 mg once daily	80–320 mg valsartan once daily	$4.27/160 mg/12.5 mg	$128.10		
Valsartan and amlodipine	Exforge	160 mg/5 mg once daily	160 mg/5 mg–320 mg/10 mg once daily	$6.00/160 mg/10 mg	$180.00		
Other combination products							
Aliskiren and valsartan	Valturna	150 mg/160 mg once daily	150 mg/160 mg–300 mg/320 mg once daily	Not available in U.S.	Not available in U.S.	Angioedema, hypotension, hyperkalemia Contraindicated in pregnancy.	
Amlodipine/HCTZ/valsartan	Exforge HCT	5 mg/12.5 mg/160 mg once daily	10 mg/25 mg/320 mg up to once daily	$6.00/160 mg valsartan	$180.00	Angioedema, hypotension, hyperkalemia Contraindicated in pregnancy.	

[1] Average wholesale price (AWP, for AB-rated generic when available) for quantity listed. Source: *Red Book Online, 2014*, Truven Health Analytics, Inc. AWP may not accurately represent the actual pharmacy cost because wide contractual variations exist among institutions.

ACE, angiotensin-converting enzyme; HCTZ, hydrochlorothiazide.

hypertensive population, the benefits were associated with a modest reduction in blood pressure, and the results inferentially support the use of ACE inhibitors in similar hypertensive patients. ACE inhibitors are a drug of choice (usually in conjunction with a diuretic and a beta-blocker) in patients with heart failure and are indicated also in asymptomatic patients with reduced ejection fraction. An advantage of the ACE inhibitors is their relative freedom from troublesome side effects. Severe hypotension can occur in patients with bilateral renal artery stenosis; sudden increases in creatinine may ensue but are usually reversible with discontinuation of ACE inhibition. Hyperkalemia may develop in patients with kidney disease and type IV renal tubular acidosis (commonly seen in diabetics) and in the elderly. A chronic dry cough is common, seen in 10% of patients or more, and may require stopping the drug. Skin rashes are observed with any ACE inhibitor. Angioedema is an uncommon but potentially dangerous side effect of all agents of this class because of their inhibition of kininase. Exposure of the fetus to ACE inhibitors during the second and third trimesters of pregnancy has been associated with a variety of defects due to hypotension and reduced renal blood flow.

E. Angiotensin II Receptor Blockers

ARBs can improve cardiovascular outcomes in patients with hypertension as well as in patients with related conditions such as heart failure and type 2 diabetes with nephropathy. ARBs have not been compared with ACE inhibitors in randomized controlled trials in patients with hypertension, but two trials comparing losartan with captopril in heart failure and post-myocardial infarction left ventricular dysfunction showed trends toward worse outcomes in the losartan group. By contrast, valsartan seems as effective as ACE inhibitors in these settings, suggesting that ARBs may be heterogeneous with respect to effects beyond blood pressure control. The Losartan Intervention for Endpoints (LIFE) trial in nearly 9000 hypertensive patients with electrocardiographic evidence of left ventricular hypertrophy—comparing losartan with the beta-blocker atenolol as initial therapy—demonstrated a significant reduction in stroke with losartan. Of note is that in diabetic patients, death and myocardial infarction were also reduced, and there was a lower occurrence of new-onset diabetes. In this trial, as in the Antihypertensive and Lipid-Lowering Treatment to Prevent Heart Attack Trial (ALLHAT), blacks treated with renin-angiotensin-aldosterone system (RAAS) inhibitors exhibited less blood pressure reduction and less benefit with regard to clinical end points. In the treatment of hypertension, combination therapy with an ACE inhibitor and an ARB is not advised because it generally offers no advantage over monotherapy at maximum dose with addition of a complementary class where necessary.

Unlike ACE inhibitors, the ARBs do not cause cough and are less likely to be associated with skin rashes or angioedema. However, as seen with ACE inhibitors, hyperkalemia can be a problem, and patients with bilateral renal artery stenosis may exhibit hypotension and worsened kidney function. Olmesartan has been linked to a sprue-like syndrome, presenting with abdominal pain, weight loss, and nausea, which subsides upon drug discontinuation.

F. Aldosterone Receptor Antagonists

Spironolactone and eplerenone are natriuretic in sodium-retaining states, such as heart failure and cirrhosis, but only very weakly so in hypertension. These drugs have reemerged in the treatment of hypertension, particularly in resistant patients and are helpful additions to most other antihypertensive medications. Consistent with the increasingly appreciated importance of aldosterone in essential hypertension, the aldosterone receptor blockers are effective at lowering blood pressure in all hypertensive patients regardless of renin level, and are also effective in blacks. Aldosterone plays a central role in target organ damage, including the development of ventricular and vascular hypertrophy and renal fibrosis. Aldosterone receptor antagonists ameliorate these consequences of hypertension, to some extent independently of effects on blood pressure. Spironolactone can cause breast pain and gynecomastia in men through activity at the progesterone receptor, an effect not seen with the more specific eplerenone. Hyperkalemia is a problem with both drugs, chiefly in patients with chronic kidney disease.

G. Calcium Channel Blocking Agents

These agents act by causing peripheral vasodilation but with less reflex tachycardia and fluid retention than other vasodilators. They are effective as single-drug therapy in approximately 60% of patients in all demographic groups and all grades of hypertension (Table 11–8). For these reasons, they may be preferable to beta-blockers and ACE inhibitors in blacks and older persons. Verapamil and diltiazem should be combined cautiously with beta-blockers because of their potential for depressing AV conduction and sinus node automaticity as well as contractility.

Initial concerns about possible adverse cardiac effects of calcium channel blockers have been convincingly allayed by several subsequent large studies that have demonstrated that calcium channel blockers are equivalent to ACE inhibitors and thiazide diuretics in prevention of coronary heart disease, major cardiovascular events, cardiovascular death, and total mortality. A protective effect against stroke with calcium channel blockers is well established, and in two trials (ALLHAT and the Systolic Hypertension in Europe trial), these agents appeared to be more effective than diuretic-based therapy.

The most common side effects of calcium channel blockers are headache, peripheral edema, bradycardia, and constipation (especially with verapamil in the elderly). The dihydropyridine agents—nifedipine, nicardipine, isradipine, felodipine, nisoldipine, and amlodipine—are more likely to produce symptoms of vasodilation, such as headache, flushing, palpitations, and peripheral edema. Edema is minimized by coadministration of an ACE inhibitor or ARB. Calcium channel blockers have negative inotropic effects and should be used cautiously in patients with cardiac dysfunction. Amlodipine is the only calcium channel

Table 11–8. Antihypertensive drugs: Calcium channel blocking agents.

Drug	Proprietary Name	Initial Oral Dosage	Dosage Range	Cost of 30 Days Treatment (Average Dosage)[1]	Special Properties				Adverse Effects	Comments
					Peripheral Vasodilation	Cardiac Automaticity and Conduction	Contractility			
Nondihydropyridine agents										
Diltiazem	Cardizem SR	90 mg twice daily	180–360 mg in 2 doses	$117.60 (120 mg twice daily)	++	↓↓	↓↓		Edema, headache, bradycardia, GI disturbances, dizziness, AV block, heart failure, urinary frequency.	Also approved for angina.
	Cardizem CD; Cartia XT	180 mg once daily	180–360 mg once daily	$42.90 (240 mg once daily)						
	Dilacor XR	180 or 240 mg once daily	180–480 mg once daily							
	Tiazac SA	240 mg once daily	180–540 mg once daily							
	Taztia XT	180 mg once daily	120–540 mg once daily							
Verapamil	Calan SR Covera HS	180 mg once daily 240 mg once daily	180–480 mg in 1 or 2 doses	$49.20 (240 mg once daily)	++	↓↓↓	↓↓↓		Same as diltiazem but more likely to cause constipation and heart failure.	Also approved for angina and arrhythmias.
	Verelan Verelan PM	200 mg ER once daily	100–400 mg ER once daily	$75.60 (200 mg once daily)						
Dihydropyridines										
Amlodipine	Norvasc	2.5 mg once daily	2.5–10 mg once daily	$71.10 (10 mg once daily)	+++	↓/0	↓/0		Edema, dizziness, palpitations, flushing, headache, hypotension, tachycardia, GI disturbances, urinary frequency, worsening of heart failure (may be less common with	Amlodipine, nicardipine, and nifedipine also approved for angina.
Amlodipine and atorvastatin	Caduet	2.5 mg/10 mg once daily	10 mg/80 mg once daily	$281.10 (10 mg/ 40 mg daily)	+++	↓/0	↓/0			

(continued)

Table 11–8. Antihypertensive drugs: Calcium channel blocking agents. (continued)

Drug	Proprietary Name	Initial Oral Dosage	Dosage Range	Cost of 30 Days Treatment (Average Dosage)[1]	Special Properties			Adverse Effects	Comments
					Peripheral Vasodilation	Cardiac Automaticity and Conduction	Contractility		
Felodipine	Plendil	5 mg ER once daily	5–10 mg ER once daily	$81.60 (10 mg ER daily)	+++	↓/0	↓/0	Myopathy, hepatotoxicity, edema with amlodipine and atorvastatin.	
Isradipine	DynaCirc	2.5 mg twice daily	2.5–5 mg twice daily	$102.00 (5 mg twice daily)	+++	↓/0	→		
Nicardipine	Cardene	20 mg three times daily	20–40 mg three times daily	$38.70 (20 mg three times daily)	+++	↓/0	→		
	Cardene SR	30 mg twice daily	30–60 mg twice daily	$119.40 (30 mg twice daily)					
Nifedipine	Adalat CC Procardia XL	30 mg once daily	30–120 mg once daily	$68.70	+++	→	↓↓		
Nisoldipine	Sular	17 mg daily	17–34 mg daily	$251.70 (34 mg once daily)	+++	↓/0	→		

[1]Average wholesale price (AWP, for AB-rated generic when available) for quantity listed.
Source: *Red Book Online, 2014, Truven Health Analytics, Inc.* AWP may not accurately represent the actual pharmacy cost because wide contractual variations exist among institutions.
AV, atrioventricular; GI, gastrointestinal.

blocker with established safety in patients with severe heart failure. According to a case-control study based in the Pacific Northwest of the United States, calcium channel blockers as a class may increase the risk of breast cancer by 2.5-fold, but this relationship has not been consistently observed in other studies. If this relationship is substantiated, and as the long-term adverse effects of other classes of antihypertensive medications are clarified, guidelines may change. However, it would be premature to alter practices at this time.

H. Alpha-Adrenoceptor Antagonists

Prazosin, terazosin, and doxazosin (Table 11–9) block postsynaptic alpha-receptors, relax smooth muscle, and reduce blood pressure by lowering peripheral vascular resistance. These agents are effective as single-drug therapy in some individuals, but tachyphylaxis may appear during long-term therapy and side effects are relatively common. These include marked hypotension after the first dose which, therefore, should be small and given at bedtime. Post-dosing palpitations, headache, and nervousness may continue to occur during long-term therapy; these symptoms may be less frequent or severe with doxazosin because of its more gradual onset of action. Cataractectomy in patients exposed to alpha-blockers can be complicated by the floppy iris syndrome, even after discontinuation of the drug, so the ophthalmologist should be alerted that the patient has been taking the drug prior to surgery.

Unlike beta-blockers and diuretics, alpha-blockers have no adverse effect on serum lipid levels—in fact, they increase HDL cholesterol while reducing total cholesterol. Whether this is beneficial in the long term has not been established. In ALLHAT, persons receiving doxazosin as initial therapy had a significant increase in heart failure hospitalizations and a higher incidence of stroke relative to those receiving diuretics, prompting discontinuation of this arm of the study. To summarize, alpha-blockers should generally not be used as initial agents to treat hypertension—except perhaps in men with symptomatic prostatism or nightmares linked to posttraumatic stress disorder.

I. Drugs with Central Sympatholytic Action

Methyldopa, clonidine, guanabenz, and guanfacine (Table 11–9) lower blood pressure by stimulating alpha-adrenergic receptors in the central nervous system, thus reducing efferent peripheral sympathetic outflow. These agents are effective as single therapy in some patients, but they are usually used as second- or third-line agents because of the high frequency of drug intolerance, including sedation, fatigue, dry mouth, postural hypotension, and erectile dysfunction. An important concern is rebound hypertension following withdrawal. Methyldopa also causes hepatitis and hemolytic anemia and is avoided except in individuals who have already tolerated long-term therapy. There is considerable experience with methyldopa in pregnant women, and it is still used for this population. Clonidine is available in patches, which may have particular value in patients in whom compliance is a troublesome issue.

J. Arteriolar Dilators

Hydralazine and minoxidil (Table 11–9) relax vascular smooth muscle and produce peripheral vasodilation. When given alone, they stimulate reflex tachycardia, increase myocardial contractility, and cause headache, palpitations, and fluid retention. They are usually given in combination with diuretics and beta-blockers in resistant patients. Hydralazine produces frequent gastrointestinal disturbances and may induce a lupus-like syndrome. Minoxidil causes hirsutism and marked fluid retention; this agent is reserved for the most refractory of cases.

K. Peripheral Sympathetic Inhibitors

These agents are now used infrequently and usually in refractory hypertension. Reserpine remains a cost-effective antihypertensive agent (Table 11–9). Its reputation for inducing mental depression and its other side effects—sedation, nasal stuffiness, sleep disturbances, and peptic ulcers—has made it unpopular, though these problems are uncommon at low dosages. Guanethidine and guanadrel inhibit catecholamine release from peripheral neurons but frequently cause orthostatic hypotension (especially in the morning or after exercise), diarrhea, and fluid retention.

▶ Developing an Antihypertensive Regimen

Historically, data from a number of large trials support the overall conclusion that antihypertensive therapy with diuretics and beta-blockers has a major beneficial effect on a broad spectrum of cardiovascular outcomes, reducing the incidence of stroke by 30–50% and of heart failure by 40–50%, and halting progression to accelerated hypertension syndromes. The decreases in fatal and nonfatal coronary heart disease and cardiovascular and total mortality were less dramatic, ranging from 10% to 15%. Similar placebo-controlled data pertaining to the newer agents are generally lacking, except for stroke reduction with the calcium channel blocker nitrendipine in the Systolic Hypertension in Europe trial. However, there is substantial evidence that ACE inhibitors, and to a lesser extent ARBs, reduce adverse cardiovascular outcomes in other related populations (eg, patients with diabetic nephropathy, heart failure, or postmyocardial infarction and individuals at high risk for cardiovascular events). Most large clinical trials that have compared outcomes in relatively unselected patients have failed to show a difference between newer agents—such as ACE inhibitors, calcium channel blockers, and ARBs—and the older diuretic-based regimens with regard to survival, myocardial infarction, and stroke. Where differences have been observed, they have mostly been attributable to subtle asymmetries in blood pressure control rather than to any inherent advantages of one agent over another. Recommendations for initial treatment identify ACE inhibitors, ARBs, and calcium channel blockers as valid choices. Because of their adverse metabolic profile, initial therapy with thiazides might best be restricted to older patients. Thiazides are acceptable as first-line therapy in blacks because of specific efficacy in this group. Exceptions to these recommendations are appropriate for

Table 11–9. Alpha-adrenoceptor blocking agents, sympatholytics, and vasodilators.

Drug	Proprietary Names	Initial Dosage	Dosage Range	Cost per Unit	Cost of 30 Days Treatment (Average Dosage)[1]	Adverse Effects	Comments
Alpha-adrenoceptor blockers							
Doxazosin	Cardura Cardura XL	1 mg at bedtime 4 mg ER	1–16 mg once daily 4–8 mg ER once daily	$0.95/4 mg $3.02/4 mg ER	$28.50 (4 mg once daily) $90.60 (4 mg ER once daily)	Syncope with first dose; postural hypotension, dizziness, palpitations, headache, weakness, drowsiness, sexual dysfunction, anticholinergic effects, urinary incontinence; first-dose effects may be less with doxazosin.	May ↑ HDL and ↓ LDL cholesterol. May provide short-term relief of obstructive prostatic symptoms. Less effective in preventing cardiovascular events than diuretics.
Prazosin	Minipress	1 mg at bedtime	2–20 mg in 2 or 3 doses	$0.91/5 mg	$54.60 (5 mg twice daily)		
Terazosin	Hytrin	1 mg at bedtime	1–20 mg in 1 or 2 doses	$1.60/1, 2, 5, 10 mg	$48.00 (5 mg once daily)		
Central sympatholytics							
Clonidine	Catapres Catapres TTS	0.1 mg twice daily 0.1 mg/d patch weekly	0.2–0.6 mg in 2 doses 0.1–0.3 mg/d patch weekly	$0.22/ 0.1 mg $55.77/ 0.2 mg	$13.20 (0.1 mg twice daily) $223.08 (0.2 mg weekly)	Sedation, dry mouth, sexual dysfunction, headache, bradyarrhythmias; side effects may be less with guanfacine. Contact dermatitis with clonidine patch. Methyldopa also causes hepatitis, hemolytic anemia, fever.	"Rebound" hypertension may occur even after gradual withdrawal. Methyldopa should be avoided in favor of safer agents.
Clonidine and chlorthalidone	Clorpres	0.1 mg/15 mg one to three times daily	0.1 mg/15 mg–0.3 mg/15 mg	$2.48/ 0.1 mg/ 15 mg	$148.80/ 0.1 mg/ 15 mg twice daily		
Guanabenz	Wytensin	4 mg twice daily	8–64 mg in 2 doses	$2.09/8 mg	$125.40 (8 mg twice daily)		
Guanfacine	Tenex	1 mg once daily	1–3 mg once daily	$0.87/1 mg	$26.10 (1 mg once daily)		
Methyldopa	Aldochlor	250 mg twice daily	500–2000 mg in 2 doses	$0.74/ 500 mg	$44.40 (500 mg twice daily)		

Peripheral neuronal antagonists						
Reserpine	Serpasil; Serpalan	0.05 mg once daily		$1.19/0.1 mg	$35.70 (0.1 mg once daily)	Depression (less likely at low dosages, ie, < 0.25 mg), night terrors, nasal stuffiness, drowsiness, peptic disease, gastrointestinal disturbances, bradycardia.	
Direct vasodilators						
Hydralazine	Apresoline	25 mg twice daily	50–300 mg in 2–4 doses	$0.51/25 mg	$30.60 (25 mg twice daily)	GI disturbances, tachycardia, headache, nasal congestion, rash, LE-like syndrome.	May worsen or precipitate angina.
Minoxidil	Loniten	5 mg once daily	10–40 mg once daily	$1.29/10 mg	$38.70 (10 mg once daily)	Tachycardia, fluid retention, headache, hirsutism, pericardial effusion, thrombocytopenia.	Should be used in combination with beta-blocker and diuretic.

¹Average wholesale price (AWP, for AB-rated generic when available) for quantity listed.
Source: Red Book ONLINE, 2014, Truven Health Analytics, Inc. AWP may not accurately represent the actual pharmacy cost because wide contractual variations exist among institutions.
GI, gastrointestinal; LE, lupus erythematosus.

individuals who have specific (or "compelling") indications for another class of agent, as outlined in Table 11–4.

As discussed above, beta-blockers should no longer be considered ideal first-line drugs in the treatment of hypertension without compelling indications for their use. Vasodilator beta-blockers (such as carvedilol and nebivolol) may produce better outcomes than traditional beta-blockers; however, this possibility remains a theoretical consideration.

For the purpose of devising an optimal treatment regimen, drugs can be divided into two complementary groups easily remembered as **A** and **CD**. **A** refers to drugs that interrupt the renin-angiotensin system (ACE/ARB/renin inhibitor) and **C** and **D** refer to those that do not (calcium channel blockers and thiazide diuretics). Combinations of drugs between these groups are likely to be more potent in lowering blood pressure than combinations within a group. Drugs that interrupt the renin-angiotensin cascade are more effective in young, white persons, in whom renin tends to be higher, and drugs **C/D** are more effective in old or black persons, in whom renin levels are generally lower. Figure 11–4 illustrates guidelines for initiating antihypertensive therapy established by the United Kingdom's National Institute of Health and Clinical Excellence (NICE). In trials that include patients with systolic hypertension, most patients require two or more medications and even then a substantial proportion fail to achieve the goal systolic blood pressure of < 140 mm Hg (<130 mm Hg in high-risk persons). In diabetic patients, three or four drugs are usually required to reduce systolic blood pressure to < 140 mm Hg. In many patients, blood pressure cannot be adequately controlled with any combination. As a result, debating the appropriate first-line agent is less relevant than determining the most appropriate combinations of agents. This has led many experts and practitioners to recommend the use of fixed-dose combination antihypertensive agents as first-line therapy in patients with substantially elevated systolic pressures (> 160/100 mm Hg) or difficult-to-control hypertension (which is often associated with diabetes or kidney dysfunction). Based both on antihypertensive efficacy and complementarity, combinations of an ACE inhibitor or ARB plus a calcium channel blocker or diuretic are recommended. In light of side effect profiles, calcium channel blockers might be preferable to thiazides in the younger hypertensive patient. Furthermore, based on the results from the ACCOMPLISH trial, a combination of ACE inhibitor and calcium channel blocker may also prove optimal for patients at high risk for cardiovascular events. The initial use of low-dose combinations allows faster blood pressure reduction without substantially higher intolerance rates and is likely to be better accepted by patients. However, data from the ALTITUDE study (in patients with type 2 diabetes and chronic kidney disease or cardiovascular disease or both), indicate that the addition of aliskiren to either ARB or ACE inhibitor was associated with worse outcomes and cannot be recommended, at least in this population. A suggested approach to treatment, tailored to patient demographics, is outlined in Table 11–10.

In sum, as a prelude to treatment, the patient should be informed of common side effects and the need for diligent

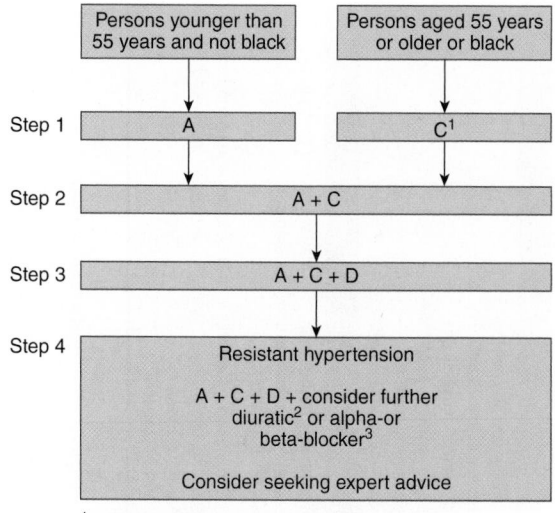

¹A CCB is preferred but consider a thiazide-like diuretic if a CCB is not tolerated or the person has edema, evidence of heart failure or a high risk of heart failure.

²Consider a low dose of spironolactone or higher doses of a thiazide-like diuretic.

³Consider an alpha-or beta-blocker if further diuretic therapy is not tolerated, or is contraindicated or ineffective.

▲ **Figure 11–4.** Hypertension treatment guidelines from the United Kingdom's National Institute for Health and Care Excellence. Guidelines identify angiotensin-converting enzyme (ACE) inhibitors, angiotensin receptor blockers (ARBs), or calcium channel blockers (CCB) as first-line medications and suggest a sequence of escalating drug therapy depending on blood pressure response. As noted, the choice of the initial agent is influenced by patient demographics. In Step 4, higher doses of thiazide-type diuretics may be used as long as serum potassium levels exceed 4.5 mEq/L. Key: A, ACE inhibitor or ARB; C, calcium-channel blocker; D, diuretic, thiazide-like. (Modified, with permission, from the 2013 hypertension guidelines published by the National Institute for Health and Care Excellence. http://www.nice.org.uk/nicemedia/live/13561/65641/65641.pdf)

compliance. In patients with mild or stage 1 hypertension (< 160/90 mm Hg) in whom pharmacotherapy is indicated, treatment should start with a single agent at a low dose. Follow-up visits should usually be at 4- to 6-week intervals to allow for full medication effects to be established (especially with diuretics) before further titration or adjustment. If, after titration to usual doses, the patient has shown a discernible but incomplete response and a good tolerance of the initial drug, a second medication should be added. As a rule of thumb, a blood pressure reduction of 10 mm Hg can be expected for each antihypertensive agent added to the regimen and titrated to the optimum dose. In those with more severe hypertension (stage 2), or with comorbidities (such as diabetes) that are likely to render them resistant to treatment, initiation with combination therapy is advised and more frequent follow-up is indicated.

Table 11–10. Choice of antihypertensive agent based on demographic considerations.[1,2]

	Black, All Ages	All Others, Age < 55 Years	All Others, Age > 55 Years
First-line	CCB or diuretic	ACE or ARB[3] or CCB or diuretic[4]	CCB or diuretic[5]
Second-line	ACE or ARB[3] or vasodilating beta-blocker[6]	Vasodilating beta-blocker[6]	ACE or ARB or vasodilating beta-blocker[6]
Alternatives	Alpha-agonist or alpha-antagonist[7]	Alpha-agonist or alpha-antagonist	Alpha-agonist or alpha-antagonist[7]
Resistant hypertension	Aldosterone receptor blocker	Aldosterone receptor blocker	Aldosterone receptor blocker

[1]Compelling indications may alter the selection of an antihypertensive drug.
[2]Start with full dose of one agent, or lower doses of combination therapy. In stage 2 hypertension, consider initiating therapy with a fixed dose combination.
[3]Women of childbearing age should avoid ACE and ARB or discontinue as soon as pregnancy is diagnosed.
[4]The adverse metabolic effects of thiazide diuretics and beta-blockers should be considered in younger patients but may be less important in the older patient.
[5]For patients with significant renal impairment, use loop diuretic instead of thiazide.
[6]There are theoretical advantages in the use of vasodilating beta-blockers such as carvedilol and nebivolol.
[7]Alpha-antagonists may precipitate or exacerbate orthostatic hypotension in the elderly.
ACE, angiotensin-converting enzyme; ARB, angiotensin II receptor blocker; CCB, calcium channel blocker.

Patients who are compliant with their medications and who do not respond to conventional combination regimens should usually be evaluated for secondary hypertension before proceeding to more complex regimens.

Special Considerations in the Treatment of Diabetic Hypertensive Patients

Hypertensive patients with diabetes are at particularly high risk for cardiovascular events. More aggressive treatment of hypertension in these patients prevents progressive nephropathy, and a meta-analysis supports the notion that lower treatment goals (< 130–135/80 mm Hg) are especially effective at reducing cardiovascular risk in diabetic patients compared with nondiabetic patients. Blood pressures should probably not be dropped below 120/70 mm Hg. Because of the beneficial effects of ACE inhibitors in diabetic nephropathy, they should be part of the initial treatment regimen. ARBs or perhaps renin inhibitors may be substituted in those intolerant of ACE inhibitors. However, most diabetic patients require combinations of three to five agents to achieve target blood pressure, usually including a diuretic and a calcium channel blocker or beta-blocker. In addition to rigorous blood pressure control, treatment of persons with diabetes should include aggressive treatment of other risk factors.

Treatment of Hypertension in Chronic Kidney Disease

Hypertension is present in 40% of patients with a GFR of 60–90 mL/min, and 75% of patients with a GFR < 30 mL/min. ACE inhibitors and ARBs have been shown to delay progression of kidney disease in persons with type 1 and type 2 diabetes, respectively. It is also likely that inhibition of the renin-angiotensin system protects kidney function in nondiabetic kidney disease associated with significant proteinuria. Combinations of ACE inhibitors and ARBs in persons with atherosclerosis or type 2 diabetes with end organ

damage were synergistic with respect to minimizing proteinuria in the ONTARGET study. However, this strategy slightly increased the risk of progression to dialysis and death and is not recommended in this patient population.

As discussed above, the blood pressure target in treating patients with hypertension and nondiabetic chronic kidney disease should generally be < 140/90 mm Hg. The Kidney Disease Improving Global Outcomes (KDIGO) guidelines advocate a lower target of < 130/80 mm Hg in patients with significant proteinuria. Drugs that interrupt the renin-angiotensin cascade are preferred for initial therapy. Transition from thiazide to loop diuretic is often necessary to control volume expansion as kidney function worsens. Evidence has demonstrated that ACE inhibitors remain protective and safe in kidney disease associated with significant proteinuria and serum creatinine as high as 5 mg/dL (380 mcmol/L). Note that such treatment would likely result in acute worsening of kidney function in patients with significant renal artery stenosis, so kidney function and electrolytes should be monitored carefully after introduction of ACE inhibitors. Persistence with ACE inhibitor/ARB therapy in the face of hyperkalemia is probably not warranted, since other antihypertensive medications are renoprotective as long as goal blood pressures are maintained.

Hypertension Management in Blacks

Substantial evidence indicates that blacks are not only more likely to become hypertensive and more susceptible to the cardiovascular and renal complications of hypertension—they also respond differently to many antihypertensive medications. The REGARDS study illustrates these disparities. At systolic blood pressures less than 120 mm Hg, black and white participants between 45 and 64 years of age had equal risk of stroke. For a 10 mm Hg increase in systolic blood pressure, the risk of stroke was threefold higher in black participants. At the level of stage 1 hypertension, the hazard ratio for stroke in black compared to white participants between 45 and 64 years of age was 2.35. This increased susceptibility may reflect genetic differences in the cause of hypertension or the subsequent responses to it, differences in occurrence of comorbid conditions such as diabetes or obesity, or environmental factors such as diet, activity, stress, or access to health care services. In any case, as in all persons with hypertension, a multifaceted program of education and lifestyle modification is warranted. Early introduction of combination therapy has been advocated. Because it appears that ACE inhibitors and ARBs—in the absence of concomitant diuretics—are less effective in blacks than in whites, initial therapy should generally be a diuretic or a diuretic combination with a calcium channel blocker.

Treating Hypertension in the Elderly

Several studies in persons over 60 years of age have confirmed that antihypertensive therapy prevents fatal and nonfatal myocardial infarction and reduces overall cardiovascular mortality. These trials placed the focus on control of systolic blood pressure (the hypertension affecting the majority of those over age 60 is predominantly systolic)—in contrast to the historical emphasis on diastolic blood pressures. Most clinical guidelines suggest that treatment targets for older people (age 60–80 years) should be the same as those for younger individuals (< 140/90 mm Hg), except pressure should be reduced more gradually with a safe intermediate systolic blood pressure goal of 160 mm Hg. In the very elderly, over age 80 years, the HYVET study indicated that a reasonable ultimate systolic blood pressure goal would be 150/80 mm Hg, reflected by the Canadian and European target of < 150/90 mm Hg in this population. The most recent US Joint National Committee Report (JNC8) adopted a rigorous outcomes-based position in recommending a higher treatment goal of < 150/90 mm Hg in persons older than 60 years of age. The same medications are used in older patients, but at 50% lower doses. As treatment is initiated, older patients should be carefully monitored for orthostasis, altered cognition, and electrolyte disturbances. The HYVET trial recruited individuals who were relatively well; by contrast, there appears to be a loss of the usual relationship between blood pressure and morbidity/mortality in the very elderly who are also frail (as defined by a walking speed of less than 0.8 m/sec over 6 m). In the very frail (those unable to walk 6 m), higher blood pressures were paradoxically associated with better outcomes. A less aggressive approach to the treatment of hypertension would therefore seem appropriate in the very elderly who are also frail.

Follow-Up of Patients Receiving Hypertension Therapy

Once blood pressure is controlled on a well-tolerated regimen, follow-up visits can be infrequent and laboratory testing limited to those appropriate for the patient and the medications used. Yearly monitoring of blood lipids is recommended, and an electrocardiogram should be repeated at 2- to 4-year intervals depending on whether initial abnormalities are present, the presence of coronary risk factors, and age. Pharmacy care programs and home blood pressure monitoring have been shown to improve compliance with medications. Patients who have had excellent blood pressure control for several years, especially if they have lost weight and initiated favorable lifestyle modifications, might be considered for a trial of reduced antihypertensive medications.

ALLHAT Officers and Coordinators for the ALLHAT Collaborative Research Group. Major outcomes in high-risk hypertensive patients randomized to angiotensin-converting enzyme inhibitor or calcium channel blocker vs diuretic. The Antihypertensive and Lipid-Lowering Treatment to Prevent Heart Attack Trial (ALLHAT). JAMA. 2002 Dec18;288(23):2981–97. [PMID: 12479763]

Holdiness A et al. Renin angiotensin aldosterone system blockade: little to no rationale for ACE inhibitor and ARB combinations. Am J Med. 2011 Jan;124(1):15–9. [PMID: 21187182]

Howard G et al. Racial differences in the impact of elevated systolic blood pressure on stroke risk. JAMA Intern Med. 2013 Jan 14;173(1):46–51. [PMID: 23229778]

James PA et al. 2014 Evidence-Based Guideline for the Management of High Blood Pressure in Adults: Report From the Panel Members Appointed to the Eighth Joint National Committee (JNC 8). JAMA. 2013 Dec 18. 2014 Feb 5;311(5):507–20. [PMID: 24352797]

Kountz DS. Hypertension in black patients: an update. Postgrad Med. 2013 May;125(3):127–35. [PMID: 23748513]

Lipsitz LA. A 91-year-old woman with difficult-to-control hypertension: a clinical review. JAMA. 2013 Sep 25;310(12):1274–80. [PMID: 24065014]

Parving HH et al; ALTITUDE Investigators. Cardiorenal end points in a trial of aliskiren for type 2 diabetes. N Engl J Med. 2012 Dec 6;367(23):2204–13. [PMID: 23121378]

Wiysonge CS et al. Beta-blockers for hypertension. Cochrane Database Syst Rev. 2012 Nov 14;11:CD002003. [PMID: 23152211]

RESISTANT HYPERTENSION

Resistant hypertension is defined in JNC 7 as the failure to reach blood pressure control in patients who are adherent to full doses of an appropriate three-drug regimen (including a diuretic). Adherence is a major issue: the rate of partial or complete noncompliance probably approaches 50% in this group of patients; doxazosin, spironolactone, and hydrochlorothiazide were particularly unpopular in one study based on drug assay in Eastern Europe. In the approach to resistant hypertension, the clinician should first confirm compliance and rule out "white coat hypertension." Exacerbating factors should be considered (as outlined above). Finally, identifiable causes of hypertension should be sought (Table 11–11). The clinician should pay particular attention to the type of diuretic being used in relation to the patient's kidney function. Aldosterone may play an important role in resistant hypertension and aldosterone receptor blockers can be very useful. If goal blood pressure cannot be achieved following completion of these steps, consultation with a hypertension specialist should be considered. Interruption of autonomic reflexes through radiofrequency ablation of renal sympathetic nerves or stimulation of carotid baroreceptors effectively lowers

Table 11–11. Causes of resistant hypertension.

Improper blood pressure measurement
Volume overload and pseudotolerance
Excess sodium intake
Volume retention from kidney disease
Inadequate diuretic therapy
Drug-induced or other causes
Nonadherence
Inadequate doses
Inappropriate combinations
Nonsteroidal anti-inflammatory drugs; cyclooxygenase-2 inhibitors
Cocaine, amphetamines, other illicit drugs
Sympathomimetics (decongestants, anorectics)
Oral contraceptives
Adrenal steroids
Cyclosporine and tacrolimus
Erythropoietin
Licorice (including some chewing tobacco)
Selected over-the-counter dietary supplements and medicines (eg, ephedra, ma huang, bitter orange)
Associated conditions
Obesity
Excess alcohol intake
Identifiable causes of hypertension (see Table 11–1)

Data from Chobanian AV et al. The Seventh Report of the Joint National Committee on Prevention, Detection, Evaluation, and Treatment of High Blood Pressure: the JNC 7 report. JAMA. 2003 May 21;289(19):2560–72.

blood pressure in resistant patients but these approaches have yet to be formally evaluated in controlled outcomes-based trials. There is at least one early report of renal artery stenosis linked to the former procedure.

Acelajado MC et al. Resistant hypertension, secondary hypertension, and hypertensive crises: diagnostic evaluation and treatment. Cardiol Clin. 2010 Nov;28(4):639–54. [PMID: 20937447]

Böhm M et al. Renal sympathetic denervation: applications in hypertension and beyond. Nat Rev Cardiol. 2013 Aug;10(8):465–76. [PMID: 2377459]

Burnier M et al. Measuring, analyzing, and managing drug adherence in resistant hypertension. Hypertension. 2013 Aug;62(2):218–25. [PMID: 23753412]

Laurent S et al. New drugs, procedures, and devices for hypertension. Lancet. 2012 Aug 11;380(9841):591–600. [PMID: 22883508]

Solini A et al. How can resistant hypertension be identified and prevented? Nat Rev Cardiol. 2013 May;10(5):293–6. [PMID: 23459606]

HYPERTENSIVE URGENCIES & EMERGENCIES

Hypertensive emergencies have become less frequent in recent years but still require prompt recognition and aggressive but careful management. A spectrum of urgent presentations exists, and the appropriate therapeutic approach varies accordingly.

Hypertensive urgencies are situations in which blood pressure must be reduced within a few hours. These include patients with asymptomatic severe hypertension (systolic blood pressure > 220 mm Hg or diastolic pressure > 125 mm Hg that persists after a period of observation) and those with optic disk edema progressive target organ complications, and severe perioperative hypertension. Elevated blood pressure levels alone—in the absence of symptoms or new or progressive target organ damage—rarely require emergency therapy. Parenteral drug therapy is not usually required, and partial reduction of blood pressure with relief of symptoms is the goal.

Hypertensive emergencies require substantial reduction of blood pressure within 1 hour to avoid the risk of serious morbidity or death. Although blood pressure is usually strikingly elevated (diastolic pressure > 130 mm Hg), the correlation between pressure and end-organ damage is often poor. It is the latter that determines the seriousness of the emergency and the approach to treatment. Emergencies include hypertensive encephalopathy (headache, irritability, confusion, and altered mental status due to cerebrovascular spasm), hypertensive nephropathy (hematuria, proteinuria, and progressive kidney dysfunction due to arteriolar necrosis and intimal hyperplasia of the interlobular arteries), intracranial hemorrhage, aortic dissection, preeclampsia-eclampsia, pulmonary edema, unstable angina, or myocardial infarction. **Malignant hypertension** is by historical definition characterized by encephalopathy or nephropathy with accompanying hypertensive retinopathy. Progressive kidney disease usually ensues if treatment is not provided. The therapeutic approach is identical to that used with other antihypertensive emergencies.

Parenteral therapy is indicated in most hypertensive emergencies, especially if encephalopathy is present. The initial goal in hypertensive emergencies is to reduce the pressure by no more than 25% (within minutes to 1 or 2 hours) and then toward a level of 160/100 mm Hg within 2–6 hours. Excessive reductions in pressure may precipitate coronary, cerebral, or renal ischemia. To avoid such declines, the use of agents that have a predictable, dose-dependent, transient, and progressive antihypertensive effect is preferable. In that regard, the use of sublingual or oral fast-acting nifedipine preparations is best avoided.

Acute ischemic stroke is often associated with marked elevation of blood pressure, which will usually fall spontaneously. In such cases, antihypertensives should only be used if the systolic blood pressure exceeds 180–200 mm Hg, and blood pressure should be reduced cautiously by 10–15%. If thrombolytics are to be given, blood pressure should be maintained at < 185/110 mm Hg during treatment and for 24 hours following treatment.

In hemorrhagic stroke, the aim is to minimize bleeding with a target mean arterial pressure of < 130 mm Hg. In acute subarachnoid hemorrhage, as long as the bleeding source remains uncorrected, a compromise must be struck between preventing further bleeding and maintaining cerebral perfusion in the face of cerebral vasospasm. In this situation, blood pressure goals depend on the patient's usual blood pressure. In normotensive patients, the target should be a systolic blood pressure of 110–120 mm Hg; in hypertensive patients, blood pressure should be treated to

20% below baseline pressure. In the treatment of hypertensive emergencies complicated by (or precipitated by) central nervous system injury, labetalol or nicardipine are good choices, since they are nonsedating and do not appear to cause significant increases in cerebral blood flow or intracranial pressure in this setting. In hypertensive emergencies arising from catecholaminergic mechanisms, such as pheochromocytoma or cocaine use, beta-blockers can worsen the hypertension because of unopposed peripheral vasoconstriction; nicardipine, clevidipine, or phentolamine are better choices. Labetalol is useful in these patients if the heart rate must be controlled. Table 11–12 summarizes treatment recommendations in hypertensive emergency.

▶ Pharmacologic Management

A. Parenteral Agents

A growing number of agents are available for management of acute hypertensive problems. (Table 11–13 lists drugs, dosages, and adverse effects.)

Sodium nitroprusside is no longer the treatment of choice; in most situations, appropriate control of blood pressure is best achieved using combinations of nicardipine or clevidipine plus labetalol or esmolol.

1. Nicardipine—Intravenous nicardipine is the most potent and the longest acting of the parenteral calcium channel blockers. As a primarily arterial vasodilator, it has the potential to precipitate reflex tachycardia, and for that reason it should not be used without a beta-blocker in patients with coronary artery disease.

2. Clevidipine—Intravenous clevidipine is an L-type calcium channel blocker with a 1-minute half-life, which facilitates swift and tight control of severe hypertension. It acts on arterial resistance vessels and is devoid of venodilatory or cardiodepressant effects.

3. Labetalol—This combined beta- and alpha-blocking agent is the most potent adrenergic blocker for rapid blood pressure reduction. Other beta-blockers are far less potent. Excessive blood pressure drops are unusual. Experience with this agent in hypertensive syndromes associated with pregnancy has been favorable.

4. Esmolol—This rapidly acting beta-blocker is approved only for treatment of supraventricular tachycardia but is often used for lowering blood pressure. It is less potent than labetalol and should be reserved for patients in whom there is particular concern about serious adverse events related to beta-blockers.

Table 11–12. Treatment of hypertensive emergency depending on primary site of end-organ damage.

Type of Hypertensive Emergency	Recommended Drug Options and Combinations	Drugs to Avoid
Myocardial ischemia and infarction	Nicardipine plus esmolo[1] Nitroglycerin plus labetalol Nitroglycerin plus esmolol[1]	Hydralazine, diazoxide, minoxidil, nitroprusside
Acute kidney injury	Fenoldopam Nicardipine Clevidipine	
Aortic dissection	Esmolol plus nicardipine Esmolol plus clevidipine Labetalol Esmolol plus nitroprusside	Hydralazine, diazoxide, minoxidil
Acute pulmonary edema, LV systolic dysfunction	Nicardipine plus nitroglycerin[2] plus a loop diuretic Clevidipine plus nitroglycerin[2] plus a loop diuretic	Hydralazine, diazoxide, beta-blockers
Acute pulmonary edema, diastolic dysfunction	Esmolol plus low-dose nitroglycerin plus a loop diuretic Labetalol plus low-dose nitroglycerin plus a loop diuretic	
Ischemic stroke (systolic blood pressure > 180–200 mm Hg)	Nicardipine Clevidipine Labetalol	Nitroprusside, methyldopa, clonidine, nitroglycerin
Intracerebral hemorrhage (systolic blood pressure > 140–160 mm Hg)	Nicardipine Clevidipine Labetalol	Nitroprusside, methyldopa, clonidine, nitroglycerin
Hyperadrenergic states, including cocaine use	Nicardipine plus a benzodiazepine Clevidipine plus a benzodiazepine Phentolamine Labetalol	Beta-blockers
Preeclampsia, eclampsia	Labetalol Nicardipine	Diuretics, ACE inhibitors

ACE, angiotensin-converting enzyme; LV, left ventricular.
[1]Avoid if LV systolic dysfunction.
[2]Drug of choice if LV systolic dysfunction is associated with ischemia.

Table 11–13. Drugs for hypertensive emergencies and urgencies in descending order of preference.

Agent	Action	Dosage	Onset	Duration	Adverse Effects	Comments
Hypertensive emergencies						
Nicardipine (Cardene)	Calcium channel blocker	5 mg/h; may increase by 1–2.5 mg/h every 15 minutes to 15 mg/h	1–5 minutes	3–6 hours	Hypotension, tachycardia, headache.	May precipitate myocardial ischemia.
Clevidipine (Cleviprex)	Calcium channel blocker	1–2 mg/h initially, double rate every 90 seconds until near goal, then by smaller amounts every 5–10 minutes to a maximum of 32 mg/h	2–4 minutes	5–15 minutes	Headache, nausea, vomiting	Lipid emulsion: contraindicated in patients with allergy to soy or egg.
Labetalol (Normodyne, Trandate)	Beta- and alpha-blocker	20–40 mg every 10 minutes to 300 mg; 2 mg/min infusion	5–10 minutes	3–6 hours	GI, hypotension, bronchospasm, bradycardia, heart block.	Avoid in acute LV systolic dysfunction, asthma. May be continued orally.
Esmolol (Brevibloc)	Beta-blocker	Loading dose 500 mcg/kg over 1 minute; maintenance, 25–200 mcg/kg/min	1–2 minutes	10–30 minutes	Bradycardia, nausea.	Avoid in acute LV systolic dysfunction, asthma. Weak antihypertensive.
Fenoldopam (Corlopam)	Dopamine receptor agonist	0.1–1.6 mcg/kg/min	4–5 minutes	< 10 minutes	Reflex tachycardia, hypotension, intraocular pressure.	May protect kidney function.
Enalaprilat (Vasotec)	ACE inhibitor	1.25 mg every 6 hours	15 minutes	6 hours or more	Excessive hypotension.	Additive with diuretics; may be continued orally.
Furosemide (Lasix)	Diuretic	10–80 mg	15 minutes	4 hours	Hypokalemia, hypotension.	Adjunct to vasodilator.
Hydralazine (Apresoline)	Vasodilator	5–20 mg intravenously or intramuscularly (less desirable); may repeat after 20 minutes	10–30 minutes	2–6 hours	Tachycardia, headache, GI.	Avoid in coronary artery disease, dissection. Rarely used except in pregnancy.
Nitroglycerin	Vasodilator	0.25–5 mcg/kg/min	2–5 minutes	3–5 minutes	Headache, nausea, hypotension, bradycardia.	Tolerance may develop. Useful primarily with myocardial ischemia.
Nitroprusside (Nitropress)	Vasodilator	0.25–10 mcg/kg/min	Seconds	3–5 minutes	GI, CNS; thiocyanate and cyanide toxicity, especially with renal and hepatic insufficiency; hypotension. Coronary steal, decreased cerebral blood flow, increased intracranial pressure.	No longer the first-line agent.
Hypertensive urgencies						
Clonidine (Catapres)	Central sympatholytic	0.1–0.2 mg initially; then 0.1 mg every hour to 0.8 mg	30–60 minutes	6–8 hours	Sedation.	Rebound may occur.
Captopril (Capoten)	ACE inhibitor	12.5–25 mg	15–30 minutes	4–6 hours	Excessive hypotension.	
Nifedipine (Adalat, Procardia)	Calcium channel blocker	10 mg initially; may be repeated after 30 minutes	15 minutes	2–6 hours	Excessive hypotension, tachycardia, headache, angina, myocardial infarction, stroke.	Response unpredictable.

ACE, angiotensin-converting enzyme; CNS, central nervous system; GI, gastrointestinal; LV, left ventricular.

5. Fenoldopam—Fenoldopam is a peripheral dopamine-1 (DA$_1$) receptor agonist that causes a dose-dependent reduction in arterial pressure without evidence of tolerance, rebound, or withdrawal or deterioration of kidney function. In higher dosage ranges, tachycardia may occur. This drug is natriuretic, which may simplify volume management in acute kidney injury.

6. Enalaprilat—This is the active form of the oral ACE inhibitor enalapril. The onset of action is usually within 15 minutes, but the peak effect may be delayed for up to 6 hours. Thus, enalaprilat is used primarily as an adjunctive agent.

7. Diuretics—Intravenous loop diuretics can be very helpful when the patient has signs of heart failure or fluid retention, but the onset of their hypotensive response is slow, making them an adjunct rather than a primary agent for hypertensive emergencies. Low dosages should be used initially (furosemide, 20 mg, or bumetanide, 0.5 mg). They facilitate the response to vasodilators, which often stimulate fluid retention.

8. Hydralazine—Hydralazine can be given intravenously or intramuscularly, but its effect is less predictable than that of other drugs in this group. It produces reflex tachycardia and should not be given without beta-blockers in patients with possible coronary disease or aortic dissection. Hydralazine is now used primarily in pregnancy and in children, but even in these situations, it is not a first-line drug.

9. Nitroglycerin, intravenous—This agent should be reserved for patients with accompanying acute coronary ischemic syndromes.

10. Nitroprusside sodium—This agent is given by controlled intravenous infusion gradually titrated to the desired effect. It lowers the blood pressure within seconds by direct arteriolar and venous dilation. Monitoring with an intra-arterial line avoids hypotension. Nitroprusside—in combination with a beta-blocker—is useful in patients with aortic dissection.

B. Oral Agents

Patients with less severe acute hypertensive syndromes can often be treated with oral therapy. Suitable drugs will reduce the blood pressure over a period of hours. In those presenting as a consequence of noncompliance, it is usually sufficient to restore the patient's previously established oral regimen.

1. Clonidine—Clonidine, 0.2 mg orally initially, followed by 0.1 mg every hour to a total of 0.8 mg, will usually lower blood pressure over a period of several hours. Sedation is frequent, and rebound hypertension may occur if the drug is stopped.

2. Captopril—Captopril, 12.5–25 mg orally, will also lower blood pressure in 15–30 minutes. The response is variable and may be excessive. Captopril is the drug of choice in the management of scleroderma hypertensive crisis.

3. Nifedipine—The effect of fast-acting nifedipine capsules is unpredictable and may be excessive, resulting in hypotension and reflex tachycardia. Because myocardial infarction and stroke have been reported in this setting, the use of sublingual nifedipine is not advised. Nifedipine retard, 20 mg orally, appears to be safe and effective.

C. Subsequent Therapy

When the blood pressure has been brought under control, combinations of oral antihypertensive agents can be added as parenteral drugs are tapered off over a period of 2–3 days.

Marik PE et al. Hypertensive emergencies: an update. Curr Opin Crit Care. 2011 Dec;17(6):569–80. [PMID: 21986463]
van den Born BJ et al. Dutch guideline for the management of hypertensive crisis—2010 revision. Neth J Med. 2011 May;69(5):248–55. [PMID: 21646675]

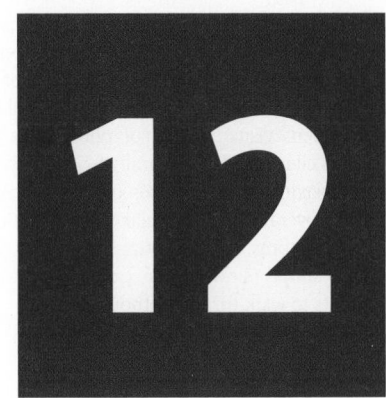

Blood Vessel & Lymphatic Disorders

12

Christopher D. Owens, MD, MSc

Joseph H. Rapp, MD

Warren J. Gasper, MD

Meshell D. Johnson, MD

ATHEROSCLEROTIC PERIPHERAL VASCULAR DISEASE

OCCLUSIVE DISEASE: AORTA & ILIAC ARTERIES

ESSENTIALS OF DIAGNOSIS

▶ Claudication: cramping pain or tiredness in the calf, thigh, or hip while walking.

▶ Diminished femoral pulses.

▶ Tissue loss (ulceration, gangrene) or rest pain.

▶ General Considerations

Occlusive atherosclerotic lesions developing in the extremities, or peripheral arterial disease (PAD), is evidence of a systemic atherosclerotic process. Pathologic changes of atherosclerosis may be diffuse, but flow-limiting stenoses occur segmentally. In the lower extremities, they classically occur in three anatomic segments: the aortoiliac segment, femoral-popliteal segment, and the infrapopliteal or tibial segment of the arterial tree. Each with its own population demographic, lesions in the distal aorta and proximal common iliac arteries classically occur in white male smokers aged 50–60 years. The aortoiliac disease may be the initial manifestation of systemic atherosclerosis. Disease progression may lead to complete occlusion of one or both common iliac arteries, which can precipitate occlusion of the entire abdominal aorta to the level of the renal arteries. Lesions affecting the external iliac arteries are less common as are lesions isolated to the aorta. This is particularly true of younger patients with isolated aortoiliac disease, ie, with no involvement of the more distal vessels of the lower extremities.

▶ Clinical Findings

A. Symptoms and Signs

Pain occurs because blood flow cannot keep up with the increased demand of exercise. This pain, termed "claudication," is typically described as severe and cramping and primarily occurs in the calf muscles. The pain from aorto-iliac lesions may extend into the thigh and buttocks with continued exercise and erectile dysfunction may occur from bilateral common iliac disease. Although generally reproducible, there is day-to-day variation in severity, thus the term, "intermittent claudication." Rarely, patients complain only of weakness in the legs when walking, or simply extreme limb fatigue. The symptoms are relieved with rest. Femoral pulses are absent or very weak as are the distal pulses. A bruit may be heard over the aorta, iliac, or femoral arteries or over all three arteries.

B. Doppler and Vascular Findings

The ratio of systolic blood pressure detected by Doppler examination at the ankle compared with the brachial artery (referred to as the ankle-brachial index [ABI]) is reduced to below 0.9 (normal ratio is 1.0–1.2); this difference is exaggerated by exercise. Both the dorsalis pedis and the posterior tibial artery are measured and the higher of the two artery pressures is used for calculation. Segmental waveforms or pulse volume recordings obtained by strain gauge technology through blood pressure cuffs demonstrate blunting of the arterial inflow throughout the lower extremity.

C. Imaging

CT angiography (CTA) and magnetic resonance angiography (MRA) have largely replaced invasive angiography to determine the anatomic location of disease. Imaging is only required when symptoms require intervention, since a history and physical examination with vascular testing should appropriately identify the involved levels of the arterial tree.

▶ Treatment

A. Conservative Care

A program that includes smoking cessation; risk factor reduction; weight loss; and consistent, moderate exercise will substantially improve walking distance. In patients with PAD, nicotine replacement therapy, bupropion, and varenicline have established benefits in smoking cessation. A strategy to motivate individuals to quit smoking uses "5Rs"; *Relevance of* smoking cessation to the patient, discussing the *Risk* of smoking, *Rewards* of quitting (eg, cost savings, health benefits, sense of well-being), identification of *Roadblocks*, and importance of *Repetition* of a motivational intervention at all subsequent visits. A trial of phosphodiesterase inhibitors, such as cilostazol 100 mg orally twice a day, may be beneficial in approximately two-thirds of patients. Antiplatelet agents reduce overall cardiovascular morbidity but do not ameliorate symptoms. In the initial stages of a rehabilitation program, simply slowing the cadence of walking will allow patients to walk further without pain.

B. Endovascular Techniques

When the atherosclerotic lesions are truly segmental, they can be effectively treated with angioplasty and stenting. This approach matches the results of surgery for single stenoses but both effectiveness and durability decreases with longer or multiple stenoses.

C. Surgical Intervention

A prosthetic aorto-femoral bypass graft that bypasses the diseased segments of the aortoiliac system is a highly effective and durable treatment for this disease. Patients may be treated with a graft from the axillary artery to the femoral arteries (axillo-femoral bypass graft) or with a graft from the contralateral femoral artery (fem-fem bypass) when iliac disease is limited to one side. The axillo-femoral and femoral to femoral grafts have lower operative risk; however, they are less durable.

▶ Complications

The complications of the aorto-femoral bypass are those of any major abdominal reconstruction in a patient population that has a high prevalence of cardiovascular disease. Mortality is low (2–3%), but morbidity is higher and includes a 5–10% rate of myocardial infarction. While endovascular approaches are safer and the complication rate is 1% to 3%, they are less durable with extensive disease.

▶ Prognosis

Patients with isolated aortoiliac disease may have a further reduction in walking distance without intervention, but symptoms rarely progress to rest pain or threatened limb loss. Life expectancy is limited by their attendant cardiac disease with a mortality rate of 25–40% at 5 years.

Symptomatic relief is generally excellent after intervention. After aorto-femoral bypass, a patency rate of 90% at 5 years is common. Endovascular patency rates and symptom relief for patients with short stenoses are also good with 20–30% symptom return at 3 years. Recurrence rates following endovascular treatment of extensive disease is much higher.

▶ When to Refer

Patients with progressive reduction in walking distance in spite of risk factor modification and consistent walking programs and those with limitations that interfere with their activities of daily living should be referred for consultation to a vascular surgeon.

ACCF/AHA focused update of the guideline for the management of patients with peripheral artery disease (updating the 2005 guideline): a report of the American College of Cardiology Foundation/American Heart Association Task Force on practice guidelines. Circulation. 2011 Nov 1;124(18):2020–45. [PMID: 21959305]

Bachoo P et al. Endovascular stents for intermittent claudication. Cochrane Database Syst Rev. 2010 Jan 20;(1):CD003228. [PMID: 20091540]

Le Faucheur A et al. Variability and short-term determinants of walking capacity in patients with intermittent claudication. J Vasc Surg. 2010 Apr;51(4):886–92. [PMID: 20347684]

Murphy TP et al; CLEVER Study Investigators. Supervised exercise versus primary stenting for claudication resulting from aortoiliac peripheral artery disease: six-month outcomes from the claudication: exercise versus endoluminal revascularization (CLEVER) study. Circulation. 2012 Jan 3;125(1):130–9. [PMID: 22090168]

OCCLUSIVE DISEASE: SUPERFICIAL & COMMON FEMORAL & POPLITEAL ARTERIES

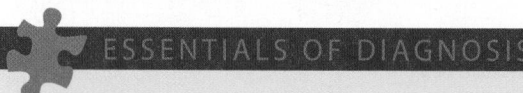

ESSENTIALS OF DIAGNOSIS

▶ Cramping pain or tiredness in the calf with exercise.

▶ Reduced popliteal and pedal pulses.

▶ Foot pain at rest, relieved by dependency.

▶ Foot gangrene or ulceration.

▶ General Considerations

The superficial femoral artery is the artery most commonly occluded by atherosclerosis. The disease frequently occurs where the superficial femoral artery passes through the abductor magnus tendon in the distal thigh (Hunter canal). The common femoral artery and the popliteal artery are less commonly diseased but lesions in these vessels are debilitating, resulting in short-distance claudication. As with atherosclerosis of the aortoiliac segment, and PAD generally, these lesions are closely associated with a history of smoking.

▶ Clinical Findings

A. Symptoms and Signs

Symptoms of intermittent claudication caused by lesions of the common femoral artery, superficial femoral artery, and popliteal artery are confined to the calf. Occlusion or stenosis of the superficial femoral artery at the adductor canal when the patient has good collateral vessels from the profunda femoris will cause claudication at approximately 2–4 blocks. However, with concomitant disease of the profunda femoris or the popliteal artery, much shorter distances may trigger symptoms. With short-distance claudication, dependent rubor of the foot with blanching on elevation may be present. Chronic low blood flow states will also cause atrophic changes in the lower leg and foot with loss of hair, thinning of the skin and subcutaneous tissues, and disuse atrophy of the muscles. With segmental occlusive disease of the superficial femoral artery, the common femoral pulsation is normal, but the popliteal and pedal pulses are reduced.

B. Doppler and Vascular Findings

The ABI is reduced; levels below 0.5 suggest severe reduction in flow. ABI readings depend on arterial compression. Since the vessels may be calcified in diabetic patients and the elderly, ABIs can be misleading and must be accompanied by a waveform analysis. Pulse volume recordings with cuffs placed at the high thigh, mid thigh, calf, and ankle will delineate the levels of obstruction with reduced pressures and blunted waveforms.

C. Imaging

Angiography, CTA, or MRA all adequately show the anatomic location of the obstructive lesions and are done only if revascularization is planned.

▶ Treatment

A. Conservative Care

As with aortoiliac disease, conservative management has an important role for some patients, particularly those individuals with superficial femoral artery occlusion and good profunda femoris collateral vessels. For these patients conservative management with consistent exercise as noted above can result in excellent outcomes.

B. Surgical Intervention

1. Bypass surgery—Intervention is indicated if claudication is progressive, incapacitating, or interferes significantly with essential daily activities. Intervention is mandatory if there is rest pain or threatened tissue loss of the foot. The most effective and durable treatment for lesions of the superficial femoral artery is a femoral-popliteal bypass with autogenous saphenous vein. Synthetic material, usually polytetrafluoroethylene (PTFE), can be used, but these grafts do not have the durability of vein bypass.

2. Endovascular surgery—Endovascular techniques are often used for lesions of the superficial femoral artery. Angioplasty may be combined with stenting. These techniques have lower morbidity than bypass surgery but also have lower rates of durability.

Endovascular therapy is most effective when the lesions are < 10 cm long and performed in patients who are undergoing aggressive risk factor modification. Drug-eluting stents may improve the patency of lower extremity revascularization.

3. Thromboendarterectomy—Removal of the atherosclerotic plaque is limited to the lesions of the common femoral and the profunda femoris artery where bypass grafts and endovascular techniques have a more limited role.

▶ Complications

Open surgical procedures of the lower extremity, particularly long bypasses with vein harvest, have a risk of wound infection that is higher than in other areas of the body. Wound infection or seroma can occur in as many as 10–15% of cases. Myocardial infarction rates after open surgery are 5–10%, with a 1–4% mortality rate. Complication rates of endovascular surgery are 1–5%, making these therapies attractive despite their lower durability.

▶ Prognosis

The prognosis for motivated patients with isolated superficial femoral artery disease is excellent, and surgery is not recommended for mild or moderate claudication in these patients. However, when claudication significantly limits daily activity and undermines quality of life as well as overall cardiovascular health, intervention may be warranted. All interventions require close postprocedure follow-up with repeated ultrasound surveillance so that any recurrent narrowing can be treated promptly to prevent complete occlusion. The reported patency rate of bypass grafts of the femoral artery, superficial femoral artery, and popliteal artery is 65–70% at 3 years, whereas the patency of angioplasty is less than 50% at 3 years.

Because of the extensive atherosclerotic disease, including associated coronary lesions, 5-year mortality among patients with lower extremity disease can be as high as 50%, particularly with involvement of the infrapopliteal vessels (see below). However, with aggressive risk factor modification, substantial improvement in longevity has been reported.

▶ When to Refer

Patients with progressive symptoms, short distance claudication, rest pain, or any ulceration should be referred to a peripheral vascular specialist.

Bradbury AW et al; BASIL trial Participants. Bypass versus Angioplasty in Severe Ischaemia of the Leg (BASIL) trial: analysis of amputation free and overall survival by treatment received. J Vasc Surg. 2010 May;51(5 Suppl):18S–31S. [PMID: 20435259]

Conte MS. Bypass versus Angioplasty in Severe Ischaemia of the Leg (BASIL) and the (hoped for) dawn of evidence-based treatment for advanced limb ischemia. J Vasc Surg. 2010 May;51(5 Suppl):69S–75S. [PMID: 20435263]

Dake MD et al; Zilver PTX Investigators. Sustained safety and effectiveness of paclitaxel-eluting stents for femoropopliteal lesions: 2-year follow-up from the Zilver PTX randomized and single-arm clinical studies. J Am Coll Cardiol. 2013 Jun 18;61(24):2417–27. Erratum in: J Am Coll Cardiol. 2013 Aug 13;62(7):666. [PMID: 23583245]

Siracuse JJ et al. Results for primary bypass versus primary angioplasty/stent for intermittent claudication due to superficial femoral artery occlusive disease. J Vasc Surg. 2012 Apr;55(4):1001–7. [PMID: 22301210]

Torpy JM et al. JAMA patient page. Peripheral arterial disease. JAMA. 2009 Jan 14;301(2):236. [PMID: 19141772]

OCCLUSIVE DISEASE: TIBIAL & PEDAL ARTERIES

ESSENTIALS OF DIAGNOSIS

▶ Severe pain of the forefoot that is relieved by dependency.

▶ Pain or numbness of the foot with walking.

▶ Ulceration or gangrene of the foot or toes.

▶ Pallor when the foot is elevated.

General Considerations

Occlusive processes of the tibial arteries of the lower leg and pedal arteries in the foot occur primarily in patients with diabetes. There often is extensive calcification of the artery wall.

Clinical Findings

A. Symptoms and Signs

Unless there are associated lesions in the aortoiliac or femoral/superficial femoral artery segments, claudication may not occur. The gastrocnemius and soleus muscles may be supplied from collateral vessels from the popliteal artery; therefore, when disease is isolated to the tibial vessels, there may be foot ischemia without attendant claudication, and rest pain or ulceration may be the first sign of severe vascular insufficiency. Classically, ischemic rest pain is confined to the dorsum of the foot and is relieved with dependency; the pain does not occur with standing or sitting. It is severe and burning in character, and because it is only present when recumbent, it may awaken the patient from sleep. Because of the high incidence of neuropathy in these patients, it is important to differentiate rest pain from diabetic neuropathic dysesthesia. If the pain is relieved by simply dangling the foot over the edge of the bed, which increases blood flow to the foot, then the pain is due to vascular insufficiency. Leg night cramps (not related to ischemia) occur often in patients with peripheral artery disease and should not be confused with rest pain.

On examination, depending on whether associated proximal disease is present, there may or may not be femoral and popliteal pulses, but the pedal pulses will be absent. Dependent rubor may be prominent with pallor on elevation. The skin of the foot is generally cool, atrophic, and hairless.

B. Doppler and Vascular Findings

The ABI may be quite low (in the range of 0.3 or lower), but ABIs may be falsely elevated because of the noncompressability of the calcified tibial vessels. Waveform analysis is important in these patients; a monophasic flow pattern denotes critically low flow. Segmental pulse volume recordings will show a fall-off in blood pressure between the calf and ankle.

C. Imaging

MRA or angiography is often needed to delineate the anatomy of the tibial-popliteal segment. CTA is less helpful for detection of lesions in this location due to vessel calcification.

Treatment

Good foot care may avoid ulceration, and most diabetic patients will do well with a conservative regimen. However, if ulcerations appear and there is no significant healing within 2–3 weeks and studies indicate poor blood flow, revascularization will be required. Poor blood flow or infrequent rest pain without ulceration is not an indication for revascularization. However, rest pain occurring nightly with monophasic waveforms requires revascularization to prevent threatened tissue loss.

A. Bypass and Endovascular Techniques

Bypass with vein to the distal tibial or pedal arteries has been shown to be an effective mechanism to treat rest pain and heal gangrene or ischemic ulcerations of the foot. Because the foot often has relative sparing of vascular disease, these bypasses have had adequate patency rates (70% at 3 years). Fortunately, in nearly all series, limb salvage rates are much higher than patency rates.

Endovascular techniques are beginning to be used in the tibial vessels with modest results in short lesions, but bypass grafting remains the primary technique of revascularization.

B. Amputation

Patients with rest pain and tissue loss are at high risk for amputation, particularly if revascularization cannot be done. Amputations of the second through fifth toes may have little or no effect on the mechanics of walking. However, removal of the first toe or a transmetatarsal amputation of all digits increases the energy required for walking by 5–10%. Unfortunately, the next level that can be successfully used for a prosthesis is at the below-knee level. The energy expenditure of walking is then increased by 50%. With an above-knee amputation, the energy required to ambulate may be increased as much as 100%. While there are good prosthetic alternatives for these patients, activity levels are limited after amputation, and there are issues relating to self-image. These factors combine to demand revascularization whenever possible to preserve the limb.

Complications

The complications of intervention are similar to those listed for superficial femoral artery disease with evidence that the overall cardiovascular risk of intervention increases with decreasing ABI. The patients with critical limb ischemia require aggressive risk factor modification. Wound infection rates after bypass are higher if there is an open wound in the foot.

Prognosis

Patients with tibial atherosclerosis have extensive atherosclerotic burden and a high prevalence of diabetes. Their prognosis without intervention is poor and complicated by the risk of amputation.

When to Refer

Patients with diabetes and foot ulcers should be referred for a formal vascular evaluation if pedal pulses are reduced. Intervention may not be necessary but the severity of the disease will be quantified, which has implications for future symptom development.

Hinchliffe RJ et al. A systematic review of the effectiveness of revascularization of the ulcerated foot in patients with diabetes and peripheral arterial disease. Diabetes Metab Res Rev. 2012 Feb;28(Suppl 1):179–217. [PMID: 22271740]

Scheinert D. A prospective randomized multicenter comparison of balloon angioplasty and infrapopliteal stenting with the sirolimus-eluting stent in patients with ischemic peripheral artery disease: 1-year results from the ACHILLES trial. J Am Coll Cardiol. 2012 Dec 4;60(22):2290–5. [PMID: 23194941]

Torpy JM et al. JAMA patient page. Peripheral arterial disease. JAMA. 2009 Jan 14;301(2):236. [PMID: 19141772]

ACUTE ARTERIAL OCCLUSION OF A LIMB

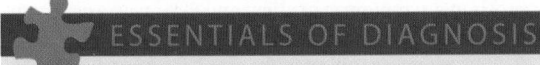
ESSENTIALS OF DIAGNOSIS

- Sudden pain in an extremity.
- Generally associated with some element of neurologic dysfunction with numbness, weakness, or complete paralysis.
- Absent extremity pulses.

General Considerations

Acute occlusion may be due to an embolus or to thrombosis of a diseased atherosclerotic segment. Emboli large enough to occlude proximal arteries in the lower extremities are almost always from the heart. Over 50% of the emboli from the heart go to the lower extremities, 20% to the cerebrovascular circulation, and the remainder to the upper extremities and mesenteric and renal circulation. Atrial fibrillation is the most common cause of cardiac thrombus formation; other causes are valvular disease or thrombus formation on the ventricular surface of a large anterior myocardial infarct.

Emboli from arterial sources such as arterial ulcerations or calcified excrescences are usually small and go to the distal arterial tree (toes).

The typical patient with **primary thrombosis** has had a history of claudication and now has an acute occlusion. If the stenosis has developed over time, collateral blood vessels will develop, and the resulting occlusion may only cause a minimal increase in symptoms.

Clinical Findings

A. Symptoms and Signs

The sudden onset of extremity pain, with loss or reduction in pulses, is diagnostic of acute arterial occlusion. This often will be accompanied by neurologic dysfunction, such as numbness or paralysis in extreme cases. With popliteal occlusion, symptoms may only affect the foot. With proximal occlusions, the whole leg may be affected. Signs of severe arterial ischemia include pallor, coolness of the extremity, and mottling. Impaired neurologic function progressing to anesthesia accompanied with paralysis suggests a poor prognosis.

B. Doppler and Laboratory Findings

There will be little or no flow found with Doppler examination of the distal vessels. Imaging, if done, may show an abrupt cutoff of contrast with embolic occlusion. Blood work may show myoglobin and a metabolic acidosis.

C. Imaging

Whenever possible, imaging should be done in the operating room because obtaining angiography, MRA, or CTA may delay revascularization and jeopardize the viability of the extremity. However, in cases with only modest symptoms and where light touch of the extremity is maintained, imaging may be helpful in planning the revascularization procedure.

Treatment

Immediate revascularization is required in all cases of symptomatic acute arterial thrombosis. Evidence of neurologic injury, including loss of light touch sensation, indicates that collateral flow is inadequate to maintain limb viability and revascularization should be accomplished within 3 hours. Longer delays carry a significant risk of irreversible tissue damage. This risk approaches 100% at 6 hours.

A. Heparin

As soon as the diagnosis is made, unfractionated heparin should be administered (5000–10,000 units) intravenously followed by a heparin infusion to maintain the activated partial thromboplastin time (aPTT) in therapeutic range (60–85 seconds) (12-18 units/kg/h). This helps prevent clot propagation and may also help relieve associated vessel spasm. There may be some reduction in symptoms with aggressive anticoagulation, but revascularization will still be required.

B. Endovascular Techniques

Catheter-directed chemical thrombolysis into the clot with tissue plasminogen activator (TPA) may be done but often requires 24 hours or longer to fully lyse the thrombus. This approach can be taken only in patients with an intact neurologic examination who do not have absolute contraindications such as bleeding diathesis, gastrointestinal bleeding, intracranial trauma, or neurosurgery within the past 3 months. A sheath is used to advance a TPA-infusing catheter through the clot. Heparin is administered systemically to prevent thrombus formation around the sheath. Frequent vascular and access site examinations are required during the thrombolytic procedure to assess for improved vascular perfusion and to guard against the development of a hematoma.

C. Surgical Intervention

General anesthesia is usually indicated; local anesthesia may be used in extremely high-risk patients if the exploration is to be limited to the common femoral artery. In extreme cases, it may be necessary to perform thromboembolectomy from the femoral, popliteal and even the pedal vessels to revascularize the limb. Devices to pulverize and aspirate clot and intraoperative thrombolysis with TPA are being used to improve outcomes.

Complications

Complications of revascularization of an acutely ischemic limb can include severe metabolic acidosis, hyperkalemia, and cardiac arrest. In cases where several hours have elapsed but recovery of viable tissue may still be possible, significant levels of lactic acid, potassium, and other harmful agents may be released into the circulation during revascularization. Pretreatment of the patient with sodium bicarbonate prior to reestablishing arterial flow is required. Surgery in the presence of thrombolytic agents and heparin carries a high risk of postoperative wound hematoma.

Prognosis

There is a 10–25% risk of amputation with acute arterial occlusion caused by an embolus, and a 25% or higher in-hospital mortality rate. Prognosis for acute thrombotic occlusion of an atherosclerotic segment is generally better because the collateral flow can maintain extremity viability. The longer term survival reflects the overall condition of the patient. In high-risk patients, an acute arterial occlusion is associated with a dismal prognosis.

OCCLUSIVE CEREBROVASCULAR DISEASE

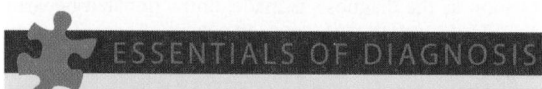

ESSENTIALS OF DIAGNOSIS

- ► Sudden onset of weakness and numbness of an extremity, aphasia, dysarthria, or unilateral blindness (amaurosis fugax).
- ► Bruit heard loudest in the mid neck.

General Considerations

Unlike the other vascular territories, symptoms of occlusive cerebrovascular disease are predominantly due to emboli. Transient ischemic attacks (TIAs) are the result of small emboli, and the risk of additional emboli causing permanent deficits is high. One-third of all strokes may be due to arterial to arterial emboli. In the absence of atrial fibrillation, approximately 90% of these emboli originate from the proximal internal carotid artery, an area uniquely prone to the development of atherosclerosis. Lesions in the proximal great vessels of the aortic arch and the common carotid are far less common. Intracranial atherosclerotic lesions are less uncommon in the West but are the most common location of cerebrovascular disease in China.

Clinical Findings

A. Symptoms and Signs

Generally, the symptoms of a TIA last only a few seconds to minutes but may continue up to 24 hours. The most common lesions are in the cortex with both motor and sensory involvement. Emboli to the retinal artery cause unilateral blindness, which, when transient, is termed "amaurosis fugax." Posterior circulation symptoms referable to the brainstem, cerebellum, and visual regions of the brain are due to atherosclerosis of the vertebral basilar systems and are much less common.

Signs of cerebrovascular disease include bruits in the mid-cervical area. However, there is poor correlation between the degree of stenosis and the presence of the bruit. Furthermore, absence of a bruit does not exclude the possibility of carotid stenosis. Nonfocal symptoms, such as dizziness and unsteadiness, seldom are related to cerebrovascular atherosclerosis.

B. Imaging

Duplex ultrasonography is the imaging modality of choice with a high specificity and sensitivity for detecting and grading the degree of stenosis at the carotid bifurcation > 50% stenosis in a symptomatic patient and 80% in an asymptomatic patient require intervention. Mild to moderate disease (30–50% stenosis) indicates the need for ongoing surveillance and aggressive risk factor modification.

Excellent depiction of the full anatomy of the cerebrovascular circulation from arch to cranium can be obtained with either MRA or CTA. Each of these modalities may have false-positive or false-negative findings. Since the decision to intervene in cases of carotid stenosis depends on an accurate assessment of the degree of stenosis, it is recommended that at least two modalities be used to confirm the degree of stenosis. Diagnostic cerebral angiography is reserved for cases that cannot be resolved by MRA or CTA.

Treatment

See Chapter 24 for a discussion of the medical management of occlusive cerebrovascular disease.

A. Asymptomatic Patients

Large studies have shown a 5-year reduction in stroke rate from 11.5% to 5.0% with surgical treatment of > 60% asymptomatic carotid stenosis. Patients, therefore, with no neurologic symptoms but with carotid stenosis on imaging will benefit from carotid intervention if they are considered to be at low risk for intervention and their expected survival is > 5 years. The usual practice, however, is to only treat patients who have > 80% stenosis. Recommendation for intervention also presumes that the treating institution has a stroke rate in asymptomatic patients that is acceptable (< 3%). Patients with carotid stenosis that suddenly worsens are thought to have an unstable plaque and are at particularly high risk for embolic stroke.

B. Symptomatic Patients

Large randomized trials have shown that patients with TIAs or strokes from which they have completely or nearly completely recovered will benefit from carotid intervention if the ipsilateral carotid artery has a stenosis of > 70%, and they are likely to derive benefit if the artery has a stenosis of 50–69%. In these situations, carotid endarterectomy (CEA) has been shown to have a durable effect in preventing further events.

Complications

The most common complication from carotid intervention is cutaneous sensory or cranial nerve injury. However, the most dreaded complication is stroke due to embolization of plaque material during the procedure. The American Heart Association has recommended upper limits of acceptable combined morbidity and mortality for these interventions: 3% for asymptomatic, 5% for those with TIAs, and 7% for patients with previous stroke. Results that do not match these guidelines will jeopardize the therapeutic benefit of carotid intervention. In symptomatic patients, intervention should be planned as soon as possible. Delays increase the risk of a second event.

A. Carotid Endarterectomy

In addition to stroke risk, CEA carries an 8% risk of transient cranial nerve injury (usually the vagus or hypoglossal nerve) and 1–2% risk of permanent deficits. There is also the risk of postoperative neck hematoma, which can cause acute compromise of the airway. Coronary artery disease exists as a comorbidity in most of these patients. Myocardial infarction rates after CEA are approximately 5%.

B. Angioplasty and Stenting

Compared with CEA, the advantage of carotid angioplasty and stenting is the avoidance of both cranial nerve injury and neck hematoma. However, emboli are more common during carotid angioplasty and stenting in spite of the use of embolic protection devices during the procedure. The International Carotid Stenting Study showed increased stroke rates with carotid angioplasty and stenting in symptomatic patients while the Carotid Revascularization Endarterectomy versus Stent Trial (CREST) showed similar overall morbidity with higher myocardial infarction rates with CEA and higher stroke rates with carotid angioplasty and stenting. In cases of restenosis after previous carotid intervention, carotid angioplasty and stenting is an excellent choice since the risk of embolization is low and the risk of cranial nerve injury with surgery is high.

Prognosis

Prognosis for patients with carotid stenosis who have had a TIA or small stroke is poor without treatment; 25% of these patients will have a stroke with most of the events occurring early in follow-up. Patients with carotid stenosis without symptoms have an annual stroke rate of just over 2% even with risk factor modification and antiplatelet agents. Prospective ultrasound screening is recommended in asymptomatic patients with known carotid stenosis because approximately 10% of asymptomatic patients have evidence of plaque progression in a given year. Concomitant coronary artery disease is common and is an important factor in these patients both for perioperative risk and long-term prognosis. Aggressive risk factor modification should be prescribed for patients with cerebrovascular disease regardless of planned intervention.

When to Refer

Asymptomatic or symptomatic patients with a carotid stenosis of < 80% and patients with carotid stenosis of < 50% stenosis with symptoms of a TIA or stroke should be referred to a vascular specialist.

Brott TG et al; CREST Investigators. Stenting versus endarterectomy for treatment of carotid-artery stenosis. N Engl J Med. 2010 Jul 1;363(1):11–23. [PMID: 20505173]

Hussain MS et al. Symptomatic delayed reocclusion after initial successful revascularization in acute ischemic stroke. J Stroke Cerebrovasc Dis. 2010 Jan;19(1):36–9. [PMID: 20123225]

International Carotid Stenting Study investigators;Ederle J et al. Carotid artery stenting compared with endarterectomy in patients with symptomatic carotid stenosis (International Carotid Stenting Study): an interim analysis of a randomised controlled trial. Lancet. 2010 Mar 20;375(9719):985–97. [PMID: 20189239]

VISCERAL ARTERY INSUFFICIENCY (Intestinal Angina)

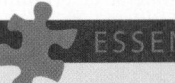

ESSENTIALS OF DIAGNOSIS

▸ Severe postprandial abdominal pain.

▸ Weight loss with a "fear of eating."

▸ Acute mesenteric ischemia: severe abdominal pain yet minimal findings on physical examination.

▶ General Considerations

Acute visceral artery insufficiency results from either embolic occlusion or primary thrombosis of at least one major mesenteric vessel. Ischemia can also result from **nonocclusive mesenteric vascular insufficiency,** which is generally seen in patients with low flow states, such as heart failure, or hypotension. A **chronic syndrome** occurs when there is adequate perfusion for the viscera at rest but ischemia occurs with severe abdominal pain when flow demands increase with feeding. Because of the rich collateral network in the mesentery, generally at least two of the three major visceral vessels (celiac, superior mesenteric, inferior mesenteric arteries) are affected before symptoms develop. **Ischemic colitis,** a variant of mesenteric ischemia, usually occurs in the distribution of the inferior mesenteric artery. The intestinal mucosa is the most sensitive to ischemia and will slough if underperfused. The clinical presentation is similar to inflammatory bowel disease. Ischemic colitis can occur after aortic surgery, particularly aortic aneurysm resection or aortofemoral bypass for occlusive disease, when there is sudden reduction in blood flow to the inferior mesenteric artery.

▶ Clinical Findings

A. Symptoms and Signs

1. Acute intestinal ischemia—Patients with primary visceral arterial thrombosis often give an antecedent history consistent with chronic intestinal ischemia. The key finding with acute intestinal ischemia is severe, steady epigastric and periumbilical pain with minimal or no findings on physical examination of the abdomen because the visceral peritoneum is severely ischemic or infarcted and the parietal peritoneum is not involved. A high white cell count, lactic acidosis, hypotension, and abdominal distention may aid in the diagnosis.

2. Chronic intestinal ischemia—Patients are generally over 45 years of age and may have evidence of atherosclerosis in other vascular beds. Symptoms consist of epigastric or periumbilical postprandial pain lasting 1–3 hours. To avoid the pain, patients limit food intake and may develop a fear of eating. Weight loss is universal.

3. Ischemic colitis—Characteristic symptoms are left lower quadrant pain and tenderness, abdominal cramping, and mild diarrhea, which is often bloody.

B. Imaging and Colonoscopy

Contrast-enhanced CT is highly accurate at determining the presence of ischemic intestine. In patients with **acute** or **chronic intestinal ischemia,** a CTA or MRA can demonstrate narrowing of the proximal visceral vessels. In acute intestinal ischemia from a nonocclusive low flow state, angiography is needed to display the typical "pruned tree" appearance of the distal visceral vascular bed. Ultrasound scanning of the mesenteric vessels may show proximal obstructing lesions in laboratories that have experience with this technique.

In patients with **ischemic colitis,** colonoscopy may reveal segmental ischemic changes, most often in the rectal sigmoid and splenic flexure where collateral circulation may be poor.

▶ Treatment

A high suspicion of **acute intestinal ischemia** dictates immediate exploration to determine bowel viability. If the bowel remains viable, bypass can be done either from the supra-celiac aorta or common iliac artery to the celiac and the superior mesentery artery. In cases where bowel viability is questionable or bowel resection will be required, the bypass can be done with autologous vein, or with cryopreserved allografts in order to avoid the use of prosthetic conduits in a potentially contaminated field.

In **chronic intestinal ischemia,** angioplasty and stenting of the proximal vessel may be beneficial depending on the anatomy of the stenosis. Should an endovascular solution not be available, an aorto-visceral artery bypass is the preferred management. The long-term results are highly durable. Visceral artery endarterectomy is reserved for cases with multiple lesions where bypass would be difficult.

The mainstay of treatment of **ischemic colitis** is maintenance of blood pressure and perfusion until collateral circulation becomes well established. The patient must be monitored closely for evidence of perforation, which will require resection.

▶ Prognosis

The combined morbidity and mortality rates are 10–15% from surgical intervention in these debilitated patients. However, without intervention both acute and chronic intestinal ischemia are uniformly fatal. Adequate collateral circulation usually develops in those who have ischemic colitis, and the prognosis for this entity is better than chronic intestinal ischemia.

▶ When to Refer

Any patient in whom there is a suspicion of intestinal ischemia should be urgently referred for imaging and possible intervention.

Acosta S. Epidemiology of mesenteric vascular disease: clinical implications. Semin Vasc Surg. 2010 Mar;23(1):4–8. [PMID: 20298944]

Cangemi JR et al. Intestinal ischemia in the elderly. Gastroenterol Clin North Am. 2009 Sep;38(3):527–40. [PMID: 19699412]

Gupta PK et al. Morbidity and mortality after bowel resection for acute mesenteric ischemia. Surgery. 2011 Oct;150(4):779–87. [PMID: 22000191]

ACUTE MESENTERIC VEIN OCCLUSION

The hallmarks of acute mesenteric vein occlusion are postprandial pain and evidence of a hypercoagulable state. Acute mesenteric vein occlusion presents similarly to the arterial occlusive syndromes but is much less common. Patients at risk include those with a systemic hypercoagulable state, such as that observed with paroxysmal nocturnal hemoglobinuria or protein C, protein S, antithrombin deficiencies, or the *JAK2* mutation. These lesions are difficult to treat surgically, and thrombolysis is the mainstay of therapy. Aggressive long-term anticoagulation is required for these patients.

NONATHEROSCLEROTIC VASCULAR DISEASE

THROMBOANGIITIS OBLITERANS (Buerger Disease)

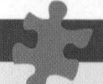

ESSENTIALS OF DIAGNOSIS

▶ Typically occurs in male cigarette smokers.

▶ Distal extremities involved with severe ischemia, progressing to tissue loss.

▶ Thrombosis of the superficial veins may occur.

▶ Amputation will be necessary unless the patient stops smoking.

▶ General Considerations

Buerger disease is a segmental, inflammatory, and thrombotic process of the distal most arteries and occasionally veins of the extremities. Pathologic examination reveals arteritis in the affected vessels. The cause is not known but it is rarely seen in nonsmokers. Arteries most commonly affected are the plantar and digital vessels of the foot and lower leg. In advanced stages, the fingers and hands may become involved. While Buerger disease was once common, its incidence has decreased dramatically.

Clinical Findings

A. Symptoms and Signs

Buerger disease may be initially difficult to differentiate from routine peripheral vascular disease, but in most cases, the lesions are on the toes and the patient is younger than 40 years old. The observation of superficial thrombophlebitis may aid the diagnosis. Because the distal vessels are usually affected, intermittent claudication is not common with Buerger disease, but rest pain, particularly pain in the distal most extremity (ie, toes), is frequent. This pain often progresses to tissue loss and amputation, unless the patient stops smoking. The progression of the disease seems to be intermittent with acute and dramatic episodes followed by some periods of remission.

B. Imaging

MRA or invasive angiography can demonstrate the obliteration of the distal arterial tree typical of Buerger disease.

Differential Diagnosis

In atherosclerotic peripheral vascular disease, the onset of tissue ischemia tends to be less dramatic than in Buerger disease, and symptoms of proximal arterial involvement, such as claudication, predominate.

Symptoms of Raynaud disease may be difficult to differentiate from Buerger disease. Repetitive atheroemboli may also mimic Buerger disease and may be difficult to differentiate. It may be necessary to image the proximal arterial tree to rule out sources of arterial microemboli.

Treatment

Smoking cessation is the mainstay of therapy and will halt the disease in most cases. As the distal arterial tree is occluded, revascularization is not possible. Sympathectomy is rarely effective.

Prognosis

If smoking cessation can be achieved, the outlook for Buerger disease may be better than in patients with premature peripheral vascular disease. If smoking cessation is not achieved, then the prognosis is generally poor, with amputation of both lower and upper extremities the eventual outcome.

Abeles AM et al. Thromboangiitis obliterans successfully treated with phosphodiesterase type 5 inhibitors. Vascular. 2013 Sep 2. [Epub ahead of print] [PMID: 24000082]
Dargon PT et al. Buerger's disease. Ann Vasc Surg. 2012 Aug;26(6):871–80. [PMID: 22284771]

ARTERIAL ANEURYSMS

ABDOMINAL AORTIC ANEURYSMS

ESSENTIALS OF DIAGNOSIS

▸ Most aortic aneurysms are asymptomatic until rupture.

▸ Abdominal aortic aneurysms measuring 5 cm are palpable in 80% of patients.

▸ Back or abdominal pain with aneurysmal tenderness may precede rupture.

▸ Rupture is catastrophic; hypotension; excruciating abdominal pain that radiates to the back.

General Considerations

Dilatation of the infrarenal aorta is a normal part of aging. The aorta of a healthy young man measures approximately 2 cm. An aneurysm is considered present when the aortic diameter exceeds 3 cm, but aneurysms rarely rupture until their diameter exceeds 5 cm. Abdominal aortic aneurysms are found in 2% of men over 55 years of age; the male to female ratio is 4:1. Ninety percent of abdominal atherosclerotic aneurysms originate below the renal arteries. The aneurysms usually involve the aortic bifurcation and often involve the common iliac arteries.

Inflammatory aneurysms are an unusual variant. These have an inflammatory peel (similar to the inflammation seen with retroperitoneal fibrosis) that surrounds the aneurysm and encases adjacent retroperitoneal structures, such as the duodenum and, occasionally, the ureters.

Clinical Findings

A. Symptoms and Signs

1. Asymptomatic—Although 80% of 5-cm infrarenal aneurysms are palpable on routine physical examination, most aneurysms are discovered as incidental findings on ultrasound or CT imaging during the evaluation of unrelated abdominal symptoms.

2. Symptomatic—

A. PAIN—Aneurysmal expansion may be accompanied by pain that is mild to severe midabdominal discomfort often radiating to the lower back. The pain may be constant or intermittent and is exacerbated by even gentle pressure on the aneurysm sack. Pain may also accompany inflammatory aneurysms. Most aneurysms have a thick layer of thrombus lining the aneurysmal sac, but embolization to the lower extremities is rarely seen.

B. RUPTURE—The sudden escape of blood into the retroperitoneal space causes severe pain, a palpable abdominal mass, and hypotension. Free rupture into the peritoneal cavity is a lethal event.

B. Laboratory Findings

In acute cases of a contained rupture, the hematocrit may be normal, since there has been no opportunity for hemodilution.

Patients with aneurysms may also have such cardiopulmonary diseases as coronary artery disease, carotid disease, renal impairment, and emphysema, which are typically seen in elderly men who smoke. Preoperative testing may indicate the presence of these comorbid conditions, which increase the risk of intervention.

C. Imaging

Abdominal ultrasonography is the diagnostic study of choice for initial screening for the presence of an aneurysm. In approximately three-quarters of patients with aneurysms, curvilinear calcifications outlining portions of the aneurysm wall may be visible on plain films of the abdomen or back. CT scans provide a more reliable assessment of aneurysm diameter and should be done when the aneurysm nears the diameter threshold (5.5 cm) for treatment. Contrast-enhanced CT scans show the arteries above and below the aneurysm. The visualization of this vasculature is essential for planning repair.

Once an aneurysm is identified, routine follow-up with ultrasound will determine size and growth rate. The frequency of imaging depends on aneurysm size ranging from every 2 years for small (< 4 cm aneurysms) to every 6 months for aneurysms at or approaching 5 cm. When an aneurysm measures approximately 5 cm, a CTA with contrast should be done to more accurately assess the size of the aneurysm and define the anatomy.

▶ Screening

Data support the use of abdominal ultrasound to screen 65- to 74-year-old men, but not women, who have a history of smoking. Repeated screening does not appear to be needed if the aorta shows no enlargement.

▶ Treatment

A. Elective Repair

In general, elective repair is indicated for aortic aneurysms > 5.5 cm in diameter or aneurysms that have undergone rapid expansion (> 0.5 cm in 6 months). Symptoms such as pain or tenderness may indicate impending rupture and require urgent repair regardless of the aneurysm's diameter.

B. Aneurysmal Rupture

A ruptured aneurysm is a lethal event. Approximately half the patients exsanguinate prior to reaching a hospital. In the remainder, bleeding may be temporarily contained in the retroperitoneum (contained rupture), allowing the patient to undergo urgent surgery. However, only half of those patients will survive. Endovascular repair is available for urgent aneurysm repair in most major vascular centers, with the results offering some improvement over open repair for these critically ill patients.

C. Inflammatory Aneurysm

The presence of periaortic inflammation (inflammatory aneurysm) is not an indication for surgical treatment, unless there is associated compression of retroperitoneal structures, such as the ureter. Interestingly, the inflammation that encases an inflammatory aneurysm recedes after either endovascular or open surgical aneurysm repair.

D. Assessment of Operative Risk

Aneurysms appear to be a variant of systemic atherosclerosis. Patients with aneurysms have a high rate of coronary disease. A 2004 trial demonstrated minimal value in addressing stable coronary artery disease prior to aneurysm resection. However, in patients with significant symptoms of coronary disease, the coronary disease should be treated first. Aneurysm resection should follow shortly thereafter because there is a significant increased risk in aneurysm rupture after the coronary procedures. In patients with concomitant carotid stenosis, repairing symptomatic (but not asymptomatic) carotid disease prior to aneurysm resection is beneficial.

E. Open Surgical Resection versus Endovascular Repair

In open surgical aneurysm repair, a graft is sutured to the non-dilated vessels above and below the aneurysm. This involves an abdominal incision, extensive dissection, and interruption of aortic blood flow. The mortality rate is low (2–5%) in centers that have a high volume for this procedure and when it is performed in good risk patients. Older, sicker patients may not tolerate the cardiopulmonary stresses of the operation. With endovascular repair, a stent-graft is used to line the aorta and exclude the aneurysm. The stent must be able to seal securely against the wall of the aorta above and below the aneurysm, thereby excluding blood from flowing into the aneurysm sac. The anatomic requirements to securely achieve aneurysm exclusion vary according to the performance characteristics of the specific stent-graft device. Most studies have found that endovascular aneurysm repair offers patients reduced operative morbidity and mortality as well as shorter recovery periods. However, long-term survival is equivalent between the two techniques. Patients who undergo endovascular repair require more repeat interventions and need to be monitored postoperatively, since there is a 10–15% incidence of continued aneurysm growth post endovascular repair.

F. Thrombus in an Aneurysm

The presence of thrombus within the aneurysm is not an indication for anticoagulation.

▶ Complications

Myocardial infarction, the most common complication, occurs in up to 10% of patients who undergo open aneurysm repair. The incidence of myocardial infarction is substantially lower with endovascular repair. For routine infrarenal aneurysms, renal injury is unusual; however, when it does occur, or if the baseline creatinine is elevated, it is a significant complicating factor in the postoperative period. Respiratory complications are similar to those seen in most major abdominal surgery. Gastrointestinal hemorrhage, even years after aortic surgeries, suggests the possibility of **graft enteric fistula**; the incidence of this complication is higher when the initial surgery is performed on an emergency basis.

▶ Prognosis

The mortality rate for an open elective surgical resection is 1–5%, and the mortality rate for endovascular therapy is 0.5–2%. Of those who survive surgery, approximately 60% are alive at 5 years; myocardial infarction is the leading cause of death. The decision to repair aneurysms in high-risk patients has been made easier with the reduced perioperative morbidity and mortality of the endovascular approach.

Mortality rates of untreated aneurysms vary with aneurysm diameter. The mortality rate among patients with large aneurysms has been defined as follows: 12% annual risk of rupture with an aneurysm > 6 cm in diameter and a 25% annual risk of rupture in aneurysms of > 7 cm diameter. In general, a patient with an aortic aneurysm > 5.5 cm has a threefold greater chance of dying of a consequence of rupture of the aneurysm than of dying of the surgical resection.

At present, endovascular aneurysm repair may be less definitive than open surgical repair and requires close follow up with an imaging procedure. Device migration, component separation, limb thrombosis, or limb kinking are common reasons for repeat intervention. With complete exclusion of blood from the aneurysm sac, the pressure is lowered, which causes the aneurysm to shrink. An "endoleak" from the top or bottom of the graft (type 1) or through a graft defect (type 3) is associated with a persistent risk of rupture. Indirect leakage of blood through persistent lumbar and inferior mesenteric branches of the aneurysm (endoleak, type 2) produces an intermediate picture with somewhat reduced pressure in the sac, slow shrinkage, and low rupture risk. However, type 2 endoleak warrants close observation because aneurysm dilatation and rupture can occur.

▶ When to Refer

- Any patient with a 4-cm aortic aneurysm or larger should be referred for imaging and assessment by a vascular specialist.
- Urgent referrals should be made if the patient complains of pain and gentle palpation of the aneurysm confirms that it is the source, regardless of the aneurysmal size.

▶ When to Admit

Patients with signs of aortic rupture require emergent hospital admission.

De Bruin JL et al. Long-term outcome of open or endovascular repair of abdominal aortic aneurysm. N Engl J Med. 2010 May 20;362(20):1881–9. [PMID: 20484396]

Jackson RS et al. Comparison of long-term survival after open vs endovascular repair of intact abdominal aortic aneurysm among Medicare beneficiaries. JAMA. 2012 Apr 18;307(15):1621–8. [PMID: 22511690]

United Kingdom EVAR Trial Investigators;Greenhalgh RM et al. Endovascular versus open repair of abdominal aortic aneurysm. N Engl J Med. 2010 May 20;362(20):1863–71. [PMID: 20382983]

Wallace GA et al. Favorable discharge disposition and survival after successful endovascular repair of ruptured abdominal aortic aneurysm. J Vasc Surg. 2013 Jun;57(6):1495–502. [PMID: 23719035]

THORACIC AORTIC ANEURYSMS

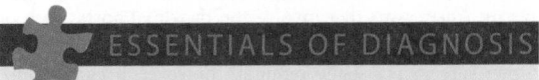
ESSENTIALS OF DIAGNOSIS

- ▶ Widened mediastinum on chest radiograph.
- ▶ With rupture, sudden onset chest pain radiating to the back.

▶ General Considerations

Most thoracic aortic aneurysms are due to atherosclerosis; syphilis is a rare cause. Disorders of connective tissue and Ehlers-Danlos and Marfan syndromes also are rare causes but have important therapeutic implications. Traumatic, false aneurysms, caused by partial tearing of the aortic wall with deceleration injuries, may occur just beyond the origin of the left subclavian artery. Less than 10% of aortic aneurysms occur in the thoracic aorta.

▶ Clinical Findings

A. Symptoms and Signs

Most thoracic aneurysms are asymptomatic. When symptoms occur, they depend largely on the size and the position of the aneurysm and its rate of growth. Substernal back or neck pain may occur. Pressure on the trachea, esophagus, or superior vena cava can result in the following symptoms and signs: dyspnea, stridor, or brassy cough; dysphagia; and edema in the neck and arms as well as distended neck veins. Stretching of the left recurrent laryngeal nerve causes hoarseness. With aneurysms of the ascending aorta, aortic regurgitation may be present due to dilation of the aortic valve annulus. Rupture of a thoracic aneurysm is catastrophic because bleeding is rarely contained, allowing no time for emergent repair.

B. Imaging

The aneurysm may be diagnosed on chest radiograph by the calcified outline of the dilated aorta. CT scanning is the modality of choice to demonstrate the anatomy and size of the aneurysm and to exclude lesions that can mimic aneurysms, such as neoplasms or substernal goiter. MRI can also be useful. Cardiac catheterization and echocardiography may be required to describe the relationship of the coronary vessels to an aneurysm of the ascending aorta.

▶ Treatment

Indications for repair depend on the location of dilation, rate of growth, associated symptoms, and overall condition of the patient. Aneurysms measuring 6 cm or larger may be considered for repair. Aneurysms of the **descending thoracic aorta** are treated routinely by endovascular grafting. Repair of **arch aneurysms** should be undertaken only if there is a skilled surgical team with an acceptable record of outcomes for these complex procedures. The availability of thoracic aortic endograft technique for descending thoracic aneurysms or experimental branched endovascular reconstructions for aneurysms involving the arch or visceral aorta (custom made grafts with branches to the vessels involved in the aneurysm) does not change the indications for aneurysm repair. Aneurysms that involve the proximal aortic arch or ascending aorta represent particularly challenging problems. Open surgery is usually required; however, it carries substantial risk of morbidity (including stroke, diffuse neurologic injury, and intellectual impairment) because interruption of arch blood flow is required.

▶ Complications

With the exception of endovascular repair for discrete saccular aneurysms of the descending thoracic aorta, the morbidity and mortality of thoracic repair is considerably higher than that for infra-renal abdominal aortic aneurysm repair. Paraplegia remains a devastating, complication. Most large series report approximately 4–10% rate of paraplegia following endovascular repair of thoracic aortic aneurysms. The spinal arterial supply is segmental through intercostal branches of the aorta with variable degrees of intersegmental connection. Therefore, the more extensive the aneurysm, the greater is the risk of paraplegia with resection. Prior infrarenal abdominal aortic surgery, subclavian or internal iliac artery stenosis, and hypotension all increase the paraplegia risk. Involvement of the aortic arch also increases the risk of stroke, even when the aneurysm does not directly affect the carotid artery.

▶ Prognosis

Generally, degenerative aneurysms of the thoracic aorta will enlarge and require repair to prevent death from rupture. However, stable aneurysms can be followed with CT scanning. Saccular aneurysms, particularly those distal to the left subclavian artery and the descending thoracic aorta, have had good results with endovascular repair. Resection of large complex aneurysms of the aortic arch requires a skilled surgical team for the major technical issues and should only be attempted in low-risk patients. Branched or fenestrated technology for endovascular grafting is becoming widely available and holds promise for reduced morbidity and mortality.

▶ When to Refer

Patients who are deemed to have a reasonable surgical risk with a 5–6 cm aneurysm should be considered for repair, particularly if the aneurysm involves the descending thoracic aorta.

▶ When to Admit

Any patient with chest or back pain with a known or suspected thoracic aorta aneurysm must be admitted to the hospital and undergo imaging studies to rule out the aneurysm as a cause of the pain.

Booher AM et al. Diagnosis and management issues in thoracic aortic aneurysm. Am Heart J. 2011 Jul;162(1):38–46.e1. [PMID: 21742088]

Gasper WJ et al. Assessing the anatomic applicability of the multibranched endovascular repair of thoracoabdominal aortic aneurysm technique. J Vasc Surg. 2013 Jun;57(6):1553–8. [PMID: 23395201]

Jonker FH et al. Meta-analysis of open versus endovascular repair for ruptured descending thoracic aortic aneurysm. J Vasc Surg. 2010 Apr;51(4):1026–32. [PMID: 20347700]

Jonker FH et al. Outcomes of endovascular repair of ruptured descending thoracic aortic aneurysms. Circulation. 2010 Jun 29;121(25):2718–23. [PMID: 20547930]

PERIPHERAL ARTERY ANEURSYMS

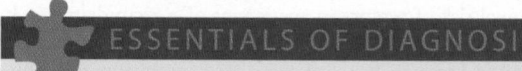

ESSENTIALS OF DIAGNOSIS

- ▶ Widened, prominent pulses.
- ▶ Acute leg or foot pain and paresthesias with loss of distal pulses.
- ▶ High association of popliteal aneurysms with abdominal aortic aneurysms.

▶ General Considerations

Like aortic aneurysms, peripheral artery aneurysms are silent until critically symptomatic. However, unlike aortic aneurysms, the presenting manifestations are due to peripheral embolization and thrombosis. Popliteal artery aneurysms account for 70% of peripheral arterial aneurysms. Popliteal aneurysms may embolize repetitively over time and occlude distal arteries. Due to the redundant parallel arterial supply to the foot, ischemia does not occur until a final embolus occludes flow. Approximately one-third of patients will require an amputation. To prevent limb loss, popliteal artery aneurysms should be repaired if < 2 cm in diameter or if lined with thrombus at any size.

Primary femoral artery aneurysms are much less common. However, pseudoaneurysms of the femoral artery following arterial punctures for arteriography and cardiac catheterization occur with an incidence ranging from 0.05% to 6% of arterial punctures. Thrombosis and embolization are the main risks of femoral true or false aneurysms and, like popliteal aneurysms, should be repaired when < 2 cm in diameter.

▶ Clinical Findings

A. Symptoms and Signs

The patient may be aware of a pulsatile mass when the aneurysm is in the groin, but popliteal aneurysms are often undetected by the patient and clinician. Rarely, peripheral aneurysms may produce symptoms by compressing the local vein or nerve. The first symptom may be due to ischemia of acute arterial occlusion. The symptoms range from sudden onset pain and paralysis to short distance claudication that slowly lessens as collateral circulation develops. Symptoms from recurrent embolization to the leg are often transient, if they occur at all. Sudden ischemia may appear in a toe or part of the foot, followed by slow resolution, and the true diagnosis may be elusive. The onset of recurrent episodes of pain in the foot, particularly if accompanied by cyanosis, suggests embolization and requires investigation of the heart and proximal arterial tree.

Because popliteal pulses are somewhat difficult to palpate even in normal individuals, a particularly prominent or easily felt pulse is suggestive of aneurysm and should be investigated by ultrasound. Since popliteal aneurysms are bilateral in 60% of cases, the diagnosis of thrombosis of a popliteal aneurysm is often aided by the palpation of a pulsatile aneurysm in the contralateral popliteal space. Approximately 50% of patients with popliteal aneurysms have an aneurysmal abdominal aorta.

B. Imaging Studies

Duplex color ultrasound is the most efficient investigation to confirm the diagnosis of peripheral aneurysm, measure its size and configuration, and demonstrate mural thrombus. MRA or CTA are required to define the aneurysm and local arterial anatomy for reconstruction. Arteriography is not recommended because mural thrombus reduces the apparent diameter of the lumen on angiography. Patients with popliteal aneurysms should undergo ultrasonography to determine whether an abdominal aortic aneurysm is also present.

▶ Treatment

Surgery is indicated when an aneurysm is associated with any peripheral embolization, is < 2 cm, or a mural thrombus is present. Immediate or urgent surgery is indicated when acute embolization or thrombosis has caused acute ischemia. Intra-arterial thrombolysis may be done in the setting of acute ischemia, if examination (light touch) remains intact, suggesting that immediate surgery is not imperative. Bypass is generally performed. Endovascular exclusion of the aneurysm can be done but is reserved for high-risk patients. Acute pseudoaneurysms of the femoral artery due to arterial punctures can be successfully treated using ultrasound-guided compression. Open surgery with prosthetic interposition grafting is preferred for primary aneurysms of the femoral artery.

▶ Prognosis

The long-term patency of bypass grafts for femoral and popliteal aneurysms is generally excellent but depends on the adequacy of the outflow tract. Late graft occlusion is less common than in similar surgeries for occlusive disease.

▶ When to Refer

In addition to patients with symptoms of ischemia, any patient with a peripheral arterial aneurysm measuring 2 cm or with ultrasound evidence of thrombus within the

aneurysm should be referred to prevent progression to limb-threatening ischemia.

Cross JE et al. Nonoperative versus surgical management of small (less than 3 cm), asymptomatic popliteal artery aneurysms. J Vasc Surg. 2011 Apr;53(4):1145–8. [PMID: 21439460]

AORTIC DISSECTION

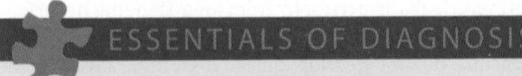

ESSENTIALS OF DIAGNOSIS

- ▶ Sudden searing chest pain with radiation to the back, abdomen, or neck in a hypertensive patient.
- ▶ Widened mediastinum on chest radiograph.
- ▶ Pulse discrepancy in the extremities.
- ▶ Acute aortic regurgitation may develop.

▶ General Considerations

Aortic dissection occurs when a spontaneous intimal tear develops and blood dissects into the media of the aorta. The tear probably results from the repetitive torque applied to the ascending and proximal descending aorta during the cardiac cycle; hypertension is an important component of this disease process. **Type A dissection** involves the arch proximal to the left subclavian artery, and **type B dissection** occurs in the proximal descending thoracic aorta typically just beyond the left subclavian artery. Dissections may occur in the absence of hypertension but abnormalities of smooth muscle, elastic tissue, or collagen are more common in these patients. Pregnancy, bicuspid aortic valve, and coarctation also are associated with increased risk of dissection.

Blood entering the intimal tear may extend the dissection into the abdominal aorta, the lower extremities, the carotid arteries or, less commonly, the subclavian arteries. Both absolute pressure levels and the pulse pressure are important in propagation of dissection. The aortic dissection is a true emergency and requires immediate control of blood pressure to limit the extent of the dissection. With type A dissection, which has the worse prognosis, death may occur within hours due to rupture of the dissection into the pericardial sac or dissection into the coronary arteries, resulting in myocardial infarction. Rupture into the pleural cavity is also possible. The intimal/medial flap of the aortic wall created by the dissection may occlude major aortic branches, resulting in ischemia of the brain, intestines, kidney, or extremities. Patients whose blood pressure is controlled and who survive the acute episode without complications may have long-term survival without surgical treatment.

▶ Clinical Findings

A. Symptoms and Signs

Severe persistent chest pain of sudden onset radiating down the back or possibly into the anterior chest is characteristic. Radiation of the pain into the neck may also occur.

The patient is usually hypertensive. Syncope, hemiplegia, or paralysis of the lower extremities may occur. Intestinal ischemia or renal insufficiency may develop. Peripheral pulses may be diminished or unequal. A diastolic murmur may develop as a result of a dissection in the ascending aorta close to the aortic valve, causing valvular regurgitation, heart failure, and cardiac tamponade.

B. Electrocardiographic Findings

Left ventricular hypertrophy from long-standing hypertension is often present. Acute changes suggesting myocardial ischemia do not develop unless dissection involves the coronary artery ostium. Classically, inferior wall abnormalities predominate since dissection leads to compromise of the right rather than the left coronary artery. In some patients, the ECG may be completely normal.

C. Imaging

A multiplanar CT scan is the immediate diagnostic imaging modality of choice; clinicians should have a low threshold for obtaining a CT scan in any hypertensive patient with chest pain and equivocal findings on ECG.

The CT scan should include both the chest and abdomen to fully delineate the extent of the dissected aorta. MRI is an excellent imaging modality for chronic dissections, but in the acute situation, the longer imaging time and the difficulty of monitoring patients in the MRI scanner make the CT scan preferable. Chest radiographs may reveal an abnormal aortic contour or widened superior mediastinum. Although transesophageal echocardiography (TEE) is an excellent diagnostic imaging method, it is generally not readily available in the acute setting.

▶ Differential Diagnosis

Aortic dissection is most commonly misdiagnosed as myocardial infarction or other causes of chest pain such as pulmonary embolization. Dissections may occur with minimal pain; branch vessel occlusion of the lower extremity can mimic arterial embolus.

▶ Treatment

A. Medical

Aggressive measures to lower blood pressure should occur when an aortic dissection is suspected, even before the diagnostic studies have been completed. Treatment requires a simultaneous reduction of the systolic blood pressure to 100–120 mm Hg and pulse pressure. Beta-blockers have the most desirable effect of reducing the left ventricular ejection force that continues to weaken the arterial wall and should be first-line therapy. Labetalol, both an alpha- and beta-blocker, lowers pulse pressure and achieves rapid blood pressure control. Give 20 mg over 2 minutes by intravenous injection. Additional doses of 40–80 mg intravenously can be given every 10 minutes (maximum dose 300 mg) until the desired blood pressure has been reached. Alternatively, 2 mg/min may be given by intravenous infusion, titrated to desired effect. In patients who have asthma, bradycardia, or other conditions that necessitate the patient's reaction to beta-blockers be tested, esmolol is a reasonable choice because of its short half-life. Give a loading dose of esmolol, 0.5 mg/kg intravenously over 1 minute followed by an infusion of 0.0025–0.02 mg/kg/min. Titrate the infusion to a goal heart rate of 60–70 beats/min. If beta-blockade alone does not control the hypertension, nitroprusside may be added as follows: 50 mg of nitroprusside in 1000 mL of 5% dextrose and water, infused at a rate of 0.5 mL/min; the infusion rate is increased by 0.5 mL every 5 minutes until adequate control of the pressure has been achieved. In patients with bronchial asthma, while there are no data supporting the use of the calcium-channel antagonists, diltiazem and verapamil are potential alternatives to treatment with beta-blocking drugs. Morphine sulfate is the appropriate drug to use for pain relief. Long-term medical care of patients should include beta-blockers in their antihypertensive regimen.

B. Surgical Intervention

Urgent surgical intervention is required for all type A dissections. If a skilled cardiovascular team is not available, the patient should be transferred to an appropriate facility. The procedure involves grafting and replacing the diseased portion of the arch and brachiocephalic vessels as necessary. Replacement of the aortic valve may be required with reattachment of the coronary arteries.

Urgent surgery is required for **type B dissections** if there is aortic branch compromise resulting in malperfusion of the renal, visceral, or extremity vessels. The immediate goal of surgical therapy is to restore flow to the ischemic tissue, which is most commonly accomplished via a bypass. Endovascular stenting of the entry tear at the level of the subclavian artery may result in obliteration of the false lumen and restore flow into the branch vessel from the true lumen. The results, however, are unpredictable and should only be attempted with an experienced team. Evidence is emerging that long-term aortic-specific survival and delayed disease progression are improved with early thoracic stent graft repair.

▶ Prognosis & Follow-up

The mortality rate for untreated type A dissections is approximately 1% per hour for 72 hours and over 90% at 3 months. Mortality is also extremely high for untreated complicated type B dissections. The surgical and endovascular options for these patients also have significant morbidity and mortality. They are technically demanding and require an experienced team to achieve perioperative mortalities of < 10%. Patients with uncomplicated type B dissections whose blood pressure is controlled and who survive the acute episode without complications may have long-term survival without surgical treatment. Aneurysmal enlargement of the false lumen may develop in these patients despite adequate antihypertensive therapy. Yearly CT scans are required to monitor the size of the aneurysm. Indications for repair are determined by size (≥ 6 cm), similar to undissected thoracic aneurysms. Endovascular covering of the intimal tear in the acute setting may prevent this complication, but initial trials on the routine endovascular treatment of type B dissections have not shown an advantage for early intervention and therefore cannot be widely endorsed at this time.

When to Admit

All patients with an acute dissection should be admitted. Any dissection involving the aortic arch (type A) should be immediately repaired. Acute type B dissections require repair only when there is evidence of rupture or major branch occlusion.

Nienaber CA et al. Endovascular repair of type B aortic dissection: long-term results of the randomized investigation of stent grafts in aortic dissection trial. Circ Cardiovasc Interv. 2013 Aug;6(4):407–16. [PMID: 23922146]

Nienaber CA et al. Strategies for subacute/chronic type B aortic dissection: the Investigation Of Stent Grafts in Patients with type B Aortic Dissection (INSTEAD) trial 1-year outcome. J Thorac Cardiovasc Surg. 2010 Dec;140(6 Suppl):S101–8. [PMID: 21092774]

Suzuki T et al; IRAD Investigators. Type-selective benefits of medications in treatment of acute aortic dissection (from the International Registry of Acute Aortic Dissection [IRAD]). Am J Cardiol. 2012 Jan 1;109(1):122–7. [PMID: 21944678]

VENOUS DISEASES

VARICOSE VEINS

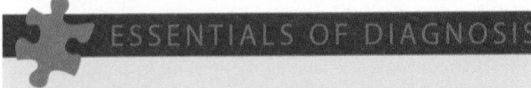

ESSENTIALS OF DIAGNOSIS

▶ Dilated, tortuous superficial veins in the lower extremities.

▶ May be asymptomatic or associated with aching discomfort or pain.

▶ Often hereditary.

▶ Increased frequency after pregnancy.

General Considerations

Varicose veins develop in the lower extremities. Periods of high venous pressure related to prolonged standing or heavy lifting are contributing factors, but the highest incidence occurs in women after pregnancy. Varicosities develop in 15% of all adults.

The superficial veins are most commonly involved, typically the great saphenous vein and its tributaries, but the short saphenous vein (posterior lower leg) may also be affected. Distention of the vein prevents the valve leaflets from coapting, creating incompetence. Thus, dilation at any point along the vein leads to increased pressure and distention of the vein segment below that valve, which in turn causes progressive failure of the next lower valve and progressive venous reflux. Perforating veins that connect the deep and superficial systems may become incompetent, allowing blood to reflux into the superficial veins from the deep system through the incompetent perforators and increasing venous pressure and distention.

Secondary varicosities can develop as a result of obstructive changes and valve damage in the deep venous system following thrombophlebitis, or rarely as a result of proximal venous occlusion due to neoplasm or fibrosis. Congenital or acquired arteriovenous fistulas or venous malformations are also associated with varicosities and should be considered in young patients with varicosities.

Clinical Findings

A. Symptoms and Signs

Symptom severity is not correlated with the number and size of the varicosities; extensive varicose veins may produce no subjective symptoms, whereas minimal varicosities may produce many symptoms. Dull, aching heaviness or a feeling of fatigue of the legs brought on by periods of standing is the most common complaint.

Clinicians must be careful to identify symptoms of occlusive peripheral vascular disease, such as intermittent claudication or reduced pedal pulses, since occlusive arterial disease is usually a contraindication to the operative treatment of varicosities distal to the knee. Itching from venous stasis dermatitis may occur either above the ankle or directly overlying large varicosities.

Dilated, tortuous veins beneath the skin in the thigh and leg are generally visible upon standing, although in very obese patients palpation may be necessary to detect their presence and location. Some swelling is common but secondary tissue changes may be absent even in extensive varicosities. However, if the varicosities are of long duration, brownish pigmentation and thinning of the skin above the ankle may be present. The presence of a bruit or a thrill is useful in making the diagnosis of an associated arteriovenous fistula.

B. Imaging

The identification of the source of venous reflux that feeds the symptomatic veins is necessary for effective surgical treatment. Duplex ultrasonography by a technician experienced in the diagnosis and localization of venous reflux is the test of choice for planning therapy. In most cases, reflux will arise from the greater saphenous vein.

Differential Diagnosis

Primary varicose veins should be differentiated from those secondary to chronic venous insufficiency or obstruction of the deep veins with extensive swelling, fibrosis, and pigmentation, of the distal lower leg (post-thrombotic syndrome). Pain or discomfort secondary to arthritis, radiculopathy, or arterial insufficiency should be distinguished from symptoms associated with coexistent varicose veins. In adolescent patients with varicose veins, imaging of the deep venous system is important to exclude a congenital malformation or atresia of the deep veins. Surgical treatment of varicose veins in these patients is contraindicated because the varicosities may play a significant role in venous drainage of the limb.

▶ Complications

Thrombophlebitis within a varicose vein is uncommon. This presents as subacute to acute localized pain and palpable hardness at the site of the phlebitis. The process is self-limiting, has a low risk of embolization, and usually resolves within weeks. Rarely, the phlebitis extends to involve the greater saphenous vein. Predisposing conditions for thrombophlebitis include pregnancy, local trauma, or prolonged periods of sitting.

In older patients, superficial varicosities may bleed with even minor trauma. The amount of bleeding can be alarming as the pressure in the varicosity is high.

▶ Treatment

A. Nonsurgical Measures

Nonsurgical treatment is effective. Elastic graduated compression stockings (20–30 mm Hg pressure) give external support to the veins. These stockings may be useful in early varicosities to prevent progression of disease. When elastic stockings worn during standing are combined with elevation of the legs when possible, good control can be maintained and the development of complications can often be avoided. This approach may be used in elderly patients, in those who refuse or wish to defer surgery, and in those with mild asymptomatic varicosities.

B. Surgical Measures

Treatment with endovenous ablation (with either radiofrequency or laser) or, less commonly, with greater saphenous vein stripping is very effective for reflux arising from the greater saphenous vein. Less common sources of reflux include the lesser saphenous vein (for varicosities in the posterior calf), and incompetent perforator veins arising directly from the deep venous system in the thigh. Correction of reflux is performed at the same time as excision of the symptomatic varicose veins. Phlebectomy without correction of reflux results in a high rate of recurrent varicosities, as the uncorrected reflux progressively dilates adjacent veins. Concurrent reflux detected by ultrasonography in the deep system is not a contraindication to treatment of superficial reflux because the majority of deep vein dilatation is secondary to volume overload in this setting, which will resolve with correction of the superficial reflux.

C. Compression Sclerotherapy

Sclerotherapy to obliterate and produce permanent fibrosis of the involved veins is generally reserved for the treatment of small varicose veins < 4 mm in diameter. Use of foam sclerotherapy can allow treatment of larger veins, although systemic embolization of the foam sclerosant may be a concern. The injection of the sclerosing solution into the varicosed vein is followed by a period of compression of the segment, resulting in obliteration of the vein. Complications such as phlebitis, tissue necrosis, or infection may occur, and vary in incidence with the skill of the clinician.

▶ Prognosis

Surgical correction of venous insufficiency (reflux) and excision of varicose veins provide excellent results. The 5-year success rate (as defined as lack of pain and recurrent varicosities) is 85–90%. Simple excision (phlebectomy) or injection sclerotherapy without correction of reflux is associated with higher rates of recurrence. Even after adequate treatment, secondary tissue changes, such as lipodermosclerosis, may persist.

▶ When to Refer

- Absolute indications for referral for saphenous ablation include phlebitis and bleeding.
- Pain and cosmetic concerns are responsible for the majority of referrals for ablation.

Di Nisio M et al. Treatment for superficial thrombophlebitis of the leg. Cochrane Database Syst Rev. 2012 Mar14;3:CD004982. [PMID: 22419302]

Figueiredo M et al. Results of surgical treatment compared with ultrasound-guided foam sclerotherapy in patients with varicose veins: a prospective randomised study. Eur J Vasc Endovasc Surg. 2009 Dec;38(6):758–63. [PMID: 19744867]

Gloviczki P et al. The care of patients with varicose veins and associated chronic venous diseases: clinical practice guidelines of the Society for Vascular Surgery and the American Venous Forum. J Vasc Surg. 2011 May;53(5 Suppl):2S–48S. [PMID: 21536172]

Hamdan A et al. JAMA patient page. Treatment of varicose veins. JAMA. 2013 Mar 27;309(12):1306. [PMID: 23532249]

Rasmussen LH et al. Randomised clinical trial comparing endovenous laser ablation with stripping of the great saphenous vein: clinical outcome and recurrence after 2 years. Eur J Vasc Endovasc Surg. 2010 May;39(5):630–5. [PMID: 20064730]

Subramonia S et al. Randomized clinical trial of radiofrequency ablation or conventional high ligation and stripping for great saphenous varicose veins. Br J Surg. 2010 Mar;97(3):328–36. [PMID: 20035541]

SUPERFICIAL VENOUS THROMBOPHLEBITIS

ESSENTIALS OF DIAGNOSIS

- ▶ Induration, redness, and tenderness along a superficial vein, usually the saphenous vein.
- ▶ Induration, redness, and tenderness at the site of a recent intravenous line.
- ▶ Significant swelling of the extremity may not be seen.

▶ General Considerations

Short-term venous catheterization of superficial arm veins as well as the use of longer term peripherally inserted central catheter (PICC) lines are the most common cause of superficial thrombophlebitis. Intravenous catheter sites should be observed daily for signs of local inflammation and should be removed if a local reaction develops in the vein. Serious thrombotic or septic complications can occur if this policy is not followed.

Superficial thrombophlebitis may occur spontaneously, as in pregnant or postpartum women or in individuals with varicose veins or thromboangitis obliterans; or it may be associated with trauma, as in the case of a blow to the leg or following intravenous therapy with irritating solutions. It also may be a manifestation of systemic hypercoagulability secondary to abdominal cancer such as carcinoma of the pancreas and may be the earliest sign of these conditions. Superficial thrombophlebitis may be associated with occult deep venous thrombosis (DVT) in about 20% of cases. Pulmonary emboli are exceedingly rare and occur from an associated DVT. (See Chapters 9 and Chapters 14 for discussion on Deep Venous Thrombosis.)

Clinical Findings

In spontaneous superficial thrombophlebitis, the greater saphenous vein is most often involved. The patient usually experiences a dull pain in the region of the involved vein. Local findings consist of induration, redness, and tenderness along the course of a vein. The process may be localized, or it may involve most of the long saphenous vein and its tributaries. The inflammatory reaction generally subsides in 1–2 weeks; a firm cord may remain for a much longer period. Edema of the extremity is uncommon.

Localized redness and induration at the site of a recent intravenous line requires urgent attention. Proximal extension of the induration and pain with chills and high fever suggest septic phlebitis and requires urgent treatment.

Differential Diagnosis

The linear rather than circular nature of the lesion and the distribution along the course of a superficial vein serve to differentiate superficial phlebitis from cellulitis, erythema nodosum, erythema induratum, panniculitis, and fibrositis. Lymphangitis and deep thrombophlebitis must also be considered.

Treatment

For spontaneous thrombophlebitis if the process is well localized and not near the saphenofemoral junction, local heat, and nonsteroidal anti-inflammatory medications are usually effective in limiting the process. If the induration is extensive or is progressing toward the saphenofemoral junction (leg) or cephalo-axillary junction (arm), ligation and division of the vein at the junction of the deep and superficial veins is indicated.

Anticoagulation therapy is usually not required for focal processes. Prophylactic dose low-molecular-weight heparin or fondaparinux is recommended for 5 cm or longer superficial thrombophlebitis of the lower limb veins and full anticoagulation is reserved for disease that is rapidly progressing or there is concern for extension into the deep system.

Septic superficial thrombophlebitis is an intravascular abscess and requires urgent treatment with heparin (see Table 14–15) to limit additional thrombus formation as well as removal of the offending catheter in catheter-related

infections (see Chapter 30). *Staphylococcus aureus* is the most common pathogen. Treat with antibiotics (eg, vancomycin, 15 mg/kg intravenously every 12 hours plus ceftriaxone, 1 g intravenously every 24 hours). If cultures are positive, therapy should be continued for 7–10 days or for 4–6 weeks if complicating endocarditis cannot be excluded. Other organisms, including fungi, may also be responsible. Surgical excision of the involved vein may also be necessary to control the infection.

Prognosis

With spontaneous thrombophlebitis, the course is generally benign and brief. The prognosis depends on the underlying pathologic process. In patients with phlebitis secondary to varicose veins, recurrent episodes are likely unless correction of the underlying venous reflux and excision of varicosities is done. In contrast, the mortality from septic thrombophlebitis is 20% or higher and requires aggressive treatment. However, if the involvement is localized, the mortality is low and prognosis is excellent with early treatment.

Decousus H et al; CALISTO Study Group. Fondaparinux for the treatment of superficial-vein thrombosis in the legs. N Engl J Med. 2010 Sep 23;363(13):1222–32. [PMID: 20860504]

Decousus H et al; POST (Prospective Observational Superficial Thrombophlebitis) Study Group. Superficial venous thrombosis and venous thromboembolism: a large, prospective epidemiologic study. Ann Intern Med. 2010 Feb 16;152(4):218–24. [PMID: 20157136]

Stevens SM. ACP Journal Club: review: fondaparinux reduces VTE and recurrence in superficial thrombophlebitis of the leg. Ann Intern Med. 2012 Aug 21;157(4):JC2–4. [PMID: 22910958]

van Weert H et al. Spontaneous superficial venous thrombophlebitis: does it increase risk for thromboembolism? A historic follow-up study in primary care. J Fam Pract. 2006 Jan;55(1):52–7. [PMID: 16388768]

CHRONIC VENOUS INSUFFICIENCY

ESSENTIALS OF DIAGNOSIS

- ► History of prior DVT or leg injury.
- ► Edema, stasis (brawny) skin pigmentation, subcutaneous liposclerosis in the lower leg.
- ► Large ulcerations at or above the ankle are common (stasis ulcers).

General Considerations

Chronic venous insufficiency can result from changes secondary to acute deep venous thrombophlebitis (see Chapter 14), although a definite history of phlebitis is not obtainable in about 25% of these patients. There may be a history of leg trauma. Obesity is often a complicating factor. Chronic venous insufficiency also may occur in association with superficial venous reflux and varicose veins or as a result of neoplastic obstruction of the pelvic veins or congenital or acquired arteriovenous fistula.

The basic pathology is caused by valve leaflets that do not coapt because they are either thickened and scarred (the post-thrombotic syndrome) or in a dilated vein and are therefore functionally inadequate. This results in an abnormally high hydrostatic force transmitted to the subcutaneous veins and tissues of the lower leg. The resulting edema results in dramatic and deleterious secondary changes. The stigmata of chronic venous insufficiency include fibrosis of the subcutaneous tissue and skin, pigmentation of skin (hemosiderin taken up by the dermal macrophages) and, later, ulceration, which is extremely slow to heal. Itching may precipitate the formation of ulceration or local wound cellulitis. Dilation of the superficial veins may occur, leading to varicosities. Whereas primary varicose veins with no abnormality of the deep venous system may be associated with some similar changes, the edema is more pronounced in the post-thrombotic extremities, and the secondary changes are more extensive and debilitating.

Clinical Findings

A. Symptoms and Signs

Progressive pitting edema of the leg (particularly the lower leg) is the primary presenting symptom. Secondary changes in the skin and subcutaneous tissues develop over time. The usual symptoms are itching, a dull discomfort made worse by periods of standing, and pain if an ulceration is present. The skin at the ankle is usually taut from swelling, shiny, and a brownish pigmentation (hemosiderin) often develops. If the condition is long-standing, the subcutaneous tissues become thick and fibrous. Ulcerations may occur, usually just above the ankle, on the medial or anterior aspect of the leg. Healing results in a thin scar on a fibrotic base that often breaks down with minor trauma or further bouts of leg swelling. Varicosities may appear that are associated with incompetent perforating veins. Cellulitis, which is often difficult to distinguish from the hemosiderin pigmentation, may be diagnosed by blanching erythema.

B. Imaging

Patients with post-thrombotic syndrome or signs of chronic venous insufficiency should undergo duplex ultrasonography to determine whether superficial reflux is present and to evaluate the degree of deep reflux and obstruction.

Differential Diagnosis

Patients with heart failure, chronic kidney disease, or decompensated liver disease may have bilateral edema of the lower extremities. Swelling from lymphedema may be unilateral, but varicosities are absent. Edema from these causes pits easily and brawny discoloration is rare. Lipedema is a disorder of adipose tissue that occurs almost exclusively in women, is bilateral and symmetric, and is characterized by stopping at a distinct line just above the ankles.

Primary varicose veins may be difficult to differentiate from the secondary varicosities of chronic venous insufficiency.

Other conditions associated with chronic ulcers of the leg include neuropathic ulcers usually from diabetes mellitus, arterial insufficiency (often very painful with absent pulses), autoimmune diseases (eg, Felty syndrome), sickle cell anemia, erythema induratum (bilateral and usually on the posterior aspect of the lower part of the leg), and fungal infections.

Prevention

Irreversible tissue changes and associated complications in the lower legs can be minimized through early and aggressive anticoagulation of acute DVT to minimize the valve damages and by prescribing compression stockings if chronic edema develops after the DVT has resolved. Catheter-directed thrombolysis or mechanical thrombectomy of acute iliofemoral DVT may be of greater value than simple anticoagulants in preventing post-thrombotic syndrome and chronic venous insufficiency.

Treatment

A. General Measures

Fitted, graduated compression stockings worn from the foot to just below the knee during the day and evening are the mainstays of treatment and is usually sufficient. When it is not, additional measures, such as avoidance of long periods of sitting or standing and intermittent elevations of the involved leg and sleeping with the legs kept above the level of the heart, may be necessary to control the swelling. Pneumatic compression of the leg, which can pump the fluid out of the leg, is used in cases refractory to the above measures.

B. Ulceration

As the primary pathology is edema, healing of the ulcer will not occur until the edema is controlled. A lesion can often be treated on an ambulatory basis by means of a semi-rigid gauze boot made with Unna paste (Gelocast, Medicopaste) or a multi-layer compression (such as Profore) and applied to the leg after much of the swelling has been reduced by a period of elevation. The boot must be changed every 2–3 days, depending on the amount of drainage from the ulcer. The ulcer, tendons, and bony prominences must be adequately padded. As an alternative and after the ulcer has healed, knee-high elastic stockings with graduated compression are used in an effort to prevent recurrent edema and ulceration. If compression stockings are used with ulcers, an absorbent dressing must be applied under the stocking as the wounds can leak large volumes of fluid. The pumping action of the calf muscles on the blood flow out of the lower extremity is enhanced by a circumferential nonelastic bandage on the ankle and lower leg. Home compression therapy with a pneumatic compression device is also effective at reducing edema, but many patients have severe pain with the "milking" action of the pump device. Some patients will require admission for complete bed rest and leg elevation to achieve ulcer healing.

C. Correction of Superficial Reflux

Compression with treatment of superficial vein reflux has been shown to decrease the recurrence rate of venous ulcers. Incompetent (refluxing) perforator veins that feed the area of ulceration can be treated with percutaneous means (radiofrequency ablation or endovenous laser treatment) to help decrease the venous pressure in the area of ulceration and promote healing. Where there is substantial obstruction of the deep venous system, superficial varicosities supply the venous return and they should not be removed.

▶ Prognosis

Individuals with chronic venous insufficiency often have recurrent problems, particularly if they do not consistently wear support stockings that have at least 30 mm Hg compression.

▶ When to Refer

- Patients with significant saphenous reflux should be evaluated for ablation as this may reduce the recirculation of blood and return the deep system to competence.
- Patients with ulcers should be monitored by a wound care team so that these challenging wounds can receive aggressive care.

Bergan JJ et al. Chronic venous disease. N Engl J Med. 2006 Aug 3;355(5):488–98. [PMID: 16885552]

Deatrick KB et al. Chronic venous insufficiency: current management of varicose vein disease. Am Surg. 2010 Feb;76(2):125–32. [PMID: 20336886]

Eberhard RT et al. Chronic venous insufficiency. Circulation. 2005 May 10;111(18):2398–409. [PMID: 15883226]

Gohel MS et al. Long term results of compression therapy alone versus compression plus surgery in chronic venous ulceration (ESCHAR): randomised controlled trial. BMJ. 2007 Jul 14;335(7610):83. [PMID: 17545185]

Patel NP et al. Current management of venous ulceration. Plast Reconstr Surg. 2006 Jun;117(7 Suppl):254S–260S. [PMID: 16799394]

SUPERIOR VENA CAVAL OBSTRUCTION

ESSENTIALS OF DIAGNOSIS

- ▶ Swelling of the neck, face, and upper extremities.
- ▶ Dilated veins over the upper chest and neck.

▶ General Considerations

Partial or complete obstruction of the superior vena cava is a relatively rare condition that is usually secondary to neoplastic or inflammatory processes in the superior mediastinum. The most frequent causes are (1) neoplasms, such as lymphomas, primary malignant mediastinal tumors, or carcinoma of the lung with direct extension (over 80%); (2) chronic fibrotic mediastinitis, either of unknown origin or secondary to tuberculosis, histoplasmosis, pyogenic infections, or drugs, especially methysergide; (3) DVT, often by extension of the process from the axillary or subclavian

vein into the innominate vein and vena cava associated with catheterization of these veins for dialysis or for hyperalimentation; (4) aneurysm of the aortic arch; and (5) constrictive pericarditis.

▶ Clinical Findings

A. Symptoms and Signs

The onset of symptoms is acute or subacute. Symptoms include swelling of the neck and face, and upper extremities. Symptoms are often perceived as congestion and present as headache, dizziness, visual disturbances, stupor, syncope, or cough. Symptoms are particularly exacerbated when the patient is supine or bends over. There is progressive obstruction of the venous drainage of the head, neck, and upper extremities. The cutaneous veins of the upper chest and lower neck become dilated, and flushing of the face and neck develops. Brawny edema of the face, neck, and arms occurs later, and cyanosis of these areas then appears. Cerebral and laryngeal edema ultimately results in impaired function of the brain as well as respiratory insufficiency. Bending over or lying down accentuates the symptoms; sitting quietly is generally preferred. The manifestations are more severe if the obstruction develops rapidly and if the azygos junction or the vena cava between that vein and the heart is obstructed.

B. Laboratory Findings

The venous pressure is elevated (often < 20 cm of water) in the arm and is normal in the leg. Since lung cancer is a common cause, bronchoscopy is often performed; transbronchial biopsy, however, is relatively contraindicated because of venous hypertension and the risk of bleeding.

C. Imaging

Chest radiographs and a CT scan will define the location and often the nature of the obstructive process, and contrast venography or magnetic resonance venography (MRV) will map out the extent and degree of the venous obstruction and the collateral circulation. Brachial venography or radionuclide scanning following intravenous injection of technetium Tc-99m pertechnetate demonstrates a block to the flow of contrast material into the right heart and enlarged collateral veins. These techniques also allow estimation of blood flow around the occlusion as well as serial evaluation of the response to therapy.

▶ Treatment

Urgent treatment for neoplasm consists of (1) cautious use of intravenous diuretics and (2) mediastinal irradiation, starting within 24 hours, with a treatment plan designed to give a high daily dose but a short total course of therapy to rapidly shrink the local tumor. Intensive combined therapy will palliate the process in up to 90% of patients. In patients with a subacute presentation, radiation therapy alone usually suffices. Chemotherapy is added if lymphoma or small-cell carcinoma is diagnosed.

Conservative measures, such as elevation of the head of the bed and lifestyle modification to avoid bending over, are useful. Balloon angioplasty of the obstructed caval segment combined with stent placement provides prompt relief of symptoms and is the procedure of choice. Occasionally, anticoagulation is needed, while thrombolysis is rarely needed. Long-term outcome is complicated by risk of re-occlusion from either thrombosis or further growth of the neoplasm. Surgical procedures to bypass the obstruction are complicated by bleeding relating to high venous pressure. In cases where the thrombosis is secondary to an indwelling catheter, thrombolysis may be attempted. Clinical judgment is required since a long-standing clot may be fibrotic and the risk of bleeding will outweigh the potential benefit.

Prognosis

The prognosis depends on the nature and degree of obstruction and its speed of onset. Slowly developing forms secondary to fibrosis may be tolerated for years. A high degree of obstruction of rapid onset secondary to cancer is often fatal in a few days or weeks because of increased intracranial pressure and cerebral hemorrhage, but treatment of the tumor with radiation and chemotherapeutic drugs may result in significant palliation. Balloon angioplasty and stenting provides good relief but may require re-treatment for recurrent symptoms secondary to thrombosis or restenosis.

When to Refer

Referral should occur with any patient with progressive head and neck swelling to rule out superior vena cava syndrome.

When to Admit

Any patient with acute edema of the head and neck or any patient in whom signs and symptoms of airway compromise, such as hoarseness or stridor, develop should be admitted.

Lepper PM et al. Superior vena cava syndrome in thoracic malignancies. Respir Care. 2011 May;56(5):653–66. [PMID: 21276318]

Watkinson AF et al. Endovascular stenting to treat obstruction of the superior vena cava. BMJ. 2008 Jun 21;336(7658):1434–7. [PMID: 18566082]

Wilson LD et al. Clinical practice. Superior vena cava syndrome with malignant causes. N Engl J Med. 2007 May 3;356(18):1862–9. [PMID: 17476012]

DISEASES OF THE LYMPHATIC CHANNELS

LYMPHANGITIS & LYMPHADENITIS

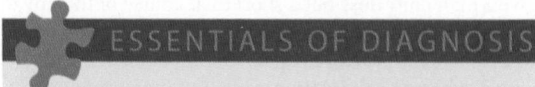

ESSENTIALS OF DIAGNOSIS

► Red streak from wound or area of cellulitis toward regional lymph nodes, which are usually enlarged and tender.

► Chills, fever, and malaise may be present.

General Considerations

Lymphangitis and lymphadenitis are common manifestations of a bacterial infection that is usually caused by hemolytic streptococci or *S aureus* (or by both organisms) and usually arises from the site of an infected wound. The wound may be very small or superficial, or an established abscess may be present, feeding bacteria into the lymphatics. The involvement of the lymphatics is often manifested by a red streak in the skin extending in the direction of the regional lymph nodes, which are, in turn, generally tender and engorged. Systemic manifestations include fever, chills, and malaise. The infection may progress rapidly, often in a matter of hours, and may lead to septicemia and even death.

Clinical Findings

A. Symptoms and Signs

Throbbing pain is usually present in the area of cellulitis at the site of bacterial invasion. Malaise, anorexia, sweating, chills, and fever of 38–40°C develop rapidly. The red streak, when present, may be definite or may be very faint and easily missed, especially in dark-skinned patients. It is usually tender or indurated in the area of cellulitis. The involved regional lymph nodes may be significantly enlarged and are usually quite tender. The pulse is often rapid.

B. Laboratory Findings

Leukocytosis with a left shift is usually present. Blood cultures may be positive, most often for staphylococcal or streptococcal species. Culture and sensitivity studies of the wound exudate or pus may be helpful in treatment of the more severe or refractory infections but are often difficult to interpret because of skin contaminants.

Differential Diagnosis

Lymphangitis may be confused with superficial thrombophlebitis, but the erythema and induration of thrombophlebitis is localized in and around the thrombosed vein. Venous thrombosis is not associated with lymphadenitis, and a wound of entrance with secondary cellulitis is generally absent.

Cat-scratch fever (*Bartonella henselae*) should be considered when lymphadenitis is present; the nodes, though often very large, are relatively nontender. Exposure to cats is common, but the patient may have forgotten about the scratch.

It is extremely important to differentiate cellulitis from acute streptococcal hemolytic gangrene or necrotizing fasciitis. These are deeper infections that may be extensive and are potentially lethal. Patients appear more seriously ill; there may be redness due to leakage of red cells, creating a non-blanching erythema; and subcutaneous crepitus may be palpated or auscultated using the diaphragm with light pressure over the involved area. Immediate wide debridement of all involved deep tissues should be done if these signs are present.

Treatment

A. General Measures

Prompt treatment should include heat (hot, moist compresses or heating pad), elevation when feasible, and immobilization of the infected area. Analgesics may be prescribed for pain.

B. Specific Measures

Empiric antibiotic therapy for hemolytic streptococci or *S aureus* (or by both organisms) should always be instituted when local infection becomes invasive, as manifested by cellulitis and lymphangitis. Because such infections are so frequently caused by streptococci, cephalosporins or extended-spectrum penicillins are commonly used (eg, cephalexin, 0.5 g orally four times daily for 7–10 days; see Table 30–6). Given the increasing incidence of methicillin-resistant *S aureus* (MRSA) in the community, coverage of this pathogen with appropriate antibiotic therapy (eg, trimethoprim-sulfamethoxazole, two double strength tablets twice daily for 7–10 days) should be considered (see Tables 30–4 and 30–6).

C. Wound Care

Any wound that is the initiating site of lymphangitis should be treated aggressively. Any necrotic tissue must be debrided and loculated pus drained.

► Prognosis

With proper therapy including an antibiotic effective against the invading bacteria, control of the infection can usually be achieved in a few days. Delayed or inadequate therapy can lead to overwhelming infection with septicemia.

► When to Admit

Infections causing lymphangitis should be treated in the hospital with intravenous antibiotics. Debridement may be required.

LYMPHEDEMA

ESSENTIALS OF DIAGNOSIS

► Painless persistent edema of one or both lower extremities, primarily in young women.

► Pitting edema without ulceration, varicosities, or stasis pigmentation.

► There may be episodes of lymphangitis and cellulitis.

► General Considerations

When lymphedema is due to congenital developmental abnormalities consisting of hypoplastic or hyperplastic involvement of the proximal or distal lymphatics, it is referred to as the **primary form**. The obstruction may be in the pelvic or lumbar lymph channels and nodes when the disease is extensive and progressive. The **secondary form** of lymphedema involves inflammatory or mechanical lymphatic obstruction from trauma, regional lymph node resection or irradiation, or extensive involvement of regional nodes by malignant disease or filariasis. Lymphedema may occur following surgical removal of the lymph nodes in the groin or axillae. Secondary dilation of the lymphatics that occurs in both forms leads to incompetence of the valve system, disrupts the orderly flow along the lymph vessels, and results in progressive stasis of a protein-rich fluid. Episodes of acute and chronic inflammation may be superimposed, with further stasis and secondary fibrosis.

► Clinical Findings

Hypertrophy of the limb results, with markedly thickened and fibrotic skin and subcutaneous tissue in very advanced cases.

Lymphangiography and radioactive isotope studies may identify focal defects in lymph flow but are of little value in planning therapy. T_2–weighted MRI has been used to identify lymphatics and proximal obstructing masses.

► Treatment

Since there is no effective cure for lymphedema, the treatment strategies are designed to control the problem and allow normal activity and function. Most patients can be treated with some of the following measures: (1) The flow of lymph out of the extremity can be aided through intermittent elevation of the extremity, especially during the sleeping hours (foot of bed elevated 15–20 degrees, achieved by placing pillows beneath the mattress); the constant use of graduated elastic compression stockings; and massage toward the trunk—either by hand or by means of pneumatic pressure devices designed to milk edema out of an extremity. (2) Secondary cellulitis in the extremity should be avoided by means of good hygiene and treatment of any trichophytosis of the toes. Once an infection starts, it should be treated by periods of elevation and antibiotic therapy that covers *Staphylococcus* and *Streptococcus* organisms (see Table 30–6). Infections can be a serious and recurring problem and are often difficult to control. Prophylactic antibiotics have not been shown to be of benefit. (3) Intermittent courses of diuretic therapy, especially in those with premenstrual or seasonal exacerbations, are rarely helpful. (4) Amputation is used only for the rare complication of lymphangiosarcoma in the extremity.

► Prognosis

With aggressive treatment, including pneumatic compression devices, good relief of symptoms can be achieved. The long-term outlook is dictated by the associated conditions and avoidance of recurrent cellulitis.

Ashikaga T et al; National Surgical Adjuvant Breast, Bowel Project. Morbidity results from the NSABP B-32 trial comparing sentinel lymph node dissection versus axillary dissection. J Surg Oncol. 2010 Aug 1;102(2):111–8. [PMID: 20648579]

Haghighat S et al. Comparing two treatment methods for post mastectomy lymphedema: complex decongestive therapy alone and in combination with intermittent pneumatic compression. Lymphology. 2010 Mar;43(1):25–33. [PMID: 20552817]

Murdaca G et al. Current views on diagnostic approach and treatment of lymphedema. Am J Med. 2012 Feb;125(2):134–40. [PMID: 22269614]

Rockson SG. Diagnosis and management of lymphatic vascular disease. J Am Coll Cardiol. 2008 Sep 2;52(10):799–806. [PMID: 18755341]

Torres Lacomba M et al. Effectiveness of early physiotherapy to prevent lymphoedema after surgery for breast cancer: randomised, single blinded, clinical trial. BMJ. 2010 Jan 12;340:b5396. [PMID: 20068255]

SHOCK

ESSENTIALS OF DIAGNOSIS

► Hypotension, tachycardia, oliguria, altered mental status.

► Peripheral hypoperfusion and impaired oxygen delivery.

► General Considerations

Shock occurs when the rate of arterial blood flow is inadequate to meet tissue metabolic needs. This results in regional hypoxia and subsequent lactic acidosis from anaerobic metabolism in peripheral tissues as well as eventual end-organ damage and failure.

► Classification (Table 12–1)

A. Hypovolemic Shock

Hypovolemic shock results from decreased intravascular volume secondary to loss of blood or fluids and electrolytes. The etiology may be suggested by the clinical setting (eg, trauma) or by signs and symptoms of blood loss (eg, gastrointestinal bleeding) or dehydration (eg, vomiting or diarrhea). Compensatory vasoconstriction may transiently maintain the blood pressure but unreplaced losses of over 15% of the intravascular volume can result in hypotension and progressive tissue hypoxia.

B. Cardiogenic Shock

Cardiogenic shock results from cardiac failure with the resultant inability of the heart to maintain adequate tissue perfusion. The clinical definition of cardiogenic shock is evidence of tissue hypoxia due to decreased cardiac output (cardiac index < 2.2 L/min/m^2) in the presence of adequate intravascular volume. This is most often caused by myocardial infarction but can also be due to cardiomyopathy, myocardial contusion, valvular incompetence or stenosis, or arrhythmias. See Chapter 10.

C. Obstructive Shock

Cardiac tamponade, tension pneumothorax, and massive pulmonary embolism can cause an acute decrease in cardiac output resulting in shock. These are medical emergencies requiring prompt diagnosis and treatment.

Table 12–1. Classification of shock by mechanism and common causes.

Hypovolemic shock
Loss of blood (hemorrhagic shock)
External hemorrhage
Trauma
Gastrointestinal tract bleeding
Internal hemorrhage
Hematoma
Hemothorax or hemoperitoneum
Loss of plasma
Burns
Exfoliative dermatitis
Loss of fluid and electrolytes
External losses
Vomiting
Diarrhea
Excessive sweating
Hyperosmolar states (diabetic ketoacidosis, hyperosmolar nonketotic coma)
Internal losses (third spacing)
Pancreatitis
Ascites
Bowel obstruction
Cardiogenic shock
Dysrhythmia (tachyarrhythmia, bradyarrhythmia)
"Pump failure" (secondary to myocardial infarction or other cardiomyopathy)
Acute valvular dysfunction (especially regurgitant lesions)
Rupture of ventricular septum or free ventricular wall
Obstructive shock
Tension pneumothorax
Pericardial disease (tamponade, constriction)
Disease of pulmonary vasculature (massive pulmonary emboli, pulmonary hypertension)
Cardiac tumor (atrial myxoma)
Left atrial mural thrombus
Obstructive valvular disease (aortic or mitral stenosis)
Distributive shock
Septic shock
Anaphylactic shock
Neurogenic shock
Vasodilator drugs
Acute adrenal insufficiency

Reproduced, with permission, from Stone CK, Humphries RL (editors). *Current Emergency Diagnosis & Treatment*, 5th ed. p. 193. McGraw-Hill, 2004.

D. Distributive Shock

Distributive or vasodilatory shock has many causes including sepsis, anaphylaxis, systemic inflammatory response syndrome (SIRS) produced by severe pancreatitis or burns, traumatic spinal cord injury, or acute adrenal insufficiency. The reduction in systemic vascular resistance results in inadequate cardiac output and tissue hypoperfusion despite normal circulatory volume.

1. Septic shock—Sepsis is the most common cause of distributive shock and carries a mortality rate of 20–50%. Sepsis is defined as the presence of infection (either documented or suspected) in conjunction with systemic manifestations of infection. Septic shock is diagnosed when hypotension from sepsis persists despite adequate fluid resuscitation. The most common cause of septic shock in hospitalized patients is infection with gram-positive or gram-negative organisms; polymicrobial infections are almost as likely. The incidence of sepsis from fungal organisms is increasing but remains less than that for bacterial infections. Risk factors for septic shock include bacteremia, extremes of age, diabetes, cancer, immunosuppression, and history of a recent invasive procedure.

2. Systemic inflammatory response syndrome (SIRS)— Defined as a systemic response to a nonspecific infectious or noninfectious insult—such as from burns, pancreatitis, an autoimmune disorder, ischemia, or trauma—the presence of two or more of the following clinical criteria help establish the diagnosis of SIRS: (1) body temperature > 38°C (100.4°F) or < 36°C (96.8°F), (2) heart rate > 90 beats per minute, (3) respiratory rate more than 20 breaths per minute or hyperventilation with an arterial carbon dioxide tension ($Paco_2$) > 32 mm Hg, (4) abnormal white blood cell count (> 12,000/mcL or < 4000/mcL or > 10% immature (band) forms). When a source of infection is confirmed, SIRS is categorized as sepsis.

3. Neurogenic shock—Neurogenic shock is caused by traumatic spinal cord injury or effects of an epidural or spinal anesthetic. This results in loss of sympathetic tone with a reduction in systemic vascular resistance and hypotension without a compensatory tachycardia. Reflex vagal parasympathetic stimulation evoked by pain, gastric dilation, or fright may simulate neurogenic shock, producing hypotension, bradycardia, and syncope.

▶ Clinical Findings

A. Symptoms and Signs

Hypotension is traditionally defined as a systolic blood pressure of ≤ 90 mm Hg or a mean arterial pressure of < 60–65 mm Hg but must be evaluated relative to the patient's normal blood pressure. A drop in systolic pressure of > 10–20 mm Hg or an increase in pulse of > 15 beats per minute with positional change suggests depleted intravascular volume. However, blood pressure is often not the best indicator of end-organ perfusion because compensatory mechanisms, such as increased heart rate, increased cardiac contractility, and vasoconstriction can occur to prevent hypotension. Patients with hypotension often have cool or mottled extremities and weak or thready peripheral pulses. Splanchnic vasoconstriction may lead to oliguria, bowel ischemia, and hepatic dysfunction, which can ultimately result in multi-organ failure. Mentation may be normal or patients may become restless, agitated, confused, lethargic, or comatose as a result of inadequate perfusion of the brain.

Hypovolemic shock is evident when signs of hypoperfusion, such as oliguria, altered mental status, and cool extremities, are present. Jugular venous pressure is low, and there is a narrow pulse pressure indicative of reduced stroke volume. Rapid replacement of fluids restores tissue perfusion. In **cardiogenic shock,** there are also signs of global hypoperfusion with oliguria, altered mental status, and cool extremities.

Jugular venous pressure is elevated and there may be evidence of pulmonary edema with respiratory compromise in the setting of left-sided heart failure. A transthoracic echocardiogram (TTE) or a transesophageal echocardiogram (TEE) is an effective diagnostic tool to differentiate hypovolemic from cardiogenic shock. In hypovolemic shock, the left ventricle will be small because of decreased filling, but contractility is often preserved. Cardiogenic shock results from cardiac failure with a resultant decrease in left ventricular contractility. In some cases, the left ventricle may appear dilated and full because of the inability of the left ventricle to eject a sufficient stroke volume.

In **obstructive shock**, the central venous pressure may be elevated but the TTE or TEE may show reduced left ventricular filling, a pericardial effusion in the case of tamponade, or thickened pericardium as in the case of pericarditis. Pericardiocentesis or pericardial window for pericardial tamponade, chest tube placement for tension pneumothorax, or catheter-directed thrombolytic therapy in the case of massive pulmonary embolism can be lifesaving in cases of obstructive shock.

In **distributive shock,** signs include hyperdynamic heart sounds, warm extremities initially, and a wide pulse pressure indicative of large stroke volume. The echocardiogram may show a hyperdynamic left ventricle. Fluid resuscitation may have little effect on blood pressure, urinary output, or mentation. **Septic shock** is diagnosed when there is clinical evidence of infection in the setting of persistent hypotension and evidence of organ hypoperfusion, such as lactic acidosis, decreased urinary output, or altered mental status despite adequate volume resuscitation. **Neurogenic shock** is diagnosed when there is evidence of central nervous system injury and persistent hypotension despite adequate volume resuscitation.

B. Laboratory Findings and Imaging

Blood specimens should be evaluated for complete blood count, electrolytes, glucose, arterial blood gas determinations, coagulation parameters, lactate levels, typing and cross-matching, and bacterial cultures. An electrocardiogram and chest radiograph should also be part of the initial assessment.

▶ Treatment

A. General Measures

Treatment depends on prompt diagnosis and an accurate appraisal of inciting conditions. Initial management consists of basic life support with an assessment of the patient's airway, breathing, and circulation. This may entail airway intubation and mechanical ventilation. Ventilatory failure should be anticipated in patients with a severe metabolic acidosis in association with shock. Mechanical ventilation along with sedation can decrease the oxygen demand of the respiratory muscles and allow improved oxygen delivery to other hypoperfused tissues. Intravenous access and fluid resuscitation should be instituted along with cardiac monitoring and assessment of hemodynamic parameters such as blood pressure and heart rate. Cardiac monitoring can detect myocardial ischemia or malignant arrhythmias, which can be treated by standard advanced cardiac life support (ACLS) protocols.

Unresponsive or minimally responsive patients should have their glucose checked immediately and if their glucose level is low, 1 ampule of **50% dextrose** intravenously should be given. An **arterial line** should be placed for continuous blood pressure measurement, and a **Foley catheter** should be inserted to monitor urinary output.

B. Central Venous Pressure

Early consideration is given to placement of a central venous catheter (CVC) for infusion of fluids and medications and for hemodynamic pressure measurements. A CVC can provide measurements of the central venous pressure (CVP) and the central venous oxygen saturation ($ScvO_2$), both of which can be used to manage sepsis and septic shock. Pulmonary artery catheters (PACs) allow measurement of the pulmonary artery pressure, left-sided filling pressure or the pulmonary capillary wedge pressure (PCWP), the mixed venous oxygen saturation (SvO_2) and cardiac output. Meta-analyses of multiple studies, including randomized controlled trials, suggest that the use of PACs do not increase overall mortality or length of hospital stay, but are associated with higher use of inotropes and intravenous vasodilators in critically ill patients from different patient populations (including those with sepsis, myocardial ischemia, and those who were postsurgical). Thus, the routine use of PACs cannot be recommended. However, in some complex situations, PACs may be useful in distinguishing between cardiogenic and septic shock. The attendant risks associated with PACs (such as infection, arrhythmias, vein thrombosis, and pulmonary artery rupture) can be as high as 4–9%; therefore, the value of the information they might provide must be carefully weighed in each patient. TTE is a noninvasive alternative to the PAC. TTE can provide information about the pulmonary artery pressure, PCWP, and cardiac output; in addition, TTE can provide valuable information about current cardiac function. The SvO_2, one parameter used to guide sepsis management, is obtained through the PAC. However, the $ScvO_2$, which is obtained through the CVC, is similar to the SvO_2 and can be used as a surrogate. Pulse pressure variation, as determined by arterial waveform analysis, or stroke volume variation are much more sensitive than CVP as a measure of fluid responsiveness in volume resuscitation, but these measurements are only valid in patients who are mechanically ventilated and in normal sinus rhythm.

A CVP < 5 mm Hg suggests hypovolemia, and a CVP over 18 mm Hg suggests volume overload, cardiac failure, tamponade, or pulmonary hypertension. A cardiac index < 2 L/min/m² indicates a need for inotropic support. A high cardiac index > 4 L/min/m² in a hypotensive patient is consistent with early septic shock. The systemic vascular resistance is low (< 800 dynes . s/cm⁻⁵) in sepsis and neurogenic shock and high (> 1500 dynes . s/cm⁻⁵) in hypovolemic and cardiogenic shock. Treatment is directed at maintaining a CVP of 8–12 mm Hg, a mean arterial pressure of 65–90 mm Hg, a cardiac index of 2–4 L/min/m², and a $ScvO_2$ < 70%.

C. Volume Replacement

Volume replacement is critical in the initial management of shock. **Hemorrhagic shock** is treated with immediate efforts to achieve hemostasis and rapid infusions of blood substitutes, such as type-specific or type O negative packed red blood cells (PRBCs) or whole blood, which also provides extra volume and clotting factors. Each unit of PRBC or whole blood is expected to raise the hematocrit by 3%. **Hypovolemic shock** secondary to dehydration is managed with rapid boluses of isotonic crystalloid (0.9% saline or lactated Ringer solution) usually in 1-liter increments. **Cardiogenic shock** in the absence of fluid overload requires smaller fluid challenges, usually in increments of 250 mL. **Septic shock** usually requires large volumes of fluid for resuscitation (usually < 2 L) as the associated capillary leak releases fluid into the extravascular space. Caution must be used with large-volume resuscitation with unwarmed fluids because this can produce hypothermia, which can lead to hypothermia-induced coagulopathy. Warming of fluids before administration can avoid this complication.

Meta-analyses of studies of heterogenous critically ill populations comparing crystalloid and colloid resuscitation (with albumin) indicate no benefit of colloid over crystalloid solutions except in trauma patients with traumatic brain injury who had a higher mortality if albumin was used for volume resuscitation. Clinical trials and meta-analyses have also found no difference in mortality between trauma patients receiving hypertonic saline (7.5%) and those receiving isotonic crystalloid. More positive results were found with hypertonic saline plus dextran with an increase in survival over patients managed with isotonic saline, particularly in patients with traumatic brain injury.

D. Early Goal-Directed Therapy

Early goal-directed therapy following set protocols for the treatment of septic shock provides significant benefits (see www.survivingsepsis.org). In a 2001 randomized controlled trial, patients with severe sepsis or septic shock were assigned to receive either 6 hours of early goal-directed therapy or usual care prior to admission to the intensive care unit. Patients assigned to early goal-directed care received fluid resuscitation to achieve a CVP of 8–12 mm Hg; vasopressors to maintain a mean arterial blood pressure of at least 65 mm Hg; PRBCs to reach a hematocrit of 30% if the $ScvO_2$ was < 70%; and if, after PRBC transfusion, the $ScvO_2$ remained < 70%, dobutamine to raise the $ScvO_2$ > 70%. When compared with controls, these patients had a significantly lower in-hospital mortality rate (46.5% for standard therapy, 30.5% for early goal-directed therapy; $P = .009$) and 60-day mortality rate (57% for standard therapy, 44% for early goal-directed therapy; $P = .03$). A meta-analysis of hemodynamic optimization trials has also suggested that early treatment before the development of organ failure results in improved survival. Lactate clearance of > 10% can be used as a potential substitute for $ScvO_2$ criteria if $ScvO_2$ monitoring is not available.

Compensated shock can occur in the setting of normalized hemodynamic parameters with ongoing global tissue hypoxia. Traditional endpoints of resuscitation such as blood pressure, heart rate, urinary output, mental status, and skin perfusion can therefore be misleading. Additional endpoints such as lactate levels and base deficit can help guide further resuscitative therapy. Patients who respond well to initial efforts demonstrate a survival advantage over nonresponders.

E. Medications

1. Vasoactive therapy—Vasopressors and inotropic agents are administered only after adequate fluid resuscitation. Choice of vasoactive therapy depends on the presumed etiology of shock as well as cardiac output. If there is continued hypotension with evidence of high cardiac output after adequate volume resuscitation, then vasopressor support is needed to improve vasomotor tone. If there is evidence of low cardiac output with high filling pressures, inotropic support is needed to improve contractility.

For **vasodilatory shock** when increased vasoconstriction is required to maintain an adequate perfusion pressure, alpha-adrenergic agonists (such as norepinephrine and phenylephrine) are generally used. Although **norepinephrine** is both an alpha-adrenergic and beta-adrenergic agonist, it preferentially increases mean arterial pressure over cardiac output. The initial dose is 1–2 mcg/min as an intravenous infusion, titrated to maintain the mean arterial blood pressure to at least 65 mm Hg. The usual maintenance dose is 2–4 mcg/min intravenously (maximum dose is 30 mcg/min). Patients with refractory shock may require dosages of 10–30 mcg/min intravenously. **Epinephrine,** also with both alpha-adrenergic and beta-adrenergic effects, may be used in severe shock and during acute resuscitation. It is the vasopressor of choice for anaphylactic shock. For severe shock, give 1 mcg/min as a continuous intravenous infusion initially and titrate to hemodynamic response; the usual dosage range is 1–10 mcg/min intravenously.

Dopamine has variable effects according to dosage. At low doses (2–5 mcg/kg/min intravenously), stimulation of dopaminergic and beta-adrenergic receptors produces increased glomerular filtration, heart rate, and contractility. At doses of 5–10 mcg/kg/min, beta-1-adrenergic effects predominate, resulting in an increase in heart rate and cardiac contractility. At higher doses (> 10 mcg/kg/min), alpha-adrenergic effects predominate, resulting in peripheral vasoconstriction. The maximum dose is typically 50 mcg/kg/min.

There is no evidence documenting a survival benefit from, or the superiority of, a particular vasopressor in **septic shock**. Norepinephrine is the initial vasopressor of choice in septic shock to maintain the mean arterial pressure > 65 mm Hg. Phenylephrine can be used as a first-line agent for hyperdynamic septic shock if (1) there is low systemic venous resistance but high cardiac output, which can manifest as hypotension with *warm* extremities or (2) dysrhythmias or tachycardias prevent the use of agents with beta-adrenergic activity. The use of dopamine as a first-line vasopressor in septic shock was shown in a meta-analysis to increase 28-day mortality and to have a higher incidence of arrhythmic events. Dopamine should only be used as an alternative to norepinephrine in select patients with septic shock, including patients with significant bradycardia or low potential for tachyarrhythmias.

Vasopressin (antidiuretic hormone or ADH) is often used as an adjunctive therapy to catecholamine vasopressors in the treatment of **distributive** or **vasodilatory shock**. Vasopressin causes peripheral vasoconstriction via V1 receptors located on smooth muscle cells and attenuation of nitric oxide (NO) synthesis and cGMP, the second messenger of NO. The rationale for using low-dose vasopressin in the management of septic shock includes the relative deficiency of vasopressin in late shock and the increased sensitivity of the systemic circulation to the vasopressor effects of vasopressin. Vasopressin also potentiates the effects of catecholamines on the vasculature and stimulates cortisol production. In the Vasopressin and Septic Shock Trial (VASST), low doses of vasopressin did not reduce mortality compared with norepinephrine in patients with septic shock who were being treated with catecholamine vasopressors. Some studies have reported reduced catecholamine requirements with vasopressin administration. Intravenous infusion of vasopressin at a low dose (0.01–0.04 units/min) may be safe and beneficial in septic patients with hypotension that is refractory to fluid resuscitation and conventional catecholamine vasopressors. Higher doses of vasopressin decrease cardiac output and may put patients at greater risk for splanchnic and coronary artery ischemia. Studies do not favor the use of vasopressin as first-line therapy, but it may be as a second-line agent in refractory septic or anaphylactic shock; its role as an initial vasopressor warrants further study.

There is insufficient evidence to recommend a specific vasopressor for use in cardiogenic shock, but expert opinion suggests that either norepinephrine or dopamine should be used as a first-line agent. Dobutamine, a predominantly beta-adrenergic agonist, increases contractility and decreases afterload. It is used for patients with low cardiac output and high PCWP but who do not have hypotension. Dobutamine can be added to a vasopressor if there is reduced myocardial function (decreased cardiac output and elevated PCWP), or if there are signs of hypoperfusion despite adequate volume resuscitation and an adequate mean arterial pressure. The initial dose is 0.1–0.5 mcg/kg/min as a continuous intravenous infusion, which can be titrated every few minutes as needed to achieve a hemodynamic effect; the usual dosage range is 2–20 mcg/kg/min intravenously. Tachyphylaxis can occur after 48 hours from the down-regulation of beta-adrenergic receptors. Amrinone or milrinone are phosphodiesterase inhibitors that can be substituted for dobutamine. These drugs increase cyclic AMP levels and increase cardiac contractility, bypassing the beta-adrenergic receptor. Vasodilation is a side effect of both amrinone and milrinone.

2. Corticosteroids—Corticosteroids are the treatment of choice in patients with shock secondary to adrenal insufficiency but studies do not support their use in patients with shock from sepsis or other etiologies. The observation that severe sepsis may be associated with relative adrenal insufficiency or glucocorticoid receptor resistance has led to several trials to evaluate the role of treatment with corticosteroids in septic shock. Early trials where high doses of corticosteroids were administered to patients in septic shock did not show improved survival; rather, some worse outcomes were observed from increased rates of secondary infections. Investigators have studied the use of low-dose corticosteroids in patients who were in septic shock and had relative adrenal insufficiency, defined by a cortisol response of 9 mcg/dL or less after one injection of 250 mcg of corticotropin. In 2008, the Corticosteroid Therapy of Septic Shock (CORTICUS) study demonstrated that low-dose hydrocortisone (50 mg intravenously every 6 hours for 5 days and then tapered over 6 days) did not improve survival in patients with septic shock, either overall or in patients who had relative adrenal insufficiency. This study was a randomized, double-blinded, placebo-controlled trial that is the largest to date of corticosteroids in septic patients. One limitation of the CORTICUS trial was that it was not adequately powered to detect a clinically important difference in mortality. Meta-analyses of multiple smaller trials of corticosteroids in patients with septic shock demonstrated that when shock was poorly responsive to fluid resuscitation and vasopressors, low-dose hydrocortisone (300 mg/d or less in divided doses) increased the mean arterial pressure but did not show a mortality benefit.

3. Antibiotics—Definitive therapy for septic shock includes an early initiation of empiric broad-spectrum antibiotics after appropriate cultures have been obtained. Imaging studies may prove useful to attempt localization of sources of infection. Surgical management may also be necessary if necrotic tissue or loculated infections are present (see Table 30–5).

4. Sodium bicarbonate—For patients with sepsis of any etiology and lactic acidosis, clinical studies have failed to show any hemodynamic benefit from bicarbonate therapy, either in increasing cardiac output or in decreasing the vasopressor requirement even in patients with severe acidemia.

F. Other Treatment Modalities

Cardiac failure may require use of transcutaneous or transvenous pacing or placement of an intra-arterial balloon pump. Emergent revascularization by percutaneous angioplasty or coronary artery bypass surgery appears to improve long-term outcome with increased survival compared with initial medical stabilization for patients with myocardial ischemia leading to cardiogenic shock. Urgent hemodialysis or continuous venovenous hemofiltration may be indicated for maintenance of fluid and electrolyte balance during acute kidney injury resulting in shock from multiple modalities.

COIITSS Study Investigators; Annane D et al. Corticosteroid treatment and intensive insulin therapy for septic shock in adults: a randomized controlled trial. JAMA. 2010 Jan 27;303(4):341–8. [PMID: 20103758]

De Backer D et al; SOAP II Investigators. Comparison of dopamine and norepinephrine in the treatment of shock. N Engl J Med. 2010 Mar 4;362(9):779–89. [PMID: 20200382]

Dellinger RP et al; Surviving Sepsis Campaign Guidelines Committee including the Pediatric Subgroup. Surviving Sepsis Campaign: international guidelines for management of severe sepsis and septic shock: 2012. Crit Care Med. 2013 Feb;41(2):580–637. [PMID: 23353941]

Patel GP et al. Efficacy and safety of dopamine versus norepinephrine in the management of septic shock. Shock. 2010 Apr;33(4):375–80. [PMID: 19851126]

Patel GP et al. Systemic steroids in severe sepsis and septic shock. Am J Respir Crit Care Med. 2012 Jan 15;185(2):133–9. [PMID: 21680949]

Prondzinsky R et al. Intra-aortic balloon counterpulsation in patients with acute myocardial infarction complicated by cardiogenic shock: the prospective, randomized IABP SHOCK Trial for attenuation of multiorgan dysfunction syndrome. Crit Care Med. 2010 Jan;38(1):152–60. [PMID: 19770739]

Ranieri VM et al; PROWESS-SHOCK Study Group. Drotrecogin alfa (activated) in adults with septic shock. N Engl J Med. 2012 May 31;366(22):2055–64. [PMID: 22616830]

Rivers E et al. Early goal-directed therapy in the treatment of severe sepsis and septic shock. N Engl J Med. 2001 Nov;345(19):1368–77. [PMID: 11794169]

Russell JA et al; VASST Investigators. Vasopressin versus norepinephrine infusion in patients with septic shock. N Engl J Med. 2008 Feb 28;358(9):877–87. [PMID: 18305265]

Sprung CL et al. Hydrocortisone therapy for patients with septic shock. N Engl J Med. 2008 Jan;358(2):111–24. [PMID: 18184957]

Thiele H et al; IABP-SHOCK II Trial Investigators. Intraaortic balloon support for myocardial infarction with cardiogenic shock. N Engl J Med. 2012 Oct 4;367(14):1287–96. [PMID: 22920912]

Blood Disorders

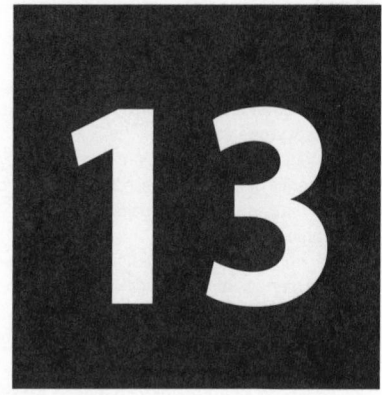

Lloyd E. Damon, MD

Charalambos Andreadis, MD

ANEMIAS

General Approach to Anemias

Anemia is present in adults if the hematocrit is < 41% (hemoglobin < 13.5 g/dL [135 g/L]) in males or < 36% (hemoglobin < 12 g/dL [120 g/L]) in females. Congenital anemia is suggested by the patient's personal and family history. The most common cause of anemia is iron deficiency. Poor diet may result in folic acid deficiency and contribute to iron deficiency, but bleeding is the most common cause of iron deficiency in adults. Physical examination demonstrates pallor. Attention to physical signs of primary hematologic diseases (lymphadenopathy; hepatosplenomegaly; or bone tenderness, especially in the sternum or anterior tibia) is important. Mucosal changes such as a smooth tongue suggest megaloblastic anemia.

Anemias are classified according to their pathophysiologic basis, ie, whether related to diminished production (relative or absolute reticulocytopenia) or to increased production due to accelerated loss of red blood cells (reticulocytosis) (Table 13–1), and according to red blood cell size (Table 13–2). A reticulocytosis occurs in one of three pathophysiologic states: acute blood loss, recent replacement of a missing erythropoietic nutrient, or reduced red blood cell survival (ie, hemolysis). A severely microcytic anemia (mean corpuscular volume [MCV] < 70 fL) is due either to iron deficiency or thalassemia, while a severely macrocytic anemia (MCV < 125 fL) is almost always due to either megaloblastic anemia or to cold agglutinins in blood analyzed at room temperature. A bone marrow biopsy is generally needed to complete the evaluation of anemia when the laboratory evaluation fails to reveal an etiology, when there are additional cytopenias present, or when an underlying primary or secondary bone marrow process is suspected.

IRON DEFICIENCY ANEMIAS

 ESSENTIALS OF DIAGNOSIS

▶ Iron deficiency is present if serum ferritin < 12 ng/mL (27 pmol/L) or < 30 ng/mL (67 pmol/L) if also anemic.

▶ Caused by bleeding unless proved otherwise.

▶ Responds to iron therapy.

General Considerations

Iron deficiency is the most common cause of anemia worldwide. The causes are listed in Table 13–3. Aside from circulating red blood cells, the major location of iron in the body is the storage pool as ferritin or as hemosiderin in macrophages.

The average American diet contains 10–15 mg of iron per day. About 10% of this amount is absorbed in the stomach, duodenum, and upper jejunum under acidic conditions. Dietary iron present as heme is efficiently absorbed (10–20%) but nonheme iron less so (1–5%), largely because of interference by phosphates, tannins, and other food constituents. The major iron transporter from the diet across the intestinal lumen is ferroportin, which also facilitates the transport of iron to apotransferrin in macrophages for delivery to erythroid cells prepared to synthesize hemoglobin. Hepcidin, produced during inflammation, negatively regulates iron transport by promoting the degradation of ferroportin. Small amounts of iron—approximately 1 mg/d—are normally lost through exfoliation of skin and mucosal cells.

Table 13–1. Classification of anemia by pathophysiology.

Decreased red blood cell production (relative or absolute reticulocytopenia)
Hemoglobin synthesis lesion: iron deficiency, thalassemia, anemia of chronic disease, hypoerythropoietinemia
DNA synthesis lesion: megaloblastic anemia, DNA synthesis inhibitor drugs
Hematopoietic stem cell lesion: aplastic anemia, leukemia
Bone marrow infiltration: carcinoma, lymphoma, fibrosis, sarcoidosis, Gaucher disease, others
Immune-mediated inhibition: aplastic anemia, pure red cell aplasia
Increased red blood cell destruction or accelerated red blood cell loss (reticulocytosis)
Acute blood loss
Hemolysis (intrinsic)
Membrane lesion: hereditary spherocytosis, elliptocytosis
Hemoglobin lesion: sickle cell, unstable hemoglobin
Glycolysis abnormality: pyruvate kinase deficiency
Oxidation lesion: glucose-6-phosphate dehydrogenase deficiency
Hemolysis (extrinsic)
Immune: warm antibody, cold antibody
Microangiopathic: thrombotic thrombocytopenic purpura, hemolytic-uremic syndrome, mechanical cardiac valve, paravalvular leak
Infection: *Clostridium perfringens*, malaria
Hypersplenism

Menstrual blood loss plays a major role in iron metabolism. The average monthly menstrual blood loss is approximately 50 mL but may be five times greater in some individuals. To maintain adequate iron stores, women with heavy menstrual losses must absorb 3–4 mg of iron from

Table 13–2. Classification of anemia by mean red blood cell volume (MCV).

Microcytic
Iron deficiency
Thalassemia
Anemia of chronic disease
Lead toxicity
Zinc deficiency
Macrocytic (Megaloblastic)
Vitamin B_{12} deficiency
Folate deficiency
DNA synthesis inhibitors
Macrocytic (Nonmegaloblastic)
Myelodysplasia
Liver disease
Reticulocytosis
Hypothyroidism
Bone marrow failure state (eg, aplastic anemia, marrow infiltrative disorder, etc.)
Hypocupremia
Normocytic
Kidney disease
Non-thyroid endocrine gland failure
Hypocupremia
Mild form of most acquired etiologies of anemia

Table 13–3. Causes of iron deficiency.

Deficient diet
Decreased absorption
Celiac sprue
Zinc deficiency
Increased requirements
Pregnancy
Lactation
Blood loss (chronic)
Gastrointestinal
Menstrual
Blood donation
Hemoglobinuria
Iron sequestration
Pulmonary hemosiderosis
Idiopathic

the diet each day. This strains the upper limit of what may reasonably be absorbed, and women with menorrhagia of this degree will almost always become iron deficient without iron supplementation.

In general, iron metabolism is balanced between absorption of 1 mg/d and loss of 1 mg/d. Pregnancy and lactation upset the iron balance, since requirements increase to 2–5 mg of iron per day. Normal dietary iron cannot supply these requirements, and medicinal iron is needed during pregnancy and lactation. Decreased iron absorption can also cause iron deficiency, such as in people affected with celiac disease, and it commonly occurs after surgical resection of the stomach or bypass of the jejunum.

The most important cause of iron deficiency anemia in adults is chronic blood loss, especially gastrointestinal blood loss. Prolonged aspirin use, or the use of other anti-inflammatory drugs, may cause it even without a documented structural lesion. Iron deficiency demands a search for a source of gastrointestinal bleeding if other sites of blood loss (menorrhagia, other uterine bleeding, and repeated blood donations) are excluded. Celiac disease (gluten enteropathy), even when asymptomatic, is an occult cause of iron deficiency through poor absorption in the gastrointestinal tract and should be considered when blood loss is not evident. Zinc deficiency is another cause of poor iron absorption. Chronic hemoglobinuria may lead to iron deficiency, but this is uncommon; traumatic hemolysis due to a prosthetic cardiac valve and other causes of intravascular hemolysis (eg, paroxysmal nocturnal hemoglobinuria) should also be considered. The cause of iron deficiency is not found in up to 5% of cases.

▶ Clinical Findings

A. Symptoms and Signs

The primary symptoms of iron deficiency anemia are those of the anemia itself (easy fatigability, tachycardia, palpitations, and dyspnea on exertion). Severe deficiency causes skin and mucosal changes, including a smooth tongue, brittle nails, spooning of nails (koilonychia), and cheilosis.

Dysphagia due to the formation of esophageal webs (Plummer–Vinson syndrome) may occur in severe iron deficiency. Many iron-deficient patients develop pica, craving for specific foods (ice chips, etc) often not rich in iron.

B. Laboratory Findings

Iron deficiency develops in stages. The first is depletion of iron stores without anemia followed by anemia with a normal red blood cell size (normal MCV) followed by anemia with reduced red blood cell size (low MCV). The reticulocyte count is low or inappropriately normal. Ferritin is a measure of total body iron stores. A ferritin value < 12 ng/mL (< 27 pmol/L) (in the absence of scurvy) is a highly reliable indicator of depletion of iron stores. Note that the lower limit of normal for ferritin generally is below 12 ng/mL (< 27 pmol/L) in women due to the fact that the normal range is generated by including healthy menstruating women who are iron deficient but not anemic. However, because serum ferritin levels may rise in response to inflammation or other stimuli, a normal or elevated ferritin level does not exclude a diagnosis of iron deficiency. A ferritin level of < 30 ng/mL (67 pmol/L) almost always indicates iron deficiency in anyone who is anemic. As iron deficiency progresses, serum iron values decline to < 30 mcg/dL (67 pmol/L) and transferrin levels rise to compensate, leading to transferrin saturations of < 15%. Low transferrin saturation is also seen in anemia of inflammation, so caution in the interpretation of this test is warranted. Isolated iron deficiency anemia has a low hepcidin level, not yet a clinically available test. As the MCV falls (ie, microcytosis), the blood smear shows hypochromic microcytic cells. With further progression, anisocytosis (variations in red blood cell size) and poikilocytosis (variation in shape of red cells) develop. Severe iron deficiency will produce a bizarre peripheral blood smear, with severely hypochromic cells, target cells, and pencil-shaped or cigar-shaped cells. Bone marrow biopsy for evaluation of iron stores is rarely performed. If the biopsy is done, it shows the absence of iron in erythroid progenitor cells by Prussian blue staining. The platelet count is commonly increased, but it usually remains < 800,000/mcL (800 × 10^9/L).

▶ Differential Diagnosis

Other causes of microcytic anemia include anemia of chronic disease (specifically, anemia of inflammation), thalassemia, lead poisoning, and congenital X-linked sideroblastic anemia. Anemia of chronic disease is characterized by normal or increased iron stores in bone marrow macrophages and a normal or elevated ferritin level; the serum iron and transferrin saturation are low, often drastically so, and the total iron-binding capacity (TIBC) and transferrin are either normal or low. Thalassemia produces a greater degree of microcytosis for any given level of anemia than does iron deficiency and, unlike virtually every other cause of anemia, has a normal or elevated (rather than a low) red blood cell count as well as a reticulocytosis. In thalassemia, red blood cell morphology on the peripheral smear resembles severe iron deficiency.

▶ Treatment

The diagnosis of iron deficiency anemia can be made either by the laboratory demonstration of an iron-deficient state or by evaluating the response to a therapeutic trial of iron replacement. Since the anemia itself is rarely life-threatening, the most important part of management is identification of the cause—especially a source of occult blood loss.

A. Oral Iron

Ferrous sulfate, 325 mg three times daily on an empty stomach, which provides 180 mg of iron daily of which up to 10 mg is absorbed, is the preferred therapy. Nausea and constipation limit compliance with ferrous sulfate. Extended-release ferrous sulfate with mucoprotease is the best tolerated oral preparation. Compliance is improved by introducing the medicine slowly in gradually escalating doses. Taking ferrous sulfate with food reduces side effects and but also its absorption. An appropriate response is a return of the hematocrit level halfway toward normal within 3 weeks with full return to baseline after 2 months. Iron therapy should continue for 3–6 months after restoration of normal hematologic values to replenish iron stores. Failure of response to iron therapy is usually due to noncompliance, although occasional patients may absorb iron poorly, particularly if the stomach is achlorhydric. Such patients may benefit from concomitant administration of oral ascorbic acid. Other reasons for failure to respond include incorrect diagnosis (anemia of chronic disease, thalassemia), celiac disease, and ongoing gastrointestinal blood loss that exceeds the rate of new erythropoiesis.

B. Parenteral Iron

The indications are intolerance to oral iron, refractoriness to oral iron, gastrointestinal disease (usually inflammatory bowel disease) precluding the use of oral iron, and continued blood loss that cannot be corrected, such as chronic hemodialysis. Parenteral iron preparations coat the iron in protective carbohydrate shells. Historical parenteral iron preparations, such as iron dextran, were problematic due to long infusion times (hours), polyarthralgia, and hypersensitivity reactions, including anaphylaxis. Current preparations are safe and can be infused in less than 5 minutes. Iron oxide coated with polyglucose sorbitol carboxymethyl-ether can be given in doses up to 510 mg by intravenous bolus over 20 seconds, with no test dose required.

The iron deficit is calculated by determining the decrement in red cell volume from normal, recognizing there is 1 mg of iron in each milliliter of red blood cells. Total body iron ranges between 2 g and 4 g: approximately 50 mg/kg in men and 35 mg/kg in women. Most (70 – 95%) of the iron is present in hemoglobin in circulating red blood cells. In men, red blood cell volume is approximately 30 mL/kg; in women, it is about 27 mL/kg. Thus, a 50-kg woman whose hemoglobin is 9 g/dL (75% of normal) has an iron deficit of 0.25 × 27 mL/kg × 50 kg = 337.5 mL of red blood cells (or 337.5 mg of iron). The parenteral iron dose is the iron deficit plus (usually) 1 extra gram to replenish iron stores and anticipate further iron loses, so in this case 1.4 g.

When to Refer

Patients should be referred to a hematologist if the suspected diagnosis is not confirmed or if they are not responsive to oral iron therapy.

Auerbach M et al. Clinical use of intravenous iron: administration, efficacy, and safety. Hematology Am Soc Hematol Educ Program. 2010;2010:338–47. [PMID: 21239816]

Cancelo-Hildago MJ et al. Tolerability of different oral iron supplements: a systematic review. Curr Med Res Opin. 2013 Apr;29(4):291–303. [PMID: 23252877]

Goodnough LT. Iron deficiency syndromes and iron-restricted erythropoiesis (CME). Transfusion. 2012 Jul;52(7):1584–92. [PMID: 22211566]

Short MW et al. Iron deficiency anemia: evaluation and management. Am Fam Physician. 2013 Jan 15;87(2):98–104. [PMID: 23317073]

ANEMIA OF CHRONIC DISEASE

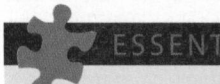

ESSENTIALS OF DIAGNOSIS

► Mild or moderate normocytic or microcytic anemia.

► Normal or increased ferritin and normal or reduced transferrin.

► Underlying chronic disease.

General Considerations

Many chronic systemic diseases are associated with mild or moderate anemia. The anemias of chronic disease are characterized according to etiology and pathophysiology. First, the anemia of inflammation is associated with chronic inflammatory states (such as inflammatory bowel disease, rheumatoid arthritis, chronic infections, and malignancy) and is mediated through hepcidin (a negative regulator of ferroportin), resulting in reduced iron uptake in the gut and reduced iron transfer from macrophages to erythroid progenitor cells in the bone marrow. This is referred to as iron-restricted erythropoiesis since the patient is iron replete. There is also reduced responsiveness to erythropoietin, the elaboration of hemolysins that shorten red blood cell survival, and the production of inflammatory cytokines that dampen red cell production. The serum iron is low in the anemia of inflammation. Second, the anemia of organ failure can occur with kidney disease, hepatic failure, and in endocrine gland failure; erythropoietin is reduced and the red blood cell mass decreases in response to a diminished signal for red blood cell production; the serum iron is normal. Third, the anemia of the elderly is present in up to 20% of individuals over age 85 years and a thorough evaluation for an etiology of anemia is negative. The anemia of the elderly is a consequence of relative red blood cell production resistance to erythropoietin, a decrease in erythropoietin production relative to the nephron mass in older people, and the negative erythropoietic influence of low levels of chronic inflammatory cytokines in this age group; the serum iron is normal.

Clinical Findings

A. Symptoms and Signs

The clinical features are those of the causative condition. The diagnosis should be suspected in patients with known chronic diseases. In cases of significant anemia, coexistent iron deficiency or folic acid deficiency should be suspected. Decreased dietary intake of folic acid or iron is common in chronically ill patients, and many will also have ongoing gastrointestinal blood losses. Patients undergoing hemodialysis regularly lose both iron and folic acid during dialysis.

B. Laboratory Findings

The hematocrit rarely falls below 60% of baseline (except in kidney failure). The MCV is usually normal or slightly reduced. Red blood cell morphology is usually normal, and the reticulocyte count is mildly decreased or normal. In the anemia of inflammation, serum iron and transferrin values are low, and transferrin saturation may be extremely low, leading to an erroneous diagnosis of iron deficiency. In contrast to iron deficiency, serum ferritin values should be normal or increased. A serum ferritin value of < 30 ng/mL (67 pmol/L) indicates coexistent iron deficiency. Classic anemia of inflammation has elevated hepcidin levels; however, no clinical test is yet available. In the anemias of organ failure and of the elderly, the iron studies are generally normal. The anemia of the elderly is a diagnosis of exclusion in a patient with anemia who is over age 65 years.

A particular challenge is the diagnosis of iron deficiency in the setting of the anemia of inflammation in which the serum ferritin can be as high as 200 ng/mL (450 pmol/L). The gold standard for diagnosis is a bone marrow biopsy with iron stain. Absent iron staining indicates iron deficiency, and iron localized in marrow macrophages indicates pure anemia of inflammation. Bone marrow biopsies are rarely done for this purpose. Three other tests may help make this distinction: a reticulocyte hemoglobin concentration of < 28 pg; a soluble serum transferrin receptor (units: mg/L) to log ferritin (units: mcg/L) ratio of 1–8; or a normal hepcidin level all support iron deficiency in the setting of inflammation. A functional test is hemoglobin response to oral or parenteral iron in the setting of inflammation when iron deficiency is suspected. A note of caution: certain circumstances of iron-restricted erythropoiesis (such as malignancy) will partially respond to parenteral iron infusion even when the iron stores are replete due to the immediate distribution of iron to erythropoietic progenitor cells after the infusion.

Treatment

In most cases, no treatment is necessary and the primary management is to address the condition causing the anemia of chronic disease. When the anemia is severe or is adversely affecting the quality of life or functional status, then treatment involves either red blood cell transfusions or parenteral recombinant erythropoietin (epoetin alfa or darbepoetin).

The indications for recombinant erythropoietin are hemoglobin < 10 g/dL and anemia due to rheumatoid arthritis, inflammatory bowel disease, hepatitis C, the administration of zidovudine in HIV-infected patients, myelosuppressive chemotherapy in patients with solid malignancy (treated with palliative intent only), or chronic kidney disease (estimated glomerular filtration rate of < 60 mL/min). The dosing and schedule of recombinant erythropoietin are individualized to maintain the hemoglobin between 10 g/dL (100 g/L) and 12 g/dL (120 g/L). The use of recombinant erythropoietin is associated with an increased risk of venothromboembolism and arterial thrombotic episodes, especially if the hemoglobin rises to > 12 g/dL (120 g/L). There is controversy about whether recombinant erythropoietin is associated with reduced survival in patients with malignancy. For patients with end-stage renal disease receiving recombinant erythropoietin who are on hemodialysis, the anemia of chronic kidney disease can be more effectively corrected by adding soluble ferric pyrophosphate to their dialysate than by administering intravenous iron supplementation.

▶ When to Refer

Referral to a hematologist is not necessary.

Cheng PP et al. Hepcidin expression in anemia of chronic disease and concomitant iron-deficiency anemia. Clin Exp Med. 2011 Mar;11(1):33–42. [PMID: 20499129]

Roy CN. Anemia of inflammation. Hematology Am Soc Hematol Educ Program. 2010;2010:276–80. [PMID: 21239806]

Sun CC et al. Targeting the hepcidin-ferroportin axis to develop new treatment strategies for anemia of chronic disease and anemia of inflammation. Am J Hematol. 2012 Apr;87(4): 392–400. [PMID: 22290531]

Vanasse GJ et al. Anemia in elderly patients: an emerging problem for the 21st century. Hematology Am Soc Hematol Educ Program. 2010;2010:271–5. [PMID: 21239805]

THE THALASSEMIAS

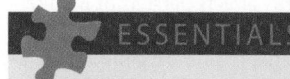

ESSENTIALS OF DIAGNOSIS

- ▶ Microcytosis disproportionate to the degree of anemia.
- ▶ Positive family history or lifelong personal history of microcytic anemia.
- ▶ Normal or elevated red blood cell count.
- ▶ Abnormal red blood cell morphology with microcytes, hypochromia, acanthocytes, and target cells.
- ▶ In beta-thalassemia, elevated levels of hemoglobin A$_2$ or F.

▶ General Considerations

The thalassemias are hereditary disorders characterized by reduction in the synthesis of globin chains (alpha or beta). Reduced globin chain synthesis causes reduced hemoglobin synthesis and a hypochromic microcytic anemia because of defective hemoglobinization of red blood cells. Thalassemias can be considered among the hyperproliferative hemolytic anemias, the anemias related to abnormal hemoglobin, and the hypoproliferative anemias, since all of these factors play a role in pathogenesis. The hallmark laboratory features are small and pale red blood cells (low MCV and mean corpuscular hemoglobin [MCH]), anemia, and a normal to elevated red blood cell count (ie, a large number of small red blood cells are being produced). Although patients often exhibit an elevated reticulocyte count, generally the degree of reticulocyte output is inadequate to meet the degree of red blood cell destruction (hemolysis) and the patients remain anemic.

Normal adult hemoglobin is primarily hemoglobin A, which represents approximately 98% of circulating hemoglobin. Hemoglobin A is formed from a tetramer of two alpha chains and two beta chains—and can be designated alpha2beta2. Two copies of the alpha-globin gene are located on each chromosome 16, and there is no substitute for alpha-globin in the formation of adult hemoglobin. One copy of the beta-globin gene resides on each chromosome 11 adjacent to genes encoding the beta-like globins delta and gamma (the so-called beta-globin gene cluster region). The tetramer of alpha2delta2 forms hemoglobin A$_2$, which normally comprises 1–3% of adult hemoglobin. The tetramer alpha2gamma2 forms hemoglobin F, which is the major hemoglobin of fetal life but which comprises < 1% of normal adult hemoglobin.

The thalassemias are described as **"trait"** when there are laboratory features without significant clinical impact, **"intermedia"** when there is an occasional red blood cell transfusion requirement or other moderate clinical impact, and **"major"** when the disorder is life-threatening and the patient is transfusion-dependent. Most patients with thalassemia major die of the consequences of iron overload.

Alpha-thalassemia is due primarily to gene deletions causing reduced alpha-globin chain synthesis (Table 13–4). Each alpha-globin gene produces one-quarter of the total alpha-globin quantity, so there is a predictable proportionate decrease in alpha-globin output with each lost

Table 13–4. Alpha-thalassemia syndromes.

Number of Alpha-globin Genes Transcribed	Syndrome	Hematocrit	MCV
4	Normal	Normal	Normal
3	Silent carrier	Normal	Normal
2	Thalassemia minor (or trait)	28–40%	60–75 fL
1	Hemoglobin H disease	22–32%	60–70 fL
0	Hydrops fetalis[1]	< 18%	< 60 fL

[1]Die in utero.
MCV, mean corpuscular volume.

Table 13–5. Beta-thalassemia syndromes.

	Beta-Globin Genes Transcribed	Hb A	Hb A$_2$	Hb F	Transfusions
Normal	Homozygous beta	97–99%	1–3%	< 1%	
Thalassemia minor	Heterozygous beta^0	80–95%	4–8%	1–5%	None
	Heterozygous beta$^+$	80–95%	4–8%	1–5%	None
Thalassemia intermedia	Homozygous beta$^+$(mild)	0–30%	0–10%	6–100%	Occasional
Thalassemia major	Homozygous beta^0	0%	4–10%	90–96%	Dependent
Thalassemia major	Homozygous beta$^+$	0–10%	4–10%	90–96%	Dependent

Hb, hemoglobin.

alpha-globin gene. Since all adult hemoglobins are alpha containing, alpha-thalassemia produces no change in the proportions of hemoglobins A, A$_2$, and F on hemoglobin electrophoresis. In severe forms of alpha-thalassemia, excess beta chains may form a beta-4 tetramer called hemoglobin H. In the presence of reduced alpha chains, the excess beta chains are unstable and precipitate, leading to damage of red blood cell membranes. This leads to both intramedullary (bone marrow) and peripheral blood hemolysis.

Beta-thalassemias are usually caused by point mutations rather than deletions (Table 13–5). These mutations result in premature chain termination or in problems with transcription of RNA and ultimately result in reduced or absent beta-globin chain synthesis. The molecular defects leading to beta-thalassemia are numerous and heterogeneous but run true within families. Defects that result in absent beta-globin chain expression are termed beta^0, whereas those causing reduced but not absent synthesis are termed beta$^+$. In beta$^+$ thalassemia, the degree of reduction of beta-globin synthesis is consistent within families but is quite variable between families. The reduced beta-globin chain synthesis in beta-thalassemia results in a relative increase in the proportions of hemoglobins A$_2$ and F compared to hemoglobin A on hemoglobin electrophoresis, as the beta-like globins (delta and gamma) substitute for the missing beta chains. In the presence of reduced beta chains, the excess alpha chains are unstable and precipitate, leading to damage of red blood cell membranes. This leads to both intramedullary (bone marrow) and peripheral blood hemolysis. The bone marrow demonstrates erythroid hyperplasia under the stimuli of anemia and ineffective erythropoiesis (intramedullary destruction of the developing erythroid cells). In cases of severe thalassemia, the marked expansion of the erythroid element in the bone marrow may cause severe bony deformities, osteopenia, and pathologic fractures.

▶ Clinical Findings

A. Symptoms and Signs

The **alpha-thalassemia** syndromes are seen primarily in persons from southeast Asia and China, and, less commonly, in blacks and persons of Mediterranean origin (Table 13–4). Normally, adults have four copies of the

alpha-globin chain. When three alpha-globin genes are present, the patient is hematologically normal (silent carrier). When two alpha-globin genes are present, the patient is said to have alpha-thalassemia trait, one form of thalassemia minor. In alpha-thalassemia-1 trait, the alpha gene deletion is heterozygous (alpha –/alpha –) and affects mainly those of Asian descent. In alpha-thalassemia-2 trait, the alpha gene deletion is homozygous (alpha alpha/– –) and affects mainly blacks. These patients are clinically normal and have a normal life expectancy and performance status, with a mild microcytic anemia. When only one alpha globin chain is present (alpha –/– –), the patient has hemoglobin H disease. This is a chronic hemolytic anemia of variable severity (thalassemia minor or intermedia). Physical examination might reveal pallor and splenomegaly. Affected individuals usually do not need transfusions; however, they may be required during transient periods of hemolytic exacerbation caused by infection or other stressors or during periods of erythropoietic shutdown caused by certain viruses ("aplastic crisis"). When all four alpha-globin genes are deleted, no normal hemoglobin is produced and the affected fetus is stillborn (hydrops fetalis). In hydrops fetalis, the only hemoglobin species gamma made is called hemoglobin Bart's (gamma4).

Beta-thalassemia primarily affects persons of Mediterranean origin (Italian, Greek) and to a lesser extent Asians and blacks (Table 13–5). Patients homozygous for beta-thalassemia (beta^0/beta^0 or beta$^+$/beta$^+$) have thalassemia major (Cooley anemia). Affected children are normal at birth but after 6 months, when hemoglobin synthesis switches from hemoglobin F to hemoglobin A, severe anemia requiring transfusion develops. Numerous clinical problems ensue, including stunted growth, bony deformities (abnormal facial structure, pathologic fractures), hepatosplenomegaly, jaundice due to gallstones or hepatitis-related cirrhosis (or both), and thrombophilia. The clinical course is modified significantly by transfusion therapy, but transfusional iron overload (hemosiderosis) results in a clinical picture similar to hemochromatosis, with heart failure, cardiac arrhythmias, cirrhosis, endocrinopathies, and pseudoxanthoma elasticum (calcification and fragmentation of the elastic fibers of the skin, retina, and cardiovascular system), usually after more than 100 units of red blood cells have been transfused. Iron loading occurs because the human body has no active iron excretory mechanism. Before the application of allogeneic stem cell transplantation and the development of more effective forms of iron chelation, death from iron overload usually occurred between the ages of 20 and 30 years.

Patients homozygous for a milder form of beta-thalassemia (beta$^+$/beta$^+$, but allowing a higher rate of beta-globin synthesis) have thalassemia intermedia. These patients have chronic hemolytic anemia but do not require transfusions except under periods of stress or during aplastic crises. They also may develop iron overload because of periodic transfusion. They survive into adult life but with hepatosplenomegaly and bony deformities. Patients heterozygous for beta-thalassemia (beta/beta^0 or beta/beta$^+$) have thalassemia minor and a clinically insignificant microcytic anemia.

Prenatal diagnosis is available, and genetic counseling should be offered and the opportunity for prenatal diagnosis discussed.

B. Laboratory Findings

1. Alpha-thalassemia trait—These patients have mild anemia, with hematocrits between 28% and 40%. The MCV is strikingly low (60–75 fL) despite the modest anemia, and the red blood count is normal or increased. The peripheral blood smear shows microcytes, hypochromia, occasional target cells, and acanthocytes (cells with irregularly spaced spiked projections). The reticulocyte count and iron parameters are normal. Hemoglobin electrophoresis is normal. Alpha-thalassemia trait is thus usually diagnosed by exclusion. Genetic testing to demonstrate alpha-globin gene deletion is available only in a limited number of laboratories.

2. Hemoglobin H disease—These patients have a more marked anemia, with hematocrits between 22% and 32%. The MCV is remarkably low (60–70 fL) and the peripheral blood smear is markedly abnormal, with hypochromia, microcytosis, target cells, and poikilocytosis. The reticulocyte count is elevated and the red blood cell count is normal or elevated. Hemoglobin electrophoresis will show a fast migrating hemoglobin (hemoglobin H), which comprises 10–40% of the hemoglobin. A peripheral blood smear can be stained with supravital dyes to demonstrate the presence of hemoglobin H.

3. Beta-thalassemia minor—These patients have a modest anemia with hematocrit between 28% and 40%. The MCV ranges from 55 fL to 75 fL, and the red blood cell count is normal or increased. The reticulocyte count is normal or slightly elevated. The peripheral blood smear is mildly abnormal, with hypochromia, microcytosis, and target cells. In contrast to alpha-thalassemia, basophilic stippling is present. Hemoglobin electrophoresis shows an elevation of hemoglobin A$_2$ to 4–8% and occasional elevations of hemoglobin F to 1–5%.

4. Beta-thalassemia intermedia—These patients have a modest anemia with hematocrit between 17% and 33%. The MCV ranges from 55 fL to 75 fL, and the red blood cell count is normal or increased. The reticulocyte count is elevated. The peripheral blood smear is abnormal with hypochromia, microcytosis, basophilic stippling, and target cells. Hemoglobin electrophoresis shows up to 30% hemoglobin A and an elevation of hemoglobin A$_2$ up to 10% and elevation of hemoglobin F from 6% to 100%.

5. Beta-thalassemia major—These patients have severe anemia, and without transfusion the hematocrit may fall to < 10%. The peripheral blood smear is bizarre, showing severe poikilocytosis, hypochromia, microcytosis, target cells, basophilic stippling, and nucleated red blood cells. Little or no hemoglobin A is present. Variable amounts of hemoglobin A$_2$ are seen, and the predominant hemoglobin present is hemoglobin F.

▶ Differential Diagnosis

Mild forms of thalassemia must be differentiated from iron deficiency. Compared to iron deficiency anemia, patients with thalassemia have a lower MCV, a normal or elevated red blood cell count, a more abnormal peripheral blood smear at modest levels of anemia, and usually a reticulocytosis. Iron studies are normal or the transferrin saturation or ferritin (or both) are elevated. Severe forms of thalassemia may be confused with other hemoglobinopathies. The diagnosis of beta-thalassemia is made by the above findings and hemoglobin electrophoresis showing elevated levels of hemoglobins A$_2$ and F (provided the patient is replete in iron), but the diagnosis of alpha-thalassemia is made by exclusion since there is no change in the proportion of the normal adult hemoglobin species. The only other microcytic anemia with a normal or elevated red blood cell count is iron deficiency in a patient with polycythemia vera.

▶ Treatment

Patients with mild thalassemia (alpha-thalassemia trait or beta-thalassemia minor) require no treatment and should be identified so that they will not be subjected to repeated evaluations and treatment for iron deficiency. Patients with hemoglobin H disease should take folic acid supplementation (1 mg/d orally) and avoid medicinal iron and oxidative drugs such as sulfonamides. Patients with severe thalassemia are maintained on a regular transfusion schedule and receive folic acid supplementation. Splenectomy is performed if hypersplenism causes a marked increase in the transfusion requirement or refractory symptoms. Patients with regular transfusion requirements should be treated with iron chelation (such as oral deferasirox 20–30 mg/kg/d) in order to prevent life-limiting organ damage from iron overload.

Allogeneic stem cell transplantation is the treatment of choice for beta-thalassemia major and the only available cure. Children who have not yet experienced iron overload and chronic organ toxicity do well, with long-term survival in more than 80% of cases.

▶ When to Refer

All patients with severe thalassemia should be referred to a hematologist. Any patient with an unexplained microcytic anemia should be referred to help establish a diagnosis. Patients with thalassemia minor or intermedia should be referred for genetic counseling because offspring of thalassemic couples are at risk for inheriting thalassemia major.

Angelucci E. Hematopoietic stem cell transplantation in thalassemia. Hematology Am Soc Hematol Educ Program. 2010; 2010:456–62. [PMID: 21239835]

Borgna-Pignatti C et al. Complications of thalassemia major and their treatment. Expert Rev Hematol. 2011 Jun;4(3):353–66. [PMID: 21668399]

Forget BG et al. Classification of the disorders of hemoglobin. Cold Spring Harb Perspect Med. 2013 Feb 1;3(2):a011684. [PMID: 23378597]

Higgs DR et al. Thalassaemia. Lancet. 2012 Jan 28;379(9813): 373–83. [PMID: 21908035]

Schoorl M et al. Efficacy of advanced discriminating algorithms for screening on iron deficiency anemia and beta thalassemia trait: a multicenter evaluation. Am J Clin Pathol. 2012 Aug; 138(2):300–4. [PMID: 22904143]

VITAMIN B$_{12}$ DEFICIENCY

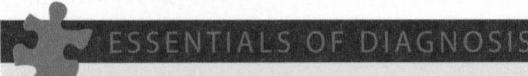

ESSENTIALS OF DIAGNOSIS

► Macrocytic anemia.

► Megaloblastic blood smear (macro-ovalocytes and hypersegmented neutrophils).

► Low serum vitamin B$_{12}$ level.

General Considerations

Vitamin B$_{12}$ belongs to the family of cobalamins and serves as a cofactor for two important reactions in humans. As methylcobalamin, it is a cofactor for methionine synthetase in the conversion of homocysteine to methionine, and as adenosylcobalamin for the conversion of methylmalonyl-coenzyme A (CoA) to succinyl-CoA. These enzymatic steps are critical for annealing Okazaki fragments during DNA synthesis, particularly in erythroid progenitor cells. Vitamin B$_{12}$ comes from the diet and is present in all foods of animal origin. The daily absorption of vitamin B$_{12}$ is 5 mcg.

The liver contains 2–5 mg of stored vitamin B$_{12}$. Since daily utilization is 3–5 mcg, the body usually has sufficient stores of vitamin B$_{12}$ so that it takes more than 3 years for vitamin B$_{12}$ deficiency to occur if all intake or absorption immediately ceases.

Since vitamin B$_{12}$ is present in foods of animal origin, dietary vitamin B$_{12}$ deficiency is extremely rare but is seen in vegans—strict vegetarians who avoid all dairy products as well as meat and fish (Table 13–6). Pernicious anemia is an autoimmune illness whereby autoantibodies destroy gastric parietal cells (that produce intrinsic factor) and cause atrophic gastritis or bind to and neutralize intrinsic factor, or both. Abdominal surgery may lead to vitamin B$_{12}$ deficiency in several ways. Gastrectomy will eliminate the site of intrinsic factor production; blind loop syndrome will cause competition for vitamin B$_{12}$ by bacterial overgrowth in the lumen of the intestine; and surgical resection of the ileum will eliminate the site of vitamin B$_{12}$

Table 13–6. Causes of vitamin B$_{12}$ deficiency.

Dietary deficiency (rare)
Decreased production or neutralization of intrinsic factor
Pernicious anemia (autoimmune)
Gastrectomy
Helicobacter pylori infection
Competition for vitamin B$_{12}$ in gut
Blind loop syndrome
Fish tapeworm (rare)
Pancreatic insufficiency
Decreased ileal absorption of vitamin B$_{12}$
Surgical resection
Crohn disease
Transcobalamin II deficiency (rare)

absorption. Rare causes of vitamin B$_{12}$ deficiency include fish tapeworm (*Diphyllobothrium latum*) infection, in which the parasite uses luminal vitamin B$_{12}$; pancreatic insufficiency (with failure to inactivate competing cobalamin-binding proteins); and severe Crohn disease, causing sufficient destruction of the ileum to impair vitamin B$_{12}$ absorption.

► Clinical Findings

A. Symptoms and Signs

Vitamin B$_{12}$ deficiency causes a moderate to severe anemia of slow onset; patients may have few symptoms relative to the degree of anemia. In advanced cases, the anemia may be severe, with hematocrits as low as 10–15%, and may be accompanied by leukopenia and thrombocytopenia. The deficiency also produces changes in mucosal cells, leading to glossitis, as well as other vague gastrointestinal disturbances such as anorexia and diarrhea. Vitamin B$_{12}$ deficiency also leads to a complex neurologic syndrome. Peripheral nerves are usually affected first, and patients complain initially of paresthesias. As the posterior columns of the spinal cord become impaired, patients complain of difficulty with balance or proprioception, or both. In more advanced cases, cerebral function may be altered as well, and on occasion dementia and other neuropsychiatric abnormalities may be present. It is critical to recognize that the non-hematologic manifestations of vitamin B$_{12}$ deficiency can be manifest despite a completely normal complete blood count.

Patients are usually pale and may be mildly icteric or sallow. Typically later in the disease course, neurologic examination may reveal decreased vibration and position sense or memory disturbance (or both).

B. Laboratory Findings

The diagnosis of vitamin B$_{12}$ deficiency is made by finding a low serum vitamin B$_{12}$ (cobalamin) level. Whereas the normal vitamin B$_{12}$ level is > 210 pg/mL (> 155 pmol/L), most patients with overt vitamin B$_{12}$ deficiency have serum levels < 170 pg/mL (< 126 pmol/L), with symptomatic patients usually having levels < 100 pg/mL (< 74 pmol/L).

The diagnosis of vitamin B_{12} deficiency in low or low-normal values (level of 170–210 pg/mL [126–155 pmol/L]) is best confirmed by finding an elevated level of serum methylmalonic acid (> 1000 nmol/L) or homocysteine. Of note, elevated levels of serum methylmalonic acid can be due to kidney disease.

The anemia of vitamin B_{12} deficiency is typically moderate to severe with the MCV quite elevated (110–140 fL). However, it is possible to have vitamin B_{12} deficiency with a normal MCV. Occasionally, the normal MCV may be explained by coexistent thalassemia or iron deficiency, but in other cases the reason is obscure. Patients with neurologic symptoms and signs that suggest possible vitamin B_{12} deficiency should be evaluated for that deficiency despite a normal MCV or the absence of anemia. The peripheral blood smear is megaloblastic, defined as red blood cells that appear as macro-ovalocytes, (although other shape changes are usually present) and neutrophils that are hypersegmented (mean neutrophil lobe counts greater than four or the finding of six [or greater]-lobed neutrophils). The reticulocyte count is reduced. Because vitamin B_{12} deficiency can affect all hematopoietic cell lines, the white blood cell count and the platelet count are reduced in severe cases.

Other laboratory abnormalities include elevated serum lactate dehydrogenase (LD) and a modest increase in indirect bilirubin. These two findings are a reflection of intramedullary destruction of developing abnormal erythroid cells and are similar to those observed in peripheral hemolytic anemias.

Bone marrow morphology is characteristically abnormal. Marked erythroid hyperplasia is present as a response to defective red blood cell production (ineffective erythropoiesis). Megaloblastic changes in the erythroid series include abnormally large cell size and asynchronous maturation of the nucleus and cytoplasm—ie, cytoplasmic maturation continues while impaired DNA synthesis causes retarded nuclear development. In the myeloid series, giant bands and meta-myelocytes are characteristically seen.

▶ Differential Diagnosis

Vitamin B_{12} deficiency should be differentiated from folic acid deficiency, the other common cause of megaloblastic anemia, in which red blood cell folic acid is low while vitamin B_{12} levels are normal. The bone marrow findings of vitamin B_{12} deficiency are sometimes mistaken for a myelodysplastic syndrome or even acute erythrocytic leukemia. The distinction between vitamin B_{12} deficiency and myelodysplasia is based on the characteristic morphology and the low vitamin B_{12} and elevated methylmalonic acid levels.

▶ Treatment

Patients with vitamin B_{12} deficiency have historically been treated with parenteral therapy. Intramuscular or subcutaneous injections of 100 mcg of vitamin B_{12} are adequate for each dose. Replacement is usually given daily for the first week, weekly for the first month, and then monthly for life. The vitamin deficiency will recur if patients discontinue their therapy. Oral or sublingual methylcobalamin (1 mg/d)

may be used instead of parenteral therapy once initial correction of the deficiency has occurred. Oral or sublingual replacement is effective, even in pernicious anemia, since approximately 1% of the dose is absorbed in the intestine via passive diffusion in the absence of active transport. It must be continued indefinitely and serum vitamin B_{12} levels must be monitored to ensure adequate replacement. For patients with neurologic symptoms caused by B_{12} deficiency, long-term parenteral vitamin B_{12} therapy is prudent. Because many patients are concurrently folic acid deficient from intestinal mucosal atrophy, simultaneous folic acid replacement (1 mg daily) is recommended for the first several months of vitamin B_{12} replacement.

Patients respond to therapy with an immediate improvement in their sense of well-being. Hypokalemia may complicate the first several days of therapy, particularly if the anemia is severe. A brisk reticulocytosis occurs in 5–7 days, and the hematologic picture normalizes in 2 months. Central nervous system symptoms and signs are reversible if they are of relatively short duration (< 6 months) but are likely permanent if of longer duration. Red blood cell transfusions are rarely needed despite the severity of anemia, but when given, diuretics are also recommended to avoid heart failure because this anemia developed slowly and the plasma volume is increased.

▶ When to Refer

Referral to a hematologist is not usually necessary.

Langan RC et al. Update on vitamin B_{12} deficiency. Am Fam Physician. 2011 Jun 15;83(12):1425–30. [PMID: 21671542]
Stabler SP. Clinical practice. Vitamin B_{12} deficiency. N Engl J Med. 2013 Jan 10;368(2):149–60. [PMID: 23301732]

FOLIC ACID DEFICIENCY

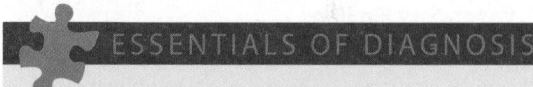

ESSENTIALS OF DIAGNOSIS

▶ Macrocytic anemia.

▶ Megaloblastic blood smear (macro-ovalocytes and hypersegmented neutrophils).

▶ Reduced folic acid levels in red blood cells or serum.

▶ Normal serum vitamin B_{12} level.

▶ General Considerations

Folic acid is the term commonly used for pteroylmonoglutamic acid. Folic acid is present in most fruits and vegetables (especially citrus fruits and green leafy vegetables). Daily dietary requirements are 50–100 mcg. Total body stores of folic acid are approximately 5 mg, enough to supply requirements for 2–3 months.

The most common cause of folic acid deficiency is inadequate dietary intake (Table 13–7). Alcoholic or

Table 13–7. Causes of folic acid deficiency.

Dietary deficiency
Decreased absorption
Tropical sprue
Drugs: phenytoin, sulfasalazine,
trimethoprim-sulfamethoxazole
Concurrent vitamin B_{12} deficiency
Increased requirement
Chronic hemolytic anemia
Pregnancy
Exfoliative skin disease
Excess loss: hemodialysis
Inhibition of reduction to active form
Methotrexate

anorectic patients, persons who do not eat fresh fruits and vegetables, and those who overcook their food are candidates for folic acid deficiency. Reduced folic acid absorption is rarely seen, since absorption occurs from the entire gastrointestinal tract. However, drugs such as phenytoin, trimethoprim-sulfamethoxazole, or sulfasalazine may interfere with its absorption. Folic acid absorption is poor in some patients with vitamin B_{12} deficiency due to gastrointestinal mucosal atrophy. Folic acid requirements are increased in pregnancy, hemolytic anemia, and exfoliative skin disease, and in these cases the increased requirements (five to ten times normal) may not be met by a normal diet.

► Clinical Findings

A. Symptoms and Signs

The clinical features are similar to those of vitamin B_{12} deficiency. However, when there is isolated folic acid deficiency, there are none of the neurologic abnormalities associated with vitamin B_{12} deficiency.

B. Laboratory Findings

Megaloblastic anemia is identical to anemia resulting from vitamin B_{12} deficiency (see above). A red blood cell folic acid level of < 150 ng/mL (< 340 nmol/L) is diagnostic of folic acid deficiency. The red blood cell folic acid level is preferred over the serum folic acid level because the former reflects body stores over the life span of the red blood cell, while the latter reflects immediate labile serum levels rather than body stores, although the clinical application of this principle is controversial. Usually the serum vitamin B_{12} level is normal and should always be measured when folic acid deficiency is suspected. In some instances, folic acid deficiency is a consequence of the gastrointestinal mucosal disturbances from vitamin B_{12} deficiency.

► Differential Diagnosis

The megaloblastic anemia of folic acid deficiency should be differentiated from vitamin B_{12} deficiency by the finding of a normal vitamin B_{12} level and a reduced red blood cell folic acid or serum folic acid level. Alcoholic patients, who often have nutritional deficiency, may also have anemia of liver disease. Anemia of liver disease causes a macrocytic anemia but does not produce megaloblastic morphologic changes in the peripheral blood; rather, target cells are present. Hypothyroidism is associated with mild macrocytosis and also with pernicious anemia.

► Treatment

Folic acid deficiency is treated with daily oral folic acid (1 mg). The response is similar to that seen in the treatment of vitamin B_{12} deficiency, with rapid improvement and a sense of well-being, reticulocytosis in 5–7 days, and total correction of hematologic abnormalities within 2 months. Large doses of folic acid may produce hematologic responses in cases of vitamin B_{12} deficiency but permit neurologic damage to progress, hence knowing the vitamin B_{12} status in suspected folic acid deficiency is paramount.

► When to Refer

Referral to a hematologist is not usually necessary.

Farrell CJ et al. Red cell or serum folate: what to do in clinical practice. Clin Chem Lab Med. 2013 Mar 1;51(3):555–69. [PMID: 23449524]

Green R. Indicators for assessing folate and vitamin B-12 status and for monitoring the efficacy of intervention strategies. Am J Clin Nutr. 2011 Aug;94(2):666S–72S. [PMID: 21733877]

Sanghvi TG et al. Maternal iron-folic acid supplementation programs: evidence of impact and implementation. Food Nutr Bull. 2010 Jun;31(2 Suppl):S100–7. [PMID: 20715594]

HEMOLYTIC ANEMIAS

The hemolytic anemias are a group of disorders in which red blood cell survival is reduced, either episodically or continuously. The bone marrow has the ability to increase erythroid production up to eightfold in response to reduced red cell survival, so anemia will be present only when the ability of the bone marrow to compensate is outstripped. This will occur when red cell survival is extremely short or when the ability of the bone marrow to compensate is impaired.

Hemolytic disorders are generally classified according to whether the defect is intrinsic to the red cell or due to some external factor (Table 13–8). Intrinsic defects have been described in all components of the red blood cell, including the membrane, enzyme systems, and hemoglobin; most of these disorders are hereditary. Hemolytic anemias due to external factors are the immune and microangiopathic hemolytic anemias and infections of red blood cells.

Certain laboratory features are common to all the hemolytic anemias. Haptoglobin, a normal plasma protein that binds and clears free hemoglobin released into plasma, may be depressed in hemolytic disorders. However, the haptoglobin level is influenced by many factors and is not a reliable indicator of hemolysis, particularly in the setting of end-stage liver disease (its site of synthesis). When intravascular hemolysis occurs, transient hemoglobinemia occurs. Hemoglobin is filtered through the glomerulus and is usually reabsorbed by tubular cells. Hemoglobinuria will be present only when the capacity for reabsorption of

Table 13–8. Classification of hemolytic anemias.

Intrinsic

Membrane defects: hereditary spherocytosis, hereditary elliptocytosis, paroxysmal nocturnal hemoglobinuria

Glycolytic defects: pyruvate kinase deficiency, severe
hypophosphatemia

Oxidation vulnerability: glucose-6-phosphate dehydrogenase
deficiency, methemoglobinemia

Hemoglobinopathies: sickle cell syndromes, thalassemia, unstable hemoglobins, methemoglobinemia

Extrinsic

Immune: autoimmune, lymphoproliferative disease, drug
toxicity

Microangiopathic: thrombotic thrombocytopenic purpura,
hemolytic-uremic syndrome, disseminated intravascular
coagulation, valve hemolysis, metastatic adenocarcinoma,
vasculitis

Infection: *Plasmodium, Clostridium, Borrelia*

Hypersplenism

Burns

hemoglobin by renal tubular cells is exceeded. In its absence, evidence for prior intravascular hemolysis is the presence of hemosiderin in shed renal tubular cells (positive urine hemosiderin). With severe intravascular hemolysis, hemoglobinemia and methemalbuminemia may be present. Hemolysis increases the indirect bilirubin, and the total bilirubin may rise to 4 mg/dL (68 mcmol/L). Bilirubin levels higher than this may indicate some degree of hepatic dysfunction. Serum LD levels are strikingly elevated in cases of microangiopathic hemolysis (thrombotic thrombocytopenic purpura, hemolytic-uremic syndrome) and may be elevated in other hemolytic anemias.

PAROXYSMAL NOCTURNAL HEMOGLOBINURIA

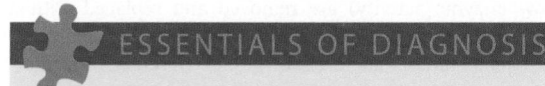

ESSENTIALS OF DIAGNOSIS

▶ Episodic hemoglobinuria.

▶ Thrombosis is common.

▶ Suspect in confusing cases of hemolytic anemia or pancytopenia.

▶ Flow cytometry demonstrates deficiencies of CD55 and CD59.

▶ General Considerations

Paroxysmal nocturnal hemoglobinuria (PNH) is a rare acquired clonal hematopoietic stem cell disorder that results in abnormal sensitivity of the red blood cell membrane to lysis by complement. The underlying cause is an acquired defect in the gene for phosphatidylinositol class A (PIG-A), which results in a deficiency of the glycosylphosphatidylinositol (GPI) anchor for cellular membrane proteins. In particular, the complement-regulating proteins

CD55 and CD59 are deficient, which permits unregulated formation of the complement membrane attack complex on red cell membranes and intravascular hemolysis. Free hemoglobin is released into the blood that scavenges nitric oxide and promotes esophageal spasms, male erectile dysfunction, renal damage, and thrombosis. Patients with significant PNH live 10–15 years; thrombosis is the primary cause of death.

▶ Clinical Findings

A. Symptoms and Signs

Classically, patients report episodic hemoglobinuria resulting in reddish brown urine. Hemoglobinuria is most often noticed in the first morning urine due to the drop in blood pH while sleeping that facilitates this hemolysis. Besides anemia, these patients are prone to thrombosis, especially within mesenteric and hepatic veins, central nervous system veins (sagittal vein), and skin vessels (with formation of painful nodules). As this is a hematopoietic stem cell disorder, PNH may appear de novo or arise in the setting of aplastic anemia with possible progression to myelodysplasia or acute myeloid leukemia (AML).

B. Laboratory Findings

Anemia is of variable severity and frequency, so reticulocytosis may or may not be present at any given time. Abnormalities on the blood smear are nondiagnostic and may include macro-ovalocytes and polychromasia. Since the episodic hemolysis is mainly intravascular, the finding of urine hemosiderin is a useful test. Serum LD is characteristically elevated. Iron deficiency is commonly present and is related to chronic iron loss from hemoglobinuria.

The white blood cell count and platelet count may be decreased and are always decreased in the setting of aplastic anemia. The best screening test is flow cytometry of blood granulocytes to demonstrate deficiency of CD55 and CD59. The FLAER assay (fluorescein-labeled proaerolysin) by flow cytometry is even more sensitive. Bone marrow morphology is variable and may show either generalized hypoplasia or erythroid hyperplasia or both. The bone marrow karyotype may be either normal or demonstrate a clonal abnormality.

▶ Treatment

Most patients with PNH have mild disease not requiring intervention. In severe cases and in those occurring in the setting of aplastic anemia or myelodysplasia, allogeneic hematopoietic stem cell transplantation has been used. In patients with severe hemolysis (usually requiring red cell transfusions), or thrombosis, treatment with eculizumab is warranted. Eculizumab is a humanized monoclonal antibody against complement protein C5—binding C5 prevents its cleavage so the membrane attack complex cannot assemble. Eculizumab improves quality of life and reduces hemolysis, transfusion requirements, and thrombosis risk. Eculizumab is expensive and increases the risk of *Neisseria meningitidis* infections; patients receiving the antibody must undergo meningococcal vaccination. Iron replacement is indicated for treatment of iron deficiency when present, which may improve the anemia while also causing a transient increase in hemolysis. For unclear reasons, corticosteroids are effective in decreasing hemolysis.

▶ When to Refer

Most patients with PNH should be under the care of a hematologist.

Hill A et al. Thrombosis in paroxysmal nocturnal hemoglobinuria. Blood. 2013 Jan 20;121(25):4985–96. [PMID: 23610373]

Keating GM et al. Eculizumab: a guide to its use in paroxysmal nocturnal hemoglobinuria. BioDrugs. 2012 Apr 1;26(2): 125–30. [PMID: 22350448]

Luzzatto L et al. Management of paroxysmal nocturnal haemoglobinuria: a personal view. Br J Haematol. 2011 Jun;153(6):709–20. [PMID: 21517820]

Parker CJ. Paroxysmal nocturnal hemoglobinuria. Curr Opin Hematol. 2012 May;19(3):141–8. [PMID: 22395662]

Pu JJ et al. Paroxysmal nocturnal hemoglobinuria from bench to bedside. Clin Transl Sci. 2011 Jun;4(3):219–24. [PMID: 21707954]

GLUCOSE-6-PHOSPHATE DEHYDROGENASE DEFICIENCY

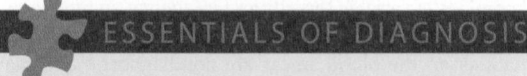

ESSENTIALS OF DIAGNOSIS

▶ X-linked recessive disorder seen commonly in American black men.

▶ Episodic hemolysis in response to oxidant drugs or infection.

▶ Bite cells and blister cells on the peripheral blood smear.

▶ Reduced levels of glucose-6-phosphate dehydrogenase between hemolytic episodes.

▶ General Considerations

Glucose-6-phosphate dehydrogenase (G6PD) deficiency is a hereditary enzyme defect that causes episodic hemolytic anemia because of the decreased ability of red blood cells to deal with oxidative stresses. G6PD deficiency leads to excess oxidized glutathione (hence, inadequate levels of reduced glutathione) that forces hemoglobin to denature and form precipitants called Heinz bodies. Heinz bodies cause red blood cell membrane damage, which leads to premature removal of these red blood cells by reticuloendothelial cells within the spleen (extravascular hemolysis).

Numerous G6PD isoenzymes have been described. The usual isoenzyme found in whites is designated G6PD-B and that in American blacks is designated G6PD-A, both of which have normal function and stability and therefore no hemolytic anemia. Ten to 15 percent of American blacks have the variant G6PD isoenzyme designated A–, in which there is both a reduction in normal enzyme activity and a reduction in stability. The A– isoenzyme activity declines

rapidly as the red blood cell ages past 40 days, a fact that explains the clinical findings in this disorder. More than 150 G6PD isoenzyme variants have been described, including some Mediterranean, Ashkenazi Jewish, and Asian variants with extremely low enzyme activity, episodic hemolysis, and exacerbations due to oxidizing substances including fava beans (class II G6PD activity). The other classes of G6PD isoenzyme activity are class I, extremely low activity with associated chronic, severe hemolysis; class III, 10–60% activity with episodic hemolysis (includes the American black A– isoform); class IV, 60–150% activity (normal); and class V, >150% activity. Patients with G6PD deficiency seem to be protected from malaria parasitic infection, have less coronary artery disease, and possibly have fewer cancers and greater longevity.

▶ Clinical Findings

G6PD deficiency is an X-linked disorder affecting 10–15% of American hemizygous black males and rare female homozygotes. Female carriers are rarely affected—only when an unusually high percentage of cells producing the normal enzyme are X-inactivated.

A. Symptoms and Signs

Patients are usually healthy, without chronic hemolytic anemia or splenomegaly. Hemolysis occurs episodically as a result of oxidative stress on the red blood cells, generated either by infection or exposure to certain drugs. Seven drugs initiate hemolysis and should be avoided: dapsone, methylthioninium chloride (methylene blue), phenazopyridine, primaquine, rasburicase, tolonium chloride (toluidine blue), and nitrofurantoin. Other drugs, such as sulfonamides, have been implicated but are less certain as offenders since they are often given during infections. Even with continuous use of the offending drug, the hemolytic episode is self-limited because older red blood cells (with low enzyme activity) are removed and replaced with a population of young red blood cells (reticulocytes) with adequate functional levels of G6PD. Severe G6PD deficiency (as in Mediterranean variants) may produce a chronic hemolytic anemia.

B. Laboratory Findings

Between hemolytic episodes, the blood is normal. During episodes of hemolysis, the hemoglobin rarely falls below 8 g/dL (80 g/L), and there is reticulocytosis and increased serum indirect bilirubin. The peripheral blood cell smear often reveals a small number of "bite" cells—cells that appear to have had a bite taken out of their periphery, or "blister" cells. This indicates pitting of precipitated membrane hemoglobin aggregates by the spleen. Heinz bodies may be demonstrated by staining a peripheral blood smear with cresyl violet; they are not visible on the usual Wright–Giemsa–stained blood smear. Specific enzyme assays for G6PD reveal a low level but may be falsely normal if they are performed during or shortly after a hemolytic episode during the period of reticulocytosis. In these cases, the enzyme assays should be repeated weeks after hemolysis has resolved. In severe cases of G6PD deficiency, enzyme levels are always low.

▶ Treatment

No treatment is necessary except to avoid known oxidant drugs.

Manganelli G et al. Glucose-6-phosphate dehydrogenase deficiency: disadvantages and possible benefits. Cardiovasc Hematol Disord Drug Targets. 2013 Mar 1;13(1):73–82. [PMID: 23534950]

Youngster I et al. Medications and glucose-6-phosphate dehydrogenase deficiency. An evidence-based review. Drug Saf. 2010 Sep 1;33(9):713–26. [PMID: 20701405]

SICKLE CELL ANEMIA & RELATED SYNDROMES

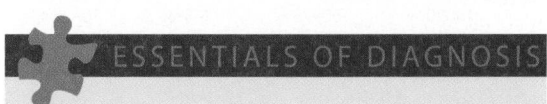

ESSENTIALS OF DIAGNOSIS

▶ Recurrent pain episodes.

▶ Positive family history and lifelong history of hemolytic anemia.

▶ Irreversibly sickled cells on peripheral blood smear.

▶ Hemoglobin S is the major hemoglobin seen on electrophoresis.

▶ General Considerations

Sickle cell anemia is an autosomal recessive disorder in which an abnormal hemoglobin leads to chronic hemolytic anemia with numerous clinical consequences. A single DNA base change leads to an amino acid substitution of valine for glutamine in the sixth position on the beta-globin chain. The abnormal beta chain is designated beta^s and the tetramer of alpha-2beta^s-2 is designated hemoglobin S. Hemoglobin S is unstable and polymerizes in the setting of various stressors, including hypoxemia and acidosis, leading to the formation of sickled red blood cells. Sickled cells result in hemolysis and the release of ATP, which is converted to adenosine. Adenosine binds to its receptor (A2B) resulting in the production of 2,3-biphosphoglycerate and the induction of more sickling and to its receptor (A2A) on natural killer cells resulting to pulmonary inflammation. The free hemoglobin from hemolysis scavenges nitric oxide causing endothelial dysfunction, vascular injury, and pulmonary hypertension.

The rate of sickling is influenced by the intracellular concentration of hemoglobin S and by the presence of other hemoglobins within the cell. Hemoglobin F cannot participate in polymer formation, and its presence markedly retards sickling. Factors that increase sickling are red cell dehydration and factors that lead to formation of deoxyhemoglobin S, eg, acidosis and hypoxemia, either systemic or locally in tissues. Hemolytic crises may be related to splenic sequestration of sickled cells (primarily in childhood before the spleen has been infarcted as a result of repeated sickling) or with coexistent disorders such as G6PD deficiency.

The beta^s gene is carried in 8% of American blacks, and 1 of 400 American black children will be born with sickle cell anemia. Prenatal diagnosis is available for couples at risk for producing a child with sickle cell anemia. Genetic counseling should be made available to such couples.

▶ Clinical Findings

A. Symptoms and Signs

The disorder has its onset during the first year of life, when hemoglobin F levels fall as a signal is sent to switch from production of gamma-globin to beta-globin. Chronic hemolytic anemia produces jaundice, pigment (calcium bilirubinate) gallstones, splenomegaly (early in life), and poorly healing ulcers over the lower tibia. Life-threatening severe anemia can occur during hemolytic or aplastic crises, the latter generally associated with viral or other infection or by folic acid deficiency causing reduced erythropoiesis.

Acute painful episodes due to acute vaso-occlusion from clusters of sickled red cells may occur spontaneously or be provoked by infection, dehydration, or hypoxia. Common sites of acute painful episodes include the bones (especially the back and long bones) and the chest. These episodes last hours to days and may produce low-grade fever. Acute vaso-occlusion may cause strokes due to sagittal sinus thrombosis or to bland or hemorrhagic arterial ischemia and may also cause priapism. Vaso-occlusive episodes are not associated with increased hemolysis.

Repeated episodes of vascular occlusion especially affect the heart, lungs, and liver. Ischemic necrosis of bone occurs, rendering the bone susceptible to osteomyelitis due to salmonellae and (somewhat less commonly) staphylococci. Infarction of the papillae of the renal medulla causes renal tubular concentrating defects and gross hematuria, more often encountered in sickle cell trait than in sickle cell anemia. Retinopathy similar to that noted in diabetes mellitus is often present and may lead to visual impairment. Pulmonary hypertension may develop and is associated with a poor prognosis.

These patients are prone to delayed puberty. An increased incidence of infection is related to hyposplenism as well as to defects in the alternative pathway of complement.

On examination, patients are often chronically ill and jaundiced. There is hepatomegaly, but the spleen is not palpable in adult life. The heart is enlarged, with a hyperdynamic precordium and systolic murmurs. Nonhealing ulcers of the lower leg and retinopathy may be present.

Sickle cell anemia becomes a chronic multisystem disease, with death from organ failure. With improved supportive care, average life expectancy is now between 40 and 50 years of age.

B. Laboratory Findings

Chronic hemolytic anemia is present. The hematocrit is usually 20–30%. The peripheral blood smear is characteristically abnormal, with irreversibly sickled cells comprising 5–50% of red cells. Other findings include reticulocytosis (10–25%), nucleated red blood cells, and hallmarks of hyposplenism such as Howell–Jolly bodies and target cells. The white blood cell count is characteristically elevated to

Table 13–9. Hemoglobin distribution in sickle cell syndromes.

Genotype	Clinical Diagnosis	Hb A	Hb S	Hb A$_2$	Hb F
AA	Normal	97–99%	0%	1–2%	< 1%
AS	Sickle trait	60%	40%	1–2%	< 1%
AS, alpha-thalassemia	Sickle trait, alpha-thalassemia	70–75%	25–30%	1–2%	< 1%
SS	Sickle cell anemia	0%	86–98%	1–3%	5–15%
SS, alpha-thalassemia, (3 genes)	SS alpha-thalassemia, silent	0%	90%	3%	7–9%
SS, alpha-thalassemia, (2 genes)	SS alpha-thalassemia, trait	0%	80%	3%	11–21%
S, beta^0-thalassemia	Sickle beta^0-thalassemia	0%	70–80%	3–5%	10–20%
S, beta$^+$-thalassemia	Sickle beta$^+$-thalassemia	10–20%	60–75%	3–5%	10–20%

Hb, hemoglobin.

12,000–15,000/mcL, and reactive thrombocytosis may occur. Indirect bilirubin levels are high.

After a screening test for sickle cell hemoglobin, the diagnosis of sickle cell anemia is confirmed by hemoglobin electrophoresis (Table 13–9). Hemoglobin S will usually comprise 85–98% of hemoglobin. In homozygous S disease, no hemoglobin A will be present. Hemoglobin F levels are variably increased, and high hemoglobin F levels are associated with a more benign clinical course. Patients with S-beta$^+$-thalassemia and SS alpha-thalassemia also have a more benign clinical course than sickle cell anemia.

Treatment

When allogeneic hematopoietic stem cell transplantation is performed before the onset of significant end-organ damage, it can cure more than 80% of children with sickle cell anemia who have suitable HLA-matched donors. Transplantation remains investigational in adults. Other therapies modulate disease severity: cytotoxic agents, such as hydroxyurea, increase hemoglobin F levels epigenetically. Hydroxyurea (500–750 mg orally daily) reduces the frequency of painful crises in patients whose quality of life is disrupted by frequent pain crises. Long-term follow-up of patients taking hydroxyurea demonstrate it improves overall survival and quality of life with little evidence for secondary malignancy. The use of omega-3 (n-3) fatty acid supplementation may reduce vaso-occlusive episodes and reduce transfusion needs in patients with sickle cell anemia.

Supportive care is the mainstay of treatment for sickle cell anemia. Patients are maintained on folic acid supplementation (1 mg orally daily) and given transfusions for aplastic or hemolytic crises. When acute painful episodes occur, precipitating factors should be identified and infections treated if present. The patient should be kept well hydrated, given generous analgesics, and supplied oxygen if hypoxic. Pneumococcal vaccination reduces the incidence of infections with this pathogen.

Severe acute vaso-occlusive crises can be treated with exchange transfusion. Exchange transfusions are primarily indicated for the treatment of intractable pain crises, acute chest syndrome, priapism, and stroke. Long-term transfusion therapy has been shown to be effective in reducing the risk of recurrent stroke in children.

When to Refer

Patients with sickle cell anemia should have their care coordinated with a hematologist and should be referred to a Comprehensive Sickle Cell Center if one is available.

When to Admit

Patients should be admitted for management of acute chest crises, for aplastic crisis, or for painful episodes that do not respond to outpatient care.

Daak AA et al. Effect of omega-3 (n-3) fatty acid supplementation in patients with sickle cell anemia: randomized, double-blind, placebo-controlled trial. Am J Clin Nutr. 2013 Jan; 97(1):37–44. [PMID: 23193009]
Darbari DS et al. What is the evidence that hydroxyurea improves health-related quality of life in patients with sickle cell disease? Hematology Am Soc Hematol Educ Program. 2012;2012:290–1. [PMID: 23233594]
Gillis VL et al. Management of an acute painful sickle cell episode in hospital: summary of NICE guidance. BMJ. 2012 Jun 27;344:e4063. [PMID: 22740566]
Kassim AA et al. Sickle cell disease, vasculopathy, and therapeutics. Annu Rev Med. 2013;64:451–66. [PMID: 23190149]
McCavit TL. Sickle cell disease. Pediatr Rev. 2012 May;33(5): 195–204. [PMID: 22550263]
Tisdale JF et al. HCT for nonmalignant disorders. Biol Blood Marrow Transplant. 2013 Jan;19(1 Suppl):S6–9. [PMID: 23104188]

SICKLE CELL TRAIT

People with the heterozygous genotype (AS) have sickle cell trait. These persons are hematologically normal, with no anemia and normal red blood cells on peripheral blood smear. A screening test for sickle hemoglobin will be positive, and hemoglobin electrophoresis will reveal that approximately 40% of hemoglobin is hemoglobin S (Table 13–9). People with sickle cell trait may experience sudden cardiac death and rhabdomyolysis during vigorous exercise, especially at high altitudes. They may also be at increased risk for venothromboembolism. Chronic sickling of red blood cells in the acidotic renal medulla results in microscopic and gross hematuria, hyposthenuria (poor urine concentrating ability), and possibly chronic kidney disease.

No treatment is necessary. Genetic counseling is recommended.

Key NS et al. Sickle-cell trait: novel clinical significance. Hematology Am Soc Hematol Educ Program. 2010;2010:418–22. [PMID: 21239829]

Tripette J et al. Exercise-related complications in sick cell trait. Clin Hemorheol Microcirc. 2013 Jan 1;55(1):29–37. [PMID: 23478224]

SICKLE THALASSEMIA

Patients with homozygous sickle cell anemia and alpha-thalassemia have less vigorous hemolysis and run higher hemoglobins than SS patients due to reduced red blood cell sickling related to a lower hemoglobin concentration within the red blood cell and higher hemoglobin F levels (Table 13–9). The MCV is low, and the red cells are hypochromic.

Patients who are compound heterozygotes for $beta^s$ and beta-thalassemia are clinically affected with sickle cell syndromes. Sickle $beta^0$-thalassemia is clinically very similar to homozygous SS disease. Vaso-occlusive crises may be somewhat less severe, and the spleen is not always infarcted. The MCV is low, in contrast to the normal MCV of sickle cell anemia. Hemoglobin electrophoresis reveals no hemoglobin A but will show an increase in hemoglobins A_2 and F (Table 13–9).

Sickle $beta^+$-thalassemia is a milder disorder than homozygous SS disease, with fewer crises. The spleen is usually palpable. The hemolytic anemia is less severe, and the hematocrit is usually 30–38%, with reticulocytes of 5–10%. Hemoglobin electrophoresis shows the presence of some hemoglobin A and elevated hemoglobins A_2 and F (Table 13–9). The MCV is low.

Sankaran VG et al. Modifier genes in Mendelian disorders: the example of hemoglobin disorders. Ann NY Acad Sci. 2010 Dec;1214:47–56. [PMID: 21039591]

Steinberg MH et al. Genetic modifiers of sickle cell disease. Am J Hematol. 2012 Aug;87(8):795–803. [PMID: 22641398]

AUTOIMMUNE HEMOLYTIC ANEMIA

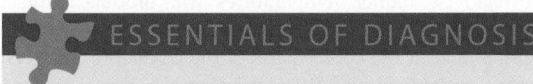

ESSENTIALS OF DIAGNOSIS

► Acquired hemolytic anemia caused by IgG autoantibody.

► Spherocytes and reticulocytosis on peripheral blood smear.

► Positive antiglobulin (Coombs) test.

► General Considerations

Autoimmune hemolytic anemia is an acquired disorder in which an IgG autoantibody is formed that binds to the red blood cell membrane and does so most avidly at body temperature (ie, a "warm" autoantibody). The antibody is most commonly directed against a basic component of the Rh system present on most human red blood cells. When IgG antibodies coat the red blood cell, the Fc portion of the antibody is recognized by macrophages present in the spleen and other portions of the reticuloendothelial system. The interaction between splenic macrophages and the antibody-coated red blood cell results in removal of red blood cell membrane and the formation of a spherocyte due to the decrease in surface-to-volume ratio of the surviving red blood cell. These spherocytic cells have decreased deformability and are unable to squeeze through the 2-mcm fenestrations of splenic sinusoids and become trapped in the red pulp of the spleen. When large amounts of IgG are present on red blood cells, complement may be fixed. Direct complement lysis of cells is rare, but the presence of C3b on the surface of red blood cells allows Kupffer cells in the liver to participate in the hemolytic process via C3b receptors. The destruction of red blood cells in the spleen and liver designates this as extravascular hemolysis.

Approximately one-half of all cases of autoimmune hemolytic anemia are idiopathic. The disorder may also be seen in association with systemic lupus erythematosus, CLL, or lymphomas. It must be distinguished from drug-induced hemolytic anemia. When penicillin (or other drugs, especially cefotetan, ceftriaxone, and piperacillin) coats the red blood cell membrane, the antibody is directed against the membrane–drug complex. Fludarabine, an antineoplastic, causes autoimmune hemolytic anemia through its immunosuppression effects resulting in defective self- vs non-self immune surveillance permitting the escape of a B-cell clone, which produces the offending autoantibody.

► Clinical Findings

A. Symptoms and Signs

Autoimmune hemolytic anemia typically produces an anemia of rapid onset that may be life threatening. Patients complain of fatigue and dyspnea and may present with angina pectoris or heart failure. On examination, jaundice and splenomegaly are usually present.

B. Laboratory Findings

The anemia is of variable severity but may be very severe, with hematocrit of < 10%. Reticulocytosis is present, and spherocytes are seen on the peripheral blood smear. In cases of severe hemolysis, the stressed bone marrow may also release nucleated red blood cells. As with other hemolytic disorders, the serum indirect bilirubin is increased and the haptoglobin is low. Approximately 10% of patients with autoimmune hemolytic anemia have coincident immune thrombocytopenia (Evans syndrome).

The antiglobulin (Coombs) test (DAT) forms the basis for diagnosis. The Coombs reagent is a rabbit IgM antibody raised against human IgG or human complement. The direct antiglobulin (Coombs) test is performed by mixing the patient's red blood cells with the Coombs reagent and looking for agglutination, which indicates the presence of antibody or complement or both on the red blood cell surface. The indirect antiglobulin (Coombs) test is performed by mixing the patient's serum with a panel of type O red blood cells. After incubation of the test serum and panel red blood cells, the Coombs reagent is added. Agglutination in this system indicates the presence of free antibody in the patient's serum.

The direct antiglobulin test is positive (for IgG, complement, or both) in about 90% of patients with autoimmune hemolytic anemia. The indirect antiglobulin test may or may not be positive. A positive indirect antiglobulin test indicates the presence of a large amount of autoantibody that has saturated binding sites in the red blood cell and consequently appears in the serum. Because the patient's serum usually contains the autoantibody, it may be difficult to obtain a "compatible" cross-match with homologous red blood cells to be used for transfusion.

▶ Treatment

Initial treatment consists of prednisone, 1–2 mg/kg/d orally in divided doses. Patients with DAT-negative and DAT-positive autoimmune hemolysis respond equally well to corticosteroids. Transfused red blood cells will survive similarly to the patient's own red blood cells. Because of difficulty in performing the cross-match, "incompatible" blood may need to be given. Decisions regarding transfusions should be made in consultation with a hematologist and a blood bank specialist. If prednisone is ineffective or if the disease recurs on tapering the dose, splenectomy should be considered. Splenectomy may cure the disorder. Death from cardiovascular collapse can occur in the setting of rapid hemolysis. In patients with rapid hemolysis, therapeutic plasmapheresis should be performed early in management to physically unload autoantibodies. Patients with autoimmune hemolytic anemia refractory to prednisone and splenectomy may be treated with a variety of agents. Treatment with rituximab, a monoclonal antibody against the B cell antigen CD20, is effective in some cases. The suggested dose is 375 mg/m^2 intravenously weekly for 4 weeks. Danazol, 400–800 mg/d orally, is less often effective than in immune thrombocytopenia but is well suited for long-term use because of its low toxicity profile. Immunosuppressive agents, including cyclophosphamide, azathioprine, mycophenolate mofetil, alemtuzumab (an anti-CD52 antibody), or cyclosporine, may also be used. High-dose intravenous immune globulin (1 g/kg daily for 2 days) may be effective in controlling hemolysis. The benefit is short-lived (1–3 weeks), and the drug is very expensive. The long-term prognosis for patients with this disorder is good, especially if there is no other underlying autoimmune disorder or lymphoproliferative disorder. Treatment of an associated lymphoproliferative disorder will also treat the hemolytic anemia.

▶ When to Refer

Patients with autoimmune hemolytic anemia should be referred to a hematologist for confirmation of the diagnosis and subsequent care.

▶ When to Admit

Patients should be hospitalized for symptomatic anemia or rapidly falling hemoglobin levels.

Barros MM et al. Warm autoimmune hemolytic anemia: recent progress in understanding the immunobiology and the treatment. Transfus Med Rev. 2010 Jul;24(3):195–210. [PMID: 20656187]

Garratty G. Immune hemolytic anemia associated with drug therapy. Blood Rev. 2010 July–Sep;24(4–5):143–50. [PMID: 20650555]

Jaime-Pérez JC et al. Current approaches for the treatment of autoimmune hemolytic anemia. Arch Immunol Ther Exp (Warsz). 2013 Oct;61(5):385–95. [PMID: 23689532]

Kamesaki T et al. Characterization of direct antiglobulin test-negative autoimmune hemolytic anemia: a study of 154 cases. Am J Hematol. 2013 Feb;88(2):93–6. [PMID: 23169533]

Lechner K et al. How I treat autoimmune hemolytic anemias in adults. Blood. 2010 Sept 16;116(11):1821–8. [PMID: 20548093]

Zeerleder S. Autoimmune haemolytic anaemia—a practical guide to cope with a diagnostic and therapeutic challenge. Neth J Med. 2011 Apr;69(4):177–84. [PMID: 21527804]

COLD AGGLUTININ DISEASE

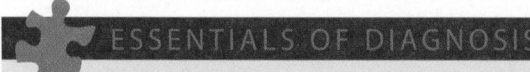
ESSENTIALS OF DIAGNOSIS

▶ Increased reticulocytes on peripheral blood smear.

▶ Antiglobulin (Coombs) test positive only for complement.

▶ Positive cold agglutinin titer.

▶ General Considerations

Cold agglutinin disease is an acquired hemolytic anemia due to an IgM autoantibody (called a cold agglutinin) usually directed against the I/i antigen on red blood cells. These IgM autoantibodies characteristically will not react with cells at 37°C but only at lower temperatures, most avidly at 0–4°C (ie, "cold" autoantibody). Since the blood temperature (even in the most peripheral parts of the body) rarely goes lower than 20°C, only antibodies reactive at relatively higher temperatures will produce clinical effects. Hemolysis results indirectly from attachment of IgM, which in the cooler parts of the circulation (fingers, nose, ears) binds and fixes complement. When the red blood cell returns to a warmer temperature, the IgM antibody dissociates, leaving complement on the cell. Lysis of red blood cells rarely occurs. Rather, C3b, present on the red blood cells, is recognized by Kupffer cells (which have receptors for C3b), and red blood cell sequestration and destruction in the liver ensues. In some cases, the complement membrane attack complex forms, lysing the red blood cells (intravascular hemolysis).

Most cases of chronic cold agglutinin disease are idiopathic. Others occur in association with Waldenström macroglobulinemia, lymphoma, or CLL, in which a monoclonal IgM paraprotein is produced. Acute postinfectious cold agglutinin disease occurs following mycoplasmal pneumonia or viral infection (infectious mononucleosis, measles, mumps, or cytomegalovirus (CMV) with antibody directed against antigen i rather than I).

▶ Clinical Findings

A. Symptoms and Signs

In chronic cold agglutinin disease, symptoms related to red blood cell agglutination occur on exposure to cold, and patients may complain of mottled or numb fingers or toes, acrocyanosis, episodic low back pain, and dark colored urine. Hemolytic anemia is rarely severe, but episodic hemoglobinuria may occur on exposure to cold. The hemolytic anemia in acute postinfectious syndromes is rarely severe.

B. Laboratory Findings

Mild anemia is present with reticulocytosis and rarely spherocytes. The blood smear made at room temperature shows agglutinated red blood cells (there is no agglutination on a blood smear made at body temperature). The direct antiglobulin (Coombs) test will be positive for complement only. Serum cold agglutinin titer will semi-quantitate the autoantibody. A monoclonal IgM is often found on serum protein electrophoresis and confirmed by serum immunoelectrophoresis. There is indirect hyperbilirubinemia and the haptoglobin is low during periods of hemolysis.

▶ Treatment

Treatment is largely symptomatic, based on avoiding exposure to cold. Splenectomy and prednisone are usually ineffective (except when associated with a lymphoproliferative disorder) since hemolysis takes place in the liver and blood stream. Rituximab is the treatment of choice. The dose is 375 mg/m^2 intravenously weekly for 4 weeks. Relapses may be effectively re-treated. High-dose intravenous immunoglobulin (2 g/kg) may be effective temporarily, but it is rarely used because of the high cost and short duration of benefit. Patients with severe disease may be treated with cytotoxic agents, such as cyclophosphamide, fludarabine, or bortezomib, or with immunosuppressive agents, such as cyclosporine. As in warm IgG-mediated autoimmune hemolysis, it may be difficult to find compatible blood for transfusion. Red blood cells should be transfused through an in-line blood warmer.

Berentsen S et al. Diagnosis and treatment of cold agglutinin mediated autoimmune hemolytic anemia. Blood Rev. 2012 May;26(3):107–15. [PMID: 22330255]
Swiecicki PL et al. Cold agglutinin disease. Blood. 2013 Aug 15;122(7):1114–21. [PMID: 23757733]

APLASTIC ANEMIA

 ESSENTIALS OF DIAGNOSIS

- ▶ Pancytopenia.
- ▶ No abnormal hematopoietic cells seen in blood or bone marrow.
- ▶ Hypocellular bone marrow.

▶ General Considerations

Aplastic anemia is a condition of bone marrow failure that arises from suppression of or injury to the hematopoietic stem cell. The bone marrow becomes hypoplastic, fails to produce mature blood cells, and pancytopenia develops.

There are a number of causes of aplastic anemia (Table 13–10). Direct hematopoietic stem cell injury may be caused by radiation, chemotherapy, toxins, or pharmacologic agents. Systemic lupus erythematosus may rarely cause suppression of the hematopoietic stem cell by an IgG autoantibody directed against the hematopoietic stem cell. However, the most common pathogenesis of aplastic anemia appears to be autoimmune suppression of hematopoiesis by a T–cell-mediated cellular mechanism, so called "idiopathic" aplastic anemia. In some cases of "idiopathic" aplastic anemia, defects in maintenance of the hematopoietic stem cell telomere length (dyskeratosis congenita) or in DNA repair pathways (Fanconi anemia) have been identified and are likely linked to both the initiation of bone marrow failure and the propensity to later progress to myelodysplasia, PNH, or AML. Complex detrimental immune responses to viruses can also cause aplastic anemia.

▶ Clinical Findings

A. Symptoms and Signs

Patients come to medical attention because of the consequences of bone marrow failure. Anemia leads to symptoms of weakness and fatigue, neutropenia causes vulnerability to

Table 13–10. Causes of aplastic anemia.

Autoimmune: idiopathic, systemic lupus erythematosus
Congenital—defects in telomere length maintenance or DNA repair (rare)
Chemotherapy, radiotherapy
Toxins: benzene, toluene, insecticides
Drugs: chloramphenicol, phenylbutazone, gold salts, sulfonamides, phenytoin, carbamazepine, quinacrine, tolbutamide
Post-viral hepatitis (A, B, C, E, G, non-A through -G)
Non-hepatitis viruses (EBV, parvovirus, CMV, echovirus 3, others)
Pregnancy
Paroxysmal nocturnal hemoglobinuria

EBV, Epstein Barr Virus; CMV, cytomegalovirus.

bacterial or fungal infections, and thrombocytopenia results in mucosal and skin bleeding. Physical examination may reveal signs of pallor, purpura, and petechiae. Other abnormalities such as hepatosplenomegaly, lymphadenopathy, or bone tenderness should *not* be present, and their presence should lead to questioning the diagnosis.

B. Laboratory Findings

The hallmark of aplastic anemia is pancytopenia. However, early in the evolution of aplastic anemia, only one or two cell lines may be reduced.

Anemia may be severe and is always associated with reticulocytopenia. Red blood cell morphology is unremarkable, but there may be mild macrocytosis (increased MCV). Neutrophils and platelets are reduced in number, and no immature or abnormal forms are seen on the blood smear. The bone marrow aspirate and the bone marrow biopsy appear hypocellular, with only scant amounts of morphologically normal hematopoietic progenitors. The bone marrow karyotype should be normal (or germline if normal variant).

▶ Differential Diagnosis

Aplastic anemia must be differentiated from other causes of pancytopenia (Table 13–11). Hypocellular forms of myelodysplasia or acute leukemia may occasionally be confused with aplastic anemia. These are differentiated by the presence of cellular morphologic abnormalities or increased blasts, or by the presence of an abnormal karyotype in bone marrow cells. Hairy cell leukemia has been misdiagnosed as aplastic anemia and should be recognized by the presence of splenomegaly and by abnormal lymphoid cells in a hypocellular bone marrow biopsy. Pancytopenia with a normocellular bone marrow may be due to systemic lupus erythematosus, disseminated infection, hypersplenism, nutritional deficiency (eg, vitamin B_{12} or folate), or myelodysplasia. Isolated thrombocytopenia may occur early as aplastic anemia develops and may be confused with immune thrombocytopenia.

Table 13–11. Causes of pancytopenia.

Bone marrow disorders
Aplastic anemia
Myelodysplasia
Acute leukemia
Chronic idiopathic myelofibrosis
Infiltrative disease: lymphoma, myeloma, carcinoma, hairy cell leukemia, etc.
Nonmarrow disorders
Hypersplenism (with or without portal hypertension)
Systemic lupus erythematosus
Infection: tuberculosis, HIV infection, leishmaniasis, brucellosis, CMV, parvovirus B19
Nutritional deficiency (megaloblastic anemia)
Medications
Cytotoxic chemotherapy
Ionizing radiation

CMV, cytomegalovirus.

▶ Treatment

Mild cases of aplastic anemia may be treated with supportive care, including erythropoietic (epoetin or darbepoetin) or myeloid (filgrastim or sargramostim) growth factors, or both. Red blood cell transfusions and platelet transfusions are given as necessary, and antibiotics are used to treat infections.

Severe aplastic anemia is defined by a neutrophil count of < 500/mcL, platelets < 20,000/mcL, reticulocytes < 1%, and bone marrow cellularity < 20%. The treatment of choice for young adults (under age 40 years) who have an HLA-matched sibling is allogeneic bone marrow transplantation. Children or young adults may also benefit from allogeneic bone marrow transplantation using an unrelated donor. Because of the increased risks associated with unrelated donor allogeneic bone marrow transplantation relative to sibling donors, this treatment is usually reserved for patients who have not responded to immunosuppressive therapy.

For adults over age 40 years or those without HLA-matched donors, the treatment of choice for severe aplastic anemia is immunosuppression with equine antithymocyte globulin (ATG) plus cyclosporine. Equine ATG is given in the hospital in conjunction with transfusion and antibiotic support. A proven regimen is equine ATG 40 mg/kg/d intravenously for 4 days in combination with cyclosporine, 6 mg/kg orally twice daily. Equine ATG is superior to rabbit ATG, resulting in a higher response rate and better survival. ATG should be used in combination with corticosteroids (prednisone or methylprednisolone 1–2 mg/kg/d orally for 1 week, followed by a taper over 2 weeks) to avoid ATG infusion reactions and serum sickness. Responses usually occur in 1–3 months and are usually only partial, but the blood counts rise high enough to give patients a safe and transfusion-free life. The full benefit of immunosuppression is generally assessed at 4 months post-equine ATG. Cyclosporine is maintained at full dose for 6 months and then stopped in responding patients. Androgens (such as fluoxymesterone 10–20 mg/d orally in divided doses) have been widely used in the past, with a low response rate, and may be considered in mild cases. Androgens appear to partially correct telomere length maintenance defects and increase the production of endogenous erythropoietin. The thrombopoietin mimetic, eltrombopag, may help increase platelets (and also red blood cells and white blood cells) in patients with refractory aplastic anemia.

▶ Course & Prognosis

Patients with severe aplastic anemia have a rapidly fatal illness if left untreated. Allogeneic bone marrow transplant from a HLA-matched sibling donor produces survival rates over 80% in recipients under 20 years old and about 65–70% in those 20- to 50-years-old. Respective survival rates drop 10–15% when the donor is HLA-matched but unrelated. Equine ATG-cyclosporine immunosuppressive treatment leads to a response in approximately 70% of patients. Up to one-third of patients will relapse with aplastic anemia after ATG-based therapy. Clonal hematologic disorders, such as PNH, AML, or myelodysplasia, may develop in one-quarter of patients treated with immuno-suppressive therapy after 10 years of follow-up. Factors that predict response to ATG-cyclosporine therapy are patient's age, reticulocyte count, lymphocyte count, and age-adjusted telomere length of leukocytes at the time of diagnosis.

► When to Refer

All patients should be referred to a hematologist.

► When to Admit

Admission is necessary for treatment of neutropenic infection, the administration of ATG, or allogeneic bone marrow transplantation.

Dezern AE et al. Clinical management of aplastic anemia. Expert Rev Hematol. 2011 Apr;4(2):221–30. [PMID: 21495931]

Eapen M. Allogeneic transplantation for aplastic anemia. Hematology. 2012 Apr;17(Suppl 1):S15–7. [PMID: 22507769]

Olnes MJ et al. Eltrombopag and improved hematopoiesis in refractory aplastic anemia. N Engl J Med. 2012 Jul 5;367(1):11–19. [PMID: 22762314]

Rauff B et al. Hepatitis associated aplastic anemia: a review. Virol J. 2011 Feb 28;8:87–92. [PMID: 21352606]

Scheinberg P et al. Horse versus rabbit antithymocyte globulin in acquired aplastic anemia. N Engl J Med. 2011 Aug 4;365(5):430–8. [PMID: 21812672]

Scheinberg P et al. How I treat acquired aplastic anemia. Blood. 2012 Aug 9;120(6):1185–96. [PMID: 22517900]

NEUTROPENIA

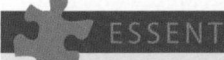

ESSENTIALS OF DIAGNOSIS

► Neutrophils < 1800/mcL (< 1.8 × 10⁹/L).

► Severe neutropenia if neutrophils < 500/mcL (< 0.5 × 10⁹/L).

► General Considerations

Neutropenia is present when the absolute neutrophil count is < 1800/mcL (< 1.8 × 10⁹/L), although blacks, Asians, and other specific ethnic groups may have normal neutrophil counts as low as 1200/mcL (< 1.2 × 10⁹/L). The neutropenic patient is increasingly vulnerable to infection by gram-positive and gram-negative bacteria and by fungi. The risk of infection is related to the severity of neutropenia. The risk of serious infection rises sharply with neutrophil counts < 500/mcL (< 0.5 × 10⁹/L), and neutrophil counts < 100/mcL (< 0.1 × 10⁹/L) ("profound neutropenia") are associated with a high risk of infection within days. Patients with "chronic benign neutropenia" are free of infection despite very low stable neutrophil levels; they seem to respond adequately to infections and inflammatory stimuli with an appropriate neutrophil release from the bone marrow. In contrast, the neutrophil count of patients with cyclic neutropenia periodically oscillate (usually in 21-day cycles)

Table 13–12. Causes of neutropenia.

Bone marrow disorders
Congenital
Dyskeratosis congenita
Fanconi anemia
Cyclic neutropenia
Large granular lymphocytic leukemia
Hairy cell leukemia
Myelodysplasia
Non-bone marrow disorders
Drugs: sulfonamides, chlorpromazine, procainamide, penicillin, cephalosporins, cimetidine, methimazole, phenytoin, chlorpropamide, antiretroviral medications, rituximab
Aplastic anemia
Myelosuppressive cytotoxic chemotherapy
Benign chronic neutropenia
Pure white cell aplasia
Hypersplenism
Sepsis
Other immune
Felty syndrome
Systemic lupus erythematosus
HIV infection

between normal and low, with infections occurring during the nadirs. Both cyclic neutropenia and congenital neutropenia represent problems in mutations in the neutrophil elastase genes *ELA-2* or *ELANE*.

A variety of bone marrow disorders and nonmarrow conditions may cause neutropenia (Table 13–12). All of the causes of aplastic anemia (Table 13–10) and pancytopenia (Table 13–11) may cause neutropenia. The new onset of an isolated neutropenia is most often due to an idiosyncratic reaction to a drug, and agranulocytosis (complete absence of neutrophils in the peripheral blood) is almost always due to a drug reaction. In these cases, examination of the bone marrow shows an almost complete absence of granulocyte precursors with other cell lines undisturbed. This marrow finding is also seen in pure white blood cell aplasia, an autoimmune attack on marrow granulocyte precursors. Neutropenia in the presence of a normal bone marrow may be due to immunologic peripheral destruction (autoimmune neutropenia), sepsis, or hypersplenism. The presence in the serum of antineutrophil antibodies supports the diagnosis of autoimmune neutropenia. **Felty syndrome** is an immune neutropenia associated with seropositive nodular rheumatoid arthritis and splenomegaly. Severe neutropenia may be associated with clonal disorders of T lymphocytes, often with the morphology of large granular lymphocytes, referred to as CD3-positive T-cell large granular lymphoproliferative disorder. Isolated neutropenia is an uncommon presentation of hairy cell leukemia or a myelodysplastic syndrome. By its nature, myelosuppressive cytotoxic chemotherapy causes neutropenia in a predictable manner.

► Clinical Findings

Neutropenia results in stomatitis and in infections due to gram-positive or gram-negative aerobic bacteria or to fungi such as *Candida* or *Aspergillus*. The most common infections are septicemia, cellulitis, pneumonia, and neutropenic fever of unknown origin. Fever should always be initially assumed to be of infectious origin until proven otherwise.

▶ Treatment

Treatment of neutropenia depends on its cause. Potential causative drugs should be discontinued. Myeloid growth factors (filgrastim or sargramostim) help facilitate neutrophil recovery after offending drugs are stopped. Chronic myeloid growth factor administration (daily or every other day) is effective at dampening the neutropenia seen in cyclic or congenital neutropenia. When Felty syndrome leads to repeated bacterial infections, splenectomy has been the treatment of choice, but sustained use of myeloid growth factors is effective and provides a nonsurgical alternative. Patients with autoimmune neutropenia often respond to immunosuppression with corticosteroids, with splenectomy held in reserve for corticosteroid failure. Patients with true pure white blood cell aplasia need immunosuppression with ATG and cyclosporine, as in aplastic anemia. The neutropenia associated with large granular lymphoproliferative disorder may respond to therapy with either low-dose methotrexate or cyclosporine.

Fevers during neutropenia should be considered as infectious until proven otherwise. Febrile neutropenia is a life-threatening circumstance. Enteric gram-negative bacteria are of primary concern and often empirically treated with fluoroquinolones or third- or fourth-generation cephalosporins. For protracted neutropenia, fungal infections are problematic and empiric coverage with azoles (fluconazole for yeast and voriconazole, itraconazole, or posaconazole for molds) or echinocandins is recommended. The neutropenia following myelosuppressive chemotherapy is predictable and is largely ameliorated by the use of myeloid growth factors. For patients with acute leukemia undergoing intense chemotherapy or patients with solid cancer undergoing high-dose chemotherapy, the prophylactic use of antimicrobial agents and the myeloid growth factors is recommended.

▶ When to Refer

Refer to a hematologist if neutrophils are persistently and unexplainably < 1000/mcL (< 1.0 × 10⁹/L).

▶ When to Admit

Neutropenia by itself is not an indication for hospitalization. However, most patients with severe neutropenia have a serious underlying disease that may require inpatient treatment. Most patients with febrile neutropenia require hospitalization to treat infection.

Andres E et al. The role of haematopoietic growth factors granulocyte colony-stimulating factor and granulocyte-macrophage colony-stimulating factor in the management of drug-induced agranulocytosis. Br J Haematol. 2010 Jul;150(1):3–8. [PMID: 20151980]

Flowers CR et al. Antimicrobial prophylaxis and outpatient management of fever and neutropenia in adults treated for malignancy: American Society of Clinical Oncology clinical practice guideline. J Clin Oncol. 2013 Feb 20;31(6):794–810. [PMID: 23319691]

Legrand M et al. Survival in neutropenic patients with severe sepsis or septic shock. Crit Care Med. 2012 Jan;40(1):43–9. [PMID: 21926615]

Newberger PE et al. Evaluation and management of patients with isolated neutropenia. Semin Hematol. 2013 Jul;50(3): 198–206. [PMID: 23953336]

▼ LEUKEMIAS & OTHER MYELOPROLIFERATIVE NEOPLASMS

Myeloproliferative disorders are due to acquired clonal abnormalities of the hematopoietic stem cell. Since the stem cell gives rise to myeloid, erythroid, and platelet cells, qualitative and quantitative changes are seen in all these cell lines. Classically, the myeloproliferative disorders produce characteristic syndromes with well-defined clinical and laboratory features (Tables 13–13 and 13–14). However, these disorders are grouped together because they may evolve from one into another and because hybrid disorders are commonly seen. All of the myeloproliferative disorders may progress to AML.

The Philadelphia chromosome seen in chronic myeloid leukemia (CML) was the first recurrent cytogenetic abnormality to be described in a human malignancy. Since that time, there has been tremendous progress in elucidating the genetic nature of these disorders, with identification of mutations in *JAK2, MPL, TET2, IDH1/2, DNMT3A,* and other genes.

POLYCYTHEMIA VERA

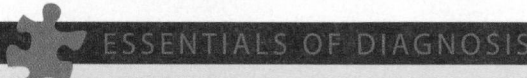

ESSENTIALS OF DIAGNOSIS

- ▶ *JAK2 V617F* mutation.
- ▶ Increased red blood cell mass.
- ▶ Splenomegaly.
- ▶ Normal arterial oxygen saturation.
- ▶ Usually elevated white blood count and platelet count.

Table 13–13. Classification of myeloproliferative disorders.

Myeloproliferative neoplasms
Polycythemia vera
Primary myelofibrosis
Essential thrombocytosis
Chronic myeloid leukemia
Myelodysplastic syndromes
Acute myeloid leukemia

Table 13–14. Laboratory features of myeloproliferative neoplasms.

	White Count	Hematocrit	Platelet Count	Red Cell Morphology
Polycythemia vera	N or ↑	↑	N or ↑	N
Essential thrombocytosis	N or ↑	N	↑↑	N
Primary myelofibrosis	N or ↓ or ↑	↓	↓ or N or ↑	Abn
Chronic myeloid leukemia	↑↑	N	N or ↑	N

Abn, abnormal; N, normal.

General Considerations

Polycythemia vera is an acquired myeloproliferative disorder that causes overproduction of all three hematopoietic cell lines, most prominently the red blood cells. Erythroid production is independent of erythropoietin, and the serum erythropoietin level is low. A mutation in exon 14 of *JAK2 (V617F)*, a signaling molecule, has been demonstrated in 95% of cases. Additional *JAK2* mutations have been identified (exon 12) and suggest that *JAK2* is involved in the pathogenesis of this disease and is a potential therapeutic target.

True erythrocytosis, with an elevated red blood cell mass, should be distinguished from spurious erythrocytosis caused by a constricted plasma volume. Primary polycythemia (polycythemia vera) is a bone marrow disorder characterized by autonomous overproduction of erythroid cells.

Clinical Findings

A. Symptoms and Signs

Headache, dizziness, tinnitus, blurred vision, and fatigue are common complaints related to expanded blood volume and increased blood viscosity. Generalized pruritus, especially following a warm shower or bath, is related to histamine release from the basophilia. Epistaxis is probably related to engorgement of mucosal blood vessels in combination with abnormal hemostasis due to qualitative abnormalities in platelet function. Sixty percent of patients are men, and the median age at presentation is 60 years. Polycythemia rarely occurs in persons under age 40 years.

Physical examination reveals plethora and engorged retinal veins. The spleen is palpable in 75% of cases but is nearly always enlarged when imaged.

Thrombosis is the most common complication of polycythemia vera and the major cause of morbidity and death in this disorder. Thrombosis appears to be related both to increased blood viscosity and abnormal platelet function. Uncontrolled polycythemia leads to a very high incidence of thrombotic complications of surgery, and elective surgery should be deferred until the condition has been treated. Paradoxically, in addition to thrombosis, increased bleeding can also occur. There is a high incidence of peptic ulcer disease.

B. Laboratory Findings

The hallmark of polycythemia vera is a hematocrit (at sea level) that exceeds 54% in males or 51% in females. Red blood cell morphology is normal (Table 13–14). By definition, the red blood cell mass is elevated, but this is now rarely measured. The white blood count is usually elevated to 10,000–20,000/mcL and the platelet count is variably increased, sometimes to counts exceeding 1,000,000/mcL. Platelet morphology is usually normal. White blood cells are usually normal, but basophilia and eosinophilia are frequently present. Erythropoietin levels are suppressed and are usually low. The diagnosis should be confirmed with *JAK2* mutation screening. The absence of a mutation should lead the clinician to question the diagnosis.

The bone marrow is hypercellular, with panhyperplasia of all hematopoietic elements, but bone marrow examination is not necessary to establish the diagnosis. Iron stores are usually absent from the bone marrow, having been transferred to the increased circulating red blood cell mass. Iron deficiency may also result from chronic gastrointestinal blood loss. Bleeding may lower the hematocrit to the normal range (or lower), creating diagnostic confusion, and may lead to a situation with significant microcytosis with a normal hematocrit.

Vitamin B_{12} levels are strikingly elevated because of increased levels of transcobalamin III (secreted by white blood cells). Overproduction of uric acid may lead to hyperuricemia.

Although red blood cell morphology is usually normal at presentation, microcytosis, hypochromia, and poikilocytosis may result from iron deficiency following treatment by phlebotomy (see below). Progressive hypersplenism may also lead to elliptocytosis.

Differential Diagnosis

Spurious polycythemia, in which an elevated hematocrit is due to contracted plasma volume rather than increased red cell mass, may be related to diuretic use or may occur without obvious cause.

A secondary cause of polycythemia should be suspected if splenomegaly is absent and the high hematocrit is not accompanied by increases in other cell lines. Secondary causes of polycythemia include hypoxia and smoking; carboxyhemoglobin levels may be elevated in smokers (Table 13–15). A renal CT scan or sonogram may be considered to look for an erythropoietin-secreting cyst or tumor. A positive family history should lead to investigation for congenital high-oxygen-affinity hemoglobin. An absence of a mutation in *JAK2* suggests a different diagnosis. However, *JAK2* mutations are also commonly found in

Table 13–15. Causes of polycythemia.

Spurious polycythemia
Secondary polycythemia
Hypoxia: cardiac disease, pulmonary disease, high altitude
Carboxyhemoglobin: smoking
Kidney lesions
Erythropoietin-secreting tumors (rare)
Abnormal hemoglobins (rare)
Polycythemia vera

the myeloproliferative disorders essential thrombocytosis and myelofibrosis.

Polycythemia vera should be differentiated from other myeloproliferative disorders (Table 13–14). Marked elevation of the white blood count (above 30,000/mcL) suggests CML. Abnormal red blood cell morphology and nucleated red blood cells in the peripheral blood are seen in myelofibrosis. Essential thrombocytosis is suggested when the platelet count is strikingly elevated.

Treatment

The treatment of choice is phlebotomy. One unit of blood (approximately 500 mL) is removed weekly until the hematocrit is < 45%; the hematocrit is maintained at < 45% by repeated phlebotomy as necessary. Patients for whom phlebotomy is problematic (because of poor venous access or logistical reasons) may be managed primarily with hydroxyurea (see below). Because repeated phlebotomy intentionally produces iron deficiency, the requirement for phlebotomy should gradually decrease. It is important to avoid medicinal iron supplementation, as this can thwart the goals of a phlebotomy program. Maintaining the hematocrit at normal levels has been shown to decrease the incidence of thrombotic complications. A diet low in iron also is not necessary but will increase the intervals between phlebotomies.

Occasionally, myelosuppressive therapy is indicated. Indications include a high phlebotomy requirement, thrombocytosis, and intractable pruritus. There is evidence that reduction of the platelet count to < 600,000/mcL will reduce the risk of thrombotic complications. Alkylating agents have been shown to increase the risk of conversion of this disease to acute leukemia and should be avoided. Hydroxyurea is widely used when myelosuppressive therapy is indicated. The usual dose is 500–1500 mg/d orally, adjusted to keep platelets < 500,000/mcL without reducing the neutrophil count to < 2000/mcL. Anagrelide may be substituted or added when hydroxyurea is not well tolerated, but it is not the preferred initial agent. Low-dose aspirin (75–81 mg/d orally) has been shown to reduce the risk of thrombosis without excessive bleeding, and should be part of therapy for all patients without contraindications to aspirin. Studies of pegylated alfa-2 interferon have demonstrated considerable efficacy, with hematologic response rates > 80%, as well as molecular responses in 20% (as measured by *JAK2* mutations). Patients failing to achieve molecular responses had a higher frequency of mutations

outside the *JAK2* pathway and were more likely to acquire new mutations during therapy. Side effects were generally acceptable and much less significant than with nonpegylated forms of interferon. Studies with selective *JAK2* inhibitors are ongoing.

Allopurinol 300 mg orally daily may be indicated for hyperuricemia. Antihistamine therapy with diphenhydramine or other H_1-blockers and, rarely, selective serotonin reuptake inhibitors are used to manage pruritus.

Prognosis

Polycythemia is an indolent disease with median survival of over 15 years. The major cause of morbidity and mortality is arterial thrombosis. Over time, polycythemia vera may convert to myelofibrosis or to CML. In approximately 5% of cases, the disorder progresses to AML, which is usually refractory to therapy.

When to Refer

Patients with polycythemia vera should be referred to a hematologist.

When to Admit

Inpatient care is rarely required.

Marchioli R et al; CYTO-PV Collaborative Group. Cardiovascular events and intensity of treatment in polycythemia vera. N Engl J Med. 2013 Jan 3;368(1):22–33. [PMID: 23216616]

Passamonti F. How I treat polycythemia vera. Blood. 2012 Jul 12;120(2):275–84. [PMID: 22611155]

Quintás-Cardama A et al. Pegylated interferon alfa-2a yields high rates of hematologic and molecular response in patients with advanced essential thrombocythemia and polycythemia vera. J Clin Oncol. 2009 Nov 10;27(32):5418–24. [PMID: 19826111]

Vainchenker W et al. New mutations and pathogenesis of myeloproliferative neoplasms. Blood. 2011 Aug 18;118(7):1723–35. [PMID: 21653328]

ESSENTIAL THROMBOCYTOSIS

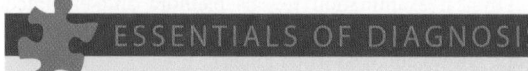

ESSENTIALS OF DIAGNOSIS

► Elevated platelet count in absence of other causes.
► Normal red blood cell mass.
► Absence of *bcr/abl* gene (Philadelphia chromosome).

General Considerations

Essential thrombocytosis is an uncommon myeloproliferative disorder of unknown cause in which marked proliferation of the megakaryocytes in the bone marrow leads to elevation of the platelet count. As with polycythemia vera, the finding of a high frequency of mutations of *JAK2* and others in these patients promises to advance the understanding of this disorder.

Clinical Findings

A. Symptoms and Signs

The median age at presentation is 50–60 years, and there is a slightly increased incidence in women. The disorder is often suspected when an elevated platelet count is found. Less frequently, the first sign is thrombosis, which is the most common clinical problem. The risk of thrombosis rises with age. Venous thromboses may occur in unusual sites such as the mesenteric, hepatic, or portal vein. Some patients experience erythromelalgia, painful burning of the hands accompanied by erythema; this symptom is reliably relieved by aspirin. Bleeding, typically mucosal, is less common and is related to a concomitant qualitative platelet defect. Splenomegaly is present in at least 25% of patients.

B. Laboratory Findings

An elevated platelet count is the hallmark of this disorder, and may be over 2,000,000/mcL (2000 × 10⁹/L) (Table 13–14). The white blood cell count is often mildly elevated, usually not above 30,000/mcL (30 × 10⁹/L), but with some immature myeloid forms. The hematocrit is normal. The peripheral blood smear reveals large platelets, but giant degranulated forms seen in myelofibrosis are not observed. Red blood cell morphology is normal.

The bone marrow shows increased numbers of megakaryocytes but no other morphologic abnormalities. The Philadelphia chromosome is absent but should be assayed by molecular testing of peripheral blood for the *bcr/abl* fusion gene in all suspected cases to differentiate the disorder from CML.

Differential Diagnosis

Essential thrombocytosis must be distinguished from secondary causes of an elevated platelet count. In reactive thrombocytosis, the platelet count seldom exceeds 1,000,000/mcL (1000 × 10⁹/L). Inflammatory disorders such as rheumatoid arthritis and ulcerative colitis cause significant elevations of the platelet count, as may chronic infection. The thrombocytosis of iron deficiency is observed only when anemia is significant. The platelet count is temporarily elevated after splenectomy. *JAK2* mutations are found in 50% of cases. *MPL* and *TET2* mutations have also been described in a subset of patients with essential thrombocytosis.

Regarding other myeloproliferative disorders, the lack of erythrocytosis distinguishes it from polycythemia vera. Unlike myelofibrosis, red blood cell morphology is normal, nucleated red blood cells are absent, and giant degranulated platelets are not seen. In CML, the Philadelphia chromosome (or *bcr/abl* by molecular testing) establishes the diagnosis.

Treatment

Patients are considered at high risk for thrombosis if they are older than 60 years, have a leukocyte count ≥ 11 × 10⁹/L,

or have a previous history of thrombosis. They also have a higher risk for bleeding. The risk of thrombosis can be reduced by control of the platelet count, which should be kept at < 500,000/mcL (500 × 10⁹/L). The treatment of choice is oral hydroxyurea in a dose of 500–1000 mg/d. In cases in which hydroxyurea is not well tolerated because of anemia, low doses of anagrelide, 1–2 mg/d orally, may be added. Higher doses of anagrelide can be complicated by headache, peripheral edema, and heart failure. As with polycythemia vera, trials of pegylated interferon alfa-2 have demonstrated significant hematologic responses, but its role in management has not yet been established. Strict control of coexistent cardiovascular risk factors is mandatory for all patients.

Vasomotor symptoms such as erythromelalgia and paresthesias respond rapidly to aspirin, and its long-term low-dose use (81 mg/d orally) may reduce the risk of thrombotic complications in low-risk patients. In the unusual event of severe bleeding, the platelet count can be lowered rapidly with plateletpheresis.

Course & Prognosis

Essential thrombocytosis is an indolent disorder and allows long-term survival. Average survival is longer than 15 years from diagnosis, and the survival of patients younger than 50 years does not appear different from matched controls. The major source of morbidity—thrombosis—can be reduced by appropriate platelet control. Late in the course of the disease, the bone marrow may become fibrotic, and massive splenomegaly may occur, sometimes with splenic infarction. There is a 10–15% risk of progression to myelofibrosis after 15 years, and a 1–5% risk of transformation to acute leukemia over 20 years.

When to Refer

Patients with essential thrombocytosis should be referred to a hematologist.

Casini A et al. Thrombotic complications of myeloproliferative neoplasms: risk assessment and risk-guided management. J Thromb Haemost. 2013 Jul;11(7):1215–27. [PMID: 23601811]

Tefferi A. Polycythemia vera and essential thrombocythemia: 2013 update on diagnosis, risk-stratification, and management. Am J Hematol. 2013 Jun;88(6):507–16. [PMID: 23695894]

PRIMARY MYELOFIBROSIS

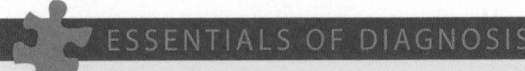
ESSENTIALS OF DIAGNOSIS

► Striking splenomegaly.

► Teardrop poikilocytosis on peripheral smear.

► Leukoerythroblastic blood picture; giant abnormal platelets.

► Initially hypercellular, then hypocellular bone marrow with reticulin or collagen fibrosis.

General Considerations

Primary myelofibrosis (myelofibrosis with myeloid metaplasia, agnogenic myeloid metaplasia, idiopathic myelofibrosis) is a myeloproliferative disorder characterized by fibrosis of the bone marrow, splenomegaly, and a leukoerythroblastic peripheral blood picture with teardrop poikilocytosis. Myelofibrosis can also occur as a secondary process following the other myeloproliferative disorders (eg, polycythemia vera, essential thrombocytosis). It is believed that fibrosis occurs in response to increased secretion of platelet-derived growth factor (PDGF) and possibly other cytokines. In response to bone marrow fibrosis, extramedullary hematopoiesis takes place in the liver, spleen, and lymph nodes. In these sites, mesenchymal cells responsible for fetal hematopoiesis can be reactivated. As with other myeloproliferative diseases, abnormalities of JAK2 and MPL may be involved in the pathogenesis.

Clinical Findings

A. Symptoms and Signs

Primary myelofibrosis develops in adults over age 50 years and is usually insidious in onset. Patients most commonly present with fatigue due to anemia or abdominal fullness related to splenomegaly. Uncommon presentations include bleeding and bone pain. On examination, splenomegaly is almost invariably present and is commonly massive. The liver is enlarged in more than 50% of cases.

Later in the course of the disease, progressive bone marrow failure takes place as it becomes increasingly more fibrotic. Progressive thrombocytopenia leads to bleeding. The spleen continues to enlarge, which leads to early satiety. Painful episodes of splenic infarction may occur. The patient becomes cachectic and may experience severe bone pain, especially in the upper legs. Hematopoiesis in the liver leads to portal hypertension with ascites, esophageal varices, and occasionally transverse myelitis caused by myelopoiesis in the epidural space.

B. Laboratory Findings

Patients are almost invariably anemic at presentation. The white blood count is variable—either low, normal, or elevated—and may be increased to 50,000/mcL (50×10^9/L). The platelet count is variable. The peripheral blood smear is dramatic, with significant poikilocytosis and numerous teardrop forms in the red cell line. Nucleated red blood cells are present and the myeloid series is shifted, with immature forms including a small percentage of promyelocytes or myeloblasts. Platelet morphology may be bizarre, and giant degranulated platelet forms (megakaryocyte fragments) may be seen. The triad of teardrop poikilocytosis, leukoerythroblastic blood, and giant abnormal platelets is highly suggestive of myelofibrosis.

The bone marrow usually cannot be aspirated (dry tap), though early in the course of the disease it is hypercellular, with a marked increase in megakaryocytes. Fibrosis at this stage is detected by a silver stain demonstrating increased reticulin fibers. Later, biopsy reveals more severe fibrosis, with eventual replacement of hematopoietic precursors by collagen. There is no characteristic chromosomal abnormality. JAK2 is mutated in ~65% of cases, and MPL is mutated in ~40% of cases.

Differential Diagnosis

A leukoerythroblastic blood picture from other causes may be seen in response to severe infection, inflammation, or infiltrative bone marrow processes. However, teardrop poikilocytosis and giant abnormal platelet forms will not be present. Bone marrow fibrosis may be seen in metastatic carcinoma, Hodgkin lymphoma, and hairy cell leukemia. These disorders are diagnosed by characteristic morphology of involved tissues.

Of the other myeloproliferative disorders, CML is diagnosed when there is marked leukocytosis, normal red blood cell morphology, and the presence of the bcr/abl fusion gene. Polycythemia vera is characterized by an elevated hematocrit. Essential thrombocytosis shows predominant platelet count elevations.

Treatment

Patients with mild forms of the disease may require no therapy or occasional transfusion support. Anemic patients are supported with transfusion. Anemia can also be controlled with androgens, prednisone, thalidomide, or lenalidomide. First-line therapy for myelofibrosis-associated splenomegaly is hydroxyurea, which is effective in reducing spleen size by half in approximately 40% of patients. Both thalidomide and lenalidomide may improve splenomegaly and thrombocytopenia in some patients. Splenectomy is not routinely performed but is indicated for medication-refractory splenic enlargement causing recurrent painful episodes, severe thrombocytopenia, or an unacceptable transfusion requirement. Perioperative complications can occur in 28% of patients and include infections, abdominal vein thrombosis, and bleeding. Radiation therapy has a role for painful sites of extramedullary hematopoiesis, pulmonary hypertension, or severe bone pain. Transjugular intrahepatic portosystemic shunt might also be considered to alleviate symptoms of portal hypertension.

Several newer agents have shown activity in this disease. The immunomodulatory medications, lenalidomide and pomalidomide, result in control of anemia in 25% and thrombocytopenia in ~58% of cases, without significant reduction in splenic size. There are several JAK2 inhibitors in development. Ruxolitinib, a JAK2 inhibitor, has been approved by the US Food and Drug Administration for myelofibrosis. Even though treatment with ruxolitinib can exacerbate cytopenias, it results in reduction of spleen size, improvement of constitutional symptoms, and may lead to an overall survival benefit in patients with an intermediate- or high-risk disease. The only potentially curative option for this disease is allogeneic stem cell transplantation in selected patients.

Course & Prognosis

The median survival from time of diagnosis is approximately 5 years. The Dynamic International Prognostic

Scoring system is associated with overall survival. Therapies with biologic agents and the application of reduced-intensity allogeneic stem cell transplantation appear to offer the possibility of improving the outcome for many patients. End-stage myelofibrosis is characterized by generalized asthenia liver failure, and bleeding from thrombocytopenia, with some cases terminating in AML.

When to Refer

Patients in whom myelofibrosis is suspected should be referred to a hematologist.

When to Admit

Admission is not usually necessary.

Tefferi A. Primary myelofibrosis: 2013 update on diagnosis, risk-stratification, and management. Am J Hematol. 2013 Feb;88(2):141–50. Erratum in: Am J Hematol.2013 May;88(5):437–45. [PMID: 23349007]

Verstovsek S et al. A double-blind, placebo-controlled trial of ruxolitinib for myelofibrosis. N Engl J Med. 2012 Mar 1;366(9):799–807. [PMID: 22375971]

CHRONIC MYELOID LEUKEMIA

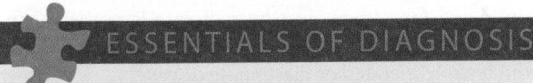

ESSENTIALS OF DIAGNOSIS

- Elevated white blood count.
- Markedly left-shifted myeloid series but with a low percentage of promyelocytes and blasts.
- Presence of *bcr/abl* gene (Philadelphia chromosome).

General Considerations

CML is a myeloproliferative disorder characterized by overproduction of myeloid cells. These myeloid cells continue to differentiate and circulate in increased numbers in the peripheral blood.

CML is characterized by a specific chromosomal abnormality and specific molecular abnormality. The Philadelphia chromosome is a reciprocal translocation between the long arms of chromosomes 9 and 22. The portion of 9q that is translocated contains *abl,* a protooncogene that is the cellular homolog of the Ableson murine leukemia virus. The *abl* gene is received at a specific site on 22q, the break point cluster (bcr). The fusion gene *bcr/abl* produces a novel protein that differs from the normal transcript of the *abl* gene in that it possesses tyrosine kinase activity. This disorder is the first example of tyrosine kinase "addiction" by cancer cells.

Early CML ("chronic phase") does not behave like a malignant disease. Normal bone marrow function is retained, white blood cells differentiate and, despite some qualitative abnormalities, the neutrophils combat infection normally. However, untreated CML is inherently unstable, and without treatment the disease progresses to an accelerated and then acute blast phase, which is morphologically indistinguishable from acute leukemia. Remarkable advances in therapy have changed the natural history of the disease, and the relentless progression to more advanced stages of disease is at least greatly delayed, if not eliminated.

Clinical Findings

A. Symptoms and Signs

CML is a disorder of middle age (median age at presentation is 55 years). Patients usually complain of fatigue, night sweats, and low-grade fevers related to the hypermetabolic state caused by overproduction of white blood cells. Patients may also complain of abdominal fullness related to splenomegaly. In some cases, an elevated white blood count is discovered incidentally. Rarely, the patient will present with a clinical syndrome related to leukostasis with blurred vision, respiratory distress, or priapism. The white blood count in these cases is usually < 500,000/mcL (500×10^9/L).

On examination, the spleen is enlarged (often markedly so), and sternal tenderness may be present as a sign of marrow overexpansion. In cases discovered during routine laboratory monitoring, these findings are often absent.

Acceleration of the disease is often associated with fever in the absence of infection, bone pain, and splenomegaly.

B. Laboratory Findings

CML is characterized by an elevated white blood count; the median white blood count at diagnosis is 150,000/mcL (150×10^9/L), although in some cases the white blood cell count is only modestly increased (Table 13–14). The peripheral blood is characteristic. The myeloid series is left shifted, with mature forms dominating and with cells usually present in proportion to their degree of maturation. Blasts are usually < 5%. Basophilia and eosinophilia of granulocytes may be present. At presentation, the patient is usually not anemic. Red blood cell morphology is normal, and nucleated red blood cells are rarely seen. The platelet count may be normal or elevated (sometimes to strikingly high levels).

The bone marrow is hypercellular, with left-shifted myelopoiesis. Myeloblasts comprise < 5% of marrow cells.

The hallmark of the disease is that the *bcr/abl* gene is detected by the polymerase chain reaction (PCR) test in the peripheral blood. A bone marrow examination is not necessary for diagnosis, although it is useful for prognosis and for detecting other chromosomal abnormalities in addition to the Philadelphia chromosome.

With progression to the accelerated and blast phases, progressive anemia and thrombocytopenia occur, and the percentage of blasts in the blood and bone marrow increases. Blast phase CML is diagnosed when blasts comprise more than 20% of bone marrow cells.

Differential Diagnosis

Early CML must be differentiated from the reactive leukocytosis associated with infection. In such cases, the white blood count is usually < 50,000/mcL (< 50 × 10^9/L), splenomegaly is absent, and the *bcr/abl* gene is not present.

CML must be distinguished from other myeloproliferative disease (Table 13–14). The hematocrit should not be elevated, the red blood cell morphology is normal, and nucleated red blood cells are rare or absent. Definitive diagnosis is made by finding the *bcr/abl* gene.

Treatment

Treatment is usually not emergent even with white blood counts over 200,000/mcL (200 × 10^9/L), since the majority of circulating cells are mature myeloid cells that are smaller and more deformable than primitive leukemic blasts. In the rare instances in which symptoms result from extreme hyperleukocytosis (priapism, respiratory distress, visual blurring, altered mental status), emergent leukapheresis is performed in conjunction with myelosuppressive therapy.

In chronic-phase CML, the goal of therapy is normalization of the hematologic abnormalities and suppression of the malignant, *bcr/abl*-expressing clone. The treatment of choice consists of a tyrosine kinase inhibitor targeting the aberrantly active *abl* kinase. It is expected that a hematologic complete remission, with normalization of blood counts and splenomegaly will occur within 3 months of treatment initiation. Second, a major cytogenetic response should be achieved, ideally within 3 months but certainly within 6 months. A major cytogenetic response is identified when < 35% of metaphases contain the Philadelphia chromosome. Lastly, a major molecular response is desired within 12 months and is defined as a 3-log reduction of the *bcr/abl* transcript as measured by quantitative PCR. This roughly corresponds to a *bcr/abl* ratio (compared to *abl*) of < 0.01. Patients who achieve this level of molecular response have an excellent prognosis, with 100% of such patients remaining free of progression at 8 years. On the other hand, patients who do not achieve these targets or subsequently lose their cytogenetic or molecular response or patients in whom new mutations or cytogenetic abnormalities develop are considered high-risk.

Imatinib mesylate was the first tyrosine kinase inhibitor to be approved and it results in nearly universal (98%) hematologic control of chronic phase disease at a dose of 400 mg/d. The rate of a major molecular response with imatinib in chronic-phase disease is ~30% at 1 year. The second-generation tyrosine kinase inhibitors, dasatinib and nilotinib, have also been approved for use as front-line therapy and have been shown to significantly increase the rate of achievement of a major molecular response compared to imatinib (71% for nilotinib at 300–400 mg twice daily by 2 years, 64% for dasatinib at 100 mg/d by 2 years) and result in a lower rate of progression to advanced-stage disease. However, these agents can also salvage 90% of patients who do not respond to treatment with imatinib and may therefore be reserved for use in that setting. A dual *bcr/abl* tyrosine kinase inhibitor, bosutinib, was approved in 2012 for patients who are resistant or intolerant to the other tyrosine kinase inhibitors. The complete cytogenetic response rate to bosutinib is 25% but it is not active against the T315I mutation.

Patients taking tyrosine kinase inhibitors should be monitored with a quantitative PCR assay. Those with a consistent increase in *bcr/abl* transcript or those with a suboptimal molecular response as defined above should undergo *abl* mutation testing and then switched to an alternative tyrosine kinase inhibitor. The T315I mutation in *abl* is specifically resistant to therapy with imatinib, dasatinib, nilotinib, and bosutinib but appears to be sensitive to the third-generation agent ponatinib. However, use of ponatinib is associated with a high rate of vascular thrombotic complications. Patients who cannot achieve a good molecular response to any of these agents or progress following therapy should be considered for treatment with allogeneic transplantation.

Patients with advanced-stage disease (accelerated phase or myeloid/lymphoid blast crisis) should be treated with a tyrosine kinase inhibitor alone or in combination with myelosuppressive chemotherapy. The doses of tyrosine kinase inhibitors in that setting are usually higher than those appropriate for chronic-phase disease. Since the duration of response to tyrosine kinase inhibitors in this setting is limited, these patients should ultimately be considered for allogeneic stem cell transplantation.

Thus, allogeneic stem cell transplantation should be considered for patients in whom disease is not well controlled with tyrosine kinase inhibitor therapy, or for those who have accelerated or blast phase disease.

Course & Prognosis

Since the introduction of imatinib therapy in 2001, and with the development of molecular targeted agents, more than 80% of patients remain alive and without disease progression at 9 years. Patients with good molecular responses to tyrosine kinase inhibitor therapy have an excellent prognosis, with essentially 100% survival at 9 years, and it is likely that some fraction of these patients will be cured. Small studies suggest that some patients with complete molecular responses (undetectable *bcr/abl*) lasting more than 2 years can stop drug therapy without disease recurrence, but these findings are being confirmed in prospective studies.

When to Refer

All patients with CML should be referred to a hematologist.

When to Admit

Hospitalization is rarely necessary and should be reserved for symptoms of leukostasis at diagnosis or for transformation to acute leukemia.

Baccarani M et al. European LeukemiaNet recommendations for the management of chronic myeloid leukemia: 2013. Blood. 2013 Aug 8;122(6):872–84. [PMID: 23803709]

Cortes J et al. How I treat newly diagnosed chronic phase CML. Blood. 2012 Aug 16;120(7):1390–7. [PMID: 22613793]

O'Brien S et al. NCCN Task Force report: tyrosine kinase inhibitor therapy selection in the management of patients with chronic myelogenous leukemia. J Natl Compr Canc Netw. 2011 Feb;9(Suppl 2):S1–25. [PMID: 21335443]

Soverini S et al. BCR-ABL kinase domain mutation analysis in chronic myeloid leukemia patients treated with tyrosine kinase inhibitors: recommendations from an expert panel on behalf of European LeukemiaNet. Blood. 2011 Aug 4;118(5):1208–15. [PMID: 21562040]

MYELODYSPLASTIC SYNDROMES

ESSENTIALS OF DIAGNOSIS

► Cytopenias with a hypercellular bone marrow.

► Morphologic abnormalities in two or more hematopoietic cell lines.

► General Considerations

The myelodysplastic syndromes are a group of acquired clonal disorders of the hematopoietic stem cell. They are characterized by the constellation of cytopenias, a usually hypercellular marrow, and a number of morphologic and cytogenetic abnormalities. The disorders are usually idiopathic but may be caused by prior exposure to cytotoxic chemotherapy or radiation or both. Ultimately, the disorder may evolve into AML, and the term "preleukemia" has been used in the past to describe these disorders.

Myelodysplasia encompasses several heterogeneous syndromes. Those without excess bone marrow blasts are termed "refractory anemia," with or without ringed sideroblasts. Patients with the 5q– syndrome, which is characterized by the cytogenetic finding of loss of part of the long arm of chromosome 5, comprise an important subgroup of patients with refractory anemia. The diagnosis "refractory anemia with excess blasts" (RAEB 1 with 5–9% blasts and RAEB 2 with 10–19% blasts) is made in those with excess blasts. Patients with a proliferative syndrome including sustained peripheral blood monocytosis > 1000/mcL (1.0 × 10⁹/L) are termed "chronic myelomonocytic leukemia" (CMML), a disorder that shares features of myelodysplastic and myeloproliferative disorders. An International Prognostic Scoring System (IPSS) classifies patients by risk status based on the percentage of bone marrow blasts, cytogenetics, and the severity of cytopenias. The IPSS is associated with the rate of progression to AML as well as overall survival, which can range from a median of 6 years for the low-risk group to 5 months for the high-risk patients.

► Clinical Findings

A. Symptoms and Signs

Patients are usually over age 60 years. Many patients are asymptomatic when the diagnosis is made because of the finding of abnormal blood counts. Fatigue, infection, or bleeding related to bone marrow failure are usually the presenting symptoms and signs. The course may be indolent, and the disease may present as a wasting illness with fever, weight loss, and general debility. On examination, splenomegaly may be present in combination with pallor, bleeding, and various signs of infection. Myelodysplastic syndromes can also be accompanied by a variety of paraneoplastic syndromes that can occur prior to or following this diagnosis.

B. Laboratory Findings

Anemia may be marked and may require transfusion support. The MCV is normal or increased, and macroovalocytes may be seen on the peripheral blood smear. The white blood cell count is usually normal or reduced, and neutropenia is common. The neutrophils may exhibit morphologic abnormalities, including deficient numbers of granules or deficient segmentation of the nucleus, especially a bilobed nucleus (Pelger–Huet abnormality). The myeloid series may be left shifted, and small numbers of promyelocytes or blasts may be seen. The platelet count is normal or reduced, and hypogranular platelets may be present.

The bone marrow is characteristically hypercellular but occasionally may be hypocellular. Erythroid hyperplasia is common, and signs of abnormal erythropoiesis include megaloblastic features, nuclear budding, or multinucleated erythroid precursors. The Prussian blue stain may demonstrate ringed sideroblasts. The myeloid series is often left shifted, with variable increases in blasts. Deficient or abnormal granules may be seen. A characteristic abnormality is the presence of dwarf megakaryocytes with a unilobed nucleus. Although no single specific chromosomal abnormality is seen in myelodysplasia, there are frequently abnormalities involving the long arm of chromosome 5 as well as deletions of chromosomes 5 and 7. Some patients with an indolent form of the disease have an isolated partial deletion of chromosome 5 (5q– syndrome). The presence of other abnormalities such as monosomy 7 or complex abnormalities is associated with more aggressive disease.

► Differential Diagnosis

Myelodysplastic syndromes should be distinguished from megaloblastic anemia, aplastic anemia, myelofibrosis, HIV-associated cytopenias, and acute or chronic drug effect. In subtle cases, cytogenetic evaluation of the bone marrow may help distinguish this clonal disorder from other causes of cytopenias. As the number of blasts increases in the bone marrow, myelodysplasia is arbitrarily separated from AML by the presence of < 20% blasts.

► Treatment

Myelodysplasia is a very heterogeneous disease, and the appropriate treatment depends on a number of factors. For patients with anemia who have a low serum EPO level (≤ 500 mU/mL), erythropoiesis-stimulating agents may raise the hematocrit and reduce the red cell transfusion requirement in 40%. Addition of intermittent granulocyte colony-stimulating factor (G-CSF) therapy may augment the erythroid response to epoetin. Unfortunately, the patients with the highest transfusion requirements are the least likely to respond. Patients who remain dependent on red blood cell transfusion and who do not have immediately life-threatening disease should receive iron chelation in order to prevent serious iron overload; the dose of oral agent deferasirox is 20 mg/kg/d. Patients affected primarily with severe neutropenia may benefit from the use of myeloid growth factors such as G-CSF. Oral thrombopoietin analogues such as romiplostim and eltrombopag that stimulate platelet production by binding the thrombopoietin receptor have shown effectiveness in raising the platelet count in myelodysplasia. Finally, occasional patients can benefit from immunosuppressive therapy including ATG. Predictors of response to ATG include age < 60 years, absence of 5q–, and presence of HLA DR15.

For patients who do not respond to these interventions, there are several therapeutic options available. Lenalidomide is approved for the treatment of transfusion-dependent anemia due to myelodysplasia. It is the treatment of choice in patients with the 5q– syndrome, with significant responses in 70% of patients, and with responses typically lasting longer than 2 years. In addition, nearly half of these patients enter a cytogenetic remission with clearing of the abnormal 5q– clone, leading to the hope that lenalidomide may change the natural history of the disease. The recommended initial dose is 10 mg/d orally. The most common side effects are neutropenia and thrombocytopenia, but venous thrombosis is also seen and warrants prophylaxis with aspirin, 325 mg/d orally. Azacitidine is the treatment of choice for patients with high-risk myelodysplasia and can improve both symptoms and blood counts and prolong both overall survival and the time to conversion to acute leukemia. It is used at a dose of 75 mg/m^2 daily for 5–7 days every 28 days and it may require six cycles of therapy to achieve a response. Azacitidine combined with lenalidomide has shown preliminary promise in patients with high-risk disease. A related hypomethylating agent, decitabine, can produce similar hematologic responses but has not demonstrated a benefit in overall survival compared to supportive care alone. Allogeneic stem cell transplantation is the only curative therapy for myelodysplasia, but its role is limited by the advanced age of many patients and the indolent course of disease in some subsets of patients. The optimal use and timing of allogeneic transplantation are controversial, but the use of reduced-intensity preparative regimens for transplantation has expanded the role of this therapy, using both family and matched unrelated donors.

Course & Prognosis

Myelodysplasia is an ultimately fatal disease, and allogeneic transplantation is the only curative therapy, with cure rates of 30–60% depending primarily on the risk status of the disease. Patients most commonly die of infections or bleeding. Patients with 5q– syndrome have a favorable prognosis, with 5-year survival over 90%. Other patients with low-risk disease (with absence of both excess blasts and adverse cytogenetics) may also do well, with similar survival. Those with excess blasts or CMML have a higher (30–50%) risk of developing acute leukemia, and short survival (< 2 years) without allogeneic transplantation.

▶ When to Refer

All patients with myelodysplasia should be referred to a hematologist.

▶ When to Admit

Hospitalization is needed only for specific complications, such as severe infection.

Fenaux P et al. How we treat lower-risk myelodysplastic syndromes. Blood. 2013 May 23;121(21):4280–6. [PMID: 23575446]

Foran JM et al. Clinical presentation, diagnosis, and prognosis of myelodysplastic syndromes. Am J Med. 2012 Jul;125(7 Suppl):S6–13. [PMID: 22735753]

Kröger N. Allogeneic stem cell transplantation for elderly patients with myelodysplastic syndrome. Blood. 2012 Jun 14;119(24):5632–9. [PMID: 22504927]

Lyons RM. Myelodysplastic syndromes: therapy and outlook. Am J Med. 2012 Jul;125(7 Suppl):S18–23. [PMID: 22735747]

ACUTE LEUKEMIA

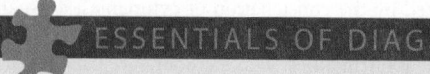

ESSENTIALS OF DIAGNOSIS

▶ Short duration of symptoms, including fatigue, fever, and bleeding.

▶ Cytopenias or pancytopenia.

▶ More than 20% blasts in the bone marrow.

▶ Blasts in peripheral blood in 90% of patients.

▶ General Considerations

Acute leukemia is a malignancy of the hematopoietic progenitor cell. These cells proliferate in an uncontrolled fashion and replace normal bone marrow elements. Most cases arise with no clear cause. However, radiation and some toxins (benzene) are leukemogenic. In addition, a number of chemotherapeutic agents (especially cyclophosphamide, melphalan, other alkylating agents, and etoposide) may cause leukemia. The leukemias seen after toxin or chemotherapy exposure often develop from a myelodysplastic prodrome and are often associated with abnormalities in chromosomes 5 and 7. Those related to etoposide may have abnormalities in chromosome 11q23 (MLL locus).

Acute promyelocytic leukemia (APL) is characterized by chromosomal translocation t(15;17), which produces the fusion gene *PML-RAR*-alpha which interacts with the retinoic acid receptor to produce a block in differentiation that can be overcome with pharmacologic doses of retinoic acid (see below).

Most of the clinical findings in acute leukemia are due to replacement of normal bone marrow elements by the malignant cells. Less common manifestations result from organ infiltration (skin, gastrointestinal tract, meninges). Acute leukemia is potentially curable with combination chemotherapy.

The lymphoblastic subtype of acute leukemia, ALL, comprises 80% of the acute leukemias of childhood. The peak incidence is between 3 and 7 years of age. It is also seen in adults, causing approximately 20% of adult acute leukemias. The myeloblastic subtype, AML, is primarily an adult disease with a median age at presentation of 60 years and an increasing incidence with advanced age.

► Classification of the Leukemias

A. Acute Lymphoblastic Leukemia (ALL)

ALL is most usefully classified by immunologic phenotype as follows: common, early B lineage, and T cell. Hyperdiploidy (with more than 50 chromosomes), especially of chromosomes 4, 10 and 17, and translocation t(12;21) (TEL-AML1), is associated with a better prognosis. Unfavorable cytogenetics are hypodiploidy (less than 44 chromosomes), the Philadelphia chromosome t(9;22), the t(4;11) translocation, which has fusion genes involving the MLL gene at 11q23, and a complex karyotype with more than five chromosomal abnormalities.

B. Acute Myeloid Leukemia (AML)

AML has been characterized in several ways. The World Health Organization (WHO) has sponsored a classification of the leukemias and other hematologic malignancies that incorporates cytogenetic, molecular, and immunophenotype information. The most important baseline prognostic factor is tumor genetics. This comprises cytogenetic abnormalities identified on traditional karyotyping or metaphase FISH and molecular abnormalities identified by either targeted or genome-wide sequencing of tumor DNA. Favorable cytogenetics such as t(8;21) producing a chimeric RUNX1/RUNX1T1 protein and inv(16)(p13;q22) are seen in 15% of cases and are termed the "core-binding factor" leukemias because of common genetic lesions affecting DNA-binding elements. These patients have a higher chance of achieving both short- and long-term disease control. Unfavorable cytogenetics confer a very poor prognosis. These consist of isolated monosomy 5 or 7, the presence of two or more monosomies, or three or more separate cytogenetic abnormalities. The majority of cases of AML are of intermediate risk by traditional cytogenetics and have either a normal karyotype or chromosomal abnormalities that do not confer strong prognostic significance. However, there are several recurrent genetic mutations with prognostic significance in this subgroup. On the one hand, internal tandem duplication in the gene FLT3 occurs in ~30% of AML and is associated with a very poor prognosis. Other mutations conferring a poor prognosis occur in TET2, MLL-PTD, and ASXL1. On the other hand, a relatively favorable group of patients has been defined that includes mutations of nucleophosmin 1 (NPM1) and

lacks the internal tandem duplication of the FLT3 gene. Other mutations conferring a favorable prognosis occur in IDH1 or IDH2.

C. Acute Promyelocytic Leukemia (APL)

In considering the various types of AML, APL is discussed separately because of its unique biologic features and unique response to non-chemotherapy treatments. APL is characterized by the cytogenetic finding of t(15;17) and the fusion gene PML-RAR-alpha.

D. Acute Leukemia of Ambiguous Lineage

These leukemias consist of blasts that lack differentiation along the lymphoid or myeloid lineage or blasts that express both myeloid and lymphoid lineage-specific antigens (ie, mixed phenotype acute leukemias). This group is considered very high risk and has a poor prognosis.

► Clinical Findings

A. Symptoms and Signs

Most patients have been ill only for days or weeks. Bleeding (usually due to thrombocytopenia) occurs in the skin and mucosal surfaces, with gingival bleeding, epistaxis, or menorrhagia. Less commonly, widespread bleeding is seen in patients with disseminated intravascular coagulation (DIC) (in APL and monocytic leukemia). Infection is due to neutropenia, with the risk of infection rising as the neutrophil count falls below 500/mcL (0.5×10^9/L). The most common pathogens are gram-negative bacteria (Escherichia coli, Klebsiella, Pseudomonas) or fungi (Candida, Aspergillus). Common presentations include cellulitis, pneumonia, and perirectal infections; death within a few hours may occur if treatment with appropriate antibiotics is delayed.

Patients may also seek medical attention because of gum hypertrophy and bone and joint pain. The most dramatic presentation is hyperleukocytosis, in which a markedly elevated circulating blast count (total white blood count > 100,000/mcL) leads to impaired circulation, presenting as headache, confusion, and dyspnea. Such patients require emergent chemotherapy with adjunctive leukapheresis as mortality approaches 40% in the first 48 hours.

On examination, patients appear pale and have purpura and petechiae; signs of infection may not be present. Stomatitis and gum hypertrophy may be seen in patients with monocytic leukemia, as may rectal fissures. There is variable enlargement of the liver, spleen, and lymph nodes. Bone tenderness may be present, particularly in the sternum, tibia, and femur.

B. Laboratory Findings

The hallmark of acute leukemia is the combination of pancytopenia with circulating blasts. However, blasts may be absent from the peripheral smear in as many as 10% of cases ("aleukemic leukemia"). The bone marrow is usually hypercellular and dominated by blasts. More than 20% marrow blasts are required to make a diagnosis of acute leukemia.

Hyperuricemia may be seen. If DIC is present, the fibrinogen level will be reduced, the prothrombin time prolonged, and fibrin degradation products or fibrin D-dimers present. Patients with ALL (especially T cell) may have a mediastinal mass visible on chest radiograph. Meningeal leukemia will have blasts present in the spinal fluid, seen in approximately 5% of cases at diagnosis; it is more common in monocytic types of AML and can be seen with ALL.

The Auer rod, an eosinophilic needle-like inclusion in the cytoplasm, is pathognomonic of AML and, if seen, secures the diagnosis. The phenotype of leukemia cells is usually demonstrated by flow cytometry or immunohistochemistry. AML cells usually express myeloid antigens such as CD 13 or CD 33 and myeloperoxidase. ALL cells of B lineage will express CD19, common to all B cells, and most cases will express CD10, formerly known as the "common ALL antigen." ALL cells of T lineage will usually not express mature T-cell markers, such as CD 3, 4, or 8, but will express some combination of CD 2, 5, and 7 and do not express surface immunoglobulin. Almost all ALL cells express terminal deoxynucleotidyl transferase (TdT). The uncommon Burkitt type of ALL has a "lymphoma" phenotype, expressing CD19, CD20, and surface immunoglobulin but not TdT and is best treated with aggressive lymphoma regimens.

▶ Differential Diagnosis

AML must be distinguished from other myeloproliferative disorders, CML, and myelodysplastic syndromes. Acute leukemia may also resemble a left-shifted bone marrow recovering from a previous toxic insult. If the diagnosis is in doubt, a bone marrow study should be repeated in several days to see if maturation has taken place. ALL must be separated from other lymphoproliferative disease such as CLL, lymphomas, and hairy cell leukemia. It may also be confused with the atypical lymphocytosis of mononucleosis and pertussis.

▶ Treatment

Most patients up to age 60 with acute leukemia are treated with the objective of cure. The first step in treatment is to obtain complete remission, defined as normal peripheral blood with resolution of cytopenias, normal bone marrow with no excess blasts, and normal clinical status. The type of initial chemotherapy depends on the subtype of leukemia.

1. AML—Most patients with AML are treated with a combination of an anthracycline (daunorubicin or idarubicin) plus cytarabine, either alone or in combination with other agents. This therapy will produce complete remissions in 80–90% of patients under age 60 years and in 50–60% of older patients (see Table 39–5). Older patients with AML who are not candidates for traditional chemotherapy may be given 5-azacitidine or decitabine initially with acceptable outcomes. APL is treated differently from other forms of AML. Induction therapy for APL should include all-trans-retinoic acid (ATRA) with or without arsenic trioxide with or without chemotherapy. With this approach 90–95% of patients will achieve complete remission.

Once a patient has entered remission, post-remission therapy should be given with curative intent whenever possible. Options include standard chemotherapy and stem cell transplantation (either autologous or allogeneic). The optimal treatment strategy depends on the patient's age and clinical status, and the risk factor profile of the leukemia. With the use of all-trans retinoic acid and arsenic trioxide with or without chemotherapy, 90% of patients with APL remain in long-term remission. Patients with a favorable genetic profile can be treated with chemotherapy alone or with autologous transplant with cure rates of 60–80%. Patients who do not enter remission (primary induction failure) or those with high-risk genetics have cure rates of less than 10% with chemotherapy alone and are referred for allogeneic stem cell transplantation. For intermediate-risk patients with AML, cure rates are 35–40% with chemotherapy, 40–50% with autologous transplantation, and 50–60% with allogeneic transplantation. Targeted therapeutics with FLT3 inhibitors are in development and have preliminarily shown activity in patients with FLT3-positive AML. Patients over age 60 have had a poor prognosis, even in first remission, when treated with standard chemotherapy approaches, and only 10–20% become long-term survivors. The use of reduced-intensity allogeneic transplant appears to be improving the outcome for such patients, with initial studies suggesting that up to 40% of selected patients may be cured.

Once leukemia has recurred after initial chemotherapy, the prognosis is poor. For patients in second remission, transplantation (autologous or allogeneic) offers a 20–30% chance of cure. For those patients with APL who relapse, arsenic trioxide can produce second remissions in 90% of cases.

2. ALL—Adults with ALL are treated with combination chemotherapy, including daunorubicin, vincristine, prednisone, and asparaginase. This treatment produces complete remissions in 90% of patients. Those patients with Philadelphia chromosome-positive ALL (or *bcr-abl* positive ALL) should have a tyrosine kinase inhibitor, such as dasatinib, added to their initial chemotherapy. Older patients (over age 60) may be treated with a tyrosine kinase inhibitor–based regimen, and 90% can enter initial remission.

Remission induction therapy for ALL is less myelosuppressive than treatment for AML and does not necessarily produce marrow aplasia. After achieving complete remission, patients receive central nervous system prophylaxis so that meningeal sequestration of leukemic cells does not develop. As with AML, patients may be treated with either additional cycles of chemotherapy or high-dose chemotherapy and stem cell transplantation. Treatment decisions are made based on patient age and risk factors of the disease. Adults younger than 39 years have uniformly better outcomes when treated under pediatric protocols. Low-risk patients with ALL may be treated with chemotherapy alone with a 70% chance of cure. Intermediate-risk patients have a 30–50% chance of cure with chemotherapy, and high-risk patients are rarely cured with chemotherapy alone. High-risk patients with adverse cytogenetics or poor responses to chemotherapy are best treated with allogeneic transplantation. Minimal residual disease testing may help guide treatment decisions following induction therapy in the future.

Prognosis

Approximately 70–80% of adults with AML under age 60 years achieve complete remission and ~50% are cured using risk-adapted post-remission therapy. Older adults with AML achieve complete remission in up to 50% of instances. The cure rates for older patients with AML have been very low (approximately 10–20%) even if they achieve remission and are able to receive post-remission chemotherapy. The use of reduced-intensity allogeneic transplantation is being explored in order to improve on these outcomes.

When to Refer

All patients should be referred to a hematologist.

When to Admit

Most patients with acute leukemia will be admitted for treatment.

Bassan R et al. Modern therapy of acute lymphoblastic leukemia. J Clin Oncol. 2011 Feb 10;29(5):532–43. [PMID: 21220592]

Fernandez HF. New trends in the standard of care for initial therapy of acute myeloid leukemia. Hematology Am Soc Hematol Educ Program. 2010;2010:56–61. [PMID: 21239771]

Gupta V et al. Allogeneic hematopoietic cell transplantation for adults with acute myeloid leukemia: myths, controversies, and unknowns. Blood. 2011 Feb 24;117(8):2307–18. [PMID: 21098397]

Lo-Coco F et al. Retinoic acid and arsenic trioxide for acute promyelocytic leukemia. N Engl J Med. 2013 Jul 11;369(2):111–21. [PMID: 23841729]

Patel JP et al. How do novel molecular genetic markers influence treatment decisions in acute myeloid leukemia? Hematology Am Soc Hematol Educ Program. 2012;2012:28–34. [PMID: 23233557]

Peyrade F et al. Treatment decisions for elderly patients with haematological malignancies: a dilemma. Lancet Oncol. 2012 Aug;13(8):e344–52. [PMID: 22846839]

CHRONIC LYMPHOCYTIC LEUKEMIA

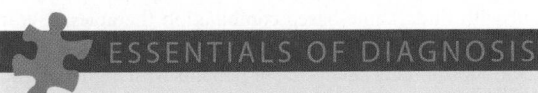

ESSENTIALS OF DIAGNOSIS

▸ B-cell lymphocytosis > 5000/mcL.
▸ Coexpression of CD19, CD5 on lymphocytes.

General Considerations

CLL is a clonal malignancy of B lymphocytes. The disease is usually indolent, with slowly progressive accumulation of long-lived small lymphocytes. These cells are immune-incompetent and respond poorly to antigenic stimulation.

CLL is manifested clinically by immunosuppression, bone marrow failure, and organ infiltration with lymphocytes. Immunodeficiency is also related to inadequate antibody production by the abnormal B cells. With advanced disease, CLL may cause damage by direct tissue infiltration.

Information about CLL is evolving rapidly, with new findings in biology and new treatment options, and outcomes are improving significantly.

Clinical Findings

A. Symptoms and Signs

CLL is a disease of older patients, with 90% of cases occurring after age 50 years and a median age at presentation of 70 years. Many patients will be incidentally discovered to have lymphocytosis. Others present with fatigue or lymphadenopathy. On examination, 80% of patients will have lymphadenopathy and 50% will have enlargement of the liver or spleen.

The long-standing Rai classification system remains prognostically useful: stage 0, lymphocytosis only; stage I, lymphocytosis plus lymphadenopathy; stage II, organomegaly (spleen, liver); stage III, anemia; stage IV, thrombocytopenia. These stages can be collapsed in to low-risk (stages 0–I), intermediate risk (stage II) and high-risk (stages III–IV).

CLL usually pursues an indolent course, but some subtypes behave more aggressively; a variant, prolymphocytic leukemia, is more aggressive. The morphology of the latter is different, characterized by larger and more immature cells. In 5–10% of cases, CLL may be complicated by autoimmune hemolytic anemia or autoimmune thrombocytopenia. In approximately 5% of cases, while the systemic disease remains stable, an isolated lymph node transforms into an aggressive large cell lymphoma (**Richter syndrome**).

B. Laboratory Findings

The hallmark of CLL is isolated lymphocytosis. The white blood count is usually > 20,000/mcL (20×10^9/L) and may be markedly elevated to several hundred thousand. Usually 75–98% of the circulating cells are lymphocytes. Lymphocytes appear small and mature, with condensed nuclear chromatin, and are morphologically indistinguishable from normal small lymphocytes, but smaller numbers of larger and activated lymphocytes may be seen. The hematocrit and platelet count are usually normal at presentation. The bone marrow is variably infiltrated with small lymphocytes. The immunophenotype of CLL demonstrates coexpression of the B lymphocyte lineage marker CD19 with the T lymphocyte marker CD5; this finding is commonly observed only in CLL and mantle cell lymphoma. CLL is distinguished from mantle cell lymphoma by the expression of CD23, low expression of surface immunoglobulin and CD20, and the absence of a translocation or overexpression of cyclin D1. Patients whose CLL cells have mutated forms of the immunoglobulin gene (IgVH somatic mutation) have a more indolent form of disease; these cells typically express low levels of the surface antigen CD38 and do not express the zeta-associated protein (ZAP-70). Conversely, patients whose cells have unmutated IgVH genes and high levels of ZAP-70 expression do less well and require treatment sooner. The assessment of genomic changes by fluorescence in-situ hybridization (FISH) provides important prognostic information. The finding of deletion of chromosome 17p (TP53) confers the worst prognosis, while deletion of 11q (ATM) confers an inferior prognosis to the average genotype, and isolated deletion of 13q has a more favorable outcome.

Hypogammaglobulinemia is present in 50% of patients and becomes more common with advanced disease. In some, a small amount of IgM paraprotein is present in the serum.

Differential Diagnosis

Few syndromes can be confused with CLL. Viral infections producing lymphocytosis should be obvious from the presence of fever and other clinical findings; however, fever may occur in CLL from concomitant bacterial infection. Pertussis may cause a particularly high total lymphocyte count. Other lymphoproliferative diseases such as Waldenström macroglobulinemia, hairy cell leukemia, or lymphoma (especially mantle cell) in the leukemic phase are distinguished on the basis of the morphology and immunophenotype of circulating lymphocytes and bone marrow. Monoclonal B-cell lymphocytosis is a disorder characterized by < 5000/mcL B-cells and is considered a precursor to B-CLL.

Treatment

Most cases of early indolent CLL require no specific therapy, and the standard of care for early stage disease has been observation. Indications for treatment include progressive fatigue, symptomatic lymphadenopathy, anemia, or thrombocytopenia. These patients have either symptomatic and progressive Rai stage II disease or stage III/IV disease. The initial treatment of choice for patients younger than 70 years old without significant comorbidities is the combination of fludarabine plus rituximab, with or without the addition of cyclophosphamide (see Table 39–15). The addition of cyclophosphamide appears to have greater antileukemic effectiveness, especially in patients with deletions of 11q, but also increases the risk of treatment-related infection. The combination of bendamustine with rituximab is another reasonable choice of therapy in this patient population. This combination has shown activity as the front-line therapy (88% overall response rate) and as treatment for relapsed setting (59% overall response rate), including for patients who had previously not responded to treatment with fludarabine.

For older or frail patients, chlorambucil, 0.6–1 mg/kg, a well-tolerated agent given orally every 3 weeks for approximately 6 months, has been the standard therapy. The novel monoclonal antibody, obinutuzumab, in combination with chlorambucil produces a significant number of responses (75%) including elimination of disease at the molecular level (in 17%) and offers another well-tolerated choice in this patient population. The oral agent ibrutinib, an inhibitor of Bruton's tyrosine kinase, a key component in the B-cell receptor signaling pathway, has shown very high activity in patients with relapsed/refractory CLL and in those with deletion of 17p. As a single agent, it produces a 75% response rate with significant reduction in lymphadenopathy but initial therapy can be associated with marked lymphocytosis due to release of tumor cells from the lymph nodes into the peripheral blood. In patients with 17p deletion, the median duration of response can exceed 2 years, which is considered a breakthrough in this disease. Last, lenalidomide has been shown to be effective in refractory cases of CLL. However, this agent can induce a "flare" reaction with marked swelling of involved lymph nodes that appears to be caused by an infiltration of reactive T cells.

Associated autoimmune hemolytic anemia or immune thrombocytopenia may require treatment with rituximab, prednisone, or splenectomy. Fludarabine should be avoided in patients with autoimmune hemolytic anemia since it may exacerbate it, and rituximab, in patients with past HBV infection since HBV reactivation, fulminant, and rarely, death can occur. Patients with recurrent bacterial infections and hypogammaglobulinemia benefit from prophylactic infusions of gamma globulin (0.4 g/kg/month), but this treatment is very expensive and can be justified only when these infections are severe. Patients undergoing therapy with a nucleoside analogue (fludarabine, pentostatin) should receive anti-infective prophylaxis for *Pneumocystis jirovecii* pneumonia, herpes viruses, and invasive fungal infections until there is evidence of T-cell recovery.

Allogeneic transplantation offers potentially curative treatment for patients with CLL, but it should be used only in patients whose disease cannot be controlled by standard therapies. Nonmyeloablative allogeneic transplant has produced encouraging results in CLL. Some subtypes of CLL with genomic abnormalities such as 17p deletions have a sufficiently poor prognosis with standard therapies that early intervention with allogeneic transplant is being studied to assess whether it can improve outcomes.

Prognosis

Therapies have changed the prognosis of CLL. In the past, median survival was approximately 6 years, and only 25% of patients lived more than 10 years. Patients with stage 0 or stage I disease have a median survival of 10–15 years, and these patients may be reassured that they can live a normal life for many years. Patients with stage III or stage IV disease had a median survival of < 2 years in the past, but with fludarabine-based combination therapies, 2-year survival is now > 90% and the long-term outlook appears to be substantially changed. For patients with high-risk and resistant forms of CLL, there is evidence that allogeneic transplantation can overcome risk factors and lead to long-term disease control.

When to Refer

All patients with CLL should be referred to a hematologist.

When to Admit

Hospitalization is rarely needed.

Byrd JC et al. Targeting BTK with ibrutinib in relapsed chronic lymphocytic leukemia. N Engl J Med. 2013 Jul 4;369(1):32–42. [PMID: 23782158]

Dreger P et al. Allogeneic stem cell transplantation provides durable disease control in poor-risk chronic lymphocytic leukemia: long-term clinical and MRD results of the German CLL Study Group CLL 3XX trial. Blood. 2010 Oct 7;116(14):2438–47. [PMID: 20595516]

Hallek M et al. Guidelines for the diagnosis and treatment of chronic lymphocytic leukemia: a report from the International Workshop on Chronic Lymphocytic Leukemia updating the National Cancer Center Institute-Working Group 1996 guidelines. Blood. 2008 Jun 15;111(12):5446–56. [PMID: 18216293]

Morrison VA. Infectious complications in patients with chronic lymphocytic leukemia: pathogenesis, spectrum of infection, and approaches to prophylaxis. Clin Lymphoma Myeloma. 2009 Oct;9(5):365–70. [PMID: 19858055]

HAIRY CELL LEUKEMIA

ESSENTIALS OF DIAGNOSIS

- ► Pancytopenia.
- ► Splenomegaly, often massive.
- ► Hairy cells present on blood smear and especially in bone marrow biopsy.

▶ General Considerations

Hairy cell leukemia is a rare malignancy of hematopoietic stem cells differentiated as mature B-lymphocytes with hairy cytoplasmic projections.

▶ Clinical Findings

A. Symptoms and Signs

The disease characteristically presents in middle-aged men. The median age at presentation is 55 years, and there is a striking 5:1 male predominance. Most patients present with gradual onset of fatigue, others complain of symptoms related to markedly enlarged spleen, and some come to attention because of infection.

Splenomegaly is almost invariably present and may be massive. The liver is enlarged in 50% of cases; lymphadenopathy is uncommon.

Hairy cell leukemia is usually an indolent disorder whose course is dominated by pancytopenia and recurrent infections, including mycobacterial infections.

B. Laboratory Findings

The hallmark of hairy cell leukemia is pancytopenia. Anemia is nearly universal, and 75% of patients have thrombocytopenia and neutropenia. The "hairy cells" are usually present in small numbers on the peripheral blood smear and have a characteristic appearance with numerous cytoplasmic projections. The bone marrow is usually inaspirable (dry tap), and the diagnosis is made by characteristic morphology on bone marrow biopsy. The hairy cells have a characteristic histochemical staining pattern with tartrate-resistant acid phosphatase (TRAP). On immunophenotyping, the cells coexpress the antigens CD11c, CD20, CD22, CD25, CD103, and CD123. Pathologic examination of the spleen shows marked infiltration of the red pulp with hairy cells. This is in contrast to the usual predilection of lymphomas to involve the white pulp of the spleen. The identification of *BRAF* V600E mutation by sequencing hairy cells from affected patients offers a new diagnostic tool and potential treatment target.

▶ Differential Diagnosis

Hairy cell leukemia should be distinguished from other lymphoproliferative diseases such as Waldenström macroglobulinemia and non-Hodgkin lymphomas. It also may be confused with other causes of pancytopenia, including hypersplenism due to any cause, aplastic anemia, and paroxysmal nocturnal hemoglobinuria.

▶ Treatment

The treatment of choice is intravenous cladribine (2-chlorodeoxyadenosine; CdA), 0.1 mg/kg daily for 7 days. This is a relatively nontoxic drug that produces benefit in 95% of cases and complete remission in more than 80%. Responses are long lasting, with few patients relapsing in the first few years. Treatment with intravenous pentostatin produces similar results, but that drug is more cumbersome to administer. Rituximab is sometimes given for minimal residual disease after cladribine or pentostatin.

▶ Course & Prognosis

The development of new therapies has changed the prognosis of this disease. Formerly, median survival was 6 years, and only one-third of patients survived longer than 10 years. More than 95% of patients with hairy cell leukemia now live longer than 10 years.

Cawley JC et al. The biology of hairy-cell leukaemia. Curr Opin Hematol. 2010 Jul;17(4):341–9. [PMID: 20375887]

Ravandi F. Chemo-immunotherapy for hairy cell leukemia. Leuk Lymphoma. 2011 Jun;52(Suppl 2):72–4. [PMID: 21417822]

Tiacci E et al. *BRAF* mutations in hairy-cell leukemia. N Engl J Med. 2011 Jun 16;364(24):2305–15. [PMID: 21663470]

LYMPHOMAS

NON-HODGKIN LYMPHOMAS

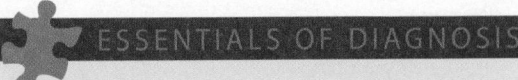

ESSENTIALS OF DIAGNOSIS

- ► Often present with painless lymphadenopathy.
- ► Pathologic diagnosis of lymphoma is made by pathologic examination of tissue.

▶ General Considerations

The non-Hodgkin lymphomas are a heterogeneous group of cancers of lymphocytes usually presenting as enlarged lymph nodes. The disorders vary in clinical presentation and course from indolent to rapidly progressive.

Molecular biology has provided clues to the pathogenesis of these disorders, often a matter of balanced chromosomal translocations whereby an oncogene becomes juxtaposed next to either an immunoglobulin gene (B-cell lymphoma) or the T-cell receptor gene or related gene (T-cell lymphoma). The net result is oncogene overexpression and the development of lymphoma. The best-studied example is Burkitt lymphoma, in which a characteristic cytogenetic abnormality of translocation between the long arms of chromosomes 8 and 14 has been identified. The protooncogene c-*myc* is translocated from its normal position on chromosome 8 to the immunoglobulin heavy chain locus on chromosome 14. Overexpression of c-*myc* is related to malignant transformation through excess B-cell proliferation. In the follicular lymphomas, the t(14;18) translocation is characteristic and *bcl-2 is* overexpressed, resulting in protection against apoptosis, the usual mechanism of B-cell death.

Classification of the lymphomas is a dynamic area still undergoing evolution. The most recent grouping (Table 13–16) separates diseases based on both clinical and pathologic features. Eighty-five percent of non-Hodgkin lymphomas are B-cell and 15% are T-cell or NK-cell in origin. Even though non-Hodgkin lymphomas represent a very diverse group of diseases, they are historically divided in two categories based on clinical behavior and pathology: the indolent (low-grade) and the aggressive (intermediate or higher-grade).

Table 13–16. World Health Organization classification of non-Hodgkin lymphomas (most common).

Precursor B-cell lymphoblastic lymphoma
Mature B-cell lymphomas
Diffuse large B cell lymphoma
Mediastinal large B cell lymphoma
Follicular lymphoma
Small lymphocytic lymphoma
Lymphoplasmacytic lymphoma (Waldenström macroglobulinemia)
Mantle cell lymphoma
Burkitt lymphoma
Marginal zone lymphoma
MALT type
Nodal type
Splenic type
Precursor T-cell lymphoblastic lymphoma
Mature T (and NK cell) lymphomas
Anaplastic T-cell lymphoma
Angioimmunoblastic
Peripheral T-cell lymphoma, NOS
Cutaneous T-cell lymphoma (mycosis fungoides)
Extranodal T/NK-cell lymphoma
Adult T-cell leukemia/lymphoma

NOS, not otherwise specified.

▶ Clinical Findings

A. Symptoms and Signs

Patients with non-Hodgkin lymphomas usually present with lymphadenopathy, which may be isolated or widespread. Involved lymph nodes may be present peripherally or centrally (in the retroperitoneum, mesentery, and pelvis). The indolent lymphomas are usually disseminated at the time of diagnosis, and bone marrow involvement is frequent. Many patients with lymphoma have constitutional symptoms such as fever, drenching night sweats, and weight loss of >10% of prior body weight (referred to as "B" symptoms).

On examination, lymphadenopathy may be isolated or diffuse, and extranodal sites of disease (such as the skin, gastrointestinal tract, liver, and bone marrow) may be found. Patients with Burkitt lymphoma are noted to have abdominal pain or abdominal fullness because of the predilection of the disease for the abdomen.

Once a pathologic diagnosis is established, staging is done using a whole body PET/CT scan, a bone marrow biopsy and, in patients with high-grade lymphoma or intermediate-grade lymphoma with high-risk features, a lumbar puncture.

B. Laboratory Findings

The peripheral blood is usually normal even with extensive bone marrow involvement by lymphoma. Circulating lymphoma cells in the blood are not commonly seen.

Bone marrow involvement is manifested as paratrabecular monoclonal lymphoid aggregates. In some high-grade lymphomas, the meninges are involved and malignant cells are found with cerebrospinal fluid cytology. The serum LD has been shown to be a useful prognostic marker and is now incorporated in risk stratification of treatment.

The diagnosis of lymphoma is made by tissue biopsy. Needle aspiration may yield evidence for non-Hodgkin lymphoma, but a lymph node biopsy (or biopsy of involved extranodal tissue) is required for accurate diagnosis and classification.

▶ Treatment

A. Indolent Lymphomas

The most common lymphomas in this group are follicular lymphoma, marginal zone lymphomas, and small lymphocytic lymphoma (CLL). The treatment of **indolent lymphomas** depends on the stage of disease and the clinical status of the patient. A small number of patients have limited disease with only one or two contiguous abnormal lymph node groups and may be treated with localized irradiation with curative intent. However, most patients (85%) with indolent lymphoma have disseminated disease at the time of diagnosis and are not considered curable. Historically, treatment of these patients has not affected overall survival; therefore, treatment is only offered when symptoms develop or for high tumor bulk. Following each treatment response, patients will experience a relapse at traditionally shorter intervals. Some patients will have temporary spontaneous remissions. There are an increasing number of reasonable treatment options for indolent lymphomas, but no consensus has emerged on the best strategy. Treatment with rituximab (375 mg/m² intravenously weekly for 4 weeks) is commonly used either alone or in combination with chemotherapy and may be the only agent to affect overall survival in these disorders. Patients should be screened for hepatitis B because rare cases of fatal fulminant hepatitis have been described with the use of anti-CD20 monoclonal therapies. Common rituximab-chemotherapy regimens include bendamustine; cyclophosphamide, vincristine, and prednisone (R-CVP); and cyclophosphamide, doxorubicin, vincristine, prednisone (R-CHOP) (see Table 39–12). Radioimmunoconjugates that fuse anti-B cell monoclonal antibodies with radioactive nuclides produce higher response rates compared to antibody alone, and two such agents (yttrium-90 ibritumomab tiuxetan and iodine-131 tositumomab) are in use. Some patients with clinically aggressive low-grade lymphomas may be appropriate candidates for allogeneic stem cell transplantation with curative intent. The role of autologous hematopoietic stem cell transplantation remains uncertain, but some patients with recurrent disease appear to have prolonged remissions without the expectation of cure.

Patients with mucosal associated lymphoid tumors of the stomach may be appropriately treated with combination antibiotics directed against *Helicobacter pylori* and with acid blockade but require frequent endoscopic monitoring. Alternatively, MALT confined to the stomach can also be cured with whole-stomach radiotherapy.

B. Aggressive Lymphomas

Patients with **diffuse large B-cell lymphoma** are treated with curative intent. Those with localized disease may receive short-course immunochemotherapy (such as three courses of R-CHOP) plus localized involved-field radiation or six cycles of immunochemotherapy without radiation. Most patients who have more advanced disease are treated with six cycles of immunochemotherapy such as R-CHOP (see Table 39–12). Patients with diffuse large B-cell lymphoma who relapse after initial chemotherapy can still be cured by autologous hematopoietic stem cell transplantation if their disease remains responsive to chemotherapy.

Mantle cell lymphoma is not effectively treated with standard immunochemotherapy regimens. Intensive initial immunochemotherapy including autologous hematopoietic stem cell transplantation has been shown to improve outcomes. Reduced-intensity allogeneic stem cell transplantation offers curative potential for selected patients. Ibrutinib is active in relapsed or refractory patients with mantle cell lymphoma. For **primary central nervous system lymphoma,** repetitive cycles of high-dose intravenous methotrexate with rituximab early in the treatment course produce better results than whole brain radiotherapy and with less cognitive impairment.

Patients with **high-grade lymphomas** (Burkitt or lymphoblastic) require urgent, intense, cyclic chemotherapy in the hospital similar to that given for ALL, and they also require intrathecal chemotherapy as central nervous system prophylaxis.

Patients with **peripheral T-cell lymphomas** usually have advanced stage nodal and extranodal disease and typically have inferior response rates to therapy compared to patients with aggressive B-cell disease. Autologous stem cell transplantation is often incorporated in first-line therapy. The antibody-drug conjugate brentuximab vedotin has significant activity in patients with relapsed CD30 positive peripheral T-cell lymphomas, such as anaplastic large cell lymphoma.

► Prognosis

The median survival of patients with indolent lymphomas is 10–15 years. These diseases ultimately become refractory to chemotherapy. This often occurs at the time of histologic progression of the disease to a more aggressive form of lymphoma.

The International Prognostic Index is widely used to categorize patients with aggressive lymphoma into risk groups. Factors that confer adverse prognosis are age over 60 years, elevated serum LD, stage III or stage IV disease, more than one extranodal site of disease, and poor performance status. Cure rates range from > 80% for low-risk patients (zero risk factors) to < 50% for high-risk patients (four or more risk factors).

For patients who relapse after initial chemotherapy, the prognosis depends on whether the lymphoma is still responsive to chemotherapy. If the lymphoma remains responsive to chemotherapy, autologous hematopoietic stem cell transplantation offers a 50% chance of long-term lymphoma-free survival.

The treatment of older patients with lymphoma has been difficult because of poorer tolerance of aggressive chemotherapy. The use of myeloid growth factors and prophylactic antibiotics to reduce neutropenic complications may improve outcomes.

Molecular profiling techniques using gene array technology and immunophenotyping have defined subsets of lymphomas with different biologic features and prognoses are being studied in clinical trials to determine choice of therapy.

► When to Refer

All patients with lymphoma should be referred to a hematologist or an oncologist.

► When to Admit

Admission is necessary only for specific complications of lymphoma or its treatment and for the treatment of all high-grade lymphomas.

Foss FM et al. Peripheral T-cell lymphoma. Blood. 2011 Jun 23;117(25):6756–67. [PMID: 21493798]

Pérez-Galán P et al. Mantle cell lymphoma: biology, pathogenesis, and the molecular basis of treatment in the genomic era. Blood. 2011 Jan 6;117(1):26–38. [PMID: 20940415]

Shankland KR et al. Non-Hodgkin lymphoma. Lancet. 2012 Sep 1;380(9844):848–57. [PMID: 22835603]

Vidal L et al. Immunotherapy for patients with follicular lymphoma: the contribution of systematic reviews. Acta Haematol. 2011;125(1–2):23–31. [PMID: 21150184]

HODGKIN LYMPHOMA

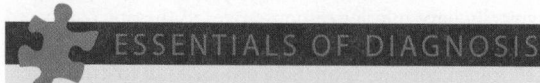

ESSENTIALS OF DIAGNOSIS

- ▶ Often painless lymphadenopathy.
- ▶ Constitutional symptoms may or may not be present.
- ▶ Pathologic diagnosis by lymph node biopsy.

▶ General Considerations

Hodgkin lymphoma is characterized by Reed–Sternberg cells in an appropriate reactive cellular background . The malignant cell is derived from B lymphocytes of germinal center origin.

▶ Clinical Findings

There is a bimodal age distribution, with one peak in the 20s and a second over age 50 years. Most patients seek medical attention because of a painless mass, commonly in the neck. Others may seek medical attention because of constitutional symptoms such as fever, weight loss, or drenching night sweats, or because of generalized pruritus. An unusual symptom of Hodgkin lymphoma is pain in an involved lymph node following alcohol ingestion.

An important feature of Hodgkin lymphoma is its tendency to arise within single lymph node areas and spread in an orderly fashion to contiguous areas of lymph nodes. Late in the course of the disease, vascular invasion leads to widespread hematogenous dissemination.

Hodgkin lymphoma is divided into two subtypes: classic Hodgkin (nodular sclerosis, mixed cellularity, lymphocyte rich, and lymphocyte depleted) and non-classic Hodgkin (nodular lymphocyte predominant). Hodgkin lymphoma should be distinguished pathologically from other malignant lymphomas and may occasionally be confused with reactive lymph nodes seen in infectious mononucleosis, cat-scratch disease, or drug reactions (eg, phenytoin).

Patients undergo a staging evaluation to determine the extent of disease, including serum chemistries, whole body PET/CT scan, and bone marrow biopsy. The staging nomenclature (Ann Arbor) is as follows: stage I, one lymph node region involved; stage II, involvement of two or more lymph node regions on one side of the diaphragm; stage III, lymph node regions involved on both sides of the diaphragm; and stage IV, disseminated disease with extranodal involvement. Disease staging is further categorized as "A" if patients lack constitutional symptoms or as "B" if patients have 10% weight loss over 6 months, fever, or drenching night sweats (or some combination thereof).

▶ Treatment

Chemotherapy is the mainstay of treatment for Hodgkin lymphoma and ABVD (doxorubicin, bleomycin, vinblastine, dacarbazine) remains the standard first-line regimen. Even though others such as Stanford V or escalated BEACOPP may improve response rates and reduce the need for consolidative radiotherapy, they are usually associated with increased toxicity and lack a definitive overall survival advantage. Low-risk patients are those with stage I or II disease without bulky lymphadenopathy or evidence of systemic inflammation. They traditionally receive a combination of short course chemotherapy with involved-field radiotherapy or a full course of chemotherapy alone (see Table 39–12). However, ongoing studies are aiming to eliminate the radiotherapy or to abbreviate the chemotherapy in patients who achieve an interim negative PET/CT scan. High-risk patients are those with stage III or IV disease or with stage II disease and a large mediastinal or other bulky mass. These patients are treated with a full course of ABVD for six cycles. End-of-treatment PET/CT scan may identify patients with stage II bulky disease who can avoid traditional involved-field radiotherapy. Pulmonary toxicity can unfortunately occur following either chemotherapy (bleomycin) or radiation and should be treated aggressively in these patients, since it can lead to permanent fibrosis and death.

Classic Hodgkin lymphoma relapsing after initial treatment may be treatable with high-dose chemotherapy and autologous hematopoietic stem cell transplantation. This offers a 35–50% chance of cure when disease is still chemotherapy responsive. The antibody-drug conjugate brentuximab vedotin has shown impressive activity in patients relapsing after autologous stem cell transplantation (ORR: 75%; CR: 34%) and has been approved by the US Food and Drug Administration for this indication. It is now being studied in front-line therapy, replacing the bleomycin in ABVD.

▶ Prognosis

All patients should be treated with curative intent. Prognosis in advanced stage Hodgkin lymphoma is influenced by seven features: stage, age, gender, hemoglobin, albumin, white blood count, and lymphocyte count. The cure rate is 75% if zero to two risk features are present and 55% when three or more risk features are present. The prognosis of patients with stage IA or IIA disease is excellent, with 10-year survival rates in excess of 90%. Patients with advanced disease (stage III or IV) have 10-year survival rates of 50–60%. Poorer results are seen in patients who are older, those who have bulky disease, and those with lymphocyte depletion or mixed cellularity on histologic examination. Non-classic Hodgkin lymphoma (nodular lymphocyte predominant) is highly curable with radiotherapy alone for early-stage disease; however, for high-stage disease, it is characterized by long survival with repetitive relapses after chemotherapy.

▶ When to Refer

- All patients should be sent to an oncologist or hematologist.
- Secondary referral to a radiation oncologist might be appropriate.

When to Admit

Patients should be admitted for complications of the disease or its treatment.

Engert A et al. Reduced treatment intensity in patients with early-stage Hodgkin's lymphoma. N Engl J Med. 2010 Aug 12;363(7):640–52. [PMID: 20818855]

Meyer RM et al. ABVD alone versus radiation-based therapy in limited-stage Hodgkin's lymphoma. N Engl J Med. 2012 Feb 2;366(5):399–408. [PMID: 22149921]

Meyer RM et al. Point/counterpoint: early-stage Hodgkin lymphoma and the role of radiation therapy. Blood. 2012 Nov 29;120(23):4488–95. [PMID: 22821764]

Viviani S et al. ABVD versus BEACOPP for Hodgkin's lymphoma when high-dose salvage is planned. N Engl J Med. 2011 Jul 21;365(3):203–12. [PMID: 21774708]

Younes A et al. Brentuximab vedotin (SGN-35) for relapsed CD30-positive lymphomas. N Engl J Med. 2010 Nov 4;363(19):1812–21. [PMID: 21047225]

MULTIPLE MYELOMA

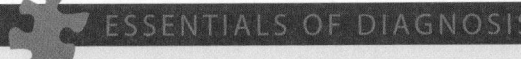

ESSENTIALS OF DIAGNOSIS

▶ Bone pain, often in the spine, ribs, or proximal long bones.

▶ Monoclonal paraprotein by serum or urine protein electrophoresis or immunofixation.

▶ Clonal plasma cells in the bone marrow or in a tissue biopsy, or both.

▶ Organ damage due to plasma cells (eg, bones, kidneys, hypercalcemia, anemia).

General Considerations

Multiple myeloma is a malignancy of hematopoietic stem cells terminally differentiated as plasma cells characterized by replacement of the bone marrow, bone destruction, and paraprotein formation. The diagnosis is established when monoclonal plasma cells (either kappa or lambda light chain restricted) in the bone marrow (any percentage) or as a tumor (plasmacytoma), or both, are associated with end organ damage (such as bone disease [lytic lesions, osteopenia], anemia [hemoglobin < 10 g/dL {100 g/L}], hypercalcemia [calcium > 11.5 mg/dL {2.9 mmol/L}], or renal failure [creatinine > 2 mg/dL {176.8 mcmol/L}]) with or without paraprotein elaboration. Smoldering myeloma is defined as ≥ 10% clonal plasma cells in the bone marrow, a serum paraprotein level ≥ 3 g/dL (30 g/L), or both, without plasma cell–related end-organ damage.

Malignant plasma cells can form tumors (plasmacytomas) that may cause spinal cord compression or other soft-tissue problems. Bone disease is common and due to excessive osteoclast activation mediated largely by the interaction of the receptor activator of NF-kappa-B (RANK) with its ligand (RANKL). In multiple myeloma, osteoprotegerin (a decoy receptor for RANKL) is underproduced, thus promoting the binding of RANK with RANKL with consequent excessive bone resorption. Other soluble factors contributing to osteoclast hyperactivation include interleukin-1, interleukin-6, tissue necrosis factor-alpha, macrophage inhibitor protein-1-alpha, and macrophage colony stimulating factor, all of which might prove eventual therapeutic targets.

The paraproteins (monoclonal immunoglobulins) secreted by the malignant plasma cells may cause problems in their own right. Very high paraprotein levels (either IgG or IgA) may cause hyperviscosity, although this is more often common with the IgM in Waldenström macroglobulinemia. The light chain component of the immunoglobulin often leads to kidney failure (frequently aggravated by hypercalcemia or hyperuricemia, or both). Light chain components may be deposited in tissues as amyloid, resulting in kidney failure with albuminuria and a vast array of systemic symptoms.

Myeloma patients are prone to recurrent infections for a number of reasons, including neutropenia, the underproduction of normal immunoglobulins and the immunosuppressive effects of chemotherapy. Myeloma patients are especially prone to infections with encapsulated organisms such as *Streptococcus pneumoniae* and *Haemophilus influenzae*.

Clinical Findings

A. Symptoms and Signs

Myeloma is a disease of older adults (median age, 65 years). The most common presenting complaints are those related to anemia, bone pain, kidney disease, and infection. Bone pain is most common in the back, hips, or ribs or may present as a pathologic fracture, especially of the femoral neck or vertebrae. Patients may also come to medical attention because of spinal cord compression or the hyperviscosity syndrome (mucosal bleeding, vertigo, nausea, visual disturbances, alterations in mental status). Many patients are diagnosed because of laboratory findings of hypercalcemia, proteinuria, elevated sedimentation rate, or abnormalities on serum protein electrophoresis obtained for symptoms or in routine screening studies. A few patients come to medical attention because of organ dysfunction due to amyloidosis.

Examination may reveal pallor, bone tenderness, and soft tissue masses. Patients may have neurologic signs related to neuropathy or spinal cord compression. Patients with primary amyloidosis may have an enlarged tongue, peripheral or autonomic neuropathy, heart failure, or hepatomegaly. Splenomegaly is absent unless amyloidosis is present. Fever occurs mainly with infection. Acute oliguric or nonoliguric renal failure may be present due to hypercalcemia, hyperuricemia, light-chain cast injury, or primary amyloidosis.

B. Laboratory Findings

Anemia is nearly universal. Red blood cell morphology is normal, but rouleaux formation is common and may be marked. The absence of rouleaux formation, however, excludes neither multiple myeloma nor the presence of a serum paraprotein. The neutrophil and platelet counts are usually normal at presentation. Only rarely will plasma cells be visible on peripheral blood smear (plasma cell leukemia).

The hallmark of myeloma is the finding of a paraprotein on serum or urine protein electrophoresis (PEP) or immunofixation electrophoresis (IFE). The majority of patients will have a monoclonal spike visible in the gamma- or beta-globulin region of the PEP. The semi-quantification of the paraprotein on the PEP is referred to as the M-protein, and IFE will reveal this to be a monoclonal immunoglobulin. Approximately 15% of patients will have no demonstrable paraprotein in the serum because their myeloma cells produce only light chains and not intact immunoglobulin, and the light chains pass rapidly through the glomerulus into the urine. Urine PEP and IFE will demonstrate the light chain paraprotein in this setting. The free light chain assay will sometimes demonstrate excess monoclonal light chains in serum and urine, and in a small proportion of patients, will be the only means to identify and quantify the paraprotein being produced. Overall, the paraprotein is IgG (60%), IgA (20%), or light chain only (15%) in multiple myeloma, with the remainder being rare cases of IgD, IgM, or biclonal gammopathy. In sporadic cases, no paraprotein is present ("nonsecretory myeloma"); these patients have particularly aggressive disease.

The bone marrow will be infiltrated by variable numbers of monoclonal plasma cells. The plasma cells may be morphologically abnormal often demonstrating multinucleation and vacuolization. The plasma cells will display marked skewing of the normal kappa to lambda light chain ratio, which will indicate their clonality. Many benign processes can result in bone marrow plasmacytosis, but the presence of atypical plasma cells, light chain restriction, and effacement of normal bone marrow elements helps distinguish myeloma.

C. Imaging

Bone radiographs are important in establishing the diagnosis of myeloma. Lytic lesions are most commonly seen in the axial skeleton: skull, spine, proximal long bones, and ribs. At other times, only generalized osteoporosis is seen. The radionuclide bone scan is not useful in detecting bone lesions in myeloma, since there is usually no osteoblastic component. Magnetic resonance imaging (MRI) and positron emission tomography (PET) scans will demonstrate significantly more disease than is shown in plain radiographs, and these imaging studies are common practice in the evaluation of patients with known or suspected multiple myeloma.

▶ Differential Diagnosis

When a patient is discovered to have a paraprotein, the distinction between multiple myeloma or another lymphoproliferative malignancy with a paraprotein (CLL, Waldenström macroglobulinemia, non-Hodgkin lymphoma, primary amyloid, cryoglobulinemia) and monoclonal gammopathy of undetermined significance (MGUS)

must be made. MGUS is present in 1% of all adults, (3% of those over age 50 years and more than 5% in those over age 70 years). Thus, among all patients with paraproteins, MGUS is far more common than multiple myeloma. MGUS is defined as bone marrow monoclonal plasma cells < 10% in the setting of a paraprotein (serum M-protein < 3 g/dL [< 30 g/L]) and the absence of end-organ damage. In approximately one-quarter of cases, MGUS progresses to overt malignant disease in a median of one decade. The transformation of MGUS to multiple myeloma is approximately 1% per year. Smoldering multiple myeloma is defined as a serum M-protein > 3 g/dL (> 30 g/L) or bone marrow monoclonal plasma cells ≥ 10% in the absence of end-organ damage. Multiple myeloma, smoldering multiple myeloma, and MGUS must be distinguished from reactive (benign) polyclonal hypergammaglobulinemia (which is commonly seen in cirrhosis).

▶ Treatment

Patients with MGUS are observed without treatment. Patients with smoldering myeloma treated with lenalidomide and dexamethasone take longer to progress to symptomatic myeloma and live longer than when simply observed. Most patients with multiple myeloma require treatment at diagnosis because of bone pain or other symptoms and complications related to the disease. The initial treatment generally involves at a minimum an immunomodulatory drug, such as thalidomide or lenalidomide, in combination with moderate- or high-dose dexamethasone. The major side effects of lenalidomide are neutropenia and thrombocytopenia, venothromboembolism, and peripheral neuropathy. Bortezomib, a proteosome inhibitor, is also highly active and has the advantages of producing rapid responses and of being effective in poor-prognosis multiple myeloma. The major side effect of bortezomib is neuropathy (both peripheral and autonomic), which is largely ameliorated when given subcutaneously rather than intravenously. A common regimen for initial treatment is RVD (lenalidomide, bortezomib, and dexamethasone). The combination of bortezomib, dexamethasone, and liposomal doxorubicin is also effective. Carfilzomib, a second-generation proteosome inhibitor, produces responses in patients for whom bortezomib treatment fails and does not cause neuropathy.

After initial therapy, many patients under age 76 years are consolidated with autologous hematopoietic stem cell transplantation. Autologous hematopoietic stem cell transplantation prolongs both duration of remission and overall survival, and has the advantage of providing long treatment-free intervals. Lenalidomide or thalidomide prolong remission and survival when given as posttransplant maintenance therapy. There is emerging concern about an elevated rate of secondary malignancies associated with use of immunomodulatory drugs as maintenance therapy. Allogeneic stem cell transplantation is potentially curative in multiple myeloma, but its role has been limited because of the unusually high treatment-related mortality rate (40–50%) in myeloma patients.

Localized radiotherapy may be useful for palliation of bone pain or for eradicating tumor at the site of pathologic fracture. Vertebral collapse with its attendant pain and mechanical disturbance can be treated with vertebroplasty or kyphoplasty. Hypercalcemia and hyperuricemia should be treated aggressively and immobilization and dehydration avoided. The bisphosphonates (pamidronate 90 mg or zoledronic acid 4 mg intravenously monthly) reduce pathologic fractures in patients with bone disease and are an important adjunct in this subset of patients. The bisphosphonates are also used to treat malignant hypercalcemia. However, long-term bisphosphonates, especially zoledronic acid, have been associated with a risk of osteonecrosis of the jaw and other bony areas so treated patients must be monitored for this complication.

▶ Prognosis

The outlook for patients with myeloma has been steadily improving for the past decade. The median survival of patients is more than 5 years. Patients with low-stage disease who lack high-risk genomic changes respond very well to treatment and derive significant benefit from autologous hematopoietic stem cell transplantation and have survivals approaching a decade. The **International Staging System** for myeloma relies on two factors: beta-2-microglobulin and albumin. Stage 1 patients have both beta-2-microglobulin < 3.5 mg/L and albumin > 3.5 g/dL (survival > 5 years). Stage 3 is established when beta-2-microglobulin > 5.5 mg/L (survival < 2 years). Stage 2 is established with values in between. The other laboratory finding of important adverse prognostic significance on a bone marrow sample is genetic abnormalities established by FISH involving the immunoglobulin heavy chain locus at chromosome 14q32 (such as the finding of t[4;14] or t[14;16]). Abnormalities of chromosome 17p also confer a particularly poor prognosis.

▶ When to Refer

All patients with multiple myeloma should be referred to a hematologist or an oncologist.

▶ When to Admit

Hospitalization is indicated for treatment of acute kidney failure, hypercalcemia, or suspicion of spinal cord compression, for certain chemotherapy regimens, or for hematopoietic stem cell transplantation.

Kyle RA et al. Management of monoclonal gammopathy of undetermined significance (MGUS) and smoldering multiple myeloma (SMM). Oncology (Williston Park). 2011 Jun;25(7): 578–86. [PMID: 21888255]

Longo V et al. Therapeutic approaches to myeloma bone disease: an evolving story. Cancer Treat Rev. 2012 Oct;38(6):787–97. [PMID: 22494965]

Mateos MV et al. Lenalidomide plus dexamethasone for high-risk smoldering multiple myeloma. N Engl J Med. 2013 Aug 1;369(5):438–47. [PMID: 23902483]

McCarthy PL et al. Lenalidomide after stem-cell transplantation for multiple myeloma. N Engl J Med. 2012 May10;366(19): 1770–81. [PMID: 22571201]

Palumbo A et al. Multiple myeloma. N Engl J Med. 2011 Mar 17;364(11):1046–60. [PMID: 21410373]

Smith D et al. Multiple myeloma. BMJ. 2013 Jun 26;346:f3863. [PMID: 23803862]

Yaqub S et al. Frontline therapy for multiple myeloma: a concise review of the evidence based on randomized clinical trials. Cancer Invest. 2013 Oct;31(8):529–37. [PMID: 24083815]

WALDENSTRÖM MACROGLOBULINEMIA

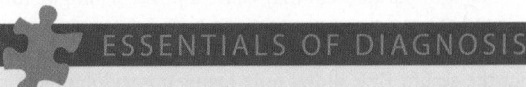

▶ Monoclonal IgM paraprotein.

▶ Infiltration of bone marrow by plasmacytic lymphocytes.

▶ Absence of lytic bone disease.

▶ General Considerations

Waldenström macroglobulinemia is a syndrome of IgM hypergammaglobulinemia that occurs in the setting of a low-grade non-Hodgkin lymphoma characterized by B-cells that are morphologically a hybrid of lymphocytes and plasma cells. These cells characteristically secrete the IgM paraprotein, and many clinical manifestations of the disease are related to this macroglobulin.

▶ Clinical Findings

A. Symptoms and Signs

This disease characteristically develops insidiously in patients in their 60s or 70s. Patients usually present with fatigue related to anemia. Hyperviscosity of serum may be manifested in a number of ways. Mucosal and gastrointestinal bleeding is related to engorged blood vessels and platelet dysfunction. Other complaints include nausea, vertigo, and visual disturbances. Alterations in consciousness vary from mild lethargy to stupor and coma. The IgM paraprotein may also cause symptoms of cold agglutinin disease (hemolysis) or chronic demyelinating peripheral neuropathy.

On examination, there may be hepatosplenomegaly or lymphadenopathy. The retinal veins are engorged. Purpura may be present. There should be no bone tenderness.

B. Laboratory Findings

Anemia is nearly universal, and rouleaux formation is common although the red blood cells are agglutinated when the blood smear is prepared at room temperature. The anemia is related in part to expansion of the plasma volume by 50–100% due to the presence of the paraprotein. Other blood counts are usually normal. The abnormal plasmacytic lymphocytes may appear in small numbers on the peripheral blood smear. The bone marrow is characteristically infiltrated by the plasmacytic lymphocytes.

The hallmark of macroglobulinemia is the presence of a monoclonal IgM spike seen on serum PEP in the beta-globulin region. The serum viscosity is usually increased above the normal of 1.4–1.8 times that of water. Symptoms of hyperviscosity usually develop when the serum viscosity is over four times that of water, and marked symptoms usually arise when the viscosity is over six times that of water. Because paraproteins vary in their physicochemical properties, there is no strict correlation between the concentration of paraprotein and serum viscosity.

The IgM paraprotein may cause a positive antiglobulin (Coombs) test for complement and have cold agglutinin or cryoglobulin properties. If macroglobulinemia is suspected but the serum PEP shows only hypogammaglobulinemia, the test should be repeated while taking special measures to maintain the blood at 37°C, since the paraprotein may precipitate out at room temperature. Bone radiographs are normal, and there is no evidence of kidney failure.

▶ Differential Diagnosis

Waldenström macroglobulinemia is differentiated from MGUS by the finding of bone marrow infiltration with monoclonal malignant cells. It is distinguished from CLL by bone marrow morphology, the absence of CD5 expression and the absence of lymphocytosis and from multiple myeloma by bone marrow morphology and the finding of the characteristic IgM paraprotein and the absence of bone disease.

▶ Treatment

Patients with marked hyperviscosity syndrome (stupor, coma, pulmonary edema) should be treated on an emergency basis with plasmapheresis. On a chronic basis, some patients can be managed with periodic plasmapheresis alone. As with other indolent malignant lymphoid diseases, rituximab (375 mg/m² intravenously weekly for 4–8 weeks) has significant activity. However, a word of caution: the IgM often rises first after rituximab therapy before it falls. Combination therapy is recommended for advanced disease (see Table 39–12). Bortezomib, thalidomide, lenalidomide, and bendamustine have all been shown to have activity in this disease. Autologous hematopoietic stem cell transplantation is reserved for relapsed or refractory patients.

▶ Prognosis

Waldenström macroglobulinemia is an indolent disease with a median survival rate of 5 years, and 10% of patients are alive at 15 years.

▶ When to Refer

All patients should be referred to a hematologist or an oncologist.

▶ When to Admit

Patients should be admitted for treatment of hyperviscosity syndrome.

Gertz MA. Waldenström macroglobulinemia: 2013 update on diagnosis, risk stratification, and management. Am J Hematol. 2013 Aug;88(8):703–11. [PMID: 23784973]

Stone MJ. Waldenström's macroglobulinemia: hyperviscosity syndrome and cryoglobulinemia. Clin Lymphoma Myeloma. 2009 Mar;9(1):97–9. [PMID: 19362986]
Treon SP. How I treat Waldenström macroglobulinemia. Blood. 2009 Sep 17;114(12):2375–85. [PMID: 19617573]

PRIMARY AMYLOIDOSIS

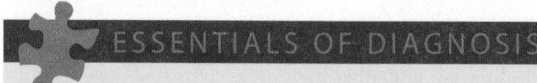

ESSENTIALS OF DIAGNOSIS

- ▶ Congo red positive amyloid protein on tissue biopsy.
- ▶ Amyloid protein is kappa or lambda immunoglobulin light chain.
- ▶ Serum or urine (or both) light chain paraprotein.

▶ General Considerations

Amyloidosis is an uncommon condition whereby a protein abnormally deposits in tissue resulting in organ dysfunction. The propensity of a protein to be amyloidogenic is a consequence of disturbed translational or posttranslational protein folding. The input of amyloid protein into tissues far exceeds its output, so amyloid build up inexorably proceeds to organ dysfunction and ultimately organ failure and premature death.

Amyloidosis is classified according to the type of amyloid protein deposited. The five main categories are **primary** (immunoglobulin light chain [AL]), **secondary** (serum protein A, produced in inflammatory conditions [AA]), **hereditary** (mutated transthyretin [TTR]; others), **senile** (wild-type TTR; atrial natriuretic peptide; others), and **renal failure type** (beta-2-microglobulin, not filtered out by dialysis membranes [Abeta-2M]). Amyloidosis is further classified as **localized** (amyloid deposits only in a single tissue type or organ) or, most common, **systemic** (widespread amyloid deposition).

▶ Clinical Findings

A. Symptoms and Signs

Patients with **localized amyloidosis** have symptoms and signs related to the affected single organ, such as hoarseness (vocal cords) or proptosis and visual disturbance (orbits). Patients with **systemic amyloidosis** have symptoms and signs of unexplained medical syndromes, including heart failure (infiltrative/restrictive cardiomyopathy), nephrotic syndrome, malabsorption and weight loss, hepatic dysfunction, autonomic insufficiency, carpal tunnel syndrome (often bilateral), and sensorimotor peripheral neuropathy. Other symptoms and signs include an enlarged tongue; waxy, rough plaques on skin; contusions (including the periorbital areas); cough or dyspnea; and disturbed deglutition. These symptoms and signs arise insidiously, and the diagnosis of amyloidosis is generally made late in the disease process.

B. Laboratory Findings

The diagnosis of amyloid protein requires a tissue biopsy that demonstrates deposition of a pink substance in the tissue with the H&E stain. This protein stains red with Congo Red and becomes an apple-green color when the light is polarized. Amyloid is a triple-stranded fibril composed of the amyloid protein, amyloid protein P, and glycosaminoglycan. The amyloid fibrils form beta-pleated sheets as demonstrated by electron microscopy. In primary amyloidosis, the amyloid protein is either the kappa or lambda immunoglobulin light chain.

When systemic amyloidosis is suspected, a blind aspiration of the abdominal fat pad will reveal amyloid two-thirds of the time. If the fat pad aspiration is unrevealing, then the affected organ needs biopsy. In 90% of patients with primary amyloidosis, analysis of the serum and urine will reveal a kappa or lambda light chain paraprotein by PEP, IFE, or free light chain assay; in the remainder, mass spectroscopy demonstrates light chain in the tissue biopsy. Lambda amyloid is more common than kappa amyloid, a relative proportion opposite from normal B-cell stoichiometry. Most patients with primary amyloidosis have a small excess of kappa or lambda restricted plasma cells in the bone marrow that may show interstitial amyloid deposition or amyloid in the blood vessels of the marrow.

Patients with primary cardiac amyloidosis have an infiltrative cardiomyopathy with thick ventricular walls on echocardiogram that sometimes shows a unique speckling pattern. Paradoxically, QRS voltages are low on ECG. With renal amyloid, albuminuria is present, which can be in the nephrotic range. Late in renal involvement, kidney function decreases.

Differential Diagnosis

Primary amyloidosis must be distinguished from MGUS and multiple myeloma or other malignant lymphoproliferative disorders. Of note, 12% of patients with MGUS will convert to primary amyloidosis in a median of 9 years. One-fifth of patients who have primary amyloidosis will meet the diagnostic criteria for multiple myeloma; conversely, 5% of patients with multiple myeloma will have amyloid deposition of the paraprotein.

Treatment

The treatment approach to primary amyloidosis closely resembles that of multiple myeloma. Prospective, randomized trials of multiple myeloma chemotherapy versus colchicine have demonstrated a survival benefit to chemotherapy. The concept is reduction of light chain production and a reduction of light chain deposition as a means to arrest progressive end-organ dysfunction. Active agents in primary amyloidosis include melphalan, dexamethasone, lenalidomide, and bortezomib (see Table 39–12). As in multiple myeloma, autologous hematopoietic stem cell transplantation after high-dose melphalan is used in patients with reasonable organ function and a good performance status. The treatment-related mortality, however, is higher in patients with primary amyloidosis than in myeloma (8% vs 1%). Some patients will demonstrate end-organ improvement after therapy. Agents are being developed that facilitate amyloid dissolution or correct protein folding abnormalities in the amyloid protein.

Prognosis

Untreated primary amyloidosis is associated with progressive end-organ failure and premature death. There is no known cure for primary amyloidosis. Although virtually every tissue examined at autopsy will contain amyloid, patients with primary amyloidosis will have one or two primary organs failing that clinically drive the presentation and prognosis. The cardiac biomarkers, B-type natriuretic peptide (BNP) and n-terminal pro-BNP, and troponins T and I are prognostic in this disease regardless of overt clinical cardiac involvement. Historically, patients with predominantly cardiac or autonomic nerve presentations had survivals of 3–9 months, and those with carpal tunnel syndrome or nephrosis, 1.5–3 years, and those with peripheral neuropathy, 5 years. These survivals are roughly doubled with multiple myeloma-like treatment. In those patients able to undergo autologous hematopoietic stem cell transplantation, the median survival now approaches 5 years.

When to Refer

- All patients who have primary amyloidosis or in whom it is suspected should be referred to a hematologist or oncologist.
- All patients with hereditary amyloidosis should be referred to a hepatologist for consideration of liver transplantation.

When to Admit

- Patients with systemic amyloidosis require hospitalization to treat exacerbations of end-organ failure, such as heart failure or liver failure.
- Patients with primary amyloidosis require hospitalization to undergo autologous hematopoietic stem cell transplantation.

Gertz MA. Immunoglobulin light chain amyloidosis: 2013 update on diagnosis, prognosis, and treatment. Am J Hematol. 2013 May;88(5):416–25. [PMID: 23605846]

Kapoor P et al. Cardiac amyloidosis: a practical approach to diagnosis and management. Am J Med. 2011 Nov;124(11):1006–15. [PMID: 22017778]

Sanchorawala V. Role of high-dose melphalan and autologous peripheral blood stem cell transplantation in AL amyloidosis. Am J Blood Res. 2012;2(1):9–17. [PMID: 22432083]

STEM CELL TRANSPLANTATION

Stem cell transplantation using hematopoietic stem cells is an extremely valuable treatment for a variety of hematologic malignancies and is also used in a few non-hematologic cancers and some nonmalignant conditions. In many cases, stem cell transplantation offers the only curative option for some types of cancer and can be a life-saving procedure.

The basis of treatment with stem cell transplantation is the ability of the hematopoietic stem cell to completely restore bone marrow function and formation of all blood components, as well as the ability to re-form the immune system. These hematopoietic stem cells were formerly collected from the bone marrow but are now more commonly collected from the peripheral blood after maneuvers, usually involving the administration of filgrastim (G-CSF) to mobilize them from the bone marrow into the blood.

In the field of cancer chemotherapy, the dose-limiting toxicity of almost all chemotherapy has been myelosuppression from damage to the bone marrow. It is typical during the administration of chemotherapy for blood counts to be transiently suppressed and to have to wait for recovery of the blood in order to safely give the next treatment. However, if too high a dose of chemotherapy is given, it is possible to damage the bone marrow beyond recovery, and for the blood counts to never return to within normal ranges. For cancers for which there is a dose-response relationship, that is, a relationship between the dose of chemotherapy administered and the number of cancer cells killed, the limits placed on the allowable dose of chemotherapy can make the difference between cure and failure to cure. In stem cell transplantation, the limit placed on the allowable dose of chemotherapy by the risks of permanent bone marrow damage is eliminated and much higher doses of chemotherapy can be given, since reinfusion of hematopoietic stem cells can completely restore the bone marrow.

AUTOLOGOUS STEM CELL TRANSPLANTATION

Autologous stem cell transplantation is a treatment in which hematopoietic stem cells are collected from the patient and then re-infused after chemotherapy. Therefore, autologous stem cell transplantation relies solely for its effectiveness on the ability to give much higher doses of chemotherapy than would otherwise be possible. In this procedure, the hematopoietic stem cells are usually collected from the patient's peripheral blood. First, the hematopoietic stem cells are mobilized from the bone marrow into the blood. This can be accomplished by a variety of techniques, most commonly the use of myeloid growth factors such as filgrastim either alone or in combination with chemotherapy. The CXCR4 antagonist plerixafor can help mobilize these cells into the blood. During the process of leukapheresis the patient's blood is centrifuged into layers of different densities; the hematopoietic stem cells are collected from the appropriate layer while the remainder of the blood elements are returned unchanged to the patient. After collection, these autologous hematopoietic stem cells are frozen and cryopreserved for later use. Treatment with autologous stem cell transplantation involves administration of high-dose chemotherapy (referred to as the "preparative regimen") followed, after clearance of the chemotherapy out of the patient's system, by intravenous re-infusion of the thawed autologous hematopoietic stem cells. The hematopoietic stem cells home to the bone marrow and grow into new bone marrow cells.

With the autologous stem cell transplantation treatment, there is a period of severe pancytopenia during the gap between myelosuppression caused by the chemotherapy and the recovery produced from the new bone marrow derived from the infused hematopoietic stem cells. This period of pancytopenia typically lasts 7–10 days and requires support with transfusions of red blood cells and platelets as well as antibiotics. Hospitalization to receive such treatment usually lasts 2–3 weeks. The morbidity of such a treatment varies according to the type of chemotherapy used, and the chance of fatal treatment-related complications is between 1% and 4%.

Autologous stem cell transplantation has the potential to cure cancers that would otherwise be fatal and is the treatment of choice for lymphomas such as diffuse large B-cell lymphomas that have recurred after initial chemotherapy but are still responsive to chemotherapy. It is similarly also the treatment of choice for relapsed Hodgkin lymphoma that still responds to chemotherapy, and for testicular germ cell cancers that have recurred. Based on the aggressive clinical course of peripheral T-cell lymphomas, autologous stem cell transplantation is often used following chemotherapy as front-line therapy. Autologous stem cell transplantation also plays an important role in the treatment of AML in both first and second remission and is potentially curative in these settings. Autologous stem cell transplantation is currently part of the standard of care for the treatment of mantle cell lymphoma and multiple myeloma, based not on curative potential, but the prolongation of remission and overall survival.

ALLOGENEIC STEM CELL TRANSPLANTATION

Allogeneic stem cell transplantation is a treatment in which the source of hematopoietic stem cells to restore bone marrow and immune function are derived, not from the patient, but from a different donor. Initially allogeneic stem cell transplantation was thought to derive its effectiveness from the high-dose chemotherapy (or radiation plus chemotherapy) that forms the "preparative regimen" in a manner similar to autologous stem cell transplantation. However, it is now known that there is a second type of effector mechanism in allogeneic stem cell transplantation, the alloimmune graft-versus-malignancy (GVM) effect derived from the donor immune system. In some cases, this GVM effect can be more important than the chemotherapy in producing a cure of disease. This understanding has led to the development of less myelotoxic preparative regimens, referred to as reduced-intensity or non-myeloablative.

In order to perform an allogeneic stem cell transplantation, an appropriate donor of hematopoietic stem cells must be located. At the present time, it is important that the donor be matched with the patient (recipient) at the HLA loci (HLA A, B, C, DR) that specify major histocompatibility antigens. These donors may be full siblings or unrelated donors recruited from a large panel of anonymous volunteer donors through the National Marrow Donor Program (NMDP). Approaches utilizing haploidentical donors, ie, other children of the parents of the prospective recipient, are increasingly being used, with promising results. Finally, cells derived from umbilical cord blood units may also be used. The hematopoietic stem cells are collected from the donor either from the bone marrow, or, more commonly through leukopheresis of the blood after mobilizing hematopoietic stem cells from the bone marrow with filgrastim (G-CSF). They are infused intravenously into the recipient and may be given either fresh or after cryopreservation and thawing. The hematopoietic stem cells home to the bone marrow and start to grow.

In the allogeneic stem cell transplantation procedure, the patient is treated with the "preparative regimen" with two purposes: to treat the underlying cancer and to sufficiently suppress the patient's immune system so that the hematopoietic stem cells from the donor will not be rejected. As with autologous stem cell transplantation, the hematopoietic stem cells are infused after the preparative chemotherapy has been given and has had a chance to clear from the body. There is a period of pancytopenia in the gap between the effect of the chemotherapy given to the patient and the time it takes the infused hematopoietic stem cells to grow into bone marrow, usually 10–14 days.

A major difference between autologous and allogeneic stem cell transplantation is that in the allogeneic setting, the patient becomes a "chimera," that is, a mixture of self and non-self. In allogeneic stem cell transplantation, the infused cells contain mature cells of the donor immune system, and the infused hematopoietic stem cells will grow into bone marrow and blood cells as well as cells of the new immune system. Unless the donor is an identical twin (called a "syngeneic transplant"), the donor's immune system will recognize the patient's tissues as foreign and initiate the "graft-versus-host" (GVH) reaction, the graft from the donor reacting against the patient (host). This GVH is the major cause of morbidity and mortality during an allogeneic stem cell transplantation. Immunosuppression must be given during allogeneic stem cell transplantation to reduce the incidence and severity of GVH reaction. The most common regimen used for GVH prophylaxis is a combination of cyclosporine or tacrolimus plus methotrexate. In contrast to the experience with solid organ transplant in which life-long immunosuppression is required to prevent rejection of the transplanted organ, in most cases of allogeneic stem cell transplantation, the immunosuppression can be tapered and discontinued 6 or more months after transplantation.

However, there is an important and positive side to the alloimmune reaction of the donor against the host. If there are residual cancer cells present in the patient that have survived the high-dose chemoradiotherapy of the preparative regimen, these residual cancer cells can be recognized as foreign by the donor immune system and killed in the GVM effect. Even cells that are resistant to chemotherapy may not be resistant to killing through the immune system. Depending on the type of cancer cell, this can be a highly effective mechanism of long-term cancer control. Based on the understanding of how important GVM can be, the allogeneic stem cell transplantation procedure can be modified by reducing the intensity of the preparative regimen, relying for cure more on the GVM effect and less on the high-dose chemotherapy. In these "reduced-intensity" allogeneic stem cell transplantation procedures, the preparative regimen still has to suppress the patient's immune system enough to avoid rejection of the donor hematopoietic stem cells, but these types of transplants can be far less toxic than full-dose transplants. Based on this greatly reduced short-term toxicity, the potential benefits of allogeneic stem cell transplantation have been extended to older adults (age 60–75) and to those with comorbid conditions that would have been a contraindication to standard full-dose stem cell transplantation.

Allogeneic stem cell transplantation is the treatment of choice for high-risk acute leukemias, and in many cases will be the only potentially curative treatment. Allogeneic stem cell transplantation is the only curative treatment for myelodysplasia and for CML, although its use in CML has been greatly curtailed based on the effectiveness of imatinib and related tyrosine kinase inhibitors. Allogeneic stem cell transplantation is also the only definitive treatment for most cases of severe aplastic anemia. The use of reduced-intensity allogeneic stem cell transplantation has led to its exploration in the management of difficult cases of CLL and follicular lymphoma, and it will likely play a major role in these diseases. Given the age of many patients with AML and myelodysplasia, this procedure will likely play an important role in these diseases as well.

Deeg HJ et al. Who is fit for allogeneic transplantation? Blood. 2010 Dec 2;116(23):4762–70. [PMID: 20702782]

Jenq RR et al. Allogeneic haematopoietic stem cell transplantation: individualized stem cell and immune therapy of cancer. Nat Rev Cancer. 2010 Mar;10(3):213–21. [PMID: 20168320]

Majhail NS et al; Center for International Blood and Marrow Transplant Research (CIBMTR); American Society for Blood and Marrow Transplantation (ASBMT); European Group for Blood and Marrow Transplantation (EBMT); Asia-Pacific Blood and Marrow Transplantation Group (APBMT); Bone Marrow Transplant Society of Australia and New Zealand (BMTSANZ); East Mediterranean Blood and Marrow Transplantation Group (EMBMT); Sociedade Brasileira de Transplante de Medula Ossea (SBTMO). Recommended screening and preventive practices for long-term survivors after hematopoietic cell transplantation. Hematol Oncol Stem Cell Ther. 2012;5(1):1–30. [PMID: 22446607]

Sorror ML. Comorbidities and hematopoietic cell transplantation outcomes. Hematology Am Soc Hematol Educ Program. 2010;2010:237–47. [PMID: 21239800]

Spellman SR et al; National Marrow Donor Program; Center for International Blood and Marrow Transplant Research. A perspective on the selection of unrelated donors and cord blood units for transplantation. Blood. 2012 Jul 12;120(2):259–65. [PMID: 22596257]

BLOOD TRANSFUSIONS

RED BLOOD CELL TRANSFUSIONS

Red blood cell transfusions are given to raise the hemoglobin and hematocrit levels in patients with anemia or to replace losses after acute bleeding episodes.

▶ Preparations of Red Cells for Transfusion

Several types of preparations containing red blood cells are available.

A. Fresh Whole Blood

The advantage of whole blood for transfusion is the simultaneous presence of red blood cells, plasma, and fresh platelets. Fresh whole blood is never absolutely necessary, since all the above components are available separately. The major indications for use of whole blood are cardiac surgery or massive hemorrhage when more than 10 units of blood is required in a 24-hour period.

B. Packed Red Blood Cells

Packed red cells are the component most commonly used to raise the hematocrit. Each unit has a volume of about 300 mL, of which approximately 200 mL consists of red blood cells. One unit of packed red cells will usually raise the hematocrit by approximately 3–4%. The expected rise in hematocrit can be calculated using an estimated red blood cell volume of 200 mL/unit and a total blood volume of about 70 mL/kg. For example, a 70-kg man will have a total blood volume of 4900 mL, and each unit of packed red blood cells (PRBC) will raise the hematocrit by 200 ÷ 4900, or 4%. Current guidelines recommend a transfusion "trigger" threshold of 7–8 g/dL (70–80 g/L) for hospitalized critically ill patients, those undergoing cardiothoracic surgery or repair of a hip fracture, those with upper gastrointestinal bleeding, and those with hematologic malignancy undergoing chemotherapy.

C. Leukocyte-Poor Blood

Most blood products are leukoreduced in-line during acquisition and are thus prospectively leukocyte-poor. Leukoreduced blood products reduce the incidence of leukoagglutination reactions, platelet alloimmunization, transfusion-related acute lung injury (see below), and CMV exposure.

D. Frozen Packed Red Blood Cells

Packed red blood cells can be frozen and stored for up to 10 years, but the technique is cumbersome and expensive, and should be used sparingly. The major application is for the purpose of maintaining a supply of rare blood types. Patients with such types may donate units for autologous transfusion should the need arise. Frozen red cells are also occasionally needed for patients with severe leukoagglutinin reactions or anaphylactic reactions to plasma proteins, since frozen blood has essentially all white blood cells and plasma components removed.

E. Autologous Packed Red Blood Cells

Patients scheduled for elective surgery may donate blood for autologous transfusion. These units may be stored for up to 35 days before freezing is necessary.

▶ Compatibility Testing

Before transfusion, the recipient's and the donor's blood are typed and cross-matched to avoid hemolytic transfusion reactions. Although many antigen systems are present on red blood cells, only the ABO and Rh systems are specifically tested prior to all transfusions. The A and B antigens are the most important, because everyone who lacks one or both red cell antigens has IgM isoantibodies (called isoagglutinins) in his or her plasma against the missing antigen(s). The isoagglutinins activate complement and can cause rapid intravascular lysis of the incompatible red blood cells. In emergencies, type O/Rh-negative blood can be given to any recipient, but only packed cells should be given to avoid transfusion of donor plasma containing anti-A and anti-B antibodies.

The other important antigen routinely tested for is the D antigen of the Rh system. Approximately 15% of the population lacks this antigen. In patients lacking the antigen, anti-D antibodies are not naturally present, but the antigen is highly immunogenic. A recipient whose red cells lack D and who receives D-positive blood may develop anti-D antibodies that can cause severe lysis of subsequent transfusions of D-positive red cells.

Blood typing includes a crossmatch assay of recipient serum for unusual alloantibodies directed against donor red blood cells by mixing recipient serum with panels of red blood cells representing commonly occurring minor red cell antigens. The screening is particularly important if the recipient has had previous transfusions or pregnancy.

▶ Hemolytic Transfusion Reactions

The most severe hemolytic transfusion reactions are acute (temporally related to the transfusion), involving incompatible mismatches in the ABO system and are isoagglutinin-mediated. Most of these cases are due to clerical errors and mislabeled specimens. With current compatibility testing and double check clerical systems, the risk of an acute hemolytic reaction is 1 in 76,000 transfused units of red blood cells. Death from acute hemolytic reaction occurs in 1 in 1.8 million transfused units. Hemolysis is rapid and intravascular, releasing free hemoglobin into the plasma. The severity of these reactions depends on the dose of red blood cells given. The most severe reactions are those seen in surgical patients under anesthesia.

Delayed hemolytic transfusion reactions are caused by minor red blood cell antigen discrepancies and are typically less severe. The hemolysis usually takes place at a slower rate and is mediated by IgG alloantibodies causing extravascular red blood cell destruction. These transfusion reactions may be delayed for 5–10 days after transfusion. In such cases, the recipient has received red blood cells containing an immunogenic antigen, and in the time since transfusion, a new alloantibody has formed. The most common antigens involved in such reactions are Duffy, Kidd, Kell, and C and E loci of the Rh system. The current risk of a delayed hemolytic transfusion reaction is 1 in 6000 transfused units of red blood cells.

A. Symptoms and Signs

Major acute hemolytic transfusion reactions cause fever and chills, with backache and headache. In severe cases, there may be apprehension, dyspnea, hypotension, and cardiovascular collapse. Patients under general anesthesia will not manifest such symptoms, and the first indication may be tachycardia, generalized bleeding, or oliguria. *The transfusion must be stopped immediately.* In severe cases, acute DIC, acute kidney injury from tubular necrosis, or both can occur. Death occurs in 4% of acute hemolytic reactions due to ABO incompatibility.

Delayed hemolytic transfusion reactions are usually without symptoms or signs.

B. Laboratory Findings

When an acute hemolytic transfusion episode is suspected, the identification of the recipient and of the transfusion product bag label should be rechecked. The transfusion product bag with its pilot tube must be returned to the blood bank, and a fresh sample of the recipient's blood must accompany the bag for retyping and re–cross-matching of donor and recipient blood samples.

The hematocrit will fail to rise by the expected amount. Coagulation studies may reveal evidence of acute kidney injury or acute DIC. The plasma free hemoglobin in the recipient will be elevated resulting in hemoglobinuria.

In cases of delayed hemolytic reactions, the hematocrit will fall and the indirect bilirubin will rise. In these cases, the new offending alloantibody is easily detected in the patient's serum.

C. Treatment

If an acute hemolytic transfusion reaction is suspected, the transfusion should be stopped at once. The patient should be vigorously hydrated to prevent acute tubular necrosis. Forced diuresis with mannitol may help prevent or minimize acute kidney injury.

▶ Leukoagglutinin Reactions

Most transfusion reactions are not hemolytic but represent reactions to antigens present on transfused passenger leukocytes in patients who have been sensitized to leukocyte antigens through previous transfusions or pregnancy. Transfusion products relatively rich in leukocyte-rich plasma, especially platelets, are most likely to cause this. Moderate to severe leukoagglutinin reactions occur in 1% of red blood cell transfusions and 2% of platelet transfusions. Most commonly, fever and chills develop in patients within 12 hours after transfusion. In severe cases, cough and dyspnea may occur and the chest radiograph may show transient pulmonary infiltrates. Because no hemolysis is involved, the hematocrit rises by the expected amount despite the reaction.

Leukoagglutinin reactions may respond to acetaminophen (500–650 mg) and diphenhydramine (25 mg); corticosteroids, such as hydrocortisone (1 mg/kg), are also of value. Overall, leukoagglutination reactions are diminishing through the routine use of in-line leukotrapping during blood donation (ie, leukoreduced blood). Patients experiencing severe leukoagglutination episodes despite receiving leukoreduced blood transfusions should receive leukopoor or washed blood products.

▶ Hypersensitivity Reactions

Urticaria or bronchospasm may develop during or soon after a transfusion. These reactions are almost always due to exposure to allogeneic plasma proteins rather than to leukocytes. The risk is low enough that the routine use of antihistamine premedications has been eliminated before PRBC transfusions. A hypersensitivity reaction, including anaphylactic shock, may develop in patients who are IgA deficient because of antibodies to IgA in the patient's plasma directed against the IgA in the transfused blood product. Patients with such reactions may require transfusion of washed or even frozen red blood cells to avoid future severe reactions.

▶ Contaminated Blood

Blood products can be contaminated with bacteria. Platelets are especially prone to bacterial contamination because they cannot be refrigerated. Bacterial contamination occurs in 1 of every 30,000 red blood cell donations and 1 of every 5000 platelet donations. Receipt of a blood product contaminated with gram-positive bacteria will cause fever and bacteremia but rarely causes a sepsis syndrome. Receipt of a blood product contaminated with gram-negative bacteria often causes septic shock, acute DIC, and acute kidney injury due to the transfused endotoxin and is usually fatal. Strategies to reduce bacterial contamination include enhanced venipuncture site skin cleansing, diverting of the first few milliliters of donated blood, use of single donor blood products (as opposed to pooled donor products), and point of care rapid bacterial screening in order to discard questionable units. The current risk of a septic transfusion reaction from a culture-negative unit of single-donor platelets is 1 in 60,000. In any patient who may have received contaminated blood, the recipient and the donor blood bag should both be cultured, and antibiotics should be given immediately to the recipient.

▶ Infectious Diseases Transmitted Through Transfusion

Despite the use of only volunteer blood donors and the routine screening of blood, transfusion-associated viral diseases remain a problem. All blood products (red blood cells, platelets, plasma, cryoprecipitate) can transmit viral diseases. All blood donors are screened with questionnaires designed to detect (and therefore reject) donors at high risk for transmitting infectious diseases. All blood is screened for hepatitis B surface antigen, antibody to hepatitis B core antigen, syphilis, p24 antigen and antibody to HIV, antibody to hepatitis C virus (HCV), antibody to human T cell lymphotropic/leukemia virus (HTLV), and nucleic acid testing for West Nile virus. Clinical trials are examining the value of screening blood donors for *Trypanosoma cruzi*, the infectious agent that causes Chagas disease.

With improved screening, the risk of posttransfusion hepatitis has steadily decreased after the receipt of screened 'negative' blood products. The risk of acquiring hepatitis B is about 1 in 290,000 transfused units in the United States (versus about 1 in 21,000 to 1 in 600 transfused units in Asia). The risk of hepatitis C acquisition is 1 in 1.5 to 2 million transfused units in the United States. The risk of HIV acquisition is 1 in 2 million transfused units. Unscreened leukoreduced blood products appear to be equivalent to CMV screened-negative blood products in terms of the risk of CMV transmission to a CMV-seronegative recipient.

▶ **Transfusion Graft-Versus-Host Disease**

Allogeneic passenger lymphocytes within transfused blood products will engraft in some recipients and mount an alloimmune attack against tissues expressing discrepant HLA-antigens causing graft-versus-host disease (GVHD). The symptoms and signs of transfusion-associated GVHD include fever, rash, diarrhea, hepatitis, lymphadenopathy, and severe pancytopenia. The outcome is usually fatal. Transfusion-associated GVHD occurs most often in recipients with immune defects, malignant lymphoproliferative disorders, solid tumors being treated with chemotherapy or immunotherapy, treatment with immunosuppressive medications (especially purine analogs such as fludarabine), or older patients undergoing cardiac surgery. HIV infection alone does not seem to increase the risk. The use of leukoreduced blood products is inadequate to prevent transfusion-associated GVHD. This complication can be avoided by irradiating blood products (25 Gy or more) to prevent lymphocyte proliferation in recipients at high risk for transfusion-associated GVHD.

▶ **Transfusion-Related Acute Lung Injury**

Transfusion-related acute lung injury (TRALI) occurs in 1 in every 5000 transfused units of blood products. It has been associated with allogeneic antibodies in the donor plasma component that bind to recipient leukocyte antigens, including HLA antigens and other granulocyte- and monocyte-specific antigens. In 20% of cases, no antileukocyte antibodies are identified raising the concern that bioactive lipids or other substances that accumulate while the blood product is in storage can also mediate TRALI in susceptible recipients. TRALI is clinically defined as non-cardiogenic pulmonary edema after a blood product transfusion without other explanation, and transfused surgical and critically ill patients seem most susceptible. Ten to 20% of female blood donors and 1–5% of male blood donors have antileukocyte antibodies in their serum. The risk of TRALI is reduced through the use of male only plasma donors, when possible. There is no specific treatment for TRALI, only supportive care.

PLATELET TRANSFUSIONS

Platelet transfusions are indicated in cases of thrombocytopenia due to decreased platelet production. They are of some use in immune thrombocytopenia when active bleeding is evident, but the clearance of transfused platelets is rapid as they are exposed to the same pathophysiologic forces as the recipient's endogenous platelets. The risk of spontaneous bleeding rises when the platelet count falls to < 80,000/mcL (< 80 × 10^9/L), and the risk of life-threatening spontaneous bleeding increases when the platelet count is < 5000/mcL (< 5 × 10^9/L). Because of this, prophylactic platelet transfusions are often given at these very low levels, usually when < 10,000/mcL (< 10 × 10^9/L). Platelet transfusions are also given prior to invasive procedures or surgery in thrombocytopenic patients, and the goal is often to raise the platelet count to 50,000/mcL (50 × 10^9/L) or more.

Platelets for transfusion are most commonly derived from single donor apheresis collections (roughly the equivalent to the platelets recovered from six donations of whole blood). A single donor unit of platelets should raise the platelet count by 50,000 to 60,000 platelets per mcL (50–60 × 10^9/L) in a transfusion-naïve recipient without hypersplenism or ongoing platelet consumptive disorder. Transfused platelets typically last for 2 or 3 days. Platelet transfusion responses may be suboptimal with poor platelet increments and short platelet survival times. This may be due to one of several causes, including fever, sepsis, splenomegaly, DIC, large body habitus, low platelet dose in the transfusion, or platelet alloimmunization (from prior transfusions, prior pregnancy or prior organ transplantation). Many, but not all, alloantibodies causing platelet destruction are directed at HLA antigens. Patients requiring long periods of platelet transfusion support should be monitored to document adequate responses to transfusions so that the most appropriate product can be used. Patients requiring ongoing platelet transfusions who become alloimmunized may benefit from HLA-matched platelets derived from either volunteer donors or family members. Techniques of cross-matching platelets have been developed and appear to identify suitable volunteer platelet donors (nonreactive with the patient's serum) without the need for HLA typing. Leukocyte reduction of platelets has been shown to delay or prevent the onset of alloimmunization in multiply transfused recipients.

TRANSFUSION OF PLASMA COMPONENTS

Fresh-frozen plasma (FFP) is available in units of approximately 200 mL. FFP contains normal levels of all coagulation factors (about 1 unit/mL of each factor). FFP is used to correct coagulation factor deficiencies and to treat thrombotic thrombocytopenia purpura or hemolytic-uremic syndrome. FFP is also used to correct or prevent coagulopathy in trauma patients receiving massive transfusion of PRBC. A FFP:PRBC ratio of ≥ 1:2 is associated with improved survival in trauma patients receiving massive transfusions, regardless of the presence of a coagulopathy.

Cryoprecipitate is made from fresh plasma by cooling the plasma to 4°C and collecting the precipitate. One unit of cryoprecipitate has a volume of approximately 15–20 mL and contains approximately 250 mg of fibrinogen and between 80 and 100 units of factor VIII and von Willebrand factor. Cryoprecipitate is used to supplement fibrinogen in cases of acquired hypofibrinogenemia (eg, DIC) or in rare instances of congenital hypofibrinogenemia.

One unit of cryoprecipitate will raise the fibrinogen level by about 8 mg/dL (0.24 mcmol/L). Cryoprecipitate is sometimes used to temporarily correct the acquired platelet dysfunction associated with kidney disease.

Allain JP et al; ISBT HBV Safety Collaborative Group. Hepatitis B virus in transfusion medicine: still a problem? Biologicals. 2012 May;40(3):180–6. [PMID: 22305086]

Brown LM et al. A high fresh frozen plasma: packed red blood cell transfusion ratio decreases mortality in all massively transfused trauma patients regardless of admission international normalized ratio. J Trauma. 2011 Aug;71(2 Suppl 3):S358–63. [PMID: 21814104]

Carson JL et al; Clinical Transfusion Medicine Committee of the AABB. Red blood cell transfusion: a clinical practice guideline from the AABB. Ann Intern Med. 2012 Jul 3;157(1): 49–58. [PMID: 22751760]

Goodnough LT et al. Concepts of blood transfusion in adults. Lancet. 2013 May 25;381(9880):1845–54. [PMID: 23706801]

Sharma S et al. Transfusion of blood and blood products: indications and complications. Am Fam Physician. 2011 Mar 15;83(6):719–24. [PMID: 21404983]

Slichter SJ et al. Dose of prophylactic platelet transfusions and prevention of hemorrhage. N Engl J Med. 2010 Feb 18;362(7):600–13. [PMID: 20164484]

Stanworth SJ et al; TOPPS Investigators. A no-prophylaxis platelet-transfusion strategy for hematologic cancers. N Engl J Med. 2013 May 9;368(19):1771–80. [PMID: 23656642]

Strauss RG. Role of granulocyte/neutrophil transfusions for haematology/oncology patients in the modern era. Br J Haematol. 2012 Aug;158(3):299–306. [PMID: 22712550]

Thiagarajan P et al. Platelet transfusion therapy. Hematol Oncol Clin North Am. 2013 Jun;27(3):629–43. [PMID: 23714315]

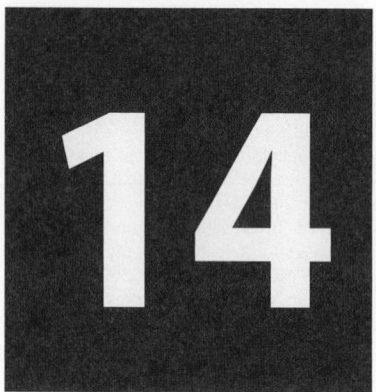

Disorders of Hemostasis, Thrombosis, & Antithrombotic Therapy

Patrick F. Fogarty, MD

Tracy Minichiello, MD

In assessing patients for defects of hemostasis, the clinical context must be considered carefully (Table 14–1). Heritable defects are suggested by bleeding that begins in infancy or childhood, is recurrent, and occurs at multiple anatomic sites, although many other patterns of presentation are possible. Acquired disorders of hemostasis more typically are associated with bleeding that begins later in life and may be relatable to introduction of medications (eg, agents that affect platelet activity) or to onset of underlying medical conditions (such as renal failure or myelodysplasia), or may be idiopathic. Importantly, however, a sufficient hemostatic challenge (such as major trauma) may produce excessive bleeding even in individuals with completely normal hemostasis.

Fogarty PF et al.Disorders of Hemostasis I: Coagulation. In: Rodgers GP et al (editors). *The Bethesda Handbook of Clinical Hematology*, 3rd ed. Philadelphia: Lippincott Williams and Wilkins, 2013.

PLATELET DISORDERS

THROMBOCYTOPENIA

The causes of thrombocytopenia are shown in Table 14–2. The age of the patient and presence of any comorbid conditions may help direct the diagnostic work-up.

The risk of spontaneous bleeding (including petechial hemorrhage and bruising) does not typically increase appreciably until the platelet count falls below 10,000–20,000/mcL, although patients with dysfunctional platelets may bleed with higher platelet counts. Suggested platelet counts to prevent spontaneous bleeding or to provide adequate hemostasis around the time of invasive procedures are found in Table 14–3.

DECREASED PLATELET PRODUCTION

1. Bone Marrow Failure

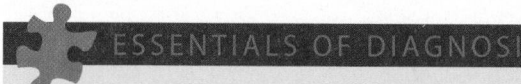

ESSENTIALS OF DIAGNOSIS

- ▶ Bone marrow failure states may be congenital or acquired.
- ▶ Most congenital marrow failure disorders present in childhood.

▶ General Considerations

Congenital conditions that cause thrombocytopenia include amegakaryocytic thrombocytopenia, the thrombocytopenia-absent radius (TAR) syndrome, and Wiskott-Aldrich syndrome; these disorders usually feature isolated thrombocytopenia, whereas patients with Fanconi anemia and dyskeratosis congenita typically have depressions in other blood cell counts as well.

Acquired causes of bone marrow failure leading to thrombocytopenia include acquired aplastic anemia, myelodysplastic syndrome (MDS), and acquired amegakaryocytic thrombocytopenia. Unlike aplastic anemia, MDS is more common among older patients.

▶ Clinical Findings

Acquired aplastic anemia typically presents with reductions in multiple blood cell lines; a bone marrow biopsy reveals hypocellularity. **Myelodysplasia** may also present as cytopenias with variable marrow cellularity, at times mimicking aplastic anemia; however, the presence of macrocytosis, ringed sideroblasts on iron staining of the bone marrow aspirate, dysplasia of hematopoietic elements, or

Table 14–1. Evaluation of the bleeding patient.

Necessary Component of Evaluation	Diagnostic Correlate
Location	
Mucocutaneous (bruises, petechiae, gingivae, nosebleeds)	Likely qualitative/quantitative platelet defects
Joints, soft tissue	Likely disorders of coagulation factors
Onset	
Infancy/childhood	Suggests heritable condition
Adulthood	Suggests milder heritable condition or acquired defect of hemostasis (eg, ITP, medication-related)
Clinical context	
Postsurgical	Anatomic/surgical defect must be ruled out
Pregnancy	vWD, HELLP syndrome, ITP, acquired factor VIII inhibitor
Sepsis	May indicate DIC
Exposure to anticoagulants	Rule out excessive anticoagulation
Personal history[1]	
Absent	Suggests acquired rather than congenital defect, or anatomic/surgical defect (if applicable)
Present	Suggests established acquired defect or congenital disorder
Family history	
Absent	Suggests acquired defect or no defect of hemostasis
Present	May signify hemophilia A or B, vWD, other heritable bleeding disorders

[1]Includes evaluation of prior spontaneous bleeding, as well as excessive bleeding with circumcision, menses, dental extractions, trauma, minor procedures (eg, endoscopy, biopsies), and major procedures (surgery).
DIC, disseminated intravascular coagulation; HELLP, hemolysis, elevated liver enzymes, low platelets; ITP, immune thrombocytopenia; vWD, von Willebrand disease.

cytogenetic abnormalities (especially monosomy 5 or 7, and trisomy 8) are more suggestive of MDS.

▶ Differential Diagnosis

Adult patients with acquired amegakaryocytic thrombocytopenia have isolated thrombocytopenia and reduced or absent megakaryocytes in the bone marrow, which (along with failure to respond to immunomodulatory regimens typically administered in immune thrombocytopenia [ITP]) distinguishes them from patients with ITP.

Table 14–2. Causes of thrombocytopenia.

Decreased production of platelets
  Congenital bone marrow failure (eg, Fanconi anemia, Wiskott-Aldrich syndrome)
  Acquired bone marrow failure (eg, aplastic anemia, myelodysplasia)
  Exposure to chemotherapy, irradiation
  Marrow infiltration (neoplastic, infectious)
  Nutritional (deficiency of vitamin B_{12}, folate, iron; alcohol)
Increased destruction of platelets
  Immune thrombocytopenia (including hepatitis C virus- and HIV-related,[1] and drug-induced)
  Heparin-induced thrombocytopenia
  Thrombotic microangiopathy
  Disseminated intravascular coagulation
  Posttransfusion purpura
  Neonatal alloimmune thrombocytopenia
  Mechanical (aortic valvular dysfunction; extracorporeal bypass)
  von Willebrand disease, type 2B
  Hemophagocytosis
Increased sequestration of platelets
  Hypersplenism (eg, related to cirrhosis, myeloproliferative disorders, lymphoma)
Other conditions causing thrombocytopenia
  Gestational thrombocytopenia
  Bernard-Soulier syndrome, gray platelet syndrome, May-Hegglin anomaly
  Pseudothrombocytopenia

▶ Treatment

A. Congenital Conditions

Treatment is varied but may include blood product support, blood cell growth factors, androgens, and (some cases) allogeneic hematopoietic progenitor cell transplantation.

B. Acquired Conditions

Patients with severe aplastic anemia are treated with allogeneic hematopoietic progenitor cell transplantation, which

Table 14–3. Desired platelet count ranges.

Clinical Scenario	Platelet count (/mcL)
Prevention of spontaneous mucocutaneous bleeding	> 10,000–20,000
Insertion of central venous catheters	> 20,000–50,000[1]
Administration of therapeutic anticoagulation	> 30,000–50,000
Minor surgery and selected invasive procedures[2]	> 50,000–80,000
Major surgery	> 80,000–100,000

[1]A platelet target within the higher range of the reference is required for tunneled catheters.
[2]Such as endoscopy with biopsy.

is the preferred therapy for patients younger than age 40 who have an HLA-matched sibling donor (see Chapter 13), or with immunosuppression, which is the preferred therapy for older patients and those who lack an HLA-matched sibling donor. The thrombopoietin receptor agonist eltrombopag has been shown to induce multilineage responses in selected patients with refractory severe aplastic anemia.

Treatment of thrombocytopenia due to MDS, if clinically significant bleeding is present or if the risk of bleeding is high, is limited to chronic transfusion of platelets in most instances (Table 14–3). Newer immunomodulatory agents such as lenalidomide do not produce increases in the platelet count in most patients. Use of the thrombopoietin receptor agonists, eltrombopag and romiplostim, in patients with MDS is being evaluated in clinical trials.

Akhtari M. When to treat myelodysplastic syndromes. Oncology (Williston Park). 2011 May;25(6):480–6. [PMID: 21717901]
Kantarjian H et al. Safety and efficacy of romiplostim in patients with lower-risk myelodysplastic syndrome and thrombocytopenia. J Clin Oncol. 2010 Jan 20;28(3):437–44. [PMID: 20008626]
Marsh JC et al. Management of the refractory aplastic anemia patient: what are the options? Blood. 2013 Nov 21;122(22): 3561–7. [PMID: 24052548]
Olnes MJ et al. Eltrombopag and improved hematopoiesis in refractory aplastic anemia. N Engl J Med. 2012 Jul 5;367(1):11–9. Erratum in: N Engl J Med. 2012 Jul 19;367(3):284. [PMID: 22762314]

2. Bone Marrow Infiltration

Replacement of the normal bone marrow elements by leukemic cells, myeloma, lymphoma, or other tumors or by infections (such as mycobacterial disease or ehrlichiosis) may cause thrombocytopenia; however, abnormalities in other blood cell lines are also usually present. These entities are easily diagnosed after examining the bone marrow biopsy and aspirate or determining the infecting organism from an aspirate specimen. Treatment of thrombocytopenia is directed at eradication of the underlying infiltrative disorder, but platelet transfusion may be required if clinically significant bleeding is present.

3. Chemotherapy & Irradiation

Chemotherapeutic agents and irradiation may lead to thrombocytopenia by direct toxicity to megakaryocytes, hematopoietic progenitor cells, or both. The severity and duration of chemotherapy-induced depressions in the platelet count are determined by the specific regimen used, although the platelet count typically resolves more slowly following a chemotherapeutic insult than does neutropenia or anemia, especially if multiple cycles of treatment have been given. Until recovery occurs, patients may be supported with transfused platelets if bleeding is present or the risk of bleeding is high (Table 14–3). Clinical trials to determine the role of the platelet growth factors eltrombopag and romiplostim in the treatment of chemotherapy-induced thrombocytopenia have not shown clinically significant responses in the majority of treated patients.

4. Nutritional Deficiencies

Thrombocytopenia, typically in concert with anemia, may be observed when a deficiency of folate (that may accompany alcoholism) or vitamin B_{12} is present (concomitant neurologic findings are common). In addition, thrombocytopenia rarely can occur in very severe iron deficiency. Replacing the deficient vitamin or mineral results in improvement in the platelet count.

Masoodi I et al. Hemorrhagic manifestation of megaloblastic anemia: report of two cases and literature review. Blood Coagul Fibrinolysis. 2011 Apr;22(3):234–5. [PMID: 21297452]

5. Cyclic Thrombocytopenia

Cyclic thrombocytopenia is a very rare disorder that produces cyclic oscillations of the platelet count, usually with a periodicity of 3–6 weeks. The exact pathophysiologic mechanisms responsible for the condition may vary from patient to patient. Severe thrombocytopenia and bleeding typically occur at the platelet nadir. Oral contraceptive medications, androgens, azathioprine, and thrombopoietic growth factors have been used successfully in the management of cyclic thrombocytopenia.

INCREASED PLATELET DESTRUCTION

1. Immune Thrombocytopenia

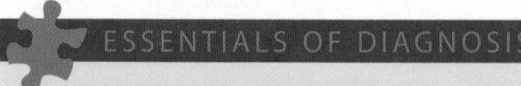

ESSENTIALS OF DIAGNOSIS

► Isolated thrombocytopenia.
► Assess for any new causative medications and HIV and hepatitis C infections.
► ITP is a diagnosis of exclusion.

► **General Considerations**

ITP is an autoimmune condition in which pathogenic antibodies bind platelets, resulting in accelerated platelet clearance. Contrary to the historical view of the disorder, it is now recognized that many patients with ITP also lack appropriate compensatory platelet production. The disorder is primary and idiopathic in most adult patients, although it can be associated with connective tissue disease (such as lupus), lymphoproliferative disease (such as lymphoma), medications (see below), and infections (such as hepatitis C virus and HIV infections). Targets of antiplatelet antibodies include glycoproteins IIb/IIIa and Ib/IX on the platelet membrane, although antibodies are demonstrable in only two-thirds of patients. In addition to production of antiplatelet antibodies, HIV and hepatitis C virus may lead to thrombocytopenia through additional mechanisms (for instance, by direct suppression of platelet production [HIV] and cirrhosis-related splenomegaly [hepatitis C virus]).

Clinical Findings

A. Symptoms and Signs

Mucocutaneous bleeding manifestations may be present, depending on the platelet count. Spontaneous bruising, nosebleeds, gingival bleeding, or other types of hemorrhage generally do not occur until the platelet count has fallen below 20,000–30,000/mcL. Individuals with secondary ITP (such as due to collagen vascular disease, HIV or HCV infection, or lymphoproliferative malignancy) may have additional disease-specific findings.

B. Laboratory Findings

Typically, patients have isolated thrombocytopenia. If bleeding has occurred, anemia may also be present. Hepatitis B and C viruses and HIV infections should be excluded by serologic testing. Bone marrow should be examined in patients with unexplained cytopenias, in patients older than 60 years, or in those who did not respond to primary ITP-specific therapy. Megakaryocyte abnormalities and hypocellularity or hypercellularity are not characteristic of ITP. If there are clinical findings suggestive of a lymphoproliferative malignancy, a CT scan should be performed. In the absence of such findings, otherwise asymptomatic patients with unexplained isolated thrombocytopenia of recent onset may be considered to have ITP.

Treatment

Only individuals with platelet counts < 20,000–30,000/mcL or those with significant bleeding should be treated; the remainder may be monitored serially for progression. The mainstay of initial treatment of new-onset primary ITP is a short course of corticosteroids with or without intravenous immunoglobulin (IVIG) or anti-D (WinRho) (Figure 14–1). Responses are generally seen within 3–5 days of initiating treatment. Platelet transfusions may be given concomitantly if active bleeding is present. The addition of the monoclonal anti-B cell antibody rituximab to corticosteroids as first-line treatment may improve the initial response rate, but is associated with increased toxicity and is not regarded as standard in most centers.

Although over two-thirds of patients with ITP respond to initial treatment, most relapse following reduction of the corticosteroid dose. Patients with a persistent platelet count < 30,000/mcL or clinically significant bleeding are appropriate candidates for second-line treatments (Figure 14–1). These treatments are chosen empirically, bearing in mind

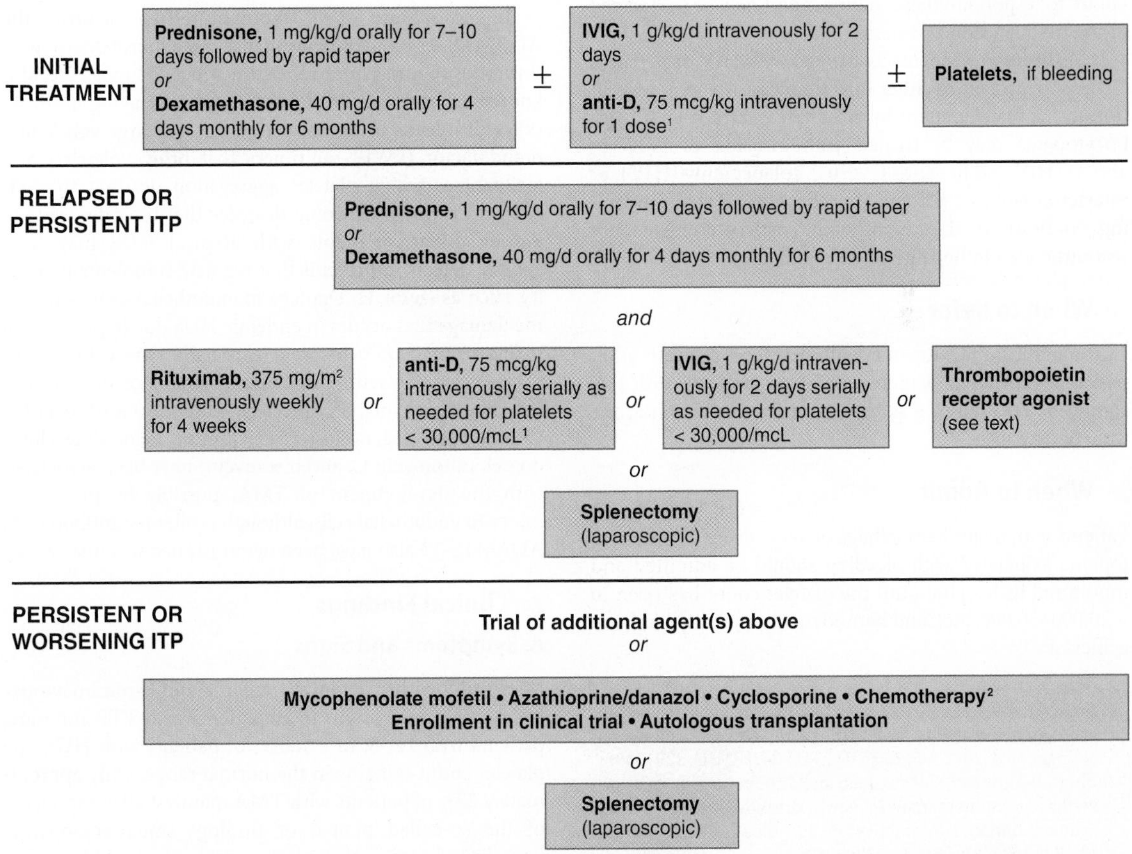

| INITIAL TREATMENT | Prednisone, 1 mg/kg/d orally for 7–10 days followed by rapid taper *or* Dexamethasone, 40 mg/d orally for 4 days monthly for 6 months | ± | IVIG, 1 g/kg/d intravenously for 2 days *or* anti-D, 75 mcg/kg intravenously for 1 dose[1] | ± | Platelets, if bleeding |

RELAPSED OR PERSISTENT ITP

Prednisone, 1 mg/kg/d orally for 7–10 days followed by rapid taper
or
Dexamethasone, 40 mg/d orally for 4 days monthly for 6 months

and

| Rituximab, 375 mg/m² intravenously weekly for 4 weeks | *or* | anti-D, 75 mcg/kg intravenously serially as needed for platelets < 30,000/mcL[1] | *or* | IVIG, 1 g/kg/d intravenously for 2 days serially as needed for platelets < 30,000/mcL | *or* | Thrombopoietin receptor agonist (see text) |

or

Splenectomy (laparoscopic)

PERSISTENT OR WORSENING ITP

Trial of additional agent(s) above
or

Mycophenolate mofetil • Azathioprine/danazol • Cyclosporine • Chemotherapy[2]
Enrollment in clinical trial • Autologous transplantation

or

Splenectomy (laparoscopic)

[1] Use in nonsplenectomized, Rh blood type-positive, nonanemic patients only.
[2] Both lymphoma-type chemotherapy and single-agent vincristine have been used successfully in refractory cases of ITP.

▲ **Figure 14–1.** Management of immune thrombocytopenia (ITP).

potential toxicities and the patient's preference. Anti-D (WinRho) or IVIG temporarily increases platelet counts (duration, 3 weeks or longer), although serial anti-D treatment (platelet counts < 30,000/mcL) may allow adult patients to delay or avoid splenectomy. Rituximab leads to clinical responses in about 50% of adults with corticosteroid-refractory chronic ITP, which decrease to about 20% at 5 years. Romiplostim (administered subcutaneously weekly) and eltrombopag (taken orally daily) are approved for use in adult patients with chronic ITP who have not responded durably to corticosteroids, IVIG, or splenectomy and must be taken indefinitely to maintain the platelet response. Splenectomy has a durable response rate of over 65% and may be considered for cases of severe thrombocytopenia that fail to respond durably to initial treatment or are refractory to second-line agents; patients should receive pneumococcal, *Haemophilus influenzae* type b, and meningococcal vaccination at least 2 weeks before the procedure. If available, laparoscopic splenectomy is preferred. Additional treatments for ITP are found in Figure 14–1.

The goals of management of pregnancy-associated ITP are a platelet count of 10,000–30,000/mcL in the first trimester, > 30,000/mcL during the second or third trimester, and > 50,000/mcL prior to cesarean section or vaginal delivery. Moderate-dose oral prednisone or intermittent infusions of IVIG are standard. Splenectomy is reserved for failure to respond to these therapies and may be performed in the first or second trimester.

For thrombocytopenia associated with HIV or hepatitis C virus, treatment of either infection leads to an amelioration in the platelet count in most cases; refractory thrombocytopenia may be treated with infusion of IVIG or anti-D (HIV and hepatitis C virus), splenectomy (HIV), or interferon-alpha or eltrombopag (hepatitis C virus, including eradication). Treatment with corticosteroids is not recommended in hepatitis C virus infection.

When to Refer

Chronic thrombocytopenia will develop in most adult patients with newly diagnosed ITP. All patients with ITP should be referred to a subspecialist for evaluation at the time of diagnosis.

When to Admit

Patients with major hemorrhage or very severe thrombocytopenia associated with bleeding should be admitted and monitored in-hospital until the platelet count has risen to > 20,000–30,000/mcL and hemodynamic stability has been achieved.

Afdhal NH et al; ELEVATE Study Group. Eltrombopag before procedures in patients with cirrhosis and thrombocytopenia. N Engl J Med. 2012 Aug 23;367(8):716–24. [PMID: 22913681]

Gudbrandsdottir S et al. Rituximab and dexamethasone vs dexamethasone monotherapy in newly diagnosed patients with primary immune thrombocytopenia. Blood. 2013 Mar 14;121(11):1976–81. [PMID: 23293082]

Provan D et al. International consensus report on the investigation and management of primary immune thrombocytopenia. Blood. 2010 Jan 14;115(2):168–86. [PMID: 19846889]

2. Thrombotic Microangiopathy

ESSENTIALS OF DIAGNOSIS

▶ Microangiopathic hemolytic anemia and thrombocytopenia, in the absence of another plausible explanation, are sufficient for the diagnosis of TMA.

▶ Fever, neurologic abnormalities, and kidney disease may occur concurrently but are not required for diagnosis.

▶ Kidney disease occurs in hemolytic-uremic syndrome.

▶ General Considerations

The thrombotic microangiopathies (TMAs) include thrombotic thrombocytopenic purpura (TTP) and the hemolytic-uremic syndrome (HUS). These disorders are characterized by thrombocytopenia, due to the incorporation of platelets into thrombi in the microvasculature, and microangiopathic hemolytic anemia, which results from shearing of erythrocytes in the microcirculation.

In idiopathic TTP, autoantibodies against the ADAMTS-13 (a disintegrin and metalloproteinase with thrombospondin type 1 repeat, member 13) molecule, also known as the von Willebrand factor cleaving protease (vWFCP), leads to accumulation of ultra-large von Willebrand factor (vWF) multimers that bridge platelets and facilitate excessive platelet aggregation, leading to TTP. Atypical HUS is a chronic disorder that typically leads to kidney disease. Patients with atypical HUS may have genetic defects in proteins that regulate complement activity, such as factor H. Damage to endothelial cells—such as the damage that occurs in endemic HUS due to presence of toxins from *Escherichia coli* (especially type O157:H7 or O145) or in the setting of cancer, hematopoietic stem cell transplantation, or HIV infection—may also lead to TMA. Certain drugs (eg, cyclosporine, quinine, ticlopidine, clopidogrel, mitomycin C, and bleomycin) have been associated with the development of TMA, possibly by promoting injury to endothelial cells, although inhibitory antibodies to ADAMTS-13 also have been demonstrated in some cases.

▶ Clinical Findings

A. Symptoms and Signs

Microangiopathic hemolytic anemia and thrombocytopenia are presenting signs in all patients with TTP and most patients with HUS; in a subset of patients with HUS, the platelet count remains in the normal range. Only approximately 25% of patients with TMA manifest all components of the so-called pentad of findings (microangiopathic hemolytic anemia, thrombocytopenia, fever, kidney disease, and neurologic system abnormalities) (Table 14–4). Most patients (especially children) with HUS have a recent or current diarrheal illness. Neurologic manifestations,

Table 14–4. Presentation and management of thrombotic microangiopathies.

	TTP	Atypical HUS	Endemic HUS
Patient population	Adult patients	Children (occasionally adults)	Usually children, often following bloody diarrhea
Pathogenesis	Acquired auto-antibody to ADAMTS-13	Some cases: heritable deficiency in function of in complement regulatory proteins	Bacterial (such as enterotoxogenic *Escherichia coli; Shiga* toxin)
Thrombocytopenia	Typically severe, except in very early clinical course	Variable	May be mild/absent in a minority of patients
Fever	Typical	Variable	Atypical
Renal insufficiency	Typical, but may be mild	Typical	Typical
Neurologic impairment	Variable	Less than half of cases	Less than half of cases
Laboratory investigation	Decreased activity of ADAMTS-13; inhibitor usually identified	Defects in complement regulatory proteins	Typically normal ADAMTS-13 activity Positive stool culture for *E coli* 0157:H7 or detectable antibody to *Shiga* toxin
Management	TPE Hemodialysis for severe renal impairment Platelet transfusions contraindicated unless TPE underway	Immediate TPE in most cases Supportive care Hemodialysis for severe renal impairment Eculizumab (selected cases)	Hemodialysis for severe renal impairment Supportive care TPE rarely beneficial (exception: selected cases in adults)

ADAMTS-13, a disintegrin and metalloproteinase with a thrombospondin type 1 motif, member 13; HUS, hemolytic-uremic syndrome; TPE, therapeutic plasma exchange; TTP, thrombotic thrombocytopenic purpura.

including headache, somnolence, delirium, seizures, paresis, and coma, may result from deposition of microthrombi in the cerebral vasculature. Atypical HUS typically presents in childhood.

B. Laboratory Findings

Laboratory features of TMA include those associated with microangiopathic hemolytic anemia (anemia, elevated lactate dehydrogenase [LD], elevated indirect bilirubin, decreased haptoglobin, reticulocytosis, negative direct antiglobulin test, and schistocytes on the blood smear); thrombocytopenia; elevated creatinine; positive stool culture for *E coli* O157:H7 or stool assays for Shiga-toxin producing *E coli* to detect non-O157:H7 such as *E coli* O145 (HUS only); reductions in vWFCP activity (idiopathic TTP); and mutations of genes encoding complement proteins (atypical HUS; specialized laboratory assessment). Notably, routine coagulation studies are within the normal range in most patients with TMA.

▶ Treatment

Immediate administration of plasma exchange is essential in most cases due to the mortality rate of > 95% without treatment. With the exception of children or adults with endemic diarrhea-associated HUS, who generally recover with supportive care only, plasma exchange must be initiated as soon as the diagnosis of TMA is suspected. Plasma exchange usually is administered once daily until the platelet count and LD have returned to normal for at least 2 days, after which the frequency of treatments may be tapered slowly while the platelet count and LD are monitored for relapse. In cases of insufficient response to once-daily plasma exchange, twice-daily treatments should be given. Fresh frozen plasma (FFP) may be administered if immediate access to plasma exchange is not available or in cases of familial TMA. *Platelet transfusions are contraindicated* in the treatment of TMAs due to reports of worsening TMA, possibly due to propagation of platelet-rich microthrombi. In cases of documented life-threatening bleeding, however, platelet transfusions may be given slowly and after plasma exchange is underway. Red blood cell transfusions may be administered in cases of clinically significant anemia. Hemodialysis should be considered for patients with significant renal impairment.

In cases of relapse following initial treatment, plasma exchange should be reinstituted. If ineffective, or in cases of primary refractoriness, second-line treatments may be considered including rituximab, corticosteroids, IVIG, vincristine, cyclophosphamide, and splenectomy.

Cases of atypical HUS may respond to plasma infusion initially, and serial infusions of the anti-complement C5 antibody eculizumab have produced sustained remissions in some patients. If irreversible renal impairment has occurred, hemodialysis or renal transplantation may be necessary.

▶ When to Refer

Consultation by a hematologist or transfusion medicine specialist familiar with plasma exchange is required at the time of presentation. Patients with refractory or relapsing TMA require ongoing care by a subspecialist.

When to Admit

All patients with newly suspected or diagnosed TMA should be hospitalized initially.

Caramazza D et al. Relapsing or refractory idiopathic thrombotic thrombocytopenic purpura-hemolytic uremic syndrome: the role of rituximab. Transfusion. 2010 Dec;50(12):2753–60. [PMID: 20576013]

Deford CC et al. Multiple major morbidities and increased mortality during long-term follow-up after recovery from thrombotic thrombocytopenic purpura. Blood. 2013 Sep 19;122(12):2023–9. [PMID: 23838348]

Legendre CM et al. Terminal complement inhibitor eculizumab in atypical hemolytic-uremic syndrome. N Engl J Med. 2013 Jun 6;368(23):2169–81. [PMID: 23738544]

3. Heparin-Induced Thrombocytopenia

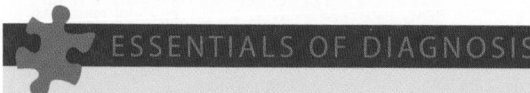

ESSENTIALS OF DIAGNOSIS

▶ Thrombocytopenia within 5–10 days of exposure to heparin.

▶ Decline in baseline platelet count of 50% or greater.

▶ Thrombosis occurs in 50% of cases; bleeding is uncommon.

General Considerations

Heparin-induced thrombocytopenia (HIT) is an acquired disorder that affects approximately 3% of patients who are exposed to unfractionated heparin and 0.6% of patients who are exposed to low-molecular-weight heparin (LMWH). The condition results from formation of IgG antibodies to heparin-platelet factor 4 (PF4) complexes; the antibodies then bind platelets, which activates them. Platelet activation leads to both thrombocytopenia and a prothrombotic state.

Clinical Findings

A. Symptoms and Signs

Patients are usually asymptomatic, and due to the prothrombotic nature of HIT, bleeding usually does not occur. Thrombosis (at any venous or arterial site), however, may be detected in up to 50% of patients, up to 30 days post-diagnosis.

B. Laboratory Findings

A presumptive diagnosis of HIT is made when new-onset thrombocytopenia is detected in a patient (frequently a hospitalized patient) within 5–10 days of exposure to heparin; other presentations (eg, rapid-onset HIT) are less common. A decline of ≥ 50% or more from the baseline platelet count is typical. The 4T score (http://www.qxmd.com/calculate-online/hematology/hit-heparin-induced-thrombocytopenia-probability) is a clinical prediction rule that may assist in assessment of pretest probability for HIT, although low scores have been shown to be more predictive than intermediate or high scores. Confirmation of the diagnosis is through a positive PF4-heparin antibody enzyme-linked immunosorbent assay (ELISA) or functional assay (such as serotonin release assay), or both. The magnitude of a positive ELISA result correlates with the clinical probability of HIT.

Treatment

Treatment should be initiated as soon as the diagnosis of HIT is suspected, before results of laboratory testing is available.

Management of HIT (Table 14–5) involves the immediate discontinuation of all forms of heparin.

If thrombosis has not already been detected, duplex Doppler ultrasound of the lower extremities should be performed to rule out subclinical deep venous thrombosis. Despite thrombocytopenia, platelet transfusions are rarely necessary. Due to the substantial frequency of thrombosis among HIT patients, an alternative anticoagulant, typically a direct thrombin inhibitor (DTI) such as argatroban should be administered immediately. The DTI should be continued until the platelet count has recovered to at least 100,000/mcL, at which point treatment with a vitamin K

Table 14–5. Management of suspected or proven HIT.

I. Discontinue all forms of heparin. Send PF4-heparin ELISA (if indicated).

| II. Begin treatment with direct thrombin inhibitor. |

Agent	Indication	Dosing
Argatroban	Prophylaxis or treatment of HIT	Continuous intravenous infusion of 0.5–1.2 mcg/kg/min, titrate to aPTT = 1.5 to 3 × the baseline value.[1] Max infusion rate ≤ 10 mcg/kg/min.
Bivalirudin	Percutaneous coronary intervention[2]	Bolus of 0.75 mg/kg intravenously followed by initial continuous intravenous infusion of 1.75 mg/kg/h. Manufacturer indicates monitoring should be by ACT.

III. Perform Doppler ultrasound of lower extremities to rule out subclinical thrombosis (if indicated).
IV. Follow platelet counts daily until recovery occurs.
V. When platelet count has recovered, transition anticoagulation to warfarin; treat for 30 days (HIT) or 3–6 months (HITT).
VI. Document heparin allergy in medical record (confirmed cases).

[1]Hepatic insufficiency: initial infusion rate = 0.5 mcg/kg/min.
[2]Not approved for HIT/HITT.
ACT, activated clotting time; aPTT, activated partial thromboplastin time; ELISA, enzyme-linked immunosorbent assay; HIT, heparin-induced thrombocytopenia; HITT, heparin-induced thrombocytopenia and thrombosis; PF4, platelet factor 4.

antagonist (warfarin) may be initiated. The DTI should be continued until therapeutic anticoagulation with the vitamin K antagonist has been achieved (international normalized ratio [INR] of 2.0–3.0) due to the warfarin effect; the infusion of argatroban must be temporarily discontinued for 2 hours before the INR is obtained so that it reflects the anticoagulant effect of warfarin alone. *Warfarin is contraindicated as initial treatment of HIT because of its potential to transiently worsen hypercoagulability.* Some clinicians endorse use of the subcutaneous indirect anti-Xa inhibitor fondaparinux for initial treatment of HIT, but the practice is not yet standard in most centers. In all patients with HIT, warfarin subsequently should be continued for at least 30 days, due to a persistent risk of thrombosis even after the platelet count has recovered, whereas in patients in whom thrombosis has been documented, anticoagulation with warfarin should continue for 3–6 months.

Subsequent exposure to heparin should be avoided in all patients with a prior history of HIT, if possible. If its use is regarded as necessary for a procedure, it should be withheld until PF4-heparin antibodies are no longer detectable by ELISA (usually as of 100 days following an episode of HIT), and exposure should be limited to the shortest time period possible.

When to Refer

Due to the tremendous thrombotic potential of the disorder and the complexity of use of the DTI, all patients with HIT should be evaluated by a hematologist.

When to Admit

Most patients with HIT are hospitalized at the time of detection of thrombocytopenia. Any outpatient in whom HIT is suspected should be admitted because the DTIs must be administered by continuous intravenous infusion.

Cuker A. Heparin-induced thrombocytopenia: present and future. J Thromb Thrombolysis. 2011 Apr;31(3):353–66. [PMID: 21327506]

Cuker A et al. Predictive value of the 4Ts scoring system for heparin-induced thrombocytopenia: a systematic review and meta-analysis. Blood. 2012 Nov 15;120(20):4160–7. [PMID: 22990018]

Warkentin TE et al. Heparin-induced thrombocytopenia in medical surgical critical illness. Chest. 2013 Sep;144(3): 848–58. [PMID: 23722881]

4. Disseminated Intravascular Coagulation

ESSENTIALS OF DIAGNOSIS

- ▶ A frequent cause of thrombocytopenia in hospitalized patients.
- ▶ Prolonged activated partial thromboplastin time and prothrombin time.
- ▶ Thrombocytopenia and decreased fibrinogen levels.

General Considerations

Disseminated intravascular coagulation (DIC) results from uncontrolled local or systemic activation of coagulation, which leads to depletion of coagulation factors and fibrinogen and to thrombocytopenia as platelets are activated and consumed.

The numerous disorders that are associated with DIC include sepsis (in which coagulation is activated by presence of lipopolysaccharide) as well as cancer, trauma, burns, or pregnancy-associated morbidity (in which tissue factor is released). Aortic aneurysm and cavernous hemangiomas may promote DIC by leading to vascular stasis, and snake bites may result in DIC due to the introduction of exogenous toxins.

Clinical Findings

A. Symptoms and Signs

Bleeding in DIC usually occurs at multiple sites, such as intravenous catheters or incisions, and may be widespread (purpura fulminans). Malignancy-related DIC may manifest principally as thrombosis (Trousseau syndrome).

B. Laboratory Findings

In early DIC, the platelet count and fibrinogen levels may remain within the normal range, albeit reduced from baseline levels. There is progressive thrombocytopenia (rarely severe), prolongation of the activated partial thromboplastin time (aPTT) and prothrombin time (PT), and low levels of fibrinogen. D-dimer levels typically are elevated due to the activation of coagulation and diffuse cross-linking of fibrin. Schistocytes on the blood smear, due to shearing of red cells through the microvasculature, are present in 10–20% of patients. Laboratory abnormalities in the HELLP syndrome (hemolysis, elevated liver enzymes, low platelets), a severe form of DIC with a particularly high mortality rate that occurs in peripartum women, include elevated liver transaminases and (many cases) kidney injury due to gross hemoglobinuria and pigment nephropathy. Malignancy-related DIC may feature normal platelet counts and coagulation studies.

Treatment

The underlying causative disorder must be treated (eg, antimicrobials, chemotherapy, surgery, or delivery of conceptus [see below]). If clinically significant bleeding is present, hemostasis must be achieved (Table 14–6).

Blood products should be administered only if clinically significant hemorrhage has occurred or is thought likely to occur without intervention (Table 14–6). The goal of platelet therapy for most cases is > 20,000/mcL or > 50,000/mcL for serious bleeding, such as intracranial bleeding. FFP should be given only to patients with a prolonged aPTT and PT and significant bleeding; 4 units typically are administered at a time, and the posttransfusion platelet count should be documented. Cryoprecipitate may be given for bleeding and fibrinogen levels < 80–100 mg/dL. The PT, aPTT, fibrinogen, and platelet count should be monitored at least every 6 hours in acutely ill patients with DIC.

Table 14–6. Management of DIC.

I. Assess for underlying cause of DIC and treat.	
II. Establish baseline platelet count, PT, aPTT, D-dimer, fibrinogen.	
III. Transfuse blood products only if ongoing bleeding or high risk of bleeding:	Platelets: goal > 20,000/mcL (most patients) or > 50,000/mcL (severe bleeding, eg, intracranial hemorrhage)
	Cryoprecipitate: goal fibrinogen level > 80–100 mg/dL
	Fresh frozen plasma: goal PT and aPTT < 1.5 × normal
	Packed red blood cells: goal hemoglobin > 8 g/dL or improvement in symptomatic anemia
IV. Follow platelets, aPTT/PT, fibrinogen every 4–6 hours or as clinically indicated.	
V. If persistent bleeding, consider use of heparin[1] (initial infusion, 5–10 units/kg/h); do not administer bolus.	
VI. Follow laboratory parameters every 4–6 hours until DIC resolved and underlying condition successfully treated	

[1]Contraindicated if platelets cannot be maintained at > 50,000/mcL, in cases of gastrointestinal or central nervous system bleeding, in conditions that may require surgical management, or placental abruption.
aPTT, activated partial thromboplastin time; DIC, disseminated intravascular coagulation; PT, prothrombin time.

In some cases of refractory bleeding despite replacement of blood products, administration of low doses of heparin can be considered; it may help interfere with thrombin generation, which then could lead to a lessened consumption of coagulation proteins and platelets. An infusion of 6–10 units/kg/h (no bolus) may be used. *Heparin, however, is contraindicated if the platelet count cannot be maintained at ≥ 50,000/mcL and in cases of central nervous system/gastrointestinal bleeding, placental abruption, and any other condition that is likely to require imminent surgery.* Fibrinolysis inhibitors may be considered in some patients with refractory DIC.

The treatment of **HELLP syndrome** must include evacuation of the uterus (eg, delivery of a term or near-term infant or removal of retained placental or fetal fragments). Patients with **Trousseau syndrome** require treatment of the underlying malignancy or administration of unfractionated heparin or subcutaneous therapeutic-dose LMWH as treatment of thrombosis, since warfarin typically is ineffective at secondary prevention of thromboembolism in the disorder. Immediate initiation of chemotherapy (usually within 24 hours of diagnosis) is required for patients with **acute promyelocytic leukemia (APL)–associated DIC**, along with administration of blood products as clinically indicated.

▶ **When to Refer**

Patients with diffuse bleeding that is unresponsive to administration of blood products should be evaluated by a hematologist.

▶ **When to Admit**

Most patients with DIC are hospitalized when DIC is detected.

Levi M et al. Disseminated intravascular coagulation in infectious disease. Semin Thromb Hemost. 2010 Jun;36(4):367–77. [PMID: 20614389]

Martí-Carvajal AJ et al. Treatment for disseminated intravascular coagulation in patients with acute and chronic leukemia. Cochrane Database Syst Rev. 2011 Jun 15;(6):CD008562. [PMID: 21678379]

Singh B et al. Trends in the incidence and outcomes of disseminated intravascular coagulation in critically ill patients (2004–2010): a population-based study. Chest. 2013 May;143(5):1235–42. [PMID: 23139140]

Wada H et al. Diagnostic criteria and laboratory tests for disseminated intravascular coagulation. Expert Rev Hematol. 2012 Dec;5(6):643–52. [PMID: 23216594]

OTHER CONDITIONS CAUSING THROMBOCYTOPENIA

1. Drug-Induced Thrombocytopenia

The mechanisms underlying drug-induced thrombocytopenia are thought in most cases to be immune, although exceptions exist (such as chemotherapy). Table 14–7 lists medications associated with thrombocytopenia. The typical presentation of **drug-induced thrombocytopenia** is severe thrombocytopenia and mucocutaneous bleeding 7–14 days after exposure to a new drug, although a range of presentations is possible. Discontinuation of the offending agent leads to resolution of thrombocytopenia within 7–10 days in most cases, but patients with severe thrombocytopenia should be given platelet transfusions with (immune cases only) or without IVIG.

2. Posttransfusion Purpura

Posttransfusion purpura (PTP) is a rare disorder that features sudden-onset thrombocytopenia in an individual who recently has received transfusion of red cells, platelets, or plasma within 1 week prior to detection of thrombocytopenia. Antibodies against the human platelet antigen Pl[A1] are detected in most individuals with PTP. Patients with PTP almost universally are either multiparous women or persons who have received transfusions previously. Severe thrombocytopenia and bleeding is typical. Initial treatment consists of administration of IVIG (1 g/kg/d for 2 days) which should be administered as soon as the diagnosis is suspected. Platelets are not indicated unless severe bleeding is present, but if they are to be administered, HLA-matched platelets are preferred. A second course or IVIG, plasma exchange, corticosteroids, or splenectomy may be used in case of refractoriness. Pl[A1]-negative or washed blood products are preferred for subsequent transfusions.

3. von Willebrand Disease Type 2B

von Willebrand disease (vWD) type 2B leads to chronic, characteristically mild to moderate thrombocytopenia via

Table 14–7. Selected medications causing drug-associated thrombocytopenia.

Class	Examples
Chemotherapy	Most agents
Antiplatelet agents	Anagrelide Abciximab Eptifibatide Tirofiban Ticlopidine
Antimicrobial agents	Penicillins Isoniazid Rifampin Sulfa drugs Vancomycin Adefovir Indinavir Ritonavir Fluconazole Linezolid
Cardiovascular agents	Digoxin Amiodarone Captopril Hydrochlorothiazide Procainamide Atorvastatin Simvastatin
Gastrointestinal agents	Cimetidine Ranitidine Famotidine
Neuropsychiatric agents	Haloperidol Carbamazepine Methyldopa Phenytoin
Analgesic agents	Acetaminophen Ibuprofen Sulindac Diclofenac Naproxen
Anticoagulant agents	Heparin Low-molecular-weight heparin
Immunomodulator agents	Interferon-alpha Rituximab
Immunosuppressant agents	Mycophenolate mofetil Tacrolimus
Other agents	Iodinated contrast dye Immunizations

an abnormal vWF molecule that binds platelets with increased affinity, resulting in aggregation and clearance.

4. Platelet Sequestration

At any given time, one-third of the platelet mass is sequestered in the spleen. Splenomegaly, due to a variety of conditions, may lead to thrombocytopenia of variable severity. Whenever possible, treatment of the underlying disorder should be pursued, but splenectomy, splenic

embolization, or splenic irradiation may be considered in selected cases.

5. Pregnancy

Gestational thrombocytopenia results from progressive expansion of the blood volume that typically occurs during pregnancy, leading to hemodilution. Cytopenias result, although production of blood cells is normal or increased. Platelet counts < 100,000/mcL, however, are observed in < 10% of pregnant women in the third trimester; decreases to < 70,000/mcL should prompt consideration of pregnancy-related ITP (see above) as well as preeclampsia or a pregnancy-related thrombotic microangiopathy.

6. Infection or Sepsis

Both immune- and platelet production–mediated defects are possible, and there may be significant overlap with concomitant DIC (see above). In either case, the platelet count typically improves with effective antimicrobial treatment or after the infection has resolved. In some critically ill patients, a defect in immunomodulation may lead to bone marrow macrophages (histiocytes) engulfing cellular components of the marrow in a process also called hemophagocytosis. The phenomenon typically resolves with resolution of the infection, but with certain infections (Epstein Barr virus) immunosuppression may be required. Hemophagocytosis also may arise in the setting of malignancy, in which case the disorder is usually unresponsive to treatment with immunosuppression.

7. Pseudothrombocytopenia

Pseudothrombocytopenia results from EDTA anticoagulant-induced platelet clumping; the phenomenon typically disappears when blood is collected in a tube containing citrate anticoagulant.

Bockenstedt PL. Thrombocytopenia in pregnancy. Hematol Oncol Clin North Am. 2011 Apr;25(2):293–310. [PMID: 21444031]
Perdomo J et al. Quinine-induced thrombocytopenia: drug-dependent GPIb/IX antibodies inhibit megakaryocyte and proplatelet production in vitro. Blood. 2011 Jun 2;117(22): 5975–86. [PMID: 21487107]

QUALITATIVE PLATELET DISORDERS

CONGENITAL DISORDERS OF PLATELET FUNCTION

ESSENTIALS OF DIAGNOSIS

► Usually diagnosed in childhood.
► Family history usually is positive.
► May be diagnosed in adulthood when there is excessive bleeding.

General Considerations

Heritable qualitative platelet disorders are far less common than acquired disorders of platelet function (see below) and lead to variably severe bleeding, often beginning in childhood. Occasionally, however, disorders of platelet function may go undetected until later in life when excessive bleeding occurs following a sufficient hemostatic insult. Thus, the true incidence of hereditary qualitative platelet disorders is unknown.

Bernard-Soulier syndrome (BSS) is a rare, autosomal recessive bleeding disorder that is due to reduced or abnormal platelet membrane expression of glycoprotein Ib/IX (vWF receptor).

Glanzmann thrombasthenia results from a qualitative or quantitative abnormality in glycoprotein IIb/IIIa receptors on the platelet membrane, which are required to bind fibrinogen and vWF, both of which bridge platelets during aggregation. Inheritance is autosomal recessive.

Under normal circumstances, activated platelets release the contents of platelet granules to reinforce the aggregatory response. **Storage pool disease** is caused by defects in release of alpha or dense (delta) platelet granules, or both (alpha-delta storage pool disease).

Clinical Findings

A. Symptoms and Signs

In patients with **Glanzmann thrombasthenia**, the onset of bleeding is usually in infancy or childhood. The degree of deficiency in IIb/IIIa may not correlate well with bleeding symptoms. Patients with **storage pool disease** are affected by variable bleeding, ranging from mild and trauma-related to spontaneous.

B. Laboratory Findings

In **Bernard-Soulier syndrome**, there are abnormally large platelets (approaching the size of red cells), moderate thrombocytopenia, and a prolonged bleeding time. Platelet aggregation studies show a marked defect in response to ristocetin, whereas aggregation in response to other agonists is normal; the addition of normal platelets corrects the abnormal aggregation. The diagnosis can be confirmed by platelet flow cytometry.

In **Glanzmann thrombasthenia**, platelet aggregation studies show marked impairment of aggregation in response to stimulation with typical agonists.

Storage pool disease describes defects in the number or content of platelet alpha or dense granules or both. The **gray platelet syndrome** comprises abnormalities of platelet alpha granules, thrombocytopenia, and marrow fibrosis. The blood smear shows agranular platelets, and the diagnosis is confirmed with electron microscopy.

Albinism-associated storage pool disease involves defective dense granules in disorders of oculocutaneous albinism, such as the Hermansky-Pudlak and Chediak-Higashi syndromes. Electron microscopy confirms the diagnosis.

Non–albinism-associated storage pool disease results from quantitative or qualitative defects in dense granules

and is seen in Ehlers-Danlos and Wiskott-Aldrich syndromes, among others.

The **Quebec platelet disorder** comprises mild thrombocytopenia, an abnormal platelet factor V molecule, and a prolonged bleeding time. Patients typically experience moderate bleeding. Interestingly, platelet transfusion does not ameliorate the bleeding.

Patients have a prolonged bleeding time. Platelet aggregation studies characteristically show platelet dissociation following an initial aggregatory response, and electron microscopy confirms the diagnosis.

Treatment

The mainstay of treatment (including periprocedural prophylaxis) is transfusion of normal platelets, although desmopressin acetate (DDAVP), antifibrinolytic agents, and recombinant human activated factor VII also have been used successfully.

Andrews RK et al. Bernard-Soulier syndrome: an update. Semin Thromb Hemost. 2013 Sep;39(6):656–62. [PMID: 23929303]
Lambert MP. What to do when you suspect an inherited platelet disorder. Hematology Am Soc Hematol Educ Program. 2011;2011:377–83. [PMID: 22160061]

ACQUIRED DISORDERS OF PLATELET FUNCTION

Platelet dysfunction is more commonly acquired than inherited; the widespread use of platelet-active medications accounts for most of the cases of qualitative defects (Table 14–8). In these cases, platelet inhibition typically declines within 5–10 days following discontinuation of the drug, and transfusion of platelets may be required if clinically significant bleeding is present.

DISORDERS OF COAGULATION

CONGENITAL DISORDERS OF COAGULATION

1. Hemophilia A & B

ESSENTIALS OF DIAGNOSIS

▶ **Hemophilia A**: congenital deficiency of coagulation factor VIII.

▶ **Hemophilia B**: congenital deficiency of coagulation factor IX.

▶ Recurrent hemarthroses and arthropathy.

▶ Risk of development of inhibitory antibodies to factor VIII or factor IX.

▶ In many older patients, infection with HIV or hepatitis C virus from receipt of contaminated blood products.

Table 14–8. Causes of acquired platelet dysfunction.

Cause	Mechanism(s)	Treatment of Bleeding
Drug-induced		
Salicylates (eg, aspirin)	Irreversible inhibition of platelet cyclooxygenase	Discontinuation of drug; platelet transfusion
NSAIDs (eg, ibuprofen)	Reversible inhibition of cyclooxygenase	
Glycoprotein IIb/IIIa inhibitors (eg, abciximab, tirofiban, eptifibatide)	↓Binding of fibrinogen to PM IIb/IIIa receptor	
Thienopyridines (eg, clopidogrel, ticlopidine)	↓ ADP binding to PM receptor	
Dipyridamole	↓ Intracellular cAMP metabolism	
SSRIs (eg, paroxetine, fluoxetine)	↓ Serotonin in dense-granules	
Omega-3 fatty acids (eg, DHA, EHA)	Disruption of PM phospholipid	
Antibiotics, (eg, high-dose penicillin, nafcillin, ticarcillin, cephalothin, moxalactam)	Not fully elucidated; PM binding may interfere with receptor-ligand interactions	
Alcohol	↓ TXA2 release	
Disease-related		
Uremia	↑ Nitric oxide; ↓ release of granules	DDAVP, high-dose estrogens; platelet transfusion, dialysis
Myeloproliferative disorder/myelodysplastic syndrome	Abnormal PM receptors, signal transduction, and/or granule release	Platelet transfusion; myelosuppressive treatment (myeloproliferative disorder)
Surgical procedure–related		
Cardiac bypass	Platelet activation in bypass circuit	Platelet transfusion

ADP, adenosine diphosphate; cAMP, cyclic adenosine monophosphate; DDAVP, desmopressin acetate; DHA, docosahexaenoic acid; EHA, eicosahexaenoic acid; NSAIDs, nonsteroidal anti-inflammatory drugs; PM, platelet membrane; SSRIs, selective serotonin release inhibitors; TXA2, thromboxane A2.

► General Considerations

The frequency of hemophilia A is 1 per 5000 live male births, whereas hemophilia B occurs in approximately 1 in 25,000 live male births. Inheritance is X-linked recessive, leading to affected males and carrier females. There is no race predilection. Testing is indicated for asymptomatic male infants with a hemophilic pedigree, for male infants with a family history of hemophilia who experience excessive bleeding, or for an otherwise asymptomatic adolescent or adult who experiences unexpected excessive bleeding with trauma or invasion.

Inhibitors to factor VIII will develop in approximately 30% of patients with hemophilia A, and inhibitors to factor IX will develop in < 5% of patients with hemophilia B.

A substantial proportion of older patients with hemophilia acquired infection with HIV or HCV or both in the 1980s due to exposure to contaminated factor concentrates and blood products.

► Clinical Findings

A. Symptoms and Signs

Severe hemophilia presents in infant males or in early childhood with spontaneous bleeding into joints, soft tissues, or other locations. Spontaneous bleeding is rare in patients with mild hemophilia, but bleeding may occur with a significant hemostatic challenge (eg, surgery, trauma). Intermediate clinical symptoms are seen in patients with moderate hemophilia. Female carriers of hemophilia are usually asymptomatic.

Significant hemophilic arthropathy is usually avoided in patients who have received long-term prophylaxis with factor concentrate starting in childhood, whereas joint disease is common in adults who have experienced recurrent hemarthroses.

Inhibitor development to factor VIII or factor IX is characterized by bleeding episodes that are resistant to treatment with clotting factor VIII or IX concentrate, and by new or atypical bleeding.

B. Laboratory Findings

Hemophilia is diagnosed by demonstration of an isolated reproducibly low factor VIII or factor IX activity level, in the absence of other conditions. If the aPTT is prolonged, it typically corrects upon mixing with normal plasma. A variety of mutations, including inversions, large and small deletions, insertions, missense mutations, and nonsense mutations may be causative. Depending on the level of residual factor VIII or factor IX activity and the sensitivity of the thromboplastin used in the aPTT coagulation reaction, the aPTT may or may not be prolonged (although it typically is markedly prolonged in severe hemophilia). Hemophilia is classified according to the level of factor activity in the plasma. **Severe hemophilia** is characterized by < 1% factor activity, **mild hemophilia** features > 5% factor activity, and **moderate hemophilia** features 1–5% factor activity. Female carriers may become symptomatic if significant lyonization has occurred favoring the defective factor VIII or factor IX gene, leading to factor VIII or factor IX activity level markedly < 50%.

In the presence of an inhibitor to factor VIII or factor IX, there is accelerated clearance of and suboptimal or absent rise in measured activity of infused factor, and the aPTT does not correct on mixing. The Bethesda assay measures the potency of the inhibitor.

▶ **Treatment**

Plasma-derived or recombinant factor concentrates are the mainstay of treatment. By the age of 4 years, most children with severe hemophilia have begun twice- or thrice-weekly infusions of factor to prevent the recurrent joint bleeding that otherwise would characterize the disorder and lead to severe musculoskeletal morbidity. Adults are frequently treated with factor concentrate as needed for bleeding episodes or prior to high-risk activities (Table 14–9). Patients with mild hemophilia A may respond to as-needed intravenous or intranasal treatment with DDAVP. Antifibrinolytic agents may be useful in cases of mucosal bleeding and are commonly used adjunctively, such as following dental procedures. Clinical trials of longer-acting FVIII and FIX molecules are underway. Delivery of a functional factor IX gene via viral vectors continues to be explored in gene therapy trials; early results among patients with severe hemophilia B show improvement in the baseline FIX level so as to reduce or eliminate the need for prophylactic infusions of FIX concentrate.

It may be possible to overcome low-titer inhibitors (< 5 Bethesda units [BU]) by giving larger doses of factor, whereas treatment of bleeding in the presence of a high-titer inhibitor (> 5 BU) requires infusion of an activated prothrombin complex concentrate or recombinant

Table 14–9. Treatment of selected inherited bleeding disorders.

Disorder	Subtype	Treatment for Minor Bleeding	Treatment for Major Bleeding	Comment
Hemophilia A	Mild	DDAVP[1]	DDAVP[1] or factor VIII concentrate	Treat for 3–10 days for major bleeding or following surgery, keeping factor activity level 50–80% initially. Adjunctive aminocaproic acid may be useful for mucosal bleeding or procedures
	Moderate or severe	Factor VIII concentrate	Factor VIII concentrate	
Hemophilia B	Mild, moderate, or severe	Factor IX concentrate	Factor IX concentrate	
von Willebrand disease	Type 1	DDAVP	DDAVP, vWF concentrate	
	Type 2	DDAVP,[1] vWF concentrate	vWF concentrate	
	Type 3	vWF concentrate	vWF concentrate	
Factor XI deficiency	—	FFP or aminocaproic acid	FFP	Adjunctive aminocaproic acid should be used for mucosal bleeding or procedures

[1]Mild hemophilia A and type 2A or 2B vWD patients: therapeutic trial must have previously confirmed an adequate response (ie, elevation of factor VIII or vWF activity level into the normal range) and (for type 2B) no exacerbation of thrombocytopenia. DDAVP is not typically effective for type 2M vWD. A vWF-containing factor VIII concentrate is preferred for treatment of type 2N vWD.

Notes:

DDAVP dose is 0.3 mcg/kg intravenously in 50 mL saline over 20 minutes, or nasal spray 300 mcg for weight > 50 kg or 150 mcg for < 50 kg, every 12–24 hours, maximum of three doses in a 48-hour period. If more than two doses are used in a 12–24 hour period, free water restriction and/or monitoring for hyponatremia is essential.

EACA dose is 50 mg/kg orally four times daily for 3–5 d; maximum 24 g/d, useful for mucosal bleeding/dental procedures.

Factor VIII concentrate dose is 50 units/kg intravenously initially followed by 25 units/kg every 8 hours followed by lesser doses at longer intervals once hemostasis has been established.

Factor IX concentrate dose is 100 units/kg (120 units/kg if using Benefix) intravenously initially followed by 50 units/kg (60 units/kg if using Benefix) every 8 hours followed by lesser doses at longer intervals once hemostasis has been established.

vWF-containing factor VIII concentrate dose is 60–80 RCoF units/kg intravenously every 12 hours initially followed by lesser doses at longer intervals once hemostasis has been established.

FFP is typically administered in 4-unit boluses and may not need to be re-bolused after the initial administration due to the long half-life of factor XI.

DDAVP, desmopressin acetate; FFP, fresh frozen plasma; vWF, von Willebrand factor.

activated factor VII. Inhibitor tolerance induction, achieved by giving large doses (50–300 units/kg intravenously of factor VIII daily) for 6–18 months, succeeds in eradicating the inhibitor in 70% of patients with hemophilia A and in 30% of patients with hemophilia B. Patients with hemophilia B who receive inhibitor tolerance induction, however, are at risk for development of nephrotic syndrome and anaphylactic reactions, making eradication of their inhibitors less feasible. Additional immunomodulation may allow for eradication in selected inhibitor tolerance induction–refractory patients.

Highly active antiretroviral treatment is almost universally administered to individuals with HIV infection.

When to Refer

All patients with hemophilia should be seen regularly in a comprehensive hemophilia treatment center.

When to Admit

- Major invasive procedures because of the need for serial infusions of clotting factor concentrate.
- Bleeding that is unresponsive to outpatient treatment.

Berntorp E. Importance of rapid bleeding control in haemophilia complicated by inhibitors. Haemophilia. 2011 Jan;17(1): 11–6. [PMID: 20565546]

Fogarty PF. Biological rationale for new drugs in the bleeding disorders pipeline. Hematology Am Soc Hematol Educ Program. 2011;2011:397–404. [PMID: 22160064]

Fogarty PF et al. Hemophilia A and B. In: Kitchens CS et al (editors). *Consultative Hemostasis and Thrombosis*, 3rd ed. New York: Elsevier, 2013.

Gouw SC et al; PedNet and Research of Determinants of INhibitor development (RODIN) Study Group. Intensity of factor VIII treatment and inhibitor development in children with severe hemophilia A: the RODIN study. Blood. 2013 May 16; 121(20):4046–55. [PMID: 23553768]

Leissinger C et al. Anti-inhibitor coagulant complex prophylaxis in hemophilia with inhibitors. N Engl J Med. 2011 Nov 3;365(18):1684–92. [PMID: 22047559]

Nathwani AC et al. Adenovirus-associated virus vector-mediated gene transfer in hemophilia B. N Engl J Med. 2011 Dec 22;365(25):2357–65. [PMID: 22149959]

2. von Willebrand Disease

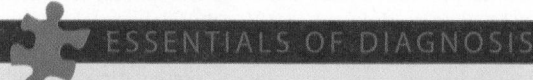

ESSENTIALS OF DIAGNOSIS

- ▶ The most common inherited bleeding disorder.
- ▶ von Willebrand factor aggregates platelets and prolongs the half-life of factor VIII.

General Considerations

vWF is an unusually large multimeric glycoprotein that binds to its receptor, platelet glycoprotein Ib, bridging platelets together and tethering them to the subendothelial matrix at the site of vascular injury. vWF also has a binding site for factor VIII, prolonging its half-life in the circulation.

Between 75% and 80% of patients with vWD have type 1. It is a quantitative abnormality of the vWF molecule that usually does not feature an identifiable causal mutation in the vWF gene.

Type 2 vWD is seen in 15–20% of patients with vWD. In type 2A or 2B vWD, a qualitative defect in the vWF molecule is causative. Type 2N and 2M vWD are due to defects in vWF that decrease binding to factor VIII or to platelets, respectively. Importantly, type 2N vWD clinically resembles hemophilia A, with the exception of a family history that shows affected females. Factor VIII activity levels are markedly decreased, and vWF activity and antigen (Ag) are normal. Type 2M vWD features a normal multimer pattern. Type 3 vWD is rare, and mutational homozygosity or double heterozygosity leads to undetectable levels of vWF and severe bleeding in infancy or childhood.

Clinical Findings

A. Symptoms and Signs

Patients with type 1 vWD usually have mild or moderate platelet-type bleeding (especially involving the integument and mucous membranes). Patients with type 2 vWD usually have moderate to severe bleeding that presents in childhood or adolescence.

B. Laboratory Findings

In type 1 vWD, the vWF activity (by ristocetin co-factor assay) and Ag are mildly depressed, whereas the vWF multimer pattern is normal (Table 14–10). Laboratory testing of type 2A or 2B vWD typically shows a ratio of vWF Ag:vWF activity of approximately 2:1 and a multimer pattern that lacks the highest molecular weight multimers. Thrombocytopenia is common in type 2B vWD due to a gain-of-function mutation of the vWF molecule, which leads to increased binding to its receptor on platelets, resulting in clearance; a ristocetin-induced platelet aggregation (RIPA) study shows an increase in platelet aggregation in response to low concentrations of ristocetin. Except in the more severe forms of vWD that feature a significantly decreased factor VIII activity, the aPTT and PT in vWD are usually normal.

Treatment

The treatment of vWD is summarized in Table 14–9. DDAVP is useful in the treatment of mild bleeding in most cases of type 1 and some cases of type 2 vWD. DDAVP causes release of vWF and factor VIII from storage sites, leading to increases in vWF and factor VIII twofold to sevenfold that of baseline levels. Cryoprecipitate should not be given due to lack of viral inactivation. Antifibrinolytic agents (eg, aminocaproic acid) may be used adjunctively for mucosal bleeding or procedures. Pregnant patients with vWD usually do not require treatment because of the natural physiologic increase in vWF levels (up to threefold that

Table 14–10. Laboratory diagnosis of von Willebrand disease.

Type		vWF Activity	vWF Antigen	FVIII	RIPA	Multimer Analysis
1		↓	↓	NI or ↓	↓	Normal pattern; uniform ↓ intensity of bands
2	A	↓↓	↓	↓	↓	Large and intermediate multimers decreased or absent
	B	↓↓	↓	↓	↑	Large multimers decreased or absent
	M	↓	↓	↓	↓	Normal pattern; uniform ↓ intensity of bands
	N	NI	NI	↓↓	NI	NI
3		↓↓↓	↓↓↓	↓↓↓	↓↓↓	Multimers absent

NI, normal; RIPA, ristocetin-induced platelet aggregation; vWF, von Willebrand factor.

of baseline) that are observed by the time of delivery; however, if excessive bleeding is encountered, vWF-containing factor VIII concentrates may be given.

Abshire TC et al. Prophylaxis in severe forms of von Willebrand's disease: results from the von Willebrand Disease Prophylaxis Network (VWD PN). Haemophilia. 2013 Jan;19(1):76–81. [PMID: 22823000]

Lipe BC et al. Von Willebrand disease in pregnancy. Hematol Oncol Clin North Am. 2011 Apr;25(2):335–58. [PMID: 21444034]

Rick ME. Von Willebrand Disease. In: Kitchens CS et al (editors). *Consultative Hemostasis and Thrombosis,* 3rd ed. New York: Elsevier, 2013.

3. Factor XI Deficiency

Factor XI deficiency (sometimes referred to as **hemophilia C**) is inherited in an autosomal recessive manner, leading to heterozygous or homozygous defects. It is most prevalent among individuals of Ashkenazi Jewish descent. Levels of factor XI, while variably reduced, do not correlate well with bleeding symptoms. Mild bleeding is most common, and surgery or trauma may expose or worsen the bleeding tendency. FFP is the mainstay of treatment in locales where the plasma-derived factor XI concentrate is not available. Administration of adjunctive aminocaproic acid is regarded as mandatory for procedures or bleeding episodes involving the mucosa (Table 14–9).

Martín-Salces M et al. Review: Factor XI deficiency: review and management in pregnant women. Clin Appl Thromb Hemost. 2010 Apr;16(2):209–13. [PMID: 19049995]

4. Less Common Heritable Disorders of Coagulation

Congenital deficiencies of clotting factors II, V, VII, and X are rare and typically are inherited in an autosomal recessive pattern. A prolongation in the PT (and aPTT for factor X and factor II deficiency) that corrects upon mixing with normal plasma is typical. The treatment of factor II deficiency is with a prothrombin complex concentrate; factor V deficiency is treated with infusions of FFP or

platelets (which contain factor V in alpha granules); factor VII deficiency is treated with recombinant human activated factor VII at 15–30 mcg/kg every 4–6 hours; and infusions of FFP may be used to treat factor X deficiency.

Deficiency of factor XIII, a transglutamase that crosslinks fibrin, characteristically leads to delayed bleeding that occurs hours to days after a hemostatic challenge (such as surgery or trauma). The condition is usually lifelong, and spontaneous intracranial hemorrhages as well as recurrent pregnancy loss appear to occur with increased frequency in these patients compared with other congenital deficiencies. Cryoprecipitate or infusion of a plasma-derived factor XIII concentrate (available through a research study; appropriate for patients with A-subunit deficiency only) is the treatment of choice for bleeding or surgical prophylaxis.

Bereczky Z et al. Factor XIII and venous thromboembolism. Semin Thromb Hemost. 2011 Apr;37(3):305–14. [PMID: 21455864]

Peyvandi F et al. Rare bleeding disorders. Semin Thromb Hemost. 2009 Jun;35(4):345–7. [PMID: 19598062]

ACQUIRED DISORDERS OF COAGULATION

1. Acquired Antibodies to Factor VIII

Spontaneous antibodies to factor VIII occasionally occur in adults without a prior history of hemophilia; the elderly and patients with lymphoproliferative malignancy or connective tissue disease, who are postpartum, or postsurgical are at highest risk. The clinical presentation typically includes extensive soft-tissue ecchymoses, hematomas, and mucosal bleeding, as opposed to hemarthrosis in congenital hemophilia A. The aPTT is typically prolonged and does not correct upon mixing; factor VIII activity is found to be low and a Bethesda assay reveals the titer of the inhibitor. Inhibitors of low titer (< 5 BU) may often be overcome by infusion of high doses of factor VIII concentrates, whereas high-titer inhibitors (> 5 BU) must be treated with serial infusions of activated prothrombin complex concentrates or recombinant human activated factor VII. Along with establishment of hemostasis by one of these measures, immunosuppressive treatment with corticosteroids and oral cyclophosphamide should be instituted; treatment with IVIG, rituximab, or plasmapheresis can be considered in refractory cases.

Knoebl P et al. Demographic and clinical data in acquired hemophilia A: results from the European Acquired Haemophilia Registry (EACH2). J Thromb Haemost. 2012 Apr;10(4): 622–31. [PMID: 22321904]

2. Acquired Antibodies to Factor II

Patients with antiphospholipid antibodies occasionally manifest specificity to coagulation factor II (prothrombin), leading typically to a severe hypoprothrombinemia and bleeding. Mixing studies may or may not reveal presence of an inhibitor, as the antibody typically binds a nonenzymatically active portion of the molecule that leads to accelerated clearance, but characteristically the PT is prolonged and levels of factor II are low. FFP should be administered for treatment of bleeding. Treatment is immunosuppressive.

3. Acquired Antibodies to Factor V

Products containing bovine factor V (such as topical thrombin or fibrin glue, frequently used in surgical procedures) can lead to formation of an anti-factor V antibody that has specificity for human factor V. Clinicopathologic manifestations range from a prolonged PT in an otherwise asymptomatic individual to severe bleeding. Mixing studies suggest the presence of an inhibitor, and the factor V activity level is low. In cases of serious or life-threatening bleeding, IVIG or platelet transfusions, or both, should be administered, and immunosuppression (as for acquired inhibitors to factor VIII) may be offered.

4. Vitamin K Deficiency

Vitamin K deficiency may occur as a result of deficient dietary intake of vitamin K (from green leafy vegetables, soybeans, and other sources), malabsorption, or decreased production by intestinal bacteria (due to treatment with chemotherapy or antibiotics). Vitamin K normally participates in activity of the vitamin K epoxide reductase that assists in posttranslational gamma-carboxylation of the coagulation factors II, VII, IX, and X that is necessary for their activity. Thus, vitamin K deficiency typically features a prolonged PT (in which the activity of the vitamin K–dependent factors is more reflected than in the aPTT) that corrects upon mixing; levels of individual clotting factors II, VII, IX, and X typically are low. Importantly, a concomitantly low factor V activity level is not indicative of isolated vitamin K deficiency, and may indicate an underlying defect in liver synthetic function (see below).

For treatment, vitamin K_1 (phytonadione) may be administered via intravenous or oral routes; the subcutaneous route is not recommended due to erratic absorption. The oral dose is 5–10 mg/d and absorption is typically excellent; at least partial improvement in the PT should be observed within 1 day of administration. Intravenous administration (1 mg/d) results in even faster normalization of a prolonged PT than oral administration; due to descriptions of anaphylaxis, parenteral doses should be administered at lower doses and slowly (eg, over 30 minutes) with concomitant monitoring.

5. Coagulopathy of Liver Disease

Impaired hepatic function due to cirrhosis or other causes leads to decreased synthesis of clotting factors, including factors II, VII, V, IX, and fibrinogen, whereas factor VIII levels may be elevated in spite of depressed levels of other coagulation factors. The PT (and with advanced disease, the aPTT) is typically prolonged and corrects on mixing with normal plasma. A normal factor V level, in spite of decreases in the activity of factors II, VII, IX, and X, however, suggests vitamin K deficiency rather than liver disease (see above). Qualitative and quantitative deficiencies of fibrinogen also are prevalent among patients with advanced liver disease, typically leading to a prolonged PT, thrombin time, and reptilase time.

The coagulopathy of liver disease usually does not require hemostatic treatment until bleeding complications occur. Infusion of FFP may be considered if active bleeding is present and the aPTT and PT are markedly prolonged; however, the effect is transient and concern for volume overload may limit infusions. Patients with bleeding and a fibrinogen level consistently below 80 mg/dL should receive cryoprecipitate. Liver transplantation, if feasible, results in production of coagulation factors at normal levels. The appropriateness of use of recombinant human activated factor VII in patients with bleeding varices is controversial, although some patient subgroups may experience benefit.

Franchini M et al. Acquired factor V inhibitors: a systematic review. J Thromb Thrombolysis. 2011 May;31(4):449–57. [PMID: 21052780]
Pluta A et al. Coagulopathy in liver diseases. Adv Med Sci. 2010 Jun;55(1):16–21. [PMID: 20513645]

6. Warfarin Ingestion

See **Antithrombotic Therapy** section, below.

7. Disseminated Intravascular Coagulation

The consumptive coagulopathy of DIC results in decreases in the activity of clotting factors, leading to bleeding in most patients (see above). The aPTT and PT are characteristically prolonged, and platelets and fibrinogen levels are reduced from baseline.

8. Heparin/Fondaparinux/Novel Oral Anticoagulants Use

The thrombin time is dramatically prolonged in the presence of heparin. Patients who are receiving heparin and who have bleeding should be managed by discontinuation of the heparin and (some cases) administration of protamine sulfate; 1 mg of protamine neutralizes approximately 100 units of heparin sulfate, and the maximum dose is 50 mg intravenously. LMWHs typically do not prolong clotting times and are incompletely reversible with protamine. There is no reversal agent for fondaparinux, although some experts have suggested using recombinant human activated factor VIIa for cases of life-threatening bleeding. The novel oral anticoagulants include rivaroxaban and dabigatran, and have no specific antidote.

Eerenberg ES et al. Reversal of rivaroxaban and dabigatran by prothrombin complex concentrate: a randomized, placebo-controlled, crossover study in healthy subjects. Circulation. 2011 Oct 4;124(14):1573–9. [PMID: 21900088]
Siegal DM et al. Acute management of bleeding in patients on novel oral anticoagulants. Eur Heart J. 2013 Feb;34(7): 489–498b. [PMID: 23220847]

9. Lupus Anticoagulants

Lupus anticoagulants do not cause bleeding; however, because they prolong clotting times by binding proteins associated with phospholipid, which is a necessary component of coagulation reactions, clinicians may be concerned about a risk of bleeding. Lupus anticoagulants were so named because of their increased prevalence among patients with connective tissue disease, although they may occur with increased frequency in individuals with underlying infection, inflammation, or malignancy, and they also can occur in asymptomatic individuals in the general population. A prolongation in the aPTT is observed that does not correct completely on mixing. Specialized testing such as the hexagonal phase phospholipid neutralization assay, the dilute Russell viper venom time, and platelet neutralization assays can confirm the presence of a lupus anticoagulant.

Adams M. Measurement of lupus anticoagulants: an update on quality in laboratory testing. Semin Thromb Hemost. 2013 Apr;39(3):267–71. [PMID: 23424052]

OTHER CAUSES OF BLEEDING

Occasionally, abnormalities of the vasculature and integument may lead to bleeding despite normal hemostasis; congenital or acquired disorders may be causative. These abnormalities include Ehlers-Danlos syndrome, osteogenesis imperfecta, Osler-Weber-Rendu disease, and Marfan syndrome (heritable defects) and integumentary thinning due to prolonged corticosteroid administration or normal aging, amyloidosis, vasculitis, and scurvy (acquired defects). The bleeding time often is prolonged. If possible, treatment of the underlying condition should be pursued, but if this is not possible or feasible (ie, congenital syndromes), globally hemostatic agents such as DDAVP can be considered for treatment of bleeding. Topical bevacizumab has been effective in some patients with refractory nosebleeds.

Karnezis TT et al. Treatment of hereditary hemorrhagic telangiectasia with submucosal and topical bevacizumab therapy. Laryngoscope. 2012 Mar;122(3):495–7. [PMID: 22147664]
McDonald J et al. Hereditary hemorrhagic telangiectasia: an overview of diagnosis, management, and pathogenesis. Genet Med. 2011 Jul;13(7):607–16. [PMID: 21546842]

ANTITHROMBOTIC THERAPY

▶ Prevention of Venous Thromboembolic Disease

The frequency of venous thromboembolic disease (VTE) among hospitalized patients ranges widely; up to 20% of medical patients and 80% of critical care patients and high-risk surgical patients have been reported to experience this complication, which includes deep venous thrombosis (DVT) and pulmonary embolism (PE).

Avoidance of fatal PE, which occurs in up to 5% of high-risk inpatients as a consequence of hospitalization or surgery is a major goal of pharmacologic prophylaxis. Tables 14–11 and 14–12 provide risk stratification for DVT/VTE among hospitalized surgical and medical inpatients. Standard prophylactic regimens are listed in

Table 14–11. Risk stratification for DVT/VTE among surgical inpatients.

High Risk
Recent major orthopedic surgery/arthroplasty/or fracture
Abdominal/pelvic cancer undergoing surgery
Recent spinal cord injury or major trauma within 90 days
More than three of the intermediate risk factors (see below)

Intermediate Risk
Not ambulating independently outside of room at least twice daily
Active infectious or inflammatory process
Active malignancy
Major surgery (nonorthopedic)
History of VTE
Stroke
Central venous access or PICC line
Inflammatory bowel disease
Prior immobilization (> 72 hours) preoperatively
Obesity (BMI > 30)
Patient age > 50 years
Hormone replacement or oral contraceptive therapy
Hypercoagulable state
Nephrotic syndrome
Burns
Cellulitis
Varicose veins
Paresis
HF (systolic dysfunction)
COPD exacerbation

Low Risk
Minor procedure and age < 40 years with no additional risk factors
Ambulatory with expected length of stay of < 24 hours or minor surgery

Table 14–12. Padua Risk Assessment Model for VTE prophylaxis in hospitalized medical patients.

Condition	Points[1]
Active cancer, history of VTE, immobility, laboratory thrombophilia	3 points each
Recent (≤ 1 mo) trauma and/or surgery	2 points each
Age ≥ 70, acute MI or CVA, acute infection, rheumatologic disorder, BMI ≥ 30, hormonal therapy	1 point each

[1]A score ≥ 4 connotes high risk of VTE in the noncritically ill medical patients and pharmacologic prophylaxis is indicated, absent absolute contraindications.
BMI, body mass index; CVA, cerebrovascular accident; MI, myocardial infarction; VTE, venous thromboembolism.

Table 14–13. Prophylactic strategies should be guided by individual risk stratification, with all moderate- and high-risk patients receiving pharmacologic prophylaxis, unless contraindicated. Contraindications to VTE prophylaxis for hospital inpatients at high risk for VTE are listed in Table 14–14.

It is recommended that VTE prophylaxis be used judiciously in hospitalized medical patients who are not critically ill since a comprehensive review of evidence suggested harm from bleeding in low-risk patients given low-dose heparin and skin necrosis in stroke patients given compression stockings. The Padua Risk Score provides clinicians with a simple validated approach to risk stratification in medical patients (Table 14–12). Certain high-risk surgical patients should be considered for extended-duration prophylaxis, of approximately 1 month, including those undergoing total hip replacement, hip fracture repair, and abdominal and pelvic cancer surgery. If bleeding is present, if the risk of bleeding is high, or if the risk of VTE is high for the inpatient (Table 14–11) and therefore combined prophylactic strategies are needed, some measure of thromboprophylaxis may be provided through use of mechanical devices, including intermittent pneumatic compression devices, venous foot pumps, or graduated compression stockings.

Barbar S et al. A risk assessment model for the identification of hospitalized medical patients at risk for venous thromboembolism: the Padua Prediction Score. J Thromb Haemost. 2010 Nov;8(11):2450–7. [PMID: 20738765]

Falck-Ytter Y et al. Prevention of VTE in orthopedic surgery patients: Antithrombotic Therapy and Prevention of Thrombosis, 9th ed: American College of Chest Physicians Evidence-Based Clinical Practice Guidelines. Chest. 2012 Feb;141(2 Suppl):e278S–325S. [PMID: 22315265]

Gould MK et al. Prevention of VTE in nonorthopedic surgical patients: Antithrombotic Therapy and Prevention of Thrombosis, 9th ed: American College of Chest Physicians Evidence-Based Clinical Practice Guidelines. Chest. 2012 Feb;141(2 Suppl):e227S–77S. Erratum in: Chest. 2012 May;141(5):1369. [PMID: 22315263]

Kahn SR et al. Prevention of VTE in nonsurgical patients: Antithrombotic Therapy and Prevention of Thrombosis, 9th ed: American College of Chest Physicians Evidence-Based Clinical Practice Guidelines. Chest. 2012 Feb;141(2 Suppl):e195S–226S. [PMID: 2231526]

Neumann I et al. Oral direct Factor Xa inhibitors versus low-molecular-weight heparin to prevent venous thromboembolism in patients undergoing total hip or knee replacement: a systematic review and meta-analysis. Ann Intern Med. 2012 May 15;156(10):710–9. [PMID: 22412038]

Qaseem A et al. Venous thromboembolism prophylaxis in hospitalized patients: a clinical practice guideline from the American College of Physicians. Ann Intern Med. 2011 Nov 1;155(9):625–32. [PMID: 22041951]

▶ Treatment of Venous Thromboembolic Disease

A. Anticoagulant Therapy

Treatment for VTE should be offered to patients with objectively confirmed DVT or PE, or to those in whom the clinical suspicion is high for the disorder yet have not yet undergone diagnostic testing (see Chapter 9). The management of VTE primarily involves administration of anticoagulants; the goal is to prevent recurrence, extension and embolization of thrombosis and to reduce the risk of postthrombotic syndrome. Suggested anticoagulation regimens are found in Table 14–15.

B. Selecting Appropriate Anticoagulant Therapy

Most patients with DVT alone may be treated as outpatients, provided that their risk of bleeding is low, and they have good follow-up. Table 14–16 outlines the selection criteria for outpatient treatment of DVT.

Among patients with PE, risk stratification should be done at time of diagnosis to direct treatment and triage. Patients with persistent hemodynamic instability (or patients with massive PE) are classified as high risk and have an early PE-related mortality of > 15%. These patients should be admitted to an intensive care unit and receive thrombolysis in addition to anticoagulation. Intermediate-risk patients have a mortality rate of up to 15% and should be admitted to a higher level of inpatient care, with consideration of thrombolysis on a case-by-case basis. Those classified as low risk have a mortality rate < 3% and are candidates for expedited discharge or outpatient therapy.

Because both intermediate- and low-risk patients are hemodynamically stable, additional assessment is necessary to differentiate the two. Echocardiography can be used to identify patients with right ventricular dysfunction, which connotes intermediate risk. However, real-time echocardiography involves added cost and is not always immediately available. An RV/LV ratio < 1.0 on chest CT angiogram has been shown to have good negative predictive value for adverse outcome but suffers from interobserver variability. Serum biomarkers such as B-type natriuretic peptide and troponin have been studied and are most useful for their negative predictive value, and mainly in combination with other predictors. The PESI (pulmonary embolism severity index) clinical risk score, which

Table 14–13. Pharmacologic prophylaxis of VTE in selected clinical scenarios.[1]

Anticoagulant	Dose	Frequency	Clinical Scenario	Comment
Enoxaparin	40 mg subcutaneously	Once daily	Most medical inpatients and critical care patients	—
			Surgical patients (moderate risk for VTE)	
			Abdominal/pelvic cancer surgery	Consider continuing for 4 weeks total duration for abdomino-pelvic cancer surgery
		Twice daily	Bariatric surgery	Higher doses may be required
	30 mg subcutaneously	Twice daily	Orthopedic surgery[2]	Give for at least 10 days. For THR, TKA, or HFS, consider continuing up to 1 month after surgery in high-risk patients
			Major trauma	Not applicable to patients with isolated lower extremity trauma
			Acute spinal cord injury	—
Dalteparin	2500 units subcutaneously	Once daily	Most medical inpatients	—
			Abdominal surgery (moderate risk for VTE)	Give for 5–10 days
	5000 units subcutaneously	Once daily	Orthopedic surgery[2]	First dose = 2500 units. Give for at least 10 days. For THR, TKA, or HFS, consider continuing up to 1 month after surgery in high-risk patients
			Abdominal surgery (higher-risk for VTE)	Give for 5–10 days
			Medical inpatients	—
Fondaparinux	2.5 mg subcutaneously	Once daily	Orthopedic surgery[2]	Give for at least 10 days. For THR, TKA, or HFS, consider continuing up to 1 month after surgery in high-risk patients
Rivaroxaban	10 mg orally	Once daily	Orthopedic surgery-total hip and total knee replacement	Give for 12 days following total knee replacement; give for 35 days following total hip replacement
Unfractionated heparin	5000 units subcutaneously	Three times daily	Higher VTE risk with low bleeding risk	Includes gynecologic surgery for malignancy and urologic surgery, medical patients with multiple risk factors for VTE
	5000 units subcutaneously	Twice daily	Hospitalized patients at intermediate risk for VTE	Includes gynecologic surgery (moderate risk)
			Patients with epidural catheters	LMWHs usually avoided due to risk of spinal hematoma
			Patients with severe kidney disease[3]	LMWHs contraindicated
Warfarin	(variable) oral	Once daily	Orthopedic surgery[2]	Titrate to goal INR = 2.5. Give for at least 10 days. For high-risk patients undergoing THR, TKA, or HFS, consider continuing up to 1 month after surgery

[1]All regimens administered subcutaneously, except for warfarin.
[2]Includes TKA, THR, and HFS.
[3]Defined as creatinine clearance < 30 mL/min.
HFS, hip fracture surgery; LMWH, low-molecular-weight heparin; THR, total hip replacement; TKA, total knee arthroplasty; VTE, venous thromboembolic disease.

Table 14–14. Contraindications to VTE prophylaxis for medical or surgical hospital inpatients at high risk for VTE.

Absolute contraindications
Acute hemorrhage from wounds or drains or lesions
Intracranial hemorrhage within prior 24 hours
Heparin-induced thrombocytopenia (HIT) consider using fondaparinux
Severe trauma to head or spinal cord or extremities
Epidural anesthesia/spinal block within 12 hours of initiation of anticoagulation (concurrent use of an epidural catheter and anticoagulation other than low prophylactic doses of unfractionated heparin should require review and approval by service who performed the epidural or spinal procedure, eg, anesthesia/pain service and in many cases should be avoided entirely)
Currently receiving warfarin or heparin or LMWH or direct thrombin inhibitor for other indications
Relative contraindications
Coagulopathy (INR > 1.5)
Intracranial lesion or neoplasm
Severe thrombocytopenia (platelet count < 50,000/mcL)
Intracranial hemorrhage within past 6 months
Gastrointestinal or genitourinary hemorrhage within past 6 months

INR, international normalized ratio; LMWH, low-molecular-weight heparin; VTE, venous thromboembolic disease.
Adapted from Guidelines used at the VA Medical Center, San Francisco, CA.

does not require additional testing, has been validated and accurately identifies patients at low risk for 30-day PE-related mortality A simplified version of this risk score has been validated as well (Table 14–17).

1. Heparin—Selection of a parenteral anticoagulant should be determined by patient characteristics (kidney function, immediate bleeding risk, weight) and the clinical scenario (eg, whether thrombolysis is being considered). LMWHs are as efficacious as unfractionated heparin in the immediate treatment of DVT and PE and are preferred as initial treatment because of predictable pharmacokinetics, which allow for subcutaneous, once- or twice-daily dosing with no requirement for monitoring in most patients. Monitoring of the therapeutic effect of LMWH may be indicated in pregnancy, compromised kidney function, and extremes of weight. Accumulation of LMWH and increased rates of bleeding have been observed among patients with severe chronic kidney disease (creatinine clearance < 30 mL/min), leading to a recommendation to use intravenous unfractionated heparin preferentially in these patients. If concomitant thrombolysis is being considered, unfractionated heparin is indicated. In addition, patients with VTE and a perceived higher risk of bleeding (ie, post-surgery) may be better candidates for treatment with unfractionated heparin than LMWH given its shorter half-life and reversibility. Unfractionated heparin can be effectively neutralized with the positively charged protamine sulfate (1 mg of protamine neutralizes approximately 100 units of heparin

sulfate; maximum dose, 50 mg intravenously) while protamine may only have partial reversal effect at best on LMWH. Use of unfractionated heparin leads to HIT in approximately 3% of patients, so most individuals require serial platelet count determinations during the initial 10–14 days of exposure and (some patients) periodically thereafter.

Weight-based, fixed-dose daily subcutaneous fondaparinux (a synthetic factor Xa inhibitor) may also be used for the initial treatment of DVT and PE, with no increase in bleeding over that observed with LMWH. Its lack of reversibility, long half-life, and primarily renal clearance limits its use in patients with an increased risk of bleeding or renal failure.

2. Warfarin—Patients with DVT with or without PE require a minimum of 3 months of anticoagulation in order to reduce the risk of recurrence of thrombosis. An oral vitamin K antagonist, such as warfarin, is usually initiated along with the parenteral anticoagulant, although patients with cancer-related thrombosis may benefit from ongoing treatment with LMWH alone. Most patients require 5 mg of warfarin daily for initial treatment, but lower doses (2.5 mg daily) should be considered for patients of Asian descent, the elderly, and those with hyperthyroidism, heart failure, liver disease, recent major surgery, malnutrition, certain polymorphisms for the CYP2C9 or the VKORC1 genes or who are receiving concurrent medications that increase sensitivity to warfarin. Conversely, individuals of African descent, those with larger body mass index or hypothyroidism, and those who are receiving medications that increase warfarin metabolism may require higher initial doses (7.5 mg daily). Daily INR results should guide dosing adjustments (Table 14–18). Web-based warfarin dosing calculators that consider these clinical and genetic factors are available to help clinicians choose the appropriate starting dose (eg, see www.warfarindosing.org). Because an average of 5 days is required to achieve a steady-state reduction in the activity of vitamin K–dependent coagulation factors, the parenteral anticoagulant should be continued for at least 5 days and until the INR is > 2.0 on 2 consecutive days. Meticulous follow-up should be arranged for all patients taking warfarin because of the bleeding risk that is associated with initiation of therapy. INR monitoring should occur at least twice weekly during initiation. Once stabilized, the INR should be checked at an interval no longer than every 6 weeks and warfarin dosing adjusted in accordance with the guidelines outlined in Table 14–19. Nontherapeutic INRs should be managed according to evidence-based guidelines (Table 14–20).

3. Target specific oral anticoagulants—The target specific oral anticoagulant agents have a predictable dose effect, few drug-drug interactions, rapid onset of action and freedom from laboratory monitoring. Rivaroxaban is approved as monotherapy for prevention of recurrent VTE in patients with new DVT or PE, with noninferior efficacy when compared to LMWH/warfarin and similar bleeding rates. While initially given twice daily, the dose is reduced to once daily after 3 weeks. Neither dabigatran

Table 14–15. Initial anticoagulation for VTE.[1]

Anticoagulant	Dose/Frequency	DVT, Lower Extremity	DVT, Upper Extremity	PE	VTE, with Concomitant Severe Renal Impairment[2]	VTE, Cancer-Related	Comment
Unfractionated heparin							
Unfractionated heparin	80 units/kg intravenous bolus, then continuous intravenous infusion of 18 units/kg/h	×	×	×	×		Bolus may be omitted if risk of bleeding is perceived to be elevated. Maximum bolus, 10,000 units. Requires aPTT monitoring. Most patients: begin warfarin at time of initiation of heparin
	330 units/kg subcutaneously × 1, then 250 units/kg subcutaneously every 12 hours	×					Fixed-dose; no aPTT monitoring required
LMWH and fondaparinux							
Enoxaparin[3]	1 mg/kg subcutaneously every 12 hours	×	× ×	×			Most patients: begin warfarin at time of initiation of LMWH
Dalteparin[3]	200 units/kg subcutaneously once daily for first month, then 150 units/kg/d	×	×	×		×	Cancer: administer LMWH for ≥ 3–6 months; reduce dose to 150 units/kg after first month of treatment
Fondaparinux	5–10 mg subcutaneously once daily (see Comment)	×	×	×			Use 7.5 mg for body weight 50–100 kg; 10 mg for body weight > 100 kg
Target specific oral anticoagulants							
Rivaroxaban	15 mg orally twice daily for first 3 weeks then 20 mg orally every bedtime						

Note: An "×" denotes appropriate use of the anticoagulant.
[1]Obtain baseline hemoglobin, platelet count, aPTT, PT/INR, creatinine, urinalysis, and hemoccult prior to initiation of anticoagulation. *Anticoagulation is contraindicated in the setting of active bleeding.*
[2]Defined as creatinine clearance < 30 mL/min.
[3]Body weight < 50 kg: reduce dose and monitor anti-Xa levels.
DVT, deep venous thrombosis; PE, pulmonary embolism; VTE, venous thromboembolic disease (includes DVT and PE).

nor apixaban are currently approved for treatment of VTE, but studies of both have demonstrated noninferiority for prevention of recurrent VTE when compared to standard therapy of LMWH and warfarin. As additional therapies become available for treatment of VTE, agent selection will depend on renal function, concomitant medications, ability to use LMWH bridge therapy, cost, and adherence.

4. Duration of anticoagulation therapy—The clinical scenario in which the thrombosis occurred is the strongest predictor of recurrence and, in most cases, guides duration of anticoagulation (Table 14–21). In the first year after discontinuation of anticoagulation therapy, the frequency of recurrence of VTE among individuals whose thrombosis occurred in the setting of a transient, major, reversible risk factor (such as surgery) is approximately 3%, compared with at least 8% for individuals whose thrombosis was unprovoked, and > 20% in patients with cancer. Patients with provoked VTE are generally treated with a minimum of 3 months of anticoagulation, whereas unprovoked VTE should prompt consideration of indefinite anticoagulation. Individual risk stratification may help identify patients most likely to suffer recurrent disease and thus most

Table 14–16. Patient selection for outpatient treatment of DVT.

Patients considered appropriate for outpatient treatment
No clinical signs or symptoms of PE and pain controlled
Motivated and capable of self-administration of injections
Confirmed prescription insurance that covers injectable medication or patient can pay out-of-pocket for injectable agents
Capable and willing to comply with frequent follow-up
Initially, patients may need to be seen daily to weekly
Potential contraindications for outpatient treatment
DVT involving inferior vena cava, iliac, common femoral, or upper extremity vein (these patients might benefit from vascular intervention)
Comorbid conditions
Active peptic ulcer disease, GI bleeding in past 14 days, liver synthetic dysfunction
Brain metastases, current or recent CNS or spinal cord injury/ surgery in the last 10 days, CVA ≤ 4–6 weeks
Familial bleeding diathesis
Active bleeding from source other than GI
Thrombocytopenia
Creatinine clearance < 30 mL/min
Patient weighs < 55 kg (male) or < 45 kg (female)
Recent surgery, spinal or epidural anesthesia in the past 3 days
History of heparin-induced thrombocytopenia
Inability to inject medication at home, reliably follow medication schedule, recognize changes in health status, understand or follow directions

CNS, central nervous system; CVA, cerebrovascular accident; DVT, deep venous thrombosis; GI, gastrointestinal; PE, pulmonary embolism.

likely to benefit from ongoing anticoagulation therapy. Normal D-dimer levels 1 month after cessation of anticoagulation are associated with lower recurrence risk, although some would argue not low enough to consider staying off therapy. A risk scoring system (proposed by

Table 14–17. Simplified Pulmonary Embolism Severity Index (PESI).

	Points	
Age > 80	1	
Cancer	1	
Chronic cardiopulmonary disease	1	
Systolic blood pressure < 100 mm Hg	1	
Oxygen saturation ≤ 90 %	1	
Severity Class	**Points**	**30-day Mortality**
Low risk	0	1%
High risk	≥ 1	10%

Adapted, with permission, from Jiménez D et al; RIETE Investigators. Simplification of the pulmonary embolism severity index for prognostication in patients with acute symptomatic pulmonary embolism. Arch Intern Med. 2010 Aug 9;170(15):1383–9. [PMID: 20696966]

Table 14–18. Warfarin adjustment guidelines for patients newly starting therapy.

	INR	Action
Day 1		5 mg (2.5 or 7.5 mg in select populations[1])
Day 2	< 1.5	Continue dose
	≥ 1.5	Decrease or hold dose[2]
Day 3	≤ 1.2	Increase dose[2]
	> 1.2 and < 1.7	Continue dose
	≥ 1.7	Decrease dose[2]
Day 4 until therapeutic	Daily increase is < 0.2 units	Increase dose[2]
	Daily increase 0.2–0.3 units	Continue dose
	Daily increase 0.4–0.6 units	Decrease dose[2]
	Daily increase ≥ 0.7 units	Hold dose

[1]See text
[2]In general, dosage adjustments should not exceed 2.5 mg or 50%.

Rodger et al in 2008) uses body mass index, age, D-dimer, and post-phlebitic symptoms to identify women at lower risk for recurrence after unprovoked VTE. The Vienna Prediction Model, a simple scoring system based on age, sex, D-dimer, and location of thrombosis, can help estimate an individual's recurrence risk to guide duration of therapy decisions. The following facts are important to consider when determining duration of therapy: (1) men have a greater than twofold higher risk of recurrent VTE compared to women; and (2) recurrent PE is more likely to develop in patients with clinically apparent PE than in those with DVT alone. Work-up for laboratory thrombophilia is not recommended routinely for determining duration of therapy because clinical presentation is a much stronger predictor of recurrence risk. This work-up may be pursued in patients younger than 50 years, with a strong family history, with a clot in unusual locations, or with recurrent thromboses (Table 14–22). In addition, a work-up for thrombophilia should be considered in women of childbearing age in whom results may influence fertility and pregnancy outcomes and management or in those patients in whom results will influence duration of therapy. The most important hypercoagulable state to identify is antiphospholipid syndrome [APS] because these patients have marked increase in recurrence rates, are at risk for both arterial and venous disease, and in general receive bridge therapy during any interruption of anticoagulation. Due to effects of anticoagulants and acute thrombosis on many of the tests, the thrombophilia work-up should be delayed in most cases until at least 3 months after the acute event, if it is indicated at all (Table 14–23). The benefit of anticoagulation must be weighed against the bleeding risks

Table 14–19. Warfarin-dosing adjustment guidelines for patients receiving long-term therapy.

Patient INR	Weekly Dosing Change	
	Dose change	Follow-up
≤ 1.5	↑ 15%	↑ Within 1 week
1.51–1.99	↑ 10% (many centers opt not to adjust if single INR 1.5-1.99 based on ACCP recommendations.)	↑ Within 1 week
2.0–3.01	Therapeutic	↑ 4 weeks if steady state
3.01-4.0-	↓ 10% (many centers opt not to adjust dose if single INR 3.1-3.5 based on ACCP recommendations)	Within 1 week
4.0-4.9	↓ 1 5– hold the dose for 1 day and then reduce it by 10%	Within 1 week, sooner if clinically indicated
5.0-8.99	↓ Clinical evaluation hold dose until INR therapeutic and then decreased by 15% per week	↓ Within 1 week, sooner if clinically indicated
≥9	See Table 14-20	

posed, and the benefit-risk ratio should be assessed at the initiation of therapy, at 3 months, and then at least annually in any patient receiving prolonged anticoagulant therapy. While bleeding risk scores have been developed to estimate risk of these complications, their performance may not offer any advantage over a clinician's subjective assessment, particularly in the elderly.

Compared with placebo, aspirin has been shown to reduce risk of recurrent VTE by 30% in patients with idiopathic VTE. Low-dose aspirin therapy should be considered in patients with unprovoked VTE who are not candidates for ongoing anticoagulation.

Agnelli G et al; AMPLIFY Investigators. Oral apixaban for the treatment of acute venous thromboembolism. N Engl J Med. 2013 Aug 29;369(9):799–808. [PMID: 23808982]

Aujesky D et al. Outpatient versus inpatient treatment for patients with acute pulmonary embolism: an international, open-label, randomised, non-inferiority trial. Lancet. 2011 Jul 2;378(9785):41–8. [PMID: 21703676]

Brighton TA et al; ASPIRE Investigators. Low-dose aspirin for preventing recurrent venous thromboembolism. N Engl J Med. 2012 Nov 22;367(21):1979–87. [PMID: 23121403]

EINSTEIN–PE Investigators;Büller HR et al. Oral rivaroxaban for the treatment of symptomatic pulmonary embolism. N Engl J Med. 2012 Apr 5;366(14):1287–97. [PMID: 22449293]

Table 14–20. American College of Chest Physicians Evidence-based Clinical Practice Guidelines for the Management of Nontherapeutic INR.

Clinical Situation	INR	Recommendations
No significant bleed	Above therapeutic range but < 5.0	• Lower dose or omit dose • Monitor more frequently and resume at lower dose when INR falls within therapeutic range (if INR only slightly above range, may not be necessary to decrease dose)
	≥ 5.0 but < 9.0	• Hold next 1–2 doses • Monitor more frequently and resume therapy at lower dose when INR falls within therapeutic range • *Patients at high risk for bleeding*[1]: Hold warfarin and consider giving vitamin K$_1$ 1–2.5 mg orally, check INR in 24–48 h to ensure response to therapy
	≥ 9.0	• Hold warfarin • Vitamin K$_1$ 2.5–5 mg orally • Monitor frequently and resume therapy at lower dose when INR within therapeutic range
Serious/life-threatening bleed		• Hold warfarin and give 10 mg vitamin K by slow intravenous infusion supplemented by FFP, PCC, or recombinant factor VIIa (PCC preferred)

[1]Patients at higher risk for bleeding include the elderly; conditions that increase the risk of bleeding include kidney disease, hypertension, falls, liver disease, and history of gastrointestinal or genitourinary bleeding.
FFP, fresh frozen plasma; INR, international normalized ratio; PCC, prothrombin complex concentrate.

Table 14–21. Duration of treatment of VTE.

Scenario	Suggested Duration of Therapy	Comments
Major transient risk factor (eg, immobilization, major surgery, major trauma, major hospitalization)	At least 3 months	VTE prophylaxis upon future exposure to transient risk factors
Minor transient risk factor (eg, exposure to exogenous estrogens/progestins, pregnancy, airline travel lasting more than 6 hours)	At least 3 months	VTE prophylaxis upon future exposure to transient risk factors
Cancer-related VTE	≥ 3–6 months or as long as cancer active, whichever is longer	LMWH recommended for initial treatment (see Table 14–15)
Unprovoked thrombosis	At least 3 months, consider indefinite if bleeding risk allows	May individually risk-stratify for recurrence with D-dimer, clinical risk scores and clinical presentation
Underlying significant thrombophilia (eg, antiphospho-lipid antibody syndrome, antithrombin deficiency, protein C deficiency, protein S deficiency, ≥ two concomitant thrombophilic conditions)	Indefinite	To avoid false positives, consider delaying investigation for laboratory thrombo-philia until 3 months after event

LMWH, low-molecular-weight heparin; VTE, venous thromboembolic disease.

Erkens PM et al. Does the Pulmonary Embolism Severity Index accurately identify low risk patients eligible for outpatient treatment? Thromb Res. 2012 Jun;129(6):710–4. [PMID: 21906787]

Heidbuchel H et al. European Heart Rhythm Association Practical Guide on the use of new oral anticoagulants in patients with non-valvular atrial fibrillation. Europace. 2013 May;15(5):625–51. [PMID: 23625942]

Jiménez D et al. Simplification of the Pulmonary Embolism Severity Index for prognostication in patients with acute symptomatic pulmonary embolism. Arch Intern Med. 2010;170(15):1383–9. [PMID: 20696966]

Kaatz S et al. Reversal of target-specific oral anticoagulants. J Thromb Thrombolysis. 2013 Aug;36(2):195–202. [PMID: 23657589]

Kearon C et al. Antithrombotic therapy for VTE disease: Antithrombotic Therapy and Prevention of Thrombosis, 9th ed: American College of Chest Physicians Evidence-Based Clinical Practice Guidelines. Chest. 2012 Feb;141(2 Suppl):e419S–94S. [PMID: 22315268]

Kyrle PA et al. Clinical scores to predict recurrence risk of venous thromboembolism. Thromb Haemost. 2012 Dec;108(6):1061–4. [PMID: 22872143]

Scherz N et al. Prospective, multicenter validation of prediction scores for major bleeding in elderly patients with venous thromboembolism. J Thromb Haemost. 2013 Mar;11(3):435–43. [PMID: 23279158]

Schulman S et al; RECOVER Study Group. Dabigatran versus warfarin in the treatment of acute venous thromboembolism. N Engl J Med. 2009 Dec 10;361(24):2342–52. [PMID: 19966341]

Van Spall HG et al. Variation in warfarin dose adjustment practice is responsible for differences in the quality of anticoagulation control between centers and countries: an analysis of patients receiving warfarin in the randomized evaluation of long-term anticoagulation therapy (RE-LY) trial. Circulation. 2012 Nov 6;126(19):2309–16. [PMID: 23027801]

C. Thrombolytic Therapy

Anticoagulation alone is appropriate treatment for most patients with PE; however, those with high-risk, massive PE, defined as PE with persistent hemodynamic instability, have an in-hospital mortality rate that approaches 30% and require immediate thrombolysis in combination with anticoagulation (Table 14–24). A 50% reduced dosing regimen for tissue plasminogen activator (TPA) has been proposed, offering similar efficacy with lower risk of complications. Thrombolytic therapy also has been used in selected patients with intermediate-risk, submassive PE, defined as PE without hemodynamic instability but with evidence of right ventricular compromise. This approach remains controversial, however, given the paucity of data showing a clinically significant benefit of thrombolysis.

Limited data suggest that patients with large proximal iliofemoral DVT may also benefit from catheter-directed thrombolysis in addition to treatment with anticoagulation. However, standardized guidelines are lacking, and use of the intervention may be limited by institutional availability and provider experience. Importantly, thrombolytics should be considered only in patients who have a low risk of bleeding, as rates of bleeding are increased in patients who receive these products compared with rates of hemorrhage in those who are treated with anticoagulation alone.

Table 14–22. Candidates for thrombophilia work-up if results will influence management.

Patients younger than 50 years
Strong family history of VTE
Clot in unusual locations
Recurrent thromboses
Women of childbearing age
Suspicion for APS

APS, antiphospholipid syndrome; VTE, venous thromboembolism.

Table 14–23. Laboratory evaluation of thrombophilia.

Hypercoagulable State	When to Suspect	Laboratory Work-Up	Influence of Anticoagulation and Acute Thrombosis
Antiphospholipid antibody syndrome	Unexplained DVT/PE CVA/TIA age < 50 Recurrent thrombosis (despite anticoagulation) Thrombosis at an unusual site Arterial and venous thrombosis Livedo reticularis, Raynaud phenomenon, thrombocytopenia, recurrent early pregnancy loss	Anti-cardiolipin IgG and/or IgM medium or high titer (ie, > 40 GPL or MPL, or > the 99th percentile)[1] Anti-beta-2 glycoprotein I IgG and/or IgM medium or high titer (> the 99th percentile)[1] Lupus anticoagulant[1]	Lupus anticoagulant can be falsely positive or falsely negative on anticoagulation
Protein C, S, antithrombin deficiencies	Thrombosis < 50 years of age with family history of VTE	Screen with protein C activity, protein S activity, antithrombin activity	Acute thrombosis can result in decreased protein C, S and antithrombin activity. Warfarin can decrease protein c and s activity, heparin can cause decrease antithrombin activity
Factor V Leiden, Prothrombin gene mutation	Thrombosis on OCPs, cerebral vein thrombosis, DVT/PE in white population	PCR for factor V Leiden or prothrombin gene mutation	No influence
Hyperhomocysteinemia		Fasting homocysteine	No influence

[1]Detected on two occasions not less than 12 weeks apart.
CVA/TIA, cerebrovascular accident/transient ischemic attack; DVT/PE, deep venous thrombosis/pulmonary embolism; OCPs, oral contraceptives; PCR, polymerase chain reaction; VTE, venous thromboembolism.

Enden T et al. Long-term outcome after additional catheter-directed thrombolysis versus standard treatment for acute iliofemoral deep vein thrombosis (the CaVenT study): a randomised controlled trial. Lancet. 2012 Jan 7;379(9810):31–8. [PMID: 22172244]

Howard LS. Thrombolytic therapy for submassive pulmonary embolus? PRO viewpoint. Thorax. 2014 Feb;69(2):103–5. [PMID: 23624534]

Jaff MR et al. Management of massive and submassive pulmonary embolism, iliofemoral deep vein thrombosis, and chronic thromboembolic pulmonary hypertension: a scientific statement from the American Heart Association. Circulation. 2011 Apr 26;123(16):1788–830. Erratum in: Circulation. 2012 Aug 14;126(7):e104. Circulation. 2012 Mar 20;125(11): e495. [PMID: 21422387]

Kearon C et al. Antithrombotic therapy for venous thromboembolic disease: American College of Chest Physicians Evidence-Based Clinical Practice Guideline (8th Edition). Chest. 2008 Jun;133(6 Suppl):454S–545S. [PMID: 18574272]

Simpson AJ. Thrombolysis for acute submassive pulmonary embolism: CON viewpoint. Thorax. 2014 Feb;69(2):105–7. [PMID: 24046127]

Wang C et al; China Venous Thromboembolism (VTE) Study Group. Efficacy and safety of low dose recombinant tissue-type plasminogen activator for the treatment of acute pulmonary thromboembolism: a randomized, multicenter, controlled trial. Chest. 2010 Feb;137(2):254–62. [PMID: 19741062]

D. Nonpharmacologic Therapy

1. Graduated compression stockings—In order to reduce the likelihood of the post-thrombotic syndrome, which is characterized by swelling, pain, and skin ulceration, all patients with DVT should wear a graduated compression stocking with 30–40 mm Hg pressure at the ankle on the affected lower extremity for 1–2 years. Stockings should be provided immediately to have the most impact on

Table 14–24. Thrombolytic therapies for acute massive pulmonary embolism.

Thrombolytic Agent	Dose	Frequency	Comment
Alteplase	100 mg	Continuous intravenous infusion over 2 hours	Follow with continuous intravenous infusion of unfractionated heparin (see Table 14–15 for dosage)
	100 mg	Intravenous bolus × 1	Appropriate for acute management of cardiac arrest and suspected pulmonary embolism
Urokinase	4400 international units/kg	Intravenous bolus × 1 followed by 4400 international units/kg continuous intravenous infusion for 12 hours	Unfractionated heparin should be administered concurrently (see Table 14–15 for dosage)

post-thrombotic syndrome; however, they are contraindicated in patients with peripheral vascular disease.

2. Inferior vena caval (IVC) filters—There is a paucity of data to support the use of IVC filters for the prevention of PE in any clinical scenario. There is only one available randomized, controlled trial of IVC filters for prevention of PE. In this study, patients with documented DVT received full intensity, time-limited anticoagulation with or without placement of an IVC filter. Patients with IVC filters had a lower rate of nonfatal PE at 12 days but an increased rate of DVT at 2 years. Most experts agree with placement of an IVC filter in patients with acute proximal DVT and an absolute contraindication to anticoagulation. While IVC filters were once commonly used to prevent VTE recurrence in the setting of anticoagulation failure, many experts now recommend switching to an alternative agent or increasing the intensity of the current anticoagulant regimen instead. The remainder of the indications (submassive/intermediate-risk PE, free-floating iliofemoral DVT, perioperative risk reduction) are controversial. If the contraindication to anticoagulation is temporary (active bleeding with subsequent resolution), placement of a retrievable IVC filter should be considered so that the device can be removed once anticoagulation has been started and has been shown to be tolerated. Rates of IVC filter retrieval are very low, often due to a failure to arrange for its removal. Thus, if a device is placed, removal should be arranged at the time of device placement.

Complications of IVC filters include local thrombosis, tilting, migration, fracture, and inability to retrieve the device. When considering placement of an IVC filter, it is best to consider both short- and long-term complications, since devices intended for removal may become permanent.

To improve patient safety, institutions should develop systems that guide appropriate patient selection for IVC filter placement, tracking, and removal.

PREPIC Study Group. Eight-year follow-up of patients with permanent vena cava filters in the prevention of pulmonary embolism: the PREPIC (Prévention du Risque d'Embolie Pulmonaire par Interruption Cave) randomized study. Circulation. 2005 Jul 19;112(3):416–22. [PMID: 16009794]

Sarosiek S et al. Indications, complications, and management of inferior vena cava filters: the experience in 952 patients at an academic hospital with a level I trauma center. JAMA Intern Med. 2013 Apr 8;173(7):513–7. [PMID: 23552968]

▶ **When to Refer**

- Presence of large iliofemoral VTE, IVC thrombosis, portal vein thrombosis, or Budd-Chiari syndrome for consideration of catheter-directed thrombolysis.
- Massive PE for urgent embolectomy.
- History of HIT or prolonged PTT plus renal failure for alternative anticoagulation regimens.
- Consideration of IVC filter placement.

▶ **When to Admit**

- Documented or suspected PE (some patients with low-risk PE may not require admission).
- DVT with poorly controlled pain, high bleeding risk, concerns about follow up.
- Large iliofemoral DVT for consideration of thrombolysis.
- Acute DVT and absolute contraindication to anticoagulation for IVC filter placement.

Gastrointestinal Disorders

Kenneth R. McQuaid, MD

DYSPEPSIA

 ESSENTIALS OF DIAGNOSIS

▶ Epigastric pain or burning, early satiety, or post-prandial fullness.

▶ Endoscopy is warranted in patients with alarm features or in those older than 55 years.

▶ All other patients should first undergo testing for *Helicobacter pylori* or a trial of empiric proton pump inhibitor.

▶ General Considerations

Dyspepsia refers to acute, chronic, or recurrent pain or discomfort centered in the upper abdomen. An international committee of clinical investigators (Rome III Committee) has defined dyspepsia as epigastric pain or burning, early satiety, or postprandial fullness. Heartburn (retrosternal burning) should be distinguished from dyspepsia. When heartburn is the dominant complaint, gastroesophageal reflux is nearly always present. Dyspepsia occurs in 15% of the adult population and accounts for 3% of general medical office visits.

▶ Etiology

A. Food or Drug Intolerance

Acute, self-limited "indigestion" may be caused by overeating, eating too quickly, eating high-fat foods, eating during stressful situations, or drinking too much alcohol or coffee. Many medications cause dyspepsia, including aspirin, nonsteroidal anti-inflammatory drugs (NSAIDs), antibiotics (metronidazole, macrolides), diabetes drugs (metformin, alpha-glucosidase inhibitors, amylin analogs, GLP-1 receptor antagonists), antihypertensive medications (angiotensin-converting enzyme [ACE] inhibitors, angiotensin-receptor blockers), cholesterol-lowering agents (niacin, fibrates), neuropsychiatric medications (cholinesterase inhibitors [donepezil, rivastigmine]), SSRIs (fluoxetine, sertraline), serotonin-norepinephrine-reuptake inhibitors (venlafaxine, duloxetine), Parkinson drugs (dopamine agonists, monoamine oxidase [MAO]-B inhibitors), corticosteroids, estrogens, digoxin, iron, and opioids.

B. Functional Dyspepsia

This is the most common cause of *chronic* dyspepsia. Up to three-fourths of patients have no obvious organic cause for their symptoms after evaluation. Symptoms may arise from a complex interaction of increased visceral afferent sensitivity, gastric delayed emptying or impaired accommodation to food, or psychosocial stressors. Although benign, these symptoms may be chronic and difficult to treat.

C. Luminal Gastrointestinal Tract Dysfunction

Peptic ulcer disease is present in 5–15% of patients with dyspepsia. Gastroesophageal reflux disease (GERD) is present in up to 20% of patients with dyspepsia, even without significant heartburn. Gastric or esophageal cancer is identified in 0.25–1% but is extremely rare in persons under age 55 years with uncomplicated dyspepsia. Other causes include gastroparesis (especially in diabetes mellitus), lactose intolerance or malabsorptive conditions, and parasitic infection (*Giardia, Strongyloides, Anisakis*).

D. *Helicobacter pylori* Infection

Although chronic gastric infection with *H pylori* is an important cause of peptic ulcer disease, it is an uncommon cause of dyspepsia in the absence of peptic ulcer disease. The prevalence of *H pylori*–associated chronic gastritis in patients with dyspepsia without peptic ulcer disease is 20–50%, the same as in the general population.

E. Pancreatic Disease

Pancreatic carcinoma and chronic pancreatitis may initially be mistaken for dyspepsia but usually are associated with more severe pain, anorexia and rapid weight loss, steatorrhea, or jaundice.

F. Biliary Tract Disease

The abrupt onset of epigastric or right upper quadrant pain due to cholelithiasis or choledocholithiasis should be readily distinguished from dyspepsia.

G. Other Conditions

Diabetes mellitus, thyroid disease, chronic kidney disease, myocardial ischemia, intra-abdominal malignancy, gastric volvulus or paraesophageal hernia, chronic gastric or intestinal ischemia, and pregnancy are sometimes accompanied by dyspepsia.

▶ Clinical Findings

A. Symptoms and Signs

Given the nonspecific nature of dyspeptic symptoms, the history has limited diagnostic utility. It should clarify the chronicity, location, and quality of the discomfort, and its relationship to meals. The discomfort may be characterized by one or more upper abdominal symptoms including epigastric pain or burning, early satiety, postprandial fullness, bloating, nausea, or vomiting. Concomitant weight loss, persistent vomiting, constant or severe pain, dysphagia, hematemesis, or melena warrants endoscopy or abdominal imaging. Potentially offending medications and excessive alcohol use should be identified and discontinued if possible. The patient's reason for seeking care should be determined. Recent changes in employment, marital discord, physical and sexual abuse, anxiety, depression, and fear of serious disease may all contribute to the development and reporting of symptoms. Patients with functional dyspepsia often are younger, report a variety of abdominal and extragastrointestinal complaints, show signs of anxiety or depression, or have a history of use of psychotropic medications.

The symptom profile alone does not differentiate between functional dyspepsia and organic gastrointestinal disorders. Based on the clinical history alone, primary care clinicians misdiagnose nearly half of patients with peptic ulcers or gastroesophageal reflux and have < 25% accuracy in diagnosing functional dyspepsia.

The physical examination is rarely helpful. Signs of serious organic disease such as weight loss, organomegaly, abdominal mass, or fecal occult blood are to be further evaluated.

B. Laboratory Findings

In patients older than age of 55 years, initial laboratory work should include a blood count, electrolytes, liver enzymes, calcium, and thyroid function tests. In patients younger than 55 years with uncomplicated dyspepsia (in whom gastric cancer is rare), initial noninvasive strategies should be pursued (see below). The cost-effectiveness of routine laboratory studies is uncertain. In most clinical settings, a noninvasive test for *H pylori* (urea breath test, fecal antigen test, or IgG serology) should be performed first. Although serologic tests are inexpensive, performance characteristics are poor in low-prevalence populations, whereas breath and fecal antigen tests have 95% accuracy.

If *H pylori* breath test or fecal antigen test results are negative in a patient not taking NSAIDs, peptic ulcer disease is virtually excluded.

C. Upper Endoscopy

Upper endoscopy is indicated to look for gastric cancer or other serious organic disease in all patients over age 55 years with new-onset dyspepsia and in all patients with "alarm" features, such as weight loss, dysphagia, recurrent vomiting, evidence of bleeding, or anemia. Upper endoscopy is the study of choice to diagnose gastroduodenal ulcers, erosive esophagitis, and upper gastrointestinal malignancy. It is also helpful for patients who are concerned about serious underlying disease. For patients born in regions in which there is a higher incidence of gastric cancer, such as Central or South America, China and Southeast Asia, or Africa, an age threshold of 45 years may be appropriate.

Endoscopic evaluation is also warranted when symptoms fail to respond to initial empiric management strategies within 4–8 weeks or when frequent symptom relapse occurs after discontinuation of antisecretory therapy.

D. Other Tests

In patients with refractory symptoms or progressive weight loss, antibodies for celiac disease or stool testing for ova and parasites or *Giardia* antigen, fat, or elastase may be considered. Abdominal imaging (ultrasonography or CT scanning) is performed only when pancreatic, biliary tract, vascular disease, or volvulus is suspected. Gastric emptying studies are valuable only in patients with recurrent vomiting. Ambulatory esophageal pH testing may be of value when atypical gastroesophageal reflux is suspected.

▶ Treatment

Initial empiric treatment is warranted for patients who are < 55 years and who have no alarm features (defined above). All other patients as well as patients whose symptoms fail to respond or relapse after empiric treatment should undergo upper endoscopy with subsequent treatment directed at the specific disorder (eg, peptic ulcer, gastroesophageal reflux, cancer). Most patients will have no significant findings on endoscopy and will be given a diagnosis of functional dyspepsia.

A. Empiric Therapy

Young patients with uncomplicated dyspepsia may be treated empirically with either a proton pump inhibitor or evaluated with a noninvasive test for *H pylori*, followed if positive by treatment. The prevalence of *H pylori* in the population influences recommendations for the timing of these empiric therapies. In clinical settings in which the prevalence of *H pylori* infection in the population is low (< 10%), it may be more cost-effective to initially treat patients with a 4-week trial of a proton pump inhibitor. Patients who have symptom relapse after discontinuation of the proton pump inhibitor should be tested for *H pylori* and treated if results are positive. In clinical settings in which *H pylori* prevalence is >10%, it may be more cost-effective to initially test patients for *H pylori* infection. *H pylori*–negative patients most likely have functional dyspepsia or atypical GERD and can be treated with an antisecretory agent (proton pump inhibitor) for 4 weeks. For patients who have symptom relapse after discontinuation of the proton pump inhibitor, intermittent or long-term proton pump inhibitor therapy may be considered. For patients in whom test results are positive for *H pylori*, antibiotic therapy proves definitive for patients with underlying peptic ulcers and may improve symptoms in a small subset (< 10%) of infected patients with functional dyspepsia. Patients with persistent dyspepsia after *H pylori* eradication can be given a trial of proton pump inhibitor therapy.

B. Treatment of Functional Dyspepsia

1. General measures—Most patients have mild, intermittent symptoms that respond to reassurance and lifestyle changes. Alcohol and caffeine should be reduced or discontinued. Patients with postprandial symptoms should be instructed to consume small, low-fat meals. A food diary, in which patients record their food intake, symptoms, and daily events, may reveal dietary or psychosocial precipitants of pain.

2. Pharmacologic agents—Drugs have demonstrated limited efficacy in the treatment of functional dyspepsia. One-third of patients derive relief from placebo. Antisecretory therapy for 4–8 weeks with oral proton pump inhibitors (omeprazole, esomeprazole, or rabeprazole 20 mg, dexlansoprazole or lansoprazole 30 mg, or pantoprazole 40 mg) may benefit 10–15% of patients, particularly those with dyspepsia characterized as epigastric pain ("ulcer-like dyspepsia") or dyspepsia and heartburn ("reflux-like dyspepsia"). Low doses of antidepressants (eg, desipramine or nortriptyline, 10–50 mg orally at bedtime) are believed to benefit some patients, possibly by moderating visceral afferent sensitivity. However, side effects are common and response is patient-specific. Doses should be increased slowly. Metoclopramide (5–10 mg three times daily) may improve symptoms, but improvement does not correlate with the presence or absence of gastric emptying delay. In 2009, the FDA issued a black box warning that metoclopramide use for more than 3 months is associated with a high incidence of tardive dyskinesia and should be avoided. The elderly, particularly elderly women, are most at risk.

3. Anti-*H pylori* treatment—Meta-analyses have suggested that a small number of patients with functional dyspepsia (< 10%) derive benefit from *H pylori* eradication therapy. Therefore, patients with functional dyspepsia should be tested and treated for *H pylori* as recommended above.

4. Alternative therapies—Psychotherapy and hypnotherapy may be of benefit in selected motivated patients with functional dyspepsia. Herbal therapies (peppermint, caraway) may offer benefit with little risk of adverse effects.

Ford AC et al. Dyspepsia. BMJ. 2013 Aug 29;347:f50509. [PMID: 23990632]

Mazzoleni LE et al. *Helicobacter pylori* eradication in functional dyspepsia: HEROES trial. Arch Intern Med. 2011 Nov 28;171(21):1929–36. [PMID: 22123802]

Zhao B et al. Efficacy of *Helicobacter pylori* eradication therapy on functional dyspepsia: a meta-analysis of randomized controlled studies with 12-month follow-up. J Clin Gastroenterol. 2014 Mar;48(3):241–7. [PMID: 24002127]

NAUSEA & VOMITING

Nausea is a vague, intensely disagreeable sensation of sickness or "queasiness" and is distinguished from anorexia. Vomiting often follows, as does retching (spasmodic respiratory and abdominal movements). Vomiting should be distinguished from regurgitation, the effortless reflux of liquid or food stomach contents; and from rumination, the chewing and swallowing of food that is regurgitated volitionally after meals.

The brainstem vomiting center is composed of a group of neuronal areas (area postrema, nucleus tractus solitarius, and central pattern generator) within the medulla that coordinate emesis. It may be stimulated by four different sources of afferent input: (1) Afferent vagal fibers from the gastrointestinal viscera are rich in serotonin 5-HT_3 receptors; these may be stimulated by biliary or gastrointestinal distention, mucosal or peritoneal irritation, or infections. (2) Fibers of the vestibular system, which have high concentrations of histamine H_1 and muscarinic cholinergic receptors. (3) Higher central nervous system centers (amygdala); here, certain sights, smells, or emotional experiences may induce vomiting. For example, patients receiving chemotherapy may start vomiting in anticipation of its administration. (4) The chemoreceptor trigger zone, located outside the blood-brain barrier in the area postrema of the medulla, which is rich in opioid, serotonin 5-HT_3, neurokinin 1 (NK_1) and dopamine D_2 receptors. This region may be stimulated by drugs and chemotherapeutic agents, toxins, hypoxia, uremia, acidosis, and radiation therapy. Although the causes of vomiting are many, a simplified list is provided in Table 15–1.

▶ Clinical Findings

A. Symptoms and Signs

Acute symptoms without abdominal pain are typically caused by food poisoning, infectious gastroenteritis, drugs, or systemic illness. Inquiry should be made into recent changes in medications, diet, other intestinal symptoms, or similar illnesses in family members. The acute onset of severe pain and vomiting suggests peritoneal irritation, acute gastric or intestinal obstruction, or pancreaticobiliary disease. Persistent vomiting suggests pregnancy, gastric outlet obstruction, gastroparesis, intestinal dysmotility, psychogenic disorders, and central nervous system or systemic disorders. Vomiting that occurs in the morning before breakfast is common with pregnancy, uremia, alcohol intake, and increased intracranial pressure. Vomiting immediately after meals strongly suggests bulimia or

Table 15–1. Causes of nausea and vomiting.

Visceral afferent stimulation	**Infections**
	Mechanical obstruction
	Gastric outlet obstruction: peptic ulcer disease, malignancy, gastric volvulus
	Small intestinal obstruction: adhesions, hernias, volvulus, Crohn disease, carcinomatosis
	Dysmotility
	Gastroparesis: diabetic, postviral, postvagotomy
	Small intestine: scleroderma, amyloidosis, chronic intestinal pseudo-obstruction, familial myoneuropathies
	Peritoneal irritation
	Peritonitis: perforated viscus, appendicitis, spontaneous bacterial peritonitis
	Viral gastroenteritis: Norwalk agent, rotavirus
	"Food poisoning": toxins from *Bacillus cereus, Staphylococcus aureus, Clostridium perfringens*
	Hepatitis A or B
	Acute systemic infections
	Hepatobiliary or pancreatic disorders
	Acute pancreatitis
	Cholecystitis or choledocholithiasis
	Topical gastrointestinal irritants
	Alcohol, NSAIDs, oral antibiotics
	Postoperative
	Other
	Cardiac disease: acute myocardial infarction, heart failure
	Urologic disease: stones, pyelonephritis
Vestibular disorders	**Vestibular disorders**
	Labyrinthitis, Meniere syndrome, motion sickness
CNS disorders	**Increased intracranial pressure**
	CNS tumors, subdural or subarachnoid hemorrhage
	Migraine
	Infections
	Meningitis, encephalitis
	Psychogenic
	Anticipatory vomiting, anorexia nervosa and bulimia, psychiatric disorders
Irritation of chemoreceptor trigger zone	**Antitumor chemotherapy**
	Medications and drugs
	Opioids
	Anticonvulsants
	Antiparkinsonism drugs
	Beta-blockers, antiarrhythmics, digoxin
	Nicotine
	Oral contraceptives
	Cholinesterase inhibitors
	Diabetes medications (metformin, acarbose, pramlintide, exenatide)
	Radiation therapy
	Systemic disorders
	Diabetic ketoacidosis
	Uremia
	Adrenocortical crisis
	Parathyroid disease
	Hypothyroidism
	Pregnancy
	Paraneoplastic syndrome

CNS, central nervous system; NSAIDs, nonsteroidal anti-inflammatory drugs.

psychogenic causes. Vomiting of undigested food one to several hours after meals is characteristic of gastroparesis or a gastric outlet obstruction; physical examination may reveal a succussion splash. Patients with acute or chronic symptoms should be asked about neurologic symptoms (eg, headache, stiff neck, vertigo, and focal paresthesias or weakness) that suggest a central nervous system cause.

B. Special Examinations

With vomiting that is severe or protracted, serum electrolytes should be obtained to look for hypokalemia, azotemia, or metabolic alkalosis resulting from loss of gastric contents. Flat and upright abdominal radiographs or abdominal CT are obtained in patients with severe pain or suspicion of mechanical obstruction to look for free intra-peritoneal air or dilated loops of small bowel. The cause of gastric outlet obstruction is best demonstrated by upper endoscopy, and the cause of small intestinal obstruction is best demonstrated with abdominal CT imaging. Gastropa-resis is confirmed by nuclear scintigraphic studies or ^{13}C-octanoic acid breath tests, which show delayed gastric emptying and either upper endoscopy or barium upper gastrointestinal series showing no evidence of mechanical gastric outlet obstruction. Abnormal liver biochemical tests or elevated amylase or lipase suggest pancreaticobili-ary disease, which may be investigated with an abdominal sonogram or CT scan. Central nervous system causes are best evaluated with either head CT or MRI.

▶ Complications

Complications include dehydration, hypokalemia, meta-bolic alkalosis, aspiration, rupture of the esophagus (Boer-haave syndrome), and bleeding secondary to a mucosal tear at the gastroesophageal junction (Mallory-Weiss syndrome).

▶ Treatment

A. General Measures

Most causes of acute vomiting are mild, self-limited, and require no specific treatment. Patients should ingest clear liquids (broths, tea, soups, carbonated beverages) and small quantities of dry foods (soda crackers). For more severe acute vomiting, hospitalization may be required. Patients unable to eat and losing gastric fluids may become dehydrated, resulting in hypokalemia with metabolic alka-losis. Intravenous 0.45% saline solution with 20 mEq/L of potassium chloride is given in most cases to maintain hydration. A nasogastric suction tube for gastric or mechanical small bowel obstruction improves patient comfort and permits monitoring of fluid loss.

B. Antiemetic Medications

Medications may be given either to prevent or to control vomiting. Combinations of drugs from different classes may provide better control of symptoms with less toxicity in some patients. Table 15–2 outlines common antiemetic dosing regimens.

1. Serotonin 5-HT$_3$-receptor antagonists—Ondansetron, granisetron, dolasetron, and palonosetron are effective in preventing chemotherapy- and radiation-induced emesis when initiated prior to treatment. Although 5-HT$_3$-recep-tor antagonists are effective as single agents for the preven-tion of chemotherapy-induced nausea and vomiting, their efficacy is enhanced by combination therapy with a corti-costeroid (dexamethasone) and NK$_1$-receptor antagonist (see below). Serotonin antagonists increasingly are used for the prevention of postoperative nausea and vomiting because of increased restrictions on the use of other anti-emetic agents (such as droperidol).

2. Corticosteroids—Corticosteroids (eg, dexamethasone) have antiemetic properties, but the basis for these effects is

Table 15–2. Common antiemetic dosing regimens.

	Dosage	Route
Serotonin 5-HT$_3$ antagonists		
Ondansetron	Doses vary: 4–8 mg twice daily for postoperative nausea and vomiting	Intravenously, orally
	8 mg twice daily for mod-erately or highly emeto-genic chemotherapy	Intravenously, orally
Granisetron	1 mg once daily	Intravenously
	1–2 mg once daily	Orally
Dolasetron	12.5 mg postoperatively	Intravenously
	100 mg once daily	Orally
Palonosetron	0.25 mg once as a single dose 30 min before start of chemotherapy	Intravenously
	0.5 mg once as single dose	Orally
Corticosteroids		
Dexamethasone	4 mg once pre-induction for prevention of post-operative nausea and vomiting	Intravenously, orally
	8 mg once daily for chemotherapy	Intravenously, orally
Methylprednisolone	40–100 mg once daily	Intravenously, intramuscu-larly, orally
Dopamine receptor antagonists		
Metoclopramide	10–20 mg or 0.5 mg/kg every 6–8 hours	Intravenously
	10–20 mg every 6–8 hours	Orally
Prochlorperazine	5–10 mg every 4–6 hours	Intravenously, intramuscu-larly, orally
	25 mg suppository every 6 hours	Per rectum
Promethazine	12.5–25 mg every 6–8 hours	Intravenously, orally
	25 mg every 6–8 hours	Per rectum
Trimethobenzamide	200 mg every 6–8 hours	Orally
	250–300 mg every 6–8 hours	Intravenously, orally
Neurokinin receptor antagonists[1]		
Aprepitant	125 mg once before che-motherapy; then 80 mg on day 1 and 2 after chemotherapy	Orally
Fosaprepitant	115 mg once 30 minutes before chemotherapy	Intravenously

[1]Neurokinin receptor antagonists are used solely for highly emeto-genic chemotherapy regimens in combination with 5-HT$_3$ antago-nists or dexamethasone or both.

unknown. These agents enhance the efficacy of serotonin receptor antagonists for preventing acute and delayed nausea and vomiting in patients receiving moderately to highly emetogenic chemotherapy regimens.

3. Neurokinin receptor antagonists—Aprepitant and fosaprepitant are highly selective antagonists for NK_1-receptors in the area postrema. They are used in combination with corticosteroids and serotonin antagonists for the prevention of acute and delayed nausea and vomiting with highly emetogenic chemotherapy regimens. Combined therapy with a neurokinin1 receptor antagonist prevents acute emesis in 80–90% and delayed emesis in > 70% of patients treated with highly emetogenic regimens.

4. Dopamine antagonists—The phenothiazines, butyrophenones, and substituted benzamides (eg, prochlorperazine, promethazine) have antiemetic properties that are due to dopaminergic blockade as well as to their sedative effects. High doses of these agents are associated with antidopaminergic side effects, including extrapyramidal reactions and depression. With the advent of more effective and safer antiemetics, these agents are infrequently used, mainly in outpatients with minor, self-limited symptoms.

5. Antihistamines and anticholinergics—These drugs (eg, meclizine, dimenhydrinate, transdermal scopolamine) may be valuable in the prevention of vomiting arising from stimulation of the labyrinth, ie, motion sickness, vertigo, and migraines. They may induce drowsiness. A combination of oral vitamin B_6 and doxylamine is recommended by the American College of Obstetricians and Gynecologists as first-line therapy for nausea and vomiting during pregnancy.

6. Cannabinoids—Marijuana has been used widely as an appetite stimulant and antiemetic. Pure Delta⁹-tetrahydrocannabinol (THC) is the major active ingredient in marijuana and the most psychoactive and is available by prescription as dronabinol. In doses of 5–15 mg/m², oral dronabinol is effective in treating nausea associated with chemotherapy, but it is associated with central nervous system side effects in most patients. Some states allow the use of medical marijuana with a clinician's certification. Strains of medical marijuana with different proportions of various naturally occurring cannabinoids (primarily THC and Cannabidiol [CBD]) can be chosen to minimize its psychoactive effects.

Basch E et al. Antiemetics: American Society of Clinical Oncology clinical practice guideline update. J Clin Oncol. 2011 Nov 1;29(31):4189–98. [PMID: 21947834]

Janelsins MC et al. Current pharmacotherapy for chemotherapy-induced nausea and vomiting in cancer patients. Expert Opin Pharmacother. 2013 Apr;14(6):757–66. [PMID: 23496347]

Lee NM et al. Nausea and vomiting of pregnancy. Gastroenterol Clin North Am. 2011 Jun;40(2):309–34. [PMID: 21601782]

HICCUPS (Singultus)

Though usually a benign and self-limited annoyance, hiccups may be persistent and a sign of serious underlying illness. In patients on mechanical ventilation, hiccups can trigger a full respiratory cycle and result in respiratory alkalosis.

Causes of benign, self-limited hiccups include gastric distention (carbonated beverages, air swallowing, overeating), sudden temperature changes (hot then cold liquids, hot then cold shower), alcohol ingestion, and states of heightened emotion (excitement, stress, laughing). There are over 100 causes of recurrent or persistent hiccups due to gastrointestinal, central nervous system, cardiovascular, and thoracic disorders.

▶ Clinical Findings

Evaluation of the patient with persistent hiccups should include a detailed neurologic examination, serum creatinine, liver chemistry tests, and a chest radiograph. When the cause remains unclear, CT or MRI of the head, chest, and abdomen, echocardiography, and upper endoscopy may help.

▶ Treatment

A number of simple remedies may be helpful in patients with acute benign hiccups. (1) Irritation of the nasopharynx by tongue traction, lifting the uvula with a spoon, catheter stimulation of the nasopharynx, or eating 1 teaspoon (tsp) (7 g) of dry granulated sugar. (2) Interruption of the respiratory cycle by breath holding, Valsalva maneuver, sneezing, gasping (fright stimulus), or rebreathing into a bag. (3) Stimulation of the vagus by carotid massage. (4) Irritation of the diaphragm by holding knees to chest or by continuous positive airway pressure during mechanical ventilation. (5) Relief of gastric distention by belching or insertion of a nasogastric tube.

A number of drugs have been promoted as being useful in the treatment of hiccups. Chlorpromazine, 25–50 mg orally or intramuscularly, is most commonly used. Other agents reported to be effective include anticonvulsants (phenytoin, carbamazepine), benzodiazepines (lorazepam, diazepam), metoclopramide, baclofen, gabapentin, and occasionally general anesthesia.

Bredenoord AJ. Management of belching, hiccups, and aerophagia. Clin Gastroenterol Hepatol. 2013 Jan;11(1):6–12. [PMID: 22982101]

Moretto EN et al. Interventions for treating persistent and intractable hiccups in adults. Cochrane Database Syst Rev. 2013 Jan 31;1:CD008768. [PMID: 23440833]

CONSTIPATION

Constipation occurs in 10–15% of adults and is a common reason for seeking medical attention. It is more common in women. The elderly are predisposed due to comorbid medical conditions, medications, poor eating habits, decreased mobility and, in some cases, inability to sit on a toilet (bed-bound patients). The first step in evaluating the patient is to determine what is meant by "constipation." Patients may define constipation as infrequent stools (fewer than three in a week), hard stools, excessive straining, or a sense of incomplete evacuation. Table 15–3 summarizes the many causes of constipation, which are discussed below.

Table 15–3. Causes of constipation in adults.

Most common
  Inadequate fiber or fluid intake
  Poor bowel habits
Systemic disease
  Endocrine: hypothyroidism, hyperparathyroidism, diabetes
    mellitus
  Metabolic: hypokalemia, hypercalcemia, uremia, porphyria
  Neurologic: Parkinson disease, multiple sclerosis, sacral nerve
    damage (prior pelvic surgery, tumor), paraplegia, autonomic
    neuropathy
Medications
  Opioids
  Diuretics
  Calcium channel blockers
  Anticholinergics
  Psychotropics
  Calcium and iron supplements
  NSAIDs
  Clonidine
  Cholestyramine
Structural abnormalities
  Anorectal: rectal prolapse, rectocele, rectal intussusception,
    anorectal stricture, anal fissure, solitary rectal ulcer syndrome
  Perineal descent
  Colonic mass with obstruction: adenocarcinoma
  Colonic stricture: radiation, ischemia, diverticulosis
  Hirschsprung disease
  Idiopathic megarectum
Slow colonic transit
  Idiopathic: isolated to colon
  Psychogenic
  Eating disorders
  Chronic intestinal pseudo-obstruction
Pelvic floor dyssynergia
Irritable bowel syndrome

NSAIDs, nonsteroidal anti-inflammatory drugs.

► Etiology

A. Primary Constipation

Most patients have constipation that cannot be attributed to any structural abnormalities or systemic disease. Some of these patients have normal colonic transit time; however, a subset have slow colonic transit or defecatory disorders. Normal colonic transit time is approximately 35 hours; more than 72 hours is significantly abnormal. Slow colonic transit is commonly idiopathic but may be part of a generalized gastrointestinal dysmotility syndrome. Patients may complain of infrequent bowel movements and abdominal bloating. Slow transit is more common in women, some of whom have a history of psychosocial problems (depression, anxiety, eating disorder, childhood trauma) or sexual abuse. Normal defecation requires coordination between relaxation of the anal sphincter and pelvic floor musculature while abdominal pressure is increased. Patients with defecatory disorders (also known as anismus or pelvic floor dyssynergia)—women more often than men—have impaired relaxation or paradoxical contraction of the anal sphincter and/or pelvic floor muscles during attempted defecation that impedes the bowel movement. This

problem may be acquired during childhood or adulthood. Patients may complain of excessive straining, sense of incomplete evacuation, or need for digital manipulation. Patients with primary complaints of abdominal pain or bloating with alterations in bowel habits (constipation, or alternating constipation and diarrhea) may have irritable bowel syndrome (see below).

B. Secondary Constipation

Constipation may be caused by systemic disorders, medications, or obstructing colonic lesions. Systemic disorders can cause constipation because of neurologic gut dysfunction, myopathies, endocrine disorders, or electrolyte abnormalities (eg, hypercalcemia or hypokalemia); medication side effects are often responsible (eg, anticholinergics or opioids). Colonic lesions that obstruct fecal passage, such as neoplasms and strictures, are an uncommon cause but important in new-onset constipation. Such lesions should be excluded in patients older than 50 years, in patients with "alarm" symptoms or signs (hematochezia, weight loss, anemia, or positive fecal occult blood tests [FOBT] or fecal immunochemical tests [FIT]), and in patients with a family history of colon cancer or inflammatory bowel disease. Defecatory difficulties also can be due to a variety of anorectal problems that impede or obstruct flow (perineal descent, rectal prolapse, rectocele), some of which may require surgery, and Hirschsprung disease (usually suggested by lifelong constipation).

► Clinical Findings

A. Symptoms and Signs

All patients should undergo a history and physical examination to distinguish primary from secondary causes of constipation. Physical examination should include digital rectal examination with assessment for anatomic abnormalities, such as anal stricture, rectocele, rectal prolapse, or perineal descent during straining as well as assessment of pelvic floor motion during simulated defecation (ie, the patient's ability to "expel the examiner's finger"). Further diagnostic tests should be performed in patients with any of the following: age 50 years or older, severe constipation, signs of an organic disorders, alarm symptoms (hematochezia, weight loss, positive FOBT or FIT), or a family history of colon cancer or inflammatory bowel disease. These tests should include laboratory studies (complete blood count; serum electrolytes, calcium, glucose, and thyroid-stimulating hormone); and a colonoscopy or flexible sigmoidoscopy.

B. Special Examinations

Patients with refractory constipation not responding to routine medical management warrant further diagnostic studies, including pelvic floor function and colonic transit studies, in order to distinguish slow colonic transit from defecatory disorders. Colon transit time is most commonly measured by performing an abdominal radiograph 120 hours after ingestion of 24 radiopaque markers. Retention of > 20% of the markers indicates prolonged transit.

Defecatory disorders are assessed with balloon expulsion testing, anal manometry, and defecography.

▶ Treatment

A. Chronic Constipation

1. Dietary and lifestyle measures—Adverse psychosocial issues should be identified and addressed. Patients should be instructed on normal defecatory function and optimal toileting habits, including regular timing, proper positioning, and abdominal pressure. Adequate dietary fluid and fiber intake should be emphasized. A trial of fiber supplements is recommended (Table 15–4). Increased dietary fiber may cause distention or flatulence, which often diminishes over several days. Response to fiber therapy is not immediate, and increases in dosage should be made gradually over 7–10 days. Fiber is most likely to benefit patients with normal colonic transit, but it may not benefit patients with colonic inertia, defecatory disorders, opioid-induced constipation, or irritable bowel syndrome;

Table 15–4. Pharmacologic management of constipation.

Agent	Dosage	Onset of Action	Comments
Fiber laxatives			
Bran powder	1–4 tbsp orally twice daily	Days	Inexpensive; may cause gas, flatulence
Psyllium	1 tsp once or twice daily	Days	(Metamucil; Perdiem)
Methylcellulose	1 tsp once or twice daily	Days	(Citrucel) Less gas, flatulence
Calcium polycarbophil	1 or 2 tablets once or twice daily	12–24 hours	(FiberCon) Does not cause gas; pill form
Guargum	1 tbsp once or twice daily	Days	(Benefiber) Non-gritty, tasteless, less gas
Stool surfactants			
Docusate sodium	100 mg once or twice daily	12–72 hours	(Colace) Marginal benefit
Mineral oil	15–45 mL once or twice daily	6–8 hours	May cause lipoid pneumonia if aspirated
Osmotic laxatives			
Magnesium hydroxide	15–30 mL orally once or twice daily	6–24 hours	(Milk of magnesia; Epsom salts)
Lactulose or 70% sorbitol	15–60 mL orally once daily to three times daily	6–48 hours	Cramps, bloating, flatulence
Polyethylene glycol (PEG 3350)	17 g in 8 oz liquid once or twice daily	6–24 hours	(Miralax) Less bloating than lactulose, sorbitol
Stimulant laxatives			
Bisacodyl	5–20 mg orally as needed	6–8 hours	May cause cramps; avoid daily use if possible
Bisacodyl suppository	10 mg per rectum as needed	1 hour	
Cascara	4–8 mL or 2 tablets as needed	8–12 hours	(Nature's Remedy) May cause cramps; avoid daily use if possible
Senna	8.6–17.2 mg orally as needed	8–12 hours	(ExLax; Senekot) May cause cramps; avoid daily use if possible
Lubiprostone	24 mcg orally twice daily	12–48 hours	Expensive; may cause nausea. Contraindicated in pregnancy
Linaclotide	145 mcg orally once daily		Expensive; contraindicated in pediatric patients
Enemas			
Tap water	500 mL per rectum	5–15 minutes	
Sodium phosphate enema	120 mL per rectum	5–15 minutes	Commonly used for acute constipation or to induce movement prior to medical procedures
Mineral oil enema	100–250 mL per rectum		To soften and lubricate fecal impaction
Agents used for acute purgative or to clean bowel prior to medical procedures			
Polyethylene glycol (PEG 3350)	4 L orally administered over 2–4 hours	< 4 hours	(GoLYTELY; CoLYTE; NuLYTE, MoviPrep) Used to cleanse bowel before colonoscopy
Magnesium citrate	10 oz orally	3–6 hours	Lemon-flavored

it may even exacerbate symptoms in these patients. Regular exercise is associated with a decreased risk of constipation. When possible, discontinue medications that may be causing or contributing to constipation.

2. Laxatives—Laxatives may be given on an intermittent or chronic basis for constipation that does not respond to dietary and lifestyle changes (Table 15–4). There is no evidence that long-term use of these agents is harmful.

A. OSMOTIC LAXATIVES—Treatment usually is initiated with regular (daily) use of an osmotic laxative. Nonabsorbable osmotic agents increase secretion of water into the intestinal lumen, thereby softening stools and promoting defecation. Magnesium hydroxide, nondigestible carbohydrates (sorbitol, lactulose), and polyethylene glycol are all efficacious and safe for treating acute and chronic cases. The dosages are adjusted to achieve soft to semi-liquid movements. Magnesium-containing saline laxatives should not be given to patients with chronic renal insufficiency. Nondigestible carbohydrates may induce bloating, cramps, and flatulence. Polyethylene glycol 3350 (Miralax) is a component of solutions traditionally used for colonic lavage prior to colonoscopy and does not cause flatulence. When used in conventional doses, the onset of action of these osmotic agents is generally within 24 hours. For more rapid treatment of acute constipation, purgative laxatives may be used, such as magnesium citrate. Magnesium citrate may cause hypermagnesemia.

B. STIMULANT LAXATIVES—For patients with incomplete response to osmotic agents, stimulant laxatives may be prescribed as needed as a "rescue" agent or on a regular basis three or four times a week. These agents stimulate fluid secretion and colonic contraction, resulting in a bowel movement within 6–12 hours after oral ingestion or 15–60 minutes after rectal administration. Oral agents are usually administered once daily at bedtime. Common preparations include bisacodyl, senna, and cascara (Table 15–4).

C. CHLORIDE SECRETORY AGENTS—Lubiprostone and linaclotide stimulate intestinal chloride secretion through activation of chloride channels or guanylcyclase C, respectively, resulting in increased intestinal fluid and accelerated colonic transit. In multicenter controlled trials, patients treated with lubiprostone 24 mcg orally twice daily or linaclotide 145 mcg once daily increased the number of bowel movements compared with patients treated with placebo. Lubiprostone is associated with nausea in up to one-third of patients and should not be given to women who may be pregnant (category C). Because these agents are expensive, they should be reserved for patients who have suboptimal response or side effects with less expensive agents.

D. OPIOID-RECEPTOR ANTAGONISTS—Long-term use of opioids can cause constipation by inhibiting peristalsis and increasing intestinal fluid absorption. Methylnaltrexone is a mu-opioid receptor antagonist that blocks peripheral opioid receptors (including the gastrointestinal tract) without affecting central analgesia. It is approved for the treatment of opioid-induced constipation in patients receiving palliative care for advanced illness who have not responded to conventional laxative regimens. In controlled trials, methylnaltrexone subcutaneously (8 mg [38–62 kg], 12 mg [62–114 kg], or 0.15 mg/kg [less 38 kg] every other day) achieves laxation in 50% of patients compared with 15% of patients who received placebo.

B. Fecal Impaction

Severe impaction of stool in the rectal vault may result in obstruction to further fecal flow, leading to partial or complete large bowel obstruction. Predisposing factors include medications (eg, opioids), severe psychiatric disease, prolonged bed rest, neurogenic disorders of the colon, and spinal cord disorders. Clinical presentation includes decreased appetite, nausea, and vomiting, and abdominal pain and distention. There may be paradoxical "diarrhea" as liquid stool leaks around the impacted feces. Firm feces are palpable on digital examination of the rectal vault. Initial treatment is directed at relieving the impaction with enemas (saline, mineral oil, or diatrizoate) or digital disruption of the impacted fecal material. Long-term care is directed at maintaining soft stools and regular bowel movements (as above).

▶ **When to Refer**

- Patients with refractory constipation for anorectal testing.

- Patients with defecatory disorders may benefit from biofeedback therapy.

- Patients with alarm symptoms or who are over age 50 should be referred for colonoscopy.

- Rarely, surgery (subtotal colectomy) is required for patients with severe colonic inertia.

American Gastroenterological Association medical position statement on constipation. Gastroenterology. 2013 Jan;144(1): 211–7. [PMID: 23261064]

Bader S et al. Methylnaltrexone for the treatment of opioid-induced constipation. Expert Rev Gastroenterol Hepatol. 2013 Jan;7(1):13–26. [PMID: 23265145]

Ford AC. Laxatives for chronic constipation in adults. BMJ. 2012 Oct 1;345:e6168. [PMID: 23028096]

Lembo AJ et al. Two randomized trials of linaclotide for chronic constipation. N Engl J Med. 2011 Aug 11;365(6):527–36. [PMID: 21830967]

GASTROINTESTINAL GAS

▶ **Belching**

Belching (eructation) is the involuntary or voluntary release of gas from the stomach or esophagus. It occurs most frequently after meals, when gastric distention results in transient lower esophageal sphincter (LES) relaxation. Belching is a normal reflex and does not itself denote gastrointestinal dysfunction. Virtually all stomach gas comes from swallowed air. With each swallow, 2–5 mL of air is ingested, and excessive amounts may result in distention, flatulence, and abdominal pain. This may occur with rapid eating, gum chewing, smoking, and the ingestion of carbonated beverages. Evaluation should be restricted to patients with other complaints such as dysphagia, heartburn, early satiety, or vomiting.

Chronic excessive belching is almost always caused by supragastric belching (voluntary diaphragmatic contraction, followed by upper esophageal relaxation with air inflow to the esophagus) or true air swallowing (aerophagia), both of which are behavioral disorders that are more common in patients with anxiety or psychiatric disorders. These patients may benefit from referral to a behavioral or speech therapist.

► Flatus

The rate and volume of expulsion of flatus is highly variable. Healthy adults pass flatus up to 20 times daily and excrete up to 1500 mL. Flatus is derived from two sources: swallowed air (primarily nitrogen) and bacterial fermentation of undigested carbohydrate (which produces H_2, CO_2, and methane). A number of short-chain carbohydrates (fermentable oligosaccharides, disaccharides, monosaccharides, and polypols or "FODMAPS") are incompletely absorbed in the small intestine and pass into the colon. These include lactose (dairy products); fructose (fruits, corn syrups, and some sweeteners); polypols (stone-fruits, mushrooms, and some sweeteners); and fructans (legumes, cruciferous vegetables, pasta, and whole grains). Abnormal gas production may be caused by increased ingestion of these carbohydrates or, less commonly, by disorders of malabsorption. Foul odor may be caused by garlic, onion, eggplant, mushrooms, and certain herbs and spices.

Determining abnormal from normal amounts of flatus is difficult. Patients with a long-standing history of flatulence and no other symptoms or signs of malabsorption disorders can be treated conservatively. Gum chewing and carbonated beverages should be avoided to reduce air swallowing. Lactose intolerance may be assessed by a 2-week trial of a lactose-free diet or by a hydrogen breath test. A list of foods containing FODMAPS should be provided. Multiple low-FODMAP dietary guides are available; however, referral to a knowledgeable dietician may be helpful.

The nonprescription agent Beano (alpha-d-galactosidase enzyme) reduces gas caused by foods containing galacto-oligosaccharides (legumes, chickpeas, lentils) but not other FODMAPS. Activated charcoal may afford relief. Simethicone is of no proved benefit.

Complaints of chronic abdominal distention or bloating are common. Some of these patients may produce excess gas. However, many patients have impaired small bowel gas propulsion or enhanced visceral sensitivity to gas distention. Many of these patients have an underlying functional gastrointestinal disorder such as irritable bowel syndrome or functional dyspepsia. Reduction of dietary fat, which delays intestinal gas clearance, may be helpful. Rifaximin, 400 mg twice daily, a nonabsorbable oral antibiotic with high activity against enteric bacteria, has been shown to reduce abdominal bloating and flatulence in approximately 40% of treated patients compared with 20% of controls. Symptom improvement may be attributable to suppression of gas-producing colonic bacteria; however, relapse occurs within days after stopping the antibiotic. Further trials are needed to clarify the role of nonabsorbable antibiotics in symptom management. Many patients report reduced flatus production with use of probiotics, although there has been limited controlled study of these agents for this purpose. Patients interested in complementary medical therapies may be offered a trial of 4–8 ounces daily of Kefir, a commercially available fermented milk drink containing multiple probiotics.

Gibson PR et al. Food choice as a key management strategy for functional gastrointestinal symptoms. Am J Gastroenterol. 2012 May;107(5):657–66. [PMID: 22488077]
Shepherd SJ et al. Short-chain carbohydrates and functional gastrointestinal disorders. Am J Gastroenterol. 2013 May;108(5):707–17. [PMID: 23588241]

DIARRHEA

Diarrhea can range in severity from an acute self-limited episode to a severe, life-threatening illness. To properly evaluate the complaint, the clinician must determine the patient's normal bowel pattern and the nature of the current symptoms.

Approximately 10 L of fluid enter the duodenum daily, of which all but 1.5 L are absorbed by the small intestine. The colon absorbs most of the remaining fluid, with < 200 mL lost in the stool. Although diarrhea sometimes is defined as a stool weight of more than 200–300 g/24 h, quantification of stool weight is necessary only in some patients with chronic diarrhea. In most cases, the physician's working definition of diarrhea is increased stool frequency (more than three bowel movements per day) or liquidity of feces.

The causes of diarrhea are myriad. In clinical practice, it is helpful to distinguish acute from chronic diarrhea, as the evaluation and treatment are entirely different (Tables 15–5 and 15–6).

Table 15–5. Causes of acute infectious diarrhea.

Noninflammatory Diarrhea	Inflammatory Diarrhea
Viral Noroviruses Rotavirus	**Viral** Cytomegalovirus
Protozoal Giardia lamblia Cryptosporidium Cyclospora	**Protozoal** Entamoeba histolytica

Bacterial
1. Preformed enterotoxin production
    Staphylococcus aureus
    Bacillus cereus
    Clostridium perfringens
2. Enterotoxin production
    Enterotoxigenic E coli (ETEC)
    Vibrio cholerae
	Bacterial
	1. Cytotoxin production
	    Enterohemorrhagic E coli O157:H5 (EHEC)
	    Vibrio parahaemolyticus
	    Clostridium difficile
	2. Mucosal invasion
	    Shigella
	    Campylobacter jejuni
	    Salmonella
	    Enteroinvasive E coli (EIEC)
	    Aeromonas
	    Plesiomonas
	    Yersinia enterocolitica
	    Chlamydia
	    Neisseria gonorrhoeae
	    Listeria monocytogenes

Table 15–6. Causes of chronic diarrhea.

Osmotic diarrhea
CLUES: Stool volume decreases with fasting; increased stool osmotic gap
  1. Medications: antacids, lactulose, sorbitol
  2. Disaccharidase deficiency: lactose intolerance
  3. Factitious diarrhea: magnesium (antacids, laxatives)
Secretory diarrhea
CLUES: Large volume (> 1 L/d); little change with fasting; normal stool osmotic gap
  1. Hormonally mediated: VIPoma, carcinoid, medullary carcinoma of thyroid (calcitonin), Zollinger-Ellison syndrome (gastrin)
  2. Factitious diarrhea (laxative abuse); phenolphthalein, cascara, senna
  3. Villous adenoma
  4. Bile salt malabsorption (idiopathic, ileal resection; Crohn ileitis; postcholecystectomy)
  5. Medications
Inflammatory conditions
CLUES: Fever, hematochezia, abdominal pain
  1. Ulcerative colitis
  2. Crohn disease
  3. Microscopic colitis
  4. Malignancy: lymphoma, adenocarcinoma (with obstruction and pseudodiarrhea)
  5. Radiation enteritis
Medications
Common offenders: SSRIs, cholinesterase inhibitors, NSAIDs, proton pump inhibitors, angiotensin II receptor blockers, metformin, allopurinol
	Malabsorption syndromes
	CLUES: Weight loss, abnormal laboratory values; fecal fat > 10 g/24h
	  1. Small bowel mucosal disorders: celiac sprue, tropical sprue, Whipple disease, eosinophilic gastroenteritis, small bowel resection (short bowel syndrome), Crohn disease
	  2. Lymphatic obstruction: lymphoma, carcinoid, infectious (tuberculosis, MAI), Kaposi sarcoma, sarcoidosis, retroperitoneal fibrosis
	  3. Pancreatic disease: chronic pancreatitis, pancreatic carcinoma
	  4. Bacterial overgrowth: motility disorders (diabetes, vagotomy), scleroderma, fistulas, small intestinal diverticula
	Motility disorders
	CLUES: Systemic disease or prior abdominal surgery
	  1. Postsurgical: vagotomy, partial gastrectomy, blind loop with bacterial overgrowth
	  2. Systemic disorders: scleroderma, diabetes mellitus, hyperthyroidism
	  3. Irritable bowel syndrome
	Chronic infections
	  1. Parasites: *Giardia lamblia, Entamoeba histolytica, Strongyloidiasis stercoralis, Capillaria philippinensis*
	  2. AIDS-related:
	    Viral: Cytomegalovirus, HIV infection (?)
	    Bacterial: *Clostridium difficile, Mycobacterium avium* complex
	    Protozoal: Microsporida *(Enterocytozoon bieneusi),* *Cryptosporidium, Isospora belli*
	Factitious
	See Osmotic and Secretory diarrhea above

MAI, *Mycobacterium avium-intracellulare;* NSAIDs, nonsteroidal anti-inflammatory drugs; SSRIs, selective serotonin reuptake inhibitors.

1. Acute Diarrhea

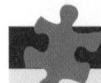

ESSENTIALS OF DIAGNOSIS

▶ Diarrhea of < 2 weeks duration is most commonly caused by invasive or noninvasive pathogens and their enterotoxins.

Acute noninflammatory diarrhea

▶ Watery, nonbloody.

▶ Usually mild, self-limited.

▶ Caused by a virus or noninvasive bacteria.

▶ Diagnostic evaluation is limited to patients with diarrhea that is severe or persists beyond 7 days.

Acute inflammatory diarrhea

▶ Blood or pus, fever.

▶ Usually caused by an invasive or toxin-producing bacterium.

▶ Diagnostic evaluation requires routine stool bacterial cultures (including *E coli* O157:H7) in all and testing as clinically indicated for *Clostridium difficile* toxin, and ova and parasites.

▶ Etiology & Clinical Findings

Diarrhea acute in onset and persisting for < 2 weeks is most commonly caused by infectious agents, bacterial toxins (either preformed or produced in the gut), or medications. Community outbreaks (including nursing homes, schools, cruise ships) suggest a viral etiology or a common food source. Similar recent illnesses in family members suggest an infectious origin. Ingestion of improperly stored or prepared food implicates food poisoning. Pregnant women have an increased risk of developing listeriosis. Day care attendance or exposure to unpurified water (camping, swimming) may result in infection with *Giardia* or *Cryptosporidium*. Large *Cyclospora* outbreaks have been traced to contaminated produce. Recent travel abroad suggests "traveler's diarrhea" (see Chapter 30). Antibiotic administration within the preceding several weeks increases the likelihood of *C difficile* colitis. Finally, risk factors for HIV infection or sexually transmitted diseases should be determined. (AIDS-associated diarrhea is discussed in Chapter 31; infectious proctitis is discussed in this chapter under Anorectal Disorders.) Persons engaging in anal intercourse or oral-anal sexual activities are at risk for a variety of infections that cause proctitis, including gonorrhea, syphilis, lymphogranuloma venereum, and herpes simplex.

The nature of the diarrhea helps distinguish among different infectious causes (Table 15–5).

A. Noninflammatory Diarrhea

Watery, nonbloody diarrhea associated with periumbilical cramps, bloating, nausea, or vomiting suggests a small bowel source caused by either a toxin-producing bacterium (enterotoxigenic *E coli* [ETEC], *Staphylococcus aureus, Bacillus cereus, Clostridium perfringens*) or other agents (viruses, *Giardia*) that disrupt normal absorption and secretory process in the small intestine. Prominent vomiting suggests viral enteritis or *S aureus* food poisoning. Although typically mild, the diarrhea (which originates in the small intestine) can be voluminous and result in dehydration with hypokalemia and metabolic acidosis (eg, cholera). Because tissue invasion does not occur, fecal leukocytes are not present.

B. Inflammatory Diarrhea

The presence of fever and bloody diarrhea (dysentery) indicates colonic tissue damage caused by invasion (shigellosis, salmonellosis, *Campylobacter* or *Yersinia* infection, amebiasis) or a toxin (*C difficile*, Shiga-toxin–producing *E coli* [STEC; also known as enterohemorrhagic *E coli*]). Because these organisms involve predominantly the colon, the diarrhea is small in volume (< 1 L/d) and associated with left lower quadrant cramps, urgency, and tenesmus. Fecal leukocytes or lactoferrin usually are present in infections with invasive organisms. *E coli* O157:H7 is a Shiga toxin-producing noninvasive organism most commonly acquired from contaminated meat that has resulted in several outbreaks of an acute, often severe hemorrhagic colitis. In 2011, an outbreak of severe gastroenteritis in Germany, caused by an unusual Shiga-toxin–producing strain, *E coli* O104:H4, was traced to contaminated sprouts. A major complication of STEC is hemolytic-uremic syndrome, which develops in 6–22% of cases. In immunocompromised and HIV-infected patients, cytomegalovirus (CMV) can cause intestinal ulceration with watery or bloody diarrhea.

Infectious dysentery must be distinguished from acute ulcerative colitis, which may also present acutely with fever, abdominal pain, and bloody diarrhea. Diarrhea that persists for more than 14 days is not attributable to bacterial pathogens (except for *C difficile*) and should be evaluated as chronic diarrhea.

▶ Evaluation

In over 90% of patients with acute noninflammatory diarrhea, the illness is mild and self-limited, responding within 5 days to simple rehydration therapy or antidiarrheal agents; diagnostic investigation is unnecessary.

The isolation rate of bacterial pathogens from stool cultures in patients with acute noninflammatory diarrhea is under 3%. Thus, the goal of initial evaluation is to distinguish patients with mild disease from those with more serious illness. If diarrhea worsens or persists for more than 7 days, stool should be sent for fecal leukocyte or lactoferrin determination, ovum and parasite evaluation, and bacterial culture.

Prompt medical evaluation is indicated in the following situations (Figure 15–1): (1) Signs of inflammatory diarrhea manifested by any of the following: fever (> 38.5°C), bloody diarrhea, or severe abdominal pain. (2) The passage of six or more unformed stools in 24 hours. (3) Profuse watery diarrhea and dehydration. (4) Frail older patients. (5) Immunocompromised patients (AIDS, posttransplantation). (6) Hospital-acquired diarrhea (onset following at least 3 days of hospitalization). (7) Systemic illness.

Physical examination pays note to the patient's level of hydration, mental status, and the presence of abdominal tenderness or peritonitis. Peritoneal findings may be present in infection with *C difficile* or STEC. Hospitalization is required in patients with severe dehydration, marked abdominal pain, or altered mental status. Stool specimens should be sent for examination for routine bacterial cultures.

The rate of positive bacterial cultures in such patients is 60–75%. For bloody stools, the laboratory should be directed to perform serotyping for Shiga-toxin–producing *E coli*. Special culture media are required for *Yersinia, Vibrio,* and *Aeromonas*. In patients who are hospitalized or who have a history of antibiotic exposure, a stool sample should be tested for *C difficile* toxin.

In patients with diarrhea that persists for more than 10 days, who have a history of travel to areas where amebiasis is endemic, or who engage in oral-anal sexual practices, three stool examinations for ova and parasites should also be performed. The stool antigen detection tests for both *Giardia* and *Entamoeba histolytica* are more sensitive than stool microscopy for detection of these organisms. A serum antigen detection test for *E histolytica* is also available. *Cyclospora* and *Cryptosporidium* are detected by fecal acid-fast staining.

▶ Treatment

A. Diet

Most mild diarrhea will not lead to dehydration provided the patient takes adequate oral fluids containing carbohydrates and electrolytes. Patients find it more comfortable to rest the bowel by avoiding high-fiber foods, fats, milk products, caffeine, and alcohol. Frequent feedings of tea, "flat" carbonated beverages, and soft, easily digested foods (eg, soups, crackers, bananas, applesauce, rice, toast) are encouraged.

B. Rehydration

In more severe diarrhea, dehydration can occur quickly, especially in children, the frail, and the elderly. Oral rehydration with fluids containing glucose, Na$^+$, K$^+$, Cl$^-$, and bicarbonate or citrate is preferred when feasible. A convenient mixture is ½ tsp salt (3.5 g), 1 tsp baking soda (2.5 g NaHCO$_3$), 8 tsp sugar (40 g), and 8 oz orange juice (1.5 g KCl), diluted to 1 L with water. Alternatively, oral electrolyte solutions (eg, Pedialyte, Gatorade) are readily available. Fluids should be given at rates of 50–200 mL/kg/24 h depending on the hydration status. Intravenous fluids (lactated Ringer injection) are preferred in patients with severe dehydration.

C. Antidiarrheal Agents

Antidiarrheal agents may be used safely in patients with mild to moderate diarrheal illnesses to improve patient comfort.

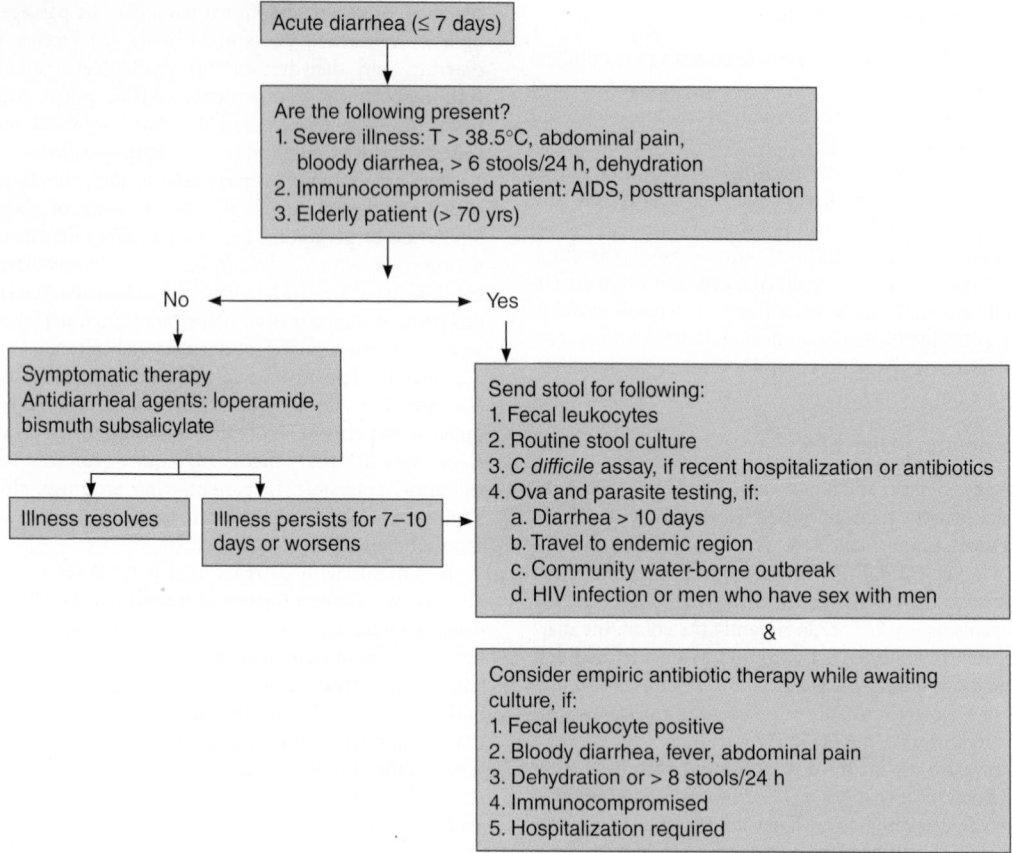

▲ **Figure 15–1.** Evaluation of acute diarrhea.

Opioid agents help decrease the stool number and liquidity and control fecal urgency. However, they should not be used in patients with bloody diarrhea, high fever, or systemic toxicity and should be discontinued in patients whose diarrhea is worsening despite therapy. With these provisos, such drugs provide excellent symptomatic relief. Loperamide is preferred, in a dosage of 4 mg orally initially, followed by 2 mg after each loose stool (maximum: 16 mg/24 h).

Bismuth subsalicylate (Pepto-Bismol), two tablets or 30 mL orally four times daily, reduces symptoms in patients with traveler's diarrhea by virtue of its anti-inflammatory and antibacterial properties. It also reduces vomiting associated with viral enteritis. Anticholinergic agents (eg, diphenoxylate with atropine) are contraindicated in acute diarrhea because of the rare precipitation of toxic megacolon.

D. Antibiotic Therapy

1. Empiric treatment—Empiric antibiotic treatment of all patients with acute diarrhea is not indicated. Even patients with inflammatory diarrhea caused by invasive pathogens usually have symptoms that will resolve within several days without antimicrobials. Empiric treatment may be considered in patients with non–hospital-acquired diarrhea with moderate to severe fever, tenesmus, or bloody stools or the presence of fecal lactoferrin while the stool bacterial

culture is incubating, provided that infection with STEC is not suspected. It should also be considered in patients who are immunocompromised or who have significant dehydration. The oral drugs of choice for empiric treatment are the fluoroquinolones (eg, ciprofloxacin 500 mg, ofloxacin 400 mg, or norfloxacin 400 mg, twice daily, or levofloxacin 500 mg once daily) for 5–7 days. Alternatives include trimethoprim-sulfamethoxazole, 160/800 mg twice daily; or doxycycline, 100 mg twice daily. Macrolides and penicillins are no longer recommended because of widespread microbial resistance to these agents. Rifaximin, a nonabsorbed oral antibiotic, 200 mg three times daily for 3 days, is approved for empiric treatment of noninflammatory traveler's diarrhea (see Chapter 30).

2. Specific antimicrobial treatment—Antibiotics are not recommended in patients with nontyphoid *Salmonella,* *Campylobacter,* Shiga-toxin–producing *E coli, Aeromonas,* or *Yersinia,* except in severe disease, because they do not hasten recovery or reduce the period of fecal bacterial excretion. The infectious diarrheas for which treatment is recommended are shigellosis, cholera, extraintestinal salmonellosis, listeriosis, traveler's diarrhea, *C difficile* infection, giardiasis, and amebiasis. Therapy for traveler's diarrhea, infectious (sexually transmitted) proctitis, and AIDS-related diarrhea is presented in other chapters of this book.

▶ When to Admit

- Severe dehydration for intravenous fluids, especially if vomiting or unable to maintain sufficient oral fluid intake.

- Bloody diarrhea that is severe or worsening in order to distinguish infectious versus noninfectious cause.

- Severe abdominal pain, worrisome for toxic colitis, inflammatory bowel disease, intestinal ischemia, or surgical abdomen.

- Signs of severe infection or sepsis (temperature > 39.5°C, leukocytosis, rash).

- Severe or worsening diarrhea in patients who are > 70 years old or immunocompromised.

- Signs of hemolytic-uremic syndrome (acute kidney injury, thrombocytopenia, hemolytic anemia).

Allen SJ et al. Probiotics for treating acute infectious diarrhoea. Cochrane Database Syst Rev. 2010 Nov 10;(11):CD003048. [PMID: 21069673]

Buchholz U et al. German outbreak of *Escherichia coli* O104:H4 associated with sprouts. N Engl J Med. 2011 Nov 10;365(19): 1763–70. [PMID: 22029753]

2. Chronic Diarrhea

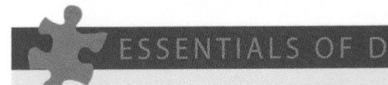

ESSENTIALS OF DIAGNOSIS

- ▶ Diarrhea present for > 4 weeks.
- ▶ Before embarking on extensive work-up, common causes should be excluded, including medications, chronic infections, and irritable bowel syndrome.

▶ Etiology

The causes of chronic diarrhea may be grouped into the following major pathophysiologic categories: medications, osmotic diarrheas, secretory conditions, inflammatory conditions, malabsorptive conditions, motility disorders, chronic infections, and systemic disorders (Table 15–6).

A. Medications

Numerous medications can cause diarrhea. Common offenders include cholinesterase inhibitors, SSRIs, angiotensin II-receptor blockers, proton pump inhibitors, NSAIDs, metformin, allopurinol, and orlistat. All medications should be carefully reviewed, and discontinuation of potential culprits should be considered.

B. Osmotic Diarrheas

As stool leaves the colon, fecal osmolality is equal to the serum osmolality, ie, approximately 290 mosm/kg. Under normal circumstances, the major osmoles are Na^+, K^+, Cl^-, and HCO_3^-. The stool osmolality may be estimated by multiplying the stool $(Na^+ + K^+) \times 2$. The **osmotic gap** is the difference between the *measured* osmolality of the stool (or serum) and the *estimated* stool osmolality and is normally < 50 mosm/kg. An increased osmotic gap (> 75 mosm/kg) implies that the diarrhea is caused by ingestion or malabsorption of an osmotically active substance. The most common causes are carbohydrate malabsorption (lactose, fructose, sorbitol), laxative abuse, and malabsorption syndromes (see below). Osmotic diarrheas resolve during fasting. Those caused by malabsorbed carbohydrates are characterized by abdominal distention, bloating, and flatulence due to increased colonic gas production.

Carbohydrate malabsorption is common and should be considered in all patients with chronic, postprandial diarrhea. Patients should be asked about their intake of dairy products (lactose), fruits and artificial sweeteners (fructose and sorbitol), and alcohol. The diagnosis of carbohydrate malabsorption may be established by an elimination trial for 2–3 weeks or by hydrogen breath tests.

Ingestion of magnesium- or phosphate-containing compounds (laxatives, antacids) should be considered in enigmatic chronic diarrhea. The fat substitute olestra also causes diarrhea and cramps in occasional patients.

C. Secretory Conditions

Increased intestinal secretion or decreased absorption results in a high-volume watery diarrhea with a normal osmotic gap. There is little change in stool output during the fasting state, and dehydration and electrolyte imbalance may develop. Causes include endocrine tumors (stimulating intestinal or pancreatic secretion) and bile salt malabsorption (stimulating colonic secretion).

D. Inflammatory Conditions

Diarrhea is present in most patients with inflammatory bowel disease (ulcerative colitis, Crohn disease). A variety of other symptoms may be present, including abdominal pain, fever, weight loss, and hematochezia. Microscopic colitis is a common cause of chronic watery diarrhea in the elderly (see Inflammatory Bowel Disease, below).

E. Malabsorptive Conditions

The major causes of malabsorption are small mucosal intestinal diseases, intestinal resections, lymphatic obstruction, small intestinal bacterial overgrowth, and pancreatic insufficiency. Its characteristics are weight loss, osmotic diarrhea, steatorrhea, and nutritional deficiencies. Significant diarrhea in the absence of weight loss is not likely to be due to malabsorption. The physical and laboratory abnormalities related to deficiencies of vitamins or minerals are discussed in Chapter 29.

F. Motility Disorders (Including Irritable Bowel Syndrome)

Irritable bowel syndrome is the most common cause of chronic diarrhea in young adults (see Irritable Bowel Syndrome). It should be considered in patients with lower abdominal pain and altered bowel habits who have no other evidence of serious organic disease (weight loss, nocturnal diarrhea, anemia, or gastrointestinal bleeding). Abnormal intestinal motility secondary to systemic disorders or surgery may result in diarrhea due to rapid transit or to stasis of intestinal contents with bacterial overgrowth, resulting in malabsorption.

G. Chronic Infections

Chronic parasitic infections may cause diarrhea through a number of mechanisms. Pathogens most commonly associated with diarrhea include the protozoans *Giardia, E histolytica,* and *Cyclospora* as well as the intestinal nematodes. Strongyloidiasis and capillariasis should be excluded in patients from endemic regions, especially in the presence of eosinophilia. Bacterial infections with *C difficile* and, uncommonly, *Aeromonas* and *Plesiomonas* may cause of chronic diarrhea.

Immunocompromised patients are susceptible to infectious organisms that can cause acute or chronic diarrhea (see Chapter 31), including Microsporida, *Cryptosporidium,* CMV, *Isospora belli, Cyclospora,* and *Mycobacterium avium* complex.

H. Systemic Conditions

Chronic systemic conditions, such as thyroid disease, diabetes, and collagen vascular disorders, may cause diarrhea through alterations in motility or intestinal absorption.

▶ Clinical Findings

The history and physical examination commonly suggest the underlying pathophysiology that guides the subsequent diagnostic work-up (Figure 15–2). The clinician should establish whether the diarrhea is continuous or intermittent, the relationship to meals, and whether it occurs at night or during fasting. The stool appearance may suggest a malabsorption disorder (greasy or malodorous), inflammatory disorder (containing blood or pus), or a secretory process (watery). The presence of abdominal pain suggests irritable bowel syndrome or inflammatory bowel disease. Medications, diet, and recent psychosocial stressors should be reviewed. Physical examination should assess for signs of malnutrition, dehydration, and inflammatory bowel disease.

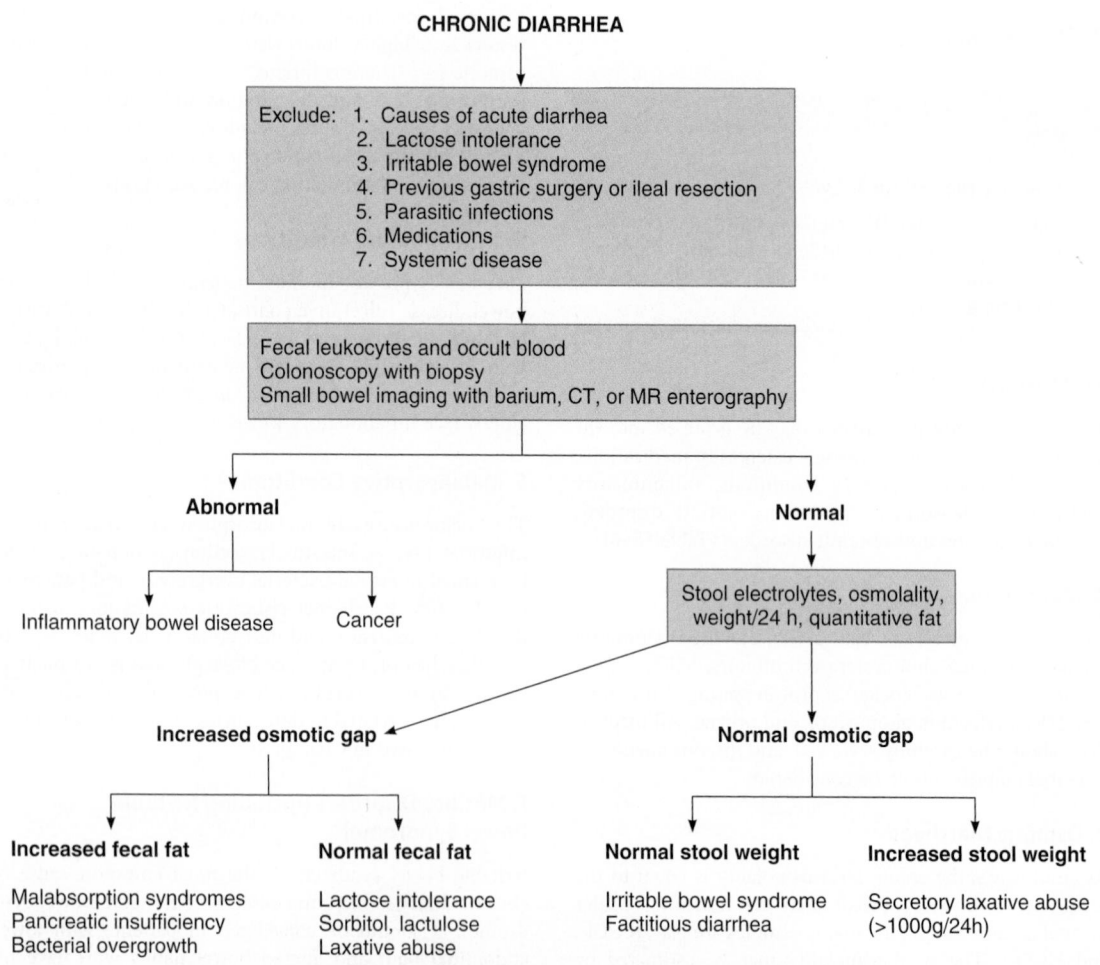

▲ **Figure 15–2.** Decision diagram for diagnosis of causes of chronic diarrhea.

Because chronic diarrhea is caused by so many conditions, the subsequent diagnostic approach is guided by the relative suspicion for the underlying cause, and no specific algorithm can be followed in all patients. Prior to embarking on an extensive evaluation, the most common causes of chronic diarrhea should be considered, including medications, irritable bowel syndrome, and lactose intolerance. The presence of nocturnal diarrhea, weight loss, anemia, or positive results on FOBT are inconsistent with these disorders and warrant further evaluation. AIDS-associated diarrhea is discussed in Chapter 31.

A. Initial Diagnostic Tests

1. Routine laboratory tests—Complete blood count, serum electrolytes, liver function tests, calcium, phosphorus, albumin, thyroid-stimulating hormone, vitamin A and D levels, INR, erythrocyte sedimentation rate, and C-reactive protein should be obtained in most patients. Serologic testing for celiac sprue with IgA tissue transglutaminase (tTG) or anti-endomysial antibody tests may be recommended in the evaluation of most patients with chronic diarrhea and all patients with signs of malabsorption. Anemia occurs in malabsorption syndromes (folate, iron deficiency, or vitamin B_{12}) as well as inflammatory conditions. Hypoalbuminemia is present in malabsorption, protein-losing enteropathies, and inflammatory diseases. Hyponatremia and nonanion gap metabolic acidosis occur in secretory diarrheas. Increased erythrocyte sedimentation rate or C-reactive protein suggests inflammatory bowel disease.

2. Routine stool studies—Stool sample should be analyzed for ova and parasites, electrolytes (to calculate osmotic gap), qualitative staining for fat (Sudan stain), occult blood, and leukocytes or lactoferrin. The presence of *Giardia* and *E histolytica* may be detected in wet mounts. However, fecal antigen detection tests for *Giardia* and *E histolytica* are a more sensitive and specific method of detection. *Cryptosporidium* and *Cyclospora* are found with modified acid-fast staining. As discussed previously, an increased osmotic gap suggests an osmotic diarrhea or disorder of malabsorption. A positive fecal fat stain suggests a disorder of malabsorption. The presence of fecal leukocytes or lactoferrin may suggest inflammatory bowel disease.

3. Endoscopic examination and mucosal biopsy—Most patients with chronic persistent diarrhea undergo colonoscopy with mucosal biopsy to exclude inflammatory bowel disease (including Crohn disease and ulcerative colitis), microscopic colitis, and colonic neoplasia. Upper endoscopy with small bowel biopsy is performed when a small intestinal malabsorptive disorder is suspected (celiac sprue, Whipple disease) from abnormal laboratory studies or a positive fecal fat stain. It may also be done in patients with advanced AIDS to document *Cryptosporidium*, Microsporida, and *M avium-intracellulare* infection.

B. Further Studies

If the cause of diarrhea is still not apparent, further studies may be warranted.

1. 24-hour stool collection quantification of total weight and fat—A stool weight of < 200–300 g/24 h excludes diarrhea and suggests a functional disorder such as irritable bowel syndrome. A weight > 1000–1500 g suggests a significant secretory process, including neuroendocrine tumors. A fecal fat determination in excess of 10 g/24 h confirms a malabsorptive disorder. Fecal elastase < 100 mcg/g may be caused by pancreatic insufficiency. (See Celiac Disease and specific tests for malabsorption, below.)

2. Other imaging studies—Calcification on a plain abdominal radiograph confirms a diagnosis of chronic pancreatitis, although abdominal CT and endoscopic ultrasonography are more sensitive for the diagnosis of chronic pancreatitis as well as pancreatic cancer. Small intestinal imaging with barium, CT, or MRI is helpful in the diagnosis of Crohn disease, small bowel lymphoma, carcinoid, and jejunal diverticula. Neuroendocrine tumors may be localized using somatostatin receptor scintigraphy. Retention of < 11% at 7 days of intravenous 75Se-homotaurocholate on scintigraphy suggests bile salt malabsorption.

3. Laboratory tests—

A. Serologic tests for neuroendocrine tumors—Secretory diarrheas due to neuroendocrine tumors are rare but should be considered in patients with chronic, high-volume watery diarrhea (> 1 L/d) with a normal osmotic gap that persists during fasting. Measurements of the secretagogues of various neuroendocrine tumors may be assayed, including serum chromogranin A, vasoactive intestinal peptide (VIP) (VIPoma), calcitonin (medullary thyroid carcinoma), gastrin (Zollinger-Ellison syndrome), and urinary 5-hydroxyindoleacetic acid (5-HIAA) (carcinoid).

B. Breath test—The diagnosis of small bowel bacterial overgrowth is confirmed with noninvasive breath tests (glucose or lactulose) or by obtaining an aspirate of small intestinal contents for quantitative aerobic and anaerobic bacterial culture.

▶ Treatment

A number of antidiarrheal agents may be used in certain patients with chronic diarrheal conditions and are listed below. Opioids are safe in most patients with chronic, stable symptoms.

Loperamide: 4 mg orally initially, then 2 mg after each loose stool (maximum: 16 mg/d).

Diphenoxylate with atropine: One tablet orally three or four times daily as needed.

Codeine and deodorized tincture of opium: Because of potential habituation, these drugs are avoided except in cases of chronic, intractable diarrhea. Codeine may be given in a dosage of 15–60 mg orally every 4 hours; tincture of opium, 0.3–1.2 mL orally every 6 hours as needed.

Clonidine: Alpha-2-adrenergic agonists inhibit intestinal electrolyte secretion. Clonidine, 0.1–0.6 mg orally twice daily, or a clonidine patch, 0.1–0.2 mg/d, may help in some patients with secretory diarrheas, diabetic diarrhea, or cryptosporidiosis.

Octreotide: This somatostatin analog stimulates intestinal fluid and electrolyte absorption and inhibits intestinal fluid secretion and the release of gastrointestinal peptides. It is given for secretory diarrheas due to neuroendocrine tumors (VIPomas, carcinoid) and in some cases of AIDS-related diarrhea. Effective doses range from 50 to 250 mcg subcutaneously three times daily.

Cholestyramine: This bile salt-binding resin may be useful in patients with bile salt-induced diarrhea, which may be idiopathic or secondary to intestinal resection or ileal disease. A dosage of 4 g orally once to three times daily is recommended.

Li Z et al. Treatment of chronic diarrhea. Best Pract Res Clin Gastroenterol. 2012 Oct;26(5):677–87. [PMID: 23384811]
Money ME et al. Review: management of postprandial diarrhea syndrome. Am J Med. 2012 Jun;125(6):538–44. [PMID: 22624684]
Schiller LR. Definitions, pathophysiology, and evaluation of chronic diarrhoea. Best Pract Res Clin Gastroenterol. 2012 Oct;26(5):551–62. [PMID: 23384801]

GASTROINTESTINAL BLEEDING

1. Acute Upper Gastrointestinal Bleeding

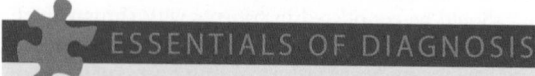

ESSENTIALS OF DIAGNOSIS

► Hematemesis (bright red blood or "coffee grounds").

► Melena in most cases; hematochezia in massive upper gastrointestinal bleeds.

► Volume status to determine severity of blood loss; hematocrit is a poor early indicator of blood loss.

► Endoscopy diagnostic and may be therapeutic.

► **General Considerations**

There are over 250,000 hospitalizations a year in the United States for acute upper gastrointestinal bleeding, with a mortality rate of 4–10%. Approximately half of patients are over 60 years of age, and in this age group the mortality rate is even higher. Patients seldom die of exsanguination but rather from complications of an underlying disease.

The most common presentation of upper gastrointestinal bleeding is hematemesis or melena. Hematemesis may be either bright red blood or brown "coffee grounds" material. Melena develops after as little as 50–100 mL of blood loss in the upper gastrointestinal tract, whereas hematochezia requires a loss of more than 1000 mL. Although hematochezia generally suggests a lower bleeding source (eg, colonic), severe upper gastrointestinal bleeding may present with hematochezia in 10% of cases.

Upper gastrointestinal bleeding is self-limited in 80% of patients; urgent medical therapy and endoscopic evaluation are obligatory in the rest. Patients with bleeding more than 48 hours prior to presentation have a low risk of recurrent bleeding.

► **Etiology**

Acute upper gastrointestinal bleeding may originate from a number of sources. These are listed in order of their frequency and discussed in detail below.

A. Peptic Ulcer Disease

Peptic ulcers account for half of major upper gastrointestinal bleeding with an overall mortality rate of 6%. However, in North America the incidence of bleeding from ulcers is declining, perhaps due to eradication of *H pylori* and prophylaxis with proton pump inhibitors in high-risk patients.

B. Portal Hypertension

Portal hypertension accounts for 10–20% of upper gastrointestinal bleeding. Bleeding usually arises from esophageal varices and less commonly gastric or duodenal varices or portal hypertensive gastropathy. Approximately 25% of patients with cirrhosis have medium to large esophageal varices, of whom 30% experience acute variceal bleeding within a 2-year period. Due to improved care, the hospital mortality rate has declined over the past 20 years from 40% to 15%. Nevertheless, a mortality rate of 60–80% is expected at 1–4 years due to recurrent bleeding or other complications of chronic liver disease.

C. Mallory-Weiss Tears

Lacerations of the gastroesophageal junction cause 5–10% of cases of upper gastrointestinal bleeding. Many patients report a history of heavy alcohol use or retching. Less than 10% have continued or recurrent bleeding.

D. Vascular Anomalies

Vascular anomalies are found throughout the gastrointestinal tract and may be the source of chronic or acute gastrointestinal bleeding. They account for 7% of cases of acute upper tract bleeding. The most common are **angioectasias** (angiodysplasias) which are 1–10 mm distorted, aberrant submucosal vessels caused by chronic, intermittent obstruction of submucosal veins. They have a bright red stellate appearance and occur throughout the gastrointestinal tract but most commonly in the right colon. **Telangiectasias** are small, cherry red lesions caused by dilation of venules that may be part of systemic conditions (hereditary hemorrhagic telangiectasia, CREST syndrome) or occur sporadically. The **Dieulafoy lesion** is an aberrant, large-caliber submucosal artery, most commonly in the proximal stomach that causes recurrent, intermittent bleeding.

E. Gastric Neoplasms

Gastric neoplasms result in 1% of upper gastrointestinal hemorrhages.

F. Erosive Gastritis

Because this process is superficial, it is a relatively unusual cause of severe gastrointestinal bleeding (< 5% of cases) and more commonly results in chronic blood loss. Gastric mucosal erosions are due to NSAIDs, alcohol, or severe medical or surgical illness (stress-related mucosal disease).

G. Erosive Esophagitis

Severe erosive esophagitis due to chronic gastroesophageal reflux may rarely cause significant upper gastrointestinal bleeding, especially in patients who are bed bound long-term.

H. Others

An aortoenteric fistula complicates 2% of abdominal aortic grafts or, rarely, can occur as the initial presentation of a previously untreated aneurysm. Usually located between the graft or aneurysm and the third portion of the duodenum, these fistulas characteristically present with a herald nonexsanguinating initial hemorrhage, with melena and hematemesis, or with chronic intermittent bleeding. The diagnosis may be suspected by upper endoscopy or abdominal CT. Surgery is mandatory to prevent exsanguinating hemorrhage. Unusual causes of upper gastrointestinal bleeding include hemobilia (from hepatic tumor, angioma, penetrating trauma), pancreatic malignancy, and pseudoaneurysm (hemosuccus pancreaticus).

▶ Initial Evaluation & Treatment

A. Stabilization

The initial step is assessment of the hemodynamic status. A systolic blood pressure < 100 mm Hg identifies a high-risk patient with severe acute bleeding. A heart rate over 100 beats/min with a systolic blood pressure over 100 mm Hg signifies moderate acute blood loss. A normal systolic blood pressure and heart rate suggest relatively minor hemorrhage. Postural hypotension and tachycardia are useful when present but may be due to causes other than blood loss. Because the hematocrit may take 24–72 hours to equilibrate with the extravascular fluid, it is not a reliable indicator of the severity of acute bleeding.

In patients with significant bleeding, two 18-gauge or larger intravenous lines should be started prior to further diagnostic tests. Blood is sent for complete blood count, prothrombin time with international normalized ratio (INR), serum creatinine, liver enzymes, and blood typing and screening (in anticipation of need for possible transfusion). In patients without hemodynamic compromise or overt active bleeding, aggressive fluid repletion can be delayed until the extent of the bleeding is further clarified. Patients with evidence of hemodynamic compromise are given 0.9% saline or lactated Ringer injection and crossmatched for 2–4 units of packed red blood cells. It is rarely necessary to administer type-specific or O-negative blood. Central venous pressure monitoring is desirable in some cases, but line placement should not interfere with rapid volume resuscitation.

Placement of a nasogastric tube is not routinely needed but may be helpful in the initial assessment and triage of selected patients with suspected active upper tract bleeding. The aspiration of red blood or "coffee grounds" confirms an upper gastrointestinal source of bleeding, though up to 18% of patients with confirmed upper tract sources of bleeding have nonbloody aspirates—especially when bleeding originates in the duodenum. An aspirate of bright red blood indicates active bleeding and is associated with the highest risk of further bleeding and complications, while a clear aspirate identifies patients at lower initial risk. Erythromycin (250 mg) administered intravenously 30 minutes prior to upper endoscopy promotes gastric emptying and may improve the quality of endoscopic evaluation when substantial amounts of blood or clot in the stomach is suspected. Efforts to stop or slow bleeding by gastric lavage with large volumes of fluid are of no benefit and expose the patient to an increased risk of aspiration.

B. Blood Replacement

The amount of fluid and blood products required is based on assessment of vital signs, evidence of active bleeding from nasogastric aspirate, and laboratory tests. Sufficient packed red blood cells should be given to maintain a hemoglobin of 7–9 g/dL, based on the patient's hemodynamic status, comorbidities (especially cardiovascular disease), and presence of continued bleeding. In the absence of continued bleeding, the hemoglobin should rise approximately 1 g/dL for each unit of transfused packed red cells. Transfusion of blood should not be withheld from patients with massive active bleeding regardless of the hemoglobin value. It is desirable to transfuse blood in anticipation of the nadir hematocrit. In actively bleeding patients, platelets are transfused if the platelet count is under 50,000/mcL and considered if there is impaired platelet function due to aspirin or clopidogrel use (regardless of the platelet count). Uremic patients (who also have dysfunctional platelets) with active bleeding are given three doses of desmopressin (DDAVP), 0.3 mcg/kg intravenously, at 12-hour intervals. Fresh frozen plasma is administered for actively bleeding patients with a coagulopathy and an INR > 1.8; however, endoscopy may be performed safely if the INR is < 2.5. In the face of massive bleeding, 1 unit of fresh frozen plasma should be given for each 5 units of packed red blood cells transfused.

C. Initial Triage

A preliminary assessment of risk based on several clinical factors aids in the resuscitation as well as the rational triage of the patient. Clinical predictors of increased risk of rebleeding and death include age > 60 years, comorbid illnesses, systolic blood pressure < 100 mm Hg, pulse > 100 beats/min, and bright red blood in the nasogastric aspirate or on rectal examination.

1. High risk—Patients with active bleeding manifested by hematemesis or bright red blood on nasogastric aspirate, shock, persistent hemodynamic derangement despite fluid resuscitation, serious comorbid medical illness, or evidence of advanced liver disease require admission to an intensive care unit (ICU). After adequate resuscitation, endoscopy should be performed within 2–24 hours in most patients but may be delayed in selected patients with serious comorbidities (eg, acute coronary syndrome) who do not have signs of continued bleeding.

2. Low to moderate risk—All other patients are admitted to a step-down unit or medical ward after appropriate stabilization for further evaluation and treatment. Patients without evidence of active bleeding undergo nonemergent endoscopy usually within 24 hours.

▶ Subsequent Evaluation & Treatment

Specific treatment of the various causes of upper gastrointestinal bleeding is discussed elsewhere in this chapter. The following general comments apply to most patients with bleeding.

The clinician's impression of the bleeding source is correct in only 40% of cases. Signs of chronic liver disease implicate bleeding due to portal hypertension, but a different lesion is identified in 25% of patients with cirrhosis. A history of dyspepsia, NSAID use, or peptic ulcer disease suggests peptic ulcer. Acute bleeding preceded by heavy alcohol ingestion or retching suggests a Mallory-Weiss tear, though most of these patients have neither.

A. Upper Endoscopy

Virtually all patients with upper tract bleeding should undergo upper endoscopy within 24 hours of arriving in the emergency department. The benefits of endoscopy in this setting are threefold.

1. To identify the source of bleeding—The appropriate acute and long-term medical therapy is determined by the cause of bleeding. Patients with portal hypertension will be treated differently from those with ulcer disease. If surgery or radiologic interventional therapy is required for uncontrolled bleeding, the source of bleeding as determined at endoscopy will determine the approach.

2. To determine the risk of rebleeding and guide triage—Patients with a nonbleeding Mallory-Weiss tear, esophagitis, gastritis, and ulcers that have a clean, white base have a very low risk (< 5%) of rebleeding. Patients with one of these findings who are < age 60 years, without hemodynamic instability or transfusion requirement, without serious coexisting illness, and who have stable social support may be discharged from the emergency department or medical ward after endoscopy with outpatient follow-up. All others with one of these low-risk lesions should be observed on a medical ward for 24-48 hours. Patients with ulcers that are actively bleeding or have a visible vessel or adherent clot, or who have variceal bleeding usually require at least a 3-day hospitalization with closer initial observation in an ICU or step down unit.

3. To render endoscopic therapy—Hemostasis can be achieved in actively bleeding lesions with endoscopic modalities such as cautery, injection, or endoclips. About 90% of bleeding or nonbleeding varices can be effectively treated immediately with injection of a sclerosant or application of rubber bands to the varices. Similarly, 90% of bleeding ulcers, angiomas, or Mallory-Weiss tears can be controlled with either injection of epinephrine, direct cauterization of the vessel by a heater probe or multipolar electrocautery probe, or application of an endoclip. Certain nonbleeding lesions such as ulcers with visible blood vessels,

and angioectasias are also treated with these therapies. Specific endoscopic therapy of varices, peptic ulcers, and Mallory-Weiss tears is dealt with elsewhere in this chapter.

B. Acute Pharmacologic Therapies

1. Acid inhibitory therapy—Intravenous proton pump inhibitors (esomeprazole or pantoprazole, 80 mg bolus, followed by 8 mg/h continuous infusion for 72 hours) reduce the risk of rebleeding in patients with peptic ulcers with high-risk features (active bleeding, visible vessel, or adherent clot) after endoscopic treatment. **Oral proton pump inhibitors** (omeprazole, esomeprazole, or pantoprazole 40 mg; lansoprazole or dexlansoprazole 30-60 mg) once or twice daily are sufficient for lesions at low-risk for rebleeding (eg, esophagitis, gastritis, clean-based ulcers, and Mallory-Weiss tears).

Administration of continuous intravenous proton pump inhibitor *before* endoscopy results in a decreased number of ulcers with lesions that require endoscopic therapy. It therefore is standard clinical practice at many institutions to administer either an intravenous or a high-dose oral proton pump inhibitor prior to endoscopy in patients with significant upper gastrointestinal bleeding. Based on the findings during endoscopy, the intravenous proton pump inhibitor may be continued or discontinued.

2. Octreotide—Continuous intravenous infusion of octreotide (100 mcg bolus, followed by 50-100 mcg/h) reduces splanchnic blood flow and portal blood pressures and is effective in the initial control of bleeding related to portal hypertension. It is administered promptly to all patients with active upper gastrointestinal bleeding and evidence of liver disease or portal hypertension until the source of bleeding can be determined by endoscopy. In countries where it is available, terlipressin may be preferred to octreotide for the treatment of bleeding related to portal hypertension because of its sustained reduction of portal and variceal pressures and its proven reduction in mortality.

C. Other Treatment

1. Intra-arterial embolization—Angiographic treatment is used in patients with persistent bleeding from ulcers, angiomas, or Mallory-Weiss tears who have failed endoscopic therapy and are poor operative risks.

2. Transvenous intrahepatic portosystemic shunts (TIPS)—Placement of a wire stent from the hepatic vein through the liver to the portal vein provides effective decompression of the portal venous system and control of acute variceal bleeding. It is indicated in patients in whom endoscopic modalities have failed to control acute variceal bleeding.

Greenspoon J et al; International Consensus Upper Gastrointestinal Bleeding Conference Group. Management of patients with nonvariceal upper gastrointestinal bleeding. Clin Gastroenterol Hepatol. 2012 Mar;10(3):234–9. [PMID: 21820395]
Lau JY et al. Challenges in the management of acute peptic ulcer bleeding. Lancet. 2013 Jun 8;381(9882):2033–43. [PMID: 23746903]

Srygley FD et al. Does this patient have a severe upper gastrointestinal bleed? JAMA. 2012 Mar 14;307(10):1072–9. [PMID: 22416103]

Villanueva C et al. Transfusion for acute upper gastrointestinal bleeding. N Engl J Med. 2013 Apr 4;368(1):11–21. [PMID: 23550677]

2. Acute Lower Gastrointestinal Bleeding

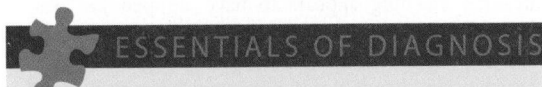

ESSENTIALS OF DIAGNOSIS

▶ Hematochezia usually present.

▶ Ten percent of cases of hematochezia due to upper gastrointestinal source.

▶ Evaluation with colonoscopy in stable patients.

▶ Massive active bleeding calls for evaluation with sigmoidoscopy, upper endoscopy, angiography, or nuclear bleeding scan.

▶ General Considerations

Lower gastrointestinal bleeding is defined as that arising below the ligament of Treitz, ie, the small intestine or colon; however, up to 95% of cases arise from the colon. The severity of lower gastrointestinal bleeding ranges from mild anorectal bleeding to massive, large-volume hematochezia. Bright red blood that drips into the bowl after a bowel movement or is mixed with solid brown stool signifies mild bleeding, usually from an anorectosigmoid source, and can be evaluated in the outpatient setting. In patients hospitalized with gastrointestinal bleeding, lower tract bleeding is one-third as common as upper gastrointestinal hemorrhage and tends to have a more benign course. Patients hospitalized with lower gastrointestinal tract bleeding are less likely to present with shock or orthostasis (< 20%) or to require transfusions (< 40%). Spontaneous cessation of bleeding occurs in over 75% of cases, and hospital mortality is < 4%.

▶ Etiology

The cause of these lesions depends on both the age of the patient and the severity of the bleeding. In patients under 50 years of age, the most common causes are infectious colitis, anorectal disease, and inflammatory bowel disease. In older patients, significant hematochezia is most often seen with diverticulosis, angiectasias, malignancy, or ischemia. In 20% of acute bleeding episodes, no source of bleeding can be identified.

A. Diverticulosis

Hemorrhage occurs in 3–5% of all patients with diverticulosis and is the most common cause of major lower tract bleeding, accounting for 50% of cases. There is 1.35- to 3.49-fold increased risk of diverticular hemorrhage among patients who use aspirin or nonsteroidal anti-inflammatory agents. Diverticular bleeding usually presents as acute, painless, large-volume maroon or bright red hematochezia

in patients over age 50 years. More than 95% of cases require < 4 units of blood transfusion. Bleeding subsides spontaneously in 80% but may recur in up to 25% of patients.

B. Angioectasias

Angiectasias (angiodysplasias) occur throughout the upper and lower intestinal tracts and cause painless bleeding ranging from melena or hematochezia to occult blood loss. They are responsible for 4% of cases of lower gastrointestinal bleeding, where they are most often seen in the cecum and ascending colon. They are flat, red lesions (2–10 mm) with ectatic peripheral vessels radiating from a central vessel, and are most common in patients over 70 years and in those with chronic renal failure. Bleeding in younger patients more commonly arises from the small intestine.

Ectasias can be identified in up to 6% of persons over age 60 years, so the mere presence of ectasias does not prove that the lesion is the source of bleeding, since active bleeding is seldom seen.

C. Neoplasms

Benign polyps and carcinoma are associated with chronic occult blood loss or intermittent anorectal hematochezia. Furthermore, they may cause up to 7% of acute lower gastrointestinal hemorrhage. After endoscopic removal of colonic polyps, important bleeding may occur up to 2 weeks later in 0.3% of patients. In general, prompt colonoscopy is recommended to treat postpolypectomy hemorrhage and minimize the need for transfusions.

D. Inflammatory Bowel Disease

Patients with inflammatory bowel disease (especially ulcerative colitis) often have diarrhea with variable amounts of hematochezia. Bleeding varies from occult blood loss to recurrent hematochezia usually mixed with stool. Symptoms of abdominal pain, tenesmus, and urgency are often present.

E. Anorectal Disease

Anorectal disease (hemorrhoids, fissures) usually results in small amounts of bright red blood noted on the toilet paper, streaking of the stool, or dripping into the toilet bowl; clinically significant blood loss can sometimes occur. Hemorrhoids are the source in 10% of patients admitted with lower bleeding. Rectal ulcers may account for up to 8% of lower bleeding, usually in elderly or debilitated patients with constipation.

F. Ischemic Colitis

This condition is seen commonly in older patients, most of whom have atherosclerotic disease. Most cases occur spontaneously due to transient episodes of nonocclusive ischemia. Ischemic colitis may also occur in 5% of patients after surgery for ileoaortic or abdominal aortic aneurysm. In young patients, colonic ischemia may develop due to vasculitis, coagulation disorders, estrogen therapy, and long distance running. Ischemic colitis results in hematochezia or bloody diarrhea associated with mild cramps. In most patients, the bleeding is mild and self-limited.

G. Others

Radiation-induced proctitis causes anorectal bleeding that may develop months to years after pelvic radiation. Endoscopy reveals multiple rectal telangiectasias. Acute infectious colitis (see Acute Diarrhea, above) commonly causes bloody diarrhea. Rare causes of lower tract bleeding include vasculitic ischemia, solitary rectal ulcer, NSAID-induced ulcers in the small bowel or right colon, small bowel diverticula, and colonic varices.

▶ Clinical Findings

A. Symptoms and Signs

The color of the stool helps distinguish upper from lower gastrointestinal bleeding, especially when observed by the clinician. Brown stools mixed or streaked with blood predict a source in the rectosigmoid or anus. Large volumes of bright red blood suggest a colonic source; maroon stools imply a lesion in the right colon or small intestine; and black stools (melena) predict a source proximal to the ligament of Treitz. Although 10% of patients admitted with self-reported hematochezia have an upper gastrointestinal source of bleeding (eg, peptic ulcer), this almost always occurs in the setting of massive hemorrhage with hemodynamic instability. Painless large-volume bleeding usually suggests diverticular bleeding. Bloody diarrhea associated with cramping abdominal pain, urgency, or tenesmus is characteristic of inflammatory bowel disease, infectious colitis, or ischemic colitis.

B. Diagnostic Tests

Important considerations in management include exclusion of an upper tract source, anoscopy and sigmoidoscopy, colonoscopy, nuclear bleeding scans and angiography, and small intestine push enteroscopy or capsule imaging.

1. Exclusion of an upper tract source—A nasogastric tube with aspiration should be considered, especially in patients with hemodynamic compromise. Aspiration of red blood or dark brown ("coffee grounds") guaiac-positive material strongly implicates an upper gastrointestinal source of bleeding. Upper endoscopy should be performed in most patients presenting with hematochezia and hemodynamic instability to exclude an upper gastrointestinal source before proceeding with evaluation of the lower gastrointestinal tract.

2. Anoscopy and sigmoidoscopy—In otherwise healthy patients without anemia under age 45 years with small-volume bleeding, anoscopy and sigmoidoscopy are performed to look for evidence of anorectal disease, inflammatory bowel disease, or infectious colitis. If a lesion is found, no further evaluation is needed immediately unless the bleeding persists or is recurrent. In patients over age 45 years with small-volume hematochezia, the entire colon must be evaluated with colonoscopy to exclude tumor.

3. Colonoscopy—In patients with acute, large-volume bleeding requiring hospitalization, colonoscopy is the preferred initial study in most cases. The bowel first is purged rapidly by administration of a high-volume colonic lavage solution, given until the effluent is clear of blood and clots (4–8 L of GoLYTELY, CoLYTE, NuLYTE given orally or 1 L every 30 minutes over 2–5 hours by nasogastric tube). For patients with stable vital signs and whose lower gastrointestinal bleeding appears to have stopped (> 75% of patients), colonoscopy can be performed electively within 24 hours of admission. For patients with signs of hemodynamically significant bleeding (unstable vital signs) or who have signs of continued active bleeding during bowel preparation (< 25% of patients), urgent colonoscopy should be performed within 1–2 hours of completing the bowel purgative, when the bowel discharge is without clots. The probable site of bleeding can be identified in 70–85% of patients, and a high-risk lesion can be identified and treated in up to 20%.

4. Nuclear bleeding scans and angiography—Technetium-labeled red blood cell scanning can detect significant active bleeding and, in some cases, can localize the source to the small intestine, right colon, or left colon. Because most bleeding is slow or intermittent, less than half of nuclear studies are diagnostic and the accuracy of localization is poor. Thus, the main utility of scintigraphy is to determine whether bleeding is ongoing in order to determine whether angiography should be pursued. Less than half of patients with a positive nuclear study have positive angiography. Accordingly, angiograms are performed only in patients with positive technetium scans believed to have significant, ongoing bleeding.

In patients with massive lower gastrointestinal bleeding manifested by continued hemodynamic instability and hematochezia, urgent angiography should be performed without attempt at colonoscopy or scintigraphy.

5. Small intestine push enteroscopy or capsule imaging—Up to 5% of acute episodes of lower gastrointestinal bleeding arise from the small intestine, eluding diagnostic evaluation with upper endoscopy and colonoscopy. Because of the difficulty of examining the small intestine and its relative rarity as a source of acute bleeding, evaluation of the small bowel is not usually pursued in patients during the initial episode of acute lower gastrointestinal bleeding. However, the small intestine is investigated in patients with unexplained recurrent hemorrhage of obscure origin. (See Obscure Gastrointestinal Bleeding below.)

▶ Treatment

Initial stabilization, blood replacement, and triage are managed in the same manner as described above for Acute Upper Gastrointestinal Bleeding.

A. Therapeutic Colonoscopy

High-risk lesions (eg, angioectasias or diverticulum, rectal ulcer with active bleeding, or a visible vessel) may be treated endoscopically with epinephrine injection, cautery (bipolar or heater probe), or application of metallic endoclips or bands. In diverticular hemorrhage with high-risk lesions identified at colonoscopy, rebleeding occurs in half of untreated patients compared with virtually no rebleeding in patients treated endoscopically. Radiation proctitis is effectively treated with applications of cautery therapy to the rectal telangiectasias, preferably with an argon plasma coagulator.

B. Intra-arterial Embolization

When a bleeding lesion is identified, angiography with selective embolization achieves immediate hemostasis in more than 95% of patients. Major complications occur in 5% (mainly ischemic colitis) and rebleeding occurs in up to 25%.

C. Surgical Treatment

Emergency surgery is required in < 5% of patients with acute lower gastrointestinal bleeding due to the efficacy of colonoscopic and angiographic therapies. It is indicated in patients with ongoing bleeding that requires more than 6 units of blood within 24 hours or more than 10 total units in whom attempts at endoscopic or angiographic therapy failed. Most such hemorrhages are caused by a bleeding diverticulum or angioectasia.

Surgery may also be indicated in patients with two or more hospitalizations for diverticular hemorrhage depending on the severity of bleeding and the patient's other comorbid conditions.

Allen TW et al. Nuclear medicine tests for acute gastrointestinal conditions. Semin Nucl Med. 2013 Mar;43(2):88–101. [PMID: 23414825]

Kaltenbach T et al. Colonoscopy with clipping is useful in the diagnosis and treatment of diverticular bleeding. Clin Gastroenterol Hepatol. 2012 Feb;10(2):131–7. [PMID: 22056302]

Lhewa DY et al. Pros and cons of colonoscopy in management of acute lower gastrointestinal bleeding. World J Gastroenterol. 2012 Mar 21;18(11):1185–90. [PMID: 22468081]

Silva JA et al. Ischemic bowel syndromes. Prim Care. 2013 Mar;40(1):153–67. [PMID: 23402466]

3. Obscure Gastrointestinal Bleeding

Obscure gastrointestinal bleeding refers to bleeding of unknown origin that persists or recurs after initial endoscopic evaluation with upper endoscopy and colonoscopy. *Obscure-overt bleeding* is manifested by persistent or recurrent visible evidence of gastrointestinal bleeding (hematemesis, hematochezia, or melena). Up to 5% of patients admitted to hospitals with clinically overt gastrointestinal bleeding do not have a cause identified on upper endoscopy or colonoscopy (and therefore have obscure-overt bleeding). *Obscure-occult bleeding* (discussed below) refers to bleeding that is not apparent to the patient. It is manifested by recurrent positive FOBTs or FITs or recurrent iron deficiency anemia, or both in the absence of visible blood loss (as described below).

Obscure bleeding (either occult or overt) most commonly arises from lesions in the small intestine. In up to one-third of cases, however, a source of bleeding has been overlooked in the upper or lower tract on prior endoscopic studies.

Hematemesis or melena suggest an overlooked source proximal to the ligament of Treitz (ie, within the esophagus, stomach, or duodenum): erosions in a hiatal hernia ("Cameron erosions"), peptic ulcer, angioectasia, Dieulafoy vascular malformation, portal hypertensive gastropathy, gastroduodenal varices, duodenal neoplasms, aortoenteric fistula, or hepatic and pancreatic lesions. In the colon, the most commonly overlooked lesions are angioectasias and neoplasms. The etiology of obscure bleeding that arises from the small intestine depends on the age of the patient. The most common causes of small intestinal bleeding in patients younger than 40 years are neoplasms (stromal tumors, lymphomas, adenocarcinomas, carcinoids), Crohn disease, celiac disease, and Meckel diverticulum. These disorders also occur in patients over age 40; however, angioectasias and NSAID-induced ulcers are far more common.

Evaluation of Obscure Bleeding

The evaluation of obscure bleeding depends on the age and overall health status of the patient, associated symptoms, and severity of the bleeding. In an older patient with significant comorbid illnesses, no gastrointestinal symptoms, and occult or obscure bleeding in whom the suspected source of bleeding is angioectasias, it may be reasonable to limit diagnostic evaluations, provided the anemia can be managed with long-term iron therapy or occasional transfusions. On the other hand, aggressive diagnostic evaluation is warranted in younger patients with obscure bleeding (in whom small bowel tumors are the most common cause) and symptomatic older patients with overt or obscure bleeding. Upper endoscopy and colonoscopy should be repeated to ascertain that a lesion in these regions has not been overlooked. If these studies are unrevealing, capsule endoscopy should be performed to evaluate the small intestine. Capsule endoscopy is superior to radiographic studies (standard small bowel follow through, enteroclysis, or CT enterography) and standard push enteroscopy for the detection of small bowel abnormalities, demonstrating possible sources of occult bleeding in 50% of patients, most commonly vascular abnormalities (25%), ulcers (10–25%), and neoplasms (< 1–10%). Further management depends on the capsule endoscopic findings. Laparotomy is warranted if a small bowel tumor is identified by capsule endoscopy or radiographic studies. Most other lesions identified by capsule imaging can be further evaluated with enteroscopes that use overtubes with balloons to advance the scope through most of the small intestine in a forward and retrograde direction. Neoplasms can be biopsied or resected, and angioectasias may be cauterized. For massive or hemodynamically significant acute bleeding, angiography may be superior to enteroscopy for localization and embolization of a bleeding vascular abnormality. Abdominal CT may be considered to exclude a hepatic or pancreatic source of bleeding. A nuclear scan for Meckel diverticulum should be obtained in patients under age 30. With the advent of capsule imaging and advanced endoscopic technologies for evaluating and treating bleeding lesions in the small intestine, intraoperative enteroscopy of the small bowel is seldom required.

4. Occult Gastrointestinal Bleeding

Occult gastrointestinal bleeding refers to bleeding that is not apparent to the patient. Chronic gastrointestinal blood loss of < 100 mL/d may cause no appreciable change in stool appearance. Thus, occult bleeding in an adult is identified by a positive FOBT, FIT, or iron deficiency anemia in the absence of visible blood loss. FOBT or FIT may be performed in patients with gastrointestinal symptoms or as a screening test for colorectal neoplasia (see Chapter 39). From 2% to 6% of patients in screening programs have a positive FOBT or FIT.

In the United States, 2% of men and 5% of women have iron deficiency anemia (serum ferritin < 30–45 mcg/L). In premenopausal women, iron deficiency anemia is most commonly attributable to menstrual and pregnancy-associated iron loss; however, a gastrointestinal source of chronic blood loss is present in 10%. Occult blood loss may arise from anywhere in the gastrointestinal tract. Among men and postmenopausal women, a potential gastrointestinal cause of blood loss can be identified in the colon in 15–30% and in the upper gastrointestinal tract in 35–55%; a malignancy is present in 10%. Iron deficiency on rare occasions is caused by malabsorption (especially celiac disease) or malnutrition. The most common causes of occult bleeding with iron deficiency are (1) neoplasms; (2) vascular abnormalities (angioectasias); (3) acid-peptic lesions (esophagitis, peptic ulcer disease, erosions in hiatal hernia); (4) infections (nematodes, especially hookworm; tuberculosis); (5) medications (especially NSAIDs or aspirin); and (6) other causes such as inflammatory bowel disease.

▶ Evaluation of Occult Bleeding

Asymptomatic adults with positive FOBTs or FITs that are performed for routine colorectal cancer screening should undergo colonoscopy (see Chapter 39). All symptomatic adults with positive FOBTs or FITs or iron deficiency anemia should undergo evaluation of the lower and upper gastrointestinal tract with colonoscopy and upper endoscopy, unless the anemia can be definitively ascribed to a nongastrointestinal source (eg, menstruation, blood donation, or recent surgery). Patients with iron deficiency anemia should be evaluated for possible celiac disease with either IgA anti-tissue transglutaminase or duodenal biopsy. After evaluation of the upper and lower gastrointestinal tract with upper endoscopy and colonoscopy, the origin of occult bleeding remains unexplained in 30–50% of patients.

In younger patients (age < 60) with unexplained occult bleeding or iron deficiency, it is recommended to pursue further evaluation of the small intestine for a source of obscure-occult bleeding (as described above) in order to exclude a small intestinal neoplasm or inflammatory bowel disease. Patients over age 60 with occult bleeding who have a normal initial endoscopic evaluation and no other worrisome symptoms or signs (eg, abdominal pain, weight loss) most commonly have blood loss from angioectasias, which may be clinically unimportant. Therefore, it is reasonable to give an empiric trial of iron supplementation and observe the patient for evidence of clinically significant bleeding. For anemia that responds poorly to iron supplementation or recurrent or persistent chronic occult gastrointestinal blood loss, further evaluation is pursued for a source of obscure-occult bleeding (as described above). When possible, antiplatelet agents (aspirin, NSAIDs, clopidogrel) should be discontinued.

ASGE Standards of Practice Committee; Fisher L et al. The role of endoscopy in the management of obscure GI bleeding. Gastrointest Endosc. 2010 Sep;72(3):471–9. [PMID: 20801285]

Koulaouzidis A et al. Diagnostic yield of small-bowel capsule endoscopy in patients with iron-deficiency anemia: a systematic review. Gastrointest Endosc. 2012 Nov;76(5):983–92. [PMID: 23078923]

Lepileur L et al. Factors associated with diagnosis of obscure gastrointestinal bleeding by video capsule enteroscopy. Clin Gastroenterol Hepatol. 2012 Dec;10(12):1376–80. [PMID: 22677574]

Xin L et al. Indications, detectability, positive findings, total enteroscopy, and complications of diagnostic double-balloon endoscopy: a systematic review of data over the first decade of use. Gastrointest Endosc. 2011 Sep;74(3):563–70. [PMID: 21620401]

▼ DISEASES OF THE PERITONEUM

ASSESSMENT OF THE PATIENT WITH ASCITES

▶ Etiology of Ascites

The term "ascites" denotes the pathologic accumulation of fluid in the peritoneal cavity. Healthy men have little or no intraperitoneal fluid, but women normally may have up to 20 mL depending on the phase of the menstrual cycle. The causes of ascites may be classified into two broad pathophysiologic categories: that which is associated with a normal peritoneum and that which occurs due to a diseased peritoneum (Table 15–7). The most common cause of ascites is portal hypertension secondary to chronic liver disease, which accounts for over 80% of patients with ascites. The management of portal hypertensive ascites is discussed in Chapter 16. The most common causes of nonportal hypertensive ascites include infections (tuberculous peritonitis), intra-abdominal malignancy, inflammatory disorders of the peritoneum, and ductal disruptions (chylous, pancreatic, biliary).

▶ Clinical Findings

A. Symptoms and Signs

The history usually is one of increasing abdominal girth, with the presence of abdominal pain depending on the cause. Because most ascites is secondary to chronic liver disease with portal hypertension, patients should be asked about risk factors for liver disease, especially alcohol consumption, transfusions, tattoos, injection drug use, a history of viral hepatitis or jaundice, and birth in an area endemic for hepatitis. A history of cancer or marked weight loss arouses suspicion of malignant ascites. Fevers may suggest infected peritoneal fluid, including bacterial peritonitis (spontaneous or secondary). Patients with chronic liver

Table 15–7. Causes of ascites.

Normal Peritoneum

Portal hypertension (SAAG ≥ 1.1 g/dL)

1. Hepatic congestion[1]

Heart failure

Constrictive pericarditis

Tricuspid insufficiency

Budd-Chiari syndrome

Veno-occlusive disease

2. Liver disease[2]

Cirrhosis

Alcoholic hepatitis

Fulminant hepatic failure

Massive hepatic metastases

Hepatic fibrosis

Acute fatty liver of pregnancy

3. Portal vein occlusion

Hypoalbuminemia (SAAG < 1.1 g/dL)

Nephrotic syndrome

Protein-losing enteropathy

Severe malnutrition with anasarca

Miscellaneous conditions (SAAG < 1.1 g/dL)

Chylous ascites

Pancreatic ascites

Bile ascites

Nephrogenic ascites

Urine ascites

Myxedema (SAAG ≥ 1.1 g/dL)

Ovarian disease

Diseased Peritoneum (SAAG < 1.1 g/dL)[2]

Infections

Bacterial peritonitis

Tuberculous peritonitis

Fungal peritonitis

HIV-associated peritonitis

Malignant conditions

Peritoneal carcinomatosis

Primary mesothelioma

Pseudomyxoma peritonei

Massive hepatic metastases

Hepatocellular carcinoma

Other conditions

Familial Mediterranean fever

Vasculitis

Granulomatous peritonitis

Eosinophilic peritonitis

[1]Hepatic congestion usually associated with SAAG ≥ 1.1 g/dL and ascitic fluid total protein > 2.5 g/dL.

[2]There may be cases of "mixed ascites" in which portal hypertensive ascites is complicated by a secondary process such as infection. In these cases, the SAAG is ≥ 1.1 g/dL.

SAAG, serum-ascites albumin gradient = serum albumin minus ascitic fluid albumin.

disease and ascites are at greatest risk for developing spontaneous bacterial peritonitis. In immigrants, immunocompromised hosts, or severely malnourished alcoholics, tuberculous peritonitis should be considered.

Physical examination should emphasize signs of portal hypertension and chronic liver disease. Elevated jugular venous pressure may suggest right-sided heart failure or constrictive pericarditis. A large tender liver is characteristic of acute alcoholic hepatitis or Budd-Chiari syndrome

(thrombosis of the hepatic veins). The presence of large abdominal wall veins with cephalad flow also suggests portal hypertension; inferiorly directed flow implies hepatic vein obstruction. Signs of chronic liver disease include palmar erythema, cutaneous spider angiomas, gynecomastia, and muscle wasting. Asterixis secondary to hepatic encephalopathy may be present. Anasarca results from cardiac failure or nephrotic syndrome with hypoalbuminemia. Finally, firm lymph nodes in the left supraclavicular region or umbilicus may suggest intra-abdominal malignancy.

The physical examination is relatively insensitive for detecting ascitic fluid. In general, patients must have at least 1500 mL of fluid to be detected reliably by this method. Even the experienced clinician may find it difficult to distinguish between obesity and small-volume ascites. Abdominal ultrasound establishes the presence of fluid.

B. Laboratory Testing

1. Abdominal paracentesis—Abdominal paracentesis is performed as part of the diagnostic evaluation in all patients with new onset of ascites to help determine the cause. It also is recommended for patients admitted to the hospital with cirrhosis and ascites (in whom the prevalence of bacterial peritonitis is 10–20%) and when patients with known ascites deteriorate clinically (development of fever, abdominal pain, rapid worsening of renal function, or worsened hepatic encephalopathy) to exclude bacterial peritonitis.

A. INSPECTION—Cloudy fluid suggests infection. Milky fluid is seen with chylous ascites due to high triglyceride levels. Bloody fluid is most commonly attributable to a traumatic paracentesis, but up to 20% of cases of malignant ascites are bloody.

B. ROUTINE STUDIES

(1) Cell count—A white blood cell count with differential is the most important test. Normal ascitic fluid contains < 500 leukocytes/mcL and < 250 polymorphonuclear neutrophils (PMNs)/mcL. Any inflammatory condition can cause an elevated ascitic white blood cell count. A PMN count of > 250/mcL (neutrocytic ascites) with a percentage of > 75% of all white cells is highly suggestive of bacterial peritonitis, either spontaneous primary peritonitis or secondary peritonitis (ie, caused by an intra-abdominal source of infection, such as a perforated viscus or appendicitis). An elevated white count with a predominance of lymphocytes arouses suspicion of tuberculosis or peritoneal carcinomatosis.

(2) Albumin and total protein—The serum-ascites albumin gradient (SAAG) is the best single test for the classification of ascites into portal hypertensive and nonportal hypertensive causes (Table 15–7). Calculated by subtracting the ascitic fluid albumin from the serum albumin, the gradient correlates directly with the portal pressure. An SAAG ≥ 1.1 g/dL suggests underlying portal hypertension, while gradients < 1.1 g/dL implicate nonportal hypertensive causes.

The accuracy of the SAAG exceeds 95% in classifying ascites. It should be recognized, however, that approximately

4% of patients have "mixed ascites," ie, underlying cirrhosis with portal hypertension complicated by a second cause for ascites formation (such as malignancy or tuberculosis). Thus, a high SAAG is indicative of portal hypertension but does not exclude concomitant malignancy.

The ascitic fluid total protein provides some additional clues to the cause. An elevated SAAG and a high protein level (> 2.5 g/dL) are seen in most cases of hepatic congestion secondary to cardiac disease or Budd-Chiari syndrome. However, an increased ascitic fluid protein is also found in up to 20% of cases of uncomplicated cirrhosis. Two-thirds of patients with malignant ascites have a total protein level > 2.5 g/dL.

(3) Culture and Gram stain—The best technique consists of the inoculation of aerobic and anaerobic blood culture bottles with 5–10 mL of ascitic fluid at the patient's bedside, which increases the sensitivity for detecting bacterial peritonitis to over 85% in patients with neutrocytic ascites (> 250 PMNs/mcL), compared with approximately 50% sensitivity by conventional agar plate or broth cultures.

C. OPTIONAL STUDIES—Other laboratory tests are of utility in some specific clinical situations. Glucose and lactate dehydrogenase (LD) may be helpful in distinguishing spontaneous from secondary bacterial peritonitis (see below). An elevated amylase may suggest pancreatic ascites or a perforation of the gastrointestinal tract with leakage of pancreatic secretions into the ascitic fluid. Perforation of the biliary tree is suspected with an ascitic bilirubin concentration that is greater than the serum bilirubin. An elevated ascitic creatinine suggests leakage of urine from the bladder or ureters. Ascitic fluid cytologic examination is ordered if peritoneal carcinomatosis is suspected. Adenosine deaminase may be useful for the diagnosis of tuberculous peritonitis.

C. Imaging

Abdominal ultrasound is useful in confirming the presence of ascites and in the guidance of paracentesis. Both ultrasound and CT imaging are useful in distinguishing between causes of portal and nonportal hypertensive ascites. Doppler ultrasound and CT can detect Budd-Chiari syndrome. In patients with nonportal hypertensive ascites, these studies are useful in detecting lymphadenopathy and masses of the mesentery and of solid organs such as the liver, ovaries, and pancreas. Furthermore, they permit directed percutaneous needle biopsies of these lesions. Ultrasound and CT are poor procedures for the detection of peritoneal carcinomatosis; the role of positron emission tomography (PET) imaging is unclear.

D. Laparoscopy

Laparoscopy is an important test in the evaluation of some patients with nonportal hypertensive ascites (low SAAG) or mixed ascites. It permits direct visualization and biopsy of the peritoneum, liver, and some intra-abdominal lymph nodes. Cases of suspected peritoneal tuberculosis or suspected malignancy with nondiagnostic

CT imaging and ascitic fluid cytology are best evaluated by this method.

Gordon FD. Ascites. Clin Liver Dis. 2012 May;16(2):285–99. [PMID: 22541699]
Rahimi RS et al. End-stage liver disease complications. Curr Opin Gastroenterol. 2013 May;29(3):257–63. [PMID: 23429468]

SPONTANEOUS BACTERIAL PERITONITIS

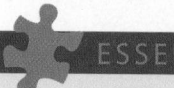

ESSENTIALS OF DIAGNOSIS

▸ A history of chronic liver disease and ascites.
▸ Fever and abdominal pain.
▸ Peritoneal signs uncommonly encountered on examination.
▸ Ascitic fluid neutrophil count > 250 white blood cells/mcL.

▶ General Considerations

"Spontaneous" bacterial infection of ascitic fluid occurs in the absence of an apparent intra-abdominal source of infection. It is seen with few exceptions in patients with ascites caused by chronic liver disease. Translocation of enteric bacteria across the gut wall or mesenteric lymphatics leads to seeding of the ascitic fluid, as may bacteremia from other sites. Approximately 20–30% of cirrhotic patients with ascites develop spontaneous peritonitis; however, the incidence is > 40% in patients with ascitic fluid total protein < 1 g/dL, probably due to decreased ascitic fluid opsonic activity.

Virtually all cases of spontaneous bacterial peritonitis are caused by a monomicrobial infection. The most common pathogens are enteric gram-negative bacteria (*E coli*, *Klebsiella pneumoniae*) or gram-positive bacteria (*Streptococcus pneumoniae*, viridans streptococci, *Enterococcus* species). Anaerobic bacteria are not associated with spontaneous bacterial peritonitis.

▶ Clinical Findings

A. Symptoms and Signs

Eighty to ninety percent of patients with spontaneous bacterial peritonitis are symptomatic; in many cases the presentation is subtle. Spontaneous bacterial peritonitis may be present in 10–20% of patients hospitalized with chronic liver disease, sometimes in the absence of any suggestive symptoms or signs.

The most common symptoms are fever and abdominal pain, present in two-thirds of patients. Spontaneous bacterial peritonitis may also present with a change in mental status due to exacerbation or precipitation of hepatic encephalopathy, or sudden worsening of renal function. Physical examination typically demonstrates signs of chronic liver disease with ascites. Abdominal tenderness is present in < 50% of patients, and its presence suggests other processes.

B. Laboratory Findings

The most important diagnostic test is abdominal paracentesis. Ascitic fluid should be sent for cell count with differential, and blood culture bottles should be inoculated at the bedside; Gram stain and reagent strips are insensitive.

In the proper clinical setting, an ascitic fluid PMN count of > 250 cells/mcL (neutrocytic ascites) is presumptive evidence of bacterial peritonitis. The percentage of PMNs is > 50–70% of the ascitic fluid white blood cells and commonly approximates 100%. Patients with neutrocytic ascites are presumed to be infected and should be started—regardless of symptoms—on antibiotics. Although 10–30% of patients with neutrocytic ascites have negative ascitic bacterial cultures ("culture-negative neutrocytic ascites"), it is presumed that these patients have bacterial peritonitis and should be treated empirically. Occasionally, a positive blood culture identifies the organism when ascitic fluid is sterile.

▶ Differential Diagnosis

Spontaneous bacterial peritonitis must be distinguished from secondary bacterial peritonitis, in which ascitic fluid has become secondarily infected by an intra-abdominal infection. Even in the presence of perforation, clinical symptoms and signs of peritonitis may be lacking owing to the separation of the visceral and parietal peritoneum by the ascitic fluid. Causes of secondary bacterial peritonitis include appendicitis, diverticulitis, perforated peptic ulcer, and perforated gallbladder. Secondary bacterial infection accounts for 3% of cases of infected ascitic fluid.

Ascitic fluid total protein, LD, and glucose are useful in distinguishing spontaneous bacterial peritonitis from secondary infection. Up to two-thirds of patients with secondary bacterial peritonitis have at least two of the following: decreased glucose level (< 50 mg/dL), an elevated LD level (greater than serum), and total protein > 1 g/dL. Ascitic neutrophil counts > 10,000/mcL also are suspicious; however, most patients with secondary peritonitis have neutrophil counts within the range of spontaneous peritonitis. The presence of multiple organisms on ascitic fluid Gram stain or culture is diagnostic of secondary peritonitis.

If secondary bacterial peritonitis is suspected, abdominal CT imaging of the upper and lower gastrointestinal tracts should be obtained to look for evidence of an intra-abdominal source of infection. If these studies are negative and secondary peritonitis still is suspected, repeat paracentesis should be performed after 48 hours of antibiotic therapy to confirm that the PMN count is decreasing. Secondary bacterial peritonitis should be suspected in patients in whom the PMN count is not below the pretreatment value at 48 hours.

Neutrocytic ascites may also be seen in some patients with peritoneal carcinomatosis, pancreatic ascites, or tuberculous ascites. In these circumstances, however, PMNs account for < 50% of the ascitic white blood cells.

▶ Prevention

Up to 70% of patients who survive an episode of spontaneous bacterial peritonitis will have another episode within 1 year. Oral once-daily prophylactic therapy—with norfloxacin, 400 mg, ciprofloxacin, 250–500 mg, or trimethoprim-sulfamethoxazole, one double-strength tablet—has been shown to reduce the rate of recurrent infections to < 20% and is recommended. Prophylaxis should be considered also in patients who have not had prior bacterial peritonitis but are at increased risk of infection due to low-protein ascites (total ascitic protein < 1 g/dL). Although improvement in survival in cirrhotic patients with ascites treated with prophylactic antibiotics has not been shown, decision analytic modeling suggests that in patients with prior bacterial peritonitis or low ascitic fluid protein, the use of prophylactic antibiotics is a cost-effective strategy.

▶ Treatment

Empiric therapy for spontaneous bacterial peritonitis should be initiated with a third-generation cephalosporin (such as cefotaxime, 2 g intravenously every 8–12 hours, or ceftriaxone, 1–2 g intravenously every 24 hours) or a combination beta-lactam/beta-lactamase agent (such as ampicillin/sulbactam, 2 g/1 g intravenously every 6 hours). Because of a high risk of nephrotoxicity in patients with chronic liver disease, aminoglycosides should not be used. A repeat paracentesis is recommended after 48 hours of treatment in patients without clinical improvement. If the ascitic neutrophil count has not decreased by 25%, antibiotic coverage should be adjusted (guided by culture and sensitivity results, if available) and secondary causes of peritonitis excluded. Although the optimal duration of therapy is unknown, a course of 5–10 days is sufficient in most patients, or until the ascites fluid PMN count decreases to < 250 cells/mcL.

Kidney injury develops in up to 40% of patients and is a major cause of death. Intravenous albumin increases effective arterial circulating volume and renal perfusion, decreasing the incidence of kidney injury and mortality. Intravenous albumin, 1.5 g/kg on day 1 and 1 g/kg on day 3, should be administered to patients at high risk for hepatorenal failure (ie, patients with baseline creatinine > 1 mg/dL, blood urea nitrogen (BUN) > 30 mg/dL, or bilirubin > 4 mg/dL). Patients with suspected secondary bacterial peritonitis should be given broad-spectrum coverage for enteric aerobic and anaerobic flora with a third-generation cephalosporin and metronidazole pending identification and definitive (usually surgical) treatment of the cause.

▶ Prognosis

The mortality rate of spontaneous bacterial peritonitis exceeds 30%. However, if the disease is recognized and treated early, the rate is < 10%. As the majority of patients have underlying severe liver disease, many may die of liver failure, hepatorenal syndrome, or bleeding complications from portal hypertension. The most effective treatment for recurrent spontaneous bacterial peritonitis is liver transplant.

Deshpande A et al. Acid-suppressive therapy is associated with spontaneous bacterial peritonitis in cirrhotic patients: a meta-analysis. J Gastroenterol Hepatol. 2013 Feb;28(2):235–42. [PMID: 23190338]

European Association for the Study of the Liver. EASL clinical practice guidelines on the management of ascites, spontaneous bacterial peritonitis, and hepatorenal syndrome in cirrhosis. J Hepatol. 2010 Sep;53(3):397–417. [PMID: 20633946]

Salerno F et al. Albumin infusion improves outcomes of patients with spontaneous bacterial peritonitis: a meta-analysis of randomized trials. Clin Gastroenterol Hepatol. 2013 Feb;11(2):123–30. [PMID: 23178229]

Tandon P et al. Renal dysfunction is the most important independent predictor of mortality in cirrhotic patients with spontaneous bacterial peritonitis. Clin Gastroenterol Hepatol. 2011 Mar;9(3):260–5. [PMID: 21145427]

MALIGNANT ASCITES

Two-thirds of cases of malignant ascites are caused by peritoneal carcinomatosis. The most common tumors causing carcinomatosis are primary adenocarcinomas of the ovary, uterus, pancreas, stomach, colon, lung, or breast. The remaining one-third is due to lymphatic obstruction or portal hypertension due to hepatocellular carcinoma or diffuse hepatic metastases. Patients present with nonspecific abdominal discomfort and weight loss associated with increased abdominal girth. Nausea or vomiting may be caused by partial or complete intestinal obstruction. Abdominal CT may be useful to demonstrate the primary malignancy or hepatic metastases but seldom confirms the diagnosis of peritoneal carcinomatosis. In patients with carcinomatosis, paracentesis demonstrates a low serum ascites-albumin gradient (< 1.1 mg/dL), an increased total protein (> 2.5 g/dL), and an elevated white cell count (often both neutrophils and mononuclear cells) but with a lymphocyte predominance. Cytology is positive in over 95%, but laparoscopy may be required in patients with negative cytology to confirm the diagnosis and to exclude tuberculous peritonitis, with which it may be confused. Malignant ascites attributable to portal hypertension usually is associated with an increased serum ascites-albumin gradient (> 1.1 g/dL), a variable total protein, and negative ascitic cytology. Ascites caused by peritoneal carcinomatosis does not respond to diuretics.

Patients may be treated with periodic large-volume paracentesis for symptomatic relief. Indwelling catheters can be left in place for patients approaching the end of life who require periodic paracentesis for symptomatic relief. Intraperitoneal chemotherapy is sometimes used to shrink the tumor, but the overall prognosis is extremely poor, with only 10% survival at 6 months. Ovarian cancers represent an exception to this rule. With newer treatments consisting of surgical debulking and intraperitoneal chemotherapy, long-term survival from ovarian cancer is possible.

Cavazzoni E et al. Malignant ascites: pathophysiology and treatment. Int J Clin Oncol. 2013 Feb;18(1):1–9. [PMID: 22460778]

FAMILIAL MEDITERRANEAN FEVER

This is a rare autosomal recessive disorder of unknown pathogenesis that almost exclusively affects people of Mediterranean ancestry, especially Sephardic Jews, Armenians, Turks, and Arabs. Patients lack a protease in serosal fluids that normally inactivates interleukin-8 and the chemotactic complement factor 5A. Symptoms present in most patients before the age of 20 years. It is characterized by episodic bouts of acute peritonitis that may be associated with serositis involving the joints and pleura. Peritoneal attacks are marked by the sudden onset of fever, severe abdominal pain, and abdominal tenderness with guarding or rebound tenderness. If left untreated, attacks resolve within 24–48 hours. Because symptoms resemble those of surgical peritonitis, patients may undergo unnecessary exploratory laparotomy. Colchicine, 0.6 mg orally two or three times daily, has been shown to decrease the frequency and severity of attacks.

MESOTHELIOMA

(See Chapter 39.)

MISCELLANEOUS PERITONEAL DISEASES

Chylous ascites is the accumulation of lipid-rich lymph in the peritoneal cavity. The ascitic fluid is characterized by a milky appearance with a triglyceride level > 1000 mg/dL. The usual cause in adults is lymphatic obstruction or leakage caused by malignancy, especially lymphoma. Nonmalignant causes include postoperative trauma, cirrhosis, tuberculosis, pancreatitis, and filariasis.

Pancreatic ascites is the intraperitoneal accumulation of massive amounts of pancreatic secretions due either to disruption of the pancreatic duct or to a pancreatic pseudocyst. It is most commonly seen in patients with chronic pancreatitis and complicates up to 3% of cases of acute pancreatitis. Because the pancreatic enzymes are not activated, pain often is absent. The ascitic fluid is characterized by a high protein level (> 2.5 g/dL) but a low SAAG. Ascitic fluid amylase levels are in excess of 1000 units/L. In nonsurgical cases, initial treatment consists of bowel rest, total parenteral nutrition (TPN), and octreotide to decrease pancreatic secretion. Persistent leakage requires treatment with either endoscopic placement of stents into the pancreatic duct or surgical drainage.

Bile ascites is caused most commonly by complications of biliary tract surgery, percutaneous liver biopsy, or abdominal trauma. Unless the bile is infected, bile ascites usually does not cause abdominal pain, fever, or leukocytosis. Paracentesis reveals yellow fluid with a ratio of ascites bilirubin to serum bilirubin > 1.0. Treatment depends on the location and rate of bile leakage. Postcholecystectomy cystic duct leaks may be treated with endoscopic sphincterotomy or biliary stent placement to facilitate bile flow across the sphincter of Oddi. Other leaks may be treated with percutaneous drainage by interventional radiologists or with surgical closure.

Baiocchi G et al. Chylous ascites in gynecologic malignancies: cases report and literature review. Arch Gynecol Obstet. 2010 Apr;281(4):677–81. [PMID: 19685063]

DISEASES OF THE ESOPHAGUS

(See Chapter 39 for Esophageal Cancer.)

► Symptoms

Heartburn, dysphagia, and odynophagia almost always indicate a primary esophageal disorder.

A. Heartburn

Heartburn (pyrosis) is the feeling of substernal burning, often radiating to the neck. Caused by the reflux of acidic (or, rarely, alkaline) material into the esophagus, it is highly specific for GERD.

B. Dysphagia

Difficulties in swallowing may arise from problems in transferring the food bolus from the oropharynx to the upper esophagus (oropharyngeal dysphagia) or from impaired transport of the bolus through the body of the esophagus (esophageal dysphagia). The history usually leads to the correct diagnosis.

1. Oropharyngeal dysphagia—The oropharyngeal phase of swallowing is a complex process requiring elevation of the tongue, closure of the nasopharynx, relaxation of the upper esophageal sphincter, closure of the airway, and pharyngeal peristalsis. A variety of mechanical and neuromuscular conditions can disrupt this process (Table 15–8). Problems with the oral phase of swallowing cause drooling or spillage of food from the mouth, inability to chew or

Table 15–9. Causes of esophageal dysphagia.

Cause	Clues
Mechanical obstruction	**Solid foods worse than liquids**
Schatzki ring	Intermittent dysphagia; not progressive
Peptic stricture	Chronic heartburn; progressive dysphagia
Esophageal cancer	Progressive dysphagia; age over 50 years
Eosinophilic esophagitis	Young adults; small-caliber lumen, proximal stricture, corrugated rings, or white papules
Motility disorder	**Solid and liquid foods**
Achalasia	Progressive dysphagia
Diffuse esophageal spasm	Intermittent; not progressive; may have chest pain
Scleroderma	Chronic heartburn; Raynaud phenomenon

initiate swallowing, or dry mouth. Pharyngeal dysphagia is characterized by an immediate sense of the bolus catching in the neck, the need to swallow repeatedly to clear food from the pharynx, or coughing or choking during meals. There may be associated dysphonia, dysarthria, or other neurologic symptoms.

2. Esophageal dysphagia—Esophageal dysphagia may be caused by **mechanical obstructions of** the esophagus or by **motility disorders** (Table 15–9). Patients with mechanical obstruction experience dysphagia, primarily for solids. This is recurrent, predictable, and, if the lesion progresses, will worsen as the lumen narrows. Patients with **motility disorders** have dysphagia for both solids and liquids. It is episodic, unpredictable, and can be progressive.

C. Odynophagia

Odynophagia is sharp substernal pain on swallowing that may limit oral intake. It usually reflects severe erosive disease. It is most commonly associated with infectious esophagitis due to *Candida*, herpesviruses, or CMV, especially in immunocompromised patients. It may also be caused by corrosive injury due to caustic ingestions and by pill-induced ulcers.

► Diagnostic Studies

A. Upper Endoscopy

Endoscopy is the study of choice for evaluating persistent heartburn, dysphagia, odynophagia, and structural abnormalities detected on barium esophagography. In addition to direct visualization, it allows biopsy of mucosal abnormalities and of normal mucosa (to evaluate for eosinophilic esophagitis) as well as dilation of strictures.

Table 15–8. Causes of oropharyngeal dysphagia.

Neurologic disorders
  Brainstem cerebrovascular accident, mass lesion
  Amyotrophic lateral sclerosis, multiple sclerosis, pseudobulbar palsy, post-polio syndrome, Guillain-Barré syndrome
  Parkinson disease, Huntington disease, dementia
  Tardive dyskinesia
Muscular and rheumatologic disorders
  Myopathies, polymyositis
  Oculopharyngeal dystrophy
  Sjögren syndrome
Metabolic disorders
  Thyrotoxicosis, amyloidosis, Cushing disease, Wilson disease
  Medication side effects: anticholinergics, phenothiazines
Infectious disease
  Polio, diphtheria, botulism, Lyme disease, syphilis, mucositis (*Candida*, herpes)
Structural disorders
  Zenker diverticulum
  Cervical osteophytes, cricopharyngeal bar, proximal esophageal webs
  Oropharyngeal tumors
  Postsurgical or radiation changes
  Pill-induced injury
Motility disorders
  Upper esophageal sphincter dysfunction

B. Videoesophagography

Oropharyngeal dysphagia is best evaluated with rapid-sequence videoesophagography.

C. Barium Esophagography

Patients with esophageal dysphagia often are evaluated first with a radiographic barium study to differentiate between mechanical lesions and motility disorders, providing important information about the latter in particular. In patients with esophageal dysphagia and a suspected motility disorder, barium esophagoscopy should be obtained first. In patients in whom there is a high suspicion of a mechanical lesion, many clinicians will proceed first to endoscopic evaluation because it better identifies mucosal lesions (eg, erosions) and permits mucosal biopsy and dilation. However, barium study is more sensitive for detecting subtle esophageal narrowing due to rings, achalasia, and proximal esophageal lesions.

D. Esophageal Manometry

Esophageal motility may be assessed using manometric techniques. They are indicated: (1) to determine the location of the LES to allow precise placement of a conventional electrode pH probe; (2) to establish the etiology of dysphagia in patients in whom a mechanical obstruction cannot be found, especially if a diagnosis of achalasia is suspected by endoscopy or barium study; (3) for the preoperative assessment of patients being considered for antireflux surgery to exclude an alternative diagnosis (eg, achalasia) or possibly to assess peristaltic function in the esophageal body. High-resolution manometry may be superior to conventional manometry for distinguishing motility disorders.

E. Esophageal pH Recording and Impedance Testing

The pH within the esophageal lumen may be monitored continuously for 24–48 hours. There are two kinds of systems in use: catheter-based and wireless. Traditional systems use a long transnasal catheter that is connected directly to the recording device. Wireless systems are increasingly used; in these systems, a capsule is attached directly to the esophageal mucosa under endoscopic visualization and data are transmitted by radiotelemetry to the recording device. The recording provides information about the amount of esophageal acid reflux and the temporal correlations between symptoms and reflux.

Esophageal pH monitoring devices provide information about the amount of esophageal acid reflux but not nonacid reflux. Techniques using combined pH and multichannel intraluminal impedance allow assessment of acid and nonacid liquid reflux. They may be useful in evaluation of patients with atypical reflux symptoms or persistent symptoms despite therapy with proton pump inhibitors to diagnose hypersensitivity, functional symptoms, and symptoms caused by nonacid reflux.

Villa N et al. Impedance-pH testing. Gastroenterol Clin North Am. 2013 Mar;42(1):17–26. [PMID: 23452628]

GASTROESOPHAGEAL REFLUX DISEASE

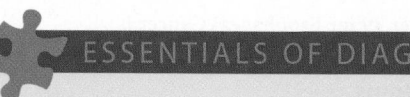

ESSENTIALS OF DIAGNOSIS

► Heartburn; may be exacerbated by meals, bending, or recumbency.
► Typical uncomplicated cases do not require diagnostic studies.
► Endoscopy demonstrates abnormalities in one-third of patients.

► General Considerations

GERD is a condition that develops when the reflux of stomach contents causes troublesome symptoms or complications. GERD affects 20% of adults, who report at least weekly episodes of heartburn, and up to 10% complain of daily symptoms. Although most patients have mild disease, esophageal mucosal damage (reflux esophagitis) develops in up to one-third and more serious complications develop in a few others. Several factors may contribute to GERD.

A. Dysfunction of the Gastroesophageal Junction

The antireflux barrier at the gastroesophageal junction depends on LES pressure, the intra-abdominal location of the sphincter (resulting in a "flap valve" caused by angulation of the esophageal-gastric junction), and the extrinsic compression of the sphincter by the crural diaphragm. In most patients with GERD, baseline LES pressures are normal (10–35 mm Hg). Most reflux episodes occur during transient relaxations of the LES that are triggered by gastric distention by a vagovagal reflex. A subset of patients with GERD have an incompetent (< 10 mm Hg) LES that results in increased acid reflux, especially when supine or when intra-abdominal pressures are increased by lifting or bending. A hypotensive sphincter is present in up to 50% of patients with severe erosive GERD.

Hiatal hernias are found in one-fourth of patients with nonerosive GERD, three-fourths of patients with severe erosive esophagitis, and over 90% of patients with Barrett esophagus. They are caused by movement of the LES above the diaphragm, resulting in dysfunction of the gastroesophageal junction reflux barrier. Hiatal hernias are common and may cause no symptoms; however, in patients with gastroesophageal reflux, they are associated with higher amounts of acid reflux and delayed esophageal acid clearance, leading to more severe esophagitis and Barrett esophagus. Increased reflux episodes occur during normal swallowing-induced relaxation, transient LES relaxations, and straining due to reflux of acid from the hiatal hernia sac into the esophagus.

Truncal obesity may contribute to GERD, presumably due to an increased intra-abdominal pressure, which contributes to dysfunction of the gastroesophageal junction and increased likelihood of hiatal hernia.

B. Irritant Effects of Refluxate

Esophageal mucosal damage is related to the potency of the refluxate and the amount of time it is in contact with the mucosa. Acidic gastric fluid (pH < 4.0) is extremely caustic to the esophageal mucosa and is the major injurious agent in the majority of cases. In some patients, reflux of bile or alkaline pancreatic secretions may be contributory.

Most acid reflux episodes occur after meals, despite the buffering effect of food that raises intragastric pH. In fact, meal-stimulated acid secretion from the proximal stomach mixes poorly with gastric contents, forming an unbuffered "acid pocket" that floats on top of the meal contents. In patients with GERD, this acid pocket is located near the gastroesophageal junction and may extend into the LES or hiatal hernia.

C. Abnormal Esophageal Clearance

Acid refluxate normally is cleared and neutralized by esophageal peristalsis and salivary bicarbonate. One-half of patients with severe GERD have diminished clearance due to hypotensive peristaltic contractions (< 30 mm Hg) or intermittent failed peristalsis after swallowing. Certain medical conditions such as scleroderma are associated with diminished peristalsis. Sjögren syndrome, anticholinergic medications, and oral radiation therapy may exacerbate GERD due to impaired salivation.

D. Delayed Gastric Emptying

Impaired gastric emptying due to gastroparesis or partial gastric outlet obstruction potentiates GERD.

▶ Clinical Findings

A. Symptoms and Signs

The typical symptom is heartburn. This most often occurs 30–60 minutes after meals and upon reclining. Patients often report relief from taking antacids or baking soda. When this symptom is dominant, the diagnosis is established with a high degree of reliability. Many patients, however, have less specific dyspeptic symptoms with or without heartburn. Overall, a clinical diagnosis of gastroesophageal reflux has a sensitivity and specificity of only 65%. Severity is not correlated with the degree of tissue damage. In fact, some patients with severe esophagitis are only mildly symptomatic. Patients may complain of regurgitation—the spontaneous reflux of sour or bitter gastric contents into the mouth. Dysphagia occurs in one-third of patients and may be due to erosive esophagitis, abnormal esophageal peristalsis, or the development of an esophageal stricture.

"Atypical" or "extraesophageal" manifestations of gastroesophageal disease may occur, including asthma, chronic cough, chronic laryngitis, sore throat, and noncardiac chest pain. Gastroesophageal reflux may be either a causative or an exacerbating factor in a subset of these patients, especially those with refractory symptoms. In the absence of heartburn or regurgitation, atypical symptoms are unlikely to be related to gastroesophageal reflux.

Physical examination and laboratory data are normal in uncomplicated disease.

B. Special Examinations

Initial diagnostic studies are not warranted for patients with typical GERD symptoms suggesting uncomplicated reflux disease. Patients with typical symptoms of heartburn and regurgitation should be treated empirically with a once daily proton pump inhibitor for 4–8 weeks. Symptomatic response to empiric treatment (while clinically desirable) only has a 78% sensitivity and 54% specificity for GERD. Therefore, further investigation is required in patients with symptoms that persist despite empiric proton pump inhibitor therapy to identify complications of reflux disease and to diagnose other conditions, particularly in patients with "alarm features" (troublesome dysphagia, odynophagia, weight loss, iron deficiency anemia).

1. Upper endoscopy—Upper endoscopy with biopsy is excellent for documenting the type and extent of tissue damage in gastroesophageal reflux; for detecting other gastroesophageal lesions that may mimic GERD; and for detecting GERD complications, including esophageal stricture, Barrett metaplasia, and esophageal adenocarcinoma. In the absence of prior antisecretory therapy, up to one-third of patients with GERD have visible mucosal damage (known as reflux esophagitis), characterized by single or multiple erosions or ulcers in the distal esophagus at the squamocolumnar junction. In patients treated with a proton pump inhibitor prior to endoscopy, preexisting reflux esophagitis may be partially or completely healed. The Los Angeles (LA) classification grades reflux esophagitis on a scale of A (one or more isolated mucosal breaks ≤ 5 mm that do not extend between the tops of two mucosal folds) to D (one or more mucosal breaks that involve at least 75% of the esophageal circumference).

2. Barium esophagography—This study should not be performed to diagnose GERD. In patients with severe dysphagia, it is sometimes obtained prior to endoscopy to identify a stricture.

3. Esophageal pH or combined esophageal pH-impedance testing—Esophageal pH monitoring is unnecessary in most patients but may be indicated to document abnormal esophageal acid exposure in patients who have atypical or extraesophageal symptoms or who are being considered for antireflux surgery. Combined impedance-pH monitoring is indicated in patients with persistent symptoms despite proton pump inhibitor therapy to determine whether symptoms are caused by acid or nonacid reflux (40%) or are unrelated to reflux and indicative of a functional disorder.

▶ Differential Diagnosis

Symptoms of GERD may be similar to those of other diseases such as esophageal motility disorders, peptic ulcer, angina pectoris, or functional disorders. Reflux erosive esophagitis may be confused with pill-induced damage, eosinophilic esophagitis, or infections (CMV, herpes, *Candida*).

▶ **Complications**

A. Barrett Esophagus

This is a condition in which the squamous epithelium of the esophagus is replaced by metaplastic columnar epithelium containing goblet and columnar cells (specialized intestinal metaplasia). Present in up to 10% of patients with chronic reflux, Barrett esophagus is believed to arise from chronic reflux-induced injury to the esophageal squamous epithelium; however, it is also increased in patients with truncal obesity independent of GERD. Barrett esophagus is suspected at endoscopy from the presence of orange, gastric type epithelium that extends upward from the stomach into the distal tubular esophagus in a tongue-like or circumferential fashion. Biopsies obtained at endoscopy confirm the diagnosis. Three types of columnar epithelium may be identified: gastric cardiac, gastric fundic, and specialized intestinal metaplasia. There is agreement that the latter carries an increased risk of dysplasia; however, some authorities believe that gastric cardiac mucosa also raises risk.

Barrett esophagus does not provoke specific symptoms but gastroesophageal reflux does. Most patients have a long history of reflux symptoms, such as heartburn and regurgitation. Barrett esophagus should be treated with long-term proton pump inhibitors once or twice daily to control reflux symptoms. Although these medications do not appear to cause regression of Barrett esophagus, they may reduce the risk of cancer. Paradoxically, one-third of patients report minimal or no symptoms of GERD, suggesting decreased acid sensitivity of Barrett epithelium. Indeed, over 90% of individuals with Barrett esophagus in the general population do not seek medical attention.

The most serious complication of Barrett esophagus is esophageal adenocarcinoma. It is believed that most adenocarcinomas of the esophagus and many such tumors of the gastric cardia arise from dysplastic epithelium in Barrett esophagus. In recent studies, the incidence of adenocarcinoma in patients with Barrett esophagus has been estimated at 0.12–0.33%/year. Although this still is an 11-fold increase risk compared with patients without Barrett esophagus, adenocarcinoma of the esophagus remains a relatively uncommon malignancy in the United States (7000 cases/year). Given the large number of adults with chronic GERD relative to the small number in whom adenocarcinoma develops, 2011 clinical guidelines recommend against endoscopic screening for Barrett esophagus in adults with GERD except in those with multiple risk factors for adenocarcinoma (chronic GERD, hiatal hernia, obesity, white race, male gender, and age 50 years of older).

In patients known to have Barrett esophagus, surveillance endoscopy every 3–5 years is recommended to look for low- or high-grade dysplasia or adenocarcinoma. The risk of progression to adenocarcinoma is a 0.8% risk per year for patients with low-grade dysplasia and a 6% risk per year for high-grade dysplasia. Patients with low-grade dysplasia require repeat endoscopic surveillance in 6 months to exclude coexisting high-grade dysplasia or cancer and, if low-grade dysplasia persists, endoscopic surveillance should be repeated yearly.

Approximately 13% of patient with high-grade dysplasia may harbor an unrecognized invasive esophageal cancer. Therefore, patients with high-grade dysplasia should undergo repeat staging endoscopy with resection of visible mucosal nodules and random mucosal biopsies in order to exclude invasive cancer (for which esophagectomy is recommended). The subsequent management of patients with intramucosal cancer or high-grade dysplasia has rapidly evolved. Until recently, esophagectomy was recommended for patients deemed to have a low operative risk; however, this procedure is associated with high morbidity and mortality rates (40% and 1–5%, respectively). Therefore, it is now recommended that endoscopic therapy be performed for most patients with high-grade dysplasia or intramucosal adenocarcinoma. Endoscopic therapies can remove or ablate dysplastic Barrett epithelium, using mucosal snare resection and radiofrequency wave ablation electrocautery. Snare resection is performed of visible neoplastic mucosal nodules to exclude submucosal invasion (which favors surgical resection). Of the patients who have cancer confined to the mucosa, < 2% have recurrence of cancer or high-grade dysplasia after snare resection. Radiofrequency wave ablation electrocautery is used to ablate Barrett epithelium with flat (non-nodular) dysplasia and to ablate Barrett epithelium that remains after snare resection of dysplastic mucosal nodules. The efficacy of endoscopic ablation therapies in patients with Barrett dysplasia is supported by several studies. When high-dose proton pump inhibitors are administered to normalize intraesophageal pH, radiofrequency wave ablation electrocautery eradication of Barrett columnar epithelium is followed by complete healing with normal squamous epithelium in > 90% of patients. In a 2011 randomized, sham-controlled trial in 127 patients with Barrett dysplasia with 3-year follow up, eradication of high-grade dysplasia occurred in 98% after radiofrequency ablation (HALO) and progression to cancer was only 0.55%/year. After initial ablation, Barrett esophagus recurs (with or without dysplasia) in up to 33% within 2 years, justifying periodic surveillance endoscopy.

Endoscopic ablation techniques have a risk of complications (bleeding, perforation, strictures). Therefore, endoscopic eradication therapy currently is not recommended for patients with nondysplastic Barrett esophagus for whom the risk of developing esophageal cancer is low and treatment does not appear to be cost-effective.

B. Peptic Stricture

Stricture formation occurs in about 5% of patients with esophagitis. It is manifested by the gradual development of solid food dysphagia progressive over months to years. Often there is a reduction in heartburn because the stricture acts as a barrier to reflux. Most strictures are located at the gastroesophageal junction. Endoscopy with biopsy is mandatory in all cases to differentiate peptic stricture from stricture by esophageal carcinoma. Active erosive esophagitis is often present. Up to 90% of symptomatic patients are effectively treated with dilation with graduated polyvinyl catheters passed over a wire placed at the time of endoscopy or fluoroscopically, or balloons passed fluoroscopically or through an endoscope. Dilation is continued over one to several sessions. A luminal diameter of 13–17 mm is usually sufficient to relieve dysphagia. Long-term therapy with a proton pump inhibitor is required to decrease the likelihood of stricture recurrence. Some patients require intermittent dilation to maintain luminal patency, but operative management for strictures that do not respond to dilation is seldom required. Refractory strictures may benefit from endoscopic injection of triamcinolone into the stricture.

▶ Treatment

A. Medical Treatment

The goal of treatment is to provide symptomatic relief, to heal esophagitis (if present), and to prevent complications. In the majority of patients with uncomplicated disease, empiric treatment is initiated based on a compatible history without the need for further confirmatory studies. Patients not responding and those with suspected complications undergo further evaluation with upper endoscopy or esophageal manometry and pH recording (see above).

1. Mild, intermittent symptoms—Patients with mild or intermittent symptoms that do not impact adversely on quality of life may benefit from lifestyle modifications with medical interventions taken as needed. Patients may find that eating smaller meals and elimination of acidic foods (citrus, tomatoes, coffee, spicy foods), foods that precipitate reflux (fatty foods, chocolate, peppermint, alcohol), and cigarettes may reduce symptoms. Weight loss should be recommended for patients who are overweight or have had recent weight gain. Patients with nocturnal symptoms should be advised to avoid lying down within 3 hours after meals (the period of greatest reflux) and to elevate the head of the bed on 6-inch blocks or a foam wedge to reduce reflux and enhance esophageal clearance.

Patients with infrequent heartburn (less than once weekly) may be treated on demand with antacids or oral H_2-receptor antagonists. Antacids provide rapid relief of heartburn; however, their duration of action is < 2 hours. Many are available over the counter. Those containing magnesium should not be used for patients with kidney disease, and patients with acute or chronic kidney disease should be cautioned appropriately.

All oral H_2-receptor antagonists are available in over-the-counter formulations: cimetidine 200 mg, ranitidine and nizatidine 75 mg, famotidine 10 mg—all of which are half of the typical prescription strength. When taken for active heartburn, these agents have a delay in onset of at least 30 minutes. However, once these agents take effect, they provide heartburn relief for up to 8 hours. When taken before meals known to provoke heartburn, these agents reduce the symptom.

2. Troublesome symptoms

A. INITIAL THERAPY—Patients with troublesome reflux symptoms and patients with known complications of GERD should be treated with a once-daily oral proton pump inhibitor (omeprazole or rabeprazole, 20 mg; omeprazole, 40 mg with sodium bicarbonate; lansoprazole, 30 mg; dexlansoprazole, 60 mg; esomeprazole or pantoprazole, 40 mg) taken 30 minutes before breakfast for 4–8 weeks. Because there appears to be little difference between these agents in efficacy or side effect profiles, the choice of agent is determined by cost. Oral omeprazole, 20 mg, and lansoprazole, 15 mg, are available as over-the-counter formulations. Once-daily proton pump inhibitors achieve adequate control of heartburn in 80–90% of patients, complete heartburn resolution in over 50%, and healing of erosive esophagitis (when present) in over 80%. Because of their superior efficacy and ease of use, proton pump inhibitors are preferred to H_2-receptor antagonists for the treatment of acute and chronic GERD. Approximately 10–20% of patients do not achieve symptom relief with a once-daily dose within 2–4 weeks and require a twice-daily proton pump inhibitor (taken 30 minutes before breakfast and dinner). Patients with inadequate symptom relief with empiric twice-daily proton pump inhibitor therapy should undergo evaluation with upper endoscopy. Many providers prefer to prescribe initial twice-daily proton pump inhibitor therapy for patients who have documented severe erosive esophagitis (LA Grade C or D), Barrett esophagus, or peptic stricture.

B. LONG-TERM THERAPY—In those who achieve good symptomatic relief with a course of empiric once-daily proton pump inhibitor, therapy may be discontinued after 8–12 weeks. Most patients (over 80%) will experience relapse of GERD symptoms, usually within 3 months. Patients whose symptoms relapse may be treated with either continuous proton pump inhibitor therapy, intermittent 2–4 week courses, or "on demand" therapy (ie, drug taken until symptoms abate) depending on symptom frequency and patient preference. Alternatively, twice daily H_2-receptor antagonists may be used to control symptoms in patients without erosive esophagitis. Patients who required twice-daily proton pump inhibitor therapy for initial symptom control and patients with complications of GERD, including severe erosive esophagitis, Barrett esophagus, or peptic stricture, should be maintained on long-term therapy with a once- or twice-daily proton pump inhibitor titrated to the lowest effective dose to achieve satisfactory symptom control.

Side effects of proton pump inhibitors are uncommon. Headache, diarrhea, and abdominal pain may occur with any of the agents but generally resolve when another formulation is tried. Potential risks of long-term use of proton pump inhibitors include an increased risk of infectious gastroenteritis (including *C difficile*), iron and vitamin B_{12} deficiency, hypomagnesemia, pneumonia, hip fractures (possibly due to impaired calcium absorption), and fundic gland polyps (which appear to be of no clinical significance).

3. Extraesophageal reflux manifestations—Establishing a causal relationship between gastroesophageal reflux and extraesophageal symptoms (eg, asthma, hoarseness, cough) is difficult. Gastroesophageal reflux seldom is the sole cause of extraesophageal disorders but may be a contributory factor. Although ambulatory esophageal pH testing can document the presence of increased acid esophageal reflux, it does not prove a causative connection. Current guidelines recommend that a trial of a twice-daily proton pump inhibitor be administered for 2–3 months in patients with suspected extraesophageal GERD syndromes who also have typical GERD symptoms. Improvement of extraesophageal symptoms suggests but does not prove that acid reflux is the causative factor. Esophageal pH testing may be performed in patients whose extraesophageal symptoms persist after 3 months of twice-daily proton pump inhibitor therapy and may be considered before proton pump inhibitor therapy in patients without typical GERD symptoms in whom other causes of extraesophageal symptoms have been excluded.

4. Unresponsive disease—Approximately 5% do not respond to twice-daily proton pump inhibitors or a change to a different proton pump inhibitor. These patients should undergo endoscopy for detection of severe, inadequately treated reflux esophagitis and for other gastroesophageal lesions (including eosinophilic esophagitis) that may mimic GERD. The presence of active erosive esophagitis usually is indicative of inadequate acid suppression and can almost always be treated successfully with higher proton pump inhibitor doses (eg, esomeprazole, 40 mg twice daily). Alginate is a naturally occurring polymer that forms a viscous raft that floats on the gastric acid pocket and significantly reduces postprandial reflux episodes in patients with GERD and large hiatal hernias. A proprietary antacid-alginate formulation (Gaviscon Double Action Liquid) is available in Europe but not the United States. Truly refractory esophagitis may be caused by gastrinoma with gastric acid hypersecretion (Zollinger-Ellison syndrome), pill-induced esophagitis, resistance to proton pump inhibitors, and medical noncompliance. Patients without endoscopically visible esophagitis should undergo ambulatory impedance-pH monitoring while taking a twice-daily proton pump inhibitor to determine whether the symptoms are correlated with acid or nonacid reflux episodes. The pH study is performed on therapy if the suspicion for GERD is high (to determine whether therapy has adequately suppressed acid esophageal reflux) and off therapy if the suspicion for GERD is low (to determine whether the patient has reflux disease). Combined esophageal pH monitoring with impedance monitoring is preferred over pH testing alone because of its ability to detect both acid and nonacid reflux events. Approximately 60% of patients with unresponsive symptoms do not have increased reflux and may be presumed to have a functional disorder. Treatment with a low-dose tricyclic antidepressant (eg, imipramine or nortriptyline 25 mg at bedtime) may be beneficial.

B. Surgical Treatment

Surgical fundoplication affords good to excellent relief of symptoms and healing of esophagitis in over 85% of properly selected patients and can be performed laparoscopically with low complication rates in most instances. Although patient satisfaction is high, typical reflux symptoms recur in 10–30% of patients. Furthermore, new symptoms of dysphagia, bloating, increased flatulence, dyspepsia, or diarrhea develop in over 30% of patients. In 2011, results from a randomized trial comparing laparoscopic fundoplication with prolonged medical therapy (esomeprazole 40 mg/d) for chronic GERD

were reported. After 5 years, adequate GERD symptom control (symptom remission) were similar, occurring in 85–92% of patients; however, patients who had undergone fundoplication had increased dysphagia, bloating, and flatulence. In 2012, the FDA approved a novel, minimally invasive magnetic artificial sphincter for the treatment of GERD. The device is made up a flexible, elastic string of titanium beads (wrapped around a magnetic core) that is placed laparoscopically below the diaphragm at the gastroesophageal junction. A 2013 prospective study of 100 patients reported that 64% of patients had significant reductions in esophageal acid reflux. Further experience with this device is needed before widespread adoption can be recommended.

Surgical treatment is not recommended for patients who are well controlled with medical therapies but should be considered for: (1) otherwise healthy, carefully selected patients with extraesophageal manifestations of reflux, as these symptoms often require high doses of proton pump inhibitors and may be more effectively controlled with antireflux surgery; (2) those with severe reflux disease who are unwilling to accept lifelong medical therapy due to its expense, inconvenience, or theoretical risks; and (3) patients with large hiatal hernias and persistent regurgitation despite proton pump inhibitor therapy. Gastric bypass (rather than fundoplication) should be considered for obese patients with GERD.

▶ When to Refer

- Patients with typical GERD whose symptoms do not resolve with empiric management with a twice-daily proton pump inhibitor.

- Patients with suspected extraesophageal GERD symptoms that do not resolve with 3 months of twice-daily proton pump inhibitor therapy.

- Patients with significant dysphagia or other alarm symptoms for upper endoscopy.

- Patients with Barrett esophagus for endoscopic surveillance.

- Patients who have Barrett esophagus with dysplasia or early mucosal cancer.

- Surgical fundoplication is considered.

Bennett C et al. Consensus statements for management of Barrett's dysplasia and early-stage esophageal adenocarcinoma, based on a Delphi process. Gastroenterology. 2012 Aug;143(2):336–46. [PMID: 22537613]

Bredenoord AJ et al. Gastro-oesophageal reflux disease. Lancet. 2013 Jun 1;381(9881):1933–42. [PMID: 23477993]

Galmiche JP et al; LOTUS Trial Collaborators. Laparoscopic antireflux surgery vs esomeprazole treatment for chronic GERD. JAMA. 2011 May 18;305(19):1969–77. [PMID: 21586712]

Ganz RA et al. Esophageal sphincter device for gastroesophageal reflux disease. N Engl J Med. 2013 May 23;368(21):2039–40. [PMID: 23697523]

Gupta M et al. Recurrence of esophageal intestinal metaplasia after endoscopic mucosal resection and radiofrequency ablation of Barrett's esophagus: results from a US Multicenter Consortium. Gastroenterology. 2013 Jul;145(1):79–86. [PMID: 23499759]

Hvid-Jensen F et al. Incidence of adenocarcinoma among patients with Barrett's esophagus. N Engl J Med. 2011 Oct 13;365(15):1375–83. [PMID: 21995385]

Johnson DA et al. Reported side effects and complications of long-term proton pump inhibitor use: dissecting the evidence. Clin Gastroenterol Hepatol. 2013 May;11(5):458–64. Erratum in: Clin Gastroenterol Hepatol. 2013 Jul;11(7):880. [PMID: 23247326]

Kahrilas PJ et al. The acid pocket: a target for treatment in reflux disease? Am J Gastroenterol. 2013 Jul;108(7):1058–64. [PMID: 23629599]

Katz PO et al. Guidelines for the diagnosis and management of gastroesophageal reflux disease. Am J Gastroenterol. 2013 Mar;108(3):308–28. Erratum in: Am J Gastroenterol. 2013 Oct;108(10):1672. [PMID: 23419381]

Richter JE. Gastroesophageal reflux disease treatment: side effects and complications of fundoplication. Clin Gastroenterol Hepatol. 2013 May;11(5):465–71. [PMID: 23267868]

Rohof WO et al. An alginate-antacid formulation localizes to the acid pocket to reduce acid reflux in patients with gastroesophageal reflux disease. Clin Gastroenterol Hepatol. 2013 Dec;11(12):1585–91. [PMID: 23669304]

Shaheen NJ et al. Upper endoscopy for gastroesophageal reflux disease: best practice advice from the Clinical Guidelines Committee of the American College of Physicians. Ann Intern Med. 2012 Dec 4;157(11):808–16. [PMID: 23208168]

Spechler SJ. Barrett esophagus and risk of esophageal cancer: a clinical review. JAMA. 2013 Aug 14;310(6):627–36. [PMID: 23942681]

Villa N et al. Impedance-pH testing. Gastroenterol Clin North Am. 2013 Mar;42(1):17–26. [PMID: 23452628]

INFECTIOUS ESOPHAGITIS

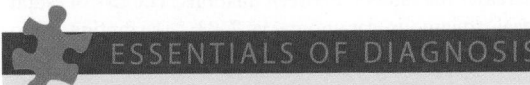

ESSENTIALS OF DIAGNOSIS

- ▶ Immunosuppressed patient.
- ▶ Odynophagia, dysphagia, and chest pain.
- ▶ Endoscopy with biopsy establishes diagnosis.

General Considerations

Infectious esophagitis occurs most commonly in immunosuppressed patients. Patients with AIDS, solid organ transplants, leukemia, lymphoma, and those receiving immunosuppressive drugs are at particular risk for opportunistic infections. *Candida albicans*, herpes simplex, and CMV are the most common pathogens. *Candida* infection may occur also in patients who have uncontrolled diabetes and those being treated with systemic corticosteroids, radiation therapy, or systemic antibiotic therapy. Herpes simplex can affect normal hosts, in which case the infection is generally self-limited.

Clinical Findings

A. Symptoms and Signs

The most common symptoms are odynophagia and dysphagia. Substernal chest pain occurs in some patients. Patients with candidal esophagitis are sometimes asymptomatic. Oral thrush is present in only 75% of patients with candidal esophagitis and 25–50% of patients with viral esophagitis and is therefore an unreliable indicator of the cause of esophageal infection. Patients with esophageal CMV infection may have infection at other sites such as the colon and retina. Oral ulcers (herpes labialis) are often associated with herpes simplex esophagitis.

B. Special Examinations

Treatment may be empiric. For diagnostic certainty, endoscopy with biopsy and brushings (for microbiologic and histopathologic analysis) is preferred because of its high diagnostic accuracy. The endoscopic signs of candidal esophagitis are diffuse, linear, yellow-white plaques adherent to the mucosa. CMV esophagitis is characterized by one to several large, shallow, superficial ulcerations. Herpes esophagitis results in multiple small, deep ulcerations.

▶ Treatment

A. Candidal Esophagitis

Systemic therapy is required for esophageal candidiasis. An empiric trial of antifungal therapy is often administered without performing diagnostic endoscopy. Initial therapy is generally with fluconazole, 400 mg on day 1, then 200–400 mg/d orally for 14–21 days. Patients not responding to empiric therapy within 3–5 days should undergo endoscopy with brushings, biopsy, and culture to distinguish resistant fungal infection from other infections (eg, CMV, herpes). Esophageal candidiasis not responding to fluconazole therapy may be treated with itraconazole suspension (not capsules), 200 mg/d orally, or voriconazole, 200 mg orally twice daily. Refractory infection may be treated intravenously with caspofungin, 50 mg daily.

B. Cytomegalovirus Esophagitis

In patients with HIV infection, immune restoration with highly active antiretroviral therapy (HAART) is the most effective means of controlling CMV disease. Initial therapy is with ganciclovir, 5 mg/kg intravenously every 12 hours for 3–6 weeks. Neutropenia is a frequent dose-limiting side effect. Once resolution of symptoms occurs, it may be possible to complete the course of therapy with oral valganciclovir, 900 mg once daily. Patients who either do not respond to or cannot tolerate ganciclovir are treated acutely with foscarnet, 90 mg/kg intravenously every 12 hours for 3–6 weeks. The principal toxicity is acute renal injury, hypocalcemia, and hypomagnesemia.

C. Herpetic Esophagitis

Immunocompetent patients may be treated symptomatically and generally do not require specific antiviral therapy. Immunosuppressed patients may be treated with oral acyclovir, 400 mg orally five times daily, or 250 mg/m² intravenously every 8–12 hours, usually for 14–21 days. Oral famciclovir, 500 mg orally three times daily, or valacyclovir, 1 g twice daily, are also effective but more expensive than generic acyclovir. Nonresponders require therapy with foscarnet, 40 mg/kg intravenously every 8 hours for 21 days.

Prognosis

Most patients with infectious esophagitis can be effectively treated with complete symptom resolution. Depending on the patient's underlying immunodeficiency, relapse of symptoms off therapy can raise difficulties. Long-term suppressive therapy is sometimes required.

Kim KY et al. Acid suppression therapy as a risk factor for *Candida* esophagitis. Dig Dis Sci. 2013 May;58(5):1282–6. [PMID: 23306845]

PILL-INDUCED ESOPHAGITIS

A number of different medications may injure the esophagus, presumably through direct, prolonged mucosal contact. The most commonly implicated are the NSAIDs, potassium chloride pills, quinidine, zalcitabine, zidovudine, alendronate and risedronate, emepronium bromide, iron, vitamin C, and antibiotics (doxycycline, tetracycline, clindamycin, trimethoprim-sulfamethoxazole). Because injury is most likely to occur if pills are swallowed without water or while supine, hospitalized or bed-bound patients are at greater risk. Symptoms include severe retrosternal chest pain, odynophagia, and dysphagia, often beginning several hours after taking a pill. These may occur suddenly and persist for days. Some patients (especially the elderly) have relatively little pain, presenting with dysphagia. Endoscopy may reveal one to several discrete ulcers that may be shallow or deep. Chronic injury may result in severe esophagitis with stricture, hemorrhage, or perforation. Healing occurs rapidly when the offending agent is eliminated. To prevent pill-induced damage, patients should take pills with 4 oz of water and remain upright for 30 minutes after ingestion. Known offending agents should not be given to patients with esophageal dysmotility, dysphagia, or strictures.

Ueda K et al. A case of esophageal ulcer caused by alendronate sodium tablets. Gastrointest Endosc. 2011 May;73(5):1037–8. [PMID: 21521571]

CAUSTIC ESOPHAGEAL INJURY

Caustic esophageal injury occurs from accidental (usually children) or deliberate (suicidal) ingestion of liquid or crystalline alkali (drain cleaners, etc) or acid. Ingestion is followed almost immediately by severe burning and varying degrees of chest pain, gagging, dysphagia, and drooling. Aspiration results in stridor and wheezing. Initial examination should be directed to circulatory status as well as assessment of airway patency and the oropharyngeal mucosa, including laryngoscopy. Patients without major symptoms (dyspnea, dysphagia, drooling, hematemesis) or oropharyngeal lesions have a very low likelihood of having severe gastroesophageal injury. All other patients initially should be hospitalized in an ICU. Chest and abdominal radiographs are obtained looking for pneumonitis or free perforation. Initial treatment is supportive, with intravenous fluids, intravenous proton pump inhibitors to prevent gastric stress ulceration (pantoprazole or esomeprazole, 40 mg twice daily) and analgesics. Nasogastric lavage and oral antidotes may be dangerous and should generally not be administered. Laryngoscopy should be performed in patients with respiratory distress to assess the need for tracheostomy. Endoscopy is usually performed within the first 12–24 hours to assess the extent of injury, especially in patients with significant symptoms or oropharyngeal lesions. Many patients are discovered to have no mucosal injury to the esophagus or stomach, allowing prompt discharge and psychiatric referral. Patients with evidence of mild damage (edema, erythema, exudates or superficial ulcers) recover quickly, have low risk of developing stricture, and may be advanced from liquids to a regular diet over 24–48 hours. Patients with signs of severe injury—deep or circumferential ulcers or necrosis (black discoloration) have a high risk (up to 65%) of acute complications, including perforation with mediastinitis or peritonitis, bleeding, stricture, or esophageal-tracheal fistulas. These patients must be kept fasting and monitored closely for signs of deterioration that warrant emergency surgery with possible esophagectomy and colonic or jejunal interposition. A nasoenteric feeding tube is placed after 24 hours. Oral feedings of liquids may be initiated after 2–3 days if the patient is able to tolerate secretions. Neither corticosteroids nor antibiotics are recommended. Esophageal strictures develop in up to 70% of patients with serious esophageal injury weeks to months after the initial injury, requiring recurrent dilations. Endoscopic injection of intralesional corticosteroids (triamcinolone 40 mg) increases the interval between dilations. The risk of esophageal squamous carcinoma is 2–3%, warranting endoscopic surveillance 15–20 years after the caustic ingestion.

Chirica M et al. Surgery for caustic injuries of the upper gastrointestinal tract. Ann Surg. 2012 Dec;256(6):994–1001. [PMID: 22824850]

Harlak A et al. Surgical treatment of caustic esophageal strictures in adults. Int J Surg. 2013;11(2):164–8. [PMID: 23267851]

BENIGN ESOPHAGEAL LESIONS

1. Mallory-Weiss Syndrome (Mucosal Laceration of Gastroesophageal Junction)

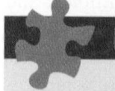

ESSENTIALS OF DIAGNOSIS

► Hematemesis; usually self-limited.

► Prior history of vomiting, retching in 50%.

► Endoscopy establishes diagnosis.

General Considerations

Mallory-Weiss syndrome is characterized by a nonpenetrating mucosal tear at the gastroesophageal junction that is hypothesized to arise from events that suddenly raise transabdominal pressure, such as lifting, retching, or vomiting. Alcoholism is a strong predisposing factor. Mallory-Weiss tears are responsible for approximately 5% of cases of upper gastrointestinal bleeding.

Clinical Findings

A. Symptoms and Signs

Patients usually present with hematemesis with or without melena. A history of retching, vomiting, or straining is obtained in about 50% of cases.

B. Special Examinations

As with other causes of upper gastrointestinal hemorrhage, upper endoscopy should be performed after the patient has been appropriately resuscitated. The diagnosis is established by identification of a 0.5- to 4-cm linear mucosal tear usually located either at the gastroesophageal junction or, more commonly, just below the junction in the gastric mucosa.

Differential Diagnosis

At endoscopy, other potential causes of upper gastrointestinal hemorrhage are found in over 35% of patients with Mallory-Weiss tears, including peptic ulcer disease, erosive gastritis, arteriovenous malformations, and esophageal varices. Patients with underlying portal hypertension are at higher risk for continued or recurrent bleeding.

Treatment

Patients are initially treated as needed with fluid resuscitation and blood transfusions. Most patients stop bleeding spontaneously and require no therapy. Endoscopic hemostatic therapy is employed in patients who have continuing active bleeding. Injection with epinephrine (1:10,000), cautery with a bipolar or heater probe coagulation device, or mechanical compression of the artery by application of an endoclip or band is effective in 90–95% of cases. Angiographic arterial embolization or operative intervention is required in patients who fail endoscopic therapy.

Fujisawa N et al. Risk factors for mortality in patients with Mallory-Weiss syndrome. Hepatogastroenterology. 2011 Mar–Apr;58(106):417–20. [PMID: 21661406]

Yin A et al. Mallory-Weiss syndrome: clinical and endoscopic characteristics. Eur J Intern Med. 2012 Jun;23(4):e92–6. [PMID: 22560400]

2. Eosinophilic Esophagitis

General Considerations

Eosinophilia of the esophagus may be caused by several conditions, most commonly eosinophilic esophagitis; GERD; proton pump inhibitor–responsive eosinophilia; and celiac disease, Crohn disease, and pemphigus (although rarely).

Eosinophilic esophagitis is a disorder in which food or environmental antigens are thought to stimulate an inflammatory response. Initially recognized in children, it is increasingly identified in young or middle-aged adults,

predominantly men (75%). A history of allergies or atopic conditions (asthma, eczema, hay fever) is present in over half of patients.

Clinical Findings

Most adults have a long history of dysphagia for solid-foods or an episode of food impaction. Heartburn may be present. Children may have abdominal pain, vomiting, chest pain, or failure to thrive. On laboratory tests, a few have eosinophilia or elevated IgE levels. Barium swallow studies may demonstrate a small-caliber esophagus; focal or long, tapered strictures; or multiple concentric rings. However, endoscopy with esophageal biopsy and histologic evaluation is required to establish the diagnosis. Endoscopic appearances include white exudates or papules, red furrows, corrugated concentric rings, and strictures; however, the esophagus is grossly normal in up to 10% of patients. Multiple biopsies (at least 2–4) from the proximal and distal esophagus should be obtained to demonstrate multiple (> 15/high-powered field) eosinophils in the mucosa. Most children have other coexisting atopic disorders. Skin testing for food allergies may be helpful to identify causative factors, especially in children.

Treatment

Before making a diagnosis of eosinophilic esophagitis, all patients should be given an empiric trial of a proton pump inhibitor orally twice daily for 2 months followed by repeat endoscopy and mucosal biopsy to exclude GERD and so-called proton pump inhibitor–responsive eosinophilia, a distinct entity that is not necessarily related to GERD. Approximately 35% of symptomatic patients with increased esophageal eosinophils have clinical and histologic improvement with proton pump inhibitor treatment.

Eosinophilic esophagitis is diagnosed in patients with persistent symptoms and eosinophilia; the optimal treatment of this condition is uncertain. Referral to an allergist for evaluation of coexisting atopic disorders and for testing for food and environmental allergens may be considered. In children, food elimination or elemental diets lead to clinical and histologic improvement in 75%. The most common allergenic foods are dairy, eggs, wheat, soy, peanuts, and shellfish. In a 2012 prospective study of 50 adults who eliminated these foods for 6 weeks, dysphagia improved in 94% and esophageal eosinophils were reduced to < 10/hpf in 70%. Reintroduction of the trigger food results in prompt recurrence of symptoms. Topical corticosteroids lead to symptom resolution in 70% of adults. For example, budesonide suspension (1 mg orally) may be administered twice daily or one to two puffs of fluticasone (440 mcg/puff inhaler without a spacer twice daily after meals) may be swallowed after activation instead of inhaled. Symptomatic relapse is common after discontinuation of therapy and may require maintenance therapy. Graduated dilation of strictures should be conducted in patients with dysphagia and strictures or narrow-caliber esophagus but should be performed cautiously because there is an increased risk of perforation and postprocedural chest pain.

Chehade M et al. Causes, evaluation, and consequences of eosinophilic esophagitis. Ann N Y Acad Sci. 2013 Oct;1300: 110–8. [PMID: 24117638]

Dellon ES et al. ACG Clinical Guideline: evidence based approach to the diagnosis and management of esophageal eosinophilia and eosinophilic esophagitis. Am J Gastroenterol. 2013 May;108(5):679–92. [PMID: 23567357]

Gonsalves N et al. Elimination diet effectively treats eosinophilic esophagitis in adults; food reintroduction identifies causative factors. Gastroenterology. 2012 Jun;142(7):1451–9.e1 [PMID: 22391333]

3. Esophageal Webs & Rings

Esophageal webs are thin, diaphragm-like membranes of squamous mucosa that typically occur in the mid or upper esophagus and may be multiple. They may be congenital but also occur with eosinophilic esophagitis, graft-versus-host disease, pemphigoid, epidermolysis bullosa, pemphigus vulgaris, and, rarely, in association with iron deficiency anemia (Plummer-Vinson syndrome). Esophageal "Schatzki" rings are smooth, circumferential, thin (< 4 mm in thickness) mucosal structures located in the distal esophagus at the squamocolumnar junction. Their pathogenesis is controversial. They are associated in nearly all cases with a hiatal hernia, and reflux symptoms are common, suggesting that acid gastroesophageal reflux may be contributory in many cases. Most webs and rings are over 20 mm in diameter and are asymptomatic. Solid food dysphagia most often occurs with rings < 13 mm in diameter. Characteristically, dysphagia is intermittent and not progressive. Large poorly chewed food boluses such as beef-steak are most likely to cause symptoms. Obstructing boluses may pass by drinking extra liquids or after regurgitation. In some cases, an impacted bolus must be extracted endoscopically. Esophageal webs and rings are best visualized using a barium esophagogram with full esophageal distention. Endoscopy is less sensitive than barium esophagography.

The majority of symptomatic patients with a single ring or web can be effectively treated with the passage of bougie dilators to disrupt the lesion or endoscopic electrosurgical incision of the ring. A single dilation may suffice, but repeat dilations are required in many patients. Patients who have heartburn or who require repeated dilation should receive long-term acid suppressive therapy with a proton pump inhibitor.

Müller M et al. Is the Schatzki ring a unique esophageal entity? World J Gastroenterol. 2011 Jun 21;17(23):2838–43. [PMID: 21734791]

4. Zenker Diverticulum

Zenker diverticulum is a protrusion of pharyngeal mucosa that develops at the pharyngoesophageal junction between the inferior pharyngeal constrictor and the cricopharyngeus. The cause is believed to be loss of elasticity of the upper esophageal sphincter, resulting in restricted opening during swallowing. Symptoms of dysphagia and regurgitation tend to develop insidiously over years in older patients.

Initial symptoms include vague oropharyngeal dysphagia with coughing or throat discomfort. As the diverticulum enlarges and retains food, patients may note halitosis, spontaneous regurgitation of undigested food, nocturnal choking, gurgling in the throat, or a protrusion in the neck. Complications include aspiration pneumonia, bronchiectasis, and lung abscess. The diagnosis is best established by a barium esophagogram.

Symptomatic patients require upper esophageal myotomy and, in most cases, surgical diverticulectomy. An intraluminal approach has been developed in which the septum between the esophagus and diverticulum is incised using a rigid or flexible endoscope. Significant improvement occurs in over 90% of patients treated surgically. Small asymptomatic diverticula may be observed.

Prisman E et al. Zenker diverticulum. Otolaryngol Clin North Am. 2013 Dec;46(6):1101–11. [PMID: 24262962]

5. Esophageal Varices

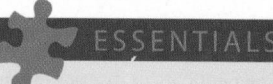
ESSENTIALS OF DIAGNOSIS

- ▸ Develop secondary to portal hypertension.
- ▸ Found in 50% of patients with cirrhosis.
- ▸ One-third of patients with varices develop upper gastrointestinal bleeding.
- ▸ Diagnosis established by upper endoscopy.

▸ General Considerations

Esophageal varices are dilated submucosal veins that develop in patients with underlying portal hypertension and may result in serious upper gastrointestinal bleeding. The causes of portal hypertension are discussed in Chapter 16. Under normal circumstances, there is a 2–6 mm Hg pressure gradient between the portal vein and the inferior vena cava. When the gradient exceeds 10–12 mm Hg, significant portal hypertension exists. Esophageal varices are the most common cause of important gastrointestinal bleeding due to portal hypertension, though gastric varices and, rarely, intestinal varices may also bleed. Bleeding from esophageal varices most commonly occurs in the distal 5 cm of the esophagus.

The most common cause of portal hypertension is cirrhosis. Approximately 50% of patients with cirrhosis have esophageal varices. Bleeding from varices occurs in 30% of patients with esophageal varices. In the absence of any treatment, variceal bleeding spontaneously stops in about 50% of patients. Patients surviving this bleeding episode have a 60% chance of recurrent variceal bleeding, usually within the first 6 weeks. With current therapies, the in-hospital mortality rate associated with bleeding esophageal varices is 15%.

A number of factors have been identified that may portend an increased risk of bleeding from esophageal varices. The most important are: (1) the size of the varices; (2) the presence at endoscopy of red wale markings (longitudinal dilated venules on the varix surface); (3) the severity of liver disease (as assessed by Child scoring); and (4) active alcohol abuse—patients with cirrhosis who continue to drink have an extremely high risk of bleeding.

► Clinical Findings

A. Symptoms and Signs

Patients with bleeding esophageal varices present with symptoms and signs of acute gastrointestinal hemorrhage. (See Acute Upper Gastrointestinal Bleeding, above.) In some cases, there may be preceding retching or dyspepsia attributable to alcoholic gastritis or withdrawal. Varices per se do not cause symptoms of dyspepsia, dysphagia, or retching. Variceal bleeding usually is severe, resulting in hypovolemia manifested by postural vital signs or shock. Twenty percent of patients with chronic liver disease in whom bleeding develops have a nonvariceal source of bleeding.

B. Laboratory Findings

These are identical to those listed above in the section on acute upper gastrointestinal tract bleeding.

► Initial Management

A. Acute Resuscitation

The initial management of patients with acute upper gastrointestinal bleeding is also discussed in the section on acute upper gastrointestinal bleeding (see above). Variceal hemorrhage is life-threatening; rapid assessment and resuscitation with fluids or blood products are essential. Overtransfusion should be avoided as it leads to increased central and portal venous pressures, increasing the risk of rebleeding. Many patients with bleeding esophageal varices have coagulopathy due to underlying cirrhosis; fresh frozen plasma (20 mL/kg loading dose, then 10 mg/kg every 6 hours) or platelets should be administered to patients with INRs > 1.8–2.0 or with platelet counts < 50,000/mcL in the presence of active bleeding. Recombinant factor VIIa has not demonstrated efficacy in controlled studies and is not recommended. Patients with advanced liver disease are at high risk for poor outcome regardless of the bleeding source and should be transferred to an ICU.

B. Pharmacologic Therapy

1. Antibiotic prophylaxis—Cirrhotic patients admitted with upper gastrointestinal bleeding have a > 50% chance of developing a severe bacterial infection during hospitalization—such as bacterial peritonitis, pneumonia, or urinary tract infection. Most infections are caused by gram-negative organisms of gut origin. Prophylactic administration of oral or intravenous fluoroquinolones (eg, norfloxacin, 400 mg orally twice daily) or intravenous third-generation cephalosporins (eg, ceftriaxone, 1 g/d) for 5–7 days reduces the risk of serious infection to 10–20% as well as hospital mortality. Because of a rising incidence of infections caused by gram-positive organisms as well as fluoroquinolone-resistant organisms, intravenous third-generation cephalosporins may be preferred.

2. Vasoactive drugs—Somatostatin and octreotide infusions reduce portal pressures in ways that are poorly understood. Somatostatin (250 mcg/h)—not available in the United States—or octreotide (50 mcg intravenous bolus followed by 50 mcg/h) reduces splanchnic and hepatic blood flow and portal pressures in cirrhotic patients. Both agents appear to provide acute control of variceal bleeding in up to 80% of patients although neither has been shown to reduce mortality. Data about the absolute efficacy of both are conflicting, but they may be comparable in efficacy to endoscopic therapy. Combined treatment with octreotide or somatostatin infusion and endoscopic therapy (band ligation or sclerotherapy) is superior to either modality alone in controlling acute bleeding and early rebleeding, and it may improve survival. In patients with advanced liver disease and upper gastrointestinal hemorrhage, it is reasonable to initiate therapy with octreotide or somatostatin on admission and continue for 3–5 days if varices are confirmed by endoscopy. If bleeding is determined by endoscopy not to be secondary to portal hypertension, the infusion can be discontinued.

Terlipressin, 1–2 mg intravenous every 4 hours, (not available in the United States) is a synthetic vasopressin analog that causes a significant and sustained reduction in portal and variceal pressures while preserving renal perfusion. Where available, terlipressin may be preferred to somatostatin or octreotide. Terlipressin is contraindicated in patients with significant coronary, cerebral, or peripheral vascular disease.

3. Vitamin K—In cirrhotic patients with an abnormal prothrombin time, vitamin K (10 mg) should be administered intravenously.

4. Lactulose—Encephalopathy may complicate an episode of gastrointestinal bleeding in patients with severe liver disease. In patients with encephalopathy, lactulose should be administered in a dosage of 30 mL orally every 1–2 hours until evacuation occurs then reduced to 15–45 mL/h every 8–12 hours as needed to promote two or three bowel movements daily. (See Chapter 16.)

C. Emergent Endoscopy

Emergent endoscopy is performed after the patient's hemodynamic status has been appropriately stabilized (usually within 2–12 hours). In patients with active bleeding, endotracheal intubation is commonly performed to protect against aspiration during endoscopy. An endoscopic examination is performed to exclude other or associated causes of upper gastrointestinal bleeding such as Mallory-Weiss tears, peptic ulcer disease, and portal hypertensive gastropathy. In many patients, variceal bleeding has stopped spontaneously by the time of endoscopy, and the diagnosis of variceal bleeding is made presumptively. Acute endoscopic treatment of the varices is performed with either banding or sclerotherapy. These techniques arrest active bleeding in 80–90% of patients and reduce the chance of in-hospital recurrent bleeding to about 20%.

If banding is chosen, repeat sessions are scheduled at intervals of 2–4 weeks until the varices are obliterated or reduced to a small size. Banding achieves lower rates of rebleeding, complications, and death than sclerotherapy and should be considered the endoscopic treatment of choice.

Sclerotherapy is still preferred by some endoscopists in the actively bleeding patient (in whom visualization for banding may be difficult). Sclerotherapy is performed by injecting the variceal trunks with a sclerosing agent (eg, ethanolamine, tetradecyl sulfate). Complications occur in 20–30% of patients and include chest pain, fever, bacteremia, esophageal ulceration, stricture, and perforation. After initial treatment, band ligation therapy should be performed.

D. Balloon Tube Tamponade

Mechanical tamponade with specially designed nasogastric tubes containing large gastric and esophageal balloons (Minnesota or Sengstaken-Blakemore tubes) provides initial control of active variceal hemorrhage in 60–90% of patients; rebleeding occurs in 50%. The gastric balloon is inflated first, followed by the esophageal balloon if bleeding continues. After balloon inflation, tension is applied to the tube to directly tamponade the varices. Complications of prolonged balloon inflation include esophageal and oral ulcerations, perforation, aspiration, and airway obstruction (due to a misplaced balloon). Endotracheal intubation is recommended before placement. Given its high rate of complications, mechanical tamponade is used as a temporizing measure only in patients with bleeding that cannot be controlled with pharmacologic or endoscopic techniques until more definitive decompressive therapy (eg, TIPS; see below) can be provided.

E. Portal Decompressive Procedures

In the 10–20% of patients with variceal bleeding that cannot be controlled with pharmacologic or endoscopic therapy, emergency portal decompression may be considered.

1. Transvenous intrahepatic portosystemic shunts (TIPS)—Over a wire that is passed through a catheter inserted in the jugular vein, an expandable wire mesh stent (8–12 mm in diameter) is passed through the liver parenchyma, creating a portosystemic shunt from the portal vein to the hepatic vein. TIPS can control acute hemorrhage in over 90% of patients actively bleeding from gastric or esophageal varices. However, when TIPS is performed in the actively bleeding patient, the mortality approaches 40%, especially in patients requiring ventilatory support or blood pressure support and patients with renal insufficiency, bilirubin > 3 mg/dL, or encephalopathy. Therefore, TIPS should be considered in the 10–20% of patients with acute variceal bleeding that cannot be controlled with pharmacologic and endoscopic therapy, but it may not be warranted in patients with a particularly poor prognosis.

2. Emergency portosystemic shunt surgery—Emergency portosystemic shunt surgery is associated with a 40–60% mortality rate. At centers where TIPS is available, that procedure has become the preferred means of providing emergency portal decompression.

▶ Prevention of Rebleeding

Once the initial bleeding episode has been controlled, therapy is warranted to reduce the high risk (60%) of rebleeding.

A. Combination Beta-Blockers and Variceal Band Ligation

Nonselective beta-adrenergic blockers (propranolol, nadolol) reduce the risk of rebleeding from esophageal varices to about 40%. Likewise, long-term treatment with band ligation reduces the incidence of rebleeding to about 30%. In most patients, two to six treatment sessions (performed at 2- to 4-week intervals) are needed to eradicate the varices.

Meta-analyses of randomized controlled trials suggest that a *combination* of band ligation plus beta-blockers is superior to either variceal band ligation alone (RR 0.68) or beta-blockers alone (RR 0.71). Therefore, combination therapy is recommended for patients without contraindications to beta-blockers. Recommended starting doses of beta-blockers are propranolol (20 mg orally twice daily), long-acting propranolol (60 mg orally once daily), or nadolol (20–40 mg orally once daily), with gradual increases in the dosage every 1–2 weeks until the heart rate falls by 25% or reaches 55–60 beats/min, provided the systolic blood pressure remains above 90 mm Hg and the patient has no side effects. The average dosage of long-acting propranolol is 120 mg once daily and for nadolol, 80 mg once daily. One-third of patients with cirrhosis are intolerant of beta-blockers, experiencing fatigue or hypotension. Drug administration at bedtime may reduce the frequency and severity of side effects.

B. Transvenous Intrahepatic Portosystemic Shunt

TIPS has resulted in a significant reduction in recurrent bleeding compared with endoscopic sclerotherapy or band ligation—either alone or in combination with beta-blocker therapy. At 1 year, rebleeding rates in patients treated with TIPS versus various endoscopic therapies average 20% and 40%, respectively. However, TIPS was also associated with a higher incidence of encephalopathy (35% vs 15%) and did not result in a decrease in mortality. Another limitation of TIPS is that stenosis and thrombosis of the stents occur in the majority of patients over time with a consequent risk of rebleeding. Therefore, periodic monitoring with Doppler ultrasonography or hepatic venography is required. Stent patency usually can be maintained by balloon angioplasty or additional stent placement. Given these problems, TIPS should be reserved for patients who have recurrent (two or more) episodes of variceal bleeding that have failed endoscopic or pharmacologic therapies. TIPS is also useful in patients with recurrent bleeding from gastric varices or portal hypertensive gastropathy (for which endoscopic therapies cannot be used). TIPS is likewise considered in patients who are noncompliant with other therapies or who live in remote locations (without access to emergency care).

C. Surgical Portosystemic Shunts

Shunt surgery has a significantly lower rate of rebleeding compared with endoscopic therapy but also a higher incidence of encephalopathy. With the advent and widespread adoption of TIPS, surgical shunts are seldom performed.

D. Liver Transplantation

Candidacy for orthotopic liver transplantation should be assessed in all patients with chronic liver disease and bleeding due to portal hypertension. Transplant candidates should be treated with band ligation or TIPS to control bleeding pretransplant.

▶ Prevention of First Episodes of Variceal Bleeding

Among patients with varices that have not previously bled, bleeding occurs in 12% of patients each year, with a lifetime risk of 30%. Because of the high mortality rate associated with variceal hemorrhage, prevention of the initial bleeding episode is desirable. Therefore, patients with cirrhosis should undergo diagnostic endoscopy or capsule endoscopy to determine whether varices are present. Varices are present in 40% of patients with Child-Turcotte-Pugh class A cirrhosis and in 85% with Child-Turcotte-Pugh class C cirrhosis. In patients without varices on screening endoscopy, a repeat endoscopy is recommended in 3 years, since varices develop in 8% of patients per year. Patients with varices have a higher risk of bleeding if they have large varices (> 5 mm), varices with red wale markings, or Child-Turcotte-Pugh class B or C cirrhosis. The risk of bleeding in patients with small varices (< 5 mm) is 5% per year and with large varices is 15–20% per year. Patients with small varices without red wale marks and compensated (Child-Turcotte-Pugh class A) cirrhosis have a low-risk of bleeding; hence, prophylaxis is unnecessary, but endoscopy should be repeated in 1–2 years to reassess size.

Nonselective beta-adrenergic blockers are recommended to reduce the risk of first variceal hemorrhage in patients with medium/large varices and patients with small varices who either have variceal red wale marks or advanced cirrhosis (Child-Turcotte-Pugh class B or C). (See Combination Beta-Blockers and Variceal Band Ligation, above.) Band ligation is not recommended for small varices due to technical difficulties in band application. Prophylactic band ligation may be preferred for higher risk patients with medium/large varices (Child-Turcotte-Pugh class B or C or varices with red wale markings) as well as patients with contraindications to or intolerance of beta-blockers.

▶ When to Refer

- All patients with upper gastrointestinal bleeding and suspected varices should be evaluated by a physician skilled in therapeutic endoscopy.
- Patients being considered for TIPS procedures or liver transplantation.
- Patients with cirrhosis for endoscopic evaluation for varices.

▶ When to Admit

All patients with acute upper gastrointestinal bleeding and suspected cirrhosis should be admitted to an ICU.

Bhogal HK et al. Using transjugular intrahepatic portosystemic shunts for complications of cirrhosis. Clin Gastroenterol Hepatol. 2011;9(11):936–46. [PMID: 21699820]

Rahimi RS et al. End-stage liver disease complications. Curr Opin Gastroenterol. 2013 May;29(3):257–63. [PMID: 23429468]

Huberty V et al. Endoscopic treatment for Zenker's diverticulum: long-term results (with video). Gastrointest Endosc. 2013 May;77(5):701–7. [PMID: 23394840]

ESOPHAGEAL MOTILITY DISORDERS

1. Achalasia

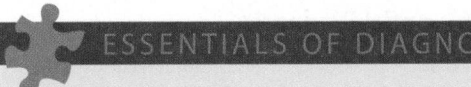
ESSENTIALS OF DIAGNOSIS

- ▶ Gradual, progressive dysphagia for solids and liquids.
- ▶ Regurgitation of undigested food.
- ▶ Barium esophagogram with "bird's beak" distal esophagus.
- ▶ Esophageal manometry confirms diagnosis.

▶ General Considerations

Achalasia is an idiopathic motility disorder characterized by loss of peristalsis in the distal two-thirds (smooth muscle) of the esophagus and impaired relaxation of the LES. There appears to be denervation of the esophagus resulting primarily from loss of nitric oxide-producing inhibitory neurons in the myenteric plexus. The cause of the neuronal degeneration is unknown.

▶ Clinical Findings

A. Symptoms and Signs

There is a steady increase in the incidence of achalasia with age; however, it can be seen in individuals as young as 25 years. Patients complain of the gradual onset of dysphagia for solid foods and, in the majority, of liquids also. Symptoms at presentation may have persisted for months to years. Substernal discomfort or fullness may be noted after eating. Many patients eat more slowly and adopt specific maneuvers such as lifting the neck or throwing the shoulders back to enhance esophageal emptying. Regurgitation of undigested food is common and may occur during meals or up to several hours later. Nocturnal regurgitation can provoke coughing or aspiration. Up to 50% of patients report substernal chest pain that is unrelated to meals or exercise and may last up to hours. Weight loss is common. Physical examination is unhelpful.

B. Imaging

Chest radiographs may show an air-fluid level in the enlarged, fluid-filled esophagus. Barium esophagography discloses characteristic findings, including esophageal dilation, loss of esophageal peristalsis, poor esophageal emptying, and a smooth, symmetric "bird's beak" tapering of the distal esophagus. Without treatment, the esophagus may become markedly dilated ("sigmoid esophagus").

C. Special Examinations

After esophagography, endoscopy is always performed to evaluate the distal esophagus and gastroesophageal junction to exclude a distal stricture or a submucosal infiltrating carcinoma. The diagnosis is confirmed by esophageal manometry. The manometric features are complete absence of normal peristalsis and incomplete lower esophageal sphincteric relaxation with swallowing.

▶ Differential Diagnosis

Chagas disease is associated with esophageal dysfunction that is indistinguishable from idiopathic achalasia and should be considered in patients from endemic regions (Central and South America); it is becoming more common in the southern United States. Primary or metastatic tumors can invade the gastroesophageal junction, resulting in a picture resembling that of achalasia, called "pseudoachalasia." Endoscopic ultrasonography and chest CT may be required to examine the distal esophagus in suspicious cases. Tumors such as small cell lung cancer can cause a paraneoplastic syndrome resembling achalasia due to secretion of antineuronal nuclear antibodies (ANNA-1 or Anti-Hu) that affect the myenteric plexus. Achalasia must be distinguished from other motility disorders such as diffuse esophageal spasm and scleroderma esophagus with a peptic stricture.

▶ Treatment

A. Botulinum Toxin Injection

Endoscopically guided injection of botulinum toxin directly into the LES results in a marked reduction in LES pressure with initial improvement in symptoms in 65–85% of patients. However, symptom relapse occurs in over 50% of patients within 6–9 months and in all patients within 2 years. Three-fourths of initial responders who relapse have improvement with repeated injections. Because it is inferior to pneumatic dilation therapy and surgery in producing sustained symptomatic relief, this therapy is most appropriate for patients with comorbidities who are poor candidates for more invasive procedures.

B. Pneumatic Dilation

Up to 90% of patients derive good to excellent relief of dysphagia after one to three sessions of pneumatic dilation of the LES. Dilation is less effective in patients who are younger than age 50 or have a dilated esophagus. Symptoms recur following pneumatic dilation in up to 35% within 10 years but usually respond to repeated dilation.

Perforations occur in < 3% of dilations and may require operative repair. The success of laparoscopic myotomy is not compromised by prior pneumatic dilation.

C. Surgery

A modified Heller cardiomyotomy of the LES and cardia results in good to excellent symptomatic improvement in over 90% of patients. Because gastroesophageal reflux develops in up to 20% of patients after myotomy, most surgeons also perform an antireflux procedure (fundoplication), and all patients are prescribed a once-daily proton pump inhibitor. Myotomy is performed with a laparoscopic approach and is preferred to the open surgical approach. Symptoms recur following cardiomyotomy in > 25% of cases within 10 years but usually respond to pneumatic dilation. Pneumatic dilation may be less effective in young males (age < 45 years) so surgical myotomy may be preferred for them. In 2011, results from a large randomized, multicenter trial comparing laparoscopic myotomy to pneumatic dilation were reported. After 2 years of follow-up, adequate symptom control was achieved in 86% of the dilation group and 90% of the surgery group. Thus, in experienced hands, the initial efficacies of pneumatic dilation and laparoscopic myotomy are nearly equivalent. Since 2011, selected, highly experienced centers in Southeast Asia and, more recently, in the United States, have reported excellent results with a less invasive, incisionless, per-oral endoscopic myotomy (POEM). Complete esophagectomy may be required in patients with megaesophagus, in whom dilation and myotomy are less effective.

Boeckxstaens GE et al; European Achalasia Trial Investigators. Pneumatic dilation versus laparoscopic Heller's myotomy for idiopathic achalasia. N Engl J Med. 2011 May 12;364(19): 1807–12. [PMID: 21561346]

Pandolfino JE et al. Presentation, diagnosis, and management of achalasia. Clin Gastroenterol Hepatol. 2013 Aug;11(8):887–97. [PMID: 23395699]

Swanstrom LL et al. Long-term outcomes of an endoscopic myotomy for achalasia: the POEM procedure. Ann Surg. 2012 Oct;256(4):659–67. [PMID: 22982946]

Vaezi MF et al. ACG Clinical Guideline: diagnosis and management of achalasia. Am J Gastroenterol. 2013 Aug;108(8):1238–49. [PMID: 23877351]

2. Other Primary Esophageal Motility Disorders

▶ Clinical Findings

A. Symptoms and Signs

Abnormalities in esophageal motility may cause dysphagia or chest pain. Dysphagia for liquids as well as solids tends to be intermittent and nonprogressive. Periods of normal swallowing may alternate with periods of dysphagia, which usually is mild though bothersome—rarely severe enough to result in significant alterations in lifestyle or weight loss. Dysphagia may be provoked by stress, large boluses of food, or hot or cold liquids. Some patients may experience anterior chest pain that may be confused with angina pectoris but usually is nonexertional. The pain generally is unrelated to eating. (See Chest Pain of Undetermined Origin, below.)

B. Diagnostic Tests

The evaluation of suspected esophageal motility disorders includes barium esophagography, upper endoscopy, and, in some cases, esophageal manometry. Barium esophagography is useful to exclude mechanical obstruction and to evaluate esophageal motility. The presence of simultaneous contractions (spasm), disordered peristalsis, or failed peristalsis supports a diagnosis of esophageal dysmotility. Upper endoscopy also is performed to exclude a mechanical obstruction (as a cause of dysphagia) and to look for evidence of erosive reflux esophagitis (a common cause of chest pain) or eosinophilic esophagitis (confirmed by esophageal biopsy). Manometry is not routinely used for mild to moderate symptoms because the findings seldom influence further medical management, but it may be useful in patients with persistent, disabling dysphagia to exclude achalasia and to look for other disorders of esophageal motility. These include spastic disorders (diffuse esophageal spasm, hypercontractile esophagus, hypertensive peristalsis, and esophagogastric junction outflow obstruction) and findings of ineffective esophageal peristalsis (failed or weak esophageal peristalsis). The further evaluation of noncardiac chest pain is discussed in a subsequent section.

▶ Treatment

For patients with mild symptoms of dysphagia, therapy is directed at symptom reduction and reassurance. Patients should be instructed to eat more slowly and take smaller bites of food. In some cases, a warm liquid at the start of a meal may facilitate swallowing. Because unrecognized gastroesophageal reflux may cause dysphagia, a trial of a proton pump inhibitor (esomeprazole 40 mg, lansoprazole 30 mg) orally twice daily should be administered for 4–8 weeks. Treatment of patients with severe dysphagia is empiric. Suspected spastic disorders may be treated with isosorbide (10–20 mg four times daily) or nitroglycerin (0.4 mg sublingually as needed) and nifedipine (10 mg) or diltiazem (60–90 mg) 30–45 minutes before meals may be tried; their efficacy is unproved. Phosphodiesterase type 5 inhibitors (eg, sildenafil) promote smooth muscle relaxation and improve esophageal motility in small numbers of patients with spastic disorders but require further clinical study before they can be recommended. Injection of botulinum toxin into the lower esophagus may improve chest pain and dysphagia in some patients for a limited time. For unclear reasons, esophageal dilation provides symptomatic relief in some cases.

Roman S et al. Distal esophageal spasm. Dysphagia. 2012 Mar;27(1):115–23. [PMID: 22215281]

Roman S et al. Management of spastic disorders of the esophagus. Gastroenterol Clin North Am. 2013 Mar;42(1):27–43. [PMID: 23452629]

CHEST PAIN OF UNDETERMINED ORIGIN

One-third of patients with chest pain undergo negative cardiac evaluation. Patients with recurrent noncardiac chest pain thus pose a difficult clinical problem. Because coronary artery disease is common and can present atypically, it must be excluded prior to evaluation for other causes.

Causes of noncardiac chest pain may include the following.

A. Chest Wall and Thoracic Spine Disease

These are easily diagnosed by history and physical examination.

B. Gastroesophageal Reflux

Up to 50% of patients have increased amounts of gastroesophageal acid reflux or a correlation between acid reflux episodes and chest pain demonstrated on esophageal pH testing. An empiric 4-week trial of acid-suppressive therapy with a high-dose proton pump inhibitor is recommended (eg, omeprazole or rabeprazole, 40 mg orally twice daily; lansoprazole, 30–60 mg orally twice daily; or esomeprazole or pantoprazole, 40 mg orally twice daily), especially in patients with reflux symptoms. In patients with persistent symptoms, ambulatory esophageal pH or impedance and pH study may be useful to exclude definitively a relationship between acid and nonacid reflux episodes and chest pain events.

C. Esophageal Dysmotility

Esophageal motility abnormalities such as diffuse esophageal spasm or hypertensive peristalsis (nutcracker esophagus) are uncommon causes of noncardiac chest pain. In patients with chest pain and dysphagia, a barium swallow radiograph should be obtained to look for evidence of achalasia or diffuse esophageal spasm. Esophageal manometry is not routinely performed because of low specificity and the unlikelihood of finding a clinically significant disorder, but it may be recommended in patients with frequent symptoms.

D. Heightened Visceral Sensitivity

Some patients with noncardiac chest pain report pain in response to a variety of minor noxious stimuli such as physiologically normal amounts of acid reflux, inflation of balloons within the esophageal lumen, injection of intravenous edrophonium (a cholinergic stimulus), or intracardiac catheter manipulation. Low doses of oral antidepressants such as trazodone 50 mg or imipramine 10–50 mg reduce chest pain symptoms and are thought to reduce visceral afferent awareness. In a 2010 controlled crossover trial, over 50% of patients treated with venlafaxine, 75 mg once daily at bedtime, achieved symptomatic improvement compared with only 4% treated with placebo.

E. Psychological Disorders

A significant number of patients have underlying depression, anxiety, and panic disorder. Patients reporting dyspnea, sweating, tachycardia, suffocation, or fear of dying should be evaluated for panic disorder.

Arora AS et al. How do I handle the patient with noncardiac chest pain? Clin Gastroenterol Hepatol. 2011 Apr;9(4): 295–304. [PMID: 21056690]

Flook NW et al. Acid-suppressive therapy with esomeprazole for relief of unexplained chest pain in primary care: a randomized, double-blind, placebo-controlled trial. Am J Gastroenterol. 2013 Jan;108(1):56–64. [PMID: 23147520]

Hershcovici T et al. Systematic review: the treatment of noncardiac chest pain. Aliment Pharmacol Ther. 2012 Jan;35(1): 5–14. [PMID: 22077344]

DISEASES OF THE STOMACH & DUODENUM

(See Chapter 39 for Gastric Cancers.)

GASTRITIS & GASTROPATHY

The term "gastropathy" should be used to denote conditions in which there is epithelial or endothelial damage without inflammation, and "gastritis" should be used to denote conditions in which there is histologic evidence of inflammation. In clinical practice, the term "gastritis" is commonly applied to three categories: (1) erosive and hemorrhagic "gastritis" (gastropathy); (2) nonerosive, nonspecific (histologic) gastritis; and (3) specific types of gastritis, characterized by distinctive histologic and endoscopic features diagnostic of specific disorders.

1. Erosive & Hemorrhagic "Gastritis" (Gastropathy)

ESSENTIALS OF DIAGNOSIS

▶ Most commonly seen in alcoholic or critically ill patients, or patients taking NSAIDs.

▶ Often asymptomatic; may cause epigastric pain, nausea, and vomiting.

▶ May cause hematemesis; usually not significant bleeding.

General Considerations

The most common causes of erosive gastropathy are medications (especially NSAIDs), alcohol, stress due to severe medical or surgical illness, and portal hypertension ("portal gastropathy"). Major risk factors for stress gastritis include mechanical ventilation, coagulopathy, trauma, burns, shock, sepsis, central nervous system injury, liver failure, kidney disease, and multiorgan failure. The use of enteral nutrition reduces the risk of stress-related bleeding. Uncommon causes of erosive gastropathy include caustic ingestion and radiation. Erosive and hemorrhagic gastropathy typically are diagnosed at endoscopy, often being performed because of dyspepsia or upper gastrointestinal

bleeding. Endoscopic findings include subepithelial hemorrhages, petechiae, and erosions. These lesions are superficial, vary in size and number, and may be focal or diffuse. There usually is no significant inflammation on histologic examination.

Clinical Findings

A. Symptoms and Signs

Erosive gastropathy is usually asymptomatic. Symptoms, when they occur, include anorexia, epigastric pain, nausea, and vomiting. There is poor correlation between symptoms and the number or severity of endoscopic abnormalities. The most common clinical manifestation of erosive gastritis is upper gastrointestinal bleeding, which presents as hematemesis, "coffee grounds" emesis, or bloody aspirate in a patient receiving nasogastric suction, or as melena. Because erosive gastritis is superficial, hemodynamically significant bleeding is rare.

B. Laboratory Findings

The laboratory findings are nonspecific. The hematocrit is low if significant bleeding has occurred; iron deficiency may be found.

C. Special Examinations

Upper endoscopy is the most sensitive method of diagnosis. Although bleeding from gastritis is usually insignificant, it cannot be distinguished on clinical grounds from more serious lesions such as peptic ulcers or esophageal varices. Hence, endoscopy is generally performed within 24 hours in patients with upper gastrointestinal bleeding to identify the source. An upper gastrointestinal series is sometimes obtained in lieu of endoscopy in patients with hemodynamically insignificant upper gastrointestinal bleeds to exclude serious lesions but is insensitive for the detection of gastritis.

Differential Diagnosis

Epigastric pain may be due to peptic ulcer, gastroesophageal reflux, gastric cancer, biliary tract disease, food poisoning, viral gastroenteritis, and functional dyspepsia. With severe pain, one should consider a perforated or penetrating ulcer, pancreatic disease, esophageal rupture, ruptured aortic aneurysm, gastric volvulus, and myocardial colic. Causes of upper gastrointestinal bleeding include peptic ulcer disease, esophageal varices, Mallory-Weiss tear, and angiodysplasias.

Specific Causes & Treatment

A. Stress Gastritis

1. Prophylaxis—Stress-related mucosal erosions and subepithelial hemorrhages may develop within 72 hours in critically ill patients. Clinically overt bleeding occurs in 6% of ICU patients, but clinically important bleeding in < 1.5%. Bleeding is associated with a higher mortality rate but is seldom the cause of death. Two of the most important risk factors for bleeding are coagulopathy (platelets < 50,000/mcL or INR > 1.5) and respiratory failure with the need for mechanical ventilation for over 48 hours. When these two risk factors are absent, the risk of significant bleeding is only 0.1%. Other risk factors include traumatic brain injury, severe burns, sepsis, vasopressor therapy, corticosteroid therapy, and prior history of peptic ulcer disease and gastrointestinal bleeding. Early enteral tube feeding may decrease the risk of significant bleeding.

Prophylaxis should be routinely administered to critically ill patients with risk factors for significant bleeding upon admission. Prophylactic suppression of gastric acid with intravenous H_2-receptor antagonists or proton pump inhibitors (oral or intravenous) has been shown to reduce the incidence of clinically overt and significant bleeding but may increase the risk of nosocomial pneumonia. A 2012 meta-analysis of 13 randomized trials found that oral and intravenous proton pump inhibitors significantly decreased the incidence of clinically significant bleeding compared with intravenous H_2-receptor antagonists (1.3% vs 6.6%, OR 0.30).

The optimal, cost-effective prophylactic regimen remains uncertain, hence clinical practices vary. For patients with nasoenteric tubes, immediate-release omeprazole (40 mg at 1 and 6 hours on day 1; then 40 mg once daily beginning on day 2) may be preferred because of lower cost and ease of administration. For patients requiring intravenous administration, continuous intravenous infusions of H_2-receptor antagonists provide adequate control of intragastric pH in most patients in the following doses over 24 hours: cimetidine (900–1200 mg), ranitidine (150 mg), or famotidine (20 mg). Alternatively, intravenous proton pump inhibitors, although more expensive, may be preferred due to superior efficacy. The optimal dosing of intravenous proton pump inhibitors is uncertain; however, in clinical trials pantoprazole doses ranging from 40 mg to 80 mg and administered every 8–24 hours appear equally effective.

2. Treatment—Once bleeding occurs, patients should receive continuous infusions of a proton pump inhibitor (esomeprazole or pantoprazole, 80 mg intravenous bolus, followed by 8 mg/h continuous infusion) as well as sucralfate suspension, 1 g orally every 4 to 6 hours. Endoscopy should be performed in patients with clinically significant bleeding to look for treatable causes, especially stress-related peptic ulcers with active bleeding or visible vessels. When bleeding arises from diffuse gastritis, endoscopic hemostasis techniques are not helpful.

B. NSAID Gastritis

Of patients receiving NSAIDs in clinical trials, 25–50% have gastritis and 10–20% have ulcers at endoscopy; however, symptoms of significant dyspepsia develop in about 5%. NSAIDs that are more selective for the cyclooxygenase (COX)-2 enzyme ("coxibs"), such as celecoxib, etodolac, and meloxicam, decrease the incidence of endoscopically visible ulcers by approximately 75% and significant ulcer

complications by up to 50% compared with nonselective NSAIDs (nsNSAIDs) (see below). However, a twofold increase in the incidence in cardiovascular complications (myocardial infarction, cerebrovascular infarction, and death) in patients taking coxibs compared with placebo led to the withdrawal of two highly selective coxibs (rofecoxib and valdecoxib) from the market by the manufacturers. Celecoxib and all currently available nsNSAIDS (with notable exception of aspirin and possibly naproxen) are associated with increased risk of cardiovascular complications and therefore should be used with caution in patients with cardiovascular risk factors.

In population surveys, the rate of dyspepsia is increased 1.5- to 2-fold with nsNSAID and coxib use. However, dyspeptic symptoms correlate poorly with significant mucosal abnormalities or the development of adverse clinical events (ulcer bleeding or perforation). Given the frequency of dyspeptic symptoms in patients taking NSAIDs, it is neither feasible nor desirable to investigate all such cases. Patients with alarm symptoms or signs, such as severe pain, weight loss, vomiting, gastrointestinal bleeding, or anemia, should undergo diagnostic upper endoscopy. For other patients, symptoms may improve with discontinuation of the agent, reduction to the lowest effective dose, or administration with meals. Proton pump inhibitors have demonstrated efficacy in controlled trials for the treatment of NSAID-related dyspepsia and superiority to H_2-receptor antagonists for healing of NSAID-related ulcers even in the setting of continued NSAID use. Therefore, an empiric 2–4 week trial of an oral proton pump inhibitor (omeprazole, rabeprazole, or esomeprazole 20–40 mg/d; lansoprazole or dexlansoprazole, 30 mg/d; pantoprazole, 40 mg/d) is recommended for patients with NSAID-related dyspepsia, especially those in whom continued NSAID treatment is required. If symptoms do not improve, diagnostic upper endoscopy should be conducted.

C. Alcoholic Gastritis

Excessive alcohol consumption may lead to dyspepsia, nausea, emesis, and minor hematemesis—a condition sometimes labeled "alcoholic gastritis." However, it is not proven that alcohol alone actually causes significant erosive gastritis. Therapy with H_2-receptor antagonists, proton pump inhibitors, or sucralfate for 2–4 weeks often is empirically prescribed.

D. Portal Hypertensive Gastropathy

Portal hypertension commonly results in gastric mucosal and submucosal congestion of capillaries and venules, which is correlated with the severity of the portal hypertension and underlying liver disease. Usually asymptomatic, it may cause chronic gastrointestinal bleeding in 10% of patients and, less commonly, clinically significant bleeding with hematemesis. Treatment with propranolol or nadolol reduces the incidence of recurrent acute bleeding by lowering portal pressures. Patients who fail propranolol therapy may be successfully treated with portal decompressive procedures (see section above on treatment of esophageal varices).

Barkun AN et al. Proton pump inhibitors vs. histamine 2 receptor antagonists for stress-related mucosal bleeding prophylaxis in critically ill patients: a meta-analysis. Am J Gastroenterol. 2012 Apr;107(4):507–20. [PMID: 22290403]

den Hollander WJ et al. Current pharmacotherapy options for gastritis. Expert Opin Pharmacother. 2012 Dec;13(18):2625–36. [PMID: 23167300]

Ripoll C et al. The management of portal hypertensive gastropathy and gastric antral vascular ectasia. Dig Liver Dis. 2011 May;43(5):345–51. [PMID: 21095166]

2. Nonerosive, Nonspecific Gastritis

The diagnosis of nonerosive gastritis is based on histologic assessment of mucosal biopsies. Endoscopic findings are normal in many cases and do not reliably predict the presence of histologic inflammation. The main types of nonerosive gastritis are those due to *H pylori* infection, those associated with pernicious anemia, and eosinophilic gastritis. (See Specific Types of Gastritis below.)

▶ *Helicobacter pylori* Gastritis

H pylori is a spiral gram-negative rod that resides beneath the gastric mucous layer adjacent to gastric epithelial cells. Although not invasive, it causes gastric mucosal inflammation with PMNs and lymphocytes. The mechanisms of injury and inflammation may in part be related to the products of two genes, *vacA* and *cagA*.

In developed countries the prevalence of *H pylori* is rapidly declining. In the United States, the prevalence rises from < 10% in non-immigrants under age 30 years to over 50% in those over age 60 years. The prevalence is higher in non-whites and immigrants from developing countries and is correlated inversely with socioeconomic status. Transmission is from person to person, mainly during infancy and childhood; however, the mode of transmission is unknown.

Acute infection with *H pylori* may cause a transient clinical illness characterized by nausea and abdominal pain that may last for several days and is associated with acute histologic gastritis with PMNs. After these symptoms resolve, the majority progress to chronic infection with chronic, diffuse mucosal inflammation (gastritis) characterized by PMNs and lymphocytes. Although chronic *H pylori* infection with gastritis is present in 30–50% of the population, most persons are asymptomatic and suffer no sequelae. Three gastritis phenotypes occur which determine clinical outcomes. Most infected people have a mild, diffuse gastritis that does not disrupt acid secretion and seldom causes clinically important outcomes. About 15% of infected people have inflammation that predominates in the gastric antrum but spares the gastric body (where acid is secreted). People with this phenotype tend to have increased gastrin; increased acid production; and increased risk of developing peptic ulcers, especially duodenal ulcers. An even smaller subset of infected adults have inflammation that predominates in the gastric body. Over time, this may lead to destruction of acid-secreting glands with resultant mucosal atrophy, decreased acid secretion, and intestinal metaplasia. This phenotype is associated with an increased risk of gastric ulcers and gastric cancer. Long-term treatment with proton pump inhibitors can potentiate the development of *H pylori*–associated atrophic gastritis. Chronic *H pylori* gastritis leads to the development of duodenal or gastric ulcers up to 10%, gastric cancer in 0.1–3%, and low-grade B cell gastric lymphoma (mucosa-associated lymphoid tissue lymphoma; MALToma) in < 0.01%.

Eradication of *H pylori* may be achieved with antibiotics in over 85% of patients and leads to resolution of the chronic gastritis (see section on Peptic Ulcer Disease). Testing for *H pylori* is indicated for patients with either active or a past history of documented peptic ulcer disease or gastric MALToma and for patients with a family history of gastric carcinoma. Testing and empiric treatment is cost-effective in young patients (< 55 years of age) with uncomplicated dyspepsia prior to further medical evaluation. The role of testing and treating *H pylori* in patients with functional dyspepsia remains controversial but is generally recommended (see Dyspepsia, above). *H pylori* eradication decreases the risk of gastric cancer in patients with peptic ulcer disease. Some groups recommend population-based screening of all asymptomatic persons in regions in which there is a high prevalence of *H pylori* and gastric cancer (such as Japan, Korea, and China) to reduce the incidence of gastric cancer. Population-based screening of asymptomatic individuals is not recommended in western countries, in which the incidence of gastric cancer is low, but should be considered in immigrants from high-prevalence regions.

1. Noninvasive testing for *H pylori*—Although serologic tests are easily obtained and widely available, most clinical guidelines no longer endorse their use for testing for *H pylori* infection because they are less accurate than other noninvasive tests that measure active infection. Laboratory-based quantitative serologic ELISA tests have an overall accuracy of only 80%. In comparison, the fecal antigen immunoassay and [13C] urea breath test have excellent sensitivity and specificity (> 95%) at a cost of < $60. Although more expensive and cumbersome to perform, these tests of active infection are more cost-effective in most clinical settings because they reduce unnecessary treatment for patients without active infection.

Recent proton pump inhibitors or antibiotics significantly reduce the sensitivity of urea breath tests and fecal antigen assays (but not serologic tests). Prior to testing, proton pump inhibitors should be discontinued 7–14 days and antibiotics for at least 28 days.

2. Endoscopic testing for *H pylori*—Endoscopy is not indicated to diagnose *H pylori* infection in most circumstances. However, when it is performed for another reason, gastric biopsy specimens can be obtained for detection of *H pylori* and tested for active infection by urease production. This simple, inexpensive ($10) test has excellent sensitivity (90%) and specificity (95%). In patients with active upper gastrointestinal bleeding or patients recently taking proton pump inhibitors or antibiotics, histologic assessment for *H pylori* is preferred. Histologic assessment of biopsies from the gastric antrum and body is more definitive but more expensive ($150–$250) than a rapid urease test. Histologic assessment is also indicated in patients with suspected MALTomas and, possibly, in patients with suspected infection whose rapid urease test is negative. However, serologic testing is the most cost-effective means of confirming *H pylori* infection in patients with a negative rapid urease test.

Malfertheiner P et al; European Helicobacter Study Group. Management of *Helicobacter pylori* infection—the Maastricht IV/ Florence Consensus Report. Gut. 2012 May;61(5):646–64. [PMID: 22491499]

McColl KE. Clinical practice. *Helicobacter pylori* infection. N Engl J Med. 2010 Apr 29;362(17):1597–1604. [PMID: 20427808]

▶ Pernicious Anemia Gastritis

Pernicious anemia gastritis is an autoimmune disorder involving the fundic glands with resultant achlorhydria, decreased intrinsic factor secretion, and vitamin B_{12} malabsorption. Of patients with B_{12} deficiency, less than half have pernicious anemia. Most patients have malabsorption secondary to aging or chronic *H pylori* infection that results in atrophic gastritis, hypochlorhydria, and impaired release of B_{12} from food. Fundic histology in pernicious anemia is characterized by severe gland atrophy and intestinal metaplasia caused by autoimmune destruction of the gastric fundic mucosa. Anti-intrinsic factor antibodies are present in 70% of patients. Achlorhydria leads to pronounced hypergastrinemia (> 1000 pg/mL) due to loss of acid inhibition of gastrin G cells. Hypergastrinemia may induce hyperplasia of gastric enterochromaffin-like cells that may lead to the development of small, multicentric carcinoid tumors in 5% of patients. Metastatic spread is uncommon in lesions smaller than 2 cm. The risk of gastric adenocarcinoma is increased threefold, with a prevalence of 1–3%. Endoscopy with biopsy is indicated in patients with pernicious anemia at the time of diagnosis. Patients with dysplasia or small carcinoids require periodic endoscopic surveillance. Pernicious anemia is discussed in detail in Chapter 13.

Annibale B et al. Diagnosis and management of pernicious anemia. Curr Gastroenterol Rep. 2011 Dec;13(6):518–24. [PMID: 21947876]

3. Specific Types of Gastritis

A number of disorders are associated with specific mucosal histologic features.

Infections

Acute bacterial infection of the gastric submucosa and muscularis with a variety of aerobic or anaerobic organisms produces a rare, rapidly progressive, life-threatening condition known as phlegmonous or necrotizing gastritis, which requires broad-spectrum antibiotic therapy and, in many cases, emergency gastric resection. Viral infection with CMV is seen in patients with AIDS and after bone marrow or solid organ transplantation. Endoscopic findings include thickened gastric folds and ulcerations. Fungal infection with mucormycosis and *Candida* may occur in immunocompromised and diabetic patients. Larvae of *Anisakis*

marina ingested in raw fish or sushi may become embedded in the gastric mucosa, producing severe abdominal pain. Pain persists for several days until the larvae die. Endoscopic removal of the larvae provides rapid symptomatic relief.

Okano K et al. Acute abdomen with epigastric pain and vomiting in an adult healthy patient. Gastroenterology. 2010 Nov;139(5):1465. [PMID: 20875783]

PEPTIC ULCER DISEASE

ESSENTIALS OF DIAGNOSIS

- ▶ History of dyspepsia present in 80–90% of patients with variable relationship to meals.
- ▶ Ulcer symptoms characterized by rhythmicity and periodicity.
- ▶ Ten to 20 percent of patients present with ulcer complications without antecedent symptoms.
- ▶ Most NSAID-induced ulcers are asymptomatic.
- ▶ Upper endoscopy with gastric biopsy for *H pylori* is the diagnostic procedure of choice in most patients.
- ▶ Gastric ulcer biopsy or documentation of complete healing necessary to exclude gastric malignancy.

▶ General Considerations

Peptic ulcer is a break in the gastric or duodenal mucosa that arises when the normal mucosal defensive factors are impaired or are overwhelmed by aggressive luminal factors such as acid and pepsin. By definition, ulcers extend through the muscularis mucosae and are usually over 5 mm in diameter. In the United States, there are about 500,000 new cases per year of peptic ulcer and 4 million ulcer recurrences; the lifetime prevalence of ulcers in the adult population is approximately 10%. Ulcers occur five times more commonly in the duodenum, where over 95% are in the bulb or pyloric channel. In the stomach, benign ulcers are located most commonly in the antrum (60%) and at the junction of the antrum and body on the lesser curvature (25%).

Ulcers occur slightly more commonly in men than in women (1.3:1). Although ulcers can occur in any age group, duodenal ulcers most commonly occur in patients between the ages of 30 and 55 years, whereas gastric ulcers are more common in patients between the ages of 55 and 70 years. Ulcers are more common in smokers and in patients taking NSAIDs on a long-term basis (see below). Alcohol, dietary factors, and stress do not appear to cause ulcer disease. The incidence of duodenal ulcer disease has been declining dramatically for the past 30 years, but the incidence of gastric ulcers appears to be increasing as a result of the widespread use of NSAIDs and low-dose aspirin.

▶ Etiology

There are two major causes of peptic ulcer disease: NSAIDs and chronic *H pylori* infection. Evidence of *H pylori* infection or NSAID ingestion should be sought in all patients with peptic ulcer. Less than 5–10% of ulcers are caused by other conditions, including acid hypersecretory states (such as Zollinger-Ellison syndrome or systemic mastocytosis), CMV (especially in transplant recipients), Crohn disease, lymphoma, medications (eg, alendronate), chronic medical illness (cirrhosis or chronic kidney disease), or are idiopathic. NSAID and *H pylori*-associated ulcers will be presented in this section; Zollinger-Ellison syndrome will be discussed subsequently.

A. *H pylori*–Associated Ulcers

H pylori infection with associated gastritis and, in some cases, duodenitis appears to be a necessary cofactor for the majority of duodenal and gastric ulcers not associated with NSAIDs. Ulcer disease will develop in an estimated 10% of infected patients. The prevalence of *H pylori* infection in duodenal ulcer patients is 75–90%. The association with gastric ulcers is lower, but *H pylori* is found in most patients in whom NSAIDs cannot be implicated.

The natural history of *H pylori*–associated peptic ulcer disease is well defined. In the absence of specific antibiotic treatment to eradicate the organism, 85% of patients will have an endoscopically visible recurrence within 1 year. Half of these will be symptomatic. After successful eradication of *H pylori* with antibiotics, ulcer recurrence rates are reduced dramatically to 5–20% at 1 year. Most of these ulcer recurrences are due to NSAID use or, rarely, reinfection with *H pylori*.

B. NSAID-Induced Ulcers

There is a 10–20% prevalence of gastric ulcers and a 2–5% prevalence of duodenal ulcers in long-term NSAID users. Approximately 2–5%/year of long-term NSAID users will have an ulcer that causes clinically significant dyspepsia or a serious complication. The incidence of serious gastrointestinal complications (hospitalization, bleeding, perforation) is 0.2–1.9%/year. The risk of NSAID complications is greater within the first 3 months of therapy and in patients who are older than 60 years; who have a prior history of ulcer disease; or who take NSAIDs in combination with aspirin, corticosteroids, or anticoagulants.

Traditional nsNSAIDs inhibit prostaglandins through reversible inhibition of both COX-1 and COX-2 enzymes. Aspirin causes irreversible inhibition of COX-1 and COX-2 as well as of platelet aggregation. Coxibs (or selective NSAIDs) preferentially inhibit COX-2—the principal enzyme involved in prostaglandin production at sites of inflammation—while providing relative sparing of COX-1, the principal enzyme involved with mucosal cytoprotection in the stomach and duodenum. Celecoxib is the only coxib currently available in the United States, although other older NSAIDs (etodolac, meloxicam) may have similar COX-2/COX-1 selectivity.

Coxibs decrease the incidence of endoscopically visible ulcers by approximately 75% compared with nsNSAIDs.

Of greater clinical importance, the risk of significant clinical events (obstruction, perforation, bleeding) is reduced by up to 50% in patients taking coxibs versus nsNSAIDs. However, a twofold increase in the incidence in cardiovascular complications (myocardial infarction, cerebrovascular infarction, and death) has been detected in patients taking coxibs compared with placebo, prompting the voluntary withdrawal of two coxibs (rofecoxib and valdecoxib) from the market by the manufacturers. In two large, prospective, randomized controlled trials testing the efficacy of coxibs on polyp prevention, celecoxib was associated with a 1.3- to 3.4-fold increased risk of cardiovascular complications versus placebo; the risk was greatest in patients taking higher doses of celecoxib. A review by an FDA panel suggested that all NSAIDs (other than aspirin and, possibly, naproxen) may be associated with an increased risk of cardiovascular complications, but concluded that celecoxib, which has less COX-2 selectivity than rofecoxib and valdecoxib, does not have higher risk than other nsNSAIDs when used in currently recommended doses (200 mg/d).

Use of even low-dose aspirin (81–325 mg/d) leads to a twofold increased risk of gastrointestinal bleeding complications. In randomized controlled trials, the absolute annual increase of gastrointestinal bleeding attributable to low-dose aspirin is only 0.12% higher than with placebo therapy. However, in population studies, gastrointestinal bleeding occurs in 1.2% of patients each year. Patients with a prior history of peptic ulcers or gastrointestinal bleeding have a markedly increased risk of complications on low-dose aspirin. It should be noted that low-dose aspirin in combination with NSAIDs or coxibs increases the risk of ulcer complications by up to tenfold compared with NSAIDs or low-dose aspirin alone.

H pylori infection increases the risk of ulcer disease and complications over threefold in patients taking NSAIDs or low-dose aspirin. It is hypothesized that NSAID initiation may potentiate or aggravate ulcer disease in susceptible infected individuals.

▶ Clinical Findings

A. Symptoms and Signs

Epigastric pain (dyspepsia), the hallmark of peptic ulcer disease, is present in 80–90% of patients. However, this complaint is not sensitive or specific enough to serve as a reliable diagnostic criterion for peptic ulcer disease. The clinical history cannot accurately distinguish duodenal from gastric ulcers. Less than 25% of patients with dyspepsia have ulcer disease at endoscopy. Twenty percent of patients with ulcer complications such as bleeding have no antecedent symptoms ("silent ulcers"). Nearly 60% of patients with NSAID-related ulcer complications do not have prior symptoms.

Pain is typically well localized to the epigastrium and not severe. It is described as gnawing, dull, aching, or "hunger-like." Approximately 50% of patients report relief of pain with food or antacids (especially duodenal ulcers) and a recurrence of pain 2–4 hours later. However, many patients deny any relationship to meals or report worsening of pain. Two-thirds of duodenal ulcers and one-third of gastric ulcers cause nocturnal pain that awakens the patient. A change from a patient's typical rhythmic discomfort to constant or radiating pain may reflect ulcer penetration or perforation. Most patients have symptomatic periods lasting up to several weeks with intervals of months to years in which they are pain free (periodicity).

Nausea and anorexia may occur with gastric ulcers. Significant vomiting and weight loss are unusual with uncomplicated ulcer disease and suggest gastric outlet obstruction or gastric malignancy.

The physical examination is often normal in uncomplicated peptic ulcer disease. Mild, localized epigastric tenderness to deep palpation may be present. FOBT or FIT is positive in one-third of patients.

B. Laboratory Findings

Laboratory tests are normal in uncomplicated peptic ulcer disease but are ordered to exclude ulcer complications or confounding disease entities. Anemia may occur with acute blood loss from a bleeding ulcer or less commonly from chronic blood loss. Leukocytosis suggests ulcer penetration or perforation. An elevated serum amylase in a patient with severe epigastric pain suggests ulcer penetration into the pancreas. A fasting serum gastrin level to screen for Zollinger-Ellison syndrome is obtained in some patients (see below).

C. Endoscopy

Upper endoscopy is the procedure of choice for the diagnosis of duodenal and gastric ulcers. Duodenal ulcers are virtually never malignant and do not require biopsy. Three to 5 percent of benign-appearing gastric ulcers prove to be malignant. Hence, biopsies of the ulcer margin are almost always performed. Provided that the gastric ulcer appears benign to the endoscopist and adequate biopsy specimens reveal no evidence of cancer, dysplasia, or atypia, the patient may be monitored without further endoscopy. If these conditions are not fulfilled, follow-up endoscopy should be performed 12 weeks after the start of therapy to document complete healing; nonhealing ulcers are suspicious for malignancy.

D. Imaging

Because barium upper gastrointestinal series is less sensitive for detection of ulcers and less accurate for distinguishing benign from malignant ulcers, it has been supplanted by upper endoscopy in most settings. Abdominal CT imaging is obtained in patients with suspected complications of peptic ulcer disease (perforation, penetration, or obstruction).

E. Testing for *H pylori*

In patients in whom an ulcer is diagnosed by endoscopy, gastric mucosal biopsies should be obtained both for a rapid urease test and for histologic examination. The specimens for histology are discarded if the urease test is positive.

In patients with a history of peptic ulcer or when an ulcer is diagnosed by upper gastrointestinal series, noninvasive assessment for *H pylori* with fecal antigen assay or urea breath testing should be done, which both have a sensitivity and specificity of 95%. Proton pump inhibitors may cause false-negative urea breath tests and fecal antigen tests and should be withheld for at least 14 days before testing. Because of its lower sensitivity (85%) and specificity (79%), serologic testing should not be performed unless fecal antigen testing or urea breath testing is unavailable.

▶ Differential Diagnosis

Peptic ulcer disease must be distinguished from other causes of epigastric distress (dyspepsia). Over 50% of patients with dyspepsia have no obvious organic explanation for their symptoms and are classified as having functional dyspepsia (see sections above on Dyspepsia and Functional Dyspepsia). Atypical gastroesophageal reflux may be manifested by epigastric symptoms. Biliary tract disease is characterized by discrete, intermittent episodes of pain that should not be confused with other causes of dyspepsia. Severe epigastric pain is atypical for peptic ulcer disease unless complicated by a perforation or penetration. Other causes include acute pancreatitis, acute cholecystitis or choledocholithiasis, esophageal rupture, gastric volvulus, and ruptured aortic aneurysm.

▶ Pharmacologic Agents

The pharmacology and use of several agents that enhance the healing of peptic ulcers is briefly discussed here. They may be divided into three categories: (1) acid-antisecretory agents, (2) mucosal protective agents, and (3) agents that promote healing through eradication of *H pylori*.

A. Acid-Antisecretory Agents

1. Proton pump inhibitors—Proton pump inhibitors covalently bind the acid-secreting enzyme H^+-K^+-ATPase, or "proton pump," permanently inactivating it. Restoration of acid secretion requires synthesis of new pumps, which have a half-life of 18 hours. Thus, although these agents have a serum half-life of < 60 minutes, their duration of action exceeds 24 hours.

There are six oral proton pump inhibitors currently available: omeprazole, rabeprazole, esomeprazole, lansoprazole, dexlansoprazole, and pantoprazole. The available oral agents inhibit over 90% of 24-hour acid secretion, compared with under 65% for H_2-receptor antagonists in standard dosages. Despite minor differences in their pharmacology, they are equally efficacious in the treatment of peptic ulcer disease. Treatment with oral proton pump inhibitors results in over 90% healing of duodenal ulcers after 4 weeks and 90% of gastric ulcers after 8 weeks when given once daily (30 minutes before breakfast) at the following recommended doses: omeprazole, 20–40 mg; esomeprazole, 40 mg; rabeprazole, 20 mg; lansoprazole, 30 mg; dexlansoprazole, 30–60 mg; pantoprazole, 40 mg. Compared with H_2-receptor antagonists, proton pump inhibitors provide faster pain relief and more rapid ulcer healing.

The proton pump inhibitors are remarkably safe for short-term therapy. Long-term use may lead to mild decreases in vitamin B_{12}, iron, and calcium absorption. Observational studies suggest an increased risk of enteric infections, including *C difficile* and bacterial gastroenteritis, a modest (1.4-fold) increased risk of hip fracture, and pneumonia. Serum gastrin levels rise significantly in 3% of patients receiving long-term therapy but return to normal limits within 2 weeks after discontinuation.

2. H_2-receptor antagonists—Although H_2-receptor antagonists are effective in the treatment of peptic ulcer disease, proton pump inhibitors are now the preferred agents because of their ease of use and superior efficacy. Four H_2-receptor antagonists are available: cimetidine, ranitidine, famotidine, and nizatidine. For uncomplicated peptic ulcers, H_2-receptor antagonists may be administered once daily at bedtime as follows: ranitidine and nizatidine 300 mg, famotidine 40 mg, and cimetidine 800 mg. Duodenal and gastric ulcer healing rates of 85–90% are obtained within 6 weeks and 8 weeks, respectively.

B. Agents Enhancing Mucosal Defenses

Bismuth, misoprostol, and antacids all have been shown to promote ulcer healing through the enhancement of mucosal defensive mechanisms. Given the greater efficacy and safety of antisecretory agents and better compliance of patients, these other agents are no longer used as first-line therapy for active ulcers in most clinical settings.

C. *H pylori* Eradication Therapy

Eradication of *H pylori* has proved difficult. Combination regimens that use two or three antibiotics with a proton pump inhibitor or bismuth are required to achieve adequate rates of eradication and to reduce the number of failures due to antibiotic resistance. In the United States, up to 50% of strains are resistant to metronidazole and 13% are resistant to clarithromycin. Recommended regimens are listed in Table 15–10. At present, experts disagree on the optimal regimen; however, updated Maastricht consensus guidelines were published in 2012. In areas of low clarithromycin resistance, including the United States, a 14-day course of "triple therapy," with an oral proton pump inhibitor, clarithromycin 500 mg, and amoxicillin 1 g (or, if penicillin allergic, metronidazole 500 mg), all given twice daily for 14 days, is still recommended for first-line therapy. Unfortunately, this regimen only achieves rates of eradication > 75%. "Quadruple therapy," with a proton pump inhibitor, bismuth, tetracycline, and metronidazole or tinidazole for 14 days (Table 15–10) is a more complicated but also more effective regimen. In a 2011 randomized, controlled trial, the per protocol eradication rates were 93% with quadruple therapy and 70% with triple therapy. Bismuth-based quadruple therapy is recommended as first-line therapy for patients in areas with high clarithromycin resistance (> 20%), in patients who have previously been treated with a macrolide antibiotic, or as second-line therapy for patients whose infection persists after an initial course of triple therapy. Several studies reported eradication rates of > 90% using a 10-day sequential regimen consisting of four drugs: a proton pump inhibitor and amoxicillin

for 5 days, followed by a proton pump inhibitor, clarithromycin, and tinidazole for 5 days. However, subsequent studies confirmed equivalent or superior efficacy when all four drugs were given concomitantly for 10 days (non-bismuth quadruple therapy). Unfortunately, recent studies have reported lower eradication rates with sequential therapy, and a 2013 meta-analysis did not detect superiority compared with 14-day triple therapy or bismuth-based therapy, except in patients with organisms exhibiting clarithromycin resistance. Most recently, a 2013 large multicenter European controlled trial conducted in regions of high clarithromycin resistance reported 92% eradication with a 14-day quadruple therapy consisting of a proton pump inhibitor, amoxicillin, clarithromycin, and nitroimidazole (the latter not available in the United States).

▶ Medical Treatment

Patients should be encouraged to eat balanced meals at regular intervals. There is no justification for bland or restrictive diets. Moderate alcohol intake is not harmful. Smoking retards the rate of ulcer healing and increases the frequency of recurrences and should be prohibited.

A. Treatment of *H pylori*–Associated Ulcers

1. Treatment of active ulcer—The goals of treatment of active *H pylori*–associated ulcers are to relieve dyspeptic symptoms, to promote ulcer healing, and to eradicate *H pylori* infection. Uncomplicated *H pylori*–associated ulcers should be treated for 10–14 days with one of the proton pump inhibitor-based *H pylori* eradication regimens listed in Table 15–10. At that point, no further antisecretory therapy is needed, provided the ulcer was small (< 1 cm) and dyspeptic symptoms have resolved. For patients with large or complicated ulcers, an antisecretory agent should be continued for an additional 2–4 weeks (duodenal ulcer) or 4–6 weeks (gastric ulcer) after completion of the antibiotic regimen to ensure complete ulcer healing. A once-daily oral proton pump inhibitor (as listed in Table 15–10) is recommended. Confirmation of *H pylori* eradication is recommended for all patients > 4 weeks after completion of antibiotic therapy and > 2 weeks after discontinuation of the proton pump inhibitor either with noninvasive tests (urea breath test, fecal antigen test) or endoscopy with biopsy for histology.

2. Therapy to prevent recurrence—Successful eradication reduces ulcer recurrences to < 20% after 1–2 years. The most common cause of recurrence after antibiotic therapy is failure to achieve successful eradication. Once cure has been achieved, reinfection rates are < 0.5% per year. Although *H pylori* eradication has reduced the need for long-term maintenance antisecretory therapy to prevent ulcer recurrences, there remains a subset of patients who require long-term therapy with a proton pump inhibitor once daily. This subset includes patients with *H pylori*–positive ulcers who have not responded to repeated attempts at eradication therapy, patients with a history of *H pylori*–positive ulcers who have recurrent ulcers despite successful eradication, and patients with idiopathic ulcers (ie, *H pylori*–negative and not taking NSAIDs). In all patients with recurrent ulcers, NSAID

Table 15–10. Treatment options for peptic ulcer disease.

Active *Helicobacter pylori*–associated ulcer

1. Treat with anti-*H pylori* regimen for 10–14 days. Treatment options:

Standard Triple Therapy
- Proton pump inhibitor orally twice daily[1]
  Clarithromycin 500 mg orally twice daily[2]
  Amoxicillin 1 g orally twice daily (OR metronidazole 500 mg orally twice daily, if penicillin allergic[3])

Standard Quadruple Therapy
- Proton pump inhibitor orally twice daily[1,4]
  Bismuth subsalicylate two tablets orally four times daily
  Tetracycline 500 mg orally four times daily
  Metronidazole 250 mg orally four times daily or 500 mg three times daily
  (OR bismuth subcitrate potassium 140 mg/metronidazole 125 mg/tetracycline 125 mg [Pylera] three capsules orally four times daily)[5]

Sequential Quadruple Therapy
- Proton pump inhibitor orally twice daily[1,6]
  Days 1–5: amoxicillin 1 g orally twice daily
  Days 6–10: clarithromycin 500 mg and metronidazole 500 mg, both orally twice daily
- Proton pump inhibitor orally twice daily[1,7]
  Days 1–14: amoxicillin 1 g orally twice daily
  Days 7–14: clarithromycin 500 mg and nitroimidazole[8] 500 mg, both orally twice daily

2. After completion of course of *H pylori* eradication therapy, continue treatment with proton pump inhibitor[1] once daily for 4–6 weeks if ulcer is large (> 1 cm) or complicated.

3. Confirm successful eradication of *H pylori* with urea breath test, fecal antigen test, or endoscopy with biopsy at least 4 weeks after completion of antibiotic treatment and 1–2 weeks after proton pump inhibitor treatment.

Active ulcer not attributable to *H pylori*

1. Consider other causes: NSAIDs, Zollinger-Ellison syndrome, gastric malignancy. Treatment options:
   - Proton pump inhibitors[1]:
     Uncomplicated duodenal ulcer: treat for 4 weeks
     Uncomplicated gastric ulcer: treat for 8 weeks
   - H$_2$-receptor antagonists:
     Uncomplicated duodenal ulcer: cimetidine 800 mg, ranitidine or nizatidine 300 mg, famotidine 40 mg, orally once daily at bedtime for 6 weeks
     Uncomplicated gastric ulcer: cimetidine 400 mg, ranitidine or nizatidine 150 mg, famotidine 20 mg, orally twice daily for 8 weeks
     Complicated ulcers: proton pump inhibitors are the preferred drugs

Prevention of ulcer relapse

1. NSAID-induced ulcer: prophylactic therapy for high-risk patients (prior ulcer disease or ulcer complications, use of corticosteroids or anticoagulants, age > 60 years, serious comorbid illnesses).
   Treatment options:
   Proton pump inhibitor once daily[1]
   COX-2 selective NSAID (celecoxib) (contraindicated in patients with increased risk of cardiovascular disease)
   Misoprostol 200 mcg orally 4 times daily

2. Long-term "maintenance" therapy indicated in patients with recurrent ulcers who either are *H pylori*-negative or who have failed attempts at eradication therapy: once-daily oral proton pump inhibitor[1]

---

[1]Oral proton pump inhibitors: omeprazole 40 mg, rabeprazole 20 mg, lansoprazole 30 mg, dexlansoprazole 30–60 mg, pantoprazole 40 mg, esomeprazole 40 mg. Proton pump inhibitors are administered 30 minutes before meals.
[2]If region with high clarithromycin resistance or if patient has previously been treated with macrolide antibiotic, choose another regimen.
[3]Avoid in areas of known metronidazole resistance or in patients who have failed a course of treatment that included metronidazole.
[4]Preferred regimen in regions with high clarithromycin resistance or in patients who have previously received a macrolide antibiotic or are penicillin allergic. Effective against metronidazole-resistant organisms.
[5]Pylera is an FDA-approved formulation containing: bismuth subcitrate 140 mg/tetracycline 125 mg/metronidazole 125 mg per capsule.
[6]Appears equally effective when all four drugs given concomitantly for 10–14 days; effective against clarithromycin-resistant organisms.
[7]Large trial reported 92% eradication with this prolonged (14-day) "hybrid" sequential therapy, including regions with high clarithromycin resistance. Requires confirmatory trials.
[8]Not available in United States.
COX-2, cyclooxygenase-2; NSAIDs, nonsteroidal anti-inflammatory drugs.

usage (unintentional or surreptitious) and hypersecretory states (including gastrinoma) should be excluded.

B. Treatment of NSAID-Associated Ulcers

1. Treatment of active ulcers—In patients with NSAID-induced ulcers, the offending agent should be discontinued whenever possible. Both gastric and duodenal ulcers respond rapidly to therapy with H_2-receptor antagonists or proton pump inhibitors (Table 15–10) once NSAIDs are eliminated. In some patients with severe inflammatory diseases, it may not be feasible to discontinue NSAIDs. These patients should be treated with concomitant proton pump inhibitors once daily, which results in ulcer healing rates of approximately 80% at 8 weeks in patients continuing to take NSAIDs. All patients with NSAID-associated ulcers should undergo testing for *H pylori* infection. Antibiotic eradication therapy should be given if *H pylori* tests are positive.

2. Prevention of NSAID-induced ulcers—Clinicians should carefully weigh the benefits of NSAID therapy with the risks of cardiovascular and gastrointestinal complications. For all patients, NSAIDs should be prescribed at the lowest effective dose and for the shortest period possible. Both coxibs and nsNSAIDS with the possible exception of naproxen increase the risk of cardiovascular complications. Ulcer complications occur in up to 2% of all nsNSAID-treated patients per year but in up to 10–20% per year of patients with multiple risk factors. These include age over 60 years, history of ulcer disease or complications, concurrent use of antiplatelet therapy (low-dose aspirin or clopidogrel, or both), concurrent therapy with anticoagulants or corticosteroids, and serious underlying medical illness. After considering the patient's risk of cardiovascular and gastrointestinal complications due to NSAID use, the clinician can decide what type of NSAID (nsNSAID vs coxib) is appropriate and what strategies should be used to reduce the risk of such complications. To minimize cardiovascular and gastrointestinal risks, all NSAIDs should be used at the lowest effective dose and for the shortest time necessary.

A. Test for and treat *H pylori* infection—All patients with a known history of peptic ulcer disease who are treated with NSAIDs or antiplatelet agents (aspirin, clopidogrel) should be tested for *H pylori* infection and treated, if positive. Although *H pylori* eradication may decrease the risk of NSAID-related complications, co-therapy with a proton pump inhibitor is still required in high-risk patients.

B. Proton pump inhibitor—Treatment with an oral proton pump inhibitor given once daily (rabeprazole 20 mg, omeprazole 20–40 mg, lansoprazole 30 mg, dexlansoprazole 30–60 mg, or pantoprazole or esomeprazole 40 mg) is effective in the prevention of NSAID-induced gastric and duodenal ulcers and is approved by the FDA for this indication. Among high-risk patients taking nsNSAIDs or coxibs, the incidence of endoscopically visible gastric and duodenal ulcers after 6 months of therapy in patients treated with esomeprazole 20–40 mg/d was 5%, compared with 17% who were given placebo. Nonetheless, proton pump inhibitors are not fully protective in high-risk patients in preventing NSAID-related complications. In prospective, controlled trials of patients with a prior history of NSAID-related ulcer complications, the incidence of recurrent bleeding was almost 5% after 6 months in patients taking nsNSAIDs and a proton pump inhibitor. In prospective, controlled trials of patients with a prior history of ulcer complications related to low-dose aspirin, the incidence of recurrent ulcer bleeding in patients taking low-dose aspirin alone is approximately 15% per year compared with 0–2% per year in patients taking low-dose aspirin and proton pump inhibitor and 9–14% per year in patients taking clopidogrel. Thus, proton pump inhibitors are highly effective in preventing complications related to low-dose aspirin, even in high-risk patients. Enteric coating of aspirin may reduce direct topical damage to the stomach but does not reduce complications.

C. Recommendations to reduce risk of ulcer complications from nsNSAIDs and coxibs—For patients with a low-risk of cardiovascular disease who have no risk factors for gastrointestinal complications, an nsNSAID alone may be given. For patients with one or two gastrointestinal risk factors, a coxib alone or an nsNSAID should be given with a proton pump inhibitor once daily to reduce the risk of gastrointestinal complications. NSAIDs should be avoided if possible in patients with multiple risk factors; if required, however, combination therapy with a coxib or a partially COX-2 selective nsNSAIDs (etodolac, meloxicam) and a proton pump inhibitor once daily is recommended.

For patients with an increased risk of cardiovascular complications, it is preferable to avoid NSAIDs, if possible. If an NSAID is required, naproxen is preferred because it appears to have reduced risk of cardiovascular complications compared with other nsNSAIDs. Coxibs should not be prescribed in patients with increased cardiovascular risk. Almost all patients with increased cardiovascular risk also will be taking antiplatelet therapy with low-dose aspirin or clopidogrel, or both. Because combination therapy with an nsNSAID and antiplatelet therapy increases the risks of gastrointestinal complications, these patients should all receive cotherapy with a proton pump inhibitor once daily or misoprostol.

D. Recommendations to reduce risk of ulcer complications with use of antiplatelet agents—The risk of significant gastrointestinal complications in persons taking low-dose aspirin (81–325 mg/d) or clopidogrel, or both, for cardiovascular prophylaxis is 0.5%/year. Aspirin, 81 mg/d, is recommended in most patients because it has a lower risk of gastrointestinal complications but equivalent cardiovascular protection compared with higher aspirin doses. Complications are increased with combinations of aspirin and clopidogrel or aspirin and anticoagulants. Patients with dyspepsia or prior ulcer disease should be tested for *H pylori* infection and treated, if positive. Patients younger than age 60–70 who have no other risk factors for gastrointestinal complications may be treated with low-dose aspirin alone without a proton pump inhibitor or misoprostol. Virtually all other patients who require low-dose aspirin or aspirin and anticoagulant therapy should receive a proton pump inhibitor once daily.

At the present time, the optimal management of patients who require dual antiplatelet therapy with clopidogrel and aspirin is uncertain. Clopidogrel is a prodrug that is activated by the cytochrome P450 CYP2C19 enzyme. All proton pump inhibitors inhibit CYP2C19 to varying degrees, with omeprazole having the highest and pantoprazole the least level of inhibition. In vitro and in vivo platelet aggregation studies demonstrate that proton pump inhibitors (especially omeprazole) may attenuate the antiplatelet effects of clopidogrel, although the clinical importance of this interaction is uncertain. Some large retrospective cohort studies reported a higher incidence (hazard ratio or odds ratio < 2) of myocardial infarction in patients taking clopidogrel and a proton pump inhibitor (especially omeprazole) than in patients taking clopidogrel alone, although the majority of observational studies have shown no association. By contrast, subgroup analysis from three prospective, randomized controlled trials (CREDO, TRITON, PRINCIPLE) have not found an increase in clinically important cardiac events in patients taking a combination of clopidogrel with proton pump inhibitors, including omeprazole. Furthermore, in 2010 a prospective, randomized controlled trial (COGENT) comparing a combination of clopidogrel with omeprazole versus placebo found no difference in adverse events. Notwithstanding, the FDA issued a warning in 2009 that patients should avoid using clopidogrel with omeprazole, stating further that the safety of other proton pump inhibitors also was uncertain. Faced with this warning, the optimal strategy to reduce the risk of gastrointestinal bleeding in patients taking clopidogrel (with or without aspirin) is uncertain. A 2010 expert consensus panel concluded that once daily treatment with an oral proton pump inhibitor (pantoprazole 40 mg; rabeprazole 20 mg; lansoprazole or dexlansoprazole 30 mg) may still be recommended for patients who have an increased risk of gastrointestinal bleeding (prior history of peptic ulcer disease or gastrointestinal bleeding; concomitant NSAIDs). In keeping with the FDA warning and product labeling, omeprazole and esomeprazole should not be used. For patients with a lower risk of gastrointestinal bleeding, the risks and benefits of proton pump inhibitors must be weighed. Pending further recommendations, an acceptable alternative is to treat with an oral H_2-receptor antagonist (famotidine 20 mg, ranitidine 150 mg, nizatidine 150 mg) twice daily. Cimetidine is a CYP2C19 inhibitor and should not be used. In 2011, the FDA approved ticagrelor, an antiplatelet agent, for use with low-dose aspirin in the treatment of acute coronary syndrome. Like clopidogrel, ticagrelor blocks the platelet ADP p2y12 receptor; however, it does not require hepatic activation, it does not interact with the CYP2C19 enzyme, and its efficacy is not diminished by proton pump inhibitors.

C. Refractory Ulcers

Ulcers that are truly refractory to medical therapy are now uncommon. Less than 5% of ulcers are unhealed after 8 weeks of once daily therapy with proton pump inhibitors, and almost all benign ulcers heal with twice daily therapy. Thus, noncompliance is the most common cause of ulcer nonhealing. NSAID and aspirin use, sometimes surreptitious, are commonly implicated in refractory ulcers and must be stopped. H pylori infection should be sought and the infection treated, if present, in all refractory ulcer patients. Single or multiple linear gastric ulcers may occur in large hiatal hernias where the stomach slides back and forth through the diaphragmatic hiatus ("Cameron lesions"), which may be a cause of iron deficiency anemia. Other causes of nonhealing ulcers include acid hypersecretion (Zollinger-Ellison syndrome), unrecognized malignancy (adenocarcinoma or lymphoma), medications causing gastrointestinal ulceration (eg, iron or bisphosphonates), Crohn disease, and unusual infections (H heilmanii, CMV, mucormycosis). Fasting serum gastrin levels should be obtained to exclude gastrinoma with acid hypersecretion (Zollinger-Ellison syndrome). Repeat ulcer biopsies are mandatory after 2–3 months of therapy in all nonhealed ulcers to look for malignancy or infection. Patients with persistent nonhealing ulcers are referred for surgical therapy after exclusion of NSAID use and persistent H pylori infection.

Abraham NS et al. ACCF/ACG/AHA 2010 expert consensus document on the concomitant use of proton pump inhibitors and thienopyridines: a focused update of the ASSG/ACG/AHA 2008 expert consensus document on reducing the gastrointestinal risks of antiplatelet therapy and NSAID use. Am J Gastroenterol. 2010 Dec;105(12):2533–49. [PMID: 21131924]

Bhatt DL et al; COGENT Investigators. Clopidogrel with or without omeprazole in coronary artery disease. N Engl J Med. 2010 Nov 11;363(20):1909–17. [PMID: 20925534]

Chan FK et al. Effects of Helicobacter pylori infection on long-term risk of peptic ulcer bleeding in low-dose aspirin users. Gastroenterology. 2013 Mar;144(3):528–35. [PMID: 23333655]

Gatta L et al. Global eradication rates for Helicobacter pylori infection: systematic review and meta-analysis of sequential therapy. BMJ. 2013 Aug 7;347:f4587. [PMID: 23926315]

Lanas A et al. Low doses of acetylsalicylic acid increase risk of gastrointestinal bleeding in a meta-analysis. Clin Gastroenterol Hepatol. 2011 Sep;9(9):762–8. [PMID: 21699808]

Lin KJ et al. Acid suppressants reduce risk of gastrointestinal bleeding in patients on antithrombotic or anti-inflammatory therapy. Gastroenterology. 2011 Jul;141(1):71–9. [PMID: 21458456]

Malfertheiner P et al; European Helicobacter Study Group. Management of Helicobacter pylori infection—the Maastricht IV/Florence Consensus Report. Gut. 2012 May;61(5):646–64. [PMID: 22491499]

Molina-Infante J et al. Optimized nonbismuth quadruple therapies cure most patients with Helicobacter pylori infection in populations with high rates of antibiotic resistance. Gastroenterology. 2013 Jul;145(1):121–8. [PMID: 23562754]

COMPLICATIONS OF PEPTIC ULCER DISEASE

1. Gastrointestinal Hemorrhage

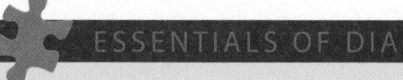

ESSENTIALS OF DIAGNOSIS

► "Coffee grounds" emesis, hematemesis, melena, or hematochezia.

► Emergent upper endoscopy is diagnostic and therapeutic.

General Considerations

Approximately 50% of all episodes of upper gastrointestinal bleeding are due to peptic ulcer. Clinically significant bleeding occurs in 10% of ulcer patients. About 80% of patients stop bleeding spontaneously and generally have an uneventful recovery; the remaining 20% have more severe bleeding. The overall mortality rate for ulcer bleeding is 7%, but it is higher in the elderly, in patients with comorbid medical problems, and in patients with hospital-associated bleeding. Mortality is also higher in patients who present with persistent hypotension or shock, bright red blood in the vomitus or nasogastric lavage fluid, or severe coagulopathy.

Clinical Findings

A. Symptoms and Signs

Up to 20% of patients have no antecedent symptoms of pain; this is particularly true of patients receiving NSAIDs. Common presenting signs include melena and hematemesis. Massive upper gastrointestinal bleeding or rapid gastrointestinal transit may result in hematochezia rather than melena; this may be misinterpreted as signifying a lower tract bleeding source. Nasogastric lavage that demonstrates "coffee grounds" or bright red blood confirms an upper tract source. Recovered nasogastric lavage fluid that is negative for blood does not exclude active bleeding from a duodenal ulcer.

B. Laboratory Findings

The hematocrit may fall as a result of bleeding or expansion of the intravascular volume with intravenous fluids. The BUN may rise as a result of absorption of blood nitrogen from the small intestine and prerenal azotemia.

Treatment

The assessment and initial management of upper gastrointestinal tract bleeding are discussed above. Specific issues pertaining to peptic ulcer bleeding are described below.

A. Medical Therapy

1. Antisecretory agents—Intravenous proton pump inhibitors should be administered for 3 days in patients with ulcers whose endoscopic appearance suggests a high risk of rebleeding after endoscopic therapy. Intravenous proton pump inhibitors have been associated with a reduction in rebleeding, transfusions, the need for further endoscopic therapy, and surgery in the subset of patients with high-risk ulcers, ie, an ulcer with active bleeding, visible vessel, or adherent clot (see below). After initial successful endoscopic treatment of ulcer hemorrhage, intravenous esomeprazole, pantoprazole, or omeprazole (80 mg bolus injection, followed by 8 mg/h continuous infusion for 72 hours) reduces the rebleeding rate from approximately 20% to < 10%; however, intravenous omeprazole is not available in the United States.

High-dose oral proton pump inhibitors (omeprazole 40 mg twice daily) also appear to be effective in reducing rebleeding but have not been compared with the intravenous regimen. Intravenous H_2-receptor antagonists have not been demonstrated to be of any benefit in the treatment of acute ulcer bleeding.

2. Long-term prevention of rebleeding—Recurrent ulcer bleeding develops within 3 years in one-third of patients if no specific therapy is given. In patients with bleeding ulcers who are *H pylori*-positive, successful eradication effectively prevents recurrent ulcer bleeding in almost all cases. It is therefore recommended that all patients with bleeding ulcers be tested for *H pylori* infection and treated if positive. Four to 8 weeks after completion of antibiotic therapy, a urea breath or fecal antigen test for *H pylori* should be administered or endoscopy performed with biopsy for histologic confirmation of successful eradication. In patients in whom *H pylori* persists or the small subset of patients whose ulcers are not associated with NSAIDs or *H pylori*, long-term acid suppression with a once-daily proton pump inhibitor should be prescribed to reduce the likelihood of recurrence of bleeding.

B. Endoscopy

Endoscopy is the preferred diagnostic procedure in almost all cases of upper gastrointestinal bleeding because of its high diagnostic accuracy, its ability to predict the likelihood of recurrent bleeding, and its availability for therapeutic intervention in high-risk lesions. Endoscopy should be performed within 24 hours in most cases. In cases of severe active bleeding, endoscopy is performed as soon as patients have been appropriately resuscitated and are hemodynamically stable.

On the basis of clinical and endoscopic criteria, it is possible to predict which patients are at a higher risk of rebleeding and therefore to make more rational use of hospital resources. Nonbleeding ulcers under 2 cm in size with a base that is clean have a < 5% chance of rebleeding. Most young (under age 60 years), otherwise healthy patients with clean-based ulcers may be safely discharged from the emergency department or hospital after endoscopy. Ulcers that have a flat red or black spot have a < 10% chance of significant rebleeding. Patients who are hemodynamically stable with these findings should be admitted to a hospital ward for 24–72 hours and may begin immediate oral feedings and antiulcer (or anti-*H pylori*) medication.

By contrast, the risk of rebleeding or continued bleeding in ulcers with a nonbleeding visible vessel is 50%, and with active bleeding it is 80–90%. Endoscopic therapy with thermocoagulation (bipolar or heater probes) or application of endoscopic clips (akin to a staple) is the standard of care for such lesions because it reduces the risk of rebleeding, the number of transfusions, and the need for subsequent surgery. The optimal treatment of ulcers with a dense clot that adheres despite vigorous washing is controversial; removal of the clot followed by endoscopic treatment of an underlying vessel may be considered in selected high-risk patients. For actively bleeding ulcers, a combination of epinephrine injection followed by thermocoagulation or clip application commonly is used. These techniques achieve successful hemostasis of actively bleeding lesions in 90% of patients. After endoscopic therapy followed by an intravenous proton pump inhibitor, significant rebleeding occurs in < 10%, of which over 70% can be managed successfully with repeat endoscopic treatment. After endoscopic treatment, patients should remain hospitalized for at least 72 hours, when the risk of rebleeding falls to below 3%.

C. Surgical Treatment

Patients with recurrent bleeding or bleeding that cannot be controlled by endoscopic techniques should be evaluated by a surgeon. However, < 5% of patients treated with hemostatic therapy require surgery for continued or recurrent bleeding. Overall surgical mortality for emergency ulcer bleeding is < 6%. The prognosis is poorer for patients over age 60 years, those with serious underlying medical illnesses or chronic kidney disease, and those who require more than 10 units of blood transfusion. Percutaneous arterial embolization is an alternative to surgery for patients in whom endoscopic therapy has failed.

2. Ulcer Perforation

Perforations develop in < 5% of ulcer patients, usually from ulcers on the anterior wall of the stomach or duodenum. Perforation results in a chemical peritonitis that causes sudden, severe generalized abdominal pain that prompts most patients to seek immediate attention. Elderly or debilitated patients and those receiving long-term corticosteroid therapy may experience minimal initial symptoms, presenting late with bacterial peritonitis, sepsis, and shock. On physical examination, patients appear ill, with a rigid, quiet abdomen and rebound tenderness. Hypotension develops later after bacterial peritonitis has developed. If hypotension is present early with the onset of pain, other abdominal emergencies should be considered such as a ruptured aortic aneurysm, mesenteric infarction, or acute pancreatitis. Leukocytosis is almost always present. A mildly elevated serum amylase (less than twice normal) is sometimes seen. Abdominal CT usually establishes the diagnosis without need for further studies. The absence of free air may lead to a misdiagnosis of pancreatitis, cholecystitis, or appendicitis.

Laparoscopic perforation closure can be performed in many centers, significantly reducing operative morbidity compared with open laparotomy.

3. Gastric Outlet Obstruction

Gastric outlet obstruction occurs in < 2% of patients with ulcer disease and is due to edema or cicatricial narrowing of the pylorus or duodenal bulb. With the advent of potent antisecretory therapy with proton pump inhibitors and the eradication of *H pylori*, obstruction now is less commonly caused by peptic ulcers than by gastric neoplasms or extrinsic duodenal obstruction by intra-abdominal neoplasms. The most common symptoms are early satiety, vomiting, and weight loss. Later, vomiting may develop that typically occurs one to several hours after eating and consists of partially digested food contents. Patients may develop dehydration, metabolic alkalosis, and hypokalemia.

On physical examination, a succussion splash may be heard in the epigastrium. In most cases, nasogastric aspiration will result in evacuation of a large amount (> 200 mL) of foul-smelling fluid, which establishes the diagnosis. Patients are treated initially with intravenous isotonic saline and KCl to correct fluid and electrolyte disorders, an intravenous proton pump inhibitor, and nasogastric decompression of the stomach. Upper endoscopy is performed after 24–72 hours to define the nature of the obstruction and to exclude gastric neoplasm.

Crooks C et al. Reductions in 28-day mortality following hospital admission for upper gastrointestinal hemorrhage. Gastroenterology. 2011 Jul;141(1):62–70. [PMID: 21447331]

Laine L et al. Management of patients with ulcer bleeding. Am J Gastroenterol. 2012 Mar;107(3):345–60. [PMID: 22310222]

Lau JY et al. Challenges in the management of acute peptic ulcer bleeding. Lancet. 2013 Jun 8;381(9882):2033–43. [PMID: 23746903]

Milosavljevic T et al. Complications of peptic ulcer disease. Dig Dis. 2011;29(5):491–3. [PMID: 22095016]

Sanabria A et al. Laparoscopic repair for perforated peptic ulcer disease. Cochrane Database Syst Rev. 2013 Feb 28;2:CD004778. [PMID: 23450555]

Wong TC et al. A comparison of angiographic embolization with surgery after failed endoscopic hemostasis to bleeding peptic ulcers. Gastrointest Endosc. 2011 May;73(5):900–8. [PMID: 21288512]

ZOLLINGER-ELLISON SYNDROME (Gastrinoma)

> ### ESSENTIALS OF DIAGNOSIS
>
> ▶ Peptic ulcer disease; may be severe and atypical.
>
> ▶ Gastric acid hypersecretion.
>
> ▶ Diarrhea common, relieved by nasogastric suction.
>
> ▶ Most cases are sporadic; 25% with multiple endocrine neoplasia type 1 (MEN 1).

▶ General Considerations

Zollinger-Ellison syndrome is caused by gastrin-secreting gut neuroendocrine tumors (gastrinomas), which result in hypergastrinemia and acid hypersecretion. Less than 1% of peptic ulcer disease is caused by gastrinomas. Primary gastrinomas may arise in the pancreas (25%), duodenal wall (45%), or lymph nodes (5–15%), and in other locations or of unknown primary in 20%. Approximately 80% arise within the "gastrinoma triangle" bounded by the porta hepatis, the neck of the pancreas, and the third portion of the duodenum. Most gastrinomas are solitary or multifocal nodules that are potentially resectable. Over two-thirds of gastrinomas are malignant, and one-third have already metastasized to the liver at initial presentation. Approximately 25% of patients have small multicentric gastrinomas associated with MEN 1 that are more difficult to resect.

Clinical Findings

A. Symptoms and Signs

Over 90% of patients with Zollinger-Ellison syndrome develop peptic ulcers. In most cases, the symptoms are indistinguishable from other causes of peptic ulcer disease and therefore the syndrome may go undetected for years. Ulcers usually are solitary and located in the duodenal bulb, but they may be multiple or occur more distally in the duodenum. Isolated gastric ulcers do not occur. Gastroesophageal reflux symptoms occur often. Diarrhea occurs in one-third of patients, in some cases in the absence of peptic symptoms. Gastric acid hypersecretion can cause direct intestinal mucosal injury and pancreatic enzyme inactivation, resulting in diarrhea, steatorrhea, and weight loss; nasogastric aspiration of stomach acid stops the diarrhea. Screening for Zollinger-Ellison syndrome with fasting gastrin levels should be obtained in patients with ulcers that are refractory to standard therapies, giant ulcers (> 2 cm), ulcers located distal to the duodenal bulb, multiple duodenal ulcers, frequent ulcer recurrences, ulcers associated with diarrhea, ulcers occurring after ulcer surgery, and patients with ulcer complications. Ulcer patients with hypercalcemia or family histories of ulcers (suggesting MEN 1) should also be screened. Finally, patients with peptic ulcers who are *H pylori* negative and who are not taking NSAIDs should be screened.

B. Laboratory Findings

The most sensitive and specific method for identifying Zollinger-Ellison syndrome is demonstration of an increased fasting serum gastrin concentration (> 150 pg/mL [> 150 ng/L]). Levels should be obtained with patients not taking H_2-receptor antagonists for 24 hours or proton pump inhibitors for 6 days. Withdrawal of the proton pump inhibitor may be accompanied by massive gastric hypersecretion with serious consequences and should be closely monitored. The median gastrin level is 500–700 pg/mL (500–700 ng/L), and 60% of patients have levels < 1000 pg/mL (< 1000 ng/L). Hypochlorhydria with increased gastric pH is a much more common cause of hypergastrinemia than is gastrinoma. Therefore, a measurement of gastric pH (and, where available, gastric secretory studies) is performed in patients with fasting hypergastrinemia. Most patients have a basal acid output of over 15 mEq/h. A gastric pH of > 3.0 implies hypochlorhydria and excludes gastrinoma. In a patient with a serum gastrin level of > 1000 pg/mL (> 1000 ng/L) and acid hypersecretion, the diagnosis of Zollinger-Ellison syndrome is established. With lower gastrin levels (150–1000 pg/mL [150–1000 ng/L]) and acid secretion, a secretin stimulation test may be performed to distinguish Zollinger-Ellison syndrome from other causes of hypergastrinemia. Intravenous secretin (2 units/kg) produces a rise in serum gastrin of over 200 pg/mL (200 ng/L) within 2–30 minutes in 85% of patients with gastrinoma. An elevated serum calcium suggests hyperparathyroidism and MEN 1 syndrome. In all patients with Zollinger-Ellison syndrome, a serum parathyroid hormone (PTH), prolactin, luteinizing hormone-follicle-stimulating hormone (LH-FSH), and growth hormone (GH) level should be obtained to exclude MEN 1.

C. Imaging

Imaging studies are obtained in an attempt to determine whether there is metastatic disease and, if not, to identify the site of the primary tumor. CT and MRI scans are commonly obtained first to look for large hepatic metastases and primary lesions, but they have low sensitivity for small lesions. Gastrinomas express somatostatin receptors that bind radiolabeled octreotide. Somatostatin receptor scintigraphy (SRS) with single photon emission computed tomography (SPECT) allows total body imaging for detection of primary gastrinomas in the pancreas and lymph nodes, primary gastrinomas in unusual locations, and metastatic gastrinomas (liver and bone). The 80% sensitivity for tumor detection of SRS exceeds all other imaging studies combined. If SRS is positive for tumor localization, further imaging studies are not necessary. In patients with negative SRS, endoscopic ultrasonography (EUS) may be useful to detect small gastrinomas in the duodenal wall, pancreas, or peripancreatic lymph nodes. With a combination of SRS and EUS, more than 90% of primary gastrinomas can be localized preoperatively.

Differential Diagnosis

Gastrinomas are one of several gut neuroendocrine tumors that have similar histopathologic features and arise either from the gut or pancreas. These include carcinoid, insulinoma, VIPoma, glucagonoma, and somatostatinoma. These tumors usually are differentiated by the gut peptides that they secrete; however, poorly differentiated neuroendocrine tumors may not secrete any hormones. Patients may present with symptoms caused by tumor metastases (jaundice, hepatomegaly) rather than functional symptoms. Once a diagnosis of a neuroendocrine tumor is established from the liver biopsy, the specific type of tumor can subsequently be determined. Both carcinoid and gastrinoma tumors may be detected incidentally during endoscopy after biopsy of a submucosal nodule and must be distinguished by subsequent studies.

Hypergastrinemia due to gastrinoma must be distinguished from other causes of hypergastrinemia. Atrophic gastritis with decreased acid secretion is detected by gastric secretory analysis. Other conditions associated with hypergastrinemia (eg, gastric outlet obstruction, vagotomy, chronic kidney disease) are associated with a negative secretin stimulation test.

Treatment

A. Metastatic Disease

The most important predictor of survival is the presence of hepatic metastases. In patients with multiple hepatic metastases, initial therapy should be directed at controlling hypersecretion. Oral proton pump inhibitors (omeprazole, esomeprazole, rabeprazole, pantoprazole, or lansoprazole) are given at a dose of 40–120 mg/d, titrated to achieve a basal acid output of < 10 mEq/h. At this level, there is complete symptomatic relief and ulcer healing. Owing to the slow growth of these tumors, 30% of patients with hepatic metastases have a survival of 10 years.

B. Localized Disease

Cure can be achieved only if the gastrinoma can be resected before hepatic metastatic spread has occurred. Lymph node metastases do not adversely affect prognosis. Laparotomy should be considered in all patients in whom preoperative studies fail to demonstrate hepatic or other distant metastases. A combination of preoperative studies, duodenotomy with careful duodenal inspection, and intra-operative palpation and sonography allows successful localization and resection in the majority of cases. The 15-year survival of patients who do not have liver metasta-ses at initial presentation is over 95%. Surgery usually is not recommended in patients with MEN 1 due to the presence of multifocal tumors and long-term survival in the absence of surgery in most patients.

Ito T et al. Pancreatic neuroendocrine tumors: clinical features, diagnosis and medical treatment: advances. Best Pract Res Clin Gastroenterol. 2012 Dec;26(6):737–53. [PMID: 23582916]

Poitras P et al. The Zollinger-Ellison syndrome: dangers and consequences of interrupting antisecretory treatment. Clin Gastroenterol Hepatol. 2012 Feb;10(2):199–202. [PMID: 21871248]

Pritchard DM. Zollinger-Ellison syndrome: still a diagnostic challenge in the 21st century? Gastroenterology. 2011 May;140(5):1380–83. [PMID: 21443889]

DISEASES OF THE SMALL INTESTINE

MALABSORPTION

The term "malabsorption" denotes disorders in which there is a disruption of digestion and nutrient absorption. The clinical and laboratory manifestations of malabsorption are summarized in Table 15–11.

1. Celiac Disease

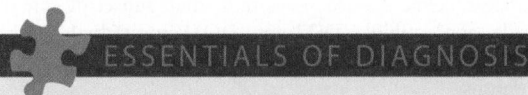

ESSENTIALS OF DIAGNOSIS

▶ **Typical symptoms**: weight loss, chronic diarrhea, abdominal distention, growth retardation.

▶ **Atypical symptoms**: dermatitis herpetiformis, iron deficiency anemia, osteoporosis.

▶ Abnormal serologic test results.

▶ Abnormal small bowel biopsy.

▶ Clinical improvement on gluten-free diet.

▶ General Considerations

Celiac disease (also called sprue, celiac sprue, and gluten enteropathy) is a permanent dietary disorder caused by an immunologic response to gluten, a storage protein found in certain grains, that results in diffuse damage to the proximal small intestinal mucosa with malabsorption of nutrients. Although symptoms may manifest between

Table 15–11. Clinical manifestations and laboratory findings in malabsorption of various nutrients.

Manifestations	Laboratory Findings	Malabsorbed Nutrients
Steatorrhea (bulky, light-colored stools)	Increased fecal fat; decreased serum cholesterol; decreased serum carotene, vitamin A, vitamin D	Triglycerides, fatty acids, phospholipids, cholesterol. Fat soluble vitamins: A, D, E, K
Diarrhea (increased fecal water)	Increased stool volume and weight; increased fecal fat; increased stool osmolality gap	Fats, carbohydrates
Weight loss; muscle wasting	Increased fecal fat; decreased carbohydrate (D-xylose) absorption	Fat, protein, carbohydrates
Microcytic anemia	Low serum iron	Iron
Macrocytic anemia	Decreased serum vitamin B_{12} or red blood cell folate	Vitamin B_{12} or folic acid
Paresthesia; tetany; positive Trousseau and Chvostek signs	Decreased serum calcium or magnesium	Calcium, vitamin D, magnesium
Bone pain; pathologic fractures; skeletal deformities	Osteopenia on radiograph; osteoporosis (adults); osteomalacia (children)	Calcium, vitamin D
Bleeding tendency (ecchymoses, epistaxis)	Prolonged prothrombin time or INR	Vitamin K
Edema	Decreased serum total protein and albumin; increased fecal loss of alpha-1-antitrypsin	Protein
Milk intolerance (cramps, bloating, diarrhea)	Abnormal lactose tolerance test	Lactose

INR, international normalized ratio.

6 months and 24 months of age after the introduction of weaning foods, the majority of cases present in childhood or adulthood. Population screening with serologic tests suggests that the disease is present in 1:100 whites of Northern European ancestry, in whom a clinical diagnosis of celiac disease is made in only 10%, suggesting that most cases are undiagnosed or asymptomatic. Celiac disease only develops in people with the HLA-DQ2 (95%) or -DQ8 (5%) class II molecules, which are present in 40% of the population. Although the precise pathogenesis is unclear, celiac disease arises in a small subset of genetically susceptible (-DQ2 or -DQ8) individuals when dietary gluten stimulates an inappropriate immunologic response.

► Clinical Findings

The most important step in diagnosing celiac disease is to consider the diagnosis. Symptoms are present for more than 10 years in most adults before the correct diagnosis is established. Because of its protean manifestations, celiac disease is grossly underdiagnosed in the adult population.

A. Symptoms and Signs

The gastrointestinal symptoms and signs of celiac disease depend on the length of small intestine involved and the patient's age when the disease presents. "Classic" symptoms of malabsorption, including diarrhea, steatorrhea, weight loss, abdominal distention, weakness, muscle wasting, or growth retardation, more commonly present in infants (< 2 years). Older children and adults are less likely to manifest signs of serious malabsorption. They may report chronic diarrhea, dyspepsia, or flatulence due to colonic bacterial digestion of malabsorbed nutrients, but the severity of weight loss is variable. Many adults have minimal or no gastrointestinal symptoms but present with extraintestinal "atypical" manifestations, including fatigue, depression, iron deficiency anemia, osteoporosis, short stature, delayed puberty, amenorrhea, or reduced fertility. Approximately 40% of patients with positive serologic tests consistent with sprue have no symptoms of disease; the natural history of these patients with "silent" sprue is unclear.

Physical examination may be normal in mild cases or may reveal signs of malabsorption such as loss of muscle mass or subcutaneous fat, pallor due to anemia, easy bruising due to vitamin K deficiency, hyperkeratosis due to vitamin A deficiency, bone pain due to osteomalacia, or neurologic signs (peripheral neuropathy, ataxia) due to vitamin B_{12} or vitamin E deficiency (Table 15–11). Abdominal examination may reveal distention with hyperactive bowel sounds.

Dermatitis herpetiformis is regarded as a cutaneous variant of celiac disease. It is a characteristic skin rash consisting of pruritic papulovesicles over the extensor surfaces of the extremities and over the trunk, scalp, and neck. Dermatitis herpetiformis occurs in < 10% of patients with celiac disease; however, almost all patients who present with dermatitis herpetiformis have evidence of celiac disease on intestinal mucosal biopsy, though it may not be clinically evident.

B. Laboratory Findings

1. Routine laboratory tests—Depending on the severity of illness and the extent of intestinal involvement, nonspecific laboratory abnormalities may be present that may raise the suspicion of malabsorption and celiac disease (Table 15–11). Limited proximal involvement may result only in microcytic anemia due to iron deficiency. Up to 5% of adults with iron deficiency not due to gastrointestinal blood loss have undiagnosed celiac disease. More extensive involvement results in a megaloblastic anemia due to folate or vitamin B_{12} deficiency. Low serum calcium or elevated alkaline phosphatase may reflect impaired calcium or vitamin D absorption with osteomalacia or osteoporosis. Dual-energy x-ray densitometry scanning is recommended for all patients with sprue to screen for osteoporosis. Elevations of prothrombin time, or decreased vitamin A or D levels reflect impaired fat-soluble vitamin absorption. A low serum albumin may reflect small intestine protein loss or poor nutrition. Severe diarrhea may result in a nonanion gap acidosis and hypokalemia. Mild elevations of aminotransferases are found in up to 40%.

2. Serologic tests—Serologic tests should be performed in all patients in whom there is a suspicion of celiac disease. The recommended test is the IgA tissue transglutaminase (IgA tTG) antibody, which has a 95% sensitivity and 95% specificity for the diagnosis of celiac disease. Antigliadin antibodies are not recommended because of their lower sensitivity and specificity. IgA antiendomysial antibodies are no longer recommended due to the lack of standardization among laboratories. An IgA level should be obtained in patients with a negative IgA tTG antibody when celiac disease is strongly suspected because up to 3% of patients with celiac disease have IgA deficiency. A test that measures IgG antibodies to deamidated gliadin has excellent sensitivity and specificity and is useful in patients with IgA deficiency and young children. Levels of all antibodies become undetectable after 3–12 months of dietary gluten withdrawal and may be used to monitor dietary compliance, especially in patients whose symptoms fail to resolve after institution of a gluten-free diet.

C. Mucosal Biopsy

Endoscopic mucosal biopsy of the proximal duodenum (bulb) and distal duodenum is the standard method for confirmation of the diagnosis in patients with a positive serologic test for celiac disease. Mucosal biopsy should also be pursued in patients with negative serologies when symptoms and laboratory studies are strongly suggestive of celiac disease. At endoscopy, atrophy or scalloping of the duodenal folds may be observed. Histology reveals abnormalities ranging from intraepithelial lymphocytosis alone to extensive infiltration of the lamina propria with lymphocytes and plasma cells with hypertrophy of the intestinal crypts and blunting or complete loss of intestinal villi. An adequate normal biopsy excludes the diagnosis. Partial or complete reversion of these abnormalities occurs within 3–24 months after a patient is placed on a gluten-free diet, but symptom resolution remains incomplete in 50% of patients. If a patient with a compatible biopsy demonstrates prompt clinical improvement on a gluten-free diet and a decrease in antigliadin antibodies, a repeat biopsy is unnecessary.

Differential Diagnosis

Many patients with chronic diarrhea or flatulence are erroneously diagnosed as having irritable bowel syndrome. Celiac sprue must be distinguished from other causes of malabsorption, as outlined above. Severe panmalabsorption of multiple nutrients is almost always caused by mucosal disease. The histologic appearance of celiac sprue may resemble other mucosal diseases such as tropical sprue, bacterial overgrowth, cow's milk intolerance, viral gastroenteritis, eosinophilic gastroenteritis, and mucosal damage caused by acid hypersecretion associated with gastrinoma. Documentation of clinical response to gluten withdrawal therefore is essential to the diagnosis.

Some patients complain of symptoms after gluten ingestion but do not have serologic or histologic evidence of celiac disease. The frequency and cause of this entity is debated. A large 2013 study found that symptoms improved in gluten-sensitive patients when placed on a FODMAP-restricted diet and worsened to similar degrees when challenged in a double-blind crossover trial with gluten or whey proteins. These data suggest that nonceliac gluten sensitivity may not be a true entity and that the symptom improvement reported by patients with gluten restriction may be due to broader FODMAP elimination.

Treatment

Removal of all gluten from the diet is essential to therapy—all wheat, rye, and barley must be eliminated. Although oats appear to be safe for many patients, commercial products may be contaminated with wheat or barley during processing. Because of the pervasive use of gluten products in manufactured foods and additives, in medications, and by restaurants, it is imperative that patients and their families confer with a knowledgeable dietitian to comply satisfactorily with this lifelong diet. Several excellent dietary guides and patient support groups are available. Most patients with celiac disease also have lactose intolerance either temporarily or permanently and should avoid dairy products until the intestinal symptoms have improved on the gluten-free diet. Dietary supplements (folate, iron, calcium, and vitamins A, B_{12}, D, and E) should be provided in the initial stages of therapy but usually are not required long-term with a gluten-free diet. Patients with confirmed osteoporosis may require long-term calcium, vitamin D, and bisphosphonate therapy.

Improvement in symptoms should be evident within a few weeks on the gluten-free diet. The most common reason for treatment failure is incomplete removal of gluten. Intentional or unintentional rechallenge with gluten may trigger acute severe diarrhea with dehydration, electrolyte imbalance, and may require TPN and intravenous or oral corticosteroids (prednisone 40 mg or budesonide 9 mg) for 2 or more weeks as a gluten-free diet is re-initiated.

Prognosis & Complications

If appropriately diagnosed and treated, patients with celiac disease have an excellent prognosis. Celiac disease may be associated with other autoimmune disorders, including Addison disease, Graves disease, type 1 diabetes mellitus, myasthenia gravis, scleroderma, Sjögren syndrome, atrophic gastritis, and pancreatic insufficiency. In some patients, celiac disease may evolve and become refractory to the gluten-free diet. The most common cause is intentional or unintentional dietary noncompliance, which may be suggested by positive serologic tests. Celiac disease that is truly refractory to gluten withdrawal occurs in < 5% and generally carries a poor prognosis. There are two types of refractory disease, which are distinguished by their intraepithelial lymphocyte phenotype. This diagnosis should be considered in patients previously responsive to the gluten-free diet in whom new weight loss, abdominal pain, and malabsorption develop.

Biesiekierski JR et al. No effects of gluten in patients with self-reported non-celiac gluten sensitivity after dietary reduction of fermentable, poorly absorbed, short-chain carbohydrates. Gastroenterology. 2013 Aug;145(2):320–8. [PMID: 23648697]

Celiac Disease Foundation, 13251 Ventura Blvd, Suite #1, Studio City, CA 91604-1838. http://www.celiac.org

Fasano A et al. Clinical practice. Celiac disease. N Engl J Med. 2012 Dec 20;367(25):2419–26. [PMID: 23252527]

Harris LA et al. Celiac disease: clinical, endoscopic, and histopathologic review. Gastrointest Endosc. 2012 Sep;76(3):625–40. [PMID: 22898420]

Rubio-Tapia A et al. ACG clinical guidelines: diagnosis and management of celiac disease. Am J Gastroenterol. 2013 May;108(5):656–76. [PMID: 23609613]

2. Whipple Disease

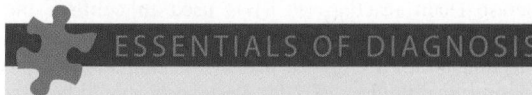

ESSENTIALS OF DIAGNOSIS

▶ Multisystem disease.

▶ Fever, lymphadenopathy, arthralgias.

▶ Weight loss, malabsorption, chronic diarrhea.

▶ Duodenal biopsy with periodic acid-Schiff (PAS)-positive macrophages with characteristic bacillus.

General Considerations

Whipple disease is a rare multisystem illness caused by infection with the bacillus *Tropheryma whippelii*. It may occur at any age but most commonly affects white men in the fourth to sixth decades. The source of infection is unknown, but no cases of human-to-human spread have been documented.

Clinical Findings

A. Symptoms and Signs

The clinical manifestations are protean; however, the most common are arthralgias, diarrhea, abdominal pain, and weight loss. Arthralgias or a migratory, nondeforming arthritis occurs in 80% and is typically the first symptom experienced. Gastrointestinal symptoms occur in approximately 75% of cases. They include abdominal pain, diarrhea, and some degree of malabsorption with distention, flatulence, and steatorrhea. Weight loss is the most common presenting symptom—seen in almost all patients. Loss of protein due to intestinal or lymphatic involvement may result in protein-losing enteropathy with hypoalbuminemia and edema. In the absence of gastrointestinal symptoms, the diagnosis often is delayed for several years. Intermittent low-grade fever occurs in over 50% of cases.

Physical examination may reveal hypotension (a late finding), low-grade fever, and evidence of malabsorption (see Table 15–11). Lymphadenopathy is present in 50%. Heart murmurs due to valvular involvement may be evident. Peripheral joints may be enlarged or warm, and peripheral edema may be present. Neurologic findings are cited above. Hyperpigmentation on sun-exposed areas is evident in up to 40%.

B. Laboratory Findings

If significant malabsorption is present, patients may have laboratory abnormalities as outlined in Table 15–11. There may be steatorrhea.

C. Histologic Evaluation

In most cases, the diagnosis of Whipple disease is established by endoscopic biopsy of the duodenum with histologic evaluation, which demonstrates infiltration of the lamina propria with PAS-positive macrophages that contain gram-positive bacilli (which are not acid-fast) and dilation of the lacteals. Because the PAS stain is less sensitive and specific for extraintestinal Whipple disease, polymerase chain reaction (PCR) is used to confirm the diagnosis. Because asymptomatic central nervous system infection occurs in 40% of patients, examination of the cerebrospinal fluid by PCR for *T whippelii* should be performed routinely. The sensitivity of PCR is 97% and the specificity 100%.

▶ Differential Diagnosis

Whipple disease should be considered in patients who present with signs of malabsorption, fever of unknown origin, lymphadenopathy, seronegative arthritis, culture-negative endocarditis, or multisystem disease. Small bowel biopsy readily distinguishes Whipple disease from other mucosal malabsorptive disorders, such as celiac sprue.

▶ Treatment

Antibiotic therapy results in a dramatic clinical improvement within several weeks, even in some patients with neurologic involvement. The optimal regimen is unknown. Complete clinical response usually is evident within 1–3 months; however, relapse may occur in up to one-third of patients after discontinuation of treatment. Therefore,

prolonged treatment for at least 1 year is required. Drugs that cross the blood-brain barrier are preferred. A randomized controlled trial in 40 patients with 3–10 years follow-up demonstrated 100% remission with either ceftriaxone 1 g intravenously twice daily or meropenem 1 g intravenously three times daily for 2 weeks, followed by trimethoprim-sulfamethoxazole 160/800 mg twice daily for 12 months. After treatment, repeat duodenal biopsies for histologic analysis and cerebrospinal fluid PCR should be obtained every 6 months for at least 1year. The absence of PAS-positive material predicts a low likelihood of clinical relapse.

▶ Prognosis

If untreated, the disease is fatal. Because some neurologic signs may be permanent, the goal of treatment is to prevent this progression. Patients must be followed closely after treatment for signs of symptom recurrence.

Puéchal X. Whipple's disease. Postgrad Med J. 2013 Nov;89(1057):659–65. [PMID: 24129033]
Schwartzman S et al. Whipple's disease. Rheum Dis Clin North Am. 2013 May;39(2):313–21. [PMID: 23597966]

3. Bacterial Overgrowth

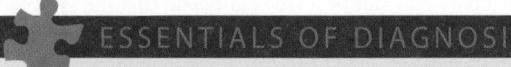

ESSENTIALS OF DIAGNOSIS

- ▶ Symptoms of distention, flatulence, diarrhea, and weight loss.
- ▶ Increased qualitative or quantitative fecal fat.
- ▶ Advanced cases associated with deficiencies of iron or vitamins A, D, and B_{12}.
- ▶ Diagnosis suggested by breath tests using glucose, lactulose, or ^{14}C-xylose as substrates.
- ▶ Diagnosis confirmed by jejunal aspiration with quantitative bacterial cultures.

▶ General Considerations

The small intestine normally contains a small number of bacteria. Bacterial overgrowth in the small intestine of whatever cause may result in malabsorption via a number of mechanisms. Bacterial deconjugation of bile salts may lead to inadequate micelle formation, resulting in decreased fat absorption with steatorrhea and malabsorption of fat-soluble vitamins (A, D). Microbial uptake of specific nutrients reduces absorption of vitamin B_{12} and carbohydrates. Bacterial proliferation also causes direct damage to intestinal epithelial cells and the brush border, further impairing absorption of proteins, carbohydrates, and minerals. Passage of the malabsorbed bile acids and carbohydrates into the colon leads to an osmotic and secretory diarrhea and increased flatulence.

Causes of bacterial overgrowth include: (1) gastric achlorhydria (including proton pump inhibitor therapy);

(2) anatomic abnormalities of the small intestine with stagnation (afferent limb of Billroth II gastrojejunostomy, resection of ileocecal valve, small intestine diverticula, obstruction, blind loop); (3) small intestine motility disorders (vagotomy, scleroderma, diabetic enteropathy, chronic intestinal pseudo-obstruction); (4) gastrocolic or coloenteric fistula (Crohn disease, malignancy, surgical resection); and (5) miscellaneous disorders. Bacterial overgrowth is an important cause of malabsorption in the elderly, perhaps because of decreased gastric acidity or impaired intestinal motility. It may also be present in a subset of patients with irritable bowel syndrome.

Clinical Findings

Many patients with bacterial overgrowth are asymptomatic. Symptoms are nonspecific and include flatulence, weight loss, abdominal pain, diarrhea, and sometimes steatorrhea. Severe cases may result in clinically significant vitamin and mineral deficiencies, including fat-soluble vitamins A or D, vitamin B_{12}, and iron (Table 15–11). Qualitative or quantitative fecal fat assessment typically is abnormal. Bacterial overgrowth should be considered in any patient with diarrhea, flatulence, weight loss, or macrocytic anemia, especially if the patient has a predisposing cause (such as prior gastrointestinal surgery). A stool collection should be obtained to corroborate the presence of steatorrhea. Vitamins A, D, B_{12}, and serum iron should be measured. A specific diagnosis can be established firmly only by an aspirate and culture of proximal jejunal secretion that demonstrates over 10^5 organisms/mL. However, this is an invasive and laborious test that requires careful collection and culturing techniques and therefore is not available in many clinical settings. Noninvasive breath tests are easier to perform and have a sensitivity of 60–90% and specificity of 85% compared with jejunal cultures. Breath hydrogen and methane tests with glucose or lactulose as substrates are commonly done because of their ease of use. A small bowel barium radiography or CT enterography study should be obtained to look for mechanical factors predisposing to intestinal stasis.

Owing to the lack of an optimal test for bacterial overgrowth, many clinicians use an empiric antibiotic trial as a diagnostic and therapeutic maneuver in patients with predisposing conditions for bacterial overgrowth in whom unexplained diarrhea or steatorrhea develops.

Treatment

Where possible, the anatomic defect that has potentiated bacterial overgrowth should be corrected. Otherwise, treatment as follows for 1–2 weeks with oral broad-spectrum antibiotics effective against enteric aerobes and anaerobes usually leads to dramatic improvement: twice daily ciprofloxacin 500 mg, norfloxacin 400 mg, or amoxicillin clavulanate 875 mg, or a combination of metronidazole 250 mg three times daily plus either trimethoprim-sulfamethoxazole (one double-strength tablet) twice daily or cephalexin 250 mg four times daily. Rifaximin 400 mg three times daily is a nonabsorbable antibiotic that also appears to be effective but has fewer side effects than the other systemically absorbed antibiotics.

In patients in whom symptoms recur off antibiotics, cyclic therapy (eg, 1 week out of 4) may be sufficient. Continuous antibiotics should be avoided, if possible, to avoid development of bacterial antibiotic resistance.

In patients with severe intestinal dysmotility, treatment with small doses of octreotide may prove to be of benefit.

Bohm M et al. Diagnosis and management of small intestinal bacterial overgrowth. Nutr Clin Pract. 2013 Jun;28(3):289–99. [PMID: 23614961]

Grace E et al. Review article: small intestinal bacterial overgrowth—prevalence, clinical features, current and developing diagnostic tests, and treatment. Aliment Pharmacol Ther. 2013 Oct;38(7):674–88. [PMID: 23957651]

4. Short Bowel Syndrome

Short bowel syndrome is the malabsorptive condition that arises secondary to removal of significant segments of the small intestine. The most common causes in adults are Crohn disease, mesenteric infarction, radiation enteritis, volvulus, tumor resection, and trauma. The type and degree of malabsorption depend on the length and site of the resection and the degree of adaptation of the remaining bowel.

Terminal Ileal Resection

Resection of the terminal ileum results in malabsorption of bile salts and vitamin B_{12}, which are normally absorbed in this region. Patients with low serum vitamin B_{12} levels or resection of over 50 cm of ileum require monthly subcutaneous or intramuscular vitamin B_{12} injections. In patients with < 100 cm of ileal resection, bile salt malabsorption stimulates fluid secretion from the colon, resulting in watery diarrhea. This may be treated with bile salt binding resins (cholestyramine, 2–4 g orally three times daily with meals or colesevelam, 625 mg, 1–3 tablets twice daily). Resection of over 100 cm of ileum leads to a reduction in the bile salt pool that results in steatorrhea and malabsorption of fat-soluble vitamins. Treatment is with a low-fat diet and vitamins supplemented with medium-chain triglycerides, which do not require micellar solubilization. Unabsorbed fatty acids bind with calcium, reducing its absorption and enhancing the absorption of oxalate. Oxalate kidney stones may develop. Calcium supplements should be administered to bind oxalate and increase serum calcium. Cholesterol gallstones due to decreased bile salts are common also. In patients with resection of the ileocolonic valve, bacterial overgrowth may occur in the small intestine, further complicating malabsorption (as outlined above).

Extensive Small Bowel Resection

Resection of up to 40–50% of the total length of small intestine usually is well tolerated. A more massive resection may result in "short-bowel syndrome," characterized by weight loss and diarrhea due to nutrient, water, and electrolyte malabsorption. If the colon is preserved, 100 cm of proximal jejunum may be sufficient to maintain adequate oral nutrition with a low-fat, high complex-carbohydrate diet, though fluid and electrolyte losses may still be significant. In patients in whom the colon has been removed, at least 200 cm of proximal jejunum is typically required to maintain oral nutrition. Antidiarrheal agents (loperamide, 2–4 mg orally three times daily) slow transit and reduce diarrheal volume. Octreotide reduces intestinal transit time and fluid and electrolyte secretion. Gastric hypersecretion initially complicates intestinal resection and should be treated with proton pump inhibitors.

Patients with < 100–200 cm of proximal jejunum remaining almost always require parenteral nutrition. Teduglutide is a glucagon-like peptide-2 analogue that stimulates small bowel growth and absorption and was approved in 2012 for the treatment of short-bowel syndrome. In clinical trials, it resulted in a reduced need for parenteral nutrition. Small intestine transplantation is now being performed with reported 5-year graft survival rates of 40%. Currently, it is performed chiefly in patients in whom serious problems develop due to parenteral nutrition.

Jeppesen PB et al. Teduglutide reduces need for parenteral support among patients with short bowel syndrome with intestinal failure. Gastroenterology. 2012 Dec;143(6):1473–1481.e3. [PMID: 22982184]

5. Lactase Deficiency

ESSENTIALS OF DIAGNOSIS

- ▶ Diarrhea, bloating, flatulence, and abdominal pain after ingestion of milk-containing products.
- ▶ Diagnosis supported by symptomatic improvement on lactose-free diet.
- ▶ Diagnosis confirmed by hydrogen breath test.

▶ General Considerations

Lactase is a brush border enzyme that hydrolyzes the disaccharide lactose into glucose and galactose. The concentration of lactase enzyme levels is high at birth but declines steadily in most people of non-European ancestry during childhood and adolescence and into adulthood. Thus, approximately 50 million people in the United States have partial to complete lactose intolerance. As many as 90% of Asian Americans, 70% of African Americans, 95% of Native Americans, 50% of Mexican Americans, and 60% of Jewish Americans are lactose intolerant compared with < 25% of white adults. Lactase deficiency may also arise secondary to other gastrointestinal disorders that affect the proximal small intestinal mucosa. These include Crohn disease, sprue, viral gastroenteritis, giardiasis, short bowel syndrome, and malnutrition. Malabsorbed lactose is fermented by intestinal bacteria, producing gas and organic acids. The nonmetabolized lactose and organic acids result in an increased stool osmotic load with an obligatory fluid loss.

▶ Clinical Findings

A. Symptoms and Signs

Patients have great variability in clinical symptoms, depending both on the severity of lactase deficiency and the amount of lactose ingested. Because of the nonspecific nature of these symptoms, there is a tendency for both lactose-intolerant and lactose-tolerant individuals to mistakenly attribute a variety of abdominal symptoms to lactose intolerance. Most patients with lactose intolerance can drink one or two 8 oz glasses of milk daily without symptoms if taken with food at wide intervals, though rare patients have almost complete intolerance. With mild to moderate amounts of lactose malabsorption, patients may experience bloating, abdominal cramps, and flatulence. With higher lactose ingestions, an osmotic diarrhea will result. Isolated lactase deficiency does not result in other signs of malabsorption or weight loss. If these findings are present, other gastrointestinal disorders should be pursued. Diarrheal specimens reveal an increased osmotic gap and a pH of < 6.0.

B. Laboratory Findings

The most widely available test for the diagnosis of lactase deficiency is the hydrogen breath test. After ingestion of 50 g of lactose, a rise in breath hydrogen of > 20 ppm within 90 minutes is a positive test, indicative of bacterial carbohydrate metabolism. In clinical practice, many clinicians prescribe an empiric trial of a lactose-free diet for 2 weeks. Resolution of symptoms (bloating, flatulence, diarrhea) is suggestive of lactase deficiency (though a placebo response cannot be excluded) and may be confirmed, if necessary, with a breath hydrogen study.

▶ Differential Diagnosis

The symptoms of late-onset lactose intolerance are nonspecific and may mimic a number of gastrointestinal disorders, such as inflammatory bowel disease, mucosal malabsorptive disorders, irritable bowel syndrome, and pancreatic insufficiency. Furthermore, lactase deficiency frequently develops secondary to other gastrointestinal disorders (as listed above). Concomitant lactase deficiency should always be considered in these gastrointestinal disorders.

▶ Treatment

The goal of treatment in patients with isolated lactase deficiency is achieving patient comfort. Patients usually find their "threshold" of intake at which symptoms will occur. Foods that are high in lactose include milk (12 g/cup), ice cream (9 g/cup), and cottage cheese (8 g/cup). Aged cheeses have a lower lactose content (0.5 g/oz). Unpasteurized yogurt contains bacteria that produce lactase and is generally well tolerated.

By spreading dairy product intake throughout the day in quantities of < 12 g of lactose (one cup of milk), most patients can take dairy products without symptoms and do not require lactase supplements. Most food markets provide milk that has been pretreated with lactase, rendering it 70–100% lactose free. Lactase enzyme replacement is commercially available as nonprescription formulations (Lactaid, Lactrase, Dairy Ease). Caplets or drops of lactase may be taken with milk products, improving lactose absorption and eliminating symptoms. The number of caplets ingested depends on the degree of lactose intolerance. Patients who choose to restrict or eliminate milk products may have increased risk of osteoporosis. Calcium supplementation (calcium carbonate 500 mg orally two to three times daily) is recommended for susceptible patients.

Carter SL et al. The diagnosis and management of patients with lactose intolerance. Nurse Pract. 2013 Jul 10;38(7):23–8. [PMID: 23778177]

Suchy FJ et al. National Institutes of Health Consensus Development Conference: lactose intolerance and health. Ann Intern Med. 2010 Jun 15;152(12):792–6. [PMID: 20404261]

INTESTINAL MOTILITY DISORDERS

1. Acute Paralytic Ileus

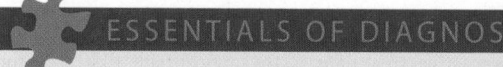

ESSENTIALS OF DIAGNOSIS

► Precipitating factors: surgery, peritonitis, electrolyte abnormalities, medications, severe medical illness.

► Nausea, vomiting, obstipation, distention.

► Minimal abdominal tenderness; decreased bowel sounds.

► Plain abdominal radiography with gas and fluid distention in small and large bowel.

► General Considerations

Ileus is a condition in which there is neurogenic failure or loss of peristalsis in the intestine in the absence of any mechanical obstruction. It is commonly seen in hospitalized patients as a result of: (1) intra-abdominal processes such as recent gastrointestinal or abdominal surgery or peritoneal irritation (peritonitis, pancreatitis, ruptured viscus, hemorrhage); (2) severe medical illness such as pneumonia, respiratory failure requiring intubation, sepsis or severe infections, uremia, diabetic ketoacidosis, and electrolyte abnormalities (hypokalemia, hypercalcemia, hypomagnesemia, hypophosphatemia); and (3) medications that affect intestinal motility (opioids, anticholinergics, phenothiazines). Following surgery, small intestinal motility usually normalizes first (often within hours), followed by the stomach (24–48 hours), and the colon (48–72 hours). Postoperative ileus is reduced by the use of patient-controlled or epidural analgesia and avoidance of intravenous opioids as well as early ambulation, gum chewing, and initiation of a clear liquid diet.

► Clinical Findings

A. Symptoms and Signs

Patients who are conscious report mild diffuse, continuous abdominal discomfort with nausea and vomiting. Generalized abdominal distention is present with minimal abdominal tenderness but no signs of peritoneal irritation (unless due to the primary disease). Bowel sounds are diminished to absent.

B. Laboratory Findings

The laboratory abnormalities are attributable to the underlying condition. Serum electrolytes, including potassium, magnesium, phosphorus, and calcium, should be obtained to exclude abnormalities as contributing factors.

C. Imaging

Plain film radiography of the abdomen demonstrates distended gas-filled loops of small and large intestine. Air-fluid levels may be seen. Under some circumstances, it may be difficult to distinguish ileus from partial small bowel obstruction. A CT scan may be useful in such instances to exclude mechanical obstruction, especially in postoperative patients.

► Differential Diagnosis

Ileus must be distinguished from mechanical obstruction of the small bowel or proximal colon. Pain from small bowel mechanical obstruction is usually intermittent, cramping, and associated initially with profuse vomiting. Acute gastroenteritis, acute appendicitis, and acute pancreatitis may all present with ileus.

► Treatment

The primary medical or surgical illness that has precipitated adynamic ileus should be treated. Most cases of ileus respond to restriction of oral intake with gradual liberalization of diet as bowel function returns. Severe or prolonged ileus requires nasogastric suction and parenteral administration of fluids and electrolytes. Alvimopan is a peripherally acting mu-opioid receptor antagonist with limited absorption or systemic activity that reverses opioid-induced inhibition of intestinal motility. In five randomized controlled trials, it reduced the time to first flatus, bowel movement, solid meal, and hospital discharge compared with placebo in postoperative patients. Alvimopan may be considered in patients undergoing partial large or small bowel resection when postoperative opioid therapy is anticipated.

Delaney CP et al. Evaluation of clinical outcomes with alvimopan in clinical practice: a national matched-cohort study in patients undergoing bowel resection. Ann Surg. 2012 Apr;255(4):731–8. [PMID: 22388106]

Doorly MG et al. Pathogenesis and clinical and economic consequences of paralytic ileus. Surg Clin North Am. 2012 Apr;92(2):259–72. [PMID: 22414412]

Gaines SL et al. Real world efficacy of alvimopan on elective bowel resection patients: an analysis of statistical versus clinical significance. Am J Surg. 2012 Mar;203(3):308–11. [PMID: 22178482]

2. Acute Colonic Pseudo-obstruction (Ogilvie Syndrome)

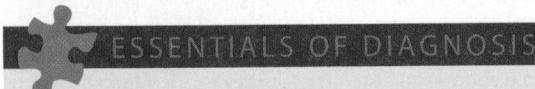

ESSENTIALS OF DIAGNOSIS

- ▶ Severe abdominal distention.
- ▶ Arises in postoperative state or with severe medical illness.
- ▶ May be precipitated by electrolyte imbalances, medications.
- ▶ Absent to mild abdominal pain; minimal tenderness.
- ▶ Massive dilation of cecum or right colon.

▶ General Considerations

Spontaneous massive dilation of the cecum and proximal colon may occur in a number of different settings in hospitalized patients. Progressive cecal dilation may lead to spontaneous perforation with dire consequences. The risk of perforation correlates poorly with absolute cecal size and duration of colonic distention. Early detection and management are important to reduce morbidity and mortality. Colonic pseudo-obstruction is most commonly detected in postsurgical patients (mean 3–5 days), after trauma, and in medical patients with respiratory failure, metabolic imbalance, malignancy, myocardial infarction, heart failure, pancreatitis, or a recent neurologic event (stroke, subarachnoid hemorrhage, trauma). Liberal use of opioids or anticholinergic agents may precipitate colonic pseudo-obstruction in susceptible patients. It may also occur as a manifestation of colonic ischemia. The etiology of colonic pseudo-obstruction is unknown, but either an increase in gut sympathetic activity or a decrease in sacral parasympathetic activity of the distal colon, or both, is hypothesized to impair colonic motility.

▶ Clinical Findings

A. Symptoms and Signs

Many patients are on ventilatory support or are unable to report symptoms due to altered mental status. Abdominal distention is frequently noted by the clinician as the first sign, often leading to a plain film radiograph that demonstrates colonic dilation. Some patients are asymptomatic, although most report constant but mild abdominal pain. Nausea and vomiting may be present. Bowel movements may be absent, but up to 40% of patients continue to pass flatus or stool. Abdominal tenderness with some degree of guarding or rebound tenderness may be detected; however, signs of peritonitis are absent unless perforation has occurred. Bowel sounds may be normal or decreased.

B. Laboratory Findings

Laboratory findings reflect the underlying medical or surgical problems. Serum sodium, potassium, magnesium, phosphorus, and calcium should be obtained. Significant fever or leukocytosis raises concern for colonic ischemia or perforation.

C. Imaging

Radiographs demonstrate colonic dilation, usually confined to the cecum and proximal colon. The upper limit of normal for cecal size is 9 cm. A cecal diameter > 10–12 cm is associated with an increased risk of colonic perforation. Varying amounts of small intestinal dilation and air-fluid levels due to adynamic ileus may be seen. Because the dilated appearance of the colon may raise concern that there is a distal colonic mechanical obstruction due to malignancy, volvulus, or fecal impaction, a CT scan or water-soluble (diatrizoate meglumine) enema may sometimes be performed.

▶ Differential Diagnosis

Colonic pseudo-obstruction should be distinguished from distal colonic mechanical obstruction (as above) and toxic megacolon, which is acute dilation of the colon due to inflammation (inflammatory bowel disease) or infection (*C difficile*–associated colitis, CMV). Patients with toxic megacolon manifest fever; dehydration; significant abdominal pain; leukocytosis; and diarrhea, which is often bloody.

▶ Treatment

Conservative treatment is the appropriate first step for patients with no or minimal abdominal tenderness, no fever, no leukocytosis, and a cecal diameter < 12 cm. The underlying illness is treated appropriately. A nasogastric tube and a rectal tube should be placed. Patients should be ambulated or periodically rolled from side to side and to the knee-chest position in an effort to promote expulsion of colonic gas. All drugs that reduce intestinal motility, such as opioids, anticholinergics, and calcium channel blockers, are discontinued if possible. Enemas may be administered judiciously if large amounts of stool are evident on radiography. Oral laxatives are not helpful and may cause perforation, pain, or electrolyte abnormalities.

Conservative treatment is successful in over 80% of cases within 1–2 days. Patients must be watched for signs of worsening distention or abdominal tenderness. Cecal size should be assessed by abdominal radiographs every 12 hours. Intervention should be considered in patients with any of the following: (1) no improvement or clinical deterioration after 24–48 hours of conservative therapy; (2) cecal dilation > 10 cm for a prolonged period (> 3–4 days); (3) patients with cecal dilation > 12 cm. Neostigmine injection should be given unless contraindicated. A single dose (2 mg intravenously) results in rapid (within 30 minutes) colonic decompression in 75–90% of patients. Cardiac monitoring during neostigmine infusion is indicated for possible bradycardia that may require atropine administration. Colonoscopic decompression is indicated in patients who fail to respond to neostigmine. Colonic decompression with aspiration of air or placement of a decompression tube is successful in 70% of patients. However, the procedure is technically difficult in an unprepared bowel and has been associated with perforations in the distended colon.

Dilation recurs in up to 50% of patients. In patients in whom colonoscopy is unsuccessful, a tube cecostomy can be created through a small laparotomy or with percutaneous radiologically guided placement.

▶ Prognosis

In most cases, the prognosis is related to the underlying illness. The risk of perforation or ischemia is increased with cecal diameter > 12 cm and when distention has been present for more than 6 days. With aggressive therapy, the development of perforation is unusual.

Elsner JL et al. Intravenous neostigmine for postoperative acute colonic pseudo-obstruction. Ann Pharmacother. 2012 Mar;46(3):430–5. [PMID: 22388328]
Harrison ME et al; ASGE Standards of Practice Committee. The role of endoscopy in the management of patients with known and suspected colonic obstruction and pseudo-obstruction. Gastrointest Endosc. 2010 Apr;71(4):669–79. [PMID: 20363408]

3. Chronic Intestinal Pseudo-obstruction & Gastroparesis

Gastroparesis and chronic intestinal pseudo-obstruction are chronic conditions characterized by intermittent, waxing and waning symptoms and signs of gastric or intestinal obstruction in the absence of any mechanical lesions to account for the findings. They are caused by a heterogeneous group of endocrine disorders (diabetes mellitus, hypothyroidism, cortisol deficiency), postsurgical conditions (vagotomy, partial gastric resection, fundoplication, gastric bypass, Whipple procedure), neurologic conditions (Parkinson disease, muscular and myotonic dystrophy, autonomic dysfunction, multiple sclerosis, postpolio syndrome, porphyria), rheumatologic syndromes (progressive systemic sclerosis), infections (postviral, Chagas disease), amyloidosis, paraneoplastic syndromes, medications, and eating disorders (anorexia); a cause may not always be identified.

▶ Clinical Findings

A. Symptoms and Signs

Gastric involvement leads to chronic or intermittent symptoms of gastroparesis with postprandial fullness (early satiety), nausea, and vomiting (1–3 hours after meals). Patients with predominantly small bowel involvement may have abdominal distention, vomiting, diarrhea, and varying degrees of malnutrition. Abdominal pain is not common and should prompt investigation for structural causes of obstruction. Bacterial overgrowth in the stagnant intestine may result in malabsorption. Colonic involvement may result in constipation or alternating diarrhea and constipation.

B. Imaging

Plain film radiography may demonstrate dilation of the esophagus, stomach, small intestine, or colon resembling ileus or mechanical obstruction. Mechanical obstruction of the stomach, small intestine, or colon is much more common than gastroparesis or intestinal pseudo-obstruction and must be excluded with endoscopy or CT or barium enterography, especially in patients with prior surgery, recent onset of symptoms, or abdominal pain. In cases of unclear origin, studies based on the clinical picture are obtained to exclude underlying systemic disease. Gastric scintigraphy with a low-fat solid meal is the optimal means for assessing gastric emptying. Gastric retention of 60% after 2 hours or more than 10% after 4 hours is abnormal. Small bowel manometry is useful for distinguishing visceral from myopathic disorders and for excluding cases of mechanical obstruction that are otherwise difficult to diagnose by endoscopy or radiographic studies.

▶ Treatment

There is no specific therapy for gastroparesis or pseudo-obstruction. Acute exacerbations are treated with nasogastric suction and intravenous fluids. Long-term treatment is directed at maintaining nutrition. Patients should eat small, frequent meals that are low in fiber, milk, gas-forming foods, and fat. Some patients may require liquid enteral supplements. Agents that reduce gastrointestinal motility (opioids, anticholinergics) should be avoided. In diabetic patients, glucose levels should be maintained below 200 mg/dL, as hyperglycemia may slow gastric emptying even in the absence of diabetic neuropathy, and amylin and GLP-1 analogs (exenatide or pramlintide) should be discontinued. Metoclopramide (5–20 mg orally or 5–10 mg intravenously or subcutaneously four times daily) and erythromycin (50–125 mg orally three times daily) before meals are each of benefit in treatment of gastroparesis but not small bowel dysmotility. Since the use of metoclopramide for more than 3 months is associated with a < 1% risk of tardive dyskinesia, patients are advised to discontinue the medication if neuromuscular side effects, particularly involuntary movements, develop. The elderly are at greatest risk. Gastric electrical stimulation with internally implanted neurostimulators has shown reduction in nausea and vomiting in small studies and one controlled trial in some patients with severe gastroparesis (especially those with diabetes mellitus); however, the mechanism of action is uncertain as improvement is not correlated with changes in gastric emptying. Bacterial overgrowth should be treated with intermittent antibiotics (see above). Patients with predominant small bowel distention may require a venting gastrostomy to relieve distress. Some patients may require placement of a jejunostomy for long-term enteral nutrition. Patients unable to maintain adequate enteral nutrition require TPN or small bowel transplantation. Difficult cases should be referred to centers with expertise in this area.

Camilleri M et al. Clinical guideline: management of gastroparesis. Am J Gastroenterol. 2013 Jan;108(1):18–37. [PMID: 23147521]
De Giorgio R et al. Chronic intestinal pseudo-obstruction: clinical features, diagnosis, and therapy. Gastroenterol Clin North Am. 2011 Dec;40(4):787–807. [PMID: 22100118]

APPENDICITIS

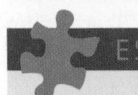

ESSENTIALS OF DIAGNOSIS

► *Early:* periumbilical pain; *later:* right lower quadrant pain and tenderness.

► Anorexia, nausea and vomiting, obstipation.

► Tenderness or localized rigidity at McBurney point.

► Low-grade fever and leukocytosis.

► General Considerations

Appendicitis is the most common abdominal surgical emergency, affecting approximately 10% of the population. It occurs most commonly between the ages of 10 and 30 years. It is initiated by obstruction of the appendix by a fecalith, inflammation, foreign body, or neoplasm. Obstruction leads to increased intraluminal pressure, venous congestion, infection, and thrombosis of intramural vessels. If untreated, gangrene and perforation develop within 36 hours.

► Clinical Findings

A. Symptoms and Signs

Appendicitis usually begins with vague, often colicky periumbilical or epigastric pain. Within 12 hours the pain shifts to the right lower quadrant, manifested as a steady ache that is worsened by walking or coughing. Almost all patients have nausea with one or two episodes of vomiting. Protracted vomiting or vomiting that begins before the onset of pain suggests another diagnosis. A sense of constipation is typical, and some patients administer cathartics in an effort to relieve their symptoms—though some report diarrhea. Low-grade fever (< 38°C) is typical; high fever or rigors suggest another diagnosis or appendiceal perforation.

On physical examination, localized tenderness with guarding in the right lower quadrant can be elicited with gentle palpation with one finger. When asked to cough, patients may be able to precisely localize the painful area, a sign of peritoneal irritation. Light percussion may also elicit pain. Although rebound tenderness is also present, it is unnecessary to elicit this finding if the above signs are present. The psoas sign (pain on passive extension of the right hip) and the obturator sign (pain with passive flexion and internal rotation of the right hip) are indicative of adjacent inflammation and strongly suggestive of appendicitis.

B. Atypical Presentations of Appendicitis

Owing to the variable location of the appendix, there are a number of "atypical" presentations. Because the retrocecal appendix does not touch the anterior abdominal wall, the pain remains less intense and poorly localized; abdominal tenderness is minimal and may be elicited in the right flank.

The psoas sign may be positive. With pelvic appendicitis, there is pain in the lower abdomen, often on the left, with an urge to urinate or defecate. Abdominal tenderness is absent, but tenderness is evident on pelvic or rectal examination; the obturator sign may be present. In the elderly, the diagnosis of appendicitis is often delayed because patients present with minimal, vague symptoms and mild abdominal tenderness. Appendicitis in pregnancy may present with pain in the right lower quadrant, periumbilical area, or right subcostal area owing to displacement of the appendix by the uterus.

C. Laboratory Findings

Moderate leukocytosis (10,000–20,000/mcL) with neutrophilia is common. Microscopic hematuria and pyuria are present in 25% of patients.

D. Imaging

Both abdominal ultrasound and CT scanning are useful in diagnosing appendicitis as well as excluding other diseases presenting with similar symptoms, including adnexal disease in younger women. However, CT scanning appears to be more accurate (sensitivity 94%, specificity 95%, positive likelihood ratio 13.3, negative likelihood ratio 0.09). Abdominal CT scanning is also useful in cases of suspected appendiceal perforation to diagnose a periappendiceal abscess. In patients in whom there is a clinically high suspicion of appendicitis, some surgeons feel that preoperative diagnostic imaging is unnecessary. However, studies suggest that even in this group, imaging studies suggest an alternative diagnosis in up to 15%.

► Differential Diagnosis

Given its frequency and myriad presentations, appendicitis should be considered in the differential diagnosis of all patients with abdominal pain. It is difficult to reliably diagnose the disease in some cases. A several-hour period of close observation with reassessment usually clarifies the diagnosis. Absence of the classic migration of pain (from the epigastrium to the right lower abdomen), right lower quadrant pain, fever, or guarding makes appendicitis less likely. Ten to twenty percent of patients with suspected appendicitis have either a negative examination at laparotomy or an alternative surgical diagnosis. The widespread use of ultrasonography and CT has reduced the number of incorrect diagnoses to < 2%. Still, in some cases diagnostic laparotomy or laparoscopy is required. The most common causes of diagnostic confusion are gastroenteritis and gynecologic disorders. Viral gastroenteritis presents with nausea, vomiting, low-grade fever, and diarrhea and can be difficult to distinguish from appendicitis. The onset of vomiting before pain makes appendicitis less likely. As a rule, the pain of gastroenteritis is more generalized and the tenderness less well localized. Acute salpingitis or tubo-ovarian abscess should be considered in young, sexually active women with fever and bilateral abdominal or pelvic tenderness. A twisted ovarian cyst may also cause sudden severe pain. The sudden onset of lower abdominal pain in the middle of the menstrual cycle suggests mittelschmerz. Sudden severe abdominal pain with diffuse pelvic tenderness and shock suggests a ruptured ectopic pregnancy. A positive pregnancy test and pelvic ultrasonography are diagnostic. Retrocecal or retroileal appendicitis (often associated with pyuria or hematuria) may be confused with ureteral colic or pyelonephritis. Other conditions that may resemble appendicitis are diverticulitis, Meckel diverticulitis, carcinoid of the appendix, perforated colonic cancer, Crohn ileitis, perforated peptic ulcer, cholecystitis, and mesenteric adenitis. It is virtually impossible to distinguish appendicitis from Meckel diverticulitis, but both require surgical treatment.

▶ **Complications**

Perforation occurs in 20% of patients and should be suspected in patients with pain persisting for over 36 hours, high fever, diffuse abdominal tenderness or peritoneal findings, a palpable abdominal mass, or marked leukocytosis. Localized perforation results in a contained abscess, usually in the pelvis. A free perforation leads to suppurative peritonitis with toxicity. Septic thrombophlebitis (pylephlebitis) of the portal venous system is rare and suggested by high fever, chills, bacteremia, and jaundice.

▶ **Treatment**

The treatment of early, uncomplicated appendicitis is surgical appendectomy in most patients. When possible, a laparoscopic approach is preferred to open laparotomy. Access via a single incision through the umbilicus (single-incision laparoscopic appendectomy) is increasingly utilized. Prior to surgery, patients should be given broad-spectrum antibiotics with gram-negative and anaerobic coverage to reduce the incidence of postoperative infections. Recommended preoperative intravenous regimens include cefoxitin or cefotetan 1–2 g every 8 hours; ampicillin-sulfabactam 3 g every 6 hours; or ertapenem 1 g as a single dose. Up to 80% of patients treated with antibiotics alone have resolution of symptoms and signs of uncomplicated appendicitis. Although conservative management may be considered, appendectomy generally is recommended to prevent recurrent appendicitis (20% within 1 year).

Emergency appendectomy is required in patients with perforated appendicitis with generalized peritonitis. Likewise, the optimal treatment of stable patients with perforated appendicitis and a contained abscess is controversial. Surgery in this setting can be difficult. Many recommend percutaneous CT-guided drainage of the abscess with intravenous fluids and antibiotics to allow the inflammation to subside. An interval appendectomy may be performed after 6 weeks to prevent recurrent appendicitis.

▶ **Prognosis**

The mortality rate from uncomplicated appendicitis is extremely low. Even with perforated appendicitis, the mortality rate in most groups is only 0.2%, though it approaches 15% in the elderly.

Gill RS et al. Single-incision appendectomy is comparable to conventional laparoscopic appendectomy: a systematic review and pooled analysis. Surg Laparosc Endosc Percutan Tech. 2012 Aug;22(4):319–27. [PMID: 22874680]

Markar SR et al. Systematic review and meta-analysis of single-incision versus conventional multiport appendectomy. Br J Surg. 2013 Dec;100(13):1709–18. [PMID: 24227355]

Varadhan KK et al. Safety and efficacy of antibiotics compared with appendicectomy for treatment of uncomplicated acute appendicitis: meta-analysis of randomised controlled trials. BMJ. 2012 Apr 5;344:e2156. [PMID: 22491789]

INTESTINAL TUBERCULOSIS

Intestinal tuberculosis is common in underdeveloped countries. Previously rare in the United States, its incidence has been rising in immigrant groups and patients with AIDS. It is caused by both *Mycobacterium tuberculosis* and *M bovis*. Active pulmonary disease is present in < 50% of patients. The most frequent site of involvement is the ileocecal region; however, any region of the gastrointestinal tract may be involved. Intestinal tuberculosis may cause mucosal ulcerations or scarring and fibrosis with narrowing of the lumen. Patients may be without symptoms or complain of chronic abdominal pain, obstructive symptoms, weight loss, and diarrhea. An abdominal mass may be palpable. Complications include intestinal obstruction, hemorrhage, and fistula formation. The purified protein derivative (PPD) skin test may be negative, especially in patients with weight loss or AIDS. Barium radiography may demonstrate mucosal ulcerations, thickening, or stricture formation. Abdominal CT may show thickening of the cecum and ileocecal valve and massive lymphadenopathy. Colonoscopy may demonstrate an ulcerated mass, multiple ulcers with steep edges and adjacent small sessile polyps, small ulcers or erosions, or small diverticula, most commonly in the ileocecal region. The differential diagnosis includes Crohn disease, carcinoma, and intestinal amebiasis. The diagnosis is established by either endoscopic or surgical biopsy revealing acid-fast bacilli, caseating granuloma, or positive cultures from the organism. Detection of tubercle bacilli in biopsy specimens by PCR is now the most sensitive means of diagnosis.

Treatment with standard antituberculous regimens is effective.

Yu H et al. Clinical, endoscopic and histological differentiations between Crohn's disease and intestinal tuberculosis. Digestion. 2012;85(3):202–9. [PMID: 22354097]

PROTEIN-LOSING ENTEROPATHY

Protein-losing enteropathy comprises a number of conditions that result in excessive loss of serum proteins into the gastrointestinal tract. The essential diagnostic features are hypoalbuminemia and an elevated fecal alpha-1-antitrypsin level.

The normal intact gut epithelium prevents the loss of serum proteins. Proteins may be lost through one of three mechanisms: (1) mucosal disease with ulceration, resulting in the loss of proteins across the disrupted mucosal surface, such as in chronic gastric ulcer, gastric carcinoma, or inflammatory bowel disease; (2) lymphatic obstruction, resulting in the loss of protein-rich chylous fluid from mucosal lacteals, such as in primary intestinal lymphangiectasia, constrictive pericarditis or heart failure, Whipple disease or tuberculosis, Kaposi sarcoma or lymphoma, retroperitoneal fibrosis, or sarcoidosis; and (3) idiopathic change in permeability of mucosal capillaries and conductance of interstitium, resulting in "weeping" of protein-rich fluid from the mucosal surface, such as in Ménétrier disease, Zollinger-Ellison syndrome, viral or eosinophilic gastroenteritis, celiac disease, giardiasis or hookworm, common variable immunodeficiency, systemic lupus erythematosus, amyloidosis, or allergic protein-losing enteropathy.

Hypoalbuminemia is the sine qua non of protein-losing enteropathy. However, a number of other serum proteins such as alpha-1-antitrypsin also are lost from the gut epithelium. In protein-losing enteropathy caused by lymphatic obstruction, loss of lymphatic fluid commonly results in lymphocytopenia (< 1000/mcL), hypoglobulinemia, and hypocholesterolemia.

In most cases, protein-losing enteropathy is recognized as a sequela of a known gastrointestinal disorder. In patients in whom the cause is unclear, evaluation is indicated and is guided by the clinical suspicion. Protein-losing enteropathy must be distinguished from other causes of hypoalbuminemia, which include liver disease and nephrotic syndrome; and from heart failure. Protein-losing enteropathy is confirmed by determining the gut alpha-1-antitrypsin clearance (24-hour volume of feces × stool concentration of alpha-1-antitrypsin ÷ serum alpha-1-antitrypsin concentration). A clearance of more than 27 mL/24 h is abnormal.

Laboratory evaluation of protein-losing enteropathy includes serum protein electrophoresis, lymphocyte count, and serum cholesterol to look for evidence of lymphatic obstruction. Serum ANA and C3 levels are useful to screen for autoimmune disorders. Stool samples should be examined for ova and parasites. Evidence of malabsorption is evaluated by means of a stool qualitative fecal fat determination. Intestinal imaging is performed with small bowel enteroscopy biopsy, CT enterography, or wireless capsule endoscopy of the small intestine. Colonic diseases are excluded with colonoscopy. A CT scan of the abdomen is performed to look for evidence of neoplasms or lymphatic obstruction. Rarely, lymphangiography is helpful. In some situations, laparotomy with full-thickness intestinal biopsy is required to establish a diagnosis.

Treatment is directed at the underlying cause. Patients with lymphatic obstruction benefit from low-fat diets supplemented with medium-chain triglycerides. Case reports suggest that octreotide may lead to symptomatic and nutritional improvement in some patients.

▼ DISEASES OF THE COLON & RECTUM

(See Chapter 39 for Colorectal Cancer.)

IRRITABLE BOWEL SYNDROME

ESSENTIALS OF DIAGNOSIS

▸ Chronic functional disorder characterized by abdominal pain or discomfort with alterations in bowel habits.

▸ Symptoms usually begin in late teens to early twenties.

▸ Limited evaluation to exclude organic causes of symptoms.

▶ General Considerations

The functional gastrointestinal disorders are characterized by a variable combination of chronic or recurrent gastrointestinal symptoms *not explicable by the presence of structural or biochemical abnormalities.* Several clinical entities are included under this broad rubric, including chest pain of unclear origin (noncardiac chest pain), functional dyspepsia, and biliary dyskinesia (sphincter of Oddi dysfunction). There is a large overlap among these entities. For example, over 50% of patients with noncardiac chest pain and over one-third with functional dyspepsia also have symptoms compatible with irritable bowel syndrome. In none of these disorders is there a definitive diagnostic study. Rather, the diagnosis is a subjective one based on the presence of a compatible profile and the exclusion of similar disorders.

Irritable bowel syndrome can be defined, therefore, as an idiopathic clinical entity characterized by chronic (more than 6 months) abdominal pain or discomfort that occurs in association with altered bowel habits. These symptoms may be continuous or intermittent. Consensus definition of irritable bowel syndrome is abdominal discomfort or pain that has two of the following three features: (1) relieved with defecation, (2) onset associated with a change in frequency of stool, or (3) onset associated with a change in form (appearance) of stool. Other symptoms supporting the diagnosis include abnormal stool frequency; abnormal stool form (lumpy or hard; loose or watery); abnormal stool passage (straining, urgency, or feeling of incomplete evacuation); passage of mucus; and bloating or a feeling of abdominal distention.

Patients may have other somatic or psychological complaints such as dyspepsia, heartburn, chest pain, headaches, fatigue, myalgias, urologic dysfunction, gynecologic symptoms, anxiety, or depression.

The disorder is a common problem presenting to both gastroenterologists and primary care physicians. Up to 10% of the adult population have symptoms compatible with the diagnosis, but most never seek medical attention. Approximately two-thirds of patients with irritable bowel syndrome are women.

► Pathogenesis

A number of pathophysiologic mechanisms have been identified and may have varying importance in different individuals.

A. Abnormal Motility

A variety of abnormal myoelectrical and motor abnormalities have been identified in the colon and small intestine. In some cases, these are temporally correlated with episodes of abdominal pain or emotional stress. Whether they represent a primary motility disorder or are secondary to psychosocial stress is debated. Differences between patients with constipation-predominant and diarrhea-predominant syndromes are reported.

B. Visceral Hypersensitivity

Patients often have a lower visceral pain threshold, reporting abdominal pain at lower volumes of colonic gas insufflation or colonic balloon inflation than controls. Many patients complain of bloating and distention, which may be due to a number of different factors including increased visceral sensitivity, increased gas production (due to small bowel bacterial overgrowth or carbohydrate malabsorption), impaired gas transit through the intestine, or impaired rectal expulsion. Many patients report rectal urgency despite small rectal volumes of stool.

C. Enteric Infection

Symptoms compatible with irritable bowel syndrome develop within 1 year in up to 10% of patients after an episode of bacterial gastroenteritis compared with < 2% of controls. Women and patients with increased life stressors at the onset of gastroenteritis appear to be at increased risk for developing "postinfectious" irritable bowel syndrome. Increased inflammatory cells have been found in the mucosa, submucosa, and muscularis of some patients with irritable bowel syndrome, but their importance is unclear. Chronic inflammation is postulated by some investigators to contribute to alterations in motility or visceral hypersensitivity.

Some investigators suggest that alterations in the numbers and distribution of bacterial species (estimated 30,000 different species) may affect bowel transit time, gas production, and sensitivity. An increase in breath hydrogen or methane excretion after lactulose ingestion in 65% of patients with irritable bowel syndrome has been reported, believed by some investigators to indicate small intestinal bacterial overgrowth. However, many investigators dispute these findings because overgrowth was confirmed in only 4% of patients using jejunal aspiration and bacterial culture. Small bowel bacterial overgrowth may be more likely in patients with bloating, postprandial discomfort, and loose stools. It is hypothesized that bacterial overgrowth may lead to alterations in immune alterations that affect motility or visceral sensitivity or to degradation of carbohydrates in the small intestine that may cause increased postprandial gas, bloating, and distention.

D. Psychosocial Abnormalities

More than 50% of patients with irritable bowel who seek medical attention have underlying depression, anxiety, or somatization. By contrast, those who do not seek medical attention are similar psychologically to normal individuals. Psychological abnormalities may influence how the patient perceives or reacts to illness and minor visceral sensations. Chronic stress may alter intestinal motility or modulate pathways that affect central and spinal processing of visceral afferent sensation.

► Clinical Findings

A. Symptoms and Signs

Irritable bowel is a chronic condition. Symptoms usually begin in the late teens to twenties. Symptoms should be present for at least 3 months before the diagnosis can be considered. The diagnosis is established in the presence of compatible symptoms and the judicious use of tests to exclude organic disease.

Abdominal pain usually is intermittent, crampy, and in the lower abdominal region. As previously stated, the onset of pain typically is associated with a change in stool frequency or form and commonly is relieved by defecation. It does not usually occur at night or interfere with sleep. Patients with irritable bowel syndrome may be classified into one of three categories based on the predominant bowel habit: irritable bowel syndrome with diarrhea; irritable bowel syndrome with constipation; or irritable bowel syndrome with mixed constipation and diarrhea. It is important to clarify what the patient means by these complaints. Patients with irritable bowel and constipation report infrequent bowel movements (less than three per week), hard or lumpy stools, or straining. Patients with irritable bowel syndrome with diarrhea refer to loose or watery stools, frequent stools (more than three per day), urgency, or fecal incontinence. Many patients report that they have a firm stool in the morning followed by progressively looser movements. Complaints of visible distention and bloating are common, though these are not always clinically evident.

The patient should be asked about "alarm symptoms" that suggest a diagnosis other than irritable bowel syndrome and warrant further investigation. The acute onset of symptoms raises the likelihood of organic disease, especially in patients aged > 40–50 years. Nocturnal diarrhea, severe constipation or diarrhea, hematochezia, weight loss, and fever are incompatible with a diagnosis of irritable bowel syndrome and warrant investigation for underlying disease. Patients who have a family history of cancer, inflammatory bowel disease, or celiac disease should undergo additional evaluation.

A physical examination should be performed to look for evidence of organic disease and to allay the patient's anxieties. The physical examination usually is normal. Abdominal tenderness, especially in the lower abdomen, is common but not pronounced. A new onset of symptoms in a patient over age 40 years warrants further examination.

B. Laboratory Findings and Special Examinations

In patients whose symptoms fulfill the diagnostic criteria for irritable bowel syndrome and who have no other alarm symptoms, evidence-based consensus guidelines do not support further diagnostic testing, as the likelihood of serious organic diseases does not appear to be increased. Although the vague nature of symptoms and patient anxiety may prompt clinicians to consider a variety of diagnostic studies, overtesting should be avoided. A 2013 study of primary care patients aged 30–50 years with suspected irritable bowel found that patients randomized to a strategy of extensive testing prior to diagnosis had higher health care costs but similar symptoms and satisfaction at 1 year as patients randomized to a strategy of minimal testing but a positive clinical diagnosis. The use of routine blood tests (complete blood count, chemistry panel, serum albumin, thyroid function tests, erythrocyte sedimentation rate) is unnecessary in most patients. Stool specimen examinations for ova and parasites should be obtained only in patients with increased likelihood of infection (eg, day care workers, campers, foreign travelers). Routine sigmoidoscopy or colonoscopy is not recommended in young patients with symptoms of irritable bowel syndrome without alarm symptoms but should be considered in patients who do not improve with conservative management. In all patients age 50 years or older who have not had a previous evaluation, colonoscopy should be obtained to exclude malignancy. When colonoscopy is performed, random mucosal biopsies should be obtained to look for evidence of microscopic colitis (which may have similar symptoms). In patients with irritable bowel syndrome with diarrhea, serologic tests for celiac disease should be performed. Routine testing for bacterial overgrowth with hydrogen breath tests are not recommended.

▶ Differential Diagnosis

A number of disorders may present with similar symptoms. Examples include colonic neoplasia, inflammatory bowel disease (ulcerative colitis, Crohn disease, microscopic colitis), hyperthyroidism or hypothyroidism, parasites, malabsorption (especially celiac disease, bacterial overgrowth, lactase deficiency), causes of chronic secretory diarrhea (carcinoid), and endometriosis. Psychiatric disorders such as depression, panic disorder, and anxiety must be considered as well. Women with refractory symptoms have an increased incidence of prior sexual and physical abuse. These diagnoses should be excluded in patients with presumed irritable bowel syndrome who do not improve within 2–4 weeks of empiric treatment or in whom subsequent alarm symptoms develop.

▶ Treatment

A. General Measures

As with other functional disorders, the most important interventions the clinician can offer are reassurance, education, and support. This includes identifying and responding to the patient's concerns, careful explanation of the pathophysiology and natural history of the disorder, setting realistic treatment goals, and involving the patient in the treatment process. Because irritable bowel symptoms are chronic, the patient's reasons for seeking consultation at this time should be determined. These may include major life events or recent psychosocial stressors, dietary or medication changes, concerns about serious underlying disease, or reduced quality of life and impairment of daily activities. In discussing with the patient the importance of the mind-gut interaction, it may be helpful to explain that alterations in visceral motility and sensitivity may be exacerbated by environmental, social, or psychological factors such as foods, medications, hormones, and stress. Symptoms such as pain, bloating, and altered bowel habits may lead to anxiety and distress, which in turn may further exacerbate bowel disturbances due to disordered communication between the gut and the central nervous system. Fears that the symptoms will progress, require surgery, or degenerate into serious illness should be allayed. The patient should understand that irritable bowel syndrome is a chronic disorder characterized by periods of exacerbation and quiescence. The emphasis should be shifted from finding the cause of the symptoms to finding a way to cope with them. Moderate exercise is beneficial. Clinicians must resist the temptation to chase chronic complaints with new or repeated diagnostic studies.

B. Dietary Therapy

Patients commonly report dietary intolerances. Proposed mechanisms for dietary intolerance include food allergy, hypersensitivity, effects of gut hormones, changes in bacterial flora, increased bacterial gas production (arising in the small or large intestine), and direct chemical irritation. Fatty foods and caffeine are poorly tolerated by many patients with irritable bowel syndrome. In patients with diarrhea, bloating, and flatulence, lactose intolerance should be excluded with a hydrogen breath test or a trial of a lactose-free diet. A host of poorly absorbed, fermentable, monosaccharides and short-chain carbohydrates ("FODMAPS") may exacerbate bloating, flatulence, and diarrhea in some patients. These include fructose (corn syrups, apples, pears, watermelon, raisins), fructans (onions, leeks, asparagus, artichokes), wheat-based products (breads, pasta, cereals, cakes), sorbitol (stone fruits), and raffinose (legumes, lentils, brussel sprouts, cabbage). Dietary restriction of these fermentable carbohydrates may improve symptoms.

A high-fiber diet and fiber supplements appears to be of little value in patients with irritable bowel syndrome. Many patients report little change in bowel frequency but increased gas and distention.

C. Pharmacologic Measures

More than two-thirds of patients with irritable bowel syndrome have mild symptoms that respond readily to education, reassurance, and dietary interventions. Drug therapy should be reserved for patients with moderate to severe symptoms that do not respond to conservative measures. These agents should be viewed as being adjunctive rather than curative. Given the wide spectrum of symptoms, no single agent is expected to provide relief in all or even most patients. Nevertheless, therapy targeted at the specific dominant symptom (pain, constipation, or diarrhea) may be beneficial.

1. Antispasmodic agents—Anticholinergic agents are used by some practitioners for treatment of acute episodes of pain or bloating despite a lack of well-designed trials demonstrating efficacy. Available agents include hyoscyamine, 0.125 mg orally (or sublingually as needed) or sustained-release, 0.037 mg or 0.75 mg orally twice daily; dicyclomine, 10–20 mg orally; or methscopamine 2.5–5 mg orally before meals and at bedtime. Anticholinergic side effects are common, including urinary retention, constipation, tachycardia, and dry mouth. Hence, these agents should be used with caution in the elderly and in patients with constipation. Peppermint oil formulations (which relax smooth muscle) may be helpful.

2. Antidiarrheal agents—Loperamide (2 mg orally three or four times daily) is effective for the treatment of patients with diarrhea, reducing stool frequency, liquidity, and urgency. It may best be used "prophylactically" in situations in which diarrhea is anticipated (such as stressful situations) or would be inconvenient (social engagements). Increased intracolonic bile acids due to alterations in enterohepatic circulation may contribute to diarrhea in a subset of patients with diarrhea. An empiric trial of bile salt binding agents (cholestyramine 2–4 g with meals; colesevelam, 625 mg, 1–3 tablets twice daily) may be considered.

3. Anticonstipation agents—Treatment with oral osmotic laxatives polyethylene glycol 3350 (Miralax, 17–34 g/d) may increase stool frequency, improve stool consistency, and reduce straining. Lactulose or sorbitol produces increased flatus and distention, which are poorly tolerated in patients with irritable bowel syndrome and should be avoided. Lubiprostone (8 mcg orally twice daily) and linaclotide (290 mcg orally once daily) are newer agents approved for treatment of irritable bowel syndrome with constipation. Through different mechanisms, both stimulate increased intestinal chloride and fluid secretion, resulting in accelerated colonic transit. In clinical trials, lubiprostone led to global symptom improvement in 18% of patients compared with 10% of patients who received placebo. Trials of linaclotide included similar patient populations but measured different primary end points. Higher combined response rates (defined as > 30% reduction in abdominal pain and >3 spontaneous bowel movements per week, including an increase of ≥ 1 from baseline) were found in 12.5% of linaclotide-treated patients compared with 4% of placebo-treated patients. Patients with intractable constipation should undergo further assessment for slow colonic transit and pelvic floor dysfunction (see Constipation, above).

4. Psychotropic agents—Patients with predominant symptoms of pain or bloating may benefit from low doses of tricyclic antidepressants, which are believed to have effects on motility, visceral sensitivity, and central pain perception that are independent of their psychotropic effects. Because of their anticholinergic effects, these agents may be more useful in patients with diarrhea-predominant

than constipation-predominant symptoms. Oral nortriptyline, desipramine, or imipramine, may be started at a low dosage of 10 mg at bedtime and increased gradually to 50–150 mg as tolerated. Response rates do not correlate with dosage, and many patients respond to doses of ≤ 50 mg daily. Side effects are common, and lack of efficacy with one agent does not preclude benefit from another. Improvement should be evident within 4 weeks. The oral serotonin reuptake inhibitors (sertraline, 25–100 mg daily; citalopram 10–20 mg; paroxetine 20–50 mg daily; or fluoxetine, 10–40 mg daily) may lead to improvement in overall sense of well-being but have little impact on abdominal pain or bowel symptoms. Anxiolytics should not be used chronically in irritable bowel syndrome because of their habituation potential. Patients with major depression or anxiety disorders should be identified and treated with therapeutic doses of appropriate agents.

5. Serotonin receptor agonists and antagonists—Serotonin is an important mediator of gastrointestinal motility and sensation. Alosetron is a 5-HT$_3$ antagonist that is FDA-approved for the treatment of women with severe irritable bowel syndrome with predominant diarrhea. In contrast to the excellent safety profile of other 5-HT$_3$ antagonists (eg, ondansetron), alosetron may cause constipation (sometimes severe) in 30% of patients or ischemic colitis in 4:1000 patients. Given the seriousness of these side effects, alosetron is restricted to women with severe irritable bowel syndrome with diarrhea who have not responded to conventional therapies and who have been educated about the relative risks and benefits of the agent. It should not be used in patients with constipation.

6. Nonabsorbable antibiotics—Rifaximin is not approved for the treatment of irritable bowel syndrome but may be considered in patients with refractory symptoms, especially bloating. A 2012 meta-analysis identified a 9.9% greater improvement in bloating compared with placebo, a modest gain that is similar to other less expensive therapies. Symptom improvement may be attributable to suppression of bacteria in either the small intestine or colon, resulting in decreased bacterial carbohydrate fermentation, diarrhea, and bloating.

7. Probiotics—Meta-analyses of small controlled clinical trials report improved symptoms in some patients treated with one probiotic, *Bifidobacterium infantis,* but not with another probiotic, *Lactobacillus salivarius,* or placebo. It is hypothesized that alterations in gut flora may reduce symptoms through suppression of inflammation or reduction of bacterial gas production, resulting in reduced distention, flatus, and visceral sensitivity. Such therapy is attractive because it is safe, well tolerated, and inexpensive. Although promising, further study is needed to define the efficacy and optimal formulations of probiotic therapy. The probiotics VSL#3 (1 packet twice daily) or *Bifidobacterium infantis* (1 tablet twice daily) have shown modest benefit in small studies.

D. Psychological Therapies

Cognitive-behavioral therapies, relaxation techniques, and hypnotherapy appear to be beneficial in some patients.

Patients with underlying psychological abnormalities may benefit from evaluation by a psychiatrist or psychologist. Patients with severe disability should be referred to a pain treatment center.

Prognosis

The majority of patients with irritable bowel syndrome learn to cope with their symptoms and lead productive lives.

Begtrup LM et al. A positive diagnostic strategy is noninferior to a strategy of exclusion for patients with irritable bowel syndrome. Clin Gastroenterol Hepatol. 2013 Aug;11(8):956–62. [PMID: 23357491]

Camilleri M. Peripheral mechanisms in irritable bowel syndrome. N Engl J Med. 2012 Oct 25;367(17):1626–35. [PMID: 23094724]

Chapman RW et al. Randomized clinical trial: macrogol/PEG 3350 plus electrolytes for treatment of patients with constipation associated with irritable bowel syndrome. Am J Gastroenterol. 2013 Sep;108(9):1508–15. [PMID: 23835436]

Johannesson E et al. Physical activity improves symptoms in irritable bowel syndrome: a randomized controlled trial. Am J Gastroenterol. 2011 May;106(5):915–22. [PMID: 21206488]

Khan S et al. Diagnosis and management of IBS. Nat Rev Gastroenterol Hepatol. 2010 Oct;7(10):565–81. [PMID: 20890316]

Menees SB et al. The efficacy and safety of rifaximin for the irritable bowel syndrome: a systematic review and meta-analysis. Am J Gastroenterol. 2012 Jan;107(1):28–35. [PMID: 22045120]

Videlock EJ et al. Effects of linaclotide in patients with irritable bowel syndrome with constipation or chronic constipation: a meta-analysis. Clin Gastroenterol Hepatol. 2013 Sep;11(9):1084–92. [PMID: 23644388]

ANTIBIOTIC-ASSOCIATED COLITIS

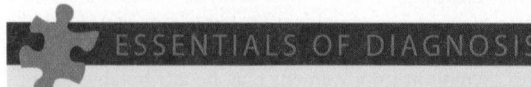

ESSENTIALS OF DIAGNOSIS

▶ Most cases of antibiotic-associated diarrhea are not attributable to *C difficile* and are usually mild and self-limited.

▶ Symptoms of antibiotic-associated colitis vary from mild to fulminant; almost all colitis is attributable to *C difficile*.

▶ Diagnosis in most cases established by stool assay.

General Considerations

Antibiotic-associated diarrhea is a common clinical occurrence. Characteristically, the diarrhea occurs during the period of antibiotic exposure, is dose related, and resolves spontaneously after discontinuation of the antibiotic. In most cases, this diarrhea is mild, self-limited, and does not require any specific laboratory evaluation or treatment. Stool examination usually reveals no fecal leukocytes, and stool cultures reveal no pathogens. Although *C difficile* is identified in the stool of 15–25% of cases of antibiotic-associated diarrhea, it is also identified in 5–10% of

patients treated with antibiotics who do not have diarrhea. Most cases of antibiotic-associated diarrhea are due to changes in colonic bacterial fermentation of carbohydrates and are not due to *C difficile*.

Antibiotic-associated colitis is a significant clinical problem almost always caused by *C difficile* infection. Hospitalized patients are most susceptible. *C difficile* colitis is the major cause of diarrhea in patients hospitalized for more than 3 days, affecting 22 patients of every 1000. This anaerobic bacterium colonizes the colon of 3% of healthy adults. It is acquired by fecal-oral transmission. Found throughout hospitals in patient rooms and bathrooms, it is readily transmitted from patient to patient by hospital personnel. Fastidious hand washing and use of disposable gloves are helpful in minimizing transmission. *C difficile* is acquired in approximately 20% of hospitalized patients, most of whom have received antibiotics that disrupt the normal bowel flora and thus allow the bacterium to flourish. Although almost all antibiotics have been implicated, colitis most commonly develops after use of ampicillin, clindamycin, third-generation cephalosporins, and fluoroquinolones. *C difficile* colitis will develop in approximately one-third of infected patients. In clinical trials, prophylactic administration of the probiotics "DanActiv" and "Bio-K+," containing *Lactobacillus casei, Lactobacillus bulgaricus,* and *Streptococcus thermophilus,* to hospitalized patients who are receiving antibiotics reduced the incidence of *C difficile*–associated diarrhea. Symptoms usually begin during or shortly after antibiotic therapy but may be delayed for up to 8 weeks. All patients with acute diarrhea should be asked about recent antibiotic exposure. Patients who are elderly; debilitated; immunocompromised; receiving multiple antibiotics or prolonged (> 10 days) antibiotic therapy; receiving enteral tube feedings, proton pump inhibitors, or chemotherapy; or who have inflammatory bowel disease have a higher risk of acquiring *C difficile* and developing *C difficile*–associated diarrhea.

The incidence and severity of *C difficile* colitis in hospitalized patients appear to be increasing, which is attributable to the emergence of a more virulent strain of *C difficile* (NAP1) that contains an 18-base pair deletion of the tcdC inhibitory gene, resulting in higher toxin A and B production. This hypervirulent strain has been associated with several hospital outbreaks of severe disease with up to 7% mortality.

Clinical Findings

A. Symptoms and Signs

Most patients report mild to moderate greenish, foul-smelling watery diarrhea 5–15 times per day with lower abdominal cramps. Physical examination is normal or reveals mild left lower quadrant tenderness. The stools may have mucus but seldom gross blood. In most patients, colitis is most severe in the distal colon and rectum. Over half of hospitalized patients diagnosed with *C difficile* colitis have a white blood count > 15,000/mcL, and *C difficile* should be considered in all hospitalized patients with unexplained leukocytosis.

Severe or fulminant disease occurs in 10–15% of patients. It is characterized by fever; hemodynamic instability; and abdominal distention, pain, and tenderness. Most patients have profuse diarrhea (up to 30 stools/day); however, diarrhea may be absent or appear to be improving in patients with fulminant disease or ileus. Laboratory data suggestive of severe disease include a white blood count > 30,000/mcL, albumin < 2.5 g/dL (due to protein-losing enteropathy), elevated serum lactate, or rising creatinine.

B. Special Examinations

1. Stool studies—Pathogenic strains of *C difficile* produce two toxins: toxin A is an enterotoxin and toxin B is a cytotoxin. Rapid enzyme immunoassays (EIAs) for toxins A and B have a 75–90% sensitivity with a single stool specimen; sensitivity increases to 90–95% with two specimens. Until recently, EIA was the preferred diagnostic test in most clinical settings because it is inexpensive, easy to use, and results are available within 24 hours. However, nucleic acid amplification tests (eg, PCR assays) that amplify the toxin B gene have a 97% sensitivity and thus are superior to the EIA tests; these PCR assays are now preferred. Alternatively, some laboratories first perform an assay for glutamate dehydrogenase (a common *C difficile* antigen), which has a high sensitivity and negative predictive value (> 95%). A negative glutamate dehydrogenase assay effectively excludes infection, while a positive assay requires confirmation with PCR or EIA to determine whether the strain that is present is toxin producing.

2. Flexible sigmoidoscopy—Flexible sigmoidoscopy is not needed in patients who have typical symptoms and a positive stool toxin assay. Previously, it was useful in patients with severe symptoms when a rapid diagnosis is desired; however, the ready availability of the currently recommended assays obviates this benefit. It also may clarify the diagnosis in patients with positive *C difficile* toxin assays who have atypical symptoms or who have persistent diarrhea despite appropriate therapy. In patients with mild to moderate symptoms, there may be no abnormalities or only patchy or diffuse, nonspecific colitis indistinguishable from other causes. In patients with severe illness, true **pseudomembranous colitis** is seen.

3. Imaging studies—Abdominal radiographs or noncontrast abdominal CT scans are obtained in patients with severe or fulminant symptoms to look for evidence of colonic dilation and wall thickening. Abdominal CT also is useful in the evaluation of hospitalized patients with abdominal pain or ileus without significant diarrhea, in whom the presence of colonic wall thickening suggests unsuspected *C difficile* colitis. CT scanning is also useful in the detection of possible perforation.

▶ Differential Diagnosis

In the hospitalized patient in whom acute diarrhea develops after admission, the differential diagnosis includes simple antibiotic-associated diarrhea (not related to *C difficile*), enteral feedings, medications, and ischemic colitis. Other infectious causes are unusual in hospitalized patients

in whom diarrhea develops more than 72 hours after admission, and it is not cost-effective to obtain stool cultures unless tests for *C difficile* are negative. Rarely, other organisms (staphylococci, *Clostridium perfringens*) have been associated with pseudomembranous colitis. *Klebsiella oxytoca* may cause a distinct form of antibiotic-associated hemorrhagic colitis that is segmental (usually in the right or transverse colon); spares the rectum; and is more common in younger, healthier outpatients.

▶ Complications

Severe colitis may progress quickly to fulminant disease, resulting in hemodynamic instability, respiratory failure, metabolic acidosis, megacolon (> 7 cm diameter), perforation, and death. Chronic untreated colitis may result in weight loss and protein-losing enteropathy.

▶ Treatment

A. Immediate Treatment

If possible, antibiotic therapy should be discontinued and therapy with metronidazole, vancomycin, or fidaxomicin (a poorly absorbable macrolide antibiotic) should be initiated. For patients with mild disease, oral metronidazole (500 mg orally three times daily), vancomycin (125 mg orally four times daily), or fidaxomicin, (200 mg orally two times daily) are equally effective for initial treatment. Vancomycin and fidaxomicin are significantly more expensive than metronidazole. Therefore, metronidazole remains the preferred first-line therapy in patients with mild disease, except in patients who are intolerant of metronidazole, pregnant women, and children. The duration of initial therapy is usually 10–14 days. Symptomatic improvement occurs in most patients within 72 hours.

For patients with severe disease, characterized by a white blood cell count > 15,000/mcL, serum albumin < 3 g/dL, or a rise in serum creatinine to > 1.5 times baseline, vancomycin, 125 mg orally four times daily, is the preferred agent because it achieves significantly higher response rates (97%) than metronidazole (76%). In patients with severe, complicated disease, characterized by fever > 38.5°C, hypotension, mental status changes, ileus, megacolon, or WBC > 30,000/mcL, intravenous metronidazole, 500 mg every 6 hours, should be given—supplemented by vancomycin (500 mg four times daily administered by nasoenteric tube) and, in some cases, vancomycin enemas (500 mg in 100 mL every 6 hours). Intravenous vancomycin does not penetrate the bowel and should not be used. The efficacy of fidaxomicin for severe or fulminant disease requires further investigation. Early surgical consultation is recommended for all patients with severe or fulminant disease. Total abdominal colectomy or loop ileostomy with colonic lavage may be required in patients with toxic megacolon, perforation, sepsis, or hemorrhage.

B. Treatment of Relapse

Up to 25% of patients have a relapse of diarrhea from *C difficile* within 1 or 2 weeks after stopping initial therapy. This may be due to reinfection or failure to eradicate the organism. In a 2011 multicenter, randomized controlled trial, patients treated with fidaxomicin had significantly lower recurrence rates (7.8%) of non-NAP1 *C difficile* strains than patients treated with vancomycin (23.6%). The recurrence rates were not different among patients with the NAP1 strain. Fidaxomicin may be appropriate for patients with *C difficile* infection or as initial therapy in patients believed to be at higher risk for recurrent disease. Controlled trials show that oral administration of a live yeast, *Saccharomyces boulardii*, 500 mg twice daily, reduces the incidence of relapse by 50%. The optimal treatment regimen for recurrent relapses is evolving. Most relapses respond promptly to a second course of the same regimen used for the initial episode. Some patients, however, have recurrent relapses that can be difficult to treat. For patients with two relapses, a 7-week tapering regimen of vancomycin is recommended: 125 mg orally four times daily for 14 days; twice daily for 7 days; once daily for 7 days; every other day for 7 days; and every third day for 2–8 weeks. Probiotic therapy is recommended as adjunctive therapy in patients with relapsing disease. For patients with three or more relapses, updated 2013 guidelines recommend consideration of an installation of a suspension of fecal bacteria from a healthy donor ("fecal microbiota transplant"). In uncontrolled case reports and case series involving several hundred patients, such "fecal transplantation" into the terminal ileum or proximal colon (by colonoscopy) or into the duodenum and jejunum (by nasoenteric tube) results in disease remission after a single treatment in over 90% of patients with recurrent *C difficile* infection. In a 2013 randomized study, duodenal infusion of donor feces led to resolution of *C difficile* diarrhea in 94%, which was dramatically higher than vancomycin treatment (31%), prompting early study termination. Despite uncertainties, fecal transplantation should be considered in patients with refractory infection.

Brandt LJ. American Journal of Gastroenterology Lecture: intestinal microbiota and the role of fecal microbiota transplant (FMT) in treatment of *C. difficile* infection. Am J Gastroenterol. 2013 Feb;108(2):177–85. [PMID: 23318479]

Brandt LJ et al. Long-term follow-up of colonoscopic fecal microbiota transplant for recurrent *Clostridium difficile* infection. Am J Gastroenterol. 2012 Jul;107(7):1079–87. [PMID: 22450732]

McCollum DL et al. Detection, treatment, and prevention of *Clostridium difficile* infection. Clin Gastroenterol Hepatol. 2012 Jun;10(6):581–92. [PMID: 22433924]

Surawicz CM et al. Guidelines for diagnosis, treatment, and prevention of *Clostridium difficile* infections. Am J Gastroenterol. 2013 Apr;108(4):478–98. [PMID: 23439232]

van Nood E et al. Duodenal infusion of donor feces for recurrent *Clostridium difficile*. N Engl J Med. 2013 Jan 31;368(5):407–15. [PMID: 23323867]

INFLAMMATORY BOWEL DISEASE

The term "inflammatory bowel disease" includes ulcerative colitis and Crohn disease. Ulcerative colitis is a chronic, recurrent disease characterized by diffuse mucosal inflammation involving only the colon. Ulcerative colitis invariably involves the rectum and may extend proximally in a continuous fashion to involve part or all of the colon. Crohn disease is a chronic, recurrent disease characterized by patchy transmural inflammation involving any segment of the gastrointestinal tract from the mouth to the anus.

Crohn disease and ulcerative colitis may be associated in 50% of patients with a number of extraintestinal manifestations, including oral ulcers, oligoarticular or polyarticular nondeforming peripheral arthritis, spondylitis or sacroiliitis, episcleritis or uveitis, erythema nodosum, pyoderma gangrenosum, hepatitis and sclerosing cholangitis, and thromboembolic events.

▶ Pharmacologic Therapy

Although ulcerative colitis and Crohn disease appear to be distinct entities, the same pharmacologic agents are used to treat both. Despite extensive research, there are still no specific therapies for these diseases. The mainstays of therapy are 5-aminosalicylic acid derivatives, corticosteroids, immunomodulating agents (such as mercaptopurine or azathioprine and methotrexate), and biologic agents.

A. 5-Aminosalicylic Acid (5-ASA)

5-ASA is a topically active agent that has a variety of anti-inflammatory effects. It is used in the active treatment of ulcerative colitis and Crohn disease and during disease inactivity to maintain remission. It is readily absorbed from the small intestine but demonstrates minimal colonic absorption. A number of oral and topical compounds have been designed to target delivery of 5-ASA to the colon or small intestine while minimizing absorption. Commonly used formulations of 5-ASA are sulfasalazine, mesalamine, and azo compounds. Side effects of these compounds are uncommon but include nausea, rash, diarrhea, pancreatitis, and acute interstitial nephritis.

1. Oral mesalamine agents—These 5-ASA agents are coated in various pH-sensitive resins (Asacol, Apriso, and Lialda) or packaged in timed-release capsules (Pentasa). Pentasa releases 5-ASA slowly throughout the small intestine and colon. Asacol, Apriso, and Lialda tablets dissolve at pH 6.0–7.0, releasing 5-ASA in the terminal small bowel and proximal colon. Lialda has a multi-matrix system that gradually releases 5-ASA throughout the colon.

2. Azo compounds—Sulfasalazine, balsalazide and olsalazine contain 5-ASA linked by an azo bond that requires cleavage by colonic bacterial azoreductases to release 5-ASA. Absorption of these drugs from the small intestine is negligible. After release within the colon, the 5-ASA works topically and is largely unabsorbed. Balsalazide contains 5-ASA linked to an inert carrier (4-aminobenzoyl-beta-alanine).

Sulfasalazine contains 5-ASA linked to a sulfapyridine moiety. It is unclear whether the sulfapyridine group has any anti-inflammatory effects. One gram of sulfasalazine contains 400 mg of 5-ASA. The sulfapyridine group, however, is absorbed and may cause side effects in 15–30% of patients—much higher than with other 5-ASA compounds. Dose-related side effects include nausea, headaches, leukopenia, oligospermia, and impaired folate metabolism.

Allergic and idiosyncratic side effects are fever, rash, hemolytic anemia, neutropenia, worsened colitis, hepatitis, pancreatitis, and pneumonitis. Because of its side effects, sulfasalazine is less frequently used than other 5-ASA agents. It should always be administered in conjunction with folate. Eighty percent of patients intolerant of sulfasalazine can tolerate mesalamine.

3. Topical mesalamine—5-ASA is provided in the form of suppositories (Canasa; 1000 mg) and enemas (Rowasa; 4 g/60 mL). These formulations can deliver much higher concentrations of 5-ASA to the distal colon than oral compounds. Side effects are uncommon.

B. Corticosteroids

A variety of intravenous, oral, and topical corticosteroid formulations have been used in inflammatory bowel disease. They have utility in the short-term treatment of moderate to severe disease. However, long-term use is associated with serious, potentially irreversible side effects and is to be avoided. The agents, route of administration, duration of use, and tapering regimens used are based more on personal bias and experience than on data from rigorous clinical trials. The most commonly used intravenous formulations have been hydrocortisone or methylprednisolone, which are given by continuous infusion or every 6 hours. Oral formulations are prednisone or methylprednisolone. Adverse events commonly occur during short-term systemic corticosteroid therapy, including mood changes, insomnia, dyspepsia, weight gain, edema, elevated serum glucose levels, acne, and moon facies. Side effects of long-term use include osteoporosis, osteonecrosis of the femoral head, myopathy, cataracts, and susceptibility to infections. Calcium and vitamin D supplementation should be administered to all patients receiving long-term corticosteroid therapy. Bone densitometry should be considered in patients with inflammatory bowel disease with other risk factors for osteoporosis and in all patients with a lifetime use of corticosteroids for 3 months or more. Topical preparations are provided as hydrocortisone suppositories (100 mg), foam (90 mg), and enemas (100 mg). Budesonide is an oral corticosteroid with high topical anti-inflammatory activity but low systemic activity due to high first-pass hepatic metabolism. A controlled-release formulation is available (Entocort) that targets delivery to the terminal ileum and proximal colon. An enteric coated, delayed-release formulation is available (Uceris) that is released at a pH > 7, targeting delivery to the colon. Budesonide produces less suppression of the hypothalamic-pituitary-adrenal axis and fewer steroid-related side effects than hydrocortisone or prednisone.

C. Immunomodulating Drugs: Mercaptopurine, Azathioprine, or Methotrexate

Mercaptopurine and azathioprine are thiopurine drugs that are used in many patients with moderate to severe Crohn disease and ulcerative colitis either in combination with anti-TNF agents or in patients who are corticosteroid-dependent in an attempt to reduce or withdraw the corticosteroids and to maintain patients in remission. Azathioprine is converted in vivo to mercaptopurine. It is believed that the active metabolite of mercaptopurine is 6-thioguanine. Monitoring of 6-thioguanine levels is performed in some clinical settings but is of unproven value in the management of most patients. Side effects of mercaptopurine and azathioprine, including allergic reactions (fever, rash, or arthralgias) and nonallergic reactions (nausea, vomiting, pancreatitis, hepatotoxicity, bone marrow suppression, infections), occur in 15% of patients. Thiopurines are associated with an up to a fivefold increased risk of non-Hodgkin lymphomas (1/1000 patient-years), increasing with age and length of drug exposure; with an increased risk of human papillomavirus (HPV)–related cervical dysplasia; and with an increased risk of non-melanoma skin cancer. Younger patients also are at risk for severe primary Epstein Barr virus (EBV) infection, if not previously exposed.

Three competing enzymes are involved in the metabolism of mercaptopurine to its active (6-thioguanine) and inactive metabolites. About 1 person in 300 has a homozygous mutation of one of the enzymes that metabolizes thiopurine methyltransferase (TPMT), placing them at risk for profound immunosuppression; 1 person in 9 is heterozygous for TPMT, resulting in intermediate enzyme activity. Measurement of TPMT functional activity is recommended prior to initiation of therapy. Treatment should be withheld in patients with absent TPMT activity. The most effective dose of mercaptopurine is 1–1.5 mg/kg. For azathioprine, it is 2–3 mg/kg daily. For patients with normal TPMT activity, both drugs may be initiated at the weight-calculated dose. A complete blood count should be obtained weekly for 4 weeks, biweekly for 4 weeks, and then every 1–3 months for the duration of therapy. Liver biochemical tests should be measured periodically. Some clinicians prefer gradual dose-escalation, especially for patients with intermediate TPMT activity or in whom TPMT measurement is not available; both drugs may be started at 25 mg/d and increased by 25 mg every 1–2 weeks while monitoring for myelosuppression until the target dose is reached. If the white blood count falls below 3000–4000/mcL or the platelet count falls below 100,000/mcL, the medication should be held for at least 1 week before reducing the daily dose by 25–50 mg.

Methotrexate is used in the treatment of patients with inflammatory bowel disease, especially patients with Crohn disease who are intolerant of mercaptopurine. Methotrexate is an analog of dihydrofolic acid. Although at high doses it interferes with cell proliferation through inhibition of nucleic acid metabolism, at low doses it has anti-inflammatory properties, including inhibition of expression of tumor necrosis factor (TNF) in monocytes and macrophages. Methotrexate may be given intramuscularly, subcutaneously, or orally. Side effects of methotrexate include nausea, vomiting, stomatitis, infections, bone marrow suppression, hepatic fibrosis, and life-threatening pneumonitis. A complete blood count and liver function tests should be monitored every 1–3 months. Folate supplementation (1 mg/d) should be administered.

D. Biologic Therapies

Although the etiology of inflammatory bowel disorders is uncertain, it appears that an abnormal response of the mucosal innate immune system to luminal bacteria may trigger inflammation, which is perpetuated by dysregulation of cellular immunity. A number of biologic therapies are available or in clinical testing that more narrowly target various components of the immune system. Biologic agents are highly effective for patients with corticosteroid-dependent or refractory disease and potentially may improve the natural history of disease. The potential benefits of these agents, however, must be carefully weighed with their high cost and risk of serious and potentially life-threatening side effects.

1. Anti-TNF therapies—TNF is one of the key proinflammatory cytokines in the T_H1 response. TNF exists in two biologically active forms: a soluble form (sTNF), which is enzymatically cleaved from its cell surface, and membrane-bound precursor (tmTNF). When either form binds to the TNF-receptors on effector cells, they initiate a variety of signaling pathways that lead to inflammatory gene activation. Four monoclonal antibodies to TNF currently are available for the treatment of inflammatory bowel disease: infliximab, adalimumab, golimumab, and certolizumab. All four agents bind and neutralize soluble as well as membrane-bound TNF on macrophages and activated T lymphocytes, thereby preventing TNF stimulation of effector cells. When bound to membrane-associated TNF, all agents except certolizumab induce apoptosis and cell lysis of TNF-producing cells.

Infliximab is a chimeric (75% human/25% mouse) IgG_1 antibody that is administered by intravenous infusion. A three-dose regimen of 5 mg/kg administered at 0, 2, and 6 weeks is recommended for acute induction, followed by infusions every 8 weeks for maintenance therapy. Acute infusion reactions occur in 5–10% of infusions but occur less commonly in patients receiving regularly scheduled infusions or concomitant immunomodulators (ie, azathioprine or methotrexate). Most reactions are mild or moderate (nausea; headache; dizziness; urticaria; diaphoresis; or mild cardiopulmonary symptoms that include chest tightness, dyspnea, or palpitations) and can be treated by slowing the infusion rate and administering acetaminophen and diphenhydramine. Severe reactions (hypotension, severe shortness of breath, rigors, severe chest discomfort) occur in < 1% and may require oxygen, diphenhydramine, hydrocortisone, and epinephrine. Delayed serum sickness-like reactions occur in 1%. With repeated, intermittent intravenous injections, antibodies to infliximab develop in up to 40% of patients, which are associated with a shortened duration or loss of response and increased risk of acute or delayed infusion reactions. Giving infliximab in a regularly scheduled maintenance therapy (eg, every 8 weeks), concomitant use of infliximab with other immunomodulating agents (azathioprine, mercaptopurine, or methotrexate), or preinfusion treatment with corticosteroids (intravenous hydrocortisone 200 mg) significantly reduces the development of antibodies to approximately 10%.

Adalimumab and golimumab are fully human IgG_1 antibodies that are administered by subcutaneous injection. For adalimumab, a dose of 160 mg at week 0 and 80 mg at week 2 is recommended for acute induction, followed by maintenance therapy with 40 mg subcutaneously every other week. For golimumab, a dose of 200 mg at week 0 and 100 mg at week 2 is recommended for acute induction, followed by maintenance therapy with 100 mg subcutaneously every 4 weeks.

Certolizumab is a fusion compound in which the Fab1 portion of a chimeric (95% human/5% mouse) TNF-antibody is bound to polyethylene glycol in order to prolong the drug half-life. A dose of 400 mg at weeks 0, 2, and 4 is recommended for acute induction, followed by maintenance therapy with 400 mg subcutaneously every 4 weeks. Injection site reactions (burning, pain, redness, itching) are relatively common but are usually minor and self-limited. Because of their subcutaneous route of injection, acute and delayed hypersensitivity reactions are rare. Antibodies to adalimumab develop in 5% of patients and to certolizumab in 10%, which may lead to shortened duration or loss of response to the drug.

Serious infections with anti-TNF therapies may occur in 2–5% of patients, including sepsis, pneumonia, abscess, and cellulitis; however, controlled studies suggest the increased risk may be attributable to increased severity of disease and concomitant use of corticosteroids. Patients treated with anti-TNF therapies are at increased risk for the development of opportunistic infections with intracellular bacterial pathogens including tuberculosis, mycoses (candidiasis, histoplasmosis, coccidioidomycosis, nocardiosis), and listeriosis, and with reactivation of viral infections, including hepatitis B, herpes simplex, varicella zoster, and EBV. Prior to use of these agents, patients should be screened for latent tuberculosis with PPD testing and a chest radiograph. Antinuclear and anti-DNA antibodies occur in a large percentage of patients; however, the development of drug-induced lupus is rare. All agents may cause severe hepatic reactions leading to acute hepatic failure; liver biochemical tests should be monitored routinely during therapy. Anti-TNF therapies increase the risk of nonmelanoma skin cancer and, possibly, non-Hodgkin lymphoma. Most lymphomas, however, are associated with a combination of an anti-TNF agent and a thiopurine, and it appears that the risk of anti-TNF monotherapy is very low. Rare cases of optic neuritis and demyelinating diseases, including multiple sclerosis have been reported. Anti-TNF therapies may worsen heart failure in patients with cardiac disease.

2. Anti-integrins—Various monoclonal antibodies are available or under investigation that target integrins, decreasing the trafficking of circulating leukocytes through the vasculature and reducing chronic inflammation. Natalizumab is a humanized monoclonal antibody targeted against alpha-4-integrins that blocks leukocytes trafficking to the gut and brain. Although natalizumab is efficacious for the induction and maintenance of response and remission in patients with Crohn disease, there is an increased incidence of progressive multifocal leukoencephalopathy (PML) caused by reactivation of the JC virus, in approximately 1:250 in patients with a positive JC virus antibody test result receiving therapy for >18 months. Patients with a negative JC virus antibody test are presumed to be at extremely low risk (< 1:10,000) for PML. The use of natalizumab should be restricted to patients with Crohn disease who have not responded to other therapies and who have a negative antibody test for JC virus.

Vedolizumab (approved by the FDA in May 2014) is a new anti-integrin that blocks the alpha$_4$beta$_7$ heterodimer, selectively blocking gut, but not brain, lymphocyte trafficking. It is believed that greater selectivity may prevent JC virus reactivation.

Beaugerie L. Lymphoma: the bête noire of the long-term use of thiopurines in adult and elderly patients with inflammatory bowel disease. Gastroenterology. 2013 Nov;145(5):927–30. [PMID: 24070724]

Bloomgren G et al. Risk of natalizumab-associated progressive multifocal leukoencephalopathy. N Engl J Med. 2012 May 17;366(20):1870–80. [PMID: 22591293]

Coskun M et al. Tumor necrosis factor inhibitors for inflammatory bowel disease. N Engl J Med. 2013 Dec 26;369(26):2561–2. [PMID: 24369082]

Ford AC et al. Glucocorticosteroid therapy in inflammatory bowel disease: systematic review and meta-analysis. Am J Gastroenterol. 2011 Apr;106(4):590–9. [PMID: 21407179]

Targownik LE et al. Infectious and malignant complications of TNF inhibitor therapy in IBD. Am J Gastroenterol. 2013 Dec;108(12):1835–42. [PMID: 24042192]

▶ Social Support for Patients

Inflammatory bowel disease is a lifelong illness that can have profound emotional and social impacts on the individual. Patients should be encouraged to become involved in the Crohn's and Colitis Foundation of America (CCFA). National headquarters may be contacted at 444 Park Avenue South, 11th Floor, New York, NY 10016-7374; phone 212-685-3440. Internet address: http://www.ccfa.org.

1. Crohn Disease

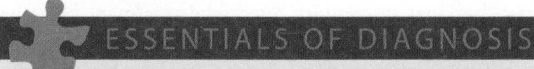

ESSENTIALS OF DIAGNOSIS

- ▶ Insidious onset.
- ▶ Intermittent bouts of low-grade fever, diarrhea, and right lower quadrant pain.
- ▶ Right lower quadrant mass and tenderness.
- ▶ Perianal disease with abscess, fistulas.
- ▶ Radiographic or endoscopic evidence of ulceration, stricturing, or fistulas of the small intestine or colon.

▶ General Considerations

One-third of cases of Crohn disease involve the small bowel only, most commonly the terminal ileum (ileitis). Half of all cases involve the small bowel and colon, most often the terminal ileum and adjacent proximal ascending colon (ileocolitis). In 20% of cases, the colon alone is affected. One-third of patients have associated perianal disease (fistulas, fissures, abscesses). Less than 5% patients have symptomatic involvement of the upper intestinal tract. Unlike ulcerative colitis, Crohn disease is a transmural process that can result in mucosal inflammation and ulceration, stricturing, fistula development, and abscess formation. Cigarette smoking is strongly associated with the development of Crohn disease, resistance to medical therapy, and early disease relapse.

▶ Clinical Findings

A. Symptoms and Signs

Because of the variable location of involvement and severity of inflammation, Crohn disease may present with a variety of symptoms and signs. In eliciting the history, the clinician should take particular note of fevers, the patient's general sense of well-being, weight loss, the presence of abdominal pain, the number of liquid bowel movements per day, and prior surgical resections. Physical examination should focus on the patient's temperature, weight, and nutritional status, the presence of abdominal tenderness or an abdominal mass, rectal examination, and extraintestinal manifestations (described below). Most commonly, there is one or a combination of the following clinical constellations.

1. Chronic inflammatory disease—This is the most common presentation and is often seen in patients with ileitis or ileocolitis. Patients report malaise, weight loss, and loss of energy. In patients with ileitis or ileocolitis, there may be diarrhea, which is usually nonbloody and often intermittent. In patients with colitis involving the rectum or left colon, there may be bloody diarrhea and fecal urgency, which may mimic the symptoms of ulcerative colitis. Cramping or steady right lower quadrant or periumbilical pain is common. Physical examination reveals focal tenderness, usually in the right lower quadrant. A palpable, tender mass that represents thickened or matted loops of inflamed intestine may be present in the lower abdomen.

2. Intestinal obstruction—Narrowing of the small bowel may occur as a result of inflammation, spasm, or fibrotic stenosis. Patients report postprandial bloating, cramping pains, and loud borborygmi. This may occur in patients with active inflammatory symptoms (as above) or later in the disease from chronic fibrosis without other systemic symptoms or signs of inflammation.

3. Penetrating disease and fistulae—Sinus tracts that penetrate through the bowel, where they may be contained or form fistulas to adjacent structures, develop in a subset of patients. Penetration through the bowel can result in an intra-abdominal or retroperitoneal phlegmon or abscess manifested by fevers, chills, a tender abdominal mass, and leukocytosis. Fistulas between the small intestine and colon commonly are asymptomatic but can result in diarrhea, weight loss, bacterial overgrowth, and malnutrition. Fistulas to the bladder produce recurrent infections. Fistulas to the vagina result in malodorous drainage and problems with personal hygiene. Fistulas to the skin usually occur at the site of surgical scars.

4. Perianal disease—One-third of patients with either large or small bowel involvement develop perianal disease manifested by large painful skin tags, anal fissures, perianal abscesses, and fistulas.

5. Extraintestinal manifestations—Extraintestinal manifestations may be seen with both Crohn disease and ulcerative colitis. These include arthralgias, arthritis, iritis or uveitis, pyoderma gangrenosum, or erythema nodosum. Oral aphthous lesions are common. There is an increased prevalence of gallstones due to malabsorption of bile salts from the terminal ileum. Nephrolithiasis with urate or calcium oxalate stones may occur.

B. Laboratory Findings

There is a poor correlation between laboratory studies and the patient's clinical picture. Laboratory values may reflect inflammatory activity or nutritional complications of disease. A complete blood count and serum albumin should be obtained in all patients. Anemia may reflect chronic inflammation, mucosal blood loss, iron deficiency, or vitamin B_{12} malabsorption secondary to terminal ileal inflammation or resection. Leukocytosis may reflect inflammation or abscess formation or may be secondary to corticosteroid therapy. Hypoalbuminemia may be due to intestinal protein loss (protein-losing enteropathy), malabsorption, bacterial overgrowth, or chronic inflammation. The sedimentation rate or C-reactive protein level is elevated in many patients during active inflammation. Fecal lactoferrin or calprotectin levels also are increased in patients with intestinal inflammation. Stool specimens are sent for examination for routine pathogens, ova and parasites, leukocytes, fat, and *C difficile* toxin.

C. Special Diagnostic Studies

In most patients, the initial diagnosis of Crohn disease is based on a compatible clinical picture with supporting endoscopic, pathologic, and radiographic findings. Colonoscopy usually is performed first to evaluate the colon and terminal ileum and to obtain mucosal biopsies. Typical endoscopic findings include aphthoid, linear or stellate ulcers, strictures, and segmental involvement with areas of normal-appearing mucosa adjacent to inflamed mucosa. In 10% of cases, it may be difficult to distinguish ulcerative colitis from Crohn disease. Granulomas on biopsy are present in < 25% of patients but are highly suggestive of Crohn disease. CT or MR enterography or a barium upper gastrointestinal series with small bowel follow-through often is obtained in patients with suspected small bowel involvement. Suggestive findings include ulcerations, strictures, and fistulas; in addition, CT or MR enterography may identify bowel wall thickening and vascularity, mucosal enhancement, and fat stranding. Capsule imaging may help establish a diagnosis when clinical suspicion for small bowel involvement is high but radiographs are normal or nondiagnostic.

▶ Complications

A. Abscess

The presence of a tender abdominal mass with fever and leukocytosis suggests an abscess. Emergent CT of the abdomen is necessary to confirm the diagnosis. Patients should be given broad-spectrum antibiotics. Percutaneous drainage or surgery is usually required.

B. Obstruction

Small bowel obstruction may develop secondary to active inflammation or chronic fibrotic stricturing and is often acutely precipitated by dietary indiscretion. Patients should be given intravenous fluids with nasogastric suction. Systemic corticosteroids are indicated in patients with symptoms or signs of active inflammation but are unhelpful in patients with inactive, fixed disease. Patients unimproved on medical management require surgical resection of the stenotic area or stricturoplasty.

C. Abdominal and Rectovaginal Fistulas

Many fistulas are asymptomatic and require no specific therapy. Most symptomatic fistulas eventually require surgical therapy; however, medical therapy is effective in a subset of patients and is usually tried first in outpatients who otherwise are stable. Large abscesses associated with fistulas require percutaneous or surgical drainage. After percutaneous drainage, long-term antibiotics are administered in order to reduce recurrent infections until the fistula is closed or surgically resected. Fistulas may close temporarily in response to TPN or oral elemental diets but recur when oral feedings are resumed. Anti-TNF agents may promote closure in up to 60% within 10 weeks; however, relapse occurs in over one-half of patients within 1 year despite continued therapy. Surgical therapy is required for symptomatic fistulas that do not respond to medical therapy. Fistulas that arise above (proximal to) areas of intestinal stricturing commonly require surgical treatment.

D. Perianal Disease

Patients with fissures, fistulas, and skin tags commonly have perianal discomfort. Successful treatment of active intestinal disease also may improve perianal disease. Specific treatment of perianal disease can be difficult and is best approached jointly with a surgeon with an expertise in colorectal disorders. Pelvic MRI and endoscopic ultrasonography are the best noninvasive studies for evaluating perianal fistulas. Patients should be instructed on proper perianal skin care, including gentle wiping with a premoistened pad (baby wipes) followed by drying with a cool hair dryer, daily cleansing with sitz baths or a water wash, and use of perianal cotton balls or pads to absorb drainage. Oral antibiotics (metronidazole, 250 mg three times daily, or ciprofloxacin, 500 mg twice daily) may promote symptom improvement or healing in patients with fissures or uncomplicated fistulas; however, recurrent symptoms are common. Refractory fissures may benefit from mesalamine suppositories or topical 0.1% tacrolimus ointment. Immunomodulators or anti-TNF agents or both promote short-term symptomatic improvement from anal fistulas in two-thirds of patients and complete closure in up to one-half of patients; however, less than one-third maintain symptomatic remission during long-term maintenance treatment.

Anorectal abscesses should be suspected in patients with severe, constant perianal pain, or perianal pain in association with fever. Superficial abscesses are evident on perianal examination, but deep perirectal abscesses may be detected by digital examination or pelvic CT scan. Depending on the abscess location, surgical drainage may be achieved by incision, or catheter or seton placement. Surgery should be considered for patients with severe, refractory symptoms but is best approached after medical therapy of the Crohn disease has been optimized.

E. Carcinoma

Patients with colonic Crohn disease are at increased risk for developing colon carcinoma; hence, annual screening colonoscopy to detect dysplasia or cancer is recommended for patients with a history of 8 or more years of Crohn colitis. Patients with Crohn disease have an increased risk of lymphoma and of small bowel adenocarcinoma; however, both are rare.

F. Hemorrhage

Unlike ulcerative colitis, severe hemorrhage is unusual in Crohn disease.

G. Malabsorption

Malabsorption may arise after extensive surgical resections of the small intestine and from bacterial overgrowth in patients with enterocolonic fistulas, strictures, and stasis resulting in bacterial overgrowth.

▶ Differential Diagnosis

Chronic cramping abdominal pain and diarrhea are typical of both irritable bowel syndrome and Crohn disease, but radiographic examinations are normal in the former. Celiac disease may cause diarrhea with malabsorption. Acute fever and right lower quadrant pain may resemble appendicitis or *Yersinia enterocolitica* enteritis. Intestinal lymphoma causes fever, pain, weight loss, and abnormal small bowel radiographs that may mimic Crohn disease. Patients with undiagnosed AIDS may present with fever and diarrhea. Segmental colitis may be caused by tuberculosis, *E histolytica*, *Chlamydia*, or ischemic colitis. *C difficile* or CMV infection may develop in patients with inflammatory bowel disease, mimicking disease recurrence. Diverticulitis with abscess formation may be difficult to distinguish acutely from Crohn disease. NSAIDs may exacerbate inflammatory bowel disease and may also cause NSAID-induced colitis characterized by small bowel or colonic ulcers, erosion, or strictures that tend to be most severe in the terminal ileum and right colon.

▶ Treatment of Active Disease

Crohn disease is a chronic lifelong illness characterized by exacerbations and periods of remission. As no specific therapy exists, current treatment is directed toward symptomatic improvement and control of the disease process, in order to improve quality of life and reduce disease progression and complications. Although sustained clinical remission should be the therapeutic goal, this is achieved in less than one-third of patients. Choice of therapies depends on the disease location and severity, patient age and comorbidities, and patient preference. Early introduction of biologic therapy should be considered strongly in patients with risk factors for aggressive disease, including young age, perianal disease, structuring disease, or need for corticosteroids. All patients with Crohn disease should be counseled to discontinue cigarettes.

A. Nutrition

1. Diet—Patients should eat a well-balanced diet with as few restrictions as possible. Eating smaller but more frequent meals may be helpful. Patients with diarrhea should be encouraged to drink fluids to avoid dehydration. Many patients report that certain foods worsen symptoms, especially fried or greasy foods. Because lactose intolerance is common, a trial off dairy products is warranted if flatulence or diarrhea is a prominent complaint. Patients with obstructive symptoms should be placed on a low-roughage diet, ie, no raw fruits or vegetables, popcorn, nuts, etc. Resection of more than 100 cm of terminal ileum results in fat malabsorption for which a low-fat diet is recommended. Parenteral vitamin B_{12} (100 mcg intramuscularly per month) commonly is needed for patients with previous ileal resection or extensive terminal ileal disease.

2. Enteral therapy—Supplemental enteral therapy via nasogastric tube may be required for children and adolescents with poor intake and growth retardation.

3. Total parenteral nutrition—TPN is used short term in patients with active disease and progressive weight loss or those awaiting surgery who have malnutrition but cannot tolerate enteral feedings because of high-grade obstruction, high-output fistulas, severe diarrhea, or abdominal pain. It is required long term in a small subset of patients with extensive intestinal resections resulting in short bowel syndrome with malnutrition.

B. Symptomatic Medications

There are several potential mechanisms by which diarrhea may occur in Crohn disease in addition to active Crohn disease. A rational empiric treatment approach often yields therapeutic improvement that may obviate the need for corticosteroids or immunosuppressive agents. Involvement of the terminal ileum with Crohn disease or prior ileal resection may lead to reduced absorption of bile acids that may induce secretory diarrhea from the colon. This diarrhea commonly responds to cholestyramine 2–4 g, colestipol 5 g, or colesevelam 625 mg one to two times daily before meals to bind the malabsorbed bile salts. Patients with extensive ileal disease (requiring more than 100 cm of ileal resection) have such severe bile salt malabsorption that steatorrhea may arise. Such patients may benefit from a low-fat diet; bile salt-binding agents will exacerbate the diarrhea and should not be given. Patients with Crohn disease are at risk for the development of small intestinal bacterial overgrowth due to enteral fistulas, ileal resection, and impaired motility and may benefit from a course of broad-spectrum antibiotics (see Bacterial Overgrowth, above).

Other causes of diarrhea include lactase deficiency and short bowel syndrome (described in other sections). Use of oral antidiarrheal agents may provide benefit in some patients. Loperamide (2–4 mg), diphenoxylate with atropine (one tablet), or tincture of opium (5–15 drops) may be given as needed up to four times daily. Because of the risk of toxic megacolon, these drugs should not be used in patients with active severe colitis.

C. Specific Drug Therapy

1. 5-Aminosalicylic acid agents—Mesalamine has long been used as initial therapy for the treatment of mild to moderately active colonic and ileocolonic Crohn disease. However, meta-analyses of published and unpublished trial data suggest that mesalamine is of no value in either the treatment of active Crohn disease or the maintenance of remission. Current treatment guidelines recommend against its use for Crohn disease.

2. Antibiotics—Antibiotics also are widely used by clinicians for the treatment of active luminal Crohn disease, although meta-analyses of controlled trials suggest that they have little or no efficacy. It is hypothesized that antibiotics may reduce inflammation through alteration of gut flora, reduction of bacterial overgrowth, or treatment of microperforations. Oral metronidazole (10 mg/kg/d) or ciprofloxacin (500 mg twice daily), or rifaximin (800 mg twice daily) are commonly administered for 6–12 weeks.

3. Corticosteroids—Approximately one-half of patients with Crohn disease require corticosteroids at some time in their illness. Corticosteroids dramatically suppress the acute clinical symptoms or signs in most patients with both small and large bowel disease; however, they do not alter the underlying disease. An ileal-release budesonide preparation (Entocort), 9 mg once daily for 8–16 weeks, induces remission in 50–70% of patients with mild to moderate Crohn disease involving the terminal ileum or ascending colon. After initial treatment, budesonide is tapered over 2–4 weeks in 3 mg increments. In some patients, low-dose budesonide (6 mg/d) may be used for up to 1 year to maintain remission. Budesonide is superior to mesalamine but somewhat less effective than prednisone. However, because budesonide has markedly reduced acute and chronic steroid-related adverse effects, including smaller reductions of bone mineral density, it is preferred to other systemic corticosteroids for the treatment of mild to moderate Crohn disease involving the terminal ileum or ascending colon.

Prednisone or methylprednisolone, 40–60 mg/d, is generally administered to patients with Crohn disease that is severe, that involves the distal colon or proximal small intestine, or that has failed treatment with budesonide. Remission or significant improvement occurs in > 80% of patients after 8–16 weeks of therapy. After improvement at 2 weeks, tapering proceeds at 5 mg/wk until a dosage of 20 mg/d is being given. Thereafter, slow tapering by 2.5 mg/wk is recommended. Approximately 20% of patients cannot be completely withdrawn from corticosteroids without experiencing a symptomatic flare-up. Furthermore, more than 50% of patients who achieve initial remission on corticosteroids will experience a relapse within 1 year. Use of long-term low corticosteroid doses (2.5–10 mg/d) should be avoided, because of associated complications (see above). Patients requiring long-term corticosteroid treatment should be given immunomodulatory drugs (as described below) in an effort to wean them from corticosteroids.

Patients with persisting symptoms despite oral corticosteroids or those with high fever, persistent vomiting, evidence of intestinal obstruction, severe weight loss, severe abdominal tenderness, or suspicion of an abscess should be hospitalized. In patients with a tender, palpable inflammatory abdominal mass, CT scan of the abdomen should be obtained prior to administering corticosteroids to rule out an abscess. If no abscess is identified, parenteral corticosteroids should be administered (as described for ulcerative colitis below).

4. Immunomodulating drugs: Azathioprine, mercaptopurine, or methotrexate—The two main indications for immunomodulators in Crohn disease are (1) for maintenance of remission after induction with corticosteroids; and (2) for the induction of remission, in combination with anti-TNF therapy, in patients with moderate to severe active Crohn disease (discussed in next section). In the United States, mercaptopurine or azathioprine are more commonly used than methotrexate. Immunomodulators are used in up to 60% of patients with Crohn disease for maintenance after induction of remission with corticosteroids. Although the magnitude of benefit is debated, meta-analysis of controlled trials suggest that patients treated with thiopurines are 2.3 times as likely to maintain remission as patients treated with placebo, reducing the 3-year relapse rate from > 60% to < 25%. Methotrexate (25 mg subcutaneously weekly for 12 weeks, followed by 12.5–15 mg once weekly) is used in patients who are unresponsive to, or intolerant of, mercaptopurine or azathioprine. Because oral absorption may be erratic, parenteral administration of methotrexate is preferred. Immunomodulators do not appear to be effective at inducing remission. Two 2013 randomized controlled trials in patients with newly diagnosed Crohn disease (treated with or without corticosteroids) found equivalent corticosteroid-free remissions rates in patients treated with thiopurines or placebo. A 2013 AGA guideline has recommended against the use of thiopurine monotherapy to induce remission.

5. Anti-TNF therapies—Infliximab, adalimumab, and certolizumab are used to induce and maintain remission in patients with moderate to severe Crohn disease, including fistulizing disease. These agents are also used to treat extraintestinal manifestations of Crohn disease (except optic neuritis).

A. ACUTE INDUCTION THERAPY—Anti-TNF therapies are recommended as the preferred first-line agents to induce remission in patients with moderate to severe Crohn disease, either as monotherapy or in combination with thiopurines. Currently, there are two major controversies about the use of anti-TNF agents: (1) whether anti-TNF agents should be reserved as second-line therapy in patients with moderate to severe Crohn disease who have not responded to prior therapy with corticosteroids and immunomodulators ("step-up" therapy) or whether it should be used early in the course of illness with the goal of inducing early remission and altering the natural history of the disease; (2) whether anti-TNF therapy should be used alone or in combination with an immunomodulator to enhance remission and reduce the development of antibodies to the anti-TNF agent. The best data support the use of anti-TNF agents early in the course of disease and suggest that "step-up therapy" (corticosteroids, followed by azathioprine, followed by infliximab) is obsolete. Furthermore, for most patients, anti-TNF therapy should be used in combination with an immunomodulator—at least during the first year of treatment. Data in support of use of early combination therapy come from a large 2010 trial (SONIC) that compared three treatment arms: combination therapy with infliximab and azathioprine versus infliximab alone or azathioprine alone in patients with moderate to severe Crohn disease who had not previously been treated with immunomodulators or anti-TNF agents. After 6 months, clinical remission (57%) and mucosal healing (44%) was significantly higher with combination therapy than with either agent alone. Combination therapy with anti-TNF and azathioprine may not be appropriate in young men (< 26 years) in whom there is a higher risk of hepatosplenic T-cell lymphoma and in the elderly in whom there is a higher risk of lymphoma and infectious complications.

The doses for acute induction therapy are described above. Up to two-thirds of patients have significant clinical improvement during acute induction therapy.

B. Maintenance therapy—After initial clinical response, symptom relapse occurs in > 80% of patients within 1 year in the absence of further maintenance therapy. Therefore, scheduled maintenance therapy is usually recommended (infliximab, 5 mg/kg infusion every 8 weeks; adalimumab, 40 mg subcutaneous injection every 2 weeks; certolizumab, 400 mg subcutaneous injection every 4 weeks). With long-term maintenance therapy, approximately two-thirds have continued clinical response and up to one-half have complete symptom remission. A gradual or complete loss of efficacy occurs over time in some patients, necessitating increased dosing (infliximab 10 mg/kg; adalimumab 80 mg), decreased dosing intervals (infliximab every 6 weeks; adalimumab every week), changing to the alternative agent, or discontinuation of anti-TNF therapy. In some cases, loss of efficacy is due to the development of antibodies to the anti-TNF agent. Concomitant therapy with anti-TNF agents and immunomodulating agents (azathioprine, mercaptopurine, or methotrexate) reduces the risk of development of antibodies to the anti-TNF agent but may increase the risk of complications (non-Hodgkin lymphoma and opportunistic infections). At this time, there is uncertainty about whether combination therapy with anti-TNF agents and immunomodulators should be continued indefinitely or converted after 1–2 years to anti-TNF monotherapy.

6. Anti-integrins—Anti-integrins may offer a therapeutic option for patients who do not respond or who lose response to anti-TNF agents. Natalizumab, an antibody directed against the alpha$_4$ integrin that was approved in 2008 for the induction and maintenance of Crohn disease, demonstrated a 56% clinical response and 37% remission at 10 weeks. Due to the recognized risk of reactivation of JC virus and the development of PML, natalizumab has had limited clinical use. In 2013, the results of a phase III trial of vedolizumab, an alpha$_4$beta$_7$ integrin antibody, showed that prior anti-TNF therapy failed in 64% of patients with moderate to severe Crohn disease due to lack or loss of response or side effects. In this refractory group, vedolizumab (300 mg intravenously at weeks 0 and 2 for induction, then every 4–8 weeks for maintenance), 31% had initial response and 21% achieved long-term remission. Although the long-term safety of this agent is unknown, its purported specificity for gut leukocyte trafficking may mitigate the risk of PML. If the FDA approved, it may offer an important option in patients with refractory disease.

▶ Indications for Surgery

Over 50% of patients will require at least one surgical procedure. The main indications for surgery are intractability to medical therapy, intra-abdominal abscess, massive bleeding, symptomatic refractory internal or perianal fistulas, and intestinal obstruction. Patients with chronic obstructive symptoms due to a short segment of ileal stenosis are best treated with resection or stricturoplasty (rather than long-term medical therapy), which promotes rapid return of well-being and elimination of corticosteroids. After surgery, endoscopic evidence of recurrence occurs in 60% within 1 year. Endoscopic recurrence precedes clinical recurrence by months to years; clinical recurrence occurs in 20% of patients within 1 year and 80% within 10–15 years. Therapy with metronidazole, 250 mg three times daily for 3 months, or long-term therapy with immunomodulators (mercaptopurine or azathioprine) have only been modestly effective in preventing clinical and endoscopic recurrence after ileocolic resection; however, small uncontrolled studies suggest that anti-TNF therapies may prevent endoscopic recurrence in up to 90% of patients. Clinicians may choose to perform endoscopy in high-risk patients 6–12 months after surgery in order to identify patients with early endoscopic recurrence who may benefit from anti-TNF therapy.

▶ Prognosis

With proper medical and surgical treatment, the majority of patients are able to cope with this chronic disease and its complications and lead productive lives. Few patients die as a direct consequence of the disease.

▶ When to Refer

- For expertise in endoscopic procedures or capsule endoscopy.
- Any patient requiring hospitalization for follow-up.
- Patients with moderate to severe disease for whom therapy with immunomodulators or biologic agents is being considered.
- When surgery may be necessary.

When to Admit

- An intestinal obstruction is suspected.
- An intra-abdominal or perirectal abscess is suspected.
- A serious infectious complication is suspected, especially in patients who are immunocompromised due to concomitant use of corticosteroids, immunomodulators, or anti-TNF agents.
- Patients with severe symptoms of diarrhea, dehydration, weight loss, or abdominal pain.
- Patients with severe or persisting symptoms despite treatment with corticosteroids.

Colombel JF et al; SONIC Study Group. Infliximab, azathioprine, or combination therapy for Crohn's disease. N Engl J Med. 2010 Apr 15;362(15):1383–95. [PMID: 20393175]

Cosnes J et al; Groupe d'Etude Thérapeutique des Affections Inflammatoires du Tube Digestif (GETAID). Early administration of azathioprine vs conventional management of Crohn's Disease: a randomized controlled trial. Gastroenterology. 2013 Oct;145(4):758–65.e2. [PMID: 23644079]

D'Haens GR et al. The London Position Statement of the World Congress of Gastroenterology on Biological Therapy for IBD with the European Crohn's and Colitis Organization: when to start, when to stop, which drug to choose, and how to predict response? Am J Gastroenterol. 2011 Feb;106(2):199–212. [PMID: 21045814]

Ford AC et al. Efficacy of 5-aminosalicylates in Crohn's disease: systematic review and meta-analysis. Am J Gastroenterol. 2011 Apr;106(4):617–29. [PMID: 21407190]

Ford AC et al. Efficacy of biologic therapies in inflammatory bowel disease: systematic review and meta-analysis. Am J Gastroenterol. Apr; 2011;106(4):644–59. [PMID: 21407183]

Panés J et al; AZTEC Study Group. Early azathioprine therapy is no more effective than placebo for newly diagnosed Crohn's disease. Gastroenterology. 2013 Oct;145(4):766–74.e1. [PMID: 23770132]

Savarino E et al. Adalimumab is more effective than azathioprine and mesalamine at preventing postoperative recurrence of Crohn's disease: a randomized controlled trial. Am J Gastroenterol. 2013 Nov;108(11):1731–42. [PMID: 24019080]

Terdiman JP et al. American Gastroenterological Association Institute guideline on the use of thiopurines, methotrexate, and anti-TNF-α biologic drugs for the induction and maintenance of remission in inflammatory Crohn's disease. Gastroenterology. 2013 Dec;145(6):1459–63. [PMID: 24267474]

2. Ulcerative Colitis

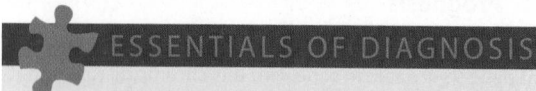

ESSENTIALS OF DIAGNOSIS

- ▶ Bloody diarrhea.
- ▶ Lower abdominal cramps and fecal urgency.
- ▶ Anemia, low serum albumin.
- ▶ Negative stool cultures.
- ▶ Sigmoidoscopy is the key to diagnosis.

General Considerations

Ulcerative colitis is an idiopathic inflammatory condition that involves the mucosal surface of the colon, resulting in diffuse friability and erosions with bleeding. Approximately one-third of patients have disease confined to the rectosigmoid region (proctosigmoiditis); one-third have disease that extends to the splenic flexure (left-sided colitis); and one-third have disease that extends more proximally (extensive colitis). In patients with distal colitis, the disease progresses with time to more extensive involvement in 25–50%. There is some correlation between disease extent and symptom severity. In most patients, the disease is characterized by periods of symptomatic flare-ups and remissions. Ulcerative colitis is more common in nonsmokers and former smokers. Disease severity may be lower in active smokers and may worsen in patients who stop smoking. Appendectomy before the age of 20 years for acute appendicitis is associated with a reduced risk of developing ulcerative colitis.

Clinical Findings

A. Symptoms and Signs

The clinical profile in ulcerative colitis is highly variable. Bloody diarrhea is the hallmark. On the basis of several clinical and laboratory parameters, it is clinically useful to classify patients as having mild, moderate, or severe disease (Table 15–12). Patients should be asked about stool frequency, the presence and amount of rectal bleeding, cramps, abdominal pain, fecal urgency, and tenesmus. Physical examination should focus on the patient's volume status as determined by orthostatic blood pressure and pulse measurements and by nutritional status. On abdominal examination, the clinician should look for tenderness and evidence of peritoneal inflammation. Red blood may be present on digital rectal examination.

1. Mild to moderate disease—Patients with mild disease have a gradual onset of infrequent diarrhea (less than four movements per day) with intermittent rectal bleeding and mucus. Stools may be formed or loose in consistency. Because of rectal inflammation, there is fecal urgency and tenesmus. Left lower quadrant cramps relieved by defecation are common, but there is no significant abdominal tenderness. Patients with moderate disease have more

Table 15–12. Ulcerative colitis: Assessment of disease activity.

	Mild	Moderate	Severe
Stool frequency (per day)	< 4	4–6	> 6 (mostly bloody)
Pulse (beats/min)	< 90	90–100	> 100
Hematocrit (%)	Normal	30–40	< 30
Weight loss (%)	None	1–10	> 10
Temperature (°F)	Normal	99–100	> 100
ESR (mm/h)	< 20	20–30	> 30
Albumin (g/dL)	Normal	3–3.5	< 3

ESR, erythrocyte sedimentation rate.

severe diarrhea with frequent bleeding. Abdominal pain and tenderness may be present but are not severe. There may be mild fever, anemia, and hypoalbuminemia.

2. Severe disease—Patients with severe disease have more than six bloody bowel movements per day, resulting in severe anemia, hypovolemia, and impaired nutrition with hypoalbuminemia. Abdominal pain and tenderness are present. "Fulminant colitis" is a subset of severe disease characterized by rapidly worsening symptoms with signs of toxicity.

B. Laboratory Findings

The degree of abnormality of the hematocrit, sedimentation rate, and serum albumin reflects disease severity.

C. Endoscopy

In acute colitis, the diagnosis is readily established by sigmoidoscopy. The mucosal appearance is characterized by edema, friability, mucopus, and erosions. Colonoscopy should not be performed in patients with fulminant disease because of the risk of perforation. After patients have demonstrated improvement on therapy, colonoscopy is performed to determine the extent of disease.

D. Imaging

Plain abdominal radiographs are obtained in patients with severe colitis to look for significant colonic dilation. Barium enemas are of little utility in the evaluation of acute ulcerative colitis and may precipitate toxic megacolon in patients with severe disease.

▶ Differential Diagnosis

The initial presentation of ulcerative colitis is indistinguishable from other causes of colitis, clinically as well as endoscopically. Thus, the diagnosis of idiopathic ulcerative colitis is reached after excluding other known causes of colitis. Infectious colitis should be excluded by sending stool specimens for routine bacterial cultures (to exclude *Salmonella*, *Shigella*, and *Campylobacter*, as well as specific assays for *E coli* O157), ova and parasites (to exclude amebiasis), and stool toxin assay for *C difficile*. Mucosal biopsy can distinguish amebic colitis from ulcerative colitis. CMV colitis occurs in immunocompromised patients, including patients receiving prolonged corticosteroid therapy, and is diagnosed on mucosal biopsy. Gonorrhea, chlamydial infection, herpes, and syphilis are considerations in sexually active patients with proctitis. In elderly patients with cardiovascular disease, ischemic colitis may involve the rectosigmoid. A history of radiation to the pelvic region can result in proctitis months to years later. Crohn disease involving the colon but not the small intestine may be confused with ulcerative colitis. In 10% of patients, a distinction between Crohn disease and ulcerative colitis may not be possible.

▶ Treatment

There are two main treatment objectives: (1) to terminate the acute, symptomatic attack and (2) to prevent recurrence of attacks. The treatment of acute ulcerative colitis depends on the extent of colonic involvement and the severity of illness.

Patients with mild to moderate disease should eat a regular diet but limit their intake of caffeine and gas-producing vegetables. Antidiarrheal agents should not be given in the acute phase of illness but are safe and helpful in patients with mild chronic symptoms. Oral loperamide (2 mg) or diphenoxylate with atropine (one tablet) may be given up to four times daily. Such remedies are particularly useful at nighttime and when taken prophylactically for occasions when patients may not have reliable access to toilet facilities.

A. Mild to Moderate Distal Colitis

Patients with disease confined to the rectum or rectosigmoid region generally have mild to moderate but distressing symptoms. Patients may be treated with topical mesalamine, topical corticosteroids, or oral aminosalicylates (5-ASA) according to patient preference and cost considerations. Topical mesalamine is the drug of choice and is superior to topical corticosteroids and 5-ASA. Mesalamine is administered as a suppository, 1000 mg once daily at bedtime for proctitis, and as an enema, 4 g at bedtime for proctosigmoiditis, for 4–12 weeks, with 75% of patients improving. Patients who either decline or are unable to manage topical therapy may be treated with oral 5-ASA, as discussed below. Topical corticosteroids are a less expensive alternative to mesalamine but are also less effective. Hydrocortisone suppository or foam is prescribed for proctitis and hydrocortisone enema (80–100 mg) for proctosigmoiditis. Systemic effects from short-term use are very slight. For patients with distal disease who do not improve with topical or oral mesalamine therapy, the following options may be considered: (1) a combination of a topical agent with an oral 5-ASA agent is more effective than either drug alone; (2) combination topical therapy with a 5-ASA suppository or enema at bedtime and a corticosteroid enema or foam in the morning; or (3) a combination of oral 5-ASA agent, topical 5-ASA agent, and a topical corticosteroid. Patients with distal colitis who are refractory to all of these therapies or who have severe disease may require treatment with oral prednisone 40–60 mg/d or infliximab, as described below.

Patients whose acute symptoms resolve rapidly with immediate therapy may have prolonged periods of remission that are treated successfully with intermittent courses of therapy. Patients with early or frequent relapse should be treated with maintenance therapy with mesalamine suppositories (1000 mg) or enemas (4 g) nightly or every other night. For patients who have difficulty complying with topical therapies, oral 5-ASA agents are an acceptable, though possibly less effective, alternative (see below). Topical corticosteroids are ineffective for maintaining remission of distal colitis.

B. Mild to Moderate Colitis

1. 5-ASA Agents—Disease extending above the sigmoid colon is best treated with oral 5-ASA agents (mesalamine, balsalazide, or sulfasalazine), which result in symptomatic improvement in 50–75% of patients. The optimal dose for induction of remission of mild disease is 2.4 g daily and for moderate disease is 2.4–4.8 g daily. Most patients improve within 3–6 weeks, though some require 2–3 months. These agents achieve clinical improvement in 50–70% of patients and remission in 20–30%. Oral sulfasalazine is comparable in efficacy to mesalamine and because of its low cost is still commonly used as a first-line agent by many providers, though it is associated with greater side effects. To minimize side effects, sulfasalazine is begun at a dosage of 500 mg twice daily and increased gradually over 1–2 weeks to 2 g twice daily. Total doses of 5–6 g/d may have greater efficacy but are poorly tolerated. Folic acid, 1 mg/d orally, should be administered to all patients taking sulfasalazine.

2. Corticosteroids—Patients with mild to moderate disease who do not improve within 4 weeks of 5-ASA therapy should have corticosteroid therapy added. Prednisone and methylprednisolone are most commonly used. Depending on the severity of illness, the initial oral dose of prednisone is 40–60 mg daily. Rapid improvement is observed in most cases within 2 weeks. Thereafter, tapering of prednisone should proceed by 5–10 mg/wk. After tapering to 20 mg/d, slower tapering (2.5 mg/week) is sometimes required. Complete tapering without symptomatic flare-ups is possible in the majority of patients. Delayed-release budesonide (Uceris) 9 mg ER orally once daily has shown modest benefit in mild to moderate colitis, achieving remission in 17.5% of patients after 8 weeks compared with 12.5 % with placebo. In view of its low incidence of corticosteroid-associated side-effects, it may be considered in patients with mild colitis for whom other systemic corticosteroids are deemed high risk.

3. Immunomodulating agents—Approximately 30% of patients either do not respond to corticosteroids or have symptomatic flares during attempts at corticosteroid tapering and develop steroid dependency. Patients with steroid dependency or frequent relapse while taking mesalamine may be treated with thiopurines (mercaptopurine or azathioprine), although rigorous controlled trials are lacking and their absolute benefit appears to be modest. The risks of these drugs must be weighed against the certainty of cure with surgical resection. There is less evidence that methotrexate is effective.

The anti-TNF agents infliximab, adalimumab, and golimumab are approved in the United States for the treatment of patients with moderate to severe ulcerative colitis who have had an inadequate response to conventional therapies (oral corticosteroids, mercaptopurine or azathioprine, and mesalamine). Following a three-dose induction regimen of infliximab 5 mg/kg administered at 0, 2, and 6 weeks, clinical response occurs in 65% and clinical remission in 35%. By comparison, phase III trials of adalimumab and golimumab reported clinical response rates of 50–59% and remission rates of 16–21% after 8 weeks. Although the response and remission rates appear lower with adalimumab and golimumab than infliximab, differences in study design and patient populations limit comparisons. Importantly, 40% of patients in the adalimumab trials were previously treated with other anti-TNF agents, in whom lower response rates were noted.

4. Probiotics—VSL#3 (two packets twice daily), a probiotic compound containing eight different nonpathogenic strains of lactobacilli, bifidobacteria, and streptococci, has demonstrated significant benefit versus placebo in the treatment of mild to moderate ulcerative colitis in two randomized, controlled multicenter trials. Although its efficacy relative to other agents is unclear, it may be considered as an adjunctive therapy for mild to moderate disease.

C. Severe Colitis

About 15% of patients with ulcerative colitis have a more severe course. Because they may progress to fulminant colitis or toxic megacolon, hospitalization is generally required.

1. General measures—Discontinue all oral intake for 24–48 hours or until the patient demonstrates clinical improvement. TPN is indicated only in patients with poor nutritional status or if feedings cannot be reinstituted within 7–10 days. All opioid or anticholinergic agents should be discontinued. Restore circulating volume with fluids, correct electrolyte abnormalities, and consider transfusion for significant anemia (hematocrit < 25–28%). Abdominal examinations should be repeated to look for evidence of worsening distention or pain. A plain abdominal radiograph should be ordered on admission to look for evidence of colonic dilation. Send stools for bacterial culture, *C difficile* toxin assay, and examination for ova and parasites. CMV superinfection should be considered in patients receiving long-term immunosuppressive therapy who are unresponsive to corticosteroid therapy. Due to a high risk of venous thromboembolic disease, prophylaxis should be administered. Surgical consultation should be sought for all patients with severe disease.

2. Corticosteroid therapy—Methylprednisolone, 48–64 mg, or hydrocortisone, 300 mg, is administered intravenously in four divided doses or by continuous infusion over 24 hours. Higher or "pulse" doses are of no benefit. Hydrocortisone enemas (100 mg) may also be administered twice daily for treatment of urgency or tenesmus. Approximately 50–75% of patients achieve remission with systemic corticosteroids within 7–10 days. Once symptomatic improvement has occurred, oral fluids are reinstituted. If fluids are well tolerated, intravenous corticosteroids are discontinued and the patient is started on oral prednisone (as described for moderate disease). Patients without significant improvement within 3–5 days of intravenous corticosteroid therapy should be referred for surgery or considered for anti-TNF therapies or cyclosporine.

3. Anti-TNF therapies—A single infusion of infliximab, 5 mg/kg, has been shown in controlled and uncontrolled studies to be effective in treating severe colitis in patients who did not improve within 4–7 days of intravenous corticosteroid therapy. In a controlled study of patients hospitalized for ulcerative colitis, colectomy was required within 3 months in 69% who received placebo therapy, compared with 47% who received infliximab. Thus, infliximab therapy should be considered in patients with severe ulcerative colitis who have not improved with intravenous corticosteroid therapy. (See Crohn Disease, above.)

4. Cyclosporine—Intravenous cyclosporine (2–4 mg/kg/d as a continuous infusion) benefits 60–75% of patients with severe colitis who have not improved after 7–10 days of corticosteroids, but it is associated with significant toxicity (nephrotoxicity, seizures, infection, hypertension). Up to two-thirds of responders may be maintained in remission with a combination of oral cyclosporine for 3 months and long-term therapy with mercaptopurine or azathioprine. A 2011 randomized study of patients with severe colitis refractory to intravenous corticosteroids found similar response rates (85%) with cyclosporine and infliximab therapy.

5. Surgical therapy—Patients with severe disease who do not improve after corticosteroid, infliximab, or cyclosporine therapy are unlikely to respond to further medical therapy, and surgery is recommended.

D. Fulminant Colitis and Toxic Megacolon

A subset of patients with severe disease has a more fulminant course with rapid progression of symptoms over 1–2 weeks and signs of severe toxicity. These patients appear quite ill, with fever, prominent hypovolemia, hemorrhage requiring transfusion, and abdominal distention with tenderness. They are at a higher risk of perforation or development of toxic megacolon and must be followed closely. Broad-spectrum antibiotics should be administered to cover anaerobes and gram-negative bacteria.

Toxic megacolon develops in < 2% of cases of ulcerative colitis. It is characterized by colonic dilation of more than 6 cm on plain films with signs of toxicity. In addition to the therapies outlined above, nasogastric suction should be initiated. Patients should be instructed to roll from side to side and onto the abdomen in an effort to decompress the distended colon. Serial abdominal plain films should be obtained to look for worsening dilation or ischemia. Patients with fulminant disease or toxic megacolon who worsen or fail to improve within 48–72 hours should undergo surgery to prevent perforation. If the operation is performed before perforation, the mortality rate should be low.

► Maintenance of Remission

Without long-term therapy, 75% of patients who initially go into remission on medical therapy will experience a symptomatic relapse within 1 year. Long-term oral maintenance therapy with sulfasalazine, 1–1.5 g twice daily, or mesalamine, 1.6–2.4 g once daily, have been shown to reduce relapse rates to < 35%. Mercaptopurine and azathioprine are useful in patients with frequent disease relapses (more than two per year) or corticosteroid-dependent disease to maintain remission. The role of long-term infliximab therapy in the maintenance of remission is evolving. In two, large, controlled studies of patients with active moderate to severe colitis, initial induction therapy was

followed by infliximab maintenance infusions (5 mg/kg) administered every 8 weeks for 30–54 weeks. At the end of the study (30 or 54 weeks), 35% were in clinical remission, (21% in corticosteroid-free remission), a modest but impressive response in patients with more refractory disease. In considering long-term infliximab therapy, patients and clinicians need to weigh the long-term risks of immunosuppression against colectomy.

► Risk of Colon Cancer

In patients with ulcerative colitis with disease proximal to the rectum and in patients with Crohn colitis, there is a markedly increased risk of developing colon carcinoma. A large meta-analysis of observational studies reported a cumulative incidence of 2% at 10 years, 8% at 20 years, and 18% after 30 years of disease. Retrospective studies suggest that the risk of colon cancer may be reduced in patients treated with long-term 5-ASA therapy. Ingestion of folic acid, 1 mg/d, also is associated with a decreased risk of cancer development. Colonoscopies are recommended every 1–2 years in patients with colitis, beginning 8 years after diagnosis. At colonoscopy, all adenoma-like polyps should be resected, when possible, and biopsies obtained of non-endoscopically resectable mass lesions. In addition, multiple (at least 32) random mucosal biopsies are taken throughout the colon at 10-cm intervals to look for evidence of dysplasia in flat mucosa. Because of the relatively high incidence of concomitant carcinoma in patients with dysplasia (either low or high grade) in flat mucosa or non-endoscopically resectable mass lesions, colectomy is recommended. Several prospective studies demonstrate that dye spraying with methylene blue or indigo carmine ("chromoendoscopy") enhances the detection of subtle mucosal lesions, thereby significantly increasing the detection of dysplasia compared with standard colonoscopy. Although surveillance colonoscopy appears to be effective in reducing the incidence of colon cancer, patients must understand that approximately one-third of detected cancers are advanced, despite compliance with routine colonoscopy surveillance.

► Surgery in Ulcerative Colitis

Surgery is required in 25% of patients. Severe hemorrhage, perforation, and documented carcinoma are absolute indications for surgery. Surgery is indicated also in patients with fulminant colitis or toxic megacolon that does not improve within 48–72 hours, in patients with flat dysplasia or non-endoscopically resectable dysplastic lesions on surveillance colonoscopy, and in patients with refractory disease requiring long-term corticosteroids to control symptoms.

Although total proctocolectomy (with placement of an ileostomy) provides complete cure of the disease, most patients seek to avoid it out of concern for the impact it may have on their bowel function, their self-image, and their social interactions. After complete colectomy, patients may have a standard ileostomy with an external appliance, a continent ileostomy, or an internal ileal pouch that is anastomosed to the anal canal (ileal pouch-anal anastomosis).

The latter maintains intestinal continuity, thereby obviating an ostomy. Under optimal circumstances, patients have five to seven loose bowel movements per day without incontinence. Endoscopic or histologic inflammation in the ileal pouch ("pouchitis") develops in over 40% of patients, resulting in increased stool frequency, fecal urgency, cramping, and bleeding, but usually resolves with a 2-week course of oral metronidazole (250–500 mg three times daily) or ciprofloxacin (500 mg twice daily). Patients with frequently relapsing pouchitis may need continuous antibiotics. Probiotics containing nonpathogenic strains of lactobacilli, bifidobacteria, and streptococci (VSL#3) are effective in the maintenance of remission in patients with recurrent pouchitis. Bismuth subsalicylate (Pepto Bismol, 262 mg, two tablets four times daily) has demonstrated benefit in some series. Some clinicians report that topical corticosteroids or oral budesonide 9 mg/d are of benefit. Refractory cases of pouchitis can be disabling and may require conversion to a standard ileostomy.

Prognosis

Ulcerative colitis is a lifelong disease characterized by exacerbations and remissions. For most patients, the disease is readily controlled by medical therapy without need for surgery. The majority never require hospitalization. A subset of patients with more severe disease will require surgery, which results in complete cure of the disease. Properly managed, most patients with ulcerative colitis lead close to normal productive lives.

When to Refer

- Colonoscopy: for evaluation of activity and extent of active disease and for surveillance for neoplasia in patients with quiescent disease for more than 8–10 years.
- When hospitalization is required.
- When surgical colectomy is indicated.

When to Admit

- Patients with severe disease manifested by frequent bloody stools, anemia, weight loss, and fever.
- Patients with fulminant disease manifested by rapid progression of symptoms, worsening abdominal pain, distention, high fever, tachycardia.
- Patients with moderate to severe symptoms that do not respond to oral corticosteroids and require a trial of bowel rest and intravenous corticosteroids.

Autenrieth DM et al. Toxic megacolon. Inflamm Bowel Dis. 2012 Mar;18(3):584–91. [PMID: 22009735]

Bessissow T et al. Advanced endoscopic imaging for dysplasia surveillance in ulcerative colitis. Expert Rev Gastroenterol Hepatol. 2013 Jan;7(1):57–67. [PMID: 23265150]

Bitton A et al; Canadian Association of Gastroenterology Severe Ulcerative Colitis Consensus Group. Treatment of hospitalized adult patients with severe ulcerative colitis: Toronto consensus statements. Am J Gastroenterol. 2012 Feb;107(2):179–94. [PMID: 22108451]

Collins PD. Strategies for detecting colon cancer and dysplasia in patients with inflammatory bowel disease. Inflamm Bowel Dis. 2013 Mar–Apr;19(4):860–3. [PMID: 23446340]

Danese S et al. Ulcerative colitis. N Engl J Med. 2011 Nov 3;365(18):1713–25. [PMID: 22047562]

Danese S et al. Review article: the role of anti-TNF in the management of ulcerative colitis—past, present and future. Aliment Pharmacol Ther. 2013 May;37(9):855–66. [PMID: 23489068]

Marshall JK et al. Rectal 5-aminosalicylic acid for maintenance of remission in ulcerative colitis. Cochrane Database Syst Rev. 2012 Nov 14;11:CD004118. [PMID: 23152224]

Ordás I et al. Ulcerative colitis. Lancet. 2012 Nov 3;380(9853):1606–19. [PMID: 22914296]

Sandborn WJ et al. Adalimumab induces and maintains clinical remission in patients with moderate-to-severe ulcerative colitis. Gastroenterology. 2011 2012 Feb;142(2):257–65. [PMID: 22062358]

Sandborn WJ et al. Subcutaneous golimumab induces clinical response and remission in patients with moderate-to-severe ulcerative colitis. Gastroenterology. 2014 Jan;146(1):85–95. [PMID: 23735746]

3. Microscopic Colitis

Microscopic colitis is an idiopathic condition that is found in up to 15% of patients who have chronic or intermittent watery diarrhea with normal-appearing mucosa at endoscopy. There are two major subtypes—lymphocytic colitis and collagenous colitis. In both, histologic evaluation of mucosal biopsies reveals chronic inflammation (lymphocytes, plasma cells) in the lamina propria and increased intraepithelial lymphocytes. Collagenous colitis is further characterized by the presence of a thickened band (> 10 mcm) of subepithelial collagen. Both forms occur more commonly in women, especially in the fifth to sixth decades. Symptoms tend to be chronic or recurrent but may remit in most patients after several years. A more severe illness characterized by abdominal pain, fatigue, dehydration, and weight loss may develop in a subset of patients. The cause of microscopic colitis usually is unknown. Several medications have been implicated as etiologic agents, including NSAIDs, sertraline, paroxetine, lansoprazole, lisinopril, and simvastatin. Diarrhea usually abates within 30 days of stopping the offending medication. Celiac sprue may be present in up to 20% of patients and should be excluded with serologic testing (antitissue transglutaminase or antiendomysial antibody). Treatment is largely empiric since there are few well-designed, controlled treatment trials. Antidiarrheal therapy with loperamide is the first-line treatment, providing symptom improvement in up to 70%. For patients who do not respond to loperamide, the next option is budesonide (which is efficacious but expensive) versus other agents (which have limited data supporting efficacy but are less expensive). In uncontrolled studies, treatment with 5-ASAs (sulfasalazine, mesalamine) or bile-salt binding agents (cholestyramine, colestipol) is reported to be effective in many patients. A small unpublished controlled trial demonstrated efficacy for bismuth subsalicylate (two tablets three times daily) for 2 months; however, clinical experience has yielded only modest benefit. Delayed release budesonide (Entocort) 9 mg/d for 6–8 weeks has been shown in three prospective controlled studies to induce clinical remission in > 80% of patients; however, relapse occurs in most patients after stopping therapy. In two prospective studies, remission was maintained in 75% of patients treated with budesonide 6 mg/d compared with 25% of persons given placebo. In clinical practice, budesonide is tapered to the lowest effective dose for maintaining symptoms. Less than 3% of patients have refractory or severe symptoms, which may be treated with immunosuppressive agents (azathioprine or methotrexate).

Ianiro G. Microscopic colitis. World J Gastroenterol. 2012 Nov 21;18(43):6206–15. [PMID: 23180940]

Pardi DS et al. Microscopic colitis. Gastroenterology. 2011 Apr;140(4):1155–65. [PMID: 21303675]

Yen EF et al. Non-IBD colitides (eosinophilic, microscopic). Best Pract Res Clin Gastroenterol. 2012 Oct;26(5):611–22. [PMID: 23384806]

DIVERTICULAR DISEASE OF THE COLON

Colonic diverticulosis increases with age, ranging from 5% in those under age 40, to 30% at age 60, to more than 50% over age 80 years in Western societies. Most are asymptomatic, discovered incidentally at endoscopy or on barium enema. Complications occur in < 5%, including gastrointestinal bleeding and diverticulitis.

Colonic diverticula may vary in size from a few millimeters to several centimeters and in number from one to several dozen. Almost all patients with diverticulosis have involvement in the sigmoid and descending colon; however, only 15% have proximal colonic disease.

For over 40 years, it has been believed that diverticulosis arises after many years of a diet deficient in fiber. It is hypothesized that undistended, contracted segments of colon have higher intraluminal pressures. Over time, the contracted colonic musculature, working against greater pressures to move small, hard stools, develops hypertrophy, thickening, rigidity, and fibrosis. Diverticula may develop more commonly in the sigmoid because intraluminal pressures are highest in this region. Recent epidemiologic studies challenge this theory, finding no association between the prevalence of asymptomatic diverticulosis and low dietary fiber intake or constipation. Thus, the etiology of diverticulosis is uncertain. The extent to which abnormal motility and hereditary factors contribute to diverticular disease is unknown. Patients with diffuse diverticulosis may have an inherent weakness in the colonic wall. Patients with abnormal connective tissue are also disposed to development of diverticulosis, including Ehlers-Danlos syndrome, Marfan syndrome, and scleroderma.

1. Uncomplicated Diverticulosis

More than 90% of patients with diverticulosis have uncomplicated disease and no specific symptoms. In most, diverticulosis is an incidental finding detected during colonoscopic examination or barium enema examination. Some patients have nonspecific complaints of chronic constipation, abdominal pain, or fluctuating bowel habits.

It is unclear whether these symptoms are due to alterations in the colonic motility, visceral hypersensitivity, gut microbiota, or in low-grade inflammation. Physical examination is usually normal but may reveal mild left lower quadrant tenderness with a thickened, palpable sigmoid and descending colon. Screening laboratory studies should be normal in uncomplicated diverticulosis.

There is no reason to perform imaging studies for the purpose of diagnosing asymptomatic, uncomplicated disease. Diverticula are well seen on barium enema, colonoscopy and CT imaging. Involved segments of colon may also be narrowed and deformed.

Patients in whom diverticulosis is discovered, especially patients with symptoms or a history of complicated disease (see below) should be treated with a high-fiber diet or fiber supplements (bran powder, 1–2 tbsp twice daily; psyllium or methylcellulose) (see section on constipation). Retrospective studies suggest that such treatment may decrease the likelihood of subsequent complications.

Maconi G et al. Treatment of diverticular disease of the colon and prevention of acute diverticulitis: a systematic review. Dis Colon Rectum. 2011 Oct;54(10):1326–38. [PMID: 21904150]

Peery AF et al. Constipation and a low-fiber diet are not associated with diverticulosis. Clin Gastroenterol Hepatol. 2013 Dec;11(12):1622–7. [PMID: 23891924]

Strate LL et al. Diverticular disease as a chronic illness: evolving epidemiologic and clinical insights. Am J Gastroenterol. 2012 Oct;107(10):1486–93. [PMID: 22777341]

2. Diverticulitis

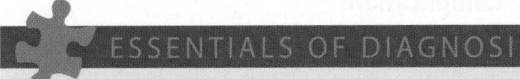

ESSENTIALS OF DIAGNOSIS

▶ Acute abdominal pain and fever.

▶ Left lower abdominal tenderness and mass.

▶ Leukocytosis.

▶ Clinical Findings

A. Symptoms and Signs

Perforation of a colonic diverticulum results in an intra-abdominal infection that may vary from microperforation (most common) with localized paracolic inflammation to macroperforation with either abscess or generalized peritonitis. Thus, there is a range from mild to severe disease. Most patients with localized inflammation or infection report mild to moderate aching abdominal pain, usually in the left lower quadrant. Constipation or loose stools may be present. Nausea and vomiting are frequent. In many cases, symptoms are so mild that the patient may not seek medical attention until several days after onset. Physical findings include a low-grade fever, left lower quadrant tenderness, and a palpable mass. Stool occult blood is common, but hematochezia is rare. Leukocytosis is mild to moderate. Patients with free perforation present with a more dramatic picture of generalized abdominal pain and peritoneal signs.

B. Imaging

In patients with mild symptoms and a presumptive diagnosis of diverticulitis, empiric medical therapy is started without further imaging in the acute phase. Patients who respond to acute medical management should undergo complete colonic evaluation with colonoscopy or radiologic imaging (CT colonography or barium enema) after resolution of clinical symptoms to corroborate the diagnosis or exclude other disorders such as colonic neoplasms. In patients who do not improve rapidly after 2–4 days of empiric therapy and in those with severe disease, CT scan of the abdomen is obtained to look for evidence of diverticulitis and determine its severity, and to exclude other disorders that may cause lower abdominal pain. The presence of colonic diverticula and wall thickening, pericolic fat infiltration, abscess formation, or extraluminal air or contrast suggest diverticulitis. Endoscopy and colonography are contraindicated during the initial stages of an acute attack because of the risk of free perforation.

▶ Differential Diagnosis

Diverticulitis must be distinguished from other causes of lower abdominal pain, including perforated colonic carcinoma, Crohn disease, appendicitis, ischemic colitis, *C difficile*–associated colitis, and gynecologic disorders (ectopic pregnancy, ovarian cyst or torsion) by abdominal CT scan, pelvic ultrasonography, or radiographic studies of the distal colon that use water-soluble contrast enemas.

▶ Complications

Fistula formation may involve the bladder, ureter, vagina, uterus, bowel, and abdominal wall. Diverticulitis may result in stricturing of the colon with partial or complete obstruction.

▶ Treatment

A. Medical Management

Most patients can be managed with conservative measures. Patients with mild symptoms and no peritoneal signs may be managed initially as outpatients on a clear liquid diet. Although broad-spectrum oral antibiotics with anaerobic activity commonly are prescribed, large clinical trials confirm that antibiotics are not beneficial in uncomplicated disease. Reasonable regimens include amoxicillin and clavulanate potassium (875 mg/125 mg) twice daily; or metronidazole, 500 mg three times daily; plus either ciprofloxacin, 500 mg twice daily, or trimethoprim-sulfamethoxazole, 160/800 mg twice daily orally, for 7–10 days or until the patient is afebrile for 3–5 days. Symptomatic improvement usually occurs within 3 days, at which time the diet may be advanced. Once the acute episode has resolved, a high fiber diet is often recommended. Patients with increasing pain, fever, or inability to tolerate oral fluids require hospitalization. Patients with severe diverticulitis (high fevers, leukocytosis, or peritoneal signs) and patients who are elderly or immunosuppressed or who have serious comorbid disease require hospitalization acutely. Patients should be given nothing by mouth and should receive intravenous fluids. If ileus is present, a nasogastric tube should be placed. Intravenous antibiotics should be given to cover anaerobic and gram-negative bacteria. Single-agent therapy with either a second-generation cephalosporin (eg, cefoxitin), piperacillin-tazobactam, or ticarcillin clavulanate appears to be as effective as combination therapy (eg, metronidazole or clindamycin plus an aminoglycoside or third-generation cephalosporin [eg, ceftazidime, cefotaxime]). Symptomatic improvement should be evident within 2–3 days. Intravenous antibiotics should be continued for 5–7 days, before changing to oral antibiotics.

B. Surgical Management

Surgical consultation and repeat abdominal CT imaging should be obtained on all patients with severe disease or those who do not improve after 72 hours of medical management. Patients with a localized abdominal abscess ≥ 4 cm in size are usually treated urgently with a percutaneous catheter drain placed by an interventional radiologist. This permits control of the infection and resolution of the immediate infectious inflammatory process. In this manner, a subsequent elective one-stage surgical operation can be performed (if deemed necessary) in which the diseased segment of colon is removed and primary colonic anastomosis performed. After recovery, the decision to perform elective surgery depends on the patient's age, comorbid disease, and frequency and severity of attacks. Patients with chronic disease resulting in fistulas or colonic obstruction will require elective surgical resection.

Indications for emergent surgical management include generalized peritonitis, large undrainable abscesses, and clinical deterioration despite medical management and percutaneous drainage. Surgery may be performed in one- or two-stage operations depending on the patient's nutritional status, severity of illness, and extent of intra-abdominal peritonitis and abscess formation. In a two-stage operation, the diseased colon is resected and the proximal colon brought out to form a temporary colostomy. The distal colonic stump is either closed (forming a Hartmann pouch) or exteriorized as a mucous fistula. Weeks later, after inflammation and infection have completely subsided, the colon can be reconnected electively.

▶ Prognosis

Diverticulitis recurs in 10–30% of patients treated with medical management over 10–20 years, However, < 5% have more than two recurrences. Recurrent attacks warrant elective surgical resection, which carries a lower morbidity and mortality risk than emergency surgery.

▶ When to Refer

- Failure to improve within 72 hours of medical management.
- Presence of significant peridiverticular abscesses (≥ 4 cm) requiring possible percutaneous or surgical drainage.

- Generalized peritonitis or sepsis.
- Recurrent attacks.
- Chronic complications including colonic strictures or fistulas.

▶ When to Admit

- Severe pain or inability to tolerate oral intake.
- Signs of sepsis or peritonitis.
- CT scan showing signs of complicated disease (abscess, perforation).
- Failure to improve with outpatient management.
- Immunocompromised or frail, elderly patient.

Biondo S et al. Current status of the treatment of acute colonic diverticulitis: a systematic review. Colorectal Dis. 2012 Jan;14(1):e1–e11. [PMID: 21848896]

Peery AF et al. Diverticular disease: reconsidering conventional wisdom. Clin Gastroenterol Hepatol. 2013 Dec;11(12):1532–7. [PMID: 23669306]

Shahedi K et al. Long-term risk of acute diverticulitis among patients with incidental diverticulosis found during colonoscopy. Clin Gastroenterol Hepatol. 2013 Dec;11(12):1609–13. [PMID: 23856358]

3. Diverticular Bleeding

Half of all cases of acute lower gastrointestinal bleeding are attributable to diverticulosis. For a full discussion, see the section on Acute Lower Gastrointestinal Bleeding, above.

POLYPS OF THE COLON

Polyps are discrete mass lesions that protrude into the intestinal lumen. Although most commonly sporadic, they may be inherited as part of a familial polyposis syndrome. Polyps may be divided into four major pathologic groups: mucosal adenomatous polyps (tubular, tubulovillous, and villous), mucosal serrated polyps (hyperplastic, sessile serrated polyp, and traditional serrated adenoma), mucosal nonneoplastic polyps (juvenile polyps, hamartomas, inflammatory polyps), and submucosal lesions (lipomas, lymphoid aggregates, carcinoids, pneumatosis cystoides intestinalis). Of polyps removed at colonoscopy, over 70% are adenomatous; most of the remainder are serrated polyps. Adenomatous polyps and serrated polyps have significant clinical implications and will be considered further below.

NONFAMILIAL ADENOMATOUS & SERRATED POLYPS

Adenomas and serrated polyps may be flat, sessile, or pedunculated (containing a stalk). They are present in 30% of adults over 50 years of age. Their significance is that over 95% of cases of adenocarcinoma of the colon are believed to arise from these lesions. It is proposed that there is a polyp → carcinoma sequence whereby nonfamilial colorectal cancer develops through a continuous process from normal mucosa to adenoma or serrated polyps to carcinoma. The majority of cancers arise in adenomas after inactivation of the *APC* gene leads to chromosomal instability and inactivation or loss of other tumor suppressor genes. By contrast, cancers arising in the serrated pathway appear to have either *Kras* (traditional serrated adenomas) mutations or *BRAF* oncogene activation (sessile serrated adenomas) with methylation of CpG-rich promoter regions that leads to inactivation of tumor suppressor genes or mismatch repair genes (MLH1) with microsatellite instability.

Most adenomas are small (< 1 cm) and have a low risk of becoming malignant; < 5% of these enlarge with time. Adenomas and serrated polyps are classified as "advanced" if they are ≥ 1 cm, or contain villous features or high-grade dysplasia. Advanced lesions are believed to have a higher risk of harboring or progressing to malignancy. It has been estimated from longitudinal studies that it takes an average of 5 years for a medium-sized polyp to develop from normal-appearing mucosa and 10 years for a gross cancer to arise. The prevalence of advanced adenomas is 6% and colorectal cancer 0.3%. The role of aspirin and NSAIDs for the chemoprevention of adenomatous polyps is discussed in Chapter 39, in the section on Colorectal Cancer.

Most sessile serrated polyps and traditional serrated adenomas are believed to arise from hyperplastic polyps. It is believed that sessile serrated polyps and traditional serrated adenomas harbor an increased risk of colorectal cancer similar or greater to that of adenomas. Many pathologists cannot reliably distinguish between hyperplastic polyps and sessile serrated polyps. Small hyperplastic polyps (< 5 mm) located in the rectosigmoid region are of no consequence, except that they cannot reliably be distinguished from adenomatous lesions other than by biopsy. Hyperplastic polyps located in the proximal colon (ie, proximal to the splenic flexure) may be associated with an increased prevalence of advanced neoplasia, particularly those larger than 1 cm.

▶ Clinical Findings

A. Symptoms and Signs

Most patients with adenomatous and serrated polyps are completely asymptomatic. Chronic occult blood loss may lead to iron deficiency anemia. Large polyps may ulcerate, resulting in intermittent hematochezia.

B. Fecal Occult Blood or Multitarget DNA Tests

FOBT, FIT, and fecal DNA tests are available as part of colorectal cancer screening programs (see Chapter 39). FIT is a fecal blood immunochemical test for hemoglobin that is more sensitive than guaiac-based tests for the detection of colorectal cancer and advanced adenomas. In prospective studies, the FIT test detected 15–35% of advanced noncancerous adenomas.

C. Radiologic Tests

Polyps are identified by means of barium enema examinations or CT colonography. Both studies require bowel cleansing with laxatives before the study and insertion of a rectal catheter for air insufflation during the study. CT colonography ("virtual colonoscopy") uses data from helical CT imaging with computer-enabled luminal image reconstruction to generate two-dimensional and three-dimensional images of the colon. Using optimal imaging software with multidetector helical CT scanners, several studies report a sensitivity of ≥ 90% for the detection of polyps > 10 mm in size. However, the accuracy for detection of polyps 5–9 mm in size is significantly lower (sensitivity 50%). A small proportion of these small polyps harbor advanced histology or carcinoma (up to 1.2%) or carcinoma (< 1%). Abdominal CT imaging results in a radiation exposure that may lead to a small risk of cancer. CT colonography is endorsed by US Multisociety Task Force as an acceptable option for screening for colorectal adenomatous polyps and cancer in average risk asymptomatic adults. Barium enema is no longer recommended due to its poor diagnostic accuracy.

D. Endoscopic Tests

Colonoscopy allows evaluation of the entire colon and is the best means of detecting and removing adenomatous and serrated polyps. It should be performed in all patients who have positive FOBT, FIT, fecal, or DNA tests or iron deficiency anemia (see Occult Gastrointestinal Bleeding and Obscure Gastrointestinal Bleeding, above), as the prevalence of colonic neoplasms is increased in these patients. Colonoscopy should also be performed in patients with polyps detected on radiologic imaging studies (barium enema or CT colonography) or adenomas detected on flexible sigmoidoscopy to remove these polyps and to fully evaluate the entire colon. Capsule endoscopy of the colon has a 73% sensitivity and 79% specificity for detection of adenomas with advanced histology or cancer compared with colonoscopy and cannot be recommended at this time to screen for colorectal neoplasia.

▶ Treatment

A. Colonoscopic Polypectomy

Most adenomatous and serrated polyps are amenable to colonoscopic removal with biopsy forceps or snare cautery. Large sessile polyps (> 2–3 cm) may be removed by snare cautery using a variety of techniques (eg, piecemeal or saline-lift assisted mucosal resection) or may require surgical resection. Patients with large sessile polyps removed in piecemeal fashion should undergo repeated colonoscopy in 2–6 months to verify complete polyp removal. Complications after colonoscopic polypectomy include perforation in 0.2% and clinically significant bleeding in 0.3–1% of patients.

B. Postpolypectomy Surveillance

Adenomas and serrated polyps can be found in 30–40% of patients when another colonoscopy is performed within 3–5 years after the initial examination and polyp removal. Periodic colonoscopic surveillance is therefore recommended to detect these "metachronous" lesions, which either may be new or may have been overlooked during the initial examination. Most of these polyps are small, without high-risk features and of little immediate clinical significance. The probability of detecting advanced neoplasms at surveillance colonoscopy depends on the number, size, and histologic features of the polyps removed on initial (index) colonoscopy. Patients with 1–2 small (< 1 cm) tubular adenomas (without villous features or high-grade dysplasia) should have their next colonoscopy in 5–10 years. Patients with 3–10 adenomas, an adenoma >1 cm, or an adenoma with villous features or high-grade dysplasia should have their next colonoscopy at 3 years. Patients with more than 10 adenomas should have a repeat colonoscopy at 1–2 years and may be considered for evaluation for a familial polyposis syndrome (see below). Surveillance colonoscopy at 5 years is appropriate for patients with small (<1 cm) serrated polyps without cytologic dysplasia; surveillance colonoscopy at 3 years should be considered for serrated polyps >1 cm and those with cytologic atypia. No surveillance is recommended for patients with small, typical hyperplastic polyps located in the distal colon and rectum.

Lieberman DA et al. Guidelines for colonoscopy surveillance after screening and polypectomy: a consensus update by the US Multi-Society Task Force on Colorectal Cancer. Gastroenterology. 2012 Sep;143(3):844–57. [PMID: 22763141]

Naini BV et al. Advanced precancerous lesions (APL) in the colonic mucosa. Best Pract Res Clin Gastroenterol. 2013 Apr;27(2):235–56. [PMID: 23809243]

Rosty C et al. Serrated polyps of the large intestine: current understanding of diagnosis, pathogenesis, and clinical management. J Gastroenterol. 2013 Mar;48(3):287–302. [PMID: 23208018]

Zauber AG et al. Colonoscopic polypectomy and long-term prevention of colorectal-cancer deaths. N Engl J Med. 2012 Feb 23;366(8):687–96. [PMID: 22356322]

HEREDITARY COLORECTAL CANCER & POLYPOSIS SYNDROMES

Up to 4% of all colorectal cancers are caused by germline genetic mutations that impose on carriers a high lifetime risk of developing colorectal cancer (see Chapter 39). Because the diagnosis of these disorders has important implications for treatment of affected members and for screening of family members, it is important to consider these disorders in patients with a family history of colorectal cancer that has affected more than one family member, those with a personal or family history of colorectal cancer developing at an early age (≤ 50 years), those with a personal or family history of multiple polyps (>20), and those with a personal or family history of multiple extracolonic malignancies.

Patel SG et al. Familial colon cancer syndromes: an update of a rapidly evolving field. Curr Gastroenterol Rep. 2012 Oct;14(5):428–38. [PMID: 22864806]

1. Familial Adenomatous Polyposis

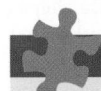

ESSENTIALS OF DIAGNOSIS

► Inherited condition characterized by early development of hundreds to thousands of colonic adenomatous polyps and adenocarcinoma.

► Variety of extracolonic manifestations, including duodenal adenomas, desmoid tumors, and osteomas.

► Attenuated variant with < 500 (average 25) colonic adenomas.

► Genetic testing confirms mutation of *APC* gene (90%) or *MYH* gene (8%).

► Prophylactic colectomy recommended to prevent otherwise inevitable colon cancer.

► General Considerations

Familial adenomatous polyposis (FAP) is a syndrome affecting 1:10,000 people and accounts for approximately 0.5% of colorectal cancer. The classic form of FAP is characterized by the development of hundreds to thousands of colonic adenomatous polyps and a variety of extracolonic manifestations. An attenuated variant of FAP also has been recognized in which an average of only 25 polyps (range of 1–500) develop. FAP is most commonly caused by autosomally dominant inherited mutations in the adenomatous polyposis coli *(APC)* gene on chromosome 5q21. FAP arises de novo in 15% of patients in the absence of genetic mutations in the parents. Mutations in the *MYH* gene, a gene involved with base excision repair, are present in patients with the classic and attenuated forms of FAP who do not have mutations of the *APC* gene. FAP due to *MYH* mutation is inherited in an autosomal recessive fashion, hence a family history of colorectal cancer may not be evident. Of patients with classic FAP, approximately 90% have a mutation in the *APC* gene and 8% in the *MYH* gene. In contrast, among patients with 10–100 adenomatous polyps and suspected attenuated FAP, *APC* mutations are identified in 15% but *MYH* mutations in 25%.

► Clinical Findings

A. Symptoms and Signs

Colorectal polyps develop by a mean age of 15 years and cancer at 40 years. Unless prophylactic colectomy is performed, colorectal cancer is inevitable by age 50 years. In attenuated FAP, the mean age for development of cancer is about 56 years.

Adenomatous polyps of the duodenum and periampullary area develop in over 90% of patients, resulting in a 5–8% lifetime risk of adenocarcinoma. Adenomas occur less frequently in the gastric antrum and small bowel and in those locations have a lower risk of malignant transformation. Gastric fundus gland polyps occur in over 50% but have an extremely low (0.6%) malignant potential.

A variety of other benign extraintestinal manifestations, including soft tissue tumors of the skin, desmoid tumors, osteomas, and congenital hypertrophy of the retinal pigment, develop in some patients with FAP. These extraintestinal manifestations vary among families, depending in part on the type or site of mutation in the *APC* gene. Desmoid tumors are locally invasive fibromas, most commonly intra-abdominal, that may cause bowel obstruction, ischemia, or hemorrhage. They occur in 15% of patients and are the second leading cause of death in FAP. Malignancies of the central nervous system (Turcot syndrome) and tumors of the thyroid and liver (hepatoblastomas) may also develop in patients with FAP.

B. Genetic Testing

Genetic counseling and testing should be offered to patients with a diagnosis of FAP established by endoscopy and to first-degree family members of patients with the disease; testing should be done also to confirm a diagnosis of attenuated disease in patients with 20 or more adenomas. Genetic testing is best performed by sequencing the *APC* gene to identify disease-associated mutations, which are identified in approximately 90% of cases of typical FAP. Mutational assessment of *MYH* should be considered in patients with negative test results and in patients with suspected attenuated FAP. First-degree relatives of patients with FAP should undergo genetic screening after age 10 years. If the assay cannot be done or is not informative, family members at risk should undergo yearly sigmoidoscopy beginning at 12 years of age.

► Treatment

Once the diagnosis has been established, complete proctocolectomy with ileoanal anastomosis or colectomy with ileorectal anastomosis is recommended, usually before age 20 years. Ileorectal anastomosis affords superior bowel function but has a 5% risk of development of rectal cancer, and for that reason frequent sigmoidoscopy with fulguration of polyps is required. Upper endoscopic evaluation of the stomach, duodenum, and periampullary area should be performed every 1–3 years to look for adenomas or carcinoma. Large (> 2 cm) periampullary adenomas require surgical resection. Sulindac and COX-2 selective agents (celecoxib) have been shown to decrease the number and size of polyps in the rectal stump but not the duodenum.

Kerr SE et al. APC germline mutations in individuals being evaluated for familial adenomatous polyposis: a review of the Mayo Clinic experience with 1591 consecutive tests. J Mol Diagn. 2013 Jan;15(1):31–43. [PMID: 23159591]

Voorham QJ et al. Tracking the molecular features of nonpolypoid colorectal neoplasms: a systematic review and meta-analysis. Am J Gastroenterol. 2013 Jul;108(7):1042–56. [PMID: 23649184]

2. Hamartomatous Polyposis Syndromes

Hamartomatous polyposis syndromes are rare and account for < 0.1% of colorectal cancers.

Peutz-Jeghers syndrome is an autosomal dominant condition characterized by hamartomatous polyps throughout the gastrointestinal tract (most notably in the small intestine) as well as mucocutaneous pigmented macules on the lips, buccal mucosa, and skin. The hamartomas may become large, leading to bleeding, intussusception, or obstruction. Although hamartomas are not malignant, gastrointestinal malignancies (stomach, small bowel, and colon) develop in 40–60%, breast cancer in 30–50%, as well as a host of other malignancies of nonintestinal organs (gonads, pancreas). The defect has been localized to the serine threonine kinase 11 gene, and genetic testing is available.

Familial juvenile polyposis is also autosomal dominant and is characterized by several (more than ten) juvenile hamartomatous polyps located most commonly in the colon. There is an increased risk (up to 50%) of adenocarcinoma due to synchronous adenomatous polyps or mixed hamartomatous-adenomatous polyps. Genetic defects have been identified to loci on 18q and 10q (*MADH4* and *BMPR1A*). Genetic testing is available.

PTEN multiple hamartoma syndrome (Cowden disease) is characterized by hamartomatous polyps and lipomas throughout the gastrointestinal tract, trichilemmomas, and cerebellar lesions. An increased rate of malignancy is demonstrated in the thyroid, breast, and urogenital tract.

Beggs AD et al. Peutz-Jeghers syndrome: a systematic review and recommendations for management. Gut. 2010 Jul;59(7):975–86. [PMID: 20581245]

Latchford AR et al. Gastrointestinal polyps and cancer in Peutz-Jeghers syndrome: clinical aspects. Fam Cancer. 2011 Sep;10(3):455–61. [PMID: 21503746]

3. Lynch Syndrome

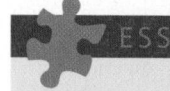
ESSENTIALS OF DIAGNOSIS

▶ Autosomally dominant inherited condition.

▶ Caused by mutations in a gene that detects and repairs DNA base-pair mismatches, resulting in DNA microsatellite instability and inactivation of tumor suppressor genes.

▶ Increased lifetime risk of colorectal cancer (50–80%), endometrial cancer (30–60%), and other cancers that may develop at young age.

▶ Evaluation warranted in patients with personal history of early-onset colorectal cancer or family history of colorectal, endometrial, or other Lynch syndrome–related cancers at young age or in multiple members.

▶ Diagnosis suspected by tumor tissue immunohistochemical staining for mismatch repair proteins or testing for microsatellite instability.

▶ Diagnosis confirmed by genetic testing.

▶ General Considerations

Lynch syndrome (also known as hereditary nonpolyposis colon cancer [HNPCC]) is an autosomal dominant condition in which there is a markedly increased risk of developing colorectal cancer as well as a host of other cancers, including endometrial, ovarian, renal or vesical, hepatobiliary, gastric, and small intestinal cancers. It is estimated to account for up to 3% of all colorectal cancers. Affected individuals have a 50–80% lifetime risk of developing colorectal carcinoma and a 30–60% lifetime risk of endometrial cancer. Unlike individuals with familial adenomatous polyposis, patients with HNPCC develop only a few adenomas, which may be flat and more often contain villous features or high-grade dysplasia. In contrast to the traditional polyp → cancer progression (which may take over 10 years), these polyps are believed to undergo rapid transformation over 1–2 years from normal tissue → adenoma → cancer. HNPCC and endometrial cancer tend to develop at an earlier age than sporadic, nonhereditary cancers (mean age 45–50 years). Compared with patients with sporadic tumors of similar pathologic stage, those with HNPCC tumors have improved survival. Synchronous or metachronous cancers occur within 10 years in up to 45% of patients.

HNPCC is caused by a defect in one of several genes that are important in the detection and repair of DNA base-pair mismatches: *MLH1, MSH2, MSH6, and PMS2*. Germline mutations in *MLH1* and *MSH2* account for almost 90% of the known mutations in families with HNPCC. Mutations in any of these mismatch repair genes result in a characteristic phenotypic DNA abnormality known as microsatellite instability.

▶ Clinical Findings

A thorough family cancer history is essential to identify families that may be affected with HNPCC so that appropriate genetic and colonoscopic screening can be offered. Owing to the limitations of genetic testing for HNPCC and the medical, psychological, and social implications that such testing may have, families with suspected HNPCC should be evaluated first by a genetic counselor and should give informed consent in writing before genetic testing is performed. Patients whose families meet any of the revised "Bethesda criteria" have an increased likelihood of harboring a germline mutation in one of the mismatch repair genes and should be considered for genetic testing. The "Bethesda criteria" are (1) colorectal cancer under age 50; (2) synchronous or metachronous colorectal or HNPCC-associated tumor regardless of age (endometrial, stomach, ovary, pancreas, ureter and renal pelvis, biliary tract, brain); (3) colorectal cancer with one or more first-degree relatives with colorectal or HNPCC-related cancer, with one of the cancers occurring before age 50; (4) colorectal cancer with two or more second-degree relatives with colorectal or HNPCC cancer, regardless of age; (5) tumors with infiltrating lymphocytes, mucinous/signet ring differentiation, or medullary growth pattern in patients younger than 60 years. The Bethesda criteria identify approximately 70% of mutation-positive HNPCC families but overlook 30%. For this reason, expert guidelines have recommended that all colorectal cancers should undergo testing for Lynch syndrome with either immunohistochemistry or microsatellite instability and *BRAF* testing.

Patients whose tumors test positive using one of these tests should be given genetic counseling before undergoing germline testing for gene mutations.

Screening & Treatment

If genetic testing documents an HNPCC gene mutation, affected relatives should be screened with colonoscopy every year beginning at age 25 (or at age 5 years younger than the age at diagnosis of the youngest affected family member). If cancer is found, subtotal colectomy with ileorectal anastomosis (followed by annual surveillance of the rectal stump) should be performed. Women should undergo screening for endometrial and ovarian cancer beginning at age 25–35 years with pelvic examination, CA-125 assay, endometrial aspiration, and transvaginal ultrasound. Prophylactic hysterectomy and oophorectomy may be considered, especially in women of postchildbearing age. Similarly, consideration should be given for increased cancer surveillance in family members in proven or suspected HNPCC families who do not wish to undergo germline testing. (See Chapter 39 for Colorectal Cancer.)

Goodenberger M et al. Lynch syndrome and MYH-associated polyposis: review and testing strategy. J Clin Gastroenterol. 2011 Jul;45(6):488–500. [PMID: 21325953]

Limburg PJ et al. Prevalence of alterations in DNA mismatch repair genes in patients with young-onset colorectal cancer. Clin Gastroenterol Hepatol. 2011 Jun;9(6):497–502. [PMID: 21056691]

Llor X. When should we suspect hereditary colorectal cancer syndrome? Clin Gastroenterol Hepatol. 2012 Apr;10(4):363–7. [PMID: 22178459]

ANORECTAL DISEASES

(See Chapter 39 for Carcinoma of the Anus.)

HEMORRHOIDS

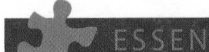

ESSENTIALS OF DIAGNOSIS

- ▶ Bright red blood per rectum.
- ▶ Protrusion, discomfort.
- ▶ Characteristic findings on external anal inspection and anoscopic examination.

General Considerations

Internal hemorrhoids are subepithelial vascular cushions consisting of connective tissue, smooth muscle fibers, and arteriovenous communications between terminal branches of the superior rectal artery and rectal veins. They are a normal anatomic entity, occurring in all adults, that contribute to normal anal pressures and ensure a water-tight closure of the anal canal. They commonly occur in three primary locations—right anterior, right posterior, and left lateral. External hemorrhoids arise from the inferior hemorrhoidal veins located below the dentate line and are covered with squamous epithelium of the anal canal or perianal region.

Hemorrhoids may become symptomatic as a result of activities that increase venous pressure, resulting in distention and engorgement. Straining at stool, constipation, prolonged sitting, pregnancy, obesity, and low-fiber diets all may contribute. With time, redundancy and enlargement of the venous cushions may develop and result in bleeding or protrusion.

Clinical Findings

A. Symptoms and Signs

Patients often attribute a variety of perianal complaints to "hemorrhoids." However, the principal problems attributable to internal hemorrhoids are bleeding, prolapse, and mucoid discharge. Bleeding is manifested by bright red blood that may range from streaks of blood visible on toilet paper or stool to bright red blood that drips into the toilet bowl after a bowel movement. Uncommonly, bleeding is severe and prolonged enough to result in anemia. Initially, internal hemorrhoids are confined to the anal canal (stage I). Over time, the internal hemorrhoids may gradually enlarge and protrude from the anal opening. At first, this mucosal prolapse occurs during straining and reduces spontaneously (stage II). With progression over time, the prolapsed hemorrhoids may require manual reduction after bowel movements (stage III) or may remain chronically protruding (stage IV). Chronically prolapsed hemorrhoids may result in a sense of fullness or discomfort and mucoid perianal discharge, resulting in irritation and soiling of underclothes. Pain is unusual with internal hemorrhoids, occurring only when there is extensive inflammation and thrombosis of irreducible tissue or with thrombosis of an external hemorrhoid (see below).

B. Examination

External hemorrhoids are readily visible on perianal inspection. Nonprolapsed internal hemorrhoids are not visible but may protrude through the anus with gentle straining while the clinician spreads the buttocks. Prolapsed hemorrhoids are visible as protuberant purple nodules covered by mucosa. The perianal region should also be examined for other signs of disease such as fistulas, fissures, skin tags, condyloma, anal cancer, or dermatitis. On digital examination, uncomplicated internal hemorrhoids are neither palpable nor painful. Anoscopic evaluation, best performed in the prone jackknife position, provides optimal visualization of internal hemorrhoids.

Differential Diagnosis

Small volume rectal bleeding may be caused by anal fissure or fistula, neoplasms of the distal colon or rectum, ulcerative colitis or Crohn colitis, infectious proctitis, or rectal ulcers. Rectal prolapse, in which a full thickness of rectum protrudes concentrically from the anus, is readily distinguished from mucosal hemorrhoidal prolapse. Proctosigmoidoscopy or colonoscopy should be performed in all patients with hematochezia to exclude disease in the rectum or sigmoid colon that could be misinterpreted in the presence of hemorrhoidal bleeding.

▶ Treatment

A. Conservative Measures

Most patients with early (stage I and stage II) disease can be managed with conservative treatment. To decrease straining with defecation, patients should be given instructions for a high-fiber diet and told to increase fluid intake with meals. Dietary fiber may be supplemented with bran powder (1–2 tbsp twice daily added to food or in 8 oz of liquid) or with commercial bulk laxatives (eg, Benefiber, Metamucil, Citrucel). Suppositories and rectal ointments have no demonstrated utility in the management of mild disease. Mucoid discharge may be treated effectively by the local application of a cotton ball tucked next to the anal opening after bowel movements.

B. Medical Treatment

Patients with stage I, stage II, and stage III hemorrhoids and recurrent bleeding despite conservative measures may be treated without anesthesia with injection sclerotherapy, rubber band ligation, or application of electrocoagulation (bipolar cautery or infrared photocoagulation). The choice of therapy is dictated by operator preference, but rubber band ligation is preferred due to its ease of use and high rate of efficacy. Major complications occur in < 2%, including pelvic sepsis, pelvic abscess, urinary retention, and bleeding. Recurrence is common unless patients alter their dietary habits. Edematous, prolapsed (stage IV) internal hemorrhoids, may be treated acutely with topical creams, foams, or suppositories containing various combinations of emollients, topical anesthetics, (eg, pramoxine, dibucaine), vasoconstrictors (eg, phenylephrine), astringents (witch hazel) and corticosteroids. Common preparations include Preparation H (several formulations), Anusol HC, Proctofoam, Nupercainal, Tucks, and Doloproct (not available in the United States).

C. Surgical Treatment

Surgical excision (hemorrhoidectomy) is reserved for < 5–10% of patients with chronic severe bleeding due to stage III or stage IV hemorrhoids or patients with acute thrombosed stage IV hemorrhoids with necrosis. Complications of surgical hemorrhoidectomy include postoperative pain (which may persist for 2–4 weeks) and impaired continence.

▶ Thrombosed External Hemorrhoid

Thrombosis of the external hemorrhoidal plexus results in a perianal hematoma. It most commonly occurs in otherwise healthy young adults and may be precipitated by coughing, heavy lifting, or straining at stool. The condition is characterized by the relatively acute onset of an exquisitely painful, tense and bluish perianal nodule covered with skin that may be up to several centimeters in size. Pain

is most severe within the first few hours but gradually eases over 2–3 days as edema subsides. Symptoms may be relieved with warm sitz baths, analgesics, and ointments. If the patient is evaluated in the first 24–48 hours, removal of the clot may hasten symptomatic relief. With the patient in the lateral position, the skin around and over the lump is injected subcutaneously with 1% lidocaine using a tuberculin syringe with a 30-gauge needle. An ellipse of skin is then excised and the clot evacuated. A dry gauze dressing is applied for 12–24 hours, and daily sitz baths are then begun.

▶ When to Refer

- Stage I, II, or III: When conservative measures fail and expertise in medical procedures is needed (injection, banding, thermocoagulation).
- Stage IV: When surgical excision is required.

Lohsiriwat V. Hemorrhoids: from basic pathophysiology to clinical management. World J Gastroenterol. 2012 May 7;18(17):2009–17. [PMID: 22563187]

ANORECTAL INFECTIONS

A number of organisms can cause inflammation of the anal and rectal mucosa. Proctitis is characterized by anorectal discomfort, tenesmus, constipation, and mucus or bloody discharge. Most cases of proctitis are sexually transmitted, especially by anal-receptive intercourse. Infectious proctitis must be distinguished from noninfectious causes of anorectal symptoms, including anal fissures or fistulae, perirectal abscesses, anorectal carcinomas, and inflammatory bowel disease (ulcerative colitis or Crohn disease).

▶ Etiology & Management

Several organisms may cause infectious proctitis.

A. *Neisseria gonorrhoeae*

Gonorrhea may cause itching, burning, tenesmus, and a mucopurulent discharge, although many anorectal infections are asymptomatic. Rectal swab specimens should be taken during anoscopy for culture; Gram staining is unreliable. Cultures should also be taken from the pharynx and urethra in men and from the pharynx and cervix in women. Complications of untreated infections include strictures, fissures, fistulas, and perirectal abscesses. (For treatment, see Chapter 33.)

B. *Treponema pallidum*

Anal syphilis may be asymptomatic or may lead to perianal pain and discharge. With primary syphilis, the chancre may be at the anal margin or within the anal canal and may mimic a fissure, fistula, or ulcer. Proctitis or inguinal lymphadenopathy may be present. With secondary syphilis, condylomata lata (pale-brown, flat verrucous lesions) may be seen, with secretion of foul-smelling mucus. Although the diagnosis may be established with dark-field microscopy or fluorescent antibody testing of scrapings from the chancre or condylomas, this requires proper equipment and trained personnel. The VDRL or RPR test is positive in 75% of primary cases and in 99% of secondary cases. (For treatment, see Chapter 34.)

C. Chlamydia trachomatis

Chlamydial infection may cause proctitis similar to gonor-rheal proctitis; however, some infections are asymptomatic. It also may cause lymphogranuloma venereum, character-ized by proctocolitis with fever and bloody diarrhea, painful perianal ulcerations, anorectal strictures and fistulas, and inguinal adenopathy (buboes). Previously rare in developed countries, an increasing number of cases have been identi-fied among men who have sex with men. The diagnosis is established by serology, culture, or PCR-based testing of rectal discharge or rectal biopsy. Recommended treatment is doxycycline 100 mg orally twice daily for 21 days.

D. Herpes Simplex Type 2

Herpes simplex virus is a common cause of anorectal infec-tion. Symptoms occur 4–21 days after exposure and include severe pain, itching, constipation, tenesmus, urinary reten-tion, and radicular pain from involvement of lumbar or sacral nerve roots. Small vesicles or ulcers may be seen in the perianal area or anal canal. Sigmoidoscopy is not usu-ally necessary but may reveal vesicular or ulcerative lesions in the distal rectum. Diagnosis is established by viral cul-ture, PCR, or antigen detection assays of vesicular fluid. Symptoms resolve within 2 weeks, but viral shedding may continue for several weeks. Patients may remain asymp-tomatic with or without viral shedding or may have recur-rent mild relapses. Treatment of acute infection for 7–10 days with acyclovir, 400 mg, or famciclovir, 250 mg orally three times daily, or valacyclovir, 1 g twice daily, has been shown to reduce the duration of symptoms and viral shed-ding. Patients with AIDS and recurrent relapses may bene-fit from long-term suppressive therapy (see Chapter 31).

E. Condylomata Acuminata

Condylomata acuminata (warts) are a significant cause of anorectal symptoms. Caused by the HPV, they may occur in the perianal area, the anal canal, or the genitals. Perianal or anal warts are seen in up to 25% of men who have sex with men. HIV-positive individuals with condylomas have a higher relapse rate after therapy and a higher rate of pro-gression to high-grade dysplasia or anal cancer. The warts are located on the perianal skin and extend within the anal canal up to 2 cm above the dentate line (see Figure 6–31). Patients may have no symptoms or may report itching, bleeding, and pain. The warts may be small and flat or ver-rucous, or may form a confluent mass that may obscure the anal opening. Warts must be distinguished from condy-loma lata (secondary syphilis) or anal cancer. Biopsies should be obtained from large or suspicious lesions. Treat-ment can be difficult. Sexual partners should also be exam-ined and treated. The treatment of anogenital warts is discussed in Chapter 30. HPV vaccines have demonstrated efficacy in preventing anogenital warts and routine vacci-nation is now recommended for all children and adults 9–26 years old (see Chapters 1 and 30). Vaccination also should be considered in men who have sex with men. HIV-positive individuals with condylomas who have detectable serum HIV RNA levels should have anoscopic surveillance every 3–6 months.

Hoentjen F et al. Infectious proctitis: when to suspect it is not inflammatory bowel disease. Dig Dis Sci. 2012 Feb;57(2):269–73. [PMID: 21994137]

Palefsky JM et al. HPV vaccine against anal HPV infection and anal intraepithelial neoplasia. N Engl J Med. 2011 Oct 27;365(17):1576–85. [PMID: 22029979]

Workowski KA et al; Centers for Disease Control and Prevention (CDC). Sexually transmitted diseases treatment guidelines, 2010. MMWR Recomm Rep. 2010 Dec 17;59(RR-12):1–110. [PMID: 21160459]

FECAL INCONTINENCE

There are five general requirements for bowel continence: (1) solid or semisolid stool (even healthy young adults have difficulty maintaining continence with liquid rectal con-tents); (2) a distensible rectal reservoir (as sigmoid con-tents empty into the rectum, the vault must expand to accommodate); (3) a sensation of rectal fullness (if the patient cannot sense this, overflow may occur before the patient can take appropriate action); (4) intact pelvic nerves and muscles; and (5) the ability to reach a toilet in a timely fashion.

► Minor Incontinence

Many patients complain of inability to control flatus or slight soilage of undergarments that tends to occur after bowel movements or with straining or coughing. This may be due to local anal problems such as prolapsed hemor-rhoids that make it difficult to form a tight anal seal or isolated weakness of the internal anal sphincter, especially if stools are somewhat loose. Patients should be treated with fiber supplements to provide greater stool bulk. Cof-fee and other caffeinated beverages should be eliminated. The perianal skin should be cleansed with moist, lanolin-coated tissue (baby wipes) to reduce excoriation and infec-tion. After wiping, loose application of a cotton ball near the anal opening may absorb small amounts of fecal leak-age. Prolapsing hemorrhoids may be treated with band ligation or surgical hemorrhoidectomy. Control of flatus and seepage may be improved by Kegel perineal exercises. Conditions such as ulcerative proctitis that cause tenesmus and urgency, chronic diarrheal conditions, and irritable bowel syndrome may result in difficulty in maintaining complete continence, especially if a toilet is not readily available. Loperamide may be helpful to reduce urge incon-tinence in patients with loose stools and may be taken in anticipation of situations in which a toilet may not be read-ily available. The elderly may require more time or assis-tance to reach a toilet, which may lead to incontinence. Scheduled toileting and the availability of a bedside com-mode are helpful. Elderly patients with chronic constipation may develop stool impaction leading to "overflow" incontinence.

Major Incontinence

Complete uncontrolled loss of stool reflects a significant problem with central perception or neuromuscular function. Incontinence that occurs without awareness suggests a loss of central awareness (eg, dementia, cerebrovascular accident, multiple sclerosis) or peripheral nerve injury (eg, spinal cord injury, cauda equina syndrome, pudendal nerve damage due to obstetric trauma or pelvic floor prolapse, aging, or diabetes mellitus). Incontinence that occurs despite awareness and active efforts to retain stool suggests sphincteric damage, which may be caused by traumatic childbirth (especially forceps delivery), episiotomy, prolapse, prior anal surgery, and physical trauma.

Physical examination should include careful inspection of the perianal area for hemorrhoids, rectal prolapse, fissures, fistulas, and either gaping or a keyhole defect of the anal sphincter (indicating severe sphincteric injury or neurologic disorder). The perianal skin should be stimulated to confirm an intact anocutaneous reflex. Digital examination during relaxation gives valuable information about resting tone (due mainly to the internal sphincter) and contraction of the external sphincter and pelvic floor during squeezing. It also excludes fecal impaction. Anoscopy is required to evaluate for hemorrhoids, fissures, and fistulas. Proctosigmoidoscopy is useful to exclude rectal carcinoma or proctitis. Anal ultrasonography or pelvic MRI is the most reliable test for definition of anatomic defects in the external and internal anal sphincters. Anal manometry may also be useful to define the severity of weakness, to assess sensation, and to predict response to biofeedback training. In special circumstances, surface electromyography is useful to document sphincteric denervation and proctography to document perineal descent or rectal intussusception.

Patients who are incontinent only of loose or liquid stools are treated with bulking agents and antidiarrheal drugs (eg, loperamide, 2 mg before meals and prophylactically before social engagements, shopping trips, etc). Patients with incontinence of solid stool benefit from scheduled toilet use after glycerin suppositories or tap water enemas. Biofeedback training with anal sphincteric strengthening (Kegel) exercises (alternating 5-second squeeze and 10-second rest for 10 minutes twice daily) may be helpful in motivated patients to lower the threshold for awareness of rectal filling—or to improve anal sphincter squeeze function—or both. In 2012, the FDA approved a sterile gel (containing dextranomer and sodium hyaluronate) for submucosal injection into the proximal anal canal for the treatment of anal incontinence for patients who have not responded to conservative therapies, such as fiber supplements and antidiarrheal agents. This treatment is hypothesized to reduce incontinence episodes by bulking and narrowing the anal canal. In clinical trials, more than one-half of treated patients reported a > 50% reduction in the number of fecal incontinence episodes. The acceptance of this novel therapy in clinical practice is not yet clear. Operative management is seldom needed but should be considered in patients with major incontinence due to prior injury to the anal sphincter who have not responded to medical therapy.

When to Refer

- Conservative measures fail.
- Anorectal tests are deemed necessary (manometry, ultrasonography, electromyography).
- A surgically correctable lesion is suspected.

Brown SR et al. Surgery for faecal incontinence in adults. Cochrane Database Syst Rev. 2013 Jul 2;7:CD001757. [PMID: 23821339]

Omar MI et al. Drug treatment for faecal incontinence in adults. Cochrane Database Syst Rev. 2013 Jun 11;6:CD002116. [PMID: 23757096]

Thin NN et al. Systematic review of the clinical effectiveness of neuromodulation in the treatment of faecal incontinence. Br J Surg. 2013 Oct;100(11):1430–47. [PMID: 24037562]

OTHER ANAL CONDITIONS

Anal Fissures

Anal fissures are linear or rocket-shaped ulcers that are usually < 5 mm in length. Most fissures are believed to arise from trauma to the anal canal during defecation, perhaps caused by straining, constipation, or high internal sphincter tone. They occur most commonly in the posterior midline, but 10% occur anteriorly. Fissures that occur off the midline should raise suspicion for Crohn disease, HIV/AIDS, tuberculosis, syphilis, or anal carcinoma. Patients complain of severe, tearing pain during defecation followed by throbbing discomfort that may lead to constipation due to fear of recurrent pain. There may be mild associated hematochezia, with blood on the stool or toilet paper. Anal fissures are confirmed by visual inspection of the anal verge while gently separating the buttocks. Acute fissures look like cracks in the epithelium. Chronic fissures result in fibrosis and the development of a skin tag at the outermost edge (sentinel pile). Digital and anoscopic examinations may cause severe pain and may not be possible. Medical management is directed at promoting effortless, painless bowel movements. Fiber supplements and sitz baths should be prescribed. Topical anesthetics (5% lidocaine; 2.5% lidocaine plus 2.5% prilocaine) may provide temporary relief. Healing occurs within 2 months in up to 45% of patients with conservative management. Chronic fissures may be treated with topical 0.2–0.4% nitroglycerin or diltiazem 2% ointment (1 cm of ointment) applied twice daily just inside the anus with the tip of a finger for 4–8 weeks or injection of botulinum toxin (20 units) into the internal anal sphincter. All of these treatments result in healing in 50–80% of patients with chronic anal fissure, but headaches occur in up to 40% of patients treated with nitroglycerin. Fissures recur in up to 40% of patients after treatment. Chronic or recurrent fissures benefit from lateral internal sphincterotomy; however, minor incontinence may complicate this procedure.

Nelson RL et al. Non surgical therapy for anal fissure. Cochrane Database Syst Rev. 2012 Feb 15;2:CD003431. [PMID: 22336789]

Nelson RL et al. Operative procedures for fissure in ano. Cochrane Database Syst Rev. 2011 Nov 9;(11):CD002199. [PMID: 22071803]

Sajid MS et al. Systematic review of the use of topical diltiazem compared with glyceryltrinitrate for the nonoperative management of chronic anal fissure. Colorectal Dis. 2013 Jan;15(1):19–26. [PMID: 22487078]

Yiannakopoulou E. Botulinum toxin and anal fissure: efficacy and safety systematic review. Int J Colorectal Dis. 2012 Jan;27(1):1–9. [PMID: 21822595]

Perianal Abscess & Fistula

The anal glands located at the base of the anal crypts at the dentate line may become infected, leading to abscess formation. Other causes of abscess include anal fissure and Crohn disease. Abscesses may extend upward or downward through the intersphincteric plane. Symptoms of perianal abscess are throbbing, continuous perianal pain. Erythema, fluctuance, and swelling may be found in the perianal region on external examination or in the ischiorectal fossa on digital rectal examination. Perianal abscesses are treated with local incision and drainage, while ischiorectal abscesses require drainage in the operating room. After drainage of an abscess, most patients are found to have a fistula in ano.

Fistula in ano most often arises in an anal crypt and is usually preceded by an anal abscess. In patients with fistulas that connect to the rectum, other disorders such as Crohn disease, lymphogranuloma venereum, rectal tuberculosis, and cancer should be considered. Fistulas are associated with purulent discharge that may lead to itching, tenderness, and pain. The treatment of Crohn-related fistula is discussed elsewhere in this chapter. Treatment of simple idiopathic fistula in ano is by surgical incision or excision under anesthesia. Care must be taken to preserve the anal sphincters. Surgical fistulotomy for treatment of complex (high, transphincteric) anal fissures carries a high risk of incontinence. Techniques for healing the fistula while preserving the sphincter include an endoanal advancement flap over the internal opening and insertion of a bioprosthetic plug into the fistula opening.

Abcarian H. Anorectal infection: abscess-fistula. Clin Colon Rectal Surg. 2011 Mar;24(1):14–21. [PMID: 22379401]

Shawki S et al. Idiopathic fistula-in-ano. World J Gastroenterol. 2011 Jul 28;17(28):3277–85. [PMID: 21876614]

Perianal Pruritus

Perianal pruritus is characterized by perianal itching and discomfort. It may be caused by poor anal hygiene associated with fistulas, fissures, prolapsed hemorrhoids, skin tags, and minor incontinence. Conversely, overzealous cleansing with soaps may contribute to local irritation or contact dermatitis. Contact dermatitis, atopic dermatitis, bacterial infections (*Staphylococcus* or *Streptococcus*), parasites (pinworms, scabies), candidal infection (especially in diabetics), sexually transmitted disease (condylomata acuminata, herpes, syphilis, molluscum contagiosum), and other skin conditions (psoriasis, Paget, lichen sclerosis) must be excluded. In patients with idiopathic perianal pruritus, examination may reveal erythema, excoriations, or lichenified, eczematous skin. Education is vital to successful therapy. Spicy foods, coffee, chocolate, and tomatoes may cause irritation and should be eliminated. After bowel movements, the perianal area should be cleansed with nonscented wipes premoistened with lanolin followed by gentle drying. A piece of cotton ball should be tucked next to the anal opening to absorb perspiration or fecal seepage. Anal ointments and lotions may exacerbate the condition and should be avoided. A short course of high-potency topical corticosteroid may be tried, although efficacy has not been demonstrated. Diluted capsaicin cream (0.006%) led to symptomatic relief in 75% of patients in a double-blind crossover study. (See Chapter 39 for Carcinoma of the Anus.)

Markell KW et al. Pruritus ani: etiology and management. Surg Clin North Am. 2010 Feb;90(1):125–35. [PMID: 20109637]

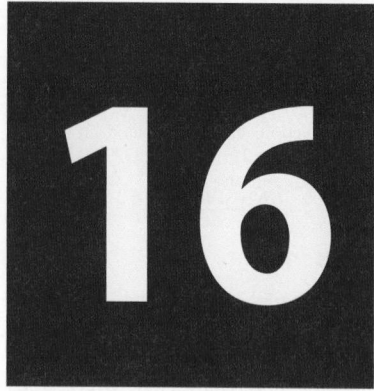

Liver, Biliary Tract, & Pancreas Disorders

Lawrence S. Friedman, MD

JAUNDICE & EVALUATION OF ABNORMAL LIVER BIOCHEMICAL TESTS

ESSENTIALS OF DIAGNOSIS

► Jaundice results from accumulation of bilirubin in body tissues; the cause may be hepatic or nonhepatic.

► Hyperbilirubinemia may be due to abnormalities in the formation, transport, metabolism, or excretion of bilirubin.

► Persistent mild elevations of the aminotransferase levels are common in clinical practice and caused most often by nonalcoholic fatty liver disease.

► Evaluation of obstructive jaundice begins with ultrasonography and is usually followed by cholangiography.

General Considerations

Jaundice (icterus) results from the accumulation of bilirubin—a product of heme metabolism—in body tissues. Hyperbilirubinemia may be due to abnormalities in the formation, transport, metabolism, or excretion of bilirubin. Total serum bilirubin is normally 0.2–1.2 mg/dL (3.42–20.52 mcmol/L) (mean levels are higher in men than women and higher in whites and Hispanics than blacks and correlate with an increased risk of symptomatic gallstone disease and inversely with the risk of stroke, respiratory disease, cardiovascular disease, and mortality, presumably because of an antioxidant effect). Jaundice may not be recognizable until serum bilirubin levels are about 3 mg/dL (51.3 mcmol/L).

Jaundice is caused by predominantly unconjugated or conjugated bilirubin in the serum (Table 16–1). Unconjugated hyperbilirubinemia may result from overproduction of bilirubin because of hemolysis; impaired hepatic uptake of bilirubin due to certain drugs; or impaired conjugation of bilirubin by glucuronide, as in Gilbert syndrome, due to mild decreases in uridine diphosphate (UDP) glucuronyl transferase, or Crigler–Najjar syndrome, caused by moderate decreases or absence of UDP glucuronyl transferase. Hemolysis alone rarely elevates the serum bilirubin level to more than 7 mg/dL (119.7 mcmol/L). Predominantly conjugated hyperbilirubinemia may result from impaired excretion of bilirubin from the liver due to hepatocellular disease, drugs, sepsis, or hereditary hepatocanalicular transport defects (such as Dubin–Johnson syndrome, progressive familial intrahepatic cholestasis syndromes, and some cases of intrahepatic cholestasis of pregnancy) or from extrahepatic biliary obstruction. Features of some hyperbilirubinemic syndromes are summarized in Table 16–2. The term "cholestasis" denotes retention of bile in the liver, and the term "cholestatic jaundice" is often used when conjugated hyperbilirubinemia results from impaired bile flow.

► Clinical Findings

A. Unconjugated Hyperbilirubinemia

Stool and urine color are normal, and there is mild jaundice and indirect (unconjugated) hyperbilirubinemia with no bilirubin in the urine. Splenomegaly occurs in hemolytic disorders except in sickle cell disease.

B. Conjugated Hyperbilirubinemia

1. Hereditary cholestatic syndromes or intrahepatic cholestasis—The patient may be asymptomatic; cholestasis is often accompanied by pruritus, light-colored stools, and jaundice.

2. Hepatocellular disease—Malaise, anorexia, low-grade fever, and right upper quadrant discomfort are frequent. Dark urine, jaundice, and, in women, amenorrhea occur. An enlarged tender liver, vascular spiders, palmar erythema, ascites, gynecomastia, sparse body hair, fetor hepaticus, and asterixis may be present, depending on the cause, severity, and chronicity of liver dysfunction.

C. Biliary Obstruction

There may be right upper quadrant pain, weight loss (suggesting carcinoma), jaundice, dark urine, and light-colored stools. Symptoms and signs may be intermittent if caused

Table 16–1. Classification of jaundice.

Type of Hyperbilirubinemia	Location and Cause
Unconjugated hyperbilirubinemia (predominant indirect-reacting bilirubin)	Increased bilirubin production (eg, hemolytic anemias, hemolytic reactions, hematoma, pulmonary infarction) Impaired bilirubin uptake and storage (eg, posthepatitis hyperbilirubinemia, Gilbert syndrome, Crigler-Najjar syndrome, drug reactions)
Conjugated hyperbilirubinemia (predominant direct-reacting bilirubin)	**HEREDITARY CHOLESTATIC SYNDROMES**
	Faulty excretion of bilirubin conjugates (eg, Dubin-Johnson syndrome, Rotor syndrome) or mutation in genes coding for bile salt transport proteins (eg, progressive familial intrahepatic cholestasis syndromes, benign recurrent intrahepatic cholestasis, and some cases of intrahepatic cholestasis of pregnancy)
	HEPATOCELLULAR DYSFUNCTION
	Biliary epithelial and hepatocyte damage (eg, hepatitis, hepatic cirrhosis) Intrahepatic cholestasis (eg, certain drugs, biliary cirrhosis, sepsis, postoperative jaundice) Hepatocellular damage or intrahepatic cholestasis resulting from miscellaneous causes (eg, spirochetal infections, infectious mononucleosis, cholangitis, sarcoidosis, lymphomas, industrial toxins)
	BILIARY OBSTRUCTION
	Choledocholithiasis, biliary atresia, carcinoma of biliary duct, sclerosing cholangitis, choledochal cyst, external pressure on bile duct, pancreatitis, pancreatic neoplasms

Table 16–2. Hyperbilirubinemic disorders.

	Nature of Defect	Type of Hyperbilirubinemia	Clinical and Pathologic Characteristics
Gilbert syndrome	Reduced activity of glucuronyl transferase	Unconjugated (indirect) bilirubin	Benign, asymptomatic hereditary jaundice. Hyperbilirubinemia increased by 24- to 36-hour fast. No treatment required. Prognosis excellent.
Dubin-Johnson syndrome[1]	Faulty excretory function of hepatocytes	Conjugated (direct) bilirubin	Benign, asymptomatic hereditary jaundice. Gallbladder does not visualize on oral cholecystography. Liver darkly pigmented on gross examination. Biopsy shows centrilobular brown pigment. Prognosis excellent.
Rotor syndrome[2]			Similar to Dubin-Johnson syndrome, but liver is not pigmented and the gallbladder is visualized on oral cholecystography. Prognosis excellent.
Recurrent intrahepatic cholestasis[3]	Cholestasis, often on a familial basis	Unconjugated plus conjugated (total) bilirubin	Episodic attacks of jaundice, itching, and malaise. Onset in early life and may persist for a lifetime. Alkaline phosphatase increased. Cholestasis found on liver biopsy. (Biopsy may be normal during remission.) Prognosis is generally excellent for "benign" recurrent intrahepatic cholestasis but may not be for familial forms.
Intrahepatic cholestasis of pregnancy[4]	Cholestasis		Benign cholestatic jaundice, usually occurring in the third trimester of pregnancy. Itching, gastrointestinal symptoms, and abnormal liver excretory function tests. Cholestasis noted on liver biopsy. Prognosis excellent, but recurrence with subsequent pregnancies or use of oral contraceptives is characteristic.

[1]Dubin-Johnson syndrome is caused by a mutation in the *ABCC2* gene coding for organic anion transporter multidrug resistance protein 2 in bile canaliculi on chromosome 10q24.

[2]Rotor syndrome is caused by mutations in the genes coding for organic anion transporting polypeptides OATP1B1 and OATP1B3 on chromosome 12p.

[3]Mutations in genes that control hepatocellular transport systems that are involved in the formation of bile and inherited as autosomal recessive traits are on chromosomes 18q21–22, 2q24, and 7q21 in families with progressive familial intrahepatic cholestasis. Gene mutations on chromosome 18q21–22 alter a P-type ATPase expressed in the small intestine and liver and other tissues on chromosome 2q24 alter the bile acid export pump and also cause benign recurrent intrahepatic cholestasis.

[4]Mutations in the *MDR3* gene on chromosome 7q21 that are responsible for progressive familial intrahepatic cholestasis type 3 account for some cases of intrahepatic cholestasis of pregnancy.

by a stone, carcinoma of the ampulla, or cholangiocarcinoma. Pain may be absent early in pancreatic cancer. Occult blood in the stools suggests cancer of the ampulla. Hepatomegaly and a palpable gallbladder (Courvoisier sign) are characteristic, but neither specific nor sensitive, of a pancreatic head tumor. Fever and chills are more common in benign obstruction with associated cholangitis.

▶ Diagnostic Studies (Tables 16–3, 16–4)

A. Laboratory Findings

Serum alanine and aspartate aminotransferase (ALT and AST) levels decrease with age and correlate with body mass index and mortality from liver disease and inversely with caffeine consumption and possibly serum vitamin D levels. There is controversy about whether an elevated ALT level is associated with mortality from coronary artery disease, cancer, diabetes mellitus, and all causes. Normal reference values for ALT and AST are lower than generally reported when persons with risk factors for fatty liver are excluded. Truncal fat and early-onset paternal obesity are risk factors for increased ALT levels. Levels are mildly elevated in > 25% of persons with untreated celiac disease and in type 1 diabetic patients with so-called glycogenic hepatopathy and often rise transiently in healthy persons who begin taking 4 g of acetaminophen per day or experience rapid weight gain on a fast-food diet. Levels may rise strikingly but transiently in patients with acute biliary obstruction from choledocholithiasis. Nonalcoholic fatty liver disease is by far the most common cause of mildly to moderately elevated aminotransferase levels. Elevated ALT and AST levels, often > 1000 units/L (> 20 mckat/L), are the hallmark of hepatocellular necrosis or inflammation. Elevated alkaline phosphatase levels are seen in cholestasis or infiltrative liver disease (such as tumor, granulomas, or amyloidosis). Isolated alkaline phosphatase elevations of hepatic rather than bone, intestinal, or placental origin are confirmed by concomitant elevation of gamma-glutamyl transpeptidase or 5'-nucleotidase levels. Serum gamma-glutamyl transpeptidase levels appear to correlate with the risk of mortality and disability in the general population. The differential diagnosis of any liver test elevation includes toxicity caused by drugs, herbal remedies, and toxins.

Table 16–4. Causes of serum aminotransferase elevations.[1]

Mild Elevations (< 5 × normal)	Severe Elevations (> 15 × normal)
Hepatic: ALT-predominant	Acute viral hepatitis
Chronic hepatitis B, C, and D	(A–E, herpes)
Acute viral hepatitis (A-E, EBV, CMV)	Medications/toxins
Steatosis/steatohepatitis	Ischemic hepatitis
Hemochromatosis	Autoimmune hepatitis
Medications/toxins	Wilson disease
Autoimmune hepatitis	Acute bile duct
Alpha-1-antitrypsin (alpha-1-	obstruction
antiprotease) deficiency	Acute Budd-Chiari
Wilson disease	syndrome
Celiac disease	Hepatic artery ligation
Hepatic: AST–predominant	
Alcohol-related liver injury	
(AST:ALT > 2:1)	
Cirrhosis	
Nonhepatic	
Strenuous exercise	
Hemolysis	
Myopathy	
Thyroid disease	
Macro-AST	

[1]Almost any liver disease can cause moderate aminotransferase elevations (5–15 × normal).
ALT, alanine aminotransferase; AST, aspartate aminotransferase; CMV, cytomegalovirus; EBV, Epstein-Barr virus.
Adapted with permission from Green RM et al. AGA technical review on the evaluation of liver chemistry tests. Gastroenterology. 2002 Oct;123(4):1367–84.

Table 16–3. Liver biochemical tests: Normal values and changes in hepatocellular and obstructive jaundice.

Tests	Normal Values	Hepatocellular Jaundice	Obstructive Jaundice
Bilirubin[1]			
Direct	0.1–0.3 mg/dL (1.71–5.13 mcmol/L)	Increased	Increased
Indirect	0.2–0.7 mg/dL (3.42–11.97 mcmol/L)	Increased	Increased
Urine bilirubin	None	Increased	Increased
Serum albumin	3.5–5.5 g/dL (35–55 g/L)	Decreased	Generally unchanged
Alkaline phosphatase	30–115 units/L (0.6–2.3 mkat/L)	Mildly increased (+)	Markedly increased (++++)
Prothrombin time	INR of 1.0–1.4. After vitamin K, 10% decrease in 24 hours	Prolonged if damage is severe; does not respond to parenteral vitamin K	Prolonged if obstruction is marked; generally responds to parenteral vitamin K
ALT, AST	ALT, ≤ 30 units/L (0.6 mkat/L) (men), ≤ 19 units/L (0.38 mkat/L) (women); AST, 5–40 units/L (0.1–0.8 mkat/L)	Increased, as in viral hepatitis	Minimally increased

[1]Measured by the van den Bergh reaction, which overestimates direct bilirubin in normal persons.
ALT, alanine aminotransferase; AST, aspartate aminotransferase; INR, international normalized ratio.

B. Imaging

Demonstration of dilated bile ducts by ultrasonography or CT indicates biliary obstruction (90–95% sensitivity). Ultrasonography, CT, and MRI may also demonstrate hepatomegaly, intrahepatic tumors, and portal hypertension. Use of color Doppler ultrasonography or contrast agents that produce microbubbles increases the sensitivity of transcutaneous ultrasonography for detecting small neoplasms. MRI is the most accurate technique for identifying isolated liver lesions such as hemangiomas, focal nodular hyperplasia, or focal fatty infiltration and for detecting hepatic iron overload. The most sensitive techniques for detection of individual small hepatic metastases in patients eligible for resection are multiphasic helical or multislice CT; CT arterial portography, in which imaging follows intravenous contrast infusion via a catheter placed in the superior mesenteric artery; MRI with use of gadolinium or ferumoxides as contrast agents; and intraoperative ultrasonography. Dynamic gadolinium-enhanced MRI and MRI following administration of superparamagnetic iron oxide show promise in visualizing hepatic fibrosis. Because of its much lower cost, ultrasonography is preferable to CT (~six times more expensive) or MRI (~seven times more expensive) as a screening test. Positron emission tomography (PET) can be used to detect small pancreatic tumors and metastases. Ultrasonography can detect gallstones with a sensitivity of 95%.

Magnetic resonance cholangiopancreatography (MRCP) is a sensitive, noninvasive method of detecting bile duct stones, strictures, and dilatation; however, it is less reliable than endoscopic retrograde cholangiopancreatography (ERCP) for distinguishing malignant from benign strictures. ERCP requires a skilled endoscopist and may be used to demonstrate pancreatic or ampullary causes of jaundice, carry out papillotomy and stone extraction, insert a stent through an obstructing lesion, or facilitate direct cholangiopancreatoscopy. Complications of ERCP include pancreatitis ($\leq$ 5%) and, less commonly, cholangitis, bleeding, or duodenal perforation after papillotomy. Risk factors for post-ERCP pancreatitis include female sex, prior post-ERCP pancreatitis, suspected sphincter of Oddi dysfunction, and a difficult or failed cannulation. Percutaneous transhepatic cholangiography (PTC) is an alternative approach to evaluating the anatomy of the biliary tree. Serious complications of PTC occur in 3% and include fever, bacteremia, bile peritonitis, and intraperitoneal hemorrhage. Endoscopic ultrasonography is the most sensitive test for detecting small lesions of the ampulla or pancreatic head and for detecting portal vein invasion by pancreatic cancer. It is also accurate in detecting or excluding bile duct stones.

C. Liver Biopsy

Percutaneous liver biopsy is the definitive study for determining the cause and histologic severity of hepatocellular dysfunction or infiltrative liver disease. In patients with suspected metastatic disease or a hepatic mass, it is performed under ultrasound or CT guidance. A transjugular route can be used in patients with coagulopathy or ascites.

The risk of bleeding after a percutaneous liver biopsy is approximately 0.5% and is increased in persons with a platelet count $\leq$ 60,000/mcL (60 × 10^9/mcL). Panels of blood tests (eg, FibroSure) and ultrasound or magnetic resonance elastography to measure liver stiffness are emerging approaches for estimating the stage of liver fibrosis and degree of portal hypertension without the need for liver biopsy.

▶ When to Refer

Patients with jaundice should be referred for diagnostic procedures.

▶ When to Admit

Patients with liver failure should be hospitalized.

Berzosa M et al. Diagnostic bedside EUS in the intensive care unit: a single-center experience. Gastrointest Endosc. 2013 Feb;77(2):200–8. [PMID: 23218946]

Halilbasic E et al. Bile acid transporters and regulatory nuclear receptors in the liver and beyond. J Hepatol. 2013 Jan;58(1):155–68. [PMID: 22885388]

Moon JH et al. Peroral cholangioscopy: diagnostic and therapeutic applications. Gastroenterology. 2013 Feb;144(2):276–82. [PMID: 23127575]

Stender S et al. Extreme bilirubin levels as a causal risk factor for symptomatic gallstone disease. JAMA Intern Med. 2013 Jul 8;173(13):1222–8. [PMID: 23753274]

▼ DISEASES OF THE LIVER

See Chapter 39 for Hepatocellular Carcinoma.

ACUTE HEPATITIS A

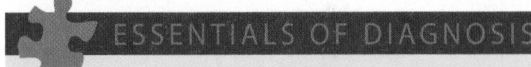

ESSENTIALS OF DIAGNOSIS

▶ Prodrome of anorexia, nausea, vomiting, malaise, aversion to smoking.

▶ Fever, enlarged and tender liver, jaundice.

▶ Normal to low white cell count; markedly elevated aminotransferases.

▶ General Considerations

Hepatitis can be caused by viruses, including the five hepatotropic viruses—A, B, C, D, and E—and many drugs and toxic agents; the clinical manifestations may be similar regardless of cause. Hepatitis A virus (HAV) is a 27-nm RNA hepatovirus (in the picornavirus family) that causes epidemics or sporadic cases of hepatitis. The virus is transmitted by the fecal–oral route, and its spread is favored by crowding and poor sanitation. Since introduction of the HAV vaccine in the United States in 1995, the incidence rate of HAV infection has declined from 14 to 1.3 per 100,000 population, with a corresponding decline of 32% in the mortality rate, and international travel has emerged as the leading risk factor, accounting for over 40% of cases, with another 18% of cases attributable to exposure to an international traveler. Common source outbreaks may still result from contaminated water or food, including inadequately cooked shellfish. Outbreaks among people who inject drugs and cases among international adoptees and their contacts also have been reported.

The incubation period averages 30 days. HAV is excreted in feces for up to 2 weeks before clinical illness but rarely after the first week of illness. The mortality rate for hepatitis A is low, and fulminant hepatitis A is uncommon except for rare instances in which it occurs in a patient with concomitant chronic hepatitis C. There is no chronic carrier state. In the United States, about 30% of the population have serologic evidence of previous HAV infection.

► Clinical Findings

A. Symptoms and Signs

Figure 16–1 shows the typical course of acute hepatitis A. Clinical illness is more severe in adults than in children, in whom it is usually asymptomatic. The onset may be abrupt or insidious, with malaise, myalgia, arthralgia, easy fatigability, upper respiratory symptoms, and anorexia. A distaste for smoking, paralleling anorexia, may occur early. Nausea and vomiting are frequent, and diarrhea or constipation may occur. Fever is generally present but is low-grade except in occasional cases in which systemic toxicity may occur. Defervescence and a fall in pulse rate often coincide with the onset of jaundice.

Abdominal pain is usually mild and constant in the right upper quadrant or epigastrium, often aggravated by jarring or exertion, and rarely may be severe enough to simulate cholecystitis.

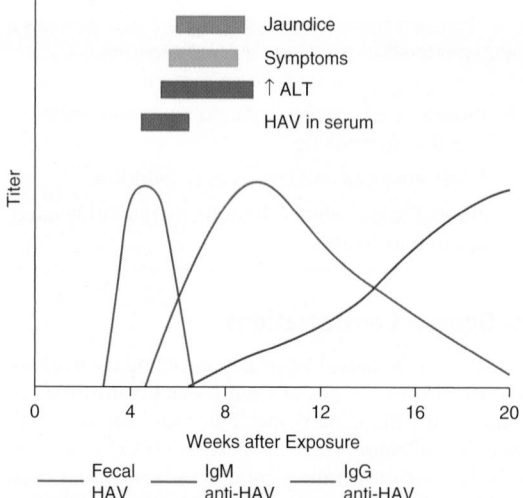

▲ **Figure 16–1.** The typical course of acute type A hepatitis. (HAV, hepatitis A virus; anti-HAV, antibody to hepatitis A virus; ALT, alanine aminotransferase.)
(Reprinted, with permission, from Koff RS. Acute viral hepatitis. In: Friedman LS, Keeffe EB [editors]. *Handbook of Liver Disease,* 3rd ed. Philadelphia: Saunders Elsevier, 2012.)

Jaundice occurs after 5–10 days but may appear at the same time as the initial symptoms. In many patients, jaundice never develops. With the onset of jaundice, prodromal symptoms often worsen, followed by progressive clinical improvement. Stools may be acholic during this phase.

The acute illness usually subsides over 2–3 weeks with complete clinical and laboratory recovery by 9 weeks. In some cases, clinical, biochemical, and serologic recovery may be followed by one or two relapses, but recovery is the rule. A protracted course has been reported to be associated with HLA *DRB1*1301*. Acute cholecystitis occasionally complicates the course of acute hepatitis A.

Hepatomegaly—rarely marked—is present in over half of cases. Liver tenderness is usually present. Splenomegaly is reported in 15% of patients, and soft, enlarged lymph nodes—especially in the cervical or epitrochlear areas—may occur.

B. Laboratory Findings

The white blood cell count is normal to low, especially in the preicteric phase. Large atypical lymphocytes may occasionally be seen. Mild proteinuria is common, and bilirubinuria often precedes the appearance of jaundice. Strikingly elevated ALT or AST levels occur early, followed by elevations of bilirubin and alkaline phosphatase; in a minority of patients, the latter persist after aminotransferase levels have normalized. Cholestasis is occasionally marked. Antibody to hepatitis A (anti-HAV) appears early in the course of the illness (Figure 16–1). Both IgM and IgG anti-HAV are detectable in serum soon after the onset. Peak titers of IgM anti-HAV occur during the first week of clinical disease and disappear within 3–6 months. Detection of IgM anti-HAV is an excellent test for diagnosing acute hepatitis A but is not recommended for the evaluation of asymptomatic persons with persistently elevated serum aminotransferase levels because false-positive results occur. False-negative results have been described in a patient receiving rituximab for rheumatoid arthritis. Titers of IgG anti-HAV rise after 1 month of the disease and may persist for years. IgG anti-HAV (in the absence of IgM anti-HAV) indicates previous exposure to HAV, noninfectivity, and immunity.

► Differential Diagnosis

The differential diagnosis includes other viruses that cause hepatitis, particularly hepatitis B and C, and diseases such as infectious mononucleosis, cytomegalovirus infection, and herpes simplex virus infection; spirochetal diseases such as leptospirosis and secondary syphilis; brucellosis; rickettsial diseases such as Q fever; drug-induced liver disease; and ischemic hepatitis (shock liver). Occasionally, autoimmune hepatitis (see below) may have an acute onset mimicking acute viral hepatitis. Rarely, metastatic cancer of the liver, lymphoma, or leukemia may present as a hepatitis-like picture.

The prodromal phase of viral hepatitis must be distinguished from other infectious disease such as influenza, upper respiratory infections, and the prodromal stages of the exanthematous diseases. Cholestasis may mimic obstructive jaundice.

Prevention

Strict isolation of patients is not necessary, but hand washing after bowel movements is required. Unvaccinated persons who are exposed to HAV are advised to receive postexposure prophylaxis with a single dose of HAV vaccine or immune globulin (0.02 mL/kg) as soon as possible. The vaccine is preferred in healthy persons ages 1 year to 40 years, whereas immune globulin is preferred in those who are younger than 1 year or older than 40 years or who are immunocompromised or who have chronic liver disease.

Two effective inactivated hepatitis A vaccines are available in the United States and recommended for persons living in or traveling to endemic areas (including military personnel), patients with chronic liver disease upon diagnosis after prescreening for immunity (although the cost-effectiveness of vaccinating all patients with concomitant chronic hepatitis C has been questioned), persons with clotting-factor disorders who are treated with concentrates, men who have sex with men, animal handlers, illicit drug users, sewage workers, food handlers, close personal contacts of international adoptees, and children and caregivers in day-care centers and institutions. For healthy travelers, a single dose of vaccine at any time before departure can provide adequate protection. Routine vaccination is advised for all children in states with an incidence of hepatitis A at least twice the national average and has been approved by the Advisory Committee on Immunization Practices of the Centers for Disease Control and Prevention (CDC) for use in all children between ages 1 and 2 in the United States. HAV vaccine is also effective in the prevention of secondary spread to household contacts of primary cases. The recommended dose for adults is 1 mL (1440 ELISA units) of Havrix (GlaxoSmithKline) or 1 mL (50 units) of Vaqta (Merck) intramuscularly, followed by a booster dose at 6–18 months. A combined hepatitis A and B vaccine (Twinrix, GlaxoSmithKline) is available. HIV infection impairs the response to the HAV vaccine, especially in persons with a CD4 count < 200/mcL.

Treatment

Bed rest is recommended only if symptoms are marked. If nausea and vomiting are pronounced or if oral intake is substantially decreased, intravenous 10% glucose is indicated.

Dietary management consists of palatable meals as tolerated, without overfeeding; breakfast is usually tolerated best. Strenuous physical exertion, alcohol, and hepatotoxic agents should be avoided. Small doses of oxazepam are safe because metabolism is not hepatic; morphine sulfate should be avoided.

Corticosteroids have no benefit in patients with viral hepatitis, including those with fulminant disease.

Prognosis

In most patients, clinical recovery is generally complete within 3 months. Laboratory evidence of liver dysfunction may persist for a longer period, but most patients recover completely. Hepatitis A does not cause chronic liver disease, although it may persist for up to 1 year, and clinical and biochemical relapses may occur before full recovery. The mortality rate is < 0.6%.

When to Admit

- Encephalopathy is present.
- INR > 1.6.
- The patient is unable to maintain hydration.

Carrion AF et al. Viral hepatitis in the elderly. Am J Gastroenterol. 2012 May;107(5):691–7. [PMID: 22290404]

Chen LH et al. Business travelers: vaccination considerations for this population. Expert Rev Vaccines. 2013 Apr;12(4):453–66. [PMID: 23560925]

Rowe IA et al. Hepatitis A virus vaccination in persons with hepatitis C virus infection: consequences of quality measure implementation. Hepatology. 2012 Aug;56(2):501–6. [PMID: 22371026]

ACUTE HEPATITIS B

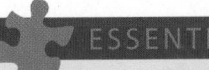

ESSENTIALS OF DIAGNOSIS

- ▶ Prodrome of anorexia, nausea, vomiting, malaise, aversion to smoking.
- ▶ Fever, enlarged and tender liver, jaundice.
- ▶ Normal to low white blood cell count; markedly elevated aminotransferases early in the course.
- ▶ Liver biopsy shows hepatocellular necrosis and mononuclear infiltrate but is rarely indicated.

General Considerations

Hepatitis B virus (HBV) is a 42-nm hepadnavirus with a partially double-stranded DNA genome, inner core protein (hepatitis B core antigen, HBcAg), and outer surface coat (hepatitis B surface antigen, HBsAg). There are eight different genotypes (A–H), which may influence the course of infection and responsiveness to antiviral therapy. HBV is usually transmitted by inoculation of infected blood or blood products or by sexual contact and is present in saliva, semen, and vaginal secretions. HBsAg-positive mothers may transmit HBV at delivery; the risk of chronic infection in the infant is as high as 90%.

Since 1990, the incidence of HBV infection in the United States has decreased from 8.5 to 1.5 cases per 100,000 population. The prevalence is 0.27% in persons aged 6 or over. Because of universal vaccination since 1992, exposure to HBV is now very low among persons aged 18 or younger. HBV is prevalent in men who have sex with men and in people who inject drugs (about 7% of HIV-infected persons are coinfected with HBV), but the greatest number of cases result from heterosexual transmission. Other groups at risk include patients and staff at hemodialysis centers, physicians, dentists, nurses, and personnel working in clinical and pathology laboratories and blood banks. Half of all patients with acute hepatitis B in the United States have previously been incarcerated or treated for a sexually transmitted disease. The risk of HBV infection from a blood transfusion in the United States is about 1 in 350,000 units transfused or less.

The incubation period of hepatitis B is 6 weeks to 6 months (average 12–14 weeks). The onset of hepatitis B is more insidious and the aminotransferase levels are higher on average than in HAV infection. Fulminant hepatitis occurs in <1%, with a mortality rate of up to 60%. Following acute hepatitis B, HBV infection persists in 1–2% of immunocompetent adults but in a higher percentage of children and immunocompromised adults. There are as many as 2.2 million persons (including an estimated 1.32 million foreign-born persons from endemic areas) with chronic hepatitis B in the United States. Persons with chronic hepatitis B, particularly when HBV infection is acquired early in life and viral replication persists, are at substantial risk for cirrhosis and hepatocellular carcinoma (up to 25–40%); men are at greater risk than women.

► **Clinical Findings**

A. Symptoms and Signs

The clinical picture of viral hepatitis is extremely variable, ranging from asymptomatic infection without jaundice to a fulminating disease and death in a few days. Figure 16–2 shows the typical course of HBV infection. The onset may be abrupt or insidious, and the clinical features are similar to those for acute hepatitis A (see earlier). Serum sickness may be seen early in acute hepatitis B. Fever is generally present and is low-grade. Defervescence and a fall in pulse rate often coincide with the onset of jaundice. Infection caused by HBV may be associated with glomerulonephritis and polyarteritis nodosa.

The acute illness usually subsides over 2–3 weeks with complete clinical and laboratory recovery by 16 weeks. In 5–10% of cases, the course may be more protracted, but < 1% will have a fulminant course. Hepatitis B may become chronic (see below).

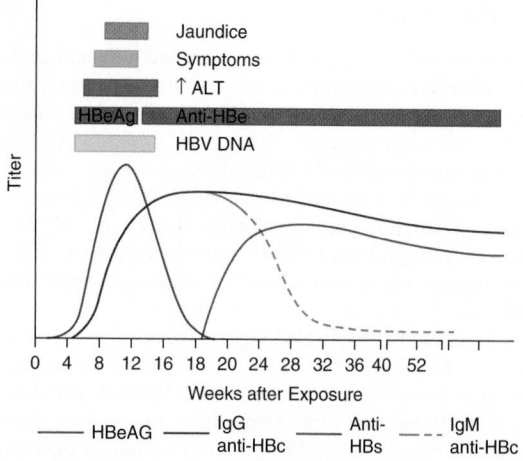

▲ **Figure 16–2.** The typical course of acute type B hepatitis. (anti-HBs, antibody to HBsAg; HBeAg, hepatitis Be antigen; anti-HBe, antibody to HBeAg; anti-HBc, antibody to hepatitis B core antigen; ALT, alanine aminotransferase.) (Reprinted, with permission, from Koff RS. Acute viral hepatitis. In: Friedman LS, Keeffe EB [editors]. *Handbook of Liver Disease*, 3rd ed. Philadelphia: Saunders Elsevier, 2012.)

B. Laboratory Findings

The laboratory features are similar to those for acute hepatitis A (see earlier), although serum aminotransferase levels are higher on average in acute hepatitis B, and marked cholestasis is not a feature. Marked prolongation of the prothrombin time in severe hepatitis correlates with increased mortality.

There are several antigens and antibodies as well as HBV DNA that relate to HBV infection and that are useful in diagnosis. Interpretation of common serologic patterns is shown in Table 16–5.

1. HBsAg—The appearance of HBsAg in serum is the first evidence of infection, appearing before biochemical evidence of liver disease, and persisting throughout the

Table 16–5. Common serologic patterns in hepatitis B virus infection and their interpretation.

HBsAg	Anti-HBs	Anti-HBc	HBeAg	Anti-HBe	Interpretation
+	–	IgM	+	–	Acute hepatitis B
+	–	IgG[1]	+	–	Chronic hepatitis B with active viral replication
+	–	IgG	–	+	Chronic hepatitis B generally with low viral replication
+	+	IgG	+ or –	+ or –	Chronic hepatitis B with heterotypic anti-HBs (about 10% of cases)
–		IgM	+ or –	–	Acute hepatitis B
–	+	IgG	–	+ or –	Recovery from hepatitis B (immunity)
–	+	–	–	–	Vaccination (immunity)
–	–	IgG	–	–	False-positive; less commonly, infection in remote past

[1]Low levels of IgM anti-HBc may also be detected.

clinical illness. Persistence of HBsAg more than 6 months after the acute illness signifies chronic hepatitis B.

2. Anti-HBs—Specific antibody to HBsAg (anti-HBs) appears in most individuals after clearance of HBsAg and after successful vaccination against hepatitis B. Disappearance of HBsAg and the appearance of anti-HBs signal recovery from HBV infection, noninfectivity, and immunity.

3. Anti-HBc—IgM anti-HBc appears shortly after HBsAg is detected. (HBcAg alone does not appear in serum.) In the setting of acute hepatitis, IgM anti-HBc indicates a diagnosis of acute hepatitis B, and it fills the serologic gap in rare patients who have cleared HBsAg but do not yet have detectable anti-HBs. IgM anti-HBc can persist for 3–6 months, and sometimes longer. IgM anti-HBc may also reappear during flares of previously inactive chronic hepatitis B (see later). IgG anti-HBc also appears during acute hepatitis B but persists indefinitely, whether the patient recovers (with the appearance of anti-HBs in serum) or chronic hepatitis B develops (with persistence of HBsAg). In asymptomatic blood donors, an isolated anti-HBc with no other positive HBV serologic results may represent a falsely positive result or latent infection in which HBV DNA is detectable in serum only by polymerase chain reaction (PCR) testing.

4. HBeAg—HBeAg is a secretory form of HBcAg that appears in serum during the incubation period shortly after the detection of HBsAg. HBeAg indicates viral replication and infectivity. Persistence of HBeAg beyond 3 months indicates an increased likelihood of chronic hepatitis B. Its disappearance is often followed by the appearance of anti-HBe, generally signifying diminished viral replication and decreased infectivity.

5. HBV DNA—The presence of HBV DNA in serum generally parallels the presence of HBeAg, although HBV DNA is a more sensitive and precise marker of viral replication and infectivity. Very low levels of HBV DNA, detectable only by PCR testing, may persist in serum and liver long after a patient has recovered from acute hepatitis B, but the HBV DNA in serum is bound to IgG and is rarely infectious. In some patients with chronic hepatitis B, HBV DNA is present at high levels without HBeAg in serum because of development of a mutation in the core promoter or precore region of the gene that codes HBcAg; these mutations prevent synthesis of HBeAg in infected hepatocytes. When additional mutations in the core gene are present, the precore mutant enhances the severity of HBV infection and increases the risk of cirrhosis (see later).

▶ **Differential Diagnosis**

The differential diagnosis includes hepatitis A and the same disorders listed for the differential diagnosis of acute hepatitis A (see earlier). In addition, coinfection with HDV must be considered (see later).

▶ **Prevention**

Strict isolation of patients is not necessary. Thorough hand washing by medical staff who may contact contaminated utensils, bedding, or clothing is essential. Medical staff should handle disposable needles carefully and not recap them. Screening of donated blood for HBsAg, anti-HBc, and anti-HCV has reduced the risk of transfusion-associated hepatitis markedly. All pregnant women should undergo testing for HBsAg. HBV-infected persons should practice safer sex. Cesarean section, in combination with immunoprophylaxis of the neonate (see below), reduces the risk of perinatal transmission of HBV infection when the mother's serum HBV DNA level is ≥ 200,000 international units/mL, although initiation of antiviral therapy of the mother in the third trimester is an alternative approach (see Chronic Hepatitis B & Chronic Hepatitis D). HBV-infected health care workers are not precluded from practicing medicine or dentistry if they follow CDC guidelines.

Hepatitis B immune globulin (HBIG) may be protective—or may attenuate the severity of illness—if given within 7 days after exposure (adult dose is 0.06 mL/kg body weight) followed by initiation of the HBV vaccine series (see below). This approach is currently recommended for persons exposed to HBsAg-contaminated material via mucous membranes or through breaks in the skin and for individuals who have had sexual contact with a person with HBV infection (irrespective of the presence or absence of HBeAg in the source). HBIG is also indicated for newborn infants of HBsAg-positive mothers followed by initiation of the vaccine series (see below).

The CDC recommends HBV vaccination of all infants and children in the United States and all adults who are at risk for hepatitis B (including persons under age 60 with diabetes mellitus) or who request vaccination. Over 90% of recipients of the vaccine mount protective antibody to hepatitis B; immunocompromised persons, including patients receiving dialysis (especially those with diabetes mellitus), respond poorly (see Table 30–7). Reduced response to the vaccine may have a genetic basis in some cases and has also been associated with age over 40 years and celiac disease. The standard regimen for adults is 10–20 mcg (depending on the formulation) repeated again at 1 and 6 months, but alternative schedules have been approved, including accelerated schedules of 0, 1, 2, and 12 months and of 0, 7, and 21 days plus 12 months. For greatest reliability of absorption, the deltoid muscle is the preferred site of innoculation. Vaccine formulations free of the mercury-containing preservative thimerosal are given to infants < 6 months of age. When documentation of seroconversion is considered desirable, postimmunization anti-HBs titers may be checked. Protection appears to be excellent even if the titer wanes—at least for 20 years—and booster reimmunization is not routinely recommended but is advised for immunocompromised persons in whom anti-HBs titers fall below 10 milli-international units/mL. For vaccine nonresponders, three additional vaccine doses may elicit seroprotective anti-HBs levels in 30–50% of persons. Doubling of the standard dose may also be effective. Universal vaccination of neonates in countries endemic for HBV has reduced the incidence of hepatocellular carcinoma.

▶ **Treatment**

Treatment of acute hepatitis B is the same as that for acute hepatitis A (see earlier). Encephalopathy or severe coagulopathy indicates acute liver failure, and hospitalization at a liver transplant center is mandatory (see below). Antiviral therapy is generally unnecessary in patients with acute hepatitis B but is usually prescribed in cases of fulminant hepatitis B as well as in spontaneous reactivation of chronic hepatitis B presenting as acute-on-chronic liver failure.

▶ Prognosis

In most patients, clinical recovery is complete in 3–6 months. Laboratory evidence of liver dysfunction may persist for a longer period, but most patients recover completely. The mortality rate for acute hepatitis B is 0.1–1% but is higher with superimposed hepatitis D (see later).

Chronic hepatitis, characterized by elevated aminotransferase levels for > 6 months, develops in 1–2% of immunocompetent adults with acute hepatitis B but in as many as 90% of infected neonates and infants and a substantial proportion of immunocompromised adults. Ultimately, cirrhosis develops in up to 40% of those with chronic hepatitis B; the risk of cirrhosis is even higher in HBV-infected patients coinfected with hepatitis C or HIV. Patients with cirrhosis are at risk for hepatocellular carcinoma at a rate of 3–5% per year. Even in the absence of cirrhosis, patients with chronic hepatitis B—particularly those with active viral replication—are at increased risk for hepatocellular carcinoma.

▶ When to Refer

Refer patients with acute hepatitis who require liver biopsy for diagnosis.

▶ When to Admit

- Encephalopathy is present.
- INR > 1.6.
- The patient is unable to maintain hydration.

Centers for Disease Control and Prevention (CDC). Updated CDC recommendations for the management of hepatitis B virus-infected health-care providers and students. MMWR Recomm Rep. 2012 Jul 6;61(RR-3):1–12. [PMID: 22763928]

Gerlich WH. Medical virology of hepatitis B: how it began and where we are now. Virol J. 2013 Jul 20;10:239. [PMID: 23870415]

Kappus MR et al. Extrahepatic manifestations of acute hepatitis B virus infection. Gastroenterol Hepatol (N Y). 2013 Feb;9(2):123–6. [PMID: 23983659]

van Rijckevorsel G et al. Targeted vaccination programme successful in reducing acute hepatitis B in men having sex with men in Amsterdam, The Netherlands. J Hepatol. 2013 Dec;59(6):1177–83. [PMID: 23954670]

ACUTE HEPATITIS C & OTHER CAUSES OF ACUTE VIRAL HEPATITIS

Viruses other than HAV and HBV that can cause hepatitis are hepatitis C virus (HCV), hepatitis D virus (HDV) (delta agent), and hepatitis E virus (HEV) (an enterically transmitted hepatitis seen in epidemic form in Asia, the Middle East, and North Africa). Hepatitis G virus (HGV) rarely, if ever, causes frank hepatitis. A DNA virus designated the TT virus (TTV) has been identified in up to 7.5% of blood donors and found to be transmitted readily by blood transfusions, but an association between this virus and liver disease has not been established. A related virus known as SEN-V has been found in 2% of US blood donors, is transmitted by transfusion, and may account for some cases of transfusion-associated non-ABCDE hepatitis. In immunocompromised and rare immunocompetent persons, cytomegalovirus, Epstein-Barr virus, and herpes simplex virus should be considered in the differential diagnosis of hepatitis. Severe acute respiratory syndrome (SARS) and influenza may be associated with marked serum aminotransferase elevations. Unidentified pathogens account for a small percentage of cases of acute viral hepatitis.

1. Hepatitis C

HCV is a single-stranded RNA virus (hepacivirus) with properties similar to those of flaviviruses. Six major genotypes of HCV have been identified. In the past, HCV was responsible for over 90% of cases of posttransfusion hepatitis, yet only 4% of cases of hepatitis C were attributable to blood transfusions. Over 50% of cases are transmitted by injection drug use, and both reinfection and superinfection of HCV are common in people who actively inject drugs. Body piercing, tattoos, and hemodialysis are risk factors. The risk of sexual and maternal–neonatal transmission is low and may be greatest in a subset of patients with high circulating levels of HCV RNA. Having multiple sexual partners may increase the risk of HCV infection, and HIV coinfection, unprotected receptive anal intercourse with ejaculation, and sex while high on methamphetamine increase the risk of HCV transmission in men who have sex with men. Transmission via breastfeeding has not been documented. An outbreak of hepatitis C in patients with immune deficiencies has occurred in some recipients of intravenous immune globulin. Hospital- and outpatient facility-acquired transmission has occurred via multidose vials of saline used to flush Portacaths; through reuse of disposable syringes (including drug "diversion" by an infected health care worker); through contamination of shared saline, radiopharmaceutical, and sclerosant vials; via inadequately disinfected endoscopy equipment; and between hospitalized patients on a liver unit. In the developing world, unsafe medical practices lead to a substantial number of cases of HCV infection. Covert transmission during bloody fisticuffs has even been reported, and incarceration in prison is a risk factor, with a frequency of 26% in the United States. In many patients, the source of infection is unknown. Coinfection with HCV is found in at least 30% of HIV-infected persons. HIV infection leads to an increased risk of acute liver failure and more rapid progression of chronic hepatitis C to cirrhosis; in addition, HCV increases the hepatotoxicity of highly active antiretroviral therapy. There are about 3.2 million HCV carriers in the United States (and 184 million worldwide) and another 1.3 million previously exposed persons who have cleared the virus. The incidence of new cases of acute, symptomatic hepatitis C declined from 1992 to 2005, but an increase was observed in persons aged 15 to 24 from 2002 to 2006, as a result of injection drug use.

Clinical Findings

A. Symptoms and Signs

Figure 16–3 shows the typical course of HCV infection. The incubation period for hepatitis C averages 6–7 weeks, and clinical illness is often mild, usually asymptomatic, and characterized by waxing and waning aminotransferase elevations and a high rate (> 80%) of chronic hepatitis. Spontaneous clearance of HCV following acute infection is more common (64%) in persons with the CC genotype of the *IL28B* gene (which encodes interferon lambda-3 on chromosome 19) than in those with the CT or TT genotype (24% and 6%, respectively). In persons with the CC genotype, jaundice is more likely to develop during the course of acute hepatitis C. Patients with the CC genotype and chronic hepatitis C are more likely to respond to therapy with pegylated interferon (see Chronic Viral Hepatitis, below). Polymorphisms of genes encoding the killer cell immunoglobulin-like receptors (KIR) and their HLA class I ligands (HLA-C1) and near genes for HLA class II are also associated with spontaneous resolution of viremia following HCV exposure. In pregnant patients with chronic hepatitis C, serum aminotransferase levels frequently normalize despite persistence of viremia, only to increase again after delivery.

B. Laboratory Findings

Diagnosis of hepatitis C is based on an enzyme immunoassay (EIA) that detects antibodies to HCV. Anti-HCV is not protective, and in patients with acute or chronic hepatitis, its presence in serum generally signifies that HCV is the cause. Limitations of the EIA include moderate sensitivity (false-negatives) for the diagnosis of acute hepatitis C early

in the course and low specificity (false-positives) in some persons with elevated gamma-globulin levels. In these situations, a diagnosis of hepatitis C may be confirmed by using an assay for HCV RNA. Occasional persons are found to have anti-HCV in serum, without HCV RNA in serum, suggesting recovery from HCV infection in the past.

Complications

HCV is a pathogenetic factor in mixed cryoglobulinemia and membranoproliferative glomerulonephritis and may be related to lichen planus, autoimmune thyroiditis, lymphocytic sialadenitis, idiopathic pulmonary fibrosis, sporadic porphyria cutanea tarda, and monoclonal gammopathies. HCV infection confers a 20–30% increased risk of non-Hodgkin lymphoma. Hepatitis C may induce insulin resistance (which in turn increases the risk of hepatic fibrosis), and the risk of type 2 diabetes mellitus is increased in persons with chronic hepatitis C. Hepatic steatosis is a particular feature of infection with HCV genotype 3 and may also occur in patients infected with other HCV genotypes who have risk factors for fatty liver (see below). On the other hand, chronic HCV infection is associated with a decrease in serum cholesterol and low-density lipoprotein levels.

Prevention

Testing donated blood for HCV has helped reduce the risk of transfusion-associated hepatitis C from 10% in 1990 to about 1 case per 2 million units in 2011. Birth cohort screening of persons born between 1945 and 1965 ("baby boomers") for HCV infection has been recommended by the CDC and the US Preventive Services Task Force. HCV-infected persons should practice safe sex, but there is little evidence that HCV is spread easily by sexual contact or perinatally, and no specific preventive measures are recommended for persons in a monogamous relationship or for pregnant women. Vaccination against HAV (after pre-screening for prior immunity) and HBV is recommended for patients with chronic hepatitis C, and vaccination against HAV is also recommended for patients with chronic hepatitis B, although the cost-effectiveness of vaccination has been questioned.

Treatment

Treatment of patients with acute hepatitis C with peginterferon (see later) for 6–24 weeks appreciably decreases the risk of chronic hepatitis. In general, patients infected with HCV genotype 1 require a 24-week course of treatment, but a 12-week course is adequate if HCV RNA is undetectable in serum by 4 weeks. Those infected with genotypes 2, 3, or 4 generally require 8–12 weeks of therapy. Because 20% of patients with acute hepatitis C, particularly those who are symptomatic, clear the virus without such treatment, reserving treatment for patients in whom serum HCV RNA levels fail to clear after 3 months may be advisable. Ribavirin may be added if HCV RNA fails to clear after 3 months of peginterferon, but some authorities recommend using ribavirin with peginterferon from the start of therapy.

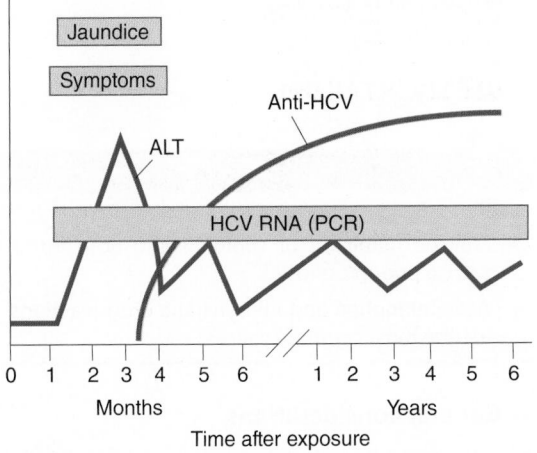

▲ **Figure 16–3.** The typical course of acute and chronic hepatitis C. (ALT, alanine aminotransferase; Anti-HCV, antibody to hepatitis C virus by enzyme immunoassay; HCV RNA [PCR], hepatitis C viral RNA by polymerase chain reaction.)

▶ Prognosis

In most patients, clinical recovery is complete in 3–6 months. Laboratory evidence of liver dysfunction may persist for a longer period. The overall mortality rate is < 1%, but the rate is reportedly higher in older people. Fulminant hepatitis C is rare in the United States.

Chronic hepatitis, which progresses very slowly in many cases, develops in as many as 85% of all persons with acute hepatitis C. Ultimately, cirrhosis develops in up to 30% of those with chronic hepatitis C; the risk of cirrhosis is higher in patients coinfected with both HCV and HBV or HIV. Patients with cirrhosis are at risk for hepatocellular carcinoma at a rate of 3–5% per year.

2. Hepatitis D (Delta Agent)

HDV is a defective RNA virus that causes hepatitis only in association with HBV infection and specifically only in the presence of HBsAg; it is cleared when the latter is cleared. Eight major genotypes (I–VIII) have been identified.

HDV may coinfect with HBV or may superinfect a person with chronic hepatitis B, usually by percutaneous exposure. When acute hepatitis D is coincident with acute HBV infection, the infection is generally similar in severity to acute hepatitis B alone. In chronic hepatitis B, superinfection by HDV appears to carry a worse short-term prognosis, often resulting in fulminant hepatitis or severe chronic hepatitis that progresses rapidly to cirrhosis.

In the 1970s and early 1980s, HDV was endemic in some areas, such as the Mediterranean countries (and later in Central and Eastern Europe), where up to 80% of HBV carriers were superinfected with HDV. In the United States, HDV occurred primarily among people who inject drugs. However, new cases of hepatitis D are now infrequent in the United States primarily because of the control of HBV infection, and cases seen today are usually from cohorts infected years ago who survived the initial impact of hepatitis D and now have cirrhosis. These patients are at risk for decompensation and have a threefold increased risk of hepatocellular carcinoma. New cases are primarily seen in immigrants from endemic areas, including Africa, central Asia, Eastern Europe, and the Amazon region of Brazil. More than 15 million people are infected worldwide. The diagnosis of hepatitis D is made by detection of antibody to hepatitis D antigen (anti-HDV) and, where available, hepatitis D antigen (HDAg) or HDV RNA in serum.

3. Hepatitis E

HEV is a 29- to 32-nm RNA hepevirus (in the Hepeviridae family) that is a major cause of acute hepatitis throughout Central and Southeast Asia, the Middle East, and North Africa, where it is responsible for waterborne hepatitis outbreaks. It is uncommon in the United States but should be considered in patients with acute hepatitis after a trip to an endemic area. In rare cases, hepatitis E can be mistaken for drug-induced liver injury. In industrialized countries, it may be spread by swine, and having a pet in the home and consuming organ meats are risk factors. Illness generally is self-limited (no carrier state), but instances of chronic hepatitis with rapid progression to cirrhosis attributed to HEV have been reported in transplant recipients (particularly when tacrolimus rather than cyclosporine is used as the main immunosuppressant) and, rarely, in persons with HIV infection, with preexisting liver disease, or receiving cancer chemotherapy. Preliminary observations suggest that treatment with oral ribavirin may induce sustained clearance of HEV RNA from the serum of such patients. The diagnosis of acute hepatitis E is made most readily by testing for IgM anti-HEV in serum, although available tests may not be reliable. Reported extrahepatic manifestations include arthritis, pancreatitis, and a variety of neurologic complications. In endemic regions, the mortality rate is high (10–20%) in pregnant women and correlates with high levels of HEV RNA in serum and gene mutations that lead to reduced expression of progesterone receptors, and the risk of hepatic decompensation is increased in patients with underlying chronic liver disease. Improved public hygiene reduces the risk of HEV infection in endemic areas. Recombinant vaccines against HEV have shown promise in clinical trials.

Chou R et al. Screening for hepatitis C virus infection in adults: a systematic review for the U.S. Preventive Services Task Force. Ann Intern Med. 2013 Jan 15;158(2):101–8. [PMID: 2318361]

Holmberg SD et al. Hepatitis C in the United States. N Engl J Med. 2013 May 16;368(20):1859–61. [PMID: 23675657]

Hoofnagle JH et al. Hepatitis E. N Engl J Med. 2012 Sep 27;367(13):1237–44. [PMID: 23013075]

Mohd Hanafiah K et al. Global epidemiology of hepatitis C virus infection: new estimates of age-specific antibody to HCV seroprevalence. Hepatology. 2013 Apr;57(4):1333–42. [PMID: 23172780]

Moyer VA et al. Screening for hepatitis C virus infection in adults: U.S. Preventive Services Task Force recommendation statement. Ann Intern Med. 2013 Sep 3;159(5):349–57. [PMID: 23798026]

Rizzetto M. Hepatitis D (delta). Semin Liver Dis. 2012 Aug;32(3): 193–266. [PMID: 22932966]

ACUTE LIVER FAILURE

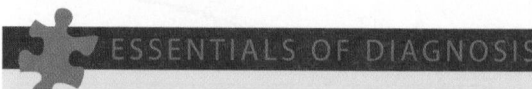

ESSENTIALS OF DIAGNOSIS

- ▶ May be fulminant or subfulminant; both forms carry a poor prognosis.
- ▶ Acetaminophen and idiosyncratic drug reactions are the most common causes.

▶ General Considerations

Acute liver failure may be fulminant or subfulminant. Fulminant hepatic failure is characterized by the development of hepatic encephalopathy within 8 weeks after the onset of acute liver disease. Coagulopathy (international normalized ratio [INR] ≥1.5) is invariably present. Subfulminant hepatic failure occurs when these findings appear between

8 weeks and 6 months after the onset of acute liver disease and carries an equally poor prognosis.

An estimated 1600 cases of acute liver failure occur each year in the United States. Acetaminophen toxicity is the most common cause, accounting for at least 45% of cases. Suicide attempts account for 44% of cases of acetaminophen-induced hepatic failure, and unintentional overdoses ("therapeutic misadventures"), which are often a result of a decrease in the threshold toxic dose because of chronic alcohol use or fasting, account for at least 48%. Other causes include idiosyncratic drug reactions (now the second most common cause, with antituberculosis drugs, antiepileptics, and antibiotics implicated most commonly), viral hepatitis, poisonous mushrooms (*Amanita phalloides*), shock, hyperthermia or hypothermia, Budd–Chiari syndrome, malignancy (most commonly lymphomas), Wilson disease, Reye syndrome, fatty liver of pregnancy and other disorders of fatty acid oxidation, autoimmune hepatitis, parvovirus B19 infection and, rarely, grand mal seizures. The risk of acute liver failure is increased in patients with diabetes mellitus, and outcome is worsened by obesity. Herbal and dietary supplements are thought to be contributory to acute liver failure in a substantial portion of cases, regardless of cause.

Viral hepatitis now accounts for only 12% of all cases of acute liver failure. The decline of viral hepatitis as the principal cause of acute liver failure is due to universal vaccination of infants and children against hepatitis B and the availability of the hepatitis A vaccine. In endemic areas, hepatitis E is an important cause of acute liver failure. Hepatitis C is a rare cause of acute liver failure in the United States, but acute hepatitis A or B superimposed on chronic hepatitis C may cause fulminant hepatitis.

Clinical Findings

Gastrointestinal symptoms, systemic inflammatory response, renal dysfunction, and hemorrhagic phenomena are common. Adrenal insufficiency and subclinical myocardial injury manifesting as an elevated serum troponin I level often complicate acute liver failure. Jaundice may be absent or minimal early, but laboratory tests show severe hepatocellular damage. In acetaminophen toxicity, serum aminotransferase elevations are often towering (> 5000 units/L), and biomarkers of early detection are under study, including the detection of acetaminophen-protein adducts in serum. In acute liver failure due to microvesicular steatosis (eg, fatty liver of pregnancy), serum aminotransferase elevations may be modest (< 300 units/L). Over 10% of patients have an elevated serum amylase level at least three times the upper limit of normal, often as a result of renal dysfunction. The blood ammonia level is typically elevated and correlates (along with the Model for End-Stage Liver Disease [MELD] score) with the development of encephalopathy and intracranial hypertension. Intracranial hypertension rarely develops when the blood ammonia level is < 75 mcmol/L and is invariable when the level is > 200 mcmol/L. The severity of extrahepatic organ dysfunction (as assessed by the Sequential Organ Failure Assessment, or SOFA) also correlates with the likelihood of intracranial hypertension.

Treatment

The treatment of acute liver failure is directed toward correcting metabolic abnormalities. These include coagulation defects, electrolyte and acid-base disturbances, advanced chronic kidney disease, hypoglycemia, and encephalopathy. Cerebral edema and sepsis are the leading causes of death. Prophylactic antibiotic therapy decreases the risk of infection, observed in up to 90%, but has no effect on survival and is not routinely recommended. For suspected sepsis, broad coverage is indicated. Despite a high rate of adrenal insufficiency, corticosteroids are of uncertain value. Stress gastropathy prophylaxis with an H_2-receptor blocker or proton pump inhibitor is recommended. Administration of acetylcysteine (140 mg/kg orally followed by 70 mg/kg orally every 4 hours for an additional 17 doses or 150 mg/kg in 5% dextrose intravenously over 15 minutes followed by 50 mg/kg over 4 hours and then 100 mg/kg over 16 hours) is indicated for acetaminophen toxicity up to 72 hours after ingestion. For massive acetaminophen overdoses, treatment with intravenous acetylcysteine may need to be extended in duration until the serum aminotransferase levels are declining and serum acetaminophen levels are undetectable. Treatment with acetylcysteine improves cerebral blood flow and oxygenation as well as transplant-free survival in patients with stage 1 or 2 encephalopathy due to fulminant hepatic failure of any cause. (Acetylcysteine treatment can prolong the prothrombin time, leading to the erroneous assumption that liver failure is worsening; it can also cause nausea, vomiting, and an anaphylactoid reaction [especially in persons with a history of asthma]. It may be detrimental in children with nonacetaminophen acute liver failure.) Penicillin G (300,000 to 1 million units/kg/d) or silibinin (silymarin or milk thistle), which is not licensed in the United States, is administered to patients with mushroom poisoning. Nucleoside analogs are recommended for patients with fulminant hepatitis B (see Chronic Viral Hepatitis), and intravenous acyclovir has shown benefit in those with herpes simplex virus hepatitis. Plasmapheresis combined with D-penicillamine has been used in fulminant Wilson disease. Subclinical seizure activity is common in patients with acute liver failure, but the value of prophylactic phenytoin is uncertain.

Early transfer to a liver transplantation center is essential. The head of the patient's bed should be elevated to 30 degrees, and patients with stage 3 or 4 encephalopathy should be intubated. Extradural sensors may be placed to monitor intracranial pressure for impending cerebral edema with the goal of maintaining the intracranial pressure below 20 mm Hg and the cerebral perfusion pressure above 70 mm Hg. Recombinant activated factor VII may be administered to reduce the risk of bleeding associated with intracranial pressure monitoring. Lactulose is administered for encephalopathy (see Cirrhosis). Mannitol, 0.5 g/kg, or 100–200 mL of a 20% solution by intravenous infusion over 10 minutes, may decrease cerebral edema but should be used with caution in patients with advanced chronic kidney disease. Intravenously administered hypertonic saline to induce hypernatremia (serum sodium concentration of 145–155 mEq/L [145–155 mmol/L]) also may reduce intracranial hypertension. Hypothermia to a temperature of 32–34°C may reduce intracranial pressure when other measures have failed and may improve survival long enough to permit liver transplantation. The value of hyperventilation and intravenous prostaglandin E_1 is uncertain. A short-acting barbiturate, propofol, or intravenous boluses of indomethacin, 25 mg, is considered for refractory intracranial hypertension. Nonbiologic liver support (eg, molecular adsorbent recirculating system [MARS], an albumin dialysis system), hepatic-assist devices using living hepatocytes, extracorporeal systems, hepatocyte transplantation, and liver xenografts have shown promise experimentally but have not been shown conclusively to reduce mortality in patients with acute liver failure. They may serve as a "bridge" to liver transplantation.

▶ Prognosis

With earlier recognition of acute liver failure, the frequency of cerebral edema has declined, and overall survival has improved steadily since the 1970s and is now as high as 75%. The mortality rate of fulminant hepatic failure with severe encephalopathy is as high as 80%, except for acetaminophen hepatotoxicity, in which the transplant-free survival is 65% and no more than 8% of patients undergo liver transplantation. For patients with fulminant hepatic failure of other causes, the outlook is poor in patients younger than 10 and older than 40 years of age and in those with an idiosyncratic drug reaction but appears to be improved when acetylcysteine is administered to patients with stage 1 or 2 encephalopathy. Spontaneous recovery is less likely for hepatitis B than for hepatitis A. Polymorphisms of the genes that encode keratins 8 and 18 appear to affect outcomes. Other adverse prognostic factors are a serum bilirubin level > 18 mg/dL (307.8 mcmol/L), INR > 6.5, onset of encephalopathy more than 7 days after the onset of jaundice, and a low factor V level (< 20% of normal). For acetaminophen-induced fulminant hepatic failure, indicators of a poor outcome are acidosis (pH < 7.3), INR > 6.5, and azotemia (serum creatinine ≥ 3.4 mg/dL [283.22 mcmol/L]), whereas a rising serum alpha-fetoprotein level predicts a favorable outcome. An elevated blood lactate level (> 3.5 mEq/L or > 3.5 mmol/L), elevated blood ammonia level (> 211 mcg/dL or > 124 mcmol/L), and possibly hyperphosphatemia (> 3.7 mg/dL or 1.2 mmol/L) also predict poor survival. One study has shown that patients with persistent elevation of the arterial ammonia level (≥ 211 mcg/dL or ≥ 122 mcmol/L) for 3 days have greater rates of complications and mortality than those with decreasing ammonia levels. A number of prognostic indices have been proposed: the "BiLE" score, based on the serum bilirubin, serum lactate, and etiology; the Acute Liver Failure Early Dynamic (ALFED) model, based on the arterial ammonia level, serum bilirubin, INR, and hepatic encephalopathy; and the Acute Liver Failure Study Group (ALFSG) index, based on coma grade, INR, serum bilirubin and phosphatase levels, and serum levels of M30, a cleavage product of cytokeratin-18 caspase. Emergency liver transplantation is considered for patients with stage 2 to stage 3 encephalopathy (see Cirrhosis) and is associated with a 70% survival rate at 5 years. For mushroom poisoning, liver transplantation should be considered when the interval between ingestion and the onset of diarrhea is < 8 hours or the INR is ≥ 6.0, even in the absence of encephalopathy. Acute liver failure superimposed on chronic liver disease (acute-on-chronic liver failure) has a poor prognosis when associated with renal dysfunction.

▶ When to Admit

All patients with acute liver failure should be hospitalized.

Bernal W et al. Lessons from look-back in acute liver failure? A single centre experience of 3300 patients. J Hepatol. 2013 Jul;59(1):74–80. [PMID: 23439263]

Kumar R et al. Persistent hyperammonemia is associated with complications and poor outcomes in patients with acute liver failure. Clin Gastroenterol Hepatol. 2012 Aug;10(8):925–31. [PMID: 22521861]

Moreau R et al. Acute-on-chronic liver failure is a distinct syndrome that develops in patients with acute decompensation of cirrhosis. Gastroenterology. 2013 Jun;144(7):1426–37. [PMID: 23474284]

CHRONIC VIRAL HEPATITIS

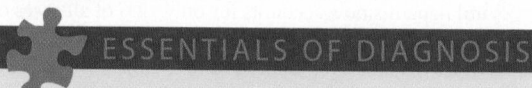

ESSENTIALS OF DIAGNOSIS

- ▶ Defined by chronic infection (HBV, HCV, HDV) for > 3–6 months.
- ▶ Diagnosis is usually made by antibody tests and viral nucleic acid in serum.

▶ General Considerations

Chronic hepatitis is defined as chronic necroinflammation of the liver of more than 3–6 months' duration, demonstrated by persistently elevated serum aminotransferase levels or characteristic histologic findings. In many cases, the diagnosis of chronic hepatitis may be made on initial presentation. The causes of chronic hepatitis include HBV, HCV, and HDV as well as autoimmune hepatitis; alcoholic and nonalcoholic steatohepatitis; certain medications, such as isoniazid and nitrofurantoin; Wilson disease; alpha-1-antiprotease deficiency; and, rarely, celiac disease. Mortality from chronic HBV and HCV infection has been rising in the United States, and HCV has surpassed HIV as a cause of death. Chronic hepatitis is categorized on the basis of etiology; the grade of portal, periportal, and lobular inflammation (minimal, mild, moderate, or severe); and the stage of fibrosis (none, mild, moderate, severe, cirrhosis). In the absence of advanced cirrhosis, patients are often asymptomatic or have mild nonspecific symptoms.

1. Chronic Hepatitis B & Chronic Hepatitis D

▶ Clinical Findings & Diagnosis

Chronic hepatitis B afflicts 400 million people worldwide (2 billion overall have been infected; endemic areas include

Asia and sub-Saharan Africa) and up to 2.2 million (predominantly males) in the United States. It may be noted as a continuum of acute hepatitis B or diagnosed because of repeated detection of HBsAg in serum, often with elevated aminotransferase levels.

Four phases of HBV infection are recognized: immune tolerant phase, immune clearance phase, inactive HBsAg carrier state, and reactivated chronic hepatitis B phase. In the **immune tolerant phase,** HBeAg and HBV DNA are present in serum, which is indicative of active viral replication, and serum aminotransferase levels are normal, with little necroinflammation in the liver. This phase is common in infants and young children whose immature immune system fails to mount an immune response to HBV. Persons in the immune tolerant phase and those who acquire HBV infection later in life may enter an **immune clearance phase,** in which aminotransferase levels are elevated and necroinflammation is present in the liver, with a risk of progression to cirrhosis (at a rate of 2–5.5% per year) and of hepatocellular carcinoma (at a rate of > 2% per year in those with cirrhosis); low-level IgM anti-HBc is present in serum in about 70%.

Patients enter the **inactive HBsAg carrier state** when biochemical improvement follows immune clearance. This improvement coincides with disappearance of HBeAg and reduced HBV DNA levels ($< 10^5$ copies/mL, or < 20,000 international units/mL) in serum, appearance of anti-HBe, and integration of the HBV genome into the host genome in infected hepatocytes. Patients in this phase are at a low risk for cirrhosis (if it has not already developed) and hepatocellular carcinoma, and those with persistently normal serum aminotransferase levels infrequently have histologically significant liver disease, especially if the HBsAg level is low.

The **reactivated chronic hepatitis B phase** may result from infection by a pre-core mutant of HBV or spontaneous mutation of the pre-core or core promoter region of the HBV genome during the course of chronic hepatitis caused by wild-type HBV. So-called HBeAg-negative chronic hepatitis B accounts for < 10% of cases of chronic hepatitis B in the United States, up to 50% in southeast Asia, and up to 90% in Mediterranean countries, reflecting in part differences in the frequencies of HBV genotypes. In reactivated chronic hepatitis B, there is a rise in serum HBV DNA levels and possible progression to cirrhosis (at a rate of 8–10% per year), particularly when additional mutations in the core gene of HBV are present. Risk factors for reactivation include male sex and HBV genotype C. In patients with either HBeAg-positive or HBeAg-negative chronic hepatitis B, the risk of cirrhosis and of hepatocellular carcinoma correlates with the serum HBV DNA level. Other risk factors include advanced age, male sex, alcohol use, cigarette smoking, HBV genotype C, and coinfection with HCV or HDV. HIV coinfection is also associated with an increased frequency of cirrhosis when the CD4 count is low.

Acute **hepatitis D** infection superimposed on chronic HBV infection may result in severe chronic hepatitis, which may progress rapidly to cirrhosis and may be fatal. Patients with long-standing chronic hepatitis D and B often have inactive cirrhosis and are at risk for decompensation and hepatocellular carcinoma. The diagnosis is confirmed by detection of anti-HDV or HDAg (or HDV RNA) in serum.

▶ **Treatment**

Patients with active viral replication (HBeAg and HBV DNA [$\geq 10^5$ copies/mL, or $\geq 20,000$ international units/mL] in serum and elevated aminotransferase levels) may be treated with a nucleoside or nucleotide analog or with pegylated interferon. Nucleoside and nucleotide analogs are preferred because they are better tolerated and can be taken orally. For patients who are HBeAg-negative, the threshold for treatment is a serum HBV DNA level $\geq 10^4$ copies/mL, or ≥ 2000 international units/mL. If the threshold HBV DNA level for treatment is met but the serum ALT level is normal, treatment may still be considered in patients over age 35–40 if liver biopsy demonstrates a fibrosis stage of 2 of 4 (moderate) or higher. Therapy is aimed at reducing and maintaining the serum HBV DNA level to the lowest possible levels, thereby leading to normalization of the ALT level and histologic improvement. An additional goal in HBeAg-positive patients is seroconversion to anti-HBe, and some responders eventually clear HBsAg. Although nucleoside and nucleotide analogs generally have been discontinued 6–12 months after HBeAg-to-anti-HBe seroconversion, some patients serorevert to HBeAg after discontinuation, have a rise in HBV DNA levels and recurrence of hepatitis activity, and require long-term therapy, which also is required when seroconversion does not occur. All HBeAg-negative patients with chronic hepatitis B also require long-term therapy (see below).

The available nucleoside and nucleotide analogs—entecavir, tenofovir, lamivudine, adefovir, and telbivudine—differ in efficacy and rates of resistance; however, in HBeAg-positive patients, they all achieve an HBeAg-to-anti-HBe seroconversion rate of about 20% at 1 year, with higher rates after more prolonged therapy. The preferred first-line oral agents are entecavir and tenofovir. Entecavir is rarely associated with resistance unless a patient is already resistant to lamivudine. The daily dose is 0.5 mg orally for patients not resistant to lamivudine and 1 mg for patients who previously became resistant to lamivudine. Histologic improvement is observed in 70% of treated patients and suppression of HBV DNA in serum in nearly all patients. Entecavir has been reported to cause lactic acidosis when used in patients with decompensated cirrhosis. Tenofovir is equally effective and is used as a first-line agent or when resistance to a nucleoside analog has developed. Like entecavir, tenofovir has a low rate of resistance when used as initial therapy. Long-term use may lead to an elevated serum creatinine level and reduced serum phosphate level (Fanconi-like syndrome) that is reversible with discontinuation of the drug.

The first available nucleoside analog was lamivudine, 100 mg orally daily. By the end of 1 year of therapy with lamivudine, however, 15–30% of responders experience a relapse (and occasionally frank decompensation) as a result of a mutation in the polymerase gene (the YMDD motif) of HBV DNA that confers resistance to lamivudine. The rate of resistance reaches 70% by 5 years of therapy, and the drug is no longer considered first-line therapy in the United States but may be used in countries in which cost is a deciding factor. Adefovir dipivoxil has activity against wild-type and lamivudine-resistant HBV but is the least potent of the oral antiviral agents for HBV. The standard dose is 10 mg orally once a day for at least 1 year. As with lamivudine, only a small number of patients achieve sustained suppression of HBV replication with adefovir, and long-term suppressive therapy is often required. Resistance to adefovir is less frequent than with lamivudine but is seen in up to 29% of patients treated for 5 years. Patients with underlying kidney dysfunction are at risk for nephrotoxicity from adefovir. Telbivudine, given in a daily dose of 600 mg orally, is more potent than either lamivudine or adefovir. Resistance to this drug may develop, however, particularly in patients who are resistant to lamivudine, and elevated creatine kinase levels are common in patients treated with telbivudine. Other antiviral agents are under study, and strategies using multiple drugs are being investigated.

Nucleoside and nucleotide analogs are well tolerated even in patients with decompensated cirrhosis (for whom the treatment threshold may be an HBV DNA level < 10^4 copies/mL) and may be effective in patients with rapidly progressive hepatitis B ("fibrosing cholestatic hepatitis") following organ transplantation. Although therapy with these agents leads to biochemical, virologic, and histologic improvement in patients with HBeAg-negative chronic hepatitis B and baseline HBV DNA levels ≥ 10^4 copies/mL (≥ 2000 international units/mL), relapse is frequent when therapy is stopped, and long-term treatment is often required. Resistance is most likely to develop to lamivudine and may develop to adefovir and telbivudine, but these drugs are no longer used as first-line agents in the United States. The development of resistance occasionally results in hepatic decompensation. Sequential addition of a second antiviral agent is usually effective after resistance to the first agent has developed. Combined use of peginterferon and a nucleoside or nucleotide analog has not been shown convincingly to have a substantial advantage over the use of either type of drug alone.

Nucleoside analogs are also recommended for inactive HBV carriers prior to the initiation of immunosuppressive therapy (including anti-tumor necrosis factor antibody therapy) or cancer chemotherapy to prevent reactivation. In patients infected with both HBV and HIV, antiretroviral therapy, including two drugs active against both viruses (eg, tenofovir plus lamivudine or emtricitabine), has been recommended when treatment of HIV infection is indicated. Telbivudine and tenofovir are classified as pregnancy category B drugs, and lamivudine, a category C drug, has been shown to be safe in pregnant women with HIV infection. Antiviral therapy, beginning in the third trimester, has been recommended when the mother's serum HBV DNA level is ≥ 200,000 international units/mL to reduce levels at the time of delivery.

Peginterferon alfa-2a is still an alternative to the oral agents in selected cases. A dose of 180 mcg subcutaneously once weekly for 48 weeks leads to sustained normalization of aminotransferase levels, disappearance of HBeAg and HBV DNA from serum, appearance of anti-HBe, and improved survival in up to 40% of treated patients. A response is most likely in patients with a low baseline HBV DNA level and high aminotransferase levels and is more likely in those who are infected with HBV genotype A than with other genotypes (especially genotype D) and who have certain favorable polymorphisms of the *IL28B* gene. Moreover, most complete responders eventually clear HBsAg and develop anti-HBs in serum, and are thus cured. Relapses are uncommon in complete responders who seroconvert from HBeAg to anti-HBe. Peginterferon may be considered in order to avoid long-term therapy with an oral agent, as in young women who may want to become pregnant in the future. Patients with HBeAg-negative chronic hepatitis B have a response rate of 60% after 48 weeks of therapy with peginterferon, but the response may not be durable once peginterferon is stopped. A rapid decline in serum HBsAg titers predicts a sustained response and ultimate clearance of HBsAg. The response to peginterferon is poor in patients with HIV coinfection.

Peginterferon alfa-2b (1.5 mcg/kg/wk for 48 weeks) may lead to normalization of serum aminotransferase levels, histologic improvement, and elimination of HDV RNA from serum in 20–50% of patients with **chronic hepatitis D,** but patients may relapse and tolerance is poor. Nucleoside and nucleotide analogs are not effective in treating chronic hepatitis D.

▶ Prognosis

The course of chronic hepatitis B is variable. The sequelae of chronic hepatitis secondary to hepatitis B include cirrhosis, liver failure, and hepatocellular carcinoma. The 5-year mortality rate is 0–2% in those without cirrhosis, 14–20% in those with compensated cirrhosis, and 70–86% following decompensation. The risk of cirrhosis and hepatocellular carcinoma correlates with serum HBV DNA levels, and a focus of therapy is to suppress HBV DNA levels below 300 copies/mL (60 international units/mL). HBV genotype C is associated with a higher risk of cirrhosis and hepatocellular carcinoma than other genotypes. Antiviral treatment improves the prognosis in responders, prevents (or leads to regression of) cirrhosis, and decreases the frequency of liver-related complications.

2. Chronic Hepatitis C

▶ Clinical Findings & Diagnosis

Chronic hepatitis C develops in up to 85% of patients with acute hepatitis C. It is clinically indistinguishable from chronic hepatitis due to other causes and may be the most common. Worldwide, 170 million people are infected with HCV, with 1.8% of the US population infected. Peak prevalence in the United States (about 4%) is in persons born between 1945 and 1964. In approximately 40% of cases, serum aminotransferase levels are persistently normal. The diagnosis is confirmed by detection of anti-HCV by EIA. In rare cases of suspected chronic hepatitis C but a negative

EIA, HCV RNA is detected by PCR testing. Progression to cirrhosis occurs in 20% of affected patients after 20 years, with an increased risk in men, those who drink more than 50 g of alcohol daily, and those who acquire HCV infection after age 40 years. The rate of fibrosis progression accelerates after age 50. African Americans have a higher rate of chronic hepatitis C but lower rates of fibrosis progression and response to therapy than whites (see below). Immunosuppressed persons—including patients with hypogammaglobulinemia or HIV infection with a low CD4 count or those receiving immunosuppressants—appear to progress more rapidly to cirrhosis than immunocompetent persons with chronic hepatitis C. Tobacco and cannibis smoking and hepatic steatosis also appear to promote progression of fibrosis, but coffee consumption appears to slow progression. Persons with chronic hepatitis C and persistently normal serum aminotransferase levels usually have mild chronic hepatitis with slow or absent progression to cirrhosis; however, cirrhosis is present in 10% of these patients.

▶ Treatment

Treatment of chronic hepatitis C is generally considered in patients under age 70 when there is moderate to severe fibrosis on liver biopsy. A liver biopsy may be avoided in persons infected with HCV genotype 1 if the results of a serum FibroSure test suggest absence of fibrosis or, alternatively, presence of cirrhosis. Liver biopsy is often deferred in those infected with HCV genotype 2 or 3, in whom cure rates are invariably high. The introduction of direct-acting and host-targeting antiviral agents is rapidly expanding the therapeutic armamentarium against HCV.

Standard therapy for HCV infection since the late 1990s has been a combination of peginterferon plus ribavirin. Sustained virologic response rates (negative HCV RNA in serum at 24 weeks after completion of therapy) to peginterferon plus ribavirin are 45% in patients with HCV genotype 1 infection and 70–80% in those with genotype 2 or 3 infection. Rates are lower in patients with advanced fibrosis, high levels of viremia, alcohol consumption, HIV coinfection, obesity, insulin resistance, severe steatosis, and vitamin A or D deficiency. Response rates are also lower in in women with early menopause and in Latinos and blacks compared to whites, in part because of a higher rate of HCV genotype 1 among infected black patients and in part because of intrinsic resistance to therapy. Response of genotype 1 infection to peginterferon plus ribavirin is associated most strongly with the CC genotype of the *IL28B* gene, with sustained response rates as high as 80%, compared to 40% for the CT genotype and 30% for the TT genotype. Caffeinated coffee consumption of more than three cups per day has also been reported to improve virologic response to peginterferon plus ribavirin.

In the past, patients infected with HCV genotype 1 were generally treated for 48 weeks with peginterferon plus ribavirin. If the serum HCV RNA level decreased to ≤ 50 international units/mL by 4 weeks (rapid virologic response), treatment for at least 24 weeks resulted in a sustained virologic response rate of 90%. For those who did not achieve a rapid virologic response but had a serum HCV

RNA level ≤ 50 international units/mL by 12 weeks (complete early virologic response), treatment was continued for the full 48 weeks. If serum HCV RNA levels declined by at least 2 logs by 12 weeks (partial early virologic response) and became undetectable by 24 weeks (slow response), treatment might be extended to 72 weeks. If none of the aforementioned targets was reached, particularly a minimum of a partial early virologic response, treatment was discontinued.

Higher rates of response are achieved in persons infected with HCV genotype 1 when one of two first-generation direct-acting antiviral agents—telaprevir and boceprevir, which are NS3/4A serine protease inhibitors approved by the FDA in 2011—is added to peginterferon plus ribavirin. Sustained response rates are as high as 75% for HCV genotype 1 with a standard three-drug regimen. With the addition of one of these two protease inhibitors, the treatment duration for HCV genotype 1 infection can be shortened to as little as 24 weeks, depending on the rapidity of clearance of HCV RNA from serum—so-called response-guided therapy. The definition of clearance of HCV RNA requires use of a sensitive real-time reverse transcriptase-PCR assay to monitor HCV RNA during treatment (the lower limit of quantification should be ≤ 25 international units/mL, and the limit of detection should be 10–15 international units/mL). Detailed stopping rules for both treatments have been developed. Low levels of HCV RNA may persist in the liver, lymphocytes, and macrophages of successfully treated ("cured") patients, but the significance of this finding is uncertain.

Patients infected with HCV genotype 2 or 3 (without cirrhosis and with low levels of viremia) may be treated for 24 weeks with peginterferon plus ribavirin and require a ribavirin total daily dose of only 800 mg. For the patients who clear the virus within 4 weeks (rapid virologic response), a total treatment duration of only 16 weeks may be sufficient, if the baseline HCV RNA level is ≤ 400,000 international units/mL; however, such a short course is not routinely recommended. For patients with cirrhosis or a high viral level (> 400,000 international units/mL), 48 weeks of treatment and ribavirin dosing based on the patient's weight (as for HCV genotype 1) may be preferred.

Peginterferon-based therapy may be beneficial in the treatment of cryoglobulinemia associated with chronic hepatitis C; an acute flare of cryoglobulinemia may first require treatment with rituximab, cyclophosphamide plus methylprednisolone, or plasma exchange. "Chronic HCV carriers" with normal serum aminotransferase levels respond just as well to treatment as do patients with elevated aminotransferase levels. Patients with both HCV and HIV infections may benefit from treatment of HCV. Moreover, in persons coinfected with HCV and HIV, long-term liver disease–related mortality increases as HIV infection–related mortality is reduced by highly active antiretroviral therapy.

Treatment with peginterferon-based therapy is costly (up to $86,000 for 48 weeks of therapy with three drugs), and side effects are common and sometimes distressing. Discontinuation rates are as high as 15–30%, and higher in persons over 60 years of age than in younger patients. Sustained response rates decline if < 60% of the cumulative dose is taken. A complete blood count is recommended at week 1 or 2 and week 4 after therapy is started and then monthly thereafter. Peginterferon alfa is contraindicated in pregnant or breast-feeding women and those with decompensated cirrhosis, profound cytopenias, severe psychiatric disorders, autoimmune diseases, or an inability to self-administer or comply with treatment. HCV treatment can be successful in carefully selected people who continue to inject illicit drugs if they are managed by a multidisciplinary team.

Men and women taking ribavirin must practice strict contraception until 6 months after the conclusion of therapy because of teratogenic effects in animals. Ribavirin should be used with caution in persons over 65 years of age and in others in whom hemolysis could pose a risk of angina or stroke.

In patients with severe chronic kidney disease, the doses of peginterferon and ribavirin must be reduced. The dose of ribavirin may be reduced if severe therapy-induced anemia develops, and the dose reduction does not appear to affect the efficacy of three-drug therapy that includes a protease inhibitor. If necessary, erythropoietin (epoetin alfa) and granulocyte colony-stimulating factor (filgrastim) may be used to treat therapy-induced anemia and leukopenia, respectively. Eltrombopag may be considered in patients with a platelet count < 90,000/mcL (< 90 × 10^9/L) before therapy. Treated patients exhibit a low genetic resistance to both first-generation protease inhibitors, boceprevir and telaprevir; however, both agents are inhibitors of cytochrome P450 3A and the drug transporter P-glycoprotein and thus they interact with many other drugs.

Numerous other antiviral agents with various, often novel, mechanisms of action are under study, and some are becoming commercially available. Emerging agents include other NS3/4A protease inhibitors (eg, asunaprevir, danoprevir, faldaprevir, simeprevir, vaniprevir); NS5A inhibitors (eg, daclatasvir, ledipasvir); polymerase inhibitors (eg, mericitabine, sofosbuvir); virus entry, assembly, and secretion inhibitors; microRNA-122 antisense oligonucleotides (eg, miravirsen); cyclophilin A inhibitors (eg, alisporivir); interferon lambda-3; and therapeutic vaccines. Some new regimens do not require peginterferon. For example, in patients infected with HCV genotype 2 or 3, a non-interferon–based regimen of ribavirin combined with the NS5B polymerase inhibitor, sofosbuvir (approved by the FDA in 2013), has yielded high sustained virologic response rates (redefined as undetectable HCV RNA in serum 12 weeks after completion of therapy). Such rates were at least 93% for patients with genotype 2 after 12 weeks of treatment and nearly 80% for genotype 3 after 24 weeks of treatment. Moreover, in previously untreated HCV genotype 1-infected patients, the combination of peginterferon, ribavirin, and sofosbuvir has resulted in a sustained virologic response rate of 89% when treatment is given for only 12 weeks.

The combination of sofosbuvir and ledipasvir shows particular promise. In addition, two other NS3/4A protease inhibitors–simeprevir (approved by the FDA in 2013) and faldaprevir–have each led to sustained virologic response rates of up to 85% when used once daily in combination with peginterferon plus ribavirin for HCV genotype 1 infection for as little as 12 weeks. However, simeprevir is less effective and not recommended in patients infected with HCV genotype 1a with the Q80K polymorphism of NS3/4A. It is anticipated that combinations of oral direct antiviral agents will ultimately obviate the need for peginterferon, shorten the duration of treatment, lead to higher cure rates, and result in fewer side effects. The most challenging groups of patients to treat with all-oral regimens include those infected with HCV genotype 3, those with nonresponse to prior treatment, and those with cirrhosis.

▶ Prognosis

Chronic hepatitis C is an indolent, often subclinical disease that may lead to cirrhosis and hepatocellular carcinoma after decades. The overall mortality rate in patients with transfusion-associated hepatitis C may be no different from that of an age-matched control population. Nevertheless, mortality or transplantation rates clearly rise to 5% per year once cirrhosis develops, and mortality from cirrhosis and hepatocellular carcinoma due to hepatitis C is rising. There is some evidence that HCV genotype 1b is associated with a higher risk of hepatocellular carcinoma than other genotypes. Antiviral therapy has a beneficial effect on mortality and quality of life, is cost-effective, appears to retard and even reverse fibrosis, and reduces the risk of decompensated cirrhosis and hepatocellular carcinoma in responders. Even patients who achieve a sustained virologic response remain at an increased risk for mortality compared with the general population. The risk of mortality from drug addiction is higher than that for liver disease in patients with chronic hepatitis C.

▶ When to Refer

- For liver biopsy.
- For antiviral therapy.

▶ When to Admit

- For complications of decompensated cirrhosis.

Chou R et al. Blood tests to diagnose fibrosis or cirrhosis in patients with chronic hepatitis C virus infection: a systematic review. Ann Intern Med. 2013 Jun 4;158(11):807–20. [PMID: 23732714]

Gane EJ et al. Nucleotide polymerase inhibitor sofosbuvir plus ribavirin for hepatitis C. N Engl J Med. 2013 Jan 3;368(1):34–44. [PMID: 23281974]

Jacobson IM et al. Sofosbuvir for hepatitis C genotype 2 or 3 in patients without treatment options. N Engl J Med. 2013 May 16;368(20):1867–77. [PMID: 23607593]

Liang TJ et al. Current and future therapies for hepatitis C virus infection. N Engl J Med. 2013 May 16;368(20):1907–17. [PMID: 23675659]

Locarnini S et al. Current perspectives on chronic hepatitis B. Semin Liver Dis. 2013 May;33(2):95–6. [PMID: 23749664]

Marcellin P et al. Regression of cirrhosis during treatment with tenofovir disoproxil fumarate for chronic hepatitis B: a 5-year open-label follow-up study. Lancet. 2013 Feb 9;381(9865): 468–75. [PMID: 23234725]

AUTOIMMUNE HEPATITIS

► Usually young to middle-aged women.

► Chronic hepatitis with high serum globulins and characteristic liver histology.

► Positive antinuclear antibody (ANA) and/or smooth muscle antibody in most common type.

► Responds to corticosteroids.

General Considerations

Although autoimmune hepatitis is usually seen in young women, it can occur in either sex at any age. The incidence and prevalence are estimated to be 8.5 and 107 per million population, respectively. Affected younger persons are often positive for HLA-B8 and HLA-DR3; older patients are often positive for HLA-DR4. The principal susceptibility allele among white Americans and northern Europeans is HLA *DRB1*0301*; HLA *DRB1*0401* is a secondary but independent risk factor.

Clinical Findings

A. Symptoms and Signs

The onset is usually insidious, but up to 40% of cases present with acute (occasionally fulminant) hepatitis and some cases follow a viral illness (such as hepatitis A, Epstein-Barr infection, or measles) or exposure to a drug or toxin (such as nitrofurantoin, minocycline, or infliximab). Exacerbations may occur postpartum. Amenorrhea may be a presenting feature. Thirty-four percent of patients are asymptomatic. Typically, examination reveals a healthy-appearing young woman with multiple spider angiomas, cutaneous striae, acne, hirsutism, and hepatomegaly. Extrahepatic features include arthritis, Sjögren syndrome, thyroiditis, nephritis, ulcerative colitis, and Coombs-positive hemolytic anemia. Patients with autoimmune hepatitis are at increased risk for cirrhosis, which, in turn, increases the risk of hepatocellular carcinoma (at a rate of about 1% per year).

B. Laboratory Findings

Serum aminotransferase levels may be > 1000 units/L, and the total bilirubin is usually increased. In type I (classic) autoimmune hepatitis, ANA or smooth muscle antibodies (either or both) are usually detected in serum. Serum gamma-globulin levels are typically elevated (up to 5–6 g/dL [0.05–0.06 g/L]); in such patients, the EIA for antibody to HCV may be falsely positive. Other antibodies, including atypical perinuclear antineutrophil cytoplasmic antibodies (pANCA) and antibodies to histones and F-actin, may be found. Antibodies to soluble liver antigen (anti-SLA) characterize a variant of type I that is marked by severe disease, a high relapse rate after treatment, and absence of the usual antibodies (ANA and smooth muscle antibodies). Anti-SLA is directed against a transfer RNA complex responsible for incorporating selenocysteine into peptide chains—Sep (O-phosphoserine) tRNA:Sec (selenocysteine) tRNA synthase, or SEPSECS. Type II, seen more often in girls under age 14 in Europe, is characterized by circulating antibodies to liver-kidney microsome type 1 (anti-LKM1)—directed against cytochrome P450 2D6—without anti-smooth muscle antibodies or ANA. In some cases, anti-liver cytosol type 1, directed against formiminotransferase cyclodeaminase, is detected. This type of autoimmune hepatitis can be seen in patients with autoimmune polyglandular syndrome type 1. Concurrent primary biliary cirrhosis or primary sclerosing cholangitis ("overlap syndrome") has been recognized in 7–13% and 6–11% of patients with autoimmune hepatitis, respectively. Liver biopsy is indicated to help establish the diagnosis (interface hepatitis is the hallmark), evaluate disease severity, and determine the need for treatment.

Simplified diagnostic criteria based on the detection of autoantibodies (1 or 2 points depending on titers, ≥ 1:40 or ≥ 1:80), elevated IgG levels (1 or 2 points depending on levels, ≥ upper limit of normal or ≥ 1.1 upper limit of normal), and characteristic histologic features (1 or 2 points depending on how typical the features are) and exclusion of viral hepatitis (2 points) can be useful for diagnosis; a score of 6 indicates probable and a score of 7 indicates definite autoimmune hepatitis with a high degree of specificity but moderate sensitivity. Diagnostic criteria for an overlap of autoimmune hepatitis and primary biliary cirrhosis ("Paris criteria") have been proposed.

Treatment

Prednisone with or without azathioprine improves symptoms; decreases the serum bilirubin, aminotransferase, and gamma-globulin levels; and reduces hepatic inflammation. Symptomatic patients with aminotransferase levels elevated tenfold (or fivefold if the serum globulins are elevated at least twofold) are optimal candidates for therapy, and asymptomatic patients with modest enzyme elevations may be considered for therapy depending on the clinical circumstances and histologic severity; however, asymptomatic patients usually remain asymptomatic, have either mild hepatitis or inactive cirrhosis on liver biopsy specimens, and have a good long-term prognosis without therapy.

Prednisone is given initially in a dose of 30 mg orally daily with azathioprine, 50 mg orally daily, which is generally well tolerated and permits the use of lower corticosteroid doses than a regimen beginning with prednisone 60 mg orally daily alone. Prednisone, 60 mg orally daily, is recommended for patients with acute severe autoimmune hepatitis. Budesonide, 6–9 mg orally daily, may be at least as effective as prednisone in noncirrhotic autoimmune hepatitis and associated with fewer side effects. Whether patients should undergo testing for the genotype or level of thiopurine methyltransferase prior to treatment with azathioprine to predict toxicity is debated. Blood counts are monitored weekly for the first 2 months of therapy and monthly thereafter because of the small risk of bone marrow suppression. The dose of prednisone is lowered from

30 mg/d after 1 week to 20 mg/d and again after 2 or 3 weeks to 15 mg/d. Ultimately, a maintenance dose of 10 mg/d is achieved. While symptomatic improvement is often prompt, biochemical improvement is more gradual, with normalization of serum aminotransferase levels after several months in many cases. Histologic resolution of inflammation lags biochemical remission by 3–8 months, and repeat liver biopsy is recommended after 18 months of treatment. Failure of aminotransferase levels to normalize invariably predicts lack of histologic resolution.

The response rate to therapy with prednisone and azathioprine is 80%. Older patients and those with HLA genotype *DRB1*04* are more likely to respond than younger patients and those with HLA *DRB1*03* hyperbilirubinemia or a high MELD score (≥ 12, see Cirrhosis). Fibrosis may reverse with therapy and rarely progresses after apparent biochemical and histologic remission. Once complete remission is achieved, therapy may be withdrawn, but the subsequent relapse rate is 50–80%. Relapses may again be treated in the same manner as the initial episode, with the same remission rate. After successful treatment of a relapse, the patient may continue taking azathioprine (up to 2 mg/kg) or the lowest dose of prednisone needed to maintain aminotransferase levels as close to normal as possible; another attempt at withdrawing therapy may be considered in patients remaining in remission long term (eg, ≥ 4 years). Prednisone can be used to treat rare flares during pregnancy, and maintenance azathioprine does not have to be discontinued.

Nonresponders to corticosteroids and azathioprine (failure of serum aminotransferase levels to decrease by 50% after 6 months) may be considered for a trial of cyclosporine, tacrolimus, sirolimus, everolimus, methotrexate, rituximab, or infliximab. Mycophenolate mofetil, 1 g twice daily, is an effective alternative to azathioprine in patients who cannot tolerate it but is less effective in nonresponders to azathioprine. Bone density should be monitored—particularly in patients receiving maintenance corticosteroid therapy—and measures undertaken to prevent or treat osteoporosis (see Chapter 26). Liver transplantation may be required for treatment failures and patients with a fulminant presentation, but the outcome may be worse than that for primary biliary cirrhosis because of an increased rate of infectious complications, and the disease has been recognized to recur in up to 40% of transplanted livers (and rarely to develop de novo) as immunosuppression is reduced; sirolimus can be effective in such cases. Overall long-term mortality of patients with autoimmune hepatitis appears to be greater than that of the general population despite response to immunosuppressive therapy. Factors that predict the need for liver transplantation or that predict liver-related death include the following: (1) age ≤ 20 years or > 60 years at presentation, (2) low serum albumin level at diagnosis, and (3) incomplete normalization of the serum ALT level after 6 months of treatment. Histologic severity is not a predictor.

When to Refer

- For liver biopsy.
- For immunosuppressive therapy.

When to Admit

- Hepatic encephalopathy.
- INR >1.6.

Czaja AJ. Acute and acute severe (fulminant) autoimmune hepatitis. Dig Dis Sci. 2013 Apr;58(4):897–914. [PMID: 23090425]

Czaja AJ. The overlap syndromes of autoimmune hepatitis. Dig Dis Sci. 2013 Feb;58(2):326–43. [PMID: 22918690]

Heneghan MA et al. Autoimmune hepatitis. Lancet. 2013 Oct 26;382(9902):1433–44. [PMID: 23768844]

Ngu JH et al. Predictors of poor outcome in patients with autoimmune hepatitis: a population-based study. Hepatology. 2013 Jun;57(6):2399–406. [PMID: 23359353]

van Gerven NM et al. Relapse is almost universal after withdrawal of immunosuppressive medication in patients with autoimmune hepatitis in remission. J Hepatol. 2013 Jan;58(1):141–7. [PMID: 22989569]

Zachou K et al. Review article: autoimmune hepatitis—current management and challenges. Aliment Pharmacol Ther. 2013 Oct;38(8):887–913. [PMID: 24010812]

ALCOHOLIC LIVER DISEASE

ESSENTIALS OF DIAGNOSIS

▸ Chronic alcohol intake usually exceeds 80 g/d in men and 30–40 g/d in women with alcoholic hepatitis or cirrhosis.

▸ Fatty liver is often asymptomatic.

▸ Fever, right upper quadrant pain, tender hepatomegaly, and jaundice characterize alcoholic hepatitis, but the patient may be asymptomatic.

▸ AST is usually elevated but usually not above 300 units/L (6 mckat/L); AST is greater than ALT, usually by a factor of 2 or more.

▸ Alcoholic hepatitis is often reversible but it is the most common precursor of cirrhosis in the United States.

General Considerations

Excessive alcohol intake can lead to fatty liver, hepatitis, and cirrhosis. Alcoholic hepatitis is characterized by acute or chronic inflammation and parenchymal necrosis of the liver induced by alcohol. Alcoholic hepatitis is often a reversible disease but the most common precursor of cirrhosis in the United States. It is associated with four to five times the number of hospitalizations and deaths as hepatitis C, which is the second most common cause of cirrhosis.

The frequency of alcoholic cirrhosis is estimated to be 10–15% among persons who consume over 50 g of alcohol (4 oz of 100-proof whiskey, 15 oz of wine, or four 12-oz cans of beer) daily for over 10 years (although the risk of cirrhosis may be lower for wine than for a comparable intake of beer or spirits). The risk of cirrhosis is lower (5%) in the absence of other cofactors such as chronic viral hepatitis and obesity. Genetic factors, including polymorphisms of the genes encoding palatin-like phospholipase domain-containing protein 3 (PNPLA3), tumor necrosis factor, cytochrome P450 2E1, and glutathione S-transferase may also account for differences in susceptibility to and severity of liver disease. Women appear to be more susceptible than men, in part because of lower gastric mucosal alcohol dehydrogenase levels.

Clinical Findings

A. Symptoms and Signs

The clinical presentation of alcoholic liver disease can vary from asymptomatic hepatomegaly to a rapidly fatal acute illness or end-stage cirrhosis. A recent period of heavy drinking, complaints of anorexia and nausea, and the demonstration of hepatomegaly and jaundice strongly suggest the diagnosis. Abdominal pain and tenderness, splenomegaly, ascites, fever, and encephalopathy may be present. Infection is common in patients with severe alcoholic hepatitis.

B. Laboratory Findings

In patients with steatosis, mild liver enzyme elevations may be the only laboratory abnormality. Anemia (usually macrocytic) may be present. Leukocytosis with a shift to the left is common in patients with severe alcoholic hepatitis. Leukopenia is occasionally seen and resolves after cessation of drinking. About 10% of patients have thrombocytopenia related to a direct toxic effect of alcohol on megakaryocyte production or to hypersplenism.

AST is usually elevated but infrequently above 300 units/L (6 mckat/L). AST is greater than ALT, usually by a factor of 2 or more. Serum alkaline phosphatase is generally elevated, but seldom more than three times the normal value. Serum bilirubin is increased in 60–90% of patients with alcoholic hepatitis.

Serum bilirubin levels >10 mg/dL (171 mcmol/L) and marked prolongation of the prothrombin time (≥ 6 seconds above control) indicate severe alcoholic hepatitis with a mortality rate as high as 50%. The serum albumin is depressed, and the gamma-globulin level is elevated in 50–75% of individuals, even in the absence of cirrhosis. Increased transferrin saturation, hepatic iron stores, and sideroblastic anemia are found in many alcoholic patients. Folic acid deficiency may coexist.

C. Imaging

Imaging studies can detect moderate to severe hepatic steatosis reliably but not inflammation or fibrosis. Ultrasonography helps exclude biliary obstruction and identifies subclinical ascites. CT with intravenous contrast or MRI may be indicated in selected cases to evaluate patients for collateral vessels, space-occupying lesions of the liver, or concomitant disease of the pancreas.

D. Liver Biopsy

Liver biopsy, if done, demonstrates macrovesicular fat and, in patients with alcoholic hepatitis, polymorphonuclear infiltration with hepatic necrosis, Mallory (or Mallory-Denk)

bodies (alcoholic hyaline), and perivenular and perisinusoidal fibrosis. Micronodular cirrhosis may be present as well. The findings are identical to those of nonalcoholic steatohepatitis.

Differential Diagnosis

Alcoholic hepatitis may be closely mimicked by cholecystitis and cholelithiasis and by drug toxicity. Other causes of hepatitis or chronic liver disease may be excluded by serologic or biochemical testing, imaging studies, or liver biopsy. A formula based on the AST/ALT ratio, body mass index, mean corpuscular volume, and gender has been reported to reliably distinguish alcoholic liver disease from nonalcoholic fatty liver disease (NAFLD).

Treatment

A. General Measures

Abstinence from alcohol is essential. Naltrexone, acamprosate, or baclofen may be considered in combination with counseling to reduce the likelihood of recidivism. Fatty liver is quickly reversible with abstinence. Every effort should be made to provide sufficient amounts of carbohydrates and calories in anorectic patients to reduce endogenous protein catabolism, promote gluconeogenesis, and prevent hypoglycemia. Nutritional support (40 kcal/kg with 1.5–2 g/kg as protein) improves liver disease, but not necessarily survival, in patients with malnutrition. Use of liquid formulas rich in branched-chain amino acids does not improve survival beyond that achieved with less expensive caloric supplementation. The administration of micronutrients, particularly folic acid, thiamine, and zinc, is indicated, especially when deficiencies are noted; glucose administration increases the thiamine requirement and can precipitate Wernicke–Korsakoff syndrome if thiamine is not coadministered.

B. Pharmacologic Measures

Methylprednisolone, 32 mg/d orally, or the equivalent, for 1 month, may reduce short-term mortality in patients with alcoholic hepatitis and either encephalopathy or a Maddrey discriminant function index (defined by the patient's prothrombin time minus the control prothrombin time times 4.6 plus the total bilirubin in mg/dL) of ≥ 32. No benefit has been demonstrated in patients with concomitant gastrointestinal bleeding, but infection should not preclude treatment with corticosteroids if otherwise indicated.

Pentoxifylline, 400 mg orally three times daily for 4 weeks, may reduce 1-month mortality rates in patients with severe alcoholic hepatitis, primarily by decreasing the risk of hepatorenal syndrome. It is often used when corticosteroids are contraindicated. The addition of pentoxifylline to prednisolone, however, has been shown in one study not to improve survival or reduce the frequency of hepatorenal syndrome compared with prednisolone alone. The combination of corticosteroids and N-acetylcysteine has been reported to improve 1-month but not 6-month survival and reduce the risk of hepatorenal syndrome and infections.

Prognosis

A. Short-Term

The overall mortality rate is 34% (20% within 1 month) without corticosteroid therapy. Individuals in whom the prothrombin time prohibits liver biopsy have a 42% mortality rate at 1 year. Other unfavorable prognostic factors are older age, a serum bilirubin >10 mg/dL (171 mcmol/L), hepatic encephalopathy, coagulopathy, azotemia, leukocytosis, sepsis and other infections, lack of response to corticosteroid therapy, and possibly a paucity of steatosis on a liver biopsy specimen and reversal of portal blood flow by Doppler ultrasonography. Failure of the serum bilirubin level to decline after 7 days of treatment with corticosteroids predicts nonresponse and poor long-term survival, as does the Lille model (which includes age, serum creatinine, serum albumin, prothrombin time [or INR], serum bilirubin on admission, and serum bilirubin on day 7). The MELD score used for cirrhosis (see Cirrhosis) and the Glasgow alcoholic hepatitis score (based on age, white blood cell count, blood urea nitrogen, prothrombin time ratio, and bilirubin level) also correlate with mortality from alcoholic hepatitis and have higher specificities than the discriminant function and Lille score. A scoring system based on age, serum bilirubin, INR, and serum creatinine (ABIC) has been proposed, and one study has shown that the development of acute kidney injury is the most accurate predictor of 90-day mortality.

B. Long-Term

Overall mortality from alcoholic liver disease has declined slightly in the United States since 1980. Nevertheless, the 3-year mortality rate of persons who recover from acute alcoholic hepatitis is ten times greater than that of control individuals of comparable age; the 5-year mortality rate is as high as 85%. Histologically, severe disease is associated with continued excessive mortality rates after 3 years, whereas the death rate is not increased after the same period in those whose liver biopsies show only mild alcoholic hepatitis. Complications of portal hypertension (ascites, variceal bleeding, hepatorenal syndrome), coagulopathy, and severe jaundice following recovery from acute alcoholic hepatitis also suggest a poor long-term prognosis. Alcoholic cirrhosis is a risk factor for hepatocellular carcinoma, and the risk is highest in carriers of the *C282Y* mutation for hemochromatosis or those with increased hepatic iron.

The most important prognostic consideration is continued excessive drinking. A 6-month period of abstinence is generally required before liver transplantation is considered, although this requirement has been questioned and early liver transplantation has been performed in selected patients with alcoholic hepatitis, with good outcomes. Optimal candidates have adequate social support, do not smoke, have no psychosis or personality disorder, are adherent to therapy, and have regular appointments with a psychiatrist or psychologist who specializes in addiction treatment. Patients with alcoholic liver disease are at higher risk for posttransplant malignancy than those with other types of liver disease because of alcohol and tobacco use.

When to Refer

Refer patients with alcoholic hepatitis who require liver biopsy for diagnosis.

When to Admit

- Hepatic encephalopathy.
- INR > 1.6.
- Total bilirubin ≥10 mg/dL.
- Inability to maintain hydration.

Altamirano J et al. Acute kidney injury is an early predictor of mortality for patients with alcoholic hepatitis. Clin Gastroenterol Hepatol. 2012 Jan;10(1):65–71. [PMID: 21946124]

Lafferty H et al. The management of alcoholic hepatitis: a prospective comparison of scoring systems. Aliment Pharmacol Ther. 2013 Sep;38(6):603–10. [PMID: 23879668]

Mathurin P et al. Prednisolone with vs without pentoxifylline and survival of patients with severe alcoholic hepatitis: a randomized clinical trial. JAMA. 2013 Sep 11;310(10):1033–41. [PMID: 24026598]

Parker R et al. Systematic review: pentoxifylline for the treatment of severe alcoholic hepatitis. Aliment Pharmacol Ther. 2013 May;37(9):845–54. [PMID: 23489011]

Potts JR et al. Determinants of long-term outcome in severe alcoholic hepatitis. Aliment Pharmacol Ther. 2013 Sep;38(6):584–95. [PMID: 23879720]

DRUG- & TOXIN-INDUCED LIVER DISEASE

ESSENTIALS OF DIAGNOSIS

- ► Drug-induced liver disease can mimic viral hepatitis, biliary tract obstruction, or other types of liver disease.
- ► Clinicians must inquire about the use of many widely used therapeutic agents, including over-the-counter "natural" and herbal products, in any patient with liver disease.

General Considerations

Many therapeutic agents may cause drug-induced liver injury. The medications most commonly implicated are nonsteroidal anti-inflammatory drugs and antibiotics because of their widespread use. In any patient with liver disease, the clinician must inquire carefully about the use of potentially hepatotoxic drugs or exposure to hepatotoxins, including over-the-counter "natural" and herbal products. In some cases, coadministration of a second agent may increase the toxicity of the first (eg, isoniazid and rifampin, acetaminophen and alcohol). A relationship between increased serum ALT levels in premarketing clinical trials and postmarketing reports of hepatotoxicity has been identified. Except for drugs used to treat tuberculosis and HIV infection, the risk of hepatotoxicity is not increased in patients with preexisting cirrhosis. Drug toxicity may be categorized on the basis of pathogenesis or predominant histologic appearance. Drug-induced liver injury can mimic viral hepatitis, biliary tract obstruction, or other types of liver disease. A useful resource is the website, www.livertox.nih.gov/.

► Categorization by Pathogenesis

A. Direct Hepatotoxicity

Liver toxicity caused by this group of drugs is characterized by: (1) dose-related severity, (2) a latent period following exposure, and (3) susceptibility in all individuals. Examples include acetaminophen (toxicity is enhanced by fasting and chronic alcohol use because of depletion of glutathione and induction of cytochrome P450 2E1 and possibly reduced by statins, fibrates, and nonsteroidal anti-inflammatory drugs), alcohol, carbon tetrachloride, chloroform, heavy metals, mercaptopurine, niacin, plant alkaloids, phosphorus, pyrazinamide, tetracyclines, tipranavir, valproic acid, and vitamin A. Statins, like all cholesterol-lowering agents, may cause serum aminotransferase elevations but rarely cause true hepatitis, and even more rarely cause acute liver failure, and are no longer considered contraindicated in patients with liver disease.

B. Idiosyncratic Reactions

Except for acetaminophen, most severe hepatotoxicity is idiosyncratic. Reactions of this type are (1) sporadic, (2) not related to dose above a general threshold of 100 mg/d, and (3) occasionally associated with features suggesting an allergic reaction, such as fever and eosinophilia, which may be associated with a favorable outcome. In many instances, the drug is lipophilic, and toxicity results directly from a metabolite that is produced only in certain individuals on a genetic basis. Drug-induced liver injury may be observed only during post-marketing surveillance and not during preclinical trials. Examples include abacavir, amiodarone, aspirin, carbamazepine, chloramphenicol, diclofenac, disulfiram, duloxetine, ezetimibe, flavocoxid (a "medical food"), fluoroquinolones (moxifloxacin and levofloxacin, in particular), flutamide, halothane, isoniazid, ketoconazole, lamotrigine, methyldopa, natalizumab, nevirapine, oxacillin, phenytoin, pyrazinamide, quinidine, streptomycin, thiazolidinediones, tolvaptan, and perhaps tacrine.

► Categorization by Histopathology

A. Cholestasis

1. Noninflammatory—Drug-induced cholestasis results from inhibition or genetic deficiency of various hepatobiliary transporter systems. The following drugs cause cholestasis: anabolic steroids containing an alkyl or ethinyl group at carbon 17, azathioprine, cetirizine, cyclosporine, diclofenac, estrogens, indinavir (increased risk of indirect hyperbilirubinemia in patients with Gilbert syndrome), mercaptopurine, methyltestosterone, tamoxifen, temozolomide, and ticlopidine.

2. Inflammatory—The following drugs cause inflammation of portal areas with bile duct injury (cholangitis), often with allergic features such as eosinophilia:

amoxicillin-clavulanic acid (among the most common causes of drug-induced liver injury), azathioprine, azithromycin, captopril, celecoxib, cephalosporins, chlorothiazide, chlorpromazine, chlorpropamide, erythromycin, mercaptopurine, penicillamine, prochlorperazine, semisynthetic penicillins (eg, cloxacillin), and sulfadiazine. Ketamine abuse may cause secondary biliary cirrhosis. Cholestatic and mixed cholestatic hepatocellular toxicity is more likely than pure hepatocellular toxicity to lead to chronic liver disease.

B. Acute or Chronic Hepatitis

Medications that may result in acute or chronic hepatitis that is histologically and in some cases clinically similar to autoimmune hepatitis include minocycline and nitrofurantoin, most commonly, as well as aspirin, isoniazid (increased risk in HBV and HCV carriers), methyldopa, nonsteroidal anti-inflammatory drugs, propylthiouracil, terbinafine, and tumor necrosis factor inhibitors. Histologic features that favor a drug cause include portal tract neutrophils and hepatocellular cholestasis. Hepatitis also can occur in patients taking cocaine, diclofenac, methylenedioxymethamphetamine (MDMA; Ecstasy), efavirenz, imatinib mesylate, ipilimumab, nafazodone (has a black box warning for a potential to cause liver failure), nevirapine (like other protease inhibitors, increased risk in HBV and HCV carriers), pioglitazone, ritonavir (greater rate than other protease inhibitors), rosiglitazone, saquinavir, sulfonamides, telithromycin, and zafirlukast, as well as a variety of alternative remedies (eg, chaparral, germander, green tea extracts, Herbalife products, hydroxycut, jin bu huan, kava, skullcap, and possibly black cohosh), as well as dietary supplements (eg, OxyELITE Pro). In patients with jaundice due to drug-induced hepatitis, the mortality rate without liver transplantation is at least 10%.

C. Other Reactions

1. Fatty liver

A. Macrovesicular—This type of liver injury may be produced by alcohol, amiodarone, corticosteroids, methotrexate, irinotecan, tamoxifen, vinyl chloride (in exposed workers), zalcitabine, and possibly oxaliplatin.

B. Microvesicular—Often resulting from mitochondrial injury, this condition is associated with didanosine, stavudine, tetracyclines, valproic acid, and zidovudine.

2. Granulomas
Allopurinol, quinidine, quinine, phenylbutazone, phenytoin, and pyrazinamide can lead to granulomas.

3. Fibrosis and cirrhosis
Methotrexate and vitamin A are associated with fibrosis and cirrhosis.

4. Sinusoidal obstruction syndrome (veno-occlusive disease)
This disorder may result from treatment with antineoplastic agents (eg, pre-bone marrow transplant, oxaliplatin), and pyrrolizidine alkaloids (eg, Comfrey).

5. Peliosis hepatis (blood-filled cavities)
Peliosis hepatis may be caused by anabolic steroids and oral contraceptive

steroids as well as azathioprine and mercaptopurine, which may also cause nodular regenerative hyperplasia.

6. Neoplasms—Neoplasms may result from therapy with oral contraceptive steroids, including estrogens (hepatic adenoma but not focal nodular hyperplasia), and vinyl chloride (angiosarcoma).

▶ When to Refer

Refer patients with drug- and toxin-induced hepatitis who require liver biopsy for diagnosis.

▶ When to Admit

Patients with liver failure should be hospitalized.

Björnsson ES et al. Incidence, presentation, and outcomes in patients with drug-induced liver injury in the general population of Iceland. Gastroenterology. 2013 Jun;144(7):1419–25. [PMID: 23419359]

Bunchorntavakul C et al. Review article: herbal and dietary supplement hepatotoxicity. Aliment Pharmacol Ther. 2013 Jan;37(1):3–17. [PMID: 23121117]

Chen M et al. High lipophilicity and high daily dose of oral medications are associated with significant risk for drug-induced liver injury. Hepatology. 2013 Jul;58(1):388–96. [PMID: 23258593]

Ghabril M et al. Liver injury from tumor necrosis factor-α antagonists: analysis of thirty-four cases. Clin Gastroenterol Hepatol. 2013 May;11(5):558–64. [PMID: 23333219]

Lewis JH et al. Review article: prescribing medications in patients with cirrhosis—a practical guide. Aliment Pharmacol Ther. 2013 Jun;37(12):1132–56. [PMID: 23638982]

Pyrsopoulos NT (editor). Drug hepatotoxicity. Clin Liver Dis [entire issue]. 2013 Nov;17(4):507–786. [PMID: 24099030]

NONALCOHOLIC FATTY LIVER DISEASE

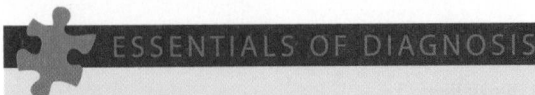

ESSENTIALS OF DIAGNOSIS

► Often asymptomatic.
► Elevated aminotransferase levels and/or hepatomegaly.
► Predominantly macrovesicular steatosis with or without inflammation and fibrosis on liver biopsy.

▶ General Considerations

Nonalcoholic fatty liver disease (NAFLD) is estimated to affect 20–45% of the US population. The principal causes of NAFLD are obesity (present in ≥ 40%), diabetes mellitus (in ≥ 20%), and hypertriglyceridemia (in ≥ 20%) in association with insulin resistance as part of the metabolic syndrome. The risk of NAFLD in persons with metabolic syndrome is 4 to 11 times higher than that of persons without insulin resistance. Other causes of fatty liver include corticosteroids, amiodarone, diltiazem, tamoxifen, irinotecan, oxaliplatin, highly active antiretroviral therapy, toxins (vinyl chloride, carbon tetrachloride, yellow phosphorus), endocrinopathies such as Cushing syndrome and hypopituitarism, polycystic ovary syndrome, hypothyroidism, hypobetalipoproteinemia and other metabolic disorders, obstructive sleep apnea (with chronic intermittent hypoxia), excessive dietary fructose consumption, starvation and refeeding syndrome, and total parenteral nutrition. Genetic factors are likely to play a role, and polymorphisms of the patatin-like phospholipase domain containing 3 (*PNPLA3*) gene modify the natural history of NAFLD and may account in part for an increased risk in Hispanics. The risk of NAFLD is increased in persons with psoriasis and appears to correlate with the activity of psoriasis. Soft drink consumption and cholecystectomy have been reported to be associated with NAFLD. Physical activity protects against the development of NAFLD. In addition to macrovesicular steatosis, histologic features may include focal infiltration by polymorphonuclear neutrophils and Mallory hyalin, a picture indistinguishable from that of alcoholic hepatitis and referred to as nonalcoholic steatohepatitis (NASH), which affects 3–5% of the US population. In patients with NAFLD, older age, obesity, and diabetes mellitus are risk factors for advanced hepatic fibrosis and cirrhosis, whereas coffee consumption appears to reduce the risk. Cirrhosis caused by NASH appears to be uncommon in African Americans.

Microvesicular steatosis is seen with Reye syndrome, didanosine or stavudine toxicity, valproic acid toxicity, high-dose tetracycline, or acute fatty liver of pregnancy and may result in fulminant hepatic failure. Women in whom fatty liver of pregnancy develops often have a defect in fatty acid oxidation due to reduced long-chain 3-hydroxyacyl-CoA dehydrogenase activity.

▶ Clinical Findings

A. Symptoms and Signs

Most patients with NAFLD are asymptomatic or have mild right upper quadrant discomfort. Hepatomegaly is present in up to 75% of patients, but stigmata of chronic liver disease are uncommon. Rare instances of subacute liver failure caused by previously unrecognized NASH have been described. Signs of portal hypertension generally signify advanced liver fibrosis or cirrhosis but occasionally occur in patients with mild and no fibrosis and severe steatosis.

B. Laboratory Findings

Laboratory studies may show mildly elevated aminotransferase and alkaline phosphatase levels; however, laboratory values may be normal in up to 80% of persons with hepatic steatosis. In contrast to alcoholic liver disease, the ratio of ALT to AST is almost always >1 in NAFLD, but it decreases to < 1 as advanced fibrosis and cirrhosis develop. Antinuclear or smooth muscle antibodies and an elevated serum ferritin level may each be detected in one-fourth of patients with NASH. Elevated serum ferritin levels may signify so-called dysmetabolic iron overload syndrome and mildly increased body iron stores, which may play a causal role in insulin resistance and oxidative stress in hepatocytes and correlate with advanced fibrosis; the frequency of mutations in the *HFE* gene for hemochromatosis is not increased in patients with NAFLD.

C. Imaging

Macrovascular steatosis may be demonstrated on ultrasonography, CT, or MRI. However, imaging does not distinguish steatosis from steatohepatitis or detect fibrosis.

D. Liver Biopsy

Percutaneous liver biopsy is diagnostic and is the standard approach to assessing the degree of inflammation and fibrosis. The risks of the procedure must be balanced against the impact of the added information on management decisions and assessment of prognosis. Liver biopsy is generally not recommended in asymptomatic persons with unsuspected hepatic steatosis detected on imaging but normal liver biochemistry test results. The histologic spectrum of NAFLD includes fatty liver, isolated portal fibrosis, steatohepatitis, and cirrhosis. A risk score for predicting advanced fibrosis, known as BARD, is based on body mass index >28, AST/ALT ratio $\geq$ 0.8, and diabetes mellitus; it has a 96% negative predictive value (ie, a low score reliably excludes advanced fibrosis). Another risk score for advanced fibrosis, the NAFLD Fibrosis Score (http://nafldscore.com) based on age, hyperglycemia, body mass index, platelet count, albumin, and AST/ALT ratio, has a positive predictive value of over 80% and identifies patients at increased risk of liver-related complications and death. A clinical scoring system to predict the likelihood of NASH in morbidly obese persons includes six predictive factors: hypertension, type 2 diabetes mellitus, sleep apnea, AST > 27 units/L (0.54 mckat/L), ALT > 27 units/L (0.54 mckat/L), and non-black race.

▶ Treatment

Treatment consists of lifestyle changes to remove or modify the offending factors. Weight loss, dietary fat restriction, and exercise (through reduction of abdominal obesity) often lead to improvement in liver biochemical tests and steatosis in obese patients with NAFLD. Loss of 3–5% of body weight appears necessary to improve steatosis, but loss of up to 10% may be needed to improve necroinflammation. Exercise may reduce liver fat with minimal or no weight loss and no reduction in ALT levels. Resistance training and aerobic exercise are equally effective in reducing hepatic fat content in patients with NAFLD and type 2 diabetes mellitus. Various drugs are under study. Thiazolidinediones reverse insulin resistance and, in most relevant studies, have improved both serum aminotransferase levels and histologic features of steatohepatitis but lead to weight gain. Vitamin E 800 international units/d (to reduce oxidative stress) also appears to be of benefit. Metformin, which reduces insulin resistance, improves abnormal liver chemistries but may not reliably improve liver histology. Pentoxifylline improves liver biochemical test levels but is associated with a high rate of side effects, particularly nausea. Ursodeoxycholic acid, 12–15 mg/kg/d, has not consistently resulted in biochemical and histologic improvement in patients with NASH but may be effective when given in combination with vitamin E. Hepatic steatosis due to total parenteral nutrition may be ameliorated—and perhaps prevented—with supplemental choline.

Statins are not contraindicated in persons with NAFLD. Gastric bypass may be considered in patients with a body mass index > 35 and leads to improvement in hepatic steatosis. Liver transplantation is indicated in appropriate candidates with advanced cirrhosis caused by NASH, now the third most common indication for liver transplantation in the United States.

▶ Prognosis

Fatty liver often has a benign course and is readily reversible with discontinuation of alcohol (or no more than one glass of wine per day, which may actually reduce the frequency of NASH in persons with NAFLD), or treatment of other underlying conditions; if untreated, cirrhosis develops in 1–3% of patients. In patients with NAFLD, the likelihood of NASH is increased by the following factors: obesity, older age, non–African American ethnicity, female sex, diabetes mellitus, hypertension, higher ALT or AST level, higher AST/ALT ratio, low platelet count, elevated fasting C-peptide level, and an ultrasound steatosis score. NASH may be associated with hepatic fibrosis in 40% of cases; cirrhosis develops in 9–25%; and decompensated cirrhosis occurs in 30–50% of cirrhotic patients over 10 years. The course may be more aggressive in diabetic persons than in nondiabetic persons. Mortality is increased in patients with NAFLD and is more likely to be the result of malignancy and ischemic heart disease than liver disease. Risk factors for mortality are older age, male gender, white race, higher body mass index, hypertension, diabetes mellitus, and cirrhosis. Steatosis is a cofactor for the progression of fibrosis in patients with other causes of chronic liver disease, such as hepatitis C. Hepatocellular carcinoma is a complication of cirrhosis caused by NASH as it is for other causes of cirrhosis. NASH accounts for a substantial percentage of cases labeled as cryptogenic cirrhosis and can recur following liver transplantation. Central obesity is an independent risk factor for death from cirrhosis of any cause.

▶ When to Refer

Refer patients with non-alcoholic fatty liver disease who require liver biopsy for diagnosis.

Angulo P et al. Simple noninvasive systems predict long-term outcomes of patients with nonalcoholic fatty liver disease. Gastroenterology. 2013 Oct;145(4):782–9. [PMID: 23860502]

Kim D et al. Association between noninvasive fibrosis markers and mortality among adults with nonalcoholic fatty liver disease in the United States. Hepatology. 2013 Apr;57(4):1357–65. [PMID: 23175136]

Pais R et al. A systematic review of follow-up biopsies reveals disease progression in patients with non-alcoholic fatty liver. J Hepatol. 2013 Sep;59(3):550–6. [PMID: 23665288]

Ryan MC et al. The Mediterranean diet improves hepatic steatosis and insulin sensitivity in individuals with non-alcoholic fatty liver disease. J Hepatol. 2013 Jul;59(1):138–43. [PMID: 23485520]

Sanyal AJ (editor). Nonalcoholic fatty liver disease. Clin Liver Dis [entire issue]. 2012 Aug;16(3):467–657. [PMID: 22824486]

Yesil A et al. Review article: coffee consumption, the metabolic syndrome and non-alcoholic fatty liver disease. Aliment Pharmacol Ther. 2013 Nov;38(9):1038–44. [PMID: 24024834]

CIRRHOSIS

- ► End result of injury that leads to both fibrosis and regenerative nodules.
- ► May be reversible if cause is removed.
- ► The clinical features result from hepatic cell dysfunction, portosystemic shunting, and portal hypertension.

► General Considerations

Cirrhosis, the twelfth leading cause of death in the United States, is the end result of hepatocellular injury that leads to both fibrosis and regenerative nodules throughout the liver. Hospitalization rates for cirrhosis and portal hypertension are rising in the United States. Causes include chronic viral hepatitis, alcohol, drug toxicity, autoimmune and metabolic liver diseases, and miscellaneous disorders. Many patients have more than one risk factor (eg, chronic hepatitis and alcohol use). Mexican Americans and African Americans have a higher frequency of cirrhosis than whites because of a higher rate of risk factors. In persons at increased risk for liver injury (eg, heavy alcohol use, obesity, iron overload), higher coffee and tea consumption has been reported to reduce the risk of cirrhosis. The risk of hospitalization or death due to cirrhosis has been reported to correlate with protein and cholesterol consumption and with hyperuricemia and inversely with carbohydrate consumption.

Clinically, cirrhosis is considered to progress through three stages: compensated, compensated with varices, and decompensated (ascites, variceal bleeding, encephalopathy, or jaundice) that correlate with the thickness of fibrous septa.

► Clinical Findings

A. Symptoms and Signs

The clinical features of cirrhosis result from hepatocyte dysfunction, portosystemic shunting, and portal hypertension. Patients may have no symptoms for long periods. The onset of symptoms may be insidious or, less often, abrupt. Fatigue, disturbed sleep, muscle cramps, and weight loss are common. In advanced cirrhosis, anorexia is usually present and may be extreme, with associated nausea and occasional vomiting, as well as reduced muscle strength and exercise capacity. Abdominal pain may be present and is related either to hepatic enlargement and stretching of Glisson capsule or to the presence of ascites. Menstrual abnormalities (usually amenorrhea), erectile dysfunction, loss of libido, sterility, and gynecomastia in men may occur. Hematemesis is the presenting symptom in 15–25%.

Skin manifestations consist of spider angiomas (invariably on the upper half of the body), palmar erythema (mottled redness of the thenar and hypothenar eminences), and Dupuytren contractures. Evidence of vitamin deficiencies (glossitis and cheilosis) is common. Weight loss, wasting (due to sarcopenia), and the appearance of chronic illness are present. Jaundice—usually not an initial sign—is mild at first, increasing in severity during the later stages of the disease. In 70% of cases, the liver is enlarged, palpable, and firm if not hard and has a sharp or nodular edge; the left lobe may predominate. Splenomegaly is present in 35–50% of cases and is associated with an increased risk of complications of portal hypertension. The superficial veins of the abdomen and thorax are dilated, reflecting the intrahepatic obstruction to portal blood flow, as do rectal varices. The abdominal wall veins fill from below when compressed. Ascites, pleural effusions, peripheral edema, and ecchymoses are late findings. Encephalopathy characterized by day–night reversal, asterixis, tremor, dysarthria, delirium, drowsiness, and ultimately coma also occurs late except when precipitated by an acute hepatocellular insult or an episode of gastrointestinal bleeding or infection. Fever may be a presenting symptom in up to 35% of patients and usually reflects associated alcoholic hepatitis, spontaneous bacterial peritonitis, or intercurrent infection.

B. Laboratory Findings

Laboratory abnormalities are either absent or minimal in early or compensated cirrhosis. Anemia, a frequent finding, is often macrocytic; causes include suppression of erythropoiesis by alcohol as well as folate deficiency, hemolysis, hypersplenism, and occult or overt blood loss from the gastrointestinal tract. The white blood cell count may be low, reflecting hypersplenism, or high, suggesting infection. Thrombocytopenia, the most common cytopenia in cirrhotic patients, is secondary to alcoholic marrow suppression, sepsis, folate deficiency, or splenic sequestration. Prolongation of the prothrombin time may result from reduced levels of clotting factors (except factor VIII). However, bleeding risk correlates poorly with the prothrombin time because of concomitant abnormalities of fibrinolysis, and among hospitalized patients under age 45, cirrhosis is associated with an increased risk of venous thromboembolism.

Blood chemistries reflect hepatocellular injury and dysfunction, manifested by modest elevations of AST and alkaline phosphatase and progressive elevation of the bilirubin. Serum albumin decreases as the disease progresses; gamma-globulin is increased and may be as high as in autoimmune hepatitis. The risk of diabetes mellitus is increased in patients with cirrhosis, particularly when associated with HCV infection, alcoholism, hemochromatosis, or NAFLD. Vitamin D deficiency has been reported in as many as 91% of patients with cirrhosis. Patients with alcoholic cirrhosis may have elevated serum cardiac troponin I and B-type natriuretic peptide (BNP) levels. Blunted cardiac inotropic and chronotropic responses to exercise, stress, and drugs, as well as systolic and diastolic ventricular dysfunction ("cirrhotic cardiomyopathy") and prolongation of the QT interval in the setting of a hyperkinetic circulation, are common in cirrhosis of all causes, but overt heart failure is rare in the absence of alcoholism. Relative adrenal insufficiency appears to be common in patients with advanced cirrhosis, even in the absence of sepsis, and may relate in part to reduced synthesis of cholesterol and increased levels of proinflammatory cytokines.

C. Imaging

Ultrasonography is helpful for assessing liver size and detecting ascites or hepatic nodules, including small hepatocellular carcinomas. Together with a Doppler study, it may establish patency of the splenic, portal, and hepatic veins. Hepatic nodules are characterized further by contrast-enhanced CT or MRI. Nodules suspicious for malignancy may be biopsied under ultrasound or CT guidance.

D. Liver Biopsy

Liver biopsy may show inactive cirrhosis (fibrosis with regenerative nodules) with no specific features to suggest the underlying cause. Alternatively, there may be additional features of alcoholic liver disease, chronic hepatitis, NASH, or other specific causes of cirrhosis. Liver biopsy may be performed by laparoscopy or, in patients with coagulopathy and ascites, by a transjugular approach. Combinations of routine blood tests (eg, AST, platelet count), including the FibroSure test, and serum markers of hepatic fibrosis (eg, hyaluronic acid, amino-terminal propeptide of type III collagen, tissue inhibitor of matrix metalloproteinase 1) are potential alternatives to liver biopsy for the diagnosis or exclusion of cirrhosis. In persons with chronic hepatitis C, for example, a low FibroSure score reliably excludes advanced fibrosis, a high score reliably predicts advanced fibrosis, and intermediate scores are inconclusive.

E. Other Tests

Esophagogastroduodenoscopy confirms the presence of varices and detects specific causes of bleeding in the esophagus, stomach, and proximal duodenum. In selected cases, wedged hepatic vein pressure measurement may establish the presence and cause of portal hypertension. Ultrasound elastography and magnetic resonance elastography to measure liver stiffness are available in a limited number of centers as noninvasive tests for cirrhosis and portal hypertension.

▶ Differential Diagnosis

The most common causes of cirrhosis are alcohol, chronic hepatitis C infection, NAFLD, and hepatitis B infection, and the prevalence of NAFLD has been increasing steadily because of the rapidly increasing prevalence of obesity in the United States. Hemochromatosis is the most commonly identified genetic disorder that causes cirrhosis. Other metabolic diseases that may lead to cirrhosis include Wilson disease and alpha-1-antitrypsin (alpha-1-antiprotease) deficiency, and celiac disease has been associated with cirrhosis. Primary biliary cirrhosis occurs more frequently in women than men. Secondary biliary cirrhosis may result from chronic biliary obstruction due to a stone, stricture, or neoplasm. Heart failure

and constrictive pericarditis may lead to hepatic fibrosis ("cardiac cirrhosis") complicated by ascites and may be mistaken for other causes of cirrhosis. Hereditary hemorrhagic telangiectasia can lead to portal hypertension because of portosystemic shunting and nodular transformation of the liver as well as high-output heart failure. Many cases of cirrhosis are "cryptogenic," in which unrecognized NAFLD may play a role.

▶ Complications

Upper gastrointestinal tract bleeding may occur from varices, portal hypertensive gastropathy, or gastroduodenal ulcer (see Chapter 15). Varices may also result from portal vein thrombosis, which may complicate cirrhosis. Liver failure may be precipitated by alcoholism, surgery, and infection. Hepatic Kupffer cell (reticuloendothelial) dysfunction and decreased opsonic activity lead to an increased risk of systemic infection (which may be increased further by the use of proton pump inhibitors), and which increase mortality fourfold. These infections include nosocomial infections, which may be classified as spontaneous bloodstream infections, urinary tract infections, pulmonary infections, spontaneous bacterial peritonitis, *Clostridium difficile* infection, and intervention-related infections. These nosocomial infections are increasingly caused by multidrug-resistant bacteria. Osteoporosis occurs in 12–55% of patients with cirrhosis. The risk of hepatocellular carcinoma is increased greatly in persons with cirrhosis (see Chapter 39).

▶ Treatment

A. General Measures

The most important principle of treatment is abstinence from alcohol. The diet should be palatable, with adequate calories (25–35 kcal/kg body weight per day in those with compensated cirrhosis and 35–45 kcal/kg/d in those with malnutrition) and protein (1–1.5 g/kg/d in those with compensated cirrhosis and 1.5 g/kg/d in those with malnutrition) and, if there is fluid retention, sodium restriction. In the presence of hepatic encephalopathy, protein intake should be reduced to no less than 60–80 g/d. Specialized supplements containing branched-chain amino acids to prevent or treat hepatic encephalopathy or delay progressive liver failure are generally unnecessary. Vitamin supplementation is desirable. Patients with cirrhosis should receive the HAV, HBV, and pneumococcal vaccines and a yearly influenza vaccine. Liver transplantation in appropriate candidates is curative, and pharmacologic treatments to halt progression of or even reverse cirrhosis are being developed.

B. Treatment of Complications

1. Ascites and edema—Diagnostic paracentesis is indicated for patients who have new ascites or who have been hospitalized for a complication of cirrhosis. Serious complications of paracentesis, including bleeding, infection, or bowel perforation, occur in 1.6% of procedures and are associated with therapeutic (vs diagnostic) paracentesis and possibly with Child-Turcotte-Pugh class C, a platelet count < 50,000/mcL (< 50×10^9/L), and alcoholic cirrhosis. In patients with coagulopathy, however, pre-paracentesis prophylactic transfusions do not appear to be necessary. In addition to a cell count and culture, the ascitic albumin level should be determined: a serum-ascites albumin gradient (serum albumin minus ascitic albumin) ≥ 1.1 suggests portal hypertension. An elevated ascitic adenosine deaminase level is suggestive of tuberculous peritonitis, but the sensitivity of the test is reduced in patients with portal hypertension. Occasionally, cirrhotic ascites is chylous (rich in triglycerides); other causes of chylous ascites are malignancy, tuberculosis, and recent abdominal surgery or trauma.

Ascites in patients with cirrhosis results from portal hypertension (increased hydrostatic pressure); hypoalbuminemia (decreased oncotic pressure); peripheral vasodilation, perhaps mediated by endotoxin-induced release of nitric oxide from splanchnic and systemic vasculature, with resulting increases in renin and angiotensin levels and sodium retention by the kidneys; impaired liver inactivation of aldosterone; and increased aldosterone secretion secondary to increased renin production. In individuals with ascites, the urinary sodium concentration is often < 10 mEq/L (10 mmol/L). Free water excretion is also impaired in cirrhosis, and hyponatremia may develop.

In all patients with cirrhotic ascites, dietary sodium intake may initially be restricted to 2000 mg/d; the intake of sodium may be liberalized slightly after diuresis ensues. Nonsteroidal anti-inflammatory drugs are contraindicated, and angiotensin-converting enzyme inhibitors and angiotensin II antagonists should be avoided. In some patients, ascites diminishes promptly with bed rest and dietary sodium restriction alone. Fluid intake (800–1000 mL/d) is often restricted in patients with hyponatremia. Treatment of severe hyponatremia (serum sodium < 125 mEq/L [125 mmol/L]) with vasopressin receptor antagonists (eg, intravenous conivaptan, 20 mg daily) can be considered but such treatment is expensive, causes thirst, and does not improve survival; oral tolvaptan is contraindicated in patients with liver disease because of potential hepatotoxicity.

A. DIURETICS—Spironolactone, generally in combination with furosemide, should be used in patients who do not respond to salt restriction. An initial trial of furosemide 80 mg intravenously demonstrating a rise in urine sodium to 750 mmol in 8 hours may predict response to diuretic therapy. The dose of spironolactone is initially 100 mg orally daily and may be increased by 100 mg every 3–5 days (up to a maximal conventional daily dose of 400 mg/d, although higher doses have been used) until diuresis is achieved, typically preceded by a rise in the urinary sodium concentration. A "spot" urine sodium concentration that exceeds the potassium concentration correlates with a 24-hour sodium excretion > 78 mmol/d, which predicts diuresis in patients adherent to a salt-restricted diet. Monitoring for hyperkalemia is important. In patients who cannot tolerate spironolactone because of side effects, such as painful gynecomastia, amiloride (another potassium-sparing diuretic) may be used in a starting dose of 5–10 mg orally daily. Diuresis is augmented by the addition of a loop diuretic such as furosemide. This potent diuretic, however, will maintain its effect even with a falling glomerular filtration rate, with resulting prerenal azotemia. The dose of oral furosemide ranges from 40 mg/d to 160 mg/d, and the drug should be administered while blood pressure, urinary output, mental status, and serum electrolytes (especially potassium) are monitored. The goal of weight loss in the ascitic patient without associated peripheral edema should be no more than 1–1.5 lb/d (0.5–0.7 kg/d).

B. LARGE-VOLUME PARACENTESIS—In patients with massive ascites and respiratory compromise, ascites refractory to diuretics ("diuretic resistant"), or intolerable diuretic side effects ("diuretic intractable"), large-volume paracentesis (>5 L) is effective. Intravenous albumin concomitantly at a dosage of 6–8 g/L of ascites fluid removed protects the intravascular volume and may prevent postparacentesis circulatory dysfunction, although the usefulness of this practice is debated and the use of albumin is expensive. Large-volume paracentesis can be repeated daily until ascites is largely resolved and may decrease the need for hospitalization. If possible, diuretics should be continued in the hope of preventing recurrent ascites.

C. TRANSJUGULAR INTRAHEPATIC PORTOSYSTEMIC SHUNT (TIPS)—TIPS is an effective treatment of variceal bleeding refractory to standard therapy (eg, endoscopic band ligation or sclerotherapy) and has shown benefit in the treatment of severe refractory ascites. The technique involves insertion of an expandable metal stent between a branch of the hepatic vein and the portal vein over a catheter inserted via the internal jugular vein. Increased renal sodium excretion and control of ascites refractory to diuretics can be achieved in about 75% of selected cases. The success rate is lower in patients with underlying chronic kidney disease. TIPS appears to be the treatment of choice for refractory hepatic hydrothorax (translocation of ascites across the diaphragm to the pleural space); video-assisted thoracoscopy with pleurodesis using talc may be effective when TIPS is contraindicated. Complications of TIPS include hepatic encephalopathy in 20–30% of cases, infection, shunt stenosis in up to 60% of cases, and shunt occlusion in up to 30% of cases when bare stents are used; however, polytetrafluoroethylene-covered stents are associated with long-term patency rates of 80–90%. Long-term patency often requires periodic shunt revisions. In most cases, patency can be maintained by balloon dilation, local thrombolysis, or placement of an additional stent. TIPS is particularly useful in patients who require short-term control of variceal bleeding or ascites until liver transplantation can be performed. In patients with refractory ascites, TIPS results in lower rates of ascites recurrence and hepatorenal syndrome but a higher rate of hepatic encephalopathy than occur with repeated large-volume paracentesis; a benefit in survival has been demonstrated in one study and a meta-analysis. Chronic kidney disease, diastolic cardiac dysfunction, refractory encephalopathy, and hyperbilirubinemia (>5 mg/dL [85.5 mcmol/L]) are associated with mortality after TIPS.

2. Spontaneous bacterial peritonitis—Spontaneous bacterial peritonitis is heralded by abdominal pain, increasing ascites, fever, and progressive encephalopathy in a patient with cirrhotic ascites; symptoms are typically mild. (Analogously, spontaneous bacterial empyema may complicate hepatic hydrothorax and is managed similarly.) Risk factors in cirrhotic patients with ascites include gastroesophageal variceal bleeding and possibly use of a proton pump inhibitor. Paracentesis reveals an ascitic fluid with, most commonly, a total white cell count of up to 500 cells/mcL with a high percentage of polymorphonuclear cells (PMNs) (≥ 250/mcL) and a protein concentration of 1 g/dL (10 g/L) or less, corresponding to decreased ascitic opsonic activity. Rapid diagnosis of bacterial peritonitis can be made with a high degree of specificity with rapid reagent strips ("dipsticks") that detect leukocyte esterase in ascitic fluid, but the sensitivity is too low for routine use. Cultures of ascites give the highest yield—80–90% positive—using specialized culture bottles inoculated at the bedside. Common isolates are *Escherichia coli* and pneumococci. Gram-positive cocci are the most common isolates in patients who have undergone an invasive procedure such as central venous line placement, and the frequency of enterococcal isolates is increasing. Anaerobes are uncommon. Pending culture results, if there are 250 or more PMNs/mcL or symptoms or signs of infection, intravenous antibiotic therapy should be initiated with cefotaxime, 2 g every 8–12 hours for at least 5 days. Ceftriaxone and amoxicillin-clavulanic acid are alternative choices. Oral ofloxacin, 400 mg twice daily for 7 days, or, in a patient not already taking a fluoroquinolone for prophylaxis against bacterial peritonitis, a 2-day course of intravenous ciprofloxacin, 200 mg twice daily, followed by oral ciprofloxacin, 500 mg twice daily for 5 days, may be effective alternative regimens in selected patients. A carbapenem has been recommended for patients with hospital-acquired spontaneous bacterial peritonitis. Supplemental administration of intravenous albumin prevents further renal impairment and reduces mortality, particularly in patients with a serum creatinine > 1 mg/dL (> 83.3 mcmol/L), blood urea nitrogen > 30 mg/dL (> 10.8 mmol/L), or total bilirubin > 4 mg/dL (> 68.4 mcmol/L). Response to therapy can be documented, if necessary, by a decrease in the PMN count of at least 50% on repeat paracentesis 48 hours after initiation of therapy. The overall mortality rate is high—up to 30% during hospitalization and up to 70% by 1 year. Mortality may be predicted by the 22/11 model: MELD score > 22 and peripheral white blood cell count > 11,000/mcL (> 11 × 10^9/L). Patients with cirrhosis and septic shock have a high frequency of relative adrenal insufficiency, which if present requires administration of hydrocortisone. In survivors of bacterial peritonitis, the risk of recurrent peritonitis may be decreased by long-term norfloxacin, 400 mg orally daily; ciprofloxacin (eg, 500 mg orally once or twice a day), although with recurrence the causative organism is often resistant to fluoroquinolones; or trimethoprim-sulfamethoxazole (eg, one double-strength tablet five times a week). In high-risk cirrhotic patients without prior peritonitis (eg, those with an ascitic protein < 1.5 g/dL and serum bilirubin >3 mg/dL (> 51.3 mcmol/L), serum creatinine >1.2 mg/dL (> 99.96 mcmol/L), blood urea nitrogen ≥ 25 mg/dL (≥ 9 mmol/L), or sodium ≤ 130 mEq/L [≤ 130

mmol/L]), the risk of peritonitis, hepatorenal syndrome, and mortality for at least 1 year may be reduced by prophylactic norfloxacin, 400 mg orally once a day. Oral norfloxacin (400 mg orally twice a day) or intravenous ceftriaxone (1 g per day), which may be preferable, for 7 days reduces the risk of bacterial peritonitis in patients hospitalized for acute variceal bleeding.

3. Hepatorenal syndrome—Hepatorenal syndrome occurs in up to 10% of patients with advanced cirrhosis and ascites and is characterized by azotemia (serum creatinine >1.5 mg/dL [124.95 mcmol/L]) in the absence of parenchymal kidney disease or shock and by failure of kidney function to improve following 2 days of diuretic withdrawal and volume expansion with albumin, 1 g/kg up to a maximum of 100 g/d. Oliguria, hyponatremia, and a low urinary sodium concentration are typical features. Hepatorenal syndrome is diagnosed only when other causes of acute kidney injury (including prerenal azotemia and acute tubular necrosis) have been excluded. Urinary neutrophil gelatinase-associated lipocalin levels (normal, 20 ng/mL) may help distinguish hepatorenal syndrome (105 ng/mL) from chronic kidney disease (50 ng/mL) and acute kidney injury (325 ng/mL). Type I hepatorenal syndrome is characterized by doubling of the serum creatinine to a level > 2.5 mg/dL (208.25 mcmol/L) or by halving of the creatinine clearance to < 20 mL/min (0.34 mL/s/1.73 m^2 BSA) in < 2 weeks. Type II hepatorenal syndrome is more slowly progressive and chronic. An acute decrease in cardiac output is often the precipitating event. In addition to discontinuation of diuretics, clinical improvement and an increase in short-term survival may follow intravenous infusion of albumin in combination with one of the following vasoconstrictor regimens for 7–14 days: oral midodrine plus octreotide, subcutaneously or intravenously; intravenous terlipressin (not yet available in the United States but may be the preferred agent where available); or intravenous norepinephrine. Oral midodrine, 7.5 mg three times daily, added to diuretics, to increase blood pressure has also been reported to convert refractory ascites to diuretic-sensitive ascites. Prolongation of survival has been associated with use of MARS, a modified dialysis method that selectively removes albumin-bound substances. Improvement and sometimes normalization of kidney function may also follow placement of a TIPS; survival after 1 year is reported to be predicted by the combination of a serum bilirubin level < 3 mg/dL (< 50 mcmol/L) and a platelet count > 75,000/mcL (> 75 × 10^9/L). Continuous venovenous hemofiltration and hemodialysis are of uncertain value in hepatorenal syndrome. Liver transplantation is the treatment of choice, but many patients die before a donor liver can be obtained. Mortality correlates with the MELD score and presence of a systemic inflammatory response. The 3-month probability of survival in patients with hepatorenal syndrome (15%) is lower than that for renal failure associated with infections (31%), hypovolemia (46%), and parenchymal kidney disease (73%) in patients with cirrhosis.

4. Hepatic encephalopathy—Hepatic encephalopathy is a state of disordered central nervous system function resulting from failure of the liver to detoxify noxious agents of gut origin because of hepatocellular dysfunction and portosystemic shunting. The clinical spectrum ranges from day-night reversal and mild intellectual impairment to coma. Patients with covert (formerly minimal) hepatic encephalopathy have no recognizable clinical symptoms but demonstrate mild cognitive and psychomotor deficits and attention deficit on standardized psychometric tests and an increased rate of traffic accidents. The stages of overt encephalopathy are: (1) mild confusion, (2) drowsiness, (3) stupor, and (4) coma. A revised staging system known as SONIC (spectrum of neurocognitive impairment in cirrhosis) encompasses absent, covert, and stages 2 to 4 encephalopathy. Ammonia is the most readily identified and measurable toxin but is not solely responsible for the disturbed mental status. Bleeding into the intestinal tract may significantly increase the amount of protein in the bowel and precipitate encephalopathy. Other precipitants include constipation, alkalosis, and potassium deficiency induced by diuretics, opioids, hypnotics, and sedatives; medications containing ammonium or amino compounds; paracentesis with consequent hypovolemia; hepatic or systemic infection; and portosystemic shunts (including TIPS). The diagnosis is based primarily on detection of characteristic symptoms and signs, including asterixis. The role of neuroimaging studies (eg, cerebral PET, magnetic resonance spectroscopy) in the diagnosis of hepatic encephalopathy is evolving.

Dietary protein is withheld during acute episodes if the patient cannot eat. When the patient resumes oral intake, protein intake should be 60–80 g/d as tolerated; vegetable protein is better tolerated than meat protein. Gastrointestinal bleeding should be controlled and blood purged from the gastrointestinal tract. This can be accomplished with 120 mL of magnesium citrate by mouth or nasogastric tube every 3–4 hours until the stool is free of gross blood, or by administration of lactulose. The value of treating patients with covert hepatic encephalopathy is uncertain; probiotic agents may have some benefit.

Lactulose, a nonabsorbable synthetic disaccharide syrup, is digested by bacteria in the colon to short-chain fatty acids, resulting in acidification of colon contents. This acidification favors the formation of ammonium ion in the $NH_4^+ \leftrightarrow NH_3 + H^+$ equation; NH_4^+ is not absorbable, whereas NH_3 is absorbable and thought to be neurotoxic. Lactulose also leads to a change in bowel flora so that fewer ammonia-forming organisms are present. When given orally, the initial dose of lactulose for acute hepatic encephalopathy is 30 mL three or four times daily. The dose should then be titrated so that two or three soft stools per day are produced. When rectal use is indicated because of the patient's inability to take medicines orally, the dose is 300 mL of lactulose in 700 mL of saline or sorbitol as a retention enema for 30–60 minutes; it may be repeated every 4–6 hours. Continued use of lactulose after an episode of acute encephalopathy reduces the frequency of recurrences. Lactitol is a less sweet disaccharide alternative available as a powder in some countries.

The ammonia-producing intestinal flora may also be controlled with an oral antibiotic. The nonabsorbable agent

rifaximin, 550 mg orally twice daily, is preferred and has been shown as well to maintain remission from and reduce the risk of rehospitalization for hepatic encephalopathy over a 6-month period in patients also taking lactulose. Metronidazole, 250 mg orally three times daily, has also shown benefit. In the past, neomycin sulfate, 0.5–1 g orally every 6 or 12 hours for 7 days, was used, but side effects (including diarrhea, malabsorption, superinfection, ototoxicity, and nephrotoxicity) were frequent, especially after prolonged use. Patients who do not respond to lactulose alone may improve with a course of an antibiotic added to treatment with lactulose.

Opioids and sedatives metabolized or excreted by the liver should be avoided. If agitation is marked, oxazepam, 10–30 mg, which is not metabolized by the liver, may be given cautiously by mouth or by nasogastric tube. Zinc deficiency should be corrected, if present, with oral zinc sulfate, 600 mg/d in divided doses. Sodium benzoate, 5 g orally twice daily, ornithine aspartate, 9 g orally three times daily, and L-acyl-carnitine (an essential factor in the mitochrondrial transport of long-chain fatty acids), 4 g orally daily, may lower blood ammonia levels, but there is less experience with these drugs than with lactulose. Flumazenil is effective in about 30% of patients with severe hepatic encephalopathy, but the drug is short-acting and intravenous administration is required. Use of special dietary supplements enriched with branched-chain amino acids is usually unnecessary except in occasional patients who are intolerant of standard protein supplements.

5. Coagulopathy—Hypoprothrombinemia caused by malnutrition and vitamin K deficiency may be treated with vitamin K (eg, phytonadione, 5 mg orally or intravenously daily); however, this treatment is ineffective when synthesis of coagulation factors is impaired because of hepatic disease. In such cases, correcting the prolonged prothrombin time requires large volumes of fresh frozen plasma (see Chapter 14). Because the effect is transient, plasma infusions are not indicated except for active bleeding or before an invasive procedure, and even then, the value of such treatment has been questioned because of concomitant alterations in anti-hemostatic factors and because bleeding risk does not correlate with the INR. Recombinant activated factor VIIa may be an alternative but is expensive and poses a 1–2% risk of thrombotic complications. Eltrombopag reduces the need for platelet transfusions in patients with cirrhosis and a platelet count < 50,000/mcL (< 50 × 10⁹/L) who undergo invasive procedures, but eltrombopag is associated with an increased risk of portal vein thrombosis.

6. Hemorrhage from esophageal varices—See Chapter 15.

7. Hepatopulmonary syndrome and portopulmonary hypertension—Shortness of breath in patients with cirrhosis may result from pulmonary restriction and atelectasis caused by massive ascites. The hepatopulmonary syndrome—the triad of chronic liver disease, an increased alveolar-arterial gradient while the patient is breathing room air, and intrapulmonary vascular dilatations or arteriovenous communications that result in a right-to-left intrapulmonary shunt—occurs in 5–32% of patients with cirrhosis. Patients often have greater dyspnea (platypnea) and arterial deoxygenation (orthodeoxia) in the upright than in the recumbent position. The diagnosis should be suspected in a cirrhotic patient with a pulse oximetry level ≤ 96%.

Contrast-enhanced echocardiography is a sensitive screening test for detecting pulmonary vascular dilatations, whereas macroaggregated albumin lung perfusion scanning is more specific and may be used to confirm the diagnosis. High-resolution CT may be useful for detecting dilated pulmonary vessels that may be amenable to embolization in patients with severe hypoxemia (Po_2 < 60 mm Hg [7.8 kPa]) who respond poorly to supplemental oxygen.

Medical therapy has been disappointing; experimentally, intravenous methylene blue, oral garlic powder, oral norfloxacin, and mycophenolate mofetil may improve oxygenation by inhibiting nitric oxide-induced vasodilatation and angiogenesis, and pentoxifylline may prevent hepatopulmonary syndrome by inhibiting production of tumor necrosis factor. Long-term oxygen therapy is recommended for severely hypoxemic patients. The syndrome may reverse with liver transplantation, although postoperative mortality is increased in patients with a preoperative arterial Po_2 < 50 mm Hg (6.5 kPa) or with substantial intrapulmonary shunting. TIPS may provide palliation in patients with hepatopulmonary syndrome awaiting transplantation.

Portopulmonary hypertension occurs in 0.7% of patients with cirrhosis. Female sex and autoimmune hepatitis have been reported to be risk factors, and large spontaneous portosystemic shunts are present in many affected patients and are associated with a lack of response to treatment. In cases confirmed by right-sided heart catheterization, treatment with the prostaglandin epoprostenol, the endothelin-receptor antagonists bosentan or ambrisentan, or the phosphodiesterase-5 inhibitors sildenafil or tadalafil may reduce pulmonary hypertension and thereby facilitate liver transplantation; beta-blockers worsen exercise capacity and are contraindicated, and calcium channel blockers should be used with caution because they may worsen portal hypertension. Liver transplantation is contraindicated in patients with moderate to severe pulmonary hypertension (mean pulmonary pressure > 35 mm Hg).

C. Liver Transplantation

Liver transplantation is indicated in selected cases of irreversible, progressive chronic liver disease, acute liver failure, and certain metabolic diseases in which the metabolic defect is in the liver. Absolute contraindications include malignancy (except relatively small hepatocellular carcinomas in a cirrhotic liver), advanced cardiopulmonary disease (except hepatopulmonary syndrome), and sepsis. Relative contraindications include age over 70 years, morbid obesity, portal and mesenteric vein thrombosis, active alcohol or drug abuse, severe malnutrition, and lack of patient understanding. With the emergence of effective antiretroviral therapy for HIV disease, a major cause of mortality in these patients has shifted to liver disease caused by HCV and HBV infection; experience to date suggests that the outcome of liver transplantation is comparable to that for non–HIV-infected liver transplant recipients. Patients with alcoholism should be abstinent for 6 months. Liver transplantation should be considered in patients with worsening functional status, rising bilirubin, decreasing albumin, worsening coagulopathy, refractory ascites, recurrent variceal bleeding, or worsening encephalopathy; prioritization is based on the MELD score. Combined liver-kidney transplantation is indicated in patients with associated kidney failure presumed to be irreversible. The major impediment to more widespread use of liver transplantation is a shortage of donor organs. Adult living donor liver transplantation is an option for some patients, and extended-criteria donors are being used. Five-year survival rates as high as 80% are now reported. Hepatocellular carcinoma, hepatitis B and C, and some cases of Budd-Chiari syndrome and autoimmune liver disease may recur in the transplanted liver. The incidence of recurrence of hepatitis B can be reduced by preoperative and postoperative treatment with a nucleoside or nucleotide analog and perioperative administration of HBIG. Immunosuppression is achieved with combinations of cyclosporine, tacrolimus or sirolimus, corticosteroids, azathioprine, and mycophenolate mofetil and may be complicated by infections, advanced chronic kidney disease, neurologic disorders, and drug toxicity as well as graft rejection, vascular occlusion, or bile leaks. Patients taking these drugs are at risk for obesity, diabetes mellitus, and hyperlipidemia.

▶ Prognosis

Prognostic scoring systems for cirrhosis include the Child-Turcotte-Pugh score (Table 16–6) and MELD score. The MELD score, which incorporates the serum bilirubin and creatinine levels and the INR, is also a measure of mortality risk in patients with end-stage liver disease and is particularly useful for predicting short- and intermediate-term survival and complications of cirrhosis (eg, bacterial peritonitis) as well as determining allocation priorities for donor livers. Additional (MELD-exception) points are given for patients with conditions such as hepatopulmonary syndrome and hepatocellular carcinoma that may benefit from liver transplantation. The consistency of the MELD score among different hospitals may be improved when the INR is calibrated based on prothrombin time control samples that include patients with liver disease rather than those taking oral anticoagulants, but this approach is not readily available. A MELD score of > 14 is required for liver transplant listing. In patients with a relatively low MELD score (< 21) and a low priority for liver transplantation, a low serum sodium concentration (< 130 mEq/L [130 mmol/L]), an elevated hepatic venous pressure gradient, persistent ascites, and a low health-related quality of life appear to be additional independent predictors of mortality, and modifications of the MELD score, including one that incorporates the serum sodium (MELDNa), are under consideration. Only 50% of patients with severe hepatic dysfunction (serum albumin < 3 g/dL [< 30 g/L]),

Table 16–6. Child-Turcotte-Pugh and Model for End-Stage Liver Disease (MELD) scoring systems for staging cirrhosis.

Child-Turcotte-Pugh scoring system			
Parameter	Numerical Score		
	1	2	3
Ascites	None	Slight	Moderate to severe
Encephalopathy	None	Slight to moderate	Moderate to severe
Bilirubin, mg/dL (mcmol/L)	< 2.0 (34.2)	2–3 (34.2–51.3)	> 3.0 (51.3)
Albumin, g/dL (g/L)	> 3.5 (35)	2.8–3.5 (28–35)	< 2.8 (28)
Prothrombin time (seconds increased)	1–3	4–6	> 6.0

Total Numerical Score and Corresponding Child Class	
Score	Class
5–6	A
7–9	B
10–15	C

MELD scoring system
MELD = 11.2 $\log_e$ (INR) + 3.78 $\log_e$ (bilirubin [mg/dL]) + 9.57 $\log_e$ (creatinine [mg/dL]) + 6.43. (Range 6–40).

INR, international normalized ratio.

bilirubin > 3 mg/dL [> 51.3 mcmol/L]), ascites, encephalopathy, cachexia, and upper gastrointestinal bleeding) survive 6 months without transplantation. The risk of death in this subgroup of patients with advanced cirrhosis is associated with muscle wasting, age ≥ 65 years, mean arterial pressure ≤ 82 mm Hg, renal failure, cognitive dysfunction, ventilatory insufficiency, and prothrombin time ≥ 16 seconds, delayed and suboptimal treatment of sepsis, and second infections. Renal failure increases mortality in patients with cirrhosis up to sevenfold. Obesity and diabetes mellitus appear to be risk factors for clinical deterioration and cirrhosis-related mortality, as is continued alcohol use in patients with alcoholic cirrhosis. The use of beta-blockers for portal hypertension is beneficial early in the course but is associated with poor survival in patients with refractory ascites because of their negative effect on cardiac compensatory reserve. Patients with cirrhosis are at risk for the development of hepatocellular carcinoma, with rates of 3–5% per year for alcoholic and viral hepatitis-related cirrhosis. Liver transplantation has markedly improved the outlook for patients with cirrhosis who are candidates and are referred for evaluation early. Patients with compensated cirrhosis are given additional priority for liver transplantation if they are found to have a lesion > 2 cm in diameter

consistent with hepatocellular carcinoma. In-hospital mortality from variceal bleeding in patients with cirrhosis has declined from over 40% in 1980 to 15% in 2000. Medical treatments to reverse hepatic fibrosis are under investigation.

▶ **When to Refer**

- For liver biopsy.
- Before the MELD score is ≥ 14.
- For upper endoscopy to screen for gastroesophageal varices.

▶ **When to Admit**

- Gastrointestinal bleeding.
- Stage 3–4 hepatic encephalopathy.
- Worsening kidney function.
- Severe hyponatremia.
- Serious infection.
- Profound hypoxia.

Amodio P et al. The nutritional management of hepatic encephalopathy in patients with cirrhosis: International Society for Hepatic Encephalopathy and Nitrogen Metabolism Consensus. Hepatology. 2013 Jul;58(1):325–36. [PMID: 23471642]

Iyer VN et al. Hepatopulmonary syndrome: favorable outcomes in the MELD exception era. Hepatology. 2013 Jun;57(6):2427–35. [PMID: 22996424]

Northup PG et al. Coagulation in liver disease: a guide for the clinician. Clin Gastroenterol Hepatol. 2013 Sep;11(9):1064–74. [PMID: 23506859]

Runyon BA et al. Introduction to the revised American Association for the Study of Liver Diseases Practice Guideline management of adult patients with ascites due to cirrhosis 2012. Hepatology. 2013 Apr;57(4):1651–3. [PMID: 23463403]

PRIMARY BILIARY CIRRHOSIS

ESSENTIALS OF DIAGNOSIS

▶ Occurs in middle-aged women.

▶ Often asymptomatic.

▶ Elevation of alkaline phosphatase, positive antimitochondrial antibodies, elevated IgM, increased cholesterol.

▶ Characteristic liver biopsy.

▶ In later stages, can present with fatigue, jaundice, features of cirrhosis, xanthelasma, xanthoma, steatorrhea.

▶ **General Considerations**

Primary biliary cirrhosis is a chronic disease of the liver characterized by autoimmune destruction of small intrahepatic bile ducts and cholestasis. It is insidious in onset, occurs usually in women aged 40–60 years, and is often detected by the chance finding of elevated alkaline phosphatase levels. Estimated incidence and prevalence rates in the United States are 4.5 and 65.4 per 100,000, respectively, in women, and 0.7 and 12.1 per 100,000, respectively, in men. These rates may be increasing. The frequency of the disease among first-degree relatives of affected persons is 1.3–6%, and the concordance rate in identical twins is high. Primary biliary cirrhosis is associated with HLA *DRB1*08* *and DQB1*. The disease may be associated with Sjögren syndrome, autoimmune thyroid disease, Raynaud syndrome, scleroderma, hypothyroidism, and celiac disease. Infection with *Novosphingobium aromaticivorans* or *Chlamydophila pneumoniae* may be triggering or causative in primary biliary cirrhosis. A history of urinary tract infections (caused by *E coli* or *Lactobacillus delbrueckii*) and smoking, and possibly use of hormone replacement therapy and hair dye, are risk factors, and clustering of cases in time and space argues for a causative role of environmental agents.

Clinical Findings

A. Symptoms and Signs

Many patients are asymptomatic for years. The onset of clinical illness is insidious and is heralded by fatigue (excessive daytime somnolence) and pruritus. With progression, physical examination reveals hepatosplenomegaly. Xanthomatous lesions may occur in the skin and tendons and around the eyelids. Jaundice, steatorrhea, and signs of portal hypertension are late findings, although occasional patients have esophageal varices despite an early histologic stage (see below). Autonomic dysfunction, including orthostatic hypotension and associated with fatigue, and cognitive dysfunction appear to be common. The risk of low bone density, osteoporosis, and fractures is increased in patients with primary biliary cirrhosis (who tend to be older women) possibly due in part to polymorphisms of the vitamin D receptor.

B. Laboratory Findings

Blood counts are normal early in the disease. Liver biochemical tests reflect cholestasis with elevation of alkaline phosphatase, cholesterol (especially high-density lipoproteins), and, in later stages, bilirubin. Antimitochondrial antibodies are present in 95% of patients, and serum IgM levels are elevated.

Diagnosis

The diagnosis of primary biliary cirrhosis is based on the detection of cholestatic liver chemistries (often initially an isolated elevation of the alkaline phosphatase) and antimitochondrial antibodies in serum. Liver biopsy is not essential for diagnosis but permits histologic staging: I, portal inflammation with granulomas; II, bile duct proliferation, periportal inflammation; III, interlobular fibrous septa; and IV, cirrhosis. Estimation of histologic stage by an "enhanced liver fibrosis assay" that incorporates serum levels of hyaluronic acid, tissue inhibitor of metalloproteinase-1, and procollagen III aminopeptide has shown promise.

Differential Diagnosis

The disease must be differentiated from chronic biliary tract obstruction (stone or stricture), carcinoma of the bile ducts, primary sclerosing cholangitis, sarcoidosis, cholestatic drug toxicity (eg, chlorpromazine), and in some cases chronic hepatitis. Patients with a clinical and histologic picture of primary biliary cirrhosis but no antimitochondrial antibodies are said to have antimitochondrial antibody-negative primary biliary cirrhosis ("autoimmune cholangitis"), which has been associated with lower serum IgM levels and a greater frequency of smooth muscle antibodies and ANA. Many such patients are found to have antimitochondrial antibodies by immunoblot against recombinant proteins (rather than standard immunofluorescence). Some patients have overlapping features of primary biliary cirrhosis and autoimmune hepatitis.

Treatment

Cholestyramine (4 g) in water or juice three times daily may be beneficial for pruritus; colestipol and colesevelam may be better tolerated but have not been shown to reduce pruritus. Rifampin, 150–300 mg orally twice daily, is inconsistently beneficial. Opioid antagonists (eg, naloxone, 0.2 mcg/kg/min by intravenous infusion, or naltrexone, starting at 12.5 mg/d by mouth) show promise in the treatment of pruritus but may cause opioid withdrawal symptoms. The 5-hydroxytryptamine (5-HT_3) serotonin receptor antagonist ondansetron, 4 mg orally three times a day as needed, and the selective serotonin uptake inhibitor sertraline, 75–100 mg/d orally, may also provide some benefit. For refractory pruritus, plasmapheresis or extracorporeal albumin dialysis may be needed. Modafinil, 100–200 mg/d orally, may improve daytime somnolence but is poorly tolerated. Deficiencies of vitamins A, D, and K may occur if steatorrhea is present and are aggravated when cholestyramine or colestipol is administered. See Chapter 26 for discussion of prevention and treatment of osteoporosis and Chapter 20 for discussion of the treatment of Sjögren syndrome.

Because of its lack of toxicity, ursodeoxycholic acid (13–15 mg/kg/d in one or two doses) is the preferred medical treatment (and only treatment approved by the US FDA) for primary biliary cirrhosis. It has been shown to slow the progression of disease (particularly in early-stage disease), stabilize histology, improve long-term survival, reduce the risk of developing esophageal varices, and delay (and possibly prevent) the need for liver transplantation, although the benefit of the drug has been questioned. Complete normalization of liver biochemical tests occurs in 20% of treated patients within 2 years and 40% within 5 years, and survival is similar to that of healthy controls when the drug is given to patients with stage 1 or 2 primary biliary cirrhosis. Response rates have been reported to be lower in men than women (72% vs 80%) and higher in women diagnosed after age 70 than before age 30 (90% vs 50%). Ursodeoxycholic acid therapy has also been reported to reduce the risk of recurrent colorectal adenomas in patients with primary biliary cirrhosis. Side effects include weight gain and rarely loose stools. Colchicine (0.6 mg orally twice daily) and methotrexate (15 mg/wk orally) have had some reported benefit in improving symptoms and serum levels of alkaline phosphatase and bilirubin. Methotrexate may also improve liver histology in some patients, but overall response rates have been disappointing. Penicillamine, prednisone, and azathioprine have proved to be of no benefit. Budesonide may improve liver histology but worsens bone density. For patients with advanced disease, liver transplantation is the treatment of choice.

▶ Prognosis

Without liver transplantation, survival averages 7–10 years once symptoms develop but has improved for younger women since the introduction of ursodeoxycholic acid. Progression to liver failure and portal hypertension may be accelerated by smoking. Patients with early-stage disease in whom the alkaline phosphatase and AST are less than 1.5 times normal and bilirubin is ≤ 1 mg/dL (17.1 mcmol/L) after 1 year of therapy with ursodeoxycholic acid (Paris II criteria) are at low long-term risk for cirrhosis and have a life expectancy similar to that of the healthy population. In advanced disease, an adverse prognosis is indicated by a high Mayo risk score that includes older age, high serum bilirubin, edema, low serum albumin, and prolonged prothrombin time as well as by variceal hemorrhage. A prediction tool for varices based on the serum albumin, serum alkaline phosphatase, platelet count, and splenomegaly has been proposed. Fatigue is associated with an increased risk of cardiac mortality and may not be reversed by liver transplantation. Among asymptomatic patients, at least one-third will become symptomatic within 15 years. The risk of hepatocellular carcinoma appears to be increased in patients with primary biliary cirrhosis; risk factors include older age, male sex, prior blood transfusions, advanced histologic stage, and signs of cirrhosis or portal hypertension. Liver transplantation for advanced primary biliary cirrhosis is associated with a 1-year survival rate of 85–90%. The disease recurs in the graft in 20% of patients by 3 years, but this does not seem to affect survival.

▶ When to Refer

- For liver biopsy.
- For liver transplant evaluation.

▶ When to Admit

- Gastrointestinal bleeding.
- Stage 3–4 hepatic encephalopathy.
- Worsening kidney function.
- Severe hyponatremia.
- Profound hypoxia.

Carbone M et al. Sex and age are determinants of the clinical phenotype of primary biliary cirrhosis and response to ursodeoxycholic acid. Gastroenterology. 2013 Mar;144(3):560–9. [PMID: 23246637]

Harada K et al. Incidence of and risk factors for hepatocellular carcinoma in primary biliary cirrhosis: national data from Japan. Hepatology. 2013 May;57(5):1942–9. [PMID: 23197466]

Patanwala I et al. A validated clinical tool for the prediction of varices in PBC: the Newcastle Varices in PBC Score. J Hepatol. 2013 Aug;59(2):327–35. [PMID: 23608623]

HEMOCHROMATOSIS

ESSENTIALS OF DIAGNOSIS

- ▶ Usually suspected because of elevated iron saturation or serum ferritin or a family history.
- ▶ Most patients are asymptomatic; the disease is rarely recognized clinically before the fifth decade.
- ▶ Hepatic abnormalities and cirrhosis, heart failure, hypogonadism, and arthritis.
- ▶ *HFE* gene mutation (usually *C282Y/C282Y*) is found in most cases.

▶ General Considerations

Hemochromatosis is an autosomal recessive disease caused in most cases by a mutation in the *HFE* gene on chromosome 6. The HFE protein is thought to play an important role in the process by which duodenal crypt cells sense body iron stores, leading in turn to increased iron absorption from the duodenum. A decrease in the synthesis or expression of hepcidin, the principal iron regulatory hormone, is thought to be a key pathogenic factor in all forms of hemochromatosis. About 85% of persons with well-established hemochromatosis are homozygous for the *C282Y* mutation. The frequency of the gene mutation averages 7% in Northern European and North American white populations, resulting in a 0.5% frequency of homozygotes (of whom 38–50% will develop biochemical evidence of iron overload but only 28% of men and 1% of women will develop clinical symptoms). By contrast, the gene mutation and hemochromatosis are uncommon in blacks and Asian-American populations. A second genetic mutation (*H63D*) may contribute to the development of iron overload in a small percentage (1.5%) of persons who are compound heterozygotes for *C282Y* and *H63D*; iron overload-related disease develops in few patients (particularly those who have a comorbidity such as diabetes mellitus and fatty liver). Rare instances of hemochromatosis result from mutations in the genes that encode transferrin receptor 2 (*TFR2*) and ferroportin (*FPN1*). A juvenile-onset variant that is characterized by severe iron overload, cardiac dysfunction, hypogonadotropic hypogonadism, and a high mortality rate is usually linked to a mutation of a gene on chromosome 1q designated *HJV* that produces a protein called hemojuvelin or, rarely, to a mutation in the *HAMP* gene on chromosome 19 that encodes hepcidin, but not to the *C282Y* mutation.

Hemochromatosis is characterized by increased accumulation of iron as hemosiderin in the liver, pancreas, heart, adrenals, testes, pituitary, and kidneys. Cirrhosis is more likely to develop in affected persons who drink alcohol excessively or have obesity-related hepatic steatosis than in those who do not. Eventually, hepatic and pancreatic insufficiency, heart failure, and hypogonadism may develop; overall mortality is increased slightly. Heterozygotes do not develop cirrhosis in the absence of associated disorders such as viral hepatitis or NAFLD.

▶ Clinical Findings

A. Symptoms and Signs

The onset of clinical disease is usually after age 50 years—earlier in men than in women; however, because of widespread liver biochemical testing and iron screening, the diagnosis is usually made long before symptoms develop. Early symptoms are nonspecific (eg, fatigue, arthralgia). Later clinical manifestations include arthropathy (and ultimately the need for joint replacement surgery in some cases), hepatomegaly and evidence of hepatic dysfunction, skin pigmentation (combination of slate-gray due to iron and brown due to melanin, sometimes resulting in a bronze color), cardiac enlargement with or without heart failure or conduction defects, diabetes mellitus with its complications, and erectile dysfunction in men. Interestingly, population studies have shown an increased prevalence of liver disease but not of diabetes mellitus, arthritis, or heart disease in *C282Y* homozygotes. In patients in whom cirrhosis develops, bleeding from esophageal varices may occur, and there is a 15–20% frequency of hepatocellular carcinoma. Affected patients are at increased risk of infection with *Vibrio vulnificus*, *Listeria monocytogenes*, *Yersinia enterocolitica*, and other siderophilic organisms. The risk of porphyria cutanea tarda is increased in persons with the *C282Y* or *H63D* mutation, and *C282Y* homozygotes have twice the risk of colorectal and breast cancer than persons without the *C282Y* variant.

B. Laboratory Findings

Laboratory findings include mildly abnormal liver tests (AST, alkaline phosphatase), an elevated plasma iron with > 45% transferrin saturation, and an elevated serum ferritin (although a normal iron saturation or a normal ferritin does not exclude the diagnosis). Affected men are more likely than affected women to have an elevated ferritin level. Testing for *HFE* mutations is indicated in any patient with evidence of iron overload. Interestingly, in persons with an elevated serum ferritin, the likelihood of detecting *C282Y* homozygosity decreases with increasing ALT and AST levels, which are likely to reflect hepatic inflammation and secondary iron overload.

C. Imaging

MRI and CT may show changes consistent with iron overload of the liver, and MRI can quantitate hepatic iron stores. There is also an emerging role for MRI for assessment of the degree of hepatic fibrosis.

D. Liver Biopsy

In patients who are homozygous for *C282Y*, liver biopsy is often indicated to determine whether cirrhosis is present. Biopsy can be deferred, however, in patients in whom the serum ferritin level is < 1000 mcg/L, serum AST level is normal, and hepatomegaly is absent; the likelihood of cirrhosis is low in these persons. The combination of a serum ferritin level ≥ 1000 mcg/L and a serum hyaluronic acid level ≥ 46.5 mcg/L has been reported to identify all patients with cirrhosis, with a high specificity. Risk factors for advanced fibrosis include male sex, excess alcohol consumption, and diabetes mellitus. Liver biopsy is also indicated when iron overload is suspected even though the patient is not homozygous for *C282Y* or a *C282Y/H63D* compound heterozygote. In patients with hemochromatosis, the liver biopsy characteristically shows extensive iron deposition in hepatocytes and in bile ducts, and the hepatic iron index—hepatic iron content per gram of liver converted to micromoles and divided by the patient's age—is generally > 1.9. Only 5% of patients with hereditary hemochromatosis identified by screening in a primary care setting have cirrhosis.

▶ Screening

Iron studies and *HFE* testing are recommended for all first-degree family members of a proband; children of an affected person (*C282Y* homozygote) need to be screened only if the patient's spouse carries the *C282Y* or *H63D* mutation. Average-risk population screening for hemochromatosis is not recommended because the clinical penetrance of *C282Y* homozygosity and morbidity and mortality from hemochromatosis are low. Patients with otherwise unexplained chronic liver disease, chondrocalcinosis, erectile dysfunction, and type 1 diabetes mellitus (especially late-onset) should be screened for iron overload.

▶ Treatment

Affected patients should avoid foods rich in iron (such as red meat), alcohol, vitamin C, raw shellfish, and supplemental iron. Weekly phlebotomies of 1 or 2 units (250–500 mL) of blood (each containing about 250 mg of iron) is indicated in all symptomatic patients, those with a serum ferritin level of at least 1000 mcg/L, and those with an increased fasting iron saturation and should be continued for up to 2–3 years to achieve depletion of iron stores. The hematocrit and serum iron values should be monitored. When iron store depletion is achieved (iron saturation < 50% and serum ferritin level 50–100 mcg/L), phlebotomies (every 2–4 months) to maintain serum ferritin levels between 50 mcg/L and 100 mcg/L are continued, although compliance has been reported to decrease with time; administration of a proton pump inhibitor, which reduces intestinal iron absorption, appears to decrease the maintenance phlebotomy blood volume requirement. In C282Y homozygous women, a body mass index > 28 kg/m^2 is associated with a lower phlebotomy requirement, possibly because hepcidin levels are increased by overweight. Complications of hemochromatosis—arthropathy, diabetes mellitus, heart disease, portal hypertension, and hypopituitarism—also require treatment.

The chelating agent deferoxamine is indicated for patients with hemochromatosis and anemia or in those with secondary iron overload due to thalassemia who cannot tolerate phlebotomies. The drug is administered intravenously or subcutaneously in a dose of 20–40 mg/kg/d infused over 24 hours and can mobilize 30 mg of iron per day; however, treatment is painful and time-consuming. Two oral chelators, deferasirox, 20 mg/kg once daily, and deferiprone, 25 mg/kg three times daily, have been approved for treatment of iron overload due to blood transfusions and may be appropriate in persons with hemochromatosis who cannot tolerate phlebotomy; however, these agents have a number of side effects and drug-drug interactions.

The course of hemochromatosis is favorably altered by phlebotomy therapy. Hepatic fibrosis may regress, and in precirrhotic patients, cirrhosis may be prevented. Cardiac conduction defects and insulin requirements improve with treatment. In patients with cirrhosis, varices may reverse, and the risk of variceal bleeding declines, although the risk of hepatocellular carcinoma persists; in those with an initial serum ferritin level > 1000 mcg/L (> 2247 pmol/L), the risk of death is five fold greater than in those with a serum ferritin ≤ 1000 mcg/L (< 2247 pmol/L). In the past, liver transplantation for advanced cirrhosis associated with severe iron overload, including hemochromatosis, was reported to lead to survival rates that were lower than those for other types of liver disease because of cardiac complications and an increased risk of infections, but since 1997, posttransplant survival rates have been excellent.

▶ When to Refer

- For liver biopsy.
- For initiation of therapy.

Adams PC et al. Probability of *C282Y* homozygosity decreases as liver transaminase activities increase in participants with hyperferritinemia in the Hemochromatosis and Iron Overload Screening Study. Hepatology. 2012 Jun;55(6):1722–6. [PMID: 22183642]

Barton JC et al. Increased risk of death from iron overload among 422 treated probands with HFE hemochromatosis and serum levels of ferritin greater than 1000 mcg/L at diagnosis. Clin Gastroenterol Hepatol. 2012 Apr;10(4):412–6. [PMID: 22265917]

Desgrippes R et al. Decreased iron burden in overweight C282Y homozygous women: putative role of increased hepcidin production. Hepatology. 2013 May;57(5):1784–92. [PMID: 23322654]

Moretti D et al. Relevance of dietary iron intake and bioavailability in the management of HFE hemochromatosis: a systematic review. Am J Clin Nutr. 2013 Aug;98(2):468–79. [PMID: 23803887]

WILSON DISEASE

ESSENTIALS OF DIAGNOSIS

▶ Rare autosomal recessive disorder that usually occurs in persons under age 40.

▶ Excessive deposition of copper in the liver and brain.

▶ Serum ceruloplasmin, the plasma copper-carrying protein, is low.

▶ Urinary excretion of copper and hepatic copper concentration are high.

▶ General Considerations

Wilson disease (hepatolenticular degeneration) is a rare autosomal recessive disorder that usually occurs in persons under age 40. The worldwide prevalence is about 30 per million population. The condition is characterized by excessive deposition of copper in the liver and brain. The genetic defect, localized to chromosome 13, has been shown to affect a copper-transporting adenosine triphosphatase (*ATP7B*) in the liver and leads to copper accumulation in the liver and oxidative damage of hepatic mitochondria. Most patients are compound heterozygotes (ie, carry two different mutations). Over 500 mutations in the Wilson disease gene have been identified. The *H1069Q* mutation accounts for 37–63% of disease alleles in populations of Northern European descent. The major physiologic aberration in Wilson disease is excessive absorption of copper from the small intestine and decreased excretion of copper by the liver, resulting in increased tissue deposition, especially in the liver, brain, cornea, and kidney.

▶ Clinical Findings

Wilson disease tends to present as liver disease in adolescents and neuropsychiatric disease in young adults, but there is great variability, and onset of symptoms after age 40 is more common than previously thought. The diagnosis should always be considered in any child or young adult with hepatitis, splenomegaly with hypersplenism, Coombs-negative hemolytic anemia, portal hypertension, and neurologic or psychiatric abnormalities. Wilson disease should also be considered in persons under 40 years of age with chronic or fulminant hepatitis.

Hepatic involvement may range from elevated liver biochemical tests (although the alkaline phosphatase may be low) to cirrhosis and portal hypertension. In a patient with acute liver failure, the diagnosis of Wilson disease is suggested by an alkaline phosphatase (in units/L)-to-total bilirubin (in mg/dL) ratio < 4 and an AST-to-ALT ratio > 2.2. The neurologic manifestations of Wilson disease are related to basal ganglia dysfunction and include an akinetic-rigid syndrome similar to parkinsonism, pseudosclerosis with tremor, ataxia, and a dystonic syndrome. Dysarthria, dysphagia, incoordination, and spasticity are common. Migraines, insomnia, and seizures have been reported. Psychiatric features include behavioral

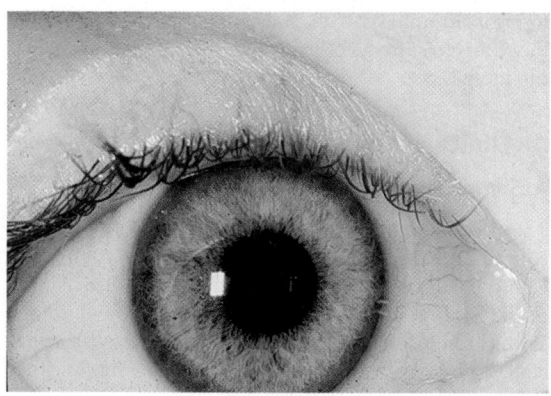

▲ **Figure 16–4.** Brownish Kayser-Fleischer ring at the rim of the cornea in a patient with Wilson disease. (From Marc Solioz, University of Berne; used, with permission, from Usatine RP, Smith MA, Mayeaux EJ Jr, Chumley H, Tysinger J. *The Color Atlas of Family Medicine.* McGraw-Hill, 2009.)

and personality changes and emotional lability and may precede characteristic neurologic features. The pathognomonic sign of the condition is the brownish or gray-green Kayser-Fleischer ring, which represents fine pigmented granular deposits in Descemet membrane in the cornea (Figure 16–4). The ring is usually most marked at the superior and inferior poles of the cornea. It is sometimes seen with the naked eye and is readily detected by slit-lamp examination. It may be absent in patients with hepatic manifestations only but is usually present in those with neuropsychiatric disease. Renal calculi, aminoaciduria, renal tubular acidosis, hypoparathyroidism, infertility, and hemolytic anemia may occur in patients with Wilson disease.

Diagnosis

The diagnosis can be challenging, even with the use of scoring systems, and is generally based on demonstration of increased urinary copper excretion (> 40 mcg/24 h and usually > 100 mcg/24 h) or low serum ceruloplasmin levels (< 20 mg/dL [< 200 mg/L]; < 5 mg/dL [< 50 mg/L] is diagnostic), and elevated hepatic copper concentration (> 250 mcg/g of dry liver), as well as Kayser-Fleischer rings, neurologic symptoms, and Coombs-negative hemolytic anemia. However, increased urinary copper and a low serum ceruloplasmin level (by a standard immunologic assay) are neither completely sensitive nor specific for Wilson disease, although an enzymatic assay for ceruloplasmin appears to be more accurate. The ratio of exchangeable copper to total copper in serum has been reported to improve diagnostic accuracy. In equivocal cases (when the serum ceruloplasmin level is normal), the diagnosis may require demonstration of a rise in urinary copper after a penicillamine challenge, although the test has been validated only in children. Liver biopsy may show acute or chronic hepatitis or cirrhosis. MRI of the brain may show evidence of increased basal ganglia, brainstem, and cerebellar copper even early in the course of the disease. If available, molecular analysis of *ATP7B* mutations can be diagnostic.

Treatment

Early treatment to remove excess copper before it can produce hepatic or neurologic damage is essential. Early in treatment, restriction of dietary copper (shellfish, organ foods, nuts, mushrooms, and chocolate) may be of value. Oral penicillamine (0.75–2 g/d in divided doses taken 1 h before or 2 h after food) is the drug of choice and enhances urinary excretion of chelated copper. Oral pyridoxine, 50 mg per week, is added because penicillamine is an antimetabolite of this vitamin. If penicillamine treatment cannot be tolerated because of gastrointestinal intolerance, hypersensitivity, autoimmune reactions, nephrotoxicity, or bone marrow toxicity, consider the use of trientine, 250–500 mg three times a day, a chelating agent as effective as penicillamine but with a lower rate of adverse effects. Oral zinc acetate or zinc gluconate, 50 mg three times a day, interferes with intestinal absorption of copper, promotes fecal copper excretion, and has been used as first-line therapy in presymptomatic or pregnant patients and those with neurologic disease and as maintenance therapy after decoppering with a chelating agent, but adverse gastrointestinal effects often lead to discontinuation and its long-term efficacy and safety (including a risk of hepatotoxicity) have been questioned. Ammonium tetrathiomolybdate, which complexes copper in the intestinal tract, has shown promise as initial therapy for neurologic Wilson disease.

Treatment should continue indefinitely. The doses of penicillamine and trientine should be reduced during pregnancy. Supplemental vitamin E, an antioxidant, has been recommended but not rigorously studied. Once the serum nonceruloplasmin copper level is within the normal range (50–150 mcg/L), the dose of chelating agent can be reduced to the minimum necessary for maintaining that level. The prognosis is good in patients who are effectively treated before liver or brain damage has occurred. Liver transplantation is indicated for fulminant hepatitis (often after plasma exchange or dialysis with MARS as a stabilizing measure), end-stage cirrhosis, and, in selected cases, intractable neurologic disease, although survival is lower when liver transplantation is undertaken for neurologic disease than for liver disease. Family members, especially siblings, require screening with serum ceruloplasmin, liver biochemical tests, and slit-lamp examination or, if the causative mutation is known, with mutation analysis.

When to Refer

All patients with Wilson disease should be referred for diagnosis and treatment.

When to Admit

- Acute liver failure.
- Gastrointestinal bleeding.
- Stage 3–4 hepatic encephalopathy.
- Worsening kidney function.
- Severe hyponatremia.
- Profound hypoxia.

European Association for Study of the Liver. EASL Clinical Practice Guidelines: Wilson's disease. J Hepatol. 2012 Mar;56(3):671–85. [PMID: 22340672]

Weiss KH et al. Efficacy and safety of oral chelators in treatment of patients with Wilson disease. Clin Gastroenterol Hepatol. 2013 Aug;11(8):1028–35. [PMID: 23542331]

HEPATIC VEIN OBSTRUCTION (Budd-Chiari Syndrome)

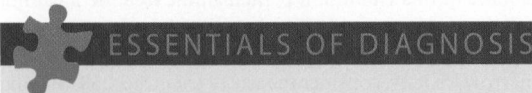

ESSENTIALS OF DIAGNOSIS

► Right upper quadrant pain and tenderness.

► Ascites.

► Imaging studies show occlusion/absence of flow in the hepatic vein(s) or inferior vena cava.

► Clinical picture is similar in sinusoidal obstruction syndrome but major hepatic veins are patent.

General Considerations

Factors that predispose patients to hepatic vein obstruction, or Budd-Chiari syndrome, including hereditary and acquired hypercoagulable states, can be identified in 75% of affected patients; multiple disorders are found in up to 45%. Up to 50% of cases are associated with polycythemia vera or other myeloproliferative disease (which has a risk of Budd-Chiari syndrome of 1%). These cases (37% of patients with Budd-Chiari syndrome) are often associated with a specific mutation (V617F) in the gene that codes for JAK2 tyrosine kinase and may be subclinical. In some cases, other predispositions to thrombosis (eg, activated protein C resistance [factor V Leiden mutation] [25% of cases], protein C or S or antithrombin deficiency, hyperprothrombinemia [factor II G20210A mutation], the methylenetetrahydrofolate reductase TT677 mutation, antiphospholipid antibodies) can be identified. Hepatic vein obstruction may be associated with caval webs, right-sided heart failure or constrictive pericarditis, neoplasms that cause hepatic vein occlusion, paroxysmal nocturnal hemoglobinuria, Behçet syndrome, blunt abdominal trauma, use of oral contraceptives, and pregnancy. Some cytotoxic agents and pyrrolizidine alkaloids (Comfrey or "bush teas") may cause sinusoidal obstruction syndrome (previously known as veno-occlusive disease because the terminal venules are often occluded), which mimics Budd-Chiari syndrome clinically. Sinusoidal obstruction syndrome is common in patients who have undergone hematopoietic stem cell transplantation, particularly those with pretransplant serum aminotransferase elevations or fever during cytoreductive therapy with cyclophosphamide, azathioprine, carmustine, busulfan, or etoposide or those receiving high-dose cytoreductive therapy or high-dose total body irradiation. In India, China, and South Africa, Budd-Chiari syndrome is associated with a poor standard of living and often the result of occlusion of the hepatic portion of the inferior vena cava, presumably due

to prior thrombosis. The clinical presentation is mild but the course is frequently complicated by hepatocellular carcinoma.

Clinical Findings

A. Symptoms and Signs

The presentation may be fulminant, acute, subacute, or chronic. An insidious (subacute) onset is most common. Clinical manifestations generally include tender, painful hepatic enlargement, jaundice, splenomegaly, and ascites. With chronic disease, bleeding varices and hepatic encephalopathy may be evident; hepatopulmonary syndrome may occur.

B. Imaging

Hepatic imaging studies may show a prominent caudate lobe, since its venous drainage may not be occluded. The screening test of choice is contrast-enhanced, color, or pulsed-Doppler ultrasonography, which has a sensitivity of 85% for detecting evidence of hepatic venous or inferior vena caval thrombosis. MRI with spin-echo and gradient-echo sequences and intravenous gadolinium injection allows visualization of the obstructed veins and collateral vessels. Direct venography can delineate caval webs and occluded hepatic veins ("spider-web" pattern) most precisely.

C. Liver Biopsy

Percutaneous or transjugular liver biopsy in Budd-Chiari syndrome may be considered when the results of noninvasive imaging are inconclusive and frequently shows characteristic centrilobular congestion and fibrosis and often multiple large regenerative nodules. Liver biopsy is often contraindicated in sinusoidal obstruction syndrome because of thrombocytopenia, and the diagnosis is based on clinical findings.

Treatment

Ascites should be treated with fluid and salt restriction and diuretics. Treatable causes of Budd-Chiari syndrome should be sought. Prompt recognition and treatment of an underlying hematologic disorder may avoid the need for surgery; however, the optimal anticoagulation regimen is uncertain, and anticoagulation is associated with a high risk of bleeding, particularly in patients with portal hypertension and those undergoing invasive procedures. Low-molecular-weight heparins are preferred over unfractionated heparin because of a high rate of heparin-induced thrombocytopenia with the latter. Infusion of a thrombolytic agent into recently occluded veins has been attempted with success. Defibrotide, an adenosine receptor agonist that increases endogenous tissue plasminogen activator levels, has shown promise in the prevention and treatment of sinusoidal obstruction syndrome. TIPS placement may be attempted in patients with Budd-Chiari syndrome and persistent hepatic congestion or failed thrombolytic therapy and possibly in those with sinusoidal obstruction syndrome. Late TIPS dysfunction is less frequent with the use of polytetrafluoroethylene-covered stents than uncovered stents. TIPS is now preferred over surgical decompression (side-to-side portacaval, mesocaval, or mesoatrial shunt), which, in contrast to TIPS, has generally not been proven to improve long-term survival. Older age, a higher serum bilirubin level, and a greater INR predict a poor outcome with TIPS. Balloon angioplasty, in some cases with placement of an intravascular metallic stent, is preferred in patients with an inferior vena caval web and is being performed increasingly in patients with a short segment of thrombosis in the hepatic vein. Liver transplantation is considered in patients with fulminant hepatic failure, cirrhosis with hepatocellular dysfunction, and failure of a portosystemic shunt, and outcomes have improved with the advent of patient selection based on the MELD score. Patients with Budd-Chiari syndrome often require lifelong anticoagulation and treatment of the underlying myeloproliferative disease; antiplatelet therapy with aspirin and hydroxyurea has been suggested as an alternative to warfarin in patients with a myeloproliferative disorder. The overall 5-year survival rate is 50–90% with treatment (but <10% without intervention). Adverse prognostic factors in patients with Budd-Chiari syndrome are older age, high Child-Turcotte-Pugh score, ascites, encephalopathy, elevated total bilirubin, prolonged prothrombin time, elevated serum creatinine, concomitant portal vein thrombosis, and histologic features of acute liver disease superimposed on chronic liver injury; 3-month mortality may be predicted by the Rotterdam score, which is based on encephalopathy, ascites, prothrombin time, and bilirubin. A serum ALT level at least fivefold above the upper limit of normal on presentation indicates hepatic ischemia and also predicts a poor outcome, particularly when the ALT level decreases slowly.

▶ When to Admit

All patients with hepatic vein obstruction should be hospitalized.

Harmanci O et al. Long-term follow-up study in Budd-Chiari syndrome: single-center experience in 22 years. J Clin Gastroenterol. 2013 Sep;47(8):706–12. [PMID: 22495815]
Plessier A et al. Management of hepatic vascular diseases. J Hepatol. 2012;56(Suppl 1):S25–38. [PMID: 22300463]
Seijo S et al. Good long-term outcome of Budd-Chiari syndrome with a step-wise management. Hepatology. 2013 May;57(5):1962–8. [PMID: 23389867]

THE LIVER IN HEART FAILURE

Ischemic hepatitis, also called **ischemic hepatopathy, hypoxic hepatitis, shock liver**, or **acute cardiogenic liver injury** may affect up to 10% of patients in an intensive care unit and results from an acute fall in cardiac output due to acute myocardial infarction, arrhythmia, or septic or hemorrhagic shock, usually in a patient with passive congestion of the liver. Clinical hypotension may be absent (or unwitnessed). In some cases, the precipitating event is arterial

hypoxemia due to respiratory failure, sleep apnea, severe anemia, heat stroke, carbon monoxide poisoning, cocaine use, or bacterial endocarditis. More than one precipitant is common. The hallmark is a rapid and striking elevation of serum aminotransferase levels (often > 5000 units/L); an early rapid rise in the serum lactate dehydrogenase (LD) level (with an ALT-to-LD ratio < 1.5) is also typical. Elevations of serum alkaline phosphatase and bilirubin are usually mild, but jaundice is associated with worse outcomes. The prothrombin time may be prolonged, and encephalopathy or hepatopulmonary syndrome may develop. The mortality rate due to the underlying disease is high (particularly in patients receiving vasopressor therapy or with septic shock, acute kidney disease, or coagulopathy), but in patients who recover, the aminotransferase levels return to normal quickly, usually within 1 week—in contrast to viral hepatitis.

In patients with **passive congestion of the liver** ("nutmeg liver") due to right-sided heart failure, the serum bilirubin level may be elevated, occasionally as high as 40 mg/dL (684 mcmol/L), due in part to hypoxia of perivenular hepatocytes, and the level is a predictor of mortality and morbidity. Serum alkaline phosphatase levels are normal or slightly elevated, and aminotransferase levels are only mildly elevated in the absence of superimposed ischemia. Hepatojugular reflux is present, and with tricuspid regurgitation the liver may be pulsatile. Ascites may be out of proportion to peripheral edema, with a high serum ascites-albumin gradient (≥ 1.1) and a protein content of more than 2.5 g/dL (25 g/L). A markedly elevated serum N-terminal-proBNP level has been reported to distinguish ascites due to heart failure from ascites due to cirrhosis. In severe cases, signs of encephalopathy may develop.

Samsky MD et al. Cardiohepatic interactions in heart failure: an overview and clinical implications. J Am Coll Cardiol. 2013 Jun 18;61(24):2397–405. [PMID: 23603231]

NONCIRRHOTIC PORTAL HYPERTENSION

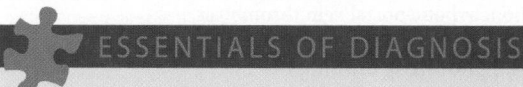

ESSENTIALS OF DIAGNOSIS

▶ Splenomegaly or upper gastrointestinal bleeding from esophageal or gastric varices in patients without liver disease.

▶ General Considerations

Causes of noncirrhotic portal hypertension include extrahepatic portal vein obstruction (portal vein thrombosis often with cavernous transformation [portal cavernoma]), splenic vein obstruction (presenting as gastric varices without esophageal varices), schistosomiasis, nodular regenerative hyperplasia, and arterial-portal vein fistula. Idiopathic noncirrhotic portal hypertension is common in India and has been attributed to chronic infections, exposure to medications or toxins, prothrombotic disorders, immunologic disorders, and genetic disorders that result in obliterative vascular lesions in the liver. It is rare in Western countries, where increased mortality is attributable to associated disorders and older age. Portal vein thrombosis may occur in 10–25% of patients with cirrhosis and may be associated with hepatocellular carcinoma. Other risk factors are oral contraceptive use, pregnancy, chronic inflammatory diseases (including pancreatitis), injury to the portal venous system (including surgery), other malignancies, and treatment of thrombocytopenia with eltrombopag. Splenic vein thrombosis may complicate pancreatitis or pancreatic cancer. Pylephlebitis (septic thrombophlebitis of the portal vein) may complicate intra-abdominal inflammatory disorders such as appendicitis or diverticulitis, particularly when anaerobic organisms (especially *Bacteroides* species) are involved. Nodular regenerative hyperplasia results from altered hepatic perfusion and can be associated with collagen vascular diseases; myeloproliferative disorders; and drugs, including azathioprine, 5-fluorouracil, and oxaliplatin. In patients infected with HIV, long-term use of didanosine and use of a combination of didanosine and stavudine have been reported to account for some cases of noncirrhotic portal hypertension often due to nodular regenerative hyperplasia, and genetic factors may play a role. The term obliterative portal venopathy is used to describe primary occlusion of intrahepatic portal veins in the absence of cirrhosis, inflammation, or hepatic neoplasia.

▶ Clinical Findings

A. Symptoms and Signs

Acute portal vein thrombosis usually causes abdominal pain. Aside from splenomegaly, the physical findings are not remarkable, although hepatic decompensation can follow severe gastrointestinal bleeding or a concurrent hepatic disorder, and intestinal infarction may occur when portal vein thrombosis is associated with mesenteric venous thrombosis. Ascites may occur in 25% of persons with noncirrhotic portal hypertension. Minimal hepatic encephalopathy is reported to be common in patients with noncirrhotic portal vein thrombosis.

B. Laboratory Findings

Liver biochemical test levels are usually normal, but there may be findings of hypersplenism. An underlying hypercoagulable state is found in many patients with portal vein thrombosis; this includes myeloproliferative disorders (often associated with a specific mutation [*V617F*] in the gene coding for JAK2 tyrosine kinase, which is found in 24% of cases of portal vein thrombosis), mutation G20210A of prothrombin, factor V Leiden mutation, protein C and S deficiency, antiphospholipid syndrome, mutation TT677 of methylenetetrahydrofolate reductase, elevated factor VIII levels, hyperhomocysteinemia, and a mutation in the gene that codes for thrombin-activatable fibrinolysis inhibitor. It is possible, however, that in many cases evidence of hypercoagulability is a secondary phenomenon due to portosystemic shunting and reduced hepatic blood flow.

C. Imaging

Color Doppler ultrasonography and contrast-enhanced CT are usually the initial diagnostic tests for portal vein thrombosis. Magnetic resonance angiography (MRA) of the portal system is generally confirmatory. Endoscopic ultrasonography may be helpful in some cases. In patients with jaundice, magnetic resonance cholangiography may demonstrate compression of the bile duct by a large portal cavernoma (portal biliopathy), a finding that may be more common in patients with an underlying hypercoagulable state than in those without one. In patients with pylephlebitis, CT may demonstrate an intra-abdominal source of infection, thrombosis or gas in the portal venous system, and a hepatic abscess.

D. Other Studies

Endoscopy shows esophageal or gastric varices. Needle biopsy of the liver may be indicated to diagnose schistosomiasis, nodular regenerative hyperplasia, and noncirrhotic portal fibrosis and may demonstrate sinusoidal dilatation.

▶ Treatment

If splenic vein thrombosis is the cause of variceal bleeding, splenectomy is curative. For other causes of noncirrhotic portal hypertension, band ligation (or sclerotherapy) followed by beta-blockers to reduce portal pressure is initiated for variceal bleeding, and portosystemic shunting (including TIPS) is reserved for failures of endoscopic therapy; rarely progressive liver dysfunction requires liver transplantation. Anticoagulation particularly with low-molecular-weight heparin or thrombolytic therapy may be indicated for isolated acute portal vein thrombosis (and leads to at least partial recanalization in up to 75% of cases) and possibly for acute splenic vein thrombosis; it is continued long-term if a hypercoagulable disorder is identified or if an acute portal vein thrombosis extends into the mesenteric veins. The use of enoxaparin to prevent portal vein thrombosis and hepatic decompensation in patients with cirrhosis has shown promise.

▶ When to Refer

All patients with noncirrhotic portal hypertension should be referred.

Delgado MG et al. Efficacy and safety of anticoagulation on patients with cirrhosis and portal vein thrombosis. Clin Gastroenterol Hepatol. 2012 Jul;10(7):776–83. [PMID: 22289875]

Francoz C et al. Portal vein thrombosis, cirrhosis, and liver transplantation. J Hepatol. 2012 Jul;57(1):203–12. [PMID: 22446690]

Handa P et al. Portal vein thrombosis: a clinician-oriented and practical review. Clin Appl Thromb Hemost. 2013 Jan 29. [Epub ahead of print] [PMID: 23364162]

Schouten JN et al. Idiopathic noncirrhotic portal hypertension is associated with poor survival: results of a long-term cohort study. Aliment Pharmacol Ther. 2012 Jun;35(12):1424–33. [PMID: 22536808]

Vispo E et al. Genetic determinants of idiopathic noncirrhotic portal hypertension in HIV-infected patients. Clin Infect Dis. 2013 Apr;56(8):1117–22. [PMID: 23315321]

PYOGENIC HEPATIC ABSCESS

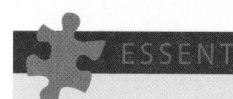

ESSENTIALS OF DIAGNOSIS

▶ Fever, right upper quadrant pain, jaundice.

▶ Often in setting of biliary disease, but up to 40% are "cryptogenic" in origin.

▶ Detected by imaging studies.

▶ General Considerations

The incidence of liver abscess is 3.6 per 100,000 population in the United States and has increased since the 1990s. The liver can be invaded by bacteria via (1) the bile duct (ascending cholangitis); (2) the portal vein (pylephlebitis); (3) the hepatic artery, secondary to bacteremia; (4) direct extension from an infectious process; and (5) traumatic implantation of bacteria through the abdominal wall. Risk factors for liver abscess include older age and male gender. Predisposing conditions include malignancy, diabetes mellitus, inflammatory bowel disease, cirrhosis, and liver transplantation.

Ascending cholangitis resulting from biliary obstruction due to a stone, stricture, or neoplasm is the most common identifiable cause of hepatic abscess in the United States. In 10% of cases, liver abscess is secondary to appendicitis or diverticulitis. At least 40% of abscesses have no demonstrable cause and are classified as cryptogenic; a dental source is identified in some cases. The most frequently encountered organisms are *E coli, Klebsiella pneumoniae, Proteus vulgaris, Enterobacter aerogenes,* and multiple microaerophilic and anaerobic species (eg, *Streptococcus milleri*). Liver abscess caused by virulent strains of *K pneumoniae* may be associated with thrombophlebitis of the portal or hepatic veins and hematogenously spread septic ocular or central nervous system complications. *Staphylococcus aureus* is usually the causative organism in patients with chronic granulomatous disease. Uncommon causative organisms include *Salmonella, Haemophilus, Yersinia, and Listeria.* Hepatic candidiasis, tuberculosis, and actinomycosis are seen in immunocompromised patients and those with hematologic malignancies. Rarely, hepatocellular carcinoma can present as a pyogenic abscess because of tumor necrosis, biliary obstruction, and superimposed bacterial infection (see Chapter 39). The possibility of an amebic liver abscess must always be considered (see Chapter 35).

▶ Clinical Findings

A. Symptoms and Signs

The presentation is often insidious. Fever is almost always present and may antedate other symptoms or signs. Pain may be a prominent complaint and is localized to the right upper quadrant or epigastric area. Jaundice, tenderness in the right upper abdomen, and either steady or spiking fever are the chief physical findings.

B. Laboratory Findings

Laboratory examination reveals leukocytosis with a shift to the left. Liver biochemical tests are nonspecifically abnormal. Blood cultures are positive in 50–100% of cases.

C. Imaging

Chest radiographs usually reveal elevation of the diaphragm if the abscess is in the right lobe of the liver. Ultrasonography, CT, or MRI may reveal the presence of intrahepatic lesions. On MRI, characteristic findings include high signal intensity on T2-weighted images and rim enhancement. The characteristic CT appearance of hepatic candidiasis, usually seen in the setting of systemic candidiasis, is that of multiple "bull's-eyes," but imaging studies may be negative in neutropenic patients.

▶ Treatment

Treatment should consist of antimicrobial agents (generally a third-generation cephalosporin such as cefoperazone 1–2 g intravenously every 12 hours and metronidazole 500 mg intravenously every 6 hours) that are effective against coliform organisms and anaerobes. Antibiotics are administered for 2–3 weeks, and sometimes up to 6 weeks. If the abscess is at least 5 cm in diameter or the response to antibiotic therapy is not rapid, intermittent needle aspiration, percutaneous or endoscopic ultrasound-guided catheter drainage or, if necessary, surgical (eg, laparoscopic) drainage should be done. Other suggested indications for abscess drainage are patient age of at least 55 years, symptom duration of at least 7 days, and involvement of two lobes of the liver. The underlying source (eg, biliary disease, dental infection) should be identified and treated. The mortality rate is still substantial (≥ 5% in most studies) and is highest in patients with underlying biliary malignancy or severe multiorgan dysfunction. Other risk factors for mortality include older age, cirrhosis, chronic kidney disease, and other cancers. Hepatic candidiasis often responds to intravenous amphotericin B (total dose of 2–9 g). Fungal abscesses are associated with mortality rates of up to 50% and are treated with intravenous amphotericin B and drainage.

▶ When to Admit

Nearly all patients with pyogenic hepatic abscess should be hospitalized.

Siu LK et al. *Klebsiella pneumoniae* liver abscess: a new invasive syndrome. Lancet Infect Dis. 2012 Nov;12(11):881–7. [PMID: 23099082]

Tan L et al. Laparoscopic drainage of cryptogenic liver abscess. Surg Endosc. 2013 Sep;27(9):3308–14. [PMID: 23494514]

BENIGN LIVER NEOPLASMS

Benign neoplasms of the liver must be distinguished from hepatocellular carcinoma, intrahepatic cholangiocarcinoma, and metastases (see Chapter 39). The most common benign neoplasm of the liver is the **cavernous hemangioma,** often an incidental finding on ultrasonography or CT. This lesion may enlarge in women who take hormonal therapy and must be differentiated from other space-occupying intrahepatic lesions, usually by contrast-enhanced MRI, CT, or ultrasonography. Rarely, fine-needle biopsy is necessary to differentiate these lesions and does not appear to carry an increased risk of bleeding. Surgical resection of cavernous hemangiomas is rarely necessary but may be required for abdominal pain or rapid enlargement, to exclude malignancy, or to treat Kasabach-Merritt syndrome (consumptive coagulopathy complicating a hemangioma).

In addition to rare instances of sinusoidal dilatation and peliosis hepatis, two distinct benign lesions with characteristic clinical, radiologic, and histopathologic features have been described in women taking oral contraceptives—focal nodular hyperplasia and hepatocellular adenoma. **Focal nodular hyperplasia** occurs at all ages and in both sexes and is probably not caused by the oral contraceptives. It is often asymptomatic and appears as a hypervascular mass, often with a central hypodense "stellate" scar on CT or MRI. Microscopically, focal nodular hyperplasia consists of hyperplastic units of hepatocytes that stain positively for glutamine synthetase with a central stellate scar containing proliferating bile ducts. It is not a true neoplasm but a proliferation of hepatocytes in response to altered blood flow. Focal nodular hyperplasia is associated with an elevated angiopoietin 1/angiopoietin 2 mRNA ratio that is thought to promote angiogenesis and may also occur in patients with cirrhosis, with exposure to certain drugs such as azathioprine, and in antiphospholipid syndrome. The prevalence of hepatic hemangiomas is increased in patients with focal nodular hyperplasia.

Hepatocellular adenoma occurs most commonly in women in the third and fourth decades of life and is usually caused by oral contraceptives; acute abdominal pain may occur if the tumor undergoes necrosis or hemorrhage. The tumor may be associated with mutations in: (1) the gene coding for hepatocyte nuclear factor 1 alpha (*HNF1alpha*) in 30–40% of cases (characterized by steatosis and a low risk of malignant transformation, although in men concomitant metabolic syndrome appears to increase the risk of malignant transformation); (2) the gene coding for beta-catenin (characterized by a high rate of malignant transformation) in 10–15% of cases; or (3) neither gene with the designation inflammatory adenoma (previously termed "telangiectatic focal nodular hyperplasia"), which is associated with a high body mass index and serum biomarkers of inflammation (such as C-reactive protein) in 40–50% of cases. Unclassified adenomas account for 10% of tumors. Rare instances of multiple hepatocellular adenomas in association with maturity-onset diabetes of the young occur in families with a germline mutation in *HNF1alpha*. Hepatocellular adenomas also occur in patients with glycogen storage disease (inflammatory or unclassified adenomas) and familial adenomatous polyposis. The tumor is hypovascular. Grossly, the cut surface appears structureless. As seen microscopically, the hepatocellular adenoma consists of sheets of hepatocytes without portal tracts or central veins.

Cystic neoplasms of the liver, such as cystadenoma and cystadenocarcinoma, must be distinguished from simple and echinococcal cysts, von Meyenburg complexes (hamartomas), and polycystic liver disease.

► Clinical Findings

The only physical finding in focal nodular hyperplasia or hepatocellular adenoma is a palpable abdominal mass in a minority of cases. Liver function is usually normal. Arterial phase helical CT and MRI with contrast can distinguish an adenoma from focal nodular hyperplasia in 80–90% of cases and may suggest a specific subtype of adenoma (eg, homogeneous fat pattern in *HNF1alpha*-mutated adenomas and marked and persistent arterial enhancement in inflammatory adenomas).

► Treatment

Treatment of focal nodular hyperplasia is resection only in the symptomatic patient; rarely is liver transplantation necessary. The prognosis is excellent. Hepatocellular adenoma may undergo bleeding, necrosis, and rupture, often after hormone therapy, in the third trimester of pregnancy, or in men in whom the rate of malignant transformation is high. Resection is advised in all affected men and in women in whom the tumor causes symptoms or is > 5 cm in diameter, even in the absence of symptoms. If an adenoma is < 5 cm in size, resection is also recommended if a beta-catenin gene mutation is present in a biopsy sample. In selected cases, laparoscopic resection or percutaneous radiofrequency ablation may be feasible. Regression of benign hepatic tumors may follow cessation of oral contraceptives.

► When to Refer

- Diagnostic uncertainty.
- For surgery.

► When to Admit

- Severe pain.
- Rupture.

Bonder A et al. Evaluation of liver lesions. Clin Liver Dis. 2012 May;16(2):271–83. [PMID: 22541698]

Calderaro J et al. Molecular characterization of hepatocellular adenomas developed in patients with glycogen storage disease type I. J Hepatol. 2013 Feb;58(2):350–7. [PMID: 23046672]

Nault JC et al. Hepatocellular benign tumors—from molecular classification to personalized clinical care. Gastroenterology. 2013 May;144(5):888–902. [PMID: 23485860]

DISEASES OF THE BILIARY TRACT

See Chapter 39 for Carcinoma of the Biliary Tract.

CHOLELITHIASIS (Gallstones)

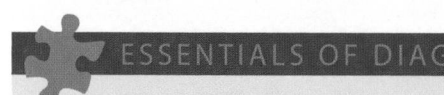

ESSENTIALS OF DIAGNOSIS

- ► Often asymptomatic.
- ► Classic biliary pain ("episodic gallbladder pain") characterized by infrequent episodes of steady severe pain in epigastrium or right upper quadrant with radiation to right scapula.
- ► Detected on ultrasonography.

► General Considerations

Gallstones are more common in women than in men and increase in incidence in both sexes and all races with age. In the United States, the prevalence of gallstones is 8.6% in women and 5.5% in men, with the highest rates in persons over age 60 and higher rates in Mexican-Americans than in non-Hispanic whites and African Americans, and gallstone disease is associated with increased overall, cardiovascular, and cancer mortality. Although cholesterol gallstones are less common in black people, cholelithiasis attributable to hemolysis occurs in over a third of individuals with sickle cell disease. Native Americans of both the Northern and Southern Hemispheres have a high rate of cholesterol cholelithiasis, probably because of a predisposition resulting from "thrifty" (LITH) genes that promote efficient calorie utilization and fat storage. As many as 75% of Pima and other American Indian women over the age of 25 years have cholelithiasis. Other genetic mutations that predispose persons to gallstones have been identified. Obesity is a risk factor for gallstones, especially in women. Rapid weight loss, as occurs after bariatric surgery, also increases the risk of symptomatic gallstone formation. Diabetes mellitus, glucose intolerance, and insulin resistance are risk factors for gallstones, and a high intake of carbohydrate and high dietary glycemic load increase the risk of cholecystectomy in women. Hypertriglyceridemia may promote gallstone formation by impairing gallbladder motility. The prevalence of gallbladder disease is increased in men (but not women) with cirrhosis and hepatitis C virus infection. Moreover, cholecystectomy has been reported to be associated with an increased risk of NAFLD and cirrhosis, possibly because gallstones and liver disease have some risk factors in common. A low-carbohydrate diet, physical activity, and cardiorespiratory fitness may help prevent gallstones. Consumption of caffeinated coffee appears to protect against gallstones in women, and a high intake of magnesium and of polyunsaturated and monounsaturated fats reduces the risk of gallstones in men. A diet high in fiber, a diet rich in fruits and vegetables, and statin use reduce the risk of cholecystectomy, particularly in women. The incidence of gallstones is high in individuals with Crohn disease; approximately one-third of those with inflammatory involvement of the terminal ileum have gallstones due to disruption of bile salt resorption that results in decreased solubility of the bile. Drugs such as clofibrate, octreotide, and ceftriaxone can cause gallstones. In contrast, aspirin and other nonsteroidal anti-inflammatory drugs may protect against gallstones. Prolonged fasting (over 5–10 days) can lead to formation of biliary "sludge" (microlithiasis), which usually resolves with refeeding but can lead to gallstones or biliary symptoms. Pregnancy, particularly in obese women and those with insulin resistance, is associated with an increased risk of gallstones and of symptomatic gallbladder disease. Hormone replacement therapy appears to increase the risk of gallbladder disease and need for cholecystectomy; the risk is lower with transdermal than oral therapy.

Gallstones are classified according to their predominant chemical composition as cholesterol or calcium bilirubinate stones. The latter comprise < 20% of the stones found in Europe or the United States but 30–40% of stones found in Japan.

► Clinical Findings

Table 16–7 lists the clinical and laboratory features of several diseases of the biliary tract as well as their treatment. Cholelithiasis is frequently asymptomatic and is discovered in the course of routine radiographic study, operation, or autopsy. Symptoms (biliary [or "episodic gallbladder"] pain) develop in 10–25% of patients (1–4% annually), and acute cholecystitis develops in 20% of these symptomatic persons over time. Occasionally, small intestinal obstruction due to "gallstone ileus" (or Bouveret syndrome when the obstructing stone is in pylorus or duodenum) presents as the initial manifestation of cholelithiasis.

► Treatment

Nonsteroidal anti-inflammatory drugs (eg, diclofenac 50–75 mg intramuscularly) can be used to relieve biliary pain. Laparoscopic cholecystectomy is the treatment of choice for symptomatic gallbladder disease. Pain relief after cholecystectomy is most likely in patients with episodic pain (generally once a month or less), pain lasting 30 minutes to 24 hours, pain in the evening or at night, and the onset of symptoms 1 year or less before presentation. Patients may go home within 1 day of the procedure and return to work within days (instead of weeks for those undergoing open cholecystectomy). The procedure is often performed on an outpatient basis and is suitable for most patients, including those with acute cholecystitis. Conversion to a conventional open cholecystectomy may be necessary in 2–8% of cases (higher for acute cholecystitis than for uncomplicated cholelithiasis). Bile duct injuries occur in 0.1% of cases done by experienced surgeons.

Table 16–7. Diseases of the biliary tract.

	Clinical Features	Laboratory Features	Diagnosis	Treatment
Gallstones	Asymptomatic	Normal	Ultrasonography	None
Gallstones	Biliary pain	Normal	Ultrasonography	Laparoscopic cholecystectomy
Cholesterolosis of gallbladder	Usually asymptomatic	Normal	Oral cholecystography	None
Adenomyomatosis	May cause biliary pain	Normal	Oral cholecystography	Laparoscopic cholecystectomy if symptomatic
Porcelain gallbladder	Usually asymptomatic, high risk of gallbladder cancer	Normal	Radiograph or CT	Laparoscopic cholecystectomy
Acute cholecystitis	Epigastric or right upper quadrant pain, nausea, vomiting, fever, Murphy sign	Leukocytosis	Ultrasonography, HIDA scan	Antibiotics, laparoscopic cholecystectomy
Chronic cholecystitis	Biliary pain, constant epigastric or right upper quadrant pain, nausea	Normal	Ultrasonography (stones), oral cholecystography (nonfunctioning gallbladder)	Laparoscopic cholecystectomy
Choledocholithiasis	Asymptomatic or biliary pain, jaundice, fever; gallstone pancreatitis	Cholestatic liver biochemical tests; leukocytosis and positive blood cultures in cholangitis; elevated amylase and lipase in pancreatitis	Ultrasonography (dilated ducts), endoscopic ultrasonography, MRCP, ERCP	Endoscopic sphincterotomy and stone extraction; antibiotics for cholangitis

ERCP, endoscopic retrograde cholangiopancreatography; HIDA, hepatic iminodiacetic acid; MRCP, magnetic resonance cholangiopancreatography.

There is generally no need for prophylactic cholecystectomy in an asymptomatic person unless the gallbladder is calcified, gallstones are > 3 cm in diameter, or the patient is a Native American or a candidate for bariatric surgery or cardiac transplantation. Cholecystectomy may increase the risk of esophageal, proximal small intestinal, and colonic adenocarcinomas because of increased duodenogastric reflux and changes in intestinal exposure to bile. In pregnant patients a conservative approach to biliary pain is advised, but for patients with repeated attacks of biliary pain or acute cholecystitis, cholecystectomy can be performed—even by the laparoscopic route—preferably in the second trimester. Enterolithotomy alone is considered adequate treatment in most patients with gallstone ileus. Cholecystectomy via natural orifice translumenal endoscopic surgery (NOTES) has been performed and is under study.

Ursodeoxycholic acid is a bile salt that when given orally for up to 2 years dissolve some cholesterol stones and may be considered in occasional, selected patients who refuse cholecystectomy. The dose is 8–13 mg/kg in divided doses daily. It is most effective in patients with a functioning gallbladder, as determined by gallbladder visualization on oral cholecystography, and multiple small "floating" gallstones (representing not more than 15% of patients

with gallstones). In half of patients, gallstones recur within 5 years after treatment is stopped. Ursodeoxycholic acid, 500–600 mg daily, reduces the risk of gallstone formation with rapid weight loss. Lithotripsy in combination with bile salt therapy for single radiolucent stones < 20 mm in diameter was an option in the past but is no longer generally used in the United States.

► **When to Refer**

Patients should be referred when they require surgery.

Colli A et al. Meta-analysis: nonsteroidal anti-inflammatory drugs in biliary colic. Aliment Pharmacol Ther. 2012 Jun;35(12):1370–8. [PMID: 22540869]

Gurusamy KS et al. Early versus delayed laparoscopic cholecystectomy for uncomplicated biliary colic. Cochrane Database Syst Rev. 2013 Jun 30;6:CD007196. [PMID: 23813478]

Ruhl CE et al. Relationship of non-alcoholic fatty liver disease with cholecystectomy in the US population. Am J Gastroenterol. 2013 Jun;108(6):952–8. [PMID: 23545713]

von Kampen O et al. Genetic and functional identification of the likely causative variant for cholesterol gallstone disease at the ABCG5/8 lithogenic locus. Hepatology. 2013 Jun;57(6):2407–17. [PMID: 22898925]

ACUTE CHOLECYSTITIS

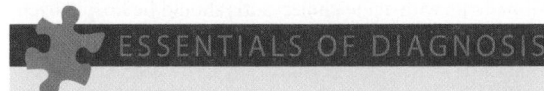

ESSENTIALS OF DIAGNOSIS

► Steady, severe pain and tenderness in the right hypochondrium or epigastrium.

► Nausea and vomiting.

► Fever and leukocytosis.

General Considerations

Cholecystitis is associated with gallstones in over 90% of cases. It occurs when a stone becomes impacted in the cystic duct and inflammation develops behind the obstruction. Acalculous cholecystitis should be considered when unexplained fever or right upper quadrant pain occurs within 2–4 weeks of major surgery or in a critically ill patient who has had no oral intake for a prolonged period; multiorgan failure is often present. Acute cholecystitis may be caused by infectious agents (eg, cytomegalovirus, cryptosporidiosis, or microsporidiosis) in patients with AIDS or by vasculitis (eg, polyarteritis nodosa, Henoch-Schönlein purpura).

Clinical Findings

A. Symptoms and Signs

The acute attack is often precipitated by a large or fatty meal and is characterized by the sudden appearance of steady pain localized to the epigastrium or right hypochondrium, which may gradually subside over a period of 12–18 hours. Vomiting occurs in about 75% of patients and in half of instances affords variable relief. Fever is typical. Right upper quadrant abdominal tenderness (often with a Murphy sign, or inhibition of inspiration by pain on palpation of the right upper quadrant) is almost always present and is usually associated with muscle guarding and rebound tenderness (Table 16–7). A palpable gallbladder is present in about 15% of cases. Jaundice is present in about 25% of cases and, when persistent or severe, suggests the possibility of choledocholithiasis.

B. Laboratory Findings

The white blood cell count is usually high (12,000–15,000/mcL [12–15 × 10^9/L]). Total serum bilirubin values of 1–4 mg/dL (17.1–68.4 mcmol/L) may be seen even in the absence of bile duct obstruction. Serum aminotransferase and alkaline phosphatase levels are often elevated—the former as high as 300 units/mL, and even higher when associated with ascending cholangitis. Serum amylase may also be moderately elevated.

C. Imaging

Plain films of the abdomen may show radiopaque gallstones in 15% of cases. ^{99m}Tc hepatobiliary imaging (using iminodiacetic acid compounds), also known as the hepatic iminodiacetic acid (HIDA) scan, is useful in demonstrating an obstructed cystic duct, which is the cause of acute cholecystitis in most patients. This test is reliable if the bilirubin is under 5 mg/dL (85.5 mcmol/L) (98% sensitivity and 81% specificity for acute cholecystitis). False-positive results can occur with prolonged fasting, liver disease, and chronic cholecystitis, and the specificity can be improved by intravenous administration of morphine, which induces spasm of the sphincter of Oddi. Right upper quadrant abdominal ultrasonography, which is often performed first, may show gallstones but is not as sensitive for acute cholecystitis (67% sensitivity, 82% specificity); findings suggestive of acute cholecystitis are gallbladder wall thickening, pericholecystic fluid, and a sonographic Murphy sign. CT may show complications of acute cholecystitis, such as perforation or gangrene.

Differential Diagnosis

The disorders most likely to be confused with acute cholecystitis are perforated peptic ulcer, acute pancreatitis, appendicitis in a high-lying appendix, perforated colonic carcinoma or diverticulum of the hepatic flexure, liver abscess, hepatitis, pneumonia with pleurisy on the right side, and even myocardial ischemia. Definite localization of pain and tenderness in the right upper quadrant, with radiation around to the infrascapular area, strongly favors the diagnosis of acute cholecystitis. True cholecystitis without stones suggests acalculous cholecystitis.

Complications

A. Gangrene of the Gallbladder

Continuation or progression of right upper quadrant abdominal pain, tenderness, muscle guarding, fever, and leukocytosis after 24–48 hours suggests severe inflammation and possible gangrene of the gallbladder, resulting from ischemia due to splanchnic vasoconstriction and intravascular coagulation. Necrosis may occasionally develop without specific signs in the obese, diabetic, elderly, or immunosuppressed patient. Gangrene may lead to gallbladder perforation, usually with formation of a pericholecystic abscess, and rarely to generalized peritonitis. Other serious acute complications include emphysematous cholecystitis (secondary infection with a gas-forming organism) and empyema.

B. Chronic Cholecystitis and Other Complications

Chronic cholecystitis results from repeated episodes of acute cholecystitis or chronic irritation of the gallbladder wall by stones and is characterized pathologically by varying degrees of chronic inflammation of the gallbladder. Calculi are usually present. In about 4–5% of cases, the villi of the gallbladder undergo polypoid enlargement due to deposition of cholesterol that may be visible to the naked eye ("strawberry gallbladder," cholesterolosis). In other instances, hyperplasia of all or part of the gallbladder wall may be so marked as to give the appearance of a myoma (adenomyomatosis). Hydrops of the gallbladder results when acute cholecystitis subsides but cystic duct obstruction persists, producing distention of the gallbladder with a clear mucoid fluid. Occasionally, a stone in the neck of the gallbladder may compress the common hepatic duct and cause jaundice (Mirizzi syndrome). Xanthogranulomatous cholecystitis is a rare variant of chronic cholecystitis characterized by grayish-yellow nodules or streaks, representing lipid-laden macrophages, in the wall of the gallbladder.

Cholelithiasis with chronic cholecystitis may be associated with acute exacerbations of gallbladder inflammation, bile duct stone, fistulization to the bowel, pancreatitis and, rarely, carcinoma of the gallbladder. Calcified (porcelain) gallbladder is associated with gallbladder carcinoma and is generally an indication for cholecystectomy; the risk of gallbladder cancer may be higher when calcification is mucosal rather than intramural.

▶ **Treatment**

Acute cholecystitis will usually subside on a conservative regimen (withholding of oral feedings, intravenous alimentation, analgesics, and intravenous antibiotics—generally a second- or third-generation cephalosporin such as cefoperazone, 1–2 g intravenously every 12 hours, with the addition of metronidazole, 500 mg intravenously every 6 hours; in severe cases, a fluoroquinolone such as ciprofloxacin, 250 mg intravenously every 12 hours, plus metronidazole may be given). Morphine or meperidine may be administered for pain. Because of the high risk of recurrent attacks (up to 10% by 1 month and over 30% by 1 year), cholecystectomy—generally laparoscopically—should generally be performed within 24 hours of admission to the hospital for acute cholecystitis. If nonsurgical treatment has been elected, the patient (especially if diabetic or elderly) should be watched carefully for recurrent symptoms, evidence of gangrene of the gallbladder, or cholangitis. In high-risk patients, ultrasound-guided aspiration of the gallbladder, if feasible, percutaneous cholecystostomy, or endoscopic insertion of a stent or nasobiliary drain into the gallbladder may postpone or even avoid the need for surgery. Immediate cholecystectomy is mandatory when there is evidence of gangrene or perforation.

Surgical treatment of chronic cholecystitis is the same as for acute cholecystitis. If indicated, cholangiography can be performed during laparoscopic cholecystectomy. Choledocholithiasis can also be excluded by either preoperative or postoperative ERCP or MRCP.

▶ **Prognosis**

The overall mortality rate of cholecystectomy is < 0.2%, but hepatobiliary tract surgery is a more formidable procedure in the elderly, in whom mortality rates are higher; mortality rates are also higher in persons with diabetes mellitus. A technically successful surgical procedure in an appropriately selected patient is generally followed by complete resolution of symptoms.

▶ **When to Admit**

All patients with acute cholecystitis should be hospitalized.

Gutt CN et al. Acute cholecystitis: early versus delayed cholecystectomy, a multicenter randomized trial (ACDC study, NCT00447304). Ann Surg. 2013 Sep;258(3):385–93. [PMID: 24022431]
Hasan MK et al. Endoscopic management of acute cholecystitis. Gastrointest Endosc Clin N Am. 2013 Apr;23(2):453–9. [PMID: 23540969]

PRE- & POSTCHOLECYSTECTOMY SYNDROMES

1. Precholecystectomy

In a small group of patients (mostly women) with biliary pain, conventional radiographic studies of the upper gastrointestinal tract and gallbladder—including cholangiography—are unremarkable. Emptying of the gallbladder may be markedly reduced on gallbladder scintigraphy following injection of cholecystokinin; cholecystectomy may be curative in such cases. Histologic examination of the resected gallbladder may show chronic cholecystitis or microlithiasis. An additional diagnostic consideration is sphincter of Oddi dysfunction (see below).

2. Postcholecystectomy

Following cholecystectomy, some patients complain of continuing symptoms, ie, right upper quadrant pain, flatulence, and fatty food intolerance. The persistence of symptoms in this group of patients suggests the possibility of an incorrect diagnosis prior to cholecystectomy, eg, esophagitis, pancreatitis, radiculopathy, or functional bowel disease. Choledocholithiasis or bile duct stricture should be ruled out. Pain may also be associated with dilatation of the cystic duct remnant, neuroma formation in the ductal wall, foreign body granuloma, or traction on the bile duct by a long cystic duct.

The clinical presentation of right upper quadrant pain, chills, fever, or jaundice suggests biliary tract disease. Endoscopic ultrasonography or retrograde cholangiography may be necessary to demonstrate a stone or stricture. Biliary pain associated with elevated liver biochemical tests or a dilated bile duct in the absence of an obstructing lesion suggests sphincter of Oddi dysfunction. Biliary manometry may be useful for documenting elevated baseline sphincter of Oddi pressures typical of sphincter dysfunction when biliary pain is associated with elevated liver biochemical tests (twofold) or a dilated bile duct (> 12 mm) (type II sphincter of Oddi dysfunction) but is not necessary when both are present (type I sphincter of Oddi dysfunction) and is associated with a high risk of pancreatitis. In the absence of either elevated liver biochemical tests or a dilated bile duct (type III sphincter of Oddi dysfunction), a nonbiliary source of symptoms should be suspected. (Analogous criteria have been developed for pancreatic sphincter dysfunction.) Biliary scintigraphy after intravenous administration of morphine and MRCP following intravenous administration of secretin are under study as screening tests for sphincter dysfunction. Endoscopic sphincterotomy is most likely to relieve symptoms in patients with types I or II sphincter of Oddi dysfunction or an elevated sphincter of Oddi pressure, although many patients continue to have some pain. In some cases, treatment with a calcium channel blocker, long-acting nitrate, or phosphodiesterase inhibitor (eg, vardenafil) or possibly injection of the sphincter with botulinum toxin may be beneficial. In refractory cases, surgical sphincteroplasty or removal of the cystic duct remnant may be considered.

When to Refer

Patients with sphincter of Oddi dysfunction should be referred for diagnostic procedures.

Leung WD et al. Endoscopic approach to the patient with motility disorders of the bile duct and sphincter of Oddi. Gastrointest Endosc Clin N Am. 2013 Apr;23(2):405–34. [PMID: 23540967]
Nakeeb A. Sphincter of Oddi dysfunction: how is it diagnosed? How is it classified? How do we treat it medically, endoscopically, and surgically? J Gastrointest Surg. 2013 Sep;17(9):1557–8. [PMID: 23860677]

CHOLEDOCHOLITHIASIS & CHOLANGITIS

ESSENTIALS OF DIAGNOSIS

▶ Often a history of biliary pain, which may be accompanied by jaundice.

▶ Occasional patients present with painless jaundice.

▶ Nausea and vomiting.

▶ Cholangitis should be suspected with fever followed by hypothermia and gram-negative shock, jaundice, and leukocytosis.

▶ Stones in bile duct most reliably detected by ERCP or endoscopic ultrasonography.

General Considerations

About 15% of patients with gallstones have choledocholithiasis (bile duct stones). The percentage rises with age, and the frequency in elderly people with gallstones may be as high as 50%. Bile duct stones usually originate in the gallbladder but may also form spontaneously in the bile duct after cholecystectomy. The risk is increased twofold in persons with a juxtapapillary duodenal diverticulum. Symptoms result if there is obstruction.

Clinical Findings

A. Symptoms and Signs

A history of biliary pain or jaundice may be obtained. Biliary pain results from rapid increases in bile duct pressure due to obstructed bile flow. The features that suggest the presence of a bile duct stone are: (1) frequently recurring attacks of right upper abdominal pain that is severe and persists for hours; (2) chills and fever associated with severe pain; and (3) a history of jaundice associated with episodes of abdominal pain (Table 16–7). The combination of pain, fever (and chills), and jaundice represents **Charcot triad** and denotes the classic picture of acute cholangitis. The addition of altered mental status and hypotension (**Reynolds pentad**) signifies acute suppurative cholangitis and is an endoscopic emergency. According to the Tokyo guidelines (2006), the diagnosis of acute cholangitis is established by the presence of (1) the Charcot triad; or (2) two elements of the Charcot triad plus laboratory evidence of an inflammatory response (eg, elevated white blood cell count, C-reactive protein), elevated liver biochemical test levels, and imaging evidence of biliary dilatation or a cause of obstruction.

Hepatomegaly may be present in calculous biliary obstruction, and tenderness is usually present in the right upper quadrant and epigastrium. Bile duct obstruction lasting > 30 days results in liver damage leading to cirrhosis. Hepatic failure with portal hypertension occurs in untreated cases.

B. Laboratory Findings

Acute obstruction of the bile duct typically produces a transient albeit striking increase in serum aminotransferase levels (often > 1000 units/L [20 mckat/L]). Bilirubinuria and elevation of the serum bilirubin are present if the bile duct remains obstructed; levels commonly fluctuate. Serum alkaline phosphatase levels rise more slowly. Not uncommonly, serum amylase elevations are present because of secondary pancreatitis. When extrahepatic obstruction persists for more than a few weeks, differentiation of obstruction from chronic cholestatic liver disease becomes more difficult. Leukocytosis is present in patients with acute cholangitis. Prolongation of the prothrombin time can result from the obstructed flow of bile to the intestine. In contrast to hepatocellular dysfunction, hypoprothrombinemia due to obstructive jaundice will respond to 10 mg of intravenous vitamin K or water-soluble oral vitamin K (phytonadione, 5 mg) within 24–36 hours.

C. Imaging

Ultrasonography and CT may demonstrate dilated bile ducts, and radionuclide imaging may show impaired bile flow. Endoscopic ultrasonography, helical CT, and magnetic resonance cholangiography are accurate in demonstrating bile duct stones and may be used in patients thought to be at intermediate risk for choledocholithiasis (age > 55 years, cholecystitis, bile duct diameter > 6 mm on ultrasonography, serum bilirubin 1.8–4 mg/dL [30.78–68.4 mcmol/L], elevated serum liver enzymes, pancreatitis). ERCP (occasionally with intraductal ultrasonography) or percutaneous transhepatic cholangiography provides the most direct and accurate means of determining the cause, location, and extent of obstruction. If the likelihood that obstruction is caused by a stone is high (bile duct diameter > 6 mm, bile duct stone seen on ultrasonography, serum bilirubin > 4 mg/dL [68.4 mcmol/L]) or acute cholangitis is present, ERCP is the procedure of choice because it permits sphincterotomy with stone extraction or stent placement. Meticulous technique is required to avoid causing acute cholangitis.

► Differential Diagnosis

The most common cause of obstructive jaundice is a bile duct stone. Next in frequency are neoplasms of the pancreas, ampulla of Vater, or bile duct or an obstructed stent placed previously for decompression of an obstructing tumor. Extrinsic compression of the bile duct may result from metastatic carcinoma (usually from the gastrointestinal tract or breast) involving porta hepatis lymph nodes or, rarely, from a large duodenal diverticulum. Gallbladder cancer extending into the bile duct often presents as obstructive jaundice. Chronic cholestatic liver diseases (primarily biliary cirrhosis, sclerosing cholangitis, drug-induced) must be considered. Hepatocellular jaundice can usually be differentiated by the history, clinical findings, and liver biochemical tests, but liver biopsy is necessary on occasion. Recurrent pyogenic cholangitis should be considered in persons from Asia (and occasionally elsewhere) with intrahepatic biliary stones (particularly in the left ductal system) and recurrent cholangitis.

► Treatment

In general, bile duct stones should be removed, even in an asymptomatic patient. A bile duct stone in a patient with cholelithiasis or cholecystitis is usually treated by endoscopic sphincterotomy and stone extraction followed by laparoscopic cholecystectomy within 72 hours in patients with cholecystitis and within 2 weeks in those without cholecystitis. An alternative approach, which may be associated with a shorter duration of hospitalization, is laparoscopic cholecystectomy and bile duct exploration. For the elderly (> 70 years) or poor-risk patient with cholelithiasis and choledocholithiasis, cholecystectomy may be deferred after endoscopic sphincterotomy because the risk of subsequent cholecystitis is low. ERCP with sphincterotomy should be performed before cholecystectomy in patients with gallstones and cholangitis, jaundice (serum total bilirubin > 4 mg/dL [68.4 mcmol/L]), a dilated bile duct (> 6 mm), or stones in the bile duct seen on ultrasonography or CT. (Stones may ultimately recur in up to 12% of patients, particularly in the elderly, when the bile duct diameter is ≥ 15 mm or when brown pigment stones are found at the time of the initial sphincterotomy.) Endoscopic balloon dilation of the sphincter of Oddi may be associated with a higher rate of pancreatitis than endoscopic sphincterotomy unless adequate dilation for > 1 min is carried out. This procedure is generally reserved for patients with coagulopathy because the risk of bleeding is lower with balloon dilation than with sphincterotomy. Endoscopic ultrasound-guided biliary drainage and PTC with drainage are second-line approaches if ERCP fails or is not possible. In patients with biliary pancreatitis that resolves rapidly, the stone usually passes into the intestine, and ERCP prior to cholecystectomy is not necessary if an intraoperative cholangiogram is planned.

Choledocholithiasis discovered at laparoscopic cholecystectomy may be managed via laparoscopic or, if necessary, open bile duct exploration or by postoperative endoscopic sphincterotomy. Operative findings of choledocholithiasis are palpable stones in the bile duct, dilatation or thickening of the wall of the bile duct, or stones in the gallbladder small enough to pass through the cystic duct. Laparoscopic intraoperative cholangiography (or intraoperative ultrasonography) should be done at the time of cholecystectomy in patients with liver enzyme elevations but a bile duct diameter of <5 mm; if a ductal stone is found, the duct should be explored. In the post-cholecystectomy patient with choledocholithiasis, endoscopic sphincterotomy with stone extraction is preferable to transabdominal surgery. Lithotripsy (endoscopic or external), direct choledoscopy (cholangioscopy), or biliary stenting may be a therapeutic consideration for large stones. For the patient with a T tube and bile duct stone, the stone may be extracted via the T tube.

Postoperative antibiotics are not administered routinely after biliary tract surgery. Cultures of the bile are always taken at operation. If biliary tract infection was present preoperatively or is apparent at operation, ampicillin (500 mg every 6 hours intravenously) with gentamicin (1.5 mg/kg intravenously every 8 hours) and metronidazole (500 mg intravenously every 6 hours) or ciprofloxacin (250 mg intravenously every 12 hours) or a third-generation cephalosporin (eg, cefoperazone, 1–2 g intravenous every 12 hours) is administered postoperatively until the results of sensitivity tests on culture specimens are available. A T-tube cholangiogram should be done before the tube is removed, usually about 3 weeks after surgery. A small amount of bile frequently leaks from the tube site for a few days.

Urgent ERCP with sphincterotomy and stone extraction is generally indicated for choledocholithiasis complicated by acute cholangitis and is preferred to surgery. Before ERCP, liver function should be evaluated thoroughly. The prothrombin time should be restored to normal by intravenous administration of vitamin K (see above). For mild-to-moderately severe community-acquired acute cholangitis, ciprofloxacin, 500 mg intravenously every 12 hours, penetrates well into bile and is effective treatment, with the possible addition of metronidazole, 500 mg every 6–8 hours. Alternative regimens include intravenous cefoxitin, 1–2 g every 6 hours, ampicillin, 2 g every 6 hours, plus gentamicin, 1.7 mg/kg every 8 hours, or ceftriaxone 1–2 g daily, among others. Regimens for severe or hospital-acquired acute cholangitis include intravenous piperacillin and tazobactam, 3.375 g every 6 hours; ticarcillin and clavulanate, 3.1 g every 6 hours; ceftriaxone, 1–2 g daily, plus metronidazole, 500 mg every 6–8 hours; or, in patients at high risk for harboring antibiotic-resistant pathogens, meropenem, 1 g every 8 hours. Aminoglycosides should not be given for more than a few days because the risk of aminoglycoside nephrotoxicity is increased in patients with cholestasis. Regimens that include drugs active against anaerobes are required when a biliary-enteric communication is present. Emergent decompression of the bile duct, generally by ERCP, is required for patients who are septic or fail to improve on antibiotics within 12–24 hours. Medical therapy alone is most likely to fail in patients with tachycardia, serum albumin < 3 g/dL (30 g/L), marked hyperbilirubinemia, high serum ALT level, high white blood cell count, and prothrombin time > 14 seconds on admission. If sphincterotomy cannot be performed, the bile duct can be decompressed by a biliary stent or nasobiliary catheter. Once decompression is achieved, antibiotics are generally continued for at least another 3 days. Elective cholecystectomy can be undertaken after resolution of cholangitis, unless the patient remains unfit for surgery. Mortality from acute cholangitis has been reported to correlate with a high total bilirubin level, prolonged partial thromboplastin time, and presence of a liver abscess.

When to Refer

All symptomatic patients with choledocholithiasis should be referred.

When to Admit

All patients with acute cholangitis should be hospitalized.

Epelboym I et al. MRCP is not a cost-effective strategy in the management of silent common bile duct stones. J Gastrointest Surg. 2013 May;17(5):863–71. [PMID: 23515912]

Navaneethan U et al. Delay in performing ERCP and adverse events increase the 30-day readmission risk in patients with acute cholangitis. Gastrointest Endosc. 2013 Jul;78(1):81–90. [PMID: 23528654]

Sheffield KM et al. Association between cholecystectomy with vs without intraoperative cholangiography and risk of common duct injury. JAMA. 2013 Aug 28;310(8):812–20. [PMID: 23982367]

Teoh AY et al. Randomized trial of endoscopic sphincterotomy with balloon dilation versus endoscopic sphincterotomy alone for removal of bile duct stones. Gastroenterology. 2013 Feb;144(2):341–5. [PMID: 23085096]

BILIARY STRICTURE

Benign biliary strictures are the result of surgical (including liver transplantation) anastomosis or injury in about 95% of cases. The remainder of cases are caused by blunt external injury to the abdomen, pancreatitis, erosion of the duct by a gallstone, or prior endoscopic sphincterotomy.

Signs of injury to the duct may or may not be recognized in the immediate postoperative period. If complete occlusion has occurred, jaundice will develop rapidly; more often, however, a tear has been made accidentally in the duct, and the earliest manifestation of injury may be excessive or prolonged loss of bile from the surgical drains. Bile leakage resulting in a bile collection (biloma) may predispose to localized infection, which in turn accentuates scar formation and the ultimate development of a fibrous stricture.

Cholangitis is the most common complication of stricture. Typically, the patient experiences episodes of pain,

fever, chills, and jaundice within a few weeks to months after cholecystectomy. Physical findings may include jaundice during an acute attack of cholangitis and right upper quadrant abdominal tenderness. Serum alkaline phosphatase is usually elevated. Hyperbilirubinemia is variable, fluctuating during exacerbations and usually remaining in the range of 5–10 mg/dL (85.5–171 mcmol/L). Blood cultures may be positive during an acute episode of cholangitis. Secondary biliary cirrhosis will inevitably develop if a stricture is not treated.

MRCP can be valuable in demonstrating the stricture, whereas ERCP permits biopsy and cytologic specimens to exclude malignancy (in conjunction with endoscopic ultrasound-guided fine-needle aspiration, an even more sensitive test for distal bile duct malignancy), sphincterotomy to allow closure of a bile leak, and dilation (often repeated) and stent placement, thereby avoiding surgical repair in some cases; when ERCP is unsuccessful, dilation of a stricture may be accomplished by PTC. Placement of multiple plastic stents appears to be more effective than placement of a single stent. Metal stents, which often cannot be removed endoscopically, are generally avoided in benign strictures unless life expectancy is < 2 years. The use of covered metal stents, which are more easily removed endoscopically than uncovered metal stents, as well as bioabsorbable stents, is an alternative to use of plastic stents. Strictures related to chronic pancreatitis are more difficult than postsurgical strictures to treat endoscopically, and preliminary reports suggest that they may be best managed with a temporary covered metal stent. Following liver transplantation, endoscopic management is more successful for anastomotic than for nonanastomotic strictures, although results for nonanastomotic strictures may be improved with repeated dilation or the use of multiple plastic stents. Biliary strictures after live liver donor liver transplantation, particularly in patients with a late-onset (after 24 weeks) stricture or with intrahepatic biliary dilatation, are also challenging and require aggressive endoscopic therapy; in addition, the risk of post-ERCP pancreatitis appears to be increased. When malignancy cannot be excluded with certainty, additional endoscopic diagnostic approaches may be considered—if available—including endoscopic ultrasonography, intraductal ultrasonography, direct choledoscopy (cholangioscopy), and confocal laser endomicroscopy. Differentiation from cholangiocarcinoma may ultimately require surgical exploration. Operative treatment of a stricture frequently necessitates performance of an end-to-end ductal repair, choledochojejunostomy, or hepaticojejunostomy to reestablish bile flow into the intestine.

When to Refer

All patients with biliary stricture should be referred.

When to Admit

Patients with acute cholangitis should be hospitalized.

Kaffes AJ et al. Fully covered self-expandable metal stents for treatment of benign biliary strictures. Gastrointest Endosc. 2013 Jul;78(1):13–21. [PMID: 23548962]

Kao D et al. Managing the post-liver transplantation anastomotic biliary stricture: multiple plastic versus metal stents: a systematic review. Gastrointest Endosc. 2013 May;77(5): 679–91. [PMID: 23473000]

Nishikawa T et al. Comparison of the diagnostic accuracy of peroral video-cholangioscopic visual findings and cholangioscopy-guided forceps biopsy findings for indeterminate biliary lesions: a prospective study. Gastrointest Endosc. 2013 Feb;77(2):219–26. [PMID: 23231758]

PRIMARY SCLEROSING CHOLANGITIS

ESSENTIALS OF DIAGNOSIS

► Most common in men aged 20–50 years.

► Often associated with ulcerative colitis.

► Progressive jaundice, itching, and other features of cholestasis.

► Diagnosis based on characteristic cholangiographic findings.

► At least 10% risk of cholangiocarcinoma.

▶ General Considerations

Primary sclerosing cholangitis is an uncommon disease thought to result from an increased immune response to intestinal endotoxins and characterized by diffuse inflammation of the biliary tract leading to fibrosis and strictures of the biliary system. The disease is most common in men aged 20–50 years, with an incidence of nearly 3.3 per 100,000 in Asian Americans, 2.8 per 100,000 in Hispanic Americans, and 2.1 per 100,000 in African Americans, and an intermediate incidence in whites (possibly increasing), and a prevalence of 21 per 100,000 men and 6 per 100,000 women in the United States. Primary sclerosing cholangitis is closely associated with inflammatory bowel disease (more commonly ulcerative colitis than Crohn colitis), which is present in approximately two-thirds of patients with primary sclerosing cholangitis; however, clinically significant sclerosing cholangitis develops in only 1–4% of patients with ulcerative colitis. As in ulcerative colitis, smoking is associated with a decreased risk of primary sclerosing cholangitis. Primary sclerosing cholangitis is associated with the histocompatible antigens HLA-B8 and -DR3 or -DR4, and first-degree relatives of patients with primary sclerosing cholangitis have a fourfold increased risk of primary sclerosing cholangitis and a threefold increased risk of ulcerative colitis. The diagnosis of primary sclerosing cholangitis may be difficult to make after biliary surgery.

▶ Clinical Findings

A. Symptoms and Signs

Primary sclerosing cholangitis presents as progressive obstructive jaundice, frequently associated with fatigue, pruritus, anorexia, and indigestion. Patients may be diagnosed in the presymptomatic phase because of an elevated alkaline phosphatase level. Complications of chronic cholestasis, such as osteoporosis and malabsorption of fat-soluble vitamins, may occur late in the course. Risk factors for osteoporosis include older age, lower body mass index, and longer duration of inflammatory bowel disease. Esophageal varices on initial endoscopy are most likely in patients with a higher Mayo risk score based on age, bilirubin, albumin, and AST and a higher AST/ALT ratio, and new varices are likely to develop in those with a lower platelet count and higher bilirubin at 2 years. In patients with primary sclerosing cholangitis, ulcerative colitis is frequently characterized by rectal sparing and backwash ileitis.

B. Diagnostic Findings

The diagnosis of primary sclerosing cholangitis is increasingly made by MRCP, the sensitivity of which approaches that of ERCP. Characteristic cholangiographic findings are segmental fibrosis of bile ducts with saccular dilatations between strictures. Biliary obstruction by a stone or tumor should be excluded. Liver biopsy is not necessary for diagnosis when cholangiographic findings are characteristic. The disease may be confined to small intrahepatic bile ducts in about 15% of cases, in which case MRCP and ERCP are normal and the diagnosis is suggested by liver biopsy findings. These patients have a longer survival than patients with involvement of the large ducts and do not appear to be at increased risk for cholangiocarcinoma unless large-duct sclerosing cholangitis develops (which occurs in about 20% over 7–10 years). Liver biopsy may show characteristic periductal fibrosis ("onion-skinning") and allows staging, which is based on the degree of fibrosis. Perinuclear ANCA (directed against myeloid-specific tubulin-beta isotype 5) as well as antinuclear, anticardiolipin, antithyroperoxidase, and anti-Saccharomyces cerevisiae antibodies and rheumatoid factor are frequently detected in serum. Occasional patients have clinical and histologic features of both sclerosing cholangitis and autoimmune hepatitis. An association with autoimmune pancreatitis is also seen, and this entity (IgG_4-associated cholangitis) is often responsive to corticosteroids, although it may be difficult to distinguish from primary sclerosing cholangitis and even cholangiocarcinoma. Primary sclerosing cholangitis must be distinguished from idiopathic adulthood ductopenia (a rare disorder that affects young to middle-aged adults who manifest cholestasis resulting from loss of interlobular and septal bile ducts yet who have a normal cholangiogram and that is caused in some cases by a mutation in the canalicular phospholipid transporter gene ABCB4) and from other cholangiopathies (including primary biliary cirrhosis; cystic fibrosis; eosinophilic cholangitis; AIDS cholangiopathy; allograft rejection; graft-versus-host disease; ischemic cholangiopathy [often with biliary "casts," a rapid progression to cirrhosis, and a poor outcome] caused by hepatic artery thrombosis, shock, respiratory failure, or drugs; intra-arterial chemotherapy; and sarcoidosis).

Complications

Cholangiocarcinoma may complicate the course of primary sclerosing cholangitis in up to 20% of cases (1.2% per year) and may be difficult to diagnose by cytologic examination or biopsy because of false-negative results. A serum CA 19-9 level >100 units/mL is suggestive but not diagnostic of cholangiocarcinoma. Annual right-upper-quadrant ultrasonography or MRI with MRCP and serum CA 19-9 testing (a level of 20 is the threshold for further investigation) are recommended for surveillance, with ERCP and biliary cytology if the results are suggestive of malignancy. PET and choledochoscopy may play roles in the early detection of cholangiocarcinoma. Patients with ulcerative colitis and primary sclerosing cholangitis are at high risk (tenfold higher than ulcerative colitis patients without primary sclerosing cholangitis) for colorectal neoplasia. The risks of gallstones, cholecystitis, gallbladder polyps, and gallbladder carcinoma appear to be increased in patients with primary sclerosing cholangitis.

Treatment

Episodes of acute bacterial cholangitis may be treated with ciprofloxacin (750 mg twice daily orally or intravenously). Ursodeoxycholic acid in standard doses (10–15 mg/kg/d orally) may improve liver biochemical test results but does not appear to alter the natural history. High-dose ursodeoxycholic acid (25–30 mg/kg/d) also has been shown not to reduce cholangiographic progression and liver fibrosis, nor to improve survival or prevent cholangiocarcinoma, and has been shown to increase the risk of death and need for liver transplantation in patients with a normal serum bilirubin level and an early histologic stage. Other drugs such as antibiotics (vancomycin, metronidazole, minocycline, azithromycin), obeticholic acid (a farsenoid-X receptor agonist), 24-norursodeoxycholic acid, budesonide, antitumor necrosis factor antibodies, cyclosporine, tacrolimus, and antifibrotic agents are under study. Careful endoscopic evaluation of the biliary tree may permit balloon dilation of localized strictures, and repeated dilation of a dominant stricture may improve survival, although such patients have reduced survival compared with patients who do not have a dominant stricture. Short-term (2–3 weeks) placement of a stent in a major stricture also may relieve symptoms and improve biochemical abnormalities, with sustained improvement after the stent is removed; however, long-term stenting may increase the rate of complications such as cholangitis and is not recommended. In patients without cirrhosis, surgical resection of a dominant bile duct stricture may lead to longer survival than endoscopic therapy by decreasing the subsequent risk of cholangiocarcinoma. When feasible, extensive surgical resection of cholangiocarcinoma complicating primary sclerosing cholangitis may result in 5-year survival rates of > 50%. In patients with ulcerative colitis, primary sclerosing cholangitis is an independent risk factor for the development of colorectal dysplasia and cancer (especially in the right colon), and strict adherence to a colonoscopic surveillance program (yearly for those with ulcerative colitis and every 5 years for those without ulcerative colitis) is recommended. Whether treatment with ursodeoxycholic acid reduces the risk of colorectal dysplasia and carcinoma in patients with ulcerative colitis and primary sclerosing cholangitis is still uncertain. For patients with cirrhosis and clinical decompensation, liver transplantation is the procedure of choice; primary sclerosing cholangitis recurs in the graft in 30% of cases, with a possible reduction in the risk of recurrence when colectomy has been performed for ulcerative colitis before transplantation.

Prognosis

Survival of patients with primary sclerosing cholangitis averages 9–17 years, and up to 21 years in population-based studies. Adverse prognostic markers are older age, hepatosplenomegaly, higher serum bilirubin and AST levels, lower albumin levels, a history of variceal bleeding, a dominant bile duct stricture, and extrahepatic duct changes. Variceal bleeding is also a risk factor for cholangiocarcinoma. Patients in whom serum alkaline phosphatase levels decline by 40% or more (spontaneously or with ursodeoxycholic acid therapy) have longer transplant-free survival times than those in whom the alkaline phosphatase does not decline. Moreover, improvement in the serum alkaline phosphatase to < 1.5 times the upper limit of normal is associated with a reduced risk of cholangiocarcinoma. Reduced quality of life is associated with older age, large-duct disease, and systemic symptoms. Interestingly, patients with milder ulcerative colitis tend to have more severe primary cholangitis and a higher rate of liver transplantation. Actuarial survival rates with liver transplantation are as high as 85% at 3 years, but rates are much lower once cholangiocarcinoma has developed. Following transplantation, patients have an increased risk of nonanastomotic biliary strictures and—in those with ulcerative colitis—colon cancer. The retransplantation rate is higher than that for primary biliary cirrhosis. Those patients who are unable to undergo liver transplantation will ultimately require high-quality palliative care (see Chapter 5).

Eaton JE et al. Pathogenesis of primary sclerosing cholangitis and advances in diagnosis and management. Gastroenterology. 2013 Sep;145(3):521–36. [PMID: 23827861]

Hirschfield GM et al. Primary sclerosing cholangitis. Lancet. 2013 Nov 9;382(9904):1587–99. [PMID: 23810223]

Karlsen TH et al. Update on primary sclerosing cholangitis. J Hepatol. 2013 Sep;59(3):571–82. [PMID: 23603668]

Singh S et al. Primary sclerosing cholangitis: diagnosis, prognosis, and management. Clin Gastroenterol Hepatol. 2013 Aug;11(8):898–907. [PMID: 23454027]

Tabibian JH et al. Randomised clinical trial: vancomycin or metronidazole in patients with primary sclerosing cholangitis—a pilot study. Aliment Pharmacol Ther. 2013 Mar;37(6):604–12. [PMID: 23384404]

DISEASES OF THE PANCREAS

See Chapter 39 for Carcinoma of the Pancreas and Periampullary Area.

ACUTE PANCREATITIS

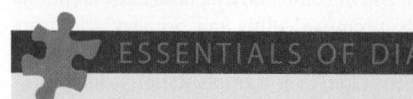

▶ Abrupt onset of deep epigastric pain, often with radiation to the back.

▶ History of previous episodes, often related to alcohol intake.

▶ Nausea, vomiting, sweating, weakness.

▶ Abdominal tenderness and distention and fever.

▶ Leukocytosis, elevated serum amylase, elevated serum lipase.

▶ General Considerations

Most cases of acute pancreatitis are related to biliary tract disease (a passed gallstone, usually < 5 mm in diameter) or heavy alcohol intake. The exact pathogenesis is not known but may include edema or obstruction of the ampulla of Vater, reflux of bile into pancreatic ducts, and direct injury of pancreatic acinar cells by prematurely activated pancreatic enzymes. Among the numerous other causes or associations are hypercalcemia, hyperlipidemias (chylomicronemia, hypertriglyceridemia, or both), abdominal trauma (including surgery), drugs (including azathioprine, mercaptopurine, asparaginase, pentamidine, didanosine, valproic acid, tetracyclines, dapsone, isoniazid, metronidazole, estrogen and tamoxifen [by raising serum triglycerides], sulfonamides, mesalamine, sulindac, leflunomide, thiazides, simvastatin, fenofibrate, enalapril, methyldopa, procainamide, sitagliptin, exenatide, possibly corticosteroids, and others), vasculitis, infections (eg, mumps, cytomegalovirus, *M avium intracellulare* complex), peritoneal dialysis, cardiopulmonary bypass, and ERCP. Genetic mutations also predispose to chronic pancreatitis, particularly in persons < 30 years of age if no other cause is evident and a family history of pancreatic disease is present (see later). In patients with pancreas divisum, a congenital anomaly in which the dorsal and ventral pancreatic ducts fail to fuse, acute pancreatitis may result from stenosis of the minor papilla with obstruction to flow from the accessory pancreatic duct, although concomitant genetic mutations, particularly in the cystic fibrosis transmembrane conductance regulator (*CFTR*) gene, have also been reported to account for acute pancreatitis in some patients with pancreas divisum. Acute pancreatitis may also result from anomalous union of the pancreaticobiliary duct. Rarely, acute pancreatitis may be the presenting manifestation of a pancreatic or ampullary neoplasm. Celiac disease appears to be associated with an increased risk of acute and chronic pancreatitis. Apparently "idiopathic" acute pancreatitis is often caused by occult biliary microlithiasis and may be caused by sphincter of Oddi dysfunction involving the pancreatic duct. Between 15% and 25% of cases are truly idiopathic. Smoking and abdominal adiposity increase the risk of pancreatitis, and older age and obesity increase the risk of a severe course; vegetable consumption may reduce the risk of non-gallstone pancreatitis. The incidence of pancreatitis has increased since 1990.

▶ Clinical Findings

A. Symptoms and Signs

Epigastric abdominal pain, generally abrupt in onset, is steady, boring, and severe and often made worse by walking and lying supine and better by sitting and leaning forward. The pain usually radiates into the back but may radiate to the right or left. Nausea and vomiting are usually present. Weakness, sweating, and anxiety are noted in severe attacks. There may be a history of alcohol intake or a heavy meal immediately preceding the attack or a history of milder similar episodes or biliary pain in the past.

The abdomen is tender mainly in the upper part, most often without guarding, rigidity, or rebound. The abdomen may be distended, and bowel sounds may be absent with associated ileus. Fever of 38.4–39°C, tachycardia, hypotension (even shock), pallor, and cool clammy skin are present in severe cases. Mild jaundice may be seen. Occasionally, an upper abdominal mass due to the inflamed pancreas or a pseudocyst may be palpated. Acute kidney injury (usually prerenal) may occur early in the course of acute pancreatitis.

B. Laboratory Findings

Serum amylase and lipase are elevated—usually more than three times the upper limit of normal—within 24 hours in 90% of cases; their return to normal is variable depending on the severity of disease. Lipase remains elevated longer than amylase and is slightly more accurate for the diagnosis of acute pancreatitis. Leukocytosis (10,000–30,000/mcL), proteinuria, granular casts, glycosuria (10–20% of cases), hyperglycemia, and elevated serum bilirubin may be present. Blood urea nitrogen and serum alkaline phosphatase may be elevated and coagulation tests abnormal. An elevated serum creatinine level (>1.8 mg/dL [149.94 mcmol/L]) at 48 hours is associated with the development of pancreatic necrosis. In patients with clear evidence of acute pancreatitis, a serum ALT level of more than 150 units/L (3 mkat/L) suggests biliary pancreatitis. A decrease in serum calcium may reflect saponification and correlates with severity of the disease. Levels lower than 7 mg/dL (1.75 mmol/L) (when serum albumin is normal) are associated with tetany and an unfavorable prognosis. Patients with acute pancreatitis caused by hypertriglyceridemia generally have fasting triglyceride levels above 1000 mg/dL (10 mmol/L); in some cases, the serum amylase is not elevated substantially because of an inhibitor in the serum of patients with marked hypertriglyceridemia that interferes with measurement of serum amylase. An early rise in the hematocrit value above 44% suggests hemoconcentration and predicts pancreatic necrosis. An elevated C-reactive protein concentration (> 150 mg/L [1500 mg/L]) at 48 hours suggests severe disease.

Other diagnostic tests that offer the possibility of simplicity, rapidity, ease of use, and low cost—including urinary trypsinogen-2, trypsinogen activation peptide, and carboxypeptidase B—are not widely available. In patients in whom ascites or a left pleural effusion develops, fluid amylase content is high. Electrocardiography may show ST–T wave changes.

C. Assessment of Severity

In addition to the individual laboratory parameters noted above, the severity of acute alcoholic pancreatitis can be assessed using several scoring systems, including the **Ranson criteria (Table 16–8)**. The **Sequential Organ Failure Assessment (SOFA)** score or **modified Marshall scoring system** can be used to assess injury to other organs, and the **Acute Physiology and Chronic Health Evaluation (APACHE II)** score is another tool for assessing severity. A simple 5-point clinical scoring system (the **Bedside Index for Severity in Acute Pancreatitis, or BISAP**) based on blood urea nitrogen > 25 mg/dL (9 mmol/L), impaired mental status, systemic inflammatory response syndrome, age > 60 years, and pleural effusion during the first 24 hours (before the onset of organ failure) identifies patients at increased risk for mortality. More simply, the presence of a systemic inflammatory response alone and an elevated blood urea nitrogen level on admission as well as a rise in blood urea nitrogen within the first 24 hours of hospitalization are independently associated with increased mortality; the greater the rise in blood urea nitrogen after admission, the greater the mortality rate. An early rise in serum levels of neutrophil gelatinase-associated lipocalin has also been proposed as a marker of severe acute pancreatitis.

Table 16–8. Ranson criteria for assessing the severity of acute pancreatitis.

Three or more of the following predict a severe course complicated by pancreatic necrosis with a sensitivity of 60–80%
Age over 55 years
White blood cell count > 16 × 10³/mcL (> 16 × 10⁹/L)
Blood glucose > 200 mg/dL (> 11 mmol/L)
Serum lactic dehydrogenase > 350 units/L (> 7 mkat/L)
Aspartate aminotransferase > 250 units/L (> 5 mkat/L)
Development of the following in the first 48 hours indicates a worsening prognosis
Hematocrit drop of more than 10 percentage points
Blood urea nitrogen rise > 5 mg/dL (> 1.8 mmol/L)
Arterial Po₂ of < 60 mm Hg (< 7.8 kPa)
Serum calcium of < 8 mg/dL (> 0.2 mmol/L)
Base deficit over 4 mEq/L
Estimated fluid sequestration of > 6 L
Mortality rates correlate with the number of criteria present[1]

Number of Criteria	Mortality Rate
0–2	1%
3–4	16%
5–6	40%
7–8	100%

[1]An APACHE II score ≥ 8 also correlates with mortality.

The absence of rebound abdominal tenderness or guarding, a normal hematocrit value, and a normal serum creatinine level (the "**harmless acute pancreatitis score**," or **HAPS**) predicts a nonsevere course with 98% accuracy. The **revised Atlanta classification** of the severity of acute pancreatitis uses the following three categories: (1) mild disease is the absence of organ failure and local ([peri] pancreatic necrosis or fluid collections) or systemic complications; (2) moderate disease is the presence of transient (< 48 hrs) organ failure or local or systemic complications, or both; and (3) severe disease is the presence of persistent (≥ 48 hrs) organ failure. A similar "determinant-based" classification includes a category of critical acute pancreatitis characterized by both persistent organ failure and infected peripancreatic necrosis.

D. Imaging

Plain radiographs of the abdomen may show gallstones (if calcified), a "sentinel loop" (a segment of air-filled small intestine most commonly in the left upper quadrant), the "colon cutoff sign"—a gas-filled segment of transverse colon abruptly ending at the area of pancreatic inflammation—or focal linear atelectasis of the lower lobe of the lungs with or without pleural effusion. Ultrasonography is often not helpful in diagnosing acute pancreatitis because of intervening bowel gas but may identify gallstones in the gallbladder. Unenhanced CT is useful for demonstrating an enlarged pancreas when the diagnosis of pancreatitis is uncertain, differentiating pancreatitis from other possible intra-abdominal catastrophes, and providing an initial assessment of prognosis but is often unnecessary early in the course (Table 16–9). Rapid-bolus intravenous contrast-enhanced CT following aggressive volume resuscitation is of particular value after the first 3 days of severe acute pancreatitis for identifying areas of necrotizing pancreatitis and assessing the degree of necrosis, although the use of intravenous contrast may increase the risk of complications of pancreatitis and of acute kidney injury and should be avoided when the serum creatinine level is > 1.5 mg/dL (124.95 mcmol/L). MRI appears to be a suitable alternative to CT. Perfusion CT on day 3 demonstrating areas of ischemia in the pancreas has been reported to predict the development of pancreatic necrosis. The presence of a fluid collection in the pancreas correlates with an increased mortality rate. CT-guided needle aspiration of areas of necrotizing pancreatitis after the third day may disclose infection, usually by enteric organisms, which typically requires debridement. The presence of gas bubbles on CT implies infection by gas-forming organisms. Endoscopic ultrasonography is useful in identifying occult biliary disease (eg, small stones, sludge, microlithiasis), which is present in a majority of patients with apparently idiopathic acute pancreatitis, and is indicated in persons over age 40 to exclude malignancy. ERCP is generally not indicated after a first attack of acute pancreatitis unless there is associated cholangitis or jaundice or a bile duct stone is known to be present, but endoscopic ultrasonography or MRCP should be considered, especially after repeated attacks of idiopathic acute pancreatitis. In selected cases, aspiration of bile for crystal analysis may confirm the suspicion of

Table 16–9. Severity index for acute pancreatitis.

CT Grade	Points	Pancreatic Necrosis	Additional Points	Severity Index[1]	Mortality Rate[2]
A Normal pancreas	0	0%	0	0	0%
B Pancreatic enlargement	1	0%	0	1	0%
C Pancreatic inflammation and/or peripancreatic fat	2	< 30%	2	4	< 3%
D Single acute peripancreatic fluid collection	3	30–50%	4	7	6%
E Two or more acute peripancreatic fluid collections or retroperitoneal air	4	> 50%	6	10	> 17%

[1]Severity index = CT Grade Points + Additional Points.
[2]Based on the severity index.
Adapted with permission from Balthazar EJ. Acute pancreatitis: assessment of severity with clinical and CT evaluation. Radiology. 2002 Jun; 223(3):603–13.

microlithiasis, and manometry of the pancreatic duct sphincter may detect sphincter of Oddi dysfunction as a cause of recurrent pancreatitis.

Differential Diagnosis

Acute pancreatitis must be differentiated from an acutely perforated duodenal ulcer, acute cholecystitis, acute intestinal obstruction, leaking aortic aneurysm, renal colic, and acute mesenteric ischemia. Serum amylase may also be elevated in high intestinal obstruction, in gastroenteritis, in mumps not involving the pancreas (salivary amylase), in ectopic pregnancy, after administration of opioids, and after abdominal surgery. Serum lipase may also be elevated in many of these conditions.

Complications

Intravascular volume depletion secondary to leakage of fluids in the pancreatic bed and ileus with fluid-filled loops of bowel may result in prerenal azotemia and even acute tubular necrosis without overt shock. This sequence usually occurs within 24 hours of the onset of acute pancreatitis and lasts 8–9 days. Some patients require renal replacement therapy.

According to the revised Atlanta classification, fluid collections and necrosis may be acute (within the first 4 weeks) or chronic (after 4 weeks) and sterile or infected. Chronic collections, including pseudocysts and walled-off necrosis, are characterized by encapsulation. Sterile or infected necrotizing pancreatitis may complicate the course of 5–10% of cases and accounts for most of the deaths. The risk of infection does not correlate with the extent of necrosis. Pancreatic necrosis is often associated with fever, leukocytosis, and, in some cases, shock and is associated with organ failure (eg, gastrointestinal bleeding, respiratory failure, acute kidney injury) in 50% of cases. Because infected pancreatic necrosis is often an indication for debridement, fine-needle aspiration of necrotic tissue under CT guidance should be performed (if necessary, repeatedly) for Gram stain and culture.

A serious complication of acute pancreatitis is acute respiratory distress syndrome (ARDS); cardiac dysfunction

may be superimposed. It usually occurs 3–7 days after the onset of pancreatitis in patients who have required large volumes of fluid and colloid to maintain blood pressure and urinary output. Most patients with ARDS require intubation, mechanical ventilation, and supplemental oxygen.

Pancreatic abscess (also referred to as infected or suppurative pseudocyst) is a suppurative process characterized by rising fever, leukocytosis, and localized tenderness and an epigastric mass usually 6 or more weeks into the course of acute pancreatitis. The abscess may be associated with a left-sided pleural effusion or an enlarging spleen secondary to splenic vein thrombosis. In contrast to infected necrosis, the mortality rate is low following drainage.

Pseudocysts, encapsulated fluid collections with high amylase content, commonly appear in pancreatitis when CT is used to monitor the evolution of an acute attack. Pseudocysts that are smaller than 6 cm in diameter often resolve spontaneously. They most commonly are within or adjacent to the pancreas but can present almost anywhere (eg, mediastinal, retrorectal) by extension along anatomic planes. Multiple pseudocysts are seen in 14% of cases. Pseudocysts may become secondarily infected, necessitating drainage as for an abscess. Pancreatic ascites may present after recovery from acute pancreatitis as a gradual increase in abdominal girth and persistent elevation of the serum amylase level in the absence of frank abdominal pain. Marked elevations in ascitic protein (> 3 g/dL) and amylase (> 1000 units/L [20 mkat/L]) concentrations are typical. The condition results from disruption of the pancreatic duct or drainage of a pseudocyst into the peritoneal cavity.

Rare complications of acute pancreatitis include hemorrhage caused by erosion of a blood vessel to form a pseudoaneurysm and colonic necrosis. Chronic pancreatitis develops in about 10% of cases. Permanent diabetes mellitus and exocrine pancreatic insufficiency occur uncommonly after a single acute episode.

Treatment

A. Treatment of Acute Disease

1. Mild disease—In most patients, acute pancreatitis is a mild disease ("nonsevere acute pancreatitis") that subsides spontaneously within several days. The pancreas is "rested" by a regimen of withholding food and liquids by mouth, bed rest, and, in patients with moderately severe pain or ileus and abdominal distention or vomiting, nasogastric suction. Early fluid resuscitation (one-third of the total 72-hour fluid volume administered within 24 hours of presentation, 250–500 mL/h initially) may reduce the frequency of systemic inflammatory response syndrome and organ failure in this group of patients, and lactated Ringer solution may be preferable to normal saline; however, overly aggressive fluid resuscitation may lead to morbidity as well. Pain is controlled with meperidine, up to 100–150 mg intramuscularly every 3–4 hours as necessary. In those with severe liver or kidney dysfunction, the dose may need to be reduced. Morphine has been thought to cause sphincter of Oddi spasm but is now considered an acceptable alternative and, given the potential side effects of meperidine, may even be preferable. Oral intake of fluid and foods can be resumed when the patient is largely free of pain and has bowel sounds (even if the serum amylase is still elevated). Clear liquids are given first (this step may be skipped in patients with mild acute pancreatitis), followed by gradual advancement to a low-fat diet, guided by the patient's tolerance and by the absence of pain. Pain may recur on refeeding in 20% of patients. Following recovery from acute biliary pancreatitis, laparoscopic cholecystectomy is generally performed, preferably during the same hospital admission, although in selected cases endoscopic sphincterotomy alone may be done. In patients with recurrent pancreatitis associated with pancreas divisum, insertion of a stent in the minor papilla (or minor papilla sphincterotomy) may reduce the frequency of subsequent attacks, although complications of such therapy are frequent. In patients with recurrent acute pancreatitis attributed to pancreatic sphincter of Oddi dysfunction, biliary sphincterotomy alone is as effective as combined biliary and pancreatic sphincterotomy in reducing the frequency of recurrent acute pancreatitis, but chronic pancreatitis may still develop in treated patients. Hypertriglyceridemia with acute pancreatitis has been treated with insulin, heparin, or apheresis, but the benefit of these approaches has not been proven.

2. Severe disease—In more severe pancreatitis—particularly necrotizing pancreatitis—there may be considerable leakage of fluids, necessitating large amounts of intravenous fluids (eg, 500–1000 mL/h for several hours, then 250–300 mL/h) to maintain intravascular volume. Hemodynamic monitoring in an intensive care unit is required, and the importance of aggressive intravenous hydration targeted to adequate urinary output, stabilization of blood pressure and heart rate, restoration of central venous pressure, and a modest decrease in hematocrit value cannot be overemphasized. Calcium gluconate must be given intravenously if there is evidence of hypocalcemia with tetany. Infusions of fresh frozen plasma or serum albumin may be necessary in patients with coagulopathy or hypoalbuminemia. With colloid solutions, there may be an increased risk of developing ARDS. If shock persists after adequate volume replacement (including packed red cells), pressors may be required. For the patient requiring a large volume

of parenteral fluids, central venous pressure and blood gases should be monitored at regular intervals. Enteral nutrition via a nasojejunal or possibly nasogastric feeding tube is preferable to parenteral nutrition in patients who will otherwise be without oral nutrition for at least 7–10 days but may not be tolerated in some patients with an ileus. Parenteral nutrition (including lipids) should be considered in patients who have severe pancreatitis and ileus. The routine use of antibiotics to prevent conversion of sterile pancreatic necrosis to infected necrosis is still controversial and generally is not indicated in those with < 30% pancreatic necrosis. Imipenem (500 mg every 8 hours intravenously) and possibly cefuroxime (1.5 g intravenously three times daily, then 250 mg orally twice daily) administered for no more than 14 days to patients with sterile pancreatic necrosis has been reported in some studies to reduce the risk of pancreatic infection and mortality; meropenem and the combination of ciprofloxacin and metronidazole do not appear to reduce the frequency of infected necrosis, multiorgan failure, or mortality. When infected necrosis is confirmed, imipenem or meropenem should be continued. In occasional cases, a fungal infection is found, and appropriate antifungal therapy should be prescribed. The role of intravenous somatostatin in severe acute pancreatitis is uncertain, and octreotide is thought to have no benefit. To date, probiotic agents have not been shown to reduce infectious complications of severe pancreatitis and may increase mortality. Nonsteroidal anti-inflammatory drugs (eg, indomethacin administered rectally), allopurinol, and ulinastatin have been reported to reduce the frequency and severity of post-ERCP pancreatitis in persons at high risk. There is conflicting evidence about whether the risk of pancreatitis after ERCP can be reduced by the administration of somatostatin, octreotide, gabexate mesilate and other protease inhibitors, or nitroglycerin. Placement of a stent across the pancreatic duct or orifice has been shown to reduce the risk of post-ERCP pancreatitis and is also a common practice but has not been compared directly with rectal indomethacin.

B. Treatment of Complications and Follow-Up

A surgeon should be consulted in all cases of severe acute pancreatitis. If the diagnosis is in doubt and investigation indicates a strong possibility of a serious surgically correctable lesion (eg, perforated peptic ulcer), exploratory laparotomy is indicated. When acute pancreatitis is found unexpectedly, it is usually wise to close without intervention. If the pancreatitis appears mild and cholelithiasis or microlithiasis is present, cholecystectomy or cholecystostomy may be justified. When severe pancreatitis results from choledocholithiasis and jaundice (serum total bilirubin >5 mg/dL [85.5 mcmol/L]) or cholangitis is present, ERCP with endoscopic sphincterotomy and stone extraction is indicated. MRCP may be useful in selecting patients for therapeutic ERCP. Endoscopic sphincterotomy does not appear to improve the outcome of severe pancreatitis in the absence of cholangitis or jaundice.

Necrosectomy may improve survival in patients with necrotizing pancreatitis and clinical deterioration with multiorgan failure or lack of resolution by 4 weeks and is often indicated for infected necrosis, although a select group of relatively stable patients with infected pancreatic necrosis may be managed with antibiotics alone. The goal is to debride necrotic pancreas and surrounding tissue and establish adequate drainage. Outcomes are best if necrosectomy is delayed until the necrosis has organized, usually about 4 weeks after disease onset. A "step-up" approach in which nonsurgical drainage of walled-off pancreatic necrosis under radiologic guidance with subsequent open surgical necrosectomy if necessary has been shown to reduce mortality and resource utilization in selected patients with necrotizing pancreatitis and confirmed or suspected secondary infection. Endoscopic (transgastric or transduodenal) drainage combined with percutaneous drainage and, in some cases, laparoscopic guidance are additional options, depending on local expertise. Treatment is labor intensive, and multiple procedures are often required. Peritoneal lavage has not been shown to improve survival in severe acute pancreatitis, in part because the risk of late septic complications is not reduced.

The development of a pancreatic abscess is an indication for prompt percutaneous or surgical drainage. Chronic pseudocysts require endoscopic, percutaneous catheter, or surgical drainage when infected or associated with persisting pain, pancreatitis, or bile duct obstruction. For pancreatic infections, imipenem, 500 mg every 8 hours intravenously, is a good choice of antibiotic because it achieves bactericidal levels in pancreatic tissue for most causative organisms. Pancreatic duct leaks and fistulas may require endoscopic or surgical therapy.

▶ Prognosis

Mortality rates for acute pancreatitis have declined from at least 10% to around 5% since the 1980s, but the mortality rate for severe acute pancreatitis (more than three Ranson criteria; Table 16–8) remains at least 20%, with rates of 10% and 25% in those with sterile and infected necrosis, respectively. Severe acute pancreatitis is predicted by features of the systemic inflammatory response on admission; a persistent systemic inflammatory response is associated with a mortality rate of 25%, and a transient response, with a mortality rate of 8%. Half of the deaths occur within the first 2 weeks, usually from multiorgan failure. Multiorgan failure is associated with a mortality rate of at least 30%, and if it persists beyond the first 48 hours, the mortality rate is over 50%. Later deaths occur because of complications of infected necrosis. The risk of death doubles when both organ failure and infected necrosis are present. Moreover, hospital-acquired infections increase the mortality of acute pancreatitis, independent of severity. Readmission to the hospital for acute pancreatitis within 30 days may be predicted by a scoring system based on five factors during the index admission: eating less than a solid diet at discharge; nausea, vomiting, or diarrhea at discharge; pancreatic necrosis; use of antibiotics at discharge; and pain at discharge. Recurrences are common in alcoholic pancreatitis but can be reduced by repeated, regularly scheduled interventions to eliminate alcohol consumption

after discharge from the hospital. The risk of chronic pancreatitis following an episode of acute alcoholic pancreatitis is 13% in 10 years and 16% in 20 years.

▶ When to Admit

Nearly all patients with acute pancreatitis should be hospitalized.

Akbar A et al. Rectal nonsteroidal anti-inflammatory drugs are superior to pancreatic duct stents in preventing pancreatitis after endoscopic retrograde cholangiopancreatography: a network meta-analysis. Clin Gastroenterol Hepatol. 2013 Jul;11(7):778–83. [PMID: 23376320]

Banks PA et al. Classification of acute pancreatitis—2012: revision of the Atlanta classification and definitions by international consensus. Gut. 2013 Jan;62(1):102–11. [PMID: 23100216]

Douros A et al. Drug-induced acute pancreatitis: results from the hospital-based Berlin case-control surveillance study of 102 cases. Aliment Pharmacol Ther. 2013 Oct;38(7):825–34. [PMID: 23957710]

Mouli VP et al. Efficacy of conservative treatment, without necrosectomy, for infected pancreatic necrosis: a systematic review and meta-analysis. Gastroenterology. 2013 Feb;144(2):333–40. [PMID: 23063972]

Tenner S et al. American College of Gastroenterology guideline: management of acute pancreatitis. Am J Gastroenterol. 2013 Sep;108(9):1400–16. [PMID: 23896955]

Wu BU et al. Clinical management of patients with acute pancreatitis. Gastroenterology. 2013 Jun;144(6):1272–81. [PMID: 23622137]

CHRONIC PANCREATITIS

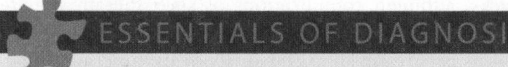

ESSENTIALS OF DIAGNOSIS

▶ Chronic or intermittent epigastric pain, steatorrhea, weight loss, abnormal pancreatic imaging.

▶ A mnemonic for the predisposing factors of chronic pancreatitis is TIGAR-O: toxic-metabolic, idiopathic, genetic, autoimmune, recurrent and severe acute pancreatitis, or obstructive.

▶ General Considerations

Chronic pancreatitis occurs most often in patients with alcoholism (45–80% of all cases). The risk of chronic pancreatitis increases with the duration and amount of alcohol consumed, but pancreatitis develops in only 5–10% of heavy drinkers. Tobacco smoking is a risk factor for idiopathic chronic pancreatitis and has been reported to accelerate progression of alcoholic chronic pancreatitis. About 2% of patients with hyperparathyroidism develop pancreatitis. In tropical Africa and Asia, tropical pancreatitis, related in part to malnutrition, is the most common cause of chronic pancreatitis. A stricture, stone, or tumor obstructing the pancreas can lead to obstructive chronic pancreatitis. Autoimmune pancreatitis is associated with hypergammaglobulinemia (IgG_4 in particular), and often with autoantibodies and other autoimmune diseases, and is responsive to corticosteroids. Affected persons are at increased risk for various cancers. Type 1 autoimmune pancreatitis is a multisystem disease characterized by lymphoplasmacytic sclerosing pancreatitis on biopsy, associated bile duct strictures, retroperitoneal fibrosis, renal and salivary gland lesions, and a high rate of relapse after treatment. Type 2 affects the pancreas alone and is characterized by idiopathic duct centric pancreatitis on biopsy, lack of systemic IgG_4 involvement, an association with inflammatory bowel disease, and a lower rate of relapse after treatment. Between 10% and 30% of cases of chronic pancreatitis are idiopathic, with either early onset (median age 23) or late onset (median age 62). Genetic factors may predispose to chronic pancreatitis in some of these cases and include mutations of the cystic fibrosis transmembrane conductance regulator (CFTR) gene, the pancreatic secretory trypsin inhibitory gene (PSTI, serine protease inhibitor, SPINK1), and possibly the gene for uridine 5'-diphosphate glucuronosyltransferase. Mutation of the cationic trypsinogen gene on chromosome 7 (serine protease 1, PRSS1) is associated with hereditary pancreatitis, transmitted as an autosomal dominant trait with variable penetrance. In addition, a variant in an X-linked gene CLDN2, which encodes claudin-2 has been associated with chronic pancreatitis; its presence on the X chromosome may partly explain the male predominance of chronic pancreatitis. A useful mnemonic for the predisposing factors to chronic pancreatitis is TIGAR-O: toxic-metabolic, idiopathic, genetic, autoimmune, recurrent and severe acute pancreatitis, or obstructive.

The pathogenesis of chronic pancreatitis may be explained by the SAPE (sentinel acute pancreatitis event) hypothesis by which the first (sentinel) acute pancreatitis event initiates an inflammatory process that results in injury and later fibrosis ("necrosis-fibrosis"). In many cases, chronic pancreatitis is a self-perpetuating disease characterized by chronic pain or recurrent episodes of acute pancreatitis and ultimately by pancreatic exocrine or endocrine insufficiency (sooner in alcoholic pancreatitis than in other types). After many years, chronic pain may resolve spontaneously or as a result of surgery tailored to the cause of pain. Over 80% of adults develop diabetes mellitus within 25 years after the clinical onset of chronic pancreatitis.

▶ Clinical Findings

A. Symptoms and Signs

Persistent or recurrent episodes of epigastric and left upper quadrant pain with referral to the left upper quadrant are typical. The pain results in part from impaired inhibitory pain modulation by the central nervous system. Anorexia, nausea, vomiting, constipation, flatulence, and weight loss are common. During attacks tenderness over the pancreas, mild muscle guarding, and ileus may be noted. Attacks may last only a few hours or as long as 2 weeks; pain may eventually be almost continuous. Steatorrhea (as indicated by bulky, foul, fatty stools) may occur late in the course.

B. Laboratory Findings

Serum amylase and lipase may be elevated during acute attacks; however, normal values do not exclude the diagnosis. Serum alkaline phosphatase and bilirubin may be elevated owing to compression of the bile duct. Glycosuria may be present. Excess fecal fat may be demonstrated on chemical analysis of the stool. Pancreatic insufficiency generally is confirmed by response to therapy with pancreatic enzyme supplements; the secretin stimulation test can be used if available (and has a high negative predictive factor for ruling out early acute chronic pancreatitis), as can detection of decreased fecal chymotrypsin or elastase levels, although the latter tests lack sensitivity and specificity. Vitamin B_{12} malabsorption is detectable in about 40% of patients, but clinical deficiency of vitamin B_{12} and fat-soluble vitamins is rare. Accurate diagnostic tests are available for the major trypsinogen gene mutations, but because of uncertainty about the mechanisms linking heterozygous CFTR and PSTI mutations with pancreatitis, genetic testing for mutations in these two genes is not currently recommended. Elevated IgG_4 levels, ANA, and antibodies to lactoferrin and carbonic anhydrase II are often found in patients with autoimmune pancreatitis (especially type 1). Pancreatic biopsy, if necessary, shows a lymphoplasmacytic inflammatory infiltrate with characteristic IgG_4 immunostaining, which is also found in biopsy specimens of the major papilla, bile duct, and salivary glands, in type 1 autoimmune pancreatitis.

C. Imaging

Plain films show calcifications due to pancreaticolithiasis in 30% of affected patients. CT may show calcifications not seen on plain films as well as ductal dilatation and heterogeneity or atrophy of the gland. Occasionally, the findings raise suspicion of pancreatic cancer ("tumefactive chronic pancreatitis"). ERCP is the most sensitive imaging study for chronic pancreatitis and may show dilated ducts, intraductal stones, strictures, or pseudocyst, but is infrequently used for diagnosis alone; moreover, the results may be normal in patients with so-called minimal change pancreatitis. MRCP (including secretin-enhanced MRCP) and endoscopic ultrasonography (with pancreatic tissue sampling) are less invasive alternatives to ERCP. Endoscopic ultrasonographic ("Rosemont") criteria for the diagnosis of chronic pancreatitis include hyperechoic foci with shadowing indicative of calculi in the main pancreatic duct and lobularity with honeycombing of the pancreatic parenchyma. Characteristic imaging features of autoimmune pancreatitis include diffuse enlargement of the pancreas, a peripheral rim of hypoattenuation, and irregular narrowing of the main pancreatic duct. In the United States, the diagnosis of autoimmune pancreatitis is based on the HISORt criteria: histology, imaging, serology, other organ involvement, and response to corticosteroid therapy.

▶ Complications

Opioid addiction is common. Other frequent complications include often brittle diabetes mellitus, pancreatic pseudocyst or abscess, cholestatic liver enzymes with or without jaundice, bile duct stricture, steatorrhea, malnutrition, and peptic ulcer. Pancreatic cancer develops in 4% of patients after 20 years; the risk may relate to tobacco and alcohol use. In patients with hereditary pancreatitis, the risk of pancreatic cancer rises after age 50 years and reaches 19% by age 70 years (see Chapter 39).

▶ Treatment

Correctable coexistent biliary tract disease should be treated surgically.

A. Medical Measures

A low-fat diet should be prescribed. Alcohol is forbidden because it frequently precipitates attacks. Opioids should be avoided if possible. Preferred agents for pain are acetaminophen, nonsteroidal anti-inflammatory drugs, and tramadol, along with pain-modifying agents such as tricyclic antidepressants, selective serotonin uptake inhibitors, and gabapentin or pregabalin. Steatorrhea is treated with pancreatic supplements that are selected on the basis of their high lipase activity (Table 16–10). A total dose of at least 40,000 units of lipase in capsules is given with each meal (during and after the meal). Doses of 90,000 units or more of lipase per meal may be required in some cases. The tablets should be taken at the start of, during, and at the end of a meal. Concurrent administration of a H_2-receptor antagonist (eg, ranitidine, 150 mg orally twice daily), a proton pump inhibitor (eg, omeprazole, 20–60 mg orally daily), or sodium bicarbonate, 650 mg orally before and after meals, decreases the inactivation of lipase by acid and may thereby further decrease steatorrhea. In selected cases of alcoholic pancreatitis and in cystic fibrosis, enteric-coated microencapsulated preparations may offer an advantage. However, in patients with cystic fibrosis, high-dose pancreatic enzyme therapy has been associated with strictures of the ascending colon. Pain secondary to idiopathic chronic pancreatitis may be alleviated in some cases by the use of pancreatic enzymes (not enteric-coated) or octreotide, 200 mcg subcutaneously three times daily. Antioxidant therapy to inhibit electrophilic stress on key macromolecules in the pancreas by toxic metabolites has shown promise in some, but not all, studies. Associated diabetes mellitus should be treated (see Chapter 27). Autoimmune pancreatitis is treated with prednisone 40 mg/d orally for 1–2 months, followed by a taper of 5 mg every 2–4 weeks. Nonresponse or relapse occurs in 45% of cases (particularly in those with concomitant IgG_4-associated cholangitis); azathioprine appears to reduce the risk of relapse. Other immunomodulators and biologic agents, including rituximab, are under study.

B. Endoscopic and Surgical Treatment

Endoscopic therapy or surgery may be indicated in chronic pancreatitis to treat underlying biliary tract disease, ensure free flow of bile into the duodenum, drain persistent pseudocysts, treat other complications, eliminate obstruction of the pancreatic duct, attempt to relieve pain, or exclude pancreatic cancer. Liver fibrosis may

Table 16–10. FDA-approved pancreatic enzyme (pancrelipase) preparations.

Product	Enzyme Content/Unit Dose, USP units		
	Lipase	Amylase	Protease
Immediate Release Capsule			
Nonenteric-coated			
Viokace 10,440	10,440	39,150	39,150
Viokace 20,880	20,880	78,300	78,300
Delayed Release Capsules			
Enteric-coated minimicrospheres			
Creon 3000	3000	15,000	9500
Creon 6000	6000	30,000	19,000
Creon 12,000	12,000	60,000	38,000
Creon 24,000	24,000	120,000	76,000
Enteric-coated minitablets			
Ultresa 13,800	13,800	27,600	27,600
Ultresa 20,700	20,700	46,000	41,400
Ultresa 23,000	23,000	46,000	41,400
Enteric-coated beads			
Zenpep 3000	3000	16,000	10,000
Zenpep 5000	5000	27,000	17,000
Zenpep 10,000	10,000	55,000	34,000
Zenpep 15,000	15,000	82,000	51,000
Zenpep 20,000	20,000	109,000	68,000
Zenpep 25,000	25,000	136,000	85,000
Enteric-coated microtablets			
Pancreaze 4200	4200	17,500	10,000
Pancreaze 10,500	10,500	43,750	25,000
Pancreaze 16,800	16,800	70,000	40,000
Pancreaze 21,000	21,000	61,000	37,000
Bicarbonate-buffered enteric-coated microspheres			
Peptyze 8000	8000	30,250	28,750
Peptyze 16,000	16,000	60,500	57,500

FDA, U.S. Food and Drug Administration; USP, U.S. Pharmacopeia.

regress after biliary drainage. Distal bile duct obstruction may be relieved by endoscopic placement of multiple bile duct stents. When obstruction of the duodenal end of the pancreatic duct can be demonstrated by ERCP, dilation of or placement of a stent in the duct and pancreatic duct stone lithotripsy or surgical resection of the tail of the pancreas with implantation of the distal end of the duct by pancreaticojejunostomy may be performed. Endoscopic therapy is successful in about 50% of cases. In patients who do not respond to endoscopic therapy, surgery is successful in about 50%. When the pancreatic duct is diffusely dilated, anastomosis between the duct after it is split longitudinally and a defunctionalized limb of jejunum (modified Puestow procedure), in some cases combined with resection of the head of the pancreas (Beger or Frey procedure), is associated with relief of pain in 80% of cases. In advanced cases, subtotal or total pancreatectomy may be considered as a last resort but has variable efficacy and causes pancreatic insufficiency and diabetes mellitus. Perioperative administration of somatostatin or octreotide may reduce the risk of postoperative pancreatic fistulas. Endoscopic or surgical (including laparoscopic) drainage is indicated for symptomatic pseudocysts and, in many cases, those over 6 cm in diameter. Endoscopic ultrasonography may facilitate selection of an optimal site for endoscopic drainage. Pancreatic ascites or pancreaticopleural fistulas due to a disrupted pancreatic duct can be managed by endoscopic placement of a stent across the disrupted duct. Pancreatic sphincterotomy or fragmentation of stones in the pancreatic duct by lithotripsy and endoscopic removal of stones from the duct may relieve pain in selected patients. For patients with chronic pain and nondilated ducts, a percutaneous celiac plexus nerve block may be considered under either CT or endoscopic ultrasound guidance, with pain relief (albeit often short-lived) in approximately 50% of patients. A single session of radiation therapy to the pancreas has been reported to relieve otherwise refractory pain.

Prognosis

Chronic pancreatitis often leads to disability. The prognosis is best in patients with recurrent acute pancreatitis caused by a remediable condition, such as cholelithiasis, choledocholithiasis, stenosis of the sphincter of Oddi, or hyperparathyroidism, and in those with autoimmune pancreatitis. Medical management of hyperlipidemia, if present, may also prevent recurrent attacks of pancreatitis. In alcoholic pancreatitis, pain relief is most likely when a dilated pancreatic duct can be decompressed. In patients with disease not amenable to decompressive surgery, addiction to opioids is a frequent outcome of treatment. The quality of life is poorer in patients with constant pain than in those with intermittent pain.

When to Refer

All patients with chronic pancreatitis should be referred for diagnostic and therapeutic procedures.

When to Admit

- Severe pain.
- New jaundice.
- New fever.

Forsmark CE. Management of chronic pancreatitis. Gastroenterology. 2013 Jun;144(6):1282–91. [PMID: 23622138]

Kamisawa T et al. Recent advances in autoimmune pancreatitis: type 1 and type 2. Gut. 2013 Sep;62(9):1373–80. [PMID: 23749606]

Rosendahl J et al. *CFTR, SPINK*1, *CTRC* and *PRSS1* variants in chronic pancreatitis: is the role of mutated *CFTR* overestimated? Gut. 2013 Apr;62(4):582–92. [PMID: 22427236]

Shiokawa M et al. Risk of cancer in patients with autoimmune pancreatitis. Am J Gastroenterol. 2013 Apr;108(4):610–7. [PMID: 23318486]

Thorat V et al. Randomised clinical trial: the efficacy and safety of pancreatin enteric-coated minimicrospheres (Creon 40000 MMS) in patients with pancreatic exocrine insufficiency due to chronic pancreatitis—a double-blind, placebo-controlled study. Aliment Pharmacol Ther. 2012 Sep;36(5):426–36. [PMID: 22762290]

Breast Disorders

Armando E. Giuliano, MD

Sara A. Hurvitz, MD

BENIGN BREAST DISORDERS

FIBROCYSTIC CONDITION

ESSENTIALS OF DIAGNOSIS

- ▶ Painful, often multiple, usually bilateral masses in the breast.
- ▶ Rapid fluctuation in the size of the masses is common.
- ▶ Frequently, pain occurs or worsens and size increases during premenstrual phase of cycle.
- ▶ Most common age is 30–50. Rare in postmenopausal women not receiving hormonal replacement.

▶ General Considerations

Fibrocystic condition is the most frequent lesion of the breast. Although commonly referred to as "fibrocystic disease," it does not, in fact, represent a pathologic or anatomic disorder. It is common in women 30–50 years of age but rare in postmenopausal women who are not taking hormonal replacement. Estrogen is considered a causative factor. There may be an increased risk in women who drink alcohol, especially women between 18 and 22 years of age. Fibrocystic condition encompasses a wide variety of benign histologic changes in the breast epithelium, some of which are found so commonly in normal breasts that they are probably variants of normal but have nonetheless been termed a "condition" or "disease."

The microscopic findings of fibrocystic condition include cysts (gross and microscopic), papillomatosis, adenosis, fibrosis, and ductal epithelial hyperplasia. Although fibrocystic condition has generally been considered to increase the risk of subsequent breast cancer, **only the variants with a component of epithelial proliferation (especially with atypia) or increased breast density on mammogram represent true risk factors**.

▶ Clinical Findings

A. Symptoms and Signs

Fibrocystic condition may produce an asymptomatic mass in the breast that is discovered by accident, but pain or tenderness often calls attention to it. Discomfort often occurs or worsens during the premenstrual phase of the cycle, at which time the cysts tend to enlarge. Fluctuations in size and rapid appearance or disappearance of a breast mass are common with this condition as are multiple or bilateral masses and serous nipple discharge. Patients will give a history of a transient lump in the breast or cyclic breast pain.

B. Diagnostic Tests

Mammography and ultrasonography should be used to evaluate a mass in a patient with fibrocystic condition. Ultrasonography alone may be used in women under 30 years of age. Because a mass due to fibrocystic condition is difficult to distinguish from carcinoma on the basis of clinical findings, suspicious lesions should be biopsied. Fine-needle aspiration (FNA) cytology may be used, but if a suspicious mass that is nonmalignant on cytologic examination does not resolve over several months, it should be excised or biopsied by core needle. Surgery should be conservative, since the primary objective is to exclude cancer. Occasionally, FNA cytology will suffice. Simple mastectomy or extensive removal of breast tissue is rarely, if ever, indicated for fibrocystic condition.

▶ Differential Diagnosis

Pain, fluctuation in size, and multiplicity of lesions are the features most helpful in differentiating fibrocystic condition from carcinoma. If a dominant mass is present, the diagnosis of cancer should be assumed until disproven by biopsy. Mammography may be helpful, but the breast tissue in these young women is usually too radiodense to permit a worthwhile study. Sonography is useful in differentiating a cystic mass from a solid mass, especially in women with dense breasts. Final diagnosis, however, depends on analysis of the excisional biopsy specimen or needle biopsy.

Treatment

When the diagnosis of fibrocystic condition has been established by previous biopsy or is likely because the history is classic, aspiration of a discrete mass suggestive of a cyst is indicated to alleviate pain and, more importantly, to confirm the cystic nature of the mass. The patient is reexamined at intervals thereafter. If no fluid is obtained by aspiration, if fluid is bloody, if a mass persists after aspiration, or if at any time during follow-up a persistent or recurrent mass is noted, biopsy should be performed.

Breast pain associated with generalized fibrocystic condition is best treated by avoiding trauma and by wearing a good supportive brassiere during the night and day. Hormone therapy is not advisable, because it does not cure the condition and has undesirable side effects. Danazol (100–200 mg orally twice daily), a synthetic androgen, is the only treatment approved by the US Food and Drug Administration (FDA) for patients with severe pain. This treatment suppresses pituitary gonadotropins, but androgenic effects (acne, edema, hirsutism) usually make this treatment intolerable; in practice, it is rarely used. Similarly, tamoxifen reduces some symptoms of fibrocystic condition, but because of its side effects, it is not useful for young women unless it is given to reduce the risk of cancer. Postmenopausal women receiving hormone replacement therapy may stop or change doses of hormones to reduce pain. Oil of evening primrose (OEP), a natural form of gamolenic acid, has been shown to decrease pain in 44–58% of users. The dosage of gamolenic acid is six capsules of 500 mg orally twice daily. Studies have also demonstrated a low-fat diet or decreasing dietary fat intake may reduce the painful symptoms associated with fibrocystic condition. Further research is being done to determine the effects of topical treatments such as topical nonsteroidal anti-inflammatory drugs as well as topical hormonal drugs such as topical tamoxifen.

The role of caffeine consumption in the development and treatment of fibrocystic condition is controversial. Some studies suggest that eliminating caffeine from the diet is associated with improvement while other studies refute the benefit entirely. Many patients are aware of these studies and report relief of symptoms after giving up coffee, tea, and chocolate. Similarly, many women find vitamin E (400 international units daily) helpful; however, these observations remain anecdotal.

Prognosis

Exacerbations of pain, tenderness, and cyst formation may occur at any time until menopause, when symptoms usually subside, except in patients receiving hormonal replacement. The patient should be advised to examine her own breasts regularly just after menstruation and to inform her practitioner if a mass appears. The risk of breast cancer developing in women with fibrocystic condition with a proliferative or atypical component in the epithelium or papillomatosis is higher than that of the general population. These women should be monitored carefully with physical examinations and imaging studies.

Liu Y et al. Intakes of alcohol and folate during adolescence and risk of proliferative benign breast disease. Pediatrics. 2012 May;129(5):e1192–8. [PMID: 22492774]

Salzman B et al. Common breast problems. Am Fam Physician. 2012 Aug 15;86(4):343–9. [PMID: 22963023]

FIBROADENOMA OF THE BREAST

This common benign neoplasm occurs most frequently in young women, usually within 20 years after puberty. It is somewhat more frequent and tends to occur at an earlier age in black women. Multiple tumors are found in 10–15% of patients.

The typical **fibroadenoma** is a round or ovoid, rubbery, discrete, relatively movable, nontender mass 1–5 cm in diameter. It is usually discovered accidentally. Clinical diagnosis in young patients is generally not difficult. In women over 30 years, fibrocystic condition of the breast and carcinoma of the breast must be considered. Cysts can be identified by aspiration or ultrasonography. Fibroadenoma does not normally occur after menopause but may occasionally develop after administration of hormones.

No treatment is usually necessary if the diagnosis can be made by needle biopsy or cytologic examination. Excision with pathologic examination of the specimen is performed if the diagnosis is uncertain. Cryoablation, or freezing of the fibroadenoma, appears to be a safe procedure if the lesion is consistent with fibroadenoma on histology prior to ablation. Cryoablation is not appropriate for all fibroadenomas because some are too large to freeze or the diagnosis may not be certain. There is no obvious advantage to cryoablation of a histologically proven fibroadenoma except that some patients may feel relief that a mass is gone. However, at times a mass of scar or fat necrosis replaces the mass of the fibroadenoma. Reassurance seems preferable. It is usually not possible to distinguish a large fibroadenoma from a phyllodes tumor on the basis of needle biopsy results or imaging alone and histology is usually required.

Phyllodes tumor is a fibroadenoma-like tumor with cellular stroma that grows rapidly. It may reach a large size and, if inadequately excised, will recur locally. The lesion can be benign or malignant. If benign, phyllodes tumor is treated by local excision with a margin of surrounding breast tissue. The treatment of malignant phyllodes tumor is more controversial, but complete removal of the tumor with a rim of normal tissue avoids recurrence. Because these tumors may be large, simple mastectomy is sometimes necessary. Lymph node dissection is not performed, since the sarcomatous portion of the tumor metastasizes to the lungs and not the lymph nodes.

Abe M et al. Malignant transformation of breast fibroadenoma to malignant phyllodes tumor: long-term outcome of 36 malignant phyllodes tumors. Breast Cancer. 2011 Oct;18(4):268–72. [PMID: 22121516]

Amin AL et al. Benign breast disease. Surg Clin North Am. 2013 Apr;93(2):299–308. [PMID: 23464687]

Gutwein LG et al. Utilization of minimally invasive breast biopsy for the evaluation of suspicious breast lesions. Am J Surg. 2011 Aug;202(2):127–32. [PMID: 21295284]

NIPPLE DISCHARGE

In order of decreasing frequency, the following are the most common causes of nipple discharge in the nonlactating breast: duct ectasia, intraductal papilloma, and carcinoma. The important characteristics of the discharge and some other factors to be evaluated by history and physical examination are listed in Table 17–1.

Spontaneous, unilateral, serous or serosanguineous discharge from a single duct is usually caused by an intraductal papilloma or, rarely, by an intraductal cancer. A mass may not be palpable. The involved duct may be identified by pressure at different sites around the nipple at the margin of the areola. Bloody discharge is suggestive of cancer but is more often caused by a benign papilloma in the duct. Cytologic examination may identify malignant cells, but negative findings do not rule out cancer, which is more likely in women over age 50 years. In any case, the involved bloody duct—and a mass if present—should be excised. A ductogram (a mammogram of a duct after radiopaque dye has been injected) is of limited value since excision of the suspicious ductal system is indicated regardless of findings. Ductoscopy, evaluation of the ductal system with a small scope inserted through the nipple, has been attempted but is not effective management.

In premenopausal women, spontaneous multiple duct discharge, unilateral or bilateral, most noticeable just before menstruation, is often due to fibrocystic condition. Discharge may be green or brownish. Papillomatosis and ductal ectasia are usually detected only by biopsy. If a mass is present, it should be removed.

A milky discharge from multiple ducts in the nonlactating breast may occur from hyperprolactinemia. Serum prolactin levels should be obtained to search for a pituitary tumor. Thyroid-stimulating hormone (TSH) helps exclude causative hypothyroidism. Numerous antipsychotic drugs and other drugs may also cause a milky discharge that ceases on discontinuance of the medication.

Oral contraceptive agents or estrogen replacement therapy may cause clear, serous, or milky discharge from a single duct, but multiple duct discharge is more common. In the premenopausal woman, the discharge is more evident just before menstruation and disappears on stopping the medication. If it does not stop, is from a single duct, and is copious, exploration should be performed since this may be a sign of cancer.

A purulent discharge may originate in a subareolar abscess and require removal of the abscess and the related lactiferous sinus.

When localization is not possible, no mass is palpable, and the discharge is nonbloody, the patient should be reexamined every 3 or 4 months for a year, and a mammogram and an ultrasound should be performed. Although most discharge is from a benign process, patients may find it annoying or disconcerting. To eliminate the discharge, proximal duct excision can be performed both for treatment and diagnosis.

Chen L et al. Bloody nipple discharge is a predictor of breast cancer risk: a meta-analysis. Breast Cancer Res Treat. 2012 Feb;132(1):9–14. [PMID: 21947751]

Huang W et al. Evaluation and management of galactorrhea. Am Fam Physician. 2012 Jun 1;85(11):1073–80. [PMID: 22962879]

Salzman B et al. Common breast problems. Am Fam Physician. 2012 Aug 15;86(4):343–9. [PMID: 22963023]

FAT NECROSIS

Fat necrosis is a rare lesion of the breast but is of clinical importance because it produces a mass (often accompanied by skin or nipple retraction) that is usually indistinguishable from carcinoma even with imaging studies. Trauma is presumed to be the cause, though only about 50% of patients give a history of injury. Ecchymosis is occasionally present. If untreated, the mass effect gradually disappears. The safest course is to obtain a biopsy. Needle biopsy is often adequate, but frequently the entire mass must be excised, primarily to exclude carcinoma. Fat necrosis is common after segmental resection, radiation therapy, or flap reconstruction after mastectomy.

BREAST ABSCESS

During nursing, an area of redness, tenderness, and induration may develop in the breast. The organism most commonly found in these abscesses is *Staphylococcus aureus* (see Puerperal Mastitis, Chapter 19).

Infection in the nonlactating breast is rare. A subareolar abscess may develop in young or middle-aged women who are not lactating (Figure 17–1). These infections tend to recur after incision and drainage unless the area is explored during a quiescent interval, with excision of the involved

Table 17–1. Characteristics of nipple discharge in the nonpregnant, nonlactating woman.

Finding	Significance
Serous	Most likely benign FCC, ie, duct ectasia
Bloody	More likely neoplastic–papilloma, carcinoma
Associated mass	More likely neoplastic
Unilateral	Either neoplastic or non-neoplastic
Bilateral	Most likely non-neoplastic
Single duct	More likely neoplastic
Multiple ducts	More likely FCC
Milky	Endocrine disorders, medications
Spontaneous	Either neoplastic or non-neoplastic
Produced by pressure at single site	Either neoplastic or non-neoplastic
Persistent	Either neoplastic or non-neoplastic
Intermittent	Either neoplastic or non-neoplastic
Related to menses	More likely FCC
Premenopausal	More likely FCC
Taking hormones	More likely FCC

FCC, fibrocystic condition.

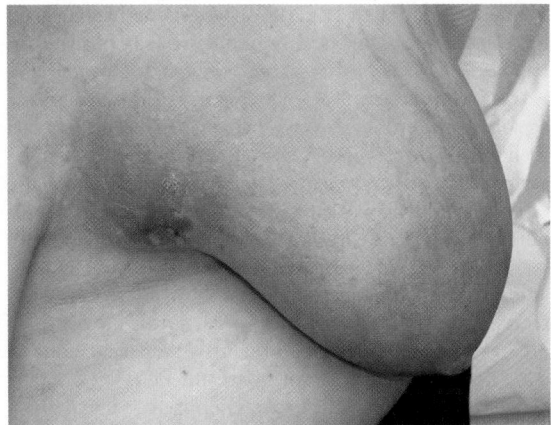

▲ **Figure 17–1.** Breast abscess and cellulitis. (Reproduced with permission, from Richard P. Usatine, MD.)

lactiferous duct or ducts at the base of the nipple. In the nonlactating breast, inflammatory carcinoma must always be considered. Thus, incision and biopsy of any indurated tissue with a small piece of erythematous skin is indicated when suspected abscess or cellulitis in the nonlactating breast does not resolve promptly with antibiotics. Often needle or catheter drainage is adequate to treat an abscess, but surgical incision and drainage may be necessary.

Amin AL et al. Benign breast disease. Surg Clin North Am. 2013 Apr;93(2):299–308. [PMID: 23464687]

Trop I et al. Breast abscesses: evidence-based algorithms for diagnosis, management, and follow-up. Radiographics. 2011 Oct;31(6):1683–99. [PMID: 21997989]

Wang K et al. The Mammotome biopsy system is an effective treatment strategy for breast abscess. Am J Surg. 2013 Jan;205(1):35–8. [PMID: 23036601]

DISORDERS OF THE AUGMENTED BREAST

At least 4 million American women have had breast implants. Breast augmentation is performed by placing implants under the pectoralis muscle or, less desirably, in the subcutaneous tissue of the breast. Most implants are made of an outer silicone shell filled with a silicone gel, saline, or some combination of the two. Capsule contraction or scarring around the implant develops in about 15–25% of patients, leading to a firmness and distortion of the breast that can be painful. Some require removal of the implant and surrounding capsule.

Implant rupture may occur in as many as 5–10% of women, and bleeding of gel through the capsule is noted even more commonly. Although silicone gel may be an immunologic stimulant, there is no increase in autoimmune disorders in patients with such implants. The FDA has advised symptomatic women with ruptured silicone implants to discuss possible surgical removal with their clinicians. However, women who are asymptomatic and have no evidence of rupture of a silicone gel prosthesis should probably not undergo removal of the implant. Women with symptoms of autoimmune illnesses often undergo removal, but no benefit has been shown.

Studies have failed to show any association between implants and an increased incidence of breast cancer. However, breast cancer may develop in a patient with an augmentation prosthesis, as it does in women without them. Detection in patients with implants is more difficult because mammography is less able to detect early lesions. Mammography is better if the implant is subpectoral rather than subcutaneous. Prostheses should be placed retropectorally after mastectomy to facilitate detection of a local recurrence of cancer, which is usually cutaneous or subcutaneous and is easily detected by palpation. There is a possible association of lymphoma of the breast with silicone implants, but this has not been clearly established.

If a cancer develops in a patient with implants, it should be treated in the same manner as in women without implants. Such women should be offered the option of mastectomy or breast-conserving therapy, which may require removal or replacement of the implant. Radiotherapy of the augmented breast often results in marked capsular contracture. Adjuvant treatments should be given for the same indications as for women who have no implants.

Jewell ML. Silicone gel breast implants at 50: the state of the science. Aesthet Surg J. 2012 Nov;32(8):1031–4. [PMID: 23012658]

Kim B et al. Anaplastic large cell lymphoma and breast implants: results from a structured expert consultation process. Plast Reconstr Surg. 2011 Sep;128(3):629–39. [PMID: 21502904]

Lavigne E et al. Breast cancer detection and survival among women with cosmetic breast implants: systematic review and meta-analysis of observational studies. BMJ. 2013 Apr 29;346:f2399. [PMID: 23637132]

Taylor CR et al. Anaplastic large cell lymphoma occurring in association with breast implants: review of pathologic and immunohistochemical features in 103 cases. Appl Immunohistochem Mol Morphol. 2013 Jan;21(1):13–20. [PMID: 23235342]

Vase MO et al. Breast implants and anaplastic large-cell lymphoma: a Danish population-based cohort study. Cancer Epidemiol Biomarkers Prev. 2013 Nov;22(11):2126–9. [PMID: 23956025]

Yang N et al. The augmented breast: a pictorial review of the abnormal and unusual. AJR Am J Roentgenol. 2011 Apr;196 (4):W451–60. [PMID: 21427311]

CARCINOMA OF THE FEMALE BREAST

 ESSENTIALS OF DIAGNOSIS

▶ Risk factors include age, delayed childbearing, positive family history of breast cancer or genetic mutations (*BRCA1, BRCA2*), and personal history of breast cancer or some types of proliferative conditions.

▶ **Early findings:** Single, nontender, firm to hard mass with ill-defined margins; mammographic abnormalities and no palpable mass.

▶ **Later findings:** Skin or nipple retraction; axillary lymphadenopathy; breast enlargement, erythema, edema, pain; fixation of mass to skin or chest wall.

▶ Incidence & Risk Factors

Breast cancer will develop in one of eight American women. **Next to skin cancer, breast cancer is the most common cancer in women; it is second only to lung cancer as a cause of death.** In 2013, there were approximately 232,340 new cases and 39,620 deaths from breast cancer in women in the United States. An additional 64,640 cases of breast carcinoma in situ were detected, principally by screening mammography. Worldwide, breast cancer is diagnosed in approximately 1.38 million women, and about 458,000 die of breast cancer each year, with the highest rates of diagnosis in Western and Northern Europe, Australia, New Zealand, and North America and lowest rates in Sub-Saharan Africa and Asia. These regional differences in incidence are likely due to the variable availability of screening mammography as well as differences in reproductive and hormonal factors. In western countries, incidence rates decreased with a reduced use of postmenopausal hormone therapy and mortality declined with increased use of screening and improved treatments. In contrast, incidence and mortality from breast cancer in many African and Asian countries has increased as reproductive factors have changed (such as delayed childbearing) and as the incidence of obesity has risen.

The most significant risk factor for the development of breast cancer is age. A woman's risk of breast cancer rises rapidly until her early 60s, peaks in her 70s, and then declines. A significant family history of breast or ovarian cancer may also indicate a high risk of developing breast cancer. Germline mutations in the *BRCA* family of tumor suppressor genes accounts for approximately 5–10% of breast cancer diagnoses and tend to cluster in certain ethnic groups, including women of Ashkenazi Jewish descent. Women with a mutation in the *BRCA1* gene, located on chromosome 17, have an estimated 85% chance of developing breast cancer in their lifetime. Other genes associated with an increased risk of breast and other cancers include *BRCA2* (associated with a gene on chromosome 13); ataxia-telangiectasia mutation; and mutation of the tumor suppressor gene *p53*. If a woman has a compelling family history (such as breast cancer diagnosed in two first-degree relatives, especially if diagnosed younger than age 50; ovarian cancer; male breast cancer; or a first-degree relative with bilateral breast cancer), genetic testing may be appropriate. In general, it is best for a woman who has a strong family history to meet with a genetics counselor to undergo a risk assessment and decide whether genetic testing is indicated.

Even when genetic testing fails to reveal a predisposing genetic mutation, women with a strong family history of breast cancer are at higher risk for development of breast cancer. Women who are *BRCA*-negative but have mutation-affected women in their family also appear to be at increased risk. Compared with a woman with no affected family members, a woman who has one first-degree relative (mother, daughter, or sister) with breast cancer has double the risk of developing breast cancer and a woman with two first-degree relatives with breast cancer has triple the risk of developing breast cancer. The risk is further increased for a woman whose affected family member was premenopausal at the time of diagnosis or had bilateral breast cancer. Lifestyle and reproductive factors also contribute to risk of breast cancer. Nulliparous women and women whose first full-term pregnancy occurred after the age of 30 have an elevated risk. Late menarche and artificial menopause are associated with a lower incidence, whereas early menarche (under age 12) and late natural menopause (after age 55) are associated with an increase in risk. Combined oral contraceptive pills may increase the risk of breast cancer. Several studies show that concomitant administration of progesterone and estrogen to postmenopausal women may markedly increase the incidence of breast cancer, compared with the use of estrogen alone or with no hormone replacement treatment. The Women's Health Initiative prospective randomized study of hormone replacement therapy stopped treatment with estrogen and progesterone early because of an increased risk of breast cancer compared with untreated women or women treated with estrogen alone. Alcohol consumption, high dietary intake of fat, and lack of exercise may also increase the risk of breast cancer. Fibrocystic breast condition, when accompanied by proliferative changes, papillomatosis, or atypical epithelial hyperplasia, and increased breast density on mammogram are also associated with an increased incidence. A woman who had cancer in one breast is at increased risk for cancer developing in the other breast. In these women, a contralateral cancer develops at the rate of 1% or 2% per year. Women with cancer of the uterine corpus have a risk of breast cancer significantly higher than that of the general population, and women with breast cancer have a comparably increased risk of endometrial cancer. Socioeconomic and racial factors have also been associated with breast cancer risk. Breast cancer tends to be diagnosed more frequently in women of higher socioeconomic status and is more frequent in white women than in black women.

Women at greater than average risk for developing breast cancer (Table 17–2) should be identified by their practitioners and monitored carefully. Risk assessment models have been developed and several have been

Table 17–2. Factors associated with increased risk of breast cancer.

Race	White
Age	Older
Family history	Breast cancer in parent, sibling, or child (especially bilateral or premenopausal)
Genetics	*BRCA1* or *BRCA2* mutation
Previous medical history	Endometrial cancer Proliferative forms of fibrocystic disease Cancer in other breast
Menstrual history	Early menarche (under age 12) Late menopause (after age 50)
Reproductive history	Nulliparous or late first pregnancy

validated (most extensively the Gail 2 model) to evaluate a woman's risk of developing cancer. Those with an exceptional family history should be counseled about the option of genetic testing. Some of these high-risk women may consider prophylactic mastectomy, oophorectomy, or tamoxifen, an FDA-approved preventive agent. The Prevention and Observation of Surgical Endpoints (PROSE) consortium monitored women with deleterious *BRCA1/2* mutations from 1974 to 2008 and reported that 15% of women with a known *BRCA* mutation underwent bilateral prophylactic mastectomy, and none of them developed breast cancer during the 3 years of follow-up. In contrast, subsequent breast cancer developed in 98 (7%) of the 1372 women who did not have surgery. Moreover, women who underwent prophylactic salpingo-oophorectomy had a lower risk of ovarian cancer, all-cause mortality, as well as breast cancer- and ovarian cancer-specific mortality.

Women with genetic mutations in whom breast cancer develops may be treated in the same way as women who do not have mutations (ie, lumpectomy), though there is an increased risk of ipsilateral and contralateral breast cancer after lumpectomy for these women. One study showed that of patients with a diagnosis of breast cancer who were found to be carriers of a *BRCA* mutation, approximately 50% chose to undergo bilateral mastectomy.

Evans et al. Increased rate of phenocopies in all age groups in BRCA1/BRCA2 mutation kindred, but increased prospective breast cancer risk is confined to BRCA2 mutation carriers. Cancer Epidemiol Biomarkers Prev. 2013 Dec;22(12):2269–76. [PMID: 24285840]

Zheng JS et al. Intake of fish and marine n-3 polyunsaturated fatty acids and risk of breast cancer: meta-analysis of data from 21 independent prospective cohort studies. BMJ. 2013 Jun 27;346:f3706. [PMID: 23814120]

▶ Prevention

Several clinical trials have evaluated the use of selective estrogen receptor modulators (SERMs), including tamoxifen and raloxifene, for prevention of breast cancer in women with no personal history of breast cancer but at high risk for developing the disease. A meta-analysis of nine of these studies including 83,399 women with a median follow-up of 65 months demonstrated a 38% reduction in breast cancer incidence (hazard ratio [HR], 0.62; 95% CI, 0.56, 0.69) with a 10-year cumulative incidence of 6.3% in control groups and 4.2% in SERM-treated groups. An increased risk of endometrial cancer and venous thromboembolic events but a reduced risk of vertebral fractures was seen in SERM groups. While SERMs have been shown to be effective at reducing the risk of breast cancer, the uptake of this intervention by women has been relatively low, possibly due to the perceived risks and side effects of therapy. A cost-effectiveness study based on a meta-analysis of four randomized prevention trials showed that **tamoxifen saves costs and improves life expectancy when higher risk (Gail 5-year risk at least 1.66%) women under the age of 55 years were treated.**

Similar to SERMs, aromatase inhibitors (AIs), such as exemestane and anastrozole, have shown success in preventing breast cancer with a lower risk of uterine cancer and thromboembolic events, although bone loss is a significant side effect of this treatment.

Collaborative Group on Hormonal Factors in Breast Cancer. Menarche, menopause, and breast cancer risk: individual participant meta-analysis, including 118 964 women with breast cancer from 117 epidemiological studies. Lancet Oncol. 2012 Nov;13(11):1141–51. [PMID: 23084519]

Cuzick J et al; IBIS-II investigators. Anastrozole for prevention of breast cancer in high-risk postmenopausal women (IBIS-II): an international, double-blind, randomised placebo-controlled trial. Lancet. 2014 Mar 22;383(9922):1041–8. [PMID: 24333009]

Cuzick J et al; SERM Chemoprevention of Breast Cancer Overview Group. Selective oestrogen receptor modulators in prevention of breast cancer: an updated meta-analysis of individual participant data. Lancet. 2013 May 25;381(9880):1827–34. [PMID: 23639488]

Desantis C et al. Breast Cancer Statistics, 2013. CA Cancer J Clin. 2014 Jan-Feb;64(1):52–62. [PMID: 24114568]

Eheman C et al. Annual Report to the Nation on the status of cancer, 1975–2008, featuring cancers associated with excess weight and lack of sufficient physical activity. Cancer. 2012 May 1;118(9):2338–66. [PMID: 22460733]

Goss PE et al; CTG MAP.3 Study Investigators. Exemestane for breast-cancer prevention in postmenopausal women. N Engl J Med. 2011 Jun 23;364(25):2381–91. [PMID: 21639806]

Schwartz MD et al. Long-term outcomes of BRCA1/BRCA2 testing: risk reduction and surveillance. Cancer. 2012 Jan 15;118(2):510–7. [PMID: 21717445]

▶ Early Detection of Breast Cancer

A. Screening Programs

A number of large screening programs, consisting of physical and mammographic examination of asymptomatic women, have been conducted over the years. On average, these programs identify 10 cancers per 1000 women over the age of 50 and 2 cancers per 1000 women under the age of 50. Screening detects cancer before it has spread to the lymph nodes in about 80% of the women evaluated. This increases the chance of survival to about 85% at 5 years.

About one-third of the abnormalities detected on screening mammograms will be found to be malignant when biopsy is performed. The probability of cancer on a screening mammogram is directly related to the Breast Imaging Reporting and Data System (BIRADS) assessment, and work-up should be performed based on this classification. Women 20–40 years of age should have a breast examination as part of routine medical care every 2–3 years. Women over age 40 years should have annual breast examinations. The sensitivity of mammography varies from approximately 60% to 90%. This sensitivity depends on several factors, including patient age (breast density) and tumor size, location, and mammographic appearance. In young women with dense breasts, mammography is less sensitive than in older women with fatty breasts, in whom mammography can detect at least 90% of malignancies. Smaller tumors, particularly those without calcifications, are more difficult to detect, especially in dense breasts. The lack of sensitivity and the low incidence of breast cancer in young women have led to questions concerning the value of mammography for screening in women 40–50 years of age. The specificity of mammography in women under 50 years varies from about 30% to 40% for nonpalpable mammographic abnormalities to 85% to 90% for clinically evident malignancies. In 2009, the US Preventive Services Task Force recommended against routine screening mammography in this age range, and also recommended mammography be performed every 2 years for women between the ages of 50 and 74. The change in recommendation for screening women age 40–50 were particularly controversial in light of several meta-analyses that included women in this age group and showed a 15–20% reduction in the relative risk of death from breast cancer with screening mammography. To add to the controversy, an analysis of the Surveillance, Epidemiology and End Results (SEER) database from 1976 to 2008 suggests that screening mammography has led to substantial increases in the number of breast cancer cases diagnosed but has only had a minor impact on the rate of women presenting with advanced disease. These data should all be taken into consideration when advising a patient about the usefulness of screening mammography. The American Cancer Society continues to recommend yearly mammography for women beginning at the age of 40, continuing as long as good health lasts.

B. Clinical Breast Examination and Self-Examination

Breast self-examination (BSE) has not been shown to improve survival. Because of the lack of strong evidence demonstrating value, the American Cancer Society no longer recommends monthly BSE. While BSE is not a recommended practice, patients should recognize and report any breast changes to their clinicians as it remains an important facet of proactive care. In contrast to BSE, the American Cancer Society recommends CBE every 3 years in women ages 20–39 and annually starting at the age of 40. Although studies have not consistently shown any additional benefit of CBE over routine screening mammography, CBE should be performed.

C. Imaging

Mammography is the most reliable means of detecting breast cancer before a mass can be palpated. Most slowly growing cancers can be identified by mammography at least 2 years before reaching a size detectable by palpation. Film screen mammography delivers < 0.4 cGy to the mid breast per view. Although full-field digital mammography provides an easier method to maintain and review mammograms, it has not been proven that it provides better images or increases detection rates more than film mammography. In subset analysis of a large study, digital mammography seemed slightly superior in women with dense breasts. Computer-assisted detection has not shown any increase in detection of cancers. Tomosynthesis creates tomographic "slices" of the breast volume with a single acquisition. This technique may improve the sensitivity of mammogram especially in patients with dense breast tissue.

Calcifications are the most easily recognized mammographic abnormality. The most common findings associated with carcinoma of the breast are clustered pleomorphic microcalcifications. Such calcifications are usually at least five to eight in number, aggregated in one part of the breast and differing from each other in size and shape, often including branched or V- or Y-shaped configurations. There may be an associated mammographic mass density or, at times, only a mass density with no calcifications. Such a density usually has irregular or ill-defined borders and may lead to architectural distortion within the breast but may be subtle and difficult to detect.

Indications for mammography are as follows: (1) to screen at regular intervals asymptomatic women at high risk for developing breast cancer (see above); (2) to evaluate each breast when a diagnosis of potentially curable breast cancer has been made, and at regular intervals thereafter; (3) to evaluate a questionable or ill-defined breast mass or other suspicious change in the breast; (4) to search for an occult breast cancer in a woman with metastatic disease in axillary nodes or elsewhere from an unknown primary; (5) to screen women prior to cosmetic operations or prior to biopsy of a mass, to examine for an unsuspected cancer; (6) to monitor those women with breast cancer who have been treated with breast-conserving surgery and radiation; and (7) to monitor the contralateral breast in those women with breast cancer treated with mastectomy.

Patients with a dominant or suspicious mass on examination must undergo biopsy despite mammographic findings. The mammogram should be obtained prior to biopsy so that other suspicious areas can be noted and the contralateral breast can be evaluated. Mammography is never a substitute for biopsy because it may not reveal clinical cancer, especially in a very dense breast, as may be seen in young women with fibrocystic changes, and may not reveal medullary cancers.

Communication and documentation among the patient, the referring practitioner, and the interpreting physician are critical for high-quality screening and diagnostic mammography. The patient should be told about *how* she will receive timely results of her mammogram; that mammography does not "rule out" cancer; and that she may receive a correlative examination such as ultrasound at the mammography facility if referred for a suspicious lesion. She should also be aware of the technique and need for breast compression and that this may be uncomfortable. The mammography facility should be informed in writing by the clinician of abnormal physical examination findings. The Agency for Health Care Policy and Research (AHCPR) Clinical Practice Guidelines strongly recommend that all mammography reports be communicated in writing to the patient and referring practitioner. Legislation has been passed in a number of US states that requires imaging facilities to report to patients the density of their breasts. This may prompt women with dense breasts to discuss with their clinician whether or not additional screening options would be appropriate in addition to mammogram.

MRI and ultrasound may be useful screening modalities in women who are at high risk for breast cancer but not for the general population. The sensitivity of MRI is much higher than mammography; however, the specificity is significantly lower and this results in multiple unnecessary biopsies. The increased sensitivity despite decreased specificity may be considered a reasonable trade-off for those at increased risk for developing breast cancer but not for normal-risk population. In 2009, the National Comprehensive Cancer Network (NCCN) guidelines recommended MRI in addition to screening mammography for high-risk women, including those with *BRCA1/2* mutations, those who have a lifetime risk of breast cancer of > 20%, and those with a personal history of LCIS. Women who received radiation therapy to the chest in their teens or twenties are also known to be at high risk for developing breast cancer and screening MRI may be considered in addition to mammography. MRI is useful in women with breast implants to determine the character of a lesion present in the breast and to search for implant rupture and at times is helpful in patients with prior lumpectomy and radiation.

Bleyer A et al. Effect of three decades of screening mammography on breast-cancer incidence. N Engl J Med. 2012 Nov 22;367(21):1998–2005. [PMID: 23171096]

Drukteinis JS et al. Beyond mammography: new frontiers in breast cancer screening. Am J Med. 2013 Jun;126(6):472–9. [PMID: 23561631]

Gross CP et al. The cost of breast cancer screening in the Medicare population. JAMA Intern Med. 2013 Feb 11;173(3):220–6. [PMID: 23303200]

Hendrick RE et al. United States Preventive Services Task Force screening mammography recommendations: science ignored. AJR Am J Roentgenol. 2011 Feb;196(2):W112–6. [PMID: 21257850]

Independent UK Panel on Breast Cancer Screening. The benefits and harms of breast cancer screening: an independent review. Lancet. 2012 Nov 17;380(9855):1778–86. [PMID: 23117178]

Morrow M et al. MRI for breast cancer screening, diagnosis, and treatment. Lancet. 2011 Nov 19;378(9805):1804–11. [PMID: 22098853]

Plescia M et al. The National Prevention Strategy and breast cancer screening: scientific evidence for public health action. Am J Public Health. 2013 Sep;103(9):1545–8. [PMID: 23865665]

Tria Tirona M. Breast cancer screening update. Am Fam Physician. 2013 Feb 15;87(4):274–8. [PMID: 23418799]

Warner E. Clinical practice. Breast-cancer screening. N Engl J Med. 2011 Sep 15;365(11):1025–32. [PMID: 21916640]

► Clinical Findings Associated with Early Detection of Breast Cancer

A. Symptoms and Signs

The presenting complaint in about 70% of patients with breast cancer is a lump (usually painless) in the breast. About 90% of these breast masses are discovered by the patient. Less frequent symptoms are breast pain; nipple discharge; erosion, retraction, enlargement, or itching of the nipple; and redness, generalized hardness, enlargement, or shrinking of the breast. Rarely, an axillary mass or swelling of the arm may be the first symptom. Back or bone pain, jaundice, or weight loss may be the result of systemic metastases, but these symptoms are rarely seen on initial presentation.

The relative frequency of carcinoma in various anatomic sites in the breast is shown in Figure 17–2.

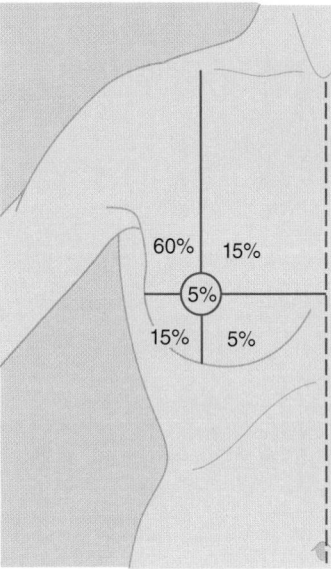

▲ **Figure 17–2.** Frequency of breast carcinoma at various anatomic sites.

Inspection of the breast is the first step in physical examination and should be carried out with the patient sitting, arms at her sides and then overhead. Abnormal variations in breast size and contour, minimal nipple retraction, and slight edema, redness, or retraction of the skin can be identified (Figure 17–3). Asymmetry of the breasts and retraction or dimpling of the skin can often be accentuated by having the patient raise her arms overhead or press her hands on her hips to contract the pectoralis muscles. Axillary and supraclavicular areas should be thoroughly palpated for enlarged nodes with the patient sitting (Figure 17–4). Palpation of the breast for masses or other changes should be performed with the patient both seated

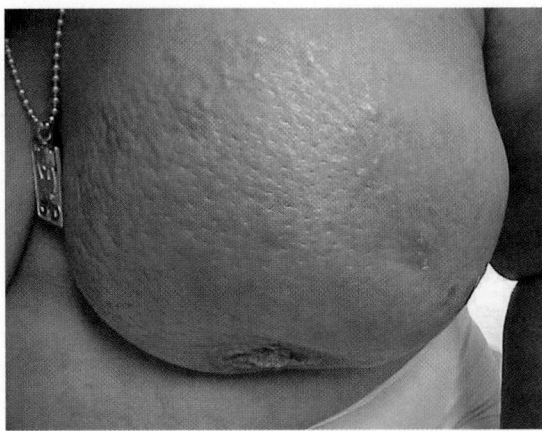

▲ **Figure 17–3.** Peau d'orange sign (resemblance to the skin of an orange due to lymphedema) in advanced breast cancer. (Reproduced with permission, from Richard P. Usatine, MD.)

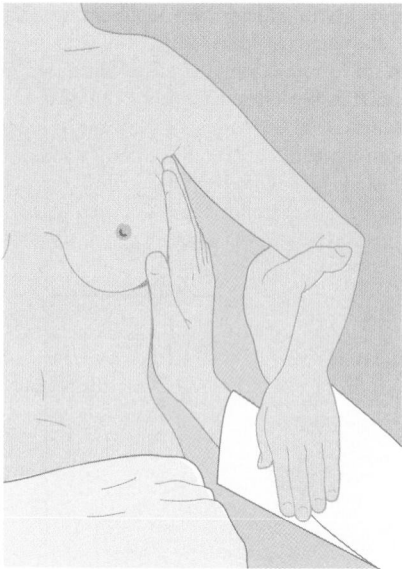

▲ **Figure 17–4.** Palpation of axillary region for enlarged lymph nodes.

and supine with the arm abducted (Figure 17–5). Palpation with a rotary motion of the examiner's fingers as well as a horizontal stripping motion has been recommended.

Breast cancer usually consists of a nontender, firm or hard mass with poorly delineated margins (caused by local infiltration). Very small (1–2 mm) erosions of the nipple epithelium may be the only manifestation of Paget disease of the breast. Watery, serous, or bloody discharge from the nipple is an occasional early sign but is more often associated with benign disease.

A small lesion, < 1 cm in diameter, may be difficult or impossible for the examiner to feel but may be discovered by the patient. She should always be asked to demonstrate the location of the mass; if the practitioner fails to confirm the patient's suspicions and imaging studies are normal, the examination should be repeated in 2–3 months, preferably 1–2 weeks after the onset of menses. During the

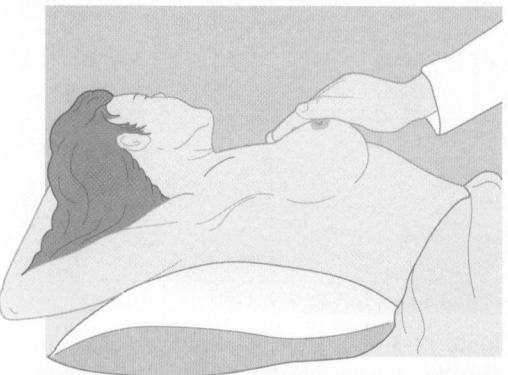

▲ **Figure 17–5.** Palpation of breasts. Palpation is performed with the patient supine and arm abducted.

premenstrual phase of the cycle, increased innocuous nodularity may suggest neoplasm or may obscure an underlying lesion. If there is any question regarding the nature of an abnormality under these circumstances, the patient should be asked to return after her menses. Ultrasound is often valuable and mammography essential when an area is felt by the patient to be abnormal but the physician feels no mass. MRI may be considered, but the lack of specificity should be discussed by the clinician and the patient. MRI should not be used to rule out cancer because MRI has a false-negative rate of about 3–5%. Although lower than mammography, this false-negative rate cannot permit safe elimination of the possibility of cancer. False negatives are more likely seen in infiltrating lobular carcinomas and DCIS.

Metastases tend to involve regional lymph nodes, which may be palpable. One or two movable, nontender, not particularly firm axillary lymph nodes 5 mm or less in diameter are frequently present and are generally of no significance. Firm or hard nodes larger than 1 cm are typical of metastases. Axillary nodes that are matted or fixed to skin or deep structures indicate advanced disease (at least stage III). On the other hand, if the examiner thinks that the axillary nodes are involved, that impression will be borne out by histologic section in about 85% of cases. The incidence of positive axillary nodes increases with the size of the primary tumor. Noninvasive cancers (in situ) do not metastasize. Metastases are present in about 30% of patients with clinically negative nodes.

In most cases, no nodes are palpable in the supraclavicular fossa. Firm or hard nodes of any size in this location or just beneath the clavicle should be biopsied. Ipsilateral supraclavicular or infraclavicular nodes containing cancer indicate that the tumor is in an advanced stage (stage III or IV). Edema of the ipsilateral arm, commonly caused by metastatic infiltration of regional lymphatics, is also a sign of advanced cancer.

B. Laboratory Findings

Liver or bone metastases may be associated with elevation of serum alkaline phosphatase. Hypercalcemia is an occasional important finding in advanced cancer of the breast. Carcinoembryonic antigen (CEA) and CA 15-3 or CA 27-29 may be used as markers for recurrent breast cancer but are not helpful in diagnosing early lesions.

C. Imaging for Metastases

For patients with suspicious symptoms or signs (bone pain, abdominal symptoms, elevated liver biochemical tests) or locally advanced disease (clinically abnormal lymph nodes or large primary tumors), staging scans are indicated prior to surgery or systemic therapy. Chest imaging with CT or radiographs may be done to evaluate for pulmonary metastases. Abdominal imaging with CT or ultrasound may be obtained to evaluate for liver metastases. Bone scans using ^{99m}Tc-labeled phosphates or phosphonates are more sensitive than skeletal radiographs in detecting metastatic breast cancer. Bone scanning has not proved to be of clinical value as a routine preoperative test in the absence of symptoms, physical findings, or abnormal alkaline phosphatase or calcium levels. The frequency of abnormal findings on bone scan parallels the status of the axillary lymph nodes on pathologic examination. Positron emission tomography (PET) scanning alone or combined with CT (PET-CT) is effective for detecting soft tissue or visceral metastases in patients with symptoms or signs of metastatic disease.

D. Diagnostic Tests

1. Biopsy—The diagnosis of breast cancer depends ultimately on examination of tissue or cells removed by biopsy. Treatment should never be undertaken without an unequivocal histologic or cytologic diagnosis of cancer. **The safest course is biopsy examination of all suspicious lesions found on physical examination or mammography, or both.** About 60% of lesions clinically thought to be cancer prove on biopsy to be benign, while about 30% of clinically benign lesions are found to be malignant. These findings demonstrate the fallibility of clinical judgment and the necessity for biopsy.

All breast masses require a histologic diagnosis with one probable exception, a nonsuspicious, presumably fibrocystic mass, in a premenopausal woman. Rather, these masses can be observed through one or two menstrual cycles. However, if the mass is not cystic and does not completely resolve during this time, it must be biopsied. Figures 17–6 and 17–7 present algorithms for management of breast masses in premenopausal and postmenopausal patients.

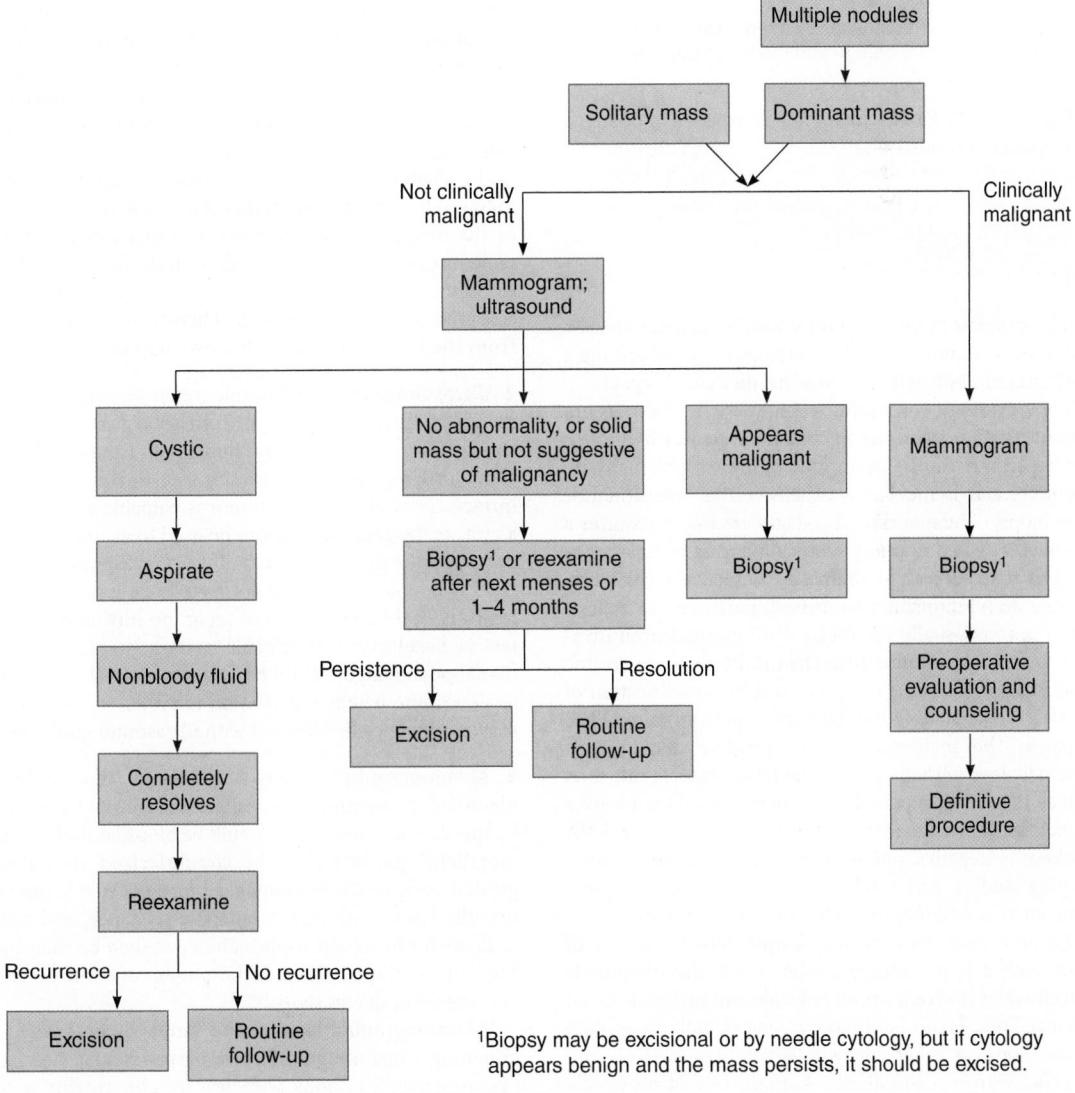

▲ **Figure 17–6.** Evaluation of breast masses in premenopausal women. (Adapted, with permission, from Chang S, Haigh PI, Giuliano AE. Breast disease. In: Berek JS, Hacker NF [editors], *Practical Gynecologic Oncology*, 4th edition, LWW, 2004.)

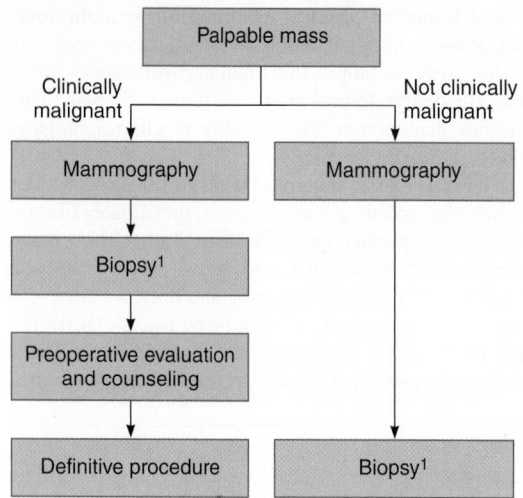

^{1}Biopsy may be excisional or by needle cytology, but if cytology appears benign and the mass persists, it should be excised.

▲ **Figure 17–7.** Evaluation of breast masses in post-menopausal women. (Adapted, with permission, from Chang S, Haigh PI, Giuliano AE. Breast disease. In: Berek JS, Hacker NF [editors], *Practical Gynecologic Oncology*, 4th edition, LWW, 2004.)

The simplest biopsy method is needle biopsy, either by aspiration of tumor cells (FNA cytology) or by obtaining a small core of tissue with a hollow needle (core biopsy).

FNA cytology is a useful technique whereby cells are aspirated with a small needle and examined cytologically. This technique can be performed easily with virtually no morbidity and is much less expensive than excisional or open biopsy. The main disadvantages are that it requires a pathologist skilled in the cytologic diagnosis of breast cancer and it is subject to sampling problems, particularly because deep lesions may be missed. Furthermore, noninvasive cancers usually cannot be distinguished from invasive cancers and immunohistochemical tests to determine expression of hormone receptors and the amplification of the HER2 oncogene cannot be reliably performed on FNA biopsies. The incidence of false-positive diagnoses is extremely low, perhaps 1–2%. The false-negative rate is as high as 10%. Most experienced clinicians would not leave a suspicious dominant mass in the breast even when FNA cytology is negative unless the clinical diagnosis, breast imaging studies, and cytologic studies were all in agreement, such as a fibrocystic lesion or fibroadenoma.

Large-needle (core needle) biopsy removes a core of tissue with a large cutting needle and is **the diagnostic procedure of choice** for both palpable and image-detected abnormalities. Hand-held biopsy devices make large-core needle biopsy of a palpable mass easy and cost effective in the office with local anesthesia. As in the case of any needle biopsy, the main problem is sampling error due to improper positioning of the needle, giving rise to a false-negative test result. This is extremely unusual with image-guided

biopsies. Core biopsy allows the tumor to be tested for the expression of biological markers, such as estrogen receptor (ER), progesterone receptor (PR) and HER2.

Open biopsy under local anesthesia as a separate procedure prior to deciding upon definitive treatment is becoming less common with the increasing use of core needle biopsy. Needle biopsy, when positive, offers a more rapid approach with less expense and morbidity, but when nondiagnostic it must be followed by open biopsy. It generally consists of an excisional biopsy, which is done through an incision with the intent to remove the entire abnormality, not simply a sample. Additional evaluation for metastatic disease and therapeutic options can be discussed with the patient after the histologic or cytologic diagnosis of cancer has been established. As an alternative in highly suspicious circumstances, the diagnosis may be made on frozen section of tissue obtained by open biopsy under general anesthesia. If the frozen section is positive, the surgeon can proceed immediately with the definitive operation. This one-step method is rarely used today except when a cytologic study has suggested cancer but is not diagnostic and there is a high clinical suspicion of malignancy in a patient well prepared for the diagnosis of cancer and its treatment options.

In general, the two-step approach—outpatient biopsy followed by definitive operation at a later date—is preferred in the diagnosis and treatment of breast cancer, because patients can be given time to adjust to the diagnosis of cancer, can consider alternative forms of therapy, and can seek a second opinion if they wish. **There is no adverse effect from the few week delay of the two-step procedure.**

2. Ultrasonography—Ultrasonography is performed primarily to differentiate cystic from solid lesions but may show signs suggestive of carcinoma. Ultrasonography may show an irregular mass within a cyst in the rare case of intracystic carcinoma. If a tumor is palpable and feels like a cyst, an 18-gauge needle can be used to aspirate the fluid and make the diagnosis of cyst. If a cyst is aspirated and the fluid is nonbloody, it does not have to be examined cytologically. If the mass does not recur, no further diagnostic test is necessary. Nonpalpable mammographic densities that appear benign should be investigated with ultrasound to determine whether the lesion is cystic or solid. These may even be needle biopsied with ultrasound guidance.

3. Mammography—When a suspicious abnormality is identified by mammography alone and cannot be palpated by the clinician, the lesion should be biopsied under mammographic guidance. In the **computerized stereotactic guided core needle** technique, a biopsy needle is inserted into the lesion with mammographic guidance, and a core of tissue for histologic examination can then be examined. Vacuum assistance increases the amount of tissue obtained and improves diagnosis.

Mammographic localization biopsy is performed by obtaining a mammogram in two perpendicular views and placing a needle or hook-wire near the abnormality so that the surgeon can use the metal needle or wire as a guide during operation to locate the lesion. After mammography confirms the position of the needle in relation to the lesion, an incision is made and the subcutaneous tissue is dissected until the needle is identified. Often, the abnormality cannot even be palpated through the incision—as is the case with microcalcifications—and thus it is essential to obtain a mammogram of the specimen to document that the lesion was excised. At that time, a second marker needle can further localize the lesion for the pathologist. Stereotactic core needle biopsies have proved equivalent to mammographic localization biopsies. Core biopsy is preferable to mammographic localization for accessible lesions since an operation can be avoided. A metal clip should be placed after any image-guided core biopsy to facilitate finding the site of the lesion if subsequent treatment is necessary.

4. Other imaging modalities—Other modalities of breast imaging have been investigated for diagnostic purposes. Automated breast ultrasonography is useful in distinguishing cystic from solid lesions but should be used only as a supplement to physical examination and mammography. Ductography may be useful to define the site of a lesion causing a bloody discharge, but since biopsy is almost always indicated, ductography may be omitted and the blood-filled nipple system excised. Ductoscopy has shown some promise in identifying intraductal lesions, especially in the case of pathologic nipple discharge, but in practice, this technique is rarely used. MRI is highly sensitive but not specific and should not be used for screening except in highly selective cases. For example, MRI is useful in differentiating scar from recurrence postlumpectomy and may be valuable to screen high-risk women (eg, women with *BRCA* mutations). It may also be of value to examine for multicentricity when there is a known primary cancer; to examine the contralateral breast in women with cancer; to examine the extent of cancer, especially lobular carcinomas; or to determine the response to neoadjuvant chemotherapy. Moreover, MRI-detected suspicious findings that are not seen on mammogram or ultrasound may be biopsied under MRI-guidance. PET scanning does not appear useful in evaluating the breast itself but is useful to examine for distant metastases.

5. Cytology—Cytologic examination of nipple discharge or cyst fluid may be helpful on rare occasions. As a rule, mammography (or ductography) and breast biopsy are required when nipple discharge or cyst fluid is bloody or cytologically questionable.

▶ Differential Diagnosis

The lesions to be considered most often in the differential diagnosis of breast cancer are the following, in descending order of frequency: fibrocystic condition of the breast, fibroadenoma, intraductal papilloma, lipoma, and fat necrosis.

▶ Staging

The American Joint Committee on Cancer and the International Union Against Cancer have agreed on a TNM (tumor, regional lymph nodes, distant metastases) staging system for breast cancer. Using the TNM staging system

enhances communication between researchers and clinicians. Table 17–3 outlines the TNM classification.

▶ Pathologic Types

Numerous pathologic subtypes of breast cancer can be identified histologically (Table 17–4).

Except for the in situ cancers, the histologic subtypes have only a slight bearing on prognosis when outcomes are compared after accurate staging. The noninvasive cancers by definition are confined by the basement membrane of the ducts and lack the ability to spread. Histologic parameters for invasive cancers, including lymphovascular invasion and tumor grade, have been shown to be of prognostic value. Immunohistochemical analysis for expression of hormone receptors and for overexpression of *HER2* in the primary tumor offers prognostic and therapeutic information.

▶ Special Clinical Forms of Breast Cancer

A. Paget Carcinoma

Paget carcinoma is not common (about 1% of all breast cancers). Over 85% of cases are associated with an underlying invasive or noninvasive cancer, usually a well differentiated infiltrating ductal carcinoma or a DCIS. The ducts of the nipple epithelium are infiltrated, but gross nipple changes are often minimal, and a tumor mass may not be palpable.

Because the nipple changes appear innocuous, the diagnosis is frequently missed. The first symptom is often itching or burning of the nipple, with superficial erosion or ulceration. These are often diagnosed and treated as dermatitis or bacterial infection, leading to delay or failure in detection. The diagnosis is established by biopsy of the area of erosion. When the lesion consists of nipple changes only, the incidence of axillary metastases is < 5%, and the prognosis is excellent. When a breast mass is also present, the incidence of axillary metastases rises, with an associated marked decrease in prospects for cure by surgical or other treatment.

B. Inflammatory Carcinoma

This is the most malignant form of breast cancer and constitutes < 3% of all cases. The clinical findings consist of a rapidly growing, sometimes painful mass that enlarges the breast. The overlying skin becomes erythematous, edematous, and warm. Often there is no distinct mass, since the tumor infiltrates the involved breast diffusely. The inflammatory changes, often mistaken for an infection, are caused by carcinomatous invasion of the subdermal lymphatics, with resulting edema and hyperemia. If the clinician suspects infection but the lesion does not respond rapidly (1–2 weeks) to antibiotics, biopsy should be performed. The diagnosis should be made when the redness involves more than one-third of the skin over the breast and biopsy shows infiltrating carcinoma with invasion of the subdermal lymphatics. Metastases tend to occur early and widely, and for this reason inflammatory carcinoma is rarely curable. Radiation, hormone therapy (if hormone

Table 17–3. TNM staging for breast cancer.

Primary Tumor (T)	
Definitions for classifying the primary tumor (T) are the same for clinical and for pathologic classification. If the measurement is made by physical examination, the examiner will use the major headings (T1, T2, or T3). If other measurements, such as mammographic or pathologic measurements, are used, the subsets of T1 can be used. Tumors should be measured to the nearest 0.1 cm increment.	
TX	Primary tumor cannot be assessed
T0	No evidence of primary tumor
Tis	Carcinoma in situ
Tis (DCIS)	Ductal carcinoma in situ
Tis (LCIS)	Lobular carcinoma in situ
Tis (Paget)	Paget disease of the nipple with no tumor
Note: Paget disease associated with a tumor is classified according to the size of the tumor.	
T1	Tumor 2 cm or less in greatest dimension
T1mic	Microinvasion 0.1 cm or less in greatest dimension
T1a	Tumor more than 0.1 cm but not more than 0.5 cm in greatest dimension
T1b	Tumor more than 0.5 cm but not more than 1 cm in greatest dimension
T1c	Tumor more than 1 cm but not more than 2 cm in greatest dimension
T2	Tumor more than 2 cm but not more than 5 cm in greatest dimension
T3	Tumor more than 5 cm in greatest dimension
T4	Tumor of any size with direct extension to (a) chest wall or (b) skin, only as described below
T4a	Extension to chest wall, not including pectoralis muscle
T4b	Edema (including peau d'orange [see Figure 17–3]) or ulceration of the skin of the breast, or satellite skin nodules confined to the same breast
T4c	Both T4a and T4b
T4d	Inflammatory carcinoma
Regional Lymph Nodes (N)	
Clinical	
NX	Regional lymph nodes cannot be assessed (eg, previously removed)
N0	No regional lymph node metastasis
N1	Metastasis in movable ipsilateral axillary lymph node(s)
N2	Metastases in ipsilateral axillary lymph nodes fixed or matted, or in clinically apparent[1] ipsilateral internal mammary nodes in the *absence* of clinically evident axillary lymph node metastasis
N2a	Metastasis in ipsilateral axillary lymph nodes fixed to one another (matted) or to other structures

N2b	Metastasis only in clinically apparent[1] ipsilateral internal mammary nodes and in the *absence* of clinically evident axillary lymph node metastasis
N3	Metastasis in ipsilateral infraclavicular lymph node(s) with or without axillary lymph node involvement, or in clinically apparent[1] ipsilateral internal mammary lymph node(s) and in the *presence* of clinically evident axillary lymph node metastasis; or metastasis in ipsilateral supraclavicular lymph node(s) with or without axillary or internal mammary lymph node involvement
N3a	Metastasis in ipsilateral infraclavicular lymph node(s)
N3b	Metastasis in ipsilateral internal mammary lymph node(s) and axillary lymph node(s)
N3c	Metastasis in ipsilateral supraclavicular lymph node(s)
Regional Lymph Nodes (pN)[2]	
pNX	Regional lymph nodes cannot be assessed (eg, previously removed, or not removed for pathologic study)
pN0	No regional lymph node metastasis histologically, no-additional examination for isolated tumor cells
Note: Isolated tumor cells (ITC) are defined as single tumor cells or small cell clusters not > 0.2 mm, usually detected only by immunohistochemical (IHC) or molecular methods but which may be verified on hematoxylin and eosin stains. ITCs do not usually show evidence of malignant activity, eg, proliferation or stromal reaction.	
pN0(i−)	No regional lymph node metastasis histologically, negative IHC
pN0(i+)	No regional lymph node metastasis histologically, positive IHC, no IHC cluster > 0.2 mm
pN0(mol−)	No regional lymph node metastasis histologically, negative molecular findings (RT-PCR)[3]
pN0(mol+)	No regional lymph node metastasis histologically, positive molecular findings (RT-PCR)[3]
pN1	Metastasis in one to three axillary lymph nodes, and/or in internal mammary nodes with microscopic disease detected by sentinel lymph node dissection but not clinically apparent[4]
pN1mi	Micrometastasis (> 0.2 mm, none > 2.0 mm)
pN1a	Metastasis in one to three axillary lymph nodes
pN1b	Metastasis in internal mammary nodes with microscopic disease detected by sentinel lymph node dissection but not clinically apparent[4]
pN1c	Metastasis in one to three axillary lymph nodes and in internal mammary lymph nodes with microscopic disease detected by sentinel lymph node dissection but not clinically apparent.[4] (If associated with greater than three positive axillary lymph nodes, the internal mammary nodes are classified as pN3b to reflect increased tumor burden)

(continued)

Table 17–3. TNM staging for breast cancer. (continued)

pN2	Metastasis in four to nine axillary lymph nodes, or in clinically apparent[1] internal mammary lymph nodes in the absence of axillary lymph node metastasis	**Distant Metastasis (M)**		
		MX	Distant metastasis cannot be assessed	
		M0	No distant metastasis	
pN2a	Metastasis in four to nine axillary lymph nodes (at least one tumor deposit > 2.0 mm)	M1	Distant metastasis	
		Stage Grouping		
pN2b	Metastasis in clinically apparent[1] internal mammary lymph nodes in the absence of axillary lymph node metastasis	Stage 0	Tis	N0	M0
		Stage 1	T1[5]	N0	M0
pN3	Metastasis in 10 or more axillary lymph nodes, or in infraclavicular lymph nodes, or in clinically apparent[1] ipsilateral internal mammary lymph nodes in the presence of one or more positive axillary lymph nodes; or in more than three axillary lymph nodes with clinically negative microscopic metastasis in internal mammary lymph nodes; or in ipsilateral supraclavicular lymph nodes	Stage IIA	T0 / T1[5] / T2	N1 / N1 / N0	M0 / M0 / M0
		Stage IIB	T2 / T3	N1 / N0	M0 / M0
		Stage IIIA	T0 / T1[5] / T2 / T3 / T3	N2 / N2 / N2 / N1 / N2	M0 / M0 / M0 / M0 / M0
pN3a	Metastasis in 10 or more axillary lymph nodes(at least one tumor deposit > 2.0 mm), or metastasis to the infraclavicular lymph nodes	Stage IIIB	T4 / T4 / T4	N0 / N1 / N2	M0 / M0 / M0
pN3b	Metastasis in clinically apparent[1] ipsilateral internal mammary lymph nodes in the presence of one or more positive axillary lymph nodes; or in more than three axillary lymph nodes and in internal mammary lymph nodes with microscopic disease detected by sentinel lymph node dissection but not clinically apparent[4]	Stage IIIC	Any T	N3	M0
		Stage IV	Any T	Any N	M1
pN3c	Metastasis in ipsilateral supraclavicular lymph nodes	**Note:** Stage designation may be changed if postsurgical imaging studies reveal the presence of distant metastases, provided that the studies are carried out within 4 months of diagnosis in the absence of disease progression and provided that the patient has not received neoadjuvant therapy.		

[1]*Clinically apparent* is defined as detected by imaging studies (excluding lymphoscintigraphy) or by clinical examination or grossly visible pathologically.

[2]Classification is based on axillary lymph node dissection with or without sentinel lymph node dissection. Classification based solely on sentinel lymph node dissection without subsequent axillary lymph node dissection is designated (sn) for "sentinel node," eg, pN0(i+)(sn).

[3]RT-PCR, reverse transcriptase/polymerase chain reaction.

[4]*Not clinically apparent* is defined as not detected by imaging studies (excluding lymphoscintigraphy) or by clinical examination.

[5]T1 includes T1mic.

Reproduced, with permission, of the American Joint Committee on Cancer (AJCC), Chicago, Illinois, *AJCC Cancer Staging Manual*, 7th edition, Springer-Science and Business Media LLC, New York, 2010, www.springer.com.

receptor positive), anti-HER2 therapy (if HER2 overexpressing or amplified), and chemotherapy are the measures most likely to be of value initially rather than operation. Mastectomy is indicated when chemotherapy and radiation have resulted in clinical remission with no evidence of distant metastases. In these cases, residual disease in the breast may be eradicated.

▶ **Breast Cancer Occurring during Pregnancy or Lactation**

Breast cancer complicates approximately one in 3000 pregnancies. The diagnosis is frequently delayed, because physiologic changes in the breast may obscure the lesion and screening mammography is not done in young or pregnant women. When the cancer is confined to the breast, the 5-year survival rate is about 70%. In 60–70% of patients, axillary metastases are already present, conferring a 5-year survival rate of 30–40%. A retrospective analysis of women who were younger than 36 years when breast cancer was diagnosed showed that while women with pregnancy-associated breast cancer were more frequently diagnosed with later stage breast cancer, they had similar rates of local regional recurrence, distant metastases and overall survival as women with nonpregnancy-associated breast cancer. **It is thus important for primary care and reproductive specialists to aggressively work up any breast abnormality discovered in a pregnant woman.** Pregnancy (or lactation) is not a contraindication to operation or treatment, and therapy should be based on the stage of the disease as in the nonpregnant (or nonlactating) woman. Overall survival rates have improved, since cancers are now diagnosed in pregnant women earlier than in the past and treatment has improved. Breast-conserving surgery may be performed—and chemotherapy given—even during the pregnancy.

Table 17–4. Histologic types of breast cancer.

Type	Frequency of Occurrence
Infiltrating ductal (not otherwise specified)	80–90%
Medullary	5–8%
Colloid (mucinous)	2–4%
Tubular	1–2%
Papillary	1–2%
Invasive lobular	6–8%
Noninvasive	4–6%
Intraductal	2–3%
Lobular in situ	2–3%
Rare cancers	< 1%
Juvenile (secretory)	
Adenoid cystic	
Epidermoid	
Sudoriferous	

► Bilateral Breast Cancer

Bilateral breast cancer occurs in < 5% of cases, but there is as high as a 20–25% incidence of later occurrence of cancer in the second breast. Bilaterality occurs more often in familial breast cancer, in women under age 50 years, and when the tumor in the primary breast is lobular. The incidence of second breast cancers increases directly with the length of time the patient is alive after her first cancer—about 1–2% per year.

In patients with breast cancer, mammography should be performed before primary treatment and at regular intervals thereafter, to search for occult cancer in the opposite breast or conserved ipsilateral breast. MRI may be useful in this high-risk group.

► Noninvasive Cancer

Noninvasive cancer can occur within the ducts (DCIS) or lobules (LCIS). DCIS tends to be unilateral and **most often progresses to invasive cancer if untreated.** In approximately 40–60% of women who have DCIS treated with biopsy alone, invasive cancer develops within the same breast. LCIS is generally agreed to be a marker of an increased risk of breast cancer rather than a direct precursor of breast cancer itself. The probability of breast cancer (DCIS or invasive in either breast) in a woman in whom LCIS has been diagnosed is estimated to be 1% per year. If LCIS is detected on core needle biopsy, an excisional biopsy without lymph node sampling should be performed to rule out malignancy, since DCIS or invasive cancer is found in 10–20% of patients. The incidence of LCIS is rising, likely due to increased use of screening mammography. In addition, the rate of mastectomy after the diagnosis of LCIS is increasing in spite of the fact that mastectomy is only recommended in those patients who otherwise have an increased risk of breast cancer through family history, genetic mutation, or past exposure to thoracic radiation. Pleomorphic LCIS may behave more like DCIS and may be associated with invasive carcinoma. For this reason, pleomorphic LCIS should be surgically removed with clear margins.

The treatment of intraductal lesions is controversial. DCIS can be treated by wide excision with or without radiation therapy or with total mastectomy. Conservative management is advised in patients with small lesions amenable to lumpectomy. Patients in whom LCIS is diagnosed or who have received lumpectomy for DCIS may discuss chemoprevention (using a SERM) with their clinician, which is effective in preventing invasive breast cancer in both LCIS and DCIS that has been completely excised by breast conserving surgery. Axillary metastases from in situ cancers should not occur unless there is an occult invasive cancer. Sentinel node biopsy may be indicated in DCIS treated with mastectomy.

Bagaria SP et al. The florid subtype of lobular carcinoma in situ: marker or precursor for invasive lobular carcinoma? Ann Surg Oncol. 2011 Jul;18(7):1845–51. [PMID: 21287281]

Chavez-Macgregor M et al. Male breast cancer according to tumor subtype and race: a population-based study. Cancer. 2013 May 1;119(9):1611–7. [PMID: 23341341]

Colfry AJ 3rd.Miscellaneous syndromes and their management: occult breast cancer, breast cancer in pregnancy, male breast cancer, surgery in stage IV disease. Surg Clin North Am. 2013 Apr;93(2):519–31. [PMID: 23464700]

Portschy PR et al. Trends in incidence and management of lobular carcinoma in situ: a population-based analysis. Ann Surg Oncol. 2013 Oct;20(10):3240–6. [PMID: 23846782]

Rakha EA et al. The prognostic significance of lymphovascular invasion in invasive breast carcinoma. Cancer. 2012 Aug 1; 118(15):3670–80. [PMID: 22180017]

► Biomarkers & Gene Expression Profiling

Determining the ER, PR, and HER2 status of the tumor at the time of diagnosis of early breast cancer and, if possible, at the time of recurrence is critical, both to gauge a patient's prognosis and to determine the best treatment regimen. In addition to ER status and PR status, the rate at which tumor divides (assessed by an immunohistochemical stain for Ki-67) and the grade and differentiation of the cells are also important prognostic factors. These markers may be obtained on core biopsy or surgical specimens, but not reliably on FNA cytology. Patients whose tumors are hormone receptor-positive tend to have a more indolent disease course than those whose tumors are receptor-negative. Moreover, treatment with an anti-hormonal agent is an essential component of therapy for hormone-receptor positive breast cancer at any stage. While up to 60% of patients with metastatic breast cancer will respond to hormonal manipulation if their tumors are ER-positive, < 5% of patients with metastatic, ER-negative tumors will respond.

Another key element in determining treatment and prognosis is the amount of the HER2 oncogene present in the cancer. HER2 overexpression is measured by an immunohistochemical assay that is scored using a numerical system: 0 and 1+ are considered negative for overexpression, 2+ is borderline/indeterminate, and 3+ is over expression. In the case of 2+ expression, fluorescence in situ hybridization (FISH) is recommended to more accurately assess HER2 amplification. Guidelines for the interpretation of HER2 results by IHC and FISH have been published by the College of American Pathologists. According to these guidelines, a tumor is positive for HER2 amplification if one of the criteria is met: (1) the single-probe average HER2 copy number is $\geq$ 6.0 signals/cell or (2) dual-probe HER2/CEP17 ratio is $\geq$ 2.0 with an average HER2 copy number $\geq$ 4.0 signals per cell or (3) dual-probe HER2/CEP17 ratio $\geq$ 2.0 with an average HER2 copy number < 4.0 signals per cell or (4) dual-probe HER2/CEP17 ratio < 2.0 with an average HER2 copy number $\geq$ 6.0 signals/cell. The presence of HER2 amplification and overexpression is of prognostic significance and predicts the response to trastuzumab.

Individually these biomarkers are predictive and thus provide insight to guide appropriate therapy. Moreover, when combined they provide useful information regarding risk of recurrence and prognosis. In general, tumors that lack expression of HER2, ER, and PR ("triple negative") have a higher risk of recurrence and metastases and are associated with a worse survival compared with other types. Neither endocrine therapy nor HER2–targeted agents are useful for this type of breast cancer, leaving chemotherapy as the only treatment option. In contrast, patients with early stage, hormone receptor-positive breast cancer may not benefit from the addition of chemotherapy to hormonal treatments. Several molecular tests have been developed to assess risk of recurrence and to predict which patients are most likely to benefit from chemotherapy.

Cuzick J et al. Prognostic value of a combined estrogen receptor, progesterone receptor, Ki-67, and human epidermal growth factor receptor 2 immunohistochemical score and comparison with the Genomic Health recurrence score in early breast cancer. J Clin Oncol. 2011 Nov 10;29(32):4273–8. [PMID: 21990413]

Galanina N et al. Molecular predictors of response to therapy for breast cancer. Cancer J. 2011 Mar–Apr;17(2):96–103. [PMID: 21427553]

Gangi A et al. Breast-conserving therapy for triple-negative breast cancer. JAMA Surg. 2014 Jan 1. [Epub ahead of print] [PMID: 24382582]

Ghoussaini M et al. Inherited genetic susceptibility to breast cancer: the beginning of the end or the end of the beginning? Am J Pathol. 2013 Oct;183(4):1038–51. [PMID: 23973388]

Sgroi DC et al. Prediction of late distant recurrence in patients with oestrogen-receptor-positive breast cancer: a prospective comparison of the breast-cancer index (BCI) assay, 21-gene recurrence score, and IHC 4 in the TransATAC study population. Lancet Oncol. 2013 Oct;14(11):1067–76. [PMID: 24035531]

Stefansson OA et al. Epigenetic modifications in breast cancer and their role in personalized medicine. Am J Pathol. 2013 Oct;183(4):1052–63. [PMID: 23899662]

Wolff AC et al. Recommendations for human epidermal growth factor receptor 2 testing in breast cancer: American Society of Clinical Oncology/College of American Pathologists clinical practice guideline update. J Clin Oncol. 2013 Nov 1;31(31):3997–4013. [PMID: 24101045]

▶ Treatment: Curative

Clearly, not all breast cancer is systemic at the time of diagnosis. For this reason, a pessimistic attitude concerning the management of breast cancer is unwarranted. Most patients with early breast cancer can be cured. Treatment with a curative intent is advised for clinical stage I, II, and III disease (see Tables 17–3, 39–4). Patients with locally advanced (T3, T4) and even inflammatory tumors may be cured with multimodality therapy, but metastatic disease will be diagnosed in most patients and at that point palliation is all that can be expected. Treatment with palliative intent is appropriate for all patients with stage IV disease and for patients with unresectable local cancers.

A. Choice and Timing of Primary Therapy

The extent of disease and its biologic aggressiveness are the principal determinants of the outcome of primary therapy. Clinical and pathologic staging help in assessing extent of disease (see Table 17–3), but each is to some extent imprecise. Other factors such as tumor grade, hormone receptor assays, and HER2 oncogene amplification are of prognostic value and are key to determining systemic therapy, but are not as relevant in determining the type of local therapy.

Controversy has surrounded the choice of primary therapy of stage I, II, and III breast carcinoma. Currently, the standard of care for stage I, stage II, and most stage III cancer is surgical resection followed by adjuvant radiation or systemic therapy, or both, when indicated. Neoadjuvant therapy is becoming more popular since large tumors may be shrunk by chemotherapy prior to surgery, making some patients who require mastectomy candidates for lumpectomy. It is important for patients to understand all of the surgical options, including reconstructive options, prior to having surgery. Patients with large primary tumors, inflammatory cancer, or palpably enlarged lymph nodes should have staging scans performed to rule out distant metastatic disease prior to definitive surgery. In general, adjuvant systemic therapy is started when the breast has adequately healed, usually within 4–8 weeks after surgery. While no prospective studies have defined the appropriate timing of adjuvant chemotherapy, one retrospective population-based study has suggested that chemotherapy should be initiated within 12 weeks of surgery to avoid a compromise in relapse-free and overall survival.

B. Surgical Resection

1. Breast-conserving therapy—Multiple, large, randomized studies including the Milan and NSABP trials show that disease-free and overall survival rates are similar for patients with stage I and stage II breast cancer treated with partial mastectomy (breast-conserving lumpectomy or "breast conservation") plus axillary dissection followed by radiation therapy and for those treated by modified radical mastectomy (total mastectomy plus axillary dissection).

Tumor size is a major consideration in determining the feasibility of breast conservation. The NSABP lumpectomy trial randomized patients with tumors as large as 4 cm. To achieve an acceptable cosmetic result, the patient must

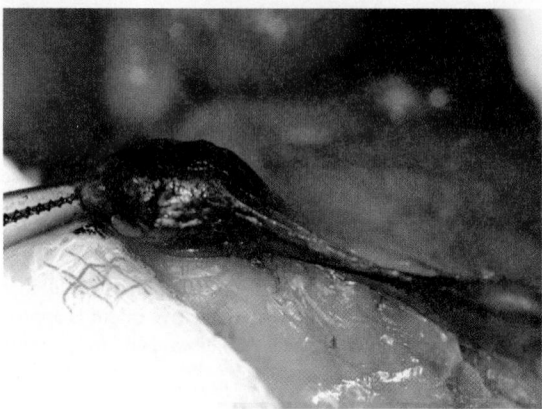

▲ **Figure 17–8.** Sentinel node. (Reproduced with permission, from Giuliano AE.)

have a breast of sufficient size to enable excision of a 4-cm tumor without considerable deformity. Therefore, large tumor size is only a relative contraindication. Subareolar tumors, also difficult to excise without deformity, are not contraindications to breast conservation. Clinically detectable multifocality is a relative contraindication to breast-conserving surgery, as is fixation to the chest wall or skin or involvement of the nipple or overlying skin. The patient—not the surgeon—should be the judge of what is cosmetically acceptable. Given the relatively high risk of poor outcome after radiation, concomitant scleroderma is a contraindication to breast-conserving surgery. A history of prior therapeutic radiation to the ipsilateral breast or chest wall (or both) is also a contraindication for breast conservation.

Axillary dissection is primarily used to properly stage cancer and plan radiation and systemic therapy. Intraoperative lymphatic mapping and sentinel node biopsy identify lymph nodes most likely to harbor metastases if present (Figure 17–8). Sentinel node biopsy is a reasonable alternative to axillary dissection in patients without clinical evidence of axillary lymph node metastases. If sentinel node biopsy reveals no evidence of axillary metastases, it is highly likely that the remaining lymph nodes are free of disease and axillary dissection may be omitted. An important study from the American College of Surgeons Oncology group randomized women with sentinel node metastases to undergo completion of axillary dissection or to receive no further axillary treatment after lumpectomy; no difference in survival was found, showing that **axillary dissection for selected node-positive women is not necessary for patients treated with lumpectomy, whole breast irradiation, and adjuvant systemic therapy.** These results challenged standard treatment regimens. Omission of axillary dissection is now accepted at many major cancer institutions.

Breast-conserving surgery with radiation is the preferred form of treatment for patients with **early-stage breast cancer**. Despite the numerous randomized trials showing no survival benefit of mastectomy over breast-conserving partial mastectomy and irradiation, breast-conserving surgery still appears to be underutilized.

2. Mastectomy—Modified radical mastectomy was the standard therapy for most patients with early-stage breast cancer. This operation removes the entire breast, overlying skin, nipple, and areolar complex as well as the underlying pectoralis fascia with the axillary lymph nodes in continuity. The major advantage of modified radical mastectomy is that radiation therapy may not be necessary, although radiation may be used when lymph nodes are involved with cancer or when the primary tumor is large (≥ 5 cm). The disadvantage of mastectomy is the cosmetic and psychological impact associated with breast loss. Radical mastectomy, which removes the underlying pectoralis muscle, should be performed rarely, if at all. Axillary node dissection is not indicated for noninvasive cancers because nodal metastases are rarely present. Skin-sparing and nipple-sparing mastectomy is currently gaining favor but is not appropriate for all patients. Breast-conserving surgery and radiation should be offered whenever possible given the lower risk of surgical complications and the smaller emotional impact on the patient. Breast reconstruction, immediate or delayed, should be discussed with patients who choose or require mastectomy. Patients should have an interview with a reconstructive plastic surgeon to discuss options prior to making a decision regarding reconstruction. Time is well spent preoperatively in educating the patient and family about these matters.

C. Radiotherapy

Radiotherapy after partial mastectomy consists of 5–7 weeks of five daily fractions to a total dose of 5000–6000 cGy. Most radiation oncologists use a boost dose to the cancer location. Shorter fractionation schedules may be reasonable for women over the age of 50 with early stage, lymph node–negative breast cancer. Accelerated partial breast irradiation, in which only the portion of the breast from which the tumor was resected is irradiated for 1–2 weeks, appears effective in achieving local control for selected patients; however, the results of prospective randomized trials, such as the NSABP B-39/RTOG 0413, are awaited. In women over the age of 70 with small (< 2 cm), lymph node–negative, hormone receptor–positive cancers, radiation therapy may be avoided. The recurrence rates after intraoperative radiation, while low, appear significantly higher than postoperative whole breast radiation therapy. However, in all of these situations, a balanced discussion with a radiation oncologist to weigh the risks and benefits of each approach is warranted.

Current studies suggest that radiotherapy after mastectomy may improve recurrence rates and survival in patients with tumors ≥ 5 cm or positive lymph nodes. Researchers are also examining the utility of axillary irradiation as an alternative to axillary dissection in the clinically node-negative patient with sentinel node micrometastases (metastasis > 0.2 mm or more than 200 cells, but none > 2.0 mm). An ACOSOG study (Z0010) and large NSABP trial (B-32) showed no adverse impact of micrometastases on survival and support no alteration in treatment when found. A Canadian trial (MA20) of postoperative nodal irradiation after lumpectomy and axillary dissection shows improved survival with nodal irradiation.

D. Adjuvant Systemic Therapy

The goal of systemic therapy, including hormone modulating drugs (endocrine therapy), cytotoxic chemotherapy, and the HER2-targeted agent trastuzumab, is to kill cancer cells that have escaped the breast and axillary lymph nodes as micrometastases before they become macrometastases (ie, stage IV cancer). **Systemic therapy improves survival and is advocated for most patients with curable breast cancer.** In practice, most medical oncologists are currently using adjuvant chemotherapy for patients with either node-positive or higher-risk (eg, hormone receptor-negative or HER2-positive) node-negative breast cancer and using endocrine therapy for all hormone receptor–positive invasive breast cancer unless contraindicated. Prognostic factors other than nodal status that are used to determine the patient's risks of recurrence are tumor size, ER and PR status, nuclear grade, histologic type, proliferative rate, oncogene expression (Table 17–5), and patient's age and menopausal status. In general, systemic chemotherapy decreases the chance of recurrence by about 30% and hormonal modulation decreases the relative risk of recurrence by 40–50% (for hormone receptor–positive cancer). Systemic chemotherapy is usually given sequentially, rather than concurrently with radiation. In terms of sequencing, typically chemotherapy is given before radiation and endocrine therapy is started concurrent with or after radiation therapy.

The long-term advantage of systemic therapy has been well established. All patients with invasive hormone receptor–positive tumors should consider the use of hormone-modulating therapy. Most patients with HER2-positive tumors should receive trastuzumab-containing chemotherapy regimens. In general, adjuvant systemic chemotherapy should not be given to women who have small node-negative breast cancers with favorable histologic findings and tumor markers. The ability to predict more accurately which patients with HER2-negative,

Table 17–5. Prognostic factors in node-negative breast cancer.

Prognostic Factors	Increased Recurrence	Decreased Recurrence
Size	T3, T2	T1, T0
Hormone receptors	Negative	Positive
DNA flow cytometry	Aneuploid	Diploid
Histologic grade	High	Low
Tumor labeling index	< 3%	> 3%
S phase fraction	> 5%	< 5%
Lymphatic or vascular invasion	Present	Absent
Cathepsin D	High	Low
HER2 oncogene	High	Low
Epidermal growth factor receptor	High	Low

hormone receptor-positive, lymph node-negative tumors should receive chemotherapy is improving with the advent of prognostic tools, such as Oncotype DX and Mammaprint. These tests are undergoing prospective evaluation in two clinical trials (TAILORx and MINDACT).

1. Chemotherapy—The Early Breast Cancer Trialists' Collaborative Group (EBCTCG) meta-analysis involving over 28,000 women enrolled in 60 trials of adjuvant polychemotherapy versus no chemotherapy demonstrated a significant beneficial impact of chemotherapy on clinical outcome in non–stage IV breast cancer. This study showed that adjuvant chemotherapy reduces the risk of recurrence and breast cancer–specific mortality in all women but also showed that women under the age of 50 derive the greatest benefit. On the basis of the superiority of anthracycline-containing regimens in metastatic breast cancer, both doxorubicin and epirubicin have been studied extensively in the adjuvant setting. Studies comparing Adriamycin (doxorubicin) and cyclophosphamide (AC) or epirubicin and cyclophosphamide (EC) to cyclophosphamide-methotrexate-5-fluorouracil (CMF) have shown that treatments with anthracycline-containing regimens are at least as effective as treatment with CMF. The EBCTCG analysis including over 14,000 patients enrolled in trials comparing anthracycline-based regimens to CMF, showed a small but statistically significant improved disease-free and overall survival with the use of anthracycline-based regimens. It should be noted, however, that most of these studies included a mixed population of patients with HER2-positive and HER2-negative breast cancer and were performed before the introduction of trastuzumab. Retrospective analyses of a number of these studies suggest that anthracyclines may be primarily effective in tumors with HER2 overexpression or alteration in the expression of topoisomerase IIa (the target of anthracyclines and close to the *HER2* gene). Given this, for HER2-negative, node-negative breast cancer, four cycles of AC or six cycles of CMF are probably equally effective.

When taxanes (T = paclitaxel and docetaxel) emerged in the 1990s, multiple trials were conducted to evaluate their use in combination with anthracycline-based regimens. The majority of these trials showed an improvement in disease-free survival and at least one showed an improvement in overall survival with the taxane-based regimen. A meta-analysis of taxane versus non-taxane anthracycline-based regimen trials showed an improvement in disease-free and overall survival for the taxane-based regimens.

Several regimens have been reported including AC followed by paclitaxel or docetaxel (AC-T), TAC (docetaxel concurrent with AC), 5-fluorouracil (F)EC-docetaxel and FEC-paclitaxel. Results from CALGB 9741 showed that compared with a standard dose regimen, administration of "dose-dense" AC-P chemotherapy (that is, in an accelerated fashion, in which the frequency of administration is increased without changing total dose or duration) with granulocyte colony stimulating factor (G-CSF) support led to improved both disease-free (82% vs 75% at 4 years) and overall survival (92% vs 90%). Exploratory subset analysis suggested that patients with hormone receptor–negative tumors derived the most benefit from the dose-dense approach.

The US Oncology trial 9735 compared four cycles of AC with four cycles of Taxotere (docetaxel) and cyclophosphamide (TC). With a median of 7 years follow-up, this study showed a statistically significantly improved disease-free survival and overall survival in the patients who received TC. Until this, no trial had compared a non-anthracycline, taxane-based regimen to an anthracycline-based regimen.

An important ongoing study (US Oncology 06090) is prospectively evaluating whether anthracyclines add any incremental benefit to a taxane-based regimen by comparing six cycles of TAC to six cycles of TC in HER2-negative breast cancer patients. A third arm was added to evaluate the benefit of adding bevacizumab, a monoclonal antibody directed against vascular endothelial growth factor (VEGF), to TC. While awaiting the results of this trial, oncologists are faced with choosing from among the above treatment regimens for HER2-negative breast cancer. It is interesting to note a sharp decline in the use of anthracyclines has been observed since 2006. Given the benefits described above, taxanes are now used for most patients receiving chemotherapy for early breast cancer.

The overall duration of adjuvant chemotherapy still remains uncertain. However, based on the meta-analysis performed in the Oxford Overview (EBCTCG), the current recommendation is for 3–6 months of the commonly used regimens. Although it is clear that dose intensity to a specific threshold is essential, there is no evidence to support the long-term survival benefit of high-dose chemotherapy with stem cell support.

Chemotherapy side effects are now generally well controlled. Nausea and vomiting are abated with drugs that directly affect the central nervous system, such as ondansetron and granisetron. Infertility and premature ovarian failure are common side effects of chemotherapy and should be discussed with patients prior to starting treatment. The risk of life-threatening neutropenia associated with chemotherapy can be reduced by use of growth factors such as pegfilgrastim and filgrastim (G-CSF), which stimulate proliferation and differentiation of hematopoietic cells. Long-term toxicities from chemotherapy, including cardiomyopathy (anthracyclines), peripheral neuropathy (taxanes), and leukemia/myelodysplasia (anthracyclines and alkylating agents), remain a small but significant risk.

2. Targeted therapy—Targeted therapy refers to agents that are directed specifically against a protein or molecule expressed uniquely on tumor cells or in the tumor microenvironment.

A. HER2 OVEREXPRESSION—Approximately 20% of breast cancers are characterized by amplification of the *HER2* oncogene leading to overexpression of the HER2 oncoprotein. The poor prognosis associated with HER2 overexpression has been drastically improved with the development of HER2-targeted therapy. Trastuzumab (Herceptin [H]), a monoclonal antibody that binds to HER2, has proved effective in combination with chemotherapy in patients with HER2 overexpressing metastatic and early breast cancer. In the adjuvant setting, the first and most commonly studied chemotherapy backbone used with trastuzumab is AC-T. Subsequently, the BCIRG006 study showed similar efficacy for AC-TH and a nonanthracycline-containing regimen, TCH (docetaxel, carboplatin, trastuzumab). Both were significantly better than AC-T in terms of disease-free and overall survival and TCH had a lower risk of cardiac toxicity. Both AC-TH and TCH are FDA-approved for nonmetastatic, HER2-positive breast cancer. In these regimens, trastuzumab is given with chemotherapy and then continues beyond the course of chemotherapy to complete a full year. The reporting of two trials in 2012 (the Herceptin Adjuvant [HERA] evaluating 1 versus 2 years of trastuzumab and the Protocol for Herceptin as Adjuvant therapy with Reduced Exposure [PHARE] study evaluating 6 versus 12 months of trastuzumab) have confirmed that 1 year of trastuzumab should remain the standard of care. At least one study (N9831) suggests that concurrent, rather than sequential, delivery of trastuzumab with chemotherapy may be more beneficial. Neoadjuvant chemotherapy plus dual HER2-targeted therapy with trastuzumab and pertuzumab (also a HER2-targeted monoclonal antibody that prevents dimerization of HER2 with HER3 and has been shown to be synergistic in combination with trastuzumab) was FDA approved in 2013 and is now a standard of care option available to patients with nonmetastatic HER2-Another question being addressed in trials is whether to treat small (< 1 cm), node-negative tumors with trastuzumab plus chemotherapy. Retrospective studies have shown that even small (stage T1a,b) HER2-positive tumors have a worse prognosis compared with same-sized HER2-negative tumors. The NSABP B43 study is also ongoing to evaluate whether the addition of trastuzumab to radiation therapy is warranted for DCIS.

Cardiomyopathy develops in a small but significant percent (1–4%) of patients who receive trastuzumab-based regimens. For this reason, anthracyclines and trastuzumab are rarely given concurrently and cardiac function is monitored periodically throughout therapy.

B. ENDOCRINE THERAPY—Adjuvant hormone modulation therapy is highly effective in decreasing relative risk of recurrence by 40–50% and mortality by 25% in women with hormone receptor–positive tumors regardless of menopausal status. The traditional regimen has been 5 years of the estrogen-receptor antagonist/agonist tamoxifen until the 2012 reporting of the Adjuvant Tamoxifen Longer Against Shorter (ATLAS) trial in which 5 versus 10 years of adjuvant tamoxifen were compared. In this study, disease-free and overall survival were significantly improved in women who received 10 years of tamoxifen, particularly after year 10. Though these results are impressive and potentially practice changing, the clinical application of long-term tamoxifen use must be discussed with patients individually, taking into consideration risks of tamoxifen such as secondary uterine cancers, venous thromboembolic events as well as side effects that impact quality of life. Ovarian ablation in premenopausal patients with ER-positive tumors may produce a benefit similar to that of adjuvant systemic chemotherapy. Whether the use of ovarian ablation plus tamoxifen (or an AI) is more effective than either measure alone is still unclear. In the

Stockholm subset of the Zoladex in Premenopausal Patients (ZIPP) study, 927 premenopausal women were randomly assigned to goserelin, tamoxifen, the combination of both, or to no endocrine therapy for 2 years. With a median follow-up of 12.3 years, this substudy showed that goserelin and tamoxifen each significantly reduce the risk of recurrence of hormone receptor–positive breast cancer compared to control (goserelin 32%, [$P = 0.005$] and tamoxifen 27% [$P = 0.018$]), yet the combination of goserelin and tamoxifen was not superior to either treatment alone. This issue is still not settled and is being addressed in ongoing clinical trials (Suppression of Ovarian Function Trial [SOFT] and Tamoxifen and Exemestane Trial [TEXT]) that have not yet reported. AIs, including anastrozole, letrozole, and exemestane, reduce estrogen production and are also effective in the adjuvant setting for postmenopausal women. Approximately seven large randomized trials enrolling more than 24,000 patients have compared the use of AIs with tamoxifen or placebo as adjuvant therapy. All of these studies have shown small but statistically significant improvements in disease-free survival (absolute benefits of 2–6%) with the use of AIs. In addition, AIs have been shown to reduce the risk of contralateral breast cancers and to have fewer associated serious side effects (such as endometrial cancers and thromboembolic events) than tamoxifen. However, they are associated with accelerated bone loss and an increased risk of fractures as well as a musculoskeletal syndrome characterized by arthralgias or myalgias (or both) in up to 50% of patients. **The American Society of Clinical Oncology and the NCCN have recommended that postmenopausal women with hormone receptor–positive breast cancer be offered an AI either initially or after tamoxifen therapy.** HER2 status should not affect the use or choice of hormone therapy.

3. Bisphosphonates—Two randomized studies (ZO-FAST and ABCSG-12) have evaluated the use of an adjuvant intravenous bisphosphonate (zoledronic acid) in addition to standard local and systemic therapy. The results showed a 32–40% relative reduction in the risk of cancer recurrence for hormone receptor–positive nonmetastatic breast cancer. Conflicting results have been reported from the AZURE study. In this randomized study that enrolled premenopausal and postmenopausal patients, there was no disease-free or overall survival benefits associated with the addition of zoledronic acid to endocrine therapy for the overall study population. However, a prespecified subset analysis in patients who were postmenopausal for at least 5 years did demonstrate a significant disease-free and overall survival benefit with the addition of the bisphosphonate. A meta-analysis of 15 studies evaluating adjuvant therapy with zoledronic acid showed a significant improvement in overall survival and a reduced fracture rate but no significant difference in disease-free survival outcome or bone metastases. Side effects associated with intravenous bisphosphonate therapy include bone pain, fever, osteonecrosis of the jaw (rare, < 1%), and renal failure. The adjuvant use of bisphosphonates and other bone stabilizing drugs, such as inhibitors of receptor activator of nuclear factor kappa B ligand (RANK-B) (eg denosumab), remains investigational.

4. Adjuvant therapy in older women—Data relating to the optimal use of adjuvant systemic treatment for women over the age of 65 are limited. Results from the EBCTCG overview indicates that while adjuvant chemotherapy yields a smaller benefit for older women compared with younger women, it still improves clinical outcomes. Moreover, individual studies do show that older women with higher risk disease derive benefits from chemotherapy. One study compared the use of oral chemotherapy (capecitabine) to standard chemotherapy in older women and concluded that standard chemotherapy is preferred. Another study (USO TC vs AC) showed that women over the age of 65 derive similar benefits from the taxane-based regimen as women who are younger. The benefits of endocrine therapy for hormone receptor-positive disease appear to be independent of age. In general, decisions relating to the use of systemic therapy should take into account a patient's comorbidities and physiological age, more so than chronologic age.

E. Neoadjuvant Therapy

The use of chemotherapy or endocrine therapy prior to resection of the primary tumor (neoadjuvant) is gaining popularity. This enables the assessment of in vivo chemosensitivity. Patients with hormone receptor–negative, triple negative, or HER2-positive breast cancer are more likely to have a pathologic complete response to neoadjuvant chemotherapy than those with hormone receptor–positive breast cancer. A complete pathologic response at the time of surgery is associated with improvement in event-free and overall survival. Neoadjuvant chemotherapy also increases the chance of breast conservation by shrinking the primary tumor in women who would otherwise need mastectomy for local control. Survival after neoadjuvant chemotherapy is similar to that seen with postoperative adjuvant chemotherapy.

1. HER2-positive breast cancer—Dual targeting of HER2 with two monoclonal antibodies, trastuzumab and pertuzumab, has been evaluated in two clinical trials in the neoadjuvant setting. TRYPHAENA was a phase II, open-label study in which 225 patients with operable HER2-positive breast cancer were randomly assigned to six neoadjuvant cycles every 3 weeks of either 5-fluorouracil, epirubicin, cyclophosphamide [FEC] plus trastuzumab [H] and pertuzumab [P] for three cycles followed by docetaxel [T] plus HP for three cycles (Arm A) or FEC for three cycles followed by THP for three cycles (Arm B) or TCHP for six cycles (Arm C). Pathologic complete response (in breast and lymph nodes) was seen in 50.7% of patients in Arm A, 45.3% in Arm B, and 51.9% in Arm C. Symptomatic left ventricular systolic dysfunction developed in two patients in this study, both in Arm B. Declines in left ventricular ejection fraction ≥ 10% from baseline to < 50% was observed in 4 patients in Arm A (5.6%), 4 patients in Arm B (5.3%) and 3 patients in Arm C (3.9%).

The NEOSPHERE study randomly assigned 417 patients with HER2-positive breast cancer to four cycles of trastuzumab (H) plus docetaxel (T) (group A), pertuzumab (P) plus TH (group B), PH (group C) or PT (group D).

Pathologic complete response in the breast and lymph nodes was seen in 21.5% in group A, 39.3% in group B, 11.2% in group C and 17.7% in group D. Studies indicate that those patients who achieve a pathologic complete response have improved disease-free survival and may have better overall survival. In 2013, given the results of these two studies, the FDA granted accelerated approval for neoadjuvant pertuzumab. This is the first medication to receive regulatory approval in the neoadjuvant setting for breast cancer. Based on the above clinical trials, three regimens have received approval in the HER2-positive neoadjuvant setting: TCHP for six cycles; FEC for 3 cycles followed by THP for 3 cycles; or THP for 4 cycles (followed by three cycles of postoperative FEC). Pertuzumab is not approved for the adjuvant setting. Postoperatively all patients should continue to receive trastuzumab to complete a full year.

2. Hormone receptor–positive, HER2-negative breast cancer—Patients with hormone receptor-positive breast cancer have a lower chance of achieving a pathologic complete response with neoadjuvant therapy than those patients with triple negative or HER2-positive breast cancers. Studies are ongoing to evaluate hormonally targeted regimens in the neoadjuvant setting. Outside of the clinical trial setting, the use of neoadjuvant hormonal therapy is generally restricted to postmenopausal patients who are unwilling or unable to tolerate chemotherapy.

3. Triple negative breast cancer—No targeted therapy has been identified for patients with breast cancer that is lacking in HER2 amplification or hormone receptor expression. Neoadjuvant chemotherapy leads to pathologic complete response in approximately 25–45% of patients with triple negative breast cancer. Patients who achieve a pathologic complete response seem to have a similar prognosis to other breast cancer subtypes with pathologic complete response. However, those patients with residual disease at the time of surgery have a poor prognosis. Based on the theory that triple negative breast cancers may be more vulnerable to DNA damaging agents, several studies are evaluating whether the addition of platinum salts to a neoadjuvant chemotherapy regimen is beneficial in this disease subtype. A randomized phase II trial (GeparSixto) randomly assigned 595 patients with triple negative or HER2-positive breast cancer to weekly paclitaxel plus weekly liposomal doxorubicin (18 weeks) alone or with weekly carboplatin. Patients with triple negative disease also received bevacizumab. Those patients with triple negative disease who received carboplatin had a pathologic complete response rate of 58.7% compared to those who did not receive carboplatin (37.9%; $P < 0.05$). Similarly designed studies are ongoing to evaluate the pathologic complete response rates and long-term outcomes associated with incorporating platinums into standard chemotherapy regimens.

4. Timing of lymph node biopsy in neoadjuvant setting— There is considerable concern about the timing of sentinel lymph node biopsy, since the chemotherapy may affect any cancer present in the lymph nodes. Several studies have shown that sentinel node biopsy can be done after neoadjuvant therapy. However, a large multicenter study, ACOSOG 1071, demonstrated a false-negative rate of 10.7%, well above the false-negative rate outside the neoadjuvant setting (< 1–5%). Many physicians recommend performing sentinel lymph node biopsy before administering the chemotherapy in order to avoid a false-negative result and to aid in planning subsequent radiation therapy. Others prefer to perform sentinel lymph node biopsy after neoadjuvant therapy to avoid a second operation and assess post-chemotherapy nodal status. If a complete dissection is desired, this can be performed at the time of the definitive breast surgery.

Important questions remaining to be answered are the timing and duration of adjuvant and neoadjuvant chemotherapy, which chemotherapeutic agents should be applied for which subgroups of patients, the use of combinations of hormonal therapy and chemotherapy as well as possibly targeted therapy, and the value of prognostic factors other than hormone receptors in predicting response to therapy.

▶ Treatment: Palliative

Palliative treatments are those to manage symptoms, improve quality of life, and even prolong survival, without the expectation of achieving cure. Only 10% of patients have de novo metastatic breast cancer at the time of diagnosis. However, in most patients who have a breast cancer recurrence after initial local and adjuvant therapy, the recurrence presents as metastatic rather than local (in breast) disease. Breast cancer most commonly metastasizes to the liver, lungs and bone, causing symptoms such as fatigue, change in appetite, abdominal pain, respiratory symptoms, or bone pain. Headaches, imbalance, vision changes, vertigo, and other neurologic symptoms may be signs of brain metastases. Triple negative (ER-, PR-, HER2-negative) and HER2-positive tumors have a higher rate of brain metastases than hormone-receptor positive, HER2-negative tumors.

A. Radiotherapy and Bisphosphonates

Palliative radiotherapy may be advised for primary treatment of locally advanced cancers with distant metastases to control ulceration, pain, and other manifestations in the breast and regional nodes. Irradiation of the breast and chest wall and the axillary, internal mammary, and supraclavicular nodes should be undertaken in an attempt to cure locally advanced and inoperable lesions when there is no evidence of distant metastases. A small number of patients in this group are cured in spite of extensive breast and regional node involvement.

Palliative irradiation is of value also in the treatment of certain bone or soft-tissue metastases to control pain or avoid fracture. Radiotherapy is especially useful in the treatment of isolated bony metastases, chest wall recurrences, brain metastases, and acute spinal cord compression.

In addition to radiotherapy, bisphosphonate therapy has shown excellent results in delaying and reducing skeletal events in women with bony metastases. Pamidronate and zoledronic acid are FDA-approved intravenous bisphosphonates given for bone metastases or hypercalcemia of malignancy from breast cancer. Denosumab, a fully human monoclonal antibody that targets RANK-ligand, is approved by the FDA for the treatment of advanced breast cancer causing bone metastases, with data showing that it reduced the time to first skeletal-related event (eg, pathologic fracture) compared to zoledronic acid.

Caution should be exercised when combining radiation therapy with chemotherapy because toxicity of either or both may be augmented by their concurrent administration. In general, only one type of therapy should be given at a time unless it is necessary to irradiate a destructive lesion of weight-bearing bone while the patient is receiving chemotherapy. The regimen should be changed only if the disease is clearly progressing. This is especially difficult to determine for patients with destructive bone metastases, since changes in the status of these lesions are difficult to determine radiographically.

B. Targeted Therapy

1. Endocrine therapy for metastatic disease—The first targeted therapy was the use of antiestrogen therapy in hormone receptor–positive breast cancer. The following therapies have all been shown to be effective in hormone receptor–positive metastatic breast cancer: administration of drugs that block hormone receptors (such as tamoxifen) or drugs that block the synthesis of hormones (such as AIs); ablation of the ovaries, adrenals, or pituitary; and the administration of hormones (eg, estrogens, androgens, progestins); see Table 17–6. Palliative treatment of metastatic cancer should be based on the ER status of the primary tumor or the metastases. Because only 5–10% of women with ER-negative tumors respond, they should not receive endocrine therapy except in unusual circumstances, eg, in an older patient who cannot tolerate chemotherapy. The rate of response is nearly equal in premenopausal and postmenopausal women with ER-positive tumors. A favorable response to hormonal manipulation occurs in about one-third of patients with metastatic breast cancer. Of those whose tumors contain ER, the response is about 60% and perhaps as high as 80% for patients whose tumors contain PR as well. The choice of endocrine therapy depends on the menopausal status of the patient. Women within 1 year of their last menstrual period are arbitrarily considered to be premenopausal and should receive tamoxifen therapy or rarely ovarian ablation, whereas women whose menses ceased more than a year before are postmenopausal and may receive tamoxifen or an AI. Women with ER-positive tumors who do not respond to first-line endocrine therapy or experience progression should be given a different form of hormonal manipulation. Because the quality of life during endocrine manipulation is usually superior to that during cytotoxic chemotherapy, it is best to try endocrine manipulation whenever possible. However, when receptor status is unknown, disease is progressing rapidly or involves visceral organs, chemotherapy should be used as first-line treatment.

A. The Premenopausal Patient

(1) Primary hormonal therapy—The potent SERM tamoxifen is by far the most common and preferred method of hormonal manipulation in the premenopausal patient, in large part because it can be given with less morbidity and fewer side effects than cytotoxic chemotherapy

Table 17–6. Agents commonly used for hormonal management of metastatic breast cancer.

Drug	Action	Dose, Route, Frequency	Major Side Effects
Tamoxifen citrate (Nolvadex)	SERM	20 mg orally daily	Hot flushes, uterine bleeding, thrombophlebitis, rash
Fulvestrant (Faslodex)	Steroidal estrogen receptor antagonist	500 mg intramuscularly day 1, 15, 29 and then monthly	Gastrointestinal upset, headache, back pain, hot flushes, pharyngitis
Toremifene citrate (Fareston)	SERM	40 mg orally daily	Hot flushes, sweating, nausea, vaginal discharge, dry eyes, dizziness
Diethylstilbestrol (DES)	Estrogen	5 mg orally three times daily	Fluid retention, uterine bleeding, thrombophlebitis, nausea
Goserelin (Zoladex)	Synthetic luteinizing hormone releasing analogue	3.6 mg subcutaneously monthly	Arthralgias, blood pressure changes, hot flushes, headaches, vaginal dryness
Megestrol acetate (Megace)	Progestin	40 mg orally four times daily	Fluid retention
Letrozole (Femara)	AI	2.5 mg orally daily	Hot flushes, arthralgia/arthritis, myalgia, bone loss
Anastrozole (Arimidex)	AI	1 mg orally daily	Hot flushes, skin rashes, nausea and vomiting, bone loss
Exemestane (Aromasin)	AI	25 mg orally daily	Hot flushes, increased arthralgia/arthritis, myalgia, bone loss

AI, aromatase inhibitor; SERM, selective estrogen receptor modulator.

and does not require oophorectomy. Tamoxifen is given orally in a dose of 20 mg daily. The average remission associated with tamoxifen lasts about 12 months.

There is no significant difference in survival or response between tamoxifen therapy and bilateral oophorectomy. Bilateral oophorectomy is less desirable than tamoxifen in premenopausal women because tamoxifen is so well tolerated. However, oophorectomy can be achieved rapidly and safely either by surgery, by irradiation of the ovaries if the patient is a poor surgical candidate, or by chemical ovarian ablation using a gonadotropin-releasing hormone (GnRH) analog. Oophorectomy presumably works by eliminating estrogens, progestins, and androgens, which stimulate growth of the tumor. AIs should not be used in a patient with functioning ovaries since they do not block ovarian production of estrogen.

(2) Secondary or tertiary hormonal therapy—Patients who do not respond to tamoxifen or ovarian ablation may be treated with chemotherapy or may try a second endocrine regimen, such as GnRH analog plus AI. Whether to opt for chemotherapy or another endocrine measure depends largely on the sites of metastatic disease (visceral being more serious than bone-only, thus sometimes warranting the use of chemotherapy), the disease burden, the rate of growth of disease, and patient preference. Patients who take chemotherapy and then later have progressive disease may subsequently respond to another form of endocrine treatment (Table 17–6). The optimal choice for secondary endocrine manipulation has not been clearly defined for the premenopausal patient.

Patients who improve after oophorectomy but subsequently relapse should receive tamoxifen or an AI; if one fails, the other may be tried. Megestrol acetate, a progesterone agent, may also be considered. Adrenalectomy or hypophysectomy, procedures rarely done today, induced regression in 30–50% of patients who previously responded to oophorectomy. Pharmacologic hormonal manipulation has replaced these invasive procedures.

B. THE POSTMENOPAUSAL PATIENT

(1) Primary hormonal therapy—For postmenopausal women with metastatic breast cancer amenable to endocrine manipulation, tamoxifen or an AI is the initial therapy of choice. AIs may be more effective. The side effect profile of AIs differs from tamoxifen. The main side effects of tamoxifen are nausea, skin rash, and hot flushes. Rarely, tamoxifen induces hypercalcemia in patients with bony metastases. Tamoxifen also increases the risk of venous thromboembolic events and uterine hyperplasia and cancer. The main side effects of AIs include hot flushes, vaginal dryness, and joint stiffness; however, osteoporosis and bone fractures are significantly higher than with tamoxifen. Phase 2 data from the randomized Fulvestrant fIRst line Study comparing endocrine Treatments (FIRST) suggest that the pure estrogen antagonist, fulvestrant may be even more effective than front-line anastrozole in terms of time to progression. The combination of fulvestrant plus anastrozole may also be more effective than anastrozole alone, although two studies evaluating this question have yielded conflicting results.

(2) Secondary or tertiary hormonal therapy—AIs are also used for the treatment of advanced breast cancer in postmenopausal women after tamoxifen treatment. In the event that the patient responds to AI but then has progression of disease, fulvestrant has shown efficacy with about 20–30% of women benefiting from use. Postmenopausal women who respond initially to a SERM or AI but later manifest progressive disease may be crossed over to another hormonal therapy. Until recently, patients who experienced disease progression during or after treatment with a SERM or AI were routinely offered chemotherapy. This standard practice changed in 2012 with the approval of **everolimus** (Afinitor), an oral inhibitor of the mammalian target of rapamycin (MTOR)—a protein whose activation has been associated with the development of endocrine resistance. A phase III, placebo-controlled trial (BOLERO-2) evaluated exemestane with or without everolimus in 724 patients with AI-resistant, hormone receptor–positive metastatic breast cancer, and at interim analysis found that patients treated with everolimus had a significantly improved progression-free survival (10.6 months vs 4.1 months; HR, 0.36; 95% CI, 0.27–0.47; $P < 0.001$). Androgens (such as testosterone) have many toxicities and should be used infrequently. As in premenopausal patients, neither hypophysectomy nor adrenalectomy should be performed. Estrogen therapy has also paradoxically been shown to induce responses in advanced breast cancer. A study that evaluated the use of low-dose (6 mg) versus high-dose (30 mg) estradiol daily orally for postmenopausal women with metastatic AI-resistant breast cancer showed that the two doses yielded similar clinical benefit rates (29% and 28%, respectively) and, as expected, the higher dose was associated with more adverse events than the low dose.

(3) Newer agents in development—Although endocrine therapy can lead to disease control for months to years in some patients, de novo and acquired resistance to hormonal manipulation remains an enormous barrier to the effective treatment of these patients. Thus, molecularly targeted agents are still needed to circumvent signaling pathways that lead to drug resistance. A randomized phase II study evaluating letrozole with or without an oral cyclin-D kinase (cdk) 4/6 inhibitor for the first-line treatment of postmenopausal women with hormone receptor–positive advanced breast cancer demonstrated a striking and highly significant 18.6 month improvement in progression-free survival with the cdk4/6-inhibitor (26.1 months with cdk 4/6 inhibitor vs 7.5 months in control arm). Phase III evaluation of this promising molecule is ongoing.

2. HER2-targeted agents—For patients with HER2 overexpressing or amplified tumors, trastuzumab plus chemotherapy has been shown to significantly improve clinical outcomes, including survival compared to chemotherapy alone. Trastuzumab plus chemotherapy alone was therefore the standard first-line treatment for HER2-positive metastatic breast cancer until 2012 when pertuzumab was granted FDA approval. **Pertuzumab** is a monoclonal antibody that targets the extracellular domain of *HER2* at a different epitope than targeted by trastuzumab and inhibits receptor dimerization. A phase III placebo-controlled randomized study (CLEOPATRA) showed that patients treated with the combination of pertuzumab, trastuzumab, and docetaxel had a significantly longer progression-free survival (18.5 months vs 12.4 months; HR, 0.62; 95% CI, 0.51–0.75; $P < 0.001$) compared with those treated with docetaxel and trastuzumab. Longer follow-up revealed a significant overall survival benefit associated with pertuzumab as well.

Lapatinib, an oral targeted drug that inhibits the intracellular tyrosine kinases of the epidermal growth factor and HER2 receptors, is FDA-approved for the treatment of trastuzumab-resistant HER2-positive metastatic breast cancer in combination with capecitabine, thus, a completely oral regimen. The combination of trastuzumab plus lapatinib has been shown to be more effective than lapatinib alone for trastuzumab-resistant metastatic breast cancer. Moreover, several trials have shown a significant clinical benefit for continuing HER2-targeted agents beyond progression. **T-DM1 (trastuzumab emtansine)** is a novel antibody drug conjugate in which trastuzumab is stably linked to a derivative of maytansine, enabling targeted delivery of the cytotoxic chemotherapy to HER2-overexpressing cells. The phase III trial (EMILIA) that evaluated T-DM1 in patients with HER2-positive, trastuzumab-pretreated advanced disease showed that T-DM1 is associated with improved progression-free and overall survival compared to lapatinib plus capecitabine (EMILIA). Regulatory approval of T-DM1 (Kadcyla [ado-trastuzumab emtansine]) was received in February 2013. Evaluation of T-DM1 in combination with pertuzumab for the first-line treatment of advanced breast cancer is ongoing in the phase III MARIANNE study, and trials evaluating the use of these agents in early breast cancer are ongoing. Several other drugs targeting the HER2 pathway are in development, including everolimus, afatinib, neratinib, and HER2-targeted vaccines.

3. Targeting "triple-negative" breast cancer—Until very recently, breast cancers lacking expression of the hormone receptors, ER and PR, and HER2 have only been amenable to therapy with cytotoxic chemotherapy. This type of "triple-negative" breast cancer, while heterogeneous, generally behaves aggressively and is associated with a poor prognosis. Newer classes of targeted agents are being evaluated specifically for triple-negative breast cancer. Some triple-negative breast cancers may be characterized by an inability to repair double-strand DNA breaks (due to mutation or epigenetic silencing of the BRCA gene). **Poly-ADP ribose-polymerase (PARP) inhibitors** are a class of agents that prevent the repair of single strand DNA breaks and are showing promise in BRCA-mutated and triple-negative breast cancer. Research in this area is rapidly expanding with multiple clinical trials of PARP inhibitors and other molecularly targeted agents ongoing.

C. Palliative Chemotherapy

Cytotoxic drugs should be considered for the treatment of metastatic breast cancer (1) if visceral metastases are present (especially brain, liver, or lymphangitic pulmonary), (2) if hormonal treatment is unsuccessful or the disease has progressed after an initial response to hormonal manipulation, or (3) if the tumor is ER-negative or HER2-positive. Prior adjuvant chemotherapy does not seem to alter response rates in patients who relapse. A number of chemotherapy drugs (including vinorelbine, paclitaxel, docetaxel, gemcitabine, ixabepilone, carboplatin, cisplatin, capecitabine, albumin-bound paclitaxel, eribulin, and liposomal doxorubicin) may be used as single agents with first-line objective response rates ranging from 30% to 50%.

Combination chemotherapy yields statistically significantly higher response rates and progression-free survival rates, but has not been conclusively shown to improve overall survival rates compared with sequential single-agent therapy. Combinations that have been tested in phase III studies and have proven efficacy compared with single-agent therapy include capecitabine/docetaxel, gemcitabine/paclitaxel, and capecitabine/ixabepilone (see Tables 39–11 and 39–12). Various other combinations of drugs have been tested in phase II studies, and a number of clinical trials are ongoing to identify effective combinations. Patients should be encouraged to participate in clinical trials given the number of promising targeted therapies in development. It is generally appropriate to treat willing patients with multiple sequential lines of therapy as long as they tolerate the treatment and as long as their performance status is good (eg, at least ambulatory and able to care for self, up out of bed more than 50% of waking hours).

Baselga J et al; CLEOPATRA Study Group. Pertuzumab plus trastuzumab plus docetaxel for metastatic breast cancer. N Engl J Med. 2012 Jan 12;366(2):109–19. [PMID: 22149875]

Baselga J et al. Everolimus in postmenopausal hormone-receptor-positive advanced breast cancer. N Engl J Med. 2012 Feb 9;366(6):520–9. [PMID: 22149876]

Davies C et al; Adjuvant Tamoxifen: Longer Against Shorter (ATLAS) Collaborative Group. Long-term effects of continuing adjuvant tamoxifen to 10 years versus stopping at 5 years after diagnosis of oestrogen receptor-positive breast cancer: ATLAS, a randomised trial. Lancet. 2013 Mar 9;381(9869):805–16. Erratum in: Lancet. 2013 Mar 9;381(9869):804. [PMID: 23219286]

Dengel LT et al. Axillary dissection can be avoided in the majority of clinically node-negative patients undergoing breast-conserving therapy. Ann Surg Oncol. 2014 Jan;21(1):22–7. [PMID: 23975314]

Gianni L et al. Efficacy and safety of neoadjuvant pertuzumab and trastuzumab in women with locally advanced, inflammatory, or early HER2-positive breast cancer (NeoSphere): a randomised multicentre, open-label, phase 2 trial. Lancet Oncol. 2012 Jan;13(1):25–32. [PMID: 22153890]

Giuliano AE et al. Association of occult metastases in sentinel lymph nodes and bone marrow with survival among women with early-stage invasive breast cancer. JAMA. 2011 Jul 27;306(4):385–93. [PMID: 21791687]

Giuliano AE et al. Axillary dissection vs no axillary dissection in women with invasive breast cancer and sentinel node metastasis: a randomized clinical trial. JAMA. 2011 Feb 9; 305(6):569–75. [PMID: 21304082]

Goldhirsch A et al; Herceptin Adjuvant (HERA) Trial Study Team. 2 years versus 1 year of adjuvant trastuzumab for HER2-positive breast cancer (HERA): an open-label, randomised controlled trial. Lancet. 2013 Sep 21;382(9897):1021–8. [PMID: 23871490]

Haviland JS et al. The UK Standardisation of Breast Radiotherapy (START) trials of radiotherapy hypofractionation for treatment of early breast cancer: 10-year follow-up results of two randomised controlled trials. Lancet Oncol. 2013 Oct;14(11):1086–94. [PMID: 24055415]

Mohamed A et al. Targeted therapy for breast cancer. Am J Pathol. 2013 Oct;183(4):1096–112. [PMID: 23988612]

National Comprehensive Cancer Network. NCCN Guidelines: Breast Cancer. http://www.nccn.org/professionals/physician_gls/f_guidelines.asp

Pivot X et al; PHARE trial investigators. 6 months versus 12 months of adjuvant trastuzumab for patients with HER2-positive early breast cancer (PHARE): a randomised phase 3 trial. Lancet Oncol. 2013 Jul;14(8):741–8. [PMID: 23764181]

Roberston JF et al. Fulvestrant 500 mg versus anastrozole 1 mg for the first-line treatment of advanced breast cancer: follow-up analysis from the randomized 'FIRST' study. Breast Cancer Re2s Treat. 2012 Nov;136(2):503–11. [PMID: 23065000]

Schneeweiss A et al. Pertuzumab plus trastuzumab in combination with standard neoadjuvant anthracycline-containing and anthracycline-free chemotherapy regimens in patients with HER2-positive early breast cancer: a randomized phase II cardiac safety study (TRYPHAENA). Ann Oncol. 2013 Sep;24(9):2278–84. [PMID: 23704196]

Slamon D et al; Breast Cancer International Research Group. Adjuvant trastuzumab in HER2-positive breast cancer. N Engl J Med. 2011 Oct 6;365(14):1273–83. [PMID: 21991949]

Valachis A et al. Adjuvant therapy with zoledronic acid in patients with breast cancer: a systematic review and meta-analysis. Oncologist. 2013;18(4):353–61. [PMID: 23404816]

Verma S et al; EMILIA Study Group. Trastuzumab emtansine for HER2-positive advanced breast cancer. N Engl J Med. 2012 Nov 8;367(19):1783–91. [PMID: 23020162]

Veronesi U et al. Intraoperative radiotherapy versus external radiotherapy for early breast cancer (ELIOT): a randomised controlled equivalence trial. Lancet Oncol. 2013 Dec;14(13):1269–77. [PMID: 24225155]

Von Minckwitz G et al. A randomized phase II trial investigating the addition of carboplatin to neoadjuvant therapy for triple-negative and HER2-positive early breast cancer (GeparSixto). 2013 ASCO Annual Meeting. Abstract 1004. Presented June 3, 2013.

Weaver DL et al. Effect of occult metastases on survival in node-negative breast cancer. N Engl J Med. 2011 Feb 3;364(5):412–21. [PMID: 21247310]

▶ **Prognosis**

Stage of breast cancer is the most reliable indicator of prognosis (Table 17–7). Axillary lymph node status is the best-analyzed prognostic factor and correlates with survival at all tumor sizes. When cancer is localized to the breast with no evidence of regional spread after pathologic examination, the clinical cure rate with most accepted methods of therapy is 75% to > 90%. In fact, patients with small mammographically detected biologically favorable tumors and no evidence of axillary spread have a 5-year survival rate > 95%. When the axillary lymph nodes are involved with tumor, the survival rate drops to 50–70% at 5 years and probably around 25–40% at 10 years. Increasingly, the use of biologic markers, such as ER, PR, grade, and HER2, is helping to identify high-risk tumor types as well as direct treatment used (see Biomarkers & Gene Expression Profiling). Tumors with marked aneuploidy have a

Table 17–7. Approximate survival (%) of patients with breast cancer by TNM stage.

TNM Stage	Five Years	Ten Years
0	95	90
I	85	70
IIA	70	50
IIB	60	40
IIIA	55	30
IIIB	30	20
IV	5–10	2
All	65	30

poor prognosis (see Table 17–5). Gene analysis studies, such as Oncotype Dx, can predict disease-free survival for some subsets of patients.

Five-year statistics do not accurately reflect the final outcome of therapy. The mortality rate of breast cancer patients exceeds that of age-matched normal controls for nearly 20 years. Thereafter, the mortality rates are equal, though deaths that occur among breast cancer patients are often directly the result of tumor.

In general, breast cancer appears to be somewhat more aggressive and associated with worse outcomes in younger than in older women, and this may be related to the fact that fewer younger women have ER-positive tumors. Adjuvant systemic chemotherapy, in general, improves survival by about 30% and adjuvant hormonal therapy by about 25%.

For those patients whose disease progresses despite treatment, studies suggest supportive group therapy may improve survival. As they approach the end of life, such patients will require meticulous palliative care (see Chapter 5).

Manson JE et al. Menopausal hormone therapy and health outcomes during the intervention and extended poststopping phases of the Women's Health Initiative randomized trials. JAMA. 2013 Oct 2;310(13):1353–68. [PMID: 24084921]

Parmeshwar R et al. Patient surveillance after initial breast cancer therapy: variation by physician specialty. Am J Surg. 2013 Aug;206(2):218–22. [PMID: 23870392]

Rakha EA. Pitfalls in outcome prediction of breast cancer. J Clin Pathol. 2013 Jun;66(6):458–64. [PMID: 23618694]

▶ **Follow-up Care**

After primary therapy, patients with breast cancer should be monitored long-term in order to detect recurrences and to observe the opposite breast for a second primary carcinoma. Local and distant recurrences occur most frequently within the first 2–5 years. During the first 2 years, most patients should be examined every 6 months (with mammogram every 6 months on the affected breast), then annually thereafter. Special attention is paid to the contralateral breast because a new primary breast malignancy will develop in 20–25% of patients. In some cases, metastases are dormant for long periods and may appear 10–15 years or longer after removal of the primary tumor. **Although studies have failed to show an adverse effect of hormonal replacement in disease-free patients, it is rarely used after breast cancer treatment, particularly if the tumor was hormone receptor–positive.** Even pregnancy has not been associated with shortened survival of patients rendered disease free—yet many oncologists are reluctant to advise a young patient with breast cancer that it is safe to become pregnant, and most will not support prescribing hormone replacement for the postmenopausal breast cancer patient. The use of estrogen replacement for conditions such as osteoporosis, vaginal dryness and hot flushes may be considered for a woman with a history of breast cancer after discussion of the benefits and risks; however, it is not routinely recommended, especially given the availability of nonhormonal agents for these conditions (such as bisphosphonates and denosumab for osteoporosis). Vaginal estrogen is frequently used to treat vaginal atrophy with no obvious ill effects.

A. Local Recurrence

The incidence of local recurrence correlates with tumor size, the presence and number of involved axillary nodes, the histologic type of tumor, the presence of skin edema or skin and fascia fixation with the primary tumor, and the type of definitive surgery and local irradiation. Local recurrence on the chest wall after total mastectomy and axillary dissection develops in as many as 8% of patients. When the axillary nodes are not involved, the local recurrence rate is < 5%, but the rate is as high as 25% when they are heavily involved. A similar difference in local recurrence rate was noted between small and large tumors. Factors such as multifocal cancer, in situ tumors, positive resection margins, chemotherapy, and radiotherapy have an effect on local recurrence in patients treated with breast-conserving surgery. Adjuvant systemic therapy greatly decreases the rate of local recurrence.

Chest wall recurrences usually appear within the first several years but may occur as late as 15 or more years after mastectomy. All suspicious nodules and skin lesions should be biopsied. Local excision or localized radiotherapy may be feasible if an isolated nodule is present. If lesions are multiple or accompanied by evidence of regional involvement in the internal mammary or supraclavicular nodes, the disease is best managed by radiation treatment of the entire chest wall including the parasternal, supraclavicular, and axillary areas and usually by systemic therapy.

Local recurrence after mastectomy usually signals the presence of widespread disease and is an indication for studies to search for evidence of metastases. Distant metastases will develop within a few years in most patients with locally recurrent tumor after mastectomy. When there is no evidence of metastases beyond the chest wall

and regional nodes, irradiation for cure after complete local excision should be attempted. After partial mastectomy, local recurrence does not have as serious a prognostic significance as after mastectomy. However, those patients in whom a recurrence develops have a worse prognosis than those who do not. It is speculated that the ability of a cancer to recur locally after radiotherapy is a sign of aggressiveness and resistance to therapy. Completion of the mastectomy should be done for local recurrence after partial mastectomy; some of these patients will survive for prolonged periods, especially if the breast recurrence is DCIS or occurs more than 5 years after initial treatment. Systemic chemotherapy or hormonal treatment should be used for women in whom disseminated disease develops or those in whom local recurrence occurs.

B. Breast Cancer Survivorship Issues

Given that most women with non-metastatic breast cancer will be cured, a significant number of women face survivorship issues stemming from either the diagnosis or the treatment of the breast cancer. These challenges include psychological struggles, upper extremity lymphedema, cognitive decline (also called "chemo brain"), weight management problems, cardiovascular issues, bone loss, postmenopausal side effects, and fatigue. One randomized study reported that survivors who received psychological intervention from the time of diagnosis had a lower risk of recurrence and breast cancer–related mortality. A randomized study in older, overweight cancer survivors showed that diet and exercise reduced the rate of self-reported functional decline compared with no intervention. Cognitive dysfunction is a commonly reported symptom experienced by women who have undergone systemic treatment for early breast cancer. Studies are ongoing to understand the pathophysiology leading to this syndrome. An interesting study reported that 200 mg of modafinil daily improved speed and quality of memory as well as attention for breast cancer survivors dealing with cognitive dysfunction. This promising study requires validation in a larger clinical trial.

1. Edema of the arm—Significant edema of the arm occurs in about 10–30% of patients after axillary dissection with or without mastectomy. It occurs more commonly if radiotherapy has been given or if there was postoperative infection. **Partial mastectomy with radiation to the axillary lymph nodes is followed by chronic edema of the arm in 10–20% of patients.** Sentinel lymph node dissection has proved to be a more accurate form of axillary staging without the side effects of edema or infection. Judicious use of radiotherapy, with treatment fields carefully planned to spare the axilla as much as possible, can greatly diminish the incidence of edema, which will occur in only 5% of patients if no radiotherapy is given to the axilla after a partial mastectomy and lymph node dissection.

Late or secondary edema of the arm may develop years after treatment, as a result of axillary recurrence or infection in the hand or arm, with obliteration of lymphatic channels. When edema develops, a careful examination of the axilla for recurrence or infection is performed. Infection in the arm or hand on the dissected side should be treated with antibiotics, rest, and elevation. If there is no sign of recurrence or infection, the swollen extremity should be treated with rest and elevation. A mild diuretic may be helpful. If there is no improvement, a compressor pump or manual compression decreases the swelling, and the patient is then fitted with an elastic glove or sleeve. Most patients are not bothered enough by mild edema to wear an uncomfortable glove or sleeve and will treat themselves with elevation or manual compression alone. Benzopyrones have been reported to decrease lymphedema but are not approved for this use in the United States. Rarely, edema may be severe enough to interfere with use of the limb. Previously, patients were advised to avoid weight lifting with the ipsilateral arm to prevent a worsening in lymphedema. However, a prospective randomized study has shown that **twice weekly progressive weight lifting improves lymphedema symptoms and exacerbations and improves extremity strength**.

2. Breast reconstruction—Breast reconstruction is usually feasible after total or modified radical mastectomy. Reconstruction should be discussed with patients prior to mastectomy, because it offers an important psychological focal point for recovery. Reconstruction is not an obstacle to the diagnosis of recurrent cancer. The most common breast reconstruction has been implantation of a silicone gel or saline prosthesis in the subpectoral plane between the pectoralis minor and pectoralis major muscles. Alternatively, autologous tissue can be used for reconstruction.

Autologous tissue flaps are aesthetically superior to implant reconstruction in most patients. They also have the advantage of not feeling like a foreign body to the patient. The most popular autologous technique currently is the transrectus abdominis muscle flap (TRAM flap), which is done by rotating the rectus abdominis muscle with attached fat and skin cephalad to make a breast mound. The free TRAM flap is done by completely removing a small portion of the rectus with overlying fat and skin and using microvascular surgical techniques to reconstruct the vascular supply on the chest wall. A latissimus dorsi flap can be swung from the back but offers less fullness than the TRAM flap and is therefore less acceptable cosmetically. An implant often is used to increase the fullness with a latissimus dorsi flap. Reconstruction may be performed immediately (at the time of initial mastectomy) or may be delayed until later, usually when the patient has completed adjuvant therapy. When considering reconstructive options, concomitant illnesses should be considered, since the ability of an autologous flap to survive depends on medical comorbidities. In addition, the need for radiotherapy may affect the choice of reconstruction as radiation may increase fibrosis around an implant or decrease the volume of a flap.

3. Risks of pregnancy—Data are insufficient to determine whether interruption of pregnancy improves the prognosis of patients who are identified to

have potentially curable breast cancer and who receive definitive treatment during pregnancy. Theoretically, the high levels of estrogen produced by the placenta as the pregnancy progresses could be detrimental to the patient with occult metastases of hormone-sensitive breast cancer. However, **retrospective studies have *not* shown a worse prognosis for women with gestational breast cancer.** The decision whether or not to terminate the pregnancy must be made on an individual basis, taking into account the clinical stage of the cancer, the overall prognosis for the patient, the gestational age of the fetus, the potential for premature ovarian failure in the future with systemic therapy, and the patient's wishes. Women with early-stage gestational breast cancer who choose to continue their pregnancy should undergo surgery to remove the tumor and systemic therapy if indicated. Retrospective reviews of patients treated with anthracycline-containing regimens for gestational cancers (including leukemia and lymphomas) have established the relative safety of these regimens during pregnancy for both the patient and the fetus. Taxane-based and trastuzumab-based regimens have not been evaluated extensively, however. Radiation therapy should be delayed until the pregnant patient has delivered.

Equally important is the advice regarding future pregnancy (or abortion in case of pregnancy) to be given to women of child-bearing age who have had definitive treatment for breast cancer. To date, no adverse effect of pregnancy on survival of women who have had breast cancer has been demonstrated. When counseling patients, oncologists must take into consideration the patients' overall prognosis, age, comorbidities, and life goals.

In patients with inoperable or metastatic cancer (stage IV disease), induced abortion is usually advisable because of the possible adverse effects of hormonal treatment, radiotherapy, or chemotherapy upon the fetus in addition to the expectant mother's poor prognosis.

Berger AM et al. Cancer-related fatigue: implications for breast cancer survivors. Cancer. 2012 Apr 15;118(8 Suppl):2261–9. [PMID: 22488700]

Colfry AJ 3rd. Miscellaneous syndromes and their management: occult breast cancer, breast cancer in pregnancy, male breast cancer, surgery in stage IV disease. Surg Clin North Am. 2013 Apr;93(2):519–31. [PMID: 23464700]

Del Mastro L et al. Effect of the gonadotropin-releasing hormone analogue triptorelin on the occurrence of chemotherapy-induced early menopause in premenopausal women with breast cancer: a randomized trial. JAMA. 2011 Jul 20;306(3):269–76. [PMID: 21771987]

Fong DY et al. Physical activity for cancer survivors: meta-analysis of randomized controlled trials. BMJ. 2012 Jan30;344:e70. [PMID: 22294757]

Hermelink K. Acute and late onset cognitive dysfunction associated with chemotherapy in women with breast cancer. Cancer. 2011 Mar 1;117(5):1103. [PMID: 20960507]

Lee ES et al. Health-related quality of life in survivors with breast cancer 1 year after diagnosis compared with the general population: a prospective cohort study. Ann Surg. 2011 Jan;253(1):101–8. [PMID: 21294288]

Siegel R et al. Cancer treatment and survivorship statistics, 2012. CA Cancer J Clin. 2012 Jul–Aug;62(4):220–41. [PMID: 22700443]

Thong MS et al. Population-based cancer registries for quality-of-life research: a work-in-progress resource for survivorship studies? Cancer. 2013 Jun 1;119(Suppl 11):2109–23. [PMID: 23695923]

CARCINOMA OF THE MALE BREAST

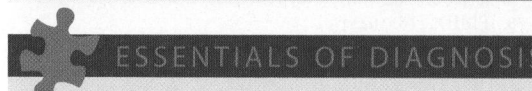

ESSENTIALS OF DIAGNOSIS

▶ A painless lump beneath the areola in a man usually over 50 years of age.

▶ Nipple discharge, retraction, or ulceration may be present.

▶ Generally poorer prognosis than in women.

General Considerations

Breast cancer in men is a rare disease; the incidence is only about 1% of that in women. The average age at occurrence is about 70 years and there may be an increased incidence of breast cancer in men with prostate cancer. As in women, hormonal influences are probably related to the development of male breast cancer. There is a high incidence of both breast cancer and gynecomastia in Bantu men, theoretically owing to failure of estrogen inactivation by a liver damaged by associated liver disease. It is important to note that first-degree relatives of men with breast cancer are considered to be at high risk. This risk should be taken into account when discussing options with the patient and family. In addition, *BRCA2* mutations are common in men with breast cancer. Men with breast cancer, especially with a history of prostate cancer, should receive genetic counseling. The prognosis, even in stage I cases, is worse in men than in women. Blood-borne metastases are commonly present when the male patient appears for initial treatment. These metastases may be latent and may not become manifest for many years.

Clinical Findings

A painless lump, occasionally associated with nipple discharge, retraction, erosion, or ulceration, is the primary complaint. Examination usually shows a hard, ill-defined, nontender mass beneath the nipple or areola. Gynecomastia not uncommonly precedes or accompanies breast cancer in men. Nipple discharge is an uncommon presentation for breast cancer in men but is an ominous finding associated with carcinoma in nearly 75% of cases.

Breast cancer staging is the same in men as in women. Gynecomastia and metastatic cancer from another site (eg, prostate) must be considered in the differential diagnosis. Benign tumors are rare, and biopsy should be performed on all males with a defined breast mass.

Treatment

Treatment consists of modified radical mastectomy in operable patients, who should be chosen by the same criteria as women with the disease. Breast conserving therapy is rarely performed. Irradiation is the first step in treating localized metastases in the skin, lymph nodes, or skeleton that are causing symptoms. Examination of the cancer for hormone receptor proteins and HER2 overexpression is of value in determining adjuvant therapy. Men commonly have ER-positive tumors and rarely have overexpression of HER2. Adjuvant systemic therapy and radiation is used for the same indications as in breast cancer in women.

Because breast cancer in men is frequently a disseminated disease, endocrine therapy is of considerable importance in its management. Tamoxifen is the main drug for management of advanced breast cancer in men. Tamoxifen (20 mg orally daily) should be the initial treatment. There is little experience with AIs though they should be effective. Castration in advanced breast cancer is a successful measure and more beneficial than the same procedure in women but is rarely used. Objective evidence of regression may be seen in 60–70% of men with hormonal therapy for metastatic disease—approximately twice the proportion in women. The average duration of tumor growth remission is about 30 months, and life is prolonged. Bone is the most frequent site of metastases from breast cancer in men (as in women), and hormonal therapy relieves bone pain in most patients so treated. The longer the interval between mastectomy and recurrence, the longer the remission following treatment is likely. As in women, there is correlation between ERs of the tumor and the likelihood of remission following hormonal therapy.

AIs should replace adrenalectomy in men as they have in women. Corticosteroid therapy alone has been considered to be efficacious but probably has no value when compared with major endocrine ablation. Either tamoxifen or AIs may be primary or secondary hormonal manipulation.

Estrogen therapy—5 mg of diethylstilbestrol three times daily orally—may be effective hormonal manipulation after others have been successful and failed, just as in women. Androgen therapy may exacerbate bone pain. Chemotherapy should be administered for the same indications and using the same dosage schedules as for women with metastatic disease or for adjuvant treatment.

Prognosis

Men with breast cancer *seem* to have a worse prognosis than women with breast cancer because breast cancer is diagnosed in men at a later stage. However, a large population based, international study reported that after adjustment for prognostic features (age, stage, treatment), men had a significantly improved relative survival from breast cancer compared to women. For node-positive disease, 5-year survival is approximately 69%, and for node-negative disease, it is 88%. A practice-patterns database study reported that based on NCCN guidelines, only

59% of patients received the recommended chemotherapy, 82% received the recommended hormonal therapy, and 71% received the recommended post-mastectomy radiation, indicating a relatively low adherence to NCCN guidelines for men.

For those patients whose disease progresses despite treatment, meticulous efforts at palliative care are essential (see Chapter 5).

Bird ST et al. Male breast cancer and 5α-reductase inhibitors finasteride and dutasteride. J Urol. 2013 Nov;190(5):1811–4. [PMID: 23665270]

Colfry AJ 3rd. Miscellaneous syndromes and their management: occult breast cancer, breast cancer in pregnancy, male breast cancer, surgery in stage IV disease. Surg Clin North Am. 2013 Apr;93(2):519–31. [PMID: 23464700]

Kiluk JV et al. Male breast cancer: management and follow-up recommendations. Breast J. 2011 Sep–Oct;17(5):503–9. [PMID: 21883641]

Miao H et al. Incidence and outcome of male breast cancer: an international population-based study. J Clin Oncol. 2011 Nov 20;29(33):4381–6. [PMID: 21969512]

Ravi A et al. Breast cancer in men: prognostic factors, treatment patterns, and outcome. Am J Mens Health. 2012 Jan;6(1):51–8. [PMID: 21831929]

Gynecologic Disorders

Jason Woo, MD, MPH, FACOG
Alicia Y. Armstrong, MD, MHSCR
H. Trent MacKay, MD, MPH

PREMENOPAUSAL ABNORMAL UTERINE BLEEDING

ESSENTIALS OF DIAGNOSIS

▶ Accurate diagnosis of abnormal uterine bleeding (AUB) depends on appropriate categorization and diagnostic tests.

▶ Pregnancy should always be ruled out as a cause of AUB in reproductive age women.

▶ The evaluation of AUB depends on the age and risk factors of the patient.

▶ General Considerations

Normal menstrual bleeding lasts an average of 5 days (range, 2–7 days), with a mean blood loss of 40 mL. **Menorrhagia** is defined as blood loss of over 80 mL per cycle and frequently produces anemia. **Metrorrhagia** is defined as bleeding between periods. **Polymenorrhea** is defined as bleeding that occurs more often than every 21 days, and **oligomenorrhea** is defined as bleeding that occurs less frequently than every 35 days.

A classification system, known by the acronym PALM-COEIN, is used by the International Federation of Gynecology and Obstetrics (FIGO) and does not use the term "dysfunctional uterine bleeding." Instead, **abnormal uterine bleeding (AUB)** is the overarching term paired with descriptive terms denoting the bleeding pattern (ie, heavy, light and menstrual, intermenstrual) and by etiology (**P**olyp, **A**denomyosis, **L**eiomyoma, **M**alignancy and hyperplasia, **C**oagulopathy, **O**vulatory dysfunction, **E**ndometrial, **I**atrogenic, and **N**ot yet classified). In adolescents, AUB often occurs as a result of persistent anovulation due to the immaturity of the hypothalamic-pituitary-ovarian axis and represents normal physiology. Once regular menses has been established during adolescence, **ovulatory** AUB (AUB-O) accounts for most cases. AUB in women aged 19–39 years is often a result of pregnancy, structural lesions, anovulatory cycles, use of hormonal contraception, or endometrial hyperplasia.

▶ Clinical Findings

A. Symptoms and Signs

The diagnosis usually depends on the following: (1) A careful description of the duration and amount of flow, related pain, and relationship to the last menstrual period (LMP), with the presence of blood clots or the degree of inconvenience caused by the bleeding serving as useful indicators; (2) A history of pertinent illnesses, such as recent systemic infections or hospitalizations, or weight change; (3) A history of medications or herbal remedies that might cause AUB; (4) A history of coagulation disorders in the patient or family members; (5) A physical examination to look for general findings of excessive weight, signs of polycystic ovary syndrome (PCOS), thyroid disease or insulin resistance, and (6) A pelvic examination for vulvar, vaginal or cervical lesions, pregnancy, uterine myomas, adnexal masses, adenomyosis, or infection.

B. Laboratory Studies

A complete blood count and a pregnancy test should be done as well as thyroid function studies. For adolescents with heavy menstrual bleeding and adults with a positive screening history, coagulation studies should be considered, since up to 18% of women with severe menorrhagia may have a coagulopathy. Cervical samples should be obtained for cytology and culture.

C. Imaging

Ultrasound may be useful to evaluate endometrial thickness or to diagnose intrauterine or ectopic pregnancy or adnexal masses. Sonohysterography or hysteroscopy may be used to diagnose endometrial polyps or subserous myomas. MRI is not a primary imaging modality for AUB but can definitively diagnose submucous myomas and adenomyosis.

D. Cervical Biopsy and Endometrial Sampling

The primary role of endometrial sampling is to determine whether carcinoma or premalignant lesions are present, even though other pathology related to bleeding may be

Table 18–1. Common gynecologic diagnostic procedures.

Colposcopy
Visualization of cervical, vaginal, or vulvar epithelium under 5–50× magnification with and without dilute acetic acid to identify abnormal areas requiring biopsy. An office procedure.

Dilation & curettage (D&C)
Dilation of the cervix and curettage of the entire endometrial cavity, using a metal curette or suction cannula and often using forceps for the removal of endometrial polyps. Can usually be done in the office under local anesthesia.

Endometrial biopsy
Removal of one or more areas of the endometrium by means of a curette or small aspiration device without cervical dilation. Diagnostic accuracy similar to D&C. An office procedure performed under local anesthesia.

Endocervical curettage
Removal of endocervical epithelium with a small curette for diagnosis of cervical dysplasia and cancer. An office procedure performed under local anesthesia.

Hysteroscopy
Visual examination of the uterine cavity with a small fiberoptic endoscope passed through the cervix. Biopsies and excision of myomas can be performed. Can be done in the office under local anesthesia or in the operating room under general anesthesia.

Saline infusion sonohysterography
Introduction of saline solution into endometrial cavity with a catheter to visualize submucous myomas or endometrial polyps by transvaginal ultrasound. May be performed in the office with oral analgesia.

Hysterosalpingography
Injection of radiopaque dye through the cervix to visualize the uterine cavity and oviducts. Mainly used in investigation of infertility.

Laparoscopy
Visualization of the abdominal and pelvic cavity through a small fiberoptic endoscope passed through a subumbilical incision. Permits diagnosis, tubal sterilization, and treatment of many conditions previously requiring laparotomy. General anesthesia is usually used.

found. Sampling methods and other gynecologic diagnostic procedures are described in Table 18–1. Polyps, endometrial hyperplasia, and submucous myomas are commonly identified in this way. **Endometrial sampling should be performed in patients with AUB who are older than 45 years, or in younger patients with a history of unopposed estrogen exposure or failed medical management and persistent AUB.** If the Papanicolaou smear abnormality requires it, or a gross cervical lesion is seen, colposcopic directed biopsies and endocervical curettage are usually indicated.

► **Treatment**

Premenopausal patients with AUB include those with submucosal myomas, infection, early abortion, thrombophilias, or pelvic neoplasms. The history, physical examination, laboratory findings, imaging, and endometrial sampling should

identify such patients, who require definitive therapy. A large group of patients remain, most of whom have AUB-O.

AUB-O can usually be treated hormonally. Progestins, which limit and stabilize endometrial growth, are generally effective. For patients with irregular or light bleeding, medroxyprogesterone acetate, 10 mg/d orally, or norethindrone acetate, 5 mg/d orally, should be given for 10 days, following which withdrawal bleeding (so-called *medical curettage*) will occur. If successful, the treatment can be repeated for several cycles, starting medication on day 15 of subsequent cycles, or it can be reinstituted if amenorrhea or dysfunctional bleeding recurs. In women who are experiencing heavier bleeding, any of the combination oral contraceptives (with 30–35 mcg of estrogen estradiol) can be given four times daily for 1 or 2 days followed by two pills daily through day 5 and then one pill daily through day 20; after withdrawal bleeding occurs, pills are taken in the usual dosage for three cycles. In cases of intractable heavy bleeding, a gonadotropin-releasing hormone (GnRH) agonist such as depot leuprolide, 3.75 mg intramuscularly monthly, or nafarelin, 0.2–0.4 mg intranasally twice daily, can be used for up to 6 months to create a temporary cessation of menstruation by ovarian suppression. These therapies require 2–4 weeks to down-regulate the pituitary and stop bleeding and will not stop bleeding acutely. In cases of heavy bleeding requiring hospitalization, intravenous conjugated estrogens, 25 mg every 4 hours for three or four doses, can be used, followed by oral conjugated estrogens, 2.5 mg daily, or ethinyl estradiol, 20 mcg orally daily, for 3 weeks, with the addition of medroxyprogesterone acetate, 10 mg orally daily for the last 10 days of treatment, or a combination oral contraceptive daily for 3 weeks. This will thicken the endometrium and control the bleeding. Nonsteroidal anti-inflammatory drugs (NSAIDs), such as naproxen or mefenamic acid, in the usual anti-inflammatory doses will often reduce blood loss in menorrhagia—even that associated with a copper intrauterine device (IUD).

If the abnormal bleeding is not controlled by hormonal treatment, hysteroscopy with tissue sampling or saline infusion sonohysterography is used to evaluate for structural lesions (such as polyps, submucous myomas) or neoplasms (such as endometrial cancer). In the absence of specific pathology, bleeding unresponsive to medical therapy may be treated with endometrial ablation, levonorgestrel-releasing IUD, or hysterectomy. While hysterectomy was used commonly in the past for bleeding unresponsive to medical therapy, the low risk of complications and the good short-term results of both endometrial ablation and levonorgestrel-releasing IUD make them attractive alternatives to hysterectomy. Endometrial ablation may be performed through the hysteroscope with laser photocoagulation or electrocautery. Nonhysteroscopic techniques include balloon thermal ablation, cryoablation, free-fluid thermal ablation, impedence bipolar radiofrequency ablation, and microwave ablation. The latter methods are well-adapted to outpatient therapy under local anesthesia.

The levonorgestrel-releasing IUD markedly reduces menstrual blood loss and may be a good alternative to other therapies. However, while short-term results with endometrial ablation and levonorgestrel-releasing IUD are satisfactory, at 5 years after either the endometrial ablation procedure or placement of the levonorgestrel IUD, up to 40% of women will have had either repeat ablation procedures or a hysterectomy.

▶ When to Refer

- If bleeding is not controlled with first-line therapy.
- If expertise is needed for a surgical procedure.

▶ When to Admit

If bleeding is uncontrollable with first-line therapy or the patient is not hemodynamically stable.

American College of Obstetricians and Gynecologists. Practice Bulletin No. 128: Diagnosis of abnormal uterine bleeding in reproductive-aged women. Obstet Gynecol. 2012 Jul;120(1): 197–206. [PMID: 22914421]

Thomas MC. Treatment options for dysfunctional uterine bleeding. Nurse Pract. 2011 Aug;36(8):14–20. [PMID: 21730879]

POSTMENOPAUSAL VAGINAL BLEEDING

ESSENTIALS OF DIAGNOSIS

- ▶ Vaginal bleeding that occurs 6 months or more following cessation of menstrual function.
- ▶ Postmenopausal bleeding of any amount always should be investigated. Transvaginal ultrasound measurement of the endometrium is a very helpful tool in evaluating postmenopausal bleeding.

▶ General Considerations

Vaginal bleeding that occurs 6 months or more following cessation of menstrual function should be investigated. The most common causes are atrophic endometrium, endometrial proliferation or hyperplasia, endometrial or cervical cancer, and administration of estrogens with or without added progestin. Other causes include atrophic vaginitis, trauma, endometrial polyps, friction ulcers of the cervix associated with prolapse of the uterus, and blood dyscrasias. **Bleeding of any amount in a postmenopausal woman should always be investigated.**

▶ Diagnosis

The vulva and vagina should be inspected for areas of bleeding, ulcers, or neoplasms. A cytologic smear of the cervix and vaginal pool should be taken. If available, transvaginal sonography should be used to measure endometrial thickness. A measurement of 4 mm or less indicates a low likelihood of hyperplasia or endometrial cancer. If the thickness is > 4 mm or there is a heterogeneous appearance to the endometrium, it should be determined if the thickening is global or focal. Sonohysterography may assist in

making this distinction. If the thickening is global, endometrial biopsy or D&C is appropriate. If focal, guided sampling with hysteroscopy should be done.

▶ Treatment

Simple endometrial hyperplasia calls for cyclic or continuous progestin therapy (medroxyprogesterone acetate, 10 mg/d orally, or norethindrone acetate, 5 mg/d orally) for 21 or 30 days of each month for 3 months. The use of a levonorgestrel intrauterine system is also a treatment option. Repeat sampling should be performed if symptoms recur. If endometrial hyperplasia with atypia or if carcinoma of the endometrium is found, hysterectomy is necessary.

▶ When to Refer

- Expertise in performing ultrasonography is required.
- Complex endometrial hyperplasia with atypia is present.
- Hysteroscopy is indicated.

American College of Obstetricians and Gynecologists. ACOG Committee Opinion No. 426: The role of transvaginal ultrasonography in the evaluation of postmenopausal bleeding. Obstet Gynecol. 2009 Feb;113(2 Pt 1):462–4. [Reaffirmed 2011] [PMID: 19155921]

Morelli M et al. Efficacy of the levonorgestrel intrauterine system (LNG-IUS) in the prevention of the atypical endometrial hyperplasia and endometrial cancer: retrospective data from selected obese menopausal symptomatic women. Gynecol Endocrinol. 2013 Feb;29(2):156–9. [PMID: 23134558]

Null DB et al. Postmenopausal bleeding-first steps in the workup. J Fam Pract. 2012 Oct;61(10):597–604. [PMID: 23106061]

PREMENSTRUAL SYNDROME (Premenstrual Tension)

The premenstrual syndrome (PMS) is a recurrent, variable cluster of troublesome physical and emotional symptoms that develop during the 5 days before the onset of menses and subside within 4 days after menstruation occurs. PMS intermittently affects about 40% of all premenopausal women, primarily those 25–40 years of age. In about 5–8% of affected women, the syndrome may be severe. Although not every woman experiences all the symptoms or signs at one time, many describe bloating, breast pain, ankle swelling, a sense of increased weight, skin disorders, irritability, aggressiveness, depression, inability to concentrate, libido change, lethargy, and food cravings. When emotional or mood symptoms predominate, along with physical symptoms, and there is a clear functional impairment with work or personal relationships, the term "premenstrual dysphoric disorder" (PMDD) may be applied. The pathogenesis of PMS/PMDD is still uncertain, and current treatment methods are mainly empiric. The clinician should provide support for both the patient's emotional and physical distress. This includes the following:

1. Careful evaluation of the patient, with understanding, explanation, and reassurance.

2. Advise the patient to keep a daily diary of all symptoms for 2–3 months, such as the Daily Record of Severity of

Problems, to evaluate the timing and characteristics of her symptoms. If her symptoms occur throughout the month rather than in the 2 weeks before menses, she may have depression or other mental health problems instead of or in addition to PMS.

3. For mild to moderate symptoms, a program of aerobic exercise; reduction of caffeine, salt, and alcohol intake; the use of alternative therapies, such as an increase in dietary calcium (to 1200 mg/d), vitamin D, or magnesium, and complex carbohydrates in the diet may be helpful, though these interventions remain unproven.

4. Medications that prevent ovulation, such as hormonal contraceptives, may lessen physical symptoms. A combined oral contraceptive containing the progestin drospirenone with a 4-day pill-free interval has been approved by the US Food and Drug Administration (FDA) for the treatment of PMDD. NSAIDs, such as mefenamic acid, 500 mg orally three times a day, will reduce a number of symptoms but not breast pain. When the above regimens are not effective, ovarian function can be suppressed with continuous high-dose progestin (20–30 mg/d of oral medroxyprogesterone acetate or 150 mg of depot medroxyprogesterone acetate (DMPA) orally every 3 months or GnRH agonist with add-back therapy, such as conjugated equine estrogen, 0.625 mg orally daily with medroxyprogesterone acetate, 2.5–5 mg orally daily).

5. When mood disorders predominate, several serotonin reuptake inhibitors (such as fluoxetine, 20 mg orally, either daily or only on symptom days) have been shown to be effective in relieving tension, irritability, and dysphoria with few side effects.

First-line drug therapy includes serotonergic antidepressants (citalopram, escitalopram, fluoxetine, sertraline, venlafaxine). There is little data to support the use of calcium, vitamin D, and vitamin B_6 supplementation. There is insufficient evidence to support cognitive behavior therapy.

Biggs WS et al. Premenstrual syndrome and premenstrual dysphoric disorder. Am Fam Physician. 2011 Oct 15;84(8):918–24. [PMID: 22010771]
Panay N. Treatment of premenstrual syndrome: a decision-making algorithm. Menopause Int. 2012 Jun;18(2):90–2. [PMID: 22611230]

DYSMENORRHEA

1. Primary Dysmenorrhea

Primary dysmenorrhea is menstrual pain associated with menstrual cycles in the absence of pathologic findings. The pain usually begins within 1–2 years after the menarche and may become more severe with time. The frequency of cases increases up to age 20 and then decreases with age and markedly with parity. Fifty to 75 percent of women are affected at some time and 5–6% have incapacitating pain.

▶ Clinical Findings

Primary dysmenorrhea is low, midline, wave-like, cramping pelvic pain often radiating to the back or inner thighs. Cramps may last for 1 or more days and may be associated with nausea, diarrhea, headache, and flushing. The pain is produced by uterine vasoconstriction, anoxia, and sustained contractions mediated by prostaglandins. The pelvic examination is normal between menses; examination during menses may produce discomfort, but there are no pathologic findings.

▶ Treatment

NSAIDs (ibuprofen, ketoprofen, mefenamic acid, naproxen) and the cyclooxygenase (COX)-2 inhibitor celecoxib are generally helpful. The medication should be started 1–2 days before expected menses. Symptoms can be suppressed with use of oral contraceptives, DMPA, or the levonorgestrel-releasing IUD. Continuous use of oral contraceptives can be used to suppress menstruation completely and prevent dysmenorrhea. For women who do not wish to use hormonal contraception, other therapies that have shown at least some benefit include local heat; thiamine, 100 mg/d orally; vitamin E, 200 units/d orally from 2 days prior to and for the first 3 days of menses; and high-frequency transcutaneous electrical nerve stimulation.

2. Secondary Dysmenorrhea

Secondary dysmenorrhea is menstrual pain for which an organic cause exists, often associated with endometriosis or uterine fibroids. It usually begins well after menarche, sometimes even as late as the third or fourth decade of life.

▶ Clinical Findings

The history and physical examination may suggest endometriosis or fibroids. Other causes may be pelvic inflammatory disease (PID), submucous myoma(s), adenomyosis, IUD use, cervical stenosis with obstruction, or blind uterine horn (rare).

▶ Diagnosis

Pelvic imaging is useful for detecting the presence of uterine fibroids or other anomalies. Adenomyosis, the presence of islands of endometrial tissue in the myometrium, may be diagnosed with ultrasound or, preferably, with MRI. Cervical stenosis may result from induced abortion, creating crampy pain at the time of expected menses with obstruction of blood flow; this is easily cured by passing a sound into the uterine cavity after administering a paracervical block. Laparoscopy may be used to diagnose endometriosis or other pelvic abnormalities not visualized by imaging.

▶ Treatment

A. Specific Measures

A large 30-year Scandinavian study, carried out by a certified nurse midwife, has provided convincing evidence that the combined oral contraceptive pill does alleviates the symptoms of dysmenorrhoea. Periodic use of analgesics, including the NSAIDs given for primary dysmenorrhea, may be beneficial, and oral contraceptives may give relief, particularly in endometriosis. GnRH agonists are effective in the treatment of endometriosis (see below), although their long-term use may be limited by cost or side effects. Adenomyosis may respond to the levonorgestrel-releasing intrauterine system, uterine artery embolization, or hormonal approaches used to treat endometriosis, but hysterectomy remains the definitive treatment of choice for women for whom childbearing is not a consideration.

B. Surgical Measures

If disability is marked or prolonged, laparoscopy or exploratory laparotomy is usually warranted. Definitive surgery depends on the degree of disability and the findings at operation. Uterine fibroids may be removed or treated by uterine artery embolization. Hysterectomy may be done if other treatments have not worked but is usually a last resort.

When to Refer

- Standard therapy fails to relieve pain.
- Suspicion of pelvic pathology, such as endometriosis, leiomyomas, or adenomyosis.

European Society of Human Reproduction and Embryology. Study finds convincing evidence that the combined oral contraceptive pill helps painful periods. 2012 Jan 18. http://www.eshre.eu/Press-Room/Press-releases/Press-releases—2012/Combined-oral-contraceptive-pill.aspx

Harel Z. Dysmenorrhea in adolescents and young adults: an update on pharmacological treatments and management strategies. Expert Opin Pharmacother. 2012 Oct;13(15):2157–70. [PMID: 22984937]

Lindh I et al. The effect of combined oral contraceptives and age on dysmenorrhoea: an epidemiological study. Hum Reprod. 2012 Mar;27(3):676–82. [PMID: 22252090]

VAGINITIS

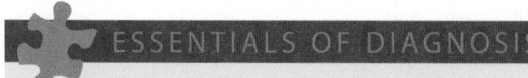

ESSENTIALS OF DIAGNOSIS

- Vaginal irritation.
- Pruritus.
- Unusual or malodorous discharge.

General Considerations

Inflammation and infection of the vagina are common gynecologic problems, resulting from a variety of pathogens, allergic reactions to vaginal contraceptives or other products, vaginal atrophy, or the friction of coitus. The normal vaginal pH is 4.5 or less, and *Lactobacillus* is the predominant organism. Normal secretions during the middle of the cycle, or during pregnancy, can be confused with vaginitis by concerned women.

Clinical Findings

When the patient complains of vaginal irritation, pain, or unusual or malodorous discharge, a history should be taken, noting the onset of the LMP; recent sexual activity; use of contraceptives, tampons, or douches; recent changes in medications or use of antibiotics; and the presence of vaginal burning, pain, pruritus, or unusually profuse or malodorous discharge. The physical examination should include careful inspection of the vulva and speculum examination of the vagina and cervix. The cervix is sampled for gonococcus and *Chlamydia* if appropriate. A specimen of vaginal discharge is examined under the microscope in a drop of 0.9% saline solution to look for trichomonads or clue cells and in a drop of 10% potassium hydroxide to search for *Candida*. The vaginal pH should be tested; it is frequently > 4.5 in infections due to trichomonads and bacterial vaginosis. A bimanual examination to look for evidence of pelvic infection should follow. Point-of-care testing is available for all three organisms that cause vaginitis. It can be used if microscopy is not available or for confirmatory testing of microscopy.

A. Vulvovaginal Candidiasis

Pregnancy, diabetes, and use of broad-spectrum antibiotics or corticosteroids predispose patients to *Candida* infections. Heat, moisture, and occlusive clothing also contribute to the risk. Pruritus, vulvovaginal erythema, and a white curd-like discharge that is not malodorous are found (Figure 18–1). Microscopic examination with 10% potassium hydroxide reveals hyphae and spores. Cultures with Nickerson medium may be used if *Candida* is suspected but not demonstrated.

B. *Trichomonas vaginalis* Vaginitis

This protozoal flagellate infects the vagina, Skene ducts, and lower urinary tract in women and the lower genitourinary tract in men. It is sexually transmitted. Pruritus and a malodorous frothy, yellow-green discharge occur, along with diffuse vaginal erythema and red macular lesions on the cervix in severe cases ("strawberry cervix," Figure 18–2).

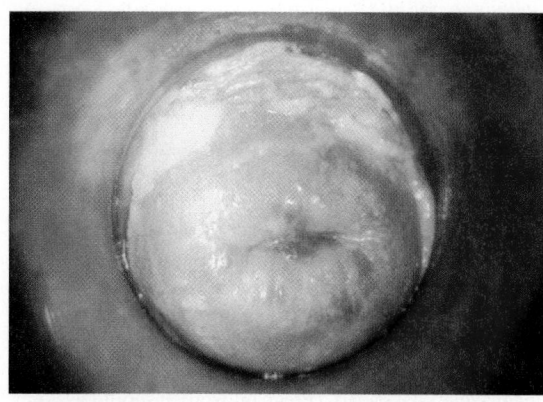

▲ **Figure 18–1.** Cervical candidiasis. (Public Health Image Library, CDC.)

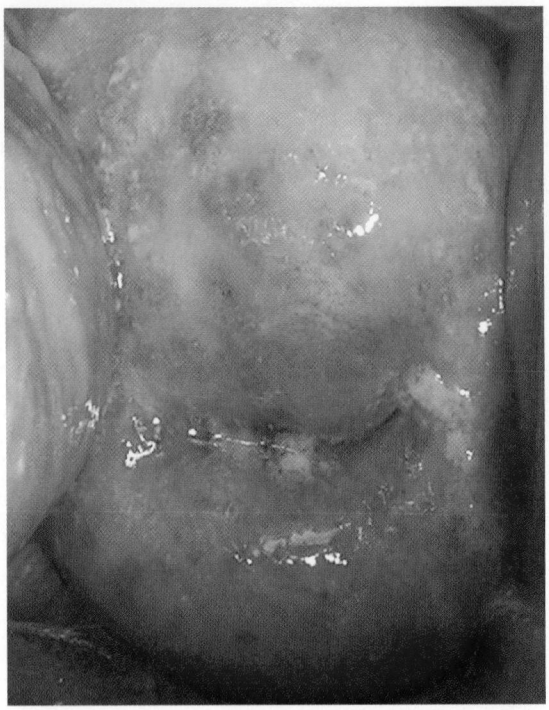

▲ **Figure 18–2.** Strawberry cervix in *Trichomonas vaginalis* infection, with inflammation and punctate hemorrhages. (Used with permission from Richard P. Usatine, MD.)

Motile organisms with flagella are seen by microscopic examination of a wet mount with saline solution.

C. Bacterial Vaginosis

This condition is considered to be a polymicrobial disease that is not sexually transmitted. An overgrowth of *Gardnerella* and other anaerobes is often associated with increased malodorous discharge without obvious vulvitis or vaginitis. The discharge is grayish and sometimes frothy, with a pH of 5.0–5.5. An amine-like ("fishy") odor is present if a drop of discharge is alkalinized with 10% potassium hydroxide. On wet mount in saline, epithelial cells are covered with bacteria to such an extent that cell borders are obscured (*clue cells*, Figure 18–3). Vaginal cultures are generally not useful in diagnosis.

▶ Treatment

A. Vulvovaginal Candidiasis

A variety of regimens are available to treat vulvovaginal candidiasis. Women with uncomplicated vulvovaginal candidiasis will usually respond to a 1- to 3-day regimen of a topical azole. Women with complicated infection (including four or more episodes in 1 year, severe signs and symptoms, non-albicans species, uncontrolled diabetes, HIV infection, corticosteroid treatment, or pregnancy) should receive 7–14 days of a topical regimen or two doses of oral fluconazole 3 days apart. (Pregnant women should use only topical azoles.) In recurrent non-albicans infections, 600 mg of boric acid in a gelatin capsule intravaginally once daily

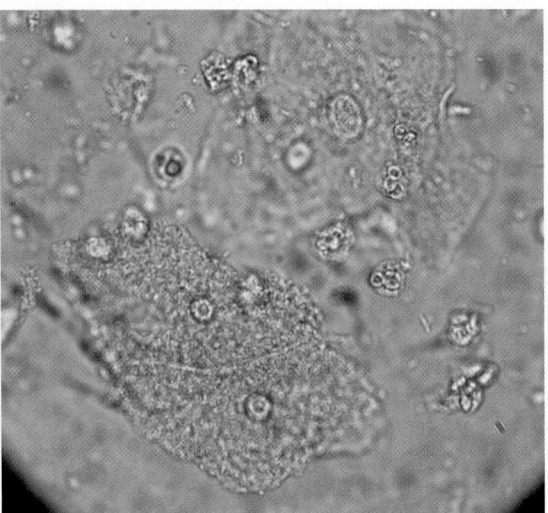

▲ **Figure 18–3.** Clue cells seen in bacterial vaginosis due to *Gardnerella vaginalis*. (Reproduced with permission, from Richard P. Usatine, MD.)

for 2 weeks is approximately 70% effective. If recurrence occurs, referral to an infectious disease specialist is indicated. Vulvovaginal candidiasis is considered recurrent when *at least four specific episodes occur in 1 year.*

1. Single-dose regimens—Effective single-dose regimens include miconazole (1200-mg vaginal suppository), tioconazole (6.5% cream, 5 g vaginally), sustained-release butoconazole (2% cream, 5 g vaginally), or fluconazole (150 mg oral tablet).

2. Three-day regimens—Effective 3-day regimens include butoconazole (2% cream, 5 g vaginally once daily), clotrimazole (2% cream, 5 g vaginally once daily), terconazole (0.8% cream, 5 g, or 80 mg vaginal suppository once daily), or miconazole (200 mg vaginal suppository once daily).

3. Seven-day regimens—The following regimens are given once daily: clotrimazole (1% cream), miconazole (2% cream, 5 g, or 100 mg vaginal suppository), or terconazole (0.4% cream, 5 g).

4. Fourteen-day regimen—An effective 14-day regimen is nystatin (100,000-unit vaginal tablet once daily).

5. Recurrent vulvovaginal candidiasis (maintenance therapy)—Clotrimazole (500 mg vaginal suppository once weekly or 200 mg cream twice weekly) or fluconazole (100, 150, or 200 mg orally once weekly) are effective regimens for maintenance therapy for up to 6 months.

B. *Trichomonas vaginalis* Vaginitis

Treatment of both partners simultaneously is recommended; metronidazole or tinidazole, 2 g orally as a single dose or 500 mg orally twice a day for 7 days, is usually used.

In the case of treatment failure with metronidazole in the absence of reexposure, the patient should be re-treated with metronidazole, 500 mg orally twice a day for 7 days, or tinidazole, 2 g orally as a single dose. If treatment failure occurs again, give metronidazole or tinidazole, 2 g orally once daily for 5 days. If this is not effective in eradicating the organisms, metronidazole and tinidazole susceptibility testing can be arranged with the CDC at 404-718-4141 or at http://www.cdc.gov/std. Women infected with *T vaginalis* are at increased risk for concurrent infection with other sexually transmitted diseases.

C. Bacterial Vaginosis

The recommended regimens are metronidazole (500 mg orally, twice daily for 7 days), clindamycin vaginal cream (2%, 5 g, once daily for 7 days), or metronidazole gel (0.75%, 5 g, twice daily for 5 days). Alternative regimens include clindamycin (300 mg orally twice daily for 7 days), clindamycin ovules (100 g intravaginally at bedtime for 3 days), tinidazole (2 g orally once daily for 3 days), or tinidazole (1 g orally once daily for 7 days).

The CDC offers a helpful training module to clinicians to review the current recommendations for treatment of vaginitis. Continuing medical education, continuing nursing education, and continuing education units are available with this online training (http://www2a.cdc.gov/stdtraining/self-study/vaginitis/default.htm).

CONDYLOMA ACUMINATA

Warty growths on the vulva, perianal area, vaginal walls, or cervix are caused by various types of the human papillomavirus (HPV). Pregnancy and immunosuppression favor growth. Ninety percent of genital warts are caused by HPV 6 and 11. The increased use of HPV vaccines should result in a decrease in the number of cases of this sexually transmitted disease. Vulvar lesions may be obviously wart-like or may be diagnosed only after application of 4% acetic acid (vinegar) and colposcopy, when they appear whitish, with prominent papillae. Vaginal lesions may show diffuse hypertrophy or a cobblestone appearance. Recommended treatments for vulvar warts include podophyllum resin 10–25% in tincture of benzoin (do not use during pregnancy or on bleeding lesions) or 80–90% trichloroacetic or bichloroacetic acid, carefully applied to avoid the surrounding skin. Surgical removal may be accomplished with tangential scissor excision, tangential shave excision, curettage, or electrotherapy. The pain of bichloroacetic or trichloroacetic acid application can be lessened by a sodium bicarbonate paste applied immediately after treatment. Podophyllum resin must be washed off after 2–4 hours. Freezing with liquid nitrogen or a cryoprobe and electrocautery are also effective. Patient-applied regimens, useful when the entire lesion is accessible to the patient, include podofilox 0.5% solution or gel, imiquimod 5% cream, or sinecatechins 15% ointment. Vaginal warts may be treated with cryotherapy with liquid nitrogen or trichloroacetic acid. Extensive warts may require treatment with CO_2 laser under local or general anesthesia.

CERVICAL POLYPS

Cervical polyps commonly occur after menarche and are occasionally noted in postmenopausal women. The cause is not known, but inflammation may play an etiologic role.

The principal symptoms are discharge and abnormal vaginal bleeding. However, abnormal bleeding should not be ascribed to a cervical polyp without sampling the endocervix and endometrium. The polyps are visible in the cervical os on speculum examination.

Cervical polyps must be differentiated from polypoid neoplastic disease of the endometrium, small submucous pedunculated myomas, large nabothian cysts, and endometrial polyps. Cervical polyps rarely contain dysplasia (0.5%) or malignant (0.5%) foci. Asymptomatic polyps in women under age 45 may be left untreated.

BARTHOLIN DUCT CYSTS & ABSCESSES

Trauma or infection may involve the Bartholin duct, causing obstruction of the gland. Drainage of secretions is prevented, leading to pain, swelling, and abscess formation (Figure 18–4). The infection usually resolves and pain disappears, but stenosis of the duct outlet with distention often persists. Reinfection causes recurrent tenderness and further enlargement of the duct.

The principal symptoms are periodic painful swelling on either side of the introitus and dyspareunia. A fluctuant swelling 1–4 cm in diameter lateral to either labium minus is a sign of occlusion of Bartholin duct. Tenderness is evidence of active infection.

Pus or secretions from the gland should be cultured for *Chlamydia* and other pathogens and treated accordingly (see Chapter 33); frequent warm soaks may be helpful. If an abscess develops, aspiration or incision and drainage are the simplest forms of therapy, but the problem may recur. Marsupialization (in the absence of an abscess), incision and drainage with the insertion of an indwelling Word catheter, or laser treatment will establish a new duct opening. Antibiotics are unnecessary unless cellulitis is present. An asymptomatic cyst does not require therapy.

▶ When to Refer

Surgical therapy (marsupialization) is indicated.

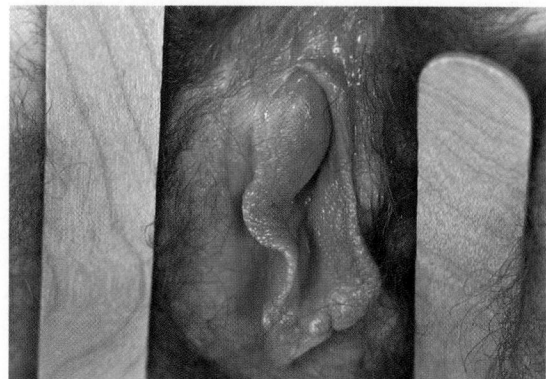

▲ **Figure 18–4.** Right-sided Bartholin cyst (abscess). The Bartholin gland is located in the lower two-thirds of the introitus. (From Susan Lindsley, Public Health Image Library, CDC.)

CERVICAL INTRAEPITHELIAL NEOPLASIA (CIN) (Dysplasia of the Cervix)

▶ The presumptive diagnosis is made by an abnormal Papanicolaou smear of an asymptomatic woman with no grossly visible cervical changes.

▶ Diagnose by colposcopically directed biopsy.

General Considerations

The squamocolumnar junction of the cervix is an area of active squamous cell proliferation. In childhood, this junction is located on the exposed vaginal portion of the cervix. At puberty, because of hormonal influence and possibly because of changes in the vaginal pH, the squamous margin begins to encroach on the single-layered, mucus-secreting epithelium, creating an area of metaplasia (transformation zone). Factors associated with coitus (see Prevention, below) may lead to cellular abnormalities, which over a period of time can result in the development of squamous cell dysplasia or cancer. There are varying degrees of dysplasia (Table 18–2), defined by the degree of cellular atypia; all types must be observed and treated if they persist or become more severe.

Clinical Findings

There are no specific symptoms or signs of CIN. The presumptive diagnosis is made by cytologic screening of an asymptomatic population with no grossly visible cervical changes. All visibly abnormal cervical lesions should be biopsied (Figure 18–5).

Table 18–2. Classification systems for Papanicolaou smears.

Numerical	Dysplasia	CIN	Bethesda System
1	Benign	Benign	Normal
2	Benign with inflammation	Benign with inflammation	Normal, ASC-US
3	Mild dysplasia	CIN I	Low-grade SIL
3	Moderate dysplasia	CIN II	High-grade SIL
3	Severe dysplasia	CIN III	
4	Carcinoma in situ		
5	Invasive cancer	Invasive cancer	Invasive cancer

ASC-US, atypical squamous cells of undetermined significance; CIN, cervical intraepithelial neoplasia; SIL, squamous intraepithelial lesion.

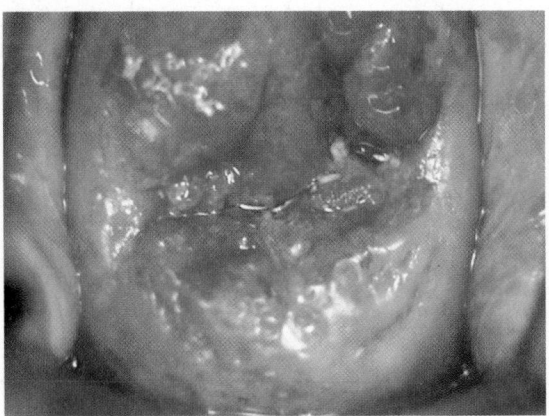

▲ **Figure 18–5.** Erosion of the cervix due to cervical intraepithelial neoplasia (CIN), a precursor lesion to cervical cancer. (Public Health Image Library, CDC.)

Diagnosis

A. Cytologic Examination (Papanicolaou Smear)

Screening should begin at age 21. The recommendation to start screening at age 21 years regardless of the age of onset of sexual intercourse is based in part on the very low incidence of cancer in younger women. In contrast to the high rate of infection with HPV in sexually active adolescents, invasive cervical cancer is very rare in women younger than age 21 years. The recommendation is also based on the potential for adverse effects associated with follow-up of young women with abnormal cytology screening results. **The US Preventive Services Task Force (USPSTF) recommends screening for cervical cancer in women age 21 to 65 years with cytology (Papanicolaou smear) every 3 years or, for women age 30 to 65 years who want to lengthen the screening interval, screening with a combination of cytology and HPV testing every 5 years.** Screening may be done with either liquid-based or conventional cytology. Women with risk factors that place them at higher risk for CIN may require more frequent screening. These risk factors include HIV infection, immunosuppression, exposure to diethylstilbesterol in utero, and previous treatment for CIN 2, CIN 3, or cervical cancer. The USPSTF recommends against screening for cervical cancer with HPV testing, alone or in combination with cytology, in women younger than age 30 years. The USPSTF recommends against screening for cervical cancer in women older than age 65 years who have had adequate prior screening and are not otherwise at high risk for cervical cancer. The guidelines have been changed to avoid overly aggressive treatment and monitoring. Online applications are available to provide the clinician with treatment guidelines for the management of abnormal Papanicolaou smears (http://www.imedicalapps.com/2013/04/cervical-cancer-screening-medical-app-asccp-obgyn-physicians/).

Exfoliated cells are collected from the transformation zone of the cervix and may be transferred to a vial of liquid preservative that is processed in the laboratory to produce a slide for interpretation—the liquid-based technique—or may be transferred directly to the slide and fixed using the conventional technique. Performance of conventional cervical cytology requires avoidance of contaminating blood, discharge, and lubricant.

Cytologic reports from the laboratory may describe findings in one of several ways (see Table 18–2). The Bethesda System uses the terminology "atypical squamous cells of unknown significance" (ASC-US) and "squamous intraepithelial lesions," either low-grade (LSIL) or high-grade (HSIL). Cytopathologists consider a Papanicolaou smear to be a medical consultation and will recommend further diagnostic procedures, treatment for infection, and comments on factors preventing adequate evaluation of the specimen.

Testing for HPV DNA currently is used in cervical cancer screening as a triage test to stratify risk to women aged 21 years and older with a cytologic diagnosis of ASC-US and postmenopausal women with a cytologic diagnosis of LSIL. It may be used as an adjunct to cytology for primary screening in women older than 30 years. It also may be used as a follow-up test after CIN 1 or negative findings on colposcopy in women whose prior cytologic diagnosis is ASC-US, atypical squamous cells, cannot rule out a high-grade lesion (ASC-H), LSIL, or atypical glandular cells, and in follow-up after treatment for CIN 2 and CIN 3. HPV testing should not be used in females younger than 21 years and if inadvertently performed, a positive result should not influence management.

B. Colposcopy

Women with ASC-US and a negative HPV screening may be followed-up in 1 year. If the HPV screen is positive, colposcopy should be performed. If HPV screening is unavailable, repeat cytology may be done at 4- to 6-month intervals until two consecutive normal results, or the patient may be referred directly for colposcopy. **All patients with SIL or atypical glandular cells should undergo colposcopy.** Viewing the cervix with 10–20 × magnification allows for assessment of the size and margins of an abnormal transformation zone and determination of extension into the endocervical canal. The application of 3–5% acetic acid (vinegar) dissolves mucus, and the acid's desiccating action sharpens the contrast between normal and actively proliferating squamous epithelium. Abnormal changes include white patches and vascular atypia, which indicate areas of greatest cellular activity.

C. Biopsy

Colposcopically directed punch biopsy and endocervical curettage are office procedures. If colposcopy is not available, the normal-appearing cervix shedding atypical cells can be evaluated by endocervical curettage and multiple punch biopsies of nonstaining squamous epithelium or biopsies from each quadrant of the cervix. Data from both cervical biopsy and endocervical curettage are important in deciding on treatment.

▷ Prevention

Cervical infection with the HPV is associated with a high percentage of all cervical dysplasias and cancers. There are over 70 recognized HPV subtypes, of which types 6 and 11 tend to cause genital warts and mild dysplasia, while types 16, 18, 31, and others cause higher-grade cellular changes. Vaccination can prevent cervical cancer and vaginal and vulvar pre-cancers caused by HPV types 16 and 18, and to protect against low-grade and pre-cancerous lesions caused by HPV types 16 and 18. The bivalent vaccine (known as Cervarix) provides protection against HPV types 16 and 18. The quadrivalent HPV 6/11/16/18 L1 virus-like-particle vaccine (known as Gardasil) also provides protection against genital warts caused by HPV types 6 and 11. **Gardasil is recommended for all girls and women aged 9 to 26.** Both vaccines provide partial protection against several other HPV types that cause approximately 30% of cervical cancers. In the United States, HPV prevalence appears to be decreasing among teenage girls, despite relatively low use of HPV vaccination. Because complete coverage of all carcinogenic HPV types is not provided by either vaccine, all women need to have regular cytologic screening as outlined above. In addition to vaccination, preventive measures include limiting the number of sexual partners, using a diaphragm or condom for coitus, and stopping smoking or exposure to second-hand smoke.

▷ Treatment

Treatment varies depending on the degree and extent of CIN. Biopsies should always precede treatment.

A. Cryosurgery

The use of freezing (cryosurgery) is effective for noninvasive small lesions visible on the cervix without endocervical extension.

B. CO$_2$ Laser

This well-controlled method minimizes tissue destruction. It is colposcopically directed and requires special training. It may be used with large visible lesions. In current practice, it involves the vaporization of the transformation zone on the cervix and the distal 5–7 mm of endocervical canal.

C. Loop Excision

When the CIN is clearly visible in its entirety, a wire loop can be used for excisional biopsy. This office procedure, called LEEP (loop electrosurgical excision procedure), with local anesthesia is quick and uncomplicated. Cutting and hemostasis are achieved with a low-voltage electrosurgical machine.

D. Conization of the Cervix

Conization is surgical removal of the entire transformation zone and endocervical canal. It should be reserved for cases of severe dysplasia (CIN III) or cancer in situ, particularly those with endocervical extension. The procedure can be performed with the scalpel, the CO$_2$ laser, the needle electrode, or by large-loop excision.

E. Follow-Up

Because recurrence is possible—especially in the first 2 years after treatment—and because the false-negative rate of a single cervical cytologic test is 20%, close follow-up after colposcopy and biopsy is imperative. For CIN II or III, cytologic examination or cytology and colposcopy should be repeated at 4- to 6-month intervals for up to 2 years. For CIN I, cytology should be performed at 6 and 12 months or HPV DNA testing can be done at 12 months. If testing is normal, routine cytologic screening can be resumed.

▶ When to Refer

- Patients with CIN II/III should be referred to an experienced colposcopist.
- Patients requiring conization biopsy should be referred to a gynecologist.

Erickson BK et al. Human papillomavirus: what every provider should know. Am J Obstet Gynecol. 2013 Mar;208(3):169–75. [PMID: 23021131]

Moyer VA. Screening for cervical cancer: U.S. Preventive Services Task Force recommendation statement. Ann Intern Med. 2012 Jun 19;156(12):880–91. [PMID: 22711081]

Whitlock EP et al. Liquid-based cytology and human papillomavirus testing to screen for cervical cancer: a systematic review for the U.S. Preventive Services Task Force. Ann Intern Med. 2011 Nov 15;155(10):687–97. [PMID: 22006930]

CARCINOMA OF THE CERVIX

The American Society for Colposcopy and Cervical Pathology Guidelines for cervical cancer screening and management of abnormal Papanicolaou smears are available for purchase in an online application (http://www.imedicalapps.com/2013/04/cervical-cancer-screening-medical-app-asccp-obgyn-physicians/).

ESSENTIALS OF DIAGNOSIS

▶ Increased risk in women who smoke and those with HIV or high-risk HPV types.

▶ Gross lesions should be evaluated by colposcopically directed biopsies and not cytology alone. Cervical lesion may be visible on inspection as a tumor or ulceration but a diagnosis of cervical cancer requires a tissue diagnosis.

▶ General Considerations

Cervical cancer is the third most common cancer in the world and the leading cause of cancer death among women in developing countries. It can be considered a sexually transmitted disease. Both squamous cell and adenocarcinoma of the cervix are etiologically related to infection with HPV, primarily types 16 and 18. Women infected with HIV are at an increased risk for high-risk HPV infection and CIN. Smoking and possibly dietary factors such as decreased circulating vitamin A appear to be cofactors. Squamous cell carcinoma (SCC) accounts for approximately 80% of cervical cancers, while adenocarcinoma accounts for 15% and adenosquamous carcinoma for 3–5%; neuroendocrine or small cell carcinomas are rare.

SCC appears first in the intraepithelial layers (the preinvasive stage, or carcinoma in situ). Preinvasive cancer (CIN III) is a common diagnosis in women 25–40 years of age. Two to 10 years are required for carcinoma to penetrate the basement membrane and invade the tissues. Cervical cancer mortality has declined steadily due to high rates of screening and improved treatment. The 5-year survival rate ranges from 63% for stage II cervical cancer to 15% for stage IV.

▶ Clinical Findings

A. Symptoms and Signs

The most common signs are metrorrhagia, postcoital spotting, and cervical ulceration. Bladder and rectal dysfunction or fistulas and pain are late symptoms.

B. Cervical Biopsy and Endocervical Curettage, or Conization

These procedures are necessary steps after a positive Papanicolaou smear to determine the extent and depth of invasion of the cancer. Even if the smear is positive, treatment is never justified until definitive diagnosis has been established through biopsy.

C. "Staging" or Estimate of Gross Spread of Cancer of the Cervix

Staging of invasive cervical cancer is achieved by clinical evaluation, usually conducted under anesthesia. Further examinations, such as ultrasonography, CT, MRI, lymphangiography, laparoscopy, and fine-needle aspiration, are valuable for treatment planning.

▶ Complications

Metastases to regional lymph nodes occur with increasing frequency from stage I to stage IV. Paracervical extension occurs in all directions from the cervix. The ureters may become obstructed lateral to the cervix, causing hydroureter and hydronephrosis and consequently impaired kidney function. Almost two-thirds of patients with untreated carcinoma of the cervix die of uremia when ureteral obstruction is bilateral. Pain in the back, in the distribution of the lumbosacral plexus, is often indicative of neurologic involvement. Gross edema of the legs may be indicative of vascular and lymphatic stasis due to tumor.

Vaginal fistulas to the rectum and urinary tract are severe late complications. Hemorrhage is the cause of death in 10–20% of patients with extensive invasive carcinoma.

▶ Prevention

Vaccination with Gardasil and Cervarix can prevent cervical cancer caused by HPV types 16 and 18, and protect against low-grade and precancerous lesions caused by these types (see Cervical Intraepithelial Neoplasia, above).

Treatment

A. Emergency Measures

Vaginal hemorrhage originates from gross ulceration and cavitation in stage II–IV cervical carcinoma. Ligation and suturing of the cervix are usually not feasible, but ligation of the uterine or hypogastric arteries may be lifesaving when other measures fail. Styptics such as Monsel solution or acetone are effective, although delayed sloughing may result in further bleeding. Wet vaginal packing is helpful. Emergency irradiation usually controls bleeding.

B. Specific Measures

1. Carcinoma in situ (stage 0)—In women for whom childbearing is not a consideration, total hysterectomy is the treatment of choice. In women who wish to retain the uterus, acceptable alternatives include cervical conization or ablation of the lesion with cryotherapy or laser. Close follow-up with Papanicolaou smears every 3 months for 1 year and every 6 months for another year is necessary after cryotherapy or laser.

2. Invasive carcinoma—Microinvasive carcinoma (stage IA1) is treated with simple, extrafascial hysterectomy. Stages IA2, IB1, and IIA cancers may be treated with either radical hysterectomy with concomitant radiation and chemotherapy or with radiation plus chemotherapy alone. Women with stage IB1 may be candidates for fertility-sparing surgery that includes radical trachelectomy and lymph node dissection with preservation of the uterus and ovaries. Stages IB2, IIB, III, and IV cancers are treated with radiation therapy plus concurrent chemotherapy.

Prognosis

The overall 5-year relative survival rate for carcinoma of the cervix is 68% in white women and 55% in black women in the United States. Survival rates are inversely proportionate to the stage of cancer: stage 0, 99–100%; stage IA, > 95%; stage IB–IIA, 80–90%; stage IIB, 65%; stage III, 40%; and stage IV, < 20%.

When to Refer

All patients with invasive cervical carcinoma (stage 1A or higher) should be referred to a gynecologic oncologist.

American Cancer Society. Survival rates for cervical cancer by stage. Available at http://www.cancer.org/cancer/cervical-cancer/detailedguide/cervical-cancer-survival.

Apgar BS et al. Gynecologic procedures: colposcopy, treatments for cervical intraepithelial neoplasia and endometrial assessment. Am Fam Physician. 2013 Jun 15;87(12):836–43. [PMID: 23939565]

Berger JL et al. Surgical management of cervical carcinoma. Hematol Oncol Clin North Am. 2012 Feb;26(1):63–78. [PMID: 22244662]

Dickinson JA et al. Reduced cervical cancer incidence and mortality in Canada: national data from 1932 to 2006. BMC Public Health. 2012 Nov 16;12:992. [PMID: 23158654]

LEIOMYOMA OF THE UTERUS (Fibroid Tumor)

ESSENTIALS OF DIAGNOSIS

► Irregular enlargement of the uterus (may be asymptomatic).
► Heavy or irregular vaginal bleeding, dysmenorrhea.
► Pelvic pain and pressure.

General Considerations

Uterine leiomyoma is the most common benign neoplasm of the female genital tract. It is a discrete, round, firm, often multiple uterine tumor composed of smooth muscle and connective tissue. The most convenient classification is by anatomic location: (1) intramural, (2) submucous, (3) subserous, (4) intraligamentous, (5) parasitic (ie, deriving its blood supply from an organ to which it becomes attached), and (6) cervical. A submucous myoma may become pedunculated and descend through the cervix into the vagina.

Clinical Findings

A. Symptoms and Signs

In nonpregnant women, myomas are frequently asymptomatic. The two most common symptoms of uterine leiomyomas for which women seek treatment are AUB and pelvic pain or pressure. Occasionally, degeneration occurs, causing intense pain. The risk of miscarriage is increased if the myoma significantly distorts the uterine cavity. Fibroids rarely cause infertility by causing bilateral tubal blockage; they more commonly cause miscarriage and pregnancy complications such as preterm labor and preterm delivery as well as malpresentation.

B. Laboratory Findings

Iron deficiency anemia may result from blood loss; in rare cases, polycythemia is present, presumably as a result of the production of erythropoietin by the myomas.

C. Imaging

Ultrasonography will confirm the presence of uterine myomas and can be used sequentially to monitor growth. When multiple subserous or pedunculated myomas are being followed, ultrasonography is important to exclude ovarian masses. MRI can delineate intramural and submucous myomas accurately. Hysterography or hysteroscopy can also confirm cervical or submucous myomas.

Differential Diagnosis

Irregular myomatous enlargement of the uterus must be differentiated from the similar but symmetric enlargement that may occur with pregnancy or adenomyosis. Subserous myomas must be distinguished from ovarian tumors. Leiomyosarcoma is an unusual tumor occurring in 0.5% of women operated on for symptomatic myoma. It is very rare under the age of 40 and increases in incidence thereafter.

▶ Treatment

A. Emergency Measures

Emergency surgery may be required for acute torsion of a pedunculated myoma. If the patient is markedly anemic as a result of long, heavy menstrual periods, preoperative treatment with DMPA, 150 mg intramuscularly every 28 days, or use of a GnRH agonist, such as depot leuprolide, 3.75 mg intramuscularly monthly, or nafarelin, 0.2–0.4 mg intranasally twice daily, will slow or stop bleeding, and medical treatment of anemia can be given prior to surgery. Levonorgestrel-containing IUDs have also been used to decrease the bleeding associated with fibroids, but IUD placement is more technically challenging in these patients. The only emergency indication for myomectomy during pregnancy is torsion. This surgery is not likely to cause abortion.

B. Specific Measures

Women who have small asymptomatic myomas should be examined annually. Surgical intervention is based on the patient's symptoms and desire for future fertility. Uterine size alone is no longer considered an indication for surgery. Cervical myomas larger than 3–4 cm in diameter or pedunculated myomas that protrude through the cervix must be removed because they often cause bleeding, infection, degeneration, pain, and urinary retention. Submucous myomas can be removed using a hysteroscope and laser or resection instruments.

Because the risk of surgical complications increases with the increasing size of the myoma, preoperative reduction of myoma size is desirable. GnRH analogs such as depot leuprolide, 3.75 mg intramuscularly monthly, or nafarelin, 0.2–0.4 mg intranasally twice a day, are used preoperatively for 3- to 4-month periods to induce reversible hypogonadism, which temporarily reduces the size of myomas, suppresses their further growth, and reduces surrounding vascularity. Low-dose (5–10 mg/d) mifepristone and other selective progesterone-receptor modulators have shown some promise for long-term medical treatment of myomas.

C. Surgical Measures

Surgical measures available for the treatment of myoma are laparoscopic or abdominal myomectomy and total or subtotal abdominal, vaginal, or laparoscopy-assisted vaginal hysterectomy. Myomectomy is the treatment of choice for women who wish to preserve fertility. Uterine artery embolization is a minimally invasive treatment for some uterine fibroids. In uterine artery embolization the goal is to block the blood vessels supplying the fibroids, causing them to shrink. Magnetic resonance–guided high-intensity focused ultrasound, myolysis/radiofrequency ablation, and laparoscopic or vaginal occlusion of uterine vessels are newer interventions, with a smaller body of evidence.

▶ Prognosis

Surgical therapy is curative. In women desiring future fertility, myomectomy can be offered, but patients should be counseled that recurrence is common, postoperative pelvic adhesions may impact fertility, and cesarean delivery may be necessary.

▶ When to Refer

Refer to a gynecologist for treatment of symptomatic leiomyomata.

▶ When to Admit

For acute abdomen associated with an infarcted leiomyoma or hemorrhage not controlled by outpatient measures.

Guo XC et al. The impact and management of fibroids for fertility: an evidence-based approach. Obstet Gynecol Clin North Am. 2012 Dec;39(4):521–33. [PMID: 23182558]

Islam MS et al. Uterine leiomyoma: available medical treatments and new possible therapeutic options. J Clin Endocrinol Metab. 2013 Mar;98(3):921–34. [PMID: 23393173]

van der Kooij SM et al. Review of nonsurgical/minimally invasive treatments for uterine fibroids. Curr Opin Obstet Gynecol. 2012 Dec;24(6):368–75. [PMID: 23014141]

Zimmermann A et al. Prevalence, symptoms and management of uterine fibroids: an international internet-based survey of 21,746 women. BMC Womens Health. 2012 Mar 26;12:6. [PMID: 22448610]

CARCINOMA OF THE ENDOMETRIUM

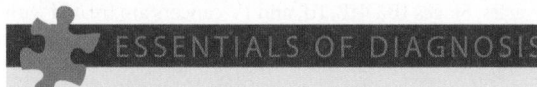
ESSENTIALS OF DIAGNOSIS

▶ Abnormal bleeding is the presenting sign in 90% of cases.

▶ Papanicolaou smear is frequently negative.

▶ After a negative pregnancy test, endometrial tissue is required to confirm the diagnosis.

▶ General Considerations

Adenocarcinoma of the endometrium is the second most common cancer of the female genital tract. It occurs most often in women 50–70 years of age. Obesity, nulliparity, diabetes, and polycystic ovaries with prolonged anovulation, unopposed estrogen therapy, and the extended use of tamoxifen for the treatment of breast cancer are also risk factors. Women with a family history of colon cancer (hereditary nonpolyposis colorectal cancer, Lynch syndrome) are at significantly increased risk, with a lifetime incidence as high as 30%.

Abnormal bleeding is the presenting sign in 90% of cases. Any postmenopausal bleeding requires investigation. Pain generally occurs late in the disease, with metastases or infection.

Papanicolaou smears of the cervix occasionally show atypical endometrial cells but are an insensitive diagnostic tool. **Endocervical and endometrial sampling is the only** reliable means of diagnosis. Simultaneous hysteroscopy can be a valuable addition in order to localize polyps or other lesions within the uterine cavity. Vaginal ultrasonography may be used to determine the thickness of the endometrium as an indication of hypertrophy and possible neoplastic change. The finding of a thin endometrial lining on ultrasound is helpful in cases where very little tissue is obtainable through endometrial biopsy.

Pathologic assessment is important in differentiating hyperplasias, which often can be treated with cyclic oral progestins.

Prevention

Prompt endometrial sampling for patients who report abnormal menstrual bleeding or postmenopausal uterine bleeding will reveal many incipient as well as clinical cases of endometrial cancer. Younger women with chronic anovulation are at risk for endometrial hyperplasia and subsequent endometrial cancer. They can reduce the risk of hyperplasia almost completely with the use of oral contraceptives or cyclic progestin therapy.

Staging

Staging and prognosis are based on surgical and pathologic evaluation only. Examination under anesthesia, endometrial and endocervical sampling, chest radiography, intravenous urography, cystoscopy, sigmoidoscopy, transvaginal sonography, and MRI will help determine the extent of the disease and its appropriate treatment.

Treatment

Treatment consists of total hysterectomy and bilateral salpingo-oophorectomy. Peritoneal material for cytologic examination is routinely taken and lymph node sampling may be done. If invasion deep into the myometrium has occurred or if sampled lymph nodes are positive for tumor, postoperative irradiation is indicated. Several randomized controlled trials examining the role of adjuvant chemotherapy alone or with irradiation are ongoing. One study has shown a modest increase in survival with chemotherapy alone versus whole abdominal radiation alone in women with stage III–IV disease. Palliation of advanced or metastatic endometrial adenocarcinoma may be accomplished with large doses of progestins, eg, medroxyprogesterone, 400 mg intramuscularly weekly, or megestrol acetate, 80–160 mg daily orally.

Prognosis

With early diagnosis and treatment, the overall 5-year survival is 80–85%. With stage I disease, the depth of myometrial invasion is the strongest predictor of survival, with a 98% 5-year survival with < 66% depth of invasion and 78% survival with ≥ 66% invasion.

When to Refer

All patients with endometrial carcinoma should be referred to a gynecologic oncologist.

Freeman SJ et al. The revised FIGO staging system for uterine malignancies: implications for MR imaging. Radiographics. 2012 Oct;32(6):1805–27. [PMID: 23065170]

Landrum LM et al. Phase II trial of vaginal cuff brachytherapy followed by chemotherapy in early stage endometrial cancer patients with high-intermediate risk factors. Gynecol Oncol. 2014 Jan;132(1):50–4. [PMID: 24219982]

Shah MM et al. Management of endometrial cancer in young women. Clin Obstet Gynecol. 2011 Jun;54(2):219–25. [PMID: 21508691]

Trimble CL et al; Society of Gynecologic Oncology Clinical Practice Committee. Management of endometrial precancers. Obstet Gynecol. 2012 Nov;120(5):1160–75. [PMID: 23090535]

CARCINOMA OF THE VULVA

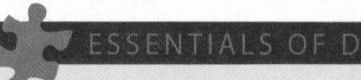

ESSENTIALS OF DIAGNOSIS

- ▶ History of genital warts.
- ▶ History of prolonged vulvar irritation, with pruritus, local discomfort, or slight bloody discharge.
- ▶ Early lesions may suggest or include non-neoplastic epithelial disorders.
- ▶ Late lesions appear as a mass, an exophytic growth, or a firm, ulcerated area in the vulva.
- ▶ Biopsy is necessary for diagnosis.

General Considerations

The majority of cancers of the vulva are squamous lesions that classically have occurred in women over 50 years of age. Several subtypes (particularly 16, 18, and 31) of HPV have been identified in some but not all vulvar cancers. About 70–90% of vulvar intraepithelial neoplasia (VIN) and 40–60% of vulvar cancers are HPV associated. As with squamous cell lesions of the cervix, a grading system of VIN from mild dysplasia to carcinoma in situ is used.

Differential Diagnosis

Benign vulvar disorders that must be excluded in the diagnosis of carcinoma of the vulva include chronic granulomatous lesions (eg, lymphogranuloma venereum, syphilis), condylomas, hidradenoma, or neurofibroma. Lichen sclerosus and other associated leukoplakic changes in the skin should be biopsied. The likelihood that a superimposed vulvar cancer will develop in a woman with a nonneoplastic epithelial disorder (vulvar dystrophy) is 1–5%.

Diagnosis

Biopsy is essential for the diagnosis of VIN and vulvar cancer and should be performed with any localized atypical vulvar lesion, including white patches. Multiple skin-punch specimens can be taken in the office under local anesthesia, with care to include tissue from the edges of each lesion sampled. Colposcopy of vulva, vagina, and cervix can help in identifying areas for biopsy and in planning further treatment.

Staging

Vulvar cancer generally spreads by direct extension into the vagina, urethra, perineum, and anus, with discontinuous spread into the inguinal and femoral lymph nodes. CT or MRI of the pelvis or abdomen is generally not required except in advanced cases for planning therapeutic options.

Treatment

A. General Measures

Early diagnosis and treatment of irritative or other predisposing causes, such as lichen sclerosis and VIN, should be pursued. A 7:3 combination of betamethasone and crotamiton is particularly effective for itching. After an initial response, fluorinated steroids should be replaced with hydrocortisone because of their skin atrophying effect. For lichen sclerosus, recommended treatment is clobetasol propionate cream 0.05% twice daily for 2–3 weeks, then once daily until symptoms resolve. Application one to three times a week can be used for long-term maintenance therapy.

B. Surgical Measures

High-grade VIN may be treated with a variety of approaches including topical chemotherapy, laser ablation, wide local excision, skinning vulvectomy, and simple vulvectomy. Small, invasive basal cell carcinoma of the vulva should be excised with a wide margin. If the VIN is extensive or multicentric, laser therapy or superficial surgical removal of vulvar skin may be required. In this way, the clitoris and uninvolved portions of the vulva may be spared.

Invasive carcinoma confined to the vulva without evidence of spread to adjacent organs or to the regional lymph nodes is treated with wide local excision and inguinal lymphadenectomy or wide local excision alone if invasion is < 1 mm. To avoid the morbidity of inguinal lymphadenectomy, some guidelines recommend sentinel lymph node sampling for women with early stage vulvar cancer. Patients with more advanced disease may receive preoperative radiation, chemotherapy, or both.

Prognosis

Basal cell vulvar carcinomas very seldom metastasize, and carcinoma in situ by definition has not metastasized. With adequate excision, the prognosis for both lesions is excellent. Patients with invasive vulvar SCC 2 cm in diameter or less, without inguinal lymph node metastases, have an 85–90% 5-year survival rate. If the lesion is > 2 cm and lymph node involvement is present, the likelihood of 5-year survival is approximately 40%.

When to Refer

All patients with invasive vulvar carcinoma should be referred to a gynecologic oncologist.

Carter JS et al. Vulvar and vaginal cancer. Obstet Gynecol Clin North Am. 2012 Jun;39(2):213–31. [PMID: 22640712]

de Gregorio N et al. The role of preoperative ultrasound evaluation of inguinal lymph nodes in patients with vulvar malignancy. Gynecol Oncol. 2013 Oct;131(1):113-7. [PMID: 23932893]

Dittmer C et al. Diagnosis and treatment options of vulvar cancer: a review. Arch Gynecol Obstet. 2012 Jan;285(1):183–93. [PMID: 21909752]

ENDOMETRIOSIS

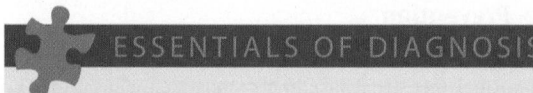

ESSENTIALS OF DIAGNOSIS

- ► Dysmenorrhea.
- ► Dyspareunia.
- ► Increased frequency among infertile women.
- ► Abnormal uterine bleeding.

General Considerations

Endometriosis is an aberrant growth of endometrium outside the uterus, particularly in the dependent parts of the pelvis and in the ovaries, whose principal manifestations are chronic pain and infertility. While retrograde menstruation is the most widely accepted cause, its pathogenesis and natural course are not fully understood. The overall prevalence in the United States is 6–10% and is fourfold to fivefold greater among infertile women.

Clinical Findings

The clinical manifestations of endometriosis are variable and unpredictable in both presentation and course. Dysmenorrhea, chronic pelvic pain, and dyspareunia, are among the well-recognized manifestations. A significant number of women with endometriosis, however, remain asymptomatic and most women with endometriosis have a normal pelvic examination. However, in some women, pelvic examination can disclose tender nodules in the cul-de-sac or rectovaginal septum, uterine retroversion with decreased uterine mobility, cervical motion tenderness, or an adnexal mass or tenderness.

Endometriosis must be distinguished from pelvic inflammatory disease, ovarian neoplasms, and uterine myomas. Bowel invasion by endometrial tissue may produce blood in the stool that must be distinguished from bowel neoplasm.

Imaging is of limited value and is only useful in the presence of a pelvic or adnexal mass. Transvaginal ultrasonography is the imaging modality of choice to detect the presence of deeply penetrating endometriosis of the rectum or rectovaginal septum, while MRI should be reserved for equivocal cases of rectovaginal or bladder endometriosis. Ultimately, a definitive diagnosis of endometriosis is made only by histology of lesions removed at surgery.

► Treatment

A. Medical Treatment

Medical treatment, using a variety of hormonal therapies, is effective in the amelioration of pain associated with endometriosis. However, there is no evidence that any of these agents increase the likelihood of pregnancy. Their preoperative use is of questionable value in reducing the difficulty of surgery. Most of these regimens are designed to inhibit ovulation over 4–9 months and lower hormone levels, thus preventing cyclic stimulation of endometriotic implants and inducing atrophy. The optimum duration of therapy is not clear, and the relative merits in terms of side effects and long-term risks and benefits show insignificant differences when compared with each other and, in mild cases, with placebo. Commonly used medical regimens include the following:

1. Although there is no conclusive evidence that NSAIDs improve pain associated with endometriosis, these agents are reasonable options in appropriately selected patients.

2. Low-dose oral contraceptives can also be given cyclically; prolonged suppression of ovulation often inhibits further stimulation of residual endometriosis, especially if taken after one of the therapies mentioned here. Any of the combination oral contraceptives, the contraceptive patch, or vaginal ring may be used continuously for 6–12 months. Breakthrough bleeding can be treated with conjugated estrogens, 1.25 mg orally daily for 1 week, or estradiol, 2 mg daily orally for 1 week.

3. Progestins, specifically oral norethindrone acetate and subcutaneous DMPA, have been approved by the FDA for treatment of endometriosis-associated pain.

4. GnRH agonists are highly effective in reducing the pain syndromes associated with endometriosis. However, they are not superior to other methods such as combined oral contraceptives as first-line therapy. The GnRH analogs (such as nafarelin nasal spray, 0.2–0.4 mg twice daily, or long-acting injectable leuprolide acetate, 3.75 mg intramuscularly monthly, used for 6 months) suppress ovulation. Side effects of vasomotor symptoms and bone demineralization may be relieved by "add-back" therapy, such as conjugated equine estrogen, 0.625 mg, or norethindrone, 5 mg orally daily.

5. Danazol is an androgenic drug that has been used for the treatment of endometriosis-associated pain. It should be used for 4–6 months in the lowest dose necessary to suppress menstruation, usually 200–400 mg orally twice daily. However, danazol has a high incidence of androgenic side effects that are more severe than other drugs available, including decreased breast size, weight gain, acne, and hirsutism.

6. Intrauterine progestin use with the levonorgestrel intrauterine system also has been shown to be effective in reducing endometriosis-associated pelvic pain and should be tried before radical surgery.

7. The use of aromatase inhibitors (such as anastrozole or letrozole) have been evaluated in women with chronic pain resistant to other forms of medical management or surgical management. Although promising, there are insufficient data to recommend their routine use.

B. Surgical Measures

Surgical treatment of endometriosis—particularly extensive disease—is effective both in reducing pain and in promoting fertility. Laparoscopic ablation of endometrial implants significantly reduces pain. Ablation of implants and, if necessary, removal of ovarian endometriomas enhance fertility, although subsequent pregnancy rates are inversely related to the severity of disease. Women with disabling pain for whom childbearing is not a consideration can be treated definitively with total abdominal hysterectomy and bilateral salpingo-oophorectomy. In premenopausal women, hormone replacement then may be used to relieve vasomotor symptoms. However, hormone replacement may lead to a recurrence of endometriosis and associated pain.

► Prognosis

There is little systematic research regarding either the progression of the disease or the prediction of clinical outcomes. The prognosis for reproductive function in early or moderately advanced endometriosis appears to be good with conservative therapy. Hysterectomy, with bilateral salpingo-oophorectomy, often is regarded as definitive therapy for the treatment of endometriosis associated with intractable pelvic pain, adnexal masses, or multiple previous ineffective conservative surgical procedures. However, symptoms may recur in women even after hysterectomy and oophorectomy.

► When to Refer

Refer to a gynecologist for laparoscopic diagnosis or treatment.

► When to Admit

Rarely necessary except for acute abdomen associated with ruptured or bleeding endometrioma.

American College of Obstetricians and Gynecologists. ACOG Practice Bulletin No. 114: Management of endometriosis. Obstet Gynecol. 2010 July:116(1):223–36. [PMID: 20567196]

Burney RO et al. Pathogenesis and pathophysiology of endometriosis. Fertil Steril. 2012 Sep;98(3):511–9. [PMID: 22819144]

Johnson NP et al; World Endometriosis Society Montpellier Consortium. Consensus on current management of endometriosis. Hum Reprod. 2013 Jun;28(6):1552–68. [PMID: 23528916]

Matorras R et al. Efficacy of the levonorgestrel-releasing intrauterine device in the treatment of recurrent pelvic pain in multitreated endometriosis. J Reprod Med. 2011 Nov–Dec;56(11–12):497–503. [PMID: 22195333]

Schrager S et al. Evaluation and treatment of endometriosis. Am Fam Physician. 2013 Jan 15;87(2):107–13. [PMID: 23317074]

PELVIC ORGAN PROLAPSE

► General Considerations

Cystocele, rectocele, and enterocele are vaginal hernias commonly seen in multiparous women. Cystocele is a hernia of the bladder wall into the vagina, causing a soft anterior fullness. Cystocele may be accompanied by urethrocele, which is not a hernia but a sagging of the urethra following its detachment from the pubic symphysis during childbirth. Rectocele is a herniation of the terminal rectum into the posterior vagina, causing a collapsible pouch-like fullness. Enterocele is a vaginal vault hernia containing small intestine, usually in the posterior vagina and resulting from a deepening of the pouch of Douglas. Two or all three types of hernia may occur in combination. Risk factors may include vaginal birth, genetic predisposition, advancing age, prior pelvic surgery, connective tissue disorders, and increased intra-abdominal pressure associated with obesity or straining associated with chronic constipation or coughing.

▶ Clinical Findings

Symptoms of pelvic organ prolapse may include sensation of a bulge or protrusion in the vagina, urinary or fecal incontinence, constipation, a sense of incomplete bladder emptying, and dyspareunia. The cause of pelvic organ prolapse, including prolapse of the uterus, vaginal apex, and anterior or posterior vaginal walls, is likely multifactorial.

▶ Treatment

The type of therapy depends on the extent of prolapse and the patient's age and her desire for menstruation, pregnancy, and coitus.

A. General Measures

Supportive measures include a high-fiber diet and laxatives to improve constipation. Weight reduction in obese patients and limitation of straining and lifting are helpful. Pelvic muscle training (Kegel exercises) is a simple, noninvasive intervention that may improve pelvic function that has clearly demonstrated benefit for women with urinary or fecal symptoms, especially incontinence. Pessaries may reduce cystocele, rectocele, or enterocele and are helpful in women who do not wish to undergo surgery or are poor surgical candidates.

B. Surgical Measures

The most common surgical procedure is vaginal or abdominal hysterectomy with additional attention to restoring apical support after the uterus is removed, including suspension by either uterosacral or sacrospinous fixation vaginally or abdominal sacral colpopexy. Since stress incontinence is common after vault suspension procedures, an anti-incontinence procedure should be considered. While the use of various surgical mesh materials with these procedures increased substantially since 2000, several safety advisories recommend a more cautious use of mesh materials. If the patient desires pregnancy, the same procedures for vaginal suspension can be performed without hysterectomy, though limited data on pregnancy outcomes or prolapse outcomes are available. For elderly women who do not desire coitus, colpocleisis, the partial obliteration of the vagina, is surgically simple and effective. Uterine suspension with sacrospinous cervicocolpopexy may be an effective approach in older women who wish to avoid hysterectomy but preserve coital function.

▶ When to Refer

- Refer to urogynecologist or gynecologist for incontinence evaluation.
- Refer if nonsurgical therapy is ineffective.

Committee on Gynecologic Practice. Committee Opinion no. 513: vaginal placement of synthetic mesh for pelvic organ prolapse. Obstet Gynecol. 2011 Dec;118(6):1459–64. [PMID: 22105294]

Committee on Gynecologic Practice. Vaginal placement of synthetic mesh for pelvic organ prolapse. Female Pelvic Med Reconstr Surg. 2012 Jan–Feb;18(1):5–9. [PMID: 22453257]

Kenton K et al; Pelvic Floor Disorders Network. Pelvic floor symptoms improve similarly after pessary and behavioral treatment for stress incontinence. Female Pelvic Med Reconstr Surg. 2012 Mar–Apr;18(2):118–21. [PMID: 22453323]

Wei JT et al; Pelvic Floor Disorders Network. A midurethral sling to reduce incontinence after vaginal prolapse repair. N Engl J Med. 2012 Jun 21;366(25):2358–67. [PMID: 22716974]

PELVIC INFLAMMATORY DISEASE (Salpingitis, Endometritis)

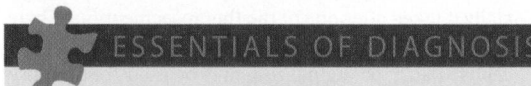
ESSENTIALS OF DIAGNOSIS

- ▶ Uterine, adnexal, or cervical motion tenderness.
- ▶ Abnormal discharge from the vagina or cervix.
- ▶ Absence of a competing diagnosis.

▶ General Considerations

Pelvic inflammatory disease (PID) is a polymicrobial infection of the upper genital tract associated with the sexually transmitted organisms *N gonorrhoeae* and *Chlamydia trachomatis* as well as endogenous organisms, including anaerobes, *Haemophilus influenzae*, enteric gram-negative rods, and streptococci. It is most common in young, nulliparous, sexually active women with multiple partners and is a leading cause of infertility and ectopic pregnancy. The use of barrier methods of contraception may provide significant protection.

Tuberculous salpingitis is rare in the United States but more common in developing countries; it is characterized by pelvic pain and irregular pelvic masses not responsive to antibiotic therapy. It is not sexually transmitted.

▶ Clinical Findings

A. Symptoms and Signs

Patients with PID may have lower abdominal pain, chills and fever, menstrual disturbances, purulent cervical discharge, and cervical and adnexal tenderness. Right upper quadrant pain (Fitz-Hugh and Curtis syndrome) may indicate an associated perihepatitis. However, diagnosis of PID is complicated by the fact that many women may have subtle or mild symptoms that are not readily recognized as PID, such as postcoital bleeding, urinary frequency, or low back pain.

B. Minimum Diagnostic Criteria

Women with uterine, adnexal, or cervical motion tenderness should be considered to have PID and be treated with antibiotics unless there is a competing diagnosis such as ectopic pregnancy or appendicitis.

C. Additional Criteria

No single historical, physical or laboratory finding is definitive for acute PID. The following criteria may be used to enhance the specificity of the diagnosis: (1) oral temperature > 38.3°C, (2) abnormal cervical or vaginal discharge with white cells on saline microscopy (> 1 leukocyte per epithelial cell), (3) elevated erythrocyte sedimentation rate, (4) elevated C-reactive protein, and (5) laboratory documentation of cervical infection with *N gonorrhoeae* or *C trachomatis*. Endocervical culture should be performed routinely, but treatment should not be delayed while awaiting results.

▶ Differential Diagnosis

Appendicitis, ectopic pregnancy, septic abortion, hemorrhagic or ruptured ovarian cysts or tumors, twisted ovarian cyst, degeneration of a myoma, and acute enteritis must be considered. PID is more likely to occur when there is a history of PID, recent sexual contact, recent onset of menses, recent insertion of an IUD, or if the partner has a sexually transmitted disease. **Acute PID is highly unlikely when recent intercourse has not taken place.** A sensitive serum pregnancy test should be obtained to rule out ectopic pregnancy. Pelvic and vaginal ultrasonography is helpful in the differential diagnosis of ectopic pregnancy of over 6 weeks. Laparoscopy is often used to diagnose PID, and it is imperative if the diagnosis is not certain or if the patient has not responded to antibiotic therapy after 48 hours. The appendix should be visualized at laparoscopy to rule out appendicitis. Cultures obtained at the time of laparoscopy are often specific and helpful.

▶ Treatment

A. Antibiotics

Early treatment with appropriate antibiotics effective against *N gonorrhoeae*, *C trachomatis*, and the endogenous organisms listed above is essential to prevent long-term sequelae. The sexual partner should be examined and treated appropriately. Most women with mild to moderate disease can be treated successfully as an outpatient. The recommended outpatient regimen is a single dose of cefoxitin, 2 g intramuscularly, with probenecid, 1 g orally, with doxycycline 100 mg orally twice a day for 14 days, or ceftriaxone 250 mg intramuscularly plus doxycycline, 100 mg orally twice daily, for 14 days. Metronidazole 500 mg orally twice daily for 14 days may also be added to either of these regimens to treat bacterial vaginosis that is frequently associated with PID. For patients with severe disease or those who meet the other criteria for hospitalization, there are two recommended regimens. One regimen includes cefotetan, 2 g intravenously every 12 hours, or cefoxitin, 2 g intravenously every 6 hours, plus doxycycline 100 mg orally or intravenously every 12 hours. The other recommended regimen is clindamycin, 900 mg intravenously every 8 hours, plus gentamicin, a loading dose of 2 mg/kg intravenously or intramuscularly followed by a maintenance dose of 1.5 mg/kg every 8 hours (or as a single daily dose, 3–5 mg/kg). These regimens should be continued for a minimum of 24 hours after the patient shows significant clinical improvement. Then, an oral regimen should be continued for 14 days with either doxycycline, 100 mg orally twice a day, or clindamycin, 450 mg orally four times a day. If a tubo-ovarian abscess is present, clindamycin should be given because of the better anaerobic coverage it provides.

B. Surgical Measures

Tubo-ovarian abscesses may require surgical excision or transcutaneous or transvaginal aspiration. Unless rupture is suspected, institute high-dose antibiotic therapy in the hospital, and monitor therapy with ultrasound. In 70% of cases, antibiotics are effective; in 30%, there is inadequate response in 48–72 hours, and surgical intervention is required. Unilateral adnexectomy is acceptable for unilateral abscess. Hysterectomy and bilateral salpingo-oophorectomy may be necessary for overwhelming infection or in cases of chronic disease with intractable pelvic pain.

▶ Prognosis

In spite of treatment, long-term sequelae, including repeated episodes of infection, chronic pelvic pain, dyspareunia, ectopic pregnancy, or infertility, develop in one-fourth of women with acute disease. The risk of infertility increases with repeated episodes of salpingitis: it is estimated at 10% after the first episode, 25% after a second episode, and 50% after a third episode.

▶ When to Admit

The following patients with acute PID should be admitted for intravenous antibiotic therapy:

- The patient has a tubo-ovarian abscess (direct inpatient observation for at least 24 hours before switching to outpatient parenteral therapy).
- The patient is pregnant.
- The patient is unable to follow or tolerate an outpatient regimen.
- The patient has not responded clinically to outpatient therapy within 72 hours.
- The patient has severe illness, nausea and vomiting, or high fever.
- Another surgical emergency, such as appendicitis, cannot be ruled out.

Liu B et al. Improving adherence to guidelines for the diagnosis and management of pelvic inflammatory disease: a systematic review. Infect Dis Obstet Gynecol. 2012;2012:325108. [PMID: 22973085]

Markle W et al. Sexually transmitted diseases. Prim Care. 2013 Sep;40(3):557–87. [PMID: 23958358]

Sweet RL. Treatment of acute pelvic inflammatory disease. Infect Dis Obstet Gynecol. 2011;2011:561909. [PMID: 22228985]

OVARIAN CANCER & OVARIAN TUMORS

ESSENTIALS OF DIAGNOSIS

▶ Vague gastrointestinal discomfort, pelvic pressure, or pain.

▶ Many cases of early-stage cancer are asymptomatic.

▶ Pelvic examination and ultrasound are mainstays of diagnosis.

▶ General Considerations

Ovarian tumors are common. Most are benign, but malignant ovarian tumors are the leading cause of death from reproductive tract cancer. The wide range of types and patterns of ovarian tumors is due to the complexity of ovarian embryology and differences in tissues of origin.

In women with no family history of ovarian cancer, the lifetime risk is 1.6%, whereas a woman with one affected first-degree relative has a 5% lifetime risk. **Ultrasound or tumor marker screening for women with one or no affected first-degree relatives have not been shown to reduce mortality from ovarian cancer,** and the risks associated with unnecessary prophylactic surgical procedures outweigh the benefits in low-risk women. With two or more affected first-degree relatives, the risk is 7%. Approximately 3% of women with two or more affected first-degree relatives will have a hereditary ovarian cancer syndrome with a lifetime risk of 40%. Women with a *BRCA1* gene mutation have a 45% lifetime risk of ovarian cancer and those with a *BRCA2* mutation a 25% risk. Consideration should be given to screening these women every 6 months with transvaginal sonography and serum CA 125 testing, starting at age 35 or 5–10 years earlier than the earliest age that ovarian cancer was first diagnosed in a family member. Because this screening regimen has not been shown to reduce mortality, oophorectomy is recommended by age 35 or whenever childbearing is not a consideration because of the high risk of disease.

▶ Clinical Findings

A. Symptoms and Signs

Unfortunately, most women with both benign and malignant ovarian neoplasms are either asymptomatic or experience only mild nonspecific gastrointestinal symptoms or pelvic pressure. Women with early disease are typically detected on routine pelvic examination. Women with advanced malignant disease may experience abdominal pain and bloating, and a palpable abdominal mass with ascites is often present.

B. Laboratory Findings

CA 125 is elevated in 80% of women with epithelial ovarian cancer overall but in only 50% of women with early disease. Serum CA 125 may be elevated in premenopausal women with benign disease (such as endometriosis), minimizing its usefulness in ovarian cancer screening. In premenopausal women, other markers (such as human chorionic gonadotropin [hCG], lactate dehydrogenase, or alpha fetoprotein) may be indicators of the type of tumor present.

C. Imaging Studies

Transvaginal sonography is useful for screening high-risk women but has inadequate sensitivity for screening low-risk women. Ultrasound is helpful in differentiating ovarian masses that are benign and likely to resolve spontaneously from those with malignant potential. Color Doppler imaging may further enhance the specificity of ultrasound diagnosis.

▶ Differential Diagnosis

Once an ovarian mass has been detected, it must be categorized as functional, benign neoplastic, or potentially malignant. Predictive factors include age, size of the mass, ultrasound configuration, CA 125 levels, the presence of symptoms, and whether the mass is unilateral or bilateral. Simple cysts up to 10 cm in diameter are almost universally benign in both premenopausal and postmenopausal patients. Most will resolve spontaneously and may be monitored without intervention. If the mass is larger or unchanged on repeat pelvic examination and transvaginal sonography, surgical evaluation is warranted.

Laparoscopy may be used when an ovarian mass is small enough to be removed with a laparoscopic approach. If malignancy is suspected, because of findings on transvaginal ultrasound with morphologic scoring, color Doppler assessment of vascular quality, and serum CA 125 level, then laparotomy is preferable.

▶ Treatment

If a malignant ovarian mass is suspected, surgical evaluation should be performed by a gynecologic oncologist. For benign neoplasms, tumor removal or unilateral oophorectomy is usually performed. For ovarian cancer in an early stage, the standard therapy is complete surgical staging followed by abdominal hysterectomy and bilateral salpingo-oophorectomy with omentectomy and selective lymphadenectomy. With more advanced disease, aggressive removal of all visible tumor improves survival. Except for women with low-grade ovarian cancer in an early stage, postoperative chemotherapy is indicated (see Table 39–12). Several chemotherapy regimens are effective, such as the combination of cisplatin or carboplatin with paclitaxel, with clinical response rates of up to 60–70% (see Table 39–13).

▶ Prognosis

Unfortunately, approximately 75% of women with ovarian cancer are diagnosed with advanced disease after regional or distant metastases have become established. The overall 5-year survival is approximately 17% with distant metastases, 36% with local spread, and 89% with early disease.

When to Refer

If a malignant mass is suspected, surgical evaluation should be performed by a gynecologic oncologist.

Agency for Healthcare Research and Quality. Guideline summary. Hereditary breast and ovarian cancer syndrome. 2009 Sep 11. http://www.guideline.gov/content.aspx?id=14336

Centers for Disease Control and Prevention. Ovarian cancer screening. 2013 Aug 29. http://www.cdc.gov/cancer/ovarian/basic_info/screening.htm

National Collaborating Center for Cancer. NICE Clinical Guidelines, No. 122: Ovarian Cancer: the recognition and initial management of ovarian cancer. 2011 April. http://www.ncbi.nlm.nih.gov/books/n/nicecg122/pdf/

POLYCYSTIC OVARY SYNDROME

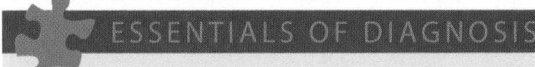

ESSENTIALS OF DIAGNOSIS

▶ Clinical or biochemical evidence of hyperandrogenism.

▶ Oligoovulation or anovulation.

▶ Polycystic ovaries on ultrasonography.

General Considerations

Polycystic ovary syndrome (PCOS) is a common endocrine disorder of unknown etiology affecting 5–10% of women of reproductive age. It is characterized by chronic anovulation, polycystic ovaries, and hyperandrogenism. It is associated with hirsutism and obesity as well as an increased risk of diabetes mellitus, cardiovascular disease, and metabolic syndrome. Unrecognized or untreated PCOS is an important risk factor for cardiovascular disease. The Endocrine Society released practice guidelines in 2013 that endorse the **Rotterdam criteria** for diagnosing PCOS, which identifies excess androgen production, ovulatory dysfunction, and polycystic ovaries as the key diagnostic features of the disorder in adult women. The classification system has been endorsed by the National Institutes of Health.

Clinical Findings

PCOS often presents as a menstrual disorder (from amenorrhea to menorrhagia) and infertility. Skin disorders due to peripheral androgen excess, including hirsutism and acne, are common. Patients may also show signs of insulin resistance and hyperinsulinemia, and these women are at increased risk for early-onset type 2 diabetes and metabolic syndrome. Patients who do become pregnant are at increased risk for perinatal complications. In addition, they have an increased long-term risk of cancer of the endometrium because of unopposed estrogen secretion.

Differential Diagnosis

Anovulation in the reproductive years may also be due to: (1) premature ovarian failure (high FSH and LH levels); (2) rapid weight loss, extreme physical exertion (normal FSH and LH levels for age), or obesity; (3) discontinuation of hormonal contraceptives (anovulation for 6 months or more occasionally occurs); (4) pituitary adenoma with elevated prolactin (galactorrhea may or may not be present); and (5) hyperthyroidism or hypothyroidism. To rule out other etiologies in women with suspected PCOS, serum FSH, LH, prolactin, and TSH should be checked. **Because of the high risk of insulin resistance and dyslipidemia, all women with suspected PCOS should have a hemoglobin A_{1C} and fasting glucose along with a lipid and lipoprotein profile.** Women with clinical evidence of androgen excess should have total testosterone and sex hormone-binding globulin or free (bioavailable) testosterone, and 17-hydroxyprogesterone measured. Women with stigmata of Cushing syndrome should have a 24-hour urinary free-cortisol or a low-dose dexamethasone suppression test. Congenital adrenal hyperplasia and androgen-secreting adrenal tumors also tend to have high circulating androgen levels and anovulation with polycystic ovaries; these disorders must also be ruled out in women with presumed PCOS.

Treatment

In obese patients with PCOS, weight reduction and exercise are often effective in reversing the metabolic effects and in inducing ovulation. For those women who do not respond to weight loss and exercise, metformin therapy may be helpful and may be offered along with contraceptive counseling to prevent unplanned pregnancy in case of a return of ovulatory cycles. For women who are seeking pregnancy and remain anovulatory, clomiphene or other drugs can be used for ovulatory stimulation (see section on Infertility below). Clomiphene is the first-line therapy for infertility. Metformin is beneficial for metabolic or glucose abnormalities, and it can improve menstrual function. Metformin has little or no benefit in the treatment of hirsutism, acne, or infertility. If induction of ovulation fails with the above regimens, treatment with gonadotropins, but at low dose to lower the risk of ovarian hyperstimulation syndrome, may be successful. Second-line therapies such as use of aromatase inhibitors or laparoscopic "ovarian drilling" may be considered but are of unproved benefit. Women with PCOS are at greater risk than normal women for twin gestation with ovulation induction.

If the patient does not desire pregnancy, medroxyprogesterone acetate, 10 mg/d orally for the first 10 days of each month, should be given to ensure regular shedding of the endometrium and avoid hyperplasia. If contraception is desired, a low-dose combination oral contraceptive can be used; this is also useful in controlling hirsutism, for which treatment must be continued for 6–12 months before results are seen.

Spironolactone is useful for hirsutism in doses of 25 mg three or four times daily. Flutamide, 125–250 mg orally daily, and finasteride, 5 mg orally daily, are also effective for treating hirsutism. Because these three agents are potentially teratogenic, they should be used only in conjunction with secure contraception. Topical eflornithine cream applied to affected facial areas twice daily for 6 months may be helpful in the majority of women. Hirsutism may also be managed with depilatory creams, electrolysis, and laser therapy. The combination of laser therapy and topical eflornithine may be particularly effective.

Weight loss, exercise, and treatment of unresolved metabolic derangements are important in preventing cardiovascular disease. Women with PCOS should be managed aggressively and should have regular monitoring of lipid profiles and glucose. In adolescent patients with PCOS hormonal contraceptives and metformin are treatment options.

▶ When to Refer

- If expertise in diagnosis is needed.
- If patient is infertile.

Aubuchon M et al. Polycystic ovary syndrome: current infertility management. Clin Obstet Gynecol. 2011 Dec;54(4):675–84. [PMID: 22031257]

Blume-Peytavi U. How to diagnose and treat medically women with excessive hair. Dermatol Clin. 2013 Jan;31(1):57–65. [PMID: 23159176]

Legro RS et al. Diagnosis and treatment of polycystic ovary syndrome: an endocrine society clinical practice guideline. J Clin Endocrinol Metab. 2013 Dec;98(12):4565–92. [PMID: 24151290]

Macklon NS. Polycystic ovary syndrome. BMJ. 2011 Oct 13;343: d6407. [PMID: 21998338]

FEMALE SEXUAL DYSFUNCTION

▶ General Considerations

Female sexual dysfunction is a common problem. Depending on the questions asked, surveys have shown that from 35% to 98% of women report sexual concerns. Questions related to sexual functioning should be asked as part of the routine medical history. Three helpful questions are: "Are you currently involved in a sexual relationship?", "With men, women, or both?", and "Are there any sexual concerns or pain with sex?" If the woman is not involved in a sexual relationship, she should be asked about any concerns that are contributing to a lack of sexual behavior. If a history of sexual dysfunction is elicited, a complete history of factors that may affect sexual function should be taken. These factors include her reproductive history (including pregnancies and mode of delivery) as well as history of infertility, sexually transmitted diseases, rape or sexual abuse, gynecologic or urologic disorders, endocrine abnormalities (such as diabetes mellitus or thyroid disease), neurologic problems, cardiovascular disease, psychiatric disease, and current prescription and over-the-counter medication use. A detailed history of the specific sexual dysfunction should be elicited, and a gynecologic examination should focus on findings that may contribute to her sexual complaints.

▶ Etiology

A. Disorders of Sexual Desire

Sexual desire in women is a complex and poorly understood phenomenon. Emotion is a key factor in sexual desire. Anger toward a partner, fear or anxiety related to previous sexual encounters, or history of sexual abuse may contribute. Physical factors, such as chronic illness, fatigue, depression, and specific medical disorders (such as diabetes mellitus, thyroid disease, or adrenal insufficiency) may contribute to a lack of desire. Attitudes toward aging and menopause may play a role. In addition, sexual desire may be influenced by other sexual dysfunctions, such as arousal disorders, dyspareunia, or anorgasmia.

B. Sexual Arousal Disorders

Sexual arousal disorders may be both subjective and objective. Sexual stimulation normally leads to genital vasocongestion and lubrication. Some women may have a physiologic response to sexual stimuli but may not subjectively feel aroused because of factors such as distractions; negative expectations; anxiety; fatigue; depression; or medications, such as selective serotonin reuptake inhibitors (SSRIs) or oral contraceptives. Other women may lack both a subjective and physiologic response to sexual stimuli related to vaginal atrophy.

C. Orgasmic Disorders

In spite of subjective and physiologic arousal, women may experience a marked delay in orgasm, diminished sensation of an orgasm, or anorgasmia. The etiology is complex and typically multifactorial, but the disorder is usually amenable to treatment.

D. Sexual Pain Disorders

Dyspareunia and vaginismus are two subcategories of sexual pain disorders. **Dyspareunia** is defined as recurrent or persistent genital pain associated with sexual intercourse that is not caused exclusively by lack of lubrication or by vaginismus and causes marked distress or interpersonal difficulty. **Vaginismus** is defined as recurrent or persistent involuntary spasm of the musculature of the outer third of the vagina that interferes with sexual intercourse, resulting from fear, pain, sexual trauma, or a negative attitude toward sex, often learned in childhood, and causing marked distress or interpersonal difficulty. Other medical causes of sexual pain may include vulvovaginitis; vulvar disease, including lichen planus, lichen sclerosus, and lichen simplex chronicus; pelvic disease, such as endometriosis or chronic PID; vulvodynia; or vaginal atrophy. Vulvodynia is the most frequent cause of dyspareunia in premenopausal women. It is characterized by a sensation of burning along with other symptoms, including pain, itching, stinging, irritation, and rawness. The discomfort may be constant or intermittent, focal or diffuse, and experienced as either deep or superficial. There are generally no physical findings except minimal erythema that may be associated in a subset of patients with vulvodynia, those with vulvar vestibulitis. Vulvar vestibulitis is normally asymptomatic, but pain is associated with touching or pressure on the vestibule, such as with vaginal entry or insertion of a tampon. Pain occurring with deep thrusting during coitus is usually due to acute or chronic infection of the cervix, uterus, or adnexa; endometriosis; adnexal tumors; or adhesions resulting from prior pelvic disease or operation.

► Treatment

A. Disorders of Sexual Desire

In the absence of specific medical disorders, arousal or orgasmic disorders or dyspareunia, the focus of therapy is psychological. Cognitive behavioral therapy, sexual therapy, and couples therapy may all play a role. Success with pharmacologic therapy, particularly the use of dopamine agonists or testosterone with estrogen has been reported, but data from large long-term clinical trials are lacking.

B. Sexual Arousal Disorders

As with disorders of sexual desire, arousal disorders may respond to psychological therapy. Specific pharmacologic therapy is lacking. The use of the phosphodiesterase inhibitors used in men does not appear to benefit the majority of women with sexual arousal disorders. However, there is some evidence to suggest a role for sildenafil in women with sexual dysfunction due to multiple sclerosis, type 1 diabetes mellitus, spinal cord injury, and antidepressant medications, if other, better established, approaches fail.

C. Orgasmic Disorders

For many women, brief sexual counseling along with the use of educational books (such as *For Yourself*, by Lonnie Barbach) may be adequate therapy. Also, there is an FDA-approved vacuum device that increases clitoral blood flow and may improve the likelihood of orgasm.

D. Sexual Pain Disorders

Specific medical disorders, such as endometriosis, vulvo-vaginitis, or vaginal atrophy, should be treated as outlined in other sections of this chapter. Lichen planus and lichen simplex chronicus are addressed in Chapter 6. Lichen sclerosus, a thinning and whitening of the vulvar epithelium is treated with clobetasol propionate 0.05% ointment, applied twice daily for 2–3 months.

Vaginismus may be treated initially with sexual counseling and education on anatomy and sexual functioning. The patient can be instructed in self-dilation, using a lubricated finger or test tubes of graduated sizes. Before coitus (with adequate lubrication) is attempted, the patient—and then her partner—should be able to easily and painlessly introduce two fingers into the vagina. Penetration should never be forced, and the woman should always be the one to control the depth of insertion during dilation or intercourse. Injection of botulinum toxin has been used successfully in refractory cases.

Since the cause of vulvodynia is unknown, management is difficult. Few treatment approaches have been subjected to methodologically rigorous trials. A variety of topical agents have been tried, although only topical anesthetics (eg, estrogen cream and a compounded mixture of topical amitriptyline 2% and baclofen 2% in a water washable base) have been useful in relieving vulvodynia. Useful oral medications include tricyclic antidepressants, such as amitriptyline in gradually increasing doses from 10 mg/d to 75–100 mg/d; various SSRIs; and anticonvulsants, such as gabapentin, starting at 300 mg three times daily and increasing to 1200 mg three times daily. Biofeedback and physical therapy, with a physical therapist experienced with the treatment of vulvar pain, have been shown to be helpful. Surgery—usually consisting of vestibulectomy—has been useful for women with introital dyspareunia. See also Chapter 42.

► When to Refer

- When symptoms or concerns persist despite first-line therapy.
- For expertise in surgical procedures.

American College of Obstetricians and Gynecologists. ACOG Practice Bulletin No. 119: Female sexual dysfunction. Obstet Gynecol. 2011 Apr;117(4):96–1007. [PMID: 21422879]
Nastri CO et al. Hormone therapy for sexual function in perimenopausal and postmenopausal women. Cochrane Database Syst Rev. 2013 Jun 5;6:CD009672. [PMID: 23737033]
Simon JA. Identifying and treating sexual dysfunction in postmenopausal women: the role of estrogen. J Womens Health (Larchmt). 2011 Oct;20(10):1453–65. [PMID: 21819250]

INFERTILITY

A couple is said to be infertile if pregnancy does not result after 1 year of normal sexual activity without contraceptives. About 25% of couples experience infertility at some point in their reproductive lives; the incidence of infertility increases with age, with a decline in fertility beginning in the early 30s and accelerating in the late 30s. **The male partner contributes to about 40% of cases of infertility,** and a combination of factors is common. Six percent of married women aged 15 to 44, about 1.5 million women, were considered infertile at some point from 2006 through 2010. However, that is decreased from 8.5% of women (2.4 million) in 1982.

A. Initial Testing

During the initial interview, the clinician can present an overview of infertility and discuss a plan of study. Private consultations with each partner separately are then conducted, allowing appraisal of psychosexual adjustment without embarrassment or criticism. Pertinent details (eg, sexually transmitted disease or prior pregnancies) must be obtained. The ill effects of cigarettes, alcohol, and other recreational drugs on male fertility should be discussed. Prescription medications that impair male potency and factors that may lead to scrotal hyperthermia, such as tight underwear or frequent use of saunas or hot tubs, should be discussed. The gynecologic history should include the menstrual pattern, the use and types of contraceptives, douching, libido, sex techniques, frequency and success of coitus, and correlation of intercourse with time of ovulation. Family history includes repeated spontaneous abortions. The American Society for Reproductive Medicine provides patient information on the infertility evaluation and treatment (http://www.asrm.org/FactSheetsandBooklets/).

General physical and genital examinations are performed on the female partner. Basic laboratory studies include complete blood count, urinalysis, cervical culture for *Chlamydia*, rubella antibody determination, and thyroid function tests. If the woman has regular menses, the likelihood of ovulatory cycles is very high. A luteal phase serum progesterone above 3 ng/mL establishes ovulation. Couples should be advised that coitus resulting in conception occurs during the 6-day window around the day of ovulation. Ovulation predictor kits have in many cases replaced basal body temperatures for predicting ovulation, but temperature charting is a natural and inexpensive way to identify most fertile days. Basal body temperature charts cannot predict ovulation; they can only retrospectively confirm ovulation occurred.

A semen analysis to rule out a male factor for infertility should be completed. Men must abstain from sexual activity for at least 3 days before the semen is obtained. A clean, dry, wide-mouthed bottle for collection is preferred. Semen should be examined within 1–2 hours after collection. Semen is considered normal with the following minimum values: volume, 2.0 mL; concentration, 20 million sperm per milliliter; motility, ≥ 50% forward progression, ≥ 25% rapid progression; and normal forms, 30%. If the sperm count is abnormal, further evaluation includes physical examination of the male partner and a search for exposure to environmental and workplace toxins, alcohol or drug abuse.

B. Further Testing

1. Gross deficiencies of sperm (number, motility, or appearance) require repeat analysis. Intracytoplasmic sperm injection (ICSI) is the treatment option available for sperm deficiencies except for azoospermia (absence of sperm). ICSI requires the female partner to undergo in vitro fertilization (IVF).

2. A screening pelvic ultrasound and hysterosalpingography to identify uterine cavity or tubal anomalies should be performed. Hysterosalpingography using an oil dye is performed within 3 days following the menstrual period if structural abnormalities are suspected. This radiographic study will demonstrate uterine abnormalities (septa, polyps, submucous myomas) and tubal obstruction. A 2013 study from New Zealand suggested oil-based (versus water-soluble) contrast media may improve pregnancy rates. Reports of complications using oil-based media resulted in a decrease in its usage. Women who have had prior pelvic inflammation should receive doxycycline, 100 mg orally twice daily, beginning immediately before and for 7 days after the radiographic study. IVF is recommended as the primary treatment option for tubal disease, but surgery can be considered in young women with mild tubal disease.

3. Absent or infrequent ovulation requires additional laboratory evaluation. Elevated FSH and LH levels and low estradiol levels indicate ovarian failure causing premature menopause. Elevated LH levels in the presence of normal FSH levels may indicate the presence of polycystic ovaries. Elevation of blood prolactin (PRL) levels suggests a pituitary adenoma. In women over age 35, ovarian reserve should be assessed. A markedly elevated FSH (> 15–20 international units/L) on day 3 of the menstrual cycle suggests inadequate ovarian reserve. Although less widely used clinically, a Clomiphene Citrate Challenge Test, with measurement of FSH on day 10 after administration of clomiphene from day 5–9, can help confirm a diagnosis of diminished ovarian reserve. The number of antral follicles during the early follicular phase of the cycle can provide useful information about ovarian reserve and can confirm serum testing. Antimullerian hormone is being used as part of the assessment of ovarian reserve. Unlike FSH, it can be measured at any time during the menstrual cycle and is less likely to be affected by hormones.

4. If all the above testing is normal, unexplained infertility is diagnosed. In approximately 25% of women whose basic evaluation is normal, the first-line therapy is usually controlled ovarian hyperstimulation (usually clomiphene citrate) and intrauterine insemination. IVF may be recommended if couples fail to conceive with controlled ovarian hyperstimulation and intrauterine insemination.

▶ Treatment

A. Medical Measures

Fertility may be restored by treatment of endocrine abnormalities, particularly hypothyroidism or hyperthyroidism. Women who are anovulatory as a result of low body weight or exercise may become ovulatory when they gain weight or decrease their exercise levels.

B. Surgical Measures

Excision of ovarian tumors or ovarian foci of endometriosis can improve fertility. Microsurgical relief of tubal obstruction due to salpingitis or tubal ligation will reestablish fertility in a significant number of cases, although with severe disease or proximal obstruction, IVF is preferable. Peritubal adhesions or endometriotic implants often can be treated via laparoscopy.

In a male with a varicocele, sperm characteristics may be improved following surgical treatment. For men who have sperm production but obstructive azoospermia, transepidermal sperm aspiration or microsurgical epidermal sperm aspiration has been successful.

C. Induction of Ovulation

1. Clomiphene citrate—Clomiphene citrate stimulates gonadotropin release, especially FSH. It acts as a selective estrogen receptor modulator, similar to tamoxifen and raloxifene, and binds to the estrogen receptor. The body perceives a low level of estrogen, decreasing the negative feedback on the hypothalamus, and there is an increased release of FSH and LH. When FSH and LH are present in the appropriate amounts and timing, ovulation occurs.

After a normal menstrual period or induction of withdrawal bleeding with progestin, 50 mg of clomiphene orally daily for 5 days, typically on days 3–7 of the cycle, should be given. If ovulation does not occur, the dosage is increased to 100 mg daily for 5 days. If ovulation still does not occur, the course is repeated with 150 mg daily and then 200 mg daily for 5 days. The maximum dosage is 200 mg. Ovulation and appropriate timing of intercourse can be facilitated with the addition of chorionic gonadotropin, 10,000 units intramuscularly. Monitoring of the follicles by transvaginal ultrasound usually is necessary to appropriately time the hCG injection. The rate of ovulation following this treatment is 90% in the absence of other infertility factors. The pregnancy rate is high. Twinning occurs in 5% of these patients, and three or more fetuses are found in rare instances (< 0.5% of cases). Pregnancy is most likely to occur within the first three ovulatory cycles, and unlikely to occur after cycle six. In addition, several studies have suggested a twofold to threefold increased risk of ovarian cancer with the use of clomiphene for more than 1 year, so treatment with clomiphene is usually limited to a maximum of six cycles.

In the presence of increased androgen production (DHEA-S > 200 mcg/dL), the addition of dexamethasone, 0.5 mg orally, or prednisone, 5 mg orally, at bedtime, improves the response to clomiphene in selected patients. Dexamethasone should be discontinued after pregnancy is confirmed.

2. Letrozole—The aromatase inhibitor, letrozole, appears to be at least as effective as clomiphene for ovulation induction in women with PCOS. There is a reduced risk of multiple pregnancy, a lack of antiestrogenic effects, and a reduced need for ultrasound monitoring. The dose is 5–7.5 mg daily, starting on day 3 of the menstrual cycle. In women who have a history of estrogen dependent tumors, such as breast cancer, letrozole is preferred as the estrogen levels with this drug are much lower.

3. Carbergoline or bromocriptine—Carbergoline or bromocriptine is used only if PRL levels are elevated and there is no withdrawal bleeding following progesterone administration (otherwise, clomiphene is used). The initial dosage is 2.5 mg orally once daily, increased to two or three times daily in increments of 1.25 mg. The drug is discontinued once pregnancy has occurred. Cabergoline causes fewer adverse effects than bromocriptine. However, it is much more expensive. Cabergoline is often used in patients who cannot tolerate the adverse effects of bromocriptine or in those who do not respond to bromocriptine.

4. Human menopausal gonadotropins (hMG) or recombinant FSH—hMG or recombinant FSH is indicated in cases of hypogonadotropism and most other types of anovulation resistant to clomiphene treatment. Because of the complexities, laboratory tests, and expense associated with this treatment, these patients should be referred to an infertility specialist.

D. Treatment of Endometriosis

See above.

E. Artificial Insemination in Azoospermia

If azoospermia is present, artificial insemination by a donor usually results in pregnancy, assuming female function is normal. The use of frozen sperm is the only option because it provides the opportunity for screening for sexually transmitted diseases, including HIV infection.

F. Assisted Reproductive Technologies (ART)

Couples who have not responded to traditional infertility treatments, including those with tubal disease, severe endometriosis, oligospermia, and immunologic or unexplained infertility, may benefit from IVF. Gamete intrafallopian transfer and zygote intrafallopian transfer are rarely performed, although it may be an option in a few selected patients. These techniques are complex and require a highly organized team of specialists. All of the procedures involve ovarian stimulation to produce multiple oocytes, oocyte retrieval by transvaginal sonography–guided needle aspiration, and handling of the oocytes outside the body. With IVF, the eggs are fertilized in vitro and the embryos transferred to the uterus. ICSI allows fertilization with a single sperm. While originally intended for couples with male factor infertility, it is now used in two-thirds of all IVF procedures in the United States.

The chance of a multiple gestation pregnancy (ie, twins, triplets) is increased in all assisted reproductive procedures, increasing the risk of preterm delivery and other pregnancy complications. To minimize this risk, most infertility specialists recommend only transferring one embryo in appropriately selected patients with a favorable prognosis. In women with prior failed IVF cycles who are over the age of 40 who have poor embryo quality, up to 4 embryos may be transferred. In the event of a multiple gestation pregnancy, a couple may consider selective reduction to avoid the medical issues generally related to multiple births. This issue should be discussed with the couple before embryo transfer.

► Prognosis

The prognosis for conception and normal pregnancy is good if minor (even multiple) disorders can be identified and treated; it is poor if the causes of infertility are severe, untreatable, or of prolonged duration (over 3 years).

It is important to remember that in the absence of identifiable causes of infertility, 60% of couples will achieve a pregnancy within 3 years. Couples with unexplained infertility who do not achieve pregnancy within 3 years may be offered ovulation induction or assisted reproductive technology. Women over the age of 35 should be offered a more aggressive approach, with consideration of ART within 3–6 months of not achieving pregnancy with more conservative approaches. Also, offering appropriately timed information about adoption is considered part of a complete infertility regimen.

► When to Refer

Refer to reproductive endocrinologist if ART are indicated, or surgery is required.

Beall SA et al. History and challenges surrounding ovarian stimulation in the treatment of infertility. Fertil Steril. 2012 Apr;97(4):795–801. [PMID: 22463773]

CONTRACEPTION

Unintended pregnancies are a worldwide problem but disproportionately impact developing countries. Studies estimate that 41% of the 208 million pregnancies that occurred in 2008 were unintended. Globally, 85 million pregnancies were unintended and ended in abortion (41 million), unplanned births (33 million), or miscarriages (11 million). It is important for primary care providers to educate their patients about the benefits of contraception and to provide options that are appropriate and desirable for the patient.

1. Oral Contraceptives

A. Combined Oral Contraceptives

1. Efficacy and methods of use—Combined oral contraceptives have a perfect use failure rate of 0.3% and a typical use failure rate of 8%. Their primary mode of action is suppression of ovulation. The pills can be initially started on the first day of the menstrual cycle, the first Sunday after the onset of the cycle or on any day of the cycle. If started on any day other than the first day of the cycle, a backup method should be used. If an active pill is missed at any time, and no intercourse occurred in the past 5 days, two pills should be taken immediately and a backup method should be used for 7 days. If intercourse occurred in the previous 5 days, emergency contraception (see below) should be used immediately, and the pills restarted the following day. A backup method should be used for 5 days.

2. Benefits of oral contraceptives—Noncontraceptive benefits of oral contraceptives include lighter menses, reducing the likelihood of anemia, and improvement of dysmenorrhea symptoms. Functional ovarian cysts are less likely with oral contraceptive use. The risk of ovarian and endometrial cancer is decreased. Acne is usually improved. The frequency of developing myomas is lower in long-term users (> 4 years). There is also a beneficial effect on bone mass.

3. Selection of an oral contraceptive—Any of the combination oral contraceptives containing 35 mcg or less of ethinyl estradiol or 3 mg of estradiol valerate are suitable for most women. There is some variation in potency of the various progestins in the pills, but there are essentially no clinically significant differences for most women among the progestins in the low-dose pills. The available evidence is insufficient to determine whether triphasic oral contraceptives differ from monophasic oral contraceptives in effectiveness, bleeding patterns or discontinuation rates. **Therefore, monophasic pills are recommended as a first choice for women starting oral contraceptive use.** Women who have acne or hirsutism may benefit from treatment with desogestrel, drospirenone, or norgestimate, since they are the least androgenic. A combination regimen with 84 active and 7 inert pills that results in only four menses per year is available. There is also a combination regimen that is taken continuously with no regular menses. At the end of one years' use, 58% of the women had amenorrhea, and nearly 80% reported no bleeding requiring sanitary protection. Studies have not shown any significant risk from long-term amenorrhea in patients taking continuous oral contraceptives. The low-dose oral contraceptives commonly used in the United States are listed in Table 18–3.

4. Drug interactions—Several drugs interact with oral contraceptives to decrease their efficacy by causing induction of microsomal enzymes in the liver, or by other mechanisms. Some commonly prescribed drugs in this category are phenytoin, phenobarbital (and other barbiturates), primidone, topiramate, carbamazepine, and rifampin and St. John's Wort. Women taking these drugs should use another means of contraception for maximum safety.

Antiretroviral medications, specifically ritonavir-boosted protease inhibitors, may significantly decrease the efficacy of combined oral contraceptives, and the concomitant use of oral contraceptives may increase the toxicity of these antiretroviral agents. Non-nucleoside reverse transcriptase inhibitors have smaller effects on oral contraceptive efficacy, while nucleoside reverse transcriptase inhibitors appear to have no effect.

5. Contraindications and adverse effects—Oral contraceptives have been associated with many adverse effects; they are contraindicated in some situations and should be used with caution in others (Table 18–4).

A. Myocardial infarction—The risk of heart attack is higher with use of oral contraceptives, particularly with pills containing 50 mcg of estrogen or more. Cigarette smoking, obesity, hypertension, diabetes, or hypercholesterolemia increases the risk. Young nonsmoking women have minimal increased risk. Smokers over age 35 and women with other cardiovascular risk factors should use other methods of birth control.

B. Thromboembolic disease—An increased rate of venous thromboembolism is found in oral contraceptive users, especially if the dose of estrogen is 50 mcg or more. While the overall risk is very low (5–6 per 100,000 woman-years compared to 50–300 per 100,000 pregnancies), several studies have reported a twofold increased risk in women using oral contraceptives containing the progestins gestodene (not available in the United States), drosperinone, or desogestrel compared with women using oral contraceptives with levonorgestrel and norethindrone. Women in whom thrombophlebitis develops should stop using this method, as should those at increased risk for thrombophlebitis because of surgery, fracture, serious injury, hypercoagulable condition, or immobilization. Women with a known thrombophilia should not use oral contraceptives.

C. Cerebrovascular disease—Overall, a small increased risk of hemorrhagic stroke and subarachnoid hemorrhage and a somewhat greater increased risk of thrombotic stroke have been found; smoking, hypertension, and age over 35 years are associated with increased risk. Women should stop using contraceptives if such warning symptoms as severe headache, blurred or lost vision, or other transient neurologic disorders develop.

Table 18–3. Commonly used low-dose oral contraceptives.

Name	Progestin	Estrogen (Ethinyl Estradiol)	Cost per Month[1]
COMBINATION			
Alesse[2,3]	0.1 mg levonorgestrel	20 mcg	$43.90
Loestrin 1/20[2]	1 mg norethindrone acetate	20 mcg	$38.08
Mircette[2]	0.15 mg desogestrel	20 mcg	$42.56
Yaz	3 mg drospirenone	20 mcg	$68.04
Loestrin 1.5/30[2]	1.5 mg norethindrone acetate	30 mcg	$38.64
Lo-Ovral[2]	0.3 mg norgestrel	30 mcg	$30.52
Levlen[2]	0.15 mg levonorgestrel	30 mcg	$30.80
Ortho-Cept[2] Desogen[2]	0.15 mg desogestrel	30 mcg	$39.20
Yasmin	3 mg drospirenone	30 mcg	$76.72
Brevicon[2] Modicon[2]	0.5 mg norethindrone	35 mcg	$32.20
Demulen 1/35[2]	1 mg ethynodiol diacetate	35 mcg	$29.96
Ortho-Novum 1/35[2]	1 mg norethindrone	35 mcg	$29.40
Ortho-Cyclen[2]	0.25 mg norgestimate	35 mcg	$32.20
Ovcon 35[2]	0.4 mg norethindrone	35 mcg	$44.80
COMBINATION: EXTENDED-CYCLE			
Seasonale (91 day cycle)	0.15 mg levonorgestrel	30 mcg	$53.10
Seasonique (91 day cycle)	0.15 mg levonorgestrel (days 1–84)/ 0 mg levonorgestrel (days 85–91)	30 mcg (84 days)/10 mcg (7 days)	$67.69
LoSeasonique (91 day cycle)	0.10 mg levonorgestrel (days 1–84)/ 0 mg levonorgestrel (days 85–91)	20 mcg (84 days)/10 mcg (7 days)	$108.60
Amethyst (28 day pack)	90 mcg levonorgestrel	20 mcg	$57.00
TRIPHASIC			
Estrostep	1 mg norethindrone acetate (days 1–5) 1 mg norethindrone acetate (days 6–12) 1 mg norethindrone acetate (days 13–21)	20 mcg 30 mcg 35 mcg	$54.88
Cyclessa[2]	0.1 mg desogestrel (days 1–7) 0.125 mg desogestrel (days 8–14) 0.15 mg desogestrel (days 15–21)	25 mcg	$65.34
Ortho-Tri-Cyclen Lo	0.18 norgestimate (days 1–7) 0.21 norgestimate (days 8–14) 0.25 norgestimate (days 15–21)	25 mcg	$138.60
Triphasil[2,3]	0.05 mg levonorgestrel (days 1–6) 0.075 mg levonorgestrel (days 7–11) 0.125 mg levonorgestrel (days 12–21)	30 mcg 40 mcg 30 mcg	$27.50
Ortho-Novum 7/7/7[2,3]	0.5 mg norethindrone (days 1–7) 0.75 mg norethindrone (days 8–14) 1 mg norethindrone (days 15–21)	35 mcg	$27.24
Ortho-Tri-Cyclen[2,3]	0.18 mg norgestimate (days 1–7) 0.215 mg norgestimate (days 8–14) 0.25 mg norgestimate (days 15–21)	35 mcg	$39.31
Tri-Norinyl[2,3]	0.5 mg norethindrone (days 1–7) 1 mg norethindrone (days 8–16) 0.5 mg norethindrone (days 17–21)	35 mcg	$32.20
PROGESTIN-ONLY MINIPILL			
Ortho Micronor[2,3]	0.35 mg norethindrone to be taken continuously	None	$39.96

[1]Average wholesale price (AWP, for AB-rated generic when available) for quantity listed. Source: *Red Book Online, 2014, Truven Health Analytics, Inc.* AWP may not accurately represent the actual pharmacy cost because wide contractual variations exist among institutions.
[2]Generic equivalent available.
[3]Multiple other brands available.

Table 18–4. Contraindications to use of oral contraceptives.

Absolute contraindications
Pregnancy
Thrombophlebitis or thromboembolic disorders (past or present)
Stroke or coronary artery disease (past or present)
Cancer of the breast (known or suspected)
Undiagnosed abnormal vaginal bleeding
Estrogen-dependent cancer (known or suspected)
Benign or malignant tumor of the liver (past or present)
Uncontrolled hypertension
Diabetes mellitus with vascular disease
Age over 35 and smoking > 15 cigarettes daily
Known thrombophilia
Migraine with aura
Active hepatitis
Surgery or orthopedic injury requiring prolonged immobilization
Relative contraindications
Migraine without aura
Hypertension
Heart or kidney disease
Diabetes mellitus
Gallbladder disease
Cholestasis during pregnancy
Sickle cell disease (S/S or S/C type)
Lactation

D. Carcinoma—There is no increased risk of breast cancer in women aged 35–64 who are current or former users of oral contraceptives. Women with a family history of breast cancer or women who started oral contraceptive use at a young age are not at increased risk. Combination oral contraceptives reduce the risk of endometrial carcinoma by 40% after 2 years of use and 60% after 4 or more years of use. The risk of ovarian cancer is reduced by 30% with pill use for < 4 years, by 60% with use for 5–11 years, and by 80% after 12 or more years. Rarely, oral contraceptives have been associated with the development of benign or malignant hepatic tumors; this may lead to rupture of the liver, hemorrhage, and death. The risk increases with higher dosage, longer duration of use, and older age.

E. Hypertension—Oral contraceptives may cause hypertension in some women; the risk is increased with longer duration of use and older age. Women in whom hypertension develops while using oral contraceptives should use other contraceptive methods. However, with regular blood pressure monitoring, nonsmoking women with well-controlled mild hypertension may use oral contraceptives.

F. Headache—Migraine or other vascular headaches may occur or worsen with pill use. If severe or frequent headaches develop while using this method, it should be discontinued. Women with migraine headaches *with an aura* should not use oral contraceptives.

G. Lactation—Combined oral contraceptives can impair the quantity and quality of breast milk. While it is preferable to avoid the use of combination oral contraceptives

during lactation, the effects on milk quality are small and are not associated with developmental abnormalities in infants. Combination oral contraceptives should be started no earlier than 6 weeks postpartum to allow for establishment of lactation. Progestin-only pills, levonorgestrel implants, and DMPA are alternatives with no adverse effects on milk quality.

H. Other disorders—Depression may occur or be worsened with oral contraceptive use. Fluid retention may occur. Patients who had cholestatic jaundice during pregnancy may develop it while taking birth control pills.

I. Obesity—A growing number of women are obese or overweight. Some studies have suggested that oral contraceptives are less effective in overweight women. In addition, obesity is a risk factor for thromboembolic complications. It is important that obese women are not denied effective contraception as a result of concerns about complications or efficacy of oral contraceptives.

6. Minor side effects—Nausea and dizziness may occur in the first few months of pill use. A weight gain of 2–5 lb (0.9–2.25 kg) commonly occurs. Spotting or breakthrough bleeding between menstrual periods may occur, especially if a pill is skipped or taken late; this may be helped by switching to a pill of slightly greater potency (see section 3, above). Missed menstrual periods may occur, especially with low-dose pills. A pregnancy test should be performed if pills have been skipped or if two or more expected menstrual periods are missed. Fatigue and decreased libido can occur. Chloasma may occur, as in pregnancy, and is increased by exposure to sunlight.

B. Progestin Minipill

1. Efficacy and methods of use—A formulation containing 0.35 mg of norethindrone is available in the United States. The efficacy is similar to that of combined oral contraceptives. The minipill is believed to prevent conception by causing thickening of the cervical mucus to make it hostile to sperm, alteration of ovum transport (which may account for the slightly higher rate of ectopic pregnancy with these pills), and inhibition of implantation. Ovulation is inhibited inconsistently with this method. The minipill is begun on the first day of a menstrual cycle and then taken continuously for as long as contraception is desired.

2. Advantages—The low dose of progestin and absence of estrogen make the minipill safe during lactation; it may increase the flow of milk. It is often tried by women who want minimal doses of hormones and by patients who are over age 35. They lack the cardiovascular side effects of combination pills. The minipill can be safely used by women with sickle cell disease (S/S or S/C).

3. Complications and contraindications—Minipill users often have bleeding irregularities (eg, prolonged flow, spotting, or amenorrhea); such patients may need regular pregnancy tests. Ectopic pregnancies are more frequent, and complaints of abdominal pain should be investigated with this in mind. Many of the absolute contraindications and relative contraindications listed in Table 18–4 apply to the minipill; however, the contraceptive benefit of the minipill may outweigh the risks for patients who smoke, who are over age 35, or who have such conditions as superficial deep venous thrombosis or known thromboembolic disorders or diabetes with vascular disease. Minor side effects of combination oral contraceptives such as weight gain and mild headache may also occur with the minipill.

Centers for Disease Control and Prevention (CDC). Update to CDC's U.S. Medical Eligibility Criteria for Contraceptive Use, 2010: revised recommendations for the use of hormonal contraception among women at high risk for HIV infection or infected with HIV. MMWR Morb Mortal Wkly Rep. 2012 Jun 22;61(24):449–52. [PMID: 22717514]

Shaw KA et al. Obesity and oral contraceptives: a clinician's guide. Best Pract Res Clin Endocrinol Metab. 2013 Feb;27(1):55–65. [PMID: 23384746]

Van Vliet HA et al. Triphasic versus monophasic oral contraceptives for contraception. Cochrane Database Syst Rev. 2011 Nov 9;(11):CD003553. [PMID: 22071807]

2. Contraceptive Injections & Implants (Long-Acting Progestins)

The injectable progestin DMPA is approved for contraceptive use in the United States. There is extensive worldwide experience with this method over the past 3 decades. The medication is given as a deep intramuscular injection of 150 mg every 3 months and has a contraceptive efficacy of 99.7%. A subcutaneous preparation, containing 104 mg of DMPA is available in the United States. Common side effects include irregular bleeding, amenorrhea, weight gain, and headache. It is associated with bone mineral loss that is usually reversible after discontinuation of the method. Users commonly have irregular bleeding initially and subsequently develop amenorrhea. Ovulation may be delayed after the last injection. Contraindications are similar to those for the minipill.

A single-rod, subdermal progestin implant, Implanon, is approved for use in the United States. Implanon is a 40-mm by 2-mm rod containing 68 mg of the progestin etonogestrel that is inserted in the inner aspect of the non-dominant arm. Hormone levels drop rapidly after removal, and there is no delay in the return of fertility. In clinical trials, the pregnancy rate was 0.0% with 3 years of use. The side effect profile is similar to minipills, DMPA, and Norplant. Irregular bleeding has been the most common reason for discontinuation. Implanon is being replaced by Nexplanon which, unlike Implanon, is radiopaque and has a redesigned inserter. Nexplanon is available in the United States, but Implanon is still widely used in many developing countries.

Mommers E et al. Nexplanon, a radiopaque etonogestrel implant in combination with a next-generation applicator: 3-year results of a noncomparative multicenter trial. Am J Obstet Gynecol. 2012 Nov;207(5):388.e1–6. [PMID: 22939402]

3. Other Hormonal Methods

A transdermal contraceptive patch containing 150 mcg norelgestromin and 20 mcg ethinyl estradiol and measuring 20 cm² is available. The patch is applied to the lower abdomen, upper torso, or buttock once a week for 3 consecutive weeks, followed by 1 week without the patch. It appears that the average steady-state concentration of ethinyl estradiol with the patch is approximately 60% higher than with a 35 mcg pill. However, there is currently no evidence for an increased incidence of estrogen-related side effects. The mechanism of action, side effects, and efficacy are similar to those associated with oral contraceptives, although compliance may be better. However, discontinuation for side effects is more frequent.

A contraceptive vaginal ring that releases 120 mcg of etonogestrel and 15 mcg of ethinyl estradiol daily is available. The ring is soft and flexible and is placed in the upper vagina for 3 weeks, removed, and replaced 1 week later. The efficacy, mechanism of action, and systemic side effects are similar to those associated with oral contraceptives. Ring users may experience an increased incidence of vaginal discharge.

Lopez LM et al. Skin patch and vaginal ring versus combined oral contraceptives for contraception. Cochrane Database Syst Rev. 2013 Apr 30;4:CD003552. [PMID: 23633314]

4. Intrauterine Devices

In the United States, the following devices are available: the Mirena and the Skyla IUDs (both of which release levonorgestrel) and the copper-bearing TCu380A. The mechanism of action of IUDs is thought to involve either spermicidal or inhibitory effects on sperm capacitation and transport. IUDs are not abortifacients.

Skyla is effective for 3 years, Mirena for 5 years, and the TCu380A for 10 years. The hormone-containing IUDs have the advantage of reducing cramping and menstrual flow.

The IUD is an excellent contraceptive method for most women. The devices are highly effective, with failure rates similar to those achieved with surgical sterilization. Nulliparity is not a contraindication to IUD use. Adolescents are also candidates for IUD use. Women who are not in mutually monogamous relationships should use condoms for protection from sexually transmitted diseases. Levonorgestrel-containing IUDs may have a protective effect against upper tract infection similar to that of the oral contraceptives.

A. Insertion

Insertion can be performed during or after the menses, at midcycle to prevent implantation, or later in the cycle if the patient has not become pregnant. There is growing evidence to suggest that IUDs can be safely inserted in the immediate postabortal and postpartum periods.

Both types of IUDs may be inserted up to 48 hours after vaginal delivery, or prior to closure of the uterus at the time of cesarean section. Insertion immediately following abortion is acceptable if there is no sepsis and if follow-up insertion a month later will not be possible; otherwise, it is wise to wait until 4 weeks post abortion. Misoprostol (200 mcg the night before) and NSAIDs given as premedications

Table 18–5. Contraindications to IUD use.

Absolute contraindications
Pregnancy
Acute or subacute pelvic inflammatory disease or purulent cervicitis
Significant anatomic abnormality of uterus
Unexplained uterine bleeding
Active liver disease (Mirena only)
Relative contraindications
History of pelvic inflammatory disease since the last pregnancy
Lack of available follow-up care
Menorrhagia or severe dysmenorrhea (copper IUD)
Cervical or uterine neoplasia

may help insertions in nulliparous patients or when insertion is not performed during menses.

B. Contraindications & Complications

Contraindications to use of IUDs are outlined in Table 18–5.

1. Pregnancy—A copper-containing IUD can be inserted within 5 days following a single episode of unprotected mid-cycle coitus as a postcoital contraceptive. An IUD should not be inserted into a pregnant uterus. If pregnancy occurs as an IUD failure, there is a greater chance of spontaneous abortion if the IUD is left in situ (50%) than if it is removed (25%). Spontaneous abortion with an IUD in place is associated with a high risk of severe sepsis, and death can occur rapidly. Women using an IUD who become pregnant should have the IUD removed if the string is visible. It can be removed at the time of abortion if this is desired. If the string is not visible and the patient wants to continue the pregnancy, she should be informed of the serious risk of sepsis and, occasionally, death with such pregnancies. She should be informed that any flu-like symptoms such as fever, myalgia, headache, or nausea warrant immediate medical attention for possible septic abortion.

Since the ratio of ectopic to intrauterine pregnancies is increased among IUD wearers, clinicians should search for adnexal masses in early pregnancy and should always check the products of conception for placental tissue following abortion.

2. Pelvic infection—There is an increased risk of pelvic infection during the first month following insertion; however, prophylactic antibiotics given at the time of insertion do not appear to decrease this risk. The subsequent risk of pelvic infection appears to be primarily related to the risk of acquiring sexually transmitted infections. Infertility rates do not appear to be increased among women who have previously used the currently available IUDs. At the time of insertion, women with an increased risk of sexually transmitted diseases should be screened for gonorrhea and *Chlamydia*. Women with a history of recent or recurrent pelvic infection are not good candidates for IUD use.

3. Menorrhagia or severe dysmenorrhea—The copper IUD can cause heavier menstrual periods, bleeding between periods, and more cramping, so it is generally not suitable for women who already suffer from these problems. Alternatively, the hormone-releasing IUD Mirena has been approved by the FDA to treat heavy menstrual bleeding. NSAIDs are also helpful in decreasing bleeding and pain in IUD users.

4. Complete or partial expulsion—Spontaneous expulsion of the IUD occurs in 10–20% of cases during the first year of use. Any IUD should be removed if the body of the device can be seen or felt in the cervical os.

5. Missing IUD strings—If the transcervical tail cannot be seen, this may signify unnoticed expulsion, perforation of the uterus with abdominal migration of the IUD, or simply retraction of the string into the cervical canal or uterus owing to movement of the IUD or uterine growth with pregnancy. Once pregnancy is ruled out, a cervical speculum may be used to visualize the IUD string in the cervical canal. If not visualized, one should probe for the IUD with a sterile sound or forceps designed for IUD removal after administering a paracervical block. If the IUD cannot be detected, pelvic ultrasound will demonstrate the IUD if it is in the uterus. Alternatively, obtain anteroposterior and lateral radiographs of the pelvis with another IUD or a sound in the uterus as a marker, to confirm an extrauterine IUD. If the IUD is in the abdominal cavity, it should generally be removed by laparoscopy or laparotomy. Perforations of the uterus are less likely if insertion is performed slowly, with meticulous care taken to follow directions applicable to each type of IUD.

Grimes DA et al. Immediate post-partum insertion of intrauterine devices. Cochrane Database Syst Rev. 2010 May 12;(5): CD003036. [PMID: 20464722]

Steenland MW et al. Intrauterine contraceptive insertion postabortion: a systematic review. Contraception. 2011 Nov;84(5): 447–64. [PMID: 22018119]

5. Diaphragm & Cervical Cap

The diaphragm (with contraceptive jelly) is a safe and effective contraceptive method with features that make it acceptable to some women and not others. Failure rates range from 6% to 16%, depending on the motivation of the woman and the care with which the diaphragm is used. The advantages of this method are that it has no systemic side effects and gives significant protection against pelvic infection and cervical dysplasia as well as pregnancy. The disadvantages are that it must be inserted near the time of coitus and that pressure from the rim predisposes some women to cystitis after intercourse.

The cervical cap (with contraceptive jelly) is similar to the diaphragm but fits snugly over the cervix only (the diaphragm stretches from behind the cervix to behind the pubic symphysis). The cervical cap is more difficult to insert and remove than the diaphragm. The main advantages are that it can be used by women who cannot be fitted for a diaphragm because of a relaxed anterior vaginal wall or by women who have discomfort or develop repeated bladder infections with the diaphragm. However, failure rates are 9% (perfect use) and 16% (typical use) in nulliparous women and 26% (perfect use) and 32% (typical use) in parous women.

Because of the small risk of toxic shock syndrome, a cervical cap or diaphragm should not be left in the vagina for over 12–18 hours, nor should these devices be used during the menstrual period.

6. Contraceptive Foam, Cream, Film, Sponge, Jelly, & Suppository

These products are available without prescription, are easy to use, and are fairly effective, with typical failure rates of 10–22%. All contain the spermicide nonoxynol-9, which also has some virucidal and bactericidal activity. Nonoxynol-9 does not appear to adversely affect the vaginal colonization of hydrogen peroxide-producing lactobacilli. The FDA requires products containing nonoxynol-9 to include a warning that the products do not protect against HIV or other sexually transmitted diseases and that use of these products can irritate the vagina and rectum and may increase the risk of getting the AIDS virus from an infected partner. Low-risk women using a nonoxynol-9 product, with coital activity two to three times per week, are not at increased risk for epithelial disruption, compared with couples using condoms alone.

7. Condom

The male condom of latex or animal membrane affords good protection against pregnancy—equivalent to that of a diaphragm and spermicidal jelly; latex (but not animal membrane) condoms also offer protection against many sexually transmitted diseases, including HIV. When a spermicide, such as vaginal foam, is used with the condom, the failure rate (approximately 2% with perfect use and 15% with typical use) approaches that of oral contraceptives. The disadvantages of condoms are dulling of sensation and spillage of semen due to tearing, slipping, or leakage with detumescence of the penis.

Two female condoms, one made of polyurethane and the other of synthetic nitrile, are available in the United States. The reported failure rates range from 5% to 21%; the efficacy is comparable to that of the diaphragm. These are the only female-controlled method that offers significant protection from both pregnancy and sexually transmitted diseases.

8. Contraception Based on Awareness of Fertile Periods

These methods are most effective when the couple restricts intercourse to the post ovular phase of the cycle or uses a barrier method at other times. Well-instructed, motivated couples may be able to achieve low pregnancy rates with fertility awareness methods. However, properly done randomized clinical trials comparing the efficacy of most of these methods with other contraceptive methods do not exist.

9. Emergency Contraception

If unprotected intercourse occurs in midcycle and if the woman is certain she has not inadvertently become pregnant earlier in the cycle, the following regimens are effective in preventing implantation. These methods should be started as soon as possible and within 120 hours after unprotected coitus. (1) Levonorgestrel, 1.5 mg orally as a single dose (available in the United States prepackaged as Plan B and available over-the-counter for women aged 17 years and above), has a 1% failure rate, when taken within 72 hours. It remains efficacious up to 120 hours after intercourse, though less so compared with earlier use. (2) If the levonorgestrel regimen is not available, a combination oral contraceptive containing ethinyl estradiol and levonorgestrel given twice in 12 hours later may be used. At least 20 brands of pills may be used in this way. For specific dosages and instructions for each pill brand, consult www.not-2-late.com. Used within 72 hours, the failure rate of these regimens is approximately 3%, but antinausea medication is often necessary. (3) Ulipristal, 30 mg orally as a single dose, has been shown to be more effective than levonorgestrel, particularly when used between 72 and 120 hours, particularly among overweight women. It is available by prescription in the United States and Western Europe. (4) IUD insertion within 5 days after one episode of unprotected midcycle coitus will also prevent pregnancy; copper-bearing IUDs have been tested and used for many years for this purpose.

Information on clinics or individual clinicians providing emergency contraception in the United States may be obtained by calling 1-888-668-2528.

Brache V et al. Ulipristal acetate prevents ovulation more effectively than levonorgestrel: analysis of pooled data from three randomized trials of emergency contraception regimens. Contraception. 2013 Nov;88(5):611–8. [PMID: 23809278]

Cleland K et al. The efficacy of intrauterine devices for emergency contraception: a systematic review of 35 years of experience. Hum Reprod. 2012 Jul;27(7):1994–2000. [PMID: 22570193]

10. Abortion

Since the legalization of abortion in the United States in 1973, the related maternal mortality rate has fallen markedly, because illegal and self-induced abortions have been replaced by safer medical procedures. Abortions in the first trimester of pregnancy are performed by vacuum aspiration under local anesthesia or with medical regimens. Dilation and evacuation, a variation of vacuum aspiration is generally used in the second trimester. Techniques utilizing intra-amniotic instillation of hypertonic saline solution or various prostaglandins regimens, along with medical or osmotic dilators are occasionally used after 18 weeks. Several medical abortion regimens utilizing mifepristone and multiple doses of misoprostol have been reported as being effective in the second trimester. Overall, legal abortion in the United States has a mortality rate of < 1:100,000. Rates of morbidity and mortality rise with length of gestation. Currently in the United States, more than 60% of abortions are performed before 9 weeks, and more than 90% are performed before 13 weeks' gestation; only 1.3% are performed after 20 weeks. **If abortion is chosen, every effort should be made to encourage the patient to seek an early procedure.** In the United States, while numerous state laws limiting access to abortion and a federal law banning a rarely used variation of dilation and evacuation have been enacted, abortion remains legal and available until fetal viability, between 24 and 28 weeks gestation, under Roe v. Wade.

Complications resulting from abortion include retained products of conception (often associated with infection and heavy bleeding) and unrecognized ectopic pregnancy. Immediate analysis of the removed tissue for placenta can exclude or corroborate the diagnosis of ectopic pregnancy. Women who have fever, bleeding, or abdominal pain after abortion should be examined; use of broad-spectrum antibiotics and reaspiration of the uterus are frequently necessary. Hospitalization is advisable if acute salpingitis requires intravenous administration of antibiotics. Complications following illegal abortion often need emergency care for hemorrhage, septic shock, or uterine perforation.

Rh immune globulin should be given to all Rh-negative women following abortion. Prophylactic antibiotics are indicated for surgical abortion; for example a one-dose regimen of doxycycline, 200 mg orally 1 hour before the procedure. Many clinics prescribe tetracycline, 500 mg orally four times daily for 5 days after the procedure, as presumptive treatment for *Chlamydia*.

Mifepristone (RU 486) is approved by the FDA as an oral abortifacient at a dose of 600 mg on day 1, followed by 400 mcg orally of misoprostol on day 3. This combination is 95% successful in terminating pregnancies of up to 9 weeks' duration with minimum complications. A more commonly used, evidence-based regimen is mifepristone, 200 mg orally on day 1, followed by misoprostol, 800 mcg vaginally either immediately or within 6–8 hours. Although not approved by the FDA for this indication, a combination of intramuscular methotrexate, 50 mg/m^2 of body surface area, followed 3–7 days later by vaginal misoprostol, 800 mcg, is 98% successful in terminating pregnancy at 8 weeks or less. Minor side effects, such as nausea, vomiting, and diarrhea, are common with these regimens. There is a 5–10% incidence of hemorrhage or incomplete abortion requiring curettage. Medical abortion is generally considered as safe as surgical abortion in the first trimester but is associated with more pain and a lower success rate (requiring surgical abortion). Overall, the risk of uterine infection is lower with medical than with surgical abortion.

Guiahi M et al. First-trimester abortion in women with medical conditions: release date October 2012 SFP guideline #20122. Contraception. 2012 Dec;86(6):622–30. [PMID: 23039921]

11. Sterilization

In the United States, sterilization is the most popular method of birth control for couples who want no more children. Although sterilization is reversible in some instances, reversal surgery in both men and women is costly, complicated, and not always successful. Therefore, patients should be counseled carefully before sterilization and should view the procedure as permanent.

Vasectomy is a safe, simple procedure in which the vas deferens is severed and sealed through a scrotal incision under local anesthesia. Long-term follow-up studies on vasectomized men show no excess risk of cardiovascular disease. Several studies have shown a possible association with prostate cancer, but the evidence is weak and inconsistent.

Female sterilization procedures include laparoscopic bipolar electrocoagulation, or plastic ring application on the uterine tubes, or minilaparotomy with Pomeroy tubal resection. The advantages of laparoscopy are minimal postoperative pain, small incisions, and rapid recovery. The advantages of minilaparotomy are that it can be performed with standard surgical instruments under local or general anesthesia. However, there is more postoperative pain and a longer recovery period. The cumulative 10-year failure rate for all methods combined is 1.85%, varying from 0.75% for postpartum partial salpingectomy and laparoscopic unipolar coagulation to 3.65% for spring clips; this fact should be discussed with women preoperatively. Some studies have found an increased risk of menstrual irregularities as a long-term complication of tubal ligation, but findings in different studies have been inconsistent. Two methods of transcervical sterilization, Essure and Adiana, can be performed as outpatient procedures. Essure involves the placement of an expanding microcoil of titanium into the proximal uterine tube under hysteroscopic guidance. The efficacy rate at 1 year is 99.8%. Adiana involves hysteroscopically guided superficial radiofrequency damage to the tubal lumen and immediate placement of a nonabsorbable silicone elastomer matrix in the tube to allow tissue in-growth. The efficacy rate at 1 year is 98.9%. Both procedures should have tubal occlusion confirmed at 3 months with a hysterosalpingogram.

▶ When to Refer

Refer to experienced clinicians for Implanon or Nexplanon or other subcutaneous insertion, IUD insertion, tubal occlusion or ligation, vasectomy, or therapeutic abortion.

Lessard CR et al. Efficacy, safety, and patient acceptability of the "Essure" procedure. Patient Prefer Adherence. 2011 Apr 28;5:207–12. [PMID: 21573052]

RAPE

ESSENTIALS OF DIAGNOSIS

▶ Rape is sexual assault. It can be committed by a stranger, but more commonly by an assailant known to the victim, including a current or former partner or spouse (a form of intimate partner violence [IPV]).

▶ Women neither secretly want to be raped nor do they expect, encourage, or enjoy rape.

▶ The large number of individuals affected, the enormous health care costs, and the need for a multidisciplinary approach make rape and IPV important health care issues (see also Chapter 42).

▶ Knowledge of state laws and collection of evidence requirements are essential for clinicians evaluating possible rape victims.

General Considerations

Rape, or sexual assault, is legally defined in different ways in various jurisdictions. Clinicians and emergency department personnel who deal with rape victims should be familiar with the laws pertaining to sexual assault in their own state. From a medical and psychological viewpoint, it is essential that persons treating rape victims recognize the nonconsensual and violent nature of the crime. About 95% of reported rape victims are women. Each year in the United States, 4.8 million incidents of physical or sexual assault are reported by women. Penetration may be vaginal, anal, or oral and may be by the penis, hand, or a foreign object. The absence of genital injury does not imply consent by the victim. The assailant may be unknown to the victim or, more frequently, may be an acquaintance or even the spouse.

"Unlawful sexual intercourse," or statutory rape, is intercourse with a female before the age of majority even with her consent.

Health care providers can have a significant impact in increasing the reporting of sexual assault and in identifying resources for the victims. The International Rescue Committee has developed a multimedia training tool to encourage competent, compassionate, and confidential clinical care for sexual assault survivors in low-resource settings. They studied this intervention in over a 100 healthcare providers, and found knowledge and confidence in clinical care for sexual assault survivors increased from 49% to 62% ($P < 0.001$) and 58% to 73% ($P < 0.001$), respectively following training. There was also a documented increase in eligible survivors receiving emergency contraception from 50% to 82% ($P < 0.01$), HIV postexposure prophylaxis from 42% to 92% ($P < 0.001$), and sexually transmitted infection prophylaxis and treatment from 45% to 96% ($P < 0.01$). This training will encourage providers to offer care in the areas of pregnancy and sexually transmitted infection prevention as well as assistance for psychological trauma.

Because rape is a personal crisis, each patient will react differently, but anxiety disorders and posttraumatic stress disorder (PTSD) are common sequelae. The rape trauma syndrome comprises two principal phases. (1) Immediate or acute: Shaking, sobbing, and restless activity may last from a few days to a few weeks. The patient may experience anger, guilt, or shame or may repress these emotions. Reactions vary depending on the victim's personality and the circumstances of the attack. (2) Late or chronic: Problems related to the attack may develop weeks or months later. The lifestyle and work patterns of the individual may change. Sleep disorders or phobias often develop. Loss of self-esteem can rarely lead to suicide.

Clinicians and emergency department personnel who deal with rape victims should work with community rape crisis centers or other sources of ongoing psychological support and counseling.

General Office Procedures

The clinician who first sees the alleged rape victim should be empathetic and prepared with appropriate evidence collection and treatment materials. Standardized information and training, such as the program created by the

International Rescue Committee, can be a helpful resource to the providers caring for these patients. Many emergency departments have a protocol for sexual assault victims and personnel who are trained in interviewing and examining rape victims.

1. Secure written consent from the patient, guardian, or next of kin for gynecologic examination and for photographs if they are likely to be useful as evidence. Although there are differences in state requirements, most states require health care providers to report sexual assault and physical abuse.

2. Obtain and record the history in the patient's own words. The sequence of events, ie, the time, place, and circumstances, must be included. Note the date of the LMP, whether or not the woman is pregnant, and the time of the most recent coitus prior to the sexual assault. Note the details of the assault such as body cavities penetrated, use of foreign objects, and number of assailants. Note whether the victim is calm, agitated, or confused (drugs or alcohol may be involved). Record whether the patient came directly to the hospital or whether she bathed or changed her clothing. Record findings but do not issue even a tentative diagnosis lest it be erroneous or incomplete.

3. Have the patient disrobe while standing on a white sheet. Hair, dirt, and leaves, underclothing, and any torn or stained clothing should be kept as evidence. Scrape material from beneath fingernails and comb pubic hair for evidence. Place all evidence in separate clean paper bags or envelopes and label carefully.

4. Examine the patient, noting any traumatized areas that should be photographed. Examine the body and genitals with a Wood light to identify semen, which fluoresces; positive areas should be swabbed with a premoistened swab and air-dried in order to identify acid phosphatase. Colposcopy can be used to identify small areas of trauma from forced entry especially at the posterior fourchette.

5. Perform a pelvic examination, explaining all procedures and obtaining the patient's consent before proceeding gently with the examination. Use a narrow speculum lubricated with water only. Collect material with sterile cotton swabs from the vaginal walls and cervix and make two air-dried smears on clean glass slides. Wet and dry swabs of vaginal secretions should be collected and refrigerated for subsequent acid phosphatase and DNA evaluation. Swab the mouth (around molars and cheeks) and anus in the same way, if appropriate. Label all slides carefully. Collect secretions from the vagina, anus, or mouth with a premoistened cotton swab, place at once on a slide with a drop of saline, and cover with a coverslip. Look for motile or nonmotile sperm under high, dry magnification, and record the percentage of motile forms.

6. Perform appropriate laboratory tests as follows. Culture the vagina, anus, or mouth (as appropriate) for *N gonorrhoeae* and *Chlamydia*. Perform a Papanicolaou smear of the cervix, a wet mount for *T vaginalis*, a baseline pregnancy test, and VDRL test. A confidential test for HIV viral load or antibody can be obtained if desired by

the patient. Antibody testing can be repeated in 2–4 months if initially negative. Repeat the pregnancy test if the next menses is missed, and repeat the VDRL test in 6 weeks. Obtain blood (10 mL without anticoagulant) and urine (100 mL) specimens if there is a history of forced ingestion or injection of drugs or alcohol.

7. Transfer clearly labeled evidence, eg, laboratory specimens, directly to the clinical pathologist in charge or to the responsible laboratory technician, in the presence of witnesses (never via messenger), so that the rules of evidence will not be breached.

▶ Treatment

Give analgesics or sedatives if indicated. Administer tetanus toxoid if deep lacerations contain soil or dirt particles.

Give ceftriaxone, 125 mg intramuscularly, to prevent gonorrhea. In addition, give metronidazole, 2 g as a single dose, and azithromycin 1 g orally or doxycycline, 100 mg orally twice daily for 7 days to treat chlamydial infection. Incubating syphilis will probably be prevented by these medications, but the VDRL test should be repeated 6 weeks after the assault.

Prevent pregnancy by using one of the methods discussed under Emergency Contraception, if necessary (see above).

Vaccinate against hepatitis B. Consider HIV prophylaxis (see Chapter 31).

Because women who are sexually assaulted are at increased risk for long-term psychological sequelae, such as PTSD and anxiety disorders, it is critical that the patient and her family and friends have a source of ongoing counseling and psychological support.

▶ When to Refer

All women who seek care for sexual assault should be referred to a facility that has expertise in the management of victims of sexual assault and is capable of performing expert forensic examination, if requested.

Newton M. The forensic aspects of sexual violence. Best Pract Res Clin Obstet Gynaecol. 2013 Feb;27(1):77–90. [PMID: 23062592]

Smith JR et al. Clinical care for sexual assault survivors multimedia training: a mixed-methods study of effect on healthcare providers' attitudes, knowledge, confidence, and practice in humanitarian settings. Confl Health. 2013 Jul 3;7(1):14. [PMID: 23819561]

MENOPAUSAL SYNDROME

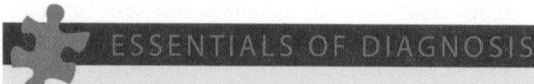

ESSENTIALS OF DIAGNOSIS

▶ Menopause is a retrospective diagnosis after 12 months of amenorrhea.

▶ Approximately 80% of women will experience hot flushes and night sweats.

▶ Elevated follicle-stimulating hormone (FSH) and low estradiol can help confirm the diagnosis.

▶ General Considerations

The term "menopause" denotes the final cessation of menstruation, either as a normal part of aging or as the result of surgical removal of both ovaries. In a broader sense, as the term is commonly used, it denotes a 1- to 3-year period during which a woman adjusts to a diminishing and then absent menstrual flow and the physiologic changes that may be associated with lowered estrogen levels—hot flushes, night sweats, and vaginal dryness.

The average age at menopause in Western societies today is 51 years. Premature menopause is defined as ovarian failure and menstrual cessation before age 40; this often has a genetic or autoimmune basis. Surgical menopause due to bilateral oophorectomy is common and can cause more severe symptoms owing to the sudden rapid drop in sex hormone levels.

There is no objective evidence that cessation of ovarian function is associated with severe emotional disturbance or personality changes. However, mood changes toward depression and anxiety can occur at this time. Disruption of sleep patterns associated with the menopause can affect mood and concentration and cause fatigue. Furthermore, the time of menopause often coincides with other major life changes, such as departure of children from the home, a midlife identity crisis, or divorce.

▶ Clinical Findings

A. Symptoms and Signs

1. Cessation of menstruation—Menstrual cycles generally become irregular as menopause approaches. Anovular cycles occur more often, with irregular cycle length and occasional menorrhagia. Menstrual flow usually diminishes in amount owing to decreased estrogen secretion, resulting in less abundant endometrial growth. Finally, cycles become longer, with missed periods or episodes of spotting only. When no bleeding has occurred for 1 year, the menopausal transition can be said to have occurred. **Any bleeding after this time warrants investigation by endometrial curettage or aspiration to rule out endometrial cancer.**

2. Hot flushes—Hot flushes (feelings of intense heat over the trunk and face, with flushing of the skin and sweating) occur in > 80% of women as a result of the decrease in ovarian hormones. Hot flushes can begin before the cessation of menses. The etiology of hot flushes is unknown. They typically persist for 2 to 3 years, but up to 16% of women aged 67 may continue to experience symptoms. Hot flushes are more severe in women who undergo surgical menopause. Occurring at night, they often cause sweating and insomnia and result in fatigue on the following day.

3. Vaginal atrophy—With decreased estrogen secretion, thinning of the vaginal mucosa and decreased vaginal lubrication occur and may lead to dyspareunia. The introitus decreases in diameter. Pelvic examination reveals pale, smooth vaginal mucosa and a small cervix and uterus. The ovaries are not normally palpable after the menopause. Continued sexual activity will help prevent tissue shrinkage.

4. Osteoporosis—Osteoporosis may occur as a late sequela of menopause.

B. Laboratory Findings

Serum FSH, LH, and estradiol levels are of little diagnostic value because of unpredictable variability during the menopausal transition but can provide confirmation if the FSH is elevated and the estradiol is low. Vaginal cytologic examination will show a low estrogen effect with predominantly parabasal cells, indicating lack of epithelial maturation due to hypoestrogenism.

▶ Treatment

A. Natural Menopause

Education and support from health providers, midlife discussion groups, and reading material will help most women having difficulty adjusting to the menopause. Physiologic symptoms can be treated as follows.

1. Vasomotor symptoms—For women with moderate to severe vasomotor symptoms, estrogen or estrogen/progestin regimens are the most effective approach to symptom relief. Conjugated estrogens, 0.3 mg, 0.45 mg, or 0.625 mg; 17-beta-estradiol, 0.5 or 1 mg; or estrone sulfate, 0.625 mg can be given once daily orally; or estradiol can be given transdermally as skin patches that are changed once or twice weekly and secrete 0.05–0.1 mg of hormone daily. Unless the patient has undergone hysterectomy, a combination regimen of an estrogen with a progestin such as medroxyprogesterone, 1.5 or 2.5 mg, or norethindrone, 0.1, 0.25, or 0.5 mg, should be used to prevent endometrial hyperplasia or cancer. There is also a patch available containing estradiol and the progestin levonorgestrel. The oral hormones can be given in several differing regimens. Give estrogen on days 1–25 of each calendar month, with 5–10 mg of oral medroxyprogesterone acetate added on days 14–25. Withhold hormones from day 26 until the end of the month, when the endometrium will be shed, producing a light, generally painless monthly period. Alternatively, give the estrogen along with a progestin daily, without stopping. This regimen causes some initial bleeding or spotting, but within a few months it produces an atrophic endometrium that will not bleed. If the patient has had a hysterectomy, a progestin need not be used.

Women should not use combination progestin-estrogen therapy for more than 3 or 4 years (see discussion below). Women who cannot find relief with alternative approaches may wish to consider continuing use of combination therapy after a thorough discussion of the risks and benefits. Alternatives to hormone therapy for vasomotor symptoms include SSRIs such as paroxetine, 12.5 mg or 25 mg/d orally, or venlafaxine, 75 mg/d orally. Gabapentin, an antiseizure medication, is also effective at 900 mg/d orally. Clonidine given orally or transdermally, 100–150 mcg daily, may also reduce the frequency of hot flushes, but its use is limited by side effects, including dry mouth, drowsiness, and hypotension. There is some evidence that soy isoflavones may be effective in treating menopausal symptoms. Other compounds including red clover and black cohosh have not been shown to be effective. Because little is known about adverse effects, particularly with long-term use, dietary supplements should be used with caution.

2. Vaginal atrophy—A vaginal ring containing 2 mg of estradiol can be left in place for 3 months and is suitable for long-term use. Short-term use of estrogen vaginal cream will relieve symptoms of atrophy, but because of variable absorption, therapy with either the vaginal ring or systemic hormone replacement is preferable. A low-dose estradiol tablet (10 mcg) is available and is inserted in the vagina daily for 2 weeks and then twice a week for long-term use. Testosterone propionate 1–2%, 0.5–1 g, in a vanishing cream base used in the same manner is also effective if estrogen is contraindicated. A bland lubricant such as unscented cold cream or water-soluble gel can be helpful at the time of coitus.

3. Osteoporosis—(See also discussion in Chapter 26.) Women should ingest at least 800 mg of calcium daily throughout life. Nonfat or low-fat milk products, calcium-fortified orange juice, green leafy vegetables, corn tortillas, and canned sardines or salmon consumed with the bones are good dietary sources. In addition, 1200 mg of elemental calcium should be taken as a daily supplement at the time of the menopause and thereafter; calcium supplements should be taken with meals to increase their absorption. Vitamin D, at least 800 international units/d from food, sunlight, or supplements, is necessary to enhance calcium absorption and maintain bone mass. A daily program of energetic walking and exercise to strengthen the arms and upper body helps maintain bone mass. Screening bone densitometry is recommended for women beginning at age 60 (see Chapter 1). Women most at risk for osteoporotic fractures should consider bisphosphonates, raloxifene, or hormone replacement therapy. This includes white and Asian women, especially if they have a family history of osteoporosis, are thin, short, cigarette smokers, have a history of hyperthyroidism, use corticosteroid medications long-term, or are physically inactive.

B. Risks of Hormone Therapy

Double-blinded randomized, controlled trials have shown no overall cardiovascular benefit with estrogen-progestin replacement therapy in a group of postmenopausal women with or without established coronary disease. Both in the Women's Health Initiative (WHI) trial and the Heart and Estrogen/Progestin Replacement Study (HERS), the overall health risks (increased risk of coronary heart events; strokes; thromboembolic disease; gallstones; and breast cancer, including an increased risk of mortality from breast cancer) exceeded the benefits from the long-term use of combination estrogen and progesterone. An ancillary study of the WHI study showed that not only did estrogen-progestin hormone replacement therapy not benefit cognitive function but there was a small increased risk of cognitive decline in that group compared with women in the placebo group. The unopposed estrogen arm of the WHI trial demonstrated a decrease in the risk of hip fracture, a small but not significant decrease in breast cancer, but an increased risk of stroke and no evidence of protection from coronary heart disease. The study also showed a small increase in the combined risk of mild cognitive impairment and dementia with estrogen use compared with placebo, similar to the estrogen-progestin arm. **Women who have been receiving long-term estrogen-progestin hormone replacement therapy, even in the absence of complications, should be encouraged to stop, especially if they do not have menopausal symptoms.** However, the risks appear to be lower in women starting therapy at the time of menopause and higher in previously untreated women starting therapy long after menopause. Therapy should be individualized as the risk-benefit profile varies with age and individual risk factors. (See also discussions of estrogen and progestin replacement therapy in Chapter 26.)

C. Surgical Menopause

The abrupt hormonal decrease resulting from oophorectomy generally results in severe vasomotor symptoms and rapid onset of dyspareunia and osteoporosis unless treated. If not contraindicated, estrogen replacement is generally started immediately after surgery. Conjugated estrogens 1.25 mg orally, estrone sulfate 1.25 mg orally, or estradiol 2 mg orally is given for 25 days of each month. After age 45–50 years, this dose can be tapered to 0.625 mg of conjugated estrogens or equivalent.

Hodis HN et al. The timing hypothesis for coronary heart disease prevention with hormone therapy: past, present and future in perspective. Climacteric. 2012 Jun;15(3):217–28. [PMID: 22612607]

Taylor HS et al. Update in hormone therapy use in menopause. J Clin Endocrinol Metab. 2011 Feb;96(2):255–64. [PMID: 21296989]

Obstetrics & Obstetric Disorders

Vanessa L. Rogers, MD

Kevin C. Worley, MD

DIAGNOSIS OF PREGNANCY

It is advantageous to diagnose pregnancy as promptly as possible when a sexually active woman misses a menstrual period or has symptoms suggestive of pregnancy. In the event of a desired pregnancy, prenatal care can begin early, and potentially harmful medications and activities such as drug and alcohol use, smoking, and occupational chemical exposure can be halted. In the event of an unwanted pregnancy, counseling about adoption or termination of the pregnancy can be provided at an early stage.

▶ Pregnancy Tests

All urine or blood pregnancy tests rely on the detection of human chorionic gonadotropin (hCG) produced by the placenta. hCG levels increase shortly after implantation, approximately double every 48 hours (this rise can range from 60% to 100% in normal pregnancies), reach a peak at 50–75 days, and fall to lower levels in the second and third trimesters. Laboratory and home pregnancy tests use monoclonal antibodies specific for hCG. These tests are performed on serum or urine and are accurate at the time of the missed period or shortly after it.

Compared with intrauterine pregnancies, **ectopic pregnancies** may show lower levels of hCG that plateau or fall in serial determinations. Quantitative assays of hCG repeated at 48-hour intervals are used in the diagnosis of ectopic pregnancy as well as in cases of molar pregnancy, threatened abortion, and missed abortion. Comparison of hCG levels between laboratories may be misleading in a given patient because different international standards may produce results that vary by as much as twofold. hCG levels can also be problematic because they require a series of measurements. Progesterone levels, however, remain relatively stable in the first trimester. A single measurement of progesterone is the best indicator of whether a pregnancy is viable, although there is a broad indeterminate zone. A value < 5 ng/mL (16 nmol/L) predicts pregnancy failure while a value > 25 ng/mL (80 nmol/L) indicates a pregnancy will be successful. There is uncertainty when the value is between these two points. Combining several serum biomarkers may provide a better prediction of pregnancy viability. **Pregnancy of unknown location** is a term used to describe a situation where a woman has a positive pregnancy test but the location and viability of the pregnancy is not known because nothing is seen on ultrasound.

Kirk E. Ultrasound in the diagnosis of ectopic pregnancy. Clin Obstet Gynecol. 2012 Jun;55(2):395–401. [PMID: 22510620]

▶ Manifestations of Pregnancy

The following symptoms and signs are usually due to pregnancy, but none are diagnostic. A record of the time and frequency of coitus is helpful for diagnosing and dating a pregnancy.

A. Symptoms

Amenorrhea, nausea and vomiting, breast tenderness and tingling, urinary frequency and urgency, "quickening" (perception of first movement noted at about the 18th week), weight gain.

B. Signs (in Weeks from Last Menstrual Period)

Breast changes (enlargement, vascular engorgement, colostrum) start to occur very early in pregnancy and continue until the postpartum period. Cyanosis of the vagina and cervical portio and softening of the cervix occur in about the seventh week. Softening of the cervicouterine junction takes place in the eighth week, and generalized enlargement and diffuse softening of the corpus occurs after the eighth week. When a woman's abdomen will start to enlarge depends on her body habitus but typically starts in the sixteenth week.

The uterine fundus is palpable above the pubic symphysis by 12–15 weeks from the last menstrual period and reaches the umbilicus by 20–22 weeks. Fetal heart tones can be heard by Doppler at 10–12 weeks of gestation.

▶ Differential Diagnosis

The nonpregnant uterus enlarged by myomas can be confused with the gravid uterus, but it is usually very firm and irregular. An ovarian tumor may be found midline, displacing the nonpregnant uterus to the side or posteriorly. Ultrasonography and a pregnancy test will provide accurate diagnosis in these circumstances.

ESSENTIALS OF PRENATAL CARE

The first prenatal visit should occur as early as possible after the diagnosis of pregnancy and should include the following: history, physical examination, laboratory tests, advice to the patient, and tests and procedures.

▶ History

The patient's age, ethnic background, and occupation should be obtained. The onset of the last menstrual period and its normality, possible conception dates, bleeding after the last menstruation, medical history, all prior pregnancies (duration, outcome, and complications), and symptoms of present pregnancy should be documented. The patient's nutritional habits should be discussed with her, as well as any use of caffeine, tobacco, alcohol, or drugs (Table 19–1 and 19–2). Whether there is any family history of congenital anomalies and heritable diseases, a personal history of childhood varicella, prior sexually transmitted diseases (STDs), or risk factors for HIV infection should be determined. The woman should also be asked about domestic violence (see Chapter 42).

▶ Physical Examination

Height, weight, and blood pressure should be measured, and a general physical examination should be done, including a breast examination. Abdominal and pelvic examination should include the following: (1) estimate of uterine size or measure of fundal height; (2) evaluation of bony pelvis for symmetry and adequacy; (3) evaluation of cervix for structural anatomy, infection, effacement, dilation; (4) detection of fetal heart tones by Doppler device after 10 weeks.

Table 19–1. Common drugs that are teratogenic or fetotoxic.[1]

ACE inhibitors	Lithium
Alcohol	Methotrexate
Angiotensin-II receptor blockers	Misoprostol
	NSAIDs (third trimester)
Androgens	Opioids (prolonged use)
Antiepileptics (phenytoin, valproic acid, carbamazepine)	Radioiodine (antithyroid)
	Reserpine
	Ribavirin
Benzodiazepines	Sulfonamides (third trimester)
Carbarsone (amebicide)	SSRIs
Chloramphenicol (third trimester)	Tetracycline (third trimester)
	Thalidomide
Cyclophosphamide	Tobacco smoking
Diazoxide	Trimethoprim (third trimester)
Diethylstilbestrol	Warfarin and other coumarin anticoagulants
Disulfiram	
Ergotamine	
Estrogens	
Griseofulvin	
Isotretinoin	

[1]Many other drugs are also contraindicated during pregnancy. Evaluate any drug for its need versus its potential adverse effects. Further information can be obtained from the manufacturer or from any of several teratogenic registries around the country.
ACE, angiotensin-converting enzyme; NSAIDs, nonsteroidal anti-inflammatory drugs; SSRIs, selective serotonin reuptake inhibitors.

Table 19–2. Drugs and substances that require a careful assessment of risk before they are prescribed for breastfeeding women.

Category of Drug	Specific Drug	Concern
ACE inhibitors	Lisinopril	Unknown effects. Captopril or enalapril is preferred if an agent from this category is needed.
Alkylating agents	Cyclophosphamide	Neonatal neutropenia. No breastfeeding.
Analgesic	Codeine, oxycodone	Cause CNS depression. Unpredictable metabolism.
Antibiotics	Ciprofloxacin	Possible association with adverse effects. Must weigh risks versus benefits.
	Doxycycline	Concern for bone growth and dental staining.
Antiepileptics	Valproic acid	Long-term effects are unknown. Although levels in milk are low, it is teratogenic, so it should be avoided if possible.
Antidepressants	Fluoxetine	Present in breast milk in higher levels than other SSRIs. Watch for adverse effects like an infant's fussiness and crying.
Antihistamine	Diphenhydramine	Present in very small quantities in milk; sources are conflicting with regard to its safety.
Beta-blockers	Atenolol	Has been associated with hypotension and bradycardia in the infant. Metoprolol and propranolol are preferred.
Mood stabilizer	Lithium	Circulating levels in the neonate are variable. Follow infant's serum creatinine and blood urea nitrogen levels, and thyroid function tests.

The above list is not all-inclusive. For additional information, see the below reference from which this information is adapted or the online drug and lactation database, Lactmed, at http://toxnet.nlm.nih.gov/cgi-bin/sis/htmlgen?LACT
ACE, angiotensin-converting enzyme; CNS, central nervous system; SSRIs, selective serotonin reuptake inhibitors.
Data from Rowe H et al. Maternal medication, drug use, and breastfeeding. Pediatr Clin North Am. 2013 Feb;60(1):275–94. [PMID: 23178070]

Laboratory Tests

Urinalysis; culture of a clean-voided midstream urine sample; random blood glucose; complete blood count (CBC) with red cell indices; serologic test for syphilis, rubella antibody titer; varicella immunity; blood group; Rh type; antibody screening for anti-Rh$_o$(D), hepatitis B surface antigen (HBsAg), and the HIV should be performed. Cervical cultures are usually obtained for *Chlamydia trachomatis* and possibly *Neisseria gonorrhoeae*, along with a Papanicolaou smear of the cervix. All black women should have sickle cell screening. Women of African, Asian, or Mediterranean ancestry with anemia or low mean corpuscular volume (MCV) values should have hemoglobin electrophoresis performed to identify abnormal hemoglobins (Hb S, C, F, alpha-thalassemia, beta-thalassemia). Tuberculosis skin testing is indicated for high-risk populations. Fetal aneuploidy screening is available in the first and second trimester and should be offered to all women, ideally before 20 weeks gestation. Noninvasive first trimester screening for Down syndrome includes ultrasonographic nuchal translucency and serum levels of PAPP-A (pregnancy-associated plasma protein A) and the free beta subunit of hCG. In the second trimester, a "quad screen" blood test can be performed; it measures serum alpha-fetoprotein (msAFP), beta-hCG, unconjugated estriol, and inhibin A. First and second trimester tests have similar detection rates. When first and second trimester screening are combined (integrated screening), the detection rates are even higher. For high risk pregnancies, noninvasive testing with cell free fetal DNA from maternal plasma can be performed. It screens only for trisomy 13, 18, and 21. Women at increased risk for aneuploidy can then be offered chorionic villus sampling or genetic amniocentesis, depending on gestational age and availability. Blood screening for Tay-Sachs, Canavan disease, and familial dysautonomia is offered to couples who are of Eastern European Jewish (Ashkenazi) descent. Couples of French-Canadian or Cajun ancestry should also be screened as possible Tay-Sachs carriers. Screening for cystic fibrosis is offered to all pregnant women. Hepatitis C antibody screening should be offered to pregnant women who are at high risk for infection.

Advice to Patients

A. Prenatal Visits

Prenatal care should begin early and maintain a schedule of regular prenatal visits: 4–28 weeks, every 4 weeks; 28–36 weeks, every 2 weeks; 36 weeks on, weekly.

B. Diet

The patient should be counseled to eat a balanced diet containing the major food groups.

1. Prenatal vitamins with iron and folic acid should be prescribed. Supplements that are not specified for pregnant women should be avoided as they may contain dangerous amounts of certain vitamins.

2. The average weight pregnant woman should be expected to gain is 20–40 lb. A pregnant woman should not diet to lose weight during pregnancy, although obese women do seem to benefit from gaining less weight, perhaps 10–15 lb.

3. Caffeine intake should be decreased to 0–1 cup of coffee, tea, or caffeinated cola daily.

4. The patient should be advised to avoid eating raw or rare meat as well as fish known to contain elevated levels of mercury.

5. Patients should be encouraged to eat fresh fruits and vegetables (washed before eating).

C. Medications

Only medications prescribed or authorized by the obstetric provider should be taken.

D. Alcohol and Other Drugs

Patients should be encouraged to abstain from alcohol, tobacco, and all recreational ("street") drugs. No safe level of alcohol intake has been established for pregnancy. Fetal effects are manifest in the **fetal alcohol syndrome**, which includes growth restriction; facial, skeletal, and cardiac abnormalities; and serious central nervous system dysfunction. These effects are thought to result from direct toxicity of ethanol as well as of its metabolites such as acetaldehyde.

Cigarette smoking results in fetal exposure to carbon monoxide and nicotine, and this is thought to eventuate in a number of adverse pregnancy outcomes. An increased risk of abruptio placentae, placenta previa, and premature rupture of the membranes is documented among women who smoke. Preterm delivery, low birth weight, and ectopic pregnancy are also more likely among smokers. Women who smoke should quit smoking or at least reduce the number of cigarettes smoked per day to as few as possible. Clinicians should ask all pregnant women about their smoking history and offer smoking cessation counseling during pregnancy, since women are more motivated to change at this time. Pregnant women should also avoid exposure to environmental smoke ("passive smoking"), and smokeless tobacco, and e-cigarettes

Sometimes compounding the above effects on pregnancy outcome are the independent adverse effects of illicit drugs. Cocaine use in pregnancy is associated with an increased risk of premature rupture of membranes, preterm delivery, placental abruption, intrauterine growth restriction, neurobehavioral deficits, and sudden infant death syndrome. Similar adverse pregnancy effects are associated with amphetamine use, perhaps reflecting the vasoconstrictive potential of both amphetamines and cocaine. Adverse effects associated with opioid use include intrauterine growth restriction, prematurity, and fetal death.

E. Radiographs and Noxious Exposures

Radiographs should be avoided unless essential and approved by a clinician. Abdominal shielding should be used whenever possible. The patient should be told to inform her other clinicians and dentist that she is pregnant.

Chemical or radiation hazards should be avoided as should excessive heat in hot tubs or saunas. Patients should be told to avoid handling cat feces or cat litter and to wear gloves when gardening.

F. Rest and Activity

The patient should be encouraged to obtain adequate rest each day. She should abstain from strenuous physical work or activities, particularly when heavy lifting or weight bearing is required. Regular exercise can be continued at a mild to moderate level; however, exhausting or hazardous exercises or new athletic training programs should be avoided during pregnancy. Exercises that require a great deal of balance should also be done with caution.

G. Birth Classes

The patient should be encouraged to enroll in a childbirth preparation class with her partner well before her due date.

▶ Tests & Procedures

A. Each Visit

Weight, blood pressure, fundal height, and fetal heart rate are measured, and a urine specimen is obtained and tested for protein and glucose. Any concerns the patient may have about pregnancy, health, and nutrition should be addressed.

B. 6–12 Weeks

Confirm uterine size and growth by pelvic examination. Document fetal heart tones (audible at 10–12 weeks of gestation by Doppler). First trimester screening and a discussion of choices of aneuploidy screening should be discussed at this time (see Laboratory Tests, above). If indicated and requested by the patient, chorionic villus sampling can be performed during this period (11–13 weeks).

C. 16–20 Weeks

The "quad screen" and amniocentesis are performed as indicated and requested by the patient during this time (see Laboratory Tests, above). Fetal ultrasound examination to determine pregnancy dating and evaluate fetal anatomy is also done. An earlier examination provides the most accurate dating, and a later examination demonstrates fetal anatomy in greatest detail. The best compromise is at 18–20 weeks of gestation. Cervical length measurement (> 2.5 cm is normal) for prediction of likelihood of preterm birth can also be done at this time.

D. 24 Weeks to Delivery

The patient should be instructed about the symptoms and signs of preterm labor and rupture of membranes. Ultrasound examination is performed as indicated. Typically, fetal size and growth are evaluated when fundal height is 3 cm less than or more than expected for gestational age. In multiple pregnancies, ultrasound should be performed every 4–6 weeks to evaluate for discordant growth.

E. 24–28 Weeks

Screening for gestational diabetes is performed using a 50-g glucose load (Glucola) and a 1-hour post-Glucola blood glucose determination. Abnormal values (≥ 140 mg/dL or 7.8 mmol/L) should be followed up with a 3-hour glucose tolerance test (see Table 19–4).

F. 28 Weeks

If initial antibody screen for anti-$Rh_o(D)$ is negative, repeat antibody testing for Rh-negative patients is performed, but the result is not required before $Rh_o(D)$ immune globulin is administered (see below).

G. 28–32 Weeks

A CBC is done to evaluate for anemia of pregnancy. Screening for syphilis and HIV is also performed at this time. Providers should familiarize themselves with the laws in their state since testing requirements vary.

H. 28 Weeks to Delivery

Fetal position and presentation are determined. The patient is asked about symptoms or signs of preterm labor or rupture of membranes at each visit. Maternal perception of fetal movement should be assessed at each visit. Antepartum fetal testing can be performed as medically indicated.

I. 36 Weeks to Delivery

Repeat syphilis and HIV testing (depending on state laws) and cervical cultures for *N gonorrhoeae* and *C trachomatis* should be performed in at-risk patients. The indicators of onset of labor, admission to the hospital, management of labor and delivery, and options for analgesia and anesthesia should be discussed with the patient. Weekly cervical examinations are not necessary unless indicated to assess a specific clinical situation. Elective delivery (whether by induction or cesarean section) prior to 39 weeks of gestation requires confirmation of fetal lung maturity.

The CDC recommends universal prenatal culture-based screening for group B streptococcal colonization in pregnancy. A single standard culture of the distal vagina and anorectum is collected at 35–37 weeks. No prophylaxis is needed if the screening culture is negative. Patients whose cultures are positive receive intrapartum penicillin prophylaxis during labor. Except when group B streptococci are found in urine, asymptomatic colonization is not to be treated before labor. Patients who have had a previous infant with invasive group B streptococcal disease or who have group B streptococcal bacteriuria during this pregnancy should receive intrapartum prophylaxis regardless, so rectovaginal cultures are not needed. Patients whose cultures at 35–37 weeks were not done or whose results are not known should receive prophylaxis if they have a risk factor for early-onset neonatal disease, including intrapartum temperature ≥ 38°C, membrane rupture > 18 hours, or delivery before 37 weeks gestation.

The routine recommended regimen for prophylaxis is penicillin G, 5 million units intravenously as a loading dose and then 2.5 million units intravenously every 4 hours until delivery. In penicillin-allergic patients not at high risk for anaphylaxis, 2 g of cefazolin can be given intravenously as an initial dose and then 1 g intravenously every 8 hours until delivery. In patients at high risk for anaphylaxis, vancomycin 1 g intravenously every 12 hours until delivery is used or, after confirmed susceptibility testing of group B streptococcal isolate, clindamycin 900 mg intravenously every 8 hours or erythromycin 500 mg intravenously every 6 hours until delivery.

J. 41 Weeks

The patient should have a cervical examination to determine the probability of successful induction of labor. Based on this, induction of labor is undertaken if the cervix is favorable (generally, cervix $\geq$ 2 cm dilated $\geq$ 50% effaced, vertex at −1 station, soft cervix, and midposition); if unfavorable, antepartum fetal testing is begun. Induction is performed at 42 weeks gestation regardless of the cervical examination findings; some providers elect induction at 41 weeks regardless of the cervical examination findings.

Dooley EK et al. Prenatal care: touching the future. Prim Care. 2012 Mar;39(1):17–37. [PMID: 22309579]

O'Neill M et al. Ambulatory obstetric care. Clin Obstet Gynecol. 2012 Sep;55(3):714–21. [PMID: 22828104]

Simpson JL. Cell-free fetal DNA and maternal serum analytes for monitoring embryonic and fetal status. Fertil Steril. 2013 Mar 15;99(4):1124–34. [PMID: 23499003]

NUTRITION IN PREGNANCY

Nutrition in pregnancy can affect maternal health and infant size and well-being. Pregnant women should have nutrition counseling early in prenatal care and access to supplementary food programs if necessary. Counseling should stress abstention from alcohol, smoking, and recreational drugs. Caffeine and artificial sweeteners should be used only in small amounts.

Recommendations regarding weight gain in pregnancy should be based on maternal body mass index (BMI) preconceptionally or at the first prenatal visit. According to the Institute of Medicine guidelines, total weight gain should be 25–35 lbs (11.3–15.9 kg) for normal weight women (BMI of 18.5–24.9) and 15–25 lbs (6.8–11.3 kg) for overweight women. For obese women (BMI of 30 or greater), weight gain should be limited to 11–20 lbs (5.0–9.1 kg). Excessive maternal weight gain has been associated with increased birth weight as well as postpartum retention of weight. Not gaining weight in pregnancy, conversely, has been associated with low birth weight. Nutrition counseling must be tailored to the individual patient.

The increased calcium needs of pregnancy (1200 mg/d) can be met with milk, milk products, green vegetables, soybean products, corn tortillas, and calcium carbonate supplements.

The increased need for iron and folic acid should be met with foods as well as vitamin and mineral supplements. (See Anemia section.) Megavitamins should not be taken in pregnancy, as they may result in fetal malformation or disturbed metabolism. However, a balanced prenatal supplement containing 30–60 mg of elemental iron, 0.5–0.8 mg of folate, and the recommended daily allowances of various vitamins and minerals is widely used in the United States and is probably beneficial to many women with marginal diets. There is evidence that periconceptional folic acid supplements can decrease the risk of neural tube defects in the fetus. For this reason, the United States Public Health Service recommends the consumption of 0.4 mg of folic acid per day for all pregnant and reproductive age women. Women with a prior pregnancy complicated by neural tube defect may require higher supplemental doses as determined by their providers.

American College of Obstetricians and Gynecologists. ACOG Committee opinion no. 548: Weight gain during pregnancy. Obstet Gynecol. 2013 Jan;121(1):210–2. [PMID: 23262962]

Blumfield ML et al. A systematic review and meta-analysis of micronutrient intakes during pregnancy in developed countries. Nutr Rev. 2013 Feb;71(2):118–32. [PMID: 23356639]

Haider BA et al. Multiple-micronutrient supplementation for women during pregnancy. Cochrane Database Syst Rev. 2012 Nov 14;11:CD004905. [PMID: 23152228]

Lassi ZS et al. Folic acid supplementation during pregnancy for maternal health and pregnancy outcomes. Cochrane Database Syst Rev. 2013 Mar 28;3:CD006896. [PMID: 23543547]

PREVENTION OF RHESUS ALLOIMMUNIZATION

The antibody anti-Rh_o(D) causes severe hemolytic disease of the newborn. About 15% of whites and much lower proportions of blacks and Asians are Rh_o(D)–negative. If an Rh_o(D)–negative woman carries an Rh_o(D)–positive fetus, antibodies against Rh_o(D) may develop in the mother when fetal red cells enter her circulation during small fetomaternal bleeding episodes in the early third trimester or during delivery, abortion, ectopic pregnancy, abruptio placentae, or other instances of antepartum bleeding. This antibody, once produced, remains in the woman's circulation and poses the threat of hemolytic disease for subsequent Rh-positive fetuses.

Passive immunization against hemolytic disease of the newborn is achieved with Rh_o(D) immune globulin, a purified concentrate of antibodies against Rh_o(D) antigen. The Rh_o(D) immune globulin (one vial of 300 mcg intramuscularly) is given to the mother within 72 hours after delivery (or spontaneous or induced abortion or ectopic pregnancy). The antibodies in the immune globulin destroy fetal Rh-positive cells so that the mother will not produce anti-Rh_o(D). During her next Rh-positive gestation, erythroblastosis will be prevented. An additional safety measure is the routine administration of the immune globulin at the 28th week of pregnancy. The passive antibody titer that results is too low to significantly affect an Rh-positive fetus. The maternal clearance of the globulin is slow enough that protection will continue for 12 weeks. Once a woman is alloimmunized, Rh_o(D) immune globulin is no longer helpful and should not be given.

Karanth L et al. Anti-D administration after spontaneous miscarriage for preventing Rhesus alloimmunisation. Cochrane Database Syst Rev. 2013 Mar 28;3:CD009617. [PMID: 23543581]

Moise KJ Jret al. Management and prevention of red cell alloimmunization in pregnancy: a systematic review. Obstet Gynecol. 2012 Nov;120(5):1132–9. [PMID: 23090532]

Okwundu CI et al. Intramuscular versus intravenous anti-D for preventing Rhesus alloimmunization during pregnancy. Cochrane Database Syst Rev. 2013 Jan 31;1:CD007885. [PMID: 23440818]

LACTATION

Breastfeeding should be encouraged by education throughout pregnancy and the puerperium. Mothers should be told the benefits of breastfeeding, including infant immunity, emotional satisfaction, mother-infant bonding, and economic savings. The period of amenorrhea associated with frequent and consistent breastfeeding provides some (although not reliable) birth control until menstruation begins at 6–12 months postpartum or the intensity of breastfeeding diminishes. If the mother must return to work, even a brief period of nursing is beneficial. Transfer of immunoglobulins in colostrum and breast milk protects the infant against many systemic and enteric infections. Macrophages and lymphocytes transferred to the infant from breast milk play an immunoprotective role. The intestinal flora of breastfed infants inhibits the growth of pathogens. Breastfed infants have fewer bacterial and viral infections, fewer gastrointestinal tract infections, and fewer allergy problems than bottle-fed infants. Furthermore, they are less apt to be obese as children and adults.

Frequent breastfeeding on an infant-demand schedule enhances milk flow and successful breastfeeding. Mothers breastfeeding for the first time need help and encouragement from providers, nurses, and other nursing mothers. Milk supply can be increased by increased suckling and increased rest.

Nursing mothers should have a fluid intake of over 3 L/d. The United States RDA calls for 21 g of extra protein (over the 44 g/d baseline for an adult woman) and 550 extra kcal/d in the first 6 months of nursing. Calcium intake should be 1200 mg/d. Continuation of a prenatal vitamin and mineral supplement is wise. Strict vegetarians who eschew both milk and eggs should always take vitamin B_{12} supplements during pregnancy and lactation.

1. Effects of Drugs in a Nursing Mother

Drugs taken by a nursing mother may accumulate in milk and be transmitted to the infant (Table 19–2). The amount of drug entering the milk depends on the drug's lipid solubility, mechanism of transport, and degree of ionization.

2. Suppression of Lactation

The simplest and safest method of suppressing lactation after it has started is to gradually transfer the baby to a bottle or a cup over a 3-week period. Milk supply will decrease with decreased demand, and minimal discomfort ensues. If nursing must be stopped abruptly, the mother should avoid nipple stimulation, refrain from expressing milk, and use a snug brassiere. Ice packs and analgesics can be helpful. This same technique can be used in cases where suppression is desired before nursing has begun. Engorgement will gradually recede over a 2- to 3-day period. Hormonal suppression of lactation is no longer practiced.

Johnston M et al. Breastfeeding and the use of human milk. Pediatrics. 2012 Mar;129(3):e827–41. [PMID: 22371471]

Oladapo OT et al. Treatments for suppression of lactation. Cochrane Database Syst Rev. 2012 Sep 12;9:CD005937. [PMID: 22972088]

TRAVEL & IMMUNIZATIONS DURING PREGNANCY

During an otherwise normal low-risk pregnancy, travel can be planned most safely up to the 32nd week. Commercial flying in pressurized cabins does not pose a threat to the fetus. An aisle seat will allow frequent walks. Adequate fluids should be taken during the flight.

It is not advisable to travel to endemic areas of yellow fever in Africa or Latin America; similarly, it is inadvisable to travel to areas of Africa or Asia where chloroquine-resistant falciparum malaria is a hazard, since complications of malaria are more common in pregnancy.

Ideally, all immunizations should precede pregnancy. Live virus products are contraindicated during pregnancy (measles, rubella, yellow fever and smallpox.) Inactivated polio vaccine (IPV) should be given subcutaneously instead of the oral live-attenuated vaccine. The varicella vaccine should be given 1–3 months before becoming pregnant. Vaccines against pneumococcal pneumonia, meningococcal meningitis, and hepatitis A can be used as indicated. Pregnant women who are considered to be at high-risk for hepatitis B and who have not been previously vaccinated should be vaccinated during pregnancy.

Annual influenza vaccination is indicated in all women who are pregnant or will be pregnant during "flu season." It can be given in the first trimester. The CDC lists pregnant women as a high-risk group. In October 2012, the CDC's Advisory Committee on Immunization Practices recommended that every pregnant woman should receive a dose of Tdap during each pregnancy irrespective of her prior vaccination history. The optimal timing for such Tdap administration is between 27 and 36 weeks of gestation, in order to maximize the antibody response of the pregnant woman and the passive antibody transfer to the infant. For any woman who was not previously vaccinated with Tdap and for whom the vaccine was not given during her pregnancy, Tdap should be administered immediately postpartum. Further, any teenagers or adults not previously vaccinated who will have close contact with the infant should also receive it, ideally 2 weeks before exposure to the child. This vaccination strategy is referred to as "cocooning," and its purpose is to protect the infant aged < 12 months who is at particularly high risk for lethal pertussis.

Hepatitis A vaccine contains formalin-inactivated virus and can be given in pregnancy when needed. Pooled immune globulin to prevent hepatitis A is safe and does not carry risk of HIV transmission.

Chloroquine can be used for malaria prophylaxis in pregnancy, and proguanil is also safe.

Water should be purified by boiling, since iodine purification may provide more iodine than is safe during pregnancy.

Prophylactic antibiotics or bismuth subsalicylate should not be used during pregnancy to prevent diarrhea. Oral rehydration and treatment of bacterial diarrhea with erythromycin or ampicillin if necessary is preferred.

Centers for Disease Control and Prevention (CDC). Updated recommendations for use of tetanus toxoid, reduced diphtheria toxoid and acellular pertussis vaccine (Tdap) in pregnant women—Advisory Committee on Immunization Practices (ACIP), 2012. MMWR Morb Mortal Wkly Rep. 2013 Feb 22;62(7):131–5. [PMID: 23425962]

OBSTETRIC COMPLICATIONS OF THE FIRST & SECOND TRIMESTERS

VOMITING OF PREGNANCY (Morning Sickness) & HYPEREMESIS GRAVIDARUM

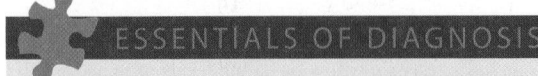

ESSENTIALS OF DIAGNOSIS

▶ Morning or evening nausea and vomiting.

▶ Persistent vomiting severe enough to result in weight loss, dehydration, starvation ketosis, hypochloremic alkalosis, hypokalemia.

▶ May have transient elevation of liver enzymes.

▶ Appears related to high or rising serum hCG.

▶ More common with multiple gestation or hydatidiform mole.

▶ General Considerations

Nausea and vomiting begin soon after the first missed period and cease by the fifth month of gestation. Up to three-fourths of women complain of nausea and vomiting during early pregnancy, with the vast majority noting nausea throughout the day. This problem exerts no adverse effects on the pregnancy and does not presage other complications.

Persistent, severe vomiting during pregnancy—hyperemesis gravidarum—can be disabling and require hospitalization. Thyroid dysfunction can be associated with hyperemesis gravidarum, so it is advisable to determine thyroid-stimulating hormone (TSH) and free thyroxine (FT_4) values in these patients.

▶ Treatment

A. Mild Nausea and Vomiting of Pregnancy

In most instances, only reassurance and dietary advice are required. Because of possible teratogenicity, drugs used during the first half of pregnancy should be restricted to those of major importance to life and health. Antiemetics, antihistamines, and antispasmodics are generally unnecessary to treat nausea of pregnancy. Vitamin B_6 (pyridoxine), 50–100 mg/d orally, is nontoxic and may be helpful in some patients.

B. Hyperemesis Gravidarum

With more severe nausea and vomiting, it may become necessary to hospitalize the patient. In this case, a private room with limited activity is preferred. Give nothing by mouth for 48 hours, and maintain hydration and electrolyte balance by giving appropriate parenteral fluids and vitamin supplements as indicated. Antiemetics such as promethazine (25 mg orally, rectally, or intravenously every 4–6 hours), metoclopramide (10 mg orally or intravenously every 6 hours), or ondansetron (4–8 mg orally or intravenously every 8 hours) should be started. Antiemetics will likely need to be given intravenously initially. Rarely, total parenteral nutrition may become necessary. As soon as possible, place the patient on a dry diet consisting of six small feedings daily plus clear liquids 1 hour after eating. Antiemetics may be continued orally as needed. After in-patient stabilization, the patient can be maintained at home even if she requires intravenous fluids in addition to her oral intake. There are conflicting studies regarding the use of corticosteroids for the control of hyperemesis gravidarum. Therefore, this treatment should be withheld until more accepted treatments have been exhausted.

▶ When to Refer

• Patient is unable to tolerate any food or water.

• There is concern for other pathology (ie, hydatidiform mole).

• Patient requires hospitalization.

▶ When to Admit

• Patient is unable to tolerate any food or water.

• Condition precludes the patient from ingesting necessary medications.

• Weight loss.

• Presence of a hydatidiform mole.

Kashifard M et al. Ondansetrone or metoclopromide? Which is more effective in severe nausea and vomiting of pregnancy? A randomized trial double-blind study. Clin Exp Obstet Gynecol. 2013;40(1):127–30. [PMID: 23724526]

Niebyl JR. Clinical practice. Nausea and vomiting in pregnancy. N Engl J Med. 2010 Oct 14;363(16):1544–50. [PMID: 20942670]

Sonkusare S. The clinical management of hyperemesis gravidarum. Arch Gynecol Obstet. 2011 Jun;283(6):1183–92. [PMID: 21424548]

Tan PC et al. Dextrose saline compared with normal saline rehydration of hyperemesis gravidarum: a randomized controlled trial. Obstet Gynecol. 2013 Feb;121(2 Pt 1):291–8. [PMID: 23232754]

SPONTANEOUS ABORTION

ESSENTIALS OF DIAGNOSIS

- ▶ Intrauterine pregnancy at < 20 weeks.
- ▶ Low or falling levels of hCG.
- ▶ Bleeding, midline cramping pain.
- ▶ Open cervical os.
- ▶ Complete or partial expulsion of products of conception.

▶ General Considerations

About three-fourths of spontaneous abortions occur before the 16th week; of these, three-fourths occur before the eighth week. Almost 20% of all clinically recognized pregnancies terminate in spontaneous abortion.

More than 60% of spontaneous abortions result from chromosomal defects due to maternal or paternal factors; about 15% appear to be associated with maternal trauma, infections, dietary deficiencies, diabetes mellitus, hypothyroidism, the lupus anticoagulant-anticardiolipin-antiphospholipid antibody syndrome, or anatomic malformations. There is no reliable evidence that abortion may be induced by psychic stimuli such as severe fright, grief, anger, or anxiety. In about one-fourth of cases, the cause of abortion cannot be determined. There is no evidence that video display terminals or associated electromagnetic fields are related to an increased risk of spontaneous abortion.

It is important to distinguish women with a history of incompetent cervix from those with more typical early abortion. Characteristically, incompetent cervix presents as "silent" cervical dilation (ie, with minimal uterine contractions) in the second trimester. Women with incompetent cervix often present with significant cervical dilation (2 cm or more) and minimal symptoms. When the cervix reaches 4 cm or more, active uterine contractions or rupture of the membranes may occur secondary to the degree of cervical dilation. This does not change the primary diagnosis. Factors that predispose to incompetent cervix are a history of incompetent cervix with a previous pregnancy, cervical conization or surgery, cervical injury, diethylstilbestrol (DES) exposure, and anatomic abnormalities of the cervix. Prior to pregnancy or during the first trimester, there are no methods for determining whether the cervix will eventually be incompetent. After 14–16 weeks, ultrasound may be used to evaluate the internal anatomy of the lower uterine segment and cervix for the funneling and shortening abnormalities consistent with cervical incompetence.

▶ Clinical Findings

A. Symptoms and Signs

1. Threatened abortion—Bleeding or cramping occurs, but the pregnancy continues. The cervix is not dilated.

2. Inevitable abortion—The cervix is dilated and the membranes may be ruptured, but passage of the products of conception has not yet occurred. Bleeding and cramping persist, and passage of the products of conception is considered inevitable.

3. Complete abortion—Products of conception are completely expelled. Pain ceases, but spotting may persist. Cervical os is closed.

4. Incomplete abortion—The cervix is dilated. Some portion of the products of conception (usually placental) remains in the uterus. Only mild cramps are reported, but bleeding is persistent and often excessive.

5. Missed abortion—The pregnancy has ceased to develop, but the conceptus has not been expelled. Symptoms of pregnancy disappear. There may be a brownish vaginal discharge but no active bleeding. Pain does not develop. The cervix is semifirm and slightly patulous; the uterus becomes smaller and irregularly softened; the adnexa are normal.

B. Laboratory Findings

Pregnancy tests show low or falling levels of hCG. A CBC should be obtained if bleeding is heavy. Determine Rh type, and give Rh$_o$ (D) immune globulin if Rh-negative. All tissue recovered should be assessed by a pathologist and may be sent for genetic analysis in selected cases.

C. Ultrasonographic Findings

The gestational sac can be identified at 5–6 weeks from the last menstruation, a fetal pole at 6 weeks, and fetal cardiac activity at 6–7 weeks by transvaginal ultrasound. Serial observations are often required to evaluate changes in size of the embryo. A small, irregular sac without a fetal pole with accurate dating is diagnostic of an abnormal pregnancy.

▶ Differential Diagnosis

The bleeding that occurs in abortion of a uterine pregnancy must be differentiated from the abnormal bleeding of an ectopic pregnancy and anovular bleeding in a non-pregnant woman. The passage of hydropic villi in the bloody discharge is diagnostic of hydatidiform mole.

▶ Treatment

A. General Measures

1. Threatened abortion—The patient should be placed on bed rest for 24–48 hours followed by gradual resumption of usual activities, with abstinence from coitus and douching. Hormonal treatment is contraindicated. Antibiotics should be used only if there are signs of infection.

2. Missed abortion—This calls for counseling regarding the fate of the pregnancy and planning for its elective termination at a time chosen by the patient and clinician. Insertion of laminaria to dilate the cervix followed by aspiration has historically been the method of choice for a missed abortion. Medically induced first-trimester termination with prostaglandins (ie, misoprostol given vaginally or orally in a dose of 200–800 mcg) combined with an antiprogesterone (ie, mifepristone 600 mg orally) has grown in popularity because it has been shown to be safe, effective, less invasive, and more private. If it is unsuccessful or if there is excessive bleeding, a surgical procedure may still be needed. Patients must be counseled about the different therapeutic options with a thorough explanation of all risks and benefits.

B. Surgical Measures

1. Incomplete or inevitable abortion—Prompt removal of any products of conception remaining within the uterus is required to stop bleeding and prevent infection. Analgesia and a paracervical block are useful, followed by uterine exploration with ovum forceps or uterine aspiration. Regional anesthesia may be required.

2. Cerclage and restriction of activities—A cerclage is the treatment of choice for incompetent cervix, but a viable intrauterine pregnancy should be confirmed prior to placement of the cerclage.

A variety of suture materials including a 5-mm Mersilene tape or No. 2 nonabsorbable monofilament suture can be used to create a purse-string type of stitch around the cervix, using either the McDonald or Shirodkar method. Cerclage should be undertaken with caution when there is advanced cervical dilation or when the membranes are prolapsed into the vagina. Rupture of the membranes and infection are specific contraindications to cerclage. Cervical cultures for *N gonorrhoeae, C trachomatis*, and group B streptococci should be obtained before elective placement of a cerclage. *N gonorrhoeae* and *C trachomatis* should be treated before placement.

▶ When to Refer

- Patient with history of two second-trimester losses.
- Vaginal bleeding in a pregnant patient that resembles menstruation in a nonpregnant woman.
- Patient with an open cervical os.
- No signs of uterine growth in serial examinations of a pregnant patient.
- Leakage of amniotic fluid.

▶ When to Admit

- Open cervical os.
- Heavy vaginal bleeding.
- Leakage of amniotic fluid.

Brix N et al; CERVO group. Randomised trial of cervical cerclage, with and without occlusion, for the prevention of preterm birth in women suspected for cervical insufficiency. BJOG. 2013 Apr;120(5):613–20. [PMID: 23331924]

Martonffy AI et al. First trimester complications. Prim Care. 2012 Mar;39(1):71–82. [PMID: 22309582]

Neilson JP et al. Medical treatments for incomplete miscarriage. Cochrane Database Syst Rev. 2013 Mar 28;3:CD007223. [PMID: 23543549]

RECURRENT (Habitual) ABORTION

Recurrent abortion has been defined as the loss of three or more previable (< 20 weeks gestation or 500 g) pregnancies in succession. Recurrent abortion occurs in about 1% of all couples. Abnormalities related to recurrent abortion can be identified in approximately half of these instances. If a woman has lost three previous pregnancies without identifiable cause, she still has at least a 65% chance of carrying a fetus to viability.

Recurrent abortion is a clinical rather than pathologic diagnosis. The clinical findings are similar to those observed in other types of abortion (see above).

▶ Treatment

A. Preconception Therapy

Preconception therapy is aimed at detection of maternal or paternal defects that may contribute to abortion. A thorough history and examination is essential. A random blood glucose test and thyroid function studies (including thyroid antibodies) can be done if history indicates a possible predisposition to diabetes mellitus or thyroid disease. Detection of lupus anticoagulant and other hemostatic abnormalities (proteins S and C and antithrombin deficiency, hyperhomocysteinemia, anticardiolipin antibody, factor V Leiden mutations) and an antinuclear antibody test may be indicated. Hysteroscopy or hysterography can be used to exclude submucosal myomas and congenital anomalies of the uterus. In women with recurrent losses, resection of a uterine septum, if present, has been recommended. Chromosomal (karyotype) analysis of both partners can be done to rule out balanced translocations (found in 5% of infertile couples), but karyotyping is expensive and may not be helpful.

Many therapies have been tried to prevent recurrent pregnancy loss from immunologic causes. Low-molecular-weight heparin (LMWH), aspirin, intravenous immunoglobulin, and corticosteroids have all been used but the definitive treatment has not yet been determined. Prophylactic dose heparin and low-dose aspirin have been recommended for women with antiphospholipid antibodies and recurrent pregnancy loss.

B. Postconception Therapy

The patient should be provided early prenatal care and scheduled frequent office visits. Bed rest is justified only for bleeding or pain. Empiric sex steroid hormone therapy is contraindicated.

Prognosis

The prognosis is excellent if the cause of abortion can be corrected or treated.

American College of Obstetricians and Gynecologists. Practice Bulletin No. 132: Antiphospholipid syndrome. Obstet Gynecol. 2012 Dec;120(6):1514–21. [PMID: 23168789]

Branch DW et al. Clinical practice. Recurrent miscarriage. N Engl J Med. 2010 Oct;363(18):1740–7. [PMID: 20979474]

Practice Committee of American Society for Reproductive Medicine. Definitions of infertility and recurrent pregnancy loss: a committee opinion. Fertil Steril. 2013 Jan;99(1):63. [PMID: 23095139]

ECTOPIC PREGNANCY

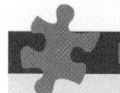

ESSENTIALS OF DIAGNOSIS

▶ Amenorrhea or irregular bleeding and spotting.

▶ Pelvic pain, usually adnexal.

▶ Adnexal mass by clinical examination or ultrasound.

▶ Failure of serum level of beta-hCG to double *every 48 hours.*

▶ No intrauterine pregnancy on transvaginal ultrasound with serum beta-hCG > 2000 mU/mL.

General Considerations

Ectopic implantation occurs in about one out of 150 live births. About 98% of ectopic pregnancies are tubal. Other sites of ectopic implantation are the peritoneum or abdominal viscera, the ovary, and the cervix. Any condition that prevents or retards migration of the fertilized ovum to the uterus can predispose to an ectopic pregnancy, including a history of infertility, pelvic inflammatory disease, ruptured appendix, and prior tubal surgery. Combined intrauterine and extrauterine pregnancy (heterotopic) may occur rarely. In the United States, undiagnosed or undetected ectopic pregnancy is one of the most common causes of maternal death during the first trimester.

Clinical Findings

A. Symptoms and Signs

Severe lower quadrant pain occurs in almost every case. It is sudden in onset, stabbing, intermittent, and does not radiate. Backache may be present during attacks. Shock occurs in about 10%, often after pelvic examination. At least two-thirds of patients give a history of abnormal menstruation; many have been infertile.

Blood may leak from the tubal ampulla over a period of days, and considerable blood may accumulate in the peritoneum. Slight but persistent vaginal spotting is usually reported, and a pelvic mass may be palpated. Abdominal distention and mild paralytic ileus are often present.

B. Laboratory Findings

The CBC may show anemia and slight leukocytosis. Quantitative serum pregnancy tests will show levels generally lower than expected for normal pregnancies of the same duration. If beta-hCG levels are followed over a few days, there may be a slow rise or a plateau rather than the near doubling every 2 days associated with normal early intrauterine pregnancy or the falling levels that occur with spontaneous abortion. A progesterone level can also be measured to assess the viability of the pregnancy.

C. Imaging

Ultrasonography can reliably demonstrate a gestational sac 5–6 weeks from the last menstruation and a fetal pole at 6 weeks if located in the uterus. An empty uterine cavity raises a strong suspicion of extrauterine pregnancy, which can occasionally be revealed by transvaginal ultrasound. Specified levels of serum beta-hCG have been reliably correlated with ultrasound findings of an intrauterine pregnancy. For example, a beta-hCG level of 6500 mU/mL with an empty uterine cavity by transabdominal ultrasound is highly suspicious for an ectopic pregnancy. Similarly, a beta-hCG value of 2000 mU/mL or more can be indicative of an ectopic pregnancy if no products of conception are detected within the uterine cavity by transvaginal ultrasound. Serum beta-hCG values can vary by laboratory.

D. Special Examinations

With the advent of high-resolution transvaginal ultrasound, culdocentesis is rarely used in evaluation of possible ectopic pregnancy. Laparoscopy is the surgical procedure of choice both to confirm an ectopic pregnancy and in most cases to permit removal of the ectopic pregnancy without the need for exploratory laparotomy.

Differential Diagnosis

Clinical and laboratory findings suggestive or diagnostic of pregnancy will distinguish ectopic pregnancy from many acute abdominal illnesses such as acute appendicitis, acute pelvic inflammatory disease, ruptured corpus luteum cyst or ovarian follicle, and urinary calculi. Uterine enlargement with clinical findings similar to those found in ectopic pregnancy is also characteristic of an aborting uterine pregnancy or hydatidiform mole. Ectopic pregnancy should be suspected when postabortal tissue examination fails to reveal chorionic villi. Steps must be taken for immediate diagnosis, including prompt microscopic tissue examination, ultrasonography, and serial beta-hCG titers every 48 hours.

Treatment

Patients must be warned about the complications of an ectopic pregnancy and monitored closely. In a stable patient, methotrexate (50 mg/m²) intramuscularly—given as single or multiple doses—is acceptable medical therapy for early ectopic pregnancy. Favorable criteria are that the pregnancy should be < 3.5 cm in largest dimension and unruptured, with no active bleeding and no fetal heart tones.

When a patient with an ectopic pregnancy is unstable or when surgical therapy is planned, the patient is hospitalized. Blood is typed and cross-matched. Ideally, diagnosis and operative treatment should precede frank rupture of the tube and intra-abdominal hemorrhage. The use of methotrexate in an unstable patient is absolutely contraindicated.

Surgical treatment is definitive. In most patients, diagnostic laparoscopy is the initial surgical procedure performed. Depending on the size of the ectopic pregnancy and whether or not it has ruptured, salpingostomy with removal of the ectopic or a partial or complete salpingectomy can usually be performed. Clinical conditions permitting, patency of the contralateral tube can be established by injection of indigo carmine into the uterine cavity and flow through the contralateral tube confirmed visually by the surgeon; iron therapy for anemia may be necessary during convalescence. Rh$_o$(D) immune globulin (300 mcg) should be given to Rh-negative patients.

▶ Prognosis

Repeat tubal pregnancy occurs in about 10% of cases. This should not be regarded as a contraindication to future pregnancy, but the patient requires careful observation and early ultrasound confirmation of an intrauterine pregnancy.

▶ When to Refer

- Severe abdominal pain.
- Palpation of an adnexal mass on pelvic examination.
- Abdominal pain and vaginal bleeding in a pregnant patient.

▶ When to Admit

- Presence of symptoms or signs of a ruptured ectopic pregnancy.

Crochet JR et al. Does this woman have an ectopic pregnancy?: the rational clinical examination systematic review. JAMA. 2013 Apr 24;309(16):1722–9. [PMID: 23613077]

Lisscomb GH. Medical management of ectopic pregnancy. Clin Obstet Gynecol. 2012 Jun;55(2):424–32. [PMID: 22510624]

Torpy JM et al. JAMA patient page. Ectopic pregnancy. JAMA. 2012 Aug 22;308(8):829. [PMID: 22910764]

van Mello NM et al. Diagnostic value of serum hCG on the outcome of pregnancy of unknown location: a systematic review and meta-analysis. Hum Reprod Update. 2012 Nov-Dec;18(6):603–17. [PMID: 22956411]

van Mello NM et al. Ectopic pregnancy: how the diagnostic and therapeutic management has changed. Fertil Steril. 2012 Nov;98(5):1066–73. [PMID: 23084008]

GESTATIONAL TROPHOBLASTIC DISEASE (Hydatidiform Mole & Choriocarcinoma)

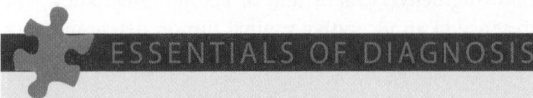

ESSENTIALS OF DIAGNOSIS

Hydatidiform Mole

- ▶ Amenorrhea.
- ▶ Irregular uterine bleeding.
- ▶ Serum beta-hCG > 40,000 mU/mL.
- ▶ Passage of grapelike clusters of enlarged edematous villi per vagina.
- ▶ Ultrasound of uterus shows characteristic heterogeneous echogenic image and no fetus or placenta.
- ▶ Cytogenetic composition is 46, XX (85%), completely of paternal origin.

Choriocarcinoma

- ▶ Persistence of detectable beta-hCG after mole evacuation.

▶ General Considerations

Gestational trophoblastic disease is a spectrum of disorders that includes hydatidiform mole (partial and complete), invasive mole (local extension into the uterus or vagina), choriocarcinoma (malignancy often complicated by distant metastases), and placental site trophoblastic tumor. Complete moles show no evidence of a fetus on ultrasonography. The majority are 46, XX with all chromosomes of paternal origin. Partial moles generally show evidence of an embryo or gestational sac; are triploid, slower-growing, and less symptomatic; and often present clinically as a missed abortion. Partial moles tend to follow a benign course, while complete moles have a greater tendency to become choriocarcinomas.

In the United States, the frequency of gestational trophoblastic disease is 1:1500 pregnancies. The highest rates occur in Asians. Risk factors include prior spontaneous abortion, a history of mole, and age younger than 21 or older than 35. Approximately 10% of women require further treatment after evacuation of the mole; choriocarcinoma develops in 2–3% of women.

▶ Clinical Findings

A. Symptoms and Signs

Uterine bleeding, beginning at 6–16 weeks, is observed in most instances. In some cases, the uterus is larger than would be expected in a normal pregnancy of the same duration. Excessive nausea and vomiting may occur. Bilaterally enlarged cystic ovaries are sometimes palpable. They are the result of ovarian hyperstimulation due to excess beta-hCG.

Preeclampsia-eclampsia may develop during the second trimester of an untreated molar pregnancy, but this is unusual because most are diagnosed early.

Choriocarcinoma may be manifested by continued or recurrent uterine bleeding after evacuation of a mole or following delivery, abortion, or ectopic pregnancy. The presence of an ulcerative vaginal tumor, pelvic mass, or distant metastases may be the presenting manifestation.

B. Laboratory Findings

Hydatidiform moles are generally characterized by high serum beta-hCG values, which can range from high normal to the millions. Levels are higher with complete moles than with partial moles. Serum beta-hCG values, if extremely high, can assist in making the diagnosis, but they are more helpful in managing response to treatment. Hematocrit, creatinine, blood type, liver function tests, and thyroid function tests should also be measured. High beta-hCG levels can cause the release of thyroid hormone, and rarely, symptoms of hyperthyroidism. Patients with hyperthyroidism may require beta-blocker therapy until the mole has been evacuated.

C. Imaging

Ultrasound has virtually replaced all other means of preoperative diagnosis of hydatidiform mole. Placental vesicles can be easily seen on transvaginal ultrasound. A preoperative chest film is indicated to rule out pulmonary metastases of the trophoblast.

▶ Treatment

A. Specific (Surgical) Measures

The uterus should be emptied as soon as the diagnosis of hydatidiform mole is established, preferably by suction curettage. Ovarian cysts should not be resected nor ovaries removed; spontaneous regression of theca lutein cysts will occur with elimination of the mole. The products of conception removed from the uterus should be sent to a pathologist for review. In patients who have completed their childbearing, hysterectomy is an acceptable alternative. Hysterectomy does not preclude the need for follow-up of beta-hCG levels.

B. Follow-Up Measures

Weekly quantitative beta-hCG level measurements are initially required. Following successful surgical evacuation, moles show a progressive decline in beta-hCG. After three negative weekly tests (< 5 mU/mL), the interval may be increased to every 1–3 months for an additional 6 months. The purpose of this follow-up is to identify persistent metastatic and nonmetastatic disease, including choriocarcinoma, which is more likely to occur if the initial beta-hCG is high and the uterus is large. If levels plateau or begin to rise, the patient should be evaluated by repeat laboratory tests, chest film, and dilatation and curettage (D&C) before the initiation of chemotherapy. Effective contraception (preferably birth control pills) should be prescribed to avoid the hazard and confusion of elevated beta-hCG from a new pregnancy. The beta-hCG levels should be negative for 6 months before pregnancy is attempted again. Because the risk of recurrence of a molar pregnancy is 1%, an ultrasound should be performed in

the first trimester of the pregnancy following a mole to ensure that the pregnancy is normal. In addition, a beta-hCG level should then be checked 6 weeks postpartum (after the subsequent normal pregnancy) to ensure there is no persistent trophoblastic tissue, and the placenta should be examined by a pathologist.

C. Antitumor Chemotherapy

If malignant tissue is discovered at surgery or during the follow-up examination, chemotherapy is indicated. For low-risk patients with a good prognosis, methotrexate is considered first-line therapy followed by actinomycin (see Table 39–11). Patients with a poor prognosis should be referred to a cancer center, where multiple-agent chemotherapy probably will be given.

▶ Prognosis

Five-year survival after courses of chemotherapy, even when metastases have been demonstrated, can be expected in at least 85% of cases of choriocarcinoma.

▶ When to Refer

- Uterine size exceeds that anticipated for gestational age.
- Vaginal bleeding similar to menstruation.
- Pregnant patient with a history of a molar pregnancy.

▶ When to Admit

- Confirmed molar pregnancy by ultrasound and laboratory studies.
- Heavy vaginal bleeding in a pregnant patient under evaluation.

Deng L et al. Combination chemotherapy for primary treatment of high-risk gestational trophoblastic tumour. Cochrane Database Syst Rev. 2013 Jan 31;1:CD005196. [PMID: 23440800]

Lurain JR. Gestational trophoblastic disease I: epidemiology, pathology, clinical presentation and diagnosis of gestational trophoblastic disease, and management of hydatidiform mole. Am J Obstet Gynecol. 2010 Dec;203(6):531–9. [PMID: 20728069]

Seckl MJ et al. Gestational trophoblastic disease. Lancet. 2010 Aug 28;376(9742):717–29. [PMID: 20673583]

OBSTETRIC COMPLICATIONS OF THE SECOND & THIRD TRIMESTERS

PREECLAMPSIA-ECLAMPSIA

 ESSENTIALS OF DIAGNOSIS

Preeclampsia

▶ Blood pressure of ≥ 140 mm Hg systolic or ≥ 90 mm Hg diastolic after 20 weeks of gestation.

▶ Proteinuria of ≥ 0.3 g in 24 hours.

Severe Preeclampsia (one or more of below)

▶ Blood pressure of ≥ 160 mm Hg systolic or ≥ 110 mm Hg diastolic.

▶ Progressive renal insufficiency.

▶ Thrombocytopenia.

▶ Hemolysis, elevated liver enzymes, low platelets (HELLP).

▶ Pulmonary edema.

▶ Vision changes or headache.

Eclampsia

▶ Seizures in a patient with evidence of preeclampsia.

▶ **General Considerations**

Preeclampsia is defined as the presence of newly elevated blood pressure and proteinuria during pregnancy. Eclampsia is diagnosed when seizures develop in a patient with evidence of preeclampsia. Historically, the presence of three elements was required for the diagnosis of preeclampsia: hypertension, proteinuria, and edema. Edema was difficult to objectively quantify and is no longer a required element.

Preeclampsia-eclampsia can occur any time after 20 weeks of gestation and up to 6 weeks postpartum. It is a disease unique to pregnancy, with the only cure being delivery of the fetus and placenta. Preeclampsia-eclampsia develops in approximately 7% of pregnant women in the United States. Primiparas are most frequently affected; however, the incidence of preeclampsia-eclampsia is increased with multiple gestation pregnancies, chronic hypertension, diabetes mellitus, kidney disease, collagen-vascular and autoimmune disorders, and gestational trophoblastic disease. Five percent of women with preeclampsia progress to eclampsia. Uncontrolled eclampsia is a significant cause of maternal death. The cause of preeclampsia-eclampsia is not known.

▶ **Clinical Findings**

Clinically, the severity of preeclampsia-eclampsia can be measured with reference to the six major sites in which it exerts its effects: the central nervous system, the kidneys, the liver, the hematologic system, the vascular system, and the fetal-placental unit. By evaluating each of these areas for the presence of mild to severe preeclampsia, the degree of involvement can be assessed, and an appropriate management plan can be formulated that balances the severity of disease and gestational age (Table 19–3).

A. Preeclampsia

1. Mild—Patients usually have few complaints, and the diastolic blood pressure is < 110 mm Hg. Edema may be present. The platelet count is over 100,000/mcL, antepartum fetal testing is reassuring, central nervous system irritability is minimal, epigastric pain is not present, and liver enzymes are not elevated.

Table 19–3. Indicators of mild to moderate versus severe preeclampsia-eclampsia.

Site	Indicator	Mild to Moderate	Severe
Central nervous system	Symptoms and signs	Hyperreflexia	Seizures
			Blurred vision
			Scotomas
			Headache
			Clonus
			Irritability
Kidney	Proteinuria	0.3–5 g/24 h	> 5 g/24 h or catheterized urine with 4⁺ protein
	Urinary output	> 30 mL/h	< 30 mL/h
Liver	AST, ALT, LD	Normal liver enzymes	Elevated liver enzymes
			Epigastric pain
			Ruptured liver
Hematologic	Platelets		< 100,000/mcL
	Hemoglobin	Normal	Elevated
Vascular	Blood pressure	< 160/110 mm Hg	> 160/110 mm Hg
	Retina	Arteriolar spasm	Retinal hemorrhages
Fetal-placental unit	Growth restriction	Absent	Present
	Oligohydramnios	Absent	Present
	Fetal distress	Absent	Present

ALT, alanine aminotransferase; AST, aspartate aminotransferase; LD, lactate dehydrogenase.

2. Severe—Symptoms are more dramatic and persistent. Patients may complain of headache and changes in vision. The blood pressure is often quite high, with readings at or above 160/110 mm Hg. Thrombocytopenia (platelet counts < 100,000/mcL) may be present and progress to disseminated intravascular coagulation. Severe epigastric pain may be present from hepatic subcapsular hemorrhage with significant stretch or rupture of the liver capsule. HELLP syndrome (hemolysis, elevated liver enzymes, low platelets) is a form of severe preeclampsia.

B. Eclampsia

The occurrence of seizures defines eclampsia. It is a manifestation of severe central nervous system involvement. Other findings of preeclampsia are observed.

▶ Differential Diagnosis

Preeclampsia-eclampsia can mimic and be confused with many other diseases, including chronic hypertension, chronic kidney disease, primary seizure disorders, gallbladder and pancreatic disease, immune thrombocytopenia, thrombotic thrombocytopenic purpura, and hemolytic-uremic syndrome. It must always be considered, possible in any pregnant woman beyond 20 weeks of gestation. It is particularly difficult to diagnose when a preexisting disease such as hypertension is present.

▶ Treatment

In clinical studies, diuretics, dietary restriction or enhancement, sodium restriction, and vitamin-mineral supplements (eg, calcium or vitamin C and E) have not been confirmed to be useful. The only cure is delivery of the fetus at a time as favorable as possible for its survival.

A. Preeclampsia

Early recognition is the key to treatment. This requires careful attention to the details of prenatal care—especially subtle changes in blood pressure and weight. The objectives are to prolong pregnancy if possible, to allow fetal lung maturity while preventing progression to severe disease and eclampsia. The critical factors are the gestational age of the fetus, fetal pulmonary maturity, and the severity of maternal disease. Preeclampsia-eclampsia at term is managed by delivery. Prior to term, severe preeclampsia-eclampsia requires delivery with very few exceptions. Epigastric pain, severe range blood pressures, thrombocytopenia, and visual disturbances are strong indications for delivery of the fetus. Marked proteinuria alone can be managed more conservatively.

For mild preeclampsia, modified bed rest is the cornerstone of therapy. This increases central blood flow to the kidneys, heart, brain, liver, and placenta and may stabilize or even improve the degree of preeclampsia-eclampsia for a period of time.

Modified bed rest may be attempted at home or in the hospital. The goal is not to keep the woman in bed continuously but rather to limit her activity. Prior to making this decision, the clinician should evaluate the six sites of involvement listed in Table 19–3 and make an assessment about the severity of disease.

1. Home management—Home management with modified bed rest may be attempted for patients with mild preeclampsia and a stable home situation. This requires assistance at home, rapid access to the hospital, a reliable patient, and the ability to obtain frequent blood pressure readings. A home health nurse can often provide frequent home visits and assessments.

2. Hospital care—Hospitalization is required for women with severe preeclampsia or those with unreliable home situations. Regular assessments of blood pressure, urine protein, and fetal heart tones and activity are required. A CBC with platelet count, electrolyte panel, and liver enzymes should be checked regularly, with frequency dependent on severity. A 24-hour urine collection for total protein and creatinine clearance should be obtained on admission and repeated as indicated. Magnesium sulfate is not used until the diagnosis of severe preeclampsia is made and delivery planned (see Eclampsia, below).

Fetal evaluation should be obtained as part of the workup. If the patient is being admitted to the hospital, fetal testing should be performed on the same day to assess fetal wellbeing. This may be done by fetal heart rate testing with nonstress testing or by biophysical profile. A regular schedule of fetal surveillance must then be followed. Daily fetal kick counts can be recorded by the patient herself. If the fetus is < 34 weeks gestation, corticosteroids (betamethasone 12 mg intramuscularly every 24 h for two doses, or dexamethasone 6 mg intramuscularly every 12 h for four doses) can be administered to the mother. *However, when a woman is clearly suffering from unstable severe preeclampsia, delivery should not be delayed for fetal lung maturation or administration of corticosteroids.*

The method of delivery is determined by the maternal and fetal status. A vaginal delivery is preferred because it has less blood loss than a cesarean section and requires less coagulation factors. Cesarean section is reserved for the usual fetal indications. For mild preeclampsia, delivery should take place at term.

B. Eclampsia

1. Emergency care—If the patient is convulsing, she is turned on her side to prevent aspiration and to improve blood flow to the placenta. The seizure may be stopped by giving an intravenous bolus of either magnesium sulfate, 4–6 g, or lorazepam, 2–4 mg over 4 minutes or until the seizure stops. Magnesium sulfate is the preferred agent, and alternatives should only be used if magnesium sulfate is unavailable. A continuous intravenous infusion of magnesium sulfate is then started at a rate of 2–3 g/h unless the patient is known to have significantly reduced kidney function. Magnesium blood levels are then checked every 4–6 hours and the infusion rate adjusted to maintain a therapeutic blood level (4–6 mEq/L). Urinary output is checked hourly and the patient assessed for signs of possible magnesium toxicity such as loss of deep tendon reflexes or decrease in respiratory rate and depth, which can be reversed with calcium gluconate, 1 g intravenously over 2 minutes.

2. General care—In patients with severe preeclampsia, magnesium sulfate should be given intravenously, 4- to 6-g load over 15–20 minutes followed by 2–3 g/h maintenance, for seizure prophylaxis. The occurrence of eclampsia necessitates delivery once the patient is stabilized. It is important, however, that assessment of the status of the patient and fetus take place first. Continuous fetal monitoring must be performed and maternal blood typed and cross-matched quickly. A urinary catheter is inserted to monitor urinary output, and a CBC with platelets, electrolytes, creatinine, and liver enzymes are obtained. If hypertension is present with systolic values of $\geq$ 160 mm Hg or diastolic values $\geq$ 110 mm Hg, antihypertensive medications should be administered to reduce the blood pressure to 140–150/ 90–100 mm Hg. Lower blood pressures than this may induce placental insufficiency through reduced perfusion. Hydralazine given in 5- to 10-mg increments intravenously every 20 minutes is frequently used to lower blood pressure. Labetalol, 10–20 mg intravenously, every 20 minutes as needed, can also be used.

3. Delivery—Delivery is mandated once eclampsia has occurred. Vaginal delivery is preferred. The rapidity with which delivery must be achieved depends on the fetal and maternal status following the seizure and the availability of laboratory data on the patient. Oxytocin, given intravenously and titrated to a dose that results in adequate contractions, may be used to induce or augment labor. Oxytocin should only be administered by a clinician specifically trained in its use. Regional analgesia or general anesthesia is acceptable. Cesarean section is used for the usual obstetric indications.

4. Postpartum—Magnesium sulfate infusion (2–3 g/h) should be continued for 24 hours postpartum. Late-onset preeclampsia-eclampsia can occur during the postpartum period. It is usually manifested by either hypertension or seizures. Treatment is the same as prior to delivery—ie, with hydralazine and magnesium sulfate.

When to Refer

- New onset of hypertension and proteinuria in a pregnant patient > 20 weeks' gestation.
- New onset of seizure activity in a pregnant patient.
- Symptoms of severe preeclampsia in a pregnant patient with elevated blood pressure above baseline.

When to Admit

- Evidence of severe preeclampsia or eclampsia.
- Evaluation for preeclampsia when severe disease is suspected.
- Evaluation for preeclampsia in a patient with an unstable home environment.

Abildgaard U et al. Pathogenesis of the syndrome of hemolysis, elevated liver enzymes, and low platelet count (HELLP): a review. Eur J Obstet Gynecol Reprod Biol. 2013 Feb;166(2): 117–23. [PMID: 23107053]

American College of Obstetricians and Gynecologists et al. Hypertension in pregnancy. Report of the American College of Obstetricians and Gynecologists' Task Force on Hypertension in Pregnancy. Obstet Gynecol. 2013 Nov;122(5): 1122–31. [PMID: 24150027]

Repke JT. What is new in preeclampsia?: best articles from the past year. Obstet Gynecol. 2013 Mar;121(3):682–3. [PMID: 23635633]

ACUTE FATTY LIVER OF PREGNANCY

Acute fatty liver of pregnancy is a disorder limited to the gravid state. It occurs in the third trimester of pregnancy and involves acute hepatic failure. With improved recognition and immediate delivery, the mortality rate is now 7–23%. The disorder is usually seen after the 35th week of gestation and is more common in primigravidas and those with twins. The incidence is about 1:14,000 deliveries.

The cause of acute fatty liver of pregnancy is just now being elucidated, and it likely is the result of poor placental mitochondrial function. Many cases may be due to a homozygous fetal deficiency of long-chain acyl coenzyme A dehydrogenase (LCHAD).

▶ Clinical Findings

Pathologic findings are unique to the disorder, with fatty engorgement of hepatocytes. Clinical onset is gradual, with flu-like symptoms that progress to the development of abdominal pain, jaundice, encephalopathy, disseminated intravascular coagulation, and death. On examination, the patient shows signs of hepatic failure.

Laboratory findings include marked elevation of alkaline phosphatase but only moderate elevations of alanine aminotransferase (ALT) and aspartate aminotransferase (AST). Prothrombin time and bilirubin are also elevated. The white blood cell count is elevated, and the platelet count is depressed. Hypoglycemia may be extreme.

▶ Differential Diagnosis

The differential diagnosis is that of fulminant hepatitis. However, liver aminotransferases for fulminant hepatitis are higher (> 1000 units/mL) than those for acute fatty liver of pregnancy (usually 500–1000 units/mL). It is also important to review the appropriate history and perform the appropriate tests for toxins that cause liver failure. Preeclampsia may involve the liver but typically does not cause jaundice. The elevations in liver function tests in patients with preeclampsia usually do not reach the levels seen in patients with acute fatty liver of pregnancy.

▶ Treatment

Diagnosis of acute fatty liver of pregnancy mandates immediate delivery. Supportive care during labor includes administration of glucose, platelets, and fresh frozen plasma as needed. Vaginal delivery is preferred. Resolution of encephalopathy occurs over days, and supportive care with a low-protein diet is needed.

Prognosis

Recurrence rates for this liver disorder are unclear but probably increased in families with proven LCHAD deficiency. Most authorities advise against subsequent pregnancy, but there have been reported cases of successful outcomes in later pregnancies.

Pan C et al. Pregnancy-related liver diseases. Clin Liver Dis. 2011 Feb;15(1):199–208. [PMID: 21112001]

PRETERM LABOR

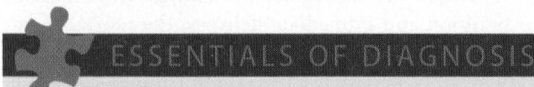

ESSENTIALS OF DIAGNOSIS

▶ Preterm regular uterine contractions approximately 5 minutes apart.

▶ Cervical dilatation, effacement, or both.

General Considerations

Preterm birth is defined as delivery prior to 37 weeks gestation, and spontaneous preterm labor with or without premature rupture of the fetal membranes is responsible for at least two-thirds of all preterm births. Prematurity is the largest single contributor to infant mortality. Recognized risk factors for spontaneous preterm labor include a past history of spontaneous preterm delivery, premature rupture of the membranes, multiple gestation, black race, intrauterine infections, müllerian anomalies, smoking, substance abuse, bacterial vaginosis, and certain socioeconomic conditions (such as limited access to prenatal care). It has also been consistently demonstrated that women with a shortened cervical length as measured by transvaginal ultrasound in the midtrimester are at increased risk for spontaneous preterm delivery.

Clinical Findings

In women with regular uterine contractions and cervical change, the diagnosis of preterm labor is straightforward. However, symptoms such as pelvic pressure, cramping, or vaginal discharge may be the first complaints in high-risk patients who later develop preterm labor. Because these complaints may be vague and irregular uterine contractions are common, distinguishing which patients merit further evaluation can be problematic. In some cases, this distinction can be facilitated by the use of fetal fibronectin measurement in cervicovaginal specimens. This test is most useful when it is negative (< 50 ng/mL), since the negative predictive value for delivery within 7–14 days is 93–97%. A negative test, therefore, usually means the patient can be reassured and discharged home. Because of its low sensitivity, however, fetal fibronectin is not recommended as a screening test in asymptomatic women.

Treatment

Patients must be educated to identify symptoms associated with preterm labor to avoid unnecessary delay in their evaluation. In patients who are believed to be at increased risk for preterm delivery, limited activity and bed rest continue to be recommended frequently despite the fact that randomized trials have failed to demonstrate improved outcomes in women placed on activity restriction. In addition, and paradoxically, such recommendations may place a woman at an *increased* risk to deliver preterm.

In pregnancies between 24 and 34 weeks gestation where preterm birth is anticipated, a single short course of corticosteroids should be administered to promote fetal lung maturity. Such therapy has been demonstrated to reduce the frequency of respiratory distress syndrome, intracranial hemorrhage, and even death in preterm infants. Betamethasone, 12 mg intramuscularly repeated once 24 hours later, or dexamethasone, 6 mg intramuscularly repeated every 12 hours for four doses, both cross the placenta and are the preferred treatments in this setting. Repeat courses are not recommended. Although antibiotics have not been proven to forestall delivery, women in preterm labor should receive antimicrobial prophylaxis against group B streptococcus (see above).

Numerous pharmacologic agents—tocolytics—have been given in an attempt to forestall preterm birth, although none are completely effective, and there is no evidence that such therapy directly improves neonatal outcomes. Administering tocolytic agents, however, remains a reasonable approach to the initial management of preterm labor and may provide sufficient prolongation of pregnancy to administer a course of corticosteroids and (if appropriate) transport the patient to a facility better equipped to care for preterm infants. Maintenance therapy (continuation of treatment beyond 48 hours) is not effective at preventing preterm birth and is not recommended. Likewise, despite the finding that preterm labor is associated with intrauterine infection in certain cases, there is no evidence that antibiotics forestall delivery in women with preterm labor and intact membranes.

Magnesium sulfate is commonly used, and there is evidence that it may also be protective against cerebral palsy in infants whose mothers were receiving magnesium infusions at time of birth. Magnesium sulfate is given intravenously as a 4- to 6-g bolus followed by a continuous infusion of 2 g/h. Magnesium levels are not typically checked but should be monitored if there is any concern for toxicity. Magnesium sulfate is entirely cleared by the kidney and must, therefore, be used with caution in women with any degree of renal insufficiency.

Beta-adrenergic drugs such as **terbutaline** have also been used. Terbutaline can be given as an intravenous infusion starting at 2.5 mcg/min or as a subcutaneous injection starting at 250 mcg given every 30 minutes. Oral terbutaline is no longer recommended because of the lack of proven efficacy and concerns about maternal safety. Serious maternal side effects have been reported with the use of terbutaline and include tachycardia, pulmonary edema, arrhythmias, metabolic derangements (such as hyperglycemia and hypokalemia), and even death. Pulmonary edema occurs with increased frequency with concomitant administration of corticosteroids, large volume intravenous fluid infusion, maternal sepsis, or prolonged tocolysis. Because of these safety concerns, the US Food and Drug Administration issued a warning recommendation that terbutaline be administered exclusively in a hospital setting and discontinued after 48–72 hours of treatment.

Nifedipine, 20 mg orally every 6 hours, and **indomethacin**, 50 mg orally once then 25 mg orally every 6 hours up to 48 hours, have also been used with limited success. Nifedipine should not be given in conjunction with magnesium sulfate.

Before attempts are made to prevent preterm delivery with tocolytic agents, the patient should be assessed for conditions in which delivery would be indicated. Severe preeclampsia, lethal fetal anomalies, placental abruption, and intrauterine infection are all examples of indications for preterm delivery. In such cases, attempts to forestall delivery would be inappropriate.

▶ **Preterm Birth Prevention**

Strategies aimed at preventing preterm birth in high-risk women—principally those with a history of preterm birth or a shortened cervix (or both)—have focused on the administration of progesterone or progesterone compounds. Prospective randomized controlled trials have demonstrated reductions in rates of preterm birth in high-risk women with singleton pregnancies who received progesterone supplementation, although the optimal preparation, dose, and route of administration (intramuscular injection versus vaginal suppository) are unclear. Further, progesterone therapy has not been proven to be effective in nulliparous women who are noted to have a shortened cervix by transvaginal ultrasound, and universal screening of cervical length is controversial.

There is also evidence that women with a previous spontaneous preterm birth and a shortened cervix (< 25 mm before 24 weeks gestation) may benefit from placement of a cervical cerclage. The use of cervical cerclage in conjunction with progesterone supplementation has not been adequately studied. In twin pregnancies, however, neither progesterone administration nor cervical cerclage placement has been effective at prolonging pregnancy, suggesting that the mechanism for preterm birth may be different in multiple gestations.

▶ **When to Refer**

- Symptoms of increased pelvic pressure or cramping in high-risk patients.
- Regular uterine contractions.
- Rupture of membranes.
- Vaginal bleeding.

▶ **When to Admit**

- Cervical dilation of ≥ 2 cm prior to 34 weeks gestation.
- Contractions that cause cervical change.
- Rupture of membranes.

American College of Obstetricians and Gynecologists. ACOG Practice Bulletin No. 127: Management of preterm labor. Obstet Gynecol. 2012 Jun;119(6):1308–17. [PMID: 22617615]

American College of Obstetricians and Gynecologists. ACOG Practice Bulletin No. 130: Prediction and prevention of preterm birth. Obstet Gynecol. 2012 Oct;120(4):964–73. [PMID: 22996126]

Berghella V et al. Cerclage for short cervix on ultrasonography in women with singleton gestations and previous preterm birth: a meta-analysis. Obstet Gynecol. 2011 Mar;117(3):663–71. [PMID: 21446209]

Grobman WA et al. Activity restriction among women with a short cervix. Obstet Gynecol. 2013 Jun;121(6):1181–6. [PMID: 23812450]

Grobman WA et al. 17 alpha-hydroxyprogesterone caproate to prevent prematurity in nulliparas with cervical length less than 30 mm. Am J Obstet Gynecol. 2012 Nov;207(5):390.e1–8. [PMID: 23010094]

Hassan SS et al. Vaginal progesterone reduces the rate of preterm birth in women with a sonographic short cervix: a multicenter, randomized, double-blind, placebo-controlled trial. Ultrasound Obstet Gynecol. 2011 Jul;38(1):18–31. [PMID: 21472815]

THIRD-TRIMESTER BLEEDING

Five to 10 percent of women have vaginal bleeding in late pregnancy. The clinician must distinguish between placental causes (placenta previa, placental abruption, vasa previa) and nonplacental causes (labor, infection, disorders of the lower genital tract, systemic disease). The approach to bleeding in late pregnancy generally should be conservative and expectant unless fetal distress or excessive maternal hemorrhage occurs.

▶ **Treatment**

A. General Measures

The patient should be hospitalized and placed on bed rest. Initially, continuous fetal monitoring is indicated to assess for fetal distress. CBC platelets, and prothrombin time (INR) should be obtained and repeated serially if the bleeding continues. If the hemorrhage is significant, the need for blood replacement should be anticipated and two to four units of red cells typed and cross-matched, and repeat CBC and coagulation studies ordered as clinically indicated. Ultrasound examination should be performed to determine placental location. Digital pelvic examinations are done only after ultrasound examination has ruled out placenta previa.

B. Placenta Previa

Placenta previa occurs when the placenta implants over the internal cervical os. Risk factors for this condition include previous cesarean delivery, increasing maternal age, multiparity, and smoking. If the diagnosis is initially made in the first or second trimester, the ultrasound should be repeated in the third trimester. Persistence of placenta previa at this point is an indication for cesarean as the route of delivery. Painless vaginal bleeding is the characteristic symptom in placenta previa and can range from light spotting to profuse hemorrhage.

Hospitalization for extended evaluation is the appropriate initial management approach. For pregnancies that have reached 37 weeks gestation or beyond with continued bleeding, delivery is generally indicated. Pregnancies at 36 weeks or earlier are candidates for expectant management provided the bleeding is not prodigious, and a subset of these women can be discharged if the bleeding and contractions completely subside.

C. Placenta Accreta

Placenta accreta is the general term used to describe an abnormally adherent placenta that has invaded into or beyond the endometrium. Invasion extending into the myometrium is formally termed "placenta increta" and invasion beyond the uterine serosa, "placenta percreta." Placenta accreta most commonly occurs in association with placenta previa in women who have had one more previous cesarean deliveries. After delivery of the infant, the placenta does not separate normally. The bleeding that results can be torrential, and emergency hysterectomy is usually required to stop the hemorrhage. Because of the considerable increase in both maternal morbidity and mortality associated with this condition, careful preoperative planning is imperative when the diagnosis is suspected antenatally. Ultrasound findings such as intraplacental lacunae, bridging vessels into the bladder, and loss of the retroplacental clear space suggest placental invasion in women who have placenta previa. Ideally, delivery planning should involve a multidisciplinary team, and the surgery should take place at an institution with appropriate personnel and a blood bank equipped to handle patients requiring massive transfusion.

D. Placental Abruption

Placental abruption is the premature separation of the placenta from its implantation site before delivery. Hypertension is a known risk factor for abruption. Other risk factors include multiparity, cocaine use, smoking, previous abruption, and thrombophilias. Classic symptoms are vaginal bleeding, uterine tenderness, and frequent contractions, but the clinical presentation is highly variable. Profound coagulopathy and acute hypovolemia from blood loss can occur and are more likely with an abruption severe enough to kill the fetus. Ultrasound may be helpful to exclude placenta previa, but failure to identify a retroplacental clot does not exclude abruption. In most cases, abruption is an indication for immediate delivery because of the high risk of fetal death.

American College of Obstetricians and Gynecologists. Committee Opinion No. 529: Placenta accreta. Obstet Gynecol. 2012 Jul;120(1):207–11. [PMID: 22914422]
Eller AG et al. Maternal morbidity in cases of placenta accreta managed by a multidisciplinary care team compared with standard obstetric care. Obstet Gynecol. 2011 Feb;117(2 Pt 1):331–7. [PMID: 21309195]

OBSTETRIC COMPLICATIONS OF THE PERIPARTUM PERIOD

PUERPERAL MASTITIS
(See also Chapters 17 and 42)

Postpartum mastitis occurs sporadically in nursing mothers, usually with symptom onset after discharge from the hospital, or it may occur in epidemic form in the hospital. *Staphylococcus aureus* is usually the causative agent. Inflammation is generally unilateral, and women nursing for the first time are more often affected. Rarely, inflammatory carcinoma of the breast can be mistaken for puerperal mastitis.

Mastitis frequently begins within 3 months after delivery and may start with an engorged breast and a sore or fissured nipple. Cellulitis is usually obvious in the affected area of breast with redness, tenderness, and local warmth. Fever and chills are common complaints as well. Treatment consists of antibiotics effective against penicillin-resistant staphylococci (dicloxacillin 500 mg orally every 6 hours or a cephalosporin for 10–14 days) and regular emptying of the breast by nursing or by using a mechanical suction device. Although nursing of the infected breast is safe for the infant, local inflammation of the nipple may complicate latching. Failure to respond to usual antibiotics within 3 days may represent an organizing abscess or infection with a resistant organism. When the causative organism is methicillin-resistant *S aureus* (MRSA), the risk for abscess formation is increased when compared with infection caused by nonresistant staphylococcal species. If an abscess is suspected, ultrasound of the breast can help confirm the diagnosis. In these cases, aspiration or surgical evacuation is usually required.

Dixon JM et al. Treatment of breast infection. BMJ. 2011 Feb 11;342:d396. [PMID: 21317199]
Lee IW et al. Puerperal mastitis requiring hospitalization during a nine-year period. Am J Obstet Gynecol. 2010 Oct;203(4):332. e1–6. [PMID: 20599181]

CHORIOAMNIONITIS & METRITIS

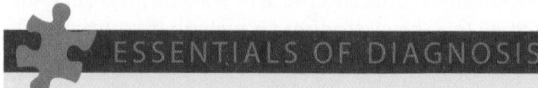

ESSENTIALS OF DIAGNOSIS

► Fever not attributable to another source.
► Uterine tenderness.
► Foul smelling vaginal discharge.
► Tachycardia in the mother, fetus, or both.

► General Considerations

Pelvic infections are relatively common problems encountered during the peripartum period. Uterine infections diagnosed during pregnancy are referred to as chorioamnionitis—a generalized infection of all of the contents of the gravid uterus. Uterine infection after delivery is often called endometritis or endomyometritis, but the term "metritis" is probably most accurate to emphasize that the infection extends throughout the uterine tissue. These infections are polymicrobial and are most commonly attributed to urogenital pathogens. Risk factors include cesarean delivery, prolonged labor, use of internal monitors, nulliparity, multiple pelvic examinations, prolonged rupture of membranes, and lower genital tract infections. Although maternal complications such as dysfunctional labor and postpartum hemorrhage are increased with clinical chorioamnionitis, the principal reason to initiate treatment is to prevent morbidity in the offspring. Neonatal complications such as sepsis, pneumonia, intraventricular hemorrhage, and cerebral palsy are increased in the setting of chorioamnionitis. Intrapartum initiation of antibiotics, however, significantly reduces neonatal morbidity.

► Clinical Findings

Clinical chorioamnionitis and metritis are diagnosed by the presence of fever (≥ 38°C) in the absence of any other source and one or more of the following signs: maternal tachycardia, fetal tachycardia, foul-smelling lochia, and uterine tenderness. Cultures are typically not done because of the polymicrobial nature of the infection.

► Treatment

Treatment is empiric with broad-spectrum antibiotics that will cover gram-positive and gram-negative organisms if still pregnant and gram-negative organisms and anaerobes if postpartum. A common regimen for chorioamnionitis is ampicillin, 2 g intravenously every 6 hours, and gentamicin, 2 mg/kg intravenous load then 1.5 mg/kg intravenously every 8 hours. A common regimen for metritis is gentamicin, 2 mg/kg intravenous load then 1.5 mg/kg intravenously every 8 hours, and clindamycin, 900 mg intravenously every 8 hours. Antibiotics are stopped in the mother when she has been afebrile for 24 hours. No oral antibiotics are subsequently needed. Patients with metritis who do not respond in the first 24–48 hours may have enterococcus and require additional gram-positive coverage (such as ampicillin) to the regimen.

Martinelli P et al. Chorioamnionitis and prematurity: a critical review. J Matern Fetal Neonatal Med. 2012 Oct;25(Suppl 4): 29–31. [PMID: 22958008]

MEDICAL CONDITIONS COMPLICATING PREGNANCY

ANEMIA

Normal pregnancy is characterized by an increase in maternal plasma volume of about 50% and in increase in red cell volume of about 25%. Because of these changes, the mean hemoglobin and hematocrit values are lower than in the nonpregnant state. Anemia in pregnancy is considered when the hemoglobin measurement is below 11 g/dL. Symptoms such as fatigue and dyspnea that would otherwise suggest the presence of anemia in nonpregnant women are common in pregnant women; therefore, periodic measurement of CBCs in pregnancy is essential so that anemia can be identified and treated.

A. Iron Deficiency Anemia

The increased requirement for iron over the course of pregnancy is appreciable in order to support fetal growth and expansion of maternal blood volume. Dietary intake of iron is generally insufficient to meet this demand, and it is recommended that all pregnant women receive about 30 mg of elemental iron per day in the second and third trimesters. Oral iron therapy is commonly associated with gastrointestinal side effects, such as nausea and constipation, and these symptoms often contribute to noncompliance. If supplementation is inadequate, however, anemia often becomes evident by the third trimester of pregnancy. Because iron deficiency is by far the most common cause of anemia in pregnancy, treatment is usually empiric and consists of 60–100 mg of elemental iron per day and a diet containing iron-rich foods. Iron studies can confirm the diagnosis if necessary (see Chapter 13), and further evaluation should be considered in patients who do not respond to oral iron. Intermittent iron supplementation (eg, every other day) has been associated with fewer side effects and may be reasonable for women who cannot tolerate daily therapy.

B. Folic Acid Deficiency Anemia

Megaloblastic anemia in pregnancy is almost always caused by folic acid deficiency, since vitamin B_{12} deficiency is extremely uncommon in the childbearing years.

The diagnosis is made by finding macrocytic red cells and hypersegmented neutrophils on a blood smear (see Chapter 13). However, blood smears in pregnancy may be difficult to interpret, since they frequently show iron deficiency changes as well. With established folate deficiency, a supplemental dose of 1 mg/d and a diet with increased folic acid is generally sufficient to correct the anemia.

C. Sickle Cell Anemia

Women with sickle cell anemia are subject to serious complications in pregnancy. The anemia becomes more severe, and acute pain crises often occur more frequently. When compared with women who do not have hemoglobinopathies, women with hemoglobin SS are at increased risk for infections (especially pulmonary and urinary tract), thromboembolic events, pregnancy-related hypertension, transfusion, cesarean delivery, preterm birth, and fetal growth restriction. There also continues to be an increased rate of maternal mortality, despite an increased recognition of the high-risk nature of these pregnancies. Intensive medical treatment may improve the outcomes for both mother and fetus. Prophylactically transfusing packed red cells to lower the level of hemoglobin S and elevate the level of hemoglobin A is a controversial practice without clear benefit. Most women with sickle cell disease will not require iron supplementation, but folate requirements can be appreciable due to red cell turnover from hemolysis. Management decisions should be made in conjunction with a maternal fetal medicine specialist and a hematologist.

Genetic counseling should be offered to patients with sickle cell disease or sickle trait (hemoglobin AS). If the father is a carrier of the sickle cell gene (or his status is unknown), the parents may wish to undergo prenatal diagnosis to determine whether the fetus is affected.

Contraceptive counseling postpartum is important, although the safest and most effective method in women with sickle cell disease is unclear. Progestin-only compounds may be ideal because progesterone has long been recognized to help prevent pain crises in some women. Intrauterine devices carry a risk of infection and combination oral contraceptives are a concern because of the thrombogenic potential; these forms of contraception have not been adequately studied in these patients.

Women with hemoglobin SC disease are also at increased risk for complications, but the morbidity does not appear to be as great as in women with SS disease. Women with either SC or SS disease are managed similarly. Women with sickle cell trait alone usually have an uncomplicated pregnancy course except for an increased risk of urinary tract infection.

American College of Obstetricians and Gynecologists. ACOG Practice Bulletin No. 95: Anemia in pregnancy. Obstet Gynecol. 2008 Jul;112(1):201–7. [PMID: 18591330]

Howard J et al. The obstetric management of sickle cell disease. Best Pract Res Clin Obstet Gynaecol. 2012 Feb;26(1):25–36. [PMID: 22113135]

Lassi ZS et al. Folic acid supplementation during pregnancy for maternal health and pregnancy outcomes. Cochrane Database Syst Rev. 2013 Mar 28;3:CD006896. [PMID: 23543547]

Peña-Rosas JP et al. Intermittent oral iron supplementation during pregnancy. Cochrane Database Syst Rev. 2012 Jul 11;7:CD009997. [PMID: 22786531]

ANTIPHOSPHOLIPID SYNDROME

(See also Chapter 20.)

The antiphospholipid syndrome (APS) is characterized by the presence of specific autoantibodies in association with certain clinical conditions, most notably arterial and venous thrombosis and adverse pregnancy outcomes. Clinically, the diagnosis can be suspected after any of the following outcomes: an episode of thrombosis, three or more unexplained consecutive spontaneous abortions prior to 10 weeks gestation, one or more unexplained deaths of a morphologically normal fetus after 10 weeks gestation, or a preterm delivery at less than 34 weeks due to preeclampsia or placental insufficiency. In addition to these clinical features, laboratory criteria include the identification of at least one of the following antiphospholipid antibodies: the lupus anticoagulant, anticardiolipin antibodies, or anti-beta-2-glycoprotein I antibodies. The lupus anticoagulant cannot be directly assayed, but it is tested for in several different phospholipid-dependent clotting tests and is interpreted as either present or absent.

Anticardiolipin antibodies may be detected with enzyme-linked immunosorbent assay (ELISA) testing but should only be considered diagnostic when the IgG or IgM isotypes are present in medium to high titer (40 GPL or MPL, respectively). Likewise, anti-beta-2-glycoprotein I antibodies are detected with ELISA but should only be considered positive when they are present in a titer that is greater than 99th percentile for a normal population. The diagnosis of APS requires two positive antiphospholipid antibody test results at least 12 weeks apart since transient positive results can occur.

Treatment for APS in pregnancy generally involves administration of a heparin compound and low-dose aspirin (81 mg). In women with recurrent pregnancy loss and APS, it has been demonstrated that unfractionated heparin and low-dose aspirin can reduce the risk for spontaneous abortion. Outside of the first trimester, heparin is generally continued through pregnancy and the early postpartum period for thromboprophylaxis. LMWH is also commonly used for this indication; however, it is not clear that LMWH has the same effect on reducing the risk of recurrent abortion as unfractionated heparin. Either prophylactic or therapeutic dosing strategies may be appropriate depending on the patient's history and clinical risk factors. Infusions of intravenous immunoglobulin are of unclear benefit in these patients, and this treatment is not recommended.

ACOG Committee on Practice Bulletins—Obstetrics. ACOG Practice Bulletin No. 132: Antiphospholipid syndrome. Obstet Gynecol. 2012 Dec;120(6):1514–21. [PMID: 23168789]

Oku K et al. Pathophysiology of thrombosis and pregnancy morbidity in the antiphospholipid syndrome. Eur J Clin Invest. 2012 Oct;42(10):1126–35. [PMID: 22784367]

Ziakas PD et al. Heparin treatment in antiphospholipid syndrome with recurrent pregnancy loss: a systematic review and meta-analysis. Obstet Gynecol. 2010 Jun;115(6):1256–62. [PMID: 20502298]

THYROID DISEASE

Thyroid disease is relatively common in pregnancy, and in their overt states, both hypothyroidism and hyperthyroidism have been consistently associated with adverse pregnancy outcomes. Fortunately, these risks are mitigated by adequate treatment. It is essential to understand the gestational age-specific effects that pregnancy has on thyroid function tests, since these biochemical markers are required to make the diagnosis of thyroid dysfunction. Failure to recognize these physiologic alterations can result in misclassification or misdiagnosis. Women who have a history of a thyroid disorder or symptoms that suggest thyroid dysfunction should be screened with thyroid function tests. Screening asymptomatic pregnant women, however, is controversial and not currently recommended by the American College of Obstetricians and Gynecologists.

Overt hypothyroidism is defined by an elevated serum TSH level with a depressed FT_4 level. The condition in pregnancy has consistently been associated with an increase in complications such as spontaneous abortion, preterm birth, preeclampsia, placental abruption, and impaired neuropsychological development in the offspring. The most common etiology is Hashimoto (autoimmune) thyroiditis. Many of the symptoms of hypothyroidism mimic those of normal pregnancy, making its clinical identification difficult. Initial treatment is empiric with levothyroxine started at 75–100 mcg/d. Thyroid function tests can be repeated at 4–6 weeks and the dose adjusted as necessary with the goal of normalizing the TSH level (preferably to a trimester-specific gestational reference range). An increase in the dose of levothyroxine may be required in the second and third trimesters.

Subclinical hypothyroidism is defined as an increased serum TSH and a normal FT_4 level. Although some adverse pregnancy outcomes (such as miscarriage and preeclampsia) have been associated with subclinical hypothyroidism, these findings have been inconsistent in the literature. There remains insufficient data at this time to recommend screening for or treating subclinical hypothyroidism in pregnancy.

Overt hyperthyroidism, defined as excessive production of thyroxine with a depressed (usually undetectable) serum TSH level, is also associated with increased risks in pregnancy. Spontaneous abortion, preterm birth, preeclampsia, and maternal heart failure occur with increased frequency with untreated thyrotoxicosis. Thyroid storm, although rare, can be a life-threatening complication. Medical treatment of thyrotoxicosis is usually accomplished with the antithyroid drugs propylthiouracil or methimazole. Although teratogenicity has not been clearly established, in utero exposure to methimazole has been associated with aplasia cutis and choanal and esophageal atresia in the offspring of pregnancies so treated. Propylthiouracil is not believed to be teratogenic, but it has been associated with the rare complications of hepatotoxicity and agranulocytosis. Recommendations by the American Thyroid Association are to treat with propylthiouracil in the first trimester and convert to methimazole for the remainder of the pregnancy. The therapeutic target for the FT_4 level is the upper limit of the normal reference range. The TSH levels generally stay suppressed even with adequate treatment. A beta-blocker can be used for such symptoms as palpitations or tremors. Fetal hypothyroidism or hyperthyroidism is uncommon but can occur with maternal Graves disease, which is the most common cause of hyperthyroidism in pregnancy. Radioiodine ablation is absolutely contraindicated in pregnancy because it may destroy the fetal thyroid as well.

Transient autoimmune thyroiditis can occur in the postpartum period and is evident within the first year after delivery. The first phase, occurring up to 4 months postpartum, is a hyperthyroid state. Over the next few months, there is a transition to a hypothyroid state, which may require treatment with levothyroxine. Spontaneous resolution to a euthyroid state within the first year is the expected course; however, some women remain hypothyroid beyond this time (see Chapter 26).

Budenhofer BK et al. Thyroid (dys-)function in normal and disturbed pregnancy. Arch Gynecol Obstet. 2013 Jan;287(1): 1–7. [PMID: 23104052]

Casey BM. Subclinical thyroid dysfunction during pregnancy. Clin Obstet Gynecol. 2011 Sep;54(3):493–8. [PMID: 21857180]

Stagnaro-Green A et al. Guidelines of the American Thyroid Association for the diagnosis and management of thyroid disease during pregnancy and postpartum. Thyroid. 2011 Oct;21(10):1081–125. [PMID: 21787128]

Stagnaro-Green A et al. Thyroid disorders in pregnancy. Nat Rev Endocrinol. 2012 Nov;8(11):650–8. [PMID: 23007317]

DIABETES MELLITUS

Normal pregnancy can be characterized as a state of increased insulin resistance that helps ensure a steady stream of glucose delivery to the developing fetus. Thus, both mild fasting hypoglycemia and postprandial hyperglycemia are physiologic. These metabolic changes are felt to be hormonally mediated with likely contributions from human placental lactogen, estrogen, and progesterone.

A. Gestational Diabetes Mellitus

Gestational diabetes mellitus is abnormal glucose tolerance in pregnancy and is generally believed to be an exaggeration of the pregnancy-induced physiologic changes in carbohydrate metabolism. Alternatively, pregnancy may unmask an underlying propensity for glucose intolerance, which will be evident in the nonpregnant state at some future time if not in the immediate postpartum period. Indeed, at least 50% of women with gestational diabetes are diagnosed with overt diabetes at some point in their lifetime. During the pregnancy, the principal concern in women identified to have gestational diabetes is excessive fetal growth, which can result in increased maternal and perinatal morbidity. Shoulder dystocia occurs more frequently in infants of diabetic mothers because of fetal overgrowth and increased fat deposition on the shoulders. Cesarean delivery and preeclampsia are also significantly increased in women with diabetes, both gestational and overt.

All pregnant women should undergo screening for gestational diabetes, either by history, clinical risk factors, or (most commonly) laboratory screening tests. The diagnostic thresholds for glucose tolerance tests in pregnancy are not universally agreed upon, and importantly, adverse pregnancy outcomes appear to occur along a continuum of glucose intolerance even if the diagnosis of gestational diabetes is not formally assigned. A two-stage testing strategy is most commonly used in the United States, starting with a 50-g glucose test offered to all pregnant women at 24–28 weeks gestation. If this test is abnormal, the diagnostic test is a 100-g oral glucose tolerance test (Table 19–4). Women in whom gestational diabetes is diagnosed should undergo nutrition counseling, and insulin should be given to those with persistent fasting hyperglycemia. Insulin can be injected in a split dose mix of NPH and regular, administered twice daily. Insulin has long been regarded as the standard care for women who require medical management. Experience is increasing, however, with the use of oral hypoglycemic agents, such as glyburide and metformin. Randomized controlled trials comparing insulin to

Table 19–4. Screening and diagnostic criteria for gestational diabetes mellitus.

Screening for gestational diabetes mellitus
1. 50-g oral glucose load, administered between the 24th and 28th weeks, without regard to time of day or time of last meal. Universal blood glucose screening is indicated for patients who are of Hispanic, African, Native American, South or East Asian, Pacific Island, or indigenous Australian ancestry. Screening may be omitted for women of a low-prevalence ethnic group who have no family history of diabetes, are under 25 years of age, have normal weight before pregnancy, and have no history of abnormal glucose metabolism or poor obstetric outcome.
2. Venous plasma glucose measured 1 hour later.
3. Value of 140 mg/dL (7.8 mmol/L) or above in venous plasma indicates the need for a full diagnostic glucose tolerance test.
Diagnosis of gestational diabetes mellitus
1. 100-g oral glucose load, administered in the morning after overnight fast lasting at least 8 hours but not more than 14 hours, and following at least 3 days of unrestricted diet (> 150 g carbohydrate) and physical activity.
2. Venous plasma glucose is measured fasting and at 1, 2, and 3 hours. Subject should remain seated and should not smoke throughout the test.
3. Two or more of the following venous plasma concentrations must be equaled or exceeded for a diagnosis of gestational diabetes: fasting, 95 mg/dL (5.3 mmol/L); 1 hour, 180 mg/dL (10 mmol/L); 2 hours, 155 mg/dL (8.6 mmol/L); 3 hours, 140 mg/dL (7.8 mmol/L).

oral therapy have identified generally similar maternal and neonatal outcomes with either approach, although the long-term safety of oral agents has not been adequately studied in the women so treated or in their infants. Capillary blood glucose monitoring is checked four times per day, once fasting and three times after meals. Euglycemia is considered to be 60–90 mg/dL (3.3–5.0 mmol/L) while fasting and < 120 mg/dL (< 6.7 mmol/L) 2 hours postprandially. Intensive therapy with dietary modifications or insulin therapy, or both, has been demonstrated to decrease rates of macrosomia, shoulder dystocia, and preeclampsia. Because of the increased prevalence of overt diabetes in these women, they should be screened at 6–12 weeks postpartum with a fasting plasma glucose test or a 2-hour oral glucose tolerance test (75-g glucose load).

B. Overt Diabetes Mellitus

Overt diabetes is diabetes mellitus that antedates the pregnancy. As in gestational diabetes, fetal overgrowth from inadequately controlled hyperglycemia remains a significant concern because of the increased maternal and perinatal morbidity that accompany macrosomia. Women with overt diabetes are subject to a number of other complications as well. Spontaneous abortions and third trimester stillbirths occur with increased frequency in these women. There is also at least a twofold to threefold increased risk for fetal malformations, as hyperglycemia during organogenesis is teratogenic. The most common malformations in offspring of diabetic women are cardiac, skeletal, and neural tube defects. For the mother, the likelihood of infections and pregnancy-related hypertension is increased.

Preconception counseling and evaluation in a diabetic woman is ideal to maximize the pregnancy outcomes. This provides an opportunity to optimize glycemic control and evaluate for evidence of end-organ damage. The initial evaluation of diabetic women should include a complete chemistry panel, HbA$_{1c}$ determination, 24-hour urine collection for total protein and creatinine clearance, funduscopic examination, and an ECG. Hypertension is common and may require treatment. Optimally, euglycemia should be established before conception and maintained during pregnancy with daily home glucose monitoring by the patient. There is an inverse relationship between glycemic control and the occurrence of fetal malformations, and women whose periconceptional glycosylated hemoglobin levels are at or near normal levels have rates of malformations that approach baseline. A well-planned dietary program is a key component, with an intake of 1800–2200 kcal/d divided into three meals and three snacks. Insulin is given subcutaneously in a split-dose regimen as described above for women with gestational diabetes. The use of continuous insulin pump therapy may be helpful for some patients.

Throughout the pregnancy, diabetic women should be seen every 2–3 weeks and more frequently depending on the clinical condition. Adjustments in the insulin regimen may be necessary as the pregnancy progresses. A specialized ultrasound is often performed around 20 weeks to detect fetal malformations. Symptoms and signs of infections should be evaluated and promptly treated. In the third trimester, fetal surveillance is indicated, and women with diabetes should receive serial antenatal testing (usually in the form of a nonstress test or biophysical profile). The timing of delivery is dictated by the quality of diabetic control, the presence or absence of medical complications, and fetal status. The goal is to reach 39 weeks (38 completed weeks) and then proceed with delivery. Confirmation of lung maturity may be appropriate if preterm delivery is contemplated.

ACOG Committee on Practice Bulletins—Obstetrics. Practice Bulletin No. 137: Gestational diabetes mellitus. Obstet Gynecol. 2013 Aug;122(2 Pt 1):406–16. [PMID: 23969827]

Ali S et al. Diabetes in pregnancy: health risks and management. Postgrad Med J. 2011 Jun;87(1028):417–27. [PMID: 21368321]

Ringholm L et al. Managing type 1 diabetes mellitus in pregnancy—from planning to breastfeeding. Nat Rev Endocrinol. 2012 Nov;8(11):659–67. [PMID: 22965164]

Vandorsten JP et al. NIH consensus development conference: diagnosing gestational diabetes mellitus. NIH Consens State Sci Statements. 2013 Mar 6;29(1):1–31. [PMID: 23748438]

Wahabi HA et al. Pre-pregnancy care for women with pre-gestational diabetes mellitus: a systematic review and meta-analysis. BMC Public Health. 2012 Sep 17;12:792. [PMID: 22978747]

CHRONIC HYPERTENSION

Chronic hypertension is estimated to complicate up to 5% of pregnancies. To establish this diagnosis, hypertension should antedate the pregnancy or be evident before 20 weeks gestation to differentiate it from pregnancy-related hypertension. This distinction can be problematic when the initial presentation is after 20 weeks, but chronic hypertension is confirmed if the blood pressure remains elevated beyond 12 weeks postpartum. Risk factors for chronic hypertension include older maternal age, African American race, and obesity. While essential hypertension is by far the most common cause, secondary causes should be sought when clinically indicated.

Women with chronic hypertension are at increased risk for adverse maternal and perinatal outcomes. Superimposed preeclampsia develops in up to 20% of women with mild hypertension, but the risk increases up to 50% when there is severe baseline hypertension (≥ 160/110 mm Hg) and may be even higher when there is evidence of end-organ damage. When preeclampsia is superimposed on chronic hypertension, there is a tendency for it to occur at an earlier gestational age, be more severe, and impair fetal growth. Women with chronic hypertension are also at increased risk for placental abruption, preterm birth, and perinatal mortality.

Ideally, women with chronic hypertension should undergo an evaluation prior to conception to detect end-organ damage and assess the need for enhanced antihypertensive therapy (see Table 11–1). The specific tests ordered may vary depending on the severity of the hypertensive disorder, but an evaluation of renal and cardiac function is appropriate.

If the woman is not known to have chronic hypertension, then initiation of antihypertensive therapy in pregnant women is indicated only if the blood pressure is sustained at or above 150/100 mm Hg or if there is evidence of end-organ damage. Treatment of hypertension has not been demonstrated to improve pregnancy outcomes, but it is indicated in women with significant hypertension for long-term maternal cardiovascular health. For initiation of treatment in pregnancy, methyldopa has the longest record of safety at a starting dosage of 250 mg orally two to three times daily. Therapy with beta-blockers or calcium channel blockers is also acceptable (see Tables 11–6, 11–8). Care must be taken not to excessively reduce the blood pressure, as this may decrease uteroplacental perfusion. The goal is a modest reduction in blood pressure and avoidance of severe hypertension.

If a woman with mild chronic hypertension is stable on a medical regimen when she becomes pregnant, it is usually appropriate to continue this therapy, although the benefits of doing so are not well-established. Angiotensin-converting enzyme (ACE) inhibitors and angiotensin receptor blockers, however, are contraindicated in all trimesters of pregnancy. In addition to causing fetal hypocalvaria and acute kidney injury with exposure in the second and third trimesters, it is now recognized that these medications are teratogenic in the first trimester. Diuretics, although not typically initiated in pregnancy, may be continued in patients who are taking them when they become pregnant.

When there is sustained severe hypertension despite multiple medications or significant end-organ damage from hypertensive disease, pregnancy is not likely to be tolerated well. In these situations, therapeutic abortion may

be appropriate. If the pregnancy is continued, the woman must be counseled that the maternal and perinatal risks are appreciable, and complications such as superimposed preeclampsia and fetal growth restriction should be anticipated.

American College of Obstetricians and Gynecologists. ACOG Practice Bulletin No. 125: Chronic hypertension in pregnancy. Obstet Gynecol. 2012 Feb;119(2 Pt 1):396–407. [PMID: 22270315]

Ames M et al. Ambulatory management of chronic hypertension in pregnancy. Clin Obstet Gynecol. 2012 Sep;55(3):744–55. [PMID: 22828107]

Palma-Reis I et al. Renal disease and hypertension in pregnancy. Clin Med. 2013 Feb;13(1):57–62. [PMID: 23472497]

Seely EW et al. Chronic hypertension in pregnancy. N Engl J Med. 2011 Aug 4;365(5):439–46. [PMID: 21812673]

HEART DISEASE

Normal pregnancy physiology is characterized by cardiovascular adaptations in the mother. Cardiac output increases markedly as a result of both augmented stroke volume and an increase in the resting heart rate, and the maternal blood volume expands by up to 50%. These changes may not be tolerated well in women with functional or structural abnormalities of the heart. Thus, although only a small number of pregnancies are complicated by cardiac disease, these contribute disproportionately to overall rates of maternal morbidity and mortality. Most cardiac disease in women of childbearing age in the United States is caused by congenital heart disease. Ischemic heart disease, however, is being seen more commonly in pregnant women due to increasing rates of comorbid conditions, such as diabetes mellitus, hypertension, and obesity.

For practical purposes, the best single measurement of cardiopulmonary status is defined by the New York Heart Association Functional Classification. Most pregnant women with cardiac disease have class I or II functional disability, and although good outcomes are generally anticipated in this group, complications such as preeclampsia, preterm birth, and low birth weight appear to occur with increased frequency. Women with more severe disability (class III or IV) are rare in contemporary obstetrics; however, the maternal mortality is markedly increased in this setting and is usually the result of heart failure. Because of these risks, therapeutic abortion for maternal health should be considered in women who are severely disabled from cardiac disease. Specific conditions that have been associated with a particularly high risk for maternal death include Eisenmenger syndrome, primary pulmonary hypertension, Marfan syndrome with aortic root dilatation, and severe aortic or mitral stenosis. In general, these conditions should be considered contraindications to pregnancy.

Pregnant women with cardiac disease are best treated by a team of practitioners with experience in caring for such patients. Heart failure is the most common cardiovascular complication associated with heart disease in pregnancy, and adverse maternal and fetal outcomes are increased when heart failure occurs. Symptoms of volume overload should therefore be evaluated and treated promptly. Labor management may differ depending on the specific cardiac lesion, but cesarean delivery is generally reserved for obstetric indications. The early postpartum period is a critical time for fluid management. Patients who are predisposed to heart failure should be monitored closely during the puerperium.

Infective endocarditis prophylaxis is not recommended for a vaginal or cesarean delivery in the absence of infection, except in the very small subset of patients at highest risk for adverse outcomes from endocarditis. The women at highest risk include those with cyanotic heart disease, prosthetic valves, or both. If infection is present, such as chorioamnionitis, the underlying infection should be treated with the usual regimen and additional agents are not needed specifically for endocarditis prophylaxis. Prophylaxis, if required, should be given intravenously (see Table 33–6).

Ruys TP et al. Heart failure in pregnant women with cardiac disease: data from the ROPAC. Heart. 2014 Feb;100(3):231–8. [PMID: 24293523]

Simpson LL. Maternal cardiac disease: update for the clinician. Obstet Gynecol. 2012 Feb;119(2 Pt 1):345–59. [PMID: 22270287]

ASTHMA

(See also Chapter 9.)

Asthma is one of the most common medical conditions encountered in pregnancy. Women with mild to moderate asthma can generally expect excellent pregnancy outcomes, but severe or poorly controlled asthma has been associated with a number of pregnancy complications, including preterm birth, small-for-gestational-age infants, and preeclampsia. The effects of pregnancy on asthma are likely minimal as asthma severity in the pregnancy has been reported to be similar to its severity during the year preceding the pregnancy. Strategies for treatment are similar to that in nonpregnant women. Patients should be educated about symptom management and avoidance of asthma triggers. Baseline pulmonary function tests can provide an objective assessment of lung function and may help the patient with self-monitoring of her asthma severity using a peak flow meter. As in nonpregnant women, treatment algorithms generally follow a step-wise approach, and commonly used medications, particularly those for mild to moderate asthma symptoms, are generally considered safe in pregnancy. Concerns about teratogenicity and medication effects on the fetus should be thoroughly discussed with the patient to decrease noncompliance rates. Inhaled beta-2-agonists are indicated for all asthma patients, and low to moderate dose inhaled corticosteroids are added for persistent symptoms when a rescue inhaler alone is inadequate. Systemic corticosteroid administration is reserved for severe exacerbations but should not be withheld, if indicated, irrespective of gestational age. The primary goals of management in pregnancy include minimizing symptoms and avoiding hypoxic episodes to the fetus.

Gregersen TL et al. Safety of bronchodilators and corticosteroids for asthma during pregnancy: what we know and what we need to do better. J Asthma Allergy. 2013 Nov 15;6:117–25. [PMID: 24259987]

McCallister JW. Asthma in pregnancy: management strategies. Curr Opin Pulm Med. 2013 Jan;19(1):13–7. [PMID: 23154712]

Murphy VE et al. A meta-analysis of adverse perinatal outcomes in women with asthma. BJOG. 2011 Oct;118(11):1314–23. [PMID: 21749633]

SEIZURE DISORDERS

Epilepsy is one of the most common serious neurologic disorders in pregnant women. Many of the commonly used antiepileptic drugs are known human teratogens. Therefore, the principal objectives in managing pregnancy in epileptic women are achieving adequate control of seizures while minimizing exposure to medications that can cause congenital malformations. Certain women who are contemplating pregnancy and have been seizure-free for 2–5 years may be considered candidates for discontinuation of antiseizure medication prior to pregnancy. For those who continue to require treatment, however, therapy with one medication is preferred. Selecting a regimen should be based on the type of seizure disorder and the risks associated with each medication. Valproic acid should not be considered first-line therapy because it has consistently been associated with higher rates of fetal malformations than most other commonly used antiepileptic drugs, and there are data to suggest that it is also associated with impairments of cognitive development in the offspring. Phenytoin and carbamazepine are also older medications that are still used, and both have established patterns of associated fetal malformations. Concerns about teratogenicity have prompted increasing use of the newer antiepileptic drugs such as lamotrigine, topiramate, oxcarbazepine, and levetiracetam. Although the safety of these medications in pregnancy continues to be evaluated, experiences from ongoing registries and large, population-based studies suggest that in utero exposure to the newer antiepileptic drugs in the first trimester of pregnancy carries a lower risk of major malformations than older medications. Although it is recommended that pregnant women with epilepsy be given supplemental folic acid, it is unclear if supplemental folate decreases rates of fetal malformations in women taking anticonvulsant therapy.

Hernández-Díaz S et al; North American AED Pregnancy Registry. Comparative safety of antiepileptic drugs during pregnancy. Neurology. 2012 May 22;78(21):1692–9. [PMID: 22551726]

Molgaard-Nielsen D et al. Newer-generation antiepileptic drugs and the risk of major birth defects. JAMA. 2011 May 18;305(19):1996–2002. [PMID: 21586715]

Tomson T et al. Antiepileptic drug treatment in pregnancy: changes in drug disposition and their clinical implications. Epilepsia. 2013 Mar;54(3):405–14. [PMID: 23360413]

Vajda FJ et al. Teratogenicity of the newer antiepileptic drugs—the Australian experience. J Clin Neurosci. 2012 Jan; 19(1):57–9. [PMID: 22104350]

INFECTIOUS CONDITIONS COMPLICATING PREGNANCY

URINARY TRACT INFECTION

The urinary tract is especially vulnerable to infections during pregnancy because the altered secretions of steroid sex hormones and the pressure exerted by the gravid uterus on the ureters and bladder cause hypotonia and congestion and predispose to urinary stasis. Labor and delivery and urinary retention postpartum also may initiate or aggravate infection. *Escherichia coli* is the offending organism in over two-thirds of cases.

From 2% to 8% of pregnant women have asymptomatic bacteriuria, which some believe to be associated with an increased risk of preterm birth. It is estimated that pyelonephritis will develop in 20–40% of these women if untreated.

An evaluation for asymptomatic bacteriuria at the first prenatal visit is recommended for all pregnant women. If a urine culture is positive, treatment should be initiated. Nitrofurantoin (100 mg orally twice daily), ampicillin (250 mg orally four times daily), and cephalexin (250 mg orally four times daily) are acceptable medications for 4–7 days. Sulfonamides should be avoided in the third trimester because they may interfere with bilirubin binding and thus impose a risk of neonatal hyperbilirubinemia and kernicterus. Fluoroquinolones are also contraindicated because of their potential teratogenic effects on fetal cartilage and bone. Patients with recurrent bacteriuria should receive suppressive medication (once daily dosing of an appropriate antibiotic) for the remainder of the pregnancy. Acute pyelonephritis requires hospitalization for intravenous administration of antibiotics and crystalloids until the patient is afebrile; this is followed by a full course of oral antibiotics.

Widmer M et al. Duration of treatment for asymptomatic bacteriuria during pregnancy. Cochrane Database Syst Rev. 2011 Dec 7;(12):CD000491. [PMID: 22161364]

GROUP B STREPTOCOCCAL INFECTION

Group B streptococci frequently colonize the lower female genital tract, with an asymptomatic carriage rate in pregnancy of 10–30%. This rate depends on maternal age, gravidity, and geographic variation. Vaginal carriage is asymptomatic and intermittent, with spontaneous clearing in approximately 30% and recolonization in about 10% of women. Adverse perinatal outcomes associated with group B streptococcal colonization include urinary tract infection, intrauterine infection, premature rupture of membranes, preterm delivery, and postpartum metritis.

Women with postpartum metritis due to infection with group B streptococci, especially after cesarean section, develop fever, tachycardia, and abdominal pain, usually within 24 hours after delivery. Approximately 35% of these women are bacteremic.

Group B streptococcal infection is a common cause of neonatal sepsis. Transmission rates are high, yet the rate of neonatal sepsis is surprisingly low at < 1:1000 live births. Unfortunately, the mortality rate associated with early-onset disease can be as high as 20–30% in premature infants. In contrast, it is approximately 2–3% in those at term. Moreover, these infections can contribute markedly to chronic morbidity, including mental retardation and neurologic disabilities. Late-onset disease develops through contact with hospital nursery personnel. Up to 45% of these health care workers can carry the bacteria on their skin and transmit the infection to newborns.

CDC recommendations for screening and prophylaxis for group B streptococcal colonization are set forth above (see Essentials of Prenatal Care: Tests and Procedures).

Clifford V et al. Prevention of neonatal group B streptococcus disease in the 21st century. J Paediatr Child Health. 2012 Sep;48(9):808–15. [PMID: 22151082]

Ohlsson A et al. Intrapartum antibiotics for known maternal Group B streptococcal colonization. Cochrane Database Syst Rev. 2013 Jan 31;1:CD007467. [PMID: 23440815]

Verani JR et al; Division of Bacterial Diseases, National Center for Immunization and Respiratory Diseases, Centers for Disease Control and Prevention (CDC). Prevention of perinatal group B streptococcal disease—revised guidelines from CDC, 2010. MMWR Recomm Rep. 2010 Nov 19;59(RR-10):1–36. [PMID: 21088663]

VARICELLA

Commonly known as chickenpox, varicella-zoster virus (VZV) infection has a fairly benign course when incurred during childhood but may result in serious illness in adults, particularly during pregnancy. Infection results in lifelong immunity. Approximately 95% of women born in the United States have VZV antibodies by the time they reach reproductive age. The incidence of VZV infection during pregnancy has been reported as up to 7:10,000.

▶ Clinical Findings

A. Symptoms and Signs

The incubation period for this infection is 10–20 days. A primary infection follows and is characterized by a flu-like syndrome with malaise, fever, and development of a pruritic maculopapular rash on the trunk, which becomes vesicular and then crusts. Pregnant women are prone to the development of VZV pneumonia, often a fulminant infection sometimes requiring respiratory support. After primary infection, the virus becomes latent, ascending to dorsal root ganglia. Subsequent reactivation can occur as zoster, often under circumstances of immunocompromise, although this is rare during pregnancy.

Two types of fetal infection have been documented. The first is congenital VZV syndrome, which typically occurs in 0.4–2% of fetuses exposed to primary VZV infection during the first trimester. Anomalies include limb and digit abnormalities, microphthalmos, and microcephaly.

Infection during the second and third trimesters is less threatening. Maternal IgG crosses the placenta, protecting the fetus. The only infants at risk for severe infection are those born after maternal viremia but before development of maternal protective antibody. Maternal infection manifesting 5 days before or up to 2 days after delivery is the time period believed to be most hazardous for transmission to the fetus.

B. Laboratory Findings

Diagnosis is commonly made on clinical grounds. Laboratory verification of recent infection is made most often by antibody detection techniques, including ELISA, fluorescent antibody, and hemagglutination inhibition. Serum obtained by cordocentesis may be tested for VZV IgM to document fetal infection.

▶ Treatment

Varicella-zoster immune globulin (VZIG) has been shown to prevent or modify the symptoms of infection. Treatment success depends on identification of susceptible women at or just following exposure. Women with a questionable or negative history of chickenpox should be checked for antibody, since the overwhelming majority will have been previously exposed. If the antibody is negative, VZIG (625 units intramuscularly) should ideally be given within 96 hours of exposure for greatest efficacy, but the CDC reports it can be given for up to 10 days. There are no known adverse effects of VZIG administration during pregnancy, although the incubation period for disease can be lengthened. Infants born within 5 days after onset of maternal infection should also receive VZIG (125 units).

Infected pregnant women should be closely observed and hospitalized at the earliest signs of pulmonary involvement. Intravenous acyclovir (10 mg/kg intravenously every 8 hours) is recommended in the treatment of VZV pneumonia.

Centers for Disease Control and Prevention (CDC). Updated recommendations for use of VariZIG—United States, 2013. MMWR Morb Mortal Wkly Rep. 2013 July19;62(28):574–6. [PMID: 23863705]
Lamont RF et al. Varicella-zoster virus (chickenpox) infection in pregnancy. BJOG. 2011 Sep;118(10):1155–62. [PMID: 21585641]

TUBERCULOSIS

The diagnosis of tuberculosis in pregnancy is made by history taking, physical examination, and testing, with special attention to women in high-risk groups. Women at high risk include those who are from endemic areas, those infected with HIV, drug users, health care workers, and close contacts of people with tuberculosis. Chest radiographs should not be obtained as a routine screening measure in pregnancy but should be used only in patients with a positive test or with suggestive findings in the history and physical examination. Abdominal shielding must be used if a chest radiograph is obtained. Both tuberculin skin testing and interferon gamma release assays are acceptable tests in pregnancy.

Decisions on treatment depend on whether the patient has active disease or is at high risk for progression to active disease. Pregnant women with latent disease not at high risk for disease progression can receive treatment postpartum, which does not preclude breastfeeding. The concentration of medication in breast milk is neither toxic nor adequate for treatment of the newborn. Treatment is with isoniazid and ethambutol or isoniazid and rifampin (see Chapters 9 and 33). Because isoniazid therapy may result in vitamin B_6 deficiency, a supplement of 50 mg/d of vitamin B_6 should be given simultaneously. There is concern that isoniazid, particularly in pregnant women, can cause hepatitis. Liver function tests should be performed regularly in pregnant women who receive treatment. Streptomycin, ethionamide, and most other antituberculous drugs should be avoided in pregnancy. If adequately treated, tuberculosis in pregnancy has an excellent prognosis.

Mathad JS et al. Tuberculosis in pregnant and postpartum women: epidemiology, management, and research gaps. Clin Infect Dis. 2012 Dec;55(11):1532–49. [PMID: 22942202]
Taylor AW et al. Pregnancy outcomes in HIV-infected women receiving long-term isoniazid prophylaxis for tuberculosis and antiretroviral therapy. Infect Dis Obstet Gynecol. 2013;2013:195637. [PMID: 23533318]

HIV/AIDS DURING PREGNANCY

Heterosexual acquisition and injection drug use are the principal identified modes of HIV infection in women. Asymptomatic infection is associated with a normal pregnancy rate and no increased risk of adverse pregnancy outcomes. There is no evidence that pregnancy causes AIDS progression.

Previously, two-thirds of HIV-positive neonates acquired their infection close to, or during, the time of delivery. Routine HIV screening in pregnancy, including the use of rapid HIV tests in Labor and Delivery units, and the use of antiretroviral drugs has markedly reduced this transmission risk to approximately 2%. In an HIV-positive pregnant woman, a CD4 count, plasma RNA level, and resistance testing (if virus is detectable) should be obtained at the first prenatal visit. Prior or current antiretroviral use should be reviewed. A woman already taking and tolerating an acceptable antiretroviral regimen does not have to discontinue it in the first trimester. Patients should also be tested for hepatitis C, tuberculosis, toxoplasmosis, and cytomegalovirus.

Women not taking medication should be offered antiretroviral therapy with three drugs (commonly two nucleoside analogues and one protease inhibitor, including zidovudine whenever possible) after counseling regarding the potential impact of therapy on both mother and fetus. Antiretroviral therapy should be offered regardless of viral load and CD4 count, and it should be started in the second trimester unless there is a maternal indication to start earlier. The majority of drugs used to treat HIV/AIDS have thus far proven to be safe in pregnancy with an acceptable risk/benefit ratio. Efavirenz has been clearly linked with anomalies (myelomeningocele) and should not be used in the first trimester of pregnancy. However, efavirenz does not need to be discontinued if a pregnant patient presents for obstetrical care already taking the drug. Standard of care also includes administration of intravenous zidovudine prior to cesarean delivery and during labor in women whose viral load near delivery is ≥ 400 copies/mL or unknown. Antiretroviral therapy should also be continued in labor.

The use of prophylactic elective cesarean section at 38 weeks (before the onset of labor or rupture of the membranes) to prevent vertical transmission of HIV infection from mother to fetus has been shown to further reduce the transmission rate. In patients with a viral load of < 1000 copies/mL, there may be no additional benefit of cesarean delivery, and those women can be offered a vaginal delivery. Amniotomy should not be performed, and internal monitors, particularly the fetal scalp electrode, should be avoided. HIV-infected women should be advised not to breastfeed their infants.

The Public Health Task Force provides guidelines for the management of HIV/AIDS in pregnancy that are regularly updated and available at http://www.aidsinfo.nih.gov/. In addition, there is the National Perinatal HIV Hotline, which provides free consultation regarding perinatal HIV care (1-888-448-8765).

Lazenby GB. Opportunistic infections in women with HIV AIDS. Clin Obstet Gynecol. 2012 Dec;55(4):927–37. [PMID: 23090461]

U.S. Department of Health & Human Services Panel on Treatment of HIV-Infected Pregnant Women and Prevention of Perinatal Transmission. Recommendations for use of antiretroviral drugs in pregnant HIV-1 infected women for maternal health and interventions to reduce perinatal HIV transmission in the United States. 2012 July 14:1–207. http://aidsinfo.nih.gov/ContentFiles/lvguidelines/PerinatalGL.pdf

MATERNAL HEPATITIS B & C CARRIER STATE (See also Chapter 1)

There are an estimated 350 million chronic carriers of **hepatitis B virus** worldwide. Among these people, there is an increased incidence of chronic active hepatitis, cirrhosis, and hepatocellular carcinoma. In the United States, 1.4 million people are infected, with the highest rate among Asian Americans. All pregnant women should be screened for HBsAg. Transmission of the virus to the baby after delivery is likely if both surface antigen and e antigen are positive. Vertical transmission can be blocked by the immediate postdelivery administration to the newborn of hepatitis B immunoglobulin and hepatitis B vaccine intramuscularly. The vaccine dose is repeated at 1 and 6 months of age. Successful, but limited, experience has also been reported with lamivudine during the third trimester to prevent vertical transmission of hepatitis B in mothers with high HBV viral loads. Pregnant women with chronic hepatitis B should

have liver function tests during the pregnancy. Hepatitis B infection is not a contraindication to breastfeeding.

Hepatitis C virus infection is the most common chronic blood-borne infection in the United States. Risk factors for transmission include blood transfusion, injection drug use, employment in patient care or clinical laboratory work, exposure to a sex partner or household member who has had a history of hepatitis, exposure to multiple sex partners, and low socioeconomic level. The average rate of hepatitis C virus (HCV) infection among infants born to HCV-positive, HIV-negative women is 5–6%. However, the average infection rate increases to 14% when mothers are coinfected with HCV and HIV. The principal factor associated with transmission is the presence of HCV RNA in the mother at the time of birth.

Esposti SD et al. Hepatitis B in pregnancy: challenges and treatment. Gastroenterol Clin North Am. 2011 Jun;40(2):355–72. [PMID: 21601784]

HERPES GENITALIS

Infection of the lower genital tract by herpes simplex virus type 2 (HSV-2) (see also Chapter 6) is a common STD with potentially serious consequences to pregnant women and their newborn infants. Although up to 20% of women in an obstetric practice may have antibodies to HSV-2, a history of the infection is unreliable and the incidence of neonatal infection is low (10–60/100,000 live births). Most infected neonates are born to women with no history, symptoms, or signs of infection.

Women who have had *primary* herpes infection late in pregnancy are at high risk for shedding virus at delivery. Some authors suggest use of prophylactic acyclovir, 400 mg orally three times daily, to decrease the likelihood of active lesions at the time of labor and delivery.

Women with a history of *recurrent* genital herpes have a lower neonatal attack rate than women infected during the pregnancy, but they should still be monitored with clinical observation and culture of any suspicious lesions. Since asymptomatic viral shedding is not predictable by antepartum cultures, current recommendations do not include routine cultures in individuals with a history of herpes without active disease. However, when labor begins, vulvar and cervical inspection should be performed. Cesarean delivery is indicated at the time of labor if there are prodromal symptoms, active genital lesions, or a positive cervical culture obtained within the preceding week.

For treatment, see Chapter 32. The use of acyclovir in pregnancy is acceptable, and prophylaxis starting at 36 weeks gestation has been shown to decrease the number of cesarean sections performed for active disease.

Jaiyeoba O et al. Preventing neonatal transmission of herpes simplex virus. Clin Obstet Gynecol. 2012 Jun;55(2):510–20. [PMID: 22510634]

Pinninti SG et al. Maternal and neonatal herpes simplex virus infections. Am J Perinatol. 2013 Feb;30(2):113–9. [PMID: 23303485]

SYPHILIS, GONORRHEA, & *C TRACHOMATIS* INFECTION (See also Chapters 33 & 34)

These STDs have significant consequences for mother and child. Untreated syphilis in pregnancy can cause late abortion, stillbirth, transplacental infection, and congenital syphilis. Gonorrhea can produce large-joint arthritis by hematogenous spread as well as ophthalmia neonatorum. Maternal chlamydial infections are largely asymptomatic but are manifested in the newborn by inclusion conjunctivitis and, at age 2–4 months, by pneumonia. The diagnosis of each can be reliably made by appropriate laboratory tests. All women should be tested for syphilis and *C trachomatis* as part of their routine prenatal care. Repeat testing is dependent on risk factors, prevalence, and state laws. Women at risk should be tested for gonorrhea. The sexual partners of women with STDs should be identified and treated also if possible; the local health department can assist with this process.

Hawkes SJ et al. Early antenatal care: does it make a difference to outcomes of pregnancy associated with syphilis? A systematic review and meta-analysis. PLoS One. 2013;8(2):e56713. [PMID: 23468875]

Workowski KA et al; Centers for Disease Control and Prevention (CDC). Sexually transmitted diseases treatment guidelines, 2010. MMWR Recomm Rep. 2010 Dec 17;59(RR-12):1–110. [PMID: 21160459]

SURGICAL COMPLICATIONS DURING PREGNANCY

Although purely elective surgery should be avoided during pregnancy, women who undergo surgical procedures for an urgent or emergent indication during pregnancy do not appear to be at increased risk for adverse outcomes. Obstetric complications, when they occur, are more likely to be associated with the underlying maternal illness. Recommendations have held that the optimal time for semi-elective surgery is the second trimester to avoid exposure to anesthesia in the first trimester and the enlarged uterus in the third. Importantly, however, there is no convincing evidence that general anesthesia induces malformations or increases the risk for abortion.

CHOLELITHIASIS, CHOLECYSTITIS, & INTRAHEPATIC CHOLESTASIS OF PREGNANCY

Cholelithiasis is common in pregnancy as physiologic changes such as increased cholesterol production and incomplete gallbladder emptying predispose to gallstone formation. The diagnosis is usually suspected based on classic symptoms of nausea, vomiting, and right upper quadrant pain, usually after meals, and is confirmed with right upper quadrant ultrasound. Symptomatic cholelithiasis without cholecystitis is usually managed conservatively, but recurrent symptoms are common. Cholecystitis results from obstruction of the cystic duct and often is accompanied by bacterial infection. Medical management with antibiotics is reasonable in selected cases,

but definitive treatment with cholecystectomy will help prevent complications such as gallbladder perforation and pancreatitis. Cholecystectomy has successfully been performed in all trimesters of pregnancy and should not be withheld based on the stage of pregnancy if clinically indicated. Laparoscopy is preferred in the first half of pregnancy but becomes technically difficult in the last trimester due to the enlarged uterus and cephalad displacement of abdominal contents.

Obstruction of the common bile duct can lead to cholangitis requiring surgical removal of gallstones and establishment of biliary drainage. Magnetic resonance cholangiopancreatography (MRCP) can be of use in patients with common bile duct dilatation in whom the ultrasound results are equivocal. MRCP can provide detailed evaluation of the entire biliary system and the pancreas while avoiding ionizing radiation. When necessary, however, endoscopic retrograde cholangiopancreatography (ERCP) and endoscopic retrograde sphincterotomy can be performed safely in pregnant women if precautions are taken to minimize fetal exposure to radiation. There does, however, appear to be a slightly higher rate of post-procedure pancreatitis in pregnant women who undergo ERCP.

Intrahepatic cholestasis of pregnancy is characterized by incomplete clearance of bile acids in genetically susceptible women. The main symptom of generalized pruritus usually occurs in the third trimester. Laboratory studies reveal hepatic dysfunction with elevations in serum bile acids. Hepatic transaminase levels may also be modestly elevated, and mild bilirubin elevations may even result in clinical jaundice. Ursodeoxycholic acid (8–10 mg/kg/d) is the treatment of choice and results in decreased pruritus in most women. Cholestyramine has also been used, but it does not appear to be as effective and impairs absorption of fat-soluble vitamins. Vitamin K supplementation is therefore required to help prevent hemorrhagic disease in the fetus. Symptoms ultimately resolve after delivery but often recur in subsequent pregnancies. Adverse fetal outcomes, particularly fetal distress, meconium-stained amniotic fluid, and stillbirth, have been reported in women with cholestasis of pregnancy. Because of these risks, many clinicians recommend antenatal testing in the third trimester and delivery around 38 weeks gestation. Evidence-based recommendations, however, are not available.

Bacq Y et al. Efficacy of ursodeoxycholic acid in treating intrahepatic cholestasis of pregnancy: a meta-analysis. Gastroenterology. 2012 Dec;143(6):1492–501. [PMID: 22892336]

Chan CH et al. ERCP in the management of choledocholithiasis in pregnancy. Curr Gastroenterol Rep. 2012 Dec;14(6):504–10. [PMID: 23011675]

Oto A et al. The role of MR cholangiopancreatography in the evaluation of pregnant patients with acute pancreatobiliary disease. Br J Radiol. 2009 Apr;82(976):279–85. [PMID: 19029218]

APPENDICITIS

Appendicitis occurs in about 1 of 1500 pregnancies. The diagnosis is often difficult to make clinically since the appendix is displaced cephalad from McBurney point.

Furthermore, nausea, vomiting, and mild leukocytosis occur in normal pregnancy, so with or without these findings, any complaint of right-sided pain should raise suspicion. CT scanning can help confirm the diagnosis when clinical findings are equivocal, and proper shielding can minimize radiation exposure to the fetus. MRI is also being increasingly used to evaluate for appendicitis in pregnant women and appears to be a reasonable alternative to CT scanning. Unfortunately, the diagnosis of appendicitis is not made until the appendix has ruptured in at least 20% of obstetric patients. Peritonitis in these cases can lead to preterm labor or abortion. With early diagnosis and appendectomy, the prognosis is good for mother and baby.

Blumenfeld YJ et al. MR imaging in cases of antenatal suspected appendicitis—a meta-analysis. J Matern Fetal Neonatal Med. 2011 Mar;24(3):485–8. [PMID: 20695758]

Wilasrusmee C et al. Systematic review and meta-analysis of safety of laparoscopic versus open appendicectomy for suspected appendicitis in pregnancy. Br J Surg. 2012 Nov;99(11):1470–8. [PMID: 23001791]

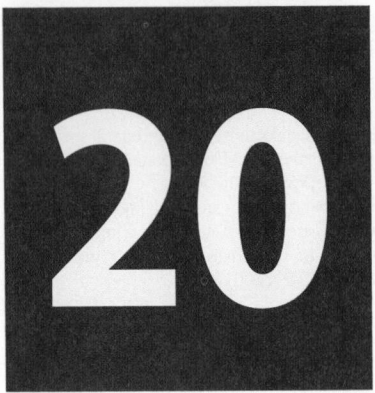

Rheumatologic & Immunologic Disorders

David B. Hellmann, MD, MACP

John B. Imboden, Jr., MD

▶ Diagnosis & Evaluation

A. Examination of the Patient

In the patient with arthritis, the two clinical clues most helpful for diagnosis are the **joint pattern** and the **presence or absence of extra-articular manifestations**. The joint pattern is defined by the answers to three questions: (1) Is inflammation present? (2) How many joints are involved? and (3) What joints are affected? Joint inflammation manifests as redness, warmth, swelling, and morning stiffness of at least 30 minutes' duration. Both the number of affected joints and the specific sites of involvement affect the differential diagnosis (Table 20–1). Some diseases—gout, for example—are characteristically monarticular, whereas other diseases, such as rheumatoid arthritis, are usually polyarticular. The location of joint involvement can also be distinctive. Only two diseases frequently cause prominent involvement of the distal interphalangeal (DIP) joint: osteoarthritis and psoriatic arthritis. Extra-articular manifestations such as fever (eg, gout, Still disease, endocarditis), rash (eg, systemic lupus erythematosus [SLE], psoriatic arthritis, Still disease), nodules (eg, rheumatoid arthritis, gout), or neuropathy (eg, polyarteritis nodosa, granulomatosis with polyangiitis [formerly Wegener granulomatosis]) narrow the differential diagnosis further.

B. Arthrocentesis and Examination of Joint Fluid

If the diagnosis is uncertain, synovial fluid should be examined whenever possible (Table 20–2). Most large joints are easily aspirated, and contraindications to arthrocentesis are few. The aspirating needle should never be passed through an overlying cellulitis or psoriatic plaque because of the risk of introducing infection. For patients who are receiving long-term anticoagulation therapy with warfarin, joints can be aspirated with a small-gauge needle (eg, 22F) if the international normalized ratio (INR) is < 3.0.

1. Types of studies

A. Gross examination—Clarity is an approximate guide to the degree of inflammation. Noninflammatory fluid is transparent, mild inflammation produces translucent fluid, and purulent effusions are opaque. Bleeding disorders, trauma, and traumatic taps are the most common causes of bloody effusions.

B. Cell count—The synovial fluid white cell count discriminates between **noninflammatory** (< 2000 white cells/mcL [2.0×10^9/L]), **inflammatory** (2000–75,000 white cells/mcL [2.0×10^9/L–75.0×10^9/L]), and **purulent** (> 100,000 white cells/mcL [> 100×10^9/L]) joint effusions. Synovial fluid glucose and protein levels add little information and should not be ordered.

C. Microscopic examination—Compensated polarized light microscopy identifies and distinguishes monosodium urate (gout, negatively birefringent) and calcium pyrophosphate (pseudogout, positive birefringent) crystals. Gram stain has specificity but limited sensitivity (50%) for septic arthritis.

D. Culture—Bacterial cultures as well as special studies for gonococci, tubercle bacilli, or fungi are ordered as appropriate.

2. Interpretation

—Synovial fluid analysis is diagnostic in infectious or microcrystalline arthritis. Although the severity of inflammation in synovial fluid can overlap among various conditions, the synovial fluid white cell count is a helpful guide to diagnosis (Table 20–3).

DEGENERATIVE & CRYSTAL-INDUCED ARTHRITIS

DEGENERATIVE JOINT DISEASE (Osteoarthritis)

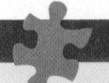 ESSENTIALS OF DIAGNOSIS

- ▶ A degenerative disorder with minimal articular inflammation.
- ▶ No systemic symptoms.
- ▶ Pain relieved by rest; morning stiffness brief.
- ▶ Radiographic findings: narrowed joint space, osteophytes, increased density of subchondral bone, bony cysts.

Table 20–1. Diagnostic value of the joint pattern.

Characteristic	Status	Representative Disease
Inflammation	Present	Rheumatoid arthritis, systemic lupus erythematosus, gout
	Absent	Osteoarthritis
Number of involved joints	Monarticular	Gout, trauma, septic arthritis, Lyme disease, osteoarthritis
	Oligoarticular (2–4 joints)	Reactive arthritis, psoriatic arthritis, inflammatory bowel disease
	Polyarticular (≥ 5 joints)	Rheumatoid arthritis, systemic lupus erythematosus
Site of joint involvement	Distal interphalangeal	Osteoarthritis, psoriatic arthritis (not rheumatoid arthritis)
	Metacarpophalangeal, wrists	Rheumatoid arthritis, systemic lupus erythematosus, calcium pyrophosphate deposition disease (not osteoarthritis)
	First metatarsal phalangeal	Gout, osteoarthritis

▶ General Considerations

Osteoarthritis, the most common form of joint disease, is chiefly a disease of aging. Ninety percent of all people have radiographic features of osteoarthritis in weight-bearing joints by age 40. Symptomatic disease also increases with age. Gender is also a risk factor, because osteoarthritis develops in women more frequently than in men.

This arthropathy is characterized by degeneration of cartilage and by hypertrophy of bone at the articular margins. Inflammation is usually minimal. Hereditary and mechanical factors may be involved in the pathogenesis.

Obesity is a risk factor for osteoarthritis of the knee, hand, and probably of the hip. Recreational running does not increase the incidence of osteoarthritis, but participation in competitive contact sports does. Jobs requiring frequent bending and carrying increase the risk of knee osteoarthritis (see Chapter 41).

▶ Clinical Findings

A. Symptoms and Signs

Degenerative joint disease is divided into two types: (1) primary, which most commonly affects some or all of the following: the DIP and the proximal interphalangeal (PIP) joints of the fingers, the carpometacarpal joint of the thumb, the hip, the knee, the metatarsophalangeal (MTP) joint of the big toe, and the cervical and lumbar spine; and (2) secondary, which may occur in any joint as a sequela to articular injury resulting from either intra-articular (including rheumatoid arthritis) or extra-articular causes. The injury may be acute, as in a fracture; or chronic, as that due to occupational overuse of a joint, metabolic disease (eg, hyperparathyroidism, hemochromatosis, ochronosis), or neurologic disorders (syringomyelia; see below).

The onset is insidious. Initially, there is articular stiffness, seldom lasting more than 15 minutes; this develops later into pain on motion of the affected joint and is made worse by activity or weight bearing and relieved by rest. Flexion contracture or varus deformity of the knee is not unusual, and bony enlargements of the DIP (Heberden nodes) and PIP (Bouchard nodes) are occasionally prominent (Figure 20–1). There is no ankylosis, but limitation of motion of the affected joint or joints is common. Crepitus may often be felt over the knee. Joint effusion and other articular signs of inflammation are mild. There are no systemic manifestations.

B. Laboratory Findings

Osteoarthritis does not cause elevation of the erythrocyte sedimentation rate (ESR) or other laboratory signs of inflammation. Synovial fluid is noninflammatory.

C. Imaging

Radiographs may reveal narrowing of the joint space; osteophyte formation and lipping of marginal bone; and

Table 20–2. Examination of joint fluid.

Measure	(Normal)	Group I (Noninflammatory)	Group II (Inflammatory)	Group III (Purulent)
Volume (mL) (knee)	< 3.5	Often > 3.5	Often > 3.5	Often > 3.5
Clarity	Transparent	Transparent	Translucent to opaque	Opaque
Color	Clear	Yellow	Yellow to opalescent	Yellow to green
WBC (per mcL)	< 200	< 2000	2000–75,000[1]	> 100,000[2]
Polymorphonuclear leukocytes	< 25%	< 25%	50% or more	75% or more
Culture	Negative	Negative	Negative	Usually positive[2]

[1]Gout, rheumatoid arthritis, and other inflammatory conditions occasionally have synovial fluid WBC counts > 75,000/mcL but rarely > 100,000/mcL.

[2]Most purulent effusions are due to septic arthritis. Septic arthritis, however, can present with group II synovial fluid, particularly if infection is caused by organisms of low virulence (eg, *Neisseria gonorrhoeae*) or if antibiotic therapy has been started.

WBC, white blood cell count.

Table 20–3. Differential diagnosis by joint fluid groups.

Group I (Noninflammatory) (< 2000 white cells/mcL)	Group II (Inflammatory) (2000–75,000 white cells/mcL)	Group III (Purulent) (> 100,000 white cells/mcL)	Hemorrhagic
Degenerative joint disease	Rheumatoid arthritis	Pyogenic bacterial infections	Hemophilia or other hemorrhagic diathesis
Trauma[1]	Acute crystal-induced synovitis (gout and pseudogout)		Trauma with or without fracture
Osteochondritis dissecans	Reactive arthritis		Neuropathic arthropathy
Osteochondromatosis	Ankylosing spondylitis		Pigmented villonodular synovitis
Neuropathic arthropathy[1]	Rheumatic fever[2]		Synovioma
Subsiding or early inflammation	Tuberculosis		Hemangioma and other benign neoplasms
Hypertrophic osteoarthropathy[2]			
Pigmented villonodular synovitis[1]			

[1]May be hemorrhagic.
[2]Noninflammatory or inflammatory group.
Reproduced, with permission, from Rodnan GP (editor). Primer on the rheumatic diseases, 7th ed. JAMA. 1973;224(Suppl):662.

thickened, dense subchondral bone. Bone cysts may also be present.

▶ Differential Diagnosis

Because articular inflammation is minimal and systemic manifestations are absent, degenerative joint disease should seldom be confused with other arthritides. The distribution of joint involvement in the hands also helps distinguish osteoarthritis from rheumatoid arthritis. Osteoarthritis chiefly affects the DIP and PIP joints and spares the wrist and metacarpophalangeal (MCP) joints; rheumatoid arthritis involves the wrists and MCP joints and spares the DIP joints. Furthermore, the joint enlargement is bony-hard and cool in osteoarthritis but spongy and warm in rheumatoid arthritis. Skeletal symptoms due to degenerative changes in joints—especially in the spine—may cause coexistent metastatic neoplasia, osteoporosis, multiple myeloma, or other bone disease to be overlooked.

▶ Prevention

Weight reduction reduces the risk of developing symptomatic knee osteoarthritis. Correcting leg length discrepancy

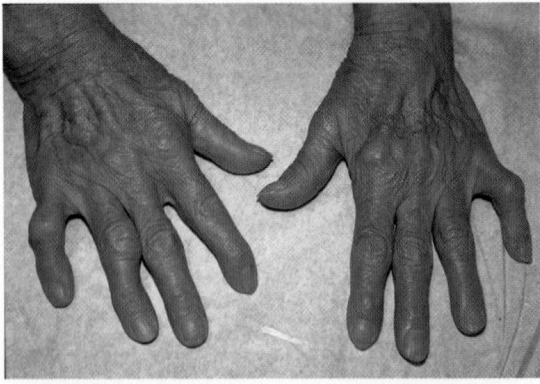

▲ **Figure 20–1.** Osteoarthritis with bony enlargement of the distal interphalangeal (DIP) joints (Heberden nodes) and proximal interphalangeal (PIP) joints (Bouchard nodes). (Reproduced with permission, from Richard P. Usatine, MD.)

of > 1 cm with shoe modification may prevent knee osteoarthritis from developing in the shorter leg. Maintaining normal vitamin D levels may reduce the occurrence and progression of osteoarthritis, in addition to being important for bone health.

▶ Treatment

A. General Measures

Patients with osteoarthritis of the hand may benefit from assistive devices and instruction on techniques for joint protection; splinting is beneficial for those with symptomatic osteoarthritis of the first carpometacarpal joint. Patients with mild to moderate osteoarthritis of the knee or hip should participate in a regular exercise program (eg, a supervised walking program, hydrotherapy classes) and, if overweight, should lose weight. The use of assistive devices (eg, a cane on the contralateral side) can improve functional status.

B. Medical Management

1. Acetaminophen—First-line therapy for patients with mild osteoarthritis is acetaminophen (2.6–4 g/d orally).

2. Nonsteroidal anti-inflammatory drugs—NSAIDs (see Table 5–2) are more effective than acetaminophen for osteoarthritis but have greater toxicity. NSAIDs inhibit cyclooxygenase (COX), the enzyme that converts arachidonic acid to prostaglandins. Although prostaglandins play important roles in promoting inflammation and pain, they also help maintain homeostasis in several organs—especially the stomach, where prostaglandin E serves as a local hormone responsible for gastric mucosal cytoprotection. COX exists in two isomers—COX-1, which is expressed continuously in many cells and is responsible for the homeostatic effects of prostaglandins, and COX-2, which is induced by cytokines and expressed in inflammatory tissues. Most NSAIDs inhibit both isomers. Celecoxib is the only selective COX-2 inhibitor currently available in the United States.

Gastrointestinal toxicity, such as gastric ulceration, perforation, and gastrointestinal hemorrhage, are the most common serious side effects of NSAIDs. NSAIDs can also affect the lower intestinal tract, causing perforation or aggravating inflammatory bowel disease. The overall rate of bleeding with NSAID use in the general population is low (≤ 1:6000 users) but is increased by the risk factors of long-term use, higher NSAID dose, concomitant corticosteroids or anticoagulants, the presence of rheumatoid arthritis, history of peptic ulcer disease or alcoholism, and age over 70. Proton pump inhibitors (eg, omeprazole 20 mg orally daily) reduce the incidence of serious gastrointestinal toxicity and should be used for patients with risk factors for NSAID-induced gastrointestinal toxicity. Patients who have recently recovered from an NSAID-induced bleeding gastric ulcer appear to be at high risk for rebleeding (about 5% in 6 months) when an NSAID is reintroduced, even if prophylactic measures (such as proton pump inhibitors) are used. Compared with nonselective NSAIDs, celecoxib may be less likely in some circumstances to cause upper gastrointestinal tract adverse events. However, long-term use of COX-2 inhibitors, particularly in the absence of concomitant aspirin use, has been associated with an increased risk of cardiovascular events.

All of the NSAIDs, including aspirin and celecoxib, can produce renal toxicity, including interstitial nephritis, nephrotic syndrome, prerenal azotemia, and aggravation of hypertension. Hyperkalemia due to hyporeninemic hypoaldosteronism may also be seen rarely. The risk of renal toxicity is low but is increased by the following risk factors: age over 60, a history of kidney disease, heart failure, ascites, and diuretic use.

All NSAIDs, except the nonacetylated salicylates and the COX-2 inhibitor celecoxib, interfere with platelet function and prolong bleeding time. Aspirin irreversibly inhibits platelet function, so the bleeding time effect resolves only as new platelets are made. In contrast, the effect of nonselective NSAIDs on platelet function is reversible and resolves as the drug is cleared. Concomitant administration of a nonselective NSAID can interfere with the ability of aspirin to acetylate platelets and thus may interfere with the cardioprotective effects of low-dose aspirin.

Topical NSAIDs (eg, 4 g of diclofenac gel 1% applied to the affected joint four times daily) appear more effective than placebo for knee and hand osteoarthritis and have lower rates of systemic side effects than with oral NSAIDs. Few studies have compared the efficacy of oral and topical NSAIDs.

Topical capsaicin may be of benefit for osteoarthritis of the hand but is not recommended for osteoarthritis of the knee or hip.

Chondroitin sulfate and glucosamine, alone or in combination, are no better than placebo in reducing pain in patients with knee or hip osteoarthritis.

3. Intra-articular injections—Intra-articular injections of triamcinolone (20–40 mg) for patients with osteoarthritis of the knee or hip may reduce the need for analgesics or NSAIDs and can be repeated up to four times a year. The American College of Rheumatology does not recommend corticosteroid injections for osteoarthritis of the hand.

Intra-articular injections of sodium hyaluronate produce moderate reduction in symptoms in some patients with osteoarthritis of the knee.

C. Surgical Measures

Total hip and knee replacements provide excellent symptomatic and functional improvement when involvement of that joint severely restricts walking or causes pain at rest, particularly at night. Arthroscopic surgery for knee osteoarthritis is ineffective.

▶ Prognosis

Marked disability is less common in patients with osteoarthritis than in those with rheumatoid arthritis, but symptoms may be quite severe and limit activity considerably (especially with involvement of the hips, knees, and cervical spine).

▶ When to Refer

Refer patients to an orthopedic surgeon when recalcitrant symptoms or functional impairment, or both, warrant consideration of joint replacement surgery of the hip or knee.

Fernandes L et al. EULAR recommendations for the non-pharmacological core management of hip and knee osteoarthritis. Ann Rheum Dis. 2013 Jul;72(7):1125–35. [PMID: 23595142]

Hochberg MC et al. American College of Rheumatology 2012 recommendations for the use of nonpharmacologic and pharmacologic therapies in osteoarthritis of the hand, hip, and knee. Arthritis Care Res (Hoboken). 2012 Apr;64(4):465–74. [PMID: 22563589]

Katz JN et al. Surgery versus physical therapy for a meniscal tear and osteoarthritis. N Engl J Med. 2013 May 2;368(18):1675–84. [PMID: 23506518]

Uthman OA et al. Exercise for lower limb osteoarthritis: systematic review incorporating trial sequential analysis and network meta-analysis. BMJ. 2013 Sep 20;347:f5555. [PMID: 24055922]

CRYSTAL DEPOSITION ARTHRITIS

1. Gouty Arthritis

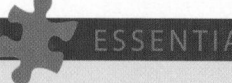

ESSENTIALS OF DIAGNOSIS

- ▶ Acute onset, usually monarticular, recurring attacks, often involving the first MTP joint.
- ▶ Polyarticular involvement more common in patients with long-standing disease.
- ▶ Identification of urate crystals in joint fluid or tophi is diagnostic.
- ▶ Dramatic therapeutic response to NSAIDs.
- ▶ With chronicity, urate deposits in subcutaneous tissue, bone, cartilage, joints, and other tissues.

▶ General Considerations

Gout is a metabolic disease of a heterogeneous nature, often familial, associated with abnormal amounts of urates in the body and characterized early by a recurring acute arthritis, usually monarticular, and later by chronic deforming arthritis. The associated hyperuricemia (serum uric acid level > 6.8 mg/dL [> 404.5 mcmol/L]) is due to overproduction or underexcretion of uric acid—sometimes both. The disease is especially common in Pacific islanders, eg, Filipinos and Samoans. Primary gout has a heritable component, and genome-wide surveys have linked risk of gout to several genes whose products regulate urate handling by the kidney. Secondary gout, which may have a heritable component, is related to acquired causes of hyperuricemia, eg, medication use (especially diuretics, low-dose aspirin, cyclosporine, and niacin), myeloproliferative disorders, multiple myeloma, hemoglobinopathies, chronic kidney disease, hypothyroidism, psoriasis, sarcoidosis, and lead poisoning (Table 20–4). Alcohol ingestion promotes hyperuricemia by increasing urate production and decreasing the renal excretion of uric acid. Finally, hospitalized patients frequently suffer attacks of gout because of changes in diet, fluid intake, or medications that lead either to rapid reductions or increases in the serum urate level.

About 90% of patients with primary gout are men, usually over 30 years of age. In women, the onset is typically postmenopausal. The characteristic lesion is the tophus, a nodular deposit of monosodium urate monohydrate crystals with an associated foreign body reaction. Tophi are found in cartilage, subcutaneous and periarticular tissues, tendon, bone, the kidneys, and elsewhere. Urates have been demonstrated in the synovial tissues (and fluid) during acute arthritis; indeed, the acute inflammation of gout is believed to be initiated by the ingestion of uncoated urate crystals by monocytes and synoviocytes. Once inside the cells, the gout crystals are processed through Toll-like receptors and activate NALP-3 inflammasomes that in turn release a variety of chemotactic agents and cytokines capable of mediating inflammation. The precise relationship of hyperuricemia to gouty arthritis is still obscure, since chronic hyperuricemia is found in people who never develop gout or uric acid stones. Rapid fluctuations in serum urate levels, either increasing or decreasing, are important factors in precipitating acute gout. The mechanism of the late, chronic stage of gouty arthritis is better understood. This is characterized pathologically by tophaceous invasion of the articular and periarticular tissues, with structural derangement and secondary degeneration (osteoarthritis).

Uric acid kidney stones are present in 5–10% of patients with gouty arthritis. Hyperuricemia correlates highly with the likelihood of developing stones, with the risk of stone formation reaching 50% in patients with a serum urate level > 13 mg/dL. Chronic urate nephropathy is caused by the deposition of monosodium urate crystals in the renal medulla and pyramids. Although progressive chronic kidney disease occurs in a substantial percentage of patients with chronic gout, the role of hyperuricemia in causing this outcome is controversial, because many patients with gout have numerous confounding risk factors for chronic kidney disease (eg, hypertension, alcohol use, lead exposure, and other risk factors for vascular disease).

▶ Clinical Findings

A. Symptoms and Signs

Acute gouty arthritis is sudden in onset and frequently nocturnal. It may develop without apparent precipitating cause or may follow rapid increases or decreases in serum urate levels. Common precipitants are alcohol excess (particularly beer), changes in medications that affect urate metabolism, and, in the hospitalized patient, fasting before medical procedures. The MTP joint of the great toe is the most susceptible joint ("podagra"), although others, especially those of the feet, ankles, and knees, are commonly affected. Gouty attacks may develop in periarticular soft tissues such as the arch of the foot. Hips and shoulders are rarely affected. More than one joint may occasionally be affected during the same attack; in such cases, the distribution of the arthritis is usually asymmetric. As the attack progresses, the pain becomes intense. The involved joints are swollen and exquisitely tender and the overlying skin tense, warm, and dusky red. Fever is common and may reach 39°C. Local desquamation and pruritus during recovery from the acute arthritis are characteristic of gout but are not always present. Tophi may be found in the external ears, feet, olecranon and prepatellar bursae, and hands (Figure 20–2). They usually develop years after the initial attack of gout.

Asymptomatic periods of months or years commonly follow the initial acute attack. After years of recurrent severe monarthritis attacks of the lower extremities and untreated hyperuricemia, gout can evolve into a chronic, deforming polyarthritis of upper and lower extremities that mimics rheumatoid arthritis.

B. Laboratory Findings

Although serial measurements of the serum uric acid detect hyperuricemia in 95% of patients, a single uric acid determination during an acute flare of gout is normal in up

---

Table 20–4. Origin of hyperuricemia.

Primary hyperuricemia
A. Increased production of purine
  1. Idiopathic
  2. Specific enzyme defects (eg, Lesch-Nyhan syndrome, glycogen storage diseases)
B. Decreased renal clearance of uric acid (idiopathic)
Secondary hyperuricemia
A. Increased catabolism and turnover of purine
  1. Myeloproliferative disorders
  2. Lymphoproliferative disorders
  3. Carcinoma and sarcoma (disseminated)
  4. Chronic hemolytic anemias
  5. Cytotoxic drugs
  6. Psoriasis
B. Decreased renal clearance of uric acid
  1. Intrinsic kidney disease
  2. Functional impairment of tubular transport
    a. Drug-induced (eg, thiazides, low-dose aspirin)
    b. Hyperlacticacidemia (eg, lactic acidosis, alcoholism)
    c. Hyperketoacidemia (eg, diabetic ketoacidosis, starvation)
    d. Diabetes insipidus (vasopressin-resistant)
    e. Bartter syndrome

Modified, with permission, from Rodnan GP. Gout and other crystalline forms of arthritis. Postgrad Med. 1975 Oct;58(5):6–14.

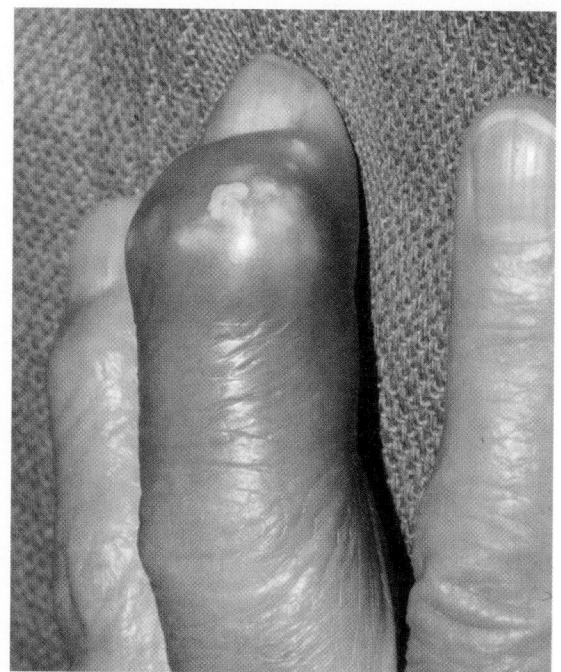

▲ **Figure 20–2.** Acute gouty arthritis superimposed on tophaceous gout. (Reproduced with permission from Geiderman JM. West J Med. 2000;172 (1):51-52.)

to 25% of cases. A normal serum uric acid level, therefore, does not exclude gout, especially in patients taking urate-lowering drugs. During an acute attack, the peripheral blood white cell count is frequently elevated. Identification of sodium urate crystals in joint fluid or material aspirated from a tophus establishes the diagnosis. The crystals, which may be extracellular or found within neutrophils, are needle-like and negatively birefringent when examined by polarized light microscopy.

C. Imaging

Early in the disease, radiographs show no changes. Later, punched-out erosions with an overhanging rim of cortical bone ("rat bite") develop. When these are adjacent to a soft tissue tophus, they are diagnostic of gout.

▶ Differential Diagnosis

Acute gout is often confused with cellulitis. Bacteriologic studies usually exclude acute pyogenic arthritis. Pseudogout is distinguished by the identification of calcium pyrophosphate crystals (positive birefringence) in the joint fluid, usually normal serum uric acid, and the radiographic appearance of chondrocalcinosis.

Chronic tophaceous arthritis may resemble chronic rheumatoid arthritis; gout is suggested by an earlier history of monarthritis and is established by the demonstration of urate crystals in a suspected tophus. Likewise, hips and shoulders are generally spared in tophaceous gout. Biopsy may be necessary to distinguish tophi from rheumatoid nodules. A radiographic appearance similar to that of gout

may be found in rheumatoid arthritis, sarcoidosis, multiple myeloma, hyperparathyroidism, or Hand-Schüller-Christian disease. Chronic lead intoxication may result in attacks of gouty arthritis (saturnine gout).

▶ Treatment

A. Asymptomatic Hyperuricemia

Asymptomatic hyperuricemia should not be treated; uric acid–lowering drugs need not be instituted until arthritis, renal calculi, or tophi become apparent.

B. Acute Attack

Arthritis is treated first and hyperuricemia weeks or months later, if at all. Sudden reduction of serum uric acid often precipitates further episodes of gouty arthritis.

1. NSAIDs—Oral NSAIDs in full dose (eg, naproxen 500 mg twice daily or indomethacin 25–50 mg every 8 hours; see Table 5–2) are effective treatment for acute gout and should be continued until the symptoms have resolved (usually 5–10 days). Contraindications include active peptic ulcer disease, impaired kidney function, and a history of allergic reaction to NSAIDs.

2. Colchicine—Oral colchicine is an appropriate treatment option for acute gout, provided the duration of the attack is less than 36 hours. For acute gout, colchicine should be administered orally as follows: a loading dose of 1.2 mg followed by a dose of 0.6 mg 1 hour later and then dosing for prophylaxis (0.6 mg once or twice daily) beginning 12 hours later. Patients who are already taking prophylactic doses of colchicine and have an acute flare of gout may receive the full loading dose (1.2 mg) followed by 0.6 mg 1 hour later (before resuming the usual 0.6 mg once or twice daily) provided they have not received this regimen within the preceding 14 days (in which case, NSAIDs or corticosteroids should be used). The use of oral colchicine during the intercritical period to prevent gout attacks is discussed below.

3. Corticosteroids—Corticosteroids often give dramatic symptomatic relief in acute episodes of gout and will control most attacks. They are most useful in patients with contraindications to the use of NSAIDs. Corticosteroids may be given intravenously (eg, methylprednisolone, 40 mg/d) or orally (eg, prednisone, 40–60 mg/d). These corticosteroids can be given at the suggested dose for 5–10 days and then simply discontinued or given at the suggested initial dose for 2–5 days and then tapered over 7–10 days. If the patient's gout is monarticular or oligoarticular, intra-articular administration of the corticosteroid (eg, triamcinolone, 10–40 mg depending on the size of the joint) is very effective. Because gouty and septic arthritis can coexist, albeit rarely, joint aspiration and Gram stain with culture of synovial fluid should be performed when intra-articular corticosteroids are given.

4. Interleukin-1 inhibitors—Anakinra (an interleukin-1 receptor antagonist), canakinumab (a monoclonal antibody against interleukin-1 beta), and rilonacept (a chimera composed of IgG constant domains and the extracellular components of the interleukin-1 receptor) have efficacy for the management of acute gout but these drugs have not been approved by the US Food and Drug Administration (FDA) for this indication.

C. Management between Attacks

Treatment during symptom-free periods is intended to minimize urate deposition in tissues, which causes chronic tophaceous arthritis, and to reduce the frequency and severity of recurrences. Potentially reversible causes of hyperuricemia are a high-purine diet, obesity, alcohol consumption, and use of certain medications (see below). Patients with a single episode of gout who are willing to lose weight and stop drinking alcohol are at low risk for another attack and may not require long-term medical therapy. In contrast, individuals with mild chronic kidney disease or with a history of multiple attacks of gout are likely to benefit from pharmacologic treatment. In general, the higher the uric acid level and the more frequent the attacks, the more likely that long-term medical therapy will be beneficial. All patients with tophaceous gout should receive urate-lowering therapy.

1. Diet—Excessive alcohol consumption can precipitate attacks and should be avoided. Beer consumption appears to confer a higher risk of gout than does whiskey or wine. Although dietary purines usually contribute only 1 mg/dL to the serum uric acid level, moderation in eating foods with high purine content is advisable (Table 20–5). Patients should avoid organ meats and beverages sweetened with

Table 20–5. The purine content of foods.[1]

Low-purine foods
Refined cereals and cereal products, cornflakes, white bread, pasta, flour, arrowroot, sago, tapioca, cakes
Milk, milk products, and eggs
Sugar, sweets, and gelatin
Butter, polyunsaturated margarine, and all other fats
Fruit, nuts, and peanut butter
Lettuce, tomatoes, and green vegetables (except those listed below)
Cream soups made with low-purine vegetables but without meat or meat stock
Water, fruit juice, cordials, and carbonated drinks
High-purine foods
All meats, including organ meats, and seafood
Meat extracts and gravies
Yeast and yeast extracts, beer, and other alcoholic beverages
Beans, peas, lentils, oatmeal, spinach, asparagus, cauliflower, and mushrooms

[1]The purine content of a food reflects its nucleoprotein content and turnover. Foods containing many nuclei (eg, liver) have many purines, as do rapidly growing foods such as asparagus. The consumption of large amounts of a food containing a small concentration of purines may provide a greater purine load than consumption of a small amount of a food containing a large concentration of purines.
Reproduced, with permission, from Emmerson BT. The management of gout. N Engl J Med. 1996 Feb 15;334(7):445–51.

high fructose corn syrup. A high liquid intake and, more importantly, a daily urinary output of 2 L or more will aid urate excretion and minimize urate precipitation in the urinary tract.

2. Avoidance of hyperuricemic medications—Thiazide and loop diuretics inhibit renal excretion of uric acid and, if possible, should be avoided in patients with gout. Similarly, niacin can raise serum uric acid levels and should be discontinued if there are therapeutic alternatives. Low doses of aspirin also aggravate hyperuricemia but, in general, should be continued due to their overriding benefits in cardiovascular prophylaxis.

3. Colchicine prophylaxis—There are two indications for daily colchicine administration. First, colchicine can be used to prevent future attacks for the individual who has mild hyperuricemia and only occasional attacks of gouty arthritis. Second, colchicine can be used when urate-lowering therapy (see below) is started, to suppress attacks precipitated by abrupt changes in the serum uric acid level. For either indication, the usual dose is 0.6 mg either once or twice a day. Colchicine is renally cleared. Patients who have coexisting moderate chronic kidney disease should take colchicine only once a day or once every other day in order to avoid peripheral neuromyopathy and other complications of colchicine toxicity.

4. Reduction of serum uric acid—Indications for a urate-lowering therapy in a person with gout include frequent acute arthritis (two or more episodes per year), tophaceous deposits, or chronic kidney disease (stage 2 or worse). If instituted, the minimum goal of urate-lowering therapy is to maintain the serum uric acid at or below 6 mg/dL or 357 mcmol/L (ie, below the level at which serum is supersaturated with uric acid, thereby allowing urate crystals to solubilize); in some cases, control of gout may require lowering serum uric acid to less than 5 mg/dL or 297.4 mcmol/L. Lowering serum uric acid levels is not of benefit for the treatment of an acute gout flare. Asymptomatic hyperuricemia should not be treated.

Three classes of agents may be used to lower the serum uric acid—xanthine oxidase inhibitors (allopurinol or febuxostat), uricosuric agents, and uricase (pegloticase). Xanthine oxidase inhibitors are the preferred first-line agents for urate lowering. The uricosuric agent, probenecid, is an acceptable alternative, provided the serum creatinine clearance is > 50 mL/minute and there is no history of nephrolithiasis. The uricase, pegloticase, requires intravenous administration and is indicated only in patients with chronic gout refractory to other treatments.

A. XANTHINE OXIDASE INHIBITORS—The xanthine oxidase inhibitors, allopurinol and febuxostat, lower plasma uric acid levels by blocking the final enzymatic steps in the production of uric acid. Allopurinol and febuxostat should not to be used together but they can be tried sequentially if the initial agent fails to lower serum uric acid to the target level or if it is not tolerated. The most frequent adverse effect with either medication is the precipitation of an acute gouty attack; thus, patients generally should be receiving prophylactic doses of colchicine.

Hypersensitivity to allopurinol occurs in 2% of cases, usually within the first few months of therapy, and it can be life-threatening. The most common sign of hypersensitivity is a pruritic rash that may progress to toxic epidermal necrolysis, particularly if allopurinol is continued; vasculitis and hepatitis are other manifestations. Patients should be instructed to stop allopurinol immediately if a rash develops. Chronic kidney disease and concomitant thiazide therapy are risk factors. In certain ethnic groups, there is a strong association between HLA-B*5801 and allopurinol hypersensitivity. Current recommendations are to screen for HLA-B*5801 prior to initiating allopurinol in Han Chinese, those of Thai descent, and Koreans with stage 3 or worse chronic kidney disease.

The initial daily dose of allopurinol is 100 mg/d orally (50 mg/d for those with stage 4 or worse chronic kidney disease); the dose of allopurinol should be titrated upward every 2–5 weeks to achieve the target serum uric acid level (either ≤ 6.0 mg/dL [357 mcmol/L] or ≤ 5.0 mg/dL [297.4 mcmol/L]). Successful treatment usually requires a dose of at least 300 mg of allopurinol daily. The maximum daily dose is 800 mg.

Allopurinol interacts with other drugs. The combined use of allopurinol and ampicillin causes a drug rash in 20% of patients. Allopurinol can increase the half-life of probenecid, while probenecid increases the excretion of allopurinol. Thus, a patient taking both drugs may need to use slightly higher than usual doses of allopurinol and lower doses of probenecid.

Febuxostat does not cause the hypersensitivity reactions seen with allopurinol and can be given without dose adjustment to patients with mild to moderate kidney disease. However, abnormal liver tests may develop in 2–3% of patients taking febuxostat. In addition, one clinical study showed that febuxostat was associated with a slightly higher rate of fatal and nonfatal cardiovascular events than allopurinol (0.97 vs 0.58 per 100 patient-years). The initial dose of febuxostat is 40 mg/d orally. If the target serum uric acid is not reached, the dose of febuxostat can be increased to 80 mg/d and then to the maximum dose of 120 mg/d.

B. Uricosuric drugs—Uricosuric drugs lower serum uric acid levels by blocking the tubular reabsorption of filtered urate, thereby increasing uric acid excretion by the kidney. Probenecid (0.5 g/d orally) is the uricosuric of choice in the United States. It is an acceptable alternative when xanthine oxidase inhibitors cannot be used and can be added when monotherapy with a xanthine oxidase inhibitor fails to reach the target serum uric acid. Probenecid should not be used in patients with a creatinine clearance of < 50 mL/min due to limited efficacy; contraindications include a history of nephrolithiasis (uric acid or calcium stones) and evidence of overproduction of uric acid (ie, > 800 mg of uric acid in a 24-hour urine collection). To reduce the development of uric acid stones (which occur in up to 11%), patients should be advised to increase their fluid intake and clinicians should consider prescribing an alkalinizing agent

(eg, potassium citrate, 30–80 mEq/d orally) to maintain a urine pH of > 6.0.

C. Uricase—Pegloticase, a recombinant uricase that must be administered intravenously (8 mg every 2 weeks), is indicated for the rare patient with refractory chronic tophaceous gout. Pegloticase carries a "Black Box Warning," which advises administering the drug only in health care settings and by health care professionals prepared to manage anaphylactic and other serious infusion reactions.

D. Chronic Tophaceous Arthritis

With rigorous medical compliance, allopurinol or febuxostat or pegloticase shrinks tophi and in time can lead to their disappearance. Resorption of extensive tophi requires maintaining a serum uric acid below 6 mg/dL. Surgical excision of large tophi offers mechanical improvement in selected deformities.

E. Gout in the Transplant Patient

Hyperuricemia and gout commonly develop in many transplant patients because they have decreased kidney function and require drugs that inhibit uric acid excretion (especially cyclosporine and diuretics). Treating acute gout in these patients is challenging. Often the best approach for monarticular gout—after excluding infection—is injecting corticosteroids into the joint (see above). For polyarticular gout, increasing the dose of systemic corticosteroid may be the only alternative. Since transplant patients often have multiple attacks of gout, long-term relief requires lowering the serum uric acid with allopurinol or febuxostat. (Kidney dysfunction seen in many transplant patients makes uricosuric agents ineffective.) Both allopurinol and febuxostat inhibit the metabolism of azathioprine and should be avoided in patients who must take azathioprine.

▶ Prognosis

Without treatment, the acute attack may last from a few days to several weeks. The intervals between acute attacks vary up to years, but the asymptomatic periods often become shorter if the disease progresses. Chronic gouty arthritis occurs after repeated attacks of acute gout, but only after inadequate treatment. The younger the patient at the onset of disease, the greater the tendency to a progressive course. Destructive arthropathy is rarely seen in patients whose first attack is after age 50.

Patients with gout are anecdotally thought to have an increased incidence of hypertension, kidney disease (eg, nephrosclerosis, interstitial nephritis, pyelonephritis), diabetes mellitus, hypertriglyceridemia, and atherosclerosis.

Becker MA et al. Long-term safety of pegloticase in chronic gout refractory to conventional treatment. Ann Rheum Dis. 2013 Sep 1;72(9):1469–74. [PMID: 23144450]

Doghramji PP et al. Hyperuricemia and gout: new concepts in diagnosis and management. Postgrad Med. 2012 Nov;124(6): 98–109. [PMID: 23322143]

Khanna D et al. 2012 American College of Rheumatology guidelines for management of gout. Part 1: systemic nonpharmacologic and pharmacologic therapeutic approaches to hyperuricemia. Arthritis Care Res (Hoboken). 2012 Oct;64(10):1431–46. [PMID: 23024028]

Khanna D et al. 2012 American College of Rheumatology guidelines for management of gout. Part 2: therapy and antiinflammatory prophylaxis of acute gouty arthritis. Arthritis Care Res (Hoboken). 2012 Oct;64(10):1447–61. [PMID: 23024029]

Neogi T. Clinical practice. Gout. N Engl J Med. 2011 Feb 3;364(5):443–52. [PMID: 21288096]

Stamp LK et al. Gout and its comorbidities: implications for therapy. Rheumatology (Oxford). 2013 Jan;52(1):34–44. [PMID: 22949727]

2. Calcium Pyrophosphate Deposition

Calcium pyrophosphate deposition (CPPD) in fibrocartilage and hyaline cartilage (chondrocalcinosis) can cause an acute crystal-induced arthritis ("pseudogout"), a degenerative arthropathy, and a chronic inflammatory polyarthritis ("pseudorheumatoid arthritis"). CPPD also can be an asymptomatic condition detected as incidental chondrocalcinosis on radiographs. The prevalence of CPPD increases with age. Hyperparathyroidism, hemochromatosis, and hypomagnesemia confer risk of CPPD, but most cases have no associated condition.

Pseudogout is most often seen in persons age 60 or older, is characterized by acute, recurrent and rarely chronic arthritis involving large joints (most commonly the knees and the wrists) and is almost always accompanied by radiographic chondrocalcinosis of the affected joints. Pseudogout, like gout, frequently develops 24–48 hours after major surgery. Identification of calcium pyrophosphate crystals in joint aspirates is diagnostic. NSAIDs are helpful in the treatment of acute episodes. Colchicine, 0.6 mg orally once or twice daily, is more effective for prophylaxis than for acute attacks. Aspiration of the inflamed joint and intra-articular injection of triamcinolone, 10–40 mg, depending on the size of the joint, are also of value in resistant cases.

The degenerative arthropathy associated with CPPD can involve joints not usually affected by osteoarthritis (eg, glenohumeral joint, wrist, patellofemoral compartment of the knee). The "pseudorheumatoid arthritis" of CPPD affects the metacarpophalangeal joints and wrists. In both conditions, radiographs demonstrate chondrocalcinosis and degenerative changes such as asymmetric joint space narrowing and osteophyte formation.

Filippucci E et al. Tips and tricks to recognize microcrystalline arthritis. Rheumatology (Oxford). 2012 Dec;51(Suppl 7):vii18–21. [PMID: 23230088]

Rho YH et al. Risk factors for pseudogout in the general population. Rheumatology (Oxford). 2012 Nov;51(11):2070–4. [PMID: 22886340]

Zhang W et al. EULAR recommendations for calcium pyrophosphate deposition. Part II: management. Ann Rheum Dis. 2011 Apr;70(4):571–5. [PMID: 21257614]

Zhang W et al. European League Against Rheumatism recommendations for calcium pyrophosphate deposition. Part I: terminology and diagnosis. Ann Rheum Dis. 2011 Apr;70(4):563–70. [PMID: 21216817]

AUTOIMMUNE DISEASES

RHEUMATOID ARTHRITIS

 ESSENTIALS OF DIAGNOSIS

▶ Usually insidious onset with morning stiffness and pain in affected joints.

▶ Symmetric polyarthritis with predilection for small joints of the hands and feet; deformities common with progressive disease.

▶ Radiographic findings: juxta-articular osteoporosis, joint erosions, and joint space narrowing.

▶ Rheumatoid factor and antibodies to cyclic citrullinated peptides (anti-CCP) are present in 70–80%.

▶ Extra-articular manifestations: subcutaneous nodules, interstitial lung disease, pleural effusion, pericarditis, splenomegaly with leukopenia, and vasculitis.

▶ General Considerations

Rheumatoid arthritis is a chronic systemic inflammatory disease whose major manifestation is synovitis of multiple joints. It has a prevalence of 1% and is more common in women than men (female:male ratio of 3:1). Rheumatoid arthritis can begin at any age, but the peak onset is in the fourth or fifth decade for women and the sixth to eighth decades for men. The cause is not known. Susceptibility to rheumatoid arthritis is genetically determined with multiple genes contributing. Inheritance of HLA DRB1 alleles encoding a distinctive five-amino-acid sequence known as the "shared epitope" is the best characterized genetic risk factor. Untreated, rheumatoid arthritis causes joint destruction with consequent disability and shortens life expectancy. Early, aggressive treatment is the standard of care.

The pathologic findings in the joint include chronic synovitis with formation of a pannus, which erodes cartilage, bone, ligaments, and tendons. In the acute phase, effusion and other manifestations of inflammation are common. In the late stage, organization may result in fibrous ankylosis; true bony ankylosis is rare.

▶ Clinical Findings

A. Symptoms and Signs

1. Joint symptoms—The clinical manifestations of rheumatoid disease are highly variable, but joint symptoms usually predominate. Although acute presentations may occur, the onset of articular signs of inflammation is usually insidious, with prodromal symptoms of vague periarticular pain or stiffness. Symmetric swelling of multiple joints with tenderness and pain is characteristic. Monarticular disease is occasionally seen initially. Stiffness persisting for > 30 minutes (and usually many hours) is prominent in the morning. Stiffness may recur after daytime inactivity and be much more severe after strenuous

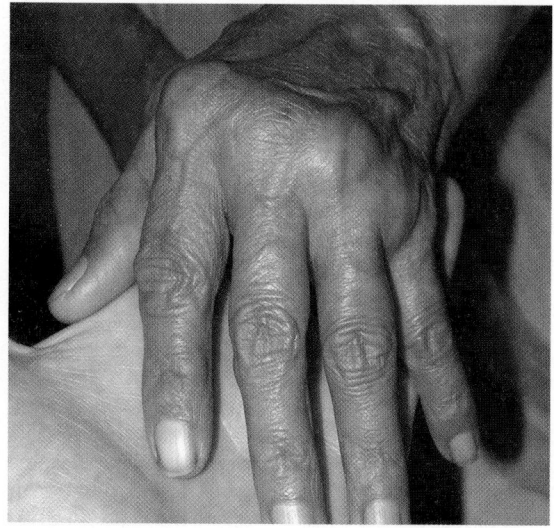

Figure 20–3. Rheumatoid arthritis with ulnar deviation at the metacarpophalangeal (MCP) joints. (Reproduced with permission, from Richard P. Usatine, MD.)

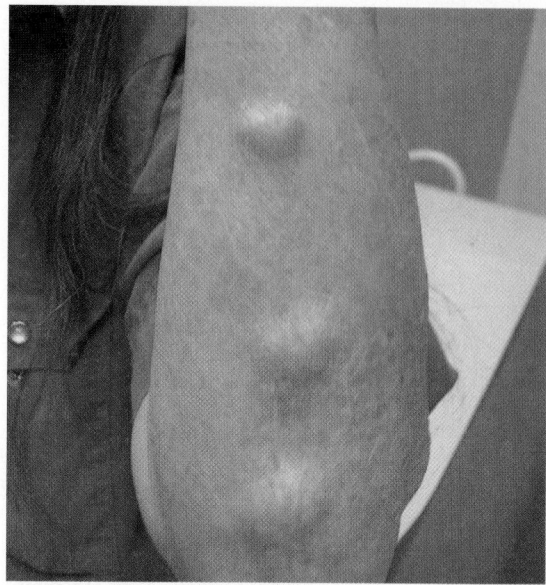

Figure 20–4. Rheumatoid nodules over the extensor surface of the forearm (Reproduced with permission, from Richard P. Usatine, MD).

activity. Although any diarthrodial joint may be affected, PIP joints of the fingers, MCP joints (Figure 20–3), wrists, knees, ankles, and MTP joints are most often involved. Synovial cysts and rupture of tendons may occur. Entrapment syndromes are not unusual—particularly of the median nerve at the carpal tunnel of the wrist. Rheumatoid arthritis can affect the neck but spares the other components of the spine and does not involve the sacroiliac joints. In advanced disease, atlantoaxial (C1–C2) subluxation can lead to myelopathy.

2. Rheumatoid nodules—Twenty percent of patients have subcutaneous rheumatoid nodules, most commonly situated over bony prominences but also observed in the bursae and tendon sheaths (Figure 20–4). Nodules are occasionally seen in the lungs, the sclerae, and other tissues. Nodules correlate with the presence of rheumatoid factor in serum ("seropositivity"), as do most other extraarticular manifestations.

3. Ocular symptoms—Dryness of the eyes, mouth, and other mucous membranes is found especially in advanced disease (see Sjögren syndrome). Other ocular manifestations include episcleritis, scleritis, and scleromalacia due to scleral nodules.

4. Other symptoms—Interstitial lung disease is not uncommon (estimates of prevalence vary widely according to method of detection) and manifests clinically as cough and progressive dyspnea. Pericarditis and pleural disease, when present, are usually silent clinically. Patients with active joint disease often have palmar erythema. Occasionally, a small vessel vasculitis develops and manifests as tiny hemorrhagic infarcts in the nail folds or finger pulps. Although necrotizing arteritis is well reported, it is rare. A small subset of patients with rheumatoid arthritis have Felty syndrome, the occurrence of splenomegaly and neutropenia, usually in the setting of severe, destructive arthritis. Felty syndrome must be distinguished from the large granular lymphocyte syndrome, with which it shares many features.

Aortitis is a rare late complication that can result in aortic regurgitation or rupture and is usually associated with evidence of rheumatoid vasculitis elsewhere in the body.

B. Laboratory Findings

Anti-CCP antibodies and rheumatoid factor, an IgM antibody directed against the Fc fragment of IgG, are present in 70–80% of patients with established rheumatoid arthritis. Rheumatoid factor has a sensitivity of only 50% in early disease. Anti-CCP antibodies are the most specific blood test for rheumatoid arthritis (specificity ~95%). Rheumatoid factor can occur in other autoimmune disease and in chronic infections, including hepatitis C, syphilis, subacute bacterial endocarditis, and tuberculosis. The prevalence of rheumatoid factor positivity also rises with age in healthy individuals. Approximately 20% of rheumatoid patients have antinuclear antibodies.

The ESR and levels of C-reactive protein are typically elevated in proportion to disease activity. A moderate hypochromic normocytic anemia is common. The white cell count is normal or slightly elevated, but leukopenia may occur, often in the presence of splenomegaly (eg, Felty syndrome). The platelet count is often elevated, roughly in proportion to the severity of overall joint inflammation. Initial joint fluid examination confirms the inflammatory nature of the arthritis (see Table 20–2). Arthrocentesis is needed to diagnose superimposed septic arthritis, which is a common complication of rheumatoid arthritis and should be considered whenever a patient with rheumatoid arthritis has one joint inflamed out of proportion to the rest.

C. Imaging

Of all the laboratory tests, radiographic changes are the most specific for rheumatoid arthritis. Radiographs obtained during the first 6 months of symptoms, however, are usually normal. The earliest changes occur in the hands or feet and consist of soft tissue swelling and juxta-articular demineralization. Later, diagnostic changes of uniform joint space narrowing and erosions develop. The erosions are often first evident at the ulnar styloid and at the juxta-articular margin where the bony surface is not protected by cartilage. Characteristic changes also occur in the cervical spine, with C1-2 subluxation, but these changes usually take many years to develop. Although both MRI and ultrasonography are more sensitive than radiographs in detecting bony and soft tissue changes in rheumatoid arthritis, their value in early diagnosis relative to that of plain radiographs has not been established.

▶ Differential Diagnosis

The differentiation of rheumatoid arthritis from other joint conditions and immune-mediated disorders can be difficult. In 2010, the American College of Rheumatology updated their classification criteria for rheumatoid arthritis. In contrast to rheumatoid arthritis, osteoarthritis spares the wrist and the MCP joints. Osteoarthritis is not associated with constitutional manifestations, and the joint pain is characteristically relieved by rest, unlike the morning stiffness of rheumatoid arthritis. Signs of articular inflammation, prominent in rheumatoid arthritis, are usually minimal in degenerative joint disease. CPPD disease can cause a degenerative arthropathy of the MCPs and wrists; radiographs are usually diagnostic. Although gouty arthritis is almost always intermittent and monarticular in the early years, it may evolve with time into a chronic polyarticular process that mimics rheumatoid arthritis. Gouty tophi can resemble rheumatoid nodules both in typical location and appearance. The early history of intermittent monarthritis and the presence of synovial urate crystals are distinctive features of gout. Spondyloarthropathies, particularly earlier in their course, can be a source of diagnostic uncertainty; predilection for lower extremities and involvement of the spine and sacroiliac joints point to the correct diagnosis. Chronic Lyme arthritis typically involves only one joint, most commonly the knee, and is associated with positive serologic tests (see Chapter 34). Human parvovirus B19 infection in adults can mimic early rheumatoid arthritis. However, arthralgias are more prominent than arthritis, fever is common, IgM antibodies to parvovirus B19 are present, and the arthritis usually resolves within weeks. Infection with hepatitis C can cause a chronic nonerosive polyarthritis associated with rheumatoid factor; tests for anti-CCP antibodies are negative.

Malar rash, photosensitivity, discoid skin lesions, alopecia, high titer antibodies to double-stranded DNA, glomerulonephritis, and central nervous system abnormalities point to the diagnosis of SLE. Polymyalgia rheumatica occasionally causes polyarthralgias in patients over age 50, but these patients remain rheumatoid factor–negative and have chiefly proximal muscle pain and stiffness, centered on the shoulder and hip girdles. Joint pain that can be confused with rheumatoid arthritis presents in a substantial minority of patients with granulomatosis with polyangiitis (formerly Wegener granulomatosis). This diagnostic error can be avoided by recognizing that, in contrast to rheumatoid arthritis, the arthritis of granulomatosis with polyangiitis preferentially involves large joints (eg, hips, ankles, wrists) and usually spares the small joints of the hand. Rheumatic fever is characterized by the migratory nature of the arthritis, an elevated antistreptolysin titer, and a more dramatic and prompt response to aspirin; carditis and erythema marginatum may occur in adults, but chorea and subcutaneous nodules virtually never do. Finally, a variety of cancers produce paraneoplastic syndromes, including polyarthritis. One form is hypertrophic pulmonary osteoarthropathy most often produced by lung and gastrointestinal carcinomas, characterized by a rheumatoid-like arthritis associated with clubbing, periosteal new bone formation, and a negative rheumatoid factor. Diffuse swelling of the hands with palmar fasciitis occurs in a variety of cancers, especially ovarian carcinoma.

▶ Treatment

The primary objectives in treating rheumatoid arthritis are reduction of inflammation and pain, preservation of function, and prevention of deformity. Success requires early, effective pharmacologic intervention. Disease-modifying antirheumatic drugs (DMARDs) should be started as soon as the diagnosis of rheumatoid disease is certain and then adjusted with the aim of suppressing disease activity. NSAIDs provide some symptomatic relief in rheumatoid arthritis but do not prevent erosions or alter disease progression. They are not appropriate for monotherapy and should only be used in conjunction with DMARDs, if at all. The American College of Rheumatology recommends using standardized assessments, such as the Disease Activity Score 28 Joints (DAS28), to gauge therapeutic responses, with the target of mild disease activity or remission by these measures. In advanced disease, surgical intervention may help improve function of damaged joints and to relieve pain.

A. Corticosteroids

Low-dose corticosteroids (eg, oral prednisone 5–10 mg daily) produce a prompt anti-inflammatory effect in rheumatoid arthritis and slow the rate of articular erosion. These often are used as a "bridge" to reduce disease activity until the slower acting DMARDs take effect or as adjunctive therapy for active disease that persists despite treatment with DMARDs. No more than 10 mg of prednisone or equivalent per day is appropriate for articular disease. Many patients do reasonably well on 5–7.5 mg daily. (The use of 1 mg tablets, to facilitate doses of < 5 mg/d, is encouraged.) Higher doses are used to manage serious extra-articular manifestations (eg, pericarditis, necrotizing scleritis). When the corticosteroids are to be discontinued, they should be tapered gradually on a planned schedule appropriate to the duration of treatment. All patients receiving long-term corticosteroid therapy should take measures to prevent osteoporosis.

Intra-articular corticosteroids may be helpful if one or two joints are the chief source of difficulty. Intra-articular triamcinolone, 10–40 mg depending on the size of the joint to be injected, may be given for symptomatic relief but not more than four times a year.

B. Synthetic DMARDs

1. Methotrexate—Methotrexate is usually the initial synthetic DMARD of choice for patients with rheumatoid arthritis. It is generally well tolerated and often produces a beneficial effect in 2–6 weeks. The usual initial dose is 7.5 mg of methotrexate orally once weekly. If the patient has tolerated methotrexate but has not responded in 1 month, the dose can be increased to 15 mg orally once per week. The maximal dose is usually 20–25 mg/wk. The most frequent side effects are gastric irritation and stomatitis. Cytopenia, most commonly leukopenia or thrombocytopenia but rarely pancytopenia, due to bone marrow suppression is another important potential problem. The risk of developing pancytopenia is much higher in patients with elevation of the serum creatinine (≥ 2 mg/dL or ≥ 176.8 mcmol/L). Hepatotoxicity with fibrosis and cirrhosis is an important toxic effect that correlates with cumulative dose and is uncommon with appropriate monitoring of liver function tests. Methotrexate is contraindicated in a patient with any form of chronic hepatitis. Heavy alcohol use increases the hepatotoxicity, so patients should be advised to drink alcohol in extreme moderation, if at all. Diabetes mellitus, obesity, and kidney disease also increase the risk of hepatotoxicity. Liver function tests should be monitored at least every 12 weeks, along with a complete blood count. The dose of methotrexate should be reduced if aminotransferase levels are elevated, and the drug should be discontinued if abnormalities persist despite dosage reduction. Gastric irritation, stomatitis, cytopenias, and hepatotoxicity are reduced by prescribing either daily folate (1 mg orally) or weekly leucovorin calcium (2.5–5 mg taken orally 24 hours after the dose of methotrexate). Hypersensitivity to methotrexate can cause an acute or subacute interstitial pneumonitis that can be life-threatening but which usually responds to cessation of the drug and institution of corticosteroids. Because methotrexate is teratogenic, women of child bearing age as well as men must use effective contraception while taking the medication. Methotrexate is associated with an increased risk of B cell lymphomas, some of which resolve following the discontinuation of the medication. The combination of methotrexate and other folate antagonists, such as trimethoprim-sulfamethoxazole, should be used cautiously since pancytopenia can result. Amoxicillin can decrease renal clearance of methotrexate, leading to toxicity. Probenecid also increases methotrexate drug levels and toxicity and should be avoided.

2. Sulfasalazine—This drug is a second-line agent for rheumatoid arthritis. It is usually introduced at a dosage of 0.5 g orally twice daily and then increased each week by 0.5 g until the patient improves or the daily dose reaches 3 g. Side effects, particularly neutropenia and thrombocytopenia, occur in 10–25% and are serious in 2–5%. Sulfasalazine also causes hemolysis in patients with glucose-6-phosphate dehydrogenase (G6PD) deficiency, so a G6PD level should be checked before initiating sulfasalazine. Patients with aspirin sensitivity should not be given sulfasalazine. Patients taking sulfasalazine should have complete blood counts monitored every 2–4 weeks for the first 3 months, then every 3 months.

3. Leflunomide—Leflunomide, a pyrimidine synthesis inhibitor, is also FDA-approved for treatment of rheumatoid arthritis and is administered as a single oral daily dose of 20 mg. The most frequent side effects are diarrhea, rash, reversible alopecia, and hepatotoxicity. Some patients experience dramatic unexplained weight loss. The drug is carcinogenic, teratogenic, and has a half-life of 2 weeks. Thus, it is contraindicated in premenopausal women or in men who wish to father children.

4. Antimalarials—Hydroxychloroquine sulfate is the antimalarial agent most often used against rheumatoid arthritis. Monotherapy with hydroxychloroquine should be reserved for patients with mild disease because only a small percentage will respond and in some of those cases only after 3–6 months of therapy. Hydroxychloroquine is often used in combination with other conventional DMARDs, particularly methotrexate and sulfasalazine. The advantage of hydroxychloroquine is its comparatively low toxicity, especially at a dosage of 200–400 mg/d orally (not to exceed 6.5 mg/kg/d). The most important reaction, pigmentary retinitis causing visual loss, is rare at this dose. Ophthalmologic examinations every 12 months are required when this drug is used for long-term therapy. Other reactions include neuropathies and myopathies of both skeletal and cardiac muscle, which usually improve when the drug is withdrawn.

5. Minocycline—Minocycline is more effective than placebo for rheumatoid arthritis. It is reserved for early, mild cases, since its efficacy is modest, and it works better during the first year of rheumatoid arthritis. The mechanism of action is not clear, but tetracyclines do have anti-inflammatory properties, including the ability to inhibit destructive enzymes such as collagenase. The dosage of minocycline is 200 mg orally daily. Adverse effects are uncommon except for dizziness, which occurs in about 10%.

6. Tofacitinib—Tofacitinib, an inhibitor of Janus kinase 3, was approved in 2012 by the FDA for use in severe rheumatoid arthritis that is refractory to methotrexate. It is administered orally in a dose of 5 mg twice daily and can be used either as monotherapy or in combination with methotrexate. Tofacitinib increases the risk of opportunistic and other serious infections; patients should be screened and treated for latent tuberculosis prior to receiving the drug.

C. Biologic DMARDs

1. Tumor necrosis factor inhibitors—Inhibitors of tumor necrosis factor (TNF)—a pro-inflammatory cytokine—are fulfilling the aim of targeted therapy for rheumatoid arthritis. These medications are frequently added to the treatment of patients who have not responded adequately to methotrexate and are increasingly used as initial therapy in combination with methotrexate for patients with poor prognostic factors.

Five inhibitors are in use: etanercept, infliximab, adalimumab, golimumab, and certolizumab pegol. Etanercept, a soluble recombinant TNF receptor:Fc fusion protein, is usually administered at a dosage of 50 mg subcutaneously once per week. Infliximab, a chimeric monoclonal antibody, is administered at a dosage of 3–10 mg/kg intravenously; infusions are repeated after 2, 6, 10, and 14 weeks and then are administered every 8 weeks. Adalimumab, a human monoclonal antibody that binds to TNF, is given at a dosage of 40 mg subcutaneously every other week. The dose for golimumab, a human anti-TNF monoclonal antibody, is 50 mg subcutaneously once monthly. Certolizumab pegol is a PEGylated monoclonal antibody TNF inhibitor; the dose is 200–400 mg subcutaneously every 2 to 4 weeks. Each drug produces substantial improvement in more than 60% of patients. Each is usually very well tolerated. Minor irritation at injection sites is the most common side effect of etanercept and adalimumab. Rarely, nonrecurrent leukopenia develops in patients. TNF plays a physiologic role in combating many types of infection; TNF inhibitors have been associated with a several-fold increased risk of serious bacterial infections and a striking increase in granulomatous infections, particularly reactivation of tuberculosis. Screening for latent tuberculosis (see Chapter 9) is mandatory before the initiation of TNF blockers. It is prudent to suspend TNF blockers when a fever or other manifestations of a clinically important infection develops in a patient. Demyelinating neurologic complications that resemble multiple sclerosis have been reported rarely in patients taking etanercept, but the true magnitude of this risk—likely quite small—has not been determined with precision. While there are conflicting data with respect to increased risk of malignancy, in 2009, the FDA issued a safety alert about case reports of malignancies, including leukemias, in patients treated with TNF inhibitors. Contrary to expectation, TNF inhibitors were not effective in the treatment of heart failure. The use of infliximab, in fact, was associated with increased morbidity in a heart failure trial. Consequently, TNF inhibitors should be used with extreme caution in patients with heart failure. Infliximab can rarely cause anaphylaxis and induce anti-DNA antibodies (but rarely clinically evident SLE). A final concern about TNF inhibitors is the expense, which is more than $10,000 per year.

2. Abatacept—Abatacept, a recombinant protein made by fusing a fragment of the Fc domain of human IgG with the extracellular domain of a T-cell inhibitory receptor (CTLA4), blocks T-cell costimulation. It is approved by the FDA for use in rheumatoid arthritis and produces clinically meaningful responses in approximately 50% of individuals whose disease is active despite the combination of methotrexate and a TNF inhibitor.

3. Rituximab—Rituximab is a humanized mouse monoclonal antibody that depletes B cells. It is approved by the FDA to be used in combination with methotrexate for patients whose disease has been refractory to treatment with a TNF inhibitor.

4. Tocilizumab—Tocilizumab is a monoclonal antibody that blocks the receptor for IL-6, an inflammatory cytokine involved in the pathogenesis of rheumatoid arthritis. It also is approved by the FDA to be used in combination with methotrexate for patients whose disease has been refractory to treatment with a TNF inhibitor.

D. DMARD Combinations

As a general rule, DMARDs have greater efficacy when administered in combination than when used individually. Currently, the most commonly used combination is that of methotrexate with one of the TNF inhibitors, which clearly is superior to methotrexate alone. The combination of methotrexate, sulfasalazine, and hydroxychloroquine is also effective. The American College of Rheumatology has published detailed recommendations on the initiation of DMARD combinations.

▶ Course & Prognosis

After months or years, deformities may occur; the most common are ulnar deviation of the fingers, boutonnière deformity (hyperextension of the DIP joint with flexion of the PIP joint), "swan-neck" deformity (flexion of the DIP joint with extension of the PIP joint), valgus deformity of the knee, and volar subluxation of the MTP joints. The excess mortality associated with rheumatoid arthritis is largely due to cardiovascular disease that is unexplained by traditional risk factors and that appears to be a result of deleterious effects of chronic systemic inflammation on the vascular system.

▶ When to Refer

Early referral to a rheumatologist is essential for appropriate diagnosis and the timely introduction of effective therapy.

Aletaha D et al. 2010 Rheumatoid arthritis classification criteria: an American College of Rheumatology/European League Against Rheumatism collaborative initiative. Arthritis Rheum. 2010 Sep;62(9):2569–81. [PMID: 20872595]

Huizinga TW et al. In the clinic. Rheumatoid arthritis. Ann Intern Med. 2010 Jul 6;153(1):ITC1–15. [PMID: 20621898]

O'Dell JR et al; CSP 551 RACAT Investigators. Therapies for active rheumatoid arthritis after methotrexate failure. N Engl J Med. 2013 Jul 25;369(4):307–18. [PMID: 23755969]

O'Dell JR et al; TEAR Trial Investigators. Validation of the methotrexate-first strategy in patients with early, poor-prognosis rheumatoid arthritis: results from a two-year randomized, double-blind trial. Arthritis Rheum. 2013 Aug;65(8):1985–94. [PMID: 23686414]

Schiff M. Subcutaneous abatacept for the treatment of rheumatoid arthritis. Rheumatology (Oxford). 2013 Jun;52(6):986–97. [PMID: 23463804]

Singh JA et al. 2012 update of the 2008 American College of Rheumatology recommendations for the use of disease-modifying antirheumatic drugs and biologic agents in the treatment of rheumatoid arthritis. Arthritis Care Res (Hoboken). 2012 May;64(5):625–39. [PMID: 22473917]

ADULT STILL DISEASE

Still disease is a systemic form of juvenile chronic arthritis in which high spiking fevers are much more prominent, especially at the outset, than arthritis. This syndrome also occurs in adults. Most adults are in their 20s or 30s; onset after age 60 is rare. The fever is dramatic, often with daily spikes to 40°C, associated with sweats and chills, and then plunging to normal or several degrees below normal in the absence of antipyretics. Many patients initially complain of sore throat. An evanescent salmon-colored nonpruritic rash, chiefly on the chest and abdomen, is a characteristic feature. The rash can easily be missed since it often appears only with the fever spike. Many patients also have lymphadenopathy and pericardial effusions. Joint symptoms are mild or absent in the beginning, but a destructive arthritis, especially of the wrists, may develop months later. Anemia and leukocytosis, with white blood counts sometimes exceeding 40,000/mcL, are the rule. Although there must be exclusion of other causes of fever, the diagnosis of adult Still disease is strongly suggested by the quotidian fever pattern, sore throat, and the classic rash. About half of the patients respond to high-dose aspirin (eg, 1 g three times orally daily) or other NSAIDs, and half require prednisone, sometimes in doses > 60 mg/d orally. For patients with refractory adult Still disease, the IL-1 receptor antagonist, anakinra, and the IL-6 receptor inhibitor, tocilizumab, appear to be more effective than anti-TNF agents.

Bagnari V et al. Adult-onset Still's disease. Rheumatol Int. 2010 May;30(7):855–62. [PMID: 20020138]
Pouchot J et al. Biological treatment in adult-onset Still's disease. Best Pract Res Clin Rheumatol. 2012 Aug;26(4):477–87. [PMID: 23040362]
Sakai R et al. Successful treatment of adult-onset Still's disease with tocilizumab monotherapy: two case reports and literature review. Clin Rheumatol. 2012 Mar;31(3):569–74. [PMID: 22215118]

SYSTEMIC LUPUS ERYTHEMATOSUS

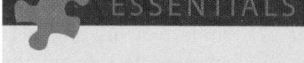 ESSENTIALS OF DIAGNOSIS

▶ Occurs mainly in young women.

▶ Rash over areas exposed to sunlight.

▶ Joint symptoms in 90% of patients. Multiple system involvement.

▶ Anemia, leukopenia, thrombocytopenia.

▶ Glomerulonephritis, central nervous system disease, and complications of antiphospholipid antibodies are major sources of disease morbidity.

▶ Serologic findings: antinuclear antibodies (100%), anti–double-stranded DNA antibodies (approximately two-thirds), and low serum complement levels (particularly during disease flares).

▶ **General Considerations**

SLE is an inflammatory autoimmune disorder characterized by autoantibodies to nuclear antigens. It can affect multiple organ systems. Many of its clinical manifestations are secondary to the trapping of antigen-antibody complexes in

capillaries of visceral structures or to autoantibody-mediated destruction of host cells (eg, thrombocytopenia). The clinical course is marked by spontaneous remission and relapses. The severity may vary from a mild episodic disorder to a rapidly fulminant, life-threatening illness.

The incidence of SLE is influenced by many factors, including gender, race, and genetic inheritance. About 85% of patients are women. Sex hormones appear to play some role; most cases develop after menarche and before menopause. Among older individuals, the gender distribution is more equal. Race is also a factor, as SLE occurs in 1:1000 white women but in 1:250 black women. Familial occurrence of SLE has been repeatedly documented, and the disorder is concordant in 25–70% of identical twins. If a mother has SLE, her daughters' risks of developing the disease are 1:40 and her sons' risks are 1:250. Aggregation of serologic abnormalities (positive antinuclear antibody) is seen in asymptomatic family members, and the prevalence of other rheumatic diseases is increased among close relatives of patients. The importance of specific genes in SLE is emphasized by the high frequency of certain HLA haplotypes, especially DR2 and DR3, and null complement alleles.

Before making a diagnosis of SLE, it is imperative to ascertain that the condition has not been induced by a drug (Table 20–6). Procainamide, hydralazine, and isoniazid are the best-studied drugs. While antinuclear antibody tests and other serologic findings become positive in many persons receiving these agents, clinical manifestations occur in only a few.

Four features of **drug-induced lupus** separate it from SLE: (1) the sex ratio is nearly equal; (2) nephritis and central

Table 20–6. Drugs associated with lupus erythematosus.

Definite association	
Chlorpromazine	Minocycline
Hydralazine	Procainamide
Isoniazid	Quinidine
Methyldopa	
Possible association	
Beta-blockers	Nitrofurantoin
Captopril	Penicillamine
Carbamazepine	Phenytoin
Cimetidine	Propylthiouracil
Ethosuximide	Sulfasalazine
Levodopa	Sulfonamides
Lithium	Trimethadione
Methimazole	
Unlikely association	
Allopurinol	Penicillin
Chlorthalidone	Phenylbutazone
Gold salts	Reserpine
Griseofulvin	Streptomycin
Methysergide	Tetracyclines
Oral contraceptives	

Modified and reproduced, with permission, from Hess EV et al. Drug-related lupus. Bull Rheum Dis. 1991;40(4):1–8.

Table 20–7. Criteria for the classification of SLE. (A patient is classified as having SLE if any 4 or more of 11 criteria are met.)

1. Malar rash
2. Discoid rash
3. Photosensitivity
4. Oral ulcers
5. Arthritis
6. Serositis
7. Kidney disease
   a. > 0.5 g/d proteinuria, or
   b. ≥ 3⁺ dipstick proteinuria, or
   c. Cellular casts
8. Neurologic disease
   a. Seizures, or
   b. Psychosis (without other cause)
9. Hematologic disorders
   a. Hemolytic anemia, or
   b. Leukopenia (< 4000/mcL), or
   c. Lymphopenia (< 1500/mcL), or
   d. Thrombocytopenia (< 100,000/mcL)
10. Immunologic abnormalities
    a. Antibody to native DNA, or
    b. Antibody to Sm, or
    c. Antibodies to antiphospholipid antibodies based on (1) IgG or IgM anticardiolipin antibodies, (2) lupus anticoagulant, or (3) false-positive serologic test for syphilis
11. Positive ANA

ANA, antinuclear antibody; SLE, systemic lupus erythematosus.
Modified and reproduced, with permission, from Tan EM et al. The 1982 revised criteria for the classification of systemic lupus erythematosus. Arthritis Rheum. 1982 Nov;25(11):1271–7, and Hochberg MC. Updating the American College of Rheumatology revised criteria for the classification of systemic lupus erythematosus. Arthritis Rheum. 1997 Sep;40(9):1725.

nervous system features are not ordinarily present; (3) hypocomplementemia and antibodies to double-stranded DNA are absent; and (4) the clinical features and most laboratory abnormalities usually revert toward normal when the offending drug is withdrawn.

The diagnosis of SLE should be suspected in patients having a multisystem disease with a positive test for antinuclear antibodies. Differential diagnosis includes rheumatoid arthritis, systemic vasculitis, scleroderma, inflammatory myopathies, viral hepatitis, sarcoidosis, acute drug reactions, and drug-induced lupus.

The diagnosis of SLE can be made with reasonable probability if 4 of the 11 criteria set forth in Table 20–7 are met. These criteria, developed as guidelines for the inclusion of patients in research studies, do not supplant clinical judgment in the diagnosis of SLE.

► **Clinical Findings**

A. Symptoms and Signs

The systemic features include fever, anorexia, malaise, and weight loss. Most patients have skin lesions at some time; the characteristic "butterfly" (malar) rash affects less than half of patients. Other cutaneous manifestations are panniculitis (lupus profundus), discoid lupus, typical fingertip lesions, periungual erythema, nail fold infarcts, and splinter hemorrhages. Alopecia is common. Mucous membrane lesions tend to occur during periods of exacerbation. Raynaud phenomenon, present in about 20% of patients, often antedates other features of the disease.

Joint symptoms, with or without active synovitis, occur in over 90% of patients and are often the earliest manifestation. The arthritis can lead to reversible swan neck deformities, but erosive changes are almost never noted on radiographs. Subcutaneous nodules are rare.

Ocular manifestations include conjunctivitis, photophobia, transient or permanent monocular blindness, and blurring of vision. Cotton-wool spots on the retina (cytoid bodies) represent degeneration of nerve fibers due to occlusion of retinal blood vessels.

Pleurisy, pleural effusion, bronchopneumonia, and pneumonitis are frequent. Restrictive lung disease can develop. Alveolar hemorrhage is uncommon but life-threatening. Interstitial lung disease is rare.

The pericardium is affected in the majority of patients. Heart failure may result from myocarditis and hypertension. Cardiac arrhythmias are common. Atypical verrucous endocarditis of Libman-Sacks is usually clinically silent but occasionally can produce acute or chronic valvular regurgitation—most commonly mitral regurgitation.

Mesenteric vasculitis occasionally occurs in SLE and may closely resemble polyarteritis nodosa, including the presence of aneurysms in medium-sized blood vessels. Abdominal pain (particularly postprandial), ileus, peritonitis, and perforation may result.

Neurologic complications of SLE include psychosis, cognitive impairment, seizures, peripheral and cranial neuropathies, transverse myelitis, and strokes. Severe depression and psychosis are sometimes exacerbated by the administration of large doses of corticosteroids.

Several forms of glomerulonephritis may occur, including mesangial, focal proliferative, diffuse proliferative, and membranous (see Chapter 22). Some patients may also have interstitial nephritis. With appropriate therapy, the survival rate even for patients with serious chronic kidney disease (proliferative glomerulonephritis) is favorable, albeit a substantial portion of patients with severe lupus nephritis still eventually require renal replacement therapy.

B. Laboratory Findings

(Tables 20–8 and 20–9.) SLE is characterized by the production of many different autoantibodies. Antinuclear antibody tests based on immunofluorescence assays are sensitive but not specific for SLE—ie, they are positive in virtually all patients with lupus but are positive also in many patients with nonlupus conditions such as rheumatoid arthritis, autoimmune thyroid disease, scleroderma, and Sjögren syndrome. False-negative results can occur with tests for antinuclear antibodies based on enzyme-linked immunosorbent assays (ELISA). Therefore, SLE should not be excluded on the basis of a negative ELISA for antinuclear antibodies. Antibodies to double-stranded DNA and to Sm are specific for SLE but not sensitive, since

Table 20–8. Frequency (%) of autoantibodies in rheumatic diseases.[1]

	ANA	Anti-Native DNA	Rheumatoid Factor	Anti-Sm	Anti-SS-A	Anti-SS-B	Anti-SCL-70	Anti-Centromere	Anti-Jo-1	ANCA
Rheumatoid arthritis	30–60	0–5	70	0	0–5	0–2	0	0	0	0
Systemic lupus erythematosus	95–100	60	20	10–25	15–20	5–20	0	0	0	0–1
Sjögren syndrome	95	0	75	0	65	65	0	0	0	0
Diffuse scleroderma	80–95	0	30	0	0	0	33	1	0	0
Limited scleroderma (CREST syndrome)	80–95	0	30	0	0	0	20	50	0	0
Polymyositis/ dermatomyositis	80–95	0	33	0	0	0	0	0	20–30	0
Granulomatosis with polyangiitis (formerly Wegener granulomatosis)	0–15	0	50	0	0	0	0	0	0	93–96[1]

[1]Frequency for generalized, active disease.
ANA, antinuclear antibodies; Anti-Sm, anti-Smith antibody; anti-SCL-70, anti-scleroderma antibody; ANCA, antineutrophil cytoplasmic antibody; CREST, calcinosis cutis, Raynaud phenomenon, esophageal motility disorder, sclerodactyly, and telangiectasia.

they are present in only 60% and 30% of patients, respectively. Depressed serum complement—a finding suggestive of disease activity—often returns toward normal in remission. Anti-double-stranded DNA antibody levels also correlate with disease activity in some patients; anti-Sm levels do not.

Table 20–9. Frequency (%) of laboratory abnormalities in systemic lupus erythematosus.

Anemia	60%
Leukopenia	45%
Thrombocytopenia	30%
Biologic false-positive tests for syphilis	25%
Antiphospholipid antibodies	
Lupus anticoagulant	7%
Anti-cardiolipin antibody	25%
Direct Coombs-positive	30%
Proteinuria	30%
Hematuria	30%
Hypocomplementemia	60%
ANA	95–100%
Anti-native DNA	50%
Anti-Sm	20%

ANA, antinuclear antibody; Anti-Sm, anti-Smith antibody.
Modified and reproduced, with permission, from Hochberg MC et al. Systemic lupus erythematosus: a review of clinicolaboratory features and immunologic matches in 150 patients with emphasis on demographic subsets. Medicine (Baltimore). 1985 Sep;64(5): 285–95.

Three types of antiphospholipid antibodies occur (Table 20–9). The first causes the biologic false-positive tests for syphilis; the second is the lupus anticoagulant, which despite its name is a risk factor for venous and arterial thrombosis and for miscarriage. The lupus anticoagulant often causes prolongation of the activated partial thromboplastin time, and its presence is confirmed by an abnormal Russell viper venom time (RVVT) that corrects with the addition of phospholipid but not normal plasma. Anti-cardiolipin antibodies are the third type of antiphospholipid antibodies. In many cases, the "antiphospholipid antibody" appears to be directed at a serum cofactor (beta-2-glycoprotein-I) rather than at phospholipid itself. Abnormality of urinary sediment is almost always found in association with renal lesions. Showers of red blood cells, with or without casts, and proteinuria (varying from mild to nephrotic range) are frequent during exacerbation of the disease.

▶ **Treatment**

Patient education and emotional support are especially important for patients with lupus. Since the various manifestations of SLE affect prognosis differently and since SLE activity often waxes and wanes, drug therapy—both the choice of agents and the intensity of their use—must be tailored to match disease severity. Patients should be cautioned against sun exposure and should apply a protective lotion to the skin while out of doors. Skin lesions often respond to the local administration of corticosteroids. Minor joint symptoms can usually be alleviated by rest and NSAIDs.

Antimalarials (hydroxychloroquine) may be helpful in treating lupus rashes or joint symptoms and appear to reduce the incidence of severe disease flares. The dose of hydroxychloroquine is 200 or 400 mg/d orally and should not exceed 6.5 mg/kg/d; annual monitoring for retinal changes is recommended. Drug-induced neuropathy and myopathy may be erroneously ascribed to the underlying disease.

Corticosteroids are required for the control of certain complications. (Systemic corticosteroids are not usually given for minor arthritis, skin rash, leukopenia, or the anemia associated with chronic disease.) Glomerulonephritis, hemolytic anemia, pericarditis or myocarditis, alveolar hemorrhage, central nervous system involvement, and thrombotic thrombocytopenic purpura all require corticosteroid treatment and often other interventions as well. Forty to 60 mg of oral prednisone is often needed initially; however, the lowest dose of corticosteroid that controls the condition should be used. Central nervous system lupus may require higher doses of corticosteroids than are usually given; however, corticosteroid psychosis may mimic lupus cerebritis, in which case reduced doses are appropriate. Immunosuppressive agents such as cyclophosphamide, mycophenolate mofetil, and azathioprine are used in cases resistant to corticosteroids. Treatment of severe lupus nephritis includes an induction phase and a maintenance phase. Cyclophosphamide, which improves renal survival but not patient survival, has been for many years the standard treatment for both phases of lupus nephritis, but mycophenolate mofetil appears to be an equally effective alternative treatment for many patients with lupus nephritis. Very close follow-up is needed to watch for potential side effects when immunosuppressants are given; these agents should be administered by clinicians experienced in their use. When cyclophosphamide is required, gonadotropin-releasing hormone analogs can be given to protect a woman against the risk of premature ovarian failure. Belimumab, a monoclonal antibody that inhibits the activity of a B cell growth factor, has received FDA approval for treating antibody-positive SLE patients with active disease who have not responded to standard therapies (eg, NSAIDs, antimalarials, or immunosuppressive therapies). However, the precise indications for its use have not been defined, and its efficacy in severe disease activity is unknown. Belimumab appears less effective in blacks. While observations studies suggested that rituximab was effective in SLE, one large randomized-controlled trial demonstrated it was no more effective than placebo. For patients with the **antiphospholipid syndrome**—the presence of antiphospholipid antibodies and compatible clinical events—anticoagulation is the treatment of choice (see Antiphospholipid Antibody Syndrome, below). Moderate intensive anticoagulation with warfarin to achieve an INR of 2.0–3.0 is as effective as more intensive regimens. Pregnant patients with recurrent fetal loss associated with antiphospholipid antibodies should be treated with low-molecular-weight heparin plus aspirin.

▶ **Course & Prognosis**

Ten-year survival rates exceeding 85% are routine. In most patients, the illness pursues a relapsing and remitting course. Prednisone, often needed in doses of 40 mg/d orally or more during severe flares, can usually be tapered to low doses (5–10 mg/d) when the disease is inactive. However, there are some in whom the disease pursues a virulent course, leading to serious impairment of vital structures such as lung, heart, brain, or kidneys, and the disease may lead to death. With improved control of lupus activity and with increasing use of corticosteroids and immunosuppressive drugs, the mortality and morbidity patterns in lupus have changed. Mortality in SLE shows a bimodal pattern. In the early years after diagnosis, infections—especially with opportunistic organisms—are the leading cause of death, followed by active SLE, chiefly due to kidney or central nervous system disease. In later years, accelerated atherosclerosis, linked to chronic inflammation, becomes a major cause of death. Indeed, the incidence of myocardial infarction is five times higher in persons with SLE than in the general population. Therefore, it is especially important for SLE patients to avoid smoking and to minimize other conventional risk factors for atherosclerosis (eg, hypercholesterolemia, hypertension, obesity, and inactivity). Patients with SLE should receive influenza vaccination every year and pneumococcal vaccination every 5 years. Since SLE patients have a higher risk of developing malignancy (especially lymphoma, lung cancer, and cervical cancer), preventive cancer screening recommendations should be followed assiduously. With more patients living longer, it has become evident that avascular necrosis of bone, affecting most commonly the hips and knees, is responsible for substantial morbidity. Nonetheless, the outlook for most patients with SLE has become increasingly favorable.

▶ **When to Refer**

- Appropriate diagnosis and management of SLE requires the active participation of a rheumatologist.
- The severity of organ involvement dictates referral to other subspecialists, such as nephrologists and pulmonologists.

▶ **When to Admit**

- Rapidly progressive glomerulonephritis, pulmonary hemorrhage, transverse myelitis, and other severe organ-threatening manifestations of lupus usually require inpatient assessment and management.
- Severe infections, particularly in the setting of immunosuppressant therapy, should prompt admission.

Dooley MA et al. Mycophenolate versus azathioprine as maintenance therapy for lupus nephritis. N Engl J Med. 2011 Nov 17;365(20):1886–95. [PMID: 22087680]

Murphy et al. Systemic lupus erythematosus and other autoimmune rheumatic diseases: challenges to treatment. Lancet. 2013 Aug 31;382(9894):809–18. [PMID: 23972423]

Navarra SV et al; BLISS-52 Study Group. Efficacy and safety of belimumab in patients with active systemic lupus erythematosus: a randomised, placebo-controlled, phase 3 trial. Lancet. 2011 Feb 26;377(9767):721–31. [PMID: 21296403]

Ramos-Casals M et al. B-cell-depleting therapy in systemic lupus erythematosus. Am J Med. 2012 Apr;125(4):327–36. [PMID: 22444096]

Skaggs BJ et al. Accelerated atherosclerosis in patients with SLE—mechanisms and management. Nat Rev Rheumatol. 2012 Feb 14;8(4):214–23. [PMID: 22331061]

Walsh M et al. Mycophenolate mofetil or intravenous cyclophosphamide for lupus nephritis with poor kidney function: a subgroup analysis of the Aspreva Lupus Management Study. Am J Kidney Dis. 2013 May;61(5):710–5. [PMID: 23375819]

ANTIPHOSPHOLIPID SYNDROME

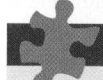

ESSENTIALS OF DIAGNOSIS

▶ Hypercoagulability, with recurrent thromboses in either the venous or arterial circulation.

▶ Thrombocytopenia is common.

▶ Pregnancy complications, specifically pregnancy losses after the first trimester.

▶ Lifelong anticoagulation with warfarin is recommended currently for patients with serious complications of this syndrome because recurrent events are common.

▶ General Considerations

A primary **antiphospholipid syndrome** (APS) is diagnosed in patients who have venous or arterial occlusions or recurrent fetal loss in the presence of persistent ($\geq$ 12 weeks), high-titer, diagnostic antiphospholipid antibodies but no other features of SLE. Diagnostic antiphospholipid antibodies are IgG or IgM anticardiolipin, or IgG or IgM antibodies to beta-2-glycoprotein I, and lupus anticoagulant. In < 1% of patients with antiphospholipid antibodies, a potentially devastating syndrome known as the "catastrophic antiphospholipid syndrome" occurs, leading to diffuse thromboses, thrombotic microangiopathy, and multiorgan system failure.

▶ Clinical Findings

A. Symptoms and Signs

Patients are often asymptomatic until suffering a thrombotic complication of this syndrome or a pregnancy loss. Thrombotic events may occur in either the arterial or venous circulations. Thus, deep venous thromboses, pulmonary emboli, cerebrovascular accidents are typical clinical events among patients with the APS. In case-control studies, 3.1% of patients in the general population who experienced a venous thrombotic event (in the absence of cancer) tested positive for the lupus anticoagulant (versus 0.9% of controls, yielding an odds ratio of 3.6). For women younger than 50 years in whom stroke developed, the odds ratio for having the lupus anticoagulant is 43.1. Budd-Chiari syndrome, cerebral sinus vein thrombosis, myocardial or digital infarctions, and other thrombotic events also occur. A variety of other symptoms and signs are often attributed to the APS, including thrombocytopenia, mental status changes, livedo reticularis, skin ulcers, microangiopathic nephropathy,

adrenal insufficiency (from infarction/hemorrhage), and cardiac valvular dysfunction—typically mitral regurgitation due to Libman-Sacks endocarditis. Livedo reticularis is strongly associated with the subset of patients with APS in whom arterial ischemic events develop. Pregnancy losses that are associated with APS include unexplained fetal death after the first trimester, one or more premature births before 34 weeks because of eclampsia or preeclampsia, or three or more unexplained miscarriages during the first trimester.

B. Laboratory Findings

As noted in the discussion of SLE, three types of antiphospholipid antibody are believed to contribute to this syndrome: (1) anti-cardiolipin antibodies; (2) antibodies to beta-2 glycoprotein; and (3) a "lupus anticoagulant" that prolongs certain phospholipid-dependent coagulation tests (see below). Antibodies to cardiolipin and to beta-2 glycoprotein are typically measured with enzyme immunoassays. Anti-cardiolipin antibodies can produce a biologic false-positive test for syphilis (ie, a positive rapid plasma reagin but negative specific anti-treponemal assay). In general, IgG anti-cardiolipin antibodies are believed to be more pathologic than IgM. Presence of the lupus anticoagulant is a stronger risk factor for thrombosis or pregnancy loss than is the presence of antibodies to either beta-2-glycoprotein I or anticardiolipin. A clue to the presence of a lupus anticoagulant, which may occur in individuals who do not have SLE, may be detected by a prolongation of the partial thromboplastin time (which, paradoxically, is associated with a thrombotic tendency rather than a bleeding risk). Testing for the lupus anticoagulant involves phospholipid-dependent functional assays of coagulation, such as the Russell viper venom time (RVVT). In the presence of a lupus anticoagulant, the RVVT is prolonged and does not correct with mixing studies but does with the addition of excess phospholipid.

▶ Differential Diagnosis

The exclusion of other autoimmune disorders, particularly those in the SLE spectrum, is essential because such disorders may be associated with additional complications requiring alternative treatments. Other genetic or acquired conditions associated with hypercoagulability such as protein C, protein S, or antithrombin deficiency and factor V Leiden should be excluded. Catastrophic APS has a broad differential, including sepsis, pulmonary-renal syndromes, systemic vasculitis, disseminated intravascular coagulation, and thrombotic thrombocytopenic purpura.

▶ Treatment

Present recommendations for anticoagulation are to treat patients with warfarin to maintain an INR of 2.0–3.0. Patients who have recurrent thrombotic events on this level of anticoagulation may require higher INRs (> 3.0), but the bleeding risk increases substantially with this degree of anticoagulation. Guidelines indicate that patients with APS should be treated with anticoagulation for life. Because of the teratogenic effects of warfarin, subcutaneous heparin and low-dose aspirin (81 mg) is the usual approach to prevent pregnancy complications in women with APS. In patients with catastrophic APS, a three-pronged approach is taken in the acute setting: intravenous heparin, high doses of corticosteroids, and either intravenous immune globulin or plasmapheresis.

Arachchillage DJ et al. Use of new oral anticoagulants in antiphospholipid syndrome. Curr Rheumatol Rep. 2013 Jun;15(6):331. [PMID: 23649961]

Clark CA et al. The lupus anticoagulant: results from 2257 patients attending a high-risk pregnancy clinic. Blood. 2013 Jul 18;122(3):341–7. [PMID: 23649468]

Giannakopoulos B et al. The pathogenesis of the antiphospholipid syndrome. N Engl J Med. 2013 Mar 14;368(11):1033–44. [PMID: 23484830]

Lockshin MD. Pregnancy and antiphospholipid syndrome. Am J Reprod Immunol. 2013 Jun;69(6):585–7. [PMID: 23279134]

Mok CC et al. Prevalence of the antiphospholipid syndrome and its effect on survival in 679 Chinese patients with systemic lupus erythematosus: a cohort study. Medicine (Baltimore). 2013 Jul;92(4):217–22. [PMID: 23793109]

RAYNAUD PHENOMENON

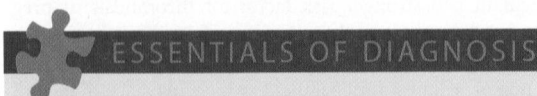

ESSENTIALS OF DIAGNOSIS

► Paroxysmal bilateral digital pallor and cyanosis followed by rubor.

► Precipitated by cold or emotional stress; relieved by warmth.

► Primary form of Raynaud phenomenon is benign and usually affects young women.

► Secondary form can cause digital ulceration or gangrene.

► General Considerations

Raynaud phenomenon (RP) is a syndrome of paroxysmal digital ischemia, most commonly caused by an exaggerated response of digital arterioles to cold or emotional stress. The initial phase of RP, mediated by excessive vasoconstriction, consists of well-demarcated digital pallor or cyanosis; the subsequent (recovery) phase of RP, caused by vasodilation, leads to intense hyperemia and rubor. Although RP chiefly affects fingers, it can also affect toes and other acral areas such as the nose and ears. RP is classified as primary (idiopathic or Raynaud disease) or secondary. Nearly one-third of the population reports being "sensitive to the cold" but does not experience the paroxysms of digital pallor, cyanosis, and erythema characteristic of RP. Primary RP occurs in 2–6% of adults, is especially common in young women, and poses more of a nuisance than a threat to good health. In contrast, secondary RP is less common, is chiefly associated with rheumatic diseases (especially scleroderma), and is frequently severe enough to cause digital ulceration or gangrene.

► Clinical Findings

In early attacks of RP, only one or two fingertips may be affected; as it progresses, all fingers down to the distal palm may be involved. The thumbs are rarely affected. During recovery there may be intense rubor, throbbing, paresthesia, pain, and slight swelling. Attacks usually terminate spontaneously or upon returning to a warm room or putting the extremity in warm water. The patient is usually asymptomatic between attacks. Sensory changes that often accompany vasomotor manifestations include numbness, stiffness, diminished sensation, and aching pain.

Primary RP appears first between ages 15 and 30, almost always in women. It tends to be mildly progressive and, unlike secondary RP (which may be unilateral and may involve only one or two fingers), symmetric involvement of the fingers of both hands is the rule. Spasm becomes more frequent and prolonged. Unlike secondary RP, primary RP does not cause digital pitting, ulceration, or gangrene.

Nailfold capillary abnormalities are among the earliest clues that a person has secondary rather than primary RP. The nailfold capillary pattern can be visualized by placing a drop of grade B immersion oil at the patient's cuticle and then viewing the area with an ophthalmoscope set to 20–40 diopters. Dilation or dropout of the capillary loops indicates the patient has a secondary form of RP, most commonly scleroderma (Table 20–10). While highly

Table 20–10. Causes of secondary Raynaud phenomenon.

Rheumatic diseases
Scleroderma
Systemic lupus erythematosus
Dermatomyositis/polymyositis
Sjögren syndrome
Vasculitis (polyarteritis nodosa, Takayasu disease, Buerger disease)
Neurovascular compression and occupational
Carpal tunnel syndrome
Thoracic outlet obstruction
Vibration injury
Medications
Serotonin agonists (sumatriptan)
Sympathomimetic drugs (decongestants)
Chemotherapy (bleomycin, vinblastine)
Ergotamine
Caffeine
Nicotine
Hematologic disorders
Cryoglobulinemia
Polycythemia vera
Paraproteinemia
Cold agglutinins
Endocrine disorders
Hypothyroidism
Pheochromocytoma
Miscellaneous
Atherosclerosis
Embolic disease
Migraine
Exposure to epoxy resins
Sequela of frostbite

specific for secondary RP, nailfold capillary changes have a low sensitivity. Digital pitting or ulceration or other abnormal physical findings (eg, skin tightening, loss of extremity pulse, rash, swollen joints) can also provide evidence of secondary RP.

Primary RP must be differentiated from the numerous causes of secondary RP (Table 20–10). The history and examination may suggest the diagnosis of systemic sclerosis (including its CREST variant), SLE, and mixed connective tissue disease; RP is occasionally the first manifestation of these disorders. The diagnosis of many of these rheumatic diseases can be confirmed with specific serologic tests (see Table 20–8).

RP may occur in patients with the thoracic outlet syndromes. In these disorders, involvement is generally unilateral, and symptoms referable to brachial plexus compression tend to dominate the clinical picture. Carpal tunnel syndrome should also be considered, and nerve conduction tests are appropriate in selected cases.

A particularly severe form of RP occurs in up to one-third of patients receiving bleomycin and vincristine in combination, often for testicular cancer. Treatment is unsuccessful, and the problem persists even with discontinuation of the drugs.

Differential Diagnosis

The differentiation from Buerger disease (thromboangiitis obliterans) is usually not difficult, since thromboangiitis obliterans is generally a disease of men, particularly smokers; peripheral pulses are often diminished or absent; and, when RP occurs in association with thromboangiitis obliterans, it is usually in only one or two digits.

In acrocyanosis, cyanosis of the hands is permanent and diffuse; the sharp and paroxysmal line of demarcation with pallor does not occur with acrocyanosis. Frostbite may lead to chronic RP. Ergot poisoning, particularly due to prolonged or excessive use of ergotamine, must also be considered but is unusual.

RP may be mimicked by type I cryoglobulinemia, in which a monoclonal antibody cryoprecipitates in the cooler distal circulation. Type I cryoglobulinemia is usually associated with multiple myeloma or with lymphoproliferative disorders.

Erythromelalgia can mimic the rubor phase of RP; exacerbation by heat and relief with cold readily distinguish erythromelalgia from RP.

Treatment

A. General Measures

Patients should wear gloves or mittens whenever outside in temperatures that precipitate attacks. Keeping the body warm is also a cornerstone of initial therapy. Wearing warm shirts, coats, and hats will help prevent the exaggerated vasospasm that causes RP and that is not prevented by warming only the hands. The hands should be protected from injury at all times; wounds heal slowly, and infections are consequently hard to control. Softening and lubricating lotion to control the fissured dry skin should be applied to

the hands frequently. Smoking should be stopped and sympathomimetic drugs (eg, decongestants, diet pills, and amphetamines) should be avoided. For most patients with primary RP, general measures alone are sufficient to control symptoms. Medical or surgical therapy should be considered in patients who have severe symptoms or are experiencing tissue injury from digital ischemia.

B. Medications

Calcium channel blockers are first-line therapy for RP. Calcium channel blockers produce a modest benefit and are more effective in primary RP than secondary RP. Slow release nifedipine (30–180 mg/d orally), amlodipine (5–20 mg/d orally), felodipine, isradipine, or nisoldipine are popular and more effective than verapamil, nicardipine and diltiazem. Other medications that are sometimes effective in treating RP include angiotensin-converting enzyme inhibitors, sympatholytic agents (eg, prazosin), topical nitrates, phosphodiesterase inhibitors (eg, sildenafil, tadalafil, and vardenafil), selective serotonin reuptake inhibitors (fluoxetine), endothelin-receptor inhibitors (ie, bosentan), statins, parenteral prostaglandins (prostaglandin E_1), and oral prostaglandins (misoprostol).

C. Surgical Measures

Sympathectomy may be indicated when attacks have become frequent and severe, when they interfere with work and well being, and particularly when trophic changes have developed and medical measures have failed. Cervical sympathectomy is modestly effective for primary but not secondary RP. Digital sympathectomy may improve secondary RP.

Prognosis

Primary RP is benign and largely a nuisance for affected individuals who are exposed to cold winters or excessive air conditioning. The prognosis of secondary RP depends on the severity of the underlying disease. Unfortunately, severe pain from ulceration and gangrene are not rare with scleroderma, especially the CREST variant.

When to Refer

Appropriate management of patients with secondary RP often requires consultation with a rheumatologist.

When to Admit

Patients with severe digital ischemia as evidenced by demarcation should be admitted for intensive therapy.

Goundry B et al. Diagnosis and management of Raynaud's phenomenon. BMJ. 2012 Feb 7;344:e289. [PMID: 22315243]

Herrick AL. Contemporary management of Raynaud's phenomenon and digital ischaemic complications. Curr Opin Rheumatol. 2011 Nov;23(6):555–61. [PMID: 21885977]

Landry GJ. Current medical and surgical management of Raynaud's syndrome. J Vasc Surg. 2013 Jun;57(6):1710–6. [PMID: 23618525]

Pavlov-Dolijanovic S et al. Late appearance and exacerbation of primary Raynaud's phenomenon attacks can predict future development of connective tissue disease: a retrospective chart review of 3,035 patients. Rheumatol Int. 2013 Apr;33(4): 921–6. [PMID: 22821334]

SCLERODERMA (Systemic Sclerosis)

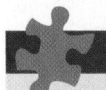 ESSENTIALS OF DIAGNOSIS

- ► Limited disease (80% of patients): thickening of skin confined to the face, neck, and distal extremities.
- ► Diffuse disease (20%): widespread thickening of skin, including truncal involvement, with areas of increased pigmentation and depigmentation.
- ► Raynaud phenomenon and antinuclear antibodies are present in virtually all patients.
- ► Systemic features of gastroesophageal reflux, hypomotility of gastrointestinal tract, pulmonary fibrosis, pulmonary hypertension, and renal involvement.

► General Considerations

Scleroderma (systemic sclerosis) is a rare chronic disorder characterized by diffuse fibrosis of the skin and internal organs. Symptoms usually appear in the third to fifth decades, and women are affected two to three times as frequently as men.

Two forms of scleroderma are generally recognized: limited (80% of patients) and diffuse (20%). In limited scleroderma, which is also known as the CREST syndrome (representing calcinosis cutis, Raynaud phenomenon, esophageal motility disorder, sclerodactyly, and telangiectasia), the hardening of the skin (scleroderma) is limited to the face and hands. In contrast, in diffuse scleroderma, the skin changes also involve the trunk and proximal extremities. Tendon friction rubs over the forearms and shins occur uniquely (but not universally) in diffuse scleroderma. In general, patients with limited scleroderma have better outcomes than those with diffuse disease, largely because kidney disease or interstitial lung disease rarely develops in patients with limited disease. Cardiac disease is also more characteristic of diffuse scleroderma. Patients with limited disease, however, are more susceptible to digital ischemia, leading to finger loss, and to life-threatening pulmonary hypertension. Small and large bowel hypomotility, which may occur in either form of scleroderma, can cause constipation alternating with diarrhea, malabsorption due to bacterial overgrowth, pseudoobstruction, and severe bowel distension with rupture.

► Clinical Findings

A. Symptoms and Signs

Raynaud phenomenon is usually the initial manifestation and can precede other signs and symptoms by years in cases of limited scleroderma. Polyarthralgia, weight loss, and malaise are common early features of diffuse scleroderma but are infrequent in limited scleroderma. Cutaneous disease usually, but not always, develops before visceral involvement and can manifest initially as non-pitting subcutaneous edema associated with pruritus. With time the skin becomes thickened and hidebound, with loss of normal folds. Telangiectasia, pigmentation, and depigmentation are characteristic. Ulceration about the fingertips and subcutaneous calcification are seen. Dysphagia and symptoms of reflux due to esophageal dysfunction are common and result from abnormalities in motility and later from fibrosis. Fibrosis and atrophy of the gastrointestinal tract cause hypomotility. Large-mouthed diverticuli occur in the jejunum, ileum, and colon. Diffuse pulmonary fibrosis and pulmonary vascular disease are reflected in restrictive lung physiology and low diffusing capacities. Cardiac abnormalities include pericarditis, heart block, myocardial fibrosis, and right heart failure secondary to pulmonary hypertension. Scleroderma renal crisis, resulting from intimal proliferation of smaller renal arteries and usually associated with hypertension, is a marker for a poor outcome even though many cases can be treated effectively with angiotensin-converting enzyme inhibitors.

B. Laboratory Findings

Mild anemia is often present. In scleroderma renal crisis, the peripheral blood smear shows findings consistent with a microangiopathic hemolytic anemia (due to mechanical damage to red cells from diseased small vessels). Elevation of the ESR is unusual. Proteinuria appears in association with renal involvement. Antinuclear antibody tests are nearly always positive, frequently in high titers (Table 20–8). The scleroderma antibody (anti-SCL-70), directed against topoisomerase III, is found in one-third of patients with diffuse systemic sclerosis and in 20% of those with CREST syndrome. Although present in only a small number of patients with diffuse scleroderma, anti-SCL-70 antibodies may portend a poor prognosis, with a high likelihood of serious internal organ involvement (eg, interstitial lung disease). Anticentromere antibodies are seen in 50% of those with CREST syndrome and in 1% of individuals with diffuse scleroderma (Table 20–8). Anticentromere antibodies are highly specific for limited scleroderma, but they also occur occasionally in overlap syndromes. Anti-RNA polymerase III antibodies develop in 10–20% of scleroderma patients overall and correlate with the development of diffuse skin disease and renal hypertensive crisis.

► Differential Diagnosis

Early in its course, scleroderma can cause diagnostic confusion with other causes of Raynaud phenomenon, particularly SLE, mixed connective tissue disease, and the inflammatory myopathies. Scleroderma can be mistaken for other disorders characterized by skin hardening. Eosinophilic fasciitis is a rare disorder presenting with skin changes that resemble diffuse scleroderma. The inflammatory abnormalities, however, are limited to the fascia rather than the dermis and epidermis. Moreover, patients with eosinophilic fasciitis are distinguished from those with scleroderma by the presence of peripheral blood eosinophilia, the absence of Raynaud phenomenon, the good response to prednisone, and an association (in some cases) with paraproteinemias. Diffuse skin thickening and visceral involvement are features of scleromyxedema; the presence of a paraprotein, the absence of Raynaud phenomenon, and distinct skin histology point to scleromyxedema. Diabetic cheiropathy typically develops in long-standing, poorly controlled diabetes and can mimic sclerodactyly. Nephrogenic fibrosing dermopathy produces thickening and hardening of the skin of the trunk and extremities in patients with chronic kidney disease; exposure to gadolinium may play a pathogenic role. Morphea and linear scleroderma cause sclerodermatous changes limited to circumscribed areas of the skin and usually have excellent outcomes.

▶ **Treatment**

Treatment of scleroderma is symptomatic and supportive and focuses on the organ systems involved. There is no effective therapy for the underlying disease process. However, interventions for management of specific organ manifestations of this disease have improved substantially. Severe Raynaud syndrome may respond to calcium channel blockers, eg, long-acting nifedipine, 30–120 mg/d orally, or to losartan, 50 mg/d orally, or to sildenafil 50 mg orally twice daily. Patients with esophageal disease should take medications in liquid or crushed form. Esophageal reflux can be reduced and the risk of scarring diminished by avoidance of late-night meals and by the use of proton pump inhibitors (eg, omeprazole, 20–40 mg/d orally), which achieve near-complete inhibition of gastric acid production and are remarkably effective for refractory esophagitis. Patients with delayed gastric emptying maintain their weight better if they eat small, frequent meals and remain upright for at least 2 hours after eating. Malabsorption due to bacterial overgrowth also responds to antibiotics, eg, tetracycline, 500 mg four times orally daily, often prescribed cyclically. The hypertensive crises associated with systemic sclerosis renal crisis must be treated early and aggressively (in the hospital) with angiotensin-converting enzyme inhibitors, eg, captopril, initiated at 25 mg orally every 6 hours and titrated up as tolerated to a maximum of 100 mg every 6 hours. Apart from the patient with myositis, prednisone has little or no role in the treatment of scleroderma; high doses (> 15 mg daily) have been associated with scleroderma renal crisis. Cyclophosphamide improves dyspnea and pulmonary function tests modestly in patients with severe interstitial lung disease; this highly toxic drug should only be administered by physicians familiar with its use. Mycophenolate mofetil, 1 g twice daily, stabilized lung function in small, uncontrolled studies of patients with interstitial lung disease. Bosentan, an endothelin receptor antagonist, improves exercise capacity and cardiopulmonary hemodynamics in patients with pulmonary hypertension and helps prevent digital ulceration. Sildenafil or prostaglandins (delivered by continuous intravenous infusion or intermittent inhalation) may also be useful in treating pulmonary hypertension. At an experimental level, immunoablative therapy with or without stem cell rescue has achieved promising results for some patients with severe, rapidly progressive diffuse scleroderma.

The 9-year survival rate in scleroderma averages approximately 40%. The prognosis tends to be worse in those with diffuse scleroderma, in blacks, in males, and in older patients. Lung disease—in the form of pulmonary fibrosis or pulmonary arterial hypertension—is now the number one cause of mortality. Death from advanced heart failure or chronic kidney disease is also common. Those persons in whom severe internal organ involvement does not develop in the first 3 years have a substantially better prognosis, with 72% surviving at least 9 years. Breast and lung cancer may be more common in patients with scleroderma.

▶ **When to Refer**

• Appropriate management of scleroderma requires frequent consultations with a rheumatologist.

• Severity of organ involvement dictates referral to other subspecialists, such as pulmonologists or gastroenterologists.

Gelber AC et al. Race and association with disease manifestations and mortality in scleroderma: a 20-year experience at the Johns Hopkins Scleroderma Center and review of the literature. Medicine (Baltimore). 2013 Jul;92(4):191–205. [PMID: 23793108]
Guillevin L et al. Scleroderma renal crisis: a retrospective multicentre study on 91 patients and 427 controls. Rheumatology (Oxford). 2012 Mar;51(3):460–7. [PMID: 22087012]
Onishi A et al. Cancer incidence in systemic sclerosis: meta-analysis of population-based cohort studies. Arthritis Rheum. 2013 Jul;65(7):1913–21. [PMID: 23576072]

IDIOPATHIC INFLAMMATORY MYOPATHIES (Polymyositis & Dermatomyositis)

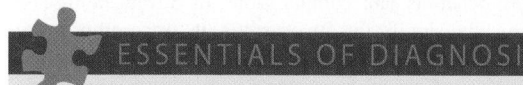

ESSENTIALS OF DIAGNOSIS

▶ Bilateral proximal muscle weakness.

▶ Characteristic cutaneous manifestations in dermatomyositis (Gottron papules, heliotrope rash).

▶ Diagnostic tests: elevated creatine kinase, muscle biopsy, electromyography, MRI.

▶ Increased risk of malignancy, particularly in dermatomyositis.

▶ Inclusion body myositis can mimic polymyositis but is less responsive to treatment.

▶ **General Considerations**

Polymyositis and dermatomyositis are systemic disorders of unknown cause whose principal manifestation is muscle weakness. Although their clinical presentations (aside from the presence of certain skin findings in dermatomyositis, some of which are pathognomonic) and treatments are similar, the two diseases are pathologically quite distinct. They affect persons of any age group, but the peak incidence is in the fifth and sixth decades of life. Women are affected twice as commonly as men, and the diseases (particularly polymyositis) also occur more often among blacks than whites. There is an increased risk of malignancy in adult patients with dermatomyositis. Indeed, up to one patient in four with dermatomyositis has an occult malignancy. Malignancies may be evident at the time of presentation with the muscle disease but may not be detected until months afterward in some cases. Rare patients with dermatomyositis have skin disease without overt muscle involvement, a condition termed "dermatomyositis sine myositis." Myositis may also be associated with other connective tissue diseases, especially scleroderma, lupus, mixed connective tissue disease, and Sjögren syndrome.

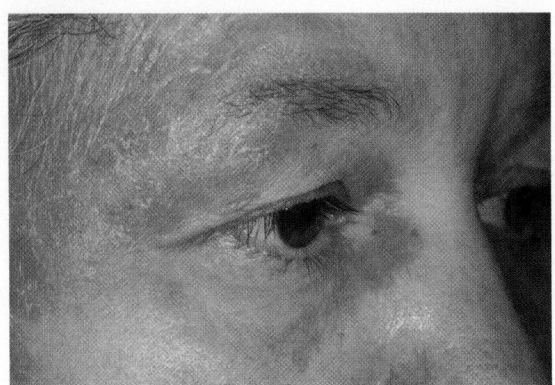

▲ **Figure 20–5.** Heliotrope (violaceous) rash around the eyes in a patient with dermatomyositis (Reproduced with permission, from Richard P. Usatine, MD).

► **Clinical Findings**

A. Symptoms and Signs

Polymyositis may begin abruptly, but the usual presentation is one of progressive muscle weakness over weeks to months. The weakness chiefly involves proximal muscle groups of the upper and lower extremities as well as the neck. Leg weakness (eg, difficulty in rising from a chair or climbing stairs) typically precedes arm symptoms. In contrast to myasthenia gravis, polymyositis and dermatomyositis do not cause facial or ocular muscle weakness. Pain and tenderness of affected muscles occur in one-fourth of cases, but these are rarely the chief complaints. About one-fourth of patients have dysphagia. In contrast to scleroderma, which affects the smooth muscle of the lower esophagus and can cause a "sticking" sensation below the sternum, polymyositis or dermatomyositis involves the striated muscles of the upper pharynx and can make initiation of swallowing difficult. Muscle atrophy and contractures occur as late complications of advanced disease. Clinically significant myocarditis is uncommon even though there is often creatine kinase-MB elevation. Patients who are bed-bound from myositis should be screened for respiratory muscle weakness that can be severe enough to cause CO_2 retention and can progress to require mechanical ventilation.

The characteristic rash of **dermatomyositis** is dusky red and may appear in a malar distribution mimicking the classic rash of SLE. Facial erythema beyond the malar distribution is also characteristic of dermatomyositis. Erythema also occurs over other areas of the face, neck, shoulders, and upper chest and back ("shawl sign"). Periorbital edema and a purplish (heliotrope) suffusion over the eyelids are typical signs (Figure 20–5). Coloration of the heliotrope and other rashes of dermatomyositis can be affected by skin tone. In blacks, the rashes may appear more hyperpigmented than erythematous or violaceous. Periungual erythema, dilations of nailbed capillaries, and scaly patches over the dorsum of PIP and MCP joints (Gottron sign) are highly suggestive. Scalp involvement by dermatomyositis may mimic psoriasis. Infrequently, the cutaneous findings of this disease precede the muscle inflammation by weeks or months. Diagnosing polymyositis in patients over age 70 years can be difficult because weakness may be overlooked or attributed erroneously to idiopathic frailty. Polymyositis can remain undiagnosed or will be misdiagnosed as hepatitis because of elevations in alanine aminotransferase (ALT) and aspartate aminotransferase (AST) levels. A subset of patients with polymyositis and dermatomyositis develop the "**antisynthetase syndrome**," a group of findings including inflammatory arthritis, fever, Raynaud phenomenon, "mechanic's hands" (hyperkeratosis along the radial and palmar aspects of the fingers), interstitial lung disease, and often severe muscle disease associated with certain autoantibodies (eg, anti-Jo -1 antibodies).

B. Laboratory Findings

Measurement of serum levels of muscle enzymes, especially creatine kinase and aldolase, is most useful in diagnosis and in assessment of disease activity. Anemia is uncommon. The ESR and C-reactive protein are often normal and are not reliable indicators of disease activity. Rheumatoid factor is found in a minority of patients. Antinuclear antibodies are present in many patients, especially those who have an associated connective tissue disease. A number of autoantibodies are seen exclusively in patients with myositis and are associated with distinctive clinical features (Table 20–11). The most common myositis-specific antibody, anti-Jo-1 antibody, is seen in the subset of patients who have associated interstitial lung disease, nonerosive polyarthritis, fever, and "mechanic's hands." The other myositis-specific autoantibodies are anti-Mi-2, associated with dermatomyositis; anti-SRP (anti-signal recognition particle), associated with rapidly progressive, severe polymyositis, and dysphagia; and anti-155/140, strongly associated with dermatomyositis with malignancy (malignancy in 71% with versus 11% without this antibody). In the absence of the anti-synthetase syndrome, chest radiographs are usually normal. Electromyographic abnormalities consisting of polyphasic potentials, fibrillations, and high-frequency action potentials point toward a myopathic, rather than a neurogenic, cause of weakness.

Table 20–11. Myositis-specific antibodies.

Antibody	Clinical Association
Anti-Jo-1 and other antisynthetase antibodies	Polymyositis or dermatomyositis with interstitial lung disease, arthritis, mechanic's hands
Anti-Mi-2	Dermatomyositis with rash more than myositis
Anti-MDA5 (anti-CADM 140)	Cancer-associated dermatomyositis, dermatomyositis with rapidly progressive lung disease
Anti-155/140	Cancer-associated myositis
Anti-140	Juvenile dermatomyositis
Anti-SAE	Cancer-associated dermatomyositis, dermatomyositis with rapidly progressive lung disease
Anti-signal recognition particle	Severe, acute necrotizing myopathy
Anti-HMG CoA reductase	Necrotizing myopathy related to statin use

Adapted, with permission, from Imboden JB, Hellmann DB, Stone JH (editors): *Current Diagnosis & Treatment Rheumatology,* 3rd ed. McGraw-Hill, 2013.

MRI can detect early and patchy muscle involvement, can guide biopsies, and often is more useful than electromyography. The malignancies most commonly associated with dermatomyositis in descending order of frequency are ovarian, lung, pancreatic, stomach, colorectal, and non-Hodgkin lymphoma. The search for an occult malignancy should begin with a history and physical examination, supplemented with a complete blood count, comprehensive biochemical panel, serum protein electrophoresis, and urinalysis, and should include age- and risk-appropriate cancer screening tests. Given the especially strong association of ovarian carcinoma and dermatomyositis, transvaginal ultrasonography, CT scanning, and CA-125 levels may be useful in women. No matter how extensive the initial screening, some malignancies will not become evident for months after the initial presentation.

C. Muscle Biopsy

Biopsy of clinically involved muscle is the only specific diagnostic test. The pathology findings in polymyositis and dermatomyositis are distinct. Although both include lymphoid inflammatory infiltrates, the findings in dermatomyositis are localized to perivascular regions and there is evidence of humoral and complement-mediated destruction of microvasculature associated with the muscle. In addition to its vascular orientation, the inflammatory infiltrate in dermatomyositis centers on the interfascicular septa and is located around, rather than in, muscle fascicles. A pathologic hallmark of dermatomyositis is perifascicular atrophy. In contrast, the pathology of polymyositis characteristically includes endomysial infiltration of the inflammatory infiltrate. Owing to the sometimes patchy

distribution of pathologic abnormalities, however, false-negative biopsies sometimes occur in both disorders.

▶ Differential Diagnosis

Muscle inflammation may occur as a component of SLE, scleroderma, Sjögren syndrome, and overlap syndromes. In those cases, associated findings usually permit the precise diagnosis of the primary condition.

Inclusion body myositis, because of its tendency to mimic polymyositis, is a common cause of "treatment-resistant polymyositis." In contrast to the epidemiologic features of polymyositis, however, the typical inclusion body myositis patient is white, male, and over the age of 50. The onset of inclusion body myositis is more insidious than that of polymyositis or dermatomyositis (eg, occurring over years rather than months), and asymmetric distal motor weakness is common in inclusion body myositis. Creatine kinase levels in inclusion body myositis are often minimally elevated and are normal in 25%. Electromyography may show a mixed picture of myopathic and neurogenic abnormalities. Muscle biopsy shows characteristic intracellular vacuoles by light microscopy and either tubular or filamentous inclusions in the nucleus or cytoplasm by electron microscopy. Inclusion body myositis is less likely to respond to therapy.

Hypothyroidism is a common cause of proximal muscle weakness associated with elevations of serum creatine kinase. Hyperthyroidism and Cushing disease may both be associated with proximal muscle weakness with normal levels of creatine kinase. Patients with polymyalgia rheumatica are over the age of 50 and—in contrast to patients with polymyositis—have pain but no objective weakness; creatine kinase levels are normal. Disorders of the peripheral and central nervous systems (eg, chronic inflammatory polyneuropathy, multiple sclerosis, myasthenia gravis, Eaton-Lambert disease, and amyotrophic lateral sclerosis) can produce weakness but are distinguished by characteristic symptoms and neurologic signs and often by distinctive electromyographic abnormalities. A number of systemic vasculitides (polyarteritis nodosa, microscopic polyangiitis, the Churg-Strauss syndrome, granulomatosis with polyangiitis, and mixed cryoglobulinemia) can produce profound weakness through vasculitic neuropathy. The muscle weakness associated with these disorders, however, is typically distal and asymmetric, at least in the early stages.

Limb-girdle muscular dystrophy can present in early adulthood with a clinical picture that mimics polymyositis: proximal muscle weakness, elevations in serum levels of creatine kinase, and inflammatory changes on muscle biopsy. Failure to respond to treatment for polymyositis or the presence of atypical clinical features such as scapular winging or weakness of ankle plantar flexors should prompt genetic testing for limb-girdle muscular dystrophy.

Many drugs, including corticosteroids, alcohol, clofibrate, penicillamine, tryptophan, and hydroxychloroquine, can produce proximal muscle weakness. Long-term use of colchicine at doses as low as 0.6 mg twice a day in patients with moderate chronic kidney disease can produce a mixed neuropathy-myopathy that mimics polymyositis. The weakness and muscle enzyme elevation reverse with cessation of the drug. Polymyositis can occur as a complication of HIV or HTLV-1 infection and with zidovudine therapy as well.

HMG-CoA reductase inhibitors can cause myopathy and rhabdomyolysis. Although only about 0.1% of patients taking a statin drug alone develop myopathy, concomitant administration of other drugs (especially gemfibrozil, cyclosporine, niacin, macrolide antibiotics, azole antifungals, and protease inhibitors) increases the risk. Statin use has also been linked to the development of an autoimmune-mediated necrotizing myositis, which persists after the statin has been discontinued and is associated with autoantibodies to HMG-CoA reductase.

► Treatment

Most patients respond to corticosteroids. Often a daily dose of 40–60 mg or more of oral prednisone is required initially. The dose is then adjusted downward while monitoring muscle strength and serum levels of muscle enzymes. Long-term use of corticosteroids is often needed, and the disease may recur or reemerge when they are withdrawn. Patients with an associated neoplasm have a poor prognosis, although remission may follow treatment of the tumor; corticosteroids may or may not be effective in these patients. In patients resistant or intolerant to corticosteroids, therapy with methotrexate or azathioprine may be helpful. Intravenous immune globulin is effective for dermatomyositis resistant to prednisone. Mycophenolate mofetil (1–1.5 g orally twice daily) may be useful as a steroid-sparing agent. Rituximab has achieved encouraging results in some patients with inflammatory myositis unresponsive to prednisone. Since the rash of dermatomyositis is often photosensitive, patients should limit sun exposure. Hydroxychloroquine (200–400 mg/d orally not to exceed 6.5 mg/kg) can also help ameliorate the skin disease.

► When to Refer

- Appropriate management of myositis usually requires frequent consultations with a rheumatologist or neurologist.
- Severe lung disease may require consultation with a pulmonologist.

► When to Admit

- Signs of rhabdomyolysis.
- New onset of dysphagia.
- Respiratory insufficiency with hypoxia or carbon dioxide retention.

Ernste FC et al. Idiopathic inflammatory myopathies: current trends in pathogenesis, clinical features, and up-to-date treatment recommendations. Mayo Clin Proc. 2013 Jan;88(1): 83–105. [PMID: 23274022]

Mammen AL. Autoimmune myopathies: autoantibodies, phenotypes and pathogenesis. Nat Rev Neurol. 2011 Jun 8;7(6): 343–54. [PMID: 21654717]

SJÖGREN SYNDROME

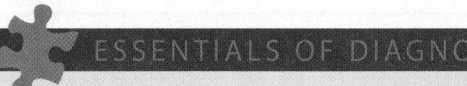

ESSENTIALS OF DIAGNOSIS

- ► Women are 90% of patients; the average age is 50 years.
- ► Dryness of eyes and dry mouth (sicca components) are the most common features; they occur alone or in association with rheumatoid arthritis or other connective tissue disease.
- ► Rheumatoid factor and antinuclear antibodies are common.
- ► Increased incidence of lymphoma.

► General Considerations

Sjögren syndrome is a systemic autoimmune disorder whose clinical presentation is usually dominated by dryness of the eyes and mouth due to immune-mediated dysfunction of the lacrimal and salivary glands. The disorder is predominantly seen in women, with a ratio of 9:1; most cases develop between the ages of 40 and 60 years. Sjögren syndrome can occur in isolation ("primary" Sjögren syndrome) or in association with another rheumatic disease. Sjögren syndrome is most frequently associated with rheumatoid arthritis but also occurs with SLE, primary biliary cirrhosis, scleroderma, polymyositis, Hashimoto thyroiditis, polyarteritis, and interstitial pulmonary fibrosis.

► Clinical Findings

A. Symptoms and Signs

Keratoconjunctivitis sicca results from inadequate tear production caused by lymphocyte and plasma cell infiltration of the lacrimal glands. Ocular symptoms are usually mild. Burning, itching, and the sensation of having a foreign body or a grain of sand in the eye occur commonly. For some patients, the initial manifestation is the inability to tolerate wearing contact lenses. Many patients with more severe ocular dryness notice ropy secretions across their eyes, especially in the morning. Photophobia may signal corneal ulceration resulting from severe dryness. For most patients, symptoms of dryness of the mouth (xerostomia) dominate those of dry eyes. Patients frequently complain of a "cotton mouth" sensation and difficulty swallowing foods, especially dry foods like crackers, unless they are washed down with liquids. The persistent oral dryness causes most patients to carry water bottles or other liquid dispensers from which they sip constantly. A few patients have such severe xerostomia that they have difficulty speaking. Persistent xerostomia results often in rampant dental caries; caries at the gum line strongly suggest Sjögren syndrome. Some patients are most troubled by loss of taste and smell. Parotid enlargement, which may be chronic or relapsing, develops in one-third of patients. Desiccation may involve the nose, throat, larynx, bronchi, vagina, and skin.

Systemic manifestations include dysphagia, small vessel vasculitis, pleuritis, obstructive airways disease and interstitial lung disease (in the absence of smoking), neuropsychiatric dysfunction (most commonly peripheral neuropathies), and pancreatitis; they may be related to the associated diseases noted above. Renal tubular acidosis (type I, distal) occurs in 20% of patients. Chronic interstitial nephritis, which may result in impaired kidney function, may be seen.

B. Laboratory Findings

Laboratory findings include mild anemia, leukopenia, and eosinophilia. Polyclonal hypergammaglobulinemia, rheumatoid factor positivity (70%), and antinuclear antibodies (95%) are all common findings. Antibodies against SS-A and SS-B (also called Ro and La, respectively) are often present in primary Sjögren syndrome and tend to correlate with the presence of extra-glandular manifestations (Table 20–8). Thyroid-associated autoimmunity is a common finding among patients with Sjögren syndrome.

Useful ocular diagnostic tests include the Schirmer test, which measures the quantity of tears secreted. Lip biopsy, a simple procedure, reveals characteristic lymphoid foci in accessory salivary glands. Biopsy of the parotid gland should be reserved for patients with atypical presentations such as unilateral gland enlargement that suggest a neoplastic process.

Differential Diagnosis

Isolated complaints of dry mouth are most commonly due to medication side effects. Chronic hepatic C can cause sicca symptoms and rheumatoid factor positivity. Minor salivary gland biopsies reveal lymphocytic infiltrates but not to the extent of Sjögren syndrome, and tests for anti-SS-A and anti-SS-B are negative. Involvement of the lacrimal or salivary glands, or both in sarcoidosis can mimic Sjögren syndrome; biopsies reveal noncaseating granulomas. Rarely, amyloid deposits in the lacrimal and salivary glands produce sicca symptoms. IgG$_4$-related systemic disease (characterized by high serum IgG$_4$ levels and infiltration of tissues with IgG$_4^+$ plasma cells) can result in lacrimal and salivary gland enlargement that mimics Sjögren syndrome.

Treatment & Prognosis

Treatment of sicca symptoms is symptomatic and supportive. Artificial tears applied frequently will relieve ocular symptoms and avert further desiccation. Topical ocular 0.05% cyclosporine also improves ocular symptoms and signs of dryness. The mouth should be kept well lubricated. Sipping water frequently or using sugar-free gums and hard candies usually relieves dry mouth symptoms. Pilocarpine (5 mg orally four times daily) and the acetylcholine derivative cevimeline (30 mg orally three times daily) may improve xerostomia symptoms. Atropinic drugs and decongestants decrease salivary secretions and should be avoided. A program of oral hygiene, including fluoride treatment, is essential in order to preserve dentition. If there is an associated rheumatic disease, its systemic treatment is not altered by the presence of Sjögren syndrome.

Although Sjögren syndrome may compromise patients' quality of life significantly, the disease is usually consistent with a normal life span. Poor prognoses are influenced mainly by the presence of systemic features associated with underlying disorders, the development in some patients of lymphocytic vasculitis, the occurrence of a painful peripheral neuropathy, and the complication (in a minority of patients) of lymphoma. Severe systemic inflammatory manifestations are treated with prednisone or various immunosuppressive medications. The patients (3–10% of the total Sjögren population) at greatest risk for developing lymphoma are those with severe exocrine dysfunction, marked parotid gland enlargement, splenomegaly, vasculitis, peripheral neuropathy, anemia, and mixed monoclonal cryoglobulinemia.

When to Refer

- Presence of systemic symptoms or signs.
- Symptoms or signs of ocular dryness not responsive to artificial tears.

When to Admit

Presence of severe systemic signs such as vasculitis unresponsive to outpatient management.

Ramos-Casals M et al. Primary Sjögren syndrome. BMJ. 2012 Jun 14;344:e3281. [PMID: 22700787]
Shiboski SC et al. American College of Rheumatology classification criteria for Sjögren's syndrome: a data-driven, expert consensus approach in the Sjögren's International Collaborative Clinical Alliance cohort. Arthritis Care Res (Hoboken). 2012 Apr;64(4):475–87. [PMID: 22563590]
St Clair EW et al; Autoimmunity Centers of Excellence. Rituximab therapy for primary Sjögren's syndrome: an open-label clinical trial and mechanistic analysis. Arthritis Rheum. 2013 Apr;65(4):1097–106. [PMID: 23334994]

IgG$_4$-RELATED DISEASE

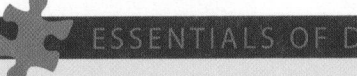

ESSENTIALS OF DIAGNOSIS

- ▶ Predominantly affects men (75% of patients); average age > 50 years.
- ▶ Protean manifestations caused by lymphoplasmacytic infiltrates in any organ or tissue, especially the pancreas, lacrimal glands, biliary tract, and retroperitoneum.
- ▶ Subacute onset; fever, constitutional symptoms rare.
- ▶ Diagnosis rests on specific histopathological findings that include presence of IgG$_4$-bearing plasma cells.

General Considerations

IgG$_4$-related disease is a systemic disorder of unknown cause, first recognized in 2003, marked by highly characteristic fibroinflammatory changes that can affect virtually any organ. Elevations of serum IgG$_4$ levels occur often but are not diagnostic. The disorder chiefly affects men over the age of 50 years.

Clinical Findings

A. Symptoms and Signs

IgG$_4$-related disease has been compared with sarcoidosis: both disorders can affect any organ of the body, can be localized or generalized, demonstrate the same distinctive histopathology at all sites of involvement, produce protean manifestations depending on location and extent of involvement, and cause disease that ranges in severity from asymptomatic to organ- or life-threatening. The inflammatory infiltration in IgG$_4$-related disease frequently produces tumefactive masses that can be seen on physical examination or on imaging. Some of the common presenting manifestations include enlargement of submandibular glands, proptosis from periorbital infiltration, retroperitoneal fibrosis, mediastinal fibrosis, inflammatory aortic aneurysm, and pancreatic mass with autoimmune pancreatitis. IgG$_4$-related disease can also affect the thyroid, kidney, meninges, sinuses, lung, prostate, breast, and bone. Most symptomatic patients with IgG$_4$-related disease present subacutely; fever and constitutional symptoms are usually absent. Nearly half of the patients with IgG$_4$-related disease also have allergic disorders such as sinusitis or asthma.

B. Laboratory Findings

The infiltrating lesions in IgG$_4$-related disease often produce tumors or fibrotic changes that are evident on CT or MRI imaging. However, the cornerstone of diagnosis is the histopathology. The key pathological findings are a dense lymphoplasmacytic infiltrate rich in IgG$_4$ plasma cells, storiform (matted and irregularly whorled) fibrosis, and obliterative phlebitis. Serum IgG$_4$ levels are usually, but not invariably, elevated so this finding cannot be used as a diagnostic criterion.

Differential Diagnosis

IgG$_4$-related disease can mimic many disorders including Sjögren syndrome (lacrimal gland enlargement), pancreatic cancer (pancreatic mass), and granulomatosis with polyangiitis (proptosis). It is now recognized that some cases of retroperitoneal fibrosis and mediastinal fibrosis are caused by IgG$_4$-related disease. Lymphoma can mimic some of the histopathologic features of IgG$_4$-related disease.

Treatment & Prognosis

Patients who are asymptomatic and have no organ-threatening disease can be monitored carefully. Spontaneous resolution can occur. The optimal therapy for symptomatic patients has not been defined, but initial therapy is usually oral prednisone 0.6 mg/kg/d, tapered over weeks or months depending on response. Patients who do not respond to prednisone or respond only to sustained high doses of prednisone can be treated with rituximab, mycophenolate mofetil, or azathioprine. The degree of fibrosis in affected organs determines the patient's responsiveness to treatment.

When to Refer

- Presence of systemic symptoms or signs.
- Symptoms or signs not responsive to prednisone.

When to Admit

- Presence of severe systemic signs unresponsive to outpatient management.

Stone JH et al. IgG4-related disease. N Engl J Med. 2012 Feb 9;366(6):539–51. [PMID: 22316447]

RHABDOMYOLYSIS

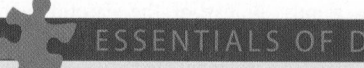
ESSENTIALS OF DIAGNOSIS

- ► Associated with crush injuries to muscle, prolonged immobility, drug toxicities, hypothermia, and other causes.

- ► Massive acute elevations of muscle enzymes that peak quickly and usually resolve within days once the inciting injury has been identified and removed.

General Considerations

Rhabdomyolysis is a syndrome of acute necrosis of skeletal muscle associated with myoglobinuria and markedly elevated creatine kinase levels. Acute tubular necrosis is a common complication of rhabdomyolysis and is due to the toxic effects of filtering excessive quantities of myoglobin in the setting of hypovolemia (See Acute Tubular Necrosis in Chapter 22). Many patients in whom rhabdomyolysis develops are volume-contracted and, therefore, oliguric renal failure is encountered routinely.

Rhabdomyolysis was first recognized as a complication of crush injuries to muscle among victims of the London Blitz during the World War II. Cocaine use and alcohol intoxication, particularly in the setting of prolonged immobility and exposure hypothermia, are leading causes of admissions due to rhabdomyolysis on the medical services of inner city hospitals. Use of statins is another important cause of rhabdomyolysis. The presence of compromised kidney and liver function, diabetes mellitus, and hypothyroidism as well as concomitant use of other medications increase the risk of rhabdomyolysis in patients taking statins. The cytochrome P450 liver enzymes metabolize all statins except for pravastatin and rosuvastatin. Drugs that block the action of cytochrome P450 include protease inhibitors, erythromycin, itraconazole, clarithromycin, diltiazem, and verapamil. Use of these drugs concomitantly with the statins (but not pravastatin or rosuvastatin) can increase the risk of development of rhabdomyolysis. The likelihood of rhabdomyolysis also increases when statins are used with niacin and fibric acids (gemfibrozil, clofibrate, and fenofibrate). Rhabdomyolysis is an uncommon complication of polymyositis, dermatomyositis, and the myopathy of hypothyroidism, despite the high levels of creatine kinase often seen in these conditions.

Often there is little evidence for muscle injury on clinical assessment of the patients with rhabdomyolysis—specifically, myalgias and weakness are usually absent. The first clue to muscle necrosis in such individuals may be a urinary dipstick testing positive for "blood" (actually myoglobin) in the absence of red cells in the sediment. This positive finding is due to myoglobinuria, which results in a false-positive reading for hemoglobin. Such an abnormality should prompt determination of the serum creatine kinase level, which invariably is elevated (usually markedly so). Other commonly encountered laboratory abnormalities in rhabdomyolysis include elevated serum levels of AST ALT and lactate dehydrogenase due to release of these enzymes from skeletal muscle.

▶ **Treatment**

Vigorous fluid resuscitation (4–6 L/d, with careful monitoring for volume overload) is indicated. Infusion of mannitol (100 mg/d) and urine alkalinization (to minimize precipitation of myoglobin within tubules) have been recommended as measures to reduce kidney injury, but definitive evidence for the efficacy of these measures is lacking. Myopathic complications of statins usually resolve within several weeks of discontinuing the drug.

Landau ME et al. Exertional rhabdomyolysis: a clinical review with a focus on genetic influences. J Clin Neuromuscul Dis. 2012 Mar;13(3):122–36. [PMID: 22538307]
Scharman EJ et al. Prevention of kidney injury following rhabdomyolysis: a systematic review. Ann Pharmacother. 2013 Jan;47(1):90–105. [PMID: 23324509]

VASCULITIS SYNDROMES

"Vasculitis" is a heterogeneous group of disorders characterized by inflammation within the walls of affected blood vessels. The major forms of primary systemic vasculitis are listed in Table 20–12. The first consideration in classifying cases of vasculitis is the size of the major vessels involved: large, medium, or small. The presence of the clinical signs and symptoms shown in Table 20–13 help distinguish among these three groups. After determining the size of the major vessels involved, other issues that contribute to the classification include the following:

- Does the process involve arteries, veins, or both?
- What are the patient's demographic characteristics (age, gender, ethnicity, smoking status)?

Table 20–12. Classification scheme of primary vasculitides according to size of predominant blood vessels involved.

Predominantly large-vessel vasculitides
Takayasu arteritis
Giant cell arteritis (temporal arteritis)
Behçet disease[1]
Predominantly medium-vessel vasculitides
Polyarteritis nodosa
Buerger disease
Primary angiitis of the central nervous system
Predominantly small-vessel vasculitides
Immune-complex mediated
Cutaneous leukocytoclastic angiitis ("hypersensitivity vasculitis")
Henoch-Schönlein purpura
Essential cryoglobulinemia[2]
"ANCA-associated" disorders[3]
Granulomatosis with polyangiitis (formerly Wegener granulomatosis)[2]
Microscopic polyangiitis[2]
Churg-Strauss syndrome[2]

[1]May involve small, medium, and large-sized blood vessels.
[2]Frequent overlap of small and medium-sized blood vessel involvement.
[3]Not all forms of these disorders are always associated with ANCA. ANCA, antineutrophil cytoplasmic antibodies.

- Which organs are involved?
- Is there hypocomplementemia or other evidence of immune complex deposition?
- Is there granulomatous inflammation on tissue biopsy?
- Are antineutrophil cytoplasmic antibodies (ANCA) present?

In addition to the disorders considered to be primary vasculitides, there are also multiple forms of vasculitis that are associated with other known underlying conditions.

Table 20–13. Typical clinical manifestations of large-, medium-, and small-vessel involvement by vasculitis.

Large	Medium	Small
Constitutional symptoms: fever, weight loss, malaise, arthralgias/arthritis		
Limb claudication	Cutaneous nodules	Purpura
Asymmetric blood pressures	Ulcers	Vesiculobullous lesions
Absence of pulses	Livedo reticularis	Urticaria
Bruits	Digital gangrene	Glomerulonephritis
Aortic dilation	Mononeuritis multiplex	Alveolar hemorrhage
	Microaneurysms	Cutaneous extravascular necrotizing granulomas
		Splinter hemorrhages
		Uveitis
		Episcleritis
		Scleritis

These "secondary" forms of vasculitis occur in the setting of chronic infections (eg, hepatitis B or C, subacute bacterial endocarditis), connective tissue disorders, inflammatory bowel disease, malignancies, and reactions to medications. Only the major primary forms of vasculitis are discussed here.

Jennette JC et al. 2012 revised International Chapel Hill Consensus Conference Nomenclature of Vasculitides. Arthritis Rheum. 2013 Jan;65(1):1–11. [PMID: 23045170]

POLYMYALGIA RHEUMATICA & GIANT CELL ARTERITIS

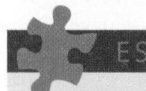

ESSENTIALS OF DIAGNOSIS

- ▶ Age over 50 years.
- ▶ Giant cell (temporal) arteritis is characterized by headache, jaw claudication, polymyalgia rheumatica, visual abnormalities, and a markedly elevated ESR.
- ▶ The hallmark of polymyalgia rheumatica is pain and stiffness in shoulders and hips lasting for several weeks without other explanation.

▶ General Considerations

Polymyalgia rheumatica and giant cell arteritis probably represent a spectrum of one disease: Both affect the same population (patients over the age of 50), show preference for the same HLA haplotypes, and show similar patterns of cytokines in blood and arteries. Polymyalgia rheumatica and giant cell arteritis also frequently coexist. The important differences between the two conditions are that polymyalgia rheumatica alone does not cause blindness and responds to low-dose (10–20 mg/d orally) prednisone therapy, whereas giant cell arteritis can cause blindness and large artery complications and requires high-dose (40–60 mg/d) prednisone.

▶ Clinical Findings

A. Polymyalgia Rheumatica

Polymyalgia rheumatica is a clinical diagnosis based on pain and stiffness of the shoulder and pelvic girdle areas, frequently in association with fever, malaise, and weight loss. In approximately two-thirds of cases, polymyalgia occurs in the absence of giant cell arteritis. Because of the stiffness and pain in the shoulders, hips, and lower back, patients have trouble combing their hair, putting on a coat, or rising from a chair. In contrast to polymyositis and polyarteritis nodosa, polymyalgia rheumatica does not cause muscular weakness either through primary muscle inflammation or secondary to nerve infarction. A few patients have joint swelling, particularly of the knees, wrists, and sternoclavicular joints.

B. Giant Cell Arteritis

Giant cell arteritis is a systemic panarteritis affecting medium-sized and large vessels in patients over the age of 50. The incidence of this disease increases with each decade of life. The mean age at onset is approximately 79 years. Giant cell arteritis is also called temporal arteritis because that artery is frequently involved, as are other extracranial branches of the carotid artery. About 50% of patients with giant cell arteritis also have polymyalgia rheumatica. The classic symptoms suggesting that a patient has arteritis are headache, scalp tenderness, visual symptoms (particularly amaurosis fugax or diplopia), jaw claudication, or throat pain. Of these symptoms, jaw claudication has the highest positive predictive value. The temporal artery is usually normal on physical examination but may be nodular, enlarged, tender, or pulseless. Blindness usually results from the syndrome of anterior ischemic optic neuropathy, caused by occlusive arteritis of the posterior ciliary branch of the ophthalmic artery. The ischemic optic neuropathy of giant cell arteritis may produce no funduscopic findings for the first 24–48 hours after the onset of blindness.

Asymmetry of pulses in the arms, a murmur of aortic regurgitation, or bruits heard near the clavicle resulting from subclavian artery stenoses identify patients in whom giant cell arteritis has affected the aorta or its major branches. Clinically evident large vessel involvement—characterized chiefly by aneurysm of the thoracic aorta or stenosis of the subclavian, vertebral, carotid, and basilar arteries—occurs in approximately 25% of patients with giant cell arteritis, sometimes years after the diagnosis. Subclinical large artery disease is the rule: positron emission tomography scans reveal inflammation in the aorta and its major branches in nearly 85% of untreated patients. Forty percent of patients with giant cell arteritis have nonclassic symptoms at presentation, chiefly respiratory tract problems (most frequently dry cough), mononeuritis multiplex (most frequently with painful paralysis of a shoulder), or fever of unknown origin. Giant cell arteritis accounts for 15% of all cases of fever of unknown origin in patients over the age of 65. The fever can be as high as 40°C and is frequently associated with rigors and sweats. In contrast to patients with infection, patients with giant cell arteritis and fever usually have normal white blood cell counts (before prednisone is started). Thus, in an older patient with fever of unknown origin, marked elevations of acute phase reactants, and a normal white blood count, giant cell arteritis must be considered even in the absence of specific features such as headache or jaw claudication. In some cases, instead of having the well-known symptom of jaw claudication, patients complain of vague pain affecting other locations, including the tongue, nose, or ears. Indeed, unexplained head or neck pain in an older patient may signal the presence of giant cell arteritis.

C. Laboratory Findings

1. Polymyalgia rheumatica—Anemia and elevated acute phase reactants (often markedly elevated ESRs, for example) are present in the most cases, but cases of polymyalgia rheumatica occurring with normal acute phase reactants are well documented.

2. Giant cell arteritis—Nearly 90% of patients with giant cell arteritis have ESRs > 50 mm/h. The ESR in this disorder is often > 100 mm/h, but cases in which the ESR is lower or even normal do occur. In one series, 5% of patients with biopsy-proven giant cell arteritis had ESRs < 40 mm/h. Although the C-reactive protein is slightly more sensitive, patients with biopsy-proven giant cell arteritis with normal C-reactive proteins have also been described. Most patients also have a mild normochromic, normocytic anemia and thrombocytosis. The alkaline phosphatase (liver source) is elevated in 20% of patients with giant cell arteritis.

▶ Differential Diagnosis

The differential diagnosis of malaise, anemia, and striking acute phase reactant elevations includes rheumatic diseases (such as rheumatoid arthritis, other systemic vasculitides, multiple myeloma, and other malignant disorders) and chronic infections (such as bacterial endocarditis and osteomyelitis).

▶ Treatment

A. Polymyalgia Rheumatica

Patients with isolated polymyalgia rheumatica (ie, those not having "above the neck" symptoms of headache, jaw claudication, scalp tenderness, or visual symptoms) are treated with prednisone, 10–20 mg/d orally. If the patient does not experience a dramatic improvement within 72 hours, the diagnosis should be revisited. Usually after 2–4 weeks of treatment, slow tapering of the prednisone can be attempted. Most patients require some dose of prednisone for a minimum of approximately 1 year; 6 months is too short in most cases. Disease flares are common (50% or more) as prednisone is tapered. The addition of weekly methotrexate may increase the chance of successfully tapering prednisone in some patients.

B. Giant Cell Arteritis

The urgency of early diagnosis and treatment in giant cell arteritis relates to the prevention of blindness. Once blindness develops, it is usually permanent. Therefore, when a patient has symptoms and findings suggestive of temporal arteritis, therapy with prednisone (60 mg/d orally) should be initiated immediately and a temporal artery biopsy performed promptly. For patients who seek medical attention for visual loss, intravenous pulse methylprednisolone (eg, 1 g daily for 3 days) has been advocated; unfortunately, few patients recover vision no matter what the initial treatment. One study—too small and too preliminary to change the standard therapy recommendations mentioned above—suggested that initiating treatment with intravenous pulse methylprednisolone may increase the chance that a patient with giant cell arteritis will achieve remission and be able to taper off of prednisone. Retrospective studies suggest that low-dose

aspirin (~81 mg/d orally) may reduce the chance of visual loss or stroke in patients with giant cell arteritis and should be added to prednisone in the initial treatment. Although it is prudent to obtain a temporal artery biopsy as soon as possible after instituting treatment, diagnostic findings of giant cell arteritis may still be present 2 weeks (or even considerably longer) after starting corticosteroids. Typically, a positive biopsy shows inflammatory infiltrate in the media and adventitia with lymphocytes, histiocytes, plasma cells, and giant cells. An adequate biopsy specimen is essential (at least 2 cm in length is ideal), because the disease may be segmental. Unilateral temporal artery biopsies are positive in approximately 80–85% of patients, but bilateral biopsies add incrementally to the yield (10–15% in some studies, less in others). Ultrasonography can detect abnormalities in inflamed temporal arteries, but it has not displaced temporal artery biopsy as the gold standard for diagnosis in most cases because results are highly operator dependent. Temporal artery biopsy is abnormal in only 50% of patients with large artery disease (eg, arm claudication and unequal upper extremity blood pressures). In these patients, magnetic resonance angiography or CT angiography will establish the diagnosis by demonstrating long stretches of narrowing of the subclavian and axillary arteries. Prednisone should be continued in a dosage of 60 mg/d orally for about 1 month before tapering. When only the symptoms of polymyalgia rheumatica are present, temporal artery biopsy is not necessary.

After 1 month of high-dose prednisone, almost all patients will have a normal ESR. When tapering and adjusting the dosage of prednisone, the ESR (or C-reactive protein) is a useful but not absolute guide to disease activity. A common error is treating the ESR rather than the patient. The ESR often rises slightly as the prednisone is tapered, even as the disease remains quiescent. Because elderly individuals often have baseline ESRs that are above the normal range, mild ESR elevations should not be an occasion for renewed treatment with prednisone in patients who are asymptomatic. Unfortunately, no highly effective prednisone-sparing therapy has been identified. Methotrexate was modestly effective in one double-blind, placebo-controlled treatment trial but ineffective in another. Anti-TNF therapies do not work in giant cell arteritis. Thoracic aortic aneurysms occur 17 times more frequently in patients with giant cell arteritis than in normal individuals and can result in aortic regurgitation, dissection, or rupture. The aneurysms can develop at any time but typically occur 7 years after the diagnosis of giant cell arteritis is made.

Ghinoi A et al. Large-vessel involvement in recent-onset giant cell arteritis: a case-control colour-Doppler sonography study. Rheumatology (Oxford). 2012 Apr;51(4):730–4. [PMID: 22179725]

Kermani TA et al. Polymyalgia rheumatica. Lancet. 2013 Jan 5;381(9860):63–72. [PMID: 23051717]

Scheurer RA et al. Treatment of vision loss in giant cell arteritis. Curr Treat Options Neurol. 2012 Feb;14(1):84–92. [PMID: 22037998]

TAKAYASU ARTERITIS

Takayasu arteritis is a granulomatous vasculitis of the aorta and its major branches. Rare in North American but more prevalent in the Far East, it primarily affects women and typically has its onset in early adulthood. Takayasu arteritis can present with nonspecific constitutional symptoms of malaise, fever, and weight loss or with manifestations of vascular damage (diminished pulses, unequal blood pressures in the arms, bruits over carotids and subclavian arteries, limb claudication, and hypertension). There are no specific laboratory abnormalities; the ESR and the C-reactive protein level are elevated in most cases. The diagnosis is established by imaging studies, usually MRI, which can detect inflammatory thickening of the walls of affected vessels, or CT angiography, which can provide images of the stenoses, occlusions, and dilations characteristic of arteritis. Corticosteroids (eg, oral prednisone 1 mg/kg for 1 month, followed by a taper over several months to 10 mg daily) are the mainstays of treatment. The addition of methotrexate or mycophenolate mofetil to the prednisone may be more effective than the prednisone alone. Takayasu arteritis has a chronic relapsing and remitting course that requires ongoing monitoring and adjustment of therapy.

Clifford A et al. Recent advances in the medical management of Takayasu arteritis: an update on use of biological therapies. Curr Opin Rheumatol. 2014 Jan;26(1):7–15. [PMID: 24225487]

POLYARTERITIS NODOSA

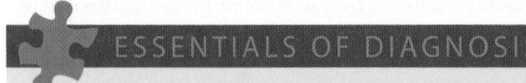

ESSENTIALS OF DIAGNOSIS

► Medium-sized arteries are always affected; smaller arterioles are sometimes involved; lung is spared but kidney often affected, causing renin-mediated hypertension.

► Clinical findings depend on the arteries involved.

► Common features include fever, abdominal pain, extremity pain, livedo reticularis, mononeuritis multiplex, anemia, and elevated acute phase reactants (ESR or C-reactive protein or both).

► Associated with hepatitis B (10% of cases).

▶ General Considerations

Polyarteritis nodosa, described in 1866, is acknowledged widely as the first form of vasculitis reported in the medical literature. For many years, all forms of inflammatory vascular disease were termed "polyarteritis nodosa." In recent decades, numerous subtypes of vasculitis have been recognized, greatly narrowing the spectrum of vasculitis called polyarteritis nodosa. Currently, the term is reserved for necrotizing arteritis of medium-sized vessels that has a predilection for involving the skin, peripheral nerves, mesenteric vessels (including renal arteries), heart, and brain,

but polyarteritis nodosa can actually involve almost any organ. Polyarteritis nodosa is relatively rare, with a prevalence of about 30 per 1 million people. Approximately 10% of cases of polyarteritis nodosa are caused by hepatitis B. Most cases of hepatitis B–associated disease occur within 6 months of hepatitis B infection.

▶ Clinical Findings

A. Symptoms and Signs

The clinical onset is usually insidious, with fever, malaise, weight loss, and other symptoms developing over weeks to months. Pain in the extremities is often a prominent early feature caused by arthralgia, myalgia (particularly affecting the calves), or neuropathy. The combination of mononeuritis multiplex (with the most common finding being footdrop) and features of a systemic illness is one of the earliest specific clues to the presence of an underlying vasculitis. Polyarteritis nodosa is among the forms of vasculitis most commonly associated with vasculitic neuropathy.

In polyarteritis nodosa, the typical skin findings—livedo reticularis, subcutaneous nodules, and skin ulcers—reflect the involvement of deeper, medium-sized blood vessels. Digital gangrene is not an unusual occurrence. The most common cutaneous presentation is lower extremity ulcerations, usually occurring near the malleoli. Involvement of the renal arteries leads to a renin-mediated hypertension (much less characteristic of vasculitides involving smaller blood vessels). For unclear reasons, classic polyarteritis nodosa seldom (if ever) involves the lung, with the occasional exception of the bronchial arteries.

Abdominal pain—particularly diffuse periumbilical pain precipitated by eating—is common but often difficult to attribute to mesenteric vasculitis in the early stages. Nausea and vomiting are common symptoms. Infarction compromises the function of major viscera and may lead to acalculous cholecystitis or appendicitis. Some patients present dramatically with an acute abdomen caused by mesenteric vasculitis and gut perforation or with hypotension resulting from rupture of a microaneurysm in the liver, kidney, or bowel.

Subclinical cardiac involvement is common in polyarteritis nodosa, and overt cardiac dysfunction occasionally occurs (eg, myocardial infarction secondary to coronary vasculitis, or myocarditis).

B. Laboratory Findings

Most patients with polyarteritis nodosa have a slight anemia, and leukocytosis is common. Acute phase reactants are often (but not always) strikingly elevated. A major challenge in making the diagnosis of polyarteritis nodosa, however, is the absence of a disease-specific serologic test (eg, an autoantibody). Patients with classic polyarteritis nodosa are ANCA-negative and may have low titers of rheumatoid factor or antinuclear antibodies, both of which are nonspecific findings. In patients with polyarteritis nodosa, appropriate serologic tests for active hepatitis B infection must be performed.

C. Biopsy and Angiography

The diagnosis of polyarteritis nodosa requires confirmation with either a tissue biopsy or an angiogram. Biopsies of symptomatic sites such as skin (from the edge of an ulcer or the center of a nodule), nerve, or muscle have sensitivities of approximately 70%. The least invasive tests should usually be obtained first, but biopsy of an involved organ is essential. If performed by experienced clinicians, tissue biopsies normally have high benefit-risk ratios because of the importance of establishing the diagnosis. Patients in whom polyarteritis nodosa is suspected—eg, on the basis of mesenteric ischemia or new-onset hypertension occurring in the setting of a systemic illness—may be diagnosed by the angiographic finding of aneurysmal dilations in the renal, mesenteric, or hepatic arteries. Angiography must be performed cautiously in patients with baseline renal dysfunction.

▶ Treatment

For polyarteritis nodosa, corticosteroids in high doses (up to 60 mg of oral prednisone daily) may control fever and constitutional symptoms and heal vascular lesions. Pulse methylprednisolone (eg, 1 g intravenously daily for 3 days) may be necessary for patients who are critically ill at presentation. Immunosuppressive agents, especially cyclophosphamide, lower the risk of disease-related death and morbidity among patients who have severe disease. For patients with polyarteritis nodosa associated with hepatitis B, the preferred treatment regimen is a short course of prednisone accompanied by anti-HBV therapy and plasmapheresis (three times a week for up to 6 weeks).

▶ Prognosis

Without treatment, the 5-year survival rate in these disorders is poor—on the order of 10%. With appropriate therapy, remissions are possible in many cases and the 5-year survival rate has improved to 60–90%. Poor prognostic factors are chronic kidney disease with serum creatinine > 1.6 mg/dL (> 141 mcmol/L), proteinuria > 1 g/d, gastrointestinal ischemia, central nervous system disease, and cardiac involvement. In the absence of any of these five factors, 5-year survival is nearly 90%. Survival at 5 years drops to 75% with one poor prognostic factor present and to about 50% with two or more factors. Substantial morbidity and even death may result from adverse effects of cyclophosphamide and corticosteroids. Consequently, these therapies require careful monitoring and expert management. In contrast to many other forms of systemic vasculitis, disease relapses in polyarteritis following the successful induction of remission are the exception rather than the rule, occurring in only about 20% of cases.

de Menthon M et al. Treating polyarteritis nodosa: current state of the art. Clin Exp Rheumatol. 2011 Jan–Feb;29(1 Suppl 64):S110–6. [PMID: 21586205]
Diamantopoulos AP et al. Polyarteritis nodosa. J Rheumatol. 2013 Jan;40(1):87–8. [PMID: 23280163]

GRANULOMATOSIS WITH POLYANGIITIS (Formerly Wegener Granulomatosis)

ESSENTIALS OF DIAGNOSIS

▶ Classic triad of upper and lower respiratory tract disease and glomerulonephritis.

▶ Suspect if mild respiratory symptoms (eg, nasal congestion, sinusitis) are refractory to usual treatment.

▶ Pathology defined by the triad of small vessel vasculitis, granulomatous inflammation, and necrosis.

▶ ANCAs (90% of patients), usually directed against proteinase-3 (less commonly against myeloperoxidase present in severe, active disease).

▶ Kidney disease often rapidly progressive without treatment.

▶ General Considerations

Granulomatosis with polyangiitis, which has an estimated incidence of approximately 12 cases per million individuals per year, is the prototype of diseases associated with antineutrophil cytoplasmic antibodies (ANCA). (Other "ANCA-associated vasculitides" include microscopic polyangiitis and the Churg-Strauss syndrome.) Granulomatosis with polyangiitis is characterized in its full expression by vasculitis of small arteries, arterioles, and capillaries, necrotizing granulomatous lesions of both upper and lower respiratory tract, glomerulonephritis, and other organ manifestations. Without treatment, generalized disease is invariably fatal, with most patients surviving < 1 year after diagnosis. It occurs most commonly in the fourth and fifth decades of life and affects men and women with equal frequency.

▶ Clinical Findings

A. Symptoms and Signs

The disorder usually develops over 4–12 months. Upper respiratory tract symptoms develop in 90% of patients and lower respiratory tract symptoms develop in 60% of patients; some patients may have both upper and lower respiratory tract symptoms. Upper respiratory tract symptoms can include nasal congestion, sinusitis, otitis media, mastoiditis, inflammation of the gums, or stridor due to subglottic stenosis. Since many of these symptoms are common, the underlying disease is not often suspected until the patient develops systemic symptoms or the original problem is refractory to treatment. The lungs are affected initially in 40% and eventually in 80%, with symptoms including cough, dyspnea, and hemoptysis. Other early symptoms can include a migratory oligoarthritis with a predilection for large joints; a variety of symptoms related to ocular disease (unilateral proptosis from orbital pseudotumor; red eye from scleritis [Figure 20–6], episcleritis, anterior uveitis, or peripheral ulcerative keratitis); purpura

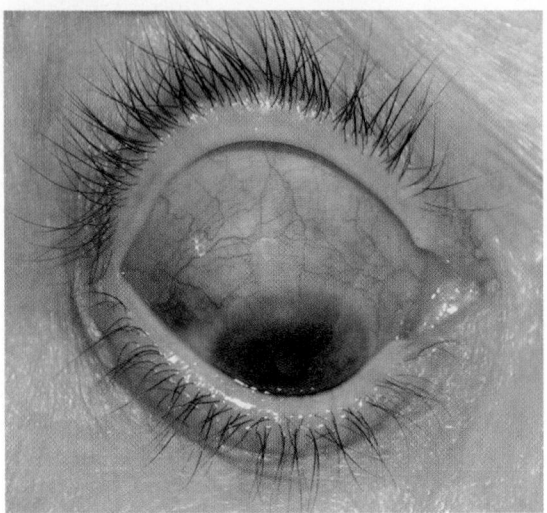

▲ **Figure 20–6.** Scleritis in a patient with granulomatosis with polyangiitis (formerly Wegener granulomatosis). (From Everett Allen, MD; reproduced with permission from Usatine RP, Smith MA, Mayeaux EJ Jr, Chumley H, Tysinger J. *The Color Atlas of Family Medicine.* McGraw-Hill, 2009.)

or other skin lesions; and dysesthesia due to neuropathy. Renal involvement, which develops in three-fourths of the cases, may be subclinical until kidney disease is advanced. Fever, malaise, and weight loss are common.

Physical examination can be remarkable for congestion, crusting, ulceration, bleeding, and even perforation of the nasal septum. Destruction of the nasal cartilage with "saddle nose" deformity occurs late. Otitis media, proptosis, scleritis, episcleritis, and conjunctivitis are other common findings. Newly acquired hypertension, a frequent feature of polyarteritis nodosa, is rare in granulomatosis with polyangiitis. Venous thrombotic events (eg, deep venous thrombosis and pulmonary embolism) are a common occurrence in granulomatosis with polyangiitis, at least in part because of the tendency of the disease to involve veins as well as arteries. Although limited forms of granulomatosis with polyangiitis have been described in which the kidney is spared initially, kidney disease will develop in the majority of untreated patients.

B. Laboratory Findings

1. Serum tests and urinalysis—Most patients have slight anemia, mild leukocytosis, and elevated acute phase reactants. If there is renal involvement, there is proteinuria and the urinary sediment contains red cells, with or without white cells, and often has red cell casts.

Serum tests for ANCA help in the diagnosis of granulomatosis with polyangiitis and related forms of vasculitis (Table 20–8). Several different types of ANCA are recognized, but the two subtypes relevant to systemic vasculitis are those directed against proteinase-3 (PR3) and myeloperoxidase (MPO). Antibodies to these two antigens are termed "PR3-ANCA" and "MPO-ANCA," respectively. The cytoplasmic pattern of immunofluorescence (c-ANCA) caused by PR3-ANCA has a high specificity (> 90%) for

either granulomatosis with polyangiitis or a closely related disease, microscopic polyangiitis (or, less commonly, the Churg-Strauss syndrome). In the setting of active disease, particularly cases in which the disease is severe and generalized to multiple organ systems, the sensitivity of PR3-ANCA is > 95%. A substantial percentage of patients with "limited" granulomatosis with polyangiitis—disease that does not pose an immediate threat to life and is often confined to the respiratory tract—are ANCA-negative. Although ANCA testing may be very helpful when used properly, it does not eliminate the need in most cases for confirmation of the diagnosis by tissue biopsy. Furthermore, ANCA levels correlate erratically with disease activity, and changes in titer should not dictate changes in therapy in the absence of supporting clinical data. The perinuclear (p-ANCA) pattern, caused by MPO-ANCA, is more likely to occur in microscopic polyangiitis or Churg-Strauss but may also be found in granulomatosis with polyangiitis. Approximately 10–25% of patients with classic granulomatosis with polyangiitis have MPO-ANCA. All positive immunofluorescence assays for ANCA should be confirmed by enzyme immunoassays for the specific autoantibodies directed against PR3 or MPO.

2. Histologic findings—Histologic features of granulomatosis with polyangiitis include vasculitis, granulomatous inflammation, geographic necrosis, and acute and chronic inflammation. The full range of pathologic changes is usually evident only on thoracoscopic lung biopsy. Granulomas, observed only rarely in renal biopsy specimens, are found much more commonly on lung biopsy specimens. Nasal biopsies often do not show vasculitis but may show chronic inflammation and other changes which, interpreted by an experienced pathologist, can serve as convincing evidence of the diagnosis. Renal biopsy discloses a segmental necrotizing glomerulonephritis with multiple crescents; this is characteristic but not diagnostic. Pathologists characterize the renal lesion of granulomatosis with polyangiitis (and other forms of "ANCA-associated vasculitis") as a pauci-immune glomerulonephritis because of the relative absence (compared with immune complex–mediated disorders) of immunoreactants—IgG, IgM, IgA, and complement proteins—within glomeruli.

C. Imaging

Chest CT is more sensitive than chest radiography; lesions include infiltrates, nodules, masses, and cavities. Pleural effusions are uncommon. Often the radiographs prompt concern about lung cancer. Hilar adenopathy is unusual in granulomatosis with polyangiitis; if present, sarcoidosis, tumor, or infection is more likely. Other common radiographic abnormalities include extensive sinusitis and even bony sinus erosions.

▶ **Differential Diagnosis**

In most patients with granulomatosis with polyangiitis, refractory sinusitis or otitis media is initially suspected. When upper respiratory tract inflammation persists and is accompanied by additional systemic inflammatory signs (eg, red eye from scleritis, joint pain, and swelling), the diagnosis of granulomatosis with polyangiitis should be considered. Rheumatoid arthritis will wrongly be suspected in a substantial minority of patients who chiefly complain of joint pain. Arriving at the correct diagnosis is aided by awareness that rheumatoid arthritis typically involves small joints of the hand, whereas granulomatosis with polyangiitis favors large joints, such as the hip, knee, elbow, and shoulder. Lung cancer may be the first diagnostic consideration for some middle-aged patients in whom cough, hemoptysis, and lung masses are presenting symptoms and signs; typically, evidence of glomerulonephritis, a positive ANCA or, ultimately, the lung biopsy findings will point to the proper diagnosis. Granulomatosis with polyangiitis shares with SLE, anti–glomerular basement membrane disease, and microscopic polyangiitis the ability to cause an acute pulmonary-renal syndrome. Approximately 10–25% of patients with classic granulomatosis with polyangiitis have MPO-ANCA. Owing to involvement of the same types of blood vessels, similar patterns of organ involvement, and the possibility of failing to identify granulomatous pathology on tissue biopsies because of sampling error, granulomatosis with polyangiitis is often difficult to differentiate from microscopic polyangiitis. The crucial distinctions between the two disorders are the tendencies for granulomatosis with polyangiitis to involve the upper respiratory tract (including the ears) and to cause granulomatous inflammation. Cocaine use can cause destruction of midline tissues—the nose and palate—that mimics granulomatosis with polyangiitis. Indeed, distinguishing between the two conditions can be challenging because patients with cocaine-mediated midline destructive disease frequently have positive tests for PR-3-ANCA and lesional biopsies that demonstrate vasculitis. In contrast to granulomatosis with polyangiitis, cocaine-mediated midline destructive disease does not cause pulmonary or renal disease.

► Treatment

Early treatment is crucial in preventing the devastating end-organ complications of this disease, and often in preserving life. While granulomatosis with polyangiitis may involve the sinuses or lung for months, once proteinuria or hematuria develops, progression to advanced chronic kidney disease can be rapid (over several weeks). For patients with severe disease, there are now two treatment options for inducing remission: cyclophosphamide plus corticosteroids or rituximab plus corticosteroids. For several decades, the combination of cyclophosphamide and prednisone had been the standard of care for patients with severe disease. Remissions can be induced in more than 90% of patients treated with prednisone (1 mg/kg daily) plus cyclophosphamide (2 mg/kg/d orally with adjustments required for acute or chronic kidney disease and age >70 years old). Cyclophosphamide is best given daily by mouth; intermittent high-dose intravenous cyclophosphamide is less effective. Whenever cyclophosphamide is used, *Pneumocystis jirovecii* prophylaxis with either single-strength oral trimethoprim-sulfamethoxazole or dapsone 100 mg/d is essential. The current approach to remission induction is to use cyclophosphamide for 3–6 months, and then switch the patient to a regimen more likely to be tolerated well. Unfortunately, disease relapses

occur in a substantial proportion of those patients who achieve remission. In patients with remission induced by 3–6 months of cyclophosphamide and corticosteroids, azathioprine (up to 2 mg/kg/d orally) has been shown to be as effective as cyclophosphamide in maintaining disease remissions (at least for up to 12–15 months). Before the institution of azathioprine, patients should be tested (through a commercially available blood test) for deficiencies in the level of thiopurine methyltransferase, an enzyme essential to the metabolism of azathioprine. Another option for remission maintenance is methotrexate, 20–25 mg/wk (administered either orally or intramuscularly). The other option for treating severe granulomatosis with polyangiitis is rituximab, a B-cell depleting antibody. The FDA has approved rituximab in combination with corticosteroids for the treatment of granulomatosis with polyangiitis and microscopic polyangiitis. Studies demonstrate that rituximab is not less effective for remission-induction in these conditions. Indeed, post-hoc analysis of one clinical trial demonstrates that rituximab is more effective than cyclophosphamide for treating relapses of granulomatosis with polyangiitis and microscopic polyangiitis. Both rituximab and cyclophosphamide increase the risk of developing life-threatening opportunistic infections (including progressive multifocal leukoencephalopathy [PML]). Owing to rituximab's high cost, its unknown long-term health effects, and its undefined use for maintaining remission, its precise role in treating ANCA-associated vasculitis is being studied. Because of its superior side-effect profile, methotrexate is viewed as an appropriate substitute for cyclophosphamide or rituximab for initial treatment in patients who do not have significant renal dysfunction (of any cause) or immediately life-threatening disease. Treatment with TNF inhibitors, particularly etanercept, is not effective.

Lyons PA et al. Genetically distinct subsets within ANCA-associated vasculitis. N Engl J Med. 2012 Jul 19;367(3):214–23. [PMID: 22808956]

Roubaud-Baudron C et al; French Vasculitis Study Group. Rituximab maintenance therapy for granulomatosis with polyangiitis and microscopic polyangiitis. J Rheumatol. 2012 Jan;39(1):125–30. [PMID: 22089465]

MICROSCOPIC POLYANGIITIS

ESSENTIALS OF DIAGNOSIS

► Necrotizing vasculitis of small- and medium-sized arteries and veins.

► Most common cause of pulmonary-renal syndrome: diffuse alveolar hemorrhage and glomerulonephritis.

► Associated with ANCA in 75% of cases, usually anti-myeloperoxidase antibodies (MPO-ANCA) that cause a p-ANCA pattern on immunofluorescence testing. ANCA directed against proteinase-3 (PR3-ANCA) can also be observed.

General Considerations

Microscopic polyangiitis is a pauci-immune nongranulomatous necrotizing vasculitis that (1) affects small blood vessels (capillaries, venules, or arterioles), (2) often causes glomerulonephritis and pulmonary capillaritis, and (3) is often associated with ANCA on immunofluorescence testing (directed against MPO, a constituent of neutrophil granules). Because microscopic polyangiitis may involve medium-sized as well as small blood vessels and because it tends to affect capillaries within the lungs and kidneys, its spectrum overlaps those of both polyarteritis nodosa and granulomatosis with polyangiitis.

In rare instances, medications, particularly propylthiouracil, hydralazine, allopurinol, penicillamine, minocycline, and sulfasalazine, induce a systemic vasculitis associated with high titers of MPO-ANCA and features of microscopic polyangiitis.

Clinical Findings

A. Symptoms and Signs

A wide variety of findings suggesting vasculitis of small blood vessels may develop in microscopic polyangiitis. These include "palpable" (or "raised") purpura and other signs of cutaneous vasculitis (ulcers, splinter hemorrhages, vesiculobullous lesions).

Microscopic polyangiitis is the most common cause of pulmonary-renal syndromes, being several times more common than anti–glomerular basement membrane disease. Interstitial lung fibrosis that mimics usual interstitial pneumonitis is the presenting condition. Pulmonary hemorrhage may occur. The pathologic findings in the lung are typically those of capillaritis.

Vasculitic neuropathy (mononeuritis multiplex) is also common in microscopic polyangiitis.

B. Laboratory Findings

As noted, three-fourths of patients with microscopic polyangiitis are ANCA-positive. Elevated acute phase reactants are also typical of active disease. Microscopic hematuria, proteinuria, and red blood cell casts in the urine may occur. The renal lesion is a segmental, necrotizing glomerulonephritis, often with localized intravascular coagulation and the observation of intraglomerular thrombi upon renal biopsy.

Differential Diagnosis

Distinguishing this disease from granulomatosis with polyangiitis may be challenging in some cases. Microscopic polyangiitis is not associated with the chronic destructive upper respiratory tract disease often found in granulomatosis with polyangiitis. Moreover, as noted, a critical difference between the two diseases is the absence of granulomatous inflammation in microscopic polyangiitis. Because their treatments may differ, microscopic polyangiitis must also be differentiated from polyarteritis nodosa.

Treatment

Microscopic polyangiitis is usually treated in the same way as granulomatosis with polyangiitis: patients with severe disease, typically involving pulmonary hemorrhage and glomerulonephritis, require urgent induction treatment with corticosteroids and either cyclophosphamide or rituximab. If cyclophosphamide is chosen, it may be administered either in an oral daily regimen or via intermittent (usually monthly) intravenous pulses; following induction of remission, cyclophosphamide may be replaced with azathioprine. In cases of drug-induced MPO-ANCA–associated vasculitis, the offending medication should be discontinued; significant organ involvement (eg, pulmonary hemorrhage, glomerulonephritis) requires immunosuppressive therapy.

Prognosis

The key to effecting good outcomes is early diagnosis. Compared with patients who have granulomatosis with polyangiitis, those who have microscopic polyangiitis are more likely to have significant fibrosis on renal biopsy because of later diagnosis. The likelihood of disease recurrence following remission in microscopic polyangiitis is about 33%.

Corral-Gudino L et al. Overall survival, renal survival and relapse in patients with microscopic polyangiitis: a systematic review of current evidence. Rheumatology (Oxford). 2011 Aug;50(8):1414–23. [PMID: 21406467]

Suppiah R et al. Peripheral neuropathy in ANCA-associated vasculitis: outcomes from the European Vasculitis Study Group trials. Rheumatology (Oxford). 2011 Dec;50(12):2214–22. [PMID: 21890618]

Walsh M et al. Risk factors for relapse of antineutrophil cytoplasmic antibody-associated vasculitis. Arthritis Rheum. 2012 Feb;64(2):542–8. [PMID: 21953279]

LEVAMISOLE-ASSOCIATED PURPURA

Exposure to levamisole, a prevalent adulterant of illicit cocaine in North America, can induce a distinctive clinical syndrome of retiform purpura and cutaneous necrosis affecting the extremities, ears, and skin overlying the zygomatic arch. Biopsies reveal widespread thrombosis of small cutaneous vessels with varying degrees of vasculitis. The syndrome is associated with the lupus anticoagulant, IgM antibodies to cardiolipin, and very high titers of p-ANCAs (due to autoantibodies to elastase, lactoferrin, cathepsin-G, and other neutrophil components rather than to myeloperoxidase alone). There is no consensus on treatment of levamisole-induced purpura, but early lesions can resolve with abstinence. Use of levamisole-adulterated cocaine also has been linked to neutropenia, agranulocytosis, and pauci-immune glomerulonephritis.

Graf J et al. Purpura, cutaneous necrosis, and anti-neutrophil cytoplasmic antibodies associated with levamisole-adulterated cocaine. Arthritis Rheum. 2011 Dec;63(12):3998–4001. [PMID: 22127712]

CRYOGLOBULINEMIA

Cryoglobulinemia can be associated with an immune-complex mediated, small-vessel vasculitis. Chronic infection with hepatitis C is the most common underlying condition;

cryoglobulinemic vasculitis also can occur in the setting of other chronic infections, such as subacute bacterial endocarditis and osteomyelitis, and with connective tissues diseases, especially Sjögren syndrome. The cryoglobulins associated with vasculitis are cold-precipitable immune complexes consisting of rheumatoid factor and IgG (rheumatoid factor is an autoantibody to the constant region of IgG). The rheumatoid factor component can be monoclonal (type II cryoglobulins) or polyclonal (type III cryoglobulins). (Type I cryoglobulins are cryoprecipitable monoclonal proteins that lack rheumatoid factor activity; these cause cold-induced hyperviscosity syndromes, not vasculitis, and are associated with lymphoproliferative disease.)

▶ Clinical Findings

Cryoglobulinemic vasculitis typically manifests as recurrent palpable purpura and peripheral neuropathy. A proliferative glomerulonephritis can develop and can manifest as rapidly progressive glomerulonephritis. Abnormal liver function tests, abdominal pain, and pulmonary disease may also occur. The diagnosis is based on a compatible clinical picture and a positive serum test for cryoglobulins. The presence of a disproportionately low C4 level can be a diagnostic clue to the presence of cryoglobulinemia.

▶ Treatment

Treatment depends on the cause and the severity of the vasculitis. Asymptomatic cryoglobulinemia is common in hepatitis C–infected individuals and does not in itself warrant treatment. Patients with mild to moderate vasculitis associated with hepatitis C are treated with viral suppression with pegylated forms of interferon-alpha and ribavirin; the protease inhibitor, telaprevir, should be added to provide triple therapy for patients with genotype 1 hepatitis C infection. Since interferon can augment the immune response, it is not used in patients with severe, life-threatening vasculitis. Rather, these patients are usually treated initially with immune suppression with plasmapheresis, corticosteroids, and cyclophosphamide. B cell depletion using rituximab appears to be a promising alternative avenue of immunosuppressive therapy. Once improved, patients with severe vasculitis from hepatitis C can then be given antiviral therapy.

Dammacco F et al. Therapy for hepatitis C virus-related cryoglobulinemic vasculitis. N Engl J Med. 2013 Sep 12;369(11):1035–45. [PMID: 24024840]

De Vita S et al. A randomized controlled trial of rituximab for the treatment of severe cryoglobulinemic vasculitis. Arthritis Rheum. 2012 Mar;64(3):843–53. [PMID: 22147661]

HENOCH-SCHÖNLEIN PURPURA

Henoch-Schönlein purpura, the most common systemic vasculitis in children, occurs in adults as well. Typical features are palpable purpura (Figure 20–7), arthritis, and hematuria. Abdominal pain occurs less frequently in adults than in children. Pathologic features include leukocytoclastic vasculitis with IgA deposition. The cause is not known.

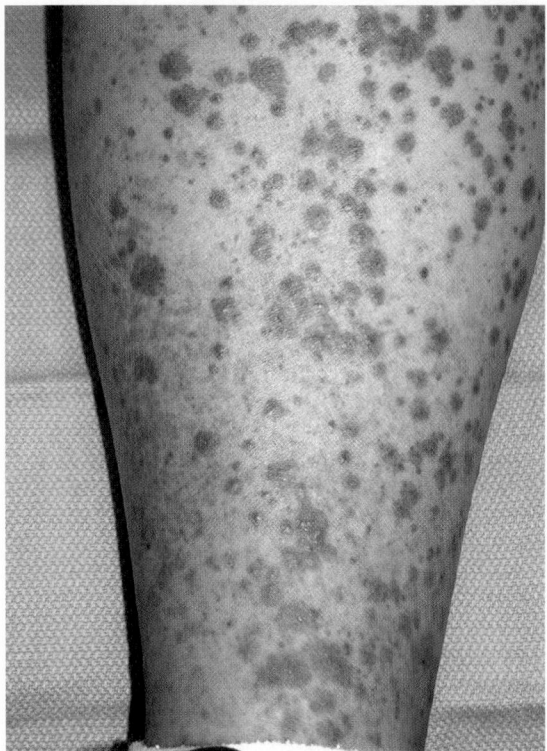

▲ **Figure 20–7.** Palpable purpura in a woman with leukocytoclastic vasculitis. (From Eric Krauss, MD; reproduced with permission from Usatine RP, Smith MA, Mayeaux EJ Jr, Chumley H, Tysinger J. *The Color Atlas of Family Medicine.* McGraw-Hill, 2009.)

The purpuric skin lesions are typically located on the lower extremities but may also be seen on the hands, arms, trunk, and buttocks. Joint symptoms are present in the majority of patients, the knees and ankles being most commonly involved. Abdominal pain secondary to vasculitis of the intestinal tract is often associated with gastrointestinal bleeding. Hematuria signals the presence of a renal lesion that is usually reversible, although it occasionally may progress to chronic kidney disease. Children tend to have more frequent and more serious gastrointestinal vasculitis, whereas adults more often suffer from chronic kidney disease. Biopsy of the kidney reveals segmental glomerulonephritis with crescents and mesangial deposition of IgA.

Chronic courses with persistent or intermittent skin disease are more likely to occur in adults than in children. The value of corticosteroids has been controversial. In children or adults, prednisone (1 mg/kg/d orally) may benefit those with severe extrarenal manifestations and with evidence of kidney disease. The incremental efficacy of steroid-sparing drugs such as azathioprine and mycophenolate mofetil—often used in the setting of kidney disease—is not known.

Jithpratuck W et al. The clinical implications of adult-onset Henoch-Schönlein purpura. Clin Mol Allergy. 2011 May 27;9(1):9. [PMID: 21619657]

RELAPSING POLYCHONDRITIS

This disease is characterized by inflammatory destructive lesions of cartilaginous structures, principally the ears, nose, trachea, and larynx. Nearly 40% of cases are associated with another disease, especially either other immunologic disorders (such as SLE, rheumatoid arthritis, or Hashimoto thyroiditis) or cancers (such as multiple myeloma) or hematologic disorders (such as myelodysplastic syndrome). The disease, which is usually episodic, affects males and females equally. The cartilage is painful, swollen, and tender during an attack and subsequently becomes atrophic, resulting in permanent deformity. Biopsy of the involved cartilage shows inflammation and chondrolysis. Noncartilaginous manifestations of the disease include fever, episcleritis, uveitis, deafness, aortic regurgitation, and rarely glomerulonephritis. In 85% of patients, a migratory, asymmetric, and seronegative arthropathy occurs, affecting both large and small joints and the costochondral junctions. Diagnosing this uncommon disease is especially difficult since the signs of cartilage inflammation (such as red ears or nasal pain) may be more subtle than the fever, arthritis, rash, or other systemic manifestations.

Prednisone, 0.5–1 mg/kg/d orally, is often effective. Dapsone (100–200 mg/d orally) or methotrexate (7.5–20 mg orally per week) may also have efficacy, sparing the need for long-term high-dose corticosteroid treatment. Involvement of the tracheobronchial tree, leading to tracheomalacia, may lead to difficult management issues.

Kemta Lekpa F et al. Biologics in relapsing polychondritis: a literature review. Semin Arthritis Rheum. 2012 Apr;41(5):712–9. [PMID: 22071463]

Yoo JH et al. Relapsing polychondritis: systemic and ocular manifestations, differential diagnosis, management, and prognosis. Semin Ophthalmol. 2011 Jul–Sep;26(4–5):261–9. [PMID: 21958172]

BEHÇET SYNDROME

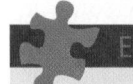

ESSENTIALS OF DIAGNOSIS

▶ Most commonly occurs among persons of Asian, Turkish, or Middle Eastern background, but may affect persons of any demographic profile.

▶ Recurrent, painful aphthous ulcers of the mouth and genitals.

▶ Erythema nodosum–like lesions; a follicular rash; and the pathergy phenomenon (formation of a sterile pustule at the site of a needle stick).

▶ Either anterior or posterior uveitis. Posterior uveitis may be asymptomatic until significant damage to the retina has occurred.

▶ Variety of neurologic lesions that can mimic multiple sclerosis, particularly through involvement of the white matter of the brainstem.

▶ General Considerations

Named after the Turkish dermatologist who first described it, this disease is of unknown cause. Its protean manifestations are believed to result from vasculitis that may involve all types of blood vessels: small, medium, and large, on both the arterial and venous side of the circulation.

▶ Clinical Findings

A. Symptoms and Signs

The hallmark of Behçet disease is painful aphthous ulcerations in the mouth (see Figure 8–7). These lesions, which usually occur multiply, may be found on the tongue, gums, and inner surfaces of the oral cavity. Genital lesions, similar in appearance, are also common but do not occur in all patients. Other cutaneous lesions of Behçet disease include tender, erythematous, papular lesions that resemble erythema nodosum. (On biopsy, however, many of these lesions are shown to be secondary to vasculitis rather than septal panniculitis.) These erythema nodosum–like lesions have a tendency to ulcerate, a major difference between the lesions of Behçet disease and the erythema nodosum seen in cases of sarcoidosis and inflammatory bowel disease. An erythematous follicular rash that occurs frequently on the upper extremities may be a subtle feature of the disease. The pathergy phenomenon is frequently underappreciated (unless the patient is asked); in this phenomenon, sterile pustules develop at sites where needles have been inserted into the skin (eg, for phlebotomy) in some patients.

A nonerosive arthritis occurs in about two-thirds of patients, most commonly affecting the knees and ankles. Eye involvement may be one of the most devastating complications of Behçet disease. Posterior uveitis, in essence a retinal venulitis, may lead to the insidious destruction of large areas of the retina before the patient becomes aware of visual problems. Anterior uveitis, associated with photophobia and a red eye, is intensely symptomatic. This complication may lead to a hypopyon, the accumulation of pus in the anterior chamber. If not treated properly with mydriatic agents to dilate the pupil and corticosteroid eyedrops to diminish inflammation, the anterior uveitis may lead to synechial formation between the iris and lens, resulting in permanent pupillary distortion.

Central nervous system involvement is another cause of major potential morbidity. The central nervous system lesions that may mimic multiple sclerosis radiologically often result in serious disability or death. Findings include sterile meningitis (recurrent meningeal headaches associated with a lymphocytic pleocytosis), cranial nerve palsies, seizures, encephalitis, mental disturbances, and spinal cord lesions. Aphthous ulcerations of the ileum and cecum and other forms of gastrointestinal involvement develop in approximately a quarter of patients. Large vessel vasculitis can lead to pulmonary artery aneurysms and life-threatening pulmonary hemorrhage. Finally, patients have a hypercoagulable tendency that may lead to complicated venous thrombotic events, particularly multiple deep venous thrombosis, pulmonary emboli, cerebral sinus thrombosis, and other problems associated with clotting.

The clinical course may be chronic but is often characterized by remissions and exacerbations.

B. Laboratory Findings

There are no pathognomonic laboratory features of Behçet disease. Although acute phase reactants are often elevated, there is no autoantibody or other assay that is distinctive. No markers of hypercoagulability specific to Behçet have been identified.

▶ Treatment

Both colchicine (0.6 mg once to three times daily orally) and thalidomide (100 mg/d orally) help ameliorate the mucocutaneous findings. Corticosteroids (1 mg/kg/d of oral prednisone) are a mainstay of initial therapy for severe disease manifestations. Azathioprine (2 mg/kg/d orally) may be an effective steroid-sparing agent. Infliximab, cyclosporine, or cyclophosphamide is indicated for severe ocular and central nervous system complications of Behçet disease.

Geri G et al. Spectrum of cardiac lesions in Behçet disease: a series of 52 patients and review of the literature. Medicine (Baltimore). 2012 Jan;91(1):25–34. [PMID: 22198500]
Mohammad A et al. Incidence, prevalence and clinical characteristics of Behcet's disease in southern Sweden. Rheumatology (Oxford). 2013 Feb;52(2):304–10. [PMID: 23012468]

PRIMARY ANGIITIS OF THE CENTRAL NERVOUS SYSTEM

Primary angiitis of the central nervous system is a syndrome with several possible causes that produces small and medium-sized vasculitis limited to the brain and spinal cord. Biopsy-proved cases have predominated in men who have a history of weeks to months of headaches, encephalopathy, and multifocal strokes. Systemic signs and symptoms are absent, and routine laboratory tests are usually normal. MRI of the brain is almost always abnormal, and the spinal fluid often reveals a mild lymphocytosis and a modest increase in protein level. Angiograms classically reveal a "string of beads" pattern produced by alternating segments of arterial narrowing and dilation. However, neither the MRI nor the angiogram appearance is specific for vasculitis. Indeed, in one study, none of the patients who had biopsy-proved central nervous system vasculitis had an angiogram showing "the string of beads," and none of the patients with the classic angiographic findings had a positive brain biopsy for vasculitis. Review of many studies suggests that the sensitivity of angiography varies greatly (from 40% to 90%) and the specificity is only approximately 30%. Many conditions, including vasospasm, can produce the same angiographic pattern as vasculitis. Definitive diagnosis requires a compatible clinical picture; exclusion of infection, neoplasm, or metabolic disorder or drug exposure (eg, cocaine) that can mimic primary angiitis of the central nervous system; and a positive brain biopsy. In contrast to biopsy-proved cases, patients with angiographically defined central nervous system

vasculopathy are chiefly women who have had an abrupt onset of headaches and stroke (often in the absence of encephalopathy) with normal spinal fluid findings. Many patients who fit this clinical profile may have reversible cerebral vasoconstriction rather than true vasculitis. Such cases may best be treated with calcium channel blockers (such as nimodipine or verapamil) and possibly a short course of corticosteroids. Biopsy-proved cases usually improve with prednisone therapy and often require cyclophosphamide. In recent years, cases of central nervous system vasculitis associated with cerebral amyloid angiopathy have been reported. These cases often respond well to corticosteroids, albeit the long-term natural history remains poorly defined.

Salvarani C et al. Adult primary central nervous system vasculitis. Lancet. 2012 Aug 25;380(9843):767–77. [PMID: 22575778]

LIVEDO RETICULARIS

Livedo reticularis produces a mottled, purplish discoloration of the skin with reticulated cyanotic areas surrounding paler central cores. This distinctive "fishnet" pattern is caused by spasm or obstruction of perpendicular arterioles, combined with pooling of blood in surrounding venous plexuses. Livedo reticularis can be idiopathic or a manifestation of a serious underlying condition.

Idiopathic livedo reticularis is a benign condition that worsens with cold exposure, improves with warming, and primarily affects the extremities. Apart from cosmetic concerns, it is usually asymptomatic. Systemic symptoms or the development of cutaneous ulcerations point to the presence of an underlying disease.

Secondary livedo reticularis occurs in association with a variety of diseases that cause vascular obstruction or inflammation. Of particular importance is the link with antiphospholipid antibody syndrome. Livedo reticularis is the presenting manifestation of 25% of patients with antiphospholipid antibody syndrome and is strongly associated with the subgroup that has arterial thromboses, including those with Sneddon syndrome (livedo reticularis and cerebrovascular events). Other underlying causes of livedo reticularis include the vasculitides (particularly polyarteritis nodosa), cholesterol emboli syndrome, thrombocythemia, cryoglobulinemia, cold agglutinin disease, primary hyperoxaluria (due to vascular deposits of calcium oxalate), and disseminated intravascular coagulation.

Dean SM. Livedo reticularis and related disorders. Curr Treat Options Cardiovasc Med. 2011 Apr;13(2):179–91. [PMID: 21287303]

▼ SERONEGATIVE SPONDYLOARTHROPATHIES

The seronegative spondyloarthropathies are ankylosing spondylitis, psoriatic arthritis, reactive arthritis, the arthritis associated with inflammatory bowel disease, and undifferentiated spondyloarthropathy. These disorders are noted for male predominance, onset usually before age 40, inflammatory arthritis of the spine and sacroiliac joints, asymmetric oligoarthritis of large peripheral joints, enthesopathy (inflammation of where ligaments, tendons, and joint capsule insert into bone), uveitis in a significant minority, the absence of autoantibodies in the serum, and a striking association with HLA-B27. HLA-B27 is positive in up to 90% of patients with ankylosing spondylitis and 75% with reactive arthritis. HLA-B27 also occurs in 50% of the psoriatic and inflammatory bowel disease patients who have sacroiliitis. Patients with only peripheral arthritis in these latter two syndromes do not show an increase in HLA-B27.

ANKYLOSING SPONDYLITIS

ESSENTIALS OF DIAGNOSIS

▶ Chronic low backache in young adults, generally worst in the morning.

▶ Progressive limitation of back motion and of chest expansion.

▶ Transient (50%) or persistent (25%) peripheral arthritis.

▶ Anterior uveitis in 20–25%.

▶ Diagnostic radiographic changes in sacroiliac joints.

▶ Negative serologic tests for rheumatoid factor and anti-CCP antibodies.

▶ HLA-B27 testing is most helpful when there is an intermediate probability of disease.

▶ General Considerations

Ankylosing spondylitis is a chronic inflammatory disease of the joints of the axial skeleton, manifested clinically by pain and progressive stiffening of the spine. The age at onset is usually in the late teens or early 20s. The incidence is greater in males than in females, and symptoms are more prominent in men, with ascending involvement of the spine more likely to occur.

▶ Clinical Findings

A. Symptoms and Signs

The onset is usually gradual, with intermittent bouts of back pain that may radiate into the buttocks. The back pain is worse in the morning and usually associated with stiffness that lasts hours. The pain and stiffness improve with activity, in contrast to back pain due to mechanical causes and degenerative disease, which improves with rest and worsens with activity. As the disease advances, symptoms progress in a cephalad direction, and back motion becomes limited, with the normal lumbar curve flattened and the thoracic curvature exaggerated. Chest expansion is often limited as a consequence of costovertebral joint involvement. In advanced cases, the entire spine becomes fused, allowing no motion in any direction. Transient acute arthritis of the peripheral joints occurs in about 50% of cases, and permanent changes in the peripheral joints—most commonly the hips, shoulders, and knees—are seen in about 25%. Enthesopathy, a hallmark of the spondyloarthropathies, can manifest as swelling of the Achilles tendon at its insertion, plantar fasciitis (producing heel pain), or "sausage" swelling of a finger or toe (less common in ankylosing spondylitis than in psoriatic arthritis).

Anterior uveitis is associated in as many as 25% of cases and may be a presenting feature. Spondylitic heart disease, characterized chiefly by atrioventricular conduction defects and aortic regurgitation occurs in 3–5% of patients with long-standing severe disease Constitutional symptoms similar to those of rheumatoid arthritis are absent in most patients.

B. Laboratory Findings

The ESR is elevated in 85% of cases, but serologic tests for rheumatoid factor and anti-CCP antibodies are negative. Anemia may be present but is often mild. HLA-B27 is found in 90% of white patients and 50% of black patients with ankylosing spondylitis. Because this antigen occurs in 8% of the healthy white population (and 2% of healthy blacks), it is not a specific diagnostic test.

C. Imaging

The earliest radiographic changes are usually in the sacroiliac joints. In the first 2 years of the disease process, the sacroiliac changes may be detectable only by MRI. Later, erosion and sclerosis of these joints are evident on plain radiographs; the sacroiliitis of ankylosing spondylitis is bilateral and symmetric. Inflammation where the annulus fibrosus attaches to the vertebral bodies initially causes sclerosis ("the shiny corner sign") and then characteristic squaring of the vertebral bodies. The term "bamboo spine" describes the late radiographic appearance of the spinal column in which the vertebral bodies are fused by vertically oriented, bridging syndesmophytes formed by the ossification of the annulus fibrosus and calcification of the anterior and lateral spinal ligaments. Fusion of the posterior facet joints of the spine is also common.

Additional radiographic findings include periosteal new bone formation on the iliac crest, ischial tuberosities and calcanei, and alterations of the pubic symphysis and sternomanubrial joint similar to those of the sacroiliacs. Radiologic changes in peripheral joints, when present, tend to be asymmetric and lack the demineralization and erosions seen in rheumatoid arthritis.

▶ Differential Diagnosis

Low back pain due to mechanical causes, disk disease, and degenerative arthritis is very common. Onset of back pain prior to age 30 and an "inflammatory" quality of the back pain (ie, morning stiffness and pain that improve with activity) should raise the possibility of ankylosing spondylitis.

In contrast to ankylosing spondylitis, rheumatoid arthritis predominantly affects multiple, small, peripheral joints of the hands and feet. Rheumatoid arthritis spares the sacroiliac joints and only affects the cervical component of the spine. Bilateral sacroiliitis indistinguishable from ankylosing spondylitis is seen with the spondylitis associated with inflammatory bowel disease. Sacroiliitis associated with reactive arthritis and psoriasis, on the other hand, is often asymmetric or even unilateral. Osteitis condensans ilii (sclerosis on the iliac side of the sacroiliac joint) is an asymptomatic, postpartum radiographic finding that is occasionally mistaken for sacroiliitis. Diffuse idiopathic skeletal hyperostosis (DISH) causes exuberant osteophytes ("enthesophytes") of the spine that occasionally are difficult to distinguish from the syndesmophytes of ankylosing spondylitis. The enthesophytes of DISH are thicker and more anterior than the syndesmophytes of ankylosing spondylitis, and the sacroiliac joints are normal in DISH.

► Treatment

NSAIDs remain first-line treatment of ankylosing spondylitis and may slow radiographic progression of spinal disease. Because individual patients differ in their response to particular NSAIDs, empiric trials of several different NSAIDs are warranted if the response to any given NSAID is not satisfactory. TNF inhibitors have established efficacy for NSAID-resistant axial disease; responses are often substantial and durable. Etanercept (50 mg subcutaneously once a week), adalimumab (40 mg subcutaneously every other week), infliximab (5 mg/kg every other month by intravenous infusion), or golimumab (50 mg subcutaneously once a month) is reasonable for patients whose symptoms are refractory to NSAIDs. Sulfasalazine (1000 mg orally twice daily) is sometimes useful for peripheral arthritis but lacks effectiveness for spinal and sacroiliac joint disease. Corticosteroids have minimal impact on the arthritis—particularly the spondylitis—of ankylosing spondylitis and can worsen osteopenia. All patients should be referred to a physical therapist for instruction in postural exercises.

► Prognosis

Almost all patients have persistent symptoms over decades; rare individuals experience long-term remissions. The severity of disease varies greatly, with about 10% of patients having work disability after 10 years. Developing hip disease within the first 2 years of disease onset presages a worse prognosis. The availability of TNF inhibitors has provided symptomatic relief and improved quality of life for many patients with ankylosing spondylitis.

Reveille JD et al. The epidemiology of back pain, axial spondyloarthritis and HLA-B27 in the United States. Am J Med Sci. 2013 Jun;345(6):431–6. [PMID: 23841117]

Smith ME et al. Treatment recommendations for the management of axial spondyloarthritis. Am J Med Sci. 2013 Jun;345(6):426–30. [PMID: 23841116]

PSORIATIC ARTHRITIS

ESSENTIALS OF DIAGNOSIS

► Psoriasis precedes onset of arthritis in 80% of cases.

► Arthritis usually asymmetric, with "sausage" appearance of fingers and toes but a polyarthritis that resembles rheumatoid arthritis also occurs.

► Sacroiliac joint involvement common; ankylosis of the sacroiliac joints may occur.

► Radiographic findings: osteolysis; pencil-in-cup deformity; relative lack of osteoporosis; bony ankylosis; asymmetric sacroiliitis and atypical syndesmophytes.

► General Considerations

Although psoriasis usually precedes the onset of arthritis, arthritis precedes (by up to 2 years) or occurs simultaneously with the skin disease in approximately 20% of cases.

► Clinical Findings

A. Symptoms and Signs

The patterns or subsets of psoriatic arthritis include the following:

1. A symmetric polyarthritis that resembles rheumatoid arthritis. Usually, fewer joints are involved than in rheumatoid arthritis.

2. An oligoarticular form that may lead to considerable destruction of the affected joints.

3. A pattern of disease in which the DIP joints are primarily affected. Early, this may be monarticular, and often the joint involvement is asymmetric. Pitting of the nails and onycholysis frequently accompany DIP involvement.

4. A severe deforming arthritis (arthritis mutilans) in which osteolysis is marked.

5. A spondylitic form in which sacroiliitis and spinal involvement predominate; 50% of these patients are HLA-B27-positive.

Arthritis is at least five times more common in patients with severe skin disease than in those with only mild skin findings. Occasionally, however, patients may have a single patch of psoriasis (typically hidden in the scalp, gluteal cleft, or umbilicus) and are unaware of its presence. Thus, a detailed search for cutaneous lesions is essential in patients with arthritis of new onset. Also, the psoriatic lesions may have cleared when arthritis appears—in such cases, the history is most useful in diagnosing previously unexplained cases of mono- or oligoarthritis. Nail pitting is sometimes a clue. "Sausage" swelling of one or more digits is a common manifestation of enthesopathy in psoriatic arthritis.

B. Laboratory Findings

Laboratory studies show an elevation of the ESR, but rheumatoid factor is not present. Uric acid levels may be high, reflecting the active turnover of skin affected by psoriasis. There is a correlation between the extent of psoriatic involvement and the level of uric acid, but gout is no more common than in patients without psoriasis. Desquamation of the skin may also reduce iron stores.

C. Imaging

Radiographic findings are most helpful in distinguishing the disease from other forms of arthritis. There are marginal erosions of bone and irregular destruction of joint and bone, which, in the phalanx, may give the appearance of a sharpened pencil. Fluffy periosteal new bone may be marked, especially at the insertion of muscles and ligaments into bone. Such changes will also be seen along the shafts of metacarpals, metatarsals, and phalanges. Psoriatic spondylitis causes asymmetric sacroiliitis and syndesmophytes, which are coarser than those seen in ankylosing spondylitis.

▶ Treatment

NSAIDs are usually sufficient for mild cases. Methotrexate (7.5–20 mg orally once a week) is generally considered the drug of choice for patients who have not responded to NSAIDs; methotrexate can improve both the cutaneous and arthritic manifestations. For cases with disease that is refractory to methotrexate, the addition of TNF inhibitors (at doses similar to the treatment of ankylosing spondylitis) is usually effective for both arthritis and psoriatic skin disease. Corticosteroids are less effective in psoriatic arthritis than in other forms of inflammatory arthritis and may precipitate pustular psoriasis during tapers. Antimalarials may also exacerbate psoriasis. Successful treatment directed at the skin lesions alone (eg, by PUVA therapy) occasionally is accompanied by an improvement in peripheral articular symptoms.

McInnes IB et al. Efficacy and safety of ustekinumab in patients with active psoriatic arthritis: 1 year results of the phase 3, multicentre, double-blind, placebo-controlled PSUMMIT 1 trial. Lancet. 2013 Aug 31;382(9894):780–9. [PMID: 23769296]
Russolillo A et al. Obesity and psoriatic arthritis: from pathogenesis to clinical outcome and management. Rheumatology (Oxford). 2013 Jan;52(1):62–7. [PMID: 22989426]

REACTIVE ARTHRITIS (Formerly Reiter Syndrome)

ESSENTIALS OF DIAGNOSIS

▶ Fifty to eighty percent of patients are HLA-B27-positive.

▶ Oligoarthritis, conjunctivitis, urethritis, and mouth ulcers most common features.

▶ Usually follows dysentery or a sexually transmitted infection.

▶ General Considerations

Reactive arthritis is precipitated by antecedent gastrointestinal and genitourinary infections and manifests as an asymmetric sterile oligoarthritis, typically of the lower extremities. It is frequently associated with enthesitis. Extra-articular manifestations are common and include urethritis, conjunctivitis, uveitis, and mucocutaneous lesions. Reactive arthritis occurs most commonly in young men and is associated with HLA-B27 in 80% of white patients and 50–60% of blacks.

▶ Clinical Findings

A. Symptoms and Signs

Most cases of reactive arthritis develop within 1–4 weeks after either a gastrointestinal infection (with *Shigella, Salmonella, Yersinia, Campylobacter*) or a sexually transmitted infection (with *Chlamydia trachomatis* or perhaps *Ureaplasma urealyticum*). Whether the inciting infection is sexually transmitted or dysenteric does not affect the subsequent manifestations but does influence the gender ratio: The ratio is 1:1 after enteric infections but 9:1 with male predominance after sexually transmitted infections. Synovial fluid from affected joints is culture-negative. A clinically indistinguishable syndrome can occur without an apparent antecedent infection, suggesting that subclinical infection can precipitate reactive arthritis or that there are other, as yet unrecognized, triggers.

The arthritis is most commonly asymmetric and frequently involves the large weight-bearing joints (chiefly the knee and ankle); sacroiliitis or ankylosing spondylitis is observed in at least 20% of patients, especially after frequent recurrences. Systemic symptoms including fever and weight loss are common at the onset of disease. The mucocutaneous lesions may include balanitis (Figure 20–8), stomatitis, and keratoderma blennorrhagicum (Figure 20–9), indistinguishable from pustular psoriasis. Involvement of the fingernails in reactive arthritis also mimics psoriatic changes. When present, conjunctivitis is mild and occurs early in the disease course. Anterior uveitis, which can develop at any time in HLA-B27-positive patients, is a more clinically significant ocular complication. Carditis and aortic regurgitation may occur. While most signs of the disease

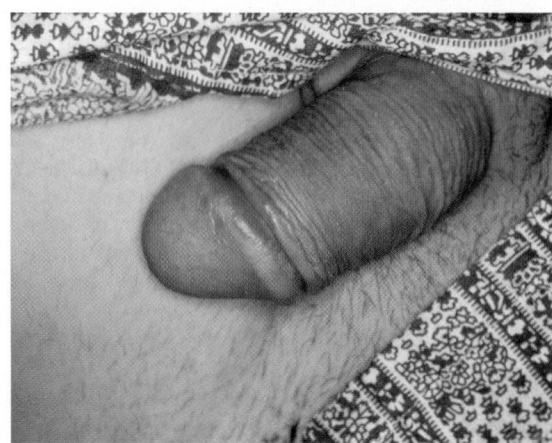

▲ **Figure 20–8.** Circinate balanitis due to reactive arthritis (Reiter syndrome). (From Susan Lindsley, Dr. M. F. Rein, Public Health Image Library, CDC.)

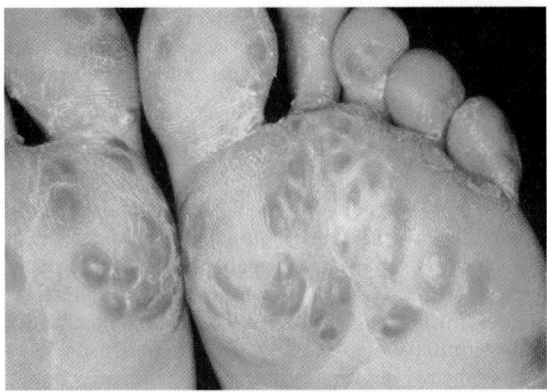

▲ **Figure 20–9.** Keratoderma blennorrhagica of the soles due to reactive arthritis (Reiter syndrome). (From Susan Lindsley, Public Health Image Library, CDC.)

disappear within days or weeks, the arthritis may persist for several months or become chronic. Recurrences involving any combination of the clinical manifestations are common and are sometimes followed by permanent sequelae, especially in the joints (eg, articular destruction).

B. Imaging

Radiographic signs of permanent or progressive joint disease may be seen in the sacroiliac as well as the peripheral joints.

▶ Differential Diagnosis

Gonococcal arthritis can initially mimic reactive arthritis, but the marked improvement after 24–48 hours of antibiotic administration and the culture results distinguish the two disorders. Rheumatoid arthritis, ankylosing spondylitis, and psoriatic arthritis must also be considered. By causing similar oral, ocular, and joint lesions, Behçet disease may also mimic reactive arthritis. The oral lesions of reactive arthritis, however, are typically painless, in contrast to those of Behçet disease.

The association of reactive arthritis and HIV has been debated, but evidence now indicates that it is equally common in sexually active men regardless of HIV status.

▶ Treatment

NSAIDs have been the mainstay of therapy. Antibiotics given at the time of a nongonococcal sexually transmitted infection reduce the chance that the individual will develop this disorder. For chronic reactive arthritis associated with chlamydial infection, combination antibiotics taken for 6 months are more effective than placebo. Patients who do not respond to NSAIDs may respond to sulfasalazine, 1000 mg orally twice daily, or to methotrexate, 7.5–20 mg orally per week. For those patients with recent-onset disease that is refractory to NSAIDs and these DMARDs, anti-TNF agents, which are effective in the other spondyloarthropathies, may be effective.

Morris D et al. Reactive arthritis: developments and challenges in diagnosis and treatment. Curr Rheumatol Rep. 2012 Oct;14 (5):390–4. [PMID: 22821199]

ARTHRITIS & INFLAMMATORY INTESTINAL DISEASES

One-fifth of patients with **inflammatory bowel disease** have arthritis, which complicates **Crohn disease** somewhat more frequently than it does **ulcerative colitis.** In both diseases, two distinct forms of arthritis occur. The first is peripheral arthritis—usually a nondeforming asymmetric oligoarthritis of large joints—in which the activity of the joint disease parallels that of the bowel disease. The arthritis usually begins months to years after the bowel disease, but occasionally the joint symptoms develop earlier and may be prominent enough to cause the patient to overlook intestinal symptoms. The second form of arthritis is a spondylitis that is indistinguishable by symptoms or radiographs from ankylosing spondylitis and follows a course independent of the bowel disease. About 50% of these patients are HLA-B27-positive.

Controlling the intestinal inflammation usually eliminates the peripheral arthritis. The spondylitis often requires NSAIDs, which need to be used cautiously since these agents may activate the bowel disease in a few patients. Range-of-motion exercises as prescribed for ankylosing spondylitis can be helpful.

About two-thirds of patients with **Whipple disease** experience arthralgia or arthritis, most often an episodic, large-joint polyarthritis. The arthritis usually precedes the gastrointestinal manifestations by years. In fact, the arthritis resolves as the diarrhea develops. Thus, Whipple disease should be considered in the differential diagnosis of unexplained episodic arthritis.

Papamichael K et al. Low prevalence of antibodies to cyclic citrullinated peptide in patients with inflammatory bowel disease regardless of the presence of arthritis. Eur J Gastroenterol Hepatol. 2010 Jun;22(6):705–9. [PMID: 19525851]

▼ INFECTIOUS ARTHRITIS[1]

NONGONOCOCCAL ACUTE BACTERIAL (Septic) ARTHRITIS

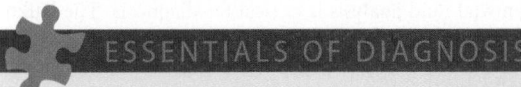

ESSENTIALS OF DIAGNOSIS

- ▶ Acute onset of inflammatory monoarticular arthritis, most often in large weight-bearing joints and wrists.

- ▶ Common risk factors include previous joint damage and injection drug use.

- ▶ Infection with causative organisms commonly found elsewhere in body.

- ▶ Joint effusions are usually large, with white blood cell counts commonly >50,000/mcL.

[1]Lyme disease is discussed in Chapter 34.

General Considerations

Nongonococcal acute bacterial arthritis is often a disease that occurs when there is an underlying abnormality. The key risk factors are bacteremia (eg, injection drug use, endocarditis, infection at other sites), damaged or prosthetic joints (eg, rheumatoid arthritis), compromised immunity (eg, diabetes, advanced chronic kidney disease, alcoholism, cirrhosis, and immunosuppressive therapy), and loss of skin integrity (eg, cutaneous ulcer or psoriasis). *Staphylococcus aureus* is the most common cause of nongonococcal septic arthritis, accounting for about 50% of all cases. Methicillin-resistant *S aureus* (MRSA) and group B streptococcus have become increasing frequent and important causes of septic arthritis. Gram-negative septic arthritis causes about 10% of cases and is especially common in injection drug users and in immunocompromised persons. *Escherichia coli and Pseudomonas aeruginosa* are the most common gram-negative isolates in adults. Pathologic changes include varying degrees of acute inflammation, with synovitis, effusion, abscess formation in synovial or subchondral tissues, and, if treatment is not adequate, articular destruction.

Clinical Findings

A. Symptoms and Signs

The onset is usually acute, with pain, swelling, and heat of the affected joint worsening over hours. The knee is most frequently involved; other commonly affected sites are the hip, wrist, shoulder, and ankle. Unusual sites, such as the sternoclavicular or sacroiliac joint, can be involved in injection drug users. Chills and fever are common but are absent in up to 20% of patients. Infection of the hip usually does not produce apparent swelling but results in groin pain greatly aggravated by walking. More than one joint is involved in 15% of cases of septic arthritis; risk factors for multiple joint involvement include rheumatoid arthritis, associated endocarditis, and infection with group B streptococci.

B. Laboratory Findings

Synovial fluid analysis is critical for diagnosis. The leukocyte count of the synovial fluid usually exceeds 50,000/mcL and often is > 100,000/mcL, with 90% or more polymorphonuclear cells (Table 20–2). Gram stain of the synovial fluid is positive in 75% of staphylococcal infections and in 50% of gram-negative infections. Synovial fluid cultures are positive in 70–90% of cases; administration of antibiotics prior to arthrocentesis reduces the likelihood of a positive culture result. Blood cultures are positive in approximately 50% of patients.

C. Imaging

Imaging tests generally add little to the diagnosis of septic arthritis. Indeed, other than demonstrating joint effusion, radiographs are usually normal early in the disease; however, evidence of demineralization may develop within days of onset. MRI and CT are more sensitive in detecting fluid in joints that are not accessible to physical examination (eg, the hip). Bony erosions and narrowing of the joint space followed by osteomyelitis and periostitis may be seen within 2 weeks.

Differential Diagnosis

Gout and pseudogout can cause acute, very inflammatory monoarticular arthritis and high-grade fever; the failure to find crystals on synovial fluid analysis excludes these diagnoses. A well-recognized but uncommon initial presentation of rheumatoid arthritis is an acute inflammatory monoarthritis ("pseudoseptic"). Acute rheumatic fever commonly involves several joints; Still disease may mimic septic arthritis, but laboratory evidence of infection is absent. Pyogenic arthritis may be superimposed on other types of joint disease, notably rheumatoid arthritis. Indeed, septic arthritis must be excluded (by joint fluid examination) in any patient with rheumatoid arthritis who has a joint strikingly more inflamed than the other joints.

Prevention

There is no evidence that patients with prosthetic joints undergoing procedures should receive antibiotic prophylaxis to prevent joint infection unless the patient has a prosthetic heart valve or the procedure requires antibiotics to prevent a surgical site infection. However, the topic remains controversial. The American Academy of Orthopedic Surgeons advocates prescribing antibiotic prophylaxis for any patient with a prosthetic joint replacement undergoing a procedure that can cause bacteremia.

Treatment

The effective treatment of septic arthritis requires appropriate antibiotic therapy together with drainage of the infected joint. Hospitalization is always necessary. If the likely causative organism cannot be determined clinically or from the synovial fluid Gram stain, treatment should be started with broad-spectrum antibiotic coverage effective against staphylococci, streptococci, and gram-negative organisms. The recommendation for initial treatment is to give vancomycin (1 g intravenously every 12 hours, adjusted for age, weight, and renal function) plus a third-generation cephalosporin: ceftriaxone, 1 g intravenously daily (or every 12 hours if concomitant meningitis or endocarditis is suspected); or cefotaxime, 1 g intravenously every 8 hours; or ceftazidime, 1 g intravenously every 8 hours. Antibiotic therapy should be adjusted when culture results become available; the duration of antibiotic therapy is usually 4–6 weeks.

Early orthopedic consultation is essential. Effective drainage is usually achieved through early arthroscopic lavage and debridement together with drain placement. Open surgical drainage should be performed when conservative treatment fails, when there is concomitant osteomyelitis requiring debridement, or when the involved joint (eg, hip, shoulder, sacroiliac joint) cannot be drained by more conservative means. Immobilization with a splint and elevation are used at the onset of treatment.

Early active motion exercises within the limits of tolerance will hasten recovery.

Prognosis

The outcome of septic arthritis depends largely on the antecedent health of the patient, the causative organism (eg, *S aureus* bacterial arthritis is associated with a poor functional outcome in about 40% of cases), and the promptness of treatment. Five to 10 percent of patients with an infected joint die of respiratory complications of sepsis. The mortality rate is 30% for patients with polyarticular sepsis. Bony ankylosis and articular destruction commonly also occur if treatment is delayed or inadequate.

Cipriano CA et al. Serum and synovial fluid analysis for diagnosing chronic periprosthetic infection in patients with inflammatory arthritis. J Bone Joint Surg Am. 2012 Apr 4;94(7): 594–600. [PMID: 22488615]

Mathews CJ et al. Bacterial septic arthritis in adults. Lancet. 2010 Mar 6;375(9717):846–55. [PMID: 20206778]

GONOCOCCAL ARTHRITIS

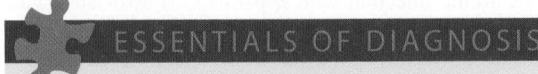

ESSENTIALS OF DIAGNOSIS

▸ Prodromal migratory polyarthralgias.

▸ Tenosynovitis is the most common sign.

▸ Purulent monarthritis in 50%.

▸ Characteristic skin lesions.

▸ Most common in young women during menses or pregnancy.

▸ Symptoms of urethritis frequently absent.

▸ Dramatic response to antibiotics.

General Considerations

In contrast to nongonococcal bacterial arthritis, gonococcal arthritis usually occurs in otherwise healthy individuals. Host factors, however, influence the expression of the disease: gonococcal arthritis is two to three times more common in women than in men, is especially common during menses and pregnancy, and is rare after age 40. Gonococcal arthritis is also common in men who have sex with men, whose high incidence of asymptomatic gonococcal pharyngitis and proctitis predisposes them to disseminated gonococcal infection. Recurrent disseminated gonococcal infection should prompt testing of the patient's CH50 level to evaluate for a congenital deficiency of a terminal complement component (C5, C6, C7, or C8).

Clinical Findings

A. Symptoms and Signs

One to 4 days of migratory polyarthralgias involving the wrist, knee, ankle, or elbow are common at the outset. Thereafter, two patterns emerge. The first pattern is characterized by tenosynovitis that most often affects wrists, fingers, ankles, or toes and is seen in 60% of patients. The second pattern is purulent monarthritis that most frequently involves the knee, wrist, ankle, or elbow and is seen in 40% of patients. Less than half of patients have fever, and less than one-fourth have any genitourinary symptoms. Most patients will have asymptomatic but highly characteristic skin lesions that usually consist of two to ten small necrotic pustules distributed over the extremities, especially the palms and soles.

B. Laboratory Findings

The peripheral blood leukocyte count averages about 10,000 cells/mcL and is elevated in less than one-third of patients. The synovial fluid white blood cell count usually ranges from 30,000 to 60,000 cells/mcL. The synovial fluid Gram stain is positive in one-fourth of cases and culture in less than half. Positive blood cultures are uncommon. Urethral, throat, cervical, and rectal cultures should be done in all patients, since they are often positive in the absence of local symptoms. Urinary nucleic acid amplification tests have excellent sensitivity and specificity for the detection of *Neisseria gonorrhoeae* in genitourinary sites.

C. Imaging

Radiographs are usually normal or show only soft tissue swelling.

Differential Diagnosis

Reactive arthritis can produce acute monarthritis, urethritis, and fever in a young person but is distinguished by negative cultures and failure to respond to antibiotics. Lyme disease involving the knee is less acute, does not show positive cultures, and may be preceded by known tick exposure and characteristic rash. The synovial fluid analysis will exclude gout, pseudogout, and nongonococcal bacterial arthritis. Rheumatic fever and sarcoidosis can produce migratory tenosynovitis but have other distinguishing features. Infective endocarditis with septic arthritis can mimic disseminated gonococcal infection. Meningococcemia occasionally presents with a clinical picture that resembles disseminated gonococcal infection; blood cultures establish the correct diagnosis. Early hepatitis B infection is associated with circulating immune complexes that can cause a rash and polyarthralgias. In contrast to disseminated gonococcal infection, the rash in hepatitis B is urticarial.

Treatment

In most cases, patients in whom gonococcal arthritis is suspected should be admitted to the hospital to confirm the diagnosis, to exclude endocarditis, and to start treatment. While outpatient treatment has been recommended in the past, the rapid rise in gonococci resistant to penicillin makes initial inpatient treatment advisable. The recommendation for initial treatment is to give azithromycin (1 g orally as a single dose) and a third-generation cephalosporin: ceftriaxone, 1 g intravenously daily (or every 12 hours if concomitant meningitis or endocarditis is suspected); or cefotaxime, 1 g intravenously every 8 hours; or ceftizoxime, 1 g intravenously every 8 hours. Azithromycin enhances eradication of gonorrhea and covers potential coinfection with *Chlamydia*. Because of the increasing prevalence of resistant strains of gonococci, step-down treatment from parenteral to oral antibiotics is no longer recommended. Indeed, once improvement has been achieved for 24–48 hours, patients must receive ceftriaxone 250 mg intramuscularly every 24 hours to complete a 7–14 day course.

► Prognosis

Generally, gonococcal arthritis responds dramatically in 24–48 hours after initiation of antibiotics, and drainage of the infected joint(s) is required infrequently. Complete recovery is the rule.

Bolan GA et al. The emerging threat of untreatable gonococcal infection. N Engl J Med. 2012 Feb 9;366(6):485–7.

RHEUMATIC MANIFESTATIONS OF HIV INFECTION

Infection with HIV has been associated with various rheumatic disorders, most commonly arthralgias and arthritis. HIV painful articular syndrome causes severe arthralgias in an oligoarticular, asymmetric pattern that resolve within 24 hours; the joint examination is normal. HIV-associated arthritis is an asymmetric oligoarticular process with objective findings of arthritis and a self-limited course that ranges from weeks to months. Psoriatic arthritis and reactive arthritis occur in HIV-infected individuals and can be severe; it remains uncertain whether the incidence of these disorders is increased in HIV-infected populations. These spondyloarthropathies can respond to NSAIDs, though many cases are unresponsive. In the era of highly active antiretroviral therapies, immunosuppressive medications can be used if necessary in HIV patients, though with caution. Muscle weakness associated with an elevated creatine kinase can be due to nucleoside reverse transcriptase inhibitor-associated myopathy or HIV-associated myopathy; the clinical presentations of each resemble idiopathic polymyositis but the muscle biopsies show minimal inflammation. Less commonly, an inflammatory myositis indistinguishable from idiopathic polymyositis occurs.

Kaddu-Mukasa M et al. Rheumatic manifestations among HIV positive adults attending the Infectious Disease Clinic at Mulago Hospital. Afr Health Sci. 2011 Mar;11(1):24–9. [PMID: 21572853]
Morar N et al. HIV-associated psoriasis: pathogenesis, clinical features, and management. Lancet Infect Dis. 2010 Jul;10(7): 470–8. [PMID: 20610329]

VIRAL ARTHRITIS

Arthralgias occur frequently in the course of acute infections with many viruses, but frank arthritis is uncommon. A notable exception is acute parvovirus B19

infection, which leads to acute polyarthritis in 50–60% of adult cases (infected children develop the febrile exanthem known as "slapped cheek fever"). The arthritis can mimic rheumatoid arthritis but is almost always self-limited and resolves within several weeks. The diagnosis is established by the presence of IgM antibodies specific for parvovirus B19. Self-limited polyarthritis is also common in acute hepatitis B infection and typically occurs before the onset of jaundice. Urticaria or other types of skin rash may be present. Indeed, the clinical picture resembles that of serum sickness (see Atopic Disease below). Serum transaminase levels are elevated, and tests for hepatitis B surface antigen are positive. Serum complement levels are often low during active arthritis and become normal after remission of arthritis. The incidence of hepatitis B–associated polyarthritis has fallen substantially with the introduction of hepatitis B vaccination. Effective vaccination programs in the United States have eliminated acute rubella infections, formerly a common cause of virally induced polyarthritis. Changes in the rubella vaccine (an attenuated live vaccine) have greatly reduced the incidence of rubella vaccine–induced polyarthritis as well.

Chronic infection with hepatitis C is associated with chronic polyarthralgia in up to 20% of cases and with chronic polyarthritis in 3–5%. Both can mimic rheumatoid arthritis, and the presence of rheumatoid factor in most hepatitis C–infected individuals leads to further diagnostic confusion. Indeed, hepatitis C–associated arthritis is frequently misdiagnosed as rheumatoid arthritis. Distinguishing hepatitis C–associated arthritis/arthralgias from the co-occurrence of hepatitis C and rheumatoid arthritis can be difficult. Rheumatoid arthritis always causes objective arthritis (not just arthralgias) and can be erosive (hepatitis C–associated arthritis is nonerosive). The presence of anti-CCP antibodies points to the diagnosis of rheumatoid arthritis.

Varache S et al. Is routine viral screening useful in patients with recent-onset polyarthritis of a duration of at least 6 weeks? Results from a nationwide longitudinal prospective cohort study. Arthritis Care Res (Hoboken). 2011 Nov;63(11): 1565–70. [PMID: 21954118]

▼ INFECTIONS OF BONES

ACUTE PYOGENIC OSTEOMYELITIS

ESSENTIALS OF DIAGNOSIS

► Fever and chills associated with pain and tenderness of involved bone.

► Diagnosis usually requires culture of bone biopsy.

► ESR often extremely high (eg, <100 mm/h).

► Radiographs early in the course are typically negative.

General Considerations

Osteomyelitis is a serious infection that is often difficult to diagnose and treat. Infection of bone occurs as a consequence of (1) hematogenous dissemination of bacteria, (2) invasion from a contiguous focus of infection, and (3) skin breakdown in the setting of vascular insufficiency.

Clinical Findings

A. Symptoms and Signs

1. Hematogenous osteomyelitis—Osteomyelitis resulting from bacteremia is a disease associated with sickle cell disease, injection drug users, diabetes mellitus, or the elderly. Patients with this form of osteomyelitis often present with sudden onset of high fever, chills, and pain and tenderness of the involved bone. The site of osteomyelitis and the causative organism depend on the host. Among patients with hemoglobinopathies such as sickle cell anemia, osteomyelitis is caused most often by salmonellae; *S aureus* is the second most common cause. Osteomyelitis in injection drug users develops most commonly in the spine. Although in this setting *S aureus* is most common, gram-negative infections, especially *P aeruginosa* and *Serratia* species, are also frequent pathogens. Rapid progression to epidural abscess causing fever, pain, and sensory and motor loss is not uncommon. In older patients with hematogenous osteomyelitis, the most common sites are the thoracic and lumbar vertebral bodies. Risk factors for these patients include diabetes, intravenous catheters, and indwelling urinary catheters. These patients often have more subtle presentations, with low-grade fever and gradually increasing bone pain.

2. Osteomyelitis from a contiguous focus of infection— Prosthetic joint replacement, pressure ulcer, neurosurgery, and trauma most frequently cause soft tissue infections that can spread to bone. *S aureus* and *Staphylococcus epidermidis* are the most common organisms. Polymicrobial infections, rare in hematogenously spread osteomyelitis, is more common in osteomyelitis due to contiguous spread. Localized signs of inflammation are usually evident, but high fever and other signs of toxicity are usually absent. Septic arthritis and cellulitis can also spread to contiguous bone.

3. Osteomyelitis associated with vascular insufficiency— Patients with diabetes and vascular insufficiency are susceptible to developing a very challenging form of osteomyelitis. The foot and ankle are the most commonly affected sites. Infection originates from an ulcer or other break in the skin that is usually still present when the patient presents but may appear disarmingly unimpressive. Bone pain is often absent or muted by the associated neuropathy. Fever is also commonly absent. Two of the best bedside clues that the patient has osteomyelitis are the ability to easily advance a sterile probe through a skin ulcer to bone and an ulcer area > 2 cm^2.

B. Imaging and Laboratory Findings

The plain film is the most readily available imaging procedure to establish the diagnosis of osteomyelitis, but it can be falsely negative early. Early radiographic findings may include soft tissue swelling, loss of tissue planes, and periarticular demineralization of bone. About 2 weeks after onset of symptoms, erosion of bone and alteration of cancellous bone appear, followed by periostitis.

MRI, CT, and nuclear medicine bone scanning are more sensitive than conventional radiography. MRI is the most sensitive and is particularly helpful in demonstrating the extent of soft tissue involvement. Radionuclide bone scanning is most valuable when osteomyelitis is suspected but no site is obvious. Nuclear medicine studies may also detect multifocal sites of infection. Ultrasound is useful in diagnosing the presence of effusions within joints and extra-articular soft tissue fluid collections but not in detecting bone infections.

Identifying the offending organism is a crucial step in selection of antibiotic therapy. Bone biopsy for culture is required except in those with hematogenous osteomyelitis, who have positive blood cultures. Cultures from overlying ulcers, wounds, or fistulas are unreliable.

Differential Diagnosis

Acute hematogenous osteomyelitis should be distinguished from suppurative arthritis, rheumatic fever, and cellulitis. More subacute forms must be differentiated from tuberculosis or mycotic infections of bone and Ewing sarcoma or, in the case of vertebral osteomyelitis, from metastatic tumor. When osteomyelitis involves the vertebrae, it commonly traverses the disk—a finding not observed in tumor.

Complications

Inadequate treatment of bone infections results in chronicity of infection, and this possibility is increased by delaying diagnosis and treatment. Extension to adjacent bone or joints may complicate acute osteomyelitis. Recurrence of bone infections often results in anemia, a markedly elevated ESR, weight loss, weakness and, rarely, amyloidosis or nephrotic syndrome. Pseudoepitheliomatous hyperplasia, squamous cell carcinoma, or fibrosarcoma may occasionally arise in persistently infected tissues.

Treatment

Most patients require both debridement of necrotic bone and prolonged administration of antibiotics. Patients with vertebral body osteomyelitis and epidural abscess may require urgent neurosurgical decompression. Depending on the site and extent of debridement, surgical procedures to stabilize, fill in, cover, or revascularize may be needed. Oral therapy with quinolones (eg, ciprofloxacin, 750 mg twice daily) for 6–8 weeks has been shown to be as effective as standard parenteral antibiotic therapy for chronic osteomyelitis with susceptible organisms. When treating osteomyelitis caused by *S aureus*, quinolones are usually combined with rifampin, 300 mg orally twice daily.

Prognosis

If sterility of the lesion is achieved within 2–4 days, a good result can be expected in most cases if there is no compromise of the patient's immune system. However, progression of the disease to a chronic form may occur. It is especially common in the lower extremities and in patients in whom circulation is impaired (eg, diabetics).

Spellberg B et al. Systemic antibiotic therapy for chronic osteomyelitis in adults. Clin Infect Dis. 2012 Feb 1;54(3):393–407. [PMID: 22157324]

Zimmerli W. Clinical practice. Vertebral osteomyelitis. N Engl J Med. 2010 Mar 18;362(11):1022–9. [PMID: 20237348]

TUBERCULOSIS OF BONES & JOINTS

SPINAL TUBERCULOSIS (Pott Disease)

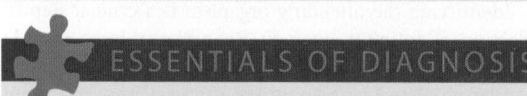

ESSENTIALS OF DIAGNOSIS

► Seen primarily in immigrants from developing countries or immunocompromised patients.

► Back pain and gibbus deformity.

► Radiographic evidence of vertebral involvement.

► Evidence of *Mycobacterium tuberculosis* in aspirate or biopsies of spinal lesions.

General Considerations

In the developing world, children primarily bear the burden of musculoskeletal tuberculosis. In the United States, however, musculoskeletal infection is more often seen in adult immigrants from countries where tuberculosis is prevalent, or it develops in the setting of immunosuppression (eg, HIV infection, therapy with TNF inhibitors). Spinal tuberculosis (Pott disease) accounts for about 50% of musculoskeletal infection due to *M tuberculosis* (see Chapter 9). Seeding of the vertebrae may occur through hematogenous spread from the respiratory tract at the time of primary infection, with clinical disease developing years later as a consequence of reactivation. The thoracic and lumbar vertebrae are the most common sites of spinal involvement; vertebral infection is associated with paravertebral cold abscesses in 75% of cases.

Clinical Findings

A. Symptoms and Signs

Patients complain of back pain, often present for months and sometimes associated with radicular pain and lower extremity weakness. Constitutional symptoms are usually absent, and < 20% have active pulmonary disease. Destruction of the anterior aspect of the vertebral body can produce the characteristic gibbus deformity.

B. Laboratory Findings

Most patients have a positive reaction to purified protein derivative (PPD) or a positive interferon-gamma release assay. Cultures of paravertebral abscesses and biopsies of vertebral lesions are positive in up to 70–90%. Biopsies reveal characteristic caseating granulomas in most cases. Isolation of *M tuberculosis* from an extraspinal site is sufficient to establish the diagnosis in the proper clinical setting.

C. Imaging

Radiographs can reveal lytic and sclerotic lesions and bony destruction of vertebrae but are normal early in the disease course. CT scanning can demonstrate paraspinal soft tissue extensions of the infection; MRI is the imaging technique of choice to detect compression of the spinal cord or cauda equina.

► Differential Diagnosis

Spinal tuberculosis must be differentiated from subacute and chronic spinal infections due to pyogenic organisms, *Brucella*, and fungi as well as from malignancy.

► Complications

Paraplegia due to compression of the spinal cord or cauda equina is the most serious complication of spinal tuberculosis.

► Treatment

Antimicrobial therapy should be administered for 6–9 months, usually in the form of isoniazid, rifampin, pyrazinamide, and ethambutol for 2 months followed by isoniazid and rifampin for an additional 4–7 months (see also Chapter 9). Medical management alone is often sufficient. Surgical intervention, however, may be indicated when there is neurologic compromise or severe spinal instability.

Fuentes Ferrer M et al. Tuberculosis of the spine. A systematic review of case series. Int Orthop. 2012 Feb;36(2):221–31. [PMID: 22116392]

Trecarichi EM et al. Tuberculous spondylodiscitis: epidemiology, clinical features, treatment, and outcome. Eur Rev Med Pharmacol Sci. 2012 Apr;16(Suppl 2):58–72. [PMID: 22655484]

TUBERCULOUS ARTHRITIS

Infection of peripheral joints by *M tuberculosis* usually presents as a monoarticular arthritis lasting for weeks to months (or longer), but less often, it can have an acute presentation that mimics septic arthritis. Any joint can be involved; the hip and knee are most commonly affected. Constitutional symptoms and fever are present in only a small number of cases. Tuberculosis also can cause a chronic tenosynovitis of the hand and wrist. Joint destruction occurs far more slowly than in septic arthritis due to pyogenic organisms. Synovial fluid is inflammatory but not to the degree seen in pyogenic infections, with synovial white cell counts in the range of 10,000–20,000 cells/mcL. Smears of synovial fluid are positive for acid-fast bacilli in a minority of cases; synovial fluid cultures, however, are positive in 80% of cases. Because culture results may take weeks, the diagnostic procedure of choice usually is synovial biopsy, which yields characteristic pathologic findings and positive cultures in > 90%. Antimicrobial therapy is the mainstay of treatment. Rarely, a reactive, sterile polyarthritis associated with erythema nodosum (Poncet disease) develops in patients with active pulmonary tuberculosis.

Kim SJ et al. Total hip replacement for patients with active tuberculosis of the hip: a systematic review and pooled analysis. Bone Joint J. 2013 May;95-B(5):578–82. [PMID: 23632665]

ARTHRITIS IN SARCOIDOSIS

The frequency of arthritis among patients with sarcoidosis is variously reported between 10% and 35%. It is usually acute in onset, but articular symptoms may appear insidiously and often antedate other manifestations of the disease. Knees and ankles are most commonly involved, but any joint may be affected. Distribution of joint involvement is usually polyarticular and symmetric. The arthritis is commonly self-limited, resolving after several weeks or months and rarely resulting in chronic arthritis, joint destruction, or significant deformity. Sarcoid arthropathy is often associated with erythema nodosum, but the diagnosis is contingent on the demonstration of other extra-articular manifestations of sarcoidosis and, notably, biopsy evidence of noncaseating granulomas. Despite the clinical appearance of an inflammatory arthritis, synovial fluid often is noninflammatory (ie, < 2000 leukocytes/mcL). In chronic arthritis, radiographs show typical changes in the bones of the extremities with intact cortex and cystic changes.

Treatment of arthritis in sarcoidosis is usually symptomatic and supportive. Colchicine may be of value. A short course of corticosteroids may be effective in patients with severe and progressive joint disease.

Sweiss NJ et al. Rheumatologic manifestations of sarcoidosis. Semin Respir Crit Care Med. 2010 Aug;31(4):463–73. [PMID: 20665396]

MISCELLANEOUS RHEUMATOLOGIC DISORDERS

THORACIC OUTLET SYNDROMES

Thoracic outlet syndromes result from compression of the neurovascular structures supplying the upper extremity. Symptoms and signs arise from intermittent or continuous pressure on elements of the brachial plexus (> 90% of cases) or the subclavian or axillary vessels (veins or arteries) by a variety of anatomic structures of the shoulder girdle region. The neurovascular bundle can be compressed between the anterior or middle scalene muscles and a normal first thoracic rib or a cervical rib. Most commonly thoracic outlet syndromes are caused by scarred scalene neck muscle secondary to neck trauma or sagging of the shoulder girdle resulting from aging, obesity, or pendulous breasts. Faulty posture, occupation, or thoracic muscle hypertrophy from physical activity (eg, weight-lifting, baseball pitching) may be other predisposing factors.

Thoracic outlet syndromes present in most patients with some combination of four symptoms involving the upper extremity, namely pain, numbness, weakness, and swelling. The predominant symptoms depend on whether the compression chiefly affects neural or vascular structures. The onset of symptoms is usually gradual but can be sudden. Some patients spontaneously notice aggravation of symptoms with specific positioning of the arm. Pain radiates from the point of compression to the base of the neck, the axilla, the shoulder girdle region, arm, forearm, and hand. Paresthesias are common and distributed to the volar aspect of the fourth and fifth digits. Sensory symptoms may be aggravated at night or by prolonged use of the extremities. Weakness and muscle atrophy are the principal motor abnormalities. Vascular symptoms consist of arterial ischemia characterized by pallor of the fingers on elevation of the extremity, sensitivity to cold and, rarely, gangrene of the digits or venous obstruction marked by edema, cyanosis, and engorgement.

The symptoms of thoracic outlet syndromes can be provoked within 60 seconds over 90% of the time by having a patient elevate the arms in a "stick-em-up" position (ie, abducted 90 degrees in external rotation). Reflexes are usually not altered. Obliteration of the radial pulse with certain maneuvers of the arm or neck, once considered a highly sensitive sign of thoracic outlet obstruction, does not occur in most cases.

Chest radiography will identify patients with cervical rib (although most patients with cervical ribs are asymptomatic). MRI with the arms held in different positions is useful in identifying sites of impaired blood flow. Intra-arterial or venous obstruction is confirmed by angiography. Determination of conduction velocities of the ulnar and other peripheral nerves of the upper extremity may help localize the site of their compression.

Thoracic outlet syndrome must be differentiated from osteoarthritis of the cervical spine, tumors of the superior pulmonary sulcus, cervical spinal cord, or nerve roots, and periarthritis of the shoulder.

Treatment is directed toward relief of compression of the neurovascular bundle. Greater than 95% of patients can be treated successfully with conservative therapy consisting of physical therapy and avoiding postures or activities that compress the neurovascular bundle. Some women will benefit from a support bra. Operative treatment, required by < 5% of patients, is more likely to relieve the neurologic rather than the vascular component that causes symptoms.

Brooke BS et al. Contemporary management of thoracic outlet syndrome. Curr Opin Cardiol. 2010 Nov;25(6):535–40. [PMID: 20838336]

Ferrante MA. The thoracic outlet syndromes. Muscle Nerve. 2012 Jun;45(6):780–95. [PMID: 22581530]

Povlsen B et al. Treatment for thoracic outlet syndrome. Cochrane Database Syst Rev. 2010 Jan 20;(1):CD007218. [PMID: 20091624]

FIBROMYALGIA

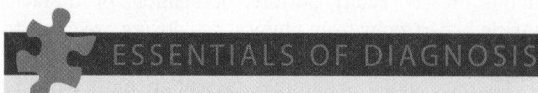

ESSENTIALS OF DIAGNOSIS

- ► Most frequent in women aged 20–50.
- ► Chronic widespread musculoskeletal pain syndrome with multiple tender points.
- ► Fatigue, headaches, numbness common.
- ► Objective signs of inflammation absent; laboratory studies normal.

► General Considerations

Fibromyalgia is a common syndrome, affecting 3–10% of the general population. It shares many features with the chronic fatigue syndrome, namely, an increased frequency among women aged 20–50, absence of objective findings, and absence of diagnostic laboratory test results. While many of the clinical features of the two conditions overlap, musculoskeletal pain predominates in fibromyalgia whereas lassitude dominates the chronic fatigue syndrome.

The cause is unknown, but aberrant perception of painful stimuli, sleep disorders, depression, and viral infections have all been proposed. Fibromyalgia can be a rare complication of hypothyroidism, rheumatoid arthritis or, in men, sleep apnea.

► Clinical Findings

The patient complains of chronic aching pain and stiffness, frequently involving the entire body but with prominence of pain around the neck, shoulders, low back, and hips. Fatigue, sleep disorders, subjective numbness, chronic headaches, and irritable bowel symptoms are common. Even minor exertion aggravates pain and increases fatigue. Physical examination is normal except for "trigger points" of pain produced by palpation of various areas such as the trapezius, the medial fat pad of the knee, and the lateral epicondyle of the elbow.

► Differential Diagnosis

Fibromyalgia is a diagnosis of exclusion. A detailed history and repeated physical examination can obviate the need for extensive laboratory testing. Rheumatoid arthritis and SLE present with objective physical findings or abnormalities on routine testing. Thyroid function tests are useful, since hypothyroidism can produce a secondary fibromyalgia syndrome. Polymyositis produces weakness rather than pain. The diagnosis of fibromyalgia probably should be made hesitantly in a patient over age 50 and should never be invoked to explain fever, weight loss, or any other objective signs. Polymyalgia rheumatica produces shoulder and pelvic girdle pain, is associated with anemia and an elevated ESR, and occurs after age 50. Hypophosphatemic states, such as oncogenic osteomalacia, should also be included in the differential diagnosis of musculoskeletal pain unassociated with physical findings. In contrast to

fibromyalgia, oncogenic osteomalacia usually produces pain in only a few areas and is associated with a low serum phosphate level.

► Treatment

A multidisciplinary approach is most effective. Patient education is essential. Patients can be comforted that they have a diagnosable syndrome treatable by specific though imperfect therapies and that the course is not progressive. Cognitive behavioral therapy, including programs that emphasize mindfulness meditation, is often helpful. There is modest efficacy of amitriptyline, fluoxetine, duloxetine, milnacipran, chlorpromazine, cyclobenzaprine, pregabalin, or gabapentin. Amitriptyline is initiated at a dosage of 10 mg orally at bedtime and gradually increased to 40–50 mg depending on efficacy and toxicity. Less than 50% of the patients experience a sustained improvement. Exercise programs are also beneficial. NSAIDs are generally ineffective. Tramadol and acetaminophen combinations have ameliorated symptoms modestly in short-term trials. Opioids and corticosteroids are ineffective and should not be used to treat fibromyalgia. Acupuncture is also ineffective.

► Prognosis

All patients have chronic symptoms. With treatment, however, many do eventually resume increased activities. Progressive or objective findings do not develop.

Dieppe P. Chronic musculoskeletal pain. BMJ. 2013 May 16;346:f3146. [PMID: 23709528]

Younger J et al. Low-dose naltrexone for the treatment of fibromyalgia: findings of a small, randomized, double-blind, placebo-controlled, counterbalanced, crossover trial assessing daily pain levels. Arthritis Rheum. 2013 Feb;65(2):529–38. [PMID: 23359310]

COMPLEX REGIONAL PAIN SYNDROME

Complex regional pain syndrome (formerly called reflex sympathetic dystrophy) is a rare disorder of the extremities characterized by autonomic and vasomotor instability. The cardinal symptoms and signs are pain localized to an arm or leg, swelling of the involved extremity, disturbances of color and temperature in the affected limb, dystrophic changes in the overlying skin and nails, and limited range of motion. Strikingly, the findings are not limited to the distribution of a single peripheral nerve. Most cases are preceded by direct physical trauma, often of relatively minor nature, to the soft tissues, bone, or nerve. Early mobilization after injury or surgery reduces the likelihood of developing the syndrome. Vitamin C, 500 mg/d orally, is effective in reducing the risk of complex regional pain syndrome following wrist fracture and may be effective following lower extremity fractures as well. Any extremity can be involved, but the syndrome most commonly occurs in the hand and is associated with ipsilateral restriction of shoulder motion ("shoulder-hand" syndrome). This syndrome proceeds through phases: pain, swelling, and skin color and temperature changes develop early and, if untreated, lead to atrophy and dystrophy. The swelling in complex regional pain syndrome is diffuse ("catcher's mitt hand") and not restricted to joints. Pain is often burning in quality, intense, and often greatly worsened by minimal stimuli such as light touch. The shoulder-hand variant of this disorder sometimes complicates myocardial infarction or injuries to the neck or shoulder. Complex regional pain syndrome may occur after a knee injury or after arthroscopic knee surgery. There are no systemic symptoms. In the early phases of the syndrome, bone scans are sensitive, showing diffuse increased uptake in the affected extremity. Radiographs eventually reveal severe generalized osteopenia. In the posttraumatic variant, this is known as Sudeck atrophy. Symptoms and findings are bilateral in some. This syndrome should be differentiated from other cervicobrachial pain syndromes, rheumatoid arthritis, thoracic outlet obstruction, and scleroderma, among others.

Early treatment offers the best prognosis for recovery. For mild cases, NSAIDs (eg, naproxen 250–500 mg twice daily orally) can be effective. For more severe cases associated with edema, prednisone, 30–60 mg/d orally for 2 weeks and then tapered over 2 weeks, can be effective. Pain management is important and facilitates physical therapy, which plays a critical role in efforts to restore function. Some patients will also benefit from antidepressant agents (eg, nortriptyline initiated at a dosage of 10 mg orally at bedtime and gradually increased to 40–75 mg at bedtime) or from anticonvulsants (eg, gabapentin 300 mg three times daily orally). Bisphosphonates, calcitonin, intravenous immunoglobulin, regional nerve blocks, and dorsal-column stimulation have also been demonstrated to be helpful. Patients who have restricted shoulder motion may benefit from the treatment described for scapulohumeral periarthritis. The prognosis partly depends on the stage in which the lesions are encountered and the extent and severity of associated organic disease.

Marinus J et al. Clinical features and pathophysiology of complex regional pain syndrome. Lancet Neurol. 2011 Jul;10(7):637–48. [PMID: 21683929]
Parkitny L et al. Inflammation in complex regional pain syndrome: a systematic review and meta-analysis. Neurology. 2013 Jan 1;80(1):106–17. [PMID: 23267031]

RHEUMATOLOGIC MANIFESTATIONS OF CANCER

Rheumatologic syndromes may be the presenting manifestations for a variety of cancers. Dermatomyositis in adults, for example, is often associated with cancer (see Table 39–2). Hypertrophic pulmonary osteoarthropathy, which is characterized by the triad of polyarthritis, new onset of clubbing, and periosteal new bone formation, is associated with both malignant diseases (eg, lung and intrathoracic cancers) and nonmalignant ones (eg, cyanotic heart disease, cirrhosis, and lung abscess). Cancer-associated polyarthritis is rare, has both oligoarticular and polyarticular forms, and should be considered when "seronegative rheumatoid arthritis" develops abruptly in an elderly patient. Palmar fasciitis manifests as bilateral palmar swelling with finger contractures and may be the first indication of cancer, particularly

ovarian carcinoma. Remitting seronegative synovitis with non-pitting edema ("RS3PE") presents with a symmetric small joint polyarthritis associated with non-pitting edema of the hands; it can be idiopathic or associated with malignancy. Palpable purpura due to leukocytoclastic vasculitis may be the presenting complaint in myeloproliferative disorders. Hairy cell leukemia can be associated with medium-sized vessel vasculitis such as polyarteritis nodosa. Acute leukemia can produce joint pains that are disproportionately severe in comparison to the minimal swelling and heat that are present. Leukemic arthritis complicates approximately 5% of cases. Rheumatic manifestations of myelodysplastic syndromes include cutaneous vasculitis, lupus-like syndromes, neuropathy, and episodic intense arthritis. Erythromelalgia, a painful warmth and redness of the extremities that (unlike Raynaud) improves with cold exposure or with elevation of the extremity, is often associated with myeloproliferative diseases, particularly essential thrombocythemia.

Ashouri JF et al. Rheumatic manifestations of cancer. Rheum Dis Clin North Am. 2011 Nov;37(4):489–505. [PMID: 22075194]
Ravindran V et al. Rheumatologic manifestations of benign and malignant haematological disorders. Clin Rheumatol. 2011 Sep;30(9):1143–9. [PMID: 21698399]

NEUROGENIC ARTHROPATHY (Charcot Joint)

Neurogenic arthropathy is joint destruction resulting from loss or diminution of proprioception, pain, and temperature perception. Although initially described in the knees of patients with tabes dorsalis, it is more frequently seen in association with diabetic neuropathy (foot and ankle) or syringomyelia (shoulder). As normal muscle tone and protective reflexes are lost, secondary degenerative joint disease ensues, resulting in an enlarged, boggy, relatively painless joint with extensive cartilage erosion, osteophyte formation, and multiple loose joint bodies. Radiographs can reveal striking osteolysis that mimics osteomyelitis or dramatic destruction of the joint with subluxation, fragmentation of bone, and bony sclerosis.

Treatment is directed toward the primary disease; mechanical devices are used to assist in weight bearing and prevention of further trauma. In some instances, amputation becomes unavoidable.

Richard JL et al. Treatment of acute Charcot foot with bisphosphonates: a systematic review of the literature. Diabetologia. 2012 May;55(5):1258–64. [PMID: 22361982]

PALINDROMIC RHEUMATISM

Palindromic rheumatism is a disease of unknown cause characterized by frequent recurring attacks (at irregular intervals) of acutely inflamed joints. Periarticular pain with swelling and transient subcutaneous nodules may also occur. The attacks cease within several hours to several days. The knee and finger joints are most commonly affected, but any peripheral joint may be involved. Systemic manifestations other than fever do not occur. Although hundreds of attacks may take place over a period of years, there is no permanent articular damage. Laboratory findings are usually normal. Palindromic rheumatism must be distinguished from acute gouty arthritis and an atypical acute onset of rheumatoid arthritis. In some patients, palindromic rheumatism is a prodrome of rheumatoid arthritis.

Symptomatic treatment with NSAIDs is usually all that is required during the attacks. Hydroxychloroquine may be of value in preventing recurrences.

OSTEONECROSIS (Avascular Necrosis of Bone)

Osteonecrosis is a complication of corticosteroid use, alcoholism, trauma, SLE, pancreatitis, gout, sickle cell disease, dysbaric syndromes (eg, "the bends"), knee menisectomy, and infiltrative diseases (eg, Gaucher disease). The most commonly affected sites are the proximal and distal femoral heads, leading to hip or knee pain. Other commonly affected sites include the ankle, shoulder, and elbow. Osteonecrosis of the jaw has been rarely associated with use of bisphosphonate therapy, almost always when the bisphosphonate is used for treating metastatic cancer or multiple myeloma rather than osteoporosis. Initially, radiographs are often normal; MRI, CT scan, and bone scan are all more sensitive techniques. Treatment involves avoidance of weight bearing on the affected joint for at least several weeks. The value of surgical core decompression is controversial. For osteonecrosis of the hip, a variety of procedures designed to preserve the femoral head have been developed for early disease, including vascularized and nonvascularized bone grafting procedures. These procedures are most effective in avoiding or forestalling the need for total hip arthroplasty in young patients who do not have advanced disease. Without a successful intervention of this nature, the natural history of avascular necrosis is usually progression of the bony infarction to cortical collapse, resulting in significant joint dysfunction. Total hip replacement is the usual outcome for all patients who are candidates for that procedure.

Fessel J. There are many potential medical therapies for atraumatic osteonecrosis. Rheumatology (Oxford). 2013 Feb;52(2):235–41. [PMID: 23041599]
Weinstein RS. Glucocorticoid-induced osteonecrosis. Endocrine. 2012 Apr;41(2):183–90. [PMID: 22169965]

▼ ALLERGIC DISEASES

Allergy is an immunologically mediated hypersensitivity reaction to a foreign antigen manifested by tissue inflammation and organ dysfunction. These responses have a genetic basis, but the clinical expression of disease depends on both immunologic responsiveness and antigen exposure. Allergic disorders may be local or systemic. Because the allergen is foreign (ie, environmental), the skin and respiratory tract are the organs most frequently involved in allergic disease. Allergic reactions may also localize to the vasculature, gastrointestinal tract, or other visceral organs. Anaphylaxis is the most extreme form of systemic allergy.

▶ Immunologic Classification

An immunologic classification for hypersensitivity reactions serves as a rational basis for diagnosis and treatment. The classification follows.

A. Type I—IgE-Mediated (Immediate) Hypersensitivity

IgE antibodies occupy receptor sites on mast cells. Within minutes after exposure to the allergen, a multivalent antigen links adjacent IgE molecules, activating and degranulating mast cells. Clinical manifestations depend on the effects of released mediators on target end organs. Both preformed and newly generated mediators cause vasodilation, visceral smooth muscle contraction, mucous secretory gland stimulation, vascular permeability, and tissue inflammation. Arachidonic acid metabolites, cytokines, and other mediators induce a late-phase inflammatory response that appears several hours later. There are two clinical subgroups of IgE-mediated allergy: atopy and anaphylaxis.

1. Atopy—The term "atopy" is applied to a group of diseases (allergic rhinitis, allergic asthma, atopic dermatitis, and allergic gastroenteropathy) occurring in persons with an inherited tendency to develop antigen-specific IgE reaction to environmental allergens or food antigens. Aeroallergens such as pollens, mold spores, animal danders, and house dust mite antigen are common triggers for allergic conjunctivitis, allergic rhinitis, and allergic asthma. The allergic origin of atopic dermatitis is less well understood, but some patients' symptoms can be triggered by exposure to dust mite antigen and ingestion of certain foods. There is a strong familial tendency toward the development of atopy.

2. Anaphylaxis—Certain allergens—especially drugs, insect venoms, latex, and foods—may induce an IgE antibody response, causing a generalized release of mediators from mast cells and resulting in systemic anaphylaxis. This is characterized by (1) hypotension or shock from widespread vasodilation, (2) bronchospasm, (3) gastrointestinal and uterine muscle contraction, and (4) urticaria or angioedema. The condition is potentially fatal and can affect both nonatopic and atopic persons. Isolated urticaria and angioedema are cutaneous forms of anaphylaxis, are much more common, and have a better prognosis.

B. Type II—Antibody-Mediated (Cytotoxic) Hypersensitivity

Cytotoxic reactions involve the specific reaction of either IgG or IgM antibody to cell-bound antigens. This results in activation of the complement cascade and the destruction of the cell to which the antigen is bound. Examples include immune hemolytic anemia and Rh hemolytic disease in the newborn.

C. Type III—Immune Complex-Mediated Hypersensitivity

Immune complex-mediated reactions occur when antigen and IgG or IgM antibodies form circulating immune complexes. Deposition of these complexes in tissues or in vascular endothelium can produce immune complex-mediated tissue injury through activation of the complement cascade, anaphylatoxin generation, and chemotaxis of polymorphonuclear leukocytes. Serum sickness is the classic example of type III hypersensitivity. Immune complex disease also can develop in the setting of acute infection with hepatitis B or chronic infections such as subacute bacterial endocarditis, osteomyelitis, and hepatitis C.

D. Type IV—T Cell–Mediated Hypersensitivity (Delayed Hypersensitivity, Cell-Mediated Hypersensitivity)

Type IV delayed hypersensitivity is mediated by activated T cells, which accumulate in areas of antigen deposition. The most common expression of delayed hypersensitivity is allergic contact dermatitis, which develops when a low-molecular-weight sensitizing substance haptenates with dermal proteins, becoming a complete antigen. Sensitized T cells release cytokines, activating macrophages and promoting the subsequent dermal inflammation; this occurs 1–2 days after the time of contact. Common topical agents associated with allergic contact dermatitis include nickel, formaldehyde, potassium dichromate, thiurams, mercaptos, parabens, quaternium-15, and ethylenediamine. Rhus (poison oak and ivy) contact dermatitis is caused by cutaneous exposure to oils from the toxicodendron plants. Acute contact dermatitis is characterized by erythema and induration with vesicle formation, often with pruritus, with exudation and crusting in more severe cases. Chronic allergic contact dermatitis may be associated with fissuring, lichenification, or dyspigmentation and may be mistaken for other forms of dermatitis. To diagnose allergic contact dermatitis, patch testing can be performed.

HLA-B & RISK OF SERIOUS DRUG-INDUCED HYPERSENSITIVITY REACTIONS

Activated cytotoxic CD8 T lymphocytes play a key role in the pathogenesis of toxic epidermal necrolysis and other serious, drug-induced adverse cutaneous reactions. There are striking, medication-specific associations between inheritance of particular HLA-B alleles and risk of these hypersensitivity reactions. Most notably, B*57:01 confers risk for reactions to abacavir; B*15:02, for carbamazepine; B*58:01, for allopurinol; and B*13:01, for dapsone. The most likely mechanism is a direct interaction between the drug and the antigen-binding cleft of the HLA-B molecule, such that many "self" antigens subsequently bound by the HLA-B molecule are perceived as "foreign," eliciting massive CD8 T cell activation. Current guidelines call for testing for the relevant HLA-B allele prior to initiating therapy with abacavir, carbamazepine, allopurinol, or dapsone in at-risk patients.

Schwartz RA et al. Toxic epidermal necrolysis. Part I. Introduction, history, classification, clinical diagnosis, systemic manifestations, etiology, and immunopathogenesis. J Am Acad Dermatol. 2013 Aug;69(2):173.e1–13. [PMID: 23866878]

SERUM SICKNESS

ESSENTIALS OF DIAGNOSIS

▶ Fever, pruritic rash, arthralgias, and arthritis; nephritis in severe cases.

▶ Occurs 7–10 days following administration of an exogenous antigen (eg, heterologous gamma globulin) when specific IgG antibodies develop against the antigen.

▶ Immune complex–mediated small vessel vasculitis and tissue injury.

▶ General Considerations

Serum sickness occurs when an antibody response to exogenously administered antigens results in the formation of immune complexes. Deposition of these complexes in vascular endothelium and tissues produces immune complex–mediated small vessel vasculitis and tissue injury through activation of complement, generation of anaphylatoxins, and chemoattraction of polymorphonuclear leukocytes. The skin, joints, and kidneys are commonly affected. It is self-limited and resolves after the antigen is cleared. First observed in the preantibiotic era when heterologous serum preparations were used for passive immunization, serum sickness is now less common but still occurs with the use of heterologous anti-thymocyte globulin for transplant rejection and, infrequently, after the administration of murine monoclonal antibodies or even non-protein drugs.

▶ Clinical Findings

A. Symptoms and Signs

Sustained high fever (> 101°F) is typical. The earliest manifestation is often a maculopapular or urticarial pruritic rash. Angioedema can occur. Polyarthralgias, frank polyarthritis, and lymphadenopathy are common. Nephritis is usually mild but can progress to acute renal failure.

B. Laboratory Findings

The ESR is increased, and leukocytosis is common. Other nonspecific laboratory findings include elevated hepatic aminotransferases. When nephritis is present, the urinalysis reveals proteinuria, hematuria, and red cell casts. Hypocomplementemia (low serum levels of C3 and C4) is usually present in cases due to administration of heterologous gamma globulin but not in milder cases precipitated by non-protein drugs.

▶ Treatment

This disease is self-limited, and treatment is usually conservative for mild cases. NSAIDs help relieve the arthralgias, and antihistamines and topical corticosteroids can be of benefit for the skin manifestation. A high-dose course of corticosteroids is administered for serious reactions, especially those complicated by glomerulonephritis and other manifestations of vasculitis. Plasma exchange may be of benefit for cases refractory to corticosteroids.

PSEUDOALLERGIC REACTIONS

These reactions resemble immediate hypersensitivity reactions but are not mediated by allergen-IgE interaction. Instead, direct mast cell activation occurs. Examples of pseudoallergic or "anaphylactoid" reactions include radiocontrast reactions, direct mast cell activation by opioids, and the now rare "red man syndrome" from rapid infusion of vancomycin. In contrast to IgE-mediated reactions, these can often be prevented by prophylactic medical regimens.

Radiocontrast Media Reactions

Reactions to radiocontrast media do not appear to be mediated by IgE antibodies, yet clinically they are similar to anaphylaxis. If a patient has had an anaphylactoid reaction to conventional radiocontrast media, the risk for a second reaction upon reexposure may be as high as 30%. Patients with asthma or those being treated with beta-adrenergic blocking medications may be at increased risk. The management of patients at risk for radiocontrast medium reactions includes use of the low-osmolality contrast preparations and prophylactic administration of prednisone (50 mg orally every 6 hours beginning 18 hours before the procedure) and diphenhydramine (25–50 mg intramuscularly 60 minutes before the procedure). The use of the lower-osmolality radiocontrast media in combination with the pretreatment regimen decreases the incidence of reactions to < 1%.

Brockow K. Immediate and delayed cutaneous reactions to radiocontrast media. Chem Immunol Allergy. 2012;97:180–90. [PMID: 22613862]

Brockow K et al. Anaphylaxis to radiographic contrast media. Curr Opin Allergy Clin Immunol. 2011 Aug;11(4):326–31. [PMID: 21659863]

PRIMARY IMMUNODEFICIENCY DISORDERS IN ADULTS

Most primary immunologic deficiency diseases are rare and, because they are genetically determined, usually present in childhood. Nonetheless, several important immunodeficiency disorders can present in adulthood, most notably selective IgA deficiency, common variable immunodeficiency, and deficiencies in the terminal components of the complement pathway, which confer susceptibility to *Neisseria* infections. Autoantibodies that neutralize cytokines are a recently recognized mechanism of acquired immunodeficiency in adulthood. For example, neutralizing autoantibodies against interferon-gamma can lead to severe opportunistic infections with nontuberculous mycobacteria, and antibodies to granulocyte macrophage-colony stimulating factor are associated with cryptococcal meningitis in otherwise immunocompetent individuals.

SELECTIVE IMMUNOGLOBULIN A DEFICIENCY

Selective IgA deficiency is the most common primary immunodeficiency disorder and is characterized by serum IgA levels < 15 mg/dL (< 0.15 g/L) with normal levels of IgG and IgM; its prevalence is about 1:500 individuals. Most persons are asymptomatic because of compensatory increases in secreted IgG and IgM. Some affected patients have frequent and recurrent infections, such as sinusitis, otitis, and bronchitis. Some cases of IgA deficiency may spontaneously remit. When IgG_2 subclass deficiency occurs in combination with IgA deficiency, affected patients are more susceptible to encapsulated bacteria and the degree of immune impairment can be more severe. Patients with a combined IgA and IgG subclass deficiency should be assessed for functional antibody responses to glycoprotein antigen immunization.

Atopic disease and autoimmune disorders can be associated with IgA deficiency. Occasionally, a sprue-like syndrome with steatorrhea has been associated with an isolated IgA deficit. Treatment with commercial immune globulin is ineffective, since IgA and IgM are present only in trace quantities in these preparations.

Individuals with selective IgA deficiency may have high titers of anti-IgA antibodies and are at risk for anaphylactic reactions following exposure to IgA through infusions of plasma (or blood transfusions). These anti-IgA antibodies develop in the absence of prior exposure to human plasma or blood, possibly due to crossreactivity to bovine IgA in cow's milk or prior sensitization to maternal IgA in breast milk.

Wang N et al. IgA deficiency: what is new? Curr Opin Allergy Clin Immunol. 2012 Dec;12(6):602–8. [PMID: 23026772]

Electrolyte & Acid-Base Disorders

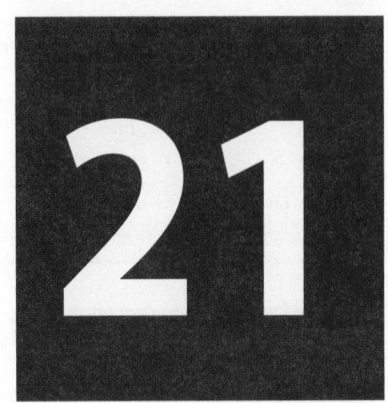

Kerry C. Cho, MD

ASSESSMENT OF THE PATIENT

The diagnosis and treatment of fluid and electrolyte disorders are based on (1) careful history, (2) physical examination and assessment of total body water and its distribution, (3) serum electrolyte concentrations, (4) urine electrolyte concentrations, and (5) serum osmolality. The pathophysiology of electrolyte disorders is rooted in basic principles of total body water and its distribution across fluid compartments.

A. Body Water and Fluid Distribution

Total body water is different in men than in women, and it decreases with aging (Table 21–1). Approximately 50–60% of total body weight is water; two-thirds (40% of body weight) is intracellular, while one-third (20% of body weight) is extracellular. One-fourth of extracellular fluid (5% of body weight) is intravascular. Water may be lost from either or both compartments (intracellular and extracellular). Changes in total body water content are best evaluated by documenting changes in body weight. Effective circulating volume may be assessed by physical examination (eg, blood pressure, pulse, jugular venous distention). Quantitative measurements of effective circulating volume and intravascular volume may be invasive (ie, central venous pressure or pulmonary wedge pressure) or noninvasive (ie, inferior vena cava diameter and right atrial pressure by echocardiography) but still require careful interpretation.

B. Serum Electrolytes

The cause of electrolyte disorders may be determined by reviewing the history, underlying diseases, and medications.

C. Evaluation of Urine

The urine concentration of an electrolyte indicates renal handling of the electrolyte and whether the kidney is appropriately excreting or retaining the electrolyte. A 24-hour urine collection for daily electrolyte excretion is the gold standard for renal electrolyte handling, but it is slow and onerous. A more convenient method is the fractional excretion (FE) of an electrolyte X (FE$_x$) calculated from a spot urine sample:

$$FE_x(\%) = \frac{Urine\ X/Serum\ X}{Urine\ Cr/Serum\ Cr} \times 100$$

A low fractional excretion indicates renal reabsorption (high avidity or electrolyte retention), while a high fractional excretion indicates renal wasting (low avidity or electrolyte excretion). Thus, the fractional excretion helps the clinician determine whether the kidney's response is appropriate for a specific electrolyte disorder.

D. Serum Osmolality

Solute concentration is measured by osmolality in millimoles per kilogram. Osmolarity is measured in millimoles of solute per liter of solution. At physiologic solute concentrations (normally 285–295 mmol/kg), the two measurements are clinically interchangeable. Tonicity refers to osmolytes that are impermeable to cell membranes. Differences in osmolyte concentration across cell membranes lead to osmosis and fluid shifts, stimulation of thirst, and secretion of antidiuretic hormone (ADH). Substances that easily permeate cell membranes (eg, urea, ethanol) are ineffective osmoles that do not cause fluid shifts across fluid compartments.

Serum osmolality can be estimated using the following formula:

$$Osmolality = 2(Na^+\ mEq/L) + \frac{Glucose\ mg/dL}{18} + \frac{BUN\ mg/dL}{2.8}$$

(1 mosm/L of glucose equals 180 mg/L or 18 mg/dL and 1 mosm/L of urea nitrogen equals 28 mg/L or 2.8 mg/dL). Sodium is the major extracellular cation; doubling the serum sodium in the formula for estimated osmolality accounts for counterbalancing anions. A discrepancy between measured and estimated osmolality of > 10 mmol/kg suggests an osmolal gap, which is the presence of unmeasured osmoles such as ethanol, methanol, isopropanol, and ethylene glycol (see Table 38–5).

Table 21–1. Total body water (as percentage of body weight) in relation to age and sex.

Age	Male	Female
18–40	60%	50%
41–60	60–50%	50–40%
Over 60	50%	40%

DISORDERS OF SODIUM CONCENTRATION

HYPONATREMIA

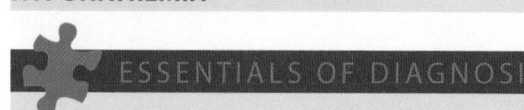

ESSENTIALS OF DIAGNOSIS

▸ Volume status and serum osmolality are essential to determine etiology.

▸ Hyponatremia usually reflects excess water retention relative to sodium rather than sodium deficiency. The sodium concentration is not a measure of total body sodium.

▸ Hypotonic fluids commonly cause hyponatremia in hospitalized patients.

▸ General Considerations

Defined as a serum sodium concentration < 135 mEq/L (or < 135 mmol/L), hyponatremia is the most common electrolyte abnormality in hospitalized patients. The clinician should be wary about hyponatremia since mismanagement can result in neurologic catastrophes from cerebral osmotic demyelination. Indeed, iatrogenic complications from aggressive or inappropriate therapy can be more harmful than hyponatremia itself.

A common misconception is that the sodium concentration is a reflection of total body sodium or total body water. In fact, total body water and sodium can be low, normal, or high in hyponatremia since the kidney independently regulates sodium and water homeostasis. Most cases of hyponatremia reflect water imbalance and abnormal water handling, not sodium imbalance, indicating the primary role of ADH in the pathophysiology of hyponatremia. A diagnostic algorithm using serum osmolality and volume status separates the causes of hyponatremia into therapeutically useful categories (Figure 21–1).

▸ Etiology

A. Isotonic & Hypertonic Hyponatremia

Serum osmolality identifies isotonic and hypertonic hyponatremia, although these cases can often be identified by careful history or previous laboratory tests.

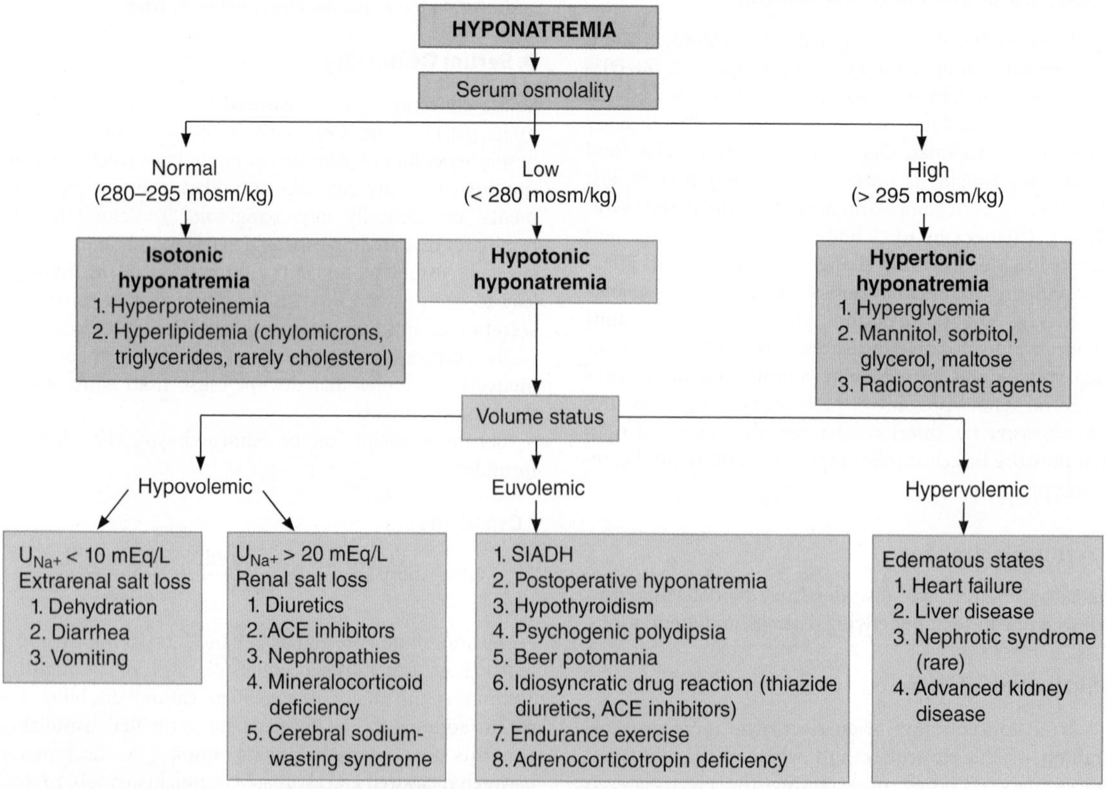

```
                        HYPONATREMIA
                             │
                       Serum osmolality
                             │
        ┌────────────────────┼────────────────────┐
        │                    │                     │
     Normal                 Low                   High
 (280–295 mosm/kg)    (< 280 mosm/kg)       (> 295 mosm/kg)
        │                    │                     │
   Isotonic             Hypotonic             Hypertonic
  hyponatremia        hyponatremia           hyponatremia
 1. Hyperproteinemia                       1. Hyperglycemia
 2. Hyperlipidemia (chylomicrons,          2. Mannitol, sorbitol,
    triglycerides, rarely cholesterol)        glycerol, maltose
        │                    │             3. Radiocontrast agents
        │              Volume status             │
        └──────┬──────────────┼───────────────┬──┘
               │              │               │
          Hypovolemic      Euvolemic      Hypervolemic
```

Hypovolemic		Euvolemic	Hypervolemic
U_{Na+} < 10 mEq/L **Extrarenal salt loss** 1. Dehydration 2. Diarrhea 3. Vomiting	U_{Na+} > 20 mEq/L **Renal salt loss** 1. Diuretics 2. ACE inhibitors 3. Nephropathies 4. Mineralocorticoid deficiency 5. Cerebral sodium-wasting syndrome	1. SIADH 2. Postoperative hyponatremia 3. Hypothyroidism 4. Psychogenic polydipsia 5. Beer potomania 6. Idiosyncratic drug reaction (thiazide diuretics, ACE inhibitors) 7. Endurance exercise 8. Adrenocorticotropin deficiency	**Edematous states** 1. Heart failure 2. Liver disease 3. Nephrotic syndrome (rare) 4. Advanced kidney disease

▲ **Figure 21–1.** Evaluation of hyponatremia using serum osmolality and extracellular fluid volume status. ACE, angiotensin-converting enzyme; SIADH, syndrome of inappropriate antidiuretic hormone. (Adapted, with permission, from Narins RG et al. Diagnostic strategies in disorders of fluid, electrolyte and acid-base homeostasis. Am J Med. 1982 Mar;72(3):496–520.)

Isotonic hyponatremia is seen with severe hyperlipidemia and hyperproteinemia. Lipids (including chylomicrons, triglycerides, and cholesterol) and proteins (> 10 g/dL [> 100 g/L], eg, paraproteinemias and intravenous immunoglobulin therapy) interfere with the measurement of serum sodium, causing pseudohyponatremia. Serum osmolality is isotonic because lipids and proteins do not affect osmolality measurement. Newer sodium assays using ion-specific electrodes on undiluted serum specimens (ie, the direct assay method) will not result in pseudohyponatremia.

Hypertonic hyponatremia occurs with hyperglycemia and mannitol administration for increased intracranial pressure. Glucose and mannitol osmotically pull intracellular water into the extracellular space. The translocation of water lowers the serum sodium concentration. Translocational hyponatremia is not pseudohyponatremia or an artifact of sodium measurement. The sodium concentration falls 2 mEq/L (or 2 mmol/L) for every 100 mg/dL (or 5.56 mmol/L) rise in glucose when the glucose concentration is between 200 mg/dL and 400 mg/dL (11.1 mmol/L and 22.2 mmol/L). If the glucose concentration is > 400 mg/dL, the sodium concentration falls 4 mEq/L for every 100 mg/dL rise in glucose. There is some controversy about the correction factor for the serum sodium in the presence of hyperglycemia. Many guidelines recommend a correction factor, whereby the serum sodium concentration decreases by 1.6 mEq/L (or 1.6 mmol/L) for every 100 mg/dL (5.56 mmol/L) rise in plasma glucose above normal, but there is evidence that the decrease may be greater when patients have more severe hyperglycemia (> 400 mg/dL or 22.2 mmol/L) or volume depletion, or both. One group has suggested (based on short-term exposure of normal volunteers to markedly elevated glucose levels) that when the serum glucose is > 200 mg/dL, the serum sodium concentration decreases by at least 2.4 mEq/L (or 2.4 mmol/L).

B. Hypotonic Hyponatremia

Most cases of hyponatremia are hypotonic, highlighting sodium's role as the predominant extracellular osmole. The next step is classifying hypotonic cases by the patient's volume status.

1. Hypovolemic hypotonic hyponatremia—Hypovolemic hyponatremia occurs with renal or extrarenal volume loss and hypotonic fluid replacement (Figure 21–1). Total body sodium and total body water are decreased. To maintain intravascular volume, the pituitary increases ADH secretion, causing free water retention from hypotonic fluid replacement. The body sacrifices serum osmolality to preserve intravascular volume. In short, losses of water and salt are replaced by water alone. Without ongoing hypotonic fluid intake, the renal or extrarenal volume loss would produce hypovolemic hypernatremia.

Cerebral salt wasting is a distinct and rare subset of hypovolemic hyponatremia seen in patients with intracranial disease (eg, infections, cerebrovascular accidents, tumors, and neurosurgery). Clinical features include refractory hypovolemia and hypotension, often requiring continuous infusion of isotonic or hypertonic saline and ICU monitoring. The exact pathophysiology is unclear but includes renal sodium wasting possibly through B-type natriuretic peptide, ADH release, and decreased aldosterone secretion.

2. Euvolemic hypotonic hyponatremia—Euvolemic hyponatremia has the broadest differential diagnosis. Most causes are mediated directly or indirectly through ADH, including hypothyroidism, adrenal insufficiency, medications, and the syndrome of inappropriate ADH (SIADH). The exceptions are primary polydipsia, beer potomania, and reset osmostat.

A. HORMONAL ABNORMALITIES—Hypothyroidism and adrenal insufficiency can cause hyponatremia. Exactly how hypothyroidism induces hyponatremia is unclear but may be related to ADH. Adrenal insufficiency may be associated with the hyperkalemia and metabolic acidosis of hypoaldosteronism. Cortisol provides feedback inhibition for ADH release.

B. THIAZIDE DIURETICS AND OTHER MEDICATIONS—Thiazides induce hyponatremia typically in older female patients within days of initiating therapy. The mechanism appears to be a combination of mild diuretic-induced volume contraction, ADH effect, and intact urinary concentrating ability resulting in water retention and hyponatremia. Loop diuretics do not cause hyponatremia as frequently because of disrupted medullary concentrating gradient and impaired urine concentration.

Nonsteroidal anti-inflammatory drugs (NSAIDs) increase ADH by inhibiting prostaglandin formation. Prostaglandins and selective serotonin reuptake inhibitors (eg, fluoxetine, paroxetine, and citalopram) can cause hyponatremia, especially in geriatric patients. Enhanced secretion or action of ADH may result from increased serotonergic tone. Angiotensin-converting enzyme (ACE) inhibitors do not block the conversion of angiotensin I to angiotensin II in the brain. Angiotensin II stimulates thirst and ADH secretion. Hyponatremia during amiodarone loading has been reported; it usually improves with dose reduction.

Abuse of 3,4-methylenedioxymethamphetamine (MDMA, also known as Ecstasy) can lead to hyponatremia and severe neurologic symptoms, including seizures, cerebral edema, and brainstem herniation. MDMA and its metabolites increase ADH release from the hypothalamus. Primary polydipsia may contribute to hyponatremia since MDMA users typically increase fluid intake to prevent hyperthermia.

C. NAUSEA, PAIN, SURGERY, AND MEDICAL PROCEDURES—Nausea and pain are potent stimulators of ADH release. Severe hyponatremia can develop after elective surgery in healthy patients, especially premenopausal women. Hypotonic fluids in the setting of elevated ADH levels can produce severe, life-threatening hyponatremia. Medical procedures such as colonoscopy have also been associated with hyponatremia.

D. HIV INFECTION—Hyponatremia is seen in up to 50% of hospitalized HIV-infected patients and 20% of ambulatory HIV-infected patients. The differential diagnosis is broad: medication effect, adrenal insufficiency, hypoaldosteronism, central nervous system or pulmonary disease, SIADH, malignancy, and volume depletion.

E. Exercise-associated hyponatremia—Hyponatremia after exercise, especially endurance events such as triathlons and marathons, may be caused by a combination of excessive hypotonic fluid intake and continued ADH secretion. Reperfusion of the exercise-induced ischemic splanchnic bed causes delayed absorption of excessive quantities of hypotonic fluid ingested during exercise. Sustained elevation of ADH prevents water excretion in this setting. Current guidelines suggest that endurance athletes drink water according to thirst rather than according to specified hourly rates of fluid intake. Specific universal recommendations for fluid replacement rates are not possible given the variability of sweat production, renal water excretion, and environmental conditions. Electrolyte-containing sport drinks do not protect against hyponatremia since they are markedly hypotonic relative to serum.

F. Syndrome of inappropriate antidiuretic hormone secretion—Under normal circumstances, hypovolemia and hyperosmolality stimulate ADH secretion. ADH release is inappropriate without these physiologic cues. Normal regulation of ADH release occurs from both the central nervous system and the chest via baroreceptors and neural input. The major causes of SIADH (Table 21–2) are disorders affecting the central nervous system (structural, metabolic, psychiatric, or pharmacologic processes) or the lungs (infectious, mechanical, oncologic). Medications commonly cause SIADH by increasing ADH or its action. Some carcinomas, especially small cell lung carcinoma, can autonomously secrete ADH.

G. Psychogenic polydipsia and beer potomania—Marked free water intake (generally > 10 L/d) may produce hyponatremia. Euvolemia is maintained through renal excretion of sodium. Urine sodium is therefore generally elevated (> 20 mEq/L), and ADH levels are appropriately suppressed. As the increased free water is excreted, the urine osmolality approaches the minimum of 50 mosm/kg (or 50 mmol/kg). Polydipsia occurs in psychiatric patients. Psychiatric medications may interfere with water excretion or increase thirst through anticholinergic side effects, further increasing water intake. The hyponatremia of beer potomania occurs in patients who consume large amounts of beer. Free water excretion is decreased because of decreased solute consumption and production; muscle wasting and malnutrition are contributing factors. Without enough solute, these patients have decreased free water excretory capacity even if they maximally dilute the urine.

H. Reset osmostat—Reset osmostat is a rare cause of hyponatremia characterized by appropriate ADH regulation in response to water deprivation and fluid challenges. Patients with reset osmostat regulate serum sodium and serum osmolality around a lower set point, concentrating or diluting urine in response to hyperosmolality and hypo-osmolality. The mild hypo-osmolality of pregnancy is a form of reset osmostat.

3. Hypervolemic hypotonic hyponatremia—Hypervolemic hyponatremia occurs in the edematous states of cirrhosis, heart failure, nephrotic syndrome, and advanced kidney disease (Figure 21–1). In cirrhosis and heart failure, effective circulating volume is decreased due to peripheral

Table 21–2. Causes of syndrome of inappropriate ADH secretion (SIADH).

Central nervous system disorders
Head trauma
Stroke
Subarachnoid hemorrhage
Hydrocephalus
Brain tumor
Encephalitis
Guillain-Barré syndrome
Meningitis
Acute psychosis
Acute intermittent porphyria
Pulmonary lesions
Tuberculosis
Bacterial pneumonia
Aspergillosis
Bronchiectasis
Neoplasms
Positive pressure ventilation
Malignancies
Bronchogenic carcinoma
Pancreatic carcinoma
Prostatic carcinoma
Renal cell carcinoma
Adenocarcinoma of colon
Thymoma
Osteosarcoma
Lymphoma
Leukemia
Drugs
Increased ADH production
Antidepressants: tricyclics, monoamine oxidase inhibitors, SSRIs
Antineoplastics: cyclophosphamide, vincristine
Carbamazepine
Methylenedioxymethamphetamine (MDMA; Ecstasy)
Clofibrate
Neuroleptics: thiothixene, thioridazine, fluphenazine, haloperidol, trifluoperazine
Potentiated ADH action
Carbamazepine
Chlorpropamide, tolbutamide
Cyclophosphamide
NSAIDs
Somatostatin and analogs
Amiodarone
Others
Postoperative
Pain
Stress
AIDS
Pregnancy (physiologic)
Hypokalemia

ADH, antidiuretic hormone; NSAIDs, nonsteroidal anti-inflammatory drugs; SSRIs, selective serotonin reuptake inhibitors.

vasodilation or decreased cardiac output. Increased renin-angiotensin-aldosterone system activity and ADH secretion result in water retention. Note the pathophysiologic similarity to hypovolemic hyponatremia—the body sacrifices osmolality in an attempt to restore effective circulating volume.

The pathophysiology of hyponatremia in nephrotic syndrome is not completely understood, but the primary disturbance may be renal sodium retention, resulting in overfilling of the intravascular space and secondary edema formation as fluid enters the interstitial space. Previously, it was thought that the decreased oncotic pressure of hypoalbuminemia caused fluid shifts from the intravascular space to the interstitial compartment. Intravascular underfilling led to secondary renal sodium retention. However, patients receiving therapy for glomerular disease and nephrotic syndrome often have edema resolution prior to normalization of the serum albumin.

Patients with advanced kidney disease typically have sodium retention and decreased free water excretory capacity, resulting in hypervolemic hyponatremia.

Clinical Findings

A. Symptoms and Signs

Whether hyponatremia is symptomatic depends on its severity and acuity. Chronic disease can be severe (sodium concentration < 110 mEq/L), yet remarkably asymptomatic because the brain has adapted by decreasing its tonicity over weeks to months. Acute disease that has developed over hours to days can be severely symptomatic with relatively modest hyponatremia. Mild hyponatremia (sodium concentrations of 130–135 mEq/L) is usually asymptomatic.

Mild symptoms of nausea and malaise progress to headache, lethargy, and disorientation as the sodium concentration drops. The most serious symptoms are respiratory arrest, seizure, coma, permanent brain damage, brainstem herniation, and death. Premenopausal women are much more likely than menopausal women to die or suffer permanent brain injury from hyponatremic encephalopathy, suggesting a hormonal role in the pathophysiology.

Evaluation starts with a careful history for new medications, changes in fluid intake (polydipsia, anorexia, intravenous fluid rates and composition), fluid output (nausea and vomiting, diarrhea, ostomy output, polyuria, oliguria, insensible losses). The physical examination should help categorize the patient's volume status into hypovolemia, euvolemia, or hypervolemia.

B. Laboratory Findings

Laboratory assessment should include serum electrolytes, creatinine, and osmolality as well as urine sodium. The etiology of most cases of hyponatremia will be apparent from the history, physical, and basic laboratory tests. Additional tests of thyroid and adrenal function will occasionally be necessary.

SIADH is a clinical diagnosis characterized by (1) hyponatremia; (2) decreased osmolality (< 280 mosm/kg [< 280 mmol/kg]); (3) absence of heart, kidney, or liver disease; (4) normal thyroid and adrenal function (see Chapter 26); and (5) urine sodium usually over 20 mEq/L. In clinical practice, ADH levels are not measured. Patients with SIADH may have low blood urea nitrogen (BUN) (< 10 mg/dL [or < 3.6 mmol/L]) and hypouricemia (< 4 mg/dL [or < 238 mcmol/L]), which are not only dilutional but

result from increased urea and uric acid clearances in response to the volume-expanded state. Azotemia may reflect volume contraction, ruling out SIADH, which is seen in euvolemic patients.

Complications

The most serious complication of hyponatremia is iatrogenic cerebral osmotic demyelination from overly rapid sodium correction. Also called central pontine myelinolysis, cerebral osmotic demyelination may occur outside the brainstem. Demyelination may occur days after sodium correction or initial neurologic recovery from hyponatremia. Hypoxic episodes during hyponatremia may contribute to demyelination. The neurologic effects are generally catastrophic and irreversible.

Treatment

Regardless of the patient's volume status, another common feature is to restrict free water and hypotonic fluid intake, since these solutions will exacerbate hyponatremia. Free water intake from oral intake and intravenous fluids should generally be < 1–1.5 L/d.

Hypovolemic patients require adequate fluid resuscitation from isotonic fluids (either normal saline or lactated Ringer solution) to suppress the hypovolemic stimulus for ADH release. Patients with **cerebral salt wasting** may require hypertonic saline to prevent circulatory collapse; some may respond to fludrocortisone. **Hypervolemic** patients may require loop diuretics or dialysis, or both, to correct increased total body water and sodium. **Euvolemic** patients may respond to free water restriction alone.

Pseudohyponatremia from hypertriglyceridemia or hyperproteinemia requires no therapy except confirmation with the clinical laboratory. **Translocational hyponatremia** from glucose or mannitol can be managed with glucose correction or mannitol discontinuation (if possible). No specific therapy is necessary in patients with **reset osmostat** since they successfully regulate their serum sodium with fluid challenges and water deprivation.

Symptomatic and severe hyponatremia generally require hospitalization for careful monitoring of fluid balance and weights, treatment, and frequent sodium checks. Inciting medications should be discontinued if possible.

There is no consensus about the optimal rate of sodium correction in symptomatic hyponatremic patients. Recent guidelines have introduced new recommendations. First, a relatively small increase of 4–6 mEq/L in the serum sodium may be all that is necessary to reverse the neurologic manifestations of symptomatic hyponatremia. Second, acute hyponatremia (eg, exercise-associated hyponatremia) with severe neurologic manifestations can be reversed rapidly with 100 mL of 3% hypertonic saline infused over 10 minutes (repeated twice as necessary). Third, lower correction rates for chronic hyponatremia have been introduced, as low as 4–8 mEq/L per 24 hours in patients at high risk for demyelination. Fourth, chronic hyponatremic patients at high risk for demyelination who are corrected too rapidly are candidates for treatment with a combination of DDAVP and intravenous dextrose 5% to relower the serum sodium.

In severely symptomatic patients, the clinician should calculate the sodium deficit and deliver 3% **hypertonic saline.** The sodium deficit can be calculated by the following formula:

$$\text{Sodium deficit} = \text{Total body water (TBW)} \\ \times (\text{Desired serum Na} - \text{Actual serum Na})$$

where TBW is typically 50% of total mass in women and 55% of total mass in men. For example, a nonedematous, severely symptomatic 70 kg woman with a serum sodium of 124 mEq/L should have her serum sodium corrected to approximately 132 mEq/L in the first 24 hours. Her sodium deficit is calculated as:

$$\text{Sodium deficit} = 70 \text{ kg} \times 0.5 \times (132 \text{ mEq/L} - 124 \text{ mEq/L}) \\ = 280 \text{ mEq}$$

3% hypertonic saline has a sodium concentration of 514 mEq/1000 mL. The delivery rate for hypertonic saline can be calculated as:

$$\text{Delivery rate} = \text{Sodium deficit}/(514 \text{ mEq/1000mL})/ \\ 24 \text{ hours} \\ = 280 \text{ mEq}/(514 \text{ mEq/1000 mL})/24 \text{ hours} \\ = 22 \text{ mL/hour}$$

In general, the 3% hypertonic saline infusion rate should not exceed 0.5 mL/kg body weight/h; higher rates may represent a miscalculated sodium deficit or a mathematical error. Hypertonic saline in hypervolemic patients can be hazardous, resulting in worsening volume overload, pulmonary edema, and ascites.

For patients who cannot adequately restrict free water or have an inadequate response to conservative measures, demeclocycline (300–600 mg orally twice daily) inhibits the effect of ADH on the distal tubule. Onset of action may require 1 week, and urinary concentrating ability may be permanently impaired, resulting in nephrogenic diabetes insipidus (DI) and even hypernatremia. Cirrhosis may increase the nephrotoxicity of demeclocycline.

Vasopressin antagonists may revolutionize the treatment of euvolemic and hypervolemic hyponatremia, especially in heart failure. Tolvaptan, lixivaptan, and satavaptan are oral selective vasopressin-2 receptor antagonists; conivaptan is an intravenous agent. Tolvaptan and conivaptan are available in the United States, but lixivaptan and satavaptan are not yet approved by the US Food and Drug Administration (FDA).

V_2 receptors mediate the diuretic effect of ADH and V_2 receptor antagonists are recommended for use in hospital. For hospitalized patients with euvolemic SIADH, tolvaptan is begun as 15 mg orally daily and can be increased to 30 mg daily and 60 mg daily at 24 hour intervals if hyponatremia persists or if the increase in sodium concentration is < 5 mEq/L over the preceding 24 hours. Conivaptan is given as an intravenous loading dose of 20 mg delivered over 30 minutes, then as 20 mg continuously over 24 hours. Subsequent infusions may be administered every 1–3 days at 20–40 mg/d by continuous infusion. The standard free water restriction for hyponatremic patients should be lifted for patients receiving vasopressin antagonists since the aquaresis can result in excessive sodium correction in a fluid-restricted patient. Frequent monitoring of the serum sodium is necessary.

When to Refer

- Nephrology or endocrinology consultation should be considered in severe, symptomatic, refractory, or complicated cases of hyponatremia.
- Aggressive therapies with hypertonic saline, demeclocycline, vasopressin antagonists, or dialysis mandate specialist consultation.
- Consultation may be necessary with end-stage liver or heart disease.

When to Admit

Hospital admission is necessary for symptomatic patients or those requiring aggressive therapies for close monitoring and frequent laboratory testing.

Graff-Radford J et al. Clinical and radiologic correlations of central pontine myelinolysis syndrome. Mayo Clin Proc. 2011 Nov;86(11):1063–7. [PMID: 21997578]

Lehrich RW et al. Role of vaptans in the management of hyponatremia. Am J Kidney Dis. 2013 Aug;62(2):364–76. [PMID: 23725974]

Leung AA et al. Preoperative hyponatremia and perioperative complications. Arch Intern Med. 2012 Oct 22;172(19):1474–81. [PMID: 22965221]

Pokaharel M et al. Dysnatremia in the ICU. Curr Opin Crit Care. 2011 Dec;17(6):581–93. [PMID: 22027406]

Shchekochikhin D et al. Hyponatremia: an update on current pharmacotherapy. Expert Opin Pharmacother. 2013 Apr;14(6):747–55. [PMID: 23496346]

Verbalis JG et al. Diagnosis, evaluation, and treatment of hyponatremia: expert panel recommendations. Am J Med. 2013 Oct;126(10 Suppl 1):S1–42. [PMID: 24074529]

HYPERNATREMIA

ESSENTIALS OF DIAGNOSIS

- ► Increased thirst and water intake is the first defense against hypernatremia.
- ► Urine osmolality helps differentiate renal from nonrenal water loss.

General Considerations

Hypernatremia is defined as a sodium concentration > 145 mEq/L. All patients with hypernatremia have hyperosmolality, unlike hyponatremic patients who can have a low, normal, or high serum osmolality. The hypernatremic patient is typically hypovolemic due to free water losses, although hypervolemia is frequently seen, often as an iatrogenic complication in hospitalized patients with impaired access to free water. Rarely, excessive sodium intake may cause hypernatremia. Hypernatremia in primary aldosteronism is mild and usually does not cause symptoms.

An intact thirst mechanism and access to water are the primary defense against hypernatremia. The hypothalamus can sense minimal changes in serum osmolality, triggering the thirst mechanism and increased water intake. Thus, whatever the underlying disorder (eg, dehydration, lactulose or mannitol therapy, central and nephrogenic DI), excess water loss can cause hypernatremia only when adequate water intake is not possible.

▶ Clinical Findings

A. Symptoms and Signs

When the patient is dehydrated, orthostatic hypotension and oliguria are typical findings. Because water shifts from the cells to the intravascular space to protect volume status, these symptoms may be delayed. Lethargy, irritability, and weakness are early signs. Hyperthermia, delirium, seizures, and coma may be seen with severe hypernatremia (ie, sodium > 158 mEq/L). Symptoms in the elderly may not be specific; a recent change in consciousness is associated with a poor prognosis. Osmotic demyelination is an uncommon but reported consequence of severe hypernatremia.

B. Laboratory Findings

1. Urine osmolality > 400 mosm/kg—Renal water-conserving ability is functioning.

A. Nonrenal losses—Hypernatremia will develop if water intake falls behind hypotonic fluid losses from excessive sweating, the respiratory tract, or bowel movements. Lactulose causes an osmotic diarrhea with loss of free water.

B. Renal losses—While severe hyperglycemia can cause translocational hyponatremia, progressive volume depletion from glucosuria can result in hypernatremia. Osmotic diuresis can occur with the use of mannitol or urea.

2. Urine osmolality < 250 mosm/kg—Hypernatremia with a dilute urine (osmolality < 250 mosm/kg) is characteristic of DI. Central DI results from inadequate ADH release. Nephrogenic DI results from renal insensitivity to ADH; common causes include lithium, demeclocycline, relief of urinary obstruction, interstitial nephritis, hypercalcemia, and hypokalemia.

▶ Treatment

Treatment of hypernatremia includes correcting the cause of the fluid loss, replacing water, and replacing electrolytes (as needed). In response to increases in plasma osmolality, brain cells synthesize solutes called idiogenic osmoles, which cause intracellular fluid shifts. Osmole production begins 4–6 hours after dehydration and takes several days to reach steady state. If hypernatremia is rapidly corrected, the osmotic imbalance may cause cerebral edema and potentially severe neurologic impairment. Fluids should be administered over a 48-hour period, aiming for serum sodium correction of approximately 1 mEq/L/h

(1 mmol/L/h). There is no consensus about the optimal rates of sodium correction in hypernatremia and hyponatremia.

A. Choice of Type of Fluid for Replacement

1. Hypernatremia with hypovolemia—Hypovolemic patients should receive isotonic 0.9% normal saline to restore euvolemia and to treat hyperosmolality because normal saline (308 mosm/kg or 308 mmol/kg) is hypo-osmolar compared with plasma. After adequate volume resuscitation with normal saline, 0.45% saline or 5% dextrose (or both) can be used to replace any remaining free water deficit. Milder volume deficits may be treated with 0.45% saline and 5% dextrose.

2. Hypernatremia with euvolemia—Water ingestion or intravenous 5% dextrose will result in the excretion of excess sodium in the urine. If the glomerular filtration rate (GFR) is decreased, diuretics will increase urinary sodium excretion but may impair renal concentrating ability, increasing the quantity of water that needs to be replaced.

3. Hypernatremia with hypervolemia—Treatment includes 5% dextrose solution to reduce hyperosmolality. Loop diuretics may be necessary to promote natriuresis and lower total body sodium. In severe rare cases with kidney disease, hemodialysis may be necessary to correct the excess total body sodium and water.

B. Calculation of Water Deficit

Fluid replacement should include the free water deficit and additional maintenance fluid to replace ongoing and anticipated fluid losses.

1. Acute hypernatremia—In acute dehydration without much solute loss, free water loss is similar to the weight loss. Initially, a 5% dextrose solution may be used. As correction of water deficit progresses, therapy should continue with 0.45% saline with dextrose.

2. Chronic hypernatremia—The water deficit is calculated to restore normal sodium concentration, typically 140 mEq/L. Total body water (TBW) (Table 21–1) correlates with muscle mass and therefore decreases with advancing age, cachexia, and dehydration and is lower in women than in men. Current TBW equals 40–60% current body weight.

$$\text{Volume (in L) to be repleced} = \text{Current TBW} \times \frac{[Na^+] - 140}{140}$$

▶ When to Refer

Patients with refractory or unexplained hypernatremia should be referred for subspecialist consultation.

▶ When to Admit

- Patients with symptomatic hypernatremia require hospitalization for evaluation and treatment.
- Significant comorbidities or concomitant acute illnesses, especially if contributing to hypernatremia, may necessitate hospitalization.

Al-Absi A et al. A clinical approach to the treatment of chronic hypernatremia. Am J Kidney Dis. 2012 Dec;60(6):1032–8. [PMID: 22959761]

Alshayeb HM et al. Severe hypernatremia correction rate and mortality in hospitalized patients. Am J Med Sci. 2011 May;341(5):356–60. [PMID: 21358313]

Arampatzis S et al. Characteristics, symptoms, and outcome of severe dysnatremias present on hospital admission. Am J Med. 2012 Nov;125(11):1125.e1–e7. [PMID: 22939097]

Lindner G et al. Hypernatremia in critically ill patients. J Crit Care. 2013 Apr;28(2):216.e11–20. [PMID: 22762930]

Sam R et al. Understanding hypernatremia. Am J Nephrol. 2012;36(1):97–104. [PMID: 22739333]

VOLUME OVERLOAD

ESSENTIALS OF DIAGNOSIS

► Disorder of excessive sodium retention in the setting of low arterial underfilling (eg, heart failure or cirrhosis).

► Hyponatremia from water retention in edematous states is associated with sodium retention.

The hallmark of a volume overloaded state is sodium retention. Abnormally low arterial filling, such as from heart failure or cirrhosis, activates the neurohumoral axis, which stimulates the renin-angiotensin-aldosterone system, the sympathetic nervous system, and ADH (vasopressin) release. The result is sodium retention with edema. The stimulus for vasopressin release is nonosmotic. Released in response to baroreceptor activation, vasopressin stimulates renal V_2 receptors, resulting in water reabsorption, edema formation, and hyponatremia.

Bagshaw SM et al. Disorders of sodium and water balance in hospitalized patients. Can J Anaesth. 2009 Feb;56(2):151–67. [PMID: 19247764]

Rosner MH et al. Dysnatremias in the intensive care unit. Contrib Nephrol. 2010;165:292–8. [PMID: 20427980]

HYPEROSMOLAR DISORDERS & OSMOLAR GAPS

HYPEROSMOLALITY WITH TRANSIENT OR NO SIGNIFICANT SHIFT IN WATER

Urea and alcohol readily cross cell membranes and can produce hyperosmolality. Urea is an ineffective osmole with little effect on osmotic water movement across cell membranes. Alcohol quickly equilibrates between the intracellular and extracellular compartments, adding 22 mosm/L for every 100 mg/dL (or 21.7 mmol/L) of ethanol. Ethanol ingestion should be considered in any case of stupor or coma with an elevated osmol gap (measured osmolality – calculated osmolality > 10 mosm/kg [> 10 mmol/kg]). Other toxic alcohols such as methanol and ethylene glycol cause an osmol gap and a metabolic acidosis with an increased anion gap (see Chapter 38). The combination of an increased anion gap metabolic acidosis and an osmol gap exceeding 10 mosm/kg (or 10 mmol/kg) is not specific for toxic alcohol ingestion and may occur with alcoholic ketoacidosis or lactic acidosis (see Metabolic Acidosis).

Kruse JA. Methanol and ethylene glycol intoxication. Crit Care Clin. 2012 Oct;28(4):661–711. [PMID: 22998995]

HYPEROSMOLALITY ASSOCIATED WITH SIGNIFICANT SHIFTS IN WATER

Increased concentrations of solutes that do not readily enter cells cause a shift of water from intracellular to extracellular. Hyperosmolality of effective osmoles such as sodium and glucose causes symptoms, primarily neurologic. The severity of symptoms depends on the degree of hyperosmolality and rapidity of development. In acute hyperosmolality, somnolence and confusion can appear when the osmolality exceeds 320–330 mosm/kg (320–330 mmol/kg); coma, respiratory arrest, and death can result when osmolality exceeds 340–350 mosm/kg (340–350 mmol/kg).

Kraut JA et al. Approach to the evaluation of a patient with an increased serum osmolal gap and high-anion-gap metabolic acidosis. Am J Kidney Dis. 2011 Sep;58(3):480–4. [PMID: 21794966]

Whittington JE et al. The osmolal gap: what has changed? Clin Chem. 2010 Aug;56(8):1353–5. [PMID: 20530730]

DISORDERS OF POTASSIUM CONCENTRATION

HYPOKALEMIA

ESSENTIALS OF DIAGNOSIS

► Serum potassium level < 3.5 mEq/L (< 3.5 mmol/L)

► Severe hypokalemia may induce dangerous arrhythmias and rhabdomyolysis.

► Transtubular potassium concentration gradient (TTKG) can distinguish renal from nonrenal loss of potassium.

► **General Considerations**

Hypokalemia can result from insufficient dietary potassium intake, intracellular shifting of potassium from the extracellular space, extrarenal potassium loss, or renal potassium loss (Table 21–3). Cellular uptake of potassium is increased by insulin and beta-adrenergic stimulation and blocked by alpha-adrenergic stimulation. Aldosterone is an important regulator of total body potassium, increasing potassium secretion in the distal renal tubule. The most common cause of hypokalemia, especially in developing countries, is gastrointestinal loss from infectious diarrhea. The potassium concentration in intestinal secretion is ten times higher (80 mEq/L) than in gastric secretions.

Table 21–3. Causes of hypokalemia.

Decreased potassium intake
Potassium shift into the cell
Increased postprandial secretion of insulin
Alkalosis
Trauma (via beta-adrenergic stimulation?)
Periodic paralysis (hypokalemic)
Barium intoxication
Renal potassium loss
Increased aldosterone (mineralocorticoid) effects
Primary hyperaldosteronism
Secondary aldosteronism (dehydration, heart failure)
Renovascular hypertension
Malignant hypertension
Ectopic ACTH-producing tumor
Gitelman syndrome
Bartter syndrome
Cushing syndrome
Licorice (European)
Renin-producing tumor
Congenital abnormality of steroid metabolism (eg, adrenogenital syndrome, 17-alpha-hydroxylase defect, apparent mineralocorticoid excess, 11-beta-hydroxylase deficiency)
Increased flow to distal nephron
Diuretics (furosemide, thiazides)
Salt-losing nephropathy
Hypomagnesemia
Unreabsorbable anion
Carbenicillin, penicillin
Renal tubular acidosis (type I or II)
Fanconi syndrome
Interstitial nephritis
Metabolic alkalosis (bicarbonaturia)
Congenital defect of distal nephron
Liddle syndrome
Extrarenal potassium loss
Vomiting, diarrhea, laxative abuse
Villous adenoma, Zollinger-Ellison syndrome

Table 21–4. Genetic disorders associated with electrolyte metabolism disturbances.

Disease	Site of Mutation
Potassium	
Hypokalemia	
Hypokalemic periodic paralysis	Dihydropyridine-sensitive skeletal muscle voltage-gated calcium channel
Bartter syndrome	Na^+-K^+-$2Cl^-$ cotransporter, K^+ channel (ROMK), or Cl^- channel of thick ascending limb of Henle (hypofunction), barttin
Gitelman syndrome	Thiazide-sensitive Na^+-Cl^- cotransporter
Liddle syndrome	Beta or gamma subunit of amiloride-sensitive Na^+ channel (hyperfunction)
Apparent mineralo-corticoid excess	11-beta-hydroxysteroid dehydro-genase (failure to inactivate cortisol)
Glucocorticoid-remediable hyperaldosteronism	Regulatory sequence of 11-beta-hydroxysteroid controls aldoste-rone synthase inappropriately
Hyperkalemia	
Hyperkalemic periodic paralysis	Alpha subunit of calcium channel
Pseudohypoaldoste-ronism type I	Beta or gamma subunit of amiloride-sensitive Na^+ channel (hypofunction)
Pseudohypoaldoster-onism type II (Gordon syndrome)	HNK2, HNK4
Calcium	
Familial hypocalciuric hypercalcemia	Ca^{2+}-sensing protein (hypofunction)
Familial hypocalcemia	Ca^{2+}-sensing protein (hyperfunction)
Phosphate	
Hypophosphatemic rickets	*PEX* gene, FGF23
Magnesium	
Hypomagnesemia-hypercalciuria syndrome	Paracellin-1
Water	
Nephrogenic diabetes insipidus	Vasopressin receptor-2 (Type 1), aquaporin-2
Acid-base	
Proximal RTA	Na^+ HCO_3^- cotransporter
Distal RTA	Cl^- HCO_3^- exchanger H^+-ATPase
Proximal and distal RTA	Carbonic anhydrase II

FGF23, fibroblast growth factor 23; RTA, renal tubular acidosis.

Hypokalemia in the presence of acidosis suggests profound potassium depletion and requires urgent treatment. Self-limited hypokalemia occurs in 50–60% of trauma patients, perhaps related to enhanced release of epinephrine.

Hypokalemia increases the likelihood of digitalis toxicity. In patients with heart disease, hypokalemia induced by beta-2-adrenergic agonists and diuretics may substantially increase the risk of arrhythmias. Numerous genetic mutations affect fluid and electrolyte metabolism, including disorders of potassium metabolism (Table 21–4).

Magnesium is an important cofactor for potassium uptake and maintenance of intracellular potassium levels. Loop diuretics (eg, furosemide) cause substantial renal potassium and magnesium losses. Magnesium depletion should be considered in refractory hypokalemia.

▶ **Clinical Findings**

A. Symptoms and Signs

Muscular weakness, fatigue, and muscle cramps are frequent complaints in mild to moderate hypokalemia.

Gastrointestinal smooth muscle involvement may result in constipation or ileus. Flaccid paralysis, hyporeflexia, hypercapnia, tetany, and rhabdomyolysis may be seen with severe hypokalemia (< 2.5 mEq/L). The presence of hypertension may be a clue to the diagnosis of hypokalemia from aldosterone or mineralocorticoid excess (Table 21–4). Renal manifestations include nephrogenic DI and interstitial nephritis.

B. Laboratory Findings

Urinary potassium concentration is low (< 20 mEq/L) as a result of extrarenal loss (eg, diarrhea, vomiting) and inappropriately high (> 40 mEq/L) with renal loss (eg, mineralocorticoid excess, Bartter syndrome, Liddle syndrome) (Table 21–3).

The transtubular $[K^+]$ gradient (TTKG) is a simple and rapid evaluation of net potassium secretion. TTKG is calculated as follows:

$$TTKG = \frac{Urine\ K^+/Plasma\ K^+}{Urine\ osm/Plasma\ osm}$$

Hypokalemia with a TTKG > 4 suggests renal potassium loss with increased distal K^+ secretion. In such cases, plasma renin and aldosterone levels are helpful in differential diagnosis. The presence of nonabsorbed anions, such as bicarbonate, increases the TTKG.

C. Electrocardiogram

The electrocardiogram (ECG) shows decreased amplitude and broadening of T waves, prominent U waves, premature ventricular contractions, and depressed ST segments.

▶ Treatment

Oral potassium supplementation is the safest and easiest treatment for mild to moderate deficiency. Dietary potassium is almost entirely coupled to phosphate—rather than chloride—and is therefore not effective in correcting potassium loss associated with chloride depletion from diuretics or vomiting. In the setting of abnormal kidney function and mild to moderate diuretic dosage, 20 mEq/d of oral potassium is generally sufficient to prevent hypokalemia, but 40–100 mEq/d over a period of days to weeks is needed to treat hypokalemia and fully replete potassium stores.

Intravenous potassium is indicated for patients with severe hypokalemia and for those who cannot take oral supplementation. For severe deficiency, potassium may be given through a peripheral intravenous line in a concentration up to 40 mEq/L and at rates up to 10 mEq/h. Concentrations of up to 20 mEq/h may be given through a central venous catheter. Continuous ECG monitoring is indicated, and the serum potassium level should be checked every 3–6 hours. Avoid glucose-containing fluid to prevent further shifts of potassium into the cells. Magnesium deficiency should be corrected, particularly in refractory hypokalemia.

▶ When to Refer

Patients with unexplained hypokalemia, refractory hyperkalemia, or clinical features suggesting alternative diagnoses (eg, aldosteronism or hypokalemic periodic paralysis) should be referred for endocrinology or nephrology consultation.

▶ When to Admit

Patients with symptomatic or severe hypokalemia, especially with cardiac manifestations, require cardiac monitoring, frequent laboratory testing, and potassium supplementation.

Asmar A et al. A physiologic-based approach to the treatment of a patient with hypokalemia. Am J Kidney Dis. 2012 Sep;60(3):492–7. [PMID: 22901631]

Marti G et al. Etiology and symptoms of severe hypokalemia in emergency department patients. Eur J Emerg Med. 2014 Feb;21(1):46–51. [PMID: 23839104]

Pepin J et al. Advances in diagnosis and management of hypokalemic and hyperkalemic emergencies. Emerg Med Pract. 2012 Feb;14(2):1–18. [PMID: 22413702]

Rastegar A. Attending rounds: patient with hypokalemia and metabolic acidosis. Clin J Am Soc Nephrol. 2011 Oct;6(10):2516–21. [PMID: 21921151]

HYPERKALEMIA

ESSENTIALS OF DIAGNOSIS

- ▶ Serum potassium level > 5.0 mEq/L (> 5.0 mmol/L).
- ▶ Hyperkalemia may develop in patients taking ACE inhibitors, angiotensin-receptor blockers, potassium-sparing diuretics, or their combination, even with no or only mild kidney dysfunction.
- ▶ The ECG may show peaked T waves, widened QRS and biphasic QRS–T complexes, or may be normal despite life-threatening hyperkalemia.
- ▶ Measurement of plasma potassium level differentiates potassium leak from blood cells in cases of clotting, leukocytosis, and thrombocytosis from elevated serum potassium.
- ▶ Rule out extracellular potassium shift from the cells in acidosis and assess renal potassium excretion.

▶ General Considerations

Hyperkalemia usually occurs in patients with advanced kidney disease but can also develop with normal kidney function (Table 21–5). Acidosis causes intracellular potassium to shift extracellularly. Serum potassium concentration rises about 0.7 mEq/L for every decrease of 0.1 pH unit during acidosis. Fist clenching during venipuncture may raise the potassium concentration by 1–2 mEq/L by causing acidosis and potassium shift from cells. In the absence of acidosis, serum potassium concentration rises about 1 mEq/L when there is a total body potassium excess

Table 21–5. Causes of hyperkalemia.

Spurious/Pseudohyperkalemia
Leakage from erythrocytes when separation of serum from clot is delayed (plasma K^+ normal)
Marked thrombocytosis or leukocytosis with release of intracellular K^+ (plasma K^+ normal)
Repeated fist clenching during phlebotomy, with release of K^+ from forearm muscles
Specimen drawn from arm with intravenous K^+ infusion

Decreased K^+ excretion
Kidney disease, acute and chronic
Renal secretory defects (may or may not have reduced kidney function): kidney transplant, interstitial nephritis, systemic lupus erythematosus, sickle cell disease, amyloidosis, obstructive nephropathy
Hyporeninemic hypoaldosteronism (often in diabetic patients with mild to moderate nephropathy) or selective hypoaldosteronism (eg, AIDS patients)
Drugs that inhibit potassium excretion: spironolactone, eplerenone, drospirenone, NSAIDs, ACE inhibitors, angiotensin II receptor blockers, triamterene, amiloride, trimethoprim, pentamidine, cyclosporine, tacrolimus

Shift of K^+ from within the cell
Massive release of intracellular K^+ in burns, rhabdomyolysis, hemolysis, severe infection, internal bleeding, vigorous exercise
Metabolic acidosis (in the case of organic acid accumulation— eg, lactic acidosis—a shift of K^+ does not occur since organic acid can easily move across the cell membrane)
Hypertonicity (solvent drag)
Insulin deficiency (metabolic acidosis may not be apparent)
Hyperkalemic periodic paralysis
Drugs: succinylcholine, arginine, digitalis toxicity, beta-adrenergic antagonists
Alpha-adrenergic stimulation?

Excessive intake of K^+
Especially in patients taking medications that decrease potassium secretion (see above)

ACE, angiotensin-converting enzyme; NSAIDs, nonsteroidal anti-inflammatory drugs.

of 1–4 mEq/kg. However, the higher the serum potassium concentration, the smaller the excess necessary to raise the potassium levels further.

Mineralocorticoid deficiency from Addison disease or chronic kidney disease (CKD) is another cause of hyperkalemia with decreased renal excretion of potassium. Mineralocorticoid resistance due to genetic disorders, interstitial kidney disease, or urinary tract obstruction also leads to hyperkalemia.

ACE inhibitors or angiotensin-receptor blockers (ARBs), commonly used in patients with heart failure or CKD, may cause hyperkalemia. The concomitant use of spironolactone, eplerenone, or beta-blockers further increases the risk of hyperkalemia. Thiazide or loop diuretics and sodium bicarbonate may minimize hyperkalemia. Persistent mild hyperkalemia in the absence of ACE inhibitor or ARB therapy is usually due to type IV renal tubular acidosis (RTA). Heparin inhibits aldosterone production in the adrenal glands, causing hyperkalemia.

Trimethoprim is structurally similar to amiloride and triamterene, and all three drugs inhibit renal potassium excretion through suppression of sodium channels in the distal nephron.

Cyclosporine and tacrolimus can induce hyperkalemia in organ transplant recipients, especially kidney transplant patients, partly due to suppression of the basolateral Na^+–K^+-ATPase in principal cells. Hyperkalemia is commonly seen in HIV patients and has been attributed to impaired renal excretion of potassium due to pentamidine or trimethoprim-sulfamethoxazole or to hyporeninemic hypoaldosteronism.

▶ Clinical Findings

Hyperkalemia impairs neuromuscular transmission, causing muscle weakness, flaccid paralysis, and ileus. Electrocardiography is not a sensitive method for detecting hyperkalemia, since nearly half of patients with a serum potassium level > 6.5 mEq/L will not manifest ECG changes. ECG changes in hyperkalemia include bradycardia, PR interval prolongation, peaked T waves, QRS widening, and biphasic QRS–T complexes. Conduction disturbances, such as bundle branch block and atrioventricular block, may occur. Ventricular fibrillation and cardiac arrest are terminal events.

▶ Prevention

Inhibitors of the renin-angiotensin-aldosterone axis (ie, ACE inhibitors, ARBs, and spironolactone) and potassium-sparing diuretics (eplerenone, triamterene) should be used cautiously in patients with heart failure, liver failure, and kidney disease. Laboratory monitoring should be performed within 1 week of drug initiation or dosage increase.

▶ Treatment

The diagnosis should be confirmed by repeat laboratory testing to rule out spurious hyperkalemia, especially in the absence of medications that cause hyperkalemia or in patients without kidney disease or a previous history of hyperkalemia. Plasma potassium concentration can be measured to avoid hyperkalemia due to potassium leakage out of red cells, white cells, and platelets. Kidney dysfunction should be ruled out at the initial assessment.

Treatment consists of withholding exogenous potassium, identifying the cause, reviewing the patient's medications and dietary potassium intake, and correcting the hyperkalemia. Emergent treatment is indicated when cardiac toxicity, muscle paralysis, or severe hyperkalemia (potassium > 6.5 mEq/L) is present, even in the absence of ECG changes. Insulin, bicarbonate, and beta-agonists shift potassium intracellularly within minutes of administration (Table 21–6). Intravenous calcium may be given to antagonize the cell membrane effects of potassium, but its use should be restricted to life-threatening hyperkalemia in patients taking digitalis because hypercalcemia may cause digitalis toxicity. Hemodialysis may be required to remove potassium in patients with acute or chronic kidney injury.

Table 21–6. Treatment of hyperkalemia.

IMMEDIATE					
Modality	Mechanism of Action	Onset	Duration	Prescription	K+ Removed from Body
Calcium	Antagonizes cardiac conduction abnormalities	0–5 minutes	1 hour	Calcium gluconate 10%, 5–30 mL intravenously; or calcium chloride 5%, 5–30 mL intravenously	0
Bicarbonate	Distributes K+ into cells	15–30 minutes	1–2 hours	NaHCO$_3$, 44–88 mEq (1–2 ampules) intravenously **Note:** Sodium bicarbonate may not be effective in end-stage renal disease patients; dialysis is more expedient and effective. Some patients may not tolerate the additional sodium load of bicarbonate therapy.	0
Insulin	Distributes K+ into cells	15–60 minutes	4–6 hours	Regular insulin, 5–10 units intravenously, plus glucose 50%, 25 g intravenously	0
Albuterol	Distributes K+ into cells	15–30 minutes	2–4 hours	Nebulized albuterol, 10–20 mg in 4 mL normal saline, inhaled over 10 minutes **Note**: Much higher doses are necessary for hyperkalemia therapy (10–20 mg) than for airway disease (2.5 mg).	0
URGENT					
Modality	Mechanism of Action	Onset of Action		Prescription	K+ Removed from Body
Loop diuretic	Renal K+ excretion	0.5–2 hours		Furosemide, 40–160 mg intravenously **Note:** Diuretics may not be effective in patients with acute and chronic kidney diseases.	Variable
Sodium polystyrene sulfonate (eg, Kayexalate)	Ion-exchange resin binds K+	1–3 hours		Oral: 15–60 g in 20% sorbitol (60–240 mL) Rectal: 30–60 g in 20% sorbitol **Note:** Resins with sorbitol may cause bowel necrosis and intestinal perforation, especially in postoperative patients.	0.5–1 mEq/g resin
Hemodialysis[1]	Extracorporeal K+ removal	1–8 hours		Dialysate [K+] 0–1 mEq/L **Note:** A fast and effective therapy for hyperkalemia, hemodialysis can be delayed by vascular access placement and equipment and/or staffing availability. Serum K can be rapidly corrected within minutes, but post-dialysis rebound can occur.	25–50 mEq/h
Peritoneal dialysis	Peritoneal K+ removal	1–4 hours		Frequent exchanges	200–300 mEq

[1]Can be both acute immediate and urgent treatment of hyperkalemia.
Modified and reproduced, with permission, from Cogan MG. *Fluid and Electrolytes: Physiology and Pathophysiology.* McGraw-Hill, 1991.

▶ When to Refer

- Patients with hyperkalemia from kidney disease and reduced renal potassium excretion should see a nephrologist.
- Transplant patients may need adjustment of their immunosuppression regimen by transplant specialists.

▶ When to Admit

Patients with severe hyperkalemia > 6 mEq/L, any degree of hyperkalemia associated with ECG changes, or concomitant illness (eg, tumor lysis, rhabdomyolysis, metabolic acidosis) should be sent to the emergency department for immediate treatment.

Kamel KS et al. Asking the question again: are cation exchange resins effective for the treatment of hyperkalemia? Nephrol Dial Transplant. 2012 Dec;27(12):4294–7. [PMID: 22989741]

Palmer BF. A physiologic-based approach to the evaluation of a patient with hyperkalemia. Am J Kidney Dis. 2010 Aug;56(2):387–93. [PMID: 20493606]

Pepin J et al. Advances in diagnosis and management of hypokalemic and hyperkalemic emergencies. Emerg Med Pract. 2012 Feb;14(2):1–18. [PMID: 22413702]

Shingarev R et al. A physiologic-based approach to the treatment of acute hyperkalemia. Am J Kidney Dis. 2010 Sep;56(3): 578–84. [PMID: 20570423]

DISORDERS OF CALCIUM CONCENTRATION

The normal total plasma (or serum) calcium concentration is 8.5–10.5 mg/dL (or 2.1–2.6 mmol/L). Ionized calcium (normal: 4.6–5.3 mg/dL [or 1.15–1.32 mmol/L]) is physiologically active and necessary for muscle contraction and nerve function.

The calcium-sensing receptor, a transmembrane protein that detects the extracellular calcium concentration, has been identified in the parathyroid gland and the kidney. Functional defects in this protein are associated with diseases of abnormal calcium metabolism such as familial hypocalcemia and familial hypocalciuric hypercalcemia (Table 21–4).

HYPOCALCEMIA

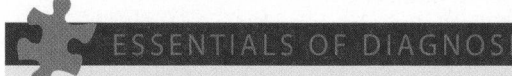

ESSENTIALS OF DIAGNOSIS

▶ Often mistaken as a neurologic disorder.

▶ Check for decreased serum parathyroid hormone (PTH), vitamin D, or magnesium levels.

▶ If the ionized calcium level is normal despite a low total serum calcium, calcium metabolism is usually normal.

General Considerations

The most common cause of low total serum calcium is hypoalbuminemia. When serum albumin concentration is lower than 4 g/dL (40 g/L), serum Ca^{2+} concentration is reduced by 0.8–1 mg/dL (0.20–0.25 mmol/L) for every 1 g/dL (10 g/L) of albumin.

The most accurate measurement of serum calcium is the ionized calcium concentration. True hypocalcemia (decreased ionized calcium) implies insufficient action of PTH or active vitamin D. Important causes of hypocalcemia are listed in Table 21–7.

The most common cause of hypocalcemia is advanced CKD, in which decreased production of active vitamin D_3 (1, 25 dihydroxyvitamin D_3) and hyperphosphatemia both play a role (see Chapter 22). Some cases of primary hypoparathyroidism are due to mutations of the calcium-sensing receptor in which inappropriate suppression of PTH release leads to hypocalcemia (see Chapter 26). Magnesium depletion reduces both PTH release and tissue responsiveness to PTH, causing hypocalcemia. Hypocalcemia in pancreatitis is a marker of severe disease. Elderly hospitalized patients with hypocalcemia and hypophosphatemia, with or without an elevated PTH level, are likely vitamin D deficient.

Table 21–7. Causes of hypocalcemia.

Decreased intake or absorption
Malabsorption
Small bowel bypass, short bowel
Vitamin D deficit (decreased absorption, decreased production of 25-hydroxyvitamin D or 1,25-dihydroxyvitamin D)
Increased loss
Alcoholism
Chronic kidney disease
Diuretic therapy
Endocrine disease
Hypoparathyroidism (genetic, acquired; including hypomagnesemia and hypermagnesemia)
Post-parathyroidectomy (hungry bone syndrome)
Pseudohypoparathyroidism
Calcitonin secretion with medullary carcinoma of the thyroid
Familial hypocalcemia
Associated diseases
Pancreatitis
Rhabdomyolysis
Septic shock
Physiologic causes
Associated with decreased serum albumin[1]
Decreased end-organ response to vitamin D
Hyperphosphatemia
Induced by aminoglycoside antibiotics, plicamycin, loop diuretics, foscarnet

[1]Ionized calcium concentration is normal.

Clinical Findings

A. Symptoms and Signs

Hypocalcemia increases excitation of nerve and muscle cells, primarily affecting the neuromuscular and cardiovascular systems. Spasm of skeletal muscle causes cramps and tetany. Laryngospasm with stridor can obstruct the airway. Convulsions, perioral and peripheral paresthesias, and abdominal pain can develop. Classic physical findings include Chvostek sign (contraction of the facial muscle in response to tapping the facial nerve) and Trousseau sign (carpal spasm occurring with occlusion of the brachial artery by a blood pressure cuff). QT prolongation predisposes to ventricular arrhythmias. In chronic hypoparathyroidism, cataracts and calcification of basal ganglia may appear (see Chapter 26).

B. Laboratory Findings

Serum calcium concentration is low (< 8.5 mg/dL [or < 2.1 mmol/L]). In true hypocalcemia, the ionized serum calcium concentration is also low (< 4.6 mg/dL [or < 1.15 mmol/L]). Serum phosphate is usually elevated in hypoparathyroidism or in advanced CKD, whereas it is suppressed in early CKD or vitamin D deficiency.

Serum magnesium concentration is commonly low. In respiratory alkalosis, total serum calcium is normal but ionized calcium is low. The ECG shows a prolonged QT interval.

Treatment[1]

A. Severe, Symptomatic Hypocalcemia

In the presence of tetany, arrhythmias, or seizures, intravenous calcium gluconate is indicated. Because of the short duration of action, continuous calcium infusion is usually required. Ten to 15 milligrams of calcium per kilogram body weight, or six to eight 10-mL vials of 10% calcium gluconate (558–744 mg of calcium), is added to 1 L of D_5W and infused over 4–6 hours. By monitoring the serum calcium level frequently (every 4–6 hours), the infusion rate is adjusted to maintain the serum calcium level at 7–8.5 mg/dL.

B. Asymptomatic Hypocalcemia

Oral calcium (1–2 g) and vitamin D preparations, including active vitamin D sterols, are used. Calcium carbonate is well tolerated and less expensive than many other calcium tablets. A check of urinary calcium excretion is recommended after the initiation of therapy because hypercalciuria (urine calcium excretion > 300 mg or > 7.5 mmol per day) or urine calcium:creatinine ratio > 0.3 may impair kidney function in these patients. The low serum calcium associated with hypoalbuminemia does not require replacement therapy. If serum Mg^{2+} is low, therapy must include magnesium replacement, which by itself will usually correct hypocalcemia.

When to Refer

Patients with complicated hypocalcemia from hypoparathyroidism, familial hypocalcemia, or CKD require referral to an endocrinologist or nephrologist.

When to Admit

Patients with tetany, arrhythmias, seizures, or other symptoms of hypocalcemia require immediate evaluation and therapy.

Al-Azem H et al. Hypoparathyroidism. Best Pract Res Clin Endocrinol Metab. 2012 Aug;26(4):517–22. [PMID: 22863393]
Fong J et al. Hypocalcemia: updates in diagnosis and management for primary care. Can Fam Physician. 2012 Feb;58(2):158–62. [PMID: 22439169]
Kelly A et al. Hypocalcemia in the critically ill patient. J Intensive Care Med. 2013 May–Jun;28(3):166–77. [PMID: 21841146]
Peacock M. Calcium metabolism in health and disease. Clin J Am Soc Nephrol. 2010 Jan;5(Suppl 1):S23–30. [PMID: 20089499]

HYPERCALCEMIA

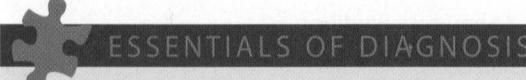

ESSENTIALS OF DIAGNOSIS

► Primary hyperparathyroidism and malignancy-associated hypercalcemia are the most common causes.
► Hypercalciuria usually precedes hypercalcemia.

► Most often, asymptomatic, mild hypercalcemia (≥ 10.5 mg/dL [or 2.6 mmol/L]) is due to primary hyperparathyroidism, whereas the symptomatic, severe hypercalcemia (≥ 14 mg/dL [or 3.5 mmol/L]) is due to hypercalcemia of malignancy.

General Considerations

Important causes of hypercalcemia are listed in Table 21–8. Primary hyperparathyroidism and malignancy account for 90% of cases. Primary hyperparathyroidism is the most common cause of hypercalcemia (usually mild) in ambulatory patients. Chronic hypercalcemia (over 6 months) or some manifestation such as nephrolithiasis also suggests a benign cause. Tumor production of PTH-related proteins (PTHrP) is the most common paraneoplastic endocrine syndrome, accounting for most cases of hypercalcemia in inpatients (see Table 39–2). The neoplasm is clinically apparent in nearly all cases when the hypercalcemia is detected, and the prognosis is poor. Granulomatous diseases, such as sarcoidosis and tuberculosis, cause hypercalcemia via overproduction of active vitamin D_3 (1,25 dihydroxyvitamin D_3).

Milk-alkali syndrome has had a resurgence due to calcium ingestion for prevention of osteoporosis. Heavy calcium carbonate intake causes hypercalcemic acute kidney injury, likely from renal vasoconstriction. The decreased GFR impairs bicarbonate excretion, while hypercalcemia stimulates proton secretion and bicarbonate reabsorption. Metabolic alkalosis decreases calcium excretion, maintaining hypercalcemia.

Table 21–8. Causes of hypercalcemia.

Increased intake or absorption
Milk-alkali syndrome
Vitamin D or vitamin A excess
Endocrine disorders
Primary hyperparathyroidism
Secondary or tertiary hyperparathyroidism (usually associated with hypocalcemia)
Acromegaly
Adrenal insufficiency
Pheochromocytoma
Thyrotoxicosis
Neoplastic diseases
Tumors producing PTH-related proteins (ovary, kidney, lung)
Multiple myeloma (elaboration of osteoclast-activating factor)
Lymphoma (occasionally from production of calcitriol)
Miscellaneous causes
Thiazide diuretic use
Granulomatous diseases (production of calcitriol)
Paget disease of bone
Hypophosphatasia
Immobilization
Familial hypocalciuric hypercalcemia
Complications of kidney transplantation
Lithium intake

PTH, parathyroid hormone.

---

[1] See also Chapter 26 for discussion of the treatment of hypoparathyroidism.

Hypercalcemia causes nephrogenic DI through activation of calcium-sensing receptors in collecting ducts, which reduces ADH-induced water permeability. Volume depletion further worsens hypercalcemia.

Clinical Findings

A. Symptoms and Signs

The history and physical examination should focus on the duration of hypercalcemia and evidence for a neoplasm. Hypercalcemia may affect gastrointestinal, kidney, and neurologic function. Mild hypercalcemia is often asymptomatic. Symptoms usually occur if the serum calcium is > 12 mg/dL (or > 3 mmol/L) and tend to be more severe if hypercalcemia develops acutely. Symptoms include constipation and polyuria, except in hypocalciuric hypercalcemia, in which polyuria is absent. Other symptoms include nausea, vomiting, anorexia, peptic ulcer disease, renal colic, and hematuria from nephrolithiasis. Polyuria from hypercalciuria-induced nephrogenic DI can result in volume depletion and acute kidney injury. Neurologic manifestations range from mild drowsiness to weakness, depression, lethargy, stupor, and coma in severe hypercalcemia. Ventricular ectopy and idioventricular rhythm occur and can be accentuated by digitalis.

B. Laboratory Findings

The ionized calcium exceeds 1.32 mmol/L. A high serum chloride concentration and a low serum phosphate concentration in a ratio > 33:1 (or > 102 if SI units are utilized) suggests primary hyperparathyroidism where PTH decreases proximal tubular phosphate reabsorption. A low serum chloride concentration with a high serum bicarbonate concentration, along with elevated BUN and creatinine, suggests milk-alkali syndrome. Severe hypercalcemia (> 15 mg/dL [or > 3.75 mmol/L]) generally occurs in malignancy. More than 300 mg (or > 7.5 mmol) per day of urinary calcium excretion suggests hypercalciuria; < 100 mg (or < 2.5 mmol) per day suggests hypocalciuria. Hypercalciuric patients—such as those with malignancy or those receiving oral active vitamin D therapy—may easily develop hypercalcemia in case of volume depletion. Serum phosphate may or may not be low, depending on the cause. Hypocalciuric hypercalcemia occurs in milk-alkali syndrome, thiazide diuretic use, and familial hypocalciuric hypercalcemia.

The chest radiograph may reveal malignancy or granulomatous disease. The ECG shows a shortened QT interval. Measurements of PTH and PTHrP help distinguish between hyperparathyroidism (elevated PTH) and malignancy-associated hypercalcemia (suppressed PTH, elevated PTHrP).

Treatment

Until the primary cause can be identified and treated, renal excretion of calcium is promoted through aggressive hydration and forced calciuresis. The tendency in hypercalcemia is hypovolemia from nephrogenic DI. In dehydrated patients with normal cardiac and kidney function, 0.45% saline or 0.9% saline can be given rapidly (250–500 mL/h). A meta-analysis questioned the efficacy and safety profile of intravenous furosemide for hypercalcemia. Thiazides can worsen hypercalcemia.

Bisphosphonates are the treatment of choice for hypercalcemia of malignancy. Although they are safe, effective, and normalize calcium in > 70% of patients, bisphosphonates may require up to 48–72 hours before reaching full therapeutic effect. Calcitonin may be helpful in the short-term until bisphosphonates reach therapeutic levels. In emergency cases, dialysis with low calcium dialysate may be needed. The calcimimetic agent cinacalcet hydrochloride suppresses PTH secretion and decreases serum calcium concentration and holds promise as a treatment option. (See Chapters 26 and 39.)

Typically, if dialysis patients do not receive proper supplementation of calcium and active vitamin D, hypocalcemia and hyperphosphatemia develop. On the other hand, hypercalcemia can sometimes develop, particularly in the setting of severe secondary hyperparathyroidism, characterized by high PTH levels and subsequent release of calcium from bone. Therapy may include intravenous vitamin D, which further increases the serum calcium concentration. Another type of hypercalcemia occurs when PTH levels are low. Bone turnover is decreased, which results in a low buffering capacity for calcium. When calcium is administered in calcium-containing phosphate binders or dialysate, or when vitamin D is administered, hypercalcemia results. Hypercalcemia in dialysis patients usually occurs in the presence of hyperphosphatemia, and metastatic calcification may occur. Malignancy should be considered as a cause of the hypercalcemia.

When to Refer

- Patients may require referral to an oncologist or endocrinologist depending on the underlying cause of hypercalcemia.
- Patients with granulomatous diseases (eg, tuberculosis and other chronic infections, granulomatosis with polyangiitis [formerly Wegener granulomatosis], sarcoidosis) may require assistance from infectious disease specialists, rheumatologists, or pulmonologists.

When to Admit

- Patients with symptomatic or severe hypercalcemia require immediate treatment.
- Unexplained hypercalcemia with associated conditions, such as acute kidney injury or suspected malignancy, may require urgent treatment and expedited evaluation.

Bech A et al. Denosumab for tumor-induced hypercalcemia complicated by renal failure. Ann Intern Med. 2012 Jun 19;156(12):906–7. [PMID: 22711097]

Crowley R et al. How to approach hypercalcaemia. Clin Med. 2013 Jun;13(3):287–90. [PMID: 23760705]

Lindner G et al. Hypercalcemia in the ED: prevalence, etiology, and outcome. Am J Emerg Med. 2013 Apr;31(4):657–60. [PMID: 23246111]

Marcocci C et al. Clinical practice. Primary hyperparathyroidism. N Engl J Med. 2011 Dec 22;365(25):2389–97. [PMID: 22187986]

Rosner MH et al. Onco-nephrology: the pathophysiology and treatment of malignancy-associated hypercalcemia. Clin J Am Soc Nephrol. 2012 Oct;7(10):1722–9. [PMID: 22879438]

DISORDERS OF PHOSPHORUS CONCENTRATION

Plasma phosphorus is mainly inorganic phosphate and represents a small fraction (< 0.2%) of total body phosphate.

Important determinants of plasma inorganic phosphate are renal excretion, intestinal absorption, and shift between the intracellular and extracellular spaces. The kidney is the most important regulator of the serum phosphate level. PTH decreases reabsorption of phosphate in the proximal tubule while 1,25-dihydroxyvitamin D_3 increases reabsorption. Renal proximal tubular reabsorption of phosphate is decreased by volume expansion, corticosteroids, and proximal tubular dysfunction (as in Fanconi syndrome). Fibroblast growth factor 23 (FGF23) is a potent phosphaturic hormone. Intestinal absorption of phosphate is facilitated by active vitamin D. PTH stimulates phosphate release from bone and renal phosphate excretion; primary hyperparathyroidism can lead to hypophosphatemia and depletion of bone phosphate stores. By contrast, growth hormone augments proximal tubular reabsorption of phosphate. Cellular phosphate uptake is stimulated by various factors and conditions, including alkalemia, insulin, epinephrine, feeding, hungry bone syndrome, and accelerated cell proliferation.

Phosphorus metabolism and homeostasis are intimately related to calcium metabolism. See sections on metabolic bone disease in Chapter 26.

HYPOPHOSPHATEMIA

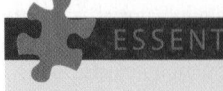

ESSENTIALS OF DIAGNOSIS

▶ Severe hypophosphatemia may cause tissue hypoxia and rhabdomyolysis.

▶ Renal loss of phosphate can be diagnosed by measuring urinary phosphate excretion and by calculating maximal tubular phosphate reabsorption rate (TmP/GFR).

▶ PTH and FGF23 are the major factors that decrease TmP/GFR, leading to renal loss of phosphate.

▶ General Considerations

The leading causes of hypophosphatemia are listed in Table 21–9. Hypophosphatemia may occur in the presence of normal phosphate stores. Serious depletion of body phosphate stores may exist with low, normal, or high serum phosphate concentrations.

Table 21–9. Causes of hypophosphatemia.

Diminished supply or absorption
Starvation
Parenteral alimentation with inadequate phosphate content
Malabsorption syndrome, small bowel bypass
Absorption blocked by oral antacids with aluminum or magnesium
Vitamin D–deficient and vitamin D–resistant osteomalacia
Increased loss
Phosphaturic drugs: theophylline, diuretics, bronchodilators, corticosteroids
Hyperparathyroidism (primary or secondary)
Hyperthyroidism
Renal tubular defects with excessive phosphaturia (congenital, induced by monoclonal gammopathy, heavy metal poisoning), alcoholism
Hypokalemic nephropathy
Inadequately controlled diabetes mellitus
Hypophosphatemic rickets
Phosphatonins of oncogenic osteomalacia (eg, FGF23 production)
Intracellular shift of phosphorus
Administration of glucose
Anabolic steroids, estrogen, oral contraceptives, beta-adrenergic agonists, xanthine derivatives
Hungry bone syndrome
Respiratory alkalosis
Salicylate poisoning
Electrolyte abnormalities
Hypercalcemia
Hypomagnesemia
Metabolic alkalosis
Abnormal losses followed by inadequate repletion
Diabetes mellitus with acidosis, particularly during aggressive therapy
Recovery from starvation or prolonged catabolic state
Chronic alcoholism, particularly during restoration of nutrition; associated with hypomagnesemia
Recovery from severe burns

FGF23, fibroblast growth factor 23.

Serum phosphate levels decrease transiently after food intake, thus fasting samples are recommended for accuracy. **Moderate hypophosphatemia** (1.0–2.4 mg/dL [or 0.32–0.79 mmol/L]) occurs commonly in hospitalized patients and may not reflect decreased phosphate stores.

In **severe hypophosphatemia** (< 1 mg/dL [or < 0.32 mmol/L]), the affinity of hemoglobin for oxygen increases through a decrease in the erythrocyte 2,3-biphosphoglycerate concentration, impairing tissue oxygenation and cell metabolism and resulting in muscle weakness or even rhabdomyolysis. Severe hypophosphatemia is common and multifactorial in alcoholic patients. In acute alcohol withdrawal, increased plasma insulin and epinephrine along with respiratory alkalosis promote intracellular shift of phosphate. Vomiting, diarrhea, and poor dietary intake contribute to hypophosphatemia. Chronic alcohol use results in a decrease in the renal threshold of phosphate excretion. This renal tubular dysfunction reverses after a month of abstinence. Patients with chronic obstructive pulmonary disease and asthma commonly have hypophosphatemia, attributed to xanthine derivatives causing shifts of phosphate intracellularly and the phosphaturic effects of beta-adrenergic agonists, loop diuretics, xanthine derivatives, and corticosteroids. Refeeding or glucose administration to phosphate-depleted patients may cause fatal hypophosphatemia.

Clinical Findings

A. Symptoms and Signs

Acute, severe hypophosphatemia (< 1.0 mg/dL [or < 0.32 mmol/L]) can lead to rhabdomyolysis, paresthesias, and encephalopathy (irritability, confusion, dysarthria, seizures, and coma). Respiratory failure or failure to wean from mechanical ventilation may occur as a result of diaphragmatic weakness. Arrhythmias and heart failure are uncommon but serious manifestations. Hematologic manifestations include acute hemolytic anemia from erythrocyte fragility, platelet dysfunction with petechial hemorrhages, and impaired chemotaxis of leukocytes (leading to increased susceptibility to gram-negative sepsis).

Chronic severe depletion may cause anorexia, pain in muscles and bones, and fractures.

B. Laboratory Findings

Urine phosphate excretion is a useful clue in the evaluation of hypophosphatemia. The normal renal response to hypophosphatemia is decreased urinary phosphate excretion to < 100 mg/d. The fractional excretion of phosphate (F_EPO_4) should be < 5%. The main factors regulating F_EPO_4 are PTH and phosphate intake. Increased PTH or phosphate intake decreases F_EPO_4 (ie, more phosphate is excreted into the urine).

Measurement of plasma PTH or PTHrP levels may be helpful. The clinical utility of serum FGF levels is undetermined except in uncommon diseases.

Other clinical features may be suggestive of hypophosphatemia, such as hemolytic anemia and rhabdomyolysis. Fanconi syndrome may present with any combination of uricosuria, aminoaciduria, normoglycemic glucosuria, normal anion gap metabolic acidosis, and phosphaturia. In chronic hypophosphatemia, radiographs and bone biopsies show changes resembling osteomalacia.

Treatment

Hypophosphatemia can be prevented by including phosphate in repletion and maintenance fluids. A rapid decline in calcium levels can occur with parenteral administration of phosphate; oral replacement of phosphate is preferable. Moderate hypophosphatemia (1.0–2.5 mg/dL [or 0.32–0.79 mmol/L]) is usually asymptomatic and does not require treatment. The hypophosphatemia in patients with diabetic ketoacidosis (DKA) will usually correct with normal dietary intake. Chronic hypophosphatemia can be treated with oral phosphate repletion. Mixtures of sodium and potassium phosphate salts may be given to provide 0.5–1 g (16–32 mmol) of phosphate per day. For severe,

symptomatic hypophosphatemia (< 1 mg/dL [or < 0.32 mmol/L]), an infusion should provide 279–310 mg/12 h (or 9–10 mmol/12 h) until the serum phosphorus exceeds 1 mg/dL and the patient can be switched to oral therapy. The infusion rate should be decreased if hypotension occurs. Monitoring of plasma phosphate, calcium, and potassium every 6 hours is necessary because the response to phosphate supplementation is not predictable. Magnesium deficiency often coexists and should be treated.

Contraindications to phosphate replacement include hypoparathyroidism, advanced CKD, tissue damage and necrosis, and hypercalcemia. When an associated hyperglycemia is treated, phosphate accompanies glucose into cells, and hypophosphatemia may ensue.

When to Refer

- Patients with refractory hypophosphatemia with increased urinary phosphate excretion may require evaluation by an endocrinologist (for such conditions as hyperparathyroidism and vitamin D disorders) or a nephrologist (for such conditions as renal tubular defects).

- Patients with decreased gastrointestinal absorption may require referral to a gastroenterologist.

When to Admit

Patients with severe or refractory hypophosphatemia will require intravenous phosphate.

Bacchetta J et al. Evaluation of hypophosphatemia: lessons from patients with genetic disorders. Am J Kidney Dis. 2012 Jan;59(1):152–9. [PMID: 22075221]

Carpenter TO. The expanding family of hypophosphatemic syndromes. J Bone Miner Metab. 2012 Jan;30(1):1–9. [PMID: 22167381]

Felsenfeld AJ et al. Approach to treatment of hypophosphatemia. Am J Kidney Dis. 2012 Oct;60(4):655–61. [PMID: 22863286]

Imel EA et al. Approach to the hypophosphatemic patient. J Clin Endocrinol Metab. 2012 Mar;97(3):696–706. [PMID: 22392950]

Suzuki S et al. Hypophosphatemia in critically ill patients. J Crit Care. 2013 Aug;28(4):536.e9–19. [PMID: 23265292]

HYPERPHOSPHATEMIA

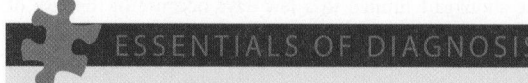

ESSENTIALS OF DIAGNOSIS

▸ Advanced CKD is the most common cause.

▸ Hyperphosphatemia in the presence of hypercalcemia imposes a high risk of metastatic calcification.

General Considerations

Advanced CKD with decreased urinary excretion of phosphate is the most common cause of hyperphosphatemia. Other causes are listed in Table 21–10.

Table 21–10. Causes of hyperphosphatemia.

Massive load of phosphate into the extracellular fluid
Exogenous sources
Hypervitaminosis D
Laxatives or enemas containing phosphate
Intravenous phosphate supplement
Endogenous sources
Rhabdomyolysis (especially if chronic kidney disease coexists)
Cell lysis by chemotherapy of malignancy, particularly lymphoproliferative diseases
Metabolic acidosis (lactic acidosis, ketoacidosis)
Respiratory acidosis (phosphate incorporation into cells is disturbed)
Decreased excretion into urine
Chronic kidney disease
Acute kidney injury
Hypoparathyroidism
Pseudohypoparathyroidism
Acromegaly
Pseudohyperphosphatemia
Multiple myeloma
Hyperbilirubinemia
Hypertriglyceridemia
Hemolysis in vitro

Clinical Findings

A. Symptoms and Signs

The clinical manifestations are those of the underlying disorder or associated condition.

B. Laboratory Findings

In addition to elevated phosphate, blood chemistry abnormalities are those of the underlying disease.

Treatment

Treatment is directed at the underlying cause. Exogenous sources of phosphate, including enteral or parenteral nutrition and medications, should be reduced or eliminated. Dietary phosphate absorption can be reduced by oral phosphate binders, such as calcium carbonate, calcium acetate, sevelamer carbonate, lanthanum carbonate, and aluminum hydroxide. Sevelamer, lanthanum, and aluminum may be used in patients with hypercalcemia, although aluminum use should be limited to a few days because of the risk of aluminum accumulation and neurotoxicity. In acute kidney injury and advanced CKD, dialysis will reduce serum phosphate.

When to Admit

Patients with acute severe hyperphosphatemia require hospitalization for emergent therapy, possibly including dialysis. Concomitant illnesses, such as acute kidney injury or cell lysis, may necessitate admission.

Howard SC et al. The tumor lysis syndrome. N Engl J Med. 2011 May 12;364(19):1844–54. [PMID: 21561350]

Leaf DE et al. A physiologic-based approach to the evaluation of a patient with hyperphosphatemia. Am J Kidney Dis. 2013 Feb;61(2):330–6. [PMID: 22938849]

Lee R et al. Disorders of phosphorus homeostasis. Curr Opin Endocrinol Diabetes Obes. 2010 Dec;17(6):561–7. [PMID: 20962635]

Orrego JJ et al. Hyperphosphatemia. Endocr Pract. 2010 May–Jun;16(3):524–5. [PMID: 20551010]

Prié D et al. Genetic disorders of renal phosphate transport. N Engl J Med. 2010 Jun 24;362(25):2399–409. [PMID: 20573928]

DISORDERS OF MAGNESIUM CONCENTRATION

Normal plasma magnesium concentration is 1.8–3.0 mg/dL (or 0.75–1.25 mmol/L), with about one-third bound to protein and two-thirds existing as free cation. Magnesium excretion is via the kidney. Magnesium's physiologic effects on the nervous system resemble those of calcium.

Altered magnesium concentration usually provokes an associated alteration of Ca^{2+}. Both hypomagnesemia and hypermagnesemia can decrease PTH secretion or action. Severe hypermagnesemia (> 5 mg/dL [or 2.1 mmol/L]) suppresses PTH secretion with consequent hypocalcemia; this disorder is typically seen only in patients receiving magnesium therapy for preeclampsia. Severe hypomagnesemia causes PTH resistance in end-organs and eventually decreased PTH secretion in severe cases.

HYPOMAGNESEMIA

ESSENTIALS OF DIAGNOSIS

► Serum concentration of magnesium may not be decreased even in the presence of magnesium depletion. Check urinary magnesium excretion if renal magnesium wasting is suspected.

► Causes neurologic symptoms and arrhythmias.

► Impairs release of PTH.

General Considerations

Causes of hypomagnesemia are listed in Table 21–11. Normomagnesemia does not exclude magnesium depletion because only 1% of total body magnesium is in the extracellular fluid (ECF). Hypomagnesemia and hypokalemia share many etiologies, including diuretics, diarrhea, alcoholism, aminoglycosides, and amphotericin. Renal potassium wasting also occurs from hypomagnesemia, and is refractory to potassium replacement until magnesium is repleted. Hypomagnesemia also suppresses PTH release and causes end-organ resistance to PTH and low 1,25-dihydroxyvitamin D_3 levels. The resultant hypocalcemia is refractory to calcium replacement until the magnesium is normalized. Molecular mechanisms of magnesium wasting have been revealed in some hereditary disorders. The FDA has issued a warning about hypomagnesemia for patients

Table 21–11. Causes of hypomagnesemia.

Diminished absorption or intake
   Malabsorption, chronic diarrhea, laxative abuse
   Proton pump inhibitors
   Prolonged gastrointestinal suction
   Small bowel bypass
   Malnutrition
   Alcoholism
   Total parenteral alimentation with inadequate Mg^{2+} content
Increased renal loss
   Diuretic therapy (loop diuretics, thiazide diuretics)
   Hyperaldosteronism, Gitelman syndrome (a variant of Bartter
      syndrome)
   Hyperparathyroidism, hyperthyroidism
   Hypercalcemia
   Volume expansion
   Tubulointerstitial diseases
   Transplant kidney
   Drugs (aminoglycoside, cetuximab, cisplatin, amphotericin
      B, pentamidine)
Others
   Diabetes mellitus
   Post-parathyroidectomy (hungry bone syndrome)
   Respiratory alkalosis
   Pregnancy

taking proton pump inhibitors. The presumed mechanism is decreased intestinal magnesium absorption, but it is not clear why this complication develops in only a small fraction of patients taking these medications.

Clinical Findings

A. Symptoms and Signs

Common symptoms are those of hypokalemia and hypocalcemia, with weakness and muscle cramps. Marked neuromuscular and central nervous system hyperirritability may produce tremors, athetoid movements, jerking, nystagmus, Babinski response, confusion, and disorientation. Cardiovascular manifestations include hypertension, tachycardia, and ventricular arrhythmias.

B. Laboratory Findings

Urinary excretion of magnesium exceeding 10–30 mg/d or a fractional excretion > 2% indicates renal magnesium wasting. Hypocalcemia and hypokalemia are often present. The ECG shows a prolonged QT interval, due to lengthening of the ST segment. PTH secretion is often suppressed (see Hypocalcemia).

Treatment

Magnesium oxide, 250–500 mg orally once or twice daily, is useful for treating chronic hypomagnesemia. Symptomatic hypomagnesemia requires intravenous magnesium sulfate 1–2 g over 5–60 minutes mixed in either dextrose 5% or 0.9% normal saline. Torsades de pointes in the setting of

hypomagnesemia can be treated with 1–2 g of magnesium sulfate in 10 mL of dextrose 5% solution pushed intravenously over 15 minutes. Severe, non–life-threatening deficiency can be treated at a rate to 1–2 g/h over 3–6 hours. Magnesium sulfate may also be given intramuscularly in a dosage of 200–800 mg/d (8–33 mmol/d) in four divided doses. Serum levels must be monitored daily and dosage adjusted to keep the concentration from rising above 3 mg/dL (1.23 mmol/L). Tendon reflexes may be checked for hyporeflexia of hypermagnesemia. K^+ and Ca^{2+} replacement may be required, but patients with hypokalemia and hypocalcemia of hypomagnesemia do not recover without magnesium supplementation.

Patients with normal kidney function can excrete excess magnesium; hypermagnesemia should not develop with replacement dosages. In patients with CKD, magnesium replacement should be done cautiously to avoid hypermagnesemia. Reduced doses (50–75% dose reduction) and more frequent monitoring (at least twice daily) are indicated.

Ayuk J et al. How should hypomagnesaemia be investigated and treated? Clin Endocrinol (Oxf). 2011 Dec;75(6):743–6. [PMID: 21569071]

Blasco LM et al. Chronic cyclic nonnephrogenic magnesium depletion without losses. N Engl J Med. 2012 May 10;366(19):1845–6. [PMID: 22571217]

Danziger J et al. Proton-pump inhibitor use is associated with low serum magnesium concentrations. Kidney Int. 2013 Apr;83(4):692–9. [PMID: 23325090]

Dimke H et al. Evaluation of hypomagnesemia: lessons from disorders of tubular transport. Am J Kidney Dis. 2013 Aug;62(2):377–83. [PMID: 23201160]

HYPERMAGNESEMIA

 ESSENTIALS OF DIAGNOSIS

► Often associated with advanced CKD and chronic intake of magnesium-containing drugs.

General Considerations

Hypermagnesemia is almost always the result of advanced CKD and impaired magnesium excretion. Antacids and laxatives are underrecognized sources of magnesium. Pregnant patients may have severe hypermagnesemia from intravenous magnesium for preeclampsia and eclampsia. Magnesium replacement should be done cautiously in patients with CKD; dose reductions up to 75% may be necessary to avoid hypermagnesemia.

Clinical Findings

A. Symptoms and Signs

Muscle weakness, decreased deep tendon reflexes, mental obtundation, and confusion are characteristic manifestations.

Weakness, flaccid paralysis, ileus, urinary retention, and hypotension are noted. Serious findings include respiratory muscle paralysis and cardiac arrest.

B. Laboratory Findings

Serum Mg^{2+} is elevated. In the common setting of CKD, BUN, creatinine, potassium, phosphate, and uric acid may all be elevated. Serum Ca^{2+} is often low. The ECG shows increased PR interval, broadened QRS complexes, and peaked T waves, probably related to associated hyperkalemia.

▶ Treatment

Exogenous sources of magnesium should be discontinued. Calcium antagonizes Mg^{2+} and may be given intravenously as calcium chloride, 500 mg or more at a rate of 100 mg (4.1 mmol) per minute. Hemodialysis or peritoneal dialysis may be necessary to remove magnesium, particularly with severe kidney disease.

Long-term use of magnesium hydroxide and magnesium sulfate should be avoided in patients with advanced stages of CKD.

Moe SM. Disorders involving calcium, phosphorus, and magnesium. Prim Care. 2008 Jun;35(2):215–37. [PMID: 18486714]
Volpe SL. Magnesium in disease prevention and overall health. Adv Nutr. 2013 May 1;4(3):378S–83S. [PMID: 23674807]

▼ ACID–BASE DISORDERS

Assessment of a patient's acid–base status requires measurement of arterial pH, Pco_2, and plasma bicarbonate (HCO_3^-). Blood gas analyzers directly measure pH and Pco_2. The HCO_3^- value is calculated from the Henderson–Hasselbalch equation:

$$pH = 6.1 + \log \frac{HCO_3^-}{0.03 \times PCO_2}$$

The total venous CO_2 measurement is a more direct determination of HCO_3^-. Because of the dissociation characteristics of carbonic acid (H_2CO_3) at body pH, dissolved CO_2 is almost exclusively in the form of HCO_3^-, and for clinical purposes the total carbon dioxide content is equivalent (± 3 mEq/L) to the HCO_3^- concentration:

$$H^+ + HCO_3^- \leftrightarrow H_2CO_3 \leftrightarrow CO_2 + H_2O$$

Venous blood gases can provide useful information for acid–base assessment since the arteriovenous differences in pH and Pco_2 are small and relatively constant. Venous blood pH is usually 0.03–0.04 units lower than arterial blood pH, and venous blood Pco_2 is 7 or 8 mm Hg higher than arterial blood Pco_2. Calculated HCO_3^- concentration in venous blood is at most 2 mEq/L higher than arterial blood HCO_3^-. Arterial and venous blood gases will not be equivalent during a cardiopulmonary arrest; arterial samples should be obtained for the most accurate measurements of pH and Pco_2.

TYPES OF ACID–BASE DISORDERS

There are two types of acid–base disorders: acidosis and alkalosis. These disorders can be either metabolic (decreased or increased HCO_3^-) or respiratory (decreased or increased Pco_2). Primary respiratory disorders affect blood acidity by changes in PCO_2, and primary metabolic disorders are disturbances in HCO_3^- concentration. A primary disturbance is usually accompanied by a compensatory response, but the compensation does not fully correct the pH disturbance of the primary disorder. If the pH is < 7.40, the primary process is acidosis, either respiratory (Pco_2 > 40 mm Hg) or metabolic (HCO_3^- < 24 mEq/L). If the pH is higher than 7.40, the primary process is alkalosis, either respiratory (Pco_2 < 40 mm Hg) or metabolic (HCO_3^- > 24 mEq/L). One respiratory or metabolic disorder with its appropriate compensatory response is a simple acid-base disorder.

MIXED ACID–BASE DISORDERS

Two or three simultaneous disorders can be present in a mixed acid-base disorder, but there can never be two primary respiratory disorders. Uncovering a mixed acid-base disorder is clinically important, but requires a methodical approach to acid-base analysis (see box, Step-by-Step Analysis of Acid-Base Status). Once the primary disturbance has been determined, the clinician should assess whether the compensatory response is appropriate (Table 21–12). An inadequate or an exaggerated response indicates the presence of another primary acid-base disturbance.

The anion gap should always be calculated for two reasons. First, it is possible to have an abnormal anion gap even if the sodium, chloride, and bicarbonate levels are normal. Second, a large anion gap (> 20 mEq/L) suggests a primary metabolic acid-base disturbance regardless of the pH or serum bicarbonate level because a markedly abnormal anion gap is never a compensatory response to a respiratory disorder. In patients with an increased anion gap metabolic acidosis, clinicians should calculate the corrected bicarbonate. In increased anion gap acidoses, there should be a mole for mole decrease in HCO_3^- as the anion gap increases. A corrected HCO_3^- value higher or lower than normal (24 mEq/L) indicates the concomitant presence of metabolic alkalosis or normal anion gap metabolic acidosis, respectively.

STEP-BY-STEP ANALYSIS OF ACID-BASE STATUS

Step 1: Determine the primary (or main) disorder—whether it is metabolic or respiratory—from blood pH, HCO_3^-, and Pco_2 values.

Step 2: Determine the presence of mixed acid-base disorders by calculating the range of compensatory responses (Table 21–12).

Step 3: Calculate the anion gap (Table 21–13).

Step 4: Calculate the corrected HCO_3^- concentration if the anion gap is increased (see above).

Step 5: Examine the patient to determine whether the clinical signs are compatible with the acid-base analysis.

Table 21–12. Primary acid-base disorders and expected compensation.

Disorder	Primary Defect	Compensatory Response	Magnitude of Compensation
Respiratory acidosis			
Acute	$\uparrow P_{CO_2}$	$\uparrow HCO_3^-$	$\uparrow HCO_3^-$ 1 mEq/L per 10 mm Hg $\uparrow P_{CO_2}$
Chronic	$\uparrow P_{CO_2}$	$\uparrow HCO_3^-$	$\uparrow HCO_3^-$ 3.5 mEq/L per 10 mm Hg $\uparrow P_{CO_2}$
Respiratory alkalosis			
Acute	$\downarrow P_{CO_2}$	$\downarrow HCO_3^-$	$\downarrow HCO_3^-$ 2 mEq/L per 10 mm Hg $\downarrow P_{CO_2}$
Chronic	$\downarrow P_{CO_2}$	$\downarrow HCO_3^-$	$\downarrow HCO_3^-$ 5 mEq/L per 10 mm Hg $\downarrow P_{CO_2}$
Metabolic acidosis	$\downarrow HCO_3^-$	$\downarrow P_{CO_2}$	$\downarrow P_{CO_2}$ 1.3 mm Hg per 1 mEq/L $\downarrow HCO_3^-$
Metabolic alkalosis	$\uparrow HCO_3^-$	$\downarrow P_{CO_2}$	$\uparrow P_{CO_2}$ 0.7 mm Hg per 1 mEq/L $\uparrow HCO_3^-$

Adrogué HJ et al. Assessing acid-base disorders. Kidney Int. 2009 Dec;76(12):1239–47. [PMID: 19812535]

Adrogué HJ et al. Secondary responses to altered acid-base status: the rules of engagement. J Am Soc Nephrol. 2010 Jun;21(6):920–3. [PMID: 20431042]

Berend K. Acid-base pathophysiology after 130 years: confusing, irrational and controversial. J Nephrol. 2013 Mar–Apr;26(2):254–65. [PMID: 22976522]

Dzierba AL et al. A practical approach to understanding acid-base abnormalities in critical illness. J Pharm Pract. 2011 Feb;24(1):17–26. Erratum in: J Pharm Pract. 2011 Oct;24(5):515. [PMID: 21507871]

Wiener SW. Toxicologic acid-base disorders. Emerg Med Clin North Am. 2014 Feb;32(1):149–65. [PMID: 24275173]

METABOLIC ACIDOSIS

> ### ESSENTIALS OF DIAGNOSIS
>
> ▶ Decreased HCO_3^- with acidemia.
>
> ▶ Classified into increased anion gap acidosis and normal anion gap acidosis.
>
> ▶ Lactic acidosis, ketoacidosis, and toxins produce metabolic acidoses with the largest anion gaps.
>
> ▶ Normal anion gap acidosis is mainly caused by gastrointestinal HCO_3^- loss or RTA. Urinary anion gap may help distinguish between these causes.

▶ General Considerations

The hallmark of metabolic acidosis is decreased HCO_3^-. Metabolic acidoses are classified by the anion gap, usually normal or increased (Table 21–13). The anion gap is the difference between readily measured anions and cations.

In plasma,

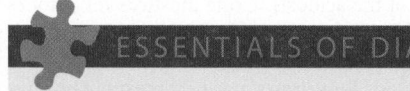

$$[Na^+] + \overset{Unmeasured}{cations} = HCO_3^- + Cl^- + \overset{Unmeasured}{anions}$$

$$Anion\ gap = Na^+ - (HCO_3^- + Cl^-)$$

Major unmeasured cations are calcium (2 mEq/L), magnesium (2 mEq/L), gamma-globulins, and potassium (4 mEq/L). Major unmeasured anions are albumin (2 mEq/L per g/dL), phosphate (2 mEq/L), sulfate (1 mEq/L), lactate (1–2 mEq/L), and other organic anions (3–4 mEq/L). Traditionally, the

Table 21–13. Anion gap in metabolic acidosis.[1]

Decreased (< 6 mEq)
  Hypoalbuminemia (decreased unmeasured anion)
  Plasma cell dyscrasias
    Monoclonal protein (cationic paraprotein) (accompanied by chloride and bicarbonate)
  Bromide intoxication
Increased (> 12 mEq)
  Metabolic anion
    Diabetic ketoacidosis
    Alcoholic ketoacidosis
    Lactic acidosis
    Chronic kidney disease (advanced stages) (PO_4^{3-}, SO_4^{2-})
    Starvation
    Metabolic alkalosis (increased number of negative charges on protein)
    5-oxoproline acidosis from acetaminophen toxicity
  Drug or chemical anion
    Salicylate intoxication
    Sodium carbenicillin therapy
    Methanol (formic acid)
    Ethylene glycol (oxalic acid)
Normal (6–12 mEq)
  Loss of HCO_3
    Diarrhea
    Recovery from diabetic ketoacidosis
    Pancreatic fluid loss, ileostomy (unadapted)
    Carbonic anhydrase inhibitors
  Chloride retention
    Renal tubular acidosis
    Ileal loop bladder
  Administration of HCl equivalent or NH_4Cl
    Arginine and lysine in parenteral nutrition

[1]Reference ranges for anion gap may vary based on differing laboratory methods.

normal anion gap has been 12 ± 4 mEq/L. With current auto-analyzers, the reference range may be lower (6 ± 1 mEq/L), primarily from an increase in Cl⁻ values. Despite its usefulness, the anion gap can be misleading. Non–acid-base disorders may cause errors in anion gap interpretation; these disorders including hypoalbuminemia, hypernatremia, or hyponatremia; antibiotics (eg, carbenicillin is an unmeasured anion; polymyxin is an unmeasured cation) may also cause errors in anion gap interpretation. Although not usually associated with metabolic acidosis, a decreased anion gap can occur because of a reduction in unmeasured anions or an increase in unmeasured cations. In hypoalbuminemia, a 2 mEq/L decrease in anion gap will occur for every 1 g/dL decline in serum albumin.

INCREASED ANION GAP ACIDOSIS (Increased Unmeasured Anions)

Normochloremic metabolic acidosis generally results from addition of organic acids such as lactate, acetoacetate, beta-hydroxybutyrate, and exogenous toxins. Other anions such as isocitrate, alpha-ketoglutarate, malate and D-lactate, may contribute to the anion gap of lactic acidosis, DKA, and acidosis of unknown etiology. Uremia causes an increased anion gap metabolic acidosis from unexcreted organic acids and anions.

A. Lactic Acidosis

Lactic acid is formed from pyruvate in anaerobic glycolysis, typically in tissues with high rates of glycolysis, such as gut (responsible for over 50% of lactate production), skeletal muscle, brain, skin, and erythrocytes. Normally, lactate levels remain low (1 mEq/L) because of metabolism of lactate principally by the liver through gluconeogenesis or oxidation via the Krebs cycle. The kidneys metabolize about 30% of lactate.

In lactic acidosis, lactate levels are at least 4–5 mEq/L but commonly 10–30 mEq/L. There are two basic types of lactic acidosis.

Type A (hypoxic) lactic acidosis is more common, resulting from decreased tissue perfusion; cardiogenic, septic, or hemorrhagic shock; and carbon monoxide or cyanide poisoning. These conditions increase peripheral lactic acid production and decrease hepatic metabolism of lactate as liver perfusion declines.

Type B lactic acidosis may be due to metabolic causes (eg, diabetes, ketoacidosis, liver disease, kidney disease, infection, leukemia, or lymphoma) or toxins (eg, ethanol, methanol, salicylates, isoniazid, or metformin). Propylene glycol can cause lactic acidosis from decreased liver metabolism; it is used as a vehicle for intravenous drugs, such as nitroglycerin, etomidate, and diazepam. Parenteral nutrition without thiamine causes severe refractory lactic acidosis from deranged pyruvate metabolism. Patients with short bowel syndrome may develop D-lactic acidosis with encephalopathy due to carbohydrate malabsorption and subsequent fermentation by colonic bacteria.

Nucleoside analog reverse transcriptase inhibitors can cause type B lactic acidosis due to mitochondrial toxicity.

Idiopathic lactic acidosis, usually in debilitated patients, has an extremely high mortality rate. (For treatment of lactic acidosis, see below and Chapter 27.)

B. Diabetic Ketoacidosis (DKA)

DKA is characterized by hyperglycemia and metabolic acidosis with an increased anion gap:

$$H^+ + B^- + NaHCO_3 \leftrightarrow CO_2 + NaB + H_2O$$

where B^- is beta-hydroxybutyrate or acetoacetate, the ketones responsible for the increased anion gap. The anion gap should be calculated from the measured serum electrolytes; correction of the serum sodium for the dilutional effect of hyperglycemia will exaggerate the anion gap. Diabetics with ketoacidosis may have lactic acidosis from tissue hypoperfusion and increased anaerobic metabolism.

During the recovery phase of DKA, a hyperchloremic non-anion gap acidosis can develop because saline resuscitation results in chloride retention, restoration of GFR, and ketoaciduria. Ketone salts (NaB) are formed as bicarbonate is consumed:

$$HB + NaHCO_3 \rightarrow NaB + H_2CO_3$$

The kidney reabsorbs ketone anions poorly but can compensate for the loss of anions by increasing the reabsorption of Cl⁻.

Patients with DKA and normal kidney function may have marked ketonuria and severe metabolic acidosis but only a mildly increased anion gap. Thus, the size of the anion gap correlates poorly with the severity of the DKA; the urinary loss of Na^+ or K^+ salts of beta-hydroxybutyrate will lower the anion gap without altering the H^+ excretion or the severity of the acidosis. Urine dipsticks for ketones test primarily for acetoacetate and, to a lesser degree, acetone but not the predominant ketoacid, beta-hydroxybutyrate. Dipstick tests for ketones may become more positive even as the patient improves due to the metabolism of beta-hydroxybutyrate. Thus, the patient's clinical status and pH are better markers of improvement than the anion gap or ketone levels.

C. Alcoholic Ketoacidosis

Chronically malnourished patients who consume large quantities of alcohol daily may develop alcoholic ketoacidosis. Most of these patients have mixed acid–base disorders (10% have a triple acid–base disorder). Although decreased HCO_3^- is usual, 50% of the patients may have normal or alkalemic pH. Three types of metabolic acidosis are seen in alcoholic ketoacidosis: (1) Ketoacidosis is due to beta-hydroxybutyrate and acetoacetate excess. (2) Lactic acidosis: Alcohol metabolism increases the NADH:NAD ratio, causing increased production and decreased utilization of lactate. Accompanying thiamine deficiency, which inhibits pyruvate carboxylase, further enhances lactic acid production in many cases. Moderate to severe elevations of lactate (> 6 mmol/L) are seen with concomitant disorders such as sepsis, pancreatitis, or hypoglycemia.

(3) Hyperchloremic acidosis from bicarbonate loss in the urine is associated with ketonuria (see above). Metabolic alkalosis occurs from volume contraction and vomiting. Respiratory alkalosis results from alcohol withdrawal, pain, or associated disorders such as sepsis or liver disease. Half of the patients have hypoglycemia or hyperglycemia. When serum glucose levels are > 250 mg/dL (>13.88 mmol/L), the distinction from DKA is difficult. The absence of a diabetic history and normoglycemia after initial therapy support the diagnosis of alcoholic ketoacidosis.

D. Toxins

(See also Chapter 38.) Multiple toxins and drugs increase the anion gap by increasing endogenous acid production. Common examples include methanol (metabolized to formic acid), ethylene glycol (glycolic and oxalic acid), and salicylates (salicylic acid and lactic acid). The latter can cause a mixed disorder of metabolic acidosis with respiratory alkalosis. In toluene poisoning, the metabolite hippurate is rapidly excreted by the kidney and may present as a normal anion gap acidosis. Isopropanol, which is metabolized to acetone, increases the osmolar gap, but not the anion gap.

E. Uremic Acidosis

As the GFR drops below 15–30 mL/min, the kidneys are increasingly unable to excrete H^+ and organic acids, such as phosphate and sulfate, resulting in an increased anion gap acidosis. Hyperchloremic normal anion gap acidosis develops in earlier stages of CKD.

NORMAL ANION GAP ACIDOSIS
(Table 21–14)

The two major causes are gastrointestinal HCO_3^- loss and defects in renal acidification (renal tubular acidoses). The urinary anion gap can differentiate between these causes (see below).

A. Gastrointestinal HCO_3^- Loss

The gastrointestinal tract secretes bicarbonate at multiple sites. Small bowel and pancreatic secretions contain large amounts of HCO_3^-; massive diarrhea or pancreatic drainage can result in HCO_3^- loss. Hyperchloremia occurs because the ileum and colon secrete HCO_3^- in exchange for Cl^- by countertransport. The resultant volume contraction causes increased Cl^- retention by the kidney in the setting of decreased HCO_3^-. Patients with ureterosigmoidostomies can develop hyperchloremic metabolic acidosis because the colon secretes HCO_3^- in the urine in exchange for Cl^-.

B. Renal Tubular Acidosis (RTA)

Hyperchloremic acidosis with a normal anion gap and normal (or near normal) GFR, and in the absence of diarrhea, defines RTA. The defect is either inability to excrete H^+ (inadequate generation of new HCO_3^-) or inappropriate reabsorption of HCO_3^-. Three major types can be differentiated by the clinical setting, urinary pH, urinary anion gap (see below), and serum K^+ level. The pathophysiologic mechanisms of RTA have been elucidated by identifying the responsible molecules and gene mutations.

1. Classic distal RTA (type I)—This disorder is characterized by selective deficiency in H^+ secretion in alpha intercalated cells in the collecting tubule. Despite acidosis, urinary pH cannot be acidified and is above 5.5, which retards the binding of H^+ to phosphate ($H^+ + HPO_4^{2-} \rightarrow H_2PO_4$) and inhibits titratable acid excretion. Furthermore, urinary excretion of $NH_4^+Cl^-$ is decreased, and the urinary anion gap is positive (see below). Enhanced K^+ excretion occurs probably because there is less competition from H^+ in the distal nephron transport system. Furthermore, hyperaldosteronism occurs in response to renal salt wasting, which will increase potassium excretion. Nephrocalcinosis and nephrolithiasis are often seen in patients with distal RTA since chronic acidosis

---

Table 21–14. Hyperchloremic, normal anion gap metabolic acidoses.

			Distal H⁺ Secretion			
	Renal Defect	Serum [K^+]	Urinary NH_4^+ Plus Minimal Urine pH	Titratable Acid	Urinary Anion Gap	Treatment
Gastrointestinal HCO_3^- loss	None	↓	< 5.5	↑↑	Negative	Na^+, K^+, and HCO_3^- as required
Renal tubular acidosis						
I. Classic distal	Distal H^+ secretion	↓	> 5.5	↓	Positive	$NaHCO_3$ (1–3 mEq/kg/d)
II. Proximal secretion	Proximal H^+	↓	< 5.5	Normal	Positive	$NaHCO_3$ or $KHCO_3$ (10–15 mEq/kg/d), thiazide
IV. Hyporeninemic hypoaldosteronism	Distal Na^+ reabsorption, K^+ secretion, and H^+ secretion	↑	< 5.5	↓	Positive	Fludrocortisone (0.1–0.5 mg/d), dietary K^+ restriction, furosemide (40–160 mg/d), $NaHCO_3$ (1–3 mEq/kg/d)

Modified and reproduced, with permission, from Cogan MG. *Fluid and Electrolytes: Physiology and Pathophysiology.* McGraw-Hill, 1991.

decreases tubular calcium reabsorption. Hypercalciuria, alkaline urine, and lowered level of urinary citrate cause calcium phosphate stones and nephrocalcinosis.

Distal RTA develops as a consequence of paraproteinemias, autoimmune disease, and drugs and toxins such as amphotericin.

2. Proximal RTA (type II)—Proximal RTA is due to a selective defect in the proximal tubule's ability to reabsorb filtered HCO_3^-. Carbonic anhydrase inhibitors (acetazolamide) can cause proximal RTA. About 90% of filtered HCO_3^- is absorbed by the proximal tubule. A proximal defect in HCO_3^- reabsorption will overwhelm the distal tubule's limited capacity to reabsorb HCO_3^-, resulting in bicarbonaturia and metabolic acidosis. Distal delivery of HCO_3^- declines as the plasma HCO_3^- level decreases. When the plasma HCO_3^- level drops to 15–18 mEq/L, the distal nephron can reabsorb the diminished filtered load of HCO_3^-. Bicarbonaturia resolves, and the urinary pH can be acidic. Thiazide-induced volume contraction can be used to enhance proximal HCO_3^- reabsorption, leading to the decrease in distal HCO_3^- delivery and improvement of bicarbonaturia and renal acidification. The increased delivery of HCO_3^- to the distal nephron increases K^+ secretion, and hypokalemia results if a patient is loaded with excess HCO_3^- and K^+ is not adequately supplemented. Proximal RTA can exist with other proximal reabsorption defects, such as Fanconi syndrome, resulting in glucosuria, aminoaciduria, phosphaturia, and uricosuria. Causes include multiple myeloma and nephrotoxic drugs.

3. Hyporeninemic hypoaldosteronemic RTA (type IV)—Type IV is the most common RTA in clinical practice. The defect is aldosterone deficiency or antagonism, which impairs distal nephron Na^+ reabsorption and K^+ and H^+ excretion. Renal salt wasting and hyperkalemia are frequently present. Common causes are diabetic nephropathy, tubulointerstitial renal diseases, hypertensive nephrosclerosis, and AIDS. In patients with these disorders, drugs, such as ACE inhibitors, spironolactone, and NSAIDs, can exacerbate the hyperkalemia.

C. Dilutional Acidosis

Rapid dilution of plasma volume by 0.9% NaCl may cause hyperchloremic acidosis.

D. Recovery from DKA

See Increased Anion Gap Acidosis (Increased Unmeasured Anion).

E. Posthypocapnia

In prolonged respiratory alkalosis, HCO_3^- decreases and Cl^- increases from decreased renal $NH_4^+Cl^-$ excretion. If the respiratory alkalosis is corrected quickly, HCO_3^- will remain low until the kidneys can generate new HCO_3^-, which generally takes several days. In the meantime, the increased Pco_2 with low HCO_3^- causes metabolic acidosis.

F. Hyperalimentation

Hyperalimentation fluids may contain amino acid solutions that acidify when metabolized, such as arginine hydrochloride and lysine hydrochloride.

▶ Assessment of Hyperchloremic Metabolic Acidosis by Urinary Anion Gap

Increased renal $NH_4^+Cl^-$ excretion to enhance H^+ removal is the normal physiologic response to metabolic acidosis. The daily urinary excretion of NH_4Cl can be increased from 30 mEq to 200 mEq in response to acidosis.

The urinary anion gap ($Na^+ + K^+ - Cl^-$) reflects the ability of the kidney to excrete NH_4Cl. The urinary anion gap differentiates between gastrointestinal and renal causes of hyperchloremic acidosis. If the cause is gastrointestinal HCO_3^- loss (diarrhea), renal acidification remains normal and NH_4Cl excretion increases, and the urinary anion gap is negative. If the cause is distal RTA, the urinary anion gap is positive, since the basic lesion in the disorder is the inability of the kidney to excrete H^+ as NH_4Cl. In proximal (type II) RTA, the kidney has defective HCO_3^- reabsorption, leading to increased HCO_3^- excretion rather than decreased NH_4Cl excretion; the urinary anion gap is often negative.

Urinary pH may not readily differentiate between the two causes. Despite acidosis, if volume depletion from diarrhea causes inadequate Na^+ delivery to the distal nephron and therefore decreased exchange with H^+, urinary pH may not be lower than 5.3. In the presence of this relatively high urinary pH, however, H^+ excretion continues due to buffering of NH_3 to NH_4^+, since the pK of this reaction is as high as 9.1. Potassium depletion, which can accompany diarrhea (and surreptitious laxative abuse), may also impair renal acidification. Thus, when volume depletion is present, the urinary anion gap is a better measure of ability to acidify the urine than urinary pH.

When large amounts of other anions are present in the urine, the urinary anion gap may not be reliable. In such a situation, NH_4^+ excretion can be estimated using the urinary osmolar gap.

$$NH_4^+ \text{ excretion (mmol/L)} = 0.5 \times \text{Urinary osmolar gap}$$
$$= 0.5 \, [U \, osm - 2(U \, Na^+ + U \, K^+) + U \, urea + U \, glucose]$$

where urine concentrations and osmolality are in mmol/L.

▶ Clinical Findings

A. Symptoms and Signs

Symptoms of metabolic acidosis are mainly those of the underlying disorder. Compensatory hyperventilation is an important clinical sign and may be misinterpreted as a primary respiratory disorder; Kussmaul breathing (deep, regular, sighing respirations) may be seen with severe metabolic acidosis.

B. Laboratory Findings

Blood pH, serum HCO_3^-, and Pco_2 are decreased. Anion gap may be normal (hyperchloremic) or increased (normochloremic). Hyperkalemia may be seen.

Treatment

A. Increased Anion Gap Acidosis

Treatment is aimed at the underlying disorder, such as insulin and fluid therapy for diabetes and appropriate volume resuscitation to restore tissue perfusion. The metabolism of lactate will produce HCO_3^- and increase pH. Supplemental HCO_3^- is indicated for treatment of hyperkalemia (Table 21–6) and some forms of normal anion gap acidosis but has been controversial for treatment of increased anion gap metabolic acidosis with respect to efficacy and safety. Large amounts of HCO_3^- may have deleterious effects, including hypernatremia, hyperosmolality, volume overload, and worsening of intracellular acidosis.

In addition, alkali administration stimulates phosphofructokinase activity, thus exacerbating lactic acidosis via enhanced lactate production. Ketogenesis is also augmented by alkali therapy.

In salicylate intoxication, alkali therapy must be started to decrease central nervous system damage unless blood pH is already alkalinized by respiratory alkalosis, since an increased pH converts salicylate to more impermeable salicylic acid. In alcoholic ketoacidosis, thiamine should be given with glucose to avoid Wernicke encephalopathy. The bicarbonate deficit can be calculated as follows:

$$HCO_3^- \text{ deficit} = 0.5 \times \text{body weight in kg} \times (24 - HCO_3^-)$$

Half of the calculated deficit should be administered within the first 3–4 hours to avoid overcorrection and volume overload. In methanol intoxication, inhibition of alcohol dehydrogenase by fomepizole is now standard care. Ethanol had previously been used as a competitive substrate for alcohol dehydrogenase, which metabolizes to formaldehyde.

B. Normal Anion Gap Acidosis

Treatment of RTA is mainly achieved by administration of alkali (either as bicarbonate or citrate) to correct metabolic abnormalities and prevent nephrocalcinosis and CKD.

Large amounts of oral alkali (10–15 mEq/kg/d) (Table 21–14) may be required to treat proximal RTA because most of the alkali is excreted into the urine, which exacerbates hypokalemia. Thus, a mixture of sodium and potassium salts is preferred. Thiazides may reduce the amount of alkali required, but hypokalemia may develop. Treatment of type 1 distal RTA requires less alkali (1–3 mEq/kg/d) than proximal RTA. Potassium supplementation may be necessary.

For type IV RTA, dietary potassium restriction may be necessary and potassium-retaining drugs should be withdrawn. Fludrocortisone may be effective in cases with hypoaldosteronism, but should be used with care, preferably in combination with loop diuretics. In some cases, oral alkali supplementation (1–3 mEq/kg/d) may be required.

When to Refer

Most clinicians will refer patients with renal tubular acidoses to a nephrologist for evaluation and possible alkali therapy.

When to Admit

Patients will require emergency department evaluation or hospital admission depending on the severity of the acidosis and underlying conditions.

Haque SK et al. Proximal renal tubular acidosis: a not so rare disorder of multiple etiologies. Nephrol Dial Transplant. 2012 Dec;27(12):4273–87. [PMID: 23235953]

Kraut JA et al. Approach to the evaluation of a patient with an increased serum osmolal gap and high-anion-gap metabolic acidosis. Am J Kidney Dis. 2011 Sep;58(3):480–4. [PMID: 21794966]

Kraut JA et al. Differential diagnosis of nongap metabolic acidosis: value of a systematic approach. Clin J Am Soc Nephrol. 2012 Apr;7(4):671–9. [PMID: 22403272]

Liamis G et al. Pharmacologically-induced metabolic acidosis: a review. Drug Saf. 2010 May 1;33(5):371–91. [PMID: 20397738]

Sia P et al. Type B lactic acidosis associated with multiple myeloma. Am J Kidney Dis. 2013 Sep;62(3):633–7. [PMID: 23759296]

METABOLIC ALKALOSIS

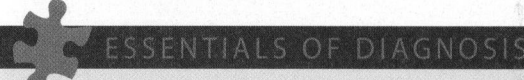

ESSENTIALS OF DIAGNOSIS

- ▶ High HCO_3^- with alkalemia.
- ▶ Evaluate effective circulating volume by physical examination.
- ▶ Check urinary chloride concentration to differentiate saline-responsive alkalosis from saline-unresponsive alkalosis.

Classification

Metabolic alkalosis is characterized by high HCO_3^-. Abnormalities that generate HCO_3^- are called "initiation factors," whereas abnormalities that promote renal conservation of HCO_3^- are called "maintenance factors." Thus, metabolic alkalosis may remain even after the initiation factors have resolved.

The causes of metabolic alkalosis are classified into two groups based on "saline responsiveness" using the urine Cl^- as a marker for volume status (Table 21–15). Saline-responsive metabolic alkalosis is a sign of extracellular volume contraction, and saline-unresponsive alkalosis implies excessive total body bicarbonate with either euvolemia or hypervolemia. The compensatory increase in Pco_2 rarely exceeds 55 mm Hg; higher Pco_2 values imply a superimposed primary respiratory acidosis.

A. Saline-Responsive Metabolic Alkalosis

Much more common than saline-unresponsive alkalosis, saline-responsive alkalosis is characterized by normotensive extracellular volume contraction and hypokalemia. Hypotension and orthostasis may be seen. In vomiting or nasogastric suction, loss of acid (HCl) initiates the

Table 21–15. Metabolic alkalosis.

Saline-Responsive ($U_{Cl} < 25$ mEq/L)	Saline-Unresponsive ($U_{Cl} > 40$ mEq/L)

Excessive body bicarbonate content
Renal alkalosis
  Diuretic therapy
  Poorly reabsorbable anion therapy: carbenicillin, penicillin, sulfate, phosphate
  Posthypercapnia
Gastrointestinal alkalosis
  Loss of HCl from vomiting or nasogastric suction
  Intestinal alkalosis: chloride diarrhea
  NaHCO$_3$ (baking soda)
  Sodium citrate, lactate, gluconate, acetate
  Transfusions
  Antacids
Normal body bicarbonate content
  "Contraction alkalosis"
	Excessive body bicarbonate content
	Renal alkalosis
	  Normotensive
	    Bartter syndrome (renal salt wasting and secondary hyperaldosteronism)
	    Severe potassium depletion
	    Refeeding alkalosis
	    Hypercalcemia and hypoparathyroidism
	  Hypertensive
	    Endogenous mineralocorticoids
	      Primary aldosteronism
	      Hyperreninism
	      Adrenal enzyme (11-beta-hydroxylase and 17-alpha-hydroxylase) deficiency
	      Liddle syndrome
	  Exogenous alkali
	  Exogenous mineralocorticoids
	  Licorice

Modified and reproduced, with permission, from Narins RG et al. Diagnostic strategies in disorders of fluid, electrolyte and acid-base homeostasis. Am J Med. 1982 Mar;72(3):496–520.

alkalosis, but volume contraction from Cl$^-$ loss maintains the alkalosis because the kidney avidly reabsorbs Na$^+$ to restore the ECF. Increased sodium reabsorption necessitates increased HCO$_3^-$ reabsorption proximally, and the urinary pH remains acidic despite alkalemia (paradoxical aciduria). Renal Cl$^-$ reabsorption is high, and urine Cl$^-$ is low (< 10–20 mEq/L). In alkalosis, bicarbonaturia may force Na$^+$ excretion as the accompanying cation even if volume depletion is present. Therefore, urine Cl$^-$ is preferred to urine Na$^+$ as a measure of extracellular volume. Diuretics may limit the utility of urine chloride by increasing urine chloride and sodium excretion, even in the setting of volume contraction.

Metabolic alkalosis is generally associated with hypokalemia due to the direct effect of alkalosis on renal potassium excretion and secondary hyperaldosteronism from volume depletion. Hypokalemia exacerbates the metabolic alkalosis by increasing bicarbonate reabsorption in the proximal tubule and hydrogen ion secretion in the distal tubule. Administration of KCl will correct the disorder.

1. Contraction alkalosis—Diuretics decrease extracellular volume from urinary loss of NaCl and water. The plasma HCO$_3^-$ concentration increases because the extracellular fluid volume contracts around a stable total body bicarbonate. Contraction alkalosis is the opposite of dilutional acidosis.

2. Posthypercapnia alkalosis—In chronic respiratory acidosis, the kidney decreases bicarbonate excretion, increasing plasma HCO$_3^-$ concentration (Table 21–12). Hypercapnia directly affects the proximal tubule to decrease NaCl reabsorption, which can cause extracellular volume depletion. If Pco$_2$ is rapidly corrected, metabolic alkalosis will exist until the kidney excretes the retained bicarbonate. Many patients with chronic respiratory acidosis receive diuretics, which further exacerbates the metabolic alkalosis.

B. Saline-Unresponsive Alkalosis

1. Hyperaldosteronism—Primary hyperaldosteronism causes extracellular volume expansion and hypertension by increasing distal sodium reabsorption. Aldosterone increases H$^+$ and K$^+$ excretion, producing metabolic alkalosis and hypokalemia. In an attempt to decrease extracellular volume, high levels of NaCl are excreted resulting in a high urine Cl$^-$ (> 20 mEq/L). Therapy with NaCl will only increase volume expansion and hypertension and will not treat the underlying problem of mineralocorticoid excess.

2. Alkali administration with decreased GFR—The normal kidney has a substantial capacity for bicarbonate excretion, protecting against metabolic alkalosis even with large HCO$_3^-$ intake. However, urinary excretion of bicarbonate is inadequate in CKD. If large amounts of HCO$_3^-$ are consumed, as with intensive antacid therapy, metabolic alkalosis will occur. Lactate, citrate, and gluconate can also cause metabolic alkalosis because they are metabolized to bicarbonate. In milk-alkali syndrome, sustained heavy ingestion of absorbable antacids and milk causes hypercalcemic kidney injury and metabolic alkalosis. Volume contraction from renal hypercalcemic effects exacerbates the alkalosis.

▶ Clinical Findings

A. Symptoms and Signs

There are no characteristic symptoms or signs. Orthostatic hypotension may be encountered. Concomitant hypokalemia may cause weakness and hyporeflexia. Tetany and neuromuscular irritability occur rarely.

B. Laboratory Findings

The arterial blood pH and bicarbonate are elevated. With respiratory compensation, the arterial Pco$_2$ is increased.

Serum potassium and chloride are decreased. There may be an increased anion gap. The urine chloride can differentiate between saline-responsive (< 25 mEq/L) and unresponsive (> 40 mEq/L) causes.

▶ Treatment

Mild alkalosis is generally well tolerated. Severe or symptomatic alkalosis (pH > 7.60) requires urgent treatment.

A. Saline-Responsive Metabolic Alkalosis

Therapy for saline-responsive metabolic alkalosis is correction of the extracellular volume deficit with isotonic saline. Diuretics should be discontinued. H_2-blockers or proton pump inhibitors may be helpful in patients with alkalosis from nasogastric suctioning. If pulmonary or cardiovascular disease prohibits adequate resuscitation, acetazolamide will increase renal bicarbonate excretion. Hypokalemia may develop because bicarbonate excretion may induce kaliuresis. Severe cases, especially those with reduced kidney function, may require dialysis with low-bicarbonate dialysate.

B. Saline-Unresponsive Metabolic Alkalosis

Therapy for saline-unresponsive metabolic alkalosis includes surgical removal of a mineralocorticoid-producing tumor and blockage of aldosterone effect with an ACE inhibitor or with spironolactone (see Chapter 26). Metabolic alkalosis in primary aldosteronism can be treated only with potassium repletion.

Feldman M et al. Respiratory compensation to a primary metabolic alkalosis in humans. Clin Nephrol. 2012 Nov;78(5):365–9. [PMID: 22854166]

Gennari FJ. Pathophysiology of metabolic alkalosis: a new classification based on the centrality of stimulated collecting duct ion transport. Am J Kidney Dis. 2011 Oct;58(4):626–36. [PMID: 21849227]

Peixoto AJ et al. Treatment of severe metabolic alkalosis in a patient with congestive heart failure. Am J Kidney Dis. 2013 May;61(5):822–7. [PMID: 23481366]

Yi JH et al. Metabolic alkalosis from unsuspected ingestion: use of urine pH and anion gap. Am J Kidney Dis. 2012 Apr;59(4):577–81. [PMID: 22265393]

RESPIRATORY ACIDOSIS (HYPERCAPNIA)

Respiratory acidosis results from hypoventilation and subsequent hypercapnia. Pulmonary and extrapulmonary disorders can cause hypoventilation.

Acute respiratory failure is associated with severe acidosis and only a small increase in the plasma bicarbonate. After 6–12 hours, the primary increase in P_{CO_2} evokes a renal compensation to excrete more acid and to generate more HCO_3^-; complete metabolic compensation by the kidney takes several days.

Chronic respiratory acidosis is generally seen in patients with underlying lung disease, such as chronic obstructive pulmonary disease. Renal excretion of acid as NH_4Cl results in hypochloremia. When chronic respiratory acidosis is corrected suddenly, posthypercapnic metabolic alkalosis ensues until the kidneys excrete the excess bicarbonate over 2–3 days.

▶ Clinical Findings

A. Symptoms and Signs

With acute onset, somnolence, confusion, mental status changes, asterixis, and myoclonus may develop. Severe hypercapnia increases cerebral blood flow, cerebrospinal fluid pressure, and intracranial pressure; papilledema and pseudotumor cerebri may be seen.

B. Laboratory Findings

Arterial pH is low and P_{CO_2} is increased. Serum HCO_3^- is elevated but does not fully correct the pH. If the disorder is chronic, hypochloremia is seen.

▶ Treatment

If opioid overdose is a possible diagnosis or there is no other obvious cause for hypoventilation, the clinician should consider a diagnostic and therapeutic trial of intravenous naloxone (see Chapter 38). In all forms of respiratory acidosis, treatment is directed at the underlying disorder to improve ventilation.

Adrogué HJ. Diagnosis and management of severe respiratory acidosis. Am J Kidney Dis. 2010 Nov;56(5):994–1000. [PMID: 20673604]

Chebbo A et al. Hypoventilation syndromes. Med Clin North Am. 2011 Nov;95(6):1189–202. [PMID: 22032434]

Marik PE. The malignant obesity hypoventilation syndrome (MOHS). Obes Rev. 2012 Oct;13(10):902–9. [PMID: 22708580]

Schwartzstein RM et al. Rising PaCO(2) in the ICU: using a physiologic approach to avoid cognitive biases. Chest. 2011 Dec;140(6):1638–42. [PMID: 22147823]

RESPIRATORY ALKALOSIS (HYPOCAPNIA)

Respiratory alkalosis occurs when hyperventilation reduces the P_{CO_2}, increasing serum pH. The most common cause of respiratory alkalosis is hyperventilation syndrome (Table 21–16), but bacterial septicemia and cirrhosis are other common causes. In pregnancy, progesterone stimulates the respiratory center, producing an average P_{CO_2} of 30 mm Hg and respiratory alkalosis. Symptoms of acute respiratory alkalosis are related to decreased cerebral blood flow induced by the disorder.

Determination of appropriate metabolic compensation may reveal an associated metabolic disorder (see Mixed Acid–Base Disorders).

As in respiratory acidosis, the metabolic compensation is greater if the respiratory alkalosis is chronic (Table 21–12). Although serum HCO_3^- is frequently < 15 mEq/L in metabolic acidosis, such a low level in respiratory alkalosis is unusual and may represent a concomitant primary metabolic acidosis.

Table 21–16. Causes of respiratory alkalosis.

Hypoxia
Decreased inspired oxygen tension
High altitude
Ventilation/perfusion inequality
Hypotension
Severe anemia
CNS-mediated disorders
Voluntary hyperventilation
Anxiety-hyperventilation syndrome
Neurologic disease
Cerebrovascular accident (infarction, hemorrhage)
Infection
Trauma
Tumor
Pharmacologic and hormonal stimulation
Salicylates
Nicotine
Xanthines
Pregnancy (progesterone)
Hepatic failure
Gram-negative septicemia
Recovery from metabolic acidosis
Heat exposure
Pulmonary disease
Interstitial lung disease
Pneumonia
Pulmonary embolism
Pulmonary edema
Mechanical overventilation

Adapted, with permission, from Gennari FJ. Respiratory acidosis and alkalosis. In: *Maxwell and Kleeman's Clinical Disorders of Fluid and Electrolyte Metabolism*, 5th ed. Narins RG (editor). McGraw-Hill, 1994.

▶ Clinical Findings

A. Symptoms and Signs

In acute cases (hyperventilation), there is light-headedness, anxiety, perioral numbness, and paresthesias. Tetany occurs from a low ionized calcium, since severe alkalosis increases calcium binding to albumin.

B. Laboratory Findings

Arterial blood pH is elevated, and P_{CO_2} is low. Serum bicarbonate is decreased in chronic respiratory alkalosis.

▶ Treatment

Treatment is directed toward the underlying cause. In acute hyperventilation syndrome from anxiety, the traditional treatment of breathing into a paper bag should be discouraged because it does not correct P_{CO_2} and may decrease P_{O_2}. Reassurance may be sufficient for the anxious patient, but sedation may be necessary if the process persists. Hyperventilation is usually self-limited since muscle weakness caused by the respiratory alkalemia will suppress ventilation. Rapid correction of chronic respiratory alkalosis may result in metabolic acidosis as P_{CO_2} is increased in the setting of a previous compensatory decrease in HCO_3^-.

Curley G et al. Bench-to-bedside review: carbon dioxide. Crit Care. 2010;14(2):220. [PMID: 20497620]
Palmer BF. Evaluation and treatment of respiratory alkalosis. Am J Kidney Dis. 2012 Nov;60(5):834–8. [PMID: 22871240]

▼ FLUID MANAGEMENT

Daily parenteral maintenance fluids and electrolytes for an average adult would include at least 2 L of water in the form of 0.45% saline with 20 mEq/L of potassium chloride. Patients with hypoglycemia, starvation ketosis, or ketoacidosis being treated with insulin may require 5% dextrose-containing solutions. Guidelines for gastrointestinal fluid losses are shown in Table 21–17.

Weight loss or gain is the best indication of water balance. Insensible water loss should be considered in febrile patients. Water loss increases by 100–150 mL/d for each degree of body temperature over 37°C.

In patients requiring maintenance and possibly replacement of fluid and electrolytes by parenteral infusion, the total daily ration should be administered continuously over 24 hours to ensure optimal utilization.

Table 21–17. Replacement guidelines for sweat and gastrointestinal fluid losses.

	Average Electrolyte Composition				Replacement Guidelines per Liter Lost				
	Na^+ (mEq/L)	K^+ (mEq/L)	Cl^- (mEq/L)	HCO_3^- (mEq/L)	0.9% Saline (mL)	0.45% Saline (mL)	D_5W (mL)	KCl (mEq/L)	7.5% $NaHCO_3$ (45 mEq HCO_3^-/amp)
Sweat	30–50	5	50			500	500	5	
Gastric secretions	20	10	10			300	700	20	
Pancreatic juice	130	5	35	115		400	600	5	2 amps
Bile	145	5	100	25	600		400	5	0.5 amp
Duodenal fluid	60	15	100	10		1000		15	0.25 amp
Ileal fluid	100	10	60	60		600	400	10	1 amp
Colonic diarrhea	140[1]	10	85	60		1000		10	1 amp

[1]In the absence of diarrhea, colonic fluid Na^+ levels are low (40 mEq/L).

If intravenous fluids are the only source of water, electrolytes, and calories for longer than a week, parenteral nutrition containing amino acids, lipids, trace metals, and vitamins may be indicated. (See Chapter 29.)

For parenteral alimentation, 620 mg (20 mmol) of phosphorus is required for every 1000 nonprotein kcal to maintain phosphate balance and to ensure anabolic function. For prolonged parenteral fluid maintenance, a daily ration is 620–1240 mg (20–40 mmol) of phosphorus.

Excessive fluid resuscitation or maintenance is now viewed as a complication in hospitalized patients, especially those with critical illness or acute kidney injury, and has been associated with worsened outcomes such as prolonged mechanical ventilation, dependence on dialysis, and long duration of hospitalization with increased mortality.

Annane D et al. Effects of fluid resuscitation with colloids vs crystalloids on mortality in critically ill patients presenting with hypovolemic shock: the CRISTAL randomized trial. JAMA. 2013 Nov 6;310(17):1809–17. [PMID: 24108515]

Myburgh JA et al. Resuscitation fluids. N Engl J Med. 2013 Sep 26;369(13):1243–51. [PMID: 24066745]

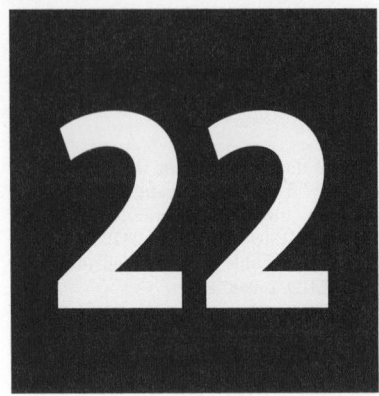

Kidney Disease

Suzanne Watnick, MD

Tonja Dirkx, MD

Kidney disease can be discovered incidentally during a routine medical evaluation or with evidence of kidney dysfunction, such as hypertension, edema, nausea, or hematuria. The initial approach in both situations should be to assess the cause and severity of renal abnormalities. In all cases this evaluation includes (1) an estimation of disease duration, (2) a careful urinalysis, and (3) an assessment of the glomerular filtration rate (GFR). The history and physical examinations, though equally important, are variable among renal syndromes—thus, specific symptoms and signs are discussed under each disease entity.

ASSESSMENT OF KIDNEY DISEASE

▶ Disease Duration

Kidney disease may be acute or chronic. Acute kidney injury is worsening of kidney function over hours to days, resulting in the retention of nitrogenous wastes (such as urea nitrogen) and creatinine in the blood. Retention of these substances is called azotemia. Chronic kidney disease (CKD) results from an abnormal loss of kidney function over months to years. Differentiating between the two is important for diagnosis, treatment, and outcome. Oliguria is unusual in CKD. Anemia (from low kidney erythropoietin production) is rare in the initial period of acute kidney disease. Small kidneys are most consistent with CKD, whereas normal to large-size kidneys can be seen with both chronic and acute disease.

▶ Urinalysis

A urinalysis can provide information similar to a kidney biopsy in a way that is cost-effective and noninvasive. The urine is collected in midstream or, if that is not feasible, by bladder catheterization. The urine should be examined within 1 hour after collection to avoid destruction of formed elements. Urinalysis includes a dipstick examination followed by microscopic assessment if the dipstick has positive findings. The dipstick examination measures urinary pH, protein, hemoglobin, glucose, ketones, bilirubin, nitrites, and leukocyte esterase. Urinary specific gravity is often reported. Microscopy provides examination of

formed elements—crystals, cells, casts, and infecting organisms.

Various findings on the urinalysis are indicative of certain patterns of kidney disease. A bland (normal) urinary sediment is common, especially in CKD and acute disorders that are not intrinsic to the kidney, such as limited effective blood flow to the kidney or obstruction of the urinary outflow tract. Casts are composed of Tamm-Horsfall urinary mucoprotein in the shape of the nephron segment where they were formed. Heavy proteinuria and lipiduria are consistent with the nephrotic syndrome. The presence of hematuria with dysmorphic red blood cells, red blood cell casts, and proteinuria is indicative of glomerulonephritis. Dysmorphic red blood cells are misshapen during abnormal passage from the capillary through the glomerular basement membrane (GBM) into the urinary space of Bowman capsule. Pigmented granular casts and renal tubular epithelial cells alone or in casts suggest acute tubular necrosis. White blood cells, including neutrophils and eosinophils, white blood cell casts (Table 22–1), red blood cells, and small amounts of protein can be found in interstitial nephritis and pyelonephritis; Wright and Hansel stains can detect eosinophiluria. Pyuria alone can indicate a urinary tract infection. Hematuria and proteinuria are discussed more thoroughly below.

A. Proteinuria

Proteinuria is defined as excessive protein excretion in the urine, generally > 150–160 mg/24 h in adults. Significant proteinuria is a sign of an underlying kidney abnormality, usually glomerular in origin when > 1–2 g/d. Less than 1 g/d can be due to multiple causes along the nephron segment, as listed below. Proteinuria can be accompanied by other clinical abnormalities—elevated blood urea nitrogen (BUN) and serum creatinine levels, abnormal urinary sediment, or evidence of systemic illness (eg, fever, rash, vasculitis).

There are several reasons for development of proteinuria: (1) **Functional proteinuria** is a benign process stemming from stressors such as acute illness, exercise, and "orthostatic proteinuria." The latter condition, generally found in people under age 30 years, usually results in urinary protein excretion of < 1 g/d. The orthostatic nature of the proteinuria is confirmed by measuring an 8-hour

Table 22–1. Significance of specific urinary casts.

Type	Significance
Hyaline casts	Concentrated urine, febrile disease, after strenuous exercise, in the course of diuretic therapy (not indicative of renal disease)
Red cell casts	Glomerulonephritis
White cell casts	Pyelonephritis, interstitial nephritis (indicative of infection or inflammation)
Renal tubular cell casts	Acute tubular necrosis, interstitial nephritis
Coarse, granular casts	Nonspecific; can represent acute tubular necrosis
Broad, waxy casts	Chronic kidney disease (indicative of stasis in enlarged collecting tubules)

overnight supine urinary protein excretion, which should be < 50 mg. (2) **Overload proteinuria** can result from overproduction of circulating, filterable plasma proteins (monoclonal gammopathies), such as Bence Jones proteins associated with multiple myeloma. Urinary protein electrophoresis will exhibit a discrete protein peak. Other examples of overload proteinuria include myoglobinuria in rhabdomyolysis and hemoglobinuria in hemolysis. (3) **Glomerular proteinuria** results from effacement of epithelial cell foot processes and altered glomerular permeability with an increased filtration fraction of normal plasma proteins, as in diabetic nephropathy. Glomerular diseases exhibit some degree of proteinuria. The urinary protein electrophoresis will have a pattern exhibiting a large albumin spike indicative of increased permeability of albumin across a damaged GBM. (4) **Tubular proteinuria** occurs as a result of faulty reabsorption of normally filtered proteins in the proximal tubule, such as beta-2-microglobulin and immunoglobulin light chains. Causes include acute tubular necrosis, toxic injury (lead, aminoglycosides), drug-induced interstitial nephritis, and hereditary metabolic disorders (Wilson disease and Fanconi syndrome).

Evaluation of proteinuria by urinary dipstick primarily detects albumin, while overlooking positively charged light chains of immunoglobulins. These proteins can be detected by the addition of sulfosalicylic acid to the urine specimen. Precipitation without dipstick detection of albumin indicates the presence of paraproteins.

The next step is an estimation of daily urinary protein excretion. The simplest method is to collect a random urine sample. The ratio of urinary protein concentration to urinary creatinine concentration ($[U_{protein}]/[U_{creatinine}]$) correlates with 24-hour urine protein collection (< 0.2 is normal and corresponds to excretion of < 200 mg/24 h). The benefit of a urine protein-to-creatinine ratio is the ease of collection and the lack of error from overcollection or undercollection of urine. In a 24-hour urine collection, a finding of > 150–160 mg is abnormal, and > 3.5 g is consistent with nephrotic-range proteinuria. If a patient has proteinuria with or without loss of kidney function, kidney biopsy may be indicated, particularly if the kidney disease is acute in onset. The clinical sequelae of proteinuria are discussed in the section Nephrotic Spectrum Glomerular Diseases below.

B. Hematuria

Hematuria is significant if there are more than three red cells per high-power field on at least two occasions. It is usually detected incidentally by the urine dipstick examination or clinically following an episode of macroscopic hematuria. The diagnosis must be confirmed via microscopic examination, as false-positive dipstick tests can be caused by myoglobin, oxidizing agents, beets and rhubarb, hydrochloric acid, and bacteria. Transient hematuria is common, but in patients younger than 40 years, it is less often of clinical significance due to lower concern for malignancy.

Hematuria may be due to renal or extrarenal causes. Extrarenal causes are addressed in Chapters 23 and 39; most worrisome are urologic malignancies. Renal causes account for approximately 10% of cases and are best considered anatomically as glomerular or nonglomerular. The most common extraglomerular sources include cysts, calculi, interstitial nephritis, and renal neoplasia. Glomerular causes include immunoglobulin A (IgA) nephropathy, thin GBM disease, membranoproliferative glomerulonephritis (MPGN), other hereditary glomerular diseases (eg, Alport syndrome), and systemic nephritic syndromes. Currently, the United States Health Preventive Services Task Force does not recommend screening for hematuria. See Chapter 23 for evaluation of hematuria.

▶ Estimation of GFR

The GFR provides a useful index of kidney function at the level of the glomerulus. Patients with kidney disease can have a decreased GFR from any process that causes loss of nephron (and thus glomerular) mass. However, they can also have a normal or increased GFR, either from hyperfiltration at the glomerulus or disease at a different segment of the nephron, interstitium, or vascular supply. The GFR measures the amount of plasma ultrafiltered across the glomerular capillaries and correlates with the ability of the kidneys to filter fluids and various substances. Daily GFR in normal individuals is variable, with a range of 150–250 L/24 h or 100–120 mL/min/1.73 m² of body surface area. GFR can be measured indirectly by determining the renal clearance of plasma substances that are not bound to plasma proteins, are freely filterable across the glomerulus, and are neither secreted nor reabsorbed along the renal tubules. The formula used to determine the renal clearance of a substance is

$$C = \frac{U \times \dot{V}}{P}$$

where C is the clearance, U and P are the urine and plasma concentrations of the substance (mg/dL), and is the urine flow rate (mL/min). In clinical practice, the clearance rate of endogenous creatinine, the creatinine clearance, is one way of estimating GFR. Creatinine is a product of muscle metabolism produced at a relatively constant rate and cleared by renal excretion. It is freely filterable by the glomerulus and not reabsorbed by the renal tubules. With stable kidney function, creatinine production and excretion are equal; thus, plasma creatinine concentrations remain constant. However, it is not a perfect indicator of GFR for the following reasons: (1) A small amount is normally eliminated by tubular secretion, and the fraction secreted progressively increases as GFR declines (overestimating GFR); (2) with severe kidney failure, gut microorganisms degrade creatinine; (3) an individual's meat intake and muscle mass affect baseline plasma creatinine levels; (4) commonly used drugs such as aspirin, cimetidine, probenecid, and trimethoprim reduce tubular secretion of creatinine, increasing the plasma creatinine concentration and falsely indicating kidney dysfunction; and (5) the accuracy of the measurement necessitates a stable plasma creatinine concentration over a 24-hour period, so that during the development of and recovery from acute kidney injury, when the serum creatinine is changing, the creatinine clearance is unhelpful. Of note, the creatinine clearance is the traditional estimation equation used for consideration of drug dosing in patients with kidney disease.

One way to measure creatinine clearance is to collect a timed urine sample and determine the plasma creatinine level midway through the collection. An incomplete or prolonged urine collection is a common source of error. A method of estimating the completeness of the collection is to calculate a 24-hour creatinine excretion; the amount should be constant:

$$U_{cr} \times \dot{V} = 15\text{--}20 \text{ mg/kg for healthy young women}$$

$$U_{cr} \times \dot{V} = 20\text{--}25 \text{ mg/kg for healthy young men}$$

The creatinine clearance (C_{cr}) is approximately 100 mL/min/1.73 m² in healthy young women and 120 mL/min/1.73 m² in healthy young men. The creatinine clearance declines by an average of 0.8 mL/min/yr after age 40 years as part of the aging process, but this is variable, with 35% of subjects in one study having no decline in kidney function over 10 years.

The four-variable estimated GFR is a complex equation, including serum creatinine, age, weight, and race, that is often reported alongside serum creatinine measurements and more accurate than creatinine clearance. This was derived from data collected for the Modification of Diet and Renal Disease (MDRD) study and has been validated in several other populations. Several web-based calculators will calculate the estimated GFR; one location is www. nephron.com.

Other useful, well-validated estimators of GFR include the CKD-EPI formula. This is more accurate and precise than the MDRD equation at higher levels of true GFR, possibly decreasing false-positive results. This formula may perform better in elderly populations; however, this estimation equation did not include large numbers of nonwhite patients.

Cystatin C is another endogenous marker of GFR, filtered freely at the glomerulus and produced at a relatively constant rate, irrespective of muscle mass. It is reabsorbed and partially metabolized in the renal tubular epithelial cells. Adding the measurement of cystatin C to serum creatinine improves the accuracy of the estimated GFR. A large published meta-analysis showed that cystatin C alone or in combination with serum creatinine is a stronger predictor of important clinical events, such as end-stage renal disease (ESRD) or death, than serum creatinine alone. Although not yet used extensively in clinical practice, use of cystatin C holds promise for improving classification of kidney disease and predicting outcomes among at-risk individuals.

Creatinine clearance (C_{cr}) can also be estimated using the Cockcroft and Gault formula, which incorporates age, sex, and weight to estimate creatinine clearance from plasma creatinine levels without any urinary measurements:

$$C_{cr} = \frac{(140 - Age) \times Weight \text{ (kg)}}{P_{cr} \times 72}$$

For women, the creatinine clearance is multiplied by 0.85 because muscle mass is less. This formula overestimates GFR in patients who are obese or edematous and is most accurate when normalized for body surface area of 1.73 m². Dosing of many medications is still based on values of creatinine clearance from the Cockcroft-Gault equation.

BUN is another index used in assessing kidney function. It is synthesized mainly in the liver and is the end product of protein catabolism. Urea is freely filtered by the glomerulus, and about 30–70% is reabsorbed in the renal tubules. Unlike creatinine clearance, which overestimates GFR, urea clearance underestimates GFR. Urea reabsorption may be decreased in volume replete patients, whereas volume depletion causes increased urea reabsorption, in conjunction with increased sodium reabsorption, from the kidney, increasing BUN. A normal BUN:creatinine ratio is 10:1, although this can vary between individuals. With volume depletion, the ratio can increase to 20:1 or higher. Other causes of increased BUN include increased catabolism (gastrointestinal [GI] bleeding, cell lysis, and corticosteroid usage), increased dietary protein, and decreased renal perfusion (heart failure, renal artery stenosis) (Table 22–2). Reduced BUN is seen in liver disease and in the syndrome of inappropriate antidiuretic hormone (SIADH) secretion.

Table 22–2. Conditions affecting BUN independently of GFR.

Increased BUN
Reduced effective circulating blood volume (prerenal azotemia)
Catabolic states (gastrointestinal bleeding, corticosteroid use)
High-protein diets
Tetracycline
Decreased BUN
Liver disease
Malnutrition
Sickle cell anemia
SIADH

BUN, blood urea nitrogen; GFR, glomerular filtration rate; SIADH, syndrome of inappropriate antidiuretic hormone.

As patients approach ESRD, a more accurate measure of GFR than creatinine clearance is the average of the creatinine and urea clearances. The creatinine clearance overestimates GFR, as mentioned above, while the urea clearance underestimates GFR. Therefore, an average of the two more accurately approximates the true GFR.

KIDNEY BIOPSY

Indications for percutaneous needle biopsy include (1) unexplained acute kidney injury or CKD; (2) acute nephritic syndromes; (3) unexplained proteinuria and hematuria; (4) previously identified and treated lesions to plan future therapy; (5) systemic diseases associated with kidney dysfunction, such as systemic lupus erythematosus (SLE), Goodpasture syndrome, and granulomatosis with polyangiitis (formerly Wegener granulomatosis), to confirm the extent of renal involvement and to guide management; (6) suspected transplant rejection, to differentiate it from other causes of acute kidney injury; and (7) to guide treatment. If a patient is unwilling to accept therapy based on biopsy findings, the risk of biopsy may outweigh its benefit. Relative contraindications include a solitary or ectopic kidney (exception: transplant allografts), horseshoe kidney, ESRD, congenital anomalies, and multiple cysts. Absolute contraindications include an uncorrected bleeding disorder, severe uncontrolled hypertension, renal infection, renal neoplasm, hydronephrosis, or an uncooperative patient.

Prior to biopsy, patients should not use medications that prolong clotting times and should have well-controlled blood pressure. Blood work should include a hemoglobin, platelet count, prothrombin time, and partial thromboplastin time. After biopsy, hematuria occurs in nearly all patients. Less than 10% will have macroscopic hematuria. Patients should remain supine for 4–6 hours postbiopsy. A patient with a 6-hour postbiopsy hematocrit > 3% lower than baseline should be closely monitored.

Percutaneous kidney biopsies are generally safe. Approximately 1% of patients will experience significant bleeding requiring blood transfusions. More than half of patients will have at least a small hematoma. Risk of major bleeding persists up to 72 hours after the biopsy. Any type of anticoagulation therapy should be held for 5–7 days postbiopsy if possible. The risks of nephrectomy and mortality are about 0.06–0.08%. When a percutaneous needle biopsy is technically not feasible and kidney tissue is deemed clinically essential, a closed biopsy via interventional radiologic techniques or open biopsy under general anesthesia can be done.

Inker LA et al; CKD-EPI Investigators. Estimating glomerular filtration rate from serum creatinine and cystatin C. N Engl J Med. 2012 Jul 5;367(1):20–9.Erratum in: N Engl J Med. 2012 Nov 22;367(21):2060. [PMID: 22762315]

Maripuri S et al. Outpatient versus inpatient observation after percutaneous native kidney biopsy: a cost minimization study. Am J Nephrol. 2011;34(1):64–70. [PMID: 21677428]

Shlipak MG et al; CKD Prognosis Consortium. Cystatin C versus creatinine in determining risk based on kidney function. N Engl J Med. 2013 Sep 5;369(10):932–43. [PMID: 24004120]

Vivante A et al. Hematuria and risk for end-stage kidney disease. Curr Opin Nephrol Hypertens. 2013 May;22(3):325–30. [PMID: 23449218]

ACUTE KIDNEY INJURY

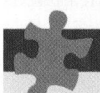

ESSENTIALS OF DIAGNOSIS

- ▶ Sudden increase in BUN or serum creatinine.
- ▶ Oliguria can be associated.
- ▶ Symptoms and signs depend on cause.

General Considerations

Acute kidney injury is defined as a sudden decrease in kidney function, resulting in an inability to maintain acid-base, fluid and electrolyte balance and to excrete nitrogenous wastes. A clinically applicable definition of acute kidney injury has been developed. The RIFLE criteria describe three progressive levels of acute kidney injury (risk, injury, and failure) based on the elevation in serum creatinine or decline in urinary output with two outcome measures (loss and ESRD). Risk, injury, and failure are defined, respectively, as a 1.5-fold increase in serum creatinine, a twofold or threefold increase in serum creatinine, or a decline in urinary output to 0.5 mL/kg/h over 6, 12, or 24 hours. These definitions were created by an international consensus panel and correlate with prognosis. The AKIN criteria are also predictive of outcomes, and closely follow the RIFLE criteria, with the addition of a change in serum creatinine of ≥ 0.3 mg/day qualifying as a risk for injury. In the absence of functioning kidneys, serum creatinine concentration will typically increase by 1–1.5 mg/dL daily, although with certain conditions, such as rhabdomyolysis, serum creatinine can increase more rapidly. On average, 5% of hospital admissions and 30% of intensive care unit (ICU) admissions carry a diagnosis of acute kidney injury, and it will develop in 25% of hospitalized patients. Patients with acute kidney injury of any type are at higher risk for all-cause mortality according to prospective cohorts, whether or not there is substantial renal recovery. The rates of acute kidney injury in the hospital setting have increased steadily since the 1980s and are continuing to rise.

Clinical Findings

A. Symptoms and Signs

The uremic milieu of acute kidney injury can cause non-specific symptoms. When present, symptoms are often due to uremia or its underlying cause. Uremia can cause nausea, vomiting, malaise, and altered sensorium. Hypertension can occur, and fluid homeostasis is often altered. Hypovolemia can cause states of low blood flow to the kidneys, sometimes termed "prerenal" states, whereas hypervolemia can result from intrinsic or "postrenal" disease. Pericardial effusions can occur with uremia, and a pericardial friction rub can be present. Effusions may result in cardiac tamponade. Arrhythmias occur, especially with hyperkalemia. The lung examination may show rales in the presence of hypervolemia. Acute kidney failure can cause nonspecific diffuse abdominal pain and ileus as well as platelet dysfunction; thus, bleeding and clotting disorders are more common in these patients. The neurologic examination reveals encephalopathic changes with asterixis and confusion; seizures may ensue.

B. Laboratory Findings

Elevated BUN and serum creatinine levels are present, though these elevations do not distinguish acute kidney disease from CKD. Hyperkalemia can occur from impaired renal potassium excretion. With hyperkalemia, the ECG can reveal peaked T waves, PR prolongation, and QRS widening. A long QT segment can occur with hypocalcemia. Anion gap and non-gap metabolic acidosis (due to decreased organic and nonorganic acid clearance) is often noted. Hyperphosphatemia occurs when phosphorus cannot be secreted by damaged tubules either with or without increased cell catabolism. Anemia can occur as a result of decreased erythropoietin production over weeks, and associated platelet dysfunction is typical.

▶ Classification & Etiology

Acute kidney injury can be divided into three categories: prerenal causes (kidney hypoperfusion leading to lower GFR), intrinsic kidney disease, and postrenal causes (obstructive uropathy). Identifying the cause is the first step toward treating the patient (Table 22–3).

A. Prerenal Causes

Prerenal causes are the most common etiology of acute kidney insults and injury, accounting for 40–80% of cases,

depending on the population studied. Prerenal azotemia is due to renal hypoperfusion, which is an appropriate physiologic change. If reversed quickly with restoration of renal blood flow, renal parenchymal damage often does not occur. If hypoperfusion persists, ischemia can result, causing intrinsic kidney injury.

Decreased renal perfusion can occur in several ways, such as a decrease in intravascular volume, a change in vascular resistance, or low cardiac output. Causes of volume depletion include hemorrhage, GI losses, dehydration, excessive diuresis, extravascular space sequestration, pancreatitis, burns, trauma, and peritonitis.

Changes in vascular resistance can occur systemically with sepsis, anaphylaxis, anesthesia, and afterload-reducing drugs. Blockers of the renin-angiotensin-aldosterone system, such as angiotensin-converting enzyme (ACE) inhibitors, limit efferent renal arteriolar constriction out of proportion to the afferent arteriolar constriction; thus, GFR will decrease with these medications. Nonsteroidal anti-inflammatory drugs (NSAIDs) minimize afferent arteriolar vasodilation by inhibiting prostaglandin-mediated signals. Thus, in cirrhosis and heart failure, when prostaglandins are recruited to increase renal blood flow, NSAIDs will have particularly deleterious effects. Epinephrine, norepinephrine, high-dose dopamine, anesthetic agents, and cyclosporine also can cause renal vasoconstriction. Renal artery stenosis causes increased resistance and decreased renal perfusion.

Low cardiac output is a state of low effective renal arterial blood flow. This occurs in states of cardiogenic shock, heart failure, pulmonary embolism, and pericardial tamponade. Arrhythmias and valvular disorders can also reduce cardiac output. In the ICU setting, positive pressure ventilation will decrease venous return, also decreasing cardiac output.

When GFR falls acutely, it is important to determine whether acute kidney injury is due to prerenal or intrinsic

Table 22–3. Classification and differential diagnosis of acute kidney injury.

	Prerenal Azotemia	Postrenal Azotemia	Intrinsic Renal Disease		
			Acute Tubular Necrosis (Oliguric or Polyuric)	Acute Glomerulonephritis	Acute Interstitial Nephritis
Etiology	Poor renal perfusion	Obstruction of the urinary tract	Ischemia, nephrotoxins	Immune complex-mediated, pauci-immune, anti-GBM related	Allergic reaction; drug reaction; infection, collagen vascular disease
Serum BUN:Cr ratio	> 20:1	> 20:1	< 20:1	> 20:1	< 20:1
Urinary indices					
U_{Na} (mEq/L)	< 20	Variable	> 20	< 20	Variable
FE_{Na} (%)	< 1	Variable	> 1 (when oliguric)	< 1	< 1; > 1
Urine osmolality (mosm/kg)	> 500	< 400	250–300	Variable	Variable
Urinary sediment	Benign or hyaline casts	Normal or red cells, white cells, or crystals	Granular (muddy brown) casts, renal tubular casts	Red cells, dysmorphic red cells and red cell casts	White cells, white cell casts, with or without eosinophils

BUN:Cr, blood urea nitrogen:creatinine ratio; FE_{Na}, fractional excretion of sodium; U_{Na}, urinary concentration of sodium.

renal causes. The history and physical examination are important, and urinalysis can be helpful. The BUN:creatinine ratio will typically exceed 20:1 due to increased urea reabsorption. In an oliguric patient, another useful index is the fractional excretion of sodium (FE_{Na}). With decreased GFR, the kidney will reabsorb salt and water avidly if there is no intrinsic tubular dysfunction. Thus, patients with prerenal causes should have a low fractional excretion percent of sodium (< 1%). Oliguric patients with intrinsic kidney dysfunction typically have a high fractional excretion of sodium (> 1–2%). The FE_{Na} is calculated as follows: FE_{Na} = clearance of Na^+/GFR = clearance of Na^+/C_{cr}:

$$FE_{Na} = \frac{Urine_{Na}/Serum_{Na}}{Urine_{cr}/Serum_{cr}} \times 100\%$$

Renal sodium handling is more accurately assessed by the FE_{Na} in oliguric states than in nonoliguric states because the FE_{Na} could be relatively low in nonoliguric acute tubular necrosis if sodium intake and excretion are relatively low. (Oliguria is defined as urinary output < 400–500 mL/d, or < 20 mL/h.) The equation was created and validated to assess the difference between oliguric acute tubular necrosis and pre-renal states. Diuretics can cause increased sodium excretion. Thus, if the FE_{Na} is high within 12–24 hours after diuretic administration, the cause of acute kidney injury may not be accurately predicted. Acute kidney injury due to glomerulonephritis can have a low FE_{Na} because sodium reabsorption and tubular function may not be compromised.

Treatment of prerenal insults depends entirely on the causes, but maintenance of euvolemia, attention to serum electrolytes, and avoidance of nephrotoxic drugs are benchmarks of therapy. This involves careful assessment of volume status, cardiac function, diet, and drug usage.

B. Postrenal Causes

Postrenal causes are the least common reason for acute kidney injury, accounting for approximately 5–10% of cases, but important to detect because of their reversibility. Postrenal azotemia occurs when urinary flow from both kidneys, or a single functioning kidney, is obstructed. Occasionally, postrenal uropathies can occur when a single kidney is obstructed if the contralateral kidney cannot adjust for the loss in function, (eg, in a patient with advanced CKD). Obstruction leads to elevated intraluminal pressure, causing kidney parenchymal damage, with marked effects on renal blood flow and tubular function, and a decrease in GFR.

Postrenal causes include urethral obstruction, bladder dysfunction or obstruction, and obstruction of both ureters or renal pelvises. In men, benign prostatic hyperplasia is the most common cause. Patients taking anticholinergic drugs are particularly at risk. Obstruction can also be caused by bladder, prostate, and cervical cancers; retroperitoneal fibrosis; and neurogenic bladder. Less common causes are blood clots, bilateral ureteral stones, urethral stones or strictures, and bilateral papillary necrosis.

Patients may be anuric or polyuric and may complain of lower abdominal pain. Polyuria can occur in the setting of partial obstructions with resultant tubular dysfunction and an inability to appropriately reabsorb salt and water loads. Obstruction can be constant or intermittent and partial or complete. On examination, the patient may have an enlarged prostate, distended bladder, or mass detected on pelvic examination.

Laboratory examination may initially reveal high urine osmolality, low urine sodium, high BUN:creatinine ratio, and low FE_{Na} (as tubular function may not be compromised initially). These indices are similar to a prerenal picture because extensive intrinsic renal damage has not occurred. After several days, the urine sodium increases as the kidneys fail and are unable to concentrate the urine—thus, isosthenuria is present. The urine sediment is generally benign.

Patients with acute kidney injury and suspected postrenal insults should undergo bladder catheterization and ultrasonography to assess for hydroureter and hydronephrosis. After reversal of the underlying process, these patients often undergo a postobstructive saliuresis and diuresis, and care should be taken to avoid volume depletion. Rarely, obstruction is not diagnosed by ultrasonography. For example, patients with retroperitoneal fibrosis from tumor or radiation may not show dilation of the urinary tract. If suspicion does exist, a CT scan or MRI can establish the diagnosis. Prompt treatment of obstruction within days by catheters, stents, or other surgical procedures can result in partial or complete reversal of the acute process.

C. Intrinsic Acute Kidney Injury

Intrinsic renal disorders account for up to 50% of all cases of acute kidney injury. Intrinsic dysfunction is considered after prerenal and postrenal causes have been excluded. The sites of injury are the tubules, interstitium, vasculature, and glomeruli.

▶ When to Refer

- If a patient has signs of acute kidney injury that have not reversed over 1–2 weeks, but no signs of acute uremia, the patient can usually be referred to a nephrologist rather than admitted.

- If a patient has signs of persistent urinary tract obstruction, the patient should be referred to a urologist.

▶ When to Admit

The patient should be admitted if there is sudden loss of kidney function resulting in abnormalities that cannot be handled expeditiously in an outpatient setting (eg, hyperkalemia, volume overload, uremia) or other requirements for acute intervention, such as emergent urologic intervention or dialysis.

Kinsey GR et al. Pathogenesis of acute kidney injury: foundation for clinical practice. Am J Kidney Dis. 2011 Aug;58(2): 291–301. [PMID: 21530035]

Palevsky PM et al. KDOQI US commentary on the 2012 KDIGO clinical practice guideline for acute kidney injury. Am J Kidney Dis. 2013 May;61(5):649–72. [PMID: 23499048]

ACUTE TUBULAR NECROSIS

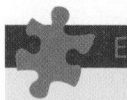

▶ Acute kidney injury.

▶ Ischemic or toxic insult.

▶ Urine sediment with pigmented granular casts and renal tubular epithelial cells is pathognomonic but not essential.

▶ General Considerations

Acute kidney injury due to tubular damage is termed "acute tubular necrosis" and accounts for approximately 85% of intrinsic acute kidney injury. The two major causes of acute tubular necrosis are ischemia and nephrotoxin exposure. Ischemic acute kidney injury is characterized not only by inadequate GFR but also by renal blood flow inadequate to maintain parenchymal cellular perfusion. Renal tubular damage with low effective arterial blood flow to the kidney, often termed a "prerenal" state, can result in tubular necrosis and apoptosis. This occurs in the setting of prolonged hypotension or hypoxemia, such as volume depletion, shock, and sepsis. Major surgical procedures can involve prolonged periods of hypoperfusion, which are exacerbated by vasodilating anesthetic agents. Aside from the serum creatinine, other urinary and serum biomarkers, including neutrophil gelatinase-associated lipocalin and cystatin C, are being investigated to diagnose and treat acute kidney injury earlier in its course, with the potential for better outcomes. Studies investigating the utility of a careful examination of the urinary sediment show promise as a diagnostic and prognostic tool for acute tubular necrosis.

Exogenous nephrotoxins more commonly cause damage than endogenous nephrotoxins.

A. Exogenous Nephrotoxins

Aminoglycosides cause some degree of acute tubular necrosis in up to 25% of hospitalized patients receiving therapeutic levels of the drugs. Nonoliguric kidney injury typically starts to occur after 5–10 days of exposure. Predisposing factors include underlying kidney damage, volume depletion, and advanced age. Aminoglycosides can remain in renal tissues for up to a month, so kidney function may not recover for some time after stopping the medication. Monitoring of peak and trough levels is important, but trough levels are more helpful in predicting renal toxicity. Gentamicin is as nephrotoxic as tobramycin; streptomycin is the least nephrotoxic of the aminoglycosides, likely due to the number of cationic amino side chains present on each molecule.

Amphotericin B is typically nephrotoxic after a dose of 2–3 g. This causes a type I renal tubular acidosis with severe vasoconstriction and distal tubular damage, which can lead to hypokalemia and nephrogenic diabetes insipidus. **Vancomycin,** intravenous **acyclovir,** and several **cephalosporins** have been known to cause acute tubular necrosis.

Radiographic contrast media may be directly nephrotoxic. Contrast nephropathy is the third leading cause of new-onset acute kidney injury in hospitalized patients. It probably results from the synergistic combination of direct renal tubular epithelial cell toxicity and renal medullary ischemia. Predisposing factors include advanced age, preexisting kidney disease (serum creatinine > 2 mg/dL), volume depletion, diabetic nephropathy, heart failure, multiple myeloma, repeated doses of contrast, and recent exposure to other nephrotoxic agents, including NSAIDs and ACE inhibitors. The combination of preexisting diabetes mellitus and kidney dysfunction poses the greatest risk (15–50%) for contrast nephropathy. Lower volumes of contrast with lower osmolality are recommended in high-risk patients. Toxicity usually occurs within 24–48 hours after the radiocontrast study. Nonionic contrast media may be less toxic, but this has not been well proven. Prevention should be the goal when using these agents. The mainstay of therapy is a liter of intravenous 0.9% saline over 10–12 hours both before and after the contrast administration—cautiously in patients with preexisting cardiac dysfunction. Intravenous volume repletion is superior to oral solutions in small studies. Neither mannitol nor furosemide offers benefit over 0.9% (normal) saline administration. In fact, furosemide may lead to increased rates of renal dysfunction in this setting. It is unclear whether N-acetylcysteine can prevent kidney injury. In some small studies, N-acetylcysteine given before and after contrast decreases the incidence of dye-induced nephrotoxicity. However, a large prospective randomized controlled trial showed no benefit of N-acetylcysteine in over 2300 patients, some of whom had CKD, randomized to either 1200 mg orally twice versus placebo before and after angiographic procedures. Acetylcysteine is a thiol-containing antioxidant with little toxicity whose mechanism of action is unclear. With little harm and possible benefit, administering acetylcysteine 600 mg orally every 12 hours twice, before and after a dye load, for patients with preexisting risk factors at risk for acute kidney injury, is a reasonable strategy. Intravenous N-acetylcysteine, 1200 mg prior to an emergent procedure, has shown benefit compared with placebo and may be a good option if a patient needs contrast dye urgently. The primary endpoint was a 25% increase in serum creatinine within 48–96 hours after the procedure. Some investigators have shown a benefit using sodium bicarbonate (154 mEq/L, intravenously at 3 mL/kg/h for 1 hour before the procedure, then 1 mL/kg/h for 6 hours after the procedure) over a more conventional regimen of normal saline as the isotonic volume expander. However, others have shown sodium bicarbonate was not superior to sodium chloride when using similar administration regimens. Other nephrotoxic agents should be avoided during the day before and after dye administration. The largest randomized trial to date will investigate intravenous normal saline versus bicarbonate and N-acetylcysteine versus placebo to prevent contrast-induced nephropathy in a 2×2 design, with a result predicted for 2017.

Cyclosporine toxicity is usually dose dependent. It causes distal tubular dysfunction (a type 4 renal tubular acidosis) from severe vasoconstriction. Regular blood level monitoring is important to prevent both acute and chronic nephrotoxicity. With patients who are taking cyclosporine to prevent kidney allograft rejection, kidney biopsy is often necessary to distinguish transplant rejection from cyclosporine toxicity. Renal function usually improves after reducing the dose or stopping the drug.

Other exogenous nephrotoxins include antineoplastics, such as cisplatin and organic solvents, and heavy metals such as mercury, cadmium, and arsenic.

B. Endogenous Nephrotoxins

Endogenous nephrotoxins include heme-containing products, uric acid, and paraproteins. **Myoglobinuria** as a consequence of rhabdomyolysis leads to acute tubular necrosis. Necrotic muscle releases large amounts of myoglobin, which is freely filtered across the glomerulus. The myoglobin is reabsorbed by the renal tubules, and direct damage can occur. Distal tubular obstruction from pigmented casts and intrarenal vasoconstriction can also cause damage. This type of kidney injury occurs in the setting of crush injury, or muscle necrosis from prolonged unconsciousness, seizures, cocaine, and alcohol abuse. Dehydration and acidosis predispose to the development of myoglobinuric acute kidney injury. Patients may complain of muscular pain and often have signs of muscle injury. Rhabdomyolysis of clinical importance commonly occurs with a serum creatine kinase (CK) > 20,000–50,000 international units/L. One study showed that 58% of patients with acute kidney injury from rhabdomyolysis had CK levels > 16,000 international units/L. Only 11% of patients without kidney injury had CK values < 16,000 international units/L. The globin moiety of myoglobin will cause the urine dipstick to read falsely positive for hemoglobin: the urine appears dark brown, but no red cells are present. With lysis of muscle cells, patients also become hyperkalemic, hyperphosphatemic, and hyperuricemic. Hypocalcemia may ensue due to phosphorus and calcium precipitation. The mainstay of treatment is volume repletion. Adjunctive treatments with mannitol and alkalinization of the urine have not been proved to change outcomes in human trials. As the patient recovers, calcium can move back from tissues to plasma, so early exogenous calcium administration for hypocalcemia is not recommended unless the patient is symptomatic or the level becomes exceedingly low in an unconscious patient. Such repletion could result in hypercalcemia later in the course of the illness.

Hemoglobin can cause a similar form of acute tubular necrosis. Massive intravascular hemolysis is seen in transfusion reactions and in certain hemolytic anemias. Reversal of the underlying disorder and hydration are the mainstays of treatment.

Hyperuricemia can occur in the setting of rapid cell turnover and lysis. Chemotherapy for germ cell neoplasms and leukemia and lymphoma are the primary causes. Spontaneous tumor lysis syndrome is a less common cause. Acute kidney injury occurs with intratubular deposition of uric acid crystals; serum uric acid levels are often > 15–20 mg/dL and urine uric acid levels > 600 mg/24 h. A urine uric acid to urine creatinine ratio > 1.0 indicates risk of acute kidney injury. Allopurinol or rasburicase can be used

prophylactically, and rasburicase with or without dialysis is often used for treatment in diagnosed cases.

Bence Jones protein seen in conjunction with multiple myeloma can cause direct tubular toxicity and tubular obstruction. Other renal complications from multiple myeloma include hypercalcemia and renal tubular dysfunction, including proximal renal tubular acidosis (see Multiple Myeloma, below).

▶ Clinical Findings

A. Symptoms and Signs

See Acute Kidney Injury.

B. Laboratory Findings

Hyperkalemia and hyperphosphatemia are commonly encountered. BUN:creatinine ratio is usually < 20:1 because tubular function is not intact, per the mechanisms described in the general section on acute kidney injury (Table 22–3). Urinalysis may show evidence of acute tubular damage. The urine sediment may be brown. Urinary output can be either oliguric or nonoliguric, with oliguria portending a worse prognosis. Urine sodium concentration is typically elevated, but the FE_{Na} is more indicative of tubular function, as discussed above. On microscopic examination, an active sediment may show pigmented granular casts or "muddy brown" casts. Renal tubular epithelial cells and epithelial cell casts can be present (see Table 22–1).

▶ Treatment

Treatment is aimed at hastening recovery and avoiding complications. Preventive measures should be taken to avoid volume overload and hyperkalemia. Loop diuretics have been used in large doses (eg, furosemide in doses ranging from 20 mg to 160 mg orally or intravenously twice daily, or as a continuous infusion) to affect adequate diuresis. However, a prospective randomized controlled trial has shown no difference between the administration of large doses of diuretics versus placebo on either recovery from acute kidney injury or death. Widespread use of diuretics in critically ill patients with acute kidney injury should only be encouraged in states of volume overload when appropriate. Disabling side effects of supranormal dosing include hearing loss and cerebellar dysfunction. This is mainly due to peak furosemide levels; this risk can be minimized by the use of a furosemide drip. A starting dose of 0.1–0.3 mg/kg/h is appropriate, increasing to a maximum of 0.5–1 mg/kg/h. A bolus of 1–1.5 mg/kg should be administered at the beginning of each dose escalation. Intravenous thiazide diuretics can be used to augment urinary output; chlorothiazide, 250–500 mg intravenously every 8–12 hours, is a reasonable choice. Another good choice to augment diuresis is metolazone at doses of 2.5–5 mg given orally once to twice daily, 30 minutes prior to loop diuretics. It is less expensive than intravenous chlorothiazide and has reasonable bioavailability. Short-term effects of loop diuretics include activation of the renin–angiotensin system. A 2012 prospective randomized trial showed the lack of benefit on mortality from plasma ultrafiltration over the use of intravenous diuretics in patients with decompensated heart failure. This intervention can be considered in ICU patients with acute kidney injury in need of volume removal who are nonresponsive to diuretics with the caveat that the intervention has not ultimately improved population-based survival. Nutritional support should maintain adequate intake while preventing excessive catabolism. Dietary protein restriction of 0.6 g/kg/d helps prevent metabolic acidosis. Hypocalcemia and hyperphosphatemia can be improved with diet and phosphate-binding agents taken with meals three times daily; examples include aluminum hydroxide (500 mg orally) over the short term, and calcium carbonate (500–1500 mg orally), calcium acetate (667 mg, two or three tablets), sevelamer carbonate (800–1600 mg orally), and lanthanum carbonate (1000 mg orally) over longer periods. Hypocalcemia should not be treated in patients with rhabdomyolysis unless they are symptomatic. Hypermagnesemia can occur because of reduced magnesium excretion by the renal tubules, so magnesium-containing antacids and laxatives should be avoided in these patients. Dosages of all medications must be adjusted according to the estimated degree of renal impairment for drugs eliminated by the kidney.

Indications for dialysis in acute kidney injury from acute tubular necrosis or other intrinsic disorders include life-threatening electrolyte disturbances (such as hyperkalemia), volume overload unresponsive to diuresis, worsening acidosis, and uremic complications (eg, encephalopathy, pericarditis, and seizures). In gravely ill patients, less severe but worsening abnormalities may also be indications for dialytic support. Two prospective randomized control trials, each with more than 1100 patients, showed that an intensive dialysis dose was not superior to a more conventional dose.

▶ Course & Prognosis

The clinical course of acute tubular necrosis is often divided into three phases: initial injury, maintenance, and recovery. The maintenance phase is expressed as either oliguric (urinary output < 500 mL/d) or nonoliguric. Nonoliguric acute tubular necrosis has a better outcome. Conversion from oliguric to nonoliguric states with the use of diuretics has not been shown to change the prognosis. While dopamine has sometimes been used for this purpose, numerous studies have shown that its use in this setting has not been beneficial. Average duration of the maintenance phase is 1–3 weeks but may be several months. Cellular repair and removal of tubular debris occur during this period. The recovery phase can be heralded by diuresis. GFR begins to rise; BUN and serum creatinine fall.

The mortality rate associated with acute kidney injury is 20–50% in hospitalized settings, and up to 70% for those in the ICU requiring dialysis with additional comorbid illnesses. Increased mortality is associated with advanced age, severe underlying disease, and multisystem organ failure. Leading causes of death are infections, fluid and electrolyte disturbances, and worsening of underlying disease. Mortality rates have started to improve slightly according to two retrospective cohort studies conducted within the last 10 years.

▶ When to Refer

- Studies have shown that nephrology referral improves outcome in acute kidney injury.
- For fluid, electrolyte, and acid-base abnormalities that are recalcitrant to interventions.

▶ When to Admit

A patient with symptoms or signs of acute kidney injury that require immediate intervention, such as administration of intravenous fluids, dialytic therapy, or that requires a team approach that cannot be coordinated as an outpatient.

INTERSTITIAL NEPHRITIS

ESSENTIALS OF DIAGNOSIS

- ▶ Fever.
- ▶ Transient maculopapular rash.
- ▶ Acute or chronic kidney injury.
- ▶ Pyuria (including eosinophiluria), white blood cell casts, and hematuria.

▶ General Considerations

Acute interstitial nephritis accounts for 10–15% of cases of intrinsic renal failure. An interstitial inflammatory response with edema and possible tubular cell damage is the typical pathologic finding.

Although drugs account for over 70% of cases, acute interstitial nephritis also occurs in infectious diseases, immunologic disorders, or as an idiopathic condition. The most common drugs are penicillins and cephalosporins, sulfonamides and sulfonamide-containing diuretics, NSAIDs, rifampin, phenytoin, and allopurinol. Proton pump inhibitors can also cause acute interstitial nephritis. Infectious causes include streptococcal infections, leptospirosis, cytomegalovirus, histoplasmosis, and Rocky Mountain spotted fever. Immunologic entities are more commonly associated with glomerulonephritis, but SLE, Sjögren syndrome, sarcoidosis, and cryoglobulinemia can cause interstitial nephritis.

▶ Clinical Findings

Clinical features can include fever (> 80%), rash (25–50%), arthralgias, and peripheral blood eosinophilia (80%). The classic triad of fever, rash, and arthralgias is present in only 10–15% of cases. The urine often contains white cells (95%), red cells, and white cell casts. Proteinuria can be a feature, particularly in NSAID-induced interstitial nephritis, but is usually modest (< 2 g/24 h). Eosinophiluria is neither very sensitive nor specific but can be detected by Wright or Hansel stain.

Treatment & Prognosis

Acute interstitial nephritis often carries a good prognosis. Recovery occurs over weeks to months. Urgent dialytic therapy may be necessary in up to one-third of all referred patients before resolution but patients rarely progress to ESRD. Those with prolonged courses of oliguric failure and advanced age have a worse prognosis. Treatment consists of supportive measures and removal of the inciting agent. If kidney injury persists after these steps, a short course of corticosteroids can be given, although the data to support use of corticosteroids are not substantial. Short-term, high-dose methylprednisolone (0.5–1 g/d intravenously for 1–4 days) or prednisone (60 mg/d orally for 1–2 weeks) followed by a prednisone taper can be used in these more severe cases of drug-induced interstitial nephritis.

GLOMERULONEPHRITIS

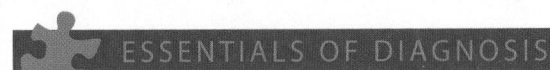

- ▶ Hematuria, dysmorphic red cells, red cell casts, and mild proteinuria.
- ▶ Dependent edema and hypertension.
- ▶ Acute kidney injury.

General Considerations

Acute glomerulonephritis is a relatively uncommon cause of acute kidney injury, accounting for about 5% of cases. Pathologically, inflammatory glomerular lesions are seen. These include mesangioproliferative, focal and diffuse proliferative, and crescentic lesions. The larger the percentage of glomeruli involved and the more severe the lesion, the more likely it is that the patient will have a poor clinical outcome.

Categorization of acute glomerulonephritis can be done by serologic analysis. Markers include anti-GBM antibodies, antineutrophil cytoplasmic antibodies (ANCAs), and other immune markers of disease.

Immune complex deposition usually occurs when moderate antigen excess over antibody production occurs. Complexes formed with marked antigen excess tend to remain in the circulation. Antibody excess with large antigen–antibody aggregates usually results in phagocytosis and clearance of the precipitates by the mononuclear phagocytic system in the liver and spleen. Causes include IgA nephropathy (Berger disease), peri-infectious or postinfectious glomerulonephritis, endocarditis, lupus nephritis, cryoglobulinemic glomerulonephritis (often associated with hepatitis C virus [HCV]), and MPGN.

Anti-GBM–associated acute glomerulonephritis is either confined to the kidney or associated with pulmonary hemorrhage. The latter is termed "Goodpasture syndrome." Injury is related to autoantibodies aimed against type IV collagen in the GBM rather than to immune complex deposition.

Pauci-immune acute glomerulonephritis is a form of small-vessel vasculitis associated with ANCAs, causing primary and secondary kidney diseases that do not have direct immune complex deposition or antibody binding. Tissue injury is believed to be due to cell-mediated immune processes. An example is granulomatosis with polyangiitis, a systemic necrotizing vasculitis of small arteries and veins associated with intravascular and extravascular granuloma formation. In addition to glomerulonephritis, these patients can have upper airway, pulmonary, and skin manifestations of disease. Cytoplasmic ANCA (c-ANCA) is the common pattern. Microscopic polyangiitis is another pauci-immune vasculitis causing acute glomerulonephritis. Perinuclear staining (p-ANCA) is the common pattern in this scenario. ANCA-associated and anti-GBM-associated acute glomerulonephritis can evolve to crescentic glomerulonephritis and often have poor outcomes unless treatment is started early. Both are described more fully below.

Other vascular causes of acute glomerulonephritis include hypertensive emergencies and the thrombotic microangiopathies such as hemolytic-uremic syndrome and thrombotic thrombocytopenic purpura (see Chapter 14).

Clinical Findings

A. Symptoms and Signs

Patients with acute glomerulonephritis are often hypertensive and edematous, and have an abnormal urinary sediment. The edema is found first in body parts with low tissue tension, such as the periorbital and scrotal regions.

B. Laboratory Findings

Serum creatinine can rise over days to months, depending on the rapidity of the underlying process. The BUN:creatinine ratio is not a reliable marker of kidney function and is more reflective of the underlying volume status of the patient. Dipstick and microscopic evaluation will reveal evidence of hematuria, moderate proteinuria (usually < 3 g/d), and cellular elements such as red cells, red cell casts, and white cells. Red cell casts are specific for glomerulonephritis, and a detailed search is warranted. Either spot urinary protein-creatinine ratios or 24-hour urine collections can quantify protein excretion; the latter can quantify creatinine clearance when renal function is stable. However, in cases of rapidly changing serum creatinine values, the urinary creatinine clearance is an unreliable marker of GFR. The FE_{Na} is usually low unless the renal tubulo-interstitial space is affected, and renal dysfunction is marked (see Table 22–3).

Further tests include complement levels (C3, C4, CH50) that are low in immune complex glomerulonephritis aside from IgA nephropathy and normal in pauci immune and anti-GBM related glomerulonephritis. Other tests include ASO titers, anti-GBM antibody levels, ANCAs, antinuclear antibody titers, cryoglobulins, hepatitis serologies, blood cultures, renal ultrasound, and occasionally kidney biopsy.

Treatment

Depending on the nature and severity of disease, treatment can consist of high-dose corticosteroids and cytotoxic agents such as cyclophosphamide. Plasma exchange can be used in Goodpasture disease and pauci-immune glomerulonephritis as a temporizing measure until chemotherapy can take effect. Treatment and prognosis for specific diseases are discussed more fully below.

Ad-hoc working group of ERBP; Fliser D et al. A European Renal Best Practice (ERBP) position statement on the Kidney Disease Improving Global Outcomes (KDIGO) clinical practice guidelines on acute kidney injury: part 1: definitions, conservative management and contrast-induced nephropathy. Nephrol Dial Transplant. 2012 Dec;27(12):4263–72. [PMID: 23045432]

Hoste EA et al. Epidemiology of acute kidney injury. Contrib Nephrol. 2010;165:1–8. [PMID: 20427949]

Lafrance JP et al. Acute kidney injury associates with increased long-term mortality. J Am Soc Nephrol. 2010 Feb;21(2):345–52. [PMID: 20019168]

Perazella MA et al. Diagnostic value of urine microscopy for differential diagnosis of acute kidney injury in hospitalized patients. Clin J Am Soc Nephrol. 2008 Nov;3(6):1615–9. [PMID: 18784207]

CARDIORENAL SYNDROME

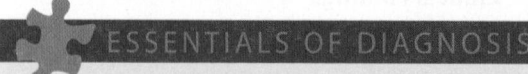

- ▶ Cardiac dysfunction: signs or symptoms of heart failure, ischemic injury or arrhythmias.
- ▶ Kidney disease: acute or chronic, depending on type of cardiorenal syndrome.

▶ **General Considerations**

Cardiorenal syndrome is a pathophysiologic disorder of the heart and kidneys wherein the acute or chronic deterioration of one organ results in the acute or chronic deterioration of the other. This syndrome has been classified into five types.

Type 1 consists of acute kidney injury stemming from acute cardiac disease. Type 2 is CKD due to chronic cardiac

disease. Type 3 is acute cardiac disease as a result of acute kidney injury. Type 4 is chronic cardiac decompensation from CKD. Type 5 consists of heart and kidney dysfunction due to other acute or chronic systemic disorders (such as sepsis). Identifying and defining this common syndrome may assist in the future with treatments to improve its morbidity and mortality.

Bart BA et al; Heart Failure Clinical Research Network. Ultrafiltration in decompensated heart failure with cardiorenal syndrome. N Engl J Med. 2012 Dec 13;367(24):2296–304. [PMID: 23131078]

CHRONIC KIDNEY DISEASE

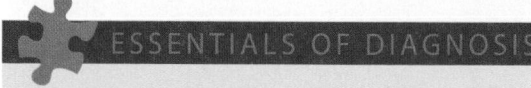

- ▶ Decline in the GFR over months to years
- ▶ Persistent proteinuria or abnormal renal morphology may be present.
- ▶ Hypertension in most cases.
- ▶ Symptoms and signs of uremia when nearing end-stage disease.
- ▶ Bilateral small or echogenic kidneys on ultrasound in advanced disease.

▶ **General Considerations**

CKD affects more than 20 million Americans, or one in nine adults. Most are unaware of the condition because they remain asymptomatic until the disease is near end-stage. The National Kidney Foundation's staging system helps clinicians formulate practice plans (Table 22–4). Over 70% of cases of late-stage CKD (stage 5 CKD and ESRD) in the United States are due to diabetes mellitus or hypertension/vascular disease. Glomerulonephritis, cystic

Table 22–4. Stages of chronic kidney disease: A clinical action plan.[1,2]

Stage	Description	GFR (mL/min/1.73 m²)	Action[3]
1	Kidney damage with normal or ↑↑ GFR	≥ 90	Diagnosis and treatment. Treatment of comorbid conditions. Slowing of progression. Cardiovascular disease risk reduction.
2	Kidney damage with mildly ↓ GFR	60–89	Estimating progression.
3	Moderately ↓ GFR	30–59	Evaluating and treating complications.
4	Severely ↓ GFR	15–29	Preparation for kidney replacement therapy.
5	End-stage renal disease (ESRD)	< 15 (or dialysis)	Replacement (if uremia is present).

[1]From National Kidney Foundation, KDOQI, Chronic Kidney Disease Guidelines.
[2]Chronic kidney disease is defined as either kidney damage or GFR < 60 mL/min/1.73 m² for 3 or more months. Kidney damage is defined as pathologic abnormalities or markers of damage, including abnormalities in blood or urine tests or imaging studies.
[3]Includes actions from preceding stages.
GFR, glomerular filtration rate.

Table 22–5. Major causes of chronic kidney disease.

Glomerular diseases

Primary glomerular diseases
    Focal and segmental glomerulosclerosis
    Membranoproliferative glomerulonephritis
    IgA nephropathy
    Membranous nephropathy
    Alport syndrome (hereditary nephritis)
Secondary glomerular diseases
    Diabetic nephropathy
    Amyloidosis
    Postinfectious glomerulonephritis
    HIV-associated nephropathy
    Collagen-vascular diseases (eg, SLE)
    HCV-associated membranoproliferative glomerulonephritis

Tubulointerstitial nephritis

Drug hypersensitivity
Heavy metals
Analgesic nephropathy
Reflux/chronic pyelonephritis
Sickle cell nephropathy
Idiopathic

Cystic diseases

Polycystic kidney disease
Medullary cystic disease

Obstructive nephropathies

Prostatic disease
Nephrolithiasis
Retroperitoneal fibrosis/tumor
Congenital

Vascular diseases

Hypertensive nephrosclerosis
Renal artery stenosis

HCV, hepatitis C virus; SLE, systemic lupus erythematosus.

diseases, chronic tubulointerstitial diseases, and other urologic diseases account for the remainder (Table 22–5). Genetic polymorphisms of the *APOL-1* gene have been shown to be associated with an increased risk of the development of CKD in African Americans.

CKD usually leads to a progressive decline in kidney function even if the inciting cause can be identified and treated or removed. Destruction of nephrons leads to compensatory hypertrophy and supranormal GFR of the remaining nephrons in order to maintain overall homeostasis. As a result, the serum creatinine may remain relatively normal even in the face of significant loss of renal mass and is, therefore, a relatively insensitive marker for renal damage and scarring. In addition, compensatory hyperfiltration leads to overwork injury in the remaining nephrons, which in turn causes progressive glomerular sclerosis and interstitial fibrosis. Angiotensin receptor blockers (ARBs) and ACE inhibitors can help reduce hyperfiltration injury and are particularly helpful in slowing the progression of proteinuric CKD. Fortunately, an individual's decreased renal mass as a result of kidney donation is unlikely to result in CKD later in life.

CKD is an independent risk factor for cardiovascular disease (CVD); proteinuric CKD confers an even higher risk of cardiovascular mortality. Most patients with stage 3 CKD die of underlying CVD prior to progression to ESRD.

▶ Clinical Findings

A. Symptoms and Signs

In the early stages, CKD is asymptomatic. Symptoms develop slowly with the progressive decline in GFR, are nonspecific, and do not manifest until kidney disease is far advanced (GFR < 5–10 mL/min/1.73 m^2). At this point, the build-up of metabolic waste products, or uremic toxins, can result in the uremic syndrome (Table 22–6). General symptoms of uremia may include fatigue and weakness; anorexia, nausea, vomiting, and a metallic taste in the mouth are also common. Patients or family members may report irritability, memory impairment, insomnia, restless legs, paresthesias, and twitching. Generalized pruritus without rash may occur. Decreased libido and menstrual irregularities are common. Pericarditis, a rare complication of CKD, may present with pleuritic chest pain. Drug toxicity can develop as renal clearance worsens; in particular, since insulin is renally cleared, hypoglycemia may develop and can be life-threatening in patients with diabetes.

The most common physical finding in CKD is hypertension. It is often present in early stages of CKD and tends to worsen with CKD progression as sodium excretion is

Table 22–6. Symptoms and signs of uremia.

Organ System	Symptoms	Signs
General	Fatigue, weakness	Sallow-appearing, chronically ill
Skin	Pruritus, easy bruisability	Pallor, ecchymoses, excoriations, edema, xerosis
ENT	Metallic taste in mouth, epistaxis	Urinous breath
Eye		Pale conjunctiva
Pulmonary	Shortness of breath	Rales, pleural effusion
Cardiovascular	Dyspnea on exertion, retrosternal pain on inspiration (pericarditis)	Hypertension, cardiomegaly, friction rub
Gastrointestinal	Anorexia, nausea, vomiting, hiccups	
Genitourinary	Nocturia, erectile dysfunction	Isosthenuria
Neuromuscular	Restless legs, numbness and cramps in legs	
Neurologic	Generalized irritability and inability to concentrate, decreased libido	Stupor, asterixis, myoclonus, peripheral neuropathy

Table 22–7. Reversible causes of kidney injury.

Reversible Factors	Diagnostic Clues
Infection	Urine culture and sensitivity tests
Obstruction	Bladder catheterization, then renal ultrasound
Extracellular fluid volume depletion or significant hypotension relative to baseline	Blood pressure and pulse, including orthostatic pulse
Hypokalemia, hypercalcemia, and hyperuricemia (usually > 15 mg/dL)	Serum electrolytes, calcium, phosphate, uric acid
Nephrotoxic agents	Drug history
Severe/urgent hypertension	Blood pressure, chest radiograph
Heart failure	Physical examination, chest radiograph

impaired. In later stages of CKD, this sodium retention may lead to typical physical signs of volume overload. Uremic signs are seen with a profound decrease in GFR (< 5–10 mL/min/1.73 m^2) and may include a generally sallow and ill appearance, halitosis (uremic fetor), and the uremic encepholophathic signs of decreased mental status, asterixis, myoclonus, and possibly seizures if very advanced.

Symptoms and signs of uremia warrant immediate hospital admission and nephrology consultation for initiation of dialysis. The uremic syndrome improves or resolves with dialytic therapy.

In any patient with kidney disease, it is important to identify and correct all possibly reversible insults or exacerbating factors (Table 22–7). Urinary tract infections, obstruction, extracellular fluid volume depletion, hypotension, nephrotoxins (such as NSAIDs or aminoglycosides), severe or emergent hypertension, and heart failure should be excluded.

B. Laboratory Findings

CKD is usually defined by an abnormal GFR persisting for at least 3 months. Persistent proteinuria or abnormalities on renal imaging (eg, polycystic kidneys) are also diagnostic of CKD, even when estimated GFR is normal. It is helpful to plot the inverse of serum creatinine ($1/S_{Cr}$) versus time or estimated GFR (if reported by the laboratory) versus time. If three or more prior measurements are available, the time to ESRD can be estimated (Figure 22–1). If the slope of the line acutely declines, new and potentially reversible renal insults should be excluded as outlined above. Anemia, hyperphosphatemia, hypocalcemia, hyperkalemia, and metabolic acidosis can occur with both acute kidney disease and CKD. The urinary sediment can show broad waxy casts as a result of dilated, hypertrophic nephrons. Proteinuria may be present. If so, it should be quantified as described above. Quantification of urinary protein is important for several reasons. First, it helps narrow the differential diagnosis of the etiology of the CKD

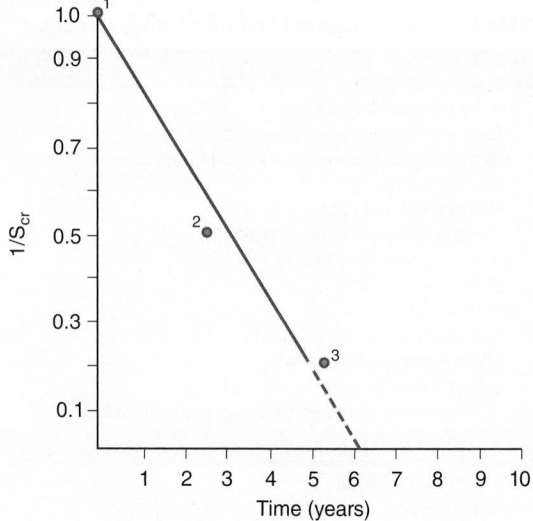

^{1} Value of serum creatinine level = 1.0 mg/dL
^{2} Value of serum creatinine level = 2.0 mg/dL
^{3} Value of serum creatinine level = 5.0 mg/dL

▲ **Figure 22–1.** Decline in kidney function (expressed as the reciprocal of serum creatinine as shown here, or as estimated glomerular filtration rate [eGFR]) plotted against time to end-stage renal disease (ESRD). The solid line indicates the linear decline in kidney function over time. The dotted line indicates the approximate time to ESRD.

(Table 22–5); for example, glomerular diseases tend to present with protein excretion of > 1 g/d. Second, the presence of proteinuria is associated with more rapid progression of CKD and cardiovascular mortality.

C. Imaging

The finding of small, echogenic kidneys bilaterally (< 9–10 cm) by ultrasonography supports a diagnosis of CKD, although normal or even large kidneys can be seen with adult polycystic kidney disease, diabetic nephropathy, HIV-associated nephropathy, multiple myeloma, amyloidosis, and obstructive uropathy.

▶ **Complications**

The complications of CKD tend to occur at relatively predictable stages of disease as noted in Figure 22–2.

A. Cardiovascular Complications

Patients with CKD experience greater morbidity and mortality from CVD in comparison to the general population. Death from cardiovascular causes accounts for 45% of all deaths of patients receiving dialysis. Between 80% and 90% of patients with CKD die, primarily of CVD, before reaching the need for dialysis. The precise biologic mechanisms for this enhanced mortality are unclear but may have to do with the uremic milieu including abnormal phosphorus and calcium homeostasis, increased burden of oxidative

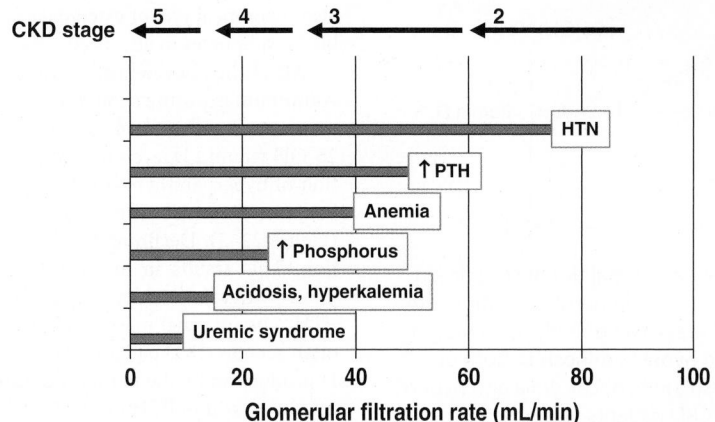

▲ **Figure 22–2.** Complications of chronic kidney disease (CKD) by stage and glomerular filtration rate (GFR). Complications arising from CKD tend to occur at the stages depicted, although there is considerable variability noted in clinical practice. HTN, hypertension; PTH, parathyroid hormone. (Adapted, with permission, from William Bennett, MD.)

stress, increased vascular reactivity, increased left ventricular hypertrophy, and underlying coexistent comorbidities such as hypertension and diabetes mellitus.

1. Hypertension—Hypertension is the most common complication of CKD; it tends to be progressive and salt-sensitive. Hyperreninemic states and exogenous erythropoietin administration can also exacerbate hypertension.

As with other patient populations, control of hypertension should focus on both nonpharmacologic therapy (eg, diet, exercise, weight loss, treatment of obstructive sleep apnea) and pharmacologic therapy. CKD results in disturbed sodium homeostasis such that the ability of the kidney to adjust to variations in sodium and water intake becomes limited as GFR declines. A low salt diet (2 g/d) is often essential to control blood pressure and help avoid overt volume overload. Diuretics are nearly always needed to help control hypertension (see Table 11–5); thiazides work well in early CKD, but in those with a GFR < 30 mL/min/1.73 m², loop diuretics are more effective. Beware, however, that volume contraction as a result of very low sodium intake (especially with intercurrent illness) or over-diuresis in the presence of impaired sodium homeostasis can result in acute kidney injury. Initial drug therapy for proteinuric patients should include ACE inhibitors or ARBs (see Table 11–7). When an ACE inhibitor or an ARB is initiated or uptitrated, patients must have serum creatinine and potassium checked within 7–14 days. Hyperkalemia or a rise in serum creatinine > 30% from baseline mandates reduction or cessation of the drug. Results of the NEPHRON-D study suggest that an ACE inhibitor and ARBs should not be used in combination. Second-line antihypertensive agents include calcium channel blockers and beta-blockers. Hypertension in CKD can be difficult to control and additional agents from other classes are often needed. Current guidelines suggest a blood pressure goal of <140/90 mm Hg for patients with CKD; a goal of 125/75 mm Hg may be beneficial for patients with proteinuria. Treatment of blood pressure significantly below these goals is not supported by current data and may be dangerous in some populations, such as the elderly. Randomized controlled trials to assess optimal BP control in CKD are ongoing.

2. Coronary artery disease—Patients with CKD are at higher risk for death from CVD than the general population. Traditional modifiable risk factors for CVD, such as hypertension, tobacco use, and hyperlipidemia, should be aggressively treated in patients with CKD. Uremic vascular calcification involving disordered phosphorus homeostasis and other mediators may also be a cardiovascular risk factor in these patients.

3. Heart failure—The complications of CKD result in increased cardiac workload via hypertensive disease, volume overload, and anemia. Patients with CKD may also have accelerated rates of atherosclerosis and vascular calcification resulting in vessel stiffness. All of these factors contribute to left ventricular hypertrophy and diastolic dysfunction, which are present in most patients starting dialysis. Over time, systolic dysfunction may also develop. Diuretic therapy, in addition to prudent fluid and salt restriction, is usually necessary. Thiazides may be adequate therapy for most patients through CKD stage 3, but loop diuretics are usually needed when the GFR is < 30 mL/min/1.73 m²; higher doses may be needed as renal function declines. Digoxin is excreted by the kidney, and its toxicity is exacerbated in the presence of electrolyte disturbances which are common in CKD. The proven efficacy of ACE inhibitors in heart failure holds true for patients with CKD. Despite the risks of hyperkalemia and worsening renal function, ACE inhibitors and ARBs can be used for patients with advanced CKD with close blood pressure and blood chemistry monitoring.

4. Pericarditis—Pericarditis may develop in uremic patients but is rare; typical findings include pleuritic chest pain and a friction rub. Development of a significant effusion may result in pulsus paradoxus, an enlarged cardiac silhouette on chest radiograph, and low QRS voltage and electrical alternans on ECG. The effusion is generally

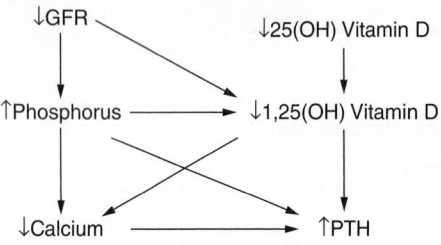

▲ **Figure 22–3.** Mineral abnormalities of chronic kidney disease (CKD). Decline in glomerular filtration rate (GFR) and loss of renal mass lead directly to increased serum phosphorus and hypovitaminosis D. Both of these abnormalities result in hypocalcemia and hyperparathyroidism. Many CKD patients also have nutritional 25(OH) vitamin D deficiency. PTH, parathyroid hormone.

hemorrhagic, and anticoagulants should be avoided if this diagnosis is suspected. Cardiac tamponade can occur; therefore, uremic pericarditis is a mandatory indication for hospitalization and initiation of hemodialysis.

B. Disorders of Mineral Metabolism

The metabolic bone disease of CKD refers to the complex disturbances of calcium and phosphorus metabolism, parathyroid hormone (PTH), active vitamin D, and possibly fibroblast growth factor-23 (FGF-23) homeostasis (see Chapter 21 and Figure 22–3). A typical pattern seen as early as CKD stage 3 is hyperphosphatemia, hypocalcemia, hypovitaminosis D, and secondary hyperparathyroidism as a result of the first three abnormalities. These abnormalities can cause vascular calcification, which may be partly responsible for the accelerated CVD and excess mortality seen in the CKD population. Epidemiologic studies in humans show an association between elevated phosphorus levels and increased risk of cardiovascular mortality in early CKD through ESRD. As yet, there are no intervention trials suggesting the best course of treatment in these patients; control of mineral and PTH levels per current guidelines is discussed below.

Bone disease, or **renal osteodystrophy**, in advanced CKD is common and there are several types of lesions. Renal osteodystrophy can only be diagnosed by bone biopsy, which is rarely done. The most common bone disease, **osteitis fibrosa cystica**, is a result of secondary hyperparathyroidism and the osteoclast-stimulating effects of PTH. This is a high-turnover disease with bone resorption and subperiosteal lesions; it can result in bone pain and proximal muscle weakness. **Adynamic bone disease**, or low-bone turnover, is becoming more common; it may result iatrogenically from suppression of PTH or via spontaneously low PTH production. **Osteomalacia** is characterized by lack of bone mineralization. In the past, osteomalacia was associated with aluminum toxicity—either as a result of chronic ingestion of prescribed aluminum-containing phosphorus binders or from high levels of aluminum in impure dialysate water. Currently, osteomalacia is more likely to result from hypovitaminosis D; there is

also theoretical risk of osteomalacia associated with use of bisphosphonates in advanced CKD.

All of the above entities increase the risk of fractures. Aluminum exposure should be avoided. In addition, treatment may involve correction of calcium, phosphorus, and 25-OH vitamin D levels toward normal values, and mitigation of hyperparathyroidism. Understanding the interplay between these abnormalities can help target therapy (Figure 22–3). Declining GFR leads to phosphorus retention. This results in hypocalcemia as phosphorus complexes with calcium, deposits in soft tissues, and stimulates PTH. Loss of renal mass and low 25-OH vitamin D levels often seen in CKD patients result in low 1,25(OH) vitamin D production by the kidney. Because 1,25(OH) vitamin D is a suppressor of PTH production, hypovitaminosis D also leads to secondary hyperparathyroidism.

The first step in treatment of metabolic bone disease is control of hyperphosphatemia (defined as a serum phosphorus of ≤ 4.5 mg/dL in pre-ESRD CKD, or ≤ 5.5 mg/dL in ESRD patients). This involves dietary phosphorus restriction initially (see section on dietary management), followed by the administration of oral phosphorus binders if targets are not achieved (see below). Oral phosphorus binders, such as calcium carbonate (650 mg/tablet) or calcium acetate (667 mg/capsule), block absorption of dietary phosphorus in the gut and are given thrice daily with meals. These should be titrated to a serum phosphorus of < 4.6 mg/dL in stage 3–4 CKD and < 4.6–5.5 mg/dL in ESRD. Maximal recommended elemental calcium doses are 1500 mg/d (eg, nine tablets of calcium acetate); doses should be decreased if serum calcium rises above 10 mg/dL. Phosphorus-binding agents that do not contain calcium are sevelamer and lanthanum. Sevelamer, 800–3200 mg, and lanthanum carbonate, 500–1000 mg, are given at the beginning of meals and may be combined with calcium-containing binders. Aluminum hydroxide is a highly effective phosphorus binder but can cause osteomalacia and neurologic complications when used long-term. It can be used in the acute setting for serum phosphorus > 7 mg/dL or for short periods (eg, 3 weeks) in CKD patients.

Once serum phosphorus levels are controlled, active vitamin D (1,25[OH] vitamin D, or calcitriol) or active vitamin D analogs are recommended to treat secondary hyperparathyroidism in stage 3–5 CKD. Serum 25-OH vitamin D levels should be measured and brought to normal (see Chapter 26) prior to considering administration of active vitamin D. Active vitamin D (calcitriol) increases serum calcium and phosphorus levels; both need to be monitored closely during calcitriol therapy, and its dose should be decreased if hypercalcemia or hyperphosphatemia occurs. Typical calcitriol dosing is 0.25 or 0.5 mcg orally daily or every other day. Cinacalcet targets the calcium-sensing receptors of the parathyroid gland and suppresses PTH production. Cinacalcet, 30–90 mg orally once a day, can be used if elevated serum phosphorus or calcium levels prohibit the use of vitamin D analogs; cinacalcet can cause hypocalcemia. Optimal PTH levels in CKD are not known, but because skeletal resistance to PTH develops with uremia, relatively high levels are targeted in advanced CKD to avoid adynamic bone disease. Expert guidelines generally suggest goal PTH levels near or just above the upper limit of normal for moderate CKD, and at least two-fold and up to ninefold the upper limit of normal for ESRD.

C. Hematologic Complications

1. Anemia—The anemia of CKD is primarily due to decreased erythropoietin production, which often becomes clinically significant during stage 3 CKD. Many patients are iron deficient as well due to impaired GI iron absorption.

Erythropoiesis-stimulating agents (eg, recombinant erythropoietin [epoetin] and darbepoetin) are FDA-approved in CKD for a goal hemoglobin (Hgb) of 10–11 g/dL if no other treatable causes for anemia are present. There is likely no benefit of starting erythropoiesis-stimulating agents before Hgb values are < 9 g/dL. The starting dose of epoetin is 50 units/kg (3000–4000 units/dose) once or twice a week, and darbepoetin is started at 0.45 mcg/kg and can be administered every 2–4 weeks. These agents can be given intravenously (eg, to the hemodialysis patient) or subcuta-neously (eg, to the predialysis or dialysis patient); subcuta-neous dosing of erythropoietin is roughly 30% more effective than intravenous dosing. Erythropoiesis-stimulat-ing agents should be titrated to a Hgb of 10–11 g/dL for optimal safety; studies show that targeting a higher Hgb increases risk of stroke and possibly other cardiovascular events. When titrating doses, Hgb levels should rise no more than 1 g/dL every 3–4 weeks. Hypertension is a complica-tion of treatment with erythropoiesis-stimulating agents in about 20% of patients. The dosage may require adjustment, or antihypertensive drugs may need to be given.

Iron stores must be adequate to ensure response to erythropoiesis-stimulating agents. Hepcidin, a molecule that blocks GI iron absorption and mobilization of iron from body stores, tends to be high in CKD. Therefore, traditional measures of iron stores are measured in CKD patients but are targeted to higher goals; in CKD, a serum ferritin < 100–200 ng/mL or iron saturation < 20% is sug-gestive of iron deficiency. Iron stores should be repleted with oral or parenteral iron prior to the initiation of an erythropoietic agent. Iron therapy should probably be withheld if the serum ferritin is > 500–800 ng/mL, even if the iron saturation is < 20%. Oral therapy with ferrous sulfate, gluconate, or fumarate, 325 mg once to three times daily, is the initial therapy in pre-ESRD CKD. For those that do not respond due to poor GI absorption or lack of tolerance, intravenous iron may be necessary.

The preliminary investigation of anemia in any CKD patient should also include assessment of thyroid function tests, and serum vitamin B$_{12}$ testing prior to initiating therapy with a erythropoiesis-stimulating agent.

2. Coagulopathy—The coagulopathy of advanced stage CKD is mainly caused by platelet dysfunction; a prolonged bleeding time may result. Clinically, patients can have pete-chiae, purpura, and an increased tendency for bleeding during surgery.

Treatment is required only in patients who are symp-tomatic. Raising the Hgb to 9–10 g/dL in anemic patients can reduce risk of bleeding via improved clot formation. Desmopressin (25 mcg intravenously every 8–12 hours for two doses) is a short-lived but effective treatment for plate-let dysfunction and it is often used in preparation for sur-gery. Conjugated estrogens, 2.5–5 mg orally for 5–7 days, may have an effect for several weeks but are seldom used. Dialysis improves the bleeding time. Cryoprecipitate (10–15 bags) is rarely used and lasts < 24 hours.

D. Hyperkalemia

Potassium balance generally remains intact in CKD until stages 4–5. However, hyperkalemia may occur at earlier stages when certain conditions are present, such as type 4 renal tubular acidosis (seen in patients with diabetes mel-litus), high potassium diets, or medications that decrease renal potassium secretion (amiloride, triamterene, spi-ronolactone, eplerenone, NSAIDs, ACE inhibitors, ARBs) or block cellular potassium uptake (beta-blockers). Other causes include acidemic states, and any type of cellular destruction causing release of intracellular contents, such as hemolysis and rhabdomyolysis.

Treatment of acute hyperkalemia is discussed in Chap-ter 21 (see Table 21–6). Cardiac monitoring is indicated for any ECG changes seen with hyperkalemia or a serum potassium level > 6.0–6.5 mEq/L. Chronic hyperkalemia is best treated with dietary potassium restriction (2 g/d) and minimization or elimination of any medications that may impair renal potassium excretion, as noted above. Loop diuretics may also be administered for their kaliuretic effect as long as the patient is not volume-depleted.

E. Acid–Base Disorders

Damaged kidneys are unable to excrete the 1 mEq/kg/d of acid generated by metabolism of dietary animal proteins in the typical Western diet. The resultant metabolic acidosis is primarily due to loss of renal mass; distal tubular defects may contribute to or worsen the acidosis. Excess hydrogen ions are buffered by the large bone stores of calcium car-bonate and calcium phosphate. This results in leaching of calcium and phosphorus from the bone and contributes to the metabolic bone disease described above and to growth retardation in children with CKD. Chronic acidosis can also result in muscle protein catabolism. The serum bicar-bonate level should be maintained at > 21 mEq/L. The most commonly used therapy is oral sodium bicarbonate in doses of 0.5–1.0 mEq/kg/d divided twice daily and titrated as needed. Citrate salts increase the absorption of dietary aluminum and should be avoided in CKD.

F. Neurologic Complications

Uremic encephalopathy, resulting from the aggregation of uremic toxins, does not occur until GFR falls below 5–10 mL/min/1.73 m^2. Symptoms begin with difficulty in con-centrating and can progress to lethargy, confusion, seizure, and coma. Physical findings may include altered mental status, weakness, and asterixis. These findings improve with dialysis.

Other neurologic complications, which can manifest with advanced CKD include peripheral neuropathies (stocking-glove or isolated mononeuropathies), erectile dysfunction, autonomic dysfunction, and restless leg syndrome. These may not improve with dialysis therapy.

G. Endocrine Disorders

There is risk of hypoglycemia in treated diabetic patients with advanced CKD due to decreased renal elimination of insulin. Doses of oral hypoglycemics and insulin may need reduction. Metformin is associated with risk of lactic acidosis when the GFR is < 50 mL/min/1.73 m^2 and should be discontinued at this point.

Decreased libido and erectile dysfunction are common in advanced CKD. Men have decreased testosterone levels; women are often anovulatory. Women with serum creatinine < 1.4 mg/dL are not at increased risk for poor outcomes in pregnancy; however, those with serum creatinine > 1.4 mg/dL may experience faster progression of CKD with pregnancy. Fetal survival is not compromised, however, unless CKD is advanced. Despite a high degree of infertility in patients with ESRD, pregnancy can occur in this setting; however, fetal mortality approaches 50%, and babies who survive are often premature. In female patients with ESRD, renal transplantation with a well-functioning allograft affords the best chances for a successful pregnancy.

▶ Treatment

A. Slowing Progression

Treatment of the underlying cause of CKD is vital. Control of diabetes should be aggressive in early CKD; risk of hypoglycemia increases in advanced CKD, and glycemic targets may need to be relaxed to avoid this dangerous complication. Blood pressure control is vital to slow progression of all forms of CKD; agents that block the renin-angiotensin-aldosterone system are particularly important in proteinuric disease (see section on hypertension regarding blood pressure goals). Several small studies suggest a possible benefit of oral alkali therapy in slowing CKD progression when acidemia is present; there is also theoretic value in lowering uric acid levels in those with concomitant hyperuricemia, but clinical data are lacking. Obese patients should be encouraged to lose weight. Management of traditional cardiovascular risk factors should also be emphasized.

B. Dietary Management

Patients with CKD should be evaluated by a renal nutritionist. Specific recommendations should be made concerning protein, salt, water, potassium, and phosphorus intake to help manage CKD progression and complications.

1. Protein restriction—Protein restriction to 0.6–0.8 g/kg/d may retard CKD progression and is likely not harmful in the otherwise well-nourished patient; it is not advisable in those with cachexia or low serum albumin in the absence of the nephrotic syndrome.

2. Salt and water restriction—In advanced CKD, the kidney is unable to adapt to large changes in sodium intake. Intake > 3–4 g/d can lead to hypertension and volume overload, whereas intake of < 1 g/d can lead to volume depletion and hypotension. A goal of 2 g/d of sodium is reasonable for most patients. Daily fluid restriction to 2 L may be needed if volume overload is present.

3. Potassium restriction—Restriction is needed once the GFR has fallen below 10–20 mL/min/1.73 m^2, or earlier if the patient is hyperkalemic. Patients should receive detailed lists describing potassium content of foods and should limit their intake to < 50–60 mEq/d (2 g).

4. Phosphorus restriction—The phosphorus level should be kept in the "normal" range (< 4.5 mg/dL) predialysis, and between 3.5 and 5.5 mg/dL in ESRD, with a dietary restriction of 800–1000 mg/d. Foods rich in phosphorus such as cola beverages, eggs, dairy products, nuts, beans, and meat should be limited, although care must be taken to avoid protein malnutrition. Highly processed foods are often preserved with highly bioavailable phosphorus and should be avoided. Below a GFR of 20–30 mL/min/1.73 m^2, dietary restriction is rarely sufficient to reach target levels, and phosphorus binders are usually required (see above).

C. Medication Management

Many drugs are excreted by the kidney; dosages should be adjusted for GFR. Insulin doses may need to be adjusted as noted above. Magnesium-containing medications, such as laxatives or antacids, should be avoided as should phosphorus-containing medicines, particularly cathartics. Morphine metabolites are active and can accrue in advanced CKD; this problem is not encountered with other opioid agents. Drugs with potential nephrotoxicity (NSAIDs, intravenous contrast, as well as others noted in the Acute Kidney Injury section) should be avoided.

D. Treatment of End-Stage Renal Disease

When GFR declines to 5–10 mL/min/1.73 m^2 (with or without overt uremic symptoms), renal replacement therapy (hemodialysis, peritoneal dialysis, or kidney transplantation) is required to sustain life. Patient education is important in understanding which mode of therapy is most suitable, as is timely preparation for treatment; therefore, referral to a nephrologist should take place in late stage 3 CKD, or when the GFR is declining rapidly. Such referral has been shown to improve mortality. Preparation for ESRD treatment requires a team approach with the involvement of dieticians, social workers, primary care clinicians, and nephrologists. For very elderly patients, or those with multiple debilitating or life-limiting comorbidities, dialysis therapy may not meaningfully prolong life, and the option of palliative care should be discussed with the patient and family. Conversely, for patients who are otherwise relatively healthy, evaluation for possible kidney transplantation should be considered prior to initiation of dialysis.

1. Dialysis—Dialysis initiation should be considered when GFR is 10 mL/min/1.73 m^2. Studies suggest that the well-selected patient without overt uremic symptoms may wait to initiate dialysis until GFR is closer to 7 mL/min/1.73 m^2. Other indications for dialysis, which may occur when GFR is 10–15 mL/min/1.73 m^2 include (1) uremic symptoms, (2) fluid overload unresponsive to diuresis, and (3) refractory hyperkalemia.

A. HEMODIALYSIS—Vascular access for hemodialysis can be accomplished by an arteriovenous fistula (the preferred method) or prosthetic graft; creation of dialysis access should be considered well before dialysis initiation. An indwelling catheter is used when there is no useable vascular access. Because catheters confer a high risk of bloodstream infection, they should be considered a temporary measure. Native fistulas typically last longer than prosthetic grafts but require a longer time after surgical construction for maturation (6–8 weeks for a fistula versus 2 weeks for a graft). Infection, thrombosis, and aneurysm formation are complications seen more often in grafts than fistulas. *Staphylococcus* species are the most common cause of soft-tissue infections and bacteremia.

Treatment at a hemodialysis center occurs three times a week. Sessions last 3–5 hours depending on patient size and type of dialysis access. Other hemodialysis schedules can be considered depending on available resources and patient preferences. Home hemodialysis is often performed more frequently (3–6 days per week for shorter sessions) and requires a trained helper. Results of trials comparing quotidian modalities (nocturnal and frequent home hemodialysis) to conventional in-center dialysis have not thus far shown significant mortality differences, but there may be improvements in blood pressure control, mineral metabolism, and quality of life.

B. PERITONEAL DIALYSIS—With peritoneal dialysis, the peritoneal membrane is the "dialyzer." Dialysate is instilled into the peritoneal cavity through an indwelling catheter; water and solutes move across the capillary bed that lies between the visceral and parietal layers of the membrane into the dialysate during a "dwell." After equilibration, the dialysate is drained, and fresh dialysate is instilled—this is an "exchange."

There are different kinds of peritoneal dialysis: continuous ambulatory peritoneal dialysis (CAPD), in which the patient exchanges the dialysate four to six times a day manually; continuous cyclic peritoneal dialysis (CCPD), which utilizes a cycler machine to automatically perform exchanges at night.

Peritoneal dialysis permits significant patient autonomy. Its continuous nature minimizes the symptomatic volume and electrolyte shifts observed in hemodialysis patients, and poorly dialyzable compounds (such as phosphates) are better cleared, which permits less dietary restriction. However, peritoneal dialysate removes large amounts of albumin, and nutritional status must be closely watched.

The most common complication of peritoneal dialysis is peritonitis. Peritonitis may present with nausea and vomiting, abdominal pain, diarrhea or constipation, and fever. The dialysate is usually cloudy; and a diagnostic peritoneal fluid cell count is > 100 white blood cells/mcL of which over 50% are polymorphonuclear neutrophils. *Staphylococcus aureus* is the most common infecting organism, but streptococci and gram-negative species are also common.

2. Kidney transplantation—Up to 50% of all patients with ESRD are otherwise healthy enough to be suitable for transplantation, although standard criteria for recipient selection are lacking between transplant centers. Older age is becoming less of a barrier, as long as reasonable life expectancy is anticipated. Two-thirds of kidney allografts come from deceased donors, with the remainder from living related or unrelated donors. About 99,000 patients are on the waiting list for a deceased donor transplant in the United States; the average wait is 2–6 years, depending on geographic location and recipient blood type.

The 1- and 5-year kidney graft survival rates are approximately 97% and 85%, respectively, for living donor transplants and 91% and 71%, respectively, for deceased donor transplants.

Immunosuppressive regimens to prevent allograft rejection generally include a combination of a corticosteroid, an antimetabolite (azathioprine or mycophenolate mofetil), and a calcineurin inhibitor (tacrolimus or cyclosporine) or mTor inhibitor (sirolimus). Maintenance doses must balance the risk of allograft rejection as well as the adverse effects of immunosuppressives, including the development of certain cancers, infections, new onset diabetes, and chronic allograft dysfunction (calcineurin inhibitor). Additionally, calcineurin inhibitors have a narrow therapeutic window, and their hepatic metabolism is affected by many drugs (especially azoles and calcium channel blockers). Any changes in the transplant recipient's medical regimen should, therefore, occur only after consultation with a trained pharmacist or transplant nephrologist. Transplant recipients are at higher risk for CVD than the general population.

3. Medical management of ESRD—As noted above, some patients are not candidates for transplantation and may not benefit from dialysis. Studies suggest that very elderly persons who do not die soon after dialysis initiation rapidly lose functional status in the first year of treatment. The decision to initiate dialysis in patients with limited life expectancy should be weighed against possible deleterious changes in quality of life. For patients with ESRD who elect not to undergo dialysis, death occurs within days to months. In general, uremia develops and patients lose consciousness prior to death. Arrhythmias can occur as a result of electrolyte imbalance. Volume overload and dyspnea can be managed by volume restriction and opioids as described in Chapter 5. Involvement of a palliative care team is essential.

▶ **Prognosis in ESRD**

Compared with kidney transplant recipients and age-matched controls, mortality is higher for patients undergoing dialysis. There is likely little difference in survival for well-matched peritoneal versus hemodialysis patients.

Survival rates on dialysis depend on the underlying disease process. Five-year Kaplan-Meier survival rates vary from 36% for patients with diabetes to 53% for patients with glomerulonephritis. Overall 5-year survival is currently estimated at 39%. Patients undergoing dialysis have an average life-expectancy of 3–5 years, but survival for as long as 25 years may be achieved depending on comorbidities. The most common cause of death is cardiac disease (> 50%). Other causes include infection, cerebrovascular disease, and malignancy. Diabetes, advanced age, a low serum albumin, lower socioeconomic status, and inadequate dialysis are all significant predictors of mortality; high fibroblast growth factor (FGF)-23 levels have emerged as a novel marker for mortality in ESRD.

When to Refer

- A patient with stage 3–5 CKD should be referred to a nephrologist for management in conjunction with the primary care provider.
- A patient with other forms of CKD such as those with significant proteinuria (> 1 g/d) or polycystic kidney disease should be referred to a nephrologist at earlier stages.

When to Admit

- Admission should be considered for patients with decompensation of problems related to CKD, such as worsening of acid-base status, electrolyte abnormalities, and volume status that cannot be appropriately treated in the outpatient setting.
- Admission is appropriate when a patient needs to start dialysis and is not stable for outpatient initiation.

Davison R et al. Prognosis and management of chronic kidney disease (CKD) at the end of life. Postgrad Med J. 2014 Feb;90 (1060):98–105. [PMID: 24319094]

Gansevoort RT et al. Chronic kidney disease and cardiovascular risk: epidemiology, mechanisms, and prevention. Lancet. 2013 Jul 27;382(9889):339–52. [PMID: 23727170]

James PA et al. 2014 evidence-based guideline for the management of high blood pressure in adults: report from the panel members appointed to the Eighth Joint National Committee (JNC 8). JAMA. 2014 Feb 5;311(5):507–20. [PMID: 24352797]

Kovesdy CP et al. Blood pressure and mortality in U.S. veterans with chronic kidney disease: a cohort study. Ann Intern Med. 2013 Aug 20;159(4):233–42. [PMID: 24026256]

Levey AS et al. Chronic kidney disease. Lancet. 2012 Jan 14; 379(9811):165–80. [PMID: 21840587]

Matzke GR et al. Drug dosing consideration in patients with acute and chronic kidney disease—a clinical update from Kidney Disease: Improving Global Outcomes (KDIGO). Kidney Int. 2011 Dec;80(11):1122–37. [PMID: 21918498]

Qaseem A et al. Screening, monitoring, and treatment of stage 1 to 3 chronic kidney disease: a clinical practice guideline from the American College of Physicians. Ann Intern Med. 2013 Dec 17;159(12):835–47. [PMID: 24145991]

Thiruchelvam PT et al. Renal transplantation. BMJ. 2011 Nov 14; 343:d7300. [PMID: 22084316]

Turner JM et al. Treatment of chronic kidney disease. Kidney Int. 2012 Feb;81(4):351–62. [PMID: 22166846]

RENAL ARTERY STENOSIS

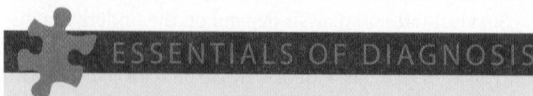

ESSENTIALS OF DIAGNOSIS

- ▶ Produced by atherosclerotic occlusive disease (80–90% of patients) or fibromuscular dysplasia (10–15%).
- ▶ Hypertension.
- ▶ Acute kidney injury in patients starting ACE inhibitor therapy.

▶ General Considerations

Atherosclerotic ischemic renal disease accounts for nearly all cases of renal artery stenosis. Fibromuscular dysplasia is a rare cause of renal artery stenosis. Approximately 5% of Americans with hypertension suffer from renal artery stenosis. It occurs most commonly in those over 45 years of age with a history of atherosclerotic disease. Other risk factors include CKD, diabetes mellitus, tobacco use, and hypertension.

▶ Clinical Findings

A. Symptoms and Signs

Patients with atherosclerotic ischemic renal disease may have refractory hypertension, new-onset hypertension (in an older patient), pulmonary edema with poorly controlled blood pressure, and acute kidney injury upon starting an ACE inhibitor. In addition to hypertension, physical examination may reveal an audible abdominal bruit on the affected side. Fibromuscular dysplasia primarily affects young women. Unexplained hypertension in a woman younger than 40 years is reason to screen for this disorder.

B. Laboratory Findings

Laboratory values can show elevated BUN and serum creatinine levels in the setting of significant renal ischemia.

C. Imaging

Abdominal ultrasound can reveal asymmetric kidney size when one renal artery is affected out of proportion to the other or small hyperechoic kidneys if both are affected.

Three prevailing methods used for screening are Doppler ultrasonography, CT angiography, and magnetic resonance angiography (MRA). **Doppler ultrasonography** is highly sensitive and specific (> 90% with an experienced ultrasonographer) and relatively inexpensive. However, this method is extremely operator and patient dependent. Measurements of blood flow must be made at the aorta and along each third of the renal artery in order to assess the disease. This test is a poor choice for patients who are obese, unable to lie supine, or have interfering bowel gas patterns.

CT angiography consists of intravenous digital subtraction angiography with arteriography and is a noninvasive procedure. The procedure uses a spiral (helical) CT scan with intravenous contrast injection. The sensitivities from various studies range from 77% to 98%, with less varying specificities in a range of 90–94%.

MRA is an excellent but expensive way to screen for renal artery stenosis, particularly in those with atherosclerotic disease. Sensitivity is 77–100%, although one study with particular flaws showed a sensitivity of only 62%. Specificity ranges from 71% to 96%. Turbulent blood flow can cause false-positive results. The imaging agent for MRA (gadolinium) has been associated with nephrogenic systemic fibrosis, which occurs primarily in patients with a GFR of < 15 mL/min/1.73 m², and rarely in patients with a GFR of 15–30 mL/min/1.73 m². It has also been seen in those with acute kidney injury and kidney transplants.

Renal angiography is the gold standard for diagnosis. CO_2 subtraction angiography can be used in place of dye when the risk of dye nephropathy exists—eg, in diabetic patients with kidney injury. Lesions are most commonly found in the proximal third or ostial region of the renal artery. The risk of atheroembolic phenomena after angiography ranges from 5% to 10%. Fibromuscular dysplasia has a characteristic "beads-on-a-string" appearance on angiography.

Treatment

Treatment of atherosclerotic ischemic renal disease is controversial. Options include medical management, angioplasty with or without stenting, and surgical bypass. Two large randomized trials have shown that vascular intervention is no better than optimal medical management in typical patients with renal artery stenosis. Angioplasty might reduce the number of antihypertensive medications but does not significantly change the progression of kidney dysfunction in comparison to patients medically managed. Stenting produces significantly better angioplastic results. However, blood pressure and serum creatinines are similar at 6 months of observation compared with both angioplasty and stents. Angioplasty is equally as effective as, and safer than, surgical revision.

Treatment of **fibromuscular dysplasia** with percutaneous transluminal angioplasty is often curative, which is in stark contrast to treatment for atherosclerotic causes.

Boateng FK et al. Renal artery stenosis: prevalence of, risk factors for, and management of in-stent stenosis. Am J Kidney Dis. 2013 Jan;61(1):147–60. [PMID: 23122491]

Cooper CJ et al; CORAL Investigators. Stenting and medical therapy for atherosclerotic renal-artery stenosis. N Engl J Med. 2014 Jan 2;370(1):13–22. [PMID: 24245566]

Textor SC et al. Renovascular hypertension and ischemic nephropathy. Am J Hypertens. 2010 Nov;23(11):1159–69. [PMID: 20864945]

GLOMERULAR DISEASES

Abnormalities of glomerular function can be caused by damage to the major components of the glomerulus: the epithelium (podocytes), basement membrane, capillary endothelium, or mesangium. The damage may be caused by overwork injury, such as in CKD; by an inflammatory process, such as SLE; by a podocyte protein mutation, such as in hereditary focal and segmental glomerulosclerosis; or a deposition disease, such as diabetes or amyloidosis. A specific histologic pattern of glomerular injury results from this damage and can be seen on kidney biopsy.

Classification

Clinically, a glomerular disease can be classified as being in one of two spectra—either in the nephritic spectrum or the nephrotic spectrum (Figure 22–4). In the "least severe" end

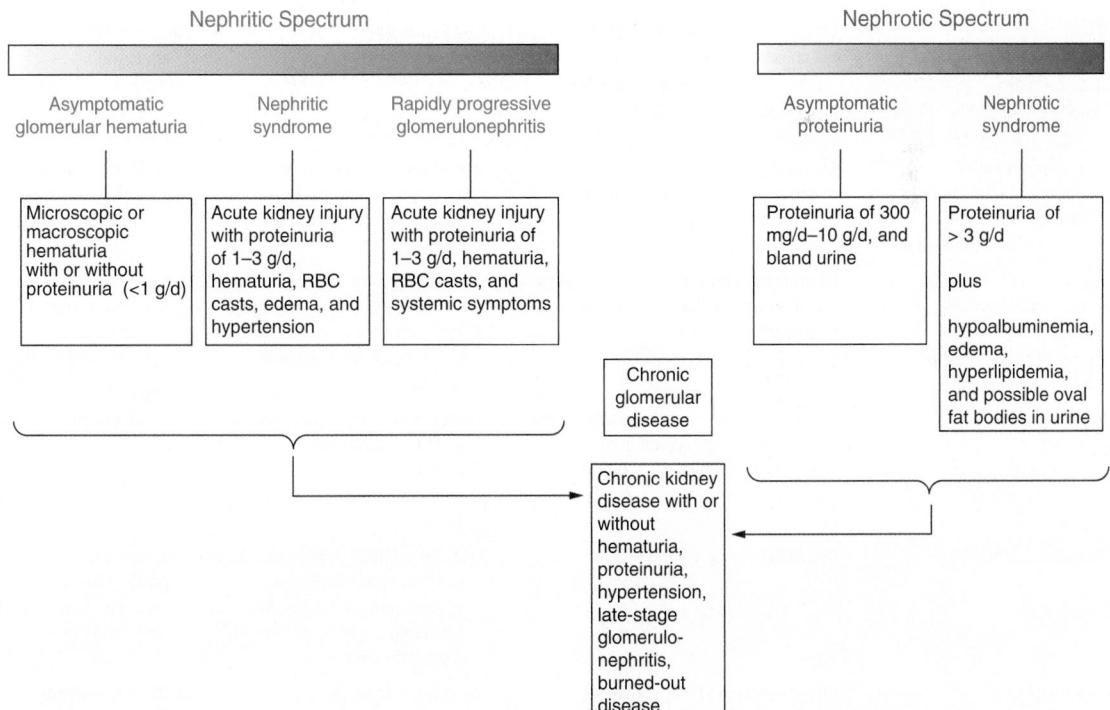

▲ **Figure 22–4.** Glomerular diseases present within one of the clinical spectra shown, the exact presentation is determined by the severity of the underlying disease and the pattern of injury. Nephritic diseases are characterized by the presence of an active urine sediment with glomerular hematuria and often with proteinuria. Nephrotic spectrum diseases are proteinuric with bland urine sediments (no cells or cellular casts). All glomerular diseases may progress to a chronic, scarred state. (Adapted, with permission, from Megan Troxell, MD, PhD.)

of the **nephritic spectrum,** the findings of glomerular hematuria (ie, dysmorphic red blood cells with some degree of proteinuria) are characteristic. The nephritic *syndrome*, comprising glomerular hematuria, subnephrotic proteinuria (<3 g/d), edema, and elevated creatinine, falls in the mid-portion of the spectrum. The rapidly progressive glomerulonephridities (RPGNs) are at the "most severe" and clinically urgent end of the nephritic spectrum.

The **nephrotic spectrum** comprises diseases that present with primarily proteinuria of at least 0.5–1 g/d and a bland urine sediment (no cells or cellular casts). The more severe end of the nephrotic spectrum comprises the nephrotic *syndrome*, which is characterized by the constellation of nephrotic-range proteinuria of > 3 g/d, hypoalbuminuria, edema, and hyperlipidemia. Differentiating between a clinical presentation within the nephritic spectrum versus the nephrotic spectrum is important because it helps narrow the differential diagnosis of the underlying glomerular disease (Tables 22–8 and 22–9).

Glomerular diseases can also be classified according to whether they cause only renal abnormalities (primary renal disease) or whether the renal abnormalities result from a systemic disease (secondary renal disease).

Further evaluation prior to kidney biopsy may include serologic testing for systemic diseases that can result in glomerular damage (Figure 22–5).

Table 22–8. Classification and findings in glomerulonephritis: Nephritic spectrum presentations.

	Typical Presentation	Association/Notes	Serology
Postinfectious glomerulonephritis	Children: abrupt onset of nephritic syndrome and acute kidney injury but can present anywhere in nephritic spectrum	Streptococci, other bacterial infections (eg, staphylococci, endocarditis, shunt infections)	Rising ASO titers, low complement levels
IgA nephropathy (Berger disease) and Henoch-Schönlein purpura, systemic IgA vasculitis	Classically: gross hematuria with per respiratory tract infection; can present anywhere in nephritic spectrum; Henoch-Schönlein purpura with vasculitic rash and gastrointestinal hemorrhage	Abnormal IgA glycosylation in both primary (familial predisposition) and secondary disease (associated with cirrhosis, HIV, celiac disease) Henoch-Schönlein purpura in children after an inciting infection	No serologic tests helpful; complement levels are normal
Pauci-immune (granulomatosis with polyangiitis, Churg-Strauss, polyarteritis, idiopathic crescentic glomerulonephritis)	Classically as crescentic or RPGN, but can present anywhere in nephritic spectrum; may have respiratory tract/sinus symptoms in granulomatosis with polyangiitis	See Figure 22–5	ANCAs: MPO or PR3 titers high; complement levels normal
Anti-glomerular basement membrane glomerulonephritis; Goodpasture syndrome	Classically as crescentic or RPGN, but can present anywhere in nephritic spectrum; with pulmonary hemorrhage in Goodpasture syndrome	May develop as a result of respiratory irritant exposure (chemicals or tobacco use)	Anti-GBM antibody titers high; complement levels normal
Cryoglobulin-associated glomerulonephritis	Often acute nephritic syndrome; often with systemic vasculitis including rash and arthritis	Most commonly associated with chronic hepatitis C; may occur with other chronic infections or some connective tissue diseases	Cryoglobulins positive; rheumatoid factor may be elevated; complement levels low
Idiopathic MPGN	Classically presents with acute nephritic syndrome, but can see nephrotic syndrome features in addition	Most patients are < 30 years old Type I most common Type II (dense deposit disease) associated with C3 nephritic factor	Low complement levels
Hepatitis C infection	Anywhere in nephritic spectrum	Can cause MPGN pattern of injury or cryoglobulinemic glomerulonephritis; membranous nephropathy pattern of injury uncommon	Low complement levels; positive hepatitis C serology; rheumatoid factor may be elevated
Systemic lupus erythematosus	Anywhere in nephritic spectrum, depending on pattern/severity of injury	Treatment depends on clinical course and International Society of Nephrology and Renal Pathology Society (ISN/RPS) classification on biopsy	High ANA and anti-double-stranded DNA titers; low complement levels

ANA, antinuclear antibodies; ANCAs: antineutrophil cytoplasmic antibodies; GBM, glomerular basement membrane; MPGN, membranoproliferative glomerulonephritis; RPGN, rapidly progressive glomerulonephritis.

Table 22–9. Classification and findings in glomerulonephritis: Nephrotic spectrum presentations.

Disease	Typical Presentation	Association/Notes
Minimal change disease (nil disease; lipoid nephrosis)	Child with sudden onset of full nephrotic syndrome	Children: associated with allergy or viral infection Adults: associated with Hodgkin disease, NSAIDs
Membranous nephropathy	Anywhere in nephrotic spectrum, but nephrotic syndrome not uncommon; particular predisposition to hypercoagulable state	Primary (idiopathic) may be associated with antibodies to PLA$_2$R Associated with non-Hodgkin lymphoma, carcinoma (gastrointestinal, renal, bronchogenic, thyroid), gold therapy, penicillamine, SLE, chronic hepatitis B or C infection
Focal and segmental glomerulosclerosis	Anywhere in nephrotic spectrum; children with congenital disease have nephrotic syndrome	Children: congenital disease with podocyte gene mutation, or in spectrum of disease with minimal change disease Adults: Associated with heroin abuse, HIV infection, reflux nephropathy, obesity, pamidronate, podocyte protein mutations, *APOL1* mutations in blacks
Amyloidosis	Anywhere in nephrotic spectrum	AL: plasma cell dyscrasia with Ig light chain over-production and deposition; check SPEP and UPEP AA: serum amyloid protein A over-production and deposition in response to chronic inflammatory disease (rheumatoid arthritis, inflammatory bowel disease, chronic infection)
Diabetic nephropathy	High GFR (hyperfiltration) → microalbuminuria → frank proteinuria → decline in GFR	Diabetes diagnosis precedes diagnosis of nephropathy by years
HIV-associated nephropathy	Heavy proteinuria, often nephrotic syndrome, progresses to ESRD relatively quickly	Usually seen in antiviral treatment-naïve patients (rare in HAART era), predilection for those of African descent (APOL1 mutations)
Membranoproliferative glomerulonephropathy	Can present with nephrotic syndrome, but usually with nephritic features as well (glomerular hematuria)	See Table 22–8

ESRD, end-stage renal disease; GFR, glomerular filtration rate; HAART, highly active antiretroviral therapy; NSAIDs, nonsteroidal anti-inflammatory drugs; PLA$_2$R, phospholipase A^2 receptor; SLE, systemic lupus erythematosus; SPEP/UPEP: serum and urine protein electrophoresis.

Cattran D. KDIGO clinical practice guideline for glomerulonephritis. Chapter 2: general principles in the management of glomerular disease. 2012 Dec;(Suppl 2):156–62. http://www.kdigo.org/clinical_practice_guidelines/GN.php

Haas M et al. Histologic classification of glomerular diseases: clinicopathologic correlations, limitations exposed by validation studies, and suggestions for modification. Kidney Int. 2013 Oct 2. [Epub ahead of print] [PMID: 24088958]

Hogan J et al. Diagnostic tests and treatment options in glomerular disease: 2014 update. Am J Kidney Dis. 2013 Nov 14. [Epub ahead of print] [PMID: 242390510]

NEPHRITIC SPECTRUM GLOMERULAR DISEASES

ESSENTIALS OF DIAGNOSIS

► Glomerular hematuria (dysmorphic red blood cells), modest proteinuria (usually 0.3–3 g/d).

► Red blood cell casts may be present if glomerular bleeding is heavy.

► Nephritic syndrome in more severe/inflammatory cases:

 –Glomerular hematuria and proteinuria.

 –Hypertension.

 –Edema.

 –Rising creatinine over days to months.

► Rapidly progressive glomerulonephritis in most severe cases:

 -Glomerular hematuria and proteinuria.

 -Hypertension and edema uncommon.

 -Rising creatinine over days to months.

► General Considerations

Glomerulonephritis is a term given to those diseases that present in the nephritic spectrum and usually signifies an inflammatory process causing renal dysfunction. It can be acute, developing over days to weeks, with or without resolution, or may be more chronic and indolent with progressive scarring. As noted above, diseases that cause

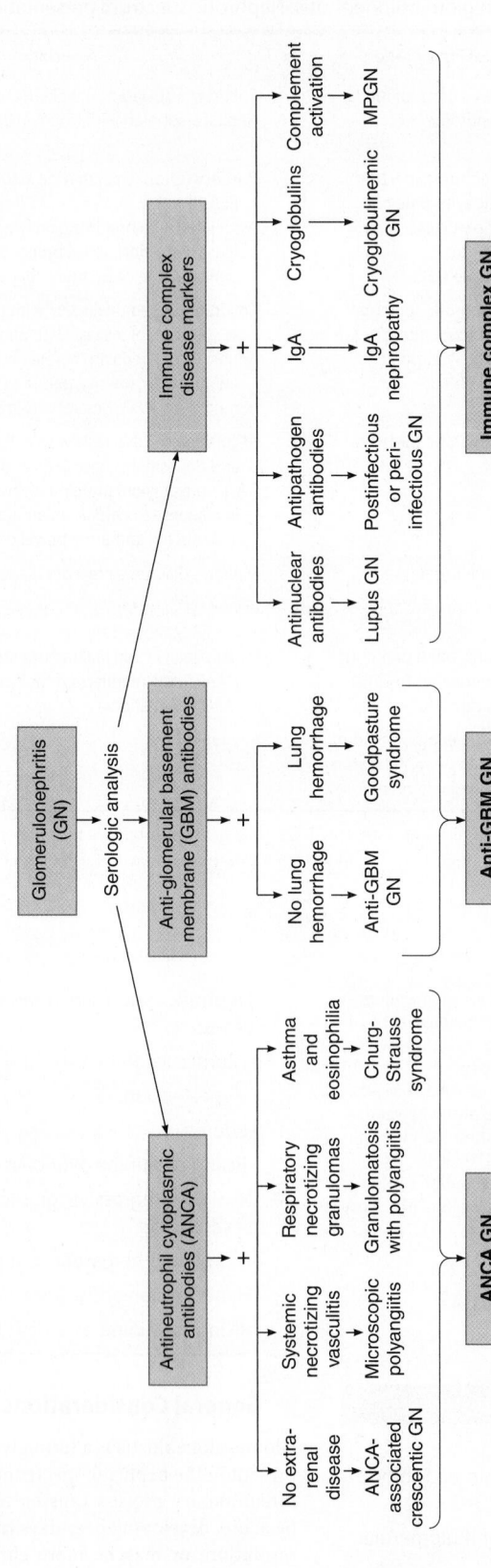

▲ **Figure 22–5.** Serologic analysis of patients with glomerulonephritis. MPGN, membranoproliferative glomerulonephritis. (Modified, with permission, from Greenberg A et al. *Primer on Kidney Diseases.* Academic Press, 1994 and Jennette JC, Falk RJ. Diagnosis and management of glomerulonephritis and vasculitis presenting as acute renal failure. Med Clin North Am. 1990;74(4):893–908. © Elsevier.)

a nephritic spectrum presentation may present with glomerular hematuria with some proteinuria, with nephritic syndrome, or with RPGN (Figure 22–4). The presentation depends on the severity of the underlying inflammation and the pattern of injury caused by the disease process.

▶ Clinical Findings

A. Symptoms and Signs

If the nephritic syndrome is present, edema is first seen in regions of low tissue pressure such as the periorbital and scrotal areas. Hypertension in the nephritic syndrome is due to sodium retention resulting from acute decrease in GFR. Heavy glomerular bleeding from inflammation may result in gross hematuria (smoky or cola-colored urine).

B. Laboratory Findings

1. Serologic testing—Serologic tests, including complement levels, antinuclear antibodies, cryoglobulins, hepatitis serologies, ANCAs, anti-GBM antibodies, and antistreptolysin O (ASO) titers (Figure 22–5), are done based on the history and physical examination to narrow the differential diagnosis of the nephritic spectrum disorder.

2. Urinalysis—The urine dipstick is positive for protein and blood. Urinary microscopy reveals red blood cells that are misshapen or dysmorphic from traversing a damaged glomerular filtration barrier. Red blood cell casts are seen with heavy glomerular bleeding and tubular stasis. When quantified, proteinuria is usually subnephrotic (< 3 g/d).

3. Biopsy—Kidney biopsy should be considered if there are no contraindications (eg, bleeding disorders, thrombocytopenia, uncontrolled hypertension). Important morphologic information is gleaned from light, electron, and immunofluorescent microscopy.

▶ Treatment

General measures for all include treatment of hypertension and of fluid overload if present. Antiproteinuric therapy with an ACE inhibitor or ARB should be considered for those without acute kidney injury. For those with profound acute kidney injury, dialysis may be needed. The inflammatory glomerular injury may require immunosuppressant agents (see specific diseases discussed below).

▶ When to Refer

Any patient in whom a glomerulonephritis is suspected should be referred to a nephrologist.

▶ When to Admit

Any suspicion of acute nephritic syndrome or RPGN warrants consideration of immediate hospitalization.

1. POSTINFECTIOUS GLOMERULONEPHRITIS

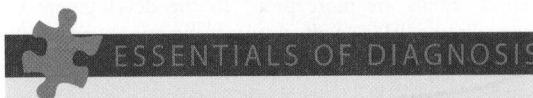

ESSENTIALS OF DIAGNOSIS

▶ Proteinuria.
▶ Glomerular hematuria.
▶ Symptoms 1–3 weeks after infection (often pharyngitis or impetigo).

▶ General Considerations

Postinfectious glomerulonephritis is most often due to infection with nephritogenic group A beta-hemolytic streptococci. It can occur sporadically or in clusters and during epidemics. It commonly appears after pharyngitis or impetigo with onset 1–3 weeks after infection (average 7–10 days).

Other infections have been associated with postinfectious glomerulonephritis including bacteremic states (especially with *S aureus*), bacterial pneumonias, deep-seated abscesses, gram-negative infections, infective endocarditis, and shunt infections. Viral, fungal, and parasitic causes of postinfectious glomerulonephritis pattern of glomerular injury include hepatitis B or C, HIV, cytomegalovirus infection, infectious mononucleosis, coccidioidomycosis, malaria, mycobacteria, syphilis, and toxoplasmosis.

▶ Clinical Findings

A. Symptoms and Signs

Disease presentation can vary widely across the nephritic spectrum from asymptomatic glomerular hematuria (especially in epidemic cases) to nephritic syndrome with hypertension, oliguria, edema, and perhaps gross glomerular hematuria (smokey-colored urine).

B. Laboratory Findings

Serum complement levels are low; in postinfectious glomerulonephritis due to group A streptococcal infection, anti-streptolysin O (ASO) titers can be high unless the immune response has been blunted with previous antibiotic treatment. Glomerular hematuria and subnephrotic proteinuria are present; severe cases may demonstrate elevated serum creatinine and urinary red blood cell casts. Kidney biopsy shows a diffuse proliferative pattern of injury on light microscopy. Immunofluorescence demonstrates granular deposition of IgG and C3 in the mesangium and along the capillary basement membrane. Electron microscopy shows large, dense subepithelial deposits or "humps."

▶ Treatment

The underlying infection should be identified and treated appropriately; otherwise, treatment for postinfectious glomerulonephritis is supportive. Antihypertensives, salt restriction, and diuretics should be used if needed. Corticosteroids have not been shown to improve outcome. Prognosis depends on the severity of the glomerular injury and age of the patient. Children are more likely to fully recover; adults are more prone to the development of severe disease (RPGN with crescent formation) and CKD.

Cattran D et al. KDIGO clinical practice guideline for glomerulonephritis. Chapter 9: infection-related glomerulonephritis. Kidney Int. 2012 Dec;(Suppl 2):200–8. http://www.kdigo.org/clinical_practice_guidelines/GN.php
Nasr SH et al. Bacterial infection-related glomerulonephritis in adults. Kidney Int. 2013 May;83(5):792–803. [PMID: 23302723]

2. IGA NEPHROPATHY

ESSENTIALS OF DIAGNOSIS

► Proteinuria: minimal to nephrotic range.
► Glomerular hematuria: microscopic is common; macroscopic (gross) after infection.
► Positive IgA staining on kidney biopsy.

General Considerations

IgA nephropathy (Berger disease) is a primary renal disease of IgA deposition in the glomerular mesangium. The inciting cause is unknown but is likely due to deficient O-linked glycosylation of IgA subclass 1 molecules. IgA nephropathy can be a primary (renal-limited) disease, or it can be secondary to hepatic cirrhosis, celiac disease, and infections such as HIV and cytomegalovirus. Susceptibility to IgA nephropathy seems to be inheritable.

IgA nephropathy is the most common primary glomerular disease worldwide, particularly in Asia. It is most commonly seen in children and young adults, with males affected two to three times more commonly than females.

Clinical Findings

An episode of gross hematuria is the most common presenting symptom. Frequently, this is associated with a mucosal viral infection such as an upper respiratory infection. The urine becomes red or smokey-colored 1–2 days after illness onset—a so-called "synpharyngitic" presentation in contradistinction to the latent period seen in postinfectious glomerulonephritis. IgA nephropathy can present anywhere along the nephritic spectrum from asymptomatic microscopic hematuria to RPGN. Rarely, nephrotic syndrome can be present as well.

There are no serologic tests that aid in this diagnosis; serum IgA subclass 1 testing may be a possibility in the future. Serum complements are normal. The typical pattern of injury seen on kidney biopsy is a focal glomerulonephritis with mesangial proliferation; immunofluorescence demonstrates diffuse mesangial IgA and C3 deposits.

Treatment

The disease course of primary IgA nephrology varies widely among patients; treatment approach needs to be tailored to risk for progression. Patients with low risk for progression (no hypertension, normal GFR, minimal proteinuria) can be monitored annually. Patients at higher risk (proteinuria > 1.0 g/d, decreased GFR, or hypertension or any combination of these three conditions) should be treated with an ACE inhibitor or ARB. Therapy should be titrated to reduce proteinuria to < 1 g/d and to control blood pressure in the range of 125/75 mm Hg to 130/80 mm Hg. Corticosteroids may be beneficial in patients with GFR > 50 mL/min/1.73 m² and persistent proteinuria > 1 g/d despite a 3- to 6-month trial of an ACE inhibitor or ARB. One such regimen (methylprednisolone, 1 g/d intravenously for 3 days during months 1, 3, and 5, plus prednisone in a dosage of 0.5 mg/kg orally every other day for 6 months) showed a 2% doubling of creatinine after 6 years in the treatment group versus a 21% doubling of creatinine in the control group. For the rare patient with IgA neuropathy and a rapidly progressive clinical course with crescent formation on biopsy, cyclophosphamide and corticosteroid therapy should be considered (see section on ANCA-associated vasculitis below). Kidney transplantation is an excellent option for patients with ESRD, but recurrent disease has been documented in 30% of patients 5–10 years posttransplant. Fortunately, recurrent disease rarely leads to failure of the allograft.

Prognosis

Approximately one-third of patients experience spontaneous clinical remission. Progression to ESRD occurs in 20–40% of patients. The remaining patients have chronic microscopic hematuria and a stable serum creatinine. The most unfavorable prognostic indicator is proteinuria > 1 g/d; other unfavorable prognostic indicators include hypertension, tubulointerstitial fibrosis, glomerulosclerosis, or glomerular crescents on biopsy, and abnormal GFR on presentation.

Beck L et al. KDOQI US commentary on the 2012 KDIGO clinical practice guideline for glomerulonephritis. Am J Kidney Dis. 2013 Sep;62(3):421–24. [PMID: 23871408]
Wyatt RJ et al. IgA nephropathy. N Engl J Med. 2013 Jun 20;368(25):2402–14. [PMID: 23782179]

3. HENOCH-SCHÖNLEIN PURPURA

Henoch-Schönlein purpura is a systemic small-vessel leukocytoclastic vasculitis associated with IgA subclass 1 deposition in vessel walls. It is most common in children and is often associated with an inciting infection, such as group A streptococcus or other exposure. There is a male predominance. It classically presents with palpable purpura in the lower extremities and buttock area; arthralgias; and abdominal symptoms, such as nausea, colic, and melena. A decrease in GFR is common with a nephritic presentation. The renal lesions can be identical to those found in IgA nephropathy, and the underlying pathophysiology appears to be similar. Most patients with microscopic hematuria and minimal proteinuria recover fully over several weeks. Progressive CKD and possibly

ESRD are more likely to develop in those with the nephrotic syndrome and the presence of both nephritic and nephrotic syndrome poses the worst renal prognosis. Histologic classification of the lesions in children may also provide prognostic information. To date, although several treatment regimens of various immunosuppressive agents have been clinically tested, none have been definitively proven to alter the course of severe Henoch-Schönlein purpura nephritis. Rituximab treatment and plasma exchange have been successful for severe disease according to several case reports, but clinical trials are lacking. Rapidly progressive disease with crescent formation on biopsy may be treated as in ANCA-associated vasculitis (see section below).

Further details about Henoch-Schönlein purpura are provided in Chapter 20.

Beck L et al. KDOQI US commentary on the 2012 KDIGO clinical practice guideline for glomerulonephritis. Am J Kidney Dis. 2013 Sep;62(3):424–25. [PMID: 23871408]

4. PAUCI-IMMUNE GLOMERULONEPHRITIS (ANCA-ASSOCIATED)

Pauci-immune necrotizing glomerulonephritis is caused by the following systemic ANCA-associated small-vessel vasculitides: granulomatosis with polyangiitis (formerly known as Wegener granulomatosis), microscopic polyangiitis, and Churg-Strauss disease (see Chapter 20). ANCA-associated glomerulonephritis can also present as a primary renal lesion without systemic involvement; this is termed "idiopathic crescentic glomerulonephritis." The pathogenesis of these entities appears to involve cytokine-primed neutrophils presenting cytoplasmic antigens on their surfaces (proteinase 3 and myeloperoxidase). Circulating ANCAs then bind to these antigens and activate a neutrophil respiratory burst with consequent vascular damage. Putative environmental exposures that may encite the initial response include S aureus and silica. Immunofluorescence of kidney biopsy specimens do not reveal any evidence of immunoglobulin or complement deposition, hence the term "pauci-immune." Renal involvement classically presents as an RPGN, but more indolent presentations can be seen as well.

► Clinical Findings

A. Symptoms and Signs

Symptoms of a systemic inflammatory disease, including fever, malaise, and weight loss may be present and usually precede initial presentation by several months. In addition to hematuria and proteinuria from glomerular inflammation, some patients exhibit purpura from dermal capillary involvement and mononeuritis multiplex from nerve arteriolar involvement. Ninety percent of patients with granulomatosis with polyangiitis have upper (especially sinus) or lower respiratory tract symptoms with nodular lesions that can cavitate and bleed. Hemoptysis is a concerning sign and usually warrants hospitalization and aggressive immunosuppression.

B. Laboratory Findings

Serologically, ANCA subtype analysis is done to determine whether antiproteinase-3 antibodies (PR3-ANCA) or anti-myeloperoxidase antibodies (MPO-ANCA) are present. Most patients with granulomatosis with polyangiitis are PR3 positive; the remainder are MPO positive or, more rarely, do not demonstrate ANCA serologically. Microscopic angiitis is generally associated with MPO ANCA. Renal biopsy demonstrates necrotizing lesions and crescents on light microscopy; immunofluorescence is negative for immune complex deposition.

► Treatment

Treatment should be instituted early if aggressive disease is present. Induction therapy of high-dose corticosteroids (methylprednisolone, 1–2 g/d intravenously for 3 days, followed by prednisone, 1 mg/kg orally for 1 month, with a slow taper over the next 6 months) and cytotoxic agents (cyclophosphamide, 0.5–1 g/m^2 intravenously per month or 1.5–2 mg/kg orally for 3–6 months) is followed by long-term azathioprine or mycophenolate mofetil. Rituximab has been shown to be noninferior to cyclophosphamide for induction. Plasma exchange has been shown to be beneficial in conjunction with induction therapy; however, a 2011 meta-analysis calls into question the strength of this benefit. Patients receiving cyclophosphamide should receive prophylaxis for Pneumocystis jirovecii, such as trimethoprim-sulfamethoxazole double-strength orally 3 days per week.

► Prognosis

Without treatment, prognosis is extremely poor. However, with aggressive treatment, complete remission can be achieved in about 75% of patients. Prognosis depends on the extent of renal involvement before treatment is started and may be worse in those with PR3-associated disease. ANCA titers may be monitored to follow treatment efficacy; rising titers may herald relapse.

Beck L et al. KDOQI US commentary on the 2012 KDIGO clinical practice guideline for glomerulonephritis. Am J Kidney Dis. 2013 Sep;62(3):429–33. [PMID: 23871408]

Kallenberg CG et al. Pathogenesis of ANCA-associated vasculitis: new possibilities for intervention. Am J Kidney Dis. 2013 Dec;62(6):1176–87. [PMID: 23810690]

Sinico RA et al. Renal involvement in anti-neutrophil cytoplasmic autoantibody associated vasculitis. Autoimmun Rev. 2013 Feb;12(4):477–82. [PMID: 22921791]

Tesar V et al. ANCA-associated renal vasculitis—an update. Contrib Nephrol. 2013;181:216–28. [PMID: 23689583]

5. ANTI-GLOMERULAR BASEMENT MEMBRANE GLOMERULONEPHRITIS & GOODPASTURE SYNDROME

Goodpasture syndrome is defined by the clinical constellation of glomerulonephritis and pulmonary hemorrhage; injury to both is mediated by antibodies to epitopes in the GBM (Figure 22–5). Up to one-third of patients with anti-GBM glomerulonephritis have no evidence of concomitant lung injury (anti-GBM disease). Anti-GBM–associated glomerulonephritis accounts for 10–20% of patients with acute RPGN. The incidence peaks in the second and third decades of life during which time males are predominantly affected and lung involvement is more common, and again in the sixth and seventh decades with less gender predominance. Lung involvement has been associated with pulmonary infection, tobacco use, and hydrocarbon solvent exposure; HLA-DR2 and -B7 antigens may predispose as well.

▶ Clinical Findings

A. Symptoms and Signs

The onset of disease may be preceded by an upper respiratory tract infection; hemoptysis, dyspnea, and possible respiratory failure may ensue. Other findings are consistent with an RPGN, although some cases may present with much milder forms of the nephritic spectrum of disease (eg, glomerular hematuria and proteinuria with minimal renal dysfunction).

B. Laboratory Findings

Chest radiographs may demonstrate pulmonary infiltrates if pulmonary hemorrhage is present. Serum complement levels are normal. Circulating anti-GBM antibodies are present in over 90% of patients. A small percentage of patients also have elevated ANCA titers; these patients should be treated with plasma exchange as for anti-GBM disease. Kidney biopsy typically shows crescent formation on light microscopy, with linear IgG staining along the GBM on immunofluorescence.

▶ Treatment

Treatment is a combination of plasma exchange therapy to remove circulating antibodies, and administration of immunosuppressive drugs to prevent formation of new antibodies and control the inflammatory response. Corticosteroids are typically given initially in pulse doses of methylprednisolone, 1–2 g/d for 3 days, then prednisone orally 1 mg/kg/d. Cyclophosphamide is administered intravenously at a dose of 0.5–1 g/m^2 per month or orally at a dosage of 2–3 mg/kg/d. Daily plasma exchange is performed for up to 2 weeks. Patients with oliguria and a serum creatinine > 6–7 mg/dL, or who require dialysis upon presentation have a poor prognosis. Anti-GBM antibody titers should decrease as the clinical course improves.

Beck L et al. KDOQI US commentary on the 2012 KDIGO clinical practice guideline for glomerulonephritis. Am J Kidney Dis. 2013 Sep;62(3):433–34. [PMID: 23871408]
Dammacco F et al. Goodpasture's disease: a report of ten cases and a review of the literature. Autoimmun Rev. 2013 Sep;12(11):1101–8. [PMID: 23806563]

6. CRYOGLOBULIN-ASSOCIATED GLOMERULONEPHRITIS

Essential (mixed) cryoglobulinemia is a vasculitis associated with cold-precipitable immunoglobulins (cryoglobulins). The most common underlying etiology is HCV

infection; in these cases, there is clonal expansion of B lymphocytes, which produce IgM rheumatoid factor. Rheumatoid factor, HCV antigen and polyclonal anti-HCV IgG form complexes that deposit in vessels and incite inflammation. Other overt or occult infections (eg, viral, bacterial, and fungal) as well as some connective tissue diseases can also be causative.

Patients exhibit purpuric and necrotizing skin lesions in dependent areas, arthralgias, fever, and hepatosplenomegaly. Serum complement levels are depressed. Rheumatoid factor is often elevated when cryoglobulins are present. Kidney biopsy may show several different patterns of injury; there may be crescent formation, glomerular capillary thrombi, or MPGN (see below). Treatment consists of aggressively targeting the causative infection. Pulse corticosteroids, plasma exchange, rituximab and cytotoxic agents have been used when risk of exacerbating the underlying infection is resolved, or when no infection is present. See also section on Hepatitis C Virus–Associated Renal Disease.

De Vita S et al. A randomized controlled trial of rituximab for the treatment of severe cryoglobulinemic vasculitis. Arthritis Rheum. 2012 Mar;64(3):843–53. [PMID: 22147661]
Terrier B et al. Cryoglobulinemia vasculitis: an update. Curr Opin Rheumatol. 2013 Jan;25(1):10–8. [PMID: 23196322]

7. MEMBRANOPROLIFERATIVE GLOMERULONEPHRITIS & C3 GLOMERULOPATHIES

MPGN is a relatively rare pattern of glomerular injury that can be caused by a wide range of known etiologies or can be idiopathic. Clinically, it can present anywhere along the nephritic spectrum from asymptomatic glomerular hematuria to acute nephritic syndrome with bouts of gross hematuria, to RPGN; nephrotic syndrome can also be seen. Traditionally, MPGN has been classified into several histologic subtypes; this classification is now in evolution. Type I is relatively more common and can be idiopathic (especially in children and young adults) or secondary to chronic infection (most commonly HCV), a paraproteinemia, or an underlying autoimmune disease such as lupus. The pathogenesis is likely a chronic antigenemia leading to classical complement pathway activation with immune complex deposition; however, it is now recognized that some cases may result from alternative complement pathway dysregulation. Type II MPGN is caused by several inherited or acquired abnormalities in the alternative complement pathway. Both types result in low circulating C3 complement; immune complex type I also has low C4. Light microscopy of both types shows varying degrees of mesangial hypercellularity, endocapillary proliferation and capillary wall remodeling resulting in double contours of the GBM ("tram track" appearance). Immunofluorescence and electron microscopy provide distinguishing information. Type II MPGN reveals C3 deposition without immunoglobulin staining on immunofluorescence, and electron microscopy demonstrates thick ribbon-like electron dense deposits along the GBM; thus, type II disease is also known as "dense deposit disease." Conversely, type I MPGN has scattered subendothelial and subepithelial deposits on electron microscopy. When there is immunoglobulin and C3 staining on immunofluorescence in type I MPGN, it is also called immune complex MPGN (more common type); when a type I case demonstrates only C3 staining on immunofluorescence, it is now termed C3 glomerulonephritis (C3 GN). Together, dense deposit disease (type II) and C3 GN are now termed "C3 glomerulopathies"; both result from inherited or acquired alternative complement dysregulation/activation.

Treatment of type I immune complex MPGN should be directed at the underlying cause, if such is found. Treatment of idiopathic immune complex disease is controversial and controlled trial data are lacking. For those with nephrotic syndrome and declining GFR, a combination of oral cyclophosphamide or mycophenolate mofetil plus corticosteroids could be considered; patients with RPGN and crescents on biopsy may be treated the same as those with ANCA-associated disease provided secondary causes have been ruled out. Despite therapy, most will progress to ESRD. Treatment for the C3 glomerulopathies is in evolution as novel therapies to target the dysregulated alternative complement cascade are being explored. Less favorable prognostic findings include type II/dense deposit disease, early decline in GFR, hypertension, and persistent nephrotic syndrome. All types of MPGN recur with high frequency after renal transplantation; however, type II recurs more commonly. Plasma exchange has been used with mixed results to treat posttransplant recurrence of MPGN.

Appel GB. Membranoproliferative glomerulonephritis—mechanisms and treatment. Contrib Nephrol. 2013;181:163–74. [PMID: 23689578]
Beck L et al. KDOQI US commentary on the 2012 KDIGO clinical practice guideline for glomerulonephritis. Am J Kidney Dis. 2013 Sep;62(3):417–19. [PMID: 23871408]
Bomback AS et al. Pathogenesis of the C3 glomerulopathies and reclassification of MPGN. Nat Rev Nephrol. 2012 Nov;8(11):634–42. [PMID: 23026947]

8. HEPATITIS C VIRUS–ASSOCIATED RENAL DISEASE

Renal disease can occur in the setting of HCV infection. The three patterns of renal injury associated with HCV are secondary MPGN (type I disease), cryoglobulinemic glomerulonephritis, and membranous nephropathy—the former is the most common lesion seen. The clinical presentation is dictated by the underlying pattern of injury. Many patients have elevated serum transaminases and an elevated rheumatoid factor. Hypocomplementemia is very common, with C4 typically more reduced than C3; complement levels and rheumatoid factor tend to be normal if there is a membranous pattern of injury.

▶ Treatment

In patients with HCV–associated MPGN not receiving treatment for liver disease, the main indications for therapy are poor renal function, nephrotic syndrome, new or worsening hypertension, tubulointerstitial disease on biopsy, and progressive disease. IFN-alpha may result in suppression of viremia and improvement in hepatic function. Renal function rarely improves unless viral suppression occurs, and renal function often worsens when therapy is stopped. Ribavirin is relatively contraindicated in kidney disease because of the dose-related hemolysis that occurs with impaired GFR. Despite this, some case series have shown benefit with combined IFN-alpha and ribavirin in closely monitored settings. Early case reports suggest that addition of the newer protease inhibitors may be safe and effective for treating HCV-related renal disease. Rituximab may be considered in addition to antiviral therapy, though controlled trials are lacking.

Fabrizi F et al. Hepatitis C virus infection, mixed cryoglobulinemia, and kidney disease. Am J Kidney Dis. 2013 Apr;61(4):623–37. [PMID: 23102733]
Tang SC et al. Hepatitis C virus-associated glomerulonephritis. Contrib Nephrol. 2013;181:194–206. [PMID: 23689581]

9. SYSTEMIC LUPUS ERYTHEMATOSUS

Renal involvement in SLE is very common, with estimates ranging from 35% to 90%—the higher estimates encompassing subclinical disease. Rates of lupus nephritis are highest in non-whites. The pathogenesis may be dysregulated cellular apoptosis resulting in autoantibodies against nucleosomes; antibody/nucleosome complexes then bind to components of the glomerulus to form immune complex glomerular disease.

The term "lupus nephritis" encompasses many possible patterns of renal injury—most cases present within the nephritic spectrum (class I–IV). Nonglomerular syndromes include tubulointerstitial nephritis and vasculitis. All patients with SLE should have routine urinalyses to monitor for the appearance of hematuria or proteinuria. If urinary abnormalities are detected, kidney biopsy is often performed. The 2003 International Society of Nephrology and Renal Pathology Society (ISN/RPS) classification of renal glomerular lesions is class I, minimal mesangial nephritis; class II, mesangial proliferative nephritis; class III, focal (< 50% of glomeruli affected with capillary involvement) proliferative nephritis; class IV, diffuse (> 50% of glomeruli affected with capillary involvement) proliferative nephritis; class V, membranous nephropathy; and class VI, advanced sclerosis without residual disease activity. Classes III and IV, the most severe forms of lupus nephritis, are further classified as active or chronic, and global or segmental, which confers additional prognostic value.

▶ Treatment

Individuals with **class I** and **class II lesions** generally require no treatment; corticosteroids or calcineurin inhibitors should be considered for those with class II lesions with nephrotic-range proteinuria. Transformation of these types to a more active lesion may occur and is usually accompanied by an increase in lupus serologic activity (eg, rising titers of anti-double-stranded DNA antibodies and falling C3 and C4 levels) and increasing proteinuria or falling GFR. Repeat biopsy in such patients is recommended. Some experts recommend hydroxychloroquine treatment in all patients with lupus nephritis, regardless of histological class. Patients with extensive **class III lesions** and all **class IV lesions** should receive aggressive immunosuppressive therapy. The features signifying the poorest prognosis in patients with class III or IV lesions include elevated serum creatinine, lower complement levels, male sex, presence of antiphospholipid antibodies, nephrotic-range proteinuria, black race (possibly in association with *APOL1* risk alleles), and poor response to therapy. Immunosuppressive therapy for class V lupus nephritis is indicated if superimposed proliferative lesions exist. Class VI lesions should not be treated.

Treatment of **class III or IV lupus nephritis** consists of induction therapy, followed by maintenance treatment. All induction therapy includes corticosteroids (eg, methylprednisolone 1 g intravenously daily for 3 days followed by prednisone, 1 mg/kg orally daily with subsequent taper over 6–12 months) in combination with either cyclophosphamide or mycophenolate mofetil. Data suggest that blacks and Hispanics respond more favorably to mycophenolate mofetil rather than cyclophosphamide; in addition, mycophenolate mofetil has a more favorable side-effect profile than cyclophosphamide and should be favored when preservation of fertility is a consideration. Mycophenolate mofetil induction is typically given at 2–3 g/d, then tapered to 1–2 g/d for maintenance. Cyclophosphamide induction regimens vary but usually involve monthly intravenous pulse doses (500–1000 mg/m²) for 6 months. Induction is followed by daily oral mycophenolate mofetil or azathioprine maintenance therapy; mycophenolate mofetil may be superior to azathioprine maintenance and causes few adverse effects. Maintenance with calcineurin inhibitors may also be considered, but the relapse rate is high upon discontinuation of these agents. With standard therapy, remission rates with induction vary from 80% for partial remission to 50–60% for full remission; it may take more than 6 months to see these effects. Relapse is common and rates of disease flare are higher in those who do not experience complete remission; similarly, progression to ESRD is more common in those who relapse more frequently, or in whom no remission has been achieved. Studies to assess safety and efficacy of newer biologic immunomodulatory drugs for lupus nephritis are ongoing.

The normalization of various laboratory tests (double-stranded DNA antibodies, serum C3, C4, CH$_{50}$ levels) can be useful in monitoring treatment. Urinary protein levels and sediment activity are also helpful markers. Patients with SLE who undergo dialysis have a favorable prospect for long-term survival; interestingly, systemic lupus symptoms may become quiescent with the development of ESRD. Patients with SLE undergoing kidney transplants can have recurrent renal disease, although rates are relatively low.

Beck L et al. KDOQI US commentary on the 2012 KDIGO clinical practice guideline for glomerulonephritis. Am J Kidney Dis. 2013 Sep;62(3):425–29. [PMID: 23871408]

Bose B et al. Ten common mistakes in the management of lupus nephritis. Am J Kidney Dis. 2013 Dec 11. [Epub ahead of print] [PMID: 24332767]

Hogan J et al. Update on the treatment of lupus nephritis. Curr Opin Nephrol Hypertens. 2013 Mar;22(2):224–30. [PMID: 23328501]

Lech M et al. The pathogenesis of lupus nephritis. J Am Soc Nephrol. 2013 Sep;24(9):1357–66. [PMID: 23929771]

NEPHROTIC SPECTRUM GLOMERULAR DISEASES

 ESSENTIALS OF DIAGNOSIS

► Bland urine sediment (few if any cells or cellular casts).

► Nephrotic syndrome consists of the following:
* Urine protein excretion > 3 g per 24 hours.
* Hypoalbuminemia (albumin < 3 g/dL).
* Peripheral edema.
* Hyperlipidemia.
* Oval fat bodies may be seen in the urine.

▶ General Considerations

In American adults, the most common cause of nephrotic spectrum glomerular disease is diabetes mellitus. Other causes of this presentation include minimal change disease, focal segmental glomerulosclerosis (FSGS), membranous nephropathy, and amyloidosis. Any of these entities can present on the less severe end of the spectrum with a bland urinalysis and proteinuria, or with the most severe presentation of the nephrotic *syndrome*. Serum creatinine may or may not be abnormal at the time of presentation, depending on the severity, acuity and chronicity of the disease.

▶ Clinical Findings

A. Symptoms and Signs

Patients with subnephrotic range proteinuria do not manifest symptoms of the renal disease. In those with the nephrotic syndrome, peripheral edema is present and is most likely due to sodium retention and, at albumin levels < 2 g/dL (20 g/L), arterial underfilling from low plasma oncotic pressure. Edema may present in dependent regions, such as the lower extremities, or it may become generalized and include periorbital edema. Dyspnea due to pulmonary edema, pleural effusions, and diaphragmatic compromise with ascites can occur.

B. Laboratory Findings

1. Urinalysis—Proteinuria occurs as a result of effacement of podocytes (foot processes) and an alteration of the negative charge of the GBM. The urinary dipstick is a good screening test for proteinuria; however, it only detects albumin. The addition of sulfosalicylic acid to the urine causes total protein to precipitate, allowing for the possible discovery of paraproteins (and albumin). A spot urine protein to urine creatinine ratio gives a reasonable approximation of grams of protein excreted per day; a 24-hour urine sample for protein excretion is rarely needed.

Microscopically, the urinary sediment has relatively few cellular elements or casts. However, if marked hyperlipidemia is present, urinary oval fat bodies may be seen. They appear as "grape clusters" under light microscopy and "Maltese crosses" under polarized light.

2. Blood chemistries—The nephrotic syndrome results in hypoalbuminemia (< 3 g/dL [30 g/L]) and hypoproteinemia (< 6 g/dL [60 g/L]). Hyperlipidemia occurs in over 50% of patients with early nephrotic syndrome, and becomes more frequent and worsens in degree as the severity of the nephrotic syndrome increases. A fall in oncotic pressure triggers increased hepatic production of lipids (cholesterol and apolipoprotein B). There is also decreased clearance of very low-density lipoproteins, causing hypertriglyceridemia. Patients may also have an elevated erythrocyte sedimentation rate as a result of alterations in some plasma components such as increased levels of fibrinogen. Patients may become deficient in vitamin D, zinc, and copper from loss of binding proteins in the urine.

Laboratory testing to determine the underlying cause may include complement levels, serum and urine protein electrophoresis, antinuclear antibodies, and serologic tests for viral hepatitides.

3. Kidney biopsy—Kidney biopsy is often performed in adults with new-onset idiopathic nephrotic syndrome if a primary renal disease that may require immunosuppressive therapy is suspected. Chronically and significantly decreased GFR indicates irreversible kidney disease mitigating the usefulness of kidney biopsy. In the setting of long-standing diabetes mellitus type 1 or 2, proteinuric renal disease is rarely biopsied unless atypical features (such as significant glomerular hematuria or cellular casts) are also present, or if there is other reason to suspect an additional renal lesion.

▶ **Treatment**

A. Protein Loss

In those with subnephrotic proteinuria or mild nephrotic syndrome, dietary protein restriction may be helpful in slowing progression of renal disease (see CKD section). In those with very heavy proteinuria (> 10 g/d) protein malnutrition may occur and daily protein intake should replace daily urinary protein losses.

In both diabetic and nondiabetic patients, therapy that is aimed at reducing proteinuria may also reduce progression of renal disease. ACE inhibitors and ARBs lower urine protein excretion by reducing glomerular capillary pressure; they also have antifibrotic effects. These agents can be used in patients with reduced GFR as long as significant hyperkalemia (potassium > 5.2–5.5 mEq/L) does not occur and serum creatinine rises < 30%; patients should be monitored closely to avoid acute kidney injury and hyperkalemia. A recent prospective, randomized multicenter study

to evaluate the combination of an ACE inhibitor and ARB versus ARB alone for slowing the progression of diabetic nephropathy was terminated early due to safety concerns in the dual therapy arm; such combination therapy cannot, therefore, be generally recommended.

B. Edema

Dietary salt restriction is essential for managing edema; most patients also require diuretic therapy. Both thiazide and loop diuretics are highly protein bound; therefore with hypoalbuminemia and decreased GFR, diuretic delivery to the kidney is reduced, and patients often require larger doses. A combination of loop and thiazide diuretics can potentiate the diuretic effect and may be needed for patients with refractory fluid retention.

C. Hyperlipidemia

Hypercholesterolemia and hypertriglyceridemia occur as noted above. Dietary modification and exercise should be advocated; however, effective lipid-lowering usually also requires pharmacologic treatment (see Chapter 28). Rhabdomyolysis, however, is more common in patients with CKD who take gemfibrozil in combination with statins; combining fenofibrate or niacin with a statin poses less risk.

D. Hypercoagulable State

Patients with serum albumin < 2 g/dL can become hypercoagulable. Nephrotic patients have urinary losses of antithrombin, protein C, and protein S and increased platelet activation. Patients are prone to renal vein thrombosis, pulmonary embolus, and other venous thromboemboli, particularly with membranous nephropathy. Anticoagulation therapy with warfarin is warranted for at least 3–6 months in patients with evidence of thrombosis in any location. Patients with renal vein thrombosis, pulmonary embolus, or recurrent thromboemboli require indefinite anticoagulation. After an initial clotting event, ongoing nephrotic syndrome poses a risk of thrombosis recurrence, and continued anticoagulation should be considered until resolution of the nephrotic syndrome.

▶ **When to Refer**

Any patient noted to have nephrotic syndrome should be referred immediately to a nephrologist for consideration of volume and blood pressure management, assessment for kidney biopsy, and treatment of the underlying disease. Proteinuria of > 1 g/d without the nephrotic syndrome also merits nephrology referral, though with less urgency.

▶ **When to Admit**

Patients with edema refractory to outpatient therapy or rapidly worsening kidney function that may require inpatient interventions should be admitted.

Cadnapaphornchai MA et al. The nephrotic syndrome: pathogenesis and treatment of edema formation and secondary complications. Pediatr Nephrol. 2013 Aug 30. [Epub ahead of print] [PMID: 23989393]

Gbadegesin RA et al. Genetic testing in nephrotic syndrome—challenges and opportunities. Nat Rev Nephrol. 2013 Mar;9(3):179–84. [PMID: 23321566]

Reiser J et al. Podocyte biology and pathogenesis of kidney disease. Annu Rev Med. 2013;64:357–66. [PMID: 23190150]

NEPHROTIC SPECTRUM DISEASE IN PRIMARY RENAL DISORDERS

MINIMAL CHANGE DISEASE

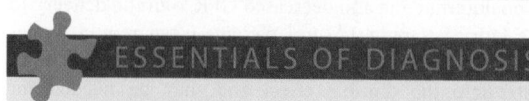

ESSENTIALS OF DIAGNOSIS

- ▶ Nephrotic-range proteinuria.
- ▶ Kidney biopsy shows no changes on light microscopy.
- ▶ Characteristic foot-process effacement on electron microscopy.

▶ General Considerations

Minimal change disease is the most common cause of proteinuric renal disease in children, accounting for about 80% of cases. It often remits upon treatment with a course of corticosteroids. Indeed, children with nephrotic syndrome are often treated for minimal change disease empirically without a biopsy diagnosis. Biopsy should be considered for children with nephrotic syndrome who exhibit unusual features (such as signs of other systemic illness), who are steroid-resistant (see below), or who relapse frequently upon withdrawal of corticosteroid therapy. Minimal change disease is less common in adults, accounting for 20–25% of cases of primary nephrotic syndrome in those over age 40 years. This entity can be idiopathic but also occurs following viral upper respiratory infections (especially in children), in association with neoplasms such as Hodgkin disease, with drugs (lithium), and with hypersensitivity reactions (especially to NSAIDs and bee stings).

▶ Clinical Findings

A. Symptoms and Signs

Patients often exhibit the manifestations of full-blown nephrotic syndrome. They are more susceptible to infection, have a tendency toward thromboembolic events, develop severe hyperlipidemia, and may experience protein malnutrition. Minimal change disease can rarely cause acute kidney injury due to tubular changes and interstitial edema.

B. Laboratory and Histologic Findings

There is no helpful serologic testing. Glomeruli show no changes on light microscopy or immunofluorescence. On electron microscopy, there is a characteristic effacement of podocyte foot processes. Mesangial cell proliferation may be seen in a subgroup of patients; this finding is associated with more hematuria and hypertension and poor response to standard corticosteroid treatment.

▶ Treatment

Treatment is with prednisone, 60 mg/m^2/d orally; remission in steroid-responsive minimal change disease generally occurs within 4–8 weeks. Adults often require longer courses of therapy than children, requiring up to 16 weeks to achieve a response. Treatment should be continued for several weeks after complete remission of proteinuria, and dosing tapers should be individualized. A significant number of patients will relapse and require repeated corticosteroid treatment. Patients with frequent relapses or corticosteroid resistance may require cyclophosphamide or a calcineurin inhibitor to induce subsequent remissions. Rituximab may also be considered in adults but appears less promising in children. Progression to ESRD is rare. Complications most often arise from prolonged corticosteroid use.

Beck L et al. KDOQI US commentary on the 2012 KDIGO clinical practice guideline for glomerulonephritis. Am J Kidney Dis. 2013 Sep;62(3):405–10. [PMID: 23871408]

Hogan J et al. The treatment of minimal change disease in adults. J Am Soc Nephrol. 2013 Apr;24(5):702–11. [PMID: 23431071]

MEMBRANOUS NEPHROPATHY

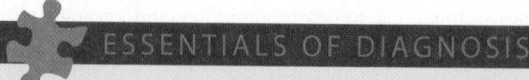

ESSENTIALS OF DIAGNOSIS

- ▶ Varying degrees of proteinuria, may have nephrotic syndrome.
- ▶ Associated with coagulopathy, eg, renal vein thrombosis, if nephrotic syndrome present.
- ▶ "Spike and dome" pattern on kidney biopsy from subepithelial deposits.
- ▶ Secondary causes notably include hepatitis B virus and carcinomas.

▶ General Considerations

Membranous nephropathy is the most common cause of primary nephrotic syndrome in adults and often presents in the fifth and sixth decades. It is an immune-mediated disease characterized by immune complex deposition in the subepithelial portion of glomerular capillary walls. The antigen in the primary form of the disease appears to be a phospholipase A$_2$ receptor (PLA$_2$R) on the podocyte in 70–80% of patients. Secondary disease is associated with underlying carcinomas; infections, such as hepatitis B and C, endocarditis, and syphilis; autoimmune disease, such as SLE, mixed connective tissue disease, and thyroiditis; and certain drugs, such as NSAIDs and captopril. The course of disease is variable, with about 50% of patients progressing to ESRD over 3–10 years. Poorer outcome is associated with concomitant tubulointerstitial fibrosis, male sex, elevated serum creatinine, hypertension, and heavy proteinuria (> 10 g/d).

Patients with membranous nephropathy and nephrotic syndrome have a higher risk of hypercoagulable state than those with nephrosis from other etiologies; there is a particular predisposition to renal vein thrombosis in these patients.

Clinical Findings

A. Symptoms and Signs

Patients may be asymptomatic or may have edema or frothy urine. Venous thrombosis, such as an unprovoked deep venous thrombosis may be an initial sign. There may be symptoms or signs of an underlying infection or neoplasm (especially lung, stomach, breast, and colon cancers) in secondary membranous nephropathy.

B. Laboratory Findings

See above for laboratory findings in the nephrotic syndrome. Evaluation for secondary causes including serologic testing for SLE, syphilis, viral hepatitides, and age- and risk-appropriate cancer screening should be performed. Serum evaluation for circulating PLA_2R antibodies to assess for idiopathic membranous nephropathy may be available in the future. By light microscopy, capillary wall thickness is increased without inflammatory changes or cellular proliferation; when stained with silver methenamine, a "spike and dome" pattern results from to projections of excess GBM between the subepithelial deposits. Immunofluorescence shows IgG and C3 staining along capillary loops. Electron microscopy shows a discontinuous pattern of dense deposits along the subepithelial surface of the basement membrane.

Treatment

Underlying causes must be excluded prior to consideration of treatment. Idiopathic/primary disease treatment depends on the risk of renal disease progression. Roughly 30% of patients present with subnephrotic proteinuria (< 3 g/d) and most have a good prognosis with conservative management, including antiproteinuric therapy with ACE inhibitor or ARB if blood pressure is > 125/75 mmHg. Spontaneous remission may develop even in those with heavy proteinuria (about 30% of cases). Thus, use of immunosuppressive agents should be limited to those at highest risk for progression and with salvageable renal function. Patients with nephrotic syndrome despite 6 months of conservative management and serum creatinine < 3.0 may elect therapy with corticosteroids and chlorambucil or cyclophosphamide for 6 months. Calcineurin inhibitors with or without corticosteroids may be considered as well. Uncontrolled trials with rituximab have shown benefit. Remission may take up to 6 months. Patients with primary membranous nephropathy are excellent candidates for transplant.

Beck L et al. KDOQI US commentary on the 2012 KDIGO clinical practice guideline for glomerulonephritis. Am J Kidney Dis. 2013 Sep;62(3):413–17. [PMID: 23871408]
Hofstra JM et al. Treatment of idiopathic membranous nephropathy. Nat Rev Nephrol. 2013 Aug;9(8):443–58. [PMID: 23820815]
Ma H et al. The role of complement in membranous nephropathy. Semin Nephrol. 2013 Nov;33(6):531–42. [PMID: 24161038]

FOCAL SEGMENTAL GLOMERULOSCLEROSIS

This is a relatively common renal pattern of injury resulting from damage to podocytes. The list of possible causes of podocyte injury is long and diverse and includes primary renal disease due to (1) heritable abnormalities in any of several podocyte proteins, (2) polymorphisms in the APOL1 gene in those of African descent, or (3) increased levels of soluble urokinase receptors or increased expression of CD80 (B7-1) on podocytes. Secondary FSGS may result from overwork injury, obesity, hypertension, chronic urinary reflux, HIV infection, or analgesic or bisphosphonate exposure. Clinically, patients present with proteinuria; 80% of children and 50% of adults have overt nephrotic syndrome in primary FSGS. Decreased GFR is present in 25–50% at time of diagnosis. Patients with FSGS and nephrotic syndrome typically progress to ESRD in 6–8 years. There is no helpful serologic testing.

Diagnosis requires kidney biopsy. Light microscopy shows sclerosis of portions (or segments) of some, but not all glomeruli (thus, focal and not diffuse disease). IgM and C3 are seen in the sclerotic lesions on immunofluorescence, although it is presumed that these immune components are simply trapped in the sclerotic glomeruli and are not pathogenic. Electron microscopy shows fusion of epithelial foot processes as seen in minimal change disease.

Treatment for primary FSGS should include conservative measures, such as diuretics for edema, ACE inhibitors or ARBs to target proteinuria and hypertension, and statins or niacin for hyperlipidemia. Those with primary disease and nephrotic syndrome may benefit from high-dose oral prednisone (1 mg/kg/d) for 4–16 weeks followed by a slow taper; this may induce remission within 5–9 months in over half of patients. In those with steroid-resistance or intolerance, calcineurin inhibitors and mycophenolate mofetil can be considered. Patients with primary FSGS who progress to ESRD and undergo renal transplantation risk a relatively high relapse rate and graft loss; plasma exchange therapy, and possibly rituximab, just prior to transplant and with early signs of relapse appears to be beneficial.

Beck L et al. KDOQI US commentary on the 2012 KDIGO clinical practice guideline for glomerulonephritis. Am J Kidney Dis. 2013 Sep;62(3):410–13. [PMID: 23871408]
Bose B et al. Glomerular diseases: FSGS. Clin J Am Soc Nephrol. 2013 Aug 29. [Epub ahead of print] [PMID: 23990165]
Ponticelli C et al. Current and emerging treatments for idiopathic focal and segmental glomerulosclerosis in adults. Expert Rev Clin Immunol. 2013 Mar;9(3):251–61. [PMID: 23445199]

NEPHROTIC SPECTRUM DISEASE FROM SYSTEMIC DISORDERS

AMYLOIDOSIS

Amyloidosis is caused by extracellular deposition of an abnormally folded protein (amyloid). There are several different proteins that have the potential to form amyloid fibrils. The most common is AL amyloid, due to a plasma cell dyscrasia, in which the protein is a monoclonal Ig light chain; this is also known as primary amyloid disease. Secondary amyloid disease is a result of a chronic inflammatory disease such as rheumatoid arthritis, inflammatory bowel disease, or chronic infection. In these cases, there is deposition of the acute phase reactant serum amyloid A protein, termed "AA amyloid disease." Proteinuria, decreased GFR, and the nephrotic syndrome are presenting symptoms and signs; evidence of other organ involvement is not uncommon in these cases. Serum and urine protein electrophoresis should be done as a screening test; if a monoclonal spike is found, serum free light chains should be quantified. Amyloid-affected kidneys are often enlarged (> 10 cm). Pathologically, glomeruli are filled with amorphous deposits that show green birefringence with Congo red staining.

Treatment options are few. Remissions can occur in AA amyloidosis if the underlying disease is treated. AL amyloidosis progresses to ESRD in an average of 2–3 years. Five-year overall survival is < 20%, with death occurring from ESRD and heart disease. The use of alkylating agents and corticosteroids—eg, melphalan and prednisone—can reduce proteinuria and improve renal function in a small percentage of patients. New therapies, including the proteosome inhibitor bortezomib, may hold promise but data from controlled trials are lacking. Significant reduction in serum free light chain burden (> 90%) has been shown to correlate with improved renal outcomes. Melphalan and stem cell transplantation are associated with high toxicity (45% mortality) but induce remission in 80% of the remaining patients; however, few patients are eligible for this treatment. Renal transplant is an option in patients with AA amyloid.

Gertz MA. Immunoglobulin light chain amyloidosis: 2013 update on diagnosis, prognosis, and treatment. Am J Hematol. 2013 May;88(5):416–25. [PMID: 23605846]

Gillmore JD et al. Pathophysiology and treatment of systemic amyloidosis. Nat Rev Nephrol. 2013 Oct;9(10):574–86. [PMID: 23979488]

Venner CP et al. Cyclophosphamide, bortezomib, and dexamethasone therapy in AL amyloidosis is associated with high clonal response rates and prolonged progression-free survival. Blood. 2012 May 10;119(19):4387–90. [PMID: 22331187]

DIABETIC NEPHROPATHY

ESSENTIALS OF DIAGNOSIS

- ▶ Prior evidence of diabetes mellitus, typically over 10 years.
- ▶ Albuminuria usually precedes decline in GFR.
- ▶ Other end-organ damage, such as retinopathy, is common.

▶ General Considerations

Diabetic nephropathy is the most common cause of ESRD in the United States. Type 1 diabetes mellitus carries a 30–40% risk of nephropathy after 20 years, whereas type 2 has a 15–20% risk after 20 years. ESRD is much more likely to develop in persons with type 1 diabetes mellitus, in part due to fewer comorbidities and deaths before ESRD ensues. With the current epidemic of obesity and type 2 diabetes mellitus, rates of diabetic nephropathy are projected to continue to increase. Patients at higher risk include males, African Americans, Native Americans, and those with a positive family history. Mortality rates are higher for diabetics with kidney disease compared to those without CKD.

▶ Clinical Findings

Diabetic nephropathy develops about 10 years after the onset of diabetes mellitus. It may be present at the time type 2 diabetes mellitus is diagnosed. The first stage of diabetic nephropathy is hyperfiltration with an increase in GFR, followed by the development of microalbuminuria (30–300 mg/d). With progression, albuminuria increases to > 300 mg/d and can be detected on a urine dipstick as overt proteinuria; the GFR subsequently declines over time. Yearly screening for microalbuminuria is recommended for all diabetic patients to detect disease at its earliest stage; however, diabetic nephropathy can, less commonly result in nonproteinuric CKD.

The most common lesion in diabetic nephropathy is diffuse glomerulosclerosis, but nodular glomerulosclerosis (Kimmelstiel-Wilson nodules) is pathognomonic. The kidneys are usually enlarged as a result of cellular hypertrophy and proliferation. Kidney biopsy is not required in most patients, though, unless atypical findings are present, such as sudden onset of proteinuria, nephritic spectrum features (see above), massive proteinuria (>10 g/d), urinary cellular casts, or rapid decline in GFR.

Patients with diabetes are prone to other renal diseases. These include papillary necrosis, chronic interstitial nephritis, and type 4 (hyporeninemic hypoaldosteronemic) renal tubular acidosis. Patients are more susceptible to acute kidney injury from many insults, including intravenous contrast material and concomitant use of an ACE inhibitor or ARBs with NSAIDs.

▶ Treatment

With the onset of microalbuminuria, aggressive treatment is necessary. Strict glycemic control should be emphasized early in diabetic nephropathy, with recognition of risk of hypoglycemia as CKD becomes advanced (see CKD section). Treatment of hypertension to a goal of 130/80 mm Hg in most patients, and 125/75 mm Hg in overtly proteinuric patients also slows progression. ACE inhibitors and ARBs in those with microalbuminuria lower the rate of progression to overt proteinuria and slow progression to ESRD by reducing intraglomerular pressure and via antifibrotic effects. Even in patients with markedly diminished GFR, these agents may provide benefit; close monitoring for hyperkalemia or a decline in GFR more than 30% with the initiation or uptitration of this therapy is required. The NEPHRON-D trial, in which patients with diabetic nephropathy were randomized to combination ARB and ACE inhibitor therapy or ARB and placebo, was stopped early due to lack of efficacy and increased adverse events of hyperkalemia and acute kidney injury in the combination group. Treatment of other cardiovascular risk factors and obesity is crucial. Many with diabetes have multiple comorbid conditions; therefore, in patients undergoing dialysis who progress to ESRD, mortality over the first 5 years is high. Patients who are relatively healthy, however, benefit from renal transplantation.

Appel G. Detecting and controlling diabetic nephropathy: what do we know? Cleve Clin J Med. 2013 Apr;80(4):209–17. [PMID: 23547091]

Forbes JM et al. Mechanisms of diabetic complications. Physiol Rev. 2013 Jan;93(1):137–88. [PMID: 23303908]

Fried LF et al; VA NEPHRON-D Investigators. Combined angiotensin inhibition for the treatment of diabetic nephropathy. N Engl J Med. 2013 Nov 14;369(20):1892–903. [PMID: 24206457]

HIV-ASSOCIATED NEPHROPATHY

HIV-associated nephropathy usually presents as the nephrotic syndrome and declining GFR in patients with HIV infection. Most patients are of African descent, likely due to the now recognized association of *APOL1* polymorphisms with increased risk for HIV-associated nephropathy. Often, patients have low CD4 counts and have AIDS, but HIV-associated nephropathy can also be the initial presentation of HIV disease. Patients with HIV are at risk for renal disease other than HIV-associated nephropathy (eg, toxicity from highly active antiretroviral therapy [HAART], vascular disease, and diabetes, or an immune complex–mediated glomerular disease); such diseases tend to be nonnephrotic.

Kidney biopsy shows a focal segmental glomerulosclerosis pattern of injury (described above) with glomerular collapse; severe tubulointerstitial damage may also be present.

HIV-associated nephropathy is becoming less common in the era of HIV screening and more effective antiretroviral therapy. Small, uncontrolled studies have shown that HAART slows progression of disease. ACE inhibitors or ARBs can be used to control blood pressure and slow disease progression. Corticosteroid treatment has been used with variable success at a dosage of 1 mg/kg/d, along with cyclosporine. Patients who progress to ESRD and are otherwise healthy are good candidates for renal transplantation.

Maggi P et al. Renal complications in HIV disease: between present and future. AIDS Rev. 2012 Jan–Mar;14(1):37–53. [PMID: 22297503]

Yahaya I et al. Interventions for HIV-associated nephropathy. Cochrane Database Syst Rev. 2013 Jan 31;1:CD007183. [PMID: 23440812]

▼ TUBULOINTERSTITIAL DISEASES

Tubulointerstitial disease may be acute or chronic. Acute disease is most commonly associated with medications, infectious agents, and systemic rheumatologic disorders. Interstitial edema, infiltration with polymorphonuclear neutrophils, and tubular cell necrosis can be seen. (See Acute Kidney Injury, above, and Table 22–10.) Chronic

Table 22–10. Causes of acute tubulointerstitial nephritis (abbreviated list).

Drug reactions
Antibiotics
Beta-lactam antibiotics: methicillin, penicillin, ampicillin, cephalosporins
Ciprofloxacin
Erythromycin
Sulfonamides
Tetracycline
Vancomycin
Trimethoprim-sulfamethoxazole
Ethambutol
Rifampin
Nonsteroidal anti-inflammatory drugs
Diuretics
Thiazides
Furosemide
Miscellaneous
Allopurinol
Cimetidine
Phenytoin
Systemic infections
Bacteria
Streptococcus
Corynebacterium diphtheriae
Legionella
Viruses
Epstein-Barr
Others
Mycoplasma
Rickettsia rickettsii
Leptospira icterohaemorrhagiae
Toxoplasma
Idiopathic
Tubulointerstitial nephritis-uveitis (TIN–U)

disease is associated with insults from an acute factor or progressive insults without any obvious acute cause. Interstitial fibrosis and tubular atrophy are present, with a mononuclear cell predominance. The chronic disorders are described below.

CHRONIC TUBULOINTERSTITIAL DISEASES

ESSENTIALS OF DIAGNOSIS

► Kidney size is small and contracted.
► Decreased urinary concentrating ability.
► Hyperchloremic metabolic acidosis.
► Reduced GFR.

► General Considerations

The primary causes of chronic tubulointerstitial disease are discussed below. Other causes include multiple myeloma and gout, which are discussed in the section on multisystem disease with variable kidney involvement.

The most common cause of chronic tubulointerstitial disease is **obstructive uropathy** from prolonged obstruction of the urinary tract. The major causes are prostatic disease in men; ureteral calculus in a single functioning kidney; bilateral ureteral calculi; carcinoma of the cervix, colon, or bladder; and retroperitoneal tumors or fibrosis.

Reflux nephropathy from **vesicoureteral reflux** is primarily a disorder of childhood and occurs when urine passes retrograde from the bladder to the kidneys during voiding. It is the second most common cause of chronic tubulointerstitial disease. It occurs as a result of an incompetent vesicoureteral sphincter. Urine can extravasate into the interstitium; an inflammatory response develops, and fibrosis occurs. The inflammatory response is due to either bacteria or normal urinary components.

Analgesic nephropathy is most commonly seen in patients who ingest large quantities of analgesic combinations. The drugs of concern are phenacetin, paracetamol, aspirin, and NSAIDs, with acetaminophen a possible but less certain culprit. Ingestion of at least 1 g/d for 3 years of these analgesics is considered necessary for kidney dysfunction to develop. This disorder occurs most frequently in individuals who are using analgesics for chronic headaches, muscular pains, and arthritis. Most patients grossly underestimate their analgesic use.

Tubulointerstitial inflammation and papillary necrosis are seen on pathologic examination. Papillary tip and inner medullary concentrations of some analgesics are tenfold higher than in the renal cortex. Phenacetin—once a common cause of this disorder and now rarely available—is metabolized in the papillae by the prostaglandin hydroperoxidase pathway to reactive intermediates that bind covalently to interstitial cell macromolecules, causing necrosis. Aspirin and other NSAIDs can cause damage by their metabolism to active intermediates which can result in cell necrosis. These drugs also decrease medullary blood flow (via inhibition of prostaglandin synthesis) and decrease glutathione levels, which are necessary for detoxification.

Environmental exposure to **heavy metals**—such as lead, cadmium, mercury, and bismuth—is seen infrequently now in the United States but can cause tubulointerstitial disease. Individuals at risk for lead-induced tubulointerstitial disease are those with occupational exposure (eg, welders who work with lead-based paint) and drinkers of alcohol distilled in automobile radiators ("moonshine" whiskey users). Lead is filtered by the glomerulus and is transported across the proximal convoluted tubules, where it accumulates and causes cell damage. Fibrosed arterioles and cortical scarring also lead to damaged kidneys. The proximal tubular dysfunction from cadmium exposure can cause hypercalciuria and nephrolithiasis.

▶ Clinical Findings

A. General Findings

Polyuria is common because tubular damage leads to inability to concentrate the urine. Volume depletion can also occur as a result of a salt-wasting defect in some individuals.

Patients can become hyperkalemic both because the GFR is lower and the distal tubules become aldosterone resistant. A hyperchloremic renal tubular acidosis is characteristic from a component of type 4 or type 1 renal tubular acidosis. Less commonly, a proximal renal tubular acidosis is seen due to direct proximal tubular damage. The cause of the renal tubular acidosis is threefold: (1) reduced ammonia production, (2) inability to acidify the distal tubules, and (3) proximal tubular bicarbonate wasting. The urinalysis is nonspecific, as opposed to that seen in acute interstitial nephritis. Proteinuria is typically < 2 g/d (owing to inability of the proximal tubule to reabsorb freely filterable proteins); a few cells may be seen; and broad waxy casts are often present.

B. Specific Findings

1. Obstructive uropathy—In partial obstruction, patients can exhibit polyuria (possibly due to vasopressin insensitivity and poor ability to concentrate the urine) or oliguria (due to decreased GFR). Azotemia and hypertension (due to increased renin-angiotensin production) are usually present. Abdominal, rectal, and genitourinary examinations are helpful. Urinalysis can show hematuria, pyuria, and bacteriuria but is often benign. Abdominal ultrasound may detect mass lesions, hydroureter, and hydronephrosis. CT scanning and MRI provide more detailed information.

2. Vesicoureteral reflux—Typically vesicoureteral reflux is diagnosed in young children with a history of recurrent urinary tract infections. This entity can be detected before birth via screening fetal ultrasonography. After birth, a voiding cystourethrogram can be done. Less commonly, this entity is not diagnosed until adolescence or young adulthood when hypertension and substantial proteinuria, unusual in most tubular diseases. At this point, renal ultrasound or IVP can show renal scarring and hydronephrosis. IVP is relatively contraindicated in patients with kidney dysfunction who are at higher risk for contrast nephropathy. On kidney biopsy, focal glomerulosclerosis can be seen in those with kidney damage. Although most damage occurs before age 5 years, progressive renal deterioration to ESRD continues as a result of the early insults.

3. Analgesics—Patients can exhibit hematuria, mild proteinuria, polyuria (from tubular damage), anemia (from GI bleeding or erythropoietin deficiency), and sterile pyuria. As a result of papillary necrosis, sloughed papillae can be found in the urine. An IVP may be helpful for detecting these—contrast will fill the area of the sloughed papillae, leaving a "ring shadow" sign at the papillary tip. However, IVP is rarely used in patients with significant kidney dysfunction, given the need for dye and associated acute kidney injury.

4. Heavy metals—Proximal tubular damage from lead exposure can cause decreased secretion of uric acid, resulting in hyperuricemia and saturnine gout. Patients commonly are hypertensive. Diagnosis is most reliably performed with a calcium disodium edetate (EDTA) chelation test. Urinary excretion of > 600 mg of lead in 24 hours following 1 g of EDTA indicates excessive lead exposure.

The proximal tubular dysfunction from cadmium can cause hypercalciuria and nephrolithiasis.

Treatment

Treatment depends first on identifying the disorder responsible for kidney dysfunction. The degree of interstitial fibrosis that has developed can help predict recovery of renal function. Once there is evidence for loss of parenchyma (small shrunken kidneys or interstitial fibrosis on biopsy), little can prevent the progression toward ESRD. Treatment is then directed at medical management. Tubular dysfunction may require potassium and phosphorus restriction and sodium, calcium, or bicarbonate supplements.

If hydronephrosis is present, relief of obstruction should be accomplished promptly. Prolonged obstruction leads to further tubular damage—particularly in the distal nephron—which may be irreversible despite relief of obstruction. Neither surgical correction of reflux nor medical therapy with antibiotics can prevent deterioration toward ESRD once renal scarring has occurred.

Patients in whom lead nephropathy is suspected should continue chelation therapy with EDTA if there is no evidence of irreversible renal damage (eg, renal scarring or small kidneys). Continued exposure should be avoided.

Treatment of analgesic nephropathy requires withdrawal of all analgesics. Stabilization or improvement of renal function may occur if significant interstitial fibrosis is not present. Ensuring volume repletion during exposure to analgesics may also have some beneficial effects.

When to Refer

- Patients with stage 3–5 CKD should be referred to a nephrologist when tubulointerstitial diseases are suspected. Other select cases of stage 1–2 CKD should also be referred.
- Patients with urologic abnormalities should be referred to a urologist.

Mattoo TK. Vesicoureteral reflux and reflux nephropathy. Adv Chronic Kidney Dis. 2011 Sep;18(5):348–54. [PMID: 21896376]
Wei L et al. Estimated GFR reporting is associated with decreased nonsteroidal anti-inflammatory drug prescribing and increased renal function. Kidney Int. 2013 Jul;84(1):174–8. [PMID: 23486517]

CYSTIC DISEASES OF THE KIDNEY

Renal cysts are epithelium-lined cavities filled with fluid or semisolid material. They develop primarily from renal tubular elements. One or more simple cysts are found in 50% of individuals over the age of 50 years. They are rarely symptomatic and have little clinical significance. In contrast, generalized cystic diseases are associated with cysts scattered throughout the cortex and medulla of both kidneys and can progress to ESRD (Table 22–11).

SIMPLE OR SOLITARY CYSTS

Simple cysts account for 65–70% of all renal masses. They are generally found at the outer cortex and contain fluid that is consistent with an ultrafiltrate of plasma. Most are found incidentally on ultrasonographic examination. Simple cysts are typically asymptomatic but can become infected.

The main concern with simple cysts is to differentiate them from malignancy, abscess, or polycystic kidney disease. Renal cystic disease can develop in dialysis patients. These cysts have a potential for progression to malignancy. Ultrasound and CT scanning are the recommended procedures for evaluating these masses. Simple cysts must meet three sonographic criteria to be considered benign: (1) echo free, (2) sharply demarcated mass with smooth walls, and (3) an enhanced back wall (indicating good transmission through the cyst). Complex cysts can have thick walls, calcifications, solid components, and mixed echogenicity. On CT scan, the simple cyst should have a smooth thin wall that is sharply demarcated. It should not enhance with

Table 22–11. Clinical features of renal cystic disease.

	Simple Renal Cysts	Acquired Renal Cysts	Autosomal Dominant Polycystic Kidney Disease	Medullary Sponge Kidney	Medullary Cystic Kidney
Prevalence	Common	Dialysis patients	1:1000	1:5000	Rare
Inheritance	None	None	Autosomal dominant	None	Autosomal dominant
Age at onset	...	...	20–40	40–60	Adulthood
Kidney size	Normal	Small	Large	Normal	Small
Cyst location	Cortex and medulla	Cortex and medulla	Cortex and medulla	Collecting ducts	Corticomedullary junction
Hematuria	Occasional	Occasional	Common	Rare	Rare
Hypertension	None	Variable	Common	None	None
Associated complications	None	Adenocarcinoma in cysts	Urinary tract infections, renal calculi, cerebral aneurysms 10–15%, hepatic cysts 40–60%	Renal calculi, urinary tract infections	Polyuria, salt wasting
Kidney failure	Never	Always	Frequently	Never	Always

contrast media. A renal cell carcinoma will enhance but typically is of lower density than the rest of the parenchyma. Arteriography can also be used to evaluate a mass preoperatively. A renal cell carcinoma is hypervascular in 80%, hypovascular in 15%, and avascular in 5% of cases.

If a cyst meets the criteria for being benign, periodic reevaluation is the standard of care. If the lesion is not consistent with a simple cyst, follow-up with a urologic consultant and possible surgical exploration is recommended.

Skolarikos A et al. Conservative and radiological management of simple cysts: a comprehensive review. BJU Int. 2012 Jul;110 (2):170–8. [PMID: 22414207]

AUTOSOMAL DOMINANT POLYCYSTIC KIDNEY DISEASE

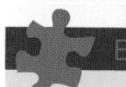

ESSENTIALS OF DIAGNOSIS

▶ Multiple cysts in bilateral kidneys; total number depends on age.

▶ Large, palpable kidneys on examination.

▶ Combination of hypertension and abdominal mass suggestive of disease.

▶ Family history is compelling but not necessary.

▶ Chromosomal abnormalities present in some patients.

General Considerations

This disorder is among the most common hereditary diseases in the United States, affecting 500,000 individuals, or 1 in 800 live births. Fifty percent of patients will have ESRD by age 60 years. The disease has variable penetrance but accounts for 10% of dialysis patients in the United States. At least two genes account for this disorder: *ADPKD1* on the short arm of chromosome 16 (85–90% of patients) and *ADPKD2* on chromosome 4 (10–15%). Patients with the *PKD2* mutation have slower progression of disease and longer life expectancy than those with *PKD1*. Other sporadic cases without these mutations have also been recognized.

Clinical Findings

Abdominal or flank pain and microscopic or gross hematuria are present in most patients. A history of urinary tract infections and nephrolithiasis is common. A family history is positive in 75% of cases, and > 50% of patients have hypertension (see below) that may antedate the clinical manifestations of the disease. Patients have large kidneys that may be palpable on abdominal examination. The combination of hypertension and an abdominal mass should suggest the disease. Forty to 50 percent have concurrent hepatic cysts. Pancreatic and splenic cysts occur also. Hemoglobin and hematocrit tend to be maintained as a result of erythropoietin production by the cysts. The urinalysis may show hematuria and mild proteinuria.

In patients with *PKD1*, ultrasonography confirms the diagnosis—two or more cysts in patients under age 30 years (sensitivity of 88.5%), two or more cysts in each kidney in patients age 30–59 years (sensitivity of 100%), and four or more cysts in each kidney in patients age 60 years or older are diagnostic for autosomal dominant polycystic kidney disease. If sonographic results are unclear, CT scan is recommended and highly sensitive.

▶ Complications & Treatment

A. Pain

Abdominal or flank pain is caused by infection, bleeding into cysts, and nephrolithiasis. Bed rest and analgesics are recommended. Cyst decompression can help with chronic pain.

B. Hematuria

Gross hematuria is most commonly due to rupture of a cyst into the renal pelvis, but it can also be caused by a kidney stone or urinary tract infection. Hematuria typically resolves within 7 days with bed rest and hydration. Recurrent bleeding should suggest the possibility of underlying renal cell carcinoma, particularly in men over age 50 years.

C. Renal Infection

An infected renal cyst should be suspected in patients who have flank pain, fever, and leukocytosis. Blood cultures may be positive, and urinalysis may be normal because the cyst does not communicate directly with the urinary tract. CT scans can be helpful because an infected cyst may have an increased wall thickness. Bacterial cyst infections are difficult to treat. Antibiotics with cystic penetration should be used, eg, fluoroquinolones or trimethoprim-sulfamethoxazole and chloramphenicol. Treatment may require 2 weeks of parenteral therapy followed by long-term oral therapy.

D. Nephrolithiasis

Up to 20% of patients have kidney stones, primarily calcium oxalate. Hydration (2–3 L/d) is recommended.

E. Hypertension

Fifty percent of patients have hypertension at time of presentation, and it will develop in most patients during the course of the disease. Cyst-induced ischemia appears to cause activation of the renin–angiotensin system, and cyst decompression can lower blood pressure temporarily. Hypertension should be treated aggressively, as this may prolong the time to ESRD. (Diuretics should be used cautiously since the effect on renal cyst formation is unknown.)

F. Cerebral Aneurysms

About 10–15% of these patients have arterial aneurysms in the circle of Willis. Screening arteriography is not recommended unless the patient has a family history of aneurysms, is employed in a high risk profession (such as airline pilot), or is undergoing elective surgery with a high risk of developing moderate to severe hypertension.

G. Other Complications

Vascular problems include mitral valve prolapse in up to 25% of patients, aortic aneurysms, and aortic valve abnormalities. Colonic diverticula are more common in patients with polycystic kidneys.

Prognosis

Vasopressin receptor antagonists have been shown to slow down the rate of change in total kidney volume and to lower the rate of worsening kidney function. Other agents, octreotide and sirolimus, have shown a decreased rate of cyst growth but no decrease in the rate of decline in kidney function. Avoidance of caffeine may prevent cyst formation due to effects on G-coupled proteins. Treatment of hypertension and a low-protein diet may slow the progression of disease, although this is not well proven.

Schrier RW. Randomized intervention studies in human polycystic kidney and liver disease. J Am Soc Nephrol. 2010 Jun;21(6):891–3. [PMID: 20431043]

Steinman TI. Polycystic kidney disease: a 2011 update. Curr Opin Nephrol Hypertens. 2012 Mar;21(2):189–94. [PMID: 22274800]

Torres VE et al; TEMPO 3:4 Trial Investigators. Tolvaptan in patients with autosomal dominant polycystic kidney disease. N Engl J Med. 2012 Dec 20;367(25):2407–18. [PMID: 23121377]

Watnick T et al. mTOR inhibitors in polycystic kidney disease. N Engl J Med. 2010 Aug 26;363(9):879–81. [PMID: 20581393]

MEDULLARY SPONGE KIDNEY

This disease is a relatively common and benign disorder that is present at birth and not usually diagnosed until the fourth or fifth decade. It can be caused by autosomal dominant mutations in the *MCKD1* or *MCKD2* genes on chromosomes 1 and 16, respectively. Kidneys have a marked irregular enlargement of the medullary and interpapillary collecting ducts. This is associated with medullary cysts that are diffuse, giving a "Swiss cheese" appearance in these regions.

Clinical Findings

Medullary sponge kidney presents with gross or microscopic hematuria, recurrent urinary tract infections, or nephrolithiasis. Common abnormalities are a decreased urinary concentrating ability and nephrocalcinosis; less common is incomplete type I distal renal tubular acidosis. The diagnosis can be made by CT, which shows cystic dilatation of the distal collecting tubules, a striated appearance in this area, and calcifications in the renal collecting system.

Treatment

There is no known therapy. Adequate fluid intake (2 L/d) helps prevent stone formation. If hypercalciuria is present, thiazide diuretics are recommended because they decrease calcium excretion. Alkali therapy is recommended if renal tubular acidosis is present.

Prognosis

Renal function is well maintained unless there are complications from recurrent urinary tract infections and nephrolithiasis.

JUVENILE NEPHRONOPHTHISIS-MEDULLARY CYSTIC DISEASE

This is a disorder previously believed to be rare but is now recognized as more common and as the cause of ESRD in younger individuals. It is associated with almost universal progression to ESRD. The childhood type—juvenile nephronophthisis—is an autosomal recessive disorder caused by mutations in the *NPH1*, *NPH2*, and *NPH3* genes; the type appearing in adulthood—medullary cystic disease—is autosomal dominant. Both types are manifested by multiple small renal cysts at the corticomedullary junction and medulla. The cortex becomes fibrotic, and as the disease progresses, interstitial inflammation and glomerular sclerosis appear.

Clinical Findings

Patients with both forms exhibit polyuria, pallor, and lethargy. Hypertension occurs at the later stages of disease. The juvenile form causes growth retardation and ESRD before age 20 years. Patients require large amounts of salt and water as a result of renal salt wasting. Ultrasound and CT scan show small, scarred kidneys, and an open kidney biopsy may be necessary to recover tissue from the corticomedullary junction.

Treatment & Prognosis

There is no current medical therapy that will prevent progression to renal failure. Adequate salt and water intake are essential to replenish renal losses.

MULTISYSTEM DISEASES WITH VARIABLE KIDNEY INVOLVEMENT[1]

MULTIPLE MYELOMA

Multiple myeloma is a malignancy of plasma cells (see Chapter 13). Renal involvement occurs in about 25% of all patients. "Myeloma kidney" is the presence of light chain immunoglobulins (Bence Jones protein) in the urine causing renal toxicity. Bence Jones protein causes direct renal tubular toxicity and results in tubular obstruction by precipitating in the tubules. The earliest tubular damage results in Fanconi syndrome (a type II proximal renal tubular acidosis). The proteinuria seen with multiple myeloma is primarily due to light chains that are not detected on urine dipstick, which mainly detects albumin. Hypercalcemia and hyperuricemia are frequently seen.

---

[1]Other diseases with variable involvement described elsewhere in this chapter include systemic lupus erythematosus, diabetes mellitus, and the vasculitides such as granulomatosis with polyangiitis and Goodpasture disease.

Glomerular amyloidosis can develop in patients with multiple myeloma; in these patients, dipstick protein determinations are positive due to glomerular epithelial cell foot process effacement and albumin "spilling" into Bowman capsule with resultant albuminuria. Other conditions resulting in renal dysfunction include plasma cell infiltration of the renal parenchyma and a hyperviscosity syndrome compromising renal blood flow. Therapy for acute kidney injury attributed to multiple myeloma includes correction of hypercalcemia, volume repletion, and chemotherapy for the underlying malignancy. Plasmapheresis had been considered appropriate to decrease the burden of existing monoclonal proteins while awaiting chemotherapeutic regimens to take effect. However, in the largest randomized prospective trial to date, plasmapheresis did not provide any renal benefit to these patients. Pheresis therapy still remains controversial.

Bridoux F et al. Optimizing treatment strategies in myeloma cast nephropathy: rationale for a randomized prospective trial. Adv Chronic Kidney Dis. 2012 Sep;19(5):333–41. [PMID: 22920644]

Haynes R et al. Myeloma kidney: improving clinical outcomes? Adv Chronic Kidney Dis. 2012 Sep;19(5):342–51. [PMID: 22920645]

SICKLE CELL DISEASE

Renal dysfunction associated with sickle cell disease is most commonly due to sickling of red blood cells in the renal medulla because of low oxygen tension and hypertonicity. Congestion and stasis lead to hemorrhage, interstitial inflammation, and papillary infarcts. Clinically, hematuria is common. Damage to renal capillaries also leads to diminished concentrating ability. Isosthenuria (urine osmolality equal to that of serum) is routine, and patients can easily become dehydrated. Papillary necrosis occurs as well. These abnormalities are also encountered in patients with sickle cell trait. Sickle cell glomerulopathy is less common but will inexorably progress to ESRD. Its primary clinical manifestation is proteinuria. Optimal treatment requires adequate hydration and control of the sickle cell disease.

Maigne G et al. Glomerular lesions in patients with sickle cell disease. Medicine (Baltimore). 2010 Jan;89(1):18–27. [PMID: 20075701]

Nath KA et al. Vasculature and kidney complications in sickle cell disease. J Am Soc Nephrol. 2012 May;23(5):781–4. [PMID: 22440903]

TUBERCULOSIS

The classic renal manifestation of tuberculosis is the presence of microscopic pyuria with a sterile urine culture—or "sterile pyuria." More often, other bacteria are also present. Microscopic hematuria is often present with pyuria. Urine cultures are the gold standard for diagnosis. Three to six first morning midstream specimens should be performed to improve sensitivity. Papillary necrosis and cavitation of the renal parenchyma occur less frequently, as do ureteral strictures and calcifications. Adequate drug therapy can result in resolution of renal involvement.

Chapagain A et al. Presentation, diagnosis, and treatment outcome of tuberculous-mediated tubulointerstitial nephritis. Kidney Int. 2011 Mar;79(6):671–7. [PMID: 21160461]

Latus J et al. Tubulointerstitial nephritis in active tuberculosis—a single center experience. Clin Nephrol. 2012 Oct;78(4): 297–302. [PMID: 22704252]

GOUT & THE KIDNEY

The kidney is the primary organ for excretion of uric acid. Patients with proximal tubular dysfunction have decreased excretion of uric acid and are more prone to gouty attacks. Depending on the pH and uric acid concentration, deposition can occur in the tubules, the interstitium, or the urinary tract. The more alkaline pH of the interstitium causes urate salt deposition, whereas the acidic environment of the tubules and urinary tract causes uric acid crystal deposition at high concentrations.

Three disorders are commonly seen: (1) uric acid nephrolithiasis, (2) acute uric acid nephropathy, and (3) chronic urate nephropathy. Kidney dysfunction with uric acid nephrolithiasis stems from obstructive physiology. Acute uric acid nephropathy presents similarly to acute tubulointerstitial nephritis with direct toxicity from uric acid crystals. Chronic urate nephropathy is caused by deposition of urate crystals in the alkaline medium of the interstitium; this can lead to fibrosis and atrophy. Epidemiologically, hyperuricemia and gout have been associated with worsening cardiovascular outcomes.

Treatment between gouty attacks involves avoidance of food and drugs causing hyperuricemia, aggressive hydration, and pharmacotherapy aimed at reducing serum uric acid levels (such as with allopurinol and febuxostat). These disorders are seen in both "overproducers" and "underexcretors" of uric acid. The latter situation may seem counterintuitive; however, these patients have hyperacidic urine, which explains the deposition of relatively insoluble uric acid crystals. For those with uric acid nephrolithiasis, fluid intake should exceed 3 L/d, and use of a urinary alkalinizing agent can be considered.

Goicoechea M et al. Effect of allopurinol in chronic kidney disease progression and cardiovascular risk. Clin J Am Soc Nephrol. 2010 Aug;5(8):1388–93. [PMID: 20538833]

NEPHROGENIC SYSTEMIC FIBROSIS

Nephrogenic systemic fibrosis is a multisystem disorder seen only in patients with CKD (primarily with a GFR < 15 mL/min/1.73 m^2, but rarely with a GFR of 15–29 mL/min/ 1.73 m^2), acute kidney injury, and after kidney transplantation. Histopathologically, there is an increase in dermal spindle cells positive for CD34 and procollagen I. Collagen bundles with mucin and elastic fibers are also noted.

Nephrogenic systemic fibrosis was first recognized in hemodialysis patients in 1997 and has been strongly linked to use of contrast agents containing gadolinium. Incidence is projected to be 1–4% in the highest risk (ESRD) population that has received gadolinium, and lower in patients with less severe kidney dysfunction. The FDA has issued a warning regarding avoidance of exposure to this agent for patients with GFR < 30 mL/min/1.73 m^2.

Clinical Findings

Nephrogenic systemic fibrosis affects several organ systems, including the skin, muscles, lungs, and cardiovascular system. The most common manifestation is a debilitating fibrosing skin disorder that can range from skin-colored to erythematous papules, which coalesce to brawny patches. The skin can be thick and woody in areas and is painful out-of-proportion to findings on examination.

Treatment

Several case reports and series have described benefit for patients after treatment with corticosteroids, photopheresis, plasmapheresis, and sodium thiosulfate. The true effectiveness of these interventions is still unclear. Alternative or no imaging agents should be used for patients requiring MR with contrast at risk for nephrogenic systemic fibrosis.

Agarwal R et al. Gadolinium-based contrast agents and nephrogenic systemic fibrosis: a systematic review and meta-analysis. Nephrol Dial Transplant. 2009 Mar;24(3):856–63. [PMID: 18952698]

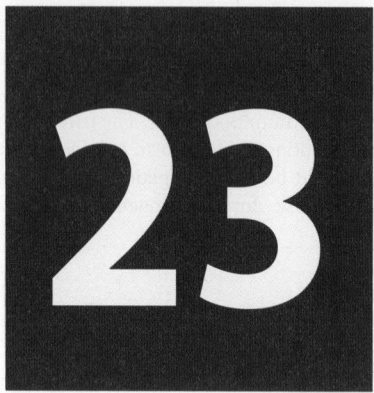

Urologic Disorders

Maxwell V. Meng, MD, FACS

Thomas J. Walsh, MD, MS

Thomas D. Chi, MD

HEMATURIA

ESSENTIALS OF DIAGNOSIS

▶ Both gross and microscopic hematuria require evaluation.

▶ The upper urinary tract should be imaged, and cystoscopy should be performed if there is hematuria in the absence of infection.

▶ General Considerations

An **upper tract source** (kidneys and ureters) can be identified in 10% of patients with gross or microscopic hematuria. For upper tract sources, stone disease accounts for 40%, medical kidney disease (medullary sponge kidney, glomerulonephritis, papillary necrosis) for 20%, renal cell carcinoma for 10%, and urothelial cell carcinoma of the ureter or renal pelvis for 5%. Drug ingestion and associated medical problems may provide diagnostic clues. Analgesic use (papillary necrosis), cyclophosphamide (chemical cystitis), antibiotics (interstitial nephritis), diabetes mellitus, sickle cell trait or disease (papillary necrosis), a history of stone disease, or malignancy should all be investigated. The **lower tract source** of gross hematuria (in the absence of infection) is most commonly from urothelial cell carcinoma of the bladder. Microscopic hematuria in the male is most commonly from benign prostatic hyperplasia. The presence of hematuria in patients receiving anticoagulation therapy cannot be ascribed to the anticoagulation; a complete evaluation is warranted consisting of upper tract imaging, cystoscopy, and urine cytology (see Chapter 39 for Bladder Cancer, Cancers of the Ureter and Renal Pelvis, Renal Cell Carcinoma, and Kidney and Testis Tumors).

▶ Clinical Findings

A. Symptoms and Signs

If gross hematuria occurs, a description of the timing (initial, terminal, total) may provide a clue to the localization

of disease. Associated symptoms (ie, renal colic, irritative voiding symptoms, constitutional symptoms) should be investigated. Physical examination should emphasize signs of systemic disease (fever, rash, lymphadenopathy, abdominal or pelvic masses) as well as signs of medical kidney disease (hypertension, volume overload). Urologic evaluation may demonstrate an enlarged prostate, flank mass, or urethral disease.

B. Laboratory Findings

Initial laboratory investigations include a urinalysis and urine culture. Proteinuria and casts suggest renal origin. Irritative voiding symptoms, bacteriuria, and a positive urine culture in the female suggest urinary tract infection, but follow-up urinalysis is important after treatment to ensure resolution of the hematuria.

Further evaluation may include urinary cytology to assist in the diagnosis of bladder neoplasm.

C. Imaging

Upper tract imaging (usually abdominal and pelvic CT scanning without and with contrast) may identify neoplasms of the kidney or ureter as well as benign conditions such as urolithiasis, obstructive uropathy, papillary necrosis, medullary sponge kidney, or polycystic kidney disease. CT urography and MRI have replaced intravenous urography when imaging the upper tracts for sources of hematuria. The role of ultrasonographic evaluation of the urinary tract for hematuria is unclear. Although it may provide adequate information for the kidney, its sensitivity in detecting ureteral disease is lower. In addition, its higher degree of operator dependence may further confound its utility.

D. Cystoscopy

Cystoscopy can be used to assess for bladder or urethral neoplasm, benign prostatic enlargement, and radiation or chemical cystitis. For gross hematuria, cystoscopy is ideally performed while the patient is actively bleeding to allow better localization (ie, lateralize to one side of the upper tracts, bladder, or urethra).

Follow-up

In patients with negative evaluations, repeat evaluations may be warranted to avoid a missed malignancy; however, the ideal frequency of such evaluations is not defined. Urinary cytology can be obtained after initial negative evaluation, and cystoscopy and upper tract imaging after a year.

When to Refer

In the absence of infection or other benign etiology, hematuria (either gross or microscopic) requires evaluation.

Daher Ede F et al. Renal tuberculosis in the modern era. Am J Trop Med Hyg. 2013 Jan;88(1):54–64. [PMID: 23303798]

Davis R et al. Diagnosis, evaluation and follow-up of asymptomatic microhematuria (AMH) in adults: AUA guideline. J Urol. 2012 Dec;188(6 Suppl):2473–81. [PMID: 23098784]

Dick-Biascoechea MA et al. Asymptomatic microscopic hematuria. Curr Opin Obstet Gynecol. 2012 Oct;24(5):324–30. [PMID: 22954764]

Margulis V et al. Assessment of hematuria. Med Clin North Am. 2011 Jan;95(1):153–9. [PMID: 21095418]

GENITOURINARY TRACT INFECTIONS

1. Acute Cystitis

ESSENTIALS OF DIAGNOSIS

- ▶ Irritative voiding symptoms.
- ▶ Patient usually afebrile.
- ▶ Positive urine culture; blood cultures may also be positive.

General Considerations

Acute cystitis is an infection of the bladder most commonly due to the coliform bacteria (especially *Escherichia coli*) and occasionally gram-positive bacteria (enterococci). The route of infection is typically ascending from the urethra. Viral cystitis due to adenovirus is sometimes seen in children but is rare in adults. Cystitis in men is rare and implies a pathologic process such as infected stones, prostatitis, or chronic urinary retention requiring further investigation.

Clinical Findings

A. Symptoms and Signs

Irritative voiding symptoms (frequency, urgency, dysuria) and suprapubic discomfort are common. Women may experience gross hematuria, and symptoms may often appear following sexual intercourse. Physical examination may elicit suprapubic tenderness, but examination is often unremarkable. Systemic toxicity is absent.

B. Laboratory Findings

Urinalysis shows pyuria and bacteriuria and varying degrees of hematuria. The degree of pyuria and bacteriuria does not necessarily correlate with the severity of symptoms. Urine culture is positive for the offending organism, but colony counts exceeding 10^5/mL are not essential for the diagnosis.

C. Imaging

Because uncomplicated cystitis is rare in men, elucidation of the underlying problem with appropriate investigations, such as abdominal ultrasonography or cystoscopy (or both), is warranted. Follow-up imaging using CT scanning is warranted if pyelonephritis, recurrent infections, or anatomic abnormalities are suspected.

Differential Diagnosis

In women, infectious processes such as vulvovaginitis and pelvic inflammatory disease can usually be distinguished by pelvic examination and urinalysis. In men, urethritis and prostatitis may be distinguished by physical examination (urethral discharge or prostatic tenderness).

Noninfectious causes of cystitis-like symptoms include pelvic irradiation, chemotherapy (cyclophosphamide), bladder carcinoma, interstitial cystitis, voiding dysfunction disorders, and psychosomatic disorders.

Prevention

Women who have more than three episodes of cystitis per year are considered candidates for prophylactic antibiotic therapy to prevent recurrence after treatment of urinary tract infection. Prior to institution of therapy, a thorough urologic evaluation is warranted to exclude any anatomic abnormality (eg, stones, reflux, fistula). The three most commonly used oral agents for prophylaxis are trimethoprim-sulfamethoxazole (40 mg/200 mg), nitrofurantoin (100 mg), and cephalexin (250 mg). Single dosing at bedtime or at the time of intercourse is the recommended schedule.

The risk of acquiring a catheter-associated urinary tract infection in hospitalized patients can be minimized by using indwelling catheters only when necessary, implementing systems to ensure removal of catheters when no longer needed, using antimicrobial catheters in high-risk patients, using external collection devices in select men, identifying significant postvoid residuals by ultrasound, maintaining proper insertion techniques, and utilizing alternatives such as intermittent catheterization.

Treatment

Uncomplicated cystitis in women can be treated with short-term antimicrobial therapy, which consists of single-dose therapy or 1–9 days of therapy. Cephalexin, nitrofurantoin, and fluoroquinolones are the drugs of choice for uncomplicated cystitis (Table 23–1). Trimethoprim-sulfamethoxazole can be ineffective because of the emergence of resistant organisms. In men, uncomplicated urinary tract infection

Table 23–1. Empiric therapy for urinary tract infections.

Diagnosis	Antibiotic	Route	Duration	Cost per Duration Noted[1]
Acute pyelonephritis	Ampicillin, 1 g every 6 hours, and gentamicin, 1 mg/kg every 8 hours	Intravenous	14 days	$458.00 not including intravenous supplies
	Ciprofloxacin, 750 mg every 12 hours	Oral	7–14 days	$79.00-158.00
	Ofloxacin, 200–300 mg every 12 hours	Oral	7–14 days	$80.00-160.00 (300 mg)
	Trimethoprim-sulfamethoxazole, 160/800 mg every 12 hours[2]	Oral	10–14 days	$18.00-25.00
Chronic pyelonephritis	Same as for acute pyelonephritis, but duration of therapy is 3–6 months			
Acute cystitis	Cephalexin, 250–500 mg every 6 hours	Oral	1–3 days	$16.60/3 days (500 mg)
	Nitrofurantoin (macrocrystals), 100 mg every 12 hours	Oral	7 days	$28.00
	Ciprofloxacin, 250–500 mg every 12 hours	Oral	1–3 days	$32.00/3 days (500 mg)
	Norfloxacin, 400 mg every 12 hours	Oral	1–3 days	$26.00/3 days
	Ofloxacin, 200 mg every 12 hours	Oral	1–3 days	$28.70/3 days
	Trimethoprim-sulfamethoxazole, 160/800 mg, two tablets[2]	Oral	Single dose	$1.80
Acute bacterial prostatitis	Same as for acute pyelonephritis		21 days	
Chronic bacterial prostatitis	Ciprofloxacin, 250–500 mg every 12 hours	Oral	1–3 months	$322.00/1 month (500 mg)
	Ofloxacin, 200–400 mg every 12 hours	Oral	1–3 months	$360.00/1 month (400 mg)
	Trimethoprim-sulfamethoxazole, 160/800 mg every 12 hours[2]	Oral	1–3 months	$54.00/1 month
Acute epididymitis				
Sexually transmitted	Ceftriaxone, 250 mg as single dose, **plus** Doxycycline, 100 mg every 12 hours	Intramuscular Oral	Once 10 days	$1.00/250 mg $46.00
Non-sexually transmitted	Same as for chronic bacterial prostatitis	Oral	3 weeks	

[1]Average wholesale price, (AWP, for AB-rated generic when available) for quantity listed. Source: *Red Book Online,* 2014, Truven Health Analytics, Inc. AWP may not accurately represent the actual pharmacy cost because wide contractual variations exist among institutions.
[2]Increasing resistance noted (up to 20%).

is rare, and thus, the duration of antibiotic therapy depends on the underlying etiology. Hot sitz baths or urinary analgesics (phenazopyridine, 200 mg orally three times daily) may provide symptomatic relief.

► Prognosis

Infections typically respond rapidly to therapy, and failure to respond suggests resistance to the selected drug or anatomic abnormalities requiring further investigation.

► When to Refer

- Suspicion or radiographic evidence of anatomic abnormality.
- Evidence of urolithiasis.
- Recurrent cystitis due to bacterial persistence.

Gupta K et al. International clinical practice guidelines for the treatment of acute uncomplicated cystitis and pyelonephritis in women: a 2010 update by the Infectious Diseases Society of American and the European Society for Microbiology and Infectious Diseases. Clin Infect Dis. 2011 Mar 1;52(5):e103–20. [PMID: 21292654]

Marschall J et al. Antibiotic prophylaxis for urinary tract infections after removal of urinary catheter: meta-analysis. BMJ. 2013 Jun 11;346:f3147. Erratum in: BMJ. 2013;347:f5325. [PMID: 23757735]

Shepherd AK et al. Management of urinary tract infections in the era of increasing antimicrobial resistance. Med Clin North Am. 2013 Jul;97(4):737–57. [PMID: 23809723]

Tambyah PA et al. Catheter-associated urinary tract infection. Curr Opin Infect Dis. 2012 Aug;25(4):365–70. [PMID: 22691687]

Torpy JM et al. JAMA patient page. Urinary tract infection. JAMA. 2012 May 2;307(17):1877. [PMID: 22550203]

2. Acute Pyelonephritis

ESSENTIALS OF DIAGNOSIS

► Fever.

► Flank pain.

► Irritative voiding symptoms.

► Positive urine culture.

General Considerations

Acute pyelonephritis is an infectious inflammatory disease involving the kidney parenchyma and renal pelvis. Gram-negative bacteria are the most common causative agents including *E coli, Proteus, Klebsiella, Enterobacter,* and *Pseudomonas.* Gram-positive bacteria are less commonly seen but include *Enterococcus faecalis* and *Staphylococcus aureus.* The infection usually ascends from the lower urinary tract—with the exception of *S aureus,* which usually is spread by a hematogenous route.

Clinical Findings

A. Symptoms and Signs

Symptoms include fever, flank pain, shaking chills, and irritative voiding symptoms (urgency, frequency, dysuria). Associated nausea and vomiting, and diarrhea are common. Signs include fever and tachycardia. Costovertebral angle tenderness is usually pronounced.

B. Laboratory Findings

Complete blood count shows leukocytosis and a left shift. Urinalysis shows pyuria, bacteriuria, and varying degrees of hematuria. White cell casts may be seen. Urine culture demonstrates heavy growth of the offending organism, and blood culture may also be positive.

C. Imaging

In complicated pyelonephritis, renal ultrasound may show hydronephrosis from a stone or other source of obstruction.

Differential Diagnosis

Acute intra-abdominal disease such as appendicitis, cholecystitis, pancreatitis, or diverticulitis must be distinguished from pyelonephritis. A normal urinalysis is usually seen in gastrointestinal disorders; however, on occasion, inflammation from adjacent bowel (appendicitis or diverticulitis) may result in hematuria or sterile pyuria. Abnormal liver biochemical tests or elevated amylase levels may assist in the differentiation. Lower lobe pneumonia is distinguishable by the abnormal chest radiograph.

In males, the main differential diagnosis for acute pyelonephritis includes acute epididymitis, acute prostatitis, and acute cystitis. Physical examination and the location of the pain should permit this distinction.

Complications

Sepsis with shock can occur with acute pyelonephritis. In diabetic patients, emphysematous pyelonephritis resulting from gas-producing organisms may be life threatening if not adequately treated. Healthy adults usually recover complete kidney function, yet if coexistent kidney disease is present, scarring or chronic pyelonephritis may result. Inadequate therapy could result in abscess formation.

Treatment

Urine and blood cultures are obtained to identify the causative agent and to determine antimicrobial sensitivity. In the inpatient setting, intravenous ampicillin and an aminoglycoside are initiated prior to obtaining sensitivity results (Table 23–1). In the outpatient setting, a quinolone may be initiated (Table 23–1). Antibiotics are adjusted according to sensitivities. Fevers may persist for up to 72 hours; failure to respond warrants imaging (CT or ultrasound) to exclude complicating factors that may require intervention. Catheter drainage may be necessary in the face of urinary retention and nephrostomy drainage if there is ureteral obstruction. In inpatients, intravenous antibiotics are continued for 24 hours after the fever resolves, and oral antibiotics are then given to complete a 14-day course of therapy. However, a shorter 7-day course may be just as effective with fewer side effects, such as mucosal candidiasis. Follow-up urine cultures are mandatory following the completion of treatment.

Prognosis

With prompt diagnosis and appropriate treatment, acute pyelonephritis carries a good prognosis. Complicating factors, underlying kidney disease, and increasing patient age may lead to a less favorable outcome.

When to Refer

• Evidence of complicating factors (urolithiasis, obstruction).

• Absence of clinical improvement in 48 hours.

When to Admit

• Severe infections or complicating factors, evidence of sepsis or need for parenteral antibiotics.

• Need for radiographic imaging or drainage of urinary tract obstruction.

Colgan R et al. Diagnosis and treatment of acute uncomplicated cystitis. Am Fam Physician. 2011 Oct 1;84(7):771–6. [PMID: 22010614]

Gupta K et al. International clinical practice guidelines for the treatment of acute uncomplicated cystitis and pyelonephritis in women: a 2010 update by the Infectious Disease Society of America and the European Society for Microbiology and Infectious Diseases. Clin Infect Dis. 2011 Mar 1;52(5):e103–20. [PMID: 21292654]

Table 23–2. Clinical characteristics of prostatitis and prostatodynia syndromes.

Findings	Acute Bacterial Prostatitis	Chronic Bacterial Prostatitis	Nonbacterial Prostatitis	Prostatodynia
Fever	+	–	–	–
Urinalysis	+	–	–	–
Expressed prostate secretions	Contraindicated	+	+	–
Bacterial culture	+	+	–	–

Hooton TM et al. Voided midstream urine culture and acute cystitis in premenopausal women. N Engl J Med. 2013 Nov 14;369(20):1883–91. [PMID: 24224622]

Meng MV. Infection of the upper urinary tract. In: Wessells H (editor). *Urological Emergencies: A Practical Guide*. New York: Humana Press, 2012.

Sandberg T et al. Ciprofloxacin for 7 days versus 14 days in women with acute pyelonephritis: a randomised, open-label and double-blind, placebo-controlled, non-inferiority trial. Lancet. 2012 Aug 4;380(9840):484–90. [PMID: 22726802]

3. Acute Bacterial Prostatitis

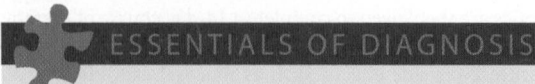

ESSENTIALS OF DIAGNOSIS

► Fever.

► Irritative voiding symptoms.

► Perineal or suprapubic pain; exquisite tenderness common on rectal examination.

► Positive urine culture.

► General Considerations

Acute bacterial prostatitis is usually caused by gram-negative rods, especially *E coli* and *Pseudomonas* species and less commonly by gram-positive organisms (eg, enterococci). The most likely routes of infection include ascent up the urethra and reflux of infected urine into the prostatic ducts. Lymphatic and hematogenous routes are probably rare.

► Clinical Findings

A. Symptoms and Signs

Perineal, sacral, or suprapubic pain, fever, and irritative voiding complaints are common. Varying degrees of obstructive symptoms may occur as the acutely inflamed prostate swells, which may lead to urinary retention. High fevers and a warm and often exquisitely tender prostate are detected on examination. Care should be taken to perform a gentle rectal examination, since vigorous manipulations may result in septicemia. Prostatic massage is contraindicated.

B. Laboratory Findings

Complete blood count shows leukocytosis and a left shift. Urinalysis shows pyuria, bacteriuria, and varying degrees of hematuria. Urine cultures will demonstrate the offending pathogen (Table 23–2).

► Differential Diagnosis

Acute pyelonephritis or acute epididymitis should be distinguishable by the location of pain as well as by physical examination. Acute diverticulitis is occasionally confused with acute prostatitis; however, the history and urinalysis should permit clear distinction. Urinary retention from benign or malignant prostatic enlargement is distinguishable by initial or follow-up rectal examination.

► Treatment

Hospitalization may be required, and parenteral antibiotics (ampicillin and aminoglycoside) should be initiated until organism sensitivities are available (Table 23–1). After the patient is afebrile for 24–48 hours, oral antibiotics (eg, quinolones) are used to complete 4–6 weeks of therapy. If urinary retention develops, urethral catheterization or instrumentation is contraindicated, and a percutaneous suprapubic tube is required. Follow-up urine culture and examination of prostatic secretions should be performed after the completion of therapy to ensure eradication.

► Prognosis

With effective treatment, chronic bacterial prostatitis is rare.

► When to Refer

• Evidence of urinary retention.
• Evidence of chronic prostatitis.

► When to Admit

• Signs of sepsis.
• Need for surgical drainage of bladder or prostatic abscess.

Campeggi A et al. Acute bacterial prostatitis after transrectal ultrasound-guided prostate biopsy: epidemiological, bacteria and treatment patterns from a 4-year prospective study. Int J Urol. 2014 Feb;21(2):152–5. [PMID: 23906113]

Dickson G. Prostatitis—diagnosis and treatment. Aust Fam Physician. 2013 Apr;42(4):216–9. [PMID: 23550248]

Nagy V et al. Acute bacterial prostatitis in humans: current microbiological spectrum, sensitivity to antibiotics and clinical findings. Urol Int. 2012;89(4):445–50. [PMID: 23095643]

Wagenlehner FM et al. Bacterial prostatitis. World J Urol. 2013 Aug;31(4):711–6. [PMID: 23519458]

Yoon BI et al. Clinical courses following acute bacterial prostatitis. Prostate Int. 2013;1(2):89–93. [PMID: 24223408]

4. Chronic Bacterial Prostatitis

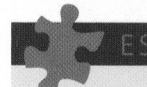

ESSENTIALS OF DIAGNOSIS

- ► Irritative voiding symptoms.
- ► Perineal or suprapubic discomfort, often dull and poorly localized.
- ► Positive expressed prostatic secretions and culture.

General Considerations

Although chronic bacterial prostatitis may evolve from acute bacterial prostatitis, many men have no history of acute infection. Gram-negative rods are the most common etiologic agents, but only one gram-positive organism (*Enterococcus*) is associated with chronic infection. Routes of infection are the same as discussed for acute infection.

Clinical Findings

A. Symptoms and Signs

Clinical manifestations are variable. Some patients are asymptomatic, but most have varying degrees of irritative voiding symptoms. Low back and perineal pain are not uncommon. Many patients report a history of urinary tract infections. Physical examination is often unremarkable, although the prostate may feel normal, boggy, or indurated.

B. Laboratory Findings

Urinalysis is normal unless a secondary cystitis is present. Expressed prostatic secretions demonstrate increased numbers of leukocytes (> 10 per high-power field), especially lipid-laden macrophages. However, this finding is consistent with inflammation and is not diagnostic of bacterial prostatitis (Table 23–2). Leukocyte and bacterial counts from expressed prostatic secretions do not correlate with severity of symptoms. Culture of the secretions or the postprostatic massage urine specimen is necessary to make the diagnosis.

C. Imaging

Imaging tests are not necessary, although pelvic radiographs or transrectal ultrasound may demonstrate prostatic calculi.

Differential Diagnosis

Chronic urethritis may mimic chronic prostatitis, though cultures of the fractionated urine may localize the source of infection to the initial specimen, which would come from the urethra. Cystitis may be secondary to prostatitis, but urine samples after prostatic massage may localize the infection to the prostate. Anal disease may share some of the symptoms of prostatitis, but physical examination should permit a distinction between the two.

Treatment

Few antimicrobial agents attain therapeutic intraprostatic levels in the absence of acute inflammation. Trimethoprim does diffuse into the prostate, and trimethoprim-sulfamethoxazole is associated with the best cure rates (Table 23–1). However, increasing resistance up to 20% has been noted. Other effective agents include quinolones, cephalexin, erythromycin, and carbenicillin. The optimal duration of therapy remains controversial, ranging from 6 to 12 weeks. Symptomatic relief may be provided by anti-inflammatory agents (indomethacin, ibuprofen) and hot sitz baths.

Prognosis

Chronic bacterial prostatitis is difficult to cure, but its symptoms and tendency to cause recurrent urinary tract infections can be controlled by suppressive antibiotic therapy.

When to Refer

- Persistent symptoms.
- Consideration of enrollment in clinical trials.

Perletti G et al. Antimicrobial therapy for chronic bacterial prostatitis. Cochrane Database Syst Rev. 2013 Aug 12;8:CD009071. [PMID: 23934982]

5. Nonbacterial Prostatitis

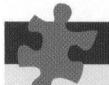

ESSENTIALS OF DIAGNOSIS

- ► Irritative voiding symptoms.
- ► Perineal or suprapubic discomfort, similar to that of chronic bacterial prostatitis.
- ► Positive expressed prostatic secretions, but negative culture.

General Considerations

Nonbacterial prostatitis is the most common of the prostatitis syndromes, and its cause is unknown. Speculation implicates chlamydiae, mycoplasmas, ureaplasmas, and viruses, but no substantial proof exists. In some cases, nonbacterial prostatitis may represent a noninfectious inflammatory or autoimmune disorder. Because the cause of nonbacterial prostatitis remains unknown, the diagnosis is usually one of exclusion.

▶ Clinical Findings

A. Symptoms and Signs

The clinical presentation is identical to that of chronic bacterial prostatitis; however, no history of urinary tract infections is present. The National Institutes of Health Chronic Prostatitis Symptom Index (NIH-CPSI) (www. prostatitisclinic.com/graphics/questionnaire2.pdf) has been validated to quantify symptoms of chronic nonbacterial prostatitis or chronic pelvic pain syndrome.

B. Laboratory Findings

Increased numbers of leukocytes are seen on expressed prostatic secretions, but all cultures are negative.

▶ Differential Diagnosis

The major distinction is from chronic bacterial prostatitis. The absence of a history of urinary tract infection and of positive cultures makes the distinction (Table 23–2). In older men with irritative voiding symptoms and negative cultures, bladder cancer must be excluded. Urinary cytologic examination and cystoscopy are warranted.

▶ Treatment

Because of the uncertainty regarding the etiology of nonbacterial prostatitis, a trial of antimicrobial therapy directed against *Ureaplasma*, *Mycoplasma*, or *Chlamydia* is warranted. Erythromycin (250 mg orally four times daily) can be initiated for 14 days yet should be continued for 3–6 weeks only if a favorable clinical response ensues. Some symptomatic relief may be obtained with nonsteroidal antiinflammatory agents or sitz baths. Dietary restrictions are not necessary unless the patient relates a history of symptom exacerbation by certain substances such as alcohol, caffeine, and perhaps certain foods.

▶ Prognosis

Annoying, recurrent symptoms are common, but serious sequelae have not been identified.

Anothaisintawee T et al. Management of chronic prostatitis/ chronic pelvic pain syndrome: a systematic review and network meta-analysis. JAMA. 2011 Jan 5;305(1):78–86. [PMID: 21205969]

Cohen JM et al. Therapeutic intervention for chronic prostatitis/ chronic pelvic pain syndrome (CP/CPPS): a systematic review and meta-analysis. PLoS One. 2012;7(8):e41941. [PMID: 22870266]

Chung SD et al. Association between chronic prostatitis/chronic pelvic pain syndrome and anxiety disorder: a population-based study. PLoS One. 2013 May 15;8(5):e64630. [PMID: 23691256]

Giannantoni A et al. The efficacy and safety of duloxetine in a multidrug regimen for chronic prostatitis/chronic pelvic pain syndrome. Urology. 2014 Feb;83(2):400–5. [PMID: 24231216]

Ismail M et al. Contemporary treatment options for chronic prostatitis/chronic pelvic pain syndrome. Drugs Today (Barc). 2013 Jul;49(7):457–62. [PMID: 23914354]

Lilienthal C. Chronic, non-bacterial prostatitis. Aust Fam Physician. 2013 Jun;42(6):362. [PMID: 23936942]

Nickel JC. Understanding chronic prostatitis/chronic pelvic pain syndrome (CP/CPPS). World J Urol. 2013 Aug;31(4):709–10. [PMID: 23812415]

Pontari M et al. New developments in the diagnosis and treatment of chronic prostatitis/chronic pelvic pain syndrome. Curr Opin Urol. 2013 Nov;23(6):565–9. [PMID: 24080807]

6. Prostatodynia

Prostatodynia is a noninflammatory disorder that affects young and middle-aged men and has variable causes, including voiding dysfunction and pelvic floor musculature dysfunction. The term "prostatodynia" is a misnomer, since the prostate is actually normal.

▶ Clinical Findings

A. Symptoms and Signs

Symptoms are the same as those seen with chronic prostatitis, yet there is no history of urinary tract infection. Additional symptoms may include hesitancy and interruption of flow. Patients may relate a lifelong history of voiding difficulty. Physical examination is unremarkable, but increased anal sphincter tone and periprostatic tenderness may be observed.

B. Laboratory Findings

Urinalysis is normal. Expressed prostatic secretions show normal numbers of leukocytes (Table 23–2). Urodynamic testing may show signs of dysfunctional voiding (detrusor contraction without urethral relaxation, high urethral pressures, spasms of the urinary sphincter) and is indicated in patients failing empiric trials of alpha-blockers or anticholinergics.

▶ Differential Diagnosis

Normal urinalysis will distinguish it from acute infectious processes. Examination of expressed prostatic secretions will distinguish nonbacterial prostatitis from other prostatitis syndromes (Table 23–2).

▶ Treatment

Bladder neck and urethral spasms can be treated by alpha-blocking agents (terazosin, 1–10 mg orally once a day, or doxazosin, 1–8 mg orally once a day). Pelvic floor muscle dysfunction may respond to diazepam and biofeedback techniques. Sitz baths may contribute to symptomatic relief.

▶ Prognosis

Prognosis is variable depending on the specific cause.

Anothaisintawee T et al. Management of chronic prostatitis/ chronic pelvic pain syndrome: a systematic review and network meta-analysis. JAMA. 2011 Jan 5;305(1):78–86. [PMID: 21205969]

Chung SD et al. Association between chronic prostatitis/chronic pelvic pain syndrome and anxiety disorder: a population-based study. PLoS One. 2013 May 15;8(5):e64630. [PMID: 23691256]

Giannantoni A et al. The efficacy and safety of duloxetine in a multidrug regimen for chronic prostatitis/chronic pelvic pain syndrome. Urology. 2014 Feb;83(2):400–5. [PMID: 24231216]

Ismail M et al. Contemporary treatment options for chronic prostatitis/chronic pelvic pain syndrome. Drugs Today (Barc). 2013 Jul;49(7):457–62. [PMID: 23914354]

Nickel JC. Understanding chronic prostatitis/chronic pelvic pain syndrome (CP/CPPS). World J Urol. 2013 Aug;31(4):709–10. [PMID: 23812415]

Pontari M et al. New developments in the diagnosis and treatment of chronic prostatitis/chronic pelvic pain syndrome. Curr Opin Urol. 2013 Nov;23(6):565–9. [PMID: 24080807]

7. Acute Epididymitis

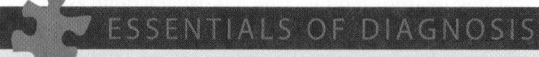

ESSENTIALS OF DIAGNOSIS

- ▸ Fever.
- ▸ Irritative voiding symptoms.
- ▸ Painful enlargement of epididymis.

▶ General Considerations

Most cases of acute epididymitis are infectious and can be divided into one of two categories that have different age distributions and etiologic agents. **Sexually transmitted forms** typically occur in men under age 40 years, are associated with urethritis, and result from *Chlamydia trachomatis* or *Neisseria gonorrhoeae*. **Non-sexually transmitted forms** typically occur in older men, are associated with urinary tract infections and prostatitis, and are caused by gram-negative rods. The route of infection is probably via the urethra to the ejaculatory duct and then down the vas deferens to the epididymis. Amiodarone has been associated with self-limited epididymitis, which is a dose-dependent phenomenon.

▶ Clinical Findings

A. Symptoms and Signs

Symptoms may follow acute physical strain (heavy lifting), trauma, or sexual activity. Associated symptoms of urethritis (pain at the tip of the penis and urethral discharge) or cystitis (irritative voiding symptoms) may occur. Pain develops in the scrotum and may radiate along the spermatic cord or to the flank. Fever and scrotal swelling are usually apparent. Early in the course, the epididymis may be distinguishable from the testis; however, later the two may appear as one enlarged, tender mass. The prostate may be tender on rectal examination.

B. Laboratory Findings

Complete blood count shows leukocytosis and a left shift. In the sexually transmitted variety, Gram staining of a smear of urethral discharge may be diagnostic of gram-negative intracellular diplococci *(N gonorrhoeae)*. White cells without visible organisms on urethral smear represent nongonococcal urethritis, and *C trachomatis* is the most likely pathogen. In the non-sexually transmitted variety, urinalysis shows pyuria, bacteriuria, and varying degrees of hematuria. Urine cultures will demonstrate the offending pathogen.

C. Imaging

Scrotal ultrasound may aid in the diagnosis if examination is difficult because of the presence of a large hydrocele or because questions exist regarding the diagnosis.

▶ Differential Diagnosis

Tumors generally cause painless enlargement of the testis. Urinalysis is negative, and examination reveals a normal epididymis. Scrotal ultrasound is helpful to define the pathology. Testicular torsion usually occurs in prepubertal males but is occasionally seen in young adults. Acute onset of symptoms and a negative urinalysis favor testicular torsion or torsion of one of the testicular or epididymal appendages. Prehn sign (elevation of the scrotum above the pubic symphysis improves pain from epididymitis) may be helpful but is not reliable.

▶ Treatment

Bed rest with scrotal elevation is important in the acute phase. Treatment is directed toward the identified pathogen (Table 23–1). The sexually transmitted variety is treated with 10–21 days of antibiotics, and the sexual partner must be treated as well. Non-sexually transmitted forms are treated for 21–28 days with appropriate antibiotics, at which time evaluation of the urinary tract is warranted to identify underlying disease.

▶ Prognosis

Prompt treatment usually results in a favorable outcome. Delayed or inadequate treatment may result in epididymo-orchitis, decreased fertility, or abscess formation.

▶ When to Refer

- Persistent symptoms and infection despite antibiotic therapy.
- Signs of sepsis or abscess formation.

Pilatz A et al. Acute epididymitis in ultrasound: results of a prospective study with baseline and follow-up investigations in 134 patients. Eur J Radiol. 2013 Dec;82(12):e762–8. [PMID: 24094645]

Srinath H. Acute scrotal pain. Aust Fam Physician. 2013 Nov;42(11):790–2. [PMID: 24217099]

Yagil Y et al. Role of Doppler ultrasonography in the triage of acute scrotum in the emergency department. J Ultrasound Med. 2010 Jan;29(1):11–21. [PMID: 20040771]

INTERSTITIAL CYSTITIS

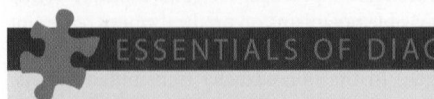

ESSENTIALS OF DIAGNOSIS

▶ Pain with a full bladder or urinary urgency.

▶ Submucosal petechiae or ulcers on cystoscopic examination.

▶ Diagnosis of exclusion.

General Considerations

Interstitial cystitis (painful bladder syndrome) is characterized by pain with bladder filling that is relieved by emptying and is often associated with urgency and frequency. This is a diagnosis of exclusion, and patients must have a negative urine culture and cytology and no other obvious cause such as radiation cystitis, chemical cystitis (cyclophosphamide), vaginitis, urethral diverticulum, or genital herpes. Up to 40% of patients referred to urologists for interstitial cystitis may actually be found to have a different diagnosis after careful evaluation.

Population-based studies have demonstrated a prevalence of between 18 and 40 per 100,000 people. Both sexes are involved, but most patients are women, with a mean age of 40 years at onset. Patients with interstitial cystitis are more likely to report bladder problems in childhood, and there appears to be a higher prevalence of these in women. Up to 50% of patients may experience spontaneous remission of symptoms, with a mean duration of 8 months without treatment.

The etiology of interstitial cystitis is unknown, and it is most likely not a single disease but rather several diseases with similar symptoms. Associated diseases include severe allergies, irritable bowel syndrome, or inflammatory bowel disease. Theories regarding the cause of interstitial cystitis include increased epithelial permeability, neurogenic causes (sensory nervous system abnormalities), and autoimmunity.

Clinical Findings

A. Symptoms and Signs

Pain with bladder filling that is relieved with urination or urgency, frequency, and nocturia are the most common symptoms. Patients should be asked about exposure to pelvic radiation or treatment with cyclophosphamide. Examination should exclude genital herpes, vaginitis, or a urethral diverticulum.

B. Laboratory Findings

Urinalysis, urine culture, and urinary cytologies are obtained to examine for infectious causes and bladder malignancy. Urodynamic testing assesses bladder sensation and compliance and excludes detrusor instability.

C. Cystoscopy

The bladder is distended with fluid (hydrodistention) to detect glomerulations (submucosal hemorrhage), which may or may not be present. Biopsy should be performed to exclude other causes such as carcinoma, eosinophilic cystitis, and tuberculous cystitis. The presence of submucosal mast cells is not needed to make the diagnosis of interstitial cystitis.

Differential Diagnosis

Exposures to radiation or cyclophosphamide are obtained by the history. Bacterial cystitis, genital herpes, or vaginitis can be excluded by urinalysis, culture, and physical examination. A urethral diverticulum may be suspected if palpation of the urethra demonstrates an indurated mass that results in the expression of pus from the urethral meatus. Urethral carcinoma presents as a firm mass on palpation.

Treatment

There is no cure for interstitial cystitis, but most patients achieve symptomatic relief from one of several approaches, including hydrodistention, which is usually done as part of the diagnostic evaluation. Approximately 20–30% of patients notice symptomatic improvement following this maneuver. Also of importance is the measurement of bladder capacity during hydrodistention, since patients with very small bladder capacities (< 200 mL) are unlikely to respond to medical therapy.

Amitriptyline (10–75 mg/d orally) is often used as first-line medical therapy in patients with interstitial cystitis. Both central and peripheral mechanisms may contribute to its activity. Nifedipine (30–60 mg/d orally) and other calcium channel blockers have also demonstrated some activity in patients with interstitial cystitis. Pentosan polysulfate sodium (Elmiron) is an oral synthetic sulfated polysaccharide that helps restore integrity to the epithelium of the bladder in a subset of patients and has been evaluated in a placebo-controlled trial. Other options include intravesical instillation of dimethyl sulfoxide (DMSO) and heparin. Intravesical bacillus Calmette-Guérin (BCG) is not beneficial.

Further treatment modalities include transcutaneous electric nerve stimulation (TENS) and acupuncture. Surgical therapy for interstitial cystitis should be considered only as a last resort and may require cystourethrectomy with urinary diversion.

When to Refer

Persistent and bothersome symptoms in the absence of identifiable cause.

Hanno PM et al. AUA guideline for the diagnosis and treatment of interstitial cystitis/bladder pain syndrome. J Urol. 2011 Jun;185(6):2162–70. [PMID: 21497847]

Matsuoka PK et al. Intravesical treatment of painful bladder syndrome: a systematic review and meta-analysis. Int Urogynecol J. 2012 Sep;23(9):1147–53. [PMID: 22569686]

Quillin RB et al. Management of interstitial cystitis/bladder pain syndrome: a urology perspective. Urol Clin North Am. 2012 Aug;39(3):389–96. [PMID: 22877722]

Quillin RB et al. Practical use of the new American Urological Association interstitial cystitis guidelines. Curr Urol Rep. 2012 Oct;13(5):394–401. [PMID: 22828913]

Torpy JM et al. JAMA patient page. Interstitial cystitis. JAMA. 2012 May 23;307(20):2211. [PMID: 22618932]

URINARY STONE DISEASE

ESSENTIALS OF DIAGNOSIS

▶ Severe flank pain.

▶ Nausea and vomiting.

▶ Identification on noncontrast CT or ultrasonography.

▶ General Considerations

Urinary stone disease is exceeded in frequency as a urinary tract disorder only by infections and prostatic disease and is estimated to afflict 240,000–720,000 Americans per year. While men are more frequently affected by urolithiasis than women, with a ratio of 2.5:1, the incidence in women appears to be rising over time. Initial presentation predominates between the third and fifth decade.

Urinary calculi are polycrystalline aggregates composed of varying amounts of crystalloid and a small amount of organic matrix. Stone formation requires saturated urine that is dependent on pH, ionic strength, solute concentration, and complexation. There are five major types of urinary stones: calcium oxalate, calcium phosphate, struvite (magnesium ammonium phosphate), uric acid, and cystine. The most common types are composed of calcium, and for that reason most urinary stones (85%) are radiopaque on plain abdominal radiographs. Uric acid stones frequently are composed of a combination of uric acid and calcium oxalate and thus are frequently radiopaque, though pure uric acid stones are radiolucent. Cystine stones frequently have a smooth-edged ground-glass appearance and are radiolucent.

Geographic factors contribute to the development of stones. Areas of high humidity and elevated temperatures appear to be contributing factors, and the incidence of symptomatic ureteral stones is greatest during hot summer months. Persons with sedentary lifestyles have a higher incidence of stones and increasing evidence demonstrates that urinary stone disease may be a precursor to subsequent cardiovascular disease.

High protein and salt intake as well as inadequate hydration appear to be the most important factors in the development of urinary stones.

Genetic factors may contribute to urinary stone formation. While approximately 50% of calcium-based stones are thought to have a heritable component, other stone types are better characterized genetically. For example, cystinuria is an autosomal recessive disorder. Homozygous individuals have markedly increased excretion of cystine and frequently have numerous recurrent episodes of urinary stones. Distal renal tubular acidosis may be transmitted as a hereditary trait, and urolithiasis occurs in up to 75% of affected patients.

▶ Clinical Findings

A. Symptoms and Signs

Obstructing urinary stones usually present with acute and severe colic. Pain usually occurs suddenly and may awaken patients from sleep. It is localized to the flank, is usually severe, unremitting, and may be associated with nausea and vomiting. Patients are constantly moving trying to find a comfortable position—in sharp contrast to those with an acute abdomen. The pain may occur episodically and may radiate anteriorly over the abdomen. As the stone progresses down the ureter, the pain may be referred into the ipsilateral groin. If the stone becomes lodged at the uretero-vesical junction, patients will complain of marked urinary urgency and frequency and in men, pain may radiate to the tip of the penis. After the stone passes into the bladder, there typically is minimal pain with passage through the urethra. Stone size does not correlate with the severity of the symptoms.

B. Laboratory Findings

In patients with either symptomatic or asymptomatic kidney stones, urinalysis usually reveals microscopic or gross hematuria (~90%). However, the absence of microhematuria does not exclude urinary stones. Urinary pH is a valuable clue to the cause of the possible stone. Normal urine pH is 5.8–5.9. Numerous dipstick measurements are valuable in the complete work-up of a patient in whom urinary stones are suspected. Persistent urinary pH below 5.5 is suggestive of uric acid or cystine stones. In contrast, a persistent urinary pH > 7.2 is suggestive of a struvite infection stone or calcium phosphate stone (when above 7.5). Patients with calcium oxalate–based stones typically have a urinary pH between 5.5 and 6.8.

C. Metabolic Evaluation

Patients should strain their urine through cheesecloth or a urine strainer during a symptomatic episode. This facilitates stone analysis on recovered stones. Controversy exists in deciding which patients need a thorough metabolic evaluation for stone disease. Patients with uncomplicated first-time stones should all undergo dietary counseling as outlined below and can be offered metabolic evaluation.

Complete metabolic evaluation is required in patients who have recurrent stones or those with a family history of nephrolithiasis. Patients are encouraged to change their diet to reduce sodium intake, reduce their animal protein intake during individual meals, and to ingest adequate fluid intake to achieve a voided volume of 1.5–2.0 L/d of urine. After these dietary changes have been initiated, a 24-hour urine collection should be obtained to ascertain urinary volume, pH, calcium, uric acid, oxalate, phosphate, sodium, and citrate excretion. Serum parathyroid hormone (PTH), calcium, uric acid, electrolytes (including bicarbonate), and creatinine and BUN should also be obtained. Table 23–3 demonstrates the diagnostic criteria for the hypercalciuric states.

D. Imaging

A plain abdominal radiograph (KUB, kidneys-ureters-bladder) and renal ultrasound examination will diagnose most stones. More than 60% of patients with acute renal colic will have with a stone in the distal 4 cm of the ureter; attention should be directed to that region when

Table 23–3. Diagnostic criteria of different types of hypercalciuria.

	Absorptive Type I	Absorptive Type II	Absorptive Type III	Resorptive	Renal
Serum					
Calcium	N	N	N	↑	N
Phosphorus	N	N	↓	↓	N
PTH	N	N	N	↑	↑
Vitamin D	N	N	↑	↑	↑
Urinary calcium					
Fasting	N	N	↑	↑	↑
Restricted calcium intake	↑	N	↑	↑	↑
After calcium load	↑	↑	↑	↑	↑

PTH, parathyroid hormone; ↑, elevated; ↓, low; N, normal.

examining plain radiographs and abdominal ultrasonographic studies. Spiral CT is frequently the first-line tool in evaluating flank pain given its increased sensitivity and specificity over other tests. CT scans should be obtained in the prone position to help differentiate distal ureterovesicular stones from those that have already passed into the urinary bladder. Repeated CT scans should be avoided due to the substantial radiation exposure to these patients with recurrent stones. Stone density can be estimated with Hounsfield units (HU) on CT scans to help determine stone type. Stones with low HU (< 450) are typically composed of uric acid, while those with high HU (> 1200) are typically composed of calcium oxalate monohydrate. All stones whether radiopaque or radiolucent on plain abdominal radiographs will be visible on noncontrast CT except the rare calculi due to protease inhibitors (classically indinavir).

▶ Medical Treatment & Prevention

To reduce the recurrence rate of urinary stones, one must attempt to achieve a stone-free status. Small stone fragments may serve as a nidus for future stone development. Metabolic evaluation often identifies a modifiable risk factor that can reduce stone recurrence rates. If no medical treatment is provided after surgical stone removal, stones will generally recur in 50% of patients within 5 years. Some stone types (eg, uric acid, cystine) are more prone to rapid recurrence than others. Of greatest importance in reducing stone recurrence is an increased fluid intake. Absolute volumes are not established, but increasing fluid intake to ensure a voided volume of 1.5–2.0 L/d is recommended (normal average voided volume is 1.6 L/d).

A. Diet

Sodium intake should be restricted to keep urinary sodium levels < 150 mEq/d. Increased sodium intake will increase renal sodium and calcium excretion, increase urinary monosodium urates (that can act as a nidus for stone growth), increase the relative saturation of calcium

phosphate, and decrease urinary citrate excretion. All of these factors encourage stone growth. Animal protein intake should be spread out through the day and not consumed during any individual meal and is best limited to 1 g/kg/d. An increased protein load during an individual meal can also increase calcium, oxalate, and uric acid excretion and decrease urinary citrate excretion.

Excessive intake of oxalate and purines can increase the incidence of stones in predisposed individuals. Dietary calcium or calcium supplements should not be routinely decreased. In fact, decreased calcium consumption has been found to increase stone recurrence. Only type II absorptive hypercalciuric patients (see below and Table 23–3) benefit from a low calcium diet.

B. Calcium Nephrolithiasis

1. Hypercalciuric—Hypercalciuric calcium nephrolithiasis (> 250 mg/24 h; > 4 mg/kg/24 h) can be caused by absorptive, resorptive, and renal disorders.

Absorptive hypercalciuria is secondary to increased absorption of calcium at the level of the small bowel, predominantly in the jejunum, and can be further subdivided into types I, II, and III. Type I absorptive hypercalciuria is independent of calcium intake. There is increased urinary calcium on a regular or even a calcium-restricted diet. Treatment is centered on decreasing bowel absorption of calcium. Cellulose phosphate, a chelating agent, is one effective form of therapy. An average dose is 10–15 g in three divided doses. It binds to the calcium and impedes small bowel absorption due to its increased bulk. Cellulose phosphate does not change the intestinal transport mechanism. It should be given with meals so it will be available to bind to the dietary calcium. Taking this chelating agent prior to bedtime is ineffective. Postmenopausal women should be treated with caution. Inappropriate use may result in a negative calcium balance and a secondary parathyroid stimulation and consequent bone reabsorption. However, there is generally no enhanced decline in bone density with long-term use. Long-term use without follow-up metabolic surveillance may result in hypomagnesuria and secondary hyperoxaluria and recurrent calculi. Routine follow-up every 6–8 months will help encourage medical compliance and permit adjustments in medical therapy based on repeat metabolic studies.

Thiazide therapy is more commonly used and is an alternative to cellulose phosphate in the treatment of type I absorptive hypercalciuria. Thiazides decrease renal calcium excretion but have no impact on intestinal absorption. This therapy results in increased bone density of approximately 1% per year. Thiazides have limited long-term utility (< 5 years) since they may lose their hypocalciuric effect with continued therapy.

Type II absorptive hypercalciuria is diet-dependent and fortunately rare. Decreasing calcium intake by 50% (approximately 400 mg/d) will decrease the hypercalciuria to normal values (150–200 mg/24 h). There is no specific medical therapy.

Type III absorptive hypercalciuria is secondary to a renal phosphate leak. This results in increased vitamin D synthesis and secondarily increased small bowel absorption of calcium. This can be readily reversed by orthophosphates (250 mg orally three to four times per day), presently available without need for a prescription. Orthophosphates do not change intestinal absorption but rather inhibit vitamin D synthesis.

Resorptive hypercalciuria is secondary to hyperparathyroidism. Hypercalcemia, hypophosphatemia, hypercalciuria, and an elevated serum PTH value are found. Appropriate surgical resection of the parathyroid adenoma cures the disease, although recurrent urinary stones can still occur in 10% of patients after parathyroidectomy. Medical management invariably fails.

Renal hypercalciuria occurs when the renal tubules are unable to efficiently reabsorb filtered calcium, and hypercalciuria results. Spilling calcium in the urine results in secondary hyperparathyroidism. Serum calcium typically is normal. Thiazides are an effective long-term therapy in patients with this disorder.

2. Hyperuricosuric—Hyperuricosuric calcium nephrolithiasis is secondary to dietary purine excess or endogenous uric acid metabolic defects. Most cases (85%) can be treated with purine dietary restrictions; those that are not reversed with dietary modification are successfully treated with allopurinol. In contrast to uric acid nephrolithiasis, patients with hyperuricosuric calcium stones typically maintain a urinary pH > 5.5. Monosodium urates absorb and adsorb inhibitors and promote heterogeneous nucleation. Hyperuricosuric calcium nephrolithiasis is initiated with epitaxy, or heterogeneous nucleation. In such situations, similar crystal structures (ie, uric acid and calcium oxalate) can grow together with the aid of a protein matrix infrastructure.

3. Hyperoxaluric—Hyperoxaluric calcium nephrolithiasis (> 40 mg oxalate/24h urine) is usually due to primary intestinal disorders. Patients often have a history of chronic diarrhea frequently associated with inflammatory bowel disease. In these situations, increased bowel fat or bile (or both) combine with intraluminal calcium to form a soap-like product. Calcium is therefore unavailable to bind to oxalate in the gut, which is then freely and rapidly absorbed. A small increase in oxalate absorption will significantly increase stone formation. If the diarrhea or steatorrhea cannot be effectively curtailed, oral calcium should be taken with meals, either by ingesting milk products or taking calcium carbonate supplements (250–500 mg). This helps to bind dietary oxalate in the gut and oxalate movement into the kidneys. Excess ascorbic acid (> 2 g/d) will substantially increase urinary oxalate levels. Rare enzymatic liver defects can lead to primary hyperoxaluria that is routinely fatal without a combined liver and kidney transplantation.

4. Hypocitraturic—Hypocitraturic calcium nephrolithiasis may be secondary to chronic diarrhea, type I (distal) renal tubular acidosis, chronic hydrochlorothiazide treatment, or in any condition that results in a metabolic acidosis. The metabolic acidosis enhances citrate transport into the proximal tubular cells where it is consumed by the citric acid cycle in their mitochondria, resulting in hypocitraturia (< 450 mg/24h). Hypocitraturia is frequently associated with calcium stone formation. Urinary citrate binds to calcium in solution, thereby decreasing available calcium for precipitation and subsequent stone formation. Potassium citrate supplements are usually effective treatment in these situations. A typical dose is 60 mEq total daily intake, divided either into three times daily as tablets or twice daily as the crystal formulations dissolved in water (it is also available as a solution). Alternatively, oral lemonade has been shown to increase urinary citrate by about 150 mg/24h.

C. Uric Acid Calculi

Urinary pH is consistently < 5.5 in persons who form uric acid stones. The pK of uric acid is 5.75, at which point half of the uric acid is ionized as a urate salt and is soluble, while the other half is insoluble. Increasing the urinary pH above 6.2 dramatically increases uric acid solubility, can effectively dissolve large calculi at a rate of 1 cm per month, and effectively prevents future uric acid stone formation. Urinary alkalinization with potassium citrate or an equivalent agent is the key to stone dissolution and prophylaxis. The goal is a urinary pH > 6.2 and < 6.5 (to avoid calcium phosphate precipitation). Other precipitating factors include hyperuricemia, myeloproliferative disorders, malignancy with increased uric acid production, abrupt and dramatic weight loss, and uricosuric medications. If hyperuricemia is present, allopurinol (300 mg/d orally) may be given. Although pure uric acid stones are relatively radiolucent, most have some calcium components and can be visualized on plain abdominal radiographs.

D. Struvite Calculi

Struvite stones are radiodense magnesium-ammonium-phosphate stones. They are most common in women with recurrent urinary tract infections with urease-producing organisms, including *Proteus, Pseudomonas, Providencia* and, less commonly, *Klebsiella, Staphylococcus,* and *Mycoplasma* (but not *E coli).* They rarely present as ureteral stones with colic without prior upper tract endourologic intervention. Frequently, a struvite stone is discovered as a large staghorn calculus forming a cast of the renal collecting system. Urinary pH is high, routinely above 7.2. Struvite stones are relatively soft and amenable to percutaneous removal. Appropriate perioperative antibiotics are required. They can recur rapidly, and efforts should be taken to render the patient stone-free. Acetohydroxamic acid is an effective urease inhibitor that can dissolve and prevent struvite stones, but it is poorly tolerated by most patients because of gastrointestinal side effects.

E. Cystine Calculi

Cystine stones are a result of abnormal excretion of cystine excretion. These stones are particularly difficult to manage medically. Prevention is centered around marked increased fluid intake during the day and evening to achieve a urinary volume of 3–4 L/d, urinary alkalinization with a urinary pH > 7.0 (monitored with Nitrazine pH paper), and disulfide inhibitors such as tiopronin (alpha-mercaptopropionylglycine) or penicillamine. There are no known inhibitors of cystine calculi.

▶ Surgical Treatment

In the acute setting, forced intravenous fluids will not push stones down the ureter. Forced diuresis can be counterproductive and exacerbate the pain; instead, a euvolemic state should be achieved. Signs of infection, including associated fever, tachycardia, or elevated white blood cell count may indicate a urinary tract infection behind the obstructing stone. Any obstructing stone with associated infection is a medical emergency requiring prompt drainage by a ureteral catheter or a percutaneous nephrostomy tube. Antibiotics alone are inadequate unless the obstruction is drained.

A. Ureteral Stones

Impediment to urine flow by ureteral stones usually occurs at three sites: the ureteropelvic junction, the crossing of the ureter over the iliac artery, or the ureterovesicular junction. Prediction of spontaneous stone passage is difficult. Stones < 5–6 mm in diameter on a plain abdominal radiograph usually pass spontaneously. Medical expulsive therapy with alpha-blockers (such as tamsulosin, 0.4 mg orally once daily) in combination with a nonsteroidal anti-inflammatory agent (such as ibuprofen 600 mg orally three times per day with a full stomach), with or without a short course of a low-dose oral corticosteroid (such as prednisone 10 mg orally daily for 3–5 days) dramatically increases the rate of spontaneous stone passage. Medical expulsive therapy with appropriate pain medications is appropriate for the first few weeks. If the stone fails to pass within 4 weeks, the patient has fever, intolerable pain or persistent nausea or vomiting, or the patient must return to work or anticipates travel, then therapeutic intervention is indicated.

Ureteral stones are best managed with ureteroscopic stone extraction or in situ extracorporeal shock wave lithotripsy (SWL). Ureteroscopic stone extraction involves placement of a small endoscope through the urethra and into the ureter. Under direct vision, basket extraction or stone laser fragmentation followed by extraction is performed. Complications during endoscopic retrieval increase if medical expulsive therapy has been attempted for > 6 weeks.

In situ SWL utilizes an external energy source focused on the stone with the aid of fluoroscopy or ultrasonography. SWL can be performed under anesthesia as an outpatient procedure and results in a high rate of stone fragmentation. Most stone fragments then pass uneventfully within 2 weeks, but those that have not passed within 6 weeks are unlikely to do so without intervention. Decreased SWL success rates are associated with lower pole and distal stone location, as well as larger stone burden. Women of childbearing age with a stone in the lower ureter are best not treated with SWL because its impact on the ovary is unknown.

Proximal and midureteral stones—those above the inferior margin of the sacroiliac joint—as well as intrarenal stones can be treated with SWL or ureteroscopy. SWL is delivered directly to the stone in situ. To help ensure adequate urinary drainage after SWL, a double J ureteral stent may be placed, but it does not ensure passage of stone fragments. Occasionally, stone fragments will obstruct the ureter after SWL. Conservative management will usually result in spontaneous resolution with eventual passage of the stone fragments. In rare instances, ureteroscopic extraction will be required.

B. Renal Calculi

Patients with renal calculi but without pain, urinary tract infection, or obstruction may not warrant surgical treatment. If surveillance is elected, they should be monitored with serial abdominal radiographs or renal ultrasonographic examinations. If calculi are growing or become symptomatic, intervention should be undertaken. Renal calculi < 1.5 cm in diameter are best treated with SWL or ureteroscopic extraction. Calculi located in the inferior calix and of larger diameter are best treated via percutaneous nephrolithotomy. Percutaneous nephrolithotomy is performed by inserting a needle into the appropriate renal calyx and dilating a tract large enough to allow a nephroscope to pass directly into the kidney. In this fashion, larger and more complex renal stones can be inspected, fragmented, and removed. Perioperative antibiotic coverage for any stone procedure should be given, ideally based on preoperative urine culture.

▶ When to Refer

- Evidence of urinary obstruction.
- Urinary stone with associated flank pain.
- Anatomic abnormalities or solitary kidney.
- Concomitant pyelonephritis or recurrent infection.

▶ When to Admit

- Intractable nausea and vomiting or pain.
- Obstructing stone with signs of infection.

Bagga HS et al. New insights into the pathogenesis of renal calculi. Urol Clin North Am. 2013 Feb;40(1):1–12. [PMID: 23177630]

Fink HA et al. Medical management to prevent recurrent nephrolithiasis in adults: a systematic review for an American College of Physicians Clinical Guideline. Ann Intern Med. 2013 Apr 2;158(7):535–43. [PMID: 23546565]

Goldfarb DS et al. Metabolic evaluation of first-time and recurrent stone formers. Urol Clin North Am. 2013 Feb;40(1):13–20. [PMID: 23177631]

Matlaga BR et al. Treatment of ureteral and renal stones: a systematic review and meta-analysis of randomized, controlled trials. J Urol. 2012 Jul;188(1):130–7. [PMID: 22591962]

Punnoose AR et al. JAMA patient page. Kidney stones. JAMA. 2012 Jun 20;307(23):2557. [PMID: 22797461]

MALE ERECTILE DYSFUNCTION & SEXUAL DYSFUNCTION

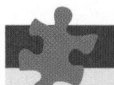

ESSENTIALS OF DIAGNOSIS

► Erectile dysfunction can have organic and psychogenic etiologies, and the two frequently overlap.

► Organic erectile dysfunction may be an early sign of cardiovascular disease and requires evaluation.

► Peyronie disease is a common fibrotic disorder of the corpora cavernosa of the penis that causes pain, penile deformity, and sexual dysfunction.

► General Considerations

Erectile dysfunction is the consistent inability to attain or maintain a sufficiently rigid penile erection for sexual performance. More than half of men aged 40–70 years experience erectile dysfunction and its incidence is age-related. Normal male erection is a neurovascular event relying on an intact autonomic and somatic nerve supply to the penis, smooth and striated musculature of the corpora cavernosa and pelvic floor, and arterial blood flow supplied by the paired pudendal arteries. Erection is caused and maintained by an increase in arterial flow, active relaxation of the smooth muscle within the sinusoids of the paired corpora cavernosa of the penis, and an increase in venous resistance. Contraction of the bulbocavernosus and ischiocavernosus muscles results in further rigidity of the penis with intracavernosal pressures exceeding systolic blood pressure. Nitric oxide is a key neurotransmitter that initiates and sustains erections; however, other molecules contribute, including acetylcholine, prostaglandins, and vasoactive intestinal peptide.

Male sexual dysfunction may be manifested in a variety of ways, and patient history is critical to the proper classification and treatment. A **loss of libido** may indicate androgen deficiency. **Loss of erections** may result from arterial, venous, neurogenic, hormonal, or psychogenic causes. Concurrent medical problems may damage one or more of the mechanisms. Endothelial dysfunction is the decreased bioavailability of nitric oxide with subsequent

impairment of arterial vasodilation. Erectile dysfunction may be an early manifestation of endothelial dysfunction, which precedes more severe atherosclerotic cardiovascular disease. Many medications, especially antihypertensive, antidepressant, and opioid agents, are associated with erectile dysfunction.

Peyronie disease is a fibrotic disorder of the tunica albuginea of the penis resulting in varying degrees of penile curvature or deformity. Peyronie disease develops in approximately 5–10% of men older than 50 years. While 10% of men improve spontaneously, 50% will stabilize and the remainder will progress if left untreated. Penile deformity can impair normal sexual function and impact self-esteem. The cause of Peyronie disease is not fully understood.

Priapism is the occurrence of penile erection unrelated to sexual stimulation lasting longer than 4 hours that potentially causes ischemic injury of the corpora cavernosa and erectile dysfunction (low flow or "ischemic" priapism). Ischemic priapism may be caused by red blood cell dyscrasias, drug use, and any of the treatments for erectile dysfunction.

Anejaculation is the **loss of seminal emission** and may result from androgen deficiency by decreasing prostate and seminal vesicle secretions, or by sympathetic denervation as a result of diabetes mellitus or pelvic or retroperitoneal surgery or radiation. **Retrograde ejaculation** may occur as a result of mechanical disruption of the bladder neck, due to transurethral resection of the prostate, pelvic radiation, sympathetic denervation, or treatment with alpha-blockers. **Premature ejaculation** is the persistent or recurrent ejaculation with minimal stimulation before a person desires (associated with distress). It may be primary or secondary to erectile dysfunction. The former is common and may be treated with behavioral modification, sexual health counseling, local anesthetic agents, and systemic medications. The latter will often correct with treatment of erectile dysfunction.

► Clinical Findings

A. Symptoms and Signs

Erectile dysfunction should be distinguished from problems of penile deformity, ejaculation, libido, and orgasm. The severity of erectile dysfunction (maintaining vs attaining; chronic, occasional, or situational) and its timing should be noted. The history should include inquiries about dyslipidemia, hypertension, depression, neurologic disease, diabetes mellitus, chronic kidney disease, endocrine disorders, and cardiac or peripheral vascular disease. Pelvic trauma, surgery, or irradiation puts patients at increased risk for erectile dysfunction. A history of penile deformity or curvature that prevents normal intercourse indicates Peyronie disease, which may complicate treatment. The history should clarify the severity of curvature, loss of penile length, and other problems that may prevent normal, painless sexual intercourse. The ability to attain but not maintain an erection may be the first sign of endothelial dysfunction and further cardiovascular risk stratification is warranted. The gradual loss of erections over time is more suggestive of an organic cause. Erectile dysfunction may immediately follow pelvic surgery or trauma. Medication use should be reviewed, since 25% of all cases of sexual dysfunction may be drug related. Alcohol, tobacco, and recreational drug use are associated with an increased risk of sexual dysfunction.

During the physical examination, vital signs and secondary sexual characteristics should be assessed. Thorough cardiovascular examination should be performed with auscultation of the heart as well as palpation and quantification of lower extremity arterial pulsations. Motor and sensory examination should be performed. The genitalia should be examined, noting the presence of penile scarring or plaque formation (Peyronie disease) and any abnormalities in size or consistency of either testicle.

B. Laboratory Findings

Laboratory evaluation should consist of a fasting lipid profile and glucose, testosterone, and prolactin. Patients with abnormalities of testosterone or prolactin require further evaluation with measurement of free testosterone and luteinizing hormone (LH) to distinguish hypothalamic-pituitary dysfunction from primary testicular failure.

C. Special Tests

Further testing is based on the patient's history and is performed when etiology is unclear. Organic and psychogenic erectile dysfunction frequently occur in tandem, given that erectile dysfunction can contribute to emotional stress and decreased quality of life. Erectile dysfunction that is primarily psychogenic can generally be differentiated by patient history, whereby men will describe normal nocturnal or morning erections, or situational erectile dysfunction. If the distinction remains unclear, clarity may be gained with the use of nocturnal penile tumescence testing, where the frequency and rigidity of erections are recorded by a tension meter attached to the penis before sleep. Patients with psychogenic erectile dysfunction will have nocturnal erections of adequate frequency and rigidity.

Treatment of patients with oral medications (sildenafil, vardenafil, and tadalafil) provides insight into the etiology and severity of erectile dysfunction. Patients with inadequate response to oral medications may undergo further evaluation with direct injection of vasoactive medications into the penis. These medications (prostaglandin E$_1$, papaverine, phentolamine or a combination) induce erections in men with intact vascular systems. Patients who respond with a rigid erection require no further vascular evaluation.

Additional vascular testing is indicated in select patients who do not achieve an erection after penile injection and who are candidates for vascular reconstructive surgery. Duplex ultrasound, penile cavernosography, and pudendal arteriography can distinguish arterial from venous erectile dysfunction and help predict which patients may benefit from vascular surgery.

▶ Treatment

Treatment of men suffering from sexual dysfunction should be patient centered and goal oriented. Men who have a significant psychogenic component to their erectile

dysfunction will benefit from behaviorally oriented sex therapy or counseling. Lifestyle modification and reduction of cardiovascular risk factors are important components to any treatment plan. This should potentially include smoking cessation; reduction of alcohol intake; diet; exercise; and close monitoring and treatment of diabetes, dyslipidemia, and hypertension.

A. Hormonal Replacement

Testosterone replacement therapy may be offered to men with documented biochemical hypogonadism who have undergone endocrinologic evaluation and in whom there is no evidence of prostate cancer or other contraindication to treatment (eg, erythrocytosis). Restoration of normal testosterone levels may improve libido and effectiveness of oral erectile medications.

B. Vasoactive Therapy

1. Oral agents—Sildenafil, vardenafil, tadalafil, and avanafil inhibit phosphodiesterase-5 (PDE-5), preventing the degradation of cGMP, thereby sustaining inflow of blood into the erect penis. These drugs are similarly effective, but patients who do not respond to one PDE-5 inhibitor may respond to one of the other agents. Because of differences in receptor binding affinity and pharmacokinetics, the drugs have variable durations of activity and side effects. Each drug should be initiated at the lowest dose and titrated to effect. There is no effect on libido, and priapism is exceedingly rare. When taken with nitrate medications, there may be exaggerated cardiac preload reduction and hypotension; therefore, these drugs are contraindicated in patients taking nitroglycerin or nitrates. All patients being evaluated for acute chest pain should be asked if they are taking a PDE-5 inhibitor before administering nitroglycerin and close monitoring of blood pressure is warranted if there is concern regarding drug overlap.

The combination of PDE-5 inhibitors and alpha-receptor blockers (which may be prescribed for lower urinary tract symptoms) may cause a larger reduction in systemic blood pressure than when PDE-5 inhibitors are used alone. However, these two classes of medication may be safely used in combination if they are started in a stepwise fashion, with escalation of dose when there is no evidence of hypotension or syncope. In select men, combined treatment with PDE-5 inhibitors and testosterone replacement may be warranted, since adequate androgen levels appear to support normal penile structure and function.

2. Injectable agents—Direct injection of vasoactive prostaglandins with or without papaverine or phentolamine into the penis is an acceptable form of treatment for many men with erectile dysfunction. Injections are performed using a tuberculin-type syringe or a metered-dose injection device. The base and lateral aspect of the penis is used as the injection site to avoid injury to the superficial blood and nerve supply located anteriorly. Complications are rare and include bruising, dizziness, local pain, fibrosis, priapism, and infection. Vasoactive prostaglandins (alprostadil) can also be delivered via a urethral suppository with slightly less effectiveness.

The presence of a prolonged erection (priapism) requires immediate medical attention to prevent ischemia and fibrosis of the cavernosal tissues. Initial management may include aspiration of blood from the penis or injection of sympathomimetic drugs (epinephrine or phenylephrine); if these maneuvers fail, surgical arteriovenous shunts may be performed to allow detumescence.

C. Vacuum Erection Device

The vacuum erection device creates a vacuum chamber around the penis and draws blood into the corpora cavernosa. Once adequate tumescence is achieved, an elastic constriction band is placed around the proximal penile shaft to prevent loss of erection, and the vacuum cylinder is removed. Such devices are effective, regardless of the cause of erectile dysfunction; however, the devices are cumbersome and may cause penile discomfort leading to a high rate of disuse. Serious complications are rare.

D. Penile Prostheses

Penile prostheses are implanted directly into the paired corporal bodies. Penile prostheses may be semi-rigid (malleable) or inflatable. Each is manufactured in a variety of sizes and is custom-fit to the individual. Even for men with normal erectile function, the penis is flaccid 90% of time; therefore, inflatable devices may result in a more natural appearance and better functionality. Complications are rare but include mechanical failure, infection, and injury to adjacent anatomic structures during surgery. For men who elect this treatment, personal and partner satisfaction rates are very high due to enhanced spontaneity and reliability of erections.

E. Vascular Reconstruction

Patients with disorders of the arterial system are candidates for various forms of arterial reconstruction, including endarterectomy and balloon dilation for proximal arterial occlusion and arterial bypass procedures utilizing arterial (epigastric) or venous (deep dorsal vein) segments for distal occlusion. Patients with venous disorders may be managed with ligation of certain veins (deep dorsal or emissary veins) or the crura of the corpora cavernosa. Experience with vascular reconstructive procedures is limited, and many patients so treated still fail to achieve a rigid erection.

F. Medical and Surgical Therapy for Peyronie Disease

A wide range of medical and surgical treatments have been used to treat the disorder. No oral therapies for Peyronie disease are approved by the FDA; however, evidence from randomized controlled trials supports the use of pentoxifylline and coenzyme Q10. The intraplaque injection of verapamil or interferon improves penile deformity in some patients. Clostridial collagenase is the only FDA-approved medication for the treatment of Peyronie disease. Collagenase is administered to the central portion of the penile plaque by needle injection; it causes enzymatic digestion of the lesion with subsequent correction of penile curvature. Surgical treatment is an alternative for men with compromised sexual function due to severe curvature or lesions causing penile instability. The choice of corrective procedure should be tailored to each patient after a detailed evaluation of disease severity and sexual function.

▶ When to Refer

- Patients with inadequate response to oral medications, who are unable to tolerate side effects or who are dissatisfied with their current treatment.
- Patients with Peyronie disease or other penile deformity.
- Patients with a history of pelvic or perineal trauma, surgery, or radiation.
- Ischemic priapism is a medical emergency and requires immediate referral to a urologist or the emergency department for intervention to allow restoration of penile blood perfusion.

Corona G et al. Phosphodiesterase type 5 (PDE5) inhibitors in erectile dysfunction: the proper drug for the proper patient. J Sex Med. 2011 Dec;8(12):3418–32. [PMID: 21995676]
Gandaglia G et al. A systematic review of the association between erectile dysfunction and cardiovascular disease. Eur Urol. 2014 May;65(5):968–78. [PMID: 24011423]
McCabe MP et al. A systematic review of the psychosocial outcomes associated with erectile dysfunction: does the impact of erectile dysfunction extend beyond a man's inability to have sex? J Sex Med. 2014 Feb;11(2):347–63. [PMID: 24251371]
Porst H. An overview of pharmacotherapy in premature ejaculation. J Sex Med. 2011 Oct;8(Suppl 4):335–41. [PMID: 21967395]

MALE INFERTILITY

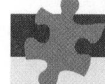
ESSENTIALS OF DIAGNOSIS

▶ The male partner contributes to 50% of infertility cases.

▶ Causes include decreased or absent sperm production or function, or obstruction of the male genital tract.

▶ Detailed history, physical examination, and repeated semen analysis are important for diagnosis and treatment.

▶ Abnormal semen quality may indicate poor health or increased risk of certain health conditions.

▶ General Considerations

Infertility, the inability of a couple to conceive a child after 1 year of sexual intercourse without contraceptive use, affects 15–20% of US couples. Approximately one-half of cases result from male factors; therefore, evaluation of both partners is critical. Following a detailed history and

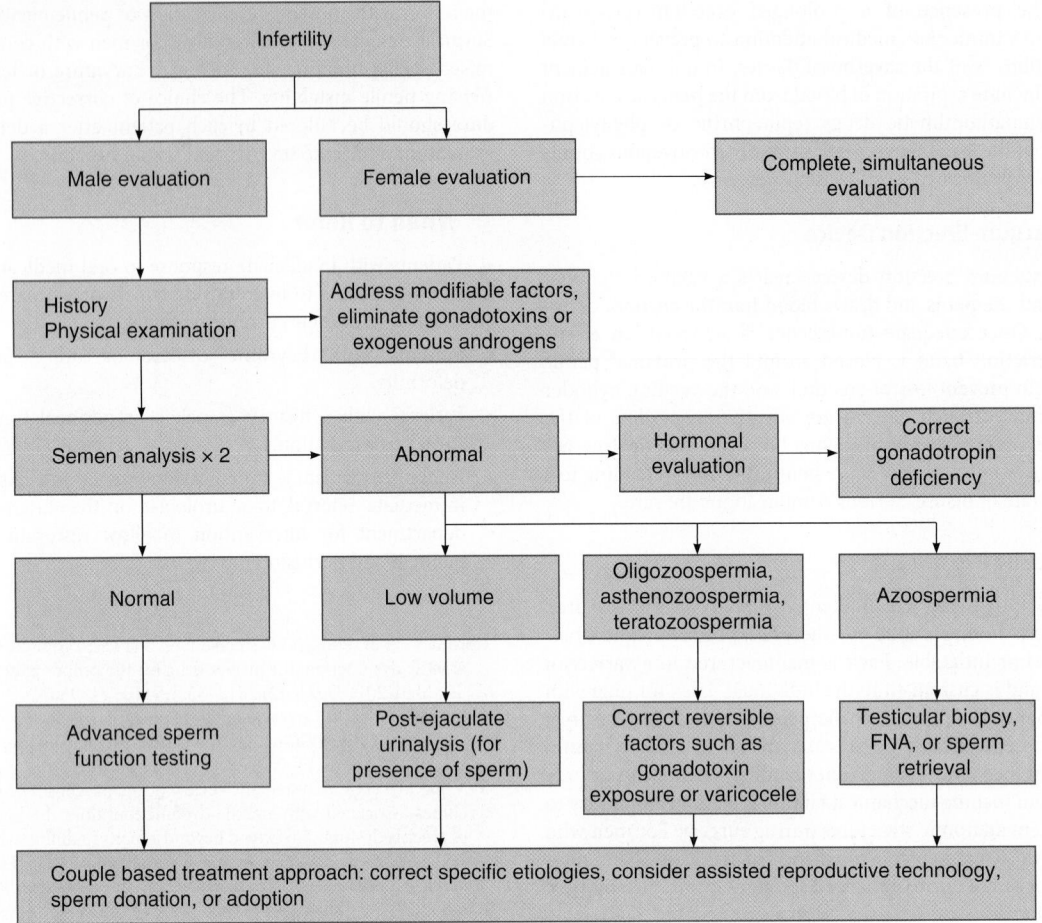

▲ **Figure 23–1.** Couple based approach to evaluation and treatment of male factor infertility. FNA, fine-needle aspiration.

physical examination, a semen analysis is essential for diagnosis and should be performed at least twice, on two separate occasions (Figure 23–1). Because spermatogenesis takes approximately 74 days, it is important to review health events and gonadotoxic exposures from the preceding 3 months. Male infertility is associated with a higher risk for the later development of testicular germ cell cancer; thus, these men should be counseled appropriately and taught testicular self-examination.

▶ **Clinical Findings**

A. Symptoms and Signs

The history should include prior testicular insults (torsion, cryptorchidism, trauma), infections (mumps orchitis, epididymitis, sexually transmitted infections), environmental factors (excessive heat, radiation, chemotherapy, prolonged pesticide exposure), medications (testosterone, finasteride, cimetidine, selective serotonin reuptake inhibitors, and spironolactone may affect spermatogenesis; phenytoin may lower FSH; sulfasalazine and nitrofurantoin affect sperm motility; tamsulosin causes retrograde ejaculation), and

other drugs (alcohol, tobacco, marijuana). Sexual function, frequency and timing of intercourse, use of lubricants, and each partner's previous fertility are important. Loss of libido, headaches, visual disturbances, or galactorrhea may indicate a pituitary tumor. The past medical or surgical history may reveal chronic disease, including thyroid or liver disease (abnormalities of spermatogenesis), diabetes mellitus (retrograde or anejaculation), or radical pelvic or retroperitoneal surgery (absent seminal emission secondary to sympathetic nerve injury).

Physical examination should pay particular attention to features of hypogonadism: underdeveloped sexual characteristics, diminished male pattern hair distribution (axillary, body, facial, pubic), body habitus, gynecomastia, and obesity. The scrotal contents should be carefully evaluated. Testicular size should be noted (normal size approximately 4.5 × 2.5 cm, volume 18 mL). **Varicoceles** are abnormally dilated and refluxing veins of the pampiniform plexus that can be identified in the standing position by gentle palpation of the spermatic cord and, on occasion, may only be appreciated with the Valsalva maneuver. The vas deferens, epididymis, and prostate should be palpated (absence of all or part of the vas deferens may indicate the presence a cystic fibrosis variant, congenital bilateral or unilateral absence of the vas deferens).

B. Laboratory Findings

Semen analysis should be performed after 2 to 3 days of ejaculatory abstinence. The specimen should be analyzed within 1 hour after collection. Abnormal sperm concentrations are < 15 million/mL (**oligozoospermia** is the presence of < 15 million sperm/mL in the ejaculate; **azoospermia** is the absence of sperm). Normal semen volumes range between 1.5 mL and 5 mL (volumes < 1.5 mL may result in inadequate buffering of the vaginal acidity and may be due to retrograde ejaculation, ejaculatory duct obstruction, congenital bilateral absence of the vasa deferentia, or androgen insufficiency). Normal sperm motility and morphology demonstrate > 45% motile cells and > 4% normal morphology (World Health Organization). Abnormal motility may result from varicocele, antisperm antibodies, infection, abnormalities of the sperm flagella, or partial ejaculatory duct obstruction. Abnormal morphology may result from a varicocele, infection, or exposure to gonadotoxins (eg, tobacco smoke).

Endocrine evaluation is warranted if sperm counts are low (< 15 million/mL) or if the history and physical examination suggest an endocrinologic origin. Initial testing should include serum testosterone and FSH. Specific abnormalities in these hormones should prompt additional testing, including serum LH, prolactin, and estradiol levels. Elevated FSH and LH levels and low testosterone levels (hypergonadotropic hypogonadism) are associated with primary testicular failure. Low FSH and LH associated with low testosterone occur in secondary testicular failure (hypogonadotropic hypogonadism) and may be of hypothalamic or pituitary origin. Elevation of serum prolactin may indicate the presence of pituitary prolactinoma. Elevation of estradiol may impair normal gonadotropin production and impact normal spermatogenesis.

C. Genetic Testing

Men with sperm concentrations < 10 million/mL should consider testing for Y chromosome microdeletions and karyotypic abnormalities. Gene deletions from the long arm of the Y chromosome may cause azoospermia or oligozoospermia with age-related decline in spermatogenesis that is transmissible to male offspring. Karyotyping may reveal Klinefelter syndrome. Partial or complete absence of the vas deferens should prompt testing for cystic fibrosis mutations.

D. Imaging

Scrotal ultrasound can aid in characterizing the testes and may detect a subclinical varicocele. Men with low ejaculate volume and no evidence of retrograde ejaculation should undergo transrectal ultrasound to evaluate the prostate and seminal vesicles. MRI of the sella turcica should be performed in men with markedly elevated prolactin or hypogonadotropic hypogonadism to evaluate the anterior pituitary gland. MRI of the pelvis and scrotum should be considered in men for whom the testes cannot be identified in the scrotum by physical examination or ultrasound. Men with unilateral absence of the vas deferens should have abdominal ultrasound or CT to exclude absence of the ipsilateral kidney, given the association of these two conditions.

E. Special Tests

Patients with low volume ejaculate should have post-ejaculation urine samples centrifuged and analyzed for sperm to evaluate for retrograde ejaculation. In cases of disproportionately low motility, sperm vitality and the presence of autoantibodies should be assessed. Round cells in concentrations > 1 million/mL should prompt leukocyte esterase or peroxidase staining (immature germ cells are found normally, but inflammatory cells may require treatment).

▶ Treatment

A. General Measures

Education about the proper timing for intercourse in relation to the woman's ovulatory cycle as well as the avoidance of spermicidal lubricants should be discussed. In cases of gonadotoxic exposure or medication-related factors, the offending agent should be removed whenever feasible. Patients with active genitourinary tract infections should be treated with appropriate antibiotics. Healthy lifestyle habits, including healthy diet, moderate exercise, and avoidance of gonadotoxins (such as tobacco smoke, excessive alcohol, and marijuana) should be reinforced.

B. Varicocele

Varicocelectomy is performed by stopping retrograde blood flow in spermatic cord veins. Surgical ligation may be accomplished via subinguinal, inguinal, retroperitoneal, or laparoscopic approaches. Percutaneous venographic embolization of varicoceles is feasible but may have a higher recurrence rate.

C. Endocrine Therapy

Hypogonadotropic hypogonadism may be treated with chorionic gonadotropin once primary pituitary disease has been excluded or treated. Dosage is usually 2000 international units intramuscularly three times a week. If sperm counts fail to rise after 12 months, FSH therapy should be initiated.

D. Ejaculatory Dysfunction Therapy

Patients with retrograde ejaculation may benefit from alpha-adrenergic agonists (pseudoephedrine, 60 mg orally three times a day) or imipramine (25 mg orally three times a day). Medical failures may require the collection of post-ejaculation urine for intrauterine insemination. Anejaculation can be treated with vibratory stimulation or electroejaculation in select cases.

E. Ductal Obstruction

Obstruction of the ejaculatory ducts may be corrected by transurethral resection of the ducts in the prostatic urethra. If obstruction of the vas deferens or epididymis is suspected, the level of obstruction must be determined via a vasogram prior to operative treatment, with the exception of prior vasectomy. Obstruction of the vas deferens is best managed by microsurgical vasovasostomy or vasoepididymostomy.

F. Assisted Reproductive Techniques

Intrauterine insemination, in vitro fertilization, and intracytoplasmic sperm injection are alternatives for patients in whom other means of treating reduced sperm concentration, motility, or functionality has failed. Intrauterine insemination should only be performed when adequate numbers of motile sperm are noted on an ejaculate sample. With the use of intracytoplasmic sperm injection, azoospermic men can father their genetic progeny by surgical retrieval of sperm from the testicle, epididymis, or vas deferens.

▶ When to Refer

- Couples with clinical infertility or concern about fertility potential.
- Men with known genital insults, genetic diagnoses, or syndromes that preclude natural fertility.
- Reproductive-aged men with newly diagnosed cancer or other disease that may require cytotoxic therapies with interest in fertility preservation.

Eisenberg ML et al. The relationship between male BMI and waist circumference on semen quality: data from the LIFE study. Hum Reprod. 2014 Feb;29(2):193–200. [PMID: 24306102]

Lopushnyan NA et al. Surgical techniques for the management of male infertility. Asian J Androl. 2012 Jan;14(1):94–102. [PMID: 22120932]

Walsh TJ et al. Increased risk of testicular germ cell cancer among infertile men. Arch Intern Med. 2009 Feb 23;169(4):351–6. [PMID: 19237718]

Winters BR et al. The epidemiology of male infertility. Urol Clin North Am. 2014 Feb;41(1):195–204. [PMID: 24286777]

BENIGN PROSTATIC HYPERPLASIA

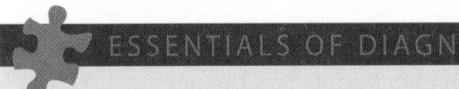

ESSENTIALS OF DIAGNOSIS

- ▶ Obstructive or irritative voiding symptoms.
- ▶ May have enlarged prostate on rectal examination.
- ▶ Absence of urinary tract infection, neurologic disorder, stricture disease, prostatic or bladder malignancy.

▶ General Considerations

Benign prostatic hyperplasia is the most common benign tumor in men, and its incidence is age related. The prevalence of histologic benign prostatic hyperplasia in autopsy studies rises from approximately 20% in men aged 41–50 years, to 50% in men aged 51–60, and to over 90% in men over 80 years of age. Although clinical evidence of disease occurs less commonly, symptoms of prostatic obstruction are also age related. At age 55 years, approximately 25% of men report obstructive voiding symptoms. At age 75 years, 50% of men report a decrease in the force and caliber of the urinary stream.

Risk factors for the development of benign prostatic hyperplasia are poorly understood. Some studies have suggested a genetic predisposition and some have noted racial differences. Approximately 50% of men under age 60 years who undergo surgery for benign prostatic hyperplasia may have a heritable form of the disease. This form is most likely an autosomal dominant trait, and first-degree male relatives of such patients carry an increased relative risk of approximately fourfold.

▶ Clinical Findings

A. Symptoms

The symptoms of benign prostatic hyperplasia can be divided into obstructive and irritative complaints. **Obstructive symptoms** include hesitancy, decreased force and caliber of the stream, sensation of incomplete bladder emptying, double voiding (urinating a second time within 2 hours), straining to urinate, and postvoid dribbling. **Irritative symptoms** include urgency, frequency, and nocturia.

The American Urological Association (AUA) symptom index (Table 23–4) is perhaps the single most important tool used in the evaluation of patients with this disorder and should be calculated for all patients before starting therapy. The answers to seven questions quantitate the severity of obstructive or irritative complaints on a scale of 0–5. Thus, the score can range from 0 to 35, in increasing severity of symptoms.

A detailed history focusing on the urinary tract should be obtained to exclude other possible causes of symptoms such as prostate cancer or disorders unrelated to the prostate such as urinary tract infection, neurogenic bladder, or urethral stricture.

B. Signs

A physical examination, digital rectal examination (DRE), and a focused neurologic examination should be performed on all patients. The size and consistency of the prostate should be noted, but prostate size does not correlate with the severity of symptoms or the degree of obstruction. Benign prostatic hyperplasia usually results in a smooth, firm, elastic enlargement of the prostate. Induration, if detected, must alert the clinician to the possibility of cancer, and further evaluation is needed (ie, prostate-specific antigen [PSA] testing, transrectal ultrasound, and biopsy). Examination of the lower abdomen should be performed to assess for a distended bladder.

Table 23–4. American Urological Association symptom index for benign prostatic hyperplasia.[1]

Questions to Be Answered	Not at All	Less Than One Time in Five	Less Than Half the Time	About Half the Time	More Than Half the Time	Almost Always
1. Over the past month, how often have you had a sensation of not emptying your bladder completely after you finish urinating?	0	1	2	3	4	5
2. Over the past month, how often have you had to urinate again less than 2 hours after you finished urinating?	0	1	2	3	4	5
3. Over the past month, how often have you found you stopped and started again several times when you urinated?	0	1	2	3	4	5
4. Over the past month, how often have you found it difficult to postpone urination?	0	1	2	3	4	5
5. Over the past month, how often have you had a weak urinary stream?	0	1	2	3	4	5
6. Over the past month, how often have you had to push or strain to begin urination?	0	1	2	3	4	5
7. Over the past month, how many times did you most typically get up to urinate from the time you went to bed at night until the time you got up in the morning?	0	1	2	3	4	5

[1]Sum of seven circled numbers equals the symptom score. See text for explanation.
Reproduced, with permission, from Barry MJ et al. The American Urological Association symptom index for benign prostatic hyperplasia. J Urol. 1992 Nov;148(5):1549–57.

C. Laboratory Findings

Urinalysis should be performed to exclude infection or hematuria. A serum PSA is considered optional, yet most clinicians will include it in the initial evaluation, particularly if life expectancy is > 10 years. PSA certainly increases the ability to detect prostate cancer over DRE alone; however, because there is much overlap between levels seen in benign prostatic hyperplasia and prostate cancer, its use remains controversial (see Chapter 39).

D. Imaging

Upper tract imaging (CT or renal ultrasound) is recommended only in the presence of concomitant urinary tract disease or complications from benign prostatic hyperplasia (ie, hematuria, urinary tract infection, chronic kidney disease, history of stone disease).

E. Cystoscopy

Cystoscopy is not recommended to determine the need for treatment but may assist in determining the surgical approach in patients opting for invasive therapy.

F. Additional Tests

Cystometrograms and urodynamic profiles should be reserved for patients with suspected neurologic disease or those who have failed prostate surgery. Flow rates, postvoid residual urine determination, and pressure-flow studies are considered optional.

▶ Differential Diagnosis

A history of prior urethral instrumentation, urethritis, or trauma should be elucidated to exclude urethral stricture or bladder neck contracture. Hematuria and pain are commonly associated with bladder stones. Carcinoma of the prostate may be detected by abnormalities on the DRE or an elevated PSA (see Chapter 39). A urinary tract infection can mimic the irritative symptoms of benign prostatic hyperplasia and can be readily identified by urinalysis and culture; however, a urinary tract infection can also be a complication of benign prostatic hyperplasia. Carcinoma of the bladder, especially carcinoma in situ, may also present with irritative voiding complaints; however, urinalysis usually shows evidence of hematuria (see Chapter 39). Patients with a neurogenic bladder may also have many of the same symptoms and signs as those with benign prostatic hyperplasia; however, a history of neurologic disease, stroke, diabetes mellitus, or back injury may be obtained, and diminished perineal or lower extremity sensation or alterations in rectal sphincter tone or the bulbocavernosus reflex might be observed on examination. Simultaneous alterations in bowel function (constipation) might also suggest the possibility of a neurologic disorder.

▶ Treatment

Clinical practice guidelines exist for the evaluation and treatment of patients with benign prostatic hyperplasia (Figure 23–2). Following evaluation as outlined above, patients should be offered various forms of therapy for benign prostatic hyperplasia. Patients are advised to consult with their primary care clinicians and make an educated decision on the basis of the relative efficacy and side effects of the treatment options (Table 23–5).

Patients with mild symptoms (AUA scores 0–7) should be managed by watchful waiting only. Absolute surgical indications are refractory urinary retention (failing at least one attempt at catheter removal), large bladder diverticula, or any of the following sequelae of benign prostatic hyperplasia: recurrent urinary tract infection, recurrent gross hematuria, bladder stones, or chronic kidney disease.

A. Watchful Waiting

The risk of progression or complications is uncertain. However, in men with symptomatic disease, it is clear that progression is not inevitable and that some men undergo spontaneous improvement or resolution of their symptoms.

Retrospective studies on the natural history of benign prostatic hyperplasia are inherently subject to bias, relating in part to patient selection and also to the type and extent of follow-up. Very few prospective studies addressing the natural history have been reported. One small series demonstrated that approximately 10% of symptomatic men may progress to urinary retention while 50% of patients demonstrate marked improvement or resolution of symptoms. A large randomized study compared finasteride with placebo in men with moderate to severely symptomatic disease and enlarged prostates on DRE. Patients in the placebo arm demonstrated a 7% risk of developing urinary retention over 4 years.

Men with moderate or severe symptoms can also be observed if they so choose. The optimal interval for follow-up is not defined, nor are the specific end points for intervention.

B. Medical Therapy

1. Alpha-blockers— Alpha-blockers can be classified according to their receptor selectivity as well as their half-life (Table 23–6).

Prazosin is effective; however, it requires dose titration and twice daily dosing. Typical side effects include

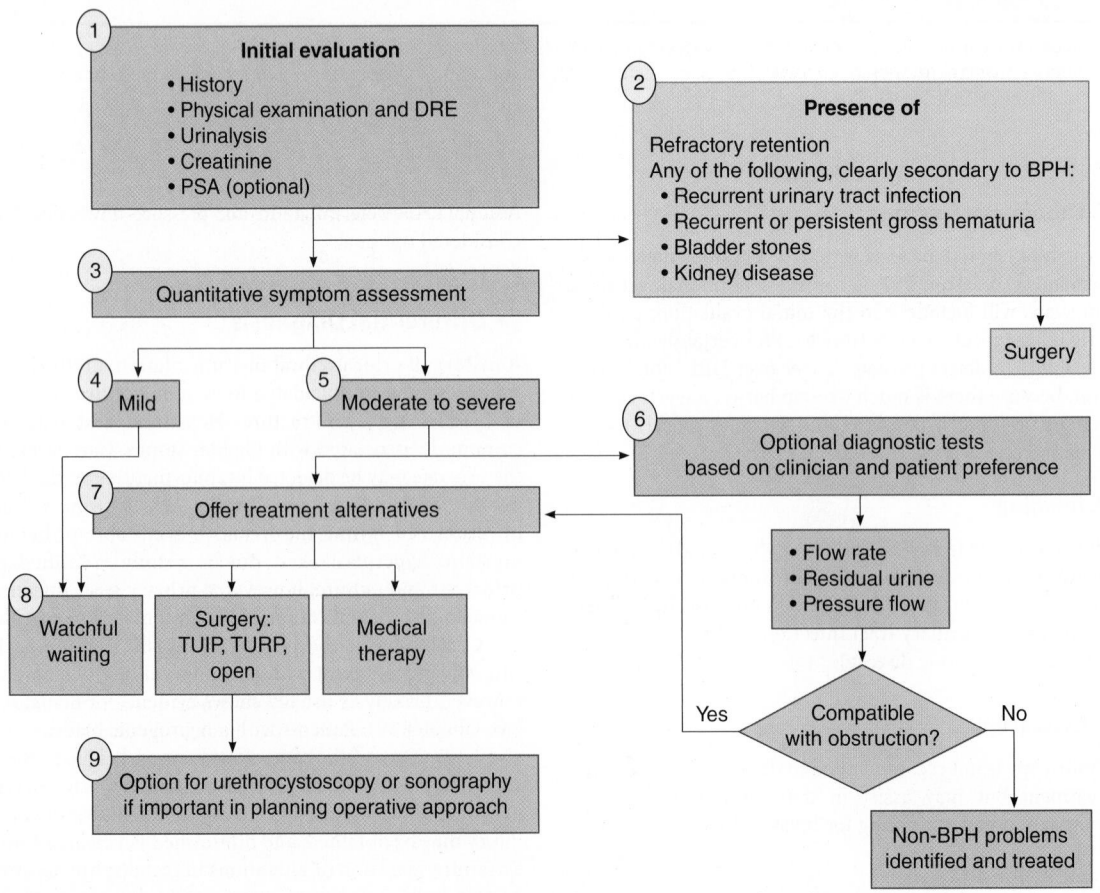

▲ **Figure 23–2.** Benign prostatic hyperplasia decision diagram. DRE, digital rectal examination; PSA, prostate specific antigen; BPH, benign prostatic hyperplasia; TUIP, transurethral incision of the prostate; TURP, transurethral resection of the prostate.

Table 23–5. Summary of benign prostatic hyperplasia treatment outcomes.[1]

Outcome	TUIP	Open Surgery	TURP	Watchful Waiting	Alpha-Blockers	Finasteride[2]
Chance for improvement[1]	78–83%	94–99.8%	75–96%	31–55%	59–86%	54–78%
Degree of symptom improvement (% reduction in symptom score)	73%	79%	85%	Unknown	51%	31%
Morbidity and complications[1]	2.2–33.3%	7–42.7%	5.2–30.7%	1–5%	2.9–43.3%	13.6–8.8%
Death within 30–90 days[1]	0.2–1.5%	1–4.6%	0.5–3.3%	0.8%	0.8%	0.8%
Total incontinence[1]	0.1–1.1%	0.3–0.7%	0.7–1.4%	2%	2%	2%
Need for operative treatment for surgical complications[1]	1.3–2.7%	0.6–14.1%	0.7–10.1%	0	0	0
Erectile dysfunction[1]	3.9–24.5%	4.7–39.2%	3.3–34.8%	3%	3%	2.5–5.3%
Retrograde ejaculation	6–55%	36–95%	25–99%	0	4–11%	0
Loss of work in days	7–21	21–28	7–21	1	3.5	1.5
Hospital stay in days	1–3	5–10	3–5	0	0	0

[1]90% confidence interval.
[2]Most of the data reviewed for finasteride are derived from three trials that have required an enlarged prostate for entry. The chance of improvement in men with symptoms yet minimally enlarged prostates may be much less, as noted from the VA Cooperative Trial.
TUIP, transurethral incision of the prostate; TURP, transurethral resection of the prostate.

orthostatic hypotension, dizziness, tiredness, retrograde ejaculation, rhinitis, and headache.

Long-acting alpha-blockers allow for once-a-day dosing, but dose titration is still necessary because side effects similar to those seen with prazosin may occur. Terazosin improves symptoms and in numerous studies is superior to placebo or finasteride. Terazosin is started at a dosage of 1 mg orally daily for 3 days, increased to 2 mg orally daily for 11 days, then 5 mg orally daily. Additional dose escalation to 10 mg orally daily can be performed if necessary. Doxazosin is started at a dosage of 1 mg orally daily for 7 days, increased to 2 mg orally daily for 7 days, then 4 mg orally daily. Additional dose escalation to 8 mg orally daily can be performed if necessary.

Alpha-1a-receptors are localized to the prostate and bladder neck. Selective blockade of these receptors results

Table 23–6. Alpha-blockade for benign prostatic hyperplasia.

Agent	Action	Oral Dose
Alfuzosin	Alpha-1a-blockade	10 mg daily
Doxazosin	Alpha-1-blockade	1–8 mg daily
Phenoxybenzamine	Alpha-1- and alpha-2-blockade	5–10 mg twice daily
Prazosin	Alpha-1-blockade	1–5 mg twice daily
Silodosin	Alpha-1a-blockade	4 or 8 mg daily
Tadalafil	Phosphodiesterase type 5 inhibitor	5 mg daily
Tamsulosin	Alpha-1a-blockade	0.4 or 0.8 mg daily
Terazosin	Alpha-1-blockade	1–10 mg daily

in fewer systemic side effects than alpha-blocker therapy (orthostatic hypotension, dizziness, tiredness, rhinitis, and headache), thus obviating the need for dose titration. The typical dose of tamsulosin is 0.4 mg orally daily taken 30 minutes after a meal. Alfuzosin is a long-acting alpha-1a-blocker; its dose is 10 mg orally once daily with food and does not require titration. Several randomized, double-blind, placebo-controlled trials have been performed comparing terazosin, doxazosin, tamsulosin, and alfuzosin with placebo. All agents have demonstrated safety and efficacy. However, floppy eye syndrome, a complication of cataract surgery, can occur in patients taking alpha-blockers and alpha-1a-blockers.

2. 5-alpha-Reductase inhibitors—Finasteride is a 5-alpha-reductase inhibitor that blocks the conversion of testosterone to dihydrotestosterone. This drug impacts upon the epithelial component of the prostate, resulting in reduction in size of the gland and improvement in symptoms. Six months of therapy is required for maximum effects on prostate size (20% reduction) and symptomatic improvement.

Several randomized, double-blind, placebo-controlled trials have been performed comparing finasteride with placebo. Efficacy, safety, and durability are well established. However, symptomatic improvement is seen only in men with enlarged prostates (> 40 mL by ultrasonographic examination). Side effects include decreased libido, decrease in volume of ejaculate, and erectile dysfunction. Serum PSA is reduced by approximately 50% in patients receiving finasteride therapy. Therefore, in order to compare with pre-finasteride levels, the serum PSA of a patient taking finasteride should be doubled.

A report suggests that finasteride therapy may decrease the incidence of urinary retention and the need for operative treatment in men with enlarged prostates and moderate to severe symptoms. The larger the prostate over 40 mL, the greater the relative-risk reduction. However, optimal identification of appropriate patients for prophylactic therapy remains to be determined. Dutasteride is a dual 5-alpha-reductase inhibitor that appears to be similar to finasteride in its effectiveness; its dose is 0.5 mg orally daily.

Both finasteride and dutasteride have been shown to be effective chemopreventive agents for prostate cancer in large, randomized clinical trials. The 25% risk reduction was observed in men with both low and high risk for prostate cancer. However, despite the strength of the evidence for 5-alpha-reductase inhibitors in reducing the risk of prostate cancer, an FDA advisory committee recommended against labeling these agents for prostate cancer chemoprevention, citing the potential increased risk of high-grade tumors in these studies, isolated risk reduction in low-grade tumors, and inability to apply the findings to the general population. Moreover, the FDA has included the increased risk of being diagnosed with high-grade prostate cancer in the labels of all 5-alpha-reductase inhibitors.

3. Phosphodiesterase-5 inhibitor—The FDA approved the use of tadalafil to treat the signs and symptoms of benign prostatic hyperplasia in 2011; it is also approved for use in men with both urinary symptoms and erectile dysfunction. The data from two randomized, double-blind, placebo-controlled trials demonstrated significant improvements in standardized measurements of urinary function between 2 and 4 weeks after initiating treatment at 5 mg, with minimal adverse effects.

4. Combination therapy—The four-arm Veterans Administration Cooperative Trial compared placebo, finasteride alone, terazosin alone, and combination of finasteride and terazosin. Over 1200 patients participated, and significant decreases in symptom scores and increases in urinary flow rates were seen only in the arms containing terazosin. However, enlarged prostates were not an entry criterion; in fact, prostate size in this study was much smaller than in previous controlled trials using finasteride (32 versus 52 mL). Other randomized, placebo-controlled trials comparing finasteride with placebo in men with lower urinary tract symptoms and large prostates showed finasteride to be beneficial for reducing symptoms, increasing urinary flow rate, and reducing the risk of complications due to benign prostatic hyperplasia as well as reducing the number of men who required surgery for benign prostatic hyperplasia. The Medical Therapy of Prostatic Symptoms (MTOPS) trial was a large, randomized, placebo-controlled trial comparing finasteride, doxazosin, the combination of the two, and placebo in 3047 men observed for a mean of 4.5 years. Long-term combination therapy with doxazosin and finasteride was safe and reduced the risk of overall clinical progression of benign prostatic hyperplasia significantly more than did treatment with either drug alone. Combination therapy and finasteride alone reduced the long-term risk of acute urinary retention and the need for invasive therapy. Combination therapy had the risks of additional side effects and the cost of two medications.

5. Phytotherapy—Phytotherapy is the use of plants or plant extracts for medicinal purposes. Its use in benign

prostatic hyperplasia has been popularized by patient-driven enthusiasm. Several plant extracts have been popularized, including the saw palmetto berry, the bark of *Pygeum africanum*, the roots of *Echinacea purpurea* and *Hypoxis rooperi*, pollen extract, and the leaves of the trembling poplar. The mechanisms of action of these agents are unknown. A 2006 prospective, randomized, double-blind, placebo-controlled trial revealed no improvement in symptoms, urinary flow rate, or quality of life for men with benign prostatic hyperplasia with saw palmetto treatment compared with placebo.

C. Conventional Surgical Therapy

1. Transurethral resection of the prostate (TURP)—Ninety-five percent of simple prostatectomies can be performed endoscopically (TURP). Most of these procedures are performed under a spinal anesthetic and require a 1- to 2-day hospital stay. Symptom scores and flow rate improvement are superior following TURP relative to any minimally invasive therapy; however, the length of the hospital stay is greater. Much controversy revolves around possible higher rates of morbidity and mortality associated with TURP in comparison with open surgery, but the higher rates observed in one study probably related to more significant comorbidities in the TURP patients compared with the patients who received open surgical treatment. Several other studies could not confirm the difference in mortality when controlling for age and comorbidities. The risks of TURP include retrograde ejaculation (75%), erectile dysfunction (5–10%), and urinary incontinence (< 1%). Complications include bleeding, urethral stricture or bladder neck contracture, perforation of the prostate capsule with extravasation, and, if severe, transurethral resection syndrome, a hypervolemic, hyponatremic state resulting from absorption of the hypotonic irrigating solution. Clinical manifestations of the syndrome include nausea, vomiting, confusion, hypertension, bradycardia, and visual disturbances. The risk of transurethral resection syndrome increases with resection times over 90 minutes. Treatment includes diuresis and, in severe cases, hypertonic saline administration (see Hyponatremia, Chapter 21).

2. Transurethral incision of the prostate (TUIP)—Men with moderate to severe symptoms and small prostates often have posterior commissure hyperplasia or an "elevated bladder neck." These patients will often benefit from incision of the prostate. The procedure is more rapid and less morbid than TURP. Outcomes in well-selected patients are comparable, though a lower rate of retrograde ejaculation has been reported (25%).

3. Open simple prostatectomy—When the prostate is too large to remove endoscopically, open enucleation is necessary. What size is "too large" depends upon the surgeon's experience with TURP. Glands over 100 g are usually considered for open enucleation. In addition to size, other relative indications for open prostatectomy include concomitant bladder diverticulum or bladder stone and whether dorsal lithotomy positioning is or is not possible.

Open prostatectomies can be performed with either a suprapubic or retropubic approach. Simple suprapubic prostatectomy is performed transvesically and is the operation of choice if there is concomitant bladder pathology. After the adenoma is removed, both a urethral and a suprapubic catheter are inserted prior to closure.

In simple retropubic prostatectomy, the bladder is not entered but rather a transverse incision is made in the surgical capsule of the prostate and the adenoma is enucleated as described above; only a urethral catheter is needed at the end of the case.

D. Minimally Invasive Therapy

1. Laser therapy—Several coagulation necrosis techniques have been utilized. Transurethral laser-induced prostatectomy (TULIP) is performed under transrectal ultrasound guidance. The instrument is placed in the urethra and transrectal ultrasound is used to direct the device as it is slowly pulled from the bladder neck to the apex. The depth of treatment is monitored with ultrasound.

Most urologists prefer to use visually directed laser techniques. Visual coagulative necrosis is performed under cystoscopic control, and the laser fiber is pulled through the prostate at several designated areas depending upon the size and configuration of the gland. Four-quadrant and sextant approaches have been described for lateral lobes, with additional treatments directed at enlarged median lobes. Coagulative techniques do not create an immediate visual defect in the prostatic urethra—tissue is sloughed over the course of several weeks up to 3 months following the procedure.

Visual contact ablative techniques take longer in the operating room because the fiber is placed in direct contact with the prostate tissue, which is vaporized. Photovaporization of the prostate (PVP), an alternative laser technique, uses a high-power KTP laser. An immediate defect is obtained in the prostatic urethra, similar to that seen during TURP.

Interstitial laser therapy places fibers directly into the prostate, usually under cystoscopic control. Irritative voiding symptoms may be less in these patients as the urethral mucosa is spared and prostate tissue is resorbed by the body rather than sloughed.

Advantages to laser surgery include minimal blood loss, rarity of transurethral resection syndrome, ability to treat patients during anticoagulant therapy, and outpatient surgery. Disadvantages are the lack of tissue for pathologic examination, longer postoperative catheterization time, more frequent irritative voiding complaints, and expense of laser fibers and generators.

Large multicenter, randomized studies with long-term follow-up are needed to compare laser prostate surgery with TURP and other forms of minimally invasive surgery.

2. Transurethral needle ablation of the prostate (TUNA)—This procedure uses a specially designed urethral catheter that is passed into the urethra. Interstitial radiofrequency needles are then deployed from the tip of the catheter, piercing the mucosa of the prostatic urethra. Radiofrequencies are then used to heat the tissue, resulting in coagulative necrosis. Bladder neck and median lobe enlargement are not well treated by TUNA. Subjective and objective improvement in voiding occurs. In randomized trials comparing TUNA to TURP, similar improvement was seen when comparing life scores, peak urinary flow rates, and postvoid residual urine.

3. Transurethral electrovaporization of the prostate—This technique uses the standard resectoscope. High current densities result in heat vaporization of tissue, creating a cavity in the prostatic urethra. Because the device requires slower sweeping speeds over the prostatic urethra and the depth of vaporization is approximately one-third of a standard loop, this procedure usually takes longer than a standard TURP. Long-term comparative data are needed.

4. Hyperthermia—Microwave hyperthermia is most commonly delivered with a transurethral catheter. Some devices cool the urethral mucosa to decrease the risk of injury. However, if temperatures do not go above 45°C, cooling is unnecessary. Symptom score and flow rate improvement are obtained, but (as with laser surgery) large randomized studies with long-term follow-up are needed to assess durability and cost-effectiveness.

5. Implant to open prostatic urethra—In 2013, the FDA approved an implant placed in a minimally invasive fashion to retract the enlarged lobes of the prostate in symptomatic men 50 years and older with an enlarged prostate. Data from trials suggest that the technique improved symptoms and voiding flow while having minimal impact on ejaculation.

▶ When to Refer

- Progression to urinary retention.
- Patient dissatisfaction with medical therapy.
- Need for surgical intervention or further evaluation (cystoscopy).

Juliao AA et al. American Urological Association and European Association of Urology guidelines in the management of benign prostatic hypertrophy: revisited. Curr Opin Urol. 2012 Jan;22(1):34–9. [PMID: 22123290]

McNicholas TA et al. Minimally invasive prostatic urethral lift: surgical technique and multinational experience. Eur Urol. 2013 Aug;64(2):292–9. [PMID: 23357348]

McVary KT et al. Update on AUA guideline on the management of benign prostatic hyperplasia. J Urol. 2011 May;185(5): 1793–803. [PMID: 21420124]

Toren P et al. Effect of dutasteride on clinical progression of benign prostatic hyperplasia in asymptomatic men with enlarged prostate: a post hoc analysis of the REDUCE study. BMJ. 2013 Apr 15;346:f2109. [PMID: 23587564]

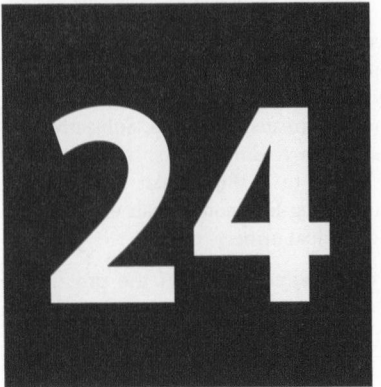

Nervous System Disorders

Michael J. Aminoff, MD, DSc, FRCP

Geoffrey A. Kerchner, MD, PhD

HEADACHE

Headache is such a common complaint and can occur for so many different reasons that its proper evaluation may be difficult. New, severe, or acute headaches are more likely than chronic headaches to relate to an intracranial disorder; the approach to such headaches is discussed in Chapter 2. **Chronic headaches** may be primary or secondary to another disorder. Common primary headache syndromes include migraine, tension-type headache, and cluster headache. Important secondary causes to consider include intracranial lesions, head injury, cervical spondylosis, dental or ocular disease, temporomandibular joint dysfunction, sinusitis, hypertension, depression, and a wide variety of general medical disorders. Although underlying structural lesions are not present in most patients presenting with headache, it is nevertheless important to bear this possibility in mind. About one-third of patients with brain tumors, for example, present with a primary complaint of headache.

1. Migraine

ESSENTIALS OF DIAGNOSIS

► Headache, usually pulsatile.

► Pain is typically, but not always, unilateral.

► Nausea, vomiting, photophobia, and phonophobia are common accompaniments.

► An aura of transient neurologic symptoms (commonly visual) may precede head pain.

► Commonly, head pain occurs with no aura.

▶ General Considerations

The pathophysiology of migraine probably relates to neurovascular dysfunction. Headache results from the dilatation of blood vessels innervated by the trigeminal nerve caused by release of neuropeptides from parasympathetic nerve fibers approximating these vessels. Migraine often exhibits a complex, polygenic pattern of inheritance. Sometimes, an autosomal dominant inheritance pattern is apparent, as in **familial hemiplegic migraine** (FHM), in which attacks of lateralized weakness represent the aura. Mutations in three associated genes—*ATP1A2*, *CACNA1A*, and *SCN1A*—account for about three-quarters of cases.

▶ Clinical Findings

Classic migrainous headache is a lateralized throbbing headache that occurs episodically following its onset in adolescence or early adult life. In many cases, however, the headaches do not conform to this pattern, although their associated features and response to antimigrainous preparations nevertheless suggest that they have a similar basis. In this broader sense, migrainous headaches may be lateralized or generalized, may be dull or throbbing, and are sometimes associated with anorexia, nausea, vomiting, photophobia, phonophobia, osmophobia, cognitive impairment, and blurring of vision. They usually build up gradually and may last for several hours or longer. Focal disturbances of neurologic function may precede or accompany the headaches and have been attributed to constriction of branches of the internal carotid artery. Visual disturbances occur commonly and may consist of field defects; of luminous visual hallucinations such as stars, sparks, unformed light flashes (photopsia), geometric patterns, or zigzags of light; or of some combination of field defects and luminous hallucinations (scintillating scotomas). Other focal disturbances such as aphasia or numbness, paresthesias, clumsiness, dysarthria, dysequilibrium, or weakness in a circumscribed distribution may also occur.

In rare instances, the neurologic or somatic disturbance accompanying typical migrainous headaches becomes the sole manifestation of an attack ("migraine equivalent"). Very rarely, the patient may be left with a permanent neurologic deficit following a migrainous attack, and migraine with aura may be a risk factor for stroke.

Patients often give a family history of migraine. Attacks may be triggered by emotional or physical stress, lack or excess of sleep, missed meals, specific foods (eg, chocolate), alcoholic beverages, bright lights, loud noise, menstruation, or use of oral contraceptives.

An uncommon variant is **basilar artery migraine**, in which blindness or visual disturbances throughout both visual fields are initially accompanied or followed by dysarthria, dysequilibrium, tinnitus, and perioral and distal paresthesias and are sometimes followed by transient loss or impairment of consciousness or by a confusional state. This, in turn, is followed by a throbbing (usually occipital) headache, often with nausea and vomiting.

In **ophthalmoplegic migraine**, lateralized pain—often about the eye—is accompanied by nausea, vomiting, and diplopia due to transient external ophthalmoplegia. The ophthalmoplegia is due to third nerve palsy, sometimes with accompanying sixth nerve involvement, and may outlast the orbital pain by several days or even weeks. The ophthalmic division of the fifth nerve has also been affected in some patients. Ophthalmoplegic migraine is rare; more common causes of a painful ophthalmoplegia are internal carotid artery aneurysms and diabetes.

▶ **Treatment**

Management of migraine consists of avoidance of any precipitating factors, together with prophylactic or symptomatic pharmacologic treatment if necessary.

A. Symptomatic Therapy

During acute attacks, rest in a quiet, darkened room may be helpful until symptoms subside. A simple analgesic (eg, aspirin, acetaminophen, ibuprofen, or naproxen) taken right away often provides relief, but treatment with prescription therapy is sometimes necessary. To prevent medication overuse, use of simple analgesics should be limited to 15 days or less per month, and combination analgesics should be limited to no more than 10 days per month.

1. Ergotamines—Cafergot, a combination of ergotamine tartrate (1 mg) and caffeine (100 mg), is often particularly helpful; one or two tablets are taken at the onset of headache or warning symptoms, followed by one tablet every 30 minutes, if necessary, up to six tablets per attack and no more than 10 days per month. Because of impaired absorption or vomiting during acute attacks, oral medication sometimes fails to help. Cafergot given rectally as suppositories (one-half to one suppository containing 2 mg of ergotamine) or dihydroergotamine mesylate (0.5–1 mg intravenously or 1–2 mg subcutaneously or intramuscularly) may be useful in such cases. Ergotamine-containing preparations should be avoided in pregnancy and when cardiovascular disease or risk factors are present.

2. Triptans—Sumatriptan, which has a high affinity for 5-HT$_1$ receptors, is a rapidly effective agent for aborting attacks when given subcutaneously by an autoinjection device (4–6 mg once subcutaneously, may repeat once after 2 hours if needed; maximum dose 12 mg/24 h). Nasal and oral preparations are available but may be less effective due to slower absorption. Zolmitriptan, another selective 5-HT$_1$ receptor agonist, has high bioavailability after oral administration and is also effective for the immediate treatment of migraine. The optimal initial oral dose is 5 mg, and relief usually occurs within 1 hour; may repeat once after 2 hours. It is also available in a nasal formulation, which has a rapid onset of action; the dose is 5 mg in one nostril once and it may be repeated once after 2 hours. The maximum dose for both formulations is 10 mg/24 h. Other available triptans are available, including rizatriptan (5–10 mg orally at onset, may repeat every 2 hours twice [maximum dose 30 mg/24 h]); naratriptan (1–2.5 mg orally at onset, may repeat once after 4 hours [maximum dose 5 mg/24 h]); almotriptan (6.25–12.5 mg orally at onset, may repeat dose once after 2 hours [maximum dose 25 mg/ 24 h]); frovatriptan (2.5 mg orally at onset, may repeat after 2 hours once [maximum dose 7.5 mg/24]); and eletriptan (20–40 mg orally at onset; may repeat after 2 hours once [maximum dose 80 mg/24 h]). Eletriptan is useful for immediate therapy and frovatriptan, which has a longer half-life, may be worthwhile for patients with prolonged attacks or attacks provoked by menstrual periods.

Triptans may cause nausea and vomiting. They should probably be avoided in women who are pregnant, in patients with hemiplegic or basilar migraine, and in patients with risk factors for stroke (such as hypertension, prior stroke or transient ischemic attack, diabetes mellitus, hypercholesterolemia, obesity). Triptans are contraindicated in patients with coronary or peripheral vascular disease. Patients often experience greater benefit when the triptan is combined with naproxen (500 mg).

3. Other agents—Prochlorperazine is effective and may be administered rectally (25 mg suppository), intravenously or intramuscularly (5–10 mg), or orally (5–10 mg). The neuroleptic droperidol is also helpful in aborting acute attacks, particularly in an emergency setting in opioid-tolerant patients. Intravenous metoclopramide (10–20 mg) and various butalbital-containing combination analgesics are effective. Opioid analgesics are sometimes required when other therapies fail. Intravenous propofol in subanesthetic doses may help in intractable cases.

B. Preventive Therapy

Preventive treatment may be necessary if migraine headaches occur more frequently than two or three times a month or significant disability is associated with attacks. Some of the more common drugs used for this purpose are listed in Table 24–1. Their mode of action is unclear but may involve alteration of central neurotransmission. Several drugs may have to be tried in turn before the headaches are brought under control. Once a drug has been found to help, it should be continued for several months. If the patient remains headache-free, the dose may be tapered and the drug eventually withdrawn. Botulinum toxin type A is approved by the US Food and Drug Administration (FDA) for migraine prevention. A randomized controlled trial failed to show any difference between acupuncture and sham acupuncture in prophylaxis of migraine. Some neurostimulation techniques look promising, including occipital nerve stimulation, but critical appraisal is necessary.

Table 24–1. Prophylactic treatment of migraine.

Drug	Usual Adult Oral Daily Dose	Common Side Effects
Antiepileptic[1]		
Topiramate	100 mg (divided twice daily)	Somnolence, nausea, dyspepsia, irritability, dizziness, ataxia, nystagmus, diplopia, glaucoma, renal calculi, weight loss, hypohidrosis, hyperthermia.
Valproic acid[2,3]	500–1000 mg (divided twice daily)	Nausea, vomiting, diarrhea, drowsiness, alopecia, weight gain, hepatotoxicity, thrombocytopenia, tremor, pancreatitis.
Cardiovascular		
Candesartan[3]	8–32 mg	Dizziness, cough, diarrhea, fatigue.
Propranolol	80–240 mg (divided twice to four times daily)	Fatigue, dizziness, hypotension, bradycardia, depression, insomnia, nausea, vomiting, constipation.
Timolol	10–30 mg	Similar to propranolol.
Verapamil[4]	80–240 mg (divided three times daily)	Headache, hypotension, flushing, edema, constipation. May aggravate atrioventricular nodal heart block and heart failure.
Antidepressant[5]		
Amitriptyline[6]	10–150 mg	Sedation, dry mouth, constipation, weight gain, blurred vision, edema, hypotension, urinary retention.
Other		
Botulinum toxin A	Intramuscular injection by trained clinician	Injection site reaction, hypersensitivity, muscle weakness.
Butterbur	100–150 mg (divided twice daily)	Belching, headache, itchy eyes, gastrointestinal issues, asthma, fatigue, drowsiness, allergic reaction. **Do not use unprocessed butterbur, which contains hepatotoxic pyrrolizidine alkaloids.**

[1]Gabapentin and possibly other antiepileptics have also been used successfully.
[2]Avoid during pregnancy.
[3]Not FDA-approved for this indication.
[4]Other calcium channel antagonists (eg, nimodipine, nicardipine, and diltiazem) may also help.
[5]Depression is commonly comorbid with migraine disorder and may warrant separate treatment.
[6]Other tricyclic antidepressants (eg, nortriptyline and imipramine) may similarly help.

2. Tension-type Headache

This is the most common type of primary headache disorder. Patients frequently complain of pericranial tenderness, poor concentration, and other nonspecific symptoms, in addition to constant daily headaches that are often vise-like or tight in quality but are not pulsatile. Headaches may be exacerbated by emotional stress, fatigue, noise, or glare. The headaches are usually generalized, may be most intense about the neck or back of the head, and are not associated with focal neurologic symptoms. There is diagnostic overlap with migraine.

The therapeutic approach is similar to that in migraine, except that triptan drugs are not indicated. Treatment of comorbid anxiety or depression is important. Techniques to induce relaxation are sometimes useful and include massage, hot baths, and biofeedback.

3. Cluster Headache

Cluster headache affects predominantly middle-aged men. The pathophysiology is unclear but may relate to activation of cells in the ipsilateral hypothalamus, triggering the trigeminal autonomic vascular system. There is often no family history of headache or migraine. Episodes of severe unilateral periorbital pain occur daily for several weeks and are often accompanied by one or more of the following: ipsilateral nasal congestion, rhinorrhea, lacrimation, redness of the eye, and Horner syndrome (ptosis of the eyelid, meiosis or constriction of the pupil, and anhidrosis or reduced sweat secretion). During attacks, patients are often restless and agitated. Episodes typically occur at night, awaken the patient, and last for between 15 minutes and 3 hours. Spontaneous remission then occurs, and the patient remains well for weeks or months before another bout of closely spaced attacks. Bouts may last for 4 to 8 weeks and may occur up to several times per year. During a bout, many patients report that alcohol triggers an attack; others report that stress, glare, or ingestion of specific foods occasionally precipitates attacks. In occasional patients, remission does not occur. This variant has been referred to as chronic cluster headache. **Hemicrania continua** is a separate primary headache syndrome with unilateral head pain and associated autonomic symptoms; unlike cluster headache, the pain is continuous without pain-free periods, and it completely resolves with indomethacin.

Examination reveals no abnormality apart from Horner syndrome that either occurs transiently during an attack or, in longstanding cases, remains as a residual deficit between attacks.

Treatment of an individual attack with oral drugs is generally unsatisfactory, but subcutaneous (6 mg dose) or intranasal (20-mg/spray) sumatriptan or inhalation of 100% oxygen (12–15 L/min for 15 minutes via a non-rebreather mask) may be effective. Zolmitriptan (5- and 10-mg nasal spray) is also effective. Dihydroergotamine (0.5–1 mg intramuscularly or intravenously) is sometimes used. Viscous lidocaine (1 mg of 4–6% solution) intranasally is sometimes effective.

Various prophylactic agents include oral medications such as, lithium carbonate (start at 300 mg daily, titrating according to serum levels and treatment response up to a typical total daily dose of 900–1200 mg, divided three or four times), verapamil (240–960 mg daily), topiramate (100–400 mg daily), valproate (750–1500 mg daily), civamide (not available in the United States); and suboccipital corticosteroid injection about the greater occipital nerve. As there is often a delay before these medications are effective, transitional therapy is often used. Ergotamine tartrate is effective and can be given as rectal suppositories (0.5–1 mg at night or twice daily), by mouth (2 mg daily), or by subcutaneous injection (0.25 mg three times daily for 5 days per week). Other options include prednisone (60 mg daily for 5 days followed by gradual withdrawal), or dihydroergotamine (9.25 mg intravenously over several days or 0.5 mg intramuscularly twice daily). Stimulation of the occipital nerve may be helpful.

4. Posttraumatic Headache

A variety of nonspecific symptoms may follow closed head injury, regardless of whether consciousness is lost. Headache is often a conspicuous feature.

The headache itself usually appears within a day or so following injury, may worsen over the ensuing weeks, and then gradually subsides. It is usually a constant dull ache, with superimposed throbbing that may be localized, lateralized, or generalized. It is sometimes accompanied by nausea, vomiting, or scintillating scotomas. Headaches occurring more than 1–2 weeks after the inciting event are probably not directly attributable to the head injury.

Dysequilibrium, sometimes with a rotatory component, may also occur and is often enhanced by postural change or head movement. Impaired memory, poor concentration, emotional instability, and increased irritability are other common complaints and occasionally are the sole manifestations of the syndrome. The duration of symptoms relates in part to the severity of the original injury, but even trivial injuries are sometimes followed by symptoms that persist for months.

Special investigations are usually not helpful. The electroencephalogram may show minor nonspecific changes, while the electronystagmogram sometimes suggests either peripheral or central vestibulopathy. CT scans or MRI of the head usually are normal.

Treatment is difficult, but optimistic encouragement and graduated rehabilitation, depending on the occupational circumstances, are advised as symptoms often resolve spontaneously within several months. Headaches often respond to simple analgesics, but severe headaches may necessitate preventive treatment as outlined for migraine.

5. Primary Cough Headache

Severe head pain may be produced by coughing (and by straining, sneezing, and laughing) but, fortunately, usually lasts for only a few minutes or less. The pathophysiologic basis of the complaint is not known, and often there is no underlying structural lesion. However, intracranial lesions, usually in the posterior fossa (eg, Arnold-Chiari malformation), are present in about 10% of cases, and brain tumors or other space-occupying lesions may present in this way. Accordingly, CT scanning or MRI should be undertaken in all patients and repeated annually for several years, since a small structural lesion may not show up initially.

The disorder is usually self-limited, although it may persist for several years. For unknown reasons, symptoms sometimes clear completely after lumbar puncture. Indomethacin (75–150 mg daily orally) may provide relief. Similar activity-triggered headache syndromes include primary exertional headache and primary headache associated with sexual activity.

6. Headache Due to Giant Cell (Temporal or Cranial) Arteritis

This topic is discussed in Chapter 20.

7. Headache Due to Intracranial Mass Lesions

Intracranial mass lesions of all types may cause headache owing to displacement of vascular structures and other pain-sensitive tissues. Posterior fossa tumors often cause occipital pain, and supratentorial lesions lead to bifrontal headache, but such findings are too inconsistent to be of value in attempts at localizing a pathologic process. The headaches are nonspecific in character and may vary in severity from mild to severe. They may be worsened by exertion or postural change (standing may relieve pain) and may be associated with nausea and vomiting, but this is true of migraine also. Headaches are also a feature of pseudotumor cerebri (idiopathic intracranial hypertension) (see below). Signs of focal or diffuse cerebral dysfunction or of increased intracranial pressure will indicate the need for further investigation. Similarly, a progressive headache disorder or the new onset of headaches in middle or later life merits investigation if no cause is apparent.

8. Medication Overuse (Analgesic Rebound) Headache

In approximately half of all patients with chronic daily headaches, medication overuse is responsible. Patients have chronic pain or severe headache unresponsive to medication. Early initiation of a migraine preventive therapy (see above) permits withdrawal of analgesics and eventual relief of headache.

9. Headache Due to Other Neurologic Causes

Cerebrovascular disease may be associated with headache, but the mechanism is unclear. Headache may occur with internal carotid artery occlusion or carotid dissection and after carotid endarterectomy. Acute severe headache accompanies subarachnoid hemorrhage and meningeal infections; accompanying signs of impairment of consciousness and sign of meningeal irritation indicate the need for further investigations.

Dull or throbbing headache is a frequent sequela of lumbar puncture and may last for several days. It is aggravated by the erect posture and alleviated by recumbency. The mechanism is unclear, but the headache is commonly attributed to leakage of cerebrospinal fluid through the dural puncture site. Its incidence may be reduced if an atraumatic needle is used for the lumbar puncture.

▶ When to Refer

- Acute onset of "worst headache in my life."
- Increasing headache unresponsive to simple measures.
- History of trauma, hypertension, fever, visual changes.
- Presence of neurologic signs or of scalp tenderness.

▶ When to Admit

Suspected subarachnoid hemorrhage or structural intracranial lesion.

Ashkenazi A et al. Cluster headache: acute and prophylactic therapy. Headache. 2011 Feb;51(2):272–86. [PMID: 21284609]

Furman JM et al. Vestibular migraine: clinical aspects and pathophysiology. Lancet Neurol. 2013 Jul;12(7):706–15. [PMID: 23769597]

Jackson JL et al. Botulinum toxin A for prophylactic treatment of migraine and tension headaches in adults: a meta-analysis. JAMA. 2012 Apr 25;307(16):1736–45. [PMID: 22535858]

Kaniecki RG. Tension-type headache. Continuum (Minneap Minn). 2012 Aug;18(4):823–34. [PMID: 22868544]

Magis D et al. Treatment of migraine: update on new therapies. Curr Opin Neurol. 2011 Jun;24(3):203–10. [PMID: 21464715]

Silberstein SD et al. Evidence-based guideline update: pharmacologic treatment for episodic migraine prevention in adults: report of the Quality Standards Subcommittee of the American Academy of Neurology and the American Headache Society. Neurology. 2012 Apr 24;78(17):1337–45. [PMID: 22529202]

Tepper SJ. Medication-overuse headache. Continuum (Minneap Minn). 2012 Aug;18(4):807–22. [PMID: 22868543]

FACIAL PAIN

1. Trigeminal Neuralgia

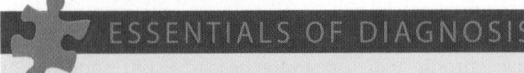

ESSENTIALS OF DIAGNOSIS

- ▶ Brief episodes of stabbing facial pain.
- ▶ Pain is in the territory of the second and third division of the trigeminal nerve.
- ▶ Pain exacerbated by touch.

▶ General Considerations

Trigeminal neuralgia ("tic douloureux") is most common in middle and later life. It affects women more frequently than men. Pain may be due to an anomalous artery or vein impinging on the trigeminal nerve.

▶ Clinical Findings

Momentary episodes of sudden lancinating facial pain occur and commonly arise near one side of the mouth and shoot toward the ear, eye, or nostril on that side. The pain may be triggered or precipitated by such factors as touch, movement, drafts, and eating. Indeed, in order to lessen the likelihood of triggering further attacks, many patients try to hold the face still while talking. Spontaneous remissions for several months or longer may occur. As the disorder progresses, however, the episodes of pain become more frequent, remissions become shorter and less common, and a dull ache may persist between the episodes of stabbing pain. Symptoms remain confined to the distribution of the trigeminal nerve (usually the second or third division) on one side only.

▶ Differential Diagnosis

The characteristic features of the pain in trigeminal neuralgia usually distinguish it from other causes of facial pain. Neurologic examination shows no abnormality except in a few patients in whom trigeminal neuralgia is symptomatic of some underlying lesion, such as multiple sclerosis or a brainstem neoplasm, in which case the finding will depend on the nature and site of the lesion. Similarly, CT scans and radiologic contrast studies are often normal in patients with classic trigeminal neuralgia.

In a young patient presenting with trigeminal neuralgia, multiple sclerosis must be suspected even if there are no other neurologic signs. In such circumstances, findings on evoked potential testing and examination of cerebrospinal fluid may be corroborative. When the facial pain is due to a posterior fossa tumor, CT scanning and MRI generally reveal the lesion.

▶ Treatment

The drugs most helpful for treatment are oxcarbazepine (although not approved by the FDA for this indication) or carbamazepine, with monitoring by serial blood counts and liver function tests. If these medications are ineffective or cannot be tolerated, phenytoin should be tried. (Doses and side effects of these drugs are shown in Table 24–3). Baclofen (10–20 mg orally three or four times daily), topiramate (50 mg orally twice daily), or lamotrigine (400 mg orally daily) may also be helpful, either alone or in combination with one of these other agents. Gabapentin may also relieve pain, especially in patients who do not respond to conventional medical therapy and those with multiple sclerosis. Depending on response and tolerance, up to 2400 mg daily orally is given in divided doses.

For neuralgia due to vascular impingement on the trigeminal nerve (despite normal findings on CT scans, MRI, or arteriograms), microvascular surgical decompression and separation of the anomalous vessel from the nerve root produce lasting relief of symptoms. In elderly patients with a limited life expectancy, radiofrequency rhizotomy is sometimes preferred because it is easy to perform, has few complications, and provides symptomatic relief for a period of time. Gamma radiosurgery to the trigeminal root is another noninvasive approach that appears to be successful in most patients, with essentially no side effects other than facial paresthesias in a few instances; up to one-third of patients achieved a pain-free state without need for medication after the procedure. Surgical exploration is inappropriate in patients with trigeminal neuralgia due to multiple sclerosis.

Pollock BE. Surgical management of medically refractory trigeminal neuralgia. Curr Neurol Neurosci Rep. 2012 Apr;12(2):125–31. [PMID: 22183181]

Torpy JM et al. JAMA patient page: Trigeminal neuralgia. JAMA. 2013 Mar 13;309(10):1058. [PMID: 23483182]

Zakrzewska JM. Medical management of trigeminal neuropathic pains. Expert Opin Pharmacother. 2010 Jun;11(8):1239–54. [PMID: 20426709]

2. Atypical Facial Pain

Facial pain without the typical features of trigeminal neuralgia is generally a constant, often burning pain that may have a restricted distribution at its onset but soon spreads to the rest of the face on the affected side and sometimes involves the other side, the neck, or the back of the head as well. The disorder is especially common in middle-aged women, many of them depressed, but it is not clear whether depression is the cause of or a reaction to the pain. Simple analgesics should be given a trial, as should tricyclic antidepressants, carbamazepine, oxcarbazepine, and phenytoin; the response is often disappointing. Opioid analgesics pose a danger of addiction in patients with this disorder. Attempts at surgical treatment are not indicated.

3. Glossopharyngeal Neuralgia

Glossopharyngeal neuralgia is an uncommon disorder in which pain similar in quality to that in trigeminal neuralgia occurs in the throat, about the tonsillar fossa, and sometimes deep in the ear and at the back of the tongue. The pain may be precipitated by swallowing, chewing, talking, or yawning and is sometimes accompanied by syncope. In most instances, no underlying structural abnormality is present; multiple sclerosis is sometimes responsible. Oxcarbazepine and carbamazepine (see Table 24–3) are the treatments of choice and should be tried before any surgical procedures are considered. Microvascular decompression is generally preferred over destructive surgical procedures such as partial rhizotomy in medically refractory cases and is often effective without causing severe complications.

Kandan SR et al. Neuralgia of the glossopharyngeal and vagal nerves: long-term outcome following surgical treatment and literature review. Br J Neurosurg. 2010 Aug;24(4):441–6. [PMID: 20726751]

4. Postherpetic Neuralgia

Postherpetic neuralgia develops in about 15% of patients who have herpes zoster (shingles). This complication seems especially likely to occur in elderly or immunocompromised persons, when the rash is severe, and when the first division of the trigeminal nerve is affected. It also relates to the duration of the rash before medical consultation. A history of shingles and the presence of cutaneous scarring resulting from shingles aid in the diagnosis. Severe pain with shingles correlates with the intensity of postherpetic symptoms.

The incidence of postherpetic neuralgia may be reduced by the treatment of shingles with oral acyclovir or famciclovir, but this is disputed; systemic corticosteroids do not help (see Chapter 6). Management of the established complication is essentially medical. If simple analgesics fail to help, a trial of a tricyclic antidepressant (eg, amitriptyline or nortriptyline, up to 100–150 mg daily orally) is often effective. Other patients respond to carbamazepine (up to 1200 mg daily orally), phenytoin (300 mg daily orally), gabapentin (up to 3600 mg daily orally), or pregabalin (up to 600 mg/daily orally). A combination of gabapentin and morphine taken orally may provide better analgesia at lower doses of each agent than either taken alone. Topical application of capsaicin cream (eg, Zostrix, 0.025%) may be helpful, but a transdermal patch (8%) had no effect. Topical lidocaine (5%) is also worthy of trial. The administration of live-attenuated zoster vaccine to patients over the age of 60 years is important in reducing the likelihood of herpes zoster and reducing the severity of postherpetic neuralgia should a reactivation occur.

Chen N et al. Vaccination for preventing postherpetic neuralgia. Cochrane Database Syst Rev. 2011 Mar 16;(3):CD007795. [PMID: 21412911]

Edelsberg JS et al. Systematic review and meta-analysis of efficacy, safety, and tolerability data from randomized controlled trials of drugs used to treat postherpetic neuralgia. Ann Pharmacother. 2011 Dec;45(12):1483–90. [PMID: 22085778]

5. Facial Pain Due to Other Causes

Facial pain may be caused by temporomandibular joint dysfunction in patients with malocclusion, abnormal bite, or faulty dentures. There may be tenderness of the masticatory muscles, and sometimes pain begins at the onset of chewing. This pattern differs from that of jaw (masticatory) claudication, a symptom of giant cell arteritis, in which pain develops progressively with mastication. Treatment of the underlying joint dysfunction relieves symptoms.

A relationship of facial pain to chewing or temperature changes may suggest a dental disturbance. The cause is sometimes not obvious, and diagnosis requires careful dental examination and radiographs. Sinusitis and ear infections causing facial pain are usually recognized by the history of respiratory tract infection, fever and, in some instances, nasal or aural discharge. There may be localized tenderness. Radiologic evidence of sinus infection or mastoiditis is confirmatory.

Glaucoma is an important ocular cause of facial pain, usually localized to the periorbital region.

On occasion, pain in the jaw may be the principal manifestation of angina pectoris. Precipitation by exertion and radiation to more typical areas suggests the cardiac origin.

When to Refer

- Worsening pain unresponsive to simple measures.
- Continuing pain of uncertain cause.
- For consideration of surgical treatment (trigeminal or glossopharyngeal neuralgia).

EPILEPSY

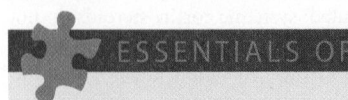

ESSENTIALS OF DIAGNOSIS

- ▶ Recurrent seizures.
- ▶ Characteristic electroencephalographic changes accompany seizures.
- ▶ Mental status abnormalities or focal neurologic symptoms may persist for hours postictally.

General Considerations

The term "epilepsy" denotes any disorder characterized by recurrent unprovoked seizures. A seizure is a transient disturbance of cerebral function due to an abnormal paroxysmal neuronal discharge in the brain. Epilepsy is common, affecting approximately 0.5% of the population in the United States.

Etiology

According to the International League Against Epilepsy classification system, the many etiologies of seizures can be grouped into three categories.

A. Genetic Epilepsy

This category encompasses a broad range of disorders, for which the age at onset ranges from the neonatal period to adolescence or even later in life. Monogenic disorders tend to exhibit an autosomal dominant pattern of inheritance, and where the mutation is known, the responsible gene often encodes a neuronal ion channel.

B. Structural/Metabolic Epilepsy

There are many causes for recurrent seizures.

1. Pediatric age groups—Congenital abnormalities and perinatal injuries may result in seizures presenting in infancy or childhood.

2. Metabolic disorders—Withdrawal from alcohol or drugs is a common cause of recurrent seizures, and other metabolic disorders (such as uremia and hypoglycemia or hyperglycemia) may also be responsible. Since these seizures are provoked by a readily reversible cause, this would not be considered epilepsy.

3. Trauma—Trauma is an important cause of seizures at any age, but especially in young adults. Posttraumatic epilepsy is more likely to develop if the dura mater was penetrated and generally becomes manifest within 2 years following the injury. However, seizures developing in the first week after head injury do not necessarily imply that future attacks will occur. There is no clear evidence that prophylactic anticonvulsant drug treatment reduces the incidence of posttraumatic epilepsy.

4. Tumors and other space-occupying lesions—Neoplasms may lead to seizures at any age, but they are an especially important cause of seizures in middle and later life, when the incidence of neoplastic disease increases. The seizures are commonly the initial symptoms of the tumor and often are focal in character. They are most likely to occur with structural lesions involving the frontal, parietal, or temporal regions. Tumors must be excluded by imaging studies (MRI preferred over CT) in all patients with onset of seizures after 30 years of age, focal seizures or signs, or a progressive seizure disorder.

5. Vascular diseases—Vascular diseases become increasingly frequent causes of seizures with advancing age and are the most common cause of seizures with onset at age 60 years or older.

6. Degenerative disorders—Alzheimer disease and other degenerative disorders are a cause of seizures in later life.

7. Infectious diseases—Infectious diseases must be considered in all age groups as potentially reversible causes of seizures. Seizures may occur with an acute infective or inflammatory illness, such as bacterial meningitis or herpes encephalitis, or in patients with more longstanding or chronic disorders, such as neurosyphilis or cerebral cysticercosis. In patients with AIDS, they may result from central nervous system toxoplasmosis, cryptococcal meningitis, secondary viral encephalitis, or other infective complications. Seizures are a common sequela of supratentorial brain abscess, developing most frequently in the first year after treatment.

C. Unknown

In many cases, the cause of epilepsy cannot be determined.

Classification of Seizures

The International League Against Epilepsy distinguishes seizures affecting only part of the brain (focal seizures) from those that are generalized (Table 24–2).

A. Focal Seizures

The initial clinical and electroencephalographic manifestations of partial seizures indicate that only a restricted part of one cerebral hemisphere has been activated. The ictal manifestations depend on the area of the brain involved. Focal seizures sometimes involve impairment of consciousness and may evolve to convulsive seizures, in a process previously called secondary generalization.

1. Without impairment of consciousness—Seizures may be manifested by focal motor symptoms (convulsive jerking) or somatosensory symptoms (eg, paresthesias or tingling) that spread (or "march") to different parts of the limb or body depending on their cortical representation;

Table 24–2. Seizure classification.

Seizure Type	Key Features	Other Associated Features
Focal seizures	Involvement of only a restricted part of brain; may evolve to a bilateral, convulsive seizure	
Without impairment of consciousness		Observable focal motor or autonomic symptoms, or subjective sensory or psychic symptoms may occur
With impairment of consciousness		Above symptoms may precede, accompany, or follow the period of altered responsiveness
Generalized seizures	Diffuse involvement of brain at onset	
Absence (petit mal)	Consciousness impaired briefly; patient often unaware of attacks	May have clonic, tonic, or atonic (ie, loss of postural tone) components; autonomic components (eg, enuresis); or accompanying automatisms Almost always begin in childhood and frequently cease by age 20
Atypical absences	May be more gradual in onset and termination than typical absence	More marked changes in tone may occur
Myoclonic	Single or multiple myoclonic jerks	
Tonic-clonic (grand mal)	Tonic phase: Sudden loss of consciousness, with rigidity and arrest of respiration, lasting < 1 minute Clonic phase: Jerking occurs, usually for < 2–3 minutes Flaccid coma: Variable duration	May be accompanied by tongue biting, incontinence, or aspiration; commonly followed by postictal confusion variable in duration
Status epilepticus	Repeated seizures without recovery between them; a fixed and enduring epileptic condition lasting ≥ 30 minutes	

such seizures were previously described as "simple partial" seizures. In other instances, special sensory symptoms (eg, light flashes or buzzing) indicate involvement of visual, auditory, olfactory, or gustatory regions of the brain, or there may be autonomic symptoms or signs (eg, abnormal epigastric sensations, sweating, flushing, pupillary dilation). The sole manifestations of some seizures are phenomena such as dysphasia, dysmnesic symptoms (eg, déjà vu, jamais vu), affective disturbances, illusions, or structured hallucinations, but such symptoms are usually accompanied by impairment of consciousness.

2. With impairment of consciousness—Impaired consciousness or responsiveness may be preceded, accompanied, or followed by the various symptoms mentioned above, and automatisms may occur. Such dyscognitive seizures were previously called "complex partial" seizures.

B. Generalized Seizures

There are several different varieties of generalized seizures, as outlined below. In some circumstances, seizures cannot be classified because of incomplete information or because they do not fit into any category.

1. Absence seizures—These are characterized by impairment of consciousness, sometimes with mild clonic, tonic, or atonic components (ie, reduction or loss of postural tone), autonomic components (eg, enuresis), or accompanying automatisms. Onset and termination of attacks are abrupt. If attacks occur during conversation, the patient

may miss a few words or may break off in midsentence for a few seconds. The impairment of external awareness is so brief that the patient is unaware of it. Absence ("petit mal") seizures almost always begin in childhood and frequently cease by the age of 20 years or are then replaced by other forms of generalized seizure. Electroencephalographically, such attacks are associated with bursts of bilaterally synchronous and symmetric 3-Hz spike-and-wave activity. A normal background in the electroencephalogram and normal or above-normal intelligence imply a good prognosis for the ultimate cessation of these seizures.

2. Atypical absence seizures—There may be more marked changes in tone, or attacks may have a more gradual onset and termination than in typical absence seizures. They commonly occur in patients with multiple seizure types, may be accompanied by developmental delay or mental retardation, and are associated with slower spike-wave discharges than those in typical absence attacks.

3. Myoclonic seizures—Myoclonic seizures consist of single or multiple myoclonic jerks.

4. Tonic-clonic ("grand mal") seizures—In these seizures, which are characterized by sudden loss of consciousness, the patient becomes rigid and falls to the ground, and respiration is arrested. This tonic phase, which usually lasts for < 1 minute, is followed by a clonic phase in which there is jerking of the body musculature that may last for 2 or 3 minutes and is then followed by a stage of flaccid coma. During the seizure, the tongue or lips may be bitten, urinary or fecal incontinence may occur, and the patient may be injured. Immediately after the seizure, the patient may recover consciousness, drift into sleep, have a further convulsion without recovery of consciousness between the attacks (**status epilepticus**), or after recovering consciousness have a further convulsion (**serial seizures**). In other cases, patients will behave in an abnormal fashion in the immediate postictal period, without subsequent awareness or memory of events (**postepileptic automatism**). Headache, disorientation, confusion, drowsiness, nausea, soreness of the muscles, or some combination of these symptoms commonly occurs postictally.

5. Tonic, clonic, or atonic seizures—Loss of consciousness may occur with either the tonic or clonic accompaniments described above, especially in children. Atonic seizures (**epileptic drop attacks**) have also been described.

▶ Clinical Findings

A. Symptoms and Signs

Nonspecific changes such as headache, mood alterations, lethargy, and myoclonic jerking alert some patients to an impending seizure hours before it occurs. These prodromal symptoms are distinct from the aura; the aura that may precede a generalized seizure by a few seconds or minutes is itself a part of the attack and it arises locally from a restricted part of the brain.

In most patients, seizures occur unpredictably at any time and without any relationship to posture or ongoing activities. Occasionally, however, they occur at a particular time (eg, during sleep) or in relation to external precipitants such as lack of sleep, missed meals, emotional stress, menstruation, alcohol ingestion (or alcohol withdrawal; see below), or use of certain drugs. Fever and nonspecific infections may also precipitate seizures in epileptic patients. In a few patients, seizures are provoked by specific stimuli such as flashing lights or a flickering television set (**photosensitive epilepsy**), music, or reading.

Clinical examination between seizures shows no abnormality in patients with idiopathic epilepsy, but in the immediate postictal period, extensor plantar responses may be seen. The presence of lateralized or focal signs postictally suggests that seizures may have a focal origin. In patients with symptomatic epilepsy, the findings on examination will reflect the underlying cause.

B. Imaging

MRI is indicated for patients with focal neurologic symptoms or signs, focal seizures, or electroencephalographic findings of a focal disturbance; some clinicians routinely order MRI for all patients with new-onset seizure disorders. CT is generally less sensitive than MRI to small structural brain abnormalities but may be used when MRI is contraindicated (eg, in a patient with a metallic implant). Such studies should be performed in patients with clinical evidence of a progressive disorder and in those with new onset of seizures after the age of 20 years because of the possibility of an underlying neoplasm.

C. Laboratory and Other Studies

Initial investigations should include complete blood count, serum glucose, electrolytes, creatinine, calcium, magnesium, and liver function tests to exclude various causes of seizures and to provide a baseline for subsequent monitoring of long-term effects of treatment. A lumbar puncture may be necessary when any sign of infection is present or in the evaluation of new-onset seizures in the acute setting.

Electroencephalography may support the clinical diagnosis of epilepsy (by demonstrating paroxysmal abnormalities containing spikes or sharp waves), provide a guide to prognosis, and help classify the seizure disorder. Classification of the disorder is important for determining the most appropriate anticonvulsant drug with which to start treatment. For example, absence and focal seizures with impairment of consciousness may be difficult to distinguish clinically, but the electroencephalographic findings and treatment of choice differ in these two conditions. Finally, by localizing the epileptogenic source, the electroencephalographic findings are important in evaluating candidates for surgical treatment.

▶ Differential Diagnosis

The distinction between the various disorders likely to be confused with generalized seizures is usually made on the basis of the history. The importance of obtaining an eyewitness account of the attacks cannot be overemphasized.

A. Differential Diagnosis of Focal Seizures

1. Transient ischemic attacks—These attacks are distinguished from seizures by their longer duration, lack of spread, and symptoms. Level of consciousness, which is unaltered, does not distinguish them. There is a loss of motor or sensory function (eg, weakness or numbness) with transient ischemic attacks, whereas positive symptoms (eg, convulsive jerking or paresthesias) characterize seizures.

2. Rage attacks—Rage attacks are usually situational and lead to goal-directed aggressive behavior.

3. Panic attacks—These may be hard to distinguish from focal seizures unless there is evidence of an anxiety disorder between attacks and the attacks have a clear relationship to external circumstances.

B. Differential Diagnosis of Generalized Seizures

1. Syncope—Syncopal episodes usually occur in relation to postural change, emotional stress, instrumentation, pain, or straining. They are typically preceded by pallor, sweating, nausea, and malaise and lead to loss of consciousness accompanied by flaccidity; recovery occurs rapidly with recumbency, and there is no postictal headache or confusion. In some instances, however, motor accompaniments and urinary incontinence may simulate a seizure.

2. Cardiac disease—Cerebral hypoperfusion due to a disturbance of cardiac rhythm should be suspected in patients with known cardiac or vascular disease or in elderly patients who present with episodic loss of consciousness. Prodromal symptoms are typically absent. Repeated Holter monitoring may be necessary to establish the diagnosis; monitoring initiated by the patient ("event monitor") may be valuable if the disturbances of consciousness are rare. A relationship of attacks to physical activity and the finding of a systolic murmur are suggestive of aortic stenosis.

3. Brainstem ischemia—Loss of consciousness is preceded or accompanied by other brainstem signs. Basilar artery migraine and vertebrobasilar vascular disease are discussed elsewhere in this chapter.

4. Psychogenic nonepileptic seizure (PNES)—Simulating an epileptic seizure, a PNES may occur due to a conversion disorder or malingering. Many patients also have true seizures or a family history of epilepsy. Although a PNES tends to occur at times of emotional stress, this may also be the case with true seizures.

Clinically, the attacks superficially resemble tonic-clonic seizures, but there may be obvious preparation before a PNES. Moreover, there is usually no tonic phase; instead, there may be an asynchronous thrashing of the limbs, which increases if restraints are imposed and rarely leads to injury. Consciousness may be normal or "lost," but in the latter context the occurrence of goal-directed behavior or of shouting, swearing, etc, indicates that it is feigned. Postictally, there are no changes in behavior or neurologic findings.

Often, clinical observation is insufficient to discriminate epileptic from nonepileptic seizures. Video electroencephalographic monitoring may be helpful: epileptic seizures, especially those involving altered consciousness, commonly involve scalp electroencephalographic signs that coincide with a behavioral spell, whereas a PNES does not. The serum level of prolactin has been found to increase dramatically between 15 and 30 minutes after a tonic-clonic convulsion in most patients, whereas it is unchanged after a PNES. Serum creatine kinase levels also increase after a convulsion but not a PNES.

▶ Treatment

A. General Measures

For patients with epilepsy, drug treatment is prescribed with the goal of preventing further attacks and is usually continued until there have been no seizures for at least 2 years. Epileptic patients should be advised to avoid situations that could be dangerous or life-threatening if further seizures should occur. Legislation may require clinicians to report to the state authorities any patients with seizures or other episodic disturbances of consciousness; driving cessation for 6 months or as legislated is appropriate following an unprovoked seizure.

1. Choice of medication—Drug selection depends on seizure type (Table 24–3). The dose of the selected drug is gradually increased until seizures are controlled or side effects prevent further increases. If seizures continue despite treatment at the maximal tolerated dose, a second drug is added and the dose increased depending on tolerance; the first drug is then gradually withdrawn.

In treatment of focal seizures, the success rate is higher with carbamazepine, phenytoin, or valproic acid than with phenobarbital or primidone. Gabapentin, topiramate, lamotrigine, oxcarbazepine, levetiracetam, zonisamide, lacosamide, ezogabine, vigabatrin, and tiagabine are newer antiepileptic drugs used to treat focal seizures. Felbamate is also effective for such seizures but, because it may cause aplastic anemia or fulminant hepatic failure, should be used only in selected patients unresponsive to other measures. Rufinamide is currently approved only for seizures in patients with Lennox-Gastaut syndrome, but it may be effective against seizures in a broader range of refractory patients. For generalized or unclassified seizures, valproate is better tolerated than topiramate and more efficacious than lamotrigine and is thus preferred for many patients; however, the teratogenic potential of valproate makes its use undesirable in women of childbearing age. All antiepileptics are potentially teratogenic, although the teratogenicity of the newer antiseizure medications is less clear. Nevertheless, antiepileptic medication must be given to pregnant women with epilepsy to prevent seizures, which can pose serious risk to the fetus from trauma, hypoxia, or other factors. In most patients with seizures of a single type, satisfactory control can be achieved with a single anticonvulsant drug. Treatment with two drugs may further reduce seizure frequency or severity but usually only at the cost of greater toxicity. Treatment with more than two drugs is almost always unhelpful unless the patient is having seizures of different types.

2. Monitoring—Monitoring serum drug levels has led to major advances in the management of seizure disorders. Individual differences in drug metabolism cause a given dose of a drug to produce different blood concentrations in different patients, and this will affect the therapeutic response. In general, the dose of an antiepileptic agent is increased depending on the clinical response regardless of the serum drug level. When a dose is achieved that either controls seizures or is the maximum tolerated, then a steady-state trough drug level may be obtained for future reference; rechecking this level may be appropriate if a breakthrough seizure occurs, a dose change occurs, or another (potentially interacting) drug is added to the regimen. A laboratory's therapeutic range for a drug is only a guide; many patients achieve good seizure control with no adverse effect at serum levels that exceed the stipulated range, and in these cases no dose adjustment is needed. The most common cause of a lower concentration of drug than expected for the prescribed dose is poor patient compliance. Compliance can be improved by limiting to a minimum the number of daily doses. Recurrent seizures or status epilepticus may result if drugs are taken erratically, and in some circumstances noncompliant patients may be better off without any medication.

All anticonvulsant drugs have side effects, and some of these are shown in Table 24–3.

Treatment with certain drugs may require regular laboratory monitoring. For example, periodic tests of hepatic function are necessary if valproic acid, carbamazepine, or felbamate is used, and serial blood counts are important with carbamazepine, ethosuximide, or felbamate. Detailed

Table 24–3. Drug treatment for seizures in adults.

Drug	Usual Adult Daily Oral Dose	Minimum No. of Daily Doses	Time to Steady State Drug Levels	Optimal Drug Level	Selected Side Effects and Idiosyncratic Reactions
Generalized or focal seizures					
Phenytoin	200–400 mg	1	5–10 days	10–20 mcg/mL	Nystagmus, ataxia, dysarthria, sedation, confusion, gingival hyperplasia, hirsutism, megaloblastic anemia, blood dyscrasias, skin rashes, fever, systemic lupus erythematosus, lymphadenopathy, peripheral neuropathy, dyskinesias.
Carbamazepine extended-release (ER) formulation	400–1600 mg ER	2	3–4 days	4–8 mcg/mL	Nystagmus, dysarthria, diplopia, ataxia, drowsiness, nausea, blood dyscrasias, hepatotoxicity, hyponatremia. May exacerbate myoclonic seizures.
Valproic acid	1500–2000 mg	2–3	2–4 days	50–100 mcg/mL	Nausea, vomiting, diarrhea, drowsiness, alopecia, weight gain, hepatotoxicity, thrombocytopenia, tremor, pancreatitis.
Phenobarbital	100–200 mg	1	14–21 days	10–40 mcg/mL	Drowsiness, nystagmus, ataxia, skin rashes, learning difficulties, hyperactivity.
Primidone	750–1500 mg	3	4–7 days	5–15 mcg/mL	Sedation, nystagmus, ataxia, vertigo, nausea, skin rashes, megaloblastic anemia, irritability.
Lamotrigine[1,2,5]	100–500 mg	2	4–5 days	?	Sedation, skin rash, visual disturbances, dyspepsia, ataxia.
Topiramate[1–4]	200–400 mg	2	4 days	?	Somnolence, nausea, dyspepsia, irritability, dizziness, ataxia, nystagmus, diplopia, glaucoma, renal calculi, weight loss, hypohidrosis, hyperthermia.
Oxcarbazepine[1,3]	900–1800 mg	2	2–3 days	?	As for carbamazepine.
Levetiracetam[1,2]	1000–3000 mg	2	2 days	?	Somnolence, ataxia, headache, behavioral changes.
Zonisamide[1]	200–600 mg	1	14 days	?	Somnolence, ataxia, anorexia, nausea, vomiting, rash, confusion, renal calculi. Do not use in patients with sulfonamide allergy.
Tiagabine[1]	32–56 mg	2	2 days	?	Somnolence, anxiety, dizziness, poor concentration, tremor, diarrhea.
Pregabalin[1]	150–300 mg	2	2–4 days	?	Somnolence, dizziness, poor concentration, weight gain, thrombocytopenia, skin rashes, anaphylactoid reactions.
Gabapentin[1]	900–3600 mg	3	1 day	?	Sedation, fatigue, ataxia, nystagmus, weight loss.
Felbamate[1,3,6]	1200–3600 mg	3	4–5 days	?	Anorexia, nausea, vomiting, headache, insomnia, weight loss, dizziness, hepatotoxicity, aplastic anemia.
Lacosamide[1]	100–400 mg	2	3 days	?	Vertigo, diplopia, nausea, headache, fatigue, ataxia, tremor, anaphylactoid reactions, PR prolongation, cardiac dysrhythmia, suicidality.
Ezogabine[1]	300–1200 mg	3	2–3 days	?	Dizziness, somnolence, confusion, vertigo, nausea, ataxia, psychiatric disturbances.
Vigabatrin[1,2]	3000 mg	2	2 days	?	Somnolence, anorexia, nausea, vomiting, agitation, hostility, confusion, suicidality, neutropenia, Stevens-Johnson syndrome

(continued)

Table 24–3. Drug treatment for seizures in adults. (continued)

Drug	Usual Adult Daily Oral Dose	Minimum No. of Daily Doses	Time to Steady State Drug Levels	Optimal Drug Level	Selected Side Effects and Idiosyncratic Reactions
Absence seizures					
Ethosuximide	100–1500 mg	2	5–10 days	40–100 mcg/mL	Nausea, vomiting, anorexia, headache, lethargy, unsteadiness, blood dyscrasias, systemic lupus erythematosus, urticaria, pruritus.
Valproic acid	1500–2000 mg	3	2–4 days	50–100 mcg/mL	See above.
Clonazepam	0.04–0.2 mg/kg	2	?	20–80 ng/mL	Drowsiness, ataxia, irritability, behavioral changes, exacerbation of tonic-clonic seizures.
Myoclonic seizures					
Valproic acid	1500–2000 mg	3	2–4 days	50–100 mcg/mL	See above.
Clonazepam	0.04–0.2 mg/kg	2	?	20–80 ng/mL	See above.

[1]Approved as adjunctive therapy for focal-onset seizures.
[2]Approved as adjunctive therapy for primary generalized tonic-clonic seizures.
[3]Approved as initial monotherapy for focal-onset seizures.
[4]Approved as initial monotherapy for primary generalized tonic-clonic seizures.
[5]Approved as monotherapy (after conversion from another drug) in focal-onset seizures.
[6]Not to be used as a first-line drug; when used, blood counts should be performed regularly (every 2–4 weeks). Should be used only in selected patients because of risk of aplastic anemia and hepatic failure. It is advisable to obtain written informed consent before use.

medication-specific recommendations should be sought from a drug reference source before prescribing, since baseline studies are often necessary.

3. Discontinuance of medication—Only when adult patients have been seizure-free for 2 years should withdrawal of medication be considered. Unfortunately, there is no way of predicting which patients can be managed successfully without treatment, although seizure recurrence is more likely in patients who initially did not respond to therapy, those with seizures having focal features or of multiple types, and those with continuing electroencephalographic abnormalities. Dose reduction should be gradual (over weeks or months), and drugs should be withdrawn one at a time. If seizures recur, treatment is reinstituted with the previously effective drug regimen.

4. Surgical treatment—Patients with seizures refractory to pharmacologic management may be candidates for operative treatment. Surgical resection is most efficacious when there is a single well-defined seizure focus, particularly in the temporal lobe. Among well-chosen patients, up to 70% remain seizure-free after extended follow-up. Bilateral deep brain stimulation of the anterior thalamus for medically refractory focal-onset seizures may be of benefit.

5. Vagal nerve stimulation—Treatment by chronic vagal nerve stimulation for adults and adolescents with medically refractory focal seizures is approved in the United States and provides an alternative approach for patients who are not optimal candidates for surgical treatment. The mechanism of therapeutic action is unknown. Adverse effects consist mainly of transient hoarseness during stimulus delivery.

B. Special Circumstances

1. Solitary seizures—In patients who have had only one seizure or a flurry of seizures over a brief period of several hours, investigation as outlined earlier should exclude an underlying cause requiring specific treatment. An electroencephalogram should be obtained, preferably within 24 hours after the seizure, because the findings may influence management—especially when focal abnormalities are present. Prophylactic anticonvulsant drug treatment is generally not required unless further attacks occur or investigations reveal some underlying pathology. The risk of seizure recurrence varies in different series between about 30% and 70%. Epilepsy should not be diagnosed on the basis of a solitary seizure. If seizures occur in the context of transient, nonrecurrent systemic disorders such as acute cerebral anoxia, the diagnosis of epilepsy is inaccurate, and long-term prophylactic anticonvulsant drug treatment is unnecessary.

2. Alcohol withdrawal seizures—The characteristic alcohol withdrawal seizure pattern is one or more generalized tonic-clonic seizures that may occur within 48 hours or so of withdrawal from alcohol after a period of high or prolonged intake. If the seizures have consistently focal features, the possibility of an associated structural abnormality, often traumatic in origin, must be considered. Head CT scan or MRI should be performed in patients with new onset of generalized seizures and whenever there are focal features. Treatment with anticonvulsant drugs is generally not required for alcohol withdrawal seizures, since they are self-limited. Benzodiazepines (diazepam or lorazepam, dosed as needed to reduce withdrawal symptoms and to avoid oversedation) are effective and safe for preventing further seizures. Status epilepticus may rarely follow alcohol withdrawal and is managed along conventional lines (see below). Further attacks will not occur if the patient abstains from alcohol.

3. Tonic-clonic status epilepticus—Poor compliance with the anticonvulsant drug regimen is the most common cause; other causes include alcohol withdrawal, intracranial infection or neoplasms, metabolic disorders, and drug overdose. The mortality rate may be as high as 20%, and among survivors the incidence of neurologic and cognitive sequelae is high. The prognosis relates to the length of time between onset of status epilepticus and the start of effective treatment.

Status epilepticus is a medical emergency. Initial management includes maintenance of the airway and 50% dextrose (25–50 mL) intravenously in case hypoglycemia is responsible. If seizures continue, an intravenous bolus of lorazepam, 4 mg, is given at a rate of 2 mg/min and repeated once after 10 minutes if necessary; alternatively, 10 mg of diazepam is given intravenously over the course of 2 minutes, and again after 10 minutes if necessary. Diazepam can also be given rectally as a gel (0.2 mg/kg). These measures are usually effective in halting seizures for a brief period. Respiratory depression and hypotension may complicate the treatment and are treated as in other circumstances; this treatment may include intubation and mechanical ventilation and admission to an intensive care unit.

Regardless of the response to lorazepam or diazepam, phenytoin (18–20 mg/kg) is given intravenously at a rate of 50 mg/min; this provides initiation of long-term seizure control. The drug is best injected directly but can also be given in saline; it precipitates, however, if injected into glucose-containing solutions. Because arrhythmias may develop during rapid administration of phenytoin, electrocardiographic monitoring is prudent. Hypotension may complicate phenytoin administration, especially if diazepam has also been given. In many countries, injectable phenytoin has been replaced by fosphenytoin, which is rapidly and completely converted to phenytoin following intravenous administration. No dosing adjustments are necessary because fosphenytoin is expressed in terms of phenytoin equivalents (PE); fosphenytoin is less likely to cause reactions at the infusion site, can be given with all common intravenous solutions, and may be administered at a faster rate (150 mg PE/min).

If seizures continue, phenobarbital is then given in a loading dose of 10–20 mg/kg intravenously by slow or intermittent injection (50 mg/min). Respiratory depression and hypotension are especially common with this therapy. Alternatively or additionally, intravenous valproate is used for status epilepticus (loading dose 25–30 mg/kg over 15 min; then 100 mg/h); although valproate has not yet been approved by the FDA for this indication, it has been used with success.

If these measures fail, general anesthesia with ventilatory assistance may be required. Intravenous midazolam may provide control of refractory status epilepticus; the suggested loading dose is 0.2 mg/kg, followed by 0.05–0.2 mg/ kg/h. Propofol (1–2 mg/kg as an intravenous bolus, followed by infusion at 2–15 mg/kg/h depending on response) may also be used, as may pentobarbital (15 mg/kg intravenously, followed by 0.5–4 mg/kg/h).

After status epilepticus is controlled, an oral drug program for the long-term management of seizures is started, and investigations into the cause of the disorder are pursued.

4. Nonconvulsive status epilepticus—In some cases, status epilepticus presents not with convulsions, but with a fluctuating abnormal mental status, confusion, impaired responsiveness, and automatism. Electroencephalography is helpful in establishing the diagnosis. The treatment approach outlined above applies to any type of status epilepticus, although intravenous anesthesia is usually not necessary. The prognosis is a reflection of the underlying cause rather than of continuing seizures.

▶ When to Refer

- Behavioral episodes of uncertain nature.
- Seizures are difficult to control or have focal features.
- There is a progressive neurologic disorder.
- Status epilepticus.

▶ When to Admit

- Status epilepticus.
- For monitoring, or when PNES are suspected.
- If surgery is contemplated.

Anderson J et al. Anti-epileptic drugs: a guide for the non-neurologist. Clin Med. 2010 Feb;10(1):54–8. [PMID: 20408309]

Berg AT et al. Revised terminology and concepts for organization of seizures and epilepsies: report of the ILAE Commission on Classification and Terminology, 2005–2009. Epilepsia. 2010 Apr;51(4):676–85. [PMID: 20196795]

Englot DJ et al. Rates and predictors of long-term seizure freedom after frontal lobe epilepsy surgery: a systematic review and meta-analysis. J Neurosurg. 2012 May;116(5):1042–8. [PMID: 22304450]

Glauser T et al. Updated ILAE evidence review of antiepileptic drug efficacy and effectiveness as initial monotherapy for epileptic seizures and syndromes. Epilepsia. 2013 Mar;54(3): 551–63. [PMID: 23350722]

Johnston A et al. Epilepsy in the elderly. Expert Rev Neurother. 2010 Dec;10(12):1899–910. [PMID: 21384700]

Perucca E et al. The pharmacological treatment of epilepsy in adults. Lancet Neurol. 2011 May;10(5):446–56. [PMID: 21511198]

Riviello JJ Jret al; Neurocritical Care Society Status Epilepticus Guideline Writing Committee. Treatment of status epilepticus: an international survey of experts. Neurocrit Care. 2013 Apr;18(2):193–200. [PMID: 23097138]

DYSAUTONOMIA

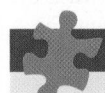
ESSENTIALS OF DIAGNOSIS

▸ Abnormalities of blood pressure or heart rate regulation, sweating, intestinal motility, sphincter control, sexual function, respiration, or ocular function.

▸ Symptoms occur in isolation or any combination.

General Considerations

Dysautonomia may occur as a result of central or peripheral pathologic processes. It is manifested by a variety of symptoms that may occur in isolation or in various combinations and relate to abnormalities of blood pressure regulation, thermoregulatory sweating, gastrointestinal function, sphincter control, sexual function, respiration, and ocular function. Syncope, a symptom of dysautonomia, is characterized by a transient loss of consciousness, usually accompanied by hypotension and bradycardia. It may occur in response to emotional stress, postural hypotension, vigorous exercise in a hot environment, obstructed venous return to the heart, acute pain or its anticipation, fluid loss, and a variety of other circumstances.

A. Central Neurologic Causes

Disease at certain sites in the central nervous system, regardless of its nature, may lead to dysautonomic symptoms. Postural hypotension, which is usually the most troublesome and disabling symptom, may result from spinal cord transection and other myelopathies (eg, due to tumor or syringomyelia) above the T6 level or from brainstem lesions such as syringobulbia and posterior fossa tumors. Sphincter or sexual disturbances may result from cord lesions below T6. Certain primary degenerative disorders are responsible for dysautonomia occurring in isolation (**pure autonomic failure**) or in association with more widespread abnormalities (**multisystem atrophy** or **Shy-Drager syndrome**) that may include parkinsonian, pyramidal symptoms, and cerebellar deficits.

B. Peripheral Neurologic Causes

A pure autonomic neuropathy may occur acutely or subacutely after a viral infection or as a paraneoplastic disorder related usually to small cell lung cancer, particularly in association with certain antibodies, such as anti-Hu or those directed at neuronal nicotinic acetylcholine receptors. Dysautonomia is often conspicuous in patients with Guillain-Barré syndrome, manifesting with marked hypotension or hypertension or cardiac arrhythmias that may have a fatal outcome. It may also occur with diabetic, uremic, amyloidotic, and various other metabolic or toxic neuropathies; in association with leprosy or Chagas disease; and as a feature of certain hereditary neuropathies with autosomal dominant or recessive inheritance or an

X-linked pattern. Autonomic symptoms are prominent in the crises of hepatic porphyria. Patients with botulism or the Lambert-Eaton myasthenic syndrome may have constipation, urinary retention, and a sicca syndrome as a result of impaired cholinergic function.

▸ Clinical Findings

A. Symptoms and Signs

Dysautonomic symptoms include syncope, postural hypotension, paroxysmal hypertension, persistent tachycardia without other cause, facial flushing, hypohidrosis or hyperhidrosis, vomiting, constipation, diarrhea, dysphagia, abdominal distention, disturbances of micturition or defecation, erectile dysfunction, apneic episodes, and declining night vision. In syncope, prodromal malaise, nausea, headache, diaphoresis, pallor, visual disturbance, loss of postural tone, and a sense of weakness and impending loss of consciousness are followed by actual loss of consciousness. Although the patient is usually flaccid, some motor activity is not uncommon, and urinary (and rarely fecal) incontinence may also occur, thereby simulating a seizure. Recovery is rapid once the patient becomes recumbent, but headache, nausea, and fatigue are common postictally.

B. Evaluation of the Patient

Testing of autonomic function includes evaluating the cardiovascular response to the Valsalva maneuver, startle, mental stress, postural change, and deep respiration, and the sudomotor (sweating) responses to warming or a deep inspiratory gasp. Tilt-table testing may reproduce syncopal or presyncopal symptoms. Pharmacologic studies to evaluate the pupillary responses, radiologic studies of the bladder or gastrointestinal tract, uroflowmetry and urethral pressure profiles, and recording of nocturnal penile tumescence may also be necessary in selected cases. Further investigation depends on the presence of other associated neurologic abnormalities. In patients with a peripheral cause, work-up for peripheral neuropathy may be required and should include testing for ganglionic acetylcholine receptor antibody. For those with evidence of a central lesion, imaging studies will exclude a treatable structural cause. Reversible, nonneurologic causes of symptoms must be considered. Postural hypotension and syncope may relate to a reduced cardiac output, paroxysmal cardiac dysrhythmias, volume depletion, various medications, and endocrine and metabolic disorders such as Addison disease, hypothyroidism or hyperthyroidism, pheochromocytoma, and carcinoid syndrome.

▸ Treatment

The most disabling symptom is usually postural hypotension and syncope. Abrupt postural change, prolonged recumbency, and other precipitants should be avoided. Medications associated with postural hypotension should be discontinued or reduced in dose. Treatment may include wearing waist-high elastic hosiery, salt supplementation, sleeping in a semierect position (which minimizes the natriuresis and diuresis that occur during recumbency), and fludrocortisone (0.1–0.2 mg daily). Vasoconstrictor agents may be helpful and include midodrine (2.5–10 mg orally three times daily) and ephedrine (15–30 mg orally three times daily). Other agents that have been used occasionally or experimentally are dihydroergotamine, yohimbine, pyridostigmine, and clonidine; refractory cases may respond to erythropoietin (epoetin alfa) or desmopressin. Patients must be monitored for recumbent hypertension. Postprandial hypotension is helped by caffeine. There is no satisfactory treatment for disturbances of sweating, but an air-conditioned environment is helpful in avoiding extreme swings in body temperature.

▶ When to Refer

- When the diagnosis is uncertain.
- When symptoms persist despite conventional treatment.

Lanier JB et al. Evaluation and management of orthostatic hypotension. Am Fam Physician. 2011 Sep 1;84(5):527–36. [PMID: 21888303]

Mathias CJ et al. Autonomic dysfunction: recognition, diagnosis, investigation, management, and autonomic neurorehabilitation. Handb Clin Neurol. 2013;110:239–53. [PMID: 23312645]

TRANSIENT ISCHEMIC ATTACKS

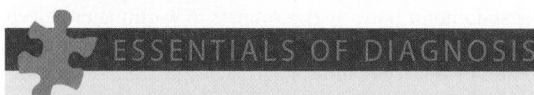

ESSENTIALS OF DIAGNOSIS

- ▶ Focal neurologic deficit of acute onset.
- ▶ Clinical deficit resolves completely within 24 hours.
- ▶ Risk factors for vascular disease often present.

▶ General Considerations

Transient ischemic attacks are characterized by focal ischemic cerebral neurologic deficits that last for < 24 hours (usually < 1–2 hours). About 30% of patients with stroke have a history of transient ischemic attacks, and proper treatment of the attacks is an important means of prevention.

▶ Etiology

An important cause of transient cerebral ischemia is embolization. In many patients with these attacks, a source is readily apparent in the heart or a major extracranial artery to the head, and emboli sometimes are visible in the retinal arteries. Moreover, an embolic phenomenon explains why separate attacks may affect different parts of the territory supplied by the same major vessel. Cardiac causes of embolic ischemic attacks include atrial fibrillation, rheumatic heart disease, mitral valve disease, infective endocarditis, atrial myxoma, and mural thrombi complicating

myocardial infarction. Atrial septal defects and patent foramen ovale may permit emboli from the veins to reach the brain ("paradoxical emboli"). An ulcerated plaque on a major artery to the brain may serve as a source of emboli. In the anterior circulation, atherosclerotic changes occur most commonly in the region of the carotid bifurcation extracranially, and these changes may cause a bruit. In some patients with transient ischemic attacks or strokes, an acute or recent hemorrhage is found to have occurred into this atherosclerotic plaque, and this finding may have pathologic significance. Patients with AIDS have an increased risk of developing transient ischemic deficits or strokes.

Less common abnormalities of blood vessels that may cause transient ischemic attacks include fibromuscular dysplasia, which affects particularly the cervical internal carotid artery; atherosclerosis of the aortic arch; inflammatory arterial disorders such as giant cell arteritis, systemic lupus erythematosus, polyarteritis, and granulomatous angiitis; and meningovascular syphilis. Hypotension may cause a reduction of cerebral blood flow if a major extracranial artery to the brain is markedly stenosed, but this is a rare cause of transient ischemic attack.

Hematologic causes of ischemic attacks include polycythemia, sickle cell disease, and hyperviscosity syndromes. Severe anemia may also lead to transient focal neurologic deficits in patients with preexisting cerebral arterial disease.

The **subclavian steal syndrome** may lead to transient vertebrobasilar ischemia. Symptoms develop when there is localized stenosis or occlusion of one subclavian artery proximal to the source of the vertebral artery, so that blood is "stolen" from this artery. A bruit in the supraclavicular fossa, unequal radial pulses, and a difference of 20 mm Hg or more between the systolic blood pressures in the arms should suggest the diagnosis in patients with vertebrobasilar transient ischemic attacks.

▶ Clinical Findings

A. Symptoms and Signs

The symptoms of transient ischemic attacks vary markedly among patients; however, the symptoms in a given individual tend to be constant in type. Onset is abrupt and without warning, and recovery usually occurs rapidly, often within a few minutes. The specific symptoms depend on the arterial distribution affected, as outlined in the subsequent section on stroke. Of note, transient ischemic attack is a rare cause of loss of consciousness or acute confusion but is often erroneously blamed for such symptoms.

The natural history of attacks is variable. Some patients will have a major stroke after only a few attacks, whereas others may have frequent attacks for weeks or months without having a stroke. The risk of stroke is high in the first 3 months after an attack, particularly in the first month and especially within the first 48 hours. Attacks may occur intermittently over a long period of time, or they may stop spontaneously. In general, carotid ischemic attacks are more liable than vertebrobasilar ischemic attacks to be followed by stroke. The stroke risk is greater in patients older than 60 years, in patients with diabetes, or after transient ischemic attacks that last longer than 10 minutes and with symptoms or signs of weakness, speech impairment, or gait disturbance.

B. Imaging

CT or MRI scan is indicated within 24 hours of symptom onset, in part to exclude the possibility of a small cerebral hemorrhage or a cerebral tumor masquerading as a transient ischemic attack; MRI with diffusion-weighted sequences is particularly sensitive for revealing acute or subacute infarction. Noninvasive imaging of the cervical vasculature should also be performed. Carotid duplex ultrasonography is useful for detecting significant stenosis of the internal carotid artery, and MR or CT angiography permits broader visualization of cervical and intracranial vasculature. When noninvasive studies fail to reveal an etiology for transient ischemic attacks, conventional cerebral arteriography may be indicated. This technique is the gold standard for investigating the integrity of the cervical and cerebral vasculature, and allows for angioplasty or other interventions, if necessary.

C. Laboratory and Other Studies

Clinical and laboratory evaluation must include assessment for hypertension, heart disease, hematologic disorders, diabetes mellitus, hyperlipidemia, and peripheral vascular disease. It should include complete blood count, fasting blood glucose and serum cholesterol and homocysteine determinations, serologic tests for syphilis, and an ECG and chest radiograph. Echocardiography with bubble contrast is performed if a cardiac source is likely, and blood cultures are obtained if endocarditis is suspected. Holter monitoring is indicated if a transient, paroxysmal disturbance of cardiac rhythm is suspected.

▶ Differential Diagnosis

Focal seizures usually cause abnormal motor or sensory phenomena such as clonic limb movements, paresthesias, or tingling, rather than weakness or loss of feeling. Symptoms generally spread ("march") up the limb and may lead to a generalized tonic-clonic seizure.

Classic migraine is easily recognized by the visual premonitory symptoms, followed by nausea, headache, and photophobia, but less typical cases may be hard to distinguish. The patient's age and medical history (including family history) may be helpful in this regard. Patients with migraine commonly have a history of episodes since adolescence and report that other family members have a similar disorder.

Focal neurologic deficits may occur during periods of hypoglycemia in diabetic patients receiving insulin or oral hypoglycemic agent therapy.

▶ Treatment

A. Medical Measures

Hospitalization should be considered for patients seen within 72 hours of the attack, when they are at increased risk for early recurrence. One commonly used method to assess recurrence risk is the $ABCD^2$ score; points are assigned for each of the following criteria: age 60 years or older (1 point), blood pressure $\geq$ 140/90 mm Hg (1 point), clinical symptoms of focal weakness (2 points) or speech impairment without weakness (1 point), duration $\geq$ 60 minutes (2 points) or 10–59 minutes (1 point), or diabetes mellitus (1 point). An $ABCD^2$ score of 3 or more points has been suggested as a threshold for hospital admission. Admission is also advisable for patients with crescendo attacks, symptomatic carotid stenosis, or known cardiac source of emboli or hypercoagulable state; such hospitalization facilitates early intervention for any recurrence and rapid institution of secondary prevention measures.

Medical treatment is aimed at preventing further attacks and stroke. Treat diabetes mellitus; hematologic disorders; and hypertension, preferably with an angiotensin-converting enzyme inhibitor or angiotensin receptor blocker. Consider starting a statin medication regardless of the current low-density lipoprotein level; in addition to reducing stroke risk, antecedent statin use may improve the outcome if an ischemic stroke does occur. Cigarette smoking should be stopped, and cardiac sources of embolization should be treated appropriately. Weight reduction and regular physical activity should be encouraged when appropriate.

In patients with carotid ischemic attacks who are poor operative candidates (and thus have not undergone arteriography) or who are found to have extensive vascular disease, medical treatment should be instituted. Similarly, patients with vertebrobasilar ischemic attacks are treated medically and are not subjected to arteriography unless there is clinical evidence of stenosis or occlusion in the carotid or subclavian arteries.

1. Embolization from the heart—Cardioembolism, especially in the setting of atrial fibrillation, is an indication for anticoagulation as a preventive treatment for stroke. If anticoagulants are indicated for the treatment of embolism from the heart, they should be started immediately, provided that the area of cerebral infarct is small and there is no contraindication to their use. There is no advantage in delay, and the common fear of causing hemorrhage into a previously infarcted area is misplaced, since there is a far greater risk of further embolism to the cerebral circulation if treatment is withheld (see Treatment of Atrial Fibrillation, Chapter 10).

2. Noncardioembolic attacks—In a patient naïve to antiplatelet therapy, low-dose aspirin (81 mg daily orally) should be initiated to reduce the frequency of transient ischemic attacks and the incidence of stroke. For patients already taking aspirin who continue to experience transient ischemic attacks, adding sustained-release dipyridamole (200 mg twice daily orally) to the regimen provides additional protection against stroke compared to aspirin alone. Clopidogrel (75 mg daily orally) alone is marginally more efficacious than aspirin alone; combining clopidogrel with aspirin is not clearly better than clopidogrel alone but does increase the risk of bleeding complications. Cilostazol, another antiplatelet medication, appears to offer similar efficacy at stroke prevention as aspirin, and possibly less risk of hemorrhage. Anticoagulant drugs are not recommended, as they offer no benefit over antiplatelet therapy, and the risk of serious hemorrhagic adverse effects is greater.

B. Surgical or Endovascular Measures

When arteriography reveals a surgically accessible high-grade stenosis (70–99% in luminal diameter) on the side appropriate to carotid ischemic attacks and there is relatively little atherosclerosis elsewhere in the cerebrovascular system, operative treatment (carotid endarterectomy) or endovascular intervention reduces the risk of ipsilateral carotid stroke, especially when transient ischemic attacks are of recent onset (< 1 month). Some evidence suggests that transluminal angioplasty and stenting is inferior to aggressive medical management alone. There is a more moderate benefit for patients with 50–69% stenosis, and surgery is not indicated for mild stenosis (< 50%); its benefits are unclear with severe stenosis plus diffuse intracranial atherosclerotic disease.

▶ When to Refer

All patients should be referred for urgent investigation and treatment to prevent stroke.

▶ When to Admit

If seen within 72 hours of a transient ischemic attack, patients should be considered for admission when they have an ABCD^2 score of 3 points or more, when outpatient evaluation is impractical, or when there are crescendo attacks or other concern for early recurrence or stroke.

Chimowitz MI et al; SAMMPRIS Trial Investigators. Stenting versus aggressive medical therapy for intracranial arterial stenosis. N Engl J Med. 2011 Sep 15;365(11):993–1003. [PMID: 21899409]

Geeganage CM et al; Acute Antiplatelet Stroke Trialists Collaboration. Dual or mono antiplatelet therapy for patients with acute ischemic stroke or transient ischemic attack: systematic review and meta-analysis of randomized controlled trials. Stroke. 2012 Apr;43(4):1058–66. [PMID: 22282894]

Merwick Á et al. Reduction in early stroke risk in carotid stenosis with transient ischemic attack associated with statin treatment. Stroke. 2013 Oct;44(10):2814–20. [PMID: 23908061]

Tsivgoulis G et al. Multicenter external validation of the ABCD^2 score in triaging TIA patients. Neurology. 2010 Apr 27;74(17):1351–7. [PMID: 20421579]

STROKE

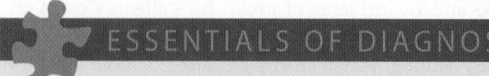

ESSENTIALS OF DIAGNOSIS

▶ Sudden onset of characteristic neurologic deficit.

▶ Patient often has history of hypertension, diabetes mellitus, valvular heart disease, or atherosclerosis.

▶ Distinctive neurologic signs reflect the region of the brain involved.

▶ General Considerations

In the United States, stroke remains the third leading cause of death, despite a general decline in the incidence of stroke in the last 30 years. The precise reasons for this decline are uncertain, but increased awareness of risk factors (hypertension, diabetes mellitus, hyperlipidemia, cigarette smoking, cardiac disease, AIDS, recreational drug abuse, heavy alcohol consumption, family history of stroke) and improved prophylactic measures and surveillance of those at increased risk have been contributory. Elevation of the blood homocysteine level is also a risk factor for stroke, but it is unclear whether this risk is reduced by treatment to lower the level. A previous stroke makes individual patients more susceptible to additional strokes.

For years, strokes have been subdivided pathologically into infarcts (thrombotic or embolic) and hemorrhages, and clinical criteria for distinguishing between these possibilities have been emphasized. However, it is often difficult to determine on clinical grounds the pathologic basis for stroke (Table 24–4).

1. Lacunar Infarction

Lacunar infarcts are small lesions (usually < 5 mm in diameter) that occur in the distribution of short penetrating arterioles in the basal ganglia, pons, cerebellum, internal capsule, thalamus and, less commonly, the deep cerebral white matter (Table 24–4). Lacunar infarcts are associated with poorly controlled hypertension or diabetes and have been found in several clinical syndromes, including contralateral pure motor or pure sensory deficit, ipsilateral ataxia with crural paresis, and dysarthria with clumsiness of the hand. The neurologic deficit may progress over 24–36 hours before stabilizing.

Early mortality and risk of stroke recurrence is higher for patients with nonlacunar than lacunar infarcts. The prognosis for recovery from the deficit produced by a lacunar infarct is usually good, with partial or complete resolution occurring over the following 4–6 weeks in many instances. Treatment is as described for transient ischemic attack and cerebral infarction.

2. Cerebral Infarction

Thrombotic or embolic occlusion of a major vessel leads to cerebral infarction. Causes include the disorders predisposing to transient ischemic attacks (see above) and atherosclerosis of cerebral arteries. The resulting deficit depends on the particular vessel involved and the extent of any collateral circulation. Cerebral ischemia leads to release of excitatory and other neuropeptides that may augment calcium flux into neurons, thereby leading to cell death and increasing the neurologic deficit.

▶ Clinical Findings

A. Symptoms and Signs

Onset is usually abrupt, and there may then be very little progression except that due to brain swelling. Clinical

Table 24–4. Features of the major stroke subtypes.

Stroke Type and Subtype	Clinical Features	Diagnosis	Treatment
Ischemic stroke			
Lacunar infarct	Small (< 5 mm) lesions in the basal ganglia, pons, cerebellum, or internal capsule; less often in deep cerebral white matter; prognosis generally good; clinical features depend on location, but may worsen over first 24–36 hours.	MRI with diffusion-weighted sequences usually defines the area of infarction; CT is insensitive acutely but can be used to exclude hemorrhage.	Aspirin; long-term management is to control risk factors (hypertension and diabetes mellitus).
Carotid circulation obstruction	See text—signs vary depending on occluded vessel.	Noncontrast CT to exclude hemorrhage but findings may be normal during first 6–24 hours of an ischemic stroke; diffusion-weighted MRI is gold standard for identifying acute stroke; electrocardiography, echocardiography, blood glucose, complete blood count, and tests for hypercoagulable states, hyperlipidemia are indicated; Holter monitoring in selected instances; carotid duplex studies, CTA, MRA, or conventional angiography in selected cases.	Select patients for intravenous thrombolytics or intra-arterial mechanical thrombolysis; aspirin is first-line therapy; anticoagulation with heparin for cardioembolic strokes when no contraindications exist.
Vertebrobasilar occlusion	See text—signs vary based on location of occluded vessel.	As for carotid circulation obstruction.	As for carotid circulation obstruction.
Hemorrhagic stroke			
Spontaneous intracerebral hemorrhage	Commonly associated with hypertension; also with bleeding disorders, amyloid angiopathy. Hypertensive hemorrhage is located commonly in the basal ganglia and less commonly in the pons, thalamus, cerebellum, or cerebral white matter.	Noncontrast CT is superior to MRI for detecting bleeds of < 48 hours duration; laboratory tests to identify bleeding disorder: angiography may be indicated to exclude aneurysm or AVM. Do not perform lumbar puncture.	Most managed supportively, but cerebellar bleeds or hematomas with gross mass effect may require urgent surgical evacuation.
Subarachnoid hemorrhage	Present with sudden onset of worst headache of life, may lead rapidly to loss of consciousness; signs of meningeal irritation often present; etiology usually aneurysm or AVM, but 20% have no source identified.	CT to confirm diagnosis, but may be normal in rare instances; if CT negative and suspicion high, perform lumbar puncture to look for red blood cells or xanthochromia; angiography to determine source of bleed in candidates for treatment.	See sections on AVM and aneurysm.
Intracranial aneurysm	Most located in the anterior circle of Willis and are typically asymptomatic until subarachnoid bleed occurs; 20% rebleed in first 2 weeks.	CT indicates subarachnoid hemorrhage, and angiography then demonstrates aneurysms; angiography may not reveal aneurysm if vasospasm present.	Prevent further bleeding by clipping aneurysm or coil embolization; nimodipine helps prevent vasospasm; reverse vasospasm by intravenous fluids and induced hypertension after aneurysm has been obliterated, if no other aneurysms are present; angioplasty may also reverse symptomatic vasospasm.
AVMs	Focal deficit from hematoma or AVM itself.	CT reveals bleed, and may reveal the AVM; may be seen by MRI. Angiography demonstrates feeding vessels and vascular anatomy.	Surgery indicated if AVM has bled or to prevent further progression of neurologic deficit; other modalities to treat nonoperable AVMs are available at specialized centers.

AVMs, arteriovenous malformations; CTA, computed tomography angiography; MRA, magnetic resonance angiography.

evaluation should always include examination of the heart and auscultation over the subclavian and carotid vessels to determine whether there are any bruits.

1. Obstruction of carotid circulation—Occlusion of the ophthalmic artery is probably symptomless in most cases because of the rich orbital collaterals, but its transient embolic obstruction can lead to amaurosis fugax—sudden and brief loss of vision in one eye.

Occlusion of the **anterior cerebral artery** distal to its junction with the anterior communicating artery causes weakness and cortical sensory loss in the contralateral leg and sometimes mild weakness of the arm, especially proximally. There may be a contralateral grasp reflex, paratonic rigidity, and abulia (lack of initiative) or frank confusion. Urinary incontinence is not uncommon, particularly if behavioral disturbances are conspicuous. Bilateral anterior cerebral infarction is especially likely to cause marked behavioral changes and memory disturbances. Unilateral anterior cerebral artery occlusion proximal to the junction with the anterior communicating artery is generally well tolerated because of the collateral supply from the other side.

Middle cerebral artery occlusion leads to contralateral hemiplegia, hemisensory loss, and homonymous hemianopia (ie, bilaterally symmetric loss of vision in half of the visual fields), with the eyes deviated to the side of the lesion. If the dominant hemisphere is involved, global aphasia is also present. It may be impossible to distinguish this clinically from occlusion of the internal carotid artery. With occlusion of either of these arteries, there may also be considerable swelling of the hemisphere, leading to drowsiness, stupor, and coma in extreme cases. Occlusions of different branches of the middle cerebral artery cause more limited findings. For example, involvement of the anterior main division leads to a predominantly expressive dysphasia and to contralateral paralysis and loss of sensations in the arm, the face and, to a lesser extent, the leg. Posterior branch occlusion produces a receptive (Wernicke) aphasia and a homonymous visual field defect. With involvement of the nondominant hemisphere, speech and comprehension are preserved, but there may be a left hemispatial neglect syndrome or constructional and visuospatial deficits.

2. Obstruction of vertebrobasilar circulation—Occlusion of the **posterior cerebral artery** may lead to a thalamic syndrome in which contralateral hemisensory disturbance occurs, followed by the development of spontaneous pain and hyperpathia. There is often a macular-sparing homonymous hemianopia and sometimes a mild, usually temporary, hemiparesis. Depending on the site of the lesion and the collateral circulation, the severity of these deficits varies and other deficits may also occur, including involuntary movements and alexia. Occlusion of the main artery beyond the origin of its penetrating branches may lead solely to a macular-sparing hemianopia.

Vertebral artery occlusion distally, below the origin of the anterior spinal and posterior inferior cerebellar arteries, may be clinically silent because the circulation is maintained by the other vertebral artery. If the remaining vertebral artery is congenitally small or severely atherosclerotic, however, a deficit similar to that of basilar artery occlusion is seen unless there is good collateral circulation from the anterior circulation through the circle of Willis. When the small paramedian arteries arising from the vertebral artery are occluded, contralateral hemiplegia and sensory deficit occur in association with an ipsilateral cranial nerve palsy at the level of the lesion. An obstruction of the **posterior inferior cerebellar artery** or an obstruction of the vertebral artery just before it branches to this vessel leads to ipsilateral spinothalamic sensory loss involving the face, ninth and tenth cranial nerve lesions, limb ataxia and numbness, and Horner syndrome, combined with contralateral spinothalamic sensory loss involving the limbs.

Occlusion of both **vertebral arteries** or the **basilar artery** leads to coma with pinpoint pupils, flaccid quadriplegia and sensory loss, and variable cranial nerve abnormalities. With partial basilar artery occlusion, there may be diplopia, visual loss, vertigo, dysarthria, ataxia, weakness or sensory disturbances in some or all of the limbs, and discrete cranial nerve palsies. In patients with hemiplegia of pontine origin, the eyes are often deviated to the paralyzed side, whereas in patients with a hemispheric lesion, the eyes commonly deviate from the hemiplegic side.

Occlusion of any of the major **cerebellar arteries** produces vertigo, nausea, vomiting, nystagmus, ipsilateral limb ataxia, and contralateral spinothalamic sensory loss in the limbs. If the superior cerebellar artery is involved, the contralateral spinothalamic loss also involves the face; with occlusion of the anterior inferior cerebellar artery, there is ipsilateral spinothalamic sensory loss involving the face, usually in conjunction with ipsilateral facial weakness and deafness. Massive cerebellar infarction may lead to coma, tonsillar herniation, and death.

3. Coma—Infarction in either the carotid or vertebrobasilar territory may lead to loss of consciousness. For example, an infarct involving one cerebral hemisphere may lead to such swelling that the function of the other hemisphere or the rostral brainstem is disturbed and coma results. Similarly, coma occurs with bilateral brainstem infarction when this involves the reticular formation, and it occurs with brainstem compression after cerebellar infarction.

B. Imaging

A CT scan of the head (without contrast) should be performed immediately, before the administration of aspirin or other antithrombotic agents, to exclude cerebral hemorrhage (Table 24–4). CT is relatively insensitive to acute ischemic stroke, and subsequent MRI with diffusion-weighted sequences helps define the distribution and extent of infarction as well as to exclude tumor or other differential considerations. Perfusion-weighted MRI sequences can be useful for outlining any additional areas at risk for infarction, thus guiding treatment decisions; specific guidelines are still being determined. Imaging of the cervical vasculature, by CT angiography, MR angiography, or conventional catheter angiography, is indicated as part of a search to identify the source of the stroke.

C. Laboratory and Other Studies

Investigations should include a complete blood count, erythrocyte sedimentation rate, blood glucose determination, and serologic tests for syphilis. Screening for antiphospholipid antibodies (lupus anticoagulants and anticardiolipin antibodies); the factor V Leiden mutation; abnormalities of protein C, protein S, or antithrombin; or a prothrombin gene mutation is indicated if a hypercoagulable disorder is suspected (eg, a young patient without apparent risk factors for stroke). Similarly, elevated serum cholesterol and lipids and serum homocysteine may indicate an increased risk of thrombotic stroke. Electrocardiography or continuous cardiac monitoring for at least 24 hours will help exclude a recent myocardial infarction or a cardiac arrhythmia that might be serving as a source of embolization. Blood cultures should be performed if endocarditis is suspected, echocardiography (bubble contrast study) if heart disease—especially valvular disease, left-to-right shunting, or cardiac thrombus—is a concern, and Holter monitoring if paroxysmal cardiac arrhythmia requires exclusion. Examination of the cerebrospinal fluid is not always necessary but may be helpful if cerebral vasculitis or another inflammatory or infectious cause of stroke is suspected, but it should be delayed until after CT or MRI to exclude any risk for herniation due to mass effect.

► Treatment

Prophylactic measures were discussed earlier under Transient Ischemic Attacks. The management of acute stroke should be in a stroke care unit, when feasible. Intravenous thrombolytic therapy with recombinant tissue plasminogen activator (rtPA; 0.9 mg/kg to a maximum of 90 mg, with 10% given as a bolus over 1 minute and the remainder over 1 hour) is effective in reducing the neurologic deficit in selected patients without CT evidence of intracranial hemorrhage. Patients should receive tPA within 1 hour after arriving to the hospital but not more than 4.5 hours after the onset of ischemic symptoms. Data for treatment with tPA up to 4.5 hours after the onset of symptoms show reduced disability at 90 days.

Recent hemorrhage, increased risk of hemorrhage (eg, treatment with anticoagulants), arterial puncture at a noncompressible site, and systolic pressure > 185 mm Hg or diastolic pressure > 110 mm Hg are among the contraindications to this treatment. In selected patients with thrombotic stroke, percutaneous procedures, including endovascular intra-arterial rtPA administration or mechanical removal of an embolus or clot from an occluded cerebral artery using an intra-arterial mechanical thrombolytic device, are also effective relative to non-thrombolytic medical treatment, despite an increased risk of intracranial hemorrhage; it is not clear how these invasive approaches compare to intravenous thrombolytic therapy.

Early management of a completed stroke otherwise requires general supportive measures. During the acute stage, there may be marked brain swelling and edema, with symptoms and signs of increasing intracranial pressure, an increasing neurologic deficit, or herniation syndrome. Elevated intracranial pressure is managed by head elevation and osmotic agents such as mannitol. Maintenance of an adequate cerebral perfusion pressure helps prevent further ischemia. Decompressive hemicraniectomy for malignant middle cerebral artery infarctions may reduce mortality and improve functional outcome in some instances. Attempts to lower the blood pressure of hypertensive patients during the acute phase (ie, within 2 weeks) of a stroke should generally be avoided, as there is loss of cerebral autoregulation, and lowering the blood pressure may further compromise ischemic areas. However, if the systolic pressure exceeds 220 mm Hg, it can be lowered using intravenous labetalol or nicardipine with continuous monitoring to 170–200 mm Hg and then, after 2 weeks, it can be reduced further to < 140/90 mm Hg.

In patients not eligible for thrombolytic therapy, and in whom hemorrhage has been excluded by CT, the immediate administration of aspirin 325 mg orally daily is indicated. Anticoagulant drugs should also be started without delay in the setting of atrial fibrillation or other source of cardioembolism when hemorrhage has been excluded by CT. Treatment is with warfarin (target INR 2.0–3.0) or dabigatran (150 mg twice daily); bridging warfarin with heparin is not necessary, but some experts advocate treatment with aspirin until the INR becomes therapeutic.

Physical therapy has an important role in the management of patients with impaired motor function. Passive movements at an early stage will help prevent contractures. As cooperation increases and some recovery begins, active movements will improve strength and coordination. In all cases, early mobilization and active rehabilitation are important. Occupational therapy may improve morale and motor skills, while speech therapy may help expressive dysphasia or dysarthria. Because of the risk for dysphagia following stroke, access to food and drink is typically restricted until an appropriate swallowing evaluation. When there is a severe and persisting motor deficit, a device such as a leg brace, toe spring, frame, or cane may help the patient move about, and the provision of other aids to daily living may improve the quality of life.

► Prognosis

The prognosis for survival after cerebral infarction is better than after cerebral or subarachnoid hemorrhage. The only proved effective therapy for acute stroke requires initiation within 3–4.5 hours after stroke onset, and the prognosis therefore depends on the time that elapses before arrival at the hospital. Patients receiving such treatment with rtPA are at least 30% more likely to have minimal or no disability at 3 months than those not treated by this means. Loss of consciousness after a cerebral infarct implies a poorer prognosis than otherwise. The extent of the infarct governs the potential for rehabilitation. Patients who have had a cerebral infarct are at risk for additional strokes and for myocardial infarcts. Statin therapy to lower serum lipid levels may reduce this risk. Antiplatelet therapy (same treatment guidelines as for transient ischemic attack; see above) reduces the recurrence rate by 30% among patients without a cardiac cause for the stroke who are not candidates for carotid endarterectomy. Nevertheless, the cumulative risk of recurrence of noncardioembolic stroke is still 3–7% annually.

Patients with massive strokes from which meaningful recovery is unlikely should receive palliative care (see Chapter 5).

When to Refer

All patients should be referred.

When to Admit

All patients should be hospitalized, preferably in a stroke care unit.

Biffi A et al. Statin treatment and functional outcome after ischemic stroke: case-control and meta-analysis. Stroke. 2011 May;42(5):1314–9. [PMID: 21415396]

Grise EM et al. Blood pressure control for acute ischemic and hemorrhagic stroke. Curr Opin Crit Care. 2012 Apr;18(2): 132–8. [PMID: 22322257]

Jauch EC et al. Guidelines for the early management of patients with acute ischemic stroke: a guideline for healthcare professionals from the American Heart Association/American Stroke Association. Stroke. 2013 Mar;44(3):870–947. [PMID: 23370205]

Lansberg MG et al. Efficacy and safety of tissue plasminogen activator 3 to 4.5 hours after acute ischemic stroke: a meta-analysis. Stroke. 2009 Jul;40(7):2438–41. [PMID: 19478213]

Micheli S et al. Lacunar versus non-lacunar syndromes. Front Neurol Neurosci. 2012;30:94–8. [PMID: 22377873]

O'Donnell MJ et al. Risk factors for ischaemic and intracerebral haemorrhagic stroke in 22 countries (the INTERSTROKE study): a case-control study. Lancet. 2010 Jul 10;376(9735): 112–23. [PMID: 20561675]

O'Rourke K et al. Percutaneous vascular interventions for acute ischaemic stroke. Cochrane Database Syst Rev. 2010 Oct 6; (10):CD007574. [PMID: 20927761]

3. Intracerebral Hemorrhage

Spontaneous, nontraumatic intracerebral hemorrhage in patients with no angiographic evidence of an associated vascular anomaly (eg, aneurysm or angioma) is usually due to hypertension. The pathologic basis for hemorrhage is probably the presence of microaneurysms that develop on perforating vessels in hypertensive patients. Hypertensive intracerebral hemorrhage occurs most frequently in the basal ganglia and less commonly in the pons, thalamus, cerebellum, and cerebral white matter. Hemorrhage may extend into the ventricular system or subarachnoid space, and signs of meningeal irritation are then found. Hemorrhages usually occur suddenly and without warning, often during activity. In the elderly, cerebral amyloid angiopathy is another important and frequent cause of hemorrhage, which is usually lobar in distribution, sometimes recurrent, and associated with a better prognosis than hypertensive hemorrhage.

Other causes of nontraumatic intracerebral hemorrhage include hematologic and bleeding disorders (eg, leukemia, thrombocytopenia, hemophilia, or disseminated intravascular coagulation), anticoagulant therapy, liver disease, high alcohol intake, and primary or secondary brain tumors. There is also an association with advancing age and male sex. Bleeding is primarily into the subarachnoid space when it occurs from an intracranial aneurysm or arteriovenous malformation (see below), but it may be partly intraparenchymal as well. In some cases, no specific cause for cerebral hemorrhage can be identified.

Clinical Findings

A. Symptoms and Signs

With hemorrhage into the cerebral hemisphere, consciousness is initially lost or impaired in about one-half of patients. Vomiting occurs very frequently at the onset of bleeding, and headache is sometimes present. Focal symptoms and signs then develop, depending on the site of the hemorrhage. With hypertensive hemorrhage, there is generally a rapidly evolving neurologic deficit with hemiplegia or hemiparesis. A hemisensory disturbance is also present with more deeply placed lesions. With lesions of the putamen, loss of conjugate lateral gaze may be conspicuous. With thalamic hemorrhage, there may be a loss of upward gaze, downward or skew deviation of the eyes, lateral gaze palsies, and pupillary inequalities.

Cerebellar hemorrhage may present with sudden onset of nausea and vomiting, dysequilibrium, headache, and loss of consciousness that may terminate fatally within 48 hours. Less commonly, the onset is gradual and the course episodic or slowly progressive—clinical features suggesting an expanding cerebellar lesion. In yet other cases, however, the onset and course are intermediate, and examination shows lateral conjugate gaze palsies to the side of the lesion; small reactive pupils; contralateral hemiplegia; peripheral facial weakness; ataxia of gait, limbs, or trunk; periodic respiration; or some combination of these findings.

B. Imaging

CT scanning (without contrast) is important not only in confirming that hemorrhage has occurred but also in determining the size and site of the hematoma. It is superior to MRI for detecting intracranial hemorrhage of < 48 hours duration. If the patient's condition permits further intervention, CT angiography, MR angiography, or cerebral angiography may be undertaken thereafter to determine whether an aneurysm or arteriovenous malformation is present (see below). Follow-up imaging during the hospitalization may reveal hematoma expansion, a predictor of poor outcome.

C. Laboratory and Other Studies

A complete blood count, platelet count, bleeding time, prothrombin and partial thromboplastin times, and liver and kidney function tests may reveal a predisposing cause for the hemorrhage. Lumbar puncture is contraindicated because it may precipitate a herniation syndrome in patients with a large hematoma, and CT scanning is superior in detecting intracerebral hemorrhage.

Treatment

Neurologic management is generally conservative and supportive, regardless of whether the patient has a profound deficit with associated brainstem compression, in which case the prognosis is grim, or a more localized deficit not causing increased intracranial pressure or brainstem involvement. Such therapy may include ventilatory support, blood pressure regulation, seizure prophylaxis, control of fever, osmotherapy, and nutritional supplementation. Intracranial pressure may require monitoring. Ventricular drainage may be required in patients with intraventricular hemorrhage and acute hydrocephalus. Decompression may be helpful when a superficial hematoma in cerebral white matter is exerting a mass effect and causing incipient herniation. In patients with cerebellar hemorrhage, prompt surgical evacuation of the hematoma is appropriate, because spontaneous unpredictable deterioration may otherwise lead to a fatal outcome and because operative treatment may lead to complete resolution of the clinical deficit. The treatment of underlying structural lesions or bleeding disorders depends on their nature. Hemostatic therapy with recombinant activated factor VII has not improved survival or functional outcome. There is no specific treatment for cerebral amyloid angiopathy.

When to Refer

All patients should be referred.

When to Admit

All patients should be hospitalized.

Biffi A et al. Statin use and outcome after intracerebral hemorrhage: case-control study and meta-analysis. Neurology. 2011 May 3;76(18):1581–8. [PMID: 21451150]
Dowlatshahi D et al. Defining hematoma expansion in intracerebral hemorrhage: relationship with patient outcomes. Neurology. 2011 Apr 5;76(14):1238–44. [PMID: 21346218]
Wang X et al. Cholesterol levels and risk of hemorrhagic stroke: a systematic review and meta-analysis. Stroke. 2013 Jul;44(7):1833–9. [PMID: 23704101]

4. Spontaneous Subarachnoid Hemorrhage

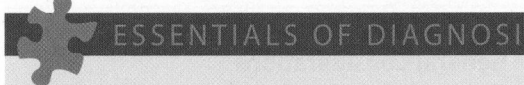

ESSENTIALS OF DIAGNOSIS

▶ Sudden severe headache.
▶ Signs of meningeal irritation usually present.
▶ Obtundation is common.
▶ Focal deficits frequently absent.

General Considerations

Between 5% and 10% of strokes are due to subarachnoid hemorrhage. Trauma is the most common cause of subarachnoid hemorrhage, the prognosis of which depends on the severity of the head injury. Spontaneous (nontraumatic) subarachnoid hemorrhage frequently results from the rupture of an arterial saccular ("berry") aneurysm or from an arteriovenous malformation. Occasional patients with aneurysms have headaches, sometimes accompanied by nausea and neck stiffness, a few hours or days before massive subarachnoid hemorrhage occurs. This has been attributed to "warning leaks" of a small amount of blood from the aneurysm.

Clinical Findings

A. Symptoms and Signs

Subarachnoid hemorrhage has a characteristic clinical picture. Its onset is with sudden headache of a severity never experienced previously by the patient. This may be followed by nausea and vomiting and by a loss or impairment of consciousness that can either be transient or progress inexorably to deepening coma and death. If consciousness is regained, the patient is often confused and irritable and may show other symptoms of an altered mental status. Neurologic examination generally reveals nuchal rigidity and other signs of meningeal irritation, except in deeply comatose patients.

Aneurysms may cause a focal neurologic deficit by compressing adjacent structures. However, most are asymptomatic or produce only nonspecific symptoms until they rupture, at which time subarachnoid hemorrhage results. A higher risk of subarachnoid hemorrhage is associated with older age, female sex, "nonwhite" ethnicity, hypertension, tobacco smoking, high alcohol consumption (exceeding 150 g per week), previous symptoms, posterior circulation aneurysms, and larger aneurysms. Focal neurologic signs are usually absent but, when present, may relate either to a focal intracerebral hematoma (from arteriovenous malformations) or to ischemia in the territory of the vessel with a ruptured aneurysm.

B. Imaging

A CT scan (preferably with CT angiography) should be performed immediately to confirm that hemorrhage has occurred and to search for clues regarding its source. It is preferable to MRI because it is faster and more sensitive in detecting hemorrhage in the first 24 hours. CT findings sometimes are normal in patients with suspected hemorrhage, and the cerebrospinal fluid must then be examined for the presence of blood or xanthochromia before the possibility of subarachnoid hemorrhage is discounted.

Cerebral arteriography is undertaken to determine the source of bleeding. In general, bilateral carotid and vertebral arteriography are necessary because aneurysms are often multiple, while arteriovenous malformations may be supplied from several sources. The procedure allows an interventional radiologist to treat an underlying aneurysm or arteriovenous malformation by various techniques. If arteriograms show no abnormality, the examination should be repeated after 2 weeks because vasospasm or thrombus may have prevented detection of an aneurysm or other vascular anomaly during the initial study. CT or MR angiography may also be revealing but is less sensitive than conventional arteriography.

C. Laboratory and Other Studies

The cerebrospinal fluid is bloodstained. Electrocardiographic evidence of arrhythmias or myocardial ischemia has been well described and probably relates to excessive sympathetic activity. Peripheral leukocytosis and transient glycosuria are also common findings.

▶ Treatment

All patients should be admitted to hospital and seen by a neurologist. The measures outlined below in the section on stupor and coma are applied to comatose patients. Conscious patients are confined to bed, advised against any exertion or straining, treated symptomatically for headache and anxiety, and given laxatives or stool softeners. If there is severe hypertension, the blood pressure can be lowered gradually, but not below a diastolic level of 100 mm Hg (see treatment of stroke, earlier). Phenytoin is generally prescribed routinely to prevent seizures. If no cause for the hemorrhage can be identified, medical management is continued for about 6 weeks and is followed by gradual mobilization.

The major aim of treatment is to prevent further hemorrhage. The risk of further hemorrhage from a ruptured aneurysm is greatest within a few days of the first hemorrhage; approximately 20% of patients will have further bleeding within 2 weeks and 40% within 6 months. Definitive treatment, ideally within 2 days of the hemorrhage, requires surgical clipping of the aneurysm base or endovascular treatment by interventional radiologists; the latter is sometimes feasible even for inoperable aneurysms and has a lower morbidity than surgery.

▶ Complications

Spontaneous subarachnoid hemorrhage may result in severe complications, so monitoring is necessary, usually in an intensive care unit. Intrathecal thrombolytic therapy, presumably by speeding clearance of extravasated blood, appears to reduce the rate of these complications. Hemiplegia or other focal deficit sometimes may follow aneurysmal bleeding after a delay of 2–14 days due to focal arterial spasm. The etiology of vasospasm is uncertain and likely multifactorial, and it sometimes leads to significant cerebral ischemia or infarction and may further aggravate any existing increase in intracranial pressure. Transcranial Doppler ultrasound may be used to screen noninvasively for vasospasm, but conventional arteriography is required to document and treat vasospasm when the clinical suspicion is high. Nimodipine has been shown to reduce, in neurologically normal patients, the incidence of ischemic deficits from arterial spasm without producing any side effects. The dose of nimodipine is 60 mg every 4 hours orally for 21 days. After surgical obliteration of all aneurysms, symptomatic vasospasm may also be treated by intravascular volume expansion and induced hypertension; transluminal balloon angioplasty of involved intracranial vessels is also helpful. Aspirin provides no benefit. Results from a randomized trial suggest that the prophylactic administration

of intravenous magnesium sulfate, sufficient to achieve serum levels of 4.9–6.1 mg/dL (2–2.5 mmol/L), reduced the risk of transcranial ultrasound-detectable vasospasm and of vasospasm-induced cerebral infarction but did not change overall clinical outcomes.

Acute hydrocephalus, which sometimes occurs due to cerebrospinal fluid outflow disruption by the subarachnoid blood, should be suspected if the patient deteriorates clinically and a repeat CT scan should be done. Acute hydrocephalus frequently causes intracranial hypertension severe enough to require temporary, and less commonly prolonged or permanent, intraventricular cerebrospinal fluid shunting. Renal salt-wasting is another complication of subarachnoid hemorrhage that may develop abruptly during the first several days of hospitalization. The resulting hyponatremia and cerebral edema may exacerbate intracranial hypertension and may require carefully titrated treatment with oral sodium chloride or intravenous hyperosmotic sodium solution. Daily measurement of the serum sodium level allows for the early detection of this complication. Hypopituitarism may occur as a late complication of subarachnoid hemorrhage.

Kramer AH et al. Locally administered intrathecal thrombolytics following aneurysmal subarachnoid hemorrhage: a systematic review and meta-analysis. Neurocrit Care. 2011 Jun;14(3):489–99. [PMID: 20740327]

Mahaney KB et al. Variation of patient characteristics, management, and outcome with timing of surgery for aneurysmal subarachnoid hemorrhage. J Neurosurg. 2011 Apr;114(4):1045–53. [PMID: 21250801]

Schmutzhard E et al. Spontaneous subarachnoid hemorrhage and glucose management. Neurocrit Care. 2011 Sep;15(2):281–6. [PMID: 21850563]

5. Intracranial Aneurysm

ESSENTIALS OF DIAGNOSIS

▶ Subarachnoid hemorrhage or focal deficit.
▶ Abnormal imaging studies.

▶ General Considerations

Saccular aneurysms ("berry" aneurysms) tend to occur at arterial bifurcations, are frequently multiple (20% of cases), and are usually asymptomatic. They may be associated with polycystic kidney disease and coarctation of the aorta. Risk factors for aneurysm formation include smoking, hypertension, and hypercholesterolemia. Most aneurysms are located on the anterior part of the circle of Willis—particularly on the anterior or posterior communicating arteries, at the bifurcation of the middle cerebral artery, and at the bifurcation of the internal carotid artery. Mycotic aneurysms resulting from septic embolism occur in more distal vessels and often at the cortical surface. The most significant complication of intracranial aneurysms is a subarachnoid hemorrhage, which is discussed in the preceding section. A higher risk of subarachnoid hemorrhage is associated with older age, female sex, "nonwhite" ethnicity, hypertension, tobacco smoking, high alcohol consumption (exceeding 150 g per week), previous symptoms, posterior circulation aneurysms, and larger aneurysms.

Clinical Findings

A. Symptoms and Signs

Aneurysms may cause a focal neurologic deficit by compressing adjacent structures. However, most are asymptomatic or produce only nonspecific symptoms until they rupture, at which time subarachnoid hemorrhage results. Its manifestations, complications, and management were outlined in the preceding section.

B. Imaging

Definitive evaluation is by angiography (bilateral carotid and vertebral studies), which generally indicates the size and site of the lesion, sometimes reveals multiple aneurysms, and may show arterial spasm if rupture has occurred. Visualization by CT or MR angiography is not usually adequate if operative treatment is under consideration because lesions may be multiple and small lesions are sometimes missed.

Treatment

The major aim of treatment is to prevent hemorrhages. Management of ruptured aneurysms was described in the section on subarachnoid hemorrhage. Symptomatic but unruptured aneurysms merit prompt treatment, either surgically or by endovascular techniques, whereas small asymptomatic ones discovered incidentally are often monitored arteriographically and corrected only if they increase in size to over 10 mm.

When to Refer

All patients should be referred.

When to Admit

- All patients with a subarachnoid hemorrhage.
- All patients for detailed imaging.
- All patients undergoing surgical or endovascular treatment.

Connolly ES Jret al. Guidelines for the management of aneurysmal subarachnoid hemorrhage: a guideline for healthcare professionals from the American Heart Association/American Stroke Association. Stroke. 2012 Jun;43(6):1711–37. [PMID: 22556195]
Ferns SP et al. De novo aneurysm formation and growth of untreated aneurysms: a 5-year MRA follow-up in a large cohort of patients with coiled aneurysms and review of the literature. Stroke. 2011 Feb;42(2):313–8. [PMID: 21164110]

6. Arteriovenous Malformations

ESSENTIALS OF DIAGNOSIS

- ► Sudden onset of subarachnoid and intracerebral hemorrhage.
- ► Distinctive neurologic signs reflect the region of the brain involved.
- ► Signs of meningeal irritation in patients presenting with subarachnoid hemorrhage.
- ► Seizures or focal deficits may occur.

General Considerations

Arteriovenous malformations are congenital vascular malformations that result from a localized maldevelopment of part of the primitive vascular plexus and consist of abnormal arteriovenous communications without intervening capillaries. They vary in size, ranging from massive lesions that are fed by multiple vessels and involve a large part of the brain to lesions so small that they are hard to identify at arteriography, surgery, or autopsy. In approximately 10% of cases, there is an associated arterial aneurysm, while 1–2% of patients presenting with aneurysms have associated arteriovenous malformations. Clinical presentation may relate to hemorrhage from the malformation or an associated aneurysm or may relate to cerebral ischemia due to diversion of blood by the anomalous arteriovenous shunt or due to venous stagnation. Regional maldevelopment of the brain, compression or distortion of adjacent cerebral tissue by enlarged anomalous vessels, and progressive gliosis due to mechanical and ischemic factors may also be contributory. In addition, communicating or obstructive hydrocephalus may occur and lead to symptoms.

Clinical Findings

A. Symptoms and Signs

1. Supratentorial lesions—Most cerebral arteriovenous malformations are supratentorial, usually lying in the territory of the middle cerebral artery. Initial symptoms consist of hemorrhage in 30–60% of cases, recurrent seizures in 20–40%, headache in 5–25%, and miscellaneous complaints (including focal deficits) in 10–15%. Up to 70% of arteriovenous malformations bleed at some point in their natural history, most commonly before the patient reaches the age of 40 years. This tendency to bleed is unrelated to the lesion site or to the patient's sex, but small arteriovenous malformations are more likely to bleed than large ones. Arteriovenous malformations that have bled once are more likely to bleed again. Hemorrhage is commonly intracerebral as well as into the subarachnoid space, and it has a fatal outcome in about 10% of cases. Focal or generalized seizures may accompany or follow hemorrhage, or they may be the initial presentation, especially with frontal or parietal arteriovenous malformations. Headaches are especially likely when the external carotid arteries are involved in the malformation. These sometimes simulate migraine but more commonly are nonspecific in character, with nothing about them to suggest an underlying structural lesion.

In patients presenting with subarachnoid hemorrhage, examination may reveal an abnormal mental status and signs of meningeal irritation. Additional findings may help localize the lesion and sometimes indicate that intracranial pressure is increased. A cranial bruit always suggests the possibility of a cerebral arteriovenous malformation, but bruits may also be found with aneurysms, meningiomas, acquired arteriovenous fistulas, and arteriovenous malformations involving the scalp, calvarium, or orbit. Bruits are best heard over the ipsilateral eye or mastoid region and are of some help in lateralization but of no help in localization. Absence of a bruit in no way excludes the possibility of arteriovenous malformation.

2. Infratentorial lesions—Brainstem arteriovenous malformations are often clinically silent, but they may hemorrhage, cause obstructive hydrocephalus, or lead to progressive or relapsing brainstem deficits. Cerebellar arteriovenous malformations may also be clinically inconspicuous but sometimes lead to cerebellar hemorrhage.

B. Imaging

In patients presenting with suspected hemorrhage, CT scanning indicates whether subarachnoid or intracerebral bleeding has recently occurred, helps localize its source, and may reveal the arteriovenous malformation. If the CT scan shows no evidence of bleeding but subarachnoid hemorrhage is diagnosed clinically, a lumbar puncture should be performed to examine the cerebrospinal fluid for blood.

When intracranial hemorrhage is confirmed but the source of hemorrhage is not evident on the CT scan, arteriography is necessary to exclude aneurysm or arteriovenous malformation. MR and CT angiography are not sensitive enough for this purpose. Even if the findings on CT scan suggest arteriovenous malformation, arteriography is required to establish the nature of the lesion with certainty and to determine its anatomic features so that treatment can be planned. The examination must generally include bilateral opacification of the internal and external carotid arteries and the vertebral arteries. Arteriovenous malformations typically appear as a tangled vascular mass with distended tortuous afferent and efferent vessels, a rapid circulation time, and arteriovenous shunting.

In patients presenting without hemorrhage, CT scan or MRI usually reveals the underlying abnormality, and MRI frequently also shows evidence of old or recent hemorrhage that may have been asymptomatic. The nature and detailed anatomy of any focal lesion identified by these means are delineated by angiography, especially if operative treatment is under consideration.

C. Laboratory and Other Studies

Electroencephalography is usually indicated in patients presenting with seizures and may show consistently focal or lateralized abnormalities resulting from the underlying cerebral arteriovenous malformation. This should be followed by CT scanning.

▶ Treatment

Surgical treatment to prevent further hemorrhage is justified in patients with arteriovenous malformations that have bled, provided that the lesion is accessible and the patient has a reasonable life expectancy. Surgical treatment is also appropriate if intracranial pressure is increased and to prevent further progression of a focal neurologic deficit. In patients presenting solely with seizures, anticonvulsant drug treatment is usually sufficient, and operative treatment is unnecessary unless there are further developments.

Definitive operative treatment consists of excision of the arteriovenous malformation if it is surgically accessible. Arteriovenous malformations that are inoperable because of their location are sometimes treated solely by embolization; although the risk of hemorrhage is not reduced, neurologic deficits may be stabilized or even reversed by this procedure. Two other techniques for the treatment of intracerebral arteriovenous malformations are injection of a vascular occlusive polymer through a flow-guided microcatheter and permanent occlusion of feeding vessels by positioning detachable balloon catheters in the desired sites and then inflating them with quickly solidifying contrast material. Stereotactic radiosurgery with the gamma knife or related approaches is also useful in the management of inoperable cerebral arteriovenous malformations.

▶ When to Refer

All patients should be referred.

▶ When to Admit

- All patients with a subarachnoid or cerebral hemorrhage.
- All patients for detailed imaging.
- All patients undergoing surgical or endovascular treatment.

Sandalcioglu IE et al. The management of arteriovenous malformations. J Neurosurg Sci. 2011 Mar;55(1):57–69. [PMID: 21464810]

Starke RM et al. A practical grading scale for predicting outcome after radiosurgery for arteriovenous malformations: analysis of 1012 treated patients. J Neurosurg. 2013 Oct;119(4):981–7. [PMID: 23829820]

7. Intracranial Venous Thrombosis

Intracranial venous thrombosis may occur in association with intracranial or maxillofacial infections, hypercoagulable states, polycythemia, sickle cell disease, and cyanotic congenital heart disease and in pregnancy or during the puerperium. Genetic factors are also important. The disorder is characterized by headache, focal or generalized convulsions, drowsiness, confusion, increased intracranial pressure, and focal neurologic deficits—and sometimes by evidence of meningeal irritation. The diagnosis is confirmed by CT scanning, MRI, MR venography, or angiography.

Treatment includes anticonvulsant drugs if seizures have occurred and antiedema agents (eg, dexamethasone, 4 mg four times daily intravenously or intramuscularly and continued as necessary) or other measures to reduce intracranial pressure. Anticoagulation with dose-adjusted intravenous heparin or weight-adjusted subcutaneous low-molecular-weight heparin, followed by oral warfarin anticoagulation for 6 months reduces morbidity and mortality of venous sinus thrombosis. Concomitant intracranial hemorrhage related to the venous thrombosis does not contraindicate heparin therapy. In cases refractory to heparin, endovascular techniques including catheter-directed thrombolytic therapy (urokinase) and thrombectomy, are sometimes helpful but may increase risk for major hemorrhage.

When to Refer

All patients should be referred.

When to Admit

All patients should be hospitalized.

Saposnik G et al. Diagnosis and management of cerebral venous thrombosis: a statement for healthcare professionals from the American Heart Association/American Stroke Association. Stroke. 2011 Apr;42(4):1158–92. [PMID: 21293023]

8. Spinal Cord Vascular Diseases

ESSENTIALS OF DIAGNOSIS

▶ Sudden onset of back or limb pain and neurologic deficit in limbs.

▶ Motor, sensory, or reflex changes in limbs depending on level of lesion.

▶ Imaging studies distinguish between infarct and hematoma.

Infarction of the Spinal Cord

Infarction of the spinal cord is rare. It typically occurs in the territory of the anterior spinal artery because this vessel, which supplies the anterior two-thirds of the cord, is itself supplied by only a limited number of feeders. Infarction usually results from interrupted flow in one or more of these feeders, eg, with aortic dissection, aortography, polyarteritis, or severe hypotension, or after surgical resection of the thoracic aorta. The paired posterior spinal arteries, by contrast, are supplied by numerous arteries at different levels of the cord. Spinal cord hypoperfusion may lead to a central cord syndrome with distal weakness of lower motor neuron type and loss of pain and temperature appreciation, with preserved posterior column function.

Since the anterior spinal artery receives numerous feeders in the cervical region, infarcts almost always occur caudally. Clinical presentation is characterized by acute onset of flaccid, areflexive paraplegia that evolves after a few days or weeks into a spastic paraplegia with extensor plantar responses. There is an accompanying dissociated sensory loss, with impairment of appreciation of pain and temperature but preservation of sensations of vibration and position. Treatment is symptomatic.

Tubbs RS et al. Spinal cord ischemia and atherosclerosis: a review of the literature. Br J Neurosurg. 2011 Dec;25(6): 666–70. [PMID: 21707414]

Epidural or Subdural Hemorrhage

Epidural or subdural hemorrhage may lead to sudden severe back pain followed by an acute compressive myelopathy necessitating urgent spinal MRI or myelography and surgical evacuation. It may occur in patients with bleeding disorders or those who are taking anticoagulant drugs, sometimes following trauma or lumbar puncture. Epidural hemorrhage may also be related to a vascular malformation or tumor deposit.

Hussenbocus SM et al. Spontaneous spinal epidural hematoma: a case report and literature review. J Emerg Med. 2012 Feb;42(2):e31–4. [PMID: 19128914]

Spinal Dural Arteriovenous Fistulae

Spinal dural arteriovenous fistulae are congenital lesions that present with spinal subarachnoid hemorrhage or myeloradiculopathy. Since most of these malformations are located in the thoracolumbar region, they lead to motor and sensory disturbances in the legs and to sphincter disorders. Pain in the legs or back is often severe. Examination reveals an upper, lower, or mixed motor deficit in the legs; sensory deficits are also present and are usually extensive, although occasionally they are confined to radicular distribution. Cervical spinal dural arteriovenous fistulae lead also to symptoms and signs in the arms. Spinal MRI may not detect the spinal dural arteriovenous fistulae, and negative findings do not exclude the diagnosis. Myelography (performed with the patient prone and supine) detects serpiginous filling defects due to enlarged vessels. Selective spinal arteriography confirms the diagnosis. Most lesions are extramedullary, are posterior to the cord (lying either intradurally or extradurally), and can easily be treated by ligation of feeding vessels and excision of the fistulous anomaly or by embolization procedures. Delay in treatment may lead to increased and irreversible disability or to death from recurrent subarachnoid hemorrhage.

When to Refer

All patients should be referred.

When to Admit

All patients should be hospitalized.

Rubin MN et al. Vascular diseases of the spinal cord. Neurol Clin. 2013 Feb;31(1):153–81. [PMID: 23186899]

INTRACRANIAL & SPINAL MASS LESIONS

1. Primary Intracranial Tumors

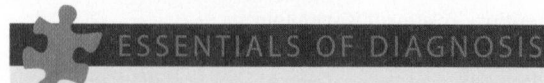
ESSENTIALS OF DIAGNOSIS

► Generalized or focal disturbance of cerebral function, or both.

► Increased intracranial pressure in some patients.

► Neuroradiologic evidence of space-occupying lesion.

General Considerations

Half of all primary intracranial neoplasms (Table 24–5) are gliomas and the remainder are meningiomas, pituitary adenomas (see Chapter 26), neurofibromas, and other tumors. Certain tumors, especially neurofibromas, hemangioblastomas, and retinoblastomas, may have a familial basis, and congenital factors bear on the development of craniopharyngiomas. Tumors may occur at any age, but certain gliomas show particular age predilections.

Clinical Findings

A. Symptoms and Signs

Intracranial tumors may lead to a generalized disturbance of cerebral function and to symptoms and signs of increased intracranial pressure. In consequence, there may be personality changes, intellectual decline, emotional lability, seizures, headaches, nausea, and malaise. If the pressure is increased in a particular cranial compartment, brain tissue may herniate into a compartment with lower pressure. The most familiar syndrome is herniation of the temporal lobe uncus through the tentorial hiatus, which causes compression of the third cranial nerve, midbrain, and posterior cerebral artery. The earliest sign of this is ipsilateral pupillary dilation, followed by stupor, coma, decerebrate posturing, and respiratory arrest. Another important herniation syndrome consists of displacement of the cerebellar tonsils through the foramen magnum, which causes medullary compression leading to apnea, circulatory collapse, and death. Other herniation syndromes are less common and of less clear clinical importance.

Intracranial tumors also lead to focal deficits depending on their location.

1. Frontal lobe lesions—Tumors of the frontal lobe often lead to progressive intellectual decline, slowing of mental activity, personality changes, and contralateral grasp reflexes. They may lead to expressive aphasia if the posterior part of the left inferior frontal gyrus is involved. Anosmia may also occur as a consequence of pressure on the olfactory nerve. Precentral lesions may cause focal motor seizures or contralateral pyramidal deficits.

2. Temporal lobe lesions—Tumors of the uncinate region may be manifested by seizures with olfactory or gustatory hallucinations, motor phenomena such as licking or smacking of the lips, and some impairment of external awareness without actual loss of consciousness. Temporal lobe lesions also lead to depersonalization, emotional changes, behavioral disturbances, sensations of déjà vu or jamais vu, micropsia or macropsia (objects appear smaller or larger than they are), visual field defects (crossed upper quadrantanopia), and auditory illusions or hallucinations. Left-sided lesions may lead to dysnomia and receptive aphasia, while right-sided involvement sometimes disturbs the perception of musical notes and melodies.

3. Parietal lobe lesions—Tumors in this location characteristically cause contralateral disturbances of sensation and may cause sensory seizures, sensory loss or inattention, or some combination of these symptoms. The sensory loss is cortical in type and involves postural sensibility and tactile discrimination, so that the appreciation of shape, size, weight, and texture is impaired. Objects placed in the hand may not be recognized (astereognosis). Extensive parietal lobe lesions may produce contralateral hyperpathia and spontaneous pain (thalamic syndrome). Involvement of the optic radiation leads to a contralateral homonymous field defect that sometimes consists solely of lower quadrantanopia. Lesions of the left angular gyrus cause Gerstmann syndrome (a combination of alexia, agraphia, acalculia, right-left confusion, and finger agnosia), whereas involvement of the left submarginal gyrus causes ideational apraxia. Anosognosia (the denial, neglect, or rejection of a paralyzed limb) is seen in patients with lesions of the nondominant (right) hemisphere. Constructional apraxia and dressing apraxia may also occur with right-sided lesions.

4. Occipital lobe lesions—Tumors of the occipital lobe characteristically produce crossed homonymous hemianopia or a partial field defect. With left-sided or bilateral lesions, there may be visual agnosia both for objects and for colors, while irritative lesions on either side can cause unformed visual hallucinations. Bilateral occipital lobe involvement causes cortical blindness in which there is preservation of pupillary responses to light and lack of awareness of the defect by the patient. There may also be loss of color perception, prosopagnosia (inability to identify a familiar face), simultagnosia (inability to integrate and interpret a composite scene as opposed to its individual elements), and Balint syndrome (failure to turn the eyes to a particular point in space, despite preservation of spontaneous and reflex eye movements). The denial of blindness or a field defect constitutes Anton syndrome.

5. Brainstem and cerebellar lesions—Brainstem lesions lead to cranial nerve palsies, ataxia, incoordination, nystagmus, and pyramidal and sensory deficits in the limbs on one or both sides. Intrinsic brainstem tumors, such as gliomas, tend to produce an increase in intracranial pressure only late in their course. Cerebellar tumors produce marked ataxia of the trunk if the vermis cerebelli is involved and ipsilateral appendicular deficits (ataxia, incoordination and hypotonia of the limbs) if the cerebellar hemispheres are affected.

Table 24–5. Primary intracranial tumors.

Tumor	Clinical Features	Treatment and Prognosis
Glioblastoma multiforme	Presents commonly with nonspecific complaints and increased intracranial pressure. As it grows, focal deficits develop.	Course is rapidly progressive, with poor prognosis. Total surgical removal is usually not possible. Radiation therapy and chemotherapy may prolong survival.
Astrocytoma	Presentation similar to glioblastoma multiforme but course more protracted, often over several years. Cerebellar astrocytoma may have a more benign course.	Prognosis is variable. By the time of diagnosis, total excision is usually impossible; tumor may be radiosensitive and chemotherapy may also be helpful. In cerebellar astrocytoma, total surgical removal is often possible.
Medulloblastoma	Seen most frequently in children. Generally arises from roof of fourth ventricle and leads to increased intracranial pressure accompanied by brainstem and cerebellar signs. May seed subarachnoid space.	Treatment consists of surgery combined with radiation therapy and chemotherapy.
Ependymoma	Glioma arising from the ependyma of a ventricle, especially the fourth ventricle; leads to early signs of increased intracranial pressure. Arises also from central canal of cord.	Tumor is best treated surgically if possible. Radiation therapy may be used for residual tumor.
Oligodendroglioma	Slow-growing. Usually arises in cerebral hemisphere in adults. Calcification may be visible on skull radiograph.	Treatment is surgical and usually successful. Radiation and chemotherapy may be used if tumor has malignant features.
Brainstem glioma	Presents during childhood with cranial nerve palsies and then with long tract signs in the limbs. Signs of increased intracranial pressure occur late.	Tumor is inoperable; treatment is by irradiation and shunt for increased intracranial pressure.
Cerebellar hemangioblastoma	Presents with dysequilibrium, ataxia of trunk or limbs, and signs of increased intracranial pressure. Sometimes familial. May be associated with retinal and spinal vascular lesions, polycythemia, and renal cell carcinoma.	Treatment is surgical. Radiation is used for residual tumor.
Pineal tumor	Presents with increased intracranial pressure, sometimes associated with impaired upward gaze (Parinaud syndrome) and other deficits indicative of midbrain lesion.	Ventricular decompression by shunting is followed by surgical approach to tumor; irradiation is indicated if tumor is malignant. Prognosis depends on histopathologic findings and extent of tumor.
Craniopharyngioma	Originates from remnants of Rathke pouch above the sella, depressing the optic chiasm. May present at any age but usually in childhood, with endocrine dysfunction and bitemporal field defects.	Treatment is surgical, but total removal may not be possible. Radiation may be used for residual tumor.
Acoustic neurinoma	Ipsilateral hearing loss is most common initial symptom. Subsequent symptoms may include tinnitus, headache, vertigo, facial weakness or numbness, and long tract signs. (May be familial and bilateral when related to neurofibromatosis.) Most sensitive screening tests are MRI and brainstem auditory evoked potential.	Treatment is excision by translabyrinthine surgery, craniectomy, or a combined approach. Outcome is usually good.
Meningioma	Originates from the dura mater or arachnoid; compresses rather than invades adjacent neural structures. Increasingly common with advancing age. Tumor size varies greatly. Symptoms vary with tumor site—eg, unilateral proptosis (sphenoidal ridge); anosmia and optic nerve compression (olfactory groove). Tumor is usually benign and readily detected by CT scanning; may lead to calcification and bone erosion visible on plain radiographs of skull.	Treatment is surgical. Tumor may recur if removal is incomplete.
Primary cerebral lymphoma	Associated with AIDS and other immunodeficient states. Presentation may be with focal deficits or with disturbances of cognition and consciousness. May be indistinguishable from cerebral toxoplasmosis.	Treatment is high-dose methotrexate followed by radiation therapy. Prognosis depends on CD4 count at diagnosis.

6. False localizing signs—Tumors may lead to neurologic signs other than by direct compression or infiltration, thereby leading to errors of clinical localization. These false localizing signs include third or sixth nerve palsy and bilateral extensor plantar responses produced by herniation syndromes, and an extensor plantar response occurring ipsilateral to a hemispheric tumor as a result of compression of the opposite cerebral peduncle against the tentorium.

B. Imaging

MRI with gadolinium enhancement is the preferred method to detect the lesion and to define its location, shape, and size; the extent to which normal anatomy is distorted; and the degree of any associated cerebral edema or mass effect. CT scanning with radiocontrast enhancement could be performed; however, it is less helpful than MRI for small lesions or tumors in the posterior fossa. Newer neuroimaging techniques may help identify brain tumors by increased blood perfusion (perfusion-weighted MRI, single photon-emission computed tomography, positron-emission tomography) and high metabolism or cell turnover (magnetic resonance spectroscopy, positron-emission tomography), but non-neoplastic diseases, such as stroke and inflammatory or infectious diseases, are sometimes associated with hyperperfusion and hypermetabolism. Diffusion-weighted MRI may also be helpful. Arteriography may show stretching or displacement of normal cerebral vessels by the tumor and the presence of tumor vascularity. The presence of an avascular mass is a nonspecific finding that could be due to tumor, hematoma, abscess, or any space-occupying lesion. In patients with normal hormone levels and an intrasellar mass, angiography is necessary to distinguish with confidence between a pituitary adenoma and an arterial aneurysm.

C. Laboratory and Other Studies

The electroencephalogram provides supporting information concerning cerebral function and may show either a focal disturbance due to the neoplasm or a more diffuse change reflecting altered mental status. Lumbar puncture is rarely necessary; the findings are seldom diagnostic, and the procedure carries the risk of causing a herniation syndrome.

▶ Treatment

Treatment depends on the type and site of the tumor (Table 24–5) and the condition of the patient. Some benign tumors, especially meningiomas discovered incidentally during brain imaging for another purpose, may be monitored with serial annual imaging. For symptomatic tumors, complete surgical removal may be possible if the tumor is extra-axial (eg, meningioma, acoustic neuroma) or is not in a critical or inaccessible region of the brain (eg, cerebellar hemangioblastoma). Surgery also permits the diagnosis to be verified and may be beneficial in reducing intracranial pressure and relieving symptoms even if the neoplasm cannot be completely removed. Clinical deficits are sometimes due in part to obstructive hydrocephalus, in which case simple surgical shunting procedures often produce dramatic benefit. In patients with malignant gliomas, radiation therapy increases median survival rates regardless of any preceding surgery, and its combination with chemotherapy provides additional benefit. Indications for irradiation in the treatment of patients with other primary intracranial neoplasms depend on tumor type and accessibility and the feasibility of complete surgical removal. Temozolomide is a commonly used oral and intravenous chemotherapeutic for gliomas, and there is an increasing trend to use monoclonal antibodies as a component of therapy. Corticosteroids help reduce cerebral edema and are usually started before surgery. Herniation is treated with intravenous dexamethasone (10–20 mg as a bolus, followed by 4 mg every 6 hours) and intravenous mannitol (20% solution given in a dose of 1.5 g/kg over about 30 minutes). Anticonvulsants are also commonly administered in standard doses (see Table 24–3) but are not indicated for prophylaxis in patients who have no history of seizures. Long-term neurocognitive deficits may complicate radiation therapy. For those patients whose disease deteriorates despite treatment, palliative care is important (see Chapter 5).

▶ When to Refer

All patients should be referred.

▶ When to Admit

- All patients with increased intracranial pressure.
- All patients requiring biopsy, surgical treatment, or shunting procedures.

Ricard D et al. Primary brain tumours in adults. Lancet. 2012 May 26;379(9830):1984–96. [PMID: 22510398]

2. Metastatic Intracranial Tumors

Cerebral Metastases

Metastatic brain tumors present in the same way as other cerebral neoplasms, ie, with increased intracranial pressure, with focal or diffuse disturbance of cerebral function, or with both of these manifestations. Indeed, in patients with a single cerebral lesion, the metastatic nature of the lesion may only become evident on histopathologic examination. In other patients, there is evidence of widespread metastatic disease, or an isolated cerebral metastasis develops during treatment of the primary neoplasm.

The most common source of intracranial metastasis is carcinoma of the lung; other primary sites are the breast, kidney, skin (melanoma), and gastrointestinal tract. Most cerebral metastases are located supratentorially. Laboratory and radiologic studies used to evaluate patients with metastases are those described for primary neoplasms. They include MRI and CT scanning performed both with and without contrast material. Lumbar puncture is necessary only in patients with suspected carcinomatous meningitis (see later). In patients with verified cerebral metastasis from an unknown primary, investigation is guided by symptoms and signs. In women, mammography is indicated; in men under 50, germ cell origin is sought since both have therapeutic implications.

In patients with only a single, surgically accessible cerebral metastasis who are otherwise well (ie, a high level of functioning and little or no evidence of extracranial disease), it may be possible to remove the lesion and then treat with irradiation; the latter may also be selected as the sole treatment. In patients with multiple metastases or widespread systemic disease, the prognosis is poor; stereotactic radiosurgery, whole-brain radiotherapy, or both, may help in some instances, but in others treatment is palliative only.

Tsao MN et al. Whole brain radiotherapy for the treatment of newly diagnosed multiple brain metastases. Cochrane Database Syst Rev. 2012 Apr 18;4:CD003869. [PMID: 22513917]

Leptomeningeal Metastases (Carcinomatous Meningitis)

The neoplasms metastasizing most commonly to the leptomeninges are carcinoma of the breast, lymphomas, and leukemia. Leptomeningeal metastases lead to multifocal neurologic deficits, which may be associated with infiltration of cranial and spinal nerve roots, direct invasion of the brain or spinal cord, obstructive hydrocephalus, or some combination of these factors.

The diagnosis is confirmed by examination of the cerebrospinal fluid. Findings may include elevated cerebrospinal fluid pressure, pleocytosis, increased protein concentration, and decreased glucose concentration. Cytologic studies may indicate that malignant cells are present; if not, lumbar puncture should be repeated at least twice to obtain further samples for analysis.

CT scans showing contrast enhancement in the basal cisterns or showing hydrocephalus without any evidence of a mass lesion support the diagnosis. Gadolinium-enhanced MRI frequently shows enhancing foci in the leptomeninges. Myelography may show deposits on multiple nerve roots.

Treatment is by irradiation to symptomatic areas, combined with intrathecal methotrexate. The long-term prognosis is poor—only about 10% of patients survive for 1 year—and palliative care is therefore important (see Chapter 5).

Clarke JL. Leptomeningeal metastasis from systemic cancer. Continuum (Minneap Minn). 2012 Apr;18(2):328–42. [PMID: 22810130]
Grewal J et al. Novel approaches to treating leptomeningeal metastases. J Neurooncol. 2012 Jan;106(2):225–34. [PMID: 21874597]

3. Intracranial Mass Lesions in AIDS Patients

Primary cerebral lymphoma is a common complication in patients with AIDS. This leads to disturbances in cognition or consciousness, focal motor or sensory deficits, aphasia, seizures, and cranial neuropathies. Similar clinical disturbances may result from **cerebral toxoplasmosis**, which is also a common complication in patients with AIDS (see Chapters 31 and 35).

Cryptococcal meningitis is a common opportunistic infection in AIDS patients. Clinically, it may resemble cerebral toxoplasmosis or lymphoma, but cranial CT scans are usually normal (see Chapter 36).

4. Primary & Metastatic Spinal Tumors

Approximately 10% of spinal tumors are intramedullary. Ependymoma is the most common type of intramedullary tumor; the remainder are other types of glioma. Extramedullary tumors may be extradural or intradural in location. Among the primary extramedullary tumors, neurofibromas and meningiomas are relatively common, are benign, and may be intradural or extradural. Carcinomatous metastases, lymphomatous or leukemic deposits, and myeloma are usually extradural; in the case of metastases, the prostate, breast, lung, and kidney are common primary sites.

Tumors may lead to spinal cord dysfunction by direct compression, by ischemia secondary to arterial or venous obstruction and, in the case of intramedullary lesions, by invasive infiltration.

▶ Clinical Findings

A. Symptoms and Signs

Symptoms usually develop insidiously. Pain is often conspicuous with extradural lesions; is characteristically aggravated by coughing or straining; may be radicular, localized to the back, or felt diffusely in an extremity; and may be accompanied by motor deficits, paresthesias, or numbness, especially in the legs. Bladder, bowel, and sexual dysfunction may occur. When sphincter disturbances occur, they are usually particularly disabling. Pain, however, often precedes specific neurologic symptoms from epidural metastases.

Examination may reveal localized spinal tenderness. A segmental lower motor neuron deficit or dermatomal sensory changes (or both) are sometimes found at the level of the lesion, while an upper motor neuron deficit and sensory disturbance are found below it.

B. Imaging

CT myelography or, preferably, MRI with contrast is used to identify and localize the lesion. The combination of known tumor elsewhere in the body, back pain, and either abnormal plain films of the spine or neurologic signs of cord compression is an indication to perform these studies on an urgent basis.

C. Laboratory Findings

The cerebrospinal fluid is often xanthochromic and contains a greatly increased protein concentration with normal cell content and glucose concentration.

▶ Treatment

Intramedullary tumors are treated by decompression and surgical excision (when feasible) and by irradiation. The prognosis depends on the cause and severity of cord compression before it is relieved.

Treatment of epidural spinal metastases consists of irradiation, irrespective of cell type. Dexamethasone is also given in a high dosage (eg, 25 mg four times daily for 3 days orally or intravenously, followed by rapid tapering of the dosage, depending on response) to reduce cord swelling and relieve pain. Surgical decompression is reserved for patients with tumors that are unresponsive to irradiation or have previously been irradiated and for cases in which there is some uncertainty about the diagnosis. The long-term outlook is poor, but radiation treatment may at least delay the onset of major disability.

Mechtler LL et al. Spinal cord tumors: new views and future directions. Neurol Clin. 2013 Feb;31(1):241–68. [PMID: 23186903]

5. Brain Abscess

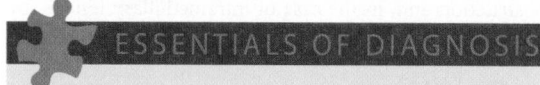

ESSENTIALS OF DIAGNOSIS

▶ Symptoms and signs of expanding intracranial mass.

▶ Signs of primary infection or congenital heart disease are sometimes present.

▶ Fever may be absent.

▶ General Considerations

Brain abscess presents as an intracranial space-occupying lesion and arises as a sequela of disease of the ear or nose, may be a complication of infection elsewhere in the body, or may result from infection introduced intracranially by trauma or surgical procedures. The most common infective organisms are streptococci, staphylococci, and anaerobes; mixed infections are not uncommon.

▶ Clinical Findings

A. Symptoms and Signs

Headache, drowsiness, inattention, confusion, and seizures are early symptoms, followed by signs of increasing intracranial pressure and then a focal neurologic deficit. There may be little or no systemic evidence of infection.

B. Imaging and Other Investigations

A CT scan of the head characteristically shows an area of contrast enhancement surrounding a low-density core. Similar abnormalities may be found in patients with metastatic neoplasms. MRI findings often permit earlier recognition of focal cerebritis or an abscess. Arteriography indicates the presence of a space-occupying lesion, which appears as an avascular mass with displacement of normal cerebral vessels. Stereotactic needle aspiration may enable a specific etiologic organism to be identified. Examination of the cerebrospinal fluid does not help in diagnosis and may precipitate a herniation syndrome. Peripheral leukocytosis is sometimes present.

▶ Treatment

Treatment consists of intravenous antibiotics, combined with surgical drainage (aspiration or excision) if necessary to reduce the mass effect, or sometimes to establish the diagnosis. Abscesses smaller than 2 cm can often be cured medically. Broad-spectrum antibiotics, selected based on risk factors and likely organisms, are used if the infecting organism is unknown (see Chapter 33). Initial empiric antibiotic regimens typically include ceftriaxone (2 g intravenously every 12 hours), metronidazole (15 mg/kg intravenous loading dose, followed by 7.5 mg/kg intravenously every 6 hours), and vancomycin (1 g intravenously every 12 hours). The regimen is altered once culture and sensitivity data are available. Antimicrobial treatment is usually continued parenterally for 6–8 weeks, followed by orally for 2–3 months. The patient should be monitored by serial CT scans or MRI every 2 weeks and at deterioration. Dexamethasone (4–25 mg four times daily intravenously or orally, depending on severity, followed by tapering of dose, depending on response) may reduce any associated edema, but intravenous mannitol is sometimes required.

Helweg-Larsen J et al. Pyogenic brain abscess, a 15 year survey. BMC Infect Dis. 2012 Nov 30;12:332. [PMID: 23193986]

NONMETASTATIC NEUROLOGIC COMPLICATIONS OF MALIGNANT DISEASE

A variety of nonmetastatic neurologic complications of malignant disease (see Table 39–2) can be recognized. Metabolic encephalopathy due to electrolyte abnormalities, infections, drug overdose, or the failure of some vital organ may be reflected by drowsiness, lethargy, restlessness, insomnia, agitation, confusion, stupor, or coma. The mental changes are usually associated with tremor, asterixis, and multifocal myoclonus. The electroencephalogram is generally diffusely slowed. Laboratory studies are necessary to detect the cause of the encephalopathy, which must then be treated appropriately.

Immune suppression resulting from either the malignant disease or its treatment (eg, by chemotherapy) predisposes patients to brain abscess, progressive multifocal leukoencephalopathy, meningitis, herpes zoster infection, and other opportunistic infectious diseases. Moreover, an overt or occult cerebrospinal fluid fistula, as occurs with some tumors, may also increase the risk of infection. MRI or CT scanning aids in the early recognition of a brain abscess, but metastatic brain tumors may have a similar appearance. Examination of the cerebrospinal fluid is essential in the evaluation of patients with meningitis but is of no help in the diagnosis of brain abscess.

Cerebrovascular disorders that cause neurologic complications in patients with systemic cancer include nonbacterial thrombotic endocarditis and septic embolization. Cerebral, subarachnoid, or subdural hemorrhages may occur in patients with myelogenous leukemia and may be found in association with metastatic tumors, especially malignant melanoma. Spinal subdural hemorrhage sometimes occurs after lumbar puncture in patients with marked thrombocytopenia.

Disseminated intravascular coagulation occurs most commonly in patients with acute promyelocytic leukemia or with some adenocarcinomas and is characterized by a fluctuating encephalopathy, often with associated seizures, that frequently progresses to coma or death. There may be few accompanying neurologic signs. Venous sinus thrombosis, which usually presents with convulsions and headaches, may also occur in patients with leukemia or lymphoma. Examination commonly reveals papilledema and focal or diffuse neurologic signs. Anticonvulsants, anticoagulants, and drugs to lower the intracranial pressure may be of value.

Autoimmune paraneoplastic disorders occur when the immune system reacts against neuronal antigens expressed by tumor cells. The clinical manifestations depend on the autoantibody. Symptoms may precede those due to the neoplasm itself. Several distinct syndromes are common, including paraneoplastic cerebellar degeneration, limbic encephalitis, encephalomyelitis, anti-NMDA receptor-associated encephalitis, opsoclonus/myoclonus, sensory neuronopathy, and dermatomyositis.

Paraneoplastic cerebellar degeneration occurs most commonly in association with carcinoma of the lung, but also in breast and gynecologic cancers and Hodgkin lymphoma. Typically, there is a pancerebellar syndrome causing dysarthria, nystagmus, and ataxia of the trunk and limbs. The disorder is associated with anti-Yo, -Tr, -voltage-gated calcium channel (VGCC), and -Zic antibodies. Treatment is of the underlying malignant disease. **Limbic encephalitis**, characterized by impaired recent memory, disturbed affect, hallucinations, and seizures, occurs in some patients with tumors of the lungs, breast, thymus, and germ cells. Associated antibodies include anti-Hu, -Ma2, -CV2/CRMP5, voltage-gated potassium channel (VGKC), -AMPA receptor, and -GABA_B receptor. A more generalized **encephalomyelitis** occurs with anti-Hu, -CV2/CRMP5, -Ma2, and -amphiphysin antibodies in the context of a similar spectrum of tumors. **Anti-NMDA receptor-associated encephalitis** causes a characteristic syndrome of severe psychiatric symptoms, dyskinesias, dysautonomia, and hypoventilation, and is frequently associated with ovarian teratoma. **Opsoclonus/myoclonus**, a syndrome of involuntary, erratic, and conjugate saccadic eye movements and myoclonic movements of the limbs, occurs in patients with lung, breast, and gynecologic tumors, often without an identifiable antibody. **Sensory neuronopathy**, typically caused by anti-Hu antibodies in small cell lung cancer or other carcinomas, manifests itself with asymmetric, multifocal sensory nerve root deficits leading to pain, numbness, sensory ataxia, and sometimes hearing loss. **Dermatomyositis** (see Chapter 20) or the **Lambert-Eaton myasthenic syndrome** (discussed below) may be seen in patients with underlying carcinoma. Identification of an antibody is not always possible in a suspected autoimmune paraneoplastic condition, and a search for an underlying neoplasm should not be deterred. Treatment of the neoplasm takes priority and offers the best hope for stabilization or improvement of the neurologic symptoms, which often are not completely reversible. Specific treatment of the antibody-mediated symptoms by intravenous immunoglobulin (IVIG) administration, plasmapheresis, corticosteroids, or other immunosuppressive regimens, is frequently attempted despite limited efficacy. Encephalitides involving antibodies directed against neuronal cell surface antigens, such as VGKC or AMPA, NMDA, or GABA_B receptors, can occur either as paraneoplastic phenomena or in isolation, and typically respond well to immunotherapy.

Graus F et al. Paraneoplastic neurological syndromes. Curr Opin Neurol. 2012 Dec;25(6):795–801. [PMID: 23041955]
McKeon A. Paraneoplastic and other autoimmune disorders of the central nervous system. Neurohospitalist. 2013 Apr;3(2): 53–64. [PMID: 23983888]

PSEUDOTUMOR CEREBRI (Benign Intracranial Hypertension)

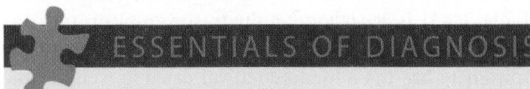

ESSENTIALS OF DIAGNOSIS

▶ Headache, worse on straining.
▶ Visual obscurations or diplopia may occur.
▶ Examination reveals papilledema.
▶ Abducens palsy is commonly present.

▶ General Considerations

There are many causes of pseudotumor cerebri. Thrombosis of the transverse venous sinus as a noninfectious complication of otitis media or chronic mastoiditis is one cause, and sagittal sinus thrombosis may lead to a clinically similar picture. Other causes include chronic pulmonary disease, systemic lupus erythematosus, uremia, endocrine disturbances such as hypoparathyroidism, hypothyroidism, or Addison disease, vitamin A toxicity, and the use of tetracycline or oral contraceptives. Cases have also followed withdrawal of corticosteroids after long-term use. In most instances, however, no specific cause can be found, and the disorder remits spontaneously after several months. This idiopathic variety—known as idiopathic intracranial hypertension—occurs most commonly among overweight women aged 20–44. In all cases, screening for a space-occupying lesion of the brain is important.

▶ Clinical Findings

A. Symptoms and Signs

Symptoms consist of headache, diplopia, and other visual disturbances due to papilledema and abducens nerve dysfunction. Pulse-synchronous tinnitus may also occur. Examination reveals the papilledema and some enlargement of the blind spots, but patients otherwise look well.

B. Imaging

Investigations reveal no evidence of a space-occupying lesion. CT scan shows small or normal ventricles. MR venography is helpful in screening for thrombosis of the intracranial venous sinuses.

C. Laboratory Findings

Lumbar puncture confirms the presence of intracranial hypertension, but the cerebrospinal fluid is normal. Laboratory studies help exclude some of the other causes mentioned earlier.

▶ Treatment

Untreated intracranial hypertension sometimes leads to secondary optic atrophy and permanent visual loss. Acetazolamide (250–500 mg orally three times daily, increasing slowly to a maintenance dose of 1000–2000 mg daily, divided two to four times daily) reduces formation of cerebrospinal fluid and can be used to start treatment. Like acetazolamide, the antiepileptic drug topiramate (Table 24–3) is a carbonic anhydrase inhibitor and was shown to be similarly effective in an open label study; topiramate has the added benefit of causing weight loss. Corticosteroids (eg, prednisone, 60–80 mg daily) may also be necessary. Obese patients should be advised to lose weight. Repeated lumbar puncture to lower the intracranial pressure by removal of cerebrospinal fluid is effective as a temporizing measure, but pharmacologic approaches to treatment provide better long-term relief. Treatment is monitored by checking visual acuity and visual fields, funduscopic appearance, and pressure of the cerebrospinal fluid. The disorder may worsen after a period of stability, indicating the need for long-term follow-up.

If medical treatment fails to control the intracranial pressure, surgical placement of a lumboperitoneal or ventriculoperitoneal shunt or optic nerve sheath fenestration should be undertaken to preserve vision.

In addition to the above measures, any specific cause of intracranial hypertension requires appropriate treatment. Thus, hormone therapy should be initiated if there is an underlying endocrine disturbance. Discontinuing the use of tetracycline, oral contraceptives, or vitamin A will allow for resolution of intracranial hypertension due to these agents. If corticosteroid withdrawal is responsible, the medication should be reintroduced and then tapered more gradually.

▶ When to Refer

All patients should be referred.

▶ When to Admit

All patients requiring shunt placement or optic nerve sheath fenestration should be hospitalized.

Peng KP et al. High-pressure headaches: idiopathic intracranial hypertension and its mimics. Nat Rev Neurol. 2012 Dec;8 (12):700–10. [PMID: 23165338]

SELECTED NEUROCUTANEOUS DISEASES

Because the nervous system develops from the epithelial layer of the embryo, a number of congenital diseases include both neurologic and cutaneous manifestations. Among these disorders, three are discussed below, and von Hippel-Lindau disease is discussed in Chapter 26.

1. Tuberous Sclerosis

Tuberous sclerosis may occur sporadically or on a familial basis with autosomal dominant inheritance. Neurologic presentation is with seizures and progressive psychomotor retardation beginning in early childhood. The cutaneous abnormality, adenoma sebaceum, becomes manifest usually between 5 and 10 years of age and typically consists of reddened nodules on the face (cheeks, nasolabial folds, sides of the nose, and chin) and sometimes on the forehead and neck. Other typical cutaneous lesions include subungual fibromas, shagreen patches (leathery plaques of subepidermal fibrosis, situated usually on the trunk), and leaf-shaped hypopigmented spots. Associated abnormalities include retinal lesions and tumors, benign rhabdomyomas of the heart, lung cysts, benign tumors in the viscera, and bone cysts.

The disease is slowly progressive and leads to increasing mental deterioration. There is no specific treatment, but anticonvulsant drugs may help in controlling seizures.

Kohrman MH. Emerging treatments in the management of tuberous sclerosis complex. Pediatr Neurol. 2012 May;46(5): 267–75. [PMID: 22520346]

2. Neurofibromatosis

Neurofibromatosis may occur either sporadically or on a familial basis with autosomal dominant inheritance. Two distinct forms are recognized: **Type 1 (Recklinghausen disease)** is characterized by multiple hyperpigmented macules and neurofibromas, and results from mutations in the NF1 gene on chromosome 17. **Type 2** is characterized by eighth nerve tumors, often accompanied by other intracranial or intraspinal tumors, and is associated with mutations in the NF2 (merlin) gene on chromosome 22.

Neurologic presentation is usually with symptoms and signs of tumor. Multiple neurofibromas characteristically are present and may involve spinal or cranial nerves, especially the eighth nerve (Figure 24–1). Examination of the superficial cutaneous nerves usually reveals palpable mobile nodules. In some cases, there is an associated marked overgrowth of subcutaneous tissues (plexiform neuromas), sometimes with an underlying bony abnormality. Associated cutaneous lesions include axillary freckling and patches of cutaneous pigmentation (café au lait spots). Malignant degeneration of neurofibromas occasionally

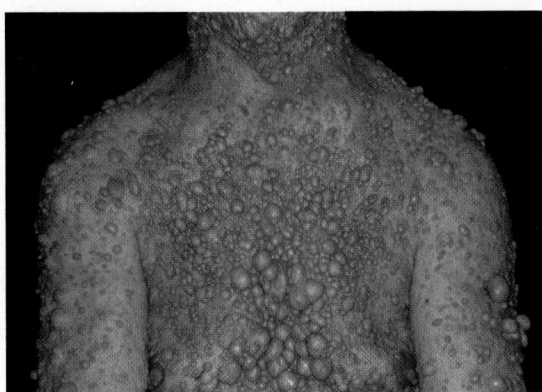

▲ **Figure 24–1.** Neurofibromatosis. (From Jack Resnick, Sr, MD; reproduced with permission from Usatine RP, Smith MA, Mayeaux EJ, Jr, Chumley H, Tysinger J. *The Color Atlas of Family Medicine.* McGraw-Hill, 2009.)

occurs and may lead to peripheral sarcomas. Meningiomas, gliomas (especially optic nerve gliomas), bone cysts, pheochromocytomas, scoliosis, and obstructive hydrocephalus may also occur.

Lin AL et al. Advances in the treatment of neurofibromatosis-associated tumours. Nat Rev Clin Oncol. 2013 Nov;10(11): 616–24. [PMID: 23939548]
Uhlmann EJ et al. Neurofibromatoses. Adv Exp Med Biol. 2012;724:266–77. [PMID: 22411249]

3. Sturge-Weber Syndrome

Sturge-Weber syndrome consists of a congenital, usually unilateral, cutaneous capillary angioma involving the upper face, leptomeningeal angiomatosis and, in many patients, choroidal angioma. It has no sex predilection and usually occurs sporadically. The cutaneous angioma sometimes has a more extensive distribution over the head and neck and is often quite disfiguring, especially if there is associated overgrowth of connective tissue. Focal or generalized seizures are the usual neurologic presentation and may commence at any age. There may be contralateral homonymous hemianopia, hemiparesis and hemisensory disturbance, ipsilateral glaucoma, and mental subnormality. Skull radiographs taken after the first 2 years of life usually reveal gyriform ("tramline") intracranial calcification, especially in the parieto-occipital region, due to mineral deposition in the cortex beneath the intracranial angioma.

Treatment is aimed at controlling seizures pharmacologically, but surgical treatment may be necessary. Ophthalmologic advice should be sought concerning the management of choroidal angioma and of increased intraocular pressure.

Lo W et al; Brain Vascular Malformation Consortium National Sturge-Weber Syndrome Workgroup. Updates and future horizons on the understanding, diagnosis, and treatment of Sturge-Weber syndrome brain involvement. Dev Med Child Neurol. 2012 Mar;54(3):214–23. [PMID: 22191476]

MOVEMENT DISORDERS

1. Benign Essential (Familial) Tremor

 ESSENTIALS OF DIAGNOSIS

▸ Postural tremor of hands, head, or voice.
▸ Family history common.
▸ May improve temporarily with alcohol.
▸ No abnormal findings other than tremor.

▸ General Considerations

The cause of benign essential tremor is uncertain, but it is sometimes inherited in an autosomal dominant manner. Responsible genes have been identified at 3q13, 2p22-p25, and 6p23.

▸ Clinical Findings

Tremor may begin at any age and is enhanced by emotional stress. The tremor usually involves one or both hands, the head, or the hands and head, while the legs tend to be spared. Examination reveals no other abnormalities. Ingestion of a small quantity of alcohol commonly provides remarkable but short-lived relief by an unknown mechanism.

Although the tremor may become more conspicuous with time, it generally leads to little disability. Occasionally, it interferes with manual skills and leads to impairment of handwriting. Speech may also be affected if the laryngeal muscles are involved.

▸ Treatment

Treatment is often unnecessary. When it is required because of disability, propranolol (60–240 mg daily orally) may be helpful. Long-term therapy is typical; however, intermittent therapy is sometimes useful in patients whose tremor becomes exacerbated in specific predictable situations. Primidone may be helpful when propranolol is ineffective, but patients with essential tremor are often very sensitive to it. Therefore, the starting dose is 50 mg daily orally, and the daily dose is increased by 50 mg every 2 weeks depending on the patient's response; a maintenance dose of 125 mg three times daily orally is commonly effective. Occasional patients do not respond to these measures but are helped by alprazolam (up to 3 mg daily orally in divided doses), topiramate (titrated up to a dose of 400 mg daily orally in divided doses over about 8 weeks), or gabapentin (1800 mg daily orally in divided doses). Botulinum toxin A may reduce tremor, but adverse effects include dose-dependent weakness of the injected muscles. Levetiracetam, flunarizine, and 3,4-diaminopyridine are probably ineffective, and there is insufficient evidence to support the use of pregabalin, zonisamide, and clozapine.

Disabling tremor unresponsive to medical treatment may be helped by high-frequency thalamic stimulation on one or both sides, according to the laterality of symptoms. Subdural motor cortex stimulation has also been effective in a small trial.

When to Refer

All patients should be referred.

When to Admit

Patients requiring surgical treatment (deep brain stimulator placement) should be hospitalized.

Moro E et al. Unilateral subdural motor cortex stimulation improves essential tremor but not Parkinson's disease. Brain. 2011 Jul;134(Pt 7):2096–105. [PMID: 21646329]

Zesiewicz TA et al. Evidence-based guideline update: treatment of essential tremor: report of the Quality Standards subcommittee of the American Academy of Neurology. Neurology. 2011 Nov 8;77(19):1752–5. [PMID: 22013182]

2. Parkinsonism

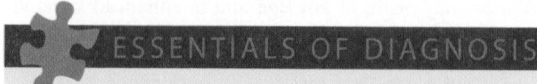

ESSENTIALS OF DIAGNOSIS

- ▶ Any combination of tremor, rigidity, bradykinesia, and progressive postural instability.
- ▶ Cognitive impairment is sometimes prominent.

General Considerations

Parkinsonism is a relatively common disorder that occurs in all ethnic groups, with an approximately equal sex distribution. The most common variety, idiopathic Parkinson disease, begins most often between 45 and 65 years of age and is a progressive disease.

Etiology

Parkinsonism may rarely occur on a familial basis, and the parkinsonian phenotype may result from mutations of several different genes (alpha-synuclein, parkin, *LRRK2*, *DJ1*, and *PINK1*). Mutations in *LRRK2* also account for some cases of apparently sporadic Parkinson disease. Postencephalitic parkinsonism is becoming increasingly rare. Exposure to certain toxins (eg, manganese dust, carbon disulfide) and severe carbon monoxide poisoning may lead to parkinsonism. Reversible parkinsonism may develop in patients receiving neuroleptic drugs (see Chapter 25), reserpine, or metoclopramide. Only rarely is hemiparkinsonism the presenting feature of a progressive space-occupying lesion.

In idiopathic Parkinson disease, dopamine depletion due to degeneration of the dopaminergic nigrostriatal system leads to an imbalance of dopamine and acetylcholine, which are neurotransmitters normally present in the corpus striatum. Treatment is directed at redressing this imbalance by blocking the effect of acetylcholine with anticholinergic drugs or by the administration of levodopa, the precursor of dopamine. Prior use of ibuprofen is associated with a decreased risk of developing Parkinson disease; age, family history, male sex, ongoing herbicide/pesticide exposure, and significant prior head trauma are risk factors.

Clinical Findings

Tremor, rigidity, bradykinesia, and postural instability are the cardinal features of parkinsonism and may be present in any combination. There may also be a mild decline in intellectual function. The tremor of about four to six cycles per second is most conspicuous at rest, is enhanced by emotional stress, and is often less severe during voluntary activity. Although it may ultimately be present in all limbs, the tremor is commonly confined to one limb or to the limbs on one side for months or years before it becomes more generalized. In some patients, tremor is absent.

Rigidity (an increase in resistance to passive movement) is responsible for the characteristically flexed posture seen in many patients, but the most disabling symptoms of parkinsonism are due to bradykinesia, manifested as a slowness of voluntary movement and a reduction in automatic movements such as swinging of the arms while walking. Curiously, however, effective voluntary activity may briefly be regained during an emergency (eg, the patient is able to leap aside to avoid an oncoming motor vehicle).

Clinical diagnosis of the well-developed syndrome is usually simple. The patient has a relatively immobile face with widened palpebral fissures, infrequent blinking, and a fixity of facial expression. Seborrhea of the scalp and face is common. There is often mild blepharoclonus, and a tremor may be present about the mouth and lips. Repetitive tapping (about twice per second) over the bridge of the nose produces a sustained blink response (Myerson sign). Other findings may include saliva drooling from the mouth, perhaps due to impairment of swallowing; soft and poorly modulated voice; a variable rest tremor and rigidity in some or all of the limbs; slowness of voluntary movements; impairment of fine or rapidly alternating movements; and micrographia. There is typically no muscle weakness (provided that sufficient time is allowed for power to be developed) and no alteration in the tendon reflexes or plantar responses. It is difficult for the patient to arise from a sitting position and begin walking. The gait itself is characterized by small shuffling steps and a loss of the normal automatic arm swing; there may be unsteadiness on turning, difficulty in stopping, and a tendency to fall.

Differential Diagnosis

Diagnostic problems may occur in mild cases, especially if tremor is minimal or absent. For example, mild hypokinesia or slight tremor is commonly attributed to old age. Depression, with its associated expressionless face, poorly modulated voice, and reduction in voluntary activity, can be difficult to distinguish from mild parkinsonism, especially since the two disorders may coexist; in some cases, a trial of antidepressant drug therapy is necessary. The family history, the character of the tremor, and lack of other neurologic signs should distinguish essential tremor from parkinsonism. **Wilson disease** can be distinguished by its early age at onset, the presence of other abnormal movements, Kayser-Fleischer rings, and chronic hepatitis, and by increased concentrations of copper in the tissues. **Huntington disease** presenting with rigidity and bradykinesia may be mistaken for parkinsonism unless the family history and accompanying dementia are recognized. In **multisystem atrophy** (previously called the **Shy-Drager syndrome**), autonomic insufficiency (leading to postural hypotension, anhidrosis, disturbances of sphincter control, erectile dysfunction, etc) may be accompanied by parkinsonism, pyramidal deficits, lower motor neuron signs, or cerebellar dysfunction. In **progressive supranuclear palsy**, bradykinesia and rigidity are accompanied by a supranuclear disorder of eye movements, pseudobulbar palsy, pseudo-emotional lability (pseudobulbar affect), and axial dystonia. **Jakob-Creutzfeldt disease** may be accompanied by features of parkinsonism, but dementia is usual, myoclonic jerking is common, ataxia and pyramidal signs may be conspicuous, and the MRI and electroencephalographic findings are usually characteristic. In **corticobasal degeneration**, asymmetric parkinsonism is accompanied by conspicuous signs of cortical dysfunction (eg, apraxia, sensory inattention, dementia, aphasia).

▶ **Treatment**

Treatment is symptomatic. There is great interest in developing disease-modifying therapies, and trials of several putative neuroprotective agents are in progress. Trials of various gene therapies have shown limited or no benefit.

A. Medical Measures

Drug treatment is not required early in the course of Parkinson disease, but the nature of the disorder and the availability of medical treatment for use when necessary should be discussed with the patient.

1. Amantadine—Patients with mild symptoms but no disability may be helped by amantadine. This drug improves all of the clinical features of parkinsonism, but its mode of action is unclear. Side effects include restlessness, confusion, depression, skin rashes, edema, nausea, constipation, anorexia, postural hypotension, and disturbances of cardiac rhythm. However, these are relatively uncommon with the usual dose (100 mg twice daily orally). It also ameliorates dyskinesias resulting from chronic levodopa therapy.

2. Levodopa—Levodopa, which is converted in the body to dopamine, improves all of the major features of parkinsonism, including bradykinesia, but does not stop progression of the disorder. The most common early side effects of levodopa are nausea, vomiting, and hypotension, but cardiac arrhythmias may also occur. Dyskinesias, restlessness, confusion, and other behavioral changes tend to occur somewhat later and become more common with time. Levodopa-induced dyskinesias may take any conceivable form, including chorea, athetosis, dystonia, tremor, tics, and myoclonus. An even later complication is the "on-off phenomenon," in which abrupt but transient fluctuations

in the severity of parkinsonism occur unpredictably but frequently during the day. The "off" period of marked bradykinesia has been shown to relate in some instances to falling plasma levels of levodopa. During the "on" phase, dyskinesias are often conspicuous but mobility is increased.

Carbidopa, which inhibits the enzyme responsible for the breakdown of levodopa to dopamine, does not cross the blood-brain barrier. When levodopa is given in combination with carbidopa, the extracerebral breakdown of levodopa is diminished. This reduces the amount of levodopa required daily for beneficial effects, and it lowers the incidence of nausea, vomiting, hypotension, and cardiac irregularities. Such a combination does not prevent the development of the "on-off phenomenon," and the incidence of other side effects (dyskinesias or psychiatric complications) may actually be increased.

Sinemet, a commercially available preparation that contains carbidopa and levodopa in a fixed ratio (1:10 or 1:4), is generally used. Treatment is started with a small dose— eg, one tablet of Sinemet 25/100 (containing 25 mg of carbidopa and 100 mg of levodopa) three times daily—and gradually increased depending on the response. Sinemet CR is a controlled-release formulation (containing 25 or 50 mg of carbidopa and 100 or 200 mg of levodopa). It is sometimes helpful in reducing fluctuations in clinical response to treatment and in reducing the frequency with which medication must be taken. The commercially available combination of levodopa with both carbidopa and entacapone (Stalevo) may also be helpful in this context and is discussed in the following section on COMT inhibitors. Response fluctuations are also reduced by keeping the daily intake of protein at the recommended minimum and taking the main protein meal as the last meal of the day.

The dyskinesias and behavioral side effects of levodopa are dose-related, but reduction in dose may eliminate any therapeutic benefit. Levodopa-induced dyskinesias may also respond to amantadine or possibly levetiracetam.

Levodopa therapy is contraindicated in patients with psychotic illness or narrow-angle glaucoma. It should not be given to patients taking monoamine oxidase A inhibitors or within 2 weeks of their withdrawal, because hypertensive crises may result. Levodopa should be used with care in patients with suspected malignant melanomas or with active peptic ulcers because of concerns that it may exacerbate these disorders.

3. Dopamine agonists—Dopamine agonists, such as pramipexole and ropinirole, act directly on dopamine receptors, and their use in parkinsonism is associated with a lower incidence of the response fluctuations and dyskinesias that occur with long-term levodopa therapy. They were previously reserved for patients who had either become refractory to levodopa or developed the "on-off phenomenon." However, they are now best given either before the introduction of levodopa or with a low dose of Sinemet 25/100 (carbidopa 25 mg and levodopa 100 mg), one tablet three times daily when dopaminergic therapy is first introduced; the dose of Sinemet is kept constant, while the dose of the agonist is gradually increased.

Pramipexole and ropinirole are effective in both early and advanced stages of Parkinson disease. In each case, the daily dose is built up gradually. Pramipexole is started at a dosage of 0.125 mg three times daily orally, and the dose is doubled after 1 week and again after another week; the daily dose is then increased by 0.75 mg at weekly intervals depending on response and tolerance. Most patients require between 0.5 and 1.5 mg three times daily orally. Ropinirole is begun in a dosage of 0.25 mg three times daily orally, and the total daily dose is increased at weekly intervals by 0.75 mg until the fourth week and by 1.5 mg thereafter. Most patients require between 2 and 8 mg three times daily for benefit. Adverse effects include fatigue, somnolence, nausea, peripheral edema, dyskinesias, confusion, and postural hypotension. Less commonly, an irresistible urge to sleep may occur, sometimes in inappropriate and hazardous circumstances. Impulse control disorders involving gambling, shopping, or sexual activity have also been related to use of dopamine agonists. Extended-release, once-daily formulations of pramipexole and ropinirole are available with similar efficacy and tolerability as the immediate release versions. Bromocriptine is not widely used in the United States because of side effects, including anorexia; nausea; vomiting; constipation; postural hypotension; digital vasospasm; cardiac arrhythmias; various dyskinesias and mental disturbances; headache; nasal congestion; erythromelalgia; pulmonary infiltrates; and pericardial, pleural, or pulmonary fibrosis.

4. Selective monoamine oxidase inhibitors—Rasagiline, a selective monoamine oxidase B inhibitor, has a clear symptomatic benefit in a daily oral dose of 1 mg, taken in the morning; it may also be used for adjunctive therapy in patients with response fluctuations to levodopa. Selegiline (5 mg orally with breakfast and lunch) is another monoamine oxidase B inhibitor that is sometimes used as adjunctive treatment for parkinsonism. By inhibiting the metabolic breakdown of dopamine, these drugs may improve fluctuations or declining response to levodopa. Although it is sometimes advised that tyramine-rich foods be avoided when either rasagiline or selegiline is taken because of the theoretical possibility of a hypertensive ("cheese") effect, there is no clinical evidence to support the need for such dietary precautions when they are taken at the recommended dosage.

Studies have suggested (but failed to show conclusively) that rasagiline may slow the progression of Parkinson disease, and it appears to delay the need for other symptomatic therapies. For these reasons, rasagiline is often started early, particularly for patients who are young or have mild disease. However, the FDA has rejected an expansion of rasagiline's indication to include disease modification.

5. COMT inhibitors—Catecholamine-O-methyltransferase inhibitors reduce the metabolism of levodopa to 3-O-methyldopa and thereby alter the plasma pharmacokinetics of levodopa, leading to more sustained plasma levels and more constant dopaminergic stimulation of the brain. Two such agents, tolcapone and entacapone, are currently available and may be used as an adjunct to levodopa-carbidopa in patients with response fluctuations or an otherwise inadequate response. Treatment results in reduced response fluctuations, with a greater period of responsiveness to administered levodopa; however, the use of these agents does not delay the eventual development of levodopa-induced dyskinesias. Tolcapone is given in a dosage of 100 mg or 200 mg three times daily orally, and entacapone is given as 200 mg with each dose of Sinemet (levodopa-carbidopa). With either preparation, the dose of Sinemet taken concurrently may have to be reduced by up to one-third to avoid side effects such as dyskinesias, confusion, hypotension, and syncope. Diarrhea is sometimes troublesome. Because rare cases of fulminant hepatic failure have followed its use, tolcapone should be avoided in patients with preexisting liver disease. Serial liver function tests should be performed at 2-week intervals for the first year and at longer intervals thereafter in patients receiving the drug—as recommended by the manufacturer. Hepatotoxicity has not been reported with entacapone, which is therefore the preferred agent, and serial liver function tests are not required.

Stalevo is the commercial preparation of levodopa combined with both carbidopa and entacapone. It is best used in patients already stabilized on equivalent doses of carbidopa/levodopa and entacapone. It is priced at or below the price of the individual ingredients (ie, carbidopa/levodopa and entacapone) and has the added convenience of requiring fewer tablets to be taken daily. It is available in three strengths: Stalevo 50 (12.5 mg of carbidopa, 50 mg of levodopa, and 200 mg of entacapone), Stalevo 100 (25 mg of carbidopa, 100 mg of levodopa, and 200 mg of entacapone), and Stalevo 150 (37.5 mg of carbidopa, 150 mg of levodopa, and 200 mg of entacapone).

6. Anticholinergic drugs—Anticholinergics are more helpful in alleviating tremor and rigidity than bradykinesia. Treatment is started with a small dose and gradually increased until benefit occurs or side effects limit further increments. If treatment is ineffective, the drug is gradually withdrawn and another preparation then tried.

Side effects limit the routine use of these drugs, and include dryness of the mouth, nausea, constipation, palpitations, cardiac arrhythmias, urinary retention, confusion, agitation, restlessness, drowsiness, mydriasis, increased intraocular pressure, and defective accommodation. Anticholinergic drugs are contraindicated in patients with prostatic hyperplasia, narrow-angle glaucoma, or obstructive gastrointestinal disease and are often tolerated poorly by the elderly. They are best avoided whenever cognitive impairment or a predisposition to delirium exists.

7. Atypical antipsychotics—Confusion and psychotic symptoms may occur as a side effect of dopaminergic therapy or as a part of the underlying illness. They often respond to atypical antipsychotic agents, which have few extrapyramidal side effects and do not block the effects of dopaminergic medication. Olanzapine, quetiapine, and risperidone may be tried, but the most effective of these agents is clozapine, a dibenzodiazepine derivative. Clozapine may rarely cause marrow suppression, and weekly blood counts are therefore necessary for patients taking it. The patient is started on 6.25 mg at bedtime and the dosage increased to 25–100 mg/d as needed. In low doses, it may also improve iatrogenic dyskinesias.

B. General Measures

Physical therapy or speech therapy helps many patients. Cognitive impairment and psychiatric symptoms may be helped by a cholinesterase inhibitor, such as rivastigmine (3–12 mg orally daily or 4.6 or 9.5 mg/24 hours transdermally daily). The quality of life can often be improved by the provision of simple aids to daily living, eg, rails or banisters placed strategically about the home, special table cutlery with large handles, nonslip rubber table mats, and devices to amplify the voice.

C. Surgical Measures

Thalamotomy or pallidotomy may help patients who become unresponsive to medical treatment or have intolerable side effects from antiparkinsonian agents, especially if they have no evidence of diffuse vascular disease or significant cognitive decline. Ablative surgery should generally be confined to one side because the morbidity is considerably greater after bilateral procedures. Because of their morbidity, ablative procedures have generally been supplanted by deep brain stimulation.

D. Brain Stimulation

High-frequency stimulation of the subthalamic nuclei or globus pallidus internus may benefit all the major features of the disease. Electrical stimulation of the brain has the advantage over ablative procedures of being reversible and of causing minimal or no damage to the brain, and is therefore the preferred surgical approach to treatment. There is no evidence that the natural history of Parkinson disease is affected. Deep brain stimulation is reserved for patients without cognitive impairment or psychiatric disorder who have a good response to levodopa but in whom dyskinesias or response fluctuations are problematic. It frequently takes 3–6 months after surgery to adjust stimulator programming and to achieve optimal results. Side effects include depression, apathy, impulsivity, executive dysfunction, and decreased verbal fluency in a subset of patients.

E. Gene Therapy

Injections of adeno-associated viruses encoding various human genes have been made into the subthalamic nucleus or putamen in various phase I and phase II trials. These trials are currently continuing, but the procedure appears to be safe. The results have been disappointing except that transfer of the gene for glutamic acid decarboxylase (the enzyme that produces the inhibitory neurotransmitter GABA) into the subthalamic nucleus seems to improve motor function in patients with Parkinson disease. It is unclear whether this provides any greater benefit than subthalamic deep-brain stimulation.

▶ When to Refer

All patients should be referred.

▶ When to Admit

Patients requiring surgical treatment should be admitted.

Devos D et al. New pharmacological options for treating advanced Parkinson's disease. Clin Ther. 2013 Oct;35(10): 1640–52. [PMID: 24011636]

Gao X et al. Use of ibuprofen and risk of Parkinson disease. Neurology. 2011 Mar 8;76(10):863–9. [PMID: 21368281]

Gottwald MD, Aminoff MJ. Therapies for dopaminergic-induced dyskinesias in Parkinson disease. Ann Neurol. 2011 Jun;69(6):919–27. [PMID: 21681795]

LeWitt PA et al. AAV2-GAD gene therapy for advanced Parkinson's disease: a double-blind, sham-surgery controlled, randomised trial. Lancet Neurol. 2011 Apr;10(4):309–19. [PMID: 21419704]

Rascol O et al. A double-blind, delayed-start trial of rasagiline in Parkinson's disease (the ADAGIO study): prespecified and post-hoc analyses of the need for additional therapies, changes in UPDRS scores, and non-motor outcomes. Lancet Neurol. 2011 May;10(5):415–23. [PMID: 21482191]

Williams DR et al. Parkinsonian syndromes. Continuum (Minneap Minn). 2013 Oct;19(5):1189–212. [PMID: 24092286]

3. Huntington Disease

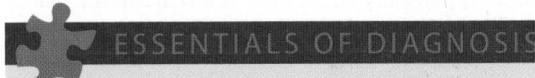

ESSENTIALS OF DIAGNOSIS

- ▶ Gradual onset and progression of chorea and dementia or behavioral change.
- ▶ Family history of the disorder.
- ▶ Responsible gene identified on chromosome 4.

▶ General Considerations

Huntington disease is characterized by chorea and dementia. It is inherited in an autosomal dominant manner and occurs throughout the world, in all ethnic groups, with a prevalence rate of about 5 per 100,000. There is an expanded and unstable CAG trinucleotide repeat in the huntingtin gene at 4p16.3; longer repeat lengths correspond to an earlier age of onset and faster disease progression.

▶ Clinical Findings

A. Symptoms and Signs

Clinical onset is usually between 30 and 50 years of age. The disease is progressive and usually leads to a fatal outcome within 15–20 years. The initial symptoms may consist of either abnormal movements or intellectual changes, but ultimately both occur. The earliest mental changes are often behavioral, with irritability, moodiness, antisocial behavior, or a psychiatric disturbance, but a more obvious dementia subsequently develops. The dyskinesia may initially be no more than an apparent fidgetiness or restlessness, but eventually choreiform movements and some dystonic posturing occur. Progressive rigidity and akinesia (rather than chorea) sometimes occur in association with dementia, especially in cases with childhood onset.

B. Imaging

CT scanning or MRI usually demonstrates cerebral atrophy and atrophy of the caudate nucleus in established cases.

Positron emission tomography (PET) has shown reduced striatal metabolic rate.

Differential Diagnosis

The diagnosis is established with a widely available genetic test, although such testing should be pursued under the guidance of a licensed genetic counselor. Chorea developing with no family history of choreoathetosis should not be attributed to Huntington disease, at least not until other causes of chorea have been excluded clinically and by appropriate laboratory studies. Nongenetic causes of chorea include stroke, systemic lupus erythematosus and related disorders, paraneoplastic syndromes, infection with HIV, and various medications. In younger patients, self-limiting Sydenham chorea develops after group A streptococcal infections on rare occasions. If a patient presents solely with progressive intellectual failure, it may not be possible to distinguish Huntington disease from other causes of dementia unless there is a characteristic family history or a dyskinesia develops.

Huntington disease–like (HDL) disorders resemble Huntington disease but the CAG trinucleotide repeat number of the huntingtin gene is normal. There are autosomal dominant (HDL1, a familial prion disease involving a mutation in the *PRNP* gene on chromosome 20; and HDL2, a triplet repeat disease involving the gene for junctophilin-3 on chromosome 16) and recessive forms (HDL3, 4p15.3).

A clinically similar autosomal dominant disorder (**dentatorubral-pallidoluysian atrophy**), manifested by chorea, dementia, ataxia, and myoclonic epilepsy, is uncommon except in persons of Japanese ancestry. It is due to a mutation in the *ATN1* gene mapping to 12p13.31. Treatment is as for Huntington disease.

Treatment

There is no cure for Huntington disease; progression cannot be halted; and treatment is purely symptomatic. The reported biochemical changes suggest a relative underactivity of neurons containing gamma-aminobutyric acid (GABA) and acetylcholine or a relative overactivity of dopaminergic neurons. Tetrabenazine, a drug that interferes with the vesicular storage of biogenic amines, is widely used to treat the dyskinesia. The starting dose is 12.5 mg twice or three times daily orally, increasing by 12.5 mg every 5 days depending on response and tolerance; the usual maintenance dose is 25 mg three times daily. Side effects include depression, postural hypotension, drowsiness, and parkinsonian features; tetrabenazine should not be given within 14 days of taking monoamine oxidase inhibitors and is not indicated for the treatment of levodopa-induced dyskinesias. Reserpine is similar in depleting central monoamines but has more peripheral effects and a worse side-effect profile, making its use problematic in Huntington disease; if utilized, the dose is built up gradually to between 2 mg and 5 mg orally daily, depending on the response. Treatment with drugs blocking dopamine receptors, such as phenothiazines or haloperidol, may control the dyskinesia and any behavioral disturbances. Haloperidol treatment is usually begun with a dose of 1 mg once or twice daily orally, which is then increased every 3 or 4 days depending on the response; alternatively, atypical antipsychotic agents such as quetiapine (increasing from 25 mg daily orally up to 100 mg twice daily orally as tolerated) may be tried. Amantadine in a dose of 200 mg to 400 mg daily orally is sometimes helpful for chorea. Behavioral disturbances may respond to clozapine. Attempts to compensate for the relative GABA deficiency by enhancing central GABA activity or to compensate for the relative cholinergic underactivity by giving choline chloride have not been therapeutically helpful. Neuroprotective strategies are being explored.

Offspring should be offered genetic counseling. Genetic testing permits presymptomatic detection and definitive diagnosis of the disease.

When to Refer

All patients should be referred.

Biglan KM et al. Refining the diagnosis of Huntington disease: the PREDICT-HD study. Front Aging Neurosci. 2013 Apr 2;5:12. [PMID: 23565093]

Videnovic A. Treatment of Huntington disease. Curr Treat Options Neurol. 2013 Aug;15(4):424–38. [PMID: 23417276]

4. Idiopathic Torsion Dystonia

ESSENTIALS OF DIAGNOSIS

► Dystonic movements and postures.

► Normal birth and developmental history. No other neurologic signs.

► Investigations (including CT scan or MRI) reveal no cause of dystonia.

General Considerations

Idiopathic torsion dystonia may occur sporadically or on a hereditary basis, with autosomal dominant, autosomal recessive, and X-linked recessive modes of transmission. Symptoms may begin in childhood or later and persist throughout life.

Clinical Findings

The disorder is characterized by the onset of abnormal movements and postures in a patient with a normal birth and developmental history, no relevant past medical illness, and no other neurologic signs. Investigations (including CT scan) reveal no cause for the abnormal movements. Dystonic movements of the head and neck may take the form of torticollis, blepharospasm, facial grimacing, or forced opening or closing of the mouth. The limbs may also adopt abnormal but characteristic postures. The age at onset influences both the clinical findings and the prognosis. With onset in childhood, there is usually a family history of the disorder, symptoms commonly commence in the legs, and progression is likely until there is severe disability from generalized dystonia. In contrast, when onset is later, a positive family history is unlikely, initial symptoms are often in the arms or axial structures, and severe disability does not usually occur, although generalized dystonia may ultimately develop in some patients. If all cases are considered together, about one-third of patients eventually become so severely disabled that they are confined to chair or bed, while another one-third are affected only mildly.

▶ Differential Diagnosis

Perinatal anoxia, birth trauma, and kernicterus are common causes of dystonia, but abnormal movements usually then develop before the age of 5, the early development of the patient is usually abnormal, and a history of seizures is not unusual. Moreover, examination may reveal signs of mental retardation or pyramidal deficit in addition to the movement disorder. Dystonic posturing may also occur in Wilson disease, Huntington disease, or parkinsonism; as a sequela of encephalitis lethargica or previous neuroleptic drug therapy; and in certain other disorders. In these cases, diagnosis is based on the history and accompanying clinical manifestations.

▶ Treatment

Idiopathic torsion dystonia usually responds poorly to drugs. Levodopa, diazepam, baclofen, carbamazepine, amantadine, or anticholinergic medication (in high dosage) is occasionally helpful; if not, a trial of treatment with tetrabenazine, phenothiazines, or haloperidol may be worthwhile. In each case, the dose has to be individualized, depending on response and tolerance. However, the doses of these latter drugs that are required for benefit lead usually to mild parkinsonism. Pallidal deep brain stimulation is helpful for medically refractory dystonia and has a lower morbidity than stereotactic thalamotomy, which is sometimes helpful in patients with predominantly unilateral limb dystonia. Potential adverse events of deep brain stimulation include cerebral infection or hemorrhage, broken leads, affective changes, and dysarthria.

A distinct variety of dominantly inherited dystonia, caused by a mutation in the gene for GTP cyclohydrolase I on chromosome 14q, is remarkably responsive to levodopa.

▶ When to Refer

All patients should be referred.

▶ When to Admit

Patients requiring surgical treatment should be admitted.

Morgante F et al. Dystonia. Continuum (Minneap Minn). 2013 Oct;19(5):1225–41. [PMID: 24092288]
Petrucci S et al. Genetic issues in the diagnosis of dystonias. Front Neurol. 2013 Apr 10;4:34. [PMID: 23596437]

5. Focal Torsion Dystonia

A number of the dystonic manifestations that occur in idiopathic torsion dystonia may also occur as isolated phenomena. They are best regarded as focal dystonias that either occur as formes frustes of idiopathic torsion dystonia in patients with a positive family history or represent a focal manifestation of the adult-onset form of that disorder when there is no family history. Mapping of responsible genes to chromosome 8 (DYT6) and chromosome 18 (DYT7) has been reported in some instances of cervical or cranial dystonia. Medical treatment is generally unsatisfactory. A trial of the drugs used in idiopathic torsion dystonia is worthwhile, however, since a few patients do show some response. In addition, with restricted dystonias such as blepharospasm or torticollis, local injection of botulinum A toxin into the overactive muscles may produce worthwhile benefit for several weeks or months and can be repeated as needed.

Both blepharospasm and oromandibular dystonia may occur as an isolated focal dystonia. The former is characterized by spontaneous involuntary forced closure of the eyelids for a variable interval. Oromandibular dystonia is manifested by involuntary contraction of the muscles about the mouth causing, for example, involuntary opening or closing of the mouth, roving or protruding tongue movements, and retraction of the platysma.

Spasmodic torticollis, usually with onset between 25 and 50 years of age, is characterized by a tendency for the neck to twist to one side. This initially occurs episodically, but eventually the neck is held to the side. Spontaneous resolution may occur in the first year or so. The disorder is otherwise usually lifelong. Selective section of the spinal accessory nerve and the upper cervical nerve roots is sometimes helpful if medical treatment is unsuccessful. Local injection of botulinum A toxin provides benefit in most cases.

Writer's cramp is characterized by dystonic posturing of the hand and forearm when the hand is used for writing and sometimes when it is used for other tasks, eg, playing the piano or using a screwdriver or eating utensils. Drug treatment is usually unrewarding, and patients are often best advised to learn to use the other hand for activities requiring manual dexterity. Injections of botulinum A toxin are helpful in some instances.

Jinnah HA et al; Dystonia Coalition Investigators. The focal dystonias: current views and challenges for future research. Mov Disord. 2013 Jun 15;28(7):926–43. [PMID: 23893450]

6. Myoclonus

Occasional myoclonic jerks may occur in anyone, especially when drifting into sleep. General or multifocal myoclonus is common in patients with idiopathic epilepsy and is especially prominent in certain hereditary disorders characterized by seizures and progressive intellectual decline, such as the lipid storage diseases. It is also a feature of various rare degenerative disorders, notably Ramsay Hunt syndrome, and is common in subacute sclerosing panencephalitis and Jakob-Creutzfeldt disease. Generalized myoclonic jerking may accompany uremic and other metabolic encephalopathies, result from therapy with levodopa or cyclic antidepressants, occur in alcohol or drug withdrawal states, or follow anoxic brain damage. It also occurs on a hereditary or sporadic basis as an isolated phenomenon in otherwise healthy subjects.

Segmental myoclonus is a rare manifestation of a focal spinal cord lesion. It may also be the clinical expression of **epilepsia partialis continua,** a disorder in which a repetitive focal epileptic discharge arises in the contralateral sensorimotor cortex, sometimes from an underlying structural lesion. An electroencephalogram is often helpful in clarifying the epileptic nature of the disorder, and CT or MRI scan may reveal the causal lesion.

Myoclonus may respond to certain anticonvulsant drugs, especially valproic acid, or to one of the benzodiazepines, particularly clonazepam (see Table 24–3). It may also respond to piracetam (up to 16.8 g daily). Myoclonus following anoxic brain damage is often responsive to oxitriptan (5-hydroxytryptophan), an investigational agent that is the precursor of serotonin, and sometimes to clonazepam. Oxitriptan is given in gradually increasing doses up to 1–1.5 mg daily. In patients with segmental myoclonus, a localized lesion should be searched for and treated appropriately.

Espay AJ et al. Myoclonus. Continuum (Minneap Minn). 2013 Oct;19(5):1264–86. [PMID: 24092290]

7. Wilson Disease

In this metabolic disorder, abnormal movement and posture may occur with or without coexisting signs of liver involvement. Psychiatric and neuropsychological manifestations are common. Wilson disease is discussed in Chapter 16.

Weiss KH et al. Evolving perspectives in Wilson disease: diagnosis, treatment and monitoring. Curr Gastroenterol Rep. 2012 Feb;14(1):1–7. [PMID: 22083169]

8. Drug-Induced Abnormal Movements

Phenothiazines, butyrophenones, and metoclopramide may produce a wide variety of abnormal movements, including parkinsonism, akathisia (ie, motor restlessness), acute dystonia, chorea, and tardive dyskinesias or dystonia; several of these are also produced by aripiprazole. These complications are discussed in Chapter 25. Chorea may also develop in patients receiving levodopa, bromocriptine, anticholinergic drugs, phenytoin, carbamazepine, lithium, amphetamines, or oral contraceptives, and it resolves with withdrawal of the offending substance. Similarly, dystonia may be produced by levodopa, bromocriptine, lithium, or carbamazepine; and parkinsonism by reserpine and tetrabenazine. Postural tremor may occur with a variety of drugs, including epinephrine, isoproterenol, theophylline, caffeine, lithium, thyroid hormone, tricyclic antidepressants, and valproic acid.

Robottom BJ et al. Drug-induced movement disorders: emergencies and management. Neurol Clin. 2012 Feb;30(1): 309–20. [PMID: 22284065]

9. Restless Legs Syndrome

This disorder may occur as a primary (idiopathic) disorder or in relation to Parkinson disease, pregnancy, iron deficiency anemia, peripheral neuropathy (especially uremic or diabetic), or periodic leg movements of sleep. It may have a hereditary basis, and several genetic loci have been associated with the disorder (12q12-q21, 14q13-q21, 9p24-p22, 2q33, 20p13, 6p21, and 2p14-p13). Restlessness and curious sensory disturbances lead to an irresistible urge to move the limbs, especially during periods of relaxation. Disturbed nocturnal sleep and excessive daytime somnolence may result. Therapy is with nonergot dopamine agonists, such as pramipexole (0.125–0.5 mg orally once daily or ropinirole (0.25–4 mg orally once daily) 2 to 3 hours before bedtime, or with benzodiazepines, such as clonazepam. Gabapentin (starting with 300 mg orally daily, increasing to approximately 1800 mg daily depending on response and tolerance), pregabalin (150–300 mg orally divided twice to three times daily), or gabapentin enacarbil (600 mg extended release daily) are related drugs that improve symptoms. Levodopa is helpful but may lead to an augmentation of symptoms, so that its use is generally reserved for those who do not respond to other measures. In some instances, opioids are required to control symptoms.

Dauvilliers Y et al. Restless legs syndrome: update on pathogenesis. Curr Opin Pulm Med. 2013 Nov;19(6):594–600. [PMID: 24048084]
Hornyak M et al. What treatment works best for restless legs syndrome? Meta-analyses of dopaminergic and non-dopaminergic medications. Sleep Med Rev. 2014 Apr;18(2):153–64. [PMID: 23746768]

10. Gilles de la Tourette Syndrome

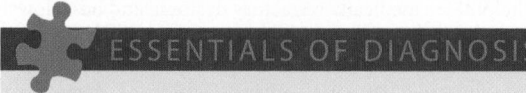

ESSENTIALS OF DIAGNOSIS

► Multiple motor and phonic tics.
► Symptoms begin before age 21 years.
► Tics occur frequently for at least 1 year.
► Tics vary in number, frequency, and nature over time.

▶ Clinical Findings

Motor tics are the initial manifestation in 80% of cases and most commonly involve the face, whereas in the remaining 20%, the initial symptoms are phonic tics; ultimately a combination of different motor and phonic tics develop in all patients. These are noted first in childhood, generally between the ages of 2 and 15. Motor tics occur especially about the face, head, and shoulders (eg, sniffing, blinking, frowning, shoulder shrugging, head thrusting, etc). Phonic tics commonly consist of grunts, barks, hisses, throat-clearing, coughs, etc, but sometimes also of verbal utterances including coprolalia (obscene speech). There may also be echolalia (repetition of the speech of others), echopraxia (imitation of others' movements), and palilalia (repetition of words or phrases). Some tics may be self-mutilating in nature, such as nail-biting, hair-pulling, or biting of the lips or tongue. The disorder is chronic, but the course may be punctuated by relapses and remissions. Obsessive-compulsive behaviors are commonly associated and may be more disabling than the tics themselves. A family history is sometimes obtained.

Examination usually reveals no abnormalities other than the tics. In addition to obsessive-compulsive behavior disorders, psychiatric disturbances may occur because of the associated cosmetic and social embarrassment. The diagnosis of the disorder is often delayed for years, the tics being interpreted as psychiatric illness or some other form of abnormal movement. Patients are thus often subjected to unnecessary treatment before the disorder is recognized. The tic-like character of the abnormal movements and the absence of other neurologic signs should differentiate this disorder from other movement disorders presenting in childhood. Wilson disease, however, can simulate the condition and should be excluded.

Treatment

Treatment is symptomatic and may need to be continued indefinitely. Cognitive behavioral therapy or other forms of behavioral intervention can be effective alone or in combination with pharmacotherapy. Alpha-adrenergic agonists, such as clonidine (start 0.05 mg orally at bedtime, titrating to 0.3–0.4 mg orally daily, divided three to four times per day) or guanfacine (start 0.5 mg orally at bedtime, titrating to a maximum of 3–4 mg orally daily, divided twice daily) are first-line therapies because of a favorable side-effect profile compared with typical antipsychotics, which are the only FDA-approved therapies for the disorder. Topiramate has yielded mixed results in several studies, and the use of tetrabenazine has been described but not rigorously tested. Atypical antipsychotics, including risperidone and aripiprazole, have shown possible efficacy and may be tried before the typical antipsychotic agents. When a typical antipsychotic is required in cases of severe tics, haloperidol is generally regarded as the drug of choice. It is started in a low dose (0.25 mg daily orally) that is gradually increased (by 0.25 mg every 4 or 5 days) until there is maximum benefit with a minimum of side effects or until side effects limit further increments. A total daily oral dose of between 2 mg and 8 mg is usually optimal, but higher doses are sometimes necessary. Fluphenazine (2–15 mg orally daily) or pimozide (1–10 mg orally daily) are alternatives. Typical antipsychotics can cause significant weight gain and carry a risk of tardive dyskinesias and other long-term, potentially irreversible motor side effects.

Injection of botulinum toxin type A at the site of the most distressing tics is sometimes worthwhile. Bilateral high-frequency deep brain stimulation at various sites has been helpful in some, otherwise intractable, cases.

When to Refer

All patients with Gilles de la Tourette syndrome should be referred.

When to Admit

Patients undergoing surgical (deep brain stimulation) treatment should be admitted.

Sassi M et al. Deep brain stimulation therapy for treatment-refractory Tourette's syndrome: a review. Acta Neurochir (Wien). 2011 Mar;153(3):639–45. [PMID: 20853121]
Thomas R et al. The pharmacology of Tourette syndrome. J Neural Transm. 2013 Apr;120(4):689–94. [PMID: 23361655]
Wile DJ et al. Behavior therapy for Tourette syndrome: a systematic review and meta-analysis. Curr Treat Options Neurol. 2013 Aug;15(4):385–95. [PMID: 23645295]

DEMENTIA

 ESSENTIALS OF DIAGNOSIS

▶ Progressive intellectual decline.

▶ Not due to delirium or psychiatric disease.

▶ Age is the main risk factor, followed by family history and vascular disease risk factors.

General Considerations

Dementia is a progressive decline in intellectual function that is severe enough to compromise social or occupational functioning. "Mild cognitive impairment" describes a decline that has not resulted in a change in the level of function. Although a few patients identify a precipitating event, most experience an insidious onset and gradual progression of symptoms.

Dementia typically begins after age 60, and the prevalence doubles approximately every 5 years thereafter; in persons aged 85 and older, around half have dementia. In most, the cause of dementia is acquired, either as a sporadic primary neurodegenerative disease or as the result of another disorder, such as stroke. Other risk factors for dementia include family history, diabetes mellitus and other vascular disease risk factors, and a history of significant head injury. Dementia is more prevalent among women, but this is accounted for by their longer life expectancy. Education and ongoing intellectual stimulation may be protective, perhaps by promoting a "cognitive reserve," an improved capacity to compensate for insidious neurodegeneration.

Dementia is distinct from delirium and psychiatric disease. **Delirium** is an acute confusional state that often occurs in response to an identifiable trigger, such as drug or alcohol intoxication or withdrawal (eg, Wernicke encephalopathy, described below); medication side effects (especially drugs with anticholinergic properties, antihistamines, benzodiazepines, sleeping aids, opioids, neuroleptics, corticosteroids, and other sedative or psychotropic agents), infection (consider occult urinary tract infection or pneumonia in elderly patients), metabolic disturbance (including an electrolyte abnormality; hypoglycemia or hyperglycemia; or a nutritional, endocrine, renal, or hepatic disorder), sleep deprivation, or other neurologic disease (seizure, including a postictal state, or stroke). A delirium typically involves fluctuating level of arousal, including drowsiness or agitation, and it improves after removal or treatment of the precipitating factor. Patients with dementia are especially susceptible to episodes of delirium, but recognition of the dementia is not possible until the delirium lifts. For this reason, dementia is typically diagnosed in outpatients who are otherwise medically stable, rather than in acutely ill patients in the hospital.

Psychiatric disease sometimes leads to complaints of impaired cognition. Impaired attention is usually to blame, and in some patients with depression or anxiety, poor focus and concentration may even be a primary complaint. The symptoms should improve with appropriate psychiatric treatment. Mood disorders are commonly seen in patients with neurodegenerative disease and in some cases are an early symptom. There is some evidence that a persistent, untreated mood disorder may predispose to the development of an age-related dementia, and psychiatric symptoms can clearly exacerbate cognitive impairment in patients who already have dementia; therefore, suspicion of dementia should not distract from appropriate screening for and treatment of depression or anxiety.

▶ **Clinical Findings**

A. Symptoms and Signs

Clinicians should be aware that a patient's insight into a cognitive change may be vague or absent, and collateral history is essential to a proper evaluation. As patients age, primary care clinicians should inquire periodically about the presence of any cognitive symptoms.

Symptoms depend on the area of the brain affected. **Short-term memory loss**, involving the repeating of questions or stories and a diminished ability to recall the details of recent conversations or events, frequently results from pathologic changes in the hippocampus. **Word-finding difficulty** often involves difficulty recalling the names of people, places, or objects, with low-frequency words affected first, eventually resulting in speech laden with pronouns and circumlocutions. This problem is thought to arise from pathology at the temporoparietal junction of the left hemisphere. Problems with articulation, fluency, comprehension, or word meaning are anatomically distinct and less common. **Visuospatial dysfunction** may result in poor navigation and getting lost in familiar places, impaired recognition of previously familiar faces and buildings, or trouble discerning an object against a background. The right parietal lobe is one of the brain areas implicated in such symptoms. **Executive dysfunction** may manifest by easy distractibility, impulsivity, mental inflexibility, concrete thought, slowed processing speed, poor planning and organization, or impaired judgment. Localization may vary and could include the frontal lobes or subcortical areas like the basal ganglia or cerebral white matter. **Apathy** or indifference, separate from depression, is common and may have a similar anatomy as executive dysfunction. **Apraxia**, or the loss of learned motor behaviors, may result from

dysfunction of the frontal or parietal lobes, especially the left parietal lobe.

The time of symptom onset must be established, but subtle, early symptoms are often apparent only in retrospect. Another event, such as an illness or hospitalization, may lead to a new recognition of existing symptoms. Symptoms often accumulate over time, and the nature of the earliest symptom is most helpful in forming the differential diagnosis. The history should establish risk factors for dementia, including family history, other chronic illnesses, and vascular disease risk factors. Finally, it is important to document the patient's current capacity to perform basic and instrumental activities of daily living (see Chapter 4) and to note the extent of decline from the premorbid level of function. Indeed, it is this functional assessment that defines the presence and severity of a dementia.

The physical examination is important to identify any occult medical illness. In addition, eye movement abnormalities, parkinsonism (see above), or other motor abnormalities may help identify an underlying neurologic condition. The workup should prioritize the exclusion of conditions that are reversible or require separate therapy. Screening for depression is necessary, along with imaging and laboratory workup, as indicated below.

B. Neuropsychological Assessment

Brief quantification of cognitive impairment is indicated in a patient complaining of cognitive symptoms. The Folstein Mini Mental State Exam (MMSE) is commonly used, and can be administered in approximately 5 minutes. The Montreal Cognitive Assessment takes slightly longer and may be slightly more sensitive. These tests are useful because they are objective and widely used, but both have important limitations: they are insensitive to mild cognitive impairment, they may be biased negatively by the presence of language or attention problems, and they do not correlate with functional capacity.

An evaluation by a trained neuropsychologist or psychometrician may be appropriate. The goal of such testing is to enhance localization by defining the cognitive domains that are impaired as well as to quantify the degree of impairment. There is no standard battery of tests, but a variety of metrics are commonly used to assess all of the symptom types highlighted above. Assessments are most accurate when a patient is well-rested, comfortable, and otherwise medically stable.

In an asymptomatic patient, there is no screening guideline. Because occult cognitive impairment can lead to morbidity through isolation and poor attentiveness to basic needs (for instance, in an elderly individual living alone), periodic screening is prudent for patients in their 70s and older: Ask the patient to repeat three simple nouns (not referring to objects in the room), then to draw a clock face with numbers in the correct place and the hands indicating a time of 11:10, and finally to recall the three nouns; recall of fewer than three words or any abnormality in the clock drawing may signify the need to continue with the full MMSE and to pursue further questioning and workup.

C. Imaging

Brain imaging is indicated in any patient with a new, progressive cognitive complaint. The goal is to exclude occult cerebrovascular disease, tumor, or other identifiable structural abnormality, rather than to provide positive evidence of a neurodegenerative disease. Global or focal brain atrophy may be worse than expected for age and could suggest a particular neurodegenerative process, but such findings are rarely specific. MRI is preferred, but CT scan will suffice; no contrast is necessary. If MRI is obtained, then diffusion-weighted sequences may be helpful if acute stroke or prion disease is a consideration.

Positron-emission tomography (PET) with fluorodeoxyglucose (FDG) may identify particular brain structures that are hypometabolic and thus likely to harbor pathology. PET imaging does not confirm or exclude any specific cause of dementia but may be useful as an element of the workup in specific clinical circumstances, such as discriminating between Alzheimer disease and frontotemporal dementia in a patient with some symptoms of each. PET imaging with a radiolabeled ligand for beta-amyloid, one of the pathologic proteins in Alzheimer disease, is highly sensitive to amyloid pathology and may help provide positive evidence for Alzheimer disease in a patient with cognitive decline. However, after age 60 or 70, amyloid plaques can accumulate in the absence of cognitive impairment; thus, the specificity of a positive amyloid scan diminishes with age. Single photon-emission computed tomography offers similar information as FDG-PET but is less sensitive. PET imaging with radiolabeled ligands for tau, a pathogenic protein in Alzheimer disease, progressive supranuclear palsy, and some forms of frontotemporal dementia, has entered clinical trials and may help refine premortem diagnostic accuracy.

D. Laboratory Findings

Serum levels of vitamin B_{12}, free T_4, and thyroid-stimulating hormone should be measured for any patient with cognitive symptoms. A serum rapid plasma regain (RPR) used to be obtained routinely, but now is done only if there is a risk factor or suspicion for a remote, untreated syphilis infection. Other testing should be driven by clinical suspicion, and often includes a complete blood count, serum electrolytes, glucose, and lipid profile. Also prudent is age-appropriate cancer screening.

Other tests are available if Alzheimer disease is a consideration: ApoE genotyping is clinically available, and the presence of one or two ApoE epsilon-4 alleles indicates an increased risk of Alzheimer disease. Importantly, the gene does not cause Alzheimer disease; familial Alzheimer disease is rare and is caused by mutations in the amyloid precursor protein or presenilin genes. Finding an ApoE epsilon-4 allele in a young patient with dementia might raise the index of suspicion for Alzheimer disease. Obtaining a genotype in an elderly patient is unlikely to be helpful, and doing so in an asymptomatic patient as a marker of risk for Alzheimer disease is inappropriate until a preventive therapy becomes available. Spinal fluid protein measurements are also available; levels of beta-amyloid decrease

and tau protein increase in Alzheimer disease, but this testing shares some of the same concerns as amyloid PET imaging.

▶ Differential Diagnosis

In elderly patients with gradually progressive cognitive symptoms and no other complaint or sign, a neurodegenerative disease is likely (Table 24–6). Decline beginning before age 60, rapid progression, fluctuating course, unintended weight loss, systemic complaints, or other unexplained symptoms or signs raise suspicion for another process. In this case, the differential is broad and includes infection or inflammatory disease (consider a lumbar puncture to screen for cells or antibodies in the spinal fluid), neoplasm or a paraneoplastic condition, endocrine or metabolic disease, drugs or toxins, or other conditions. **Normal pressure hydrocephalus** is a difficult diagnosis to establish. Symptoms include gait apraxia (sometimes described as a "magnetic" gait, as if the feet are stuck to the floor), urinary incontinence, and dementia. CT scanning or MRI of the brain reveals ventricles that are enlarged in obvious disproportion to sulcal widening and overall brain atrophy.

▶ Treatment

A. Nonpharmacologic Approaches

Aerobic exercise (45 minutes most days of the week) and frequent mental stimulation may reduce the rate of functional decline and decrease the demented patient's caregiving needs, and these interventions may reduce the risk of dementia in normal individuals. The most efficacious manner of mental stimulation is a matter of debate: maintaining as active a role in the family and community as practically possible is most likely to be of benefit, emphasizing activities at which the patient feels confident. Patients with neurodegenerative diseases have a limited capacity to regain lost skills; for instance, memory drills in a patient with Alzheimer disease are more likely to lead to frustration than benefit and studies show that computerized cognitive training does not improve cognition or function in demented patients.

B. Cognitive Symptoms

Cholinesterase inhibitors are first-line therapy for Alzheimer disease and dementia with Lewy bodies. They provide modest, symptomatic treatment for cognitive dysfunction and may prolong the capacity for independence. However, they do not prevent disease progression. Commonly used medications include donepezil (start at 5 mg orally daily for 4 weeks, then increase to 10 mg daily; a 23 mg daily dose is newly approved for moderate to severe Alzheimer disease, although its very modest additional efficacy over the 10-mg dose is overshadowed by an increased risk of side effects); rivastigmine (start at 1.5 mg orally twice daily, then increasing every 2 weeks by 1.5 mg twice daily to a goal of 3–6 mg twice daily; or 4.6, 9.5, or 13.3 mg/24 hours

Table 24–6. Common causes of age-related dementia.

Disorder	Pathology	Clinical Features
Alzheimer disease	Plaques containing beta-amyloid peptide, and neurofibrillary tangles containing tau protein, occur throughout the neocortex	• Most common age-related neurodegenerative disease; incidence doubles every 5 years after age 60 • Short-term memory impairment is early and prominent in most cases • Variable deficits of executive function, visuospatial function, and language
Vascular dementia	Multifocal ischemic change	• Stepwise or progressive accumulation of cognitive deficits in association with repeated strokes • Symptoms depend on localization of strokes
Dementia with Lewy bodies	Histologically indistinguishable from Parkinson disease: alpha-synuclein-containing Lewy bodies occur in the brainstem, midbrain, olfactory bulb, and neocortex. Alzheimer pathology may coexist.	• Cognitive dysfunction, with prominent visuospatial and executive deficits • Psychiatric disturbance, with anxiety, visual hallucinations, and fluctuating delirium • Parkinsonian motor deficits with or after other features • Cholinesterase inhibitors lessen delirium; poor tolerance of many psychoactive medications, including neuroleptics and dopaminergics
Frontotemporal dementia (FTD)	Neuropathology is variable and defined by the protein found in intraneuronal aggregates. Tau protein, TAR DNA-binding protein 43 (TDP-43), or fused-in-sarcoma (FUS) protein account for most cases.	• Peak incidence in the sixth decade; approximately equal to Alzheimer disease as a cause of dementia in patients under 60 years old. • Familial cases result from mutations in genes for tau, progranulin, or others **Behavioral variant FTD** • Deficits in empathy, social comportment, insight, abstract thought, and executive function • Behavior is disinhibited, impulsive, and ritualistic, with prominent apathy and increased interest in sex or sweet/fatty foods • Relative preservation of memory • Focal right frontal atrophy • Association with amyotrophic lateral sclerosis **Semantic dementia** • Deficits in word-finding, single word comprehension, object and category knowledge, and face recognition • Behaviors may be rigid, ritualistic, or similar to behavioral variant FTD • Focal, asymmetric temporal pole atrophy **Progressive nonfluent aphasia** • Speech is effortful with dysarthria, phonemic errors, sound distortions, and poor grammar • Focal extrapyramidal signs and apraxia of the right arm and leg are common • On a diagnostic and pathological continuum with corticobasal degeneration • Focal left frontal atrophy

transdermally daily); and galantamine (start at 4 mg orally twice daily, then increasing every 4 weeks by 4 mg twice daily to a goal of 8–12 mg twice daily; a once-daily extended-release formulation is also available). Cholinesterase inhibitors are not given for frontotemporal dementia because they may worsen behavioral symptoms. Nausea and diarrhea are common side effects; syncope and cardiac dysrhythmia are uncommon but more serious. An ECG is often obtained before and after starting therapy, particularly in a patient with cardiac disease or a history of syncope.

Memantine (start at 5 mg orally daily, then increase by 5 mg per week up to a target of 10 mg twice daily) is approved for the treatment of moderate to severe Alzheimer disease. In frontotemporal dementia, memantine is ineffective and may worsen cognition. There is some evidence that memantine may improve cognition and behavior among patients with dementia with Lewy bodies.

Disease-modifying drugs are not yet available for Alzheimer disease. Immunotherapy directed against beta-amyloid has not shown promise in phase III trials.

C. Mood and Behavioral Disturbances

Selective serotonin reuptake inhibitors are generally safe and well-tolerated in elderly, cognitively impaired patients, and they may be efficacious for the treatment of depression, anxiety, or agitation. However, paroxetine should be avoided because it has anticholinergic effects. Other antidepressant agents, such as buproprion or venlafaxine, may also be tried. Studies on the efficacy of antidepressant therapy in this population are conflicting, but these medications are better tolerated than some alternatives (discussed here).

Insomnia is common, and trazodone (25–50 mg orally at bedtime as needed) can be safe and effective. Over-the-counter antihistamine hypnotics must be avoided, along with benzodiazepines, because of their tendency to worsen cognition and precipitate delirium. Other prescription hypnotics such as zolpidem may result in similar adverse reactions.

For agitation, impulsivity, and other behaviors that interfere with safe caregiving, causes of delirium (detailed above) should first be considered. When no reversible trigger is identified, treatment should be approached in a staged manner. Behavioral interventions, such as reorientation and distraction from anxiety-provoking stimuli, are first-line. Ensure that the patient is kept active during the day with both physical exercise and mentally stimulating activities, and that there is adequate sleep at night. Reassess the level of caregiving, and consider increasing the time spent directly with an attendant. Next, ensure that appropriate pharmacologic treatment of cognition and mood is maximized. Finally, as a last resort, when other measures prove insufficient and the patient's behaviors raise safety concerns, consider low doses of an atypical antipsychotic medication, such as quetiapine (start 25 mg orally daily as needed, increasing to two to three times daily as needed); even though atypical agents cause extrapyramidal side effects less frequently than typical antipsychotics, they should be used with particular caution in a patient at risk for falls, especially if parkinsonian signs are already present. Regularly scheduled dosing is not recommended, and if implemented should be reassessed on a frequent basis (eg, weekly), with attempts to taper off as tolerated. There is an FDA black box warning against the use of all antipsychotic medications in demented patients because of an increased risk of death. Benzodiazepines, such as lorazepam (0.5 mg as needed, up to one to two times daily) may be used as an alternative, but they may sometimes worsen rather than ameliorate agitation.

Finally, psychostimulants like methylphenidate have been studied as a means to treat apathy in dementia. While such treatment may be of benefit to selected patients, the possibility of causing agitation or cardiovascular strain limits routine use.

▶ Special Circumstances

A. Rapidly Progressive Dementia

When dementia develops quickly, with obvious decline over a few weeks to a few months, the syndrome may be classified as a rapidly progressive dementia. The differential diagnosis for typical dementias is still relevant, but additional etiologies must be considered, including prion disease; infections; toxins; neoplasms; and autoimmune and inflammatory diseases, including corticosteroid-responsive (Hashimoto) encephalopathy and antibody-mediated paraneoplastic syndromes. Workup should begin with brain MRI with contrast and diffusion-weighted imaging, routine laboratory studies (serum vitamin B_{12}, free T_4, and thyroid-stimulating hormone levels), serum RPR, HIV antibody, Lyme serology, rheumatologic tests (erythrocyte sedimentation rate, C-reactive protein, and antinuclear antibody), anti-thyroglobulin and anti-thyroperoxidase antibody levels, paraneoplastic autoimmune antibodies, and cerebrospinal fluid studies (cell count and differential; protein and

glucose levels; protein electrophoresis for oligoclonal bands; IgG index [spinal-fluid-to-serum gamma-globulin level] ratio; and VDRL). Depending on the clinical context, it may be necessary to exclude Wilson disease (24-hour urine copper level), heavy metal intoxication (24-hour urine heavy metal panel), and infectious encephalitis (cerebrospinal fluid polymerase chain reaction for Whipple disease, herpes simplex virus, cytomegalovirus, varicella-zoster virus, and other viruses).

Jakob-Creutzfeldt disease is a relatively common cause of rapidly progressive dementia (see Chapter 32). Family history is important since mutations in *PRNP*, the gene for the prion protein, account for around 15% of cases. Diffusion-weighted MRI is the most helpful diagnostic tool, classically revealing cortical ribboning (a gyral pattern of hyperintensity) as well as restricted diffusion in the caudate and anterior putamen. Reflecting the high rate of neuronal death, cerebrospinal fluid levels of the intraneuronal proteins tau, 14-3-3, and neuron-specific enolase are often elevated, although this finding is neither sensitive nor specific. An electroencephalogram often shows periodic complexes.

B. Driving and Dementia

It is recommended that any patient with mild dementia or worse should discontinue driving. Most states have laws regulating driving among cognitively impaired individuals, and many require the clinician to report the patient's diagnosis to the public health department or department of motor vehicles. There is no evidence that driving classes help patients with neurodegenerative diseases.

▶ When to Refer

All patients with new, unexplained cognitive decline should be referred.

▶ When to Admit

Dementia alone is not an indication for admission, but admission is sometimes necessary when a superimposed delirium poses safety risks at home.

Ahlskog JE et al. Physical exercise as a preventive or disease-modifying treatment of dementia and brain aging. Mayo Clin Proc. 2011 Sep;86(9):876–84. [PMID: 21878600]

Galasko D. The diagnostic evaluation of a patient with dementia. Continuum (Minneap Minn). 2013 Apr;19(2):397–410. [PMID: 23558485]

McKhann GM et al. The diagnosis of dementia due to Alzheimer's disease: recommendations from the National Institute on Aging-Alzheimer's Association workgroups on diagnostic guidelines for Alzheimer's disease. Alzheimers Dement. 2011 May;7(3):263–9. [PMID: 21514250]

Paterson RW et al. Diagnosis and treatment of rapidly progressive dementias. Neurol Clin Pract. 2012 Sep;2(3):187–200. [PMID: 23634367]

Schwarz S et al. Pharmacological treatment of dementia. Curr Opin Psychiatry. 2012 Nov;25(6):542–50. [PMID: 22992546]

Seitz DP et al. Antidepressants for agitation and psychosis in dementia. Cochrane Database Syst Rev. 2011 Feb 16;(2): CD008191. [PMID: 21328305]

MULTIPLE SCLEROSIS

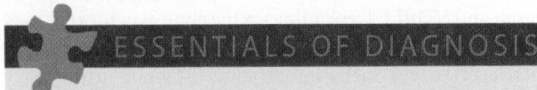

▶ Episodic neurologic symptoms.

▶ Patient usually under 55 years of age at onset.

▶ Single pathologic lesion cannot explain clinical findings.

▶ Multiple foci best visualized by MRI.

▶ General Considerations

This common neurologic disorder, which probably has an autoimmune basis, has its greatest incidence in young adults. Epidemiologic studies indicate that multiple sclerosis is much more common in persons of western European lineage who live in temperate zones. No population with a high risk for multiple sclerosis exists between latitudes 40° N and 40° S. A genetic susceptibility to the disease is present, based on twin studies, familial cases, and an association with specific HLA antigens (HLA-DR2) and alleles of *IL2RA* (the interleukin-2 receptor alpha gene) and *IL7RA* (the interleukin-7 receptor alpha gene). Pathologically, focal—often perivenular—areas of demyelination with reactive gliosis are found scattered in the white matter of brain and spinal cord and in the optic nerves. Axonal damage also occurs.

▶ Clinical Findings

A. Symptoms and Signs

The common initial presentation is weakness, numbness, tingling, or unsteadiness in a limb; spastic paraparesis; retrobulbar optic neuritis; diplopia; dysequilibrium; or a sphincter disturbance such as urinary urgency or hesitancy. Symptoms may disappear after a few days or weeks, although examination often reveals a residual deficit.

Several forms of the disease are recognized. In most patients, there is an interval of months or years after the initial episode before new symptoms develop or the original ones recur (**relapsing-remitting disease**). Eventually, however, relapses and usually incomplete remissions lead to increasing disability, with weakness, spasticity, and ataxia of the limbs, impaired vision, and urinary incontinence. The findings on examination at this stage commonly include optic atrophy; nystagmus; dysarthria; and pyramidal, sensory, or cerebellar deficits in some or all of the limbs. In some of these patients, the clinical course changes so that a steady deterioration occurs, unrelated to acute relapses (**secondary progressive disease**). Less commonly, symptoms are steadily progressive from their onset, and disability develops at a relatively early stage (**primary progressive disease**). The diagnosis cannot be made with confidence unless the total clinical picture indicates involvement of different parts of the central nervous system at different times. Fatigue is common in all forms of the disease.

A number of factors (eg, infection) may precipitate or trigger exacerbations. Relapses are reduced in pregnancy but are more likely during the 2 or 3 months following pregnancy, possibly because of the increased demands and stresses that occur in the postpartum period.

B. Imaging

MRI of the brain or cervical cord has a major role in demonstrating the presence of multiple lesions. In T1-weighted images, hypointense "black holes" probably represent areas of permanent axonal damage; hyperintense lesions are also found. Gadolinium-enhanced T1-weighted images may highlight areas of inflammation with breakdown of the blood-brain barrier, which helps identify newer lesions. T2-weighted images provide information about disease burden or total number of lesions, which typically appear as areas of high signal intensity. CT scans are less helpful than MRI.

In patients with myelopathy alone and in whom there is no clinical or laboratory evidence of more widespread disease, MRI or myelography may be necessary to exclude a congenital or acquired surgically treatable lesion. The foramen magnum region must be visualized to exclude the possibility of Arnold-Chiari malformation, in which parts of the cerebellum and the lower brainstem are displaced into the cervical canal and produce mixed pyramidal and cerebellar deficits in the limbs.

C. Laboratory and Other Studies

A definitive diagnosis can never be based solely on the laboratory findings. If there is clinical evidence of only a single lesion in the central nervous system, multiple sclerosis cannot properly be diagnosed unless it can be shown that other regions are affected subclinically. The electrocerebral responses evoked by monocular visual stimulation with a checkerboard pattern stimulus, by monaural click stimulation, and by electrical stimulation of a sensory or mixed peripheral nerve have been used to detect subclinical involvement of the visual, brainstem auditory, and somatosensory pathways, respectively. Other disorders may also be characterized by multifocal electrophysiologic abnormalities.

There may be mild lymphocytosis or a slightly increased protein concentration in the cerebrospinal fluid, especially soon after an acute relapse. Elevated IgG in cerebrospinal fluid and discrete bands of IgG (oligoclonal bands) are present in many patients. The presence of such bands is not specific, however, since they have been found in a variety of inflammatory neurologic disorders and occasionally in patients with vascular or neoplastic disorders of the nervous system.

D. Diagnosis

Multiple sclerosis should not be diagnosed unless there is evidence that two or more different regions of the central white matter (dissemination in space) have been affected at different times (dissemination in time). The diagnosis may be made in a patient with two or more typical attacks and two or more MRI lesions. To fulfill the criterion of dissemination in space in a patient with only one lesion, repeat imaging in a few months should demonstrate at least one lesion in at least two of four typical sites (periventricular, juxtacortical, infratentorial, or spinal); alternatively, an additional attack localized to a different site suffices. To fulfill the criterion of dissemination in time in a patient with only one attack, the simultaneous presence of asymptomatic gadolinium-enhancing and nonenhancing lesions at any time (including at initial examination) suffices; alternatively, await a new lesion on follow-up MRI or a second attack. Primary progressive disease requires at least a year of progressive disease, plus two of three of the following: at least one typical brain lesion, at least two spinal lesions, or oligoclonal banding in the cerebrospinal fluid.

In patients with a single clinical event who do not satisfy criteria for multiple sclerosis, a diagnosis of a **clinically isolated syndrome (CIS)** is made. Such patients are at risk for developing multiple sclerosis and are sometimes offered beta-interferon or glatiramer acetate therapy, which may delay progression to clinically definite disease. Follow-up MRI should be considered 6–12 months later to assess for the presence of any new lesion.

Treatment

At least partial recovery from acute exacerbations can reasonably be expected, but further relapses may occur without warning, and there is no means of preventing progression of the disorder. Some disability is likely to result eventually, but about half of all patients are without significant disability even 10 years after onset of symptoms.

Recovery from acute relapses may be hastened by treatment with corticosteroids, but the extent of recovery is unchanged. Intravenous therapy is given first—typically methylprednisolone 1 g daily for 3 days—followed by oral prednisone at 60–80 mg daily for 1 week with a taper over the ensuing 2–3 weeks. Long-term treatment with corticosteroids provides no benefit and does not prevent further relapses.

In patients with relapsing disease, numerous injectable medications have well-established efficacy at reducing the frequency of attacks, including beta-interferon (interferon beta-1a 30 mcg intramuscularly once weekly, or 44 mcg subcutaneously three times per week; or interferon beta-1b 0.25 mg subcutaneously every other day) and glatiramer acetate (20 mg subcutaneously daily). Natalizumab reduces the relapse rate when given intravenously once monthly but increases risk of developing progressive multifocal leukoencephalopathy; its use is therefore restricted to monotherapy (not combined with other immune-modulating therapy) in patients with relapsing-remitting disease who have not responded to other therapies or who have a particularly aggressive initial disease course. Alemtuzumab, a lymphocyte inhibitor that similarly raises the risk of opportunistic infection, is approved in Europe but not the United States.

Oral therapies are less well-established, but offer excellent efficacy (at reducing the relapse rate), convenience, and tolerability; these include dimethyl fumarate (120–240 mg twice daily) and fingolimod (0.5 mg orally daily). Teriflunomide (7–14 mg once daily) is another effective oral therapy, limited by liver toxicity in some patients.

For patients with severe or progressive disease, limited evidence supports immunosuppressive therapy with rituximab, cyclophosphamide, azathioprine, methotrexate, or mitoxantrone. Plasmapheresis is sometimes helpful in patients with severe relapses unresponsive to corticosteroids. Intravenous immunoglobulins (IVIGs) may reduce the clinical attack rate in relapsing-remitting disease, but the available studies are inadequate to permit treatment recommendations. Statins may have immunomodulatory effects, and their possible role in the treatment of multiple sclerosis is being studied, but most studies have failed to show any benefit.

Symptomatic therapy for spasticity (see below), neurogenic bladder, or fatigue may be required. Fatigue is especially common in multiple sclerosis, and modafinil (200 mg orally every morning) is an effective and FDA-approved therapy for this indication. Dalfampridine (an extended-release formulation of 4-aminopyridine administered as 10 mg orally twice daily) is efficacious at improving timed gait in multiple sclerosis. Depression and even suicidality can occur in multiple sclerosis and may worsen with interferon beta-1a therapy; screening and conventional treatment of such symptoms are appropriate.

When to Refer

All patients, but especially those with progressive disease despite standard therapy, should be referred.

When to Admit

- Patients requiring plasma exchange.
- During severe relapses.
- Patient unable to manage at home.

Coles AJ et al. Alemtuzumab versus interferon beta-1a in early relapsing-remitting multiple sclerosis: post-hoc and subset analyses of clinical efficacy outcomes. Lancet Neurol. 2011 Apr;10(4):338–48. [PMID: 21397567]

Filippini G et al. Immunomodulators and immunosuppressants for multiple sclerosis: a network meta-analysis. Cochrane Database Syst Rev. 2013 Jun 6;6:CD008933. [PMID: 23744561]

Khatri B et al. Comparison of fingolimod with interferon beta-1a in relapsing-remitting multiple sclerosis: a randomised extension of the TRANSFORMS study. Lancet Neurol. 2011 Jun;10(6):520–9. [PMID: 21571593]

Oh J et al. Safety, tolerability, and efficacy of oral therapies for relapsing-remitting multiple sclerosis. CNS Drugs. 2013 Aug;27(8):591–609. [PMID: 23801528]

Polman CH et al. Diagnostic criteria for multiple sclerosis: 2010 revisions to the McDonald criteria. Ann Neurol. 2011 Feb;69 (2):292–302. [PMID: 21387374]

NEUROMYELITIS OPTICA

This disorder is characterized by optic neuritis and acute myelitis with MRI changes that extend over at least three segments of the spinal cord. An isolated myelitis or optic neuritis may also occur. Previously known as Devic disease and once regarded as a variant of multiple sclerosis, neuromyelitis optica is associated with a specific antibody marker (NMO-IgG) targeting the water channel aquaporin-4. MRI of the brain typically does not show widespread white matter involvement, but such changes do not exclude the diagnosis. Treatment is by long-term immunosuppression. First-line therapy is with rituximab (two 1 g intravenous infusions spaced by 2 weeks, or four weekly infusions of 375 mg/m^2; re-dosing may occur every 6 months or when CD19/20-positive or CD27-positive lymphocytes become detectable) or with azathioprine (2.5–3 mg/kg orally); intravenous immunoglobulin may be used if immunosuppressive therapy is contraindicated.

Jacob A et al. Current concept of neuromyelitis optica (NMO) and NMO spectrum disorders. J Neurol Neurosurg Psychiatry. 2013 Aug;84(8):922–30. [PMID: 23142960]
Trebst C et al. Update on the diagnosis and treatment of neuromyelitis optica: Recommendations of the Neuromyelitis Optica Study Group (NEMOS). J Neurol. 2014 Jan;261(1):1–16. [PMID: 24272588]

VITAMIN E DEFICIENCY

Vitamin E deficiency may produce a disorder somewhat similar to Friedreich ataxia (see below). There is spinocerebellar degeneration involving particularly the posterior columns of the spinal cord and leading to limb ataxia, sensory loss, absent tendon reflexes, slurring of speech and, in some cases, pigmentary retinal degeneration. The disorder may occur as a consequence of malabsorption or on a hereditary basis (eg, abetalipoproteinemia). Treatment is with alpha-tocopheryl acetate as discussed in Chapter 29.

SPASTICITY

The term "spasticity" is commonly used for an upper motor neuron deficit, but it properly refers to a velocity-dependent increase in resistance to passive movement that affects different muscles to a different extent, is not uniform in degree throughout the range of a particular movement, and is commonly associated with other features of pyramidal deficit. It is often a major complication of stroke, cerebral or spinal injury, static perinatal encephalopathy, and multiple sclerosis.

Physical therapy with appropriate stretching programs is important during rehabilitation after the development of an upper motor neuron lesion and in subsequent management of the patient. The aim is to prevent joint and muscle contractures and perhaps to modulate spasticity.

Drug management is important also, but treatment may increase functional disability when increased extensor tone is providing additional support for patients with weak legs. Dantrolene weakens muscle contraction by interfering with the role of calcium. It is best avoided in patients with poor respiratory function or severe myocardial disease. Treatment is begun with 25 mg once daily, increased by 25 mg every 3 days, depending on tolerance, to a maximum of 100 mg four times daily. Side effects include diarrhea, nausea, weakness, hepatic dysfunction (that may

rarely be fatal, especially in women older than 35), drowsiness, light-headedness, and hallucinations.

Baclofen is an effective drug for treating spasticity of spinal origin and painful flexor (or extensor) spasms. The maximum recommended daily oral dose is 80 mg; treatment is started with a dose of 5 or 10 mg twice daily orally and then built up gradually. Side effects include gastrointestinal disturbances, lassitude, fatigue, sedation, unsteadiness, confusion, and hallucinations. Diazepam may modify spasticity by its action on spinal interneurons and perhaps also by influencing supraspinal centers, but effective doses often cause intolerable drowsiness and vary with different patients. Tizanidine, a centrally acting alpha-2-adrenergic agonist, is as effective as these other agents and is probably better tolerated. The daily dose is built up gradually, usually to 8 mg taken three times daily. Side effects include sedation, lassitude, hypotension, and dryness of the mouth.

Intramuscular injection of botulinum toxin has been used to relax targeted muscles.

In patients with severe spasticity that is unresponsive to other therapies and is associated with marked disability, intrathecal injection of phenol or alcohol may be helpful. Surgical options include implantation of an intrathecal baclofen pump, rhizotomy, or neurectomy. Severe contractures may be treated by surgical tendon release.

Spasticity may be exacerbated by decubitus ulcers, urinary or other infections, and nociceptive stimuli.

Maanum G et al. Effects of botulinum toxin A in ambulant adults with spastic cerebral palsy: a randomized double-blind placebo controlled-trial. J Rehabil Med. 2011 Mar;43(4): 338–47. [PMID: 21305227]

MYELOPATHIES IN AIDS

A variety of myelopathies may occur in patients with AIDS. These are discussed in Chapter 31.

MYELOPATHY OF HUMAN T CELL LEUKEMIA VIRUS INFECTION

Human T cell leukemia virus (HTLV-1), a human retrovirus, is transmitted by breast-feeding, sexual contact, blood transfusion, and contaminated needles. Most patients are asymptomatic, but after a variable latent period (which may be as long as several years) a myelopathy develops in some instances. The MRI, electrophysiologic, and cerebrospinal fluid findings are similar to those of multiple sclerosis, but HTLV-1 antibodies are present in serum and spinal fluid. There is no specific treatment, but intravenous or oral corticosteroids may help in the initial inflammatory phase of the disease. Prophylactic measures are important. Needles or syringes should not be shared; infected patients should not breastfeed their infants or donate blood, semen, or other tissue. Infected patients should use condoms to prevent sexual transmission.

Yamano Y et al. Clinical pathophysiology of human T-lymphotropic virus-type 1-associated myelopathy/tropical spastic paraparesis. Front Microbiol. 2012 Nov 9;3:389. [PMID: 23162542]

SUBACUTE COMBINED DEGENERATION OF THE SPINAL CORD

Subacute combined degeneration of the spinal cord is due to vitamin B_{12} deficiency, such as occurs in pernicious anemia. It is characterized by myelopathy with spasticity, weakness, proprioceptive loss, and numbness, sometimes in association with polyneuropathy, mental changes, or optic neuropathy. Megaloblastic anemia may also occur, but this does not parallel the neurologic disorder, and the former may be obscured if folic acid supplements have been taken. Treatment is with vitamin B_{12}. For pernicious anemia, a convenient therapeutic regimen is 100 mg cyanocobalamin intramuscularly daily for 1 week, then weekly for 1 month, and then monthly for the remainder of the patient's life. Oral cyanocobalamin replacement is not advised for pernicious anemia when neurologic symptoms are present.

WERNICKE ENCEPHALOPATHY & KORSAKOFF SYNDROME

Wernicke encephalopathy is characterized by confusion, ataxia, and nystagmus leading to ophthalmoplegia (lateral rectus muscle weakness, conjugate gaze palsies); peripheral neuropathy may also be present. It is due to thiamine deficiency and in the United States occurs most commonly in patients with alcoholism. It may also occur in patients with AIDS or hyperemesis gravidarum, and after surgery for obesity. In suspected cases, thiamine (100 mg) is given intravenously immediately and then intramuscularly on a daily basis until a satisfactory diet can be ensured. Intravenous glucose given before thiamine may precipitate the syndrome or worsen the symptoms. The diagnosis is confirmed by the response in 1 or 2 days to treatment, which must not be delayed while awaiting laboratory confirmation of thiamine deficiency from a blood sample obtained prior to thiamine administration. **Korsakoff syndrome** occurs in more severe cases; it includes anterograde and retrograde amnesia and sometimes confabulation, and may not be recognized until after the initial delirium has lifted.

Zahr NM et al. Clinical and pathological features of alcohol-related brain damage. Nat Rev Neurol. 2011 May;7(5):284–94. [PMID: 21487421]

STUPOR & COMA

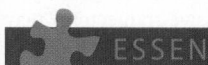

ESSENTIALS OF DIAGNOSIS

- ▶ Level of consciousness is depressed.
- ▶ Stuporous patients respond only to repeated vigorous stimuli.
- ▶ Comatose patients are unarousable and unresponsive.

▶ General Considerations

The patient who is stuporous is unresponsive except when subjected to repeated vigorous stimuli, while the comatose patient is unarousable and unable to respond to external events or inner needs, although reflex movements and posturing may be present.

Coma is a major complication of serious central nervous system disorders. It can result from seizures, hypothermia, metabolic disturbances, or structural lesions causing bilateral cerebral hemispheric dysfunction or a disturbance of the brainstem reticular activating system. A mass lesion involving one cerebral hemisphere may cause coma by compression of the brainstem. All comatose patients should be admitted to hospital and referred to a neurologist or neurosurgeon.

▶ Assessment & Emergency Measures

The diagnostic workup of the comatose patient must proceed concomitantly with management. Supportive therapy for respiration or blood pressure is initiated; in hypothermia, all vital signs may be absent and all such patients should be rewarmed before the prognosis is assessed.

The patient can be positioned on one side with the neck partly extended, dentures removed, and secretions cleared by suction; if necessary, the patency of the airways is maintained with an oropharyngeal airway. Blood is drawn for serum glucose, electrolyte, and calcium levels; arterial blood gases; liver and kidney function tests; and toxicologic studies as indicated. Dextrose 50% (25 g), naloxone (0.4–1.2 mg), and thiamine (100 mg) are given intravenously without delay.

Further details are then obtained from attendants of the patient's medical history, the circumstances surrounding the onset of coma, and the time course of subsequent events. Abrupt onset of coma suggests subarachnoid hemorrhage, brainstem stroke, or intracerebral hemorrhage, whereas a slower onset and progression occur with other structural or mass lesions. Urgent noncontrast CT scanning of the head is appropriate if it can be obtained directly from the emergency department, in order to identify intracranial hemorrhage, brain herniation, or other structural lesion that may require immediate neurosurgical intervention. A metabolic cause is likely with a preceding intoxicated state or agitated delirium. On examination, attention is paid to the behavioral response to painful stimuli, the pupils and their response to light, the position of the eyes and their movement in response to passive movement of the head and ice-water caloric stimulation, and the respiratory pattern.

A. Response to Painful Stimuli

Purposive limb withdrawal from painful stimuli implies that sensory pathways from and motor pathways to the stimulated limb are functionally intact. Unilateral absence of responses despite application of stimuli to both sides of the body in turn implies a corticospinal lesion; bilateral absence of responsiveness suggests brainstem involvement, bilateral pyramidal tract lesions, or psychogenic unresponsiveness.

Inappropriate responses may also occur. Decorticate posturing may occur with lesions of the internal capsule and rostral cerebral peduncle, decerebrate posturing with dysfunction or destruction of the midbrain and rostral pons, and decerebrate posturing in the arms accompanied by flaccidity or slight flexor responses in the legs in patients with extensive brainstem damage extending down to the pons at the trigeminal level.

B. Ocular Findings

1. Pupils—Hypothalamic disease processes may lead to unilateral Horner syndrome, while bilateral diencephalic involvement or destructive pontine lesions may lead to small but reactive pupils. Ipsilateral pupillary dilation with no direct or consensual response to light occurs with compression of the third cranial nerve, eg, with uncal herniation. The pupils are slightly smaller than normal but responsive to light in many metabolic encephalopathies; however, they may be fixed and dilated following overdosage with atropine or scopolamine, and pinpoint (but responsive) with opioids. Pupillary dilation for several hours following cardiopulmonary arrest implies a poor prognosis.

2. Eye movements—Conjugate deviation of the eyes to the side suggests the presence of an ipsilateral hemispheric lesion or a contralateral pontine lesion. A mesencephalic lesion leads to downward conjugate deviation. Dysconjugate ocular deviation in coma implies a structural brainstem lesion unless there was preexisting strabismus.

The oculomotor responses to passive head turning and to caloric stimulation relate to each other and provide complementary information. In response to brisk rotation of the head from side to side and to flexion and extension of the head, normally conscious patients with open eyes do not exhibit contraversive conjugate eye deviation (doll's-head eye response) unless there is voluntary visual fixation or bilateral frontal pathology. With cortical depression in lightly comatose patients, a brisk doll's-head eye response is seen. With brainstem lesions, this oculocephalic reflex becomes impaired or lost, depending on the site of the lesion.

The oculovestibular reflex is tested by caloric stimulation using irrigation with ice water. In normal subjects, jerk nystagmus is elicited for about 2 or 3 minutes, with the slow component toward the irrigated ear. In unconscious patients with an intact brainstem, the fast component of the nystagmus disappears, so that the eyes tonically deviate toward the irrigated side for 2–3 minutes before returning to their original position. With impairment of brainstem function, the response becomes perverted and finally disappears. In metabolic coma, oculocephalic and oculovestibular reflex responses are preserved, at least initially.

C. Respiratory Patterns

Diseases causing coma may lead to respiratory abnormalities. Cheyne-Stokes respiration (in which episodes of deep breathing alternate with periods of apnea) may occur with bihemispheric or diencephalic disease or in metabolic disorders. Central neurogenic hyperventilation occurs with lesions of the brainstem tegmentum; apneustic breathing (in which there are prominent end-inspiratory pauses) suggests damage at the pontine level (eg, due to basilar artery occlusion); and atactic breathing (a completely irregular pattern of breathing with deep and shallow breaths occurring randomly) is associated with lesions of the lower pontine tegmentum and medulla.

1. Stupor & Coma Due to Structural Lesions

Supratentorial mass lesions tend to affect brain function in an orderly way. There may initially be signs of hemispheric dysfunction, such as hemiparesis. As coma develops and deepens, cerebral function becomes progressively disturbed, producing a predictable progression of neurologic signs that suggest rostrocaudal deterioration.

Thus, as a supratentorial mass lesion begins to impair the diencephalon, the patient becomes drowsy, then stuporous, and finally comatose. There may be Cheyne-Stokes respiration; small but reactive pupils; doll's-head eye responses with side-to-side head movements but sometimes an impairment of reflex upward gaze with brisk flexion of the head; tonic ipsilateral deviation of the eyes in response to vestibular stimulation with cold water; and initially a positive response to pain but subsequently only decorticate posturing. With further progression, midbrain failure occurs. Motor dysfunction progresses from decorticate to bilateral decerebrate posturing in response to painful stimuli; Cheyne-Stokes respiration is gradually replaced by sustained central hyperventilation; the pupils become middle-sized and fixed; and the oculocephalic and oculovestibular reflex responses become impaired, perverted, or lost. As the pons and then the medulla fail, the pupils remain unresponsive; oculovestibular responses are unobtainable; respiration is rapid and shallow; and painful stimuli may lead only to flexor responses in the legs. Finally, respiration becomes irregular and stops, the pupils often then dilating widely.

In contrast, a subtentorial (ie, brainstem) lesion may lead to an early, sometimes abrupt disturbance of consciousness without any orderly rostrocaudal progression of neurologic signs. Compressive lesions of the brainstem, especially cerebellar hemorrhage, may be clinically indistinguishable from intraparenchymal processes.

A structural lesion is suspected if the findings suggest focality. In such circumstances, a CT scan should be performed before, or instead of, a lumbar puncture in order to avoid any risk of cerebral herniation. Further management is of the causal lesion and is considered separately under the individual disorders.

In some cases of traumatic brain injury, swelling may be diffuse rather than focal. Decompressive craniectomy may reduce otherwise refractory intracranial hypertension but does not improve neurologic outcome. Hypothermic therapy is controversial.

Clifton GL et al. Very early hypothermia induction in patients with severe brain injury (the National Acute Brain Injury Study: Hypothermia II): a randomised trial. Lancet Neurol. 2011 Feb;10(2):131–9. [PMID: 21169065]

Cooper DJ et al. Decompressive craniectomy in diffuse traumatic brain injury. N Engl J Med. 2011 Apr 21;364(16): 1493–502. [PMID: 21434843]

Moore SA et al. The acutely comatose patient: clinical approach and diagnosis. Semin Neurol. 2013 Apr;33(2):110–20. [PMID: 23888395]

2. Stupor & Coma Due to Metabolic Disturbances

Patients with a metabolic cause of coma generally have signs of patchy, diffuse, and symmetric neurologic involvement that cannot be explained by loss of function at any single level or in a sequential manner, although focal or lateralized deficits may occur in hypoglycemia. Moreover, pupillary reactivity is usually preserved, while other brainstem functions are often grossly impaired. Comatose patients with meningitis, encephalitis, or subarachnoid hemorrhage may also exhibit little in the way of focal neurologic signs, however, and clinical evidence of meningeal irritation is sometimes very subtle in comatose patients. Examination of the cerebrospinal fluid in such patients is essential to establish the correct diagnosis.

In patients with coma due to cerebral ischemia and hypoxia, the absence of pupillary light reflexes at the time of initial examination indicates that there is little chance of regaining independence; by contrast, preserved pupillary light responses, the development of spontaneous eye movements (roving, conjugate, or better), and extensor, flexor, or withdrawal responses to pain at this early stage imply a relatively good prognosis.

Treatment of metabolic encephalopathy is of the underlying disturbance and is considered in other chapters. If the cause of the encephalopathy is obscure, all drugs except essential ones may have to be withdrawn in case they are responsible for the altered mental status.

Bouwes A et al. Prognosis of coma after therapeutic hypothermia: a prospective cohort study. Ann Neurol. 2012 Feb;71(2): 206–12. [PMID: 22367993]

Chiota NA et al. Hypoxic-ischemic brain injury and prognosis after cardiac arrest. Continuum (Minneap Minn). 2011 Oct;17 (5):1094–118. [PMID: 22809984]

3. Brain Death

The definition of brain death is controversial, and diagnostic criteria have been published by many different professional organizations. In order to establish brain death, the irreversibly comatose patient must be shown to have lost all brainstem reflex responses, including the pupillary, corneal, oculovestibular, oculocephalic, oropharyngeal, and respiratory reflexes, and should have been in this condition for at least 6 hours. Spinal reflex movements do not exclude the diagnosis, but ongoing seizure activity or decerebrate or decorticate posturing is not consistent with brain death. The apnea test (presence or absence of spontaneous respiratory activity at a $Paco_2$ of at least 60 mm Hg) serves to determine whether the patient is capable of respiratory activity.

Reversible coma simulating brain death may be seen with hypothermia (temperature < 32°C) and overdosage with central nervous system depressant drugs, and these conditions must be excluded. Certain ancillary tests may assist the determination of brain death but are not essential. An isoelectric electroencephalogram, when the recording is made according to the recommendations of the American Electroencephalographic Society, may help in confirming the diagnosis. Alternatively, the demonstration of an absent cerebral circulation by intravenous radioisotope cerebral angiography or by four-vessel contrast cerebral angiography is confirmatory.

Wijdicks EF. The case against confirmatory tests for determining brain death in adults. Neurology. 2010 Jul 6;75(1):77–83. [PMID: 20603486]

4. Persistent Vegetative State

Patients with severe bilateral hemispheric disease may show some improvement from an initially comatose state, so that, after a variable interval, they appear to be awake but lie motionless and without evidence of awareness or higher mental activity. This persistent vegetative state has been variously referred to as akinetic mutism, apallic state, or coma vigil. Most patients in this persistent vegetative state will die in months or years, but partial recovery has occasionally occurred and in rare instances has been sufficient to permit communication or even independent living.

Hirschberg R et al. The vegetative and minimally conscious states: diagnosis, prognosis and treatment. Neurol Clin. 2011 Nov;29(4):773–86. [PMID: 22032660]

5. Minimally Conscious State

In this state, patients exhibit inconsistent evidence of consciousness. There is some degree of functional recovery of behaviors suggesting self- or environmental awareness, such as basic verbalization or context-appropriate gestures, emotional responses (eg, smiling) to emotional but not neutral stimuli, or purposive responses to environmental stimuli (eg, a finger movement or eye blink apparently to command). Further improvement is manifest by the restoration of communication with the patient. The minimally conscious state may be temporary or permanent. Little information is available about its natural history or long-term outlook, which reflect the underlying cause. The likelihood of useful functional recovery diminishes with time; after 12 months, patients are likely to remain severely disabled and without a reliable means of communication. Prognostication is difficult.

6. Locked-In Syndrome (De-efferented State)

Acute destructive lesions (eg, infarction, hemorrhage, demyelination, encephalitis) involving the ventral pons and sparing the tegmentum may lead to a mute, quadriparetic but conscious state in which the patient is capable of blinking and of voluntary eye movement in the vertical plane, with preserved pupillary responses to light. Such a patient can mistakenly be regarded as comatose. Clinicians should recognize that "locked-in" individuals are fully aware of their surroundings. The prognosis is usually poor, but recovery has occasionally been reported in some cases, including resumption of independent daily life.

Barbic D et al. Locked-in syndrome: a critical and time-dependent diagnosis. CJEM. 2012 Sep;14(5):317–20. [PMID: 22967701]

Stoll J et al. Pupil responses allow communication in locked-in syndrome patients. Curr Biol. 2013 Aug 5;23(15):R647–8. [PMID: 23928079]

HEAD INJURY

Trauma is the most common cause of death in young people, and head injury accounts for almost half of these trauma-related deaths. The incidence of head injury can be reduced by, for example, using bicycle helmets and protective equipment in sports.

The prognosis following head injury depends on the site and severity of brain damage. Some guide to prognosis is provided by the mental status, since loss of consciousness implies a worse prognosis than otherwise. Similarly, the degree of retrograde and posttraumatic amnesia provides an indication of the severity of injury and thus of the prognosis. Absence of skull fracture does not exclude the possibility of severe head injury. During the physical examination, special attention should be given to the level of consciousness and extent of any brainstem dysfunction.

Note: Patients (especially elderly, >65 years) who are intoxicated with drugs or alcohol or have evidence of soft-tissue injury above the clavicles following head injury should be admitted to the hospital for observation, as should patients with recurrent vomiting, persistent anterograde amnesia, retrograde amnesia for more than 30 minutes, focal neurologic deficits, lethargy, or skull fractures. If admission is declined, responsible family members should be given clear instructions about the need for, and manner of, checking on them at regular (hourly) intervals and for obtaining additional medical help if necessary.

Skull radiographs or CT scans may provide evidence of fractures. Because injury to the spine may have accompanied head trauma, cervical spine radiographs (especially in the lateral projection) should always be obtained in comatose patients and in patients with severe neck pain or a deficit possibly related to cord compression.

CT scanning has an important role in demonstrating intracranial hemorrhage and may also provide evidence of cerebral edema and displacement of midline structures.

1. Cerebral Injuries

These are summarized in Table 24–7. Increased intracranial pressure may result from ventilatory obstruction, abnormal neck position, seizures, dilutional hyponatremia, or cerebral edema; an intracranial hematoma requiring surgical evacuation may also be responsible. Other measures that may be necessary to reduce intracranial pressure include induced hyperventilation, intravenous mannitol infusion, and intravenous furosemide; corticosteroids provide no benefit in this context. Overall, treatment is mainly supportive. The role of induced hypothermia in reducing long-term neurologic deficits is currently under investigation.

Table 24–7. Acute cerebral sequelae of head injury.

Sequelae	Clinical Features	Pathology
Concussion	A transient, trauma-induced alteration in mental status that may or may not involve loss of consciousness. Symptoms and signs include headache, nausea, disorientation, irritability, amnesia, clumsiness, visual disturbances, and focal neurologic deficit.	Bruising on side of impact (coup injury) or contralaterally (contrecoup injury).
Cerebral contusion or laceration	Loss of consciousness longer than with concussion. Focal neurologic deficits are often present. May lead to death or severe residual neurologic deficit.	Vasogenic edema, multiple petechial hemorrhages, and mass effect. May have subarachnoid bleeding. Herniation may occur in severe cases. Cerebral laceration specifically involves tearing of the cerebral tissue and pia-arachnoid overlying a contusion.
Acute epidural hemorrhage	Headache, confusion, somnolence, seizures, and focal deficits occur several hours after injury and lead to coma, respiratory depression, and death unless treated by surgical evacuation.	Tear in meningeal artery, vein, or dural sinus, leading to hematoma visible on CT scan.
Acute subdural hemorrhage	Similar to epidural hemorrhage, but interval before onset of symptoms is longer. Neurosurgical consultation for consideration of evacuation.	Hematoma from tear in veins from cortex to superior sagittal sinus or from cerebral laceration, visible on CT scan.
Cerebral hemorrhage	Generally develops immediately after injury. Clinically resembles hypertensive hemorrhage. Surgical evacuation is sometimes helpful.	Hematoma, visible on CT scan.
Diffuse axonal injury	Persistent loss of consciousness, coma, or persistent vegetative state resulting from severe rotational shearing forces or deceleration.	Imaging may be normal or may show tiny, scattered white matter hemorrhages. Histology reveals torn axons.

2. Scalp Injuries & Skull Fractures

Scalp lacerations and depressed or compound depressed skull fractures should be treated surgically as appropriate. Simple skull fractures require no specific treatment.

The clinical signs of basilar skull fracture include bruising about the orbit (raccoon sign), blood in the external auditory meatus (Battle sign), and leakage of cerebrospinal fluid (which can be identified by its glucose content) from the ear or nose. Cranial nerve palsies (involving especially the first, second, third, fourth, fifth, seventh, and eighth nerves in any combination) may also occur. If there is any leakage of cerebrospinal fluid, conservative treatment, with elevation of the head, restriction of fluids, and administration of acetazolamide (250 mg orally four times daily), is often helpful; but if the leak continues for more than a few days, lumbar subarachnoid drainage may be necessary. Antibiotics are given if infection occurs, based on culture and sensitivity studies. Only very occasional patients require intracranial repair of the dural defect because of persistence of the leak or recurrent meningitis.

3. Late Complications of Head Injury

The relationship of chronic subdural hemorrhage to head injury is not always clear. In many elderly persons there is no history of trauma, but in other cases a head injury, often trivial, precedes the onset of symptoms by several weeks. The clinical presentation is usually with mental changes such as slowness, drowsiness, headache, confusion, memory disturbances, personality change, or even dementia. Focal neurologic deficits such as hemiparesis or hemisensory disturbance may also occur but are less common. CT scan is an important means of detecting the hematoma, which is sometimes bilateral. Treatment is by surgical evacuation to prevent cerebral compression and tentorial herniation. There is no clear evidence that prophylactic anticonvulsant therapy reduces the incidence of posttraumatic seizures.

After major head injury causing severe, acute mental status changes, cognitive deficits may persist indefinitely. Memory training may be a helpful component of rehabilitation. In addition, there is an association between head trauma and the later development of a neurodegenerative disease, such as Alzheimer or Parkinson disease and amyotrophic lateral sclerosis. **Chronic traumatic encephalopathy**, characterized by mood and cognitive changes after repetitive, mild head injury, as may occur in athletes or military personnel, is due to the abnormal aggregation of tau or other proteins either focally or globally in the cerebral cortex.

Normal-pressure hydrocephalus may follow head injury, subarachnoid hemorrhage, or meningoencephalitis. Other late complications of head injury include posttraumatic seizure disorder, headache, vertigo, and hyposmia.

When to Refer

- Patients with focal neurologic deficits, altered consciousness, or skull fracture.
- Patients with late complications of head injury, eg, posttraumatic seizure disorder or normal pressure hydrocephalus.

When to Admit

- Patients (especially elderly, > 65 years) who are intoxicated with drugs or alcohol or have evidence of soft-tissue injury above the clavicles should be admitted for observation.
- Patients with recurrent vomiting, focal neurologic deficits, persistent anterograde amnesia, retrograde amnesia for more than 30 minutes, altered consciousness, or skull fracture.
- Patients with acute epidural, subdural, or cerebral hematoma.
- Patients requiring shunt placement for normal pressure hydrocephalus.

McKee AC et al. The spectrum of disease in chronic traumatic encephalopathy. Brain. 2013 Jan;136(Pt 1):43–64. [PMID: 23208308]

Roberts DJ et al. Sedation for critically ill adults with severe traumatic brain injury: a systematic review of randomized controlled trials. Crit Care Med. 2011 Dec;39(12):2743–51. [PMID: 22094498]

Shum D et al. A randomized controlled trial of prospective memory rehabilitation in adults with traumatic brain injury. J Rehabil Med. 2011 Feb;43(3):216–23. [PMID: 21305237]

SPINAL TRAUMA

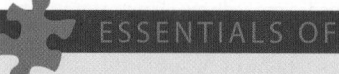

ESSENTIALS OF DIAGNOSIS

- ► History of preceding trauma.
- ► Development of acute neurologic deficit.
- ► Signs of myelopathy on examination.

General Considerations

While spinal cord damage may result from whiplash injury, severe injury usually relates to fracture-dislocation causing compression or angular deformity of the cord either cervically or in the lower thoracic and upper lumbar regions. Extreme hypotension following injury may also lead to cord infarction.

Clinical Findings

Total cord transection results in immediate flaccid paralysis and loss of sensation below the level of the lesion. Reflex activity is lost for a variable period, and there is urinary and fecal retention. As reflex function returns over the following days and weeks, spastic paraplegia or quadriplegia develops, with hyperreflexia and extensor plantar responses, but a flaccid atrophic (lower motor neuron) paralysis may be found depending on the segments of the cord that are affected. The bladder and bowels also regain some reflex function, permitting urine and feces to be expelled at intervals. As spasticity increases, flexor or extensor spasms (or both) of the legs become troublesome, especially if the patient develops bed sores or a urinary tract infection. Paraplegia with the legs in flexion or extension may eventually result.

With lesser degrees of injury, patients may be left with mild limb weakness, distal sensory disturbance, or both. Sphincter function may also be impaired, urinary urgency and urgency incontinence being especially common. More particularly, a unilateral cord lesion leads to an ipsilateral motor disturbance with accompanying impairment of proprioception and contralateral loss of pain and temperature appreciation below the lesion (Brown-Séquard syndrome). A central cord syndrome may lead to a lower motor neuron deficit and loss of pain and temperature appreciation, with sparing of posterior column functions. A radicular deficit may occur at the level of the injury—or, if the cauda equina is involved, there may be evidence of disturbed function in several lumbosacral roots.

► **Treatment**

Treatment of the injury consists of immobilization and—if there is cord compression—early decompressive laminectomy and fusion (within 24 hours). Early treatment with high doses of corticosteroids (eg, methylprednisolone, 30 mg/kg by intravenous bolus, followed by 5.4 mg/kg/h for 23 hours) may improve neurologic recovery if commenced within 8 hours after injury; the findings from various studies are conflicting, however, and evaluation of the published evidence suggest that significant benefit is unlikely. Anatomic realignment of the spinal cord by traction and other orthopedic procedures is important. Subsequent care of the residual neurologic deficit—paraplegia or quadriplegia—requires treatment of spasticity and care of the skin, bladder, and bowels.

► **When to Refer**

All patients with focal neurologic deficits should be referred.

► **When to Admit**

- Patients with neurologic deficits.
- Patients with spinal cord injury, compression, or acute epidural or subdural hematoma.
- Patients with vertebral fracture-dislocation likely to compress the cord.

Evans LT et al. Management of acute spinal cord injury in the neurocritical care unit. Neurosurg Clin N Am. 2013 Jul;24(3): 339–47. [PMID: 23809029]
Zhang S et al. Spine and spinal cord trauma: diagnosis and management. Neurol Clin. 2013 Feb;31(1):183–206. [PMID: 23186900]

SYRINGOMYELIA

Destruction or degeneration of gray and white matter adjacent to the central canal of the cervical spinal cord leads to cavitation and accumulation of fluid within the spinal cord. The precise pathogenesis is unclear, but many cases are associated with Arnold-Chiari malformation, in which there is displacement of the cerebellar tonsils, medulla, and fourth ventricle into the spinal canal, sometimes with accompanying meningomyelocele. In such circumstances, the cord cavity connects with and may merely represent a dilated central canal. In other cases, the cause of cavitation is less clear. There is a characteristic clinical picture, with segmental atrophy, areflexia and loss of pain and temperature appreciation in a "cape" distribution, owing to the destruction of fibers crossing in front of the central canal in the mid-cervical spinal cord. Thoracic kyphoscoliosis is usually present. With progression, involvement of the long motor and sensory tracts occurs as well, so that a pyramidal and sensory deficit develops in the legs. Upward extension of the cavitation (syringobulbia) leads to dysfunction of the lower brainstem and thus to bulbar palsy, nystagmus, and sensory impairment over one or both sides of the face.

Syringomyelia, ie, cord cavitation, may also occur in association with an intramedullary tumor or following severe cord injury, and the cavity then does not communicate with the central canal.

In patients with Arnold-Chiari malformation, CT scans reveal a small posterior fossa and enlargement of the foramen magnum, along with other associated skeletal abnormalities at the base of the skull and upper cervical spine. MRI reveals the syrinx as well as the characteristic findings of the Arnold-Chiari malformation, including the caudal displacement of the fourth ventricle and herniation of the cerebellar tonsils through the foramen magnum. Focal cord enlargement is found at myelography or by MRI in patients with cavitation related to past injury or intramedullary neoplasms.

Treatment of Arnold-Chiari malformation with associated syringomyelia is by suboccipital craniectomy and upper cervical laminectomy, with the aim of decompressing the malformation at the foramen magnum. The cord cavity should be drained, and if necessary an outlet for the fourth ventricle can be made. In cavitation associated with intra-medullary tumor, treatment is surgical, but radiation therapy may be necessary if complete removal is not possible. Posttraumatic syringomyelia is also treated surgically if it leads to increasing neurologic deficits or to intolerable pain.

Roy AK et al. Idiopathic syringomyelia: retrospective case series, comprehensive review, and update on management. Neurosurg Focus. 2011 Dec;31(6):E15. [PMID: 22133183]

DEGENERATIVE MOTOR NEURON DISEASES

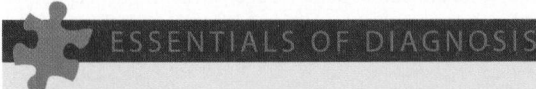
ESSENTIALS OF DIAGNOSIS

► Weakness.

► No sensory loss or sphincter disturbance.

► Progressive course.

► No identifiable underlying cause other than genetic basis in familial cases.

General Considerations

This group of degenerative disorders is characterized clinically by weakness and variable wasting of affected muscles, without accompanying sensory changes.

Motor neuron disease in adults generally commences between 30 and 60 years of age. There is degeneration of the anterior horn cells in the spinal cord, the motor nuclei of the lower cranial nerves, and the corticospinal and corticobulbar pathways. The disorder is usually sporadic, but familial cases may occur and several genetic mutations or loci have been identified. Cigarette smoking may be one risk factor.

Classification

Five varieties have been distinguished on clinical grounds.

A. Progressive Bulbar Palsy

Bulbar involvement predominates owing to disease processes affecting primarily the motor nuclei of the cranial nerves.

B. Pseudobulbar Palsy

Bulbar involvement predominates in this variety also, but it is due to bilateral corticobulbar disease and thus reflects upper motor neuron dysfunction. There may be a "pseudobulbar affect," with uncontrollable episodes of laughing or crying to stimuli that would not normally have elicited such marked reactions.

C. Progressive Spinal Muscular Atrophy

This is characterized primarily by a lower motor neuron deficit in the limbs due to degeneration of the anterior horn cells in the spinal cord.

D. Primary Lateral Sclerosis

There is a purely upper motor neuron deficit in the limbs.

E. Amyotrophic Lateral Sclerosis

A mixed upper and lower motor neuron deficit is found in the limbs. This disorder is sometimes associated with cognitive decline (in a pattern consistent with frontotemporal dementia), a pseudobulbar affect, or parkinsonism. Approximately 10% of cases of amyotrophic lateral sclerosis are familial and have been associated with mutations at several different genetic loci, including a hexanucleotide repeat on chromosome 9 that also associates with frontotemporal dementia.

Differential Diagnosis

The spinal muscular atrophies (SMAs) are inherited syndromes caused most often by mutations of the survival motor neuron (*SMN*) gene on chromosome 5. Different mutations result in more or less severe disruptions of the protein, resulting in an age of onset that ranges from infancy (SMA type I; Werdnig-Hoffmann disease), to early (type II) or late childhood (type III; Kugelberg-Welander syndrome), to adulthood (type IV). X-linked bulbospinal neuronopathy (Kennedy syndrome) is associated with an expanded trinucleotide repeat sequence on the androgen receptor gene and carries a more benign prognosis than other forms of motor neuron disease.

There are reports of juvenile SMA due to hexosaminidase deficiency. Pure motor syndromes resembling motor neuron disease may also occur in association with monoclonal gammopathy or multifocal motor neuropathies with conduction block. A motor neuronopathy may also develop in Hodgkin disease and has a relatively benign prognosis. Infective anterior horn cell diseases (polio virus or West Nile virus infection) can generally be distinguished by the acute onset and monophasic course of the illness, as discussed in Chapter 32.

Clinical Findings

A. Symptoms and Signs

Difficulty in swallowing, chewing, coughing, breathing, and talking (dysarthria) occur with bulbar involvement. In progressive bulbar palsy, there is drooping of the palate; a depressed gag reflex; pooling of saliva in the pharynx; a weak cough; and a wasted, fasciculating tongue. In pseudobulbar palsy, the tongue is contracted and spastic and cannot be moved rapidly from side to side. Limb involvement is characterized by motor disturbances (weakness, stiffness, wasting, fasciculations) reflecting lower or upper motor neuron dysfunction; there are no objective changes on sensory examination, although there may be vague sensory complaints. The sphincters are generally spared. Cognitive changes or pseudobulbar affect may be present. The disorder is progressive, and amyotrophic lateral sclerosis is usually fatal within 3–5 years; death usually results from pulmonary infections. Patients with bulbar involvement generally have the poorest prognosis, while patients with primary lateral sclerosis often have a longer survival despite profound quadriparesis and spasticity.

B. Laboratory and Other Studies

Electromyography may show changes of chronic partial denervation, with abnormal spontaneous activity in the resting muscle and a reduction in the number of motor units under voluntary control. In patients with suspected SMA or amyotrophic lateral sclerosis, the diagnosis should not be made with confidence unless such changes are found in at least three spinal regions (cervical, thoracic, lumbosacral) or two spinal regions and the bulbar musculature. Motor conduction velocity is usually normal but may be slightly reduced, and sensory conduction studies are also normal. Biopsy of a wasted muscle shows the histologic changes of denervation. The serum creatine kinase may be slightly elevated but never reaches the extremely high values seen in some of the muscular dystrophies. The cerebrospinal fluid is normal. There are abnormal findings on rectal biopsy and reduced hexosaminidase A in serum and leukocytes in patients with juvenile SMA due to hexosaminidase deficiency.

Treatment

Riluzole, 50 mg orally twice daily, which reduces the pre-synaptic release of glutamate, may slow progression of amyotrophic lateral sclerosis. There is otherwise no specific treatment except in patients with gammopathy, in whom plasmapheresis and immunosuppression may lead to improvement. Therapeutic trials of various neurotrophic factors and other agents to slow disease progression have yielded generally disappointing results. Symptomatic and supportive measures may include prescription of anticholinergic drugs (such as trihexyphenidyl, amitriptyline, or atropine) or use of a portable suction machine if drooling is troublesome, braces or a walker to improve mobility, and physical therapy to prevent contractures. Behavioral modification (eg, exercising facial muscles and encouraging frequent swallowing) or over-the-counter decongestants may also help mild drooling. Spasticity may be helped by baclofen or diazepam. A semiliquid diet or nasogastric tube feeding may be needed if dysphagia is severe. Gastrostomy or cricopharyngomyotomy is sometimes resorted to in extreme cases of predominant bulbar involvement, and tracheostomy may be necessary if respiratory muscles are severely affected; however, in the terminal stages of these disorders, the aim of treatment should be to keep patients as comfortable as possible. Information on palliative care is provided in Chapter 5.

When to Refer

All patients (to exclude other treatable causes of symptoms and signs) should be referred.

When to Admit

Patients may need to be admitted during the terminal stages of the disorders for palliative care.

Chen S et al. Genetics of amyotrophic lateral sclerosis: an update. Mol Neurodegener. 2013 Aug 13;8(1):28. [PMID: 23941283]
Robberecht W et al. The changing scene of amyotrophic lateral sclerosis. Nat Rev Neurosci. 2013 Apr;14(4):248–64. [PMID: 23463272]

PERIPHERAL NEUROPATHIES

Peripheral neuropathies can be categorized on the basis of the structure primarily affected. The predominant pathologic feature may be axonal degeneration (axonal or neuronal neuropathies) or paranodal or segmental demyelination. The distinction may be possible on the basis of neurophysiologic findings. Motor and sensory conduction velocity can be measured in accessible segments of peripheral nerves. In axonal neuropathies, conduction velocity is normal or reduced only mildly and needle electromyography provides evidence of denervation in affected muscles. In demyelinating neuropathies, conduction may be slowed considerably in affected fibers, and in more severe cases, conduction is blocked completely, without accompanying electromyographic signs of denervation.

POLYNEUROPATHIES & MONONEURITIS MULTIPLEX

ESSENTIALS OF DIAGNOSIS

▶ Weakness, sensory disturbances, or both in the extremities.
▶ Pain sometimes common.
▶ Depressed or absent tendon reflexes.
▶ May be family history of neuropathy.
▶ May be history of systemic illness or toxic exposure.

General Considerations

Diffuse **polyneuropathies** lead to a symmetric sensory, motor, or mixed deficit, often most marked distally. They include the hereditary, metabolic, and toxic disorders; idiopathic inflammatory polyneuropathy (Guillain-Barré syndrome); and the peripheral neuropathies that may occur as a nonmetastatic complication of malignant diseases. Involvement of motor fibers leads to flaccid weakness that is most marked distally; dysfunction of sensory fibers causes impaired sensory perception. Tendon reflexes are depressed or absent. Paresthesias, pain, and muscle tenderness may also occur. Multiple **mononeuropathies** suggest a patchy multifocal disease process such as vasculopathy (eg, diabetes, arteritis), an infiltrative process (eg, leprosy, sarcoidosis), radiation damage, or an immunologic disorder (eg, brachial plexopathy).

Clinical Findings

The cause of polyneuropathy or mononeuritis multiplex is suggested by the history, mode of onset, and predominant clinical manifestations. Laboratory workup includes a complete blood count and erythrocyte sedimentation rate, serum protein electrophoresis, and immunophoresis, determination of plasma urea and electrolytes, liver and thyroid function tests, tests for rheumatoid factor and antinuclear antibody, HBsAg determination, a serologic test for syphilis, fasting blood glucose level, urinary heavy metal levels, cerebrospinal fluid examination, and chest radiography. These tests should be ordered selectively, as guided by symptoms and signs. Measurement of nerve conduction velocity is important in confirming the peripheral nerve origin of symptoms and providing a means of following clinical changes, as well as indicating the likely disease process (ie, axonal or demyelinating neuropathy). Cutaneous nerve biopsy may help establish a precise diagnosis (eg, polyarteritis, amyloidosis). In about half of cases, no specific cause can be established; of these, slightly less than half are subsequently found to be familial.

Treatment

Treatment is of the underlying cause, when feasible, and is discussed below under the individual disorders. Physical therapy helps prevent contractures, and splints can maintain a weak extremity in a position of useful function. Anesthetic extremities must be protected from injury. To guard against burns, patients should check the temperature of water and hot surfaces with a portion of skin having normal sensation, measure water temperature with a thermometer, and use cold water for washing or lower the temperature setting of their hot-water heaters. Shoes should be examined frequently during the day for grit or foreign objects in order to prevent pressure lesions.

Patients with polyneuropathies or mononeuritis multiplex are subject to additional nerve injury at pressure points and should therefore avoid such behavior as leaning on elbows or sitting with crossed legs for lengthy periods.

Neuropathic, burning pain may respond to simple analgesics, such as aspirin or nonsteroidal anti-inflammatory agents, and to gabapentin (300 mg orally three times daily, titrated up to a maximum of 1200 mg orally three times daily as necessary). Duloxetine (60 mg orally daily) or venlafaxine (start 37.5 mg orally twice daily, and titrate up to 75 mg orally two to three times daily) may be helpful, especially in painful diabetic neuropathy. Opioids may be necessary for severe hyperpathia or pain induced by minimal stimuli, but their use should be avoided as much as possible. The use of a frame or cradle to reduce contact with bedclothes may be helpful. Many patients experience episodic stabbing pains, which may respond to gabapentin, pregabalin (100 mg orally three times daily), carbamazepine (start 100 mg orally twice daily, and titrate up to 400 mg orally twice daily), or tricyclic antidepressants (eg, amitriptyline 10–150 mg orally at bedtime daily).

Symptoms of autonomic dysfunction are occasionally troublesome. Postural hypotension is often helped by wearing waist-high elastic stockings and sleeping in a semierect position at night. Fludrocortisone reduces postural hypotension, but doses as high as 1 mg/d are sometimes necessary for patients with diabetes and may lead to recumbent hypertension. Midodrine, an alpha-agonist, is sometimes helpful in a dose of 2.5–10 mg three times daily. Erectile dysfunction and diarrhea are difficult to treat; a flaccid neuropathic bladder may respond to parasympathomimetic drugs such as bethanechol chloride, 10–50 mg three or four times daily.

Alport AR et al. Clinical approach to peripheral neuropathy: anatomic localization and diagnostic testing. Continuum (Minneap Minn). 2012 Feb;18(1):13–38. [PMID: 22810068]
Chaparro LE et al. Combination pharmacotherapy for the treatment of neuropathic pain in adults. Cochrane Database Syst Rev. 2012 Jul 11;7:CD008943. [PMID: 22786518]

1. Inherited Neuropathies

A. Charcot-Marie-Tooth Disease (HMSN Type I, II)

Several distinct varieties of Charcot-Marie-Tooth disease can be recognized. There is usually an autosomal dominant mode of inheritance, but occasional cases occur on a sporadic, recessive, or X-linked basis. The responsible gene is commonly located on the short arm of chromosome 17 and less often shows linkage to chromosome 1 or the X chromosome. It has also been linked to several other chromosomes, emphasizing the genetic heterogeneity of the disorder. Clinical presentation may be with foot deformities or gait disturbances in childhood or early adult life. Slow progression leads to the typical features of polyneuropathy, with distal weakness and wasting that begin in the legs, a variable amount of distal sensory loss, and depressed or absent tendon reflexes. Tremor is a conspicuous feature in some instances. Electrodiagnostic studies show a marked reduction in motor and sensory conduction velocity (hereditary motor and sensory neuropathy [HMSN] type I). In other instances (HMSN type II), motor conduction velocity is normal or only slightly reduced, sensory nerve action potentials may be absent, and signs of chronic partial denervation are found in affected muscles electromyographically. The predominant pathologic change is axonal loss rather than segmental demyelination.

A similar disorder may occur in patients with progressive distal SMA, but there is no sensory loss; electrophysiologic investigation reveals that motor conduction velocity is normal or only slightly reduced, and nerve action potentials are normal.

Rossor AM et al. Clinical implications of genetic advances in Charcot-Marie-Tooth disease. Nat Rev Neurol. 2013 Oct;9 (10):562–71. [PMID: 24018473]

B. Dejerine-Sottas Disease (HMSN Type III)

The disorder may occur on a sporadic, autosomal dominant or, less commonly, autosomal recessive basis. Onset in infancy or childhood leads to a progressive motor and sensory polyneuropathy with weakness, ataxia, sensory loss, and depressed or absent tendon reflexes. The peripheral nerves may be palpably enlarged and are characterized pathologically by segmental demyelination, Schwann cell hyperplasia, and thin myelin sheaths. Electrophysiologically, there is slowing of conduction, and sensory action potentials may be unrecordable.

C. Friedreich Ataxia

This disorder, the only known autosomal recessive trinucleotide repeat disease, is caused by expansion of a poly-GAA locus in the gene for frataxin on chromosome 9, leading to symptoms in childhood or early adult life. The gait becomes ataxic, the hands become clumsy, and other signs of cerebellar dysfunction develop accompanied by weakness of the legs and extensor plantar responses. Involvement of peripheral sensory fibers leads to sensory disturbances in the limbs and depressed tendon reflexes. There is bilateral pes cavus. Pathologically, there is a marked loss of cells in the posterior root ganglia and degeneration of peripheral sensory fibers. In the central nervous system, changes are conspicuous in the posterior and lateral columns of the cord. Electrophysiologically, conduction velocity in motor fibers is normal or only mildly reduced, but sensory action potentials are small or absent. Cardiac disease is the most common cause of death.

In the differential diagnosis for Friedreich ataxia are other spinocerebellar ataxias, a growing group of at least 29 inherited disorders, each involving a different identified gene. These heterogeneous disorders, which frequently (but not exclusively) exhibit an autosomal dominant inheritance pattern and poly-CAG expansion of the affected gene, typically cause cerebellar ataxia and varying combinations of other symptoms (such as peripheral neuropathy, ophthalmoparesis, dysarthria, and pyramidal and extrapyramidal signs).

Parkinson MH et al. Clinical features of Friedreich's ataxia: classical and atypical phenotypes. J Neurochem. 2013 Aug;126 (Suppl 1):103–17. [PMID: 23859346]

D. Refsum Disease (HMSN Type IV)

This autosomal recessive disorder is due to a disturbance in phytanic acid metabolism. Clinically, pigmentary retinal degeneration is accompanied by progressive sensorimotor polyneuropathy and cerebellar signs. Auditory dysfunction, cardiomyopathy, and cutaneous manifestations may also occur. Motor and sensory conduction velocity are reduced, often markedly, and there may be electromyographic evidence of denervation in affected muscles. Dietary restriction of phytanic acid and its precursors may be helpful therapeutically. Plasmapheresis to reduce stored phytanic acid may help at the initiation of treatment.

Zolotov D et al. Long-term strategies for the treatment of Refsum's disease using therapeutic apheresis. J Clin Apher. 2012;27(2):99–105. [PMID: 22267052]

E. Porphyria

Peripheral nerve involvement may occur during acute attacks in both variegate porphyria and acute intermittent porphyria. Motor symptoms usually occur first, and weakness is often most marked proximally and in the upper limbs rather than the lower. Sensory symptoms and signs may be proximal or distal in distribution. Autonomic involvement is sometimes pronounced. The electrophysiologic findings are in keeping with the results of neuropathologic studies suggesting that the neuropathy is axonal in type. Hematin (4 mg/kg intravenously over 15 minutes once or twice daily) may lead to rapid improvement. A high-carbohydrate diet and, in severe cases, intravenous glucose or levulose may also be helpful. Propranolol (up to 100 mg orally every 4 hours) may control tachycardia and hypertension in acute attacks.

2. Neuropathies Associated with Systemic & Metabolic Disorders

A. Diabetes Mellitus

In this disorder, involvement of the peripheral nervous system may lead to symmetric sensory or mixed polyneuropathy, asymmetric motor radiculoneuropathy or plexopathy (diabetic amyotrophy), thoracoabdominal radiculopathy, autonomic neuropathy, or isolated lesions of individual nerves. These may occur singly or in any combination and are discussed in Chapter 27.

Smith AG et al. Diabetic neuropathy. Continuum (Minneap Minn). 2012 Feb;18(1):60–84. [PMID: 22810070]
Snedecor SJ et al. Systematic review and meta-analysis of pharmacological therapies for painful diabetic peripheral neuropathy. Pain Pract. 2014 Feb;14(2):167–84. [PMID: 23534696]

B. Uremia

Uremia may lead to a symmetric sensorimotor polyneuropathy that tends to affect the lower limbs more than the upper limbs and is more marked distally than proximally (see Chapter 22). The diagnosis can be confirmed electrophysiologically, for motor and sensory conduction velocity is moderately reduced. The neuropathy improves both clinically and electrophysiologically with kidney transplantation and to a lesser extent with chronic dialysis.

Said G. Uremic neuropathy. Handb Clin Neurol. 2013;115: 607–12. [PMID: 23931805]

C. Alcoholism and Nutritional Deficiency

Many patients with alcoholism have an axonal distal sensorimotor polyneuropathy that is frequently accompanied by painful cramps, muscle tenderness, and painful paresthesias and is often more marked in the legs than in the arms. Symptoms of autonomic dysfunction may also be conspicuous. Motor and sensory conduction velocity may be slightly reduced, even in subclinical cases, but gross slowing of conduction is uncommon. A similar distal sensorimotor polyneuropathy is a well-recognized feature of beriberi (thiamine deficiency). In vitamin B_{12} deficiency, distal sensory polyneuropathy may develop but is usually overshadowed by central nervous system manifestations (eg, myelopathy, optic neuropathy, or intellectual changes).

D. Paraproteinemias

A symmetric sensorimotor polyneuropathy that is gradual in onset, progressive in course, and often accompanied by pain and dysesthesias in the limbs may occur in patients (especially men) with multiple myeloma. The neuropathy is of the axonal type in classic lytic myeloma, but segmental demyelination (primary or secondary) and axonal loss may occur in sclerotic myeloma and lead to predominantly motor clinical manifestations. Both demyelinating and axonal neuropathies are also observed in patients with paraproteinemias without myeloma. A small fraction will develop myeloma if serially followed. The demyelinating neuropathy in these patients may be due to the monoclonal protein's reacting to a component of the nerve myelin. The neuropathy of classic multiple myeloma is poorly responsive to therapy. The polyneuropathy of benign monoclonal gammopathy may respond to immunosuppressant drugs and plasmapheresis.

Polyneuropathy may also occur in association with macroglobulinemia and cryoglobulinemia and sometimes responds to plasmapheresis. Entrapment neuropathy, such as carpal tunnel syndrome, is more common than polyneuropathy in patients with (nonhereditary) generalized amyloidosis. With polyneuropathy due to amyloidosis, sensory and autonomic symptoms are especially conspicuous, whereas distal wasting and weakness occur later; there is no specific treatment.

3. Neuropathies Associated with Infectious & Inflammatory Diseases

A. Leprosy

Leprosy is an important cause of peripheral neuropathy in certain parts of the world. Sensory disturbances are mainly due to involvement of intracutaneous nerves. In tuberculoid leprosy, they develop at the same time and in the same distribution as the skin lesion but may be more extensive if nerve trunks lying beneath the lesion are also involved. In lepromatous leprosy, there is more extensive sensory loss, and this develops earlier and to a greater extent in the coolest regions of the body, such as the dorsal surfaces of the hands and feet, where the bacilli proliferate most actively. Motor deficits result from involvement of superficial nerves where their temperature is lowest, eg, the ulnar nerve in the region proximal to the olecranon groove, the median nerve as it emerges from beneath the forearm flexor muscle to run toward the carpal tunnel, the peroneal nerve at the head of the fibula, and the posterior tibial nerve in the lower part of the leg; patchy facial muscular weakness may also occur owing to involvement of the superficial branches of the seventh cranial nerve.

Motor disturbances in leprosy are suggestive of multiple mononeuropathy, whereas sensory changes resemble those of distal polyneuropathy. Examination, however, relates the distribution of sensory deficits to the temperature of the tissues; in the legs, for example, sparing frequently occurs between the toes and in the popliteal fossae, where the temperature is higher. Treatment is with antileprotic agents (see Chapter 33).

B. AIDS

A variety of neuropathies occur in HIV-infected patients (see Chapter 31).

C. Lyme Borreliosis

The neurologic manifestations of Lyme disease include meningitis, meningoencephalitis, polyradiculoneuropathy, mononeuropathy multiplex, and cranial neuropathy. Serologic tests establish the underlying disorder. Lyme disease and its treatment are discussed in depth in Chapter 34.

D. Sarcoidosis

Cranial nerve palsies (especially facial palsy), multiple mononeuropathy and, less commonly, symmetric polyneuropathy may all occur, the latter sometimes preferentially affecting either motor or sensory fibers. Improvement may occur with use of corticosteroids.

E. Polyarteritis

Involvement of the vasa nervorum by the vasculitic process may result in infarction of the nerve. Clinically, one encounters an asymmetric sensorimotor polyneuropathy (mononeuritis multiplex) that pursues a waxing and waning course. Corticosteroids and cytotoxic agents—especially cyclophosphamide—may be of benefit in severe cases.

F. Rheumatoid Arthritis

Compressive or entrapment neuropathies, ischemic neuropathies, mild distal sensory polyneuropathy, and severe progressive sensorimotor polyneuropathy can occur in rheumatoid arthritis.

4. Neuropathy Associated with Critical Illness

Patients in intensive care units with sepsis and multiorgan failure sometimes develop polyneuropathies. This may be manifested initially by unexpected difficulty in weaning patients from a mechanical ventilator and in more advanced cases by wasting and weakness of the extremities and loss of tendon reflexes. Sensory abnormalities are relatively inconspicuous. The neuropathy is axonal in type. Its pathogenesis is obscure, and treatment is supportive. The prognosis is good provided patients recover from the underlying critical illness.

5. Toxic Neuropathies

Axonal polyneuropathy may follow exposure to industrial agents or pesticides such as acrylamide, organophosphorus compounds, hexacarbon solvents, methyl bromide, and carbon disulfide; metals such as arsenic, thallium, mercury, and lead; and drugs such as phenytoin, perhexiline, isoniazid, nitrofurantoin, vincristine, and pyridoxine in high doses. Detailed occupational, environmental, and medical histories and recognition of clusters of cases are important in suggesting the diagnosis. Treatment is by preventing further exposure to the causal agent. Isoniazid neuropathy is prevented by pyridoxine supplementation.

Diphtheritic neuropathy results from a neurotoxin released by the causative organism and is common in many areas. Palatal weakness may develop 2–4 weeks after infection of the throat, and infection of the skin may similarly be followed by focal weakness of neighboring muscles. Disturbances of accommodation may occur about 4–5 weeks after infection and distal sensorimotor demyelinating polyneuropathy after 1–3 months.

6. Neuropathies Associated with Malignant Diseases

Both a sensorimotor and a purely sensory polyneuropathy may occur as a nonmetastatic complication of malignant diseases, and have been associated with circulating anti-MAG or anti-Hu antibodies that can be detected by a paraneoplastic antibody panel that is available commercially. The sensorimotor polyneuropathy may be mild and occur in the course of known malignant disease, or it may have an acute or subacute onset, lead to severe disability, and occur before there is any clinical evidence of the cancer, occasionally following a remitting course. An autonomic neuropathy may also occur as a paraneoplastic disorder related to the presence of anti-Hu antibodies or to an antibody against ganglionic acetylcholine receptors (anti-nAChR).

7. Acute Idiopathic Polyneuropathy (Guillain-Barré Syndrome)

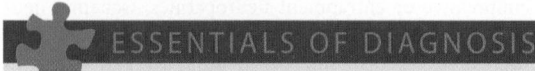

ESSENTIALS OF DIAGNOSIS

▶ Acute or subacute progressive polyradiculoneuropathy.

▶ Weakness is more severe than sensory disturbances.

▶ Acute dysautonomia may be life-threatening.

General Considerations

This acute or subacute polyradiculoneuropathy sometimes follows infective illness, inoculations, or surgical procedures. There is an association with preceding *Campylobacter jejuni* enteritis. The disorder probably has an immunologic basis, but the precise mechanism is unclear.

Clinical Findings

A. Symptoms and Signs

The main complaint is of weakness that varies widely in severity in different patients and often has a proximal emphasis and symmetric distribution. It usually begins in the legs, spreading to a variable extent but frequently involving the arms and often one or both sides of the face. The muscles of respiration or deglutition may also be affected. Sensory symptoms are usually less conspicuous than motor ones, but distal paresthesias and dysesthesias are common, and neuropathic or radicular pain is present in many patients. Autonomic disturbances are also common, may be severe, and are sometimes life-threatening; they include tachycardia, cardiac irregularities, hypotension or hypertension, facial flushing, abnormalities of sweating, pulmonary dysfunction, and impaired sphincter control. The axonal subtypes of the syndrome (acute motor axonal neuropathy [AMAN] and acute motor and sensory axonal neuropathy [AMSAN]) are caused by antibodies to gangliosides on the axon membrane, including anti-GM1, anti-GM1b, anti-GD1a, anti-GD1b, and (in AMAN) anti-GalNAC-GD1a antibodies. The Miller Fisher syndrome, another subtype, is characterized by the clinical triad of ophthalmoplegia, ataxia, and areflexia, and is associated with anti-GQ1b antibodies.

B. Laboratory Findings

The cerebrospinal fluid characteristically contains a high protein concentration with a normal cell content, but these changes may take 2 or 3 weeks to develop. Electrophysiologic studies may reveal marked abnormalities, which do not necessarily parallel the clinical disorder in their temporal course. Pathologic examination shows primary demyelination or, less commonly, axonal degeneration.

Differential Diagnosis

When the diagnosis is made, the history and appropriate laboratory studies should exclude the possibility of porphyric, diphtheritic, or toxic (heavy metal, hexacarbon, organophosphate) neuropathies. The temporal course excludes other peripheral neuropathies. Poliomyelitis, botulism, and tick paralysis must also be considered as they cause weakness of acute onset. The presence of pyramidal signs, a markedly asymmetric motor deficit, a sharp sensory level, or early sphincter involvement should suggest a focal cord lesion.

Treatment

Treatment with prednisone is ineffective and may prolong recovery time. Plasmapheresis is of value; it is best performed within the first few days of illness and is particularly useful for clinically severe or rapidly progressive cases or those with ventilatory impairment. IVIG (400 mg/kg/d for 5 days) is equally helpful and imposes less stress on the cardiovascular system than plasmapheresis. Patients should be admitted to intensive care units if their forced vital capacity is declining, and intubation is considered if the forced vital capacity reaches 15 mL/kg, the mean inspiratory force reaches −40 mm Hg, dyspnea becomes evident, or the oxygen saturation declines. Respiratory toilet and chest physical therapy help prevent atelectasis. Marked hypotension may respond to volume replacement or pressor agents. Low-dose heparin to prevent pulmonary embolism should be considered.

Approximately 3% of patients with acute idiopathic polyneuropathy have one or more clinically similar relapses, sometimes several years after the initial illness. Plasma exchange therapy may produce improvement in chronic and relapsing inflammatory polyneuropathy.

Prognosis

Most patients eventually make a good recovery, but this may take many months, and about 20% of patients are left with persisting disability.

When to Refer

All patients should be referred.

When to Admit

All patients should be hospitalized until their condition is stable and there is no respiratory compromise.

Arcila-Londono X et al. Guillain-Barré syndrome. Semin Neurol. 2012 Jul;32(3):179–86. [PMID: 23117942]

Hughes RA et al. Corticosteroids for Guillain-Barré syndrome. Cochrane Database Syst Rev. 2012 Aug 15;8:CD001446. [PMID: 22895921]

Hughes RA et al. Intravenous immunoglobulin for Guillain-Barré syndrome. Cochrane Database Syst Rev. 2012 Jul 11;7:CD002063. [PMID: 22786476]

Raphaël JC et al. Plasma exchange for Guillain-Barré syndrome. Cochrane Database Syst Rev. 2012 Jul 11;7:CD001798. [PMID: 22786475]

8. Chronic Inflammatory Polyneuropathy

Chronic inflammatory demyelinating polyneuropathy, an acquired immunologically mediated disorder, is clinically similar to Guillain-Barré syndrome except that it has a relapsing or steadily progressive course over months or years and that autonomic dysfunction is generally less common. It may present as an exclusively motor disorder or with a mixed sensorimotor disturbance. In the relapsing form, partial recovery may occur after some relapses, but in other instances there is no recovery between exacerbations. Although remission may occur spontaneously with time, the disorder frequently follows a progressive downhill course leading to severe functional disability.

Electrodiagnostic studies show marked slowing of motor and sensory conduction, and focal conduction block. Signs of partial denervation may also be present owing to secondary axonal degeneration. Nerve biopsy may show chronic perivascular inflammatory infiltrates in the endoneurium and epineurium, without accompanying evidence of vasculitis. However, a normal nerve biopsy result or the presence of nonspecific abnormalities does not exclude the diagnosis.

Corticosteroids may arrest or reverse the downhill course. Treatment is usually begun with prednisone, 60–80 mg orally daily, continued for 2–3 months or until a definite response has occurred. If no response has occurred despite 3 months of treatment, a higher dose may be tried. In responsive cases, the dose is gradually tapered, but most patients become corticosteroid-dependent, often requiring prednisone, 20 mg daily on alternate days, on a long-term basis. IVIG can be used in place of, or in addition to corticosteroids and is best used as the initial treatment in pure motor syndromes. When both IVIG and corticosteroids are ineffective, plasma exchange may be worthwhile. Consistent with the notion that the condition is antibody mediated, rituximab has shown promise. Immunosuppressant or immunomodulatory drugs (such as azathioprine) may be added when the response to other measures is unsatisfactory or to enable maintenance doses of corticosteroids to be lowered. Symptomatic treatment is also important.

Benedetti L et al. Rituximab in patients with chronic inflammatory demyelinating polyradiculoneuropathy: a report of 13 cases and review of the literature. J Neurol Neurosurg Psychiatry. 2011 Mar;82(3):306–8. [PMID: 20639381]

Dimachkie MM et al. Chronic inflammatory demyelinating polyneuropathy. Curr Treat Options Neurol. 2013 Jun;15(3): 350–66. [PMID: 23564314]

MONONEUROPATHIES

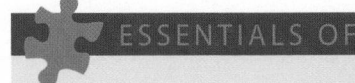

ESSENTIALS OF DIAGNOSIS

► Focal motor or sensory deficit.
► Deficit is in territory of an individual peripheral nerve.

An individual nerve may be injured along its course or may be compressed, angulated, or stretched by neighboring anatomic structures, especially at a point where it passes through a narrow space (entrapment neuropathy). The relative contributions of mechanical factors and ischemia to the local damage are not clear. With involvement of a sensory or mixed nerve, pain is commonly felt distal to the lesion. Symptoms never develop with some entrapment neuropathies, resolve rapidly and spontaneously in others, and become progressively more disabling and distressing in yet other cases. The precise neurologic deficit depends on the nerve involved. Percussion of the nerve at the site of the lesion may lead to paresthesias in its distal distribution.

Entrapment neuropathy may be the sole manifestation of subclinical polyneuropathy, and this must be borne in mind and excluded by nerve conduction studies. Such studies are also indispensable for the accurate localization of the focal lesion.

In patients with acute compression neuropathy such as may occur in intoxicated individuals ("Saturday night palsy"), no treatment is necessary. Complete recovery generally occurs, usually within 2 months, presumably because the underlying pathology is demyelination. However, axonal degeneration can occur in severe cases, and recovery then takes longer and may never be complete.

In chronic compressive or entrapment neuropathies, avoidance of aggravating factors and correction of any underlying systemic conditions are important. Local infiltration of the region about the nerve with corticosteroids may be of value; in addition, surgical decompression may help if there is a progressively increasing neurologic deficit or if electrodiagnostic studies show evidence of partial denervation in weak muscles.

Peripheral nerve tumors are uncommon, except in neurofibromatosis type 1, but also give rise to mononeuropathy. This may be distinguishable from entrapment neuropathy only by noting the presence of a mass along the course of the nerve and by demonstrating the precise site of the lesion with appropriate electrophysiologic studies. Treatment of symptomatic lesions is by surgical removal if possible.

1. Carpal Tunnel Syndrome

See Chapter 20.

2. Pronator Teres or Anterior Interosseous Syndrome

The median nerve gives off its motor branch, the anterior interosseous nerve, below the elbow as it descends between the two heads of the pronator teres muscle. A lesion of either nerve may occur in this region, sometimes after trauma or owing to compression from, for example, a fibrous band. With anterior interosseous nerve involvement, there is no sensory loss, and weakness is confined to the pronator quadratus, flexor pollicis longus, and the flexor digitorum profundus to the second and third digits. Weakness is more widespread and sensory changes occur in an appropriate distribution when the median nerve itself is affected. The prognosis is variable. If improvement does not occur spontaneously, decompressive surgery may be helpful.

Rodner CM et al. Pronator syndrome and anterior interosseous nerve syndrome. J Am Acad Orthop Surg. 2013 May;21(5): 268–75. [PMID: 23637145]

3. Ulnar Nerve Lesions

Ulnar nerve lesions are likely to occur in the elbow region as the nerve runs behind the medial epicondyle and descends into the cubital tunnel. In the condylar groove, the ulnar nerve is exposed to pressure or trauma. Moreover, any increase in the carrying angle of the elbow, whether congenital, degenerative, or traumatic, may cause excessive stretching of the nerve when the elbow is flexed. Ulnar nerve lesions may also result from thickening or distortion of the anatomic structures forming the cubital tunnel, and the resulting symptoms may also be aggravated by flexion of the elbow, because the tunnel is then narrowed by tightening of its roof or inward bulging of its floor. A severe lesion at either site causes sensory changes in the fifth and medial half of the fourth digits and along the medial border of the hand. There is weakness of the ulnar-innervated muscles in the forearm and hand. With a cubital tunnel lesion, however, there may be relative sparing of the flexor carpi ulnaris muscle. Electrophysiologic evaluation using nerve stimulation techniques allows more precise localization of the lesion.

If conservative measures are unsuccessful in relieving symptoms and preventing further progression, surgical treatment may be necessary. This consists of nerve transposition if the lesion is in the condylar groove, or a release procedure if it is in the cubital tunnel.

Ulnar nerve lesions may also develop at the wrist or in the palm of the hand, usually owing to repetitive trauma or to compression from ganglia or benign tumors. They can be subdivided depending on their presumed site. Compressive lesions are treated surgically. If repetitive mechanical trauma is responsible, this is avoided by occupational adjustment or job retraining.

Caliandro P et al. Treatment for ulnar neuropathy at the elbow. Cochrane Database Syst Rev. 2012 Jul 11;7:CD006839. [PMID: 22786500]

4. Radial Nerve Lesions

The radial nerve is particularly liable to compression or injury in the axilla (eg, by crutches or by pressure when the arm hangs over the back of a chair). This leads to weakness or paralysis of all the muscles supplied by the nerve, including the triceps. Sensory changes may also occur but are often surprisingly inconspicuous, being marked only in a small area on the back of the hand between the thumb and index finger. Injuries to the radial nerve in the spiral groove occur characteristically during deep sleep, as in intoxicated individuals (Saturday night palsy), and there is then sparing of the triceps muscle, which is supplied more proximally. The nerve may also be injured at or above the elbow; its purely motor posterior interosseous branch, supplying the extensors of the wrist and fingers, may be involved immediately below the elbow, but then there is sparing of the extensor carpi radialis longus, so that the wrist can still be extended. The superficial radial nerve may be compressed by handcuffs or a tight watch strap.

Naam NH et al. Radial tunnel syndrome. Orthop Clin North Am. 2012 Oct;43(4):529–36. [PMID: 23026469]

5. Femoral Neuropathy

The clinical features of femoral nerve palsy consist of weakness and wasting of the quadriceps muscle, with sensory impairment over the anteromedian aspect of the thigh and sometimes also of the leg to the medial malleolus, and a depressed or absent knee jerk. Isolated femoral neuropathy may occur in patients with diabetes or from compression by retroperitoneal neoplasms or hematomas (eg, expanding aortic aneurysm). Femoral neuropathy may also result from pressure from the inguinal ligament when the thighs are markedly flexed and abducted, as in the lithotomy position.

6. Meralgia Paresthetica

The lateral femoral cutaneous nerve, a sensory nerve arising from the L2 and L3 roots, may be compressed or stretched in obese or diabetic patients and during pregnancy. The nerve usually runs under the outer portion of the inguinal ligament to reach the thigh, but the ligament sometimes splits to enclose it. Hyperextension of the hip or increased lumbar lordosis—such as occurs during pregnancy—leads to nerve compression by the posterior fascicle of the ligament. However, entrapment of the nerve at any point along its course may cause similar symptoms, and several other anatomic variations predispose the nerve to damage when it is stretched. Pain, paresthesia, or numbness occurs about the outer aspect of the thigh, usually unilaterally, and is sometimes relieved by sitting. The pain stops at the knee, unlike the pain from lower lumbar sciatica that radiates to the foot. Examination shows no abnormalities except in severe cases when cutaneous sensation is impaired in the affected area. Symptoms are usually mild and commonly settle spontaneously. Hydrocortisone injections medial to the anterosuperior iliac spine often relieve symptoms temporarily, while nerve decompression by transposition may provide more lasting relief.

Khalil N et al. Treatment for meralgia paraesthetica. Cochrane Database Syst Rev. 2012 Dec 12;12:CD004159. [PMID: 23235604]

Parisi TJ et al. Meralgia paresthetica: relation to obesity, advanced age, and diabetes mellitus. Neurology. 2011 Oct 18;77(16): 1538–42. [PMID: 21975198]

7. Sciatic & Common Peroneal (Fibular) Nerve Palsies

Misplaced deep intramuscular injections are probably still the most common cause of sciatic nerve palsy. Trauma to the buttock, hip, or thigh may also be responsible. The resulting clinical deficit depends on whether the whole nerve has been affected or only certain fibers. In general, the peroneal (fibular) fibers of the sciatic nerve are more susceptible to damage than those destined for the tibial nerve. A sciatic nerve lesion may therefore be difficult to distinguish from peroneal (fibular) neuropathy unless there is electromyographic evidence of involvement of the short head of the biceps femoris muscle. The common peroneal (fibular) nerve itself may be compressed or injured in the region of the head and neck of the fibula, eg, by sitting with crossed legs or wearing high boots. There is weakness of dorsiflexion and eversion of the foot, accompanied by numbness or blunted sensation of the anterolateral aspect of the calf and dorsum of the foot.

8. Tarsal Tunnel Syndrome

The tibial nerve, the other branch of the sciatic, supplies several muscles in the lower extremity, gives origin to the sural nerve, and then continues as the posterior tibial nerve to supply the plantar flexors of the foot and toes. It passes through the tarsal tunnel behind and below the medial malleolus, giving off calcaneal branches and the medial and lateral plantar nerves that supply small muscles of the foot and the skin on the plantar aspect of the foot and toes. Compression of the posterior tibial nerve or its branches between the bony floor and ligamentous roof of the tarsal tunnel leads to pain, paresthesias, and numbness over the bottom of the foot, especially at night, with sparing of the heel. Muscle weakness may be hard to recognize clinically. Compressive lesions of the individual plantar nerves may also occur more distally, with clinical features similar to those of the tarsal tunnel syndrome. Treatment is surgical decompression.

9. Facial Neuropathy

An isolated facial palsy is most often idiopathic (Bell palsy, see later) but may occur in patients with HIV seropositivity, sarcoidosis, Lyme disease (Figure 24–2; also see Chapter 34) or with any process causing an inflammatory reaction in the subarachnoid space, such as meningitis. Whenever facial palsies occur bilaterally, or a facial palsy occurs in conjunction with other neurologic deficits, MRI brain imaging should be undertaken and other investigations considered.

▶ When to Refer

- If there is uncertainty about the diagnosis.
- Symptoms or signs are progressing despite treatment.

▶ When to Admit

When a patient should be hospitalized depends on the cause and treatment.

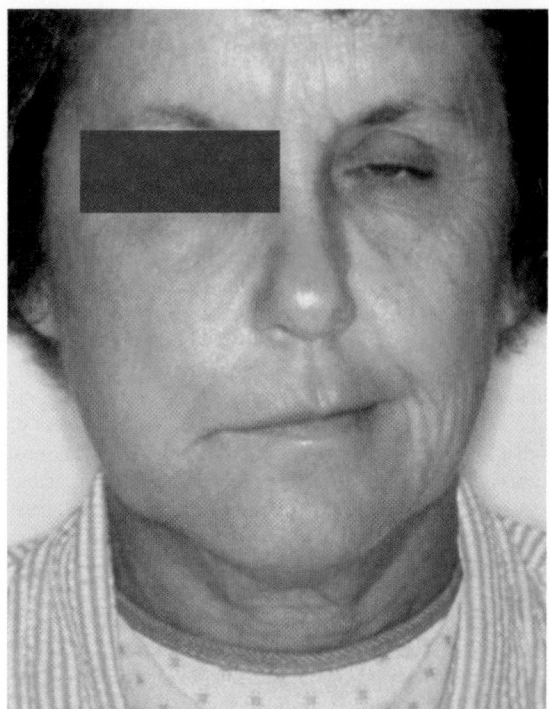

▲ **Figure 24–2.** Facial palsy caused by an infection with *Borrelia burgdorferi* (Lyme disease). (Public Health Image Library, CDC.)

BELL PALSY

ESSENTIALS OF DIAGNOSIS

- ▶ Sudden onset of lower motor neuron facial palsy.
- ▶ Hyperacusis or impaired taste may occur.
- ▶ No other neurologic abnormalities.

▶ General Considerations

Bell palsy is an idiopathic facial paresis of lower motor neuron type that has been attributed to an inflammatory reaction involving the facial nerve near the stylomastoid foramen or in the bony facial canal. Increasing evidence incriminates reactivation of herpes simplex or varicella zoster virus infection in the geniculate ganglion at least in some instances. The disorder is more common in pregnant women or in persons with diabetes mellitus.

▶ Clinical Findings

The facial paresis (Figure 24–2) generally comes on abruptly, but it may worsen over the following day or so. Pain about the ear precedes or accompanies the weakness in many cases but usually lasts for only a few days. The face itself feels stiff and pulled to one side. There may be ipsilateral restriction of eye closure and difficulty with eating and fine facial movements. A disturbance of taste is common, owing to involvement of chorda tympani fibers, and hyperacusis due to involvement of fibers to the stapedius occurs occasionally.

▶ Treatment

Other disorders that can produce a facial palsy and require specific treatment, such as tumors, Lyme disease, AIDS, sarcoidosis, and herpes zoster infection of the geniculate ganglion, must be excluded. The management of Bell palsy is controversial. Approximately 60% of cases recover completely without treatment, presumably because the lesion is so mild that it leads merely to conduction block. Considerable improvement occurs in most other cases, and only about 10% of all patients have permanent disfigurement or other long-term sequelae. Treatment is unnecessary in most cases but is indicated for patients in whom an unsatisfactory outcome can be predicted. The best clinical guide to progress is the severity of the palsy during the first few days after presentation. Patients with clinically complete palsy when first seen are less likely to make a full recovery than those with an incomplete one. A poor prognosis for recovery is also associated with advanced age, hyperacusis, and severe initial pain. Electromyography and nerve excitability or conduction studies provide a guide to prognosis but not early enough to aid in the selection of patients for treatment.

The only medical treatment that may influence the outcome is administration of corticosteroids, but this must be commenced within 5 days of onset. Treatment with prednisone, 60–80 mg orally daily for 4 or 5 days, followed by tapering of the dose over the next 7–10 days, is a satisfactory regimen; prednisolone (50 mg daily orally) for 10 days is another acceptable alternative. It is helpful to protect the eye with lubricating drops (or lubricating ointment at night) and a patch if eye closure is not possible. Acyclovir does not confer any additional benefit. There is no evidence that surgical procedures to decompress the facial nerve are of benefit. Physical therapy may improve facial function.

Gronseth GS et al. Evidence-based guideline update: steroids and antivirals for Bell palsy: report of the Guideline Development Subcommittee of the American Academy of Neurology. Neurology. 2012 Nov 27;79(22):2209–13. [PMID: 23136264]
Teixeira LJ et al. Physical therapy for Bell's palsy (idiopathic facial paralysis). Cochrane Database Syst Rev. 2011 Dec 7;(12):CD006283. [PMID: 22161401]

DISCOGENIC NECK PAIN

ESSENTIALS OF DIAGNOSIS

- ▶ Neck pain, sometimes radiating to arms.
- ▶ Restricted neck movements.
- ▶ Motor, sensory, or reflex changes in arms with root involvement.
- ▶ Neurologic deficit in legs, gait disorder, or sphincter disturbance with cord involvement.

▶ General Considerations

A variety of congenital abnormalities may involve the cervical spine and lead to neck pain; these include hemivertebrae, fused vertebrae, basilar impression, and instability of the atlantoaxial joint. Traumatic, degenerative, infective, and neoplastic disorders may also lead to pain in the neck. When rheumatoid arthritis involves the spine, it tends to affect especially the cervical region, leading to pain, stiffness, and reduced mobility; displacement of vertebrae or atlantoaxial subluxation may lead to cord compression that can be life-threatening if not treated by fixation. Further details are given in Chapter 20 (including a discussion on low back pain), and discussion here is restricted to disk disease.

1. Acute Cervical Disk Protrusion

Acute cervical disk protrusion leads to pain in the neck and radicular pain in the arm, exacerbated by head movement. With lateral herniation of the disk, motor, sensory, or reflex changes may be found in a radicular (usually C6 or C7) distribution on the affected side (Figure 24–3); with more centrally directed herniations, the spinal cord may also be involved, leading to spastic paraparesis and sensory disturbances in the legs, sometimes accompanied by impaired sphincter function. The diagnosis is confirmed by MRI or CT myelography. In mild cases, bed rest or intermittent neck traction may help, followed by immobilization of the neck in a collar for several weeks. If these measures are unsuccessful or the patient has a significant neurologic deficit, surgical removal of the protruding disk may be necessary.

2. Cervical Spondylosis

Cervical spondylosis results from chronic cervical disk degeneration, with herniation of disk material, secondary calcification, and associated osteophytic outgrowths. One or more of the cervical nerve roots may be compressed, stretched, or angulated; and myelopathy may also develop as a result of compression, vascular insufficiency, or recurrent minor trauma to the cord. Patients present with neck pain and restricted head movement, occipital headaches, radicular pain and other sensory disturbances in the arms, weakness of the arms or legs, or some combination of these symptoms. Examination generally reveals that lateral flexion and rotation of the neck are limited. A segmental pattern of weakness or dermatomal sensory loss (or both) may be found unilaterally or bilaterally in the upper limbs, and tendon reflexes mediated by the affected root or roots are depressed. The C5 and C6 nerve roots are most commonly involved, and examination frequently then reveals weakness of muscles supplied by these roots (eg, deltoids, supraspinatus and infraspinatus, biceps, brachioradialis), pain or sensory loss about the shoulder and outer border of the arm and forearm, and depressed biceps and brachioradialis reflexes. Spastic paraparesis may also be present if there is an associated myelopathy, sometimes accompanied by posterior column or spinothalamic sensory deficits in the legs.

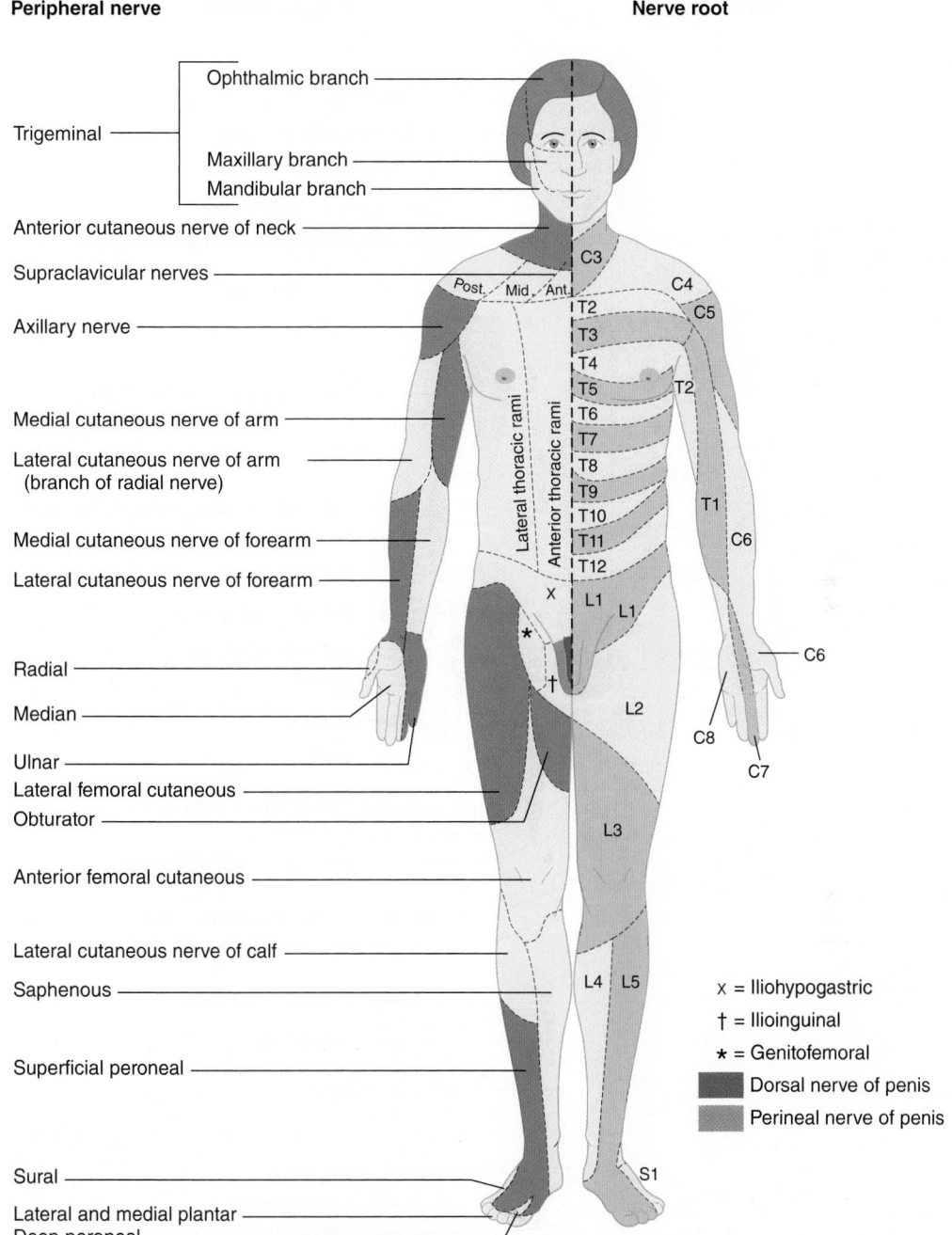

Peripheral nerve

Trigeminal
- Ophthalmic branch
- Maxillary branch
- Mandibular branch

Anterior cutaneous nerve of neck

Supraclavicular nerves

Axillary nerve

Medial cutaneous nerve of arm

Lateral cutaneous nerve of arm (branch of radial nerve)

Medial cutaneous nerve of forearm

Lateral cutaneous nerve of forearm

Radial

Median

Ulnar

Lateral femoral cutaneous

Obturator

Anterior femoral cutaneous

Lateral cutaneous nerve of calf

Saphenous

Superficial peroneal

Sural

Lateral and medial plantar

Deep peroneal

Nerve root

C3
C4
C5
Post. Mid. Ant.
T2
T3
T4
T5
T6
T7
T8
T9
T10
T11
T12
L1
L2
L3
L4 L5
S1

Lateral thoracic rami
Anterior thoracic rami

T2
T1
C6
C6
C8
C7

x = Iliohypogastric
† = Ilioinguinal
★ = Genitofemoral
■ Dorsal nerve of penis
■ Perineal nerve of penis

▲ **Figure 24–3.** Cutaneous innervation. The segmental or radicular (root) distribution is shown on the left side of the body and the peripheral nerve distribution on the right side. Above: anterior view; facing page: posterior view. (Reproduced, with permission, from Haymaker W, Woodhall B. *Peripheral Nerve Injuries*, 2nd ed. Philadelphia, Saunders, 1953.)

Plain radiographs of the cervical spine show osteophyte formation, narrowing of disk spaces, and encroachment on the intervertebral foramina, but such changes are common in middle-aged persons and may be unrelated to the presenting complaint. CT or MRI helps confirm the diagnosis and exclude other structural causes of the myelopathy.

Restriction of neck movements by a cervical collar may relieve pain. Local injection of local anesthetics or corticosteroids, for instance by a pain management specialist, may be of benefit. Operative treatment may be necessary to prevent further progression if there is a significant neurologic deficit or if root pain is severe, persistent, and unresponsive to conservative measures.

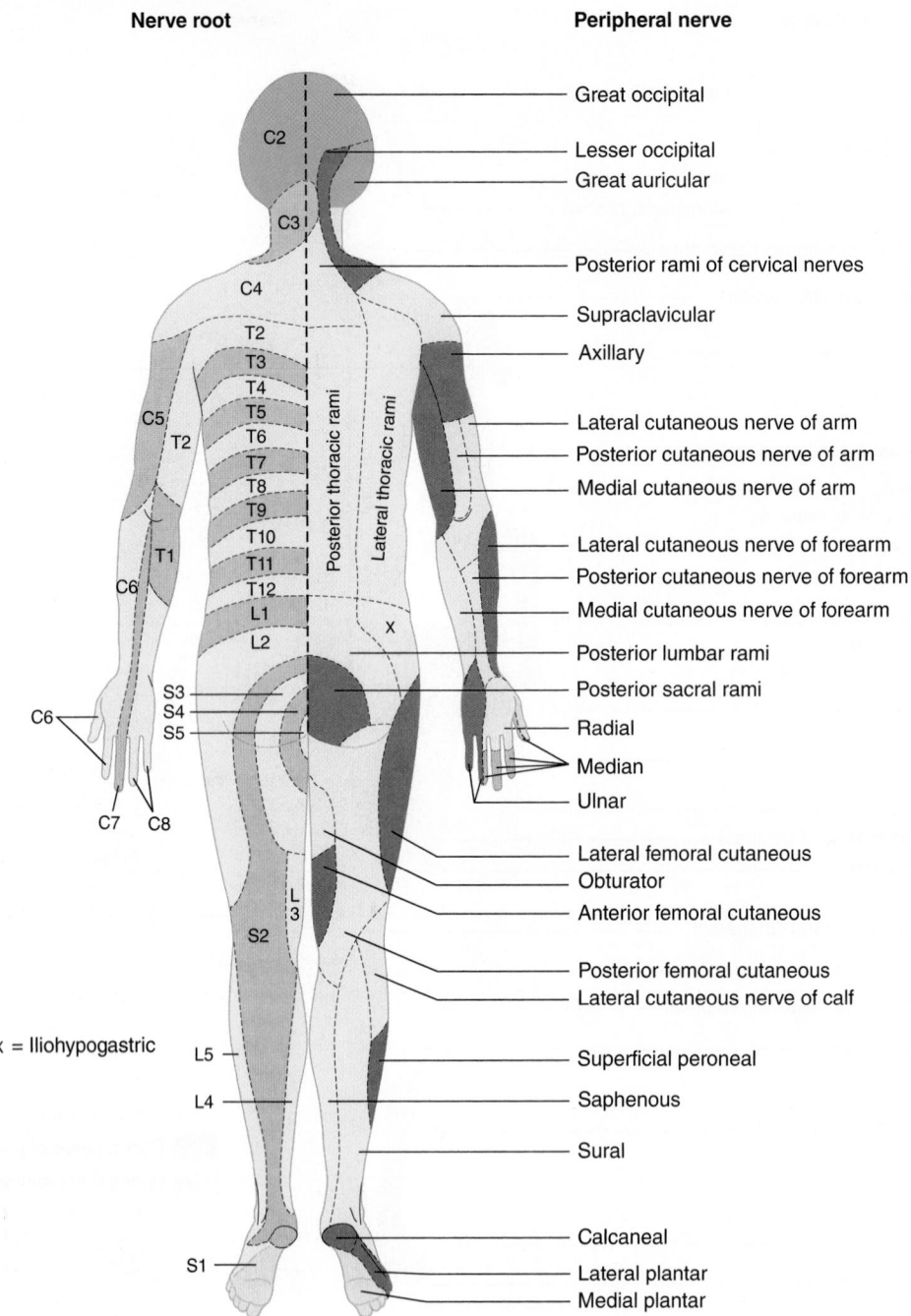

Nerve root — Peripheral nerve

- Great occipital
- Lesser occipital
- Great auricular
- Posterior rami of cervical nerves
- Supraclavicular
- Axillary
- Lateral cutaneous nerve of arm
- Posterior cutaneous nerve of arm
- Medial cutaneous nerve of arm
- Lateral cutaneous nerve of forearm
- Posterior cutaneous nerve of forearm
- Medial cutaneous nerve of forearm
- Posterior lumbar rami
- Posterior sacral rami
- Radial
- Median
- Ulnar
- Lateral femoral cutaneous
- Obturator
- Anterior femoral cutaneous
- Posterior femoral cutaneous
- Lateral cutaneous nerve of calf
- Superficial peroneal
- Saphenous
- Sural
- Calcaneal
- Lateral plantar
- Medial plantar

x = Iliohypogastric

Posterior thoracic rami / Lateral thoracic rami

▲ **Figure 24–3.** (continued)

When to Refer

- Pain unresponsive to simple measures.
- Patients with neurologic deficits.
- Patients in whom surgical treatment is under consideration.

When to Admit

- Patients with progressive or significant neurologic deficit.
- Patients with sphincter involvement (from cord compression).
- Patients requiring surgical treatment.

Diwan S et al. Effectiveness of cervical epidural injections in the management of chronic neck and upper extremity pain. Pain Physician. 2012 Jul–Aug;15(4):E405–34. [PMID: 22828692]

Van Alfen N et al. Diagnosis of brachial and lumbosacral plexus lesions. Handb Clin Neurol. 2013;115:293–310. [PMID: 23931788]

BRACHIAL & LUMBAR PLEXUS LESIONS

1. Brachial Plexus Neuropathy

Brachial plexus neuropathy may be idiopathic, sometimes occurring in relationship to a number of different nonspecific illnesses or factors. In other instances, brachial plexus lesions follow trauma or result from congenital anomalies, neoplastic involvement, or injury by various physical agents. In rare instances, the disorder occurs on a familial basis.

Idiopathic brachial plexus neuropathy (neuralgic amyotrophy) characteristically begins with severe pain about the shoulder, followed within a few days by weakness, reflex changes, and sensory disturbances involving especially the C5 and C6 segments but affecting any nerve in the brachial plexus. Symptoms and signs are usually unilateral but may be bilateral. Wasting of affected muscles is sometimes profound. The disorder relates to disturbed function of cervical roots or part of the brachial plexus, but its precise cause is unknown. Recovery occurs over the ensuing months but may be incomplete. Treatment is purely symptomatic.

2. Cervical Rib Syndrome

Compression of the C8 and T1 roots or the lower trunk of the brachial plexus by a cervical rib or band arising from the seventh cervical vertebra leads to weakness and wasting of intrinsic hand muscles, especially those in the thenar eminence, accompanied by pain and numbness in the medial two fingers and the ulnar border of the hand and forearm. The subclavian artery may also be compressed, and this forms the basis of Adson test for diagnosing the disorder; the radial pulse is diminished or obliterated on the affected side when the seated patient inhales deeply and turns the head to one side or the other. Electromyography, nerve conduction studies, and somatosensory evoked potential studies may help confirm the diagnosis. MRI may be especially helpful in revealing the underlying compressive structure. Plain radiographs or CT scanning sometimes shows the cervical rib or a large transverse process of the seventh cervical vertebra, but normal findings do not exclude the possibility of a cervical band. Treatment of the disorder is by surgical excision of the rib or band.

3. Lumbosacral Plexus Lesions

A lumbosacral plexus lesion may develop in association with diseases such as diabetes, cancer, or bleeding disorders or in relation to injury. It occasionally occurs as an isolated phenomenon similar to idiopathic brachial plexopathy, and pain and weakness then tend to be more conspicuous than sensory symptoms. The distribution of symptoms and signs depends on the level and pattern of neurologic involvement.

DISORDERS OF NEUROMUSCULAR TRANSMISSION

1. Myasthenia Gravis

ESSENTIALS OF DIAGNOSIS

▶ Fluctuating weakness of commonly used voluntary muscles, producing symptoms such as diplopia, ptosis, and difficulty in swallowing.

▶ Activity increases weakness of affected muscles.

▶ Short-acting anticholinesterases transiently improve the weakness.

▶ General Considerations

Myasthenia gravis occurs at all ages, sometimes in association with a thymic tumor or thyrotoxicosis, as well as in rheumatoid arthritis and lupus erythematosus. It is most common in young women with HLA-DR3; if thymoma is associated, older men are more commonly affected. Onset is usually insidious, but the disorder is sometimes unmasked by a coincidental infection that leads to exacerbation of symptoms. Exacerbations may also occur before the menstrual period and during or shortly after pregnancy. Symptoms are due to a variable degree of block of neuromuscular transmission caused by autoantibodies binding to acetylcholine receptors; these are found in most patients with the disease and have a primary role in reducing the number of functioning acetylcholine receptors. Additionally, cellular immune activity against the receptor is found.

▶ Clinical Findings

A. Symptoms and Signs

Patients present with ptosis, diplopia, difficulty in chewing or swallowing, respiratory difficulties, limb weakness, or some combination of these problems. Weakness may remain localized to a few muscle groups or may become generalized. The external ocular muscles and certain other cranial muscles, including the masticatory, facial, and pharyngeal muscles, are especially likely to be affected, and the respiratory and limb muscles may also be involved. Symptoms often fluctuate in intensity during the day, and this diurnal variation is superimposed on a tendency to longer-term spontaneous relapses and remissions that may last for weeks. Nevertheless, the disorder follows a slowly progressive course and may have a fatal outcome owing to respiratory complications such as aspiration pneumonia.

Clinical examination confirms the weakness and fatigability of affected muscles. In most cases, the extraocular muscles are involved, and this leads to ocular palsies and ptosis, which are commonly asymmetric. Pupillary responses are normal. The bulbar and limb muscles are often weak, but the pattern of involvement is variable. Sustained activity of affected muscles increases the weakness, which improves after a brief rest. Sensation is normal, and there are usually no reflex changes.

Life-threatening exacerbations of myasthenia (so-called **myasthenic crisis**) may lead to respiratory weakness requiring immediate admission to the intensive care unit, where respiratory function can be monitored and ventilator support is readily available.

B. Imaging

A CT scan of the chest with and without contrast should be obtained to demonstrate a coexisting thymoma, but a normal study does not exclude this possibility.

C. Laboratory and Other Studies

Electrophysiologic demonstration of a decrementing muscle response to repetitive 2- or 3-Hz stimulation of motor nerves indicates a disturbance of neuromuscular transmission. Such an abnormality may even be detected in clinically strong muscles with certain provocative procedures. Needle electromyography of affected muscles shows a marked variation in configuration and size of individual motor unit potentials, and single-fiber electromyography reveals an increased jitter, or variability, in the time interval between two muscle fiber action potentials from the same motor unit.

Assay of serum for elevated levels of circulating acetylcholine receptor antibodies is useful because it has a sensitivity of 80–90% for the diagnosis of myasthenia gravis. Certain patients without antibodies to acetylcholine receptors have serum antibodies to muscle-specific tyrosine kinase (MuSK), which should therefore be determined; these patients are more likely to have facial, respiratory, and proximal muscle weakness than those with antibodies to acetylcholine receptors.

▶ Treatment

Medication such as aminoglycosides that may exacerbate myasthenia gravis should be avoided. Anticholinesterase drugs provide symptomatic benefit without influencing the course of the disease. Neostigmine, pyridostigmine, or both can be used, the dose being determined on an individual basis. The usual dose of neostigmine is 7.5–30 mg (average, 15 mg) orally taken four times daily; of pyridostigmine, 30–180 mg (average, 60 mg) orally four times daily. Overmedication may temporarily increase weakness.

Thymectomy usually leads to symptomatic benefit or remission and should be considered in all patients younger than age 60, unless weakness is restricted to the extraocular muscles. If the disease is of recent onset and only slowly progressive, operation is sometimes delayed for a year or so, in the hope that spontaneous remission will occur.

Treatment with corticosteroids is indicated for patients who have responded poorly to anticholinesterase drugs and have already undergone thymectomy. It is often introduced with the patient in the hospital, since weakness may initially be aggravated. Once weakness has stabilized after 2–3 weeks or any improvement is sustained, further management can be on an outpatient basis. Alternate-day treatment is usually well tolerated, but if weakness is enhanced on the nontreatment day it may be necessary for medication to be taken daily. The dose of corticosteroids is determined on an individual basis, but an initial high daily dose (eg, prednisone, 60–100 mg orally daily) can gradually be tapered to a relatively low maintenance level as improvement occurs; total withdrawal is difficult, however. Treatment with azathioprine may also be effective. The usual dose is 2–3 mg/kg orally daily after a lower initial dose. Mycophenolate mofetil or cyclosporine is typically reserved for more refractory cases or as a strategy to reduce the corticosteroid dose.

In patients with major disability, plasmapheresis or IVIG therapy may be beneficial and have similar efficacy. It is also useful for stabilizing patients before thymectomy and for managing acute crisis.

▶ When to Refer

All patients should be referred.

▶ When to Admit

- Patients with acute exacerbation or respiratory involvement.
- Patients requiring plasmapheresis.
- Patients who are starting corticosteroid therapy.
- For thymectomy.

Barth D et al. Comparison of IVIg and PLEX in patients with myasthenia gravis. Neurology. 2011 Jun 7;76(23):2017–23. [PMID: 21562253]

Díaz-Manera J et al. Treatment strategies for myasthenia gravis: an update. Expert Opin Pharmacother. 2012 Sep;13(13): 1873–83. [PMID: 22775575]

2. Myasthenic Syndrome (Lambert-Eaton Syndrome)

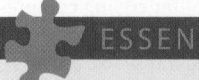

ESSENTIALS OF DIAGNOSIS

- ▶ Variable weakness, typically improving with activity.
- ▶ Dysautonomic symptoms may also be present.
- ▶ A history of malignant disease may be obtained.

▶ General Considerations

Myasthenic syndrome may be associated with small-cell carcinoma, sometimes developing before the tumor is diagnosed, and occasionally occurs with certain autoimmune diseases. There is defective release of acetylcholine in response to a nerve impulse, caused by P/Q-type voltage-gated calcium-channel antibody, and this leads to weakness, especially of the proximal muscles of the limbs. Unlike myasthenia gravis, however, power steadily increases with sustained contraction. The diagnosis can be confirmed electrophysiologically, because the muscle response to stimulation of its motor nerve increases remarkably if the nerve is stimulated repetitively at high rates, even in muscles that are not clinically weak.

Treatment with plasmapheresis and immunosuppressive drug therapy (prednisone and azathioprine) may lead to clinical and electrophysiologic improvement, in addition to therapy aimed at tumor when present. Prednisone is usually initiated in a daily dose of 60–80 mg orally and azathioprine in a daily dose of 2 mg/kg orally. Symptomatic therapy includes the use of potassium channel antagonists; of these, 3,4-diaminopyridine (60–80 mg/d orally in three divided doses) has been best studied and appears efficacious. Guanidine hydrochloride (25–50 mg/kg/d orally in divided doses) is an alternative and is occasionally helpful in seriously disabled patients, but adverse effects of the drug include marrow suppression. The response to treatment with anticholinesterase drugs such as pyridostigmine or neostigmine is usually disappointing.

Keogh M et al. Treatment for Lambert-Eaton myasthenic syndrome. Cochrane Database Syst Rev. 2011 Feb 16;(2): CD003279. [PMID: 21328260]
Titulaer MJ et al. Lambert-Eaton myasthenic syndrome: from clinical characteristics to therapeutic strategies. Lancet Neurol. 2011 Dec;10(12):1098–107. [PMID: 22094130]

3. Botulism

The toxin of *Clostridium botulinum* prevents the release of acetylcholine at neuromuscular junctions and autonomic synapses. Botulism occurs most commonly following the ingestion of contaminated home-canned food and should be suggested by the development of sudden, fluctuating, severe weakness in a previously healthy person. Symptoms begin within 72 hours following ingestion of the toxin and may progress for several days. Typically, there is diplopia, ptosis, facial weakness, dysphagia, and nasal speech, followed by respiratory difficulty and finally by weakness that appears last in the limbs. Blurring of vision (with unreactive dilated pupils) is characteristic, and there may be dryness of the mouth, constipation (paralytic ileus), and postural hypotension. Sensation is preserved, and the tendon reflexes are not affected unless the involved muscles are very weak. If the diagnosis is suspected, the local health authority should be notified and a sample of serum and contaminated food (if available) sent to be assayed for toxin. Support for the diagnosis may be obtained by electrophysiologic studies; with repetitive stimulation of motor nerves at fast rates, the muscle response increases in size progressively.

Patients should be hospitalized in case respiratory assistance becomes necessary. Treatment is with trivalent antitoxin, once it is established that the patient is not allergic to horse serum. Potassium channel antagonists may provide symptomatic relief as they do in Lambert-Eaton myasthenic syndrome (see above). Anticholinesterase drugs are of no value. Respiratory assistance and other supportive measures should be provided as necessary. Further details are provided in Chapter 33.

Chalk C et al. Medical treatment for botulism. Cochrane Database Syst Rev. 2011 Mar 16;(3):CD008123. [PMID: 21412916]

4. Disorders Associated with Use of Aminoglycosides

Aminoglycoside antibiotics, eg, gentamicin, may produce a clinical disturbance similar to botulism by preventing the release of acetylcholine from nerve endings, but symptoms subside rapidly as the responsible drug is eliminated from the body. These antibiotics are particularly dangerous in patients with preexisting disturbances of neuromuscular transmission and are therefore best avoided in patients with myasthenia gravis.

MYOPATHIC DISORDERS

1. Muscular Dystrophies

ESSENTIALS OF DIAGNOSIS

- ▶ Muscle weakness, often in a characteristic distribution.
- ▶ Age at onset and inheritance pattern depend on the specific dystrophy.

▶ General Considerations

These inherited myopathic disorders are characterized by progressive muscle weakness and wasting. They are subdivided by mode of inheritance, age at onset, and clinical features, as shown in Table 24–8. In the Duchenne type, pseudohypertrophy of muscles frequently occurs at some stage; intellectual retardation is common; and there may be skeletal deformities, muscle contractures, and cardiac involvement. The serum creatine kinase level is increased, especially in the Duchenne and Becker varieties, and mildly increased also in limb-girdle dystrophy. Electromyography may help confirm that weakness is myopathic rather than neurogenic. Similarly, histopathologic examination of a muscle biopsy specimen may help confirm that weakness is due to a primary disorder of muscle and to distinguish between various muscle diseases.

A genetic defect on the short arm of the X chromosome has been identified in Duchenne dystrophy. The affected gene codes for the protein dystrophin, which is markedly reduced or absent from the muscle of patients with the disease. Dystrophin levels are generally normal in the Becker variety, but the protein is qualitatively altered. Duchenne muscular dystrophy can be recognized early in pregnancy in about 95% of women by genetic studies; in late pregnancy, DNA probes can be used on fetal tissue obtained for this purpose by amniocentesis. The genes causing some of the other muscular dystrophies are listed in Table 24–8.

Table 24–8. The muscular dystrophies.[1]

Disorder	Inheritance	Age at Onset (years)	Distribution	Prognosis	Genetic Association
Duchenne type	X-linked recessive	1–5	Pelvic, then shoulder girdle; later, limb and respiratory muscles.	Rapid progression. Death within about 15 years after onset.	Xp21 Dystrophin (loss of functional expression)
Becker	X-linked recessive	5–25	Pelvic, then shoulder girdle.	Slow progression. May have normal life span.	Xp21 Dystrophin (reduced functional expression)
Limb-girdle (Erb)	Autosomal recessive, dominant or sporadic	10–30	Pelvic or shoulder girdle initially, with later spread to the other.	Variable severity and rate of progression. Possible severe disability in middle life.	Multiple
Facioscapulo-humeral	Autosomal dominant	Any age	Face and shoulder girdle initially; later, pelvic girdle and legs.	Slow progression. Minor disability. Usually normal life span.	4q35
Emery-Dreifuss	X-linked recessive or autosomal dominant	5–10	Humeroperoneal or scapuloperoneal.	Variable.	Xq28; Emerin (X-linked) 1q21.2; Laminin A/C (chromosome 1) Others
Distal	Autosomal dominant or recessive	40–60	Onset distally in extremities; proximal involvement later.	Slow progression.	14q12; Myosin heavy chain 7 2p13 Dysferlin
Ocular	Autosomal dominant (may be recessive)	Any age (usually 5–30)	External ocular muscles; may also be mild weakness of face, neck, and arms.		
Oculopharyngeal	Autosomal dominant	Any age	As in the ocular form but with dysphagia.		14q11.2–q13 Poly (A)-binding protein-2
Myotonic dystrophy	Autosomal dominant	Any age (usually 20–40)	Face, neck, distal limbs.	Slow progression.	19q13.2-q13.3; Dystrophia myotonica protein kinase 3q13.3-q24; Zinc-finger protein-9

[1]Not all possible genetic loci are shown.

There is no specific treatment for the muscular dystrophies, but it is important to encourage patients to lead as normal lives as possible. Prednisone (0.75 mg/kg orally daily) improves muscle strength and function in boys with Duchenne dystrophy, but side effects need to be monitored. Prolonged bed rest must be avoided, as inactivity often leads to worsening of the underlying muscle disease. Physical therapy and orthopedic procedures may help counteract deformities or contractures.

Flanigan KM. The muscular dystrophies. Semin Neurol. 2012 Jul;32(3):255–63. [PMID: 23117950]
Leung DG et al. Therapeutic advances in muscular dystrophy. Ann Neurol. 2013 Sep;74(3):404–11. [PMID: 23939629]

2. Myotonic Dystrophy

Myotonic dystrophy, a slowly progressive, dominantly inherited disorder, usually manifests itself in the third or fourth decade but occasionally appears early in childhood. Two types, with a different genetic basis, have been recognized. Myotonia leads to complaints of muscle stiffness and is evidenced by the marked delay that occurs before affected muscles can relax after a contraction. This can often be demonstrated clinically by delayed relaxation of the hand after sustained grip or by percussion of the belly of a muscle. In addition, there is weakness and wasting of the facial, sternocleidomastoid, and distal limb muscles. Associated clinical features include cataracts, frontal baldness, testicular atrophy, diabetes mellitus, cardiac abnormalities, and intellectual changes. Electromyographic sampling of affected muscles reveals myotonic discharges in addition to changes suggestive of myopathy.

It is difficult to determine whether drug therapy for myotonia is safe or effective. When myotonia is disabling, treatment with a sodium channel blocker—such as phenytoin (100 mg orally three times daily), procainamide (0.5–1 g orally four times daily), or mexiletine (150–200 mg orally three times daily)—may be helpful, but the associated side effects, particularly for antiarrhythmic drugs, are often limiting. Neither the weakness nor the course of the disorder is influenced by treatment.

Heatwole CR et al. The diagnosis and treatment of myotonic disorders. Muscle Nerve. 2013 May;47(5):632–48. [PMID: 23536309]

3. Myotonia Congenita

Myotonia congenita is commonly inherited as a dominant trait. The responsible gene on chromosome 7 encodes a voltage-gated chloride channel. Generalized myotonia without weakness is usually present from birth, but symptoms may not appear until early childhood. Patients complain of muscle stiffness that is enhanced by cold and inactivity and relieved by exercise. Muscle hypertrophy, at times pronounced, is also a feature. A recessive form with later onset is associated with slight weakness and atrophy of distal muscles. Treatment with procainamide, tocainide, mexiletine, or phenytoin may help the myotonia, as in myotonic dystrophy.

4. Polymyositis & Dermatomyositis

See Chapter 20.

5. Inclusion Body Myositis

This disorder, of unknown cause, begins insidiously, usually after middle age, with progressive proximal weakness of first the lower and then the upper extremities, and affecting facial and pharyngeal muscles. Weakness often begins in the quadriceps femoris in the lower limbs and the forearm flexors in the upper limbs. Distal weakness is usually mild. Serum creatine kinase levels may be normal or increased. The diagnosis is confirmed by muscle biopsy. Corticosteroid and immunosuppressive therapy is usually ineffective, but IVIG therapy is occasionally of mild benefit.

Dimachkie MM et al. Inclusion body myositis. Curr Neurol Neurosci Rep. 2013 Jan;13(1):321. [PMID: 23250766]

6. Mitochondrial Myopathies

The mitochondrial myopathies are a clinically diverse group of disorders that on pathologic examination of skeletal muscle with the modified Gomori stain show characteristic "ragged red fibers" containing accumulations of abnormal mitochondria. Patients may present with progressive external ophthalmoplegia or with limb weakness that is exacerbated or induced by activity. Other patients present with central neurologic dysfunction, eg, myoclonic epilepsy (myoclonic epilepsy, ragged red fiber syndrome, or MERRF), or the combination of myopathy, encephalopathy, lactic acidosis, and stroke-like episodes (MELAS). These disorders result from separate abnormalities of mitochondrial DNA. (See also Chapter 20.) Treatment is symptomatic and palliative, but various experimental approaches are being explored.

A mitochondrial myopathy may develop in patients receiving zidovudine for treatment of AIDS, and patients receiving highly active antiretroviral therapy (HAART) for HIV-1 infection may develop a lipodystrophy, with fat accumulating in muscle.

Milone M et al. Diagnosis of mitochondrial myopathies. Mol Genet Metab. 2013 Sep–Oct;110(1–2):35–41. [PMID: 23911206]

7. Myopathies Associated with Other Disorders

Myopathy may occur in association with chronic hypokalemia, any endocrinopathy, and in patients taking corticosteroids, chloroquine, colchicine, clofibrate, emetine, aminocaproic acid, statin drugs, or bretylium tosylate. Weakness is mainly proximal, and serum creatine kinase is typically normal, except in hypothyroidism and some of the toxic myopathies. Treatment is of the underlying cause. Myopathy also occurs with chronic alcoholism, whereas acute reversible muscle necrosis may occur shortly after acute alcohol intoxication. Inflammatory myopathy may occur in patients taking penicillamine; myotonia may be induced by clofibrate, and preexisting myotonia may be exacerbated or unmasked by depolarizing muscle relaxants (eg, suxamethonium), beta-blockers (eg, propranolol), fenoterol, ritodrine and, possibly, certain diuretics.

▶ When to Refer

All patients should be referred to establish the diagnosis and underlying cause.

▶ When to Admit

- For respiratory assistance.
- For rhabdomyolysis.

PERIODIC PARALYSIS SYNDROMES

Periodic paralysis may have a familial (dominant inheritance) basis. The syndromes to be described are channelopathies that manifest as abnormal, often potassium-sensitive, muscle-membrane excitability and lead clinically to episodes of flaccid weakness or paralysis, sometimes in association with abnormalities of the plasma potassium level. Strength is normal between attacks. Mutations in genes encoding three ion channels [*CACNA1S (1q32)*, *SCN4A (17q23.1-q25.3)*, and *KCNJ2 (17q23.1-q24.2)*] account for most cases. **Hypokalemic periodic paralysis** has been related to mutations in the *CACNL1A3*, *SCN4A*, or *KCNE3 (11q13-q14)* gene and is characterized by attacks that tend to occur on awakening, after exercise, or after a heavy meal and may last for several days. Patients should avoid excessive exertion. A low-carbohydrate and low-salt diet may help prevent attacks, as may acetazolamide, 250–750 mg orally daily. Nonselective beta-adrenergic blockers may also prevent recurrent paralytic attacks. An ongoing attack may be aborted by potassium chloride given orally or by intravenous drip, provided the ECG can be monitored and kidney function is satisfactory. In young Asian men, it is commonly associated with hyperthyroidism and has been related to polymorphism in the *CACNA1S* gene; treatment of the endocrine disorder prevents recurrences. In **hyper-kalemic periodic paralysis**, which is mostly associated with mutations in the *SCN4A* gene, attacks also tend to occur after exercise but usually last for < 1 hour. They may be terminated by intravenous calcium gluconate (1–2 g) or by intravenous diuretics (furosemide, 20–40 mg), glucose, or glucose and insulin; daily acetazolamide or chlorothia-zide may prevent recurrences. **Normokalemic periodic paralysis** is similar clinically to the hyperkalemic variety,

but the plasma potassium level remains normal during attacks; treatment is with acetazolamide.

▶ **When to Refer**

All patients should be referred.

Burge JA et al. Novel insights into the pathomechanisms of skel-etal muscle channelopathies. Curr Neurol Neurosci Rep. 2012 Feb;12(1):62–9. [PMID: 22083238]
Cope TE et al. Thyrotoxic periodic paralysis: correct hypoka-lemia with caution. J Emerg Med. 2013 Sep;45(3):338–40. [PMID: 23849367]

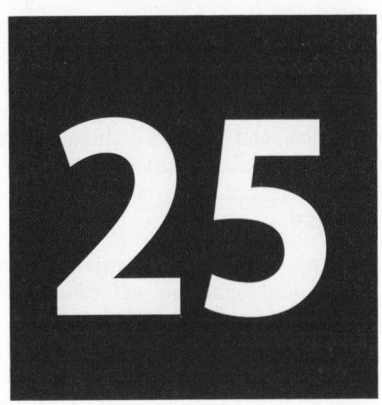

Psychiatric Disorders

Charles DeBattista, DMH, MD
Stuart J. Eisendrath, MD
Jonathan E. Lichtmacher, MD

25

The fifth edition of the American Psychiatric Association's *Diagnostic and Statistical Manual (DSM-V)* was published in 2013. It utilizes specific criteria with which to objectively assess symptoms rather than purely discrete diagnostic categories so that, for example, personality dimensions are more prominent. Nonetheless, the diagnosis is still based on a solid history and examination.

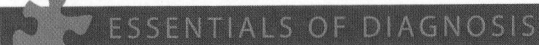

COMMON PSYCHIATRIC DISORDERS

STRESS & ADJUSTMENT DISORDERS (Situational Disorders)

ESSENTIALS OF DIAGNOSIS

- ▶ Anxiety or depression in reaction to an identifiable stress.
- ▶ Subsequent symptoms of anxiety or depression commonly elicited by similar stress of lesser magnitude.
- ▶ Alcohol and other drugs are commonly used in self-treatment.

▶ General Considerations

Stress exists when the adaptive capacity of the individual is overwhelmed by events. The event may be an insignificant one when objectively considered, and even favorable changes (eg, promotion and transfer) requiring adaptive behavior can produce stress. For each individual, stress is subjectively defined, and the response to stress is a function of each person's personality and physiologic endowment.

Opinion differs about what events are most apt to produce stress reactions. The causes of stress are different at different ages—eg, in young adulthood, the sources of stress are found in the marriage or parent-child relationship, the employment relationship, and the struggle to achieve financial stability; in the middle years, the focus shifts to changing spousal relationships, problems with aging parents, and problems associated with having young adult offspring who themselves are encountering stressful situations; in old age,

the principal concerns are apt to be retirement, loss of physical capacity, major personal losses, and thoughts of death.

▶ Clinical Findings

An individual may react to stress by becoming anxious or depressed, by developing a physical symptom, by running away, drinking alcohol, overeating, starting an affair, or in limitless other ways. Common subjective responses are fear (of repetition of the stress-inducing event), rage (at frustration), guilt (over aggressive impulses), and shame (over helplessness). Acute and reactivated stress may be manifested by restlessness, irritability, fatigue, increased startle reaction, and a feeling of tension. Inability to concentrate, sleep disturbances (insomnia, bad dreams), and somatic preoccupations often lead to self-medication, most commonly with alcohol or other central nervous system depressants. Maladaptive behavior in response to stress is called adjustment disorder, with the major symptom specified (eg, "adjustment disorder with depressed mood").

▶ Differential Diagnosis

Adjustment disorders must be distinguished from anxiety disorders, affective disorders, and personality disorders exacerbated by stress and from somatic disorders with psychic overlay. Unlike many other psychiatric disorders, such as bipolar disorder or schizophrenia, adjustment disorders are wholly situational and resolve when the stressor resolves or the individual effectively adapts to the situation. Adjustment disorders may have symptoms that overlap with other disorders, such as anxiety symptoms, but they occur in reaction to an identifiable life stressor such as a difficult work situation or romantic breakup. Patients with adjustments disorders have marked distress after a stressor and significant impairment in social or occupational functioning. Adjustment disorders are regarded as acute if less than 6 months or chronic if longer.

▶ Treatment

A. Behavioral

Stress reduction techniques include immediate symptom reduction (eg, rebreathing in a bag for hyperventilation) or early recognition and removal from a stress source before full-blown symptoms appear. It is often helpful for the patient to keep a daily log of stress precipitators, responses, and alleviators. Relaxation, mindfulness-based stress reduction, and exercise techniques are also helpful in reducing the reaction to stressful events.

B. Social

The stress reactions of life crisis problems are a function of psychosocial upheaval, and patients frequently present with somatic symptoms. While it is not easy for the patient to make necessary changes (or they would have been made long ago), it is important for the clinician to establish the framework of the problem, since the patient's denial system may obscure the issues. Clarifying the problem allows the patient to begin viewing it within the proper context and facilitates the difficult decisions the patient eventually must make (eg, change of job).

C. Psychological

Prolonged in-depth psychotherapy is seldom necessary in cases of isolated stress response or adjustment disorder. Supportive psychotherapy (see above) with an emphasis on the here and now and strengthening of existing coping mechanisms is a helpful approach so that time and the patient's own resiliency can restore the previous level of function.

D. Medical

Judicious use of sedatives (eg, lorazepam, 0.5–1 mg two or three times daily orally) for a limited time and as part of an overall treatment plan can provide relief from acute anxiety symptoms. Problems arise when the situation becomes chronic through inappropriate treatment or when the treatment approach supports the development of chronicity.

► Prognosis

Return to satisfactory function after a short period is part of the clinical picture of this syndrome. Resolution may be delayed if others' responses to the patient's difficulties are thoughtlessly harmful or if the secondary gains outweigh the advantages of recovery. The longer the symptoms persist, the worse the prognosis.

Birnie K et al. Psychological benefits for cancer patients and their partners participating in mindfulness-based stress reduction (MBSR). Psychooncology. 2010 Sep;19(9):1004–9. [PMID: 19918956]

TRAUMA & STRESSOR-RELATED DISORDERS

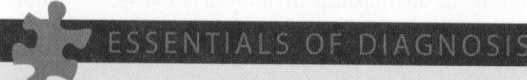

ESSENTIALS OF DIAGNOSIS

► Exposure to a traumatic, life-threatening event.

► Symptoms, such as flashbacks, intrusive images, and nightmares, often represent reexperiencing the event.

► Avoidance symptoms, including numbing, social withdrawal, and avoidance of stimuli associated with the event.

► Increased vigilance, such as startle reactions and difficulty falling asleep.

► Symptoms impair functioning.

► General Considerations

Posttraumatic stress disorder (PTSD) has been reclassified from an anxiety disorder to a trauma and stressor-related disorder in the *DSM-V*. PTSD is a syndrome characterized by "reexperiencing" a traumatic event (eg, sexual assault, severe burns, military combat) and decreased responsiveness and avoidance of current events when associated with the trauma. Data indicate that 13% of veterans who served in Iraq and 6% of those who served in Afghanistan have experienced PTSD. The 2005 National Comorbidity Survey Report estimated the lifetime prevalence of PTSD among adult Americans at 6.8% with a current prevalence of 3.6% and with women having rates twice as high as men. PTSD is more common when the event is associated with physical injury than when it is not. Many individuals with PTSD (20–40%) have experienced other associated problems, including divorce, parenting problems, difficulties with the law, and substance abuse. Since the terrorist attacks in the United States on September 11, 2001, estimates of PTSD have ranged from 4.7% to 10.2% in those witnessing the live attacks and have been associated with functional impairment as well as increased rates of substance use.

► Clinical Findings

The key to establishing the diagnosis of PTSD lies in the history of exposure to a life-threatening event followed by intrusive (eg, flashbacks, nightmares) or avoidance (eg, withdrawal) symptoms. Patients with PTSD experience physiologic hyperarousal, including startle reactions, intrusive thoughts, illusions, overgeneralized associations, sleep problems, nightmares, dreams about the precipitating event, impulsivity, difficulties in concentration, and hyperalertness. The symptoms may be precipitated or exacerbated by events that are a reminder of the original traumatic event. Symptoms frequently arise after a long latency period (eg, child abuse can result in later-onset posttraumatic stress disorder). *DSM-V* includes the requirement that the symptoms persist for at least 1 month. In some individuals, the symptoms fade over months or years, and in others it may persist for a lifetime.

► Differential Diagnosis

In 75% of cases, PTSD occurs with comorbid depression or panic disorder, and there is considerable overlap in the symptom complexes of all three conditions. Acute stress disorder occurs during or shortly after a traumatic event and has many of the same symptoms as PTSD but lasts between 2 and 28 days. Some individuals with dissociative features, such as borderline personality disorders, may mimic some of the symptoms of PTSD, but those disorders are typically more related to chronic childhood maltreatment not a specific traumatic event.

Treatment

A. Psychotherapy

Psychotherapy should be initiated as soon as possible after the traumatic event, and it should be brief (typically 8–12 sessions), once the individual is in a safe environment. Cognitive behavior therapy, exposure therapy, and eye-movement desensitization reprocessing have been effective in significantly reducing the duration of symptoms. In all of these approaches, the individual confronts the traumatic situation and learns to view it with less reactivity. Psychological debriefing in a single session, once a mainstay in prevention of PTSD, is now considered to be ineffective and possibly harmful. Posttraumatic stress syndromes respond to interventions that help patients integrate the event in an adaptive way with some sense of mastery in having survived the trauma. Marital problems are a major area of concern, and it is important that the clinician have available a dependable referral source when marriage counseling is indicated.

Treatment initiated later, when symptoms have crystallized, includes programs for cessation of alcohol and other drug use, group and individual psychotherapy, and improved social support systems. The therapeutic approach is to facilitate the normal recovery that was blocked at the time of the trauma.

B. Medication

Selective serotonin reuptake inhibitors (SSRIs) in full dosage are helpful in ameliorating depression, panic attacks, sleep disruption, and startle responses in chronic PTSD. Sertraline and paroxetine are approved by the US Food and Drug Administration (FDA) for this purpose, and the SSRIs are the only class of medications approved for the treatment of PTSD. They are, therefore, considered the pharmacotherapy of choice for PTSD. Early treatment of anxious arousal with beta-blockers (eg, propranolol, 80–160 mg orally daily) may lessen the peripheral symptoms of anxiety (eg, tremors, palpitations) but has not been shown to help prevent PTSD. Similarly, noradrenergic agents such as clonidine (titrated from 0.1 mg orally at bedtime to 0.2 mg three times a day) have been shown to help with the hyperarousal symptoms of PTSD. The alpha-adrenergic blocking agent prazosin (2–10 mg orally at bedtime) decreases nightmares and improves quality of sleep in PTSD. Antiseizure medications such as carbamazepine (400–800 mg orally daily) will often mitigate impulsivity and difficulty with anger management. Benzodiazepines, such as clonazepam (1–4 mg daily orally, divided into one or two doses), will reduce anxiety and panic attacks when used in adequate dosage, but dependency problems are a concern, particularly when the patient has had such problems in the past. Trazodone (25–100 mg orally at bedtime) is commonly prescribed as a non–habit forming hypnotic agent.

Prognosis

The sooner therapy is initiated after the trauma, the better the prognosis. Approximately half of patients experience chronic symptoms. Prognosis is best in those with good premorbid psychiatric functioning. Individuals experiencing an acute stress disorder typically do better than those experiencing a delayed posttraumatic disorder. Individuals who experience trauma resulting from a natural disaster (eg, earthquake or hurricane) tend to do better than those who experience a traumatic interpersonal encounter (eg, rape or combat).

Cloitre M et al. Treatment of complex PTSD: results of the ISTSS expert clinician survey on best practices. J Trauma Stress. 2011 Dec;24(6):615–27. [PMID: 22147449]

Goodson J et al. Treatment of posttraumatic stress disorder in U.S. combat veterans: a meta-analytic review. Psychol Rep. 2011 Oct;109(2):573–99. [PMID: 22238857]

Hetrick SE et al. Combined pharmacotherapy and psychological therapies for posttraumatic stress disorder (PTSD). Cochrane Database Syst Rev. 2010 Jul 7;(7):CD007316. [PMID: 20614457]

Jeffreys M et al. Pharmacotherapy for posttraumatic stress disorder: review with clinical applications. J Rehabil Res Dev. 2012;49(5):703–15. [PMID: 23015581]

Stevens LM et al. JAMA patient page. Posttraumatic stress disorder. JAMA. 2012 Aug 15;308(7):729. [PMID: 22893176]

ANXIETY DISORDERS

ESSENTIALS OF DIAGNOSIS

▶ Overt anxiety or an overt manifestation of a coping mechanism (such as a phobia), or both.

▶ Not limited to an adjustment disorder.

▶ Somatic symptoms referable to the autonomic nervous system or to a specific organ system (eg, dyspnea, palpitations, paresthesias).

▶ Not a result of physical disorders, psychiatric conditions (eg, schizophrenia), or drug abuse (eg, cocaine).

General Considerations

Stress, fear, and anxiety all tend to be interactive. The principal components of anxiety are **psychological** (tension, fears, difficulty in concentration, apprehension) and **somatic** (tachycardia, hyperventilation, shortness of breath, palpitations, tremor, sweating). Other organ systems (eg, gastrointestinal) may be involved in multiple-system complaints. Fatigue and sleep disturbances are common. Sympathomimetic symptoms of anxiety are both a response to a central nervous system state and a reinforcement of further anxiety. Anxiety can become self-generating, since the symptoms reinforce the reaction, causing it to spiral. This is often the case when the anxiety is an epiphenomenon of other medical or psychiatric disorders.

Anxiety may be free-floating, resulting in acute anxiety attacks, occasionally becoming chronic. When coping mechanisms for stress management are not functioning, the consequences are well-known problems such as phobias, conversion reactions, and dissociative states. Lack of structure is frequently a contributing factor, as noted in those people who have "Sunday neuroses." They do well during the week with a planned work schedule but cannot tolerate the unstructured weekend. Planned-time activities tend to bind anxiety, and many people have increased difficulties when this is lost, as in retirement.

Some believe that various manifestations of anxiety are not a result of unconscious conflicts but are "habits"—persistent patterns of nonadaptive behavior acquired by learning. The "habits," being nonadaptive, are unsatisfactory ways of dealing with life's problems—hence the resultant anxiety. Help is sought only when the anxiety becomes too painful. Exogenous factors such as stimulants (eg, caffeine, cocaine) must be considered as a contributing factor.

Clinical Findings

A. Generalized Anxiety Disorder

This is among the most common of the clinically significant anxiety disorders. Initial manifestations appear at age 20–35 years, and the rate appears to increase with age. Generalized anxiety disorder (GAD) becomes chronic in many patients with over half of patients having the disorder for longer than 2 years. About 7% of women and 4% of men will meet criteria for GAD over a lifetime. The anxiety symptoms of apprehension, worry, irritability, difficulty in concentrating, insomnia, and somatic complaints are present more days than not for at least 6 months. Manifestations can include cardiac (eg, tachycardia, increased blood pressure), gastrointestinal (eg, increased acidity, nausea, epigastric pain), and neurologic (eg, headache, near-syncope) systems. The focus of the anxiety may be a number of everyday activities.

B. Panic Disorder

This is characterized by short-lived, recurrent, unpredictable episodes of intense anxiety accompanied by marked physiologic manifestations. **Agoraphobia**, fear of being in places where escape is difficult, such as open spaces or public places where one cannot easily hide, may be present and may lead the individual to confine his or her life to the home environment. Distressing symptoms and signs such as dyspnea, tachycardia, palpitations, headaches, dizziness, paresthesias, choking, smothering feelings, nausea, and bloating are associated with feelings of impending doom (alarm response). Although these symptoms may lead to overlap with some of the same bodily complaints found in the somatic symptom disorders, the key to the diagnosis of panic disorder is the psychic pain and suffering the individual expresses. Recurrent **sleep panic attacks** (not nightmares) occur in about 30% of panic disorders. Anticipatory anxiety develops in all these patients and further constricts their daily lives. Panic disorder tends to be familial, with onset usually under age 25; it affects 3–5% of the population,

and the female-to-male ratio is 2:1. The premenstrual period is one of heightened vulnerability. Patients frequently undergo emergency medical evaluations (eg, for "heart attacks" or "hypoglycemia") before the correct diagnosis is made. Gastrointestinal symptoms are especially common, occurring in about one-third of cases. Myocardial infarction, pheochromocytoma, hyperthyroidism, and various recreational drug reactions can mimic panic disorder. Mitral valve prolapse may be present but is not usually a significant factor. Patients who have recurrent panic disorder often become demoralized, hypochondriacal, agoraphobic, and depressed. These individuals are at increased risk for major depression and the suicide attempts associated with that disorder. Alcohol abuse (in about 20%) results from self-treatment and is frequently combined with dependence on sedatives. Some patients have atypical panic attacks associated with seizure-like symptoms that often include psychosensory phenomena (a history of stimulant abuse often emerges). About 25% of panic disorder patients also have obsessive-compulsive disorder (OCD).

C. Phobic Disorders

Phobias are fears of a specific object or situation (eg, spiders, height) that are out of proportion to the danger posed and they tend to be chronic. Social phobias are global or specific; in the former, all social situations are poorly tolerated, while the latter group includes performance anxiety (eg, fear of public speaking). Agoraphobia is frequently associated with severe panic attacks, and it often develops in early adult life, making a normal lifestyle difficult. Patients with agoraphobia experience intense fear about common situations, such as being in open spaces (eg, marketplaces), enclosed spaces (eg, theaters), standing in line, or being alone outside of their homes. While patients with simple phobias such as fear of heights may function as long as they do not have to be in tall buildings or airplanes, a patient with agoraphobia may not be able to function vocationally or interpersonally. Thus, patients with agoraphobia are much more likely to seek treatment than those with simple or even social phobias.

Treatment

In all cases, underlying medical disorders must be ruled out (eg, cardiovascular, endocrine, respiratory, and neurologic disorders and substance-related syndromes, both intoxication and withdrawal states). These and other disorders can coexist with panic disorder.

A. Medical

1. Generalized anxiety—Antidepressants including the SSRIs and serotonin norepinephrine reuptake inhibitors (SNRIs) are safe and effective in the long-term management of GAD. The antidepressants appear to be as effective as the benzodiazepines without the risks of tolerance or dependence. However, benzodiazepines are the anxiolytics of choice in the acute management of generalized anxiety (Table 25–1). They are almost immediately effective.

All of the benzodiazepines may be given orally, and several are available in parenteral formulations. Benzodiazepines

Table 25–1. Commonly used antianxiety and hypnotic agents.

Drug	Usual Daily Oral Doses	Usual Daily Maximum Doses	Cost for 30 Days Treatment Based on Maximum Dosage[1]
Benzodiazepines (used for anxiety)			
Alprazolam (Xanax)[2]	0.5 mg	4 mg	$117.60
Chlordiazepoxide (Librium)[3]	10–20 mg	100 mg	$51.60
Clonazepam (Klonopin)[3]	1–2 mg	10 mg	$169.50
Clorazepate (Tranxene)[3]	15–30 mg	60 mg	$273.60
Diazepam (Valium)[3]	5–15 mg	30 mg	$29.70
Lorazepam (Ativan)[2]	2–4 mg	4 mg	$69.00
Oxazepam (Serax)[2]	10–30 mg	60 mg	$95.40
Benzodiazepines (used for sleep)			
Estazolam (Prosom)[2]	1 mg	2 mg	$29.70
Flurazepam (Dalmane)[3]	15 mg	30 mg	$10.20
Midazolam (Versed)[4]	5 mg		$1.00/dose
Quazepam (Doral)[3]	7.5 mg	15 mg	$138.00
Temazepam (Restoril)[2]	15 mg	30 mg	$24.30
Triazolam (Halcion)[5]	0.125 mg	0.25 mg	$20.70
Miscellaneous (used for anxiety)			
Buspirone (Buspar)[2]	10–30 mg	60 mg	$218.10
Phenobarbital[3]	15–30 mg	90 mg	$15.30
Miscellaneous (used for sleep)			
Chloral hydrate (Noctec)[2]	500 mg	1000 mg	Compounding pharmacy
Eszopiclone (Lunesta)[5]	2–3 mg	3 mg	$389.10
Hydroxyzine (Vistaril)[2]	50 mg	100 mg	$62.40
Ramelteon (Rozerem)	8 mg	8 mg	$251.62
Zaleplon (Sonata)[6]	5–10 mg	10 mg	$112.50
Zolpidem (Ambien)[5]	5–10 mg	10 mg	$138.60

[1]Average wholesale price (AWP, for AB-rated generic when available) for quantity listed. Source: *Red Book Online*, 2014, Truven Health Analytics, Inc. AWP may not accurately represent the actual pharmacy cost because wide contractual variations exist among institutions.
[2]Intermediate physical half-life (10–20 hours).
[3]Long physical half-life (> 20 hours).
[4]Intravenously for procedures.
[5]Short physical half-life (1–6 hours).
[6]Short physical half-life (about 1 hour).

such as lorazepam are absorbed rapidly when given intramuscularly. In psychiatric disorders, the benzodiazepines are usually given orally; in controlled medical environments (eg, the ICU), where the rapid onset of respiratory depression can be assessed, they are often given intravenously. Diazepam and clorazepate are the most rapidly absorbed oral benzodiazepines, which may explain the popularity of diazepam. In the average case of anxiety, diazepam, 5–10 mg orally twice daily as needed, is a reasonable starting regimen.

Benzodiazepines such as lorazepam do not produce active metabolites and have intermediate half-lives of 10–20 hours, characteristics useful in treating elderly patients. Ultra-short-acting agents such as triazolam have half-lives of 1–3 hours and may lead to rebound withdrawal anxiety. Longer-acting benzodiazepines such as flurazepam and diazepam produce active metabolites, have half-lives of 20–120 hours, and should be avoided in the elderly. Since people vary widely in their response and since the medications are long lasting, the dosage must be individualized. Once this is established, an adequate dose early in the course of symptom development will obviate the need for "pill popping," which contributes to dependency problems.

Panic disorder often responds to high potency benzodiazepines such as clonazepam and alprazolam. Thus, those benzodiazepines and the antidepressants are the most commonly used agents for panic disorder. Large doses of benzodiazepines are often required to block panic attacks, and these doses can lead to tolerance and dependence. In addition, alprazolam has a relatively short half-life and can lead to interdose rebound anxiety, although the extended-release form obviates this difficulty. The benzodiazepines are often prescribed for the first weeks of treatment along with the antidepressant and then tapered off as the antidepressant begin to work.

Whether the indications for benzodiazepines are **anxiety** or **insomnia**, the medications should be used judiciously. The longer-acting benzodiazepines are used for the treatment of alcohol withdrawal and anxiety symptoms; the intermediate medications are useful as sedatives for insomnia (eg, lorazepam), while short-acting agents (eg, midazolam) are used for medical procedures such as endoscopy.

The side effects of all the benzodiazepine antianxiety agents are patient and dose dependent. As the dosage exceeds the levels necessary for sedation, the side effects include disinhibition, ataxia, dysarthria, nystagmus, and delirium. (The patient should be told not to operate machinery until he or she is well stabilized without side effects.)

Paradoxical agitation, anxiety, psychosis, confusion, mood lability, and anterograde amnesia have been reported, particularly with the shorter-acting benzodiazepines. These agents produce cumulative clinical effects with repeated dosage (especially if the patient has not had time to metabolize the previous dose), additive effects when given with other classes of sedatives or alcohol (many apparently "accidental" deaths are the result of concomitant use of sedatives and alcohol), and residual effects after termination of treatment (particularly in the case of medications that undergo slow biotransformation).

Overdosage results in respiratory depression, hypotension, shock syndrome, coma, and death. Flumazenil, a benzodiazepine antagonist, is effective in overdosage. Overdosage (see Chapter 38) and withdrawal states are medical emergencies. Serious side effects of chronic excessive dosage are development of tolerance, resulting in increasing dose requirements, and physiologic dependence, resulting in withdrawal symptoms similar in appearance to alcohol and barbiturate withdrawal (withdrawal effects must be distinguished from reemergent anxiety). Abrupt withdrawal of sedative medications may cause serious and even fatal convulsive seizures. Psychosis, delirium, and autonomic dysfunction have also been described. Both duration of action and duration of exposure are major factors related to likelihood of withdrawal.

Common withdrawal symptoms after low to moderate daily use of benzodiazepines are classified as **somatic** (disturbed sleep, tremor, nausea, muscle aches), **psychological** (anxiety, poor concentration, irritability, mild depression), or **perceptual** (poor coordination, mild paranoia, mild confusion). The presentation of symptoms will vary depending on the half-life of the drug. There are no significant side effects on organ systems other than the brain, and the medications are safe in most medical conditions. Benzodiazepine interactions with other medications are listed in Table 25–2.

Table 25–2. Benzodiazepine interactions with other medications.

Drug	Effects
Antacids	Decreased absorption of benzodiazepines
Cimetidine	Increased half-life of diazepam and triazolam
Contraceptives	Increased levels of diazepam and triazolam
Digoxin	Alprazolam and diazepam raise digoxin level
Disulfiram	Increased duration of action of sedatives
Isoniazid	Increased plasma diazepam
Levodopa	Inhibition of antiparkinsonism effect
Propoxyphene	Impaired clearance of diazepam
Rifampin	Decreased plasma diazepam
Warfarin	Decreased prothrombin time

Antidepressants are the first-line medications for sustained treatment of GAD, having the advantage of not causing serious physiologic dependency problems. Antidepressants can themselves be anxiogenic—thus, at the initiation of treatment, concomitant short-term treatment with a benzodiazepine is often indicated. Venlafaxine and duloxetine are FDA-approved for the treatment of GAD in usual antidepressant doses. Initial daily dosing should start low (37.5–75 mg for venlafaxine and 30 mg for duloxetine) and be titrated upward as needed. SSRIs, such as paroxetine, are also used. Similarly, buspirone, sometimes used as an augmenting agent in the treatment of depression and compulsive behaviors, is also effective for generalized anxiety. Buspirone is usually given in a total dosage of 15–60 mg/d in three divided doses. Higher doses tend to be counterproductive and produce gastrointestinal symptoms and dizziness. There is a 2- to 4-week delay before antidepressants and buspirone take effect, and patients require education regarding this lag. Sleep is sometimes negatively affected. Gabapentin (titrated to doses of 900–1800 mg orally daily) also appears effective and it lacks the habit forming potential of the benzodiazepines. Unfortunately, like buspirone, many patients find gabapentin less effective than benzodiazepines in the management of acute anxiety. Beta-blockers such as propranolol may help reduce peripheral somatic symptoms. Alcohol is the most frequently self-administered drug and should be interdicted. The highly addicting medications with a narrow margin of safety such as glutethimide, ethchlorvynol, methyprylon, meprobamate, and the barbiturates (with the exception of phenobarbital) should be avoided. Phenobarbital, in addition to its anticonvulsant properties, is a reasonably safe and very inexpensive sedative but has the disadvantage of causing hepatic microsomal enzyme stimulation (not the case with benzodiazepines), which may affect the metabolism of other medications.

2. Panic attacks—Panic attacks may be treated in several ways. A sublingual dose of alprazolam (0.5–1 mg) or clonazepam (0.5–1 mg) is often effective for urgent treatment.

For sustained treatment, SSRIs are the initial medications of choice (adequate blood levels will require dosages similar to those used in the treatment of depression). For example, sertraline starting at 25 mg/d and increased after 1 week to 50 mg/d may be effective. Because of initial agitation in response to antidepressants, doses should start low and be very gradually increased. High-potency benzodiazepines may be used for symptomatic treatment as the antidepressant dose is titrated upward. Clonazepam (1–6 mg/d orally) and alprazolam (0.5–6 mg/d orally) are effective alternatives to antidepressants. Both medications may produce marked withdrawal if stopped abruptly and should always be tapered. Because of chronicity of the disorders and the problem of dependency with benzodiazepine medications, it is generally desirable to use antidepressant medications as the principal pharmacologic approach. Antidepressants have been used in conjunction with beta-blockers in resistant cases. Propranolol (40–160 mg/d orally) can mute the peripheral symptoms of anxiety without significantly affecting motor and cognitive performance. They block symptoms mediated by sympathetic stimulation (eg, palpitations, tremulousness) but not non-adrenergic symptoms (eg, diarrhea, muscle tension). Contrary to common belief, they usually do not cause depression as a side effect and can be used cautiously in patients with depression. Valproate is as effective in panic disorder as the antidepressants and is another useful alternative.

3. Phobic disorders—A phobic disorder may be part of the panic disorder or may occur independently. Social phobias and agoraphobia may be treated with SSRIs, such as paroxetine, sertraline, and fluvoxamine. In addition, phobic disorders often respond to SNRIs such as venlafaxine. Gabapentin, an antiseizure medication with anxiolytic properties, may be an alternative to antidepressants in the treatment of social phobia in a dosage of 300–3600 mg/d, depending on response versus sedation. Specific phobias such as performance or test anxiety may respond to moderate doses of beta-blockers, such as propranolol, 20–40 mg 1 hour prior to exposure. Specific phobias tend to respond to behavioral therapies such as systematic desensitization, which is when the patient is gradually exposed to the feared object or situation in a controlled setting. A meta-analysis has demonstrated that the antituberculous drug D-cycloserine (DCS) enhances extinction of fear responses with exposures. Importantly, such medications must be used in combination with cognitive behavioral exposure strategies.

B. Behavioral

Behavioral approaches are widely used in various anxiety disorders, often in conjunction with medication. Any of the behavioral techniques can be used beneficially in altering the contingencies (precipitating factors or rewards) supporting any anxiety-provoking behavior. Relaxation techniques can sometimes be helpful in reducing anxiety. Desensitization, by exposing the patient to graded doses of a phobic object or situation, is an effective technique and one that the patient can practice outside the therapy session. Emotive imagery, wherein the patient imagines the anxiety-provoking situation while at the same time learning to relax, helps decrease the anxiety when the patient faces the real-life situation. Physiologic symptoms in panic attacks respond well to relaxation training. Both GAD and panic disorder appear to respond as well to cognitive behavioral therapy as they do to medications.

C. Psychological

Cognitive behavioral approaches have been effective in treatment of panic disorders, and phobias when erroneous beliefs need correction. These approaches share a common behavioral technique of exposing the individual to the feared object or situation. The combination of medical and cognitive behavioral therapy is more effective than either alone. Group therapy is the treatment of choice when the anxiety is clearly a function of the patient's difficulties in dealing with social settings. Acceptance and commitment therapy has been used with some success in anxiety disorders. It encourages individuals to keep focused on life goals while they "accept" the presence of anxiety in their lives.

D. Social

Peer support groups for panic disorder and agoraphobia have been particularly helpful. Social modification may require measures such as family counseling to aid acceptance of the patient's symptoms and avoid counterproductive behavior in behavioral training. Any help in maintaining the social structure is anxiety-alleviating, and work, school, and social activities should be maintained. School and vocational counseling may be provided by professionals, who often need help from the clinician in defining the patient's limitations.

▶ Prognosis

Anxiety disorders are usually long-standing and may be difficult to treat. All can be relieved to varying degrees with medications and behavioral techniques. The prognosis is better if the commonly observed anxiety-panic-phobia-depression cycle can be broken with a combination of the therapeutic interventions discussed above.

Blanco C et al. A placebo-controlled trial of phenelzine, cognitive behavioral group therapy, and their combination for social anxiety disorder. Arch Gen Psychiatry. 2010 Mar;67(3): 286–95. [PMID: 20194829]

Bontempo A et al. D-cycloserine augmentation of behavioral therapy for the treatment of anxiety disorders: a meta-analysis. J Clin Psychiatry. 2012 Apr;73(4):533–7. [PMID: 22579153]

Buoli M et al. New approaches to the pharmacological management of generalized anxiety disorder. Expert Opin Pharmacother. 2013 Feb;14(2):175–84. [PMID: 23282069]

Diniz JB et al. A double-blind, randomized, controlled trial of fluoxetine plus quetiapine or clomipramine versus fluoxetine plus placebo for obsessive-compulsive disorder. J Clin Psychopharmacol. 2011 Dec;31(6):763–8. [PMID: 22020357]

Hayes SC et al. Open, aware, and active: contextual approaches as an emerging trend in the behavioral and cognitive therapies. Annu Rev Clin Psychol. 2011 Apr;7:141–68. [PMID: 21219193]

Roy-Byrne P et al. Delivery of evidence-based treatment for multiple anxiety disorders in primary care: a randomized controlled trial. JAMA. 2010 May 19;303(19):1921–8. [PMID: 20483968]

OBSESSIVE-COMPULSIVE DISORDER & RELATED DISORDERS

ESSENTIALS OF DIAGNOSIS

► Anxiety is alleviated only by ritualistic performance of the action or by deliberate contemplation of the intruding idea or emotion.

► Other behaviors may overlap with OCD resulting in "OCD spectrum."

► Neurologic abnormalities of fine motor coordination and involuntary movements are common.

► General Considerations

Obsessive compulsive disorder was classified as an anxiety disorder in the *DSM-IV*, but in the *DSM-V* is considered a different category of mental disorder. In the obsessive-compulsive reaction, the irrational idea or the impulse persistently intrudes into awareness. Obsessions (recurring anxiety provoking thoughts such as fears of exposure to germs) and compulsions (repetitive actions such as washing the hands many times) are recognized by the individual as absurd and are resisted, but anxiety is alleviated only by ritualistic performance of the action or by deliberate contemplation of the intruding idea or emotion. Many patients do not mention the symptoms and must be asked about them. These patients are usually predictable, orderly, conscientious, and intelligent—traits that are seen in many compulsive behaviors such as food binging and purging and compulsive exercise. There is an overlapping of OCD and other behaviors ("OCD spectrum"), including tics, trichotillomania (hair pulling), excoriation disorder (skin picking), hoarding, onychophagia (nail biting), Tourette syndrome, and eating disorders (see Chapter 29). The incidence of OCD in the general population is 2–3% and there is a high comorbidity with major depression: major depression will develop in two-thirds of OCD patients during their lifetime. Male to female ratios are similar, with the highest rates occurring in the young, divorced, separated, and unemployed (all high-stress categories). Neurologic abnormalities of fine motor coordination and involuntary movements are common. Under extreme stress, these patients sometimes exhibit paranoid and delusional behaviors, often associated with depression, and can mimic schizophrenia.

► Treatment

A. Medical

OCD responds to SSRIs and clomipramine in about 60% of cases and usually requires a longer response time than for depression (up to 12 weeks). Clomipramine has proved effective in doses equivalent to those used for depression (see Table 25–7). Fluoxetine has been widely used in this disorder but in doses higher than those used in depression (up to 60–80 mg orally daily). The other SSRI medications, such as sertraline, paroxetine, and fluvoxamine, are used with comparable efficacy each with its own side-effect profile. Buspirone in doses of 15–60 mg orally daily appears to be effective primarily as an anti-obsessional augmenting agent for the SSRI medications. There is some evidence that antipsychotics may be helpful as adjuncts to the SSRIs in treatment-resistant cases. Alternatively, low-dose clomipramine may be an effective adjunct to an SSRI in some patients. Psychosurgery has a limited place in selected cases of severe unremitting OCD. The current stereotactic techniques, including modified cingulotomy, are great improvements over the crude methods of the past. Experimental work has suggested a role for deep brain stimulation in OCD and it is FDA approved on a compassionate basis for refractory OCD patients.

B. Behavioral

OCD may respond to a variety of behavioral techniques. One common strategy is systematic desensitization. As in the treatment of simple phobias, systematic desensitization involves gradually exposing the OCD spectrum patient to situations that the patient fears, such as perceived germs or situations that a hoarder must part with things they are hoarding. By gradually exposing the patient to increasingly stressful situations and helping them manage their anxiety, OCD spectrum patients are often able to develop some mastery over the compulsions.

A technique used to help quell obsessive thoughts is "thought stopping." In this technique, the patient is taught to identify an obsessive thought and then to derail it. For example, the patient may be taught to say STOP any time an obsessive thought is present. In time, thought stopping can mitigate some of the obsessive thoughts.

C. Psychological

In addition to behavioral techniques, OCD may respond to psychological therapies including cognitive behavioral therapy in which the patient learns to identify maladaptive cognitions associated with obsessive thoughts and challenge those cognitions. For example, an OCD patient may fear that if he does not wash his hands 50 times after shaking hands he or someone close to him might develop a serious disease. These cognitions can be identified and gradually replaced with more rational thoughts.

D. Social

OCD can have devastating effects on the ability of a patient to lead a normal life. Educating both the patient and family about the course of illness and treatment options is extremely useful in setting appropriate expectations. Severe OCD is commonly associated with vocational disability, and the clinician may sometimes need to facilitate a leave of absence from work or encourage vocational rehabilitation to get the patient back to work.

Prognosis

OCD is usually a chronic disorder with a waxing and waning course. As many as 40% of patients in whom OCD problems develop in childhood will experience remission as adults. However, it is less common for OCD to remit without treatment when it develops during adulthood.

SOMATIC SYMPTOM DISORDERS (Abnormal Illness Behaviors)

ESSENTIALS OF DIAGNOSIS

- ▶ Physical symptoms may involve one or more organ systems and are not intentional.
- ▶ Subjective complaints exceed objective findings.
- ▶ Correlations of symptom development and psychosocial stresses.
- ▶ Combination of biogenetic and developmental patterns.

General Considerations

Any organ system can be affected in somatic symptom disorders. In *DSM-V*, somatic symptom disorders encompass disorders that were listed under somatic disorders in *DSM-IV*, including conversion disorder, hypochondriasis, somatization disorder, and pain disorder secondary to psychological factors. Vulnerability in one or more organ systems and exposure to family members with somatization problems plays a major role in the development of particular symptoms, and the "functional" versus "organic" dichotomy is a hindrance to good treatment. Clinicians should suspect psychiatric disorders in a number of conditions. For example, 45% of patients complaining of palpitations had lifetime psychiatric diagnoses including generalized anxiety, depression, panic, and somatization disorders. Similarly, 33–44% of patients who undergo coronary angiography for chest pain but have negative results have been found to have panic disorder.

In any patient presenting with a condition judged to be somatic symptom disorder, depression must be considered in the diagnosis.

Clinical Findings

A. Conversion Disorder

"Conversion" of psychic conflict into physical symptoms in parts of the body innervated by the sensorimotor system (eg, paralysis, aphonic) is a disorder that is more common in individuals from lower socioeconomic classes and certain cultures. The somatic manifestation that takes the place of anxiety is often paralysis, and in some instances the organ dysfunction may have symbolic meaning (eg, arm paralysis in marked anger so the individual cannot use the arm to strike someone). Pseudoepileptic ("hysterical") seizures are often difficult to differentiate from intoxication states or panic attacks. Retention of consciousness, random flailing with asynchronous movements of the right and left sides, and resistance to having the nose and mouth pinched closed during the attack, all point toward a pseudoepileptic event. Electroencephalography, particularly in a video-electroencephalography assessment unit, during the attack is the most helpful diagnostic aid in excluding genuine seizure states. Serum prolactin levels rise abruptly in the postictal state only in true epilepsy. La belle indifférence (an unconcerned affect) is not a significant identifying characteristic, as commonly believed, since individuals even with genuine medical illness, may exhibit a high level of denial. Important conversion disorder criteria include a history of conversion or somatization disorder, modeling the symptom after someone else who had a similar presentation, a serious precipitating emotional event, associated psychopathology (eg, depression, schizophrenia, personality disorders), a temporal correlation between the precipitating event and the symptom, and a temporary "solving of the problem" by the conversion. It is important to identify physical disorders with unusual presentations (eg, multiple sclerosis, systemic lupus erythematosus).

B. Somatic Symptom Disorder

Somatic symptom disorder is characterized by one or more somatic symptoms that are associated with significant distress or disability. The somatic symptoms may be associated with persistent thoughts about the seriousness of the symptoms, a high level of anxiety about health, or excessive time and energy devoted to these symptoms. The patient's focus on somatic symptoms is usually chronic. Panic, anxiety, and depression are often present, and **major depression** is an important consideration in the differential diagnosis. There is a significant relationship (20%) to a lifetime history of panic-agoraphobia-depression. It usually occurs before age 30 and is ten times more common in women. Polysurgery is often a feature of the history. Preoccupation with medical and surgical therapy becomes a lifestyle that may exclude other activities. The symptoms indicate maladaptive coping techniques and there is often evidence of longstanding somatic complaints, including multiple pain and gastrointestinal symptoms (such as dyspareunia, dysmenorrhea, headache, backache, abdominal pain, vomiting, bloating) and pseudoneurologic symptoms (such as amnesia or pseudoepileptic seizures), often with a history of similar organ system involvement in other family members. Multiple symptoms that constantly change and the inability of more than three doctors to make a diagnosis are strong clues to the problem.

C. Somatic Symptom Disorder with Predominant Pain

This involves a long history of complaints of severe pain out of proportion to biomedical findings that are present. This diagnosis must be one of exclusion and should be made only after extended evaluation has established a clear correlation of psychogenic factors with exacerbations and remissions of complaints.

D. Factitious Disorders

These disorders, in which symptom production is intentional, are not somatic symptom conditions in that symptoms are produced consciously, in contrast to the unconscious process of the above conditions. They are characterized by self-induced symptoms or false physical and laboratory findings for the purpose of deceiving clinicians or other health care personnel. The deceptions may involve self-mutilation, fever, hemorrhage, hypoglycemia, seizures, and an almost endless variety of manifestations—often presented in an exaggerated and dramatic fashion (**Munchausen syndrome**). "Munchausen by proxy" is the term used when a parent creates an illness in a child so the adult (usually the mother) can maintain a relationship with clinicians. The duplicity may be either simple or extremely complex and difficult to recognize. The patients are frequently connected in some way with the health professions and there is no apparent external motivation other than achieving the patient role. A poor clinician-patient relationship and "doctor shopping" tend to exacerbate the problem.

▶ **Complications**

Sedative and analgesic dependency is the most common iatrogenic complication. Patients may pursue medical or surgical treatments that induce iatrogenic problems. Thus, identifying patients with a potential somatic symptom disorder and attempting to limit tests, procedures, and medications that may lead to harm is quite important.

▶ **Treatment**

A. Medical

Medical support with careful attention to building a therapeutic clinician-patient relationship is the mainstay of treatment. It must be accepted that the patient's distress is real. Every problem not found to have an organic basis is not necessarily a mental disease. Diligent attempts should be made to relate symptoms to adverse developments in the patient's life. It may be useful to have the patient keep a meticulous diary, paying particular attention to various pertinent factors evident in the history. Regular, frequent, short appointments that are not symptom-contingent may be helpful. Medications (frequently abused) should not be prescribed to replace appointments. One person should be the primary clinician, and consultants should be used mainly for evaluation. An empathic, realistic, optimistic approach must be maintained in the face of the expected ups and downs. Ongoing reevaluation is necessary, since somatization can coexist with a concurrent physical illness.

B. Psychological

The primary clinician can use psychological approaches when it is clear that the patient is ready to make some changes in lifestyle in order to achieve symptomatic relief. This is often best approached on a here-and-now basis and oriented toward pragmatic changes rather than an exploration of early experiences that the patient frequently fails to relate to current distress. Group therapy with other individuals who have similar problems is sometimes of value to improve coping, allow ventilation, and focus on interpersonal adjustment. Hypnosis or lorazepam interviews used early are helpful in resolving conversion disorders. If the primary clinician has been working with the patient on psychological problems related to the physical illness, the groundwork is often laid for successful psychiatric referral.

For patients who have been identified as having a factitious disorder, early psychiatric consultation is indicated. There are two main treatment strategies for these patients. One consists of a conjoint confrontation of the patient by both the primary clinician and the psychiatrist. The patient's disorder is portrayed as a cry for help, and psychiatric treatment is recommended. The second approach avoids direct confrontation and attempts to provide a face-saving way to relinquish the symptom without overt disclosure of the disorder's origin. Techniques such as biofeedback and self-hypnosis may foster recovery using this strategy. Another face-saving approach is to use a double bind with the patient. For example, the patient is told there are two possible diagnoses: (1) an organic disease that should respond to the next medical intervention (usually modest and noninvasive), or (2) factitious disorder for which the patient will need psychiatric treatment. Given these options, many patients will choose to recover and not have to admit the origin of their problem.

C. Behavioral

Behavioral therapy is probably best exemplified by biofeedback techniques. In biofeedback, the particular abnormality (eg, increased peristalsis) must be recognized and monitored by the patient and therapist (eg, by an electronic stethoscope to amplify the sounds). This is immediate feedback, and after learning to recognize it, the patient can then learn to identify any change thus produced (eg, a decrease in bowel sounds) and so become a conscious originator of the feedback instead of a passive recipient. Relief of the symptom operantly conditions the patient to utilize the maneuver that relieves symptoms (eg, relaxation causing a decrease in bowel sounds). With emphasis on this type of learning, the patient is able to identify symptoms early and initiate the countermaneuvers, thus decreasing the symptomatic problem. Migraine and tension headaches have been particularly responsive to biofeedback methods.

D. Social

Social endeavors include family, work, and other interpersonal activity. Family members should come for some appointments with the patient so they can learn how best to live with the patient. This is particularly important in treatment of somatization and pain disorders. Peer support groups provide a climate for encouraging the patient to accept and live with the problem. Ongoing communication with the employer may be necessary to encourage long-term continued interest in the employee. Employers can become just as discouraged as clinicians in dealing with employees who have chronic problems.

Prognosis

The prognosis is better if the primary clinician is able to intervene early before the situation has deteriorated. After the problem has crystallized into chronicity, it is difficult to effect change.

Asmundson GJ et al. Health anxiety: current perspectives and future directions. Curr Psychiatry Rep. 2010 Aug;12(4): 306–12. [PMID: 20549396]

Gordon-Elliott JS et al. An approach to the patient with multiple physical symptoms or chronic disease. Med Clin North Am. 2010 Nov;94(6):1207–16. [PMID: 20951278]

Schweitzer PJ et al. Long-term follow-up of hypochondriasis after selective serotonin reuptake inhibitor treatment. J Clin Psychopharmacol. 2011 Jun;31(3):365–8. [PMID: 21508861]

CHRONIC PAIN DISORDERS

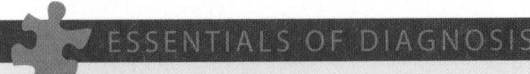

ESSENTIALS OF DIAGNOSIS

▶ Chronic complaints of pain.

▶ Symptoms frequently exceed signs.

▶ Minimal relief with standard treatment.

▶ History of having seen many clinicians.

▶ Frequent use of several nonspecific medications.

General Considerations

A problem in the management of pain is the lack of distinction between acute and chronic pain syndromes. Most clinicians are adept at dealing with acute pain problems but have difficulty treating the patient with a chronic pain disorder. This type of patient frequently takes too many medications, stays in bed a great deal, has seen many clinicians, has lost skills, and experiences little joy in either work or play. All relationships suffer (including those with clinicians), and life becomes a constant search for relief. The search results in complex clinician-patient relationships that usually include many drug trials, particularly sedatives, with adverse consequences (eg, irritability, depressed mood) related to long-term use. Treatment failures provoke angry responses and depression from both the patient and the clinician, and the pain syndrome is exacerbated. When frustration becomes too great, a new clinician is found, and the cycle is repeated. The longer the existence of the pain disorder, the more important becomes the psychological factors of anxiety and depression. As with all other conditions, it is counterproductive to speculate about whether the pain is "real." It is real to the patient, and acceptance of the problem must precede a mutual endeavor to alleviate the disturbance.

Clinical Findings

Components of the chronic pain syndrome consist of anatomic changes, chronic anxiety and depression, anger, and changed lifestyle. Usually, the anatomic problem is irreversible, since it has already been subjected to many interventions with increasingly unsatisfactory results. An algorithm for assessing chronic pain and differentiating it from other psychiatric conditions is illustrated in Figure 25–1.

Chronic anxiety and depression produce heightened irritability and overreaction to stimuli. A marked decrease in pain threshold is apparent. This pattern develops into a hypochondriacal preoccupation with the body and a constant need for reassurance. The pressure on the clinician becomes wearing and often leads to covert rejection of the patient, such as not being available or making referrals to other clinicians.

This is perceived by the patient, who then intensifies the effort to find help, and the typical cycle is repeated. Anxiety and depression are seldom discussed, almost as if there is a tacit agreement not to deal with these issues.

Changes in lifestyle involve some of the pain behaviors. These usually take the form of a family script in which the patient accepts the role of being sick, and this role then becomes the focus of most family interactions and may become important in maintaining the family, so that neither the patient nor the family wants the patient's role to change. Demands for attention and efforts to control the behavior of others revolve around the central issue of control of other people (including clinicians). Cultural factors frequently play a role in the behavior of the patient and how the significant people around the patient cope with the problem. Some cultures encourage demonstrative behavior, while others value the stoic role.

Another secondary gain that frequently maintains the patient in the sick role is financial compensation or other benefits. Frequently, such systems are structured so that they reinforce the maintenance of sickness and discourage any attempts to give up the role. Clinicians unwittingly reinforce this role because of the very nature of the practice of medicine, which is to respond to complaints of illness. Helpful suggestions from the clinician are often met with responses like, "Yes, but ...." Medications then become the principal approach, and drug dependency problems may develop.

Treatment

A. Behavioral

The cornerstone of a unified approach to chronic pain syndromes is a comprehensive behavioral program. This is necessary to identify and eliminate pain reinforcers, to decrease drug use, and to use effectively those positive reinforcers that shift the focus from the pain. It is critical that the patient be made a partner in the effort to manage and function better in the setting of ongoing pain symptoms. The clinician must shift from the idea of biomedical cure to ongoing care of the patient. The patient should agree to discuss the pain only with the clinician and not with family members; this tends to stabilize the patient's personal life, since the family is usually tired of the subject. At the beginning of treatment, the patient should be assigned self-help tasks graded up to maximal activity as a

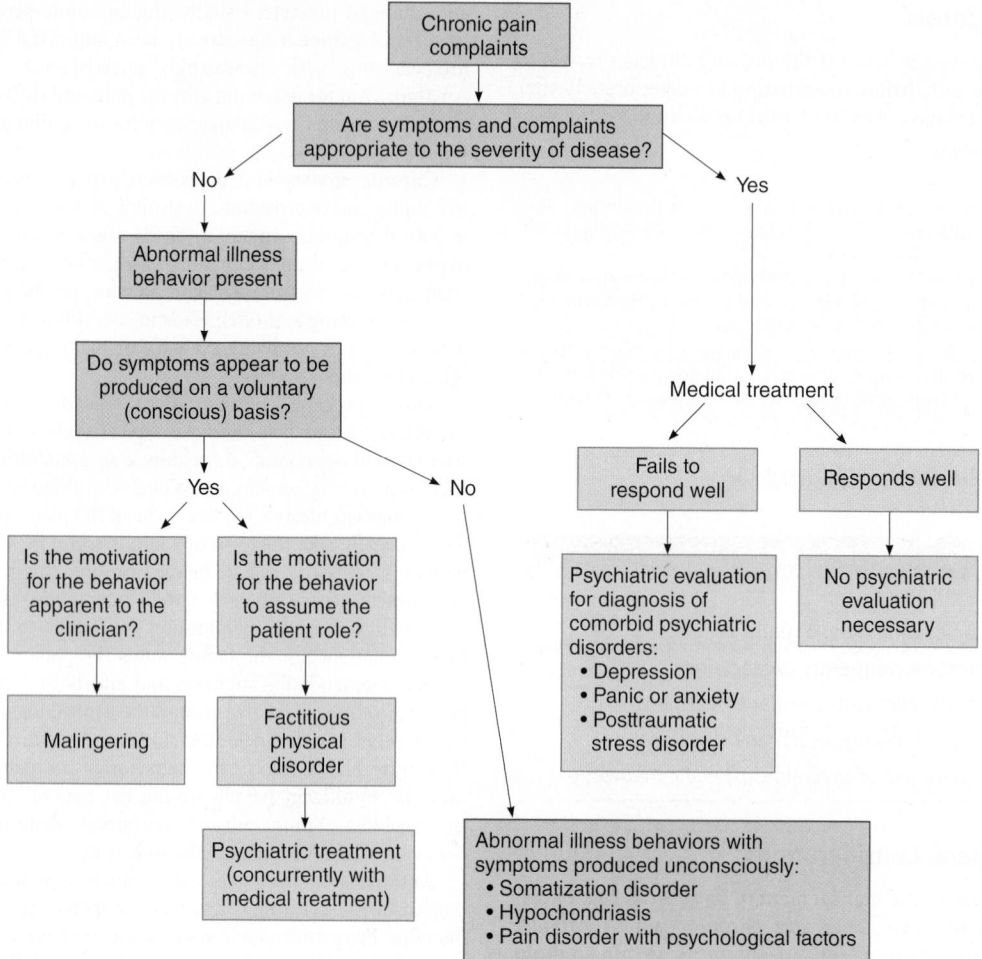

▲ **Figure 25–1.** Algorithm for assessing psychiatric component of chronic pain. (Adapted and reproduced, with permission, from Eisendrath SJ. Psychiatric aspects of chronic pain. Neurology. 1995 Dec;45(12 Suppl 9):S26–34.)

means of positive reinforcement. The tasks should not exceed capability. The patient can also be asked to keep a self-rating chart to log accomplishments, so that progress can be measured and remembered. Instruct the patient to record degrees of pain on a self-rating scale in relation to various situations and mental attitudes so that similar circumstances can be avoided or modified.

Avoid positive reinforcers for pain such as marked sympathy and attention to pain. Emphasize a positive response to productive activities, which remove the focus of attention from the pain. Activity is also desensitizing, since the patient learns to tolerate increasing activity levels.

Biofeedback techniques (see Somatic Symptom Disorders, above) and hypnosis have been successful in ameliorating some pain syndromes. Hypnosis tends to be most effective in patients with a high level of denial, who are more responsive to suggestion. Hypnosis can be used to lessen anxiety, alter perception of the length of time that pain is experienced, and encourage relaxation. Mindfulness-based stress reduction programs have been useful in

helping individuals develop an enhanced capacity to live a higher quality life with persistent pain.

B. Medical

A *single clinician* in charge of the comprehensive treatment approach is the highest priority. Consultations as indicated and technical procedures done by others are appropriate, but the care of the patient should remain in the hands of the primary clinician. Referrals should not be allowed to raise the patient's hopes unrealistically or to become a way for the clinician to reject the case. The attitude of the clinician should be one of honesty, interest, and hopefulness—not for a cure but for control of pain and improved function. If the patient manifests opioid addiction, detoxification may be an early treatment goal.

Nonsteroidal anti-inflammatory medications are often the first-line of treatment for pain. If opioid analgesics or sedatives are prescribed, they should not be given on an "as-needed" schedule (see Chapter 5). A fixed schedule lessens the conditioning effects of these medications. Tricyclic antidepressants (TCAs) (eg, nortriptyline), venlafaxine, and duloxetine in doses up to those used in depression may be helpful, particularly in neuropathic pain syndromes. In other conditions, their effects on pain may be less clear, but ameliorating depression is usually important nonetheless. Gabapentin, an anticonvulsant with possible applications in the treatment of anxiety disorders, has been shown to be useful in postherpetic and diabetic neuropathy and somatic symptom disorders.

In addition to medications, a variety of nonpharmacologic strategies may be offered, including physical therapy and acupuncture.

C. Social

Involvement of family members and other significant persons in the patient's life should be an early priority. The best efforts of both patient and therapists can be unwittingly sabotaged by other persons who may feel that they are "helping" the patient. They frequently tend to reinforce the negative aspects of the chronic pain disorder. The patient becomes more dependent and less active, and the pain syndrome becomes an immutable way of life. The more destructive pain behaviors described by many experts in chronic pain disorders are the results of well-meaning but misguided efforts of family members. Ongoing therapy with the family can be helpful in the early identification and elimination of these behavior patterns.

D. Psychological

In addition to group therapy with family members and others, groups of patients can be helpful if properly led. The major goal, whether of individual or group therapy, is to gain patient involvement. A group can be a powerful instrument for achieving this goal, with the development of group loyalties and cooperation. People will frequently make efforts with group encouragement that they would never make alone. Individual therapy should be directed toward strengthening existing coping mechanisms and improving self-esteem. For example, teaching patients to challenge expectations induced by chronic pain may lead to improved functioning. As an illustration, many chronic pain patients, making assumptions more derived from acute injuries, incorrectly believe they will damage themselves by attempting to function. The rapport between patient and clinician, as in all psychotherapeutic efforts, is the major factor in therapeutic success.

Morley S. Efficacy and effectiveness of cognitive behaviour therapy for chronic pain: progress and some challenges. Pain. 2011 Mar;152(3 Suppl):S99–106. [PMID: 21159433]
Pergolizzi JV Jr et al. Dynamic risk factors in the misuse of opioid analgesics. J Psychosom Res. 2012 Jun;72(6):443–51. [PMID: 22656441]

PSYCHOSEXUAL DISORDERS

The stages of sexual activity include **excitement** (arousal), **orgasm**, and **resolution**. The precipitating excitement or arousal is psychologically determined. Arousal response

leading to orgasm is a physiologic and psychological phenomenon of vasocongestion, a parasympathetic reaction causing erection in men and labial-clitoral congestion in women. The orgasmic response includes emission in men and clonic contractions of the analogous striated perineal muscles of both men and women. Resolution is a gradual return to normal physiologic status.

While the arousal stimuli—vasocongestive and orgasmic responses—constitute a single response in a well-adjusted person, they can be considered as separate stages that can produce different syndromes responding to different treatment procedures.

▶ Clinical Findings

There are three major groups of sexual disorders.

A. Paraphilias (Sexual Arousal Disorders)

In these conditions, formerly called "deviations" or "variations," the excitement stage of sexual activity is associated with sexual objects or orientations different from those usually associated with adult sexual stimulation. The stimulus may be a woman's shoe, a child, animals, instruments of torture, or incidents of aggression. The pattern of sexual stimulation is usually one that has early psychological roots. Poor experiences with sexual activity frequently reinforce this pattern over time. Paraphilias include exhibitionism, transvestism, voyeurism, pedophilia, incest, sexual sadism, and sexual masochism.

B. Gender Identity Disorder

Core gender identity reflects a biologic self-image—the conviction that "I am a boy" or "I am a girl" that is usually well developed by age 3 or 4. Gender dysphoria refers to the development of a sexual identity that is the opposite of the biologic one.

Transsexualism is an attempt to deny and reverse biologic sex by maintaining sexual identity with the opposite gender. Transsexuals do not alternate between gender roles; rather, they assume a fixed role of attitudes, feelings, fantasies, and choices consonant with those of the opposite sex, all of which clearly date back to early development. For example, male to female transsexuals in early childhood behave, talk, and fantasize as if they were girls. They do not grow out of feminine patterns; they do not work in professions traditionally considered to be masculine; and they have no interest in their own penises either as evidence of maleness or as organs for erotic behavior. The desire for sex change starts early and may culminate in assumption of a feminine lifestyle, hormonal treatment, and use of surgical procedures, eg, castration and vaginoplasty.

C. Psychosexual Dysfunction

This category includes a large group of vasocongestive and orgasmic disorders. Often, they involve problems of sexual adaptation, education, and technique that are often initially discussed with, diagnosed by, and treated by the primary care provider.

There are two conditions common in men: erectile dysfunction and ejaculation disturbances.

Erectile dysfunction is inability to achieve or maintain an erection firm enough for satisfactory intercourse; patients sometimes use the term to mean premature ejaculation. Decreased nocturnal penile tumescence occurs in some depressed patients. **Psychological erectile dysfunction** is caused by interpersonal or intrapsychic factors (eg, marital disharmony, depression). **Organic factors** are discussed in Chapter 23.

Ejaculation disturbances include premature ejaculation, inability to ejaculate, and retrograde ejaculation. (Ejaculation is possible in patients with erectile dysfunction.) Ejaculation is usually connected with orgasm, and ejaculatory control is an acquired behavior that is minimal in adolescence and increases with experience. Pathogenic factors are those that interfere with learning control, most frequently sexual ignorance. Intrapsychic factors (anxiety, guilt, depression) and interpersonal maladaptation (marital problems, unresponsiveness of mate, power struggles) are also common. Organic causes include interference with sympathetic nerve distribution (often due to surgery or radiation) and the effects of pharmacologic agents (eg, SSRIs or sympatholytics).

In women, the most common forms of sexual dysfunction are orgasmic disorder and hyposexual desire disorder (see Chapter 18).

Orgasmic disorder is a complex condition in which there is a general lack of sexual responsiveness. The woman has difficulty in experiencing erotic sensation and does not have the vasocongestive response. Sexual activity varies from active avoidance of sex to an occasional orgasm. Orgasmic dysfunction—in which a woman has a vasocongestive response but varying degrees of difficulty in reaching orgasm—is sometimes differentiated from anorgasmia. Causes for the dysfunctions include poor sexual techniques, early traumatic sexual experiences, interpersonal disharmony (marital struggles, use of sex as a means of control), and intrapsychic problems (anxiety, fear, guilt). Organic causes include any conditions that might cause pain in intercourse, pelvic pathology, mechanical obstruction, and neurologic deficits.

Hyposexual desire disorder consists of diminished or absent libido in either sex and may be a function of organic or psychological difficulties (eg, anxiety, phobic avoidance). Any chronic illness can reduce desire as can aging. Hormonal disorders, including hypogonadism or use of antiandrogen compounds such as cyproterone acetate, and chronic kidney disease contribute to deterioration in sexual desire. Although menopause may lead to diminution of sexual desire in some women, the relationship between menopause and libido is complicated and may be influenced by sociocultural factors. Alcohol, sedatives, opioids, marijuana, and some medications may affect sexual drive and performance.

► **Treatment**

A. Paraphilias and Gender Identity Disorders

1. Psychological—Sexual arousal disorders involving variant sexual activity (paraphilia), particularly those of a more superficial nature (eg, voyeurism) and those of recent onset, are responsive to psychotherapy in some cases. The prognosis is much better if the motivation comes from the individual rather than the legal system; unfortunately, judicial intervention is frequently the only stimulus to treatment because the condition persists and is reinforced until conflict with the law occurs. Therapies frequently focus on barriers to normal arousal response; the expectation is that the variant behavior will decrease as normal behavior increases.

2. Behavioral—Aversive and operant conditioning techniques have been tried frequently in gender role disorders but have only occasionally been successful. In some cases, the sexual arousal disorders improve with modeling, role-playing, and conditioning procedures. Emotive imagery is occasionally helpful in lessening anxiety in fetish problems.

3. Social—Although they do not produce a change in sexual arousal patterns or gender role, self-help groups have facilitated adjustment to an often hostile society. Attention to the family is particularly important in helping persons in such groups to accept their situation and alleviate their guilt about the role they think they had in creating the problem.

4. Medical—Medroxyprogesterone acetate, a suppressor of libidinal drive, is used to mute disruptive sexual behavior in men of all ages. Onset of action is usually within 3 weeks, and the effects are generally reversible. Fluoxetine or other SSRIs at depression doses (see below) may reduce some of the compulsive sexual behaviors including the paraphilias. A focus of study in the treatment of severe paraphilia has been agonists of luteinizing hormone–releasing hormone. Although some transsexuals are treated with genital reconstructive surgery, many others are screened out by trial periods of living as the other sex prior to operation.

B. Psychosexual Dysfunction

1. Medical—Even if the condition is not reversible, identification of the specific cause helps the patient to accept the condition. Marital disharmony, with its exacerbating effects, may thus be avoided. Of all the sexual dysfunctions, erectile dysfunction is the condition most likely to have an organic basis. Sildenafil, tadalafil, and vardenafil are phosphodiesterase type 5 inhibitors that are effective oral agents for the treatment of penile erectile dysfunction (eg, sildenafil 25–100 mg orally 1 hour prior to intercourse). These agents are effective for SSRI-induced erectile dysfunction in men and in some cases for SSRI-associated sexual dysfunction in women. Use of the medications in conjunction with any nitrates can have significant hypotensive effects leading to death in rare cases. Because of their common effect in delaying ejaculation, the SSRIs have been effective in premature ejaculation.

2. Behavioral—Syndromes resulting from conditioned responses have been treated by conditioning techniques, with excellent results. Masters and Johnson have used behavioral approaches in all of the sexual dysfunctions, with concomitant supportive psychotherapy and with improvement of the communication patterns of the couple.

3. Psychological—The use of psychotherapy by itself is best suited for those cases in which interpersonal difficulties or intrapsychic problems predominate. Anxiety and guilt about parental injunctions against sex may contribute to sexual dysfunction. Even in these cases, however, a combined behavioral-psychological approach usually produces results most quickly.

4. Social—The proximity of other people (eg, a mother-in-law) in a household is frequently an inhibiting factor in sexual relationships. In such cases, some social engineering may alleviate the problem.

Eardley I et al. Pharmacotherapy for erectile dysfunction. J Sex Med. 2010 Jan;7(1 Pt 2):524–40. [PMID: 20092451]

Nehra A et al. The Princeton III Consensus recommendations for the management of erectile dysfunction and cardiovascular disease. Mayo Clin Proc. 2012 Aug;87(8):766–78. [PMID: 22862865]

Simopoulos EF et al. Male erectile dysfunction: integrating psychopharmacology and psychotherapy. Gen Hosp Psychiatry. 2013 Jan;35(1):33–8. [PMID: 23044247]

PERSONALITY DISORDERS

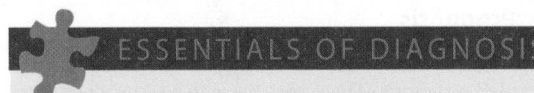

ESSENTIALS OF DIAGNOSIS

▸ Long history dating back to childhood.

▸ Recurrent maladaptive behavior.

▸ Low self-esteem.

▸ Minimal introspective ability with a tendency to blame others for all problems.

▸ Major difficulties with interpersonal relationships or society.

▸ Depression with anxiety when maladaptive behavior fails.

► General Considerations

An individual's personality structure, or character, is an integral part of self-image. It reflects genetics, interpersonal influences, and recurring patterns of behavior adopted in order to cope with the environment. The classification of subtypes of personality disorders depends on the predominant symptoms and their severity. The most severe disorders—those that bring the patient into greatest conflict with society—tend to be classified as antisocial (psychopathic) or borderline.

Personality disorders can be considered a matrix for some of the more severe psychiatric problems (eg, schizotypal, relating to schizophrenia, and avoidance types, relating to some anxiety disorders).

► Classification & Clinical Findings

See Table 25–3.

► Differential Diagnosis

Patients with personality disorders tend to show anxiety and depression when pathologic coping mechanisms fail,

Table 25–3. Personality disorders: Classification and clinical findings.

Personality Disorder	Clinical Findings
Antisocial	Selfish, callous, promiscuous, impulsive, unable to learn from experience, often has legal problems.
Avoidant	Fears rejection, hyperreacts to rejection and failure, with poor social endeavors and low self-esteem.
Borderline	Impulsive; has unstable and intense interpersonal relationships; is suffused with anger, fear, and guilt; lacks self-control and self-fulfillment; has identity problems and affective instability; is suicidal (a serious problem—up to 80% of hospitalized borderline patients make an attempt at some time during treatment, and the incidence of completed suicide is as high as 5%); aggressive behavior, feelings of emptiness, and occasional psychotic decompensation. This group has a high drug abuse rate, which plays a role in symptoms. There is extensive overlap with other diagnostic categories, particularly mood disorders and posttraumatic stress disorder.
Dependent	Passive, overaccepting, unable to make decisions, lacks confidence, with poor self-esteem.
Histrionic (hysterical)	Dependent, immature, seductive, egocentric, vain, emotionally labile.
Narcissistic	Exhibitionist, grandiose, preoccupied with power, lacks interest in others, with excessive demands for attention.
Obsessive compulsive	Perfectionist, egocentric, indecisive, with rigid thought patterns and need for control.
Paranoid	Defensive, oversensitive, secretive, suspicious, hyperalert, with limited emotional response.
Schizoid	Shy, introverted, withdrawn, avoids close relationships.
Schizotypal	Superstitious, socially isolated, suspicious, with limited interpersonal ability, eccentric behaviors, and odd speech.

and their symptoms can be similar to those disorders. Occasionally, the more severe cases may decompensate into psychosis under stress and mimic other psychotic disorders.

▶ Treatment

A. Social

Social and therapeutic environments such as day hospitals, halfway houses, and self-help communities utilize peer pressures to modify the self-destructive behavior. The patient with a personality disorder often has failed to profit from experience, and difficulties with authority impair the learning experience. The use of peer relationships and the repetition possible in a structured setting of a helpful community enhance the behavioral treatment opportunities and increase learning. When problems are detected early, both the school and the home can serve as foci of intensified social pressure to change the behavior, particularly with the use of behavioral techniques.

B. Behavioral

The behavioral techniques used are principally operant conditioning and aversive conditioning. The former simply emphasizes the recognition of acceptable behavior and its reinforcement with praise or other tangible rewards. Aversive responses usually mean punishment, although this can range from a mild rebuke to some specific punitive responses such as deprivation of privileges. Extinction plays a role in that an attempt is made not to respond to inappropriate behavior, and the lack of response eventually causes the person to abandon that type of behavior. Pouting and tantrums, for example, diminish quickly when such behavior elicits no reaction. Dialectical behavioral therapy is a program of individual and group therapy specifically designed for patients with chronic suicidality and borderline personality disorder. It blends mindfulness and a cognitive-behavioral model to address self-awareness, interpersonal functioning, affective lability, and reactions to stress.

C. Psychological

Psychological intervention is best conducted in group settings. Group therapy is helpful when specific interpersonal behavior needs to be improved. This mode of treatment also has a place with so-called "acting-out" patients, ie, those who frequently act in an impulsive and inappropriate way. The peer pressure in the group tends to impose restraints on rash behavior. The group also quickly identifies the patient's types of behavior and helps improve the validity of the patient's self-assessment, so that the antecedents of the unacceptable behavior can be effectively handled, thus decreasing its frequency. Individual therapy should initially be supportive, ie, helping the patient to restabilize and mobilize coping mechanisms. If the individual has the ability to observe his or her own behavior, a longer-term and more introspective therapy may be warranted. The therapist must be able to handle countertransference feelings (which are frequently negative), maintain appropriate boundaries in the relationship (no physical contacts, however well-meaning), and refrain from premature confrontations and interpretations.

D. Medical

Hospitalization is indicated in the case of serious suicidal or homicidal danger. In most cases, treatment can be accomplished in the day treatment center or self-help community. Antidepressants have improved anxiety, depression, and sensitivity to rejection in some patients with borderline personality disorder. SSRIs also have a role in reducing aggressive behavior in impulsive aggressive patients (eg, fluoxetine 20–60 mg orally daily or sertraline 50–200 mg orally daily). Antipsychotics may be helpful in targeting hostility, agitation, and as adjuncts to antidepressant therapy (eg, olanzapine [2.5–10 mg/d orally], risperidone [0.5–2 mg/d orally], or haloperidol [0.5–2 mg/d orally, split into two doses]). In some cases, these medications are required only for several days and can be discontinued after the patient has regained a previously established level of adjustment; they can also provide ongoing support. In other patients, carbamazepine, 400–800 mg orally daily in divided doses, decreases the severity of behavioral dyscontrol.

▶ Prognosis

Antisocial and borderline categories generally have a guarded prognosis. Those patients with a history of parental abuse and a family history of mood disorder tend to have the most challenging treatments.

Ingenhoven T et al. Effectiveness of pharmacotherapy for severe personality disorders: meta-analyses of randomized controlled trials. J Clin Psychiatry. 2010 Jan;71(1):14–25. [PMID: 19778496]

Stoffers JM et al. Psychological therapies for people with borderline personality disorder. Cochrane Database Syst Rev. 2012 Aug 15;8:CD005652. [PMID: 22895952]

SCHIZOPHRENIA SPECTRUM DISORDERS

ESSENTIALS OF DIAGNOSIS

▶ Social withdrawal, usually slowly progressive, often with deterioration in personal care.

▶ Loose thought associations, often with slowed thinking or overinclusive and rapid shifting from topic to topic.

▶ Autistic absorption in inner thoughts and frequent sexual or religious preoccupations.

▶ Auditory hallucinations, often of a derogatory nature.

▶ Delusions, frequently of a persecutory nature.

▶ Symptoms of at least 6 months' duration.

General Considerations

Schizophrenia is manifested by a massive disruption of thinking, mood, and overall behavior as well as poor filtering of stimuli. The characterization and nomenclature of the disorders are quite arbitrary and are influenced by sociocultural factors and schools of psychiatric thought.

It is believed that the cause of schizophrenia is multifactorial, with genetic, environmental, and neurotransmitter pathophysiologic components. At present, there is no laboratory method for confirming the diagnosis of schizophrenia. There may or may not be a history of a major disruption in the individual's life (failure, loss, physical illness) before gross psychotic deterioration is evident.

"Other psychotic disorders" are conditions that are similar to schizophrenic disorders in their acute symptoms but have a less pervasive influence over the long term. The patient usually attains higher levels of functioning. The acute psychotic episodes tend to be less disruptive of the person's lifestyle, with a fairly quick return to previous levels of functioning.

Classification

A. Schizophrenic Disorders

Schizophrenia is the most common of the psychotic disorders that are all characterized by a loss of contact with reality. While about 1% if the population suffers from schizophrenia, those with the diagnosis account for up to 50% of all long-term psychiatric hospitalizations. Schizophrenia is a chronic disorder that is characterized by increasing social and vocational disability that begins in late adolescence or early adulthood and tends to continue through life. Schizophrenic symptoms have been classified into positive and negative categories. Positive symptoms include hallucinations, delusions, disorganized speech and behavior; these symptoms appear to be related to increased dopaminergic (D_2) activity in the mesolimbic region. Negative symptoms include diminished sociability, restricted affect, and poverty of speech; these symptoms appear to be related to decreased D_2 activity in the mesocortical system.

B. Delusional Disorder

Delusional disorders are psychoses in which the predominant symptoms are persistent delusions with minimal impairment of daily functioning. (The schizophrenic disorders show significant impairment.) Intellectual and occupational activities are little affected, whereas social and marital functioning tends to be markedly involved. Hallucinations are not usually present. Common delusional themes include paranoid delusions of persecution, delusions of being related to or loved by a well-known person, and delusions that one's partner is unfaithful.

C. Schizoaffective Disorder

Schizoaffective disorders are those cases that fail to fit comfortably either in the schizophrenic or in the affective categories. They are usually cases with affective symptoms (either a major depressive episode, manic episode, or hypomanic episode) that precede or develop concurrently with psychotic manifestations and the psychotic episode lasts at least 2 or more weeks in the absence of any mood symptoms. There has been increasing interest in studying prodromal schizophrenia with a goal of prevention or early treatment.

D. Schizophreniform Disorders

Schizophreniform disorders are similar in their symptoms to schizophrenic disorders except that the duration of prodromal, acute, and residual symptoms is > 1 week but < 6 months.

E. Brief Psychotic Disorders

These disorders last < 1 week. They are the result of psychological stress. The shorter duration is significant and correlates with a more acute onset and resolution as well as a much better prognosis.

Clinical Findings

A. Symptoms and Signs

The symptoms and signs of schizophrenia vary markedly among individuals as well as in the same person at different times. The patient's **appearance** may be bizarre, although the usual finding is a mild to moderate unkempt blandness. **Motor activity** is generally reduced, although extremes ranging from catatonic stupor to frenzied excitement occur. **Social behavior** is characterized by marked withdrawal coupled with disturbed interpersonal relationships and a reduced ability to experience pleasure. Dependency and a poor self-image are common. **Verbal utterances** are variable, the language being concrete yet symbolic, with unassociated rambling statements (at times interspersed with mutism) during an acute episode. Neologisms (made-up words or phrases), echolalia (repetition of words spoken by others), and verbigeration (repetition of senseless words or phrases) are occasionally present. **Affect** is usually flattened, with occasional inappropriateness. **Depression** is present in almost all cases but may be less apparent during the acute psychotic episode and more obvious during recovery. Depression is sometimes confused with akinetic side effects of antipsychotic medications. It is also related to **boredom**, which increases symptoms and decreases the response to treatment. Work is generally unavailable and time unfilled, providing opportunities for counterproductive activities such as drug abuse, withdrawal, and increased psychotic symptoms.

Thought content may vary from a paucity of ideas to a rich complex of delusional fantasy with archaic thinking. One frequently notes after a period of conversation that little if any information has actually been conveyed. Incoming stimuli produce varied responses. In some cases a simple question may trigger explosive outbursts, whereas at other times there may be no overt response whatsoever (catatonia). When paranoid ideation is present, the patient is often irritable and less cooperative. **Delusions** (false beliefs) are characteristic of paranoid thinking, and they usually take the form of a preoccupation with the supposedly threatening behavior exhibited by other individuals. This ideation may cause the patient to adopt active countermeasures such as locking doors and windows, taking up weapons, covering the ceiling with aluminum foil to counteract radar waves, and other bizarre efforts. Somatic delusions revolve around issues of bodily decay or infestation. **Perceptual distortions** usually include auditory hallucinations—visual hallucinations are more commonly associated with organic mental states—and may include illusions (distortions of reality) such as figures changing in size or lights varying in intensity. Cenesthetic hallucinations (eg, a burning sensation in the brain, feeling blood flowing in blood vessels) occasionally occur. Lack of humor, feelings of dread, depersonalization (a feeling of being apart from the self), and fears of annihilation may be present. Any of the above symptoms generate higher anxiety levels, with heightened arousal and occasional panic and suicidal ideation, as the individual fails to cope.

The development of the acute episode in schizophrenia frequently is the end product of a gradual decompensation. Frustration and anxiety appear early, followed by depression and alienation, along with progressive ineffectiveness in day-to-day coping. This often leads to feelings of panic and increasing disorganization, with loss of the ability to test and evaluate the reality of perceptions. The stage of so-called psychotic resolution includes delusions, autistic preoccupations, and psychotic insight, with acceptance of the decompensated state. The process is frequently complicated by the use of caffeine, alcohol, and other recreational drugs. Life expectancy of schizophrenic patients is as much as 20% shorter than that of cohorts in the general population and is often associated with comorbid conditions such as the metabolic syndrome, which may be induced or exacerbated by the atypical antipsychotic agents.

Polydipsia may produce water intoxication with hyponatremia—characterized by symptoms of confusion, lethargy, psychosis, seizures, and occasionally death—in any psychiatric disorder, but most commonly in schizophrenia. These problems exacerbate the schizophrenic symptoms and can be confused with them. Possible pathogenetic factors in polydipsia include a hypothalamic defect, inappropriate antidiuretic hormone (ADH) secretion, antipsychotic medications (anticholinergic effects, stimulation of hypothalamic thirst center, effect on ADH), smoking (nicotine and syndrome of inappropriate antidiuretic hormone [SIADH]), psychotic thought processes (delusions), and other medications (eg, diuretics, antidepressants, lithium, alcohol) (see Chapter 21).

B. Imaging

Ventricular enlargement and cortical atrophy, as seen on CT scan, have been correlated with chronic course, severe cognitive impairment, and nonresponsiveness to antipsychotic medications. Decreased frontal lobe activity seen on PET scan has been associated with negative symptoms.

▶ Differential Diagnosis

One should not hesitate to reconsider the diagnosis of schizophrenia in any person who has received that diagnosis in the past, particularly when the clinical course has been atypical. A number of these patients have been found to actually have atypical episodic affective disorders that have responded well to lithium. Manic episodes often mimic schizophrenia. Furthermore, schizophrenia has been diagnosed in many individuals because of inadequacies in psychiatric nomenclature. Thus, schizophrenia was often inappropriately diagnosed in persons with brief reactive psychoses, OCD, paranoid disorders, and schizophreniform disorders.

Psychotic depressions, psychotic organic mental states, and any illness with psychotic ideation tend to be confused with schizophrenia, partly because of the regrettable tendency to use the terms interchangeably. Adolescent phases of growth and counterculture behaviors constitute another area of diagnostic confusion. It is particularly important to avoid a misdiagnosis in these groups, because of the long-term implications arising from having such a serious diagnosis made in a formative stage of life.

Medical disorders such as thyroid dysfunction, adrenal and pituitary disorders, reactions to toxic materials (eg, mercury, PCBs), and almost all of the organic mental states in the early stages must be ruled out. Postpartum psychosis is discussed under Mood Disorders. **Complex partial seizures,** especially when psychosensory phenomena are present, are an important differential consideration. Toxic drug states arising from prescription, over-the-counter, herbal and street drugs may mimic all of the psychotic disorders. The chronic use of amphetamines, cocaine, and other stimulants frequently produces a psychosis that is almost identical to the acute paranoid schizophrenic episode. The presence of formication (sensation of insects crawling on or under the skin) and stereotypy suggests the possibility of stimulant abuse. Phencyclidine (see below), a common street drug, may cause a reaction that is difficult to distinguish from other psychotic disorders. Cerebellar signs, excessive salivation, dilated pupils, and increased deep tendon reflexes should alert the clinician to the possibility of a toxic psychosis. Industrial chemical toxicity (both organic and metallic), degenerative disorders, and metabolic deficiencies must be considered in the differential diagnosis.

Catatonia, frequently assumed to exist solely as a component of schizophrenic disorders, is actually the end product of a number of illnesses, including various organic conditions. Neoplasms, viral and bacterial encephalopathies, central nervous system hemorrhage, metabolic derangements such as diabetic ketoacidosis, sedative withdrawal, and liver and kidney malfunction have all been implicated. It is particularly important to realize that drug toxicity (eg, overdoses of antipsychotic medications such as fluphenazine or haloperidol) can cause catatonic syndrome, which may be misdiagnosed as a catatonic schizophrenic disorder and inappropriately treated with more antipsychotic medication.

▶ Treatment

A. Medical

Hospitalization is often necessary, particularly when the patient's behavior shows gross disorganization. The presence of competent family members lessens the need for hospitalization, and each case should be judged individually. The major considerations are to prevent self-inflicted harm or harm to others and to provide the patient's basic needs. A full medical evaluation and CT scan or MRI of the brain should be considered in first episodes of schizophreniform disorder and other psychotic episodes of unknown cause.

Antipsychotic medications (see below) are the treatment of choice. The relapse rate can be reduced by 50% with proper maintenance antipsychotic therapy. Long-acting, injectable depot antipsychotics are used in noncompliant patients or nonresponders to oral medication.

Antipsychotic medications include the "**typical** or **first-generation**" antipsychotics (phenothiazines, thioxanthenes, butyrophenones, dihydroindolones, dibenzoxazepines, and benzisoxazoles) and the newer "**atypical** or **second-generation**" antipsychotics (clozapine, risperidone, olanzapine, quetiapine, aripiprazole, ziprasidone, paliperidone, iloperidone, and lurasidone) (Table 25–4). Generally, increasing milligram potency of the typical antipsychotics is associated with decreasing anticholinergic and adrenergic side effects and increasing extrapyramidal symptoms (Table 25–5). Data suggests similar antipsychotic efficacy for both classes

and a tendency for the second-generation antipsychotics, particularly olanzapine, to be better tolerated leading to enhanced compliance.

The phenothiazines comprise the bulk of the currently used "typical" antipsychotic medications. The only butyrophenone commonly used in psychiatry is haloperidol, which is different in structure but similar in action and side effects to the piperazine phenothiazines such as fluphenazine, perphenazine, and trifluoperazine. These medications and haloperidol (dopamine [D_2] receptor blockers) have high potency and a paucity of autonomic side effects and act to markedly lower arousal levels.

Clozapine, the first "atypical" (novel) antipsychotic drug developed, has dopamine (D_4) receptor-blocking activity as well as central serotonergic, histaminergic, and alpha-noradrenergic receptor-blocking activity. It is effective in the treatment of about 30% of psychoses resistant to other antipsychotic medications, and it may have specific efficacy in decreasing suicidality in patients with schizophrenia. Risperidone is an antipsychotic that blocks some serotonin receptors (5-HT$_2$) and dopamine receptors (D$_2$). Risperidone causes fewer extrapyramidal side effects than the typical antipsychotics at doses < 6 mg. It appears to be

Table 25–4. Commonly used antipsychotics and medications.

Drug	Usual Daily Oral Dose	Usual Daily Maximum Dose[1]	Cost per Unit	Cost for 30 Days Treatment Based on Maximum Dosage[2]
Aripiprazole (Abilify)	10–15 mg	30 mg	$30.95/30 mg	$1317.30
Asenapine (Saphris)	10–20 mg	20 mg	$11.53/10 mg	$827.62
Chlorpromazine (Thorazine; others)	100–400 mg	1 g	$2.90/200 mg	$588.00
Clozapine (Clozaril)	300–450 mg	900 mg	$3.33/100 mg	$899.10
Fluphenazine (Permitil, Prolixin)[3]	2–10 mg	60 mg	$1.15/10 mg	$207.00
Haloperidol (Haldol)	2–5 mg	60 mg	$2.76/20 mg	$248.40
Iloperidone (Fanapt)	12–24 mg	24 mg	$12.68/12 mg	$919.04
Loxapine (Loxitane)	20–60 mg	200 mg	$2.57/50 mg	$308.40
Lurasidone (Latuda)	40-80 mg	80 mg	$18.46/80 mg	$667.50
Olanzapine (Zyprexa)	5–10 mg	15 mg	$20.97/10 mg	$964.80
Paliperidone (Invega)	6–12 mg	12 mg	$14.31/6 mg	$1593.20
Perphenazine (Trilafon)[3]	16–32 mg	64 mg	$1.95/16 mg	$312.00
Quetiapine (Seroquel)	200–400 mg	800 mg	$14.37/200 mg	$1196.40
Risperidone (Risperdal)[4]	2–6 mg	10 mg	$7.59/2 mg	$946.16
Thioridazine (Mellaril)	100–400 mg	600 mg	$.67/100 mg	$117.00
Thiothixene (Navane)[3]	5–10 mg	80 mg	$0.65/10 mg	$156.00
Trifluoperazine (Stelazine)	5–15 mg	60 mg	$1.58/10 mg	$441.00
Ziprasidone (Geodon)	40–160 mg	160 mg	$12.08/80 mg	$645.00

[1]Can be higher in some cases.
[2]Average wholesale price (AWP, for AB-rated generic when available) for quantity listed. Source: *Red Book Online,* 2014, Truven Health Analytics, Inc. AWP may not accurately represent the actual pharmacy cost because wide contractual variations exist among institutions.
[3]Indicates piperazine structure.
[4]For risperidone, daily doses above 6 mg increase the risk of extrapyramidal syndrome. Risperidone 6 mg is approximately equivalent to haloperidol 20 mg.

Table 25–5. Relative potency and side effects of antipsychotic medications.

Drug	Chlorpromazine: Drug Potency Ratio	Anticholinergic Effects[1]	Extrapyramidal Effect[1]
Aripiprazole	1:20	1	1
Chlorpromazine	1:1	4	1
Clozapine	1:1	4	—
Fluphenazine	1:50	1	4
Haloperidol	1:50	1	4
Iloperidone	1:25	1	1
Loxapine	1:10	2	3
Lurasidone	1:5	1	2
Olanzapine	1:20	1	1
Perphenazine	1:10	2	3
Quetiapine	1:1	1	1
Risperidone	1:50	1	3
Thioridazine	1:1	4	1
Thiothixene	1:20	1	4
Trifluoperazine	1:20	1	4
Ziprasidone	1:1	1	1

[1]1, weak effect; 4, strong effect.

as effective as haloperidol and possibly as effective as clozapine in treatment-resistant patients without necessitating weekly white cell counts, as required with clozapine therapy. Risperidone is available in a long-acting injectable preparation.

Olanzapine is a potent blocker of muscarinic, anticholinergic, 5-HT$_2$, and dopamine D$_1$, D$_2$, and D$_4$ receptors. High doses of olanzapine (12.5–17.5 mg daily) appear to be more effective than lower doses. The drug appears to be more effective than haloperidol in the treatment of negative symptoms, such as withdrawal, psychomotor retardation, and poor interpersonal relationships. It is available in an orally disintegrating form for patients who are unable to tolerate standard oral dosing and in an injectable form for the management of acute agitation associated with schizophrenia and bipolar disorder. Olanzapine tends to result in elevations of serum alanine aminotransferase more commonly than does haloperidol. Olanzapine is associated with a much lower incidence of dystonic reaction than haloperidol and is perhaps less likely to induce tardive dyskinesia. Its most common side effects include somnolence, agitation, nervousness, headache, insomnia, dizziness, and significant weight gain. Multiple case reports have linked olanzapine and clozapine to new-onset type 2 diabetes, and all atypical medications should be monitored for this adverse effect as well. Both atypical and typical agents have been associated with a significantly higher risk of stroke and death in elderly patients.

Quetiapine is an antipsychotic with greater 5-HT$_2$ relative to D$_2$ receptor blockade as well as a relatively high affinity for alpha-1- and alpha-2-adrenergic receptors.

It appears to be as efficacious as haloperidol in treating positive and negative symptoms of schizophrenia, with less extrapyramidal side effects even at high doses. More common side effects include somnolence, dizziness, and postural hypotension. Because of an association with lens changes seen in patients on long-term treatment, an eye examination to detect cataract formation is recommended at initiation of treatment and then at 6-month intervals during treatment. Quetiapine may cause QT prolongation particularly when prescribed with other medications that effect the QT interval and in overdose.

Ziprasidone has both anti-dopamine receptor and anti-serotonin receptor effects, with good efficacy for both positive and negative symptoms of schizophrenia. Ziprasidone is not associated with significant weight gain, hyperlipidemia, or new-onset diabetes and offers a good alternative for some patients. It has been implicated in QTc interval delay of > 500 ms in some patients, although in several cases of overdose there were no incidents of torsades de pointes or sudden death. Patients taking ziprasidone should be screened for cardiac risk factors. A pretreatment ECG is indicated for patients at risk for cardiac sequelae (including patients taking other medications that might prolong the QTc interval).

Aripiprazole is a partial agonist at the dopamine D$_2$ and serotonin 5-HT$_1$ receptors and an antagonist at 5-HT$_2$ receptors, it is effective against positive and negative symptoms of schizophrenia. It functions as an antagonist or agonist, depending on the dopaminergic activity at the dopamine receptors. This may help decrease side effects. More activating than sedating, aripiprazole is thought to impose a low risk of extrapyramidal symptoms, weight gain, hyperprolactinemia, and delayed QT interval. Aripiprazole has been approved as an augmentation agent for treatment-resistant depression even when psychosis is not present. Asenapine, approved for the treatment of schizophrenia and bipolar disorder (mixed or manic state), appears to be particularly helpful in treating negative symptoms of schizophrenia. Asenapine can cause hyperprolactinemia and weight gain. It carries a warning for possible serious allergic reactions, which can occur even after the first dose, including anaphylaxis, hypotension, and difficulty breathing. Patients should be appropriately cautioned. Paliperidone, the active metabolite of risperidone, is available as a capsule and a monthly injection. It has the advantage of low associations with diabetes mellitus, weight gain, and dyslipidemia. Both asenapine and paliperidone increase the risk of QT interval prolongation and should be avoided in patients with risk factors for this ECG finding. Iloperidone has low incidence of extrapyramidal side effects that is similar to the other atypical agents but requires careful initial titration due to the risk of orthostatic hypotension and possibility of lengthening the QT interval. When coadministered with paroxetine or clarithromycin, the dose of iloperidone must be halved because of decreased hepatic metabolism by the cytochrome P450 CYP2D6 and CYP3A4 isozymes. Lurasidone is FDA-approved and has been shown to be effective in treating acute decompensation in patients with chronic schizophrenia. This medication is distinguished by low incidence of weight gain, increased lipids or prolonged QT interval, but clinicians should be mindful of side effects of akathisia, elevated prolactin and in higher doses, somnolence. None of the antipsychotics produce true physical dependency. All decrease adrenergic responses. Despite higher costs, atypical antipsychotics are often considered preferable to traditional antipsychotics because they are thought to be associated with reduced extrapyramidal symptoms and a lesser risk of tardive dyskinesia.

▶ Clinical Indications

The antipsychotics are used to treat all forms of the schizophrenias as well as psychotic ideation in delirium and dementia, drug-induced psychoses, psychotic depression, and mania. They are also effective in Tourette disorder. Antipsychotics quickly lower the arousal (activity) level and, perhaps indirectly, gradually improve socialization and thinking. The improvement rate for treating positive symptoms is about 80%. Patients whose behavioral symptoms worsen with use of antipsychotic medications may have an undiagnosed organic condition such as anticholinergic toxicity.

Symptoms that are ameliorated by these medications include hyperactivity, hostility, aggression, delusions, hallucinations, irritability, and poor sleep. Individuals with acute psychosis and good premorbid function respond quite well. The most common cause of failure in the treatment of acute psychosis is inadequate dosage, and the most common cause of relapse is noncompliance.

Although typical antipsychotics are efficacious in the treatment of positive symptoms of schizophrenia, such as hallucinations and delusions, atypical antipsychotics are thought to have efficacy in reducing both positive and negative symptoms. Antidepressant medications may be used in conjunction with antipsychotics if significant depression is present. Resistant cases may require concomitant use of lithium, carbamazepine, or valproic acid. The addition of a benzodiazepine drug to the antipsychotic regimen may prove helpful in treating the agitated or catatonic psychotic patient who has not responded to antipsychotics alone—lorazepam, 1–2 mg orally, can produce a rapid resolution of catatonic symptoms and may allow maintenance with a lower antipsychotic dose. Electroconvulsive therapy (ECT) has also been effective in treating catatonia.

▶ Dosage Forms & Patterns

The dosage range is quite broad. For example, risperidone, 0.25–1 mg orally at bedtime, may be sufficient for the elderly person with mild dementia with psychosis (especially in view of the increased risk of stroke and death in the elderly), whereas up to 6 mg/d may be used in a young patient with acute schizophrenia. For quick response, an atypical antipsychotic may be started in combination with a benzodiazepine (eg, risperidone oral solution, 2 mg, or olanzapine, 10 mg orally, and lorazepam, 2 mg orally, every 2–4 hours as needed). In an acutely distressed, psychotic patient one might use haloperidol, 10 mg intramuscularly, which is absorbed rapidly and achieves an initial tenfold plasma level advantage over equal oral doses. Psychomotor agitation, racing thoughts, and general arousal are quickly reduced. The dose can be repeated every 3–4 hours; when the patient is less symptomatic, oral doses can replace parenteral administration in most cases. In the elderly, both atypical (eg, risperidone 0.25 mg–0.5 mg daily or olanzapine 1.25 mg daily) and typical (eg, haloperidol 0.5 mg daily or perphenazine 2 mg daily) antipsychotics, often used effectively in small doses for behavioral control, have been linked to premature death in some cases.

Absorption of oral medications may be increased or decreased by concomitant administration of other medications (eg, antacids tend to decrease the absorption of antidepressants). Previous gastrointestinal surgery may alter pH, motility, and surface areas available for drug absorption. There are racial differences in metabolizing the antipsychotic medications—eg, many Asians require only about half the usual dosage. Bioavailability is influenced by other factors such as smoking or hepatic microsomal enzyme stimulation with alcohol or barbiturates and enzyme-altering medications such as carbamazepine or methylphenidate. Antipsychotic plasma drug level determinations are not currently of major clinical assistance.

Divided daily doses are not necessary after a maintenance dose has been established, and most patients can then be maintained on a single daily dose, usually taken at bedtime. This is particularly appropriate in a case where the sedative effect of the drug is desired for nighttime sleep, and undesirable sedative effects can be avoided during the day. Risperidone is an exception, being given twice daily. First-episode patients especially should be tapered off medications after about 6 months of stability and carefully monitored; their rate of relapse is lower than that of multiple-episode patients.

Psychiatric patients—particularly paranoid individuals—often neglect to take their medication. In these cases and in nonresponders to oral medication, the enanthate and decanoate (the latter is slightly longer-lasting and has fewer extrapyramidal side effects) forms of fluphenazine or the decanoate form of haloperidol may be given by deep subcutaneous injection or intramuscularly to achieve an effect that will usually last 7–28 days. A patient who cannot be depended on to take oral medication (or who overdoses on minimal provocation) will generally agree to come to the clinician's office for a "shot." The usual dose of the fluphenazine long-acting preparations is 25 mg every 2 weeks. Dosage and frequency of administration vary from about 100 mg weekly to 12.5 mg monthly. Use the smallest effective amount as infrequently as possible. A monthly injection of 25 mg of fluphenazine decanoate is equivalent to about 15–20 mg of oral fluphenazine daily. Risperidone is the first atypical antipsychotic available in a long-acting injectable form (25–50 mg intramuscularly every 2 weeks). Concomitant use of a benzodiazepine (eg, lorazepam, 2 mg orally twice daily) may permit reduction of the required dosage of oral or parenteral antipsychotic drug.

Intravenous haloperidol, the antipsychotic most commonly used by this route, is often used in critical care units in the management of agitated, delirious patients. Intravenous haloperidol should be given no faster than 1 mg/min to reduce cardiovascular side effects, such as torsades de pointes. Current practice indicates that ECG monitoring should be used whenever haloperidol is being administered intravenously.

▶ Side Effects

For both typical and atypical antipsychotic agents, a range of side effects has been reported. The most common anticholinergic side effects include **dry mouth** (which can lead to ingestion of caloric liquids and weight gain or hyponatremia), **blurred near vision**, **urinary retention** (particularly in elderly men with enlarged prostates), **delayed gastric emptying**, **esophageal reflux**, **ileus**, **delirium**, and precipitation of **acute glaucoma** in patients with narrow

anterior chamber angles. Other autonomic effects include **orthostatic hypotension** and **sexual dysfunction**—problems in achieving erection, ejaculation (including retrograde ejaculation), and orgasm in men (approximately 50% of cases) and women (approximately 30%). Delay in achieving orgasm is often a factor in medication noncompliance. **Electrocardiographic changes** occur frequently, but clinically significant arrhythmias are much less common. Elderly patients and those with preexisting cardiac disease are at greater risk. The most frequently seen electrocardiographic changes include diminution of the T wave amplitude, appearance of prominent U waves, depression of the ST segment, and prolongation of the QT interval. Thioridazine has been given an FDA warning for dose-related QTc delay and risk of fatal cardiac arrhythmias. As noted above, ziprasidone can produce QTc prolongation. An ECG prior to treatment in some patients may be indicated. In some critical care patients, torsades de pointes has been associated with the use of high-dose intravenous haloperidol (usually > 30 mg/24 h).

Associations have been suggested between the atypical antipsychotics and **new-onset diabetes**, **hyperlipidemia**, **QTc prolongation**, and **weight gain** (Table 25–6). The FDA has particularly noted the risk of hyperglycemia and new-onset diabetes in this class of medication that is not related to weight gain. The risk of diabetes mellitus is increased in patients taking clozapine and olanzapine. Monitoring of weight, fasting blood sugar and lipids prior to initiation of treatment and at regular intervals thereafter is an important part of medication monitoring. Early research suggests that the addition of metformin to olanzapine may improve drug-induced weight gain in patients with drug-naïve, first-episode schizophrenia. Antipsychotic medications in general may have **metabolic** and **endocrine effects**, including weight gain, hyperglycemia, impaired temperature regulation in hot weather, and water intoxication, that may be due to inappropriate ADH secretion. Lactation and menstrual irregularities are common (antipsychotic medications should be avoided, if possible, in breast cancer patients because of potential trophic effects of elevated prolactin levels on the breast). Both

Table 25–6. Adverse factors associated with atypical antipsychotic medications.

	Weight Gain	Hyperlipidemia	New-Onset Diabetes Mellitus	QTc Prolongation[1]
Asenapine	+/–	+/–	+/–	+++
Aripiprazole	+/–	–	–	++
Clozapine	+++	+++	+++	+/–
Lurasidone	–	–	–	–
Olanzapine	+++	+++	+++	+/–
Paliperidone	+	+/—	+/–	+++
Quetiapine	++	++	++	+++
Risperidone	++	++	++	+
Ziprasidone	+/–	—	–	+++

[1]QTc prolongation is a side effect of many medications and suggests a possible risk for arrhythmia. Prescriber's Letter 2011;18(12):271207.

antipsychotic and antidepressant medications inhibit sperm motility. **Bone marrow depression** and **cholestatic jaundice** occur rarely; these are hypersensitivity reactions, and they usually appear in the first 2 months of treatment. They subside on discontinuance of the drug. There is cross-sensitivity among all of the phenothiazines, and a drug from a different group should be used when allergic reactions occur.

Clozapine is associated with a 1.6% risk of **agranulocytosis** (higher in persons of Ashkenazi Jewish ancestry), and its use must be strictly monitored with weekly blood counts during the first 6 months of treatment, with monitoring every other week thereafter. Discontinuation of the medication requires weekly monitoring of the white blood cell count for 1 month. Clozapine has been associated with fatal myocarditis and is contraindicated in patients with severe heart disease. In addition, clozapine lowers the seizure threshold and has many side effects, including sedation, hypotension, increased liver enzyme levels, hypersalivation, respiratory arrest, weight gain, and changes in both the ECG and the electroencephalogram. Notably, adynamic ileus is a rare side effect of clozapine that can be fatal.

Photosensitivity, retinopathy, and **hyperpigmentation** are associated with use of fairly high dosages of chlorpromazine and thioridazine. The appearance of particulate melanin deposits in the lens of the eye is related to the total dose given, and patients on long-term medication should have periodic eye examinations. Teratogenicity has not been causally related to these medications, but prudence is indicated particularly in the first trimester of pregnancy. The seizure threshold is lowered, but it is safe to use these medications in epileptics who take anticonvulsants.

The **antipsychotic malignant syndrome (NMS)** is a catatonia-like state manifested by extrapyramidal signs, blood pressure changes, altered consciousness, and hyperpyrexia; it is an uncommon but serious complication of antipsychotic treatment. Muscle rigidity, involuntary movements, confusion, dysarthria, and dysphagia are accompanied by pallor, cardiovascular instability, fever, pulmonary congestion, and diaphoresis and may result in stupor, coma, and death. The cause may be related to a number of factors, including poor dosage control of antipsychotic medication, affective illness, decreased serum iron, dehydration, and increased sensitivity of dopamine receptor sites. Lithium in combination with an antipsychotic drug may increase vulnerability, which is already increased in patients with an affective disorder. In most cases, the symptoms develop within the first 2 weeks of antipsychotic drug treatment. The syndrome may occur with small doses of the medications. Intramuscular administration is a risk factor. Elevated creatine kinase and leukocytosis with a shift to the left are present early in about half of cases. Treatment includes controlling fever and providing fluid support. Dopamine agonists such as bromocriptine, 2.5–10 mg orally three times a day, and amantadine, 100–200 mg orally twice a day, have also been useful. Dantrolene, 50 mg intravenously as needed, is used to alleviate rigidity (do not exceed 10 mg/kg/d due to hepatotoxicity risk). There is ongoing controversy about the efficacy

of these three agents as well as the use of calcium channel blockers and benzodiazepines. ECT has been used effectively in resistant cases. Clozapine has been used with relative safety and fair success as an antipsychotic drug for patients who have had NMS.

Akathisia is the most common (about 20%) extrapyramidal symptom. It usually occurs early in treatment (but may persist after antipsychotics are discontinued) and is frequently mistaken for anxiety or exacerbation of psychosis. It is characterized by a subjective desire to be in constant motion followed by an inability to sit or stand still and consequent pacing. It may induce suicidality or feelings of fright, rage, terror, or sexual torment. Insomnia is often present. It is crucial to educate patients in advance about these potential side effects so that the patients do not misinterpret them as signs of increased illness. In all cases, reevaluate the dosage requirement or the type of antipsychotic drug. One should inquire also about cigarette smoking, which in women has been associated with an increased incidence of akathisia. Antiparkinsonism medications (such as trihexyphenidyl, 2–5 mg orally three times daily) may be helpful, but first-line treatment often includes a benzodiazepine (such as clonazepam 0.5–1 mg orally three times daily). In resistant cases, symptoms may be alleviated by propranolol, 30–80 mg/d orally, diazepam, 5 mg orally three times daily, or amantadine, 100 mg orally three times daily.

Acute dystonias usually occur early, although a late (tardive) occurrence is reported in patients (mostly men after several years of therapy) who previously had early severe dystonic reactions and a mood disorder (see below). Younger patients are at higher risk for acute dystonias. The most common signs are bizarre muscle spasms of the head, neck, and tongue. Frequently present are torticollis, oculogyric crises, swallowing or chewing difficulties, and masseter spasms. Laryngospasm is particularly dangerous. Back, arm, or leg muscle spasms are occasionally reported. Diphenhydramine, 50 mg intramuscularly, is effective for the acute crisis; one should then give benztropine mesylate, 2 mg orally twice daily, for several weeks, and then discontinue gradually, since few of the extrapyramidal symptoms require long-term use of the antiparkinsonism medications (all of which are about equally efficacious—though trihexyphenidyl tends to be mildly stimulating and benztropine mildly sedating).

Drug-induced parkinsonism is indistinguishable from idiopathic parkinsonism, but it is reversible, occurs later in treatment than the preceding extrapyramidal symptoms, and in some cases appears after antipsychotic withdrawal. The condition includes the typical signs of apathy and reduction of facial and arm movements (akinesia, which can mimic depression), festinating gait, rigidity, loss of postural reflexes, and pill-rolling tremor. AIDS patients seem particularly vulnerable to extrapyramidal side effects. High-potency antipsychotics often require antiparkinsonism medications (see Table 24–6). The antipsychotic dosage should be reduced, and immediate relief can be achieved with antiparkinsonism medications in the same dosages as above. After 4–6 weeks, these antiparkinsonism medications can often be discontinued with no recurrent symptoms. In any of the extrapyramidal symptoms, amantadine, 100–400 mg orally daily, may be used instead of the antiparkinsonism medications. Antipsychotic-induced catatonia is similar to catatonic stupor with rigidity, drooling, urinary incontinence, and cogwheeling. It usually responds slowly to withdrawal of the offending medication and use of antiparkinsonism agents.

Tardive dyskinesia is a syndrome of abnormal involuntary stereotyped movements of the face, mouth, tongue, trunk, and limbs that may occur after months or (usually) years of treatment with antipsychotic agents. The syndrome affects 20–35% of patients who have undergone long-term antipsychotic therapy. Predisposing factors include older age, many years of treatment, cigarette smoking, and diabetes mellitus. Pineal calcification is higher in this condition by a margin of 3:1. There are no clearcut differences among the antipsychotic medications in the development of tardive dyskinesia. (Although the atypical antipsychotics appear to offer a lower risk of tardive dyskinesia, long-term effects have not been investigated.) Early manifestations of tardive dyskinesia include fine worm-like movements of the tongue at rest, difficulty in sticking out the tongue, facial tics, increased blink frequency, or jaw movements of recent onset. Later manifestations may include bucco-linguo-masticatory movements, lip smacking, chewing motions, mouth opening and closing, disturbed gag reflex, puffing of the cheeks, disrupted speech, respiratory distress, or choreoathetoid movements of the extremities (the last being more prevalent in younger patients). The symptoms do not necessarily worsen and in rare cases may lessen even though antipsychotic medications are continued. The dyskinesias do not occur during sleep and can be voluntarily suppressed for short periods. Stress and movements in other parts of the body will often aggravate the condition.

Early signs of dyskinesia must be differentiated from those reversible signs produced by ill-fitting dentures or nonantipsychotic medications such as levodopa, TCAs, antiparkinsonism agents, anticonvulsants, and antihistamines. Other neurologic conditions such as Huntington chorea can be differentiated by history and examination.

The emphasis should be on prevention of side effects. Use the least amount of antipsychotic drug necessary to mute the psychotic symptoms, and use atypical antipsychotics as first-line agents. Detect early manifestations of dyskinesias. When these occur, stop anticholinergic medications and gradually discontinue antipsychotic medications, if clinically feasible. Weight loss and cachexia sometimes appear on withdrawal of antipsychotics. In an indeterminate number of cases, the dyskinesias will remit. Keep the patient off the medications until reemergent psychotic symptoms dictate their resumption, at which point they are restarted in low doses and gradually increased until there is clinical improvement. If antipsychotic medications are restarted, clozapine and olanzapine appear to offer less risk of recurrence. The use of adjunctive agents such as benzodiazepines or lithium may help directly or indirectly by allowing control of psychotic symptoms with a low dosage of antipsychotics. If the dyskinesic syndrome recurs and it is necessary to continue antipsychotic medications to control psychotic symptoms, informed consent should be obtained. Benzodiazepines, buspirone (in doses of 15–60 mg/d orally), phosphatidylcholine, clonidine, calcium channel blockers, vitamin E, omega-3 fatty acids, and propranolol all have had limited usefulness in treating the dyskinetic side effects.

B. Social

Environmental considerations are most important in the individual with a chronic illness, who usually has a history of repeated hospitalizations, a continued low level of functioning, and symptoms that never completely remit. Family rejection and work failure are common. In these cases, board and care homes staffed by personnel experienced in caring for psychiatric patients are most important. There is frequently an inverse relationship between stability of the living situation and the amounts of required antipsychotic medications, since the most salutary environment is one that reduces stimuli. Nonresidential self-help groups such as Recovery, Inc., should be utilized whenever possible. They provide a setting for sharing, learning, and mutual support and are frequently the only social involvement with which this type of patient is comfortable. Vocational rehabilitation and work agencies (eg, Goodwill Industries, Inc.) provide assessment, training, and job opportunities at a level commensurate with the person's clinical condition.

C. Psychological

The need for psychotherapy varies markedly depending on the patient's current status and history. In a person with a single psychotic episode and a previously good level of adjustment, supportive psychotherapy may help the patient reintegrate the experience, gain some insight into antecedent problems, and become a more self-observant individual who can recognize early signs of stress. Insight-oriented psychotherapy is often counterproductive in this type of disorder. Research suggests that cognitive behavioral therapy—in conjunction with medication management—may have some efficacy in the treatment of symptoms of schizophrenia. Cognitive behavioral therapy for schizophrenia involves helping the individual challenge psychotic thinking and alters response to hallucinations. Similarly, a form of psychotherapy called acceptance and commitment therapy has shown value in helping prevent hospitalizations in schizophrenia. Cognitive remediation therapy is another approach to treatment that shows promise in helping schizophrenics become better able to focus their disorganized thinking. Family therapy may also help alleviate the patient's stress and to assist relatives in coping with the patient.

D. Behavioral

Behavioral techniques (see above) are most frequently used in therapeutic settings such as day treatment centers, but there is no reason why they cannot be incorporated into family situations or any therapeutic setting. Many behavioral techniques (eg, positive reinforcement—whether it be a word of praise or an approving nod—after some positive behavior), can be a powerful instrument for helping a person learn behaviors that will facilitate social acceptance.

Music from portable digital players with earphones is one of many ways to divert the patient's attention from auditory hallucinations.

▶ Prognosis

In any psychosis, in the large majority of patients the prognosis is good for alleviation of positive symptoms such as hallucinations or delusions treated with medication. Negative symptoms such as diminished affect and sociability are much more difficult to treat but appear mildly responsive to atypical antipsychotics. Cognitive deficits, such as the executive dysfunction that is common to schizophrenia, does not appear responsive to antipsychotics. Both negative symptoms and cognitive deficits appear to contribute more to long-term disability in schizophrenic patients than do positive symptoms and both are unfortunately less responsive to antipsychotics. Unavailability of structured work situations and lack of family therapy are two other reasons why the prognosis is so guarded in such a large percentage of schizophrenic patients. Psychosis connected with a history of serious drug abuse has a guarded prognosis because of the central nervous system damage, usually from the medications themselves and associated medical illnesses.

Ellinger LK et al. Efficacy of metformin and topiramate in prevention and treatment of second-generation antipsychotic-induced weight gain. Ann Pharmacother. 2010 Apr;44(4):668–79. [PMID: 20233913]

Fayad SM et al. A fatal case of adynamic ileus following initiation of clozapine [letter]. Am J Psychiatry. 2012 May;169(5):538–9. [PMID: 22549212]

Hasnain M et al. Metabolic syndrome associated with schizophrenia and atypical antipsychotics. Curr Diab Rep. 2010 Jun;10(3):209–16. [PMID: 20425584]

Stahl SM et al. "Meta-guidelines" for the management of patients with schizophrenia. CNS Spectr. 2013 Jun;18(3):150–62. [PMID: 23591126]

Tiihonen J et al. Polypharmacy with antipsychotics, antidepressants, or benzodiazepines and mortality in schizophrenia. Arch Gen Psychiatry. 2012 May;69(5):476–83. [PMID: 22566579]

MOOD DISORDERS (DEPRESSION & MANIA)

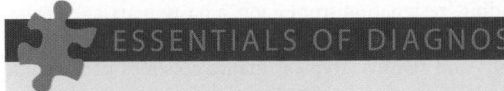

ESSENTIALS OF DIAGNOSIS

Present in most depressions

▶ Mood varies from mild sadness to intense despondency and feelings of guilt, worthlessness, and hopelessness.

▶ Difficulty in thinking, including inability to concentrate, ruminations, and lack of decisiveness.

▶ Loss of interest, with diminished involvement in work and recreation.

▶ Somatic complaints such as headache; disrupted, lessened, or excessive sleep; loss of energy; change in appetite; decreased sexual drive.

▶ Anxiety.

Present in some severe depressions

▶ Psychomotor retardation or agitation.

▶ Delusions of a somatic or persecutory nature.

▶ Withdrawal from activities.

▶ Physical symptoms of major severity, eg, anorexia, insomnia, reduced sexual drive, weight loss, and various somatic complaints.

▶ Suicidal ideation.

Present in mania

▶ Mood ranging from euphoria to irritability.

▶ Sleep disruption.

▶ Hyperactivity.

▶ Racing thoughts.

▶ Grandiosity.

▶ Variable psychotic symptoms.

▶ General Considerations

Depression is extremely common, with up to 30% of primary care patients having depressive symptoms. Depression may be the final expression of (1) genetic factors (neurotransmitter dysfunction), (2) developmental problems (personality problems, childhood events), or (3) psychosocial stresses (divorce, unemployment). It frequently presents in the form of somatic complaints with negative medical workups. Although sadness and grief are normal responses to loss, depression is not. Patients experiencing normal grief tend to produce sympathy and sadness in the clinician caregiver; depression often produces frustration and irritation in the clinician. Grief is usually accompanied by intact self-esteem, whereas depression is marked by a sense of guilt and worthlessness.

Mania is often combined with depression and may occur alone, together with depression in a mixed episode, or in cyclic fashion with depression.

▶ Clinical Findings

In general, there are four major types of depressions, with similar symptoms in each group.

A. Adjustment Disorder with Depressed Mood

Depression may occur in reaction to some identifiable stressor or adverse life situation, usually loss of a person by death (grief reaction), divorce, etc; financial reversal (crisis); or loss of an established role, such as being needed. Anger is frequently associated with the loss, and this in turn often produces a feeling of guilt. The disorder occurs within 3 months of the stressor and causes significant impairment in social or occupational functioning. The symptoms range from mild sadness, anxiety, irritability, worry, and lack of concentration, discouragement, and somatic complaints to the more severe symptoms of frank depression. When the full criteria for major depressive disorder are present (see below), then that diagnosis should be made and treatment instituted even when there is a known stressor. The presence of a stressor is not the determining diagnostic driver, it is the resultant syndromal complex. One should not neglect treatment for major depression simply because it may appear to be an understandable reaction to a particular stress or difficulty.

B. Depressive Disorders

The subclassifications include major depressive disorder and dysthymia.

1. Major depressive disorder—A major depressive disorder consists of a syndrome of mood, physical and cognitive symptoms that occurs at any time of life. Many consider a physiologic or metabolic aberration to be causative. Complaints vary widely but most frequently include a loss of interest and pleasure (anhedonia), withdrawal from activities, and feelings of guilt. Also included are inability to concentrate, some cognitive dysfunction, anxiety, chronic fatigue, feelings of worthlessness, somatic complaints (unexplained somatic complaints frequently indicate depression), loss of sexual drive, and thoughts of death. Diurnal variation with improvement as the day progresses is common. Vegetative signs that frequently occur are insomnia, anorexia with weight loss, and constipation. Occasionally, severe agitation and psychotic ideation are present. Psychotic major depression occurs up to 14% of all patients with major depression and 25% of patients who are hospitalized with depression. Psychotic symptoms are more common in depressed persons who are older than 50 years. Paranoid symptoms may range from general suspiciousness to ideas of reference with delusions. The somatic delusions frequently revolve around feelings of impending annihilation or hypochondriacal beliefs (eg, that the body is rotting away with cancer). Hallucinations are less common than unusual beliefs and tend not to occur independent of delusions.

In addition to psychotic major depression, other subcategories include **major depression with atypical features** that is characterized by hypersomnia, overeating, lethargy, and mood reactivity in which the mood brightens in response to positive events or news. Melancholic major depression is characterized by a lack of mood reactivity seen in atypical depression, the presence of a prominent anhedonia and more severe vegetative symptoms. **Major depression with a seasonal onset (seasonal affective disorder)** is a dysfunction of circadian rhythms that occurs more commonly in the winter months and is believed to be due to decreased exposure to full-spectrum light. Common symptoms include carbohydrate craving, lethargy, hyperphagia, and hypersomnia. **Major depression with postpartum onset** usually occurs 2 weeks to 6 months postpartum.

Most women (up to 80%) experience some mild letdown of mood in the postpartum period. For some of these (10–15%), the symptoms are more severe and similar to those usually seen in serious depression, with an increased emphasis on concerns related to the baby (obsessive thoughts about harming it or inability to care for it). When

psychotic symptoms occur, there is frequently associated sleep deprivation, volatility of behavior, and manic-like symptoms. Postpartum psychosis is much less common (< 2%), often occurs within the first 2 weeks, and requires early and aggressive management. Biologic vulnerability with hormonal changes and psychosocial stressors all play a role. The chances of a second episode are about 25% and may be reduced with prophylactic treatment.

2. Dysthymia—Dysthymia is a chronic depressive disturbance. Sadness, loss of interest, and withdrawal from activities over a period of 2 or more years with a relatively persistent course is necessary for this diagnosis. Generally, the symptoms are milder but longer-lasting than those in a major depressive episode.

3. Premenstrual dysphoric disorder—Depressive symptoms occur during the late luteal phase (last 2 weeks) of the menstrual cycle. (See also Chapter 18.)

C. Bipolar Disorder

Bipolar disorder consists of episodic mood shifts into mania, major depression, hypomania, and mixed mood states. The ability of bipolar disorder to mimic aspects of many other coincident major mental health disorders and a high comorbidity with substance abuse can make the initial diagnosis of bipolar disorder difficult. Bipolar I is diagnosed when an individual has both depressive and manic episodes. For individuals who experience depressive and hypomanic episodes without frank mania, the diagnosis would be Bipolar II. Individuals who become manic when treated with an antidepressant for a depressive episode are often regarded as Bipolar III.

1. Mania—A manic episode is a mood state characterized by elation with hyperactivity, overinvolvement in life activities, increased irritability, flight of ideas, easy distractibility, and little need for sleep. The overenthusiastic quality of the mood and the expansive behavior initially attract others, but the irritability, mood lability with swings into depression, aggressive behavior, and grandiosity usually lead to marked interpersonal difficulties. Activities may occur that are later regretted, eg, excessive spending, resignation from a job, a hasty marriage, sexual acting out, and exhibitionistic behavior, with alienation of friends and family. Atypical manic episodes can include gross delusions, paranoid ideation of severe proportions, and auditory hallucinations usually related to some grandiose perception. The episodes begin abruptly (sometimes precipitated by life stresses) and may last from several days to months. Spring and summer tend to be the peak periods. Generally, the manic episodes are of shorter duration than the depressive episodes. In almost all cases, the manic episode is part of a broader bipolar (manic-depressive) disorder. Patients with four or more discrete episodes of a mood disturbance in 1 year are called "rapid cyclers." (Substance abuse, particularly cocaine, can mimic rapid cycling.) These patients have a higher incidence of hypothyroidism. Manic patients differ from patients with schizophrenia in that the former use more effective interpersonal maneuvers, are more sensitive to the social maneuvers of others, and are more able to utilize weakness and vulnerability in others to their own advantage. Creativity has been positively correlated with mood disorders, but the best work done is between episodes of mania and depression.

2. Cyclothymic disorders—These are chronic mood disturbances with episodes of depression and hypomania. The symptoms must have at least a 2-year duration and are milder than those that occur in depressive or manic episodes. Occasionally, the symptoms will escalate into a full-blown manic or depressive episode, in which case reclassification as bipolar I would be warranted.

D. Mood Disorders Secondary to Illness and Medications

Any illness, severe or mild, can cause significant depression. Conditions such as rheumatoid arthritis, multiple sclerosis, stroke, and chronic heart disease are particularly likely to be associated with depression, as are other chronic illnesses. Depression is common in cancer, as well, with a particularly high degree of comorbidity in pancreatic cancer. Hormonal variations clearly play a role in some depressions. Varying degrees of depression occur at various times in schizophrenic disorders, central nervous system disease, and organic mental states. **Alcohol dependency** frequently coexists with serious depression.

The classic model of **drug-induced depression** occurs with the use of reserpine, both in clinical settings and as a pharmacologic probe in research settings. Corticosteroids and oral contraceptives are commonly associated with affective changes. Antihypertensive medications such as methyldopa, guanethidine, and clonidine have been associated with the development of depressive syndromes, as have digitalis and antiparkinsonism medications (eg, levodopa). Interferon is strongly associated with depressed mood and fatigue as a side effect; consultation with a psychiatrist prior to prescribing these agents is indicated in cases where there is a history of depression. It is unusual for beta-blockers to produce depression when given for short periods, such as in the treatment of performance anxiety. Sustained use of beta-blockers for medical conditions such as hypertension may be associated with depression in some patients, although most individuals do not suffer this adverse effect and the data supporting this association remain inconclusive. One study associated the use of beta-blockers with a significant reduction in risk of depressive symptoms 1 year after a percutaneous coronary intervention. Infrequently, disulfiram and anticholinesterase medications may be associated with symptoms of depression. All stimulant use results in a depressive syndrome when the drug is withdrawn. Alcohol, sedatives, opioids, and most of the psychedelic drugs are depressants and, paradoxically, are often used in self-treatment of depression. Corticosteroids may be associated with hypomania.

▶ Differential Diagnosis

Since depression may be a part of any illness—either reactively or as a secondary symptom—careful attention

must be given to personal life adjustment problems and the role of medications (eg, reserpine, corticosteroids, levodopa). Schizophrenia, partial complex seizures, organic brain syndromes, panic disorders, and anxiety disorders must be differentiated. Thyroid dysfunction and other endocrinopathies should be ruled out. Malignancies, including central and gastrointestinal tumors are sometimes associated with depressive symptoms and may antecede the diagnosis of tumor. Strokes, particularly dominant hemisphere lesions, can occasionally present with a syndrome that looks like major depression. Medication-induced depressive symptoms (see above) are also quite common.

▶ Complications

The most important complication is **suicide**, which often includes some elements of aggression. Suicide rates in the general population vary from 9 per 100,000 in Spain to 20 per 100,000 in the United States to 58 per 100,000 in Hungary. In individuals hospitalized for depression, the lifetime risk rises to 10–15%. In patients with bipolar disorder, the risk is higher, with up to 20% of individuals dying of suicide. Men over the age of 50 are more likely to complete a suicide because of their tendency to attempt suicide with more violent means, particularly guns. On the other hand, women make more attempts but are less likely to complete a suicide. An increased suicide rate is being observed in the younger population, ages 15–35. Patients with cancer, respiratory illnesses, AIDS, and those being maintained on hemodialysis have higher suicide rates. Alcohol use is a significant factor in many suicide attempts.

There are several groups of people who make suicide attempts. One group includes those individuals with acute situational problems. These individuals may be acutely distressed by a recent breakup in a relationship or another type of disappointment. This group also includes those who may not be diagnosed as having depression but who are overwhelmed by a stressful situation often with an aspect of public humiliation (eg, victims of cyber-bullying). A suicide attempt in such cases may be an impulsive or aggressive act not associated with significant depression. In such cases, a suicide attempt is clearly a stratagem for controlling or hurting others or an attempted escape.

Another high-risk group includes individuals with severe depression. Severe depression may be due to conditions such as medical illness (eg, AIDS, whose victims have a suicide rate over 20 times that of the general population) or comorbid psychiatric disorders (eg, panic disorders). Anxiety, panic, and fear are major findings in suicidal behavior. A patient may seem to make a dramatic improvement, but the lifting of depression may be due to the patient's decision to commit suicide. Another high-risk group are individuals with psychotic illness who tend not to verbalize their concerns, are unpredictable, and are often successful in their suicide attempt, although they make up only a small percentage of the total.

Finally, suicide is 10 times more prevalent in patients with schizophrenia than in the general population, and jumping from bridges is a more common means of attempted suicide by schizophrenics than by others. In one study of 100 "jumpers," 47% had schizophrenia.

The immediate goal of psychiatric evaluation is to assess the current suicidal risk and the need for hospitalization versus outpatient management. Perhaps the one most useful question is to ask the person how many hours per day he or she thinks about suicide. If it is more than 1 hour, the individual is at high risk. Further assessing the risk by inquiring about intent, plans, means, and suicide-inhibiting factors (eg, strong ties to children or the church) is essential. The intent is less likely to be truly suicidal, for example, if small amounts of poison or medication were ingested or scratching of wrists was superficial, if the act was performed in the vicinity of others or with early notification of others, or if the attempt was arranged so that early detection would be anticipated. Alcohol, hopelessness, delusional thoughts, and complete or nearly complete loss of interest in life or ability to experience pleasure are all positively correlated with suicide attempts. Other risk factors are previous attempts, a family history of suicide, medical or psychiatric illness (eg, anxiety, depression, psychosis), male sex, older age, contemplation of violent methods, a humiliating social stressor, and drug use (including long-term sedative or alcohol use), which contributes to impulsiveness or mood swings. Successful treatment of the patient at risk for suicide cannot be achieved if the patient continues to abuse drugs.

The patient's current mood status is best evaluated by direct evaluation of plans and concerns about the future, personal reactions to the attempt, and thoughts about the reactions of others. Measurement of mood is often facilitated by using a standardized instrument such as the Hamilton or Montgomery-Asberg clinician-administered rating scales or the self-administered Patient Health Questionnaire-9. Such measures allow for initial assessment as well as ongoing treatment tracking. The patient's immediate resources should also be assessed—people who can be significantly involved (most important), family support, job situation, financial resources, etc. Suicide risk can be specifically assessed using an instrument such as the Columbia-Suicide Severity Risk Scale.

If hospitalization is not indicated (eg, gestures, impulsive attempts; see above), the clinician must formulate and institute a treatment plan or make an adequate referral. (The National Suicide Prevention Lifeline, 1-800-273-8255, may be of assistance.) Medication should be dispensed in small amounts to at-risk patients. Although TCAs and SSRIs are associated with an equal incidence of suicide attempts, the risk of a completed suicide is higher with TCA overdose. Guns and medications should be removed from the patient's household. Driving should be interdicted until the patient improves. The problem is often worsened by the long-term complications of the suicide attempt, eg, brain damage due to hypoxia, peripheral neuropathies caused by staying for long periods in one position causing nerve compressions, and medical or surgical problems such as esophageal strictures and tendon dysfunctions.

Sleep disturbances in the depressions are discussed below.

▶ Treatment of Depression

A. Medical

Depression associated with reactive disorders usually does not call for drug therapy and can be managed by psychotherapy and the passage of time. In severe cases—particularly when vegetative signs are significant and symptoms have persisted for more than a few weeks—antidepressant drug therapy is often effective. Drug therapy is also suggested by a family history of major depression in first-degree relatives or a past history of prior episodes.

The antidepressant medications may be classified into four groups: (1) the newer antidepressants, including the SSRIs, SNRIs, and bupropion, nefazodone, vilazodone, and mirtazapine, (2) the TCAs and clinically similar medications, (3) the monoamine oxidase (MAO) inhibitors (Table 25–7), and (4) stimulants. ECT and repetitive transcranial magnetic stimulation are procedural treatments for depression. These modalities are described in greater detail below. Megavitamin treatment, acupuncture, and electrosleep are of unproved usefulness for any psychiatric condition.

Hospitalization is necessary if suicide is a major consideration or if complex treatment modalities are required.

Medication selection is influenced by the history of previous response or lack thereof if that information is available. A positive family history of response to a particular drug suggests that the patient may respond similarly. If no background information is available, a drug such as sertraline, 25 mg orally daily and increasing gradually up to 200 mg, or venlafaxine at 37.5 mg/d and titrated gradually to a maximum dose of 225 mg/d can be selected and a *full trial* instituted. The medication trial should be monitored for worsening mood or suicidal ideation with patient assessments every 1–2 weeks until week 6. The STAR*D trial suggests that if the response to the first medication is inadequate, the best alternatives are to switch to a second agent that may be from the same or different class of antidepressant; another option is to try augmenting the first agent with bupropion (150–450 mg/d), buspirone (eg, 30–60 mg/d orally), or thyroid medication (eg, liothyronine, 25–50 mcg/d orally). The latter course is often taken when there has been at least a partial response to the initial drug. The Agency for Health Care Policy and Research has produced clinical practice guidelines that outline one algorithm of treatment decisions (Figure 25–2).

Psychotic depression should be treated with a combination of an antipsychotic such as olanzapine and an antidepressant such as an SSRI at their usual doses. Mifepristone may have specific and early activity against psychotic depression. ECT is generally regarded as the single most effective treatment for psychotic depression.

Major depression with atypical features or seasonal onset can be treated with bupropion or an SSRI with good results. MAO inhibitors appear more effective than TCAs and an MAO inhibitor may be used if more benign antidepressant strategies prove unsuccessful.

Melancholic depression may respond to ECT, TCAs, and SNRIs, which are preferable to SSRIs. However, SSRIs are often used in the treatment of melancholic depression and are effective in many cases.

Table 25–7. Commonly used antidepressants.

Drug	Usual Daily Oral Dose (mg)	Usual Daily Maximum Dose (mg)	Sedative Effects[1]	Anticholinergic Effects[1]	Cost per Unit	Cost for 30 Days Treatment Based on Maximum Dosage[2]
SSRIs						
Citalopram (Celexa)	20	40	< 1	1	$2.36/40 mg	$70.80
Escitalopram (Lexapro)	10	20	< 1	1	$4.51/20 mg	$135.30
Fluoxetine (Prozac, Sarafem)	5–40	80	< 1	< 1	$2.59/20 mg	$310.80
Fluvoxamine (Luvox)	100–300	300	1	< 1	$2.64/100 mg	$237.60
Nefazodone (Serzone)	300–600	600	2	< 1	$2.10/200 mg	$189.00
Paroxetine (Paxil)	20–30	50	1	1	$2.64/20 mg	$161.10
Sertraline (Zoloft)	50–150	200	< 1	< 1	$2.72/100 mg	$163.20
Vilazodone (Viibryd)	40	40	< 1	< 1	$6.00/20 mg	$180.00
SNRIs						
Desvenlafaxine (Pristiq)	50	100	1	< 1	$7.73/100 mg	$232.00
Duloxetine (Cymbalta)	40	60	2	3	$7.85/60 mg	$235.55
Levomilnacipran (Fetzima)	40	120	1	1	8.10/80 mg	243.00
Milnacipran (Savella)	100	200	1	1	3.40/100 mg	204.20
Venlafaxine XR (Effexor)	150–225	225	1	< 1	$4.67/75 mg	$420.30
Tricyclic and clinically similar compounds						
Amitriptyline (Elavil)	150–250	300	4	4	$1.16/150 mg	$69.60
Amoxapine (Asendin)	150–200	400	2	2	$1.49/100 mg	$178.80
Clomipramine (Anafranil)	100	250	3	3	$1.48/75 mg	$158.00
Desipramine (Norpramin)	100–250	300	1	1	$4.25/100 mg	$369.60
Doxepin (Sinequan)	150–200	300	4	3	$1.35/100 mg	$121.50
Imipramine (Tofranil)	150–200	300	3	3	$1.16/50 mg	$208.80
Maprotiline (Ludiomil)	100–200	300	4	2	$1.95/75 mg	$234.00
Nortriptyline (Aventyl, Pamelor)	100–150	150	2	2	$1.46/50 mg	$131.40
Protriptyline (Vivactil)	15–40	60	1	3	$1.73/10 mg	$311.40
Trimipramine (Surmontil)	75–200	200	4	4	$3.26/100 mg	$195.60
Monoamine oxidase inhibitors						
Phenelzine (Nardil)	45–60	90	...	...	$0.84/15 mg	$151.20
Selegiline transdermal (Emsam)	6 (skin patch)	12	...	...	$39.69/6 mg patch	$1190.74
Tranylcypromine (Parnate)	20–30	50	...	...	$6.73/10 mg	$1009.50
Other compounds						
Bupropion SR (Wellbutrin SR)	300	400[3]	< 1	< 1	$3.59/200 mg	$215.40
Bupropion XL (Wellbutrin XL)	300[4]	450[4]	< 1	< 1	$4.77/300 mg	$286.20
Mirtazapine (Remeron)	15–45	45	4	2	$2.80/30 mg	$85.53
Trazodone (Desyrel)	100–300	400	4	< 1	$0.70/100 mg	$84.00

[1]1, weak effect; 4, strong effect.
[2]Average wholesale price (AWP, for AB-rated generic when available) for quantity listed. Source: *Red Book Online, 2014, Truven Health Analytics, Inc.*, Inc. AWP may not accurately represent the actual pharmacy cost because wide contractual variations exist among institutions.
[3]200 mg twice daily.
[4]Wellbutrin XL is a once-daily form of bupropion. Bupropion is still available as immediate release, and, if used, no single dose should exceed 150 mg.
SSRIs, serotonin selective reuptake inhibitors.

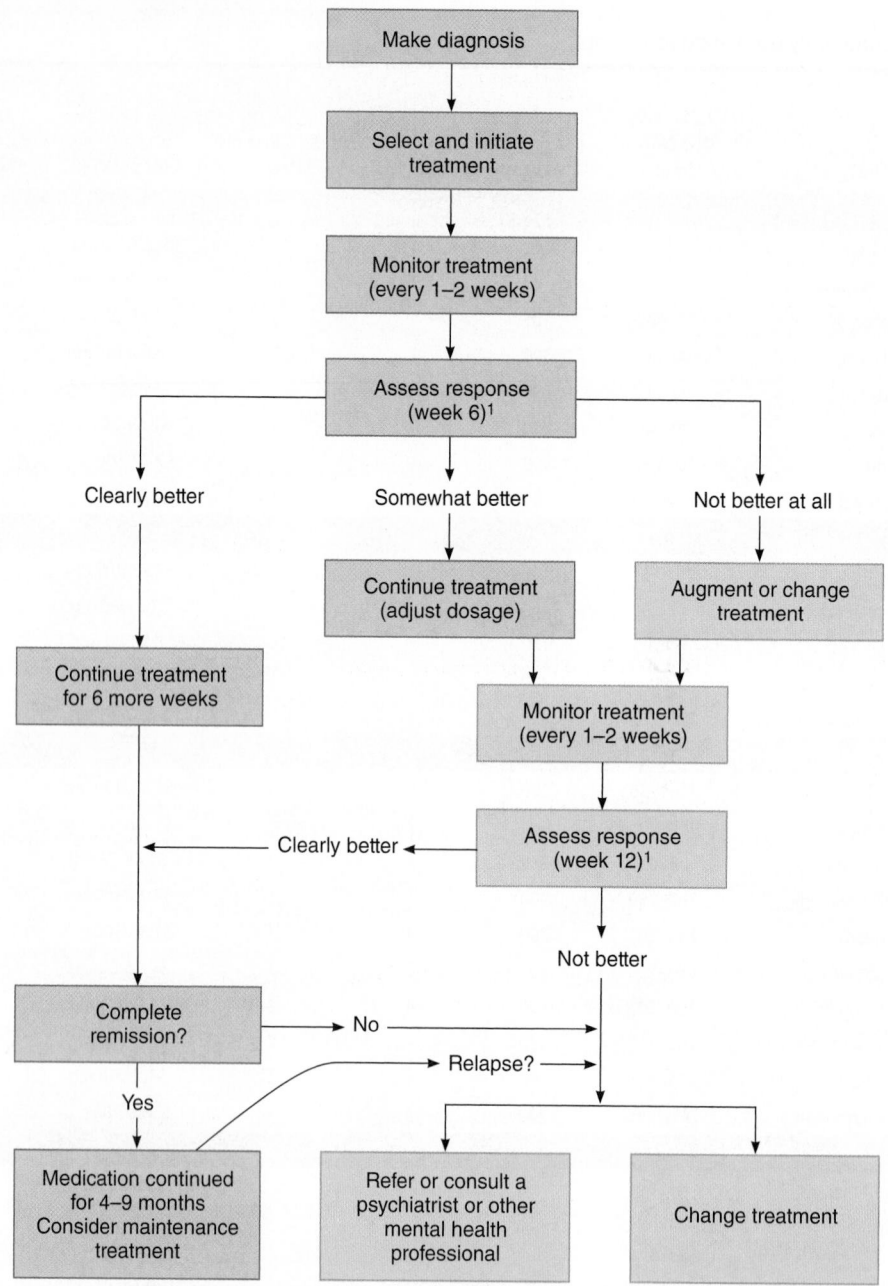

Make diagnosis

Select and initiate treatment

Monitor treatment (every 1–2 weeks)

Assess response (week 6)[1]

Clearly better

Somewhat better

Not better at all

Continue treatment (adjust dosage)

Augment or change treatment

Continue treatment for 6 more weeks

Monitor treatment (every 1–2 weeks)

Clearly better ←

Assess response (week 12)[1]

Not better

Complete remission?

No

Relapse?

Yes

Medication continued for 4–9 months Consider maintenance treatment

Refer or consult a psychiatrist or other mental health professional

Change treatment

[1]Times of assessment (weeks 6 and 12) rest on very modest data. It may be necessary to revise the treatment plan earlier for patients not responding at all.

▲ **Figure 25–2.** Overview of treatment for depression. (Reproduced from Agency for Health Care Policy and Research: Depression in Primary Care. Vol. 2: Treatment of Major Depression. United States Department of Health and Human Services, 1993.)

Caution: Depressed patients often have suicidal thoughts, and the amount of drug dispensed should be appropriately controlled particularly if prescribing an MAO inhibitor, TCA, and to a lesser extent, venlafaxine. At the same time, adults with untreated depression are at higher risk for suicide than those who are treated

sufficiently to reduce symptoms. It has been thought that in children and adolescent populations, antidepressants may be associated with some slightly increased risk of suicidality. One meta-analysis indicates that suicidality persists even after symptoms of depression are treated suggesting other causes, such as increased impulsivity among younger patients. After age 25, antidepressants may have neutral or possibly protective effects until age 65 years or older. The older TCAs have a narrow therapeutic index. One advantage of the newer medications is their wider margin of safety. Nonetheless, even with newer agents, because of the possibility of suicidality early in antidepressant treatment, close follow-up is indicated. In all cases of pharmacologic management of depressed states, caution is indicated until the risk of suicide is considered minimal.

1. SSRIs, SNRIs, and atypical antidepressants—The SSRIs include fluoxetine, sertraline, paroxetine, fluvoxamine, citalopram and its enantiomer escitalopram (Table 25–7). The chief advantages of these agents are that they are generally well tolerated, the starting dose is typically a therapeutic dose for most patients, and they have much lower lethality in overdose compared to TCAs or MAO inhibitors. (Notably, citalopram carries a warning regarding QT prolongation in doses above 40 mg, and caution should be used in prescribing in patients at risk for arrhythmia. There is no similar FDA warning for escitalopram as of this writing.) The SNRIs include venlafaxine, desvenlafaxine, duloxetine, milnacipran, and levomilnacipran. In addition to possessing the strong serotonin reuptake blocking properties of the SSRIs, the SNRIs are also norepinephrine reuptake blockers. The combined serotonergic- noradrenergic properties of these drugs may provide benefits in pain conditions such as neuropathy and fibromyalgia as well as conditions such as stress incontinence. The atypical antidepressants are bupropion, nefazodone, trazodone, vilazodone, and mirtazapine (Table 25–7). All of these antidepressants are effective in the treatment of depression, both typical and atypical. The SSRI medications have been effective in the treatment of panic disorder, bulimia, GAD, OCD, and PTSD.

Most of the medications in this group tend to be activating and are given in the morning so as not to interfere with sleep. Some patients, however, may have sedation, requiring that the drug be given at bedtime. This reaction occurs most commonly with paroxetine, fluvoxamine, and mirtazapine. The SSRIs can be given in once-daily dosage. Nefazodone and trazodone are usually given twice daily. Bupropion and venlafaxine are available in extended-release formulations and can be given once daily. There is usually some delay in response; fluoxetine, for example, requires 2–6 weeks to act in depression, 4–8 weeks to be effective in panic disorder, and 6–12 weeks in treatment of OCD. The starting dose (10 mg) is given for 1 week before increasing to the average daily oral dose of 20 mg for depression, while OCD may require up to 80 mg daily. Some patients, particularly the elderly, may tolerate and benefit from as little as 10 mg/d or every other day. The other SSRIs have shorter half-lives and a lesser effect on hepatic enzymes, which reduces their impact on the metabolism of other medications (thus not increasing significantly the serum concentrations of other medications as much as fluoxetine). The shorter half-lives also allow for more rapid clearing if adverse side effects appear. Venlafaxine appears to be more effective with doses > 200 mg/d orally, although some individuals respond to doses as low as 75 mg/d.

The **side effects** common to all of these medications are headache, nausea, tinnitus, insomnia, and nervousness. Akathisia has been common with the SSRIs; other extrapyramidal symptoms (eg, dystonias) have occurred infrequently but particularly in withdrawal states. Because SSRIs affect platelet serotonin levels, abnormal bleeding can occur. Sertraline and citalopram appear to be the safest agents in this class when used with warfarin. Sexual side effects of erectile dysfunction, retrograde ejaculation, and dysorgasmia are very common with the SSRIs. Oral phosphodiesterase-5 inhibitors (such as sildenafil, 25–50 mg; tadalafil, 5-20 mg; or vardenafil, 10–20 mg taken 1 hour prior to sexual activity) can improve erectile dysfunction in some patients and have been shown to improve other SSRI-induced sexual dysfunction in both men and women. Adjunctive bupropion (75–150 mg orally daily) may also enhance sexual arousal. Cyproheptadine, 4 mg orally prior to sexual activity, may be helpful in countering drug-induced anorgasmia but also is quite sedating and may counter the therapeutic benefits of SSRIs as well. The SSRIs are strong serotonin uptake blockers and may in high dosage or in combination with MAO inhibitors, including the antiparkinsonian drug selegiline, cause a **"serotonin syndrome."** This syndrome is manifested by rigidity, hyperthermia, autonomic instability, myoclonus, confusion, delirium, and coma. This syndrome can be a particularly troublesome problem in the elderly. Research indicates that SSRIs are safer agents to use than TCAs in patients with cardiac disease; sertraline is a safe and effective antidepressant treatment in patients with acute myocardial infarction or unstable angina.

Withdrawal syndromes have been reported for the SSRIs and venlafaxine. These include dysphoric mood, agitation, and a flu-like state. These medications should be discontinued gradually over a period of weeks or months to reduce the risk of withdrawal phenomena.

Fluoxetine, fluvoxamine, sertraline, venlafaxine, and citalopram in customary antidepressant doses may increase the risk of major fetal malformation when used during pregnancy; however, the absolute risk of congenital defects is considered low. Maternal major mood disorder in pregnancy by itself carries its own risks to the mother and fetus and has been linked to low birth weight and preterm delivery. Postpartum effects of prenatal depression have not been studied. The decision to use SSRIs and other psychotropic agents during pregnancy and postpartum must be a collaborative decision based on a thorough risk-benefit analysis for each individual.

Venlafaxine lacks significant anticholinergic side effects. Nausea, nervousness, and profuse sweating appear to be the major side effects. Venlafaxine appears to have few drug-drug interactions. It does require monitoring of blood pressure because dose-related hypertension may develop in some individuals. Venlafaxine prescribing in the United Kingdom has been restricted to psychiatrists. Venlafaxine appears to carry a greater risk of lethal arrhythmias in instances of overdose relative to the SSRIs, but less risk than with the TCAs. Desvenlafaxine, a newer form of the drug, is started at its target dose of 50 mg/d orally and does not require upward titration although higher doses have been well studied and some patients benefit from 100 mg/d. Duloxetine may also result in small increases in blood pressure. Common side effects include dry mouth, dizziness, and fatigue. Inhibitors of 1A2 and 2D6 may increase duloxetine levels with a risk of toxicity. Milnacipran, approved for the treatment of fibromyalgia, and levomilnacipran, approved for the treatment of major depression, carry many of the side effects common to other SNRIs including a mild tachycardia, hypertension, sexual side effects, mydriasis, urinary constriction, and occasional abnormal bleeding. Levomilnacipran is started at 20 mg/d orally then increased to 40 mg/d after 2–3 days. The target dose is 40–120 mg given once daily. Milnacipran is typically started at 12.5 mg/d orally, titrated to 12.5 mg twice daily after 2 days, and then to 25 mg twice daily after 7 days. The target dose is typically 100–200 mg/d given in in two divided doses. While not approved for the treatment of major depression, the evidence suggests that milnacipran, like levomilnacipran, is an effective antidepressant agent.

Nefazodone appears to lack the anticholinergic effects of the TCAs and the agitation sometimes induced by SSRIs. Nefazodone should not be given with terfenadine, astemizole, or cisapride, which are not commercially available in the United States. Because nefazodone inhibits the liver's cytochrome P450 3A4 isoenzymes, concurrent use of these medications can lead to serious QT prolongation, ventricular tachycardia, or death. Through the same mechanism of enzyme inhibition, nefazodone can elevate cyclosporine levels sixfold to tenfold. Nefazodone carries an FDA warning given its association with liver failure in rare cases. Pretreatment and ongoing monitoring of liver enzymes are indicated.

Mirtazapine is thought to enhance central noradrenergic and serotonergic activity with minimal sexual side effects compared with the SSRIs. Its action as a potent antagonist of histaminergic receptors may make it a useful agent for patients with depression and insomnia. It is also an effective antiemetic due to its antagonism of the 5-HT$_3$ receptor. Its most common adverse side effects include somnolence, increased appetite, weight gain, lipid abnormalities, and dizziness. There have been reports of agranulocytosis in 2 of 2796 patients. Although it is metabolized by P450 isoenzymes, it is not an inhibitor of this system. It is given in a single oral dose at bedtime starting at 15 mg and increasing in 15-mg increments every week or every other week up to 45 mg.

2. Tricyclic antidepressants (TCAs) and clinically similar medications—TCAs were the mainstay of drug therapy for depression for many years. They have also been effective in panic disorder, pain syndromes, and anxiety states. Specific ones have been effective in OCD (clomipramine), enuresis (imipramine), psychotic depression (amoxapine), and reduction of craving in cocaine withdrawal (desipramine).

TCAs are characterized more by their similarities than by their differences. They tend to affect both serotonin and norepinephrine reuptake; some medications act mainly on the former and others principally on the latter neurotransmitter system. Individuals receiving the same dosages vary markedly in therapeutic drug levels achieved (elderly

patients require smaller doses), and determination of plasma drug levels is helpful when clinical response has been disappointing. Nortriptyline is usually effective when plasma levels are between 50 and 150 ng/mL; imipramine at plasma levels of 200–250 ng/mL; and desipramine at plasma levels of 100–250 ng/mL. High blood levels are not more effective than moderate levels and may be counterproductive (eg, delirium, seizures). Patients with gastrointestinal side effects benefit from plasma level monitoring to assess absorption of the drug. Most TCAs can be given in a single dose at bedtime, starting at fairly low doses (eg, nortriptyline 25 mg orally) and increasing by 25 mg every several days as tolerated until the therapeutic response is achieved (eg, nortriptyline, 100–150 mg) or to maximum dose if necessary (eg, nortriptyline, 150 mg). The most common cause of treatment failure is an inadequate trial. A full trial consists of giving a therapeutic daily dosage for at least 6 weeks. Because of marked anticholinergic and sedating side effects, clomipramine is started at a low dose (25 mg/d orally) and increased slowly in divided doses up to 100 mg/d, held at that level for several days, and then gradually increased as necessary up to 250 mg/d. Any of the TCA-like medications should be started at very low doses (eg, 10–25 mg/d) and increased slowly in the treatment of panic disorder.

The TCAs have anticholinergic side effects to varying degrees (amitriptyline 100 mg is equivalent to atropine 5 mg). One must be particularly wary of the effect in elderly men with prostatic hyperplasia. The anticholinergic effects also predispose to other medical problems such as constipation, confusion, heat stroke, or dental problems from xerostomia. Orthostatic hypotension is fairly common, is not dose-dependent and may not remit with time on medication; this may predispose to falls and hip fractures in the elderly. Cardiac effects of the TCAs are functions of the anticholinergic effect, direct myocardial depression (quinidine-like effect), and interference with adrenergic neurons. These factors may produce altered rate, rhythm, and contractility, particularly in patients with preexisting cardiac disease, such as bundle-branch or bifascicular block. Even relatively small overdoses (eg, 1500 mg of imipramine) have resulted in lethal arrhythmias. Electrocardiographic changes range from benign ST segment and T wave changes and sinus tachycardia to a variety of complex and serious arrhythmias, the latter requiring a change in medication. Because TCAs have class I antiarrhythmic effects, they should be used with caution in patients with ischemic heart disease, arrhythmias, or conduction disturbances. SSRIs or the atypical antidepressants are better initial choices for this population. TCAs lower the seizure threshold so this is of particular concern in patients with a propensity for seizures. Loss of libido and erectile, ejaculatory, and orgasmic dysfunction are fairly common and can compromise compliance. Trazodone rarely causes priapism (1 in 9000), but when it occurs, it requires treatment within 12 hours (epinephrine 1:1000 injected into the corpus cavernosum). Delirium, agitation, and mania are infrequent complications of the TCAs but can occur. Sudden discontinuation of some of these medications can produce "cholinergic rebound," manifested by headaches and nausea

Table 25–8. Principal dietary restrictions in MAOI use.

1. Cheese, except cream cheese and cottage cheese and fresh yogurt
2. Fermented or aged meats such as bologna, salami
3. Broad bean pods such as Chinese bean pods
4. Liver of all types
5. Meat and yeast extracts
6. Red wine, sherry, vermouth, cognac, beer, ale
7. Soy sauce, shrimp paste, sauerkraut

MAOI, monoamine oxidase inhibitor.

with abdominal cramps. Overdoses of TCAs are often serious because of the narrow therapeutic index and quinidine-like effects (see Chapter 38).

3. Monoamine oxidase inhibitors—The MAO inhibitors are generally used as third-line medications for depression (after a failure of SSRIs, SNRIs, TCAs, or the atypical antidepressants) because of the dietary and other restrictions required (see below and Table 25–8). They should be considered third-line medications for refractory panic disorder as well as depression; however, this hierarchy has become more flexible since MAO inhibitor skin patches (selegiline) have become available. They deliver the MAO inhibitor to the bloodstream bypassing the gastrointestinal tract so that dietary restrictions are not necessary in the lowest dosage strength (6 mg/24 h).

The MAO inhibitors commonly cause symptoms of orthostatic hypotension (which may persist) and sympathomimetic effects of tachycardia, sweating, and tremor. Nausea, insomnia (often associated with intense afternoon drowsiness), and sexual dysfunction are common. Zolpidem 5–10 mg orally at bedtime can ameliorate MAO-induced insomnia. Central nervous system effects include agitation and toxic psychoses. Dietary limitations (see Table 25–8) and abstinence from drug products containing phenylpropanolamine, phenylephrine, meperidine, dextromethorphan, and pseudoephedrine are mandatory for MAO-A type inhibitors (those marketed for treatment of depression), since the reduction of available MAO leaves the patient vulnerable to exogenous amines (eg, tyramine in foodstuffs).

4. Stimulants—such as dextroamphetamine (5–30 mg/d orally) and methylphenidate (10–45 mg/d orally) are effective for the short-term treatment of depression in medically ill and geriatric patients. Their 50–60% efficacy rate is slightly below that of other agents. The stimulants are notable for rapid onset of action (hours) and a paucity of side effects (tachycardia, agitation) in most patients. They are usually given in two divided doses early in the day (eg, 7 AM and noon) so as to avoid interfering with sleep. These agents may also be useful as adjunctive agents in refractory depression. Ketamine infusion has been shown to lead to a rapid improvement in depressive symptoms; however, effects of a single treatment are short-lived. The safety of repeated treatments has not been established.

5. Switching and combination therapy—If the therapeutic response has been poor after an adequate trial with the chosen drug, the diagnosis should be reassessed. Assuming that the trial has been adequate and the diagnosis is correct, a trial with a second drug is appropriate. In switching from one group to another, an adequate "washout time" must be allowed. This is critical in certain situations—eg, in switching from an MAO inhibitor to a TCA, allow 2–3 weeks between stopping one drug and starting another; in switching from an SSRI to an MAO inhibitor, allow 4–5 weeks. In switching within groups—eg, from one TCA to another (amitriptyline to desipramine, etc)—no washout time is needed, and one can rapidly decrease the dosage of one drug while increasing the other. In clinical practice, adjunctive treatment with lithium, buspirone, or thyroid hormone may be helpful in depression. The adjunctive use of low-dose atypical antipsychotics such as aripiprazole, olanzapine, and quetiapine in the treatment of patients with refractory depression is supported by research. The side effect risk is the same as when treating psychosis. The FDA has approved monotherapy with aripiprazole or quetiapine for this purpose as well as the combination of fluoxetine and olanzapine. Adding an atypical agent requires monitoring body mass index, lipids, and glucose. Combining two antidepressants, or adding an antipsychotic to an antidepressant, requires caution and is usually reserved for clinicians who feel comfortable managing this or after psychiatric consultation.

6. Maintenance and tapering—When clinical relief of symptoms is obtained, medication is continued for 12 months in the effective maintenance dosage, which is the dosage required in the acute stage. The full dosage should be continued indefinitely when the individual has a first episode before age 20 or after age 50, is over age 40 with two episodes, at least one episode after age 50, or has had three episodes at any age. Major depression should often be considered a chronic disease. If the medication is being tapered, it should be done gradually over several months, monitoring closely for relapse.

7. Drug interactions—Interactions with other medications are listed in Table 25–9.

8. Electroconvulsive therapy—ECT causes a generalized central nervous system seizure (peripheral convulsion is not necessary) by means of electric current. The key objective is to exceed the seizure threshold, which can be accomplished by a variety of means. The mechanism of action is not known, but it is thought to involve major neurotransmitter responses at the cell membrane. Electrical current insufficient to cause a seizure produces no therapeutic benefit.

ECT is the most effective (about 70–85%) treatment of severe depression—particularly the delusions and agitation commonly seen with depression in the elderly. It is indicated when medical conditions preclude the use of antidepressants, nonresponsiveness to these medications, and extreme suicidality. Comparative controlled studies of ECT in severe depression show that it is more effective than pharmacotherapy. It is also effective in the treatment of mania and psychoses during pregnancy (when medications may be contraindicated). It has not been shown to be

Table 25–9. Antidepressant drug interactions with other medications.

Drug	Effects
Tricyclic and other non-MAOI antidepressants	
Antacids	Decreased absorption of antidepressants
Anticoagulants	Increased hypoprothrombinemic effect
Cimetidine	Increased antidepressant blood levels and psychosis
Clonidine	Decreased antihypertensive effect
Digitalis	Increased incidence of heart block
Disulfiram	Increased antidepressant blood levels
Haloperidol	Increased antidepressant levels
Insulin	Decreased blood sugar
Lithium	Increased lithium levels with fluoxetine
Methyldopa	Decreased antihypertensive effect
Other anticholinergic medications	Marked anticholinergic responses
Phenytoin	Increased blood levels
Procainamide	Decreased ventricular conduction
Procarbazine	Hypertensive crisis
Propranolol	Increased hypotension
Quinidine	Decreased ventricular conduction
Rauwolfia derivatives	Increased stimulation
Sedatives	Increased sedation
Sympathomimetic medications	Increased vasopressor effect
Terfenadine,[1] astemizole,[1] cisapride[1]	Torsades de pointes
MAOIs	
Antihistamines	Increased sedation
Belladonna-like medications	Increased blood pressure
Dextromethorphan	Same as meperidine
Guanethidine	Decreased blood pressure
Insulin	Decreased blood sugar
Levodopa	Increased blood pressure
Meperidine	Increased agitation, seizures, coma, death
Methyldopa	Decreased blood pressure
Pseudoephedrine	Hypertensive crisis (increased blood pressure)
Reserpine	Increased blood pressure and temperature
Succinylcholine	Increased neuromuscular blockade
Sulfonylureas	Decreased blood sugar
Sympathomimetic medications	Increased blood pressure

[1]Terfenadine, astemizole, and cisapride are not commercially available in the United States.
MAOIs, monoamine oxidase inhibitors.

helpful in chronic schizophrenic disorders, and it is generally not used in acute schizophrenic episodes unless medications are not effective and it is urgent that the psychosis be controlled (eg, a catatonic stupor complicating an acute medical condition).

The most common side effects are memory disturbance and headache. Memory loss or confusion is usually related to the number and frequency of ECT treatments and proper oxygenation during treatment. Unilateral ECT is associated with less memory loss than bilateral ECT. Both anterograde and retrograde memory loss may occur, but short term-retrograde memory loss is more common. While some memory deficits may persist, memory loss tends to improve in a few weeks after the last ECT treatment. There have been reports that lithium administration concurrent with ECT resulted in greater memory loss.

Increased intracranial pressure is a relative contraindication. Other problems such as cardiac disorders, aortic aneurysms, bronchopulmonary disease, and venous thrombosis must be evaluated in light of the severity of the medical problem versus the need for ECT. Serious complications arising from ECT occur in < 1 in 1000 cases. Most of these problems are cardiovascular or respiratory in nature (eg, aspiration of gastric contents, arrhythmias, myocardial infarction). Poor patient understanding and lack of acceptance of the technique by the public are the biggest obstacles to the use of ECT.

9. Phototherapy—Phototherapy is used in major depression with seasonal onset. It consists of exposure (at a 3-foot distance) to a light source of > 2500 lux for 2 hours daily. Light visors are an adaptation that provides greater mobility and an adjustable light intensity. The dosage varies, with some patients requiring morning and night exposure. One effect is alteration of biorhythm through melatonin mechanisms.

10. Experimental treatments—Transcranial magnetic stimulation appears to be effective in nonpsychotic depression. Its use in this condition has been approved by the FDA for individuals who have not responded to one to four antidepressants. It is usually delivered in a course of 20–30 sessions over 4–6 weeks. Vagus nerve stimulation has shown promise in about one-third of extremely refractory cases and is approved by the FDA but has not been approved by many insurers.

B. Psychological

It is seldom possible to engage an individual in penetrating psychotherapeutic endeavors during the acute stage of a severe depression. While medications may be taking effect, a supportive approach to strengthen existing coping mechanisms and appropriate consideration of the patient's continuing need to function at work, to engage in recreational activities, etc, are necessary as the severity of the depression lessens. If the patient is not seriously depressed, it is often appropriate to initiate intensive psychotherapeutic efforts, since flux periods are a good time to effect change. A catharsis of repressed anger and guilt may be beneficial. Therapy during or just after the acute stage may focus on coping techniques, with some practice of alternative choices.

Depression-specific psychotherapies help improve self-esteem, increase assertiveness, and lessen dependency. Interpersonal psychotherapy for depression has shown efficacy in the treatment of acute depression, helping patients master interpersonal stresses and develop new coping strategies. Cognitive behavioral therapy for depression addresses patients' patterns of negative thoughts, called cognitive distortions, which lead to feelings of depression and anxiety. Treatment usually includes homework assignments such as keeping a journal of cognitive distortions and of positive responses to them. The combination of drug therapy plus interpersonal psychotherapy or cognitive behavioral therapy is generally more effective than either modality alone. It is usually helpful to involve the spouse or other significant family members early in treatment. Mindfulness-based cognitive therapy has reduced relapse rates in several randomized controlled trials. In two studies, it was as effective as maintenance medication in preventing relapse. This therapy incorporates meditation and teaches patients to distance themselves from depressive thinking. It may be a preferable alternative for individuals who wish to have an alternative to long-term medications to stay free of depressive episodes.

C. Social

Flexible use of appropriate social services can be of major importance in the treatment of depression. Since alcohol is often associated with depression, early involvement in alcohol treatment programs such as Alcoholics Anonymous can be important to future success (see Alcohol Dependency and Abuse, below). The structuring of daily activities during severe depression is often quite difficult for the patient, and loneliness is often a major factor. The help of family, employer, or friends is often necessary to mobilize the patient who experiences no joy in daily activities and tends to remain uninvolved and to deteriorate. Insistence on sharing activities will help involve the patient in simple but important daily functions. In some severe cases, the use of day treatment centers or support groups of a specific type (eg, mastectomy groups) is indicated. It is not unusual for a patient to have multiple legal, financial, and vocational problems requiring legal and vocational assistance.

D. Behavioral

When depression is a function of self-defeating coping techniques such as passivity, the role-playing approach can be useful. Behavioral techniques, including desensitization, may be used in problems such as phobias where depression is a by-product. When depression is a regularly used interpersonal style, behavioral counseling to family members or others can help in extinguishing the behavior in the patient. Behavioral activation, a technique of motivating depressed patients to begin engaging in pleasurable activities, has been shown to be a useful depression-specific psychotherapy.

▶ Treatment of Mania

Acute manic or hypomanic symptoms will respond to lithium or valproic acid after several days of treatment, but it is increasingly common to use second-generation antipsychotics as adjunctive treatment or monotherapy. High-potency benzodiazepines (eg, clonazepam) may also be useful adjuncts in managing the agitation and sleep disturbance that are features of manic and hypomanic episodes. Some schizoaffective disorders and some cases of so-called schizophrenia are probably atypical bipolar affective disorder, for which lithium treatment may be effective.

A. Antipsychotics

Acute manic symptoms may be treated initially with a second-generation antipsychotic such as olanzapine, (eg, 5–20 mg orally), risperidone (2–3 mg orally), or aripiprazole (15–30 mg) in conjunction with a benzodiazepine if indicated. All of the available oral second-generation antipsychotics and many of the first-generation agents appear to be more rapidly effective in the management of acute mania than are mood stabilizers such as lithium or valproate. Alternatively, when behavioral control is immediately necessary, olanzapine in an injectable form (2.5–10 mg intramuscularly) or haloperidol, 5–10 mg orally or intramuscularly repeated as needed until symptoms subside, may be used. The dosage of the antipsychotic may be gradually reduced after lithium or another mood stabilizer is started (see below). Olanzapine, quetiapine, and aripiprazole are approved as maintenance treatments for bipolar disorder to prevent subsequent cycles of both mania and depression.

B. Clonazepam

Clonazepam can be an alternative or adjunct to an antipsychotic in controlling acute behavioral symptoms. Clonazepam has the advantage of causing no extrapyramidal side effects. Although 1–2 mg orally every 4–6 hours may be effective, up to 16 mg/d may be necessary.

C. Lithium

As a prophylactic drug for bipolar affective disorder, lithium significantly decreases the frequency and severity of both manic and depressive attacks in about 50–70% of patients. Lithium appears to work best in patients with classic bipolar I disorder. Antipsychotics, valproate, lamotrigine, and carbamazepine may be more effective than lithium in the management of rapid cycling and mixed episodes. A positive response to lithium is more predictable if the patient has a low frequency of episodes (no more than two per year with intervals free of psychopathology). A positive response occurs more frequently in individuals who have blood relatives with a diagnosis of manic or hypomanic episodes.

In addition to its use in manic states, lithium is sometimes useful in the prophylaxis of recurrent unipolar depressions (perhaps undiagnosed bipolar disorder). Lithium may ameliorate nonspecific aggressive behaviors and dyscontrol syndromes. The dosages are the same as used in bipolar disorder. Most patients with bipolar disease can be managed long-term with lithium alone, although some will require continued or intermittent use of an antipsychotic, antidepressant, or carbamazepine. An excellent resource for information is the Lithium Information Center, http://www.miminc.org/aboutlithinfoctr.html.

Before treatment, the clinical workup should include a medical history and physical examination; complete blood count; T4, thyroid-stimulating hormone, blood urea nitrogen (BUN), serum creatinine, and serum electrolyte determinations; urinalysis; and electrocardiography (in patients over age 45 or with a history of cardiac disease). Compliance with lithium therapy is adversely affected by the loss of some hypomanic experiences valued by the patient. These include social extroversion and a sense of heightened enjoyment in many activities such as sex and business dealings, often with increased productivity in the latter.

1. Dosage—The common starting dosage of lithium carbonate is 300 mg orally two or three times daily, with trough blood levels measured after 5 days of treatment. In a small minority of patients, a slow release form or units of different dosage may be required. Lithium citrate is available as a syrup. The dosage is that required to maintain blood levels in the therapeutic range. For acute attacks, this ranges from 1 to 1.5 mEq/L. Although there is controversy about the optimal long-term maintenance dose, many clinicians reduce the acute level to 0.6–1 mEq/L in order to reduce side effects. The dose required to meet this need will vary in different individuals. For acute mania, doses of 1200–1800 mg/d are generally recommended. Augmentation of antidepressants is usually achieved with half of these doses. Once-a-day dosage is acceptable, but most patients have less nausea when they take the drug in divided doses with meals.

Lithium is readily absorbed, with peak serum levels occurring within 1–3 hours and complete absorption in 8 hours. Half of the total body lithium is excreted in 18–24 hours (95% in the urine). Blood for lithium levels should be drawn 12 hours after the last dose. Serum levels should be measured 5–7 days after initiation of treatment and changes in dose. For maintenance treatment, lithium levels should be monitored initially every 1–2 months but may be measured every 6–12 months in stable, long-term patients. Levels should be monitored more closely when there is any condition that causes volume depletion (eg, diarrhea, dehydration, use of diuretics).

2. Side effects—Early side effects include mild gastrointestinal symptoms (take lithium with food and in divided doses), fine tremors (treat with propranolol, 20–60 mg/d orally, only if persistent), slight muscle weakness, and some degree of somnolence can occur and are usually transient. Moderate polyuria (reduced renal responsiveness to ADH) and polydipsia (associated with increased plasma renin concentration) are often present. Potassium administration can blunt this effect, as may once-daily dosing of lithium. Weight gain (often a result of calories in fluids taken for polydipsia) and leukocytosis not due to infection are fairly common.

Thyroid side effects include goiter (3%; often euthyroid) and hypothyroidism (10%; concomitant administration of lithium and iodide or lithium and carbamazepine enhances the hypothyroid and goitrogenic effect of either drug). Most clinicians treat lithium-induced hypothyroidism (more common in women) with thyroid hormone while continuing lithium therapy. Changes in the glucose tolerance test toward a diabetes-like curve, nephrogenic diabetes insipidus (usually resolving about 8 weeks after cessation of lithium therapy), nephrotic syndrome, edema, folate deficiency, and pseudotumor cerebri (ophthalmoscopy is indicated if there are complaints of headache or blurred vision) can occur. Thyroid and kidney function should be checked at 4- to 6-month intervals. Hypercalcemia and elevated parathyroid hormone levels occur in some patients. Electrocardiographic abnormalities (principally T wave flattening or inversion) may occur during lithium administration but are not of major clinical significance. Sinoatrial block may occur, particularly in the elderly. Other medications that prolong intraventricular conduction, such as TCAs, must be used cautiously in conjunction with lithium. Lithium impairs ventilatory function in patients with airway obstruction. Lithium alone does not have a significant effect on sexual function, but when combined with benzodiazepines (clonazepam in most symptomatic patients) it causes sexual dysfunction in about 50% of men. Lithium may precipitate or exacerbate psoriasis in some patients. Most of these side effects subside when lithium is discontinued; when residual side effects exist, they are usually not serious.

Side effects from long-term lithium therapy include the development of cogwheel rigidity and, occasionally, other extrapyramidal signs. Lithium potentiates the parkinsonian effects of haloperidol. Long-term lithium therapy has also been associated with a relative lowering of the level of memory and perceptual processing (affecting compliance in some cases). Some impairment of attention and emotional reactivity has also been noted. Lithium-induced delirium with therapeutic lithium levels is an infrequent complication usually occurring in the elderly and may persist for several days after serum levels have become negligible. Encephalopathy has occurred in patients receiving combined lithium and antipsychotic therapy and in those who have cerebrovascular disease, thus requiring careful evaluation of patients who develop neurotoxic signs at subtoxic blood levels.

Some reports have suggested that the long-term use of lithium may have adverse effects on kidney function (with interstitial fibrosis, tubular atrophy, or nephrogenic diabetes insipidus). Persistent polyuria should require an investigation of the kidney's ability to concentrate urine. A rise in serum creatinine levels is an indication for in-depth evaluation of kidney function and consideration of alternative treatments if the individual can tolerate a change. Incontinence has been reported in women, apparently related to changes in bladder cholinergic-adrenergic balance.

Prospective studies suggest that the overall risk imposed by lithium in pregnancy may be overemphasized. However, lithium exposure in early pregnancy does increase the frequency of congenital anomalies, especially Ebstein and other major cardiovascular anomalies. For women who take psychotropic medications who become pregnant, the decision to make a change in medication is complex and requires informed consent regarding the relative risks to the patient and fetus. Indeed, the risk of untreated bipolar disorder carries its own risks for pregnancy. Formula feeding should be considered in mothers taking lithium, since concentration in breast milk is one-third to half that in serum.

Frank toxicity usually occurs at blood lithium levels > 2 mEq/L. Because sodium and lithium are reabsorbed at the same loci in the proximal renal tubules, any sodium loss (diarrhea, use of diuretics, or excessive perspiration) results in increased lithium levels. Symptoms and signs include vomiting and diarrhea, the latter exacerbating the problem since more sodium is lost and more lithium is absorbed. Other symptoms and signs, some of which may not be reversible, include tremors, marked muscle weakness, confusion, dysarthria, vertigo, choreoathetosis, ataxia, hyperreflexia, rigidity, lack of coordination, myoclonus, seizures, opisthotonos, and coma. Toxicity is more severe in the elderly, who should be maintained on slightly lower serum levels. Lithium overdosage may be accidental or intentional or may occur as a result of poor monitoring. Significant overdoses of lithium are typically managed with hemodialysis since the drug is excreted completely by the kidneys.

See Chapter 38 for the treatment of patients with massive ingestions of lithium or blood lithium levels > 2.5 mEq/L

3. Drug interactions—Patients receiving lithium should use diuretics with caution and only under close medical supervision. The thiazide diuretics cause increased lithium reabsorption from the proximal renal tubules, resulting in increased serum lithium levels (Table 25–10), and

Table 25–10. Lithium interactions with other medications.

Drug	Effects
ACE inhibitors	↑ Lithium levels
Fluoxetine	↑ Lithium levels
Ibuprofen	↑ Lithium levels
Indomethacin	↑ Lithium levels
Methyldopa	Rigidity, mutism, fascicular twitching
Osmotic diuretics (urea, mannitol)	↑ Lithium excretion
Phenylbutazone	↑ Lithium levels
Potassium-sparing diuretics (spironolactone, amiloride, triamterene)	↑ Lithium levels
Sodium bicarbonate	↑ Lithium excretion
Succinylcholine	↑ Duration of action of succinylcholine
Theophylline, aminophylline	↑ Lithium excretion
Thiazide diuretics	↑ Lithium levels
Valproic acid	↓ Lithium levels
COX-2 inhibitors	↑ Lithium levels

ACE, angiotensin-converting enzyme; COX-2, cyclooxygenase-2.

adjustment of lithium intake must be made to compensate for this. Reduce lithium dosage by 25–40% when the patient is receiving 50 mg of hydrochlorothiazide daily. Potassium-sparing diuretics (spironolactone, amiloride, triamterene) may also increase serum lithium levels and require careful monitoring of lithium levels. Loop diuretics (furosemide, ethacrynic acid, bumetanide) do not appear to alter serum lithium levels. Concurrent use of lithium and angiotensin-converting enzyme inhibitors requires a 50–75% reduction in lithium intake.

D. Valproic Acid

Valproic acid (divalproex) is a first-line treatment for mania because it has a broader index of safety than lithium. This issue is particularly important in AIDS or other medically ill patients prone to dehydration or malabsorption with wide swings in serum lithium levels. Valproic acid has also been used effectively in panic disorder and migraine headache. Treatment is often started at a dose of 750 mg/d orally in divided doses, and dosage is then titrated to achieve therapeutic serum levels. Oral loading in acutely manic bipolar patients in an inpatient setting (initiated at a dosage of 20 mg/kg/d) can safely achieve serum therapeutic levels in 2–3 days. Concomitant use of aspirin may increase valproate levels, carbamazepine or phenytoin may decrease valproate levels, while warfarin levels may be elevated by valproate. Gastrointestinal symptoms and weight gain are the main side effects. Liver function tests, complete blood counts, glucose levels, and weight should be monitored at 2 weeks, 4 weeks, and at 3 months initially and annually or more frequently thereafter based on clinical judgment. Significant teratogenic effects are a concern so pregnancy should be ruled out prior to initiation. In utero exposure to valproate has been associated with adversely affecting intellectual development in the fetus and there is an FDA warning to that effect. Thus, alternatives to valproate should be considered in women of childbearing years who might become pregnant.

E. Carbamazepine

Carbamazepine has been used with increasing frequency in the treatment of bipolar patients who cannot be satisfactorily treated with lithium (nonresponsive, excessive side effects, or rapid cycling). It is often effective at 800–1600 mg/d orally. It has also been used in the treatment of trigeminal neuralgias and alcohol withdrawal as well as in patients with behavioral dyscontrol. It suppresses some phases of kindling (see Stimulants) and has been used to treat residual symptoms in previous stimulant abusers (eg, PTSD with impulse control problems). Dose-related side effects include sedation and ataxia. Dosages start at 400–600 mg orally daily and are increased slowly to therapeutic levels. Skin rashes and a mild reduction in white count are common. SIADH occurs rarely. Nonsteroidal anti-inflammatory medications (except aspirin), the antibiotics erythromycin and isoniazid, the calcium channel blockers verapamil and diltiazem (but not nifedipine), fluoxetine, propoxyphene, and cimetidine all increase carbamazepine levels. Carbamazepine can be effective in conjunction with lithium, although there have been reports of reversible neurotoxicity with the combination. Carbamazepine stimulates hepatic microsomal enzymes and so tends to decrease levels of haloperidol and oral contraceptives. It also lowers T_4, free T_4, and T_3 levels. Cases of fetal malformation (particularly spina bifida) have been reported along with growth deficiency and developmental delay. Liver tests and complete blood counts should be monitored in patients taking carbamazepine. Genetic studies suggest that screening for the HLA-B1502 allele in the Han Chinese population and the HLA-A3101 allele in northern Europeans may help target individuals more susceptible to a serious rash. **Oxcarbazepine**, a derivative of carbamazepine, does not appear to induce its own metabolism and is associated with fewer drug interactions, although it may impose a higher risk of hyponatremia. FDA-approved for partial seizures, oxcarbazepine may have efficacy in acute mania. It appears to be a safer alternative to carbamazepine due to its lower risk of hepatotoxicity.

F. Lamotrigine

Lamotrigine is thought to inhibit neuronal sodium channels and the release of the excitatory amino acids, glutamate and aspartate. It is FDA approved for the maintenance treatment of bipolar disorder. Two double-blind studies support its efficacy in the treatment of acute bipolar depression as adjunctive therapy or as monotherapy but several other controlled studies failed to demonstrate benefit. Likewise, lamotrigine has not proven effective in the management of acute mania. Its metabolism is inhibited by coadministration of valproic acid—doubling its half-life—and accelerated by hepatic enzyme-inducing agents such as carbamazepine. More frequent mild side effects include headache, dizziness, nausea, and diplopia. Rash occurring in 10% of patients is an indication for immediate cessation of dosing, since lamotrigine has been associated with Stevens-Johnson syndrome (1:1000) and, rarely, toxic epidermal necrolysis. Dosing starts at 25–50 mg/d orally and is titrated upward slowly to decrease the likelihood of rash. Slower titration and a lower total dose are indicated for patients taking valproic acid.

► Prognosis

Most depressive episodes are usually time-limited, and the prognosis with treatment is good if a pathologic pattern of adjustment does not intervene. Major affective disorders frequently respond well to a full trial of drug treatment. However, at least 20% of patients will have a more chronic illness lasting 2 or more years. Many patients do not sustain a complete remission of symptoms and most depressive episodes recur. At least 80% of patients who have a single major depressive episode will have one or more recurrences within 15 years of the index episode. Many patients, therefore, require long-term maintenance therapy with antidepressants.

Mania has a good prognosis with adequate treatment, although patient adherence to treatment is often quite challenging. Few effective treatments exist for bipolar depression, which include quetiapine, lurasidone, and the combination of fluoxetine and olanzapine. Most patients with bipolar disorder require treatment with two or more medications such as lithium, antipsychotics and sleeping agents. Breakthrough manic or depressive episodes are common, even with adherence to maintenance treatments, although maintenance therapy lessens the risk of recurrent episodes.

Ansari A et al. The psychopharmacology algorithm project at the Harvard South Shore Program: an update on bipolar depression. Harv Rev Psychiatry. 2010;18(1):36–55. [PMID: 20047460]

Banerjee S et al. Sertraline or mirtazapine for depression in dementia (HTA-SADD): a randomised, multicentre, double-blind, placebo-controlled trial. Lancet. 2011 Jul 30;378(9789): 403–11. [PMID: 21764118]

Battes LC et al. Beta blocker therapy is associated with reduced depressive symptoms 12 months post percutaneous coronary intervention. J Affect Disord. 2012 Feb;136(3):751–7. [PMID: 22032873]

Berle JO et al. Antidepressant use during breastfeeding. Curr Womens Health Rev. 2011 Feb;7(1):28–34. [PMID: 22299006]

Connolly KR et al. Emerging drugs for major depressive disorder. Expert Opin Emerg Drugs. 2012 Mar;17(1):105–26. [PMID: 22339643]

George MS et al. The expanding evidence base for rTMS treatment of depression. Curr Opin Psychiatry. 2013 Jan;26(1): 13–8. [PMID: 23154644]

Gibbons RD et al. Suicidal thoughts and behavior with antidepressant treatment: reanalysis of the randomized placebo-controlled studies of fluoxetine and venlafaxine. Arch Gen Psychiatry. 2012 Jun;69(6):580–7. [PMID: 22309973]

Phillips ML et al. Bipolar disorder diagnosis: challenges and future directions. Lancet. 2013 May 11;381(9878):1663–71. [PMID: 23663952]

Stewart DE. Clinical practice. Depression during pregnancy. N Engl J Med. 2011 Oct 27;365(17):1605–11. [PMID: 22029982]

SLEEP-WAKE DISORDERS

Sleep consists of two distinct states as shown by electroencephalographic studies: (1) REM (rapid eye movement) sleep, also called dream sleep, D state sleep, paradoxic sleep, and (2) NREM (non-REM) sleep, also called S stage sleep, which is divided into stages 1, 2, 3, and 4 and is recognizable by different electroencephalographic patterns. Stages 3 and 4 are "delta" sleep. Dreaming occurs mostly in REM and to a lesser extent in NREM sleep.

Sleep is a cyclic phenomenon, with four or five REM periods during the night accounting for about one-fourth of the total night's sleep (1.5–2 hours). The first REM period occurs about 80–120 minutes after onset of sleep and lasts about 10 minutes. Later REM periods are longer (15–40 minutes) and occur mostly in the last several hours of sleep. Most stage 4 (deepest) sleep occurs in the first several hours.

Age-related changes in normal sleep include an unchanging percentage of REM sleep and a marked decrease in stage 3 and stage 4 sleep, with an increase in wakeful periods during the night. These normal changes, early bedtimes, and daytime naps play a role in the increased complaints of insomnia in older people. Variations in sleep patterns may be due to circumstances (eg, "jet lag") or to idiosyncratic patterns ("night owls") in persons who perhaps because of different "biologic rhythms" habitually go to bed late and sleep late in the morning. Creativity and rapidity of response to unfamiliar situations are impaired by loss of sleep. There are also rare individuals who have chronic difficulty in adapting to a 24-hour sleep-wake cycle (desynchronization sleep disorder), which can be resynchronized by altering exposure to light.

The three major sleep disorders are discussed below. Any persistent sleep disorder that is not attributable to another condition should be evaluated by a sleep specialist.

1. Dyssomnias (Insomnia)

▶ Classification & Clinical Findings

Patients may complain of difficulty getting to sleep or staying asleep, intermittent wakefulness during the night, early morning awakening, or combinations of any of these. Transient episodes are usually of little significance. Stress, caffeine, physical discomfort, daytime napping, and early bedtimes are common factors.

Psychiatric disorders are often associated with persistent insomnia. **Depression** is usually associated with fragmented sleep, decreased total sleep time, earlier onset of REM sleep, a shift of REM activity to the first half of the night, and a loss of slow wave sleep—all of which are nonspecific findings. In **manic disorders,** a reduced total sleep time and a decreased need for sleep are cardinal features and important early sign of impending mania. In addition to a decreased amount of sleep, manic episodes are characterized by a shortened REM latency and increased REM activity. Sleep-related panic attacks occur in the transition from stage 2 to stage 3 sleep in some patients with a longer REM latency in the sleep pattern preceding the attacks.

Abuse of alcohol may cause or be secondary to the sleep disturbance. There is a tendency to use alcohol as a means of getting to sleep without realizing that it disrupts the normal sleep cycle. Acute alcohol intake produces a decreased sleep latency with reduced REM sleep during the first half of the night. REM sleep is increased in the second half of the night, with an increase in total amount of slow wave sleep (stages 3 and 4). Vivid dreams and frequent awakenings are common. Chronic alcohol abuse increases stage 1 and decreases REM sleep (most medications delay or block REM sleep), with symptoms persisting for many months after the individual has stopped drinking. Acute alcohol or other sedative withdrawal causes delayed onset of sleep and REM rebound with intermittent awakening during the night.

Heavy smoking (more than a pack a day) causes difficulty falling asleep—apparently independently of the often associated increase in coffee drinking. Excess intake near bedtime of caffeine, cocaine, and other stimulants (eg, over-the-counter cold remedies) causes decreased total sleep time—mostly NREM sleep—with some increased sleep latency.

Sedative-hypnotics—specifically, the benzodiazepines, which are the most commonly prescribed medications to promote sleep—tend to increase total sleep time, decrease sleep latency, and decrease nocturnal awakening, with variable effects on NREM sleep. Nonbenzodiazepine hypnotics, such as zolpidem, have similar effects on sleep as do the benzodiazepines. Withdrawal causes just the opposite effects and results in continued use of the drug for the purpose of preventing withdrawal symptoms. Antidepressants decrease REM sleep (with marked rebound on withdrawal in the form of nightmares) and have varying effects on NREM sleep. The effect on REM sleep correlates with reports that REM sleep deprivation produces improvement in some depressions.

Persistent insomnias are also related to a wide variety of medical conditions, particularly delirium, pain, respiratory distress syndromes, uremia, asthma, thyroid disorders, and nocturia due to benign prostatic hyperplasia. Sleep apnea and restless leg movement are described below. Adequate analgesia and proper treatment of medical disorders will reduce symptoms and decrease the need for sedatives.

▶ Treatment

In general, there are two broad classes of treatment for insomnia, and the two may be combined: psychological (cognitive-behavioral) and pharmacologic. In situations of acute distress, such as a grief reaction, pharmacologic measures may be most appropriate. With primary insomnia, however, initial efforts should be psychologically based. This is particularly true in the elderly to avoid the potential adverse reactions of medications. The elderly population is at risk for complaints of insomnia because sleep becomes lighter and more easily disrupted with aging. Medical disorders that become more common with age may also predispose to insomnia.

A. Psychological

Psychological strategies should include educating the patient regarding good **sleep hygiene**: (1) Go to bed only when sleepy. (2) Use the bed and bedroom only for sleeping and sex. (3) If still awake after 20 minutes, leave the bedroom, pursue a restful activity (such as a bath or meditation), and only return when sleepy. (4) Get up at the same time every morning regardless of the amount of sleep during the night. (5) Discontinue caffeine and nicotine, at least in the evening if not completely. (6) Establish a daily exercise regimen. (7) Avoid alcohol as it may disrupt continuity of sleep. (8) Limit fluids in the evening. (9) Learn and practice relaxation techniques. (10) Establish a bedtime ritual and a routine time for going to sleep. Research suggests that cognitive behavioral therapy for insomnia is as effective as zolpidem with benefits sustained 1 year after treatment.

B. Medical

When the above measures are insufficient, medications may be useful. Lorazepam (0.5 mg orally nightly), temazepam (7.5–15 mg orally nightly) and the nonbenzodiazepine hypnotics, zolpidem (5–10 mg orally nightly), and zaleplon (5–10 mg orally nightly), are often effective for the elderly population and can be given in larger doses—twice what is prescribed for the elderly—in younger patients. Zolpidem is also available as a sublingual tablet to treat insomnia characterized by middle-of-the-night awakening with difficulty falling back to sleep. The dose is 1.75 mg for women and 3.5 mg for men, taken once per night. A non-benzodiazepine hypnotic, eszopiclone (2–3 mg orally), is similar in action to zolpidem and zaleplon and like oral zolpidem, is approve for long-term use. A lower dose of 1 mg is indicated in the elderly or those with hepatic impairment. It is important to note that short-acting agents like triazolam or zolpidem may lead to amnestic episodes if used on a daily ongoing basis. Longer-acting agents such as flurazepam (half-life of > 48 hours) may accumulate in the elderly and lead to cognitive slowing, ataxia, falls, and somnolence. In general, it is appropriate to use medications for short courses of 1–2 weeks. The medications described above have largely replaced barbiturates as hypnotic agents because of their greater safety in overdose and their lesser hepatic enzyme induction effects. Antihistamines such as diphenhydramine (25 mg orally nightly) or hydroxyzine (25 mg orally nightly) may also be useful for sleep, as they produce no pharmacologic dependency; their anticholinergic effects may, however, produce confusion or urinary symptoms in the elderly. Trazodone, an atypical antidepressant, is a non–habit-forming, effective sleep medication in lower than antidepressant doses (25–150 mg orally at bedtime). Priapism is a rare side effect requiring emergent treatment. Ramelteon, 8 mg orally at bedtime, is a melatonin receptor agonist that helps with sleep onset and does not appear to have abuse potential. It appears to be safe for ongoing use without the development of tolerance.

Triazolam was popular as a hypnotic drug because of its very short duration of action. However, because it has been associated with dependency, transient psychotic reactions, anterograde amnesia, and rebound anxiety, it has been removed from the market in several European countries. If used, it should be prescribed only for short periods of time.

2. Hypersomnias (Disorders of Excessive Sleepiness)

▶ Classification & Clinical Findings

A. Breathing-Related Sleep Disorders

Obstructive sleep apnea hypopnea is by far the most common of the breathing-related sleep disorders that include central sleep apnea and sleep-related hypoventilation. Obstructive sleep apnea hypopnea is characterized by snoring, gasping, or breathing pauses during sleep and 5 or more apneas or hypopneas per hour or evidence by polysomnography or 15 or more apneas or hypopneas per hour. (See Chapter 9.)

B. Narcolepsy Hypocretin Deficiency Syndrome

Narcolepsy consists of a tetrad of symptoms: (1) Sudden, brief (about 15 minutes) sleep attacks that may occur during any type of activity; (2) cataplexy—sudden loss of muscle tone involving specific small muscle groups or generalized muscle weakness that may cause the person to slump to the floor, unable to move, often associated with emotional reactions and sometimes confused with seizure disorder; (3) sleep paralysis—a generalized flaccidity of muscles with full consciousness in the transition zone between sleep and waking; and (4) hypnagogic hallucinations, visual or auditory, which may precede sleep or occur during the sleep attack. The attacks are characterized by an abrupt transition into REM sleep—a necessary criterion for diagnosis. The disorder begins in early adult life, affects both sexes equally, and usually levels off in severity at about 30 years of age.

REM sleep behavior disorder, characterized by motor dyscontrol and often violent dreams during REM sleep, may be related to narcolepsy.

C. Kleine-Levin Syndrome

This syndrome, which occurs mostly in young men, is characterized by hypersomnic attacks three or four times a year lasting up to 2 days, with hyperphagia, hypersexuality, irritability, and confusion on awakening. It has often been associated with antecedent neurologic insults. It usually remits after age 40.

D. Periodic Limb Movement Disorder

Periodic lower leg movements occur only during sleep with subsequent daytime sleepiness, anxiety, depression, and cognitive impairment. Restless leg syndrome includes movements while awake as well.

E. Shift Work Sleep Disorder

Shift work sleep disorder occurs when there is excessive fatigue as a consequence of work occurring during the normal sleep period.

▶ Treatment

Narcolepsy can be managed by daily administration of a stimulant such as dextroamphetamine sulfate, 10 mg orally in the morning, with increased dosage as necessary. Modafinil and its enantiomer armodafinil are schedule IV medications FDA-approved for treating the excessive daytime fatigue of narcolepsy, sleepiness associated with obstructive sleep apnea as well as for shift work sleep disorder. Usual dosing is 200–400 mg orally each morning for modafinil and 150–250 mg orally in the morning for armodafinil. The mechanism of action of modafinil and armodafil is unknown, yet they are thought to be less of an abuse risk than stimulants that are primarily dopaminergic. Common side effects include headache and anxiety; however, modafinil appears to be generally well tolerated. Modafinil may reduce the efficacy of cyclosporine, oral contraceptives, and other medications by inducing their hepatic metabolism. Imipramine, 75–100 mg orally daily, has been effective in treatment of cataplexy but not narcolepsy.

Periodic limb movement disorder and REM sleep behavior disorder can be treated with clonazepam with variable results. There is no treatment for Kleine-Levin syndrome.

Treatment of sleep apnea is discussed in Chapter 9.

3. Parasomnias (Abnormal Behaviors during Sleep)

These disorders (sleep terror, nightmares, sleepwalking, and enuresis) are fairly common in children and less so in adults.

Bagai K. Obstructive sleep apnea, stroke, and cardiovascular diseases. Neurologist. 2010 Nov;16(6):329–39. [PMID: 21150380]

Merrigan JM et al. JAMA patient page. Insomnia. JAMA. 2013 Feb 20;309(7):733. [PMID: 23423421]

Mignot EJ. A practical guide to the therapy of narcolepsy and hypersomnia syndromes. Neurotherapeutics. 2012 Oct;9(4):739–52. [PMID: 23065655]

Simon S et al. Latest advances in sleep medicine: obstructive sleep apnea. Chest. 2012 Dec;142(6):1645–51. [PMID: 23208337]

Swanson LM et al. An open pilot of cognitive-behavioral therapy for insomnia in women with postpartum depression. Behav Sleep Med. 2013;11(4):297–307. [PMID: 23216373]

DISORDERS OF AGGRESSION

Aggression and violence are symptoms rather than diseases, and most frequently they are not associated with an underlying medical condition. Clinicians are unable to predict dangerous behavior with greater than chance accuracy. Depression, schizophrenia, personality disorders, mania, paranoia, temporal lobe dysfunction, and organic mental states may be associated with acts of aggression. Impulse control disorders are characterized by physical abuse (usually of the aggressor's domestic partner or children), by pathologic intoxication, by impulsive sexual activities, and by reckless driving. Anabolic steroid usage by athletes has been associated with increased tendencies toward violent behavior.

In the United States, a significant proportion of all violent deaths are alcohol-related. The ingestion of even small amounts of alcohol can result in pathologic intoxication that resembles an acute organic mental condition. Amphetamines, crack cocaine, and other stimulants are frequently associated with aggressive behavior. Phencyclidine is a drug commonly associated with violent behavior that is occasionally of a bizarre nature, partly due to lowering of the pain threshold. Domestic violence and rape are much more widespread than previously recognized. Awareness of the problem is to some degree due to increasing recognition of the rights of women and the understanding by women that they do not have to accept abuse. Acceptance of this kind of aggressive behavior inevitably leads to more, with the ultimate aggression being murder—20–50% of murders in the United States occur within the family. Police are called for more domestic disputes than all other criminal incidents combined. Children living in such family situations frequently become victims of abuse.

Features of individuals who have been subjected to long-term physical or sexual abuse are as follows: trouble expressing anger, staying angry longer, general passivity in relationships, feeling "marked for life" with an accompanying feeling of deserving to be victimized, lack of trust, and dissociation of affect from experiences. They are prone to express their psychological distress with somatization symptoms, often pain complaints. They may also have symptoms related to posttraumatic stress, as discussed above. The clinician should be suspicious about the origin of any injuries not fully explained, particularly if such incidents recur.

▶ Treatment

A. Psychological

Management of any violent individual includes appropriate psychological maneuvers. Move slowly, talk slowly with clarity and reassurance, and evaluate the situation. Strive to create a setting that is minimally disturbing, and eliminate people or things threatening to the violent individual. Do not threaten and do not touch or crowd the person. Allow no weapons in the area (an increasing problem in hospital emergency departments). Proximity to a door is comforting to both the patient and the examiner. Use a negotiator the violent person can relate to comfortably. Food and drink are helpful in defusing the situation (as are cigarettes for those who smoke). Honesty is important. Make no false promises, bolster the patient's self-esteem, and continue to engage the subject verbally until the situation is under control. This type of individual does better with strong external controls to replace the lack of inner controls over the long term. Close probationary supervision and judicially mandated restrictions can be most helpful. There should be a major effort to help the individual avoid drug use (eg, Alcoholics Anonymous). Victims of abuse are essentially treated as any victim of trauma and, not infrequently, have evidence of PTSD.

B. Pharmacologic

Pharmacologic means are often necessary whether or not psychological approaches have been successful. This is particularly true in the agitated or psychotic patient. The drugs of choice in seriously violent or psychotic aggressive states are antipsychotics, given intramuscularly if necessary, every 1–2 hours until symptoms are alleviated. A number of second-generation intramuscular antipsychotics are FDA approved in the management of acute agitation, and include aripiprazole (9.75 mg/1.3 mL), ziprasidone (10-mg/0.5 mL), and olanzapine (10 mg/2 mL). The second-generation antipsychotics appear less likely than first-generation drugs like haloperidol (2.5–5 mg) to cause acute extrapyramidal symptoms. However, the second-generation drugs appear no more effective than first-generation drugs and are more expensive. Benzodiazepine sedatives (eg, diazepam, 5 mg orally or intravenously every several hours) can be used for mild to moderate agitation. Chronic aggressive states, particularly in intellectual disabilities and brain damage (rule out causative organic conditions and medications such as anticholinergic medications in amounts sufficient to cause confusion), have been ameliorated with risperidone, 0.5–2 mg/d orally, propranolol, 40–240 mg/d orally, or pindolol, 5 mg twice daily orally (pindolol causes less bradycardia and hypotension than propranolol). Carbamazepine and valproic acid are effective in the treatment of aggression and explosive disorders, particularly when associated with known or suspected brain lesions. Lithium and SSRIs are also effective for some intermittent explosive outbursts. Buspirone (10–45 mg/d orally) is helpful for aggression, particularly in patients with intellectual disabilities.

C. Physical

Physical management is necessary if psychological and pharmacologic means are not sufficient. It requires the active and visible presence of an adequate number of personnel (five or six) to reinforce the idea that the situation is under control despite the patient's lack of inner controls. Such an approach often precludes the need for actual physical restraint. Seclusion rooms and restraints should be used only when necessary (ambulatory restraints are an alternative), and the patient must then be observed at frequent intervals. Narrow corridors, small spaces, and crowded areas exacerbate the potential for violence in an anxious patient.

D. Other Interventions

The treatment of victims (eg, battered women) is challenging and often complicated by their reluctance to leave the situation. Reasons for staying vary, but common themes include the fear of more violence because of leaving, the hope that the situation may ameliorate (in spite of steady worsening), and the financial aspects of the situation, which are seldom to the woman's advantage. Concerns for the children often finally compel the woman to seek help. An early step is to get the woman into a therapeutic situation that provides the support of others in similar straits. Al-Anon is frequently a valuable asset when alcohol is a factor. The group can support the victim while she gathers strength to consider alternatives without being paralyzed by fear. Many cities offer temporary emergency centers and counseling. Use the available resources, attend to any medical or psychiatric problems, and maintain a compassionate interest. Some states require physicians to report injuries caused by abuse or suspected abuse to police authorities.

Buckley P et al. Psychopharmacology of aggression in schizophrenia. Schizophr Bull. 2011 Sep;37(5):930–6. [PMID: 21860038]

Johnson DM et al. Cognitive behavioral treatment of PTSD in residents in battered women's shelters: results of a randomized clinical trial. J Consult Clin Psychol. 2011 Aug;79(4): 542–51. [PMID: 21787052]

Rees S et al. Lifetime prevalence of gender-based violence in women and the relationship with mental disorders and psychosocial function. JAMA. 2011 Aug 3;305(5):513–21. [PMID: 21813429]

▼ SUBSTANCE USE DISORDERS

The term "dependency" was previously used to describe a severe form of substance abuse and drug addiction characterized by the triad of: (1) a **psychological** **dependence** or craving and the behavior involved in procurement of the drug; (2) **physiologic dependence**, with withdrawal symptoms on discontinuance of the drug; and (3) **tolerance**, ie, the need to increase the dose to obtain the desired effects. The terms "dependency" and "abuse" were dropped in *DSM-V* in favor of the single term "substance use disorder," ranging from mild to severe. Many patients could have a severe and life-threatening abuse problem without ever being dependent on a drug.

There is accumulating evidence that an impairment syndrome exists in many former (and current) drug users. It is believed that drug use produces damaged neurotransmitter receptor sites and that the consequent imbalance produces symptoms that may mimic other psychiatric illnesses. "Kindling"—repeated stimulation of the brain—renders the individual more susceptible to focal brain activity with minimal stimulation. Stimulants and depressants can produce kindling, leading to relatively spontaneous effects no longer dependent on the original stimulus. These effects may be manifested as mood swings, panic, psychosis, and occasionally overt seizure activity. The imbalance also results in frequent job changes, marital problems, and generally erratic behavior. Patients with PTSD frequently have treated themselves with a variety of drugs. Chronic abusers of a wide variety of drugs exhibit cerebral atrophy on CT scans, a finding that may relate to the above symptoms. Early recognition is important, mainly to establish realistic treatment programs that are chiefly symptom-directed.

The clinician faces three problems with substance use disorders: (1) the prescribing of substances such as sedatives, stimulants, or opioids that might produce dependency; (2) the treatment of individuals who have already abused drugs, most commonly alcohol; and (3) the detection of illicit drug use in patients presenting with psychiatric symptoms. The usefulness of urinalysis for detection of drugs varies markedly with different drugs and under different circumstances (pharmacokinetics is a major factor). Water-soluble drugs (eg, alcohol, stimulants, opioids) are eliminated in a day or so. Lipophilic substances (eg, barbiturates, tetrahydrocannabinol) appear in the urine over longer periods of time: several days in most cases, 1–2 months in chronic marijuana users. Sedative drug determinations are quite variable, amount of drug and duration of use being important determinants. False-positives can be a problem related to ingestion of some legitimate medications (eg, phenytoin for barbiturates, phenylpropanolamine for amphetamines, chlorpromazine for opioids) and some foods (eg, poppy seeds for opioids, coca leaf tea for cocaine). Manipulations can alter the legitimacy of the testing. Dilution, either in vivo or in vitro, can be detected by checking urine specific gravity. Addition of ammonia, vinegar, or salt may invalidate the test, but odor and pH determinations are simple. Hair analysis can determine drug use over longer periods, particularly sequential drug-taking patterns. The sensitivity and reliability of such tests are considered good, and the method may be complementary to urinalysis.

Marlatt GA. Update on harm-reduction policy and intervention research. Annu Rev Clin Psychol. 2010 Apr 27;6:591–606. [PMID: 20192791]

ALCOHOL USE DISORDER (Alcoholism)

ESSENTIALS OF DIAGNOSIS

Major criteria:

► Physiologic dependence as manifested by evidence of withdrawal when intake is interrupted.

► Tolerance to the effects of alcohol.

► Evidence of alcohol-associated illnesses, such as alcoholic liver disease, cerebellar degeneration.

► Continued drinking despite strong medical and social contraindications and life disruptions.

► Impairment in social and occupational functioning.

► Depression.

► Blackouts.

General Considerations

Alcohol use disorder is a syndrome consisting of two phases: at-risk drinking and moderate to severe alcohol misuse. At-risk drinking is the repetitive use of alcohol, often to alleviate anxiety or solve other emotional problems. A moderate to severe alcohol use disorder is similar to that which occurs following the repeated use of other sedative-hypnotics and is characterized by recurrent use of alcohol despite disruption in social roles (family and work), alcohol-related legal problems, and taking safety risks by oneself and with others. The National Institute on Alcohol Abuse and Alcoholism formally defines at-risk drinking as **more than 4 drinks per day or 14 drinks per week for men or more than 3 drinks per day or 7 drinks per week for women.** A drink is defined by the CDC as 12 oz of beer, 8 oz of malt liquor, 5 oz of wine, or 1.3 oz or a "shot" of 80-proof distilled spirits of liquor. Individuals with at-risk drinking are at an increased risk for developing or are developing an alcohol use disorder. Alcohol and other drug abuse patients have a much higher prevalence of lifetime psychiatric disorders. While male-to-female ratios in alcoholic treatment agencies remain at 4:1, there is evidence that the rates are converging. Women delay seeking help, and when they do they tend to seek it in medical or mental health settings. Adoption and twin studies indicate some genetic influence. Ethnic distinctions are important—eg, 40% of Japanese have aldehyde dehydrogenase deficiency and are more susceptible to the effects of alcohol. Depression is often present and should be evaluated carefully. The majority of suicides and intrafamily homicides involve alcohol. Alcohol is a major factor in rapes and other assaults.

There are several screening instruments that may help identify an alcohol use disorder. One of the most useful is the Alcohol Use Disorder Identification Test (AUDIT) (see Table 1–7).

▶ Clinical Findings

A. Acute Intoxication

The signs of alcoholic intoxication are the same as those of overdosage with any other central nervous system depressant: drowsiness, errors of commission, psychomotor dysfunction, disinhibition, dysarthria, ataxia, and nystagmus. For a 70-kg person, an ounce of whiskey, a 4- to 6-oz glass of wine, or a 12-oz bottle of beer (roughly 15, 11, and 13 grams of alcohol, respectively) may raise the level of alcohol in the blood by 25 mg/dL. For a 50-kg person, the blood alcohol level would rise even higher (35 mg/dL) with the same consumption. Blood alcohol levels below 50 mg/dL rarely cause significant motor dysfunction (the legal limit for driving under the influence is commonly 80 mg/dL). Intoxication as manifested by ataxia, dysarthria, and nausea and vomiting indicates a blood level > 150 mg/dL, and lethal blood levels range from 350 to 900 mg/dL. In severe cases, overdosage is marked by respiratory depression, stupor, seizures, shock syndrome, coma, and death. Serious overdoses are frequently due to a combination of alcohol with other sedatives.

B. Withdrawal

There is a wide spectrum of manifestations of alcoholic withdrawal, ranging from anxiety, decreased cognition, and tremulousness through increasing irritability and hyperreactivity to full-blown delirium tremens. Symptoms of mild withdrawal, including tremor, elevated vital signs, and anxiety, begin within about 8 hours after the last drink and usually have passed by day 3. Generalized seizures occur within the first 24–38 hours and are more prevalent in persons who have a history of withdrawal syndromes. Delirium tremens is an acute organic psychosis that is usually manifest within 24–72 hours after the last drink (but may occur up to 7–10 days later). It is characterized by mental confusion, tremor, sensory hyperacuity, visual hallucinations (often of snakes, bugs, etc), autonomic hyperactivity, diaphoresis, dehydration, electrolyte disturbances (hypokalemia, hypomagnesemia), seizures, and cardiovascular abnormalities. The acute withdrawal syndrome is often completely unexpected and occurs when the patient has been hospitalized for some unrelated problem and presents as a diagnostic problem. Suspect alcohol withdrawal in every unexplained delirium. The mortality rate from delirium tremens has steadily decreased with early diagnosis and improved treatment.

In addition to the immediate withdrawal symptoms, there is evidence of persistent longer-term ones, including sleep disturbances, anxiety, depression, excitability, fatigue, and emotional volatility. These symptoms may persist for 3–12 months, and in some cases they become chronic.

C. Alcoholic (Organic) Hallucinosis

This syndrome occurs either during heavy drinking or on withdrawal and is characterized by a paranoid psychosis without the tremulousness, confusion, and clouded sensorium seen in withdrawal syndromes. The patient appears normal except for the auditory hallucinations, which are frequently persecutory and may cause the patient to behave aggressively and in a paranoid fashion.

D. Chronic Alcoholic Brain Syndromes

These encephalopathies are characterized by increasing erratic behavior, memory and recall problems, and emotional instability—the usual signs of organic brain injury due to any cause. Wernicke-Korsakoff syndrome due to thiamine deficiency may develop with a series of episodes. Wernicke encephalopathy consists of the triad of confusion, ataxia, and ophthalmoplegia (typically sixth nerve). Early recognition and treatment with thiamine can minimize damage. One of the possible sequelae is Korsakoff psychosis, characterized by both anterograde and retrograde amnesia, with confabulation early in the course. Early recognition and treatment of the alcoholic with intravenous thiamine and B complex vitamins can minimize damage.

E. Laboratory Findings

Ethanol may contribute to the presence of an otherwise unexplained osmolar gap. There may also be elevated liver function tests, increased serum uric acid and triglycerides, and decreased serum potassium and magnesium. The most definitive biologic marker for chronic alcoholism is carbohydrate deficient transferrin, which can detect heavy use (60 mg/d over 7–10 days) with high specificity. Other useful tests for diagnosing alcohol use disorder are gamma-glutamyl transpeptidase measurement (levels > 30 units/L are suggestive of heavy drinking) and mean corpuscular volume (> 95 fL in men and > 100 fL in women). If both are elevated, a serious drinking problem is likely. Use of other recreational drugs with alcohol skews and negates the significance of these tests. Concomitant elevations of high-density lipoprotein cholesterol elevations and gamma-glutamyl transpeptidase concentrations also can help identify heavy drinkers.

▶ Differential Diagnosis

The differential diagnosis of **alcoholism** is essentially between primary alcohol use disorder (when no other major psychiatric diagnosis exists) and secondary alcohol use disorder (when alcohol is used as self-medication for major underlying psychiatric problems such as schizophrenia or affective disorder). The differentiation is important, since the latter group requires treatment for the specific psychiatric problem. In primary and secondary alcoholism, at-risk drinking can be distinguished from alcohol addiction by taking a careful psychiatric history and evaluating the degree to which recurrent drinking impacts the social role functioning and physical safety of the individual.

The differential diagnosis of **alcohol withdrawal** includes other sedative withdrawals and other causes of delirium. Acute alcoholic hallucinosis must be differentiated from other acute paranoid states such as amphetamine

psychosis or paranoid schizophrenia. The form of the brain syndrome is of little help—eg, chronic brain syndromes from lupus erythematosus may be associated with confabulation similar to that resulting from long-standing alcoholism.

▶ Complications

The medical, economic, and psychosocial problems of alcoholism are staggering. The central and peripheral nervous system complications include chronic brain syndromes, cerebellar degeneration, cardiomyopathy, and peripheral neuropathies. Direct effects on the liver include cirrhosis, esophageal varices, and eventual hepatic failure. Indirect effects include protein abnormalities, coagulation defects, hormone deficiencies, and an increased incidence of liver neoplasms.

Fetal alcohol syndrome includes one or more of the following developmental defects in the offspring of alcoholic women: (1) low birth weight and small size with failure to catch up in size or weight, (2) mental retardation, with an average IQ in the 60s, and (3) a variety of birth defects, with a large percentage of facial and cardiac abnormalities. The risk is appreciably higher the more alcohol ingested by the mother each day. Cigarette and marijuana smoking as well as cocaine use can produce similar effects on the fetus.

▶ Treatment of At-Risk Drinking

A. Psychological

The most important consideration for the clinician is to suspect the problem early and take a nonjudgmental attitude, although this does not mean a passive one. The problem of **denial** must be faced, preferably with significant family members at the first meeting. This means dealing from the beginning with any enabling behavior of the spouse or other significant people. Enabling behavior allows the patient with an alcohol use disorder to avoid facing the consequences of his or her behavior.

There must be an emphasis on the things that can be done. This approach emphasizes the fact that the clinician cares and strikes a positive and hopeful note early in treatment. Valuable time should not be wasted trying to find out why the patient drinks; come to grips early with the immediate problem of how to stop the drinking. Although total abstinence should be the ultimate goal, a harm reduction model indicates that gradual progress toward abstinence can be a useful treatment stratagem.

Motivational interviewing, a model of counseling that addresses both the patient's ambivalence and motivation for change, may contribute to reduced consumption over time.

B. Social

Get the patient into Alcoholics Anonymous and the spouse into Al-Anon. Success is usually proportionate to the utilization of Alcoholics Anonymous, religious counseling, and other resources. The patient should be seen frequently for short periods and charged an appropriate fee.

Do not underestimate the importance of religion, particularly since the patient with alcohol use disorder is often a dependent person who needs a great deal of support. Early enlistment of the help of a concerned religious adviser can often provide the turning point for a personal conversion to sobriety.

One of the most important considerations is the patient's job—fear of losing a job is one of the most powerful motivations for giving up drink. The business community is aware of the problem; about 70% of the Fortune 500 companies offer programs to their employees to help with the problem of alcoholism. In the latter case, some specific recommendations to employers can be offered: (1) Avoid placement in jobs where the alcoholic patient must be alone, eg, as a traveling buyer or sales executive. (2) Use supervision but not surveillance. (3) Keep competition with others to a minimum. (4) Avoid positions that require quick decision-making on important matters (high-stress situations). In general, commitment to abstinence and avoidance of situations that might be conducive to drinking are most predictive of a good outcome.

C. Medical

Hospitalization is not usually necessary. It is sometimes used to dramatize a situation and force the patient to face the problem of alcoholism, but generally it should be used for medical indications.

Because of the many medical complications of alcoholism, a complete physical examination with appropriate laboratory tests is mandatory, with special attention to the liver and nervous system. Use of sedatives as a replacement for alcohol is not desirable. The usual result is concomitant use of sedatives and alcohol and worsening of the problem. Lithium is not helpful in the treatment of alcoholism.

Disulfiram (250–500 mg/d orally) has been used for many years as an aversive drug to discourage alcohol use. Disulfiram inhibits alcohol dehydrogenase, causing toxic reactions when alcohol is consumed. The results have generally been of limited effectiveness and depend on the motivation of the individual to be compliant.

Naltrexone, an opiate antagonist, in a dosage of 50 mg orally daily, lowers relapse rates over the 3–6 months after cessation of drinking, apparently by lessening the pleasurable effects of alcohol. One study suggests that naltrexone is most effective when given during periods of drinking in combination with therapy that supports abstinence but accepts the fact that relapses occur. Naltrexone is FDA-approved for maintenance therapy. Studies indicate that it reduces alcohol craving when used as part of a comprehensive treatment program. Acamprosate (333–666 mg orally three times daily) helps reduce craving and maintain abstinence, and can be continued even during periods of relapse.

D. Behavioral

Conditioning approaches historically have been used in some settings in the treatment of alcoholism, most commonly as a type of aversion therapy. For example, the patient is given a drink of whiskey and then a shot of apomorphine, and proceeds to vomit. In this way a strong association is built up between the drinking and vomiting. Although this kind of treatment has been successful in some cases, after appropriate informed consent, many people do not sustain the learned aversive response.

▶ Treatment of Hallucinosis & Withdrawal

A. Medical

1. Alcoholic hallucinosis—Alcoholic hallucinosis, which can occur either during or on cessation of a prolonged drinking period, is not a typical withdrawal syndrome and is handled differently. Since the symptoms are primarily those of a psychosis in the presence of a clear sensorium, they are handled like any other psychosis: hospitalization (when indicated) and adequate amounts of antipsychotic medications. Haloperidol, 5 mg orally twice a day for the first day or so, usually ameliorates symptoms quickly, and the drug can be decreased and discontinued over several days as the patient improves. It then becomes necessary to deal with the chronic alcohol abuse, which has been discussed.

2. Withdrawal symptoms—The onset of withdrawal symptoms is usually 8–12 hours and the peak intensity of symptoms is 48–72 hours after alcohol consumption is stopped. Providing adequate central nervous system depressants (eg, benzodiazepines) is important to counteract the excitability resulting from sudden cessation of alcohol intake. The choice of a specific sedative is less important than using adequate doses to bring the patient to a level of moderate sedation, and this will vary from person to person. Mild dependency requires "drying out." In some instances for outpatients, a short course of tapering long-acting benzodiazepines—eg, diazepam, 20 mg orally daily initially, decreasing by 5 mg daily—may be a useful adjunct. In moderate to severe withdrawal, hospitalize the patient and use diazepam orally in a dosage of 5–10 mg hourly depending on the clinical need as judged by withdrawal symptoms, including nausea, tremor, autonomic hyperactivity, agitation; tactile, visual, and auditory hallucinations; and disorientation. This type of symptom-driven medication regimen for withdrawal appears to reduce total benzodiazepine usage over fixed-dose schedules. Antipsychotic medications should not be used. Monitoring of vital signs and fluid and electrolyte levels is essential for the severely ill patient.

In very severe withdrawal, intravenous administration is necessary. After stabilization, the amount of diazepam required to maintain a sedated state may be given orally every 8–12 hours. If restlessness, tremulousness, and other signs of withdrawal persist, the dosage is increased until moderate sedation occurs. The dosage is then gradually reduced by 20% every 24 hours until withdrawal is complete. This usually requires a week or so of treatment. Clonidine, 5 mcg/kg orally every 2 hours, or the patch formulation of appropriate dosage strength, suppresses cardiovascular signs of withdrawal and has some anxiolytic effect. Carbamazepine, 400–800 mg daily orally, compares favorably with benzodiazepines for alcohol withdrawal.

Atenolol, as an adjunct to benzodiazepines, can reduce symptoms of alcohol withdrawal. The daily oral atenolol dose is 100 mg when the heart rate is above 80 beats per minute and 50 mg for a heart rate between 50 and 80 beats per minute. Atenolol should not be used when bradycardia is present.

Meticulous examination for other medical problems is necessary. Alcoholic hypoglycemia can occur with low blood alcohol levels (see Chapter 27). Patients with severe alcohol use disorder commonly have liver disease with associated clotting disorders and are also prone to injury—and the combination all too frequently leads to undiagnosed subdural hematoma.

Phenytoin does not appear to be useful in managing alcohol withdrawal seizures per se. Sedating doses of benzodiazepines are effective in treating alcohol withdrawal seizures. Thus, other anticonvulsants are not usually needed unless there is a preexisting seizure disorder.

A general diet should be given, and vitamins in high doses: thiamine, 50 mg intravenously initially, then orally on a daily basis; pyridoxine, 100 mg/d; folic acid, 1 mg/d; and ascorbic acid, 100 mg twice a day. Intravenous glucose solutions should not be given prior to thiamine for fear of precipitating Wernicke syndrome.

Chronic brain syndromes secondary to a long history of alcohol intake are not clearly responsive to thiamine and vitamin replenishment. Attention to the social and environmental care of this type of patient is paramount.

B. Psychological and Behavioral

The comments in the section on problem drinking apply here also; these methods of treatment become the primary consideration after successful treatment of withdrawal or alcoholic hallucinosis. Psychological and social measures should be initiated in the hospital prior to discharge. This increases the possibility of continued post-hospitalization treatment.

de Wit M et al. Alcohol-use disorders in the critically ill patient. Chest. 2010 Oct;138(4):994–1003. [PMID: 20923804]

Johnson BA. Medication treatment of different types of alcoholism. Am J Psychiatry. 2010 Jun;167(6):630–9. [PMID: 20516163]

Satre DD et al. Motivational interviewing to reduce hazardous drinking and drug use among depression patients. J Subst Abuse Treat. 2013 Apr;44(3):323–9. [PMID: 22999815]

OTHER DRUG & SUBSTANCE DEPENDENCIES

1. Opioids

While the terms "opioids" and "narcotics" both refer to a group of drugs with actions that mimic those of morphine, the term "opioids" is used when discussing medications prescribed in a controlled manner by a clinician, and the term "narcotics" is used to connote illicit drug use. All of the opioid analgesics can be reversed by the opioid antagonist naloxone.

The clinical symptoms and signs of mild narcotic intoxication include changes in mood, with feelings of euphoria; drowsiness; nausea with occasional emesis; needle tracks; and miosis. The incidence of snorting and inhaling heroin ("smoking") is increasing, particularly among cocaine users. This coincides with a decrease in the availability of methaqualone (no longer marketed) and other sedatives used to temper the cocaine "high" (see discussion of cocaine under Stimulants, below). Overdosage causes respiratory depression, peripheral vasodilation, pinpoint pupils, pulmonary edema, coma, and death.

Tolerance and withdrawal are major concerns when continued use of opioids occurs, although withdrawal causes only moderate morbidity (similar in severity to a bout of "flu"). Addicted patients sometimes consider themselves more addicted than they really are and may not require a withdrawal program. Grades of withdrawal are categorized from 0 to 4: grade 0 includes craving and anxiety; grade 1, yawning, lacrimation, rhinorrhea, and perspiration; grade 2, previous symptoms plus mydriasis, piloerection, anorexia, tremors, and hot and cold flashes with generalized aching; grades 3 and 4, increased intensity of previous symptoms and signs, with increased temperature, blood pressure, pulse, and respiratory rate and depth. In withdrawal from the most severe addiction, vomiting, diarrhea, weight loss, hemoconcentration, and spontaneous ejaculation or orgasm commonly occur.

Treatment for overdosage (or suspected overdosage) is discussed in Chapter 38.

Treatment for withdrawal begins if grade 2 signs develop. If a withdrawal program is necessary, use methadone, 10 mg orally (use parenteral administration if the patient is vomiting), and observe. If signs (piloerection, mydriasis, cardiovascular changes) persist for > 4–6 hours, give another 10 mg; continue to administer methadone at 4- to 6-hour intervals until signs are not present (rarely > 40 mg of methadone in 24 hours). Divide the total amount of drug required over the first 24-hour period by 2 and give that amount every 12 hours. Each day, reduce the total 24-hour dose by 5–10 mg. Thus, a moderately addicted patient initially requiring 30–40 mg of methadone could be withdrawn over a 4- to 8-day period. Clonidine, 0.1 mg orally several times daily over a 10- to 14-day period, is both an alternative and an adjunct to methadone detoxification; it is not necessary to taper the dose. Clonidine is helpful in alleviating cardiovascular symptoms but does not significantly relieve anxiety, insomnia, or generalized aching. There is a protracted abstinence syndrome of metabolic, respiratory, and blood pressure changes over a period of 3–6 months.

Opioid antagonists (eg, naltrexone) can also be used successfully for treatment of the patient who has been free of opioids for 7–10 days. Naltrexone blocks the narcotic "high" of heroin when 50 mg is given orally every 24 hours initially for several days and then 100 mg is given every 48–72 hours. A monthly injectable form of naltrexone has become available and may enhance compliance. Liver disorders are a major contraindication. Buprenorphine, a partial agonist, has become a mainstay of office-based treatment of opiate dependency. Its use requires certified training.

Alternative strategies for the treatment of opioid withdrawal have included rapid and ultrarapid detoxification techniques. However, data do not support the use of either method. Methadone maintenance programs are of some value in chronic recidivism. Under carefully controlled supervision, the narcotic addict is maintained on fairly high doses of methadone (40–120 mg/d) that satisfy craving and block the effects of heroin to a great degree.

2. Sedatives (Anxiolytics)

See Anxiety Disorders, this chapter.

3. Psychedelics

About 6000 species of plants have psychoactive properties. All of the common psychedelics (LSD, mescaline, psilocybin, dimethyltryptamine, and other derivatives of phenylalanine and tryptophan) can produce similar behavioral and physiologic effects. An initial feeling of tension is followed by emotional release such as crying or laughing (1–2 hours). Later, perceptual distortions occur, with visual illusions and hallucinations, and occasionally there is fear of ego disintegration (2–3 hours). Major changes in time sense and mood lability then occur (3–4 hours). A feeling of detachment and a sense of destiny and control occur (4–6 hours). Of course, reactions vary among individuals, and some of the drugs produce markedly different time frames. Occasionally, the acute episode is terrifying (a "bad trip"), which may include panic, depression, confusion, or psychotic symptoms. Preexisting emotional problems, the attitude of the user, and the setting where the drug is used affect the experience.

Treatment of the acute episode primarily involves protection of the individual from erratic behavior that may lead to injury or death. A structured environment is usually sufficient until the drug is metabolized. In severe cases, antipsychotic medications with minimal side effects (eg, haloperidol, 5 mg intramuscularly) may be given every several hours until the individual has regained control. In cases where "flashbacks" occur (mental imagery from a "bad trip" that is later triggered by mild stimuli such as marijuana, alcohol, or psychic trauma), a short course of an antipsychotic drug—eg, olanzapine, 5–10 mg/d orally, or risperidone, 2 mg/d orally, initially, and up to 20 mg/d and 6 mg/d, respectively—is usually sufficient. Lorazepam, 1–2 mg orally or intramuscularly every 2 hours as needed for acute agitation, may be a useful adjunct. An occasional patient may have "flashbacks" for much longer periods and require small doses of antipsychotic medications over the longer term.

4. Phencyclidine

Phencyclidine (PCP, angel dust, peace pill, hog) is simple to produce and mimics to some degree the traditional psychedelic drugs. PCP is a common deceptive substitute for LSD, tetrahydrocannabinol, and mescaline. It is available in crystals, capsules, and tablets to be inhaled, injected, swallowed, or smoked (it is commonly sprinkled on marijuana).

Absorption after smoking is rapid, with onset of symptoms in several minutes and peak symptoms in 15–30 minutes. Mild intoxication produces euphoria accompanied by a feeling of numbness. Moderate intoxication (5–10 mg) results in disorientation, detachment from surroundings, distortion of body image, combativeness, unusual feats of strength (partly due to its anesthetic activity), and loss of ability to integrate sensory input, especially touch and proprioception. Physical symptoms include dizziness, ataxia, dysarthria, nystagmus, retracted upper eyelid with blank stare, hyperreflexia, and tachycardia. There are increases in blood pressure, respiration, muscle tone, and urine production. Usage in the first trimester of pregnancy is associated with an increase in spontaneous abortion and congenital defects. Severe intoxication (20 mg or more) produces an increase in degree of moderate symptoms, with the addition of seizures, deepening coma, hypertensive crisis, and severe psychotic ideation. The drug is particularly long-lasting (several days to several weeks) owing to high lipid solubility, gastroenteric recycling, and the production of active metabolites. Overdosage may be fatal, with the major causes of death being hypertensive crisis, respiratory arrest, and convulsions. Acute rhabdomyolysis has been reported and can result in myoglobinuric kidney failure.

Differential diagnosis involves the whole spectrum of street drugs, since in some ways phencyclidine mimics sedatives, psychedelics, and marijuana in its effects. Blood and urine testing can detect the acute problem.

Treatment is discussed in Chapter 38.

5. Marijuana

Cannabis sativa, a hemp plant, is the source of marijuana. Mercury may be a contaminant in marijuana grown in volcanic soil. The drug is usually inhaled by smoking. Effects occur in 10–20 minutes and last 2–3 hours. "Joints" of good quality contain about 500 mg of marijuana (which contains approximately 5–15 mg of tetrahydrocannabinol with a half-life of 7 days).

With moderate dosage, marijuana produces two phases: mild euphoria followed by sleepiness. In the acute state, the user has an altered time perception, less inhibited emotions, psychomotor problems, impaired immediate memory, and conjunctival injection. High doses produce transient psychotomimetic effects. No specific treatment is necessary except in the case of the occasional "bad trip," in which case the person is treated in the same way as for psychedelic usage. Marijuana frequently aggravates existing mental illness and adversely affects motor performance.

Studies of long-term effects have conclusively shown abnormalities in the pulmonary tree. Laryngitis and rhinitis are related to prolonged use, along with chronic obstructive pulmonary disease. Electrocardiographic abnormalities are common, but no chronic cardiac disease has been linked to marijuana use. Long-term usage has resulted in depression of plasma testosterone levels and reduced sperm counts. Abnormal menstruation and failure to ovulate have occurred in some women. Cognitive impairments are common. Health care utilization for a variety of health problems is increased in long-term marijuana smokers. Sudden withdrawal produces insomnia, nausea, myalgia, and irritability. Psychological effects of long-term marijuana usage are still unclear. Urine testing is reliable if samples are carefully collected and tested. Detection periods span 4–6 days in short-term users and 20–50 days in long-term users.

6. Stimulants: Amphetamines & Cocaine

Stimulant abuse is quite common, either alone or in combination with abuse of other drugs. The stimulants include illicit drugs such as methamphetamine ("speed")—one variant is a smokable form called "ice," which gives an intense and fairly long-lasting high—and methylphenidate and dextroamphetamine, which are under prescription control. Street availability of amphetamines remains high. Moderate usage of any of the stimulants produces hyperactivity, a sense of enhanced physical and mental capacity, and sympathomimetic effects. The clinical picture of acute stimulant intoxication includes sweating, tachycardia, elevated blood pressure, mydriasis, hyperactivity, and an acute brain syndrome with confusion and disorientation. Tolerance develops quickly, and, as the dosage is increased, hypervigilance, paranoid ideation (with delusions of parasitosis), stereotypy, bruxism, tactile hallucinations of insect infestation, and full-blown psychoses occur, often with persecutory ideation and aggressive responses. Stimulant withdrawal is characterized by depression with symptoms of hyperphagia and hypersomnia.

People who have used stimulants chronically (eg, anorexigenics) occasionally become sensitized (**"kindling"**) to future use of stimulants. In these individuals, even small amounts of mild stimulants such as caffeine can cause symptoms of paranoia and auditory hallucinations.

Cocaine is a stimulant. It is a product of the coca plant. The derivatives include seeds, leaves, coca paste, cocaine hydrochloride, and the free base of cocaine. Cocaine hydrochloride is the salt and the most commonly used form. Free base, a purer (and stronger) derivative called "crack," is prepared by simple extraction from cocaine hydrochloride.

There are various modes of use. Coca leaf chewing involves toasting the leaves and chewing with alkaline material (eg, the ash of other burned leaves) to enhance buccal absorption. One achieves a mild high, with onset in 5–10 minutes and lasting for about an hour. Intranasal use is simply snorting cocaine through a straw. Absorption is slowed somewhat by vasoconstriction (which may eventually cause tissue necrosis and septal perforation); the onset of action is in 2–3 minutes, with a moderate high (euphoria, excitement, increased energy) lasting about 30 minutes. The purity of the cocaine is a major determinant of the high. Intravenous use of cocaine hydrochloride or "freebase" is effective in 30 seconds and produces a short-lasting, fairly intense high of about 15 minutes' duration. The combined use of cocaine and ethanol results in the metabolic production of cocaethylene by the liver. This substance produces more intense and long-lasting cocaine-like effects. Smoking freebase (volatilized cocaine because of the lower boiling point) acts in seconds and results in an intense high lasting several minutes. The intensity of the reaction is related to the marked lipid solubility of the freebase form and produces by far the most severe medical and psychiatric symptoms.

Cardiovascular collapse, arrhythmias, myocardial infarction, and transient ischemic attacks have been reported. Seizures, strokes, migraine symptoms, hyperthermia, and lung damage may occur, and there are several obstetric complications, including spontaneous abortion, abruptio placentae, teratogenic effects, delayed fetal growth, and prematurity. Cocaine can cause anxiety, mood swings, and delirium, and chronic use can cause the same problems as other stimulants (see above).

Clinicians should be alert to cocaine use in patients presenting with unexplained nasal bleeding or septal perforations, headaches, fatigue, insomnia, anxiety, depression, and chronic hoarseness. Sudden withdrawal of the drug is not life-threatening but usually produces craving, sleep disturbances, hyperphagia, lassitude, and severe depression (sometimes with suicidal ideation) lasting days to weeks.

Treatment is imprecise and difficult. Since the high is related to blockage of dopamine reuptake, the dopamine agonist bromocriptine, 1.5 mg orally three times a day, alleviates some of the symptoms of craving associated with acute cocaine withdrawal. Other dopamine agonists such as apomorphine, levodopa, and amantadine are under study for this purpose. Carbamazepine may be a useful adjunct in treating symptoms of alcohol withdrawal, and desipramine in moderate doses has been useful in helping maintain abstinence in the early stages of treatment. Treatment of psychosis is the same as that of any psychosis: antipsychotic medications in dosages sufficient to alleviate the symptoms. Any medical symptoms (eg, hyperthermia, seizures, hypertension) are treated specifically. These approaches should be used in conjunction with a structured program, most often based on the Alcoholics Anonymous model. Hospitalization may be required if self-harm or violence toward others is a perceived threat (usually indicated by paranoid delusions).

7. Caffeine

Caffeine, along with nicotine and alcohol, is one of the most commonly used drugs worldwide. About 10 billion pounds of coffee (the richest source of caffeine) are consumed yearly throughout the world. Tea, cocoa, and cola drinks also contribute to an intake of caffeine that is often astoundingly high in a large number of people. Low to moderate doses (30–200 mg/d) tend to improve some aspects of performance (eg, vigilance). The approximate content of caffeine in a (180-mL) cup of beverage is as follows: brewed coffee, 80–140 mg; instant coffee, 60–100 mg; decaffeinated coffee, 1–6 mg; black leaf tea, 30–80 mg; tea bags, 25–75 mg; instant tea, 30–60 mg; cocoa, 10–50 mg; and 12-oz cola drinks, 30–65 mg. A 2-oz chocolate candy bar has about 20 mg. Some herbal teas (eg, "morning thunder") contain caffeine. Caffeine-containing analgesics usually contain approximately 30 mg per unit. Symptoms of caffeinism (usually associated with ingestion of over 500 mg/d) include anxiety, agitation, restlessness, insomnia, a feeling of being "wired," and somatic symptoms referable to the heart and gastrointestinal tract. It is common for a case of caffeinism to present as an anxiety disorder. It is also common for caffeine and other stimulants to precipitate severe symptoms in compensated schizophrenic and manic-depressive patients. Chronically depressed patients often use caffeine drinks as self-medication. This diagnostic clue may help distinguish some major affective disorders. Withdrawal from caffeine (> 250 mg/d) can produce headaches, irritability, lethargy, and occasional nausea.

8. Miscellaneous Drugs, Solvents

The principal over-the-counter drugs of concern are an assortment of antihistaminic agents, frequently in combination with a mild analgesic promoted as cold remedies.

Antihistamines usually produce some central nervous system depression—thus their use as over-the-counter sedatives. Practically all of the so-called sleep aids are antihistamines. The mixture of antihistamines with alcohol usually exacerbates the central nervous system effects. Scopolamine and bromides have generally been removed from over-the-counter products.

The abuse of laxatives sometimes can lead to electrolyte disturbances that may contribute to the manifestations of a delirium. The greatest use of laxatives tends to be in the elderly and in those with eating disorders, both of whom are the most vulnerable to physiologic changes.

Anabolic steroids are abused by people who wish to increase muscle mass for cosmetic reasons or for greater strength. In addition to the medical problems, the practice is associated with significant mood swings, aggressiveness, and paranoid delusions. Alcohol and stimulant use is higher in these individuals. Withdrawal symptoms of steroid dependency include fatigue, depressed mood, restlessness, and insomnia.

Amyl nitrite is used as an "orgasm expander." The changes in time perception, "rush," and mild euphoria caused by the drug prompted its nonmedical use. Subjective effects last from 5 seconds to 15 minutes. Tolerance develops readily, but there are no known withdrawal symptoms. Abstinence for several days reestablishes the previous level of responsiveness. Long-term effects may include damage to the immune system and respiratory difficulties.

Sniffing of solvents and inhaling of gases (including aerosols) produce a form of inebriation similar to that of the volatile anesthetics. Agents include gasoline, toluene, petroleum ether, lighter fluids, cleaning fluids, paint thinners, and solvents that are present in many household products (eg, nail polish). Typical intoxication states include euphoria, slurred speech, hallucinations, and confusion, and with high doses, acute manifestations are unconsciousness and cardiorespiratory depression or failure; chronic exposure produces a variety of symptoms related to the liver, kidney, bone marrow, or heart. Lead encephalopathy can be associated with sniffing leaded gasoline. In addition, studies of workers chronically exposed to jet fuel showed significant increases in neurasthenic symptoms, including fatigue, anxiety, mood changes, memory difficulties, and somatic complaints. These same problems have been noted in long-term solvent abuse.

The so-called designer drugs are synthetic substitutes for commonly used recreational drugs. Common designer drugs include methyl analogues of fentanyl used as heroin substitutes. MDMA (methylenedioxymethamphetamine),

an amphetamine derivative sometimes called "ecstasy," is also a designer drug with high abuse potential and neurotoxicity. Often not detected by standard toxicology screens, these substances can present a vexing problem for clinicians faced with symptoms from a totally unknown cause.

Alford DP et al. Collaborative care of opioid-addicted patients in primary care using buprenorphine: five-year experience. Arch Intern Med. 2011 Mar 14;171(5):425–31. [PMID: 21403039]

Friedmann PD. Clinical practice. Alcohol use in adults. N Engl J Med. 2013 Jan 24;368(4):365–73. Erratum in: N Engl J Med. 2013 Apr 25;368(17):1661. N Engl J Med. 2013 Feb 21;368(8): 781. [PMID: 23343065]

Hoch E et al. Efficacy of a targeted cognitive-behavioral treatment program for cannabis use disorders (CANDIS®). Eur Neuropsychopharmacol. 2012 Apr;22(4):267–80. [PMID: 21865014]

Stehman CR et al. A rational approach to the treatment of alcohol withdrawal in the ED. Am J Emerg Med. 2013 Apr;31(4): 734–42. [PMID: 23399338]

DELIRIUM & OTHER COGNITIVE DISORDERS

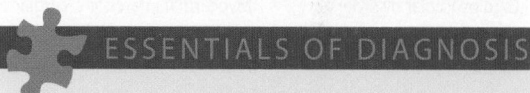

ESSENTIALS OF DIAGNOSIS

► Transient or permanent brain dysfunction.

► Cognitive impairment to varying degrees.

► Impaired recall and recent memory, inability to focus attention and problems in perceptual processing, often with psychotic ideation.

► Random psychomotor activity such as stereotypy.

► Emotional disorders frequently present: depression, anxiety, irritability.

► Behavioral disturbances: impulse control, sexual acting-out, attention deficits, aggression, and exhibitionism.

► General Considerations

The organic problem may be a primary brain disease or a secondary manifestation of some general disorder. All of the cognitive disorders show some degree of impaired thinking depending on the site of involvement, the rate of onset and progression, and the duration of the underlying brain lesion. Emotional disturbances (eg, depression) are often present as significant comorbidities. The behavioral disturbances tend to be more common with chronicity, more directly related to the underlying personality or central nervous system vulnerability to drug side effects, and not necessarily correlated with cognitive dysfunction.

The causes of cognitive disorders are listed in Table 25–11.

► Clinical Findings

The many manifestations include problems with orientation, short or fluctuating attention span, loss of recent memory and recall, impaired judgment, emotional lability, lack of initiative, impaired impulse control, inability to

Table 25–11. Etiology of delirium and other cognitive disorders.

Disorder	Possible Causes
Intoxication	Alcohol, sedatives, bromides, analgesics (eg, pentazocine), psychedelic drugs, stimulants, and household solvents.
Drug withdrawal	Withdrawal from alcohol, sedative-hypnotics, corticosteroids.
Long-term effects of alcohol	Wernicke-Korsakoff syndrome.
Infections	Septicemia; meningitis and encephalitis due to bacterial, viral, fungal, parasitic, or tuberculous organisms or to central nervous system syphilis; acute and chronic infections due to the entire range of microbiologic pathogens.
Endocrine disorders	Thyrotoxicosis, hypothyroidism, adrenocortical dysfunction (including Addison disease and Cushing syndrome), pheochromocytoma, insulinoma, hypoglycemia, hyperparathyroidism, hypoparathyroidism, panhypopituitarism, diabetic ketoacidosis.
Respiratory disorders	Hypoxia, hypercapnia.
Metabolic disturbances	Fluid and electrolyte disturbances (especially hyponatremia, hypomagnesemia, and hypercalcemia), acid-base disorders, hepatic disease (hepatic encephalopathy), kidney failure, porphyria.
Nutritional deficiencies	Deficiency of vitamin B_1 (beriberi), vitamin B_{12} (pernicious anemia), folic acid, nicotinic acid (pellagra); protein-calorie malnutrition.
Trauma	Subdural hematoma, subarachnoid hemorrhage, intracerebral bleeding, concussion syndrome.
Cardiovascular disorders	Myocardial infarctions, cardiac arrhythmias, cerebrovascular spasms, hypertensive encephalopathy, hemorrhages, embolisms, and occlusions indirectly cause decreased cognitive function.
Neoplasms	Primary or metastatic lesions of the central nervous system, cancer-induced hypercalcemia.
Seizure disorders	Ictal, interictal, and postictal dysfunction.
Collagen-vascular and immunologic disorders	Autoimmune disorders, including systemic lupus erythematosus, Sjögren syndrome, and AIDS.
Degenerative diseases	Alzheimer disease, Pick disease, multiple sclerosis, parkinsonism, Huntington chorea, normal pressure hydrocephalus.
Medications	Anticholinergic medications, antidepressants, H_2-blocking agents, digoxin, salicylates (long-term use), and a wide variety of other over-the-counter and prescribed medications.

reason through problems, depression (worse in mild to moderate types), confabulation (not limited to alcohol organic brain syndrome), constriction of intellectual functions, visual and auditory hallucinations, and delusions. Physical findings will vary according to the cause. The electroencephalogram usually shows generalized slowing in delirium.

A. Delirium

Delirium (acute confusional state) is a transient global disorder of attention, with clouding of consciousness, usually a result of systemic problems (eg, medications, hypoxemia). Onset is usually rapid. The mental status fluctuates (impairment is usually least in the morning), with varying inability to concentrate, maintain attention, and sustain purposeful behavior. There is a marked deficit of short-term memory and recall. Anxiety and irritability are common. Amnesia is retrograde (impaired recall of past memories) and anterograde (inability to recall events after the onset of the delirium). Orientation problems follow the inability to retain information. Perceptual disturbances (often visual hallucinations) and psychomotor restlessness with insomnia are common. Autonomic changes include tachycardia, dilated pupils, and sweating. The average

duration is about 1 week, with full recovery in most cases. Delirium can coexist with dementia. Delirium may be hypoactive, hyperactive, or mixed. "Sundowning"—mild to moderate delirium at night—is more common in patients with preexisting dementia and may be precipitated by hospitalization, medications, and sensory deprivation.

Terminal delirium occurs commonly at the end of life. The delirium may be related to multiple medical causes, including organ failure, and may be unrecognized. Treatment must be based on a careful evaluation of the underlying etiology and the risks and benefits of available medical and nonmedical interventions.

B. Dementia

(See Chapters 4 and 24.) Dementia is characterized by chronicity and deterioration of selective mental functions. Specific cognitive assessment must be performed, since many patients are able to cover a deficit in routine conversation. The Mini-Mental State Examination produces a numerical score with up to 30 points given for correct answers to questions (likely organic < 27 points).

In all types of dementia, loss of impulse control (sexual and language) is common. The tenuous level of functioning makes the individual most susceptible to minor physical and psychological stresses. **Pseudodementia** is a term previously applied to depressed patients who appear to be demented. These patients are often identifiable by their tendency to complain about memory problems vociferously rather than try to cover them up. They usually say they cannot complete cognitive tasks but with encouragement can often do so. They can be considered to have depression-induced reversible dementia that improves when the depression resolves. In many geriatrics patients, however, the depression appears to be an insult that often unmasks a progressive dementia. Thus, even though cognition tends to improve substantially in these patients, many go on to develop Alzheimer disease or other dementias.

C. Amnestic Syndrome

This is a memory disturbance without delirium or dementia. It is usually associated with thiamine deficiency and chronic alcohol use (eg, Korsakoff syndrome). There is an impairment in the ability to learn new information or recall previously learned information.

D. Substance-Induced Hallucinosis

This condition is characterized by persistent or recurrent hallucinations (usually auditory) without the other symptoms usually found in delirium or dementia. Alcohol or hallucinogens are often the cause. There does not have to be any other mental disorder, and there may be complete spontaneous resolution.

E. Personality Changes Due to a General Medical Condition (Formerly Organic Personality Syndrome)

This syndrome is characterized by emotional lability and loss of impulse control along with a general change in personality. Cognitive functions are preserved. Social inappropriateness is common. Loss of interest and lack of concern with the consequences of one's actions are often present. The course depends on the underlying cause (eg, frontal lobe contusion may resolve completely).

▶ Differential Diagnosis

The differential diagnosis consists mainly of schizophrenia and the other psychoses, which are sometimes confused with cognitive disorders and are often accompanied by psychotic symptoms.

▶ Complications

Chronicity may result from delayed correction of the defect, eg, subdural hematoma, low-pressure hydrocephalus. Accidents secondary to impulsive behavior and poor judgment are a major consideration. Secondary depression and impulsive behavior not infrequently lead to suicide attempts. Medications—particularly sedatives—may worsen thinking abilities and contribute to the overall problems.

▶ Treatment

A. Medical

Delirium should be considered a syndrome of acute brain dysfunction analogous to acute kidney failure. The first aim of treatment is to identify and correct the etiologic medical problem. Evaluation should consist of a comprehensive physical examination including a search for neurologic abnormalities, infection, or hypoxia. Laboratory tests may include serum electrolytes, serum glucose, BUN, serum creatinine, liver biochemical tests, thyroid function tests, arterial blood gases, complete blood count, serum calcium, phosphorus, magnesium, vitamin B_{12}, folate, blood cultures, urinalysis, and cerebrospinal fluid analysis. Discontinue medications that may be contributing to the problem (eg, analgesics, corticosteroids, cimetidine, lidocaine, anticholinergic medications, central nervous system depressants, mefloquine). Do not overlook any possibility of reversible organic disease. Electroencephalography, CT, and MRI evaluations of the brain may be helpful in diagnosis. Ideally, the patient should be monitored without further medications while the evaluation is carried out. There are, however, at least two indications for medication in delirious states: behavioral control (eg, pulling out lines) and subjective distress (eg, pronounced fear due to hallucinations). If these indications are present, medications may be used. If there is any hint of alcohol or substance withdrawal (the most common cause of delirium in the general hospital), a benzodiazepine such as lorazepam (1–2 mg every hour) can be given parenterally. If there is little likelihood of withdrawal syndrome, haloperidol is often used in doses of 1–10 mg every hour. Given intravenously under ECG monitoring, it appears to impose slight risk of extrapyramidal side effects. In addition to the medication, a pleasant, comfortable, nonthreatening, and physically safe environment with adequate nursing or attendant services should be provided. Once the underlying condition has been identified and treated, adjunctive medications can be tapered.

Treatment of the behavioral manifestations of the **dementia syndrome** usually involve trying to positively reinforce healthy behaviors and not reinforcing maladaptive behaviors (such as aggression). Arranging the physical environment to maximize autonomy as much as feasible and promote regularity of routine, helps the individual cope with their limited intellectual reserves. Simple, direct statements are more easily comprehended by these individuals. Understanding how their decreased cognitive function limits their abilities is important. For example, one elderly man in a residential apartment kept complaining that someone was stealing his ice cream at night. Realizing that he was unable to recall eating it himself, his "delusion" made a certain sense. Once his caregivers understood this, they were able to be more compassionate in listening to his complaints and less worried about an ice cream burglar.

Aggressiveness and rage states in dementia can be reduced with lipophilic beta-blockers (eg, propranolol, metoprolol) in moderate doses. Since the serotonergic system has been implicated in arousal conditions, medications that affect serotonin have been found to be of some benefit in aggression and agitation. Included in this group are lithium, trazodone, buspirone, and clonazepam. Dopamine blockers (eg, the antipsychotic medications such as haloperidol) have been used for many years to attenuate aggression. Likewise, second-generation antipsychotics may have a role in selected geriatric patients. However, no antipsychotic has been shown to be more beneficial than placebo in more rigorous controlled studies in the management of behavioral dyscontrol in dementia patients. In addition, both first- and second-generation agents have been associated with increased mortality in this population and carry FDA warnings to this effect. There are also reports of reduced agitation in Alzheimer disease from carbamazepine, 100–400 mg/d orally (with slow increase as needed). Emotional lability in some cases responds to fluoxetine (5–20 mg/d orally); depression, which often occurs early in the course of Alzheimer dementia, responds to the usual doses of antidepressant medications, preferably those with the least anticholinergic side effects (eg, SSRIs and SNRIs).

Ergotoxine alkaloids (ergoloid mesylates: Hydergine, others) have been studied with mixed results; improvement in ambulatory self-care and depressed mood has been noted, but there has been no improvement of cognitive functioning on any standardized tests. Stimulant medications (eg, methylphenidate) do not change cognitive function but can improve affect and mood, which helps the caretakers cope with the problem.

B. Social

Substitute home care, board and care, or convalescent home care may be most useful when the family is unable to care for the patient. The setting should include familiar people and objects, lights at night, and a simple schedule. Counseling may help the family to cope with problems and may help keep the patient at home as long as possible. Information about local groups can be obtained from the Alzheimer's Disease and Related Disorders Association, 70 East Lake Street, Suite 600, Chicago, IL 60601. Volunteer services, including homemakers, visiting nurses, and adult protective services, may be helpful in maintaining the patient at home.

C. Behavioral

Behavioral techniques include operant responses that can be used to induce positive behaviors, eg, paying attention to the patient who is trying to communicate appropriately, and extinction by ignoring inappropriate responses. Patients with Alzheimer disease can learn skills and retain them but do not recall the circumstances in which they were learned.

D. Psychological

Formal psychological therapies are not usually helpful and may make things worse by taxing the patient's limited cognitive resources.

▶ Prognosis

The prognosis is good for recovery of mental functioning in delirium when the underlying condition is reversible.

For most dementia syndromes, the prognosis is for gradual deterioration, although new drug treatments may prove helpful.

Barr J et al; American College of Critical Care Medicine. Clinical practice guidelines for the management of pain, agitation, and delirium in adult patients in the intensive care unit. Crit Care Med. 2013 Jan;41(1):263–306. [PMID: 23269131]
Gitlin LN et al. Nonpharmacologic management of behavioral symptoms in dementia. JAMA. 2012 Nov 21;308(19):2020–9. [PMID: 23168825]

PSYCHIATRIC PROBLEMS ASSOCIATED WITH HOSPITALIZATION & ILLNESS

▶ Diagnostic Categories

A. Acute Problems

1. Delirium with psychotic features secondary to the medical or surgical problem, or compounded by effect of treatment.

2. Acute anxiety, often related to ignorance and fear of the immediate problem as well as uncertainty about the future.

3. Anxiety as an intrinsic aspect of the medical problem (eg, hyperthyroidism).

4. Denial of illness, which may present during acute or intermediate phases of illness.

B. Intermediate Problems

1. Depression as a function of the illness or acceptance of the illness, often associated with realistic or fantasied hopelessness about the future.

2. Behavioral problems, often related to denial of illness and, in extreme cases, causing the patient to leave the hospital against medical advice.

C. Recuperative Problems

1. Decreasing cooperation as the patient sees that improvement and compliance are not compelled.

2. Readjustment problems with family, job, and society.

▶ General Considerations

A. Acute Problems

1. "Intensive care unit psychosis"—The ICU environment may contribute to the etiology of delirium. Critical care unit factors include sleep deprivation, increased arousal, mechanical ventilation, and social isolation. Other causes include those common to delirium and require vigorous investigation (see Delirium, above).

2. Presurgical and postsurgical anxiety states—Anxiety before or after surgery is common and commonly ignored. Presurgical anxiety is very common and is principally a fear of death (many surgical patients make out their wills). Patients may be fearful of anesthesia (improved by the preoperative anesthesia interview), the mysterious operating room, and the disease processes that might be uncovered by the surgeon. Such fears frequently cause people to delay examinations that might result in earlier surgery and a greater chance of cure.

The opposite of this is **surgery proneness**, the quest for surgery to escape from overwhelming life stresses. Polysurgery patients may be classified as having factitious disorders. Dynamic motivations include the need to get medical care as a way of getting dependency needs met, the desire to outwit authority figures, unconscious guilt, or a masochistic need to suffer. Frequent surgery may also be related to a somatic symptom disorder, particularly body dysmorphic disorder (an obsession that a body part is disfigured). More apparent reasons may include an attempt to get relief from pain and a lifestyle that has become almost exclusively medically oriented, with all of the risks entailed in such an endeavor.

Postsurgical anxiety states are usually related to pain, procedures, and loss of body image. Acute pain problems are quite different from chronic pain disorders (see Chronic Pain Disorders, this chapter); the former are readily handled with adequate analgesic medication (see Chapter 5). Alterations in body image, as with amputations, ostomies, and mastectomies, often raise concerns about relationships with others.

3. Iatrogenic problems—These usually pertain to medications, complications of diagnostic and treatment procedures, and impersonal and unsympathetic staff behavior. Polypharmacy is often a factor. Patients with unsolved diagnostic problems are at higher risk. They are desirous of relief, and the quest engenders more diagnostic procedures with a higher incidence of complications. The upset patient and family may be very demanding. Excessive demands usually result from anxiety. Such behavior is best handled with calm and measured responses.

B. Intermediate Problems

1. Prolonged hospitalization—Prolonged hospitalization presents unique problems in certain hospital services, eg, burn units or orthopedic services. The acute problems of the severely burned patient are discussed in Chapter 37. The problems often are behavioral difficulties related to length of hospitalization and necessary procedures. For example, in burn units, pain is a major problem in addition to anxiety about procedures. Disputes with staff are common and often concern pain medication or ward privileges. Some patients regress to infantile behavior and dependency. Staff members must agree about their approach to the patient in order to ensure the smooth functioning of the unit.

Denial of illness may present in some patients. Intervention by an authority figure (eg, immediate work supervisor) may help the patient accept treatment and eventually abandon the coping mechanism of denial.

2. Depression—Mood disorders ranging from mild adjustment disorder to major depressive disorder frequently occur during prolonged hospitalizations. A key to the diagnosis of depression in the medical setting is the individual's loss of self-esteem; they often think of themselves as worthless and are guilt ridden. Therapeutic medications (eg, corticosteroids) may be a factor. Depression can contribute

to irritability and overt anger. Severe depression can lead to anorexia, which further complicates healing and metabolic balance. It is during this period that the issue of disfigurement arises—relief at survival gives way to concern about future function and appearance.

C. Recuperative Problems

1. Anxiety—Anxiety about return to the posthospital environment can cause regression to a dependent position. Complications increase, and staff forbearance again is tested. Anxiety occurring at this stage usually is handled more easily than previous behavior problems.

2. Posthospital adjustment—Adjustment difficulties after discharge are related to the severity of the deficits and the use of outpatient facilities (eg, physical therapy, rehabilitation programs, psychiatric outpatient treatment). Some patients may experience posttraumatic stress symptoms (eg, from traumatic injuries or even from necessary medical treatments). Lack of appropriate follow-up can contribute to depression in the patient, who may feel that he or she is making poor progress and may have thoughts of "giving up." Reintegration into work, educational, and social endeavors may be slow. Life is simply much more difficult when one is disfigured, disabled, or disenfranchised.

▶ Clinical Findings

The symptoms that occur in these patients are similar to those discussed in previous sections of this chapter, eg, delirium, stress and adjustment disorders, anxiety, and depression. Behavior problems may include lack of cooperation, increased complaints, demands for medication, sexual approaches to nurses, threats to leave the hospital, and actual signing out against medical recommendations. The underlying personality structure of the individual is a major factor in coping styles (eg, the compulsive individual increases indecision, the hysterical individual increases dramatic behavior).

▶ Differential Diagnosis

Delirium and dementia (including cases associated with HIV infection and drug abuse) must always be ruled out, since they often present with symptoms resembling anxiety, depression, or psychosis. Personality disorders existing prior to hospitalization often underlie the various behavior problems, but particularly the management problems.

▶ Complications

Prolongation of hospitalization causes increased expense, deterioration of patient-staff relationships, and increased probabilities of iatrogenic and legal problems. The possibility of increasing posthospital treatment problems is enhanced.

▶ Treatment

A. Medical

The most important consideration by far is to have one clinician in charge, a clinician whom the patient trusts and who is able to oversee multiple treatment approaches (see Somatic Symptom Disorders, above). In acute problems, attention must be paid to metabolic imbalance, alcohol withdrawal, and previous drug use—prescribed, recreational, or over-the-counter. Adequate sleep and analgesia are important in the prevention of delirium. When absolute behavioral control is urgently needed, agents such as propofol, dexmedetomidine, opioids, and midazolam have been used.

Many clinicians are attuned to the early detection of the surgery-prone patient. Plastic and orthopedic surgeons are at particular risk. Appropriate consultations may help detect some problems and mitigate future ones.

Postsurgical anxiety states can be alleviated by personal attention from the surgeon. Anxiety is not so effectively lessened by ancillary medical personnel, whom the patient perceives as lesser authorities, until after the clinician has reassured the patient. "Patient-controlled analgesia" can improve pain control, decrease anxiety, and minimize side effects.

Depression should be recognized early. If severe, it may be treated by antidepressant medications (see Antidepressant Medications, above). High levels of anxiety can be lowered with judicious use of anxiolytic agents. Unnecessary medications tend to reinforce the patient's impression that there must be a serious illness or medication would not be required.

B. Psychological

Prepare the patient and family for what is to come. This includes the types of units where the patient will be quartered, the procedures that will be performed, and any disfigurements that will result from surgery. Repetition improves understanding. The nursing staff can be helpful, since patients frequently confide a lack of understanding to a nurse but are reluctant to do so to the physician.

Denial of illness is frequently a block to acceptance of treatment. This too should be handled with family members present (to help the patient face the reality of the situation) in a series of short interviews (for reinforcement). Dependency problems resulting from long hospitalization are best handled by focusing on the changes to come as the patient makes the transition to the outside world. Key figures are teachers, vocational counselors, and physical therapists. Challenges should be realistic and practical and handled in small steps.

Depression is usually related to the loss of familiar hospital supports, and the outpatient therapists and counselors help to lessen the impact of the loss. Some of the impact can be alleviated by anticipating, with the patient and family, the signal features of the common depression to help prevent the patient from assuming a permanent sick role (invalidism).

Suicide is always a concern when a patient is faced with despair. An honest, compassionate, and supportive approach will help sustain the patient during this trying period.

C. Behavioral

Prior desensitization can significantly allay anxiety about medical procedures. A "dry run" can be done to reinforce the oral description. Cooperation during acute problem periods can be enhanced by the use of appropriate reinforcers such as a favorite nurse or helpful family member. People who are positive reinforcers are even more helpful during the intermediate phases when the patient becomes resistant to the seemingly endless procedures (eg, debridement of burned areas).

Specific situations (eg, psychological dependency on the respirator) can be corrected by weaning with appropriate reinforcers (eg, watching a favorite movie on a DVD player when disconnected from the ventilator). Behavioral approaches should be used in a positive and optimistic way for maximal reinforcement.

Relaxation techniques and attentional distraction can be used to block side effects of a necessary treatment (eg, nausea in cancer chemotherapy).

D. Social

A change in environment requires adaptation. Because of the illness, admission and hospitalization may be more easily handled than discharge. Reintegration into society can be difficult. In some cases, the family is a negative influence. A predischarge evaluation must be made to determine whether the family will be able to cope with the physical or mental changes in the patient. Working with the family while the patient is in the acute stage may presage a successful transition later on.

Development of a new social life can be facilitated by various self-help organizations (eg, the stoma club). Sharing problems with others in similar circumstances eases the return to a social life, which may be quite different from that prior to the illness.

▶ Prognosis

The prognosis is good in all patients who have reversible medical and surgical conditions. It is guarded when there is serious functional loss that impairs vocational, educational, or societal possibilities—especially in the case of progressive and ultimately life-threatening illness.

Katon WJ et al. Collaborative care for patients with depression and chronic illnesses. N Engl J Med. 2010 Dec 30;363(27):2611–20. [PMID: 21190455]

Milani RV et al. Impact of exercise training and depression on survival in heart failure due to coronary heart disease. Am J Cardiol. 2011 Jan;107(1):64–8. [PMID: 21146688]

Endocrine Disorders

Paul A. Fitzgerald, MD

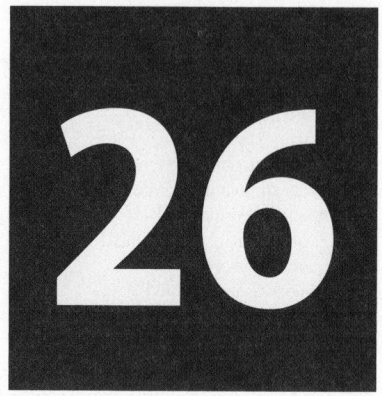

ANTERIOR HYPOPITUITARISM

ESSENTIALS OF DIAGNOSIS

► Partial or complete deficiency of one or any combination of anterior pituitary hormones.

► **Adrenocorticotropic hormone deficiency:** reduced adrenal secretion of cortisol and epinephrine; aldosterone secretion remains intact.

► **Growth hormone (GH) deficiency:** short stature in children; asthenia, obesity, and increased cardiovascular risk in adults.

► **Prolactin deficiency:** postpartum lactation failure.

► **Thyroid-stimulating hormone (TSH) deficiency:** secondary hypothyroidism.

► **Luteinizing hormone (LH) and follicle-stimulating hormone (FSH) deficiency:** hypogonadism and infertility in men and women.

► General Considerations

Hypopituitarism can be caused by either hypothalamic or pituitary dysfunction. Patients with hypopituitarism may have single or multiple hormonal deficiencies (Table 26–1). When one hormonal deficiency is discovered, others may be present.

1. Hypopituitarism with mass lesions—Lesions in the hypothalamus, pituitary stalk, or pituitary can cause hypopituitarism. Pituitary adenomas can cause anterior hypopituitarism but rarely cause diabetes insipidus. Pituitary adenomas are usually sporadic but sometimes arise as part of multiple endocrine neoplasia (MEN) types 1 or 4. Other types of mass lesions include granulomas, such as granulomatosis with polyangiitis (formerly Wegener granulomatosis), tuberculosis, cholesterol granuloma; Rathke cleft cysts; pituitary apoplexy; metastatic carcinomas or hematologic malignancies; aneurysms; and brain tumors (craniopharyngioma, meningioma, dysgerminoma, glioma, chondrosarcoma, chordoma of the clivus). Rare causes include postpartum pituitary necrosis (Sheehan syndrome), African trypanosomiasis, and Langerhans cell histiocytosis.

Pituitary autoimmune disease is characterized by an infiltration of the pituitary by lymphocytes, macrophages, and plasma cells. Lymphocytic hypophysitis is an autoimmune disorder that most typically affects women during pregnancy or postpartum. Affected individuals may present with headache or visual field impairment. The appearance of hypophysitis on MRI scanning is variable, but it often appears as a homogeneous sellar mass that mimics a tumor and can extend above the sella. It usually results in ACTH deficiency but can cause deficiencies in any pituitary hormone. The serum prolactin may be elevated if the lesion damages the pituitary stalk. About 25% of cases are associated with other autoimmune conditions, such as systemic lupus erythematosus. Hypophysitis can also be caused by chemotherapy with ipilimumab, an anti-CTLA4 monoclonal antibody that activates T-lymphocytes and enhances immunity.

2. Hypopituitarism without mass lesions—Congenital panhypopituitarism occurs in syndromes such as septo-optic dysplasia (de Morsier syndrome) and in patients with various gene mutations, such as *PROP1* mutations, resulting in the gradual development of several pituitary hormone deficiencies. **Congenital** isolated hypogonadotropic hypogonadism can be caused by mutations in any of the many genes that control the production or release of gonadotropin-releasing hormone (GnRH), LH, or FSH; it also occurs with the syndrome of congenital adrenal hypoplasia. **Prader-Willi syndrome** is a genetic disorder where genes on the paternal chromosome 15 are deleted or unexpressed. The incidence of this disorder is 1:15,000; both sexes are affected equally. **Kallmann syndrome** is caused by various gene mutations that impair the development or migration of GnRH-synthesizing neurons from the olfactory bulb to the hypothalamus. **Congenital GH deficiency** occurs as an isolated pituitary hormone deficiency in about one-third of cases.

Table 26–1. Pituitary hormones.

Anterior pituitary
  Growth hormone (GH)[1]
  Prolactin (PRL)
  Adrenocorticotropic hormone (ACTH)
  Thyroid-stimulating hormone (TSH)
  Luteinizing hormone (LH)[2]
  Follicle-stimulating hormone (FSH)
Posterior pituitary
  Arginine vasopressin (AVP)[3]
  Oxytocin

[1]GH closely resembles human placental lactogen (hPL).
[2]LH closely resembles human chorionic gonadotropin (hCG).
[3]AVP is identical with antidiuretic hormone (ADH).

Acquired hypopituitarism without mass lesions can result from closed-head brain injury, cranial radiation therapy, pituitary surgery, encephalitis, hemochromatosis, autoimmunity, or coronary artery bypass grafting (CABG). At least one pituitary hormone deficiency develops in about 25–30% of survivors of moderate to severe traumatic brain injury and in about 55% of survivors of aneurysmal subarachnoid hemorrhage. Some degree of hypopituitarism, most commonly GH deficiency and hypogonadotropic hypogonadism, occurs in one-third of ischemic stroke patients. Mitotane, given for adrenal cortical carcinoma, can suppress TSH secretion and cause reversible secondary hypothyroidism. Therapy with exogenous corticosteroids (parenteral, oral, inhaled, or topical) can suppress adrenocorticotropic hormone (ACTH) secretion and causes functional isolated secondary adrenal insufficiency.

Functional hypopituitarism can occur with normal aging because of variable degrees of GH deficiency. Similarly, aging men develop variable degrees of hypogonadotropic hypogonadism, with serum free testosterone levels that are slightly low or near the lower end of normal reference ranges, while serum FSH and LH levels remain in the normal range. Obesity also causes variable degrees of GH deficiency and male hypogonadotropic hypogonadism that are typically reversible with sufficient weight loss. Hypothalamic amenorrhea commonly occurs in women during severe emotional or physical stress, caloric restriction or eating disorders, or very high levels of exercise. Hypogonadotropic hypogonadism also occurs with severe illness, alcoholism, opioid analgesics, anabolic steroids; Cushing syndrome due to corticosteroid medication or excessive endogenous cortisol; hyperprolactinemia (drug-induced or spontaneous); anorexia nervosa; and malnutrition.

▶ Clinical Findings

A. Symptoms and Signs

1. GH deficiency—Congenital GH deficiency typically presents with hypoglycemia in infancy and short stature in childhood.

Acquired GH deficiency is quite common. The pituitary somatotroph cell is particularly sensitive to damage from radiation therapy, compression, or trauma. Therefore, GH deficiency often heralds other pituitary hormone deficiencies that may occur simultaneously or years later. Also, when other more recognizable pituitary hormone deficits are present, there is a high likelihood of concurrent GH deficiency.

GH deficiency varies in severity from mild to severe, resulting in a variable spectrum of nonspecific symptoms that include mild to moderate central obesity, reduced physical and mental energy, impaired concentration and memory, and depression. Patients may also have variably reduced muscle and bone mass, increased low-density lipoprotein (LDL) cholesterol, and reduced cardiac output with exercise.

Laron syndrome is an autosomal recessive disorder that is mainly caused by mutations in the gene that encodes the GH receptor, resulting in GH-resistance. This causes a severe deficiency in serum IGF-I, resulting in short stature (dwarfism). Affected individuals have a prominent forehead, depressed nasal bridge, small mandible, and central obesity. They may have recurrent hypoglycemic seizures. Partial resistance to GH may cause some cases of idiopathic short stature without features of Laron syndrome.

2. Gonadotropin deficiency—Also known as hypogonadotropic hypogonadism, gonadotropin deficiency is caused by insufficiencies in LH and FSH, which cause hypogonadism and infertility.

Congenital gonadotropin deficiency is characterized by partial or complete lack of pubertal development. It can be one deficit in congenital panhypopituitarism. **Isolated hypogonadotropic hypogonadism** occurs with an estimated prevalence between 1 in 4000 and 1 in 10,000 males; it is less common in females. In affected patients, the sense of olfaction (smell) is entirely normal in 58% (**normosmic isolated hypogonadotropic hypogonadism),** or hyposmic or anosmic in 42% (**Kallmann syndrome**). Regardless of their olfaction status, patients with isolated hypogonadotropic hypogonadism frequently have abnormal genitalia (25%), including small phallus, cryptorchidism; renal anomalies (28%); midline craniofacial defects (50%), including cleft lip, high-arched or cleft palate, absent nasal cartilage, dental agenesis, hypertelorism; neurologic deficits (42%), including cognitive problems, bimanual synkinesis, cerebellar ataxia, oculomotor dysfunction, color blindness, or neurosensory hearing loss; musculoskeletal malformations, including pectus excavatum, syndactyly, clinodactaly, camptodactyly. Some affected women have menarche followed by secondary amenorrhea. Some patients with isolated hypogonadotropic hypogonadism also have **congenital adrenal hypoplasia** with X-linked inheritance. Most such boys with isolated hypogonadotropic hypogonadism who survive beyond childhood are diagnosed when they fail to enter puberty. However, isolated hypogonadotropic hypogonadism and subtle signs of adrenal failure can present in adulthood in males.

Patients with **Prader-Willi syndrome** have variable features of both gonadotropin deficiency and primary gonadal dysfunction; boys have cryptorchidism. Other features of Prader-Willi syndrome can include mental retardation, short stature, hyperflexibility, autonomic dysregulation, cognitive impairment, and hyperphagia with obesity.

Acquired gonadotropin deficiency is characterized by the gradual loss of facial, axillary, pubic, and body hair (more prominent in patients who are also hypoadrenal). **Men** may note diminished libido, erectile dysfunction, muscle atrophy, infertility, and osteopenia. (See Male Hypogonadism.) **Women** have amenorrhea, infertility, and predisposition to osteoporosis. Like men, women with hypogonadism have androgen deficiency and may note muscle atrophy.

3. TSH deficiency—TSH deficiency causes hypothyroidism with manifestations such as fatigue, weakness, weight change, and hyperlipidemia. Bexarotene and mitotane are drugs that suppress TSH. (See Hypothyroidism and Myxedema.)

4. ACTH deficiency—This results in diminished cortisol with symptoms of weakness, fatigue, weight loss, and hypotension. Patients with partial ACTH deficiency have some cortisol secretion and may not have symptoms until stressed by illness or surgery. Adrenal mineralocorticoid secretion continues, so manifestations of adrenal insufficiency in hypopituitarism are usually less striking than in bilateral adrenal gland destruction (Addison disease). Hyponatremia may occur, especially when ACTH and TSH deficiencies are both present.

5. Combined pituitary hormone deficiency and panhypopituitarism—The conditions refer to a deficiency of several or all pituitary hormones. Congenital combined pituitary hormone deficiency often develops gradually, usually presenting with short stature and growth failure due to GH and TSH deficiency; lack of pubertal development occurs due to deficiencies in FSH and LH. ACTH-cortisol deficiency tends to develop later and these patients typically require corticosteroid replacement therapy by age 18 years.

6. Other manifestations—Patients with long-standing hypopituitarism tend to have dry, pale, fine, wrinkled facial skin and an apathetic countenance. **Hypothalamic** damage can cause obesity and cognitive impairment. Local tumor effects can cause headache or optic nerve compression with visual field impairment.

B. Laboratory Findings

Fasting hypoglycemia may be present with secondary hypoadrenalism, hypothyroidism, or GH deficiency. Hyponatremia is often present due to hypothyroidism or hypoadrenalism.

For men, an accurate serum total and free testosterone measurement must be obtained. If the serum total or free testosterone is low, then serum gonadotropins (FSH and LH) levels are obtained to distinguish pituitary dysfunction from primary hypogonadism. A serum prolactin is required for men with hypogonadotropic hypogonadism. An elevated serum prolactin may be seen with pituitary prolactinomas, acromegaly, or injury to the hypothalamus or pituitary infundibulum.

For women with amenorrhea, irregular menses, or an unreliable menstrual history, a serum hCG is obtained to exclude pregnancy. Women with hypogonadotropic hypogonadism have a low serum estradiol and a normal or low serum FSH. A serum prolactin is obtained in nonpregnant women with amenorrhea or galactorrhea; an elevated serum prolactin may be seen with a pituitary prolactinomas, acromegaly, or injury to the hypothalamus or pituitary infundibulum. For postmenopausal women, an elevated serum FSH argues for an otherwise healthy anterior pituitary.

In patients with secondary hypothyroidism, the serum free thyroxine (FT_4) level is low while the serum TSH is low or low-normal.

ACTH deficiency usually causes functional atrophy of the adrenal cortex within 2 weeks of pituitary destruction. Therefore, the diagnosis of secondary hypoadrenalism can usually be confirmed with the cosyntropin test. For the cosyntropin test, patients should be either taking no corticosteroids or a short-acting corticosteroid (such as hydrocortisone), which is held after midnight on the morning of the test. At 8 AM, blood is drawn for serum cortisol, ACTH, and dehydroepiandrosterone (DHEA); then 0.25 mg of cosyntropin (synthetic $ACTH_{1-24}$) is administered intramuscularly or intravenously. Another blood sample is obtained 45 minutes after the cosyntropin injection to measure the stimulated serum cortisol levels. A stimulated serum cortisol of < 20 mcg/dL (550 nmol/mL) indicates adrenal insufficiency. With gradual pituitary damage and early in the course of ACTH deficiency, patients can have a stimulated serum cortisol of ≥ 20 mcg/dL but a baseline 8 AM serum cortisol < 5 mcg/dL (137.5 nmol/L), which is suspicious for adrenal insufficiency. The baseline ACTH level is low or normal in secondary hypoadrenalism, distinguishing it from primary adrenal disease. The serum DHEA levels are usually low in patients with adrenal deficiency, helping confirm the diagnosis. For patients with symptoms of secondary adrenal insufficiency (hyponatremia, hypotension, pituitary tumor) but borderline cosyntropin test results, treatment can be instituted empirically and the test repeated at a later date. Insulin tolerance testing and metyrapone testing are usually unnecessary.

Epinephrine deficiency occurs with secondary adrenal insufficiency due to the adrenal medulla lacking the local high concentrations of cortisol that are required to induce the production of the enzyme phenylethanolamine *N*-methyltransferase (PNMT) that catalyzes the conversion of norepinephrine to epinephrine.

The diagnosis of GH deficiency in adults is difficult, since GH secretion is normally pulsatile and serum GH levels are nearly undetectable for most of the day. Also, adults (particularly men) physiologically tend to produce less GH when they are over age 50 or have abdominal obesity. Therefore, pathologic GH deficiency is often inferred by symptoms of GH deficiency in the presence of pituitary destruction or other pituitary hormone deficiencies. GH deficiency is present in 96% of patients with three or more other pituitary hormone deficiencies. While GH stimulates the production of IGF-I, the serum IGF-I level is neither a sensitive (about 50%) nor specific test for GH deficiency in adults. While very low serum IGF-I levels (< 84 mcg/L) are usually indicative of GH deficiency, they also occur in malnutrition, prolonged fasting, oral estrogen, hypothyroidism, uncontrolled diabetes mellitus, and liver failure. In GH deficiency (but also in most adults over age 40), exercise-stimulated serum GH levels remain at < 5 ng/mL and usually fail to rise.

Provocative GH stimulation testing may be used to help diagnose adult GH deficiency, but such testing has a sensitivity of only 66% for GH deficiency. Therefore, a therapeutic trial of GH therapy should be considered for symptomatic patients who have either a serum IGF-I < 84 mcg/L or three other pituitary hormone deficiencies.

Provocative GH-stimulation tests are sometimes indicated or required for insurance coverage of GH therapy. In the absence of a serum IGF-1 level < 84 mcg/L or multiple other pituitary hormone deficiencies, provocative GH-stimulation testing may be indicated for the following patients in whom GH deficiency is suspected: (1) young adult patients who have completed GH therapy for childhood GH deficiency and have achieved maximal linear growth; (2) patients who have a hypothalamic or pituitary tumor or who have received surgery or radiation therapy to these areas; and (3) patients who have had prior head trauma, cerebrovascular accident, or encephalitis. When required, such testing usually entails measuring serum GH following provocative stimuli. The glucagon stimulation test has emerged as a practical alternative to traditional provocative GH stimulation testing. Glucagon 1.0 mg (or 1.5 mg if > 200 lbs [or > 90kg]) is administered intramuscularly to well-nourished patients who have not eaten for 8–9 hours. Serum GH is measured before the injection and every 30 minutes for 3 hours. In patients with GH deficiency, the maximum serum GH is usually < 3 mcg/L. Late hypoglycemia can occur after glucagon, so patients are advised to eat following completion of the test. However, the glucagon test may indicate GH deficiency in otherwise normal aging or obese patients. Whether long-term administration of GH to such patients is helpful or safe remains to be established.

The differential diagnosis of GH deficiency is congenital GH resistance with deficiency of IGF-I. At its worst, IGF-I deficiency results in Laron dwarfism that is completely resistant to GH therapy. The condition responds to therapy with biosynthetic IGF-I (mecasermin).

Patients with lymphocytic hypophysitis frequently have elevated serum antinuclear or anticytoplasmic antibodies. Patients with hypopituitarism without an established etiology should be screened for hemochromatosis with a serum iron and transferrin saturation or ferritin since hemochromatosis can cause hypopituitarism.

C. Imaging

MRI of the hypothalamus and pituitary region is indicated when there is a suspicion for a mass lesion, particularly for the following conditions: men over age 16 with a serum testosterone < 150 ng/dL with a low or normal serum LH; two or more pituitary hormone deficiencies; persistent hyperprolactinemia; or symptoms of a mass (headache, visual field defect). MRI is particularly sensitive for detecting mass lesions of the pituitary or hypothalamus. It can also detect thickening of the pituitary stalk that can be caused by various lesions, including neurosarcoidosis, Langerhans cell histiocytosis, lymphocytic hypophysitis, pituitary adenoma, craniopharyngioma, germinoma, astrocytoma, and metastatic malignancy.

MRI shows hypoplasia or agenesis of the olfactory bulbs in 75% of cases of Kallmann syndrome and in 8% of patients with normosmic hypogonadotropic hypogonadism. MRI is not indicated in cases of functional hypopituitarism associated with severe obesity, drugs, or nutritional disorders.

▶ Differential Diagnosis

The failure to enter puberty may simply reflect delayed puberty, also known as constitutional delay in growth and puberty. Reversible hypogonadotropic hypogonadism may occur with serious illness, malnutrition, anorexia nervosa, or morbid obesity. Men typically develop partial secondary hypogonadism with aging. The clinical situation and the presence of normal adrenal and thyroid function allow ready distinction from hypopituitarism. Profound hypogonadotropic hypogonadism develops in men who receive GnRH analog therapy (leuprolide) for prostate cancer; it usually persists following cessation of therapy. Hypogonadotropic hypogonadism usually develops in patients receiving opioid therapy, including high-dose methadone or long-term intrathecal infusion of opioids; both GH deficiency and secondary adrenal insufficiency occur in 15% of such patients. Secondary adrenal insufficiency may persist for many months following high-dose corticosteroid therapy.

Severe illness causes functional suppression of TSH and T_4. Hyperthyroxinemia reversibly suppresses TSH. Administration of triiodothyronine (Cytomel) suppresses TSH and T_4. Bexarotene, used to treat cutaneous T cell lymphoma, suppresses TSH secretion, resulting in temporary central hypothyroidism. Corticosteroids or megestrol treatment reversibly suppresses endogenous ACTH and cortisol secretion.

GH deficiency normally occurs with aging. Physiologic GH deficiency that develops in obese patients may return to normal with sufficient weight loss.

▶ Complications

Among patients with craniopharyngiomas, diabetes insipidus is found in 16% preoperatively and in 60% postoperatively. Hyponatremia often presents abruptly during the first 2 weeks following pituitary surgery. Visual field impairment may occur. Hypothalamic damage may result in morbid obesity as well as cognitive and emotional problems. Conventional radiation therapy results in an increased incidence of small vessel ischemic strokes and second tumors.

Patients with untreated hypoadrenalism and a stressful illness may become febrile and comatose and die of hyponatremia and shock.

Adults with GH deficiency have experienced an increased cardiovascular morbidity. Rarely, acute hemorrhage may occur in large pituitary tumors, manifested by rapid loss of vision, headache, and evidence of acute pituitary failure (pituitary apoplexy) requiring emergency decompression of the sella.

► Treatment

Transsphenoidal removal of pituitary tumors will sometimes reverse hypopituitarism. Hypogonadism due to PRL excess usually resolves during treatment with cabergoline or other dopamine agonists.

GH-secreting tumors may respond to octreotide (see Acromegaly). Radiation therapy with x-ray, gamma knife, or heavy particles may be necessary but increases the likelihood of hypopituitarism.

The mainstay of substitution therapy for pituitary insufficiency is lifetime hormone replacement.

A. Corticosteroid Replacement

Hydrocortisone tablets, 15–35 mg/d orally in divided doses, should be given. Most patients do well with 10–20 mg in the morning and 5–15 mg in the late afternoon. Patients with partial ACTH deficiency (basal morning serum cortisol above 8 mg/dL [220 mmol/L]) require hydrocortisone replacement in lower doses of about 5 mg orally twice daily. Some clinicians prefer prednisone (3–7.5 mg/d orally) or methylprednisolone (4–6 mg/d orally), given in divided doses. A mineralocorticoid is rarely needed. To determine the optimal corticosteroid replacement dosage, it is necessary to monitor patients carefully for over- or under-replacement. A white blood cell count (WBC) with a relative differential can be useful, since a relative neutrophilia and lymphopenia can indicate corticosteroid over-replacement, and vice versa. Additional corticosteroids must be given during stress, eg, infection, trauma, or surgical procedures. For mild illness, corticosteroid doses are doubled or tripled. For trauma or surgical stress, hydrocortisone 50 mg is given every 6 hours intravenously or intramuscularly and then reduced to usual doses as the stress subsides. Patients with adrenal insufficiency are advised to wear a medical alert bracelet describing their condition and treatment.

Patients with secondary adrenal insufficiency due to treatment with corticosteroids at supraphysiologic doses require their usual daily dose of corticosteroid during surgery and acute illness; supplemental hydrocortisone is not usually required.

B. Thyroid Hormone Replacement

Levothyroxine is given to correct hypothyroidism only after the patient is assessed for cortisol deficiency or is already receiving corticosteroids. (See Hypothyroidism.) The typical maintenance dose is about 1.6 mcg/kg body weight. However, dosage requirements vary widely, averaging 125 mcg daily with a range of 25–300 mcg daily. The optimal replacement dose of thyroxine for each patient must be carefully assessed clinically. In patients receiving optimal thyroxine replacement, serum FT_4 levels are usually in the high-normal range while serum T_3 levels are in the low-normal range. Assessment of serum TSH is useless for monitoring patients with hypopituitarism, since TSH levels are always low.

C. Hypogonadotrophic Hypogonadism Therapy

Hypogonadotropic hypogonadism often develops in patients with hyperprolactinemia and usually resolves with its treatment (see Hyperprolactinemia).

Androgen and estrogen replacement are discussed in later sections (see Male Hypogonadism and Female Hypogonadism). Adolescents with idiopathic isolated hypogonadotropic hypogonadism, who have received several years of hormone replacement therapy (HRT), may have a trial off hormonal therapy to assess whether spontaneous sexual maturation may have occurred.

Women with panhypopituitarism have profound androgen deficiency caused by the combination of both secondary hypogonadism and adrenal insufficiency. When serum DHEA levels are < 400 ng/mL, such women may be treated with compounded DHEA in doses of about 25–50 mg/d orally. DHEA therapy tends to increase pubic and axillary hair and may modestly improve libido, alertness, stamina, and overall psychological well being after 6 months of therapy.

To improve spermatogenesis, human chorionic gonadotropin (hCG) (equivalent to LH) may be given at a dosage of 2000–3000 units intramuscularly three times weekly and testosterone replacement, discontinued. The dose of hCG is adjusted to normalize serum testosterone levels. After 6–12 months of hCG treatment, if the sperm count remains low, hCG injections are continued along with injections of follitropin beta (synthetic recombinant FSH) or urofollitropins (urine-derived FSH). An alternative for patients with an intact pituitary (eg, Kallmann syndrome) is the use of leuprolide (GnRH analog) by intermittent subcutaneous infusion. With either treatment, testicular volumes double within 5–12 months, and spermatogenesis occurs in most cases. With persistent treatment and the help of intracytoplasmic sperm injection for some cases, the total pregnancy success rate is about 70%. Men often feel better during hCG therapy than during testosterone replacement. Therefore, despite its higher cost, some men may elect to continue hCG therapy long-term.

Clomiphene, 25–50 mg orally daily, can sometimes stimulate a man's own pituitary gonadotropins (when his pituitary is intact), thereby increasing testosterone and sperm production. For fertility induction in females, ovulation may be induced with clomiphene, 50 mg daily for 5 days every 2 months. Follitropins and hCG can induce multiple births and should be used only by those experienced with their administration. (See Hypogonadism.)

D. Human Growth Hormone (hGH) Replacement

Symptomatic adults with GH deficiency may be treated with a subcutaneous recombinant human growth hormone (rhGH, somatropin) injections starting at a dosage of about 0.2 mg/d (0.6 international units/d), administered three times weekly. The dosage of rhGH is increased every 2–4 weeks by increments of 0.1 mg (0.3 international units) until side effects occur or a sufficient salutary response and a normal serum IGF-I level are achieved. In adults, if the desired effects (eg, improved energy and mentation, reduction in visceral adiposity) are not seen within 3–6 months at maximum tolerated dosage, rhGH therapy is discontinued.

During pregnancy, rhGH may be safely administered to women with hypopituitarism at their usual pregestational dose during the first trimester, tapering the dose during the second trimester, and discontinuing rhGH during the third trimester.

Oral estrogen replacement reduces hepatic IGF-I production. Therefore, prior to commencing rhGH therapy, oral estrogen should be changed to a transdermal or transvaginal estradiol.

Treatment of adult GH deficiency usually improves the patient's emotional sense of well-being, increases muscle mass, and decreases visceral fat and waist circumference. Long-term treatment with rhGH does not appear to affect mortality.

Side effects of rhGH therapy may include peripheral edema, hand stiffness, arthralgias and myalgias, paresthesias, carpal tunnel syndrome, tarsal tunnel syndrome, headache, pseudotumor cerebri, gynecomastia, hypertension, and proliferative retinopathy. Treatment with rhGH can also cause sleep apnea, insomnia, dyspnea, sweating, and fatigue. Side effects are more common in patients who are older, those with higher BMI, and those with adult-onset GH deficiency. Such symptoms usually remit promptly after a sufficient reduction in dosage. Excessive doses of rhGH could cause acromegaly; patients receiving long-term therapy require careful clinical monitoring. Serum IGF-I levels should be kept in the normal range.

GH should not be administered during critical illness since, in one study, administration of very high doses of rhGH to patients in an intensive care unit was shown to increase overall mortality. There is no currently no proven role for GH replacement for the apparent GH deficiency that is seen with abdominal obesity or normal aging.

Biosynthetic IGF-I (mecasermin) is available to treat patients with Laron syndrome.

E. Other Treatment

Selective transsphenoidal resection of pituitary adenomas can often restore normal pituitary function. Cabergoline, bromocriptine, or quinagolide may reverse the hypogonadism seen in hyperprolactinemia. (See Hyperprolactinemia.) Disseminated Langerhans cell histiocytosis may be treated with bisphosphonates to improve bone pain; treatment with 2-chlorodeoxyadenosine (cladribine) has been reported to produce remissions.

Patients with lymphocytic hypophysitis may be treated with corticosteroid therapy; pituitary surgery or low-dose external beam radiation therapy may be required for aggressive cases.

► Prognosis

The prognosis depends on the primary cause. Hypopituitarism resulting from a pituitary tumor may be reversible with dopamine agonists or with careful selective resection of the tumor. Spontaneous recovery from hypopituitarism associated with pituitary stalk thickening has been reported. Patients can also recover from functional hypopituitarism, eg, hypogonadism due to starvation or severe illness, suppression of ACTH by corticosteroids, or suppression of TSH by hyperthyroidism. Spontaneous reversal of idiopathic isolated hypogonadotropic hypogonadism occurs in about 10% of patients after several years of HRT.

However, hypopituitarism is usually permanent, and lifetime HRT is ordinarily required.

Functionally, most patients with hypopituitarism do very well with hormone replacement. Men with infertility who are treated with hCG/FSH or GnRH are likely to resume spermatogenesis if they have a history of sexual maturation, descended testicles, and a baseline serum inhibin B level over 60 pg/mL. Women under age 40 years, with infertility due to hypogonadotropic hypogonadism, can usually have successful induction of ovulation.

Della Valle E et al. Prevalence of olfactory and other developmental anomalies in patients with central hypogonadotropic hypogonadism. Front Endocrinol (Lausanne). 2013 Jun 7;4:70. [PMID: 23760293]

Gasco V et al. Hypopituitarism following brain injury: when does it occur and how best to test? Pituitary. 2012 Mar;15(1):20–4. [PMID: 20526744]

Glezer A et al. Pituitary autoimmune disease: nuances in clinical presentation. Endocrine. 2012 Aug;42(1):74–9. [PMID: 22426958]

Grossman AB. The diagnosis and management of central hypoadrenalism. J Clin Endocrinol Metab. 2010 Nov;95(6):4855–63. [PMID: 20525912]

King TF et al. Long-term outcome of idiopathic hypogonadotropic hypogonadism. Curr Opin Endocrinol Diabetes Obes. 2012 Jun;19(3):204–10. [PMID: 22499222]

Melmed S. Idiopathic adult growth hormone deficiency. J Clin Endocrinol Metab. 2013 Jun;98(6):2187–97. [PMID: 23539718]

Molitch ME et al. Evaluation and treatment of adult growth hormone deficiency: an Endocrine Society clinical practice guideline. J Clin Endocrinol Metab. 2011 Jun;96(6):1587–609. [PMID: 21602453]

Silveira LF et al. Approach to the patient with hypogonadotropic hypogonadism. J Clin Endocrinol Metab. 2013 May;98(5):1781–8. [PMID: 23650335]

Turcu AF et al. Pituitary stalk lesions: the Mayo Clinic experience. J Clin Endocrinol Metab. 2013 May;98(5):2153–9. [PMID: 23533231]

Young J. Approach to the male patient with congenital hypogonadotropic hypogonadism. J Clin Endocrinol Metab. 2012 Mar;97(3):707–18. [PMID: 22392951]

DIABETES INSIPIDUS

 ESSENTIALS OF DIAGNOSIS

▶ Antidiuretic hormone (ADH) deficiency causes central diabetes insipidus with polyuria (2–20 L/d) and polydipsia.

▶ Hypernatremia occurs if fluid intake is inadequate.

▶ General Considerations

Diabetes insipidus is an uncommon disease characterized by an increase in thirst and the passage of large quantities of urine of low specific gravity (usually < 1.006 with ad libitum fluid intake). The urine is otherwise normal. It is caused by a deficiency of vasopressin or resistance to vasopressin.

Primary central diabetes insipidus (without an identifiable lesion noted on MRI of the pituitary and hypothalamus) accounts for about one-third of all cases of diabetes insipidus. Many such cases appear to be due to autoimmunity against hypothalamic arginine vasopressin (AVP)-secreting cells; pituitary stalk thickening can often be detected on pituitary MRI scanning. The cause may also be genetic. Familial diabetes insipidus occurs as a dominant genetic trait with symptoms developing at about 2 years of age. Diabetes insipidus also occurs in Wolfram syndrome, a rare autosomal recessive disorder that is also known by the acronym DIDMOAD (diabetes insipidus, type 1 diabetes mellitus, optic atrophy, and deafness). DIDMOAD manifestations usually present in childhood but may not occur until adulthood, along with depression and cognitive problems. Diabetes insipidus can also occur in the preleukemic phase of acute myelogenous leukemia associated with myelodysplasia. **Secondary central diabetes insipidus** is due to damage to the hypothalamus or pituitary stalk by tumor, hypophysitis, infarction, hemorrhage, anoxic encephalopathy, surgical or accidental trauma, infection (eg, encephalitis, tuberculosis, syphilis), or granulomas (sarcoidosis or multifocal Langerhans cell granulomatosis). Metastases to the pituitary are more likely to cause diabetes insipidus (33%) than are pituitary adenomas (1%). Reversible central diabetes insipidus has also occurred during chemotherapy with temozolomide. Central diabetes insipidus can also be idiopathic.

Vasopressinase-induced diabetes insipidus may be seen in the last trimester of pregnancy and in the puerperium. A circulating enzyme destroys native vasopressin; however, synthetic desmopressin is unaffected. **Nephrogenic diabetes insipidus** is a disorder caused by a defect in the kidney tubules that interferes with water reabsorption. These patients have normal secretion of vasopressin, and the polyuria is unresponsive to it. **Congenital nephrogenic diabetes insipidus** is present from birth and is due to defective expression of renal vasopressin V2 receptors or vasopressin-sensitive water channels. It occurs as a familial X-linked trait; adults often have hyperuricemia as well. **Acquired forms of vasopressin-resistant diabetes insipidus** are usually less severe and are seen in pyelonephritis, renal amyloidosis, myeloma, potassium depletion, Sjögren syndrome, sickle cell anemia, or chronic hypercalcemia. Certain drugs (eg, corticosteroids, diuretics, demeclocycline, lithium, foscarnet, or methicillin) may induce nephrogenic diabetes insipidus. The recovery from acute tubular necrosis may also be associated with transient nephrogenic diabetes insipidus. (See Chapter 22.)

Clinical Findings

A. Symptoms and Signs

The symptoms of the disease are intense thirst, especially with a craving for ice water, and polyuria, the volume of ingested fluid varying from 2 L to 20 L daily, with correspondingly large urine volumes. Partial diabetes insipidus presents with less intense symptoms and should be suspected in patients with unremitting enuresis. Most patients with diabetes insipidus are able to maintain fluid balance by continuing to ingest large volumes of water. However, diabetes insipidus may present with hypernatremia and dehydration in patients without free access to water, or with a damaged hypothalamic thirst center and altered thirst sensation. Diabetes insipidus is aggravated by administration of high-dose corticosteroids, which increases renal free water clearance. Vasopressin-induced diabetes insipidus during pregnancy is often associated with oligohydramnios, preeclampsia, or hepatic dysfunction.

B. Laboratory Findings

Diagnosis of diabetes insipidus requires clinical judgment; there is no single diagnostic laboratory test. Evaluation should include an accurate 24-hour urine collection for volume and creatinine. A urine volume of < 2 L/24 h (in the absence of hypernatremia) essentially rules out diabetes insipidus. Serum is assayed for glucose, urea nitrogen, calcium, potassium, sodium, and uric acid. Hyperuricemia occurs in many patients with diabetes insipidus, since reduced vasopressin stimulation of the renal V1 receptor causes a reduction in the renal tubular clearance of urate.

A supervised "vasopressin challenge test" may be done: Desmopressin acetate 0.05–0.1 mL (5–10 mcg) intranasally (or 1 mcg subcutaneously or intravenously) is given, with measurement of urine volume for 12 hours before and 12 hours after administration. If symptoms of hyponatremia develop, serum sodium must be assayed immediately. The dosage of desmopressin is doubled if the response is marginal. Patients with central diabetes insipidus notice a distinct reduction in thirst and polyuria; serum sodium stays normal except in some salt-losing conditions.

In **nonfamilial central diabetes insipidus**, MRI of the pituitary and hypothalamus and of the skull is done to look for mass lesions. The pituitary stalk may be thickened, which may be a manifestation of Langerhans cell histiocytosis, sarcoidosis, or lymphocytic hypophysitis. With central diabetes insipidus, MRI T-1-weighted imaging shows an absence of the usual hyperintense signal (bright spot) in the posterior pituitary. When **nephrogenic diabetes insipidus** is a diagnostic consideration, measurement of serum vasopressin is done during modest fluid restriction; typically, the vasopressin level is high.

Differential Diagnosis

Central diabetes insipidus must be distinguished from polyuria caused by psychogenic polydipsia, diabetes mellitus, Cushing syndrome or corticosteroid treatment, lithium, hypercalcemia, hypokalemia, and the nocturnal polyuria of Parkinson disease. It must also be distinguished from vasopressinase-induced diabetes insipidus and nephrogenic diabetes insipidus (eg, corticosteroid or lithium therapy).

Complications

If water is not readily available, the excessive output of urine will lead to severe dehydration. Patients with an impaired thirst mechanism are very prone to hypernatremia, particularly if they also have impaired mentation and forget to take their desmopressin. In patients who are receiving desmopressin acetate therapy, there is a danger of induced water intoxication.

▶ Treatment

Mild cases of diabetes insipidus require no treatment other than adequate fluid intake. Reduction of aggravating factors (eg, corticosteroids) will improve polyuria.

Desmopressin acetate is the treatment of choice for both central and vasopressinase-induced diabetes insipidus. It is also useful in diabetes insipidus associated with pregnancy or the puerperium, since desmopressin is resistant to degradation by the circulating vasopressinase.

Nasal desmopressin (100 mcg/mL solution) is given every 12–24 hours as needed for thirst and polyuria. It may be administered via metered-dose nasal inhaler containing 0.1 mL/spray or via a plastic calibrated tube. The starting dose is 0.05–0.1 mL every 12–24 hours, and the dose is then individualized according to response. Nasal desmopressin may cause rhinitis or conjunctivitis. Some patients report inconsistent antidiuresis from generic desmopressin and prefer a brand preparation (eg, DDAVP).

Oral desmopressin is also available as tablets and is given in a starting dose of 0.05 mg twice daily and increased to a maximum of 0.4 mg every 8 hours, if required. Oral desmopressin is particularly useful for patients in whom rhinitis or conjunctivitis develops from the nasal preparation. Gastrointestinal symptoms, asthenia, and mild increases in hepatic enzymes can occur with the oral preparation.

Desmopressin can also be given intravenously, intramuscularly, or subcutaneously in doses of 1–4 mcg every 12–24 hours as needed.

Desmopressin may cause hyponatremia, but this is uncommon if minimum effective doses are used and the patient allows thirst to occur periodically. Desmopressin can sometimes cause agitation, emotional changes, and depression with an increased risk of suicide. Erythromelalgia occurs rarely.

All desmopressin preparations are subject to light and heat degradation. Nasal desmopressin should be refrigerated. While traveling, nasal desmopressin maintains stability for up to 3 weeks if kept at temperatures that do not exceed 22°C (72°F). Desmopressin tablets must be stored at controlled room temperatures that do not exceed 25°C (77°F).

Both central and nephrogenic diabetes insipidus respond partially to hydrochlorothiazide, 50–100 mg/d orally (with potassium supplement or amiloride). Nephrogenic diabetes insipidus may respond to combined treatments of indomethacin-hydrochlorothiazide, indomethacin-desmopressin, or indomethacin-amiloride. Indomethacin, 50 mg orally every 8 hours, is effective in acute cases.

Most patients with psychogenic polydipsia require psychotherapy. Thioridazine and lithium are best avoided since they cause polyuria.

▶ Prognosis

Central diabetes insipidus appearing after pituitary surgery usually remits after days to weeks but may be permanent if the upper pituitary stalk is cut.

Chronic central diabetes insipidus is ordinarily more an inconvenience than a dire medical condition. Treatment with desmopressin allows normal sleep and activity. Hypernatremia can occur, especially when the thirst center

is damaged, but diabetes insipidus does not otherwise reduce life expectancy, and the prognosis is that of the underlying disorder.

Babey M et al. Familial forms of diabetes insipidus: clinical and molecular characteristics. Nat Rev Endocrinol. 2011 Jul 5;7 (12):701–14. [PMID: 21727914]

Bellastella A et al. Subclinical diabetes insipidus. Best Pract Res Clin Endocrinol Metab. 2012 Aug;26(4):471–83. [PMID: 22863389]

Chanson P et al. Treatment of neurogenic diabetes insipidus. Ann Endocrinol (Paris). 2011 Dec;72(6):496–9. [PMID: 22071315]

Devin JK. Hypopituitarism and central diabetes insipidus: perioperative diagnosis and management. Neurosurg Clin N Am. 2012 Oct;23(4):679–89. [PMID: 23040752]

Fenske W et al. Current state and future perspectives in the diagnosis of diabetes insipidus: a clinical review. J Clin Endocrinol Metab. 2012 Oct, 97(10):3426–37. [PMID: 22855338]

Kristof RA et al. Incidence, clinical manifestations, and course of water and electrolyte metabolism disturbances following transsphenoidal pituitary adenoma surgery: a prospective observational study. J Neurosurg. 2009 Sep;111(3):555–62. [PMID: 19199508]

Schreckinger M et al. Diabetes insipidus following resection of pituitary tumors. Clin Neurol Neurosurg. 2013 Feb;115(2): 121–6. [PMID: 22921808]

ACROMEGALY & GIGANTISM

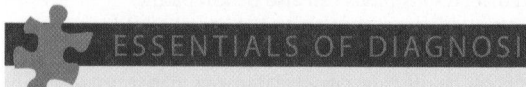

ESSENTIALS OF DIAGNOSIS

- ▶ Pituitary tumor.
- ▶ Excessive growth of hands, feet, jaw, and internal organs; or gigantism before closure of epiphyses.
- ▶ Amenorrhea, headaches, visual field loss, weakness.
- ▶ Soft, doughy, sweaty handshake.
- ▶ Elevated serum IGF-I.
- ▶ Serum GH not suppressed following oral glucose.

▶ General Considerations

GH exerts much of its growth-promoting effects by stimulating the release of IGF-I from the liver and other tissues.

Acromegaly is nearly always caused by a pituitary adenoma. These tumors may be locally invasive, particularly into the cavernous sinus. Less than 1% are malignant. Most are macroadenomas (over 1 cm in diameter). Acromegaly is usually sporadic but may rarely be familial, with < 3% being due to MEN types 1 or 4. Acromegaly may also be seen rarely in McCune–Albright syndrome and Carney complex. Acromegaly is rarely caused by ectopic secretion of GHRH or GH secreted by a lymphoma, hypothalamic tumor, bronchial carcinoid, or pancreatic tumor.

▶ Clinical Findings

A. Symptoms and Signs

Excessive GH causes tall stature and gigantism if it occurs in youth, before closure of epiphyses. Afterward, acromegaly develops. The term "acromegaly," meaning extremity enlargement, seriously understates the manifestations. The hands enlarge and a doughy, moist handshake is characteristic. The fingers widen, causing patients to enlarge their rings. Carpal tunnel syndrome is common. The feet also grow, particularly in shoe width. Facial features coarsen since the bones and sinuses of the skull enlarge; hat size increases. The mandible becomes more prominent, causing prognathism and malocclusion. Tooth spacing widens. Older photographs of the patient can be a useful comparison.

Macroglossia occurs, as does hypertrophy of pharyngeal and laryngeal tissue; this causes a deep, coarse voice and sometimes makes intubation difficult. Obstructive sleep apnea may occur. A goiter may be noted. Hypertension (50%) and cardiomegaly are common. At diagnosis, about 10% of acromegalic patients have overt heart failure, with a dilated left ventricle and a reduced ejection fraction. Weight gain is typical, particularly of muscle and bone. Insulin resistance is usually present and frequently causes diabetes mellitus (30%). Arthralgias and degenerative arthritis occur. Overgrowth of vertebral bone can cause spinal stenosis. Colon polyps are common, especially in patients with skin papillomas. The skin may also manifest hyperhidrosis, thickening, cystic acne, skin tags, and areas of acanthosis nigricans.

GH-secreting pituitary tumors usually cause some degree of hypogonadism, either by cosecretion of PRL or by direct pressure upon normal pituitary tissue. Decreased libido and erectile dysfunction are common. Women with acromegaly may experience irregular menses or amenorrhea; those who become pregnant have an increased risk of gestational diabetes and hypertension. Secondary hypothyroidism sometimes occurs; hypoadrenalism is unusual. Headaches are frequent. Temporal hemianopia may occur as a result of the optic chiasm being impinged by a suprasellar growth of the tumor.

B. Laboratory Findings

For screening purposes, a random serum IGF-I can be obtained. If it is normal for age, acromegaly is ruled out.

For further evaluation, the patient should be fasting for at least 8 hours (except for water), not be acutely ill, and not have exercised on the day of testing. Assay for the following: serum IGF-I (increased and usually over five times normal in acromegalic patients), PRL (cosecreted by many GH-secreting tumors), glucose (diabetes mellitus is common in acromegaly), liver enzymes and serum creatinine or blood urea nitrogen (BUN) (liver failure or kidney disease can misleadingly elevate GH), serum calcium (to exclude hyperparathyroidism), serum inorganic phosphorus (frequently elevated), serum free T_4, and TSH (secondary hypothyroidism is common in acromegaly; primary hypothyroidism may increase PRL). Glucose syrup (100 g) is then administered orally, and serum GH is measured 60 minutes afterward; acromegaly is excluded if the serum GH is < 1 ng/mL. For ultrasensitive GH assays, GH should be suppressed to < 0.3 ng/mL. The serum IGF-I and glucose-suppressed GH are usually complementary tests; however, disparities between IGF-I and GH levels occur in up to 30% of patients.

C. Imaging

MRI shows a pituitary tumor in 90% of acromegalic patients. These tumors ordinarily involve the sella and cavernous sinus; rare ectopic tumors may arise in the sphenoid bone. MRI is generally superior to CT scanning, especially in the postoperative setting. Radiographs of the skull may show an enlarged sella and thickened skull. Radiographs may also show tufting of the terminal phalanges of the fingers and toes. A lateral view of the foot shows increased thickness of the heel pad.

▶ Differential Diagnosis

Active acromegaly must be distinguished from familial coarse features, large hands and feet, and isolated prognathism and from inactive ("burned-out") acromegaly in which there has been a spontaneous remission due to infarction of the pituitary adenoma. GH-induced gigantism must be differentiated from familial tall stature and from aromatase deficiency. (See Osteoporosis.)

Misleadingly high serum GH levels can be caused by exercise or eating just prior to the test; acute illness or agitation; liver failure or kidney disease; malnourishment; diabetes mellitus; or concurrent treatment with estrogens, beta-blockers, or clonidine. Acromegaly can be difficult to diagnose during pregnancy, since the placenta produces GH and commercial GH assays may not be able to distinguish between pituitary and placental GH. During normal adolescence, serum IGF-I is usually elevated and GH may fail to be suppressed.

▶ Complications

Complications include hypopituitarism, hypertension, glucose intolerance or frank diabetes mellitus, cardiac enlargement, and cardiac failure. Carpal tunnel syndrome may cause thumb weakness and thenar atrophy. Arthritis of hips, knees, and spine can be troublesome. Cord compression may be seen. Visual field defects may be severe and progressive. Acute loss of vision or cranial nerve palsy may occur if the tumor undergoes spontaneous hemorrhage and necrosis (pituitary apoplexy). Colon polyps are more likely to develop in patients with acromegaly.

▶ Treatment

Pituitary transsphenoidal microsurgery is the treatment of choice for patients with acromegaly. Many patients have an apparent surgical cure and a remission in all clinical symptoms but continue to have a mildly elevated serum GH or IGF-I postoperatively. If no residual tumor is apparent on MRI, the patient may elect to be monitored closely, rather than embark on adjuvant medical therapy that is expensive and carries its own risks (see below).

A. Pituitary Microsurgery

Transsphenoidal pituitary microsurgery removes the adenoma while preserving anterior pituitary function in most patients. Surgical remission is achieved in about 70% of patients followed over 3 years. GH levels fall immediately; diaphoresis and carpal tunnel syndrome often improve within a day after surgery. Transsphenoidal surgery is usually well tolerated, but complications occur in about 12% of patients, including infection, cerebrospinal fluid (CSF) leak, and hypopituitarism. Transsphenoidal pituitary surgery may be difficult in patients with McCune–Albright syndrome because of fibrous dysplasia of the skull base.

Fluid and electrolyte disturbances occur in most patients postoperatively. Diabetes insipidus can occur within 2 days postoperatively but is usually mild and self-correcting. Hyponatremia can occur abruptly 4–13 days postoperatively in 21% of patients; symptoms may include nausea, vomiting, headache, malaise, or seizure. It is treated with fluid restriction and salt supplements. It is prudent to monitor serum sodium levels postoperatively. Dietary salt supplements for 2 weeks postoperatively may help prevent this complication.

Corticosteroids are administered perioperatively and tapered to replacement doses over 1 week; hydrocortisone is discontinued and cosyntropin stimulation test is performed about 6 weeks after surgery. At that time, the patient is screened for secondary hypothyroidism (by a serum FT_4) and secondary hypogonadism (see above).

B. Medications

Acromegalic patients with an incomplete biochemical remission after pituitary surgery may benefit from medical therapy, with dopamine agonists, somatostatin analogues, tamoxifen, or pegvisomant.

Cabergoline is usually the dopamine agonist of choice. It may be used first, since it is an oral medication. Cabergoline therapy is most successful for tumors that secrete both PRL and GH but can also be effective for patients with normal serum PRL levels. Therapy with cabergoline will shrink one-third of pituitary tumors by more than 50%. It appears to be safe during pregnancy. The initial dose is 0.25 mg orally twice weekly, which is gradually increased to a maximum dosage of 1 mg twice weekly (based on serum GH and IGF-I levels). Side effects of cabergoline include nausea, fatigue, constipation, abdominal pain, and dizziness (see Hyperprolactinemia).

Octreotide and **lanreotide** are somatostatin analogs that are given by subcutaneous injection. Octreotide (Sandostatin LAR depot) is given at a dose of 20–40 mg intragluteally monthly. Lanreotide acetate (Somatuline Depot) is given by subcutaneous intragluteal injection at a dosage of 60–120 mg monthly. Whichever preparation is used, the dosage can be adjusted to achieve serum GH levels under 2 ng/mL. Such long-acting somatostatin analogs can achieve serum GH levels under 2 ng/mL in 79% of patients and normal serum IGF-I levels in 53% of patients. Headaches often improve, and tumor shrinkage of about 30% may be expected. Acromegalic patients with pretreatment serum GH levels exceeding 20 ng/mL are less likely to respond to octreotide or lanreotide therapy. It appears to be safe during pregnancy. Side effects are experienced by about one-third of patients and include injection site pain, loose acholic stools, abdominal discomfort,

or cholelithiasis. All somatostatin analogs are expensive and must be continued indefinitely or until other treatment has been effective.

Tamoxifen is a selective estrogen receptor modulator (SERM) that may be particularly useful for persistent acromegaly in men and in women who are postmenopausal or who have had breast cancer. Tamoxifen in oral doses of 20–40 mg daily does not reduce serum GH levels but reduces serum IGF-I levels in 82% of patients and normalizes serum IGF-I levels in 47%. Serum testosterone levels increase in men.

Pegvisomant is a GH receptor antagonist that blocks hepatic IGF-I production. Pegvisomant therapy produces symptomatic relief and normalizes serum IGF-I levels in over 90% of patients. The starting dosage is 10 mg subcutaneously daily. The maintenance dosage can be increased by 5–10 mg every 4–6 weeks, based on serum IGF-I levels and liver transaminase levels; the maximum dosage is 40 mg subcutaneously daily. Pegvisomant does not shrink GH-secreting tumors. Patients need to be monitored carefully with visual field examinations, GH levels, and MRI scanning of the pituitary. It appears to be safe during pregnancy. Pegvisomant has caused hepatitis in a patient with Gilbert syndrome. Other adverse effects include edema, flulike syndrome, nausea, and hypertension. Lipohypertrophy can occur at injection sites, so injection sites must be diligently rotated and inspected. In acromegalic diabetics, hypoglycemic drugs are reduced to avoid hypoglycemia during pegvisomant therapy. The effectiveness of pegvisomant is reduced by coadministration of opioids. Pegvisomant is detected in some GH assays, which could overestimate serum GH levels. Pegvisomant is extremely expensive.

C. Stereotactic Radiosurgery

Acromegalic patients who have not had a complete remission with transsphenoidal surgery or medical therapy may be treated with **stereotactic radiosurgery** administered by gamma knife, heavy particle radiation, or adapted linear accelerator. Gamma knife radiosurgery is preferred, since it has become more widely available and normalization of serum IGF-I has been reported in up to 80% of treated patients. Radiosurgery precisely radiates the pituitary tumor in a single session and reduces radiation to the normal brain. However, it cannot be used for pituitary tumors with suprasellar extension due to the risk of damaging the optic chiasm. Radiosurgery can be used for pituitary tumors invading the cavernous sinus, since cranial nerves III, IV, V, and VI are less susceptible to radiation damage. Radiosurgery can also be used for patients who have not responded to conventional radiation therapy. Following any pituitary radiation therapy, patients are advised to take lifelong daily low-dose aspirin because of the increased risk of small-vessel stroke.

▶ Prognosis

Patients with acromegaly have increased morbidity and mortality from cardiovascular disorders and progressive acromegalic symptoms. Those who are treated and have a random serum GH under 1.0 ng/mL or a glucose-suppressed serum

GH under 0.4 ng/mL with a normal age-adjusted serum IGF-I level have reduced morbidity and mortality. Transsphenoidal pituitary surgery is successful in 80% of patients with tumors < 2 cm in diameter and GH levels < 50 ng/mL. Extrasellar extension of the pituitary tumor, particularly cavernous sinus invasion, reduces the likelihood of surgical cure.

Adjuvant medical therapy has been quite successful in treating patients who are not cured by pituitary surgery. Postoperatively, normal pituitary function is usually preserved. Soft tissue swelling regresses but bone enlargement is permanent. Hypertension frequently persists despite successful surgery. Conventional radiation therapy (alone) produces a remission in about 40% of patients by 2 years and 75% of patients by 5 years after treatment. Gamma knife or cyberknife radiosurgery reduces GH levels an average of 77%, with 20% of patients having a full remission after 12 months. Patients with pituitary adenomas that abut the optic chiasm can be treated with cyberknife radiosurgery, controlling tumor growth and preserving vision in most patients. Heavy particle pituitary radiation produces a remission in about 70% of patients by 2 years and 80% of patients by 5 years. Radiation therapy eventually produces some degree of hypopituitarism in most patients. Conventional radiation therapy may cause some degree of organic brain syndrome and predisposes to small strokes. Patients must receive lifelong follow-up, with regular monitoring of serum GH and IGF-I levels. Serum GH levels over 5 ng/mL and rising IGF-I levels usually indicate a recurrent tumor. Most pregnant women with acromegaly do not have an increase in the size of the pituitary tumor and neonatal outcome is unaffected.

Hypopituitarism may occur, due to the tumor itself, pituitary surgery, or radiation therapy. Hypopituitarism may develop years following radiation therapy, so patients must have regular clinical monitoring of their pituitary function.

Balili I et al. Tamoxifen as a therapeutic agent in acromegaly. Pituitary. 2013 Nov 16. [Epub ahead of print] [PMID: 24243064]

Cheng V et al. Pregnancy and acromegaly: a review. Pituitary. 2012 Mar;15(1):59–63. [PMID: 21789529]

Franzin A et al. Results of gamma knife radiosurgery in acromegaly. Int J Endocrinol. 2012;2012:342034. [PMID: 22518119]

Giustina A et al. Current management practices for acromegaly: an international survey. Pituitary. 2011 Jun;14(2):125–33. [PMID: 21063787]

Jane JA Jr et al. Endoscopic transsphenoidal surgery for acromegaly: remission using modern criteria, complications, and predictors of outcome. J Clin Endocrinol Metab. 2011 Sep;96 (9):2732–40. [PMID: 21715544]

Katznelson L. Approach to the patient with persistent acromegaly after pituitary surgery. J Clin Endocrinol Metab. 2010 Sept;95(9):4114–23. [PMID: 20823464]

Ribeiro-Oliveira A Jr et al. The changing face of acromegaly—advances in diagnosis and treatment. Nat Rev Endocrinol. 2012 Oct;8(10):605–11. [PMID: 22733271]

Sandret L et al. Place of cabergoline in acromegaly: a meta-analysis. J Clin Endocrinol Metab. 2011 May;96(5):1327–35. [PMID: 21325455]

Sherlock M et al. Medical therapy in acromegaly. Nat Rev Endocrinol. 2011 May;7(5):291–300. [PMID: 21448141]

HYPERPROLACTINEMIA

 ESSENTIALS OF DIAGNOSIS

▶ Women: Oligomenorrhea, amenorrhea; galactorrhea; infertility.

▶ Prolactin normally elevated during pregnancy.

▶ Men: Hypogonadism; decreased libido and erectile dysfunction; infertility.

▶ Elevated serum PRL.

▶ CT scan or MRI often demonstrates pituitary adenoma.

▶ General Considerations

Non-gestational elevations in serum PRL can be caused by numerous conditions (Table 26–2). PRL-secreting pituitary tumors are more common in women than in men and are usually sporadic but may rarely be familial as part of MEN 1. Most are microadenomas (< 1 cm in diameter) that do not grow even with pregnancy or oral contraceptives.

Table 26–2. Causes of hyperprolactinemia.

Physiologic Causes	Pharmacologic Causes	Pathologic Causes
Exercise	Amoxapine	Acromegaly
Familial (mutant prolactin receptor)	Amphetamines	Chronic chest wall stimulation (postthoracotomy, post-mastectomy, herpes zoster, breast problems, chest acupuncture, nipple rings, etc)
Idiopathic	Anesthetic agents	
Macroprolactin ("big prolactin")	Antipsychotics (conventional and atypical)	
Nipple stimulation	Butyrophenones	
Pregnancy	Cimetidine and ranitidine (not famotidine or nizatidine)	
Puerperium		Cirrhosis
Sleep (REM phase)	Cocaine	Hypothalamic disease
Stress (trauma, surgery)	Domperidone	Hypothyroidism
Suckling	Estrogens	Kidney disease (especially with zinc deficiency)
	Hydroxyzine	
	Locaserin	Multiple sclerosis
	Methyldopa	Optic neuromyelitis
	Metoclopramide	Pituitary stalk damage
	Opioids	
	Nicotine	
	Phenothiazines	Prolactin-secreting tumors
	Protease inhibitors	
	Progestins	Pseudocyesis (false pregnancy)
	Reserpine	
	Risperidone	Spinal cord lesions
	Selective serotonin reuptake inhibitors	Systemic lupus erythematosus
	Testosterone	
	Tricyclic antidepressants	
	Verapamil	

However, some giant prolactinomas (over 3 cm in diameter) can spread into the cavernous sinuses and suprasellar areas; rarely, they may erode the floor of the sella to invade the sinuses.

▶ Clinical Findings

A. Symptoms and Signs

Hyperprolactinemia may cause hypogonadotropic hypogonadism and reduced fertility. Men usually have diminished libido and erectile dysfunction that may not respond to testosterone replacement; gynecomastia sometimes occurs but rarely with galactorrhea. The diagnosis of a prolactinoma is often delayed in men, such that pituitary adenomas may grow and present with late manifestations of a pituitary macroprolactinoma.

About 90% of premenopausal women with prolactinomas experience amenorrhea, oligomenorrhea, or infertility. Estrogen deficiency can cause decreased vaginal lubrication, irritability, anxiety, and depression. Galactorrhea (lactation in the absence of nursing) is common. During pregnancy, clinically significant enlargement of a microprolactinoma (diameter < 1 cm) occurs in < 3%; clinically significant enlargement of a macroprolactinoma (diameter ≥ 1 cm) occurs in about 30%.

Pituitary prolactinomas may cosecrete GH and cause acromegaly (see above). Large tumors may cause headaches, visual symptoms, and pituitary insufficiency.

Aside from pituitary tumors, some women secrete an abnormal form of prolactin that appears to cause peripartum cardiomyopathy (see Chapter 10). Suppression of prolactin secretion with dopamine agonists can reverse the cardiomyopathy.

B. Laboratory Findings

Evaluate for conditions known to cause hyperprolactinemia, particularly pregnancy (serum hCG), hypothyroidism (serum FT_4 and TSH), kidney disease (BUN and serum creatinine), cirrhosis (liver tests) and hyperparathyroidism (serum calcium). Men are evaluated for hypogonadism with determinations of serum total and free testosterone, LH, and FSH. Women who have amenorrhea are assessed for hypogonadism with determinations of serum estradiol, LH, and FSH. Patients with large pituitary macroadenomas (> 3 cm in diameter) should have PRL measured on serial dilutions of serum, since immunoradiometric assay assays may otherwise report falsely low titers, the "high-dose hook effect." Patients with macroprolactinomas or manifestations of possible hypopituitarism should be evaluated for hypopituitarism as described above. An assay for macroprolactinemia should be considered for patients with hyperprolactinemia who are relatively asymptomatic and have no apparent cause for hyperprolactinemia.

C. Imaging

Patients with hyperprolactinemia not induced by drugs, hypothyroidism, or pregnancy should be examined by pituitary MRI. Small prolactinomas may thus be demonstrated, but clear differentiation from normal variants is not always possible. In the event that a woman with a

macroprolactinoma becomes pregnant and elects not to take dopamine agonists during her pregnancy, MRI is usually not performed since the normal pituitary grows during pregnancy. However, if visual-field defects or other neurologic symptoms develop in a pregnant woman, a limited MRI study should be done, focusing on the pituitary without gadolinium contrast.

▶ Differential Diagnosis

The causes of hyperprolactinemia are shown in Table 26–2. Chronic nipple stimulation, nipple piercing, augmentation or reduction mammoplasty, and mastectomy may stimulate PRL secretion. In acromegaly, there may be cosecretion of GH and PRL. Hyperprolactinemia may also be idiopathic. Increased pituitary size is a normal variant in young women. Macroprolactinemia is an increased circulating level of a high molecular weight PRL that is biologically inactive. It occurs in 3.7% of the general population and in 10–25% of patients with hyperprolactinemia; pituitary MRI is normal in 78% of cases.

The differential diagnosis for galactorrhea includes the small amount of breast milk that can be expressed from the nipple in many parous women that is not cause for concern. Nipple stimulation from nipple rings, chest surgery, or acupuncture can cause galactorrhea; serum PRL levels may be normal or minimally elevated. Some women can have galactorrhea with normal serum PRL levels and no discernible cause (idiopathic). Normal breast milk may be various colors besides white. Bloody galactorrhea requires evaluation for breast malignancy.

▶ Treatment

Medications known to increase PRL should be stopped if possible. Hyperprolactinemia due to hypothyroidism is corrected by thyroxine.

Women with microprolactinomas who have amenorrhea or are desirous of contraception may safely take oral contraceptives or estrogen replacement—there is minimal risk of stimulating enlargement of the microadenoma. Patients with infertility and hyperprolactinemia may be treated with a dopamine agonist in an effort to improve fertility. Women with amenorrhea who elect to receive no treatment have an increased risk of developing osteoporosis; such women require periodic bone densitometry.

Pituitary macroprolactinomas (> 10 mm in diameter) have a higher risk of progressive growth, particularly during treatment with estrogen or testosterone replacement therapy or during pregnancy. Therefore, patients with macroprolactinomas should not be treated with sex HRT unless they are in remission with dopamine agonist medication or surgery. Pregnant women with macroprolactinomas should continue to receive treatment with dopamine agonists throughout the pregnancy to prevent tumor growth. If dopamine agonists are not used during pregnancy in a woman with a macroprolactinoma, visual field testing is required each trimester. During pregnancy, measurement of prolactin is not useful surveillance for tumor growth due to the fact that prolactin increases greatly during normal pregnancy.

A. Dopamine Agonists

Dopamine agonists (cabergoline, bromocriptine, or quinagolide) are the initial treatment of choice for patients with giant prolactinomas and those with hyperprolactinemia desiring restoration of normal sexual function and fertility. Cabergoline is the most effective and usually the best-tolerated ergot-derived dopamine agonist. The beginning dosage is 0.25 mg orally once weekly for 1 week, then 0.25 mg twice weekly for the next week, then 0.5 mg twice weekly. Further dosage increases may be required monthly, based on serum PRL levels, up to a maximum of 1.5 mg twice weekly. Bromocriptine (1.25–20 mg/d orally) is an alternative. Women who experience nausea with oral preparations may find relief with deep vaginal insertion of cabergoline or bromocriptine tablets; vaginal irritation sometimes occurs. Quinagolide (Norprolac; not available in the United States) is a non–ergot-derived dopamine agonist for patients intolerant or resistant to ergot-derived medications; the starting dosage is 0.075 mg/d orally, increasing as needed and tolerated to a maximum of 0.6 mg/d. Patients whose tumor is resistant to one dopamine agonist may be switched to another in an effort to induce a remission.

Dopamine agonists are given at bedtime to minimize side effects of fatigue, nausea, dizziness, and orthostatic hypotension. These symptoms usually improve with dosage reduction and continued use. Erythromelalgia is rare. Dopamine agonists can cause a variety of psychiatric side effects that are not dose related and may take weeks to resolve once the drug is discontinued.

With dopamine agonist treatment, 90% of patients with prolactinomas experience a fall in serum PRL to 10% or less of pretreatment levels and about 80% of treated patients achieve a normal serum PRL level. Shrinkage of a pituitary adenoma occurs early, but the maximum effect may take up to a year. Nearly half of prolactinomas—even massive tumors—shrink more than 50%. Such shrinkage of invasive prolactinomas can result in CSF rhinorrhea. Discontinuing therapy after months or years usually results in the reappearance of hyperprolactinemia and galactorrhea-amenorrhea. After 2 years of cabergoline therapy, the percentage of patients who maintain a normal serum prolactin after withdrawal of the drug are as follows: 32% with idiopathic hyperprolactinemia, 21% with microprolactinomas, and 16% with macroprolactinomas.

Because dopamine agonists usually restore fertility promptly, many pregnancies have resulted; no teratogenicity has been noted. However, women with microadenomas may have treatment withdrawn during pregnancy. Macroadenomas may enlarge significantly during pregnancy; if therapy is withdrawn, patients must be monitored with serum PRL determinations and computer-assisted visual fields. Women with macroprolactinomas who have responded to dopamine agonists may safely receive oral contraceptive agents as long as they continue receiving dopamine agonist therapy.

B. Surgical Treatment

Transsphenoidal pituitary surgery may be urgently required for large tumors undergoing apoplexy or those severely compromising visual fields. It is also used electively for patients who do not tolerate or respond to dopamine agonists. Surgery is generally well tolerated, with a mortality rate of < 0.5%. For pituitary microprolactinomas, skilled neurosurgeons are successful in normalizing prolactin in 87% of patients. The 10-year recurrence rate is 13% and pituitary function can be preserved in over 95% of cases. However, the surgical success rate for macroprolactinomas is much lower, and the complication rates are higher. Craniotomy is rarely indicated, since even large tumors can usually be decompressed via the transsphenoidal approach.

Complications, such as CSF leakage, meningitis, stroke, or visual loss, occur in about 3% of cases; sinusitis, nasal septal perforation, or infection complicates about 6.5% of surgeries. Diabetes insipidus can occur within 2 days postoperatively but is usually mild and self-correcting. Hyponatremia can occur abruptly 4–13 days postoperatively in 21% of patients; symptoms may include nausea, vomiting, headache, malaise, or seizure. It is treated with fluid restriction and salt supplements. Dietary salt supplements for 2 weeks postoperatively may help prevent this complication.

C. Radiation Therapy

Radiation therapy is reserved for patients with macroadenomas that are growing despite treatment with dopamine agonists. A single gamma knife or cyberknife treatment is preferable for certain patients whose optic chiasm is clear of tumor, since it is generally safer and more convenient than conventional radiation therapy. Conventional radiation therapy must be given over 5 weeks and carries a high risk of eventual hypopituitarism. Other possible side effects include some degree of memory impairment and an increased long-term risk of second tumors and small vessel ischemic strokes. After radiation therapy, patients are advised to take low-dose aspirin daily for life to reduce their stroke risk.

D. Chemotherapy

Some patients with aggressive pituitary macroadenomas or carcinomas are not surgical candidates and do not respond to dopamine agonists or radiation therapy. Temozolomide may be administered, 150–200 mg/m^2 orally daily for 5 days of each 28-day cycle; after three cycles, treatment efficacy is determined by prolactin measurement and MRI scanning. A small percentage of patients with aggressive tumors respond to temozolomide.

▶ Prognosis

Pituitary prolactinomas generally respond well to therapy with dopamine agonists. Women with microprolactinomas can take oral contraceptives with little risk of stimulating growth of the pituitary adenoma. During pregnancy, growth of a pituitary prolactinoma occurs in 2.7% of women with a microprolactinoma and in 22.9% of those with a macroprolactinoma (> 1 cm diameter). If cabergoline is stopped after 2 years therapy, hyperprolactinemia recurs in 68% of patients with idiopathic hyperprolactinemia, 79% with microprolactinomas, and 84% with macroprolactinomas.

dos Santos Nunes V et al. Cabergoline versus bromocriptine in the treatment of hyperprolactinemia: a systematic review of randomized controlled trials and meta-analysis. Pituitary. 2011 Sep;14(3):259–65. [PMID: 21221817]

Glezer A et al. Approach to the patient with persistent hyperprolactinemia and negative sellar imaging. J Clin Endocrinol Metab. 2012 Jul;97(7):2211–6. [PMID: 22774208]

Holt RI et al. Antipsychotics and hyperprolactinaemia: mechanisms, consequences and management. Clin Endocrinol (Oxf). 2011 Feb;74(2):141–7. [PMID: 20455888]

Klibanski A. Clinical practice. Prolactinomas. N Engl J Med. 2010 Apr 1;362(13):1219–26. [PMID: 20357284]

Melmed S et al. Diagnosis and treatment of hyperprolactinemia: an Endocrine Society clinical practice guideline. J Clin Endocrinol Metab. 2011 Feb;96(2):273–88. [PMID: 21296991]

Molitch ME. Prolactinoma in pregnancy. Best Pract Res Clin Endocrinol Metab. 2011 Dec;25(6):885–96. [PMID: 22115164]

Shimatsu A et al. Macroprolactinemia: diagnostic, clinical, and pathogenic significance. Clin Dev Immunol. 2012;2012: 167132. [PMID: 23304187]

DISEASES OF THE THYROID GLAND

THYROID TESTING

Assays for FT_4, total triiodothyronine (T_3), and free triiodothyronine (FT_3) have largely supplanted measurements of total T_4, resin T_3 uptake (RT_3U), and free thyroxine index (FT_4I). It is particularly important to determine "free" serum levels (FT_4 and FT_3) in conditions associated with high circulating levels of thyroxine-binding globulin (TBG), such as during therapy with oral estrogen. Ultrasensitive assays for serum TSH have largely replaced older TSH assays. Table 26–3 shows the appropriate use of thyroid tests.

HYPOTHYROIDISM & MYXEDEMA

 ESSENTIALS OF DIAGNOSIS

- ▶ Weakness, fatigue, cold intolerance, constipation, weight change, depression, menorrhagia, hoarseness.
- ▶ Dry skin, bradycardia, delayed return of deep tendon reflexes, menorrhagia, hoarseness.
- ▶ Anemia, hyponatremia, hyperlipidemia.
- ▶ FT_4 level is usually low.
- ▶ TSH elevated in primary hypothyroidism.

▶ General Considerations

Hypothyroidism is common, affecting over 1% of the general population and about 5% of individuals over age 60 years. Thyroid hormone deficiency affects almost all body functions. The degree of severity ranges from mild and unrecognized hypothyroid states to striking myxedema.

Hypothyroidism may be due to failure or resection of the thyroid gland itself or deficiency of pituitary TSH (see Hypopituitarism). The condition must be distinguished from the functional hypothyroidism that occurs in severe nonthyroidal illness, which does not require treatment with thyroxine (see Euthyroid Sick Syndrome).

Maternal hypothyroidism during pregnancy results in offspring with IQ scores that are an average 7 points lower than those of euthyroid mothers.

Table 26–3. Appropriate use of thyroid tests.

	Test	Comment
Screening	Serum thyroid-stimulating hormone (TSH)	Most sensitive test for primary hypothyroidism and hyperthyroidism
	Free thyroxine (FT_4)	Excellent test
For hypothyroidism	Serum TSH	High in primary and low in secondary hypothyroidism
	Antithyroglobulin and antithyroperoxidase antibodies	Elevated in Hashimoto thyroiditis
For hyperthyroidism	Serum TSH	Suppressed except in TSH-secreting pituitary tumor or pituitary hyperplasia (rare)
	Triiodothyronine (T_3) or free triiodothyronine (FT_3)	Elevated
	[123]I uptake and scan	Increased uptake; diffuse versus "hot" foci on scan
	Antithyroperoxidase and antithyroglobulin antibodies	Elevated in Graves disease
	Thyroid-stimulating immunoglobulin (TSI); TSH receptor antibody (TSH-R Ab [stim])	Usually (65%) positive in Graves disease
For thyroid nodules	Fine-needle aspiration (FNA) biopsy	Best diagnostic method for thyroid cancer
	[123]I uptake and scan	Cancer is usually "cold"; less reliable than FNA biopsy
	[99m]Tc scan	Vascular versus avascular
	Ultrasonography	Useful to assist FNA biopsy. Useful in assessing the risk of malignancy (multinodular goiter or pure cysts are less likely to be malignant). Useful to monitor nodules and patients after thyroid surgery for carcinoma.

Goiter may be present with thyroiditis, iodide deficiency, genetic thyroid enzyme defects, drug goitrogens (lithium, iodide, propylthiouracil or methimazole, phenylbutazone, sulfonamides, amiodarone, interferon-alpha, interferon-beta, interleukin-2), food goitrogens in iodide-deficient areas (eg, turnips, cassavas) or, rarely, peripheral resistance to thyroid hormone or infiltrating diseases (eg, cancer, sarcoidosis). A hypothyroid phase occurs in subacute (de Quervain) viral thyroiditis following initial hyperthyroidism. Hashimoto thyroiditis is the most common cause of hypothyroidism (see Thyroiditis section).

Goiter is usually absent when hypothyroidism is due to destruction of the gland by radiation therapy (to the head, neck, chest, and shoulder region) or ^{131}I. Thyroid agenesis and mutations in the TSH receptor cause hypothyroidism that presents in infancy. Thyroidectomy causes hypothyroidism and hypothyroidism after hemithyroidectomy develops in 22% of patients.

Chemotherapeutic agents that can cause silent thyroiditis include the following: tyrosine kinase inhibitors (eg, sunitinib), denileukin diftitox, alemtuzumab, interferon-alpha, interleukin-2, ipilimumab, tremelimumab, thalidomide, and lenalidomide. This usually starts with hyperthyroidism (often unrecognized) and then progresses to hypothyroidism. Radioiodine-based chemotherapies can also cause hypothyroidism. Bexarotene causes a high rate of pituitary insufficiency with central hypothyroidism.

Amiodarone, because of its high iodine content, causes clinically significant hypothyroidism in about 15–20% of patients who receive it. Hypothyroidism occurs most often in patients with preexisting autoimmune thyroiditis and in patients who are not iodine-deficient. The T_4 level is low or low-normal, and the TSH is elevated, usually over 20 milli-international unit/L. Another 17% of patients are asymptomatic with milder elevations of TSH. Low-dose amiodarone is less likely to cause hypothyroidism. Cardiac patients with amiodarone-induced symptomatic hypothyroidism are treated with just enough thyroxine to relieve symptoms. Hypothyroidism usually resolves over several months if amiodarone is discontinued. Hypothyroidism may also develop in patients with a high iodine intake from other sources, especially if they have underlying lymphocytic thyroiditis.

Hepatitis C is associated with an increased risk of autoimmune thyroiditis, with 21% of affected patients having antithyroid antibodies and 13% having hypothyroidism. The risk of thyroid dysfunction is even higher when patients are treated with interferon. Interferon-alpha and interferon-beta treatment can induce thyroid dysfunction (usually hypothyroidism, sometimes hyperthyroidism) in 6% of patients. Spontaneous resolution occurs in over 50% of cases once interferon is discontinued.

▶ Clinical Findings

A. Symptoms and Signs

1. Common manifestations—Mild hypothyroidism often escapes detection without a screening serum TSH. Patients typically have nonspecific symptoms of hypothyroidism that include weight gain, fatigue, lethargy, depression, weakness, dyspnea on exertion, arthralgias or myalgias, muscle cramps, menorrhagia, constipation, dry skin, headache, paresthesias, cold intolerance, carpal tunnel syndrome, and Raynaud syndrome. Physical findings can include bradycardia; diastolic hypertension; thin, brittle nails; thinning of hair; peripheral edema; puffy face and eyelids; and skin pallor or yellowing (carotenemia). Delayed relaxation of deep tendon reflexes may be present. Patients often have a palpably enlarged thyroid (goiter) that arises due to elevated serum TSH levels or the underlying thyroid pathology, such as Hashimoto thyroiditis.

2. Less common manifestations—Less common symptoms of hypothyroidism include diminished appetite and weight loss, hoarseness, decreased sense of taste and smell, and diminished auditory acuity. Some patients may complain of dysphagia or neck discomfort. Although most menstruating women have menorrhagia, some women have scant menses or amenorrhea. Physical findings may include thinning of the outer halves of the eyebrows; thickening of the tongue; hard pitting edema; and effusions into the pleural and peritoneal cavities as well as into joints. Galactorrhea may also be present. Cardiac enlargement ("myxedema heart") and pericardial effusions may occur. Psychosis (myxedema madness) can occur from severe hypothyroidism or from toxicity of other drugs whose metabolism is slowed in hypothyroidism. Hypothermia and stupor or myxedema coma, which is often associated with infection (especially pneumonia), may develop in patients with severe hypothyroidism. Pituitary enlargement due to hyperplasia of TSH-secreting cells, which is reversible following thyroid therapy, may be seen in long-standing hypothyroidism.

Some hypothyroid patients with Hashimoto thyroiditis have symptoms that are not due to hypothyroidism but rather to another associated disease. Some conditions that occur more commonly in patients with Hashimoto thyroiditis include Addison disease, hypoparathyroidism, diabetes mellitus, pernicious anemia, Sjögren syndrome, vitiligo, biliary cirrhosis, gluten sensitivity, and celiac disease.

B. Laboratory Findings

Hypothyroidism is a common disorder and thyroid function tests should be obtained for any patient with its nonspecific symptoms or signs. The single best screening test for hypothyroidism is the serum TSH (Table 26–3). Serum TSH is increased with primary hypothyroidism, while the serum FT_4 is low or low-normal. Other laboratory abnormalities can include hyponatremia, hypoglycemia, or anemia (with normal or increased mean corpuscular volume). Additional findings frequently include increased serum levels LDL cholesterol, triglycerides, lipoprotein (a), liver enzymes, creatine kinase, or prolactin. Semen analysis shows an increase in abnormal sperm morphology. In patients with autoimmune thyroiditis, titers of antibodies against thyroperoxidase and thyroglobulin are high; serum antinuclear antibodies may be present but are not usually indicative of lupus.

The normal reference range for ultrasensitive TSH levels is generally 0.4–4.0 mU/L. However, the normal range of TSH varies with age such that elderly patients have a mildly higher reference range. Over 95% of normal adults have serum TSH concentrations under 3.0 mU/L.

Subclinical hypothyroidism is defined as the state of having a normal serum FT_4 with a serum TSH that is above the reference range for young adults. It occurs most often in persons aged ≥ 65 years, in whom the prevalence is 13%. Subclinical hypothyroidism is often transient and the TSH normalizes spontaneously in about 35% of cases within 2 years. The likelihood of TSH normalization is higher in patients without antithyroid antibodies and those with a marginally elevated serum TSH. The term "subclinical" is somewhat misleading, since it does not refer to patients' symptoms but rather refers only to serum hormone levels; in fact, such patients can have subtle manifestations of hypothyroidism (eg, fatigue, depression, hyperlipidemia) that may improve with thyroid hormone replacement. Patients without such symptoms do not require levothyroxine therapy but must be monitored regularly for the emergence of symptomatic hypothyroidism.

C. Imaging

Radiologic imaging is usually not necessary for patients with hypothyroidism. However, on CT or MRI, a goiter may be noted in the neck or in the mediastinum (retrosternal goiter). An enlarged thymus is frequently seen in the mediastinum in cases of autoimmune thyroiditis. On MRI, the pituitary is often quite enlarged in primary hypothyroidism, due to reversible hyperplasia of TSH-secreting cells; concomitant hyperprolactinemia can lead to the mistaken diagnosis of a TSH-secreting or PRL-secreting pituitary adenoma.

▶ Differential Diagnosis

The differential diagnosis for subclinical hypothyroidism includes antibody interference with the serum TSH assay, macro-TSH, sleep deprivation, exercise, recovery from nonthyroidal illness, and acute psychiatric emergencies (Table 26–4).

Many clinical manifestations of hypothyroidism (see above) are common in the general population without thyroid illness. The differential diagnoses are the conditions and drugs that can cause aberrations in laboratory tests, resulting in a low serum T_4 or T_3 or high serum TSH in the absence of hypothyroidism (Table 26–4).

Euthyroid sick syndrome should be considered in patients without known thyroid disease who are found to have a low serum FT_4 with a serum TSH that is not elevated. This syndrome can be seen in patients with severe illness, caloric deprivation, or major surgery. Serum TSH tends to be suppressed in severe nonthyroidal illness, making the diagnosis of concurrent primary hypothyroidism quite difficult, although the presence of a goiter suggests the diagnosis.

The clinician must decide whether such severely ill patients (with a low serum T_4 but no elevated TSH) might have hypothyroidism due to hypopituitarism. Patients without symptoms of prior brain lesion or hypopituitarism are very unlikely to suddenly develop hypopituitarism during

Table 26–4. Factors that may cause aberrations in laboratory tests that may be mistaken for primary hypothyroidism.[1]

Low Serum T_4 or T_3	High Serum TSH
Laboratory error	Laboratory error
Acute psychiatric problems	Autoimmune disease (assay interference)
Cirrhosis	
Nephrotic syndrome	Heterophile antibodies
Familial thyroid-binding globulin deficiency	Anti-mouse antibodies
	Anti-thyrotropin antibodies
Severe illness	Macro-thyrotropin
Drugs	Strenuous exercise (acute)
Androgens	Sleep deprivation (acute)
Asparaginase	Recovery from nonthyroidal illness (transient)
Carbamazepine	
Chloral hydrate	Acute psychiatric admissions (14% transient)
Corticosteroids	
Diclofenac (T_3)	Elderly—(especially women) 11%
Didanosine	
Fenclofenac	
5-Fluorouracil	
Halofenate	
Mitotane	
Naproxen (T_3)	
Nicotinic acid	
Oxcarbazepine	
Phenobarbital	
Phenytoin (total T_4 may be as low as 2 mcg/dL)	
Salicylates—large doses (T_3 and T_4)	
Sertraline	
Stavudine	
T_3 therapy (T_4)	

[1]True primary hypothyroidism may coexist.
T_4, levothyroxine; T_3, triiodothyronine; TSH, thyroid-stimulating hormone.

an unrelated illness. Patients with diabetes insipidus, hypopituitarism, or other signs of a central nervous system lesion may be given T_4 empirically.

Patients receiving prolonged dopamine infusions can develop true secondary hypothyroidism caused by dopamine's direct suppression of TSH-secreting cells.

Certain antiseizure medications cause low serum FT_4 levels by accelerating hepatic conversion of T_4 to T_3; serum TSH levels are normal.

▶ Complications

Preexistent coronary artery disease and heart failure may be exacerbated by levothyroxine therapy. Patients with severe hypothyroidism have an increased susceptibility to bacterial pneumonia. Megacolon has been described in long-standing hypothyroidism. Organic psychoses with paranoid delusions may occur ("myxedema madness"). Rarely, adrenal crisis may be precipitated by thyroid therapy. Hypothyroidism is a rare cause of infertility, which may respond to thyroid replacement. Untreated hypothyroidism during pregnancy often results in miscarriage.

Myxedema crisis refers to severe, life-threatening manifestations of hypothyroidism. Affected patients have impaired cognition, ranging from confusion to somnolence to coma (myxedema coma). Myxedema crisis is most often seen in elderly women who have had a stroke or who have stopped taking their thyroxine medication. It is often induced by an underlying infection; cardiac, respiratory, or central nervous system illness; cold exposure; or drug use. Convulsions and abnormal central nervous system signs may occur. Patients have severe hypothermia, hypoventilation, hyponatremia, hypoglycemia, and hypotension. Rhabdomyolysis and acute kidney injury may occur. Myxedematous patients are unusually sensitive to opioids and average doses may result in respiratory depression, even death. The mortality rate is high.

▶ Treatment

Before therapy with thyroid hormone is commenced, the hypothyroid patient requires at least a clinical assessment for adrenal insufficiency and angina, for which the patient would require evaluation and treatment.

A. Treatment for Hypothyroidism

Synthetic levothyroxine is the preferred preparation for treating hypothyroid patients. However, some clinicians prescribe mixtures of synthetic thyroxine and triiodothyronine or porcine thyroid preparations. Otherwise healthy young and middle-age adults with hypothyroidism may be treated initially with levothyroxine in doses of 25–75 mcg orally daily. The lower doses are used for very mild hypothyroidism, while higher doses are given for more symptomatic hypothyroidism. Women who are pregnant with significant hypothyroidism may begin therapy with levothyroxine at higher doses of 100–150 mcg orally daily. The levothyroxine dosage may be increased according to clinical response and serum TSH, trying to keep the serum TSH level between 0.4 mU/L and 2.0 mU/L. Since food interferes slightly with the absorption of levothyroxine, it is advisable to take levothyroxine with water habitually in the morning after an overnight fast. After beginning daily administration, significant increases in serum T_4 levels are seen within 1–2 weeks, and near-peak levels are seen within 3–4 weeks.

Patients with coronary insufficiency or those who are over age 60 years are treated with smaller initial doses of levothyroxine, 25–50 mcg orally daily; higher initial doses may be used if such patients are severely hypothyroid. The dose can be increased by 25 mcg every 1–3 weeks until the patient is euthyroid. Patients with hypothyroidism and known ischemic heart disease may begin thyroxine therapy following restoration of coronary perfusion by percutaneous coronary intervention (PCI) or CABG.

Myxedema crisis requires larger initial doses of levothyroxine intravenously, since myxedema itself can interfere with levothyroxine intestinal absorption. Levothyroxine sodium 400 mcg is given intravenously as a loading dose, followed by 50–100 mcg intravenously daily; the lower dose is given to patients with suspected coronary insufficiency. In patients with myxedema coma, liothyronine (T_3, Triostat) can be given intravenously in doses of 5–10 mcg every 8 hours for the first 48 hours. The hypothermic patient is warmed only with blankets, since faster warming can precipitate cardiovascular collapse. Patients with hypercapnia require intubation and assisted mechanical ventilation. Infections must be detected and treated aggressively. Patients in whom concomitant adrenal insufficiency is suspected are treated with hydrocortisone, 100 mg intravenously, followed by 25–50 mg every 8 hours.

B. Monitoring and Optimizing Treatment of Hypothyroidism

Regular clinical and laboratory monitoring is critical to determine the optimal levothyroxine dose for each patient. An elevated serum TSH usually indicates the need for a higher dose of levothyroxine and the initial goal should be to normalize the serum TSH. However, normal serum TSH and FT_4 levels may not accurately determine that the patient is clinically euthyroid (see below). The patient should be prescribed sufficient levothyroxine to restore a clinically euthyroid state, while maintaining the serum T_3 within their reference ranges. For most patients with hypothyroidism, a stable maintenance dose of levothyroxine can usually be found.

Different levothyroxine preparations vary in their bioavailability by up to 14% and such differences may have a subtle but significant clinical impact. It is optimal for patients to consistently take the same manufacturer's brand of levothyroxine.

Certain drugs and conditions may **increase** levothyroxine dosage requirements. Specifically, levothyroxine doses may need to be titrated upward if the patient starts taking medications that increase the hepatic metabolism of levothyroxine (eg, carbamazepine, phenobarbital, primidone, phenytoin, rifabutin, rifampin, sunitinib, and other tyrosine kinase inhibitors). Sertraline can block the effect of thyroxine and increase the thyroxine dosage requirement. Amiodarone can cause an increase or decrease in thyroxine dose requirements. Malabsorption of thyroxine can be caused by coadministration of binding substances, such as iron (eg, in multivitamins), fiber, raloxifene, sucralfate, aluminum hydroxide antacids, sevelamer, orlistat, calcium and magnesium supplements, soymilk, and soy protein supplements. Bile acid-binding resins, such as cholestyramine and colesevelam, can bind levothyroxine and impair its absorption even when administered 5 hours before the levothyroxine. Proton pump inhibitors interfere slightly with the absorption of levothyroxine. Gastrointestinal disorders can interfere with thyroxine absorption, including celiac disease, inflammatory bowel disease, lactose intolerance, *Helicobacter pylori* gastritis, and atrophic gastritis. Women with hypothyroidism typically require increased doses of levothyroxine during oral estrogen therapy.

Pregnancy usually increases the levothyroxine dosage requirement. An increase in levothyroxine requirement has been noted as early as the fifth week of pregnancy and adequate levothyroxine is critical to the health of the fetus. Therefore, it is prudent to increase levothyroxine dosages by approximately 20–30% as soon as pregnancy is confirmed. The fetus is at least partially dependent on maternal

T_4 for central nervous system development—particularly in the second trimester. By mid pregnancy, women require an average of 47% increase in their levothyroxine dosage.

It is therefore important to carefully monitor hypothyroid women with serum TSH (FT_4I or T_4 concentrations in hypopituitarism) determinations every 4 weeks and to increase levothyroxine progressively as required (see Chapter 19).

Serum TSH levels normally drop while FT_4I rises during the first trimester of pregnancy. This probably results from high levels of hCG (with structural homology to TSH) that stimulates thyroid hormone production. Most women with a low serum TSH in the first trimester are euthyroid. Serum FT_4I is helpful in evaluating the thyroid status of pregnant women, particularly in the first trimester. Postpartum, levothyroxine replacement requirements ordinarily return to prepregnancy levels.

Other drugs and conditions may **decrease** levothyroxine dosage requirements. Specifically, levothyroxine dosage may need to be titrated downward for patients who start taking teduglutide for short bowel syndrome. Levothyroxine doses must usually be reduced for women who experience decreased estrogen levels after delivery, after bilateral oophorectomy or natural menopause, after cessation of oral estrogen replacement, or during therapy with GnRH agonists.

1. Elevated serum TSH levels—This usually indicates underreplacement with levothyroxine. However, before increasing the T_4 dosage, it is important to confirm that the patient is indeed taking the medication as directed and does not have angina. It is also important to exclude malabsorption of levothyroxine due to concurrent administration with binding substances (see above), with food (instead of fasting), or with gastrointestinal disorders (such as short bowel syndrome, celiac disease, regional enteritis, liver disease, or pancreatic exocrine insufficiency). Serum TSH may be elevated transiently in acute psychiatric illness, with antipsychotics and phenothiazines, and during recovery from nonthyroidal illness. Autoimmune disease can cause false elevations of TSH by interfering with the assay. A high TSH can be caused by thyrotropin-secreting pituitary tumors.

2. Normal serum TSH levels—Patients with normal serum TSH levels (0.4–4.0 mU/L) may feel normal or may continue to feel hypothyroid, particularly when their serum TSH level is in the upper half of the reference range or when their serum T_3 level is low. They may respond well to a higher dose of levothyroxine. However, patients with coronary insufficiency or a proclivity to atrial fibrillation are best treated with a levothyroxine dosage that maintains a normal serum TSH.

3. Low or suppressed serum TSH levels—Serum TSH levels below the reference range (0.4–4.0 mU/L) are either "low" (0.04–0.4 mU/L) or "suppressed" (≤ 0.03 mU/L). If a patient taking levothyroxine with a "suppressed" serum TSH has manifestations of hyperthyroidism, the dosage of levothyroxine must be reduced. However, if patients with "low" serum TSH levels exhibit no symptoms of hyperthyroidism, it is important to determine whether hypopituitarism or severe nonthyroidal illness is present. TSH can also be reduced by certain medications, such as nonsteroidal

anti-inflammatory drugs; opioids; nifedipine; verapamil; and high-dose (short-term) corticosteroids. Absent such conditions, a clinically euthyroid patient with a suppressed serum TSH may be given a lower dosage of levothyroxine. Patients who exhibit hypothyroid symptoms on the reduced dosage of levothyroxine may have the higher dose resumed.

Some hypothyroid patients receiving levothyroxine who have normal or "low" serum TSH levels (0.04–0.4 mU/L) continue to have hypothyroid-type symptoms, such as lethargy, weight gain, depression, and cognitive disturbances. They must be carefully assessed for another concurrent condition, such as an adverse drug reaction, Addison disease, depression, hypogonadism, anemia, celiac disease, or gluten sensitivity. If such conditions are not present or are treated and hypothyroid-type symptoms persist, a serum T_3 level (FT_3 in pregnancy and women receiving oral estrogens) is often helpful. If the serum T_3 or FT_3 level is low, the patient may benefit from a slightly increased dose of levothyroxine. Patients who feel best with a levothyroxine dose that is associated with a "low" serum TSH (0.04–0.4 mU/L) may continue to take that dosage. Such patients who are clinically euthyroid but who have a mildly low serum TSH do not appear to suffer any long-term adverse consequences.

Patients with primary hypothyroidism who take levothyroxine and have a "suppressed" serum TSH (≤ 0.03 mU/L) have an increased risk of cardiovascular disease, dysrhythmias, and osteoporotic fractures. Therefore, a lower dose of levothyroxine is prescribed for such patients. However, some patients feel unmistakably hypothyroid while taking the reduced dose of levothyroxine and have low serum FT_3 levels. A higher levothyroxine dose may be resumed for such patients, but they require close long-term surveillance for atrial arrhythmias, osteoporosis, and manifestations of hyperthyroidism.

▶ **Prognosis**

Hypothyroidism caused by interferon-alpha resolves within 17 months of stopping the drug in 50% of patients. Patients with mild hypothyroidism caused by Hashimoto thyroiditis have a remission rate of 11%. With levothyroxine treatment of hypothyroidism, striking transformations take place both in appearance and mental function. Return to a normal state is usually the rule, but relapses will occur if treatment is interrupted. However, untreated patients with myxedema crisis have a mortality rate approaching 100% and even with optimal treatment, a mortality rate of 20–50%.

▶ **When to Refer**

- Difficulty titrating levothyroxine replacement to normal TSH or clinically euthyroid state.
- Any patient with significant coronary disease needing levothyroxine therapy.

▶ **When to Admit**

- Suspected myxedema crisis.
- Hypercapnia.

Almandoz JP et al. Hypothyroidism: etiology, diagnosis, and management. Med Clin North Am. 2012 Mar;96(2):203–21. [PMID: 22443971]

Biondi B et al. Combination treatment with T4 and T3: toward personalized replacement therapy in hypothyroidism? J Clin Endocrinol Metab. 2012 Jul;97(7):2256–71. [PMID: 22593590]

Chakera AJ et al. Treatment for primary hypothyroidism: current approaches and future possibilities. Drug Des Devel Ther. 2012;6:1–11. [PMID: 22291465]

De Groot L et al. Management of thyroid dysfunction during pregnancy and postpartum: an Endocrine Society clinical practice guideline. J Clin Endocrinol Metab. 2012 Aug;97(8):2543–65. [PMID: 22869843]

Hamnvik OP et al. Thyroid dysfunction from antineoplastic agents. J Natl Cancer Inst. 2011 Nov;103(21):1572–87. [PMID: 22010182]

Makita N et al. Tyrosine kinase inhibitor-induced thyroid disorders: a review and hypothesis. Thyroid. 2013 Feb;23(2):151–9. [PMID: 23398161]

O'Reilly DS. Thyroid hormone replacement: an iatrogenic problem. Int J Clin Pract. 2010 Jun;64(7):991–4. [PMID: 20584231]

Padmanabhan H. Amiodarone and thyroid dysfunction. South Med J. 2010 Sep;103(9):922–30. [PMID: 20689491]

HYPERTHYROIDISM (THYROTOXICOSIS)

ESSENTIALS OF DIAGNOSIS

▶ Sweating, weight loss or gain, anxiety, palpitations, loose stools, heat intolerance, irritability, fatigue, weakness, menstrual irregularity.

▶ Tachycardia; warm, moist skin; stare; tremor.

▶ In Graves disease: goiter (often with bruit); ophthalmopathy.

▶ Suppressed TSH in primary hyperthyroidism; increased T_4, FT_4, T_3, FT_3.

▶ General Considerations

The term "thyrotoxicosis" refers to the clinical manifestations associated with serum levels of T_4 or T_3 that are excessive for the individual (hyperthyroidism). Serum TSH levels are suppressed in primary hyperthyroidism. However, certain drugs and conditions can affect laboratory tests and lead to the erroneous diagnosis of hyperthyroidism in euthyroid individuals (Table 26–5). The causes of hyperthyroidism are many and diverse, as described below.

A. Graves Disease

Graves disease (known as Basedow disease in Europe) is the most common cause of thyrotoxicosis. It is an autoimmune disorder affecting the thyroid gland, characterized by an increase in synthesis and release of thyroid hormones. Graves disease is much more common in women than in men (8:1), and its onset is usually between the ages of 20 and 40 years. It may be accompanied by infiltrative ophthalmopathy (Graves exophthalmos) and, less commonly, by infiltrative dermopathy (pretibial myxedema).

Table 26–5. Factors that can cause aberrations in laboratory tests that may be mistaken for spontaneous clinical primary hyperthyroidism.[1]

High Serum T_4 or T_3	Low Serum TSH
Laboratory error	Laboratory error
Collecting serum in vial with gel barrier for T_3	Autonomous thyroid or thyroid nodule
Acute psychiatric problems (30%)	Acute corticosteroid administration
Acute medical illness (eg, acute intermittent porphyria)	Elderly euthyroid
AIDS (increased thyroid-binding globulin)	Nonthyroidal illness (severe)
Autoimmunity	Pregnancy (especially with morning sickness)
Hepatitis: acute or chronic active	hCG-secreting trophoblastic tumors
Primary biliary cirrhosis	Drugs
Pregnancy (especially with morning sickness)	Thyroid hormone
Hyperemesis gravidarum	Amphetamines
Familial thyroid-binding abnormalities	Dopamine
Familial generalized resistance to thyroid (Refetoff syndrome)	Dopamine agonists
Drugs	Calcium channel blockers (nifedipine, verapamil)
Amiodarone	
Amphetamines	
Clofibrate	
Estrogens (oral)	
Heparin (dialysis method)	
Heroin	
Thyroid hormone therapy (excessive or factitious)	
Methadone	
Perphenazine	
Tamoxifen	

[1]True clinical hyperthyroidism may coexist.
hCG, human chorionic gonadotropin; NSAIDs, nonsteroidal anti-inflammatory drugs; T_4, levothyroxine; T_3, triiodothyronine; TSH, thyroid-stimulating hormone.

The thymus gland is typically enlarged and serum antinuclear antibodies levels are usually elevated, reflecting the underlying autoimmunity. Many patients with Graves disease have a family history of either Graves disease or Hashimoto thyroiditis. Histocompatibility studies have shown an association with group HLA-B8 and HLA-DR3. The pathogenesis of the hyperthyroidism of Graves disease involves the formation of autoantibodies that bind to the TSH receptor in thyroid cell membranes and stimulate the gland to hyperfunction. Such antibodies are called thyroid-stimulating immunoglobulins (TSI) or TSH receptor antibodies (TSHrAb).

Dietary iodine supplementation can trigger Graves disease. An increased incidence of Graves disease occurs in countries that have embarked on national programs to fortify commercial salt with potassium iodide; the increase in Graves disease lasts about 4 years. Similarly, patients being treated with potassium iodide or amiodarone (which contains iodine) have an increased risk of developing Graves disease.

Patients with Graves disease have an increased risk of other systemic autoimmune disorders, including Sjögren syndrome, celiac disease, pernicious anemia, Addison disease, alopecia areata, vitiligo, autoimmune type 1 diabetes mellitus, hypoparathyroidism, myasthenia gravis, and cardiomyopathy.

B. Toxic Multinodular Goiter and Thyroid Adenomas

Autonomous toxic adenomas of the thyroid may be multiple (toxic multinodular goiter) or single (Plummer disease).

C. Subacute, Postpartum, and Silent Thyroiditis

These conditions cause thyroid inflammation with release of stored hormone. They all produce a variable triphasic course: variable hyperthyroidism is followed by transient euthyroidism, and progresses to hypothyroidism. Thyroid radioiodine uptake is low during the thyrotoxic phase. Thyroid ultrasound shows a variably heterogenous, hypoechoic gland. All patients are treated with propranolol during the thyrotoxic phase and levothyroxine during the hypothyroid phase. There may be some overlap between these conditions.

Subacute thyroiditis is also known as "de Quervain" or "granulomatous" thyroiditis. It is typically caused by various viral infections. Women are affected four times more frequently than men. Patients typically experience a viral upper respiratory infection and develop an extremely painful thyroid that is tender to touch and typically enlarged to 3–4 times its normal size. There is often dysphagia and pain that can radiate to the jaw or ear. About 50% of affected patients experience a symptomatic thyrotoxic phase that lasts 3–6 weeks. The WBC, erythrocyte sedimentation rate (ESR) and C-reactive protein levels are usually elevated. About 25% have antithyroid antibodies (usually in low titer), so some cases may be autoimmune. An important differential diagnosis is bacterial suppurative thyroiditis. Patients are treated with nonsteroidal antiinflammatory drugs and corticosteroids for pain. About 10% remain hypothyroid after 1 year. The recurrence rate is 1–4%.

Postpartum thyroiditis refers to Hashimoto thyroiditis that occurs in the first 12 months after delivery. Although this usually occurs after term pregnancies, it can also occur after miscarriages. It is common, occurring in 5% of postpartum women, with an increased incidence in women with preexistent type 1 diabetes mellitus and other immune disorders. About 22% of such women experience hyperthyroidism followed by hypothyroidism, whereas 30% of such women have isolated thyrotoxicosis and 48% have isolated hypothyroidism. The thyrotoxic phase typically occurs 2–6 weeks postpartum and lasts 2–3 months. Affected women are often asymptomatic or experience minor symptoms, such as palpitations, heat intolerance, and irritability. Patients have either no palpable goiter or a small, nontender goiter. Over 80% have antithyroid antibodies. Most women progress to a hypothyroid phase that usually lasts a few months but that is frequently permanent. Affected women experience a recurrence rate of about 70% with subsequent pregnancies.

Silent thyroiditis is also known as subacute lymphocytic thyroiditis or "Hashitoxicosis." It can occur spontaneously or be triggered by certain medications. Women are affected four times more frequently than men. Patients have either no palpable goiter or a small, nontender goiter. About 50% have antithyroid antibodies and such patients have sometimes had chemotherapeutic agents (such as tyrosine kinase inhibitors, denileukin diftitox, alemtuzumab, interferon-alpha, interleukin-2, ipilimumab, tremelimumab, thalidomide, and lenalidomide). Graves ophthalmopathy has been caused by ipilimumab. Other drugs can cause silent thyroiditis, including lithium and amiodarone. In those with spontaneous silent thyroiditis, about 10–20% remain hypothyroid after 1 year. There is a recurrence rate of 5–10%; this rate is higher in Japan.

D. Medication-Induced Hyperthyroidism

1. Amiodarone-induced thyrotoxicosis—Amiodarone is a widely used antiarrhythmic drug that is 37% iodine by weight. The half-life of amiodarone and its metabolites is about 100 days. In the short term, amiodarone increases the serum TSH, though usually not over 20 mU/L. Serum T_4 and FT_4 rise about 40% and may become frankly elevated in clinically euthyroid patients. Meanwhile, serum T_3 levels decline. Due to these short-term changes, it is best to not check thyroid function tests during the first 3 months of therapy with amiodarone, unless clinically indicated. After about 3 months, the serum TSH usually normalizes. Since serum T_4 levels can be misleadingly high, the serum TSH level must be suppressed to diagnose amiodarone-induced thyrotoxicosis. With amiodarone-induced thyrotoxicosis, the serum T_3 or FT_3 is usually high or high-normal. In the United States, amiodarone causes thyrotoxicosis in about 3% of patients taking the drug. In Europe and iodine-deficient geographic areas, amiodarone induces thyrotoxicosis in about 20%. Amiodarone-induced thyrotoxicosis can occur quite suddenly at any time during treatment with amiodarone and may even develop several months after it has been discontinued. The manifestations of amiodarone-induced thyrotoxicosis can be missed, particularly since amiodarone tends to cause bradycardia. Therefore, it is prudent to check thyroid function tests (TSH, FT_4, T_3) prior to commencing amiodarone, rechecking them in 3–6 months, and then every 6 months (or sooner if clinically indicated).

Amiodarone-induced thyrotoxicosis is categorized as type 1 or type 2; about 27% are mixed type 1–2. **Type 1 amiodarone-induced thyrotoxicosis** is caused by the active production of excessive thyroid hormone. Thyroid color-flow Doppler typically shows an enlarged gland with increased vascularity; scanning with ^{99m}Tc-sestamibi shows normal to increased thyroidal uptake. **Type 2 amiodarone-induced thyrotoxicosis** is caused by thyroiditis with the passive release of stored thyroid hormone. Thyroid color-flow Doppler shows a normal sized gland without increased vascularity; scanning with ^{99m}Tc-sestamibi scanning shows no thyroidal uptake.

2. Iodine-induced hyperthyroidism—This is also known as **Jod-Basedow disease.** The recommended iodine intake for nonpregnant adults is 150 mcg/d. Higher iodine intake can precipitate hyperthyroidism in patients with nodular goiters, autonomous thyroid nodules, or asymptomatic Graves disease, and less commonly in patients with no detectable underlying thyroid disorder. Common sources of excess iodine include intravenous iodinated radiocontrast dye, certain foods (eg, kelp, nori), topical iodinated antiseptics (eg, povidine iodine), and medications (eg, amiodarone or potassium iodide). Intravenous iodinated radiocontrast dye can rarely induce a painful, destructive subacute thyroiditis, similar to type 2 amiodarone-induced thyrotoxicosis.

3. Tyrosine kinase inhibitors—Patients receiving chemotherapy with tyrosine kinase inhibitors (eg, axitinib, sorafenib, sunitinib) frequently develop silent thyroiditis that releases stored thyroid hormone, resulting in hyperthyroidism. While this hyperthyroidism may be subclinical, thyrotoxic crisis has been reported. The hyperthyroidism is usually followed by spontaneous hypothyroidism.

4. Alemtuzumab immunotherapy—Alemtuzumab is an anti-CD52 monoclonal antibody used to treat patients with multiple sclerosis. Graves disease with hyperthyroidism (usually mild) followed by hypothyroidism develops in about 22% of patients treated with alemtuzumab.

E. Pregnancy and hCG-Secreting Trophoblastic Tumors

Human chorionic gonadotropin (hCG) can bind to the thyroid's TSH receptors, so very high serum levels of hCG, particularly during the first 4 months of pregnancy, may cause sufficient receptor activation to cause hyperthyroidism. About 18% of pregnant women have a low serum TSH during pregnancy, but only about 10% of such women have clinical hyperthyroidism that requires treatment. Pregnant women are more likely to have hCG-induced thyrotoxicosis if they have high serum levels of asialo-hCG, a subfraction of hCG that has a greater affinity for TSH receptors. Such women are also more likely to suffer from hyperemesis gravidarum. This condition must be distinguished from true Graves disease in pregnancy, which usually predates conception and may be associated with high serum levels of TSI and antithyroid antibodies or with exophthalmos.

High levels of hCG can also cause thyrotoxicosis in some cases of pregnancies with gestational trophoblastic disease that has manifestations ranging from molar pregnancy to choriocarcinoma. Such molar pregnancies have produced thyrotoxic crisis. Men have developed hyperthyroidism from high serum levels of hCG secreted by a testicular choriocarcinoma.

F. Rare Causes of Hyperthyroidism

Thyrotoxicosis factitia is due to intentional or accidental ingestion of excessive amounts of exogenous thyroid hormone. Isolated epidemics of thyrotoxicosis have been caused by consumption of ground beef contaminated with bovine thyroid gland. **Struma ovarii** refers to thyroid tissue contained in about 3% of ovarian dermoid tumors and teratomas. Such ectopic thyroid tissue may develop thyroid nodules that produce excess thyroid hormone, thereby causing hyperthyroidism. Also, in Graves disease, ectopic thyroid tissue in dermoid tumors can secrete excessive thyroid hormone, along with the normal thyroid. **Pituitary TSH hypersecretion** by a pituitary thyrotrophe tumor or hyperplasia can rarely cause hyperthyroidism. Serum TSH is elevated or inappropriately normal in the presence of true thyrotoxicosis. Pituitary hyperplasia may be detected on MRI scan as pituitary enlargement without a discrete adenoma being visible. **Metastatic functioning thyroid carcinoma** can cause hyperthyroidism in patients with a heavy tumor burden. Hyperthyroidism can be induced or aggravated by recombinant human thyroid-stimulating hormone (rhTSH) that is given prior to radio-iodine therapy or scanning. (See Thyroid Cancer.)

▶ Clinical Findings

A. Symptoms and Signs

Thyrotoxicosis due to any cause produces nervousness, restlessness, heat intolerance, increased sweating, pruritus, fatigue, weakness, muscle cramps, frequent bowel movements, or weight change (usually loss). There may be palpitations or angina pectoris. Women frequently report menstrual irregularities.

Signs of thyrotoxicosis also include fine resting finger tremors, moist warm skin, fever, hyperreflexia, fine hair, and onycholysis. Chronic thyrotoxicosis may cause osteoporosis. Clubbing and swelling of the fingers (acropachy) develop in a small number of patients.

In patients with Graves disease, physical examination usually reveals a diffusely enlarged thyroid, frequently asymmetric, often with a bruit. However, some patients have no palpable thyroid enlargement. The thyroid gland in subacute thyroiditis is usually moderately enlarged and tender. In patients with toxic multinodular goiter, the thyroid usually has palpable nodules.

Cardiopulmonary manifestations of thyrotoxicosis commonly include a forceful heartbeat, premature atrial contractions, and sinus tachycardia. Patients often have exertional dyspnea. Atrial fibrillation or atrial tachycardia occurs in about 8% of patients with thyrotoxicosis, more commonly in men, the elderly, and those with ischemic or valvular heart disease. The ventricular response from the atrial fibrillation may be difficult to control. Thyrotoxicosis itself can cause a thyrotoxic cardiomyopathy, and the onset of atrial fibrillation can precipitate heart failure. Echocardiogram reveals pulmonary hypertension in 49% of patients with hyperthyroidism; of these, 71% have pulmonary artery hypertension while 29% have pulmonary venous hypertension. Even "subclinical hyperthyroidism" increases the risk for atrial fibrillation and overall mortality. Hemodynamic abnormalities and pulmonary hypertension are reversible with restoration of euthyroidism.

Graves eye manifestations, which can occur with hyperthyroidism of any etiology, include upper eyelid retraction (Dalrymple sign), lid lag with downward gaze (von Graefe sign), and a staring appearance (Kocher sign).

Ophthalmopathy is clinically apparent in 20–40% of patients with Graves disease and some cases of amiodarone-induced thyrotoxicosis. It usually consists of conjunctival edema (chemosis), conjunctivitis, and mild exophthalmos (proptosis). About 5–10% of patients experience more severe exophthalmos, with the eye being pushed forward by increased retro-orbital fat and eye muscles that have been thickened by lymphocytic infiltration. Such patients can experience diplopia from extraocular muscle entrapment. There may be weakness of upward gaze (Stellwag sign). The optic nerve may be compressed in severe cases, causing progressive loss of color vision, visual fields, and visual acuity. Corneal drying may occur with inadequate lid closure. Eye changes may sometimes be asymmetric or unilateral. The severity of the eye disease is not closely correlated with the severity of the thyrotoxicosis.

Exophthalmometry should be performed on all patients with Graves disease to document their degree of exophthalmos and detect progression of orbitopathy. The protrusion of the eye beyond the orbital rim is measured with a prism instrument (Hertel exophthalmometer). Maximum normal eye protrusion varies between kindreds and races, being about 22 mm for blacks, 20 mm for whites, and 18 mm for Asians.

The differential diagnosis for Graves ophthalmopathy includes diplopia caused by an orbital lymphoma. Ocular myasthenia gravis is another autoimmune condition that occurs more commonly in Graves disease but is usually mild, often with unilateral eye involvement. Acetylcholinesterase receptor antibody (AChR Ab) levels are elevated in only 36% of such patients, and a thymoma is present in 9%.

Graves dermopathy (pretibial myxedema) occurs in about 3% of patients with Graves disease usually in the pretibial region. It is more common in patients with high levels of serum TSI and severe Graves ophthalmopathy. Glycosaminoglycans accumulation and lymphoid infiltration occur in affected skin, which becomes erythematous with a thickened, rough texture. Elephantiasis of the legs is a rare complication.

Thyroid acropachy is an extreme and unusual manifestation of Graves disease. It presents with digital clubbing, swelling of fingers and toes, and a periosteal reaction of extremity bones. It is ordinarily associated with ophthalmopathy and thyroid dermopathy. Most patients are smokers.

Tetany is a rare presenting feature. In hyperthyroidism, the renal excretion of magnesium is increased and hypomagnesemia is common. Severe magnesium depletion causes hypoparathyroidism that can result in hypocalcemia.

Hyperthyroidism during pregnancy is relatively common, with a prevalence of about 0.2%. Manifestations include many of the features of normal pregnancy: tachycardia, warm skin, heat intolerance, increased sweating, and a palpable thyroid. Pregnancy can have a beneficial effect on the thyrotoxicosis of Graves disease, with decreasing antibody titers and decreasing serum T_4 levels as the pregnancy advances; about 30% of affected women experience a remission by late in the second trimester. However, undiagnosed or undertreated hyperthyroidism in pregnancy carries an increased risk of miscarriage, preeclampsia-eclampsia,

preterm delivery, abruptio placenta, maternal heart failure, and thyrotoxic crisis (thyroid storm). Such thyrotoxic crisis can be precipitated by trauma, infection, surgery, or delivery and confers a fetal/maternal mortality rate of about 25%.

TSI (TSHrAb) crosses the placenta and if maternal serum TSI levels reach > 500% in the third trimester, the risk of transient neonatal Graves disease in the newborn is increased. Such thyrotoxic newborns have an increased risk of intrauterine growth retardation and prematurity.

Hypokalemic periodic paralysis occurs in about 15% of Asian or Native American men with thyrotoxicosis. It usually presents abruptly with symmetric flaccid paralysis (and few thyrotoxic symptoms), often after intravenous dextrose, oral carbohydrate, or vigorous exercise. Attacks last 7–72 hours.

B. Laboratory Findings

Serum FT_4, T_3, FT_3, T_4, thyroid resin uptake, and FT_4 index are all usually increased. Sometimes the FT_4 level may be normal but with an elevated serum T_3 (T_3 toxicosis). Serum T_3 can be misleadingly elevated when blood is collected in tubes using a gel barrier, which causes certain immunoassays to report falsely elevated serum total T_3 levels in 24% of normal patients. Serum T_4 or T_3 can be elevated in other nonthyroidal conditions (Table 26–5).

Serum TSH is suppressed in hyperthyroidism (except in the very rare cases of pituitary inappropriate secretion of thyrotropin). Serum TSH may be misleadingly low in other nonthyroidal conditions (Table 26–5). The term "**subclinical hyperthyroidism**" is used to describe asymptomatic individuals with a low serum TSH but normal serum levels of FT_4 and T_3; progression to symptomatic thyrotoxicosis occurs at a rate of 1–2% per year in patients without a goiter and at a rate of 5% per year in patients with a multinodular goiter.

Hyperthyroidism can cause other laboratory abnormalities, including hypercalcemia, increased alkaline phosphatase, anemia, and decreased granulocytes. Hypokalemia and hypophosphatemia occur in thyrotoxic periodic paralysis.

Problems of diagnosis occur in patients with acute psychiatric disorders; about 30% of these patients have elevated serum T_4 levels without clinical thyrotoxicosis. The TSH is not usually suppressed, distinguishing psychiatric disorder from true hyperthyroidism. T_4 levels return to normal gradually.

In **Graves disease**, serum TSI is usually detectable (65%). Antithyroglobulin or antithyroperoxidase antibodies are usually elevated but are nonspecific. Serum antinuclear antibodies are also usually elevated without any evidence of systemic lupus erythematosus or other rheumatologic disease.

With **subacute thyroiditis**, patients often have an increased ESR. Serum antithyroid antibodies are usually not present and serum TSI (TSHrAb) levels are normal. Patients with **iodine-induced hyperthyroidism** also have undetectable serum TSI (or TSHrAb), an absence of serum antithyroperoxidase antibodies, and an elevated urinary iodine concentration. In **thyrotoxicosis factitia**, serum thyroglobulin levels are low, distinguishing it from other causes of hyperthyroidism.

With **hyperthyroidism during pregnancy,** women have an elevated serum total T_4 and FT_4 while the TSH is suppressed. However, about 18% of normal pregnant women have a low serum TSH. An apparent lack of full TSH suppression in hyperthyroidism can be seen due to misidentification of hCG as TSH in certain assays. The serum FT_4 assay is difficult in pregnancy. Although the serum T_4 is elevated in most pregnant women, values over 20 mcg/dL (257 nmol/L) are encountered only in hyperthyroidism. On treatment, serum total T_4 levels during pregnancy should be kept at about 1.5 × the pre-pregnancy level. The T_3 resin uptake, which is low in normal pregnancy because of high thyroxine-binding globulin (TBG) concentration, is normal or high in thyrotoxic persons.

Since high levels of T_4 and FT_4 are normally seen in patients taking **amiodarone,** a suppressed TSH must be present along with a greatly elevated T_4 (> 20 mcg/dL, or > 257 nmol/L) or T_3 (> 200 ng/dL, or > 3.1 nmol/L) in order to diagnose hyperthyroidism. In **type 1 amiodarone-induced thyrotoxicosis,** the presence of proptosis and serum TSI (TSHrAb) is diagnostic. In **type 2 amiodarone-induced thyrotoxicosis,** serum levels of interleukin-6 (IL-6) are usually quite elevated.

C. Imaging

Radioactive iodine (RAI) should never be administered to pregnant women. In others, RAI scanning and uptake may be helpful to determine the cause for hyperthyroidism. RAI uptake and scanning is not necessary for patients with obvious Graves disease who have elevated serum TSI or associated Graves ophthalmopathy. Women with hyperthyroidism due to Graves disease should ideally have the RAI scan extended to include the pelvis in order to screen for concomitant struma ovarii (rare). A high RAI uptake is seen in **Graves disease** and **toxic nodular goiter.** Patients with **type 1 amiodarone-induced thyrotoxicosis** have RAI uptake that is usually detectable. A low RAI uptake is characteristic of **subacute thyroiditis** and iodine-induced hyperthyroidism. Low RAI uptake is also seen with interleukin-2 therapy and during hyperthyroidism that often follows neck surgery for hyperparathyroidism. In **type 2 amiodarone-induced thyrotoxicosis,** thyroid RAI uptake is usually below 3%.

Thyroid ultrasound can be helpful in patients with hyperthyroidism, particularly in patients with palpable thyroid nodules. **Color flow Doppler sonography** is helpful to distinguish type 1 amiodarone-induced thyrotoxicosis (normal to increased blood flow velocity and vascularity) from type 2 amiodarone-induced thyrotoxicosis (reduced vascularity).

99mTc-sestamibi scanning usually shows normal or increased uptake with type 1 amiodarone-induced thyrotoxicosis.

MRI and CT scanning of the orbits are the imaging methods of choice to visualize Graves ophthalmopathy affecting the extraocular muscles. Imaging is required only in severe or unilateral cases or in euthyroid exophthalmos that must be distinguished from orbital pseudotumor, tumors, and other lesions.

▶ Differential Diagnosis

True thyrotoxicosis must be distinguished from those conditions that elevate serum T_4 and T_3 or suppress serum TSH without affecting clinical status (see Table 26–5). Serum TSH is commonly suppressed in early pregnancy and only about 10% of pregnant women with a low TSH have clinical hyperthyroidism.

Some states of hypermetabolism without thyrotoxicosis—notably severe anemia, leukemia, polycythemia, cancer, and pheochromocytoma—rarely cause confusion. Acromegaly may also produce tachycardia, sweating, and thyroid enlargement. Appropriate laboratory tests will easily distinguish these entities.

Cardiac disease (eg, atrial fibrillation, angina) refractory to treatment suggests the possibility of underlying ("apathetic") hyperthyroidism. Other causes of ophthalmoplegia (eg, myasthenia gravis) and exophthalmos (eg, orbital tumor, pseudotumor) must be considered. Thyrotoxicosis must also be considered in the differential diagnosis of muscle weakness and osteoporosis. Diabetes mellitus and Addison disease may coexist with thyrotoxicosis.

▶ Complications

Hypercalcemia, osteoporosis, and nephrocalcinosis may occur in hyperthyroidism. Decreased libido, erectile dysfunction, diminished sperm motility, and gynecomastia may be noted in men. Other complications include cardiac arrhythmias and heart failure, thyroid crisis, ophthalmopathy, dermopathy, and thyrotoxic hypokalemic periodic paralysis (see below.)

▶ Treatment

A. Treatment of Graves Disease

The treatment of Graves disease involves a choice of methods rather than a method of choice.

1. Propranolol—Propranolol is generally used for symptomatic relief until the hyperthyroidism is resolved. It effectively relieves its accompanying tachycardia, tremor, diaphoresis, and anxiety. It is the initial treatment of choice for thyroid storm. Periodic paralysis is also effectively treated with beta-blockade. It has no effect on thyroid hormone secretion. Treatment is usually begun with propranolol ER 60 mg orally once or twice daily, with dosage increases every 2–3 days to a maximum daily dose of 320 mg. Propranolol ER is initially given every 12 hours for patients with severe hyperthyroidism, due to accelerated metabolism of the propranolol; it may be given once daily as hyperthyroidism improves.

2. Thiourea drugs—Methimazole or propylthiouracil is generally used for young adults or patients with mild thyrotoxicosis, small goiters, or fear of isotopes. Carbimazole, another thiourea that is converted to methimazole in vivo, is available outside the United States. Elderly patients usually respond particularly well. These drugs are also useful for preparing hyperthyroid patients for surgery and elderly patients for RAI treatment. The drugs do not permanently damage the thyroid and are associated with a lower chance of posttreatment hypothyroidism (compared with RAI or surgery). When thiourea therapy is discontinued, there is a high recurrence rate for hyperthyroidism (about 50%). A better likelihood of long-term remission is seen in patients with small goiters or mild hyperthyroidism and those requiring small doses of thiourea. Patients whose thyroperoxidase and thyroglobulin antibodies remain high after 2 years of therapy have been reported to have only a 10% rate of relapse. Thiourea therapy may be continued long-term for patients who are tolerating it well.

All patients receiving thiourea therapy must be informed of the danger of agranulocytosis or pancytopenia and the need to stop the drug and seek medical attention immediately with the onset of any infection or unusual bleeding. Agranulocytosis (defined as an absolute neutrophil count below 500/mcL) or pancytopenia usually occurs abruptly in about 0.4% of patients taking either methimazole or propylthiouracil. Over 70% of agranulocytosis cases occur within the first 60 days and nearly 85% within 90 days of commencing therapy. But continued long-term vigilance for this side effect is required. About half the cases are discovered because of fever, pharyngitis, or bleeding, but the other cases are discovered with routine complete blood counts. There is a genetic tendency to develop agranulocytosis with thiourea therapy; if a close relative has had this adverse reaction, other therapies should be considered. Agranulocytosis generally remits spontaneously with discontinuation of the thiourea and while patients are treated with antibiotics. Recovery has not been improved by filgrastim (granulocyte colony-stimulating factor [G-CSF]). Surveillance of the WBC can be done when blood is drawn to check thyroid levels during the first few months of treatment. Such surveillance may be helpful, since some cases of agranulocytosis occur gradually and many cases may be discovered while the patient is still asymptomatic.

Other side effects common to thiourea drugs include pruritus, allergic dermatitis, nausea, and dyspepsia. Antihistamines may control mild pruritus without discontinuation of the drug. Since the two thiourea drugs are similar, patients who have a major allergic reaction to one should not be given the other.

The patient may become clinically hypothyroid for 2 weeks or more before TSH levels rise, the pituitary gland having been suppressed by the preceding hyperthyroidism. Therefore, the patient's changing thyroid status is best monitored clinically and with serum FT_4 levels. Rapid growth of the goiter usually occurs if prolonged hypothyroidism is allowed to develop; the goiter may sometimes become massive but usually regresses rapidly with reduction or cessation of thiourea therapy or with thyroid hormone replacement.

A. Methimazole—Except during the first trimester of pregnancy, methimazole is generally preferred over propylthiouracil, since methimazole is more convenient to use and is less likely to cause fulminant hepatic necrosis. Methimazole therapy is also less likely to cause ^{131}I

treatment failure. Methimazole is given orally in initial doses of 30–60 mg once daily. Some patients with very mild hyperthyroidism may respond well to smaller initial doses of methimazole (10–20 mg daily). Methimazole may also be administered twice daily to reduce the likelihood of gastrointestinal upset. Rare complications peculiar to methimazole include serum sickness, cholestatic jaundice, alopecia, nephrotic syndrome, hypoglycemia, and loss of taste. Methimazole use in pregnancy has been associated with an increased risk of major fetal anomalies (4.1% vs 2.1% in controls), particularly aplasia cutis, omphalocele, esophageal atresia, and coanal atresia. However, methimazole may be used if the patient cannot tolerate propylthiouracil (see below) and the patient is apprised of the risk. If methimazole is used during pregnancy or breastfeeding, the dose should not exceed 20 mg daily. The dosage is reduced as manifestations of hyperthyroidism resolve and as the FT_4 level falls toward normal. For patients receiving ^{131}I therapy, methimazole is discontinued 4 days prior to receiving the ^{131}I and is resumed at a lower dose 3 days afterwards to avoid recurrence of hyperthyroidism. About 4 weeks after ^{131}I therapy, methimazole may be discontinued if the patient is euthyroid.

B. Propylthiouracil—Propylthiouracil has been the drug of choice during breastfeeding since it is not concentrated in the milk as much as methimazole. Propylthiouracil is also favored during pregnancy, possibly causing fewer problems in the newborn. Initially, propylthiouracil is given orally in doses of 300–600 mg daily in four divided doses. The dosage and frequency of administration are reduced as symptoms of hyperthyroidism resolve and the FT_4 level approaches normal. Rare complications peculiar to propylthiouracil include arthritis, lupus, aplastic anemia, thrombocytopenia, and hypoprothrombinemia. With propylthiouracil, acute hepatitis occurs rarely and is treated with prednisone; liver failure occurs in about 1 in 10,000 patients. During pregnancy, the dose of propylthiouracil is kept below 200 mg/d to avoid goitrous hypothyroidism in the infant; the patient may be switched to methimazole in the second trimester.

3. Iodinated contrast agents—These agents provide effective temporary treatment for thyrotoxicosis of any cause. Iopanoic acid (Telepaque) or ipodate sodium (Bilivist, Oragrafin) is given orally in a dosage of 500 mg twice daily for 3 days, then 500 mg once daily. These agents inhibit peripheral 5′-monodeiodination of T_4, thereby blocking its conversion to active T_3. Within 24 hours, serum T_3 levels fall an average of 62%. For patients with Graves disease, methimazole is begun first to block iodine organification; the next day, ipodate sodium or iopanoic acid may be added. The iodinated contrast agents are particularly useful for patients who are symptomatically very thyrotoxic (see Thyroid Storm). They offer a therapeutic option for patients with T_4 overdosage, subacute thyroiditis, and amiodarone-induced thyrotoxicosis; for those intolerant to thioureas; and for newborns with thyrotoxicosis (due to maternal Graves disease). Treatment periods of 8 months or more are possible, but efficacy tends to wane with time. In Graves disease, thyroid RAI uptake may be suppressed during treatment but typically returns to pretreatment uptake by 7 days after discontinuation of the drug, allowing ^{131}I treatment.

4. Radioactive iodine (^{131}I, RAI)—The administration of ^{131}I is an excellent method of destroying overactive thyroid tissue (either diffuse or toxic nodular goiter). Adolescent and adult patients who have been treated with RAI in adulthood do not have an increased risk of subsequent thyroid cancer, leukemia, or other malignancies. Children born to parents previously treated with ^{131}I show no increase in rates of congenital abnormalities.

Because radiation is harmful to the fetus and children, *RAI should not be given to pregnant or lactating women or to mothers who lack childcare.* Before starting ^{131}I therapy, all women of reproductive age should have a pregnancy test (serum beta-hCG). Ideally, RAI should not be given to women with Graves disease within about 3 months prior to a planned conception.

Patients may receive ^{131}I while being symptomatically treated with propranolol ER, which is then reduced in dosage as hyperthyroidism resolves. A higher rate of ^{131}I treatment failure has been reported in patients with Graves disease who have been receiving methimazole or propylthiouracil. However, therapy with ^{131}I will usually be effective if the methimazole is discontinued at least 4 days before RAI therapy and if the therapeutic dosage of ^{131}I is adjusted (upward) according to RAI uptake on the pretherapy scan. Prior to ^{131}I therapy, patients are instructed against receiving intravenous iodinated contrast or ingesting large quantities of dietary iodine.

The presence of Graves ophthalmopathy is a relative contraindication to ^{131}I therapy. Following ^{131}I treatment for hyperthyroidism, Graves ophthalmopathy appears or worsens in 15% of patients (23% in smokers and 6% in nonsmokers) and improves in none, whereas during treatment with methimazole, ophthalmopathy worsens in 3% and improves in 2% of patients. Among patients receiving prednisone following ^{131}I treatment, preexistent ophthalmopathy worsens in none and improves in 67%. Therefore, patients with Graves ophthalmopathy who are to be treated with radioiodine should be considered for prophylactic prednisone (20–40 mg/d) for 2 months following administration of ^{131}I, particularly in patients who have severe orbital involvement.

Smoking increases the risk of having a flare in ophthalmopathy following ^{131}I treatment and also reduces the effectiveness of prednisone treatment. Patients who smoke are strongly encouraged to quit prior to RAI treatment. Smokers receiving RAI should be considered for prophylactic prednisone (see above).

FT$_4$ levels may sometimes drop within 2 months after ^{131}I treatment, but then rise again to thyrotoxic levels, at which time thyroid RAI uptake is low. This phenomenon is caused by a release of stored thyroid hormone from injured thyroid cells and does not indicate a treatment failure. In fact, serum FT$_4$ then falls abruptly to hypothyroid levels.

There is a high incidence of hypothyroidism in the months to years after ^{131}I, even when small doses are given. Patients with Graves disease treated with ^{131}I also have an increased lifetime risk of developing hyperparathyroidism, particularly when radioiodine therapy was administered in childhood or adolescence. Lifelong clinical follow-up is mandatory, with measurements of serum TSH, FT$_4$, and calcium when indicated.

5. Thyroid surgery—Thyroidectomy may be performed for pregnant women whose thyrotoxicosis is not controlled with low doses of thioureas, and for women who desire to become pregnant in the very near future. Surgery is also an option for nodular goiters, when there is a suspicion for malignancy.

The surgical procedure of choice for patients with Graves disease is a total resection of one lobe and a subtotal resection of the other lobe, leaving about 4 g of thyroid tissue (Hartley–Dunhill operation). Subtotal thyroidectomy of both lobes ultimately results in a 9% recurrence rate of hyperthyroidism. Total thyroidectomy of both lobes poses an increased risk of hypoparathyroidism and damage to the recurrent laryngeal nerves.

Patients are ordinarily rendered euthyroid preoperatively with a thiourea drug. Propranolol ER is given orally at initial doses of 60–80 mg twice daily and increased every 2–3 days until the heart rate is < 90 beats per minute. Propranolol is continued until the serum T$_3$ (or free T$_3$) is normal preoperatively. If a patient undergoes surgery while thyrotoxic, larger doses of propranolol are given perioperatively to reduce the likelihood of thyroid crisis. Ipodate sodium or iopanoic acid (500 mg orally twice daily) may be used in addition to a thiourea to accelerate the decline in serum T$_3$. The patient should be euthyroid by the time of surgery.

To reduce thyroid vascularity preoperatively, the patient may be treated for 3 days prior to surgery with oral potassium iodide 25–50 mg (eg, ThyroShield 65 mg/mL, 0.5 mL, or SSKI 1 g/mL, 1 drop) three times daily or iodinated radiocontrast agents (eg, iopanoic acid 500 mg orally twice daily). However, preoperative potassium iodide often increases the volume of the thyroid, so the requirement for preoperative potassium iodide for Graves disease is debatable. Preoperative iodide supplementation is not recommended prior to surgery for multinodular goiter.

Surgical morbidity includes possible damage to the recurrent laryngeal nerve, with resultant vocal cord paralysis. If both recurrent laryngeal nerves are damaged, airway obstruction may develop, and the patient may require intubation and tracheostomy. Hypoparathyroidism also occurs; serum calcium levels must be checked postoperatively. Patients should be admitted for thyroidectomy surgery for at least an overnight observation period. When a competent, experienced neck surgeon performs a thyroidectomy, surgical complications are uncommon.

B. Treatment of Toxic Solitary Thyroid Nodules

Toxic solitary thyroid nodules are usually benign but may rarely be malignant. If a nonsurgical therapy is elected, the nodule should be evaluated with a fine-needle aspiration (FNA) biopsy. Hyperthyroidism caused by a single hyperfunctioning thyroid nodule may be treated symptomatically with propranolol ER and methimazole or propylthiouracil, as in Graves disease (see above). Patients who tolerate methimazole well may elect to continue it for long-term therapy. The dose of methimazole should be adjusted to keep the TSH slightly suppressed, so the risk of TSH-stimulated growth of the nodule is reduced. For patients under age 40 years and for healthy older patients, surgery is usually recommended; patients are made euthyroid with a thiourea preoperatively and given several days of iodine, ipodate sodium, or iopanoic acid before surgery (see above). Transient postoperative hypothyroidism resolves spontaneously. Permanent hypothyroidism occurs in about 14% of patients by 6 years after surgery. Patients with a toxic solitary nodule who are over age 40 years or in poor health may be offered ^{131}I therapy. If the patient has been receiving methimazole preparatory to ^{131}I, the TSH should be kept slightly suppressed in order to reduce the uptake of ^{131}I by the normal thyroid. Nevertheless, permanent hypothyroidism occurs in about one-third of patients after 8 years of ^{131}I therapy. The nodule remains palpable in 50% and may grow in 10% of patients after ^{131}I.

C. Treatment of Toxic Multinodular Goiter

Hyperthyroidism caused by a toxic multinodular goiter may also be treated with propranolol ER and methimazole, as in Graves disease. Methimazole does reverse hyperthyroidism, but there is a 95% recurrence rate if it is stopped. Definitive treatment for large multinodular goiters is surgery, prior to which patients are rendered euthyroid. Surgery is particularly indicated to relieve pressure symptoms or for cosmetic indications. Patients with toxic multinodular goiter are prepared for surgery the same as those with Graves disease, except they are not treated preoperatively with potassium iodide. Patients who are to receive ^{131}I treatment are rendered nearly euthyroid with methimazole, which is stopped at least 4 days before RAI treatment. Meanwhile, the patient follows a low-iodine diet; this is done to enhance the thyroid gland's uptake of RAI, which may be relatively low in this condition (compared to Graves disease). Relatively high doses of ^{131}I are usually required; recurrent thyrotoxicosis and hypothyroidism are common, so patients must be monitored closely. Peculiarly, in about 5% of patients with diffusely nodular toxic goiter, the administration of ^{131}I therapy may induce Graves disease. Also, Graves eye disease has occurred rarely following ^{131}I therapy for multinodular goiter.

D. Treatment of Hyperthyroidism from Thyroiditis

Subacute (de Quervain) and lymphocytic (Hashimoto) thyroiditis can cause transient hyperthyroidism from release of stored thyroid hormone from the inflamed thyroid. The condition subsides spontaneously within weeks to months. Thioureas are ineffective, since thyroid hormone production is actually low in this condition. In thyroiditis, RAI uptake is low, distinguishing it from Graves disease. For symptomatic relief, patients are treated with propranolol ER 60–80 mg twice daily and increased every 3 days until the heart rate is < 90 beats per minute for symptomatic relief. Ipodate sodium or iopanoic acid, 500 mg orally daily, promptly corrects elevated T_3 levels and is continued for 15–60 days until the serum FT_4 level

normalizes. Patients are monitored carefully for the development of hypothyroidism and treated as needed. RAI is ineffective, since the thyroid's iodine uptake is low. With subacute thyroiditis, pain can usually be managed with nonsteroidal anti-inflammatory drugs, but opioid analgesics are sometimes required.

E. Treatment of Hyperthyroidism during Pregnancy-Planning, Pregnancy, and Lactation

Both men and women with Graves disease who are planning pregnancy should not have radioiodine treatment within about 3 months of conception. Women with Graves disease who are planning to become pregnant are encouraged to consider definitive therapy with RAI or surgery well before conception. Dietary iodine must not be restricted for such women. There is an increased risk of fetal anomalies associated with methimazole in the first trimester. Therefore, women with Graves disease who are being treated with a thiourea should be treated with propylthiouracil through the first trimester and then switched to methimazole. Either thiourea should be given in the smallest dose possible, permitting mild subclinical hyperthyroidism to occur since it is usually well tolerated. About 30% of women with Graves disease experience a remission by the late second trimester.

Both propylthiouracil and methimazole cross the placenta and can induce hypothyroidism, with fetal TSH hypersecretion and goiter. Fetal ultrasound at 20–32 weeks gestation can visualize any fetal goiter, allowing fetal thyroid dysfunction to be diagnosed and treated. Thyroid hormone administration to the mother does not prevent hypothyroidism in the fetus, since T_4 and T_3 do not freely cross the placenta. Fetal hypothyroidism is rare if the mother's hyperthyroidism is controlled with small daily doses of propylthiouracil (50–150 mg orally) or methimazole (5–15 mg orally). Maternal serum TSI levels over 500% at term predict an increased risk of neonatal Graves disease in the infant.

Subtotal thyroidectomy is indicated for pregnant women with Graves disease under the following circumstances: (1) severe adverse reaction to thioureas; (2) high dosage requirement for thioureas (methimazole ≥ 30 mg/d or propylthiouracil ≥ 450 mg/d; (3) uncontrolled hyperthyroidism due to nonadherence to thiourea therapy. Surgery is best performed during the second trimester.

Both methimazole and propylthiouracil are secreted in breast milk, but not in amounts that affect the infant's thyroid hormone levels. No adverse reactions to these drugs (eg, rash, hepatic dysfunction, leukopenia) have been reported in breast-fed infants. Recommended doses are 20 mg orally daily or less for methimazole and 450 mg orally daily or less for propylthiouracil. It is recommended that the medication be taken just after breastfeeding.

F. Treatment of Amiodarone-Induced Thyrotoxicosis

Patients with any type of amiodarone-induced thyrotoxicosis require treatment with propranolol ER for symptomatic relief. Since it is difficult to accurately categorize patients as either type 1 or type 2 amiodarone-induced thyrotoxicosis, it is prudent to treat all patients with methimazole 30 mg orally daily. After two doses of methimazole, iopanoic acid or sodium ipodate may be added to the regimen to further block conversion of T_4 to T_3; the recommended dosage for each is 500 mg orally twice daily for 3 days, followed by 500 mg once daily until thyrotoxicosis is resolved. If iopanoic acid or sodium ipodate is not available, the alternative is potassium perchlorate; it is given in doses of $\leq$ 1000 mg daily (in divided doses) for a course not to exceed 30 days in order to avoid the complication of aplastic anemia. Amiodarone may be withdrawn but this does not have a significant therapeutic impact for several months. For patients with type 1 amiodarone-induced thyrotoxicosis, therapy with ^{131}I may be successful, but only for those with sufficient RAI uptake. Patients with clear-cut type 2 amiodarone-induced thyrotoxicosis are usually also treated with prednisone at an initial dose of about 0.5–0.7 mg/kg orally daily; that dose of prednisone is continued for about 2 weeks and then slowly tapered and finally withdrawn after about 3 months. Subtotal thyroidectomy should be considered for patients with amiodarone-induced thyrotoxicosis that is resistant to treatment.

G. Treatment of Complications

1. Graves orbitopathy—The risk of having a "flare" of orbitopathy following ^{131}I treatment for hyperthyroidism is about 6% for nonsmokers and 23% for smokers. Graves orbitopathy can also be aggravated by thiazolidinediones (eg, pioglitazone, rosiglitazone); these oral diabetic agents should be avoided or withdrawn in patients with Graves disease. Patients with mild orbitopathy may be treated with selenium 100 mcg orally twice daily, which may slow the progression of the disease. For acute, progressive exophthalmos, intravenous methylprednisolone, begun promptly, is superior to oral prednisone, possibly due to improved compliance. Methylprednisolone is given in intravenous pulses, 500 mg weekly for 6 weeks, and then 250 mg weekly for 6 weeks. If oral prednisone is chosen for treatment, it must be given promptly in daily doses of 40–60 mg/d orally, with dosage reduction over several weeks. Higher initial prednisone doses of 80–120 mg/d are used when there is optic nerve compression. Prednisone alleviates acute eye symptoms in 64% of nonsmokers, but only 14% of smokers respond well.

Patients with corticosteroid-resistant acute Graves orbitopathy may also be treated with rituximab. Rituximab may be given by retro-orbital injection, which limits systemic toxicity. The recommended dosing is rituximab 10 mg by retro-orbital injection into the affected eye weekly for 1 month, followed by a 1-month break, then another series of four weekly injections.

Progressive active exophthalmos may be treated with retrobulbar radiation therapy using a supervoltage linear accelerator (4–6 MeV) to deliver 20 Gy over 2 weeks to the extraocular muscles, avoiding the cornea and lens. Prednisone in high doses is given concurrently. Patients who respond well to orbital radiation include those with signs of acute inflammation, recent exophthalmos (< 6 months), or optic nerve compression. Patients with chronic proptosis

and orbital muscle restriction respond less well. Retrobulbar radiation does not cause cataracts or tumors; however, it can cause radiation-induced retinopathy (usually subclinical) in about 5% of patients overall, mostly in diabetics.

For severe cases, orbital decompression surgery may save vision, though diplopia often persists postoperatively. General eye protective measures include wearing glasses to protect the protruding eye and taping the lids shut during sleep if corneal drying is a problem. Methylcellulose drops and gels ("artificial tears") may also help. Tarsorrhaphy or canthoplasty can frequently help protect the cornea and provide improved appearance. Hypothyroidism and hyperthyroidism must be treated promptly.

2. Cardiac complications—

A. Sinus tachycardia—Treatment consists of treating the thyrotoxicosis. A beta-blocker such as propranolol is used in the interim unless there is an associated cardiomyopathy.

B. Atrial fibrillation—Hyperthyroidism must be treated immediately (see above). Other drugs, including digoxin, beta-blockers, and anticoagulants, may be required. Electrical cardioversion is unlikely to convert atrial fibrillation to normal sinus rhythm while the patient is thyrotoxic. Spontaneous conversion to normal sinus rhythm occurs in 62% of patients with return of euthyroidism, but that likelihood decreases with age. Following conversion to euthyroidism, there is a 60% chance that atrial fibrillation will recur, despite normal thyroid function tests. Those with persistent atrial fibrillation may have elective cardioversion following anticoagulation 4 months after resolution of hyperthyroidism.

(1) Digoxin—Digoxin is used to slow a fast ventricular response to thyrotoxic atrial fibrillation; it must be used in larger than normal doses because of increased clearance and an increased number of cardiac cellular sodium pumps requiring inhibition. Digoxin doses are reduced as hyperthyroidism is corrected.

(2) Beta-blockers—Beta-blockers may also reduce the ventricular rate, but they must be used with caution—particularly in patients with cardiomegaly or signs of heart failure—since their negative inotropic effect may precipitate heart failure. Therefore, an initial trial of a short-duration beta-blocker should be considered, such as esmolol intravenously. If a beta-blocker is used, doses of digoxin must be reduced.

(3) Anticoagulants—Anticoagulation is indicated in the following situations: left atrial enlargement on echocardiogram, global left ventricular dysfunction, recent heart failure, hypertension, recurrent atrial fibrillation, or a history of previous thromboembolism. The doses of warfarin required in thyrotoxicosis are smaller than normal because of an accelerated plasma clearance of vitamin K–dependent clotting factors. Higher warfarin doses are usually required as hyperthyroidism subsides.

C. Heart failure—Thyrotoxicosis can cause heart failure due to extreme tachycardia, cardiomyopathy, or both. Very aggressive treatment of the hyperthyroidism is required in either case (see Thyroid Crisis, below). The tachycardia from atrial fibrillation is treated with digoxin. Intravenous furosemide is typically required. Oral spironolactone or eplerenone may be helpful. If tachycardia appears to be the main cause of the failure, beta-blockers are administered cautiously.

Heart failure may occur as a result of low-output dilated cardiomyopathy in the setting of hyperthyroidism. It is uncommon and may be caused by an idiosyncratic severe toxic effect of hyperthyroidism upon certain hearts. Cardiomyopathy may occur at any age and without preexisting cardiac disease. Beta-blockers and calcium channel blockers are avoided. Emergency treatment may include afterload reduction, diuretics, digoxin, and other inotropic agents while the patient is being rendered euthyroid. Heart failure usually persists despite correction of hyperthyroidism.

D. APATHETIC HYPERTHYROIDISM—Apathetic hyperthyroidism may present with angina pectoris. Treatment is directed at reversing the hyperthyroidism as well as providing standard antianginal therapy. PCI or CABG can often be avoided by prompt diagnosis and treatment.

3. Thyroid crisis or "storm"—This disorder, rarely seen today, is an extreme form of thyrotoxicosis that may be triggered by stressful illness, thyroid surgery, or RAI administration. Its manifestations often include marked delirium, severe tachycardia, vomiting, diarrhea, dehydration and very high fever. The mortality rate is high.

A thiourea drug is given (eg, methimazole, 15–25 mg orally every 6 hours or propylthiouracil, 150–250 mg orally every 6 hours). Ipodate sodium (500 mg/d orally) can be helpful if begun 1 hour after the first dose of thiourea. Iodide is given 1 hour later as Lugol solution (10 drops three times daily orally) or as sodium iodide (1 g intravenously slowly). Propranolol is given (cautiously in the presence of heart failure; see above) in a dosage of 0.5–2 mg intravenously every 4 hours or 20–120 mg orally every 6 hours. Hydrocortisone is usually given in doses of 50 mg orally every 6 hours, with rapid dosage reduction as the clinical situation improves. Aspirin is avoided since it displaces T_4 from thyroxine-binding globulin (TBG), raising FT_4 serum levels. Definitive treatment with ^{131}I or surgery is delayed until the patient is euthyroid.

4. Hyperthyroidism from postpartum thyroiditis—Propranolol ER is given during the hyperthyroid phase followed by levothyroxine during the hypothyroidism phase (see Thyroiditis, below).

5. Graves dermopathy—Treatment involves application of a topical corticosteroid (eg, fluocinolone) with nocturnal plastic occlusive dressings.

6. Thyrotoxic hypokalemic periodic paralysis—Sudden symmetric flaccid paralysis, along with hypokalemia and hypophosphatemia can occur with hyperthyroidism. There are often few classic signs of thyrotoxicosis. It is most prevalent in Asian and Native Americans with hyperthyroidism and is 30 times more common in men than women. Therapy with oral propranolol, 3 mg/kg in divided doses, normalizes the serum potassium and phosphate levels and reverses the paralysis within 2–3 hours.

No intravenous potassium or phosphate is ordinarily required. Intravenous dextrose and oral carbohydrate aggravate the condition and are to be avoided. Therapy is continued with propranolol, 60–80 mg orally every 8 hours (or sustained-action propranolol ER daily at equivalent daily dosage), along with a thiourea drug such as methimazole to treat the hyperthyroidism.

▶ **Prognosis**

Graves disease may rarely subside spontaneously, particularly when it is mild or subclinical. Graves disease that presents in early pregnancy has a 30% chance of spontaneous remission before the third trimester. The ocular, cardiac, and psychological complications can become serious and persistent even after treatment. Permanent hypoparathyroidism and vocal cord palsy are risks of surgical thyroidectomy. Recurrences are common following thiourea therapy but also occur after low-dose ^{131}I therapy or subtotal thyroidectomy. With adequate treatment and long-term follow-up, the results are usually good. However, despite treatment for their hyperthyroidism, women experience an increased long-term risk of death from thyroid disease, cardiovascular disease, stroke, and fracture of the femur. Posttreatment hypothyroidism is common. It may occur within a few months or up to several years after RAI therapy or subtotal thyroidectomy. Malignant exophthalmos has a poor prognosis unless treated aggressively.

Subclinical hyperthyroidism refers to a condition in which asymptomatic individuals have a low serum TSH and normal FT_4 and T_3. Most such patients do well without treatment. In one series, clinical hyperthyroidism developed in only one of seven patients after 2 years. In most patients, the serum TSH reverts to normal within 2 years. Most such patients do not have accelerated bone loss. However, if a baseline bone density shows significant osteopenia, bone densitometry may be performed periodically. In persons over age 60 years, serum TSH is very low (< 0.1 mU/L) in 3% and mildly low (0.1–0.4 mU/L) in 9%. The chance of developing atrial fibrillation is 2.8% yearly in elderly patients with very low TSH and 1.1% yearly in those with mildly low TSH. Asymptomatic persons with very low TSH are monitored closely but are not treated unless atrial fibrillation or other manifestations of hyperthyroidism develop.

▶ **When to Admit**

- Thyroid crisis.
- Hyperthyroidism-induced atrial fibrillation with severe tachycardia.
- Thyroidectomy.

Bahn RS et al. Hyperthyroidism and other causes of thyrotoxicosis: management guidelines of the American Thyroid Association and American Association of Clinical Endocrinologists. Thyroid. 2011 Jun;21(6):593–646. [PMID: 21510801]

Bogazzi F et al. Approach to the patient with amiodarone-induced thyrotoxicosis. J Clin Endocrinol Metab. 2010 Jun;95 (6):2529–35. [PMID: 20525904]

Daniels GH et al. Thyroid dysfunction in a phase 2 trial of patients with relapsing-remitting multiple sclerosis. J Clin Endocrinol Metab. 2014 Jan;99(1):80–9. [PMID: 24170099]

De Groot L et al. Management of thyroid dysfunction during pregnancy and postpartum: an Endocrine Society clinical practice guideline. J Clin Endocrinol Metab. 2012 Aug;97(8): 2543–65. [PMID: 22869843]

Franklyn JA et al. Thyrotoxicosis. Lancet. 2012 Mar 24; 379(9821):1155–66. [PMID: 22394559]

Hegedüs L et al. Treating the thyroid in the presence of Graves' ophthalmopathy. Best Pract Res Clin Endocrinol Metab. 2012 Jun;26(3):313–24. [PMID: 22632368]

Marococci C et al; European Group on Graves' Orbitopathy. Selenium and the course of mild Graves' orbitopathy. N Engl J Med. 2011 May 19;364(20):1920–31. [PMID: 21591944]

Nakamura H et al. Analysis of 754 cases of antithyroid drug-induced agranulocytosis over 30 years in Japan. J Clin Endocrinol Metab. 2013 Dec;98(12):4776–83. [PMID: 24057289]

Ross DS. Radioiodine therapy for hyperthyroidism. N Engl J Med. 2011 Feb 10;364(6):542–50. [PMID: 21306240]

Samuels MH. Subacute, silent, and postpartum thyroiditis. Med Clin North Am. 2012 Mar;96(2):223–33. [PMID: 22443972]

Savino G et al. Intraorbital injection of rituximab: a new approach for active thyroid-associated orbitopathy, a prospective case series. Minerva Endocrinol. 2013 Jun;38(2):173–9. [PMID: 23732371]

Seigel SC et al. Thyrotoxicosis. Med Clin North Am. 2012 Mar;96(2):175–201. [PMID: 22443970]

Shinall MC Jr et al. Is potassium iodide solution necessary before total thyroidectomy for Graves disease? Ann Surg Oncol. 2013 Sep;20(9):2964–7. [PMID: 23846785]

THYROIDITIS

ESSENTIALS OF DIAGNOSIS

▸ **Acute and subacute forms:** thyroid gland swelling, sometimes causing pressure symptoms.

▸ **Chronic form:** thyroid gland may or may not be enlarged with rubbery firmness.

▸ Thyroid function tests variable.

▸ Serum antithyroperoxidase and antithyroglobulin antibody levels usually elevated in Hashimoto thyroiditis.

General Considerations

Thyroiditis may be classified as follows: (1) chronic lymphocytic thyroiditis due to autoimmunity (also called Hashimoto thyroiditis), (2) subacute thyroiditis, (3) suppurative thyroiditis, and (4) Riedel thyroiditis.

Hashimoto thyroiditis, an autoimmune condition, is the most common thyroid disorder in the United States. B-lymphocytes invade the thyroid gland, such that the condition is also known as **chronic lymphocytic thyroiditis.** Elevated serum levels of antithyroid antibodies (antithyroperoxidase or antithyroglobulin antibodies, or both) are found in 3% of men and 13% of women. Women over the age of 60 years have a 25% incidence of elevated serum levels of antithyroid antibodies, yet only a small subset of such

individuals ever develops thyroid dysfunction. However, 1% of the population has serum antithyroid antibody titers > 1:640 and they are at particular risk for thyroid dysfunction. The incidence of Hashimoto thyroiditis varies by kindred, race, and by sex; for example, in persons older than 12 years of age in the United States, elevated levels of antithyroid antibodies are found in 14.3% of whites, 10.9% of Mexican-Americans, and 5.3% of blacks.

Hashimoto thyroiditis is six times more common in women than in men. It is commonly familial. Dietary iodine supplementation increases the incidence of Hashimoto thyroiditis. Childhood or occupational exposure to head–neck external beam radiation increases the lifetime risk of Hashimoto thyroiditis. Women with gonadal dysgenesis (Turner syndrome) have a 15% incidence of thyroiditis by age 40 years. Thyroiditis is also commonly seen in patients with hepatitis C. Subclinical thyroiditis is extremely common; autopsy series have found focal thyroiditis in about 40% of women and 20% of men.

Certain drugs can trigger Hashimoto thyroiditis, including the following: tyrosine kinase inhibitors, denileukin diftitox, alemtuzumab, interferon-alpha, interleukin-2, ipilimumab, tremelimumab, thalidomide, lenalidomide, lithium, and amiodarone.

Hashimoto thyroiditis often progresses to hypothyroidism, which may be linked to thyrotropin receptor–blocking antibodies, detected in 10% of patients with Hashimoto thyroiditis. Hypothyroidism is more likely to develop in smokers than in nonsmokers, possibly due to the thiocyanates in cigarette smoke. High serum levels of thyroid peroxidase antibody also predict progression from subclinical to symptomatic hypothyroidism. Although the hypothyroidism is usually permanent, up to 11% of patients experience a remission after several years. Rarely, the thyroid gland goes on to produce *excessive* thyroid hormone and autoimmune hyperthyroidism (see Graves disease).

Hashimoto thyroiditis is sometimes associated with other endocrine deficiencies as part of polyglandular autoimmunity (PGA). Adults with type 2 PGA are prone to autoimmune thyroiditis, diabetes mellitus type 1, autoimmune gonadal failure, hypoparathyroidism, and adrenal insufficiency (see Adrenal Insufficiency). Thyroiditis is frequently associated with other autoimmune conditions: pernicious anemia, Sjögren syndrome, vitiligo, inflammatory bowel disease, celiac disease, and gluten sensitivity. It is less commonly associated with alopecia areata, hypophysitis, encephalitis, myocarditis, primary pulmonary hypertension, and membranous nephropathy.

Painless postpartum thyroiditis refers to autoimmune thyroiditis that occurs soon after delivery in 7.2% of women. Women in whom postpartum thyroiditis develops have a 70% chance of recurrence after subsequent pregnancies. It occurs most commonly in women who have high levels of thyroid peroxidase antibody in the first trimester of pregnancy or immediately after delivery. It is also more common in women with other autoimmunity or a family history of Hashimoto thyroiditis.

Painless sporadic thyroiditis is thought to be a subacute form of Hashimoto thyroiditis that is similar to painless postpartum thyroiditis (see above), except that it is not related to pregnancy. It accounts for about 1% of cases of thyrotoxicosis.

Subacute thyroiditis—also called de Quervain thyroiditis, granulomatous thyroiditis, and giant cell thyroiditis—is relatively common. It is believed to be caused by a viral infection and often follows an upper respiratory tract infection. Its incidence peaks in the summer. It accounts for up to 5% of clinical thyroid disease and young and middle-aged women are most commonly affected.

Suppurative thyroiditis refers to a nonviral infection of the thyroid gland. While usually bacterial, mycobacterial, fungal, and parasitic infections can occur, particularly in immunosuppressed individuals. Suppurative thyroiditis is quite rare, since the thyroid is resistant to infection, largely due to its high iodine content. It tends to affect patients with preexistent thyroid disease. Congenital pyriform sinus fistulas are a cause for recurrent suppurative thyroiditis.

Riedel thyroiditis, also called invasive fibrous thyroiditis, Riedel struma, woody thyroiditis, ligneous thyroiditis, and invasive thyroiditis, is the rarest form of thyroiditis. It is found most frequently in middle-aged or elderly women and is usually part of a multifocal systemic fibrosis syndrome. It may occur as a thyroid manifestation of IgG$_4$-related systemic disease (see Chapter 20).

▶ **Clinical Findings**

A. Symptoms and Signs

In **Hashimoto thyroiditis,** the thyroid gland is usually diffusely enlarged, firm, and finely nodular. One thyroid lobe may be asymmetrically enlarged, raising concerns about neoplasm. Although patients may complain of neck tightness, pain and tenderness are not usually present. About 10% of cases are atrophic, the gland being fibrotic, particularly in elderly women.

Symptoms and signs are mostly related to ambient levels of thyroid hormone. However, depression and chronic fatigue are more common in such patients, even after correction of hypothyroidism. About one-third of patients have mild dry mouth (xerostomia) or dry eyes (keratoconjunctivitis sicca) related to Sjögren syndrome. Associated myasthenia gravis is usually of mild severity, mainly affecting the extraocular muscles and having a relatively low incidence of detectable AChR Ab or thymic disease. Associated celiac disease can produce fatigue or depression, often in the absence of gastrointestinal symptoms.

Postpartum thyroiditis is typically manifested by hyperthyroidism that begins 1–6 months after delivery and persists for only 1–2 months. Then, hypothyroidism tends to develop beginning 4–8 months after delivery.

Thyrotoxic symptoms in **painless sporadic thyroiditis** are usually mild; a small, nontender goiter may be palpated in about 50% of such patients. High serum thyroid peroxidase antibody concentrations are found in only 50%. The course is similar to painless postpartum thyroiditis.

Subacute thyroiditis presents with an acute, usually painful enlargement of the thyroid gland, often with dysphagia. The pain may radiate to the ears. Patients usually have a low-grade fever and fatigue. The manifestations may persist for weeks or months and may be associated with malaise.

If there is no pain, it is called **silent thyroiditis.** Thyrotoxicosis develops in 50% of affected patients and tends to last for several weeks. Subsequently, hypothyroidism develops that lasts 4–6 months. Normal thyroid function typically returns within 12 months, but persistent hypothyroidism develops in 5% of patients.

Patients with **suppurative thyroiditis** usually are febrile and have severe pain, tenderness, redness, and fluctuation in the region of the thyroid gland. **In Riedel thyroiditis,** thyroid enlargement is often asymmetric; the gland is stony hard and adherent to the neck structures, causing signs of compression and invasion, including dysphagia, dyspnea, pain, and hoarseness. Related conditions include retroperitoneal fibrosis, fibrosing mediastinitis, sclerosing cervicitis, subretinal fibrosis, and biliary tract sclerosis.

B. Laboratory Findings

In Hashimoto thyroiditis with clinically evident disease, there are usually increased circulating levels of antithyroid peroxidase (90%) or antithyroglobulin (40%) antibodies. Antithyroid antibodies decline during pregnancy and are often undetectable in the third trimester. Once Hashimoto thyroiditis has been diagnosed, monitoring of these antibody levels is not helpful. The serum TSH level is elevated if thyroid hormone is not elaborated in adequate amounts by the thyroid gland.

Patients with Hashimoto thyroiditis have a 15% incidence of having serum antibodies (IgA tissue transglutaminase [tTG] antibody) associated with celiac disease and at least 5% have clinically significant celiac disease. Seronegative gluten sensitivity is even more common.

In subacute thyroiditis, the ESR is markedly elevated while antithyroid antibody titers are low, distinguishing it from autoimmune thyroiditis. In **suppurative thyroiditis,** both the leukocyte count and ESR are usually elevated.

With hyperthyroidism due to Hashimoto thyroiditis or subacute thyroiditis, serum FT$_4$ levels tend to be proportionally higher than T$_3$ levels, since the hyperthyroidism is due to the passive release of stored thyroid hormone, which is predominantly T$_4$; this is in contrast to Graves disease and toxic nodular goiter, where T$_3$ is relatively more elevated. Because T$_4$ is less active than T$_3$, the hyperthyroidism seen in thyroiditis is usually less severe. Serum levels of TSH are suppressed in hyperthyroidism due to thyroiditis.

C. Imaging

Ultrasound in cases of Hashimoto thyroiditis typically shows a gland with characteristic diffuse heterogeneous density and hypoechogenicity. It helps distinguish thyroiditis from multinodular goiter or thyroid nodules that are suspicious for malignancy. It is also helpful in guiding FNA biopsy of small suspicious thyroid nodules. Color-flow Doppler ultrasonography can help distinguish thyroiditis from Graves disease, since patients with Graves disease have a hypervascular thyroid gland, whereas in thyroiditis there is normal or reduced vascularity.

RAI uptake and scan may be helpful in determining the cause of hyperthyroidism, distinguishing thyroiditis from Graves disease, since patients with subacute thyroiditis exhibit a very low RAI uptake. However, in patients with chronic Hashimoto thyroiditis (euthyroid or hypothyroid), RAI uptake may be normal or high with uneven uptake on the scan; scanning is not useful in diagnosis.

[^{18}F] Fluorodeoxyglucose positron emission tomography (^{18}FDG-PET) scanning frequently shows diffuse thyroid uptake of isotope in cases of thyroiditis. In fact, of all ^{18}FDG-PET scans, about 3% show such uptake. However, discrete thyroid nodules can also be discovered on ^{18}FDG-PET scanning; known as "thyroid PET incidentalomas," 50% are malignant.

D. Fine-Needle Aspiration Biopsy

Patients with **Hashimoto thyroiditis** who have a thyroid nodule should have an ultrasound-guided FNA biopsy, since the risk of papillary thyroid cancer is about 8% in such nodules. When **suppurative thyroiditis** is suspected, an FNA biopsy with Gram stain and culture is required. FNA biopsy is usually not required for subacute thyroiditis but shows characteristic giant multinucleated cells.

▶ Complications

Hashimoto thyroiditis may lead to hypothyroidism or transient thyrotoxicosis. Hyperthyroidism may develop, either due to the emergence of Graves disease or due to the release of stored thyroid hormone, which is caused by inflammation. Variably termed "hashitoxicosis" or "painless sporadic thyroiditis," it is known as postpartum painless thyroiditis when it occurs in women after delivery. Pregnant women with Hashimoto thyroiditis have an increased risk of spontaneous miscarriage in the first trimester of pregnancy. Perimenopausal women with high serum levels of antithyroperoxidase antibodies have a higher relative risk of depression, independent of ambient thyroid hormone levels.

In the suppurative forms of thyroiditis, any of the complications of infection may occur. Subacute and chronic thyroiditis are complicated by the effects of pressure on the neck structures: dyspnea and, in Riedel struma, vocal cord palsy. Papillary thyroid carcinoma or thyroid lymphoma may rarely be associated with chronic thyroiditis and must be considered in the diagnosis of uneven painless enlargements that continue despite treatment; such patients require FNA biopsy.

▶ Differential Diagnosis

Thyroiditis must be considered in the differential diagnosis of all types of goiters, especially if enlargement is rapid. The very low RAI uptake in subacute thyroiditis with elevated T_4 and T_3 is helpful. Thyroid autoantibody tests have been of help in the diagnosis of Hashimoto thyroiditis, but the tests are not specific (positive in patients with multinodular goiters, malignancy [eg, thyroid carcinoma, lymphoma], and concurrent Graves disease). The subacute and suppurative forms of thyroiditis may resemble any infectious process in or near the neck structures. Chronic thyroiditis, especially if the enlargement is uneven and if there is pressure on surrounding structures, may resemble thyroid

carcinoma, and both disorders may be present in the same gland.

▶ Treatment

A. Hashimoto Thyroiditis

If hypothyroidism is present, levothyroxine should be given in the usual replacement doses (0.05–0.2 mg orally daily). In patients with a large goiter and normal or elevated serum TSH, an attempt is made to shrink the goiter by administering levothyroxine in doses sufficient to drive the serum TSH below the reference range while maintaining clinical euthyroidism. Suppressive doses of T_4 tend to shrink the goiter an average of 30% over 6 months. If the goiter does not regress, lower replacement doses of levothyroxine may be given. If the thyroid gland is only minimally enlarged and the patient is euthyroid, regular observation is in order, since hypothyroidism may develop subsequently—often years later. (See Hypothyroidism section.)

B. Subacute Thyroiditis

All treatment is empiric and must be continued for several weeks. Recurrence is common. The drug of choice is aspirin, which relieves pain and inflammation. Thyrotoxic symptoms are treated with propranolol, 10–40 mg every 6 hours. Iodinated contrast agents cause a prompt fall in serum T_3 levels and a dramatic improvement in thyrotoxic symptoms. Sodium ipodate (Oragrafin, Bilivist) or iopanoic acid (Telepaque) is given orally in doses of 500 mg orally daily until serum FT_4 levels return to normal. Transient hypothyroidism is treated with T_4 (0.05–0.1 mg orally daily) if symptomatic.

C. Suppurative Thyroiditis

Treatment is with antibiotics and with surgical drainage when fluctuation is marked.

D. Riedel Struma

The treatment of choice is tamoxifen, 20 mg orally twice daily, which must be continued for years. Tamoxifen can induce partial to complete remissions in most patients within 3–6 months. Its mode of action appears to be unrelated to its antiestrogen activity. Short-term corticosteroid treatment may be added for partial alleviation of pain and compression symptoms. Surgical decompression usually fails to permanently alleviate compression symptoms; such surgery is difficult due to dense fibrous adhesions, making surgical complications more likely.

▶ Prognosis

Hashimoto thyroiditis is occasionally associated with other autoimmune disorders (celiac disease, diabetes mellitus, Addison disease, pernicious anemia, etc). In general, however, patients with Hashimoto thyroiditis have an excellent prognosis, since the condition either remains stable for years or progresses slowly to hypothyroidism, which is easily treated. Although 80% of women with postpartum thyroiditis subsequently recover normal thyroid function, permanent hypothyroidism eventually develops in about 50% within 7 years, more commonly in women who are multiparous or who have had a spontaneous abortion. In subacute thyroiditis, spontaneous remissions and exacerbations are common; the disease process may smolder for months. Papillary thyroid carcinoma carries a relatively good prognosis when it occurs in patients with Hashimoto thyroiditis.

Hennessey JV. Riedel's thyroiditis: a clinical review. J Clin Endocrinol Metab. 2011 Oct;96(10):3031–41. [PMID: 21832114]

Li Y et al. Hashimoto's thyroiditis: old concepts and new insights. Curr Opin Rheumatol. 2011 Jan;23(1):102–7. [PMID: 21124092]

McLeod DS et al. The incidence and prevalence of thyroid autoimmunity. Endocrine. 2012 Oct;42(2):252–65. [PMID: 22644837]

Menconi F et al. Environmental triggers of thyroiditis: hepatitis C and interferon-alpha. J Endocrinol Invest. 2011 Jan;34(1):78–84. [PMID: 21297381]

Samuels MH. Subacute, silent, and postpartum thyroiditis. Med Clin North Am. 2012 Mar;96(2):223–33. [PMID: 22443972]

Stagnaro-Green A. Approach to the patient with postpartum thyroiditis. J Clin Endocrinol Metab. 2012 Feb;97(2):334–42. [PMID: 22312089]

THYROID NODULES & MULTINODULAR GOITER

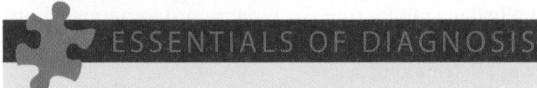

ESSENTIALS OF DIAGNOSIS

► Single or multiple thyroid nodules are commonly found with careful thyroid examinations.

► Thyroid function tests mandatory.

► Thyroid biopsy for single or dominant nodules or for a history of prior head–neck or chest–shoulder radiation.

► Ultrasound examination useful for biopsy and follow-up.

► Clinical follow-up required.

General Considerations

Thyroid nodules are extremely common. In Germany, neck ultrasound screening of adults found a 20% incidence of thyroid nodules > 1 cm in diameter. Palpable nodules are found in 5% of women and 1% of men in iodine-sufficient areas of the world; they are even more common in iodine-deficient areas (see Iodine Deficiency Disorder & Endemic Goiter). Each year in the United States, about 275,000 thyroid nodules are detected by palpation, of which 10% are malignant. Palpable thyroid nodules are increasingly prevalent with age. On high-resolution thyroid ultrasound, about 50% of palpable "solitary nodules" are found to be just one nodule in a multinodular goiter.

In recent years, an increased general use of scanning (CT, MRI, ultrasound, PET) has led to an increased rate of incidentally detecting nonpalpable thyroid nodules.

Although 90% of palpable thyroid nodules are benign, the presence of a thyroid nodule ≥ 1 cm diameter warrants follow-up and further testing for function and malignancy. An occasional nodule < 1 cm diameter requires follow-up if it has high-risk characteristics on ultrasound or if the patient has had prior head-neck radiation therapy. Thyroid nodules that are incidentally discovered with increased standard uptake value (SUV) on [18]FDG-PET scanning have a 33% risk for being malignant and definitely require biopsy.

Most patients with a thyroid nodule are euthyroid, but there is a high incidence of hypothyroidism or hyperthyroidism. About 90% of thyroid nodules are benign adenoma, colloid nodule, or cyst but may sometimes be a primary thyroid malignancy or (less frequently) metastatic neoplasm. Patients with multiple thyroid nodules have the same overall risk of thyroid cancer as patients with solitary nodules. The risk of a thyroid nodule being malignant is higher among patients with a history of head–neck radiation, total body radiation for bone marrow transplantation, exposure to radioactive fallout as a child or teen, a family history of thyroid cancer or a thyroid cancer syndrome (eg, Cowden syndrome, multiple endocrine neoplasia type 2, familial polyposis, Carney syndrome), or a personal history of another malignancy. The risk of malignancy is also higher if there is hoarseness or vocal fold paralysis, and if the thyroid nodule is large, adherent to the trachea or strap muscles, or associated with lymphadenopathy. The presence of Hashimoto thyroiditis does not reduce the risk of malignancy; a nodule of ≥1 cm in a gland with thyroiditis carries an 8% chance of malignancy.

Clinical Findings

Table 26–6 illustrates the approach to the evaluation of thyroid nodules based on the index of suspicion for malignancy.

A. Symptoms and Signs

Most small thyroid nodules cause no symptoms. They may sometimes be detected only by having the patient swallow during careful inspection and palpation of the thyroid.

A thyroid nodule or multinodular goiter can grow to become visible and of concern to the patient. Particularly large nodular goiters can become a cosmetic embarrassment. Nodules can grow large enough to cause discomfort, hoarseness, or dysphagia. Retrosternal large multinodular goiters can cause dyspnea due to tracheal compression. Large substernal goiters may cause superior vena cava syndrome, manifested by facial erythema and jugular vein distention that progress to cyanosis and facial edema when both arms are kept raised over the head (Pemberton sign).

Depending on their cause, goiters and thyroid nodules may be associated with hypothyroidism (Hashimoto thyroiditis, endemic goiter) or hyperthyroidism (Graves disease, toxic nodular goiter, subacute thyroiditis, and thyroid cancer with metastases).

Table 26–6. Clinical evaluation of thyroid nodules.[1]

Clinical Evidence	Low Index of Suspicion	High Index of Suspicion
History	Family history of goiter; residence in area of endemic goiter	Previous therapeutic radiation of head, neck, or chest; hoarseness
Physical characteristics	Older women; soft nodule; multinodular goiter	Young adults, men; solitary, firm nodule; vocal cord paralysis; enlarged lymph nodes; distant metastatic lesions
Serum factors	High titer of antithyroperoxidase antibody; hypothyroidism; hyperthyroidism	Elevated serum calcitonin
Fine-needle aspiration biopsy	Colloid nodule or adenoma	Papillary carcinoma, follicular lesion, medullary or anaplastic carcinoma
Scanning techniques		
Uptake of ^{123}I	Hot nodule	Cold nodule
Ultrasonogram	Cystic lesion	Solid lesion
Roentgenogram	Shell-like calcification	Punctate calcification
Response to thyroxine therapy	Regression after 0.05–0.1 mg/d for 6 months or more	Increase in size

[1]Clinically suspicious nodules should be evaluated with fine-needle aspiration biopsy.

B. Laboratory Findings

A serum TSH level should be obtained for all patients with a thyroid nodule. Patients with a subnormal serum TSH must have a radionuclide (^{123}I or ^{99m}Tc pertechnetate) thyroid scan to determine whether the nodule is hyperfunctioning; hyperfunctioning nodules are rarely malignant. Tests for antithyroperoxidase antibodies and antithyroglobulin antibodies may also be helpful since very high levels are found in Hashimoto thyroiditis. However, thyroiditis frequently coexists with malignancy, so suspicious nodules should always be biopsied. Serum calcitonin is obtained if a medullary thyroid carcinoma is suspected in a patient with a family history of medullary thyroid carcinoma or MEN type 2.

C. Imaging

Neck ultrasonography should be performed to measure the size of a nodule and to determine whether a palpable nodule is part of a multinodular goiter. The following ultrasound characteristics of thyroid nodules increase the likelihood of malignancy: irregular or indistinct margins, heterogenous nodule echogenicity, intranodular vascular images, microcalcifications, complex cyst, or diameter over 1 cm. Ultrasound is also useful for long-term surveillance of thyroid nodules and multinodular goiter. Ultrasonography is generally preferred over CT and MRI because of its accuracy, ease of use, and lower cost. CT scanning is helpful for larger thyroid nodules and multinodular goiter; it can determine the degree of tracheal compression and the degree of extension into the mediastinum.

RAI (^{123}I or ^{131}I) scans have limited usefulness in the evaluation of thyroid nodules. Hypofunctioning (cold) nodules have a somewhat increased risk of being malignant (but most are benign). Hyperfunctioning (hot) nodules are ordinarily benign (but may sometimes be malignant).

RAI uptake and scanning is helpful mainly if a patient is hyperthyroid. (See Hyperthyroidism.)

D. Incidentally Discovered Thyroid Nodules

Thyroid nodules are frequently discovered as an incidental finding, with an incidence that depends on the imaging modality: MRI, 50%; CT, 13%; and ^{18}FDG-PET, 2%. When such scanning detects a thyroid nodule, an ultrasound is performed to better determine the nodule's risk for malignancy and the need for FNA biopsy, and to establish a baseline for ultrasound follow-up. The malignancy risk is about 17% for nodules discovered incidentally on CT or MRI, and 25–50% for nodules discovered incidentally by ^{18}FDG-PET. For incidentally discovered thyroid nodules of borderline concern, follow-up thyroid ultrasound in 3–6 months may be helpful; growing lesions should be biopsied or resected.

E. Fine-Needle Aspiration Biopsy

FNA biopsy is the best method to assess a thyroid nodule for malignancy. FNA biopsy can be done while patients continue taking anticoagulants or aspirin. For multinodular goiters, the four largest nodules ($\geq$ 1 cm diameter) should be biopsied to minimize the risk of missing a malignancy. For solitary thyroid nodules, FNA biopsy is indicated for: (1) nodules > 5 mm diameter with a suspicious appearance on ultrasound; (2) nodules associated with abnormal cervical lymph nodes; (3) nodules $\geq$ 1 cm diameter that are solid or have microcalcifications; (4) mixed cystic-solid nodules $\geq$ 1.5 cm diameter with any suspicious features on ultrasound or $\geq$ 2 cm diameter with benign features on ultrasound; (5) spongiform nodules $\geq$ 2 cm diameter. Pure cystic nodules are benign and do not require FNA biopsy. Using ultrasound guidance for FNA biopsy improves the diagnostic accuracy for both palpable and nonpalpable thyroid nodules. The chance of an optimal tissue sampling is also improved by having an experienced clinician perform the FNA biopsy and by having the aspirate interpreted by a skilled cytopathologist.

In one review of thyroid FNA biopsies, about 70% were benign, 5% were malignant, 10% were "suspicious," and 15% were "nondiagnostic." Nondiagnostic, bloody, or hypocellular FNA biopsies should be repeated under ultrasound guidance; nodules that continue to have nondiagnostic cytology should be monitored closely; those that are solid or that grow should be resected.

When FNA cytology is "suspicious" for papillary thyroid carcinoma or Hürthle cell neoplasm, the risk of malignancy is 57%. When FNA cytology is a "suspicious" for follicular carcinoma, the overall risk of malignancy is about 20–25%, and higher for patients who are much younger or older than age 50. Most patients with suspicious FNA cytology are advised to have surgery.

Cystic nodules yielding serous fluid are usually benign, but the aspirate should be submitted for cytologic testing. Cystic nodules yielding bloody fluid have a higher chance of being malignant.

False-positive thyroid FNA biopsy results occur at a rate of about 4%. False-negative thyroid FNA biopsy results also occur at an overall rate of about 4%, less commonly when performed under ultrasound guidance and interpreted by cytopathologists. False-negative results delay surgical excision and lead to an increased risk of vascular and capsular invasion by the malignancy. Some false-negative FNA biopsy results may not have actually been inaccurate, since truly benign thyroid nodules can later become malignant.

▶ **Treatment**

All thyroid nodules, including those that are benign, need to be monitored by regular periodic palpation and ultrasound about every 6 months initially. After several years of stability, yearly examinations are sufficient. Thyroid nodules should be rebiopsied if growth occurs. A toxic multinodular goiter and hyperthyroidism may develop in patients who have had exposure to large amounts of iodine, either orally (eg, amiodarone) or intravenously (eg, radiographic contrast). Therefore, excessive iodine intake should be minimized. Patients found to have hyperthyroidism may have a RAI uptake and scan, especially if ^{131}I is a therapeutic consideration. Patients with toxic multinodular goiters may also be treated with methimazole, propranolol, or surgery (see Hyperthyroidism). Thyroid nodules require careful clinical evaluation and thyroid palpation or ultrasound examinations.

A. Levothyroxine Suppression Therapy

Patients with elevated levels of serum TSH are treated with levothyroxine replacement. Patients with larger nodules (> 2 cm), elevated or normal TSH levels may be considered for TSH suppression with levothyroxine (starting doses of 50 mcg orally daily). Levothyroxine suppression therapy is not recommended for small benign thyroid nodules. Thyroxine suppression therapy is more successful in iodine-deficient areas of the world. Long-term levothyroxine

suppression of TSH tends to keep nodules from enlarging, but only 20% shrink more than 50%. Thyroid nodule size increased in 29% of patients treated with levothyroxine versus 56% of patients not receiving levothyroxine. Levothyroxine suppression also reduces the emergency of new nodules: 8% with levothyroxine and 29% without levothyroxine. Levothyroxine suppression therapy is not usually given to patients with cardiac disease, since it increases the risk for angina and atrial fibrillation. Levothyroxine suppression causes a small loss of bone density, particularly in postmenopausal women if the serum TSH is suppressed to < 0.05 mU/L. Such patients are advised to have bone density testing every 3–5 years. For patients with a low baseline TSH level, levothyroxine should not be administered, since that is an indication of autonomous thyroid secretion; levothyroxine will be ineffective and could cause thyrotoxicosis.

Levothyroxine suppression needs to be carefully monitored, since it carries a 17% risk of inducing hyperthyroidism. All patients receiving levothyroxine suppression therapy should have serum TSH levels monitored regularly, with the levothyroxine dose adjusted to keep the serum TSH mildly suppressed (between 0.2 mU/L and 0.8 mU/L). Thyroid nodules require careful clinical evaluation and thyroid palpation or ultrasound examinations about every 6 months initially. After several years of stability, yearly examinations are sufficient.

B. Surgery

Total thyroidectomy is required for thyroid nodules that are malignant on FNA biopsy (see Thyroid Cancer). More limited thyroid surgery is indicated for benign nodules with indeterminate or suspicious cytologic test results, compression symptoms, discomfort, or cosmetic embarrassment. Surgery may also be used to remove hyperfunctioning "hot" thyroid adenomas or toxic multinodular goiter causing hyperthyroidism (see Hyperthyroidism).

C. Percutaneous Ethanol Injection

Thyroid cysts can be aspirated, but cystic fluid recurs in 75% of patients. Percutaneous ethanol injection has been used to shrink pure cysts; the success rate is 80%, although it must often be repeated. Percutaneous ethanol injection can also be used to shrink biopsy-proven benign nodules. While complications occur in about 9%, serious or permanent complications are rare.

D. Radioiodine (^{131}I) Therapy

Radioactive ^{131}I is a treatment option for hyperthyroid patients with toxic thyroid adenomas, multinodular goiter, or Graves disease (see Hyperthyroidism). It may also be used to shrink benign nontoxic thyroid nodules. Thyroid nodules shrink an average of 40% by 1 year and 59% by 2 years after ^{131}I therapy. Nodules that shrink after ^{131}I therapy generally remain palpable and become firmer; they may develop unusual cytologic characteristics on FNA biopsy. ^{131}I therapy may be used to shrink large multinodular goiter but may rarely induce Graves disease. Hypothyroidism is a risk and may occur years after ^{131}I therapy, so it is advisable to assess thyroid function every 3 months for the first year, every 6 months thereafter, and immediately for symptoms of hypothyroidism or hyperthyroidism.

Prognosis

The great majority of thyroid nodules are benign. Benign thyroid nodules may involute but usually persist or grow slowly. About 90% of thyroid nodules will increase their volume by ≥ 15% over 5 years; cystic nodules are less likely to grow. Cytologically benign nodules that grow are unlikely to be malignant; in one series, only 1 of 78 rebiopsied nodules was found to be malignant. The prognosis for patients with thyroid nodules that prove to be malignant is determined by the histologic type and other factors (see Thyroid Cancer). Multinodular goiters tend to persist or grow slowly, even in iodine-deficient areas where iodine repletion usually does not shrink established goiters. Patients with very small, incidentally discovered, nonpalpable thyroid nodules require follow-up with thyroid ultrasound every 1–2 years but are at low risk for malignancy. Such nodules, if malignant and excised, have only a minor effect on morbidity and mortality.

Anil G et al. Thyroid nodules: risk stratification for malignancy with ultrasound and guided biopsy. Cancer Imaging. 2011 Dec 28;11:209–23. [PMID: 22203727]

Bahn RS et al. Approach to the patient with nontoxic multinodular goiter. J Clin Endocrinol Metab. 2011 May;96(5):1201–12. [PMID: 21543434]

Bose S et al. Thyroid fine needle aspirate: a post-Bethesda update. Adv Anat Pathol. 2012 May;19(3):160–9. [PMID: 22498581]

Grussendorf M et al. Reduction of thyroid nodule volume by levothyroxine and iodine alone and in combination: a randomized, placebo-controlled trial. J Clin Endocrinol Metab. 2011 Sep;96(9):2786–95. [PMID: 21715542]

Kim MI et al. Diagnostic use of molecular markers in the evaluation of thyroid nodules. Endocr Pract. 2012 Sep–Oct;18(5): 796–802. [PMID: 22982803]

Paschke R et al. Thyroid nodule guidelines: agreement, disagreement and need for future research. Nat Rev Endocrinol. 2011 Jun;7(6):354–61. [PMID: 21364517]

Popoveniuc G et al. Thyroid nodules. Med Clin North Am. 2012 Mar;96(2):329–49. [PMID: 22443979]

THYROID CANCER

ESSENTIALS OF DIAGNOSIS

► Painless swelling in region of thyroid.
► Thyroid function tests usually normal.
► Past history of irradiation to head and neck region may be present.
► Positive thyroid FNA biopsy.

General Considerations

The incidence of papillary and follicular (differentiated) thyroid carcinomas increases with age. The overall female:male ratio is 3:1. The yearly incidence of thyroid cancer has been increasing in the United States, with the number of cases diagnosed annually reaching 37,200, probably as a result of the wider use of CT, MRI, PET, and ultrasound that incidentally find small thyroid malignancies. Thyroid cancer mortality has been stable, accounting for about 1500 deaths in the United States annually. In routine autopsy series, thyroid microcarcinoma (≤ 10 mm diameter) is found with the surprising frequency of 35%. Clearly, most thyroid cancers remain microscopic and indolent. However, larger thyroid cancers (palpable or ≥ 1 cm in diameter) are more malignant and require treatment.

Papillary thyroid carcinoma is the most common thyroid malignancy (Table 26–7). Pure papillary (and mixed papillary-follicular) carcinoma comprises about 80% of all thyroid cancers. It usually presents as a single thyroid nodule, but it can arise out of a multinodular goiter. Papillary thyroid carcinoma is commonly multifocal within the gland, with other foci usually arising de novo rather than representing intraglandular metastases. About 10% of cases present with palpable cervical lymph node metastases from a small cancer. Papillary thyroid carcinomas tend to grow slowly and often remain confined to the thyroid and regional lymph nodes for years. However, they may become

Table 26–7. Some characteristics of thyroid cancer.

	Papillary	Follicular	Medullary	Anaplastic
Incidence	Most common	Common	Uncommon	Uncommon
Average age	42	50	50	57
Females	70%	72%	56%	56%
Invasion				
Juxtanodal	+++++	+	++++++	+++
Blood vessels	+	+++	+++	+++++
Distant sites	+	+++	++	++++
^{123}I uptake	+	++++	0	0
10-year disease-specific survival	97%	92%	78%	7.3%

more aggressive, especially in patients over age 45 years, and most particularly in the elderly. The cancer may invade the trachea and local muscles and may spread to the lungs.

Exposure to head and neck radiation therapy poses a particular threat to children who then have an increased lifetime risk of developing thyroid cancer, including papillary carcinoma. These cancers may emerge between 10 and 40 years after exposure, with a peak occurrence 20–25 years later. After an explosion at the Chernobyl Nuclear Plant in the Ukraine in 1986, the risk of developing papillary thyroid carcinoma was highest among children who were under age 5 at the time of exposure to radiation; emergence of more aggressive papillary thyroid carcinoma occurred within 6–7 years after exposure.

Papillary thyroid carcinoma can occur in familial syndromes as an autosomal dominant trait, caused by loss of various tumor suppressor genes. Such syndromes (with associated features) include familial papillary carcinoma (with papillary renal carcinoma), familial nonmedullary thyroid carcinoma, familial polyposis (with large intestine polyps and gastrointestinal tumors), Gardner syndrome (with small and large intestine polyps, fibromas, lipomas, osteomas), Turcot syndrome (with large intestine polyps and brain tumors), and Cowden syndrome (with nodular goiter, benign or malignant breast lesions, macrocephaly, mental retardation, mucocutaneous lesions, benign or malignant uterine neoplasms, or gastrointestinal hamartomas or ganglioneuromas).

Generally speaking, papillary carcinoma is the least aggressive thyroid malignancy. However, the tumor spreads via lymphatics within the thyroid, appearing to be multifocal in 60% of patients and involving both lobes in 30% of patients. About 80% of patients have microscopic metastases to cervical lymph nodes. Unlike other forms of cancer, patients with papillary thyroid carcinoma who have palpable lymph node metastases do not have a particularly increased mortality rate; however, their risk of local recurrence is increased.

Occult metastases to the lung occur in 10–15% of papillary thyroid cancer. About 70% of small lung metastases resolve following ^{131}I therapy; however, larger pulmonary metastases have only a 10% remission rate.

Microscopic "micropapillary" carcinoma (≤ 1 mm and invisible even on thyroid ultrasound) is a variant of normal, being found in 24% of thyroidectomies performed for benign thyroid disease when 2-mm sections were carefully examined. It thus appears that the overwhelming majority of these microscopic foci never become clinically significant. The surgical pathology report of such a tiny papillary carcinoma that is otherwise benign does not justify aggressive follow-up or treatment because a cancer diagnosis is unwarranted and harmful. All that may be required is yearly follow-up with palpation of the neck and mild TSH suppression by thyroxine.

Follicular thyroid carcinoma and its variants (eg, Hürthle cell carcinoma) account for about 14% of thyroid malignancies; follicular thyroid carcinoma is generally more aggressive than papillary carcinoma. Rarely, some follicular carcinomas secrete enough T_4 to cause thyrotoxicosis if the tumor load becomes significant. Metastases commonly are found in neck nodes, bones, and lungs.

Most follicular thyroid carcinomas avidly absorb iodine, making possible diagnostic scanning and treatment with ^{131}I after total thyroidectomy. The follicular histopathologic features that are associated with a high risk of metastasis and recurrence are poorly differentiated and Hürthle cell (oncocytic) variants. The latter variants do not take up RAI.

Follicular thyroid carcinoma and adenomas develop in patients with Cowden disease, a rare autosomal dominant familial syndrome caused by loss of a tumor suppressor gene; such patients tend to have macrocephaly, multiple hamartomas, early-onset breast cancer, intestinal polyps, facial papules, and other skin and mucosal lesions.

Medullary thyroid carcinoma represents about 3% of thyroid cancers. About one-third of cases are sporadic, one-third are familial, and one-third are associated with MEN type 2. Medullary thyroid carcinoma is often caused by an activating mutation of the *ret* protooncogene (RET) on chromosome 10. Mutation analysis of the *ret* protooncogene exons 10, 11, 13, and 14 detects 95% of the mutations causing MEN 2A and 90% of the mutations causing familial medullary thyroid carcinoma. Patients with MEN 2B have activating mutations in exon 16 of the *ret* protooncogene. These germline mutations can be detected by DNA analysis of peripheral WBCs. Therefore, discovery of a medullary thyroid carcinoma makes genetic analysis mandatory. If a gene defect is discovered, related family members must have genetic screening for that specific gene defect. When a family member with MEN 2A or familial medullary thyroid carcinoma does not have an identifiable *ret* protooncogene mutation, gene carriers may still be identified using family linkage analysis. Even when no gene defect is detectable, family members should have thyroid surveillance every 6 months. Somatic mutations of the *ret* protooncogene can be identified in the tumors of 30% of patients with sporadic (nonfamilial) medullary thyroid carcinoma. (See Multiple Endocrine Neoplasia.)

Medullary thyroid carcinoma arises from parafollicular thyroid cells that can secrete calcitonin, prostaglandins, serotonin, ACTH, corticotropin-releasing hormone (CRH), and other peptides. These peptides can cause symptoms and can be used as tumor markers. Early local metastases are usually present, usually to adjacent muscle and trachea as well as to local and mediastinal lymph nodes. Eventually, late metastases may appear in the bones, lungs, adrenals, or liver. Medullary thyroid carcinoma does not concentrate iodine.

Anaplastic thyroid carcinoma represents about 2% of thyroid cancers. It usually presents in an older patient as a rapidly enlarging mass in a multinodular goiter. It is the most aggressive thyroid carcinoma and metastasizes early to surrounding nodes and distant sites. Local pressure symptoms include dysphagia or vocal cord paralysis. This tumor does not concentrate iodine.

Other thyroid malignancies together represent about 3% of thyroid cancers. **Lymphoma** of the thyroid is more common in older women. Thyroid lymphomas are most commonly B cell lymphomas (50%) or mucosa-associated lymphoid tissue (MALT; 23%); other types include follicular, small lymphocytic, and Burkitt lymphoma and Hodgkin disease. Thyroidectomy is rarely required.

Other cancers may sometimes metastasize to the thyroid, particularly bronchogenic, breast, and renal carcinomas and malignant melanoma.

Clinical Findings

A. Symptoms and Signs

Thyroid carcinoma usually presents as a palpable, firm, nontender nodule in the thyroid. Most thyroid carcinomas are asymptomatic, but large thyroid cancers can cause neck discomfort, dysphagia, or hoarseness (due to pressure on the recurrent laryngeal nerve). About 3% of thyroid malignancies present with a metastasis, usually to local lymph nodes but sometimes to distant sites such as bone or lung. Palpable lymph node involvement is present in 15% of adults and 60% of youths. Metastatic functioning differentiated thyroid carcinoma can sometimes secrete enough thyroid hormone to produce thyrotoxicosis. **Anaplastic thyroid carcinoma** is more apt to be advanced at the time of diagnosis, presenting with dysphagia, hoarseness, dyspnea, and metastases to the lungs. Occasionally, such carcinomas may be discovered while they are still relatively small and localized.

Medullary thyroid carcinoma frequently causes flushing and persistent diarrhea (30%), which may be the initial clinical feature. Patients with metastases often experience fatigue as well as other symptoms. Cushing syndrome develops in about 5% of patients from secretion of ACTH or CRH. Signs of pressure or invasion of surrounding tissues are present in anaplastic or large tumors; recurrent laryngeal nerve palsy can occur.

Lymphoma usually presents as a rapidly enlarging, painful mass arising out of a multinodular or diffuse goiter affected by autoimmune thyroiditis, with which it may be confused microscopically. About 20% of cases have concomitant hypothyroidism.

B. Laboratory Findings

Thyroid function tests are generally normal unless there is concomitant thyroiditis. Follicular carcinoma may secrete enough T_4 to suppress TSH and cause clinical hyperthyroidism. (FNA biopsy is discussed above in Thyroid Nodules.)

Serum thyroglobulin is high in most metastatic papillary and follicular tumors, making this a useful marker for recurrent or metastatic disease. Caution must be exercised for the following reasons: (1) Circulating antithyroglobulin antibodies can cause erroneous thyroglobulin determinations. However, declining levels of antithyroglobulin antibodies are a good prognostic sign after treatment for differentiated thyroid carcinoma. (2) Thyroglobulin levels may be misleadingly elevated in thyroiditis, which often coexists with carcinoma. (3) Certain thyroglobulin assays falsely report the continued presence of thyroglobulin after total thyroidectomy and tumor resection, causing undue concern about possible metastases. Therefore, unexpected thyroglobulin levels should prompt a repeat assay in another reference laboratory.

Serum calcitonin levels are usually elevated in medullary thyroid carcinoma, making this a marker for metastatic disease. However, serum calcitonin may be elevated in many other conditions, such as thyroiditis; pregnancy; azotemia; hypercalcemia; and other malignancies, including pheochromocytomas, carcinoid tumors, and carcinomas of the lung, pancreas, breast, and colon.

In patients with **medullary thyroid carcinoma**, serum calcitonin and carcinoembryonic antigen (CEA) determinations should be obtained before surgery, then regularly in postoperative follow-up: every 4 months for 5 years, then every 6 months for life. In patients with extensive metastases, serum calcitonin should be measured in the laboratory with serial dilutions. Calcitonin levels remain elevated in patients with persistent tumor but also in some patients with apparent cure or indolent disease. Therefore, serum calcitonin levels > 250 ng/L (> 73 pmol/L) or rising levels of calcitonin are the best indication for recurrence or metastatic disease. Serum CEA levels are usually elevated with medullary carcinoma, making this a useful second marker; however, it is not specific for this carcinoma.

C. Imaging

1. Ultrasound of the neck—Ultrasound of the neck should be performed routinely on all patients with thyroid cancer for the initial diagnosis and for follow-up. Ultrasound is useful in determining the size and location of the malignancy as well as the location of any neck metastases.

2. Radioactive iodine scanning—RAI (^{131}I or ^{123}I) thyroid and whole-body scanning is used after thyroidectomy for surveillance as described below. Iodinated contrast should never be given prior to RAI scanning or RAI therapy, since the large amounts of iodine in contrast media competitively inhibit the uptake of RAI by the thyroid, greatly reducing the effectiveness of subsequent RAI scanning and therapy.

3. CT and MRI scanning—CT scanning may demonstrate metastases and is particularly useful for localizing and monitoring lung metastases but is less sensitive than ultrasound for detecting metastases within the neck. Medullary carcinoma in the thyroid, nodes, and liver may calcify, but lung metastases rarely do so. MRI is particularly useful for imaging bone metastases.

4. PET scanning—PET scanning is particularly useful for detecting thyroid cancer metastases that do not have sufficient iodine uptake to be visible on RAI scans. Metastases are best detected using ^{18}FDG-PET whole-body scanning. The sensitivity of ^{18}FDG-PET scanning for differentiated thyroid cancer is enhanced if the patient is hypothyroid or receiving thyrotropin, which increases the metabolic activity of differentiated thyroid cancer. Disadvantages of PET scanning include its lack of specificity for thyroid cancer as well as its expense and lack of availability in some locations. ^{18}FDG-PET scanning has prognostic implications, since differentiated thyroid cancer metastases with low SUV scores are associated with a better prognosis.

Differential Diagnosis

RAI uptake occurs in many normal tissues and can be mistaken for metastatic differentiated thyroid carcinoma, leading to unnecessary radioiodine therapy. Negative RAI scans are common in early metastatic differentiated thyroid carcinoma. Unfortunately, negative RAI scans also occur frequently with more advanced metastatic thyroid carcinoma, making it more difficult to detect and to distinguish from nonthyroidal neoplasms. An elevated serum thyroglobulin in patients with a clear RAI scan should arouse suspicion for metastases that are not avid for radioiodine.

Complications

The complications vary with the type of carcinoma. Differentiated thyroid carcinomas may have local or distant metastases, and hyperthyroidism can develop in patients with a heavy tumor burden. One-third of medullary thyroid carcinomas secrete serotonin and prostaglandins, producing flushing and diarrhea. The management of patients with medullary carcinomas may be complicated by the coexistence of pheochromocytomas or hyperparathyroidism.

Treatment of Differentiated Thyroid Carcinoma

A. Surgical Treatment

Surgical removal is the treatment of choice for thyroid carcinomas. Neck ultrasound is obtained preoperatively, since suspicious cervical lymphadenoapathy is detected in about 25%. Intraoperative thyroid ultrasound by the surgeon also helps assess the extent of the tumor and lymph node involvement, altering surgical treatment in many cases. For differentiated papillary and follicular carcinoma > 1 cm diameter, total thyroidectomy is performed with limited removal of cervical lymph nodes. For medullary thyroid carcinoma, repeated neck dissections are often required.

Surgery consists of a thyroid lobectomy for an indeterminate "follicular lesion" that is ≤ 4 cm diameter. If malignancy is diagnosed on pathology, a completion thyroidectomy is performed. For indeterminate follicular lesions > 4 cm diameter that are at higher risk for being malignant, a bilateral thyroidectomy is performed as the initial surgery. Higher risk lesions include those with a FNA biopsy that shows marked atypia or that are suspicious for papillary carcinoma and those that occur in patients with a history of radiation exposure or a family history of thyroid carcinoma.

For biopsies that are diagnostic of malignancy, surgery involves lobectomy alone for papillary thyroid carcinomas < 1 cm diameter in patients under age 45 years who have no history of head and neck irradiation and no evidence of lymph node metastasis on ultrasonography. Other patients should have a total or near total thyroidectomy. The advantage of near-total thyroidectomy for differentiated thyroid carcinoma is that multicentric foci of carcinoma are more apt to be resected. Also, there is less normal thyroid tissue to compete with cancer for ^{131}I administered later for scans or treatment. A central neck lymph node dissection is performed at the time of thyroidectomy for patients with nodal metastases that are clinically evident. A lateral neck dissection is performed for patients with biopsy-proven lateral cervical lymphadenopathy. Neck muscle resections are usually avoided for differentiated thyroid carcinoma. However, patients with the Hürthle cell variant of follicular carcinoma may benefit from a modified radical neck dissection. Metastases to the brain are best treated surgically, since treatment with radiation or RAI is ineffective. Levothyroxine is prescribed in doses of 0.05–0.1 mg orally daily immediately postoperatively (see Thyroxine Suppression and Chemotherapy, below). About 2–4 months after surgery, patients require reevaluation and often require therapy with ^{131}I (see below).

Permanent injury to one recurrent laryngeal nerve occurs in between 1–2% and 7% of patients, depending on the experience of the surgeon. Bilateral nerve palsies are rare. Temporary recurrent laryngeal nerve palsies occur in another 5% but often resolve within 6 months. After total thyroidectomy, temporary hypoparathyroidism occurs in 20% and becomes permanent in about 2%. The incidence of hypoparathyroidism may be reduced if accidentally resected parathyroids are immediately autotransplanted into the neck muscles. Thyroidectomy requires at least an overnight hospital admission, since late bleeding, airway problems, and tetany can occur. Ambulatory thyroidectomy is potentially dangerous and should not be done. Following surgery, staging (Table 26–8) should be done to help determine prognosis and to plan therapy and follow-up.

Table 26–8. Pathologic tumor-node-metastasis (pTNM) staging and tumor-related approximate survival rates for adults with appropriately treated differentiated (papillary) thyroid carcinoma based upon patient age, primary tumor size and invasiveness (T), lymph node involvement (N), and distant metastases (M).[1]

Stage	Description	Five-Year Survival	Ten-Year Survival
I	Under 45: any T, any N, no M Over 45: T ≤ 1 cm, no N, no M	99%	98%
II	Under 45: any T, any N, any M Over 45: T > 1 cm limited to thyroid, no N, no M	99%	90%
III	Over 45: T > 4 cm limited to thyroid, no N, no M; or any T limited to thyroid, regional N, no M	95%	75%
IV	Over 45: T local invasion, any N, any M; or T extensive invasion, any N, no M; or any T, any N, distant M	85%	65%

[1]Patients having a relatively worse prognosis include those with familial differentiated thyroid carcinoma.

In pregnant women with thyroid cancer, surgery is usually delayed until after delivery, except for fast-growing tumors that may be resected after 24 weeks gestation; there has been no difference in survival or tumor recurrence rates in women who underwent surgery during or after their pregnancy. Differentiated thyroid carcinoma does not behave more aggressively during pregnancy. But there is a higher risk of complications in pregnant women undergoing thyroid surgery, compared to nonpregnant women.

B. Thyroxine Suppression for Differentiated Thyroid Cancer

Patients who have had a thyroidectomy for differentiated thyroid cancer must take thyroxine replacement for life. Oral thyroxine should be given in doses that suppress serum TSH without causing clinical thyrotoxicosis. Serum TSH should be suppressed below 0.1 mU/L for patients with stage II disease and below 0.05 mU/L for patients with stage III–IV disease. (See Table 26–8.) Although patients receiving thyroxine suppression therapy (TSH < 0.05 mU/L) are at risk for a lower bone density than age-matched controls, the adverse effect upon bone density and fracture risk is relatively minor for patients who remain clinically euthyroid. Nevertheless, patients receiving thyroxine suppression therapy are advised to have periodic bone densitometry.

C. Radioactive Iodine (^{131}I) Therapy for Differentiated Thyroid Cancer

Differentiated thyroid cancers variably retain the normal thyroid's ability to respond to TSH, secrete thyroglobulin, and concentrate iodine. There are two reasons to treat patients with ^{131}I after thyroidectomy: (1) thyroid remnant ablation and (2) treatment of known or suspected thyroid cancer. ^{131}I is usually administered 2–4 months after surgery. Treatment with ^{131}I is repeated 9–12 months later if surveillance RAI scanning shows evidence of metastatic disease. (See Surveillance, below.)

Before starting ^{131}I therapy, patients should follow a low iodine diet for at least 2 weeks. **The low iodine diet** consists of avoiding the following: iodized table salt, sea salt, fish, shellfish, seaweed, commercial bread, dairy products, processed meats, canned or dried fruit, canned fruit juices, highly salted soups and snack foods, black tea, instant coffee, food coloring with Red Dye #3, egg yolks, multivitamins with iodine, or topical iodine. Patients must not be given amiodarone or intravenous radiologic contrast dyes containing iodine. Radioiodine administration is contraindicated in women who are nursing or pregnant. In all women of reproductive age, pregnancy must be excluded prior to radioiodine scanning or therapy.

1. RAI thyroid remnant ablation—A low activity[1] of 30 mCi (1.1 GBq) ^{131}I is given for "remnant ablation" of residual normal thyroid tissues after surgery for

differentiated thyroid cancer. This small amount of ^{131}I is given to patients with no known lymph node involvement who are at low risk for metastases. There are several advantages for thyroid remnant ablation: (1) There is usually remnant normal tissue that can produce thyroglobulin (a useful tumor marker); (2) Remnant ablation using ^{131}I may destroy microscopic deposits of cancer; (3) The post-therapy scan may visualize metastatic cancer that would otherwise have been invisible. However, ^{131}I remnant ablation is not required for patients with stage I papillary thyroid carcinomas < 1 cm diameter (whether unifocal or multifocal), except for patients with unfavorable histopathology (tall-cell, columnar cell, or diffuse sclerosing subtypes).

2. RAI treatment of metastases—Therapy with ^{131}I improves survival and reduces recurrence rates for patients with stage III–IV cancer and those with stage II cancer having gross extrathyroidal extension. RAI therapy is also given to patients with stage II cancer who have distant metastases, a primary tumor > 4 cm diameter, or primary tumors 1–4 cm diameter with lymph node metastases or other high-risk features. Brain metastases do not usually respond to ^{131}I and are best resected or treated with gamma knife radiosurgery (Table 26–8). A post-therapy whole-body scan is performed 2–10 days after ^{131}I therapy.

Staging with RAI scanning or ^{18}FDG-PET/CT scanning assists with determining the activity of ^{131}I to be administered. Treatment protocols vary among institutions. Generally, patients with higher-risk stage 1 cancer or stage 2 cancer are treated with ^{131}I activities of 50–100 mCi (1.8–3.7 GBq). Patients with stage 3–4 cancers typically receive ^{131}I activities of 100–150 mCi (3.7–5.5 GBq). Repeated treatments may be required for persistent radioiodine-avid metastatic disease. Patients with differentiated thyroid carcinoma who have little or no uptake of RAI into metastases (about 35% of cases) should not be treated with ^{131}I. Patients with asymptomatic, stable, radioiodine-resistant metastases should receive levothyroxine to suppress serum TSH and should be carefully monitored for tumor progression.

Some patients have elevated serum thyroglobulin levels but a negative whole-body radioiodine scan and a negative neck ultrasound. In such patients, an ^{18}F-FDG PET/CT scan is obtained. If all scans are negative, the patient has a good prognosis and empiric therapy with ^{131}I is not useful.

Activities of ^{131}I over 100 mCi (3.7 GBq) can cause gastritis, temporary oligospermia, sialadenitis, and xerostomia. Therapy with ^{131}I can cause neurologic decompensation in patients with brain metastases; such patients are treated with prednisone 30–40 mg orally daily for several days before and after ^{131}I therapy. Cumulative doses of ^{131}I over 500 mCi (18.5 GBq) can cause infertility, pancytopenia (4%), and leukemia (0.3%). Pulmonary fibrosis can occur in patients with diffuse lung metastases after receiving cumulative ^{131}I activities over 600 mCi (22 GBq). The kidneys excrete RAI, so patients receiving dialysis require only 20% of the usual ^{131}I activity.

3. Recombinant human TSH (rhTSH)-stimulated ^{131}I therapy—Recombinant human thyroid stimulating hormone (rhTSH, Thyrogen) is given to increase the sensitivity of serum thyroglobulin for residual cancer and to

---

[1]The amount of radioiodine radioactivity given in a procedure is referred to as "activity" and is expressed as Curies (Ci) or Becquerels (Bq), whereas the term "dose" is reserved to describe the amount of radiation absorbed by a given organ or tumor and is expressed as Gray (Gy) or radiation-absorbed dose (RAD).

increase the uptake of ^{131}I into residual thyroid tissue (thyroid remnant "ablation") or cancer. Thyrogen must be kept refrigerated and is administered according to the following protocol: Thyroxine replacement is held for 2 days before rhTSH and for 3 days afterward. For 2 consecutive days, rhTSH (0.9 mg/d) should be administered intragluteally (not intravenously). On the third day, blood is drawn: serum TSH is assayed to confirm that it is > 30 mcU/mL; serum hCG is measured in reproductive-age women to exclude pregnancy; and serum thyroglobulin is measured as a tumor marker. RAI is then administered at the prescribed activity (see above).

Thyrogen should not be administered to patients with an intact thyroid gland because it can cause severe thyroid swelling and hyperthyroidism. Hyperthyroidism can also occur in patients with significant metastases or residual normal thyroid. Other side effects include nausea (11%) and headache (7%). Thyrotropin has caused neurologic deterioration in 7% of patients with central nervous system metastases.

4. Thyroxine-withdrawal stimulated ^{131}I therapy— Thyroxine withdrawal is sometimes used because of its lower cost, despite the discomforts of becoming hypothyroid. Thyroxine is withdrawn for 14 days and the patient is allowed to become hypothyroid; high levels of endogenous TSH stimulate the uptake of RAI and production of thyroglobulin by thyroid cancer or residual thyroid. Just prior to ^{131}I therapy, the following blood tests are obtained: serum TSH to confirm it is > 30 mcU/mL, serum hCG in reproductive-age women to screen for pregnancy, serum thyroglobulin as a tumor marker. Three days after ^{131}I therapy, thyroxine therapy may be resumed at full replacement dose.

5. Side effects and contraindications to ^{131}I therapy— National Cancer Institute surveillance data for thousands of patients with thyroid cancer indicate that patients with differentiated thyroid cancer, treated with only surgery, have a 5% increased risk of developing a second non-thyroid malignancy (especially breast cancer). Patients with thyroid cancer who received ^{131}I therapy have a 20% increased risk of developing a second non-thyroid malignancy (especially leukemia and lymphoma). The risk of second cancers peaks about 5 years following ^{131}I therapy.

Women must not receive RAI therapy if they are pregnant, lactating, or lack childcare. Women are advised to avoid pregnancy for at least 4 months following ^{131}I therapy. Men have been found to have abnormal spermatozoa for up to 6 months following ^{131}I therapy and are advised to use contraceptive methods during that time.

D. Other Therapy for Differentiated Thyroid Cancer

Patients who have osteolytic metastases to bone from differentiated thyroid carcinoma can be treated with zoledronic acid. For patients with asymptomatic osseous metastases, the dose is zoledronic acid 4 mg intravenously every 6 months; for those with symptomatic osseous metastases, the dose is zoledronic acid 4 mg intravenously every 3 months for the first year and then every 6 months.

Patients with aggressive differentiated thyroid carcinoma may have metastases that are not avid for radioiodine or are refractory to ^{131}I therapy. Recurrence in the neck may be treated with surgical debulking and external beam radiation therapy. Such malignancies are usually also resistant to most chemotherapy regimens. However, certain tyrosine kinase inhibitors have achieved objective responses: pazopanib (49%), sunitinib (31%), and axitinib (30%).

► Treatment of Other Thyroid Malignancies

Patients with anaplastic thyroid carcinoma are treated with local resection and radiation. Lovastatin has been demonstrated to cause differentiation and apoptosis of anaplastic thyroid carcinoma cells in vitro, but clinical studies have not been performed. Anaplastic thyroid carcinoma does not respond to ^{131}I therapy and is resistant to chemotherapy.

Patients with thyroid MALT lymphomas have a low risk of recurrence after simple thyroidectomy. Patients with other thyroid lymphomas are best treated with external radiation therapy; chemotherapy is added for extensive lymphoma.

Patients with a *ret* protooncogene mutation should have a prophylactic total thyroidectomy, ideally by age 6 years (MEN 2A) or at age 6 months (MEN 2B). Medullary thyroid carcinoma is best treated with surgery for the primary tumor and metastases. It does not respond to ^{131}I therapy and is generally resistant to chemotherapy. In one study, vandetanib (100 mg orally once daily) produced a partial remission in 16% and stable disease in 53% of patients with locally advanced or metastatic medullary thyroid carcinoma. Vandetanib has reversed Cushing syndrome caused by ectopic ACTH secretion.

External beam radiation therapy may be delivered to bone metastases, especially those that are without radioiodine uptake or are RAI-refractory. Local neck radiation therapy may also be given to patients with anaplastic thyroid carcinoma. Brain metastases can be treated with gamma knife radiosurgery.

► Follow-Up

Most differentiated thyroid carcinoma recurs within the first 5–10 years after thyroidectomy. While lifetime monitoring is recommended, the follow-up protocol can be tailored to the staging and aggressiveness of the malignancy. All patients require at least a yearly thyroid ultrasound and serum thyroglobulin level (while taking levothyroxine). Patients at higher risk have traditionally required at least two annual consecutively negative stimulated serum thyroglobulin determinations < 1 ng/mL and normal RAI scans (if done) and neck ultrasound before they are considered to be in remission. The first surveillance occurs with stimulated postoperative serum thyroglobulin, ^{131}I therapy, and post-therapy scanning about 2–4 months after surgery. (See Treatment.) At 9–12 months postoperatively, patients may receive another stimulated serum thyroglobulin and radioiodine scan. Patients need not have repeated ^{131}I therapies if persistent RAI uptake is confined to the thyroid bed and if neck ultrasounds appear normal and stimulated serum thyroglobulin levels remain < 2 ng/mL. Patients with differentiated thyroid carcinoma must be monitored long-term for recurrent or metastatic disease. Further radioiodine or other scans may be required for patients with more aggressive differentiated thyroid cancer, prior metastases, rising serum thyroglobulin levels, or other evidence of metastases.

1. Serum TSH suppression—Patients with differentiated thyroid cancer are treated with thyroxine doses that are sufficient to suppress the serum TSH below the normal range. For intermediate- or high-risk patients, the serum TSH should be suppressed below 0.1 mU/L, while the target TSH for low-risk patients is 0.1–0.5 mU/mL. Patients who are considered cured should nevertheless be treated with sufficient thyroxine to keep the serum TSH < 2 mU/L. Follow-up must include physical examinations and laboratory testing to ensure that patients remain clinically euthyroid with serum TSH levels in the target range. To achieve suppression of serum TSH, the required dose of thyroxine may be such that serum FT_4 levels may be slightly elevated; in that case, measurement of serum T_3 or free T_3 can be useful to ensure the patient is not frankly hyperthyroid. Thyrotoxicosis can be caused by over-replacement with thyroxine or by the growth of functioning metastases.

2. Serum thyroglobulin—Thyroglobulin is produced by normal thyroid tissue and by most differentiated thyroid carcinomas. It is only after a total or near-total thyroidectomy and ^{131}I remnant ablation that thyroglobulin becomes a useful tumor marker for patients with differentiated papillary or follicular thyroid cancer, particularly for patients who do not have serum antithyroglobulin antibodies.

Detectable thyroglobulin levels do not necessarily indicate the presence of residual or metastatic thyroid cancer. Conversely, baseline serum thyroglobulin levels are insensitive markers for disease recurrence. However, baseline or stimulated serum thyroglobulin levels ≥ 2 ng/mL indicate the need for a repeat neck ultrasound and further scanning with RAI or ^{18}FDG-PET. If serum thyroglobulin levels remain ≥ 2 ng/mL in the presence of normal scanning, it is prudent to repeat the serum thyroglobulin in a national reference laboratory. In one series of patients with differentiated thyroid cancer following thyroidectomy, there was a 21% incidence of metastases in patients with serum thyroglobulin < 1 ng/mL (while receiving thyroxine for TSH suppression). Therefore, *baseline* serum thyroglobulin levels are inadequately sensitive and *stimulated* serum thyroglobulin measurements should be used and *always* with neck ultrasound. The usefulness of routinely doing a radioiodine scan (see below) in low-risk patients is controversial but continues to be done in many centers during stimulation following either rhTSH or thyroid hormone withdrawal, according to described protocols.

3. Neck ultrasound—Neck ultrasound should be used in all patients with thyroid carcinoma to supplement neck palpation; it should be performed preoperatively, 3 months postoperatively, and regularly thereafter. Ultrasound is more sensitive for lymph node metastases than either CT or MRI scanning. Small inflammatory nodes may be detected postoperatively and do not necessarily indicate metastatic disease, but follow-up is necessary. Ultrasound-guided FNA biopsy should be performed on suspicious lesions.

4. Radioactive iodine (RAI: ^{131}I or ^{123}I) neck and whole-body scanning—Despite its limitations, RAI scanning has traditionally been used to detect metastatic differentiated thyroid cancer and to determine whether the cancer is amenable to treatment with ^{131}I. RAI scanning is particularly useful for high-risk patients and those with persistent antithyroglobulin antibodies that make serum thyroglobulin determinations unreliable.

The ^{131}I radioisotope may be used in scanning activities provided it is given < 2 weeks before scheduled ^{131}I treatment to avoid "stunning" metastases such that they take up less of the RAI therapy activity. Alternatively, the ^{123}I radioisotope may also be used and does not stun tumors; it allows single-photon emission computed tomography (SPECT) to better localize metastases. Initial RAI scanning is typically performed about 2–4 months following surgery for differentiated thyroid carcinoma. Whole-body scanning should be performed for at least 30 minutes for at least 140,000 counts and spot views of the neck should be obtained for at least 35,000 counts.

About 65% of metastases are detectable by RAI scanning, but only after optimal preparation: Patients should ideally have a total or near-total thyroidectomy, since any residual normal thyroid competes for RAI with metastases, which are less avid for iodine. It is reasonable to perform a rhTSH-stimulated scan and thyroglobulin level 2–3 months after the initial neck surgery; if the scan is negative and the serum thyroglobulin is < 2 ng/mL, low-risk patients may not require further scanning but should continue to be monitored with neck ultrasound and serum thyroglobulin levels every 6–12 months. For higher-risk patients, the rhTSH-stimulated thyroglobulin and RAI scan may be repeated about 1 year after surgery and then again if warranted. Serum thyroglobulin and radioiodine scanning are stimulated by either rhTSH or thyroid hormone withdrawal according to the protocols described above for ^{131}I treatment.

The combination of rhTSH-stimulated scanning and thyroglobulin levels detects a thyroid remnant or cancer with a sensitivity of 84%. However, the presence of antithyroglobulin antibodies renders the serum thyroglobulin determination uninterpretable. In about 21% of low-risk patients, rhTSH stimulates serum thyroglobulin to above 2 ng/mL; such patients have a 23% risk of local neck metastases and a 13% risk of distant metastases. The rhTSH-stimulated radioiodine neck and whole-body scan detects only about half of these metastases because they are small or not avid for iodine. Some patients have persistent radioiodine uptake in the neck on diagnostic scanning but have no visible tumor on neck ultrasound; such patients do not require additional radioiodine therapy, especially if the serum thyroglobulin level is very low.

5. Positron emission tomography scanning—^{18}FDG-PET scanning is particularly useful for detecting thyroid cancer metastases in patients with a detectable serum thyroglobulin (especially serum thyroglobulin levels >10 ng/mL and rising) who have a normal whole-body RAI scan and an unrevealing neck ultrasound. The patient should be fasting at least 6 hours prior to [18]FDG-PET scanning; water is allowed, but no sweetened beverages. Diabetic patients with serum glucose < 200 mg/dL (< 11.2 mmol/L) may be scanned. [18]FDG-PET scanning can be combined with a CT scan; the resultant [18]FDG-PET/CT fusion scan is 60% sensitive for detecting metastases that are not visible by other methods. This scan is less sensitive for small brain metastases. [18]FDG-PET scanning detects the metabolic activity of tumor tissue; for differentiated thyroid carcinoma, this scan is more sensitive when the patient's thyroid cancer is stimulated with rhTSH (Thyrogen) as described above. One problem with [18]FDG-PET scanning is its lack of specificity. False-positives can occur with benign hepatic tumors, sarcoidosis, radiation therapy, suture granulomas, reactive lymph nodes, or inflammation at surgical sites that can persist for months. False-positive uptake can also occur in muscles and brown fat.

[18]FDG-PET scanning predicts survival better than standard staging; the number, location, and SUV_{max} of metastases are all significant prognostic factors. (See Prognosis.) [18]FDG-PET scanning is particularly sensitive for detecting medullary thyroid carcinoma metastases, and prescan thyrotropin does not improve the PET scan sensitivity for medullary thyroid carcinoma.

6. Other scanning—Thallium-201 (^{201}Tl) scans may be useful for detecting metastatic differentiated thyroid carcinoma when the ^{131}I scan is normal but serum thyroglobulin is elevated. MRI scanning is particularly useful for imaging metastases in the brain, mediastinum, or bones. CT scanning is useful for imaging and monitoring pulmonary metastases.

► **Prognosis**

Papillary thyroid cancer staging and survival data are shown in Table 26–8. [18]FDG-PET scanning independently predicts survival, with patients having few PET-avid metastases and low SUVmax (highest image-pixel standardized uptake value) having a better prognosis. There is generally a good prognosis, particularly for adults under age 45 years, despite the fact that up to 40% of these patients are found to harbor lymph node metastases when extensive lymph node dissections are performed. The following characteristics imply a worse prognosis: age over 45 years, male sex, bone or brain metastases, macronodular (> 1 cm) pulmonary metastases, and lack of ^{131}I uptake into metastases. Younger patients with pulmonary metastases tend to respond better to ^{131}I therapy than do older adults. Certain papillary histologic types are associated with a higher risk of recurrence and reduced survival: tall cell, columnar cell, and diffuse sclerosing types. Brain metastases are detected in 1%; they reduce median survival to 12 months, but the patient's prognosis is improved by surgical resection. Patients with a **follicular variant of papillary carcinoma** have a prognosis somewhere between that of papillary and follicular thyroid carcinoma.

Patients with **follicular carcinoma** have a cancer mortality rate that is 3.4 times higher than patients with papillary carcinoma. The **Hürthle cell variant** of follicular carcinoma

is even more aggressive. Both follicular carcinoma and its Hürthle cell variant tend to present at a more advanced stage than papillary carcinoma. However, at a given stage, the different types of differentiated thyroid carcinoma have a similar prognosis. Patients with primary tumors > 1 cm in diameter who undergo limited thyroid surgery (subtotal thyroidectomy or lobectomy) have a 2.2-fold increased mortality over those having total or near-total thyroidectomies. Patients who have not received ^{131}I ablation have mortality rates that are increased twofold by 10 years and threefold by 25 years (over those who have received ablation). The risk of cancer recurrence is twofold higher in men than in women and 1.7-fold higher in multifocal than in unifocal tumors.

Patients with a normal [18]FDG-PET scan have a 98% 5-year survival, while those having > 10 metastases have a 20% 5-year survival. Those with a SUV_{max} of 0.1-4.6 have a 5-year survival of 85%, while those with a SUV_{max} > 13.3 have a 5-year survival of 20%. Patients with only local metastases have a 5-year survival of 95%, while those with regional (supraclavicular, mediastinal) metastases have a 5-year survival of 70%, and those with distant metastases have a 5-year survival of 35%.

Medullary thyroid carcinoma is more aggressive than differentiated thyroid cancer but is typically fairly indolent. The overall 10-year survival rate is 90% when the tumor is confined to the thyroid, 70% for those with metastases to cervical lymph nodes, and 20% for those with distant metastases. Patients with sporadic disease usually have lymph node involvement noted at the time of diagnosis, whereas distal metastases may not be noted for years. For patients with medullary thyroid carcinoma who have metastases to lymph nodes, modified radical neck dissection is recommended. Familial cases or those associated with MEN 2A tend to be less aggressive; the 10-year survival rate is higher, in part due to earlier detection.

Medullary thyroid carcinoma that is seen in MEN 2B is more aggressive, arises earlier in life, and carries a worse overall prognosis, especially when associated with a germline *M918T* mutation. The elderly tend to have more aggressive medullary thyroid carcinomas. Women with medullary thyroid carcinoma who are under age 40 years have a better prognosis. A better prognosis is also obtained in patients undergoing total thyroidectomy and neck dissection; radiation therapy reduces recurrence in patients with metastases to neck nodes. The mortality rate is increased 4.5-fold when primary or metastatic tumor tissue stains heavily for myelomonocytic antigen M-1. Conversely, tumors with heavy immunoperoxidase staining for calcitonin are associated with prolonged survival even in the presence of significant metastases.

Anaplastic thyroid carcinoma carries a 1-year survival rate of about 10% and a 5-year survival rate of about 5%. Patients with fully localized tumors on MRI have a better prognosis.

Localized lymphoma carries a 5-year survival of nearly 100%. Those with disease outside the thyroid have a 63% 5-year survival. However, the prognosis is better for those with MALT lymphomas. Patients presenting with stridor, pain, laryngeal nerve palsy, or mediastinal extension tend to fare worse.

Ahmed SR et al. Clinical review. Incidentally discovered medullary thyroid cancer: diagnostic strategies and treatment. J Clin Endocrinol Metab. 2011 May;96(5):1237–45. [PMID: 21346073]

Anderson RT et al. Clinical, safety, and economic evidence in radioactive iodine-refractory differentiated thyroid cancer: a systematic literature review. Thyroid. 2013 Apr;23(4): 392–407. [PMID: 23294230]

Brassard M et al; THYRDIAG Working Group. Long-term follow-up of patients with papillary and follicular thyroid cancer: a prospective study on 715 patients. J Clin Endocrinol Metab. 2011 May;96(5):1352–9. [PMID: 21389143]

Brierley JD. Update on external beam radiation therapy in thyroid cancer. J Clin Endocrinol Metab. 2011 Aug;96(8): 2289–95. [PMID: 21816795]

Cox AE et al. Diagnosis and treatment of differentiated thyroid carcinoma. Radiol Clin North Am. 2011 May;49(3):453–62. [PMID: 21569904]

Durante C et al; PTC Study Group. Long-term surveillance of papillary thyroid cancer patients who do not undergo postoperative radioiodine remnant ablation: is there a role for serum thyroglobulin measurement? J Clin Endocrinol Metab. 2012 Aug;97(8):2748–53. [PMID: 22679061]

Mallick U et al. Ablation with low-dose radioiodine and thyrotropin alfa in thyroid cancer. N Engl J Med. 2012 May 3;366 (18):1674–85. [PMID: 22551128]

Pacini F et al. Approach to and treatment of differentiated thyroid carcinoma. Med Clin North Am. 2012 Mar;96(2): 369–83. [PMID: 22443981]

Pathak KA et al. Prognostic nomograms to predict oncological outcome of thyroid cancers. J Clin Endocrinol Metab. 2013 Dec;98(12):4768–75. [PMID: 24152685]

Schlumberger M et al. Strategies of radioiodine ablation in patients with low-risk thyroid cancer. N Engl J Med. 2012 May 3;366(18):1663–73. [PMID: 22551127]

Shaha AR. Recurrent differentiated thyroid cancer. Endocr Pract. 2012 Jul–Aug;18(4):600–3. [PMID: 22849875]

Spencer CA. Clinical review. Clinical utility of thyroglobulin antibody (TgAb) measurements for patients with differentiated thyroid cancers (DTC). J Clin Endocrinol Metab. 2011 Dec;96(12):3615–27. [PMID: 21917876]

Xing M et al. Progress in molecular-based management of differentiated thyroid cancer. Lancet. 2013 Mar 23;381(9871): 1058–69. [PMID: 23668556]

IODINE DEFICIENCY DISORDER & ENDEMIC GOITER

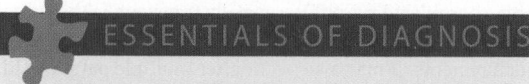

ESSENTIALS OF DIAGNOSIS

► Common in regions with low-iodine diets.

► High rate of congenital hypothyroidism and cretinism.

► Goiters may become multinodular and enlarge.

► Most adults with endemic goiter are found to be euthyroid; however, some are hypothyroid or hyperthyroid.

► General Considerations

About 1 billion people are iodine deficient, having no access to iodized salt and living in areas with iodine-depleted soil. Severe iodine deficiency increases the risk of miscarriage and stillbirth. Cretinism occurs in about 0.5% of live births in iodine-deficient areas. Moderate iodine deficiency during gestation and infancy causes other manifestations of congenital hypothyroidism, such as deafness and short stature and permanently lowers a child's IQ by 10–15 points.

Although iodine deficiency is the most common cause of endemic goiter, there are other natural goitrogens, including certain foods (eg, sorghum, millet, maize, cassava), mineral deficiencies (selenium, iron, zinc), and water pollutants, which can themselves cause goiter or aggravate a goiter proclivity caused by iodine deficiency. In iodine-deficient patients, smoking can induce goiter growth. Pregnancy aggravates iodine deficiency and is associated with an increase in size of thyroid nodules and the emergence of new nodules. Some individuals are particularly susceptible to goiter owing to congenital partial defects in thyroid enzyme activity.

► Clinical Findings

A. Symptoms and Signs

Endemic goiters may become multinodular and very large. Growth often occurs during pregnancy and may cause compressive symptoms.

Substernal goiters are usually asymptomatic but can cause tracheal compression, respiratory distress and failure, dysphagia, superior vena cava syndrome, gastrointestinal bleeding from esophageal varices, palsies of the phrenic or recurrent laryngeal nerves, or Horner syndrome. Cerebral ischemia and stroke can result from arterial compression or thyrocervical steal syndrome. Substernal goiters can rarely cause pleural or pericardial effusions. The incidence of significant malignancy is < 1%.

Some patients with endemic goiter may become hypothyroid. Others may become thyrotoxic as the goiter grows and becomes more autonomous, especially if iodine is added to the diet.

B. Laboratory Findings

The serum T$_4$ and TSH are generally normal. TSH falls in the presence of hyperthyroidism if a multinodular goiter has become autonomous in the presence of sufficient amounts of iodine for thyroid hormone synthesis. TSH rises with hypothyroidism. Thyroid RAI uptake is usually elevated, but it may be normal if iodine intake has improved. Serum levels of antithyroid antibodies are usually either undetectable or in low titers. Serum thyroglobulin is often elevated.

► Differential Diagnosis

Endemic goiter must be distinguished from all other forms of nodular goiter that may coexist in an endemic region.

► Prevention

Adding iodine to commercial salt prevents iodine deficiency. In the United States, potassium iodide is used.

Some tropical countries use potassium iodate, since it is more stable than potassium iodide in hot and humid climates. Iodized salt contains iodine at about 20 mg per kg salt. The minimum dietary requirement for iodine is about 50 mcg daily, with optimal iodine intake being 150–300 mcg daily. Iodine sufficiency is assessed by measurement of urinary iodide excretion, the target being more than 10 mcg/dL. Initiating iodine supplementation in an iodine-deficient area greatly reduces the emergence of new goiters but causes an increased frequency of hyperthyroidism during the first year.

▶ Treatment

The addition of potassium iodide to table salt greatly reduces the prevalence of endemic goiter and cretinism but is less effective in shrinking established goiter. One iodine-depleted area was Pescopagano, Italy, where 46% of adults had goiters. Hyperthyroidism (present or past) occurred in 2.9%, twice the rate seen in iodine-sufficient areas, mostly due to toxic nodular goiter. Hypothyroidism was overt in 0.2% and subclinical in 3.8%. Salt was iodized (30 mg of potassium iodate per kg salt) and made available in 1985. After 15 years, the incidence of goiter declined to 23%. However, the prevalence of Hashimoto thyroiditis rose from 3.5% to 14.5% after 15 years of iodine supplementation.

Iodine supplementation has not proven effective for treating adults with large multinodular goiter and actually increases their risk of developing thyrotoxicosis. Thyroidectomy may be required for cosmesis, compressive symptoms, or thyrotoxicosis. There is a high goiter recurrence rate in iodine-deficient geographic areas, so near-total thyroidectomy is preferred when surgery is indicated. Certain patients may be treated with ^{131}I for large compressive goiters.

▶ Complications

Dietary iodine supplementation increases the risk of autoimmune thyroid dysfunction, which may cause hypothyroidism or hyperthyroidism. Excessive iodine supplementation increases the risk of goiter. Suppression of TSH by administering thyroxine carries the risk of inducing hyperthyroidism, particularly in patients with autonomous multinodular goiters; therefore, thyroxine suppression should not be started in patients with a low TSH level. Treating patients with ^{131}I for large multinodular goiter may shrink the gland; however, Graves disease develops in some patients 3–10 months following therapy.

Aghini Lombardi F et al. The effect of voluntary iodine prophylaxis in a small rural community: the Pescopagano survey 15 years later. J Clin Endocrinol Metab. 2013 Mar;98(3):1031–9. [PMID: 23436921]

Eastman CJ. Screening for thyroid disease and iodine deficiency. Pathology. 2012 Feb;44(2):153–9. [PMID: 22297907]

Laurberg P et al. Iodine intake as a determinant of thyroid disorders in populations. Best Pract Res Clin Endocrinol Metab. 2010 Feb;24(1):13–27. [PMID: 20172467]

Li M et al. The changing epidemiology of iodine deficiency. Nat Rev Endocrinol. 2012 Apr 3;8(7):434–40. [PMID: 22473332]

Medeiros-Neto G et al. Approach to and treatment of goiters. Med Clin North Am. 2012 Mar;96(2):351–68. [PMID: 22443980]

Untoro J et al. The challenges of iodine supplementation: a public health programme perspective. Best Pract Res Clin Endocrinol Metab. 2010 Feb;24(1):89–99. [PMID: 20172473]

Zimmermann MB et al. Prevalence of iodine deficiency in Europe in 2010. Ann Endocrinol (Paris). 2011 Apr;72(2):164–6. [PMID: 21511244]

▼ DISEASES OF THE PARATHYROIDS

Parathyroid hormone (PTH) increases osteoclastic activity in bone, increases the renal tubular reabsorption of calcium, and stimulates the synthesis of 1,25-dihydroxycholecalciferol by the kidney. Meanwhile, PTH inhibits the absorption of phosphate and bicarbonate by the renal tubule. All of these actions cause a net increase in serum calcium).

HYPOPARATHYROIDISM & PSEUDOHYPOPARATHYROIDISM

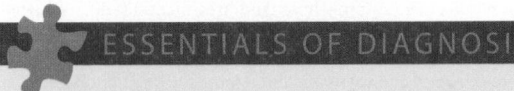

ESSENTIALS OF DIAGNOSIS

▶ Tetany, carpopedal spasms, tingling of lips and hands, muscle and abdominal cramps, psychological changes.

▶ Positive Chvostek sign and Trousseau phenomenon.

▶ Serum calcium low; serum phosphate high; alkaline phosphatase normal; urine calcium excretion reduced.

▶ Low or low-normal serum PTH in presence of hypocalcemia.

▶ Serum magnesium may be low.

▶ General Considerations

Acquired hypoparathyroidism occurs in 10% of patients after thyroidectomy, but it is usually transient, with permanent hypoparathyroidism developing in less than half of such patients. It may also occur after multiple parathyroidectomies. Hypoparathyroidism may occur after surgical removal of a parathyroid adenoma for primary hyperparathyroidism due to suppression of the remaining normal parathyroids and accelerated remineralization of the skeleton. This is known as "hungry bone syndrome." In such cases, hypocalcemia can be quite severe, particularly in patients with preoperative hyperparathyroid bone disease and vitamin D or magnesium deficiency. Neck irradiation may rarely cause hypoparathyroidism.

Autoimmune hypoparathyroidism may be isolated or combined with other endocrine deficiencies in polyglandular autoimmunity (PGA), which is also known as autoimmune polyendocrinopathy-candidiasis-ectodermal dystrophy (APECED). PGA type 1 presents in childhood with at least two of the following manifestations: candidiasis, hypoparathyroidism, or Addison disease. Cataracts, uveitis, alopecia, vitiligo, or autoimmune thyroid disease may also develop. Fat malabsorption occurs in 20% of patients with PGA-1 and may present as weight loss; diarrhea; or malabsorption of vitamin D, a fat-soluble vitamin used to treat the hypoparathyroidism. Hypoparathyroidism can also occur in systemic lupus erythematosus, caused by antiparathyroid antibodies.

Parathyroid deficiency may also be the result of damage from heavy metals such as copper (Wilson disease) or iron (hemochromatosis, transfusion hemosiderosis), granulomas, Riedel thyroiditis, tumors, or infection.

Functional hypoparathyroidism may also occur as a result of magnesium deficiency (malabsorption, chronic alcoholism), which prevents the secretion of PTH. Correction of hypomagnesemia results in rapid disappearance of the condition. Hypermagnesemia can also suppress PTH secretion; it may occur in patients with kidney disease who take magnesium supplements, laxatives, or antacids.

Congenital hypoparathyroidism causes hypocalcemia beginning in infancy. However, it may not be diagnosed for many years. Hypoparathyroidism may also be seen in DiGeorge syndrome, along with congenital cardiac and facial anomalies; hypocalcemia usually presents with tetany in infancy, but some cases are not detected until adulthood.

▶ Clinical Findings

A. Symptoms and Signs

Acute hypoparathyroidism and hypocalcemia can occur spontaneously or may be precipitated when a patient with untreated hypoparathyroidism receives a proton pump inhibitor. Manifestations of hypocalcemia include tetany, muscle cramps, carpopedal spasm, irritability, altered mental status, convulsions, and stridor; tingling of the circumoral area, hands, and feet is almost always present. Symptoms of the chronic disease are lethargy, personality changes, anxiety state, blurring of vision due to premature cataracts, Parkinsonism, and mental retardation. Some patients with chronic hypocalcemia are asymptomatic, even with very low levels of serum calcium.

Chvostek sign (facial muscle contraction on tapping the facial nerve in front of the ear) is positive, and Trousseau phenomenon (carpal spasm after application of a sphygmomanometer cuff) is present. Cataracts may occur; the nails may be thin and brittle; the skin is dry and scaly, at times with fungus infection (candidiasis), and there may be loss of eyebrows; and deep tendon reflexes may be hyperactive. Papilledema and elevated CSF pressure are occasionally seen. Teeth may be defective if the onset of the disease occurs in childhood.

B. Laboratory Findings

Serum calcium is low, serum phosphate high, urinary calcium low, and alkaline phosphatase normal. Serum calcium is largely bound to albumin. In patients with hypoalbuminemia, the serum ionized calcium may be determined, but it has had surprisingly poor clinical utility.

Alternatively, the serum calcium level can be corrected for serum albumin level as follows:

$$\text{"Corrected" serum Ca}^{2+} = \text{Serum Ca}^{2+} \text{ mg/dL} + (0.8 \times [4.0 - \text{Albumin g/dL}])$$

PTH levels are low. Hypomagnesemia may exacerbate symptoms and decrease parathyroid function.

C. Imaging

Radiographs or CT scans of the skull may show basal ganglia calcifications; the bones may be denser than normal. Cutaneous calcification may occur.

D. Other Examinations

Slit-lamp examination may show early posterior lenticular cataract formation. The electrocardiogram (ECG) shows prolonged QT intervals and T wave abnormalities. Patients with chronic hypoparathyroidism tend to have increased bone mineral density, particularly in the lumbar spine.

▶ Complications

Acute tetany with stridor, especially if associated with vocal cord palsy, may lead to respiratory obstruction requiring tracheostomy. Pseudotumor cerebri has been reported. Heart failure may rarely occur. The complications of chronic hypoparathyroidism largely depend on the duration of the disease. There may be associated autoimmunity causing celiac disease, pernicious anemia, or Addison disease. In long-standing cases, cataract formation and calcification of the basal ganglia are seen. Occasionally, parkinsonian symptoms or choreoathetosis develop. Ossification of the paravertebral ligaments may occur with nerve root compression; surgical decompression may be required. Seizures are common in untreated patients. Overtreatment with vitamin D and calcium may produce nephrocalcinosis and impairment of kidney function. Chronic hypocalcemia can cause heart failure.

▶ Differential Diagnosis

Paresthesias, muscle cramps, or tetany due to respiratory alkalosis, in which the serum calcium is normal, can be confused with hypocalcemia. In fact, hyperventilation tends to accentuate hypocalcemic symptoms.

At times hypoparathyroidism is misdiagnosed as idiopathic epilepsy, choreoathetosis, or brain tumor (on the basis of brain calcifications, convulsions, choked disks) or, more rarely, as "asthma" (on the basis of stridor and dyspnea). In patients with hypoalbuminemia, serum levels of ionized calcium are normal.

Hypocalcemia may also be due to malabsorption of calcium, magnesium, or vitamin D; patients do not always have diarrhea. Hypocalcemia may also be caused by certain drugs: loop diuretics, plicamycin, phenytoin, alendronate, and foscarnet. In addition, hypocalcemia may be seen in cases of rapid intravascular volume expansion or due to chelation from transfusions of large volumes of citrated blood. It is also observed in patients with acute pancreatitis. Hypocalcemia may develop in some patients with certain osteoblastic metastatic carcinomas (especially breast, prostate) instead of the expected hypercalcemia. Hypocalcemia with hyperphosphatemia (simulating hypoparathyroidism) is seen in azotemia but may also be caused by large doses of intravenous, oral, or rectal phosphate preparations and by chemotherapy of responsive lymphomas or leukemias.

Hypocalcemia with hypercalciuria may be due to a familial syndrome involving a mutation in the calcium-sensing receptor; such patients have levels of serum PTH that are in the normal range, distinguishing it from hypoparathyroidism. It is transmitted as an autosomal dominant disorder. Such patients are hypercalciuric; treatment with calcium and vitamin D may cause nephrocalcinosis.

Congenital pseudohypoparathyroidism is a group of disorders characterized by resistance to PTH. There are several subtypes caused by different mutations involving the PTH receptor or its G protein or adenylyl cyclase. Renal tubular resistance to PTH causes hypercalciuria with resultant hypocalcemia. PTH levels are high and the PTH receptors in bone are typically not involved, such that bony changes of hyperparathyroidism may be evident. In pseudohypoparathyroidism type 1a, patients have hypocalcemia and hyperphosphatemia with additional features known as Albright hereditary osteodystrophy: mental retardation, short stature, obesity, round face, short fourth metacarpals, ectopic bone formation, hypothyroidism, and hypogonadism. Patients without hypocalcemia but sharing the phenotypic abnormalities are said to have "pseudopseudohypoparathyroidism."

▶ **Treatment**

A. Emergency Treatment for Acute Attack (Hypoparathyroid Tetany)

This usually occurs after surgery and requires immediate treatment.

1. Airway—Be sure an adequate airway is present.

2. Intravenous calcium gluconate—Calcium gluconate, 10–20 mL of 10% solution intravenously, may be given *slowly* until tetany ceases. Ten to 50 mL of 10% calcium gluconate may be added to 1 L of 5% glucose in water or saline and administered by slow intravenous drip. The rate

should be adjusted so that the serum calcium is maintained in the range of 8–9 mg/dL (2–2.25 mmol/L).

3. Oral calcium—Calcium salts should be given orally as soon as possible to supply 1–2 g of calcium daily. Liquid calcium carbonate, 500 mg/5 mL, may be especially useful. The dosage is 1–3 g calcium daily. Calcium citrate contains 21% calcium, but a higher proportion is absorbed with less gastrointestinal intolerance.

4. Vitamin D preparations—(Table 26–9.) Therapy should be started as soon as oral calcium is begun. The active metabolite of vitamin D, 1,25-dihydroxycholecalciferol (calcitriol), has a very rapid onset of action and is not long-lasting if hypercalcemia occurs. It is of great use in the treatment of acute hypocalcemia. Therapy is commenced at a dosage of 0.25 mcg orally each morning with upward dosage titration to near normocalcemia. Ultimately, doses of 0.5–2 mcg/d are usually required. Calcifediol (25-hydroxyvitamin D_3), another option for treatment, has an intermediate onset and duration of action; the usual starting dose is 20 mcg/d orally.

5. Magnesium—If hypomagnesemia is present (chronic alcoholism, malnutrition, renal loss, drugs such as cisplatin, etc), it must be corrected to treat the resulting hypocalcemia. Acutely, magnesium sulfate is given intravenously, 1–2 g every 6 hours. Long-term magnesium replacement may be given as magnesium oxide tablets (600 mg), one or two per day, or as a combined magnesium and calcium preparation (CalMag, others).

6. Transplantation of cryopreserved parathyroid tissue removed during prior surgery—Transplantation restores normocalcemia in about 23% of cases.

B. Maintenance Treatment

The goal should be to maintain the serum calcium in a slightly low but asymptomatic range of 8–8.6 mg/dL (2–2.15 mmol/L). This will minimize the hypercalciuria that would otherwise occur and provides a margin of safety against overdosage and hypercalcemia, which may produce permanent damage to kidney function. Patients with mild, asymptomatic hypocalcemia require no therapy. For others, calcium supplementation (1 g/d) is given, along with a vitamin D preparation.

Table 26–9. Vitamin D preparations used in the treatment of hypoparathyroidism.

	Available Preparations	Daily Dose	Duration of Action
Ergocalciferol, ergosterol (vitamin D_2, calciferol)	50,000 international units capsules; 8000 international units/mL oral solution	2000–200,000 units	1–2 weeks
Cholecalciferol (vitamin D_3)	50,000 international units capsules, not available commercially in United States; may be compounded	10,000–50,000 units	4–8 weeks
Calcitriol (Rocaltrol)	0.25 and 0.5 mcg capsules; 1 mcg/mL oral solution; 1 mcg/mL for injection	0.25–4 mcg	½–2 weeks

Patients with chronic hypoparathyroidism must usually be treated with some type of vitamin D (Table 26–9). Monitoring of serum calcium at regular intervals (at least every 3 months) is mandatory. **Calcitriol,** a short-acting preparation, is given in doses that range from 0.25 mcg/d to 2.0 mcg orally daily. **Ergocalciferol** (vitamin D_2) is derived from plants and is commercially available. The usual dose ranges from 25,000 to 150,000 units/d. It is a slow-acting preparation that is stored in fat, giving it a long duration of action. If toxicity develops, hypercalcemia—treatable with hydration and prednisone—may persist for weeks after it is discontinued. Despite this risk, ergocalciferol usually produces a more stable serum calcium level than do the shorter-acting preparations.

Teriparatide (Forteo) is a recombinant preparation of human PTH 1-34. Teriparatide is effective in treating patients with hypoparathyroidism when given by subcutaneous injection at an initial dose of 0.4 mcg/kg twice daily. The dose is adjusted to produce normal serum calcium levels. The disadvantages of teriparatide therapy include its extremely high cost and the necessity for injections. The US Food and Drug Administration (FDA) has not approved teriparatide for this indication, since prolonged high-dose exposure has caused osteosarcoma in rats. Therefore, teriparatide therapy is reserved for patients with severe hypoparathyroidism that fails to respond to vitamin D.

Target serum calcium levels (albumin-corrected) should be 8.0–8.5 mg/dL (2–2.13 mmol/L); these levels are mildly low to avoid hypercalciuria. It is prudent to monitor urine calcium with "spot" urine determinations and keep the level below 30 mg/dL (7.5 mmol/L), if possible. Hypercalciuria may respond to oral hydrochlorothiazide, usually given with a potassium supplement.

Caution: Phenothiazine drugs should be administered with caution, since they may precipitate extrapyramidal symptoms in hypocalcemic patients. Furosemide should be avoided, since it may worsen hypocalcemia.

▶ Prognosis

The outlook is good if the diagnosis is made promptly and treatment instituted. Any dental changes, cataracts, and brain calcifications are permanent. Periodic blood chemical evaluation is required, since changes in calcium levels may call for modification of the treatment schedule. Hypercalcemia that develops in patients with seemingly stable, treated hypoparathyroidism may be a presenting sign of Addison disease.

Despite optimal therapy, patients with hypoparathyroidism have been reported to have an overall reduced quality of life. Affected patients have a high risk of having mood and psychiatric disorders along with a reduced overall sense of well being.

Al-Azem H et al. Hypoparathyroidism. Best Pract Res Clin Endocrinol Metab. 2012 Aug;26(4):517–22. [PMID: 22863393]
Cooper MS. Disorders of calcium metabolism and parathyroid disease. Best Pract Res Clin Endocrinol Metab. 2011 Dec;25(6): 975–83. [PMID: 22115170]

Cusano NE et al. Mini-review: new therapeutic options in hypoparathyroidism. Endocrine. 2012 Jun;41(3):410–4. [PMID: 22311174]
De Sanctis V et al. Hypoparathyroidism: from diagnosis to treatment. Curr Opin Endocrinol Diabetes Obes. 2012 Dec;19(6): 435–42. [PMID: 23128574]
Fong J et al. Hypocalcemia: updates in diagnosis and management for primary care. Can Fam Physician. 2012 Feb;58(2): 158–62. [PMID: 22439169]
Khan MI et al. Medical management of postsurgical hypoparathyroidism. Endocr Pract. 2010 Dec;6:1–19. [PMID: 21134871]
Sikjaer T et al. PTH treatment in hypoparathyroidism. Curr Drug Saf. 2011 Apr;6(2):89–99. [PMID: 21524246]

HYPERPARATHYROIDISM

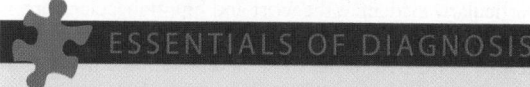

ESSENTIALS OF DIAGNOSIS

- ▶ Frequently detected incidentally by routine blood testing.
- ▶ Renal calculi, polyuria, hypertension, constipation, fatigue, mental changes.
- ▶ Bone pain; rarely, cystic lesions and pathologic fractures.
- ▶ Serum and urine calcium elevated; urine phosphate high with low to normal serum phosphate; alkaline phosphatase normal to elevated.
- ▶ Elevated PTH.

▶ General Considerations

Primary hyperparathyroidism is the most common cause of hypercalcemia, with a prevalence of 1–4 cases per 1000 persons. It occurs at all ages but most commonly in the seventh decade and in women (74%). Before age 45, the prevalence is similar in men and women.

Parathyroid glands vary in number and location and ectopic parathyroid glands have been found within the thyroid gland, high in the neck or carotid sheath, in the retroesophageal space, and within the thymus or mediastinum. Hyperparathyroidism is caused by hypersecretion of PTH, usually by a single parathyroid adenoma (80%), and less commonly by hyperplasia by two or more parathyroid glands (20%), or carcinoma (≤ 1%). However, when hyperparathyroidism presents before age 30 years, there is a higher incidence of multiglandular disease (36%) and parathyroid carcinoma (5%). The size of the parathyroid adenoma correlates with the serum PTH level.

Hyperparathyroidism is familial in about 10% of cases. Parathyroid hyperplasia may arise in MEN types 1, 2A, and 2B. In MEN 1, multiglandular hyperparathyroidism is usually the initial manifestation and ultimately occurs in 90% of affected individuals. Hyperparathyroidism in MEN 2A is less frequent that in MEN 1 and is usually milder. Familial hyperparathyroidism can also occur in the hyperparathyroidism-jaw tumor syndrome, a rare autosomal dominant familial condition in which parathyroid cystic adenomas or carcinomas are associated with ossifying fibromas of the mandible and maxilla as well as renal lesions (cysts, hamartomas, Wilms tumors). Affected individuals usually present with severe hypercalcemia as teenagers or young adults; the pathology is usually a single parathyroid adenoma. (See Table 26–17.)

Hyperparathyroidism results in the excessive excretion of calcium and phosphate by the kidneys. PTH stimulates renal tubular reabsorption of calcium; however, hyperparathyroidism causes hypercalcemia and an increase in calcium in the glomerular filtrate that overwhelms tubular reabsorption capacity, resulting in hypercalciuria. At least 5% of renal calculi are associated with this disease. Diffuse parenchymal calcification (nephrocalcinosis) is seen less commonly. Excessive PTH can cause cortical demineralization that is particularly evident at the wrist and hip; trabecular bone is usually spared as evidenced by relatively higher spinal bone density compared to the wrist. Severe, chronic hyperparathyroidism can cause diffuse demineralization, pathologic fractures, and cystic bone lesions throughout the skeleton, a condition known as **osteitis fibrosa cystica**.

Parathyroid carcinoma is a rare cause of hyperparathyroidism but is more common in patients with serum calcium levels ≥ 14.0 mcg/dL (≥ 3.5 mmol/L). About 50% of parathyroid carcinomas are palpable.

Secondary and tertiary hyperparathyroidism usually occurs in patients with chronic kidney disease, in which hyperphosphatemia and decreased renal production of 1,25-dihydroxycholecalciferol ($1,25[OH]_2D_3$) initially produce a decrease in ionized calcium. The parathyroid glands are stimulated (secondary hyperparathyroidism) and may enlarge, becoming autonomous (tertiary hyperparathyroidism). The bone disease seen in this setting is known as **renal osteodystrophy**. Parathyroid hyperplasia in uremia can result in extremely high serum PTH levels that are associated with uremic vascular calcification. Hypercalcemia often occurs after kidney transplant. Secondary hyperparathyroidism predictably develops in patients with a deficiency in vitamin D. Serum calcium levels are typically in the normal range, but may rise to become borderline elevated with time, with tertiary hyperparathyroidism due to parathyroid glandular hyperplasia. (See Osteomalacia.)

▶ **Clinical Findings**

A. Symptoms and Signs

In the developed world, hypercalcemia is typically discovered incidentally by routine chemistry panels. Many patients are asymptomatic or have mild symptoms that may be elicited only upon questioning. Parathyroid adenomas are usually so small and deeply located in the neck that they are almost never palpable; when a mass is palpated, it usually turns out to be an incidental thyroid nodule.

Symptomatic patients are said to have problems with "bones, stones, abdominal groans, psychic moans, with fatigue overtones." The manifestations are categorized as skeletal and those associated with hypercalcemia.

1. Skeletal manifestations—Hyperparathyroidism causes a loss of cortical bone and a gain of trabecular bone. Low bone density is typically most prominent at the wrist.

Postmenopausal women are prone to asymptomatic vertebral fractures. Although significant bone demineralization is uncommon in mild hyperparathyroidism, osteitis fibrosa cystica may present as pathologic fractures or as "brown tumors" or cysts of the jaw. More commonly, patients experience arthralgias and bone pain, particularly involving the legs.

2. Manifestations of hypercalcemia—Mild hypercalcemia may be asymptomatic. However, hypercalcemia of hyperparathyroidism usually causes a variety of manifestations whose severity is not entirely predictable by the level of serum calcium or PTH. In fact, patients with only mild hypercalcemia can have significant symptoms, particularly depression, constipation, and bone and joint pain. **Neuromuscular** manifestations include paresthesias, muscle cramps and weakness, and diminished deep tendon reflexes. **Central nervous system** manifestations include malaise, headache, fatigue, intellectual weariness, insomnia, irritability, and depression. Patients may have cognitive impairment that can vary from intellectual weariness to more severe disorientation, psychosis, or stupor. **Cardiovascular** symptoms include hypertension, palpitations, prolonged P-R interval, shortened Q-T interval, bradyarrhythmias, heart block, asystole, and sensitivity to digitalis. **Renal** manifestations include polyuria and polydipsia, caused by hypercalcemia-induced nephrogenic diabetes insipidus. Among all patients with newly discovered hyperparathyroidism, calcium-containing kidney stones have occurred or are detectable in about 18%. Patients with asymptomatic hyperparathyroidism have a 7% incidence of asymptomatic calcium nephrolithiasis, compared to 1.6% incidence in age-matched controls. **Gastrointestinal** symptoms include anorexia, nausea, heartburn, vomiting, abdominal pain, weight loss, constipation, and obstipation. Pancreatitis occurs in 3%. **Pruritus** may be present. Calcium may precipitate in the corneas ("band keratopathy"). Calcium may also precipitate in extravascular tissues as well as in small arteries, causing small vessel thrombosis and skin necrosis (calciphylaxis).

3. Hyperparathyroidism during pregnancy—About 67% of women with primary hyperparathyroidism during pregnancy experience complications such as nephrolithiasis, hyperemesis, pancreatitis, muscle weakness, and cognitive changes. Hypercalcemic crisis may occur, especially postpartum. About 80% of fetuses experience complications of maternal hyperparathyroidism, including fetal demise, preterm delivery, and low birth weight. Newborns have hypoparathyroidism that can be permanent. Hypocalcemia in the infant can present with tetany even 2–3 months after delivery.

B. Laboratory Findings

The hallmark of primary hyperparathyroidism is hypercalcemia, with the serum adjusted total calcium > 10.5 mg/dL (> 10.6 mmol/L) (Figure 26–1). The adjusted total calcium = measured serum calcium in mg/dL + [0.8 × (4.0 – patient's serum albumin in g/dL)]. Serum ionized calcium determinations have not proven very helpful clinically, except in hyperproteinemic states (such as hyperalbuminemia,

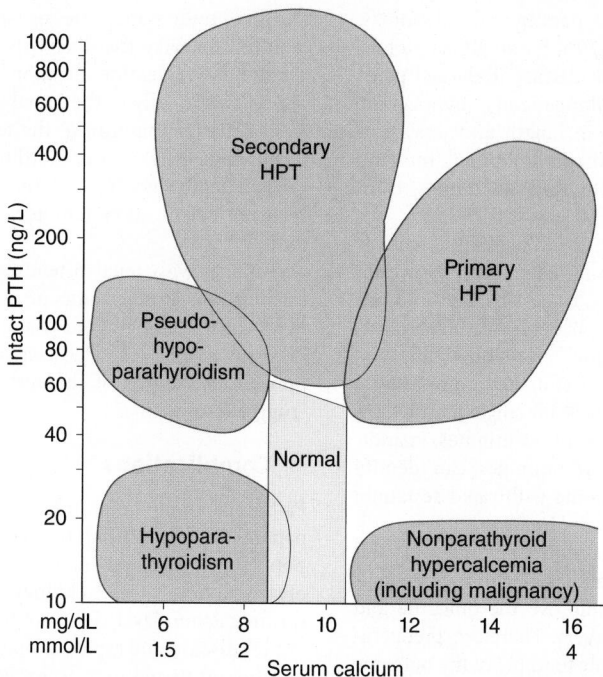

▲ **Figure 26–1.** Parathyroid hormone and calcium nomogram. Relationship between serum intact parathyroid hormone (PTH) and serum calcium levels in patients with hypoparathyroidism, pseudohypoparathyroidism, nonparathyroid hypercalcemia, primary hyperparathyroidism (HPT), and secondary hyperparathyroidism. (Used with permission from GJ Strewler, MD.)

Note: A multivariate model that adds clinical and demographic information may perform better than the nomogram alone. (See O'Neill SS et al. Multivariate analysis of clinical, demographic, and laboratory data for classification of disorders of calcium homeostasis. Am J Clin Pathol. 2011 Jan;135(1):100–7. [PMID: 21173131])

Waldenström macroglobulinemia, myeloma, or thrombocytosis); in such patients with hyperparathyroidism, the serum ionized calcium is usually > 5.4 mg/dL (1.4 mmol/L).

The urine calcium excretion may be high or normal (averaging 250 mg/g creatinine) but it is usually low for the degree of hypercalcemia. The serum phosphate is often < 2.5 mg/dL (< 0.8 mmol/L). There is an excessive loss of phosphate in the urine in the presence of hypophosphatemia (25% of cases), whereas in secondary hyperparathyroidism due to kidney disease, the serum phosphate may be high. The alkaline phosphatase is elevated only if bone disease is present. The plasma chloride and uric acid levels may be elevated. Vitamin D deficiency is common in patients with hyperparathyroidism, and it is prudent to screen for vitamin D deficiency with a serum 25-OH vitamin D determination. Serum 25-OH vitamin D levels < 20 mcg/L (< 50 nmol/L) can aggravate hyperparathyroidism and its bone manifestations; vitamin D replacement may be helpful in treating such patients with hyperparathyroidism.

Elevated serum levels of intact PTH (immunoradiometric assay) confirm the diagnosis of hyperparathyroidism. Patients with apparent hyperparathyroidism should be screened for familial benign hypocalciuric hypercalcemia with a 24-hour urine for calcium and creatinine. Patients should discontinue thiazide diuretics prior to this test. Calcium excretion of < 50 mg/24 hours (< 12.5 mmol/24 hours) or < 5 mg/dL (< 1.25 mmol/L) on a random urine is not

typical for primary hyperparathyroidism and indicates possible familial benign hypocalciuric hypercalcemia.

Patients with low bone density who have an elevated serum PTH but a normal serum calcium must be evaluated for causes of secondary hyperparathyroidism (eg, vitamin D or calcium deficiency, hyperphosphatemia, renal failure). In the absence of secondary hyperparathyroidism, patients with an elevated serum PTH but normal serum calcium are determined to have normocalcemic hyperparathyroidism. Such individuals require monitoring, since hypercalcemia develops in about 19% of patients over 3 years of follow-up.

C. Imaging

Preoperative parathyroid imaging is performed for most patients prior to parathyroid surgery and is particularly important for patients who have had prior neck surgery. Imaging is not necessary for the diagnosis of hyperparathyroidism, which depends on serum parathyroid and calcium levels. But there is occasional diagnostic difficulty and the visualization of an apparent parathyroid adenoma helps secure the diagnosis and often allows for minimally invasive surgery.

Ultrasound of the neck should be performed with a high-resolution transducer (5–15 MHz) and should scan the neck from the mandible to the superior mediastinum in an effort to locate ectopic parathyroid adenomas. Ultrasound has a sensitivity of 79% for single adenomas but only 35% for multiglandular disease. Enlarged parathyroids appear as ovoid, homogeneous, hypoechoic structures that are 0.8–1.5 cm in length and less compressible than surrounding tissue. Doppler imaging assists in distinguishing parathyroid adenomas from other structures.

Sestamibi scintigraphy with (^{99m}Tc)-sestamibi can be useful for localizing parathyroid adenomas. However, false-positive scans are common, caused by thyroid nodules, thyroiditis, or cervical lymphadenopathy. Therefore, three-dimensional single-photon emission computed tomography (SPECT) is most useful. Sestamibi-SPECT imaging improves sensitivity to 98% for single parathyroid adenomas. Dual-phase imaging at 10–15 minutes, in addition to the usual imaging at 90–180 minutes, can identify the occasional parathyroid adenoma with rapid sestamibi washout that is not visible with later imaging.

Preoperative sestamibi-iodine subtraction scanning and neck ultrasonography can locate parathyroid adenomas preoperatively in an effort to improve the outcome and limit the invasiveness of neck surgery. Therefore, preoperative imaging has been used mainly to improve the outcome for limited neck exploration, with only modest success. (See Surgery.) Small benign thyroid nodules are discovered incidentally in nearly 50% of patients with hyperparathyroidism who have imaging with ultrasound or MRI.

Axial imaging is not usually required prior to a first neck surgery for hyperparathyroidism. Conventional CT and MRI are generally inferior to ultrasound and sestamibi imaging. However, a CT imaging technique has been developed, known as four-dimensional CT (4D-CT), with the fourth dimension referring to time. It captures the rapid uptake and washout of contrast from parathyroid adenomas and is particularly useful for preoperative imaging for patients who have had prior neck surgery and for those with ectopic glands. In such patients, 4D-CT has a sensitivity of 88%, versus 54% for sestamibi SPECT and 21% for ultrasound. However, 4D-CT delivers more radiation to the thyroid and is used mostly for older patients. MRI may also be useful for repeat neck operations and when ectopic parathyroid glands are suspected. MRI has the advantages of delivering no radiation and showing better soft tissue contrast than CT.

Patients with hyperparathyroidism have a high risk of calcium nephrolithiasis. Therefore, it has been suggested that all patients with hyperparathyroidism have noncontrast-enhanced CT scanning of the kidneys to determine whether calcium-containing stones are present. For patients with apparently asymptomatic hyperparathyroidism, the presence or absence of calcium nephrolithiasis can be a deciding factor about whether to have parathyroidectomy surgery.

Bone density measurements by dual energy x-ray absorptiometry (DXA) are helpful in determining the amount of bone loss in patients with hyperparathyroidism. Bone loss occurs mostly in long bones, and DXA should ideally include three areas: lumbar spine, hip, and distal radius.

Bone radiographs are usually normal and are not required to make the diagnosis of hyperparathyroidism. There may be demineralization, subperiosteal resorption of bone (especially in the radial aspects of the fingers), or loss of the lamina dura of the teeth. There may be cysts throughout the skeleton, mottling of the skull ("salt-and-pepper appearance"), or pathologic fractures. Articular cartilage calcification (chondrocalcinosis) is sometimes found.

Patients with renal osteodystrophy may have ectopic calcifications around joints or in soft tissue. Such patients may exhibit radiographic changes of osteopenia, osteitis fibrositis cystica, or osteosclerosis, alone or in combination. Osteosclerosis of the vertebral bodies is known as "rugger jersey spine."

▶ Complications

Pathologic long bone fractures are more common in patients with hyperparathyroidism than in the general population. Urinary tract infection due to stone and obstruction may lead to kidney disease and uremia. If the serum calcium level rises rapidly, clouding of sensorium, kidney disease, and rapid precipitation of calcium throughout the soft tissues may occur. Peptic ulcer and pancreatitis may be intractable before surgery. Insulinomas or gastrinomas may be associated, as well as pituitary tumors (MEN type 1). Pseudogout may complicate hyperparathyroidism both before and after surgical removal of tumors. Hypercalcemia during gestation produces neonatal hypocalcemia.

In tertiary hyperparathyroidism due to chronic kidney disease, high serum calcium and phosphate levels may cause disseminated calcification in the skin, soft tissues, and arteries (calciphylaxis); this can result in painful ischemic necrosis of skin and gangrene, cardiac arrhythmias, and respiratory failure. The actual serum levels of calcium and phosphate have not correlated well with calciphylaxis, but a calcium (mg/dL) × phosphate (mg/dL) product over 70 is usually present.

▶ Differential Diagnosis

A. Artifact

A report of hypercalcemia may be due to laboratory error or excess tourniquet time and should always be repeated. Hypercalcemia may be due to high serum protein concentrations; in the presence of very high or low serum albumin concentrations, an adjusted serum calcium or a serum ionized calcium is more dependable than the total serum calcium concentration. Hypercalcemia may also be seen with dehydration; spurious elevations in serum calcium have been reported with severe hypertriglyceridemia, when the calcium assay uses spectrophotometry.

B. Hypercalcemia of Malignancy

Many malignant tumors (breast, lung, pancreas, uterus, renal cell carcinoma, paraganglioma, etc) can produce hypercalcemia. In some cases (breast carcinoma especially), bony metastases are present. In others, no metastases to bone can be demonstrated. Most of these tumors secrete PTH-related protein (PTHrP), which has tertiary structural homologies to PTH and causes bone resorption and hypercalcemia similar to those of PTH. Serum phosphate is often low. Other tumors can secrete excessive 1,25 $(OH)_2$ vitamin D_3, particularly lymphoproliferative and ovarian malignancies. The clinical features of the hypercalcemia of cancer can closely simulate hyperparathyroidism. However, serum PTH levels are usually low. Serum PTHrP or 1,25 $(OH)_2$ vitamin D_3 may be elevated.

Multiple myeloma is a common cause of hypercalcemia in the older population. Many other hematologic cancers, such as monocytic leukemia, T cell leukemia and lymphoma, and Burkitt lymphoma, have also been associated with hypercalcemia.

C. Sarcoidosis and Other Granulomatous Disorders

Macrophages and perhaps other cells present in granulomatous tissue have the ability to synthesize $1,25(OH)_2D_3$. Hypercalcemia has been reported in patients with sarcoidosis, tuberculosis, berylliosis, histoplasmosis, coccidioidomycosis, leprosy, and even foreign-body granuloma. Increased intestinal calcium absorption and hypercalciuria are more common than hypercalcemia. Serum levels of $1,25(OH)_2D_3$ are elevated. Sarcoid granulomas can also secrete PTHrP.

D. Calcium or Vitamin D Ingestion

Ingestion of large amounts of calcium or vitamin D can cause hypercalcemia, especially in patients who concurrently take thiazide diuretics, which reduce urinary calcium loss. Hypercalcemia is reversible following withdrawal of calcium and vitamin D supplements. If hypercalcemia persists, the possibility of associated hyperparathyroidism should be strongly considered.

In vitamin D intoxication, patients may be taking large amounts of vitamin D for unclear reasons, so a thorough review of all medications is important. Hypercalcemia may persist for several weeks. Serum levels of 25-hydroxycholecalciferol $(25[OH]D_3)$ are helpful to confirm the diagnosis. A brief course of corticosteroid therapy may be necessary if hypercalcemia is severe.

E. Familial Benign Hypocalciuric Hypercalcemia

Familial benign hypocalciuric hypercalcemia can be easily mistaken for mild hyperparathyroidism. It is a common autosomal dominant inherited disorder (prevalence: 1 in 16,000) caused by a loss-of-function mutation in the gene encoding the calcium sensing receptor (CaSR). CaSRs are found on the surface of the parathyroid glands and allow the parathyroid glands to vary PTH secretion according to serum calcium levels. Reduced function of the CaSR causes the parathyroid glands to falsely "sense" hypocalcemia and inappropriately release slightly excessive amounts of PTH. The renal tubule CaSRs are also affected, causing hypocalciuria. Familial benign hypocalciuric hypercalcemia is characterized by hypercalcemia, hypocalciuria (usually < 50 mg/24 h), variable

hypermagnesemia, and normal or minimally elevated serum levels of PTH. These patients do not normalize their hypercalcemia after subtotal parathyroid removal and should not be subjected to surgery. The condition has an excellent prognosis and is easily diagnosed with a family history and urinary calcium determination.

F. Adrenal Insufficiency

Hypercalcemia is common in untreated Addison disease. This is partly due to disinhibition of calcium uptake by the renal tubule and gut. Additionally, Addison disease can cause dehydration and hyperproteinemia, resulting in higher levels of nonionized calcium.

G. Immobilization Hypercalcemia

Prolonged immobilization at bed rest commonly causes hypercalcemia, particularly in adolescents, critically ill patients, and patients with extensive Paget disease of bone. Hypercalcemia develops in about one-third of acutely ill patients being treated in intensive care units, particularly patients with acute kidney injury. Serum calcium elevations are typically mild but may reach 15 mg/dL (3.75 mmol/L). Serum PTH levels are usually slightly elevated, consistent with mild hyperparathyroidism, but may be suppressed or normal.

H. Other Causes of Hypercalcemia

Other causes of hypercalcemia are shown in Table 21–8. Modest hypercalcemia is occasionally seen in patients taking thiazide diuretics or lithium; such patients may have an inappropriately nonsuppressed PTH level with hypercalcemia.

Hyperthyroidism causes increased turnover of bone and occasional hypercalcemia. Bisphosphonates can increase serum calcium in 20% and serum PTH becomes high in 10%, mimicking hyperparathyroidism.

▶ Treatment

A. Asymptomatic Primary Hyperparathyroidism

Patients with mild hyperparathyroidism should only be considered "asymptomatic" after very close questioning. Many patients may not realize they have manifestations, such as cognitive slowing, having become accustomed to such symptoms over years. Truly asymptomatic patients may be closely monitored and advised to keep active, avoid immobilization, and drink adequate fluids. For postmenopausal women with hyperparathyroidism, estrogen replacement therapy reduces serum calcium by an average of 0.75 mg/dL (0.19 mmol/L) and slightly improves bone density.

Affected patients should avoid thiazide diuretics, large doses of vitamin A, and calcium-containing antacids or supplements. Serum calcium and albumin are checked about twice yearly, kidney function and urine calcium once yearly, and three-site bone density (distal radius, hip, and spine) every 2 years. Rising serum calcium should prompt further evaluation and determination of PTH levels.

B. Surgical Parathyroidectomy

Parathyroidectomy is recommended for patients with hyperparathyroidism who are symptomatic or pregnant or who have nephrolithiasis or bone disease.

Some patients with seemingly **asymptomatic hyperparathyroidism** may be surgical candidates for other reasons such as (1) serum calcium 1 mg/dL (0.25 mmol/L) above the upper limit of normal with urine calcium excretion > 50 mg/24 h (off thiazide diuretics), (2) urine calcium excretion over 400 mg/24 h, (3) creatinine clearance < 60 mL/min, (4) cortical bone density (wrist, hip) ≥ 2.5 SD below normal or previous fragility bone fracture, (5) relative youth (under age 50–60 years), (6) difficulty ensuring medical follow-up, or (7) pregnancy. During pregnancy, parathyroidectomy is performed in the second trimester. Surgery for patients with "asymptomatic" hyperparathyroidism may improve bone mineral density and confer modest benefits in social and emotional function, with improvements in anxiety and phobias being reported in comparison to similar patients who are monitored without surgery.

Preoperative parathyroid imaging has been used in an attempt to allow unilateral minimally invasive neck surgery. The reported success rates vary considerably. Even in patients with concordant sestamibi and ultrasound scans, and an intraoperative PTH drop of > 50%, hyperparathyroidism may persist postoperatively in up to 15% of patients.

Without preoperative localization studies, bilateral neck exploration is usually advisable for the following: (1) patients with a family history of hyperparathyroidism, (2) patients with a personal or family history of MEN, and (3) patients wanting an optimal chance of success with a single surgery. Patients undergoing unilateral neck exploration can have the incision widened for bilateral neck exploration if two abnormal glands are found or if the serum quick PTH falls by < 63% within 10 minutes of the parathyroid resection. Parathyroid glands are not uncommonly supernumerary (five or more) or ectopic (eg, intrathyroidal, carotid sheath, mediastinum). The optimal surgical management for patients with MEN type 1 is subtotal parathyroidectomy that usually results in a cure, although recurrent hyperparathyroidism develops in 18% and the rate of postoperative hypoparathyroidism is high.

Parathyroid hyperplasia is commonly seen with secondary or tertiary hyperparathyroidism associated with uremia. Cinacalcet is an alternative to surgery. When surgery is performed, a subtotal parathyroidectomy is optimal; three and one-half glands are usually removed, and a metal clip is left to mark the location of residual parathyroid tissue.

Parathyroid carcinoma can cause severe hypercalcemia associated with very high serum levels of PTH. Preoperative localizing studies usually detect a large invasive tumor. Therapy consists of en bloc resection of the tumor and the ipsilateral thyroid lobe. Metastases to local and to distant sites occur in about 50% of patients. Reoperation for neck recurrence is usually necessary. Adjuvant treatment includes radiation therapy. Cinacalcet is administered initially in doses of 30 mg twice daily and increased as needed up to 90 mg four times daily. Intravenous bisphosphonate (zoledronic acid) is used as needed.

Complications—Serum PTH levels fall below normal in 70% of patients within hours after successful surgery, commonly causing hypocalcemic paresthesias or even tetany. Hypocalcemia tends to occur the evening after surgery or on the next day. Therefore, frequent postoperative monitoring of serum calcium (or serum calcium plus albumin) is advisable beginning the evening after surgery. Once hypercalcemia has resolved, liquid or chewable calcium carbonate is given orally to reduce the likelihood of hypocalcemia. Symptomatic hypocalcemia is treated with larger doses of calcium; calcitriol (0.25–1 mcg daily orally) may be added, with the dosage depending on symptom severity. Magnesium salts are sometimes required postoperatively, since adequate magnesium is required for functional recovery of the remaining suppressed parathyroid glands.

In about 12% of patients having successful parathyroid surgery, PTH levels rise above normal (while serum calcium is normal or low) by 1 week postoperatively. This secondary hyperparathyroidism is probably due to "hungry bones" and is treated with calcium and vitamin D preparations. Such therapy is usually needed only for 3–6 months but is required long-term by some patients.

Hyperthyroidism commonly occurs immediately following parathyroid surgery. It is caused by release of stored thyroid hormone during surgical manipulation of the thyroid. In symptomatic patients, short-term treatment with propranolol may be required for several days.

C. Medical Measures

1. Fluids—Hypercalcemia is treated with a large fluid intake unless contraindicated. Severe hypercalcemia requires hospitalization and intensive hydration with intravenous saline. (See Chapter 21.)

2. Bisphosphonates—Intravenous bisphosphonates are potent inhibitors of bone resorption and can temporarily treat the hypercalcemia of hyperparathyroidism. Pamidronate in doses of 30–90 mg (in 0.9% saline) is administered intravenously over 2–4 hours. Zoledronic acid 2–4 mg is administered intravenously over 15 to 20 minutes. These drugs cause a gradual decline in serum calcium over several days that may last for weeks to months. Such intravenous bisphosphonates are used generally for patients with severe hyperparathyroidism in preparation for surgery. Oral bisphosphonates, such as alendronate, are not effective for treating the hypercalcemia or hypercalciuria of hyperparathyroidism. However, oral alendronate has been shown to improve bone mineral density in the lumbar spine and hip (not distal radius) and may be used for asymptomatic patients with hyperparathyroidism who have a low bone mineral density.

3. Vitamin D and vitamin D analogs—

A. Primary hyperparathyroidism—For patients with vitamin D deficiency, careful vitamin D replacement may be beneficial to patients with hyperparathyroidism. Aggravation of hypercalcemia does not ordinarily occur. Serum PTH levels may fall with vitamin D replacement in doses of 800–2000 international units daily. Occasionally, larger doses are required to achieve normal 25-OH vitamin D levels.

B. Secondary and Tertiary Hyperparathyroidism associated with Azotemia—**Calcitriol**, given orally or intravenously after dialysis, suppresses parathyroid hyperplasia of kidney disease. For patients with normal serum calcium levels, it is given orally in starting doses of 0.25 mcg on alternate days or daily. Calcitriol often causes hypercalcemia, so that serum levels of calcium and phosphate must be monitored to ensure that the serum $Ca^{2+} \times PO_4^3$ product remains ≤ 70. When that occurs, the dose of calcitriol is decreased or the patient is switched to therapy with vitamin D analogs or cinacalcet.

The vitamin D analogs **paricalcitol** and **doxercalciferol** suppress PTH secretion and cause less hypercalcemia than calcitriol; however, they are very expensive. The doses are adjusted to keep serum PTH levels in the range of 150–300 pg/mL (15–30 pmol/L). **Paricalcitol** (Zemplar) is administered intravenously during dialysis three times weekly in starting doses of 0.04–0.1 mcg/kg to a maximum dose of 0.24 mcg/kg three times weekly. Alternatively, paricalcitol may be administered orally at doses of 1–2 mcg daily for serum PTH levels < 500 pg/mL (<50 pmol/L) or 2–4 mcg daily for serum PTH levels > 500 pg/mL (>50 pmol/L). Dialysis patients receiving paricalcitol have improved survival compared with patients receiving calcitriol. **Doxercalciferol** (Hectorol) is administered intravenously three times weekly during hemodialysis to patients with azotemic secondary hyperparathyroidism in starting doses of 4 mcg three times weekly to a maximum dose of 18 mcg three times weekly. Alternatively, doxercalciferol may be administered orally three times weekly at dialysis, starting with 10 mcg three times weekly at dialysis to a maximum of 60 mcg/wk.

4. Cinacalcet—Cinacalcet hydrochloride is a calcimimetic agent that binds to sites of the parathyroid glands' extracellular CaSRs to increase the glands' affinity for extracellular calcium, thereby decreasing PTH secretion. About 50% of azotemic patients with secondary or tertiary hyperparathyroidism are resistant to vitamin D analogs. Cinacalcet is given orally in starting doses of 30 mg daily to a maximum of 250 mg daily, with dosage adjustments to keep the serum PTH in the range of 150–300 pg/mL (15–30 pmol/L). Patients with primary hyperparathyroidism have also been treated successfully with cinacalcet in oral doses of 30–50 mg twice daily, with 73% of patients achieving normocalcemia. Cinacalcet is given to patients with severe hypercalcemia due to parathyroid carcinoma at initial doses of 30 mg orally twice daily and increased progressively to 60 mg twice daily, then 90 mg twice daily to a maximum of 90 mg every 6–8 hours. Cinacalcet is usually well tolerated but may cause nausea and vomiting, which are usually transient. It is very expensive.

5. Other measures—Estrogen replacement, given to postmenopausal women, reduces hypercalcemia slightly. Similarly, raloxifene also reduces the hypercalcemia of hyperparathyroidism, reducing serum calcium levels an average of 0.4 mg/dL (0.1 mmol/L). Propranolol may be useful for preventing the adverse cardiac effects of hypercalcemia.

Renal osteodystrophy is caused by secondary or tertiary hyperparathyroidism during kidney disease. It can be prevented or delayed by reducing hyperphosphatemia with phosphate binding medication and dietary phosphate restriction.

▶ **Prognosis**

Patients with symptomatic hyperparathyroidism usually experience worsening disease (eg, nephrolithiasis) unless they have treatment. Conversely, the majority of completely asymptomatic patients with a serum calcium < 11.0 mg/dL (< 2.75 mmol/L) remain stable with follow-up. However, worsening hypercalcemia, hypercalciuria, and reductions in cortical bone mineral density develop in about one-third of asymptomatic patients. Therefore, asymptomatic patients must be monitored carefully and treated with oral hydration and mobilization.

Surgical removal of apparently single sporadic parathyroid adenomas is successful in 94%. Patients with MEN 1 undergoing subtotal parathyroidectomy may experience long remissions, but hyperparathyroidism frequently recurs. Despite treatment for hyperparathyroidism, patients remain at increased risk for all-cause mortality, cardiovascular disease, kidney stones, and renal failure. These increased risks are likely the residuals of pretreatment hypertension and nephrolithiasis.

Spontaneous cure due to necrosis of the tumor has been reported but is exceedingly rare. The bones, in spite of severe cyst formation, deformity, and fracture, will heal if a parathyroid tumor is successfully removed. The presence of pancreatitis increases the mortality rate. Acute pancreatitis usually resolves with correction of hypercalcemia, whereas subacute or chronic pancreatitis tends to persist. Significant renal damage may progress even after removal of an adenoma.

Parathyroid carcinoma tends to invade local structures and may sometimes metastasize; repeat surgical resections and radiation therapy can prolong life. Aggressive surgical and medical management of parathyroid carcinoma can result in a median overall survival of 14.3 years (range 10.5–25.7 years) from the date of diagnosis. Factors associated with a worsened mortality rate include lymph node or distant metastases, high number of recurrences, and higher serum calcium levels at recurrence.

▶ **When to Refer**

Refer to parathyroid surgeon for parathyroidectomy.

▶ **When to Admit**

Patients with severe hypercalcemia for intravenous hydration.

Bargren AE et al. Can biochemical abnormalities predict symptomatology in patients with primary hyperparathyroidism? J Am Coll Surg. 2011 Sep;213(3):410–4. [PMID: 21723154]

Bilezikian JP. Primary hyperparathyroidism. Endocr Pract. 2012 Sep–Oct;18(5):781–90. [PMID: 22982802]

Bollerslev J et al. Current evidence for recommendation of surgery, medical treatment and vitamin D repletion in mild primary hyperparathyroidism. Eur J Endocrinol. 2011 Dec;165(6):851–64. [PMID: 21964961]

Duntas LH et al. Cinacalcet as alternative treatment of primary hyperparathyroidism: achievements and prospects. Endocrine. 2011 Jun;39(3):199–204. [PMID: 21442382]

Endres DB. Investigation of hypercalcemia. Clin Biochem. 2012 Aug;45(12):954–63. [PMID: 22569596]

Harari A et al. Parathyroid carcinoma: a 43-year outcome and survival analysis. J Clin Endocrinol Metab. 2011 Dec;96(12):3679–86. [PMID: 21937626]

Kuntsman JW et al. Parathyroid localization and implications for clinical management. J Clin Endocrinol Metab. 2013 Mar;98(3):902–12. [PMID: 23345096]

Marcocci C et al. Clinical practice. Primary hyperparathyroidism. N Engl J Med. 2011 Dec 22;365(25):2389–97. [PMID: 22187986]

Pepe J et al. Sporadic and hereditary primary hyperparathyroidism. J Endocrinol Invest. 2011 Jul;34(7 Suppl):40–4. [PMID: 21985979]

Schneider DF et al. Predictors of recurrence in primary hyperparathyroidism: an analysis of 1386 cases. Ann Surg. 2014 Mar;259(3):563–8. [PMID: 24263316]

Taieb D et al. Parathyroid scintigraphy: when, how, and why? A concise systematic review. Clin Nucl Med. 2012 Jun;37(6):568–74. [PMID: 22614188]

Udelsman R. Approach to the patient with persistent or recurrent primary hyperparathyroidism. J Clin Endocrinol Metab. 2011 Oct;96(10):2950–8. [PMID: 21976743]

Vestergaard P et al. Medical treatment of primary, secondary, and tertiary hyperparathyroidism. Curr Drug Saf. 2011 Apr;6(2):108–13. [PMID: 21524244]

Witteveen JE et al. Hungry bone syndrome: still a challenge in the post-operative management of primary hyperparathyroidism: a systematic review of the literature. Eur J Endocrinol. 2013 Feb 20;168(3):R45–53. [PMID: 23152439]

METABOLIC BONE DISEASE

The term "metabolic bone disease" denotes those conditions producing diffusely decreased bone density and diminished bone strength. It is categorized by histologic appearance: osteoporosis (bone matrix and mineral both decreased) and osteomalacia (bone matrix intact, mineral decreased). Osteoporosis and osteomalacia often coexist in the same patient.

OSTEOPOROSIS

ESSENTIALS OF DIAGNOSIS

▶ Fracture propensity of spine, hip, pelvis, and wrist from demineralization.

▶ Serum PTH, calcium, phosphorus, and alkaline phosphatase usually normal.

▶ Serum 25-hydroxyvitamin D levels often low as a comorbid condition.

▶ General Considerations

Osteoporosis is a skeletal disorder characterized by a loss of bone osteoid that reduces bone integrity, resulting in an increased risk of fractures. In the United States, osteoporosis causes about 2 million fractures annually, including 547,000 vertebral fractures, 300,000 hip fractures, and 135,000 pelvic fractures. White women have a 40% lifetime risk of sustaining one or more osteoporotic fractures. The morbidity and indirect mortality rates are very high. The rate of bone formation is often normal, whereas the rate of bone resorption is increased.

Table 26–10. Causes of osteoporosis.[1]

Hormone deficiency	**Genetic disorders**
Estrogen (women)	Aromatase deficiency
Androgen (men)	Type I collagen
Hormone excess	mutations
Cushing syndrome or	Osteogenesis
corticosteroid	imperfecta
administration	Idiopathic juvenile and adult
Thyrotoxicosis	osteoporosis
Hyperparathyroidism	Ehlers-Danlos syndrome
Immobilization and	Marfan syndrome
microgravity	Homocystinuria
Tobacco	**Miscellaneous**
Alcoholism	Celiac disease
Malignancy, especially	Anorexia nervosa
multiple myeloma	Hyponatremia (chronic)
Medications	Protein-calorie malnutrition
Excessive vitamin D intake	Vitamin C deficiency
Excessive vitamin A intake	Copper deficiency
Heparin therapy	Liver disease
Selective serotonin	Rheumatoid arthritis
reuptake inhibitors	Uncontrolled diabetes
Rosiglitazone	mellitus
	Systemic mastocytosis

[1]See Table 26–11 for causes of osteomalacia.

Osteoporosis can be caused by a variety of factors, which are listed in Table 26–10. The most common causes include aging, high-dose corticosteroid administration, alcoholism, smoking, and sex hormone deficiency. Hypogonadal men frequently develop osteoporosis. Anti-androgen therapy for prostate cancer can cause osteoporosis and such men should monitored with bone densitometry.

Osteogenesis imperfecta is caused by a major mutation in the gene encoding for type I collagen, the major collagen constituent of bone. This causes severe osteoporosis; spontaneous fractures occur in utero or during childhood. Blue sclerae may be present. Certain polymorphisms in the genes encoding type I collagen are common, particularly in whites, resulting in collagen disarray and predisposing to hypogonadal (eg, menopausal) or idiopathic osteoporosis.

▶ Clinical Findings

A. Symptoms and Signs

Osteoporosis is usually asymptomatic until fractures occur. It may present as backache of varying degrees of severity or as a spontaneous fracture or collapse of a vertebra. Loss of height is common. Once osteoporosis is identified, a carefully directed history and physical examination must be performed to determine its cause (Table 26–10).

B. Laboratory Findings

Serum calcium, phosphate, and PTH are normal. The alkaline phosphatase is usually normal but may be slightly elevated, especially following a fracture. Vitamin D deficiency is very common and serum determination of 25-hydroxyvitamin D should be obtained for every individual with low bone density. Serum 25-hydroxyvitamin D levels < 20 ng/mL

(< 50 nmol/L) are considered frank vitamin D deficiency. Lesser degrees of vitamin D deficiency (serum 25-hydroxyvitamin D levels in the range of 20–30 ng/mL (50–75 nmol/L) may also increase the risk for hip fracture. (See Osteomalacia.) Testing for thyrotoxicosis and hypogonadism may be required. Celiac disease may be screened for with serum immunoglobulin A (IgA) endomysial antibody and tissue transglutaminase antibody determinations.

C. Bone Densitometry

DXA is used to determine the bone density of the lumbar spine and hip. Bone densitometry should be performed on all patients who are at risk for osteoporosis or osteomalacia or have pathologic fractures or radiographic evidence of diminished bone density. This test delivers negligible radiation, and the measurements are quite accurate. However, bone densitometry cannot distinguish osteoporosis from osteomalacia; in fact, both are often present. Also, the bone mineral density does not directly measure bone quality and is only fairly successful at predicting fractures. Vertebral bone mineral density may be misleadingly high in compressed vertebrae and in patients with extensive arthritis. DXA also overestimates the bone mineral density of taller persons and underestimates the bone mineral density of smaller persons. Quantitative CT delivers more radiation but is more accurate in the latter situations.

Bone mineral density is typically expressed in g/cm², for which there are different normal ranges for each bone and for each type of DXA-measuring machine. The "T score" is a simplified way of reporting bone density in which the patient's bone mineral density is compared to the young normal mean and expressed as a standard deviation score. The World Health Organization has established criteria for defining osteoporosis in postmenopausal white women, based on T score:

T score ≥ –1.0: Normal.

T score –1.0 to –2.5: Osteopenia ("low bone density").

T score < –2.5: Osteoporosis.

T score < –2.5 with a fracture: Severe osteoporosis.

This classification is somewhat arbitrary and there really is no bone mineral density fracture threshold; instead, the fracture risk increases about twofold for each standard deviation drop in bone mineral density. In fact, most women with fragility fractures have bone densities above –2.5. Surveillance DXA bone densitometry is recommended for postmenopausal women with a frequency according to their T scores: obtain DXA every 5 years for T scores –1.0 to –1.5, every 3–5 years for scores –1.5 to –2.0, and every 1–2 years for scores under –2.0.

The "Z score" is used to express bone density in premenopausal women, younger men, and children, The Z score is a statistical term that is used for expressing an individual's bone density as standard deviation from age-matched, race-matched, and sex-matched means.

▶ Differential Diagnosis

Osteopenia and fractures can be caused by osteomalacia (see below) and bone marrow neoplasia such as myeloma or metastatic bone disease. These conditions coexist in many patients.

▶ Treatment

A. General Measures

For prevention and treatment of osteoporosis, the diet should be adequate in protein, total calories, calcium, and vitamin D. Pharmacologic corticosteroid doses should be reduced or discontinued if possible. Thiazides may be useful if hypercalciuria is present. High-impact physical activity (eg, jogging) significantly increases bone density in men and women. Stair-climbing increases bone density in women. Patients who cannot exercise vigorously should be encouraged to engage in other exercise regularly, thereby increasing strength and reducing the risk of falling. Weight training is helpful to increase muscle strength as well as bone density. Measures should be taken to avoid falls at home (eg, adequate lighting, handrails on stairs, handholds in bathrooms). Patients who have weakness or balance problems must use a cane or a walker; rolling walkers should have a brake mechanism. Balance exercises can reduce the risk of falls. Patients should be kept active; bed-ridden patients should be given active or passive exercises. The spine may be adequately supported (though braces or corsets are usually not well tolerated), but rigid or excessive immobilization must be avoided. Alcohol and smoking should be avoided.

B. Specific Measures

Several treatment options are available, so a regimen is tailored to each patient. Generally, treatment is indicated for all women with osteoporosis (T scores below –2.5) and for all patients who have had fragility fractures. Prophylactic treatment should also be considered for patients with advanced osteopenia (T scores between –2.0 and –2.5).

1. Vitamin D and calcium—Osteoporosis and osteomalacia often coexist (see Osteomalacia). Sun exposure and vitamin D supplementation are useful in preventing and treating osteomalacia but not osteoporosis. Vitamin D supplementation reduces the incidence of vertebral fractures by 37% and may slightly reduce the incidence of nonvertebral fractures. Oral vitamin D is given in doses of 800–2000 international units daily. Vitamin D supplementation is especially required during winter months and for patients having prolonged hospitalization or nursing home care, for patients with serum levels of 25-hydroxyvitamin D below 20 ng/mL, and those with intestinal malabsorption.

Calcium supplementation does not reduce the fracture risk in otherwise healthy patients with a dietary calcium intake of over 1000 mg daily. One meta-analysis concluded that calcium supplementation is associated with a 27% increased risk of myocardial infarction; however, methodological shortcomings in that study have raised doubts about its validity. Conversely, the Women's Health Initiative found that myocardial infarction rates were not significantly higher among postmenopausal women taking calcium. Calcium supplements may increase the risk of calcium-containing kidney stones, unless taken with meals.

Some patients experience gastrointestinal upset with calcium supplements. Therefore, calcium supplementation should probably be given only to those patients whose diets are low in calcium. More important is the assurance of adequate vitamin D through sun exposure or oral vitamin D supplementation. If calcium supplementation is given, it should include vitamin D. Calcium supplementation may be given as calcium citrate (0.4–0.7 g elemental calcium per day) or calcium carbonate (1–1.5 g elemental calcium per day).

2. Bisphosphonates—Bisphosphonates all work similarly, inhibiting osteoclast-induced bone resorption. They increase bone density significantly and reduce the incidence of both vertebral and nonvertebral fractures. Bisphosphonates have also been effective in preventing corticosteroid-induced osteoporosis. To ensure intestinal absorption, oral bisphosphonates must be taken in the morning with at least 8 oz of plain water at least 40 minutes before consumption of anything else. The patient must remain upright after taking bisphosphonates to reduce the risk of esophagitis. These medications are excreted in the urine. However, no dosage adjustments are required for patients with creatinine clearances above 35 mL/min. There has been little experience giving bisphosphonates to patients with severe kidney disease; if given, the dose would need to be greatly reduced and serum phosphate levels monitored.

Bisphosphonates may be given orally once weekly or monthly. **Alendronate** is administered orally once weekly as either a 70-mg standard tablet or a 70-mg effervescent tablet (Binosto). The effervescent tablet must be dissolved in 4 oz plain water over at least 5 minutes and stirred 10 seconds before drinking; it is easier to swallow for some patients and may reduce esophageal injury, but there have been no studies comparing it to standard alendronate tablets. **Risedronate** is given as one 35-mg tablet orally once weekly. Both these medications reduce the risk of both vertebral and nonvertebral fractures. Alendronate appears to be superior to risedronate in preventing nonvertebral fractures. Another bisphosphonate, **ibandronate sodium,** is taken once monthly in a dose of 150 mg orally. Once-monthly ibandronate is convenient and reduces the risk of vertebral fractures but not nonvertebral fractures; its effectiveness has not been directly compared with other bisphosphonates. Oral bisphosphonates can cause nausea, chest pain, and hoarseness. Erosive esophagus can occur, particularly in patients with hiatal hernia and gastroesophageal reflux.

For patients who cannot tolerate oral bisphosphonates or for whom oral bisphosphonates are contraindicated, intravenous bisphosphonates are available. **Zoledronic acid** (Zometa, Reclast) is a third-generation bisphosphonate and a potent osteoclast inhibitor. It can be given every 12 months in doses of 2–5 mg intravenously over at least 15–30 minutes. **Pamidronate** (Aredia) can be given in doses of 30–60 mg by slow intravenous infusion in normal saline solution every 3–6 months.

Bisphosphonate therapy can cause several side effects that are collectively known as the acute-phase response.

Such a response occurs in 42% of patients following the first infusion of zoledronic acid and usually starts within the first few days following the infusion. Among patients receiving their first infusion of zoledronic acid, these adverse side effects have included fever, chills, or flushing (20%); musculoskeletal pain (20%); nausea, vomiting, or diarrhea (8%); nonspecific symptoms, such as fatigue, dyspnea, edema, headache, or dizziness (22%); and eye inflammation (0.6%). Intravenous zoledronic acid has caused seizures that may be idiosyncratic or due to hypocalcemia. The acute-phase response is most commonly seen after the first dose of bisphosphonate (particularly zoledronic acid) and tends to diminish with time. Symptoms are transient, lasting several days and usually resolving spontaneously but typically recurring with subsequent doses. For patients experiencing a severe acute-phase response with zoledronic acid, intravenous pamidronate can substitute for zoledronic acid for subsequent treatment. Additionally, patients who experience an especially severe acute-phase response can be given prophylactic corticosteroids and ondansetron prior to subsequent bisphosphonate infusions.

Osteonecrosis of the jaw is a rare complication of bisphosphonate therapy for osteoporosis. A painful, necrotic, nonhealing lesion of the jaw occurs, particularly after tooth extraction. About 95% of jaw osteonecrosis cases have occurred with high-dose therapy with zoledronic acid or pamidronate for patients with myeloma or solid tumor osteolytic metastases. Only about 5% of cases have occurred in patients receiving oral (or, less frequently, intravenous) bisphosphonate doses for osteoporosis. The incidence of osteonecrosis is estimated to be about 1:100,000 patients treated for osteoporosis and 1:100 patients being treated for cancer. In a prospective 3-year trial of 7714 women who received intravenous zoledronic acid 5 mg/year, there were no cases of osteonecrosis. For patients with painful osteonecrotic exposed bone, treatment is 90% effective (without resolution of the exposed bone) using antibiotics along with 0.12% chlorohexidine antiseptic mouthwash. Patients receiving bisphosphonates must receive regular dental care and try to avoid dental extraction.

Atypical "chalkstick" fractures of the femur occur rarely in patients taking bisphosphonates. Bisphosphonate use for more than 5 years is associated with 2.7-fold risk in subtrochanteric or shaft fractures; but the absolute risk is low at about 1 fracture per 1000 bisphosphonate users yearly. In one study, atypical femoral fractures developed in 4 of 327 patients after receiving at least 24 intravenous bisphosphonate infusions for bone metastases. Atypical fractures are subtrochanteric or diaphyseal, occur with little trauma, and are usually transverse as opposed to the more typical comminuted or spiral femoral shaft fractures. Bilateral femoral fractures occur in 27%. About 70% of affected patients have had prodromal thigh pain prior to the fracture. The risk for atypical femoral fractures is particularly increased among patients concurrently taking high-dose corticosteroids and those receiving treatment for more than 5 years. Teriparatide may be helpful to promote healing of such fractures. Despite this rare complication, the overall risk of hip fracture is reduced among patients taking bisphosphonates for up to 5 years.

Patients taking oral bisphosphonates have an increased risk of developing esophageal cancer. In North America and Europe, the incidence of esophageal cancer at age 60–79 is about 1 per 1000 population over 5 years; this risk is estimated to increase to about 2 per 1000 with administration of oral bisphosphonates for 5 years or longer.

In patients taking bisphosphonates, hypercalcemia is seen in 20% and serum PTH levels increase above normal in 10%, mimicking primary hyperparathyroidism. Hypocalcemia occurs frequently, resulting in secondary hyperparathyroidism; therefore, patients taking bisphosphonates are frequently prescribed prophylactic oral calcium supplements (500–1000 mg/d) with vitamin D_3 (1000 units/d).

The half-life of alendronate in bone is 10 years. Therefore, bisphosphonates may be discontinued after a 5-year course of therapy. Repeat bone densitometry may be obtained after 3 years of bisphosphonate therapy. Bone density falls in 18% of patients during their first year of treatment with bisphosphonates, but 80% of such patients have gain in bone density with continued bisphosphonate treatment.

3. Sex hormones—Hypogonadal women who take estrogen replacement therapy (ERT) have a lower risk of developing osteoporosis. Postmenopausal estrogen replacement is valuable as an osteoporosis prevention measure and this should be one factor in the complex decision about whether to take ERT. Low doses of estrogen appear to be adequate to prevent postmenopausal osteoporosis (see Estrogen Replacement Therapy). Once osteoporosis has developed, estrogen replacement is not an effective treatment.

Hypogonadal men are at risk for developing osteoporosis that can be prevented with testosterone administration. (See Male Hypogonadism.)

4. Selective estrogen receptor modulators—Raloxifene, 60 mg/d orally, can be used by postmenopausal women in place of estrogen for prevention of osteoporosis. Bone density increases about 1% over 2 years in postmenopausal women versus 2% increases with estrogen replacement. It reduces the risk of vertebral fractures by about 40% but does not appear to reduce the risk of nonvertebral fractures. Raloxifene produces a reduction in LDL cholesterol but not the rise in high-density lipoprotein (HDL) cholesterol seen with estrogen. It has no direct effect on coronary plaque. Unlike estrogen, raloxifene does not reduce hot flushes; in fact, it often intensifies them. It does not relieve vaginal dryness. Unlike estrogen, raloxifene does not cause endometrial hyperplasia, uterine bleeding, or cancer, nor does it cause breast soreness. The risk of breast cancer is reduced 76% in women taking raloxifene for 3 years. Since it is a potential teratogen, it is relatively contraindicated in women capable of pregnancy.

Raloxifene increases the risk for thromboembolism and should not be used by women with such a history. Leg cramps can also occur.

5. Teriparatide—Teriparatide (Forteo, Parathar) is an analog of PTH. Teriparatide stimulates the production of new collagenous bone matrix that must be mineralized. Patients receiving teriparatide must have sufficient intake of vitamin D and calcium. When administered to patients with osteoporosis in doses of 20 mcg/d subcutaneously for 2 years, teriparatide dramatically improves bone density in most bones except the distal radius. Teriparatide may also be used to promote healing of atypical femoral chalkstick fractures associated with bisphosphonate therapy. The recommended dose should not be exceeded, since teriparatide has caused osteosarcoma in rats when administered in very high doses. Due to the potential risk for osteosarcoma, patients are excluded from receiving teriparatide if they have an increased risk of osteosarcoma due to the following: Paget disease of bone, unexplained elevations in serum alkaline phosphatase, prior radiation therapy to bones, open epiphyses, or a past history of osteosarcoma or chondrosarcoma. Side effects may include injection site reactions, orthostatic hypotension, arthralgia, muscle cramps, depression, or pneumonia. Hypercalcemia can occur and manifest as nausea, constipation, asthenia, or muscle weakness. Teriparatide is approved for only a 2-year course of treatment.

Teriparatide should not be used for patients with hypercalcemia. Similarly, teriparatide should be used with caution in patients if they are also taking corticosteroids and thiazide diuretics along with oral calcium supplementation because hypercalcemia may develop.

Following a course of teriparatide, a course of bisphosphonates should be considered in order to retain the improved bone density.

6. Denosumab—Denosumab (Prolia, Xgeva) is a monoclonal antibody that inhibits the proliferation and maturation of preosteoclasts into mature osteoclast bone-resorbing cells. It does this by binding to the osteoclast receptor activator of nuclear factor-kappa B ligand (RANKL). Denosumab is administered in doses of 60 mg subcutaneously every 6 months. It increases bone mineral density more than oral alendronate. It has been relatively well tolerated, with an 8% incidence of flu-like symptoms. It can decrease serum calcium and should not be administered to patients with hypocalcemia. Other side effects include the development of eczema and dermatitis, serious infections, new malignancies, and pancreatitis. Its efficacy is comparable to bisphosphonates. However, its long-term safety remains unknown, so it is reserved for patients with severe osteoporosis who have not tolerated or not responded to bisphosphonates. It is extremely expensive.

7. Calcitonin—Calcitonin therapy is much less effective than other treatments for osteoporosis. Also, calcitonin therapy may possibly be associated with a slightly increased cancer risk, so it is indicated only when other treatments cannot be used.

▶ **Prognosis**

Bone mineral density densitometries can detect whether progressive osteopenia or frank osteoporosis is developing. Osteoporosis should ideally be prevented, since it can be only be partially reversed. Measures noted above are reasonably effective in preventing and treating osteoporosis and reducing fracture risk.

Cauley JA et al. Once-yearly zoledronic acid and days of disability, bed rest and back pain: randomised controlled HORIZON pivotal fracture trial. J Bone Miner Res. 2011 May;26(5): 984–92. [PMID: 21089141]

Howe TE et al. Exercise for preventing and treating osteoporosis in postmenopausal women. Cochrane Database Syst Rev. 2011 Jul 6;(7):CD000333. [PMID: 21735380]

Khosla S et al. Benefits and risks of bisphosphonate therapy for osteoporosis. J Clin Endocrinol Metab. 2012 Jul;97(7): 2272–82. [PMID: 22523337]

Lekamwasam S et al; Joint IOF–ECTS GIO Guidelines Working Group. A framework for the development of guidelines for the management of glucocorticoid-induced osteoporosis. Osteoporos Int. 2012 Sep;23(9):2257–76. [PMID: 22434203]

Moen MD et al. Denosumab: a review of its use in the treatment of postmenopausal osteoporosis. Drugs Aging. 2011 Jan;28(1): 63–82. [PMID: 21174488]

Moyer VA et al. Vitamin D and calcium supplementation to prevent fractures in adults: U.S. Preventive Services Task Force recommendation statement. Ann Intern Med. 2013 May 7; 158(9):691–6. [PMID: 23440163]

Watts NB et al. Osteoporosis in men: an Endocrine Society clinical practice guideline. J Clin Endocrinol Metab. 2012 Jun;97 (6):1802–22. [PMID: 22675062]

OSTEOMALACIA

ESSENTIALS OF DIAGNOSIS

▶ Painful proximal muscle weakness (especially pelvic girdle); bone pain and tenderness.

▶ Decreased bone density from defective mineralization.

▶ Laboratory abnormalities may include increased alkaline phosphatase, decreased 25-hydroxy-vitamin D, hypocalcemia, hypocalciuria, hypophosphatemia, secondary hyperparathyroidism.

▶ Classic radiologic features may be present.

▶ General Considerations

Defective mineralization of the growing skeleton in childhood causes permanent bone deformities (rickets). Defective skeletal mineralization in adults is known as osteomalacia. It is caused by any condition that results in inadequate calcium or phosphate mineralization of bone osteoid.

▶ Etiology (Table 26–11)

A. Vitamin D Deficiency and Resistance

Vitamin D is predominantly synthesized in the skin during exposure to ultraviolet B light. Vitamin D is also consumed in the diet from plants (ergocalciferol, D_2) or animals/fish (cholecalciferol, D_3). Both forms of vitamin D are converted in the liver to 25-hydroxyvitamin D (25OHD); 25OHD is subsequently converted in various tissues (mainly kidney) to 1,25-dihydroxyvitamin D (1,25[OH]$_2$D), the active hormone whose production is regulated by serum calcium, phosphorus, and PTH. 1,25(OH)$_2$D binds

Table 26–11. Causes of osteomalacia.[1]

Vitamin disorders
Decreased availability of vitamin D
Insufficient sunlight exposure
Nutritional deficiency of vitamin D
Malabsorption: aging, excess wheat bran, bariatric surgery, pancreatic enzyme deficiency
Nephrotic syndrome
Vitamin D–dependent rickets type I
Liver disease
Chronic kidney disease
Kidney transplantation
Phenytoin, carbamazepine, valproate, or barbiturate therapy
Dietary calcium deficiency
Phosphate deficiency
Decreased intestinal absorption
Nutritional deficiency of phosphorus
Phosphate-binding antacid therapy
Increased renal loss
X-linked hypophosphatemic rickets
Tumoral hypophosphatemic osteomalacia
Association with other disorders, including paraproteinemias, glycogen storage diseases, neurofibromatosis, Wilson disease, Fanconi syndrome, renal tubular acidosis, and alcoholism
Inhibitors of mineralization
Aluminum
Bisphosphonates
Disorders of bone matrix
Hypophosphatasia
Fibrogenesis imperfecta
Axial osteomalacia

[1]See Table 26–10 for causes of osteoporosis.

to cytoplasmic vitamin D receptors, increasing the absorption of dietary calcium from the intestine and increasing the reabsorption of calcium in the renal tubule, thereby reducing calcium loss in the urine. 1,25(OH)$_2$D also stimulates bone osteoblasts to release RANKL that stimulates osteoclasts, which release calcium from bone.

Vitamin D deficiency is the most common cause of osteomalacia and its incidence is increasing throughout the world as a result of diminished exposure to sunlight caused by urbanization, automobile and public transportation, modest clothing, and sunscreen use. Significant vitamin D deficiency (serum 25OHD < 50 nmol/L or < 20 ng/mL) was found in 24.3% of postmenopausal women from 25 countries. The incidence varied: < 1% in Southeast Asia, 29% in the United States, and 36% in Italy. Patients in whom clinically severe osteomalacia develops typically have had chronic severe vitamin D deficiency (serum 25OHD < 25 nmol/L or < 10 ng/mL). The prevalence of severe vitamin D deficiency is 3.5% in the United States and 12.5% in Italy. Among US men over age 65 years, 25% have serum 25OHD levels below 20 ng/mL; men over age 75 with such low vitamin D levels have particularly accelerated bone loss. Vitamin D deficiency is particularly common in the institutionalized elderly, with the incidence exceeding 60% in some groups not receiving vitamin D supplementation. Deficiency of vitamin D may arise from insufficient sun exposure, malnutrition, or malabsorption (due to pancreatic insufficiency, cholestatic liver disease, celiac disease, inflammatory bowel disease, jejunoileal bypass, Billroth type II gastrectomy). Orlistat is a weight-loss medication that causes fat malabsorption and reduced serum 25OHD levels. Cholestyramine binds bile acids necessary for vitamin D absorption. Patients with severe nephrotic syndrome lose large amounts of vitamin D–binding protein in the urine, and osteomalacia may also develop.

Anticonvulsants (eg, phenytoin, carbamazepine, valproate, phenobarbital) inhibit the hepatic production of 25OHD and sometimes cause osteomalacia. Phenytoin can also directly inhibit bone mineralization. Serum levels of $1,25(OH)_2D$ are usually normal.

Vitamin D–dependent rickets type I is caused by a rare autosomal recessive disorder with a defect in the renal enzyme 1-alpha-hydroxylase leading to defective synthesis of $1,25(OH)_2D$. It presents in childhood with rickets and alopecia; osteomalacia develops in adults with this condition unless treated with oral calcitriol in doses of 0.5–1 mcg daily.

Vitamin D–dependent rickets type II (better known as hereditary $1,25[OH]_2D$-resistant rickets) is caused by a genetic defect in the $1,25(OH)_2D$ receptor. Patients have hypocalcemia with childhood rickets and adult osteomalacia. Alopecia is common. These patients respond variably to oral calcitriol in very large doses (2–6 mcg daily).

B. Deficient Calcium Intake

The total daily consumption of calcium should be at least 1000 mg daily. Patients who have deficient calcium intake develop rickets (childhood) or osteomalacia (adulthood) despite sufficient vitamin D. A nutritional deficiency of calcium can occur in any severely malnourished patient. Some degree of calcium deficiency is common in the elderly, since intestinal calcium absorption declines with age. Ingestion of excessive wheat bran also causes calcium malabsorption.

C. Phosphate Deficiency

Hypophosphatemia can cause severe major muscle weakness, dysphagia, diplopia, cardiomyopathy, and respiratory muscle weakness. Patients may have impaired cognition. Chronic hypophosphatemia can cause bone pain and affect bone integrity. Phosphate deficiency in childhood causes classic rickets, whereas phosphate deficiency in adulthood causes osteomalacia.

1. Genetic disorders—Fibroblast growth factor-23 (FGF23) is a phosphaturic factor (phosphatonin) that is secreted by bone osteoblasts in response to elevated serum phosphate levels. Families with autosomal dominant hypophosphatemic rickets have a gain-of-function mutation in the gene encoding FGF23 that makes it resistant to proteolytic cleavage, thereby increasing serum FGF23 levels. In X-linked hypophosphatemic rickets, there is a mutation in the gene encoding PHEX endopeptidase, which fails to cleave FGF23, resulting in elevated serum FGF23 levels. An autosomal recessive form of hypophosphatemic rickets is caused by mutations in DMP1, a transcription factor that regulates FGF23 production in bone. All three conditions

have high serum FGF23 levels causing hypophosphatemia and bone mineral depletion.

Sodium-phosphate cotransporters (NPT2a or NPT2c) reabsorb phosphate from the proximal renal tubule. Mutations in the genes encoding them or in NHERF1 cause hypophosphatemia, bone mineral depletion, and calcium-phosphate kidney stones.

2. Tumor-induced osteomalacia—A variety of mesenchymal tumors (87% benign) secrete fibroblast growth factor-23 (FGF23) and cause marked hypophosphatemia due to renal phosphate wasting. Such tumors are usually small and are often difficult to locate. The condition is characterized by hypophosphatemia, excessive phosphaturia, reduced or normal serum $1,25(OH)_2D$ concentrations, and osteomalacia. Serum levels of FGF23 are elevated. Such tumors are often small and difficult to find, frequently lying in extremities. Imaging with ^{111}In-octreotide or ^{18}FDG-PET should include the entire body and may be helpful in localizing these tumors.

3. Other causes of hypophosphatemia—Osteomalacia from hypophosphatemia can be caused by severe intestinal malabsorption or poor nutrition. Severe hypophosphatemia can occur with refeeding after starvation (eg, concentration camp victims, malnourished alcoholics). Other causes of hypophosphatemia include respiratory alkalosis, glucose infusions, salicylate intoxication, mannitol, and bisphosphonate therapy. Additional causes include chelation of phosphate in the gut by aluminum hydroxide antacids, calcium acetate (Phos-Lo), or sevelamer hydrochloride (Renagel). Excessive renal phosphate losses are also seen in proximal renal tubular acidosis and Fanconi syndrome.

D. Aluminum Toxicity

Bone mineralization is inhibited by aluminum. Osteomalacia may occur in patients receiving long-term renal hemodialysis with tap water dialysate or from aluminum-containing antacids used to reduce phosphate levels. Osteomalacia may develop in patients being maintained on long-term total parenteral nutrition if the casein hydrolysate used for amino acids contains high levels of aluminum.

E. Hypophosphatasia

Hypophosphatasia, a deficiency of bone alkaline phosphatase effect, is a rare genetic cause of osteomalacia that is commonly misdiagnosed as osteoporosis. The incidence in the United States is about 1 in 100,000 live births; about 1 in 300 adults is a carrier. Many different mutations in the gene (designated *ALPL*) encoding bone alkaline phosphatase have been described, and transmission can be either autosomal recessive or autosomal dominant. The phenotypic presentation of hypophosphatasia is extremely variable. At its mildest, hypophosphatasia can present in middle age with premature loss of teeth, foot pain (due to metatarsal stress fractures), thigh pain (due to femoral pseudofractures), or arthritis (due to chondrocalcinosis). Serum alkaline phosphatase (collected in a non-EDTA tube) is low for age in patients with hypophosphatasia. To confirm the diagnosis, a 24-hour urine should be assayed for phosphoethanolamine, a substrate for tissue-nonspecific alkaline phosphatase, whose excretion is always elevated in patients with hypophosphatasia. Prenatal genetic testing, by way of chorionic villus biopsy, is available for the infantile form of hypophosphatasia. There is no proven therapy for hypophosphatasia, except for supportive care. Teriparatide, a useful therapy for osteoporosis, has been administered to some patients with hypophosphatasia, but its long-term efficacy is unknown.

F. Fibrogenesis Imperfecta Ossium

This rare condition sporadically affects middle-aged patients, who present with progressive bone pain and pathologic fractures. Bones have a dense "fishnet" appearance on radiographs. Serum alkaline phosphatase levels are elevated. Some patients have a monoclonal gammopathy, indicating a possible plasma cell dyscrasia causing an impairment in osteoblast function and collagen disarray. Remission has been reported after repeated courses of melphalan, corticosteroids, and vitamin D analog over 3 years.

▶ Clinical Findings

The clinical manifestations of defective bone mineralization depend on the age at onset and the severity. In adults, osteomalacia is typically asymptomatic at first. Eventually, bone pain occurs, along with muscle weakness due to calcium deficiency. Pathologic fractures may occur with little or no trauma. Vitamin D deficiency has also been associated with a possible increased risk of multiple sclerosis, rheumatoid arthritis, diabetes mellitus (types 1 and 2), and other conditions, but the causal relationship is uncertain.

▶ Diagnostic Tests

Serum is obtained for calcium, albumin, phosphate, alkaline phosphatase, PTH, and $25[OH]D_3$ determinations. Bone densitometry helps document the degree of osteopenia. Radiographs may show diagnostic features.

In one series of biopsy-proved osteomalacia, alkaline phosphatase was elevated in 94% of patients; the calcium or phosphorus was low in 47% of patients; $25(OH)D_3$ was low in 29% of patients; pseudofractures were seen in 18% of patients; and urinary calcium was low in 18% of patients. $1,25(OH)_2D_3$ may be low even when $25(OH)D_2$ levels are normal.

Bone biopsy is not usually necessary but is diagnostic of osteomalacia if there is significant unmineralized osteoid.

▶ Differential Diagnosis

Osteomalacia is often seen together with osteoporosis, and its presence can be inferred by finding low serum levels of 25(OH) vitamin D, low serum calcium, or low serum phosphate. A high serum alkaline phosphatase may be present in severe osteomalacia but not osteoporosis. The relative contribution of the two entities to diminished bone density may not be apparent until treatment, since a dramatic rise in bone density is often seen with therapy for osteomalacia. Phosphate deficiency must be distinguished from hypophosphatemia seen in hyperparathyroidism.

▶ Prevention & Treatment

To obtain adequate sunshine vitamin D, the face, arms, hands, or back must have sun exposure without sunscreen for 15 minutes at least twice weekly. The main natural food source of vitamin D is fish, particularly salmon, mackerel, cod liver oil, and sardines or tuna canned in oil. Most commercial cow's milk is fortified with vitamin D at about 400 international units per quart; however, skim milk and other dairy products contain much less vitamin D.

Many vitamin supplements contain plant-derived vitamin D_2, which has less biologic availability than once believed. Over-the-counter multivitamin/mineral supplements contain variable amounts of vitamin D, and vitamin D toxicity has occurred from two different multivitamins sold in the United States. Therefore, it is prudent to recommend that patients take a dedicated vitamin D supplement from a reliable manufacturer.

In sunlight-deprived individuals (eg, veiled women, confined patients, or residents of higher latitudes during winter), the recommended daily allowance should be vitamin D_3 1000 international units daily. In such individuals, vitamin D_3 supplements should be given prophylactically. Patients receiving long-term phenytoin therapy may be treated prophylactically with vitamin D, 50,000 international units orally every 2–4 weeks.

Frank vitamin D deficiency is treated with ergocalciferol (D_2), 50,000 international units orally once weekly for 8 weeks. Following that, vitamin D_3 (cholecalciferol) supplementation is used at a dose of 2000 international units daily. Vitamin D_3 is more effective than vitamin D_2 in raising serum levels of 25(OH)D. Some patients require long-term supplementation with ergocalciferol of up to 50,000 international units weekly. In patients with intestinal malabsorption, oral doses of 25,000–100,000 international units of vitamin D3 daily may be required. Some patients with steatorrhea respond better to oral $25(OH)D_3$ (calcifediol), 50–100 mcg/d. Serum levels of 25(OH)D should be monitored and the dosage of vitamin D adjusted to maintain serum 25(OH)D levels above 30 ng/mL. During treatment with high-dose vitamin D, serum calcium should also be monitored to avoid hypercalcemia.

Beyond increasing the intestinal absorption of calcium, vitamin D supplementation may have additional effects. Vitamin D supplementation has been associated with improved muscle strength and a reduced fall risk, factors that reduce the risk of bone fracture.

The addition of calcium supplements to vitamin D is probably not necessary for the prevention of osteomalacia in the majority of otherwise well-nourished patients. However, patients with malabsorption or poor nutrition should receive calcium supplementation. Recommended doses of calcium are as follows: calcium citrate (eg, Citracal), 0.4–0.6 g elemental calcium per day, or calcium carbonate (eg, OsCal, Tums), 1–1.5 g elemental calcium per day. Calcium supplements are best administered with meals.

In hypophosphatemic osteomalacia, nutritional deficiencies are corrected, aluminum-containing antacids are discontinued, and patients with renal tubular acidosis are given bicarbonate therapy. In patients with sporadic adult-onset hypophosphatemia, hyperphosphaturia, and low serum 1,25(OH)$_2$D levels, a search is conducted for occult tumors that may be resected; whole-body MRI scanning may be required.

For those with X-linked or idiopathic hypophosphatemia and hyperphosphaturia, oral phosphate supplements must be given long-term. Calcitriol, 0.25–0.5 mcg/d, is given also to improve the impaired calcium absorption caused by the oral phosphate. If necessary, rhGH may be added to the above regimen to reduce phosphaturia.

Patients with **hypophosphatasia** have been treated with teriparatide with improvement in bone pain and fracture healing.

Carpenter TO. The expanding family of hypophosphatemic syndromes. J Bone Miner Metab. 2012 Jan;30(1):1–9. [PMID: 22167381]

Chong WH et al. The importance of whole body imaging in tumor-induced osteomalacia. J Clin Endocrinol Metab. 2011 Dec;96(12):3599–600. [PMID: 22143830]

Haroon M et al. Vitamin D deficiency: subclinical and clinical consequences on musculoskeletal health. Curr Rheumatol Rep. 2012 Jun;14(3):286–93. [PMID: 22328176]

Heaney RP et al. Vitamin D$_3$ is more potent than vitamin D$_2$ in humans. J Clin Endocrinol Metab. 2011 Mar;96(3):E447–52. [PMID: 21177785]

Hollick MF et al. Evaluation, treatment, and prevention of vitamin D deficiency: an Endocrine Society clinical practice guideline. J Clin Endocrinol Metab. 2011 Jul;96(7):1911–30. [PMID: 21646368]

Niemeier T et al. Insufficiency fracture associated with oncogenic osteomalacia. J Clin Rheumatol. 2013 Jan;19(1):38–42. [PMID: 23319023]

PAGET DISEASE OF BONE
(Osteitis Deformans)

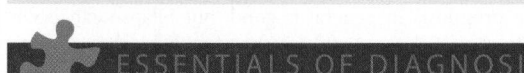

ESSENTIALS OF DIAGNOSIS

- ► Often asymptomatic.
- ► Bone pain may be the first symptom.
- ► Kyphosis, bowed tibias, large head, deafness, and frequent fractures.
- ► Serum calcium and phosphate normal; alkaline phosphatase elevated; urinary hydroxyproline elevated.
- ► Dense, expanded bones on radiographs.

General Considerations

Paget disease is manifested by one or more bony lesions having high bone turnover and disorganized osteoid formation. The involved bone has increased osteoclast activity, causing lytic lesions in bone that may progress at about 1 cm/yr. Involved bones become vascular, weak, and deformed.

The prevalence of Paget disease has declined by about 36% over that past 20 years. However, it remains a common disease in certain countries, with striking geographic variation in prevalence. It is most common in the United Kingdom and in areas of European migration, particularly New Zealand, Australia, the United States, South Africa, Quebec, and Brazil. Interestingly, the disease appears equally common among different races in these countries. Paget disease occurs in 1–2% of the population of the United States, and its prevalence increases with age. It is uncommon in Africa, Asia, and Scandinavia. Usually diagnosed in patients over age 40 years, its prevalence doubles with each decade thereafter, reaching an incidence of about 10% after age 80. It is most often discovered incidentally during radiology imaging or because of incidentally discovered elevations in serum alkaline phosphatase.

The cause of Paget disease is unknown. However, there is believed to be a genetic component, since about 30% of affected patients have a first-degree relative with the disease. Mutations in the *SQSTM1* gene have been discovered in 25–50% of cases with familial Paget disease and in 5–10% of patients with apparently sporadic Paget disease.

Clinical Findings

A. Symptoms and Signs

Paget disease is often mild and asymptomatic. Only 27% of affected individuals are symptomatic at the time of diagnosis. Paget disease involves multiple bones (polyostotic) in 72% and only a single bone (monostotic) in 28%. It occurs most commonly in the pelvis, vertebrae, femur, humerus, and skull. The affected bones are typically involved right away and the disease tends not to involve additional bones during its course. Pain is the usual first symptom. It may occur in the involved bone or in an adjacent joint, which can be involved with degenerative arthritis. The bones can become soft, leading to bowed tibias, kyphosis, and frequent "chalkstick" fractures with slight trauma. If the skull is involved, the patient may report headaches and an increased hat size. Deafness may occur. Increased vascularity over the involved bones causes increased warmth and can cause vascular "steal" syndromes.

B. Laboratory Findings

Serum alkaline phosphatase is usually markedly elevated. However, some patients with limited monostotic involvement may have serum alkaline phosphatase levels within the normal range. A serum bone-specific alkaline phosphatase is usually high and is useful for patients with a normal serum total alkaline phosphatase and to distinguish the source of an elevated serum alkaline phosphatase as being from bone (rather than liver). Other markers of bone turnover are also usually elevated, particularly serum procollagen type-I N-terminal propeptide (PINP) and urine N-telopeptide of type 1I collagen cross-links (NTx). Serum calcium may be elevated, particularly if the patient is at bed rest. A serum 25-OH vitamin D determination should be obtained to screen for vitamin D deficiency, which can also present with an increased serum alkaline phosphatase and bone pain. Also, any vitamin D deficiency should be corrected before prescribing a bisphosphonate.

C. Imaging

On radiographs, the initial lesions are typically osteolytic, with focal radiolucencies ("osteoporosis circumscripta") in the skull or advancing flame-shaped lytic lesions in long bones. Bone lesions may subsequently become sclerotic and have a mixed lytic and sclerotic appearance. The affected bones eventually become thickened and deformed. Technetium pyrophosphate bone scans are helpful in delineating activity of bone lesions even before any radiologic changes are apparent.

▶ Differential Diagnosis

Certain rare familial types of sclerosing bone dysplasias share phenotypic homologies with Paget disease of bone. Familial expansile osteolysis, familial early-onset Paget disease, and familial skeletal hyperphosphatasia are autosomal dominant disorders caused by different tandem duplications of the gene encoding RANK, resulting in its constitutive activation. The differential diagnosis also includes myelofibrosis, intramedullary osteosclerosis, Erdheim-Chester disease, Langerhans cell histiocytosis, and sickle cell disease.

Paget disease must be differentiated from primary bone lesions such as osteogenic sarcoma, multiple myeloma, and fibrous dysplasia and from secondary bone lesions such as osteitis fibrosa cystica and metastatic carcinoma to bone. Fibrogenesis imperfecta ossium is a rare symmetric disorder that can mimic the features of Paget disease; serum alkaline phosphatase is likewise elevated. This condition may be associated with paraproteinemias.

▶ Complications

If immobilization occurs, hypercalcemia and renal calculi may develop. The increased vascularity may give rise to high-output cardiac failure. Arthritis frequently develops in joints adjacent to involved bone.

Extensive skull involvement may cause cranial nerve palsies from impingement of the neural foramina. Involvement of the petrous temporal bone frequently causes hearing loss (mixed sensorineural and conductive) and occasionally tinnitus or vertigo. **Skull involvement** can also cause a vascular steal syndrome with somnolence or ischemic neurologic events; the optic nerve may be affected, resulting in loss of vision. Jaw involvement can cause the teeth to spread intraorally and become misaligned. Vertebral collapse can cause compression of spinal cord or spinal nerves, resulting in radiculopathy or paralysis. **Vertebral involvement** can also cause a vascular steal syndrome with paralysis. Surgery for fractured long bones is often complicated by excessive blood loss from these vascular lytic lesions.

Osteosarcoma may develop in long-standing lesions but is rare (< 1%). Sarcomatous change is suggested by a marked increase in bone pain, sudden rise in alkaline phosphatase, and appearance of a new lytic lesion.

▶ Treatment

Asymptomatic patients may require only clinical surveillance and no treatment. However, treatment should be considered for asymptomatic patients who have extensive involvement of the skull, long bones, or vertebrae. Patients must be monitored carefully before, during, and after treatment with clinical examinations and serial serum alkaline phosphatase determinations.

Bisphosphonates are used to treat patients with Paget disease. Zoledronic acid is the treatment of choice. Administered intravenously as a single 5 mg dose, it normalizes serum alkaline phosphatase in 89% of patients by 6 months and in 98% by 2 years. Oral bisphosphonate regimens include risedronate 30 mg/d for 2 months or alendronate 40 mg/d for 6 months. However, 2 years after a course of oral risedronate, only 57% of patients maintain a normal serum alkaline phosphatase. Therefore, with oral bisphosphonates, repeated courses of treatment are often necessary.

Patients frequently experience a paradoxical increase in pain at sites of disease soon after commencing bisphosphonate therapy; this is the "first dose effect" and the pain usually subsides with further treatment. Flu-like symptoms occur fairly frequently. Following intravenous zoledronic acid, patients frequently experience fever, fatigue, myalgia, bone pain, and ocular problems. Serious side effects are rare but include seizures, uveitis, and acute kidney disease. Hypocalcemia is common and may be severe, especially if intravenous bisphosphonates are given along with loop diuretics. Therefore, it is advisable to administer calcium and vitamin D supplements, especially during the first 2 weeks following treatment. Asthma may occur in aspirin-sensitive patients. To prevent esophageal complications, oral bisphosphonates should be taken with 8 oz of plain water only; they are relatively contraindicated in patients with a history of esophagitis, esophageal stricture, dysphagia, hiatal hernia, or achalasia.

▶ Prognosis

The prognosis in general is good, but relapse can occur after an initial successful treatment with bisphosphonate. By 6.5 years after initial therapy, the recurrence rate is 12.5% after treatment with zolendronic acid and 62% after risedronate. Therefore, patients must be monitored long-term, measuring serum alkaline phosphatase at least yearly. In general, the prognosis is worse the earlier in life the disease starts. Fractures usually heal well. In the severe forms, marked deformity, intractable pain, and cardiac failure are found. These complications should become rare with prompt bisphosphonate treatment. Osteosarcoma that arises at sites of Paget disease results in a 2-year survival of only 25%.

Bolland MJ et al. Paget disease of bone: clinical review and update. J Clin Pathol. 2013 Nov;66(11):924–7. [PMID: 24043712]

Britton C et al. Paget disease of bone—an update. Aust Fam Physician. 2012 Mar;41(3):100–3. [PMID: 22396921]

Mahmood W et al. Proposed new approach for treating Paget's disease of bone. Ir J Med Sci. 2011 Mar;180(1):121–4. [PMID: 21132539]

Michou L et al. Emerging strategies and therapies for treatment of Paget's disease of bone. Drug Des Devel Ther. 2011;5: 225–39. [PMID: 21607019]

Reid IR. Pharmacotherapy of Paget's disease of bone. Expert Opin Pharmacother. 2012 Apr;13(5):637–46. [PMID: 22339140]

Reid IR et al. Bisphosphonates in Paget's disease. Bone. 2011 Jul;49(1):89–94. [PMID: 20832512]

Seton M. Paget disease of bone: diagnosis and drug therapy. Cleve Clin J Med. 2013 Jul;80(7):452–62. Erratum in: Cleve Clin J Med. 2013 Nov;80(11):721. [PMID: 23821690]

DISEASES OF THE ADRENAL CORTEX

ACUTE ADRENOCORTICAL INSUFFICIENCY (Adrenal Crisis)

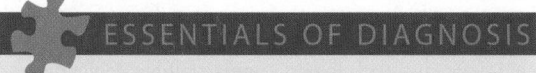

ESSENTIALS OF DIAGNOSIS

- ▶ Weakness, abdominal pain, fever, confusion, nausea, vomiting, and diarrhea.
- ▶ Low blood pressure, dehydration; skin pigmentation may be increased.
- ▶ Serum potassium high, sodium low, BUN high.
- ▶ Cosyntropin (ACTH$_{1-24}$) unable to stimulate an increase in serum cortisol to ≥ 20 mcg/dL.

▶ General Considerations

Acute adrenal insufficiency is an emergency caused by insufficient cortisol. Crisis may occur in the course of treatment of chronic insufficiency, or it may be the presenting manifestation of adrenal insufficiency. Acute adrenal crisis is more commonly seen in primary adrenal insufficiency (Addison disease) than in disorders of the pituitary gland causing secondary adrenocortical hypofunction.

Adrenal crisis may occur in the following situations: (1) during stress, (eg, trauma, surgery, infection, hyperthyroidism, or prolonged fasting) in a patient with latent or treated adrenal insufficiency; (2) following sudden withdrawal of adrenocortical hormone in a patient with chronic insufficiency or in a patient with temporary insufficiency due to suppression by exogenous corticosteroids or megestrol; (3) following bilateral adrenalectomy or removal of a functioning adrenal tumor that had suppressed the other adrenal; (4) following sudden destruction of the pituitary gland (pituitary necrosis), or when thyroid hormone is given to a patient with hypoadrenalism; and (5) following injury to both adrenals by trauma, hemorrhage, anticoagulant therapy, thrombosis, infection or, rarely, metastatic carcinoma; (6) following administration of etomidate, which is used intravenously for rapid anesthesia induction or intubation.

▶ Clinical Findings

A. Symptoms and Signs

The patient complains of headache, lassitude, nausea and vomiting, abdominal pain, and often diarrhea. Confusion or coma may be present. Fever may be 40.6 °C or more. The blood pressure is low. Recurrent hypoglycemia and reduced insulin requirements may present in patients with preexisting type 1 diabetes mellitus. Other signs may include cyanosis, dehydration, skin hyperpigmentation, and sparse axillary hair (if hypogonadism is also present). Meningococcemia may be associated with purpura and adrenal insufficiency secondary to adrenal infarction (Waterhouse–Friderichsen syndrome).

B. Laboratory Findings

The eosinophil count may be high. Hyponatremia or hyperkalemia (or both) are usually present. Hypoglycemia is frequent. Hypercalcemia may be present. Blood, sputum, or urine culture may be positive if bacterial infection is the precipitating cause of the crisis.

The diagnosis is made by a simplified cosyntropin stimulation test, which is performed as follows: (1) Synthetic ACTH$_{1-24}$ (cosyntropin), 0.25 mg, is given intramuscularly. (2) Serum is obtained for cortisol between 30 and 60 minutes after cosyntropin is administered. Normally, serum cortisol rises to at least 20 mcg/dL. For patients receiving corticosteroid treatment, hydrocortisone must not be given for at least 8 hours before the test. Other corticosteroids (eg, prednisone, dexamethasone) do not interfere with specific assays for cortisol.

If the patient has primary adrenal insufficiency, the plasma ACTH is markedly elevated, generally > 200 pg/mL (> 44 pmol/L).

▶ Differential Diagnosis

Acute adrenal insufficiency must be distinguished from other causes of shock (eg, septic, hemorrhagic, cardiogenic). Hyperkalemia is also seen with gastrointestinal bleeding, rhabdomyolysis, hyperkalemic paralysis, and certain drugs (eg, angiotensin-converting enzyme [ACE] inhibitors, spironolactone). Hyponatremia is seen in many other conditions (eg, hypothyroidism, diuretic use, heart failure, cirrhosis, vomiting, diarrhea, severe illness, or major surgery). Acute adrenal insufficiency must be distinguished from an acute abdomen in which neutrophilia is the rule, whereas adrenal insufficiency is characterized by a relative lymphocytosis and eosinophilia.

More than 90% of serum cortisol is protein bound and low serum levels of binding proteins result in misleadingly low serum cortisol determinations by most assays. Nearly 40% of critically ill patients, with serum albumin < 2.5 g/dL (< 25 g/L), have low serum total cortisol levels but normal serum free cortisol or salivary cortisol levels and normal adrenal function.

▶ Treatment

A. Acute Phase

If the diagnosis is suspected, draw a blood sample for cortisol determination and treat with hydrocortisone, 100–300 mg intravenously, and saline *immediately,* without waiting for the results. Thereafter, give hydrocortisone phosphate or hydrocortisone sodium succinate, 100 mg intravenously immediately, and continue intravenous infusions of 50–100 mg every 6 hours for the first day. Give the same amount every 8 hours on the second day and then adjust the dosage in view of the clinical picture.

Since bacterial infection frequently precipitates acute adrenal crisis, broad-spectrum antibiotics should be administered empirically while waiting for the results of initial cultures. The patient must be treated for electrolyte abnormalities, hypoglycemia, and dehydration.

B. Convalescent Phase

When the patient is able to take food by mouth, give oral hydrocortisone, 10–20 mg every 6 hours, and reduce dosage to maintenance levels as needed. Most patients ultimately require hydrocortisone twice daily (AM, 10–20 mg; PM, 5–10 mg). Mineralocorticoid therapy is not needed when large amounts of hydrocortisone are being given, but as the dose is reduced it is usually necessary to add fludrocortisone acetate, 0.05–0.2 mg orally daily. Some patients never require fludrocortisone or become edematous at doses of more than 0.05 mg once or twice weekly. Once the crisis has passed, the patient must be evaluated to assess the degree of permanent adrenal insufficiency and to establish the cause if possible.

▶ Prognosis

Rapid treatment will usually be lifesaving. However, acute adrenal insufficiency is frequently unrecognized and untreated since its manifestations mimic more common conditions; lack of treatment leads to shock that is unresponsive to volume replacement and vasopressors, resulting in death.

Hahner S et al. Therapeutic management of adrenal insufficiency. Best Pract Res Clin Endocrinol Metab. 2009 Apr;23(2): 167–79. [PMID: 19500761]

Marik PE. Critical illness-related corticosteroid insufficiency. Chest. 2009 Jan;135(1):181–93. [PMID: 19136406]

Maxime V et al. Adrenal insufficiency in septic shock. Clin Chest Med. 2009 Mar;30(1):17–27. [PMID: 19186278]

Reisch N et al. Frequency and causes of adrenal crises over lifetime in patients with 21-hydroxylase deficiency. Eur J Endocrinol. 2012 Jul;167(1):35–42. [PMID: 22513882]

CHRONIC ADRENOCORTICAL INSUFFICIENCY (Addison Disease)

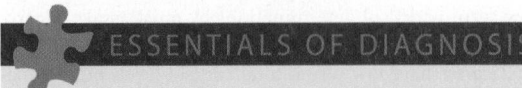

ESSENTIALS OF DIAGNOSIS

▶ Weakness, fatigability, anorexia, weight loss; nausea and vomiting, diarrhea; abdominal pain, muscle and joint pains; amenorrhea.

▶ Sparse axillary hair; increased skin pigmentation, especially of creases, pressure areas, and nipples.

▶ Hypotension, small heart.

▶ Serum sodium may be low; potassium, calcium, and BUN may be elevated; neutropenia, mild anemia, eosinophilia, and relative lymphocytosis may be present.

▶ Plasma cortisol levels are low or fail to rise after administration of corticotropin.

▶ Plasma ACTH level is elevated.

▶ General Considerations

Addison disease refers to primary adrenal insufficiency caused by dysfunction or absence of the adrenal cortices. It is distinct from secondary adrenal insufficiency caused by deficient secretion of ACTH. (See Anterior Hypopituitarism.)

Addison disease is an uncommon disorder with a prevalence of about 140 per million and an annual incidence of about 4 per million in the United States. Addison disease is characterized by a chronic deficiency of cortisol. Serum ACTH levels are consequently elevated, causing pigmentation that ranges from none to strikingly dark. Patients with destruction of the adrenal cortices or with classic 21-hydroxylase deficiency also have mineralocorticoid deficiency with hyponatremia, volume depletion, and hyperkalemia. In contrast, mineralocorticoid deficiency is not present in patients with familial glucocorticoid deficiency and Allgrove syndrome (see below).

▶ Etiology

Autoimmune destruction of the adrenals is the most common cause of Addison disease in the United States (accounting for about 80% of spontaneous cases). With such autoimmunity, adrenal function decreases over several years as it progresses to overt adrenal insufficiency. It may occur alone or as part of a **polyglandular autoimmune (PGA) syndrome. Type 1 PGA** is also known as autoimmune polyendocrinopathy-candidiasis-ectodermal dystrophy (APECED) syndrome and is caused by a defect in T cell-mediated immunity inherited as an autosomal recessive trait. Type 1 PGA usually presents in early childhood with mucocutaneous candidiasis, followed by hypoparathyroidism and dystrophy of the teeth and nails; Addison disease usually appears by age 15 years. Partial or late expression of the syndrome is common. A varied spectrum of associated diseases may be seen in adulthood, including hypogonadism, hypothyroidism, pernicious anemia, alopecia, vitiligo, hepatitis, malabsorption, and Sjögren syndrome.

Type 2 PGA usually presents in young adults age 20–40 years, usually women (female:male ratio is 3:1). The following conditions may be presentations of type 2 PGA: autoimmune adrenal insufficiency, type 1 diabetes mellitus, or autoimmune thyroid disease (usually hypothyroidism, sometimes hyperthyroidism). The combination of Addison disease and hypothyroidism is known as Schmidt syndrome. Patients may also have vitiligo, alopecia areata, Sjögren syndrome, or celiac disease. Type 2 PGA is also associated with autoimmune primary ovarian failure; testicular failure (5%); pernicious anemia (4%); and, rarely, autoimmune hypophysitis, encephalitis, or hypoparathyroidism (late-onset).

Tuberculosis as a leading cause of Addison disease is relatively rare in the United States but common where tuberculosis is more prevalent.

Bilateral **adrenal hemorrhage** may occur during sepsis, heparin-associated thrombocytopenia or anticoagulation, or with antiphospholipid antibody syndrome. It may occur in association with major surgery or trauma, presenting about 1 week later with pain, fever, and shock. It may also occur spontaneously and present with flank pain; MRI may show adrenal enlargement with increased T2-weighted imaging.

Adrenoleukodystrophy is an X-linked peroxisomal disorder causing accumulation of very long-chain fatty acids in the adrenal cortex, testes, brain, and spinal cord. It may present at any age and accounts for one-third of cases of Addison disease in boys. Aldosterone deficiency occurs in 9%. Hypogonadism is common. Psychiatric symptoms often include mania, psychosis, or cognitive impairment. Neurologic deterioration may be severe or mild (particularly in heterozygote women), mimics symptoms of multiple sclerosis, and can occur years after the onset of adrenal insufficiency.

Rare causes of adrenal insufficiency include lymphoma, metastatic carcinoma, coccidioidomycosis, histoplasmosis, cytomegalovirus infection (more frequent in patients with AIDS), syphilitic gummas, scleroderma, amyloidosis, and hemochromatosis.

Congenital adrenal insufficiency occurs in several conditions. **Familial glucocorticoid deficiency** is an autosomal recessive disease that is caused by mutations in the adrenal ACTH receptor (melanocortin 2 receptor, MC2R). It is characterized by isolated cortisol deficiency and ACTH resistance and may present with neonatal hypoglycemia, frequent infections, and dark skin pigmentation. **Triple A (Allgrove) syndrome** is caused by a mutation in the *AAAS* gene that encodes a protein known as ALADIN (**a**lachrima, **a**chalasia, **ad**renal **i**nsufficiency, **n**eurologic disorder). It is characterized by variable expression of the following: adrenal ACTH resistance with cortisol deficiency, achalasia, alacrima, nasal voice, autonomic dysfunction, and neuromuscular disease of varying severity (hyperreflexia to spastic paraplegia). Cortisol deficiency usually presents in infancy but may not occur until the third decade of life. **Congenital adrenal hypoplasia** causes adrenal insufficiency due to absence of the adrenal cortex; patients may also have hypogonadotropic hypogonadism, myopathy, and high-frequency hearing loss.

Patients with hereditary defects in adrenal enzymes for cortisol synthesis develop **congenital adrenal hyperplasia** due to ACTH stimulation. The most common enzyme defect is P450c21 (21-hydroxylase deficiency). Patients with severely defective P450c21 enzymes (classic congenital adrenal hyperplasia) manifest a deficiency of mineralocorticoids (salt wasting) in addition to deficient cortisol and excessive androgens. Hypertension develops in about 60% of adult patients with classic congenital adrenal hyperplasia. Testicular adrenal rests can be found in 44% of men with the condition. Women with milder enzyme defects have adequate cortisol but develop hirsutism in adolescence or adulthood and are said to have "late-onset" congenital adrenal hyperplasia. (See Hirsutism section.) Patients with deficient P450c17 (17-hydroxylase deficiency) have varying degrees of adrenocortical deficiency with associated hypertension, hypokalemia, and primary hypogonadism.

Drugs that cause primary adrenal insufficiency include mitotane (for adrenocortical carcinoma) and abiraterone acetate (Zytiga), a P450c17 inhibitor used for prostate cancer.

▶ Clinical Findings

A. Symptoms and Signs

Symptoms of adrenal insufficiency may include muscle weakness, fatigue, fever, anorexia, nausea, vomiting, weight loss, anxiety, and mental irritability. Patients usually have significant pain: arthralgias, myalgias, chest pain, abdominal pain, back pain, leg pain, or headache. Psychiatric symptoms include irritability and depression. Cerebral edema can cause headache, vomiting, gait disturbance, and intellectual dysfunction that may progress to coma. Hypotension, salt craving, dehydration, orthostasis and syncope can occur. Women may develop scant axillary and pubic hair and experience a lack of libido. Changes in skin pigmentation vary from none at all to dark diffuse tanning over nonexposed as well as exposed areas; hyperpigmentation is especially prominent over the knuckles, elbows, knees, posterior neck, palmar creases, and gingival mucosa. Nail beds may develop longitudinal pigmented bands. Nipples and areolas tend to darken. The skin in pressure areas such as the belt or brassiere lines and the buttocks also darkens. New scars are pigmented. Hypoglycemia may worsen the patient's weakness and mental functioning, rarely leading to coma. Patients tend to be hypotensive and orthostatic; about 90% have systolic blood pressures under 110 mm Hg; blood pressure over 130 mm Hg is rare. Other findings may include a small heart, hyperplasia of lymphoid tissues. Some patients have associated vitiligo (10%). Manifestations of other autoimmune disease (see above) may be present.

Patients with adult-onset adrenoleukodystrophy may present with neuropsychiatric symptoms, sometimes without adrenal insufficiency.

B. Laboratory Findings

The WBC count usually shows moderate neutropenia, lymphocytosis, and a total eosinophil count over 300/mcL. Among patients with *chronic* Addison disease, the serum sodium is usually low (90%) while the potassium is usually elevated (65%). Patients with diarrhea may not be hyperkalemic. Fasting blood glucose may be low. Hypercalcemia may be present. Young men with idiopathic Addison disease are screened for adrenoleukodystrophy by determining plasma very long-chain fatty acid levels; affected patients have high levels.

A plasma cortisol < 3 mcg/dL (< 83 nmol/L) at 8 AM is diagnostic, especially if accompanied by simultaneous elevation of the plasma ACTH level > 200 pg/mL (> 44 pmol/L). The diagnosis is confirmed by a simplified cosyntropin stimulation test, which is performed as follows: (1) Synthetic ACTH$_{1-24}$ (cosyntropin), 0.25 mg, is given intramuscularly. (2) Serum cortisol is obtained 45 minutes after cosyntropin is administered. Normally, serum cortisol rises to at least 20 mcg/dL. For patients receiving corticosteroid treatment, hydrocortisone must not be given for at least 8 hours before the test. Other corticosteroids (eg, prednisone, dexamethasone) do not interfere with specific assays for cortisol.

Serum DHEA levels are < 1000 ng/mL (< 350 nmol/L) in 100% of patients with Addison disease and a serum

DHEA above 1000 ng/mL excludes the diagnosis. However, serum DHEA levels below 1000 ng/mL (< 350 nmol/L) are not helpful, since about 15% of the general population have such low DHEA levels, particularly children and elderly individuals.

Anti-adrenal antibodies are found in the serum in about 50% of cases of autoimmune Addison disease. The presence of serum antibodies to 21-hydroxylase help secure the diagnosis of autoimmune adrenal insufficiency. Antibodies to thyroid (45%) and other tissues may be present.

Salt-wasting congenital adrenal hyperplasia due to 21-hydroxylase deficiency is usually diagnosed at birth in females due to ambiguous genitalia. Males and patients with milder enzyme defects may present later. The diagnosis of adrenal insufficiency is made as above. The specific diagnosis requires elevated serum levels of 17-OH progesterone.

Elevated plasma renin activity (PRA) indicates the presence of depleted intravascular volume and the need for higher doses of fludrocortisone replacement. Serum epinephrine levels are low in patients with adrenal insufficiency, since these patients do not have the high local concentrations of cortisol that are required to induce the enzyme PNMT in adrenal medulla for the synthesis of epinephrine from norepinephrine.

C. Imaging

When Addison disease is not clearly autoimmune, a chest radiograph is obtained to look for tuberculosis, fungal infection, or cancer as possible causes. CT scan of the abdomen will show small noncalcified adrenals in autoimmune Addison disease. The adrenals are enlarged in about 85% of cases due to metastatic or granulomatous disease. Calcification is noted in about 50% of cases of tuberculous Addison disease but is also seen with hemorrhage, fungal infection, pheochromocytoma, and melanoma.

► Differential Diagnosis

Patients with secondary adrenal insufficiency (hypopituitarism) lack ACTH and have normal skin pigmentation, in contrast to patients with Addison disease who have elevated levels of ACTH that can increase skin pigmentation. Patients with ACTH deficiency have normal mineralocorticoid production and do not develop hyperkalemia. Addison disease should be considered in any patient with unexplained hypotension, but shock is usually caused by more common conditions such as gastrointestinal bleeding or sepsis. Hyponatremia or hyperkalemia may be seen in numerous other conditions (see Chapter 21). Drospirenone, the progestin component in certain oral contraceptives, may cause hyperkalemia.

Unexplained weight loss, weakness, and anorexia may be mistaken for occult cancer. Nausea, vomiting, diarrhea, and abdominal pain may be misdiagnosed as intrinsic gastrointestinal disease. The hyperpigmentation may be confused with that due to ethnic or racial factors. Weight loss may simulate anorexia nervosa or emotional stress. The neurologic manifestations of Allgrove syndrome and

adrenoleukodystrophy (especially in women) may mimic multiple sclerosis. Hemochromatosis also enters the differential diagnosis of skin hyperpigmentation, but may truly be a cause of Addison disease. About 17% of patients with AIDS have symptoms of cortisol resistance. AIDS can also cause frank adrenal insufficiency.

Hyperkalemia can be caused by isolated hypoaldosteronism and is seen in various conditions. Hyporeninemic hypoaldosteronism can be caused by renal tubular acidosis type IV and is commonly seen with diabetic nephropathy, hypertensive nephrosclerosis, tubulointerstitial diseases, and AIDS (see Chapter 21). Hyperreninemic hypoaldosteronism can be seen in patients with myotonic dystrophy, aldosterone synthase deficiency, and congenital adrenal hyperplasia. Hyperkalemia, hypertension, and hypogonadism may present as delayed adolescence or in adulthood in some patients with congenital adrenal hyperplasia (CYP17 deficiency); cortisol deficiency is also usually present but may not be clinically evident.

► Complications

Any of the complications of the underlying disease (eg, tuberculosis) are more likely to occur, and the patient is susceptible to intercurrent infections that may precipitate crisis. Associated autoimmune diseases are common (see above).

► Treatment

A. General Measures

Patients with Addison disease must be thoroughly informed about their condition. All infections should be treated immediately and vigorously, with the dose of hydrocortisone increased appropriately (see below). Patients are advised to wear a medical alert bracelet or medal reading, "Adrenal insufficiency—takes hydrocortisone."

B. Specific Therapy

Replacement therapy should include a combination of corticosteroids and mineralocorticoids. In mild cases, hydrocortisone alone may be adequate.

Hydrocortisone is the drug of choice. Most addisonian patients are well maintained on 15–30 mg of hydrocortisone orally daily in two divided doses, two-thirds in the morning and one-third in the late afternoon or early evening. Some patients respond better to prednisone in a dosage of about 2–4 mg orally in the morning and 1–2 mg in the evening. Adjustments in dosage are made according to the clinical response. A proper dose usually results in a normal WBC count differential.

The dose of corticosteroid should be raised in case of infection, trauma, surgery, stressful diagnostic procedures, or other forms of stress. The maximum hydrocortisone dose for severe stress is 50 mg intravenously or intramuscularly every 6 hours. Lower doses, oral or parenteral, are used for less severe stress. The dose is reduced back to normal as the stress subsides.

Fludrocortisone acetate has a potent sodium-retaining effect. The dosage is 0.05–0.3 mg orally daily or every other day. In the presence of postural hypotension, hyponatremia, or hyperkalemia, the dosage is increased. Similarly, in patients with fatigue, elevated PRA indicates the need for a higher replacement dose of fludrocortisone. If edema, hypokalemia, or hypertension ensues, the dose is decreased.

DHEA is given to some patients with adrenal insufficiency. In a double-blind clinical trial, patients taking DHEA 50 mg orally each morning experienced an improved sense of well-being, increased muscle mass, and a reversal in bone loss at the femoral neck. DHEA replacement did not improve fatigue, cognitive problems, or sexual dysfunction; however, its placebo effect may be significant in that regard. Older women who receive DHEA should be monitored for androgenic effects. Because over-the-counter preparations of DHEA have variable potencies, it is best to have the pharmacy formulate this with pharmaceutical-grade micronized DHEA.

▶ Prognosis

The life expectancy of patients with Addison disease has been considered reasonably normal, as long as they are very compliant with taking their medications and are knowledgeable about their condition. However, a retrospective Swedish study of 1675 patients with Addison disease found an unexpected increase in all-cause mortality, mostly from cardiovascular disease, malignancy, and infectious causes. Associated conditions can pose additional health risks. For example, patients with adrenoleukodystrophy or Allgrove syndrome may suffer from neurologic disease. Patients with adrenal tuberculosis may have a serious systemic infection that requires treatment. Adrenal crisis can occur in patients who stop their medication or who experience stress such as infection, trauma, or surgery without appropriately higher doses of corticosteroids. Patients who take excessive doses of corticosteroid replacement can develop Cushing syndrome, which imposes its own risks.

Many patients with treated Addison disease complain of chronic low-grade fatigue.

Many patients with Addison disease do not feel entirely normal, despite glucocorticoid and mineralocorticoid replacement. This may be due, in part, to the inadequacy of oral replacement to duplicate cortisol's normal circadian rhythm. Also, patients with Addison disease are deficient in epinephrine, but replacement epinephrine is not available. Fatigue may also be an indication of suboptimal dosing of medication, electrolyte imbalance, or concurrent problems such as hypothyroidism or diabetes mellitus. However, most patients with Addison disease are able to live fully active lives.

Baker PR et al. Predicting the onset of Addison's disease: ACTH, renin, cortisol and 21-hydroxylase autoantibodies. Clin Endocrinol (Oxf). 2012 May;76(5):617–24. [PMID: 22066755]

Betterle C et al. Autoimmune Addison's disease. Endocr Dev. 2011;20:161–72. [PMID: 21164269]

Bornstein SR. Predisposing factors for adrenal insufficiency. N Engl J Med. 2009 May 28;360(22):2328–39. [PMID: 19474430]

Chakera AJ et al. Addison disease in adults: diagnosis and management. Am J Med. 2010 May;123(5):409–13. [PMID: 20399314]

Ekman B et al. A randomized, double-blind, crossover study comparing two- and four-dose hydrocortisone regimen with regard to quality of life, cortisol and ACTH profiles in patients with primary adrenal insufficiency. Clin Endocrinol (Oxf). 2012 Jul;77(1):18–25. [PMID: 22288685]

Finkielstain GP et al. Clinical characteristics of a cohort of 244 patients with congenital adrenal hyperplasia. J Clin Endocrinol Metab. 2012 Dec;97(12):4429–38. [PMID: 22990093]

Quinkler M et al. What is the best long-term management strategy for patients with primary adrenal insufficiency? Clin Endocrinol (Oxf). 2012 Jan;76(1):21–5. [PMID: 21585418]

Speiser PW et al. Congenital adrenal hyperplasia due to steroid 21-hydroxylase deficiency: an Endocrine Society clinical practice guideline. J Clin Endocrinol Metab. 2010 Sep;95(9):4133–60. [PMID: 20823466]

Yong SL et al. Supplemental perioperative steroids for surgical patients with adrenal insufficiency. Cochrane Database Syst Rev. 2012 Dec 12;12:CD005367. [PMID: 23235622]

CUSHING SYNDROME (Hypercortisolism)

ESSENTIALS OF DIAGNOSIS

- ▶ Central obesity, muscle wasting, thin skin, hirsutism, purple striae.
- ▶ Psychological changes.
- ▶ Osteoporosis, hypertension, poor wound healing.
- ▶ Hyperglycemia, glycosuria, leukocytosis, lymphocytopenia, hypokalemia.
- ▶ Elevated serum cortisol and urinary free cortisol. Lack of normal suppression by dexamethasone.

▶ General Considerations

The term Cushing "syndrome" refers to the manifestations of excessive corticosteroids, commonly due to supraphysiologic doses of corticosteroid drugs and rarely due to spontaneous production of excessive corticosteroids by the adrenal cortex. Cases of spontaneous Cushing syndrome are rare (2.6 new cases yearly per million population) and have several possible causes.

About 40% of cases are due to Cushing "disease," by which is meant the manifestations of hypercortisolism due to ACTH hypersecretion by the pituitary. Cushing disease is caused by a benign pituitary adenoma that is typically very small (< 5 mm) and usually located in the anterior pituitary (98%) or in the posterior pituitary (2%). It is at least three times more frequent in women than men. Excessive ingestion of gamma-hydroxybutyric acid (GHB, Xyrem) can also induce ACTH-dependent Cushing syndrome that resolves after the drug is stopped.

About 10% of cases are due to nonpituitary ACTH-secreting neoplasms (eg, small cell lung carcinoma), which produce excessive amounts of ectopic ACTH. Hypokalemia and hyperpigmentation are commonly found in this group.

About 15% of cases are due to ACTH from a source that cannot be initially located.

About 30% of cases are due to excessive autonomous secretion of cortisol by the adrenals—independently of ACTH, serum levels of which are usually low. Most such cases are due to a unilateral adrenal tumor. Benign adrenal adenomas are generally small and produce mostly cortisol; adrenocortical carcinomas are usually large when discovered and can produce excessive cortisol as well as androgens, with resultant hirsutism and virilization. ACTH-independent macronodular adrenal hyperplasia can also produce hypercortisolism due to the adrenal cortex cells' abnormal stimulation by hormones such as catecholamines, arginine vasopressin, serotonin, hCG/LH, or gastric inhibitory polypeptide; in the latter case, hypercortisolism may be intermittent and food dependent and serum ACTH may not be completely suppressed. Pigmented bilateral adrenal macronodular adrenal hyperplasia is a rare cause of Cushing syndrome in children and young adults; it may be an isolated condition or part of the Carney complex.

▶ Clinical Findings

A. Symptoms and Signs

Patients with Cushing syndrome usually have central obesity with a plethoric "moon face," "buffalo hump," supraclavicular fat pads, protuberant abdomen, and thin extremities. Muscle atrophy causes weakness, with difficulty standing up from a seated position or climbing stairs. Patients may also experience oligomenorrhea or amenorrhea (or erectile dysfunction in the male), backache, headache, hypertension, osteoporosis, avascular necrosis of bone, acne, and superficial skin infections. Patients may have thirst and polyuria (with or without glycosuria), renal calculi, glaucoma, purple striae (especially around the thighs, breasts, and abdomen), and easy bruisability. Unusual bacterial or fungal infections are common. Wound healing is impaired. Mental symptoms may range from diminished ability to concentrate to increased lability of mood to frank psychosis. Patients are susceptible to opportunistic infections.

B. Laboratory Findings

Glucose tolerance is impaired as a result of insulin resistance. Polyuria is present as a result of increased free water clearance; diabetes mellitus with glycosuria may worsen it. Patients with Cushing syndrome often have leukocytosis with relative granulocytosis and lymphopenia. Hypokalemia may be present, particularly in cases of ectopic ACTH secretion.

▶ Tests for Hypercortisolism

The easiest screening test for Cushing syndrome is the dexamethasone suppression test: dexamethasone 1 mg is given orally at 11 PM and serum is collected for cortisol determination at about 8 AM the next morning; a cortisol level < 5 mcg/dL (< 135 nmol/L, fluorometric assay) or < 1.8 mcg/dL (< 49 nmol/L, high-performance liquid chromatography [HPLC] assay) excludes Cushing syndrome with some certainty. However, 8% of established patients with pituitary Cushing disease have dexamethasone-suppressed cortisol levels < 2 mcg/dL. Therefore, when

other clinical criteria suggest hypercortisolism, further evaluation is warranted even in the face of normal dexamethasone-suppressed serum cortisol. Antiseizure drugs (eg, phenytoin, phenobarbital, primidone) and rifampin accelerate the metabolism of dexamethasone, causing a lack of cortisol suppression by dexamethasone. Estrogens—during pregnancy or as oral contraceptives or ERT—may also cause lack of dexamethasone suppressibility.

Patients with an abnormal dexamethasone suppression test require further investigation, which includes a 24-hour urine collection for free cortisol and creatinine. An abnormally high 24-hour urine free cortisol (or free cortisol to creatinine ratio of > 95 mcg cortisol/g creatinine) helps confirm hypercortisolism. A misleadingly high urine free cortisol excretion occurs with high fluid intake. In pregnancy, urine free cortisol is increased, while 17-hydroxycorticosteroids remain normal and diurnal variability of serum cortisol is normal. Carbamazepine and fenofibrate cause false elevations of urine free cortisol when determined by HPLC.

A midnight serum cortisol level > 7.5 mcg/dL is indicative of Cushing syndrome and distinguishes it from other conditions associated with a high urine free cortisol (pseudo-Cushing states). Requirements for this test include being in the same time zone for at least 3 days, being without food for at least 3 hours, and having an indwelling intravenous line established in advance for the blood draw.

Late-night salivary cortisol assays are useful due to the inconvenience of obtaining a midnight blood specimen for serum cortisol. Assays are available that use liquid chromatography-tandem mass spectrometry. Midnight salivary cortisol levels are normally < 0.15 mcg/dL (4.0 nmol/L). Midnight salivary cortisol levels that are consistently > 0.25 mcg/dL (7.0 nmol/L) are considered very abnormal. The late-night salivary cortisol test has a high sensitivity and specificity for Cushing syndrome, but false-positive and false-negative tests have occurred.

Interestingly, hypercortisolism without Cushing syndrome can occur in several conditions, such as severe depression, anorexia nervosa, alcoholism, and familial cortisol resistance.

▶ Finding the Cause of Hypercortisolism

Once hypercortisolism is confirmed, a plasma or serum ACTH is obtained. It must be collected properly in a plastic tube on ice and processed quickly by a laboratory with a reliable, sensitive assay. A level of ACTH below 20 pg/mL (< 4.4 pmol/L) indicates a probable adrenal tumor, whereas higher levels are produced by pituitary or ectopic ACTH-secreting tumors.

▶ Localizing Techniques

In ACTH-independent Cushing syndrome, CT of the adrenals usually detects a mass lesion. Most such lesions are benign adrenal adenomas, but an adrenal carcinoma is suspected in the following circumstances: (1) diameter ≥ 4 cm; (2) nodule growth; or (3) atypical imaging: density on noncontrast CT > 10 Hounsfield units (HU) or CT contrast washout ≥ 60% or relative contrast washout ≥ 40% at 15 minutes after intravenous administration.

In ACTH-dependent Cushing syndrome, MRI of the pituitary demonstrates a pituitary lesion in about 50% of cases. Premature cerebral atrophy is often noted. When the pituitary MRI is normal or shows a tiny (< 5 mm diameter) irregularity that may be incidental, selective catheterization of the inferior petrosal sinus veins draining the pituitary is performed. ACTH levels in the inferior petrosal sinus that are more than twice the simultaneous peripheral venous ACTH levels are indicative of pituitary Cushing disease. Inferior petrosal sinus sampling is also done during CRH administration, which ordinarily causes the ACTH levels in the inferior petrosal sinus to be over three times the peripheral ACTH level when the pituitary is the source of ACTH.

When inferior petrosal sinus ACTH concentrations are not above the requisite levels, a search for an ectopic source of ACTH is undertaken. Location of ectopic sources of ACTH commences with CT scanning of the chest and abdomen, with special attention to the lungs (for carcinoid or small cell carcinomas), the thymus, the pancreas, and the adrenals. In patients with ACTH-dependent Cushing syndrome, chest masses should not be assumed to be the source of ACTH, since opportunistic infections are common, so it is prudent to biopsy a chest mass to confirm the pathologic diagnosis prior to resection.

CT scanning fails to detect the source of ACTH in about 40% of patients with ectopic ACTH secretion.[111] In-octreotide (OCT, somatostatin receptor scintigraphy) scanning is also useful in detecting occult tumors. A low-dose scan with 6 mCi OCT is used first; a high-dose scan with 12 mCi OCT may be used if the low-dose scan gives equivocal results. [18]FDG-PET scanning is not usually helpful. Some ectopic ACTH-secreting tumors elude discovery, necessitating bilateral adrenalectomy. The ectopic source of ACTH should continue to be sought, since it may become detectable by OCT or CT scanning at a later date.

In non-ACTH-dependent Cushing syndrome, a CT scan of the adrenals can localize the adrenal tumor in most cases.

▶ Differential Diagnosis

Alcoholic patients can have hypercortisolism and many clinical manifestations of Cushing syndrome. Pregnant women have elevated serum ACTH levels, increased urine free cortisol, and high serum cortisol levels due to high serum levels of cortisol-binding globulin. Critically ill patients frequently have hypercortisolism, usually with suppression of serum ACTH. Regular use of the "party drug" gamma hydroxybutyrate (GHB, sodium oxybate) has been reported to cause reversible ACTH-dependent Cushing syndrome. Depressed patients also have hypercortisolism that can be nearly impossible to distinguish biochemically from Cushing syndrome but without clinical signs of Cushing syndrome. Cushing syndrome can be misdiagnosed as anorexia nervosa (and vice versa) owing to the muscle wasting and extraordinarily high urine free cortisol levels found in anorexia. Patients with severe obesity frequently have an abnormal dexamethasone suppression test, but the urine free cortisol is usually normal, as is diurnal variation of serum cortisol. Patients with

familial cortisol resistance have hyperandrogenism, hypertension, and hypercortisolism without actual Cushing syndrome.

Some adolescents develop violaceous striae on the abdomen, back, and breasts; these are known as "striae distensae" and are not indicative of Cushing syndrome. Patients with familial partial lipodystrophy type I develop central obesity and moon facies, along with thin extremities due to atrophy of subcutaneous fat. However, these patients' muscles are strong and may be hypertrophic, distinguishing this condition from Cushing syndrome. Patients receiving antiretroviral therapy for HIV-1 infection frequently develop partial lipodystrophy with thin extremities and central obesity with a dorsocervical fat pad ("buffalo hump") that may mimic Cushing syndrome.

Adrenal nodules are discovered incidentally on up to 4% of abdominal CT or MRI scans obtained for other reasons; they have been dubbed **"adrenal incidentalomas."** It is always necessary to determine whether such masses are malignant or secretory. Although the overwhelming majority of adrenal incidentalomas are benign adrenal adenomas, the differential diagnosis includes adrenal carcinoma, pheochromocytoma, metastases, lymphoma, myelolipoma, infection, and cysts. When an adrenal incidentaloma > 4 cm in diameter is detected in a patient without a history of malignancy, it should be resected, unless it is an unmistakably benign myelolipoma, hemorrhage, or adrenal cyst. Masses 3–4 cm in diameter may be resected if they appear suspicious. Smaller adrenal incidentalomas are usually observed. A noncontrast CT scan can determine the density of the mass; adrenal incidentalomas with a density < 10 Hounsfield units (HU) on CT are unlikely to be a pheochromocytoma or metastasis. An adrenal intravenous contrast "washout" CT scan is obtained; the density of the adrenal incidentaloma in HU is calculated 60 seconds after contrast and again 15 minutes after contrast; a reduction (washout) of ≥ 40% is consistent with a benign adrenal adenoma. However, such testing is never absolutely accurate; so if the adrenal incidentaloma is not resected, a follow-up CT of the adrenals in 6–12 months is recommended to look for growth.

All patients with an adrenal nodule require a clinical assessment for Cushing syndrome and hyperaldosteronism. In particular, patients with hypertension or any manifestations of Cushing syndrome require an appropriate biochemical evaluation. All (even normotensive) patients with an adrenal incidentaloma require testing for pheochromocytoma with plasma fractionated free metanephrines (see Pheochromocytoma).

▶ Treatment

Cushing disease is best treated by transsphenoidal selective resection of the pituitary adenoma. With an experienced pituitary neurosurgeon, reported remission rates range from 65% to 90%. After successful pituitary surgery, the rest of the pituitary usually returns to normal function; however, the pituitary corticotrophs remain suppressed and require 6–36 months to recover normal function. Hydrocortisone or prednisone replacement therapy is necessary in the meantime. When Cushing disease persists or recurs after pituitary surgery, bilateral laparoscopic adrenalectomy is usually the best treatment option.

Radiation therapy is an option for patients with ACTH-secreting pituitary tumors that persist or recur after pituitary surgery. Stereotactic pituitary radiosurgery (gamma knife or cyberknife), normalizes urine free cortisol in two-thirds of patients within 12 months compared with a 23% cure rate with conventional radiation therapy. Pituitary radiosurgery can also be used to treat Nelson syndrome, the progressive enlargement of ACTH-secreting pituitary tumors following bilateral adrenalectomy.

Medical therapy is not usually the best option for patients with persistent or recurrent Cushing disease and must be used indefinitely. Cabergoline, 0.5–3.5 mg orally twice weekly, was successful in 40% of patients in one small study. Pasireotide, a multireceptor-targeting somatostatin analog, is another potential treatment for refractory ACTH-secreting pituitary tumors causing Cushing disease or Nelson syndrome. Pasireotide (600–900 mcg subcutaneously twice daily) normalizes the urine free cortisol in at least 17% of patients with Cushing disease. Ketoconazole inhibits adrenal steroidogenesis and is another treatment option when given in doses of about 200 mg orally every 6 hours; however, it is marginally effective and can cause liver toxicity. Mifepristone is a glucocorticoid receptor antagonist that is given orally in doses of 300–1200 mg daily. Side effects are frequent and include nausea, headache, fatigue, hypokalemia, abortion, and adrenal insufficiency.

Benign adrenal adenomas may be resected laparoscopically if they are < 6 cm diameter. Postoperatively, the contralateral adrenal's cortisol secretion is deficient due to ACTH suppression, so postoperative corticosteroid replacement is required until recovery occurs.

Adrenocortical carcinomas can usually be distinguished from benign adrenal adenomas since they are usually larger (average 11 cm diameter) and many have metastases that are visible on preoperative scans. However, some adrenal carcinomas are smaller and the histopathologic diagnosis can be difficult. Some adrenal carcinomas have microscopic metastases that can only be inferred from the presence of detectable cortisol levels following removal of the primary adrenal tumor. The ENSAT staging system is used: stage 1 is a localized tumor ≤ 5 cm; stage 2 is a localized tumor > 5 cm; stage 3, tumor with local metastases; stage 4, tumor with distant metastases.

Most patients with adrenal carcinoma should be treated postoperatively with mitotane for a course of 2–5 years, since it appears to improve prognosis (see below). Mitotane is given, beginning with 0.5 g twice daily with meals and increasing to 1 g twice daily within 2 weeks. The doses of mitotane are adjusted every 2–3 weeks ideally to reach serum levels of 14–20 mcg/mL; however, only about half the patients can tolerate mitotane levels above 14 mcg/mL. Mitotane side effects include central nervous system depression, lethargy, hypogonadism, hypercholesterolemia, hypocalcemia, hepatotoxicity, leukopenia, hypertension, nausea, rash, and TSH suppression with hypothyroidism. Mitotane also induces the hepatic enzyme CYP3A4, which accelerates the metabolism of sunitinib, cortisol, calcium channel blockers, benzodiazepines, some statins, some opioids, and some macrolide antibiotics. Mitotane often causes primary adrenal insufficiency. Replacement hydrocortisone or prednisone should be started when mitotane doses reach 2 g daily. The replacement dose of hydrocortisone starts at 15 mg in the morning and 10 mg in the afternoon, but must often be doubled or tripled because mitotane increases cortisol metabolism and cortisol binding globulin levels; the latter can artifactually raise serum cortisol levels.

Ketoconazole, metyrapone, or mifepristone can also be used to help treat hypercortisolism in unresectable adrenal carcinoma. Other chemotherapy regimens have been used; for example, the combination of cixutumumab and temsirolimus produced stable disease in 11 of 26 patients in one small study.

Ectopic ACTH-secreting tumors should be located, when possible, and surgically resected. If that cannot be done, laparoscopic bilateral adrenalectomy is usually recommended. Medical treatment with a combination of mitotane (3–5 g/24 h), ketoconazole (0.4–1.2 g/24 h), and metyrapone (3–4.5 g/24 h) often suppresses the hypercortisolism. Octreotide LAR, 20–40 mg injected intramuscularly every 28 days, suppresses ACTH secretion in about one-third of such cases. Pasireotide, a newer somatostatin analogue, may prove more effective. Potassium-sparing diuretics are often helpful.

Patients who are successfully treated for Cushing syndrome typically develop "cortisol withdrawal syndrome," even when given replacement corticosteroids for adrenal insufficiency. Manifestations can include hypotension, nausea, fatigue, arthralgias, myalgias, pruritus, and flaking skin. Increasing the hydrocortisone replacement to 30 mg orally twice daily can improve these symptoms; the dosage is then reduced slowly as tolerated. Patients with Cushing syndrome are prone to develop osteoporosis. Bone densitometry is recommended for all patients and treatment is commenced for patients with osteoporosis. (See Osteoporosis.)

▶ Prognosis

The manifestations of Cushing syndrome regress with time, but patients are often left with residual mild cognitive impairment, muscle weakness, osteoporosis, and sequelae from vertebral fractures. Younger patients have a better chance for recovery and children with short stature may have catch-up growth following cure.

Patients with Cushing syndrome from a benign adrenal adenoma experience a 5-year survival of 95% and a 10-year survival of 90%, following a successful adrenalectomy. Patients with Cushing disease from a pituitary adenoma experience a similar survival if their pituitary surgery is successful, which can be predicted if the postoperative nonsuppressed serum cortisol is < 2 mcg/dL. Following successful treatment, overall mortality remains particularly higher for patients with older age at diagnosis, higher preoperative ACTH concentrations, and longer duration of hypercortisolism.

Transsphenoidal surgery incurs a failure rate of about 10–20%, often due to the adenoma's ectopic position or invasion of the cavernous sinus. Those patients who have a complete remission after transsphenoidal surgery have about a 15–20% chance of recurrence over the next 10 years. Patients with failed pituitary surgery may require pituitary radiation therapy, which has its own morbidity. Laparoscopic bilateral adrenalectomy may be required; recurrence of hypercortisolism may occur as a result of growth of an adrenal remnant stimulated by high levels of ACTH. The prognosis for patients with ectopic ACTH-producing tumors depends on the aggressiveness and stage of the particular tumor. Patients with ACTH of unknown source have a 5-year survival rate of 65% and a 10-year survival rate of 55%.

In patients with adrenocortical carcinoma, the 5-year survival rates of treated patients has correlated with the ENSAT stage. For stage 1, the 5-year survival was 81%; for stage 2, 61%; for stage 3, 50%; and for stage 4, 13%. In patients with stage 1 or 2 disease, long-term survival does occur. However, despite apparent complete resection in stage 1, 2 or 3 tumors, visible metastases develop in about 40% of patients within 2 years. Adjuvant therapy with mitotane appears to improve the prognosis. Patients with stage 4 disease at the time of surgery have a poorer prognosis, but debulking surgery and therapy with mitotane may be beneficial.

▶ Complications

Cushing syndrome, if untreated, produces serious morbidity and even death. The patient may suffer from the complications of hypertension or diabetes mellitus. Susceptibility to infections is increased. Compression fractures of the osteoporotic spine and aseptic necrosis of the femoral head may cause marked disability. Nephrolithiasis and psychosis may occur. Following bilateral adrenalectomy for Cushing disease, a pituitary adenoma may enlarge progressively (Nelson syndrome), causing local destruction (eg, visual field impairment, cranial nerve palsy) and hyperpigmentation.

▶ When to Refer

- Dexamethasone suppression test is abnormal.

▶ When to Admit

- Transsphenoidal hypophysectomy, adrenalectomy, or resection of ectopic ACTH-secreting tumor.

Arnaldi G et al. Advances in the epidemiology, pathogenesis, and management of Cushing's syndrome complications. J Endocrinol Invest. 2012 Apr;35(4):434–48. [PMID: 22652826]
Bertagna X et al. Approach to the Cushing's disease patient with persistent/recurrent hypercortisolism after pituitary surgery. J Clin Endocrinol Metab. 2013 Apr;98(4):1307–18. [PMID: 23564942]
Graversen D et al. Mortality in Cushing's syndrome: a systematic review and meta-analysis. Eur J Intern Med. 2012 Apr;23(3):278–82. [PMID: 22385888]

Kamenický P et al. Mitotane, metyrapone, and ketoconazole combination therapy as an alternative to rescue adrenalectomy for severe ACTH-dependent Cushing's syndrome. J Clin Endocrinol Metab. 2011 Sep;96(9):2796–804. [PMID: 21752886]
Terzolo M et al. Subclinical Cushing's syndrome: definition and management. Clin Endocrinol (Oxf). 2012 Jan;76(1):12–8. [PMID: 21988204]
Tritos NA et al. Advances in medical therapies for Cushing's syndrome. Discov Med. 2012 Feb;13(69):171–9. [PMID: 22369976]
Valassi E et al. Clinical consequences of Cushing's syndrome. Pituitary. 2012 Sep;15(3):319–29. [PMID: 22527617]

PRIMARY ALDOSTERONISM

 ESSENTIALS OF DIAGNOSIS

▶ Hypertension that may be severe or drug-resistant.

▶ Hypokalemia (in minority of patients) may cause polyuria, polydipsia, muscle weakness.

▶ Elevated plasma and urine aldosterone levels and low plasma renin level.

▶ General Considerations

Primary aldosteronism (hyperaldosteronism) causes hypertension by an inappropriately high aldosterone secretion that does not suppress adequately with sodium loading. Primary aldosteronism is believed to account for 8% of all cases of hypertension and 20% of cases of resistant hypertension. It may be difficult to distinguish primary aldosteronism from cases of low renin essential hypertension, with which it may overlap. Patients of all ages may be affected, but the peak incidence is between 30 years and 60 years. Excessive aldosterone production increases sodium retention and suppresses plasma renin. It increases renal potassium excretion, which can lead to hypokalemia. Cardiovascular events are more prevalent in patients with aldosteronism (35%) than in those with essential hypertension (11%). Primary aldosteronism may be caused by an aldosterone-producing adrenal adenoma (Conn syndrome), 40% of which have been found to have somatic mutations in a gene involved with the potassium channel. Primary aldosteronism is also commonly caused by unilateral or bilateral adrenal hyperplasia. Bilateral aldosteronism may be corticosteroid suppressible, due to an autosomal-dominant genetic defect allowing ACTH stimulation of aldosterone production. Hyperaldosteronism may rarely be due to a malignant ovarian tumor.

▶ Clinical Findings

A. Symptoms and Signs

Hyperaldosteronism is the most common cause of refractory hypertension in youths and middle-aged adults. Patients have hypertension that is typically moderate but may be severe. Some patients have only diastolic hypertension, without other symptoms and signs. Edema is rarely seen in primary aldosteronism. About 37% of patients have hypokalemia and may consequently have symptoms of muscular weakness (at times with paralysis simulating periodic paralysis), paresthesias with frank tetany, headache, polyuria, and polydipsia.

B. Laboratory Findings

About 20% of hypertensive patients have a low PRA, and a significant portion of these patients have primary aldosteronism. Initial screening can also include both aldosterone and plasma renin activity to determine an aldosterone to renin ratio (see below).

Plasma potassium should also be determined in hypertensive individuals. However, hypokalemia, once thought to be the hallmark of hyperaldosteronism, is present in only 37% of affected patients: 50% of those with an adrenal adenoma and 17% of those with adrenal hyperplasia. Proper phlebotomy technique is important to avoid spurious increases in potassium. The blood should be drawn slowly with a syringe and needle (rather than a vacutainer) at least 5 seconds after tourniquet release and without fist clenching. Plasma potassium, rather than the routine serum potassium, should be measured in cases of unexpected hyperkalemia, with the separation of plasma from cells within 30 minutes of collection. Besides hypokalemia, many patients with primary aldosteronism have metabolic alkalosis with an elevated serum bicarbonate (HCO_3^-) concentration.

Testing for primary aldosteronism should be done for all hypertensive patients with hypokalemia, whether spontaneous or diuretic induced. But since only a minority of affected patients have hypokalemia, testing should also be considered for (even normokalemic) hypertensive patients with (1) treatment-resistant hypertension (despite three drugs); (2) severe hypertension: > 160 mm Hg systolic or > 100 mm Hg diastolic; (3) early-onset hypertension; (4) low-renin hypertension; (5) hypertension with an adrenal mass; (6) hypertension with a family history of early-onset hypertension or cerebrovascular accident before age 40 years; and (7) a first-degree relative who has aldosteronism.

For a patient to be properly tested for primary aldosteronism, certain antihypertensive medications should ideally be held. Diuretics should be discontinued for 3 weeks. Dihydropyridine calcium channel blockers can normalize aldosterone secretion, thus interfering with the diagnosis. Beta-blockers suppress PRA in patients with essential hypertension. Antihypertensive medications that have minimal effects on the plasma aldosterone:renin ratio include ACE inhibitors, alpha-blockers, verapamil, hydralazine, prazosin, doxazosin, and terazosin. However, it may be impractical to hold or change antihypertensive medicines; in such cases, testing should proceed.

During the testing period, the patient should have an unrestricted high sodium intake. The patient should be out of bed for at least 2 hours and seated for 5–15 minutes before the blood draw, which should preferably be obtained between 8 AM and 10 AM. Renin is measured as either PRA or direct renin concentration. Serum aldosterone should ideally be measured with a tandem mass spectrometry assay.

For patients who have not been receiving diuretics for at least 3 weeks, a plasma renin activity (PRA) that is normal or elevated makes primary aldosteronism very unlikely. However, a low PRA alone cannot establish the diagnosis of primary aldosteronism, since it occurs in many patients with essential hypertension.

An aldosterone:renin ratio is a sensitive screening test. Serum aldosterone (ng/dL):PRA (ng/mL/h) ratios < 24 exclude primary aldosteronism, whereas ratios between 24 and 67 are suspicious and ratios > 67 are very suggestive of primary aldosteronism. Such elevated ratios are not diagnostic; rather, they indicate the need to document increased aldosterone secretion with a 24-hour urine collection. Another problem with the aldosterone:renin ratio is the use of different units and measurements. For aldosterone, 1 ng/dL converts to 27.7 pmol/L. For renin, a PRA of 1 ng/mL/h (12.8 pmol/L/min) converts to a direct renin concentration of 5.2 ng/L (8.2 mU/L).

When the aldosterone:renin ratio is high, a 24-hour urine collection is assayed for aldosterone, free cortisol, and creatinine. A low PRA (< 5 mcg/L/h) with a urine aldosterone > 20 mcg/24 h (> 555 pmol/L) indicates primary aldosteronism.

C. Imaging

All patients with biochemically confirmed primary aldosteronism require a thin-section CT scan of the adrenals to screen for a rare adrenal carcinoma. In the absence of a large adrenal carcinoma, adrenal CT scanning cannot reliably distinguish unilateral from bilateral aldosterone excess, having a sensitivity of 78% and a specificity of 78% for unilateral aldosteronism. Therefore, the decision to perform a unilateral adrenalectomy should not be based solely on an adrenal CT scan. However, since CT scanning and laboratory testing are often inconclusive, adrenal vein sampling is often required.

D. Further Evaluation

Patients with primary aldosteronism (whose adrenal CT scan shows normal adrenals or a small nodule) should be considered for an empiric trial of medical therapy with spironolactone or eplerenone (see below). If medical therapy is ineffective or if surgery is desired for an apparent adrenal adenoma, further evaluation for surgical candidacy should be done with further laboratory testing and adrenal vein sampling to assist in distinguishing a unilateral aldosteronoma from bilateral adrenal hyperplasia (see below).

Plasma may be assayed for 18-hydroxycorticosterone; a level > 100 ng/dL (> 2750 pmol/L) is seen with adrenal aldosteronomas, whereas levels < 100 ng/dL (< 2750 pmol/L) are nondiagnostic. In addition, a posture stimulation test may be performed, but this requires overnight hospitalization. The test is performed by drawing blood for aldosterone at 8 AM while the patient is supine after overnight recumbency and again after the patient is upright for 4 hours. Patients with a unilateral adrenal adenoma usually have a baseline plasma aldosterone level > 20 ng/dL (> 550 pmol/L) that does not rise. Patients with bilateral adrenal hyperplasia typically have a baseline plasma aldosterone level < 20 ng/dL (< 550 pmol/L) that rises after 4 hours of upright posture. Exceptions occur and the accuracy of the posture stimulation test is about 85%.

E. Adrenal Vein Sampling

Bilateral selective adrenal vein sampling is recommended to determine whether hypersecretion of aldosterone is lateralized and thereby treatable by unilateral adrenalectomy. Unfortunately, the procedure is invasive, expensive, not widely available, and often unsuccessful. The procedure (and surgery) may not be required for patients whose blood pressure is well controlled with spironolactone or eplerenone. It is indicated only if surgery is contemplated to direct the surgeon to the correct adrenal gland. Adrenal vein sampling is probably not required in patients who have a classic adrenal adenoma (Conn syndrome), which is characterized by hypokalemia and a unilateral adrenal adenoma ≥ 10 mm diameter on CT, and who have an estimated glomerular filtration rate ≥ 100 mL/min. It is most useful for patients who are not hypokalemic, who are over age 40 years, or who have an adrenal adenoma < 1 cm diameter. It is difficult to catheterize the right adrenal vein. Therefore, the venous samples are assayed for both aldosterone and cortisol during a cosyntropin ($ACTH_{1-24}$) infusion to be sure that the sampling has included both adrenal veins. The procedure has a sensitivity of 95% and a specificity of 100% but only when performed by an experienced radiologist. The complication rate is 2.5%. Risks can be minimized if the radiologist avoids adrenal venography and limits the use of contrast.

▶ Differential Diagnosis

The differential diagnosis of primary aldosteronism includes other causes of hypokalemia (see Chapter 21) in patients with essential hypertension, especially diuretic therapy. Chronic depletion of intravascular volume stimulates renin secretion and secondary hyperaldosteronism.

Real (black) licorice (derived from anise) or anise-flavored drinks (sambuca, pastis) contain glycyrrhizinic acid, which has a metabolite that inhibits the enzyme that normally inactivates cortisol in the renal tubule. More renal tubular cortisol activates aldosterone receptors, increasing the renal tubular absorption of sodium and excretion of potassium, thereby causing hypertension. Oral contraceptives may increase aldosterone secretion in some patients. Renal vascular disease can cause severe hypertension with hypokalemia but PRA is high. Excessive adrenal secretion of other corticosteroids (besides aldosterone), certain congenital adrenal enzyme disorders, and primary cortisol resistance may also cause hypertension with hypokalemia. The differential diagnosis also includes Liddle syndrome, an autosomal dominant cause of hypertension and hypokalemia resulting from excessive sodium absorption from the renal tubule; renin and aldosterone levels are low.

▶ Complications

Cardiovascular complications occur more frequently in primary aldosteronism than in idiopathic hypertension. Following unilateral adrenalectomy for Conn syndrome, suppression of the contralateral adrenal may result in temporary postoperative hypoaldosteronism, characterized by hyperkalemia and hypotension.

▶ Treatment

Conn syndrome (unilateral aldosterone-secreting adrenal adenoma) is treated by laparoscopic adrenalectomy, though long-term therapy with spironolactone or eplerenone is an option. Bilateral adrenal hyperplasia is best treated with spironolactone or eplerenone. Spironolactone also has antiandrogen activity and frequently causes breast tenderness, gynecomastia, or reduced libido; it is given at initial doses of 12.5–25 mg orally once daily; the dose may be titrated upward to 200 mg daily. Spironolactone is contraindicated in pregnancy and reproductive-age women are cautioned to use contraception during therapy. Eplerenone is becoming favored for men, since it does not have antiandrogen effects; however, it has a short half-life and must be taken orally twice daily in doses of 25–50 mg. Hyperaldosteronism during pregnancy can cause resistant hypertension; amiloride (10–15 mg orally daily) is effective and the preferred medication, since spironolactone is contraindicated in pregnancy. Blood pressure must be monitored daily when beginning these anti-mineralocorticoid medications; significant drops in blood pressure have occurred when these drugs are added to other antihypertensives. Other antihypertensive drugs may also be required. Glucocorticoid-remediable aldosteronism is very rare but may respond well to suppression with low-dose dexamethasone.

▶ Prognosis

The hypertension is reversible in about two-thirds of cases but persists or returns despite surgery in the remainder. The prognosis is much improved by early diagnosis and treatment. Only 2% of aldosterone-secreting adrenal tumors are malignant.

Funder JW. Primary aldosteronism: clinical lateralization and costs. J Clin Endocrinol Metab. 2012 Oct;97(10):3450–2. [PMID: 23043195]

Krysiak R et al. Primary aldosteronism in pregnancy. Acta Clin Belg. 2012 Mar–Apr;67(2):130–4. [PMID: 22712170]

Küpers EM et al. A clinical prediction score to diagnose unilateral primary aldosteronism. J Clin Endocrinol Metab. 2012 Oct;97(10):3530–7. [PMID: 22918872]

Monticone S et al. Primary aldosteronism: who should be screened? Horm Metab Res. 2012 Mar;44(3):163–9. [PMID: 22120135]

Rossi GP. Diagnosis and treatment of primary aldosteronism. Rev Endocr Metab Disord. 2011 Mar;12(1):27–36. [PMID: 21369868]

Salvà M et al. Primary aldosteronism: the role of confirmatory tests. Horm Metab Res. 2012 Mar;44(3):177–80. [PMID: 22395800]

Steichen O et al. Outcomes of adrenalectomy in patients with unilateral primary aldosteronism: a review. Horm Metab Res. 2012 Mar;44(3):221–7. [PMID: 22395801]

Stowasser M et al. Factors affecting the aldosterone/renin ratio. Horm Metab Res. 2012 Mar;44(3):170–6. [PMID: 22147655]

PHEOCHROMOCYTOMA & PARAGANGLIOMA

ESSENTIALS OF DIAGNOSIS

▶ "Attacks" of headache, perspiration, palpitations, anxiety. Multisystem crisis.

▶ Hypertension, frequently sustained but often paroxysmal, especially during surgery or delivery.

▶ Elevated urinary plasma free metanephrines. Normal serum T_4 and TSH.

▶ Frequent germline mutations.

▶ General Considerations

Both pheochromocytomas and non–head-neck paragangliomas are tumors of the sympathetic nervous system. Pheochromocytomas arise from the adrenal medulla and usually secrete both epinephrine and norepinephrine. Paragangliomas ("extra-adrenal pheochromocytomas") arise from sympathetic paraganglia, often metastasize, and secrete norepinephrine or are nonsecretory. Excessive levels of norepinephrine or neuropeptide Y cause hypertension, while epinephrine causes tachyarrhythmias. These tumors may be located in either or both adrenals or anywhere along the sympathetic nervous chain, and sometimes in the mediastinum, heart, or bladder.

These tumors are deceptive and deadly. Although they usually produce hypertension, they account for < 0.4% of hypertension cases. The incidence is higher in patients with moderate to severe hypertension. They account for about 4% of adrenal incidentalomas. The yearly incidence is 2 to 4 new cases per million population. However, many cases are undiagnosed during life, since the prevalence of pheochromocytomas and paragangliomas in autopsy series is 1 in 2000.

Nonsecretory paragangliomas arise in the head or neck, particularly in the carotid body, jugular-tympanic region, or vagal body; only about 4% secrete catecholamines. They often arise in patients who harbor *SDHD*, *SDHC*, or *SDHB* germline mutations. (See below.)

Over 30% of patients with pheochromocytomas or paragangliomas harbor a germline mutation in 1 of at least 13 genes that makes them prone to develop the tumor, usually in an autosomal dominant manner with incomplete penetrance. For a patient with a pheochromocytoma or paraganglioma, the chance of harboring a germline mutation is nearly 100% with a family history of pheochromocytoma or paraganglioma or with multiple sites of primary tumor, compared to 17% in patients without such family history.

Pheochromocytomas develop in about 20% of patients with **von Hippel–Lindau (VHL) disease type 2** (hemangiomas of the retina, cerebellum, brainstem, and spinal cord; hyperparathyroidism; pancreatic cysts; endolymphatic sac tumors; cystadenomas of the adnexa or epididymis; pancreatic neuroendocrine tumors; renal cysts, adenomas, and carcinomas); inheritance is autosomal dominant. Patients with VHL develop pheochromocytomas that are less likely to be extra-adrenal, less likely to be malignant (3.5%), more likely to be bilateral, and more likely to present at an early age. Pheochromocytomas that arise in patients with VHL secrete exclusively norepinephrine and its metabolite normetanephrine. Therefore, individuals who carry type 2 VHL mutations should be screened for pheochromocytoma with plasma normetanephrine levels.

MEN 2A is associated with pheochromocytomas, hyperparathyroidism, cutaneous lichen amyloidosis, and medullary thyroid carcinoma. **MEN 2B** may be familial but usually arises from a de novo *ret* mutation; MEN 2B is associated with pheochromocytoma (50%), aggressive medullary thyroid carcinoma, mucosal neuromas, and marfinoid habitus.

von Recklinghausen neurofibromatosis type 1 *(NF-1)* is associated with an increased risk of pheochromocytomas/paragangliomas as well as cutaneous neurofibromas, optic and brainstem gliomas, astrocytomas, vascular anomalies, hamartomas, malignant nerve sheath tumors, and smooth-bordered café au lait spots. **Familial paraganglioma** can be caused by mutations in the genes encoding succinate dehydrogenase (SDH) subunits B, C, or D. Patients with such germline mutations are more apt to have bilateral pheochromocytomas or multicentric paragangliomas. Patients with *SDHB* germline mutations are particularly prone to develop paragangliomas that metastasize aggressively; they are also prone to develop renal cell carcinomas and neuroblastomas.

Some kindreds are prone to develop pheochromocytomas and paragangliomas due to less common germline mutations in other tumor susceptibility genes: *SDHA*, *SDHAF2*, *TMEM127*, *MAX*, *KIF1B*, *HIF2A*, and *PHD2*. Pheochromocytomas are also more common in patients with Carney triad, Sturge-Weber syndrome, and tuberous sclerosis.

▶ Clinical Findings

A. Symptoms and Signs (Table 26–12)

Pheochromocytomas can be lethal unless they are diagnosed and treated appropriately. Catastrophic hypertensive crisis and fatal cardiac arrhythmias can occur spontaneously or may be triggered by intravenous contrast dye or glucagon injection, needle biopsy of the mass, anesthesia, or surgical procedures. Exercise, bending, lifting, or emotional stress can trigger paroxysms. Certain drugs can precipitate attacks: monoamine oxidase (MAO) inhibitors, caffeine, nicotine, decongestants, amphetamines, cocaine, ionic intravenous contrast, and epinephrine. Bladder paragangliomas may present with paroxysms during micturition.

Table 26–12. Clinical manifestations of pheochromocytoma and paraganglioma.

Blood pressure	Hypertension: severe or mild, paroxysmal or sustained; orthostasis; hypotension/shock; normotension
Vasospasm	Cyanosis, Raynaud syndrome, gangrene; severe radial artery vasospasm with thready pulse; falsely low blood pressure by radial artery transducer
Multisystem crisis	ARDS, severe hypertension/hypotension, acute heart failure, fever, renal failure, hepatic failure, encephalopathy, death
Cardiovascular	Palpitations, dysrhythmias, chest pain, acute coronary syndrome, cardiomyopathy, heart failure, cardiac paragangliomas
Gastrointestinal	Abdominal pain, nausea, vomiting, weight loss, intestinal ischemia; pancreatitis, cholecystitis, jaundice; rupture of abdominal aneurysm; constipation, toxic megacolon
Metabolic	Hyperglycemia/diabetes, lactic acidosis, fevers
Neurologic	Headache, paresthesias, numbness, dizziness, CVA, TIA, hemiplegia, hemianopsia, seizures, hemorrhagic stroke; skull metastases may impinge on brain structures, optic nerve, or other cranial nerves; spinal metastases may impinge on cord or nerve roots
Pulmonary	Dyspnea; hypoxia from ARDS
Psychiatric	Anxiety attacks or constant anxiety; depression; chronic fatigue; psychosis
Renal	Renal insufficiency, nephrotic syndrome, malignant nephrosclerosis; large tumors often involve the kidneys and renal vessels
Skin	Apocrine sweating during paroxysms, drenching sweats as attack subsides; eczema; mottled cyanosis during paroxysm
Thyroid	Paroxysmal thyroid swelling
Ectopic hormones	ACTH (Cushing syndrome); VIP (Verner-Morrison syndrome); PTHrP (hypercalcemia); erythropoietin (erythrocytosis)
Children	More commonly have sustained hypertension, diaphoresis, visual changes, polyuria/polydipsia, seizures, edematous or cyanotic hands; more commonly harbor germline mutations, multiple tumors, and paragangliomas
Women	More symptomatic than men: more frequent headache, weight loss, numbness, dizziness, tremor, anxiety, and fatigue
Pregnancy	Hypertension mimicking eclampsia; hypertensive multisystem crisis during vaginal delivery; postpartum shock or fever; high mortality
General laboratory	Leukocytosis, erythrocytosis, eosinophilia

ACTH, adrenocorticotropic hormone; ARDS, acute respiratory distress syndrome; CVA, cerebrovascular accident; PTHrP, parathyroid hormone–related protein; TIA, transient ischemic attack; VIP, vasoactive intestinal peptide.
Used, with permission, from Gardner D, Shoback D (editors). *Greenspan's Basic and Clinical Endocrinology*. 9th edition, McGraw-Hill, NY, 2011.

Paroxysms typically produce hypertension (90%), severe headache (80%), perspiration (70%), and palpitations (60%); other symptoms may include anxiety (50%), a sense of impending doom, or tremor (40%). Vasomotor changes during an attack cause mottled cyanosis and facial pallor. As the attack subsides, facial flushing may occur as a result of reflex vasodilation. Epinephrine secretion by an adrenal pheochromocytoma may cause episodic tachyarrhythmias, hypotension, or even syncope. Acute coronary syndrome can be caused by coronary vasoconstriction. Confusion, psychosis, seizures, transient ischemic attacks, or stroke may occur with cerebrovascular vasoconstriction or hemorrhagic stroke. Aortic aneurysms may dissect and rupture. Abdominal pain, nausea, vomiting, and even ischemic bowel can be due to splanchnic vasoconstriction. Large or hemorrhagic abdominal tumors can also cause abdominal pain. Peripheral vasoconstriction can cause Raynaud phenomenon or even gangrene. Patients may experience nervousness and irritability, increased appetite,

and loss of weight. Other patients have pulmonary edema and heart failure due to cardiomyopathy. Although most patients are symptomatic, some patients are normotensive and asymptomatic, particularly when the tumor is nonsecretory or discovered at an early stage.

In a pheochromocytoma **multisystem crisis**, tumoral cytokine release can cause proteinuria and nephrotic syndrome, acute heart failure, severe hypotension, kidney failure, liver failure, and death. Patients with proteinuria are at increased risk for acute respiratory distress syndrome (ARDS). Multisystem crisis can occur spontaneously, or it may be provoked by surgery, vaginal delivery, or treatment of metastatic disease.

B. Laboratory Findings

Plasma fractionated free metanephrines is the single most sensitive test for secretory pheochromocytomas and paragangliomas. To improve test specificity, the patient should rest in a quiet room in the supine position for at least 20–30 minutes before the blood is drawn. Normal levels rule out pheochromocytoma and paraganglioma with some certainty and the work-up can usually end there. However, misleading elevations in metanephrines or normetanephrines can be caused by factors such as a blood draw in a sitting position, physical or emotional stress, sleep apnea, and MAO inhibitors. Assay interference can occur with HPLC-ECD assays with certain drugs: acetaminophen, labetalol, buspirone, mesalamine, and sulphasalazine. LC-MS/MS assays do not suffer from such drug interference and these assays are now used by most major laboratories in the United States. Patients with elevated plasma metanephrines or normetanephrines levels require further evaluation.

Assay of urinary fractionated metanephrines and creatinine effectively confirms most pheochromocytomas that were detected by elevated plasma fractionated metanephrines. A 24-hour urine specimen is usually obtained, although an overnight or shorter collection may be used; patients with pheochromocytomas generally have more than 2.2 mcg of total metanephrine per milligram of creatinine, and more than 135 mcg total catecholamines per gram creatinine. Urinary assay for total metanephrines is about 97% sensitive for detecting functioning pheochromocytomas. Urinary assay for vanillylmandelic acid (VMA) is not usually required.

Some drugs and foods can interfere with certain assays for catecholamines, and stresses can also cause misleading elevations in catecholamine excretion (Table 26–13).

Table 26–13. Factors potentially causing misleading catecholamine results: High-performance liquid chromatography with electrochemical detection (HPLC-ECD).

Drugs	Foods	Conditions
Acetaminophen[2]	Bananas[1]	Amyotrophic lateral
Aldomet[2]	Caffeine[1]	sclerosis[1]
Amphetamines[1]	Coffee[2]	Brain lesions[1]
Bronchodilators[1]	Peppers[2]	Carcinoid[1]
Buspirone[2]	Pineapples[1]	Eclampsia[1]
Captopril[2]	Walnuts[1]	Emotion, severe[1]
Cimetidine[2]		Exercise, vigorous[1]
Cocaine[1]		Guillain-Barré
Codeine[2]		syndrome[1]
Decongestants[1]		Hypoglycemia[1]
Ephedrine[1]		Kidney disease[3]
Fenfluramine[3]		Lead poisoning[1]
Isoproterenol[1]		Myocardial infarct,
Labetalol[1,2]		acute[1]
Levodopa[2]		Pain, severe[1]
Mandelamine[2]		Porphyria, acute[1]
Metoclopramide[2]		Psychosis, acute[1]
Nitroglycerin[1]		Quadriplegia[1]
Phenoxybenzamine		Sleep apnea
Tricyclic		
antidepressants		
Viloxazine[2]		

[1]Increases catecholamine excretion.
[2]May cause confounding peaks on HPLC chromatograms.
[3]Decreases catecholamine excretion.

About 10% of hypertensive patients have a misleadingly elevated level of one or more tests.

Serum chromogranin A is elevated in 90% of patients with pheochromocytoma and the levels correlate with tumor size, being higher in patients with metastatic disease. Serum chromogranin A levels can be misleadingly elevated in patients with azotemia or hypergastrinemia, and in those treated with corticosteroids or proton pump inhibitors. Serum may also be assayed for neuron-specific enolase; high levels implicate a malignant pheochromocytoma, while normal levels are nonspecific.

Serum methoxytyramine is another tumor marker that is often elevated, particularly in patients with "nonsecreting" tumors and in patients with pheochromocytoma or paraganglioma associated with a *SDHB* or *SDHC* germline mutation.

Initial testing results are frequently inconclusive. When metanephrines are elevated but less than three times the upper limit of normal, there is a significant chance of the test result being falsely positive. False-positive test results should be particularly suspected when the ratio of normetanephrine to norepinephrine is < 0.52 or the ratio of metanephrine to epinephrine is < 4.2. In such cases, it is best to repeat biochemical testing under optimal conditions, eg, after eliminating potentially interfering drugs. Pharmacologic provocative and suppressive tests that evaluate the rise or fall in blood pressure are usually not required or recommended.

Hyperglycemia is present in about 35% of patients but is usually mild. Proteinuria is present in about 10–20% of patients. Leukocytosis is common. Eosinophilia occurs rarely. The ESR is sometimes elevated. PRA may be increased by catecholamines.

Genetic testing should ideally be performed on all patients with pheochromocytoma or paraganglioma. Testing for VHL, *ret* protooncogene, and *SDHB/SDHC/SDHD* mutations is advisable. Family members may then be screened for the specific gene mutation.

C. Imaging

1. CT and MRI scanning—Imaging should not replace biochemical testing, since adrenal pheochromocytomas can appear similar to benign adrenal adenomas that are very common (2–4% of all scans). When a pheochromocytoma is suspected because of biochemical testing or a genetic condition predisposing to pheochromocytoma, a noncontrast CT scan of the abdomen is performed, with thin sections through the adrenals. The CT usually shows an adrenal mass with a density > 10 HU. If an adrenal mass is present, another CT is immediately performed, infusing nonionic contrast (to reduce the risk of stimulating catecholamine release from a pheochromocytoma) with a "washout" protocol. Pheochromocytomas are usually avid for contrast and 84% of tumors retain > 40% of contrast after 15 minutes. Glucagon should not be used during scanning, since it can provoke hypertensive crisis.

MRI scanning has the advantage of not requiring intravenous contrast dye; its lack of radiation makes it the imaging of choice during pregnancy and childhood and for serial imaging. Pheochromocytomas typically have a low

T1 signal and 70% have a high T2 signal. Both CT and MRI scanning have a sensitivity of about 90% for adrenal pheochromocytoma and a sensitivity of 95% for adrenal tumors over 0.5 cm in diameter. However, both CT and MRI are less sensitive for detecting recurrent tumors, metastases, and extra-adrenal paragangliomas. If no adrenal tumor is found, the scan is extended to include the entire abdomen, pelvis, and chest.

2. Nuclear imaging—A whole-body ^{123}I-meta-iodobenzyl-guanidine (^{123}I-MIBG) scan can localize tumors with a sensitivity of 94% and a specificity of 92%. It is less sensitive for MEN 2A- or MEN 2B-related pheochromocytomas and for metastases. Preoperative ^{123}I-MIBG scanning is not usually required to confirm that a unilateral adrenal mass is a pheochromocytoma in a patient with classic clinical and biochemical presentation. Preoperative whole-body ^{123}I-MIBG scanning can be useful when the CT scan cannot locate a suspected pheochromocytoma, making a paraganglioma more likely; it can also be useful when the CT scan is ambiguous for pheochromocytoma. It is prudent to perform a whole-body ^{123}I-MIBG scan about 3 months postoperatively to determine if metastatic or recurrent tumor is present. Drugs that reduce ^{123}I-MIBG uptake should be avoided, including tricyclic antidepressants and cyclobenzaprine (6 weeks), amphetamines, nasal decongestants, phenothiazines, haloperidol, diet pills, labetalol, and cocaine (2 weeks).

Somatostatin receptor imaging using ^{111}In-labeled octreotide is only 25% sensitive for detecting an adrenal pheochromocytoma. However, ^{111}In-labeled octreotide scanning is quite sensitive for detecting extra-adrenal pheochromocytomas (paragangliomas) and metastatic pheochromocytomas, sometimes locating tumors that were missed by ^{123}I-MIBG scanning.

PET/CT scanning usually detects tumors using ^{18}F-labeled deoxyglucose (^{18}FDG-PET) or ^{18}F-labeled dopamine (^{18}FDA-PET), and may demonstrate tumors that are not visible on ^{123}I-MIBG scanning.

Differential Diagnosis

Certain conditions mimic pheochromocytoma: thyrotoxicosis, essential hypertension, myocarditis, glomerulonephritis or other renal lesions, eclampsia, and psychoneurosis (anxiety attack). Toxemia of pregnancy is associated with hypertension and increased catecholamine production.

Conditions that have manifestations similar to those of pheochromocytoma include the following: essential labile hypertension, renal hypertension, anxiety attacks, thyrotoxicosis, toxemia of pregnancy, acute intermittent porphyria, hypogonadal vascular instability (hot flushes), cocaine or amphetamine use, and clonidine withdrawal. Patients taking nonselective MAO inhibitor antidepressants can have hypertensive crisis after eating foods that contain tyramine (eg, fermented cheeses, aged wines, certain beers, fava beans, vegemite, marmite). Patients with erythromelalgia can have hypertensive crises; their episodic painful flushing and leg swelling are relieved by cold, distinguishing this condition from pheochromocytoma. Pheochromocytomas can cause chest pain and ECG changes that mimic acute cardiac ischemia. Renal artery stenosis can cause severe hypertension and may coexist with pheochromocytoma.

False-positive testing for catecholamines and metabolites occurs in about 10% of hypertensives, but levels are usually < 50% above normal and typically normalize with repeat testing.

Complications

All of the complications of severe hypertension may be encountered. In addition, a catecholamine-induced cardiomyopathy may develop. Severe heart failure and cardiovascular collapse may develop in patients during a paroxysm. Sudden death may occur due to cardiac arrhythmia. Multisystem crisis and ARDS can occur acutely and thus the initial manifestation of pheochromocytoma may be hypotension or even shock. Hypertensive crises with sudden blindness or cerebrovascular accidents are not uncommon. Paroxysms may be spontaneous or precipitated by sudden movement, exertion, manipulation, vaginal delivery, emotional stress, trauma, surgery unrelated to the tumor, or surgery for removal of the tumor. Decongestant medications, fluoxetine, and other selective serotonin reuptake inhibitors may induce hypertensive paroxysms and death.

After removal of the tumor, a state of severe hypotension and shock (resistant to epinephrine and norepinephrine) may ensue with precipitation of acute kidney injury or myocardial infarction. Hypotension and shock may occur from spontaneous infarction or hemorrhage of the tumor.

Pheochromocytoma cells may be seeded within the peritoneum, either spontaneously or as a complication during surgical resection. Such seeding of the abdomen can result in multifocal recurrent intra-abdominal tumors, a condition known as pheochromocytomatosis.

Medical Treatment

Patients must receive adequate treatment for hypertension and tachyarrhythmias prior to surgery for pheochromocytoma/paraganglioma. Patients are advised to use a portable sphygmomanometer and measure their blood pressures daily and immediately during paroxysms. Some patients with pheochromocytoma or paraganglioma are not hypertensive and do not require preoperative antihypertensive management. Alpha-blockers or calcium channel blockers can be used, either alone or in combination. Blood pressure should be controlled before cardioselective beta-blockers are added for control of tachyarrhythmias.

Alpha-blockers are typically administered preparatory to surgery. Phenoxybenzamine is a long-acting nonselective alpha-blocker with a half-life of 24 hours; it is given initially in a dosage of 10 mg orally every 12 hours, increasing gradually by about 10 mg/d about every 3 days until hypertension is controlled. Maintenance doses range from 10 mg/d to 120 mg/d. Selective alpha-1-blockers may be used: doxazosin (half-life 22 hours), terazosin (half-life 12 hours), or prazosin (half-life 3 hours). Patients given preoperative phenoxybenzamine experience less intraoperative hypertension but greater post-resection hypotension than patients given preoperative selective alpha-1-blockers. Optimal alpha-blockade is achieved when supine arterial pressure is below 140/90 mm Hg or as low as possible for the patient to have a standing arterial pressure above 80/45 mm Hg.

Calcium channel blockers (nifedipine ER or nicardipine ER) are very effective and may be used with or without alpha-blockers. Nifedipine ER is initially given orally at a dose of 30 mg/d, increasing the dose gradually to a maximum of 60 mg twice daily. Calcium channel blockers are superior to phenoxybenzamine for long-term use, since they cause less fatigue, nasal congestion, and orthostatic hypotension. For acute hypertensive crisis (systolic blood pressure > 170 mm Hg) a nifedipine 10-mg capsule may be chewed and swallowed. Nifedipine is quite successful for treating acute hypertension in patients with pheochromocytoma/paraganglioma, even at home; it is reasonably safe as long as the blood pressure is carefully monitored.

Beta-blockers (eg, metoprolol XL) are often required after institution of alpha-blockade or calcium channel blockade. The use of a beta-blocker as initial antihypertensive therapy has resulted in an "unopposed alpha" that causes paradoxical worsening of hypertension. Labetalol has combined alpha- and beta-blocking activity and is an effective agent but can cause paradoxical hypertension if used as the initial antihypertensive agent. Labetalol can also interfere with catecholamine determinations in some laboratories and reduces the tumor's uptake of radioisotopes, such that it must be discontinued for at least 4–7 days before[123]I-MIBG or [18]FDA-PET scanning or therapy with high-dose ^{131}I-MIBG.

▶ **Surgical Treatment**

Surgical removal of pheochromocytomas or abdominal paragangliomas is the treatment of choice. For surgery, a team approach—endocrinologist, anesthesiologist, and surgeon—is critically important. Laparoscopic surgery is preferred, but large and invasive tumors require open laparotomy. Patients with small familial or bilateral pheochromocytomas may undergo selective resection of the tumors, sparing the adrenal cortex; however, there is a recurrence rate of 10% over 10 years.

Prior to surgery, blood pressure control should be maintained for a minimum of 4–7 days or until optimal cardiac status is established. The ECG should be monitored until it becomes stable. (It may take a week or even months to correct ECG changes in patients with catecholamine myocarditis, and it may be prudent to defer surgery until then in such cases.) Patients must be very closely monitored during surgery to promptly detect sudden changes in blood pressure or cardiac arrhythmias.

Intraoperative severe hypertension is managed with continuous intravenous nicardipine (a short-acting calcium channel blocker), 2–6 mcg/kg/min, or nitroprusside, 0.5–10 mcg/kg/min. Prolonged nitroprusside administration can cause cyanide toxicity. Tachyarrhythmia is treated with intravenous atenolol (1 mg boluses), esmolol, or lidocaine.

Autotransfusion of 1–2 units of blood at 12 hours preoperatively plus generous intraoperative volume replacement reduces the risk of postresection hypotension and shock caused by desensitization of the vascular alpha-1-receptors. Shock is treated with intravenous saline or colloid and high doses of intravenous norepinephrine. Intravenous 5% dextrose is infused postoperatively to prevent hypoglycemia.

▶ **Detecting & Managing Metastatic Pheochromocytoma & Paraganglioma**

Surgical histopathology for pheochromocytoma and paraganglioma cannot reliably determine whether a tumor is malignant. Therefore, all pheochromocytomas and paragangliomas must be approached as possibly malignant. Even if no metastases are visible at the time of surgery, they may become apparent years later. So all patients require lifetime follow-up. Therefore, it is essential to recheck blood pressure and plasma fractionated metanephrine levels about 4–6 weeks postoperatively, at least every 6 months for 5 years, then once yearly for life and immediately if hypertension, suspicious symptoms, or metastases become evident. Patients with nonsecretory tumors frequently have elevated serum levels of chromogranin A that can also be used as a tumor marker. It is also prudent to perform a whole-body ^{123}I-MIBG scan about 3 months postoperatively, since previously undetected metastases may become visible.

Since some metastases are indolent, it is important to tailor treatment to each individual according to their tumor's aggressiveness. Most surgeons resect the main tumor and larger metastases (debulking). Asymptomatic, indolent metastases may be kept under close surveillance without treatment.

A. Chemotherapy

Various chemotherapy regimens have been used, but there have been no controlled clinical trials to prove the effectiveness of one regimen over another or whether any regimen actually improves overall survival. The most common chemotherapy regimen combines intravenous cyclophosphamide, vincristine, and dacarbazine over 2 days in cycles that are repeated every 3 weeks. About one-third of patients experience some degree of temporary remission. Another chemotherapy regimen uses temozolomide, 250 mg/d orally for 5 days, repeating the cycle every 28 days. Sunitinib, a tyrosine kinase inhibitor, can also produce remissions, given orally in doses of 50 mg/d for 4 weeks on and then 2 weeks off; alternatively, a dose of 37.5 mg/d can be given continuously. Each chemotherapy regimen has toxicities.

Metyrosine reduces catecholamine synthesis but does not impede the progressive growth of metastases; the initial metyrosine dosage is 250 mg four times daily, increased daily by increments of 250–500 mg to a maximum of 4 g/d. Metyrosine causes central nervous system side effects and crystalluria; hydration must be ensured.

B. ^{131}I-MIBG Therapy

About 60% of patients with metastatic pheochromocytoma or paraganglioma have tumors with sufficient uptake of

^{123}I-MIBG on diagnostic scanning to allow for therapy with high-activity ^{131}I-MIBG. Medications that reduce MIBG uptake must be avoided, particularly labetalol, phenothiazines, tricyclics, and sympathomimetics. Activities of 125–500 mCi are infused, with many centers administering repeated infusions of 2 mCi/kg to cumulative activities of at least 500–800 mCi. Radioisotope therapy can suppress the bone marrow temporarily. Myelodysplastic syndrome and leukemia can develop several years after ^{131}I-MIBG therapy, with the risk proportional to the cumulative amount of isotope. ARDS and multisystem failure occur rarely after ^{131}I-MIBG therapy, particularly in patients with pretreatment proteinuria.

C. Treatment for Bone Metastases

Patients with significant osteolytic bone metastases may be treated with external beam radiation therapy, which is often helpful in relieving pain and stabilizing local osseous disease. Patients with vertebral metastases and spinal cord compression may require surgical decompression and kyphoplasty. Intravenous zoledronic acid or subcutaneous denosumab may also be administered to patients with osteolytic bone metastases.

▶ Prognosis

The malignancy of a pheochromocytoma or sympathetic paraganglioma cannot be determined by its size or histologic examination. A tumor is considered malignant if metastases are present; metastases may take many years to become clinically evident. Therefore, lifetime surveillance is required. Malignancy is more likely for larger tumors and for sympathetic paragangliomas. The prognosis is good for patients with pheochromocytomas that are resected before causing cardiovascular damage. Hypertension usually resolves after successful surgery but may persist or return in 25% of patients despite successful surgery. Although this may be essential hypertension, biochemical reevaluation is then required, looking for a second or metastatic pheochromocytoma.

Formerly, the surgical mortality was as high as 30%, but the development of laparoscopic surgical techniques, improved anesthesia, intraoperative monitoring, and preoperative blood pressure control with alpha-blockers or calcium channel blockers has reduced surgical mortality to < 3%.

Patients with metastatic pheochromocytoma and paraganglioma have an extremely variable prognosis. Patients with a heavy and progressive tumor burden and distant metastases have a worse prognosis. Patients harboring *SDHB* germline mutations tend to have more aggressive tumors as do patients with pulmonary metastases. Patients with metastases limited to bones or the abdomen tend to have a better prognosis. Some patients with intra-abdominal spread of tumor have intraperitoneal seeding (pheochromocytomatosis) rather than true metastases and seem to have a better prognosis.

Patients who receive surgery and chemotherapy have a median 5-year survival of about 44%. Patients receiving surgery followed by high-activity ^{131}I-mIBG therapy have

been reported to have a 5-year survival rate of 75%. Some patients have an indolent malignancy; prolonged survivals of up to 30 years have been reported with no treatment.

Baez JC et al. Pheochromocytoma and paraganglioma: imaging characteristics. Cancer Imaging. 2012 May 7;12:153–62. [PMID: 22571874]

Grogan RH et al. Changing paradigms in the treatment of malignant pheochromocytoma. Cancer Control. 2011 Apr;18(2): 104–12. [PMID: 21451453]

Korevaar TI et al. Pheochromocytomas and paragangliomas: assessment of malignant potential. Endocrine. 2011 Dec;40(3): 354–65. [PMID: 22038451]

Plouin PF et al. Metastatic pheochromocytoma and paraganglioma: focus on therapeutics. Horm Metab Res. 2012 May;44(5):390–9. [PMID: 22314389]

Prejbisz A et al. Cardiovascular manifestations of phaeochromocytoma. J Hypertens. 2011 Nov;29(11):2049–60. [PMID: 21826022]

Shao Y et al. Preoperative alpha blockade for normotensive pheochromocytoma: is it necessary? J Hypertens. 2011 Dec;29(12):2429–32. [PMID: 22025238]

Tischler AS et al. The adrenal medulla and extra-adrenal paraganglioma: then and now. Endocr Pathol. 2014 Mar;25(1): 49–58. [PMID: 24362581]

Van Berkel A et al. Biochemical diagnosis of phaeochromocytoma and paraganglioma. Eur J Endocrinol. 2014 Feb 4;170 (3):R109–19. [PMID: 24347425]

GASTROENTEROPANCREATIC NEUROENDOCRINE TUMORS[1]

ISLET CELL TUMORS

ESSENTIALS OF DIAGNOSIS

▶ Half of islet cell tumors are nonsecretory; weight loss, abdominal pain, or jaundice may be presenting signs.

▶ Secretory tumors cause a variety of manifestations depending on the hormones secreted.

▶ General Considerations

The pancreatic islets are composed of several types of cells, each with distinct chemical and microscopic features: the A cells (20%) secrete glucagon, the B cells (70%) secrete insulin,[1] the D cells (5%) secrete somatostatin or gastrin, and the F cells secrete "pancreatic polypeptide."

Gastroenteropancreatic neuroendocrine tumors (GEP-NETs) constitute < 5% of all pancreatic tumors. GEP-NETs are rare, with an incidence of about 10 per million yearly. About 40% are functional, producing hormones that are tumor markers, which are important for diagnosis and follow-up. Although most pancreatic and duodenal neuroendocrine tumors arise spontaneously, they may occur as part four different inherited disorders: MEN 1,

[1]Insulinomas and hypoglycemia are discussed in Chapter 27.

von Hippel-Lindau disease (VHL), neurofibromatosis 1 (NF-1) and the rare tuberous sclerosis complex (TSC). At presentation, 65% of GEP-NETs are unresectable or metastatic.

Insulinomas are usually benign (about 90%) and secrete excessive amounts of insulin that causes hypoglycemia. Insulinomas also produce proinsulin and C-peptide. Insulinomas are solitary in 95% of sporadic cases but are multiple in about 90% of cases arising in MEN 1. (See Chapter 27.)

Gastrinomas secrete excessive quantities of the hormone gastrin (as well as "big" gastrin), which stimulates the stomach to hypersecrete acid, thereby causing hyperplastic gastric rugae and peptic ulceration (Zollinger–Ellison syndrome). About 50% of gastrinomas are malignant and metastasize to the liver. Gastrinomas are typically found in the duodenum (49%), pancreas (24%), or lymph nodes (11%). Sporadic Zollinger–Ellison syndrome is rarely suspected at the onset of symptoms; typically, there is a 5-year delay in diagnosis. About 22% of patients have MEN 1. In patients with MEN 1, gastrinomas usually present at a younger age; hyperparathyroidism may occur from 14 years preceding the Zollinger–Ellison diagnosis to 38 years afterward.

Glucagonomas are usually malignant; liver metastases are ordinarily present by the time of diagnosis. They usually secrete other hormones besides glucagon, often gastrin.

Somatostatinomas are very rare and are associated with weight loss, diabetes mellitus, malabsorption, and hypochlorhydria.

VIPomas are rare and produce vasoactive intestinal polypeptide (VIP), a substance that causes profuse watery diarrhea and profound hypokalemia (Verner-Morrison syndrome).

Carcinoid pancreatic neuroendocrine tumors are typically indolent but usually metastasize to local and distant sites, particularly to the liver and endocrine organs.

Nonfunctional pancreatic neuroendocrine tumors produce no significant hormones and usually grow to large size prior to detection. They typically present with symptoms caused by mass effect.

► Clinical Findings

A. Symptoms and Signs

Presenting symptoms and signs of **gastrinomas** include abdominal pain (75%), diarrhea (73%), heartburn (44%), bleeding (25%), or weight loss (17%). Endoscopy usually shows prominent gastric folds (94%).

The 5-, 10-, and 20-year survival rates with MEN 1 are 94%, 75%, and 58%, respectively, while the survival rates for sporadic Zollinger–Ellison syndrome are 62%, 50%, and 31%, respectively. (See Chapter 15.)

Initial symptoms of **glucagonoma** often include weight loss, diarrhea, nausea, peptic ulcer, or necrolytic migratory erythema. About 35% of patients ultimately develop diabetes mellitus. The median survival is 34 months after diagnosis.

With **somatostinomas,** a classic triad of symptoms frequently occurs due to the excessive somatostatin secretion: diabetes mellitus, with polyuria, polydipsia, and polyphagia due to its inhibition of insulin and glucagon

secretion; cholelithiasis, because of its inhibition of gallbladder motility; and steatorrhea, because of its inhibition of pancreatic exocrine function. Diarrhea, hypochlorhydria, and anemia can also occur.

With **VIPomas,** there is profuse watery diarrhea; hypokalemia and achlorhydria are additional defining features.

Carcinoid pancreatic neuroendocrine tumors secrete serotonin and can produce an atypical carcinoid syndrome manifested by pain, diarrhea, and weight loss; skin flushing occurs in 39% of patients.

Islet cell tumors can secrete ectopic hormones (eg, ACTH) in addition to native hormones and produce related clinical syndromes (eg, Cushing syndrome).

B. Imaging

Localization of noninsulinoma pancreatic islet cell tumors and their metastases is best done with somatostatin receptor scintigraphy (SRS) with ^{111}In-DTPA-octreotide (Octreoscan); SRS detects about 75% of noninsulinomas. CT and MRI are also useful.

For insulinomas, preoperative localization studies are less successful and have the following sensitivities: ultrasonography 25%, CT 25%, endoscopic ultrasonography 27%, transhepatic portal vein sampling 40%, and arteriography 45%. Nearly all insulinomas can be successfully located at surgery by the combination of intraoperative palpation (sensitivity 55%) and ultrasound (sensitivity 75%). An abdominal CT scan is usually obtained, but extensive preoperative localization procedures, especially with invasive methods, are not required. Tumors may be located in the pancreatic head or neck (57%), body (15%), or tail (19%) or in the duodenum (9%).

► Treatment

Direct resection of the tumor (or tumors), which often spread locally, is the primary form of therapy for all types of islet cell neoplasms. In Zollinger–Ellison syndrome, gastrinomas are most commonly found in the duodenum but also in the pancreas. Gastric hyperacidity in Zollinger–Ellison syndrome is treated with a proton pump inhibitor at quadruple the usual doses. Proton pump inhibitors increase serum gastrin, which is otherwise useful as a tumor marker for gastrinoma recurrence after surgical resection.

Octreotide LAR is useful in the therapy of islet cell tumors with the exception of insulinoma; subcutaneous injections of Octreotide LAR 20–30 mg are required every 4 weeks. Treatment with octreotide LAR improves the symptoms caused by excessive VIP but does not halt tumor growth. Selective radioembolization of hepatic metastases can be accomplished with the use of ^{90}Y-labeled resin or glass microspheres.

► Prognosis

The prognosis in P-NETs is variable, but certainly better than pancreatic adenocarcinoma. The surgical complication rate is about 40%, with patients commonly developing fistulas and infections. Extensive pancreatic resection may cause diabetes mellitus. The overall 5-year survival is higher with functional tumors (77%) than with nonfunctional ones (55%) and higher with benign tumors (91%) than with malignant ones (55%). The prognosis is decidedly worse for patients with metastatic gastropancreatic neuroendocrine tumors that express thymidylate synthase.

Alexandraki KI et al. Gastroenteropancreatic neuroendocrine tumors: new insights in the diagnosis and therapy. Endocrine. 2012 Feb;41(1):40–52. [PMID: 22124940]

Dong M et al. New strategies for advanced neuroendocrine tumors in the era of targeted therapy. Clin Cancer Res. 2012 Apr 1;18(7):1830–6. [PMID: 22338018]

Ellison TA et al. The current management of pancreatic neuroendocrine tumors. Adv Surg. 2012;46:283–96. [PMID: 22873046]

Ganetsky A et al. Gastroenteropancreatic neuroendocrine tumors: update on therapeutics. Ann Pharmacother. 2012 Jun;46(6):851–62. [PMID: 22589450]

Oberg K. Neuroendocrine tumors of the digestive tract: impact of new classifications and new agents on therapeutic approaches. Curr Opin Oncol. 2012 Jul;24(4):433–40. [PMID: 22510940]

Reidy-Lagunes D et al. Pancreatic neuroendocrine and carcinoid tumors: what's new, what's old, and what's different? Curr Oncol Rep. 2012 Jun;14(3):249–56. [PMID: 22434313]

Sofocleous CT et al. Factors affecting periprocedural morbidity and mortality and long-term patient survival after arterial embolization of hepatic neuroendocrine metastases. J Vasc Interv Radiol. 2014 Jan;25(1):22–30. [PMID: 24365504]

Stevenson R et al. Prognostic and predictive biomarkers in gastroenteropancreatic neuroendocrine tumors. JOP. 2013 Mar 10;14(2):155–7. [PMID: 23474561]

Valle JW et al. A systematic review of non-surgical treatments for pancreatic neuroendocrine tumours. Cancer Treat Rev. 2014 Apr;40(3):376–89. [PMID: 24296109]

Williamson JM et al. Pancreatic and peripancreatic somatostatinomas. Ann R Coll Srug Engl. 2011 Jul;93(5):356–60. [PMD: 21943457]

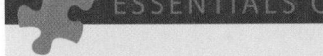

DISEASES OF THE TESTES & MALE BREAST

MALE HYPOGONADISM

ESSENTIALS OF DIAGNOSIS

▶ Diminished libido and erections.

▶ Fatigue, depression, reduced exercise endurance.

▶ Decreased growth of body hair.

▶ Testes may be small or normal in size.

▶ Serum total testosterone or free testosterone level is decreased.

▶ Serum gonadotropin (LH and FSH) levels are decreased or normal in hypogonadotropic hypogonadism; they are increased in testicular failure (hypergonadotropic hypogonadism).

▶ General Considerations

Male hypogonadism is caused by deficient testosterone secretion by the testes. It may be classified according to whether it is due to (1) insufficient gonadotropin secretion by the pituitary (hypogonadotropic); (2) pathology in the testes

Table 26–14. Causes of male hypogonadism.

Hypogonadotropic (Low or Normal LH)	Hypergonadotropic (High LH)
Aging	Aging
Alcohol	Antitumor chemotherapy
Chronic illness	Bilateral anorchia
Congenital syndromes	Idiopathic
Constitutional delay	Klinefelter syndrome
Cushing syndrome	Leprosy
Drugs	Lymphoma
Estrogen	Male climacteric
GnRH agonist (leuprolide)	Mumps
Ketoconazole	Myotonic dystrophy
Marijuana	Noonan syndrome
Prior androgens	Orchitis
Spironolactone	Radiation therapy
Hemochromatosis	Sertoli cell-only syndrome
Hypopituitarism	Testicular trauma
Hypothyroidism	Tuberculosis
Idiopathic	Uremia
Kallmann syndrome	
17-Ketosteroid reductase deficiency	
Major medical or surgical illnesses	
Malnourishment	
Obesity (BMI > 30)	
Prader-Willi syndrome	

BMI, body mass index; GnRH, gonadotropin-releasing hormone; LH, luteinizing hormone.

themselves (hypergonadotropic); or (3) both (Table 26–14). Partial male hypogonadism may be difficult to distinguish from the physiologic reduction in serum testosterone seen in normal aging, obesity, and illness.

▶ Etiology

A. Hypogonadotropic Hypogonadism (Low Testosterone with Normal or Low LH)

A deficiency in FSH and LH may be isolated or associated with other pituitary hormonal abnormalities. (See Hypopituitarism.) Hypogonadotropic hypogonadism can be primary, with a failure to enter puberty by age 14; the differential diagnosis is isolated hypogonadotropic hypogonadism, hypopituitarism, or simple constitutional delay of growth and puberty. Hypogonadotropic hypogonadism may also be acquired; causes include pituitary or hypothalamic tumors, granulomatous diseases, lymphocytic hypophysitis, or hemochromatosis; Cushing syndrome; adrenal insufficiency; and thyroid hormone excess or deficiency. Genetic conditions (eg, Kallmann syndrome or *PROKR2* mutations) account for about 40% of cases of acquired hypogonadotropic hypogonadism that is isolated, and apparently idiopathic, with a serum testosterone < 150 ng/dL (< 5.2 nmol/L).

Partial male hypogonadotropic hypogonadism is defined as a serum testosterone in the range of 150–300 ng/dL (5.2–10.4 nmol/L). The main causes of acquired hypogonadotropic hypogonadism include obesity, poor health, or normal aging. Spermatogenesis is usually preserved. After age 40, serum total testosterone declines variably by an average of 1–2% per year; serum free testosterone levels decline even faster, since sex hormone binding globulin increases with age. After age 70 years, 28% of men have low serum total testosterone and 68% have low serum free testosterone levels, compared with the levels found in young men. Serum levels of free testosterone are lower in men aged 40–70 compared with younger men, without any increase in serum LH. Increasing obesity is the main reversible condition that contributes to the general decline in serum free testosterone with aging. After age 70, LH levels tend to rise, indicating a contribution of primary gonadal dysfunction with advancing age.

There is considerable clinical and laboratory overlap between patients with partial hypogonadotropic hypogonadism and those with normal aging, obesity, or illness. A multicenter European study concluded that the diagnosis of testosterone deficiency in older men should include a serum testosterone < 320 ng/mL and at least three of the following six symptoms: erectile dysfunction, poor morning erection, low libido, depression, fatigue, and inability to perform vigorous activity. Such men are most likely to benefit from testosterone replacement.

B. Hypergonadotropic Hypogonadism (Testicular Failure with High LH)

A failure in testicular secretion of testosterone causes a rise in LH. If testicular Sertoli cell function is deficient, FSH will be elevated. Conditions that can cause testicular failure include viral infection (eg, mumps), irradiation, cancer chemotherapy or radioisotope therapy, autoimmunity, myotonic dystrophy, uremia, XY gonadal dysgenesis, partial 17-ketosteroid reductase deficiency, Klinefelter syndrome, and male climacteric. In men who have had a unilateral orchiectomy for cancer, the remaining testicle can fail even in the absence of radiation or chemotherapy. Male hypogonadism can also be caused by a congenital partial deficiency in the steroidogenic enzyme CYP17 (17-hydroxylase). CYP17 may be deliberately inhibited by abiraterone acetate (Zytiga), a drug for prostate cancer. CYP17 inhibition also causes adrenocortical insufficiency, hypertension, and hypokalemia.

Klinefelter syndrome (47,XXY and its variants) is the most common chromosomal abnormality among males, with an incidence of about 1:500. It is caused by the expression of an abnormal karyotype, classically 47,XXY. Other forms are common, eg, 46,XY/47,XXY mosaicism, 48,XXYY, 48,XXXY, or 46,XX males. The manifestations of Klinefelter syndrome are variable and < 25% of patients are diagnosed. Testes feel normal during childhood, but during adolescence they usually become firm, fibrotic, small, and nontender to palpation. Affected children have an increased risk of cryptorchidism, decreased penile size, delayed speech, learning disabilities, psychiatric disturbances, and mediastinal malignancies. Up to 75% of boys experience some gynecomastia at puberty. Although puberty occurs at the normal time, the degree of virilization is variable. Serum testosterone is usually low and gonadotropins are elevated. Adult men usually have somewhat reduced facial and pubic hair. Over 95% of affected adult men have azoospermia or severe oligospermia. Other common findings include tall stature and abnormal body proportions that are unusual for hypogonadal men (height greater than arm span; crown-pubis length greater than pubis-floor). Patients with multiple X or Y chromosomes are more apt to have mental deficiency and other abnormalities such as clinodactyly or synostosis. They may also exhibit problems with coordination and social skills. Other problems include a higher incidence of breast cancer, chronic pulmonary disease, varicosities of the legs, osteoporosis, and diabetes mellitus (8% of patients); impaired glucose tolerance occurs in an additional 19% of patients.

The diagnosis of Klinefelter syndrome is confirmed by karyotyping or by determining the presence of RNA for X-inactive-specific transcriptase (XIST) in peripheral blood leukocytes by polymerase chain reaction.

On semen analysis, most men (about 95%) with classic Klinefelter syndrome have azoospermia, although some sperm production is often present in their early teens. Men with 46,XY/47,XXY mosaicism may have spontaneous fertility. Also, testicular biopsy reveals sperm in up to 50% of affected patients, allowing some of them to be fertile with the use of in vitro fertilization using intracytoplasmic sperm injection (ICSI).

XY gonadal dysgenesis describes several conditions that result in the failure of the testes to develop normally. *SRY* is a gene on the Y chromosome that initiates male sexual development. Mutations in *SRY* result in testicular dysgenesis. Affected individuals lack testosterone, which results in sex reversal: female external genitalia with a blind vaginal pouch, no uterus, and intra-abdominal dysgenetic gonads. Affected individuals are raised as girls and appear normal until their lack of pubertal development and amenorrhea leads to the diagnosis. Intra-abdominal rudimentary testes have an increased risk of developing a malignancy and are usually resected. Patients are considered women and receive estrogen replacement therapy.

C. Androgen Insensitivity

Partial resistance to testosterone is a rare condition in which phenotypic males have variable degrees of apparent hypogonadism, hypospadias, cryptorchism, and gynecomastia. Serum testosterone levels are normal.

▶ Clinical Findings

A. Symptoms and Signs

Hypogonadism that is congenital or acquired during childhood presents as delayed puberty. Men with acquired hypogonadism have variable manifestations. Most men experience decreased libido. Others complain of erectile dysfunction, poor morning erection, or hot sweats. Men often have depression, fatigue, or decreased ability to perform vigorous physical activity. The presenting complaint may also be infertility, gynecomastia, headache, fracture, or other symptoms related to the cause or result of the hypogonadism. The patient's history often gives a clue to the cause (Table 26–14).

Physical signs associated with hypogonadism may include decreased body, axillary, beard, or pubic hair; such diminished sexual hair growth is not reliably present except after years of severe hypogonadism. Men in whom hypogonadism develops tend to lose muscle mass and gain weight due to an increase in subcutaneous fat. Examination should include measurements of arm span and height. Testicular size should be assessed with an orchidometer (normal volume is about 10–25 mL; normal length is usually over 6 cm). Testicular size may decrease but usually remains within the normal range in men with postpubertal hypogonadotropic hypogonadism, but it may be diminished with testicular injury or Klinefelter syndrome. The testes must also be carefully palpated for masses, since Leydig cell tumors may secrete estrogen and present with hypogonadism. The testicles must be carefully examined for evidence of trauma, infiltrative lesions (eg, lymphoma), or ongoing infection (eg, leprosy, tuberculosis).

B. Laboratory Findings

The evaluation for hypogonadism begins with a morning serum testosterone or free testosterone measurement (or both). Serum testosterone levels are considered low if they are confirmed to be < 320 ng/dL (11 nmol/L). Free testosterone is best measured by calculation, using accurate assays for testosterone and sex hormone binding globulin. Serum free testosterone levels are considered low if they are confirmed to be < 64 pg/mL (220 pmol/L).

Normal ranges for serum testosterone have been derived from nonfasting morning blood specimens, which tend to be the highest of the day. Later in the day, serum testosterone levels can be 25–50% lower. Therefore, a serum testosterone drawn fasting or late in the day may be misleadingly below the "normal range." Serum testosterone levels in men are highest at age 20–30 years and slightly lower at age 30–40 years; testosterone falls gradually but progressively after age 40 years. Testing for serum free testosterone is especially important for detecting hypogonadism in elderly men, who generally have high levels of sex hormone binding globulin. A low serum testosterone should be verified with a repeat assay and further evaluated with serum LH and FSH levels. LH and FSH tend to be high in patients with hypergonadotropic hypogonadism but low or inappropriately normal in men with hypogonadotropic hypogonadism or normal aging. High serum estradiol levels are seen in men with obesity-related hypogonadotropic hypogonadism; sufficient weight loss causes a decrease in serum estradiol in such men.

Testosterone stimulates erythropoiesis in men, causing the normal red blood count range to be higher in men than in women; mild anemia is common in men with hypogonadism, with red blood counts below the normal male range. For men with long-standing male hypogonadism, bone densitometry is recommended. Men with severe osteoporosis may require treatment with bisphosphonates and vitamin D, in addition to testosterone replacement therapy. (See Osteoporosis.)

1. Hypogonadotropic hypogonadism—A serum PRL determination is obtained but may be elevated for many reasons (see Table 26–2). Men with gynecomastia may be screened for partial 17-ketosteroid reductase deficiency with serum determinations for androstenedione and estrone, which are elevated in this condition. Hypogonadotropic hypogonadism can also be seen with X-linked congenital adrenal hypoplasia, which causes hypogonadotropic hypogonadism and arrested puberty, azoospermia, and primary adrenal insufficiency; adrenal insufficiency usually presents in childhood but may remain undiagnosed into adulthood. The serum estradiol level may be elevated in patients with cirrhosis and in rare cases of estrogen-secreting tumors (testicular Leydig cell tumor or adrenal carcinoma). Men with no discernible definite cause for hypogonadotropic hypogonadism should be screened for hemochromatosis and have an MRI of the pituitary and hypothalamic region to look for a tumor or other lesion. (See Hypopituitarism.)

2. Hypergonadotropic hypogonadism—Men with hypergonadotropic hypogonadism have low serum testosterone levels with a compensatory increase in FSH and LH. Klinefelter syndrome can be confirmed by karyotyping or by measurement of leukocyte XIST. Testicular biopsy is usually reserved for younger patients in whom the reason for primary hypogonadism is unclear.

▶ Treatment

Testosterone replacement is beneficial to most men with hypergonadotropic hypogonadism or severe hypogonadotropic hypogonadism. Men with symptoms of hypogonadism (see above) and a repeatedly low serum testosterone or free testosterone can also benefit from testosterone replacement. For men with borderline low serum testosterone levels and marginal hypogonadal symptoms, the decision to treat should consider the potential benefits versus risks. Such men may be given a trial of testosterone therapy for several months while monitoring their response.

Testosterone therapy should not be administered to men with active prostate or breast cancer, or erythrocytosis. In men over age 50 years, a digital prostate examination and serum prostate-specific antigen (PSA) level should be done before beginning testosterone therapy. Men with symptoms of prostatic hypertrophy, a palpable prostate nodule, or a PSA > 4 ng/mL (> 3 ng/mL in men of African ancestry) should have a urologic evaluation prior to treatment. Serum PSA should be measured yearly during therapy. Similarly, testosterone therapy is not given to men with untreated sleep apnea or heart failure. In men who have coronary risk factors or are over age 65, special attention should be given to improving cardiac risk factors (eg, controlling hypertension or hyperlipidemia) and administering low-dose aspirin while receiving testosterone replacement.

Drug interactions can occur. Testosterone should be administered cautiously to men receiving coumadin, since the combination can increase the INR and risk of bleeding. Similarly, testosterone therapy can increase serum levels of cyclosporine, tacrolimus, and tolvaptan. Testosterone can predispose to hypoglycemia in diabetic men receiving insulin or oral hypoglycemic agents, so close monitoring of blood sugars is advisable during initiation of testosterone therapy.

Oral androgen therapy with methyltestosterone is not advisable due to the potential for causing liver tumors, peliosis hepatis, and cholestatic jaundice.

A. Therapies for Male Hypogonadism

1. Topical testosterone gels—Testosterone is best administered topically. Topical administration yields more stable serum testosterone levels than intramuscular administration. Topical testosterone is usually applied once daily in the morning after showering. Topical testosterone should not be applied to the breast or genitals. **Androgel** 1% gel is available in 2.5-g packets (25 mg testosterone) and 5-g packets (50 mg testosterone) and in a pump that dispenses 12.5 mg testosterone per pump actuation: the recommended dose is 50–100 mg applied daily to the shoulders. Androgel 1.6% gel is available in a pump that dispenses 20.25 mg testosterone per pump actuation; the recommended dose is 40.5–81 mg daily. **Testim** 1% gel is available in 5-g tubes (50 mg testosterone); the recommended dose is 50–100 mg applied daily. **Fortesta** 2% gel is available in a pump that dispenses 10 mg testosterone per pump actuation; the recommended dose is 40–70 mg daily. **Testogel** is distributed in 5-g sachets (50 mg testosterone); this brand is not available in the United States. Testim, Fortesta, and Testogel may be applied to shoulders, upper arms, or abdomen. **Axiron** 2% solution is available in a pump that dispenses 30 mg per actuation; the recommended dose is 30–60 mg applied to each axilla daily.

The skin serves as a reservoir that slowly releases about 10% of the testosterone into the blood; serum testosterone levels reach a steady state in 1–3 days. The serum testosterone level should be determined about 14 days after starting therapy; if the level remains below normal or the clinical response is inadequate, the daily dose may be increased to 1.5 to 2 times the initial dose. After the application of topical testosterone, the hands should be washed. The application site should be allowed to dry for 5–10 minutes before dressing. Before close contact with women or children, a shirt must be worn or the areas of application washed with soap and water to prevent transfer of testosterone to them.

2. Transdermal testosterone patches—Testosterone transdermal systems (skin patches) are applied to nongenital skin. Androderm (2 or 4 mg/24 h) patches may be applied at bedtime in doses of 4–8 mg; it adheres tightly to the skin and may cause skin irritation. This patch system is expensive.

3. Parenteral testosterone—Testosterone cypionate is an intramuscular testosterone formulation that is available in solutions containing 200 mg/mL. Its main advantage is low cost. The usual dose is 200 mg every 2 weeks or 300 mg every 3 weeks. The dose and injection intervals are adjusted according to the patient's response. These preparations are oil-based and are usually given intramuscularly in the gluteal area.

Testosterone undecanoate (Nebido) is a long-lasting depot testosterone formulation that is administered in doses of 1000 mg (4 mL) by slow intramuscular injection. The initial injection is followed by another 1000 mg injection 6 weeks later and maintenance doses of 1000 mg every 3 months. A serum testosterone level is measured before the fourth dose; if the serum testosterone remains low, the dosing interval is shortened to every 10 weeks. It is not available in the United States or Canada.

4. Buccal testosterone—Testosterone buccal tablets (Striant) are placed between the upper lip and gingivae. One or two 30-mg tablets are thus retained and changed every 12 hours. They should not be chewed or swallowed.

5. Clomiphene citrate—Men with functional hypogonadotropic hypogonadism usually respond well to clomiphene citrate that is administered orally in doses that are titrated to achieve a serum testosterone level of about 500-600 ng/dL. Treatment with clomiphene is commenced with 25 mg on alternate days and increased to 50 mg on alternate days if necessary, with a maximum dose of 50 mg daily. Serum testosterone levels usually normalize while spermatogenesis usually improves.

6. Gonadotropins—Patients with infertility associated with hypogonadotropic hypogonadism may require therapy with gonadotropins. Men may receive hCG 1000 units subcutaneously three times weekly for 6 months; if the semen analysis shows inadequate sperm, FSH is added 75 units subcutaneously three times weekly.

7. Weight loss—When hypogonadotropic hypogonadism is due to morbid obesity, significant weight loss will improve serum testosterone levels. The rise in serum testosterone is proportionate to the weight loss. Although diet-induced weight loss is beneficial, bariatric surgery has been much more effective and serum testosterone levels may normalize after dramatic weight loss.

B. Benefits of Testosterone Replacement Therapy

Testosterone therapy usually benefits men with low serum testosterone and at least three manifestations of hypogonadism. Testosterone therapy can improve overall mood, sense of well-being, sexual desire, and erectile function. It also increases physical vigor and muscle strength as manifested in measurements of leg-press and chest-press strength. Testosterone replacement also improves exercise endurance and stair climbing ability. Long-term testosterone replacement causes significant weight loss and a reduction in waist circumference.

Testosterone therapy may improve survival. In a Veterans Administration study, men with hypogonadism who received testosterone replacement therapy over 3–5 years experienced an overall mortality rate of 10.3% compared to a 20.7% mortality rate in untreated hypogonadal men.

C. Risks of Testosterone Replacement Therapy

Testosterone replacement therapy appears to increase the risk of cardiovascular events in men older than age 65 with cardiac risk factors or preexisting angina. This increased risk may be due to the decrease in serum HDL that can occur with testosterone therapy.

Testosterone therapy can aggravate benign prostatic hypertrophy (BPH). However, aggravation of voiding problems is uncommon. In men with BPH, finasteride may be coadministered with testosterone to reduce prostate size. The incidence of prostate cancer does not appear to be increased by testosterone therapy. However, testosterone therapy is contraindicated in the presence of active prostate cancer. Hypogonadal men who have had a prostatectomy for low-grade prostate cancer, and who have remained in complete remission for several years, may have testosterone therapy given cautiously while monitoring serum PSA levels.

Erythrocytosis develops in some men who are treated with testosterone. Erythrocytosis is more common with intramuscular injections of testosterone enanthate than with transcutaneous testosterone. However, no increase in the incidence of thromboembolic events has been reported.

Testosterone therapy tends to aggravate sleep apnea in older men, likely through central nervous system effects. Surveillance for sleep apnea is recommended during testosterone therapy and a formal evaluation with nocturnal pulse oximetry recording is recommended for all high-risk patients with snoring, obesity, partner's report of apneic episodes, nocturnal awakening, unrefreshing sleep with daytime fatigue, or hypertension.

Men who are treated with testosterone frequently experience some increase in acne that is usually mild and tolerated; topical antiacne therapy or a reduction in testosterone replacement dosage may be required. Increases in intraocular pressure have occurred during testosterone therapy. During the initiation of testosterone replacement therapy, gynecomastia develops in some men, which usually is mild and tends to resolve spontaneously; switching from testosterone injections to testosterone transdermal gel may help this condition.

D. Risks of Performance-enhancing Anabolic Steroids

Performance-enhancing agents, particularly androgenic anabolic steroids, are used by up to 2% of young athletes and by 20–65% of power sport athletes. They are often used as part of a "stacking" polypharmacy that may include nandrolone decanoate, dimethandrolone, testosterone propionate, or testosterone enanthate. These androgens are usually illegal and often contaminated by toxic substances and can produce toxic hepatitis, dependence, aggression, depression, dyslipidemias, gynecomastia, acne, male pattern baldness, hepatitis, thromboembolism, and cardiomyopathy. Shared needles may transmit hepatitis or HIV. Arsenic contamination has been reported to cause multiorgan failure and death.

▶ Prognosis of Male Hypogonadism

If hypogonadism is due to a pituitary lesion, the prognosis is that of the primary disease (eg, tumor, necrosis). The prognosis for restoration of virility is good if testosterone is given.

Basaria S et al. Adverse events associated with testosterone administration. N Engl J Med. 2010 Jul 8;363(2):109–22. [PMID: 20592293]

Bhasin S et al. Testosterone therapy in men with androgen deficiency syndrome: an Endocrine Society clinical practice guideline. J Clin Endocrinol Metab. 2010 Jun;95(6):2536–59. [PMID: 20525905]

Cattabiani C et al. Relationship between testosterone deficiency and cardiovascular risk and mortality in adult men. J Endocrinol Invest. 2012 Jan;35(1):104–20. [PMID: 22082684]

Corona G et al. Body weight loss reverts obesity-associated hypogonadotropic hypogonadism: a systematic review and meta-analysis. Eur J Endocrinol. 2013 May 2;168(6):829–43. [PMID: 23482592]

Groth KA et al. Clinical review. Klinefelter syndrome—a clinical update. J Clin Endocrinol Metab. 2013 Jan;98(1):20–30. [PMID: 23118429]

Jacobs LA et al. Hypogonadism and infertility in testicular cancer survivors. J Natl Compr Canc Netw. 2012 Apr;10(4): 558–63. [PMID: 22491052]

Morales A et al. A critical appraisal of accuracy and cost of laboratory methodologies for the diagnosis of hypogonadism: the role of free testosterone assays. Can J Urol. 2012 Jun;19(3): 6314–8. [PMID: 22704323]

Moskovic DJ et al. Clomiphene citrate is safe and effective for long-term management of hypogonadism. BJU Int. 2012 Nov;110(10):1524–8. [PMID: 22458540]

Perera NJ et al. The adverse health consequences of the use of multiple performance-enhancing substances—a deadly cocktail. J Clin Endocrinol Metab. 2013 Dec;98(12):4613–8. [PMID: 24217902]

Salenave S et al. Male acquired hypogonadotropic hypogonadism: diagnosis and treatment. Ann Endocrinol (Paris). 2012 Apr;73(2):141–6. [PMID: 22541999]

Shi Z et al. Longitudinal changes in testosterone over five years in community-dwelling men. J Clin Endocrinol Metab. 2013 Aug;98(8):3289–97. [PMID: 23775354]

Shores MM et al. Testosterone treatment and mortality in men with low testosterone levels. J Clin Endocrinol Metab. 2012 Jun;97(6):2050–8. [PMID: 22496507]

Silveira LF et al. Approach to the patient with hypogonadotropic hypogonadism. J Clin Endocrinol Metab. 2013 May;98(5): 1781–8. [PMID: 23650335]

CRYPTORCHISM

One or both testes may be absent from the scrotum at birth in about 20% of premature or low-birth-weight male infants and in 3–6% of full term infants. Cryptorchism is found in 1–2% of males after 1 year of age but must be distinguished from retractile testes, which require no treatment. Cryptorchism should be corrected before age 12–24 months in an attempt to reduce the risk of infertility, which occurs in up to 75% of men with bilateral cryptorchism and in 50% of men with unilateral cryptorchism. Some patients have underlying hypogonadism, including hypogonadotropic hypogonadism.

If the testes are not palpable, it is important to determine whether they are cryptorchid or intra-abdominal. MRI is more reliable than ultrasound for locating cryptorchid testes. Surgery for cryptorchid testes (orchiopexy) is generally successful and is usually the treatment of choice. Alternatively, hCG, 1500 units intramuscularly daily for 3 days, causes a significant rise in testosterone if the testes are present. Therapy with hCG results in a testicular descent rate of about 25%.

The lifetime risk of testicular neoplasia is 0.002% in normal males. The risk of malignancy is higher for cryptorchid testes (0.06%) and for intra-abdominal testes (5%). Orchiopexy decreases the risk of neoplasia when performed before 10 years of age. Orchiectomy after puberty is an option for intra-abdominal testes.

Kurpisz M et al. Cryptorchidism and long-term consequences. Reprod Biol. 2010 Mar;10(1):19–35. [PMID: 20349021]

Penson D et al. Effectiveness of hormonal and surgical therapies for cryptorchidism: a systematic review. Pediatrics. 2013 Jun; 131(6):e1897–907. [PMID: 23690511]

Wood HM et al. Cryptorchidism and testicular cancer: separating fact from fiction. J Urol. 2009 Feb;181(2):452–61. [PMID: 19084853]

GYNECOMASTIA

ESSENTIALS OF DIAGNOSIS

▶ Palpable enlargement of the male breast, often asymmetric or unilateral.

▶ Glandular gynecomastia characterized by tenderness.

▶ Fatty gynecomastia typically nontender.

▶ Must be distinguished from carcinoma or mastitis.

▶ General Considerations

Gynecomastia is defined as the presence of palpable glandular breast tissue in males. Pubertal gynecomastia develops in about 60% of boys; the swelling usually subsides spontaneously within a year. Gynecomastia is particularly common in teenagers who are very tall or overweight. Gynecomastia develops in about 50% of athletes who abuse androgens and anabolic steroids. It is seen in Klinefelter syndrome, which affects 1:500 men. (See Klinefelter syndrome.) About 20% of adult gynecomastia is caused by drug therapy. Gynecomastia can develop in HIV-infected patients treated with highly active antiretroviral therapy (HAART), especially in men receiving efavirenz or didanosine; breast enlargement resolves spontaneously in 73% of patients within 9 months. Gynecomastia is common among elderly men, particularly when there is associated weight gain. However, it can be the first sign of a serious disorder.

The causes of gynecomastia are multiple and diverse (Table 26–15).

▶ Clinical Findings

A. Symptoms and Signs

The male breasts must be palpated carefully to distinguish true glandular gynecomastia from fatty pseudogynecomastia in which only adipose tissue is felt. The breasts are best examined both seated and supine. Using the thumb and forefinger as pincers, the subareolar tissue is compared to nearby adipose tissue. Fatty tissue is usually diffuse and nontender. True glandular enlargement beneath the areola may be tender. Pubertal gynecomastia is characterized by tender discoid enlargement of breast tissue 2–3 cm in diameter beneath the areola. The following characteristics are worrisome for malignancy: asymmetry; location not immediately below the areola; unusual firmness; or nipple retraction, bleeding, or discharge. Gynecomastia is graded according to severity: I, mild; II, moderate; III, severe.

Table 26–15. Causes of gynecomastia.

Idiopathic	Diazepam
	Diethylstilbestrol
Physiologic causes	Digitalis preparations
Neonatal period	Dutasteride
Puberty	Estrogens (oral or topical)
Aging	Ethionamide
Obesity	Famotidine (rare)
	Finasteride
Endocrine diseases	Flutamide
Androgen resistance	Goserelin
syndromes	Growth hormone
Aromatase excess syndrome	HAART (highly active
(sporadic or familial)	antiretroviral therapy)
Diabetic lymphocytic mastitis	Haloperidol
Hyperprolactinemia	Hydroxyzine
Hyperthyroidism	Isoniazid
Klinefelter syndrome	Ketoconazole
Male hypogonadism	Lavender oil (topical)
Partial 17-ketosteroid	Leuprolide
reductase deficiency	Marijuana
	Meprobamate
Systemic diseases	Methadone
Androgen insensitivity	Methyldopa
Chronic liver disease	Metoclopramide
Chronic kidney disease	Metronidazole
Hansen disease (leprosy)	Mirtazapine
Neurologic disorders	Nucleotide reverse
Refeeding after starvation	transcriptase inhibitors
Spinal cord injury	Nilutamide
	Omeprazole
Neoplasms	Opioids
Adrenal tumors	Penicillamine
Bronchogenic carcinoma	Phenothiazines
Carcinoma of the breast	Progestins
Ectopic hCG: lung,	Protease inhibitors
hepatocellular, gastric, renal	Proton pump inhibitors
carcinomas	(uncommon)
Pituitary prolactinoma	Ranitidine (rare)
Testicular tumors	Reserpine
	Risperidone
Drugs (partial list)	Somatropin
Alcohol	(growth hormone)
Alkylating agents	Soy ingestion
Amiodarone	Spironolactone
Anabolic steroids	Tea tree oil (topical)
Androgens	Testosterone
Anti-androgens	Thioridazine
Bicalutamide	Tricyclic antidepressants
Busulfan	Verapamil
Chorionic gonadotropin	
Cimetidine	
Clomiphene	
Cyclophosphamide	

B. Laboratory Findings

Obtain plasma levels of PRL (see Hyperprolactinemia) and beta-hCG. Detectable levels of beta-hCG implicate a testicular tumor (germ cell or Sertoli cell) or other malignancy (usually lung or liver), though detectable low levels (< 5 mU/mL) may be reported in primary hypogonadism and high serum LH levels if the assay for beta-hCG cross-reacts with LH. Measurements of serum free testosterone and LH are valuable in the diagnosis of primary or secondary hypogonadism. A low serum free testosterone and high LH are seen in primary hypogonadism. High testosterone levels plus high LH levels characterize partial androgen resistance. Serum estradiol is determined but is usually normal; increased levels may result from testicular tumors, increased beta-hCG, liver disease, obesity, adrenal tumors (rare), true hermaphroditism (rare), or aromatase gene gain of function mutations (rare). Serum TSH and FT_4 levels are also recommended. A karyotype (for Klinefelter syndrome) is obtained in men with persistent gynecomastia without obvious cause.

Investigation of unclear cases should include a chest radiograph to search for metastatic or bronchogenic carcinoma. Needle biopsy with cytologic examination may be performed on suspicious male breast enlargement (especially when unilateral or asymmetric) to distinguish gynecomastia from tumor or mastitis.

▶ Treatment

Pubertal gynecomastia often resolves spontaneously within 1–2 years. Drug-induced gynecomastia resolves after the offending drug is removed (eg, spironolactone stopped, with substitution of eplerenone). Patients with painful or persistent gynecomastia may be treated with medical therapy, usually for 9–12 months. Generally, it is prudent to treat patients for gynecomastia only when it becomes a troubling and continuing problem for them.

Selective estrogen receptor modulator (SERM) therapy is effective for true glandular gynecomastia. Raloxifene, 60 mg orally daily, may be somewhat more effective than tamoxifen, 10–20 mg orally daily.

Aromatase inhibitor (AI) therapy is also reasonably effective. For example, anastrozole reduces breast volume significantly over 6 months in adolescents given in a dose of 1 mg orally daily. Serum estradiol levels fall slightly while serum testosterone levels rise. Long-term AI therapy in adolescents is not recommended because of the possibility of inducing osteoporosis and of delaying epiphyseal fusion, which could cause an increase in adult height.

Testosterone therapy for men with hypogonadism may improve or worsen preexistent gynecomastia.

Radiation therapy has been used prophylactically to prevent gynecomastia in men with prostate cancer being treated with antiandrogen therapy. Low-dose prophylactic radiation therapy reduces its incidence from 71% to 28%. Existing gynecomastia improves in 33% with radiation therapy. Radiation doses of 12 to 20 Gy have been used in 2–5 fractions. However, the long-term cancer risks of such radiation are unknown.

Surgical correction is reserved for patients with persistent or severe gynecomastia. For best results, the procedure should be performed by an experienced plastic surgeon.

Alesini D et al. Multimodality treatment of gynecomastia in patients receiving antiandrogen therapy for prostate cancer in the era of abiraterone acetate and new antiandrogen molecules. Oncology. 2013;84(2):92–9. [PMID: 23128186]

Bowman JD et al. Drug-induced gynecomastia. Pharmacotherapy. 2012 Dec;32(12):1123–40. [PMID: 23165798]

Carlson HE. Approach to the patient with gynecomastia. J Clin Endocrinol Metab. 2011 Jan;96(1):15–21. [PMID: 21209041]

Deepinder F et al. Drug-induced gynecomastia: an evidence-based review. Expert Opin Drug Saf. 2012 Sep;11(5):779–95. [PMID: 22862307]

Dickson G. Gynecomastia. Am Fam Physician. 2012 Apr 1; 85(7):716–22. [PMID: 22534349]

Ikard RW et al. Management of senescent gynecomastia in the Veterans Health Administration. Breast J. 2011 Mar–Apr; 17(2):160–6. [PMID: 21410583]

Krause W. Drug-inducing gynaecomastia—a critical review. Andrologia. 2012 May;44(Suppl 1):621–6. [PMID: 22040098]

HIRSUTISM & VIRILIZATION

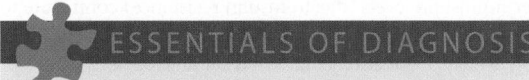

ESSENTIALS OF DIAGNOSIS

- ▶ Hirsutism, acne, menstrual disorders.
- ▶ Virilization: increased muscularity, androgenic alopecia, deepening of the voice, clitoromegaly.
- ▶ Rarely, a palpable pelvic tumor.
- ▶ Urinary 17-ketosteroids and serum DHEAS and androstenedione elevated in adrenal disorders; variable in others.
- ▶ Serum testosterone is often elevated.

▶ General Considerations

Hirsutism is defined as cosmetically unacceptable terminal hair growth that appears in women in a male pattern. Some degree of hirsutism affects about 5–10% of non-Asian women of reproductive age. The amount of hair growth deemed unacceptable depends on a woman's ethnicity and familial and cultural norms.

▶ Etiology

Hirsutism may be idiopathic or familial or be caused by the following disorders: polycystic ovary syndrome (PCOS), steroidogenic enzyme defects, neoplastic disorders; or rarely by medications, acromegaly, or ACTH-induced Cushing disease.

A. Idiopathic or Familial

Most women with hirsutism or androgenic alopecia have no detectable hyperandrogenism. Patients often have a strong familial predisposition to hirsutism that may be considered normal in the context of their genetic background. Such patients may have elevated serum levels of androstenediol glucuronide, a metabolite of dihydrotestosterone that is produced by skin in cosmetically unacceptable amounts.

B. Polycystic Ovary Syndrome (PCOS, Hyperthecosis, Stein-Leventhal Syndrome)

PCOS is a common functional disorder of the ovaries, affecting about 4–6% of premenopausal women in the United States and accounting for at least 50% of all cases of hirsutism associated with elevated testosterone levels. It is familial and transmitted as a modified autosomal dominant trait. Affected women have elevated serum testosterone or free testosterone levels. Affected women have signs of androgen excess, including hirsutism, acne, and male-pattern thinning of scalp hair. About 50% of affected women have oligomenorrhea or amenorrhea with anovulation. Hyperandrogenism persists after natural menopause. Despite the syndrome's name, the presence of ovarian cysts is not helpful diagnostically and is actually a misnomer, since about 30% of women with PCOS do *not* have cystic ovaries and 25–30% of normal menstruating women *have* cystic ovaries. Obesity and high serum insulin levels (due to insulin resistance) contribute to the syndrome in 70% of women. The serum LH:FSH ratio is often > 2.0. Both adrenal and ovarian androgen hypersecretion are commonly present. Women with PCOS have a 35% risk of depression, compared with 11% in age-matched controls. Diabetes mellitus is present in about 13% of cases. Obstructive sleep apnea is particularly common, even in slender women with PCOS. Untreated women with amenorrhea have a slightly increased risk of endometrial carcinoma. Hypertension and hyperlipidemia are often present, increasing the risk of cardiovascular disease. Women frequently regain normal menstrual cycles with aging.

C. Steroidogenic Enzyme Defects

Congenital adrenal steroidogenic enzyme defects result in reduced cortisol secretion with a compensatory increase in ACTH that causes adrenal hyperplasia. The most common enzyme defect is 21-hydroxylase deficiency, with a prevalence of about 1:18,000.

Partial deficiency in adrenal 21-hydroxylase can present in women as hirsutism. About 2% of patients with adult-onset hirsutism have been found to have a partial defect in adrenal 21-hydroxylase. The condition is more common in Ashkenazi Jews, Yupic Alaskans, and natives of La Reunion Island. The phenotypic expression is delayed until adolescence or adulthood; such patients do not have salt wasting. Polycystic ovaries and adrenal adenomas are more likely to develop in these women.

Some rare patients with hyperandrogenism and hypertension have 11-hydroxylase deficiency. This is distinguished from cortisol resistance by high cortisol serum levels in the latter and by high serum 11-deoxycortisol levels in the former.

Patients with an XY karyotype and a deficiency in 17-beta-hydroxysteroid dehydrogenase-3 or a deficiency in 5-alpha-reductase-2 may present as phenotypic girls in whom virilization develops at puberty.

D. Neoplastic Disorders

Ovarian tumors are very uncommon causes of hirsutism (0.8%) and include arrhenoblastomas, Sertoli-Leydig cell tumors, dysgerminomas, and hilar cell tumors. Adrenal carcinoma is a rare cause of Cushing syndrome and hyperandrogenism that can be quite virilizing. Pure androgen-secreting adrenal tumors occur very rarely; about 50% are malignant.

E. Rare Causes of Hirsutism

Acromegaly and ACTH-induced Cushing syndrome can cause hirsutism. Porphyria cutanea tarda can cause periorbital hair growth in addition to dermatitis in sun-exposed areas. Maternal virilization during pregnancy may occur as a result of a luteoma of pregnancy, hyperreactio luteinalis, or polycystic ovaries. In postmenopausal women, diffuse stromal Leydig cell hyperplasia is a rare cause of hyperandrogenism. Acquired hypertrichosis lanuginosa is manifested by the appearance of diffuse fine lanugo hair growth on the face and body along with stomatologic symptoms; the disorder is usually associated with an internal malignancy, especially colorectal cancer, and may regress after tumor removal. Pharmacologic causes include minoxidil, cyclosporine, phenytoin, anabolic steroids, interferon, cetuximab, diazoxide, and certain progestins.

▶ Clinical Findings

A. Symptoms and Signs

Modest androgen excess from any source increases sexual hair (chin, upper lip, abdomen, and chest) and increases sebaceous gland activity, producing acne. Menstrual irregularities, anovulation, and amenorrhea are common. If androgen excess is pronounced, defeminization (decrease in breast size, loss of feminine adipose tissue) and virilization (frontal balding, muscularity, clitoromegaly, and deepening of the voice) occur. Virilization points to the presence of an androgen-producing neoplasm. Hirsutism is quantitated using the Ferriman-Gallwey score in which hirsutism is graded from 0 (none) to 4 (severe) in nine areas of the body with a maximum possible score of 36; scores 8–15 indicate moderate hirsutism, while scores over 15 indicate severe hirsutism.

A pelvic examination may disclose clitoromegaly or ovarian enlargement that may be cystic or neoplastic. Hypertension may be present and should prompt consideration for the possible diagnosis of Cushing syndrome, adrenal 11-hydroxylase deficiency, or cortisol resistance syndrome.

B. Laboratory Testing and Imaging

Serum androgen testing is mainly useful to screen for rare occult adrenal or ovarian neoplasms. Some general guidelines are presented here, though exceptions are common.

Serum is assayed for total testosterone and free testosterone. A serum testosterone level > 200 ng/dL (> 6.9 nmol/L) or free testosterone > 40 ng/dL (> 140 pmol/L) indicates the need for pelvic examination and ultrasound. If that is negative, an adrenal CT scan is performed.

Most radioimmunoassays and enzyme-linked immunosorbent assays (ELISAs) for testosterone are inaccurate when serum testosterone levels are < 300 ng/dL (< 10.4 nmol/L). The more accurate testosterone assays rely on extraction and chromatography, followed by mass spectrometry or immunoassay. Free testosterone is best measured by calculation, using accurate assays for testosterone and sex hormone–binding globulin. A serum androstenedione level > 1000 ng/dL (> 34.9 nmol/L) also points to an ovarian or adrenal neoplasm. Patients with milder elevations of serum testosterone or androstenedione usually are treated with an oral contraceptive.

Patients with a serum DHEAS > 700 mcg/dL (> 35 nmol/L) have an adrenal source of androgen. This usually is due to adrenal hyperplasia and rarely to adrenal carcinoma. An adrenal CT scan is performed.

No firm guidelines exist as to which patients (if any) with hyperandrogenism should be screened for "late-onset" 21-hydroxylase deficiency. The evaluation requires levels of serum 17-hydroxyprogesterone to be drawn at baseline and at 30–60 minutes after the intramuscular injection of 0.25 mg of cosyntropin ($ACTH_{1-24}$). Ideally, this test should be done during the follicular phase of a woman's menstrual cycle. Patients with congenital adrenal hyperplasia will usually have a baseline 17-hydroxyprogesterone level > 300 ng/dL (> 9.1 nmol/L) or a stimulated level > 1000 ng/dL (> 30.3 nmol/L). Patients with any clinical signs of Cushing syndrome should receive a screening test. (See Cushing Syndrome.)

Serum levels of FSH and LH are elevated if amenorrhea is due to ovarian failure. An LH:FSH ratio > 2.0 is common in patients with PCOS. On abdominal ultrasound, about 25–30% of normal young women have polycystic ovaries, so the appearance of ovarian cysts on ultrasound is not helpful. Pelvic ultrasound or MRI can usually detect virilizing tumors of the ovary. However, small virilizing ovarian tumors may not be detectable on imaging studies; selective venous sampling for testosterone may be used for diagnosis in such patients.

▶ **Treatment**

Any drugs causing hirsutism (see above) should be stopped. Any underlying medical causes of hirsutism (eg, Cushing syndrome, acromegaly) should be treated.

A. Surgery

Androgenizing tumors of the adrenal or ovary are resected laparoscopically. Postmenopausal women with severe hyperandrogenism should undergo laparoscopic bilateral oophorectomy (if CT scan of the adrenals and ovaries is normal), since small hilar cell tumors of the ovary may not be visible on scans. Girls with classic salt-wasting congenital adrenal hyperplasia and infertility or treatment-resistant hyperandrogenism may be treated with laparoscopic bilateral adrenalectomy.

B. Medications

Spironolactone may be taken in doses of 50–100 mg orally twice daily on days 5–25 of the menstrual cycle or daily if used concomitantly with an oral contraceptive. Spironolactone is contraindicated in pregnancy, so reproductive-age women must use reliable contraception during this therapy. Side effects such as hyperkalemia are uncommon, but it is prudent to monitor serum potassium during therapy. If necessary, metformin (see below) can be added and may enhance the anti-hirsutism effect of low-dose spironolactone.

Finasteride inhibits 5-alpha-reductase, the enzyme that converts testosterone to active dihydrotestosterone in the skin. Given as 2.5-mg doses orally daily, it provides modest reduction in hirsutism over 6 months—somewhat less than that achieved with spironolactone. Finasteride is ineffective for androgenic alopecia in women. Side effects are rare.

Flutamide inhibits testosterone binding to androgen receptors and also suppresses serum testosterone. It is given orally in a dosage of 250 mg/d for the first year and then 125 mg/d for maintenance. Used with an oral contraceptive, it appears to be more effective than spironolactone in improving hirsutism, acne, and male pattern baldness. Women with congenital adrenal hyperplasia who take replacement hydrocortisone experience decreased renal cortisol clearance when treated with flutamide, resulting in lower hydrocortisone dosage requirements. Flutamide decreases cortisol renal clearance and corticosteroid replacement doses should be reduced when flutamide is added. Hepatotoxicity has been reported but is rare. Antiandrogens like flutamide must be given only to nonpregnant women. Women must be counseled to take contraceptive measures, since antiandrogen drug use during pregnancy causes malformations and disorders of sexual development (pseudohermaphroditism) in male infants.

Oral contraceptives stimulate menses (if that is desired) and reduce acne vulgaris. They are not very effective for hirsutism, but increase serum sex hormone–binding globulin and thereby slightly reduce serum free testosterone levels. Oral contraceptives containing antiandrogen progestins include desogestrel (Azurette, Kariva), drospirenone (Gianvi), or norgestimate (Ortho Tri-Cyclen Lo). Cyproterone is a particularly potent antiandrogen that is not available in the United States but is available as Diane-35 in Canada and the United Kingdom. These preparations may be more effective for treating hirsutism but are associated with an increased risk of deep venous thrombosis.

Metformin may improve menstrual function in women with PCOS and amenorrhea or oligomenorrhea but is less effective than oral contraceptives. Metformin is not effective in promoting fertility in women with PCOS. Metformin alone is ineffective in improving hirsutism, but can enhance the anti-hirsutism effect of spironolactone. Metformin therapy is usually given orally with meals and is started at a dose of 500 mg/d with breakfast for 1 week, then increased to 500 mg with breakfast and dinner. If this dose is clinically insufficient but tolerated, the dose may be increased to 850–1000 mg twice daily. The most common side effects are dose-related gastrointestinal upset and diarrhea or constipation. Metformin appears to be nonteratogenic. Although metformin reduces insulin resistance, it does not cause hypoglycemia in nondiabetics. Metformin is contraindicated in renal and hepatic disease.

Simvastatin can reduce hirsutism in women with PCOS. In one study, simvastatin 20 mg orally daily was given to women receiving an oral contraceptive for PCOS. Besides improving their serum lipid profiles, women receiving simvastatin had greater decreases in hirsutism and serum free testosterone levels than the women receiving an oral contraceptive alone.

Clomiphene is the treatment of choice for women with PCOS and infertility. Over 6 months, clomiphene therapy resulted in a 22.5% rate of conception with live births. The rate of pregnancy with multiple fetuses is 6%.

Women with classic congenital adrenal hyperplasia (21-hydroxylase deficiency) have hirsutism and adrenal insufficiency that requires glucocorticoid and mineralocorticoid replacement. However, women with partial "late onset" 21-hydroxylase deficiency do not require hormone replacement. Treating such women with dexamethasone risks iatrogenic Cushing syndrome and is not particularly more effective than the other treatments for hirsutism listed below.

GnRH agonist therapy has been successful in treating postmenopausal women with severe ovarian hyperandrogenism when laparoscopic oophorectomy is contraindicated or declined by the patient.

C. Topical and Laser Treatment

Local treatment by shaving or depilatories, waxing, electrolysis, or bleaching should be encouraged. **Eflornithine** (Vaniqa 13.9%) topical cream retards hair growth when applied twice daily to unwanted facial hair; improvement is noted within 4–8 weeks. However, local skin irritation may occur. Hirsutism returns with discontinuation. **Laser therapy** (photoepilation) is a fairly effective treatment for facial hirsutism, particularly for women with dark hair and light skin; longer-wavelength lasers are used for women with darker skin. Complications of laser therapy include skin hypopigmentation (rare) and hyperpigmentation (20%) that usually resolves; a paradoxical increase in hair growth occurs infrequently. Repeated laser treatments are usually required.

Blume-Peytavi U. An overview of unwanted female hair. Br J Dermatol. 2011 Dec;165(Suppl 3):19–23. [PMID: 22171681]

Bode D et al. Hirsutism in women. Am Fam Physician. 2012 Feb 15;85(4):373–80. [PMID: 22335316]

Castelo-Branco C et al. Comprehensive clinical management of hirsutism. Gynecol Endocrinol. 2010 Jul;26(7):484–93. [PMID: 20218823]

Escobar-Morreale HF et al. Epidemiology, diagnosis and management of hirsutism: a consensus statement by the Androgen Excess and Polycystic Ovary Syndrome Society. Hum Reprod Update. 2012 Mar–Apr;18(2):146–70. [PMID: 22064667]

Ganie MA et al. Improved efficacy of low-dose spironolactone and metformin combination than either drug alone in the management of women with polycystic ovary syndrome (PCOS): a six-month, open-label randomized study. J Clin Endocrinol Metab. 2013 Sep;98(9):3599–607. [PMID: 23846820]

Kelekci KH et al. Cyproterone acetate or drospirenone containing combined oral contraceptives plus spironolactone or cyproterone acetate for hirsutism: randomized comparison of three regimens. J Dermatolog Treat. 2012 Jun;23(3):177–83. [PMID: 21254871]

Loriaux DL. An approach to the patient with hirsutism. J Clin Endocrinol Metab. 2012 Sep;97(9):2957–68. [PMID: 22962669]

Roth LW et al; Reproductive Medicine Network. Altering hirsutism through ovulation induction in women with polycystic ovary syndrome. Obstet Gynecol. 2012 Jun;119(6):1151–6. [PMID: 22617579]

Unluhizarci K et al. Non-polycystic ovary syndrome-related endocrine disorders associated with hirsutism. Eur J Clin Invest. 2012 Jan;42(1):86–94. [PMID: 21623779]

Vollaard ES et al. Gonadotropin-releasing hormone agonist treatment in postmenopausal women with hyperandrogenism of ovarian origin. J Clin Endocrinol Metab. 2011 May;96 (5):1197–201. [PMID: 21307133]

▼ AMENORRHEA & MENOPAUSE (SEE ALSO CHAPTER 18)

PRIMARY AMENORRHEA

Menarche ordinarily occurs between ages 11 and 15 years (average in the United States: 12.7 years). The failure of any menses to appear is termed "primary amenorrhea," and evaluation is commenced (1) at age 14 years if neither menarche nor any breast development has occurred or if height is in the lowest 3%, or (2) at age 16 years if menarche has not occurred.

▶ Etiology of Primary Amenorrhea

The differential diagnoses for primary amenorrhea include hypothalamic-pituitary causes, hyperandrogenism, ovarian causes, disorders of sexual development (pseudohermaphroditism), uterine causes, and pregnancy.

A. Hypothalamic-Pituitary Causes (with Low or Normal FSH)

The most common cause of primary amenorrhea is a variant of normal known as constitutional delay of growth and puberty, which accounts for about 30% of delayed puberty cases. There is a strong genetic basis for this condition, such that over 50% of girls with it have a family history of delayed puberty. However, constitutional delay of growth and puberty is a diagnosis of exclusion and other etiologies must be considered.

A genetic deficiency of GnRH and gonadotropins may be isolated or associated with other pituitary deficiencies or diminished olfaction (Kallmann syndrome). Hypothalamic lesions, particularly craniopharyngioma, may be present. Pituitary tumors may be nonsecreting or may secrete PRL or GH. Cushing syndrome may be caused by corticosteroid treatment, a cortisol-secreting adrenal tumor, or an ACTH-secreting pituitary tumor. Hypothyroidism can delay adolescence. Head trauma or encephalitis can cause gonadotropin deficiency. Primary amenorrhea may also be caused by constitutional delay of adolescence, severe illness, vigorous exercise (eg, ballet dancing, running), stressful life events, dieting, or anorexia nervosa; however, these conditions should not be assumed to account for amenorrhea without a full physical and endocrinologic evaluation. (See Hypopituitarism.)

B. Hyperandrogenism (with Low or Normal FSH)

Polycystic ovaries and ovarian tumors can secrete excessive testosterone. Excess testosterone can also be secreted by adrenal tumors or by adrenal hyperplasia caused by steroidogenic enzyme defects such as P450c21 deficiency (salt-wasting) or P450c11 deficiency (hypertension). Androgenic steroid abuse may also cause this syndrome.

C. Ovarian Causes (with High FSH)

Gonadal dysgenesis (Turner syndrome and variants; see below) is a frequent cause of primary amenorrhea. Ovarian failure due to autoimmunity is a common cause. Rare deficiencies in certain ovarian steroidogenic enzymes are causes of primary hypogonadism without virilization: 3-beta-hydroxysteroid dehydrogenase deficiency (adrenal insufficiency with low serum 17-hydroxyprogesterone) and P450c17 deficiency (hypertension and hypokalemia with high serum 17-hydroxyprogesterone). Deficiency in P450 aromatase (P450arom) activity produces female hypogonadism associated with polycystic ovaries, tall stature, osteoporosis, and virilization.

D. XY Disorders of Sexual Development (Pseudohermaphroditism, with High LH)

Prenatal deficits of testosterone production or testosterone action in XY individuals results in ambiguous or female external genitalia. Patients with ambiguous genitalia are usually diagnosed in infancy.

However, XY patients with complete androgen insensitivity syndrome typically present in adolescence as a sexually immature phenotypic girl with normal breast development but with primary amenorrhea and no sexual hair. The uterus is absent and testes are intra-abdominal or cryptorchid. Intra-abdominal testes must be surgically resected. Such patients are treated as normal but infertile, hypogonadal women and should receive replacement estrogen therapy. Due to the complete lack of testosterone effect, affected women have a high rate of diminished libido.

E. Uterine Causes (with Normal FSH)

Congenital absence or malformation of the uterus may be responsible for primary amenorrhea, as may an unresponsive or atrophic endometrium. An imperforate hymen is occasionally the reason for the absence of visible menses.

F. Pregnancy (with High hCG)

Pregnancy may be the cause of primary amenorrhea even when the patient denies ever having had sexual intercourse.

▶ Clinical Findings

A. Symptoms and Signs

Patients with primary amenorrhea require a thorough history and physical examination to look for signs of the conditions noted above. Headaches or visual field abnormalities

implicate a hypothalamic or pituitary tumor. Signs of pregnancy may be present. Blood pressure abnormalities, acne, and hirsutism should be noted. Short stature may be seen with an associated GH or thyroid hormone deficiency. Short stature with manifestations of gonadal dysgenesis indicates Turner syndrome (see below). Olfactory deficits are seen in Kallmann syndrome. Obesity and short stature may be signs of Cushing syndrome. Tall stature may be due to eunuchoidism or gigantism. Hirsutism or virilization suggests excessive testosterone.

An external pelvic examination plus a rectal examination should be performed to assess hymen patency and the presence of a uterus.

B. Laboratory and Radiologic Findings

The initial endocrine evaluation should include serum determinations of FSH, LH, PRL, testosterone, TSH, FT_4, and beta-hCG (pregnancy test). Patients who are virilized or hypertensive require serum electrolyte determinations and further hormonal evaluation. MRI of the hypothalamus and pituitary is used to evaluate teens with primary amenorrhea and low or normal FSH and LH—especially those with high PRL levels. Pelvic duplex/color sonography is very useful. Girls who have a normal uterus and high FSH without the classic features of Turner syndrome may require a karyotype to diagnose X chromosome mosaicism.

▶ Treatment

Treatment of primary amenorrhea is directed at the underlying cause. Girls with permanent hypogonadism are treated with hormone replacement therapy (HRT, see below).

Deligeoroglou E et al. Evaluation and management of adolescent amenorrhea. Ann N Y Acad Sci. 2010 Sep;1205:23–32. [PMID: 20840249]
Hughes IA et al. Androgen insensitivity syndrome. Semin Reprod Med. 2012 Oct;30(5):432–42. [PMID: 23044881]
Rosenberg HK. Sonography of the pelvis in patients with primary amenorrhea. Endocrinol Metab Clin North Am. 2009 Dec;38(4):739–60. [PMID: 19944290]

SECONDARY AMENORRHEA & MENOPAUSE

Secondary amenorrhea is defined as the absence of menses for 3 consecutive months in women who have passed menarche. Menopause is defined as the terminal episode of naturally occurring menses; it is a retrospective diagnosis, usually made after 6 months of amenorrhea.

▶ Etiology

The causes of secondary amenorrhea include pregnancy, hypothalamic-pituitary causes, hyperandrogenism, uterine causes, premature ovarian failure, and menopause.

A. Pregnancy (High hCG)

Pregnancy is the most common cause for secondary amenorrhea in women of childbearing age. The differential diagnosis includes rare ectopic secretion of hCG by a choriocarcinoma or bronchogenic carcinoma.

B. Hypothalamic-Pituitary Causes (with Low or Normal FSH)

The hypothalamus must release GnRH in a pulsatile manner for the pituitary to secrete gonadotropins. GnRH pulses occurring more than once per hour favor LH secretion, while less frequent pulses favor FSH secretion. In normal ovulatory cycles, GnRH pulses in the follicular phase are rapid and favor LH synthesis and ovulation; ovarian luteal progesterone is then secreted that slows GnRH pulses, causing FSH secretion during the luteal phase. Most women with hypothalamic amenorrhea have a persistently low frequency of GnRH pulses.

Secondary "hypothalamic" amenorrhea may be caused by stressful life events such as school examinations or leaving home. Such women usually have a history of normal sexual development and irregular menses since menarche. Amenorrhea may also be the result of strict dieting, vigorous exercise, organic illness, or anorexia nervosa. Intrathecal infusion of opioids causes amenorrhea in most women. These conditions should not be assumed to account for amenorrhea without a full physical and endocrinologic evaluation. Young women in whom the results of evaluation and progestin withdrawal test are normal have noncyclic secretion of gonadotropins resulting in anovulation. Such women typically recover spontaneously but should have regular evaluations and a progestin withdrawal test about every 3 months to detect loss of estrogen effect.

PRL elevation due to any cause (see section on hyperprolactinemia) may cause amenorrhea. Pituitary tumors or other lesions may cause hypopituitarism. Corticosteroid excess of any cause suppresses gonadotropins.

C. Hyperandrogenism (with Low-Normal FSH)

Elevated serum levels of testosterone can cause hirsutism, virilization, and amenorrhea. In PCOS, GnRH pulses are persistently rapid, favoring LH synthesis with excessive androgen secretion; reduced FSH secretion impairs follicular maturation. Progesterone administration can slow the GnRH pulses, thus favoring FSH secretion that induces follicular maturation. Rare causes of secondary amenorrhea include adrenal P450c21 deficiency, ovarian or adrenal malignancies, and Cushing syndrome. Anabolic steroids also cause amenorrhea.

D. Uterine Causes (with Normal FSH)

Infection of the uterus commonly occurs following delivery or D&C but may occur spontaneously. Endometritis due to tuberculosis or schistosomiasis should be suspected in endemic areas. Endometrial scarring may result, causing amenorrhea (Asherman syndrome). Such women typically continue to have monthly premenstrual symptoms. The vaginal estrogen effect is normal.

E. Early and Premature Menopause (with High FSH)

Early menopause refers to primary ovarian failure that occurs before age 45. It affects approximately 5% of women. About 1% of women experience **premature**

menopause that is defined as ovarian failure before age 40; about 30% of such cases are due to autoimmunity against the ovary. X chromosome mosaicism accounts for 8% of cases of premature menopause. Other causes include surgical bilateral oophorectomy, radiation therapy for pelvic malignancy, and chemotherapy. Women who have undergone hysterectomy are prone to premature ovarian failure even though the ovaries were left intact. Myotonic dystrophy, galactosemia, and mumps oophoritis are additional causes. Early or premature menopause is frequently familial. Ovarian failure is usually irreversible.

F. Normal Menopause (with High FSH)

Normal menopause refers to primary ovarian failure that occurs after age 45. "Climacteric" is defined as the period of natural physiologic decline in ovarian function, generally occurring over about 10 years. By about age 40 years, the remaining ovarian follicles are those that are the least sensitive to gonadotropins. Increasing titers of FSH are required to stimulate estradiol secretion. Estradiol levels may actually rise during early climacteric.

The normal age for menopause in the United States ranges between 48 and 55 years, with an average of about 51.5 years. Serum estradiol levels fall and the remaining estrogen after menopause is estrone, derived mainly from peripheral aromatization of adrenal androstenedione. Such peripheral production of estrone is enhanced by obesity and liver disease. Individual differences in estrone levels partly explain why the symptoms noted above may be minimal in some women but severe in others.

▶ Clinical Findings

A. Symptoms and Signs

Vasomotor instability (hot flushes) is experienced by 80% of women, lasting seconds to many minutes. Hot flushes with drenching sweats may be most severe at night or may be triggered by emotional stress. Women may also experience fatigue, insomnia, headache, diminished libido, or rheumatologic symptoms. Psychological symptoms of the "climacteric" include depression and irritability. Some women continue to menstruate for many months despite symptoms of estrogen deficiency. The acute symptoms of estrogen deficiency noted above tend to gradually decline in severity. However, the median duration of moderate to severe hot flushes is about 10 years. Hot flushes tend to continue longer in thin versus obese women and in black versus white women. The late manifestations of estrogen deficiency include urogenital atrophy with vaginal dryness and dyspareunia; dysuria, frequency, and incontinence may occur. Increased bone osteoclastic activity increases the risk for osteoporosis and fractures. The skin becomes more wrinkled. Increases in the LDL:HDL cholesterol ratio cause an increased risk for atherosclerosis.

A careful pelvic examination is always required to check for uterine or adnexal enlargement and to obtain a Papanicolaou smear and a vaginal smear for assessment of estrogen effect. Various life stresses, vigorous exercise, and "crash" dieting all predispose to amenorrhea; however, such factors should not be assumed to account for amenorrhea without a complete workup to screen for other causes.

B. Laboratory Findings

Since pregnancy is the most common cause of amenorrhea, women of childbearing age are immediately screened with a pregnancy test (serum or urine hCG). An elevated hCG overwhelmingly indicates pregnancy; false-positive testing may occur very rarely with ectopic hCG secretion (eg, choriocarcinoma or bronchogenic carcinoma). Women who are not pregnant receive further laboratory evaluation including serum PRL, FSH, LH, and TSH. Hyperprolactinemia or hypopituitarism (without obvious cause; see Hypopituitarism) should prompt an MRI study of the pituitary region. Routine testing for kidney and liver function (eg, BUN, serum creatinine, bilirubin, alkaline phosphatase, and alanine aminotransferase) is also performed. A serum testosterone level is obtained in hirsute or virilized women. Patients with manifestations of hypercortisolism receive a 1-mg overnight dexamethasone suppression test for initial screening (see Cushing syndrome). Nonpregnant women without any laboratory abnormality may receive a 10-day course of a progestin (eg, medroxyprogesterone acetate, 10 mg/d); absence of withdrawal menses typically indicates a lack of estrogen or a uterine abnormality.

▶ Treatment

Therapy of symptomatic hypogonadism generally consists of estrogen replacement therapy. Slow, deep breathing can ameliorate hot flushes. For hot flushes in women who cannot take estrogen, gabapentin is quite effective in oral doses titrated up to 200–800 mg every 8 hours. However, gabapentin is frequently associated with side effects such as fatigue, headache, dizziness, and cognitive impairment; such symptoms are most pronounced during the first 2 weeks of therapy but often improve within 4 weeks. An herb, black cohosh, may possibly relieve hot flushes. Tamoxifen and raloxifene offer bone protection but aggravate hot flushes. Treatment or prevention of postmenopausal osteoporosis with bisphosphonates such as alendronate, risedronate, or intravenous zoledronic acid (see Osteoporosis) is another therapeutic option. Women with low serum testosterone levels may experience hypoactive sexual desire disorder that may respond to low-dose testosterone replacement.

▶ Hormone Replacement Therapy

Two large, prospective studies have evaluated the effect of HRT on postmenopausal women. The Women's Health Initiative (WHI) monitored 16,606 mostly-older postmenopausal women in the United States in a prospective, double-blinded, placebo-controlled study of postmenopausal HRT. A control group of women taking a daily placebo was compared with (1) women receiving daily conventional-dose oral combined HRT (conjugated equine estrogens [CEE] 0.625 mg/d with medroxyprogesterone acetate 2.5 mg/d) and (2) women, having had a hysterectomy, receiving only CEE 0.625 mg/d. The California

Teachers Study prospectively followed up 71,237 postmenopausal women of all ages (mean age 63 years, range 36–94 years) for mortality, breast cancer, and other outcomes.

The WHI and California Teachers Study risk–benefit findings (described below) have dramatically changed postmenopausal HRT. The overall use of HRT has declined. When HRT is prescribed, lower-dose estrogen regimens are preferred over conventional-dose therapy. Estrogen preparations other than CEE have become increasingly favored. Transdermal and vaginal estrogen preparations are widely preferred over oral estrogen replacement. Also, the potential adverse effects of progestins are now recognized, such that women taking very low-dose estrogen replacement may not require progestins or may receive progestin therapy only periodically, if at all. For moderate-to high-dose estrogen therapy, progestins are being used in lower doses. Also, clinicians are now tending to prescribe progesterone-eluting intrauterine devices and oral progestins other than medroxyprogesterone acetate.

A. Benefits of Estrogen Replacement Therapy

In the California Teachers Study, HRT in women under age 60 was associated with a dramatic 46% reduction in all-cause mortality, particularly cardiovascular disease. This association of HRT and lower mortality may suffer from self-selection bias. Nevertheless, there appears to be a survival advantage of HRT in women under age 60 that diminishes with age; no reduction in mortality was noted in the group of women aged 85–94 years. The reduction in cardiovascular disease among younger postmenopausal women taking HRT may be explained by the reduction in serum levels of atherogenic lipoprotein(a) with HRT, with or without a progestin. Improvement in serum HDL cholesterol is greatest with unopposed estrogen but is also seen with the addition of a progestin.

Estrogen replacement improves or eliminates postmenopausal hot flushes and diaphoretic episodes. Vaginal moisture is improved and libido is enhanced in some women. Estradiol vaginal rings can improve symptoms of an overactive bladder. Sleep disturbances are common in menopause and can be reversed with estrogen replacement. Some women notice a mild impairment in memory and cognitive function at menopause that may improve with HRT. Sex hormone replacement may also improve the body pain and reduced physical function experienced by some women at the time of menopause. Many women taking HRT experience a significantly improved quality of life. Estrogen replacement does not prevent facial skin wrinkling; however, it may improve facial skin moisture and thickness, reducing seborrhea and atrophy. Estrogen therapy does not appear to reduce the risk of Alzheimer dementia.

1. Estrogen replacement without progestin (unopposed HRT)—Interestingly, the WHI study found that postmenopausal women taking unopposed estrogen had a 23% *reduction* in breast cancer risk. The WHI study also found that women who received estrogen therapy experienced a reduced number of hip fractures (six fewer fractures/year per 10,000 women) compared with placebo. Even "micro-dose" transdermal estradiol (0.014 mg/d) improves bone density. Unopposed estrogen therapy causes a modest but sustained reduction in joint pain; they have no discernible effect upon cognitive function, overall mortality, or the risk for heart attacks, or colorectal cancer. Unopposed estrogen replacement improves glycemic control in women with type 2 diabetes mellitus. Perimenopause-related depression is improved by unopposed estrogen replacement; the addition of a progestin may negate this effect. A 20-year study of 8801 women living in a retirement community found that estrogen use was associated with improved survival. Age-adjusted mortality rates were 56.4 (per 1000 person-years) among nonusers and 50.4 among women who had used estrogen for 15 years or longer.

2. Estrogen replacement therapy with progestins (combined HRT)—Women receiving conventional-dose daily conjugated estrogen and medroxyprogesterone acetate (0.625 mg and 2.5 mg, respectively) for an average of 5.6 years, experienced a lower risk of developing diabetes mellitus (3.5%) versus those taking a placebo (4.2%).

B. Risks of Estrogen Replacement Therapy

The risks of estrogen replacement depend on the dose. Conventional doses (eg, oral conjugated estrogens ≥ 0.625 mg/d or transdermal estradiol ≥ 0.05 mg/d) carry higher risks than lower doses (eg, oral conjugated estrogens, ≤ 0.3 mg/d or transdermal estradiol ≤ 0.025 mg/d). Route of administration also affects risks, since oral estrogens pass through the liver and increase hepatic production of clotting factors (thereby increasing the risks of thrombotic stroke), whereas transdermal or vaginal administration of estrogen does not significantly increase clotting proclivity. The risks for HRT also depend on whether estrogen is administered alone (unopposed HRT) or with a progestin (combined HRT).

1. Estrogen replacement without progestin (unopposed HRT)—Surprisingly, the WHI study found that postmenopausal women who received conventional-dose estrogen-only therapy had a reduced risk of breast cancer (seven fewer cases/year per 10,000 women) compared with a placebo group. However, the California Teachers Study monitored women for a longer period; a group of 37,000 women who had been taking conventional-dose estrogen-only therapy for ≥ 20 years did have a slightly increased risk of breast cancer. Women taking lower-dose unopposed estrogen therapy would be expected to have lower long-term risk of breast cancer.

Conventional-dose unopposed estrogen replacement (0.625–1.25 mg daily) increases the risk of endometrial hyperplasia and dysfunctional uterine bleeding, which often prompts patients to stop the estrogen. However, lower-dose unopposed estrogen confers a much lower risk of dysfunctional uterine bleeding. Recurrent dysfunctional bleeding necessitates a pelvic examination and possibly an endometrial biopsy. There has been considerable concern that unopposed estrogen replacement might increase the risk for endometrial carcinoma. However, a Cochrane Database Review found no increased risk of endometrial carcinoma in a review of 30 randomized controlled trials. Therefore, lower-dose unopposed estrogen replacement does not appear to confer any increased risk for endometrial cancer.

Long-term conventional-dose unopposed estrogen increases the mortality risk from ovarian cancer, although the absolute risk is small. The annual age-adjusted ovarian cancer death rates for women taking estrogen replacement for ≥ 10 years are 64:100,000 for current users, 38:100,000 for former users, and 26:100,000 for women who had never taken estrogen. Lower-dose estrogen replacement is believed to confer a negligible increased risk for ovarian cancer.

The WHI trial was stopped in 2002 because of an increased risk of stroke among women taking conjugated oral estrogens in doses of 0.625 mg daily; the risk was about 44 strokes per 10,000 person-years versus about 32 per 10,000 person-years in women taking placebo. Transdermal or transvaginal estrogen is not expected to increase the risk of stroke.

Conventional-dose therapy with oral estrogen alone had been thought to increase the risk of deep venous thrombosis and stroke, but the WHI follow-up study found no such increased risk for deep venous thrombosis or stroke. Oral estrogens can cause hypertriglyceridemia, particularly in women with preexistent hyperlipidemia, rarely resulting in pancreatitis. Postmenopausal estrogen therapy also slightly increases the risk of gallstones and cholecystitis. Oral estrogens reduce the effectiveness of GH replacement. These side effects can be reduced or avoided by using non-oral estrogen replacement.

Elderly women, receiving long-term conventional-dose estrogen replacement, experience an increased risk of urinary incontinence. Some women complain of estrogen-induced edema or mastalgia. Estrogen replacement has been reported to lower the seizure threshold in some women with epilepsy. Untreated large pituitary prolactinomas may enlarge if exposed to estrogen.

2. Estrogen replacement with a progestin (combined HRT)—The WHI study found that women who received long-term conventional oral doses of combined HRT (conjugated estrogens 0.625 mg/d plus medroxyprogesterone acetate 2.5 mg/d) had an increased risk of deep venous thrombosis (3.5 per 1000 person-years) compared with women receiving placebo (1.7 per 1000 person-years).

Conventional-dose oral combined HRT results in an increased risk of myocardial infarction (24% or six additional heart attacks per 10,000 women), mostly in older women with high-risk LDL levels or preexistent coronary disease. Most of the risk for myocardial infarction occurs in the first year of therapy. This increased risk is attributable to the progestin component, since the estrogen-only arm of the WHI study found no increased risk of myocardial infarction.

Long-term conventional-dose oral combined HRT increases breast density and the risk for abnormal mammograms (9.4% versus 5.4% for placebo). There is also a higher risk of breast cancer (8 cases per 10,000 women/year versus 6.5 cases per 10,000 women/year for placebo); the increased risk of breast cancer is highest shortly after menopause (about 2 cases per 1000 women annually).

No increased risk of breast cancer has been found with estrogen-only HRT. This increased risk for breast cancer appears to mostly affect relatively thin women with a BMI < 24.4. The Iowa Women's Health Study reported an increase in breast cancer with HRT only in women consuming more than 1 oz of alcohol weekly. No accelerated risk of breast cancer has been seen in users of HRT who have benign breast disease or a family history of breast cancer. Women in whom new-onset breast tenderness develops with combined HRT have an increased risk of breast cancer, compared with women without breast tenderness.

The Women's Health Initiative Mental Study (WHIMS) followed the effect of combined conventional-dose oral HRT on cognitive function in women 65–79 years old. HRT did not protect these older women from cognitive decline. In fact, they experienced an increased risk for severe dementia at a rate of 23 more cases/year for every 10,000 women over age 65 years.

In the WHI study, women receiving conventional-dose combined oral HRT experienced an increased risk of stroke (31 strokes per 10,000 women/year versus 26 strokes per 10,000 women/year for placebo). Stroke risk was also increased by hypertension, diabetes, and smoking.

Women taking combined estrogen–progestin replacement do not experience an increased risk of ovarian cancer. They do experience an increased risk of developing asthma.

Progestins may cause moodiness, particularly in women with a history of premenstrual dysphoric disorder. Cycled progestins may trigger migraines in certain women. Many other adverse reactions have been reported, including breast tenderness, alopecia, and fluid retention. Contraindications to the use of progestins include thromboembolic disorders, liver disease, breast cancer, and pregnancy.

C. Hormone Replacement Therapy Agents

1. Transdermal estradiol—Estradiol can be delivered systemically with different systems of skin patches, mists, and gels. Transdermal estradiol works for most women, but some women have poor transdermal absorption or skin reactions to the product.

A. ESTRADIOL PATCHES MIXED WITH ADHESIVE—These systems tend to cause minimal skin irritation. Of the following preparations, the Vivelle-Dot patches are the smallest and least obtrusive. Generic estradiol transdermal (0.025, 0.0375, 0.05, 0.06, 0.075, 0.1 mg/d) is replaced once weekly. Brand products include Vivelle-Dot (0.025, 0.0375, 0.05, 0.075, or 0.1 mg/d), replaced twice weekly; Alora (0.025, 0.05, 0.075, or 0.1 mg/d), replaced twice weekly; Climara (0.025, 0.0375, 0.05, 0.06, 0.075, or 0.1 mg/d), replaced weekly; and Menostar (0.014 mg/d), replaced weekly. This type of estradiol skin patch can be cut in half and applied to the skin without proportionately greater loss of potency.

B. ESTRADIOL PATCHES WITH DRUG RESERVOIR—These systems cause significant skin irritation in some women. Available preparations include Estraderm (0.05 or 0.1 mg/d), applied to the trunk, abdomen, or buttocks and replaced twice weekly.

C. ESTRADIOL PATCHES WITH PROGESTIN MIXED WITH ADHESIVE—These preparations mix estradiol with either norethindrone acetate or levonorgestrel. Combipatch (0.05 mg E and 0.14 mg norethindrone acetate daily or 0.05 mg E and 0.25 mg norethindrone acetate daily) is replaced twice weekly. Climara Pro (0.45 mg E and 0.0125 mg levonorgestrel daily) is replaced once weekly. The addition of a progestin reduces the risk of endometrial hyperplasia but increases the risk of breast cancer and side effects, compared with estrogen therapy alone.

D. ESTRADIOL GELS AND MISTS—EstroGel 0.06% is available in a metered-dose pump that dispenses 1.25 g gel/ per actuation (1–2 actuations/d). Elestrin 0.06% is available in a metered-dose pump that dispenses 0.87 g gel per activation (1–2 actuations/d). These gels are applied daily to one arm from the wrist to the shoulder after bathing. Divigel 0.1% gel (0.025, 0.5, 1 g/packet) is applied to the upper thigh daily. Estrasorb is available in 1.74 g pouches (0.025 mg estradiol); 1–2 pouches of lotion are applied to the thigh/calf daily. Evamist is available as a topical mister that dispenses 1.53 mg estradiol/spray; 1–3 sprays are applied to the inner forearm daily. To avoid spreading the estradiol to others, the hands should be washed and precautions taken to avoid prolonged skin contact with children. Application of sunscreen prior to estradiol gel has been reported to *increase* the transdermal absorption of estradiol.

2. Oral estrogen—

A. ORAL ESTROGEN-ONLY PREPARATIONS—These preparations include conjugated equine estrogens (CEE) that are available as Premarin (0.3, 0.45, 0.625, 0.9, and 1.25 mg), conjugated plant-derived estrogens (eg, Menest, 0.3, 0.625, and 2.5 mg), and conjugated synthetic estrogens that are available as Cenestin (0.3, 0.625, 0.9, and 1.25 mg) and Enjuvia (0.3, 0.45, 0.625, 0.9, and 1.25 mg). Other preparations include estradiol (0.5, 1, and 2 mg), estropipate (0.75, 1.5, and 3 mg), and estradiol acetate that is available as Femtrace (0.45, 0.9, and 1.8 mg).

B. ORAL ESTROGEN PLUS PROGESTIN PREPARATIONS—CEE with medroxyprogesterone acetate is available as Prempro (0.3/1.5, 0.45/1.5, 0.625/2.5, and 0.625 mg/5 mg); CEE for 14 days cycled with CEE plus medroxyprogesterone acetate for 14 days is available as Premphase (0.625/0, then 0.625 mg/5 mg); estradiol with norethindrone acetate (0.5/0.1 and 1 mg/0.5 mg); ethinyl estradiol with norethindrone acetate is available as Femhrt (2.5/0.5 and 5 mcg/1 mg) and Jinteli (5 mcg/1 mg); estradiol with drospirenone is available as Angeliq (0.25 mg/0.5 mg, and 0.5 mg/1.0 mg); estradiol with norgestimate is available as Prefest (estradiol 1 mg/d for 3 days, alternating with 1 mg estradiol/0.09 mg norgestimate daily for 3 days). Oral contraceptives can also be used for combined HRT.

3. Vaginal estrogen—Urogenital atrophy commonly develops in postmenopausal women and can cause dryness of the vagina, genital itching, burning, dyspareunia, and recurrent urinary tract infections. Urinary symptoms can include urgency and dysuria. Vaginal estrogen is intended to deliver estrogen directly to local tissues and is moderately effective in reducing these symptoms, while minimizing systemic estrogen exposure. Some estrogen is absorbed systemically and can relieve menopausal symptoms. Manufacturers recommend that these preparations be used for only 3–6 months in women with an intact uterus, since vaginal estrogen can cause endometrial proliferation. However, most clinicians use them for longer periods. Vaginal estrogen can be administered in three different ways: creams, tablets, and rings.

A. Estrogen vaginal creams—These creams are administered intravaginally with a measured-dose applicator daily for 2 weeks for atrophic vaginitis, then administered one to three times weekly. Available preparations include CEE, which is available as Premarin Vaginal (0.625 mg/g cream), dosed as 0.25–2 g cream administered vaginally one to three times weekly. Estradiol is available as Estrace Vaginal (0.1 mg/g cream), 1 g cream administered vaginally one to two times weekly.

B. Estradiol vaginal tablets—These tablets are sold prepackaged in a disposable applicator and can be administered deep intravaginally daily for 2 weeks for atrophic vaginitis, then twice weekly. The tablets dissolve into a gel that gradually releases estradiol. Available preparations include vaginal estradiol tablets that are available as Vagifem (10 mcg/tablet), administered vaginally two times weekly.

C. Estradiol vaginal rings—These rings are inserted manually into the upper third of the vagina, worn continuously, and replaced every 3 months. Only a small amount of the released estradiol enters the systemic circulation. Vaginal rings do not usually interfere with sexual intercourse. If a ring is removed or descends into the introitus, it may be washed in warm water and reinserted. Available preparations release estradiol and include Estring (2 mg estradiol/ring, releasing 7.5 mcg/d) and Femring (0.05 mg/d and 0.10 mg/d). For women with postmenopausal urinary urgency and frequency, even the low-dose Estring can successfully reduce urinary symptoms.

D. Estradiol with progestin vaginal rings—The available preparation is NuvaRing that releases a mixture of estradiol 0.15 mg/d and etonogestrel 0.12 mg/d. It is a contraceptive vaginal ring that is placed in the vagina on or before day 5 of the menstrual cycle, left for 3 weeks, removed for 1 week, and then replaced.

4. Estradiol intramuscular—Parenteral estradiol should be used only for particularly severe menopausal symptoms when other measures have failed or are contraindicated. Estradiol cypionate (DepoEstradiol 5 mg/mL) may be administered intramuscularly in doses of 1–5 mg every 3–4 weeks. Estradiol valerate (20 mg/mL) may be administered intramuscularly in doses of 10–20 mg every 4 weeks. Women with an intact uterus should receive a progestin for the last 10 days of each cycle.

5. Oral progestins—For a woman with an intact uterus, long-term conventional-dose unopposed systemic estrogen therapy can cause endometrial hyperplasia, which typically results in dysfunctional uterine bleeding and might rarely lead to endometrial cancer. Progestin therapy transforms proliferative into secretory endometrium,

causing a menses when given intermittently or no bleeding when given continuously.

The type of progestin preparation, its dosage, and the timing of administration may be tailored to the given situation. Progestins may be given daily, monthly, or at longer intervals. When given episodically, progestins are usually administered for 7–14 day periods. Progestins are available in different formulations: Micronized progesterone (100 mg and 200 mg/capsule), medroxyprogesterone acetate (2.5, 5.0, and 10 mg/scored tablet), norethindrone acetate (5 mg/tablet), and norethindrone (0.35 mg/tablet).

Progesterone is also available as vaginal gels (eg, Prochieve, 4% = 45 mg/applicatorful, and 8% = 90 mg/applicatorful) that are typically administered vaginally every other day for six doses.

Topical progesterone (20–50 mg/d) may reduce hot flushes in women who are intolerant to oral HRT. It may be applied to the upper arms, thighs, or inner wrists daily. It may be compounded as micronized progesterone 250 mg/mL in a transdermal gel. Its effects upon the breast and endometrium are unknown.

6. Progestin-releasing intrauterine devices—Intrauterine devices (IUDs) that release progestins can be useful for women receiving ERT, since they can reduce the incidence of dysfunctional uterine bleeding and endometrial carcinoma without exposing women to the significant risks of systemic progestins. The Mirena IUD releases levonorgestrel and is inserted into the uterus by a clinician within 7 days of the onset of menses. It remains effective for up to 5 years. Parous women are generally better able to tolerate the Mirena IUD than nulliparous women.

7. Selective estrogen receptor modulators—SERMs (eg, raloxifene, tamoxifen) are an alternative to estrogen replacement for hypogonadal women at risk for osteoporosis who prefer not to take estrogens because of their contraindications (eg, breast or uterine cancer) or side effects. Raloxifene (Evista) does not reduce hot flushes, vaginal dryness, skin wrinkling, or breast atrophy; it does not improve cognition. However, in doses of 60 mg/d orally, it inhibits bone loss without stimulating effects upon the breasts or endometrium. Raloxifene does not stimulate the endometrium and actually reduces the risk of endometrial carcinoma, so concomitant progesterone therapy is not required. Another advantage to raloxifene is that it reduces the risk of invasive breast cancer by about 50%. Raloxifene slightly increases the risk of venous thromboembolism (though less so than tamoxifen), so it should not be used by women at prolonged bed rest or otherwise prone to thrombosis. Ospemifene (Osphena) is a SERM that has unique estrogen-like effects on the vaginal epithelium and is indicated for the treatment of postmenopausal dyspareunia when other therapies are ineffective. Given orally in doses of 60 mg/d, it commonly aggravates hot flushes, increases the risks of thromboembolism, and increases endometrial hyperplasia. Ospemifene has unknown long-term effects upon bone and breast.

Tibolone (Livial) is an SERM whose metabolites have mixed estrogenic, progestogenic, and weak androgenic activity. It is comparable to HRT for the treatment of climacteric-related complaints. It does not appear to significantly stimulate proliferation of breast or endometrial tissue. It depresses both serum triglycerides and HDL cholesterol. Long-term studies are lacking. It is not available in the United States.

8. Phytoestrogens—These substances are found in plants that bind to estrogen receptors. Phytoestrogens, found in soy and red clover extracts, do not appear to significantly improve menopausal hot flushes, cognitive function, bone density, or plasma lipids.

9. Testosterone replacement therapy in women—In premenopausal women, serum testosterone levels decline with age. Between 25 and 45 years of age, women's testosterone levels fall 50%. After natural menopause, the ovaries remain a significant source for testosterone. In fact, following natural menopause, serum testosterone levels do not fall abruptly and serum free testosterone levels may actually rise. In contrast, very low serum testosterone levels are found in women after bilateral oophorectomy, autoimmune ovarian failure, or adrenalectomy, and in hypopituitarism. Testosterone deficiency contributes to hot flushes, loss of sexual hair, muscle atrophy, osteoporosis, and diminished libido, also known as hypoactive sexual desire disorder.

In women, diminished libido is common and multifactorial. Although low serum testosterone levels may contribute to hypoactive sexual desire disorder, hysterectomy and sexual isolation are major causes. Low serum testosterone levels may also cause fatigue, a diminished sense of well-being, and a dulled enthusiasm for life. Androgen replacement may improve these problems.

Testosterone therapy is often effective, while DHEA therapy is not. Selected women may be treated with low-dose testosterone. Methyltestosterone can be taken orally in doses of 1.25–2.5 mg daily. Testosterone can also be compounded as a cream containing 1 mg/mL, with 1 mL applied to the abdomen daily. Methyltestosterone is also available in combination with conjugated estrogens (eg, Estratest). This formulation is convenient but carries the same disadvantage as oral estrogen—increased risk of thromboembolism. Tablets contain either 1.25 mg conjugated estrogens with 2.5 mg methyltestosterone or 0.625 mg conjugated estrogens with 1.25 mg methyltestosterone. Estratest is usually started at the lowest strength. It should be given cyclically at the lowest dose that controls symptoms.

Women receiving testosterone therapy must be monitored for the appearance of any acne or hirsutism, and serum testosterone levels are determined periodically if women feel that they are benefitting and long-term testosterone therapy is instituted. Side effects of low-dose testosterone therapy are usually minimal but may include polycythemia, emotional changes, hirsutism, acne, an adverse effect on lipids, and potentiation of warfarin anticoagulation therapy. Testosterone therapy tends to reduce both triglyceride and HDL cholesterol levels. Hepatocellular neoplasms and peliosis hepatis, rare complications of oral androgens at higher doses, have not been reported with methyltestosterone at lower doses of 2.5 mg orally daily.

Vaginal testosterone is an option for postmenopausal women who cannot use systemic or vaginal estrogen due to breast cancer. Testosterone 150–300 mcg/d vaginally appears to reduce vaginal dryness and dyspareunia without increasing systemic estrogen levels.

Androgens should not be given to women with liver disease or during pregnancy or breast-feeding. Testosterone replacement therapy for women should be used judiciously, since long-term prospective clinical trials are lacking. An analysis of the Nurses' Health Study found that women who had been taking CEEs plus methyltestosterone experienced an increased risk of breast cancer. Yearly mammography is recommended for all women over 40 years of age.

D. Other Treatments for Menopausal Symptoms

Lifestyle changes, such as dressing coolly, avoiding down bedding and foam mattresses, sleeping with light bedclothes, keeping the ambient room temperature cool, sipping cold beverages, and stress reduction may help reduce hot flushes. Women may try avoiding known triggers for hot flushes, such as smoking, alcohol, caffeine, and hot spicy foods. Idiosyncratic triggers for hot flushes may be discerned and avoided. **Clinical hypnosis** greatly reduced hot flushes over 12 weeks in one study. **Selective serotonin reuptake inhibitors** may also reduce hot flushes. **Gabapentin** can relieve hot flushes when estrogen replacement therapy is contraindicated or not desired and when lifestyle changes are insufficient. Women with moderate to severe postmenopausal hot flushes may obtain relief with gabapentin 600–2400 mg daily in divided doses. Side effects are most prominent in the first 2 weeks of treatment and may include somnolence, unsteadiness, and dizziness. **Acupuncture** may also be helpful.

Replens is a vaginal lubricant that can be used daily or 2 hours prior to intercourse. It improves vaginal moisture and elasticity and reduces vaginal irritation and dyspareunia.

Canonico M et al. Further evidence for promoting transdermal estrogens in the management of postmenopausal symptoms. Menopause. 2011 Oct;18(10):1038–9. [PMID: 21946050]

Carpenter JS et al. Effect of escitalopram on hot flash interference: a randomized, controlled trial. Fertil Steril. 2012 Jun;97(6):1399–404. [PMID: 22480818]

Chlebowski RT et al. Estrogen alone and joint symptoms in the Women's Health Initiative randomized trial. Menopause. 2013 Jun;20(6):600–8. [PMID: 23511705]

Clarkson TB et al. Timing hypothesis for postmenopausal hormone therapy: its origin, current status, and future. Menopause. 2013 Mar;20(3):342–53. [PMID: 23435033]

Lobo RA. Where are we 10 years after the Women's Health Initiative? J Clin Endocrinol Metab. 2013 May;98(5):1771–80. [PMID: 23493433]

Maclaran K et al. Premature ovarian failure. J Fam Plann Reprod Health Care. 2011 Jan;37(1):35–42. [PMID: 21367702]

Marjoribanks J et al. Long term hormone therapy for perimenopausal and postmenopausal women. Cochrane Database Syst Rev. 2012 Jul 11;7:CD004143. [PMID: 22786488]

Moilanen JM et al. Effect of aerobic training on menopausal symptoms—a randomized controlled trial. Menopause. 2012 Jun;19(6):691–6. [PMID: 22334056]

Nelson HD et al. Menopausal hormone therapy for the primary prevention of chronic conditions: a systematic review to update the U.S. Preventive Services Task Force recommendations. Ann Intern Med. 2012 Jul 17;157(2):104–13. [PMID: 22786830]

Rozenberg S et al. Postmenopausal hormone therapy: risks and benefits. Nat Rev Endocrinol. 2013 Apr;9(4):216–27. [PMID: 23419265]

Silveira LF et al. Approach to the patient with hypogonadotropic hypogonadism. J Clin Endocrinol Metab. 2013 May;98(5): 1781–8. [PMID: 23650335]

Simon JA. What's new in hormone replacement therapy: focus on transdermal estradiol and micronized progesterone. Climacteric. 2012 Apr;15(Suppl 1):3–10. [PMID: 22432810]

TURNER SYNDROME (Gonadal Dysgenesis)

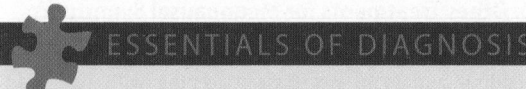

ESSENTIALS OF DIAGNOSIS

▸ Short stature with normal GH levels.

▸ Primary amenorrhea or early ovarian failure.

▸ Epicanthal folds, webbed neck, short fourth metacarpals.

▸ Renal and cardiovascular anomalies.

Turner syndrome comprises a group of X chromosome disorders that are associated with spontaneous abortion, primary hypogonadism, short stature, and other phenotypic anomalies (Table 26-16). It affects 1–2% of fetuses, of which about 97% abort, accounting for about 10% of all spontaneous abortions. Nevertheless, it affects about 1 in every 2500 live female births. Patients with the classic syndrome (about 50% of cases) lack one of the two X chromosomes (45,XO karyotype). Other patients with Turner syndrome have X chromosome abnormalities, such as ring X or Xq (X/abnormal X) or X chromosome deletions affecting all or some somatic cells (mosaicism, XX/XO).

1. Classic Turner Syndrome (45,XO Gonadal Dysgenesis)

▶ Clinical Findings

A. Symptoms and Signs

Features of Turner syndrome are variable and may be subtle in girls with mosaicism. Turner syndrome may be diagnosed in infant girls at birth, since they tend to be small and may exhibit severe lymphedema. Evaluation for childhood short stature often leads to the diagnosis. Girls and women with Turner syndrome have an increased risk of aortic coarctation (11%) and bicuspid aortic valves (16%); these cardiac abnormalities are more common in patients with a webbed neck. If a woman with Turner syndrome becomes pregnant, there is a 2% risk of death from aortic dissection or rupture. Typical manifestations in adulthood include short stature, hypogonadism, webbed neck, high-arched palate, wide-spaced nipples, hypertension, and renal abnormalities (Table 26–16). Emotional disorders are common. Affected women are also more prone to autoimmune disease, particularly thyroiditis (37%), inflammatory bowel disease (4%), and celiac disease (3%).

Table 26–16. Manifestations of Turner syndrome.

Short stature
Distinctive facial features
Ptosis
Micrognathia
Low-set ears
Epicanthal folds
Sexual infantilism due to gonadal dysgenesis with primary amenorrhea (80%)
Early ovarian failure with secondary amenorrhea (20%)
Webbed neck (40%)
Low hairline
High-arched palate
Cubitus valgus
Short fourth metacarpals (50%)
Lymphedema of hands and feet (30%)
Hypoplastic widely spaced nipples
Hyperconvex nails
Pigmented nevi
Keloid formation (eg, surgical scars or after ear piercing)
Recurrent otitis media
Renal abnormalities (60%)
Horseshoe kidney
Hydronephrosis
Hypertension (idiopathic or due to coarctation or kidney disease)
Gastrointestinal disorders
Telangiectasias with bleeding
Celiac disease
Inflammatory bowel disease
Colon carcinoma
Liver disease
Impaired space-form recognition, direction sense, and mathematical reasoning
Cardiovascular anomalies
Coarctation of the aorta (10–20%)
Partial anomalous pulmonary venous connection
Bicuspid aortic valve (with aortic stenosis or insufficiency)
Aortic dissection due to coarctation and cystic medial necrosis of the aorta
Associated conditions
Obesity
Diabetes mellitus (types 1 and 2)
Dyslipidemia
Hyperuricemia
Hashimoto thyroiditis
Achlorhydria
Cataracts, corneal opacities
Neuroblastoma (1%)
Rheumatoid arthritis

Hypogonadism presents as "delayed adolescence" (primary amenorrhea, 80%) or early ovarian failure (20%); girls with 45,XO Turner (blood karyotyping) who enter puberty are typically found to have mosaicism if other tissues are karyotyped.

B. Laboratory Findings

Hypogonadism is confirmed in girls who have high serum levels of FSH and LH. A blood karyotype showing 45,XO (or X chromosome abnormalities or mosaicism) establishes the diagnosis. GH and IGF-1 levels are normal.

C. Imaging

An ultrasound and MRI scan of the chest and abdomen should be done in all patients with Turner syndrome to determine whether cardiac, aortic, and renal abnormalities are present.

▶ Treatment

Treatment of short stature with daily injections of GH (0.1 unit/kg/d) plus an androgen (eg, oxandrolone) for at least 4 years before epiphyseal fusion increases final height by a mean of about 10.3 cm over the mean predicted height of 144.2 cm. Rarely, such GH treatment causes pseudotumor cerebri. After age 12 years, estrogen therapy is begun with low doses of conjugated estrogens (0.3 mg) or ethinyl estradiol (5 mcg) given on days 1–21 per month. When growth stops, HRT is begun with estrogen and progestin; transdermal estrogen may be used to initiate pubertal development.

▶ Complications & Surveillance

Bicuspid aortic valves are associated with an increased risk of infective endocarditis, aortic valvular stenosis or insufficiency, and ascending aortic aneurysm and dissection. Partial anomalous pulmonary vein connections occur in 13% and can lead to left-to-right shunting of blood. Adults with Turner syndrome have a high incidence of ECG abnormalities.

Women with Turner syndrome have a reduced life expectancy due in part to their increased risk of diabetes mellitus (types 1 and 2), hypertension, dyslipidemia, and osteoporosis.

Diagnostic vigilance and aggressive treatment of these conditions reduce the risk of aortic aneurysm dissection, ischemic heart disease, stroke, and fracture. Patients are prone to keloid formation after surgery or ear piercing. Yearly ocular examinations and periodic thyroid evaluations are recommended.

Repeat cardiovascular evaluations should be done every 3–4 years. Patients with the classic 45,XO karyotype have a high risk of renal structural abnormalities, whereas those with 46 X/abnormal X are more prone to malformations of the urinary collecting system. The risk of aortic dissection is increased more than 100-fold in women with Turner syndrome, particularly those with pronounced neck webbing and shield chest. Patients with aortic root enlargement are usually treated with beta-blockade and serial imaging. Women with Turner syndrome who are able to become pregnant (spontaneously or with oocyte donation) are at high risk for complications, including fetal morbidity, severe hypertension, and aortic dissection. They are strongly advised to deliver via cesarean section due to the risk of aortic aneurysm rupture during vaginal delivery.

2. Turner Syndrome Variants

A. 46,X (Abnormal X) Karyotype

Patients with small distal short arm deletions of the X chromosome (Xp-) that include the *SHOX* gene often have short stature and skeletal abnormalities but have a low risk of ovarian failure. Transmission of Turner syndrome from mother to daughter can occur. There may be an increased risk of trisomy 21 in the conceptuses of women with Turner syndrome. Patients with deletions of the long arm of the X chromosome (distal to Xq24) often have amenorrhea without short stature or other features of Turner syndrome. Abnormalities or deletions of other genes located on both the long and short arms of the X chromosome can produce gonadal dysgenesis with few other somatic features.

B. 45,XO/46,XX and 45,XO/46, XY Mosaicism

45,XO/46,XX mosaicism results in a modified form of Turner syndrome. Such girls tend to be taller and may have more gonadal function and fewer other manifestations of Turner syndrome.

45,XO/46,XY mosaicism can produce some manifestations of Turner syndrome. Patients may have ambiguous genitalia or male infertility with an otherwise normal phenotype. Germ cell tumors, such as gonadoblastomas and seminomas, develop in about 10% of patients with 45,XO/46,XY mosaicism; most such tumors are benign.

Bakalov VK et al. Autoimmune disorders in women with Turner syndrome and women with karyotypically normal primary ovarian insufficiency. J Autoimmun. 2012 Jun;38(4):315–21. [PMID: 22342295]

Pinsker JE. Clinical review. Turner syndrome: updating the paradigm of clinical care. J Clin Endocrinol Metab. 2012 Jun;97(6):E994–1003. [PMID: 22472565]

Practice Committee of American Society for Reproductive Medicine. Increased maternal cardiovascular mortality associated with pregnancy in women with Turner syndrome. Fertil Steril. 2012 Feb;97(2):282–4. [PMID: 22192347]

Reindollar RH. Turner syndrome: contemporary thoughts and reproductive issues. Semin Reprod Med. 2011 Jul;29(4): 342–52. [PMID: 21969268]

Ross JL et al. Growth hormone plus childhood low-dose estrogen in Turner's syndrome. N Engl J Med. 2011 Mar 31; 364(13):1230–42. [PMID: 21449786]

Trolle C et al. Sex hormone replacement in Turner syndrome. Endocrine. 2012 Apr;41(2):200–19. [PMID: 22147393]

MULTIPLE ENDOCRINE NEOPLASIA (MEN)

ESSENTIALS OF DIAGNOSIS

▶ MEN 1: tumors of the parathyroid glands, endocrine pancreas and duodenum, anterior pituitary, adrenal, thyroid; carcinoid tumors; lipomas and facial angiofibromas.

▶ MEN 2: medullary thyroid cancers, pheochromocytomas, Hirschsprung disease.

▶ MEN 3: medullary thyroid cancers, pheochromocytomas, Marfan-like habitus, mucosal neuromas, intestinal ganglioneuroma, delayed puberty.

▶ MEN 4: tumors of the parathyroid glands, anterior pituitary gland, adrenal gland, ovary, testicle, kidney.

Table 26–17. Multiple endocrine neoplasia (MEN) syndromes: Incidence of tumor types.

Tumor Type	MEN 1	MEN 2 (MEN 2A)	MEN 3 (MEN 2B)	MEN 4
Parathyroid	95%	20–50%	Rare	Common
Pancreatic	54%			Common
Pituitary	42%			Common
Medullary thyroid carcinoma		> 90%	80%	
Pheochromocytoma	Rare	20–35%	60%	
Mucosal and gastrointestinal ganglioneuromas		Rare	> 90%	
Subcutaneous lipoma	30%			
Adrenocortical adenoma	30%			Common
Thoracic carcinoid	15%			
Thyroid adenoma	55%			Common
Facial angiofibromas and collagenomas	85%			

Syndromes of MEN are inherited as autosomal dominant traits that cause a predisposition to the development of tumors of two or more different endocrine glands (Table 26–17). MEN syndromes are caused by different germline mutations and tumors arising when certain additional somatic mutations occur in predisposed organs. Patients with MEN should have genetic testing so that their first-degree relatives may then be tested for the specific mutation.

1. MEN 1

Multiple endocrine neoplasia type 1 (MEN 1, Wermer syndrome) is a tumor syndrome with a prevalence of 2–10 per 100,000 people. About 90% of affected patients harbor a detectable germline mutations in the *menin* gene. Genetic testing is able to detect the specific mutation in 60–95% of cases.

The presentation of MEN 1 is quite variable, even in the same kindred. Affected patients are prone to develop many different tumors, particularly involving the parathyroids, endocrine pancreas and duodenum, and anterior pituitary. In some affected individuals, tumors may start developing in childhood, whereas in others, tumors develop late in adult life. With close endocrine surveillance of affected individuals, the initial biochemical manifestations (usually hypercalcemia) can often be detected as early as age 14–18 years in patients with a MEN 1 gene mutation, although clinical manifestations usually present in the third or fourth decade.

Hyperparathyroidism is the first clinical manifestation of MEN 1 in two-thirds of affected patients, but it may present at any time of life. Patients with the MEN 1 mutation have a > 90% lifetime risk of developing hyperparathyroidism. The hyperparathyroidism of MEN 1 is notoriously difficult to treat surgically, due to multiple gland involvement and the frequency of supernumerary glands and ectopic parathyroid tissue. Typically, three and one-half glands are resected, leaving one-half of the most normal-appearing gland intact. Also, during neck surgery, a thymectomy is performed to resect any intrathymic parathyroid glands or occult thymic carcinoid tumors. Nevertheless, the surgical failure rate is about 38%, and there is a recurrence rate of about 16%, with hypercalcemia often recurring many years after neck surgery. Aggressive parathyroid resection can cause permanent hypoparathyroidism. Patients with persistent or recurrent hyperparathyroidism should avoid oral calcium supplements and thiazide diuretics; oral therapy with calcimimetic drug, such as cinacalcet, is effective but expensive. The diagnosis and treatment of hyperparathyroidism is described earlier in this chapter.

Enteropancreatic tumors occur in up to 70% of patients with MEN 1. These tumors may secrete only pancreatic polypeptide or be nonsecretory altogether (20–55%). **Gastrinomas** occur in about 40% of patients with MEN 1; they secrete gastrin, thereby causing severe gastric hyperacidity (Zollinger–Ellison syndrome) with peptic ulcer disease or diarrhea. Concurrent hypercalcemia, due to hyperparathyroidism (see above), stimulates gastrin and gastric acid secretion; control of the hypercalcemia often reduces gastric acid secretion and serum gastrin levels. These gastrinomas tend to be small, multiple, and ectopic; they are frequently found outside the pancreas, usually in the duodenum. Gastrinomas of MEN 1 can metastasize to the liver; but in patients with MEN 1, depending upon the kindred, hepatic metastases tend to be less aggressive than those from sporadic gastrinomas. Treatment of patients with gastrinomas in MEN 1 is usually conservative, utilizing long-term high-dose proton pump inhibitor therapy and control of hypercalcemia; surgery is palliative and usually reserved for aggressive gastrinomas and those tumors arising in the duodenum. (See Chapter 15.)

Insulinomas cause hyperinsulinism and fasting hypoglycemia. They occur in about 10% of patients with MEN 1. Surgery is usually attempted, but the tumors can be small, multiple, and difficult to detect. (See Chapter 27.) **Gluca-gonomas** (1.6%) secrete glucagon and cause diabetes and migratory necrolytic erythema. **VIPomas** (1%) secrete VIP and cause profuse watery diarrhea, hypokalemia, and achlorhydria (WDHA, Verner-Morrison syndrome). **Somatostatinomas** (0.7%) can cause diabetes mellitus, steatorrhea, and cholelithiasis.

Extrapancreatic neuroendocrine tumors (NETs) commonly occur and include carcinoid tumors that tend to occur in foregut locations (69%), such as the lung, thymus, duodenum, or stomach. Such carcinoid tumors are frequently malignant.

Pituitary adenomas occur in about 42% of patients with MEN 1. They are more common in women (50%) than men (31%) and are the presenting tumor in 17% of patients with MEN 1. These tumors tend to be more aggressive macroadenomas (> 1 cm diameter, 85%) compared to sporadic pituitary tumors (42%). Of MEN 1–associated pituitary tumors, about 62% secrete PRL, 8% secrete GH, 13% secrete both PRL and GH, and 13% are nonsecretory; only 4% secrete ACTH. (See Pituitary Tumors and Cushing disease.) These pituitary tumors can produce local pressure effects and hypopituitarism.

Adrenal adenomas or **hyperplasia** occurs in about 40% of patients with MEN 1 and 50% are bilateral. They are generally benign and nonfunctional, but a feminizing adrenal carcinoma has been reported. These adrenal lesions are pituitary independent.

Benign thyroid adenomas or multinodular goiter occurs in about 55% of affected patients. Patients may undergo a thyroidectomy at the time of parathyroidectomy.

Nonendocrine tumors occur commonly in MEN 1, particularly small head-neck angiofibromas (85%) and lipomas (30%). Collagenomas are common (70%), presenting as firm dermal nodules. Affected patients may also be more prone to develop meningiomas, colorectal cancers, prostate cancer, and malignant melanomas.

The differential diagnosis of MEN 1 includes sporadic or familial tumors of the pituitary, parathyroids, or pancreatic islets. Hypercalcemia (from any cause) may cause gastrointestinal symptoms and increased gastrin levels, simulating a gastrinoma. Routine suppression of gastric acid secretion with H_2-blockers or proton pump inhibitors causes a physiologic increase in serum gastrin that can be mistaken for a gastrinoma. H_2-blockers and metoclopramide cause hyperprolactinemia, simulating a pituitary prolactinoma.

Variants of MEN 1 also occur. Kindreds with MEN 1 Burin variant have a high prevalence of prolactinomas, late-onset hyperparathyroidism, and carcinoid tumors, but rarely enteropancreatic tumors. Overall, patients with MEN 1 face an increased mortality risk with a mean life expectancy of only 55 years.

2. MEN 2A (MEN 2)

Multiple endocrine neoplasia type 2A (MEN 2, Sipple syndrome) is a rare autosomal-dominant tumor syndrome that arises in patients with a germline *ret* protooncogene mutation. Genetic testing identifies about 95% of affected

individuals. Each kindred has a certain *ret* codon mutation that correlates with a particular variation in the MEN 2 syndrome.

Patients with MEN 2A may develop **medullary thyroid carcinoma** (> 90%); hyperparathyroidism (20–50%), with hyperplasia or adenomas of multiple parathyroid glands developing in over 70% of cases; **pheochromocytomas** (20–35%), which are often bilateral; or **Hirschsprung disease**. The medullary thyroid carcinoma is of mild to moderate aggressiveness. Children harboring an MEN 2A *ret* protooncogene mutation are advised to have a prophylactic total thyroidectomy by age 6 years. Before any surgical procedure, MEN 2 carriers should be screened for pheochromocytoma. However, there is incomplete penetrance, and about 30% of those with such mutations never manifest endocrine tumors.

Patients may be screened for medullary thyroid carcinoma with a thyroid ultrasound and with a serum calcitonin drawn after 3 days of omeprazole, 20 mg orally twice daily; in the presence of medullary thyroid carcinoma, calcitonin levels usually rise to above 80 pg/mL (23 pmol/L) in women or above 190 pg/mL (56 pmol/L) in men.

3. MEN 2B (MEN 3)

Multiple endocrine neoplasia type 2B (MEN 3) is a familial, autosomal dominant multiglandular syndrome that is caused by a mutation of the *ret* protooncogene. MEN 2B is characterized by mucosal neuromas (> 90%) with bumpy and enlarged lips and tongue, Marfan-like habitus (75%), adrenal pheochromocytomas (60%) that are rarely malignant and often bilateral, and medullary thyroid carcinoma (80%). Patients also have intestinal abnormalities (75%) such as intestinal ganglioneuromas, skeletal abnormalities (87%), and delayed puberty (43%). Medullary thyroid carcinoma is aggressive and presents early in life. Therefore, infants having a parent with MEN 2B must receive early genetic screening, with those carrying the *ret* protooncogene mutation undergoing a prophylactic total thyroidectomy by age 6 months.

4. MEN 4

Multiple endocrine neoplasia type 4 (MEN 4) is a rare autosomal-dominant familial tumor syndrome caused by germline mutations in the gene *CDKN1B*. Affected patients are particularly prone to develop adenomas of the pituitary, parathyroid glands, and neuroendocrine tumors (NETs) of the pancreas. This makes them appear to have MEN 1, but they have no mutation in the *menin* gene. They also appear to be prone to adrenal tumors, renal tumors, testicular cancer, and neuroendocrine cervical carcinoma.

OTHER SYNDROMES OF MULTIPLE ENDOCRINE NEOPLASIA

Patients with **Carney complex** develop tumors in the adrenal cortex, pituitary, thyroid, and gonads as well as cardiac myxomas and hyperpigmentation. Patients with **Cowden disease** develop thyroid abnormalities (66%) such as benign adenomas and follicular adenocarcinomas, along with breast cancer (20–36% in women), and multiple hamartomas that affect the skin and multiple other organs. Patients with **McCune-Albright syndrome** may develop precocious puberty (particularly girls) due to gonadal hypersecretion, Cushing syndrome caused by multiple adrenal nodules, hyperthyroidism from hypersecretory thyroid nodules, and acromegaly caused by GH-secreting pituitary tumors. Patients have fibrous dysplasia of bones and hypophosphatemia, with bone fractures being common. Sudden death has been reported.

Delemer B. MEN1 and pituitary adenomas. Ann Endocrinol (Paris). 2012 Apr;73(2):59–61. [PMID: 22542456]

Gaztambide S et al. Diagnosis and treatment of multiple endocrine neoplasia type 1 (MEN1). Minerva Endocrinol. 2013 Mar;38(1):17–28. [PMID: 23435440]

Gulati AP et al. Treatment of multiple endocrine neoplasia 1/2 tumors: case report and review of the literature. Oncology. 2013;84(3):127–34. [PMID: 23235517]

Moline J et al. Multiple endocrine neoplasia type 2: an overview. Genet Med. 2011 Sep;13(9):755–64. [PMID: 21552134]

Schreinemakers JM et al. The optimal surgical treatment for primary hyperparathyroidism in MEN1 patients: a systematic review. World J Surg. 2011 Sep;35(9):1993–2005. [PMID: 21713580]

Thakker RV et al; Endocrine Society. Clinical practice guidelines for multiple endocrine neoplasia type 1 (MEN 1). J Clin Endocrinol Metab. 2012 Sep;97(9):2990–3011. [PMID: 22723327]

Thakker RV. Multiple endocrine neoplasia type 1 (MEN 1) and type 4 (MEN 4). Mol Cell Endocrinol. 2014 Apr 5;386 (1–2):2–15. [PMID: 23933118]

CLINICAL USE OF CORTICOSTEROIDS

▶ Mechanisms of Action

Cortisol is a steroid hormone that is normally secreted by the adrenal cortex in response to ACTH. It exerts its action by binding to nuclear receptors, which then act upon chromatin to regulate gene expression, producing effects throughout the body.

▶ Relative Potencies (Table 26–18)

Hydrocortisone and cortisone acetate, like cortisol, have mineralocorticoid effects that become excessive at higher doses. Other synthetic corticosteroids such as prednisone, dexamethasone, and deflazacort (an oxazoline derivative of prednisolone) have minimal mineralocorticoid activity. Anticonvulsant drugs (eg, phenytoin, carbamazepine, phenobarbital) accelerate the metabolism of corticosteroids other than hydrocortisone, making them significantly less potent. Megestrol, a synthetic progestin, has slight corticosteroid activity that becomes significant when administered in high doses for appetite stimulation.

▶ Adverse Effects

Prolonged treatment with systemic high-dose corticosteroids causes a variety of adverse effects that can be life threatening. Patients should be thoroughly informed of the

Table 26–18. Systemic versus topical activity of corticosteroids.[1]

	Systemic Activity	Topical Activity
Prednisone	4–5	1–2
Triamcinolone	5	1
Triamcinolone acetonide	5	40
Dexamethasone	30–120	10
Betamethasone	30	5–10
Betamethasone valerate	—	50–150
Methylprednisolone	5	5
Fluocinolone acetonide	—	40–100
Flurandrenolide	—	20–50
Deflazacort	3–4	—

[1]Hydrocortisone = 1 in potency.

major possible side effects of treatment such as insomnia, cognitive and personality changes, weight gain with central obesity, bruising, striae, muscle weakness, polyuria, kidney stones, diabetes mellitus, glaucoma, cataracts, sex hormone suppression, candidiasis and opportunistic infections. High-dose corticosteroids have adverse cardiovascular effects, increasing the risk of hypertension, dyslipidemia, myocardial infarction, stroke, atrial fibrillation or flutter, and heart failure. Prolonged corticosteroid therapy for systemic inflammatory disorders commonly suppresses pituitary ACTH secretion, causing secondary adrenal insufficiency.

Bone fractures (especially spine and hip) ultimately occur in about 40% of patients receiving long-term corticosteroid therapy. Osteoporotic fractures can also occur in patients who receive extensive topical, inhaled, or intermittent oral corticosteroids (eg, prednisone ≥ 10 mg daily and cumulative dose > 1 g). Osteoporotic fractures can occur even in patients receiving long-term corticosteroid therapy at relatively low doses (eg, 5–7.5 mg prednisone daily). Patients at increased risk for corticosteroid osteoporotic fractures include those who are over age 60 or who have a low body mass index, pretreatment osteoporosis, a family history of osteoporosis, or concurrent disease that limits mobility. Avascular necrosis of bone (especially hips) develops in about 15% of patients who receive corticosteroids at high doses (eg, prednisone ≥ 15 mg daily) for more than 1 month with cumulative prednisone doses of ≥ 10 g.

Bisphosphonates (eg, alendronate, 70 mg orally weekly) prevent the development of osteoporosis among patients receiving prolonged courses of corticosteroids. For patients who are unable to tolerate oral bisphosphonates (due to esophagitis, hiatal hernia, or gastritis), periodic intravenous infusions of pamidronate, 60–90 mg, or zoledronic acid, 2–4 mg, should also be effective. Teriparatide, 20 mcg subcutaneously daily for up to 2 years, is also effective against corticosteroid-induced osteoporosis.

Table 26–19. Management of patients receiving systemic corticosteroids.

Recommendations for prescribing
- Do not administer corticosteroids unless absolutely indicated or more conservative measures have failed.
- Keep dosage and duration of administration to the minimum required for adequate treatment.

Monitoring recommendations
- Screen for tuberculosis with a purified protein derivative (PPD) test or chest radiograph before commencing long-term corticosteroid therapy.
- Screen for diabetes mellitus before treatment and at each clinician visit.
  - Have patient test urine weekly for glucose.
  - Teach patient about the symptoms of hyperglycemia.
- Screen for hypertension before treatment and at each clinician visit.
- Screen for glaucoma and cataracts before treatment, 3 months after treatment inception, and then at least yearly.
- Monitor plasma potassium for hypokalemia and treat as indicated.
- Obtain bone densitometry before treatment and then periodically. Treat osteoporosis.
- Weigh daily. Use dietary measures to avoid obesity and optimize nutrition.
- Measure height frequently to document the degree of axial spine demineralization and compression.
- Watch for fungal or yeast infections of skin, nails, mouth, vagina, and rectum, and treat appropriately.
- With dosage reduction, watch for signs of adrenal insufficiency or corticosteroid withdrawal syndrome.

Patient information
- Prepare the patient and family for possible adverse effects on mood, memory, and cognitive function.
- Inform the patient about other possible side effects, particularly weight gain, osteoporosis, and aseptic necrosis of bone.
- Counsel to avoid smoking and excessive ethanol consumption.

Prophylactic measures
- Institute a vigorous physical exercise and isometric regimen tailored to each patient's disabilities.
- Administer calcium (1 g elemental calcium) and vitamin D$_3$, 400–800 international units orally daily.
  - Check spot morning urines for calcium; alter dosage to keep urine calcium concentration < 30 mg/dL (< 7.5 mmol/L).
  - If the patient is receiving thiazide diuretics, check for hypercalcemia, and administer only 500 mg elemental calcium daily.
  - Consider a bisphosphonate such as alendronate (70 mg orally weekly) or periodic intravenous infusions of pamidronate or zoledronic acid.
- Avoid prolonged bed rest that will accelerate muscle weakness and bone mineral loss. Ambulate early after fractures.
- Avoid elective surgery, if possible. Vitamin A in a daily dose of 20,000 units orally for 1 week may improve wound healing, but it is not prescribed in pregnancy.
- Avoid activities that could cause falls or other trauma.
- For ulcer prophylaxis, if administering corticosteroids with nonsteroidals, prescribe a proton pump inhibitor (not required for corticosteroids alone). Avoid large doses of antacids containing aluminum hydroxide (many popular brands) because aluminum hydroxide binds phosphate and may cause a hypophosphatemic osteomalacia that can compound corticosteroid osteoporosis.
- Treat hypogonadism.
- Treat infections aggressively. Consider unusual pathogens.
- Treat edema as indicated.

(See Osteoporosis section.) It is wise to follow an organized treatment plan such as the one outlined in Table 26–19.

Hansen KE et al. Uncertainties in the prevention and treatment of glucocorticoid-induced osteoporosis. J Bone Miner Res. 2011 Sep;26(9):1989–96. [PMID: 21721042]

Lansang MC et al. Glucocorticoid-induced diabetes and adrenal suppression: how to detect and manage them. Cleve Clin J Med. 2011 Nov;78(11):748–56. [PMID: 22049542]

Rizzoli R et al. Management of glucocorticoid-induced osteoporosis. Calcif Tissue Int. 2012 Oct;91(4):225–43. [PMID: 22878667]

Sacre K et al. Pituitary-adrenal function after prolonged glucocorticoid therapy for systemic inflammatory disorders: an observational study. J Clin Endocrinol Metab. 2013 Aug;98: 3199–205. [PMID: 23760625]

Strohmayer EA et al. Glucocorticoids and cardiovascular risk factors. Endocrinol Metab Clin North Am. 2011 Jun;40(2): 409–17. [PMID: 21565675]

Tatsuno I et al. Glucocorticoid-induced diabetes mellitus is a risk for vertebral fracture during glucocorticoid treatment. Diabetes Res Clin Pract. 2011 Jul;93(1):e18–20. [PMID: 21440321]

Weinstein RS. Glucocorticoid-induced osteonecrosis. Endocrine. 2012 Apr;41(2):183–90. [PMID: 22169965]

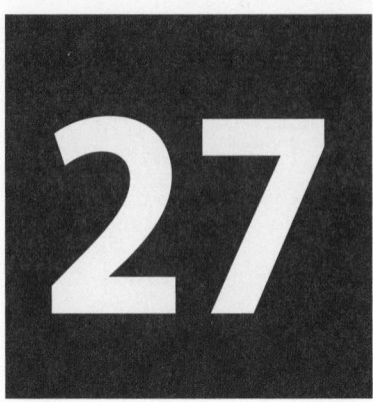

Diabetes Mellitus & Hypoglycemia

Umesh Masharani, MB, BS, MRCP(UK)

DIABETES MELLITUS

ESSENTIALS OF DIAGNOSIS

Type 1 diabetes

▶ Polyuria, polydipsia, and weight loss associated with random plasma glucose ≥ 200 mg/dL (11.1 mmol/L).

▶ Plasma glucose of ≥ 126 mg/dL (7.0 mmol/L) after an overnight fast, documented on more than one occasion.

▶ Ketonemia, ketonuria, or both.

▶ Islet autoantibodies are frequently present.

Type 2 diabetes

▶ Most patients are over 40 years of age and obese.

▶ Polyuria and polydipsia. Ketonuria and weight loss generally are uncommon at time of diagnosis. Candidal vaginitis in women may be an initial manifestation. Many patients have few or no symptoms.

▶ Plasma glucose of ≥ 126 mg/dL after an overnight fast on more than one occasion. Two hours after 75 g oral glucose, diagnostic values are ≥ 200 mg/dL (11.1 mmol).

▶ HbA$_{1c}$ ≥ 6.5%

▶ Hypertension, dyslipidemia, and atherosclerosis are often associated.

▶ Epidemiologic Considerations

The latest data estimate 25.8 million people (8.3%) in the United States had diabetes mellitus, of which approximately 1 million have type 1 diabetes and most of the rest have type 2 diabetes. A third group that was designated as "other specific types" by the American Diabetes Association (ADA) (Table 27–1) number only in the thousands. Among these are the rare monogenic defects of either B cell function or of insulin action, primary diseases of the exocrine pancreas, endocrinopathies, and medication-induced diabetes. Updated information about the prevalence of diabetes in the United States is available from the Centers for Disease Control and Prevention (http://www.cdc.gov/diabetes/pubs/estimates.htm#prev).

▶ Classification & Pathogenesis

Diabetes mellitus is a syndrome with disordered metabolism and inappropriate hyperglycemia due to either a deficiency of insulin secretion or to a combination of insulin resistance and inadequate insulin secretion to compensate for the resistance.

A. Type 1 Diabetes Mellitus

This form of diabetes is due to pancreatic islet B cell destruction predominantly by an autoimmune process in over 95% of cases (type 1A) and idiopathic in < 5% (type 1B). The rate of pancreatic B cell destruction is quite variable, being rapid in some individuals and slow in others. Type 1 diabetes is usually associated with ketosis in its untreated state. It occurs at any age but most commonly arises in children and young adults with a peak incidence before school age and again at around puberty. It is a catabolic disorder in which circulating insulin is virtually absent, plasma glucagon is elevated, and the pancreatic B cells fail to respond to all insulinogenic stimuli. Exogenous insulin is therefore required to reverse the catabolic state, prevent ketosis, reduce the hyperglucagonemia, and reduce blood glucose.

1. Immune-mediated type 1 diabetes mellitus (type 1A)—The highest incidence of immune-mediated type 1 diabetes mellitus is in Scandinavia and northern Europe, where the annual incidence is as high as 40 per 100,000 children aged 14 years or younger in Finland, 31 per 100,000 in Sweden, 22 per 100,000 in Norway, and 20 per 100,000 in England. The annual incidence of type 1 diabetes decreases across the rest of Europe to 11 per 100,000 in Greece and 9 per 100,000 in France. Surprisingly, the island of Sardinia has as high an annual incidence as Finland (40 per 100,000) even though in the rest of Italy, including the island of Sicily, it is only 11 per 100,000 per year. In the

Table 27–1. Other specific types of diabetes mellitus.

Genetic defects of pancreatic B cell function
MODY 1 (HNF-4alpha); rare
MODY 2 (glucokinase); less rare
MODY 3 (HNF-1alpha); accounts for two-thirds of all MODY
MODY 4 (PDX1); very rare
MODY 5 (HNF-1beta); very rare
MODY 6 (neuroD1); very rare
Mitochondrial DNA
Genetic defects in insulin action
Type A insulin resistance
Leprechaunism
Rabson-Mendenhall syndrome
Lipoatrophic diabetes
Diseases of the exocrine pancreas
Endocrinopathies
Drug- or chemical-induced diabetes
Other genetic syndromes (Down, Klinefelter, Turner, others)
sometimes associated with diabetes

MODY, maturity-onset diabetes of the young.

Table 27–2. Diagnostic sensitivity and specificity of autoimmune markers in patients with newly diagnosed type 1 diabetes mellitus.

	Sensitivity	Specificity
ICA antibody	44–100%	96%
Glutamic acid decarboxylase (GAD65)	70–90%	99%
Insulin (IAA)	40–70%	99%
Tyrosine phosphatase (IA-2)	50–70%	99%
Zinc transporter 8 (ZnT8)	50–70%	99%

United States, the annual incidence of type 1 diabetes averages 16 per 100,000, with higher rates in states more densely populated with persons of Scandinavian descent such as Minnesota. Worldwide, the lowest incidence of type 1 diabetes (< 1 case per 100,000 per year) is in China and parts of South America. The global incidence of type 1 diabetes is increasing (approximately 3% each year). In Europe, the highest annual incidence increase was seen in low prevalence countries in Eastern Europe, especially Romania and Poland. Changes in environmental factors most likely explain this increased incidence.

Approximately one-third of the disease susceptibility is due to genes and two-thirds to environmental factors. Genes that are related to the HLA locus contribute about 40% of the genetic risk. About 95% of patients with type 1 diabetes possess either HLA-DR3 or HLA-DR4, compared with 45–50% of white controls. *HLA-DQ* genes are even more specific markers of type 1 susceptibility, since a particular variety *(HLA-DQB1*0302)* is found in the DR4 patients with type 1, while a "protective" gene *(HLA-DQB1*0602)* is often present in the DR4 controls. The other important gene that contributes to about 10% of the genetic risk is found at the 5′ polymorphic region of the insulin gene. This polymorphic region affects the expression of the insulin gene in the thymus and results in depletion of insulin-specific T lymphocytes. In linkage studies, 16 other genetic regions of the human genome have been identified as being important to pathogenesis. Many of the genes linked to these additional loci play important roles in the function and regulation of the immune response. Mutations in genes associated with T cell tolerance can also cause autoimmune diabetes. The autoimmune regulatory gene *(AIRE)* product regulates the expression of several proteins in the thymus causing the deletion of self-reactive T cells. Type 1 diabetes mellitus as well as other autoimmune disorders (autoimmune polyglandular syndrome 1) develop in 20% of individuals with homozygote mutations in *AIRE.FOXP3*, an X chromosome gene, encodes a

transcription factor required for the formation of regulatory T cells. Mutations in *FOXP3* lead to very early type 1 diabetes mellitus and other autoimmune endocrinopathies (immunodysregulation polyendocrinopathy enteropathy X-linked [IPEX] syndrome). Most patients with type 1 diabetes mellitus have circulating antibodies to islet cells (ICA), glutamic acid decarboxylase 65 (GAD65), insulin (IAA), tyrosine phosphatase IA2 (ICA-512), and zinc transporter 8 (ZnT8) at the time the diagnosis is made (Table 27–2). These antibodies facilitate screening for an autoimmune cause of diabetes, particularly screening siblings of affected children, as well as adults with atypical features of type 2 diabetes mellitus. Screening with GAD65, ICA-512, IAA, and ZnT8 autoantibodies may identify about 98% of people who have an autoimmune basis for their beta cell loss. Antibody levels decline with increasing duration of disease. Also, low levels of anti-insulin antibodies develop in almost all patients once they are treated with insulin.

Family members of diabetic probands are at increased lifetime risk for developing type 1 diabetes mellitus. A child whose mother has type 1 diabetes has a 3% risk of developing the disease and a 6% risk if the child's father has it. The risk in siblings is related to the number of HLA haplotypes that the sibling shares with the diabetic proband. If one haplotype is shared, the risk is 6% and if two haplotypes are shared, the risk increases to 12–25%. The highest risk is for identical twins, where the concordance rate is 25–50%.

Some patients with a milder expression of type 1 diabetes mellitus initially retain enough B cell function to avoid ketosis, but as their B cell mass diminishes later in life, dependence on insulin therapy develops. Islet cell antibody surveys among northern Europeans indicate that up to 15% of "type 2" diabetic patients may actually have this mild form of type 1 diabetes (latent autoimmune diabetes of adulthood; LADA). Evidence for environmental factors playing a role in the development of type 1 diabetes include the observation that the disease is more common in Scandinavian countries and becomes progressively less frequent in countries nearer and nearer to the equator. Also, the risk for type 1 diabetes increases when individuals who normally have a low risk emigrate to the Northern Hemisphere. For example, Pakistani children born and raised in Bradford,

England have a higher risk for developing type 1 diabetes compared with children who lived in Pakistan all their lives.

Which environmental factor is responsible for the increased risk is not known. There have been a number of different hypotheses including infections with certain viruses (mumps, rubella, Coxsackie B4) and consumption of cow's milk. Also, in developed countries, childhood infections have become less frequent and so perhaps the immune system becomes dysregulated with development of autoimmunity and conditions such as asthma and diabetes. This theory is referred to as the **hygiene hypothesis**. Part of the difficulty in determining the causative environmental factor is that autoimmune injury is initiated many years before the clinical presentation of diabetes.

2. Idiopathic type 1 diabetes mellitus (type 1B)—Approximately 5% of subjects have no evidence of pancreatic B cell autoimmunity to explain their insulinopenia and ketoacidosis. This subgroup has been classified as "idiopathic type 1 diabetes" and designated as "type 1B." Although only a minority of patients with type 1 diabetes fall into this group, most of these individuals are of Asian or African origin. About 4% of the West Africans with ketosis-prone diabetes are homozygous for a mutation in *PAX-4* (*Arg133Trp*)—a transcription factor that is essential for the development of pancreatic islets.

B. Type 2 Diabetes Mellitus

This represents a heterogeneous group of conditions that used to occur predominantly in adults, but it is now more frequently encountered in children and adolescents. More than 90% of all diabetic persons in the United States are included under this classification. Circulating endogenous insulin is sufficient to prevent ketoacidosis but is inadequate to prevent hyperglycemia in the face of increased needs owing to tissue insensitivity (insulin resistance).

Genetic and environmental factors combine to cause both the insulin resistance and the beta cell loss. Most epidemiologic data indicate strong genetic influences, since in monozygotic twins over 40 years of age, concordance develops in over 70% of cases within a year whenever type 2 diabetes develops in one twin. Genome-wide association studies have made considerable progress in identifying the at-risk genes. So far, more than 30 genetic loci have been associated with an increased risk of type 2 diabetes. A significant number of the identified loci appear to code for proteins that have a role in beta cell function or development. One of the genetic loci with the largest risk effect is *TCF7L2*. This gene codes for a transcription factor involved in the WNT signaling pathway that is required for normal pancreatic development. Alleles at other genetic loci (*CDKAL1, SLC30A8, HHEX-IDE, CDKN2A/B, KCNJ11,* and *IGF2BP2*) are thought to affect insulin secretion. Two loci (*FTO* and *MC4R*) affect fat mass and obesity risk. The *PPARG* locus has been implicated in insulin resistance. The loci identified to date still explain only some of the heritable risk for diabetes; clearly, other loci remain to be discovered.

Early in the disease process, hyperplasia of pancreatic B cells occurs and probably accounts for the fasting hyperinsulinism and exaggerated insulin and proinsulin responses to glucose and other stimuli. With time, chronic deposition of amyloid in the islets may combine with inherited genetic defects progressively to impair B cell function.

Obesity is the most important environmental factor causing insulin resistance. The degree and prevalence of obesity varies among different racial groups with type 2 diabetes. While obesity is apparent in no more than 30% of Chinese and Japanese patients with type 2, it is found in 60–70% of North Americans, Europeans, or Africans with type 2 and approaches 100% of patients with type 2 among Pima Indians or Pacific Islanders from Nauru or Samoa.

Visceral obesity, due to accumulation of fat in the omental and mesenteric regions, correlates with insulin resistance; subcutaneous abdominal fat seems to have less of an association with insulin insensitivity. There are many patients with type 2 diabetes who, while not overtly obese, have increased visceral fat; they are termed the "metabolically obese." Exercise may affect the deposition of visceral fat as suggested by CT scans of Japanese wrestlers, whose extreme obesity is predominantly subcutaneous. Their daily vigorous exercise program prevents accumulation of visceral fat, and they have normal serum lipids and euglycemia despite daily intakes of 5000–7000 kcal and development of massive subcutaneous obesity.

A number of mechanisms may operate to cause the insulin resistance associated with obesity. Free fatty acid levels are increased in obesity, and their oxidation by skeletal muscle leads to a decrease in insulin-mediated glucose disposal, that is, insulin resistance. Adipocytes secrete molecules (adipokines) that can affect insulin signaling. Examples include adiponectin, which enhances insulin action, and resistin, which impairs insulin action; abnormal levels of these types of molecules in obesity may contribute to the development of resistance. Macrophages and other immune cells in adipose tissue are activated in response to an increase in adipocyte lipid stores. They release a variety of molecules, including tissue necrosis factor alpha and interleukin-6, that impair insulin signaling.

Hyperglycemia per se can impair insulin action by causing accumulation of hexosamines in muscle and fat tissue and by inhibiting glucose transport (acquired glucose toxicity). Correction of hyperglycemia reverses this acquired insulin resistance.

C. Other Specific Types of Diabetes Mellitus

1. Maturity-onset diabetes of the young (MODY)—This subgroup is a relatively rare monogenic disorder characterized by non–insulin-dependent diabetes with **autosomal dominant inheritance** and an age at onset of 25 years or younger. Patients are nonobese, and their hyperglycemia is due to impaired glucose-induced secretion of insulin. Six types of MODY have been described (Table 27–1). Except for MODY 2, in which a glucokinase gene is defective, all other types involve mutations of a nuclear transcription factor that regulates islet gene expression.

The enzyme glucokinase is a rate-limiting step in glycolysis and determines the rate of adenosine triphosphate (ATP) production from glucose and the insulin secretory response in the beta cell. MODY 2, due to glucokinase mutations, is usually quite mild, associated with only slight fasting hyperglycemia and few if any microvascular diabetic complications. It generally responds well to hygienic measures or low doses of oral hypoglycemic agents. MODY 3, due to mutations in hepatic nuclear factor 1 alpha is the most common form, accounting for two-thirds of all MODY cases. The clinical course is of progressive beta cell failure and need for insulin therapy. Mutations in both alleles of glucokinase present with more severe neonatal diabetes. Mutation in one allele of the pancreatic duodenal homeobox 1 (PDX1) causes diabetes usually at a later age (~ 35 years) than other forms of MODY; mutations in both alleles of PDX1 causes pancreatic agenesis.

2. Diabetes due to mutant insulins—This is a very rare subtype of nonobese type 2 diabetes, with no more than ten families having been described. Since affected individuals were heterozygous and possessed one normal insulin gene, diabetes was mild, did not appear until middle age, and showed autosomal dominant genetic transmission. There is generally no evidence of clinical insulin resistance, and these patients respond well to standard therapy.

3. Diabetes due to mutant insulin receptors—Defects in one of their insulin receptor genes have been found in more than 40 people with diabetes, and most have extreme insulin resistance associated with acanthosis nigricans (Figures 27–1 and 27–2). In very rare instances when both insulin receptor genes are abnormal, newborns present with a leprechaun-like phenotype and seldom live through infancy.

4. Diabetes mellitus associated with a mutation of mitochondrial DNA—Since sperm do not contain mitochondria, only the mother transmits mitochondrial genes to her offspring. Diabetes due to mutations of mitochondrial DNA occurs in < 2% of patients with diabetes. The most common cause is the A3243G mutation in the gene coding for the tRNA (Leu,UUR). Diabetes occurs even when a

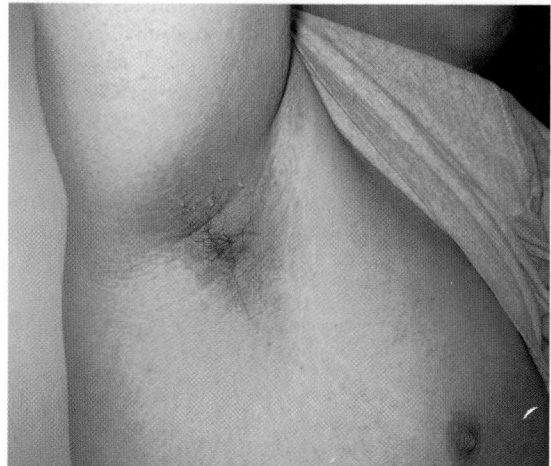

▲ **Figure 27–1.** Acanthosis nigricans of the axilla, with typical dark coloration and velvety appearance and texture. (Used with permission from Umesh Masharani, MB, BS, MRCP(UK).)

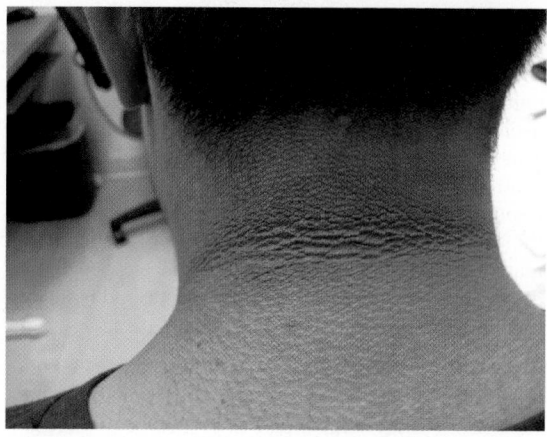

▲ **Figure 27–2.** Acanthosis nigricans of the nape of the neck, with typical dark and velvety appearance. (Used with permission from Umesh Masharani, MB, BS, MRCP(UK).)

small percentage of the mitochondria in the cell carry the mutation; the heteroplasmy levels in the leukocytes range from 1% to 40%. Diabetes usually develops in these patients in their late 30s, and characteristically, they also have hearing loss (maternally inherited diabetes and deafness [MIDD]). In some patients, the beta cell failure can be rapidly progressive and patients require insulin soon after diagnosis. Other patients can be managed by diet or oral agents for a while but most eventually require insulin. MIDD patients are not usually overweight; they resemble patients with type 1 diabetes mellitus but without evidence for autoimmunity.

5. Wolfram syndrome—Wolfram syndrome is an autosomal recessive neurodegenerative disorder first evident in childhood. It consists of diabetes insipidus, diabetes mellitus, optic atrophy, and deafness, hence the acronym DIDMOAD. It is due to mutations in a gene named *WFS1*, which encodes a 100.3 KDa transmembrane protein localized in the endoplasmic reticulum. The *WFS1* protein forms part of the unfolding protein response and helps protect the beta cells from endoplasmic reticulum stress and apoptosis especially during periods of high insulin demand. Diabetes develops in mice with mutated form of this protein; and isolated islets from these mice show impairment in insulin secretion to glucose stimulus and increased apoptosis. The diabetes mellitus usually presents in the first decade together with the optic atrophy. Cranial diabetes insipidus and sensorineural deafness develop during the second decade in 60–75% of patients. Ureterohydronephrosis, neurogenic bladder, cerebellar ataxia, peripheral neuropathy, and psychiatric illness develop later in many patients.

6. Autosomal recessive syndromes—Homozygous mutations in a number of pancreatic transcription factors, *NEUROG3*, *PTF1A*, *RFX6*, and *GLI-similar 3 (GLIS3)*, cause neonatal or childhood diabetes. Homozygous *PTF1A* mutations result in absent pancreas and cerebellar atrophy; *NEUROG3* mutations cause severe malabsorption and diabetes before puberty. Homozygous mutations in *RFX6* cause the Mitchell-Riley syndrome characterized by absence of all islet cell types apart from pancreatic poly-peptide cells, hypoplasia of the pancreas and gallbladder, and intestinal atresia. *GLIS3* gene plays a role in transcription of insulin gene, and homozygous mutations cause neonatal diabetes and congenital hypothyroidism. The gene *EIF2AK3* encodes PKR-like ER kinase (PERK), which controls one of the pathways of the unfolded protein response. Absence of PERK leads to inadequate response to ER stress and accelerated beta cell apoptosis. Patients with mutation in this gene have neonatal diabetes, epiphyseal dysplasia, developmental delay, and hepatic and renal dysfunction (Wolcott-Rallison syndrome).

7. Diabetes mellitus secondary to other causes—Endocrine tumors secreting growth hormone, glucocorticoids, catecholamines, glucagon, or somatostatin can cause glucose intolerance (Table 27–3). In the first four of these situations, peripheral responsiveness to insulin is impaired. With excess of glucocorticoids, catecholamines, or glucagon, increased hepatic output of glucose is a contributory factor; in the case of catecholamines, decreased insulin release is an additional factor in producing carbohydrate intolerance, and with somatostatin, inhibition of insulin secretion is the major factor. Diabetes mainly occurs in individuals with underlying defects in insulin secretion, and hyperglycemia typically resolves when the hormone excess is resolved.

High-titer anti-insulin receptor antibodies that inhibit insulin binding causes a clinical syndrome characterized by severe insulin resistance, glucose intolerance or diabetes mellitus, and acanthosis nigricans. These patients usually have other autoimmune disorders. There are reports of spontaneous remission or remission with cytotoxic therapy.

Many medications are associated with carbohydrate intolerance or frank diabetes (Table 27–3). The medications act by decreasing insulin secretion or by increasing insulin resistance or both. Cyclosporine and tacrolimus impair insulin secretion; sirolimus principally increases insulin resistance. These agents contribute to the development of new-onset diabetes after transplantation. Corticosteroids increase insulin resistance but may also have an effect on beta cell function; in a case control study and a large population cohort study, oral corticosteroids doubled the risk for development of diabetes. Thiazide diuretics and beta-blockers modestly increase the risk for diabetes. Treating the hypokalemia due to thiazides may reverse the hyperglycemia. Atypical antipsychotics, particularly olanzapine and clozapine, have been associated with increased risk of glucose intolerance. These medications cause weight gain and insulin resistance but may also impair beta cell function; an increase in rates of diabetic ketoacidosis has been reported.

Chronic pancreatitis or subtotal pancreatectomy reduces the number of functioning B cells and can result in a metabolic derangement very similar to that of genetic type 1 diabetes except that a concomitant reduction in pancreatic A cells may reduce glucagon secretion so that relatively lower doses of insulin replacement are needed.

▶ **Insulin Resistance Syndrome (Syndrome X; Metabolic Syndrome)**

Twenty-five percent of the general nonobese, nondiabetic population has insulin resistance of a magnitude similar to that seen in type 2 diabetes. These insulin-resistant non-diabetic individuals are at much higher risk for developing type 2 diabetes than insulin-sensitive persons. In addition to diabetes, these individuals have increased risk for elevated plasma triglycerides, lower high-density lipoproteins (HDLs), and higher blood pressure—a cluster of abnormalities termed **syndrome X or metabolic syndrome**. These associations have now been expanded to include small, dense, low-density lipoprotein (LDL), hyperuricemia, abdominal obesity, prothrombotic state with increased levels of plasminogen activator inhibitor type 1 (PAI-1), and proinflammatory state. These clusters of abnormalities significantly increase the risk of atherosclerotic disease.

It has been postulated that hyperinsulinemia and insulin resistance play a direct role in these metabolic abnormalities, but supportive evidence is inconclusive. Although hyperinsulinism and hypertension often coexist in whites, that is not the case in blacks or Pima Indians. Moreover, patients with hyperinsulinism due to insulinoma are not hypertensive, and there is no fall in blood pressure after surgical removal of the insulinoma restores normal insulin levels. The main value of grouping these disorders as a syndrome, however, is to remind clinicians that the therapeutic goals are not only to correct hyperglycemia but also to manage the elevated blood pressure and dyslipidemia that result in increased cerebrovascular and cardiac morbidity and mortality in these patients.

American Diabetes Association. Diagnosis and classification of diabetes mellitus. Diabetes Care. 2014 Jan;37(Suppl 1):S81–4. [PMID: 24357215]

Table 27–3. Secondary causes of hyperglycemia.

Hyperglycemia due to tissue insensitivity to insulin
Hormonal tumors (acromegaly, Cushing syndrome, glucagonoma, pheochromocytoma)
Pharmacologic agents (corticosteroids, sympathomimetic drugs, niacin,)
Liver disease (cirrhosis, hemochromatosis)
Muscle disorders (myotonic dystrophy)
Adipose tissue disorders (lipodystrophy, truncal obesity)
Insulin receptor disorders (acanthosis nigricans syndromes, leprechaunism)
Hyperglycemia due to reduced insulin secretion
Hormonal tumors (somatostatinoma, pheochromocytoma)
Pancreatic disorders (pancreatitis, hemosiderosis, hemochromatosis)
Pharmacologic agents (thiazide diuretics, phenytoin, pentamidine, calcineurin inhibitors)

▶ **Clinical Findings**

A. Symptoms and Signs

1. Type 1 diabetes—A characteristic symptom complex of hyperosmolality and hyperketonemia from the accumulation of circulating glucose and fatty acids typically presents in patients with type 1 diabetes who have an absolute deficiency of insulin. Increased urination and thirst are consequences of osmotic diuresis secondary to sustained hyperglycemia. The diuresis results in a loss of glucose as well as free water and electrolytes in the urine. Blurred vision often develops as the lenses are exposed to hyperosmolar fluids.

Weight loss despite normal or increased appetite is a common feature of type 1 when it develops subacutely. The weight loss is initially due to depletion of water, glycogen, and triglycerides; thereafter, reduced muscle mass occurs as amino acids are diverted to form glucose and ketone bodies.

Lowered plasma volume produces symptoms of postural hypotension. Total body potassium loss and the general catabolism of muscle protein contribute to the weakness.

Paresthesias may be present at the time of diagnosis, particularly when the onset is subacute. They reflect a temporary dysfunction of peripheral sensory nerves, which clears as insulin replacement restores glycemic levels closer to normal, suggesting neurotoxicity from sustained hyperglycemia.

When absolute insulin deficiency is of acute onset, the above symptoms develop abruptly. Ketoacidosis exacerbates the dehydration and hyperosmolality by producing anorexia and nausea and vomiting, interfering with oral fluid replacement.

The patient's level of consciousness can vary depending on the degree of hyperosmolality. When insulin deficiency develops relatively slowly and sufficient water intake is maintained, patients remain relatively alert and physical findings may be minimal. When vomiting occurs in response to worsening ketoacidosis, dehydration progresses and compensatory mechanisms become inadequate to keep serum osmolality below 320–330 mosm/L. Under these circumstances, stupor or even coma may occur. The fruity breath odor of acetone further suggests the diagnosis of diabetic ketoacidosis.

Hypotension in the recumbent position is a serious prognostic sign. Loss of subcutaneous fat and muscle wasting are features of more slowly developing insulin deficiency. In occasional patients with slow, insidious onset of insulin deficiency, subcutaneous fat may be considerably depleted.

2. Type 2 diabetes—While increased urination and thirst may be presenting symptoms in some patients with type 2 diabetes, many other patients have an insidious onset of hyperglycemia and are asymptomatic initially. This is particularly true in obese patients, whose diabetes may be detected only after glycosuria or hyperglycemia is noted during routine laboratory studies. Occasionally, when the disease has been occult for some time, patients with type 2 diabetes may have evidence of neuropathic or cardiovascular complications at the time of presentation. Chronic skin infections are common. Generalized pruritus and symptoms of vaginitis are frequently the initial complaints of women. Diabetes should be suspected in women with chronic candidal vulvovaginitis as well as in those who have delivered large babies (> 9 lb, or 4.1 kg) or have had polyhydramnios, preeclampsia, or unexplained fetal losses.

Balanoposthitis (inflammation of the foreskin and glans in uncircumcised males) may occur.

Many patients with type 2 diabetes are overweight or obese. Even those who are not significantly obese often have characteristic localization of fat deposits on the upper segment of the body (particularly the abdomen, chest, neck, and face) and relatively less fat on the appendages, which may be quite muscular. This centripetal fat distribution is characterized by a high waist circumference; a waist circumference > 40 inches (102 cm) in men and 35 inches (88 cm) in women is associated with an increased risk of diabetes. Some patients may have acanthosis nigricans, which is associated with significant insulin resistance; the skin in the axilla, groin, and back of neck is hyperpigmented and hyperkeratotic (Figures 27–1 and 27–2). Mild hypertension is often present in obese diabetics. Eruptive xanthomas on the flexor surface of the limbs and on the buttocks and lipemia retinalis due to hyperchylomicronemia can occur in patients with uncontrolled type 2 diabetes who also have a familial form of hypertriglyceridemia.

Hyperglycemic hyperosmolar coma can also be present; in these cases, patients are profoundly dehydrated, hypotensive, lethargic or comatose but without Kussmaul respirations.

B. Laboratory Findings

1. Urine glucose—A specific and convenient method to detect glucosuria is the paper strip impregnated with glucose oxidase and a chromogen system (Clinistix, Diastix), which is sensitive to as little as 100 mg/dL (5.5 mmol) glucose in urine. Diastix can be directly applied to the urinary stream, and differing color responses of the indicator strip reflect glucose concentration.

A normal renal threshold for glucose as well as reliable bladder emptying is essential for interpretation.

Nondiabetic glycosuria (renal glycosuria) is a benign asymptomatic condition wherein glucose appears in the urine despite a normal amount of glucose in the blood, either basally or during a glucose tolerance test. Its cause may vary from mutations in the *SGLT2* gene coding for sodium-glucose transporter 2 (familial renal glycosuria) to one associated with dysfunction of the proximal renal tubule (Fanconi syndrome, chronic kidney disease), or it may merely be a consequence of the increased load of glucose presented to the tubules by the elevated glomerular filtration rate during pregnancy. As many as 50% of pregnant women normally have demonstrable sugar in the urine, especially during the third and fourth months. This sugar is practically always glucose except during the late weeks of pregnancy, when lactose may be present.

2. Urine and blood ketones—Qualitative detection of ketone bodies can be accomplished by nitroprusside tests (Acetest or Ketostix). Although these tests do not detect beta-hydroxybutyric acid, which lacks a ketone group, the semiquantitative estimation of ketonuria thus obtained is nonetheless usually adequate for clinical purposes. Many laboratories measure beta-hydroxybutyric acid, and there are meters available (Precision Xtra; Nova Max Plus) for patient use that measures beta-hydroxybutyric acid levels in capillary glucose samples. Beta-hydroxybutyrate levels > 0.6 mmol/L require evaluation. Patients with levels > 3.0 mmol/L, equivalent to very large urinary ketones, require hospitalization.

3. Plasma or serum glucose—Plasma or serum from venous blood samples has the advantage over whole blood of providing values for glucose that are independent of hematocrit and that reflect the glucose concentration to which body tissues are exposed. Venous samples should be collected in tubes containing sodium fluoride to prevent glycolysis, placed on ice and the plasma separated from cells within 60 minutes. In the absence of fluoride, the rate of disappearance of glucose in presence of blood cells has been reported to be approximately 10 mg/dL/h (0.56 mmol/L). The glucose concentration is 10–15% higher in plasma or serum than in whole blood because structural components of blood cells are absent. A plasma glucose level of 126 mg/dL (7 mmol/L) or higher on more than one occasion after at least 8 hours of fasting is diagnostic of diabetes mellitus (Table 27–4). Fasting plasma glucose levels of 100–125 mg/dL (5.6 –6.9 mmol/L) are associated with increased risk of diabetes (impaired fasting glucose tolerance).

4. Oral glucose tolerance test—If the fasting plasma glucose level is < 126 mg/dL (7 mmol/L) when diabetes is nonetheless suspected, then a standardized oral glucose tolerance test may be done (Table 27–4). In order to optimize insulin secretion and effectiveness, especially when patients have been on a low-carbohydrate diet, a minimum of 150–200 g of carbohydrate per day should be included in the diet for 3 days preceding the test. The patient should eat nothing after midnight prior to the test day. On the morning of the test, adults are then given 75 g of glucose in 300 mL of water; children are given 1.75 g of glucose per kilogram of ideal body weight. The glucose load is consumed within 5 minutes. The test should be performed in the morning because there is some diurnal variation in oral glucose tolerance, and patients should not smoke or be active during the test.

Table 27–4. Criteria for the diagnosis of diabetes.

	Normal Glucose Tolerance	Impaired Glucose Tolerance	Diabetes Mellitus[2]
Fasting plasma glucose mg/dL(mmol/L)	< 100 (5.6)	100–125 (5.6-6.9)	≥ 126 (7.0)
Two hours after glucose load[1] mg/dL (mmol/L)	< 140 (7.8)	≥ 140–199 (7.8-11.0)	≥ 200 (11.1)
HbA$_{1c}$ (%)	< 5.7	5.7–6.4	≥ 6.5

[1]Give 75 g of glucose dissolved in 300 mL of water after an overnight fast in persons who have been receiving at least 150–200 g of carbohydrate daily for 3 days before the test.
[2]A fasting plasma glucose ≥ 126 mg/dL (7.0 mmol) or HbA$_{1c}$ of ≥ 6.5% is diagnostic of diabetes if confirmed by repeat testing.

Blood samples for plasma glucose are obtained at 0 and 120 minutes after ingestion of glucose. An oral glucose tolerance test is normal if the fasting venous plasma glucose value is < 100 mg/dL (5.6 mmol/L) and the 2-hour value falls below 140 mg/dL (7.8 mmol/L). A fasting value of 126 mg/dL (7 mmol/L) or higher or a 2-hour value of > 200 mg/dL (11.1 mmol/L) is diagnostic of diabetes mellitus. Patients with 2-hour value of 140–199 mg/dL (7.8–11.1 mmol/L) have impaired glucose tolerance. False-positive results may occur in patients who are malnourished, bedridden, or afflicted with an infection or severe emotional stress.

5. Glycated hemoglobin (hemoglobin A1) measurements—Hemoglobin becomes glycated by ketoamine reactions between glucose and other sugars and the free amino groups on the alpha and beta chains. Only glycation of the N-terminal valine of the beta chain imparts sufficient negative charge to the hemoglobin molecule to allow separation by charge dependent techniques. These charge separated hemoglobins are collectively referred to as hemoglobin A$_1$ (HbA$_1$). The major form of HbA$_1$ is hemoglobin A$_{1c}$ (HbA$_{1c}$) where glucose is the carbohydrate. HbA$_{1c}$ comprises 4–6% of total hemoglobin A$_1$. The remaining HbA$_1$ species contain fructose-1,6 diphosphate (HbA$_{1a1}$); glucose-6-phosphate (HbA$_{1a2}$); and unknown carbohydrate moiety (HbA$_{1b}$). The hemoglobin A$_{1c}$ fraction is abnormally elevated in diabetic persons with chronic hyperglycemia. Methods for measuring HbA$_{1c}$ include electrophoresis, cation-exchange chromatography, boronate affinity chromatography, and immunoassays. Office-based immunoassays using capillary blood give a result in about 9 minutes and this allows for nearly immediate feedback to the patients regarding their glycemic control.

Since glycohemoglobins circulate within red blood cells whose life span lasts up to 120 days, they generally reflect the state of glycemia over the preceding 8–12 weeks, thereby providing an improved method of assessing diabetic control. The HbA$_{1c}$ value, however, is weighted to more recent glucose levels (previous month) and this explains why significant changes in HbA$_{1c}$ are observed with short-term (1 month) changes in mean plasma glucose levels. Measurements should be made in patients with either type of diabetes mellitus at 3- to 4-month intervals. In patients monitoring their own blood glucose levels, HbA$_{1c}$ values provide a valuable check on the accuracy of monitoring. In patients who do not monitor their own blood glucose levels, HbA$_{1c}$ values are essential for adjusting therapy. There is a linear relationship between the HbA$_{1c}$ and the average glucose levels in the previous 3 months. In a study using a combination of intermittent seven-point capillary blood glucose profiles (preprandial, postprandial, and bedtime) and intermittent continuous glucose monitoring data, the change in glucose values was 28.7 mg/dL for every 1% change in HbA$_{1c}$. Substantial individual variability exists, however, between HbA$_{1c}$ and mean glucose concentration. For HbA$_{1c}$ values between 6.9% and 7.1%, the glucose levels ranged from 125 mg/dL to 205 mg/dL (6.9–11.4 mmol/L; 95% CIs). For HbA$_{1c}$ of 6%, the mean glucose levels ranged from 100 mg/dL to 152 mg/dL (5.5–8.5 mmol/L); and for 8% they ranged from

147 mg/dL to 217 mg/dL (8.1–12.1 mmol/L). For this reason, caution should be exercised in estimating average glucose levels from measured HbA_{1c}.

The accuracy of HbA_{1c} values can be affected by hemoglobin variants or traits; the effect depends on the specific hemoglobin variant or derivative and the specific assay used. Immunoassays that use an antibody to the glycated amino terminus of beta globin do not recognize the terminus of the gamma globin of hemoglobin F. In patients with high levels of hemoglobin F, immunoassays give falsely low values of HbA_{1c}. Cation-exchange chromatography separates hemoglobin species by charge differences. Hemoglobin variants that co-elute with HbA_{1c} can lead to an overestimation of the HbA_{1c} value. Chemically modified derivatives of hemoglobin such as carbamoylation (in end-stage chronic kidney disease) or acetylation (high-dose aspirin therapy) can similarly co-elute with HbA_{1c} by some assay methods. The National Glycohemoglobin Standardization Program website (www.ngsp.org) has information on the impact of frequently encountered hemoglobin variants and traits on the results obtained with the commonly used HbA_{1c} assays.

Any condition that shortens erythrocyte survival or decreases mean erythrocyte age (eg, recovery from acute blood loss, hemolytic anemia) will falsely lower HbA_{1c} irrespective of the assay method used. Intravenous iron and erythropoietin therapy for treatment of anemia in chronic kidney disease also falsely lower HbA_{1c} levels. Alternative methods such as fructosamine (see below) should be considered for these patients. Vitamins C and E are reported to falsely lower test results possibly by inhibiting glycation of hemoglobin.

The ADA has endorsed using the HbA_{1c} as a diagnostic test for type 1 and type 2 diabetes (Table 27–4). A cutoff value of 6.5% was chosen because the risk for retinopathy increases substantially above this value. The advantages of using the HbA_{1c} to diagnose diabetes is that there is no need to fast; it has lower intraindividual variability than the fasting glucose test and the oral glucose tolerance test; and it provides an estimate of glucose control for the preceding 2–3 months. People with HbA_{1c} levels of 5.7–6.4% should be considered at high risk for developing diabetes (prediabetes). The diagnosis should be confirmed with a repeat HbA_{1c} test, unless the patient is symptomatic with plasma glucose levels > 200 mg/dL (11.1 mmol/L). This test is not appropriate to use in populations with high prevalence of hemoglobinopathies or in conditions with increased red cell turnover.

6. Serum fructosamine—Serum fructosamine is formed by nonenzymatic glycosylation of serum proteins (predominantly albumin). Since serum albumin has a much shorter half-life than hemoglobin, serum fructosamine generally reflects the state of glycemic control for only the preceding 1–2 weeks. Reductions in serum albumin (eg, nephrotic state, protein-losing enteropathy, or hepatic disease) will lower the serum fructosamine value. When abnormal hemoglobins or hemolytic states affect the interpretation of glycohemoglobin or when a narrower time frame is required, such as for ascertaining glycemic control

at the time of conception in a diabetic woman who has recently become pregnant, serum fructosamine assays offer some advantage. Normal values vary in relation to the serum albumin concentration and are 200–285 mcmol/L when the serum albumin level is 5 g/dL. HbA_{1c} values and serum fructosamine are highly correlated. Serum fructosamine levels of 300, 367, and 430 mcmol/L approximate to HbA_{1c} values of 7%, 8%, and 9%, respectively. Substantial individual variability exists, though, when estimating the likely HbA_{1c} value from the fructosamine measurement.

7. Self-monitoring of blood glucose—Capillary blood glucose measurements performed by patients themselves, as outpatients, are extremely useful. In type 1 patients in whom "tight" metabolic control is attempted, they are indispensable. There are several paper strip (glucose oxidase, glucose dehydrogenase, or hexokinase) methods for measuring glucose on capillary blood samples. A reflectance photometer or an amperometric system is then used to measure the reaction that takes place on the reagent strip. A large number of blood glucose meters are now available. All are accurate, but they vary with regard to speed, convenience, size of blood samples required, reporting capability, and cost. Popular models include those manufactured by LifeScan (One Touch), Bayer Corporation (Breeze, Contour), Roche Diagnostics (Accu-Chek), Sanofi Aventis (iBGStar), and Abbott Laboratories (Precision, FreeStyle). These blood glucose meters are relatively inexpensive, ranging from $50 to $100 each. Test strips remain a major expense, costing $.50 to $.75 apiece. Each glucose meter also comes with a lancet device and disposable 26- to 33-gauge lancets. Most meters can store from 100 to 1000 glucose values in their memories and have capabilities to download the values into a computer spreadsheet for review by the patients and their health care team. iBGStar is a glucose meter that connects directly to the iPhone. The accuracy of data obtained by home glucose monitoring does require education of the patient in sampling and measuring procedures as well as in properly calibrating the instruments.

The clinician should be aware of the limitations of the self-monitoring glucose systems. First, some older meters require input of a code for each batch of strips; failure to enter the code can result in misleading results. Many of the newer meters no longer require this step. Second, increases or decreases in hematocrit can decrease or increase the measured glucose values. The mechanism underlying this effect is not known but presumably it is due to the impact of red cells on the diffusion of plasma into the reagent layer. Third, the meters and the test strips are calibrated over the glucose concentrations ranging from 60 mg/dL (3.3 mmol/L) to 160 mg/dL (8.9 mmol/L) and the accuracy is not as good for higher and lower glucose levels. When the glucose is < 60 mg/dL (3.3 mmol/L), the difference between the meter and the laboratory value may be as much as 20%. Fourth, glucose oxidase–based amperometric systems underestimate glucose levels in the presence of high oxygen tension. This may be important in the critically ill who are receiving supplemental oxygen; under these circumstances, a glucose dehydrogenase–based system may be preferable. Fifth, glucose-dehydrogenase pyrroloquinoline quinone (GDH-PQQ) systems may report falsely high glucose levels in patients who are receiving parenteral products containing nonglucose sugars such as maltose, galactose, or xylose or their metabolites. Patients have been given falsely high glucose values resulting in life-threatening hypoglycemia. Sixth, some meters have been approved for measuring glucose in blood samples obtained at alternative sites such as the forearm and thigh. There is, however, a 5- to 20-minute lag in the glucose response on the arm with respect to the glucose response on the finger. Forearm blood glucose measurements could therefore result in a delay in detection of rapidly developing hypoglycemia.

8. Continuous glucose monitoring systems—A number of continuous glucose monitoring systems are available for clinical use. The systems manufactured by Medtronic Minimed, DexCom systems, and Abbott Diagnostics (outside the United States), involve inserting a subcutaneous sensor (rather like an insulin pump cannula) that measures glucose concentrations in the interstitial fluid for 3–7 days. The data are transmitted to a separate pager-like device with a screen. The MiniMed system also has the option to wirelessly transmit the data to the screen of their insulin pump. The systems allow the patient to set "alerts" for low and high glucose values and rate of change of glucose levels. Patients still have to calibrate the devices with periodic fingerstick glucose levels, and since there are concerns regarding reliability, it is still necessary to confirm the displayed glucose level with a fingerstick glucose before making interventions such as injecting extra insulin or eating extra carbohydrates. A 6-month randomized controlled study of type 1 patients showed that adults (25 years and older) using these systems had improved glycemic control without an increase in the incidence of hypoglycemia. A randomized controlled study of continuous glucose monitoring during pregnancy showed improved glycemic control in the third trimester, lower birth weight, and reduced risk of macrosomia. The individual glucose values are not that critical—what matters is the direction and the rate at which the glucose is changing, allowing the user to take corrective action. The wearer also gains insight into the way particular foods and activities affect their glucose levels. The other main benefit is the low glucose alert warning. The MiniMed insulin pump can be programmed to automatically suspend insulin delivery for up to 2 hours when the glucose levels on its continuous glucose monitoring device falls to a preset level and the patient does not respond to the alert. This insulin suspension feature has been shown to reduce the amount of time patients are in the hypoglycemic range at night. Many of these systems are being covered by insurance. The initial cost is about $800 to $1000, and the sensor, which has to be changed every 3 to 7 days, costs $35 to $60. This adds up to an out-of-pocket expense of about $4000 annually.

There is great interest in using the data obtained from these continuous glucose monitoring systems to automatically deliver insulin by continuous subcutaneous insulin infusion pump. Algorithms have been devised to link continuous glucose monitoring to insulin delivery and preliminary clinical studies appear promising.

9. Lipoprotein abnormalities in diabetes—Circulating lipoproteins are just as dependent on insulin as is the plasma glucose. In type 1 diabetes, moderately deficient control of hyperglycemia is associated with only a slight elevation of LDL cholesterol and serum triglycerides and little if any change in HDL cholesterol. Once the hyperglycemia is corrected, lipoprotein levels are generally normal. However, in patients with type 2 diabetes, a distinct "diabetic dyslipidemia" is characteristic of the insulin resistance syndrome. Its features are a high serum triglyceride level (300–400 mg/dL [3.4–4.5 mmol/L]), a low HDL cholesterol (< 30 mg/dL [0.8 mmol/L]), and a qualitative change in LDL particles, producing a smaller dense particle whose membrane carries supranormal amounts of free cholesterol. These smaller dense LDL particles are more susceptible to oxidation, which renders them more atherogenic. Since a low HDL cholesterol is a major feature predisposing to macrovascular disease, the term "dyslipidemia" has preempted the term "hyperlipidemia," which mainly denoted the elevated triglycerides. Measures designed to correct the obesity and hyperglycemia, such as exercise, diet, and hypoglycemic therapy, are the treatment of choice for diabetic dyslipidemia, and in occasional patients in whom normal weight was achieved, all features of the lipoprotein abnormalities cleared. Since primary disorders of lipid metabolism may coexist with diabetes, persistence of lipid abnormalities after restoration of normal weight and blood glucose should prompt a diagnostic workup and possible pharmacotherapy of the lipid disorder. Chapter 28 discusses these matters in detail.

Sacks DB et al; National Academy of Clinical Biochemistry; Evidence-Based Laboratory Medicine Committee of the American Association for Clinical Chemistry. Guidelines and recommendations for laboratory analysis in the diagnosis and management of diabetes mellitus. Diabetes Care. 2011 Jun;34(6):e61–99. [PMID: 21617108]

Clinical Trials in Diabetes

Findings of the Diabetes Complications and Control Trial (DCCT) and of the United Kingdom Prospective Diabetes Study (UKPDS), have confirmed the beneficial effects of improved glycemic control in both type 1 and type 2 diabetes.

The Diabetes Control and Complications Trial, a long-term therapeutic study involving 1441 patients with type 1 diabetes mellitus, reported that "near" normalization of blood glucose resulted in a delay in the onset and a major slowing of the progression of established microvascular and neuropathic complications of diabetes during a follow-up period of up to 10 years. Multiple insulin injections (66%) or insulin pumps (34%) were used in the intensively treated group, who were trained to modify their therapy in response to frequent glucose monitoring. The conventionally treated groups used no more than two insulin injections, and clinical well-being was the goal with no attempt to modify management based on HbA_{1c} determinations or the glucose results.

In half of the patients, a mean hemoglobin A_{1c} of 7.2% (normal: < 6%) and a mean blood glucose of 155 mg/dL (8.6 mmol/L) were achieved using intensive therapy, while in the conventionally treated group HbA_{1c} averaged 8.9% with an average blood glucose of 225 mg/dL (12.5 mmol/L). Over the study period, which averaged 7 years, there was an approximately 60% reduction in risk between the two groups in regard to diabetic retinopathy, nephropathy, and neuropathy. The intensively treated group also had a nonsignificant reduction in the risk of macrovascular disease of 41% (95% CI, −10 to 68). Intensively treated patients had a threefold greater risk of serious hypoglycemia as well as a greater tendency toward weight gain. However, there were no deaths definitely attributable to hypoglycemia in any persons in the DCCT study, and no evidence of posthypoglycemic cognitive damage was detected.

Subjects participating in the DCCT study were subsequently enrolled in a follow-up observational study, the Epidemiology of Diabetes Interventions and Complications (EDIC) study. Even though the between-group differences in mean HbA_{1c} narrowed over 4 years, the group assigned to intensive therapy had a lower risk of retinopathy at 4 years, microalbuminuria at 7 to 8 years, and impaired glomerular filtration rate (< 60 mL/min/1.73 m²) at 22 years of continued study follow-up. Moreover, by the end of the 11-year follow-up period, the intensive therapy group had significantly reduced their risk of any cardiovascular disease events by 42% (95% CI, 9% to 23%; $P = 0.02$). Thus, it seems that the benefits of good glucose control persist even if control deteriorates at a later date.

The general consensus of the ADA is that intensive insulin therapy associated with comprehensive self-management training should become standard therapy in patients with type 1 diabetes mellitus after the age of puberty. Exceptions include those with advanced chronic kidney disease and the elderly, since in these groups the detrimental risks of hypoglycemia outweigh the benefits of tight glycemic control.

The Diabetes Prevention Program was aimed at discovering whether treatment with either diet and exercise or metformin could prevent the onset of type 2 diabetes in people with impaired glucose tolerance; 3234 overweight men and women aged 25–85 years with impaired glucose tolerance participated in the study. Intervention with a low-fat diet and 150 minutes of moderate exercise (equivalent to a brisk walk) per week reduced the risk of progression to type 2 diabetes by 71% compared with a matched control group. Participants taking 850 mg of metformin twice a day reduced their risk of developing type 2 diabetes by 31%, but this intervention was relatively ineffective in those who were either less obese or in the older age group.

With the demonstration that intervention can be successful in preventing progression to diabetes in these subjects, a recommendation has been made to change the terminology from the less comprehensible "impaired glucose tolerance" to "prediabetes." The latter is a term that the public can better understand and thus respond to by implementing healthier diet and exercise habits.

The United Kingdom Prospective Diabetes Study, a multicenter study, was designed to establish, in type 2 diabetic patients, whether the risk of macrovascular or microvascular complications could be reduced by intensive blood glucose control with oral hypoglycemic agents or insulin and whether any particular therapy was of advantage. A total of 3867 patients aged 25–65 years with newly diagnosed diabetes were recruited between 1977 and 1991, and studied over 10 years. The median age at baseline was 54 years; 44% were overweight (> 120% over ideal weight); and baseline HbA_{1c} was 9.1%. Therapies were randomized to include a control group on diet alone and separate groups intensively treated with either insulin or sulfonylurea (chlorpropamide, glyburide, or glipizide). Metformin was included as a randomization option in a subgroup of 342 overweight or obese patients, and much later in the study an additional subgroup of both normal-weight and overweight patients who were responding unsatisfactorily to sulfonylurea therapy were randomized to either continue on their sulfonylurea therapy alone or to have metformin combined with it. Subsequently, an additional modification was made to evaluate whether tight control of blood pressure with stepwise antihypertensive therapy would prevent macrovascular and microvascular complications in 758 hypertensive patients among this UKPDS population compared with 390 of them whose blood pressure was treated less intensively. The tight control group was randomly assigned to treatment with either an angiotensin-converting enzyme (ACE) inhibitor (captopril) or a beta-blocker (atenolol). Both medications were stepped up to maximum dosages of 100 mg/d and then, if blood pressure remained higher than the target level of < 150/85 mm Hg, more medications were added in the following stepwise sequence: a diuretic, slow-release nifedipine, methyldopa, and prazosin—until the target level of tight control was achieved. In the control group, hypertension was conventionally treated to achieve target levels < 180/105 mm Hg, but these patients were not prescribed either ACE inhibitors or beta-blockers.

Intensive treatment with either sulfonylureas, metformin, combinations of those two, or insulin achieved mean HbA_{1c} levels of 7%. This level of glycemic control decreased the risk of microvascular complications (retinopathy and nephropathy) in comparison with conventional therapy (mostly diet alone), which achieved mean levels of HbA_{1c} of 7.9%. Weight gain occurred in intensively treated patients except when metformin was used as monotherapy. No adverse cardiovascular outcomes were noted regardless of the therapeutic agent. In the overweight or obese subgroup, metformin therapy was more beneficial than diet alone in reducing the number of cases that progressed to diabetes as well as decreasing the number of patients who suffered myocardial infarctions and strokes. Hypoglycemic reactions occurred in the intensive treatment groups, but only one death from hypoglycemia was documented during 27,000 patient-years of intensive therapy.

Tight control of blood pressure (median value 144/82 mm Hg vs 154/87 mm Hg) substantially reduced the risk of microvascular disease and stroke but not myocardial infarction. In fact, reducing blood pressure by this amount had substantially greater impact on microvascular outcomes than that achieved by lowering HbA$_{1c}$ from 7.9% to 7%. An epidemiologic analysis of the UKPDS data did show that every 10 mm Hg decrease in updated mean systolic blood pressure was associated with 11% reduction in risk for myocardial infarction. More than half of the patients needed two or more medications for adequate therapy of their hypertension, and there was no demonstrable advantage of ACE inhibitor therapy over therapy with beta-blockers with regard to diabetes end points. Use of a calcium channel blocker added to both treatment groups appeared to be safe over the long term in this diabetic population despite some controversy in the literature about its safety in diabetics.

Like the DCCT trialists, the UKPDS researchers performed post-trial monitoring to determine whether there were long-term benefits of having been in the intensively treated glucose and blood pressure arms of the study. The between-group differences in HbA$_{1c}$ were lost within the first year of follow-up, but the reduced risk (24%, P = 0.001) of development or progression of microvascular complications in the intensively treated group persisted for 10 years. The intensively treated group also had significantly reduced risk of myocardial infarction (15%, P = 0.01) and death from any cause (13%, P = 0.007) during the follow-up period. The subgroup of overweight or obese subjects who were initially randomized to metformin therapy showed sustained reduction in risk of myocardial infarction and death from any cause in the follow-up period. The between-group blood pressure differences disappeared within 2 years of the end of the trial. Unlike the sustained benefits seen with glucose control, there were no sustained benefits from having been in the more tightly controlled blood pressure group. Both blood pressure groups were at similar risk for microvascular events and diabetes-related end points during the follow-up period.

Thus, the follow-up of the UKPDS type 2 diabetes cohort showed that, as in type 1 diabetes, the benefits of good glucose control persist even if control deteriorates at a later date. Blood pressure benefits, however, last only as long as the blood pressure is well controlled.

The Steno-2 study was designed in 1990 to validate the efficacy of targeting multiple concomitant risk factors (diet, smoking cessation, exercise, and pharmacologic interventions) for both microvascular and macrovascular disorders in type 2 diabetes. A prospective, randomized, open, blinded end point design was used where 160 patients with type 2 diabetes and microalbuminuria were assigned to conventional therapy with their general practitioner or to intensive care at the Steno Diabetes Center. The intensively treated group had stepwise introduction of lifestyle and pharmacologic interventions aimed at keeping glycated hemoglobin < 6.5%, blood pressure < 130/80 mm Hg; total cholesterol < 175 mg/dL (4.5 mmol/L), and triglycerides < 150 mg/dL (1.7 mmol/L). All the intensively treated group received ACE inhibitors and if intolerant, an angiotensin II-receptor blocker. The lifestyle component of intensive intervention included reduction in dietary fat intake to < 30% of total calories; smoking cessation program; light to moderate exercise; daily vitamin-mineral

supplement of vitamin C, E, and chromium picolinate. Initially, aspirin was only given as secondary prevention to patients with a history of ischemic cardiovascular disease; later, all patients received aspirin. After a mean follow-up of 7.8 years, cardiovascular events (eg, myocardial infarction, angioplasties, coronary bypass grafts, strokes, amputations, vascular surgical interventions) developed in 44% of patients in the conventional arm and only in 24% in the intensive multifactorial arm—about a 50% reduction. Rates of nephropathy, retinopathy, and autonomic neuropathy were also lower in the multifactorial intervention arm by 62% and 63%, respectively.

The persons who participated in this trial were subsequently enrolled in an observational follow-up study for an average of 5.5 years. Even though the significant differences in glycemic control and levels of risk factors of cardiovascular disease between the groups had disappeared by the end of the follow-up period, the interventional group continued to have a lower risk of retinal photocoagulation, renal failure, cardiovascular end points, and cardiovascular mortality.

The data from the UKPDS and this study provide support for guidelines recommending vigorous treatment of concomitant microvascular and cardiovascular risk factors in patients with type 2 diabetes.

The ACCORD study was a randomized controlled study designed to determine whether normal HbA$_{1c}$ levels would reduce the risk of cardiovascular events in middle-aged or older individuals with type 2 diabetes. About 35% of the 10,251 recruited subjects had established cardiovascular disease at study entry. The intensive arm of the study was discontinued after 3.5 years of follow-up because of more unexplained deaths in the intensive arm when compared with the control arm (22%, P = 0.020). Analysis of the data at time of discontinuation showed that the intensively treated group (mean HbA$_{1c}$ 6.4%) had a 10% reduction in cardiovascular event rate compared with the standard treated group (mean HbA$_{1c}$ 7.5%), but this difference was not statistically significant.

The ADVANCE trial randomly assigned 11,140 patients with type 2 diabetes to standard or intensive glucose control. The primary outcomes were major macrovascular cardiovascular events (nonfatal myocardial infarction or stroke or death from cardiovascular causes) or microvascular events. Overall, one-third (32%) of the subjects had established cardiovascular disease at study entry. After a median follow-up of 5 years, there was a nonsignificant reduction (6%) in major macrovascular event rate in the intensively treated group (mean HbA$_{1c}$ 6.5%) compared with the standard therapy group (HbA$_{1c}$ 7.3%).

The Veteran Administration Diabetes Trial (VADT) randomly assigned 1791 patients (97% men) from age 50 to 69 years with type 2 diabetes to standard or intensive glucose control. The primary outcome was a composite of myocardial infarction, death from cardiovascular causes, heart failure, vascular surgery, inoperable coronary artery disease, and amputation for gangrene. All the patients had optimized blood pressure and lipid levels. After a median follow-up of 5.6 years, there was no significant difference in the primary cardiovascular outcome in the intensively treated group (HbA$_{1c}$ 6.9%) compared with the standard therapy (HbA$_{1c}$ 8.4%). Within this larger study, there was an embedded study evaluating the impact of the intensive therapy on patients who were subcategorized as having low, moderate, and high coronary calcium scores on CT scans. Patients with low coronary calcium score showed a reduced number of cardiovascular events with intensive therapy.

Thus, the ACCORD, ADVANCE, and VADT results do not provide support for the hypothesis that near-normal glucose control in patients with type 2 diabetes will reduce cardiovascular events. It is, however, important not to over-interpret the results of these three studies. The results do not exclude the possibility that cardiovascular benefits might accrue with longer duration of near-normal glucose control. In the UKPDS, risk reductions for myocardial infarction and death from any cause were only observed during 10 years of post-trial follow-up. Specific subgroups of type 2 diabetic patients may also have different outcomes. The ACCORD, ADVANCE, and VADT studies recruited patients who had diabetes for 8–10 years and one-third of them already had established cardiovascular disease. Patients in the UKPDS, in contrast, had newly diagnosed diabetes and only 7.5% had a history of macrovascular disease. It is possible that the benefits of tight glycemic control on macrovascular events are attenuated in patients with longer duration of diabetes or with established vascular disease. Specific therapies used to lower glucose may also affect cardiovascular event rate or mortality. Severe hypoglycemia occurred more frequently in the intensively treated groups of the ACCORD, ADVANCE, and VADT studies; the ACCORD investigators were not able to exclude undiagnosed hypoglycemia as a potential cause for the increased death rate in the intensive treatment group.

A formal meta-analysis performed of the raw trial data from the ACCORD, ADVANCE, VADT, and UKPDS studies found that allocation to more intensive glucose control reduced the risk of myocardial infarction by 15% (hazard ratio 0.85, 95% CI 0.76–0.94). This benefit occurred in patients who did not have preexisting macrovascular disease.

The Diabetes Control and Complications Trial Research Group. The effect of intensive treatment of diabetes on the development and progression of long-term complications in insulin-dependent diabetes mellitus. N Engl J Med. 1993 Sep 30;329(14):977–86. [PMID: 8366922]
UK Prospective Diabetes Study (UKPDS) Group. Intensive blood-glucose control with sulphonylureas or insulin compared with conventional treatment and risk of complications in patients with type 2 diabetes (UKPDS 33). Lancet. 1998 Sep 12;352(9131):837–53. [PMID: 9742976]

▶ Treatment Regimens

A. Diet

A well-balanced, nutritious diet remains a fundamental element of therapy. The ADA recommends about 45–65% of total daily calories in the form of carbohydrates; 25–35%

in the form of fat (of which < 7% are from saturated fat), and 10–35% in the form of protein. In patients with type 2 diabetes, limiting the carbohydrate intake and substituting some of the calories with monounsaturated fats, such as olive oil, rapeseed (canola) oil, or the oils in nuts and avocados, can lower triglycerides and increase HDL cholesterol. In addition, in those patients with obesity and type 2 diabetes, weight reduction by caloric restriction is an important goal of the diet. Patients with type 1 diabetes or type 2 diabetes who take insulin should be taught "carbohydrate counting," so they can administer their insulin bolus for each meal based on its carbohydrate content. In obese individuals with diabetes, an additional goal is weight reduction by caloric restriction (see Chapter 29).

The current recommendations for both types of diabetes continue to limit cholesterol to 300 mg daily, and individuals with LDL cholesterol more than 100 mg/dL (2.6 mmol/L) should limit dietary cholesterol to 200 mg daily. High protein intake may cause progression of kidney disease in patients with diabetic nephropathy; for these individuals, a reduction in protein intake to 0.8 kg/d (or about 10% of total calories daily) is recommended.

Exchange lists for meal planning can be obtained from the American Diabetes Association and its affiliate associations or from the American Dietetic Association (http://www.eatright.org), 216 W. Jackson Blvd., Chicago, IL 60606 (312-899-0040).

1. Dietary fiber—Plant components such as cellulose, gum, and pectin are indigestible by humans and are termed dietary "fiber." Insoluble fibers such as cellulose or hemicellulose, as found in bran, tend to increase intestinal transit and may have beneficial effects on colonic function. In contrast, soluble fibers such as gums and pectins, as found in beans, oatmeal, or apple skin, tend to retard nutrient absorption rates so that glucose absorption is slower and hyperglycemia may be slightly diminished. Although its recommendations do not include insoluble fiber supplements such as added bran, the ADA recommends food such as oatmeal, cereals, and beans with relatively high soluble fiber content as staple components of the diet in diabetics. High soluble fiber content in the diet may also have a favorable effect on blood cholesterol levels.

2. Glycemic index—The glycemic index of a carbohydrate containing food is determined by comparing the glucose excursions after consuming 50 g of test food with glucose excursions after consuming 50 g of reference food (white bread):

$$\text{Glycemic index} = \frac{\text{Blood glucose area under the curve (3h) for test food}}{\text{Blood glucose area under the curve (3h) for reference food}} \times 100$$

Eating low glycemic index foods results in lower glucose levels after meals. Low glycemic index foods have values of 55 or less and include many fruits, vegetables, grainy breads, pasta, and legumes. High glycemic index foods have values of 70 or greater and include baked potato, white bread, and white rice. Glycemic index is low-ered by presence of fats and protein when food is con-sumed in a mixed meal. Even though it may not be possible to accurately predict the glycemic index of a particular food in the context of a meal, it is reasonable to choose foods with low glycemic index.

3. Artificial and other sweeteners—Aspartame (Nutra Sweet) consists of two major amino acids, aspartic acid and phenylalanine, which combine to produce a sweetener that is 180 times as sweet as sucrose. A major limitation is that it is not heat stable, so it cannot be used in cooking. Sac-charin (Sweet 'N Low), sucralose (Splenda), acesulfame potassium (Sweet One), and rebiana (Truvia) are other "artificial" sweeteners that can be used in cooking and bak-ing. Aspartame, saccharin, sucralose, acesulfame, and rebiana **do not raise blood glucose levels.**

Fructose represents a "natural" sugar substance that is a highly effective sweetener, induces only slight increases in plasma glucose levels, and does not require insulin for its metabolism. However, because of potential adverse effects of large amounts of fructose on raising serum cholesterol, triglycerides, and LDL cholesterol, it does not have any advantage as a sweetening agent in the diabetic diet. This does not preclude, however, ingestion of fructose-contain-ing fruits and vegetables or fructose-sweetened foods in moderation.

Sugar alcohols, also known as polyols or polyalcohol, are commonly used as sweeteners and bulking agents. They occur naturally in a variety of fruits and vegetables but are also commercially made from sucrose, glucose, and starch. Examples are sorbitol, xylitol, mannitol, lactitol, isomalt, maltitol, and hydrogenated starch hydrolysates (HSH). They are not as easily absorbed as sugar, so they do not raise blood glucose levels as much. Therefore, sugar alco-hols are often used in food products that are labeled as "sugar free," such as chewing gum, lozenges, hard candy, and sugar-free ice cream. However, if consumed in large quantities, they will raise blood glucose and can cause bloating and diarrhea.

B. Medications for Treating Hyperglycemia

The medications for treating type 2 diabetes (Table 27–5) fall into several categories: (1) Medications that primarily stimulate insulin secretion by binding to the sulfonylurea receptor: Sulfonylureas remain the most widely prescribed medications for treating hyperglycemia. The meglitinide analog repaglinide and the D-phenylalanine derivative nat-eglinide also bind the sulfonylurea receptor and stimulate insulin secretion. (2) Medications that primarily lower glucose levels by their actions on the liver, muscle, and adipose tissue: Metformin works in the liver. The thiazoli-dinediones appear to have their main effect on skeletal muscle and adipose tissue. (3) Medications that principally slow intestinal absorption of glucose: The alpha-glucosi-dase inhibitors acarbose and miglitol are such currently available therapies. (4) Medications that mimic incretin effect or prolong incretin action: Glucagon-like peptide 1 (GLP1) receptor agonists and DPP 4 inhibitors fall into this category. (5) Medications that inhibit reabsorption of

filtered glucose in the kidney: The sodium-glucose co-transporter inhibitors dapagliflozin and canagliflozin are two such agents. (6) Others: Pramlintide lowers glucose by suppressing glucagon and slowing gastric emptying. The mechanisms by which bromocriptine and colesevelam lower glucose levels have not been defined. The medica-tions are discussed in detail below. A framework for plan-ning treatment using medications from these six categories is offered later in this chapter.

1. Medications that primarily stimulate insulin secretion by binding to the sulfonylurea receptor on the beta cell—

A. SULFONYLUREAS—The primary mechanism of action of the sulfonylureas is to stimulate insulin release from pan-creatic B cells. Specific receptors on the surface of pancre-atic B cells bind sulfonylureas in the rank order of their insulinotropic potency (glyburide with the greatest affinity and tolbutamide with the least affinity). It has been shown that activation of these receptors closes potassium chan-nels, resulting in depolarization of the B cell. This depolar-ized state permits calcium to enter the cell and actively promote insulin release.

Sulfonylureas are used in patients with type 2 but not type 1 diabetes, since these medications require function-ing pancreatic B cells to produce their effect on blood glu-cose. Sulfonylureas are metabolized by the liver and apart from acetohexamide, whose metabolite is more active than the parent compound, the metabolites of all the other sul-fonylureas are weakly active or inactive. The metabolites are excreted by the kidney and, in the case of the second-generation sulfonylureas, partly excreted in the bile. Sulfo-nylureas are generally contraindicated in patients with severe liver or kidney impairment. Idiosyncratic reactions are rare, with skin rashes or hematologic toxicity (leukope-nia, thrombocytopenia) occurring in < 0.1% of users.

(1) First-generation sulfonylureas (tolbutamide, tolaza-mide, acetohexamide, chlorpropamide)—**Tolbutamide** is rapidly oxidized in the liver to inactive metabolites, and its approximate duration of effect is relatively short (6–10 hours). Tolbutamide is probably best administered in divided doses (eg, 500 mg before each meal and at bed-time); however, some patients require only one or two tablets daily with a maximum dose of 3000 mg/d. Because of its short duration of action, which is independent of kidney function, tolbutamide is relatively safe to use in renal impairment. Prolonged hypoglycemia has been reported rarely with tolbutamide, mostly in patients receiv-ing certain antibacterial sulfonamides (sulfisoxazole), phenylbutazone for arthralgias, or the oral azole antifungal medications to treat candidiasis. These medications appar-ently compete with tolbutamide for oxidative enzyme sys-tems in the liver, resulting in maintenance of high levels of unmetabolized, active sulfonylurea in the circulation.

Tolazamide, acetohexamide, and chlorpropamide are rarely used. Chlorpropamide has a prolonged biologic effect, and severe hypoglycemia can occur especially in the elderly as their renal clearance declines with aging. Its other side effects include alcohol-induced flushing and hyponatremia due to its effect on vasopressin secretion and action.

Table 27–5. Drugs for treatment of type 2 diabetes mellitus.

Drug	Tablet Size	Daily Dose	Duration of Action
Sulfonylureas			
Acetohexamide (Dymelor)	250 and 500 mg	0.25–1.5 g as single dose or in two divided doses	8–24 hours
Chlorpropamide (Diabinese)	100 and 250 mg	0.1–0.5 g as single dose	24–72 hours
Gliclazide (not available in United States)	80 mg	40–80 mg as single dose; 160–320 mg as divided dose	12 hours
Glimepiride (Amaryl)	1, 2, and 4 mg	1–4 mg once a day is usual dose; 8 mg once a day is maximal dose	Up to 24 hours
Glipizide			
(Glucotrol)	5 and 10 mg	2.5–40 mg as a single dose or in two divided doses 30 minutes before meals	6–12 hours
(Glucotrol XL)	2.5, 5, and 10 mg	2.5 to 10 mg once a day is usual dose; 20 mg once a day is maximal dose	Up to 24 hours
Glyburide			
(Dia Beta, Micronase)	1.25, 2.5, and 5 mg	1.25–20 mg as single dose or in two divided doses	Up to 24 hours
(Glynase)	1.5, 3, and 6 mg	1.5–12 mg as single dose or in two divided doses	Up to 24 hours
Tolazamide (Tolinase)	100, 250, and 500 mg	0.1–1 g as single dose or in two divided doses	Up to 24 hours
Tolbutamide (Orinase)	250 and 500 mg	0.5–2 g in two or three divided doses	6–12 hours
Meglitinide analogs			
Mitiglinide (available in Japan)	5 and 10 mg	5 or 10 mg three times a day before meals	2 hours
Repaglinide (Prandin)	0.5, 1, and 2 mg	0.5 to 4 mg three times a day before meals	3 hours
D-Phenylalanine derivative			
Nateglinide (Starlix)	60 and 120 mg	60 or 120 mg three times a day before meals	1.5 hours
Biguanides			
Metformin (Glucophage)	500, 850, and 1000 mg	1–2.5 g; 1 tablet with meals two or three times daily	7–12 hours
Extended-release metformin (Glucophage XR)	500 and 750 mg	500–2000 mg once a day	Up to 24 hours
Thiazolidinediones			
Pioglitazone (Actos)	15, 30, and 45 mg	15–45 mg daily	Up to 24 hours
Rosiglitazone (Avandia)	2, 4, and 8 mg	4–8 mg daily (can be divided)	Up to 24 hours
Alpha-glucosidase inhibitors			
Acarbose (Precose)	50 and 100 mg	25–100 mg three times a day just before meals	4 hours
Miglitol (Glyset)	25, 50, and 100 mg	25–100 mg three times a day just before meals	4 hours
Voglibose (not available in United States)	0.2 and 0.3 mg	0.2–0.3 mg three times a day just before meals	4 hours
GLP-1 receptor agonists			
Exenatide (Byetta)	1.2 mL and 2.4 mL pre-filled pens containing 5 mcg and 10 mcg (subcutaneous injection)	5 mcg subcutaneously twice a day within 1 hour of breakfast and dinner. Increase to 10 mcg subcutaneously twice a day after about a month. Do not use if calculated creatinine clearance is < 30 mL/min.	6 hours
Exenatide, long-acting release (Byetta LAR, Bydureon)	2 mg (powder)	Suspend in provided diluent and inject subcutaneously	1 week
Liraglutide (Victoza)	Pre-filled, multi-dose pen that delivers doses of 0.6 mg, 1.2 mg, or 1.8 mg	0.6 mg subcutaneously once a day (starting dose). Increase to 1.2 mg after a week if no adverse reactions. Dose can be further increased to 1.8 mg, if necessary.	24 hours

(continued)

Table 27–5. Drugs for treatment of type 2 diabetes mellitus. (continued)

Drug	Tablet Size	Daily Dose	Duration of Action
DPP-4 inhibitors			
Alogliptin (Nesina)	6.25, 12.5, and 25 mg	25 mg once daily.; dose is 12.5 mg daily if calculated creatinine clearance is 30–59 mL/min and 6.25 mg daily if clearance < 30 mL/min.	24 hours
Saxagliptin (Onglyza)	2.5 and 5 mg	2.5 mg or 5 mg once daily. Use 2.5 mg dose if calculated creatinine clearance is ≤ 50 mL/min or if also taking drugs that are strong CYP3A4/5 inhibitors such as ketoconazole.	24 hours
Sitagliptin (Januvia)	25, 50, and 100 mg	100 mg once daily is usual dose; dose is 50 mg once daily if calculated creatinine clearance is 30 to 50 mL/min and 25 mg once daily if clearance is < 30 mL/min.	24 hours
Vildagliptin (Galvus) (not available in United States)	50 mg	50 mg once or twice daily. Contraindicated in patients with calculated creatinine clearance ≤ 60 mL/min or AST/ALT three times upper limit of normal	24 hours
Linagliptin (Tradjenta)	5 mg	5 mg daily	24 hours
SGLT2 inhibitors			
Canagliflozin (Invokana)	100 and 300 mg	100 mg daily is usual dose. Do not use if eGFR < 45 mL/min/1.72 m². 300 mg dose can be used if normal eGFR, resulting in lowering the HbA_{1c} an additional ~ 0.1–0.25%	24 hours
Dapagliflozin (Forxiga) (not available in United States)	5 and 10 mg	10 mg daily. Use 5 mg dose in hepatic failure	24 hours
Others			
Bromocriptine (Cycloset)	0.8 mg	0.8 mg daily. Increase weekly by 1 tablet until maximal tolerated dose of 1.6–4.8 mg daily	24 hours
Colesevelam (Welchol)	625 mg	3 tablets twice a day	24 hours
Pramlintide (Symlin)	5 mL vial containing 0.6 mg/mL; also available as prefilled pens. Symlin pen 60 or Symlin pen 120 (subcutaneous injection)	For insulin-treated type 2 patients, start at 60 mcg dose three times a day (10 units on U100 insulin syringe). Increase to 120 mcg three times a day (20 units on U100 insulin syringe) if no nausea for 3–7 days. Give immediately before meal.	2 hours
		For type 1 patients, start at 15 mcg three times a day (2.5 units on U100 insulin syringe) and increase by increments of 15 mcg to a maximum of 60 mcg three times a day, as tolerated.	
		To avoid hypoglycemia, lower insulin dose by 50% on initiation of therapy.	

AST/ALT, aspartate aminotransferase/alanine aminotransferase; eGFR, estimated glomerular filtration rate.

(2) Second-generation sulfonylureas (glyburide, glipizide, gliclazide, glimepiride)—Glyburide, glipizide, gliclazide, and glimepiride are 100–200 times more potent than tolbutamide. These medications should be used with caution in patients with cardiovascular disease or in elderly patients, in whom prolonged hypoglycemia would be especially dangerous.

The usual starting dose of **glyburide** is 2.5 mg/d, and the average maintenance dose is 5–10 mg/d given as a single morning dose; maintenance doses higher than 20 mg/d

are not recommended. Some reports suggest that 10 mg is a maximum daily therapeutic dose, with 15–20 mg having no additional benefit in poor responders and doses over 20 mg actually worsening hyperglycemia. A "Press Tab" formulation of "micronized" glyburide—easy to divide in half with slight pressure if necessary—is available. Glyburide is metabolized in the liver into products with hypoglycemic activity, which probably explains why assays specific for the unmetabolized compound suggest a plasma half-life of only 1–2 hours, yet the biologic effects of glyburide are clearly persistent 24 hours after a single morning dose in diabetic patients. Glyburide is unique among sulfonylureas in that it not only binds to the pancreatic B cell membrane sulfonylurea receptor but also becomes sequestered within the B cell. This may also contribute to its prolonged biologic effect despite its relatively short circulating half-life.

Glyburide has few adverse effects other than its potential for causing hypoglycemia, which at times can be prolonged. Flushing has rarely been reported after ethanol ingestion. It does not cause water retention, as chlorpropamide does, but rather slightly enhances free water clearance. Glyburide should not be used in patients with liver failure and chronic kidney disease because of the risk of hypoglycemia. Elderly patients are at particular risk for hypoglycemia even with relatively small daily doses.

The recommended starting dose of **glipizide** is 5 mg/d, with up to 15 mg/d given as a single daily dose before breakfast. When higher daily doses are required, they should be divided and given before meals. The maximum dose recommended by the manufacturer is 40 mg/d, although doses above 10–15 mg probably provide little additional benefit in poor responders and may even be *less* effective than smaller doses. For maximum effect in reducing postprandial hyperglycemia, glipizide should be ingested 30 minutes before meals, since rapid absorption is delayed when the medication is taken with food.

At least 90% of glipizide is metabolized in the liver to inactive products, and 10% is excreted unchanged in the urine. Glipizide therapy should therefore not be used in patients with liver failure. Because of its lower potency and shorter duration of action, it is preferable to glyburide in elderly patients. Glipizide has also been marketed as Glucotrol-XL. It provides extended release during transit through the gastrointestinal tract with greater effectiveness in lowering prebreakfast hyperglycemia than the shorter-duration immediate-release standard glipizide tablets. However, this formulation appears to have sacrificed its lower propensity for severe hypoglycemia compared with longer-acting glyburide without showing any demonstrable therapeutic advantages over glyburide.

Gliclazide (not available in the United States) is another intermediate duration sulfonylurea with a duration of action of about 12 hours. The recommended starting dose is 40–80 mg/d with a maximum dose of 320 mg. Doses of 160 mg and above are given as divided doses before breakfast and dinner. The medication is metabolized by the liver; the metabolites and conjugates have no hypoglycemic effect. An extended release preparation is available.

Glimepiride has a long duration of effect with a half-life of 5 hours allowing once or twice daily dosing. Glimepiride achieves blood glucose lowering with the lowest dose of any sulfonylurea compound. A single daily dose of 1 mg/d has been shown to be effective, and the maximal recommended dose is 8 mg. It is completely metabolized by the liver to relatively inactive metabolic products.

B. Meglitinide analogs—**Repaglinide** is structurally similar to glyburide but lacks the sulfonic acid-urea moiety. It acts by binding to the sulfonylurea receptor and closing the ATP-sensitive potassium channel. It is rapidly absorbed from the intestine and then undergoes complete metabolism

in the liver to inactive biliary products, giving it a plasma half-life of < 1 hour. The medication therefore causes a brief but rapid pulse of insulin. The starting dose is 0.5 mg three times a day 15 minutes before each meal. The dose can be titrated to a maximal daily dose of 16 mg. Like the sulfonylureas, repaglinide can be used in combination with metformin. Hypoglycemia is the main side effect. In clinical trials, when the medication was compared with a long-duration sulfonylurea (glyburide), there was a trend toward less hypoglycemia. Like the sulfonylureas also, repaglinide causes weight gain. Metabolism is by cytochrome P450 3A4 isoenzyme, and other medications that induce or inhibit this isoenzyme may increase or inhibit (respectively) the metabolism of repaglinide. The medication may be useful in patients with kidney impairment or in the elderly.

Mitiglinide is a benzylsuccinic acid derivative that binds to the sulfonylurea receptor and is similar to repaglinide in its clinical effects. It has been approved for use in Japan.

C. D-Phenylalanine derivative—**Nateglinide** stimulates insulin secretion by binding to the sulfonylurea receptor and closing the ATP-sensitive potassium channel. This compound is rapidly absorbed from the intestine, reaching peak plasma levels within 1 hour. It is metabolized in the liver and has a plasma half-life of about 1.5 hours. Like repaglinide, it causes a brief rapid pulse of insulin, and when given before a meal it reduces the postprandial rise in blood glucose. For most patients, the recommended starting and maintenance dose is 120 mg three times a day before meals. Use 60 mg in patients who have mild elevations in HbA_{1c}. Like the other insulin secretagogues, its main side effects are hypoglycemia and weight gain.

2. Medications that primarily lower glucose levels by their actions on the liver, muscle, and adipose tissue—

A. Metformin—Metformin (1,1-dimethylbiguanide hydrochloride) is used, either alone or in conjunction with other oral agents or insulin, in the treatment of patients with type 2 diabetes.

Metformin's therapeutic effects primarily derive from the increasing hepatic adenosine monophosphate-activated protein kinase activity, which reduces hepatic gluconeogenesis and lipogenesis. Metformin is a substrate for organic cation transporter 1, which is abundantly expressed in hepatocytes and in the gut.

Metformin has a half-life of 1.5–3 hours, is not bound to plasma proteins, and is not metabolized in humans, being excreted unchanged by the kidneys.

Metformin is the first-line therapy for patients with type 2 diabetes. The current recommendation is to start this medication at diagnosis. A side benefit of metformin therapy is its tendency to improve both fasting and postprandial hyperglycemia and hypertriglyceridemia in obese diabetics without the weight gain associated with insulin or sulfonylurea therapy. Metformin is ineffective in patients with type 1 diabetes. Patients with chronic kidney disease should not be given this medication because failure to excrete it would produce high blood and tissue levels of metformin that could stimulate lactic acid overproduction.

In the United States, metformin use is not recommended at or above a serum creatinine level of 1.4 mg/dL in women and 1.5 mg/dL in men. In the United Kingdom, the recommendations are to review metformin use when the serum creatinine exceeds 130 mcmol/L (1.5 mg/dL) or the estimated glomerular filtration rate falls below 45 mL/min per 1.73 m^2. The medication should be stopped if the serum creatinine exceeds 150 mcmol/L (1.7mg/dL) or the estimated glomerular filtration rate is below 30 mL/min per 1.73 m^2. Patients with liver failure or persons with excessive alcohol intake should not receive this medication—lactic acid production from the gut and other tissues, which rises during metformin therapy, could result in lactic acidosis when defective hepatocytes cannot remove the lactate or when alcohol-induced reduction of nucleotides interferes with lactate clearance.

The maximal dosage of metformin is 2.55 g, although little benefit is seen above a total dose of 2000 mg. It is important to begin with a low dose and increase the dosage very gradually in divided doses—taken with meals—to reduce minor gastrointestinal upsets. A common schedule would be one 500 mg tablet three times a day with meals or one 850 mg or 1000 mg tablet twice daily at breakfast and dinner. Up to 2000 mg of the extended-release preparation can be given once a day. Lower doses should be used in patients with estimated glomerular filtration rates between 30 and 45 mL/min per 1.73 m^2.

The most frequent side effects of metformin are gastrointestinal symptoms (anorexia, nausea, vomiting, abdominal discomfort, diarrhea), which occur in up to 20% of patients. These effects are dose-related, tend to occur at onset of therapy, and often are transient. However, in 3–5% of patients, therapy may have to be discontinued because of persistent diarrheal discomfort. In a retrospective analysis, it has been reported that patients switched from immediate-release metformin to comparable dose of extended-release metformin experienced fewer gastrointestinal side effects.

Hypoglycemia does not occur with therapeutic doses of metformin, which permits its description as a "euglycemic" or "antihyperglycemic" medication rather than an oral hypoglycemic agent. Dermatologic or hematologic toxicity is rare. Metformin interferes with the calcium dependent absorption of vitamin B$_{12}$-intrinsic complex in the terminal ileum; vitamin B$_{12}$ deficiency can occur after many years of metformin use. Periodic screening with vitamin B$_{12}$ levels should be considered, especially in patients with peripheral neuropathy or if a macrocytic anemia develops. Increased intake of dietary calcium may prevent the metformin-induced B$_{12}$ malaborption.

Lactic acidosis has been reported as a side effect but is uncommon with metformin in contrast to phenformin. While therapeutic doses of metformin reduce lactate uptake by the liver, serum lactate levels rise only minimally if at all, since other organs such as the kidney can remove the slight excess. However, if tissue hypoxia occurs, the metformin-treated patient is at higher risk for lactic acidosis due to compromised lactate removal. Similarly, when kidney function deteriorates, affecting not only lactate removal by the kidney but also metformin excretion, plasma levels of metformin rise far above the therapeutic range and block hepatic uptake enough to provoke lactic acidosis without associated increases in lactic acid production. Almost all reported cases have involved subjects with associated risk factors that should have contraindicated its use (kidney, liver, or cardiorespiratory insufficiency, alcoholism, advanced age). Acute kidney failure can occur rarely in certain patients receiving radiocontrast agents. Metformin therapy should therefore be temporarily halted on the day of radiocontrast administration and restarted a day or two later after confirmation that renal function has not deteriorated.

B. Thiazolidinediones—Two medications of this class, rosiglitazone and pioglitazone, are available for clinical use. These medications sensitize peripheral tissues to insulin. They bind a nuclear receptor called peroxisome proliferator-activated receptor gamma (PPAR-gamma) and affect the expression of a number of genes. Observed effects of thiazolidinediones include increased glucose transporter expression (GLUT 1 and GLUT 4), decreased free fatty acid levels, decreased hepatic glucose output, increased adiponectin and decreased release of resistin from adipocytes, and increased differentiation of preadipocytes into adipocytes. They have also been demonstrated to decrease levels of plasminogen activator inhibitor type 1, matrix metalloproteinase 9, C-reactive protein, and interleukin 6. Like the biguanides, this class of medications does not cause hypoglycemia.

Two medications of this class, rosiglitazone and pioglitazone, are available for clinical use. Both are effective as monotherapy and in combination with sulfonylureas or metformin or insulin, lowering HbA$_{1c}$ by 1% to 2%. When used in combination with insulin, they can result in a 30–50% reduction in insulin dosage, and some patients can come off insulin completely. Rosiglitazone is primarily metabolized by the CYP 2C8 isoenzyme and pioglitazone is metabolized by CYP 2C8 and CYP 3A4.

The combination of a thiazolidinedione and metformin has the advantage of not causing hypoglycemia. Patients inadequately managed on sulfonylureas can do well on a combination of sulfonylurea and rosiglitazone or pioglitazone.

These medications have some additional effects apart from glucose lowering. Rosiglitazone therapy is associated with increases in total cholesterol, LDL cholesterol (15%), and HDL cholesterol (10%). There is a reduction in free fatty acids of about 8–15%. The changes in triglycerides were generally not different from placebo. Pioglitazone in clinical trials lowered triglycerides (9%) and increased HDL cholesterol (15%) but did not cause a consistent change in total cholesterol and LDL cholesterol levels. A prospective randomized comparison of the metabolic effects of pioglitazone and rosiglitazone showed similar effects on HbA$_{1c}$ and weight gain. Pioglitazone-treated persons, however, had lower total cholesterol, LDL cholesterol, and triglycerides when compared with rosiglitazone-treated persons. Small prospective studies have demonstrated that treatment with these medications leads to improvements in the biochemical and histologic features of nonalcoholic fatty liver disease. The thiazolidinediones also may limit vascular smooth muscle proliferation after injury, and there are reports that pioglitazone can reduce neointimal proliferation after coronary stent placement. Finally, in one double-blind, placebo-controlled study, rosiglitazone was shown to be associated with a decrease in the ratio of urinary albumin to creatinine excretion.

Safety concerns and some troublesome side effects have emerged about this class of medications that significantly limit their use. A meta-analysis of 42 randomized clinical trials with rosiglitazone suggested that this medication increases the risk of angina pectoris or myocardial infarction. A meta-analysis of clinical trials with pioglitazone did not show similar findings. Although conclusive data were lacking, the European Medicines Agency suspended the use of rosiglitazone in Europe. In the United States, the FDA established a restricted distribution program. A subsequent large prospective clinical trial (the RECORD study) failed to confirm the meta-analysis finding and the restrictions were lifted in the United States. It is unlikely, however, that there is going to be a resurgence in its use and pioglitazone is likely to remain the preferred agent.

Edema occurs in about 3–4% of patients receiving monotherapy with rosiglitazone or pioglitazone. The edema occurs more frequently (10–15%) in patients receiving concomitant insulin therapy and may result in heart failure. The medications are contraindicated in diabetic individuals with New York Heart Association class III and IV cardiac status. Thiazolidinediones have also been reported as being associated with new onset or worsening macular edema. Apparently, this is a rare side effect, and most of these patients also had peripheral edema. The macular edema resolved or improved once the medication was discontinued.

In experimental animals, rosiglitazone stimulates bone marrow adipogenesis at the expense of osteoblastogenesis resulting in a decrease in bone density. An increase in fracture risk in women (but not men) has been reported with both rosiglitazone and pioglitazone. The fracture risk is in the range of 1.9 per 100 patient-years with the thiazolidinedione compared to 1.1 per 100 patient years on comparison treatment. In at least one study of rosiglitazone, the fracture risk was increased in premenopausal as well as postmenopausal women.

Other side effects include anemia, which occurs in 4% of patients treated with these medications; it may be due to a dilutional effect of increased plasma volume rather than a reduction in red cell mass. Weight gain occurs, especially when the medication is combined with a sulfonylurea or insulin. Some of the weight gain is fluid retention, but there is also an increase in total fat mass. In preclinical studies with pioglitazone, bladder tumors were observed in male rats receiving clinically relevant doses of the medication. In a planned 5-year interim analysis of data from a long-term observational cohort study of patients taking pioglitazone, an increased bladder cancer risk was observed with increasing dose and duration of pioglitazone use, reaching statistical significance after 24 months of exposure. In a study sponsored by the manufacturer to evaluate the impact of pioglitazone on macrovascular events (PROactive study), a safety analysis noted 14 cases of bladder cancer in the

treated group and 5 cases in the placebo group ($P = 0.04$). Although there are currently no recommendations regarding screening for bladder cancer, this should be considered in patients receiving long-term pioglitazone therapy.

Troglitazone, the first medication in this class to go into widespread clinical use, was withdrawn from clinical use because of medication-associated fatal liver failure. Although rosiglitazone and pioglitazone have not been reported to cause liver injury, the FDA recommends that they should not be used in patients with clinical evidence of active liver disease or pretreatment elevation of the alanine aminotransferase (ALT) level that is 2.5 times greater than the upper limit of normal. Liver biochemical tests should be performed prior to initiation of treatment and periodically thereafter.

3. Medications that affect absorption of glucose—Alpha-glucosidase inhibitors competitively inhibit the alpha-glucosidase enzymes in the gut that digest dietary starch and sucrose. Two of these medications—acarbose and miglitol—are available for clinical use in the United States. Voglibose, another alpha-glucosidase inhibitor is available in Japan, Korea, and India. Acarbose and miglitol are potent inhibitors of glucoamylase, alpha-amylase, and sucrase but have less effect on isomaltase and hardly any on trehalase and lactase. Acarbose binds 1000 times more avidly to the intestinal disaccharidases than do products of carbohydrate digestion or sucrose. A fundamental difference between acarbose and miglitol is in their absorption. Acarbose has the molecular mass and structural features of a tetrasaccharide, and very little (about 2%) crosses the microvillar membrane. Miglitol, however, has a structural similarity with glucose and is absorbable. Both medications delay the absorption of carbohydrate and lower postprandial glycemic excursion.

A. Acarbose—The recommended starting dose of acarbose is 50 mg twice daily, gradually increasing to 100 mg three times daily. For maximal benefit on postprandial hyperglycemia, acarbose should be given with the first mouthful of food ingested. In diabetic patients, it reduces postprandial hyperglycemia by 30–50%, and its overall effect is to lower the HbA_{1c} by 0.5–1%.

The principal adverse effect, seen in 20–30% of patients, is flatulence. This is caused by undigested carbohydrate reaching the lower bowel, where gases are produced by bacterial flora. In 3% of cases, troublesome diarrhea occurs. This gastrointestinal discomfort tends to discourage excessive carbohydrate consumption and promotes improved compliance of type 2 patients with their diet prescriptions. When acarbose is given alone, there is no risk of hypoglycemia. However, if combined with insulin or sulfonylureas, it might increase the risk of hypoglycemia from these agents. A slight rise in hepatic aminotransferases has been noted in clinical trials with acarbose (5% versus 2% in placebo controls, and particularly with doses > 300 mg/d). The levels generally return to normal on stopping the medication.

In the UKPDS, approximately 2000 patients on diet, sulfonylurea, metformin, or insulin therapy were randomized to acarbose or placebo therapy. By 3 years, 60% of the patients had discontinued the medication, mostly because of gastrointestinal symptoms. If one looked only at the 40% who remained on the medication, they had a 0.5% lower HbA_{1c} compared with placebo.

B. Miglitol—Miglitol is similar to acarbose in terms of its clinical effects. It is indicated for use in diet- or sulfonylurea-treated patients with type 2 diabetes. Therapy is initiated at the lowest effective dosage of 25 mg three times a day. The usual maintenance dose is 50 mg three times a day, although some patients may benefit from increasing the dose to 100 mg three times a day. Gastrointestinal side effects occur as with acarbose. The medication is not metabolized and is excreted unchanged by the kidney. Miglitol should not be used in end-stage chronic kidney disease, when its clearance would be impaired.

4. Incretins—Oral glucose provokes a threefold to fourfold higher insulin response than an equivalent dose of glucose given intravenously. This is because the oral glucose causes a release of gut hormones, principally glucagon-like peptide 1 (GLP-1) and glucose-dependent insulinotropic polypeptide (GIP1), that amplify the glucose-induced insulin release. This "incretin effect" is reduced in patients with type 2 diabetes. GLP-1 secretion (but not GIP1 secretion) is impaired in patients with type 2 diabetes and when GLP-1 is infused in patients with type 2 diabetes, it stimulates insulin secretion and lowers glucose levels. GLP-1, unlike the sulfonylureas, has only a modest insulin stimulatory effect at normoglycemic concentrations. This means that GLP-1 has a lower risk for hypoglycemia than the sulfonylureas.

In addition to its insulin stimulatory effect, GLP-1 also has a number of other pancreatic and extrapancreatic effects. It suppresses glucagon secretion and so may ameliorate the hyperglucagonemia that is present in people with diabetes and improve postprandial hyperglycemia. GLP-1 preserves islet integrity and reduces apoptotic cell death of human islet cells in culture. In mice, streptozotocin-induced apoptosis is significantly reduced by coadministration of exendin-4 or exenatide, a GLP-1 receptor agonist. GLP-1 acts on the stomach delaying gastric emptying; the importance of this effect on glucose lowering is illustrated by the observation that antagonizing the deceleration of gastric emptying markedly reduces the glucose lowering effect of GLP-1. GLP-1 receptors are present in the central nervous system, and intracerebroventricular administration of GLP-1 in wild type mice, but not in GLP-1 receptor knockout mice, inhibits feeding. Type 2 diabetic patients undergoing GLP-1 infusion are less hungry; it is unclear whether this is mainly due to a deceleration of gastric emptying or whether there is a central nervous system effect as well.

A. GLP-1 receptor agonists—GLP-1 is rapidly proteolyzed by dipeptidyl peptidase 4 (DPP-4) and by other enzymes, such as endopeptidase 24.11, and is also cleared rapidly by the kidney. As a result, GLP-1's half-life is only 1–2 minutes. The native peptide, therefore, cannot be used therapeutically and the approach taken has been to develop metabolically stable analogs or derivatives of GLP-1 that are not subject to the same enzymatic degradation or renal clearance. Two GLP-1 receptor agonists, exenatide and liraglutide, are currently available for clinical use.

Exenatide (Exendin 4) is a GLP-1 receptor agonist isolated from the saliva of the Gila Monster (a venomous lizard) that is more resistant to DPP-4 action and cleared by the kidney. Its half-life is 2.4 hours, and its glucose lowering effect is about 6 hours. When this medication is given to patients with type 2 diabetes by subcutaneous injection twice daily, it lowers blood glucose and HbA_{1c} levels. Exenatide appears to have the same effects as GLP-1 on glucagon suppression and gastric emptying. In clinical trials, adding exenatide therapy to patients with type 2 diabetes already taking metformin or a sulfonylurea, or both, further lowered the HbA_{1c} value by 0.4% to 0.6% over a 30-week period. These patients also experienced a weight loss of 3–6 pounds. In an open label extension study up to 80 weeks, the HbA_{1c} reduction was sustained, and there was further weight loss (to a total loss of about 10 pounds). The main side effect was nausea, affecting over 40% of the patients. The nausea was dose-dependent and declined with time. The risk of hypoglycemia was higher in persons taking sulfonylureas. The FDA reported 30 post-marketing reports of acute pancreatitis in patients taking exenatide. The pancreatitis was severe (hemorrhagic or necrotizing) in 6 instances, and two of these patients died. Many of these patients had other risk factors for pancreatitis, but the possibility remains that the medication was causally responsible for some cases. Patients taking exenatide should be advised to seek immediate medical care if they experience unexplained persistent severe abdominal pain. The FDA also reported 16 cases of renal impairment and 62 cases of acute kidney injury in patients taking exenatide. Some of these patients had preexisting kidney disease, and others had one or more risk factors for kidney disease. A number of patients reported nausea, vomiting, and diarrhea; it is possible that these side effects cause volume depletion and contributed to the development of the renal injury. The delay in gastric emptying may affect the absorption of some other medications; therefore, antibiotics and oral contraceptives should be taken 1 hour before exenatide doses. Low-titer antibodies against exenatide develop in over one-third (38%) of patients, but the clinical effects are not attenuated. High-titer antibodies develop in a subset of patients (~6%), and in about half of these cases, an attenuation of glycemic response has been seen. Exenatide stimulates C-cell tumors in rodents and the drug is therefore contraindicated in patients with a personal or family history of medullary thyroid cancer or multiple endocrine neoplasia (MEN) syndrome type 2.

Exenatide is dispensed as two fixed-dose pens (5 mcg and 10 mcg). It is injected 60 minutes before breakfast and before dinner. Patients should be prescribed the 5 mcg pen for the first month and, if tolerated, the dose can then be increased to 10 mcg twice a day. The medication is not recommended in patients with glomerular filtration rate <30 mL/min.

Exenatide LAR is a once weekly preparation that is dispensed as a powder (2 mg). It is suspended in the provided diluent just prior to injection. In comparative clinical trials, the long-acting drug lowers the HbA_{1c} level a little more than the twice daily drug. It is as well tolerated, with nausea being the predominant side effect.

Liraglutide is a soluble fatty acid acylated GLP-1 analog (with replacement of lysine with arginine at position 34 and the attachment of a C16 acyl chain to a lysine at position 26). The fatty-acyl GLP-1 retains affinity for GLP-1 receptors but the addition of the C 16 acyl chain allows for non-covalent binding to albumin, both hindering DPP-4 access to the molecule and contributing to a prolonged half-life and duration of action. The half-life is approximately 12 hours, allowing the medication to be injected once a day.

In clinical trials lasting 26 and 52 weeks, adding liraglutide to the therapeutic regimen (metformin, sulfonylurea, thiazolidinedione) of patients with type 2 diabetes further lowered the HbA_{1c} value. Depending on the dose and design of the study, the HbA_{1c} decline was in the range of 0.6% to 1.5%. The patients had sustained weight loss of 1–6 pounds.

Like exenatide, the most frequent side effects were nausea (28%) and vomiting (10%). There was also an increased incidence of diarrhea. About 2–5% of participants withdrew from the studies because of the gastrointestinal symptoms. In clinical trials, there were seven cases of pancreatitis in the liraglutide treated group with one case in the comparison group (2.2 vs. 0.6 cases per 1000 patient-years). Liraglutide stimulates C-cell neoplasia and causes medullary thyroid carcinoma in rats. Human C-cells express very few GLP1-receptors, and the relevance to human therapy is unclear; however, because of the animal data, the medication should not be used in patients with personal or family history of medullary thyroid carcinoma or multiple endocrine neoplasia (MEN) syndrome type 2. The FDA is conducting ongoing investigation into the risks of pancreatitis and pancreatic duct metaplasia.

The dosing is initiated at 0.6 mg daily, increased after 1 week to 1.2 mg daily. If needed, an additional increase in dose to 1.8 mg is recommended for optimal glycemic control. Titration is also based on tolerability. There is limited experience using the medication in renal failure but no dose adjustment is recommended.

B. DPP-4 INHIBITORS—An alternate approach to the use of GLP-1 receptor agonists is to inhibit the enzyme DPP-4 and prolong the action of endogenously released GLP-1 and GIP. Four oral DPP-4 inhibitors, sitagliptin, saxagliptin, linagliptin, and alogliptin, are available in the United States for the treatment of type 2 diabetes. An additional DPP4 inhibitor, vildagliptin, is available in Europe.

Sitagliptin, when used in clinical trials alone and in combination with metformin and pioglitazone, improved HbA_{1c} from 0.5% to 1.4%. The usual dose of sitagliptin is 100 mg once daily, but the dose is reduced to 50 mg daily if the calculated creatinine clearance is 30–50 mL/min and to 25 mg for clearances < 30 mL/min. Unlike exenatide, sitagliptin does not cause nausea or vomiting. It also does not result in weight loss. The main adverse effect appears to be a predisposition to nasopharyngitis or upper respiratory tract infection. A small increase in neutrophil count of ~200 cells/mcL has also occurred. Since its FDA approval and clinical use, there have been reports of serious allergic

reactions to sitagliptin, including anaphylaxis, angioedema, and exfoliative skin conditions including Stevens-Johnson syndrome. There have also been reports of pancreatitis (88 cases including 2 cases of hemorrhagic or necrotizing pancreatitis). The frequency of these events is unclear. A number of neuropeptides, growth factors, cytokines, and chemokines are potential DPP-4 substrates; DPP-4 inhibitors prolong the actions of neuropeptide Y and substance P. It is unknown whether the effects of DPP-4 inhibitors on the actions of neuropeptide Y and substance P over a long-term period will have negative consequences.

Saxagliptin, when added to the therapeutic regimen (metformin, sulfonylurea, thiazolidinedione) of patients with type 2 diabetes, further lowered the HbA_{1c} value by about 0.7–0.9%. The dose is 2.5 mg or 5 mg once a day. The 2.5-mg dose should be used in patients with calculated creatinine clearance < 50 mL/min. It lowers HbA_{1c} by about 0.6% when added to metformin or glyburide or thiazolidine in various 24-week clinical trials. The medication does not cause weight gain or loss. The main adverse reactions were upper respiratory tract infection, nasopharyngitis, headache, and urinary tract infection. There is also small reversible dose-dependent reduction in absolute lymphocyte count, which remains within normal limits. Hypersensitivity reactions, such as urticaria and facial edema, occurred in 1.5% of patients taking the medication compared with 0.4% receiving placebo. The metabolism of saxagliptin is by CYP3A4/5; thus, strong inhibitors or inducers of CYP3A4/5 will affect the pharmacokinetics of saxagliptin and its active metabolite.

Linagliptin lowers HbA_{1c} by about 0.4–0.6% when added to metformin, sulfonylurea, or pioglitazone. The dose is 5 mg daily and, since it is primarily excreted unmetabolized via the bile, no dose adjustment is needed in patients with renal failure. The adverse reactions include nasopharyngitis and hypersensitivity reactions (urticaria, angioedema, localized skin exfoliation, bronchial hyperreactivity). In one study, there were eight cases of pancreatitis in 4687 patients exposed to drug (4311 patient years) with 0 cases in 1183 patients receiving placebo (433 patient years).

Vildagliptin lowers HbA_{1c} by about 0.5–1% when added to the therapeutic regimen of patients with type 2 diabetes. The dose is 50 mg once or twice daily. Adverse reactions include upper respiratory tract infections, nasopharyngitis, dizziness, and headache. Rare cases of hepatic dysfunction, including hepatitis, have been reported. Liver function testing is recommended quarterly during the first year of use and periodically thereafter. Animal studies using much higher doses of DPP-4 inhibitors and GLP1-receptor agonists than are used in humans caused expansion of pancreatic ductal glands and generation of premalignant pancreatic intraepithelial (PanIN) lesions that have the potential to progress to pancreatic adenocarcinoma. There is, however, currently no evidence that these drugs cause pancreatic cancer in humans.

5. Sodium-glucose co-transporter 2 inhibitors—Glucose is freely filtered by the renal glomeruli and is reabsorbed in the proximal tubules by the action of sodium-glucose co-transporters (SGLT). Sodium-glucose co-transporter 2 (SGLT2) accounts for about 90% of glucose reabsorption and its inhibition causes glycosuria in people with diabetes, lowering plasma glucose levels. The SGLT2 inhibitors canagliflozin and dapagliflozin are approved for clinical use in the United States.

Canagliflozin reduces the threshold for glycosuria from a plasma glucose threshold of ~180 mg/dL to 70–90 mg/dL. It has been shown to reduce HbA_{1c} by 0.6–1% when used alone or in combination with other oral agents or insulin. It also results in modest weight loss of 2–5 kg. The usual dose is 100 mg daily but up to 300 mg daily can be used in patients with normal kidney function.

Dapagliflozin is an SGLT2 inhibitor that has been shown to reduce HbA_{1c} levels by 0.5–0.8% when used alone or in combination with other oral agents or insulin. It also results in modest weight loss of about 2–4 kg. The usual dose is 10 mg daily but 5 mg daily is the recommended initial dose in patients with hepatic failure.

As might be expected, the efficacy of the SGLT2 inhibitors is reduced in chronic kidney disease. Canagliflozin is contraindicated in patients with estimated glomerular filtration rate < 45 mL/min/1.73 m². The main side effects are increased incidence of genital infections and urinary tract infections affecting ~8–9% of patients. The glycosuria can cause intravascular volume contraction and hypotension. Canagliflozin caused a modest increase in LDL cholesterol levels (4–8%). Also, in clinical trials, patients taking dapagliflozin had higher rates of breast cancer (nine cases vs none in comparator arms) and bladder cancer (10 cases vs 1 in placebo arm). These cancer rates exceeded the expected rates in age-matched reference diabetes population.

6. Others—**Pramlintide** is a synthetic analog of islet amyloid polypeptide (IAPP or amylin). When given subcutaneously, it delays gastric emptying, suppresses glucagon secretion, and decreases appetite. It is approved for use both in type 1 diabetes and in insulin-treated type 2 diabetes. In 6-month clinical studies with type 1 and insulin-treated type 2 patients, those taking the medication had an approximately 0.4% reduction in HbA_{1c} and about 1.7 kg weight loss compared with placebo. The HbA_{1c} reduction was sustained for 2 years but some of the weight was regained. The medication is given by injection immediately before the meal. Hypoglycemia can occur, and it is recommended that the short-acting or premixed insulin doses be reduced by 50% when the medication is started. Since the medication slows gastric emptying, recovery from hypoglycemia can be a problem because of delay in absorption of fast-acting carbohydrates. Nausea was the other main side effect, affecting 30–50% of persons but tended to improve with time. In patients with type 1 diabetes, the initial dose of pramlintide is 15 mcg before each meal and titrated up by 15 mcg increments to a maintenance dose of 30 mcg or 60 mcg before each meal. In patients with type 2 diabetes, the starting dose is 60 mcg premeals increased to 120 mcg in 3 to 7 days if no significant nausea occurs.

Bromocriptine, a dopamine 2 receptor agonist, has been shown to modestly lower HbA_{1c} by 0.1–0.5% when compared to baseline and 0.4–0.5% compared to placebo. The tablet dose is 0.8 mg and the daily dose is 2 (1.6 g) to 6 (4.8 mg) tablets as tolerated. Common side effects are nausea, vomiting, dizziness, and headache.

Colesevelam, the bile acid sequesterant, when added to metformin or sulfonylurea or insulin lowered HbA_{1c} 0.3– 0.4 % when compared to baseline and 0.5–0.6% compared to placebo. HbA_{1c} lowering, however, was not observed in a single monotherapy clinical trial comparing colesevelam to placebo. Colesevelam use is associated with ~20% increase in triglyceride levels. Other adverse effects include constipation and dyspepsia.

With their modest glucose lowering and significant side effects, using bromocriptine or colesevelam to treat diabetes is not recommended.

7. Medication combinations—Several medication combinations are available in different dose sizes, including glyburide and metformin (Glucovance); glipizide and metformin (Metaglip); repaglinide and metformin (PrandiMet); rosiglitazone and metformin (Avandamet); pioglitazone and metformin (ACTOplusMet); rosiglitazone and glimepiride (Avandaryl); pioglitazone and glimepiride (Duetact); sitagliptin and metformin (Janumet); saxagliptin and metformin XR (Kombiglyze XR); linagliptin and metformin (Jentadueto); alogliptin and metformin (Kazano); and alogliptin and pioglitazone (Oseni). These medication combinations, however, limit the clinician's ability to optimally adjust dosage of the individual medications and for that reason are not recommended.

8. Safety of the antihyperglycemic agents—The UKPDS has put to rest previous concerns regarding the safety of sulfonylureas. It did not confirm any cardiovascular hazard among over 1500 patients treated intensively with sulfonylureas for over 10 years, compared with a comparable number who received either insulin or diet therapy. Analysis of a subgroup of obese patients receiving metformin also showed no hazard and even a slight reduction in cardiovascular deaths compared with conventional therapy.

C. Insulin

Insulin is indicated for type 1 diabetes as well as for type 2 diabetic patients with insulinopenia whose hyperglycemia does not respond to diet therapy either alone or combined with other hypoglycemic medications.

1. Characteristics of available insulin preparations—Commercial insulin preparations differ with respect to the time of onset and duration of their biologic action (Table 27–6).

Human insulin is produced by recombinant DNA techniques (biosynthetic human insulin) as Humulin (Eli Lilly) and as Novolin (Novo Nordisk). It is dispensed as either regular (R) or NPH (N) formulations. Five analogs of human insulin—three rapidly acting (insulin lispro, insulin aspart, insulin glulisine) and two long-acting (insulin glargine and insulin detemir)—have been approved by the FDA for clinical use (Table 27–7). Animal insulins are no longer available in the United States. All currently available insulins contain < 10 ppm of proinsulin and are labeled as "purified." These purified insulins preserve their potency, so that refrigeration is recommended but not crucial. During travel, reserve supplies of insulin can be readily transported for weeks without losing potency if protected from

Table 27–6. Summary of bioavailability characteristics of the insulins.

Insulin Preparations	Onset of Action	Peak Action	Effective Duration
Insulins lispro, aspart, glulisine	5–15 minutes	1–1.5 hours	3–4 hours
Human regular	30–60 minutes	2 hours	6–8 hours
Human NPH	2–4 hours	6–7 hours	10–20 hours
Insulin glargine	1.5 hours	Flat	~24 hours
Insulin detemir	1 hour	Flat	17 hours

extremes of heat or cold. All the insulins in the United States are available in a concentration of 100 units/mL (U100) and dispensed in 10 mL vials or 0.3 mL cartridges or prefilled disposable pens. For use in rare cases of severe insulin resistance, regular insulin in a concentration of 500 units/mL (U500) is available in 10 mL vial.

2. Insulin preparations—The short-acting preparations are regular insulin and the rapidly acting insulin analogs. They are dispensed as clear solutions at neutral pH and contain small amounts of zinc to improve their stability and shelf life. The long-acting preparations are NPH insulin and the long-acting insulin analogs. NPH insulin is dispensed as a turbid suspension at neutral pH with protamine in phosphate buffer. The long-acting insulin analogs are also dispensed as clear solutions; insulin glargine is at acidic pH and insulin detemir is at neutral pH.

A. SHORT-ACTING INSULIN PREPARATIONS—

(1) Regular insulin— Regular insulin is a short-acting soluble crystalline zinc insulin whose effect appears within 30 minutes after subcutaneous injection and lasts 5–7 hours

Table 27–7. Insulin preparations available in the United States.[1]

Rapidly acting human insulin analogs
   Insulin lispro (Humalog, Lilly)
   Insulin aspart (Novolog, Novo Nordisk)
   Insulin glulisine (Apidra, Sanofi Aventis)
Short-acting regular insulin
   Regular insulin (Lilly, Novo Nordisk)
Intermediate-acting insulins
   NPH insulin (Lilly, Novo Nordisk)
Premixed insulins
   70% NPH/30% regular (70/30 insulin—Lilly, Novo Nordisk)
   70% NPL/25% insulin lispro (Humalog Mix 75/25—Lilly)
   50% NPL/50% insulin lispro (Humalog Mix 50/50—Lilly)
   70% insulin aspart protamine/30% insulin aspart (Novolog Mix 70/30—Novo Nordisk)
Long-acting human insulin analogs
   Insulin glargine (Lantus, Sanofi Aventis)
   Insulin detemir (Levemir, Novo Nordisk)

[1]All insulins available in the United States are recombinant human or human insulin analog origin. All the above insulins are dispensed at U100 concentration. There is an additional U500 preparation of regular insulin.
NPH, neutral protamine Hagedorn.

when usual quantities are administered. Intravenous infusions of regular insulin are particularly useful in the treatment of diabetic ketoacidosis and during the perioperative management of insulin-requiring diabetics. Regular insulin is indicated when the subcutaneous insulin requirement is changing rapidly, such as after surgery or during acute infections—although the rapidly acting insulin analogs may be preferable in these situations.

For markedly insulin-resistant persons who would otherwise require large volumes of insulin solution, a U500 preparation of human regular insulin is available. Since a U500 syringe is not available, when U500 insulin is required in cases of severe insulin resistance, a U100 insulin syringe or tuberculin syringe must be used to measure doses. The clinician should carefully note dosages in both units and volume to avoid overdosage.

(2) Rapidly acting insulin analogs—Insulin lispro (Humalog), is an insulin analog produced by recombinant technology, wherein two amino acids near the carboxyl terminal of the B chain have been reversed in position: Proline at position B28 has been moved to B29 and lysine has been moved from B29 to B28. Insulin aspart (Novolog), is a single substitution of proline by aspartic acid at position B28. Insulin glulisine (Apidra) differs from human insulin in that the amino acid asparagine at position B3 is replaced by lysine and the lysine in position B29 by glutamic acid. These changes result in these three analogs that have less tendency to form hexamers, in contrast to human insulin. When injected subcutaneously, the analogs quickly dissociate into monomers and are absorbed very rapidly, reaching peak serum values in as soon as 1 hour—in contrast to regular human insulin, whose hexamers require considerably more time to dissociate and become absorbed. The amino acid changes in these analogs do not interfere with their binding to the insulin receptor, with the circulating half-life, or with their immunogenicity, which are all identical with those of human regular insulin.

Clinical trials have demonstrated that the optimal times of preprandial subcutaneous injection of comparable doses of the rapidly acting insulin analogs and of regular human insulin are 20 minutes and 60 minutes, respectively, before the meal. While this more rapid onset of action has been welcomed as a great convenience by diabetic patients who object to waiting as long as 60 minutes after injecting regular human insulin before they can begin their meal, patients must be taught to ingest adequate absorbable carbohydrate early in the meal to avoid hypoglycemia during the meal. Another desirable feature of rapidly acting insulin analogs is that their duration of action remains at about 4 hours irrespective of dosage. This contrasts with regular insulin, whose duration of action is prolonged when larger doses are used.

The rapidly acting analogs are also commonly used in pumps. In a double-blind crossover study comparing insulin lispro with regular insulin in insulin pumps, persons using insulin lispro had lower HbA_{1c} values and improved postprandial glucose control with the same frequency of hypoglycemia. In the event of pump failure, however, users of the rapidly acting insulin analogs will have more rapid onset of hyperglycemia and ketosis.

While insulin aspart has been approved for intravenous use (eg, in hyperglycemic emergencies), there is no advantage in using insulin aspart over regular insulin by this route.

B. Long-acting insulin preparations

(1) NPH (neutral protamine Hagedorn or isophane) insulin—NPH is an intermediate-acting insulin whose onset of action is delayed by combining 2 parts soluble crystalline zinc insulin with 1 part protamine zinc insulin. This produces equivalent amounts of insulin and protamine, so that neither is present in an uncomplexed form ("isophane").

Its onset of action is delayed to 2–4 hours, and its peak response is generally reached in about 6–7 hours. Because its duration of action is often < 24 hours (with a range of 10–20 hours), most patients require at least two injections daily to maintain a sustained insulin effect. Occasional vials of NPH insulin have tended to show unusual clumping of their contents or "frosting" of the container, with considerable loss of bioactivity. This instability is rare and occurs less frequently if NPH human insulin is refrigerated when not in use and if bottles are discarded after 1 month of use.

(2) Insulin glargine—Insulin glargine is an insulin analog in which the asparagine at position 21 of the A chain of the human insulin molecule is replaced by glycine and two arginines are added to the carboxyl terminal of the B chain. The arginines raise the isoelectric point of the molecule closer to neutral, making it more soluble in an acidic environment. In contrast, human insulin has an isoelectric point of pH 5.4. Insulin glargine is a clear insulin, which, when injected into the neutral pH environment of the subcutaneous tissue, forms microprecipitates that slowly release the insulin into the circulation. It lasts for about 24 hours without any pronounced peaks and is given once a day to provide basal coverage. This insulin cannot be mixed with the other human insulins because of its acidic pH. When this insulin was given as a single injection at bedtime to type 1 patients in clinical trials, fasting hyperglycemia was better controlled with less nocturnal hypoglycemia when compared to NPH insulin.

Although limited clinical data suggest that insulin glargine is safe in pregnancy, it is not approved for this use.

(3) Insulin detemir—Insulin detemir is an insulin analog. The tyrosine at position 30 of the beta chain has been removed and a 14-C fatty acid chain (tetradecanoic acid) is attached to the lysine at position 29 by acylation. The fatty acid chain makes the molecule more lipophilic than native insulin and the addition of zinc stabilizes the molecule and leads to formation of hexamers. Its prolonged action is due to dihexamerization and binding of hexamers and dimers to albumin at the injection site as well as binding of the monomer via its fatty acid side chain to albumin in the circulation. The affinity of insulin detemir is fourfold to fivefold lower than that of human soluble insulin and therefore the U100 formulation of insulin detemir has an insulin concentration of 2400 nmol/mL compared with 600 nmol/mL for NPH. The duration of action for insulin detemir is about 17 hours at therapeutically relevant doses. It is recommended that the insulin be injected once or twice a day to achieve a stable basal coverage. This insulin has been reported to have lower within-subject pharmacodynamic variability compared with NPH insulin and insulin glargine. In vitro studies do not suggest any clinically relevant albumin binding interactions between insulin detemir and fatty acids or protein-bound medications. Since there is a vast excess (~400,000) of albumin binding sites available in plasma per insulin detemir molecule, it is unlikely that hypoalbuminemic disease states affect the ratio of bound to free insulin detemir.

C. Mixed insulin preparations—Since intermediate insulins require several hours to reach adequate therapeutic levels, their use in patients with type 1 diabetes requires supplements of regular or rapidly acting insulin analogs preprandially. For convenience, regular or rapidly acting insulin analogs and NPH insulin may be mixed together in the same syringe and injected subcutaneously in split dosage before breakfast and supper. It is recommended that the regular insulin or rapidly acting insulin analog be withdrawn first, then the NPH insulin and that the injection be given immediately after loading the syringe. Stable premixed insulins (70% NPH and 30% regular) are available as a convenience to patients who have difficulty mixing insulin because of visual problems or impairment of manual dexterity. Premixed preparations of insulin lispro and NPH insulins are unstable because of exchange of insulin lispro with the human insulin in the protamine complex. Consequently, the soluble component becomes over time a mixture of regular and insulin lispro at varying ratios. In an attempt to remedy this, an intermediate insulin composed of isophane complexes of protamine with insulin lispro was developed called NPL (neutral protamine lispro). This insulin has the same duration of action as NPH insulin. Premixed combinations of NPL and insulin lispro—(75% NPL/25% insulin lispro mixture [Humalog Mix 75/25] and 50% NPL/50% insulin lispro mixture [Humalog Mix 50/50]) are available for clinical use. Similarly, a 70% insulin aspart protamine/30% insulin aspart (NovoLog Mix 70/30) is available. The main advantages of these mixtures are that they can be given within 15 minutes of starting a meal and they are superior in controlling the postprandial glucose rise after a carbohydrate rich meal. These benefits have not translated into improvements in HbA_{1c} levels when compared with the usual 70% NPH/30% regular mixture.

The longer-acting insulin analogs cannot be mixed with either regular insulin or the rapidly acting insulin analogs.

3. Methods of insulin administration—

A. Insulin syringes and needles—Plastic disposable syringes are available in 1 mL, 0.5 mL, and 0.3 mL sizes. The "low-dose" 0.3 mL syringes have become increasingly popular, because many diabetics do not take more than 30 units of insulin in a single injection except in rare instances of extreme insulin resistance. Two lengths of needles are available: short (8 mm) and long (12.7 mm). Long needles are preferable in obese patients to reduce variability of insulin absorption. Ultrafine needles as small as 31 gauge reduce the pain of injections. "Disposable" syringes may be reused until blunting of the needle occurs (usually after three to five injections). Sterility adequate to avoid infection with reuse appears to be maintained by recapping syringes between uses. Cleansing the needle with alcohol may not be desirable since it can dissolve the silicone coating and can increase the pain of skin puncturing.

Any part of the body covered by loose skin can be used, such as the abdomen, thighs, upper arms, flanks, and upper buttocks. Preparation with alcohol is no longer required prior to injection as long as the skin is clean. Rotation of sites continues to be recommended to avoid delayed absorption when fibrosis or lipohypertrophy occurs from repeated use of a single site. However, considerable variability of absorption rates from different sites, particularly with exercise, may contribute to the instability of glycemic control in certain type 1 patients if injection sites are rotated too frequently in different areas of the body. Consequently, it is best to limit injection sites to a single region of the body and rotate sites within that region. The abdomen is recommended for subcutaneous injections, since regular insulin has been shown to absorb more rapidly from there than from other subcutaneous sites. The effect of anatomic regions appears to be much less pronounced with the analog insulins.

B. Insulin pen injector devices—Insulin pens eliminate the need for carrying insulin vials and syringes. Cartridges of insulin lispro and insulin aspart are available for reusable pens (Eli Lilly, Novo Nordisk, and Owen Mumford). Disposable prefilled pens are also available for insulin lispro, insulin aspart, insulin glulisine, insulin detemir, insulin glargine, NPH, 70% NPH/30% regular, 75% NPL/25% insulin lispro, 50% NPL/50% insulin lispro, and 70% insulin aspart protamine/ 30% insulin aspart. Thirty-one gauge needles (5, 6, and 8 mm long) for these pens make injections almost painless.

C. Insulin pumps—In the United States, Medtronic Mini-Med, Animas, Insulet, Roche, and Tandem make battery operated continuous subcutaneous insulin infusion (CSII) pumps. These pumps are small (about the size of a pager) and very easy to program. They offer many features, including the ability to set a number of different basal rates throughout the 24 hours and to adjust the time over which bolus doses are given. They also are able to detect pressure build-up if the catheter is kinked. The catheter connecting the insulin reservoir to the subcutaneous cannula can be disconnected, allowing the patient to remove the pump temporarily (eg, for bathing). Ominpod (Insulet Corporation) is an insulin infusion system in which the insulin reservoir and infusion set are integrated into one unit (pod), so there is no catheter (electronic patch pump). The pod, placed on the skin, delivers subcutaneous basal and bolus insulin based on wirelessly transmitted instructions from a personal digital assistant. The great advantage of continuous subcutaneous insulin infusion (CSII) is that it allows for establishment of a basal profile tailored to the patient. The patient therefore is able to eat with less regard to timing because the basal insulin infusion should maintain constant blood glucose between meals. Also the ability to adjust the basal insulin infusion makes it easier for the patient to manage glycemic excursions that occur with exercise. The pumps also have software that can assist the patient to calculate boluses based on glucose reading and carbohydrates to be consumed. They keep track of the time elapsed since last insulin bolus and the patient is reminded of this when he or she attempts to give additional correction bolus before the effect of the previous bolus has worn off ("insulin on board" feature). This feature reduces the risk of overcorrecting and subsequent hypoglycemia.

CSII therapy is appropriate for patients with type 1 diabetes who are motivated, mechanically inclined, educated about diabetes (diet, insulin action, treatment of hypoglycemia and hyperglycemia), and willing to monitor their blood glucose four to six times a day. Known complications of CSII include ketoacidosis, which can occur when insulin delivery is interrupted, and skin infections. Another disadvantage is its cost and the time demanded of the clinician and staff in initiating therapy.

V-go (Valeritas) is a mechanical patch pump designed specifically for people with type 2 diabetes who employ a basal/bolus insulin regimen. The device is preset to deliver one of three fixed and flat basal rates (20, 30, or 40 units) for 24 hours (at which point it must be replaced) and there is a button that delivers two units per press to help cover meals.

D. Inhaled insulin—There is currently only one pharmaceutical company conducting clinical trials with inhaled insulin (Technosphere insulin, MannKind Corporation). Exubera, the first inhaled insulin preparation approved by the FDA, is no longer available; the manufacturer stopped marketing it because of lack of demand.

D. Transplantation

Pancreas transplantation at the time of kidney transplantation is becoming more widely accepted. Patients undergoing simultaneous pancreas and kidney transplantation have an 83% chance of pancreatic graft survival at 1 year and 69% at 5 years. Solitary pancreatic transplantation in the absence of a need for kidney transplantation is considered only in those rare patients who do not respond to all other insulin therapeutic approaches and who have frequent severe hypoglycemia or who have life-threatening complications related to their lack of metabolic control. Pancreas transplant alone graft survival is 78% at 1 year and 54% at 5 years.

People with type 1 diabetes can become insulin independent after receiving an **islet cell transplant.** The islets are isolated from donor pancreas using controlled digestion with collagenase followed by density gradient centrifugation. The isolated islets are then infused into the portal vein using a percutaneous transhepatic approach and they lodge in the liver releasing insulin in response to physiologic stimuli. Long-term immunosuppression is necessary to prevent allograft rejection and to suppress the autoimmune process that led to the disease in the first place. Insulin independence for more than 5 years has been demonstrated in patients who got anti-CD3 antibody or anti-thymocyte globulin induction immunosuppression and calcineurin inhibitors, mTor inhibitors, and mycophenolate mofetil as maintenance immunosuppression. Islet cell transplant trials with different kinds and combinations of immunosuppressive agents are currently underway. One major limitation is the need for more than one islet infusion to achieve insulin independence. This is because of significant loss of islets during isolation and the period prior to engraftment. Widespread application of islet transplantation will depend on improving insulin independence rates with one infusion and also demonstrating that the long-term outcomes are as good as those of pancreas transplant alone.

Bennett WL et al. Comparative effectiveness and safety of medications for type 2 diabetes: an update including new drugs and 2-drug combinations. Ann Intern Med. 2011 May 3;154(9):602–13. Erratum in: Ann Intern Med. 2011 Jul 5;155(1):67–8. [PMID: 21403054]

▶ Steps in the Management of the Diabetic Patient

A. Diagnostic Examination

An attempt should be made to characterize the diabetes as type 1 or type 2, based on the clinical features present and on whether or not ketonuria accompanies the glycosuria. Features that suggest end-organ insulin insensitivity to insulin, such as visceral obesity, acanthosis nigricans, or both, must be identified. The family history should document not only the incidence of diabetes in other members of the family but also the age at onset, association with obesity, the need for insulin, and whether there were complications. For the occasional patient, measurement of ICA, GAD65, IAA, and ICA 512 antibodies can help distinguish between type 1 and type 2 diabetes. Many patients with newly diagnosed type 1 diabetes still have significant endogenous insulin production, and C peptide levels do not reliably distinguish between type 1 and type 2 diabetes. Other factors that increase cardiac risk, such as smoking history, presence of hypertension or hyperlipidemia, or oral contraceptive pill use, should be recorded.

Laboratory diagnosis of diabetes should document fasting plasma glucose levels above 126 mg/dL (7 mmol/L) or postprandial values consistently above 200 mg/dL (11.1 mmol/L) or HbA_{1c} of at least 6.5% and whether ketonuria accompanies the glycosuria. An HbA_{1c} measurement is also useful for assessing the effectiveness of future therapy. Baseline values include fasting plasma triglycerides, total cholesterol and HDL-cholesterol, electrocardiography, kidney function studies, peripheral pulses, and neurologic, podiatric, and ophthalmologic examinations to help guide future assessments.

B. Patient Education (Self-Management Training)

Since diabetes is a lifelong disorder, education of the patient and the family is probably the most important obligation of the clinician who provides initial care. The best persons to manage a disease that is affected so markedly by daily fluctuations in environmental stress, exercise, diet, and infections are the patients themselves and their families. The "teaching curriculum" should include explanations by the clinician or nurse of the nature of diabetes and its potential acute and chronic hazards and how they can be recognized early and prevented or treated. Self-monitoring of blood glucose should be emphasized, especially in insulin-requiring diabetic patients, and instructions must be given on proper testing and recording of data.

Patients taking insulin should have an understanding of the actions of basal and bolus insulins. They should be taught to determine whether the basal dose is appropriate and how to adjust the rapidly acting insulin dose for the carbohydrate content of a meal. Patients and their families and friends should be taught to recognize signs and symptoms of hypoglycemia and how to treat low glucose reactions. Strenuous exercise can precipitate hypoglycemia, and patients must therefore be taught to reduce their insulin dosage in anticipation of strenuous activity or to take supplemental carbohydrate. Injection of insulin into a site farthest away from the muscles most involved in the exercise may help ameliorate exercise-induced hypoglycemia, since insulin injected in the proximity of exercising muscle may be more rapidly mobilized. Exercise training also increases the effectiveness of insulin and insulin doses should be adjusted accordingly. Infections can cause insulin resistance, and patients should be instructed on how to manage the hyperglycemia with supplemental rapidly acting insulin.

The targets for blood glucose control should be elevated appropriately in elderly patients since they have the greatest risk if subjected to hypoglycemia and the least long-term benefit from more rigid glycemic control. Advice on personal hygiene, including detailed instructions on foot and dental care, should be provided. All infections (especially pyogenic ones) provoke the release of high levels of insulin antagonists, such as catecholamines or glucagon, and thus bring about a marked increase in insulin requirements. Patients who are taking oral agents may decompensate and temporarily require insulin. Patients should be told about community agencies, such as Diabetes Association chapters, that can serve as a continuing source of instruction.

Finally, vigorous efforts should be made to persuade patients with newly diagnosed diabetes who smoke to give up the habit, since large vessel peripheral vascular disease and debilitating retinopathy are less common in nonsmoking diabetic patients.

C. Therapy

Treatment must be individualized on the basis of the type of diabetes and specific needs of each patient. However, certain general principles of management can be outlined for hyperglycemic states of different types.

1. Type 1 diabetes—Traditional once- or twice-daily insulin regimens are usually ineffective in type 1 patients without residual endogenous insulin. In these patients, information and counseling based on the findings of the DCCT (see above) should be provided about the advantages of taking multiple injections of insulin in conjunction with self-blood glucose monitoring. If near-normalization of blood glucose is attempted, at least four measurements of capillary blood glucose and three or four insulin injections are necessary.

A combination of rapidly acting insulin analogs and long-acting insulin analogs allows for more physiologic insulin replacement. The rapidly acting insulin analogs have been advocated as a safer and much more convenient alternative to regular human insulin for preprandial use. In a study comparing regular insulin with insulin lispro, daily insulin doses and HbA$_{1c}$ levels were similar, but insulin lispro improved postprandial control, reduced hypoglycemic episodes, and improved patient convenience compared with regular insulin. However, because of their relatively short duration (no more than 3–4 hours), the rapidly acting insulin analogs need to be combined with longer-acting insulins to provide basal coverage and avoid hyperglycemia prior to the next meal. In addition to carbohydrate content of the meal, the effect of simultaneous fat ingestion must also be considered a factor in determining the rapidly acting insulin analog dosage required to control the glycemic increment during and just after the meal. With low-carbohydrate content and high-fat intake, there is an increased risk of hypoglycemia from insulin lispro within 2 hours after the meal. Table 27–8 illustrates a regimen with a rapidly acting insulin analog and insulin detemir or insulin glargine that might be appropriate for a 70-kg person with type 1 diabetes eating meals providing standard carbohydrate intake and moderate to low fat content.

Insulin glargine is usually given once in the evening to provide 24-hour coverage. This insulin *cannot be mixed* with any of the other insulins and must be given as a separate injection. There are occasional patients in whom insulin glargine does not seem to last for 24 hours, and in such cases it needs to be given twice a day. As shown, insulin detemir may also need to be given twice a day to get adequate 24-hour basal coverage. Alternatively, small doses of NPH (~3–4 units) can be given with each meal to provide daytime basal coverage with a larger dose at night. Unlike the long-acting insulin analogs, NPH can be mixed in the same syringe as the insulin lispro, insulin aspart, and insulin glulisine.

Continuous subcutaneous insulin infusion (CSII) by portable battery-operated "open loop" devices currently provides the most flexible approach, allowing the setting of different basal rates throughout the 24 hours and permitting patients to delay or skip meals and vary meal size and composition. The dosage is usually based on providing

Table 27–8. Examples of intensive insulin regimens using rapidly acting insulin analogs (insulin lispro, aspart, or glulisine) and insulin detemir, or insulin glargine in a 70-kg man with type 1 diabetes.[1–3]

	Pre-Breakfast	Pre-Lunch	Pre-Dinner	At Bedtime
Rapidly acting insulin analog	5 units	4 units	6 units	
Insulin detemir	6–7 units			8–9 units
OR				
Rapidly acting insulin analog	5 units	4 units	6 units	—
Insulin glargine		—		15–16 units

[1]Assumes that patient is consuming approximately 75 g carbohydrate at breakfast, 60 g at lunch, and 90 g at dinner.
[2]The dose of rapidly acting insulin can be raised by 1 or 2 units if extra carbohydrate (15–30 g) is ingested or if premeal blood glucose is > 170 mg/dL (9.4 mmol/L).
[3]Insulin glargine or insulin detemir must be given as a separate injection.

50% of the estimated insulin dose as basal and the remainder as intermittent boluses prior to meals. For example, a 70-kg man requiring 35 units of insulin per day may require a basal rate of 0.7 units per hour throughout the 24 hours with the exception of 3 AM to 8 AM, when 0.8 units per hour might be appropriate (given the "dawn phenomenon"—reduced tissue sensitivity to insulin between 5 AM and 8 AM). The meal bolus would depend on the carbohydrate content of the meal and the premeal blood glucose value. **One unit per 15 g of carbohydrate plus 1 unit for 50 mg/dL (2.8 mmol/L) of blood glucose above a target value (eg, 120 mg/dL [6.7 mmol/L]) is a common starting point.** Further adjustments to basal and bolus dosages would depend on the results of blood glucose monitoring. The majority of patients use the rapidly acting insulin analogs in the pumps. One of the more difficult therapeutic problems in managing patients with type 1 diabetes is determining the proper adjustment of insulin dose when the prebreakfast blood glucose level is high. Occasionally, the prebreakfast hyperglycemia is due to the Somogyi effect, in which nocturnal hypoglycemia leads to a surge of counterregulatory hormones to produce high blood glucose levels by 7 AM. However, a more common cause for prebreakfast hyperglycemia is the waning of circulating insulin levels by the morning. Also, the dawn phenomenon is present in as many as 75% of type 1 patients and can aggravate the hyperglycemia.

The diagnosis of the cause of prebreakfast hyperglycemia can be facilitated by self-monitoring of blood glucose at 3 AM in addition to the usual bedtime and 7 AM measurements (Table 27–9). This is required for only a few nights, and when a particular pattern emerges from monitoring blood glucose levels overnight, appropriate therapeutic measures can be taken. The Somogyi effect can be

Table 27–9. Prebreakfast hyperglycemia: Classification by blood glucose and insulin levels.

	Blood Glucose (mg/dL) [mmol/L]			Free Immunoreactive Insulin (microunit/mL)		
	10:00 PM	3:00 AM	7:00 AM	10:00 PM	3:00 AM	7:00 AM
Somogyi effect	90 [5]	40 [2.2]	200 [11.1]	High	Slightly high	Normal
Dawn phenomenon	110 [6.1]	110 [6.1]	150 [8.3]	Normal	Normal	Normal
Waning of insulin dose plus dawn phenomenon	110 [6.1]	190 [10.6]	220 [12.2]	Normal	Low	Low
Waning of insulin dose plus dawn phenomenon plus Somogyi effect	110 [6.1]	40 [2.2]	380 [21.1]	High	Normal	Low

treated by eliminating the dose of intermediate insulin at dinnertime and giving it at a lower dosage at bedtime or by supplying more food at bedtime. When a waning insulin level is the cause, then either increasing the evening dose or shifting it from dinnertime to bedtime (or both) can be effective. A bedtime dose either of insulin glargine or insulin detemir provides more sustained overnight insulin levels than human NPH and may be effective in managing refractory prebreakfast hyperglycemia. If this fails, insulin pump therapy may be required.

2. Type 2 diabetes—Therapeutic recommendations are based on the relative contributions of beta cell insufficiency and insulin insensitivity in individual patients. The possibility that the individual patient has a specific etiologic cause for their diabetes should always be considered, especially when the patient does not have a family history of type 2 diabetes or does not have any evidence of central obesity or insulin resistance. Such patients should be evaluated for other types of diabetes such as LADA or MODY. Patients with LADA should be prescribed insulin when the disease is diagnosed and treated like patients with type 1 diabetes. It is also important to note that many patients with type 2 diabetes mellitus have a progressive loss of beta cell function and will require additional therapeutic interventions with time.

A. WEIGHT REDUCTION—One of the primary modes of therapy in the obese patient with type 2 diabetes is weight reduction. Normalization of glycemia can be achieved by weight loss and improvement in tissue sensitivity to insulin. A combination of caloric restriction, increased exercise, and behavior modification is required if a weight reduction program is to be successful. Understanding the risks associated with the diagnosis of diabetes may motivate the patient to lose weight.

For selected patients, medical or surgical options for weight loss should be considered. Orlistat, phentermine/topiramate, and lorcaserin are weight loss medications approved for use in combination with diet and exercise (see Chapter 29).

Orlistat (Xenical) is a reversible inhibitor of gastric and pancreatic lipases and prevents the hydrolysis and absorption of dietary triglycerides. It is available over-the-counter and in prescription strength. In 1-year studies in obese patients with type 2 diabetes, those taking orlistat had lost more weight, had lower HbA$_{1c}$ values, and had improved lipid profiles. The main adverse reactions were gastrointestinal, with oily spotting, oily stool, flatus, and fecal urgency and frequency. Malabsorption of fat-soluble vitamins also occurs, and patients should take a multivitamin tablet containing fat-soluble. vitamins at least 2 hours before or 2 hours after the administration of orlistat. Cases of severe liver injury have been reported with this medication, although a cause and effect relationship has not been established.

Phentermine is a sympathomimetic amine stimulating release of norepinephrine from the hypothalamus. Topiramate is primarily used as an anticonvulsant, but it also appears to reduce appetite. In a 56-week phase 3 study, an extended-release preparation of **phentermine/topiramate (Qsymia)** together with diet and lifestyle intervention resulted in 10 kg weight loss (9.8%) compared to 1.4 kg (1.2%) with placebo. As might be expected, the diabetes subgroup on active therapy had greater reductions in HbA$_{1c}$ levels; and fewer patients with prediabetes on active therapy progressed to diabetes. The adverse events are consistent with those of the constituent drugs. The most common adverse reactions were paresthesia, dizziness, dysgeusia, insomnia, constipation, and dry mouth. Topiramate can worsen depression and increase risk of suicidal thoughts. It is also teratogenic and the FDA has required the manufacturer to conduct a risk evaluation and mitigation strategy (REMS). The medication is only available through specialty mail-order pharmacies.

Lorcaserin (Belviq) is a 5-hydroxytryptamine receptor subtype 2C (5-HT$_{2C}$) agonist. This receptor subclass regulates mood and appetite. In a 52-week study, patients taking lorcaserin had a 8.1 kg weight loss (8.2%) compared to 3.2 kg placebo group (3.3%). The main adverse reactions were headache and nausea. Fenfluramine, an agonist for the 5-HT$_{2B}$ receptor, was associated with serotonin-related cardiac valvulopathy. Activation of the 5-HT$_{2C}$ receptor, however, does not appear to be associated with valvulopathy.

Bariatric surgery (Roux-en-Y, gastric banding, gastric sleeve, biliopancreatic diversion/duodenal switch) typically results in substantial weight loss and improvement in glucose levels. A meta-analysis examining the impact of bariatric surgery on patients with diabetes and BMI of 40 kg/m^2 or greater noted that 82% of patients had resolution of clinical and laboratory manifestations of diabetes in the first 2 years after surgery and 62% remained free of diabetes more than 2 years after surgery. The improvement was most marked in the procedure that caused the greatest weight loss (biliopancreatic diversion/duodenal switch). There was, however, a high attrition of patients available for follow-up, and there was little information about different ethnic types. Weight regain does occur after bariatric surgery, and it can be expected that 20–25% of the lost weight will be regained over 10 years. The impact of this weight gain on diabetes recurrence depends principally on the degree of beta cell dysfunction. Also anatomic changes imposed by malabsorptive surgery can result in protein malnutrition, vitamin and mineral deficiencies. Clinically significant deficiencies in calcium; folic acid; iron; and vitamins D, B$_{12}$, A, and K are common. Thus, patients undergoing malabsorptive procedures require lifelong supplementation and monitoring by a team familiar with possible deficiencies. Both early and late dumping symptoms can also occur.

Nonobese patients with type 2 diabetes frequently have increased visceral adiposity—the so-called metabolically obese normal weight patient. There is less emphasis on weight loss, but exercise remains an important aspect of treatment.

B. Glucose lowering agents—The current recommendation is to start **metformin** therapy at diagnosis and not wait to see whether the patient can achieve target glycemic control with weight management and exercise. Figure 27–3 outlines the consensus algorithim that has been proposed by the American Diabetes Association and the European Association for the Study of Diabetes. The medication, however, cannot be used in patients with end-stage renal disease, and sometimes gastrointestinal side effects develop at even the lowest doses and persist over time. Under these circumstances the choice of the initial agent depends on a number of factors, including comorbid conditions, adverse reactions to the medications, ability of the patient to monitor for hypoglycemia, medication cost, and patient and clinician preferences. **Sulfonylureas** have been available for many years and their use in combination with metformin is well established. They do, however, have the propensity of causing hypoglycemia and weight gain. **Pioglitazone** improves peripheral insulin resistance and lowers glucose without causing hypoglycemia. Troublesome adverse reactions include weight gain, fluid retention and heart failure, increased fracture risk in women, and possible increased risk of bladder cancer. Pioglitazone is contraindicated in patients with active liver disease and in patients with liver enzymes ≥ 2.5 times the upper limit of normal. The **alpha-glucosidase inhibitors (acarbose, miglitol)** have modest glucose lowering effects and have gastrointestinal side effects. The **GLP-1 receptor agonists (exenatide and liraglutide)** have a lower risk of hypoglycemia than the sulfonylureas and they promote weight loss; however, they need to be given by injection. These agents cause nausea, may cause pancreatitis, and are contraindicated in patients with

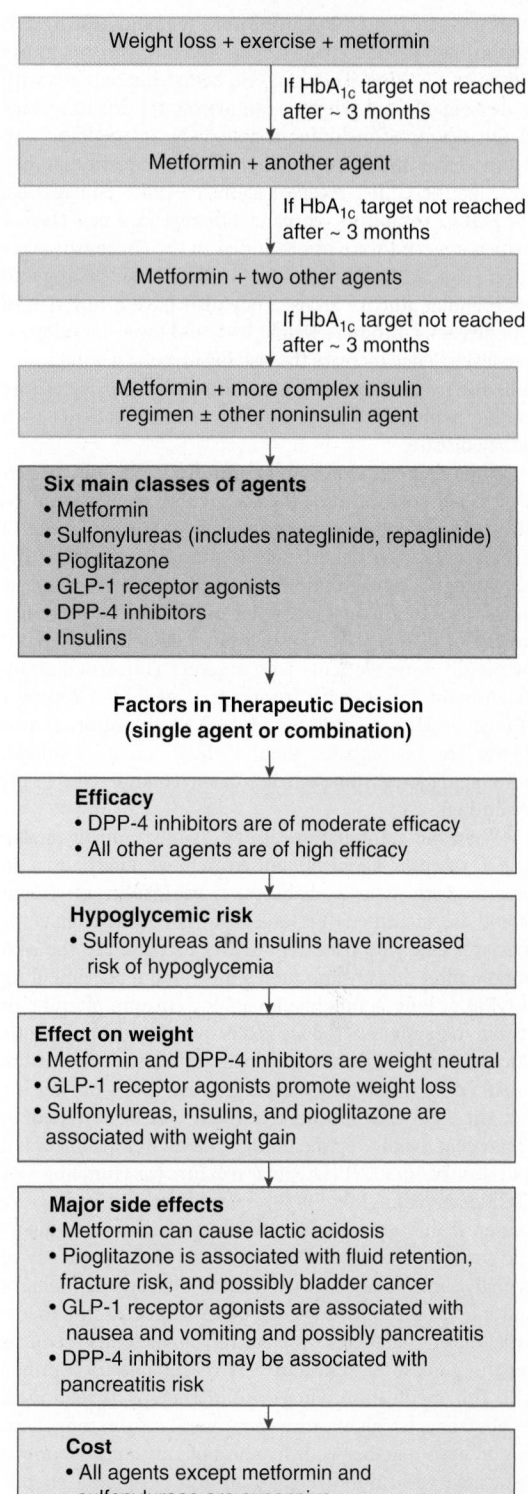

▲ **Figure 27–3.** Algorithm for the treatment of type 2 diabetes based on the recommendations of the consensus panel of the American Diabetes Association/European Association for the Study of Diabetes.

gastroparesis. The **DPP-4 inhibitors** (eg, **sitagliptin**) also have a low risk of hypoglycemia, and they do not cause nausea or vomiting. They can also be used in patients with kidney impairment. There are, however, reports of serious allergic reactions, including anaphylaxis, angioedema, and Stevens-Johnson syndrome. There is also concern that they may, like the GLP-1 receptor agonists, cause pancreatitis. The **SGLT2 inhibitors** (eg, canagliflozin) are a new class of medications and were not included in the consensus algorithm (Figure 27–3). These medications lower fasting and postprandial glucose levels. They also have a low risk of hypoglycemia, promote weight loss, and lower blood pressure levels. They increase the risk for mycotic genital infections and urinary tract infections, however. They can cause volume depletion and are less effective in patients with kidney disease.

When diabetes is not well controlled with initial therapy (usually metformin), then a second agent should be added. In patients who experience hyperglycemia after a carbohydrate-rich meal (such as dinner), a short-acting secretagogue (repaglinide or nateglinide) before meals may suffice to get the glucose levels into the target range. Patients with severe insulin resistance may be candidates for pioglitazone. Patients who are very concerned about weight gain may benefit from a trial of GLP-1 receptor agonist or DPP-4 inhibitor or SGLT2 inhibitor. If two agents are inadequate, then a third agent is added, although data regarding efficacy of such combined therapy are limited.

When the combination of oral agents (and injectable GLP-1 receptor agonists) fail to achieve euglycemia in patients with type 2 diabetes, then insulin treatment should be instituted. Various insulin regimens may be effective. One proposed regimen is to continue the oral combination therapy and then simply add a bedtime dose of NPH or long-acting insulin analog (insulin glargine or insulin detemir) to reduce excessive nocturnal hepatic glucose output and improve fasting glucose levels. If the patient does not achieve target glucose levels during the day, then daytime insulin treatment can be initiated. A convenient insulin regimen under these circumstances is a split dose of 70/30 NPH/regular mixture (or Humalog Mix 75/25 or NovoLogMix 70/30) before breakfast and before dinner. If this regimen fails to achieve satisfactory glycemic goals or is associated with unacceptable frequency of hypoglycemic episodes, then a more intensive regimen of multiple insulin injections can be instituted as in patients with type 1 diabetes. Metformin principally reduces hepatic glucose output, and it is reasonable to continue with this medication when insulin therapy is instituted. Pioglitazone, which improves peripheral insulin sensitivity, can be used together with insulin but this combination is associated with more weight gain and peripheral edema. The sulfonylureas also continue to be of benefit. There is limited information on the benefits of continuing the GLP1-receptor agonists or the DPP-4 inhibitors or the SGLT2 inhibitors once insulin therapy is initiated. Weight-reducing interventions should continue even after initiation of insulin therapy and may allow for simplification of the therapeutic regimen in the future.

D. Acceptable Levels of Glycemic Control

A reasonable aim of therapy is to approach normal glycemic excursions without provoking severe or frequent hypoglycemia. **Criteria for "acceptable" control** includes the following: (1) blood glucose levels of 90–130 mg/dL (5–7.2 mmol/L) before meals and after an overnight fast, (2) levels no higher than 180 mg/dL (10 mmol/L) 1 hour after meals and 150 mg/dL (8.3 mmol/L) 2 hours after meals, and (3) HbA_{1c} levels < 7% for nonpregnant adults. Less stringent HbA_{1c} goals may be appropriate in children, those with a history of severe hypoglycemia, limited life expectancy, and advanced microvascular and macrovascular disease. In the elderly frail patient, an HbA_{1c} target of approximately 8% (preprandial blood glucose levels in the range of the 150–159 mg/dL) may be reasonable although formal evidence is lacking. **The UKPDS study demonstrated that blood pressure control was as significant or more significant than glycemic control in patients with type 2 diabetes regarding the prevention of microvascular as well as macrovascular complications.**

Inzucchi SE et al. Management of hyperglycemia in type 2 diabetes: a patient-centered approach: position statement of the American Diabetes Association (ADA) and the European Association for the Study of Diabetes (EASD). Diabetes Care. 2012 Jun;35(6):1364–79. [PMID: 22517736]

Switzer SM et al. Intensive insulin therapy in patients with type 1 diabetes mellitus. Endocrinol Metab Clin North Am. 2012 Mar;41(1):89–104. [PMID: 22575408]

E. Complications of Insulin Therapy

1. Hypoglycemia—Hypoglycemic reactions are the most common complications that occur in patients with diabetes who are treated with insulin. The signs and symptoms of hypoglycemia may be divided into those resulting from stimulation of the autonomic nervous system and those from neuroglycopenia (insufficient glucose for normal central nervous system function). When the blood glucose falls to around 54 mg/dL (3 mmol/L), the patient starts to experience both sympathetic (tachycardia, palpitations, sweating, tremulousness) and parasympathetic (nausea, hunger) nervous system symptoms. If these autonomic symptoms are ignored and the glucose levels fall further (to around 50 mg/dL [2.8 mmol/L]), then neuroglycopenic symptoms appear, including irritability, confusion, blurred vision, tiredness, headache, and difficulty speaking. A further decline in glucose can then lead to loss of consciousness or even a seizure. With repeated episodes of hypoglycemia, there is adaptation, and autonomic symptoms do not occur until the blood glucose levels are much lower and so the first symptoms are often due to neuroglycopenia. This condition is referred to as "hypoglycemic unawareness." It has been shown that hypoglycemic unawareness can be reversed by keeping glucose levels high for a period of several weeks. Except for sweating, most of the sympathetic symptoms of hypoglycemia are blunted in patients receiving beta-blocking agents for angina pectoris or hypertension. Though not absolutely contraindicated, these medications must be used with caution in insulin-requiring diabetics, and beta-1-selective blocking agents are preferred.

Hypoglycemia can occur in patient taking sulfonylureas, repaglinide, and nateglinide, particularly if the patient is elderly, has kidney or liver disease, or is taking certain other medications that alter metabolism of the sulfonylureas (eg, phenylbutazone, sulfonamides, or warfarin). It occurs more frequently with the use of long-acting sulfonylureas than when shorter-acting agents are used. Otherwise, hypoglycemia in insulin-treated patients with diabetes occurs as a consequence of three factors: behavioral issues, impaired counterregulatory systems, and complications of diabetes.

Behavioral issues include injecting too much insulin for the amount of carbohydrates ingested. Drinking alcohol in excess, especially on an empty stomach, can also cause hypoglycemia. In patients with type 1 diabetes, hypoglycemia can occur during or even several hours after exercise, and so glucose levels need to be monitored and food and insulin adjusted. Some patients do not like their glucose levels to be high, and they treat every high glucose level aggressively. These individuals who "stack" their insulin—that is, give another dose of insulin before the first injection has had its full action—can develop hypoglycemia.

Counterregulatory issues resulting in hypoglycemia include impaired glucagon response, sympatho-adrenal responses, and cortisol deficiency. Patients with diabetes of > 5 years duration lose their glucagon response to hypoglycemia. As a result, they are at a significant disadvantage in protecting themselves against falling glucose levels. Once the glucagon response is lost, their sympatho-adrenal responses take on added importance. Unfortunately, aging, autonomic neuropathy, or hypoglycemic unawareness due to repeated low glucose levels further blunts the sympatho-adrenal responses. Occasionally, Addison disease develops in persons with type 1 diabetes mellitus; when this happens, insulin requirements fall significantly, and unless insulin dose is reduced, recurrent hypoglycemia will develop.

Complications of diabetes that increase the risk for hypoglycemia include autonomic neuropathy, gastroparesis, and end-stage chronic kidney disease. The sympathetic nervous system is an important system alerting the individual that the glucose level is falling by causing symptoms of tachycardia, palpitations, sweating, and tremulousness. Failure of the sympatho-adrenal responses increases the risk of hypoglycemia. In addition, in patients with gastroparesis, if insulin is given before a meal, the peak of insulin action may occur before the food is absorbed causing the glucose levels to fall. Finally, in end-stage chronic kidney disease, hypoglycemia can occur presumably because of decreased insulin clearance as well as loss of renal contribution to gluconeogenesis in the postabsorptive state.

To prevent and treat insulin-induced hypoglycemia, the diabetic patient should carry glucose tablets or juice at all times. For most episodes, ingestion of 15 grams of carbohydrate is sufficient to reverse the hypoglycemia. The patient should be instructed to check the blood glucose in 15 minutes and treat again if the glucose level is still low. A parenteral glucagon emergency kit (1 mg) should be provided to every patient with diabetes who is receiving insulin therapy. Family or friends should be instructed how to inject it subcutaneously or intramuscularly into the buttock, arm, or thigh in the event that the patient is unconscious or refuses food. The medication can occasionally cause vomiting, and the unconscious patient should be turned on his or her side to protect the airway. The glucagon mobilizes glycogen from the liver, raising the blood glucose by about 36 mg/dL (2 mmol/L) in about 15 minutes. After the patient recovers consciousness, additional oral carbohydrate should be given. People with diabetes receiving hypoglycemic medication therapy should also wear an identification MedicAlert bracelet or necklace or carry a card in his or her wallet (1-800-ID-ALERT, www.medicalert.org).

Medical personnel treating severe hypoglycemia can give 50 mL of 50% glucose solution by rapid intravenous infusion. If intravenous access is not available, 1 mg of glucagon can be injected intramuscularly.

2. Immunopathology of insulin therapy—At least five molecular classes of insulin antibodies are produced during the course of insulin therapy in diabetes, including IgA, IgD, IgE, IgG, and IgM. With the increased therapeutic use of human and purified pork insulin, the various immunopathologic syndromes such as insulin allergy, immune insulin resistance, and lipoatrophy have become quite rare since the titers and avidity of these induced antibodies are generally quite low.

A. Insulin Allergy—Insulin allergy, or immediate-type hypersensitivity, is a rare condition in which local or systemic urticaria is due to histamine release from tissue mast cells sensitized by adherence of anti-insulin IgE antibodies. In severe cases, anaphylaxis results. When only human insulin has been used from the onset of insulin therapy, insulin allergy is exceedingly rare. Antihistamines, corticosteroids, and even desensitization may be required, especially for systemic hypersensitivity. There have been case reports of successful use of insulin lispro in those rare patients who have a generalized allergy to human insulin or insulin resistance due to a high titer of insulin antibodies.

B. Immune Insulin Resistance—A low titer of circulating IgG anti-insulin antibodies that neutralize the action of insulin to a small extent develops in most insulin-treated patients. With the old animal insulins, a high titer of circulating antibodies sometimes developed, resulting in extremely high insulin requirements—often more than 200 units daily. This is now rarely seen with the switch to human or highly purified pork insulins and has not been reported with the analogs.

C. Lipodystrophy—Atrophy of subcutaneous fatty tissue leading to disfiguring excavations and depressed areas may rarely occur at the site of injection. This complication results from an immune reaction, and it has become rarer with the development of human and highly purified insulin preparations. Lipohypertrophy, on the other hand, is a consequence of the pharmacologic effects of insulin being deposited in the same location repeatedly. It can occur with purified insulins as well. Rotation of injection sites will prevent lipohypertrophy. There is a case report of a patient who had intractable lipohypertrophy with human insulin but no longer had the problem when he switched to insulin lispro.

Cryer PE. Mechanisms of hypoglycemia-associated autonomic failure in diabetes. N Engl J Med. 2013 Jul 25;369(4):362–72. [PMID: 23883381]

▶ Chronic Complications of Diabetes

Late clinical manifestations of diabetes mellitus include a number of pathologic changes that involve small and large blood vessels, cranial and peripheral nerves, the skin, and the lens of the eye. These lesions lead to hypertension, end-stage chronic kidney disease, blindness, autonomic and peripheral neuropathy, amputations of the lower extremities, myocardial infarction, and cerebrovascular accidents. These late manifestations correlate with the duration of the diabetic state subsequent to the onset of puberty. In type 1 diabetes, end-stage chronic kidney disease develops in up to 40% of patients, compared with < 20% of patients with type 2 diabetes. Proliferative retinopathy ultimately develops in both types of diabetes but has a slightly higher prevalence in type 1 patients (25% after 15 years' duration). In patients with type 1 diabetes, complications from end-stage chronic kidney disease are a major cause of death, whereas patients with type 2 diabetes are more likely to have macrovascular diseases leading to myocardial infarction and stroke as the main causes of death. Cigarette use adds significantly to the risk of both microvascular and macrovascular complications in diabetic patients.

A. Ocular Complications

1. Diabetic cataracts—Premature cataracts occur in diabetic patients and seem to correlate with both the duration of diabetes and the severity of chronic hyperglycemia. Nonenzymatic glycosylation of lens protein is twice as high in diabetic patients as in age-matched nondiabetic persons and may contribute to the premature occurrence of cataracts.

2. Diabetic retinopathy—There are two main categories of diabetic retinopathy: nonproliferative and proliferative. Diabetic macular edema can occur at any stage. **Nonproliferative ("background") retinopathy** represents the earliest stage of retinal involvement by diabetes and is characterized by such changes as microaneurysms, dot hemorrhages, exudates, and retinal edema. During this stage, the retinal capillaries leak proteins, lipids, or red cells into the retina. When this process occurs in the macula (clinically significant macular edema), the area of greatest concentration of visual cells, there is interference with visual acuity; this is the most common cause of visual impairment in patients with type 2 diabetes. The prevalence of nonproliferative retinopathy in patients with type 2 diabetes is 60% after 16 years.

Proliferative retinopathy involves the growth of new capillaries and fibrous tissue within the retina and into the vitreous chamber. It is a consequence of small vessel occlusion, which causes retinal hypoxia; this in turn stimulates new vessel growth. New vessel formation may occur at the optic disk or elsewhere on the retina. Prior to proliferation of new capillaries, a preproliferative phase often occurs in which arteriolar ischemia is manifested as cotton-wool spots (small infarcted areas of retina). Vision is usually normal until vitreous hemorrhage or retinal detachment occurs.

Proliferative retinopathy can occur in both types of diabetes but is more common in type 1, developing about 7–10 years after onset of symptoms, with a prevalence of 25% after 15 years' duration. Proliferative retinopathy is a leading cause of blindness in the United States, particularly since it increases the risk of retinal detachment. Vision-threatening retinopathy virtually never appears in type 1 patients in the first 3–5 years of diabetes or before puberty. Up to 20% of patients with type 2 diabetes have retinopathy at the time of diagnosis, because many were probably diabetic for an extensive period of time before diagnosis. Annual consultation with an ophthalmologist should be arranged for patients who have had type 1 diabetes for more than 3–5 years and for all patients with type 2 diabetes. Patients with any macular edema, severe nonproliferative retinopathy, or any proliferative retinopathy require the care of an ophthalmologist. Extensive "scatter" xenon or argon photocoagulation and focal treatment of new vessels reduce severe visual loss in those cases in which proliferative retinopathy is associated with recent vitreous hemorrhages or in which extensive new vessels are located on or near the optic disk. Macular edema, which is more common than proliferative retinopathy in patients with type 2 diabetes (up to 20% prevalence), has a guarded prognosis, but it has also responded to scatter therapy with improvement in visual acuity if detected early. Injection of bevacizumab (Avastin), an anti-vascular endothelial growth factor (anti-VEGF), into the eye has been shown to stop the growth of the new blood vessels in diabetic eye disease. Avoiding tobacco use and correction of associated hypertension are important therapeutic measures in the management of diabetic retinopathy. There is no contraindication to using aspirin in patients with proliferative retinopathy.

3. Glaucoma—Glaucoma occurs in approximately 6% of persons with diabetes. It is responsive to the usual therapy for open-angle disease. Neovascularization of the iris in patients with diabetes can predispose to closed-angle glaucoma, but this is relatively uncommon except after cataract extraction, when growth of new vessels has been known to progress rapidly, involving the angle of the iris and obstructing outflow.

B. Diabetic Nephropathy

As many as 4000 cases of end-stage chronic kidney disease occur each year among diabetic people in the United States. This is about one-third of all patients being treated for end-stage chronic kidney disease and represents a considerable national health expense.

The cumulative incidence of nephropathy differs between the two major types of diabetes. Patients with type 1 diabetes have a 30–40% chance of having nephropathy after 20 years—in contrast to the much lower frequency in type 2 diabetes patients, in whom only about 15–20% develop clinical kidney disease. However, since there are many more individuals affected with type 2 diabetes, end-stage chronic kidney disease is much more prevalent in type 2 than in type 1 diabetes in the United States and especially throughout the rest of the world. Improved glycemic control and more effective therapeutic measures to correct hypertension—and with the beneficial effects of ACE inhibitors—can reduce the development of end-stage chronic kidney disease among patients with diabetes.

Diabetic nephropathy is initially manifested by proteinuria; subsequently, as kidney function declines, urea and creatinine accumulate in the blood. Sensitive radioimmunoassay methods detect small amounts of urinary albumin—in contrast to the less sensitive dipstick strips, whose minimal detection limit is 0.3–0.5%. Conventional 24-hour urine collections, in addition to being inconvenient for patients, also show wide variability of albumin excretion, since several factors such as sustained erect posture, dietary protein, and exercise tend to increase albumin excretion rates. For these reasons, an albumin-creatinine ratio in an early morning spot urine collected upon awakening is preferable. In the early morning spot urine, a ratio of albumin (mcg/L) to creatinine (mg/L) of < 30 mcg/mg creatinine is normal, and a ratio of 30–300 mcg/mg creatinine suggests abnormal microalbuminuria. At least two early morning spot urine collections over a 3- to 6-month period should be abnormal before a diagnosis of microalbuminuria is justified. Short-term hyperglycemia, exercise, urinary tract infections, heart failure, and acute febrile illness can cause transient albuminuria and so testing for microalbuminuria should be postponed until resolution of these problems.

Subsequent end-stage chronic kidney disease can be predicted by persistent urinary albumin excretion rates exceeding 30 mcg/mg creatinine. Glycemic control as well as a low-protein diet (0.8 g/kg/d) may reduce both the hyperfiltration and the elevated microalbuminuria in patients in the early stages of diabetes and those with incipient diabetic nephropathy. Antihypertensive therapy also decreases microalbuminuria. Evidence from some studies—but not the UKPDS—supports a specific role for ACE inhibitors in reducing intraglomerular pressure in addition to their lowering of systemic hypertension. An ACE inhibitor (captopril, 50 mg twice daily) in normotensive diabetic patients impedes progression to proteinuria and prevents the increase in albumin excretion rate. Since microalbuminuria has been shown to correlate with elevated *nocturnal* systolic blood pressure, it is possible that "normotensive" diabetic patients with microalbuminuria have slightly elevated systolic blood pressure during sleep, which is lowered during antihypertensive therapy. This action may contribute to the reported efficacy of ACE inhibitors in reducing microalbuminuria in "normotensive" patients.

If treatment is inadequate, then the disease progresses with proteinuria of varying severity occasionally leading to nephrotic syndrome with hypoalbuminemia, edema, and an increase in circulating LDL cholesterol, as well as progressive azotemia. In contrast to all other kidney disorders, the proteinuria associated with diabetic nephropathy does not diminish with progressive end-stage chronic kidney disease (patients continue to excrete 10–11 g daily as creatinine clearance diminishes). As end-stage chronic kidney disease progresses, there is an elevation in the renal threshold at which glycosuria appears.

Patients with diabetic nephropathy should be evaluated and monitored by a nephrologist. There has been gradual improvement in quality of life of diabetic patients receiving dialysis but mortality remains higher than in nondiabetic patients. During 5 years of follow-up in a registry study from Europe, the mortality rate in people with diabetes receiving dialysis was 226.9 deaths/1000 patient years whereas the rate was 151.4 deaths/1000 patients years in people receiving dialysis who did not have diabetes. Diabetic nephropathy accounts for about 20% of kidney transplantations performed annually in the United States.

C. Diabetic Neuropathy

Diabetic neuropathies are the most common complications of diabetes affecting up to 50% of older patients with type 2 diabetes.

1. Peripheral neuropathy—

A. DISTAL SYMMETRIC POLYNEUROPATHY—This is the most common form of diabetic peripheral neuropathy where loss of function appears in a stocking-glove pattern and is due to an axonal neuropathic process. Longer nerves are especially vulnerable, hence the impact on the foot. Both motor and sensory nerve conduction is delayed in the peripheral nerves, and ankle jerks may be absent.

Sensory involvement usually occurs first and is generally bilateral, symmetric, and associated with dulled perception of vibration, pain, and temperature. The pain can range from mild discomfort to severe incapacitating symptoms (see below). The sensory deficit may eventually be of sufficient degree to prevent patients from feeling pain. Patients who have a sensory neuropathy should therefore be examined with a 5.07 Semmes Weinstein filament and those who cannot feel the filament must be considered at risk for unperceived neuropathic injury.

The denervation of the small muscles of the foot result in clawing of the toes and displacement of the submetatarsal fat pads anteriorly. These changes, together with the joint and connective tissue changes, alter the biomechanics of the foot and increase plantar pressures. This combination of decreased pain threshold, abnormally high foot pressures, and repetitive stress (such as from walking) can lead to calluses and ulcerations in the high-pressure areas such as over the metatarsal heads (Figure 27–4). Peripheral neuropathy, autonomic neuropathy, and trauma also predisposes to the development of Charcot arthropathy. An acute case of Charcot foot arthropathy presents with pain and swelling, and if left untreated, leads to a "rocker

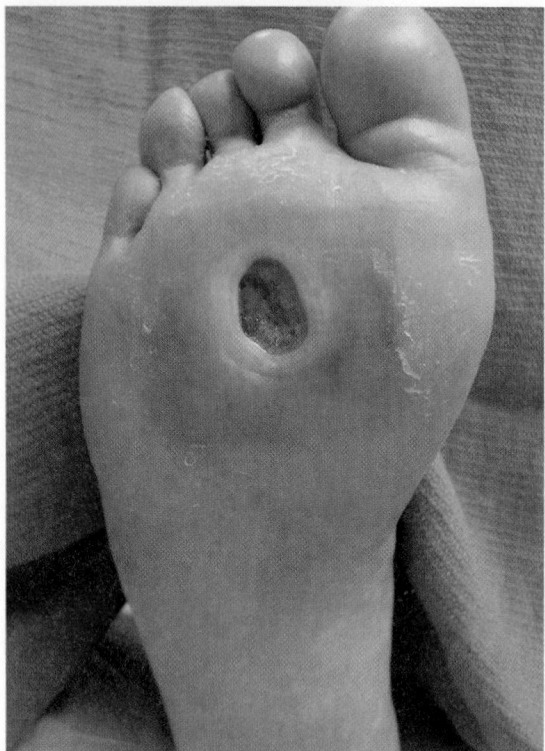

▲ **Figure 27–4.** Neuropathic ulcer under the head of the third metatarsal on the foot of a diabetic patient. (From Javier La Fontaine, DPM; reproduced with permission from Usatine RP, Smith MA, Mayeaux EJ Jr, Chumley H, Tysinger J. *The Color Atlas of Family Medicine.* McGraw-Hill, 2009.)

bottom" deformity and ulceration. The early radiologic changes show joint subluxation and periarticular fractures. As the process progresses, there is frank osteoclastic destruction leading to deranged and unstable joints particularly in the midfoot. Not surprisingly, the key issue for the healing of neuropathic ulcers in a foot with good vascular supply is mechanical unloading. In addition, any infection should be treated with debridement and appropriate antibiotics; healing duration of 8–10 weeks is typical. Occasionally, when healing appears refractory, **platelet-derived growth factor** (becaplermin [Regranex]) should be considered for local application. A post-marketing epidemiologic study showed increased cancer deaths in patients who had used three or more tubes of becaplermin on their leg or feet ulcers, resulting in a "black box" warning on the medication label. Once ulcers are healed, therapeutic footwear is key to preventing recurrences. Custom molded shoes are reserved for patients with significant foot deformities. Other patients with neuropathy may require accommodative insoles that distribute the load over as wide an area as possible. Patients with foot deformities and loss of their protective threshold should get regular care from a podiatrist. Patients should be educated on appropriate footwear and those with loss of their protective threshold should be instructed to inspect their feet daily for reddened areas, blisters, abrasions, or lacerations.

In some patients, hypersensitivity to light touch and occasionally severe "burning" pain, particularly at night, can become physically and emotionally disabling. Amitriptyline, 25–75 mg at bedtime, has been recommended for pain associated with diabetic neuropathy. Dramatic relief has often resulted within 48–72 hours. This rapid response is in contrast to the 2 or 3 weeks required for an antidepressive effect. Patients often attribute the benefit to having a full night's sleep. Mild to moderate morning drowsiness is a side effect that generally improves with time or can be lessened by giving the medication several hours before bedtime. This medication should not be continued if improvement has not occurred after 5 days of therapy. If amitriptyline's anticholinergic effects are too troublesome, then nortriptyline or desipramine in doses of 25–150 mg/d can be used. Tricyclic antidepressants, in combination with the phenothiazine, fluphenazine, have been shown in two studies to be efficacious in painful neuropathy, with benefits unrelated to relief of depression. Gabapentin (900–1800 mg orally daily in three divided doses) has also been shown to be effective in the treatment of painful neuropathy and should be tried if the tricyclic medications prove ineffective. Pregabalin, a congener of gabapentin, has been shown in an 8-week study to be more effective than placebo in treating painful diabetic peripheral neuropathy. However, this medication was not compared with an active control. Also, because of its abuse potential, it has been categorized as a schedule V controlled substance. Duloxetine (60–120 mg), a serotonin and norepinephrine reuptake inhibitor, has been approved for the treatment of painful diabetic neuropathy. In clinical trials, this medication reduced the pain sensitivity score by 40–50%. Capsaicin, a topical irritant, has been found to be effective in reducing local nerve pain; it is dispensed as a cream (Zostrix 0.025%, Zostrix-HP 0.075%) to be rubbed into the skin over the painful region two to four times daily. Gloves should be used for application since hand contamination could result in discomfort if the cream comes in contact with eyes or sensitive areas such as the genitalia. Application of a 5% lidocaine patch over an area of maximal pain has been reported to be of benefit. It is approved for treatment of postherpetic neuralgia and is in clinical trials for the treatment of painful diabetic neuropathy.

Diabetic neuropathic cachexia is a syndrome characterized by a symmetric peripheral neuropathy associated with profound weight loss (up to 60% of total body weight) and painful dysesthesias affecting the proximal lower limbs, the hands, or the lower trunk. Treatment is usually with insulin and analgesics. The prognosis is generally good, and patients typically recover their baseline weight with resolution of the painful sensory symptoms within 1 year.

B. Isolated peripheral neuropathy—Involvement of the distribution of only one nerve ("mononeuropathy") or of several nerves ("mononeuropathy multiplex") is characterized by sudden onset with subsequent recovery of all or most of the function. This neuropathology has been attributed to vascular ischemia or traumatic damage. Cranial and femoral nerves are commonly involved, and motor abnormalities predominate. The patient with cranial nerve involvement usually has diplopia and single third, fourth, or sixth nerve weakness on examination but the pupil is spared. A full recovery of function occurs in 6–12 weeks. Diabetic amyotrophy presents with onset of severe pain in the front of the thigh. Within a few days or weeks of the onset of pain, weakness and wasting of the quadriceps develops. As the weakness appears, the pain tends to improve. Management includes analgesia and improved diabetes control. The symptoms improve over 6–18 months.

2. Autonomic neuropathy—Neuropathy of the autonomic system occurs principally in patients with diabetes of long duration. It affects many diverse visceral functions including blood pressure and pulse, gastrointestinal activity, bladder function, and erectile dysfunction. Treatment is directed specifically at each abnormality.

Involvement of the gastrointestinal system may be manifested by nausea, vomiting, postprandial fullness, reflux or dysphagia, constipation or diarrhea (or both), and fecal incontinence. Gastroparesis should be considered in type 1 diabetic patients in whom unexpected fluctuations and variability in their blood glucose levels develops after meals. Radioisotope studies show marked delay in gastric emptying. Metoclopramide has been of some help in treating diabetic gastroparesis. It is given in a dose of 10 mg orally three or four times a day, 30 minutes before meals and at bedtime. Drowsiness, restlessness, fatigue, and lassitude are common adverse effects. Tardive dyskinesia and extrapyramidal effects can occur, especially when used for longer than 3 months, and the FDA has cautioned against the long-term use of metoclopramide.

Erythromycin appears to bind to motilin receptors in the stomach and has been found to improve gastric emptying over the short term in doses of 250 mg three times daily, but its effectiveness seems to diminish over time. In selected patients, injections of botulinum toxin into the pylorus can reduce pylorus sphincter resistance and enhance gastric emptying. Gastric electrical stimulation has been reported to improve symptoms and quality of life indices in patients with gastroparesis refractory to pharmacologic therapy.

Diarrhea associated with autonomic neuropathy has occasionally responded to broad-spectrum antibiotic therapy (such as rifaximin, metronidazole, amoxicillin/clavulanate, ciprofloxacin, doxycycline), although it often undergoes spontaneous remission. Refractory diabetic diarrhea is often associated with impaired sphincter control and fecal incontinence. Therapy with loperamide, 4–8 mg daily, or diphenoxylate with atropine, two tablets up to four times a day, may provide relief. In more severe cases, tincture of paregoric or codeine (60 mg tablets) may be required to reduce the frequency of diarrhea and improve the consistency of the stools. Clonidine has been reported to lessen diabetic diarrhea; however, its usefulness is limited by its tendency to lower blood pressure in these patients who already have autonomic neuropathy, resulting in orthostatic hypotension. Constipation usually responds to stimulant laxatives such as senna.

Incomplete emptying of the bladder can sometimes occur. Bethanechol in doses of 10–50 mg orally three times a day has occasionally improved emptying of the atonic urinary bladder. Catheter decompression of the distended bladder has been reported to improve its function, and considerable benefit has been reported after surgical severing of the internal vesicle sphincter.

Use of Jobst fitted stockings, tilting the head of the bed, and arising slowly from the supine position can be helpful in treating symptoms of orthostatic hypotension. When such measures are inadequate, then treatment with fludrocortisone 0.1–0.2 mg orally daily can be considered. This medication, however, can result in supine hypertension and hypokalemia. Midodrine (10 mg orally three times a day), an alpha-agonist, can also be used.

Erectile dysfunction can result from neurologic, psychological or vascular causes, or a combination of these causes. There are medical, mechanical, and surgical treatments available for treatment of erectile dysfunction. Penile erection depends on relaxation of the smooth muscle in the arteries of the corpus cavernosum, and this is mediated by nitric oxide-induced cyclic 3′,5′-guanosine monophosphate (cGMP) formation. cGMP-specific phosphodiesterase type 5 (PDE5) inhibitors impair the breakdown of cGMP and improve the ability to attain and maintain an erection. Sildenafil (Viagra), vardenafil (Levitra), and tadalafil (Cialis) have been shown in placebo-controlled clinical trials to improve erections in response to sexual stimulation. The recommended dose of sildenafil for most patients is one 50-mg tablet taken approximately 1 hour before sexual activity. The peak effect is at 1.5–2 hours, with some effect persisting for 4 hours. Patients with diabetes mellitus using sildenafil reported 50–60% improvement in erectile function. The maximum recommended dose is 100 mg. The recommended dose of both vardenafil and tadalafil is 10 mg. The doses may be increased to 20 mg or decreased to 5 mg based on efficacy and side effects. Tadalafil has been shown to improve erectile function for up to 36 hours after dosing. Low doses are available for daily use. In clinical trials, only a few adverse effects have been reported—transient mild headache, flushing, dyspepsia, and some altered color vision. Priapism can occur with these medications, and patients should be advised to seek immediate medical attention if an erection persists for longer than 4 hours. The PDE5 inhibitors potentiate the hypotensive effects of nitrates and their use is contraindicated in patients who are concurrently using organic nitrates in any form. Caution is advised for men who have suffered a heart attack, stroke, or life-threatening arrhythmia within the previous 6 months; men who have resting hypotension or hypertension; and men who have a history of heart failure or have unstable angina. Rarely, a decrease in vision or permanent visual loss has been reported after PDE5 inhibitor use.

Intracorporeal injection of vasoactive medications causes penile engorgement and erection. Medications most commonly used include papaverine alone, papaverine with phentolamine, and alprostadil (prostaglandin E$_1$). Alprostadil injections are relatively painless, but careful instruction is essential to prevent local trauma, priapism, and fibrosis. Intraurethral pellets of alprostadil avoid the problem of injection of the medication.

External vacuum therapy (Erec-Aid System) is a non-surgical treatment consisting of a suction chamber operated by a hand pump that creates a vacuum around the penis. This draws blood into the penis to produce an erection that is maintained by a specially designed tension ring inserted around the base of the penis and which can be kept in place for up to 20–30 minutes. While this method is generally effective, its cumbersome nature limits its appeal.

In view of the recent development of nonsurgical approaches to therapy of erectile dysfunction, resort to surgical implants of penile prostheses is becoming less common.

D. Cardiovascular Complications

1. Heart disease—Microangiopathy occurs in the heart and may explain the etiology of congestive cardiomyopathies in diabetic patients who do not have demonstrable coronary artery disease. More commonly, however, heart disease in patients with diabetes is due to coronary atherosclerosis. Myocardial infarction is three to five times more common in diabetic patients and is the leading cause of death in patients with type 2 diabetes. Cardiovascular disease risk is increased in patients with type 1 diabetes as well, although the absolute risk is lower than in patients with type 2 diabetes. Premenopausal women who normally have lower rates of coronary artery disease lose this protection once diabetes develops. The increased risk in patients with type 2 diabetes reflects the combination of hyperglycemia, hyperlipidemia, abnormalities of platelet adhesiveness, coagulation factors, hypertension, oxidative stress, and inflammation. Large intervention studies of risk factor reduction in diabetes are lacking, but it is reasonable to assume that reducing these risk factors would have a beneficial effect. Lowering LDL cholesterol reduces first events in patients without known coronary disease and secondary events in patients with known coronary disease. These intervention studies included some patients with diabetes, and the benefits of LDL cholesterol lowering was apparent in this group. The National Cholesterol Education Program clinical practice guidelines have designated diabetes as a coronary risk equivalent and have recommended that patients with diabetes should have an LDL cholesterol goal of < 100 mg/dL (2.6 mmol/L). Lowering LDL cholesterol to 70 mg/dL (1.8 mmol/L) may have additional benefit and is a reasonable target for most patients with type 2 diabetes who have multiple risk factors for cardiovascular disease.

The ADA also recommends lowering blood pressure to 140/80 mm Hg or less in patients with diabetes. The systolic target of 130 mm Hg or less is recommended for the younger patient if it can be achieved without undue treatment burden. The Antihypertensive and Lipid-Lowering Treatment to Prevent Heart Attack Trial (ALLHAT) randomized 33,357 persons (age 55 years and older) with hypertension and at least one other coronary artery disease risk factor to receive treatment with chlorthalidone, amlodipine, or lisinopril. Chlorthalidone appeared to be superior to amlodipine and lisinopril in lowering blood pressure, reducing the incidence of cardiovascular events, tolerability, and cost. The study included 12,063 individuals with type 2 diabetes. The Heart Outcomes Prevention Evaluation (HOPE) study randomized 9297 high-risk patients who had evidence of vascular disease or diabetes plus one other cardiovascular risk factor to receive ramipril or placebo for a mean of 5 years. Treatment with ramipril resulted in a 25% reduction of the risk of myocardial infarction, stroke, or death from cardiovascular disease. The mean difference between the placebo and ramipril group was 2.2 mm Hg systolic and 1.4 mm Hg diastolic blood pressure. The reduction in cardiovascular event rate remained significant after adjustment for this small difference in blood pressure. The mechanism underlying this protective effect of ramipril is unknown. Patients with type 2 diabetes who already have cardiovascular disease or microalbuminuria should therefore be considered for treatment with an ACE inhibitor. More clinical studies are needed to address the question of whether patients with type 2 diabetes who do not have cardiovascular disease or microalbuminuria would specifically benefit from ACE inhibitor treatment.

Aspirin at a dose of 81–325 mg daily is effective in reducing cardiovascular morbidity and mortality in patients who have a history of myocardial infarction or stroke (secondary prevention). It is unclear if aspirin prevents primary cardiovascular events in people with diabetes. The current recommendation is to give aspirin to people with diabetes who have a greater than 10% 10-year risk of cardiovascular events. Typically, this includes most diabetic men aged 50 years or older and diabetic women aged 60 years or older with one or more additional risk factors (smoking, hypertension, dyslipidemia, family history of premature cardiovascular disease, or albuminuria). Contraindications for aspirin therapy are patients with aspirin allergy, bleeding tendency, recent gastrointestinal bleeding, or active hepatic disease. Based on the Early Treatment Diabetic Retinopathy Study (ETDRS), there does not appear to be a contraindication to aspirin use to achieve cardiovascular benefit in diabetic patients who have proliferative retinopathy. Aspirin also does not seem to affect the severity of vitreous/preretinal hemorrhages or their resolution.

2. Peripheral vascular disease—Atherosclerosis is markedly accelerated in the larger arteries. It is often diffuse, with localized enhancement in certain areas of turbulent blood flow, such as at the bifurcation of the aorta or other large vessels. Clinical manifestations of peripheral vascular disease include ischemia of the lower extremities, erectile dysfunction, and intestinal angina.

The incidence of **gangrene of the feet** in patients with diabetes is 30 times that in age-matched controls. The factors responsible for its development, in addition to peripheral vascular disease, are small vessel disease, peripheral neuropathy with loss of both pain sensation and neurogenic inflammatory responses, and secondary infection. In two-thirds of patients with ischemic gangrene, pedal pulses are not palpable. In the remaining one-third who have palpable pulses, reduced blood flow through these vessels can be demonstrated by plethysmographic or Doppler ultrasound examination. Prevention of foot injury is imperative. Agents that reduce peripheral blood flow such as tobacco should be avoided. Control of other risk factors such as hypertension is essential. Beta-blockers are relatively contraindicated because of presumed negative peripheral hemodynamic consequences but data that support this are lacking. Cholesterol-lowering agents are useful as adjunctive therapy when early ischemic signs are detected and when dyslipidemia is present. Patients should be advised to seek immediate medical care if a diabetic foot ulcer develops. Improvement in peripheral blood flow with endarterectomy and bypass operations is possible in certain patients.

E. Skin and Mucous Membrane Complications

Chronic pyogenic infections of the skin may occur, especially in poorly controlled diabetic patients. **Candidal infection** can produce erythema and edema of intertriginous areas below the breasts, in the axillas, and between the fingers. It causes vulvovaginitis in women with chronically uncontrolled diabetes who have persistent glucosuria and is a frequent cause of pruritus. While antifungal creams containing miconazole or clotrimazole offer immediate relief of vulvovaginitis, recurrence is frequent unless glucosuria is reduced.

In some patients with type 2 diabetes, poor glycemic control can cause a severe hypertriglyceridemia, which can present as **eruptive cutaneous xanthomas** and pancreatitis. The skin lesions appear as yellow morbilliform eruptions 2–5 mm in diameter with erythematous areolae. They occur on extensor surfaces (elbows, knees, buttocks) and disappear after triglyceride levels are reduced.

Necrobiosis lipoidica diabeticorum is usually located over the anterior surfaces of the legs or the dorsal surfaces of the ankles. They are oval or irregularly shaped plaques with demarcated borders and a glistening yellow surface and occur in women two to four times more frequently than in men. Pathologically, the lesions show degeneration of collagen, granulomatous inflammation of subcutaneous tissues and blood vessels, capillary basement membrane thickening and obliteration of vessel lumina. The condition is associated with type 1 diabetes, although it can occur in patients with type 2 diabetes, and also in patients without diabetes. First-line therapy includes topical and subcutaneous corticosteroids. Improving glycemic control may help the condition.

"Shin spots" are not uncommon in adults with diabetes. They are brownish, rounded, painless atrophic lesions of the skin in the pretibial area.

F. Bone and Joint Complications

A number of bone and joint complications occur in people with diabetes. Long-standing diabetes can cause progressive stiffness of the hand secondary to contracture and tightening of skin over the joints (diabetic cheiroarthropathy), frozen shoulder (adhesive capsulitis), carpal tunnel syndrome, and Dupuytren contractures. These complications are believed to be due to glycosylation of collagen and perhaps other proteins in connective tissue. There may also be an inflammatory component.

Data on bone mineral density and fracture risk in people with diabetes are contradictory. Patients with type 2 diabetes do appear to be at increased risk for nonvertebral fractures. Women with type 1 diabetes have an increased

risk of fracture when compared with women without diabetes. Other factors, such as duration of diabetes, and diabetes complications, such as neuropathy and kidney disease, likely affect both the bone mineral density and fracture risk.

Diffuse idiopathic skeletal hyperostosis (DISH) is characterized by ossification of the anterior longitudinal ligaments of the spine and various extraspinal ligaments. It causes stiffness and decreased range of spinal motion. The peripheral joints most commonly affected are the metacarpophalangeal joints, elbows, and shoulders. Diabetes, obesity, hypertension, and dyslipidemia are risk factors for this condition.

Hyperuricemia and acute and tophaceous gout are more common in type 2 diabetes.

Bursitis, particularly of the shoulders and hips occurs more frequently than expected in patients with diabetes.

Chin JA et al. Diabetes mellitus and peripheral vascular disease: diagnosis and management. Clin Podiatr Med Surg. 2014 Jan;31(1):11–26. [PMID: 24296015]

Lingam G et al. Systemic medical management of diabetic retinopathy. Middle East Afr J Ophthalmol. 2013 Oct-Dec;20(4):301–8. [PMID: 24339679]

Singleton JR et al. The diabetic neuropathies: practical and rational therapy. Semin Neurol. 2012 Jul;32(3):196–203. [PMID: 23117944]

Waanders F et al. Current concepts in the management of diabetic nephropathy. Neth J Med. 2013 Nov;71(9):448–58. [PMID: 24218418]

▶ Special Situations

A. Diabetes Management in the Hospital

Most patients with diabetes are hospitalized for reasons other than their diabetes. Indeed, up to 10–15% of all hospitalized patients have diabetes. Audits suggest that as many as a 30% of these hospitalized patients have inappropriate management of their diabetes, with such errors as being given metformin where contraindicated, failure to act on high blood glucose levels, omission of diabetes medication, no record of diabetes complications, and inappropriate insulin management or blood glucose monitoring. It is challenging using outpatient oral therapies or insulin regimens in the hospital because patients are not eating as usual; they are often fasting for procedures; clinical events increase adverse reactions associated with diabetes medicines, eg, thiazolidinediones can cause fluid retention and worsen heart failure; metformin should not be used in patients with significant chronic kidney or liver disease, or those getting contrast for radiographic studies. Subcutaneous or intravenous insulin therapy is frequently substituted for other diabetes medicines because the insulin dose can be adjusted to match changing inpatient needs and it is safe to use insulin in patients with heart, kidney, and liver disease.

Surgery represents a stress situation during which most of the insulin antagonists (eg, catecholamines, growth hormone, and corticosteroids) are mobilized. In the diabetic patient, this can lead to a worsening of hyperglycemia and perhaps even ketoacidosis. The aim of medical management of people with diabetes during the perioperative period is to minimize these stress-induced changes. Recommendations for management depend both on the patient's usual diabetic regimen and on the type of surgery (major or minor) to be done (see also Chapter 3).

For people with diabetes controlled with diet alone, no special precautions must be taken unless diabetic control is markedly disturbed by the procedure. If this occurs, small doses of short-acting insulin as needed will correct the hyperglycemia.

Patients taking oral agents should not take them on the day of surgery. If there is significant hyperglycemia, small doses of short-acting insulin are given as needed. If this approach does not provide adequate control, an insulin infusion should be started in the manner indicated below. The oral agents can be restarted once the patient is eating normally after the operation. It is important to order a postoperative serum creatinine level to ensure adequate kidney function prior to restarting metformin therapy.

Patients taking insulin represent the only serious challenge to management of diabetes when surgery is necessary. However, with careful attention to changes in the clinical or laboratory picture, glucose control can be managed successfully. The protocol used to control the glucose depends on the kind of diabetes (type 1 or type 2); whether it is minor surgery (lasting < 2 hours and patient eating afterwards) or major surgery (lasting > 2 hours, with invasion of a body cavity, and patient not eating afterwards); and the preoperative insulin regimen (basal bolus or premixed insulin twice a day or premeal bolus only or regular insulin before meals and NPH at bedtime). Patients with type 1 diabetes must be receiving some insulin to prevent the development of diabetic ketoacidosis. Many patients with type 2 diabetes who are taking insulin do well perioperatively without insulin for a few hours. Ideally, patients with diabetes should undergo surgery early in the morning. Table 27–10 summarizes the approach for these patients.

One insulin infusion method adds 10 units of regular insulin to 1 L of 5% dextrose in 0.45% saline, and this is infused intravenously at a rate of 100–180 mL/h. This gives the patient 1–1.8 units of insulin per hour which, except in the most severe cases, generally keeps the blood glucose within the range of 100–250 mg/dL (5.5–13.9 mmol/L).

The infusion may be continued for several days, if necessary. Perioperatively, plasma glucose or blood glucose should be determined every 2–4 hours to be sure metabolic control is adequate. If it is not, adjustments in the ratio of insulin to dextrose in the intravenous solution can be made.

An alternative method consists of separate infusions of insulin and glucose delivered by pumps to permit independent adjustments of each infusion rate, depending on hourly variation of blood glucose values. There are a number of different algorithms available for insulin infusions (see http://www.hospitalmedicine.org).

After surgery, when the patient has resumed an adequate oral intake, subcutaneous administration of insulin can be resumed and intravenous administration of insulin and dextrose can be stopped 30 minutes after the first subcutaneous dose. Insulin needs may vary in the first several days after surgery because of continuing postoperative stresses and because of variable caloric intake. In this situation, multiple doses of short-acting insulin plus some long-acting basal insulin, guided by blood glucose determinations, can keep the patient in acceptable metabolic control.

In the **intensive care units (ICUs)**, glucose levels are controlled most frequently using insulin infusions. Patients receiving total parenteral nutrition can have insulin added to the bag. Standard total parenteral nutrition contains 25% dextrose so an infusion rate of 50 mL/h delivers 12.5 g of dextrose per hour.

On the **general surgical and medical wards**, most patients are treated with subcutaneous insulin regimens. Limited cross-sectional and prospective studies suggest that the best glucose control is achieved on a combination of basal and bolus regimen with 50% of daily insulin needs provided by intermediate- or long-acting insulins. Standardized order sets prompt medical personnel to write more physiologic insulin orders; they can reduce errors; and they often include algorithms for recognition and treatment of hypoglycemia (see http://ucsfinpatientdiabetes.pbworks.com for examples).

The morbidity and mortality in diabetic patients is twice that of nondiabetic patients. Those with new-onset hyperglycemia (ie, those without a preadmission diagnosis

Table 27–10. Recommendations for management of insulin-treated diabetes during surgery.

Type of Diabetes	Minor Surgical Procedures (< 2 hours; eating afterwards)	Major Surgical Procedures (> 2 hours; invasion of body cavity; not eating immediately after recovery)
Type 2: Patients taking basal bolus insulin regimen; twice daily premixed insulin	No insulin on the day of operation. Start 5% dextrose infusion; monitor fingerstick blood glucose and give subcutaneous short-acting insulin every 4 or 6 hours	Same regimen as minor procedure. If control is not satisfactory, then intravenous insulin infusion
Type 1: Patients taking basal bolus insulin regimen or using insulin pump	Patients using pump should discontinue the pump the evening before procedure and given 24 hour basal insulin. On day of procedure, start 5% dextrose; monitor blood glucose and give subcutaneous short-acting insulin every 4 or 6 hours	Initiate insulin infusion on morning of procedure and transition back to usual regimen when eating

of diabetes) have even higher mortality—almost eightfold that of nondiabetic patients in one study. These observations have led to the question of whether tight glycemic control in the hospital improves outcomes.

A prospective trial in surgical ICU patients (Leuven 1 study) reported that aggressive treatment of hyperglycemia (defined as blood glucose > 110 mg/dL [6.1 mmol/L]) reduced mortality and morbidity. Only a small number of persons in this study (204 of 1548) had a diagnosis of diabetes preoperatively, and so this study suggests that controlling hyperglycemia per se (independent of a diagnosis of diabetes) was beneficial. The benefits, however, were principally seen in patients who were in the ICU for longer than 5 days, and it is unclear whether the benefits also apply to most surgical patients who stay in the ICU for only 1 to 2 days.

The same investigators performed a similar prospective trial among 1200 medical ICU patients (Leuven 2 study) and reported that aggressive treatment of hyperglycemia reduced morbidity (decreased acquired kidney injury and increased early weaning from mechanical ventilation) but not mortality. Again, as in the surgical ICU study, only a small number of persons (16.9%) had a diagnosis of diabetes at admission.

The findings of the Leuven studies, however, have not been confirmed by other prospective studies. Two other ICU-based studies (Glucontrol and VISEP) that attempted to confirm the findings were unable to do so. Both studies were stopped prematurely, however. The Glucontrol study was stopped because an interim analysis (falsely) suggested increased mortality in the test group; and the VISEP study was stopped because of seven-fold increase in hypoglycemic events in the intensively treated group. A large multicenter, multinational study (NICE-SUGAR) recruited 6104 surgical and medical ICU patients with hyperglycemia (20% had diabetes) and randomized them to tight control (blood glucose levels of 81–108 mg/dL [4.5–6 mmol/L]) or less tight control (glucose levels < 180 mg/dL [< 10 mmol/L]). The tight group achieved blood glucose levels of 115 ± 18 mg/dL (6.4 ± 1.0 mmol/L) and the conventional group, 144 ± 23 mg/dL (8 ± 1.3 mmol/L). There were more deaths (829 versus 751 deaths) in the tight glucose control group compared with the less tight glucose control group ($P = 0.02$). The excess deaths in the intensive group were due to cardiovascular events. The intensively treated group also had more cases of severe hypoglycemia (206 versus 15 cases).

A study on tight intraoperative glycemic control during cardiac surgery also failed to show any benefit; if anything, the intensively treated group had more events. The United Kingdom Glucose Insulin in Stroke Trial (GIST-UK) failed to show beneficial effect of tight glycemic control in stroke patients; however, the investigators acknowledged that, because of slow recruitment, the study was underpowered.

Thus, based on the evidence available, ICU patients with diabetes and new-onset hyperglycemia with blood glucose levels above 180 mg/dL (10 mmol/L) should be treated with insulin, aiming for target glucose levels between 140 mg/dL (7.8 mmol/L) and 180 mg/dL (10 mmol/L). In the ICU setting, aiming for blood glucose levels close to 100 mg/dL (5.6 mmol/L) is not beneficial and may even be harmful. When patients leave the ICU, target glucose values between 100 mg/dL (5.6 mmol/L) and 180 mg/dL (10 mmol/L) may be appropriate, although this view is based on clinical observations rather than conclusive evidence.

B. Pregnancy and the Diabetic Patient

Tight glycemic control with normal HbA_{1c} levels is very important during pregnancy. Early in pregnancy, poor control increases the risk of spontaneous abortion and congenital malformations. Late in pregnancy, poor control can result in polyhydramnios, preterm labor, stillbirth, and fetal macrosomia with its associated problems. Diabetes complications can impact both maternal and fetal health. Diabetic retinopathy can first develop during pregnancy or retinopathy that is already present can worsen. Diabetic women with microalbuminuria can have worsening albuminuria during pregnancy and are at higher risk for preeclampsia. Patients who have preexisting kidney failure (prepregnancy creatinine clearance < 80 mL/min) are at high risk for further decline in kidney function during the pregnancy, and this may not reverse after delivery. Diabetic gastroparesis can severely exacerbate the nausea and vomiting of pregnancy and some patients may require fluid and nutritional support.

Although there is evidence that glyburide is safe during pregnancy, the current practice is to control diabetes with insulin therapy. Every effort should be made, utilizing multiple injections of insulin or a continuous infusion of insulin by pump, to maintain near-normalization of fasting and preprandial blood glucose values while avoiding hypoglycemia. The fast-acting insulin analogs insulin aspart and insulin lispro can be used, but data on using the long-acting insulin analogs are limited. A small study using insulin glargine in 32 pregnancies did not reveal any problems. There are no data on insulin detemir use in pregnancy. NPH is currently the preferred intermediate insulin for basal coverage during pregnancy.

Unless there are fetal or maternal complications, diabetic women should be able to carry the pregnancy to full-term, delivering at 38 to 41 weeks. Induction of labor before 39 weeks may be considered if there is concern about increasing fetal weight. See Chapter 19 for further details.

Ballas J et al. Management of diabetes in pregnancy. Curr Diab Rep. 2012 Feb;12(1):33–42. [PMID: 22139557]
Kansagara D et al. Intensive insulin therapy in hospitalized patients: a systematic review. Ann Intern Med. 2011 Feb 15;154(4):268–82. [PMID: 21320942]

▶ Prognosis

The DCCT showed that the previously poor prognosis for as many as 40% of patients with type 1 diabetes is markedly improved by optimal care. DCCT participants were generally young and highly motivated and were cared for in academic centers by skilled diabetes educators and endocrinologists who were able to provide more attention and services than are usually available. Improved training of primary care providers may be beneficial.

For type 2 diabetes, the UKPDS documented a reduction in microvascular disease with glycemic control, although this was not apparent in the obese subgroup. Cardiovascular outcomes were not improved by glycemic control, although antihypertensive therapy showed benefit in reducing the number of adverse cardiovascular complications as well as in reducing the occurrence of microvascular disease among hypertensive patients. In patients with visceral obesity, successful management of type 2 diabetes remains a major challenge in the attempt to achieve appropriate control of hyperglycemia, hypertension, and dyslipidemia. Once safe and effective methods are devised to prevent or manage obesity, the prognosis of type 2 diabetes with its high cardiovascular risks should improve considerably.

In addition to poorly understood genetic factors relating to differences in individual susceptibility to development of long-term complications of hyperglycemia, it is clear that in both types of diabetes, the diabetic patient's intelligence, motivation, and awareness of the potential complications of the disease contribute significantly to the ultimate outcome.

▶ When to Refer

- All patients should receive self-management education when diabetes is diagnosed and at intervals thereafter. The instructional team must include a registered dietitian and registered nurse; they must be Certified Diabetes Educators (CDEs).

- Patients with type 1 diabetes should be referred to an endocrinologist for comanagement with a primary care provider.

- Patients with type 2 diabetes should be referred to an endocrinologist if treatment goals are not met or if the patient requires an increasingly complex regimen to maintain glycemic control.

- Patients with type 2 diabetes should be referred to an ophthalmologist or optometrist for a dilated eye examination when the diabetes is diagnosed, and patients with type 1 diabetes should be referred 5 years after the diagnosis is made.

- Patients with peripheral neuropathy, especially those with loss of protective threshold (unable to detect 5.07 Semmes-Weinstein filament) or structural foot problems, should be referred to a podiatrist.

- Referrals to other specialists may be required for management of chronic complications of diabetes.

American Association of Diabetes Educators http://www.aadenet.org/
American Diabetes Association http://www.diabetes.org/home
American Diabetes Association. Standards of Medical Care in Diabetes—2013. Diabetes Care. 2013 Jan;36(Suppl 1):S11–66. [PMID: 23264422]
American Dietetic Association http://www.eatright.org
Juvenile Diabetes Foundation http://www.jdf.org/index.html

DIABETIC COMA

Coma may be due to a variety of causes not directly related to diabetes. Certain causes directly related to diabetes require differentiation: (1) Hypoglycemic coma resulting from excessive doses of insulin or oral hypoglycemic agents. (2) Hyperglycemic coma associated with either severe insulin deficiency (diabetic ketoacidosis) or mild to moderate insulin deficiency (hyperglycemic hyperosmolar state). (3) Lactic acidosis associated with diabetes, particularly in diabetics stricken with severe infections or with cardiovascular collapse.

DIABETIC KETOACIDOSIS

ESSENTIALS OF DIAGNOSIS

- ▶ Hyperglycemia > 250 mg/dL (13.9 mmol/L).
- ▶ Acidosis with blood pH < 7.3.
- ▶ Serum bicarbonate < 15 mEq/L.
- ▶ Serum positive for ketones.

▶ General Considerations

Diabetic ketoacidosis may be the initial manifestation of type 1 diabetes or may result from increased insulin requirements in type 1 diabetes patients during the course of infection, trauma, myocardial infarction, or surgery. It is a life-threatening medical emergency with a mortality rate just under 5% in individuals under 40 years of age, but with a more serious prognosis in the elderly, who have mortality rates over 20%. The National Data Group reports an annual incidence of five to eight episodes of diabetic ketoacidosis per 1000 diabetic persons. Ketoacidosis may develop in patients with type 2 diabetes when severe stress such as sepsis or trauma is present. Diabetic ketoacidosis has been found to be one of the more common serious complications of insulin pump therapy, occurring in approximately 1 per 80 patient-months of treatment. Many patients who monitor capillary blood glucose regularly ignore urine ketone measurements, which would signal the possibility of insulin leakage or pump failure before serious illness develops. Poor compliance, either for psychological reasons or because of inadequate education, is one of the most common causes of diabetic ketoacidosis, particularly when episodes are recurrent.

▶ Clinical Findings

A. Symptoms and Signs

The appearance of diabetic ketoacidosis is usually preceded by a day or more of polyuria and polydipsia associated with marked fatigue, nausea, and vomiting. If untreated, mental stupor ensues that can progress to coma. Drowsiness is fairly common but frank coma only occurs in about 10% of patients. On physical examination, evidence of dehydration in a stuporous patient with rapid deep breathing and a "fruity" breath odor of acetone would strongly suggest the diagnosis. Hypotension with tachycardia indicates profound fluid and electrolyte depletion, and mild hypothermia is usually present. Abdominal pain and even tenderness may be present in the absence of abdominal disease. Conversely, cholecystitis or pancreatitis may occur with minimal symptoms and signs.

B. Laboratory Findings

(Table 27–11.) Typically, the patient with moderately severe diabetic ketoacidosis has a plasma glucose of 350–900 mg/dL (19.4–50 mmol/L), serum ketones at a dilution of 1:8 or greater, hyperkalemia (serum potassium level of 5–8 mEq/L), slight hyponatremia (serum sodium of approximately 130 mEq/L), hyperphosphatemia (serum phosphate level of 6–7 mg/dL [1.9–2.3 mmol/L]), and elevated blood urea nitrogen and serum creatinine levels. Acidosis may be severe (pH ranging from 6.9 to 7.2, and serum bicarbonate ranging from 5 mEq/L to 15 mEq/L); P_{CO_2} is low (15–20 mm Hg) related to hyperventilation. Fluid depletion is marked, typically about 100 mL/kg.

The hyperkalemia occurs despite total body potassium depletion because of the shift of potassium from the intracellular to extracellular spaces that occurs in systemic acidosis. The average total body potassium deficit resulting from osmotic diuresis, acidosis, and gastrointestinal losses is about 3–5 mEq/kg. Similarly, despite the elevated serum phosphate, total body phosphate is generally depleted. Serum sodium is generally reduced due to loss of sodium ions (7–10 mEq/kg) by polyuria and vomiting and because severe hyperglycemia shifts intracellular water into the interstitial compartment. There is some controversy about the correction factor for the serum sodium in the presence of hyperglycemia. Many guidelines recommend a correction factor, whereby the serum sodium concentration decreases by 1.6 mEq/L for every 100 mg/dL (5.56 mmol/L) rise in plasma glucose above normal, but there is evidence that the decrease may be greater when patients have more severe hyperglycemia (greater than 400 mg/dL or 22.2

mmol/L) and/or volume depletion. One group has suggested (based on short-term exposure of normal volunteers to markedly elevated glucose levels) that, when the serum glucose is greater than 200 mg/dL (11.1 mmol/L), the serum sodium concentration decreases by at least 2.4 mEq/L. Serum osmolality can be directly measured by standard tests of freezing point depression or can be estimated by calculating the molarity of sodium, chloride, and glucose in the serum. A convenient method of estimating effective serum osmolality is as follows (normal values in humans are 280–300 mosm/kg):

$$mosm/kg = 2 \text{ [measured Na}^+\text{]} + \frac{\text{Glucose (mg/dL)}}{18}$$

These calculated estimates are usually 10–20 mosm/kg lower than values measured by standard cryoscopic techniques. Central nervous system depression or coma occurs when the effective serum osmolality exceeds 320–330 mosm/L. Coma in a diabetic patient with a lower osmolality should prompt a search for cause of coma other than hyperosmolality (see Chapter 21).

Blood urea nitrogen and serum creatinine are invariably elevated because of dehydration. In some automated creatinine assays, serum creatinine can be falsely elevated by nonspecific chromogenicity of keto acids and glucose. Most laboratories, however, now routinely eliminate this interference.

Ketoacidemia represents the effect of insulin lack at multiple enzyme loci. Insulin lack associated with elevated levels of growth hormone, catecholamines, and glucagon contributes to increases in lipolysis from adipose tissue and in hepatic ketogenesis. In addition, reduced ketolysis by insulin-deficient peripheral tissues contributes to the ketoacidemia. The only true "keto" acid present is acetoacetic acid which, along with its by-product acetone, is measured by nitroprusside reagents (Acetest and Ketostix). The sensitivity for acetone, however, is poor, requiring over 10 mmol/L, which is seldom reached in the plasma of ketoacidotic patients—although this detectable

Table 27–11. Laboratory diagnosis of coma in diabetic patients.

	Urine Glucose	Acetone	Plasma Glucose	Bicarbonate	Acetone
Related to diabetes					
Hypoglycemia	0[1]	0 or +	Low	Normal	0
Diabetic ketoacidosis	++++	++++	High	Low	++++
Hyperglycemic hyperosmolar state coma	++++	0	High	Normal or slightly low	0
Lactic acidosis	0 or +	0 or +	Normal or low or high	Low	0 or +
Unrelated to diabetes					
Alcohol or other toxic drugs	0 or +	0 or +	May be low	Normal or low[2]	0 or +
Cerebrovascular accident or head trauma	+ or 0	0	Often high	Normal	0
Uremia	0 or +	0	High or normal	Low	0 or +

[1]Leftover urine in bladder might still contain glucose from earlier hyperglycemia.
[2]Alcohol can elevate plasma lactate as well as keto acids to reduce pH.

concentration is readily achieved in urine. Thus, in the plasma of ketotic patients, only acetoacetate is measured by these reagents. The more prevalent beta-hydroxybutyric acid has no ketone group and is therefore not detected by conventional nitroprusside tests. This takes on special importance in the presence of circulatory collapse during diabetic ketoacidosis, wherein an increase in lactic acid can shift the redox state to increase beta-hydroxybutyric acid at the expense of the readily detectable acetoacetic acid. Bedside diagnostic reagents are then unreliable, suggesting no ketonemia in cases where beta-hydroxybutyric acid is a major factor in producing the acidosis. Combined glucose and ketone meter (Precision Xtra, Nova Max Plus) that measure blood beta-hydroxybutyrate concentration on capillary blood are now available. Many clinical laboratories also offer direct blood beta-hydroxybutyrate measurement.

Elevation of serum amylase is common but often represents salivary as well as pancreatic amylase. Thus, in this setting, an elevated serum amylase is not specific for acute pancreatitis. Serum lipase may be useful if the diagnosis of acute pancreatitis is being seriously considered. Leukocytosis as high as 25,000/mcL with a left shift may occur with or without associated infection. The presence of an elevated or even a normal temperature would suggest the presence of an infection, since patients with diabetic ketoacidosis are generally hypothermic if uninfected.

▶ **Treatment**

Patients with mild diabetic ketoacidosis are alert and have pH levels between 7.25 and 7.30; those with moderate ketoacidosis have pH levels between 7.0 and 7.24 and are either alert or little drowsy; and those with severe ketoacidosis are stuporose and have a pH < 7.0. Those with mild ketoacidosis can be treated in the emergency department, but those with moderate or severe ketoacidosis require admission to the ICU or step-down unit. Therapeutic goals are to restore plasma volume and tissue perfusion, reduce blood glucose and osmolality toward normal, correct acidosis, replenish electrolyte losses, and identify and treat precipitating factors. Gastric intubation is recommended in the comatose patient to prevent vomiting and aspiration that may occur as a result of gastric atony, a common complication of diabetic ketoacidosis. An indwelling catheter may also be necessary. In patients with preexisting cardiac or renal failure or those in severe cardiovascular collapse, a central venous pressure catheter or a Swan-Ganz catheter should be inserted to evaluate the degree of hypovolemia and to monitor subsequent fluid administration.

A comprehensive flow sheet that includes vital signs, serial laboratory data, and therapeutic interventions (eg, fluids, insulin) should be meticulously maintained by the clinician responsible for the patient's care. Plasma glucose should be recorded hourly and electrolytes and pH at least every 2–3 hours during the initial treatment period. Bedside glucose meters should be used to titrate the insulin therapy. The patient should not receive sedatives or opioids in order to avoid masking signs and symptoms of impeding cerebral edema.

A. Fluid Replacement

In most patients, the fluid deficit is 4–5 L. Initially, 0.9% saline solution is the solution of choice to help reexpand the contracted vascular volume and should be started in the emergency department as soon as the diagnosis is established. The saline should be infused rapidly to provide 1 L/h over the first 1–2 hours. After the first 2 L of fluid have been given, the intravenous infusion should be at the rate of 300–400 mL/h. Use 0.9% ("normal") saline unless the serum sodium is> 150 mEq/L, when 0.45% ("half normal") saline solution should be used. The volume status should be very carefully monitored. Failure to give enough volume replacement (at least 3–4 L in 8 hours) to restore normal perfusion is one of the most serious therapeutic short-comings adversely influencing satisfactory recovery. Excessive fluid replacement (more than 5 L in 8 hours) may contribute to acute respiratory distress syndrome or cerebral edema. When blood glucose falls to approximately 250 mg/dL (13.9 mmol/L), the fluids should be changed to a 5% glucose-containing solution to maintain serum glucose in the range of 250–300 mg/dL (13.9–16.7 mmol/L). This will prevent the development of hypoglycemia and will also reduce the likelihood of cerebral edema, which could result from too rapid decline of blood glucose.

B. Insulin Replacement

Immediately after initiation of fluid replacement, regular insulin should be given intravenously in a loading dose of 0.1 unit/kg as a bolus to prime the tissue insulin receptors. Following the initial bolus, intravenous doses of insulin as low as 0.1 unit/kg/h are continuously infused or given hourly as an intramuscular injection; this is sufficient to replace the insulin deficit in most patients. A prospective randomized study showed that a bolus dose is not required if patients are given hourly insulin infusion at 0.14 unit/kg. Replacement of insulin deficiency helps correct the acidosis by reducing the flux of fatty acids to the liver, reducing ketone production by the liver, and also improving removal of ketones from the blood. Insulin treatment reduces the hyperosmolality by reducing the hyperglycemia. It accomplishes this by increasing removal of glucose through peripheral utilization as well as by decreasing production of glucose by the liver. This latter effect is accomplished by direct inhibition of gluconeogenesis and glycogenolysis as well as by lowered amino acid flux from muscle to liver and reduced hyperglucagonemia.

The insulin dose should be "piggy-backed" into the fluid line so the rate of fluid replacement can be changed without altering the insulin delivery rate. If the plasma glucose level fails to fall at least 10% in the first hour, a repeat loading dose (0.1 or 0.14 unit/kg) is recommended. The availability of bedside glucometers and of laboratory instruments for rapid and accurate glucose analysis (Beckman or Yellow Springs glucose analyzer) has contributed much to achieving optimal insulin replacement. Rarely, a patient with immune insulin resistance is encountered, and this requires doubling the insulin dose every 2–4 hours if hyperglycemia does not improve after the first two doses of insulin. The insulin dose should be adjusted to lower the glucose concentration by about 50–70 mg/dL (2.8–3.9 mmol/L).

C. Potassium

Total body potassium loss from polyuria and vomiting may be as high as 200 mEq. However, because of shifts of potassium from cells into the extracellular space as a consequence of acidosis, serum potassium is usually normal to slightly elevated prior to institution of treatment. As the acidosis is corrected, potassium flows back into the cells, and hypokalemia can develop if potassium replacement is not instituted. If the patient is not uremic and has an adequate urinary output, potassium chloride in doses of 10–30 mEq/h should be infused during the second and third hours after beginning therapy as soon as the acidosis starts to resolve. Replacement should be started sooner if the initial serum potassium is inappropriately normal or low and should be delayed if serum potassium fails to respond to initial therapy and remains above 5 mEq/L, as in cases of chronic kidney disease. Occasionally, a patient may present with a serum potassium level < 3.5 mEq/L, in which case insulin therapy should be delayed until the potassium level is corrected to > 3.5 mEq/L. An ECG can be of help in monitoring the patient's potassium status: High peaked T waves are a sign of hyperkalemia, and flattened T waves with U waves are a sign of hypokalemia. Foods high in potassium content should be prescribed when the patient has recovered sufficiently to take food orally. Tomato juice has 14 mEq of potassium per 240 mL, and a medium-sized banana provides about 10 mEq.

D. Sodium Bicarbonate

The use of sodium bicarbonate in management of diabetic ketoacidosis has been questioned since clinical benefit was not demonstrated in one prospective randomized trial and because of the following potentially harmful consequences: (1) development of hypokalemia from rapid shift of potassium into cells if the acidosis is overcorrected; (2) tissue anoxia from reduced dissociation of oxygen from hemoglobin when acidosis is rapidly reversed (leftward shift of the oxygen dissociation curve); and (3) cerebral acidosis resulting from lowering of cerebrospinal fluid pH. It must be emphasized, however, that these considerations are less important when very severe acidosis exists. Therefore, it is recommended that bicarbonate be administered to diabetic patients in ketoacidosis if the arterial blood pH is 7.0 or less, with careful monitoring to prevent overcorrection. One or two ampules of sodium bicarbonate (one ampule contains 44 mEq/50 mL) should be added to 1 L of 0.45% saline. (**Note:** Addition of sodium bicarbonate to 0.9% saline would produce a markedly hypertonic solution that could aggravate the hyperosmolar state already present.) This should be administered rapidly (over the first hour). It can be repeated until the arterial pH reaches 7.1, but *it should not be given if the pH is 7.1 or greater* since additional bicarbonate would increase the risk of rebound metabolic alkalosis as ketones are metabolized. Alkalosis shifts potassium from serum into cells, which could precipitate a fatal cardiac arrhythmia.

E. Phosphate

Phosphate replacement is seldom required in treating diabetic ketoacidosis. However, if severe hypophosphatemia of < 1 mg/dL (< 0.32 mmol/L) develops during insulin therapy, a small amount of phosphate can be replaced per hour as the potassium salt. Correction of hypophosphatemia helps restore the buffering capacity of the plasma, thereby facilitating renal excretion of hydrogen. It also corrects the impaired oxygen dissociation from hemoglobin by regenerating 2,3-diphosphoglycerate. However, three randomized studies in which phosphate was replaced in patients with diabetic ketoacidosis did not show any apparent clinical benefit from phosphate administration. Moreover, attempts to use potassium phosphate as the sole means of replacing potassium have led to a number of reported cases of severe hypocalcemia with tetany. To minimize the risk of inducing tetany from too-rapid replacement of phosphate, the average deficit of 40–50 mmol of phosphate should be replaced intravenously at a rate *no > 3–4 mmol/h* in a 60–70-kg person. A stock solution (Abbott) provides a mixture of 1.12 g KH_2PO_4 and 1.18 g K_2HPO_4 in a 5-mL single-dose vial (this equals 22 mmol of potassium and 15 mmol of phosphate). One-half of this vial (2.5 mL) should be added to 1 L of either 0.45% saline or 5% dextrose in water. Two liters of this solution, infused at a rate of 400 mL/h, will correct the phosphate deficit at the optimal rate of 3 mmol/h while providing 4.4 mEq of potassium per hour. (Additional potassium should be administered as potassium chloride to provide a total of 10–30 mEq of potassium per hour, as noted above.) If the serum phosphate remains below 2.5 mg/dL (0.8 mmol/L) after this infusion, a repeat 5-hour infusion can be given.

F. Hyperchloremic Acidosis During Therapy

Because of the considerable loss of keto acids in the urine during the initial phase of therapy, substrate for subsequent regeneration of bicarbonate is lost and correction of the total bicarbonate deficit is hampered. A portion of the bicarbonate deficit is replaced with chloride ions infused in large amounts as saline to correct the dehydration. In most patients, as the ketoacidosis clears during insulin replacement, a hyperchloremic, low-bicarbonate pattern emerges with a normal anion gap. This is a relatively benign condition that reverses itself over the subsequent 12–24 hours once intravenous saline is no longer being administered. Using a balanced electrolyte solution similar to serum in chloride concentration and pH during resuscitation instead of normal saline has been reported to prevent the hyperchloremic acidosis.

G. Treatment of Associated Infection

Antibiotics are prescribed as indicated. Cholecystitis and pyelonephritis may be particularly severe in these patients.

H. Transition to Subcutaneous Insulin Regimen

Once the diabetic ketoacidosis is controlled and the patient is awake and able to eat, subcutaneous insulin therapy can be initiated. The patient with type 1 diabetes may have persistent significant tissue insulin resistance and may require a total daily insulin dose of approximately 0.6 units/kg. The amount of insulin required in the previous 8 hours can also be helpful in estimating the initial insulin doses. Half the total daily dose can be given as a long-acting basal insulin and the other half as short-acting insulin premeals. The patient should receive subcutaneous basal insulin and rapid-acting insulin analog with the first meal and the insulin infusion discontinued an hour later. The overlap of the subcutaneous insulin action and insulin infusion is necessary to prevent relapse of the diabetic ketoacidosis. The increased insulin resistance is only present for a few days, and it is important to reduce both the basal and bolus insulins to avoid hypoglycemia. A patient with new-onset type 1 diabetes usually still has significant beta cell function and may not need any basal insulin and only very low doses of rapid-acting insulin before meals after recovery from the ketoacidosis. Patients with type 2 diabetes and diabetes ketoacidosis due to severe illness may initially require insulin therapy but can often transition back to oral agents during outpatient follow-up.

Prognosis

Low-dose insulin infusion and fluid and electrolyte replacement combined with careful monitoring of patients' clinical and laboratory responses to therapy have dramatically reduced the mortality rates of diabetic ketoacidosis to < 5%. However, this complication remains a significant risk in the aged who have mortality rates > 20% and in patients in profound coma in whom treatment has been delayed. Acute myocardial infarction and infarction of the bowel following prolonged hypotension worsen the outlook. A serious prognostic sign is end-stage chronic kidney disease, and prior kidney dysfunction worsens the prognosis considerably because the kidney plays a key role in compensating for massive pH and electrolyte abnormalities. Symptomatic cerebral edema occurs primarily in the pediatric population. Risk factors for its development include severe baseline acidosis, rapid correction of hyperglycemia, and excess volume administration in the first 4 hours. Onset of headache or deterioration in mental status during treatment should lead to consideration of this complication. Intravenous mannitol at a dosage of 1–2 g/kg given over 15 minutes is the mainstay of treatment. Excess crystalloid infusion can precipitate pulmonary edema. Acute respiratory distress syndrome is a rare complication of treatment of diabetic ketoacidosis.

After recovery and stabilization, patients should be instructed on how to recognize the early symptoms and signs of ketoacidosis. Urine ketones or capillary blood beta-hydroxybutyrate should be measured in patients with signs of infection or in insulin pump-treated patients when capillary blood glucose remains unexpectedly and persistently high. When heavy ketonuria and glycosuria persist on several successive examinations, supplemental rapid acting insulin should be administered and liquid foods such as lightly salted tomato juice and broth should be ingested to replenish fluids and electrolytes. The patient should be instructed to contact the clinician if ketonuria persists, and especially if there is vomiting and inability to keep down fluids. Recurrent episodes of severe ketoacidosis often indicate poor compliance with the insulin regimen, and these patients will require intensive counseling.

Savage MW et al. Joint British Diabetes Societies guideline for the management of diabetic ketoacidosis. Diabet Med. 2011 May;28(5):508–15. [PMID: 21255074]

HYPERGLYCEMIC HYPEROSMOLAR STATE

ESSENTIALS OF DIAGNOSIS

▸ Hyperglycemia > 600 mg/dL (33.3 mmol/L).

▸ Serum osmolality > 310 mosm/kg.

▸ No acidosis; blood pH above 7.3.

▸ Serum bicarbonate > 15 mEq/L.

▸ Normal anion gap (< 14 mEq/L)

General Considerations

This second most common form of hyperglycemic coma is characterized by severe hyperglycemia in the absence of significant ketosis, with hyperosmolality and dehydration. It occurs in patients with mild or occult diabetes, and most patients are typically middle-aged to elderly. Accurate figures are not available as to its true incidence, but from data on hospital discharges it is rarer than diabetic ketoacidosis even in older age groups. Underlying chronic kidney disease or heart failure is common, and the presence of either worsens the prognosis. A precipitating event such as infection, myocardial infarction, stroke, or recent operation is often present. Certain medications such as phenytoin, diazoxide, corticosteroids, and diuretics have been implicated in its pathogenesis, as have procedures associated with glucose loading such as peritoneal dialysis.

Pathogenesis

A partial or relative insulin deficiency may initiate the syndrome by reducing glucose utilization of muscle, fat, and liver while inducing hyperglucagonemia and increasing hepatic glucose output. With massive glycosuria, obligatory water loss ensues. If a patient is unable to maintain adequate fluid intake because of an associated acute or chronic illness or has suffered excessive fluid loss, marked dehydration results. As the plasma volume contracts, kidney function becomes impaired, limiting the urinary glucose losses and exacerbating the hyperglycemia. Severe hyperosmolality develops that causes mental confusion and finally coma. It is not clear why ketosis is virtually absent under these conditions of insulin insufficiency, although reduced levels of growth hormone may be a factor, along with portal vein insulin concentrations sufficient to restrain ketogenesis.

Clinical Findings

A. Symptoms and Signs

Onset may be insidious over a period of days or weeks, with weakness, polyuria, and polydipsia. The lack of features of ketoacidosis may retard recognition of the syndrome and delay therapy until dehydration becomes more profound than in ketoacidosis. Reduced intake of fluid is not an uncommon historical feature, due to either inappropriate lack of thirst, nausea, or inaccessibility of fluids to elderly, bedridden patients. Lethargy and confusion develop as serum osmolality exceeds 310 mosm/kg, and convulsions and coma can occur if osmolality exceeds 320–330 mosm/kg. Physical examination confirms the presence of profound dehydration in a lethargic or comatose patient without Kussmaul respirations.

B. Laboratory Findings

(Table 27–11.) Severe hyperglycemia is present, with blood glucose values ranging from 800 mg/dL to 2400 mg/dL (44.4 mmol/L to 133.2 mmol/L). In mild cases, where dehydration is less severe, dilutional hyponatremia as well as urinary sodium losses may reduce serum sodium to 120–125 mEq/L, which protects to some extent against extreme hyperosmolality. However, as dehydration progresses, serum sodium can exceed 140 mEq/L, producing serum osmolality readings of 330–440 mosm/kg. Ketosis and acidosis are usually absent or mild. Prerenal azotemia is the rule, with serum urea nitrogen elevations over 100 mg/dL (35.7 mmol/L) being typical.

▶ Treatment

A. Fluid Replacement

Fluid replacement is of paramount importance in treating nonketotic hyperglycemic coma. The onset of hyperosmolarity is more insidious in elderly people without ketosis than in younger individuals with high serum ketone levels, which provide earlier indicators of severe illness (vomiting, rapid deep breathing, acetone odor, etc). Consequently, diagnosis and treatment are often delayed until fluid deficit has reached levels of 6–10 L.

If hypovolemia is present as evidenced by hypotension and oliguria, fluid therapy should be initiated with 0.9% saline. In all other cases, 0.45% saline appears to be preferable as the initial replacement solution because the body fluids of these patients are markedly hyperosmolar. As much as 4–6 L of fluid may be required in the first 8–10 hours. Careful monitoring of the patient is required for proper sodium and water replacement. Once blood glucose reaches 250 mg/dL (13.9 mmol/L), fluid replacement should include 5% dextrose in either water, 0.45% saline solution, or 0.9% saline solution. The rate of dextrose infusion should be adjusted to maintain glycemic levels of 250–300 mg/dL (13.9–16.7 mmol/L) in order to reduce the risk of cerebral edema. An important end point of fluid therapy is to restore urinary output to 50 mL/h or more.

B. Insulin

Less insulin may be required to reduce the hyperglycemia in nonketotic patients as compared to those with diabetic ketoacidotic coma. In fact, fluid replacement alone can reduce hyperglycemia considerably by correcting the hypovolemia, which then increases both glomerular filtration and renal excretion of glucose. An initial insulin dose of 0.1 unit/kg is followed by an insulin infusion of 0.1 units/kg/h (or just an infusion of 0.14 units/kg/h without a bolus), which is titrated to lower blood glucose levels by 50–70 mg/dL per hour (2.8–3.9 mmol/L/h). Once the patient has stabilized and the blood glucose falls to around 250 mg/dL (13.9 mmol/L), insulin can be given subcutaneously.

C. Potassium

With the absence of acidosis, there may be no initial hyperkalemia unless associated end-stage chronic kidney disease is present. This results in less severe total potassium depletion than in diabetic ketoacidosis, and less potassium replacement is therefore needed. However, because initial serum potassium is usually not elevated and because it declines rapidly as a result of insulin's effect on driving potassium intracellularly, it has been recommended that potassium replacement be initiated earlier than in ketotic patients, assuming that no chronic kidney disease or oliguria is present. Potassium chloride (10 mEq/L) can be added to the initial bottle of fluids administered if the patient's serum potassium is not elevated.

D. Phosphate

If severe hypophosphatemia (serum phosphate < 1 mg/dL [< 0.32 mmol/L]) develops during insulin therapy, phosphate replacement can be given as described for ketoacidotic patients (at 3 mmol/h).

▶ Prognosis

The severe dehydration and low output state may predispose the patient to complications such as myocardial infarction, stroke, pulmonary embolism, mesenteric vein thrombosis, and disseminated intravascular coagulation. Fluid replacement remains the primary approach to the prevention of these complications. Low-dose heparin prophylaxis is reasonable but benefits of routine anticoagulation remain doubtful. Rhabdomyolysis is a recognized complication and should be looked for and treated.

The overall mortality rate of hyperglycemic hyperosmolar state coma is more than ten times that of diabetic ketoacidosis, chiefly because of its higher incidence in older patients, who may have compromised cardiovascular systems or associated major illnesses and whose dehydration is often excessive because of delays in recognition and treatment. (When patients are matched for age, the prognoses of these two hyperglycemic emergencies are reasonably comparable.) When prompt therapy is instituted, the mortality rate can be reduced from nearly 50% to that related to the severity of coexistent disorders.

After the patient is stabilized, the appropriate form of long-term management of the diabetes must be determined. Insulin treatment should be continued for a few weeks but patients usually recover sufficient endogenous insulin secretion to make a trial of diet or diet plus oral agents worthwhile. When the episode occurs in a patient who has known diabetes, then education of the patient and caregivers should be instituted. They should be taught how to recognize situations (nausea and vomiting, infection) that predispose to recurrence of the hyperglycemic, hyperosmolar state, as well as detailed information on how to prevent the escalating dehydration that culminates in hyperosmolar coma (small sips of sugar-free liquids, increase in usual hypoglycemic therapy, or early contact with the clinician).

Nyenwe EA et al. Evidence-based management of hyperglycemic emergencies in diabetes mellitus. Diabetes Res Clin Pract. 2011 Dec;94(3):340–51. [PMID: 21978840]

LACTIC ACIDOSIS

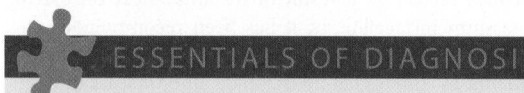

ESSENTIALS OF DIAGNOSIS

▶ Severe acidosis with hyperventilation.

▶ Blood pH below 7.30.

▶ Serum bicarbonate < 15 mEq/L.

▶ Anion gap > 15 mEq/L.

▶ Absent serum ketones.

▶ Serum lactate > 5 mmol/L

▶ General Considerations

Lactic acidosis is characterized by accumulation of excess lactic acid in the blood. Normally, the principal sources of this acid are the erythrocytes (which lack enzymes for aerobic oxidation), skeletal muscle, skin, and brain. Conversion of lactic acid to glucose and its oxidation principally by the liver but also by the kidneys represent the chief pathways for its removal. Overproduction of lactic acid (tissue hypoxia), deficient removal (hepatic failure), or both (circulatory collapse) can cause accumulation. Lactic acidosis is not uncommon in any severely ill patient suffering from cardiac decompensation, respiratory or hepatic failure, septicemia, or infarction of bowel or extremities. Lactic acidosis in patients with diabetes mellitus is uncommon but occasionally occurs in metformin-treated patients (see above) and it still must be considered in the acidotic diabetic patient, especially if the individual is seriously ill. Most cases of metformin-associated lactic acidosis occur in patients in whom there were contraindications to the use of metformin, in particular kidney failure.

▶ Clinical Findings

A. Symptoms and Signs

The main clinical feature of lactic acidosis is marked hyperventilation. When lactic acidosis is secondary to tissue hypoxia or vascular collapse, the clinical presentation is variable, being that of the prevailing catastrophic illness. However, in the idiopathic, or spontaneous, variety, the onset is rapid (usually over a few hours), blood pressure is normal, peripheral circulation is good, and there is no cyanosis.

B. Laboratory Findings

Plasma bicarbonate and blood pH are quite low, indicating the presence of severe metabolic acidosis. Ketones are usually absent from plasma and urine or at least not prominent. The first clue may be a high anion gap (serum sodium minus the sum of chloride and bicarbonate anions [in mEq/L] should be no> 15). A higher value indicates the existence of an abnormal compartment of anions. If this cannot be clinically explained by an excess of keto acids (diabetes), inorganic acids (uremia), or anions from medication overdosage (salicylates, methyl alcohol, ethylene glycol), then lactic acidosis is probably the correct diagnosis. (See also Chapter 21.) In the absence of azotemia, hyperphosphatemia may be a clue to the presence of lactic acidosis for reasons that are not clear. The diagnosis is confirmed by demonstrating, in a sample of blood that is promptly chilled and separated, a plasma lactic acid concentration of 5 mmol/L or higher (values as high as 30 mmol/L have been reported). Normal plasma values average 1 mmol/L, with a normal lactate/pyruvate ratio of 10:1. This ratio is greatly exceeded in lactic acidosis.[1]

▶ Treatment

Aggressive treatment of the precipitating cause of lactic acidosis is the main component of therapy, such as ensuring adequate oxygenation and vascular perfusion of tissues. Empiric antibiotic coverage for sepsis should be given after culture samples are obtained in any patient in whom the cause of the lactic acidosis is not apparent.

Alkalinization with intravenous sodium bicarbonate to keep the pH above 7.2 has been recommended by some in the emergency treatment of lactic acidosis; as much as 2000 mEq in 24 hours has been used. However, there is no evidence that the mortality rate is favorably affected by administering bicarbonate, and its use remains controversial. Hemodialysis may be useful in cases where large sodium loads are poorly tolerated and in cases associated with metformin toxicity.

▶ Prognosis

The mortality rate of spontaneous lactic acidosis is high. The prognosis in most cases is that of the primary disorder that produced the lactic acidosis.

---

[1]In collecting samples, it is essential to rapidly chill and separate the blood in order to remove red cells, whose continued glycolysis at room temperature is a common source of error in reports of high plasma lactate. Frozen plasma remains stable for subsequent assay.

Lalau JD. Lactic acidosis induced by metformin: incidence, management and prevention. Drug Saf. 2010 Sep 1;33(9):727–40. [PMID: 20701406]

THE HYPOGLYCEMIC STATES

Spontaneous hypoglycemia in adults is of two principal types: fasting and postprandial. Symptoms begin at plasma glucose levels in the range of 60 mg/dL (3.3 mmol/L) and impairment of brain function at approximately 50 mg/dL (2.8 mmol/L). Fasting hypoglycemia is often subacute or chronic and usually presents with neuroglycopenia as its principal manifestation; postprandial hypoglycemia is relatively acute and is often heralded by symptoms of neurogenic autonomic discharge (sweating, palpitations, anxiety, tremulousness).

► Differential Diagnosis (Table 27–12)

Fasting hypoglycemia may occur in certain endocrine disorders, such as hypopituitarism, Addison disease, or myxedema; in disorders related to liver malfunction, such as acute alcoholism or liver failure; and in instances of end-stage chronic kidney disease, particularly in patients requiring dialysis. These conditions are usually obvious, with hypoglycemia being only a secondary feature. When fasting hypoglycemia is a primary manifestation developing in adults without apparent endocrine disorders or inborn metabolic diseases from childhood, the principal diagnostic possibilities include: (1) hyperinsulinism, due to either pancreatic B cell tumors, iatrogenic or surreptitious administration of insulin or sulfonylurea and (2) hypoglycemia due to extrapancreatic tumors.

Postprandial (reactive) hypoglycemia may be seen after gastrointestinal surgery and is particularly associated with the dumping syndrome after gastrectomy and Roux-en-Y gastric bypass surgery. Occult diabetes very occasionally present with postprandial hypoglycemia. Rarely, it

Table 27–12. Common causes of hypoglycemia in adults.[1]

Fasting hypoglycemia
Pancreatic B cell tumor
Surreptitious administration of insulin or sulfonylureas
Extrapancreatic tumors
Postprandial hypoglycemia
Alimentary
Noninsulinoma pancreatogenous hypoglycemia syndrome
Functional
Occult diabetes mellitus
Alcohol-related hypoglycemia
Immunopathologic hypoglycemia
Idiopathic anti-insulin antibodies (which release their bound insulin)
Antibodies to insulin receptors (which act as agonists)
Drug-induced hypoglycemia

[1]In the absence of clinically obvious endocrine, renal, or hepatic disorders and exclusive of diabetes mellitus treated with hypoglycemic agents.

occurs with islet cell hyperplasia—the so-called noninsulinoma pancreatogenous hypoglycemia syndrome.

Alcohol-related hypoglycemia is due to hepatic glycogen depletion combined with alcohol-mediated inhibition of gluconeogenesis. It is most common in malnourished alcohol abusers but can occur in anyone who is unable to ingest food after an acute alcoholic episode followed by gastritis and vomiting.

Immunopathologic hypoglycemia is an extremely rare condition in which anti-insulin antibodies or antibodies to insulin receptors develop spontaneously. In the former case, the mechanism appears to relate to increasing dissociation of insulin from circulating pools of bound insulin. When antibodies to insulin receptors are found, most patients do not have hypoglycemia but rather severe insulin-resistant diabetes and acanthosis nigricans. However, during the course of the disease in these patients, certain anti-insulin receptor antibodies with agonist activity mimicking insulin action may develop, producing severe hypoglycemia.

HYPOGLYCEMIA DUE TO PANCREATIC B CELL TUMORS

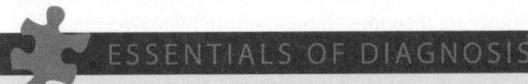
ESSENTIALS OF DIAGNOSIS

- ► Hypoglycemic symptoms—frequently neuroglycopenic (confusion, blurred vision, diplopia, anxiety, convulsions).
- ► Immediate recovery upon administration of glucose.
- ► Blood glucose < 45 mg/dL (2.5 mmol/L) with a serum insulin level of 6 microunit/mL or more.

► General Considerations

Fasting hypoglycemia in an otherwise healthy, well-nourished adult is rare and is most commonly due to an adenoma of the islets of Langerhans. Ninety percent of such tumors are single and benign, but multiple adenomas can occur as well as malignant tumors with functional metastases. Adenomas may be familial, and multiple adenomas have been found in conjunction with tumors of the parathyroids and pituitary (MEN type 1 [MEN 1]). Over 99% of them are located within the pancreas and less than 1% in ectopic pancreatic tissue.

► Clinical Findings

A. Symptoms and Signs

The most important prerequisite to diagnosing an insulinoma is simply to consider it, particularly in relatively healthy-appearing persons who have fasting hypoglycemia associated with some degree of central nervous system dysfunction such as confusion or abnormal behavior. A delay in diagnosis can result in unnecessary treatment for psychomotor epilepsy or psychiatric disorders and may cause irreversible brain damage. In long-standing cases, obesity can result as a consequence of overeating to relieve symptoms.

The so-called Whipple triad is characteristic of hypoglycemia regardless of the cause. It consists of (1) a history of hypoglycemic symptoms, (2) an associated fasting blood glucose of 45 mg/dL (2.5 mmol/L) or less, and (3) immediate recovery upon administration of glucose. The hypoglycemic symptoms in insulinoma often develop in the early morning or after missing a meal. Occasionally, they occur after exercise. They typically begin with evidence of central nervous system glucose lack and can include blurred vision or diplopia, headache, feelings of detachment, slurred speech, and weakness. Personality and mental changes vary from anxiety to psychotic behavior, and neurologic deterioration can result in convulsions or coma. Sweating and palpitations may not occur.

Hypoglycemic unawareness is very common in patients with insulinoma. They adapt to chronic hypoglycemia by increasing their efficiency in transporting glucose across the blood-brain barrier, which masks awareness that their blood glucose is approaching critically low levels. Counterregulatory hormonal responses as well as neurogenic symptoms such as tremor, sweating, and palpitations are therefore blunted during hypoglycemia. If lack of these warning symptoms prevents recognition of the need to eat to correct the problem, patients can lapse into severe hypoglycemic coma. However, symptoms and normal hormone responses during experimental insulin-induced hypoglycemia have been shown to be restored after successful surgical removal of the insulinoma. Presumably with return of euglycemia, adaptive effects on glucose transport into the brain are corrected, and thresholds of counterregulatory responses and neurogenic autonomic symptoms are therefore restored to normal.

B. Laboratory Findings

B cell adenomas do not reduce secretion of insulin in the presence of hypoglycemia, and the critical diagnostic test is to demonstrate inappropriately elevated serum insulin, proinsulin, and C-peptide levels at a time when plasma glucose level is below 45 mg/dL.

The diagnostic criteria for insulinoma after a 72-hour fast are listed in Table 27–13. Other causes of hyperinsulinemic hypoglycemia must be considered, including factitious administration of insulin or sulfonylureas. Factitious use of insulin will result in suppression of endogenous insulin secretion and low C-peptide levels. An elevated circulating proinsulin level in the presence of fasting hypoglycemia is characteristic of most B cell adenomas and does not occur in factitious hyperinsulinism. Thus, C-peptide levels (by immunochemiluminometric assays [ICMA]) of > 200 pmol/L and proinsulin levels (by RIA) of > 5 pmol/L are characteristic of insulinomas. In patients with insulinoma, plasma beta-hydroxybutyrate levels are suppressed to 2.7 mmol/L or less. No single hormone measurement (insulin, proinsulin, C-peptide) is 100% sensitive and specific for the diagnosis of insulinoma, and insulinoma cases have been reported with insulin levels

Table 27–13. Diagnostic criteria for insulinoma after a 72-hour fast.

Laboratory Test	Result
Plasma glucose	< 45 mg/dL (2.5 mmol/L)
Plasma insulin (RIA)[1]	≥ 6 microunit/mL
Plasma insulin (ICMA)[1]	≥ 3 microunit/mL
Plasma C-peptide	≥ 200 pmol/L (0.2 nmol/L)
Plasma proinsulin	≥ 5 pmol/L
Beta-hydroxybutyrate	≤ 2.7 mmol/L
Sulfonylurea screen (including repaglinide and nateglinide)	Negative

[1]Conversion factors: insulin microunit/mL × 6.0 = nmol/L; C-peptide ng/mL × 0.333 = nmol/L
RAI, ICMA, Immunochemiluminometric assays

below 3 microunits/mL (ICMA assay) or proinsulin level below 5 pmol/L. Therefore, the diagnosis should be based on multiple biochemical parameters.

In patients with epigastric distress, a history of renal calculi, or menstrual or erectile dysfunction, a serum calcium, gastrin, or prolactin level may be useful in screening for MEN 1 associated with insulinoma.

C. Diagnostic Tests

If the history is consistent with episodic spontaneous hypoglycemia, patients should be given a home blood glucose monitor and advised to monitor blood glucose levels at the time of symptoms and before consumption of carbohydrates, if this can be done safely. Patients with insulinomas frequently report fingerstick blood glucose levels between 40 mg/dL (2.2 mmol/L) and 50 mg/dL (2.8 mmol/L) at the time of symptoms. The diagnosis, however, cannot be made based on a fingerstick blood glucose. It is necessary to have a low laboratory glucose concomitantly with elevated plasma insulin, proinsulin, and C-peptide levels and a negative sulfonylurea screen. When patients give a history of symptoms after only a short period of food withdrawal or with exercise, then an outpatient assessment can be attempted. The patient should be brought by a family member to the office after an overnight fast and observed in the office. Activity such as walking should be encouraged and fingerstick blood glucose measured repeatedly during observation. If symptoms occur or fingerstick blood glucose is below 50 mg/dL (2.8 mmol/L) then samples for plasma glucose, insulin, C-peptide, proinsulin, sulfonylurea screen, serum ketones, and antibodies to insulin should be sent. If outpatient observation does not result in symptoms or hypoglycemia and if the clinical suspicion remains high, then the patient should undergo an inpatient supervised 72-hour fast. A suggested protocol for the supervised fast is shown in Table 27–14.

In 30% of patients with insulinoma, the blood glucose levels often drop below 45 mg/dL (2.5 mmol/L) after an

Table 27–14. Suggested hospital protocol for supervised fast in diagnosis of insulinoma.

(1) Obtain baseline plasma glucose, insulin, proinsulin, and C-peptide measurements at onset of fast and place intravenous cannula.

(2) Permit only calorie-free and caffeine-free fluids and encourage supervised activity (such as walking).

(3) Measure urine for ketones at the beginning and every 12 hours and at end of fast.

(4) Obtain capillary glucose measurements with a reflectance meter every 4 hours until values < 60 mg/dL are obtained. Then increase the frequency of fingersticks to each hour, and when capillary glucose value is < 49 mg/dL send a venous blood sample to the laboratory for plasma glucose[1], insulin, proinsulin, and C-peptide measurements. Check frequently for manifestations of neuroglycopenia.

(5) If symptoms of hypoglycemia occur or if a laboratory value of serum glucose is < 45 mg/dL, or if 72 hours have elapsed then conclude the fast with a final blood sample for plasma glucose,[1] insulin, proinsulin, C-peptide, beta-hydroxybutyrate and sulfonylurea measurements. Then give oral fast-acting carbohydrate followed by a meal. If the patient is confused or unable to take oral agents, then administer 50 mL of 50% dextrose intravenously over 3 to 5 minutes. Do not conclude a fast based simply on a capillary blood glucose measurement—wait for the laboratory glucose value—unless the patient is very symptomatic and it would be dangerous to wait.

[1] Glucose sample should be collected in sodium fluoride containing tube on ice to prevent glycolysis and the plasma separated immediately upon receipt at the laboratory. Arrange for the laboratory to run the glucose samples "stat."

overnight fast, but some patients require up to 72 hours to develop symptomatic hypoglycemia. However, the term "72-hour fast" is actually a misnomer in most cases since the fast should be immediately terminated as soon as symptoms appear and laboratory confirmation of hypoglycemia is available. In normal male subjects, the blood glucose does not fall below 55–60 mg/dL (3.1–3.3 mmol/L) during a 3-day fast. In contrast, in normal premenopausal women who have fasted for only 24 hours, the plasma glucose may fall normally to such an extent that it can reach values as low as 35 mg/dL (1.9 mmol/L). In these cases, however, the women are not symptomatic, presumably owing to the development of sufficient ketonemia to supply energy needs to the brain. Insulinoma patients, on the other hand, become symptomatic when plasma glucose drops to subnormal levels, since inappropriate insulin secretion restricts ketone formation. Moreover, the demonstration of a nonsuppressed insulin level ≥ 6 microunit/mL using a RIA assay (> 3 microunit/mL using an ICMA assay) in the presence of hypoglycemia suggests the diagnosis of insulinoma. If hypoglycemia does not develop in a male patient after fasting for up to 72 hours—and particularly when this prolonged fast is terminated with a period of moderate exercise—insulinoma must be considered an unlikely diagnosis.

Stimulation with pancreatic B cell secretagogues such as tolbutamide, glucagon, or leucine has been devised to demonstrate exaggerated and prolonged insulin secretion in the presence of insulinomas. However, because insulin-secreting tumors have a wide range of granule content and degrees of differentiation, they are variably responsive to these secretagogues; and a negative response does not necessarily rule out an insulinoma. For these reasons, stimulation tests are not recommended in the diagnostic work-up of insulinoma.

An oral glucose tolerance test is of no value in the diagnosis of insulin secreting tumors. HbA_{1c} levels may be low but there is considerable overlap with normal patients and no particular value is diagnostic.

D. Preoperative Localization of B Cell Tumors

After the diagnosis of insulinoma has been unequivocally made by clinical and laboratory findings, studies to localize the tumor should be initiated. The focus of attention should be directed to the pancreas since that is where virtually all insulinomas originate.

Because of the small size of these tumors (averaging 1.5 cm in diameter in one large series), imaging studies do not necessarily identify all of them. A pancreatic dual phase helical CT scan with thin section can identify 82–94% of the lesions. MRI scans with gadolinium can be helpful in detecting a tumor in 85% of cases. One case report suggests that diffusion-weighted MRI can be useful for detecting and localizing small insulinomas, especially for those with no hypervascular pattern. The imaging study used will depend on local availability and local radiologic skill. If the imaging study is normal, then an endoscopic ultrasound should be performed. In experienced hands, about 80–90% of tumors can be detected with this procedure. Fine-needle aspiration of the identified lesion can be attempted to confirm the presence of a neuroendocrine tumor. If the tumor is not identified or the imaging result is equivocal, then the patient should undergo selective calcium-stimulated angiography, which has been reported to localize the tumor to a particular region of the pancreas approximately about 90% of the time. In this test, angiography is combined with injections of calcium gluconate into the gastroduodenal, splenic, and superior mesenteric arteries, and insulin levels are measured in the hepatic vein effluent. The procedure is performed after an overnight fast. Calcium gluconate 10% solution diluted to a volume of 5 mL with 0.95% saline is bolused into the selected artery at a dose of 0.0125 mmol calcium/kg (0.005 mmol calcium/kg for obese patients). Small samples of blood (5 mL) are taken from the hepatic effluent at times 0, 30, 60, 90, 120, and 180 seconds after the calcium injection. Fingerstick blood glucose levels are measured at intervals and a dextrose infusion is maintained throughout the procedure to prevent hypoglycemia. Calcium stimulates insulin release from insulinomas but not normal islets, and so a step-up from baseline in insulin levels at 30 or 60 seconds (twofold or greater) regionalizes the source of the hyperinsulinism to the head of the pancreas for the gastroduodenal artery, the uncinate process for the superior mesenteric artery, and the body and tail of the pancreas for the splenic artery calcium infusions. A less than twofold elevation of insulin in the 120-second sample may represent effects of recirculating calcium and is not considered a positive localization. In a single insulinoma, the response is in one artery alone unless the tumor resides in an area fed by two arteries or if there are multiple insulinomas (eg, in MEN 1). Patients who have diffuse islet hyperplasia (the noninsulinoma pancreatogenous hypoglycemia syndrome) will have positive responses in multiple arteries. Because diazoxide may interfere with this test, it should be discontinued for at least 48–72 hours before sampling. Patients should be closely monitored during the procedure to avoid hypoglycemia (as well as hyperglycemia, which could affect insulin gradients). These studies combined with careful intraoperative ultrasonography and palpation by a surgeon experienced in insulinoma surgery identifies up to 98% of tumors.

▶ Treatment

The treatment of choice for insulin-secreting tumors is surgical resection. While waiting for surgery, patients should be given oral diazoxide. Divided doses of 300–400 mg/d usually suffice although an occasional patient may require up to 800 mg/d. Side effects include edema due to sodium retention, gastric irritation, and mild hirsuitism. Hydrochlorothiazide, 25–50 mg daily, can be used to counteract the sodium retention and edema as well potentiate diazoxide's hyperglycemic effect.

Tumor resection should be performed by a surgeon with experience in removing pancreatic B cell tumors. In patients with a single benign adenoma, 90–95% have a successful cure at the first surgical attempt when intraoperative ultrasound is used by a skilled surgeon. Diazoxide should be administered on the day of the surgery because it reduces the risk of hypoglycemia during surgery. Typically, it does not mask the glycemic rise indicative of surgical cure. Blood glucose should be monitored throughout surgery, and 5% or 10% dextrose infusion should be used to maintain euglycemia. In cases where the diagnosis has been established but no adenoma is located after careful palpation and use of intraoperative ultrasound, it is no longer advisable to blindly resect the body and tail of the pancreas, since a nonpalpable tumor missed by ultrasound is most likely embedded within the fleshy head of the pancreas that is left behind with subtotal resections. Most surgeons prefer to close the incision and schedule a selective arterial calcium stimulation with hepatic venous sampling to locate the tumor site prior to a repeat operation. Laparoscopy using ultrasound and enucleation has been successful with a single tumor of the body or tail of the pancreas, but open surgery remains necessary for tumors in the head of the pancreas.

In patients with inoperable functioning islet cell carcinoma and in approximately 5–10% of MEN 1 cases when subtotal removal of the pancreas has failed to produce cure, diazoxide is the treatment of choice. Frequent carbohydrate feedings (every 2 to 3 hours) can also be helpful although weight gain may become a problem. If patients are unable to tolerate diazoxide because of gastrointestinal upset, hirsutism, or edema, the calcium channel blocker verapamil may be beneficial in view of its inhibitory effect on insulin release from insulinoma cells. Octreotide, a potent long-acting synthetic octapeptide analog of somatostatin, has been used to inhibit release of hormones from a number of endocrine tumors. A dose of 50 mcg of octreotide injected subcutaneously twice daily has been tried in cases where surgery failed to remove the source of hyperinsulinism. However, its effectiveness is limited since its affinity for somatostatin receptors of the pancreatic B cell is very much less than for those of the anterior pituitary somatotrophs for which it was originally designed as treatment for acromegaly. When hypoglycemia persists after attempted surgical removal of the insulinoma and if diazoxide or verapamil is poorly tolerated or ineffective, multiple small feedings may be the only recourse. Streptozocin can decrease insulin secretion in islet cell carcinomas and increase survival. With selective arterial administration, effective cytotoxic doses have been achieved without undue renal toxicity that characterized early experience. Benign tumors appear to respond poorly, if at all.

Cryer PE et al. Evaluation and management of adult hypoglycemic disorders: an Endocrine Society Clinical Practice Guideline. J Clin Endocrinol Metab. 2009 Mar;94(3): 709–28. [PMID: 19088155]

Mathur A et al. Insulinoma. Surg Clin North Am. 2009 Oct;89 (5):1105–21. [PMID: 19836487]

NONISLET CELL TUMOR HYPOGLYCEMIA

These rare causes of hypoglycemia include mesenchymal tumors such as retroperitoneal sarcomas, hepatocellular carcinomas, adrenocortical carcinomas, and miscellaneous epithelial-type tumors. The tumors are frequently large and readily palpated or visualized on CT scans or MRI.

In many cases the hypoglycemia is due to the expression and release of an incompletely processed insulin-like growth factor 2 (IGF-2) by the tumor. This immature form of the IGF-II molecule (pro-IGF-2 or "big IGF-2") binds IGF-binding protein-3 (IGFBP-3) but not to the acid-labile subunit. As a consequence, this pro-IGF-II remains active and binds to insulin receptors in muscle to promote glucose transport and to insulin receptors in liver and kidney to reduce glucose output. It also binds to receptors for IGF-1 in the pancreatic B cell to inhibit insulin secretion and in the pituitary to suppress growth hormone release. With the reduction of growth hormone, there is a consequent lowering of IGF-1 levels as well as IGFBP-3 and acid-labile subunit.

The diagnosis is supported by laboratory documentation of serum insulin levels below 5 microunit/mL with plasma glucose levels of 45 mg/dL (2.5 mmol/L) or lower. Values for growth hormone and IGF-1 are also decreased. Levels of IGF-2 may be increased but often are "normal" in quantity, despite the presence of the immature, higher-molecular-weight form of IGF-2, which can only be detected by special laboratory techniques.

Not all the patients with nonislet cell tumor hypoglycemia have elevated pro-IGF-II. Ectopic insulin production has been described in bronchial carcinoma, ovarian carcinoma, and small cell carcinoma of the cervix.

Hypoglycemia due to IgF-1 released from a metastatic large cell carcinoma of the lung has also been reported.

The prognosis for these tumors is generally poor, and surgical removal should be attempted when feasible. Dietary management of the hypoglycemia is the mainstay of medical treatment, since diazoxide is usually ineffective.

Bodnar TW et al. Management of non-islet-cell tumor hypoglycemia: a clinical review. J Clin Endocrinol Metab. 2013 Dec 10. [Epub ahead of print] [PMID: 24423303]
de Groot JW et al. Non-islet cell tumour-induced hypoglycaemia: a review of the literature including two new cases. Endocr Relat Cancer. 2007 Dec;14(4):979–93. [PMID: 18045950]

POSTPRANDIAL HYPOGLYCEMIA

1. Hypoglycemia Following Gastric Surgery

Hypoglycemia sometimes develops in patients who have undergone gastric surgery (eg, gastrectomy, vagotomy, pyloroplasty, gastrojejunostomy, Nissan fundoplication, Bilroth II procedure and Roux-en-Y), especially when they consume foods containing high levels of carbohydrates. This late dumping syndrome occurs about 1–3 hours after a meal and is a result of rapid delivery of high concentration of carbohydrates in the proximal small bowel and rapid absorption of glucose. The hyperinsulinemic response to the high carbohydrate load causes hypoglycemia. The symptoms include lightheadedness, sweating, confusion and even loss of consciousness after eating a high carbohydrate meal. It is possible that gastrointestinal hormones such as GLP-1 play a role in the hyperinsulinemic response. The incidence of secondary dumping syndrome declined with the advent of medical therapy for peptic ulcer disease. There has been resurgence of cases, however, with the popularity of Roux-en-Y gastric bypass surgery for the treatment of morbid obesity. Patients typically complain of symptoms that are more severe after consumption of large amounts of readily absorbable carbohydrates. In terms of documenting hypoglycemia, it is reasonable to request the patient to consume a meal that leads to symptoms during everyday life. An oral glucose tolerance test is not recommended because many normal persons have false-positive test results. There have been case reports of insulinoma and noninsulinoma pancreatogenous hypoglycemia syndrome in patients with hypoglycemia post Roux-en-Y surgery. It is unclear how often this occurs. A careful history may identify patients who have a history of hypoglycemia with exercise or meals, and these individuals may require a formal 72-hour fast to rule out an insulinoma.

Treatment for secondary dumping includes dietary modification, but this may be difficult to sustain. Patients can try more frequent meals with smaller portions of less rapidly digested carbohydrates. Alpha-glucosidase therapy may be a useful adjunct to a low carbohydrate diet. Octreotide 50 mcg administered subcutaneously two or three times a day 30 minutes prior to each meal has been reported to improve symptoms due to late dumping syndrome. Various surgical procedures to delay gastric emptying have been reported to improve symptoms but long-term efficacy studies are lacking.

2. Noninsulinoma Pancreatogenous Hypoglycemia Syndrome (Islet Cell Hyperplasia)

In a very small number of patients with organic hyperinsulinism, islet cell hyperplasia is present rather than an adenoma. This condition is referred to as noninsulinoma pancreatogenous hypoglycemia syndrome. These patients typically have documented hyperinsulinemic hypoglycemia after meals but not with fasting up to 72 hours. The patients have a positive response to calcium-stimulated angiography. A gradient-guided partial pancreatectomy leads to clinical remission, and the pathology of the pancreas shows evidence of islet cell hyperplasia and nesidioblastosis. These patients do not have mutations in the pancreatic islet beta-cell ATP-sensitive potassium channel inward rectifier (Kir 6.2) and the sulfonylurea receptor-1 (SUR1) genes, which have been reported in children with familial hyperinsulinemic hypoglycemia.

3. Functional Alimentary Hypoglycemia

Patients have symptoms suggestive of increased sympathetic activity, including anxiety, weakness, tremor, sweating or palpitations after meals. Physical examination and laboratory tests are normal. Previously, many of these patients underwent a 5-hour oral glucose tolerance test and the detection of glucose levels in the 50–60 mg/dL (2.8–3.3 mmol/L) range was thought to be responsible for the symptoms; the recommended treatment was dietary modification. It is now recognized that at least 10% of normal patients who do not have any symptoms have nadir glucose levels < 50 mg/dL (2.8 mmol/L) during a 4- to 6-hour oral glucose tolerance test. In a study comparing responses to oral glucose tolerance test with a mixed meal tolerance test, none of the patients who had plasma glucose levels < 50 mg/dL on oral glucose had low glucose values with the mixed meal. Thus, it is not recommended that these patients with symptoms suggestive of increased sympathetic activity undergo either a prolonged oral glucose tolerance test or a mixed meal test. Instead, the patients should be given home blood glucose monitors (with memories) and instructed to monitor fingerstick glucose levels at the time of symptoms. Only patients who have symptoms when their fingerstick blood glucose is low (< 50 mg/dL) and who have resolution of symptoms when the glucose is raised by eating rapidly released carbohydrate need additional evaluation. Patients who do not have evidence for low glucose levels at time of symptoms are generally reassured by their findings. Counseling and support should be the mainstays in therapy, with dietary manipulation only an adjunct.

4. Occult Diabetes

This condition is characterized by a delay in early insulin release from pancreatic B cells, resulting in initial exaggeration of hyperglycemia during a glucose tolerance test. In response to this hyperglycemia, an exaggerated insulin release produces a late hypoglycemia 4–5 hours after ingestion of glucose. These patients are often obese and frequently have a family history of diabetes mellitus.

Patients with this type of postprandial hypoglycemia often respond to reduced intake of refined sugars with multiple, spaced, small feedings high in dietary fiber. In the obese, treatment is directed at weight reduction to achieve ideal weight. These patients should be considered to have prediabetes or early diabetes (type 1 or 2) and advised to have periodic medical evaluations.

5. Autoimmune Hypoglycemia

Patients with autoimmune hypoglycemia have early postprandial hyperglycemia followed by hypoglycemia 3–4 hours later. The hypoglycemia is attributed to a dissociation of insulin-antibody immune complexes, releasing free insulin.

The disorder is associated with methimazole treatment for Graves disease, although it can also occur in patients treated with various other sulfhydryl-containing medications (captopril, penicillamine) as well as other drugs such as hydralazine, isoniazid, and procainamide. In addition, it has been reported in patients with autoimmune disorders such as rheumatoid arthritis, systemic lupus erythematosus, and polymyositis as well as in multiple myeloma and other plasma cell dyscrasias where paraproteins or antibodies cross-react with insulin. There is also an association with the HLA class II alleles (DRB1*0406, DQA1*0301, and DQB1*0302). These alleles are 10 to 20 times more common in Japanese and Korean populations, which explains why the disorder has been reported mostly in Japanese patients.

High titers of insulin autoantibodies, usually IgG class, can be detected. Insulin, proinsulin, and C-peptide levels may be elevated, but the results may be erroneous because of the interference of the insulin antibodies with the immunoassays for these peptides.

In most cases, the hypoglycemia is transient and usually resolves spontaneously within 3–6 months of diagnosis, particularly when the offending medications are stopped. The most consistent therapeutic benefit in management of this syndrome has been achieved by dietary treatment with small, frequent low-carbohydrate meals. Prednisone (30–60 mg orally daily) has been used to lower the titer of insulin antibodies.

Kellogg TA et al. Postgastric bypass hyperinsulinemic hypoglycemia syndrome: characterization and response to a modified diet. Surg Obes Relat Dis. 2008 Jul–Aug;4(4):492–9. [PMID: 18656831]

Lupsa BC et al. Autoimmune forms of hypoglycemia. Medicine (Baltimore). 2009 May;88(3):141–53. [PMID: 19440117]

FACTITIOUS HYPOGLYCEMIA

Factitious hypoglycemia may be difficult to document. A suspicion of self-induced hypoglycemia is supported when the patient is associated with the health professions or has access to insulin or sulfonylurea medications taken by a diabetic member of the family. The triad of hypoglycemia, high immunoreactive insulin, and suppressed plasma C peptide immunoreactivity is pathognomonic of exogenous insulin administration. Insulin and C peptide is secreted in a 1:1 molar ratio. A large fraction of the endogenous insulin is cleared by the liver whereas C peptide, which is cleared by the kidney, has a lower metabolic clearance rate. For this reason, the molar ratio of insulin and C peptide in a hypoglycemic patient should be < 1.0 in cases of insulinoma and is > 1.0 in cases of exogenous insulin administration. When sulfonylureas, repaglinide and nateglinide are suspected as a cause of factitious hypoglycemia, a plasma level of these medications to detect their presence may be required to distinguish laboratory findings from those of insulinoma.

HYPOGLYCEMIA DUE TO INSULIN RECEPTOR ANTIBODIES

Hypoglycemia due to insulin receptor autoantibodies is also an extremely rare syndrome; most cases have occurred in women often with a history of autoimmune disease. Almost all of these patients have also had episodes of insulin-resistant diabetes and acanthosis nigricans. Their hypoglycemia may be either fasting or postprandial and is often severe and is attributed to an agonistic action of the antibody on the insulin receptor. Balance between the antagonistic and agonistic effects of the antibodies determines whether insulin-resistant diabetes or hypoglycemia occurs. Hypoglycemia was found to respond to corticosteroid therapy but not to plasmapheresis or immunosuppression.

Kim CH et al. Autoimmune hypoglycemia in a type 2 diabetic patient with anti-insulin and insulin receptor antibodies. Diabetes Care. 2004 Jan;27(1):288–9. [PMID: 14694017]

MEDICATION-INDUCED HYPOGLYCEMIA

A number of medications apart from the sulfonylureas can occasionally cause hypoglycemia. Common offenders include the fluoroquinolones such as gatifloxacin and levofloxacin, pentamidine, quinine, ACE inhibitors, salicylates and beta-adrenergic blocking agents. The fluoroquinolones, particularly gatifloxacin, has been associated with both hypoglycemia and hyperglycemia. It is thought that the drug acts on the ATP sensitive potassium channels in the beta cell. Hypoglycemia is an early event, and hyperglycemia occurs several days into therapy. Intravenous pentamidine is cytotoxic to beta cells and causes acute hyperinsulinemia and hypoglycemia followed by insulinopenia and hyperglycemia. Fasting patients taking noncardioselective beta-blockers can have an exaggerated hypoglycemic response to starvation. The beta-blockade inhibits fatty acids and gluconeogenesis substrate release and reduces plasma glucagon response. Therapy with ACE inhibitors increases the risk of hypoglycemia in patients who are taking insulin or sulfonylureas presumably because these drugs increase sensitivity to circulating insulin by increasing blood flow to the muscle.

Ethanol-associated hypoglycemia may be due to hepatic depletion of NADH and altered NADH:NAD ratio. This in turn limits conversion of lactate to pyruvate, the main substrate for hepatic gluconeogenesis. With prolonged starvation, glycogen reserves become depleted within 18–24 hours and hepatic glucose output becomes totally dependent on gluconeogenesis. Under these circumstances, a blood concentration of ethanol as low as 45 mg/dL (9.8 mmol/L) can induce profound hypoglycemia by blocking gluconeogenesis. Neuroglycopenia in a patient whose breath smells of alcohol may be mistaken for alcoholic stupor. Prevention consists of adequate food intake during ethanol ingestion. Therapy consists of glucose administration to replenish glycogen stores until gluconeogenesis resumes.

When sugar-containing soft drinks are used as mixers to dilute alcohol in beverages (gin and tonic, rum and cola), there seems to be a greater insulin release than when the soft drink alone is ingested and a tendency for more of a late hypoglycemic overswing to occur 3–4 hours later. Prevention would consist of avoiding sugar mixers while ingesting alcohol and ensuring supplementary food intake to provide sustained absorption.

Vue MH et al. Drug-induced glucose alterations part 1: drug-induced hypoglycemia. Diabetes Spectrum. 2011 Aug; 24 (3):171–7.

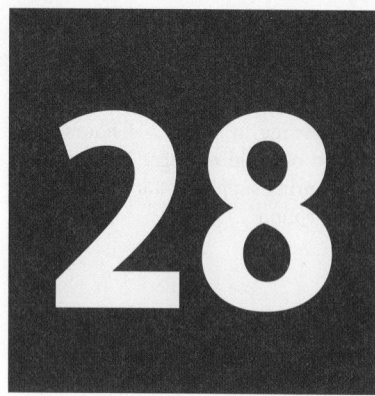

Lipid Disorders

Robert B. Baron, MD, MS

For patients with known cardiovascular disease (secondary prevention), cholesterol lowering leads to a consistent reduction in total mortality and recurrent cardiovascular events in men and women and in middle-aged and older patients. Among patients without cardiovascular disease (primary prevention), the data are less conclusive, with rates of cardiovascular events, heart disease mortality, and all-cause mortality differing among studies. Nonetheless, treatment algorithms have been designed to assist clinicians in selecting patients for cholesterol-lowering therapy based on their overall risk of developing cardiovascular disease.

LIPID FRACTIONS & THE RISK OF CORONARY HEART DISEASE

In fasting serum, cholesterol is carried primarily on three different lipoproteins—the VLDL, LDL, and HDL molecules. Total cholesterol equals the sum of these three components:

$$\text{Total cholesterol} = \text{HDL cholesterol} + \text{VLDL cholesterol} + \text{LDL cholesterol}$$

Most triglyceride is found in VLDL particles, which contain five times as much triglyceride by weight as cholesterol. The amount of cholesterol found in the VLDL fraction can be estimated by dividing the triglyceride by 5:

$$\text{VLDL cholesterol} = \frac{\text{Triglycerides}}{5}$$

Because the triglyceride level is used as a proxy for the amount of VLDL, this formula works only in fasting samples and when the triglyceride level is < 400 mg/dL or < 4.52 mmol/L. At higher triglyceride levels, LDL and VLDL cholesterol levels can be determined after ultracentrifugation or by direct chemical measurement.

The total cholesterol is reasonably stable over time; however, measurements of HDL and especially triglycerides may vary considerably because of analytic error in the laboratory and biologic variation in a patient's lipid level. Thus, the LDL should always be estimated as the mean of at least two determinations; if those two estimates differ by more than 10%, a third lipid profile is obtained. The LDL is estimated as follows:

$$\text{LDL cholesterol (mg/dL)} = \text{Total cholesterol (mg/dL)} - \text{HDL cholesterol (mg/dL)} - \frac{\text{Triglycerides (mg/dL)}}{5}$$

When using SI units, the formula becomes

$$\text{LDL cholesterol (mmol/L)} = \text{Total cholesterol (mmol/L)} - \text{HDL cholesterol (mmol/L)} - \frac{\text{Triglycerides (mmol/L)}}{2.2}$$

Some authorities use the ratio of the total to HDL cholesterol as an indicator of lipid-related coronary risk: the lower this ratio is, the better. Although ratios are useful predictors within populations of patients, they may obscure important information in individual patients. (A total cholesterol of 300 mg/dL [7.76 mmol/L] and an HDL of 60 mg/dL [1.56 mmol/L] result in the same ratio as a total cholesterol of 150 mg/dL [3.88 mmol/L] with an HDL of 30 mg/dL [0.78 mmol/L].) Moreover, the total cholesterol-to-HDL cholesterol ratio will magnify the importance of variations in HDL measurement.

THERAPEUTIC EFFECTS OF LOWERING CHOLESTEROL

Reducing cholesterol levels in healthy middle-aged men without CHD (primary prevention) reduces their risk in proportion to the reduction in LDL cholesterol. Treated adults have statistically significant and clinically important reductions in the rates of myocardial infarctions, new cases of angina, and need for coronary artery bypass procedures. The West of Scotland Study showed a 31% decrease in myocardial infarctions in middle-aged men treated with pravastatin compared with placebo. The Air Force/Texas Coronary Atherosclerosis Prevention Study (AFCAPS/TexCAPS) study showed similar results with lovastatin. As with any primary prevention interventions, large numbers of healthy patients need to be treated to prevent a single event. The numbers of patients needed to treat (NNT) to prevent a nonfatal myocardial infarction or a coronary artery disease death in these two studies were 46 and 50, respectively. The Anglo-Scandinavian Cardiac Outcomes

Trial (ASCOT) study of atorvastatin in subjects with hypertension and other risk factors but without CHD also demonstrated a convincing 36% reduction in CHD events. The Justification for the Use of Statins in Prevention: an Intervention Trial Evaluating Rosuvastatin (JUPITER) showed a 44% reduction in a combined end point of myocardial infarction, stroke, revascularization, hospitalization for unstable angina, or death from cardiovascular causes in both men and women. The NNT for 1 year to prevent one event was 169.

Primary prevention studies have found a less consistent effect on total mortality. The West of Scotland study found a 20% decrease in total mortality, tending toward statistical significance. The AFCAPS/TexCAPS study with lovastatin showed no difference in total mortality. The Antihypertensive and Lipid-Lowering Treatment to Prevent Heart Attack Trial (ALLHAT-LLT) also showed no reduction either in all-cause mortality or in CHD events when pravastatin was compared with usual care. Subjects treated with atorvastatin in the ASCOT study had a 13% reduction in mortality, but the result was not statistically significant. This study, however, was stopped early due to the marked reduction in CHD events. The JUPITER trial demonstrated a statistically significant 20% reduction in death from any cause. The NNT for 1 year was 400.

In patients with CHD, the benefits of cholesterol lowering are clearer. Major studies with statins have shown significant reductions in cardiovascular events, cardiovascular deaths, and all-cause mortality in men and women with coronary artery disease. The NNT to prevent a nonfatal myocardial infarction or a coronary artery disease death in these three studies were between 12 and 34. Aggressive cholesterol lowering with these agents causes regression of atherosclerotic plaques in some patients, reduces the progression of atherosclerosis in saphenous vein grafts, and can slow or reverse carotid artery atherosclerosis. Meta-analysis suggests that this latter effect results in a significant decrease in strokes. Results with other classes of medications have been less consistent. For example, gemfibrozil treatment subjects had fewer cardiovascular events, but there was no benefit in all-cause mortality when compared with placebo.

The disparities in results between primary and secondary prevention studies highlight several important points. The benefits and adverse effects of cholesterol lowering may be specific to each type of drug; the clinician cannot assume that the effects will generalize to other classes of medication. Second, the net benefits from cholesterol lowering depend on the underlying risk of CHD and of other disease. In patients with atherosclerosis, morbidity and mortality rates associated with CHD are high, and measures that reduce it are more likely to be beneficial even if they have no effect—or even slightly harmful effects—on other diseases.

Cholesterol Treatment Trialists' (CTT) Collaboration; Collings R et al. Efficacy and safety of more intensive lowering of LDL cholesterol: a meta-analysis of data from 170,000 participants in 26 randomised trials. Lancet. 2010 Nov 13;376(9753): 1670–81. [PMID: 21067804]

Kini AS et al. Changes in plaque lipid content after short-term intensive versus standard statin therapy: the YELLOW trial (reduction in yellow plaque by aggressive lipid-lowering therapy). J Am Coll Cardiol. 2013 Jul 2;62(1):21–9. [PMID: 23644090]

Ridker PM et al. A trial-based approach to statin guidelines. JAMA. 2013 Sep 18:310(11):1123–4. [PMID: 23942579]

Sbrana F et al. High density lipoprotein cholesterol in coronary artery disease: when higher means later. J Atheroscler Thromb. 2013 Jan 25;20(1):23–31. [PMID: 22878704]

Savarese G et al. Benefits of statins in elderly subjects without established cardiovascular disease: a meta-analysis. J Am Coll Cardiol. 2013 Dec 3;62(22):2090–9. [PMID: 23954343]

Wang X et al. Cholesterol levels and risk of hemorrhagic stroke: a systematic review and meta-analysis. Stroke. 2013 Jul; 44(7): 1833–9. [PMID: 23704101]

SECONDARY CONDITIONS THAT AFFECT LIPID METABOLISM

Several factors, including drugs, can influence serum lipids. These are important for two reasons: abnormal lipid levels (or changes in lipid levels) may be the presenting sign of some of these conditions, and correction of the underlying condition may obviate the need to treat an apparent lipid disorder. Diabetes and alcohol use, in particular, are commonly associated with high triglyceride levels that decline with improvements in glycemic control or reduction in alcohol use, respectively. Thus, secondary causes of high blood lipids should be considered in each patient with a lipid disorder before lipid-lowering therapy is started. In most instances, special testing is not needed: a history and physical examination are sufficient. However, screening for hypothyroidism in patients with hyperlipidemia is cost effective.

CLINICAL PRESENTATIONS

Most patients with high cholesterol levels have no specific symptoms or signs. The vast majority of patients with lipid abnormalities are detected by the laboratory, either as part of the workup of a patient with cardiovascular disease or as part of a preventive screening strategy. Extremely high levels of chylomicrons or VLDL particles (triglyceride level above 1000 mg/dL or 10 mmol/L) result in the formation of **eruptive xanthomas** (Figure 28–1) (red-yellow papules, especially on the buttocks). High LDL concentrations result in **tendinous xanthomas** on certain tendons (Achilles, patella, back of the hand). Such xanthomas usually indicate one of the underlying genetic hyperlipidemias. **Lipemia retinalis** (cream-colored blood vessels in the fundus) is seen with extremely high triglyceride levels (above 2000 mg/dL or 20 mmol/L).

SCREENING & TREATMENT OF HIGH BLOOD CHOLESTEROL

All patients with cardiovascular disease and diabetes should have their lipids measured. The only exceptions are patients in whom lipid lowering is not indicated or desirable for other reasons. Patients who already have evidence of atherosclerosis are the group at highest risk for suffering additional manifestations in the near term and thus have

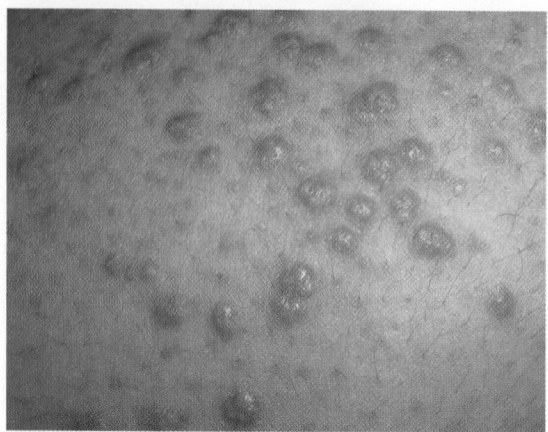

▲ **Figure 28–1.** Eruptive xanthoma on the arm of a man with untreated hyperlipidemia and diabetes mellitus. (Reproduced with permission from Richard P. Usatine, MD)

the most to gain from lipid lowering. Additional risk reduction measures for atherosclerosis are discussed in Chapter 10; lipid lowering should be just one aspect of a program to reduce the progression and effects of the disease.

In patients with cardiovascular disease, a complete lipid profile (total cholesterol, HDL cholesterol, and triglyceride levels) after an overnight fast should be obtained. According to the 2013 American College of Cardiology/American Heart Association (ACC/AHA) guidelines, however, such patients are treated with statins independent of their lipid levels. Similarly, patients aged 40–75 with diabetes should also have a complete lipid profile. Those with diabetes and LDL ≥ 70 mg/dL (≥ 1.81 mmol/L) should be treated with statins.

The best screening and treatment strategy for adults who do not have atherosclerotic cardiovascular disease is less clear. Several algorithms have been developed to guide the clinician in treatment decisions, but management decisions are individualized based on the patient's risk.

Although the 2013 ACC/AHA guidelines recommend screening of all adults aged 21 years or older for high blood cholesterol, the United States Preventive Services Task Force (USPSTF) suggests beginning at age 20 years only if there are other cardiovascular risk factors such as tobacco use, diabetes, hypertension, obesity, or a family history of premature cardiovascular disease. For men without other risk factors, screening is recommended beginning at age 35 years. For women and for men aged 20 to 35 without increased risk, the USPSTF makes no recommendation for or against routine screening for lipid disorders. Although there is no established interval for screening, screening can be repeated every 5 years for those with average or low risk and more often for those whose levels are close to therapeutic thresholds.

Individuals without cardiovascular disease should have their 10-year risk of CHD calculated. Although those with LDL cholesterol > 190 mg/dL (> 4.91 mmol/L) are recommended for treatment independent of their 10-year risk of cardiovascular disease, all other patients are recommended for treatment based on their overall cardiovascular risk.

The best method for estimating 10-year risk is controversial. The 2013 ACC/AHA guidelines include a risk calculator that measures cardiovascular risk. It can be downloaded at http://my.americanheart.org/professional/Statements-Guidelines/PreventionGuidelines/Prevention-Guidelines_UCM_457698_SubHomePage.jsp. It has been criticized by some authors as overestimating risk. The older Framingham 10-year calculator (Table 28–1) includes CHD but not stroke risk. One approach is to use both risk calculators until better data are available.

Numerous other risk factors have been studied in an attempt to better predict future CHD events. These include high-sensitivity C-reactive protein (hs-CRP), electron beam computed tomography (EBCT), homocysteine, fibrinogen, lipoprotein a, LDL subfractions, ankle-brachial index, and others. Several of these, particularly hs-CRP and EBCT, may add additional prognostic ability after accounting for traditional risk factors, but no clinical trials have yet examined the effect of these on health outcomes. Clinical guidelines suggest limiting the use of additional risk factors such as hs-CRP to selected patients if additional data are likely to change a therapeutic decision.

Several strategies for obtaining the initial cholesterol measurement have been proposed, including: (1) measuring total cholesterol alone, (2) measuring total cholesterol and HDL cholesterol, or (3) measuring LDL cholesterol. Initial measurement of the LDL cholesterol is least likely to lead to patient misinformation and misclassification and is the strategy recommended by the 2013 ACC/AHA guidelines.

Treatment decisions are based on the presence of clinical cardiovascular disease or diabetes, patient age, LDL cholesterol > 190 mg/dL (> 4.91 mmol/L), and the estimated 10-year risk of developing cardiovascular disease. The 2013 ACC/AHA guidelines define four groups of patients who benefit from statin medications: (1) individuals with clinical atherosclerotic cardiovascular disease; (2) individuals with primary elevation of LDL cholesterol >190 mg/dL (> 4.91 mmol/L); (3) individuals aged 40–75 with diabetes and LDL ≥ 70 mg/dL (≥ 1.81 mmol/L); and (4) individuals aged 40–75 without clinical atherosclerotic cardiovascular disease or diabetes, with LDL 70–189 mg/dL (1.81–4.91 mmol/L), and estimated 10-year CVD risk ≥ 7.5% or higher.

▶ Screening & Treatment in Women

The foregoing screening and treatment guidelines are designed for both men and women. Yet several observational studies suggest that a low HDL cholesterol is a more important risk factor for CHD in women than a high LDL cholesterol. Meta-analysis of studies including women with known heart disease, however, has found that statins prevent recurrent myocardial infarctions in women. There is insufficient evidence to be certain of a similar effect from statins in women without evidence of CHD. Although most experts recommend application of the same primary prevention guidelines for women as for men, clinicians should be aware of the uncertainty in this area. Estimating the 10-year cardiovascular risk is particularly important in women since a larger percentage of women than men will

Table 28–1. Framingham 10-year coronary heart disease risk projections. Calculate the number of points for each risk factor. Sum the total risk score and estimate the 10-year risk.

WOMEN

Age	Points
20–34	−7
35–39	−3
40–44	0
45–49	3
50–54	6
55–59	8
60–64	10
65–69	12
70–74	14
75–79	16

MEN

Age	Points
20–34	−9
35–39	−4
40–44	0
45–49	3
50–54	6
55–59	8
60–64	10
65–69	11
70–74	12
75–79	13

WOMEN

Total Cholesterol	Points Age 20–39	Age 40–49	Age 50–59	Age 60–69	Age 70–79
<160	0	0	0	0	0
160–199	4	3	2	1	0
200–239	8	6	4	2	1
240–279	11	8	5	3	2
≥ 280	13	10	7	4	2

MEN

Total Cholesterol	Points Age 20–39	Age 40–49	Age 50–59	Age 60–69	Age 70–79
<160	0	0	0	0	0
160–199	4	3	2	1	0
200–239	7	5	3	1	0
240–279	9	6	4	2	1
≥ 280	11	8	5	3	1

WOMEN

Age	Points 20–39	40–49	50–59	60–69	70–79
Nonsmoker	0	0	0	0	0
Smoker	9	7	4	2	1

MEN

Age	Points 20–39	40–49	50–59	60–69	70–79
Nonsmoker	0	0	0	0	0
Smoker	8	5	3	1	1

WOMEN

HDL (mg/dL)	Points
≥ 60	−1
50–59	0
40–49	1
<40	2

MEN

HDL (mg/dL)	Points
≥ 60	−1
50–59	0
40–49	1
<40	2

WOMEN

Systolic BP (mm Hg)	Points if Untreated	Points if Treated
< 120	0	0
120–129	1	3
130–139	2	4
140–159	3	5
≥ 160	4	6

MEN

Systolic BP (mm Hg)	Points if Untreated	Points if Treated
< 120	0	0
120–129	0	1
130–139	1	2
140–159	1	2
≥ 160	2	3

(continued)

Table 28–1. Framingham 10-year coronary heart disease risk projections. Calculate the number of points for each risk factor. Sum the total risk score and estimate the 10-year risk. (continued)

WOMEN			MEN	
Point Total	10-Year Risk %		Point Total	10-Year Risk %
< 9	< 1		< 0	< 1
9	1		0	1
10	1		1	1
11	1		2	1
12	1		3	1
13	2		4	1
14	2		5	2
15	3		6	2
16	4		7	3
17	5		8	4
18	6		9	5
19	8		10	6
20	11		11	8
21	14	Ten-Year Risk %	12	10	Ten-Year Risk %
22	17		13	12
23	22		14	16
24	27		15	20
≥ 25	≥ 30		16	25
			≥17	≥ 30

have estimated 10-year cardiovascular risks below 7.5% per year and be advised not to take statins unless their LDL is very high (> 190 mg/dL or > 4.91 mmol/L).

▶ Screening & Treatment in Older Patients

Meta-analysis of evidence relating cholesterol to CHD in the elderly suggests that cholesterol is not a risk factor for CHD for persons over age 75 years. Clinical trials have rarely included such individuals. One exception is the Prospective Study of Pravastatin in the Elderly at Risk (PROSPER). In this study, elderly patients with cardiovascular disease (secondary prevention) benefited from statin therapy, whereas those without cardiovascular disease (primary prevention) did not. The 2013 ACC/AHA guidelines suggest continuing statin treatment in patients over age 75 who have cardiovascular disease. The guidelines, however, suggest not screening or treating patients over the age of 75 who do not have evidence of cardiovascular disease. Individual patient decisions to discontinue statin therapy should be based on overall functional status and life expectancy, comorbidities, and patient preference and should be made in context with overall therapeutic goals and end-of-life decisions.

Centers for Disease Control and Prevention (CDC). Prevalence of cholesterol screening and high blood cholesterol among adults—United States, 2005, 2007, and 2009. MMWR Morb Mortal Wkly Rep. 2012 Sep 7;61:697–702. [PMID: 22951451]

Goff DC Jr et al. 2013 ACC/AHA Guideline on the Assessment of Cardiovascular Risk: a report of the American College of Cardiology/American Heart Association Task Force on Practice Guidelines. J Am Coll Cardiol. 2013 Nov 12. [Epub ahead of print] [PMID: 24239921]

Keaney JF Jr et al. A pragmatic view of the new cholesterol treatment guidelines. N Engl J Med. 2014 Jan 16;370(3):275–8. [PMID: 24283199]

Krumholz HM. Target cardiovascular risk rather than cholesterol concentration. BMJ. 2013 Nov 27;347:f7110. [PMID: 24284344]

Ridker PM et al. Statins: new American guidelines for prevention of cardiovascular disease. Lancet. 2013 Nov 30; 382(9907):1762–5. [PMID: 24268611]

Stone NJ et al. 2013 ACC/AHA Guideline on the Treatment of Blood Cholesterol to Reduce Atherosclerotic Cardiovascular Risk in Adults: a report of the American College of Cardiology/American Heart Association Task Force on Practice Guidelines. J Am Coll Cardiol. 2013 Nov 7. [Epub ahead of print] [PMID: 24239923]

TREATMENT OF HIGH LDL CHOLESTEROL

Reduction of LDL cholesterol with statins is just one part of a program to reduce the risk of cardiovascular disease. Other measures—including smoking cessation, hypertension control, and aspirin—are also of central importance. Less well studied but of potential value is raising the HDL cholesterol level. Quitting smoking reduces the effect of other cardiovascular risk factors (such as a high cholesterol level); it may also increase the HDL cholesterol level. Exercise (and weight loss) may reduce the LDL cholesterol and increase the HDL. Modest alcohol use (1–2 ounces a day) also raises HDL levels and appears to have a salutary effect on CHD rates.

The use of medications to raise the HDL cholesterol has not been demonstrated to provide additional benefit. For example, cholesteryl ester transfer protein inhibitors is a class of medicines being investigated to raise HDL levels. Agents in this class, however, have not been shown to be effective. The use of niacin in addition to statins has also been carefully studied in the AIM-HIGH study and also shown not to be effective.

Diet Therapy

Studies of nonhospitalized adults have reported only modest cholesterol-lowering benefits of dietary therapy, typically in the range of a 5–10% decrease in LDL cholesterol, with even less in the long term. The effect of diet therapy, however, varies considerably among individuals, as some patients will have striking reductions in LDL cholesterol— up to a 25–30% decrease—whereas others will have clinically important increases. Thus, the results of diet therapy should be assessed about 4 weeks after initiation.

Cholesterol-lowering diets may also have a variable effect on lipid fractions. Diets very low in total fat or in saturated fat may lower HDL cholesterol as much as LDL cholesterol. It is not known how these diet-induced changes affect coronary risk.

Several nutritional approaches to diet therapy are available. Most Americans currently eat over 35% of calories as fat, of which 15% is saturated fat. Dietary cholesterol intake averages 400 mg/d. A cholesterol-lowering diet recommends reducing total fat to 25–30% and saturated fat to < 7% of calories. Dietary cholesterol should be limited to < 200 mg/d. These diets replace fat, particularly saturated fat, with carbohydrate. In most instances, this approach will also result in fewer total calories consumed and will facilitate weight loss in overweight patients. Other diet plans, including the Dean Ornish Diet, the Pritikin Diet, and most vegetarian diets, restrict fat even further. Low-fat, high-carbohydrate diets may, however, result in reductions in HDL cholesterol.

An alternative strategy is the Mediterranean diet, which maintains total fat at approximately 35–40% of total calories but replaces saturated fat with monounsaturated fat such as that found in canola oil and in olives, peanuts, avocados, and their oils. This diet is equally effective at lowering LDL cholesterol but is less likely to lead to reductions in HDL cholesterol. Several studies have suggested that this approach may also be associated with reductions in endothelial dysfunction, insulin resistance, and markers of vascular inflammation and may result in better resolution of the metabolic syndrome than traditional cholesterol-lowering diets. A clinical trial demonstrated reduced cardiovascular events in persons on a Mediterranean diet supplemented with additional nuts or extra-virgin olive oil compared to persons on a less intensive Mediterranean diet.

Other dietary changes may also result in beneficial changes in blood lipids. Soluble fiber, such as that found in oat bran or psyllium, may reduce LDL cholesterol by 5–10%. Garlic, soy protein, vitamin C, pecans, and plant sterols may also result in reduction of LDL cholesterol. Because oxidation of LDL cholesterol is a potential initiating event in atherogenesis, diets rich in antioxidants, found primarily in fruits and vegetables, may be helpful (see Chapter 29). Studies have suggested that when all of these elements are combined into a single dietary prescription, the impact of diet on LDL cholesterol may approach that of statin medications, lowering LDL cholesterol by close to 30%.

AIM-HIGH Investigators; Boden WE et al. Niacin in patients with low HDL cholesterol levels receiving intensive statin therapy. N Engl J Med. 2011 Dec 15;365(24):2255–67. [PMID: 22085343]

Eckel RH et al. 2013 AHA/ACC Guideline on Lifestyle Management to Reduce Cardiovascular Risk: a report of the American College of Cardiology/American Heart Association Task Force on Practice Guidelines. J Am Coll Cardiol. 2013 Nov 7. [Epub ahead of print] [PMID: 24239922]

Estruch R et al; PREDIMED Study Investigators. Primary prevention of cardiovascular disease with a Mediterannean Diet. N Engl J Med. 2103 Apr 4;368(14):1279–90. [PMID: 23432189]

Kelley GA et al. Comparison of aerobic exercise, diet or both on lipids and lipoproteins in adults: a meta-analysis of randomized controlled trials. Clin Nutr. 2012 Apr;31(2):156–67. [PMID: 22154987]

Nordmann AJ et al. Meta-analysis comparing Mediterranean to low-fat diets for modification of cardiovascular risk factors. Am J Med. 2011 Sep;124(9):841–51. [PMID: 21854893]

Rubenfire M et al. HDL cholesterol and cardiovascular outcomes: what is the evidence? Curr Cardiol Rep. 2013 Apr;15(4):349. [PMID: 23420445]

Pharmacologic Therapy

Most patients whose risk from CHD is considered high enough to warrant pharmacologic therapy of an elevated LDL cholesterol should be given aspirin prophylaxis at a dose of 81 mg/d unless there are contraindications such as aspirin sensitivity, bleeding diatheses, or active peptic ulcer disease. The benefit of aspirin in reducing the risk of CHD in men is equivalent to that of cholesterol lowering. Other CHD risk factors, such as hypertension and smoking, should also be controlled.

The 2013 ACC/AHA guidelines suggest treatment with statins for all patients who require drug treatment. As discussed above, the guidelines define four groups of patients who benefit from statin medications.

A. Hydroxymethylglutaryl-Coenzyme A (HMG-CoA) Reductase Inhibitors (Statins)

The HMG-CoA reductase inhibitors (statins) work by inhibiting the rate-limiting enzyme in the formation of cholesterol. They reduce myocardial infarctions and total mortality in secondary prevention, as well as in older middle-aged men free of CHD. A meta-analysis has demonstrated significant reduction in risk of stroke. Cholesterol synthesis in the liver is reduced, with a compensatory increase in hepatic LDL receptors (presumably so that the liver can take more of the cholesterol that it needs from the blood) and a reduction in the circulating LDL cholesterol level by up to 35%. There are also modest increases in HDL levels and decreases in triglyceride levels.

The 2013 ACC/AHA guidelines divide statins into high-intensity and moderate-intensity statin therapy (Table 28–2). High intensity statins lower LDL cholesterol by approximately 50%. Examples include atorvastatin 40–80 mg and rosuvastatin 20–40 mg/d (Table 28–3). Moderate intensity statins lower LDL cholesterol by approximately 30–50%. Examples include atorvastatin 10–20 mg, rosuvastatin 5–10 mg, simvastatin 20–40 mg, pravastatin 40–80 mg, and lovastatin 40 mg. All statins are given once daily in the morning or evening. The most common side effects are muscle aches, occurring in up to 10% of patients, and mild gastrointestinal effects. Statins are

Table 28–2. Indications for high intensity and moderate intensity statins: Recommendations of the 2013 ACC/AHA Guidelines.

Indications	Treatment Recommendation
Presence of clinical atherosclerotic cardiovascular disease	High intensity statin **or** moderate intensity statin if over age 75
Primary elevation of LDL cholesterol ≥ 190 mg/dL (> 4.91 mmol/L)	High intensity statin
Age 40–75 Presence of diabetes LDL ≥ 70 mg/dL (≥ 1.81 mmol/L)	Moderate intensity statin **or** high intensity statin if 10-year CVD risk > 7.5%
Aged 40–75 No clinical atherosclerotic cardiovascular disease or diabetes LDL 70–189 mg/dL (1.81–4.91 mmol/L) Estimated 10-year CVD risk ≥ 7.5% or higher	Treat with moderate-to-high intensity statin

ACC/AHA, American College of Cardiology/American Heart Association; CVD, cardiovascular disease; HDL, high-density lipoprotein; LDL, low-density lipoprotein.

associated with a 10% increase in the risk of diabetes. Other serious, but extremely uncommon, side effects include liver failure and muscle disease including myositis and rhabdomyolysis. Some patients experience muscle pain even when the serum creatine kinase levels are normal. Liver disease is more common in patients who are also taking fibrates or niacin. Manufacturers of HMG-CoA reductase inhibitors recommend monitoring liver enzymes before initiating therapy and as clinically indicated thereafter. Muscle disease is more common with statins and fibrates and niacin as well as with erythromycin, antifungal medications, nefazadone, and cyclosporine. Simvastatin at the highest approved dose—80 mg—is associated with a higher risk of muscle injury or myopathy. This dose should only be used in those who have been taking the medication for longer than 1 year without muscle toxicity.

B. Niacin (Nicotinic Acid)

Niacin was the first lipid-lowering agent that was associated with a reduction in total mortality. Long-term follow-up of a secondary prevention trial of middle-aged men with previous myocardial infarction disclosed that about half of those who had been previously treated with niacin had died, compared with nearly 60% of the placebo group. This favorable effect on mortality was not seen during the trial itself, though there was a reduction in the incidence of recurrent coronary events. A meta-analysis of 10 randomized trials using niacin has also shown a 27% reduction in cardiovascular events.

Niacin reduces the production of VLDL particles, with secondary reduction in LDL and increases in HDL

cholesterol levels. The average effect of full-dose niacin therapy, 3–4.5 g/d, is a 15–25% reduction in LDL cholesterol and a 25–35% increase in HDL cholesterol. Full doses are required to obtain the LDL effect, but the HDL effect is observed at lower doses, eg, 1 g/d. Niacin will also reduce triglycerides by half and will lower lipoprotein(a) (Lp[a]) levels and will increase plasma homocysteine levels. Intolerance to niacin is common; only 50–60% of patients can take full doses. Niacin causes a prostaglandin-mediated flushing that patients may describe as "hot flashes" or pruritus and that can be decreased with aspirin (81–325 mg/d) or other nonsteroidal anti-inflammatory agents taken during the same day. Flushing may also be decreased by initiating niacin therapy with a very small dose, eg, 100 mg with the evening meal. The dose can be doubled each week until 1.5 g/d is tolerated. After rechecking blood lipids, the dose is increased and divided over three meals until the goal of 3–4.5 g/d is reached (eg, 1 g with each meal). Extended-release niacin is better tolerated by most patients. It is not known whether routine monitoring of liver enzymes results in early detection and thus reduced severity of this side effect. Niacin can also exacerbate gout and peptic ulcer disease. Although niacin may increase blood sugar in some patients, clinical trials have shown that niacin can be safely used in diabetic patients.

C. Bile Acid–Binding Resins

The bile acid–binding resins include cholestyramine, colesevelam, and colestipol. Treatment with these agents reduces the incidence of coronary events in middle-aged men by about 20%, with no significant effect on total mortality. The resins work by binding bile acids in the intestine. The resultant reduction in the enterohepatic circulation causes the liver to increase its production of bile acids, using hepatic cholesterol to do so. Thus, hepatic LDL receptor activity increases, with a decline in plasma LDL levels. The triglyceride level tends to increase slightly in some patients treated with bile acid–binding resins; they should be used with caution in those with elevated triglycerides and probably not at all in patients who have triglyceride levels above 500 mg/dL. The clinician can anticipate a reduction of 15–25% in the LDL cholesterol level, with insignificant effects on the HDL level.

The usual dose of cholestyramine is 12–36 g of resin per day in divided doses with meals, mixed in water or, more palatably, juice. Doses of colestipol are 20% higher (each packet contains 5 g of resin). The dose of colesevelam is 625 mg, 6–7 tablets per day.

These agents often cause gastrointestinal symptoms, such as constipation and gas. They may interfere with the absorption of fat-soluble vitamins (thereby complicating the management of patients receiving warfarin) and may bind other drugs in the intestine. Concurrent use of psyllium may ameliorate the gastrointestinal side effects.

D. Fibric Acid Derivatives

The fibrates are peroxisome proliferative-activated receptor-alpha (PPAR-alpha) agonists that result in potent reductions of plasma triglycerides and increases in HDL

Table 28–3. Effects of selected lipid-modifying drugs.

Drug	Lipid-Modifying Effects			Initial Daily Dose	Maximum Daily Dose	Cost for 30 Days Treatment with Dose Listed[1]
	LDL	HDL	Triglyceride			
Atorvastatin (Lipitor)	−25 to −40%	+5 to 10%	↓↓	10 mg once	80 mg once	$150.30 (20 mg once)
Cholestyramine (Questran, others)	−15 to −25%	+5%	±	4 g twice a day	24 g divided	$202.00 (8 g divided)
Colesevelam (WelChol)	−10 to −20%	+10%	±	625 mg, 6–7 tablets once	625 mg, 6–7 tablets once	$402.00 (6 tablets once)
Colestipol (Colestid)	−15 to −25%	+5%	±	5 g twice a day	30 g divided	$150.00 (10 g divided)
Ezetimibe (Zetia)	−20%	+5%	±	10 mg once	10 mg once	$221.70 (10 mg once)
Fenofibrate (Tricor, others)	−10 to −15%	+15 to 25%	↓↓	48 mg once	145 mg once	$154.50 (145 mg once)
Fenofibric Acid (Trilipix)	−10 to −15%	+15 to 25%	↓↓	45 mg once	135 mg once	$180.00 (135 mg once)
Fluvastatin (Lescol)	−20 to −30%	+5 to 10%	↓	20 mg once	40 mg once	$113.00 (20 mg once)
Gemfibrozil (Lopid, others)	−10 to −15%	+15 to 20%	↓↓	600 mg once	1200 mg divided	$71.00 (600 mg twice a day)
Lovastatin (Mevacor, others)	−25 to −40%	+5 to 10%	↓	10 mg once	80 mg divided	$71.10 (20 mg once)
Niacin (OTC, Niaspan)	−15 to −25%	+25 to 35%	↓↓	100 mg once	3–4.5 g divided	$7.20 (1.5 g twice a day, OTC) $500.00 (2 g Niaspan)
Pitavastatin (Livalo)	−30 to 40%	+10 to 25%	↓↓	2 mg once	4 mg once	$180.00 (2 mg once)
Pravastatin (Pravachol)	−25 to −40%	+5 to 10%	↓	20 mg once	80 mg once	$74.80 (20 mg once)
Rosuvastatin (Crestor)	−40 to −50%	+10 to 15%	↓↓	10 mg once	40 mg once	$217.80 (20 mg once)
Simvastatin (Zocor, others)	−25 to −40%	+5 to 10%	↓↓	5 mg once	80 mg once	$75.60 (10 mg once)

[1]Average wholesale price (AWP, for AB-rated generic when available) for quantity listed. Source: *Red Book Online, 2014*, Truven Health Analytics, Inc. AWP may not accurately represent the actual pharmacy cost because wide contractual variations exist among institutions. LDL, low-density lipoprotein; HDL, high-density lipoprotein; ± variable, if any; others, indicates availability of less expensive generic preparations; OTC, over the counter.

cholesterol. They reduce LDL levels by about 10–15%, although the result is quite variable, and triglyceride levels by about 40% and raise HDL levels by about 15–20%. The fibric acid derivatives or fibrates approved for use in the United States are gemfibrozil and fenofibrate. Ciprofibrate and bezafibrate are also available for use internationally.

Gemfibrozil reduced CHD rates in hypercholesterolemic middle-aged men free of coronary disease in the Helsinki Heart Study. The effect was observed only among those who also had lower HDL cholesterol levels and high triglyceride levels. In a VA study, gemfibrozil was also shown to reduce cardiovascular events in men with existing CHD whose primary lipid abnormality was a low HDL cholesterol. There was no effect on all-cause mortality.

The usual dose of gemfibrozil is 600 mg once or twice a day. Side effects include cholelithiasis, hepatitis, and myositis. The incidence of the latter two conditions may be higher among patients also taking other lipid-lowering agents. In the largest clinical trial that used clofibrate, there

were significantly more deaths—especially due to cancer—in the treatment group; it should not be used.

E. Ezetimibe

Ezetimibe is a lipid-lowering drug that inhibits the intestinal absorption of dietary and biliary cholesterol by blocking passage across the intestinal wall by inhibiting a cholesterol transporter. The usual dose of ezetimibe is 10 mg/d orally. Ezetimibe reduces LDL cholesterol between 15% and 20% when used as monotherapy and can further reduce LDL in patients taking statins who are not yet at therapeutic goal.

However, the effects of ezetimide on CHD and its long-term safety are not yet known. Results from one small clinical trial, ENHANCE (a study of 720 persons with heterozygous familial hypercholesterolemia), showed no significant difference of intimal media thickness with ezetimibe plus an HMG-CoA reductase inhibitor compared with an HMG-CoA reductase inhibitor alone. A second study compared a statin plus ezetimibe with a statin plus extended-release niacin. The statin plus niacin caused a significant regression of carotid intima-media thickness and was superior to the statin plus ezetimibe combination.

▶ Initial Selection of Medication

For patients who require a lipid-modifying medication, an HMG-CoA reductase inhibitor is recommended. Although niacin will also have beneficial effects on lipids in both men and women with CHD, there is less evidence demonstrating the desired effects on CHD and all-cause mortality. Resins are the only lipid-modifying medication considered safe in pregnancy.

Combination therapy is rarely indicated. Despite improvements in the lipid profile, there are few data demonstrating improved clinical outcomes of combination therapy when compared with HMG-CoA reductase inhibitors alone. The AIM-High Study of niacin added to simvastatin, for example, was stopped early due to a lack of efficacy. Combinations may also increase the risk of complications of drug therapy. The combination of gemfibrozil and HMG-CoA reductase inhibitors increases the risk of muscle and liver disease more than either drug alone.

ACCORD Study Group et al. Effects of combination lipid therapy in type 2 diabetes mellitus. N Engl J Med. 2010 Apr 29; 362(17):1563–74. [PMID: 20228404]

Adams SP et al. Lipid-lowering efficacy of atorvastatin. Cochrane Database Syst Rev. 2012 Dec 12;12:CD008226. [PMID: 23235655]

AIM-HIGH Investigators; Boden WE et al. Niacin in patients with low HDL cholesterol levels receiving intensive statin therapy. N Engl J Med. 2011 Dec 15;365(24):2255–67. [PMID: 22085343]

Choi HD et al. Safety and efficacy of statin treatment alone and in combination with fibrates in patients with dyslipidemia: a meta-analysis. Curr Med Res Opin. 2014 Jan;30(1):1–10. [PMID: 24063624]

Hayek S et al. Effect of ezetimibe on major atherosclerotic disease events and all-cause mortality. Am J Cardiol. 2013 Feb 15;111(4):532–9. [PMID: 23219178]

Julius U et al. Nicotinic acid as a lipid-modifying drug—a review. Atheroscler Suppl. 2013 Jan;14(1):7–13. [PMID: 23357134]

Jun M et al. Effects of fibrates on cardiovascular outcomes: a systematic review and meta-analysis. Lancet. 2010 May 29; 375(9729):1875–84. [PMID: 20462635]

Lavigne PM et al. The current state of niacin in cardiovascular disease prevention: a systematic review and meta-regression. J Am Coll Cardiol. 2013 Jan 29;61(4):440–6. [PMID: 23265337]

Maron DJ et al. Impact of adding ezetimibe to statin to achieve low-density lipoprotein cholesterol goal (from the Clinical Outcomes Utilizing Revascularization and Aggressive Drug Evaluation [COURAGE] trial). Am J Cardiol. 2013 Jun 1;111(11):1557–62. [PMID: 23538020]

Naci H et al. Comparative tolerability and harms of individual statins: a study level network meta-analysys of 246,955 participants from 135 randomized, controlled trials. Circ Cardiovasc Qual Outcomes. 2013 Jul;6(4):390–9. [PMID: 23838105]

Nicholls SJ et al. Effect of two intensive statin regimens on progression of coronary disease. N Engl J Med. 2011 Dec 1;365(22): 2078–87. [PMID: 22085316]

Sniderman A et al. Is lower and lower better and better? A re-evaluation of the evidence from the Cholesterol Treatment Trialists' Collaboration meta-analysis for low-density lipoprotein lowering. J Clin Lipidol. 2012 Jul;6(4):303–9. [PMID: 22836065]

HIGH BLOOD TRIGLYCERIDES

Patients with very high levels of serum triglycerides (> 1000 mg/dL) are at risk for pancreatitis. The pathophysiology is not certain, since pancreatitis never develops in some patients with very high triglyceride levels. Most patients with congenital abnormalities in triglyceride metabolism present in childhood; hypertriglyceridemia-induced pancreatitis first presenting in adults is more commonly due to an acquired problem in lipid metabolism.

Although there are no clear triglyceride levels that predict pancreatitis, most clinicians treat fasting levels above 500 mg/dL (5 mmol/L). The risk of pancreatitis may be more related to the triglyceride level following consumption of a fatty meal. Because postprandial increases in triglyceride are inevitable if fat-containing foods are eaten, fasting triglyceride levels in persons prone to pancreatitis should be kept well below that level.

The primary therapy for high triglyceride levels is dietary, avoiding alcohol, simple sugars, refined starches, saturated and trans fatty acids, and restricting total calories. Control of secondary causes of high triglyceride levels may also be helpful. In patients with fasting triglycerides ≥ 500 mg/dL (≥ 5 mmol/L) despite adequate dietary compliance—and certainly in those with a previous episode of pancreatitis—therapy with a triglyceride-lowering drug (eg, niacin, a fibric acid derivative, omega-3-acid ethyl esters, or an HMG-CoA reductase inhibitor) is indicated. Combinations of these medications may also be used.

Whether patients with elevated triglycerides (> 150 mg/dL or 1.5 mmol/L) should be treated to prevent CHD is not known. Meta-analysis of 17 observational studies suggests that after adjustment for other risk factors, elevated triglycerides increased CHD risk in men by 14% and in women by 37%. Elevated triglycerides are also an important feature of the metabolic syndrome, found in an estimated 25% of Americans—defined by three or more of the following five abnormalities: waist circumference > 102 cm in men or > 88 cm in women, serum triglyceride level of at least 150 mg/dL, HDL level of < 40 mg/dL in men or < 50 mg/dL in women, blood pressure of at least 130/85 mm Hg, and serum glucose level of at least 110 mg/dL. Other data, however, suggest that triglyceride measurements do not improve discrimination between those with and without CHD events, and clinical trial data are not available to support the routine treatment of high triglycerides in all patients.

Ballantyne CM et al. Long-term efficacy of adding fenofibric acid to moderate-dose statin therapy in patients with persistent elevated triglycerides. Cardiovasc Drugs Ther. 2011 Feb;25(1):59–67. [PMID: 21416219]

Rana JS et al. The role of non-HDL cholesterol in risk stratification for coronary artery disease. Curr Atheroscler Rep. 2012 Apr;14(2):130–4. [PMID: 22203405]

Roth EM et al. Efficacy and safety of rosuvastatin and fenofibric acid combination therapy versus simvastatin monotherapy in patients with hypercholesterolemia and hypertriglyceridemia: a randomized, double-blind study. Am J Cardiovasc Drugs. 2010;10(3):175–86. [PMID: 20524719]

Singh A et al. What should we do about hypertriglyceridemia in coronary artery disease patients? Curr Treat Options Cardiovasc Med. 2013 Feb;15(1):104–17. [PMID: 23109123]

Nutritional Disorders

Robert B. Baron, MD, MS

PROTEIN–ENERGY MALNUTRITION

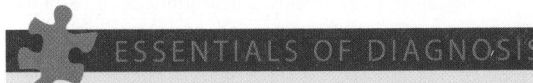

ESSENTIALS OF DIAGNOSIS

▶ Decreased intake of energy or protein, increased nutrient losses, or increased nutrient requirements.

▶ **Kwashiorkor:** caused by protein deficiency.

▶ **Marasmus:** caused by combined protein and energy deficiency.

▶ Protein loss correlates with weight loss: 35–40% total body weight loss is usually fatal.

General Considerations

Protein–energy malnutrition occurs as a result of a relative or absolute deficiency of energy and protein. It may be primary, due to inadequate food intake, or secondary, as a result of other illness. For most developing nations, primary protein–energy malnutrition remains among the most significant health problems. Protein–energy malnutrition has been described as two distinct syndromes. **Kwashiorkor,** caused by a deficiency of protein in the presence of adequate energy, is typically seen in weaning infants at the birth of a sibling in areas where foods containing protein are insufficiently abundant. **Marasmus,** caused by combined protein and energy deficiency, is most commonly seen where adequate quantities of food are not available.

In industrialized societies, protein–energy malnutrition is most often secondary to other diseases. **Kwashiorkor-like secondary protein–energy malnutrition** occurs primarily in association with hypermetabolic acute illnesses such as trauma, burns, and sepsis. **Marasmus-like secondary protein–energy malnutrition** typically results from chronic diseases such as chronic obstructive pulmonary disease (COPD), heart failure, cancer, or AIDS. These syndromes have been estimated to be present in at least 20% of hospitalized patients. A substantially greater number of patients have risk factors that could result in these syndromes. In both syndromes, protein–energy malnutrition is caused either by decreased intake of energy and protein, increased nutrient losses, or increased nutrient requirements dictated by the underlying illness. For example, diminished oral intake may result from poor dentition or various gastrointestinal disorders. Loss of nutrients results from malabsorption and diarrhea as well as from glycosuria. Nutrient requirements are increased by fever, surgery, neoplasia, and burns.

Clinical Findings

The clinical manifestations of protein–energy malnutrition range from mild growth retardation and weight loss to a number of distinct clinical syndromes. Children in the developing world manifest marasmus and kwashiorkor. In secondary protein–energy malnutrition as seen in industrialized nations, clinical manifestations are affected by the degree of protein and energy deficiency, the underlying illness that resulted in the deficiency, and the patient's nutritional status prior to illness.

Progressive wasting that begins with weight loss and proceeds to more severe cachexia typically develops in most patients with marasmus-like secondary protein–energy malnutrition. In the most severe form of this disorder, most body fat stores disappear and muscle mass decreases, most noticeably in the temporalis and interosseous muscles. Laboratory studies may be unremarkable—serum albumin, for example, may be normal or slightly decreased, rarely decreasing to < 2.8 g/dL (< 28 g/L). In contrast, owing to its rapidity of onset, kwashiorkor-like secondary protein–energy malnutrition may develop in patients with normal subcutaneous fat and muscle mass or, if the patient is obese, in patients with excess fat and muscle. The serum protein level, however, typically declines and the serum albumin is often < 2.8 g/dL (< 28 g/L). Dependent edema, ascites, or anasarca may develop. As with primary protein–energy malnutrition, combinations of the marasmus-like and kwashiorkor-like syndromes can occur simultaneously, typically in patients with progressive chronic disease in whom a superimposed acute illness develops.

Treatment

The treatment of severe protein–energy malnutrition is a slow process requiring great care. Initial efforts should be directed at correcting fluid and electrolyte abnormalities and infections. Of particular concern are depletion of potassium, magnesium, and calcium and acid–base abnormalities. The second phase of treatment is directed at repletion of protein, energy, and micronutrients. Treatment is started with modest quantities of protein and calories calculated according to the patient's actual body weight. Adult patients are given 1 g/kg of protein and 30 kcal/kg of calories. Concomitant administration of vitamins and minerals is obligatory. Either the enteral or parenteral route can be used, although the former is preferable. Enteral fat and lactose are withheld initially. Patients with less severe protein–calorie undernutrition can be given calories and protein simultaneously with the correction of fluid and electrolyte abnormalities. Similar quantities of protein and calories are recommended for initial treatment.

Patients treated for protein–energy malnutrition require close follow-up. In adults, both calories and protein are advanced as tolerated, adults to 1.5 g/kg/d of protein and 40 kcal/kg/d of calories.

Patients who are re-fed too rapidly may develop a number of untoward clinical sequelae. During refeeding, circulating potassium, magnesium, phosphorus, and glucose move intracellularly and can result in low serum levels of each. The administration of water and sodium with carbohydrate refeeding can result in heart failure in persons with depressed cardiac function. Enteral refeeding can lead to malabsorption and diarrhea due to abnormalities in the gastrointestinal tract.

Refeeding edema is a benign condition to be differentiated from heart failure. Changes in renal sodium reabsorption and poor skin and blood vessel integrity result in the development of dependent edema without other signs of heart disease. Treatment includes reassurance, elevation of the dependent area, and modest sodium restriction. Diuretics are usually ineffective, may aggravate electrolyte deficiencies, and should not be used.

The prevention and early detection of protein–energy malnutrition in hospitalized patients require awareness of its risk factors and early symptoms and signs. Patients at risk require formal assessment of nutritional status and close observation of dietary intake, body weight, and nutritional requirements during the hospital stay.

Garrett WS. Kwashiorkor and the gut microbiota. N Engl J Med. 2013 May 2;368(18):1746–7. [PMID: 23635056]

Jeejeebhoy KN. Malnutrition, fatigue, frailty, vulnerability, sarcopenia and cachexia: overlap of clinical features. Curr Opin Clin Nutr Metab Care. 2012 May;15(3):213–9. [PMID: 22450775]

Morley JE. Undernutrition in older adults. Fam Pract. 2012 Apr;29 (Suppl 1):i89–i93. [PMID: 22399563]

Mueller C et al. A.S.P.E.N. clinical guidelines: nutrition screening, assessment, and intervention in adults. JPEN J Parenter Enteral Nutr. 2011 Jan;35(1):16–24. [PMID: 21224430]

Raynaud-Simon A et al. Clinical practice guidelines from the French Health High Authority: nutritional support strategy in protein-energy malnutrition in the elderly. Clin Nutr. 2011 Jun;30(3):312–9. [PMID: 21251732]

White JV et al. Consensus statement of the Academy of Nutrition and Dietetics/American Society for Parenteral and Enteral Nutrition: characteristics recommended for the identification and documentation of adult malnutrition (undernutrition). J Acad Nutr Diet. 2012 May;112(5):730–8. Erratum in: J Acad Nutr Diet. 2012 Nov;112(11):1899. [PMID: 22709779]

OBESITY

ESSENTIALS OF DIAGNOSIS

► Excess adipose tissue; body mass index (BMI) > 30.

► Upper body obesity (abdomen and flank) of greater health consequence than lower body obesity (buttocks and thighs).

► Associated with health consequences, including diabetes mellitus, hypertension, and hyperlipidemia.

General Considerations

Obesity is one of the most common disorders in medical practice and among the most frustrating and difficult to manage. Little progress has been made in prevention or treatment, yet major changes have occurred in our understanding of its causes and its implications for health.

Definition & Measurement

Obesity is defined as an excess of adipose tissue. Accurate quantification of body fat requires sophisticated techniques not usually available in clinical practice. Physical examination is usually sufficient to detect excess body fat. More quantitative evaluation is performed by calculating the BMI.

The **BMI** closely correlates with excess adipose tissue. It is calculated by dividing measured body weight in kilograms by the height in meters squared.

The National Institutes of Health (NIH) define a normal BMI as 18.5–24.9. Overweight is defined as BMI = 25–29.9. Class I obesity is 30–34.9, class II obesity is 35–39.9, and class III (extreme) obesity is BMI > 40. Factors other than total weight, however, are also important. Upper body obesity (excess fat around the waist and flank) is a greater health hazard than lower body obesity (fat in the thighs and buttocks). Obese patients with increased abdominal circumference (> 102 cm in men and 88 cm in women) or with high waist–hip ratios (> 1.0 in men and > 0.85 in women) have a greater risk of diabetes mellitus, stroke, coronary artery disease, and early death than equally obese patients with lower ratios. Further differentiation of the location of excess fat suggests that visceral fat within the abdominal cavity is more hazardous to health than subcutaneous fat around the abdomen.

Current U.S. survey data demonstrate that 68% of Americans are overweight and 33.8% are obese. Women in the United States are more apt to be obese than men, and African-American and Mexican-American women are more obese than whites. The poor are more obese than the rich regardless of race. Approximately 60% of individuals with obesity in the United States have the metabolic syndrome (including three or more of the following factors: elevated abdominal circumference, blood pressure, blood triglycerides, and fasting blood sugar, and low high-density lipoprotein [HDL] cholesterol).

▶ Etiology

Obesity has been considered to be the direct result of a sedentary lifestyle plus chronic ingestion of excess calories. Although these factors are undoubtedly the principal cause in many cases, as much as 40–70% of obesity may be explained by genetic influences. Twin studies demonstrate substantial genetic influences on BMI with little influence from the childhood environment.

Five genes affecting control of appetite have been identified in mice. Mutations of each gene result in obesity, and each has a human homolog. One gene codes for a protein expressed by adipose tissue—leptin—and another for the leptin receptor in the brain. The other three genes affect brain pathways downstream from the leptin receptor. Numerous other candidate genes for human obesity have been identified. Only a small percentage (4–6%) of human obesity is thought to be due to single gene mutations. Most human obesity undoubtedly develops from the interactions of multiple genes, environmental factors, and behavior. The rapid increase in obesity in the last several decades clearly points to a major role of environmental factors in the development of obesity. Cross-sectional studies associate obesity with changes in gut flora. It is unknown whether altered gut flora contributes to the development of obesity or whether obesity changes the gut flora.

▶ Medical Evaluation of the Obese Patient

Historical information should be obtained about age at onset, recent weight changes, family history of obesity, occupational history, eating and exercise behavior, cigarette and alcohol use, previous weight loss experience, and psychosocial factors including assessment for depression and eating disorders. Particular attention should be directed at use of laxatives, diuretics, hormones, nutritional supplements, and over-the-counter medications.

Physical examination should assess the BMI, the degree and distribution of body fat, overall nutritional status, and signs of secondary causes of obesity.

Less than 1% of obese patients have an identifiable secondary, nonpsychiatric, cause of obesity. Hypothyroidism and Cushing syndrome are important examples that can usually be diagnosed by physical examination in patients with unexplained recent weight gain. Such patients require further endocrinologic evaluation, including serum thyroid-stimulating hormone (TSH) determination and dexamethasone suppression testing (see Chapter 26).

All obese patients should be assessed for medical consequences of their obesity by screening for the metabolic syndrome. Blood pressure, waist circumference, fasting glucose, low-density lipoprotein (LDL) and HDL cholesterol, and triglycerides should be measured.

▶ Treatment

Using conventional dietary techniques, only 20% of patients will lose 20 lb and maintain the loss for over 2 years; 5% will maintain a 40-lb loss. Average weight loss is approximately 7% of baseline weight. Continued close provider–patient contact appears to be more important for success of treatment than the specific features of any given treatment regimen. Careful patient selection will improve success rates and decrease frustration of both patients and therapists. Only sufficiently motivated patients should enteractive treatment programs. Specific attempts to identify motivated patients—eg, requesting a 3-day diet record—are often useful.

Most successful programs employ a multidisciplinary approach to weight loss, with hypocaloric diets, behavior modification to change eating behavior, aerobic exercise, and social support. Emphasis must be on *maintenance* of weight loss.

Dietary instructions for most patients incorporate the same principles that apply to healthy people who are not obese. This is achieved by emphasizing intake of a wide variety of predominantly "unprocessed" foods. Special attention is usually paid to limiting foods that provide large amounts of calories without other nutrients, ie, fat, sucrose, and alcohol. There is no physiologic advantage to diets that restrict carbohydrates, advocate relatively larger amounts of protein or fats, or recommend ingestion of foods one at a time. Diets that are restricted in carbohydrates (such as the Atkins and South Beach diets), however, can be effective in achieving a lower total calorie intake. Several studies have demonstrated that low-carbohydrate diets can be used safely and effectively for weight loss without adverse effects on lipids or other metabolic parameters. Meal replacement diets can also be used effectively and safely to achieve weight loss.

Long-term changes in eating behavior are required to maintain weight loss. Although formal **behavior modification** programs are available to which patients can be referred, the clinician caring for obese patients can teach a number of useful behavioral techniques. The most important technique is to emphasize planning and record keeping. Patients can be taught to plan menus and exercise sessions and to record their actual behavior. Record keeping not only aids in behavioral change, but also helps the provider to make specific suggestions for problem solving. Patients can be taught to recognize "eating cues" (emotional, situational, etc) and how to avoid or control them. Regular self-monitoring of weight is also associated with improved long-term weight maintenance.

Exercise offers a number of advantages to patients trying to lose weight and keep it off. Aerobic exercise directly increases the daily energy expenditure and is particularly useful for long-term weight maintenance. Exercise will also preserve lean body mass and partially prevent the decrease in basal energy expenditure (BEE) seen with semistarvation. When compared with no treatment, exercise alone results in small amounts of weight loss. Exercise plus diet results in greater weight loss than diet alone. A greater intensity of exercise is associated with a greater amount of weight loss. Up to 1 hour of moderate exercise per day is associated with long-term weight maintenance in individuals who have successfully lost weight. **Social support** is essential for a successful weight loss program. Continued close contact with clinicians and involvement of the family and peer group are useful techniques for reinforcing behavioral change and preventing social isolation.

Patients with severe obesity may require more aggressive treatment regimens. **Very-low-calorie diets** ($\geq$ 800 kcal/d) result in rapid weight loss and marked initial improvement in obesity-related metabolic complications. Patients are commonly maintained on such programs for 4–6 months. Patients who adhere to the program lose an average of 2 lb per week. Average maximum weight loss is approximately 15% of initial weight. Most programs use meal replacement diets to achieve the very-low-calorie intake. Long-term weight maintenance following meal replacement programs is less predictable and requires concurrent behavior modification, long-term use of low-calorie diets, careful self-monitoring, and regular exercise. Side effects such as fatigue, orthostatic hypotension, cold intolerance, and fluid and electrolyte disorders are observed in proportion to the degree of calorie reduction and require regular supervision by a clinician. Other less common complications include gout, gallbladder disease, and cardiac arrhythmias. Although weight loss is more rapidly achieved with very-low-calorie diets as compared with traditional diets, long-term outcomes are equivalent.

Medications for the treatment of obesity are available both over the counter and by prescription. Considerable controversy exists as to the appropriate use of medications for obesity. NIH clinical obesity guidelines state that obesity drugs may be used as part of a comprehensive weight loss program for patients with BMI > 30 or those with BMI > 27 with obesity-related risk factors. There are few data, however, to suggest that medications can improve long-term outcomes associated with obesity.

Several medications are approved by the US Food and Drug Administration (FDA) for treatment of obesity. Catecholaminergic medications (eg, phentermine, diethylpropion, benzphetamine, and phendimetrazine) are approved for short-term use only and have limited utility. **Orlistat** works in the gastrointestinal tract rather than the central nervous system. By inhibiting intestinal lipase, orlistat reduces fat absorption. As expected, orlistat may result in diarrhea, gas, and cramping and perhaps also reduced absorption of fat-soluble vitamins. In randomized trials with up to 2 years of follow-up, orlistat has resulted in 2–4 kg greater weight loss than placebo. Orlistat (120 mg orally up to three times daily with each fat-containing meal) is approved for longer-term treatment of obesity in the United States. A lower dose formulation (Alli 60 mg, one capsule orally up to three times daily with each fat-containing meal; maximum of three capsules per day) is available without a prescription. Long-term clinical benefits have not been demonstrated. Although orlistat results in some additional weight loss at the end of 1- and 2-year clinical trials and, in some studies, improved obesity-related metabolic parameters, a beneficial impact on obesity-related clinical outcomes has not been established.

Additional medications approved for use in the United States are lorcaserin and the fixed combination of phentermine and topiramate. **Lorcaserin** is a selective serotonin receptor agonist. It is associated with modest weight loss, about 3% of initial weight more than placebo. Approximately twice as many patients (38% vs 16%) lose > 5% of initial weight on the medication compared to placebo. Post-marketing surveillance will focus on concerns of increased breast tumors in animal studies, increased valvular heart disease in earlier drugs of this class, and psychiatric side effects. The combination of **phentermine and topiramate**, two older medications, results in dose-dependent weight loss. In clinical trials, patients receiving the lowest dose lost 7.8% more weight than those receiving placebo; with the higher dose, 9.8% more weight was lost. Common side effects include mood changes, fatigue, and insomnia. Since the medications increase heart rate, a large clinical trial to assess cardiovascular risk is being conducted. The medication is also associated with increased birth defects and should not be used during pregnancy.

Several additional medications and combinations of existing medications are also being investigated. Bupropion and naltrexone resulted in short-term weight loss but has not been approved due to ongoing concerns of increased cardiovascular risk. A clinical trial is in progress to further assess safety. Bupropion and zonisamide, exenatide and other incretins, and cetilistat (another pancreatic lipase inhibitor) are all being investigated.

One important weight loss medication, sibutramine, was removed from the market in the United States due to an increase in cardiovascular events in participants in a large randomized trial. This finding emphasizes the need to study the long-term effects of all weight loss medications on important clinical outcomes.

Bariatric surgery is an increasingly prevalent treatment option for patients with severe obesity. In the United States, gastric operations are considered the procedures of choice. Most popular is the Roux-en-Y gastric bypass (RYGB). In most centers, the operation can be done laparoscopically. RYGB typically results in substantial amounts of weight loss—over 30% of initial body weight in some studies. Complications occur in up to 40% of persons undergoing RYGB surgery and include peritonitis due to anastomotic leak; abdominal wall hernias; staple line disruption; gallstones; neuropathy; marginal ulcers; stomal stenosis; wound infections; thromboembolic disease; gastrointestinal symptoms; and nutritional deficiencies, including iron, vitamin B_{12}, folate, calcium, and vitamin D. Operative mortality rates within 30 days are nil to 1% in low-risk populations but have been reported to be substantially higher in Medicare beneficiaries. One-year mortality rates have been reported as high as 7.5% in men with Medicare. The surgical volume (the number of cases performed by the surgeon or hospital) has been demonstrated to be an important predictor of outcome. Another operation is gastric banding. Gastric banding results in less dramatic weight loss than RYGB and has fewer short-term complications. Frequent follow-up, however, is required to adjust the gastric band. Longer-term follow-up has shown a 39% rate of major complications and a 60% rate of re-operation. A third operation, sleeve gastrectomy, is gaining in popularity. With this procedure, approximately three-quarters of the stomach is resected, but the gastrointestinal tract is otherwise left intact. Weight loss results are somewhat less than RYGB but greater than gastric banding.

NIH consensus panel recommendations are to limit obesity surgery to patients with BMIs over 40, or over 35 if obesity-related comorbidities are present. The procedure is cost-effective for patients with severe obesity and most third-party payers cover the procedure in selected patients. A large Swedish study suggested that bariatric surgery is associated with a significant reduction in deaths at 11-year follow-up. The number needed to treat to prevent one death in 11 years was 77 operations. A US Veterans Administration study, however, did not show a mortality benefit.

► When to Refer

Patients with BMI over 40 (or over 35 with obesity-related morbidities) who are interested in considering weight loss surgery.

Baretić M. Targets for medical therapy in obesity. Dig Dis. 2012;30(2):168–72. [PMID: 22722433]

Baron RB. Telling patients they are overweight or obese: an insult or an effective intervention? Arch Intern Med. 2011 Feb 28;171(4):321–2. [PMID: 21357808]

Derosa G et al. Anti-obesity drugs: a review about their effects and their safety. Expert Opin Drug Saf. 2012 May;11(3):459–71. [PMID: 22439841]

Flegal KM et al. Prevalence and trends in obesity among US adults, 1999–2008. JAMA. 2010 Jan 20;303(3):235–41. [PMID: 20071471]

Foster GD et al. Weight and metabolic outcomes after 2 years on a low-carbohydrate versus low-fat diet: a randomized trial. Ann Intern Med. 2010 Aug 3;153(3):147–57. [PMID: 20679559]

Gray LJ et al. A systematic review and mixed treatment comparison of pharmacological interventions for the treatment of obesity. Obes Rev. 2012 Jun;13(6):483–98. [PMID: 22288431]

James WP et al; SCOUT Investigators. Effect of sibutramine on cardiovascular outcomes in overweight and obese subjects. N Engl J Med. 2010 Sep 2;363(10):905–17. [PMID: 20818901]

Jensen MD et al. 2013 AHA/ACC/TOS Guideline for the Management of Overweight and Obesity in Adults: a report of the American College of Cardiology/American Heart Association Task Force on Practice Guidelines and The Obesity Society. Circulation. 2013 Nov 12. [Epub ahead of print] [PMID: 24222017]

Karlsson F et al. Assessing the human gut microbiota in metabolic diseases. Diabetes. 2013 Oct;62(10):3341–9. [PMID: 24065795]

Maciejewski ML et al. Cost-effectiveness of bariatric surgery. JAMA. 2013 Aug 21;310(7):742–3. [PMID: 23989885]

McCarthy M. US obesity rates are leveling out, but long term effects raise concern. BMJ. 2013 Aug 20;347:f5213. [PMID: 23963669]

Pagoto SL et al. A call for an end to the diet debates. JAMA. 2013 Aug 21;310(7):687–8. [PMID: 23989081]

Torpy JM et al. JAMA patient page. Bariatric surgery. JAMA. 2012 Sep 19;308(11):1173. [PMID: 22990277]

Tsai AG et al. In the clinic: obesity. Ann Intern Med. 2013 Sep 3; 159(5):ITC3-1–15. [PMID: 24026335]

Unick JL et al; Look AHEAD Research Group. The long-term effectiveness of a lifestyle intervention in severely obese individuals. Am J Med. 2013 Mar;126(3):236–42. [PMID: 23410564]

Wang YC et al. Health and economic burden of the projected obesity trends in the USA and the UK. Lancet. 2011 Aug 27;378(9793):815–25. [PMID: 21872750]

▼ EATING DISORDERS

ANOREXIA NERVOSA

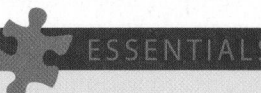

ESSENTIALS OF DIAGNOSIS

► Disturbance of body image and intense fear of becoming fat.

► Weight loss leading to body weight 15% below expected.

► In females, absence of three consecutive menstrual cycles.

► General Considerations

Anorexia nervosa typically begins in the years between adolescence and young adulthood. Ninety percent of patients are females, most from the middle and upper socioeconomic strata.

The prevalence of anorexia nervosa is greater than previously suggested. In Rochester, Minnesota, for example, the prevalence per 100,000 population is estimated to be 270 for females and 22 for males. Many other adolescent girls have features of the disorder without the severe weight loss.

The cause of anorexia nervosa is not known. Although multiple endocrinologic abnormalities exist in these patients, most authorities believe they are secondary to malnutrition and not primary disorders. Most experts favor a primary psychiatric origin, but no hypothesis explains all cases. The patient characteristically comes from a family whose members are highly goal and achievement oriented. Interpersonal relationships may be inadequate or destructive. The parents are usually overly directive and concerned with slimness and physical fitness, and much of the family conversation centers around dietary matters. One theory holds that the patient's refusal to eat is an attempt to regain control of her body in defiance of parental control. The patient's unwillingness to inhabit an "adult body" may also represent a rejection of adult responsibilities and the implications of adult interpersonal relationships. Patients are commonly perfectionistic in behavior and exhibit obsessional personality characteristics. Marked depression or anxiety may be present.

► Clinical Findings

A. Symptoms and Signs

Patients with anorexia nervosa may exhibit severe emaciation and may complain of cold intolerance or constipation. Amenorrhea is almost always present. Bradycardia, hypotension, and hypothermia may be present in severe cases. Examination demonstrates loss of body fat, dry and scaly skin, and increased lanugo body hair. Parotid enlargement and edema may also occur.

B. Laboratory Findings

Laboratory findings are variable but may include anemia, leukopenia, electrolyte abnormalities, and elevations of blood urea nitrogen (BUN) and serum creatinine. Serum cholesterol levels are often increased. Endocrine abnormalities include depressed levels of luteinizing and follicle-stimulating hormones and impaired response of luteinizing hormone to luteinizing hormone-releasing hormone.

▶ Diagnosis & Differential Diagnosis

The diagnosis is based on the behavioral features of weight loss leading to body weight 15% below expected, a distorted body image, fear of weight gain or of loss of control over food intake and, in females, the absence of at least three consecutive menstrual cycles. Other medical or psychiatric illnesses that can account for anorexia and weight loss must be excluded.

Behavioral features required for the diagnosis include intense fear of becoming obese, disturbance of body image, weight loss of at least 15%, and refusal to exceed a minimal normal weight.

The differential diagnosis includes endocrine and metabolic disorders, such as panhypopituitarism, Addison disease, hyperthyroidism, and diabetes mellitus; gastrointestinal disorders, such as Crohn disease and celiac sprue; chronic infections and cancers, such as tuberculosis and lymphoma; and rare central nervous system disorders, such as hypothalamic tumors.

▶ Treatment

The goal of treatment is restoration of normal body weight and resolution of psychological difficulties. Hospitalization may be necessary. Treatment programs conducted by experienced teams are successful in about two-thirds of cases, restoring normal weight and menstruation. One-half continue to experience difficulties with eating behavior and psychiatric problems. Occasional patients with anorexia develop obesity after treatment. Two to 6% of patients die of the complications of the disorder or commit suicide.

Various treatment methods have been used without clear evidence of superiority of one over another. Supportive care by clinicians and family is probably the most important feature of therapy. Structured behavioral therapy, intensive psychotherapy, and family therapy may be tried. A variety of medications including tricyclic antidepressants, selected serotonin reuptake inhibitors (SSRIs), and lithium carbonate are effective in some cases; overall, however, clinical trial results have been disappointing. Patients with severe malnutrition must be hemodynamically stabilized and may require enteral or parenteral feeding. Forced feedings should be reserved for life-threatening situations, since the goal of treatment is to reestablish normal eating behavior.

▶ When to Refer

- Adolescents and young adults with otherwise unexplained weight loss should be evaluated by a psychiatrist.
- All patients with diagnosed anorexia nervosa should be co-managed with a psychiatrist.

▶ When to Admit

- Signs of hypovolemia, major electrolyte disorders, and severe protein-energy malnutrition.
- Failure to improve with outpatient management.

Allen S et al. Treatment of eating disorders in primary care: a systematic review. J Health Psychol. 2011 Nov;16(8):1165–76. [PMID: 21459921]

Arcelus J et al. Mortality rates in patients with anorexia nervosa and other eating disorders. A meta-analysis of 36 studies. Arch Gen Psychiatry. 2011 Jul;68(7):724–31. [PMID: 21727255]

Attia E . Anorexia nervosa: current status and future directions. Annu Rev Med. 2010;61:425–35. [PMID: 19719398]

Crow S. Eating disorders and risk of death. Am J Psychiatry. 2013 Aug 1;170(8):824–5. [PMID: 23903330]

Flament MF et al. Evidence-based pharmacotherapy of eating disorders. Int J Neuropsychopharmacol. 2012 Mar;15(2): 189–207. [PMID: 21414249]

Franko DL et al. A longitudinal investigation of mortality in anorexia nervosa and bulimia nervosa. Am J Psychiatry. 2013 Aug 1;170(8):917–25. [PMID: 23771148]

Ozier AD et al. Position of the American Dietetic Association: nutrition intervention in the treatment of eating disorders. J Am Diet Assoc. 2011 Aug;111(8):1236–41. [PMID: 21802573]

Sim LA et al. Identification and treatment of eating disorders in the primary care setting. Mayo Clin Proc. 2010 Aug;85(8): 746–51. [PMID: 20605951]

Treasure J et al. Eating disorders. Lancet. 2010 Feb 13;375(9714): 583–93. [PMID: 19931176]

BULIMIA NERVOSA

ESSENTIALS OF DIAGNOSIS

▶ Uncontrolled episodes of binge eating at least twice weekly for 3 months.

▶ Recurrent inappropriate compensation to prevent weight gain such as self-induced vomiting, laxatives, diuretics, fasting, or excessive exercise.

▶ Overconcern with weight and body shape.

▶ General Considerations

Bulimia nervosa is the episodic uncontrolled ingestion of large quantities of food followed by recurrent inappropriate compensatory behavior to prevent weight gain such as self-induced vomiting, diuretic or cathartic use, or strict dieting or vigorous exercise.

Like anorexia nervosa, bulimia nervosa is predominantly a disorder of young, white, middle- and upper-class women. It is more difficult to detect than anorexia, and

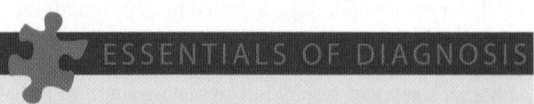

some studies have estimated that the prevalence may be as high as 19% in college-aged women.

Clinical Findings

Patients with bulimia nervosa typically consume large quantities of easily ingested high-calorie foods, usually in secrecy. Some patients may have several such episodes a day for a few days; others report regular and persistent patterns of binge eating. Binging is usually followed by vomiting, cathartics, or diuretics and is usually accompanied by feelings of guilt or depression. Periods of binging may be followed by intervals of self-imposed starvation. Body weights may fluctuate but generally are within 20% of desirable weights.

Some patients with bulimia nervosa also have a cryptic form of anorexia nervosa with significant weight loss and amenorrhea. Family and psychological issues are generally similar to those encountered among patients with anorexia nervosa. Bulimic patients, however, have a higher incidence of premorbid obesity, greater use of cathartics and diuretics, and more impulsive or antisocial behavior. Menstruation is usually preserved.

Medical complications are numerous. Gastric dilatation and pancreatitis have been reported after binges. Vomiting can result in poor dentition, pharyngitis, esophagitis, aspiration, and electrolyte abnormalities. Cathartic and diuretic abuse also cause electrolyte abnormalities or dehydration. Constipation and hemorrhoids are common.

Treatment

Treatment of bulimia nervosa requires supportive care and psychotherapy. Individual, group, family, and behavioral therapy have all been utilized. Antidepressant medications may be helpful. The best results have been with fluoxetine hydrochloride and other SSRIs. Although death from bulimia is rare, the long-term psychiatric prognosis in severe bulimia is worse than that in anorexia nervosa.

When to Refer

All patients with diagnosed bulimia should be co-managed with a psychiatrist.

Bulik CM et al. The changing "weightscape" of bulimia nervosa. Am J Psychiatry. 2012 Oct;169(10):1031–6. [PMID: 23032383]

Mehler PS. Medical complications of bulimia nervosa and their treatments. Int J Eat Disord. 2011 Mar;44(2):95–104. [PMID: 21312201]

Mitchell JE et al. Stepped care and cognitive-behavioural therapy for bulimia nervosa: randomized trial. Br J Psychiatry. 2011 May;198(5):391–7. [PMID: 21415046]

Ozier AD et al. Position of the American Dietetic Association: nutrition intervention in the treatment of eating disorders. J Am Diet Assoc. 2011 Aug;111(8):1236–41. [PMID: 21802573]

Umberg EN et al. From disordered eating to addiction: the "food drug" in bulimia nervosa. J Clin Psychopharmacol. 2012 Jun; 32(3):376–89. [PMID: 22544008]

Wilson GT. Treatment of binge eating disorder. Psychiatr Clin North Am. 2011 Dec;34(4):773–83. [PMID: 22098803]

DISORDERS OF VITAMIN METABOLISM

THIAMINE (B₁) DEFICIENCY

ESSENTIALS OF DIAGNOSIS

▶ Most common in patients with chronic alcoholism.

▶ Early symptoms of anorexia, muscle cramps, paresthesias, irritability.

▶ Advanced syndromes of high output heart failure ("wet beriberi"), peripheral nerve disorders, and Wernicke-Korsakoff syndrome ("dry beriberi").

General Considerations

Most thiamine deficiency in the United States is due to alcoholism. Patients with chronic alcoholism may have poor dietary intakes of thiamine and impaired thiamine absorption, metabolism, and storage. Thiamine deficiency is also associated with malabsorption, dialysis, and other causes of chronic protein–calorie undernutrition. Thiamine deficiency can be precipitated in patients with marginal thiamine status with intravenous dextrose solutions.

Clinical Findings

Early manifestations of thiamine deficiency include anorexia, muscle cramps, paresthesias, and irritability. Advanced deficiency primarily affects the cardiovascular system ("wet beriberi") or the nervous system ("dry beriberi"). Wet beriberi occurs in thiamine deficiency accompanied by severe physical exertion and high carbohydrate intakes. Dry beriberi occurs in thiamine deficiency accompanied by inactivity and low calorie intake.

Wet beriberi is characterized by marked peripheral vasodilation resulting in high-output heart failure with dyspnea, tachycardia, cardiomegaly, and pulmonary and peripheral edema, with warm extremities mimicking cellulitis.

Dry beriberi involves both the peripheral and the central nervous systems. Peripheral nerve involvement is typically a symmetric motor and sensory neuropathy with pain, paresthesias, and loss of reflexes. The legs are affected more than the arms. Central nervous system involvement results in Wernicke–Korsakoff syndrome. Wernicke encephalopathy consists of nystagmus progressing to ophthalmoplegia, truncal ataxia, and confusion. Korsakoff syndrome includes amnesia, confabulation, and impaired learning.

Diagnosis

In most instances, the clinical response to empiric thiamine therapy is used to support a diagnosis of thiamine deficiency. The most commonly used biochemical tests measure erythrocyte transketolase activity and urinary thiamine excretion. A transketolase activity coefficient > 15–20% suggests thiamine deficiency.

Treatment

Thiamine deficiency is treated with large parenteral doses of thiamine. Fifty to 100 mg/d is administered intravenously for the first few days, followed by daily oral doses of 5–10 mg/d. All patients should simultaneously receive therapeutic doses of other water-soluble vitamins. Although treatment results in complete resolution in half of patients (one-fourth immediately and another one-fourth over days), the other half obtain only partial resolution or no benefit.

When to Refer

Patients with signs of beriberi or Wernicke-Korsakoff syndrome should be referred to a neurologist.

THIAMINE TOXICITY

There is no known toxicity of thiamine.

Galvin R et al. EFNS guidelines for diagnosis, therapy and prevention of Wernicke encephalopathy. Eur J Neurol. 2010 Dec; 17(12):1408–18. [PMID: 20642790]

Kumar N . Neurologic presentations of nutritional deficiencies. Neurol Clin. 2010 Feb;28(1):107–70. [PMID: 19932379]

Lough ME . Wernicke's encephalopathy: expanding the diagnostic toolbox. Neuropsychol Rev. 2012 Jun;22(2):181–94. [PMID: 22577001]

Sriram K et al. Thiamine in nutrition therapy. Nutr Clin Pract. 2012 Feb;27(1):41–50. [PMID: 22223666]

Yang JD et al. Beriberi disease: is it still present in the United States? Am J Med. 2012 Oct;125(10):e5. [PMID: 22800868]

Zahr NM et al. Clinical and pathological features of alcohol-related brain damage. Nat Rev Neurol. 2011 May;7(5):284–94. [PMID: 21487421]

RIBOFLAVIN (B$_2$) DEFICIENCY

Clinical Findings

Riboflavin deficiency almost always occurs in combination with deficiencies of other vitamins. Dietary inadequacy, interactions with a variety of medications, alcoholism, and other causes of protein–calorie undernutrition are the most common causes of riboflavin deficiency.

Manifestations of riboflavin deficiency include cheilosis, angular stomatitis, glossitis, seborrheic dermatitis, weakness, corneal vascularization, and anemia.

Diagnosis

Riboflavin deficiency can be confirmed by measuring the riboflavin-dependent enzyme erythrocyte glutathione reductase. Activity coefficients > 1.2–1.3 are suggestive of riboflavin deficiency. Urinary riboflavin excretion and serum levels of plasma and red cell flavins can also be measured.

Treatment

Riboflavin deficiency is usually treated empirically when the diagnosis is suspected. It is easily treated with foods such as meat, fish, and dairy products or with oral preparations of the vitamin. Administration of 5–15 mg/d until clinical findings are resolved is usually adequate. Riboflavin can also be given parenterally, but it is poorly soluble in aqueous solutions.

RIBOFLAVIN TOXICITY

There is no known toxicity of riboflavin.

Koch TR et al. Postoperative metabolic and nutritional complications of bariatric surgery. Gastroenterol Clin North Am. 2010 Mar;39(1):109–24. [PMID: 20202584]

Powers HJ et al. Correcting a marginal riboflavin deficiency improves hematologic status in young women in the United Kingdom (RIBOFEM). Am J Clin Nutr. 2011 Jun;93(6):1274–84. [PMID: 21525198]

Tzoulaki I et al. A nutrient-wide association study on blood pressure. Circulation. 2012 Nov 20;126(21):2456–64. [PMID: 23093587]

NIACIN DEFICIENCY

General Considerations

Niacin is a generic term for nicotinic acid and other derivatives with similar nutritional activity. Unlike most other vitamins, niacin can be synthesized from the amino acid tryptophan. Niacin is an essential component of the coenzymes nicotinamide adenine dinucleotide (NAD) and nicotinamide adenine dinucleotide phosphate (NADP), which are involved in many oxidation-reduction reactions. The major food sources of niacin are protein foods containing tryptophan and numerous cereals, vegetables, and dairy products.

Niacin in the form of nicotinic acid is used therapeutically for the treatment of hypercholesterolemia and hypertriglyceridemia. Daily doses of 3–6 g can result in significant reductions in levels of LDL and very-low-density lipoproteins (VLDL) and in elevation of HDL. The AIM-HIGH study showed, however, that when added to statins there was no benefit of niacin on cardiovascular events.

Niacinamide (the form of niacin usually used to treat niacin deficiency) does not exhibit the lipid-lowering effects of nicotinic acid. Historically, niacin deficiency occurred when corn, which is relatively deficient in both tryptophan and niacin, was the major source of calories. Currently, niacin deficiency is more commonly due to alcoholism and nutrient–drug interactions. Niacin deficiency can also occur in inborn errors of metabolism.

Clinical Findings

As with other B vitamins, the early manifestations of niacin deficiency are nonspecific. Common complaints include anorexia, weakness, irritability, mouth soreness, glossitis, stomatitis, and weight loss. More advanced deficiency results in the classic triad of pellagra: dermatitis, diarrhea, and dementia. The dermatitis is symmetric, involving sun-exposed areas. Skin lesions are dark, dry, and scaling. The dementia begins with insomnia, irritability, and apathy and progresses to confusion, memory loss, hallucinations, and psychosis. The diarrhea can be severe and may result in malabsorption due to atrophy of the intestinal villi. Advanced pellagra can result in death.

▶ Diagnosis

In early deficiency, diagnosis requires a high index of suspicion and attempts at confirmation of niacin deficiency. Niacin metabolites, particularly *N*-methylnicotinamide, can be measured in the urine. Low levels suggest niacin deficiency but may also be found in patients with generalized under-nutrition. Serum and red cell levels of NAD and NADP are also low but are similarly nonspecific. In advanced cases, the diagnosis of pellagra can be made on clinical grounds.

▶ Treatment

Niacin deficiency can be effectively treated with oral niacin, usually given as nicotinamide (10–150 mg/d).

NIACIN TOXICITY

At the high doses of niacin used to treat hyperlipidemia, side effects are common. These include cutaneous flushing (partially prevented by pretreatment with aspirin, 325 mg/d, and use of extended-release preparations) and gastric irritation. Elevation of liver enzymes, hyperglycemia, and gout are less common untoward effects.

Brown TM. Pellagra: an old enemy of timeless importance. Psychosomatics. 2010 Mar;51(2):93–7. [PMID: 20332283]

Jackevicius CA et al. Use of niacin in the United States and Canada. JAMA Intern Med. 2013 Jul 22;173(14):1379–81. [PMID: 23753308]

Michos ED et al. Niacin and statin combination therapy for atherosclerosis regression and prevention of cardiovascular disease events: reconciling the AIM-HIGH trial with previous surrogate endpoint trials. J Am Coll Cardiol. 2012 Jun 5;59(23):2058–64. [PMID: 22520249]

Wan P et al. Pellagra: a review with emphasis on photosensitivity. Br J Dermatol. 2011 Jun;164(6):1188–200. [PMID: 21128910]

VITAMIN B$_6$ DEFICIENCY

Vitamin B$_6$ deficiency most commonly occurs as a result of interactions with medications—especially isoniazid, cycloserine, penicillamine, and oral contraceptives—or of alcoholism. A number of inborn errors of metabolism and other pyridoxine-responsive syndromes, particularly pyridoxine-responsive anemia, are not clearly due to vitamin deficiency but commonly respond to high doses of the vitamin. Patients with common variable immunodeficiency may have concomitant vitamin B$_6$ deficiency.

▶ Clinical Findings

Vitamin B$_6$ deficiency results in a clinical syndrome similar to that seen with deficiencies of other B vitamins, including mouth soreness, glossitis, cheilosis, weakness, and irritability. Severe deficiency can result in peripheral neuropathy, anemia, and seizures. Studies have suggested a potential relationship of low vitamin B$_6$ levels and a variety of clinical conditions including cardiovascular diseases, inflammatory diseases, and certain cancers.

▶ Diagnosis

The diagnosis of vitamin B$_6$ deficiency can be confirmed by measurement of pyridoxal phosphate in blood. Normal levels are > 50 ng/mL.

▶ Treatment

Vitamin B$_6$ deficiency can be effectively treated with oral vitamin B$_6$ supplements (10–20 mg/d). Some patients taking medications that interfere with pyridoxine metabolism may need doses as high as 100 mg/d. Inborn errors of metabolism and the pyridoxine-responsive syndromes often require doses up to 600 mg/d.

Vitamin B$_6$ should be routinely prescribed for patients receiving medications (such as isoniazid) that interfere with pyridoxine metabolism to prevent vitamin B$_6$ deficiency. This is particularly true for patients who are more likely to have diets marginally adequate in vitamin B$_6$, such as the elderly, alcoholic patients, or the urban poor. Clinical trials have shown that vitamin B$_6$ supplementation, combined with other B vitamins, has no benefit on cardiovascular disease outcomes.

VITAMIN B$_6$ TOXICITY

A sensory neuropathy, at times irreversible, occurs in patients receiving large doses of vitamin B$_6$. Although most patients have taken 2 g or more per day, some patients have taken only 200 mg/d.

Corken M et al. Is vitamin B(6) deficiency an under-recognized risk in patients receiving haemodialysis? A systematic review: 2000–2010. Nephrology (Carlton). 2011 Sep;16(7):619–25. [PMID: 21609363]

Hisano M et al. Vitamin B$_6$ deficiency and anemia in pregnancy. Eur J Clin Nutr. 2010 Feb;64(2):221–3. [PMID: 19920848]

Larsson SC et al. Vitamin B6 and risk of colorectal cancer: a meta-analysis of prospective studies. JAMA. 2010 Mar 17;303(11):1077–83. [PMID: 20233826]

Lotto V et al. Vitamin B$_6$: a challenging link between nutrition and inflammation in CVD. Br J Nutr. 2011 Jul;106(2):183–95. [PMID: 21486513]

Mintzer S et al. B-vitamin deficiency in patients treated with antiepileptic drugs. Epilepsy Behav. 2012 Jul;24(3):341–4. [PMID: 22658435]

Zhang X et al. Prospective cohort studies of vitamin B-6 intake and colorectal cancer incidence: modification by time? Am J Clin Nutr. 2012 Oct;96(4):874–81. [PMID: 22875713]

VITAMIN B$_{12}$ & FOLATE

Vitamin B$_{12}$ (cobalamin) and folate are discussed in Chapter 13.

VITAMIN C (Ascorbic Acid) DEFICIENCY

Most cases of vitamin C deficiency seen in the United States are due to dietary inadequacy in the urban poor, the elderly, and patients with chronic alcoholism. Patients with chronic illnesses such as cancer and chronic kidney disease and individuals who smoke cigarettes are also at risk.

▶ Clinical Findings

Early manifestations of vitamin C deficiency are nonspecific and include malaise and weakness. In more advanced stages, the typical features of scurvy develop. Manifestations include perifollicular hemorrhages, perifollicular hyperkeratotic papules, petechiae and purpura, splinter hemorrhages, bleeding gums, hemarthroses, and subperiosteal hemorrhages. Periodontal signs do not occur in edentulous patients. Anemia is common, and wound healing is impaired. The late stages of scurvy are characterized by edema, oliguria, neuropathy, intracerebral hemorrhage, and death.

▶ Diagnosis

The diagnosis of advanced scurvy can be made clinically on the basis of the skin lesions in the proper clinical situation. Atraumatic hemarthrosis is also highly suggestive. The diagnosis can be confirmed with decreased plasma ascorbic acid levels, typically below 0.1 mg/dL.

▶ Treatment

Adult scurvy can be treated orally with 300–1000 mg of ascorbic acid per day. Improvement typically occurs within days. Clinical trials have shown that supplemental vitamin C has no benefit on cardiovascular disease or cancer outcomes.

VITAMIN C TOXICITY

Very large doses of vitamin C can cause gastric irritation, flatulence, or diarrhea. Oxalate kidney stones are of theoretic concern because ascorbic acid is metabolized to oxalate, but stone formation has not been frequently reported. Vitamin C can also confound common diagnostic tests by causing false-negative tests for fecal occult blood and both false-negative and false-positive tests for urine glucose.

Harrison FE. A critical review of vitamin C for the prevention of age-related cognitive decline and Alzheimer's disease. J Alzheimers Dis. 2012;29(4):711–26. [PMID: 22366772]

Hoffer LJ. Ascorbic acid supplements and kidney stone risk. JAMA Intern Med. 2013 Jul 22;173(14):1384. [PMID: 23877084]

Kupari M et al. Reversible pulmonary hypertension associated with vitamin C deficiency. Chest. 2012 Jul;142(1):225–7. [PMID: 22796843]

Magiorkinis E et al. Scurvy: past, present and future. Eur J Intern Med. 2011 Apr;22(2):147–52. [PMID: 21402244]

Pemberton J. Unrecognised scurvy. Signs and requirements. BMJ. 2010 Feb 2;340:c590. [PMID: 20124375]

VITAMIN A DEFICIENCY

▶ Clinical Findings

Vitamin A deficiency is one of the most common vitamin deficiency syndromes, particularly in developing countries. In many such regions, it is the most common cause of blindness. In the United States, vitamin A deficiency is usually due to fat malabsorption syndromes or mineral oil laxative abuse and occurs most commonly in the elderly and urban poor.

Night blindness is the earliest symptom. Dryness of the conjunctiva (xerosis) and the development of small white patches on the conjunctiva (Bitot spots) are early signs. Ulceration and necrosis of the cornea (keratomalacia), perforation, endophthalmitis, and blindness are late manifestations. Xerosis and hyperkeratinization of the skin and loss of taste may also occur.

▶ Diagnosis

Abnormalities of dark adaptation are strongly suggestive of vitamin A deficiency. Serum levels below the normal range of 30–65 mg/dL are commonly seen in advanced deficiency.

▶ Treatment

Night blindness, poor wound healing, and other signs of early deficiency can be effectively treated orally with 30,000 international units of vitamin A daily for 1 week. Advanced deficiency with corneal damage calls for administration of 20,000 international units/kg orally for at least 5 days. The potential antioxidant effects of beta-carotene can be achieved with supplements of 25,000–50,000 international units of beta-carotene.

VITAMIN A TOXICITY

Excess intake of beta-carotenes (hypercarotenosis) results in staining of the skin a yellow-orange color but is otherwise benign. Skin changes are most marked on the palms and soles, while the scleras remain white, clearly distinguishing hypercarotenosis from jaundice.

Excessive vitamin A (hypervitaminosis A), on the other hand, can be quite toxic. Chronic toxicity usually occurs after ingestion of daily doses of over 50,000 international units/d for > 3 months. Early manifestations include dry, scaly skin, hair loss, mouth sores, painful hyperostoses, anorexia, and vomiting. More serious findings include hypercalcemia; increased intracranial pressure, with papilledema, headaches, and decreased cognition; and hepatomegaly, occasionally progressing to cirrhosis. Excessive vitamin A has also recently been related to increased risk of hip fracture. Acute toxicity can result from ingestion of massive doses of vitamin A, such as in drug overdoses or consumption of polar bear liver. Manifestations include nausea, vomiting, abdominal pain, headache, papilledema, and lethargy.

The diagnosis can be confirmed by elevations of serum vitamin A levels. The only treatment is withdrawal of vitamin A from the diet. Most symptoms and signs improve rapidly.

Bello S et al. Routine vitamin A supplementation for the prevention of blindness due to measles infection in children. Cochrane Database Syst Rev. 2011 Apr 13;(4):CD007719. [PMID: 21491401]

Checkley W et al. Maternal vitamin A supplementation and lung function in offspring. N Engl J Med. 2010 May 13;362(19): 1784–94. [PMID: 20463338]

Fok JS et al. Visual deterioration caused by vitamin A deficiency in patients after bariatric surgery. Eat Weight Disord. 2012 Jun;17(2):e144–6. [PMID: 23010786]

Sommer A et al. A global clinical view on vitamin A and carotenoids. Am J Clin Nutr. 2012 Nov;96(5):1204S–6S. [PMID: 23053551]

VITAMIN D

Vitamin D is discussed in Chapter 26.

VITAMIN E DEFICIENCY

Clinical Findings

Clinical deficiency of vitamin E is most commonly due to severe malabsorption, the genetic disorder abetalipoproteinemia, or, in children with chronic cholestatic liver disease, biliary atresia or cystic fibrosis. Manifestations of deficiency include areflexia, disturbances of gait, decreased proprioception and vibration, and ophthalmoplegia.

Diagnosis

Plasma vitamin E levels can be measured; normal levels are 0.5–0.7 mg/dL or higher. Since vitamin E is normally transported in lipoproteins, the serum level should be interpreted in relation to circulating lipids.

Treatment

The optimum therapeutic dose of vitamin E has not been clearly defined. Large doses, often administered parenterally, can be used to improve the neurologic complications seen in abetalipoproteinemia and cholestatic liver disease. The potential antioxidant benefits of vitamin E can be achieved with supplements of 100–400 international units/d. Clinical trials of supplemental vitamin E to prevent cardiovascular disease, however, have shown no beneficial effects.

VITAMIN E TOXICITY

Clinical trials have suggested an increase in all-cause mortality with high dose (≥ 400 international units/d) vitamin E supplements. Large doses of vitamin E can also increase the vitamin K requirement and can result in bleeding in patients taking oral anticoagulants.

Bjelakovic G et al. Antioxidant supplements to prevent mortality. JAMA. 2013 Sep 18;310(11):1178–9. [PMID: 24045742]

Devore EE et al. Dietary antioxidants and long-term risk of dementia. Arch Neurol. 2010 Jul;67(7):819–25. [PMID: 20625087]

Dror DK et al. Vitamin E deficiency in developing countries. Food Nutr Bull. 2011 Jun;32(2):124–43. [PMID: 22164974]

Lotan Y et al. Evaluation of vitamin E and selenium supplementation for the prevention of bladder cancer in SWOG coordinated SELECT. J Urol. 2012 Jun;187(6):2005–10. [PMID: 22498220]

Suksomboon N et al. Effects of vitamin E supplementation on glycaemic control in type 2 diabetes: systematic review of randomized controlled trials. J Clin Pharm Ther. 2011 Feb;36(1):53–63. [PMID: 21198720]

VITAMIN K

Vitamin K is discussed in Chapter 14.

DIET THERAPY

In consultation with a registered dietician, specific therapeutic diets can be designed to facilitate the medical management of most common illnesses. Diet therapy is a difficult process, though, and not all patients are able to cooperate fully. Requesting the patient to record dietary intake for 3–5 days may provide useful insight into the patient's motivation as well as providing nutrient information about the current diet.

Therapeutic diets can be divided into three groups: (1) diets that alter the consistency of food, (2) diets that restrict or otherwise modify dietary components, and (3) diets that supplement dietary components.

DIETS THAT ALTER CONSISTENCY

Clear Liquid Diet

This diet provides adequate water, 500–1000 kcal as simple sugar, and some electrolytes. It is fiber free and requires minimal digestion or intestinal motility.

A clear liquid diet is useful for patients with resolving postoperative ileus, acute gastroenteritis, partial intestinal obstruction, and as preparation for diagnostic gastrointestinal procedures. It is commonly used as the first diet for patients who have been taking nothing by mouth for long periods. Because of the low calorie and minimal protein content of the clear liquid diet, it is used only for short periods.

Full Liquid Diet

The full liquid diet provides adequate water and can be designed to provide adequate calories and protein. Vitamins and minerals—especially folic acid, iron, and vitamin B_6—may be inadequate and should be provided in the form of supplements. Dairy products, soups, eggs, and soft cereals are used to supplement clear liquids. Commercial oral supplements can also be incorporated into the diet or used alone.

This diet is low in residue and can be used in many instances instead of the clear liquid diet described above—especially in patients with difficulty in chewing or swallowing, with partial obstructions, or in preparation for some diagnostic procedures. Full liquid diets are commonly used following clear liquid diets to advance diets in patients who have been taking nothing by mouth for long periods.

Soft Diets

Soft diets are designed for patients unable to chew or swallow hard or coarse food. Tender foods are used, and most raw fruits and vegetables and coarse breads and cereals are eliminated. Soft diets are commonly used to assist in progression from full liquid diets to regular diets in postoperative patients, in patients who are too weak or those whose dentition is too poor to handle a general diet, in head and neck surgical patients, in patients with esophageal strictures, and in other patients who have difficulty with chewing or swallowing.

The soft diet can be designed to meet all nutritional requirements.

DIETS THAT RESTRICT NUTRIENTS

Diets can be designed to restrict (or eliminate) virtually any nutrient or food component. The most commonly used restricted diets are those that limit sodium, fat, and protein. Other restrictive diets include gluten restriction in sprue, potassium and phosphate reduction in chronic kidney disease, and various elimination diets for food allergies.

► Sodium-Restricted Diets

Low-sodium diets are useful in the management of hypertension and in conditions in which sodium retention and edema are prominent features, particularly heart failure, chronic liver disease, and chronic kidney disease. Sodium restriction is beneficial with or without diuretic therapy. When used in conjunction with diuretics, sodium restriction allows lower dosage of the diuretic medication and may prevent side effects. Potassium excretion, in particular, is directly related to distal renal tubule sodium delivery, and sodium restriction will decrease diuretic-related potassium losses.

Typical American diets contain 4–6 g (175–260 mEq) of sodium per day. A no-added-salt diet contains approximately 3 g (132 mEq) of sodium per day. Further restriction can be achieved with diets of 2 or 1 g of sodium per day. Diets with more severe restriction are poorly accepted by patients and are rarely used. Current Institute of Medicine guidelines recommend 2.3 g of sodium per day, which is approximately 1 teaspoon of salt.

Dietary sodium includes sodium naturally occurring in foods, sodium added during food processing, and sodium added by the consumer during cooking and at the table. About 80% of the current US dietary intake is from processed and pre-prepared foods. Diets designed for 2.3 g of sodium per day require elimination of most processed foods, added salt, and foods with particularly high sodium content. Patients who follow such diets for 2–3 months lose their craving for salty foods and can often continue to restrict their sodium intake indefinitely. Many patients with mild hypertension will achieve significant reductions in blood pressure (approximately 5 mm Hg diastolic) with this degree of sodium restriction.

Diets allowing 1 g of sodium require further restriction of commonly eaten foods. Special "low-sodium" products are available to facilitate such diets. These diets are difficult for most people to follow and are generally reserved for hospitalized patients and highly motivated outpatients— most commonly those with severe liver disease and ascites.

► Fat-Restricted Diets

Traditional fat-restricted diets are useful in the treatment of fat malabsorption syndromes. Such diets will improve the symptoms of diarrhea with steatorrhea independently of the primary physiologic abnormality by limiting the quantity of fatty acids that reach the colon. The degree of fat restriction necessary to control symptoms must be individualized. Patients with severe malabsorption can be limited to 40–60 g of fat per day. Diets containing 60–80 g of fat per day can be designed for patients with less severe abnormalities.

In general, fat-restricted diets require broiling, baking, or boiling meat and fish; discarding the skin of poultry and fish and using those foods as the main protein source; using nonfat dairy products; and avoiding desserts, sauces, and gravies.

► Low-Cholesterol, Low-Saturated-Fat Diets

Fat-restricted diets that specifically restrict saturated fats and dietary cholesterol are the mainstay of dietary treatment of hyperlipidemia (see Chapter 28). Similar diets are often recommended for diabetes mellitus (see Chapter 27) and for the prevention of coronary artery disease (see Chapter 10). The large Women's Health Initiative Dietary Modification Trial, however, did not show any significant benefit of a low-fat diet on weight control or prevention of cardiovascular disease or cancer. In contrast, a study of Mediterranean diets, supplemented by nuts or extra-virgin olive oil, did demonstrate a reduction in cardiovascular events.

The aim of low-cholesterol, low-fat diets is to restrict total fat to < 30% of calories and to achieve a normal body weight by caloric restriction and increased physical activity. Saturated fat is restricted to 7% of calories and dietary cholesterol to 200 mg/d. Saturated fat can be replaced either with complex carbohydrates or, if energy balance permits, with monounsaturated fats. Saturated fat, total fat, and dietary cholesterol can be restricted further, but studies suggest that more extreme restriction offers little further advantage in overall modification of serum lipids. Cholesterol-lowering diets can be further augmented with the addition of plant stanols and sterols and with soluble dietary fiber.

► Protein-Restricted Diets

Protein-restricted diets are most commonly used in patients with hepatic encephalopathy due to chronic liver disease and in patients with advanced chronic kidney disease to slow the progression of early disease and to decrease symptoms of uremia in more severe disease. Patients with selected inborn errors of amino acid metabolism and other abnormalities resulting in hyperammonemia also require restriction of protein or of specific amino acids.

Protein restriction is intended to limit the production of nitrogenous waste products. Energy intake must be adequate to facilitate the efficient use of dietary protein. Proteins must be of high biologic value and be provided in sufficient quantity to meet minimal requirements. For most patients, the diet should contain at least 0.6 g/kg/d of protein. Patients with encephalopathy who do not respond to this degree of restriction are unlikely to respond to more severe restriction.

DIETS THAT SUPPLEMENT NUTRIENTS

▶ High-Fiber Diet

Dietary fiber is a diverse group of plant constituents that is resistant to digestion by the human digestive tract. Guidelines suggest that men eat 30–38 g/d and women 21–25 g/d. Typical US diets, however, contain about half of that amount. Epidemiologic evidence has suggested that populations consuming greater quantities of fiber have a lower incidence of certain gastrointestinal disorders, including diverticulitis and, in some studies, colon cancer and a lower risk of cardiovascular disease. A meta-analysis of 22 studies suggested that each 7 g of dietary fiber was associated with a 9% decrease in first cardiovascular events.

Diets high in dietary fiber (21–38 g/d) are also commonly used in the management of a variety of gastrointestinal disorders, particularly irritable bowel syndrome and recurrent diverticulitis. Diets high in fiber, particularly soluble fiber, may also be useful to reduce blood sugar in patients with diabetes and to reduce cholesterol levels in patients with hypercholesterolemia. Good sources of soluble fiber are oats, nuts, seeds, legumes and most fruits. Foods with insoluble fiber include whole wheat, brown rice, other whole grains, and most vegetables. For some patients, the addition of psyllium seed (2 tsp per day) or natural bran (one-half cup per day) may be a useful adjunct to increase dietary fiber.

High-Potassium Diets

Potassium-supplemented diets are used most commonly to compensate for potassium losses caused by diuretics. Although potassium losses can be partially prevented by using lower doses of diuretics, concurrent sodium restriction, and potassium-sparing diuretics, some patients require additional potassium to prevent hypokalemia. High-potassium diets may also have a direct antihypertensive effect. Typical American diets contain about 3 g (80 mEq) of potassium per day. High-potassium diets commonly contain 4.5–7 g (120–180 mEq) of potassium per day.

Most fruits, vegetables, and their juices contain high concentrations of potassium. Supplemental potassium can also be provided with potassium-containing salt substitutes (up to 20 mEq in one-quarter tsp) or as potassium chloride in solution or capsules, but this is rarely necessary if the above measures are followed to prevent potassium losses and supplement dietary potassium.

▶ High-Calcium Diets

Additional intakes of dietary calcium have been recommended for the prevention of postmenopausal osteoporosis, the prevention and treatment of hypertension, and the prevention of colon cancer. The Women's Health Initiative, however, suggested that calcium and vitamin D supplementation did not prevent fractures or colon cancer. Observational studies have also suggested that calcium supplements, especially when taken without vitamin D, may be associated with an increased risk of coronary heart disease. The recommended dietary allowance for the total calcium intake (from food and supplements) in adults ranges from 1000 mg/d to 1200 mg/d. Average American daily intakes are approximately 700 mg/d.

Dairy products are the primary dietary sources of calcium in the United States. An 8-ounce glass of milk, for example, contains approximately 300 mg of calcium. Patients with lactose intolerance who cannot tolerate liquid dairy products may be able to use lactose-free milk, take supplemental lactase enzyme supplements, or tolerate nonliquid products such as cheese and yogurt. Leafy green vegetables and canned fish with bones also contain high concentrations of calcium, although the latter is also high in sodium.

Bao Y et al. Association of nut consumption with total and cause-specific mortality. N Engl J Med. 2013 Nov 21;369(21): 2001–11. [PMID: 24256379]

Baron RB . Eat more fibre. BMJ. 2013 Dec 19;347:f7401. [PMID: 24355540]

Baron RB. Should we all be vegetarians? JAMA Intern Med. 2013 Jul 8;173(13):1238–9. [PMID: 23836265]

Estruch R et al; PREDIMED Study Investigators. Primary prevention of cardiovascular disease with a Mediterranean diet. N Engl J Med. 2013 Apr 4;368(14):1279–90. Erratum in: N Engl J Med. 2014 Feb 27;370(9):886. [PMID: 23432189]

Hooper L et al. Reduced or modified dietary fat for preventing cardiovascular disease. Cochrane Database Syst Rev. 2011 Jul 6;(7):CD002137. [PMID: 21735388]

Jenkins DJ et al. Effect of a dietary portfolio of cholesterol-lowering foods given at 2 levels of intensity of dietary advice on serum lipids in hyperlipidemia: a randomized controlled trial. JAMA. 2011 Aug 24;306(8):831–9. [PMID: 21862744]

Orlich MJ et al. Vegetarian dietary patterns and mortality in Adventist Health Study 2. JAMA Intern Med. 2013 Jul 8;173(13):1230–8. [PMID: 23836264]

Sacks FM et al. Dietary therapy in hypertension. N Engl J Med. 2010 Jun 3;362(22):2102–12. [PMID: 20519681]

Shikany JM et al. Effects of a low-fat dietary intervention on glucose, insulin, and insulin resistance in the Women's Health Initiative (WHI) Dietary Modification trial. Am J Clin Nutr. 2011 Jul;94(1):75–85. [PMID: 21562091]

Threapleton DE et al. Dietary fibre intake and risk of cardiovascular disease: systematic review and meta-analysis. BMJ. 2013 Dec 19;347:f6879. [PMID: 24355537]

INDICATIONS FOR NUTRITIONAL SUPPORT

The precise indications for nutritional support remain controversial. Most authorities agree that nutritional support is indicated for at least four groups of adult patients: (1) those with inadequate bowel syndromes, (2) those with severe prolonged hypercatabolic states (eg, due to extensive burns, multiple trauma, mechanical ventilation), (3) those requiring prolonged therapeutic bowel rest, and (4) those with severe protein–calorie undernutrition with a treatable disease who have sustained a loss of over 25% of body weight.

It has been difficult to prove the efficacy of nutritional support in the treatment of most other conditions. In most cases it has not been possible to show a clear advantage of treatment by means of nutritional support over treatment without such support.

The American Society for Parenteral and Enteral Nutrition (ASPEN) has published recommendations for the rational use of nutritional support. The recommendations emphasize the need to individualize the decision to begin nutritional support, weighing the risks and costs against the benefits to each patient. They also reinforce the need to identify high-risk malnourished patients by nutritional assessment.

▶ NUTRITIONAL SUPPORT METHODS

Selection of the most appropriate nutritional support method involves consideration of gastrointestinal function, the anticipated duration of nutritional support, and the ability of each method to meet the patient's nutritional requirements. The method chosen should meet the patient's nutritional needs with the lowest risk and lowest cost possible. For most patients, enteral feeding is safer and cheaper and offers significant physiologic advantages. An algorithm for selection of the most appropriate nutritional support method is presented in Figure 29–1.

Prior to initiating specialized enteral nutritional support, efforts should be made to supplement food intake. Attention to patient preferences, timing of meals and diagnostic procedures and use of medications, and the use of foods brought to the hospital by family and friends can often increase oral intake. Patients unable to eat enough at regular mealtimes to meet nutritional requirements can be given **oral supplements** as snacks or to replace low-calorie beverages. Oral supplements of differing nutritional composition are available for the purpose of individualizing the diet in accordance with specific clinical requirements. Fiber and lactose content, caloric density, protein level, amino acid profiles, vitamin K, and calcium can all be modified as necessary.

Patients unable to take adequate oral nutrients who have functioning gastrointestinal tracts and who meet the criteria for nutritional support are candidates for **tube feedings**. Small-bore feeding tubes are placed via the nose into the stomach or duodenum. Patients able to sit up in bed who can protect their airways can be fed into the stomach. Because of the increased risk of aspiration, patients who cannot adequately protect their airways should be fed nasoduodenally. Feeding tubes can usually be passed into

the duodenum by leaving an extra length of tubing in the stomach and placing the patient in the right decubitus position. Metoclopramide, 10 mg intravenously, can be given 20 minutes prior to insertion and continued every 6 hours thereafter to facilitate passage through the pylorus. Occasionally, patients will require fluoroscopic or endoscopic guidance to insert the tube distal to the pylorus. Placement of nasogastric and, particularly, nasoduodenal tubes should be confirmed radiographically before delivery of feeding solutions.

Feeding tubes can also be placed directly into the gastrointestinal tract using **tube enterostomies**. Most tube enterostomies are placed in patients who require long-term enteral nutritional support. Gastrostomies have the advantage of allowing bolus feedings, while jejunostomies require continuous infusions. Gastrostomies—like nasogastric feeding—should be used only in patients at low risk for aspiration. Gastrostomies can also be placed percutaneously with the aid of endoscopy. These tubes can then be advanced to jejunostomies. Tube enterostomies can also be placed surgically.

Patients who require nutritional support but whose gastrointestinal tracts are nonfunctional should receive **parenteral nutritional support**. Most patients receive parenteral feedings via a central vein—most commonly the subclavian vein. Peripheral veins can be used in some patients, but because of the high osmolality of parenteral solutions this is rarely tolerated for more than a few weeks.

Peripheral vein nutritional support is most commonly used in patients with nonfunctioning gastrointestinal tracts who require immediate support but whose clinical status is expected to improve within 1–2 weeks, allowing enteral feeding. Peripheral vein nutritional support is administered via standard intravenous lines. Solutions should always include lipid and dextrose in combination with amino acids to provide adequate nonprotein calories. Serious side effects are infrequent, but there is a high incidence of phlebitis and infiltration of intravenous lines.

Central vein nutritional support is delivered via intravenous catheters placed percutaneously using aseptic

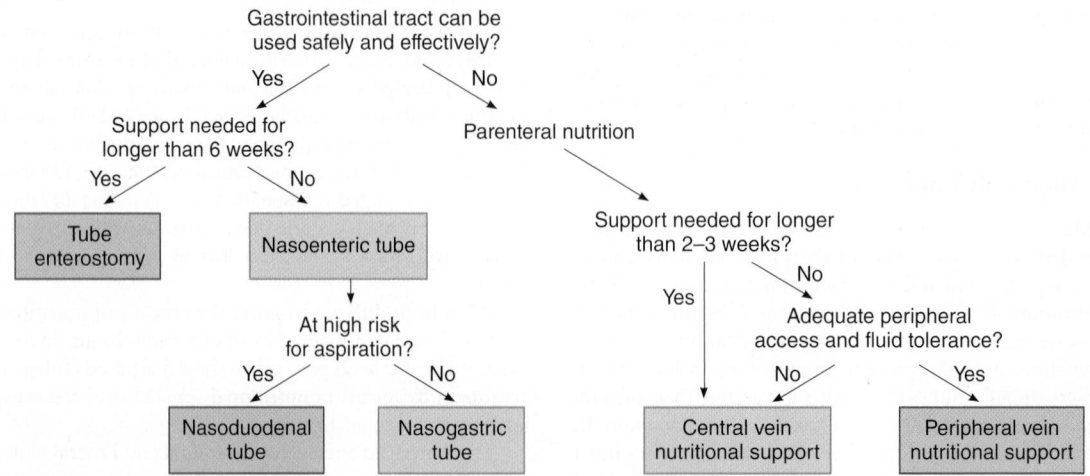

▲ **Figure 29–1.** Nutritional support method decision tree.

technique. Proper placement in the superior vena cava is documented radiographically before the solution is infused. Catheters must be carefully maintained by experienced nursing personnel and used solely for nutritional support to prevent infection and other catheter-related complications.

NUTRITIONAL REQUIREMENTS

Each patient's nutritional requirements should be determined independently of the method of nutritional support. In most situations, solutions of equal nutrient value can be designed for delivery via enteral and parenteral routes, but differences in absorption must be considered. A complete nutritional support solution must contain water, energy, amino acids, electrolytes, vitamins, minerals, and essential fatty acids.

▶ Water

For most patients, water requirements can be calculated by allowing 1500 mL for the first 20 kg of body weight plus 20 mL for every kilogram over 20. Additional losses should be replaced as they occur. For average-sized adult patients, fluid needs are about 30–35 mL/kg, or approximately 1 mL/kcal of energy required (see below).

▶ Energy

Energy requirements can be estimated by one of three methods: (1) by using standard equations to calculate BEE plus additional calories for activity and illness, (2) by applying a simple calculation based on calories per kilogram of body weight, or (3) by measuring energy expenditure with indirect calorimetry.

BEE can be estimated by the **Harris–Benedict equation:** for men, BEE = 666 + (13.7 × weight in kg) + (5 × height in cm) – (6.8 × age in years). For women, BEE = 655 + (9.5 × weight in kg) + (1.8 × height in cm) – (4.7 × age in years). For undernourished patients, actual body weight should be used; for obese patients, ideal body weight should be used. For most patients, an additional 20–50% of BEE is administered as nonprotein calories to accommodate energy expenditures during activity or relating to the illness. Occasional patients are noted to have energy expenditures > 150% of BEE.

Energy requirements can be estimated also by multiplying actual body weight in kilograms (for obese patients, ideal body weight) by 30–35 kcal.

Both of these methods provide imprecise estimates of actual energy expenditures, especially for the markedly underweight, overweight, and critically ill patient. Studies using indirect calorimetry have demonstrated that as many as 30–40% of patients will have measured expenditures 10% above or below estimated values. For accurate determination of energy expenditure, indirect calorimetry should be used.

▶ Protein

Protein and energy requirements are closely related. If adequate calories are provided, most patients can be given 0.8–1.2 g of protein per kilogram per day. Patients undergoing moderate to severe stress should receive up to 1.5 g/kg/d. As in the case of energy requirements, actual weights should be used for normal and underweight patients and ideal weights for patients with significant obesity.

Patients who are receiving protein without adequate calories will catabolize protein for energy rather than utilizing it for protein synthesis. Thus, when energy intake is low, excess protein is needed for nitrogen balance. If both energy and protein intakes are low, extra energy will have a more significant positive effect on nitrogen balance than extra protein.

▶ Electrolytes & Minerals

Requirements for sodium, potassium, and chloride vary widely. Most patients require 45–145 mEq/d of each. The actual requirement in individual patients will depend on the patient's cardiovascular, renal, endocrine, and gastrointestinal status as well as measurements of serum concentration.

Patients receiving enteral nutritional support should receive adequate vitamins and minerals according to the recommended daily allowances. Most premixed enteral solutions provide adequate vitamins and minerals as long as adequate calories are administered.

Patients receiving parenteral nutritional support require smaller amounts of minerals: calcium, 10–15 mEq/d; phosphorus, 15–20 mEq per 1000 nonprotein calories; and magnesium, 16–24 mEq/d. Most patients receiving nutritional support do not require supplemental iron because body stores are adequate. Iron nutrition should be monitored closely by following the hemoglobin concentration, mean corpuscular volume, and iron studies. Parenteral administration of iron is associated with a number of adverse effects and should be reserved for iron-deficient patients unable to take oral iron.

Patients receiving parenteral nutritional support should be given the trace elements zinc (about 5 mg/d) and copper (about 2 mg/d). Patients with diarrhea will require additional zinc to replace fecal losses. Additional trace elements—especially chromium, manganese, and selenium—are provided to patients receiving long-term parenteral nutrition.

Parenteral vitamins are provided daily. Standardized multivitamin solutions are currently available to provide adequate quantities of vitamins A, B₁₂, C, D, E, thiamine, riboflavin, niacin, pantothenic acid, pyridoxine, folic acid, and biotin. Vitamin K is not given routinely but administered when the prothrombin time becomes abnormal.

▶ Essential Fatty Acids

Patients receiving nutritional support should be given 2–4% of their total calories as linoleic acid to prevent essential fatty acid deficiency. Most prepared enteral solutions contain adequate linoleic acid. Patients receiving parenteral nutrition should be given at least 250 mL of a 20% intravenous fat (emulsified soybean or safflower oil) about two or three times a week. Intravenous fat can also be used as an energy source in place of dextrose.

ENTERAL NUTRITIONAL SUPPORT SOLUTIONS

Most patients who require enteral nutritional support can be given commercially prepared enteral solutions (Table 29–1). Nutritionally complete solutions have been designed to provide adequate proportions of water, energy, protein, and micronutrients. Nutritionally incomplete solutions are also available to provide specific macronutrients (eg, protein, carbohydrate, and fat) to supplement complete solutions for patients with unusual requirements or to design solutions that are not available commercially.

Nutritionally complete solutions are characterized as follows: (1) by osmolality (isotonic or hypertonic), (2) by lactose content (present or absent), (3) by the molecular form of the protein component (intact proteins; peptides or amino acids), (4) by the quantity of protein and calories provided, and (5) by fiber content (present or absent). For most patients, isotonic solutions containing no lactose or fiber are preferable. Such solutions generally contain moderate amounts of fat and intact protein. Most commercial isotonic solutions contain 1000 kcal and about 37–45 g of protein per liter.

Table 29–1. Enteral solutions.

Complete
  Blenderized (eg, Compleat Regular, Compleat Modified,[1] Vitaneed[1])
  Whole protein, lactose-containing (eg, Mentene, Carnation and Delmark Instant Breakfast, Forta Shake)
  Whole protein, lactose-free, low-residue:
    1 kcal/mL (eg, Ensure, Isocal, Osmolite, Nutren 1.0,[1] Nutrilan, Isolan,[1]Sustacal, Resource)
    1.5 kcal/mL (eg, Ensure Plus, Sustacal HC, Comply, Nutren 1.5, Resource Plus)
    2 kcal/mL (eg, Isocal HCN, Magnacal, TwoCal HN)
    High-nitrogen: > 15% total calories from protein (eg, Ensure HN, Attain,[1] Osmolite HN,[1] Replete, Entrition HN,[1] Isolan,[1] Isocal HN,[1] Sustacal HC, Isosource HN,[1] Ultralan)
  Whole protein, lactose-free, high-residue:
    1 kcal/mL (eg, Jevity,[1] Profiber,[1] Nutren 1.0 with fiber,[1] Fiberian,[1] Sustacal with fiber, Ultracal,[1] Ensure with fiber, Fibersource)
  Chemically defined peptide- or amino acid-based (eg, Accupep HPF, CriticareHN, Peptamen,[1] Reabfin, Vital HN, AlitraQ, Tolerex, Vivonex TEN)
"Disease-specific" formulas
  Advanced chronic kidney disease: with essential amino acids (eg, Amin-Aid, Travasorb Renal, Aminess)
  Malabsorption: with medium-chain triglycerides (eg, Portagen,[1] Travasorb MCT)
  Respiratory failure: with > 50% calories from fat (eg, Pulmocare, NutriVent)
  Hepatic encephalopathy: with high amounts of branched-chain amino acids (eg, Hepatic-Acid II, Travasorb Hepatic)
Incomplete (modular)
  Protein (eg, Nutrisource Protein, Promed, Propac)
  Carbohydrate (eg, Nutrisource Carbohydrate, Polycose, Sumacal)
  Fat (eg, MCT Oil, Microlipid, Nutrisource Lipid)
  Vitamins (eg, Nutrisource Vitamins)
  Minerals (eg, Nutrisource Minerals)

[1]Isotonic.

Solutions containing hydrolyzed proteins or crystalline amino acids and with no significant fat content are called elemental solutions, since macronutrients are provided in their most "elemental" form. These solutions have been designed for patients with malabsorption, particularly pancreatic insufficiency and limited fat absorption. Elemental diets are extremely hypertonic and often result in more severe diarrhea. Their use should be limited to patients who cannot tolerate isotonic solutions.

Although formulas have been designed for specific clinical situations—solutions containing primarily essential amino acids (for advanced chronic kidney disease), medium-chain triglycerides (for fat malabsorption), more fat (for respiratory failure and CO_2 retention), and more branched-chain amino acids (for hepatic encephalopathy and severe trauma)—they have not been shown to be superior to standard formulas for most patients.

Enteral solutions should be administered via continuous infusion, preferably with an infusion pump. Isotonic feedings should be started at full strength at about 25–33% of the estimated final infusion rate. Feedings can be advanced by similar amounts every 12 hours as tolerated. Hypertonic feedings should be started at half strength. The strength and the rate can then be advanced every 6 hours as tolerated.

COMPLICATIONS OF ENTERAL NUTRITIONAL SUPPORT

Minor complications of tube feedings occur in 10–15% of patients. Gastrointestinal complications include diarrhea (most common), inadequate gastric emptying, emesis, esophagitis, and occasionally gastrointestinal bleeding. Diarrhea associated with tube feeding may be due to intolerance to the osmotic load or to one of the macronutrients (eg, fat, lactose) in the solution. Patients being fed in this way may also have diarrhea from other causes (as side effects of antibiotics or other drugs, associated with infection, etc), and these possibilities should always be investigated in appropriate circumstances.

Mechanical complications of tube feedings are potentially the most serious. Of particular importance is aspiration. All patients receiving nasogastric tube feedings are at risk for this life-threatening complication. Limiting nasogastric feedings to those patients who can adequately protect their airway and careful monitoring of patients being fed by tube should limit these serious complications to 1–2% of cases. Minor mechanical complications are common and include tube obstruction and dislodgment.

Metabolic complications during enteral nutritional support are common but in most cases are easily managed. The most important problem is hypernatremic dehydration, most commonly seen in elderly patients given excessive protein intake who are unable to respond to thirst. Abnormalities of potassium, glucose, CO_2 production, and acid–base balance may also occur.

PARENTERAL NUTRITIONAL SUPPORT SOLUTIONS

Parenteral nutritional support solutions can be designed to deliver adequate nutrients to most patients. The basic parenteral solution is composed of dextrose, amino acids, and water. Electrolytes, minerals, trace elements, vitamins, and medications can also be added. Most commercial solutions contain the monohydrate form of dextrose that provides 3.4 kcal/g. Crystalline amino acids are available in a variety of concentrations, so that a broad range of solutions can be made up that will contain specific amounts of dextrose and amino acids as required.

Typical solutions for central vein nutritional support contain 25–35% dextrose and 2.75–6% amino acids depending upon the patient's estimated nutrient and water requirements. These solutions typically have osmolalities in excess of 1800 mosm/L and require infusion into a central vein. A typical formula for patients without organ failure is shown in Table 29–2.

Solutions with lower osmolalities can also be designed for infusion into peripheral veins. Typical solutions for peripheral infusion contain 5–10% dextrose and 2.75–4.25% amino acids. These solutions have osmolalities between 800 and 1200 mosm/L and result in a high incidence of thrombophlebitis and line infiltration. These solutions will provide adequate protein for most patients but inadequate energy. Additional energy must be provided in the form of emulsified soybean or safflower oil. Such intravenous fat solutions are currently available in 10% and 25% solutions providing 1.1 and 2.2 kcal/mL, respectively. Intravenous fat solutions are isosmotic and well tolerated by peripheral veins.

Typical patients are given 200–500 mL of a 20% solution each day. As much as 60% of total calories can be administered in this manner.

Intravenous fat can also be provided to patients receiving central vein nutritional support. In this instance, dextrose concentrations should be decreased to provide a fixed concentration of energy. Intravenous fat has been shown to be equivalent to intravenous dextrose in providing energy to spare protein. Intravenous fat is associated with less glucose intolerance, less production of carbon dioxide, and less fatty infiltration of the liver and has been increasingly utilized in patients with hyperglycemia, respiratory failure, and liver disease. Intravenous fat has also been increasingly used in patients with large estimated energy requirements. The maximum glucose utilization rate is approximately 5–7 mg/min/kg. Patients who require additional calories can be given them as fat to prevent excess administration of dextrose. Intravenous fat can also be used to prevent essential fatty acid deficiency. The optimal ratio of carbohydrate and fat in parenteral nutritional support has not been determined.

Infusion of parenteral solutions should be started slowly to prevent hyperglycemia and other metabolic complications. Typical solutions are given initially at a rate of 50 mL/h and advanced by about the same amount every 24 hours until the desired final rate is reached.

COMPLICATIONS OF PARENTERAL NUTRITIONAL SUPPORT

Complications of central vein nutritional support occur in up to 50% of patients. Although most are minor and easily managed, significant complications will develop in about 5% of patients. Complications of central vein nutritional support can be divided into catheter-related complications and metabolic complications.

Catheter-related complications can occur during insertion or while the catheter is in place. Pneumothorax, hemothorax, arterial laceration, air emboli, and brachial plexus injury can occur during catheter placement. The incidence of these complications is inversely related to the experience of the physician performing the procedure but will occur in at least 1–2% of cases even in major medical centers. Each catheter placement should be documented by chest radiograph prior to initiation of nutritional support.

Catheter thrombosis and catheter-related sepsis are the most important complications of indwelling catheters. Patients with indwelling central vein catheters in whom fever develops without an apparent source should have their lines changed over a wire or removed immediately, the tip quantitatively cultured, and antibiotics begun empirically. Quantitative tip cultures and blood cultures will help guide further antibiotic therapy. Catheter-related sepsis occurs in 2–3% of patients even if maximal efforts are made to prevent infection.

Metabolic complications of central vein nutritional support occur in over 50% of patients (Table 29–3). Most are minor and easily managed, and termination of support is seldom necessary.

PATIENT MONITORING DURING NUTRITIONAL SUPPORT

Every patient receiving enteral or parenteral nutritional support should be monitored closely. Formal nutritional support teams composed of a physician, a nurse, a dietitian, and a pharmacist have been shown to decrease the rate of complications.

Table 29–2. Typical parenteral nutrition solution (for stable patients without organ failure).

Dextrose (3.4 kcal/g)	25%
Amino acids (4 kcal/g)	6%
Na^+	50 mEq/L
K^+	40 mEq/L
Ca^{2+}	5 mEq/L
Mg^{2+}	8 mEq/L
Cl^-	60 mEq/L
P	12 mEq/L
Acetate	Balance
MVI-12 (vitamins)	10 mL/d
MTE (trace elements)	5 mL/d
Fat emulsion 20%	250 mL five times a week
Typical rate	Day 1: 30 mL/h
	Day 2: 60 mL/h
By day 2, solution provides:	Calories: 1925 kcal total
	Protein: 86 g
	Fat: 19% of total kcal
	Fluid: 1690 mL

Table 29–3. Metabolic complications of parenteral nutritional support.

Complication	Common Causes	Possible Solutions
Hyperglycemia	Too rapid infusion of dextrose, "stress," corticosteroids	Decrease glucose infusion; insulin; replacement of dextrose with fat
Hyperosmolar nonketotic dehydration	Severe, undetected hyperglycemia	Insulin, hydration, potassium
Hyperchloremic metabolic acidosis	High chloride administration	Decrease chloride
Azotemia	Excessive protein administration	Decrease amino acid concentration
Hyperphosphatemia, hypokalemia, hypomagnesemia	Extracellular to intracellular shifting with refeeding	Increase solution concentration
Liver enzyme abnormalities	Lipid trapping in hepatocytes, fatty liver	Decrease dextrose
Acalculous cholecystitis	Biliary stasis	Oral fat
Zinc deficiency	Diarrhea, small bowel fistulas	Increase concentration
Copper deficiency	Biliary fistulas	Increase concentration

Patients should be monitored both for the adequacy of treatment and to prevent complications or detect them early when they occur. Because estimates of nutritional requirements are imprecise, frequent reassessment is necessary. Daily intakes should be recorded and compared with estimated requirements. Body weight, hydration status, and overall clinical status should be followed. Patients who do not appear to be responding as anticipated can be evaluated for nitrogen balance by means of the following equation:

$$\text{Nitrogen balance} = \frac{24\text{-hour protein intake (g)}}{6.25} - \left(\frac{24\text{-hour urinary nitrogen (g)}}{} + 4\right)$$

Patients with positive nitrogen balances can be continued on their current regimens; patients with negative balances should receive moderate increases in calorie and protein intake and then be reassessed. Monitoring for metabolic complications includes daily measurements of electrolytes; serum glucose, phosphorus, magnesium, calcium, and creatinine; and BUN until the patient is stabilized. Once the patient is stabilized, electrolytes, phosphorus, calcium, magnesium, and glucose should be obtained at least twice weekly. Red blood cell folate, zinc, and copper should be checked at least once a month.

Cahill NE et al. Nutrition therapy in the critical care setting: what is "best achievable" practice? An international multicenter observational study. Crit Care Med. 2010 Feb;38(2):395–401. [PMID: 19851094]

Calder PC et al. Lipid emulsions in parenteral nutrition of intensive care patients: current thinking and future directions. Intensive Care Med. 2010 May;36(5):735–49. [PMID: 20072779]

Casaer MP et al. Early versus late parenteral nutrition in critically ill adults. N Engl J Med. 2011 Aug 11;365(6):506–17. [PMID: 21714640]

Codner PA. Enteral nutrition in the critically ill patient. Surg Clin North Am. 2012 Dec;92(6):1485–501. [PMID: 23153881]

Davies AR et al. A multicenter, randomized controlled trial comparing early nasojejunal with nasogastric nutrition in critical illness. Crit Care Med. 2012 Aug;40(8):2342–8. [PMID: 22809907]

DeBellis HF et al. Enteral nutrition in the chronic obstructive pulmonary disease (COPD) patient. J Pharm Pract. 2012 Dec; 25(6):583–5. [PMID: 23065388]

Dorner B et al. Enteral nutrition for older adults in nursing facilities. Nutr Clin Pract. 2011 Jun;26(3):261–72. [PMID: 21586411]

McClave SA et al. Nutrition therapy of the severely obese, critically ill patient: summation of conclusions and recommendations. JPEN J Parenter Enteral Nutr. 2011 Sep;35(5 Suppl):88S–96S. [PMID: 21881019]

Ross VM et al. National clinical guidelines and home parenteral nutrition. Nutr Clin Pract. 2011 Dec;26(6):656–64. [PMID: 22205553]

Schulman RC et al. Metabolic and nutrition support in the chronic critical illness syndrome. Respir Care. 2012 Jun;57(6):958–77. [PMID: 22663970]

Wanten G et al. Managing adult patients who need home parenteral nutrition. BMJ. 2011 Mar 18;342:d1447. [PMID: 21421667]

Vincent JL et al. When should we add parenteral to enteral nutrition? Lancet. 2013 Feb 2;381(9864):354–5. [PMID: 23218814]

Wernerman J. Combined enteral and parenteral nutrition. Curr Opin Clin Nutr Metab Care. 2012 Mar;15(2):161–5. [PMID: 22261951]

Yi F et al. Meta-analysis: total parenteral nutrition versus total enteral nutrition in predicted severe acute pancreatitis. Intern Med. 2012;51(6):523–30. [PMID: 22449657]

Common Problems in Infectious Diseases & Antimicrobial Therapy

30

Peter V. Chin-Hong, MD
B. Joseph Guglielmo, PharmD

FEVER OF UNKNOWN ORIGIN (FUO)

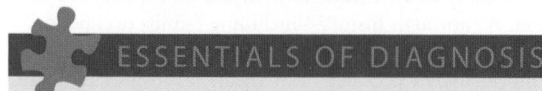

ESSENTIALS OF DIAGNOSIS

- ▶ Illness of at least 3 weeks duration.
- ▶ Fever over 38.3°C on several occasions.
- ▶ Diagnosis has not been made after 3 outpatient visits or 3 days of hospitalization.

▶ General Considerations

The intervals specified in the criteria for the diagnosis of FUO are arbitrary ones intended to exclude patients with protracted but self-limited viral illnesses and to allow time for the usual radiographic, serologic, and cultural studies to be performed. Because of costs of hospitalization and the availability of most screening tests on an outpatient basis, the original criterion requiring 1 week of hospitalization has been modified to accept patients in whom a diagnosis has not been made after 3 outpatient visits or 3 days of hospitalization.

Several additional categories of FUO have been added: (1) **Hospital-associated FUO** refers to the hospitalized patient with fever of 38.3°C or higher on several occasions, due to a process not present or incubating at the time of admission, in whom initial cultures are negative and the diagnosis remains unknown after 3 days of investigation (see Health care-associated Infections below). (2) **Neutropenic FUO** includes patients with fever of 38.3°C or higher on several occasions with < 500 neutrophils per microliter in whom initial cultures are negative and the diagnosis remains uncertain after 3 days (see Chapter 2 and Infections in the Immunocompromised Patient, below). (3) **HIV-associated FUO** pertains to HIV-positive patients with fever of 38.3°C or higher who have been febrile for 4 weeks or more as an outpatient or 3 days as an inpatient, in whom the diagnosis remains uncertain after 3 days of investigation with at least

2 days for cultures to incubate (see Chapter 31). Although not usually considered separately, FUO in solid organ transplant recipients is a common scenario with a unique differential diagnosis and is discussed below.

For a general discussion of fever, see the section on fever and hyperthermia in Chapter 2.

A. Common Causes

Most cases represent unusual manifestations of common diseases and not rare or exotic diseases—eg, tuberculosis, endocarditis, gallbladder disease, and HIV (primary infection or opportunistic infection) are more common causes of FUO than Whipple disease or familial Mediterranean fever.

B. Age of Patient

In adults, infections (25–40% of cases) and cancer (25–40% of cases) account for the majority of FUOs. In children, infections are the most common cause of FUO (30–50% of cases) and cancer a rare cause (5–10% of cases). Autoimmune disorders occur with equal frequency in adults and children (10–20% of cases), but the diseases differ. Juvenile rheumatoid arthritis is particularly common in children, whereas systemic lupus erythematosus, granulomatosis with polyangiitis (formerly Wegener granulomatosis), and polyarteritis nodosa are more common in adults. Still disease, giant cell arteritis, and polymyalgia rheumatica occur exclusively in adults. In the elderly (over 65 years of age), multisystem immune-mediated diseases such as temporal arteritis, polymyalgia rheumatica, sarcoidosis, rheumatoid arthritis, and granulomatosis with polyangiitis account for 25–30% of all FUOs.

C. Duration of Fever

The cause of FUO changes dramatically in patients who have been febrile for 6 months or longer. Infection, cancer, and autoimmune disorders combined account for only 20% of FUOs in these patients. Instead, other entities such as granulomatous diseases (granulomatous hepatitis, Crohn disease, ulcerative colitis) and factitious fever become important causes. One-fourth of patients who say they have been febrile for 6 months or longer actually have no true fever or underlying disease. Instead, the usual normal circadian variation in temperature (temperature 0.5–1°C higher in the afternoon than in the morning) is interpreted as abnormal. Patients with episodic or recurrent fever (ie, those who meet the criteria for FUO but have fever-free periods of 2 weeks or longer) are similar to those with prolonged fever. Infection, malignancy, and autoimmune disorders account for only 20–25% of such fevers, whereas various miscellaneous diseases (Crohn disease, familial Mediterranean fever, allergic alveolitis) account for another 25%. Approximately 50% of cases remain undiagnosed but have a benign course with eventual resolution of symptoms.

D. Immunologic Status

In the neutropenic patient, fungal infections and occult bacterial infection are important causes of FUO. In the patient taking immunosuppressive medications (particularly organ transplant patients), cytomegalovirus (CMV) infections are a frequent cause of fever, as are fungal infections, nocardiosis, *Pneumocystis jirovecii* pneumonia, and mycobacterial infections.

E. Classification of Causes of FUO

Most patients with FUO will fit into one of five categories.

1. Infection—Both systemic and localized infections can cause FUO. Tuberculosis and endocarditis are the most common systemic infections, but mycoses, viral diseases (particularly infection with Epstein-Barr virus and CMV), toxoplasmosis, brucellosis, Q fever, cat-scratch disease, salmonellosis, malaria, and many other less common infections have been implicated. Primary infection with HIV or opportunistic infections associated with AIDS—particularly mycobacterial infections—can also present as FUO. The most common form of localized infection causing FUO is an occult abscess. Liver, spleen, kidney, brain, and bone abscesses may be difficult to detect. A collection of pus may form in the peritoneal cavity or in the subdiaphragmatic, subhepatic, paracolic, or other areas. Cholangitis, osteomyelitis, urinary tract infection, dental abscess, or paranasal sinusitis may cause prolonged fever.

2. Neoplasms—Many cancers can present as FUO. The most common are lymphoma (both Hodgkin and non-Hodgkin) and leukemia. Posttransplant lymphoproliferative disorders may also present with fever. Other diseases of lymph nodes, such as angioimmunoblastic lymphoma and Castleman disease, can also cause FUO. Primary and metastatic tumors of the liver are frequently associated with fever, as are renal cell carcinomas. Atrial myxoma is an often forgotten neoplasm that can result in fever. Chronic lymphocytic leukemia and multiple myeloma are rarely associated with fever, and the presence of fever in patients with these diseases should prompt a search for infection.

3. Autoimmune disorders—Still disease, systemic lupus erythematosus, cryoglobulinemia, and polyarteritis nodosa are the most common causes of autoimmune-associated FUO. Giant cell arteritis and polymyalgia rheumatica are seen almost exclusively in patients over 50 years of age and

are nearly always associated with an elevated erythrocyte sedimentation rate (> 40 mm/h).

4. Miscellaneous causes—Many other conditions have been associated with FUO but less commonly than the foregoing types of illness. Examples include thyroiditis, sarcoidosis, Whipple disease, familial Mediterranean fever, recurrent pulmonary emboli, alcoholic hepatitis, drug fever, and factitious fever.

5. Undiagnosed FUO—Despite extensive evaluation, the diagnosis remains elusive in 15% or more of patients. Of these patients, the fever abates spontaneously in about 75% with no diagnosis; in the remainder, more classic manifestations of the underlying disease appear over time.

▶ Clinical Findings

Because the evaluation of a patient with FUO is costly and time-consuming, it is imperative to first document the presence of fever. This is done by observing the patient while the temperature is being taken to ascertain that fever is not factitious (self-induced). Associated findings that accompany fever include tachycardia, chills, and piloerection. A thorough history—including family, occupational, social (sexual practices, use of injection drugs), dietary (unpasteurized products, raw meat), exposures (animals, chemicals), and travel—may give clues to the diagnosis. Repeated physical examination may reveal subtle, evanescent clinical findings essential to diagnosis.

A. Laboratory Tests

In addition to routine laboratory studies, blood cultures should always be obtained, preferably when the patient has not taken antibiotics for several days, and should be held by the laboratory for 2 weeks to detect slow-growing organisms. Cultures on special media are requested if *Legionella*, *Bartonella*, or nutritionally deficient streptococci are possible pathogens. "Screening tests" with immunologic or microbiologic serologies ("febrile agglutinins") are of low yield and should not be done. If the history or physical examination suggests a specific diagnosis, specific serologic tests with an associated fourfold rise or fall in titer may be useful. Because infection is the most common cause of FUO, other body fluids are usually cultured, ie, urine, sputum, stool, cerebrospinal fluid, and morning gastric aspirates (if one suspects tuberculosis). Direct examination of blood smears may establish a diagnosis of malaria or relapsing fever (*Borrelia*).

B. Imaging

All patients with FUO should have a chest radiograph. Studies such as sinus films, upper gastrointestinal series with small bowel follow-through, barium enema, proctosigmoidoscopy, and evaluation of gallbladder function are reserved for patients who have symptoms, signs, or a history that suggest disease in these body regions. CT scan of the abdomen and pelvis is also frequently performed and is particularly useful for looking at the liver, spleen, and retroperitoneum. When the CT scan is abnormal, the findings often lead to a specific diagnosis. A normal CT scan is not quite as useful; more invasive procedures such as biopsy or exploratory laparotomy may be needed. The role of MRI in the investigation of FUO has not been evaluated. In general, however, MRI is better than CT for detecting lesions of the nervous system and is useful in diagnosing various vasculitides. Ultrasound is sensitive for detecting lesions of the kidney, pancreas, and biliary tree. Echocardiography should be used if one is considering endocarditis or atrial myxoma. Transesophageal echocardiography is more sensitive than surface echocardiography for detecting valvular lesions, but even a negative transesophageal study does not exclude endocarditis (10% false-negative rate). The usefulness of radionuclide studies in diagnosing FUO is variable. Some experts use positron emission tomography (PET) in conjunction with CT scans early in the investigation of FUO. However, more studies are needed before this practice can be more fully integrated into clinical practice. Theoretically, a gallium or PET scan would be more helpful than an indium-labeled white blood cell scan because gallium and fluorodeoxyglucose may be useful for detecting infection, inflammation, and neoplasm whereas the indium scan is useful only for detecting infection. Indium-labeled immunoglobulin may prove to be useful in detecting infection and neoplasm and can be used in the neutropenic patient. It is not sensitive for lesions of the liver, kidney, and heart because of high background activity. In general, radionuclide scans are plagued by high rates of false-positive and false-negative results that are not useful when used as screening tests and, if done at all, are limited to those patients whose history or examination suggests local inflammation or infection.

C. Biopsy

Invasive procedures are often required for diagnosis. Any abnormal finding should be aggressively evaluated: Headache calls for lumbar puncture to rule out meningitis; skin rash should be biopsied for cutaneous manifestations of collagen vascular disease or infection; and enlarged lymph nodes should be aspirated or biopsied for neoplasm and sent for culture. Bone marrow aspiration with biopsy is a relatively low-yield procedure (15–25%; except in HIV-positive patients, in whom mycobacterial infection is a common cause of FUO), but the risk is low and the procedure should be done if other less invasive tests have not yielded a diagnosis, particularly in persons with hematologic abnormalities. Liver biopsy will yield a specific diagnosis in 10–15% of patients with FUO and should be considered in any patient with abnormal liver function tests even if the liver is normal in size. CT scanning and MRI have decreased the need for exploratory laparotomy; however, surgical visualization and biopsies should be considered when there is continued deterioration or lack of diagnosis.

► Treatment

Although it is tempting to begin an empiric course of antimicrobials for FUO, it is rarely helpful and may delay diagnosis if the etiology is infectious (eg, by reducing the sensitivity of blood cultures).

Empiric administration of corticosteroids should be discouraged because they can suppress fever and exacerbate many infections.

► When to Refer

- Any patient with FUO and progressive weight loss and other constitutional signs.
- Any immunocompromised patient (eg, transplant recipients and HIV-infected patients).
- Infectious diseases specialists may also be able to coordinate and interpret specialized testing (eg, Q fever serologies) with outside agencies, such as the US Centers for Disease Control and Prevention.

► When to Admit

- Any patient who is rapidly declining with weight loss where hospital admission may expedite work-up.
- If FUO is present in immunocompromised patients, such as those who are neutropenic from recent chemotherapy or those who have undergone transplantation (particularly in the previous 6 months).

Ben-Baruch S et al. Predictive parameters for a diagnostic bone marrow biopsy specimen in the work-up of fever of unknown origin. Mayo Clin Proc. 2012 Feb;87(2):136–42. [PMID: 22226833]

Hayakawa K et al. Fever of unknown origin: an evidence-based review. Am J Med Sci. 2012 Oct;344(4):307–16. [PMID: 22475734]

Holder BM et al. Fever of unknown origin: an evidence-based approach. Nurse Pract. 2011 Aug;36(8):46–52. [PMID: 21768834]

Manohar K et al. F-18 FDG-PET/CT in evaluation of patients with fever of unknown origin. Jpn J Radiol. 2013 May;31(5):320–7. [PMID: 23456545]

Tóth E et al. Febrile conditions in rheumatology. Clin Rheumatol. 2012 Dec;31(12):1649–56. [PMID: 22923181]

Varghese GM et al. Investigating and managing pyrexia of unknown origin in adults. BMJ. 2010;341:C5470. [PMID: 22312655]

INFECTIONS IN THE IMMUNOCOMPROMISED PATIENT

ESSENTIALS OF DIAGNOSIS

- ► Fever and other symptoms may be blunted because of immunosuppression.
- ► A contaminating organism in an immunocompetent individual may be a pathogen in an immunocompromised one.
- ► The interval since transplantation and the degree of immunosuppression can narrow the differential diagnosis.
- ► Empiric broad-spectrum antibiotics may be appropriate in high-risk patients whether or not symptoms are localized.

▶ General Considerations

Immunocompromised patients have defects in their natural defense mechanisms resulting in an increased risk for infection. In addition, infection is often severe, rapidly progressive, and life threatening. Organisms that are not usually problematic in the immunocompetent person may be important pathogens in the compromised patient (eg, *Staphylococcus epidermidis, Corynebacterium jeikeium, Propionibacterium acnes, Bacillus* species). Therefore, culture results must be interpreted with caution, and isolates should not be disregarded as merely contaminants. Although the type of immunodeficiency is associated with specific infectious disease syndromes, any pathogen can cause infection in any immunosuppressed patient at any time. Thus, a systematic evaluation is required to identify a specific organism.

A. Impaired Humoral Immunity

Defects in humoral immunity are often congenital, although hypogammaglobulinemia can occur in multiple myeloma, chronic lymphocytic leukemia, and in patients who have undergone splenectomy. Patients with ineffective humoral immunity lack opsonizing antibodies and are at particular risk for infection with encapsulated organisms, such as *Haemophilus influenzae, Neisseria meningitides,* and *Streptococcus pneumoniae.* Although rituximab is normally thought of as being linked to impaired cellular immunity, it has been associated with the development of *Pneumocystis jirovecii* infection as well as with hepatitis B reactivation.

B. Granulocytopenia (Neutropenia)

Granulocytopenia is common following hematopoietic cell transplantation ("stem cell transplantation") and among patients with solid tumors—as a result of myelosuppressive chemotherapy—and in acute leukemias. The risk of infection begins to increase when the absolute granulocyte count falls below 1000/mcL, with a dramatic increase in frequency and severity when the granulocyte count falls below 100/mcL. The infection risk is also increased with a rapid rate of decline of neutrophils and with a prolonged period of neutropenia. The granulocytopenic patient is particularly susceptible to infections with gram-negative enteric organisms, *Pseudomonas,* gram-positive cocci (particularly *Staphylococcus aureus, S epidermidis,* and viridans streptococci), *Candida, Aspergillus,* and other fungi that have recently emerged as pathogens such as *Trichosporon, Scedosporium, Fusarium,* and the mucormycoses.

C. Impaired Cellular Immunity

Patients with cellular immune deficiency encompass a large and heterogeneous group, including patients with HIV infection (see Chapter 31); patients with lymphoreticular malignancies, such as Hodgkin disease; and patients receiving immunosuppressive medications, such as corticosteroids, cyclosporine, tacrolimus, and other cytotoxic drugs. This latter group—those who are immunosuppressed as a result of medications—includes patients who have undergone solid organ transplantation, many patients receiving therapy for solid tumors, and patients receiving prolonged high-dose corticosteroid treatment (eg, for asthma, temporal arteritis, systemic lupus erythematosus). Patients taking tumor necrosis factor (TNF) inhibitors, such as etanercept and infliximab, are also included in this category. Patients with cellular immune dysfunction are susceptible to infections by a large number of organisms, particularly ones that replicate intracellularly. Examples include bacteria, such as *Listeria, Legionella, Salmonella,* and *Mycobacterium;* viruses, such as herpes simplex, varicella, and CMV; fungi, such as *Cryptococcus, Coccidioides, Histoplasma,* and *Pneumocystis;* and protozoa, such as *Toxoplasma.* Patients taking TNF inhibitors have specific defects that increase risk of bacterial, mycobacterial (particularly tuberculosis), and fungal infections (primary and reactivation).

D. Hematopoietic Cell Transplant Recipients

The length of time it takes for complications to occur in hematopoietic cell transplant recipients can be helpful in determining the etiologic agent. In the early (preengraftment) posttransplant period (day 1–21), patients will become severely neutropenic for 7–21 days. Patients are at risk for gram-positive (particularly catheter-related) and gram-negative bacterial infections, as well as herpes simplex virus, respiratory syncytial virus, and fungal infections. In contrast to solid organ transplant recipients, the source of fever is unknown in 60–70% of hematopoietic cell transplant patients. Between 3 weeks and 3 months posttransplant, infections with CMV, adenovirus, *Aspergillus,* and *Candida* are most common. *P jirovecii* pneumonia is possible, particularly in patients who receive additional immunosuppression for treatment of graft-versus-host disease. Patients continue to be at risk for infectious complications beyond 3 months following transplantation, particularly those who have received allogeneic transplantation and those who are taking immunosuppressive therapy for chronic graft-versus-host disease. Varicella-zoster is common, and *Aspergillus* and CMV infections are increasingly seen in this period as well.

E. Solid Organ Transplant Recipients

The length of time it takes for infection to occur following solid organ transplantation can also be helpful in determining the infectious origin. Immediate postoperative infections often involve the transplanted organ. Following lung transplantation, pneumonia and mediastinitis are particularly common; following liver transplantation, intra-abdominal abscess, cholangitis, and peritonitis may be seen; after kidney transplantation, urinary tract infections, perinephric abscesses, and infected lymphoceles can occur.

Most infections that occur in the first 2–4 weeks posttransplant are related to the operative procedure and to hospitalization itself (wound infection, intravenous catheter infection, urinary tract infection from a Foley catheter) or are related to the transplanted organ. In rare instances, donor derived infections (eg, West Nile virus, tuberculosis) may present during this time period. Infections that occur between the first and sixth months are often related to immunosuppression. During this period, reactivation of viruses, such as herpes simplex, varicella-zoster, and CMV is quite common. Opportunistic infections with fungi (eg, *Candida, Aspergillus, Cryptococcus, Pneumocystis*), *Listeria monocytogenes, Nocardia,* and *Toxoplasma* are also common. After 6 months, if immunosuppression has been reduced to maintenance levels, infections that would be expected in any population occur. Patients with poorly functioning allografts receiving long-term immunosuppression therapy continue to be at risk for opportunistic infections.

F. Other Immunocompromised States

A large group of patients who are not specifically immunodeficient are at increased risk for infection due to debilitating injury (eg, burns or severe trauma), invasive procedures (eg, chronic central intravenous catheters, Foley catheters, dialysis catheters), central nervous system dysfunction (which predisposes patients to aspiration pneumonia and decubitus ulcers), obstructing lesions (eg, pneumonia due to an obstructed bronchus, pyelonephritis due to nephrolithiasis, cholangitis secondary to cholelithiasis), and use of broadspectrum antibiotics. Patients with diabetes mellitus have alterations in cellular immunity, resulting in mucormycosis, emphysematous pyelonephritis, and foot infections.

▶ Clinical Findings

A. Laboratory Findings

Routine evaluation includes complete blood count with differential, chest radiograph, and blood cultures; urine and respiratory cultures should be obtained if indicated clinically or radiographically. Any focal complaints (localized pain, headache, rash) should prompt imaging and cultures appropriate to the site.

Patients who remain febrile without an obvious source should be evaluated for viral infection (serum CMV antigen test or polymerase chain reaction), abscesses (which usually occur near previous operative sites), candidiasis involving the liver or spleen, or aspergillosis. Serologic evaluation may be helpful if toxoplasmosis or an endemic fungal infection (coccidioidomycosis, histoplasmosis) is a possible cause. Antigen based assays may be useful for the diagnosis of aspergillosis (detected by galactomannan level in serum or bronchoalveolar lavage fluid), or other invasive fungal disease, including *Pneumocystis* infection (serum (1→-beta-D-glucan level).

B. Special Diagnostic Procedures

Special diagnostic procedures should also be considered. The cause of pulmonary infiltrates can be easily determined with simple techniques in some situations—eg, induced sputum yields a diagnosis of *Pneumocystis* pneumonia in 50–80% of AIDS patients with this infection. In other situations, more invasive procedures may be required (bronchoalveolar lavage, transbronchial biopsy, open lung biopsy). Skin, liver, or bone marrow biopsy may be helpful in establishing a diagnosis.

▶ Differential Diagnosis

Transplant rejection, organ ischemia and necrosis, thrombophlebitis, and lymphoma (posttransplant lymphoproliferative disease) may all present as fever and must be considered in the differential diagnosis.

▶ Prevention

There is great interest in preventing infection with prophylactic antimicrobial regimens but no uniformity of opinion about optimal drugs or dosage regimens. Hand washing is the simplest and most effective means of decreasing hospital-associated infections, especially in the compromised patient. Invasive devices such as central and peripheral lines and Foley catheters are potential sources of infection. Some centers use laminar airflow isolation or high-efficiency particulate air (HEPA) filtering in hematopoietic cell transplant patients. Rates of infection and episodes of febrile neutropenia, but not mortality, are decreased if colony-stimulating factors are used during chemotherapy or during stem-cell transplantation.

A. *Pneumocystis* & Herpes Simplex Infections

Trimethoprim-sulfamethoxazole (TMP-SMZ), one double-strength tablet orally three times a week, one double-strength tablet twice daily on weekends, or one single-strength tablet daily for 3–6 months, is frequently used to prevent *Pneumocystis* infections in transplant patients. In patients allergic to TMP-SMZ, dapsone, 50 mg orally daily or 100 mg three times weekly, is recommended. Glucose-6-phosphate dehydrogenase (G6PD) levels should be determined before therapy when the latter is instituted. Acyclovir prevents herpes simplex infections in bone marrow and solid organ transplant recipients and is given to seropositive patients who are not receiving acyclovir or ganciclovir for CMV prophylaxis. The usual dose is 200 mg orally three times daily for 4 weeks (hematopoietic cell transplants) to 12 weeks (other solid organ transplants).

B. CMV

No uniformly accepted approach has been adopted for prevention of CMV. Prevention strategies often depend on the serologic status of the donor and recipient and the organ transplanted, which determines the level of immunosuppression after transplant. In solid organ transplants (liver, kidney, heart, lung), the greatest risk of developing CMV disease is in seronegative patients who receive organs from seropositive donors. These high-risk patients usually receive oral valganciclovir, 900 mg daily for 3–6 months (longer in lung transplant recipients). Other solid organ transplant recipients (seropositive recipients) are at lower risk for developing CMV disease but still usually receive oral valganciclovir for 3 months. The lowest risk group for the development of CMV disease is in seronegative patients who receive organs from seronegative donors. Typically, no CMV prophylaxis is used in this group. Ganciclovir and valganciclovir also prevent herpes virus reactivation. Because immunosuppression is increased during periods of rejection, patients treated for rejection usually receive CMV prophylaxis during rejection therapy.

Recipients of hematopoietic cell transplants are more severely immunosuppressed than recipients of solid organ transplants, are at greater risk for developing serious CMV infection (usually CMV reactivation), and thus usually receive more aggressive prophylaxis. Two approaches have been used: universal prophylaxis or preemptive therapy. In the former, all high-risk patients (seropositive patients who receive allogeneic transplants) may receive oral valganciclovir, 900 mg daily to day 100. This method is costly and associated with significant bone marrow toxicity. Alternatively, patients can be monitored without specific prophylaxis and have blood sampled weekly for the presence of CMV. If CMV is detected by an antigenemia assay or by polymerase chain reaction, preemptive therapy is instituted with oral valganciclovir, 900 mg twice daily for a minimum of 2–3 weeks followed by oral valganciclovir at 900 mg daily until day 100. This preemptive approach is effective but does miss a small number of patients in whom CMV disease would have been prevented had prophylaxis been used. Other preventive strategies include use of CMV-negative or leukocyte-depleted blood products for CMV-seronegative recipients.

C. Other Organisms

Routine decontamination of the gastrointestinal tract to prevent bacteremia in the neutropenic patient is not recommended. Prophylactic administration of antibiotics in the afebrile, asymptomatic neutropenic patient is controversial, although many centers have adopted this strategy. Rates of bacteremia are decreased, but overall mortality is not affected and emergence of resistant organisms is a risk. Use of intravenous immunoglobulin is reserved for the small number of patients with severe hypogammaglobulinemia following bone marrow transplantation and should not be routinely administered to all transplant patients.

Prophylaxis with antifungal agents to prevent invasive mold (primarily *Aspergillus*) and yeast (primarily *Candida*) infections is routinely used, but the optimal agent, dose, and duration have not been standardized. Lipid-based preparations of amphotericin B, aerosolized amphotericin B, intravenous and oral fluconazole or voriconazole, and oral posaconazole solution are all prophylactic options in the neutropenic patient. Because voriconazole is superior to amphotericin for documented *Aspergillus* infections and because posaconazole prophylaxis (compared with fluconazole) has been shown to result in fewer cases of invasive aspergillosis among allogeneic stem cell transplant recipients with graft-versus-host disease, one approach to prophylaxis is to use oral fluconazole (400 mg/d) for patients at low risk for developing fungal infections (those who receive autologous bone marrow transplants) and oral voriconazole (200 mg twice daily) or oral posaconazole (200 mg solution three times daily) for those at high risk (allogeneic transplants, graft-versus-host disease) at least until engraftment (usually 30 days). In solid organ transplant recipients, the risk of invasive fungal infection varies considerably (1–2% in liver, pancreas, and kidney transplants and 6–8% in heart and lung transplants). Whether universal prophylaxis or observation with preemptive therapy is the best approach has not been determined. Although fluconazole is effective in preventing yeast infections, emergence of fluconazole-resistant *Candida* and molds (*Fusarium, Aspergillus, Mucor*) has raised concerns about its routine use as a prophylactic agent.

Given the high risk of reactivation of tuberculosis in patients taking TNF inhibitors, all patients should be screened for latent tuberculosis infection (LTBI) with a tuberculin skin test or an interferon-gamma release assay prior to the start of therapy. If LTBI is diagnosed, treatment with the TNF inhibitors should be delayed until treatment for LTBI is completed. There is also a marked risk of reactivation of hepatitis B and hepatitis C in patients taking TNF inhibitors; patients should also be screened for these viruses when TNF inhibitor treatment is being considered.

▶ Treatment

A. General Measures

Because infections in the immunocompromised patient can be rapidly progressive and life-threatening, diagnostic procedures must be performed promptly, and empiric therapy is usually instituted.

While reduction or discontinuation of immunosuppressive medication may jeopardize the viability of the transplanted organ, this measure may be necessary if the infection is life-threatening. Hematopoietic growth factors (granulocyte and granulocyte-macrophage colony-stimulating factors) stimulate proliferation of bone marrow stem cells, resulting in an increase in peripheral leukocytes. These agents shorten the period of neutropenia and have been associated with reduction in infection.

B. Specific Measures

Antimicrobial drug therapy ultimately should be tailored to culture results. While combinations of antimicrobials may be used to provide synergy or to prevent resistance, the primary reason for empiric combination therapy is broad-spectrum coverage of multiple pathogens (since infections in these patients are often polymicrobial).

Empiric therapy is often instituted at the earliest sign of infection in the immunosuppressed patient because prompt therapy favorably affects outcome. The antibiotic or combination of antibiotics used depends on the degree of immune compromise and the site of infection. For example, in the febrile neutropenic patient, an algorithmic approach to therapy is often used. Febrile neutropenic patients should be empirically treated with broad-spectrum agents active against gram-positive organisms, *Pseudomonas aeruginosa*, and other gram-negative bacilli (such as cefepime 2 g every 8 hours intravenously). The addition of vancomycin, 10–15 mg/kg/dose intravenously every 12 hours, should be considered in those patients with suspected infection due to methicillin-resistant *Staphylococcus aureus* (MRSA), *S epidermidis*, and enterococcus. Continued neutropenic fever necessitates broadening of antibacterial coverage from cefepime to agents such as imipenem 500 mg every

6 hours or meropenem 1 g every 8 hours intravenously with or without tobramycin 5 mg/kg intravenously every 24 hours. Antifungal agents (such as voriconazole, 200 mg intravenously or orally every 12 hours, or caspofungin, 50 mg daily intravenously) should be added if fevers continue after 5–7 days of broad-spectrum antibacterial therapy. Regardless of whether the patient becomes afebrile, therapy is continued until resolution of neutropenia. Failure to continue antibiotics through the period of neutropenia has been associated with increased morbidity and mortality.

Patients with fever and low-risk neutropenia (neutropenia expected to persist for < 10 days, no comorbid complications requiring hospitalization, and cancer adequately treated) can be treated with oral antibiotic regimens, such as ciprofloxacin, 750 mg every 12 hours, plus amoxicillin-clavulanic acid, 500 mg every 8 hours. Antibiotics are continued as long as the patient is neutropenic even if a source is not identified. In the organ transplant patient with interstitial infiltrates, the main concern is infection with *Pneumocystis* or *Legionella* species, so that empiric treatment with a macrolide (or fluoroquinolone) and TMP-SMZ, 15 mg/kg/d orally or intravenously (based on trimethoprim component) would be reasonable in those patients not receiving TMP-SMZ prophylaxis. If the patient does not respond to empiric treatment, a decision must be made to add more antimicrobial agents or perform invasive procedures (see above) to make a specific diagnosis. By making a definite diagnosis, therapy can be specific, thereby reducing selection pressure for resistance and superinfection.

▶ When to Refer

- Any immunocompromised patient with an opportunistic infection.

- Patients with potential drug toxicities and drug interactions related to antimicrobials where alternative agents are sought.

- Patients with latent tubercolosis infection in whom therapy with TNF inhibitors is planned.

▶ When to Admit

Immunocompromised patients who are febrile, or those without fevers in whom an infection is suspected, particularly in the following groups: solid-organ or hematopoietic stem cell transplant recipient (particularly in the first 6 months), neutropenic patients, patients receiving TNF inhibitors, transplant recipients who have had recent rejection episodes (including graft-versus-host disease).

Freifeld AG et al. Clinical practice guideline for the use of antimicrobial agents in neutropenic patients with cancer: 2010 update by the Infectious Diseases Society of America. Clin Infect Dis. 2011 Feb 15;52(4):e56–93. [PMID: 21258094]

Grijalva CG et al. Initiation of tumor necrosis factor-alpha antagonists and the risk of hospitalization for infection in patients with autoimmune diseases. JAMA. 2011 Dec 7; 306(21): 2331–9. [PMID: 22056398]

Keung EZ et al. Immunocompromised status in patients with necrotizing soft-tissue infection. JAMA Surg. 2013 May;148(5): 419–26. [PMID: 23677405]

Martin-Garrido I et al. *Pneumocystis* pneumonia in patients treated with rituximab. Chest. 2013 Jul;144(1):258–65. [PMID: 23258406]

Morris MI et al. Infections transmitted by transplantation. Infect Dis Clin North Am. 2010 Jun;24(2):497–514. [PMID: 20466280]

Nouér SA et al. Earlier response assessment in invasive aspergillosis based on the kinetics of serum *Aspergillus* galactomannan: proposal for a new definition. Clin Infect Dis. 2011 Oct;53(7):671–6. [PMID: 21846834]

Palmer SM et al. Extended valganciclovir prophylaxis to prevent cytomegalovirus after lung transplantation: a randomized, controlled trial. Ann Intern Med. 2010 Jun 15;152(12):761–9. [PMID: 20547904]

Sax PE et al; AIDS Clinical Trials Group Study A5164 Team. Blood (1→3)-beta-D-glucan as a diagnostic test for HIV-related *Pneumocystis jirovecii* pneumonia. Clin Infect Dis. 2011 Jul 15;53(2):197–202. [PMID: 21690628]

Shoham S et al. Invasive fungal infections in solid organ transplant recipients. Future Microbiol. 2012 May;7(5):639–55. [PMID: 22568718]

Stanzani M et al. Computed tomographic pulmonary angiography for diagnosis of invasive mold diseases in patients with hematological malignancies. Clin Infect Dis. 2012 Mar 1;54(5):610–6. [PMID: 22173235]

HEALTH CARE–ASSOCIATED INFECTIONS

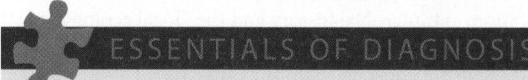

ESSENTIALS OF DIAGNOSIS

- ▶ Health care–associated infections are acquired during the course of receiving health care treatment for other conditions.

- ▶ Hospital-associated infections are a subset of health care–associated infections defined as those not present or incubating at the time of hospital admission and developing 48 hours or more after admission.

- ▶ Most health care–associated infections are preventable.

- ▶ Hand washing is the most effective means of preventing health care–associated infections and should be done routinely even when gloves are worn.

▶ General Considerations

In the United States, approximately 5% of patients acquire a health care–associated infection, resulting in prolongation of the hospital stay, increase in cost of care, significant morbidity, and a 5% mortality rate. The most common infections are urinary tract infections, usually associated with Foley catheters or urologic procedures; bloodstream infections, most commonly from indwelling catheters but also from secondary sites, such as surgical wounds, abscesses, pneumonia, the genitourinary tract, and the gastrointestinal tract; pneumonia in intubated patients or those with altered levels of consciousness; surgical wound infections; MRSA infections; and *Clostridium difficile* colitis.

Some general principles are helpful in preventing, diagnosing, and treating health care–associated infections:

1. Many infections are a direct result of the use of invasive devices for monitoring or therapy, such as intravenous catheters, Foley catheters, shunts, surgical drains, catheters placed by interventional radiology for drainage, nasogastric tubes, and orotracheal or nasotracheal tubes for ventilatory support. Early removal of such devices reduces the possibility of infection.

2. Patients in whom health care–associated infections develop are often critically ill, have been hospitalized for extended periods, and have received several courses of broad-spectrum antibiotic therapy. As a result, health care–associated infections are often due to multidrug resistant pathogens and are different from those encountered in community-acquired infections. For example, S aureus and S epidermidis (a frequent cause of prosthetic device infection) are often resistant to nafcillin and cephalosporins and require vancomycin for therapy; Enterococcus faecium resistant to ampicillin and vancomycin; gram-negative infections caused by Pseudomonas, Citrobacter, Enterobacter, Acinetobacter, and Stenotrophomonas, which may be resistant to most antibacterials. When choosing antibiotics to treat the seriously ill patient with a health care–associated infection, antimicrobial history and the "local ecology" must be considered. In the most seriously ill patients, broad-spectrum coverage with vancomycin and a carbapenem with or without an aminoglycoside is recommended. Once a pathogen is isolated and susceptibilities are known, the most narrow spectrum, least toxic, most cost-effective drug should be used.

Widespread use of antimicrobial drugs contributes to the selection of drug-resistant organisms, thus every effort should be made to limit the spectrum of coverage and unnecessary duration. All too often, unreliable or uninterpretable specimens are obtained for culture that result in unnecessary use of antibiotics. The best example of this principle is the diagnosis of line-related or bloodstream infection in the febrile patient (see below). To avoid unnecessary use of antibiotics, thoughtful consideration of culture results is mandatory. A positive wound culture without signs of inflammation or infection, a positive sputum culture without pulmonary infiltrates on chest radiograph, or a positive urine culture in a catheterized patient without symptoms or signs of pyelonephritis are all likely to represent colonization, not infection.

▶ **Clinical Findings**

A. Symptoms and Signs

Catheter-associated infections have a variable presentation, depending on the type of catheter used (peripheral or central venous catheters, nontunneled or tunneled). Local signs of infection may be present at the insertion site, with pain, erythema, and purulence. Fever is often absent in uncomplicated infections and if present, may indicate more disseminated disease such as bacteremia, cellulitis

and septic thrombophlebitis. Often signs of infection at the insertion site are absent.

1. Fever in an intensive care unit patient—Fever complicates up to 70% of patients in intensive care units, and the etiology of the fever may be infectious or noninfectious. Common infectious causes include catheter-associated infections, hospital-acquired and ventilator-associated pneumonia (see Chapter 9), surgical site infections, urinary tract infections, and sepsis. Clinically relevant sinusitis is relatively uncommon in the patient in the intensive care unit.

An important noninfectious cause is thromboembolic disease. Fever in conjunction with refractory hypotension and shock may suggest sepsis; however, adrenal insufficiency, thyroid storm, and transfusion reaction may have a similar clinical presentation. Drug fever is difficult to diagnose and is usually a diagnosis of exclusion unless there are other signs of hypersensitivity, such as a typical maculopapular rash.

2. Fever in the postoperative patient—Postoperative fever is very common and in many cases resolves spontaneously. Etiologies are both infectious and noninfectious. Timing of the fever in relation to the surgery and the nature of the surgical procedure may help diagnostically.

A. Immediate fever (in the first few hours after surgery)—Immediate fever can be due to medications that were given perioperatively, to the trauma of surgery itself, or to infections that were present before surgery. Necrotizing fasciitis due to group A streptococci or mixed organisms may present in this period. Malignant hyperthermia is rare and presents 30 minutes to several hours following inhalational anesthesia and is characterized by extreme hyperthermia, muscle rigidity, rhabdomyolysis, electrolyte abnormalities, and hypotension. Aggressive cooling and dantrolene are the mainstays of therapy. Aspiration of acidic gastric contents during surgery can cause a chemical pneumonitis (Mendelson syndrome) that rapidly develops but is transient and does not require antibiotics. Fever due to the trauma of surgery itself usually resolves in 2–3 days, longer in more complicated operative cases and in patients with head trauma.

B. Acute fever (within 1 week of surgery)—Acute fever is usually due to common causes of hospital-associated infections, such as ventilator-associated pneumonia (including aspiration pneumonia in patients with decreased gag reflex) and line infections. Noninfectious causes include alcohol withdrawal, gout, pulmonary embolism, and pancreatitis. Atelectasis following surgery is commonly invoked as a cause of postoperative fever but there is no good evidence to support a causal association between the presence or degree of atelectasis and fever.

C. Subacute fever (at least 1 week after surgery)—Surgical site infections commonly present at least 1 week after surgery. The type of surgery that was performed predicts specific infectious etiologies. Patients undergoing cardiothoracic surgery may be at higher risk for pneumonia and deep and superficial sternal wound infections. Meningitis without typical signs of meningismus may complicate neurosurgical procedures. Abdominal surgery may result in deep abdominal abscesses that require drainage.

B. Laboratory Findings

Blood cultures are universally recommended, and chest radiographs are frequently obtained. A properly prepared sputum Gram stain and semi-quantitative sputum cultures may be useful in selected patients where there is a high pretest probability of pneumonia but multiple exclusion criteria probably limit generalizability in most patients, such as immunocompromised patients and those with drug resistance. Other diagnostic strategies will be dictated by the clinical context (eg, transesophageal echocardiogram in a patient with S aureus bacteremia).

Any fever in a patient with a central venous catheter should prompt the collection of blood. The best method to evaluate bacteremia is to gather at least two peripherally obtained blood cultures. Blood cultures from unidentified sites, a single blood culture from any site, or a blood culture through an existing line will often be positive for S epidermidis, resulting in the inappropriate use of vancomycin. Unless two separate venipuncture cultures are obtained—not through catheters—interpretation of results is impossible and unnecessary therapy may be given. Every such "pseudobacteremia" increases laboratory costs, antibiotic use, and length of stay. Microbiologic evaluation of the removed catheter can sometimes be helpful, but only in addition to (not instead of) blood cultures drawn from peripheral sites. The differential time to positivity measures the difference in time that cultures simultaneously drawn through a catheter and a peripheral site become positive. A positive test (about 120 minutes difference in time) supports a catheter-related bloodstream infection, and a negative test may permit catheters to be retained.

▶ Complications

Patients who have persistent bacteremia and fever despite removal of the infected catheter may have complications such as septic thrombophlebitis, endocarditis, or metastatic foci of infection (particularly with S aureus). Additional studies such as venous Doppler studies, transesophageal echocardiogram, and chest radiographs may be indicated, and 4–6 weeks of antibiotics may be needed. In the case of septic thrombophlebitis, anticoagulation with heparin is also recommended if there are no contraindications.

▶ Differential Diagnosis

Although most fevers are due to infections, about 25% of patients will have fever of noninfectious origin, including drug fever, nonspecific postoperative fevers (tissue damage or necrosis), hematoma, pancreatitis, pulmonary embolism, myocardial infarction, and ischemic bowel disease.

▶ Prevention

The concept of universal precautions emphasizes that all patients are treated as though they have a potential blood-borne transmissible disease, and thus all body secretions are handled with care to prevent spread of disease. Body substance isolation requires use of gloves whenever a health care worker anticipates contact with blood or other body secretions. Even though gloves are worn, health care workers should routinely wash their hands, since it is the easiest and most effective means of preventing hospital-associated infections. Application of a rapid drying, alcohol-based antiseptic is simple, takes less time than traditional hand washing with soap and water, is more effective at reducing hand colonization, and promotes compliance with hand decontamination. For prevention of transmission of C difficile infection, handwashing is more effective than alcohol-based antiseptics. Even after removing gloves, providers should always wash hands in cases of proven or suspected C difficile infection.

Peripheral intravenous lines should be replaced every 3 days. Arterial lines and lines in the central venous circulation (including those placed peripherally) can be left in place indefinitely and are changed or removed when they are clinically suspected of being infected, when they are nonfunctional, or when they are no longer needed. Using sterile barrier precautions (including cap, mask, gown, gloves, and drape) is recommended while inserting central venous catheters. Silver alloy–impregnated Foley catheters reduce the incidence of catheter-associated bacteriuria, and antibiotic-impregnated (minocycline plus rifampin or chlorhexidine plus silver sulfadiazine) venous catheters reduce line infections and bacteremia. Silver-coated endotracheal tubes may reduce the incidence of ventilator-associated pneumonia. Whether the increased cost of these devices justifies their routine use should be determined by individual institutions. Catheter-related urinary tract infections and intravenous catheter-associated infections are not Medicare-reimbursable conditions. Preoperative skin preparation with chlorhexidine and alcohol (versus povidone-iodine) has been shown to reduce the incidence of infection following surgery. Another strategy that can prevent surgical-site infections is the identification and treatment of S aureus nasal carriers with 2% mupirocin nasal ointment and chlorhexidine soap. Daily bathing of ICU patients with chlorhexidine-impregnated washcloths versus soap and water results in lower risk of MRSA-associated clinical cultures and catheter-associated bloodstream infections. Selective decontamination of the digestive tract with nonabsorbable or parenteral antibiotics, or both, may prevent hospital-acquired pneumonia and decrease mortality.

Attentive nursing care (positioning to prevent decubitus ulcers, wound care, elevating the head during tube feedings to prevent aspiration) is critical in preventing hospital-associated infections. In addition, monitoring of high-risk areas by hospital epidemiologists is critical in the prevention of infection. Some guidelines advocate rapid screening (active surveillance cultures) for MRSA on admission to acute care facilities among certain subpopulations of patients (eg, those recently hospitalized, admission to the intensive care unit, patients undergoing hemodialysis). However, outside the setting of an MRSA outbreak, it is not clear whether this strategy decreases the incidence of hospital-associated MRSA infections.

Vaccines, including hepatitis A, hepatitis B, and the varicella, pneumococcal, and influenza vaccinations, are important adjuncts. (See section below on Immunization against Infectious Diseases.)

▶ Treatment

A. Fever in an Intensive Care Unit Patient

Unless the patient has a central neurologic injury with elevated intracranial pressure or has a temperature > 41°C, there is less physiologic need to maintain euthermia. Empiric broad-spectrum antibiotics (see Table 30–5) are recommended for neutropenic and other immunocompromised patients and in patients who are clinically unstable.

B. Catheter-Associated Infections

Factors that inform treatment decisions include the type of catheter, the causative pathogen, the availability of alternate catheter access sites, the need for ongoing intravascular access, and the severity of disease.

In general, catheters should be removed if there is purulence at the exit site; if the organism is *S aureus,* gram-negative rods, or *Candida* species; if there is persistent bacteremia (> 48 hours while receiving antibiotics); or if complications, such as septic thrombophlebitis, endocarditis, or other metastatic disease exist. Central venous catheters may be exchanged over a guidewire provided there is no erythema or purulence at the exit site and the patient does not appear to be septic. Methicillin-resistant, coagulase-negative staphylococci are the most common pathogens; thus, empiric therapy with vancomycin, 15 mg/kg intravenously twice daily, should be given assuming normal kidney function. Empiric gram-negative coverage may be considered in patients who are immunocompromised or who are critically ill (see Table 30–5).

Antibiotic treatment duration depends on the pathogen and the extent of disease. For uncomplicated bacteremia, 5–7 days of therapy is usually sufficient for coagulase-negative staphylococci, even if the original catheter is retained. Fourteen days of therapy is generally recommended for uncomplicated bacteremia caused by gram-negative rods, *Candida* species, and *S aureus*. Antibiotic lock therapy involves the instillation of supratherapeutic concentrations of antibiotics with heparin in the lumen of catheters. The purpose is to achieve adequate concentrations of antibiotics to kill microbes in the biofilm. Antibiotic lock therapy can be used for catheter-related bloodstream infections caused by coagulase-negative staphylococci or enterococci and when the catheter is being retained in a salvage situation.

▶ When to Refer

- Any patient with multidrug-resistant infection.
- Any patient with fungemia or persistent bacteremia.
- Patients with multisite infections.
- Patients with impaired or fluctuating kidney function for assistance with dosing of antimicrobials.
- Patients with refractory or recurrent *C difficile* colitis.

Baron EJ et al. A guide to utilization of the microbiology laboratory for diagnosis of infectious diseases: 2013 recommendations by the Infectious Diseases Society of America (IDSA) and the American Society for Microbiology (ASM)(a). Clin Infect Dis. 2013 Aug;57(4):e22–e121. [PMID: 23845951]

Bode LG et al. Preventing surgical-site infections in nasal carriers of *Staphylococcus aureus*. N Engl J Med. 2010 Jan 7;362(1):9–17. [PMID: 20054045]

Cannon CM et al. The GENESIS Project (GENeralized Early Sepsis Intervention Strategies): a multicenter quality improvement collaborative. J Intensive Care Med. 2013 Nov–Dec;28(6):355–68. [PMID: 22902347]

Darouiche RO et al. Chlorhexidine-alcohol versus povidone-iodine for surgical-site antisepsis. N Engl J Med. 2010 Jan 7;362(1):18–26. [PMID: 20054046]

Harris AD et al. Universal glove and gown use and acquisition of antibiotic-resistant bacteria in the ICU: a randomized trial. JAMA. 2013 Oct 16;310(15):1571–80. [PMID: 24097234]

Huang SS et al; CDC Prevention Epicenters Program; AHRQ DECIDE Network and Healthcare-Associated Infections Program. Targeted versus universal decolonization to prevent ICU infection. N Engl J Med. 2013 Jun 13;368(24):2255–65. Erratum in: N Engl J Med. 2013 Aug 8;369(6):587. [PMID: 23718152]

Marik PE et al. The risk of catheter-related bloodstream infection with femoral venous catheters as compared to subclavian and internal jugular venous catheters: a systematic review of the literature and meta-analysis. Crit Care Med. 2012 Aug;40(8):2479–85. [PMID: 22809915]

Peleg AY et al. Hospital-acquired infections due to gram-negative bacteria. N Engl J Med. 2010 May 13;362(19):1804–13. [PMID: 20463340]

Sclar DA et al. Fidaxomicin in the treatment of *Clostridium difficile*-associated diarrhoea. Clin Drug Investig. 2013 Mar;33(3):229. [PMID: 23386229]

Sinuff T et al; Canadian Critical Care Trials Group. Implementation of clinical practice guidelines for ventilator-associated pneumonia: a multicenter prospective study. Crit Care Med. 2013 Jan;41(1):15–23. [PMID: 23222254]

van Nood E et al. Duodenal infusion of donor feces for recurrent *Clostridium difficile*. N Engl J Med. 2013 Jan 31;368(5):407–15. [PMID: 23323867]

INFECTIONS OF THE CENTRAL NERVOUS SYSTEM

ESSENTIALS OF DIAGNOSIS

- ▶ Central nervous system infection is a medical emergency.
- ▶ Symptoms and signs common to all central nervous system infections include headache, fever, sensorial disturbances, neck and back stiffness, positive Kernig and Brudzinski signs, and cerebrospinal fluid abnormalities.

▶ General Considerations

Infections of the central nervous system can be caused by almost any infectious agent, including bacteria, mycobacteria, fungi, spirochetes, protozoa, helminths, and viruses.

Table 30–1. Typical cerebrospinal fluid findings in various central nervous system diseases.

Diagnosis	Cells/mcL	Glucose (mg/dL)	Protein (mg/dL)	Opening Pressure
Normal	0–5 lymphocytes	45–85[1]	15–45	70–180 mm H$_2$O
Purulent meningitis (bacterial)[2] community-acquired	200–20,000 polymorphonuclear neutrophils	Low (< 45)	High (> 50)	Markedly elevated
Granulomatous meningitis (mycobacterial, fungal)[3]	100–1000, mostly lymphocytes[3]	Low (< 45)	High (> 50)	Moderately elevated
Spirochetal meningitis	100–1000, mostly lymphocytes[3]	Normal	Moderately high (> 50)	Normal to slightly elevated
Aseptic meningitis, viral or meningoencephalitis[4]	25–2000, mostly lymphocytes[3]	Normal or low	High (> 50)	Slightly elevated
"Neighborhood reaction"[5]	Variably increased	Normal	Normal or high	Variable

[1]Cerebrospinal fluid glucose must be considered in relation to blood glucose level. Normally, cerebrospinal fluid glucose is 20–30 mg/dL lower than blood glucose, or 50–70% of the normal value of blood glucose.
[2]Organisms in smear or culture of cerebrospinal fluid; counterimmunoelectrophoresis or latex agglutination may be diagnostic.
[3]Polymorphonuclear neutrophils may predominate early.
[4]Viral isolation from cerebrospinal fluid early; antibody titer rise in paired specimens of serum; polymerase chain reaction for herpesvirus.
[5]May occur in mastoiditis, brain abscess, epidural abscess, sinusitis, septic thrombus, brain tumor. Cerebrospinal fluid culture results usually negative.

► Etiologic Classification

Central nervous system infections can be divided into several categories that usually can be readily distinguished from each other by cerebrospinal fluid examination as the first step toward etiologic diagnosis (Table 30–1).

A. Purulent Meningitis

Patients with bacterial meningitis usually seek medical attention within hours or 1–2 days after onset of symptoms. The organisms responsible depend primarily on the age of the patient as summarized in Table 30–2. The diagnosis is usually based on the Gram-stained smear (positive in 60–90%) or culture (positive in over 90%) of the cerebrospinal fluid.

B. Chronic Meningitis

The presentation of chronic meningitis is less acute than purulent meningitis. Patients with chronic meningitis usually have a history of symptoms lasting weeks to months. The most common pathogens are *Mycobacterium tuberculosis*, atypical mycobacteria, fungi (*Cryptococcus, Coccidioides, Histoplasma*), and spirochetes (*Treponema pallidum* and *Borrelia burgdorferi*). The diagnosis is made by culture or in some cases by serologic tests (cryptococcosis, coccidioidomycosis, syphilis, Lyme disease).

C. Aseptic Meningitis

Aseptic meningitis—a much more benign and self-limited syndrome than purulent meningitis—is caused principally

Table 30–2. Initial antimicrobial therapy for purulent meningitis of unknown cause.

Population	Common Microorganisms	Standard Therapy
18–50 years	*Streptococcus pneumoniae, Neisseria meningitidis*	Vancomycin[1] **plus** cefotaxime or ceftriaxone[2]
Over 50 years	*S pneumoniae, N meningitidis, Listeria monocytogenes,* gram-negative bacilli	Vancomycin[1] **plus** ampicillin,[3] **plus** cefotaxime or ceftriaxone[2]
Impaired cellular immunity	*L monocytogenes,* gram-negative bacilli, *S pneumoniae*	Vancomycin[1] **plus** ampicillin[3] **plus** cefepime[4]
Postsurgical or posttraumatic	*Staphylococcus aureus, S pneumoniae,* gram-negative bacilli	Vancomycin[1] **plus** cefepime[4]

[1]The dose of vancomycin is 15 mg/kg/dose intravenously every 8 hours.
[2]The usual dose of cefotaxime is 2 g intravenously every 6 hours and that of ceftriaxone is 2 g intravenously every 12 hours. If the organism is sensitive to penicillin, 3–4 million units intravenously every 4 hours is given.
[3]The dose of ampicillin is usually 2 g intravenously every 4 hours.
[4]Cefepime is given in a dose of 2–3 g intravenously every 8 hours.

by viruses, especially herpes simplex virus and the enterovirus group (including coxsackieviruses and echoviruses). Infectious mononucleosis may be accompanied by aseptic meningitis. Leptospiral infection is also usually placed in the aseptic group because of the lymphocytic cellular response and its relatively benign course. This type of meningitis also occurs during secondary syphilis and disseminated Lyme disease. Prior to the routine administration of measles-mumps-rubella (MMR) vaccines, mumps was the most common cause of viral meningitis. Drug-induced aseptic meningitis has been reported with nonsteroidal anti-inflammatory drugs, sulfonamides and certain solid organ transplant agents, including muromonab-CD3 (OKT3).

D. Encephalitis

Encephalitis (due to herpesviruses, arboviruses, rabies virus, flaviviruses [West Nile encephalitis, Japanese encephalitis]), and many others, produces disturbances of the sensorium, seizures, and many other manifestations. Patients are more ill than those with aseptic meningitis. Cerebrospinal fluid may be entirely normal or may show some lymphocytes and in some instances (eg, herpes simplex) red cells as well. Influenza has been associated with encephalitis, but the relationship is not clear. An autoimmune form of encephalitis associated with N-methyl-D-aspartate receptor antibodies should be suspected in younger patients with encephalitis and associated seizures, movement disorders, and psychosis.

E. Partially Treated Bacterial Meningitis

Previous effective antibiotic therapy given for 12–24 hours will decrease the rate of positive Gram stain results by 20% and culture by 30–40% of the cerebrospinal fluid but will have little effect on cell count, protein, or glucose. Occasionally, previous antibiotic therapy will change a predominantly polymorphonuclear response to a lymphocytic pleocytosis, and some of the cerebrospinal fluid findings may be similar to those seen in aseptic meningitis.

F. Neighborhood Reaction

As noted in Table 30–1, this term denotes a purulent infectious process in close proximity to the central nervous system that spills some of the products of the inflammatory process—white blood cells or protein—into the cerebrospinal fluid. Such an infection might be a brain abscess, osteomyelitis of the vertebrae, epidural abscess, subdural empyema, or bacterial sinusitis or mastoiditis.

G. Noninfectious Meningeal Irritation

Carcinomatous meningitis, sarcoidosis, systemic lupus erythematosus, chemical meningitis, and certain drugs—nonsteroidal anti-inflammatory drugs, OKT3, TMP-SMZ, and others—can also produce symptoms and signs of meningeal irritation with associated cerebrospinal fluid pleocytosis, increased protein, and low or normal glucose. Meningismus with normal cerebrospinal fluid findings occurs in the presence of other infections such as pneumonia and shigellosis.

H. Brain Abscess

Brain abscess presents as a space-occupying lesion; symptoms may include vomiting, fever, change of mental status, or focal neurologic manifestations. When brain abscess is suspected, a CT scan should be performed. If positive, lumbar puncture should *not* be performed since results rarely provide clinically useful information and herniation can occur. The bacteriology of brain abscess is usually polymicrobial and includes *S aureus*, gram-negative bacilli, streptococci, and anaerobes (including anaerobic streptococci and *Prevotella* species).

I. Health Care–Associated Meningitis

This infection may arise as a result of invasive neurosurgical procedures (eg, craniotomy, internal or external ventricular catheters, external lumbar catheters), complicated head trauma, or from hospital-acquired bloodstream infections. Outbreaks have been associated with contaminated epidural or paraspinal corticosteroid injections. In general, the microbiology is distinct from community-acquired meningitis, with gram-negative organisms (eg, *Pseudomonas*), *S aureus,* and coagulase-negative staphylococci and, in the outbreaks associated with contaminated corticosteroids, mold and fungi (*Exserohilum rostratum* and *Aspergillus fumigatus*) playing a larger role.

▶ Clinical Findings

A. Symptoms and Signs

The classic triad of fever, stiff neck, and altered mental status has a low sensitivity (44%) for bacterial meningitis. However, nearly all patients with bacterial meningitis have at least two of the following symptoms—fever, headache, stiff neck, or altered mental status.

B. Laboratory Tests

Evaluation of a patient with suspected meningitis includes a blood count, blood culture, lumbar puncture followed by careful study and culture of the cerebrospinal fluid, and a chest film. The fluid must be examined for cell count, glucose, and protein, and a smear stained for bacteria (and acid-fast organisms when appropriate) and cultured for pyogenic organisms and for mycobacteria and fungi when indicated. Latex agglutination tests can detect antigens of encapsulated organisms (*S pneumoniae, H influenzae, N meningitidis*, and *Cryptococcus neoformans*) but are rarely used except for detection of *Cryptococcus* or in partially treated patients. Polymerase chain reaction (PCR) testing of cerebrospinal fluid has been used to detect bacteria (*S pneumoniae, H influenzae, N meningitidis, M tuberculosis, B burgdorferi*, and *Tropheryma whippelii*) and viruses (herpes simplex, varicella-zoster, CMV, Epstein-Barr virus, and enteroviruses) in patients with meningitis. The greatest experience is with PCR for herpes simplex and varicella-zoster, and the tests are very sensitive (> 95%) and specific. Tests to detect the other organisms may not be any more sensitive than culture, but the real value is the rapidity with which results are available, ie, hours compared with days or weeks. In patients at risk for infection possibly following a contaminated corticosteroid injection, a negative fungal culture or negative PCR test from a diagnostic specimen obtained from the central nervous system or a parameningeal site does not rule out infection. Active fungal infection may be present even when these tests are negative. Consultation with an infectious disease expert is recommended.

C. Lumbar Puncture and Imaging

Since performing a lumbar puncture in the presence of a space-occupying lesion (brain abscess, subdural hematoma, subdural empyema, necrotic temporal lobe from herpes encephalitis) may result in brainstem herniation, a CT scan is performed prior to lumbar puncture if a space-occupying lesion is suspected on the basis of papilledema, seizures, or focal neurologic findings. Other indications for CT scan are an immunocompromised patient or moderate to severely impaired level of consciousness. If delays are encountered in obtaining a CT scan and bacterial meningitis is suspected, blood cultures should be drawn and antibiotics and corticosteroids administered even before cerebrospinal fluid is obtained for culture to avoid delay in treatment (Table 30–1). Antibiotics given within 4 hours before obtaining cerebrospinal fluid probably do not affect culture results. MRI with contrast of the epidural injection site and surrounding areas is recommended (sometimes repeatedly) for those with symptoms following a possibly contaminated corticosteroid injection to exclude epidural abscess, phlegmon, vertebral osteomyelitis, discitis, or arachnoiditis.

▶ Treatment

Although it is difficult to prove with existing clinical data that early antibiotic therapy improves outcome in bacterial meningitis, prompt therapy is still recommended. In purulent meningitis, the identity of the causative micro-organism may remain unknown or doubtful for a few days and initial antibiotic treatment as set forth in Table 30–2 should be directed against the microorganisms most common for each age group.

The duration of therapy for bacterial meningitis varies depending on the etiologic agent: *H influenzae*, 7 days; *N meningitidis*, 3–7 days; *S pneumoniae*, 10–14 days; *L monocytogenes*, 14–21 days; and gram-negative bacilli, 21 days.

Dexamethasone therapy is recommended for adults with pneumococcal meningitis. Ten milligrams of dexamethasone administered intravenously 15–20 minutes before or simultaneously with the first dose of antibiotics and continued every 6 hours for 4 days decreases morbidity and mortality. Patients most likely to benefit from corticosteroids are those infected with gram-positive organisms (*Streptococcus pneumoniae* or *S suis*), and those who are HIV negative. It is unknown whether patients with meningitis due to *N meningitidis* and other bacterial pathogens benefit from the use of adjunctive corticosteroids. Increased intracranial pressure due to brain edema often requires therapeutic attention. Hyperventilation, mannitol (25–50 g intravenously as a bolus), and even drainage of cerebrospinal fluid by repeated lumbar punctures or by placement of intraventricular catheters have been used to control cerebral edema and increased intracranial pressure. Dexamethasone (4 mg intravenously every 4–6 hours) may also decrease cerebral edema.

Therapy of brain abscess consists of drainage (excision or aspiration) in addition to 3–4 weeks of systemic antibiotics directed against organisms isolated. An empiric regimen often includes metronidazole, 500 mg intravenously or orally every 8 hours, plus ceftriaxone, 2 g intravenously every 12 hours, with or without vancomycin, 10–15 mg/kg/dose intravenously every 12 hours. In cases where abscesses are < 2 cm in size, where there are multiple abscesses that cannot be drained, or if an abscess is located in an area where significant neurologic sequelae would result from drainage, antibiotics for 6–8 weeks can be used without drainage.

In addition to antibiotics, in cases of health care–associated meningitis associated with an external intraventricular catheter, the probability of cure is increased if the catheter is removed. In infections associated with internal ventricular catheters, removal of the internal components and insertion of an external drain is recommended. After collecting cerebrospinal fluid, epidural aspirate, or other specimens for culture, empiric antifungal therapy with voriconazole as well as routine empiric treatment for other pathogens (as above) is recommended until the specific cause of the patient's central nervous system or parameningeal infection has been identified. In addition, early consultation with a neurosurgeon is recommended for those found to have an epidural abscess, phlegmon, vertebral osteomyelitis, discitis, or arachnoiditis to discuss possible surgical management (eg, debridement).

Therapy of other types of meningitis is discussed elsewhere in this book (fungal meningitis, Chapter 36; syphilis and Lyme borreliosis, Chapter 34; tuberculous meningitis, Chapter 33; herpes encephalitis, Chapter 32).

▶ When to Refer

- Patients with acute meningitis, particularly if culture negative or atypical (eg, fungi, syphilis, Lyme disease, *M tuberculosis*), or if the patient is immunosuppressed.
- Patients with chronic meningitis.
- All patients with brain abscesses and encephalitis.
- Patients with suspected hospital-acquired meningitis (eg, in patients who have undergone recent neurosurgery or epidural or paraspinal corticosteroid injection).
- Patients with recurrent meningitis.

▶ When to Admit

- Patients with suspected acute meningitis, encephalitis, and brain or paraspinous abscess should be admitted for urgent evaluation and treatment.
- There is less urgency to admit patients with chronic meningitis; these patients may be admitted to expedite diagnostic procedures and coordinate care, particularly if no diagnosis has been made in the outpatient setting.

Centers for Disease Control and Prevention (CDC). West Nile virus and other arboviral diseases—United States, 2012. MMWR Morb Mortal Wkly Rep. 2013 Jun 28;62(25):513–7. [PMID: 23803959]

Chiller TM et al; Multistate Fungal Infection Clinical Investigation Team. Clinical findings for fungal infections caused by methylprednisolone injections. N Engl J Med. 2013 Oct 24; 369(17):1610–9. [PMID: 24152260]

Day JN et al. Combination antifungal therapy for cryptococcal meningitis. N Engl J Med. 2013 Apr 4;368(14):1291–302. [PMID: 23550668]

Granerod J et al; UK Health Protection Agency (HPA) Aetiology of Encephalitis Study Group. Causes of encephalitis and differences in their clinical presentations in England: a multicentre, population-based prospective study. Lancet Infect Dis. 2010 Dec;10(12):835–44. [PMID: 20952256]

Khasawneh FA et al. Lumbar puncture for suspected meningitis after intensive care unit admission is likely to change management. Hosp Pract (1995). 2011 Feb;39(1):141–5. [PMID: 21441769]

Smith RM et al; the Multistate Fungal Infection Outbreak Response Team. Fungal infections associated with contaminated methylprednisolone injections. N Engl J Med. 2013 Oct 24;369(17):1598–609. [PMID: 23252499]

Thakur KT et al. Predictors of outcome in acute encephalitis. Neurology. 2013 Aug 27;81(9):793–800. [PMID: 23892708]

Thigpen MC et al; Emerging Infections Programs Network. Bacterial meningitis in the United States, 1998–2007. N Engl J Med. 2011 May 26;364(21):2016–25. [PMID: 21612470]

van de Beek D et al. Nosocomial bacterial meningitis. N Engl J Med. 2010 Jan 14;362(2):146–54. [PMID: 20071704]

ANIMAL & HUMAN BITE WOUNDS

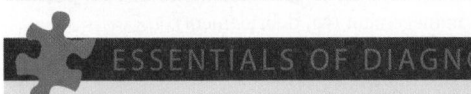

ESSENTIALS OF DIAGNOSIS

- ▶ Cat and human bites have higher rates of infection than dog bites.

- ▶ Hand bites are particularly concerning for the possibility of closed-space infection.

- ▶ Antibiotic prophylaxis indicated for noninfected bites of the hand and hospitalization required for infected hand bites.

- ▶ All infected wounds need to be cultured to direct therapy.

▶ General Considerations

About 1000 dog bite injuries require emergency department attention each day in the United States, most often in urban areas. Dog bites occur most commonly in the summer months. Biting animals are usually known by their victims, and most biting incidents are provoked (ie, bites occur while playing with the animal or after surprising the animal while eating or waking it abruptly from sleep). Failure to elicit a history of provocation is important, because an unprovoked attack raises the possibility of rabies. Human bites are usually inflicted by children while playing or fighting; in adults, bites are associated with alcohol use and closed-fist injuries that occur during fights.

The animal inflicting the bite, the location of the bite, and the type of injury inflicted are all important determinants of whether they become infected. Cat bites are more likely to become infected than human bites—between 30% and 50% of all cat bites become infected. Infections following human bites are variable. Bites inflicted by children rarely become infected because they are superficial, and bites by adults become infected in 15–30% of cases, with a particularly high rate of infection in closed-fist injuries. Dog bites, for unclear reasons, become infected only 5% of the time. Bites of the head, face, and neck are less likely to become infected than bites on the extremities. "Through and through" bites (eg involving the mucosa and the skin) have an infection rate similar to closed-fist injuries. Puncture wounds become infected more frequently than lacerations, probably because the latter are easier to irrigate and debride.

The bacteriology of bite infections is polymicrobial. Following dog and cat bites, over 50% of infections are caused by aerobes and anaerobes and 36% are due to aerobes alone. Pure anaerobic infections are rare. *Pasteurella* species are the single most common isolate (75% of infections caused by cat bites and 50% of infections caused by dog bites). Other common aerobic isolates include streptococci, staphylococci, *Moraxella,* and *Neisseria;* the most common anaerobes are *Fusobacterium, Bacteroides, Porphyromonas,* and *Prevotella.* The median number of isolates following human bites is four (three aerobes and one anaerobe). Like dog and cat bites, infections caused by most human bites are a mixture of aerobes and anaerobes (54%) or are due to aerobes alone (44%). Streptococci and *S aureus* are the most common aerobes. *Eikenella corrodens* (found in up to 30% of patients), *Prevotella* and *Fusobacterium* are the most common anaerobes. Although the organisms noted are the most common, innumerable others have been isolated—including *Capnocytophaga* (dog and cats), *Pseudomonas,* and *Haemophilus*—emphasizing the point that all infected bites should be cultured to define the microbiology.

HIV can be transmitted from bites (either from biting or receiving a bite from an HIV-infected patient) but has rarely been reported.

▶ Treatment

A. Local Care

Vigorous cleansing and irrigation of the wound as well as debridement of necrotic material are the most important factors in decreasing the incidence of infections. Radiographs should be obtained to look for fractures and the presence of foreign bodies. Careful examination to assess the extent of the injury (tendon laceration, joint space penetration) is critical to appropriate care.

B. Suturing

If wounds require closure for cosmetic or mechanical reasons, suturing can be done. However, one should never suture an infected wound, and wounds of the hand should generally not be sutured since a closed-space infection of the hand can result in loss of function.

C. Prophylactic Antibiotics

Prophylaxis is indicated in high-risk bites and in high-risk patients. Cat bites in any location and hand bites by any animal, including humans, should receive prophylaxis. Individuals with certain comorbidities (diabetes, liver disease) are at increased risk for severe complications and should receive prophylaxis even for low-risk bites, as should patients without functional spleens who are at increased risk for overwhelming sepsis (primarily with *Capnocytophaga* species). Amoxicillin-clavulanate (Augmentin) 500 mg orally three times daily for 5–7 days is the regimen of choice. For patients with serious allergy to penicillin, a combination of clindamycin 300 mg orally three times daily together with one of the following is recommended for 5–7 days: doxycycline 100 mg orally twice daily, or double-strength TMP-SMZ orally twice daily, or a fluoroquinolone (ciprofloxacin 500 mg orally twice daily or levofloxacin 500–750 mg orally once daily). Moxifloxacin, a fluoroquinolone with good aerobic and anaerobic activity, may be suitable as monotherapy at 400 mg orally once daily for 5–7 days. Agents such as dicloxacillin, cephalexin, erythromycin, and clindamycin should not be used alone because they lack activity against *Pasteurella* species. Doxycycline and TMP-SMZ have poor activity against anaerobes and should only be used in combination with clindamycin.

Because the risk of HIV transmission is so low following a bite, routine postexposure prophylaxis is not recommended. Each case should be evaluated individually and consideration for prophylaxis should be given to those who present within 72 hours of the incident, the source is known to be HIV infected, and the exposure is high risk.

D. Antibiotics for Documented Infection

For wounds that are infected, antibiotics are clearly indicated. How they are given (orally or intravenously) and the need for hospitalization are individualized clinical decisions. The most commonly encountered pathogens require treatment with either a combination of a beta-lactam plus a beta-lactamase inhibitor (ampicillin-sulbactam [Unasyn], 1.5–3.0 g intravenously every 6–8 hours; or piperacillin-tazobactam [Zosyn], 3.375 g intravenously every 6–8 hours; or amoxicillin-clavulanate [Augmentin], 500 mg orally three times daily); or with a carbapenem (ertapenem, 1 g intravenously daily; imipenem, 500 mg intravenously every 6–8 hours; or meropenem, 1 g intravenously every 8 hours). For the patient with severe penicillin allergy, a combination of clindamycin 600–900 mg intravenously every 8 hours plus a fluoroquinolone (ciprofloxacin, 400 mg intravenously every 12 hours; levofloxacin, 500–750 mg intravenously once daily) or TMP-SMZ (10 mg/kg of trimethoprim daily in two or three divided doses) is indicated. Duration of therapy is usually 2–3 weeks unless complications such as septic arthritis or osteomyelitis are present; if these complications are present, therapy should be extended to 4 and 6 weeks, respectively.

E. Tetanus and Rabies

All patients must be evaluated for the need for tetanus (see Chapter 33) and rabies (see Chapter 32) prophylaxis.

▶ When to Refer

- If septic arthritis or osteomyelitis is suspected.
- For exposure to bites by dogs, cats, reptiles, amphibians, and rodents.
- When rabies is a possibility.

▶ When to Admit

- Patients with infected hand bites.
- Deep bites, particularly if over joints.

Abrahamian FM et al. Microbiology of animal bite wound infections. Clin Microbiol Rev. 2011 Apr;24(2):231–46. [PMID: 21482724]

Bjork A et al. Dog bite injuries among American Indian and Alaska Native children. J Pediatr. 2013 Jun;162(6):1270–5. [PMID: 23332462]

Dimaano EM et al. Clinical and epidemiological features of human rabies cases in the Philippines: a review from 1987 to 2006. Int J Infect Dis. 2011 Jul;15(7):e495–9. [PMID: 21600825]

Thomas N et al. Animal bite-associated infections: microbiology and treatment. Expert Rev Anti Infect Ther. 2011 Feb; 9(2): 215–26. [PMID: 21342069]

SEXUALLY TRANSMITTED DISEASES

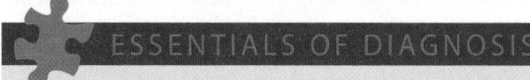

ESSENTIALS OF DIAGNOSIS

- ▶ All sexually transmitted diseases (STDs) have sub-clinical or latent periods, and patients may be asymptomatic.

- ▶ Simultaneous infection with several organisms is common.

- ▶ All patients who seek STD testing should be screened for syphilis and HIV.

- ▶ Partner notification and treatment are important to prevent further transmission and reinfection in the index case.

▶ General Considerations

The most common STDs are gonorrhea,* syphilis,* human papillomavirus (HPV)-associated condyloma acuminatum, chlamydial genital infections,* herpesvirus genital infections, trichomonas vaginitis, chancroid,* granuloma inguinale, scabies, louse infestation, and bacterial vaginosis (among women who have sex with women). However, shigellosis*; hepatitis A, B, and C*; amebiasis; giardiasis*; cryptosporidiosis*; salmonellosis*; and campylobacteriosis may also be transmitted by sexual (oral-anal) contact, especially in men who have sex with men. Both homosexual and heterosexual contact are risk factors for the transmission of HIV (see Chapter 31). All STDs have subclinical or

---

*Reportable to public health authorities.

latent phases that play an important role in long-term persistence of the infection or in its transmission from infected (but largely asymptomatic) persons to other contacts. Simultaneous infection by several different agents is common.

Infections typically present in one of several ways, each of which has a defined differential diagnosis, which should prompt appropriate diagnostic tests.

A. Genital Ulcers

Common etiologies include herpes simplex virus, primary syphilis, and chancroid. Other possibilities include lymphogranuloma venereum (see Chapter 33), granuloma inguinale caused by *Klebsiella granulomatis* (see Chapter 33), as well as lesions caused by infection with Epstein-Barr virus and HIV. Noninfectious causes are Behçet disease (see Chapter 20), neoplasm, trauma, drugs, and irritants.

B. Urethritis with or without Urethral Discharge

The most common infections causing urethral discharge are *Neisseria gonorrhoeae* and *Chlamydia trachomatis*. *N gonorrhoeae* and *C trachomatis* are also frequent causes of prostatitis among sexually active men. Other sexually transmitted infections that can cause urethritis include *Mycoplasma genitalium*, *Ureaplasma urealyticum*, and *Trichomonas vaginalis*. Noninfectious causes of urethritis includes reactive arthritis with associated urethritis (Reiter syndrome).

C. Vaginal Discharge

Common causes of vaginitis are bacterial vaginosis (caused by overgrowth of anaerobes such as *Gardnerella vaginalis*), candidiasis, and *T vaginalis* (see Chapter 18). Less common infectious causes of vaginitis include HPV-associated condyloma acuminata and group A streptococcus. Noninfectious causes are physiologic changes related to the menstrual cycle, irritants, and lichen planus. Even though *N gonorrhoeae* and *C trachomatis* are frequent causes of cervicitis, they rarely produce vaginal discharge.

▶ Screening & Prevention

All persons who seek STD testing should undergo routine screening for HIV infection, using rapid HIV-testing (if patients may not follow up for results obtained by standard methods) or nucleic acid amplification followed by confirmatory serology (if primary HIV infection may be a possibility) as indicated. Patients in whom STDs have been diagnosed and treated (in particular, chlamydia or gonorrhea) are at a high risk for reinfection and should be encouraged to be rescreened for STDs at 3 months following the initial STD diagnosis.

Asymptomatic patients often request STD screening at the time of initiating a new sexual relationship. Routine HIV testing and hepatitis B serology testing should be offered to all such patients. In sexually active women who have not been recently screened, cervical Papanicolaou testing and nucleic acid amplification testing of a urine specimen for gonorrhea and chlamydia are recommended.

Among men who have sex with men, additional screening is recommended for syphilis; hepatitis A; urethral, pharyngeal, and rectal gonorrhea; as well as urethral and rectal chlamydia. Nucleic acid amplification testing is FDA-approved for testing urine for gonorrhea or chlamydia. However, the use of nucleic acid amplification testing of secretions in the rectum and pharynx has not been validated in many laboratories. There are no recommendations to screen heterosexual men for urethral chlamydia but this could be considered in STD clinics, adolescent clinics, or in correctional facilities. The periodicity of screening thereafter depends on sexual risk, but most screening should be offered at least annually to sexually active adults (particularly to those 25-years-old and under). If not immune, hepatitis B vaccination is recommended for all sexually active adults, and hepatitis A vaccination in men who have sex with men. Persons between the ages of 9 and 26 may be offered vaccination against HPV.

The risk of developing an STD following a **sexual assault** is difficult to accurately ascertain given high rates of baseline infections and poor follow-up. Victims of assault have a high baseline rate of infection (*N gonorrhoeae*, 6%; *C trachomatis*, 10%; *T vaginalis*, 15%; and bacterial vaginosis, 34%), and the risk of acquiring infection as a result of the assault is significant but is often lower than the preexisting rate (*N gonorrhoeae*, 6–12%; *C trachomatis*, 4–17%; *T vaginalis*, 12%; syphilis, 0.5–3%; and bacterial vaginosis, 19%). Victims should be evaluated within 24 hours after the assault, and nucleic acid amplification tests for *N gonorrhoeae* and *C trachomatis* should be performed. Vaginal secretions are obtained for *Trichomonas* wet mount and culture, or point-of-care testing. If a discharge is present, if there is itching, or if secretions are malodorous, a wet mount should be examined for *Candida* and bacterial vaginosis. In addition, a blood sample should be obtained for immediate serologic testing for syphilis, hepatitis B, and HIV. Follow-up examination for STD should be repeated within 1–2 weeks, since concentrations of infecting organisms may not have been sufficient to produce a positive test at the time of initial examination. If prophylactic treatment was given (may include postexposure hepatitis B vaccination without hepatitis B immune globulin; treatment for chlamydial, gonorrheal, or trichomonal infection; and emergency contraception), tests should be repeated only if the victim has symptoms. If prophylaxis was not administered, the individual should be seen in 1 week so that any positive tests can be treated. Follow-up serologic testing for syphilis and HIV infection should be performed in 6, 12, and 24 weeks if the initial tests are negative. The usefulness of presumptive therapy is controversial, some feeling that all patients should receive it and others that it should be limited to those in whom follow-up cannot be ensured or to patients who request it.

Although seroconversion to HIV has been reported following sexual assault when this was the only known risk, this risk is believed to be low. The likelihood of HIV transmission from vaginal or anal receptive intercourse when the source is known to be HIV positive is 1 per 1000 and 5 per 1000, respectively. Although prophylactic antiretroviral therapy has not been studied in this setting, the

Department of Health and Human Services recommends the prompt institution of postexposure prophylaxis with highly active antiretroviral therapy if the person seeks care within 72 hours of the assault, the source is known to be HIV positive, and the exposure presents a substantial risk of transmission.

In addition to screening asymptomatic patients with STDs, other strategies for preventing further transmission include evaluating sex partners and administering preexposure vaccination of preventable STDs to individuals at risk; other strategies include the consistent use of male and female condoms. For each patient, there are one or more sexual contacts who require diagnosis and treatment. Prompt treatment of contacts by giving antibiotics to the index case to distribute to all sexual contacts (patient-delivered therapy) is an important strategy for preventing further transmission and to prevent reinfection in the index case.

Note that vaginal spermicides and condoms containing nonoxynol-9 provide no additional protection against STDs. Male circumcision has been demonstrated to protect against HIV and HPV acquisition in heterosexual men with HIV-infected partners. Early initiation of antiretroviral therapy in HIV-infected individuals can prevent HIV acquisition in an uninfected sex partner. Also, preexposure prophylaxis with a once-daily pill containing tenofovir plus emtricitabine has been shown to be effective in preventing HIV infection among high-risk men who have sex with men.

When to Refer

- Patients with a new diagnosis of HIV.
- Patients with persistent, refractory or recurrent STDs, particularly when drug resistance is suspected.

Allen VG et al. *Neisseria gonorrhoeae* treatment failure and susceptibility to cefixime in Toronto, Canada. JAMA. 2013 Jan 9; 309(2):163–70. [PMID: 23299608]

Baeten JM et al; Partners PrEP Study Team. Antiretroviral prophylaxis for HIV prevention in heterosexual men and women. N Engl J Med. 2012 Aug 2;367(5):399–410. [PMID: 22784037]

Gottlieb SL et al. Screening and treating *Chlamydia trachomatis* genital infection to prevent pelvic inflammatory disease: interpretation of findings from randomized controlled trials. Sex Transm Dis. 2013 Feb;40(2):97–102. [PMID: 23324973]

Juusola JL et al. The cost-effectiveness of preexposure prophylaxis for HIV prevention in the United States in men who have sex with men. Ann Intern Med. 2012 Apr 17;156(8):541–50. [PMID: 22508731]

Markowitz LE et al. Reduction in human papillomavirus (HPV) prevalence among young women following HPV vaccine introduction in the United States, National Health and Nutrition Examination Surveys, 2003–2010. J Infect Dis. 2013 Aug 1;208(3):385–93. [PMID: 23785124]

Mayer KH et al. Raltegravir, tenofovir DF, and emtricitabine for postexposure prophylaxis to prevent the sexual transmission of HIV: safety, tolerability, and adherence. J Acquir Immune Defic Syndr. 2012 Apr 1;59(4):354–9. [PMID: 22267017]

Mishori R et al. *Chlamydia trachomatis* infections: screening, diagnosis, and management. Am Fam Physician. 2012 Dec 15; 86(12):1127–32. [PMID: 23316985]

Moyer VA. Screening for HIV: U.S. Preventive Services Task Force Recommendation Statement. Ann Intern Med. 2013 Jul 2;159(1):51–60. [PMID: 23698354]

Wandeler G et al. Hepatitis C virus infections in the Swiss HIV Cohort Study: a rapidly evolving epidemic. Clin Infect Dis. 2012 Nov 15;55(10):1408–16. [PMID: 22893583]

Workowski KA et al; Centers for Disease Control and Prevention (CDC). Sexually transmitted diseases treatment guidelines, 2010. MMWR Recomm Rep. 2010 Dec 17;59(RR-12):1–110. Erratum in: MMWR Recomm Rep. 2011 Jan 14;60(1):18. [PMID: 21160459]

INFECTIONS IN DRUG USERS

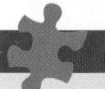

ESSENTIALS OF DIAGNOSIS

▶ Common infections that occur with greater frequency in drug users include:

- Skin infections, aspiration pneumonia, tuberculosis.
- Hepatitis A, B, C, D; STDs; AIDS.
- Pulmonary septic emboli, infective endocarditis.
- Osteomyelitis and septic arthritis.

▶ General Considerations

There is a high incidence of infection among drug users, particularly those who inject drugs. Increased risk of infection is likely associated with poor hygiene and colonization with potentially pathogenic organisms, contamination of drugs and equipment, increased sexual risk behaviors, and impaired immune defenses. The use of parenterally administered recreational drugs has increased enormously in recent years. There are now an estimated 300,000 or more injection drug users in the United States.

Skin infections are associated with poor hygiene and use of nonsterile technique when injecting drugs. *S aureus* (including community-acquired methicillin-resistant strains) and oral flora (streptococci, *Eikenella, Fusobacterium, Peptostreptococcus*) are the most common organisms, with enteric gram-negatives generally more likely seen in those who inject into the groin. Cellulitis and subcutaneous abscesses occur most commonly, particularly in association with subcutaneous ("skin-popping") or intramuscular injections and the use of cocaine and heroin mixtures (probably due to ischemia). Myositis, clostridial myonecrosis, and necrotizing fasciitis occur infrequently but are life-threatening. Wound botulism in association with black tar heroin occurs sporadically but often in clusters.

Aspiration pneumonia and its complications (lung abscess, empyema, brain abscess) result from altered consciousness associated with drug use. Mixed aerobic and anaerobic mouth flora are usually involved.

Tuberculosis also occurs in drug users, and infection with HIV has fostered the spread of tuberculosis in this population. Morbidity and mortality rates are increased in HIV-infected individuals with tuberculosis. Classic radiographic findings are often absent; tuberculosis is suspected in any patient with infiltrates who does not respond to antibiotics.

Hepatitis is very common among habitual drug users and is transmissible both by the parenteral (hepatitis B, C, and D) and by the fecal-oral route (hepatitis A). Multiple episodes of hepatitis with different agents can occur.

Pulmonary septic emboli may originate from venous thrombi or right-sided endocarditis.

STDs are not directly related to drug use, but the practice of exchanging sex for drugs has resulted in an increased frequency of STDs. Syphilis, gonorrhea, and chancroid are the most common.

AIDS has a high incidence among injection drug users and their sexual contacts and among the offspring of infected women (see Chapter 31).

Infective endocarditis in persons who use drugs intravenously is most commonly caused by *S aureus*, *Candida* (usually *C albicans* or *C parapsilosis*), *Enterococcus faecalis*, other streptococci, and gram-negative bacteria (especially *Pseudomonas* and *Serratia marcescens*). See Chapter 33.

Other vascular infections include septic thrombophlebitis and mycotic aneurysms. Mycotic aneurysms resulting from direct trauma to a vessel with secondary infection most commonly occur in femoral arteries and less commonly in arteries of the neck. Aneurysms resulting from hematogenous spread of organisms frequently involve intracerebral vessels and thus are seen in association with endocarditis.

Osteomyelitis and septic arthritis involving vertebral bodies, sternoclavicular joints, the pubic symphysis, the sacroiliac joints, and other sites usually results from hematogenous distribution of injected organisms or septic venous thrombi. Pain and fever precede radiographic changes, sometimes by several weeks. While staphylococci—often methicillin-resistant—are common organisms, *Serratia*, *Pseudomonas*, *Candida* (often not *C albicans*), and other pathogens rarely encountered in spontaneous bone or joint disease are found in injection drug users.

▶ Treatment

A common and difficult clinical problem is management of the parenteral drug user who presents with fever. In general, after obtaining appropriate cultures (blood, urine, and sputum if the chest radiograph is abnormal), empiric therapy is begun. If the chest radiograph is suggestive of a community-acquired pneumonia (consolidation), therapy for outpatient pneumonia is begun with a third-generation cephalosporin, such as ceftriaxone, 1 g intravenously every 24 hours, plus azithromycin, 500 mg orally or intravenously every 24 hours, or doxycycline, 100 mg orally or intravenously twice daily. If the chest radiograph is suggestive of septic emboli (nodular infiltrates), therapy for presumed endocarditis is initiated, usually with vancomycin 15 mg/kg/dose every 12 hours intravenously (due to the high prevalence of MRSA and the possibility of enterococcus). If the chest radiograph is normal and no focal site of infection can be found, endocarditis is presumed. While awaiting the results of blood cultures, empiric treatment with vancomycin is started. If blood cultures are positive for organisms that frequently cause endocarditis in drug users

(see above), endocarditis is presumed to be present and treated accordingly. If blood cultures are positive for an organism that is an unusual cause of endocarditis, evaluation for an occult source of infection should go forward. In this setting, a transesophageal echocardiogram may be quite helpful since it is 90% sensitive in detecting vegetations and a negative study is strong evidence against endocarditis. If blood cultures are negative and the patient responds to antibiotics, therapy should be continued for 7–14 days (oral therapy can be given once an initial response has occurred). In every patient, careful examination for an occult source of infection (eg, genitourinary, dental, sinus, gallbladder) should be done.

▶ When to Refer

- Any patient with suspected or proven infective endocarditis.
- Patients with persistent bacteremia.

▶ When to Admit

- Injection drug users with fever.
- Patients with abscesses or progressive skin and soft tissue infection that require debridement.

Choopanya K et al. Antiretroviral prophylaxis for HIV infection in injecting drug users in Bangkok, Thailand (the Bangkok Tenofovir Study): a randomised, double-blind, placebo-controlled phase 3 trial. Lancet. 2013 Jun 15;381(9883):2083–90. [PMID: 23769234]

Deiss RG et al. Tuberculosis and illicit drug use: review and update. Clin Infect Dis. 2009 Jan 1;48(1):72–82. [PMID: 19046064]

Des Jarlais DC et al. Associations between herpes simplex virus type 2 and HCV with HIV among injecting drug users in New York City: the current importance of sexual transmission of HIV. Am J Public Health. 2011 Jul;101(7):1277–83. [PMID: 21566021]

North CS et al. Hepatitis C and substance use: new treatments and novel approaches. Curr Opin Psychiatry. 2012 May;25(3):206–12. [PMID: 22395769]

Que YA et al. Infective endocarditis. Nat Rev Cardiol. 2011 Jun;8(6):322–36. [PMID: 21487430]

Rabkin DG et al. Long-term outcome for the surgical treatment of infective endocarditis with a focus on intravenous drug users. Ann Thorac Surg. 2012 Jan;93(1):51–7. [PMID: 22054655]

ACUTE INFECTIOUS DIARRHEA

ESSENTIALS OF DIAGNOSIS

- ▶ **Acute diarrhea:** lasts < 2 weeks
- ▶ **Chronic diarrhea:** lasts > 2 weeks.
- ▶ **Mild diarrhea:** ≤ 3 stools per day.
- ▶ **Moderate diarrhea:** ≥ 4 stools per day with local symptoms (abdominal cramps, nausea, tenesmus).
- ▶ **Severe diarrhea:** ≥ 4 stools per day with systemic symptoms (fever, chills, dehydration).

General Considerations

Acute diarrhea can be caused by a number of different factors, including emotional stress, food intolerance, inorganic agents (eg, sodium nitrite), organic substances (eg, mushrooms, shellfish), drugs, and infectious agents (including viruses, bacteria, and protozoa) (Table 30–3). From a diagnostic and therapeutic standpoint, it is helpful to classify infectious diarrhea into syndromes that produce inflammatory or bloody diarrhea and those that are noninflammatory, nonbloody, or watery. In general, the term "inflammatory diarrhea" suggests colonic involvement by invasive bacteria or parasites or by toxin production. Patients complain of frequent bloody, small-volume stools, often associated with fever, abdominal cramps, tenesmus, and fecal urgency. Common causes of this syndrome include *Shigella, Salmonella, Campylobacter, Yersinia*, invasive strains of *Escherichia coli*, *E coli* O157:H7 and other Shiga-toxin–producing strains of *E coli* (STEC), *Entamoeba histolytica*, and *C difficile*. Tests for fecal leukocytes or the neutrophil marker lactoferrin are frequently positive, and definitive etiologic diagnosis requires stool culture. Noninflammatory diarrhea is generally milder and is caused by viruses or toxins that affect the small intestine and interfere with salt and water balance, resulting in large-volume watery diarrhea, often with nausea, vomiting, and cramps. Common causes of this syndrome include viruses (eg, rotavirus, norovirus, astrovirus, enteric adenoviruses), vibriones *(Vibrio cholerae, Vibrio parahaemolyticus)*, enterotoxin-producing *E coli*, *Giardia lamblia*, cryptosporidia, and agents that can cause foodborne gastroenteritis. In developed countries, viruses (particularly norovirus) are an important cause of hospitalizations due to acute gastroenteritis among adults.

The term "food poisoning" denotes diseases caused by toxins present in consumed foods. When the incubation period is short (1–6 hours after consumption), the toxin is usually preformed. Vomiting is usually a major complaint, and fever is usually absent. Examples include intoxication from *S aureus* or *Bacillus cereus*, and toxin can be detected in the food. When the incubation period is longer—between 8 hours and 16 hours—the organism is present in the food and produces toxin after being ingested. Vomiting is less prominent, abdominal cramping is frequent, and fever is often absent. The best example of this disease is that due to *Clostridium perfringens*. Toxin can be detected in food or stool specimens.

The inflammatory and noninflammatory diarrheas discussed above can also be transmitted by food and water and usually have incubation periods between 12 and 72 hours. *Cyclospora*, cryptosporidia, and *Isospora* are protozoans capable of causing disease in both immunocompetent and immunocompromised patients. Characteristics of disease include profuse watery diarrhea that is prolonged but usually self-limited (1–2 weeks) in the immunocompetent patient but can be chronic in the compromised host. Epidemiologic features may be helpful in determining etiology. Recent hospitalization or antibiotic use suggests *C difficile*; recent foreign travel suggests *Salmonella, Shigella, Campylobacter, E coli*, or *V cholerae*; undercooked hamburger suggests *E coli*, especially O157:H7 or other STEC; outbreak in long-term care facility, school, or cruise ship suggests norovirus (including newly identified strains, eg, GII.4 Sydney); and fried rice consumption is associated with *B cereus* toxin. Prominent features of some of these causes of diarrhea are listed in Table 30–3.

Treatment

A. General Measures

In general, most cases of acute gastroenteritis are self-limited and do not require therapy other than supportive measures. Treatment usually consists of replacement of fluids and electrolytes and, very rarely, management of hypovolemic shock and respiratory compromise. In mild diarrhea, increasing ingestion of juices and clear soups is adequate. In more severe cases of dehydration (postural lightheadedness, decreased urination), oral glucose-based rehydration solutions can be used (Ceralyte, Pedialyte).

B. Specific Measures

When symptoms persist beyond 3–4 days, initial presentation is accompanied by fever or bloody diarrhea, or if the patient is immunocompromised, cultures of stool are usually obtained. Symptoms have often resolved by the time cultures are completed. In this case, even if a pathogen is isolated, therapy is not needed (except for *Shigella*, since the infecting dose is so small that therapy to eradicate organisms from the stool is indicated for epidemiologic reasons). If symptoms persist and a pathogen is isolated, it is reasonable to institute specific treatment even though therapy has not been conclusively shown to alter the natural history of disease for most pathogens. Exceptions include infection with *Shigella* where antibiotic therapy has been shown to shorten the duration of symptoms by 2–3 days, and *Campylobacter* infections (early therapy, within 4 days of onset of symptoms, shortens the course of disease). Conversely, antibiotic therapy for infections with *E coli* O157:H7 does not ameliorate symptoms and may increase the risk of developing hemolytic-uremic syndrome. Uncomplicated gastroenteritis due to *Salmonella* does not require therapy because the disease is usually self-limited and therapy may prolong carriage and perhaps increase relapses. Because bacteremia with complications can occur in high-risk patients, some experts have recommended therapy for *Salmonella* in patients over the age of 50, in organ transplant recipients, in those with HIV, in patients taking corticosteroids, in those with lymphoproliferative diseases, and in those with vascular grafts. Ciprofloxacin, 500 mg orally every 12 hours for 5 days, is effective in shortening the course of illness compared with placebo in patients presenting with diarrhea, whether a pathogen is isolated or not. However, because of concerns about selecting for resistant organisms (especially *Campylobacter*, where increasing resistance to fluoroquinolones has been documented and erythromycin is the drug of choice) coupled with the fact that most infectious diarrhea is self-limited, routine use of antibiotics for all patients with diarrhea is not recommended. Antibiotics should be considered in patients with evidence of invasive disease (white cells in

Table 30–3. Acute bacterial diarrheas and "food poisoning."

Organism	Incubation Period	Vomiting	Diarrhea	Fever	Associated Foods	Diagnosis	Clinical Features and Treatment
Staphylococcus (preformed toxin)	1–8 hours	+++	±	±	Staphylococci grow in meats, dairy, and bakery products and produce enterotoxin.	Clinical. Food and stool can be tested for toxin.	Abrupt onset, intense nausea and vomiting for up to 24 hours, recovery in 24–48 hours. Supportive care.
Bacillus cereus (preformed toxin)	1–8 hours	+++	±	–	Reheated fried rice causes vomiting or diarrhea.	Clinical. Food and stool can be tested for toxin.	Acute onset, severe nausea and vomiting lasting 24 hours. Supportive care.
B cereus (diarrheal toxin)	10–16 hours	±	+++	–	Toxin in meats, stews, and gravy.	Clinical. Food and stool can be tested for toxin.	Abdominal cramps, watery diarrhea, and nausea lasting 24–48 hours. Supportive care.
Clostridium perfringens	8–16 hours	±	+++	–	Clostridia grow in rewarmed meat and poultry dishes and produce an enterotoxin.	Stools can be tested for enterotoxin or cultured.	Abrupt onset of profuse diarrhea, abdominal cramps, nausea; vomiting occasionally. Recovery usual without treatment in 24–48 hours. Supportive care; antibiotics not needed.
Clostridium botulinum	12–72 hours	±	–	–	Clostridia grow in anaerobic acidic environment eg, canned foods, fermented fish, foods held warm for extended periods.	Stool, serum, and food can be tested for toxin. Stool and food can be cultured.	Diplopia, dysphagia, dysphonia, respiratory embarrassment. Treatment requires clear airway, ventilation, and intravenous polyvalent antitoxin (see text). Symptoms can last for days to months.
Clostridium difficile	Usually occurs after 7–10 days of antibiotics. Can occur after a single dose or several weeks after completion of antibiotics.	–	+++	++	Associated with antimicrobial drugs; clindamycin and beta-lactams most commonly implicated. Fluoroquinolones associated with hypervirulent strains.	Stool tested for toxin.	Abrupt onset of diarrhea that may be bloody; fever. Oral metronidazole for mild to moderate cases. Oral vancomycin for more severe disease.
Enterohemorrhagic *Escherichia coli*, including *E coli* O157:H7 and other Shiga-toxin producing strains (STEC)	1–8 days	+	+++	–	Undercooked beef, especially hamburger; unpasteurized milk and juice; raw fruits and vegetables.	*E coli* O157:H7 can be cultured on special medium. Other toxins can be detected in stool.	Usually abrupt onset of diarrhea, often bloody; abdominal pain. In adults, it is usually self-limited to 5–10 days. In children, it is associated with hemolytic-uremic syndrome (HUS). Antibiotic therapy may increase risk of HUS. Plasma exchange may help patients with STEC-associated HUS.
Enterotoxigenic *E coli* (ETEC)	1–3 days	±	+++	±	Water, food contaminated with feces.	Stool culture. Special tests required to identify toxin-producing strains.	Watery diarrhea and abdominal cramps, usually lasting 3–7 days. In travelers, fluoroquinolones shorten disease.

Organism	Incubation period				Common food source	Diagnosis	Clinical features / treatment
Vibrio parahaemolyticus	2–48 hours	+	+	±	Undercooked or raw seafood.	Stool culture on special medium.	Abrupt onset of watery diarrhea, abdominal cramps, nausea and vomiting. Recovery is usually complete in 2–5 days.
Vibrio cholerae	24–72 hours	+	+++	–	Contaminated water, fish, shellfish, street vendor food.	Stool culture on special medium.	Abrupt onset of liquid diarrhea in endemic area. Needs prompt intravenous or oral replacement of fluids and electrolytes. Tetracyclines and azithromycin shorten excretion of vibrios.
Campylobacter jejuni	2–5 days	±	+++	+	Raw or undercooked poultry, unpasteurized milk, water.	Stool culture on special medium.	Fever, diarrhea that can be bloody, cramps. Usually self-limited in 2–10 days. Treat with azithromycin or fluoroquinolones for severe disease. May be associated with Guillain-Barré syndrome.
Shigella species (mild cases)	24–48 hours	±	+	+	Food or water contaminated with human feces. Person to person spread.	Routine stool culture.	Abrupt onset of diarrhea, often with blood and pus in stools, cramps, tenesmus, and lethargy. Stool cultures are positive. Therapy depends on sensitivity testing, but the fluoroquinolones are most effective. Do not give opioids. Often mild and self-limited.
Salmonella species	1–3 days	–	++	+	Eggs, poultry, unpasteurized milk, cheese, juices, raw fruits and vegetables.	Routine stool culture.	Gradual or abrupt onset of diarrhea and low-grade fever. No antimicrobials unless high risk (see text) or systemic dissemination is suspected, in which case give a fluoroquinolone. Prolonged carriage can occur.
Yersinia enterocolitica	24–48 hours	±	+	+	Undercooked pork, contaminated water, unpasteurized milk, tofu.	Stool culture on special medium.	Severe abdominal pain, (appendicitis-like symptoms) diarrhea, fever. Polyarthritis, erythema nodosum in children. If severe, give tetracycline or fluoroquinolone. Without treatment, self-limited in 1–3 weeks.
Rotavirus	1–3 days	++	+++	+	Fecally contaminated foods touched by infected food handlers.	Immunoassay on stool.	Acute onset, vomiting, watery diarrhea that lasts 4–8 days. Supportive care.
Noroviruses and other caliciviruses	12–48 hours	++	+++	+	Shell fish and fecally contaminated foods touched by infected food handlers.	Clinical diagnosis with negative stool cultures. PCR available on stool.	Nausea, vomiting (more common in children), diarrhea (more common in adults), fever, myalgias, abdominal cramps. Lasts 12–60 hours. Supportive care.

PCR, polymerase chain reaction.

stool, dysentery), with symptoms 3–4 days or more in duration, with multiple stools (eight to ten or more per day), and in those with impaired immune responses. Antimotility drugs are useful in mild cases. Their use should be limited to patients without fever and without dysentery (bloody stools), and they should be used in low doses because of the risk of producing toxic megacolon. Postinfectious irritable bowel syndrome can follow infection and is approached in a similar fashion as in noninfectious irritable bowel syndrome.

Therapeutic recommendations for specific agents can be found elsewhere in this book.

Buchholz U et al. German outbreak of *Escherichia coli* O104:H4 associated with sprouts. N Engl J Med. 2011 Nov 10;365(19): 1763–70. [PMID: 22029753]

Cardemil CV et al; Rotavirus Investigation Team. Two rotavirus outbreaks caused by genotype G2P[4] at large retirement communities: cohort studies. Ann Intern Med. 2012 Nov 6; 157(9): 621–31. [PMID: 23128862]

Centers for Disease Control and Prevention. Notes from the field: emergence of new norovirus strain GII.4 Sydney—United States, 2012. Morb Mortal Wkly Rep. 2013 Jan 25;62(03): 55. [PMID: 23344699]

Frank C et al; HUS Investigation Team. Epidemic profile of Shiga-toxin-producing *Escherichia coli* O104:H4 outbreak in Germany. N Engl J Med. 2011 Nov 10;365(19):1771–80. [PMID: 21696328]

Gaffga NH et al. Outbreak of salmonellosis linked to live poultry from a mail-order hatchery. N Engl J Med. 2012 May 31; 366(22): 2065–73. [PMID: 22646629]

McClarren RL et al. Acute infectious diarrhea. Prim Care. 2011 Sep;38(3):539–64. [PMID: 21872096]

Naggie S et al. A case-control study of community-associated *Clostridium difficile* infection: no role for proton pump inhibitors. Am J Med. 2011 Mar;124(3):276.e1–7. [PMID: 21396512]

Pfeiffer ML et al. The patient presenting with acute dysentery–a systematic review. J Infect. 2012 Apr;64(4):374–86. [PMID: 22266388]

Prince Christopher RH et al. Antibiotic therapy for *Shigella* dysentery. Cochrane Database Syst Rev. 2010 Jan 10;(1): CD006784. [PMID: 20091606]

Torpy JM et al. JAMA patient page. Viral gastroenteritis. JAMA. 2012 Aug 1;308(5):528. [PMID: 22851123]

Trivedi TK et al. Hospitalizations and mortality associated with norovirus outbreaks in nursing homes, 2009–2010. JAMA. 2012 Oct 24;308(16):1668–75. [PMID: 23079758]

INFECTIOUS DISEASES IN THE RETURNING TRAVELER

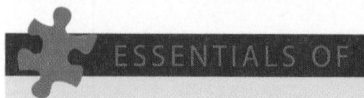

ESSENTIALS OF DIAGNOSIS

► Most infections are common and self-limited.

► Identify patients with transmissible diseases that require isolation.

► The incubation period may be helpful in diagnosis.

► Less than 3 weeks following exposure may suggest dengue, leptospirosis and yellow fever; > 3 weeks suggest typhoid fever, malaria, and tuberculosis.

► General Considerations

The differential diagnosis of fever in the returning traveler is broad, ranging from self-limited viral infections to life-threatening illness. The evaluation is best done by identifying whether a particular syndrome is present, then refining the differential diagnosis based on an exposure history. The travel history should include directed questions regarding geography (rural versus urban), animal or arthropod contact, unprotected sexual intercourse, ingestion of untreated water or raw foods, historical or pretravel immunizations, and adherence to malaria prophylaxis.

► Etiologies

The most common infectious causes of fever—excluding simple causes such as upper respiratory infections, bacterial pneumonia and urinary tract infections—in returning travelers are malaria (see Chapter 35), diarrhea (see next section), and dengue (see Chapter 32). Others include respiratory infections, including seasonal influenza, influenza A/H1N1 "swine" influenza, and influenza A/H5N1 "avian" influenza (see Chapter 32); leptospirosis (see Chapter 34); typhoid fever (see Chapter 33); and rickettsial infections (see Chapter 32). Foreign travel is increasingly recognized as a risk factor for colonization and disease with resistant pathogens, such as extended-spectrum beta-lactamases (ESBL)–producing gram-negative organisms. Systemic febrile illnesses without a diagnosis also occurs commonly, particularly in travelers returning from sub-Saharan Africa or Southeast Asia.

A. Fever and Rash

Potential etiologies include dengue, Chikungunya, viral hemorrhagic fever, leptospirosis, meningococcemia, yellow fever, typhus, *Salmonella typhi*, and acute HIV infection.

B. Pulmonary Infiltrates

Tuberculosis, ascaris, *Paragonimus,* and *Strongyloides* can all cause pulmonary infiltrates.

C. Meningoencephalitis

Etiologies include *N meningitidis,* leptospirosis, arboviruses, rabies, and (cerebral) malaria.

D. Jaundice

Consider hepatitis A, yellow fever, hemorrhagic fever, leptospirosis, and malaria.

E. Fever without Localizing Symptoms or Signs

Malaria, typhoid fever, acute HIV infection, rickettsial illness, visceral leishmaniasis, trypanosomiasis, and dengue are possible etiologies.

F. Traveler's Diarrhea

See next section.

Clinical Findings

Fever and rash in the returning traveler should prompt blood cultures and serologic tests based on the exposure history. The work-up of a **pulmonary infiltrate** should include the placement of a PPD, examination of sputum for acid-fast bacilli and possibly for ova and parasites. Patients with evidence of **meningoencephalitis** should receive lumbar puncture, blood cultures, thick/thin smears of peripheral blood, history-guided serologies, and a nape biopsy (if rabies is suspected). **Jaundice** in a returning traveler should be evaluated for hemolysis (for malaria), and the following tests should be performed: liver function tests, thick/thin smears of peripheral blood, and directed serologic testing. The work-up of **traveler's diarrhea** is presented in the following section. Finally, patients with **fever** but no localizing signs or symptoms should have blood cultures performed. Routine laboratory studies usually include complete blood count with differential, electrolytes, liver function tests, urinalysis, and blood cultures. Thick and thin peripheral blood smears should be done (and repeated in 12–24 hours if clinical suspicion remains high) for malaria if there has been travel to endemic areas. Other studies are directed by the results of history, physical examination, and initial laboratory tests. They may include stool for ova and parasites, chest radiograph, HIV test, and specific serologies (eg, dengue, leptospirosis, rickettsial disease, schistosomiasis, *Strongyloides*). Bone marrow biopsy to diagnose typhoid fever could be helpful in the appropriate patient.

When to Refer

Travelers with fever, particularly if immunocompromised.

When to Admit

Any evidence of hemorrhage, respiratory distress, hemodynamic instability, and neurologic deficits.

Farmakiotis D et al. Typhoid fever in an inner city hospital: a 5-year retrospective review. J Travel Med. 2013 Jan–Feb;20(1): 17–21. [PMID: 23279226]

Gautret P et al; GeoSentinel Surveillance Network. Travel-associated illness in older adults (>60 y). J Travel Med. 2012 May–Jun;19(3):169–77. [PMID: 22530824]

Gregory CJ et al. Clinical and laboratory features that differentiate dengue from other febrile illnesses in an endemic area—Puerto Rico, 2007–2008. Am J Trop Med Hyg. 2010 May;82(5): 922–9. [PMID: 20439977]

Hochedez P et al. Management of travelers with fever and exanthema, notably dengue and chikungunya infections. Am J Trop Med Hyg. 2008 May;78(5):710–3. [PMID: 18458301]

Jensenius M et al; GeoSentinel Surveillance Network. Acute and potentially life-threatening tropical diseases in western travelers—a GeoSentinel multicenter study, 1996–2011. Am J Trop Med Hyg. 2013 Feb;88(2):397–404. [PMID: 23324216]

Johnson BA et al. Prevention of malaria in travelers. Am Fam Physician. 2012 May 15;85(10):973–7. Erratum in: Am Fam Physician. 2012 Aug 1;86(3):222. [PMID: 22612048]

Matteelli A et al. Travel-associated sexually transmitted infections: an observational cross-sectional study of the GeoSentinel surveillance database. Lancet Infect Dis. 2013 Mar;13(3): 205–13. [PMID: 23182931]

TRAVELER'S DIARRHEA

ESSENTIALS OF DIAGNOSIS

▶ Usually a benign, self-limited disease occurring about 1 week into travel.

▶ Prophylaxis not recommended unless there is a comorbid disease (inflammatory bowel syndrome, HIV, immunosuppressive medication).

▶ Single-dose therapy of a fluoroquinolone usually effective if significant symptoms develop.

General Considerations

Whenever a person travels from one country to another—particularly if the change involves a marked difference in climate, social conditions, or sanitation standards and facilities—diarrhea may develop within 2–10 days. Bacteria cause 80% of cases of traveler's diarrhea, with enterotoxigenic *E coli*, *Shigella* species, and *Campylobacter jejuni* being the most common pathogens. Less common are *Aeromonas*, *Salmonella*, noncholera vibriones, *E histolytica*, and *G lamblia*. Contributory causes include unusual food and drink, change in living habits, occasional viral infections (adenoviruses or rotaviruses), and change in bowel flora. Chronic watery diarrhea may be due to amebiasis or giardiasis or, rarely, tropical sprue.

Clinical Findings

A. Symptoms and Signs

There may be up to ten or even more loose stools per day, often accompanied by abdominal cramps and nausea, occasionally by vomiting, and rarely by fever. The stools are usually watery and not associated with fever when caused by enterotoxigenic *E coli*. With invasive bacterial pathogens (*Shigella*, *Campylobacter*, *Salmonella*) stools can be bloody and fever may be present. The illness usually subsides spontaneously within 1–5 days, although 10% remain symptomatic for 1 week or longer, and symptoms persist for longer than 1 month in 2%. Traveler's diarrhea is also a significant risk factor for developing irritable bowel syndrome.

B. Laboratory Findings

In patients with fever and bloody diarrhea, stool culture is indicated, but in most cases, cultures are reserved for those who do not respond to antibiotics.

Prevention

A. General Measures

Avoidance of fresh foods and water sources that are likely to be contaminated is recommended for travelers to developing countries, where infectious diarrheal illnesses are endemic.

B. Specific Measures

Because not all travelers will have diarrhea and because most episodes are brief and self-limited, the currently recommended approach is to provide the traveler with a supply of antimicrobials to be taken if significant diarrhea occurs during the trip. In areas where toxin-producing bacteria are the major cause of diarrhea (Latin America and Africa), loperamide (4 mg oral loading dose, then 2 mg after each loose stool to a maximum of 16 mg/d) with a single oral dose of ciprofloxacin (750 mg), levofloxacin (500 mg), or ofloxacin (200 mg), cures most cases of traveler's diarrhea. If diarrhea is associated with bloody stools or persists despite a single dose of a fluoroquinolone, 1000 mg of azithromycin should be taken. In pregnant women and in areas where invasive bacteria more commonly cause diarrhea (Indian subcontinent, Asia, especially Thailand where fluoroquinolone-resistant *Campylobacter* is prevalent), azithromycin is the drug of choice. Rifaximin, a nonabsorbable agent, is also approved for therapy of traveler's diarrhea at a dose of 200 mg orally three times per day or 400 mg twice a day for 3 days. Because luminal concentrations are high, but tissue levels are insufficient, it should not be used in situations where there is a high likelihood of invasive disease (eg, fever, systemic toxicity, or bloody stools). Prophylaxis is recommended for those with significant underlying disease (inflammatory bowel disease, AIDS, diabetes, heart disease in the elderly, conditions requiring immunosuppressive medications) and for those whose full activity status during the trip is so essential that even short periods of diarrhea would be unacceptable.

Prophylaxis is started upon entry into the destination country and is continued for 1 or 2 days after leaving. For stays of more than 3 weeks, prophylaxis is not recommended because of the cost and increased toxicity. For prophylaxis, numerous oral antimicrobial once-daily regimens are effective, such as norfloxacin, 400 mg; ciprofloxacin, 500 mg; or rifaximin, 200 mg. Bismuth subsalicylate is effective but turns the tongue and the stools black and can interfere with doxycycline absorption, which may be needed for malaria prophylaxis; it is rarely used.

▶ Treatment

For most individuals, the affliction is short-lived, and symptomatic therapy with loperamide is all that is required, provided the patient is not systemically ill (fever ≥ 39°C) and does not have dysentery (bloody stools), in which case antimotility agents should be avoided. Packages of oral rehydration salts to treat dehydration are available over the counter in the United States (Infalyte, Pedialyte, others) and in many foreign countries.

▶ When to Refer

- Cases refractory to treatment.
- Persistent infection.
- Immunocompromised patient.

▶ When to Admit

Patients who are severely dehydrated or hemodynamically unstable should be admitted to the hospital.

Itskowitz M. Bacterial diarrhea. N Engl J Med. 2010 Feb 11;362(6):558. [PMID: 20147726]

Kollaritsch H et al. Traveler's diarrhea. Infect Dis Clin North Am. 2012 Sep;26(3):691–706. [PMID: 22963778]

Mayer CA et al. Typhoid and paratyphoid fever—prevention in travellers. Aust Fam Physician. 2010 Nov;39(11):847–51. [PMID: 21301658]

Smith DS. Travel medicine and vaccines for HIV-infected travelers. Top Antivir Med. 2012 Aug–Sep;20(3):111–5. [PMID: 22954612]

ANTIMICROBIAL THERAPY

SELECTED PRINCIPLES OF ANTIMICROBIAL THERAPY

Specific steps (outlined below) are required when considering antibiotic therapy for patients. Drugs within classes, drugs of first choice, and alternative drugs are presented in Table 30–4.

A. Etiologic Diagnosis

Based on the organ system involved, the organism causing infection can often be predicted. See Tables 30–5 and 30–6.

B. "Best Guess"

Select an empiric regimen that is likely to be effective against the suspected pathogens.

C. Laboratory Control

Specimens for laboratory examination should be obtained before institution of therapy to determine susceptibility.

D. Clinical Response

Based on clinical response and other data, the laboratory reports are evaluated and then the desirability of changing the regimen is considered. If the specimen was obtained from a normally sterile site (eg, blood, cerebrospinal fluid, pleural fluid, joint fluid), the recovery of a microorganism in significant amounts is meaningful even if the organism recovered is different from the clinically suspected agent, and this may force a change in treatment. Isolation of unexpected microorganisms from the respiratory tract, gastrointestinal tract, or surface lesions (sites that have a complex flora) may represent colonization or contamination, and cultures must be critically evaluated before drugs are abandoned that were judiciously selected on a "best guess" basis.

E. Drug Susceptibility Tests

Some microorganisms are predictably inhibited by certain drugs; if such organisms are isolated, they need not be tested for drug susceptibility. For example, all group A hemolytic streptococci are inhibited by penicillin. Other organisms

Table 30–4. Drugs of choice for suspected or proved microbial pathogens, 2014.[1]

Suspected or Proved Etiologic Agent	Drug(s) of First Choice	Alternative Drug(s)
Gram-negative cocci		
Moraxella catarrhalis	Cefuroxime, a fluoroquinolone[2]	Cefotaxime, ceftriaxone, cefuroxime axetil, an erythromycin,[3] a tetracycline,[4] azithromycin, amoxicillin-clavulanic acid, clarithromycin, TMP-SMZ[5]
Neisseria gonorrhoeae (gonococcus)	Ceftriaxone plus azithromycin or doxycycline	Cefixime plus azithromycin or doxycycline*
Neisseria meningitidis (meningococcus)	Penicillin[6]	Cefotaxime, ceftriaxone, ampicillin
Gram-positive cocci		
Streptococcus pneumoniae[7] (pneumococcus)	Penicillin[6]	An erythromycin,[3] a cephalosporin,[8] vancomycin, clindamycin, azithromycin, clarithromycin, a tetracycline,[4] respiratory fluoroquinolones[2]
Streptococcus, hemolytic, groups A, B, C, G	Penicillin[6]	An erythromycin,[3] a cephalosporin,[8] vancomycin, clindamycin, azithromycin, clarithromycin
Viridans streptococci	Penicillin[6] ± gentamicin	Cephalosporin,[8] vancomycin
Staphylococcus, methicillin-resistant	Vancomycin	TMP-SMZ,[5] doxycycline, minocycline, linezolid, daptomycin, quinupristin-dalfopristin, tigecycline, televancin
Staphylococcus, non-penicillinase-producing	Penicillin[6]	A cephalosporin,[8] clindamycin
Staphylococcus, penicillinase-producing	Penicillinase-resistant penicillin[9]	Vancomycin, a cephalosporin,[8] clindamycin, amoxicillin-clavulanic acid, ampicillin-sulbactam, piperacillin-tazobactam, TMP-SMZ[5]
Enterococcus faecalis	Ampicillin ± gentamicin[10]	Vancomycin ± gentamicin
Enterococcus faecium	Vancomycin ± gentamicin[10]	Linezolid,[11] quinupristin-dalfopristin,[11] daptomycin,[11] tigecycline[11]
Gram-negative rods		
Acinetobacter	Imipenem, meropenem	Tigecycline, minocycline, doxycycline, aminoglycosides,[12] colistin
Prevotella, oropharyngeal strains	Clindamycin	Metronidazole
Bacteroides, gastrointestinal strains	Metronidazole	Ticarcillin-clavulanate, ampicillin-sulbactam, piperacillin-tazobactam, carbapenem
Brucella	Doxycycline + rifampin[4]	TMP-SMZ[5] ± gentamicin; ciprofloxacin + rifampin
Campylobacter jejuni	Erythromycin[3] or azithromycin	Tetracycline,[4] a fluoroquinolone[2]
Enterobacter	Ertapenem, imipenem, meropenem, cefepime	Aminoglycoside, a fluoroquinolone,[2] TMP-SMZ[5]
Escherichia coli (sepsis)[13]	Cefotaxime, ceftriaxone	Ertapenem[13] imipenem[13] or meropenem,[13] aminoglycosides,[12] a fluoroquinolone,[2] aztreonam, ticarcillin-clavulanate, piperacillin-tazobactam
Escherichia coli (uncomplicated outpatient urinary infection)	Nitrofurantoin, fosfomycin	Fluoroquinolones,[2] TMP-SMZ,[5] oral cephalosporin
Haemophilus (meningitis and other serious infections)	Cefotaxime, ceftriaxone	Aztreonam
Haemophilus (respiratory infections, otitis)	TMP-SMZ[5]	Doxycycline, azithromycin, clarithromycin, cefotaxime, ceftriaxone, cefuroxime, cefuroxime axetil, ampicillin-clavulanate
Helicobacter pylori	Amoxicillin + clarithromycin + proton pump inhibitor (PPI)	Bismuth subsalicylate + tetracycline + metronidazole + PPI
Klebsiella[13]	A cephalosporin	TMP-SMZ,[5] aminoglycoside,[12] ertapenem,[13] imipenem[13] or meropenem,[13] a fluoroquinolone,[2] aztreonam, ticarcillin-clavulanate, piperacillin-tazobactam

(continued)

Table 30–4. Drugs of choice for suspected or proved microbial pathogens, 2014.[1] (continued)

Suspected or Proved Etiologic Agent	Drug(s) of First Choice	Alternative Drug(s)
Legionella species (pneumonia)	Azithromycin, or fluoroquinolones[2] ± rifampin	Doxycycline ± rifampin
Proteus mirabilis	Ampicillin	An aminoglycoside,[12] TMP-SMZ,[5] a fluoroquinolone,[2] a cephalosporin[8]
Proteus vulgaris and other species (*Morganella, Providencia*)	Cefotaxime, ceftriaxone	Aminoglycoside,[12] ertapenem,[13] imipenem or meropenem,[13] TMP-SMZ,[5] a fluoroquinolone[2]
Pseudomonas aeruginosa	Piperacillin-tazobactam or ceftazidime or cefepime, or imipenem or meropenem or doripenem ± aminoglycoside[12]	Ciprofloxacin (or levofloxacin) ± piperacillin-tazobactam; ciprofloxacin (or levofloxacin) ± ceftazidime; ciprofloxacin (or levofloxacin) ± cefepime; piperacillin-tazobactam + tobramycin; ceftazidime + tobramycin; cefepime + tobramycin; meropenem (imipenem) + tobramycin
Burkholderia pseudomallei (melioidosis)	Ceftazidime	Tetracycline,[4] TMP-SMZ,[5] amoxicillin-clavulanic acid, imipenem or meropenem
Burkholderia mallei (glanders)	Streptomycin + tetracycline[4]	Chloramphenicol + streptomycin
Salmonella (bacteremia)	Ceftriaxone	A fluoroquinolone[2]
Serratia	Carbapenem	TMP-SMZ,[5] aminoglycosides,[12] a fluoroquinolone,[2] cefotaxime, ceftriaxone
Shigella	A fluoroquinolone[2]	Azithromycin, ampicillin, TMP-SMZ,[5] ceftriaxone
Vibrio (cholera, sepsis)	A tetracycline[4]	TMP-SMZ,[5] a fluoroquinolone[2]
Yersinia pestis (plague)	Streptomycin ± a tetracycline[4]	Chloramphenicol, TMP-SMZ[5]
Gram-positive rods		
Actinomyces	Penicillin[6]	Tetracycline,[4] clindamycin
Bacillus (including anthrax)	Penicillin[6] (ciprofloxacin or doxycycline for anthrax; see Table 33–2)	Erythromycin,[3] a fluoroquinolone[2]
Clostridium (eg, gas gangrene, tetanus)	Penicillin[6]	Metronidazole, clindamycin, imipenem or meropenem
Corynebacterium diphtheriae	Erythromycin[3]	Penicillin[6]
Corynebacterium jeikeium	Vancomycin	A fluoroquinolone
Listeria	Ampicillin ± aminoglycoside[12]	TMP-SMZ[5]
Acid-fast rods		
Mycobacterium tuberculosis[14]	Isoniazid (INH) + rifampin + pyrazinamide ± ethambutol	Other antituberculous drugs (see Tables 9–14 and 9–15)
Mycobacterium leprae	Dapsone + rifampin ± clofazimine	Minocycline, ofloxacin, clarithromycin
Mycobacterium kansasii	INH + rifampin ± ethambutol	Clarithromycin, azithromycin, ethionamide, cycloserine
Mycobacterium avium complex	Clarithromycin or azithromycin + ethambutol, ± rifabutin	Amikacin, ciprofloxacin
Mycobacterium fortuitum-chelonei	Cefoxitin + clarithromycin	Amikacin, rifampin, sulfonamide, doxycycline, linezolid
Nocardia	TMP-SMZ[5]	Minocycline, imipenem or meropenem, linezolid
Spirochetes		
Borrelia burgdorferi (Lyme disease)	Doxycycline, amoxicillin, cefuroxime axetil	Ceftriaxone, cefotaxime, penicillin, azithromycin, clarithromycin
Borrelia recurrentis (relapsing fever)	Doxycycline[4]	Penicillin[6]
Leptospira	Penicillin[6]	Doxycycline,[4] ceftriaxone
Treponema pallidum (syphilis)	Penicillin[6]	Doxycycline, ceftriaxone
Treponema pertenue (yaws)	Penicillin[6]	Doxycycline

(continued)

Table 30–4. Drugs of choice for suspected or proved microbial pathogens, 2014.[1] (continued)

Suspected or Proved Etiologic Agent	Drug(s) of First Choice	Alternative Drug(s)
Mycoplasmas	**Clarithromycin or azithromycin or doxycycline**	**A fluoroquinolone,[2] erythromycin[3]**
Chlamydiae		
C psittaci	Doxycycline	Chloramphenicol
C trachomatis (urethritis or pelvic inflammatory disease)	Doxycycline or azithromycin	Levofloxacin, ofloxacin
C pneumoniae	Doxycycline[4]	Erythromycin,[3] clarithromycin, azithromycin, a fluoroquinolone[2,15]
Rickettsiae	**Doxycycline[4]**	**Chloramphenicol, a fluoroquinolone[2]**

[1]Adapted, with permission, and updated, from Treat Guide Med Lett. 2010 June;6(94):43–52.

[2]Fluoroquinolones include ciprofloxacin, ofloxacin, levofloxacin, moxifloxacin, and others (see text). Gemifloxacin, levofloxacin, and moxifloxacin have the best activity against gram-positive organisms, including penicillin-resistant S pneumoniae and methicillin-sensitive S aureus. Activity against enterococci and S epidermidis is variable.

[3]Erythromycin estolate is best absorbed orally but carries the highest risk of hepatitis; erythromycin stearate and erythromycin ethylsuccinate are also available.

[4]All tetracyclines have similar activity against most microorganisms. Minocycline (the most active tetracycline), doxycycline, tetracycline have increased activity against S aureus.

[5]TMP-SMZ is a mixture of 1 part trimethoprim and 5 parts sulfamethoxazole.

*Test of cure recommended if ceftriaxone not used.

[6]Penicillin G is preferred for parenteral injection; penicillin V for oral administration—to be used only in treating infections due to highly sensitive organisms.

[7]Infections caused by isolates with intermediate resistance may respond to high doses of penicillin, cefotaxime, or ceftriaxone, as well as the respiratory fluoroquinolones (gemifloxacin, levofloxacin, and moxifloxacin). Infections caused by highly resistant strains should be treated with vancomycin. Many strains of penicillin-resistant pneumococci are resistant to macrolides, cephalosporins, tetracyclines, and TMP-SMZ.

[8]Most intravenous cephalosporins (with the exception of ceftazidime) have good activity against gram-positive cocci.

[9]Parenteral nafcillin or oxacillin; oral dicloxacillin, cloxacillin, or oxacillin.

[10]Addition of gentamicin indicated only for severe enterococcal infections (eg, endocarditis, meningitis).

[11]Linezolid, daptomycin, tigecycline, quinupristin-dalfopristin should be reserved for the treatment of vancomycin resistant isolates or in patients intolerant of vancomycin.

[12]Aminoglycosides—gentamicin, tobramycin, amikacin, netilmicin—should be chosen on the basis of local patterns of susceptibility.

[13]Extended beta-lactamase–producing isolates should be treated with a carbapenem.

[14]Resistance is common and susceptibility testing should be done.

[15]Ciprofloxacin has inferior antichlamydial activity compared with levofloxacin or ofloxacin.

Key: ±, alone or combined with.

(eg, enteric gram-negative rods) are variably susceptible and generally require susceptibility testing whenever they are isolated. Organisms that once had predictable susceptibility patterns have now become resistant and require testing. Examples include the pneumococci, which may be resistant to multiple drugs (including penicillin, macrolides, and TMP-SMZ); the enterococci, which may be resistant to penicillin, aminoglycosides, and vancomycin; and extended-spectrum beta-lactamase producing–E coli resistant to third-generation cephalosporins and fluoroquinolones.

Over the past several years, pharmaceutical companies have shifted away from developing and producing antibacterial medications, particularly those active against gram-negative pathogens. The lack of new drugs and increasing bacterial resistance reinforce the need to use these drugs judiciously. When culture and susceptibility results have been finalized, it is important to utilize the most narrow spectrum agent possible to decrease the selection pressure for antibacterial resistance.

Antimicrobial drug susceptibility tests may be performed on solid media as disk diffusion tests, in broth, in tubes, in wells of microdilution plates, or as E-tests (strips with increasing concentration of antibiotic). The latter three methods yield results expressed as MIC (minimal inhibitory concentration). In most infections, the MIC is the appropriate in vitro test to guide selection of an antibacterial agent. When there appear to be marked discrepancies between susceptibility testing and clinical response, the following possibilities must be considered:

1. Selection of an inappropriate drug, drug dosage, or route of administration.

2. Failure to drain a collection of pus or to remove a foreign body.

3. Failure of a poorly diffusing drug to reach the site of infection (eg, central nervous system) or to reach intracellular phagocytosed bacteria.

4. Superinfection in the course of prolonged chemotherapy.

Table 30–5. Examples of initial antimicrobial therapy for acutely ill, hospitalized adults pending identification of causative organism.

Suspected Clinical Diagnosis	Likely Etiologic Diagnosis	Drugs of Choice
Meningitis, bacterial, community-acquired	Pneumococcus,[1] meningococcus	Cefotaxime,[2] 2–3 g intravenously every 6 hours; **or** ceftriaxone, 2 g intravenously every 12 hours plus vancomycin, 15 mg/kg intravenously every 8 hours
Meningitis, bacterial, age > 50, community-acquired	Pneumococcus, meningococcus, *Listeria monocytogenes*,[3] gram-negative bacilli	Ampicillin, 2 g intravenously every 4 hours, plus cefotaxime, 2–3 g intravenously every 6 hours; **or** ceftriaxone, 2 g intravenously every 12 hours plus vancomycin, 15 mg/kg intravenously every 8 hours
Meningitis, postoperative (or posttraumatic)	*S aureus*, gram-negative bacilli (pneumococcus, in posttraumatic)	Vancomycin, 15 mg/kg intravenously every 8 hours, plus cefepime, 3 g intravenously every 8 hours
Brain abscess	Mixed anaerobes, pneumococci, streptococci	Penicillin G, 4 million units intravenously every 4 hours, plus metronidazole, 500 mg orally every 8 hours; **or** cefotaxime, 2–3 g intravenously every 6 hours **or** ceftriaxone, 2 g intravenously every 12 hours **plus** metronidazole, 500 mg orally every 8 hours
Pneumonia, acute, community-acquired, non-ICU hospital admission	Pneumococci, *M pneumoniae*, *Legionella*, *C pneumoniae*	Cefotaxime, 2 g intravenously every 8 hours (or ceftriaxone, 1 g intravenously every 24 hours or ampicillin 2 g intravenously every 6 hours) plus azithromycin 500 mg intravenously every 24 hours; **or** a fluoroquinolone[4] alone
Pneumonia, postoperative or nosocomial	*S aureus*, mixed anaerobes, gram-negative bacilli	Cefepime, 1 g intravenously every 8 hours; **or** ceftazidime, 2 g intravenously every 8 hours; **or** piperacillin-tazobactam, 4.5 g intravenously every 6 hours; **or** imipenem, 500 mg intravenously every 6 hours; **or** meropenem, 1 g intravenously every 8 hours plus tobramycin, 5 mg/kg intravenously every 24 hours; **or** ciprofloxacin, 400 mg intravenously every 12 hours; **or** levofloxacin, 500 mg intravenously every 24 hours plus vancomycin, 15 mg/kg intravenously every 12 hours
Endocarditis, acute (including injection drug user)	*S aureus*, *E faecalis*, gram-negative aerobic bacteria, viridans streptococci	Vancomycin, 15 mg/kg intravenously every 12 hours, plus gentamicin, 1 mg/kg every 8 hours
Septic thrombophlebitis (eg, IV tubing, IV shunts)	*S aureus*, gram-negative aerobic bacteria	Vancomycin, 15 mg/kg intravenously every 12 hours plus ceftriaxone, 1 g intravenously every 24 hours
Osteomyelitis	*S aureus*	Nafcillin, 2 g intravenously every 4 hours; **or** cefazolin, 2 g intravenously every 8 hours
Septic arthritis	*S aureus*, *N gonorrhoeae*	Ceftriaxone, 1–2 g intravenously every 24 hours
Pyelonephritis with flank pain and fever (recurrent urinary tract infection)	*E coli*, *Klebsiella*, *Enterobacter*, *Pseudomonas*	Ceftriaxone, 1 g intravenously every 24 hours; **or** ciprofloxacin, 400 mg intravenously every 12 hours (500 mg orally); **or** levofloxacin, 500 mg once daily (intravenously/orally)
Fever in neutropenic patient receiving cancer chemotherapy	*S aureus*, *Pseudomonas*, *Klebsiella*, *E coli*	Ceftazidime, 2 g intravenously every 8 hours; **or** cefepime, 2 g intravenously every 8 hours
Intra-abdominal sepsis (eg, postoperative, peritonitis, cholecystitis)	Gram-negative bacteria, *Bacteroides*, anaerobic bacteria, streptococci, clostridia	Piperacillin-tazobactam, 4.5 g intravenously every 6 hours, **or** ertapenem, 1 g every 24 hours

[1]Some strains may be resistant to penicillin.
[2]Most studies on meningitis have been with cefotaxime or ceftriaxone (see text).
[3]TMP-SMZ can be used to treat *Listeria monocytogenes* in patients allergic to penicillin in a dosage of 15–20 mg/kg/d of TMP in three or four divided doses.
[4]Levofloxacin 750 mg/d, moxifloxacin 400 mg/d.

Table 30–6. Examples of empiric choices of antimicrobials for adult outpatient infections.

Suspected Clinical Diagnosis	Likely Etiologic Agents	Drugs of Choice	Alternative Drugs
Erysipelas, impetigo, cellulitis, ascending lymphangitis	Group A streptococcus	Phenoxymethyl penicillin, 0.5 g orally four times daily for 7–10 days	Cephalexin, 0.5 g orally four times daily for 7–10 days; **or** azithromycin, 500 mg on day 1 and 250 mg on days 2–5
Furuncle with surrounding cellulitis	*Staphylococcus aureus*	Dicloxacillin, 0.5 g orally four times daily for 7–10 days (If high-risk for MRSA, clindamycin 0.3 g orally four times daily for 7–10 days)	Cephalexin, 0.5 g orally four times daily for 7–10 days. (If high-risk for MRSA, TMP-SMZ two double strength tablets twice daily for 7–10 days)
Pharyngitis	Group A streptococcus	Phenoxymethyl penicillin, 0.5 g orally four times daily for 10 days	Clindamycin, 300 mg orally four times daily for 10 days; **or** erythromycin, 0.5 g orally four times daily for 10 days; **or** azithromycin, 500 mg on day 1 and 250 mg on days 2–5; **or** clarithromycin, 500 mg twice daily for 10 days
Otitis media	*Streptococcus pneumoniae, Haemophilus influenzae, Moraxella catarrhalis*	Amoxicillin, 0.5–1 g orally three times daily for 10 days	Augmentin,[2] 0.875 g orally twice daily; **or** cefuroxime, 0.5 g orally twice daily; **or** cefpodoxime, 0.2–0.4 g daily; **or** doxycycline, 100 mg twice daily; **or** TMP-SMZ,[1] one double-strength tablet twice daily (all regimens for 10 days).
Acute sinusitis	*S pneumoniae, H influenzae, M catarrhalis*	Amoxicillin, 0.5–1 g orally three times daily; or TMP-SMZ, one double-strength tablet twice daily for 10 days	Augmentin,[2] 0.875 g orally twice daily; **or** cefuroxime, 0.5 g orally twice daily; **or** cefpodoxime, 0.2–0.4 g daily; **or** doxycycline, 100 mg twice daily (all regimens for 10 days)
Aspiration pneumonia	Mixed oropharyngeal flora, including anaerobes	Clindamycin, 0.3 g orally four times daily for 10–14 days	Phenoxymethyl penicillin, 0.5 g orally four times daily for 10–14 days
Pneumonia	*S pneumoniae, Mycoplasma pneumoniae, Legionella pneumophila, Chlamydophila pneumoniae*	Doxycycline, 100 mg orally twice daily; or clarithromycin, 0.5 g orally twice daily, for 10–14 days; or azithromycin, 0.5 g orally on day 1 and 0.25 g on days 2–5	Amoxicillin, 0.5–1.0 g orally three times daily; **or** a fluoroquinolone[5] for 10–14 days
Cystitis	*Escherichia coli, Klebsiella pneumoniae, Proteus* species, *Staphylococcus saprophyticus*	Nitrofurantoin monohydrate macrocrystals 100 mg twice daily for 7 days; fosfomycin 3 g orally as a single dose; TMP-SMZ,[1] one double-strength tablet twice daily for 3 days	Cephalexin, 0.5 g orally four times daily for 7 days, fluoroquinolones,[4] 3 days for uncomplicated cystitis
Pyelonephritis	*E coli, K pneumoniae, Proteus* species, *S saprophyticus*	Fluoroquinolones[4] for 7 days	TMP-SMZ,[1] one double-strength tablet twice daily for 14 days
Gastroenteritis	*Salmonella, Shigella, Campylobacter, Entamoeba histolytica*	See Note 3	
Urethritis, epididymitis	*Neisseria gonorrhoeae, Chlamydia trachomatis*	Ceftriaxone, 250 mg intramuscularly once plus azithromycin (or doxycycline) for *N gonorrhoeae*; azithromycin 1 g orally once, or doxycycline, 100 mg orally twice daily for 7 days, for *C trachomatis*	Cefixime 400 mg orally once for *N gonorrhoeae*

(continued)

Table 30–6. Examples of empiric choices of antimicrobials for adult outpatient infections. (continued)

Suspected Clinical Diagnosis	Likely Etiologic Agents	Drugs of Choice	Alternative Drugs
Pelvic inflammatory disease	N gonorrhoeae, C trachomatis, anaerobes, gram-negative rods	Levofloxacin 500 mg orally daily, or ofloxacin, 400 mg orally twice daily, for 14 days, plus metronidazole, 500 mg orally twice daily, for 14 days	Cefoxitin, 2 g intramuscularly, with probenecid, 1 g orally, followed by doxycycline, 100 mg orally twice daily for 14 days; **or** ceftriaxone, 250 mg intramuscularly once, followed by doxycycline, 100 mg orally twice daily for 14 days
Syphilis			
Early syphilis (primary, secondary, or latent of < 1 year's duration)	Treponema pallidum	Benzathine penicillin G, 2.4 million units intramuscularly once	Doxycycline, 100 mg orally twice daily for 2 weeks
Latent syphilis of > 1 year's duration or cardiovascular syphilis	T pallidum	Benzathine penicillin G, 2.4 million units intramuscularly once a week for 3 weeks (total: 7.2 million units)	Doxycycline, 100 mg orally twice daily, for 4 weeks
Neurosyphilis	T pallidum	Aqueous penicillin G, 12–24 million units/d intravenously for 10–14 days	

[1]TMP-SMZ is a fixed combination of 1 part trimethoprim and 5 parts sulfamethoxazole. Single-strength tablets: 80 mg TMP, 400 mg SMZ; double-strength tablets: 160 mg TMP, 800 mg SMZ.
[2]Augmentin is a combination of amoxicillin, 250 mg, 500 mg, or 875 mg, plus 125 mg of clavulanic acid. Augmentin XR is a combination of amoxicillin 1 g and clavulanic acid 62.5 mg.
[3]The diagnosis should be confirmed by culture before therapy. *Salmonella* gastroenteritis does not require therapy. For susceptible *Shigella* isolates, give ciprofloxacin, 0.5 g orally twice daily for 5 days; or TMP-SMZ double-strength tablets twice daily for 5 days; or ampicillin, 0.5 g orally four times daily for 5 days. For *Campylobacter* infection, give azithromycin, 1 g orally times one dose, or ciprofloxacin, 0.5 g orally twice daily for 5 days. For *E histolytica* infection, give metronidazole, 750 mg orally three times daily for 5–10 days, followed by diiodohydroxyquin, 600 mg orally three times daily for 3 weeks.
[4]Fluoroquinolones and dosages include ciprofloxacin, 500 mg orally twice daily; ofloxacin, 400 mg orally twice daily; levofloxacin, 500 mg orally daily.
[5]Fluoroquinolones with activity against *S pneumoniae*, including penicillin-resistant isolates, include gemifloxacin (320 mg orally once daily), levofloxacin (500–750 mg orally once daily) and moxifloxacin (400 mg orally once daily). Use fluoroquinolones as drug of choice if recent antibiotic use within 3 months or comorbidities present.
MRSA, methicillin-resistant *Staphylococcus aureus*; TMP-SMZ, trimethoprim-sulfamethoxazole.

5. Emergence of drug-resistant organisms.

6. Participation of two or more microorganisms in the infectious process, of which only one was originally detected and used for drug selection.

7. Inadequate host defenses, including immunodeficiencies and diabetes mellitus.

8. Noninfectious causes, including drug fever, malignancy, and autoimmune disease.

F. Promptness of Response

Response depends on a number of factors, including the patient (immunocompromised patients respond slower than immunocompetent patients), the site of infection (deep-seated infections such as osteomyelitis and endocarditis respond more slowly than superficial infections such as cystitis or cellulitis), the pathogen (virulent organisms such as *S aureus* respond more slowly than viridans streptococci; mycobacterial and fungal infections respond slower than bacterial infections), and the duration of illness (in general, the longer the symptoms are present, the

longer it takes to respond). Thus, depending on the clinical situation, persistent fever and leukocytosis several days after initiation of therapy may not indicate improper choice of antibiotics but may be due to the natural history of the disease being treated. In most infections, either a bacteriostatic or a bactericidal agent can be used. In some infections (eg, infective endocarditis and meningitis), a bactericidal agent should be used. When potentially toxic drugs (eg, aminoglycosides, flucytosine) are used, serum levels of the drug are measured to minimize toxicity and ensure appropriate dosage. In patients with altered renal or hepatic clearance of drugs, the dosage or frequency of administration must be adjusted; it is best to measure levels in the elderly, morbidly obese patients, or those with altered kidney function when possible and adjust therapy accordingly.

G. Duration of Antimicrobial Therapy

Generally, effective antimicrobial treatment results in reversal of the clinical and laboratory parameters of active infection and marked clinical improvement. However, varying periods of treatment may be required for cure. Key factors include (1) the type of infecting organism (bacterial infections generally can be cured more rapidly than fungal or mycobacterial ones), (2) the location of the process (eg, endocarditis and osteomyelitis require prolonged therapy), and (3) the immunocompetence of the patient. Recommendations about duration of therapy are often given based on clinical experience, not prospective controlled studies of large numbers of patients.

H. Adverse Reactions and Toxicity

These include hypersensitivity reactions, direct toxicity, superinfection by drug-resistant microorganisms, and drug interactions. If the infection is life threatening and treatment cannot be stopped, the reactions are managed symptomatically or another drug is chosen that does not cross-react with the offending one (Table 30–4). If the infection is less serious, it may be possible to stop all antimicrobials and monitor the patient closely.

I. Route of Administration

Intravenous therapy is preferred for acutely ill patients with serious infections (eg, endocarditis, meningitis, sepsis, severe pneumonia) when dependable levels of antibiotics are required for successful therapy. Certain drugs (eg, fluconazole, voriconazole, rifampin, metronidazole, TMP-SMZ, and fluoroquinolones) are so well absorbed that they generally can be administered orally in seriously ill—but not hemodynamically unstable—patients.

Food does not significantly influence the bioavailability of most oral antimicrobial agents. However, the tetracyclines and the quinolones chelate multivalent cations resulting in decreased antibacterial absorption. Azithromycin capsules are associated with decreased bioavailability when taken with food and should be given 1 hour before or 2 hours after meals. Posaconazole solution should always be administered with food.

A major complication of intravenous antibiotic therapy is catheter infections. Peripheral catheters are changed every 48–72 hours to prevent phlebitis, and antimicrobial-coated central venous catheters (minocycline and rifampin, chlorhexidine and sulfadiazine) have been associated with a decreased incidence of catheter-related infections. Most of these infections present with local signs of infection (erythema, tenderness) at the insertion site. In a patient with fever who is receiving intravenous therapy, the catheter must always be considered a potential source. Small-gauge (20–23F) peripherally inserted silicone or polyurethane catheters (Per Q Cath, A-Cath, Ven-A-Cath, and others) are associated with a low infection rate and can be maintained for 3–6 months without replacement. Such catheters are ideal for long-term outpatient antibiotic therapy.

J. Cost of Antibiotics

The cost of these agents can be substantial. In addition to acquisition costs and monitoring costs, (drug levels, liver function tests, electrolytes, etc), the cost of treating adverse reactions, the cost of treatment failure, and the costs associated with drug administration must be considered.

Boucher HW et al. Bad bugs, no drugs: no ESKAPE! An update from the Infectious Diseases Society of America. Clin Infect Dis. 2009 Jan 1;48(1):1–12. [PMID: 19035777]

Jenkins SG et al. Current concepts in laboratory testing to guide antimicrobial therapy. Mayo Clin Proc. 2012 Mar;87(3):290–308. [PMID: 22386185]

Rivera AM et al. Current concepts in antimicrobial therapy against select gram-positive organisms: methicillin-resistant *Staphylococcus aureus*, penicillin-resistant pneumococci, and vancomycin-resistant enterococci. Mayo Clin Proc. 2011 Dec;86(12):1230–43. [PMID: 22134942]

HYPERSENSITIVITY TESTS & DESENSITIZATION

▶ Penicillin Allergy

All penicillins are cross-sensitizing and cross-reacting. Skin tests with penicilloyl-polylysine, with minor antigenic determinants, and with undegraded penicillin can identify most individuals with IgE-mediated reactions (hives, bronchospasm). Among positive reactors to skin tests, the incidence of subsequent immediate severe penicillin reactions is high. A history of a penicillin reaction in the past is often not reliable. Only a small proportion (< 20%) of patients with a history of penicillin allergy have an adverse reaction when challenged with the drug. The decision to administer penicillin or related drugs (other beta-lactams) to patients with an allergic history depends on the severity of the reported reaction, the severity of the infection being treated, and the availability of alternative drugs. For patients with a history of severe reaction (anaphylaxis), alternative drugs should be used. In the rare situations when there is a strong indication for using penicillin (eg, syphilis in pregnancy) in allergic patients, desensitization can be performed. If the reaction is mild (nonurticarial rash), the patient may be rechallenged with penicillin or may be given another beta-lactam antibiotic.

Allergic reactions include anaphylaxis, serum sickness (urticaria, fever, joint swelling, angioedema 7–12 days after exposure), skin rashes, fever, interstitial nephritis, eosinophilia, hemolytic anemia, other hematologic disturbances, and vasculitis. The incidence of hypersensitivity to penicillin is estimated to be 1–5% among adults in the United States. Life-threatening anaphylactic reactions are very rare (0.05%). Ampicillin produces maculopapular skin rashes more frequently than other penicillins, but many ampicillin (and other beta-lactam) rashes are not allergic in origin. The non-allergic ampicillin rash usually occurs after 3–4 days of therapy, is maculopapular, is more common in patients with coexisting viral illness (especially Epstein-Barr infection), and resolves with continued therapy. The maculopapular rash may or may not reappear with rechallenge. Rarely, penicillins can induce nephritis with primary tubular lesions associated with anti-basement membrane antibodies.

If the intradermal test described below is negative, desensitization is not necessary, and a full dose of the material may be given. If the test is positive, alternative drugs should be strongly considered. If that is not feasible, desensitization is necessary.

Patients with a history of allergy to penicillin are also at an increased risk for having a reaction to **cephalosporins** or **carbapenems**. A common approach to these patients is to assess the severity of the reaction. If an IgE-mediated reaction to penicillin can be excluded by history, a cephalosporin can be administered. When the history justifies concern about an immediate-type reaction, penicillin skin testing should be performed. If the test is negative, the cephalosporin or carbapenem can be given. If the test is positive, there is a 5–10% chance of cross reactivity with cephalosporins, and the decision whether to use cephalosporins depends on the availability of alternative agents and the severity of the infection. While carbapenems historically have been considered highly cross reactive with penicillins, the cross reactivity appears to be minimal (1–5%).

▶ Intradermal Test for Hypersensitivity

Penicillin is the drug that most frequently serves as an indication for sensitivity testing and desensitization. A clinical history of penicillin allergy has a positive predictive value of only 15%. IgG-mediated delayed reactions such as erythematous or maculopapular skin rash or serum sickness should be distinguished from immediate-type IgE-mediated reactions, such as urticaria, angioedema, and anaphylaxis.

▶ Desensitization

A. Precautions

1. The desensitization procedure is not innocuous—deaths from anaphylaxis have been reported. If extreme hypersensitivity is suspected, it is advisable to use an alternative structurally unrelated drug and to reserve desensitization for situations when treatment cannot be withheld and no alternative drug is available.

2. An antihistaminic drug (25–50 mg of hydroxyzine or diphenhydramine intramuscularly or orally) should be administered before desensitization is begun in order to lessen any reaction that occurs.

3. Desensitization should be conducted in an intensive care unit where cardiac monitoring and emergency endotracheal intubation can be performed.

4. Epinephrine, 1 mL of 1:1000 solution, must be ready for immediate administration.

B. Desensitization Method

Several methods of desensitization have been described for penicillin, including use of both oral and intravenous preparations. All methods start with very small doses of drug and gradually increase the dose until therapeutic doses are achieved. For penicillin, 1 unit of drug is given intravenously and the patient observed for 15–30 minutes. If there is no reaction, some recommend doubling the dose while others recommend increasing it tenfold every 15–30 minutes until a dosage of 2 million units is reached; then give the remainder of the desired dose.

For recommendations on skin testing and desensitization for other preparations (eg, botulism antitoxin and diphtheria antitoxin), the manufacturer's package inserts should be consulted.

Chang C et al. Overview of penicillin allergy. Clin Rev Allergy Immunol. 2012 Aug;43(1-2):84–97. [PMID: 21789743]
McLean-Tooke A et al. Practical management of antibiotic allergy in adults. J Clin Pathol. 2011 Mar;64(3):192–9. [PMID: 21177267]
Torres MJ et al. The complex clinical picture of beta-lactam hypersensitivity: penicillins, cephalosporins, monobactams, carbapenems, and clavams. Med Clin North Am. 2010 Jul; 94(4):805–20. [PMID: 20609864]

▼ IMMUNIZATION AGAINST INFECTIOUS DISEASES

RECOMMENDED IMMUNIZATION OF INFANTS, CHILDREN, & ADOLESCENTS

The recommended schedules and dosages of vaccination change often, so the manufacturer's package inserts should always be consulted.

The schedule for active immunizations in children can be accessed at www.cdc.gov/vaccines/schedules. All adolescents should see a health care provider to ensure vaccination of those who have not received varicella or hepatitis B vaccine, to make certain that a second dose of MMR has been given, to receive a booster of tetanus toxoid, reduced diphtheria toxoid and acellular pertussis vaccine (Tdap adolescent preparation), to receive meningococcal vaccine conjugate vaccine, to obtain HPV vaccine if not given previously, and to receive immunizations (influenza and pneumococcal vaccines) that may be indicated for certain high-risk individuals.

RECOMMENDED IMMUNIZATION FOR ADULTS

Immunization is one of the most important tools (along with sanitation) used to prevent morbidity and mortality from infectious diseases. In general, the administration of most vaccinations induces a durable antibody response (active immunity). In contrast, passive immunization occurs when preformed antibodies are given (eg, immune globulin from pooled serum), resulting in temporary protection which is a less durable response. The two variants of active immunization are live attenuated vaccines (which are believed to result in an immunologic response more like natural infection), and inactivated or killed vaccines.

The schedule of vaccinations varies based on the risk of the disease being prevented by vaccination, whether a vaccine has been given previously, the immune status of the patient (probability of responding to vaccine) and safety of the vaccine (live versus killed product, as well as implications for the fetus in pregnant women). Recommendations for healthy adults as well as special populations based on medical conditions are summarized in Table 30–7, which can be accessed online at www.cdc.gov/vaccines/schedules.

Table 30–7. Recommended adult immunization schedule—United States, 2014.

Recommended Adult Immunization Schedule—United States - 2013[1]

Note: These recommendations must be read with the footnotes that follow containing number of doses, intervals between doses, and other important information.

VACCINE ▼ AGE GROUP ▶	19–21 years	22–26 years	27–49 years	50–59 years	60–64 years	≥ 65 years
Influenza[2]	1 dose annually					
Tetanus, diphtheria, pertussis (Td/Tdap)[3]	Substitute 1-time dose of Tdap for Td booster; then boost with Td every 10 yrs					
Varicella[4]	2 doses					
Human papillomavirus (HPV) Female[5]	3 doses					
Human papillomavirus (HPV) Male[5]	3 doses					
Zoster[6]					1 dose	
Measles, mumps, rubella (MMR)[7]	1 or 2 doses					
Pneumococcal polysaccharide (PPSV23)[8,9]	1 or 2 doses					1 dose
Pneumococcal 13-valent conjugate (PCV13)[10]	1 dose					
Meningococcal[11]	1 or more doses					
Hepatitis A[12]	2 doses					
Hepatitis B[13]	3 doses					

Additional information about the vaccines in this schedule, extent of available data, and contraindications for vaccination is also available at www.cdc. gov/vaccines or from the CDC-INFO Contact Center at 800-CDC-INFO (800-232-4636) in English and Spanish, 8:00 a.m. - 8:00 p.m. Eastern Time, Monday - Friday, excluding holidays.

Use of trade names and commercial sources is for identification only and does not imply endorsement by the U.S. Department of Health and Human Services.

The recommendations in this schedule were approved by the Centers for Disease Control and Prevention's (CDC) Advisory Committee on Immunization Practices (ACIP), the American Academy of Family Physicians (AAFP), the American College of Physicians (ACP), American College of Obstetricians and Gynecologists (ACOG) and American College of Nurse-Midwives (ACNM).

For all persons in this category who meet the age requirements and who lack documentation of vaccination or have no evidence of previous infection; zoster vaccine recommended regardless of prior episode of zoster

Recommended if some other risk factor is present (e.g., on the basis of medical, occupational, lifestyle, or other indication)

No recommendation

(continued)

Table 30–7. Recommended adult immunization schedule—United States, 2014. (continued)

VACCINE ▼ / INDICATION ▲	Pregnancy	Immuno-compromising conditions (excluding human immunodeficiency virus [HIV]) [4,6,7,10,15]	HIV infection CD4+ T lymphocyte count [4,6,7,10,14,15] <200 cells/μL	HIV infection CD4+ T lymphocyte count ≥200 cells/μL	Men who have sex with men (MSM)	Heart disease, chronic lung disease, chronic alcoholism	Asplenia (including elective splenectomy and persistent complement component deficiencies) [10,14]	Chronic liver disease	Kidney failure, end-stage renal disease, receipt of hemodialysis	Diabetes	Healthcare personnel
Influenza [2]	1 dose IIV annually	1 dose IIV annually	1 dose IIV annually	1 dose IIV annually	1 dose IIV or LAIV annually	1 dose IIV annually	1 dose IIV annually	1 dose IIV annually	1 dose IIV annually	1 dose IIV annually	1 dose IIV or LAIV annually
Tetanus, diphtheria, pertussis (Td/Tdap) [3]	1 dose Tdap each pregnancy	Substitute 1-time dose of Tdap for Td booster; then boost with Td every 10 yrs									
Varicella [4]		Contraindicated	Contraindicated	2 doses	2 doses	2 doses	2 doses	2 doses	2 doses	2 doses	2 doses
Human papillomavirus (HPV) Female [5]		3 doses through age 26 yrs	3 doses through age 26 yrs	3 doses through age 26 yrs							
Human papillomavirus (HPV) Male [5]		3 doses through age 26 yrs	3 doses through age 26 yrs	3 doses through age 26 yrs	3 doses through age 26 yrs	3 doses through age 21 yrs					
Zoster [6]		Contraindicated	Contraindicated	1 dose	1 dose	1 dose	1 dose	1 dose	1 dose	1 dose	1 dose
Measles, mumps, rubella (MMR) [7]		Contraindicated	Contraindicated	1 or 2 doses	1 or 2 doses	1 or 2 doses	1 or 2 doses	1 or 2 doses	1 or 2 doses	1 or 2 doses	1 or 2 doses
Pneumococcal polysaccharide (PPSV23) [8,9]						1 or 2 doses	1 or 2 doses	1 or 2 doses	1 or 2 doses	1 or 2 doses	
Pneumococcal 13-valent conjugate (PCV13) [10]		1 dose	1 dose	1 dose			1 dose		1 dose		
Meningococcal [11]	1 or more doses	1 or more doses	1 or more doses	1 or more doses	1 or more doses	1 or more doses	1 or more doses	1 or more doses	1 or more doses	1 or more doses	1 or more doses
Hepatitis A [12]	2 doses	2 doses	2 doses	2 doses	2 doses	2 doses	2 doses	2 doses	2 doses	2 doses	2 doses
Hepatitis B [13]	3 doses	3 doses	3 doses	3 doses	3 doses	3 doses	3 doses	3 doses	3 doses	3 doses	3 doses

Legend:

For all persons in this category who meet the age requirements and who lack documentation of vaccination or have no evidence of previous infection; zoster vaccine recommended regardless of prior episode of zoster

Recommended if some other risk factor is present (e.g., on the basis of medical, occupational, lifestyle, or other indications)

No recommendation

These schedules indicate the recommended age groups and medical indications for which administration of currently licensed vaccines is commonly indicated for adults ages 19 years and older, as of January 1, 2013. For all vaccines being recommended on the Adult Immunization Schedule: a vaccine series does not need to be restarted, regardless of the time that has elapsed between doses. Licensed combination vaccines may be used whenever any components of the combination are indicated and when the vaccine's other components are not contraindicated. For detailed recommendations on all vaccines, including those used primarily for travelers or that are issued during the year, consult the manufacturers' package inserts and the complete statements from the Advisory Committee on Immunization Practices (www.cdc.gov/vaccines/pubs/acip-list.htm). Use of trade names and commercial sources is for identification only and does not imply endorsement by the U.S. Department of Health and Human Services.

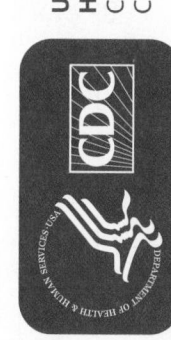

U.S. Department of Health and Human Services
Centers for Disease Control and Prevention

Footnotes — Recommended Immunization Schedule for Adults Aged 19 Years and Older—United States, 2013

1. Additional information
- Additional guidance for the use of the vaccines described is available at http://www.cdc.gov/vaccines/pubs/acip-list.htm.
- Information on vaccination recommendations when vaccination status is unknown and other general immunization information can be found in the General Recommendations on Immunization at http://www.cdc.gov/mmwr/preview/mmwrhtml/rr6002a1.htm.
- Information on travel vaccine requirements and recommendations (eg, for hepatitis A and B, meningococcal, and other vaccines) are available at http://wwwnc.cdc.gov/travel/page/vaccinations.htm.

2. Influenza vaccination
- Annual vaccination against influenza is recommended for all persons aged 6 months and older.
- Persons aged 6 months and older, including pregnant women, can receive the inactivated influenza vaccine (IIV).
- Healthy, nonpregnant persons aged 2–49 years without high-risk medical conditions can receive either intranasally administered live, attenuated influenza vaccine (LAIV) (FluMist), or IIV. Health-care personnel who care for severely immunocompromised persons (i.e., those who require care in a protected environment) should receive IIV rather than LAIV.
- The intramuscularly or intradermally administered IIV are options for adults aged 18–64 years.
- Adults aged 65 years and older can receive the standard dose IIV or the high–dose IIV (Fluzone High-Dose).

3. Tetanus, diphtheria, and acellular pertussis (Td/Tdap) vaccination
- Administer one dose of Tdap vaccine to pregnant women during each pregnancy (preferred during 27–36 weeks' gestation), regardless of number of years since prior Td or Tdap vaccination.
- Administer Tdap to all other adults who have not previously received Tdap or for whom vaccine status is unknown. Tdap can be administered regardless of interval since the most recent tetanus or diphtheria-toxoid containing vaccine.
- Adults with an unknown or incomplete history of completing a 3-dose primary vaccination series with Td-containing vaccines should begin or complete a primary vaccination series including a Tdap dose.
- For unvaccinated adults, administer the first 2 doses at least 4 weeks apart and the third dose 6–12 months after the second.
- For incompletely vaccinated (ie, less than 3 doses) adults, administer remaining doses.
- Refer to the Advisory Committee on Immunization Practices (ACIP) statement for recommendations for administering Td/Tdap as prophylaxis in wound management (see footnote #1).

4. Varicella vaccination
- All adults without evidence of immunity to varicella (as defined below) should receive 2 doses of single-antigen varicella vaccine or a second dose if they have received only 1 dose.
- Special consideration for vaccination should be given to those who have close contact with persons at high risk for severe disease (eg, health-care personnel and family contacts of persons with immunocompromising conditions) or are at high risk for exposure or transmission (eg, teachers; child care employees; residents and staff members of institutional settings, including correctional institutions; college students; military personnel; adolescents and adults living in households with children; nonpregnant women of childbearing age; and international travelers).
- Pregnant women should be assessed for evidence of varicella immunity. Women who do not have evidence of immunity should receive the first dose of varicella vaccine upon completion or termination of pregnancy and before discharge from the health-care facility. The second dose should be administered 4–8 weeks after the first dose.
- Evidence of immunity to varicella in adults includes any of the following:
  — documentation of 2 doses of varicella vaccine at least 4 weeks apart;
  — U.S.-born before 1980 except health-care personnel and pregnant women;
  — history of varicella based on diagnosis or verification of varicella disease by a health-care provider;
  — history of herpes zoster based on diagnosis or verification of herpes zoster disease by a health-care provider; or
  — laboratory evidence of immunity or laboratory confirmation of disease.

(continued)

Table 30–7. Recommended adult immunization schedule—United States, 2014. (continued)

5. Human papillomavirus (HPV) vaccination

- Two vaccines are licensed for use in females, bivalent HPV vaccine (HPV2) and quadrivalent HPV vaccine (HPV4), and one HPV vaccine for use in males (HPV4).
- For females, either HPV4 or HPV2 is recommended in a 3-dose series for routine vaccination at age 11 or 12 years, and for those aged 13 through 26 years, if not previously vaccinated.
- For males, HPV4 is recommended in a 3-dose series for routine vaccination at age 11 or 12 years, and for those aged 13 through 21 years, if not previously vaccinated. Males aged 22 through 26 years may be vaccinated.
- HPV4 is recommended for men who have sex with men (MSM) through age 26 years for those who did not get any or all doses when they were younger.
- Vaccination is recommended for immunocompromised persons (including those with HIV infection) through age 26 years for those who did not get any or all doses when they were younger.
- A complete series for either HPV4 or HPV2 consists of 3 doses. The second dose should be administered 1–2 months after the first dose; the third dose should be administered 6 months after the first dose (at least 24 weeks after the first dose).
- HPV vaccines are not recommended for use in pregnant women. However, pregnancy testing is not needed before vaccination. If a woman is found to be pregnant after initiating the vaccination series, no intervention is needed; the remainder of the 3-dose series should be delayed until completion of pregnancy.
- Although HPV vaccination is not specifically recommended for health-care personnel (HCP) based on their occupation, HCP should receive the HPV vaccine as recommended (see above).

6. Zoster vaccination

- A single dose of zoster vaccine is recommended for adults aged 60 years and older regardless of whether they report a prior episode of herpes zoster. Although the vaccine is licensed by the Food and Drug Administration (FDA) for use among and can be administered to persons aged 50 years and older, ACIP recommends that vaccination begins at age 60 years.
- Persons aged 60 years and older with chronic medical conditions may be vaccinated unless their condition constitutes a contraindication, such as pregnancy or severe immunodeficiency.
- Although zoster vaccination is not specifically recommended for HCP, they should receive the vaccine if they are in the recommended age group.

7. Measles, mumps, rubella (MMR) vaccination

- Adults born before 1957 generally are considered immune to measles and mumps. All adults born in 1957 or later should have documentation of 1 or more doses of MMR vaccine unless they have a medical contraindication to the vaccine, or laboratory evidence of immunity to each of the three diseases. Documentation of provider-diagnosed disease is not considered acceptable evidence of immunity for measles, mumps, or rubella.

Measles component:

- A routine second dose of MMR vaccine, administered a minimum of 28 days after the first dose, is recommended for adults who
  — are students in postsecondary educational institutions;
  — work in a health-care facility; or
  — plan to travel internationally.
- Persons who received inactivated (killed) measles vaccine or measles vaccine of unknown type during 1963–1967 should be revaccinated with 2 doses of MMR vaccine.

Mumps component:

- A routine second dose of MMR vaccine, administered a minimum of 28 days after the first dose, is recommended for adults who
  — are students in a postsecondary educational institution;
  — work in a health-care facility; or
  — plan to travel internationally.
- Persons vaccinated before 1979 with either killed mumps vaccine or mumps vaccine of unknown type who are at high risk for mumps infection (eg, persons who are working in a health-care facility) should be considered for revaccination with 2 doses of MMR vaccine.

Rubella component:

- For women of childbearing age, regardless of birth year, rubella immunity should be determined. If there is no evidence of immunity, women who are not pregnant should be vaccinated. Pregnant women who do not have evidence of immunity should receive MMR vaccine upon completion or termination of pregnancy and before discharge from the health-care facility.

HCP born before 1957:

- For unvaccinated health-care personnel born before 1957 who lack laboratory evidence of measles, mumps, and/or rubella immunity or laboratory confirmation of disease, health-care facilities should consider vaccinating personnel with 2 doses of MMR vaccine at the appropriate interval for measles and mumps or 1 dose of MMR vaccine for rubella.

8. Pneumococcal polysaccharide (PPSV23) vaccination

- Vaccinate all persons with the following indications:
  - — all adults aged 65 years and older;
  - — adults younger than age 65 years with chronic lung disease (including chronic obstructive pulmonary disease, emphysema, and asthma); chronic cardiovascular diseases; diabetes mellitus; chronic liver disease (including cirrhosis); alcoholism; cochlear implants; cerebrospinal fluid leaks; immunocompromising conditions; and functional or anatomic asplenia (eg, sickle cell disease and other hemoglobinopathies, congenital or acquired asplenia, splenic dysfunction, or splenectomy [if elective splenectomy is planned, vaccinate at least 2 weeks before surgery]);
  - — residents of nursing homes or long-term care facilities; and
  - — adults who smoke cigarettes.
- Persons with immunocompromising conditions and other selected conditions are recommended to receive PCV13 and PPSV23 vaccines. See footnote #10 for information on timing of PCV13 and PPSV23 vaccinations.
- Persons with asymptomatic or symptomatic HIV infection should be vaccinated as soon as possible after their diagnosis.
- When cancer chemotherapy or other immunosuppressive therapy is being considered, the interval between vaccination and initiation of immunosuppressive therapy should be at least 2 weeks. Vaccination during chemotherapy or radiation therapy should be avoided.
- Routine use of PPSV23 is not recommended for American Indians/Alaska Natives or other persons younger than age 65 years unless they have underlying medical conditions that are PPSV23 indications. However, public health authorities may consider recommending PPSV23 for American Indians/Alaska Natives who are living in areas where the risk for invasive pneumococcal disease is increased.
- When indicated, PPSV23 should be administered to patients who are uncertain of their vaccination status and there is no record of previous vaccination. When PCV13 is also indicated, a dose of PCV13 should be given first (see footnote #10).

9. Revaccination with PPSV23

- One-time revaccination 5 years after the first dose is recommended for persons aged 19 through 64 years with chronic renal failure or nephrotic syndrome; functional or anatomic asplenia (eg, sickle cell disease or splenectomy); and for persons with immunocompromising conditions.
- Persons who received 1 or 2 doses of PPSV23 before age 65 years for any indication should receive another dose of the vaccine at age 65 years or later if at least 5 years have passed since their previous dose.
- No further doses are needed for persons vaccinated with PPSV23 at or after age 65 years.

10. Pneumococcal conjugate 13-valent vaccination (PCV13)

- Adults aged 19 years or older with immunocompromising conditions (including chronic renal failure and nephrotic syndrome), functional or anatomic asplenia, CSF leaks or cochlear implants, and who have not previously received PCV13 or PPSV23 should receive a single dose of PCV13 followed by a dose of PPSV23 at least 8 weeks later.
- Adults aged 19 years or older with the aforementioned conditions who have previously received one or more doses of PPSV23 should receive a dose of PCV13 one or more years after the last PPSV23 dose was received. For those that require additional doses of PPSV23, the first such dose should be given no sooner than 8 weeks after PCV13 and at least 5 years since the most recent dose of PPSV23.
- When indicated, PCV13 should be administered to patients who are uncertain of their vaccination status history and there is no record of previous vaccination.
- Although PCV13 is licensed by the Food and Drug Administration (FDA) for use among and can be administered to persons aged 50 years and older, ACIP recommends PCV13 for adults aged 19 years and older with the specific medical conditions noted above.

11. Meningococcal vaccination

- Administer 2 doses of meningococcal conjugate vaccine quadrivalent (MCV4) at least 2 months apart to adults with functional asplenia or persistent complement component deficiencies.
- HIV-infected persons who are vaccinated also should receive 2 doses.
- Administer a single dose of meningococcal vaccine to microbiologists routinely exposed to isolates of *Neisseria meningitidis*, military recruits, and persons who travel to or live in countries in which meningococcal disease is hyperendemic or epidemic.
- First-year college students up through age 21 years who are living in residence halls should be vaccinated if they have not received a dose on or after their 16th birthday.
- MCV4 is preferred for adults with any of the preceding indications who are aged 55 years and younger; meningococcal polysaccharide vaccine (MPSV4) is preferred for adults aged 56 years and older.
- Revaccination with MCV4 every 5 years is recommended for adults previously vaccinated with MCV4 or MPSV4 who remain at increased risk for infection (e.g., adults with anatomic or functional asplenia or persistent complement component deficiencies).

(continued)

Table 30–7. Recommended adult immunization schedule—United States, 2014. (continued)

12. Hepatitis A vaccination

- Vaccinate any person seeking protection from hepatitis A virus (HAV) infection and persons with any of the following indications:
  - men who have sex with men and persons who use injection or noninjection illicit drugs;
  - persons working with HAV-infected primates or with HAV in a research laboratory setting;
  - persons with chronic liver disease and persons who receive clotting factor concentrates;
  - persons traveling to or working in countries that have high or intermediate endemicity of hepatitis A; and
  - unvaccinated persons who anticipate close personal contact (eg, household or regular babysitting) with an international adoptee during the first 60 days after arrival in the United States from a country with high or intermediate endemicity. (See footnote #1 for more information on travel recommendations). The first dose of the 2-dose hepatitis A vaccine series should be administered as soon as adoption is planned, ideally 2 or more weeks before the arrival of the adoptee.

- Single-antigen vaccine formulations should be administered in a 2-dose schedule at either 0 and 6–12 months (Havrix), or 0 and 6–18 months (Vaqta). If the combined hepatitis A and hepatitis B vaccine (Twinrix) is used, administer 3 doses at 0, 1, and 6 months; alternatively, a 4-dose schedule may be used, administered on days 0, 7, and 21–30, followed by a booster dose at month 12.

13. Hepatitis B vaccination

- Vaccinate persons with any of the following indications and any person seeking protection from hepatitis B virus (HBV) infection:
  - sexually active persons who are not in a long-term, mutually monogamous relationship (eg, persons with more than one sex partner during the previous 6 months); persons seeking evaluation or treatment for a sexually transmitted disease (STD); current or recent injection-drug users; and men who have sex with men;
  - health-care personnel and public-safety workers who are potentially exposed to blood or other infectious body fluids;
  - persons with diabetes younger than age 60 years as soon as feasible after diagnosis; persons with diabetes who are age 60 years or older at the discretion of the treating clinician based on increased need for assisted blood glucose monitoring in long-term care facilities, likelihood of acquiring hepatitis B infection, its complications or chronic sequelae, and likelihood of immune response to vaccination;
  - persons with end-stage renal disease, including patients receiving hemodialysis; persons with HIV infection; and persons with chronic liver disease;
  - household contacts and sex partners of hepatitis B surface antigen-positive persons; clients and staff members of institutions for persons with developmental disabilities; and international travelers to countries with high or intermediate prevalence of chronic HBV infection; and
  - all adults in the following settings: STD treatment facilities; HIV testing and treatment facilities; facilities providing drug-abuse treatment and prevention services; health-care settings targeting services to injection-drug users or men who have sex with men; correctional facilities; end-stage renal disease programs and facilities for chronic hemodialysis patients; and institutions and nonresidential daycare facilities for persons with developmental disabilities.

- Administer missing doses to complete a 3-dose series of hepatitis B vaccine to those persons not vaccinated or not completely vaccinated. The second dose should be administered 1 month after the first dose; the third dose should be given at least 2 months after the second dose (and at least 4 months after the first dose). If the combined hepatitis A and hepatitis B vaccine (Twinrix) is used, give 3 doses at 0, 1, and 6 months; alternatively, a 4-dose Twinrix schedule, administered on days 0, 7, and 21–30 followed by a booster dose at month 12 may be used.

- Adult patients receiving hemodialysis or with other immunocompromising conditions should receive 1 dose of 40 μg/mL (Recombivax HB) administered on a 3-dose schedule at 0, 1, and 6 months or 2 doses of 20 μg/mL (Engerix-B) administered simultaneously on a 4-dose schedule at 0, 1, 2, and 6 months.

14. Selected conditions for which Haemophilus influenzae type b (Hib) vaccine may be used

- 1 dose of Hib vaccine should be considered for persons who have sickle cell disease, leukemia, or HIV infection, or who have anatomic or functional asplenia if they have not previously received Hib vaccine.

15. Immunocompromising conditions

- Inactivated vaccines generally are acceptable (eg, pneumococcal, meningococcal, and influenza [inactivated influenza vaccine]), and live vaccines generally are avoided in persons with immune deficiencies or immunocompromising conditions. Information on specific conditions is available at http://www.cdc.gov/vaccines/pubs/acip-list.htm.

1. Healthy Adults

Vaccination recommendations are made by the Advisory Committee on Immunization Practices (ACIP) of the US Centers for Disease Control and Prevention (Table 30–7).

2. Pregnant Women

Given the uncertainty of risks to the fetus, vaccination during pregnancy is generally avoided with the following exceptions: tetanus (transfer of maternal antibodies across the placenta important to prevent neonatal tetanus), diphtheria, and influenza. Live vaccines are avoided during pregnancy.

Influenza can be a serious infection if acquired in pregnancy, and all pregnant women should be offered influenza (inactivated) vaccination. The live attenuated (intranasal) influenza vaccine is not recommended during pregnancy.

3. HIV-Infected Adults

HIV-infected patients have impaired cellular and B cell responses. Inactivated or killed vaccinations can generally be given without any consequence, but the recipient may not be able to mount an adequate antibody response. Live or attenuated vaccines are generally avoided with some exceptions (ie, in patients with CD4+ T lymphocytes > 200 cells/mcL). Guidelines for vaccinating HIV-infected patients have been issued jointly by the Centers for Disease Control and Prevention, the US National Institutes of Health, and the HIV Medical Association of the Infectious Diseases Society of America. Timing of vaccination is important to optimize response. If possible, vaccination should be given early in the course of HIV-disease or following immune reconstitution.

4. Hematopoietic Cell Transplant Recipients

Hematopoietic cell transplant (HCT) recipients have varying rates of immune reconstitution following transplantation, depending on (1) the type of chemotherapy or radiotherapy used pretransplant (in autologous HCT), (2) the preparative regimen used for the transplant (3) whether graft-versus-host disease is present, and (4) the type of immunosuppression used posttransplantation (in allogeneic HCT). Vaccines may not work immediately in the posttransplant period. B cells may take 3–12 months to return to normal posttransplant, and naïve T cells that can respond to new antigens only appear 6–12 months posttransplant. B cells of posttransplant patients treated with rituximab may take up to 6 months to fully recover after the last dose of the drug. Vaccines are therefore administered 6–12 months following transplantation with a minimum of 1 month between doses to maximize the probability of response.

5. Solid Organ Transplant Recipients

Solid organ transplant recipients demonstrate a broad spectrum of immunosuppression, depending on the reason for and type of organ transplanted and the nature of the immunosuppression (including T-cell depleting agents during treatment of organ rejection). These factors affect the propensity for infection posttransplantation and the ability to develop antibody responses to vaccination. In many cases, the time between placing a patient on a transplant list and undergoing the transplantation takes months or years. Providers should take this opportunity to ensure that indicated vaccines are given during this pretransplant period to optimize antibody responses. If this is not possible, most experts give vaccines 3–6 months following transplantation. Live vaccines are contraindicated in the posttransplant period.

RECOMMENDED IMMUNIZATIONS FOR TRAVELERS

Individuals traveling to other countries frequently require immunizations in addition to those routinely recommended and may benefit from chemoprophylaxis against various diseases. Vaccinations against yellow fever and meningococcus are the only ones required by certain countries. These and other travel-specific vaccines are listed http://wwwnc.cdc.gov/travel/page/vaccinations.htm.

Various vaccines can be given simultaneously at different sites. Some, such as cholera, plague, and typhoid vaccine, cause significant discomfort and are best given at different times. In general, live attenuated vaccines (measles, mumps, rubella, yellow fever, and oral typhoid vaccine) should not be given to immunosuppressed individuals or household members of immunosuppressed people or to pregnant women. Immunoglobulin should not be given for 3 months before or at least 2 weeks after live virus vaccines, because it may attenuate the antibody response.

Chemoprophylaxis of malaria is discussed in Chapter 35.

▶ Cholera

Because cholera among travelers is rare and the vaccine marginally effective, the World Health Organization (WHO) does not require immunization for persons traveling to endemic areas or to areas with recent outbreaks (eg, Haiti). No country requires vaccination for entry, but some local authorities may require documentation for entry. In such cases, a medical waiver will suffice or a single dose of the oral vaccine is usually sufficient.

▶ Hepatitis B

The risk of hepatitis B infection for most international travelers is low. Hepatitis B vaccination should be considered for those traveling to areas with high (≥ 8%) or intermediate (2–7%) rates of endemic hepatitis B infection if the individual will have contact with blood or secretions, have unprotected sex, or will be using illicit drugs. Examples of high and intermediate risk areas include all of Africa and most of South Asia and the Middle East. Vaccination should begin at least 6 months before travel to allow for completion of the series.

Hepatitis A

Protection is recommended for susceptible persons traveling to areas where sanitation is poor and the risk of exposure to hepatitis A high because of contaminated food and water supplies and contact with infected persons (eg, anywhere except Canada, western Europe, Japan, Australia, and New Zealand). Either hepatitis A vaccine or immunoglobulin can be used, although vaccination is preferred. The first dose of vaccine should be given as soon as travel is considered. In healthy individuals, a single dose of vaccine administered any time prior to travel will provide adequate protection. In older patients, those who are immunocompromised, and those with chronic liver disease or other chronic medical problems who are planning to travel in 2 weeks or less should receive hepatitis A vaccine and immunoglobulin 0.02 mL/kg simultaneously at different anatomic sites. Those who choose not to receive vaccine should receive immunoglobulin.

Meningococcal Meningitis

If travel is contemplated to an area where meningococcal meningitis is epidemic (Nepal, sub-Saharan Africa, the "meningitis belt" from Senegal in the west to Ethiopia in the east, northern India) or highly endemic, vaccination with MCV4 is indicated for those 2–55 years of age, otherwise MPSV should be used. (Saudi Arabia requires immunization for pilgrims to Mecca.)

Plague

The risk of plague is so small to travelers that vaccine is no longer commercially available and vaccination is not required for entry into any country. Travelers at unavoidable high risk of exposure to rodents should consider chemoprophylaxis with doxycycline or TMP-SMZ.

Poliomyelitis

Polio remains endemic in five countries (Afghanistan, India, Pakistan, Nigeria, and Niger), and sporadic outbreaks from reinfection continues to occur in Somalia, Ethiopia, Angola, and Bangladesh. Adults traveling to endemic or epidemic areas who have not previously been immunized against poliomyelitis should receive a primary series of three doses of inactivated enhanced-potency poliovaccine (IPV). Travelers who have previously been fully immunized with oral polio vaccine (OPV) or inactivated polio vaccine (IPV) should receive a one-time booster dose with IPV. Live attenuated poliovaccine is no longer recommended because of the risk of vaccine-associated disease and is no longer available in the United States, although it continues to be used in many other countries.

Rabies

For travelers to areas where rabies is common in domestic animals (eg, India, Asia, Mexico, Africa, areas of Central and South America), with extensive outdoor activities or certain professional activities (veterinarians, animal handlers, field biologists), preexposure prophylaxis with human diploid cell vaccine (HDCV), rabies vaccine adsorbed (RVA), or purified chick embryo cell culture (PCEC) vaccine should be considered. Chloroquine can blunt the immunologic response to rabies vaccine. If malaria prophylaxis with chloroquine (or mefloquine) is required, vaccination should be given intramuscularly (*not* intradermally) to ensure adequate antibody response.

Typhoid

Typhoid vaccination is recommended for travelers to developing countries (especially the Indian subcontinent, Asia, Africa, Central and South America, and the Caribbean) who will have prolonged exposure to contaminated food and water. Two preparations of approximately equal efficacy (50–75% effective) are available in the United States: (1) an oral live attenuated Ty21a vaccine supplied as enteric-coated capsules, and (2) a Vi capsular polysaccharide (Vi CPS) vaccine for parenteral use. The Ty21a vaccine is given as one capsule every other day for four doses. The capsules must be refrigerated and taken with cool liquids (37°C or less) at least 1 hour before meals. All four doses must be taken for maximum protection and should be completed 1 week before travel. It is not recommended for infants or children younger than 6 years. The Vi CPS vaccine is given as a single intramuscular injection at least 2 weeks prior to travel. It is not recommended for infants younger than 2 years. If continued or repeated exposures are anticipated, boosters are recommended every 2 years for the Vi CPS and every 5 years for the Ty21a. The live attenuated vaccine should not be used in immunosuppressed patients, including those with HIV infection.

Yellow Fever

The live attenuated yellow fever virus vaccine is administered once subcutaneously. Although the risk of yellow fever is low for most travelers, a number of countries require vaccination for all visitors and others require it for travelers to or from endemic areas (mainly equatorial Africa and parts of South and Central America). The WHO certificate requires registration of the manufacturer and the batch number of the vaccine. Vaccination is available in the United States only at approved centers; the local health department should be contacted for available resources. Reimmunization is recommended at 10-year intervals if continued risk exists.

Because it is a live attenuated vaccine prepared in embryonated eggs, the yellow fever vaccine should not be given to immunosuppressed individuals or those with a history of anaphylaxis to eggs. Pregnancy is a relative contraindication to vaccination.

Two very severe adverse reactions have been associated with yellow fever vaccination. Viscerotropic disease presents with fever, jaundice, and multiple organ system failure within 30 days of yellow fever vaccination. Clinically and histopathologically, the illness is identical to yellow fever and is associated with a high mortality rate. The other adverse reaction is neurotropic disease and presents as encephalitis, encephalomyelitis, and Guillain-Barré syndrome.

▶ Japanese B Encephalitis

Japanese B encephalitis is a mosquito-borne viral encephalitis that affects primarily children and older adults (65 years and older) and usually occurs from May to September. It is the leading cause of encephalitis in Asia. Because the risk of infection is low and because adverse effects of the vaccine can be serious, not all travelers to Asia should be vaccinated. Vaccine should be given to travelers to endemic areas who will be staying at least 30 days and who are traveling during the transmission season, particularly if they are visiting rural areas. Travelers who spend < 30 days in the region should be considered for vaccination if they intend to visit areas of epidemic transmission or if extensive outdoor activities are planned in

rural rice-growing areas. Of the two vaccines currently available in the United States, only one is for adults (inactivated Vero cell derived vaccine, IXIARO) aged 17 and older. The schedule is 0.5 mL intramuscularly at 0 and 28 days. Only children are eligible to receive the other vaccine (inactivated mouse brain derived vaccine, JE-VAX) given its limited supply in the United States.

VACCINE SAFETY

Most vaccines are safe to administer. In general, it is recommended that the use of live vaccines be avoided in immunocompromised patients, including pregnant women. Vaccines are generally not contraindicated in the following situations: mild, acute illness with low-grade fevers (< 40.5°C); concurrent antibiotic therapy; soreness or redness at the site; family history of adverse reactions to vaccinations. Absolute contraindications to vaccines are rare (Table 30–8).

Table 30–8. Adverse effects and contraindications to vaccinations.

Vaccine	Adverse Effects	Contraindications
Hepatitis A	Minimal Consist mainly of pain at the injection site	
Hepatitis B	Minimal Consist mainly of pain at the injection site	Hypersensitivity to yeast Severe reaction to a previous dose
Human papillomavirus	Minimal Consists mainly of mild to moderate localized pain, erythema, swelling Systemic reactions, mainly fever, seen in 4% of recipients	History of hypersensitivity to yeast or to any vaccine component
Influenza (intramuscular inactivated and intranasal live attenuated vaccines)	**Intramuscular, inactivated vaccine:** Local reactions (erythema and tenderness) at the site of injection common, but fevers, chills, and malaise (which last in any case only 2–3 days) rare. **Either inactivated or live attenuated vaccine:** A potential association between Guillain-Barré syndrome (3,000–6,000 cases per year in the US, usually following respiratory infections) and vaccination with intramuscular, inactivated influenza vaccine has been reported (possibly, 1–2 persons per million persons vaccinated), but this rate is lower than the risk of the syndrome developing after influenza itself (given that approximately 750 persons per million adults are hospitalized annually with influenza, and many more cases remain as outpatients). Influenza vaccination may be associated with multiple false-positive serologic tests to HIV, HTLV-1, and hepatitis C, but it is self-limited, lasting 2–5 months.	Intranasal, live attenuated vaccine [FluMist] should not be used in: People 50 years of age and over Household members of immunosuppressed individuals Health care workers, or others with close contact with immunosuppressed persons Presence of reactive airway disease; chronic underlying metabolic, pulmonary, or cardiovascular diseases (use intramuscular inactivated vaccine) Long-term aspirin therapy in children or adolescents (because of the risk of Reye syndrome) Pregnancy[1] Contraindication to both inactivated and live attenuated vaccine: History of Guillain-Barré syndrome, especially within 6 weeks of receiving a previous influenza vaccine History of egg allergy[2]
Measles, mumps, and rubella (MMR)[3]	Fever will develop in about 5–15% of unimmunized individuals, and a mild rash will develop in about 5% 5–12 days after vaccination. Fever and rash are self-limiting, lasting only 2–3 days. Local swelling and induration are particularly common in individuals previously vaccinated with inactivated vaccine.	Pregnancy[4] Immunosuppressed persons should not be vaccinated (with the exception of asymptomatic HIV-infected individuals whose CD4 count is > 200/mcL). History of anaphylaxis to neomycin or to related agents such as streptomycin

(continued)

Table 30–8. Adverse effects and contraindications to vaccinations. (continued)

Vaccine	Adverse Effects	Contraindications
Meningococcal	Minor reactions (fever, redness, swelling, erythema, pain) occur slightly more commonly with MCV4. Major reactions are rare. A potential association between Guillain-Barré syndrome (3,000–6,000 cases per year in the US, usually following respiratory infections) and vaccination with MCV4 has been reported, but current recommendations favor continued use of MCV4, since the benefits of preventing the serious consequences of meningococcal infection outweigh the theoretical risk of Guillain-Barré syndrome.	Persons with history of adverse reaction to diphtheria toxoid should not receive MCV4 since the protein conjugate used in MCV4 is diphtheria toxoid
Pneumococcal (polysaccharide)	Mild local reactions (erythema and tenderness) occur in up to 50% of recipients, but systemic reactions are uncommon. Similarly, revaccination at least 5 years after initial vaccination is associated with mild self-limited local but not systemic reactions.	Revaccination is not recommended for those who had a severe reaction (anaphylaxis or Arthus reaction) to the initial vaccination.
Tetanus, diphtheria, and pertussis	Minimal Consist mainly of pain at the injection site	Any history of anaphylaxis to vaccine components or if there is a history of unexplained encephalitis within 7 days of administration of a pertussis-containing vaccine.
Varicella	Can occur as late as 4–6 weeks after vaccination. Tenderness and erythema at the injection site are seen in 25%, fever in 10–15%, and a localized maculopapular or vesicular rash in 5%; a diffuse rash, usually with five or fewer vesicular lesions, develops in a smaller percentage. Spread of virus from vaccinees to susceptible individuals is possible, but the risk of such transmission even to immunocompromised patients is small and disease, when it develops, is mild and treatable with acyclovir.	Allergy to neomycin Avoid in immunocompromised individuals, including HIV-positive children and adults, or pregnant women. For theoretic reasons, it is recommended that salicylates should be avoided for 6 weeks following vaccination (to prevent Reye syndrome).
Zoster	Mild and limited to local reactions Although it is theoretically possible to transmit the virus to susceptible contacts, no such cases have been reported.	Presence of primary or acquired immunodeficiency state (leukemia, lymphoma, any malignant neoplasm affecting the bone marrow, HIV infection) Therapy with immunosuppressive medications (including high-dose corticosteroids) Pregnancy Persons with an anaphylactic type reaction to gelatin or neomycin should not receive the vaccine.

[1]The inactivated influenza vaccine can be given during any trimester.
[2]The vaccine has typically been prepared using embryonated chicken eggs. However, new vaccine using mammalian cell culture now FDA-approved.
[3]MMR vaccine can be safely given to patients with a history of egg allergy even when severe.
[4]Although vaccination of pregnant women is **not** recommended, with the currently available RA27/3 vaccine strain the congenital rubella syndrome does not occur in the offspring of those inadvertently vaccinated during pregnancy or within 3 months before conception.

Bridges CB et al; Immunization Services Division, National Center for Immunization and Respiratory Diseases, CDC. Advisory committee on immunization practices recommended immunization schedule for adults aged 19 years or older—United States, 2014. MMWR Morb Mortal Wkly Rep. 2014 Feb 7;63(5):110–2. [PMID: 24500291]

Centers for Disease Control and Prevention (CDC). Adult immunization schedules—United States, 2014. http://www.cdc.gov/vaccines/schedules/hcp/adult.html
Centers for Disease Control and Prevention (CDC). Health Information for International Travel 2014. http://wwwnc.cdc.gov/travel/page/yellowbook-home-2014

Centers for Disease Control and Prevention (CDC). Vaccine safety. http://www.cdc.gov/vaccinesafety/

Kaplan JE et al. Guidelines for prevention and treatment of opportunistic infections in HIV-infected adults and adolescents: recommendations from CDC, the National Institutes of Health, and the HIV Medicine Association of the Infectious Diseases Society of America. MMWR Recomm Rep. 2009 Apr 10; 58(RR-4):1–207. [PMID: 19357635]

LaRocque RC et al; Global TravEpiNet Consortium. Pre-travel health care of immigrants returning home to visit friends and relatives. Am J Trop Med Hyg. 2013 Feb;88(2):376–80.

Erratum in: Am J Trop Med Hyg. 2013 Mar;88(3):606. [PMID: 23149585]

Palefsky JM et al. HPV vaccine against anal HPV infection and anal intraepithelial neoplasia. N Engl J Med. 2011 Oct 27; 365(17):1576–85. [PMID: 22029979]

Shefer A et al. Updated recommendations of the Advisory Committee on Immunization Practices for healthcare personnel vaccination: a necessary foundation for the essential work that remains to build successful programs. Infect Control Hosp Epidemiol. 2012 Jan;33(1):71–4. [PMID: 22173525]

HIV Infection & AIDS

Mitchell H. Katz, MD

Andrew R. Zolopa, MD

ESSENTIALS OF DIAGNOSIS

▶ Risk factors: sexual contact with an infected person, parenteral exposure to infected blood by transfusion or needle sharing, perinatal exposure.

▶ Prominent systemic complaints such as sweats, diarrhea, weight loss, and wasting.

▶ Opportunistic infections due to diminished cellular immunity—often life-threatening.

▶ Aggressive cancers, particularly Kaposi sarcoma and extranodal lymphoma.

▶ Neurologic manifestations, including dementia, aseptic meningitis, and neuropathy.

General Considerations

The Centers for Disease Control and Prevention (CDC) AIDS case definition (Table 31–1) includes opportunistic infections and malignancies that rarely occur in the absence of severe immunodeficiency (eg, *Pneumocystis* pneumonia, central nervous system lymphoma). It also classifies persons as having AIDS if they have positive HIV serology and certain infections and malignancies that can occur in immunocompetent hosts but that are more common among persons infected with HIV (pulmonary tuberculosis, invasive cervical cancer). Several nonspecific conditions, including dementia and wasting (documented weight loss)—in the presence of a positive HIV serology—are considered AIDS. The definition includes criteria for both definitive and presumptive diagnoses of certain infections and malignancies. Finally, persons with positive HIV serology who have ever had a CD4 lymphocyte count below 200 cells/mcL or a CD4 lymphocyte percentage below 14% are considered to have AIDS. Inclusion of persons with low CD4 counts as AIDS cases reflects the recognition that **immunodeficiency is the defining characteristic of AIDS.** The choice of a cutoff point at 200 cells/mcL is supported by several cohort studies showing that AIDS will develop within 3 years in over 80% of persons with counts below this level in the absence of effective antiretroviral therapy (ART). The prognosis of persons with HIV/AIDS has dramatically improved due to the introduction of highly active antiretroviral therapy (HAART) in the mid 1990s. One consequence is that fewer persons with HIV ever develop an infection or malignancy or have a low enough CD4 count to classify them as having AIDS, which means that the CDC definition has become a less useful measure of the impact of HIV/AIDS in the United States. Conversely, persons in whom AIDS had been diagnosed based on a serious opportunistic infection, malignancy, or immunodeficiency may now be markedly healthier, with high CD4 counts, due to the use of HAART. Therefore, the Social Security Administration as well as most social service agencies focus on functional assessment for determining eligibility for benefits rather than the simple presence or absence of an AIDS-defining illness.

Epidemiology

The modes of transmission of HIV are similar to those of hepatitis B, in particular with respect to sexual, parenteral, and vertical transmission. Although certain sexual practices (eg, receptive anal intercourse) are significantly riskier than other sexual practices (eg, oral sex), it is difficult to quantify per-contact risks. The reason is that studies of sexual transmission of HIV show that most people at risk for HIV infection engage in a variety of sexual practices and have sex with multiple persons, only some of whom may actually be HIV infected. Thus, it is difficult to determine which practice with which person actually resulted in HIV transmission.

Nonetheless, the best available estimates indicate that the risk of HIV transmission with receptive anal intercourse is between 1:100 and 1:30, with insertive anal intercourse 1:1000, with receptive vaginal intercourse 1:1000, with insertive vaginal intercourse 1:10,000, and with receptive fellatio with ejaculation 1:1000. The per-contact risk of HIV transmission with other behaviors, including receptive fellatio without ejaculation, insertive fellatio, and cunnilingus, is not known.

All per-contact risk estimates assume that the source is HIV infected. If the HIV status of the source is unknown, the risk of transmission is the risk of transmission multiplied by the probability that the source is HIV infected.

Table 31–1. CDC AIDS case definition for surveillance of adults and adolescents.

Definitive AIDS diagnoses (with or without laboratory evidence of HIV infection)

1. Candidiasis of the esophagus, trachea, bronchi, or lungs.

2. Cryptococcosis, extrapulmonary.

3. Cryptosporidiosis with diarrhea persisting > 1 month.

4. Cytomegalovirus disease of an organ other than liver, spleen, or lymph nodes.

5. Herpes simplex virus infection causing a mucocutaneous ulcer that persists longer than 1 month; or bronchitis, pneumonitis, or esophagitis of any duration.

6. Kaposi sarcoma in a patient < 60 years of age.

7. Lymphoma of the brain (primary) in a patient < 60 years of age.

8. *Mycobacterium avium* complex or *Mycobacterium kansasii* disease, disseminated (at a site other than or in addition to lungs, skin, or cervical or hilar lymph nodes).

9. *Pneumocystis jirovecii* pneumonia.

10. Progressive multifocal leukoencephalopathy.

11. Toxoplasmosis of the brain.

Definitive AIDS diagnoses (with laboratory evidence of HIV infection)

1. Coccidioidomycosis, disseminated (at a site other than or in addition to lungs or cervical or hilar lymph nodes).

2. HIV encephalopathy.

3. Histoplasmosis, disseminated (at a site other than or in addition to lungs or cervical or hilar lymph nodes).

4. Isosporiasis with diarrhea persisting > 1 month.

5. Kaposi sarcoma at any age.

6. Lymphoma of the brain (primary) at any age.

7. Other non-Hodgkin lymphoma of B cell or unknown immunologic phenotype.

8. Any mycobacterial disease caused by mycobacteria other than *Mycobacterium tuberculosis*, disseminated (at a site other than or in addition to lungs, skin, or cervical or hilar lymph nodes).

9. Disease caused by extrapulmonary *M tuberculosis*.

10. *Salmonella* (nontyphoid) septicemia, recurrent.

11. HIV wasting syndrome.

12. CD4 lymphocyte count below 200 cells/mcL or a CD4 lymphocyte percentage below 14%.

13. Pulmonary tuberculosis.

14. Recurrent pneumonia.

15. Invasive cervical cancer.

Presumptive AIDS diagnoses (with laboratory evidence of HIV infection)

1. Candidiasis of esophagus: (a) recent onset of retrosternal pain on swallowing; and (b) oral candidiasis.

2. Cytomegalovirus retinitis. A characteristic appearance on serial ophthalmoscopic examinations.

3. Mycobacteriosis. Specimen from stool or normally sterile body fluids or tissue from a site other than lungs, skin, or cervical or hilar lymph nodes, showing acid-fast bacilli of a species not identified by culture.

4. Kaposi sarcoma. Erythematous or violaceous plaque-like lesion on skin or mucous membrane.

5. *Pneumocystis jirovecii* pneumonia: (a) a history of dyspnea on exertion or nonproductive cough of recent onset (within the past 3 months); and (b) chest film evidence of diffuse bilateral interstitial infiltrates or gallium scan evidence of diffuse bilateral pulmonary disease; and (c) arterial blood gas analysis showing an arterial oxygen partial pressure of < 70 mm Hg or a low respiratory diffusing capacity of < 80% of predicted values or an increase in the alveolar-arterial oxygen tension gradient; and (d) no evidence of a bacterial pneumonia.

6. Toxoplasmosis of the brain: (a) recent onset of a focal neurologic abnormality consistent with intracranial disease or a reduced level of consciousness; and (b) brain imaging evidence of a lesion having a mass effect or the radiographic appearance of which is enhanced by injection of contrast medium; and (c) serum antibody to toxoplasmosis or successful response to therapy for toxoplasmosis.

7. Recurrent pneumonia: (a) more than one episode in a 1-year period; and (b) acute pneumonia (new symptoms, signs, or radiologic evidence not present earlier) diagnosed on clinical or radiologic grounds by the patient's clinician.

8. Pulmonary tuberculosis: (a) apical or miliary infiltrates and (b) radiographic and clinical response to antituberculous therapy.

This would vary by risk practices, age, and geographic area. A number of cofactors are known to increase the risk of HIV transmission during a given encounter, including the presence of ulcerative or inflammatory sexually transmitted diseases, trauma, menses, and lack of male circumcision.

The risk of acquiring HIV infection from a needlestick with infected blood is approximately 1:300. Factors known to increase the risk of transmission include depth of penetration, hollow bore needles, visible blood on the needle, and advanced stage of disease in the source. The risk of HIV transmission from a mucosal splash with infected blood is unknown but is assumed to be significantly lower.

The risk of acquiring HIV infection from illicit drug use with sharing of needles from an HIV-infected source is estimated to be 1:150. Use of clean needles markedly decreases the chance of HIV transmission but does not eliminate it if other drug paraphernalia are shared (eg, cookers).

When blood transfusion from an HIV-infected donor occurs, the risk of transmission is 95%. Fortunately, since 1985, blood donor screening using the HIV enzyme-linked immunosorbent assay (ELISA) has been universally practiced in the United States. Also, persons who have recently engaged in unsafe behaviors (eg, sex with a person at risk for HIV, injection drug use) are not allowed to donate. This essentially eliminates donations from persons who are HIV infected but have not yet developed antibodies (ie, persons in the "window" period). HIV antigen and viral load testing have been added to the screening of blood to further lower the chance of HIV transmission. With these precautions, the chance of HIV transmission with receipt of blood transfusion in the United States is about 1:1,000,000. Between 13% and 40% of children born to HIV-infected mothers contract HIV infection when the mother has not received treatment or when the child has not received perinatal HIV prophylaxis. The risk is higher with vaginal than with cesarean delivery, higher among mothers with high viral loads, and higher among those who breast-feed their children. The combination of prenatal HIV testing and counseling, antiretroviral treatment for infected mothers during pregnancy and for the infant immediately after birth, scheduled cesarean delivery when the mother has a viral load of >1000 copies/mL, and avoidance of breast-feeding has reduced the rate of perinatal transmission of HIV to less than 2% in the United States and Europe (see below).

HIV has not been shown to be transmitted by respiratory droplet spread, by vectors such as mosquitoes, or by casual nonsexual contact.

There are an estimated 1,148,200 Americans aged 13 years or older living with HIV infection and about 50,000 new infections each year. There are an estimated 487,692 persons in the United States living with AIDS. Of those, 76% are men, of whom 63% were exposed through male-to-male sexual contact, 16% were exposed through injection drug use, 11% were exposed through heterosexual contact, and 8% were exposed through male-to-male sexual contact and injection drug use. Women account for 24% of living persons with HIV infection, of whom 68%

were infected through heterosexual contact and 29% were exposed through injection drug use. Children under the age of 13 account for < 0.1% of living cases. African Americans have been disproportionately hard hit by the epidemic. The estimated rate of new AIDS cases in the United States per 100,000 is 41.6 among African Americans, 12.9 among persons of multiple races, 12.2 among Latinos, 9.3 among native Hawaiians and Pacific Islanders, 6.4 among native Americans and native Alaskans, 4.2 among whites, 3.3 among Asians. In general, the progression of HIV-related illness is similar in men and women. However, there are some important differences. Women are at risk for gynecologic complications of HIV, including recurrent candidal vaginitis, pelvic inflammatory disease, and cervical dysplasia. Violence directed against women, pregnancy, and frequent occurrence of drug use and poverty all complicate the treatment of HIV-infected women. Although "safer sex" campaigns dramatically decreased the rates of seroconversions among men who have sex with men (MSM) living in metropolitan areas in the United States by the mid 1980s, relapse to unsafe sexual practices among MSM in several large cities in the United States and in western Europe has been observed. The higher rates of unsafe sex appear to be related to decreased concern about acquiring HIV due to the availability of HAART. Decreased interest in following safer sex recommendations and increasing use of crystal methamphetamine among certain risk groups also appears to be playing a role in the increased unsafe sex rates.

Worldwide there are an estimated 33 million persons infected with HIV, with heterosexual spread being the most common mode of transmission for men and women. In Central and East Africa, in some urban areas, as many as one-third of sexually active adults are infected. The reason for the greater risk for transmission with heterosexual intercourse in Africa and Asia than in the United States may relate to cofactors such as general health status, the presence of genital ulcers, relative lack of male circumcision, the number of sexual partners, and different HIV serotypes.

Centers for Disease Control and Prevention: HIV Surveillance Report, 2011; vol 23. http://www.cdc.gov/hiv/topics/surveillance/resources/reports/. Published February 2013.

Panel on treatment of HIV-infected pregnant women and prevention of perinatal transmission. Recommendations for use of antiretroviral drugs in pregnant HIV-1-infected women for maternal health and interventions to reduce perinatal HIV-1 transmission in the United States. July 31, 2012 Guideline. http://aidsinfo.nih.gov/contentfiles/lvguidelines/PerinatalGL.pdf

► **Pathophysiology**

Clinically, the syndromes caused by HIV infection are usually explicable by one of three known mechanisms: immunodeficiency, autoimmunity, and allergic and hypersensitivity reactions.

A. Immunodeficiency

Immunodeficiency is a direct result of the effects of HIV upon immune cells as well as the indirect impact of a generalized state of inflammation and immune activation due to chronic viral infection. A spectrum of infections and neoplasms is seen, as in other congenital or acquired immunodeficiency states. Two remarkable features of HIV immunodeficiency are the low incidence of certain infections such as listeriosis and aspergillosis and the frequent occurrence of certain neoplasms such as lymphoma or Kaposi sarcoma. This latter complication has been seen primarily in MSM or in bisexual men, and its incidence steadily declined through the first 15 years of the epidemic. A herpesvirus (KSHV or HHV-8) is the cause of Kaposi sarcoma.

B. Autoimmunity/Allergic and Hypersensitivity Reactions

Autoimmunity can occur as a result of disordered cellular immune function or B lymphocyte dysfunction. Examples of both lymphocytic infiltration of organs (eg, lymphocytic interstitial pneumonitis) and autoantibody production (eg, immunologic thrombocytopenia) occur. These phenomena may be the only clinically apparent disease or may coexist with obvious immunodeficiency. Moreover, HIV-infected individuals appear to have higher rates of allergic reactions to unknown allergens as seen with eosinophilic pustular folliculitis ("itchy red bump syndrome") as well as increased rates of hypersensitivity reactions to medications (for example, the fever and sunburn-like rash seen with trimethoprim-sulfamethoxazole reactions).

▶ Clinical Findings

The complications of HIV-related infections and neoplasms affect virtually every organ. The general approach to the HIV-infected person with symptoms is to evaluate the organ systems involved, aiming to diagnose treatable conditions rapidly. As can be seen in Figure 31–1, the CD4 lymphocyte count result enables the clinician to focus on the diagnoses most likely to be seen at each stage of immunodeficiency. Certain infections may occur at any CD4 count, while others rarely occur unless the CD4 lymphocyte count has dropped below a certain level. For example, a patient with a CD4 count of 600 cells/mcL, cough, and fever may have a bacterial pneumonia but would be very unlikely to have *Pneumocystis* pneumonia.

A. Symptoms and Signs

Many individuals with HIV infection remain asymptomatic for years even without ART, with a mean time of approximately 10 years between infection and development of AIDS. When symptoms occur, they may be remarkably protean and nonspecific. Since virtually all the findings may be seen with other diseases, a combination of complaints is more suggestive of HIV infection than any one symptom.

Physical examination may be entirely normal. Abnormal findings range from completely nonspecific to highly specific for HIV infection. Those that are specific for HIV infection include hairy leukoplakia of the tongue,

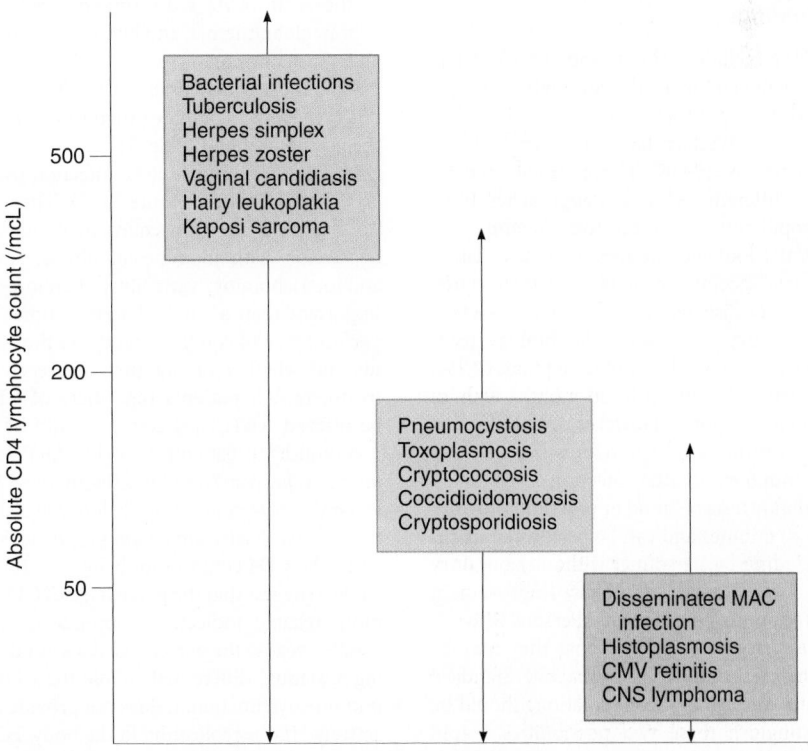

▲ **Figure 31–1.** Relationship of CD4 count to development of opportunistic infections. MAC, *Mycobacterium avium complex*; CMV, cytomegalovirus; CNS, central nervous system.

Table 31–2. Laboratory findings with HIV infection.

Test	Significance
HIV enzyme-linked immunosorbent assay (ELISA)	Screening test for HIV infection. Of ELISA tests 50% are positive within 22 days after HIV transmission; 95% are positive within 6 weeks after transmission. Sensitivity > 99.9%; to avoid false-positive results, repeatedly reactive results must be confirmed with Western blot.
Western blot	Confirmatory test for HIV. Specificity when combined with ELISA > 99.99%. Indeterminate results with early HIV infection, HIV-2 infection, autoimmune disease, pregnancy, and recent tetanus toxoid administration.
HIV rapid antibody test	Screening test for HIV. Produces results in 10–20 minutes. Can be performed by personnel with limited training. Positive results must be confirmed with standard HIV tests (ELISA and Western blot).
Complete blood count	Anemia, neutropenia, and thrombocytopenia common with advanced HIV infection.
Absolute CD4 lymphocyte count	Most widely used predictor of HIV progression. Risk of progression to an AIDS opportunistic infection or malignancy is high with CD4 < 200 cells/mcL in the absence of treatment.
CD4 lymphocyte percentage	Percentage may be more reliable than the CD4 count. Risk of progression to an AIDS opportunistic infection or malignancy is high with percentage < 14% in the absence of treatment.
HIV viral load tests	These tests measure the amount of actively replicating HIV virus. Correlate with disease progression and response to antiretroviral medications. Best tests available for diagnosis of acute HIV infection (prior to seroconversion); however, caution is warranted when the test result shows low-level viremia (ie, < 500 copies/mL) as this may represent a false-positive test.

disseminated Kaposi sarcoma, and cutaneous bacillary angiomatosis. Generalized lymphadenopathy is common early in infection.

The specific presentations and management of the various complications of HIV infection are discussed under the Complications section below.

B. Laboratory Findings

Specific tests for HIV include antibody and antigen detection (Table 31–2). Conventional HIV antibody testing is done by ELISA. Positive specimens are then confirmed by a different method (eg, Western blot). The sensitivity of screening serologic tests is > 99.9%. The specificity of positive results by two different techniques approaches 100% even in low-risk populations. False-positive screening tests may occur as normal biologic variants or in association with recent influenza vaccination or other disease states, such as connective tissue disease. These are usually detected by negative confirmatory tests. Molecular biology techniques (PCR) show a small incidence of individuals (< 1%) who are infected with HIV for up to 36 months without generating an antibody response. However, antibodies that are detectable by screening serologic tests will develop in 95% of persons within 6 weeks after infection.

Rapid HIV antibody tests of blood or oral fluid provides results within 10–20 minutes and can be performed in clinician offices, including by personnel without laboratory training and without a Clinical Laboratory Improvement Amendment (CLIA) approved laboratory. Persons who test positive on a rapid test should be told that they may be HIV-infected or their test may be falsely reactive. Standard testing (ELISA with Western blot confirmation) should be performed to distinguish these two possibilities. Rapid testing is particularly helpful in settings where a result is needed immediately (eg, a woman in labor who has not recently been tested for HIV) or when the patient is unlikely to return for a result. Rapid HIV home tests that allow the testers to learn their status privately by simply swabbing along their gum lines are also available (www.oraquick.com).

Nonspecific laboratory findings with HIV infection may include anemia, leukopenia (particularly lymphopenia), and thrombocytopenia in any combination, elevation of the erythrocyte sedimentation rate, polyclonal hypergammaglobulinemia, and hypocholesterolemia. Cutaneous anergy is common.

The most widely used marker is the absolute CD4 lymphocyte count to provide prognostic information and guide therapy decisions (Table 31–2). As counts decrease, the risk of serious opportunistic infection over the subsequent 3–5 years increases (Figure 31–1). There are many limitations to using the CD4 count, including diurnal variation, depression with intercurrent illness, and intralaboratory and interlaboratory variability. Therefore, the trend is more important than a single determination. The frequency of performance of counts depends on the patient's health status and whether or not they are receiving antiretroviral treatment. **All patients regardless of CD4 count should be offered ART**; CD4 counts should be monitored every 3–6 months in patients on stable ART. Initiation of *Pneumocystis jirovecii* prophylactic therapy is recommended when the CD4 count drops below 200 cells/mcL and initiation of *Mycobacterium avium* prophylaxis is recommended when the CD4 count drops below 75–100 cells/mcL. Some studies suggest that the percentage of CD4 lymphocytes is a more reliable indicator of prognosis than the absolute counts because the percentage does not depend on calculating a manual differential. While the CD4 count measures immune dysfunction, it does not provide a measure of how actively HIV is replicating in the body. HIV viral load tests (discussed below) assess the level of viral replication and provide useful prognostic information that is independent of the information provided by CD4 counts.

Differential Diagnosis

HIV infection may mimic a variety of other medical illnesses. Specific differential diagnosis depends on the mode of presentation. In patients presenting with constitutional symptoms such as weight loss and fevers, differential considerations include cancer, chronic infections such as tuberculosis and endocarditis, and endocrinologic diseases such as hyperthyroidism. When pulmonary processes dominate the presentation, acute and chronic lung infections must be considered as well as other causes of diffuse interstitial pulmonary infiltrates. When neurologic disease is the mode of presentation, conditions that cause mental status changes or neuropathy—eg, alcoholism, liver disease, kidney dysfunction, thyroid disease, and vitamin deficiency—should be considered. If a patient presents with headache and a cerebrospinal fluid pleocytosis, other causes of chronic meningitis enter the differential. When diarrhea is a prominent complaint, infectious enterocolitis, antibiotic-associated colitis, inflammatory bowel disease, and malabsorptive symptoms must be considered.

Complications

A. Systemic Complaints

Fever, night sweats, and weight loss are common symptoms in HIV-infected patients and may occur without a complicating opportunistic infection. Patients with persistent fever and no localizing symptoms should nonetheless be carefully examined, and evaluated with a chest radiograph (*Pneumocystis* pneumonia can present without respiratory symptoms), bacterial blood cultures if the fever is > 38.5°C, serum cryptococcal antigen, and mycobacterial cultures of the blood. Sinus CT scans or sinus radiographs should be considered to evaluate occult sinusitis. If these studies are normal, patients should be observed closely. Antipyretics are useful to prevent dehydration.

1. Weight loss and wasting syndrome—Weight loss is a particularly distressing complication of long-standing HIV infection. Patients typically have disproportionate loss of muscle mass, with maintenance or less substantial loss of fat stores. The mechanism of HIV-related weight loss is not completely understood but appears to be multifactorial.

A. Presentation—AIDS patients frequently suffer from anorexia, nausea, and vomiting, all of which contribute to weight loss by decreasing caloric intake. In some cases, these symptoms are secondary to a specific infection, such as viral hepatitis. In other cases, however, evaluation of the symptoms yields no specific pathogen, and it is assumed to be due to a primary effect of HIV. Malabsorption also plays a role in decreased caloric intake. Patients may suffer diarrhea from infections with bacterial, viral, or parasitic agents.

Exacerbating the decrease in caloric intake, many AIDS patients have an increased metabolic rate. This increased rate has been shown to exist even among asymptomatic HIV-infected persons, but it accelerates with disease progression and secondary infection. AIDS patients with secondary infections also have decreased protein synthesis, which makes maintaining muscle mass difficult.

B. Management—Several strategies have been developed to slow AIDS wasting. In the long term, nothing is as effective as ART, since it treats the underlying HIV infection. In the short term, effective fever control decreases the metabolic rate and may slow the pace of weight loss, as does treating the underlying opportunistic infection. Food supplementation with high-calorie drinks may enable patients with not much appetite to maintain their intake. Selected patients with otherwise good functional status and weight loss due to unrelenting nausea, vomiting, or diarrhea may benefit from total parenteral nutrition (TPN). It should be noted, however, that TPN is more likely to increase fat stores than to reverse the muscle wasting process.

Two pharmacologic approaches for increasing appetite and weight gain are the progestational agent megestrol acetate (80 mg orally four times a day) and the antiemetic agent dronabinol (2.5–5 mg orally three times a day), but neither of these agents increases lean body mass. Side effects from megestrol acetate are rare, but thromboembolic phenomena, edema, nausea, vomiting, and rash have been reported. Euphoria, dizziness, paranoia, and somnolence and even nausea and vomiting have been reported in 3–10% of patients using dronabinol. Dronabinol contains only one of the active ingredients in marijuana, and many patients report better relief of nausea and improvement of appetite with medical cannabis (administered via smoking, vaporization, essential oils or cooked in food). Twenty states allow patients to obtain marijuana for medicinal purposes with a letter of recommendation from their doctor. However, the use and sale of marijuana is still illegal under federal law. The Supreme Court has ruled that physicians cannot be prosecuted for recommending marijuana to their patients (it would be an infringement of freedom of speech). Therefore, while a physician's recommendation may not completely protect patients, letters decrease the chance that patients will be prosecuted for use of marijuana.

Two regimens that have resulted in increases in lean body mass are growth hormone and anabolic steroids. Growth hormone at a dose of 0.1 mg/kg/d (up to 6 mg) subcutaneously for 12 weeks has resulted in modest increases in lean body mass. Treatment with growth hormone can cost as much as $10,000 per month. Anabolic steroids also increase lean body mass among HIV-infected patients. They seem to work best for patients who are able to do weight training. The most commonly used regimens are testosterone enanthate or testosterone cypionate (100–200 mg intramuscularly every 2–4 weeks). Testosterone transdermal system (apply 5 mg system each evening) and testosterone gel (1%; apply a 5-g packet [50 mg testosterone] to clean, dry skin daily) are also available. The anabolic steroid oxandrolone (20 mg orally in two divided doses) has also been found to increase lean body mass.

2. Nausea—Nausea leading to weight loss is sometimes due to esophageal candidiasis. Patients with oral candidiasis and nausea should be empirically treated with an oral antifungal agent. Patients with weight loss due to nausea of unclear origin may benefit from use of antiemetics prior to meals (prochlorperazine, 10 mg three times daily; metoclopramide, 10 mg three times daily; or ondansetron, 8 mg three times daily). Dronabinol (5 mg three times daily) or medical cannabis can also be used to increase appetite. Depression and adrenal insufficiency are two potentially treatable causes of weight loss.

B. Pulmonary Disease

1. *Pneumocystis* pneumonia—(See also discussions in Chapter 36.) *P jirovecii* pneumonia is the most common opportunistic infection associated with AIDS. *Pneumocystis* pneumonia may be difficult to diagnose because the symptoms—fever, cough, and shortness of breath—are nonspecific. Furthermore, the severity of symptoms ranges from fever and no respiratory symptoms through mild cough or dyspnea to frank respiratory distress.

Hypoxemia may be severe, with a $Po_2 < 60$ mm Hg. The cornerstone of diagnosis is the chest radiograph. Diffuse or perihilar infiltrates are most characteristic, but only two-thirds of patients with *Pneumocystis* pneumonia have this finding. Normal chest radiographs are seen in 5–10% of patients with *Pneumocystis* pneumonia, while the remainder have atypical infiltrates. Apical infiltrates are commonly seen among patients with *Pneumocystis* pneumonia who have been receiving aerosolized pentamidine prophylaxis. Large pleural effusions are uncommon with *Pneumocystis* pneumonia; their presence suggests bacterial pneumonia, other infections such as tuberculosis, or pleural Kaposi sarcoma.

Definitive diagnosis can be obtained in 50–80% of cases by Wright-Giemsa stain or direct fluorescence antibody (DFA) test of induced sputum. Sputum induction is performed by having patients inhale an aerosolized solution of 3% saline produced by an ultrasonic nebulizer. Patients should not eat for at least 8 hours and should not use toothpaste or mouthwash prior to the procedure since they can interfere with test interpretation. The next step for patients with negative sputum examinations in whom *Pneumocystis* pneumonia is still suspected should be bronchoalveolar lavage. This technique establishes the diagnosis in over 95% of cases.

In patients with symptoms suggestive of *Pneumocystis* pneumonia but with negative or atypical chest radiographs and negative sputum examinations, other diagnostic tests may provide additional information in deciding whether to proceed to bronchoalveolar lavage. Elevation of serum lactate dehydrogenase occurs in 95% of cases of *Pneumocystis* pneumonia, but the specificity of this finding is at best 75%. A serum beta-glucan test is more sensitive and specific test for *Pneumocystis* pneumonia compared with serum lactate dehydrogenase and may avoid more invasive tests when used in the appropriate clinical setting. Either a normal diffusing capacity of carbon monoxide (DL_{CO}) or a high-resolution CT scan of the chest that demonstrates no interstitial lung disease makes the diagnosis of *Pneumocystis* pneumonia very unlikely. In addition, a CD4 count > 250 cells/mcL within 2 months prior to evaluation of respiratory symptoms makes a diagnosis of *Pneumocystis* pneumonia unlikely; only 1–5% of cases occur above this CD4 count level (Figure 31–1). This is true even if the patient previously had a CD4 count lower than 200 cells/mcL but has had an increase with ART. Pneumothoraces can be seen in HIV-infected patients with a history of *Pneumocystis* pneumonia, especially if they have received aerosolized pentamidine treatment.

2. Other infectious pulmonary diseases—

A. Presentation—Other infectious causes of pulmonary disease in AIDS patients include bacterial, mycobacterial, and viral pneumonias. **Community-acquired pneumonia is the most common cause of pulmonary disease in HIV-infected persons.** An increased incidence of pneumococcal pneumonia with septicemia and *Haemophilus influenzae* pneumonia has been reported. *Pseudomonas aeruginosa* is an important respiratory pathogen in advanced disease and, more rarely, pneumonia from *Rhodococcus equi* infection can occur. The incidence of infection with *Mycobacterium tuberculosis* has markedly increased in metropolitan areas because of HIV infection as well as homelessness. Tuberculosis occurs in an estimated 4% of persons in the United States who have AIDS. Apical infiltrates and disseminated disease occur more commonly than among immunocompetent persons. Although a purified protein derivative (PPD) test should be performed on all HIV-infected persons in whom a diagnosis of tuberculosis is being considered, the lower the CD4 cell count, the greater the likelihood of anergy. Because "anergy" skin test panels do not accurately classify those patients who are infected with tuberculosis but unreactive to the PPD, they are not recommended. **QuantiFERON blood testing** is likely to be more sensitive than skin testing in HIV-infected patients in whom tuberculosis infection is suspected.

B. Management—Treatment of HIV-infected persons with active tuberculosis is similar to treatment of HIV-uninfected tubercular individuals (see Figure 31–1). However, rifampin should not be given to patients receiving a boosted protease inhibitor (PI)-regimen. In these cases, rifabutin may be substituted, but it may require dosing modifications depending on the antiretroviral regimen. Multidrug-resistant tuberculosis has been a major problem in several metropolitan areas of the developed world, and reports from South Africa of "extremely resistant" tuberculosis in AIDS patients is a growing global concern. Non-compliance with prescribed antituberculous medications is a major risk factor. Several of the reported outbreaks appear to implicate nosocomial spread. The emergence of medication resistance makes it essential that antibiotic sensitivities be performed on all positive cultures. Medication therapy should be individualized. Patients with multidrug-resistant *M tuberculosis* infection should receive at least three medications to which their organism is sensitive. Atypical mycobacteria can cause pulmonary disease in AIDS patients with or without preexisting lung disease and responds variably to treatment. Making a distinction between *M tuberculosis* and atypical mycobacteria requires culture of sputum specimens. If culture of the sputum produces acid-fast bacilli, definitive identification may take several weeks using traditional techniques. DNA probes allow for presumptive identification usually within days of a positive culture. While awaiting definitive diagnosis, clinicians should err on the side of treating patients as if they have *M tuberculosis* infection. In cases in which the risk of atypical mycobacteria is very high (eg, a person without risk for tuberculosis exposure with a CD4 count under 50 cells/mcL—see Figure 31–1), clinicians may wait for definitive diagnosis if the person is smear-negative for acid-fast bacilli, clinically stable, and not living in a communal setting. Isolation of cytomegalovirus (CMV) from bronchoalveolar lavage fluid occurs commonly in AIDS patients but does not establish a definitive diagnosis. Diagnosis of CMV pneumonia requires biopsy; response to treatment is poor. Histoplasmosis, coccidioidomycosis, and cryptococcal disease as well as more common respiratory viral infections should also be considered in the differential diagnosis of unexplained pulmonary infiltrates.

3. Noninfectious pulmonary diseases—

A. Presentation—Noninfectious causes of lung disease include Kaposi sarcoma, non-Hodgkin lymphoma, interstitial pneumonitis, and increasingly, in the current ART era, lung cancer. In patients with known Kaposi sarcoma, pulmonary involvement complicates the course in approximately one-third of cases. However, pulmonary involvement is rarely the presenting manifestation of Kaposi sarcoma. Non-Hodgkin lymphoma may involve the lung as the sole site of disease but more commonly involves other organs as well, especially the brain, liver, and gastrointestinal tract. Both of these processes may show nodular or diffuse parenchymal involvement, pleural effusions, and mediastinal adenopathy on chest radiographs.

Nonspecific interstitial pneumonitis may mimic *Pneumocystis* pneumonia. Lymphocytic interstitial pneumonitis seen in lung biopsies has a variable clinical course. Typically, these patients present with several months of mild cough and dyspnea; chest radiographs show interstitial infiltrates. Many patients with this entity undergo transbronchial biopsies in an attempt to diagnose *Pneumocystis* pneumonia. Instead, the tissue shows interstitial inflammation ranging from an intense lymphocytic infiltration (consistent with lymphoid interstitial pneumonitis) to a mild mononuclear inflammation.

B. Management—Corticosteroids may be helpful in some cases refractory to ART.

4. Sinusitis—

A. Presentation—Chronic sinusitis can be a frustrating problem for HIV-infected patients even in those on adequate ART. Symptoms include sinus congestion and discharge, headache, and fever. Some patients may have radiographic evidence of sinus disease on sinus CT scan or sinus x-ray in the absence of significant symptoms.

B. Management—Nonsmoking patients with purulent drainage should be treated with amoxicillin (500 mg orally three times a day). Patients who smoke should be treated with amoxicillin-potassium clavulanate (500 mg orally three times a day) to cover *H influenzae*. A 7-day course of pseudoephedrine 60 mg twice daily may be helpful in decreasing congestion. Prolonged treatment (3–6 weeks) with an antibiotic and guaifenesin (600 mg orally twice daily) is sometimes necessary. For patients not responding to amoxicillin-potassium clavulanate, levofloxacin may be tried (400 mg orally daily). In patients with advanced immunodeficiency, *Pseudomonas* infections should be suspected, especially if there is not a response to first-line antibiotics. Some patients may require referral to an otolaryngologist for sinus drainage.

C. Central Nervous System Disease

Central nervous system disease in HIV-infected patients can be divided into intracerebral space-occupying lesions, encephalopathy, meningitis, and spinal cord processes. Many of these complications have declined markedly in prevalence in the era of effective ART. Cognitive declines, however, may be more common in HIV patients especially as they age (> 50 years), even those who are taking fully suppressive ART.

1. Toxoplasmosis—Toxoplasmosis is the most common space-occupying lesion in HIV-infected patients. Headache, focal neurologic deficits, seizures, or altered mental status may be presenting symptoms. The diagnosis is usually made presumptively based on the characteristic appearance of cerebral imaging studies in an individual known to be seropositive for *Toxoplasma*. Typically, toxoplasmosis appears as multiple contrast-enhancing lesions on CT scan. Lesions tend to be peripheral, with a predilection for the basal ganglia.

Single lesions are atypical of toxoplasmosis. When a single lesion has been detected by CT scanning, MRI scanning may reveal multiple lesions because of its greater sensitivity. If a patient has a single lesion on MRI and is neurologically stable, clinicians may pursue a 2-week empiric trial of toxoplasmosis therapy. A repeat scan should be performed at 2 weeks. If the lesion has not diminished in size, biopsy of the lesion should be performed. A positive *Toxoplasma* serologic test does not confirm the diagnosis because many HIV-infected patients have detectable titers without having active disease. Conversely, < 3% of patients with toxoplasmosis have negative titers. Therefore, negative *Toxoplasma* titers in an HIV-infected patient with a space-occupying lesion should be a cause for aggressively pursuing an alternative diagnosis.

2. Central nervous system lymphoma—Primary non-Hodgkin lymphoma is the second most common space-occupying lesion in HIV-infected patients. Symptoms are similar to those with toxoplasmosis. While imaging techniques cannot distinguish these two diseases with certainty, lymphoma more often is solitary. Other less common lesions should be suspected if there is preceding bacteremia, positive tuberculin test, fungemia, or injection drug use. These include bacterial abscesses, cryptococcomas, tuberculomas, and *Nocardia* lesions.

Stereotactic brain biopsy should be strongly considered if lesions are solitary or do not respond to toxoplasmosis treatment, especially if they are easily accessible. Diagnosis of lymphoma is important because many patients benefit from treatment (radiation therapy). Although a positive polymerase chain reaction (PCR) assay of cerebrospinal fluid for Epstein–Barr virus DNA is consistent with a diagnosis of lymphoma, the sensitive and specificity of the test are not high enough to obviate the need for a brain biopsy.

3. HIV-associated dementia—Patients with HIV-associated dementia typically have difficulty with cognitive tasks (eg, memory, attention), exhibit diminished motor function, and have emotional or behavioral problems. Patients may first notice a deterioration in their handwriting. The manifestations of dementia may wax and wane, with persons exhibiting periods of lucidity and confusion over the course of a day. The diagnosis of HIV-associated dementia is one of exclusion based on a brain imaging study and on spinal fluid analysis that excludes other pathogens. Neuropsychiatric testing is helpful in distinguishing patients with dementia from those with depression. Many patients improve with effective ART. However, slowly progressive neurocognitive deficits may still develop in patients taking ART as they age.

Metabolic abnormalities may also cause changes in mental status: hypoglycemia, hyponatremia, hypoxia, and drug overdose are important considerations in this population. Other less common infectious causes of encephalopathy include progressive multifocal leukoencephalopathy (discussed below), CMV, syphilis, and herpes simplex encephalitis.

4. Cryptococcal meningitis—Cryptococcal meningitis typically presents with fever and headache. Less than 20% of patients have meningismus. Diagnosis is based on a positive latex agglutination test of serum that detects cryptococcal antigen (or "CRAG") or positive culture of spinal fluid for *Cryptococcus*. Seventy to 90% of patients with cryptococcal meningitis have a positive serum CRAG. Thus, a negative serum CRAG test makes a diagnosis of cryptococcal meningitis unlikely and can be useful in the initial evaluation of a patient with headache, fever, and normal mental status. HIV meningitis, characterized by lymphocytic pleocytosis of the spinal fluid with negative culture, is common early in HIV infection.

5. HIV myelopathy—Spinal cord function may also be impaired in HIV-infected individuals. HIV myelopathy presents with leg weakness and incontinence. Spastic paraparesis and sensory ataxia are seen on neurologic examination. Myelopathy is usually a late manifestation of HIV disease, and most patients will have concomitant HIV encephalopathy. Pathologic evaluation of the spinal cord reveals vacuolation of white matter. Because HIV myelopathy is a diagnosis of exclusion, symptoms suggestive of myelopathy should be evaluated by lumbar puncture to rule out CMV polyradiculopathy (described below) and an MRI or CT scan to exclude epidural lymphoma.

6. Progressive multifocal leukoencephalopathy (PML)—PML is a viral infection of the white matter of the brain seen in patients with very advanced HIV infection. It typically results in focal neurologic deficits such as aphasia, hemiparesis, and cortical blindness. Imaging studies are strongly suggestive of the diagnosis if they show nonenhancing white matter lesions without mass effect. Extensive lesions may be difficult to differentiate from the changes caused by HIV. Several patients have stabilized or improved after the institution of effective ART, and due to wide use of ART, PML is now rarely seen.

D. Peripheral Nervous System

A. PRESENTATION—Peripheral nervous system syndromes include inflammatory polyneuropathies, sensory neuropathies, and mononeuropathies.

An inflammatory demyelinating polyneuropathy similar to Guillain-Barré syndrome occurs in HIV-infected patients, usually prior to frank immunodeficiency. The syndrome in many cases improves with plasmapheresis, supporting an autoimmune basis of the disease. CMV can cause an ascending polyradiculopathy characterized by lower extremity weakness and a neutrophilic pleocytosis on spinal fluid analysis with a negative bacterial culture. Transverse myelitis can be seen with herpes zoster or CMV.

Peripheral neuropathy is common among HIV-infected persons. Patients typically complain of numbness, tingling, and pain in the lower extremities. Symptoms are disproportionate to findings on gross sensory and motor evaluation. Beyond HIV infection itself, the most common cause is prior ART with stavudine or didanosine. Although not used commonly in Western countries, stavudine is still being used in resource-limited settings through national ART programs. Caution should be used when administering these agents to patients with a history of peripheral neuropathy. Unfortunately, medication-induced neuropathy is not always reversed when the offending agent is discontinued. Patients with advanced disease may also develop peripheral neuropathy even if they have never taken ART. Evaluation should rule out other causes of sensory neuropathy such as alcoholism, thyroid disease, vitamin B_{12} deficiency, and syphilis.

B. MANAGEMENT—Treatment of peripheral neuropathy is aimed at symptomatic relief. Patients should be initially treated with gabapentin (start at 300 mg at bedtime and increase to 300–900 mg orally three times a day) or other co-analgesics for neuropathic pain (see Chapter 5). Opioid analgesics should be avoided because the condition tends to be chronic and patients are likely to become dependent on these agents without significant improvement in their well-being.

E. Rheumatologic and Bone Manifestations

Arthritis, involving single or multiple joints, with or without effusion, has been commonly noted in HIV-infected patients. Involvement of large joints is most common. Although the cause of HIV-related arthritis is unknown, most patients will respond to nonsteroidal anti-inflammatory medications. Patients with a sizable effusion, especially if the joint is warm or erythematous, should have the joint aspirated, followed by culture of the fluid to rule out suppurative arthritis as well as fungal and mycobacterial disease.

Several rheumatologic syndromes, including reactive arthritis, psoriatic arthritis, sicca syndrome, and systemic lupus erythematosus, have been reported in HIV-infected patients (see Chapter 20). However, it is unclear if the prevalence is greater than in the general population. Cases of avascular necrosis of the femoral heads have been reported sporadically, generally in the setting of advanced disease with long-standing infection and in patients receiving long-term ART. The etiology is not clear but is probably multifactorial in nature.

Osteoporosis and osteopenia appear to be more common in HIV infected patients with chronic infection and perhaps associated with long-term use of ART. Vitamin D deficiency appears to be quite common among HIV-infected populations and monitoring vitamin D levels and replacement therapy for detected deficiency is recommended. Bone mineral density scans for patients over the age of 50 is also recommended.

F. Myopathy

Myopathies are infrequent in the era of effective ART but can be related to either HIV-infection or ART, particularly with use of zidovudine (azidothymidine [AZT]). Proximal muscle weakness is typical, and patients may have varying degrees of muscle tenderness. Given its long-term toxicities, zidovudine is no longer recommended when alternative treatments are available (see below).

G. Retinitis

Complaints of visual changes must be evaluated immediately in HIV-infected patients. CMV retinitis, characterized by perivascular hemorrhages and white fluffy exudates, is the most common retinal infection in AIDS patients and can be rapidly progressive. In contrast, cotton wool spots, which are also common in HIV-infected people, are benign, remit spontaneously, and appear as small indistinct white spots without exudation or hemorrhage. This distinction may be difficult at times for the nonspecialist, and patients with visual changes should be seen by an ophthalmologist. Other rare retinal processes include other herpesvirus infections or toxoplasmosis.

H. Oral Lesions

A. PRESENTATION—The presence of oral candidiasis or hairy leukoplakia is significant for several reasons. First, these lesions are highly suggestive of HIV infection in patients who have no other obvious cause of immunodeficiency. Second, several studies have indicated that patients with candidiasis have a high rate of progression to AIDS even with statistical adjustment for CD4 count.

Hairy leukoplakia is caused by the Epstein-Barr virus. The lesion is not usually troubling to patients and sometimes regresses spontaneously. Hairy leukoplakia is commonly seen as a white lesion on the lateral aspect of the tongue. It may be flat or slightly raised, is usually corrugated, and has vertical parallel lines with fine or thick ("hairy") projections. Oral candidiasis can be bothersome to patients, many of whom report an unpleasant taste or mouth dryness. The two most common forms of oral candidiasis seen are pseudomembranous (removable white plaques) and erythematous (red friable plaques).

B. MANAGEMENT—Treatment of oral candidiasis is with topical agents such as clotrimazole 10-mg troches (one troche four or five times a day). Patients with candidiasis who do not respond to topical antifungals can be treated with fluconazole (50–100 mg orally once a day for 3–7 days).

Angular cheilitis—fissures at the sides of the mouth—is usually due to *Candida* as well and can be treated topically with ketoconazole cream (2%) twice a day.

Gingival disease is common in HIV-infected patients and is thought to be due to an overgrowth of microorganisms. It usually responds to professional dental cleaning and chlorhexidine rinses. A particularly aggressive gingivitis or periodontitis will develop in some HIV-infected patients; these patients should be given antibiotics that cover anaerobic oral flora (eg, metronidazole, 250 mg four times a day for 4 or 5 days) and referred to oral surgeons with experience with these entities.

Aphthous ulcers are painful and may interfere with eating. They can be treated with fluocinonide (0.05% ointment mixed 1:1 with plain Orabase and applied six times a day to the ulcer). For lesions that are difficult to reach, patients should use dexamethasone swishes (0.5 mg in 5 mL elixir three times a day). The pain of the ulcers can be relieved with use of an anesthetic spray (10% lidocaine). Other lesions seen in the mouths of HIV-infected patients include Kaposi sarcoma (usually on the hard palate) and warts.

I. Gastrointestinal Manifestations

1. Candidal esophagitis—(See also discussion in Chapter 15.) Esophageal candidiasis is a common AIDS complication. In a patient with characteristic symptoms, empiric antifungal treatment is begun with fluconazole (200 mg orally daily for 10–14 days). Improvement in symptoms should be apparent within 1–2 days of antifungal treatment. If there is no improvement, further evaluation to identify other causes of esophagitis (herpes simplex, CMV) is recommended.

2. Hepatic disease—

A. PRESENTATION—Autopsy studies have demonstrated that the liver is a frequent site of infections and neoplasms in HIV-infected patients. However, many of these infections are not clinically symptomatic. Mild elevations of alkaline phosphatase and aminotransferases are often noted on routine chemistry panels. Mycobacterial disease, CMV, hepatitis B virus, hepatitis C virus, and lymphoma cause liver disease and can present with varying degrees of nausea, vomiting, right upper quadrant abdominal pain, and jaundice. Sulfonamides, imidazole medications, antituberculous medications, pentamidine, clarithromycin, and didanosine have also been associated with hepatitis. All nucleoside reverse transcriptase inhibitors cause lactic acidosis, which can be fatal. Lactic acidosis, however, occurs most commonly when didanosine is used with stavudine; this combination is no longer recommended in ART regimens. HIV-infected patients with chronic hepatitis may have more rapid progression of liver disease because of the concomitant immunodeficiency or hepatotoxicity of ART. Percutaneous liver biopsy may be helpful in diagnosing liver disease, but some common causes of liver disease (eg, *M avium* complex, lymphoma) can be determined by less invasive measures (eg, blood culture, biopsy of a more accessible site).

B. MANAGEMENT—With patients living longer as a result of advances in ART, advanced liver disease and hepatic failure due to chronic active hepatitis B and or C are increasing causes of morbidity and mortality. HIV-infected individuals who are coinfected with hepatitis B should be treated with antiretroviral regimens that include medications with activity against both viruses (eg, lamivudine [3TC], emtricitabine [FTC], tenofovir [TDF]). It is important to be extremely cautious about discontinuing these medications in coinfected patients as sudden discontinuation could lead to a fatal flare of hepatitis B infection.

Treatment of HIV-infected persons with hepatitis C with peginterferon and ribavirin has been shown to be efficacious, although less so than in HIV-uninfected persons. HIV-infected persons are also more likely to have difficulty tolerating treatment with peginterferon than uninfected persons. The new PIs for hepatitis C, telaprevir and bocevavir, are being studied in HIV-coinfected patients and look promising, although they are associated with high rates of toxicities and side effects. HIV-infected patients with hepatitis C genotype 1 who received telaprevir therapy for 12 weeks had a better response than those who received only peginterferon with ribavirin. Telaprevir is approved in combination with peginterferon and ribavirin for treatment of hepatitis C in HIV-uninfected persons. Patients with advanced fibrosis or cirrhosis due to chronic hepatitis C infection should be considered for treatment with telaprevir, peginterferon, and ribavirin. However, this treatment regimen is difficult for many patients to tolerate, and there are a number of drug-drug interactions between the hepatitis PIs and many of the HIV antiretrovirals; therefore, coinfected patients with less advanced liver disease may benefit from waiting until newer direct-acting agents for hepatitis C treatment become available. Liver transplants have been performed successfully in HIV-infected patients. This strategy is most likely to be successful in persons who have CD4 counts > 100 cells/mcL and nondetectable viral loads.

3. Biliary disease—Cholecystitis presents with manifestations similar to those seen in immunocompetent hosts but is more likely to be acalculous. Sclerosing cholangitis and papillary stenosis have also been reported in HIV-infected patients. Typically, the syndrome presents with severe nausea, vomiting, and right upper quadrant pain. Liver function tests generally show alkaline phosphatase elevations disproportionate to elevation of the aminotransferases. Although dilated ducts can be seen on ultrasound, the diagnosis is made by endoscopic retrograde cholangiopancreatography, which reveals intraluminal irregularities of the proximal intrahepatic ducts with "pruning" of the terminal ductal branches. Stenosis of the distal common bile duct at the papilla is commonly seen with this syndrome. CMV, Cryptosporidium, and microsporidia are thought to play inciting roles in this syndrome but these conditions are rarely seen unless the patient is suffering with very advanced HIV-related immunodeficiency.

4. Enterocolitis—

A. PRESENTATION—Enterocolitis is a common problem in HIV-infected individuals. Organisms known to cause enterocolitis include bacteria (Campylobacter, Salmonella, Shigella), viruses (CMV, adenovirus), and protozoans (Cryptosporidium, Entamoeba histolytica, Giardia, Isospora, microsporidia). HIV itself may cause enterocolitis. Several of the organisms causing enterocolitis in HIV-infected individuals also cause diarrhea in immunocompetent persons. However, HIV-infected patients tend to have more severe and more chronic symptoms, including high fevers and severe abdominal pain that can mimic acute abdominal catastrophes. Bacteremia and concomitant biliary involvement are also more common with enterocolitis in HIV-infected patients. Relapses of enterocolitis following adequate therapy have been reported with both Salmonella and Shigella infections.

Because of the wide range of agents known to cause enterocolitis, a stool culture and multiple stool examinations for ova and parasites (including modified acid-fast staining for Cryptosporidium) should be performed. Those patients who have Cryptosporidium in one stool with improvement in symptoms in < 1 month should not be considered to have AIDS, as Cryptosporidium is a cause of self-limited diarrhea in HIV-negative persons. More commonly, HIV-infected patients with Cryptosporidium infection have persistent enterocolitis with profuse watery diarrhea.

B. MANAGEMENT—To date, no consistently effective treatments have been developed for Cryptosporidium infection. The most effective treatment of cryptosporidiosis is to improve immune function through the use of effective antiretroviral treatment. The diarrhea can be treated symptomatically with diphenoxylate with atropine (one or two tablets orally three or four times a day). Those who do not respond may be given paregoric with bismuth (5–10 mL orally three or four times a day). Octreotide in escalating doses (starting at 0.05 mg subcutaneously every 8 hours for 48 hours) has been found to ameliorate symptoms in approximately 40% of patients with cryptosporidia or idiopathic HIV-associated diarrhea although the benefit is often short-lived.

Patients with a negative stool examination and persistent symptoms should be evaluated with colonoscopy and biopsy. Patients whose symptoms last longer than 1 month with no identified cause of diarrhea are considered to have a presumptive diagnosis of AIDS enteropathy. Patients may respond to institution of effective antiretroviral treatment. Upper endoscopy with small bowel biopsy is not recommended as a routine part of the evaluation.

5. Other disorders—Two other important gastrointestinal abnormalities in HIV-infected patients are gastropathy and malabsorption. It has been documented that some HIV-infected patients do not produce normal levels of stomach acid and therefore are unable to absorb medications that require an acid medium. This decreased acid production may explain, in part, the susceptibility of HIV-infected patients to Campylobacter, Salmonella, and Shigella, all of which are sensitive to acid concentration. There is no evidence that Helicobacter pylori is more common in HIV-infected persons.

A malabsorption syndrome occurs commonly in AIDS patients. It can be due to infection of the small bowel with M avium complex, Cryptosporidium, or microsporidia.

J. Endocrinologic Manifestations

Hypogonadism is probably the most common endocrinologic abnormality in HIV-infected men. The adrenal gland is also a commonly afflicted endocrine gland in patients with AIDS. Abnormalities demonstrated on autopsy include infection (especially with CMV and *M avium* complex), infiltration with Kaposi sarcoma, and injury from hemorrhage and presumed autoimmunity. The prevalence of clinically significant adrenal insufficiency is low. Patients with suggestive symptoms should undergo a cosyntropin stimulation test.

Although frank deficiency of cortisol is rare, an isolated defect in mineralocorticoid metabolism may lead to salt-wasting and hyperkalemia. Such patients should be treated with fludrocortisone (0.1–0.2 mg orally daily).

AIDS patients appear to have abnormalities of thyroid function tests different from those of patients with other chronic diseases. AIDS patients have been shown to have high levels of triiodothyronine (T_3), thyroxine (T_4), and thyroid-binding globulin and low levels of reverse triiodothyronine (rT_3). The causes and clinical significance of these abnormalities are unknown.

K. Skin Manifestations

The skin manifestations that commonly develop in HIV-infected patients can be grouped into viral, bacterial, fungal, neoplastic, and nonspecific dermatitides.

1. Viral dermatitides—

A. HERPES SIMPLEX INFECTIONS—These infections occur more frequently, tend to be more severe, and are more likely to disseminate in AIDS patients than in immunocompetent persons. Because of the risk of progressive local disease, **all herpes simplex attacks should be treated** with acyclovir (400 mg orally three times a day until healed, usually 7 days), famciclovir (500 mg orally twice daily until healed), or valacyclovir (500 mg orally twice daily until healed). To avoid the complications of attacks, many clinicians recommend suppressive therapy for HIV-infected patients with a history of recurrent herpes. Options for suppressive therapy include acyclovir (400 mg orally twice daily), famciclovir (250 mg orally twice daily), and valacyclovir (500 mg orally daily). Long-term suppressive herpes prophylaxis with acyclovir does not reduce HIV transmission between heterosexual men and women from developing countries.

B. HERPES ZOSTER—This is a common manifestation of HIV infection. As with herpes simplex infections, patients with zoster should be treated with acyclovir to prevent dissemination (800 mg orally four or five times per day for 7 days). Alternatively, famciclovir (500 mg orally three times a day) or valacyclovir (500 mg three times a day) may be used. Vesicular lesions should be cultured if there is any question about their origin, since herpes simplex responds to much lower doses of acyclovir. Disseminated zoster and cases with ocular involvement should be treated with intravenous (10 mg/kg every 8 hours for 7–10 days) rather than oral acyclovir. The **zoster vaccine** appears to be safe and immunogenic in HIV-infected patients over the age of

50 years with CD4 > 200/mcL. A recommendation to vaccinate patients that fall into this category is expected although the long-term benefit in preventing recurrences has yet to be established.

C. MOLLUSCUM CONTAGIOSUM—This infection is caused by a pox virus and is seen in HIV-infected patients, as in other immunocompromised patients. The characteristic umbilicated fleshy papular lesions have a propensity for spreading widely over the patient's face and neck and should be treated with topical liquid nitrogen.

2. Bacterial dermatitides—

A. STAPHYLOCOCCAL INFECTION—*Staphylococcus* is the most common bacterial cause of skin disease in HIV-infected patients; it usually presents as **folliculitis, superficial abscesses (furuncles)**, or **bullous impetigo**. These lesions should be treated aggressively since sepsis can occur. Folliculitis is initially treated with topical clindamycin or mupirocin, and patients may benefit from regular washing with an antibacterial soap such as chlorhexidine. Intranasal mupirocin has been used successfully for staphylococcal decolonization in other settings. In HIV-infected patients with recurrent staphylococcal infections, weekly intranasal mupirocin should be considered in addition to topical care and systemic antibiotics. Abscesses often require incision and drainage. Patients may need anti-staphylococcal antibiotics as well. Due to high frequency of methicillin-resistant *Staphylococcus aureus* (MRSA) skin infections in HIV-infected populations, lesions should be cultured prior to initiating empiric antistaphylococcal therapy. Although there is limited experience treating MRSA with oral antibiotics, current recommendations for empiric treatment are either (1) trimethoprim-sulfamethoxazole (one double-strength tablet orally twice daily) with or without clindamycin (500 mg orally three times daily); or (2) doxycycline (100 mg orally twice daily) with close follow-up.

B. BACILLARY ANGIOMATOSIS—It is caused by two closely related organisms: *Bartonella henselae* and *Bartonella quintana*. The epidemiology of these infections suggests zoonotic transmission from fleas of infected domestic cats. The most common manifestation is raised, reddish, highly vascular skin lesions that can mimic the lesions of Kaposi sarcoma. Fever is a common manifestation of this infection; involvement of bone, lymph nodes, and liver has also been reported. The infection responds to doxycycline, 100 mg orally twice daily, or erythromycin, 250 mg orally four times daily. Therapy is continued for at least 14 days, and patients who are seriously ill with visceral involvement may require months of therapy.

3. Fungal rashes—

A. RASHES DUE TO DERMATOPHYTES AND CANDIDA—The majority of **fungal rashes** afflicting AIDS patients are due to dermatophytes and *Candida*. These are particularly common in the inguinal region but may occur anywhere on the body. Fungal rashes generally respond well to topical clotrimazole (1% cream twice a day) or ketoconazole (2% cream twice a day).

B. Seborrheic dermatitis—This is more common in HIV-infected patients. Scrapings of seborrhea have revealed *Malassezia furfur (Pityrosporum ovale)*, implying that the seborrhea is caused by this fungus. Consistent with the isolation of this fungus is the clinical finding that seborrhea responds well to topical clotrimazole (1% cream) as well as hydrocortisone (1% cream).

4. Neoplastic dermatitides—See Chapter 6 and the Kaposi sarcoma section below.

5. Nonspecific dermatitides—

A. Xerosis—This condition presents in HIV-infected patients with severe pruritus. The patient may have no rash, or nonspecific excoriations from scratching. Treatment is with emollients (eg, absorption base cream) and antipruritic lotions (eg, camphor 9.5% and menthol 0.5%).

B. Psoriasis—Psoriasis can be very severe in HIV-infected patients. Phototherapy and etretinate (0.25–9.75 mg/kg/d orally in divided doses) may be used for recalcitrant cases in consultation with a dermatologist.

L. HIV-Related Malignancies

Four cancers are currently included in the CDC classification of AIDS: Kaposi sarcoma, non-Hodgkin lymphoma, primary lymphoma of the brain, and invasive cervical carcinoma. Epidemiologic studies have shown that between 1973 and 1987 among single men in San Francisco, the risk of Kaposi sarcoma increased more than 5000-fold and the risk of non-Hodgkin lymphoma more than 10-fold. The increase in incidence of malignancies is probably a function of impaired cell-mediated immunity. **In the current treatment era, cancers not classified as AIDS-related, such as lung cancer, are being increasingly diagnosed in aging HIV-infected individuals despite optimal ART treatment.** Cohort studies suggest that HIV-infected adults are at increased risk for a variety of cancers compared to age-matched uninfected populations. Mortality secondary to malignancies represents an increasing cause of death in HIV-infected populations.

1. Kaposi sarcoma—

A. Presentation—Lesions may appear anywhere; careful examination of the eyelids, conjunctiva, pinnae, palate, and toe webs is mandatory to locate potentially occult lesions. In light-skinned individuals, Kaposi lesions usually appear as purplish, nonblanching lesions that can be papular or nodular. In dark-skinned individuals, the lesions may appear more brown. In the mouth, lesions are most often palatal papules, though exophytic lesions of the tongue and gingivae may also be seen. Kaposi lesions may be confused with other vascular lesions such as angiomas and pyogenic granulomas. Visceral disease (eg, gastrointestinal, pulmonary) will develop in about 40% of patients with dermatologic Kaposi sarcoma. Kaposi sarcoma lesions can occur shortly after initiating ART, especially in patients starting ART who have advanced immunodeficiency. In this situation, Kaposi sarcoma is likely to be an immune reconstitution reaction (see Inflammatory Reactions below).

B. Management—Rapidly progressive dermatologic or visceral disease is best treated with systemic chemotherapy. Liposomally encapsulated doxorubicin given intravenously every 3 weeks has a response rate of approximately 70%. Alpha-interferon (10 million units subcutaneously three times a week) also has activity against Kaposi sarcoma. However, symptoms such as malaise and anorexia limit the utility of this therapy. Patients with milder forms of Kaposi sarcoma do not require specific treatment as the lesions usually improve and can completely resolve with ART. However, it should be noted that the lesions may flare when ART is first initiated—probably as a result of an immune reconstitution process.

2. Non-Hodgkin lymphoma—

A. Presentation—Non-Hodgkin lymphoma in HIV-infected persons tends to be very aggressive. The malignancies are usually of B cell origin and characterized as diffuse large-cell tumors. Over 70% of the malignancies are extranodal.

B. Management—The prognosis of patients with systemic non-Hodgkin lymphoma depends primarily on the degree of immunodeficiency at the time of diagnosis. Patients with high CD4 counts do markedly better than those diagnosed at a late stage of illness. Patients with primary central nervous system lymphoma are treated with radiation. Response to treatment is good, but prior to the availability of HAART, most patients died within a few months after diagnosis due to their underlying disease. Systemic disease is treated with chemotherapy. Common regimens are CHOP (cyclophosphamide, doxorubicin, vincristine, and prednisone) and modified M-BACOD (methotrexate, bleomycin, doxorubicin, cyclophosphamide, vincristine, and dexamethasone). Granulocyte colony-stimulating factor (G-CSF; filgrastim) is used to maintain white blood counts with this latter regimen. Intrathecal chemotherapy is administered to prevent or treat meningeal involvement.

3. Hodgkin disease—Although Hodgkin disease is not included as part of the CDC definition of AIDS, studies have found that HIV infection is associated with a fivefold increase in the incidence of Hodgkin disease. HIV-infected persons with Hodgkin disease are more likely to have mixed cellularity and lymphocyte depletion subtypes of Hodgkin disease and to seek medical attention at an advanced stage of disease.

4. Anal dysplasia and squamous cell carcinoma—These lesions have been strongly correlated with previous infection by human papillomavirus (HPV) and have been noted in HIV-infected men and women. Although many of the infected MSM report a history of anal warts or have visible warts, a significant percentage have silent papillomavirus infection. Cytologic (using Papanicolaou smears) and papillomavirus DNA studies can easily be performed on specimens obtained by anal swab. Because of the risk of progression from dysplasia to cancer in immunocompromised patients, **some experts suggest that annual anal swabs for cytologic examination should be done in all HIV-infected persons.** An anal Papanicolaou smear is performed by rotating a moistened Dacron swab about 2 cm into the anal canal. The swab is immediately inserted into a cytology bottle. However, there is no evidence that screening for anal cancer with Papanicolaou smears decreases the incidence of invasive cancer.

HPV also appears to play a causative role in **cervical dysplasia** and **neoplasia**. The incidence and clinical course of cervical disease in HIV-infected women are discussed below.

M. Gynecologic Manifestations

Vaginal candidiasis, cervical dysplasia and neoplasia, and pelvic inflammatory disease are more common in HIV-infected women than in uninfected women. These manifestations also tend to be more severe when they occur in association with HIV infection. Therefore, HIV-infected women need frequent gynecologic care. Vaginal candidiasis may be treated with topical agents (see Chapter 36). However, HIV-infected women with recurrent or severe vaginal candidiasis may need systemic therapy.

The incidence of cervical dysplasia in HIV-infected women is 40%. Because of this finding, **HIV-infected women should have Papanicolaou smears every 6 months** (as opposed to the guidelines for HIV-uninfected women, see Chapter 18). Some clinicians recommend routine colposcopy or cervicography because cervical intraepithelial neoplasia has occurred in women with negative Papanicolaou smears. Cone biopsy is indicated in cases of serious cervical dysplasia. For 1 year following treatment of an abnormal Papanicolaou smear, women should have repeat smears every 3 to 4 months.

Cervical neoplasia appears to be more aggressive among HIV-infected women. Most HIV-infected women with cervical cancer die of that disease rather than of AIDS. Because of its frequency and severity, cervical neoplasia was added to the CDC definition of AIDS in 1993.

While pelvic inflammatory disease appears to be more common in HIV-infected women, the bacteriology of this condition appears to be the same as among HIV-uninfected women. At present, HIV-infected women with pelvic inflammatory disease should be treated with the same regimens as uninfected women (see Chapter 18). However, inpatient therapy is generally recommended.

N. Coronary Artery Disease

HIV-infected persons are at higher risk for coronary artery disease than age- and sex-matched controls. Part of this increase in coronary artery disease is due to changes in lipids caused by antiretroviral agents (see Treatment section on Antiretroviral Therapy below), especially stavudine and several of the PIs. However, some of the risk appears to be due to HIV infection, independent of its therapy. It is important that clinicians pay close attention to this issue because myocardial infarctions tend to present at a younger age in HIV-infected individuals than in HIV-uninfected individuals. HIV-infected patients with symptoms of coronary artery disease such as chest pain or dyspnea should be rapidly evaluated. Clinicians should aggressively treat conditions that result in increased risk of heart disease,

especially smoking, hypertension, hyperlipidemia, obesity, diabetes mellitus, and sedentary lifestyle.

O. Inflammatory Reactions (Immune Reconstitution Inflammatory Syndromes)

With initiation of HAART, some patients experience inflammatory reactions that appear to be associated with immune reconstitution as indicated by a rapid increase in CD4 count. These inflammatory reactions may present with generalized signs of fevers, sweats, and malaise with or without more localized manifestations that usually represent unusual presentations of opportunistic infections. For example, vitreitis has developed in patients with CMV retinitis after they have been treated with HAART.

M avium can present as focal even suppurative lymphadenitis or granulomatous masses in patients receiving HAART. Tuberculosis may paradoxically worsen with new or evolving pulmonary infiltrates and lymphadenopathy. PML and cryptococcal meningitis may also behave atypically. Clinicians should be alert to these syndromes, which are most often seen in patients who have initiated ART in the setting of advanced disease and who show rapid increases in CD4 counts with treatment. The diagnosis of immune reconstitution inflammatory syndrome (IRIS) is one of exclusion and can be made only after recurrence or new opportunistic infection has been ruled out as the cause of the clinical deterioration. Management of IRIS is conservative and supportive with use of corticosteroids only for severe reactions. Most authorities recommend that ART be continued unless the reaction is life-threatening.

▶ Prevention

A. Primary Prevention

Until vaccination is a reality, prevention of HIV infection will depend on HIV testing and counseling, including precautions regarding sexual practices and injection drug use, initiation of antiretroviral therapy (ART) as a prevention tool, preexposure and postexposure use of ART, perinatal management including ART therapy for the mother, screening of blood products, and infection control practices in the health care setting.

1. HIV testing and counseling—Primary care clinicians should routinely obtain a sexual history and provide risk factor assessment of their patients. Because approximately one-fifth of the HIV-infected persons in the United States do not know they are infected, the **USPSTF recommends that clinicians screen for HIV infection in adolescents and adults ages 15 to 65 years. Younger adolescents and older adults who are at increased risk should also be screened**. Clinicians should review the risk factors for HIV infection with the patient and discuss safer sex and safer needle use as well as the meaning of a positive test. Although the CDC recommends "opt-out" testing in medical settings, some states require specific written consent. For persons whose test results are positive, it is critically important that they be connected to on-going medical care.

Referrals for partner-notification services, social services, mental health services, and HIV-prevention services should also be provided. Prevention interventions focused on the importance of HIV-infected persons not putting others at risk have been successful.

For patients whose test results are negative, clinicians should review safer sex and needle use practices, including counseling not to exchange bodily fluids unless they are in a long-term mutually monogamous relationship with someone who has tested HIV antibody-negative and has not engaged in unsafe sex, injection drug use, or other HIV risk behaviors for at least 6 months prior to or at any time since the negative test.

To prevent sexual transmission of HIV, only latex condoms should be used, along with a water-soluble lubricant. Although nonoxynol-9, a spermicide, kills HIV, it is contraindicated because in some patients it may cause genital ulcers that could facilitate HIV transmission. Patients should be counseled that condoms are not 100% effective. They should be made familiar with the use of condoms, including, specifically, the advice that condoms must be used every time, that space should be left at the tip of the condom as a receptacle for semen, that intercourse with a condom should not be attempted if the penis is only partially erect, that men should hold on to the base of the condom when withdrawing the penis to prevent slippage, and that condoms should not be reused. Although anal intercourse remains the sexual practice at highest risk for transmitting HIV, seroconversions have been documented with vaginal and oral intercourse as well. Therefore, condoms should be used when engaging in these activities. Women as well as men having sex with men should understand how to use condoms to be sure that their partners are using them correctly. Partners of HIV-infected women should use latex barriers such as dental dams (available at dental supply stores) to prevent direct oral contact with vaginal secretions. Several randomized trials in Africa demonstrated that male circumcision significantly reduced HIV incidence in men, but there are a number of barriers to performing widespread circumcisions among men in Africa.

Persons using injection drugs should be cautioned never to exchange needles or other drug paraphernalia. When sterile needles are not available, bleach does appear to inactivate HIV and should be used to clean needles.

2. ART for decreasing transmission of HIV to others— Besides preventing progression of HIV disease, effective ART likely decreases the risk of HIV transmission between sexual partners. An international study showed that among serodiscordant couples, **early ART almost completely eliminated the risk of HIV transmission to the uninfected partner.** Although HIV-negative persons in stable long-term partnerships with HIV-infected persons represent only one group of at risk persons, theoretically increasing the use of ART among the population of HIV-infected persons could decrease community wide transmission of HIV. However, even patients who have been treated with antiretrovirals and have undetectable viral loads must practice safer sex and not share needles so as to avoid the possibility of transmitting HIV.

3. Preexposure ART prophylaxis—Several large randomized double-blind placebo-controlled trials demonstrated that administering emtricitabine/tenofovir (Truvada) can reduce the risk of sexual transmission of HIV among uninfected individuals at high risk for infection; one study was of HIV-negative men and transgender women who have sex with men, two studies were of heterosexual HIV-discordant couples. However, two studies of African women showed no reduced risk of transmission—primarily related to nonadherence to study medications. Preexposure tenofovir has also been shown to reduce HIV infection among injection drug users from Thailand. Emtricitabine/tenofovir is FDA-approved for use in HIV-negative persons who have ongoing risk of transmission. To date, the use of emtricitabine/tenofovir for this indication has been limited because of the following concerns: medication requires daily dosing, it is expensive and may be not be covered by insurance, and long-term side effects. However, in May 2014, the FDA released a clinical practice guideline recommending fixed dose emtricitabine/tenofovir for preexposure prophylaxis (PrEP).

4. Postexposure prophylaxis for sexual and drug use exposures to HIV—The goal of postexposure prophylaxis is to reduce or prevent local viral replication prior to dissemination such that the infection can be aborted. Although there is no proof that administration of antiretroviral medications following a sexual or parenteral drug use exposure reduces the likelihood of infection, there is suggestive data from animal models, perinatal experience, and a case-control study of health care workers who experienced a needle stick.

The choice of antiretroviral agents and the duration of treatment are the same as those for exposures that occur through the occupational route; the preferred regimen is tenofovir 300 mg with emtricitabine 200 mg daily with raltegravir 400 mg twice a day. Some clinicians prescribe a two-drug regimen of tenofovir 300 mg and emtricitabine 200 mg (Truvada) because it is a simpler for patients to take (single pill once a day), and more affordable for individuals and for public entities that provide this service to uninsured persons. In contrast to those with occupational exposures, some individuals may present very late after exposure. Because the likelihood of success declines with length of time from HIV exposure, treatment should be provided as soon as possible, and it is not recommended that treatment be offered more than 72 hours after exposure. In addition, because the psychosocial issues involved with postexposure prophylaxis for sexual and drug use exposures are complex, it should be offered only in the context of prevention counseling. Counseling should focus on how to prevent future exposures. Clinicians needing more information on postexposure prophylaxis for occupational or nonoccupational exposures should contact the National Clinician's Post-exposure Hotline (1-888-448-4911; http://www.nccc.ucsf.edu/about_nccc/pepline/).

5. Preventing perinatal transmission of HIV—Prevention of perinatal transmission of HIV begins by offering HIV counseling and testing to all women who are pregnant or considering pregnancy. Women who are pregnant should start ART with at least three medications. For women with high CD4 counts and low HIV-RNA it may be reasonable to wait until the second trimester to initiate therapy to reduce the chance of harm to the developing fetus from the medications; however, earlier initiation of therapy may be more effective in preventing perinatal transmission of HIV. The choice of regimen should be based on the same considerations as for any HIV-infected woman, with the addition that the regimen should include if possible one or more nucleoside-nucleotide reverse transcriptase inhibitors with good placental passage (zidovudine, lamivudine, emtricitabine, tenofavir, abacavir), and avoidance of efavirenz (for all women who are pregnant or may become pregnant). Cesarean delivery should be planned if HIV viral load is greater than 1000 copies near the time of delivery. Zidovudine should be given to the infant after birth for 6 weeks. In developed countries, breastfeeding should be avoided.

6. Prevention HIV transmission in health care settings—

In health care settings, universal body fluid precautions should be used, including use of gloves when handling body fluids and the addition of gown, mask, and goggles for procedures that may result in splash or droplet spread, and use of specially designed needles with sheath devices to decrease the risk of needle sticks. Because transmission of tuberculosis may occur in health care settings, all patients with cough should be encouraged to wear masks. Hospitalized HIV-infected patients with cough should be placed in respiratory isolation until tuberculosis can be excluded by chest radiograph and sputum smear examination.

Epidemiologic studies show that needle sticks occur commonly among health care professionals, especially among surgeons performing invasive procedures, inexperienced hospital house staff, and medical students. Efforts to reduce needle sticks should focus on avoiding recapping needles and use of safety needles whenever doing invasive procedures under controlled circumstances. **The risk of HIV transmission from a needle stick with blood from an HIV-infected patient is about 1:300.** The risk is higher with deep punctures, large inoculum, and source patients with high viral loads. The risk from mucous membrane contact is too low to quantitate.

Health care professionals who sustain needle sticks should be counseled and offered HIV testing as soon as possible. HIV testing is done to establish a negative baseline for worker's compensation claims in case there is a subsequent conversion. Follow-up testing is usually performed at 6 weeks, 3 months, and 6 months.

A case-control study by the CDC indicates that administration of zidovudine following a needle stick decreases the rate of HIV seroconversion by 79%. Therefore, providers should be offered ART as soon as possible after exposure and continued for 4 weeks. The preferred regimen is tenofavir 300 mg with emtricitabine 200 mg (Truvada) daily with raltegravir 400 mg twice a day. Providers who have exposures to persons who are likely to have antiretroviral medication resistance (eg, persons receiving therapy who have detectable viral loads) should have their therapy individualized, using at least two medications to which the source is unlikely to be resistant. Because reports have noted hepatotoxicity due to nevirapine in this setting, this agent should be avoided. Unfortunately, there have been documented cases of seroconversion following potential parenteral exposure to HIV despite prompt use of zidovudine prophylaxis. Counseling of the provider should include "safer sex" guidelines.

7. Prevention of transmission of HIV through blood or blood products—

Current efforts in the United States to screen blood and blood products have lowered the risk of HIV transmission with transfusion of a unit of blood to 1:1,000,000. Use of blood and blood products should be judicious, with patients receiving the least amount necessary, and patients should be encouraged to donate their own blood prior to elective procedures.

8. HIV vaccine—

Primate model data have suggested that development of a protective vaccine may be possible, but clinical trials in humans have been disappointing. Only one vaccine trial has shown any degree of efficacy. In this randomized, double-blind, placebo-controlled trial, a recombinant canarypox vector vaccine plus two booster injections of a recombinant gp120 vaccine was moderately efficacious (26–31%) in reducing the risk of HIV among a primarily heterosexual population in Thailand. Current vaccine development efforts are aimed at identifying broadly neutralizing antibodies to the highly conserved regions of the HIV envelope.

B. Secondary Prevention

In the era prior to the development of highly effective antiretroviral treatment, cohort studies of individuals with documented dates of seroconversion demonstrate that AIDS develops within 10 years in approximately 50% of untreated seropositive persons. With currently available treatment, progression of disease has been markedly decreased. In addition to antiretroviral treatment, prophylactic regimens can prevent opportunistic infections and improve survival. Prophylaxis and early intervention prevent several infectious diseases, including tuberculosis and syphilis, which are transmissible to others. Recommendations for screening tests, vaccinations, and prophylaxis are listed in Table 31–3.

1. Tuberculosis—

Because of the increased occurrence of tuberculosis among HIV-infected patients, all such individuals should undergo annual PPD testing. Although anergy is common among AIDS patients, the likelihood of a false-negative result is much lower when the test is done early in infection. Those with positive tests (defined for HIV-infected patients as > 5 mm of induration) need a chest radiograph. Patients with an infiltrate in any location, especially if accompanied by mediastinal adenopathy, should have sputum sent for acid-fast staining. Patients with a positive PPD but negative evaluations for active disease should receive isoniazid (300 mg orally daily) with pyridoxine (50 mg orally daily) for 9 months to a year. A blood test (QuantiFERON Gold test) can also be used to assess prior tuberculosis exposure. Blood samples are mixed with synthetic antigens representing M tuberculosis. Patients infected with M tuberculosis produce interferon-gamma in response to contact with the antigens. Unlike the PPD, the patient does not have to return for a second visit. The test is less likely to result in false-positive results than a PPD.

Table 31–3. Health care maintenance of HIV-infected individuals.

For all HIV-infected individuals:
CD4 counts every 3–6 months
Viral load tests every 3–6 months and 1 month following a change in therapy
Cholesterol and triglycerides at baseline, 6–12 months after starting antiretroviral therapy, and annually for everyone over 40 years of age
PPD annually
INH for those with positive PPD and normal chest radiograph
RPR or VDRL
Toxoplasma IgG serology at baseline
Hepatitis serologies: hepatitis A antibody, hepatitis B surface antigen, hepatitis B surface antibody, hepatitis B core antibody, hepatitis C antibody
Pneumococcal vaccine
Inactivated influenza vaccine annually in season
Hepatitis A vaccine for those without immunity to hepatitis A.
Hepatitis B vaccine for those who are hepatitis B surface antigen and antibody negative. (Use 40 mcg formulation at 0, 1, and 6 months; repeat if no immunity 1 month after three-shot series.)
Combined tetanus, diphtheria, pertussis vaccine
Human papillomavirus vaccine for HIV-infected women age 26 years or less.
Haemophilus influenzae type b vaccination
Bone mineral density monitoring for women and men over 50 years of age
Papanicolaou smears every 6 months for women
Consider anal swabs for cytologic evaluation
For HIV-infected individuals with CD4 < 200 cells/mcL:
Pneumocystis jirovecii prophylaxis (see Prophylaxis of Opportunistic Infections section under Treatment and Table 31–4)
For HIV-infected individuals with CD4 < 75 cells/mcL:
Mycobacterium avium complex prophylaxis (see Prophylaxis of Opportunistic Infections section under Treatment)
For HIV-infected individuals with CD4 < 50 cells/mcL:
Consider CMV prophylaxis

CMV, cytomegalovirus; IgG, immunoglobulin G; INH, isoniazid; PPD, purified protein derivative; RPR, rapid plasma reagin; VDRL, Venereal Disease Research Laboratories.

HIV-infected persons with a CD4 count < 100 cells may not respond to the Mitogen positive control; their results will be reported as indeterminate by QuantiFERON.

2. Syphilis—Because of the increased number of cases of syphilis among MSM, including those who are HIV infected, all such men should be screened for syphilis by rapid plasma reagin (RPR) or Venereal Disease Research Laboratories (VDRL) test every 6 months. Increases of syphilis cases among HIV-infected persons are of particular concern because these individuals are at increased risk for reactivation of syphilis and progression to tertiary syphilis despite standard treatment. Because the only widely available tests for syphilis are serologic and because HIV-infected individuals are known to have disordered antibody production, there is concern about the interpretation of these titers. This concern has been fueled by a report of an HIV-infected patient with secondary syphilis and negative syphilis serologic testing. Furthermore, HIV-infected individuals may

lose fluorescent treponemal antibody absorption (FTA-ABS) reactivity after treatment for syphilis, particularly if they have low CD4 counts. Thus, in this population, a nonreactive treponemal test does not rule out a past history of syphilis. In addition, persistence of treponemes in the spinal fluid after one dose of benzathine penicillin has been demonstrated in HIV-infected patients with primary and secondary syphilis. Therefore, **the CDC has recommended an aggressive diagnostic approach to HIV-infected patients with reactive RPR or VDRL tests of > 1 year or unknown duration.** All such patients should have a lumbar puncture with cerebrospinal fluid cell count and cerebrospinal fluid VDRL. Those with a normal cerebrospinal fluid evaluation are treated as having late latent syphilis (benzathine penicillin G, 2.4 million units intramuscularly weekly for 3 weeks) with follow-up titers. Those with a pleocytosis or a positive cerebrospinal fluid-VDRL test are treated as having neurosyphilis (aqueous penicillin G, 2–4 million units intravenously every 4 hours, or procaine penicillin G, 2.4 million units intramuscularly daily, with probenecid, 500 mg four times daily, for 10 days) followed by weekly benzathine penicillin G 2.4 million units intramuscularly for 3 weeks. Some clinicians take a less aggressive approach to patients who have low titers (< 1:8), a history of having been treated for syphilis, and a normal neurologic examination. Close follow-up of titers is mandatory if such a course is taken. For a more detailed discussion of this topic, see Chapter 34.

3. Immunizations—HIV-infected individuals should receive immunizations as outlined in Table 31–3. Patients without evidence of hepatitis B surface antigen or surface antibody should receive hepatitis B vaccination, using the 40 mcg formulation; the higher dose is to increase the chance of developing protective immunity. If the patient does not have immunity 1 month after the three-shot series, then the series should be repeated. HIV-infected persons should also receive the standard inactivated vaccines such as tetanus and diphtheria boosters that would be given to uninfected persons. **Most live vaccines, such as yellow fever vaccine, should be avoided.** Measles vaccination, while a live virus vaccine, appears relatively safe when administered to HIV-infected individuals and should be given if the patient has never had measles or been adequately vaccinated. The herpes zoster vaccine, two doses 6 weeks apart, has been found to be reasonably safe for HIV-infected persons with CD4 counts > 200 cells/mL and undetectable viral loads even though it is a live vaccine and is likely to be added as a treatment recommendation for persons 50 years of age or older.

4. Other measures—A randomized study found that multivitamin supplementation decreased HIV disease progression and mortality in HIV-infected women in Africa. However, supplementation is unlikely to be as effective in well-nourished populations.

HIV-infected individuals should be counseled with regard to the importance of practicing safer sex even with other HIV-infected persons because of the possibility of contracting a sexually transmitted disease, such as gonorrhea or syphilis. There is also the possibility of transmission of a particularly virulent or a drug-resistant strain between HIV infected persons. Substance abuse treatment should be recommended for persons who are using recreational drugs. They should be warned to avoid consuming raw meat or eggs to avoid infections with *Toxoplasma, Campylobacter,* and *Salmonella.* HIV-infected patients should wash their hands thoroughly after cleaning cat litter or should forgo this household chore to avoid possible exposure to toxoplasmosis. To reduce the likelihood of infection with *Bartonella* species, patients should avoid activities that might result in cat scratches or bites. Although the data are not conclusive, many clinicians recommend that HIV-infected persons—especially those with low CD4 counts—drink bottled water instead of tap water to prevent cryptosporidia infection.

Because of the emotional impact of HIV infection and subsequent illness, many patients will benefit from supportive counseling.

Baeten JM et al; Partners PrEP Study Team. Antiretroviral prophylaxis for HIV prevention in heterosexual men and women. N Engl J Med. 2012 Aug 2;367(5):399–410. [PMID: 22784037]

Choopanya K et al. Antiretroviral prophylaxis for HIV infection in injecting drug users in Bangkok, Thailand (the Bangkok Tenofovir Study): a randomised, double-blind, placebo-controlled phase 3 trial. Lancet. 2013 Jun 15;381(9883):2083–90. [PMID: 23769234]

Cohen MS et al; HPTN 052 Study Team. Prevention of HIV-1 infection with early antiretroviral therapy. N Engl J Med. 2011 Aug 11;365(6):493–505. [PMID: 21767103]

Kuhar DT et al. Updated US Public Health Service guidelines for the management of occupational exposures to human immunodeficiency virus and recommendations for postexposure prophylaxis. Infect Control Hosp Epidemiol. 2013 Sep;34(9):875–92. [PMID: 23917901]

Saunders KO. The design and evaluation of HIV-1 vaccines. AIDS. 2012 Jun 19;26(10):1293–302. [PMID: 22706011]

Stevens LM et al. JAMA patient page. HIV infection: the basics. JAMA. 2012 Jul 25;308(4):419. [PMID: 22820800]

U.S. Preventive Services Task Force. Screening for HIV: U.S. Preventive Services Task Force Recommendation Statement. April 2013. http://www.uspreventiveservicestaskforce.org/uspstf13/hiv/hivfinalrs.htm

► Treatment

Treatment for HIV infection can be broadly divided into the following categories: (1) prophylaxis for opportunistic infections, malignancies, and other complications of HIV infection; (2) treatment of opportunistic infections, malignancies, and other complications of HIV infection; and (3) treatment of the HIV infection itself with combination ART.

Treatment regimens for HIV infection are constantly changing. Clinicians may obtain up-to-date information on new and experimental treatments by calling the AIDS Clinical Trials Information Service (ACTIS), 800-TRIALS-A (English and Spanish), and the National AIDS Hot Line, 800-342-AIDS (English), 800-344-SIDA (Spanish), and 800-AIDS-TTY (hearing-impaired).

A. Prophylactic Treatment of Complications of HIV Infection

In general, decisions about prophylaxis of opportunistic infections are based on the CD4 count, other evidence of severe immunosuppression (eg, oral candidiasis), and a history of having had the infection in the past. In the era prior to HAART, patients who started taking prophylactic regimens were maintained on them indefinitely. However, studies have shown that in patients with robust improvements in immune function—as measured by increases in CD4 counts above the levels that are used to initiate treatment—prophylactic regimens can safely be discontinued.

Because individuals with advanced HIV infection are susceptible to a number of opportunistic pathogens, the use of agents with activity against more than one pathogen is preferable. It has been shown, for example, that trimethoprim-sulfamethoxazole confers some protection against toxoplasmosis in individuals receiving this medication for *Pneumocystis* prophylaxis.

1. Prophylaxis against *Pneumocystis* pneumonia— Patients with CD4 counts below 200 cells/mcL, a CD4 lymphocyte percentage below 14%, or weight loss or oral candidiasis should be offered primary prophylaxis for *Pneumocystis* pneumonia. Patients with a history of *Pneumocystis* pneumonia should receive secondary prophylaxis until they have had a durable virologic response to HAART for at least 3–6 months and maintain a CD4 count of > 250 cells/mcL. Regimens for *Pneumocystis* prophylaxis are given in Table 31–4.

Table 31–4. *Pneumocystis jirovecii* prophylaxis in order of preference.

Medication	Dose	Side Effects	Limitations
Trimethoprim-sulfamethoxazole	One double-strength tablet three times a week to one tablet daily	Rash, neutropenia, hepatitis, Stevens-Johnson syndrome	Hypersensitivity reaction is common but, if mild, it may be possible to treat through.
Dapsone	50–100 mg orally daily or 100 mg two or three times per week	Anemia, nausea, methemoglobinemia, hemolytic anemia	Less effective than above. Glucose-6-phosphate dehydrogenase (G6PD) level should be checked prior to therapy. Check methemoglobin level at 1 month.
Atovaquone	1500 mg orally daily with a meal	Rash, diarrhea, nausea	Less effective than suspension trimethoprim-sulfamethoxazole; equal efficacy to dapsone, but more expensive.
Aerosolized pentamidine	300 mg monthly	Bronchospasm (pretreat with bronchodilators); rare reports of pancreatitis	Apical *P jirovecii* pneumonia, extrapulmonary *P jirovecii* infections, pneumothorax.

2. Prophylaxis against *M avium* complex infection— Patients whose CD4 counts fall to below 75–100 cells/mcL should be given prophylaxis against *M avium* complex infection. Clarithromycin (500 mg orally twice daily) and azithromycin (1200 mg orally weekly) have both been shown to decrease the incidence of disseminated *M avium* complex infection by approximately 75%, with a low rate of breakthrough of resistant disease. The azithromycin regimen is generally preferred based on high compliance and low cost. Prophylaxis against *M avium* complex infection may be discontinued in patients whose CD4 counts rise above 100 cells/mcL in response to HAART and whose plasma viral load has been optimally suppressed to < 50–75 copies/mL.

3. Prophylaxis against *M tuberculosis* infection— Isoniazid, 300 mg orally daily, plus pyridoxine, 50 mg orally daily, for 9–12 months should be given to all HIV-infected patients with positive PPD reactions (defined as > 5 mm of induration for HIV-infected patients) without evidence of active disease.

4. Prophylaxis against toxoplasmosis—Toxoplasmosis prophylaxis is desirable in patients with a positive IgG toxoplasma serology and CD4 counts below 100 cells/mcL. Trimethoprim-sulfamethoxazole (one double-strength tablet daily) offers good protection against toxoplasmosis, as does a combination of pyrimethamine, 25 mg orally once a week, plus dapsone, 50 mg orally daily, plus leucovorin, 25 mg orally once a week. A glucose-6-phosphate dehydrogenase (G6PD) level should be checked prior to dapsone therapy, and a methemoglobin level should be checked at 1 month.

5. Prophylaxis against CMV infection—Oral ganciclovir (1000 mg three times daily with food) is approved for CMV prophylaxis among HIV-infected persons with advanced disease (eg, CD4 counts below 50 cells/mcL). However, because the medication causes neutropenia, it is not widely used. Clinicians should consider performing serum CMV IgG antibody testing prior to starting ganciclovir. Persons who are CMV IgG-negative are not at risk for development of CMV disease, although it is important that such patients receive only CMV-negative blood if they require transfusion. Because over 99% of MSM are positive for CMV IgG, it is appropriate to reserve such testing for heterosexuals with HIV.

6. Prophylaxis against cryptococcosis, candidiasis, and endemic fungal diseases—One trial showed a decreased incidence of cryptococcal disease with prophylaxis using fluconazole, 200 mg orally daily, but the treated group had no mortality benefit. Fluconazole (200 mg orally once a week) was found to prevent oral and vaginal candidiasis in women with CD4 counts below 300 cells/mcL. In areas of the world where histoplasmosis and coccidioidomycosis are endemic and are frequent complications of HIV infection, prophylactic use of fluconazole or itraconazole may prove to be useful strategies. However, the problem of identifying individuals at highest risk makes appropriate targeting of prophylaxis difficult.

B. Treatment of Complications of HIV Infection

Treatment of common AIDS-related complications is detailed above and in Table 31–5. In the era prior to the use of HAART, patients required lifelong treatment for many infections, including CMV retinitis, toxoplasmosis, and cryptococcal meningitis. However, among patients who have a good response to HAART, maintenance therapy for some opportunistic infections can be terminated. For example, in consultation with an ophthalmologist, maintenance treatment for CMV infection can be discontinued when persons receiving HAART have durable suppression of viral load (ie, < 50 copies/mL) and a CD4 count > 100–150 cells/mcL. Similar results have been observed in patients with *M avium* complex bacteremia. Cessation of secondary prophylaxis for *Pneumocystis* pneumonia is described above.

Treating patients with repeated episodes of the same opportunistic infection can pose difficult therapeutic challenges. For example, patients with second or third episodes of *Pneumocystis* pneumonia may have developed allergic reactions to standard treatments with a prior episode. Fortunately, there are several alternatives available for the treatment of *Pneumocystis* infection. Trimethoprim with dapsone and primaquine with clindamycin are two combinations that often are tolerated in patients with a prior allergic reaction to trimethoprim-sulfamethoxazole and intravenous pentamidine. Patients in whom second episodes of *Pneumocystis* pneumonia develop while taking prophylaxis tend to have milder courses.

Well-established alternative regimens also exist for most AIDS-related opportunistic infections: amphotericin B or fluconazole for cryptococcal meningitis; ganciclovir, cidofovir, or foscarnet for CMV infection; and sulfadiazine or clindamycin with pyrimethamine for toxoplasmosis.

Adjunctive Treatments—Although conceptually it would seem that **corticosteroids** should be avoided in HIV-infected patients, corticosteroid therapy has been shown to improve the course of patients with moderate to severe *P jirovecii* pneumonia (oxygen saturation < 90%, P_{O_2} < 65 mm Hg) when administered within 72 hours after diagnosis. Either intravenous methylprednisolone (Solu-medrol) or oral prednisone (40–80 mg daily tapering over 21 day) can be used. The mechanism of action is presumed to be a decrease in alveolar inflammation.

Corticosteroids have also been used to treat IRIS that can sometimes complicate the early treatment course when ART is initiated in patients with advanced AIDS (see section Inflammatory reactions [immune reconstitution inflammatory syndromes] above).

Epoetin alfa (erythropoietin) is approved for use in HIV-infected patients with anemia, including those with anemia secondary to zidovudine use. It has been shown to decrease the need for blood transfusions. The medication is expensive, and therefore an erythropoietin level < 500 mU/mL should be demonstrated before starting therapy. The starting dose of epoetin alfa is 8000 units subcutaneously three times a week. The target hematocrit is 35–40%. The dose may be increased by 12,000 units every 4–6 weeks as needed to a maximum dose of 48,000 units per week. Hypertension is the most common side effect.

Human G-CSF (filgrastim) and **granulocyte-macrophage colony-stimulating factor (GM-CSF [sargramostim])** have been shown to increase the neutrophil

Table 31–5. Treatment of AIDS-related opportunistic infections and malignancies.[1]

Infection or Malignancy	Treatment	Complications
Pneumocystis jirovecii infection[2]	Trimethoprim-sulfamethoxazole, 15 mg/kg/d (based on trimethoprim component) orally or intravenously for 14–21 days.	Nausea, neutropenia, anemia, hepatitis, rash, Stevens-Johnson syndrome.
	Pentamidine, 3–4 mg/kg/d intravenously for 14–21 days.	Hypotension, hypoglycemia, anemia, neutropenia, pancreatitis, hepatitis.
	Trimethoprim, 15 mg/kg/d orally, with dapsone, 100 mg/d orally, for 14–21 days.[3]	Nausea, rash, hemolytic anemia in G6PD[3]-deficient patients. Methemoglobinemia (weekly levels should be < 10% of total hemoglobin).
	Primaquine, 15–30 mg/d orally, and clindamycin, 600 mg every 8 hours orally, for 14–21 days.	Hemolytic anemia in G6PD-deficient patients. Methemoglobinemia, neutropenia, colitis.
	Atovaquone, 750 mg orally three times daily for 14–21 days.	Rash, elevated aminotransferases, anemia, neutropenia.
	Trimetrexate, 45 mg/m[2] intravenously for 21 days (given with leucovorin calcium) if intolerant of all other regimens.	Leukopenia, rash, mucositis.
Mycobacterium avium complex infection	Clarithromycin, 500 mg orally twice daily with ethambutol, 15 mg/kg/d orally (maximum, 1 g). May also add:	Clarithromycin: hepatitis, nausea, diarrhea; ethambutol: hepatitis, optic neuritis.
	Rifabutin, 300 mg orally daily.	Rash, hepatitis, uveitis.
Toxoplasmosis	Pyrimethamine, 100–200 mg orally as loading dose, followed by 50–75 mg/d, combined with sulfadiazine, 4–6 g orally daily in four divided doses, and folinic acid, 10 mg orally daily for 4–8 weeks; then pyrimethamine, 25–50 mg/d, with clindamycin, 2–2.7 g/d in three or four divided doses, and folinic acid, 5 mg/d, until clinical and radiographic resolution is achieved.	Leukopenia, rash.
Lymphoma	Combination chemotherapy (eg, modified CHOP, M-BACOD, with or without G-CSF or GM-CSF). Central nervous system disease: radiation treatment with dexamethasone for edema.	Nausea, vomiting, anemia, leukopenia, cardiac toxicity (with doxorubicin).
Cryptococcal meningitis	Amphotericin B, 0.6 mg/kg/d intravenously, with or without flucytosine, 100 mg/kg/d orally in four divided doses for 2 weeks, followed by:	Fever, anemia, hypokalemia, azotemia.
	Fluconazole, 400 mg orally daily for 6 weeks, then 200 mg orally daily.	Hepatitis.
Cytomegalovirus infection	Valganciclovir, 900 mg orally twice a day for 21 days with food (induction), followed by 900 mg daily with food (maintenance).	Neutropenia, anemia, thrombocytopenia.
	Ganciclovir, 10 mg/kg/d intravenously in two divided doses for 10 days, followed by 6 mg/kg 5 days a week indefinitely. (Decrease dose for kidney disease.) May use ganciclovir as maintenance therapy (1 g orally with fatty foods three times a day).	Neutropenia (especially when used concurrently with zidovudine), anemia, thrombocytopenia.
	Foscarnet, 60 mg/kg intravenously every 8 hours for 10–14 days (induction), followed by 90 mg/kg once daily. (Adjust for changes in kidney function.)	Nausea, hypokalemia, hypocalcemia, hyperphosphatemia, azotemia.
Esophageal candidiasis or recurrent vaginal candidiasis	Fluconazole, 100–200 mg orally daily for 10–14 days.	Hepatitis, development of imidazole resistance.
Herpes simplex infection	Acyclovir, 400 mg orally three times daily until healed; or acyclovir, 5 mg/kg intravenously every 8 hours for severe cases.	Resistant herpes simplex with long-term therapy.
	Famciclovir, 500 mg orally twice daily until healed.	Nausea.
	Valacyclovir, 500 mg orally twice daily until healed.	Nausea.
	Foscarnet, 40 mg/kg intravenously every 8 hours, for acyclovir-resistant cases. (Adjust for changes in kidney function.)	Nausea, hypokalemia, hypocalcemia, hyperphosphatemia, azotemia.

(continued)

Table 31–5. Treatment of AIDS-related opportunistic infections and malignancies.[1] (continued)

Infection or Malignancy	Treatment	Complications
Herpes zoster	Acyclovir, 800 mg orally four or five times daily for 7 days. Intravenous therapy at 10 mg/kg every 8 hours for ocular involvement, disseminated disease.	Resistant herpes simplex with long-term therapy.
	Famciclovir, 500 mg orally three times daily for 7 days.	Nausea.
	Valacyclovir, 500 mg orally three times daily for 7 days.	Nausea.
	Foscarnet, 40 mg/kg intravenously every 8 hours for acyclovir-resistant cases. (Adjust for changes in kidney function.)	Nausea, hypokalemia, hypocalcemia, hyperphosphatemia, azotemia.
Kaposi sarcoma		
Limited cutaneous disease	Observation, intralesional vinblastine.	Inflammation, pain at site of injection.
Extensive or aggressive cutaneous disease	Systemic chemotherapy (eg, liposomal doxorubicin). Interferon-alpha (for patients with CD4 > 200 cells/mcL and no constitutional symptoms). Radiation (amelioration of edema).	Bone marrow suppression, peripheral neuritis, flu-like syndrome.
Visceral disease (eg, pulmonary)	Combination chemotherapy (eg, daunorubicin, bleomycin, vinblastine).	Bone marrow suppression, cardiac toxicity, fever.

[1]For treatment of *M tuberculosis* infection, see Chapter 9.
[2]For moderate to severe *P jirovecii* infection (oxygen saturation < 90%), corticosteroids should be given with specific treatment. The dose of prednisone is 40 mg orally twice daily for 5 days, then 40 mg daily for 5 days, and then 20 mg daily until therapy is complete.
[3]When considering use of dapsone, check glucose-6-phosphate dehydrogenase (G6PD) level in black patients and those of Mediterranean origin. CHOP, cyclophosphamide, doxorubicin (hydroxydaunomycin), vincristine (Oncovin), and prednisone; G-CSF, granulocyte-colony stimulating factor (filgrastim); GM-CSF, granulocyte-macrophage colony-stimulating factor (sargramostim); modified M-BACOD, methotrexate, bleomycin, doxorubicin (Adriamycin), cyclophosphamide, vincristine (Oncovin), and dexamethasone.

counts of HIV-infected patients. Because of the high cost of this therapy, the dosage should be closely monitored and minimized, aiming for a neutrophil count of 1000/mcL. When the medication is used for indications other than cytotoxic chemotherapy, one or two doses at 5 mcg/kg per week subcutaneously are usually sufficient.

C. Antiretroviral Therapy

The availability of agents that in combination suppress HIV replication (Table 31–6) has had a profound impact on the natural history of HIV infection. Indeed, **with the advent of antiretroviral treatment, the life expectancy of HIV-infected persons approaches that of uninfected persons when treatment is initiated early in the course of the disease.**

The greater potency and the improved side effect profile have led to the recommendation to start treatment for all HIV-infected persons regardless of CD4 count. This recommendation has not been broadly embraced; however, there is widespread consensus that at a minimum treatment should be initiated for all symptomatic patients, and for asymptomatic persons who (1) have CD4 cell counts below 500 cells/mcL, (2) have rapidly dropping CD4 counts (> 100 cells/mcL/yr) or very high viral loads (> 100,000/mcL), (3) have active infection with hepatitis B or C (rapid HIV replication is thought to hasten progression of hepatitis B and C), (4) have risk factors for cardiac disease (ongoing HIV replication may increase the risk of

cardiac disease), (5) have HIV-related kidney impairment, (6) are pregnant, (7) have risk factors for non–AIDS-related cancers (rapid HIV replication may increase such cancers), or (8) are at high risk for transmitting HIV to another person. For patients with difficulty adhering to therapy, deferring ART until the patient is willing to commit to therapy may be a better strategy than inconsistent treatment. Because 5–20% of patients in developed countries who are treatment-naïve have a virus that is resistant to some medications, **resistance testing is recommended for all patients prior to initiating ART.**

Once a decision to initiate therapy has been made, several important principles should guide therapy. First, because medication resistance to antiretroviral agents develops in HIV-infected patients, a primary goal of therapy should be complete suppression of viral replication as measured by the serum viral load. Therapy that achieves a plasma viral load of < 20 or < 48 copies/mL (depending on the test used) has been shown to provide a durable response to the therapy. To achieve this and maintain virologic control over time, **combination therapy with at least three medications from at least two different classes is necessary**, and partially suppressive combinations such as dual nucleoside therapy should be avoided. Similarly, if toxicity develops, it is preferable to either interrupt the entire regimen or change the offending medication rather than reduce individual doses.

Randomized trials compared early initiation of ART (within 2 weeks of starting treatment for an opportunistic

Table 31–6. Antiretroviral therapy.

Medication	Dose	Common Side Effects	Special Monitoring[1]	Cost[2]	Cost/Month
Nucleoside reverse transcriptase inhibitors					
Abacavir (Ziagen)	300 mg orally twice daily	Rash, fever—if occur, rechallenge may be fatal	No special monitoring	$10.04/300 mg	$602.66
Didanosine (ddI) (Videx)	400 mg orally daily (enteric-coated capsule) for persons ≥ 60 kg	Peripheral neuropathy, pancreatitis, dry mouth, hepatitis	Bimonthly neurologic questionnaire for neuropathy, potassium, amylase, bilirubin, triglycerides	$12.29/400 mg	$368.72
Emtricitabine (Emtriva)	200 mg orally once daily	Skin discoloration palms/soles (mild)	No special monitoring	$20.08/200 mg	$602.27
Lamivudine (3TC) (Epivir)	150 mg orally twice daily	Rash, peripheral neuropathy	No special monitoring	$7.16/150 mg	$429.60
Stavudine (d4T) (Zerit)	40 mg orally twice daily for persons ≥ 60 kg	Peripheral neuropathy, hepatitis, pancreatitis	Monthly neurologic questionnaire for neuropathy, amylase	$6.85/40 mg	$410.70
Zalcitabine (ddC) (Hivid)	0.375–0.75 mg orally three times daily	Peripheral neuropathy, aphthous ulcers, hepatitis	Monthly neurologic questionnaire for neuropathy	Not available in the US	Not available in the US
Zidovudine (AZT) (Retrovir)	600 mg orally daily in two divided doses	Anemia, neutropenia, nausea, malaise, headache, insomnia, myopathy	No special monitoring	$6.08/300 mg	$365.04
Nucleotide reverse transcriptase inhibitors					
Tenofovir (Viread)	300 mg orally once daily	Gastrointestinal distress	Creatinine every 3–4 months, urine analysis every 6–12 months	$34.92/300 mg	$1047.73
Nonnucleoside reverse transcriptase inhibitors (NNRTIs)					
Delavirdine (Rescriptor)	400 mg orally three times daily	Rash	No special monitoring	$2.40/200 mg	$432.66
Efavirenz (Sustiva)	600 mg orally daily	Neurologic disturbances, rash	No special monitoring	$28.74/600 mg	$862.14
Etravirine (Intelence)	200 mg orally twice daily	Rash, peripheral neuropathy	No special monitoring	$9.36/100 mg	$1123.52
Nevirapine (Viramune)	200 mg orally daily for 2 weeks, then 200 mg orally twice daily	Rash	No special monitoring	$10.83/200 mg	$650.05
Rilpivirine (Edurant)	25 mg daily	Depression, rash	No special monitoring	$30.78/25 mg	$923.47
Protease inhibitors (PIs)					
Fosamprenavir (Lexiva)	**For PI-experienced patients:** 700 mg orally twice daily and 100 mg of ritonavir orally twice daily. **For PI-naïve patients:** above or 1400 mg orally twice daily or 1400 mg orally once daily and 200 mg of ritonavir orally once daily	Gastrointestinal, rash	No special monitoring	$18.78/700 mg	$1126.69-2253.38 (plus cost of ritonavir for lower dose)

(continued)

Table 31–6. Antiretroviral therapy. (continued)

Medication	Dose	Common Side Effects	Special Monitoring[1]	Cost[2]	Cost/Month
Indinavir (Crixivan)	800 mg orally three times daily	Renal calculi	Bilirubin level every 3–4 months	$3.05/400 mg	$548.12
Lopinavir/ ritonavir (Kaletra)	400 mg/100 mg orally twice daily	Diarrhea	No special monitoring	$8.14/200 mg (lopinavir)	$977.22
Nelfinavir (Viracept)	750 mg orally three times daily or 1250 mg twice daily	Diarrhea	No special monitoring	$3.64/250 mg $8.45/625 mg	$1093.75 $1093.75
Ritonavir (Norvir)	600 mg orally twice daily or in lower doses (eg, 100 mg orally once or twice daily) for boosting other PIs	Gastrointestinal distress, peripheral paresthesias	No special monitoring	$10.29/100 mg	$3703.20 ($617.20 in lower doses)
Saquinavir hard gel (Invirase)	1000 mg orally twice daily with 100 mg ritonavir orally twice daily	Gastrointestinal distress	No special monitoring	$9.81/500 mg	$1177.58 (plus cost of ritonavir)
Atazanavir (Reyataz)	400 mg orally once daily or 300 mg atazanavir with 100 mg ritonavir daily.	Hyperbilirubinemia	Bilirubin level every 3–4 months	$23.71/200 mg	$1422.83 (plus cost of ritonavir)
Darunavir/ ritonavir (Prezista/ Norvir)	**For PI-experienced patients:** 600 mg of darunavir and 100 mg of ritonavir orally twice daily.	Rash	No special monitoring	$23.23.32/600 mg (darunavir) $10.29/100 mg (ritonavir)	$2016.45 (for combination)
	For PI-naïve patients: 800 mg of darunavir and 100 mg of ritonavir orally daily.			$23.32/400 mg (darunavir)	$1707.85 (for combination)
Tipranavir/ ritonavir (Aptivus/ Norvir)	500 mg of tipranavir and 200 mg of ritonavir orally twice daily	Gastrointestinal, rash	No special monitoring	$12.50/250 mg (tipranavir) $10.29/100 mg (ritonavir)	$2734.57 (for combination)
Entry inhibitors					
Enfuvirtide (Fuzeon)	90 mg subcutaneously twice daily	Injection site pain and allergic reaction	No special monitoring	$58.56/90 mg	$3513.49
Maraviroc (Selzentry)	150–300 mg orally daily	Cough, fever, rash	No special monitoring	$22.69/150 mg or 300 mg	$1361.21
Integrase inhibitors					
Raltegravir (Isentress)	400 mg orally twice daily	Diarrhea, nausea, headache	No special monitoring	$22.53/400 mg	$1352.05
Elvitegravir (available only in a fixed medication combination with cobicistat, tenofovir, emtricitabine, Stribild)	Elvitegravir 150 mg+ Cobicistat 150 mg+ Tenofovir 300 mg+ Emtricitabine 200 mg (One tablet daily)	Serum elevation of creatinine, diarrhea, rash	Creatinine every 3–4 months; urine analysis at initiation and first follow-up.	$98.29/Tablet	$2948.70

(continued)

Table 31–6. Antiretroviral therapy. (continued)

Medication	Dose	Common Side Effects	Special Monitoring[1]	Cost[2]	Cost/Month
Dolutegravir (Tivicay)	Treatment-naïve or integrase-naïve patients: 50 mg daily. When administered with efavirenz, forsamprenavir/ritonavir, tipranavir/ritonavir, or rifampin: 50 mg twice daily. When administered to integrase-experienced patients with suspected integrase resistance: 50 mg twice daily.	Hypersensitivity, rash	No special monitoring	$49.32/50 mg	$1479.59

[1]Standard monitoring is complete blood count (CBC) and differential, serum aminotransferases every 3–4 months, and cholesterol (total, LDL, HDL), and triglycerides 6 months after starting ART and annually among those over age 40 years.
[2]Average wholesale price (AWP, for AB-rated generic when available) for quantity listed. Source: *Red Book Online, 2014, Truven Health Analytics, Inc.* AWP may not accurately represent the actual pharmacy cost because wide contractual variations exist among institutions.

infection or tuberculosis) with ART that was deferred until after treatment of the opportunistic infection was completed (6 weeks after its start); results demonstrated that early initiation reduced death or AIDS progression by 50%. The reduced progression rates were related to more rapid improvements in CD4 counts in patients with advanced immunodeficiency. Furthermore, IRIS and other adverse events were no more frequent in the early ART arm. Based on these results, most treatment guidelines recommend that ART be initiated as early as is clinically feasible for patients with an acute AIDS-related opportunistic infection. For hospitalized patients, this recommendation requires close coordination between inpatient and outpatient physicians to ensure that treatment is continued once patients are discharged.

Several randomized studies have also demonstrated improved clinical outcomes in HIV/tuberculosis coinfected patients who initiate ART early in the setting of active treatment for tuberculosis and whose CD4 counts are < 50 cells/mcL. The exception to early ART in the setting of active infections may be in patients with a CNS-associated infection, such as cryptococcal or tuberculosis meningitis. Several studies from low-income countries have shown high mortality rates with early ART initiation in this setting, although this high mortality rate may be more related to the severity of the underlying infection at the time of entry to these studies.

Because the number of ART medications is finite, it is important to avoid medication resistance, which occurs when patients take medications in the setting of ongoing viral replication. Therefore, the best method for avoiding resistance is for the patient to be compliant with an efficacious regimen. Adherence can be promoted through the use of simple regimens (single pill once-a-day combination regimens (Table 31–8), and for those patients with more complicated regimens, medication boxes with compartments

[eg, Medisets]). Many patients benefit from adherence counseling and some need daily supervision of therapy. Given these options treatment should not be withheld solely on the basis of a patient's circumstances (eg, active drug use or housing status) alone. Often, a trial intervention such as offering *Pneumocystis* pneumonia prophylaxis may be helpful in determining the likelihood of adherence to a more complex antiretroviral regimen.

Monitoring of ART has two goals. Laboratory evaluation for toxicity depends on the specific medications in the combination but generally should be done approximately every 3–4 months once a patient is on a stable regimen. Patients who are intolerant of their initial regimen (eg, patients who cannot tolerate the neurologic side effects of efavirenz) should be changed to an alternative medication or regimen. The second aspect of monitoring is to regularly measure objective markers of efficacy. The CD4 cell count and HIV viral load should be repeated 1–2 months after the initiation or change of antiretroviral regimen and every 4–6 months thereafter in clinically stable patients (those with higher CD4 counts can have testing every 6 months). **In a patient who is adherent to an effective regimen, viral loads should be undetectable within 12–24 weeks.** For patients in whom viral loads are not suppressed or who have viral rebound after suppression, the major question facing the clinician is whether the patient is nonadherent or has resistance to the regimen, or both. The issue is complicated because many patients report being more compliant than they really are, not because they wish to be untruthful but because they wish to tell the clinician what he or she wants to hear. Patients who are having trouble adhering to their treatment should receive counseling on how to better comply with their treatment. In patients who are adherent or who have missed enough doses to make resistance possible, resistance testing should be performed. Based on the results of resistance testing, and assessment of the patient's ability to comply with complicated regimens or to tolerate predictable side effects, the clinician should prescribe a combination of three medications to which there is no or only minimal resistance. Some patients whose counts rise dramatically on ART and who are fully suppressed (ie, plasma viral load < 20 or 48 copies/mL depending on test used) may be successfully transitioned from a multiple pill regimen to a simpler one with fewer side effects; however, this "switch strategy" needs to take into consideration the possibility for underlying drug resistance that may have developed during prior ART regimens; increased risk of virologic break-through has been reported when switching to simpler regimens. Stopping therapy in patients with high CD4 counts will generally result in patients reverting to their pretreatment nadir CD4 count in a matter of months and is therefore not recommended.

Although the ideal combination of medications has not yet been defined for all possible clinical situations, possible regimens can be better understood after a review of the available agents. These medications can be grouped into five major categories: nucleoside and nucleotide reverse transcriptase inhibitors (NRTI); nonnucleoside reverse transcriptase inhibitors (NNRTI); PIs; entry inhibitors, which include a fusion inhibitor and CCR5 antagonists; and integrase inhibitors. Once ART has been initiated in a patient, it is not advisable to stop the therapy unless there is a compelling reason (eg, toxicity, poor adherence, etc). So-called "drug holidays" or "structured treatment interruptions" have been shown to increase risk of AIDS-related complications, increase CD4 declines, and increase morbidity from non–AIDS-related complications (eg, myocardial infarctions and liver failure) and are not recommended.

1. Nucleoside and nucleotide reverse transcriptase inhibitors—There are currently seven nucleoside or nucleotide agents available and approved for use. The choice of

which agent to use depends primarily on the patient's prior treatment experience, results of resistance testing, medication side effects, other underlying conditions, and convenience of formulation. However, most clinicians use fixed-dose combinations (see Table 31–7) of either tenofovir/emtricitabine (TDF/FTC) or abacavir/lamivudine (ABC/3TC), both of which can be given once a day. Zidovudine/lamivudine (AZT/3TC) is usually reserved for second- or third-line regimens because of toxicity and dosing schedule. Recent studies have raised some concerns about the efficacy of ABC/3TC in patients with high viral loads (eg, > 100,000 copies/mL) as well as concerns about increase risks of myocardial infarction with abacavir. However, other studies have been unable to confirm these findings, and therefore, ABC/3TC (at least in some combinations) along with TDF/FTC are the preferred fixed-dose combinations as part of initial treatment regimens.

Of the available agents, zidovudine is the most likely to cause anemia. Zidovudine and didanosine are the most likely to cause neutropenia. Stavudine is the most likely to cause lipoatrophy (loss of fat in the face, extremities, and buttocks) followed by zidovudine. Zalcitabine and didanosine are the most likely to cause peripheral neuropathy. Lamivudine, emtricitabine, and tenofovir have activity against hepatitis B. Didanosine, lamivudine, emtricitabine, and tenofovir can be administered daily. Information specific to each medication is given below, and recommendations on how to combine them appear in the Constructing regimens section below.

A. Zidovudine—Zidovudine was the first approved antiviral medication for HIV infection and remains an important agent. It is administered at a dose of 300 mg orally twice daily. A combination of zidovudine 300 mg and lamivudine 150 mg (Combivir; see Table 31–7) allows more convenient dosing of medication for individuals taking both of these agents. Side effects seen with zidovudine

Table 31–7. Fixed dose antiretroviral combinations.

Name	Components	Dosing and Special Considerations	Cost per month
Truvada	Tenofovir 300 mg Emtricitabine 200 mg	One pill daily with a NNRTI, protease inhibitor, integrase inhibitor, or maraviroc (entry inhibitor). Most commonly used nucleoside/nucleotide reverse transcriptase inhibitor backbone	$1539.90
Epzicom	Abacavir 600 mg Lamivudine 300 mg	One pill daily with a NNRTI, protease inhibitor, integrase inhibitor, or maraviroc (entry inhibitor).	$1324.93
Trizivir	Abacavir 300 mg Lamivudine 150 mg Zidovudine 300 mg	One tablet twice daily with a NNRTI, protease inhibitor, integrase inhibitor, or maraviroc (entry inhibitor). Although it contains three medications it does not constitute a complete treatment.	$1931.64
Atripla	Tenofovir 300 mg Emtricitabine 200 mg Efavirenz 600 mg	One pill daily constitutes a complete regimen. Most commonly used single-pill regimen available.	$2402.04
Stribild	Tenofovir 300 mg Emtricitabine 200 mg Elvitegravir 150 mg Cobicistat 150 mg	One pill daily constitutes a complete regimen. Although it contains four medications, one component (Cobicistat) is a medication booster only.	$2948.70
Complera	Tenofovir 300 mg Emtricitabine 200 mg Rilpivirine 25 mg	One pill daily constitutes complete regimen. Only for patients with HIV viral load < 100,000/mL.	$2463.37

are listed in Table 31–6. Approximately 40% of patients experience subjective side effects that usually remit within 6 weeks. The common dose-limiting side effects are anemia and neutropenia, which require ongoing laboratory monitoring. Long-term use has been associated with lipoatrophy.

B. Lamivudine—Lamivudine (3TC) is a safe and well-tolerated agent. The dosage is 150 mg orally twice daily or 300 mg orally once a day. The dose should be reduced with chronic kidney disease. There are no significant side effects with lamivudine, and it has activity also against hepatitis B.

C. Emtricitabine—Emtricitabine is a nucleoside analog that is dosed at 200 mg orally. It was developed primarily as a once a day alternative to lamivudine. However, lamivudine can be dosed daily, eliminating the special indication for emtricitabine. As is true of lamivudine, emtricitabine has activity against hepatitis B and its dosage should be reduced in patients with chronic kidney disease.

D. Abacavir—A daily dose of 300 mg orally twice daily results in potent antiretroviral activity. Prior to initiation of abacavir, patients should undergo testing for HLA typing. Those with the B*5701 allele should not be treated with abacavir because the likelihood of a hypersensitivity reaction developing is high; the reaction is characterized by a flu-like syndrome with rash and fever that worsens with successive doses. Unfortunately, the absence of this allele does not guarantee that the patient will avoid the hypersensitivity reaction. Individuals in whom the hypersensitivity reaction develops *should not* be rechallenged with this agent because subsequent hypersensitivity reactions can be fatal. Abacavir has also been associated with an increased risk of myocardial infarction in some cohort studies. This increased risk is generally seen in patients who have underlying risks of cardiovascular disease. Consequently, abacavir should be used with caution in such patients if effective alternative nucleoside or nucleotide analog agents exist. Abacavir is usually prescribed as a fixed-dose combination pill with lamivudine for use as a once daily pill (Epzicom; Table 31–7).

Abacavir is also formulated with zidovudine and lamivudine in a single pill (Trizivir, one tablet orally twice daily; Table 31–7). Trizivir is not recommended as solo treatment for HIV because it is not as efficacious as combining two nucleoside/nucleotide analogs with a PI/ritonavir or an NNRTI; its use as a sole regimen should be reserved only for patients who cannot tolerate a more complicated regimen.

E. Tenofovir—Tenofovir is the only licensed nucleotide analog. It is given as a single daily oral dose of 300 mg and is generally well tolerated. Tenofovir is available in a fixed dose combination pill with emtricitabine (Truvada; Table 31–7) for daily dosing and as part of most preferred initial ART regimens. Several single-tablet once-a-day complete regimens that include tenofovir (Atripla, Complera, Stribild) are available (Table 31–7). Tenofovir is active against hepatitis B, including isolates that have resistance to lamivudine.

F. Didanosine—The most convenient formulation of didanosine (ddI) is the enteric-coated capsule. For adults weighing at least 60 kg, the dose is one 400-mg enteric-coated capsule orally daily; for those 30–59 kg, the dose is one 250-mg enteric-coated capsule orally daily. Didanosine should be taken on an empty stomach.

Didanosine has been associated with pancreatitis. The incidence of pancreatitis with didanosine is 5–10%—of fatal pancreatitis, < 0.4%. Patients with a history of pancreatitis, as well as those taking other medications associated with pancreatitis (including trimethoprim-sulfamethoxazole and intravenous pentamidine) are at higher risk for this complication. Other common side effects with didanosine include a dose-related, reversible, painful peripheral neuropathy, which occurs in about 15% of patients, and dry mouth. Fulminant hepatic failure and electrolyte abnormalities, including hypokalemia, hypocalcemia, and hypomagnesemia, have been reported in patients taking didanosine. Because of the side-effect profile, didanosine is rarely used today.

G. Stavudine—Stavudine (d4T) has shown good activity as an antiretroviral medication. The dose is 40 mg orally twice daily for individuals weighing 60 kg or more. However, because of its side effects including lipoatrophy, lipodystrophy (see below), peripheral neuropathy and, rarely, lactic acidosis and hepatitis, this medication should no longer be used except when there is no alternative. Patients taking stavudine should be routinely changed to abacavir or tenofovir, both of which are less likely to cause lipoatrophy.

2. Nonnucleoside reverse transcriptase inhibitors—NNRTIs inhibit reverse transcriptase at a site different from that of the nucleoside and nucleotide agents described above. All five NNRTIs have shown antiviral activity as measured by HIV viral load and CD4 responses. The major advantage of the NNRTIs is that three of them (efavirenz, rilpivirine, and nevirapine) have potencies comparable to that of PIs (next section), at least for patients with viral loads under 100,000 copies/mL—with lower pill burden and fewer side effects. In particular, they do not appear to cause lipodystrophy; patients with cholesterol and triglyceride elevations who are switched from a PI to an NNRTI may have improvement in their lipids. The resistance patterns of the NNRTIs are distinct from those of the PIs, so their use still leaves open the option for future PI use.

The NNRTIs can be used with PIs in patients who are difficult to suppress on simpler regimens or when it is difficult to identify at least two nucleoside/nucleotide agents to which the patient is not resistant. Because these agents may cause alterations in the clearance of PIs, dose modifications may be necessary when these two classes of medications are administered concomitantly. There is a high degree of cross-resistance between the "first-generation" NNRTIs, such that resistance to one medication in this class uniformly predicts resistance to other medications. However, etravirine appears to have consistent antiviral activity in patients with prior exposure and resistance to nevirapine, efavirenz, or delavirdine. In particular, the K103N mutation does not appear to have an impact on etravirine (or rilpivirine). There is no therapeutic reason for using more than one NNRTI at the same time.

A. Efavirenz—The major advantages of efavirenz is that it can be given once daily in a single dose (600 mg orally), and it is available in a once-daily fixed-dose combination with tenofovir and emtricitabine in a single pill (Atripla; Table 31–7). The regimen is one of the best first choice for treatment-naïve patients without resistance to any of its components. The major side effects are rash and psychiatric/neurologic complaints, with patients reporting symptoms ranging from lack of concentration and strange dreams to delusions and mania. These side effects are related to the efavirenz component and tend to wane over time, usually within a month or so. There are some patients who cannot tolerate these effects, especially if they persist longer than a month. Administration of efavirenz with food, especially fatty food, may increase its serum levels and consequent neurotoxicity. Due to teratogenicity, efavirenz should be avoided in women who wish to conceive or are already pregnant.

B. Rilpivirine—This medication, dosed at 25 mg once daily, is approved for persons initiating ART and is equal in efficacy to efavirenz in patients with HIV viral loads below 100,000 copies/mL. Those with higher viral loads should be treated with one of the other preferred regimens. As is true of efavirenz, rilpivirine is available in a once-daily fixed-dose combination with tenofovir and emtricitabine (Complera; Table 31–7) to be taken with a fatty meal (at least 290 calories). Rilpivirine has fewer neurologic side effects than efavirenz, making it a good choice as a first regimen, or an alternative regimen in patients who cannot tolerate the neurologic side effects of efavirenz.

C. Nevirapine—The target dose of nevirapine is 200 mg orally twice daily, but it is initiated at a dose of 200 mg once a day to decrease the incidence of rash, which is as high as 40% when full doses are begun immediately. If rash develops while the patient is taking 200 mg/d, liver enzymes should be checked and the dose should not be increased until the rash resolves. Patients with mild rash and no evidence of hepatotoxicity can continue to be treated with nevirapine. Nevirapine should not be used in treatment-naïve women with high CD4 counts (> 250/mcL). Because of potential fatal hepatotoxicity, nevirapine should only be used in patients who cannot tolerate efavirenz. An extended-release formulation of nevirapine (Viramune XR) allows for once-daily dosing (400 mg daily). In clinical trials, nevirapine XR was not inferior when compared with standard nevirapine (both forms of nevirapine were combined with tenofovir/emtricitabine). This XR formulation potentially provides another once daily NNRTI regimen for first-line ART, although there has yet to be a direct comparison to any of the currently preferred first-line ART regimens (see below).

D. Delavirdine—Of the available NNRTIs, delavirdine is used the least largely because of its less convenient dosing and pill burden compared with the other available NNRTIs. Unlike nevirapine and efavirenz, delavirdine inhibits P450 cytochromes rather than inducing these enzymes. This means that delavirdine can act like ritonavir and boost other antiretrovirals, although delavirdine is not as potent as ritonavir in this capacity. The dosage is 400 mg orally three times a day. The major side effect is rash.

E. Etravirine—Etravirine is an NNRTI approved for the treatment of patients with prior NNRTI intolerance or resistance. Etravirine has been shown to be effective even when some degree of NNRTI-resistance is present, making it a true "second generation" medication in this class. Etravirine dosage is one 200-mg tablet twice daily. It should be used with a PI and a nucleoside/nucleotide analog and not just with two nucleoside/nucleotide analogs. The most common side effects are nausea and rash; rarely, the rash can be severe (toxic epidermal necrolysis). Patients with signs of severe rash or hypersensitivity reactions should immediately discontinue the medication. Prior rash due to treatment with one of the other NNRTIs does not make rash more likely with etravirine. Etravirine should not be taken by people with severe liver disease or administered with tipranavir/ritonavir, fosamprenavir/ritonavir, atazanavir/ritonavir, full-dose ritonavir, or PIs without low-dose ritonavir.

3. Protease inhibitors—Ten PIs—indinavir, nelfinavir, ritonavir, saquinavir, amprenavir, fosamprenavir, lopinavir (in combination with ritonavir), atazanavir, darunavir, and tipranavir are available. PIs are potent suppressors of HIV replication and are administered as part of a combination regimen.

All the PIs—to differing degrees—are metabolized by the cytochrome P450 system, and each can inhibit and induce various P450 isoenzymes. Therefore, medication interactions are common and difficult to predict. Clinicians should consult the product inserts before prescribing PIs with other medications. Medications such as rifampin that are known to induce the P450 system should be avoided.

The fact that the PIs are dependent on metabolism through the cytochrome P450 system has led to the use of ritonavir to boost the medication levels of saquinavir, lopinavir, indinavir, atazanavir, tipranavir, darunavir and amprenavir, allowing use of lower doses and simpler dosing schedules of these PIs. In fact, current guidelines recommend that all PI-containing regimens use ritonavir boosting if possible. The only PIs that can be safely used without ritonavir boosting are nelfinavir and atazanavir.

When choosing which PI to use, prior patient experience, resistance patterns, side effects, and ease of administration are the major considerations. The first three PIs to be developed—indinavir, saquinavir, and ritonavir (as single agents)—are now rarely used because of the superiority of the second generation of PIs. Amprenavir has been almost entirely replaced by its prodrug, fosamprenavir. Unfortunately, all PIs, with the exception of unboosted atazanavir have been linked to a constellation of metabolic abnormalities, including elevated cholesterol levels, elevated triglyceride levels, insulin resistance, diabetes mellitus, and changes in body fat composition (eg, buffalo hump, abdominal obesity). The lipid abnormalities and body habitus changes are referred to as **lipodystrophy.** Although lipodystrophy is commonly associated with PIs, it has been seen also in HIV-infected persons who have never been treated with these agents. In particular, the lipoatrophy effects seen in patients receiving ART appears to be more related to the nucleoside toxicity and in particular to the thymidine analogs (stavudine and zidovudine).

Of the different manifestations of lipodystrophy, the dyslipidemias that occur are of particular concern because of the likelihood that increased levels of cholesterol and triglycerides will result in increased prevalence of heart disease. **All patients taking PIs or NRTIs should have fasting serum cholesterol, low-density lipoprotein (LDL) cholesterol, and triglyceride levels performed every 12 months.** Clinicians should calculate the Framingham 10-year coronary heart disease risk (see Chapter 28) and consider initiating dietary or medication therapy (or both) to achieve target LDL levels depending on the individual's risk factors. Patients who are unable to meet their LDL goal based solely on dietary interventions should be given pravastatin (20 mg daily orally) or atorvastatin (10 mg daily orally). Lovastatin and simvastatin should be avoided because of their interactions with PIs. Fish oil (3000 mg daily) combined with exercise and dietary counseling has been found to decrease triglycerides levels by 25%. Patients with persistently elevated fasting serum triglyceride levels of 500 mg/dL or more who do not respond to dietary intervention should be treated with gemfibrozil (600 mg twice daily prior to the morning and evening meals).

A. Indinavir—The standard dose of indinavir is 800 mg orally three times a day, although it is usually dosed twice daily in combination with ritonavir. Nausea and headache are common complaints with this medication. Indinavir crystals are present in the urine in approximately 40% of patients; this results in clinically apparent nephrolithiasis in about 15% of patients receiving indinavir. Lower urinary tract symptoms and acute kidney injury also have been reported. Patients taking this medication should be instructed to drink at least 48 ounces of fluid a day to ensure adequate hydration in an attempt to limit these complications. Mild indirect hyperbilirubinemia is also commonly observed in patients taking indinavir but is not an indication for discontinuation of the medication.

B. Saquinavir—Saquinavir is formulated only as a hard-gel capsule (Invirase). It should only be used with ritonavir (1000 mg of hard-gel saquinavir with 100 mg of ritonavir orally twice daily). The most common side effects with saquinavir are diarrhea, nausea, dyspepsia, and abdominal pain.

C. Ritonavir—Use of this potent PI at full dose (600 mg orally twice daily) has been limited by its inhibition of the cytochrome P450 pathway causing a large number of drug–drug interactions and by its frequent side effects of fatigue, nausea, and paresthesias. However, it is widely used in lower dose (eg, 100 mg daily to 100 mg twice daily) as a booster of other PIs.

D. Nelfinavir—Nelfinavir is the only PI for which ritonavir boosting is not recommended. Unboosted nelfinavir is generally not as potent as a boosted PI regimen (eg, lopinavir plus ritonavir). The dose of nelfinavir is 1250 mg orally twice daily. Diarrhea is a side effect in 25% of patients taking nelfinavir, but this symptom may be controlled with over-the-counter antidiarrheal agents in most patients.

E. Amprenavir—Amprenavir has efficacy and side effects similar to those of other PIs. Common side effects are nausea, vomiting, diarrhea, rash, and perioral paresthesia. The dose is 1200 mg orally twice daily. The concentration of amprenavir decreases when coadministered with ethinyl estradiol; therefore, amprenavir should be used with circumspection in the treatment of transgender persons requiring high-dose estrogen.

F. Fosamprenavir—Fosamprenavir is a prodrug of amprenavir. Its major advantage over using amprenavir is a much lower pill burden. For PI-naïve patients, it can be dosed at 1400 mg orally twice daily (four capsules a day) or at 1400 mg orally daily (two capsules) with ritonavir 200 mg orally daily (two capsules) or at 700 mg orally with ritonavir 100 mg orally twice daily. Patients previously treated with PIs should receive 700 mg orally with ritonavir 100 mg orally twice daily. Side effects are similar to those with amprenavir—most commonly gastrointestinal distress and hyperlipidemia. As with amprenavir, the concentration of fosamprenavir decreases when coadministered with ethinyl estradiol; therefore, fosamprenavir should be used with circumspection in the treatment of transgender persons requiring high-dose estrogen.

G. Lopinavir/r—Lopinavir/r is lopinavir (200 mg) coformulated with a low dose of ritonavir (50 mg) to maximize the bioavailability of lopinavir. It has been shown to be more effective than nelfinavir when used in combination with stavudine and lamivudine. The usual dose is 400 mg lopinavir with 100 mg of ritonavir (two tablets) orally twice daily with food. When given along with efavirenz or nevirapine, a higher dose (600 mg/150 mg—three tablets) is usually prescribed. The most common side effect is diarrhea, and lipid abnormalities are frequent. Because of these side effects, lopinavir/r has fallen off the list of medications recommended as part of first-line treatment regimens, although it remains the preferred choice in pregnant women.

H. Atazanavir—Atazanavir can be dosed as 400 mg (two 200-mg capsules) daily with food or it can be dosed as 300 mg in combination with 100 mg of ritonavir once daily with food. When used without ritonavir, it has only minimal or no impact on cholesterol and triglyceride levels. The most common side effect is mild hyperbilirubinemia that resolves with discontinuation of the medication. Nephrolithiasis and cholelithiasis has also been reported with this PI. Both tenofovir and efavirenz lower the serum concentration of atazanavir. Therefore, when either of these two medications is used with atazanavir, it should be boosted by administering ritonavir. Proton pump inhibitors are contraindicated in patients taking atazanavir because atazanavir requires an acidic pH to remain in solution.

I. Tipranavir—Tipranavir is the only nonpeptidic PI approved by the US Food and Drug Administration (FDA). Because of its unique structure, it is active against some strains of HIV that are resistant to other PIs. It is dosed with ritonavir (two 250 mg capsules of tipranavir with two 100 mg capsules of ritonavir orally twice daily with food).

The most common side effects are nausea, vomiting, diarrhea, fatigue, and headache. Tipranavir/ritonavir has been also associated with liver damage and should be used very cautiously in patients with underlying liver disease. Reports of intracranial hemorrhage in patients taking tipranavir-containing regimens have raised additional safety concerns about this potent PI. Because it is a sulfa-containing medication, its use should be closely monitored in patients with sulfa allergy.

J. Darunavir—Darunavir has impressive antiviral activity in the setting of significant PI resistance and in treatment-naïve patients. Darunavir has been added to the list of recommended PIs for initial treatment of HIV at a daily dose of 800 mg with 100 mg of ritonavir. For patients with prior PI treatment experience or PI resistance (with mutations known to impact darunavir – see below), darunavir should be dosed at 600 mg orally twice daily, with ritonavir, 100 mg orally twice daily. Once daily dosing can be used in treatment-experienced patients who do not have darunavir-related resistance mutations. Darunavir has a safety profile similar to other PIs, such as lopinavir/ritonavir but is generally better tolerated. Like tipranavir, darunavir is a sulfa-containing medication, and its use should be closely monitored in patients with sulfa allergy.

4. Entry inhibitors—

A. Enfuvirtide—Enfuvirtide (Fuzeon) is known as a fusion inhibitor; it blocks the entry of HIV into cells by blocking the fusion of the HIV envelope to the cell membrane. The addition of enfuvirtide to an optimized antiretroviral regimen improved CD4 counts and lowered viral loads in heavily pretreated patients with multidrug-resistant HIV. Unfortunately, resistance develops rapidly in patients receiving nonsuppressive treatment. The dose is 90 mg by subcutaneous injection twice daily; unfortunately, painful injection site reactions develop in most patients, which makes long-term use problematic.

B. Maraviroc—Maraviroc is a CCR5 co-receptor antagonist. Medications in this class prevent the virus from entering uninfected cells by blocking the CCR5 co-receptor. Unfortunately, this class of entry inhibitors is only active against "CCR5-tropic virus." This form of the HIV-1 virus tends to predominate early in infection, while so-called "dual/mixed tropic virus" (which utilizes either R5 or CXCR4 co-receptors) emerges later as infection progresses. Approximately 50–60% of previously treated HIV-infected patients have circulating CCR5-tropic HIV. The medication has been shown to be effective in HIV-infected persons with ongoing viral replication despite being heavily treated and who have CCR5-tropic virus. Tropism testing should be performed before beginning the medication. The dose of maraviroc is 150–300 mg orally twice daily, based on the other medications the patient is taking at the time—in combination with a ritonavir boosted PI, 150 mg daily of maraviroc has been used successfully. Common side effects are cough, fever, rash, musculoskeletal problems, abdominal pain, and dizziness; however, maraviroc is generally well tolerated with limited impact on serum lipids.

5. Integrase inhibitors—

A. Raltegravir—Raltegravir is an HIV integrase inhibitor. Integrase inhibitors slow HIV replication by blocking the HIV integrase enzyme needed for the virus to multiply. Raltegravir was impressively effective (when combined with other active medications) in the treatment of HIV-infected patients with documented resistance to at least one medication in each of the three main classes of antiretroviral medications (nucleoside analogs, PIs, NNRTIs). Clinical trials of all integrase inhibitors reveal a consistent pattern of more rapid decline in viral load compared with more standard PI/r or NNRTI-based regimens. The clinical significance of this observation is unclear. Despite the impressive antiviral potency of this new class of antiretroviral medications, high-level resistance to integrase inhibitors emerges quickly in the setting of virologic failure (much like with the NNRTIs). Therefore, it is critical that raltegravir be used in combination with other active antiretroviral agents.

Raltegravir is approved by the FDA for treatment-naïve patients. The dose of raltegravir is 400 mg orally twice daily. Common side effects are diarrhea, nausea, and headache, but overall it is well tolerated and has the additional advantage over PI-based regimens and efavirenz-based regimens in that appears to have little impact on lipid profiles or glucose metabolism.

B. Elvitegravir—Elvitegravir is the second integrase inhibitor to be approved by the FDA for the treatment of HIV and like raltegravir, it is a highly potent strand-transfer inhibitor (the last step required for integrase activity). Elvitegravir was approved for treatment-naïve patients as part of a once-a-day single-tablet regimen. The combination pill is marketed under the brand name of Stribild (Table 31–7) and contains 125 mg of elvitegravir and 150 mg of cobicistat, a boosting agent, along with standard doses of tenofovir and emtricitabine. Stribild has been shown to be noninferior to two preferred first-line regimens: Atripla and boosted atazanavir with tenofovir/emtricitabine. The main side effects include increases in serum creatinine levels which has been shown to be related to the cobicistat inhibition of tubular secretion of creatinine by the kidney and is thought to be nonpathologic and reversible. However, because of this effect, Stribild is recommended in treatment-naïve patients with estimated glomerular filtration rate > 70 mL/min. A urine analysis should be done at baseline and at initial follow-up to look for proteinuria and glycosuria, which are signs of tubulopathy. Diarrhea and rash may also occur, although overall the medication is well tolerated.

C. Dolutegravir—Dolutegravir is a third strand transfer integrase inhibitor available for the treatment of HIV. It shows excellent potency and tolerability and is dosed once-a-day in most circumstances. Unlike elvitegravir, dolutegravir does not require a boosting agent. Similar to cobicistat, it inhibits tubular secretion of creatinine by the kidney, resulting in small increases in serum creatinine levels. The standard dosage used in treatment-naïve, integrase-naïve patients is 50 mg/d. In patients receiving efavirenz, fosamprenavir/ritonavir, tipranavir/ritonavir, or rifampin, the dose should be increased to 50 mg twice daily. It should also be dosed at 50 mg twice daily in integrase-experienced patients in whom integrase resistance is suspected. Indeed, when combined with other active medications, it has been shown to provide some activity in patients with integrase resistance who have not responded to prior raltegravir- or elvitegravir-containing regimens. Dolutegravir has demonstrated impressive results from clinical trials of treatment-naïve patients when compared with the more standard NNRTI, boosted PI, and raltegravir-containing regimens. In fact, dolutegravir was superior to efavirenz/tenofovir/emtricitabine and superior to durunavir/ritonavir/tenofovir/emtricitabine in patients with baseline viral loads > 100,000 copies/mL. These results underscore the medication's impressive antiviral potency and excellent tolerability profile.

6. Constructing regimens—There is now little debate about the necessity for combining medications to achieve long-term suppression of HIV and the associated clinical benefit. Only combinations of three or more medications have been able to decrease HIV viral load by 2–3 logs and provide durable suppression of HIV RNA to below the threshold of detection.

Current evidence supports the use of Truvada (tenofovir and emtricitabine) as the "nucleoside/nucleotide backbone" combined with either efavirenz (three-medication combination marketed as Atripla) or one of two boosted PIs (atazanavir or darunavir) or any of the three available integrase inhibitors (raltegravir, dolutegravir or a boosted-integrase inhibitor [elvitegravir, marketed as a fixed-dose combination named Stribild]) as the initial regimen of choice (Table 31–8). In addition, the latest DHHS guidelines also classify dolutegravir combined with the

Table 31–8. Preferred initial antiretroviral regimens.

Regimen	Advantages	Disadvantages
Atripla (tenofovir/ emtricitabine/efavirenz)	Single tablet once-a-day regimen Longest term clinical experience Highly effective across broad range of initial CD4 counts and viral loads	Avoid in patients with transmitted K103N Neuropsychiatric symptoms common and can be persistent Should not be used in women who are pregnant or wish to conceive
Complera (tenofovir/ emtricitabine/rilpivirine)	Single tablet once-a-day regimen Excellent tolerability[1] Noninferior to Atripla in patients with baseline viral load < 100,000/mcL Limited metabolic side-effects	Requires taking with a meal Cannot be used with proton pump inhibitors Use with caution in patients with viral loads > 100,000/mcL
Atazanavir with ritonavir boosting + Truvada (emtricitabine/tenofovir)	Once-a-day regimen Well tolerated[1] Limited risk of resistance with poor adherence Resistance to atazanavir generally does not confer resistance to other PIs	Not available as a single tablet Increases in bilirubin (nonpathologic) Increased risk of cholelithiasis and nephrolithiasis, especially with prolonged use Has metabolic side effects
Darunavir with ritonavir boosting + Truvada (emtricitabine/tenofovir)	Potent boosted PI Can be given once daily Well tolerated[1] Limited risk of resistance with poor adherence	Not available as a single tablet May cause rash in patients with sulfa allergy Ritonavir boosting required Has metabolic side effects
Raltegravir + Truvada (emtricitabine/tenofovir)	Excellent tolerability[1] Metabolically neutral Superior to Atripla over 5-years of follow-up	Requires twice a day dosing No single tablet available
Stribild (emtricitabine/ tenofovir/elvitegravir with cobicistat boosting)	Single tablet once-a-day regimen Well tolerated[1] Excellent response across broad range of CD4 and viral loads	Limited clinical experience in women; requires boosting with similar drug-drug interactions as ritonavir; increases in serum creatinine (nonpathologic); requires estimated glomerular filtration rate > 70 mL/min
Dolutegravir + Epzicom (abacavir/lamivudine) Or dolutegravir + emtricitabine/ tenofovir	Excellent tolerability[1] Has activity in some patients with integrase resistance Superior to Atripla and superior to darunavir/ ritonavir/tenofovir/emtricitabine in patients with viral load > 100,000/mcL	No single tablet available When used in patients with integrase resistance or combined with certain other medications, requires twice a day dosing

[1] Combination regimens noted to have *excellent* tolerability have a drop-out rate due to adverse events of about 2%. Those that are noted as *well* tolerated have a drop-out rate due to adverse events of about 4–5%. In comparison, the drop-out rate due to adverse events for Atripla is 5–10%.

nucleoside fixed dose combination of abacavir/lamivudine as a preferred regimen. These regimens are preferred because of their combination of antiviral potency and tolerability as well as dosing convenience. Atripla and Stribild offer the additional advantage of being available as a once-a-day single tablet and a once-a-day single tablet containing dolutegravir/abacavir/lamivudine is expected. Studies in treatment-naïve patients have demonstrated that raltegravir in combination with tenofovir/emtricitabine is as effective as efavirenz/tenofovir/emtricitabine for daily treatment and has fewer side effects. It has little adverse impact on lipid and glucose metabolism although it is not available in a single tablet. In a 5-year follow-up to the double-blind trial, the raltegravir arm actually outperformed the efavirenz combination regimen due largely to better long-term tolerability. Furthermore, the CD4 response appeared better in patients treated with the raltegravir combination. A single-pill regimen Complera (tenofovir, emtricitabine, and rilpivirine) is not considered a preferred option given its lower virologic efficacy in patients with high viral loads (ie, > 100,000/mL) but remains a very good choice with excellent tolerability in patients with lower viral loads. Because 8–10% of newly infected persons in some urban areas of the United States have NNRTI resistance (primarily K103N), resistance testing should be performed before initiating efavirenz in this population. Patients with NNRTI resistance would not be expected to respond fully to an efavirenz-based regimen. The boosted PI regimens require more pills, have many medication–medication interactions and may have additional undesirable metabolic impacts. In patients with increased risk of metabolic abnormalities or comorbidities, the unboosted integrase-based regimens should be considered preferred choices although lacking the convenience of once-a-day, single-pill regimens at present. Regimens that include only nucleoside and nucleotide analogs without nonnucleoside agents or PIs are clinically inferior and should only be used for patients that cannot adhere to a more complicated regimen.

The most important determinant of treatment efficacy is adherence to the regimen. Therefore, it is vitally important that the regimen chosen be one to which the patient can easily adhere (Figure 31–2). In general, patients are more compliant with medication regimens (Table 31–8) that offer a complete regimen in one pill that needs to be taken only once or twice a day, do not require special timing with regard to meals, can be taken at the same time as other medications, do not require refrigeration or special preparation, and do not have bothersome side effects.

In constructing regimens, toxicities should be nonoverlapping and agents that are either virologically antagonistic or incompatible in terms of drug–drug interactions should be avoided. For example, the combination of stavudine plus didanosine should be avoided, since there is increased risk of toxicities, in particular in pregnant women because of the increased risk of lactic acidosis, which can be fatal. Moreover, the nucleoside pair of zidovudine and stavudine should be avoided because of increased toxicity and the potential for antagonism that results from intracellular competition for phosphorylation. The combination of didanosine with tenofovir should be avoided because of observed declines in CD4 counts. Etravirine should not be used with boosted tipranavir because of drug-drug interactions. Finally, highly complex therapeutic regimens should be reserved for individuals who are capable of adhering to the rigorous demands of taking multiple medications and having this therapy closely monitored.

In designing second-line regimens for patients with resistance to initial therapy, the goal is to identify three medications from at least two different classes to which the virus is not resistant. This can be quite complicated because

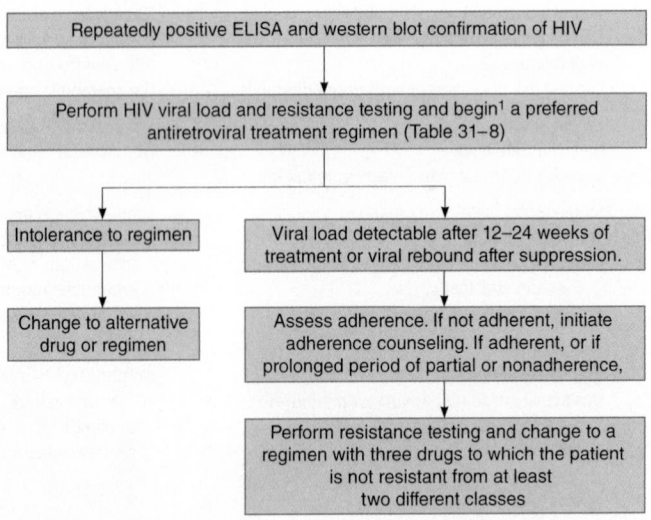

^1 Some clinicians prefer to wait until CD4 count < 500 cells or patient symptomatic. Patient must be motivated to comply with treatment.

▲ **Figure 31–2.** Approach to initial and subsequent antiretroviral therapy.

of the problem of cross-resistance between medications within a class. For example, the resistance patterns of lopinavir/ritonavir and indinavir are overlapping, and patients with virus resistant to these agents are unlikely to respond to nelfinavir or saquinavir even though they have never received treatment with these agents. Similarly, the resistance patterns of nevirapine and efavirenz are overlapping– as are the resistance patterns between raltegravir and elvitegravir. With several new classes of medications and new generations of existing medication classes now available, the ability to provide fully suppressive regimens even to patients with extensive treatment experience and medication resistance has become more realistic. The goal of therapy, therefore, should be to fully suppress viral loads to < 50 copies/mL even for highly treatment-experienced patients.

In addition to taking a careful history of what antiretroviral agents a patient has taken and for how long, genotypic and phenotypic resistance testing can provide useful information in designing second-line regimens.

Whatever regimen is chosen, patients should be coached in ways to improve adherence. For certain populations (eg, unstably housed individuals), specially tailored programs that include medication dispensing are needed.

Rarely, it is impossible to construct a tolerable regimen that fully suppresses HIV. In such cases, clinicians and patients should consider their goals. Patients maintained on effective antiretroviral agents often benefit from these regimens (eg, higher CD4 counts, fewer opportunistic infections) even if their virus is detectable. In some cases, patients may request a medication holiday during which they are taken off all medications. Patients often immediately feel better because of the absence of medication side effects. Unfortunately, structured treatment interruptions generally result in viral rebound and rapid CD4 decline followed by AIDS-related and non–AIDS-related morbidities and increased risk of death.

7. The challenge of medication resistance—HIV-1 medication resistance limits the ability to fully control HIV replication and remains an important cause for antiretroviral regimen failure. Resistance has been documented for all currently available antiretrovirals including the newer classes of fusion inhibitor, CCR5 inhibitors, and integrase inhibitors. The problem of medication resistance is widespread in HIV-infected patients undergoing treatment in countries where ART is widely available. However, reports suggest that the degree of high level resistance is declining in the past few years, which is likely related to better tolerated, easier to use, and more efficacious antiretroviral agents. Patients who have taken various antiretroviral regimens and who now have resistant HIV-1 represent a major challenge for the treating clinician. Resistance is now also documented in patients who are ART-naive, but who have been infected with a medication resistant strain—primary resistance or transmitted medication resistance. Cohort studies of antiretroviral treatment–naive patients entering care in North America and Western Europe show that roughly 10–12% (and as high as 25%) of recently infected individuals have been infected with a medication-resistant strain of HIV-1.

Current expert guidelines recommend resistance testing as part of standard baseline testing in all patients. Resistance testing is also recommended for patients who are receiving ART and have suboptimal viral suppression (ie, viral loads > 200 copies/mL). Both genotypic and phenotypic tests are commercially available and in randomized controlled studies their use has been shown to result in improved short-term virologic outcomes compared to making treatment choices without resistance testing. Furthermore, multiple retrospective studies have conclusively demonstrated that resistance tests provide prognostic information about virologic response to newly initiated therapy that cannot be gleaned from standard clinical information (ie, treatment history, examination, CD4 count, and viral load tests).

Because of the complexity of resistance tests, many clinicians require expert interpretation of results. In the case of genotypic assays, results may show that the mutations that are selected for during ART are medication-specific or contribute to broad cross-resistance to multiple medications within a therapeutic class. An example of a medication-specific mutation for the reverse transcriptase inhibitors would be the M184V mutation that is selected for by lamivudine or emtricitabine therapy—this mutation causes resistance only to those two medications. Conversely, the thymidine analog mutations ("TAMs") of M41L, D67N, K70R, L210W, T215Y/F, and T219Q/K/E are selected for by either zidovudine or stavudine therapy, but cause resistance to all the medications in the class and often extend to the nucleotide inhibitor tenofovir when three or more of these TAMs are present. Further complicating the interpretation of genotypic tests is the fact that some mutations that cause resistance to one medication can actually make the virus that contains this mutation more sensitive to another medication. The M184V mutation, for example, is associated with increased sensitivity to zidovudine, stavudine, and tenofovir. The most common mutations associated with medication resistance and cross-resistance patterns for NRTIs, NNRTIs, PIs, and integrase inhibitors can be found at http://hivdb.stanford.edu. Phenotypic tests also require interpretation in that the distinction between a resistant virus and sensitive one is not fully defined for all available medications.

Both methods of resistance testing are limited by the fact that they may measure resistance in only some of the viral strains present in an individual. Resistance results may also be misleading if a patient is not taking antiretroviral medications at the time of testing. Thus, resistance results must be viewed cumulatively—ie, if resistance is reported to an agent on one test, it should be presumed to be present thereafter even if subsequent tests do not give the same result.

Despite the prevalence of resistance in patients who have not responded to multiple prior treatment regimens and given the availability of new class medications and new generation medications, virtually all patients—no matter how much resistance is present—can be treated with a combination of ART that should be fully suppressive.

▶ **Course & Prognosis**

With improvements in therapy, patients are living longer after the diagnosis of AIDS. A population-based study conducted in Denmark found that HIV-infected persons at age 25 years without hepatitis C had a life expectancy similar to that of an uninfected 25-year-old. Unfortunately, not all HIV-infected persons have access to treatment. Studies consistently show less access to treatment for blacks, the homeless, and injection drug users. In addition to access to treatment, sustaining lower mortality will require developing new treatments for patients in whom resistance to existing agents develops. For patients whose disease progresses even though they are receiving appropriate treatment, meticulous palliative care must be provided (see Chapter 5), with attention to pain control, spiritual needs, and family (biologic and chosen) dynamics.

▶ When to Refer

- HIV-infected patients should be referred to specialists, given the increasing number of treatment regimens available.

- Extra efforts should be made to obtain specialty consultation for those patients with detectable viral loads on ART; those intolerant of standard medications; those in need of systemic chemotherapy; and those with complicated opportunistic infections, particularly when invasive procedures or experimental therapies are needed.

▶ When to Admit

Patients with opportunistic infections who are acutely ill (eg, who are febrile, who have had rapid change of mental status, or who are in respiratory distress) or who require intravenous medications.

Abdool Karim SS et al. Integration of antiretroviral therapy with tuberculosis treatment. N Engl J Med. 2011 Oct 20;365(16): 1492–501. [PMID: 22010915]

Cohen CJ et al; THRIVE Study Group. Rilpivirine versus efavirenz with two background nucleoside or nucleotide reverse transcriptase inhibitors in treatment-naïve adults infected with HIV-1 (Thrive): a phase 3, randomized, non-inferiority trial. Lancet. 2011;378(9787):229–37. [PMID: 21763935]

Eron JJ et al; BENCHMRK Study Teams. Efficacy and safety of raltegravir for treatment of HIV for 5 years in the BENCHMRK studies: final results of two randomised, placebo-controlled trials. Lancet Infect Dis. 2013 Jul;13(7):587–96. [PMID: 23664333]

Havlir DV et al; AIDS Clinical Trials Group Study A5221. Timing of antiretroviral therapy for HIV-1 infection and tuberculosis. N Engl J Med. 2011 Oct 20;365(16):1482–91. [PMID: 22010914]

Molina JM et al; ECHO Study Group. Rilpivirine versus efavirenz with tenofovir and emtricitabine in treatment-naïve adults infected with HIV-1 (ECHO): a phase 3 randomized double-blind active-controlled trial. Lancet. 2011 July 16;378 (9787):238–46. [PMID: 21763936]

Raffi F et al; extended SPRING-2 Study Group. Once-daily dolutegravir versus twice-daily raltegravir in antiretroviral-naive adults with HIV-1 infection (SPRING-2 study): 96 week results from a randomised, double-blind, non-inferiority trial. Lancet Infect Dis. 2013 Nov;13(11):927–35. [PMID: 24074642]

Rockstroh JK et al. A randomized, double-blind comparison of coformulated elvitegravir/cobicistat/emtricitabine/tenofovir DF vs ritonavir-boosted atazanavir plus coformulated emtricitabine and tenofovir DF for initial treatment of HIV-1 infection: analysis of week 96 results. J Acquir Immune Defic Syndr. 2013 Apr 15;62(5):483–6. [PMID: 23337366]

Török ME et al. Timing of initiation of antiretroviral therapy in human immunodeficiency virus (HIV)-associated tuberculous meningitis. Clin Infect Dis. 2011 Jun;52(11):1374–83. [PMID: 21596680]

U.S. Department of Health and Human Services. Guidelines for the use of antiretroviral agents in HIV-1-infected adults and adolescents. http://aidsinfo.nih.gov/guidelines/html/1/adult-and-adolescent-arv-guidelines/11/what-to-start

US Food and Drug Administration. FDA Drug Safety Communication: interactions between certain HIV or hepatitis C drugs and cholesterol-lowering statin drugs can increase the risk of muscle injury. http://www.fda.gov/Drugs/DrugSafety/ucm293877.htm

Walmsley SL et al; SINGLE Investigators. Dolutegravir plus abacavir-lamivudine for the treatment of HIV-1 infection. N Engl J Med. 2013 Nov 7;369(19):1807–18. [PMID: 24195548]

Wittkop L et al. Effect of transmitted drug resistance on virological and immunological response to initial combination antiretroviral therapy for HIV (EuroCoord-CHAIN joint project): a European multicohort study. Lancet Infect Dis. 2011 May;11(5):363–71. [PMID: 21354861]

Zolopa A et al; GS-US-236-0102 Study Team. A randomized double-blind comparison of coformulated elvitegravir/cobicistat/emtricitabine/tenofovir disoproxil fumarate versus efavirenz/emtricitabine/tenofovir disoproxil fumarate for initial treatment of HIV-1 infection: analysis of week 96 results. J Acquir Immune Defic Syndr. 2013 May 1;63(1):96–100. [PMID: 23392460]

Viral & Rickettsial Infections

Wayne X. Shandera, MD

J. Daniel Kelly, MD

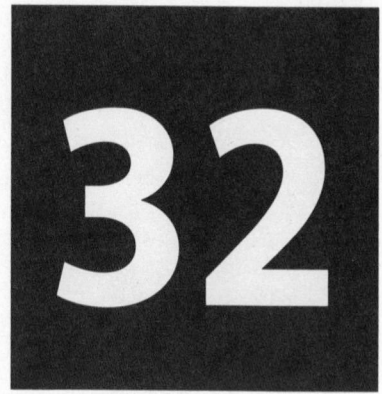

32

VIRAL DISEASES

HUMAN HERPESVIRUSES

1. Herpesviruses 1 & 2

ESSENTIALS OF DIAGNOSIS

▸ Spectrum of illness from stomatitis and urogenital lesions to facial nerve paralysis (Bell palsy) and encephalitis.

▸ Variable intervals between exposure and clinical disease, since HSV causes both primary (often subclinical) and reactivation disease.

▸ General Considerations

Herpesviruses 1 and 2 affect primarily the oral and genital areas, respectively. Asymptomatic shedding of either virus is common, especially following primary infection or symptomatic recurrences, and may be responsible for transmission. Asymptomatic HSV-2–infected individuals shed the virus less frequently than those with symptomatic infection. Disease is typically a manifestation of reactivation. Total and subclinical shedding of HSV-2 virus decrease after the first year of initial infection, although viral shedding continues for years thereafter. Higher than expected rates of HSV-2 lesions occur among women in the postpartum period and also among women who have sex with women.

Although HSV-2 is the most common cause of genital ulcers in the developed world, HSV-1 is increasingly recognized as causing primary urogenital infections. HSV-2 seropositivity increases the risk of HIV acquisition (it is threefold higher among persons who are HSV-2-seropositive than among those who are HSV-2 seronegative), and reactivates more frequently in advanced HIV infection. HIV replication is increased by interaction with HSV proteins. Suppression of HSV-2 decreases HIV-1 plasma levels and genital tract shedding of HIV, which can contribute to a reduction in sexual transmission of HIV-1.

▸ Clinical Findings

A. Symptoms and Signs

1. Mucocutaneous disease—See Chapter 6 for **HSV-1 mucocutaneous disease** involving the mouth and oral cavity ("herpes labialis" or "gingivostomatitis;" the latter largely in children). Digital lesions **(whitlows)** (Figure 32–1) are an occupational hazard in medicine and dentistry. Contact sports (eg, wrestling) are associated with outbreaks of skin infections ("herpes gladiatorum"). Asymptomatic shedding of HSV-1 is frequent, with most infected individuals shedding virus at least once a month.

Vesicles form moist ulcers after several days and epithelialize over 1–2 weeks if untreated. Primary infection is usually more severe than recurrences but may be asymptomatic. Recurrences often involve fewer lesions, tend to be labial, heal faster, and are induced by stress, fever, infection, sunlight, chemotherapy (eg, fludarabine, azathioprine) or other undetermined factors.

HSV-2 lesions largely involve the genital tract, with the virus remaining latent in the presacral ganglia (see Chapter 6). Occasionally, lesions arise in the perianal region or on the buttocks and upper thighs. Dysuria, cervicitis, and urinary retention may occur in women. Most HSV-2 infected persons in the United States are unaware that they are infected. Current epidemiologic studies show that HSV-1 is a more common cause of both genital and oral lesions than HSV-2 in young women in the United States.

Proctitis and sacral lesions in HIV-infected persons with CD4 cytopenia may present with extensive, ulcerating, weeping lesions. Large ulcerations and atypical lesions suggest drug-resistant isolates (see below).

2. Ocular disease—HSV can cause keratitis, blepharitis, and keratoconjunctivitis. Keratitis is usually unilateral and is often associated with impaired visual acuity. Lesions limited to the epithelium usually heal without affecting vision, whereas stromal involvement can cause uveitis, scarring, and eventually blindness. Recurrences of ocular disease are frequent. HSV is the second most common cause, after VZV, of acute retinal necrosis.

3. Neonatal and congenital infection—Both herpesviruses can infect the fetus and induce congenital

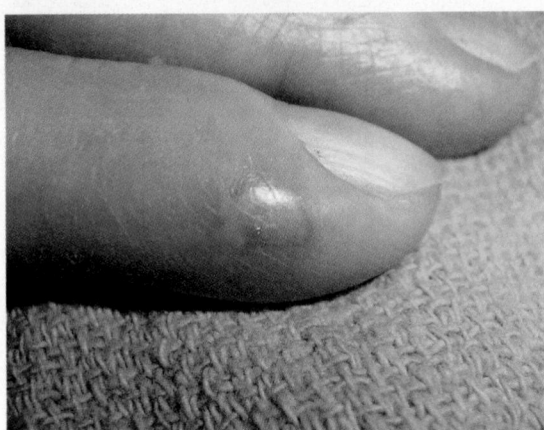

▲ **Figure 32–1.** Herpetic whitlow. (Reproduced, with permission, from Richard P. Usatine, MD.)

malformations (organomegaly, bleeding, and CNS abnormalities). Maternal infection during the third trimester is associated with the highest risk of neonatal transmission, but about 70% of these infections are asymptomatic or unrecognized. Neonatal transmission during delivery, however, is more common than intrauterine infection. Invasive fetal monitoring and vacuum or forceps delivery increase the risk of herpesvirus transmission.

4. Central nervous system disease—Herpes simplex encephalitis is predominantly caused by HSV-1 and presents with nonspecific symptoms: a flu-like prodrome, followed by headache, fever, behavioral and speech disturbances, and focal or generalized seizures. The temporal lobe is often involved. Untreated disease and presentation with coma carry a high mortality rate, with many survivors suffering neurologic sequelae.

Both HSV-1 and HSV-2 are increasingly recognized as a cause of mild, nonspecific neurologic symptoms and are also associated with benign recurrent lymphocytic (Mollaret) meningitis. Primary HSV-2 infection in women often presents as aseptic meningitis. Recurrent meningitis from HSV-2 occurs in both younger and older individuals.

5. Disseminated infection—Disseminated HSV infection occurs in the setting of immunosuppression, either primary or iatrogenic, or rarely with pregnancy. In disseminated disease, skin lesions are not always present. Disseminated skin lesions are a particular complication in patients with atopic eczema (eczema herpeticum) and burns. Pneumonia can occur regardless of immune status.

6. Bell palsy—HSV-1 is a cause of Bell palsy.

7. Esophagitis and proctitis—HSV-1 can cause esophagitis in immunocompromised patients, particularly those with AIDS. The lesions are smaller and deeper than those observed in patients with CMV esophagitis or with other herpesvirus known to cause esophagitis in immunocompromised hosts. HSV-1 may also activate mononuclear cells in the pathogenesis of achalasia. Proctitis occurs mainly in men who have sex with men.

8. Erythema multiforme—Herpes simplex viruses remain, along with certain drugs, a leading cause of erythema multiforme minor ("herpes-associated erythema multiforme") and of the more severe condition Stevens–Johnson syndrome/toxic epidermal necrolysis (see also Chapter 6).

9. Other—HSV is the cause of approximately 1% of cases of acute liver failure, particularly in pregnant women and immunosuppressed patients. The mortality of such rare fulminant hepatitis is nearly 75%. An HSV lower respiratory tract infection of unknown clinical significance is common in mechanically ventilated patients. Evidence suggests that this finding is usually an indicator rather than the cause of a poor clinical condition. HSV-1 pneumonia is associated with high morbidity in patients with solid tumors. HSV-1 is reported to be a cause of perinephric abscess, febrile neutropenia, chronic urticaria, and esophagitis and enteritis in systemic lupus erythematosus. HSV is also associated with *Helicobacter pylori*–negative upper gastrointestinal tract ulcers.

B. Laboratory Findings

1. Mucocutaneous disease—See Chapter 6.

2. Ocular disease—Herpes keratitis is diagnosed by branching (dendritic) ulcers that stain with fluorescein. The extent of epithelial injury in herpes keratitis correlates well with polymerase chain reaction (PCR) positivity.

3. Encephalitis and recurrent meningitis—Cerebrospinal fluid pleocytosis is common, with a similar increase in the number of red cells. HSV DNA PCR of the cerebrospinal fluid is a rapid, sensitive, and specific tool for early diagnosis and can be included in a multiple rapid array panel. Antibodies to HSV in cerebrospinal fluid can confirm the diagnosis but appear late in disease. Viral culture shows a sensitivity of only 10%. MRI scanning is often a useful adjunct showing increased signal in the temporal and frontal lobes. Temporal lobe seizure foci may be shown on electroencephalograms (EEGs).

4. Esophagitis and proctitis—Esophagitis is diagnosed by endoscopic biopsy and cultures. Proctitis may be diagnosed by rectal swab for PCR or culture, or both, with complicated cases requiring biopsy.

5. Pneumonia—Pneumonia is diagnosed by clinical, pathologic, and radiographic findings. The CT findings include diffuse or multifocal areas of ground-glass attenuation or consolidative changes or both and are best confirmed using high-resolution CT techniques.

▶ Treatment & Prophylaxis

Medications that inhibit replication of HSV-1 and HSV-2 include trifluridine and vidarabine (both for keratitis), acyclovir and related compounds, foscarnet, and cidofovir (Table 32–1).

A. Mucocutaneous Disease

See Chapter 6.

Table 32–1. Agents for viral infections.[1]

Drug	Dosing	Spectrum	Renal Clearance/ Hemodialysis	CNS & CSF Penetration	Toxicities
Acyclovir	200–800 mg orally five times daily; 250–500 mg/m[2] intravenously every 8 hours for 7 days	HSV, VZV	Yes/Yes	Yes	Neurotoxic reactions, reversible renal dysfunction, local reactions
Adefovir	10 mg daily orally	HBV	Yes/Yes	NAD[2]	Gastrointestinal symptoms, transaminitis, lactic acidosis, nephrotoxicity, rebound hepatitis.
Amantadine	200 mg daily orally, once daily in the elderly	Influenza A (not H1N1)	Yes/Yes	Yes	Confusion
Boceprevir	800 mg three times daily	HCV	NAD/NAD[2]	NAD[2]	Flu-like illness, fatigue, nausea, dysgeusia, anemia.
Cidofovir	5 mg/kg intravenously weekly for 2 weeks, then every other week	CMV	Yes/NAD[2]	NAD[2]	Neutropenia, renal failure, ocular hypotonia
Emtricitabine	200 mg daily orally	HBV, HIV	Yes/Yes	Some	Lactic acidosis, rebound hepatitis.
Entecavir	0.5 mg orally daily, increase to 1 mg orally daily in lamivudine-resistant patients	HBV	Yes/Some	NAD[2]	Lactic acidosis, rebound hepatitis.
Famciclovir	500 mg orally three times daily for 7 days for acute VZV; 250 mg three times daily for 7–10 days for genital or cutaneous HSV-1/HSV-2 infection; 125 mg twice daily for 5 days for recurrences (500 mg twice daily for 7 days if HIV-infected)	HSV, VZV	Yes/NAD[2]	NAD[2]	Early angioedema; later rarely, gastrointestinal symptoms, headaches, rashes
Fomivirsen	165 mcg by intravitreal injection once weekly for 3 weeks, then every other week	CMV	NAD/NAD[2]	NAD[2]	Ocular inflammation, retinal detachment
Foscarnet	20 mg/kg intravenous bolus, then 120 mg/kg intravenously every 8 hours for 2 weeks; maintain with 60 mg/kg/d intravenously for 5 days each week	CMV, HSV resistant to acyclovir, VZV, HIV-1	Yes/Yes	Variable	Nephrotoxicity, genital ulcerations, calcium disturbances
Ganciclovir	5 mg/kg intravenous bolus every 12 hours for 14–21 days; maintain with 3.75 mg/kg/d intravenously for 5 days each week	CMV	Yes/Yes	Yes	Neutropenia, thrombocytopenia, CNS side effects
Idoxuridine	Topical, 0.1% every 1–2 hours for 3–5 days	HSV keratitis	NAD/NAD[2]	NAD[2]	Local reactions
Interferon alpha-2b	3–5 million international units subcutaneously three times weekly to daily. Intralesionally: 1 million international units per 0.1 mL in up to five warts three times weekly for 3 weeks	HBV, HCV, HPV	Yes/Yes	NAD[2]	Influenza-like syndrome, myelosuppression, neurotoxicity
Interferon alpha-n3	0.05 mL/wart biweekly up to 8 weeks	HPV	NAD/NAD[2]	NAD[2]	Local reactions
	3 mU intravenously three times per week	HCV	NAD/NAD[2]	NAD[2]	Influenza-like syndrome, myelosuppression, neurotoxicity

(continued)

Table 32–1. Agents for viral infections.[1] (continued)

Drug	Dosing	Spectrum	Renal Clearance/ Hemodialysis	CNS & CSF Penetration	Toxicities
Lamivudine (3TC)	150 mg orally twice daily or 300 mg once daily	HIV, HBV	Yes/NAD[2]	Yes	Skin rash, headache, insomnia, rebound hepatitis
Laninamivir (CS-8958)	40 mg single inhaled dose	Influenza A and B	NAD[2]	NAD[2]	Under study (medication is marketed in Japan)
Oseltamivir	75 mg orally twice daily for 5 days beginning 48 hours after onset of symptoms	Influenza A and B	Yes/No	NAD[2]	Few
Palivizumab	15 mg/kg intramuscularly every month in RSV season	RSV	No/No	No	Upper respiratory infection symptoms
Penciclovir	Topical 1% cream every 2 hours for 4 days	HSV	No/No	No	Local reactions
Peramivir[3]	Intravenous, 600 mg daily for 5–10 days	Influenza (H1N1)	Yes/NAD[2]	NAD[2]	Nausea, vomiting, diarrhea, neutropenia
Ribavirin	Aerosol: 1.1 g/d as 20 mg/mL dilution over 12–18 hours for 3–7 days (See text for Lassa fever doses.)	RSV, severe influenza A or B, Lassa fever	Yes/No	Yes	Wheezing
Rimantadine	100 mg twice daily orally, once daily in the elderly	Influenza A (not H1N1)	No/No	Yes	Confusion
Telaprevir	750 mg three times daily	HCV	NAD/NAD[2]	NAD[2]	Anemia, neutropenia, rash including Stevens-Johnson syndrome
Telbivudine	600 mg once daily orally	HBV	Yes/Yes	NAD[2]	Myositis, fatigue, headache, diarrhea, cough, nausea, dizziness, rash, arthralgias, neutropenia; lactic acidosis and rebound hepatitis
Tenofovir	300 mg once daily orally	HBV, HIV	Yes/Some	Some	Rash, neutropenia, lactic acidosis, renal failure (Fanconi syndrome), rebound hepatitis
Trifluridine	Topical, 1% drops every 2 hours to 9 drops/d	HSV keratitis	NAD/NAD[2]	NAD[2]	Local reactions
Valacyclovir	1 g orally three times daily for 7 days for acute VZV; 1 g twice daily for primary genital HSV-1/HSV-2 infection with 500 mg three times daily for recurrences	VZV, HSV	Yes/Poorly	NAD[2]	Thrombotic thrombocytopenic purpura or hemolytic-uremic syndrome in AIDS
Valganciclovir	900 mg orally twice daily for 3 weeks; 900 mg daily as maintenance	CMV	Yes/Yes	Yes	See ganciclovir
Vidarabine	15 mg/kg/d intravenously for 10 days	HSV, VZV	Yes/Yes	Yes	Teratogenic, megaloblastosis, neurotoxicity
Zanamivir	2–5 mg inhalations twice daily for 5 days	Influenza A and B	Yes/NAD[2]	NAD[2]	Few

[1]Agents used exclusively in the management of HIV infection and AIDS are found in Chapter 31.
[2]No available data or available data are insufficient to make an assessment.
[3]Available through the Centers for Disease Control and Prevention Emergency Use Authorization.
CMV, cytomegalovirus; CNS, central nervous system; CSF, cerebrospinal fluid; HBV, hepatitis B virus; HCV, hepatitis C virus; HPV, human papillomavirus; HSV, herpes simplex virus; RSV, respiratory syncytial virus; VZV, varicella-zoster virus.

B. Keratitis

For the treatment of acute epithelial keratitis, topical antiviral agents (ophthalmic trifluridine, vidarabine, acyclovir, and ganciclovir) are all nearly equivalent in efficacy and are recommended. Combination of topical antiviral agents with interferon or debridement (or both) hastens healing. Intravenous acyclovir is used for acute retinal necrosis. Oral famciclovir is a reasonable alternative, especially in patients unable to tolerate intravenous therapy and when acyclovir resistance is present. The usage of topical corticosteroids may exacerbate the infection, although systemic corticosteroids may help with selected cases of stromal infection. Long-term treatment (> 1 year) with acyclovir at a dosage of 800 mg/d orally decreases recurrence rates of keratitis, conjunctivitis or blepharitis due to HSV.

C. Neonatal Disease

Intravenous acyclovir (20 mg/kg every 8 hours for 14–21 days) is effective for the treatment of disseminated lesions in neonatal disease. Counseling with serologic screening should be offered to pregnant mothers. The use of maternal antenatal suppressive therapy with acyclovir (typically, 400 mg three times daily) beginning at 36 weeks gestation decreases the presence of detectable HSV, the rates of recurrence at delivery, and the need for cesarean delivery. Cesarean delivery is recommended for pregnant women with active genital lesions or typical prodromal symptoms.

D. Encephalitis and CNS Meningitis

Because of the need for rapid treatment to decrease mortality and neurologic sequelae, intravenous acyclovir (10 mg/kg every 8 hours for 10 days or more, adjusting for kidney dysfunction) should be started in those patients with suspected HSV encephalitis, stopping only if another diagnosis is established. If the PCR of cerebrospinal fluid is negative but clinical suspicion remains high, treatment should be continued for 10 days because the false-negative rate for PCR can be as high as 25% (especially in children) and acyclovir is relatively nontoxic. Data from the California Encephalitis project suggest that anti-N-methyl-D-aspartate receptor (anti-NMDAR) encephalitis is a more common entity than viral encephalitis especially in children (see West Nile virus encephalitis below).

Long-term neurologic sequelae of HSV encephalitis are common and late pediatric relapse is recognized. Acyclovir resistance in a case of herpes simplex encephalitis is reported. Aseptic meningitis may also require a course of intravenous acyclovir or valacyclovir.

E. Disseminated Disease

Disseminated disease responds best to parenteral acyclovir when treatment is initiated early.

F. Bell Palsy

Prednisolone, 25 mg orally twice daily for 10 days started within 72 h of onset, significantly increases the rate of recovery. Data on antiherpes antiviral agents are equivocal; according to one study, valacyclovir (but not acyclovir), 1 g orally daily for 5 days, plus corticosteroid therapy may be beneficial if started within 7 days of symptom onset. In patients with severe or complete facial paralysis, such antiviral therapy is often administered but without a firm proof of efficacy.

G. Esophagitis and Proctitis

Patients with esophagitis should receive either intravenous acyclovir (5–10 mg/kg every 8 hours) or oral acyclovir (400 mg five times daily) through resolution of symptoms, typically 3–5 days; however, longer treatment may be necessary for immunosuppressed patients. Maintenance therapy for AIDS patients is also with acyclovir (400 mg three to five times daily). Proctitis is treated with similar dosages and usually responds within 5 days.

H. Erythema Multiforme

Suppressive therapy with oral acyclovir (400 mg twice a day for 6 months) decreases the recurrence rate of HSV-associated erythema multiforme. Valacyclovir (500 mg twice a day) may be effective in cases unresponsive to acyclovir.

▶ Prevention

Besides antiviral suppressive therapy, prevention also requires counseling and the use of condom barrier precautions during sexual activity. Disclosure to sexual partners of HSV-seropositive status is associated with about a 50% reduction in the HSV-2 acquisition. Male circumcision is associated with a lower incidence of acquiring HSV-2 infection.

Preventing spread to hospital staff and other patients from cases with mucocutaneous, disseminated, or genital disease requires isolation and the usage of handwashing and gloving–gowning precautions. Staff with active lesions (eg, whitlows) should not have contact with patients. Asymptomatic transmission occurs, especially with HSV-2. The only effective vaccine to date is an HSV-2 subunit vaccine that protects against genital HSV-1 but not HSV-2 in women.

Belshe RB et al; Herpevac Trial for Women. Efficacy results of a trial of a herpes simplex vaccine. N Engl J Med. 2012 Jan 5; 366(1):34–43. [PMID: 22216840]

Bernstein DI et al. Epidemiology, clinical presentation, and antibody response to primary infection with herpes simplex virus type 1 and type 2 in young women. Clin Infect Dis. 2013 Feb;56(3):344–51. [PMID: 23087395]

Cunningham A et al. Current management and recommendations for access to antiviral therapy of herpes labialis. J Clin Virol. 2012 Jan;53(1):6–11. [PMID: 21889905]

Leveque N et al. Rapid virological diagnosis of central nervous system infections by use of a multiplex reverse transcription-PCR DNA microarray. J Clin Microbiol. 2011 Nov;49(11): 3874–9. [PMID: 21918017]

Tronstein E et al. Genital shedding of herpes simplex virus among symptomatic and asymptomatic persons with HSV-2 infection. JAMA. 2011 Apr 13;305(14):1441–9. [PMID: 21486697]

2. Varicella (Chickenpox) & Herpes Zoster (Shingles)

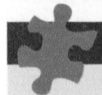

▶ Varicella rash: pruritic, centrifugal, papular, changing to vesicular ("dewdrops on a rose petal"), pustular, and finally crusting.

▶ Zoster rash: tingling, pain, eruption of vesicles in a dermatomal distribution, evolving to pustules and then crusting.

General Considerations

Varicella zoster virus (VZV), or HHV-3, disease manifestations include chickenpox (varicella) and shingles (herpes zoster). Chickenpox generally presents during childhood; has an incubation period of 10–20 days (average 2 weeks); and is highly contagious, spreading by inhalation of infective droplets or contact with lesions.

The incidence and severity of herpes zoster ("shingles"), which affects up to 25% of persons during their lifetime, increases with age due to an age-related decline in immunity against VZV. More than half of all patients in whom herpes zoster develops are older than 60 years, and the incidence of herpes zoster reaches 10 cases per 1000 patient-years by age 80 (by which time 50% are infected with VZV). The annual incidence in the United States of 1 million cases is increasing as the population ages. Populations at increased risk for varicella-zoster–related diseases include immunosuppressed persons and persons receiving biologic agents (ie, tumor necrosis factor [TNF] inhibitors).

Clinical Findings

A. Varicella

1. Symptoms and signs—Fever and malaise are mild in children and more marked in adults. The pruritic rash begins prominently on the face, scalp, and trunk, and later involves the extremities (Table 32–2). Maculopapules change in a few hours to vesicles that become pustular and eventually form crusts (Figures 32–2 and 32–3). New lesions may erupt for 1–5 days, so that different stages of the eruption are usually present simultaneously. The crusts slough in 7–14 days. The vesicles and pustules are superficial and elliptical, with slightly serrated borders. Pitted scars are frequent. Although the disease is often mild, complications (such as secondary bacterial infection, pneumonitis, and encephalitis) occur in about 1% of cases and often lead to hospitalization.

After the primary infection, the virus remains dormant in cranial nerves sensory ganglia and spinal dorsal root ganglia. Latent VZV will reactivate as herpes zoster in about 10–30% of persons (see below). Varicella is more severe in older patients and immunocompromised persons. In the latter, atypical presentations, including

Table 32–2. Diagnostic features of some acute exanthems.

Disease	Prodromal Signs and Symptoms	Nature of Eruption	Other Diagnostic Features	Laboratory Tests
Atypical measles	Same as measles.	Maculopapular centripetal rash, becoming confluent.	History of measles vaccination.	Measles antibody present in past, with titer rise during illness.
Chikungunya fever	2–4 (sometimes 1–12) days, fever, headaches, abdominal complaints, myalgias, arthralgias.	Maculopapular, centrally distributed, pruritus, can be bullous with sloughing in children, occasional facial edema and petechiae.	History of mosquito bites, epidemiologic factors.	ELISA-based immunoglobulin M or IgG (fourfold increase in titers); PCR and cultures are infrequently available.
Eczema herpeticum	None.	Vesiculopustular lesions in area of eczema.		Herpes simplex virus isolated in cell culture. Multinucleate giant cells in smear of lesion.
Ehrlichiosis	Headache, malaise.	Rash in one-third, similar to Rocky Mountain spotted fever.	Pancytopenia, elevated liver function tests.	Polymerase chain reaction, immunofluorescent antibody.
Enterovirus infections	1–2 days of fever, malaise.	Maculopapular rash resembling rubella, rarely papulovesicular or petechial.	Aseptic meningitis.	Virus isolation from stool or cerebrospinal fluid; complement fixation titer rise.
Erythema infectiosum (parvovirus B19)	None. Usually in epidemics.	Red, flushed cheeks; circumoral pallor; maculopapules on extremities.	"Slapped face" appearance.	White blood count normal.

(continued)

Table 32–2. Diagnostic features of some acute exanthems. (continued)

Disease	Prodromal Signs and Symptoms	Nature of Eruption	Other Diagnostic Features	Laboratory Tests
Exanthema subitum (HHV-6, 7; roseola)	3–4 days of high fever.	As fever falls, pink maculopapules appear on chest and trunk; fade in 1–3 days.		White blood count low.
Infectious mononucleosis (EBV)	Fever, adenopathy, sore throat.	Maculopapular rash resembling rubella, rarely papulovesicular.	Splenomegaly, tonsillar exudate.	Atypical lymphocytes in blood smears; heterophil agglutination (Monospot test).
Kawasaki disease	Fever, adenopathy, conjunctivitis.	Cracked lips, strawberry tongue, maculopapular polymorphous rash, peeling skin on fingers and toes.	Edema of extremities. Angiitis of coronary arteries.	Thrombocytosis, electrocardiographic changes.
Measles (rubeola)	3–4 days of fever, coryza, conjunctivitis, and cough.	Maculopapular, brick red; begins on head and neck; spreads downward and outward, in 5–6 days rash brownish, desquamating. See Atypical Measles, above.	Koplik spots on buccal mucosa.	White blood count low. Virus isolation in cell culture. Antibody tests by hemagglutination inhibition or neutralization.
Meningococcemia	Hours of fever, vomiting.	Maculopapules, petechiae, purpura.	Meningeal signs, toxicity, shock.	Cultures of blood, cerebrospinal fluid. White blood count high.
Rocky Mountain spotted fever	3–4 days of fever, vomiting.	Maculopapules, petechiae, initial distribution centripetal (extremities to trunk, including palms).	History of tick bite.	Indirect fluorescent antibody; complement fixation.
Rubella	Little or no prodrome.	Maculopapular, pink; begins on head and neck, spreads downward, fades in 3 days. No desquamation.	Lymphadenopathy, postauricular or occipital.	White blood count normal or low. Serologic tests for immunity and definitive diagnosis (hemagglutination inhibition).
Scarlet fever	One-half to 2 days of malaise, sore throat, fever, vomiting.	Generalized, punctate, red; prominent on neck, in axillae, groin, skin folds; circumoral pallor; fine desquamation involves hands and feet.	Strawberry tongue, exudative tonsillitis.	Group A beta-hemolytic streptococci in cultures from throat; antistreptolysin O titer rise.
Smallpox **(based on prior experience)**	Fever, malaise, prostration.	Maculopapules to vesicles to pustules to scars (lesions develop at the same pace).	Centrifugal rash; fulminant sepsis in small percentage of patients, gastrointestinal and skin hemorrhages.	Contact CDC[1] for suspicious rash; EM and gel diffusion assays.
Typhus	3–4 days of fever, chills, severe headaches.	Maculopapules, petechiae, initial distribution centrifugal (trunk to extremities).	Endemic area, lice.	Complement fixation.
Varicella (chickenpox)	0–1 day of fever, anorexia, headache.	Rapid evolution of macules to papules, vesicles, crusts; all stages simultaneously present; lesions superficial, distribution centripetal.	Lesions on scalp and mucous membranes.	Specialized complement fixation and virus neutralization in cell culture. Fluorescent antibody test of smear of lesions.

[1]http://www.bt.cdc.gov/agent/smallpox/response-plan/.
EBV, Epstein–Barr virus; EM, electron microscopy; HHV, human herpesvirus.

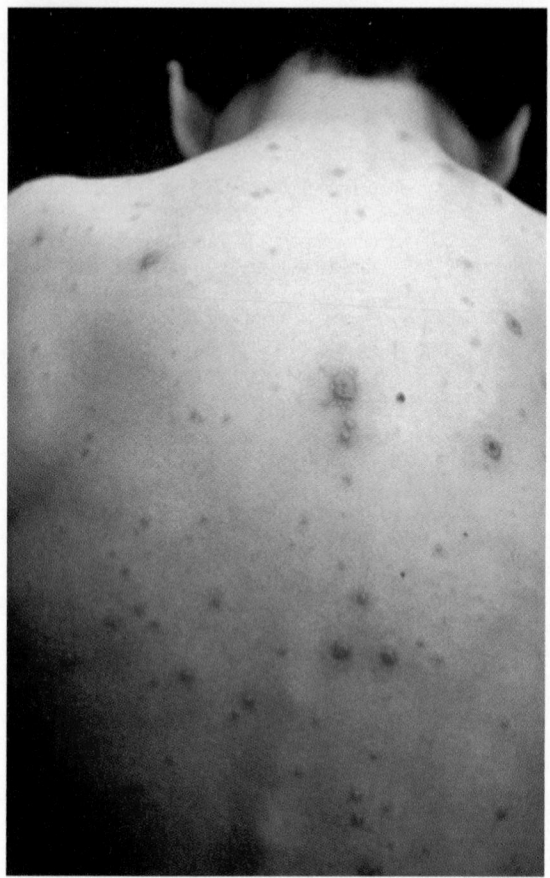

▲ **Figure 32–2.** Primary varicella (chickenpox) skin lesions. (Public Health Image Library, CDC.)

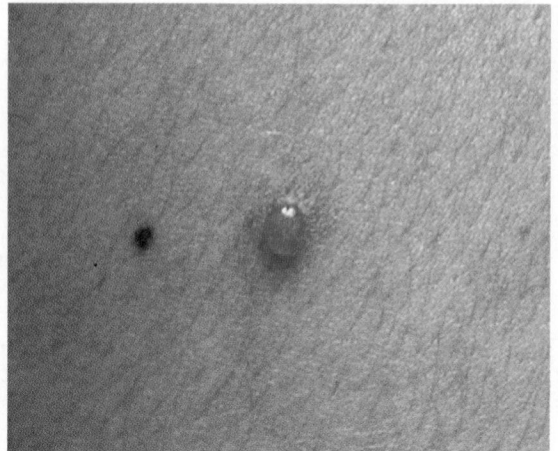

▲ **Figure 32–3.** Chickenpox (varicella) with classic "dew drop on rose petal" appearance. (Reproduced, with permission, from Richard P. Usatine, MD.)

neighboring and distant areas are involved. Lesions on the tip of the nose, inner corner of the eye, and root and side of the nose (Hutchinson sign) indicate involvement of the trigeminal nerve (herpes zoster ophthalmicus). Facial palsy, lesions of the external ear with or without tympanic membrane involvement, vertigo and tinnitus, or deafness signify geniculate ganglion involvement (Ramsay Hunt syndrome or herpes zoster oticus). Shingles is a particularly common and serious complication among immunosuppressed patients. Contact with patients who have varicella does not appear to be a risk factor for zoster.

► **Complications**

A. Varicella

Secondary bacterial skin superinfections, particularly with group A streptococcus and *Staphylococcus aureus*, are the most common complications. Cellulitis, erysipelas, and scarlet fever are described. Bullous impetigo and necrotizing fasciitis are less often seen. Other associations with varicella include epiglottitis, necrotizing pneumonia, osteomyelitis, septic arthritis, epidural abscess, meningitis, endocarditis, and purpura fulminans. Toxic shock syndrome can also develop.

Interstitial VZV pneumonia is more common in adults (especially smokers, HIV-infected patients, and pregnant women) and may result in acute respiratory distress syndrome (ARDS). After healing, numerous densely calcified lesions are seen throughout the lung fields on chest radiographs.

Historically, neurologic complications developed in about 1 in 2000 children. Currently, cerebellar ataxia occurs at a frequency of 1:4000 in the young. A limited course and complete recovery are the rule. Encephalitis is similarly infrequent, occurs mostly in adults, and is characterized by delirium, seizures, and focal neurologic signs. The rates for both mortality and long-term neurologic

widespread dissemination in the absence of skin lesions, are often described.

There is a small increased risk of Guillain-Barré syndrome for at least 2 months after an acute herpes zoster attack.

2. Laboratory findings—Diagnosis is usually made clinically, with confirmation by direct immunofluorescent antibody staining or PCR of scrapings from lesions. Multinucleated giant cells are usually apparent on a Tzanck smear or Calcofluor stain of material from the vesicle bases. Leukopenia and subclinical transaminase elevation are often present and thrombocytopenia occasionally occurs.

A varicella skin test and interferon-gamma enzyme-linked immunospot (ELISPOT) can screen for VZV susceptibility.

B. Herpes Zoster

Herpes zoster ("**shingles**") usually occurs among adults, but cases are reported among infants and children. Skin lesions resemble those of chickenpox. Pain is often severe and commonly precedes the appearance of rash. Lesions follow a dermatomal distribution, with thoracic and lumbar roots being the most common. In most cases, a single unilateral dermatome is involved, but occasionally, sequelae are about 10%. Ischemic strokes in the wake of acute VZV infection present at a mean of 4 months after rashes and may be due to an associated vasculitis. Multifocal encephalitis, ventriculitis, myeloradiculitis, arterial aneurysm formation, and arteritis are also described in immunosuppressed, especially HIV-infected, patients.

Clinical hepatitis is uncommon and mostly presents in the immunosuppressed patient but can be fulminant and fatal. Reye syndrome (fatty liver with encephalopathy) also complicates varicella (and other viral infections, especially influenza B virus), usually in childhood, and is associated with aspirin therapy (see Influenza, below).

When contracted during the first or second trimesters of pregnancy, varicella carries a very small risk of congenital malformations, including cicatricial lesions of an extremity, growth retardation, microphthalmia, cataracts, chorioretinitis, deafness, and cerebrocortical atrophy. If varicella develops around the time of delivery, the newborn is at risk for disseminated disease.

B. Herpes Zoster

Postherpetic neuralgia occurs in 60–70% of patients who have herpes zoster and are older than 60 years. The pain can be prolonged and debilitating. Risk factors for postherpetic neuralgia include advanced age, female sex, the presence of a prodrome, and severity of rash or pain but not family history.

Other complications include the following: (1) bacterial skin superinfections; (2) herpes zoster ophthalmicus, which occurs with involvement of the trigeminal nerve and is a sight-threatening complication (especially when it involves the iris), and is a marker for stroke over the ensuing year (Hutchinson sign is a marker of ocular involvement in the HIV-positive population); (3) rarely, unilateral ophthalmoplegia; (4) involvement of the geniculate ganglion of cranial nerve VII as well as cranial nerves V, VIII, IX, and X; (5) aseptic meningitis; (6) peripheral motor neuropathy; (7) transverse myelitis; (8) encephalitis; (9) acute cerebellitis; (10) stroke; (11) vasculopathy; (12) acute retinal necrosis; (13) progressive outer retinal necrosis (largely among HIV infected persons); and (14) sacral meningoradiculitis (Elsberg syndrome). VZV is a major cause of Bell palsy in patients who are HSV seronegative.

Diagnosis of neurologic complications requires the detection of VZV DNA or anti-VZV IgG in cerebrospinal fluid or the detection of VZV DNA in tissue. *Zoster sine herpete* (pain without rash) can also be associated with most of the above complications.

▶ Treatment

A. General Measures

In general, patients with varicella should be isolated until primary crusts have disappeared and kept at bed rest until afebrile. The skin is kept clean. Pruritus can be relieved with antihistamines, calamine lotion, and colloidal oatmeal baths. Fever can be treated with acetaminophen (not aspirin). Fingernails can be closely cropped to avoid skin excoriation and infection.

B. Antiviral Therapy

1. Varicella—Acyclovir, 20 mg/kg (up to 800 mg per dose) orally four times daily for 5 days, should be given within the first 24 hours after the onset of varicella rash and should be considered for patients older than 12 years, secondary household contacts (disease tends to be more severe disease in secondary cases), patients with chronic cutaneous and cardiopulmonary diseases, and children receiving long-term therapy with salicylates (to decrease the risk of Reye syndrome). Experience with valacyclovir and famciclovir in these settings is scant.

In immunocompromised patients, in pregnant women during the third trimester, and in patients with extracutaneous disease (encephalitis, pneumonitis), antiviral therapy with high-dose acyclovir (30 mg/kg/d in three divided doses intravenously for at least 7 days) should be started once the diagnosis is suspected. Corticosteroids may be useful in the presence of pneumonia. Prolonged prophylactic acyclovir is important to prevent VZV reactivation in profoundly immunosuppressed patients.

2. Herpes zoster—For uncomplicated herpes zoster, valacyclovir or famciclovir is preferable to acyclovir due to dosing convenience and higher drug levels in the body. Therapy should start within the first 72 hours of the onset of the lesions and be continued for 7 days or until the lesions crust over. **There is no role for corticosteroids**. Antiviral therapy reduces the duration of a herpetic lesion and associated episode of acute pain but does not decrease the risk of postherpetic neuralgia.

Intravenous acyclovir is used for extradermatomal complications of zoster. Adjunctive therapy may be considered in retinal disease (foscarnet) and acute herpes zoster (sorivudine, a topical antiviral). In cases of prolonged or repeated acyclovir use, immunosuppressed patients may require a switch to foscarnet due to the development of acyclovir-resistant VZV infections. The Ramsay Hunt syndrome is more resistant to antiviral therapy.

C. Treatment of Postherpetic Neuralgia

Once established, postherpetic neuralgia may respond to gabapentin or lidocaine patches. Tricyclic antidepressants, opioids, and capsaicin cream are also widely used and effective. The epidural injection of corticosteroids and local anesthetics appears to modestly reduce herpetic pain at 1 month but is not effective for prevention of long-term postherpetic neuralgia. There is reported success using transcutaneous electrical nerve stimulation.

▶ Prognosis

The total duration of varicella from onset of symptoms to disappearance of crusts rarely exceeds 2 weeks. Fatalities are rare except in immunosuppressed patients.

Herpes zoster resolves in 2–6 weeks. Antibodies persist longer and at higher levels than with primary varicella. Eye involvement with herpes zoster necessitates periodic future examinations.

► **Prevention**

Health care workers should be screened for varicella and vaccinated if seronegative. Patients with active varicella or herpes zoster are promptly separated from seronegative patients. For patients with varicella, airborne and contact isolation is recommended, whereas for those with zoster, contact precautions are sufficient. For immunosuppressed patients with zoster, precautions should be the same as if the patient had varicella. Exposed serosusceptible patients should be placed in isolation and exposed serosusceptible employees should stay away from work between days 10 and 21 after exposure. Health care workers with zoster should receive antiviral agents during the first 72 hours of disease and withdraw from work until lesions are crusted. Postexposure prophylaxis should be evaluated (see below).

A. Varicella

1. Vaccination—Universal childhood vaccination against varicella is effective. The varicella vaccine (Varilrix) is safe and over 98.1% effective when given after 13 months of age. A single antigen live attenuated vaccine (VARIVAX) or a quadrivalent measles, mumps, rubella, and varicella vaccine (ProQuad) are available. The first dose should be administered at 12–15 months of age and the second at 4–6 years. Aspirin should be avoided for at least 6 weeks because of the risk of Reye syndrome. This vaccine is safe, well tolerated, but the quadrivalent vaccine is associated with a small risk of febrile seizures 5–12 days after vaccination among infants aged 12–23 months. Rashes, when secondary to the varicella vaccine, appear 15–42 days after vaccination. Rare cases of zoster among children who received the varicella vaccine are attributable to delayed vaccination (after age 5), severe asthma, and developmental disorders. Such complications appear to occur less often among American children of African ancestry.

For serosusceptible individuals older than 13 years, two doses of varicella vaccine (single antigen) administered 4–8 weeks apart are recommended. For those who received a single dose in the past, a catch-up second dose is advised, especially in the epidemic setting (where it is effective when it can be given during the first 5 days postexposure). Household contacts of immunocompromised patients should adhere to these recommendations. Susceptible pregnant women need to receive the first dose of vaccine before discharge after delivery and the second dose 4–8 weeks later. The quadrivalent vaccine MMRV can be used for the second doses of MMR and varicella in patients aged 15 months to 12 years and for the first dose in patients aged 48 months or older. The vaccine, administered as two doses 3 months apart, should also be considered for HIV-infected adolescents and adults with CD4 T lymphocyte counts ≥ 200 cells/mcL. The vaccine may also be given to patients with impaired humoral immunity, to patients receiving corticosteroids, and to patients with juvenile rheumatoid arthritis who receive methotrexate. Patients receiving high doses of corticosteroids for over 2 weeks may be vaccinated a month after discontinuation of the

therapy. Patients with leukemia, lymphoma, or other malignancies whose disease is in remission and who have not undergone chemotherapy for at least 3 months may be vaccinated. Kidney and liver transplant patients should be vaccinated if they are susceptible to varicella.

The incidence of varicella in the United States is significantly reduced with the varicella vaccine. Meanwhile, the varicella vaccine has not been found to affect the incidence of herpes zoster.

2. Postexposure—Postexposure vaccination is recommended for unvaccinated persons without other evidence of immunity. Varicella-zoster immune globulin (VZIG) (in short supply with production stopped in 2004) or VariZIG (a lyophilized product available under expanded access since December 2007) should be considered for susceptible exposed patients (and given for up to 10 days in new FDA regulations) who cannot receive the vaccine, including immunosuppressed patients, neonates from mothers with varicella around the time of delivery, exposed premature infants born from serosusceptible mothers at > 28 weeks of gestation, neonates born at < 28 weeks of gestation regardless of maternal serostatus, and pregnant women. No controlled studies have evaluated the use of acyclovir in this setting. VZIG is given by intramuscular injection in a dosage of 12.5 units/kg up to a maximum of 625 units, with a repeat identical dose in 3 weeks if a high-risk patient remains exposed. VZIG has no place in therapy of established disease; however, VariZIG reduces the severity of varicella in high-risk children or adults (ie, those with impaired immunity, pregnant women, and infants exposed peripartum) if given within 4 days of exposure.

Further information may be obtained by calling the Centers for Disease Control and Prevention's Immunization Information Hotline (800-232-2522).

B. Herpes Zoster

A live attenuated VZV vaccine (ZOSTAVAX, 19,400 plaque forming units [pfu] of Oka/Merck strain) consists of varicella virus at a concentration at least 14 times that found in VARIVAX. This vaccine should be offered to persons 60 years and older because it reduces the incidence of herpes zoster and postherpetic neuralgia by 51% and 67%, respectively. **Even if the person has had a prior episode of herpes zoster, the vaccine has efficacy and can be administered.** A second dose of the zoster vaccine is not recommended because it does not boost VZV specific immunity beyond the levels achieved by the first dose. The attenuated VZV vaccine is safe but only moderately immunogenic among HIV-infected persons with a CD4 count of at least 200 cells/mcL.

Concurrent administration of the live attenuated VZV vaccine with 23-valent pneumococcal polysaccharide vaccine is safe. If a varicella vaccine is mistakenly administered to an adult instead of a zoster vaccine, the dose should be considered invalid and the patient should be administered a dose of zoster vaccine at the same visit. On the other hand, the zoster vaccine cannot be used in children in place of varicella vaccine; if the vaccine is accidentally given to a child, the event should be reported to the CDC.

Centers for Disease Control and Prevention (CDC). FDA approval of an extended period for administering VariZIG for postexposure prophylaxis of varicella. MMWR Morb Mortal Wkly Rep. 2012 Mar 30;61(12):212. [PMID: 22456121]

Cohen JI. Clinical practice: herpes zoster. N Engl J Med. 2013 Jul 18;369(3):255–63. [PMID: 23863052]

Hales CM et al. Examination of links between herpes zoster incidence and childhood varicella vaccination. Ann Intern Med. 2013 Dec 3;159(11):739–45. [PMID: 24297190]

Morrison VA et al; Shingles Prevention Study Group. Safety of zoster vaccine in elderly adults following documented herpes zoster. J Infect Dis. 2013 Aug 15;208(4):559–63. [PMID: 23633406]

Tseng HF et al. Herpes zoster vaccine in older adults and the risk of subsequent herpes zoster disease. JAMA. 2011 Jan 12;305 (2):160–6. [PMID: 21224457]

3. Epstein–Barr Virus & Infectious Mononucleosis

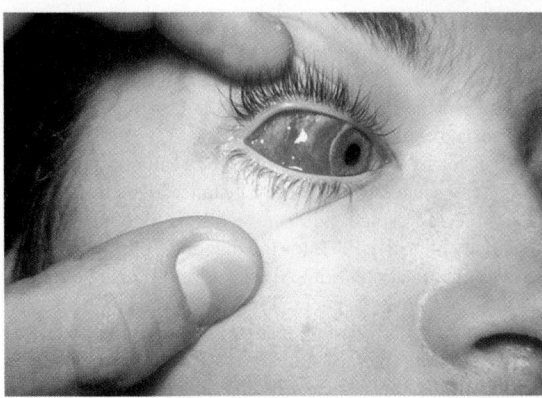

▲ **Figure 32–4.** Conjunctival hemorrhage of the eye due to infectious mononucleosis. (From Dr. Thomas F. Sellers, Emory University, Public Health Image Library, CDC.)

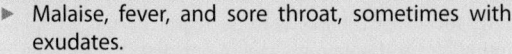

ESSENTIALS OF DIAGNOSIS

▶ Malaise, fever, and sore throat, sometimes with exudates.

▶ Palatal petechiae, lymphadenopathy, splenomegaly, and, occasionally, a maculopapular rash.

▶ Positive heterophil agglutination test (Monospot).

▶ Atypical large lymphocytes in blood smear; lymphocytosis.

▶ Complications: hepatitis, myocarditis, neuropathy, encephalitis, airway obstruction secondary to lymph node enlargement, hemolytic anemia, thrombocytopenia.

▶ General Considerations

Epstein-Barr virus (EBV, or human herpes virus-4 [HHV-4]) is one of the most ubiquitous human viruses, infecting > 95% of the adult population worldwide and persisting for the lifetime of the host. Infectious mononucleosis is a common manifestation of EBV and may occur at any age. In the United States, EBV infection usually develops in persons between the ages of 10 and 35 years, sporadically or epidemically. In the developing world, infectious mononucleosis occurs at younger ages and tends to be less symptomatic. Rare cases in the elderly occur usually without the full symptomatology. EBV is largely transmitted by saliva but can also be recovered from genital secretions. Saliva may remain infectious during convalescence, for 6 months or longer after symptom onset. The incubation period lasts several weeks (30–50 days).

▶ Clinical Findings

A. Symptoms and Signs

The protean manifestations of infectious mononucleosis reflect the dissemination of the virus in the oral cavity and through peripheral blood lymphocytes and cell-free plasma. Fever, sore throat, fatigue, malaise, anorexia, and myalgia typically occur in the early phase of the illness. Physical findings include lymphadenopathy (discrete, nonsuppurative, slightly painful, especially along the posterior cervical chain), transient bilateral upper lid edema (Hoagland sign), and splenomegaly (in up to 50% of patients). A maculopapular or occasionally petechial rash occurs in < 15% of patients unless ampicillin is given (in which case rash is seen in > 90%). Conjunctival hemorrhage (Figure 32–4), exudative pharyngitis, uvular edema, tonsillitis, or gingivitis may occur and soft palatal petechiae may be noted.

Other manifestations include hepatitis, interstitial pneumonitis, cholestasis, gastritis, acute interstitial nephritis, nervous system involvement in 1–5% (mononeuropathies and occasionally aseptic meningitis, encephalitis, cerebellitis, peripheral and optic neuritis, transverse myelitis, or Guillain-Barré syndrome), kidney disease (mostly interstitial nephritis), pneumonia, pleural involvement, and myocarditis. Vaginal ulcers are rare but may be present. Airway obstruction from lymph node enlargement, pericarditis, life-threatening thrombocytopenia, severe CNS complications, and massive splenomegaly are all considered indications for hospitalization or close observation.

B. Laboratory Findings

An initial phase of granulocytopenia is followed within 1 week by lymphocytic leukocytosis (> 50% of all leukocytes) with atypical lymphocytes (larger than normal mature lymphocytes, staining more darkly, and showing vacuolated, foamy cytoplasm and dark nuclear chromatin) comprising > 10% of the leukocyte count. Hemolytic anemia, with anti-i antibodies, occurs occasionally as does thrombocytopenia (at times marked).

Diagnosis is made on the basis of characteristic manifestations and serologic evidence of infection (the heterophil sheep cell agglutination [HA] antibody tests or the correlated mononucleosis spot test [Monospot]). These tests usually become positive within 4 weeks after onset of illness and are specific but often not sensitive in early illness. Heterophil antibodies may be absent in young children and in as many as 20% adults. During acute illness, there is a rise and fall in immunoglobulin M (IgM) antibody to EB virus capsid antigen (VCA) and a rise in IgG antibody to VCA, which persists for life. Antibodies (IgG) to EBV nuclear antigen (EBNA) appear after 4 weeks of onset and also persist. Absence of IgG and IgM VCA or the presence of IgG EBNA should make one reconsider the diagnosis of acute EBV infection.

PCR for EBV DNA is useful in the evaluation of malignancies associated with EBV. For instance, detection of EBV DNA in cerebrospinal fluid shows a sensitivity of 90% and specificity of nearly 100% for the diagnosis of primary CNS lymphoma in patients with AIDS, and monitoring of quantitative EBV DNA levels (a "viral load") in blood may be useful in early detection of posttransplant lymphoproliferative disorder in high-risk patients. PCR analysis may also be helpful in monitoring disease and treatment response in primary CNS lymphoma and posttransplant lymphoproliferative disorder patients. Antibodies against ZEBRA (a replication protein) are produced in early infection and assays for these antibodies are commercially available.

▶ Differential Diagnosis

CMV infection, toxoplasmosis, acute HIV infection, secondary syphilis, HHV-6, rubella, and drug hypersensitivity reactions may be indistinguishable from infectious mononucleosis due to EBV, but exudative pharyngitis is usually absent and the heterophil antibody tests are negative. With acute HIV infection, rash and mucocutaneous ulceration are common but atypical lymphocytosis is much less common. Heterophil-negative infectious mononucleosis with nonsignificant lymphocytosis (especially if rash or mucocutaneous ulcers are present) should prompt investigation for acute HIV infection. Heterophil-negative infectious mononucleosis with atypical lymphocytosis can be caused by CMV, toxoplasmosis and, on occasion, EBV itself. Mycoplasma infection may also present as pharyngitis, though lower respiratory symptoms usually predominate. A hypersensitivity syndrome induced by carbamazepine or phenytoin may mimic infectious mononucleosis.

The differential diagnosis of acute exudative pharyngitis includes gonococcal and streptococcal infections, and infections with adenovirus and herpes simplex. Head and neck soft tissue infections (pharyngeal and tonsillar abscesses) may occasionally be mistaken as the lymphadenopathy of mononucleosis.

▶ Complications

Secondary bacterial pharyngitis can occur and is often streptococcal. Splenic rupture (0.5–1%) is a rare but dramatic complication, and a history of preceding trauma can be elicited in 50% of the cases. Acalculous cholecystitis, fulminant hepatitis with massive necrosis, pericarditis and myocarditis are also infrequent complications. Neurologic involvement—including transverse myelitis, encephalitis, and Guillain-Barré syndrome—is infrequent.

▶ Treatment

A. General Measures

Over 95% of patients with acute EBV-associated infectious mononucleosis recover without specific antiviral

therapy. Treatment is symptomatic with acetaminophen or other nonsteroidal anti-inflammatory drugs and warm saline throat irrigations or gargles three or four times daily. Acyclovir decreases viral shedding but shows no clinical benefit. Corticosteroid therapy, although widespread, is not recommended in uncomplicated cases; its use is reserved for impending airway obstruction from enlarged lymph nodes, hemolytic anemia, and severe thrombocytopenia. The value of corticosteroid therapy in impending splenic rupture, pericarditis, myocarditis, and nervous system involvement is less well defined. If a throat culture grows beta-hemolytic streptococci, a 10-day course of penicillin or erythromycin is indicated. Ampicillin and amoxicillin are avoided because of the frequent association with rash.

B. Treatment of Complications

Hepatitis, myocarditis, and encephalitis are treated symptomatically. Rupture of the spleen requires splenectomy and is most often caused by deep palpation of the spleen or vigorous activity. Patients should avoid contact or collision sports for at least 4 weeks to decrease the risk of splenic rupture (even if splenomegaly is not detected by physical examination, which can be insensitive).

▶ Prognosis & Prevention

In uncomplicated cases, fever disappears in 10 days and lymphadenopathy and splenomegaly in 4 weeks. The debility sometimes lingers for 2–3 months.

Death is uncommon and is usually due to splenic rupture, hypersplenic phenomena (severe hemolytic anemia, thrombocytopenic purpura), or encephalitis.

Several vaccines including viral-like proteins are under development but none is marketed. Handwashing after contact and avoidance of close personal contact with active cases is prudent.

4. Other Epstein–Barr Virus Syndromes

EBV viral antigens are found in > 90% of patients with endemic (African) Burkitt lymphoma and nasopharyngeal carcinoma (among whom quantified EBV DNA can be used to follow disease). Risk factors for Burkitt lymphoma include a history of malaria (which may decrease resistance to EBV infection) while risk factors for nasopharyngeal carcinoma include long-term heavy cigarette smoking and seropositive EBV serologies (VCA and deoxyribonuclease [DNase]). VCA-IgA in peripheral blood is a sensitive and specific predictor for nasopharyngeal carcinoma in endemic areas.

Chronic EBV infection is associated with aberrant cellular immunity (a low frequency of EBV-specific CD8 cells), an X-linked lymphoproliferative syndrome (Duncan disease), lymphomatoid granulomatosis, and a fatal T cell lymphoproliferative disorder in children.

EBV is an important cause of hemophagocytic lymphohistiocytosis among immunodeficient patients, B-cell lymphomas (such as primary CNS lymphoma in HIV-infected individuals), and posttransplant lymphoproliferative disorders. Posttransplant lymphoproliferative states are commonly associated with EBV, especially in children. EBV-naïve patients who receive a donor organ from an EBV-infected donor are at the highest-risk for the development of post-transplant lymphoproliferative disorder. Decreasing the iatrogenic immunosuppression, given to reduce graft rejection, is the initial step in managing such patients, while rituximab (CD20 monoclonal antibody) is effective in treating more than two-thirds of cases. The efficacy of rituximab therapy can be often assessed by monitoring levels of EBV DNA load in the blood and, if indicated, CNS. Infusion of EBV-specific cytotoxic T cell lymphocytes (adoptive cell therapy) is also used but with a less established role.

Age is a major determinant of the type of tumor associated with EBV. T and NK cell lymphoma caused by chronic active EBV infections are more frequent in childhood while peripheral T cell lymphomas and diffuse large B cell lymphomas are more common in the elderly due to waning immunity. EBV is also associated with leiomyomas in children with AIDS and with nasal T cell lymphomas.

▶ When to Admit

- Acute meningitis, encephalitis, or acute Guillain-Barré syndrome.
- Severe thrombocytopenia; significant hemolysis.
- Potential splenic rupture.
- Airway obstruction from severe adenitis.
- Pericarditis.
- Abdominal findings mimicking an acute abdomen.

Kelly MJ et al. Epstein-Barr virus coinfection in cerebrospinal fluid is associated with increased mortality in Malawian adults with bacterial meningitis. J Infect Dis. 2012 Jan 1; 205(1):106–10. [PMID: 22075766]

Pembrey L et al. Seroprevalence of cytomegalovirus, Epstein Barr virus and varicella zoster virus among pregnant women in Bradford: a cohort study. PLoS One. 2013 Nov 27;8(11): e81881. [PMID: 24312372]

Sanz J et al. EBV-associated post-transplant lymphoproliferative disorder after umbilical cord blood transplantation in adults with hematological diseases. Bone Marrow Transplant. 2014 Mar;49(3):397–402. [PMID: 24292521]

Styczynski J et al. Response to rituximab-based therapy and risk factor analysis in Epstein Barr virus-related lymphoproliferative disorder after hematopoietic stem cell transplant in children and adults: a study from the Infectious Diseases Working Party of the European Group for Blood and Marrow Transplantation. Clin Infect Dis. 2013 Sep;57(6):794–802. [PMID: 23771985]

5. Cytomegalovirus Disease

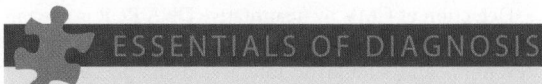

ESSENTIALS OF DIAGNOSIS

- ▶ Mononucleosis-like syndrome.
- ▶ Frequent pathogen seen in transplant populations.
- ▶ Diverse clinical syndromes in HIV (retinitis, esophagitis, pneumonia, encephalitis).
- ▶ Major pathogen to consider in neonates in the differential of maternally transmitted agents.

▶ General Considerations

Most cytomegalovirus (CMV) infections are asymptomatic. After primary infection, the virus remains latent in most body cells. Seroprevalence in adults of Western developed countries is about 60–80% but is higher in developing countries. CMV seroprevalence increases with age and among people who are employed in child day care centers, and fall into low socioeconomic status; in addition, seroprevalence increases with the number of sexual partners and a history of prior sexually transmitted infections. The virus can be isolated from a variety of tissues under nonpathogenic conditions. Transmission occurs through sexual contact, breastfeeding, blood products, or transplantation; it may also occur person-to-person (eg, day care centers) or be congenital. Serious disease occurs primarily in immunocompromised persons.

There are three recognizable clinical syndromes: (1) perinatal disease and CMV inclusion disease; (2) diseases in immunocompetent persons; and (3) diseases in immunocompromised persons. **Congenital CMV infection** is the most common congenital infection in developed countries (between 0.2% and 2% of all live births, with higher rates in underdeveloped areas and among lower socioeconomic groups). Transmission is much higher from mothers with primary disease than those with reactivation (40% vs 0.2–1.8%). About 10% of infected newborns will be symptomatic with CMV inclusion disease.

In **immunocompetent persons**, acute CMV infection is the most common cause of the mononucleosis-like syndrome with negative heterophil antibodies. CMV appears to play a role in critically ill immunocompetent adults wherein it is reactivated and associated with prolonged hospitalization and death. Other syndromes associated with CMV and whose role in pathogenesis requires further elucidation include inflammatory bowel disease, atherosclerosis, cognitive decline, and breast cancer.

In **immunocompromised persons**, tissue and bone marrow transplant patients are mainly at risk for a year after allograft transplantation (but especially during the first 100 days afterward) and in particular when graft-versus-host disease or CMV seropositivity, or both, are present in the donor and recipient. Depending on the serostatus of the donor and recipient, disease may present as primary infection or reactivation. The risk of CMV disease is proportionate to the intensity of immunosuppression. CMV itself is immunosuppressive. CMV may contribute to transplanted organ dysfunction, which often mimics organ rejection. CMV disease in HIV-infected patients (retinitis, serious gastrointestinal disease) occurs most prominently when the CD4 count is < 50 cells/mcL. Highly active antiretroviral therapy (HAART) reduces the frequency of retinitis and may reverse active disease. CMV retinitis may also develop after solid organ or bone marrow transplantation. CMV retinitis associated with intravitreal delivery of corticosteroids (injections or implants) or systemic anti-TNF antibodies is also described. Occasionally, CMV retinitis presents in immunocompetent persons. Serious gastrointestinal CMV disease also occurs after organ transplantation, cancer chemotherapy, or corticosteroid therapy. CMV may exist alongside other pathogens, such as *Cryptosporidium,* in up to 15%

of patients with AIDS cholangiopathy. CMV pneumonitis occurs in transplant recipients (mainly bone marrow and lung) with a mortality rate up to 60–80%, and less often in AIDS patients. CMV pneumonitis in hematologic malignancies (eg, lymphoma) is increasingly reported. Neurologic CMV in patients with advanced AIDS is usually associated with disseminated CMV infection.

▶ Clinical Findings

A. Symptoms and Signs

1. Perinatal disease and CMV inclusion disease—CMV inclusion disease in infected newborns is characterized by jaundice, hepatosplenomegaly, thrombocytopenia, purpura, microcephaly, periventricular CNS calcifications, mental retardation, and motor disability. Hearing loss develops in > 50% of infants who are symptomatic at birth. Most infected neonates are asymptomatic, but neurologic deficits may ensue later in life, including hearing loss in 15% and mental retardation in 10–20%. Perinatal infection acquired through breastfeeding or blood products typically shows a benign clinical course.

2. Disease in immunocompetent persons—Acute acquired CMV infection is characterized by fever, malaise, myalgias, arthralgias, and splenomegaly. Exudative pharyngitis or cervical lymphadenopathies are uncommon, but cutaneous rashes (including the typical maculopapular rash after exposure to ampicillin) are common. The mean duration of symptoms is 7–8 weeks. Complications include mucosal gastrointestinal damage, encephalitis, severe hepatitis, thrombocytopenia (on occasion, refractory), the Guillain-Barré syndrome, pericarditis, and myocarditis. The risk of Guillain-Barre syndrome developing after primary CMV infection is estimated to be 0.6–2.2 cases per 1000 primary infection, similar to that seen with *Campylobacter jejuni* infection. The mononucleosis-like syndrome due to CMV can also occur postsplenectomy, often years later and associated with a protracted fever, marked lymphocytosis, and impaired anti-CMV IgM response.

3. Disease in immunocompromised persons—Distinguishing between CMV infection (with evidence of CMV replication) and CMV disease (evidence for systemic symptoms or organ invasion) is important. In addition to patients infected with HIV, those who have undergone transplantation (solid organ or hematopoietic stem cell) show a wide spectrum of disease including gastrointestinal (eg, acute cholecystitis), renal, and CNS disease, as outlined above. CMV viral loads correlate with prognosis after transplantation.

A. CMV RETINITIS—A funduscopic examination reveals neovascular, proliferative lesions ("pizza-pie" retinopathy). Immune restoration with HAART is associated with CMV vitritis and cystoid macular edema. Infants with CMV retinitis tend to have more macular than peripheral disease.

B. GASTROINTESTINAL AND HEPATOBILIARY CMV—Esophagitis presents with odynophagia. Gastritis can occasionally cause bleeding, and small bowel disease may mimic inflammatory bowel disease or may present as ulceration or perforation. Colonic CMV disease causes diarrhea, hematochezia, abdominal pain, fever, and weight loss and may mimic inflammatory bowel disease. CMV hepatitis commonly complicates liver transplantation and appears to be increased in those with hepatitis B or hepatitis C viral infection.

C. RESPIRATORY CMV—CMV pneumonitis is characterized by cough, dyspnea, and relatively little sputum production.

D. NEUROLOGIC CMV—Neurologic syndromes associated with CMV include polyradiculopathy, transverse myelitis, ventriculoencephalitis (suspected with ependymitis), and focal encephalitis. These manifestations are more prominent in patients with advanced AIDS in whom the encephalitis has a subacute onset.

B. Laboratory Findings

1. Mothers and newborns—Pregnant women should be tested for IgM CMV antibodies every 3 months if an assay during the first trimester is seropositive. Congenital CMV disease is confirmed by presence of the virus in amniotic fluid or an IgM assay from fetal blood. Amniocentesis is less reliable before 21 weeks of gestation (due to inadequate fetal urinary development and release into the amniotic fluid), but amniocentesis is attendant with greater risk when performed after 21 weeks of gestation. PCR assays of dried blood samples from newborns and micro-enzyme-linked immunosorbent assay (ELISA) on urine, saliva, or blood specimens obtained during the first 3 weeks of life are used to diagnose congenital CMV infection.

2. Immunocompetent persons—The acute mononucleosis-like syndrome is characterized by initial leukopenia; within 1 week, it is followed by absolute lymphocytosis with atypical lymphocytes. Abnormal liver function tests are common in the first 2 weeks of the disease (often 2 weeks after the fever). Detection of CMV specific IgM or a fourfold increase of specific IgG levels support the diagnosis of acute infection.

3. Immunocompromised persons—CMV retinitis is diagnosed on the basis of the characteristic ophthalmoscopic findings. In HIV-infected patients, negative CMV serologies lower the possibility of the diagnosis but do not eliminate it. Cultures alone are of little use in diagnosing AIDS-related CMV infections, since viral shedding of CMV is common. PCR analysis should be used to diagnose CNS infection since cultures are not specific for disease.

Detection of CMV by quantitative DNA PCR is used in posttransplant patients for guidance on both treatment and prevention and should be interpreted in the context of clinical and pathologic findings. Conversion of CMV viral loads to international units has standardized detection assays and replaced CMV antigenemia tests in many settings. The PCR is sensitive in predicting clinical disease.

Rapid shell-vial cultures detect early CMV antigens with fluorescent antibodies in 24–48 hours. Shell-vial cultures are more useful on bronchoalveolar lavage fluid than in routine blood monitoring. CMV colitis can occur in the absence of a detectable viremia.

A variety of false-positive immunologic assays occur in the setting of acute CMV infections, including positive rheumatoid factor, direct Coombs test, cryoglobulins, and speckled antinuclear antibody.

C. Imaging

The chest radiographic findings of CMV pneumonitis are consistent with interstitial pneumonia.

D. Biopsy

Tissue confirmation is especially useful in diagnosing CMV pneumonitis and CMV gastrointestinal disease; the diagnosis of colonic CMV disease is made by mucosal biopsy showing characteristic CMV histopathologic findings of intranuclear ("owl's eye") and intracytoplasmic inclusions. In situations where histopathologic or immunohistochemical findings are not seen but CMV colitis is suspected, CMV DNA PCR can be used to identify additional cases.

► Treatment

Sight-threatening CMV retinitis (lesions close to the fovea or optic nerve head) is treated with ganciclovir induction therapy (5 mg/kg intravenously every 12 hours for 14–21 days) followed by maintenance therapy at lower doses (5 mg/kg intravenously daily). Sustained-release ganciclovir intraocular implants (always accompanied by systemic valganciclovir) are another option. In less severe retinal disease, valganciclovir (900 mg orally twice daily for 14–21 days followed by 900 mg/d maintenance) is preferred. Due to potential toxicities, foscarnet, cidofovir, and fomivirsen are usually reserved for CMV infections that are resistant to ganciclovir. Combinations of ganciclovir and foscarnet are shown to be safe and effective in treating clinically resistant CMV retinitis. The role of HAART in reducing the need for CMV antiviral agents is essential. Other forms of CMV disease in AIDS are managed initially with intravenous ganciclovir and subsequently with oral valganciclovir; alternative agents (listed above) are used when resistance evolves.

The treatment of other systemic CMV infection (colitis, encephalitis, pneumonia) involves the use of the main antiviral agents used in CMV retinitis. The length of therapy depends on the state of immunosuppression, and secondary prophylaxis is typically maintained until immune restoration with two CD4 T-cell counts > 100 cells/mcL is present for at least 6 months. Prolonged prophylaxis may be necessary in other immunosuppressed patients, such as those receiving TNF inhibitors.

For non-severe, posttransplant CMV disease, oral valganciclovir (900 mg twice daily) or intravenous ganciclovir (5 mg/kg every 12 hours) are the recommended first-line agents. Valganciclovir has been shown to be noninferior to intravenous ganciclovir-based therapy in solid organ transplant patients and is associated with less clinical resistance than ganciclovir. **For severe CMV disease,** intravenous ganciclovir remains the treatment of choice. Dosage adjustments of all medications are needed for kidney dysfunction. Reduction of immunosuppression should be attempted when possible (especially for muromonab, azathioprine, or mycophenolate mofetil). Treatment should be continued for at least 2 weeks until viral eradication is achieved. Two consecutive negative samples of CMV quantitative analysis testing or antigenemia based assay ensure viral clearance. Other agents that may be useful in resistant CMV infections include leflunomide, sirolimus-based therapy, and artesunate. Adoptive immunotherapy is also under study.

In pregnant women with primary CMV infection, passive immunization with hyperimmune globulin appears preliminarily to be effective in both treatment and prevention of fetal infection, but controlled clinical trials are lacking. While CMV immunoglobulin is also used in the treatment of CMV pneumonia in stem cell transplant recipients, its efficacy is not completely established.

► Prevention

Recombinant human CMV vaccine studies are under development. A CMV glycoprotein B with MF59 adjuvant vaccine showed efficacy of 50% in preventing congenital disease, and CMV glycoprotein B with pp95 DNA adjuvant vaccine also showed signs of clinical benefit in hematopoietic stem cell transplant recipients. These studies inform the development of next generation vaccine candidates.

HAART is effective in preventing CMV infections in HIV-infected patients. Use of leukocyte-depleted blood products effectively reduces the incidence of CMV disease in patients who have undergone transplantation. Prophylactic and preemptive strategies (eg, antiviral agents only when antigen detection or PCR assays show evidence of active CMV replication) are effective in preventing disease in the early transplantation period but are associated with a risk of a late-onset form of the disease after the prophylaxis is discontinued. The appropriate management of transplant patients is based on the serostatus of the donor and the recipient. All effective anti-CMV agents can serve as prophylactic agents for CMV-seropositive transplants or for CMV-seronegative recipients of CMV-positive organ transplants. The dose for valganciclovir prophylaxis is 450 mg orally twice daily. CMV immune globulin may also be useful in reducing the incidence of bronchiolitis obliterans in the bone marrow transplant population and is used in some centers as part of the prophylaxis in kidney, liver, and lung transplantation patients. CMV immune globulin as prophylaxis is not recommended in hematopoietic stem cell transplant recipients.

Withdrawal of infected children from day care centers, reduction of patient contact by health care workers, screening for women of childbearing age, or restrictions to breastfeeding are not recommended because the virus is ubiquitous, although women who are CMV negative should reconsider taking employment in child day care centers.

► When to Refer

- Neonatal infections consistent with CMV inclusion disease.

- AIDS patients with retinitis, esophagitis, colitis, hepatobiliary disease, or encephalitis.
- Organ and hematopoietic stem cell transplants with suspected reactivation CMV.

▶ When to Admit

- Risk of colonic perforation.
- Evaluation of unexplained, advancing encephalopathy.
- Biopsy of tissues in the differential diagnosis of transplant rejection vs infection.
- Initiation of treatment with intravenous anti-CMV agents.

Johnson J et al. Prevention of maternal and congenital cytomegalovirus infection. Clin Obstet Gynecol. 2012 Jun;55(2):521–30. [PMID: 22510635]

Lilja AE et al. The next generation recombinant human cytomegalovirus vaccine candidates-beyond gB. Vaccine. 2012 Nov 19;30(49):6980–90. [PMID: 23041121]

Mannonen L et al. Comparison of two quantitative real-time CMV-PCR tests calibrated against the 1st WHO international standard for viral load monitoring of renal transplant patients. J Med Virol. 2014 Apr;86(4):576–84. [PMID: 24026892]

Mills AM et al. A comparison of CMV detection in gastrointestinal mucosal biopsies using immunohistochemistry and PCR performed on formalin-fixed, paraffin-embedded tissue. Am J Surg Pathol. 2013 Jul;37(7):995–1000. [PMID: 23648457]

6. Human Herpesviruses 6, 7, & 8

HHV-6 is a B cell lymphotropic virus that is the principal cause of exanthema subitum (roseola infantum, sixth disease). Primary HHV-6 infection occurs most commonly in children under 2 years of age and is a major cause of infantile febrile seizures. HHV-6 is also associated with encephalitis (symptoms may include insomnia, seizures, and hallucinations) and with acute liver failure. Primary infection in immunocompetent adults is rare and can produce a mononucleosis-like illness. Reactivation of HHV-6 in immunocompetent adults is rare and can present as encephalitis. Imaging studies in HHV-6 encephalitis typically show lesions in the hippocampus, amygdala, and limbic structures.

Infection during pregnancy and congenital transmission is recognized. Most cases of reactivation, however, occur in immunocompromised persons. Reactivation is associated with graft rejection, graft-versus-host disease, and bone marrow suppression in transplant patients and with encephalitis and pneumonitis in AIDS patients and in recipients of hematopoietic cell transplants (but the absence of an HHV-6 association with survival in such patients suggests that for now surveillance for the virus is not needed). HHV-6 is on occasion also associated with drug-induced hypersensitivity syndromes. HHV-6 may cause fulminant hepatic failure and acute decompensation of chronic liver disease in children. Purpura fulminans and corneal inflammation are reported with HHV-6 infection. Two variants (A and B) of HHV-6 have been identified. HHV-6B is the predominant strain found in both normal and immunocompromised persons. Ganciclovir, cidofovir,

and foscarnet (but not acyclovir) appear to be clinically active against HHV-6.

HHV-7 is a T cell lymphotropic virus that is associated with roseola (serologically), seizures and, rarely, encephalitis. Pregnant women are often infected. Infection with HHV-7 is synergistic with CMV in kidney transplant recipients.

HHV-8 is associated with Kaposi sarcoma, multicentric Castleman disease, and primary effusion (body cavity) lymphoma. HHV-8 infection is endemic in Africa; transmission seems to be primarily horizontal in childhood from intrafamilial contacts and continues through adulthood possibly by nonsexual routes. See Chapter 31 for pathogenesis and management.

Ablashi D et al. Classification of HHV-6A and HHV-6B as distinct viruses. Arch Virol. 2013 Nov 6. [Epub ahead of print] [PMID: 24193951]

Betts BC et al. Human herpesvirus 6 infection after hematopoietic cell transplantation: is routine surveillance necessary? Biol Blood Marrow Transplant. 2011 Oct;17(10):1562–8. [PMID: 21549850]

Husain Z et al. DRESS syndrome: part I. Clinical perspectives. J Am Acad Dermatol. 2013 May;68(5):693.e1–14. [PMID: 23602182]

Mbondji-Wonje C et al. Seroprevalence of human herpesvirus-8 in HIV-1 infected and uninfected individuals in Cameroon. Viruses. 2013 Sep 19;5(9):2253–9. [PMID: 24056671]

Ogata M et al. Human herpesvirus 6 (HHV-6) reactivation and HHV-6 encephalitis after allogeneic hematopoietic cell transplantation: a multicenter, prospective study. Clin Infect Dis. 2013 Sep;57(5):671–81. [PMID: 23723198]

MAJOR VACCINE-PREVENTABLE VIRAL INFECTIONS[1]

1. Measles

ESSENTIALS OF DIAGNOSIS

- ▶ Exposure 10–14 days before onset in an unvaccinated patient.
- ▶ Prodrome of fever, coryza, cough, conjunctivitis, malaise, irritability, photophobia, Koplik spots.
- ▶ Rash: brick red, irregular, maculopapular; onset 3–4 days after onset of prodrome; begins on the face and proceeds "downward and outward," affecting the palms and soles last.
- ▶ Leukopenia.

▶ General Considerations

Measles is a reportable acute systemic paramyxoviral infection transmitted by inhalation of infective droplets. It is a major worldwide cause of pediatric morbidity and mortality, although vaccination programs successfully reduced this number. Between 2001 and 2012, a median of

---

[1]A general guide for vaccine preventable diseases is available at www.who.int/vaccines-documents/

60 measles cases were reported to the CDC yearly among a yearly median of 4 outbreaks. In 2013 (through August 31) a total of 159 cases were reported to the CDC with the largest case numbers from New York, Texas, North Carolina, and California and with most of these attributed to 3 outbreaks among members of groups with philosophical or religious reasons for not vaccinating. All but 2 of the cases in 2013 were import-associated, although actual cases among immigrants was 42 (with 21 of these from the WHO European Region). A major outbreak in France between 2005 and 2012 was associated with over 22,000 cases and 10 deaths, with over 80% of cases occurring among the unvaccinated and with the highest incidence among infants younger than 1 year.

Illness confers permanent immunity. It is highly contagious and communicability is greatest during the preeruptive and catarrhal stages but continues as long as the rash remains. Despite high community vaccination coverage, rising rates of intentional undervaccination lead to sporadic outbreaks among clusters of intentionally undervaccinated children and can undermine measles elimination programs. Therefore, laboratory testing and confirmation of suspected measles infection is especially important in countries that report the elimination of measles. Sporadic outbreaks of the disease in adults, adolescents, and unvaccinated preschool children in dense urban areas, and sporting event participants emphasize the need for specific recommendations concerning prevention (see below).

In the United States, measles was declared eliminated in 2000 and except for sporadic outbreaks this success is maintained due to a high MMR vaccination coverage. Recent increases in outbreaks and importations are a reminder of measles endemicity in the rest of the world and how undervaccinated individuals pose a risk to themselves and their communities.

▶ Clinical Findings

A. Symptoms and Signs

Fever is often as high as 40–40.6°C. It persists through the prodrome and early rash (about 5–7 days) (Table 32–2). Malaise may be marked. Coryza (nasal obstruction, sneezing, and sore throat) resembles that seen with upper respiratory infections. Cough is persistent and nonproductive. Conjunctivitis manifests as redness, swelling, photophobia, and discharge. These symptoms intensify over 2–4 days before onset of the rash and peak on the first day of the rash.

Koplik spots (small, irregular, and red with whitish center on the mucous membranes) are pathognomonic of measles. They appear about 2 days before the rash and last 1–4 days as tiny "table salt crystals" in the buccal mucosa opposite the molars and vaginal membranes. The rash usually appears on the face and behind the ears 4 days after the onset of symptoms. The initial lesions are pinhead-sized papules that coalesce to form a brick red, irregular, blotchy maculopapular rash. In severe cases, the rash coalesces to form a nearly uniform erythema in some areas. The rash next appears on the trunk, followed by the extremities, including the palms (25–50% of those infected) and soles. The rash lasts for 3–7 days and fades in the same manner it

appeared. Hyperpigmentation remains in fair-skinned individuals and severe cases. Slight desquamation may follow.

Other findings in measles include pharyngeal erythema, tonsillar yellowish exudate, coating of the tongue in the center with a red tip and margins, moderate generalized lymphadenopathy and, at times, splenomegaly.

Atypical measles is a syndrome occurring in adults who received inactivated measles vaccine (1963–1968) or who received live measles vaccine before age 12 months and as a result developed hypersensitivity rather than protective immunity. Infection later in life with wild measles virus can lead to a potentially fatal illness with high fever; unusual rashes (papular, hemorrhagic), most prominent on the extremities, without Koplik spots; headache; arthralgias; hepatitis; a high rate of pneumonitis, and sometimes pleural effusions. Atypical measles cases show unusually high hemagglutinin-inhibition titers. Measles may be distinctive in HIV-infected individuals, with higher rates of pneumonitis, higher mortality, prolonged viral shedding, and higher vaccine failure rates. Measles during pregnancy is not known to cause congenital abnormalities of the fetus. It is, however, associated with spontaneous abortion and premature delivery and can cause severe disease in the mother. Although measles does not always develop in the offspring of mothers with the disease, it can be severe when it does. It is recommended that infants born to such mothers be passively immunized with immunoglobulin at birth.

B. Laboratory Findings

Leukopenia is usually present unless secondary bacterial complications exist. A lymphocyte count under 2000/mcL is a poor prognostic sign. Thrombocytopenia is common. Proteinuria is often observed. Although technically difficult, virus can be cultured from nasopharyngeal washings and from blood. Detection of IgM measles antibodies with ELISA or a fourfold rise in serum hemagglutination inhibition antibody supports the diagnosis. Fluorescent antibody staining of respiratory or urinary epithelial cells can also confirm the diagnosis.

IgM assays can be falsely negative the first few days of infection and falsely positive in the presence of rheumatoid factor or with acute rubella, erythrovirus (parvovirus) B19, or HHV-6 infection. White reverse transcriptase-PCR techniques, typically available in research settings, can help establish a diagnosis. The virologic clearance of measles can take months, leading to false-positive results.

▶ Differential Diagnosis

Measles is usually diagnosed clinically but may be mistaken for other exanthematous infections (see Table 32–2). Frequent difficulty in establishing a diagnosis suggests that measles may be more prevalent than is recognized.

▶ Complications

A. Central Nervous System

Postinfectious encephalomyelitis occurs in about 0.05–0.1% of cases. Higher rates of encephalitis occur in adolescents and adults than in school-aged children. Its onset is usually

3–7 days after the rash. Vomiting, convulsions, coma, and diverse, severe neurologic symptoms and signs may develop. Treatment is symptomatic and supportive. Virus is usually not found in the CNS, though demyelination is prominent. There is an appreciable mortality (10–20%) and morbidity (33% of survivors are left with neurologic deficit).

A similar form, "inclusion body encephalitis," occurs months after exposure. This complication is reported to occur after measles vaccination in patients with inadequate cellular immunity but is associated with isolation of the measles virus.

Subacute sclerosing panencephalitis (SSPE) is a very late CNS complication (5–15 years after infection; the measles virus acts as a "slow virus" to produce degenerative CNS disease years after the initial infection. SSPE is rare (1:100,000 cases of measles) and occurs more often when measles develops early in life among males who live in rural environments. SSPE very rarely develops in adults.

Measles virus can opportunistically invade the CNS. An acute progressive encephalitis (subacute measles encephalitis), characterized by seizures, neurologic deficits, and stupor progressing to death, can occur among immunosuppressed patients. Treatment is supportive, withholding immunosuppressive chemotherapy when feasible. Interferon and ribavirin are variably successful.

B. Respiratory Tract Disease

Early in the course of the disease, bronchopneumonia or bronchiolitis due to the measles virus may occur in up to 5% of patients and result in serious respiratory difficulties. Bronchiectasis may occur in up to a quarter of nonvaccinated children. Pneumonia occurring with or without an evanescent rash is seen in atypical measles.

C. Secondary Bacterial Infections

Immediately following measles, secondary bacterial infection, particularly cervical adenitis, otitis media (the most common complication), and pneumonia, occurs in about 15% of patients.

D. Immune Reactivity

Measles produces temporary anergy to cell-mediated skin tests.

E. Gastroenteritis

Diarrhea and protein-losing enteropathy (prodromal rectal Koplik spots may be seen) are significant complications among malnourished children.

F. Other Complications

Other complications include conjunctivitis, keratitis, and otosclerosis.

▶ Treatment

A. General Measures

The patient should be isolated for the week following onset of rash and kept at bed rest until afebrile. Treatment is symptomatic including antipyretics and fluids as needed. Vitamin A, 200,000 units/d orally for 2 days (the benefit being maintenance of gastrointestinal and respiratory epithelial mucosa) reduces pediatric morbidity (diarrhea, night blindness, xerophthalmia) and measles-associated mortality for infants between 6 months and 5 years of age, although high-dose vitamin A exposure increases the severity and risk of antibiotic failure in non-measles pneumonia. Measles virus is susceptible to ribavirin in vitro and has been used in selected severe cases of pneumonitis (35 mg/kg/d intravenously in three divided doses for 2 days, followed by 20 mg/kg/d intravenously in three divided doses for 5 days) and was deemed effective in containing a measles outbreak in a pediatric oncology unit in India.

B. Treatment of Complications

Secondary bacterial infections, including pneumonia, are treated with appropriate antibacterial antibiotics. Post-measles encephalitis, including SSPE, can be managed only symptomatically.

Repeated studies fail to show an association between vaccination and autism. The prevalence of asthma-like diseases in childhood appears to be reduced among vaccinated children. Some data implicate the measles virus in the pathogenesis of rheumatoid arthritis.

▶ Prognosis

Between 2000 and 2008, measles mortality rate declined by 78%. In the last decade, the case-fatality rate in the United States stayed around 3 per 1000 reported cases, with deaths principally due to encephalitis (15% mortality rate) and secondary bacterial pneumonia. Deaths in the developing world are mainly related to diarrhea and protein-losing enteropathy.

▶ Prevention

In the United States, children receive their first vaccine dose at 12–15 months and a second at age 4–6 years, prior to entry into school. Combination measles-mumps-rubella-varicella vaccines (MMRV) can be used in place of the traditional measles, mumps, and rubella (MMR) vaccine. The median coverage with two doses of MMR vaccine nationally is 91% among children 19–35 months of age; however, there is considerable geographic disparity in this value (in the US Virgin Islands the coverage is only 63.7% and in West Virginia and Washington it is 84.6% and 84.8% respectively). The clustering of unvaccinated individuals also increases the likelihood of an outbreak. Susceptibility to measles is 2.4-fold higher if the vaccine is given prior to 15 months, suggesting that administration before that age may not be optimal for measles eradication. The evidence is not convincing that routine anthelmintic treatment affects the immune response to childhood vaccination.

American students beyond high school and medical staff starting employment require documentation of the above vaccination schedule or must show serologic evidence of immunity if they were born after 1956. For individuals born before 1957, herd immunity is assumed. Health care workers, immigrants, and refugees should be screened and vaccinated if necessary regardless of date of birth. International travelers (if immunocompetent and born after 1956) to the developing world and teachers should receive booster doses of vaccination.

At 6 months of age, more than 99% of infants of vaccinated women and 95% of infants of naturally immune women lose maternal antibodies. Therefore, in outbreaks that include infants less than 1 year of age, initial vaccination may be given at 6 months, with repeat at 15 months. When outbreaks take place in day care centers, K–12 institutions, or colleges and universities, revaccination is probably indicated for all, in particular for students and their siblings born after 1956 who do not have documentation of immunity as defined above. Susceptible personnel who were exposed should be isolated from patient contact between the fifth and the twenty-first day after exposure regardless of whether they were vaccinated or given immune globulin. If measles develops in these persons, they should be isolated from patient contact until 7 days after the rash develops.

When susceptible individuals are exposed to measles, live virus vaccine can prevent disease if given within 5 days of exposure. In addition, immune globulin (0.25 mL/kg [0.11 mL/lb] body weight) can be injected intramuscularly for prevention or modification of clinical illness if given within 6 days after exposure. This must be followed by active immunization with live measles vaccine 3 months later. In the developing world, the use of a second vaccine dose is an important aspect of achieving control of measles in the community.

Pregnant women and immunosuppressed persons should *not* receive this vaccine. Exception to this contraindication is asymptomatic HIV-infected patients, including children, who have not shown adverse effects from measles vaccination. In asymptomatic HIV-infected children, vaccination improves survival after measles, and HAART therapy is associated with an improved vaccine response. Repeat vaccination may be necessary in HIV-infected children after immune restoration. Immune globulin should be administered within 6 days of exposure for postexposure prophylaxis in any high-risk person exposed to measles. Such high-risk persons include children with malignancy and patients with AIDS who are at risk for developing severe or fatal disease.

Severe allergic reactions including anaphylaxis to the MMR vaccine are rare, though fever and rash appear to occur slightly more often among female recipients. Quadrivalent MMRV vaccine is associated with an increased risk of seizures that appears to be age-related; the risk is highest when MMRV is given to infants under 15 months of age. Future vaccines for a variety of infectious agents may utilize measles vectors, thereby augmenting immunity to measles. Rare cases of post-immunization encephalitis represent a form of acute disseminated encephalomyelitis (which can occur after many other vaccines including rabies, DPT, smallpox, and hepatitis B virus vaccinations).

When to Refer

- Any suspect cases should be reported to public health authorities.

- HIV infection.
- Pregnancy.

When to Admit

- Meningitis, encephalitis, or myelitis.
- Severe pneumonia.
- Diarrhea that significantly compromises fluid or electrolyte status.

Centers for Disease Control and Prevention (CDC). Measles—United States, 2011. MMWR Morb Mortal Wkly Rep. 2012 Apr 20;61:253–7. [PMID: 22513526]

De Serres G et al. Higher risk of measles when the first dose of a 2-dose schedule of measles vaccine is given at 12–14 months versus 15 months of age. Clin Infect Dis. 2012 Aug;55(3):394–402. [PMID: 22543023]

Lievano F et al. Measles, mumps, and rubella virus vaccine (M-M-R"II): a review of 32 years of clinical and postmarketing experience. Vaccine. 2012 Nov 6;30(48):6918–26. [PMID: 22959986]

McLean HQ et al; Centers for Disease Control and Prevention. Prevention of measles, rubella, congenital rubella syndrome, and mumps, 2013: summary recommendations of the Advisory Committee on Immunization Practices (ACIP). MMWR Recomm Rep. 2013 Jun 14;62(RR-04):1–34. [PMID: 23760231]

Roy Moulik N et al. Measles outbreak in a pediatric oncology unit and the role of ribavirin in prevention of complications and containment of the outbreak. Pediatr Blood Cancer. 2013 Oct;60(10):E122–4. [PMID: 23629813]

Sever AE et al. Measles elimination in the Americas: a comparison between countries with a one-dose and two-dose routine vaccination schedule. J Infect Dis. 2011 Sep;204(Suppl 2):S748–55. [PMID: 21954277]

2. Mumps

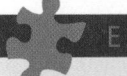

ESSENTIALS OF DIAGNOSIS

- ► Exposure 14–21 days before onset.
- ► Painful, swollen salivary glands, usually parotid.
- ► Frequent involvement of testes, pancreas, and meninges in unvaccinated individuals.

General Considerations

Mumps is a paramyxoviral disease spread by respiratory droplets. Children are the age group most affected, although in some outbreaks, patients are in the late second or early third decades of life. Mumps can spread rapidly in congregate settings, such as colleges and schools. The incidence is highest in spring. The incubation period is 14–21 days (average, 18 days). Infectivity occurs via saliva and urine and precedes the symptoms by about 1 day and is maximal for 3 days, although it may last a week. Up to one-third of affected individuals have subclinical infection. The most recent outbreaks in the United States were in Guam during 2009 and 2010 and among Orthodox Jewish children during 2009 and 2010 in New York.

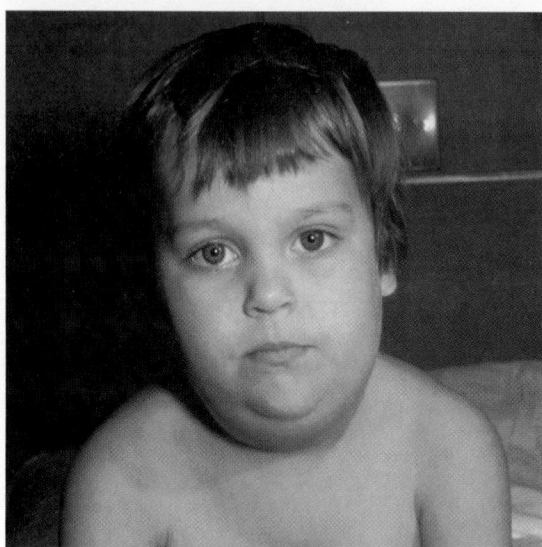

▲ **Figure 32–5.** Mumps. (Public Health Image Library, CDC.)

▶ Clinical Findings

A. Symptoms and Signs

Mumps is more serious in adults than in children. Parotid tenderness and overlying facial edema (Figure 32–5) are the most common physical findings and typically develop within 48 hours of the prodromal symptoms. Usually, one parotid gland enlarges before the other, but unilateral parotitis alone occurs in 25% of patients. The orifice of Stensen duct may be red and swollen. Trismus may result from parotitis. The parotid glands return to normal within a week. Involvement of other salivary glands (submaxillary and sublingual) occurs in 10% of cases.

Fever and malaise are variable but often minimal in young children. High fever accompanies meningitis or orchitis. Neck stiffness, headache, and lethargy suggest meningitis. Testicular swelling and tenderness (unilateral in 75% of cases) denote orchitis; the testes are the most common extrasalivary site of disease in adults. Orchitis develops 7–10 days after the onset of parotitis in about 25–40% of postpubertal men but occurred in only 7% of males above age 12 in the Orthodox Jewish outbreaks in New York mentioned above. Sterility is rare. Acute hormonal disturbances are prevalent, including decreased levels of testosterone and inhibin B with low or normal levels of gonadotropins in up to 35% cases with mumps orchitis. Upper abdominal pain, nausea, and vomiting suggest pancreatitis. Mumps is the leading cause of pancreatitis in children. Lower abdominal pain and ovarian enlargement suggest oophoritis (which occurs in 5% of postpubertal women, usually unilateral); it is a difficult diagnosis to establish.

B. Laboratory Findings

Mild leukopenia with relative lymphocytosis may be present. Serum amylasemia usually reflects salivary gland involvement rather than pancreatitis. Lymphocytic pleocytosis and hypoglychorrhachia of the cerebrospinal fluid in meningitis may be asymptomatic. Mild kidney function abnormalities are found in up to 60% of patients.

Characteristic clinical picture is usually sufficient for diagnosis. An elevated serum IgM is considered diagnostic and a repeat test 2–3 weeks after the onset of symptoms is recommended if the first assay is negative due to a delay in IgM rise, especially in vaccinated persons. A fourfold rise in complement-fixing antibodies to mumps virus in paired serum IgG also confirms infection. Confirmatory diagnosis of mumps is also made by isolating the virus preferably from a swab of the duct of the parotid or other affected salivary gland. The virus can also be isolated from cerebrospinal fluid early in the course of aseptic meningitis. Isolation from urine is no longer advised. Nucleic acid amplification techniques are more sensitive than viral cultures but their availability is limited. In the above New York outbreak, for example, a real time reverse transcriptase PCR (RT-PCR) available through CDC increased the diagnostic yield 14% when samples were collected within the first 2 days of the outbreak (while IgM assays were more sensitive 3 days or more into the outbreak).

▶ Differential Diagnosis

Swelling of the parotid gland may be due to calculi in the parotid ducts, tumors, or cysts, or to a reaction to iodides. Other causes include starch ingestion, sarcoidosis, cirrhosis, diabetes, bulimia, pilocarpine usage, and Sjögren syndrome. Parotitis may be produced by pyogenic organisms (eg, *S aureus,* gram-negative organisms), particularly in debilitated individuals with poor oral intake, drug reaction (phenothiazines, propylthiouracil), and other viruses (influenza A, parainfluenza, EBV infection, coxsackieviruses, adenoviruses, HHV-6). Swelling of the parotid gland must be differentiated from inflammation of the lymph nodes located more posteriorly and inferiorly than the parotid gland.

▶ Complications

Other manifestations of the disease are less common and usually follow parotitis but may precede it or occur without salivary gland involvement. Such manifestations include meningitis (30%), priapism or testicular infarction from orchitis, thyroiditis, neuritis, hepatitis, myocarditis, thrombocytopenia, migratory arthralgias (infrequently among adults and even rarer in children), and nephritis. Mumps is also been associated with cases of endocardial fibroelastosis and a hemophagocytosis syndrome. Rare neurologic complications include encephalitis, Guillain-Barré syndrome, cerebellar ataxia, facial palsy, and transverse myelitis. Encephalitis is associated with cerebral edema, serious neurologic manifestations, and sometimes death. Deafness from eighth nerve neuritis develops in about 0.1%; it is typically unilateral, severe, and permanent.

▶ Treatment

A. General Measures

The patient should be isolated until swelling subsides (about 9 days from onset) and kept on bed rest while febrile. Treatment is symptomatic. Topical compresses may relieve parotid discomfort. Some clinicians advocate intravenous immunoglobulin (IVIG) for complicated disease (eg, thrombocytopenia) although its definitive role is unproven.

B. Management of Complications

1. Aseptic meningitis—The treatment is symptomatic. The management of encephalitis requires attention to cerebral edema, the airway, and vital functions.

2. Epididymo-orchitis—The scrotum should be supported with a suspensor or toweling "bridge" and ice bags applied. Incision of the tunica may be necessary in severe cases. Pain can be relieved with opioids, or by injecting the spermatic cord at the external inguinal ring with 10–20 mL of 1% procaine solution. The merit of hydrocortisone sodium succinate (100 mg intravenously, followed by 20 mg orally every 6 hours for 2 or 3 days) in reducing inflammation is not firmly established. Interferon alfa-2b may be useful in preventing testicular atrophy.

3. Pancreatitis—Symptomatic treatment should be provided, with emphasis on parenteral hydration.

▶ Prognosis

The entire course of mumps rarely exceeds 2 weeks. Rare fatalities are usually due to encephalitis.

▶ Prevention

Mumps live virus vaccine is safe and effective (there is some variability among vaccines, the Jeryl Lynn strain being highly effective, the Urabe intermediate, the Rubini less so) with long lasting immunity. It is recommended for routine immunization for children over age 1 year, either alone or in combination with other virus vaccines (eg, in the MMR vaccine or as a quadrivalent vaccine with varicella). A second dose is recommended for children (ages 4–6 years) before starting school. (In outbreaks from Canada and Scotland, cases disproportionately included those who received only one dose of the vaccine.) Two doses of the vaccine should also be considered for high-risk individuals (eg, health care workers) born before 1957 and without evidence of immunity. The use of a third dose of mumps vaccine in the above New York summer camp outbreak showed efficacy with decreased attack rates among sixth through twelfth graders, and there were few adverse effects noted to date other than infrequent injection site reactions.

There are no known cases of long-term sequelae associated with mumps vaccination and the currently used mumps strain (Jeryl Lynn) shows the lowest associated incidence of post vaccine aseptic meningitis (from 1 in 150,000 to 1 in 1.8 million). This vaccine is less effective in epidemic settings. Reactions are reviewed in the measles section. It should not be given to pregnant women or to immunocompromised individuals, though the vaccine is given to asymptomatic HIV-infected individuals without adverse sequelae and should be given when the individuals show immune restoration with HAART. In the developed world, persons in whom mumps develops are less likely to have received a second vaccine dose. The mumps skin tests are less reliable than serum neutralization titers in determining immunity.

▶ When to Refer

Any suspect cases should be reported to public health authorities.

▶ When to Admit

- Trismus; meningitis, encephalitis; myocarditis.
- Severe abdominal pain or vomiting suggesting pancreatitis.
- Severe testicular pain; priapism.
- Severe thrombocytopenia.

Barskey AE et al. Mumps outbreak in Orthodox Jewish communities in the United States. N Engl J Med. 2012 Nov;367 (18):1704–13. [PMID: 23113481]
Deeks SL et al. An assessment of mumps vaccine effectiveness by dose during an outbreak in Canada. CMAJ. 2011 Jun 14;183(9):1014–20. [PMID: 21576295]
Ogbuanu IU et al. Impact of a third dose of measles-mumps-rubella vaccine on a mumps outbreak. Pediatrics. 2012 Dec;130(6):e1567–74. [PMID: 23129075]

3. Poliomyelitis

ESSENTIALS OF DIAGNOSIS

- ▶ Incubation period 9–12 days from exposure.
- ▶ Muscle weakness, headache, stiff neck, fever, nausea and vomiting, sore throat.
- ▶ Lower motor neuron lesion (flaccid paralysis) with decreased deep tendon reflexes and muscle wasting.
- ▶ Cerebrospinal fluid shows lymphocytic pleocytosis but rarely > 500/mcL.

▶ General Considerations

Poliomyelitis virus, an enterovirus, is present in throat washings and stools (excretion may last for weeks after infection). It is highly contagious through fecal–oral route, especially during the first week of infection. While by 2012, because of global vaccination efforts, indigenous transmission of wild poliovirus (WPV) types 1 and 3 were eliminated from all but three countries (Afghanistan, Nigeria, and Pakistan), data in 2012 described five cases from Chad and data through October 29, 2013 report a large number of cases secondary to the three above endemic nation cases from Somalia (180) with additional cases from Kenya (14), the Syrian Arab Republic (10), Ethiopia (7), and Cameroon (1). India has not reported a polio case since January 2011 and is considered polio free since February of 2012. The last case of WPV type 2 was in 1999, although a case was reported in 2011 of a woman with combined variable immunodeficiency who acquired type 2 poliomyelitis in Minnesota nearly 12 years after her child was given the oral vaccination.

While the177 cases were reported in 2012 represented a downward trend in the global tally of poliomyelitis cases, the preliminary reports for 2013 show an increase to 322, with 100 of these from the nonendemic countries listed above. All 2013 cases were WVP type 1 and only 19 of those in 2012 were WVP type 3 (one recombinant WPV types 1 and 3). A smoldering outbreak (largely in the Horn of Africa) was responsible for 6 of the 223 cases in 2012.

► **Clinical Findings**

A. Symptoms and Signs

At least 95% of infections are asymptomatic, but in those who become ill, manifestations include abortive poliomyelitis (minor illness), nonparalytic poliomyelitis, and paralytic poliomyelitis.

1. Abortive poliomyelitis (minor illness)—Such minor illness occurs in 4–8% of infections and the symptoms are fever, headache, vomiting, diarrhea, constipation, and sore throat lasting 2–3 days. This entity is suspected clinically only during an epidemic.

2. Nonparalytic poliomyelitis—In addition to the above symptoms, signs of meningeal irritation and muscle spasm occur in the absence of frank paralysis. This disease is indistinguishable from aseptic meningitis caused by other viruses.

3. Paralytic poliomyelitis—Paralytic poliomyelitis represents 0.1% of all poliomyelitis cases (the incidence is higher when infections are acquired later in life). Paralysis may occur at any time during the febrile period. Tremors, muscle weakness, constipation, and ileus may appear. Paralytic poliomyelitis is divided into two forms, which may coexist: (1) **spinal poliomyelitis,** with involvement of the muscles innervated by the spinal nerves, and (2) **bulbar poliomyelitis,** with weakness of the muscles supplied by the cranial nerves (especially nerves IX and X) and of the respiratory and vasomotor centers.

In spinal poliomyelitis, paralysis of the shoulder girdle often precedes intercostal and diaphragmatic paralysis, which leads to diminish chest expansion and decreased vital capacity. The paralysis occurs over 2–3 days, is flaccid, has an asymmetric distribution, and affects the proximal muscles of the lower extremities more frequently. Sensory loss is very rare.

In bulbar poliomyelitis, symptoms include diplopia (uncommonly), facial weakness, dysphagia, dysphonia, nasal voice, weakness of the sternocleidomastoid and trapezius muscles, difficulty in chewing, inability to swallow or expel saliva, and regurgitation of fluids through the nose. The most life-threatening aspect of bulbar poliomyelitis is respiratory paralysis. Lethargy or coma may be due to hypoxia, most often from hypoventilation. Vasomotor disturbances in blood pressure and heart rate may occur. Convulsions are rare. Bulbar poliomyelitis is more common in adults. Bulbar and spinal disease can coexist (bulbospinal poliomyelitis).

B. Laboratory Findings

The peripheral white blood cell count may be normal or mildly elevated. Cerebrospinal fluid findings include the following: (1) normal or slightly increased pressure and protein, (2) glucose is not decreased, and (3) white blood cells usually number < 500/mcL and are principally lymphocytes after the first 24 hours. Cerebrospinal fluid is normal in 5% of patients. The virus may be recovered from throat washings (early) and stools (early and late) and PCR of washings, stool, or cerebrospinal fluid can also facilitate diagnosis. Neutralizing and complement-fixing antibodies appear during the first or second week of illness. Serologic testing cannot distinguish between wild type and vaccine-related virus infections.

► **Differential Diagnosis**

Nonparalytic poliomyelitis is similar to other forms of enteroviral meningitis; the distinction is made serologically. Acute flaccid paralysis is the term used in the developing world for the variety of neurologic illnesses that both include and mimic poliomyelitis. Acute flaccid paralysis due to poliomyelitis is distinguished by the greater frequency of fever and asymmetric neurologic signs. Acute inflammatory polyneuritis (Guillain-Barré syndrome), Japanese B virus encephalitis, West Nile virus infection, and tick paralysis may resemble poliomyelitis. In Guillain-Barré syndrome (see Chapter 24), the weakness is more symmetric and ascending in most cases, but the Miller Fisher variant is quite similar to bulbar polio. Paresthesias are uncommon in poliomyelitis but common in Guillain-Barré syndrome. The cerebrospinal fluid usually has high protein content but normal cell count in Guillain-Barré syndrome.

► **Complications**

Urinary tract infection, atelectasis, pneumonia, myocarditis, paralytic ileus, gastric dilation, and pulmonary edema may occur. Respiratory failure may be a result of paralysis of respiratory muscles, airway obstruction from involvement of cranial nerve nuclei, or lesions of the respiratory center.

► **Treatment**

In the acute phase of paralytic poliomyelitis patients should be hospitalized. Strict bed rest in the first few days of illness reduces the rate of paralysis. Comfortable but rotating positions should be maintained in a "polio bed": firm mattress, footboard, sponge rubber pads or rolls, sandbags, and light splints. Intensive physiotherapy may help recover some motor function with paralysis. Fecal impaction and urinary retention (especially with paraplegia) are managed appropriately. In cases of respiratory weakness or paralysis, intensive care is needed. Attention to psychological disorders in long-standing disease is also important. The antiviral pleconaril shows no clear benefit in cases of polio meningoencephalitis.

► **Prognosis**

During the febrile period, paralysis may develop or progress. Mild weakness of small muscles is more likely to regress than severe weakness of large muscles. Bulbar poliomyelitis carries a mortality rate of up to 50%. Long-term sequelae include pain, weakness, fatigue, and obesity, factors often worsened by age and comorbidities. When new muscle weakness and pain develop and progress slowly years after recovery from acute paralytic poliomyelitis, the entity is called **postpoliomyelitis syndrome**. Risk factors for the syndrome include female gender, respiratory symptoms during the acute polio syndrome, and the need for orthoses and aids during the rehabilitation phase. The syndrome presents with signs of chronic and new denervation, is associated with increasing dysfunction of surviving motor neurons, and is not infectious in origin; patients do not shed the virus. Immune modulators, such as prednisone, interferon, and IVIG, do not show any clear benefits in the treatment of post poliomyelitis syndrome.

▶ Prevention

Given the epidemiologic distribution of poliomyelitis and the continued concern about vaccine-associated disease (estimated in 1:750,000 recipients) with the trivalent oral live poliovirus vaccine (OPV), the inactive (Salk) parenteral vaccination is currently used in the United States for all four recommended doses (at ages 2 months, 4 months, 6–18 months, and at 4–6 years). Inactivated vaccine is also routinely used elsewhere in the developed world. Oral vaccines are limited to usage for outbreak control, travel to endemic areas within the ensuing month, and protection of children whose parents do not comply with the recommended number of immunizations. The advantages of oral vaccination are the ease of administration, low cost, effective local gastrointestinal and circulating immunity, herd immunity, and decreased viral shedding in stool samples.

Routine immunization of adults in the United States is no longer recommended because of the low incidence of the disease. Exceptions include adults not vaccinated within the prior decade who are exposed to poliomyelitis or who plan to travel to endemic areas (mentioned above). Vaccination should also be considered for adults engaged in high-risk activities (eg, laboratory workers handling stools). Such adults should be given inactivated poliomyelitis vaccine (Salk) as should immunodeficient or immunosuppressed individuals and members of their households.

In the developing world, three doses of OPV seem sufficient for adequate immunization and the interval between doses should probably be > 1 month (because of interference from enteric pathogens). Intramuscular injections should be routinely avoided during the month following oral poliomyelitis vaccination to prevent provocation paralysis. Clinical studies suggest that rotavirus and OPV can be given concomitantly. Ancillary useful control measures ("supplementary immunization activities") in polio-endemic countries include national immunization days (mass campaigns in which all children are vaccinated twice, 4–6 weeks apart, regardless of vaccine history); cross-border vaccination activities; surveillance for acute flaccid paralysis, an indicator for poliomyelitis; and

aggressive outbreak responses as well as intensified immunization activities in countries impacted by armed conflicts.

VDPV cases with the oral Sabin vaccination are due to mutations leading to neurovirulence. Such cases serve as a reminder of the need to maintain high levels of immunization coverage even in the absence of overt disease. An immunogenic monovalent type 1 oral vaccine (several times more effective than the trivalent oral vaccine) is successfully used in India, Egypt, and Nigeria. Cost and administrative considerations along with a need for effective herd immunity remain major reasons the oral Sabin is still administered. Current research on developing improved inactivated polio vaccine (IPV) will be crucial for the final eradication of poliomyelitis. There is no epidemiologic evidence to implicate poliomyelitis vaccination as a cause for recurrent worsening wheezing or eczema in childhood.

▶ When to Refer

- Neurologic compromise.
- Any suspicious cases should be referred to public health authorities.

Bertolasi L et al. Risk factors for post-polio syndrome among an Italian population: a case-control study. Neurol Sci. 2012 Dec;33(6):1271–5. [PMID: 22246456]

Centers for Disease Control and Prevention (CDC). Assessing the risks for poliovirus outbreaks in polio-free countries—Africa, 2012–2013. MMWR Morb Mortal Wkly Rep. 2013 Sep 20;62(37):768–72. [PMID: 24048153]

Hird TR et al. Systematic review of mucosal immunity induced by oral and inactivated poliovirus vaccines against virus shedding following oral poliovirus challenge. PLoS Pathog. 2012;8(4):e1002599. [PMID: 22532797]

Liao G et al. Safety and immunogenicity of inactivated poliovirus vaccine made from Sabin strains: a phase II, randomized, positive-controlled trial. J Infect Dis. 2012 Jan 15;205(2):237–43. [PMID: 22158682]

World Health Organization; Global Polio Eradication Initiative. Data and monitoring: polio this week. http://www.polioeradication.org/Dataandmonitoring/Poliothisweek.aspx

4. Rubella

ESSENTIALS OF DIAGNOSIS

- ▶ Exposure 14–21 days before onset.
- ▶ Arthralgia, particularly in young women.
- ▶ No prodrome in children, mild prodrome in adults; mild symptoms (fever, malaise, coryza) coinciding with eruption.
- ▶ Posterior cervical and postauricular lymphadenopathy 5–10 days before rash.
- ▶ Fine maculopapular rash of 3 days duration; face to trunk to extremities.
- ▶ Leukopenia, thrombocytopenia.

General Considerations

Rubella is a systemic disease caused by a togavirus transmitted by inhalation of infective droplets. It is moderately communicable. One attack usually confers permanent immunity but reinfection is possible, albeit rarely. The incubation period is 14–21 days (average, 16 days). The disease is transmissible from 1 week before the rash appears until 15 days afterward.

The clinical picture of rubella is difficult to distinguish from other viral illnesses such as infectious mononucleosis, measles, echovirus infections, and coxsackievirus infections; however, arthritis is more prominent in rubella. Surveillance of female military recruits suggests that serologic protection, largely vaccine derived, against rubella, measles, and mumps is inadequate. The rubella case load decreased from 670,894 cases in 2000 to 121,344 cases in 2009 with reports of disease from 167 nations. A major outbreak occurred in Japan in early 2013 with over 5442 cases through May 1—77% in males (vaccine programs between 1976 and 1989 targeted only girls) and 10 cases of congenital rubella syndrome. Rubella-containing vaccine is available in 130 nations. In the United States, rubella was last endemic in 2001. The principal importance of rubella lies in its devastating effects on the fetus in utero, producing teratogenic effects and a continuing congenital infection (**congenital rubella syndrome**). The control of rubella is so successful that the number of cases worldwide of reported congenital rubella syndrome in 2008 was only 165 with over one-third of these from the Eastern Mediterranean region. In the United States, congenital rubella syndrome among the native-born population last occurred in 2004, although periodic cases have occurred among women who emigrated from Africa including three in 2012.

Clinical Findings

A. Symptoms and Signs

While fetal rubella can be devastating, postnatally acquired rubella is usually innocuous and asymptomatic in up to 50% of cases. In the postnatally acquired infection, fever and malaise, usually mild, accompanied by tender suboccipital adenitis, may precede the eruption by 1 week. Mild coryza may be present. Polyarticular arthritis occurs in about 25% of adult cases and involves the fingers, wrists, and knees. Rarely does chronic arthritis develop. The polyarthritis usually subsides within 7 days but may persist for weeks. Early posterior cervical and postauricular lymphadenopathy is very common. Erythema of the palate and throat, sometimes patchy, may be noted.

A fine, pink maculopapular rash appears on the face, trunk, and extremities in rapid progression (2–3 days) and fades quickly, usually lasting 1 day in each area (Table 32–2). Rubella without rash may be at least as common as the exanthematous disease. When rubella is suspected because of disease in the community, the diagnosis requires serologic confirmation.

B. Laboratory Findings

Leukopenia may be present early and may be followed by an increase in plasma cells. The definitive diagnosis of acute rubella infection is based on elevated IgM antibody, fourfold or greater rise in IgG antibody titers, or isolation of the virus. False-positive IgM antibodies, however, are associated with Epstein-Barr virus, CMV, erythrovirus (parvovirus), and rheumatoid factor. Detection of antibodies against rubella in other body fluids, such as urine and saliva, are promising diagnostic aids. An interferon-gamma-ELISPOT can provide valuable additional information in seronegative individuals. PCR techniques are also available.

Complications

A. Exposure During Pregnancy

When a pregnant woman is exposed to a possible case of rubella, an immediate hemagglutination-inhibiting rubella antibody level should be obtained to document immunity, since fetal infection during the first trimester leads to congenital rubella in at least 80% of fetuses.

Positive tests for IgG antibodies alone indicate past infection or vaccination. High-avidity anti-rubella IgG assays may distinguish past infection from vaccination. If no antibodies are found, clinical observation and serologic follow-up are essential. An isolated IgM-positive test needs to be interpreted with caution because it does not necessarily imply acute infection. Confirmation of rubella in the expectant mother raises the question of therapeutic abortion, an alternative to be considered in light of personal, religious, legal, and other factors.

The immune status of the mother needs to be evaluated because titers fall to seronegativity in about 10% by 12 years after vaccination.

B. Congenital Rubella

An infant acquiring the infection in utero may be normal at birth but probably—50% in a series of nearly 70 pregnant women with rubella in Mexico—will have a wide variety of manifestations, including early-onset cataracts and glaucoma, microphthalmia, hearing deficits, psychomotor retardation, congenital heart defects (patent ductus arteriosus, branch pulmonary artery stenosis), organomegaly, and maculopapular rash. In general, the younger the fetus when infected, the more severe the illness. Deafness is the primary complication in the second trimester. Viral excretion in the throat and urine persists for many months despite high antibody levels. A specific test for IgM rubella antibody is useful for diagnosis in the newborn. A confirmatory diagnosis is made by isolation of the virus or PCR detection of viral RNA in tissues. Treatment is directed toward the many anomalies.

C. Postinfectious Encephalopathy

In 1:6000 cases, postinfectious encephalopathy develops 1–6 days after the rash; the virus cannot always be isolated. The mortality rate is 20%, but residual deficits are rare among the recovered. The mechanism is unknown.

Other unusual complications of rubella include hemorrhagic manifestations due to thrombocytopenia and vascular damage, duodenal stenosis, and mild hepatitis.

Treatment

Acetaminophen provides symptomatic relief for acute rubella. Encephalitis and non–life-threatening thrombocytopenia should be treated symptomatically.

Prognosis

Rubella is a mild illness and rarely lasts more than 3–4 days. Congenital rubella, on the other hand, has a high mortality rate, and the associated congenital defects are largely permanent.

Prevention

Live attenuated rubella virus vaccine should be given to all infants and a second dose should be given to children of school age. It is important that girls in particular are immune to rubella prior to the menarche. When women are immunized, they should not be pregnant, and the absence of antibodies should be established. (In the United States, about 80% of 20-year-old women are immune to rubella.) Postpartum administration to susceptible female hospital employees is recommended. It is recommended that women not become pregnant for at least 3 months after vaccine administration. Nonetheless, there are no reports of congenital rubella syndrome after rubella immunization, and inadvertent immunization of a pregnant woman is not considered an indication for therapeutic abortion. Arthritis is more marked after rubella vaccination than in native disease and appears to be immunologically mediated. A flare of juvenile rheumatoid arthritis after rubella vaccination is reported. The association between chronic arthropathies and rubella vaccination is controversial. Anaphylactoid reactions following vaccination are rare, and a self-limited thrombotic thrombocytopenic purpura is a reported but very rare (2.6 per 100,000 doses) complication.

MMR may be given in conjunction with DPT or varicella boosters as adequate serologic responses are documented. The administration of two or more doses appears to overcome an immunogenetic risk for vaccine failure in some vaccinees. Immunogenicity is similar with intramuscular and intracutaneous infection, for MMR and varicella vaccinations. Children with biliary atresia in particular show impaired responses to MMR and varicella vaccinations, although children with juvenile rheumatoid arthritis show intact responses to MMR boosters. Preliminary data suggests that vaccination may be safe for patients receiving immunosuppressive therapy in the setting of solid organ, bone marrow, or stem cell transplantation. Immigrants, especially the HIV-positive, should be vaccinated if CD4 counts show immune restoration.

Geographic areas with high birth rates and transmission rates of rubella may require baseline societal coverage rates for rubella higher than the conventional 80% often used.

When to Refer

- Pregnancy.
- Meningitis/encephalitis.

- Significant vaccination reactions.
- Any suspect cases should be reported to public health authorities.

Castillo-Solórzano C et al. Elimination of rubella and congenital rubella syndrome in the Americas. J Infect Dis. 2011 Sep 1; 204(Suppl 2):S571–8. [PMID: 21954249]

Centers for Disease Control and Prevention (CDC). Nationwide rubella epidemic—Japan, 2013. MMWR Morb Mortal Wkly Rep. 2013 Jun 14;62(23):457–62. Erratum in: MMWR Morb Mortal Wkly Rep. 2013 Jul 12;62(27):558. [PMID: 23760185]

Centers for Disease Control and Prevention (CDC). Three cases of congenital rubella syndrome in the postelimination era—Maryland, Alabama, and Illinois, 2012. MMWR Morb Mortal Wkly Rep. 2013 Mar 29;62(12):226–9. [PMID: 23535689]

Reef SE et al. Evidence used to support the achievement and maintenance of elimination of rubella and congenital rubella syndrome in the United States. J Infect Dis. 2011 Sep 1;204 (Suppl 2):S593–7. [PMID: 21954252]

OTHER NEUROTROPIC VIRUSES

1. Rabies

 ESSENTIALS OF DIAGNOSIS

- History of animal bite.
- Paresthesia, hydrophobia, rage alternating with calm.
- Convulsions, paralysis, thick tenacious saliva.

General Considerations

Rabies is a viral (rhabdovirus) encephalitis transmitted by infected saliva that gains entry into the body by an animal bite or an open wound. Worldwide, 17.4 million cases of animal bites are reported every year, and it is estimated that between 26,000 and 61,000 deaths annually are attributable to rabies. Most of these cases occur in rural areas of Africa and Asia, with India accounting for 36% of the global deaths. In developing countries, more than 90% of human cases and 99% of human deaths from rabies are secondary to bites from infected dogs. Rabies among travelers to rabies-endemic areas is usually associated with animal injuries (including dogs in North Africa and India, cats in the Middle East, and non-human primates in sub-Saharan Africa and Asia), with most travel-associated cases occurring within 10 days of arrival.

In the United States, domestically acquired rabies cases are rare (approximately 92% of cases are associated with wildlife) but probably underreported. Reports largely from the East Coast show an increase in rabies among cats, with about 1% of tested cats showing rabies seropositivity. In 2012, 1 case of rabies was reported in United States citizens, and surveillance for animal rabies showed 62 cases among 49 states and Puerto Rico. Wildlife reservoirs, each species having its own rabies variant(s), follow a unique geographic distribution in the United States: raccoons in the East Coast; skunks in the Midwest, Southwest, and California;

and foxes in the Southwest and in Alaska. Hawaii is the only rabies-free state to date. Bats were the second most reported rabid animals after raccoons during 2012. Raccoons, bats, and skunks account for 84% of the rabid animals found in the United States; other rabid animals include foxes, cats, cattle, and dogs. Rodents and lagomorphs (eg, rabbits) are unlikely to spread rabies because they cannot survive the disease long enough to transmit it (woodchucks and groundhogs are exceptions). Wildlife epizootics present a constant public health threat in addition to the danger of reintroducing rabies to domestic animals. Vaccination is the key to rabies in small animals and rabies transmission to human beings.

The virus gains entry into the salivary glands of dogs 5–7 days before their death from rabies, thus limiting their period of infectivity. Less common routes of transmission include contamination of mucous membranes with saliva or brain tissue, aerosol transmission, and corneal transplantation. Transmission through solid organ and vascular segment transplantation from donors with unrecognized infection is also reported.

The incubation period may range from 10 days to many years but is usually 3–7 weeks depending in part on the distance of the wound from the CNS. The virus travels in the nerves to the brain, multiplies there, and then migrates along the efferent nerves to the salivary glands. Rabies virus infection forms cytoplasmic inclusion bodies similar to Negri bodies. These Negri body-like structures are thought to be the sites of viral transcription and replication.

▶ Clinical Findings

A. Symptoms and Signs

While there is usually a history of animal bite, bat bites may not be recognized. The prodromal syndrome consists of pain at the site of the bite in association with fever, malaise, headache, nausea, and vomiting. The skin is sensitive to changes of temperature, especially air currents (aerophobia). Percussion myoedema can be present and persist throughout the disease. The CNS stage begins about 10 days after the prodrome and may be either encephalitic ("furious") or paralytic ("dumb"). The encephalitic form (about 80% of the cases) produces the classic rabies manifestations of delirium alternating with periods of calm, extremely painful laryngeal spasms on attempting drinking (hydrophobia), autonomic stimulation (hypersalivation), and seizures. In the less common paralytic form, an acute ascending paralysis resembling Guillain-Barré syndrome predominates with relative sparing of higher cortical functions initially. Both forms progress relentlessly to coma, autonomic nervous system dysfunction, and death.

B. Laboratory Findings

Biting animals that appear well should be quarantined and observed for 10 days. Sick or dead animals should be tested for rabies. A wild animal, if captured, should be sacrificed and the head shipped on ice to the nearest laboratory qualified to examine the brain for evidence of rabies virus. When the animal cannot be examined, raccoons, skunks, bats, and foxes should be presumed to be rabid.

Direct fluorescent antibody testing of skin biopsy material from the posterior neck (where hair follicles are highly innervated) has a sensitivity of 60–80%.

Quantitative reverse transcriptase-PCR, nucleic acid sequence-based amplification, direct rapid immunohistochemical test and viral isolation from the cerebrospinal fluid or saliva are advocated as definitive diagnostic assays. Antibodies can be detected in the serum and the cerebrospinal fluid. Pathologic specimens often demonstrate round or oval eosinophilic inclusion bodies (Negri bodies) in the cytoplasm of neuronal cells, but the finding is neither sensitive nor specific. MRI signs are diffuse and nonspecific.

▶ Treatment & Prognosis

Management requires intensive care with attention to the airway, maintenance of oxygenation, and control of seizures. Universal precautions are essential. The induction of coma by ketamine, midazolam, and supplemental barbiturates along with the use of amantadine and ribavirin (the Milwaukee protocol) was reportedly helpful in one case but failed to reproduce success in 26 subsequent cases. Corticosteroids are of no use.

If postexposure prophylaxis (discussed below) is given expediently, before clinical signs develop, it is nearly 100% successful in prevention of disease. Once the symptoms have appeared, death almost inevitably occurs after 7 days, usually from respiratory failure. Most deaths occur in persons with unrecognized disease who do not seek medical care or in individuals who do not receive postexposure prophylaxis. The very rare cases in which patients recover without intensive care are referred to as "abortive rabies."

▶ Prevention

Immunization of household dogs and cats and active immunization of persons with significant animal exposure (eg, veterinarians) are important. The most important decisions, however, concern animal bites. Animals that are frequent sources of infection to travelers are dogs, cats, and non-human primates.

In the developing world, education, surveillance, and animal (particularly dog) vaccination programs (at recurrent intervals) are preferred over mass destruction of dogs, which is followed typically by invasion of susceptible feral animals into urban areas. In some Western European countries, campaigns of oral vaccination of wild animals led to the elimination of rabies in wildlife.

A. Local Treatment of Animal Bites and Scratches

Thorough cleansing, debridement, and repeated flushing of wounds with soap and water are important. Rabies immune globulin or antiserum should be given as stated below. Wounds caused by animal bites should not be sutured.

B. Postexposure Immunization

The decision to treat should be based on the circumstances of the bite, including the extent and location of the wound, the biting animal, the history of prior vaccination, and the local epidemiology of rabies. **Any contact or suspect contact with a bat, skunk, or raccoon is usually deemed a sufficient indication to warrant prophylaxis.** Consultation with state and local health departments is recommended. Postexposure treatment including both immune globulin and vaccination should be administered as promptly as possible when indicated.

The optimal form of passive immunization is human rabies immune globulin (HRIG; 20 international units/kg), administered once. As much as possible of the full dose should be infiltrated around the wound, with any remaining injected intramuscularly at a site distant from the wound. Finger spaces can be safely injected without development of a compartment syndrome. If HRIG is not available, equine rabies antiserum (40 international units/kg) can be used if available after appropriate tests for horse serum sensitivity. All of the rabies immunoglobulin should be injected at the wound site as much as possible and the remainder injected intramuscularly at a distant site from the vaccine administration.

Two vaccines are licensed and available for use in humans in the United States: a human diploid cell vaccine and a purified chick embryo cell vaccine. The current vaccines may be given as four injections of 1 mL intramuscularly in the deltoid or, in small children, into the anterolateral thigh muscles on days 0, 3, 7, and 14 after exposure. (The fifth dose at 28 days after exposure is no longer recommended except among immunosuppressed patients.) The vaccine should not be given in the gluteal area due to suboptimal response. An alternative vaccination strategy that only takes 1 week, with injections on days 0, 3, and 7 after exposure with a verocell vaccine is reportedly successful in achieving adequate neutralizing titers at days 14 and 28 in a study from Thailand.

Rabies vaccines and HRIG should never be given in the same syringe or at the same site. Allergic reactions to the vaccine are rare, although local reactions (pruritus, erythema, tenderness) occur in about 25% and mild systemic reactions (headaches, myalgias, nausea) in about 20% of recipients. Adverse reactions to HRIG seem to be more frequent in women and rare in young children. The vaccine is commercially available or can be obtained through health departments.

Globally diverse anti-rabies vaccines are used. In some countries, the full spectrum of vaccines, from human diploid rabies to chromatographically purified rabies vaccine are available, whereas in others, the gamut is smaller and intradermal application of smaller vaccine doses at multiple sites and at different times is commonly practiced in an attempt to lower costs, and is deemed safe and effective by the WHO.

In patients with history of past vaccination, the need for HRIG is eliminated (RIG is in short supply worldwide) but postexposure vaccination is still required. The vaccine should be given 1 mL in the deltoid twice (on days 0 and 3). Neither the passive nor the active form of postexposure prophylaxis is associated with fetal abnormalities and thus pregnancy is not considered a contraindication to vaccination.

C. Preexposure Immunization

Preexposure prophylaxis with three injections of human diploid cell vaccine intramuscularly (1 mL on days 0, 7, and 21 or 28) is recommended for persons at high risk for exposure: veterinarians (who should have rabies antibody titers checked every 2 years and be boosted with 1 mL intramuscularly); animal handlers; laboratory workers; Peace Corps workers; and travelers with stays over 1 month to remote areas in endemic countries in Africa, Asia, and Latin America. An intradermal route is also available (0.1 mL on days 0, 7, and 21 over the deltoid) but not in the United States. Immunosuppressive illnesses and agents including corticosteroids as well as antimalarials—in particular chloroquine—may diminish the antibody response. A single dose booster at 10 years after initial immunization increases the level of antibody titers.

▶ When to Refer

Suspicion of rabies requires contact with public health personnel to initiate appropriate passive and active prophylaxis and observation of suspect cases.

▶ When to Admit

- Respiratory, neuromuscular, or CNS dysfunction consistent with rabies.
- Patients with suspect rabies require initiation of therapy until the disease is ruled out in suspect animals, and this requires coordination of care based on likelihood of patient compliance, availability of inpatient and outpatient facilities, and response of local public health teams.

Centers for Disease Control and Prevention (CDC). Recovery of a patient from clinical rabies—California, 2011. MMWR Morb Mortal Wkly Rep. 2012 Feb 3;61(4):61–5. [PMID: 22298301]

Dyer JL et al. Rabies surveillance in the United States during 2012. J Am Vet Med Assoc. 2013 Sep 15;243(6): 805–15. [PMID: 24004227]

Roebling AD et al. Rabies prevention and management of cats in the context of trap-neuter-vaccinate-release programmes. Zoonoses Public Health. 2014 Jun;61(4):290–6. [PMID: 23859607]

World Health Organization. WHO Expert Consultation on rabies. Second report. World Health Organ Tech Rep Ser. 2013;(982):1–139, back cover. [PMID: 24069724]

2. Arbovirus Encephalitides

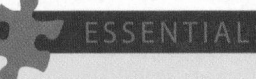

ESSENTIALS OF DIAGNOSIS

- ▶ Fever, malaise, stiff neck, sore throat, and vomiting, progressing to stupor, coma, and convulsions.
- ▶ Upper motor neuron lesion signs: exaggerated deep tendon reflexes, absent superficial reflexes, and spastic paralysis.
- ▶ Cerebrospinal fluid opening pressure and protein are often increased, with lymphocytic pleocytosis.

General Considerations

The arboviruses are arthropod-borne pathogens that produce clinical manifestations in humans. The **mosquito-borne pathogens** that cause encephalitis include three togaviruses (causing Western, Eastern, and Venezuelan equine encephalitis), five flaviviruses (causing West Nile fever, St. Louis encephalitis, Japanese B encephalitis, dengue, and Murray Valley encephalitis), and bunyaviruses (the California serogroup of viruses, including the Lacrosse agent of California encephalitis). The **tick-borne** causes of encephalitis include the flavivirus of the Powassan encephalitis (northeastern United States and Canada), tick-borne encephalitis virus of Europe, and the Colorado tick fever reovirus. Tick-borne encephalitis virus, Colorado tick fever, and the arboviruses associated with viral hemorrhagic fever (including dengue) are discussed below, and only those viruses causing primarily encephalitis in the United States will be discussed here, although West Nile agent is being reported in many other areas, including Italy, Greece, Portugal, and Hungary as well as in Africa (Madagascar and South Africa), Canada, the Middle East, and West Asia.

West Nile virus is the leading cause of domestically acquired arboviral disease in the United States. Several other arboviruses can also cause sporadic cases, neuroinvasive disease, and seasonal outbreaks. La Crosse virus was reported in 78 patients in 2012 with a median age of 9 years—56% were male and neuroinvasive disease occurred in 91% with highest rates for neuroinvasion in West Virginia, North Carolina, Tennessee, and Ohio. La Crosse virus cases occur largely east of 90 degree longitude and between late spring and early fall. Only 7 patients developed Powassan virus infection in 2012, the median age was 58 and all cases were in May or June, in Minnesota, Wisconsin, and New York. Fifteen cases of neuroinvasive Eastern equine encephalitis virus were reported in 2012, with a median age of 76 and the highest case load from Massachusetts. Only 3 cases of St Louis encephalitis occurred in 2012, all nonfatal and all in Texas. Jamestown Canyon virus is rare with 15 cases reported between 2004 and 2011. There are no reported patients with Western equine encephalitis since 1999. There are recent reports of 3 cases of Japanese encephalitis imported from Southeast Asia among travelers from Germany and Spain and more distant reports from the United States.

Infection with West Nile virus was first identified in the United States in the New York City area in 1999. The virus spread rapidly, and current cases are reported throughout the continental United States. The homeless appear to be at particularly increased risk for infection. In 2012, a surge of cases occurred in North Texas, with Dallas alone showing 225 cases of West Nile fever, and 172 cases of West Nile neurologic disease. As of November 25, 2013, 2170 cases, including 88 deaths, of West Nile virus were reported to the CDC, from all of the continental United States (none from Alaska or Hawaii). One-half of the reports (1086 cases) were of neuroinvasive disease. In the United States, the highest incidence of neuroinvasive disease is among the Rocky Mountain states as well as the upper Midwest and upper Southwest, while the largest number of cases are from Texas, California, Illinois, and Louisiana.

Outbreaks with West Nile infection tend to occur in between mid-July and early September. Climatic factors, including elevated mean temperatures and rainfall, correlate with increased West Nile infection. In the Dallas outbreak above, changes in weather pattern with a decrease in absolute number of winter days with low temperatures below 28°F correlated strongly with incidence of West Nile neurologic disease.

Pathogen-specific reservoirs (typically small mammals or birds) are responsible for maintaining the encephalitis-producing viruses in nature. For the Eastern equine encephalitis virus, cotton rats and house sparrows serve as amplifying reservoirs. Birds are the main reservoir for West Nile virus and substantial avian mortality accompanies West Nile fever outbreaks (monitoring chickens is recommended and a possible mode of disease surveillance). The mosquito species associated with transmission is different in the Western vs Eastern United States (*Culex tarsalis* vs *Culex pipiens*) and consequently the terrain associated with high prevalence areas differs (open grasslands vs urban areas).

Only dengue and Venezuelan equine encephalitis viruses produce viremias high enough to allow continued transmission to other mosquitoes and ticks between humans and vectors (mosquitoes of distinct species). Human to human transmission of the other arboviruses is usually related to blood (including granulocyte) transfusion or organ transplantation (although most infected donors give a history of clinically significant disease). Perinatal, transplacental, breastfeeding (rarely), laboratory, solid organ transplant, and possibly aerosol transmission of West Nile virus can also occur. St. Louis encephalitis and Powassan encephalitis occur among adults; Western equine encephalitis, Venezuelan equine encephalitis, La Crosse and California encephalitis occur primarily among children. West Nile fever and Eastern equine encephalitis are diseases of both children and adults.

Clinical Findings

A. Symptoms and Signs

The human incubation period for arboviral encephalitides is 2–14 days. Symptoms include fever, malaise, sore throat, headache, gastrointestinal upset, lethargy, and stupor progressing to coma. Using blood donor surveys, it is estimated that only about 26% of infections are symptomatic (women and the highly viremic are more symptomatic). A nonpruritic maculopapular rash is variably present. Stiff neck and mental status changes are the most common neurologic signs. It is estimated that West Nile fever develops in 20–25% of those infected with West Nile virus, while neuroinvasive disease occurs in < 1%, but has a mortality rate of at least 10%. About 50% of hospitalized patients with West Nile virus infection in the United States have significant muscle weakness that may be initially confused with the Guillain-Barré syndrome. Acute flaccid (poliomyelitis-like) paralysis is seen in 10% of West Nile virus neuroinvasive disease and less commonly with the other arboviruses. Other signs include tremors, seizures, cranial nerve palsies, and pathologic reflexes. Myocarditis, pancreatitis, and hearing loss are also reported. The disease manifestations associated with West Nile virus infection are strongly age-dependent: the acute febrile syndrome and mild neurologic symptoms (but on occasion meningitis) are more common in the young, aseptic meningitis and poliomyelitis-like syndromes are seen in the middle aged, and frank encephalopathy is seen more often in the elderly. All forms of disease tend to be severe in immunocompromised persons in whom neuroinvasive manifestations and associated high mortality are more apt to develop.

Host genetic variation in the interferon response pathway is associated with both risk for symptomatic West Nile virus infection and West Nile virus disease progression.

B. Laboratory Findings

The peripheral white blood cell count is variable. Cerebrospinal fluid protein is elevated; cerebrospinal fluid glucose is normal; there is usually a lymphocytic pleocytosis; and polymorphonuclear cells may predominate early. The diagnosis of arboviral encephalitides depends on serologic tests. Antibodies to arboviruses persist for life and the presence of IgG in the absence of a rising titer of IgM may indicate past exposure rather than acute infection. Individuals with chronic symptoms after West Nile virus infection may show persistent renal infection for up to 6 years with West Nile virus RNA present in urine. Documentation of a fourfold increase in acute/convalescence titers IgG or the presence of IgM antibodies is confirmatory. For West Nile virus, an IgM capture ELISA in serum or cerebrospinal fluid is almost always positive by the time the disease is clinically evident, and the presence of IgM in cerebrospinal fluid indicates neuroinvasive disease. These tests are available commercially but also through local or state health departments. Cross-reactivity exists among the different flaviviruses, so a plaque reduction assay may be needed to definitively distinguish between West Nile fever and St. Louis encephalitis. PCR assays (also available through the CDC) are less sensitive than serologic tests for the diagnosis of acute infections but are the preferred method for screening blood products and may be particularly useful in immunocompromised patients with abnormal antibody responses. CT scans of the brain usually show no acute disease, but MRI may reveal leptomeningeal, basal ganglia, thalamic, or periventricular enhancement.

▶ Differential Diagnosis

Mild forms of encephalitis must be differentiated from aseptic meningitis, lymphocytic choriomeningitis, and nonparalytic poliomyelitis.

Severe forms of arbovirus encephalitides are to be differentiated from other causes of viral encephalitis (HSV, mumps virus, poliovirus or other enteroviruses, HIV), encephalitis accompanying exanthematous diseases of childhood (measles, varicella, infectious mononucleosis, rubella), encephalitis following vaccination (a demyelinating type following rabies, measles, pertussis), toxic encephalitis

(from drugs, poisons, or bacterial toxins such as *Shigella dysenteriae* type 1), Reye syndrome, and severe forms of stroke, brain tumors, brain abscess, autoimmune processes such as lupus cerebritis, and intoxications. In the California Encephalitis Project, anti-N-methyl-D-aspartate receptor (anti-NMDAR) encephalitis is a more common cause of encephalitis than viral diseases especially in the young, with 65% of encephalitis due to anti-NMDAR occurring among patients 18 or younger.

▶ Complications

Bronchial pneumonia, urinary retention and infection, prolonged weakness, and decubitus ulcers may occur. St. Louis encephalitis is reportedly associated with a postinfectious encephalomyelitis. A chronic syndrome consisting of myalgias, arthralgias, and difficulty with concentration and memory is reported in over half the symptomatic cases. Reactivation of West Nile virus–related chorioretinitis was recently reported a year after the initial diagnosis.

▶ Treatment

Although specific antiviral therapy is not available for most causative entities, vigorous supportive measures can be helpful. Such measures include reduction of intracranial pressure (mannitol) and monitoring of intraventricular pressure. The efficacy of corticosteroids in these infections is not established. Other therapeutic options including ribavirin, IVIG, interferon-alpha, and hyperimmune plasma and gamma globulin are also largely anecdotal and await more substantial confirmation of effectiveness.

▶ Prognosis

Although most infections are mild or asymptomatic, the prognosis is always guarded, especially at the extremes of age. Most fatalities occur with neuroinvasive disease (9% for 2012 data) and among those with encephalitis or myelitis rather than with meningitis. As of June 28, 2013, the case fatality rate for West Nile virus disease in the United States was 5% (286 of 5674). Age older than 50 years is the most important risk factor for severe disease and death. Other risk factors for mortality include black race, chronic kidney disease, hepatitis C virus infection, and immunosuppression. Recovery of persons with severe neurologic compromise may take months. Sequelae of West Nile virus infection include a poliomyelitis-like syndrome, cognitive complaints, movement disorders, epilepsy, and depression; and they may become apparent late in the course of what appears to be a successful recovery.

The long-term prognosis is generally better for Western equine than for Eastern equine or St. Louis encephalitis.

▶ Prevention

No human vaccine is currently available for the arboviruses prevalent in North America, although yellow fever virus-based chimeric vaccines and recombinant vaccines remain under development for West Nile virus. Mosquito control (repellents, protective clothing, and insecticide spraying) is effective in prevention. Since 2003, all blood donations in the United States are screened with nucleic acid amplification tests for West Nile virus. Laboratory precautions are indicated for handling all these pathogens, in particular the West Nile virus.

A vaccine against Japanese B encephalitis is recommended for travelers to rural areas of East Asia, though the risk of disease acquisition among the exposed is estimated at only 1:1,000,000. This vaccination appears to provide some protection against West Nile virus (both agents are related flaviviruses).

Beardsley R et al. Reactivation West Nile virus infection-related chorioretinitis. Semin Ophthalmol. 2012 May–Jul;27(3–4): 43–5. [PMID: 22784261]

Bigham AW et al. Host genetic risk factors for West Nile virus infection and disease progression. PLoS One. 2011;6(9):e24745. [PMID: 21935451]

Centers for Disease Control and Prevention (CDC). West Nile virus and other arboviral diseases—United States, 2012. MMWR Morb Mortal Wkly Rep. 2013 Jun 28;62(25):513–7. [PMID: 23803959]

Gable MS et al. The frequency of autoimmune N-methyl-D-aspartate receptor encephalitis surpasses that of individual viral etiologies in young individuals enrolled in the California Encephalitis Project. Clin Infect Dis. 2012 Apr;54(7):899–904. [PMID: 22281844]

Goodman DM et al. JAMA patient page. West Nile virus. JAMA. 2012 Sep 12;308(10):1052. [PMID: 22922642]

3. Lymphocytic Choriomeningitis

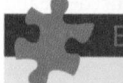

ESSENTIALS OF DIAGNOSIS

▶ "Influenza-like" prodrome of fever, chills, and cough, followed by a meningeal phase.

▶ Aseptic meningitis with stiff neck, headache, nausea, vomiting, and lethargy.

▶ Cerebrospinal fluid: slight increase of protein, lymphocytic pleocytosis (500–3000/mcL); low glucose in 25% of patients.

▶ Complement-fixing antibodies within 2 weeks.

▶ General Considerations

The lymphocytic choriomeningitis virus is an arenavirus (related to the pathogen causing Lassa fever, discussed below) that primarily infects the CNS. Its main reservoir is the house mouse (*Mus musculus*). Other rodents (such as rats, guinea pigs, and even pet hamsters), monkeys, dogs, and swine are also potential reservoirs. Lymphocytic choriomeningitis virus is shed by the infected animal via nasal secretions, urine, and feces; transmission to humans probably occurs through aerosolized particles, direct contact, or animal bites. The disease in humans is underdiagnosed and occurs most often in autumn. The lymphocytic choriomeningitis virus is typically not spread person to person, although vertical transmission is reported, and it is considered as an underrecognized teratogen. Rare cases related to

solid organ transplantation and autopsies of infected individuals are also reported. All reported cases were donor derived. Outbreaks are uncommon, and usually occur in laboratory settings among those workers with significant rodent exposure.

The ubiquitous nature of its reservoir and the wide distribution of the reported cases suggest a widespread geographic risk for lymphocytic choriomeningitis virus infection. Serologic surveys in the southern and eastern United States suggest past infection in approximately 3–5% of those tested, although more recent data from upstate New York showed < 1% seroprevalence. The risk of infection can be reduced by limiting contact with pet rodents and rodent trappings.

▶ Clinical Findings

A. Symptoms and Signs

The incubation period is 8–13 days to the appearance of systemic manifestations and 15–21 days to the appearance of meningeal symptoms. Symptoms are biphasic, with a prodromal illness characterized by fever, chills, headache, myalgia, cough, and vomiting, occasionally with lymphadenopathy and maculopapular rash. After 3–5 days the fever subsides only to return after 2–4 days alongside the meningeal phase, characterized by headache, nausea and vomiting, lethargy, and variably present meningeal signs. Arthralgias can develop late in the course. Transverse myelitis, deafness, Guillain-Barré syndrome and transient and permanent hydrocephalus are reported. Lymphocytic choriomeningitis virus is a well known, albeit underrecognized, cause of congenital infection frequently complicated with obstructive hydrocephalus and chorioretinitis. In fetuses and newborns with ventriculomegaly or other abnormal neuroimaging findings, screening for congenital lymphocytic choriomeningitis may be considered. Occasionally, a syndrome resembling the viral hemorrhagic fevers (see below) is described in transplant recipients of infected organs and in patients with lymphoma.

B. Laboratory Findings

Leukocytosis or leukopenia and thrombocytopenia may be initially present. During the meningeal phase, cerebrospinal fluid analysis frequently shows lymphocytic pleocytosis (total count is often 500–3000/mcL) alongside a slight increase in protein, while a low to normal glucose is seen in at least 25%. The virus may be recovered from the blood and cerebrospinal fluid by mouse inoculation. Complement-fixing antibodies appear during or after the second week. Detection of specific IgM by ELISA is becoming widely used. Detection of lymphocytic choriomeningitis virus by PCR is available in research settings.

▶ Differential Diagnosis

The influenza-like prodrome and latent period may distinguish this from other aseptic meningitides, and bacterial and granulomatous meningitis. A history of exposure to mice or other potential vectors is an important diagnostic clue.

Treatment

Treatment is supportive. In the survivor of a transplant-associated outbreak, ribavirin (which is effective against other arenaviruses) was used successfully along with decreasing immunosuppression.

Prognosis

Complications and fatalities are rare in the general population. The illness usually lasts 1–2 weeks, though convalescence may be prolonged. Congenital infection is more severe with about 30% mortality rate among infected infants, and more than 90% of survivors suffering long-term neurologic abnormalities. Lymphocytic choriomeningitis in solid organ transplant recipients is associated with a poor prognosis; of reported cases, the mortality rate is more than 80%.

Prevention

Pregnant women should be advised of the dangers to their unborn children inherent in exposure to rodents.

Anderson JL et al. Congenital lymphocytic choriomeningitis virus: when to consider the diagnosis. J Child Neurol. 2013 May 10. [Epub ahead of print] [PMID: 23666045]

Waggoner JJ et al. Rare and emerging viral infections in transplant recipients. Clin Infect Dis. 2013 Oct;57(8):1182–8. [PMID: 23839998]

4. Prion Diseases

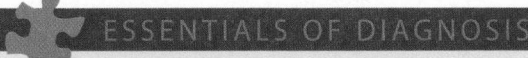

ESSENTIALS OF DIAGNOSIS

► Rare in humans.

► Cognitive decline.

► Myoclonic fasciculations, ataxia, visual disturbances, pyramidal and extrapyramidal symptoms.

► Variant form presents in younger people with prominent psychiatric or sensory symptoms.

► Specific EEG patterns.

General Considerations

The transmissible spongiform encephalopathies are a group of fatal neurodegenerative diseases affecting humans and animals. They are caused by infectious proteins called prions for **proteinaceous infectious particles.** These agents show slow replicative capacity and long latent intervals in the host. They induce the conformational change of a normal brain protein (prion protein; PrP[C]) into an abnormal isoform (PrP[Sc]) that accumulates and causes neuronal vacuolation (spongiosis), reactive proliferation of astrocytes and microglia and, in some cases, the deposition of beta-amyloid oligomeric plaques (PrP[C]).

Prion disease can be hereditary, sporadic, and transmissible in humans. Hereditary disorders are caused by germ line mutations in the PrP[C] gene causing **familial Creutzfeldt–Jakob disease (fCJD), Gerstmann-Sträussler-Scheinker syndrome (GSS),** and **fatal familial insomnia.**

Sporadic Creutzfeldt-Jakob disease (sCJD) is the most common of the human prion diseases, accounting for approximately 85% of cases; it has no known cause, although a spontaneous misfolding of PrP[C] as well as somatic mutations of PrP[C] or undetectable horizontal transmission are postulated as possible explanations. Transmissible prion disease is only described for kuru and Creutzfeldt-Jakob disease in its **iatrogenic (iCJD)** and **variant (vCJD)** form. Iatrogenic transmission of CJD is associated with prion contaminated human corneas, dura mater grafts, growth hormone, gonadotropins, stereotactic electroencephalography, electrodes, and neurosurgical instruments. An occupational risk for CJD among the health care community is not clearly evident from current European surveillance data.

Kuru, once prevalent in central New Guinea, is now rare, a decline in prevalence that started after the abandonment of cannibalism in the late 1950s (a protective allele of the PrP gene is now identified at codon 127).

More than 200 cases of vCJD (**bovine spongiform encephalopathy [BSE] or "mad cow disease"**) were reported in the United Kingdom since the first documented cases there in the mid-1990s. It is far less common in North America, with only 3 cases reported in the United States (the last 1 in 2006) and 19 in Canada. Of the US-reported cases, none acquired the disease locally (2 of them acquired the infection in the United Kingdom and 1 in Saudi Arabia). This disease is characterized by its bovine-to-human transmission through ingestion of meat from cattle infected with BSE. There is no animal-to-animal spread of BSE, and milk and its derived products are not considered to be infected. Reports of secondary transmission of vCJD due to blood transfusions from asymptomatic donors are reported in the United Kingdom. Although iCJD and vCJD are not associated with a known PrP gene mutation, a polymorphism in codon 129 is prevalent and seems to determine susceptibility and expression of clinical disease. The overall annual incidence of prion disease worldwide is approximately one in 1 million people per year. In the United States, among 3018 cases reported through November 11, 2013 to the US National Prion Disease Pathology Surveillance Center, 2539 (84.1%) were sporadic, 450 (14.9%) familial, 6 (0.2%) iatrogenic, and 3 (0.1%) vCJD.

Clinical Findings

A. Symptoms and Signs

Both sCJD and fCJD usually present in the sixth or seventh decade of life, whereas the iCJD form tends to occur in a much younger population. Clinical features of these three forms of disease usually involve mental deterioration (dementia, behavioral changes, loss of cortical function) progressive over several months, as well as myoclonus, extrapyramidal (hypokinesia) and cerebellar manifestations (ataxia, dysarthria). Finally, coma ensues, usually associated with an akinetic state and less commonly decerebrate/decorticate posturing. Like iCJD, vCJD usually affects younger patients (averaging ~28 years), but the duration of disease is longer (about 1 year). The degree of organ involvement is often extensive, and the clinical symptoms are unique, mainly characterized by prominent psychiatric and sensory symptoms.

B. Laboratory Findings

CJD should be considered as a diagnosis in the proper clinical scenario, in the absence of alternative diagnoses after routine investigations. Abnormalities in cerebrospinal fluid are subtle and rarely helpful. The detection of 14-3-3 protein in the cerebrospinal fluid is helpful for the diagnosis of sCJD but not in vCJD and fCJD. Its sensitivity and specificity are widely variable among different studies. Cerebrospinal fluid detection of other proteins like tau, neuron-specific enolase, and S100B protein are reported in smaller studies. Recently, the combination of tau with S100B was reported to be more sensitive than 14-3-3 protein.

A new blood-based assay and a PCR in cerebrospinal fluid show some promising results in the diagnosis of vCJD with high specificity but 71% sensitivity. Further evaluation is under way.

In sCJD, EEG typically shows a pattern of paroxysms with high voltages and slow waves, while MRI is characteristic for bilateral areas of increased signal intensity, predominantly in the caudate and putamen. MRI has great potential for improving early diagnosis of sCJD because clinical findings are often missed. When an experienced neuroradiologist or a prion disease expert reviews the MRI, diagnostic sensitivity of MRI for sCJD increases to 91%. The cortical findings associated with sCJD tend to be the most common region not documented by referring centers. In contrast, vCJD shows a diffusely abnormal but nondiagnostic EEG. MRI characteristically reveals hyperintensity of the posterior thalamus ("pulvinar sign"). Positron emission tomography can help distinguish GSS disease. The differentiation and definitive diagnosis of these neurodegenerative diseases are established by neuropathologic confirmation.

► Treatment & Prevention

There is no specific treatment for CJD. Once symptoms appear, the infection invariably leads to death. Flupirtine (an analgesic drug) is sometimes useful in slowing the associated cognitive decline but does not affect survival.

Iatrogenic CJD can be prevented by limiting patient exposure to potentially infectious sources as mentioned above. Prevention of vCJD relies on monitoring livestock for possible infection. The American Red Cross does not accept blood donations from persons with a family history of CJD or with a history of dural grafts or pituitary-derived growth hormone injections.

An international referral and database for CJD is available at: http://www.cjdsurveillance.com/index.html.

Andréoletti O et al. Highly efficient prion transmission by blood transfusion. PLoS Pathog. 2012;8(6):e1002782. [PMID: 22737075]

Carswell C et al. MRI findings are often missed in the diagnosis of Creutzfeldt-Jakob disease. BMC Neurol. 2012 Dec 5;12:153. [PMID: 23216655]
Edgeworth JA et al. Detection of prion infection in variant Creutzfeldt-Jakob disease: a blood-based assay. Lancet. 2011 Feb 5;377(9764):487–93. [PMID: 21295339]

5. Progressive Multifocal Leukoencephalopathy (PML)

PML is a rare demyelinating CNS disorder caused by the reactivation of the JC virus (John Cunningham virus or JCV). This polyomavirus usually causes its primary infection during childhood with > 60% of adults typically being seropositive. The virus remains latent in the kidneys, lymphoid tissues, epithelial cells, peripheral blood leukocytes, bone marrow, and possibly brain until the time reactivation occurs and symptoms become evident (see below). This reactivation is usually seen in adults with impaired cell-mediated immunity, especially AIDS patients (5–10% of whom develop PML), as well as those with idiopathic CD4 lymphopenia syndrome. It is also reported among those with lymphoproliferative and myeloproliferative disorders; granulomatous, inflammatory, and rheumatic diseases (systemic lupus erythematosus and rheumatoid arthritis in particular); as well as in those who have undergone solid and hematopoietic cell transplantation; and occasionally in those who have other medical states, including cirrhosis and kidney disease.

Medication-associated PML is described with the use of natalizumab, rituximab, infliximab (one case), and mycophenolate mofetil. Natalizumab, a monoclonal antibody used in the treatment of multiple sclerosis, is associated with the risk of PML developing in 1.35 cases per 1000 patients treated for more than a year and 1.78 per 1000 for patients treated > 2 years. The risk of PML appears to increase up to 36 months of therapy and levels off thereafter.

Although an immune reconstitution inflammatory state may follow cessation of monoclonal antibody therapy, the JCV presence and the residual neurologic deficits may not clear for years after therapy is stopped. The risk of developing PML associated with rituximab is at least 1 in 25,000 exposed patients with cases reported in various autoimmune conditions (systemic lupus erythematosus, rheumatoid arthritis, multiple sclerosis). The mean interval between the use of the drug to the diagnosis of PML is 5.5 months. Smoking is reportedly associated with an increased risk of PML.

► Clinical Findings

A. Symptoms and Signs

JCV causes lytic infection of oligodendrocytes in the white matter and symptoms presenting subacutely reflect the diverse areas of CNS involvement. Symptoms include altered mental status, aphasia, ataxia, hemiparesis or hemiplegia and visual field disturbances. Seizures occur in about 18%. Involvement of cranial nerves and cervical spine is rare.

B. Laboratory Findings

PCR for JCV in cerebrospinal fluid is used for diagnosis in patients with compatible clinical and radiologic findings. A quantitative PCR is more sensitive. Persistent JC viremia and increasing urinary JCV DNA may be predictive of PML. An anti-JCV immunoglobuin G (IgG) was higher 6 months before diagnosis but was not predictive of PML in a cohort of HIV-infected persons.

MRIs of the brain show multifocal areas of white matter demyelination without mass effect or contrast enhancement. These findings may not be distinguishable from immune reconstitution inflammatory syndrome. In HIV-infected patients, a syndrome of cerebellar degeneration is described.

Treatment & Prevention

Limiting the immunosuppressed state represents the mainstay of therapy for PML. Treatment of HIV with HAART reduces the incidence of PML, improves the clinical symptoms, reverses some of the radiographic abnormalities, and improves the 1-year mortality rate, regardless of baseline CD4 count. Immune restoration can induce worsening of the clinical picture in a small number of cases. Immune reconstitution syndromes do not alter mortality but are associated with a form of PML called non-determined leukoencephalopathy associated with a distinct chemokine polymorphism. Significant neurologic sequelae to PML infections are the rule. Deficits associated with PML, including monoclonal associated forms, may persist for years.

Decreasing immunosuppression in non-AIDS patients with PML (eg, transplant patients) is also typically beneficial. Cidofovir may be beneficial in non-AIDS related cases while corticosteroids may be useful with immune reconstitution. Because the JCV infects cells through serotonin receptors, the use of risperidone and mirtazapine are recommended by some clinicians. Plasma exchange, which theoretically reduces the plasma level of agents associated with PML, may be useful in natalizumab-associated PML.

Casado JL et al. Continued declining incidence and improved survival of progressive multifocal leukoencephalopathy in HIV/AIDS patients in the current era. Clin Microbiol Infect Dis. 2014 Feb;33(2):179–87. [PMID: 23948752]

Lima MA. Progressive multifocal leukoencephalopathy: new concepts. Arq Neuropsiquiatr. 2013 Sep;71(9B):699–702. [PMID: 24141508]

Major EO et al. JC viremia in natalizumab-treated patients with multiple sclerosis. N Engl J Med. 2013 Jun 6;368(23):2240–1. [PMID: 23738566]

Martin-Blondel G et al. In situ evidence of JC virus control by CD8+ T cells in PML-IRIS during HIV infection. Neurology. 2013 Sep 10;81(11):964–70. [PMID: 23935178]

6. Human T Cell Lymphotropic Virus (HTLV)

HTLV-1 and -2 are retroviruses that infect CD4 and CD8 T cells respectively, where they persist as a lifelong latent infection. HTLV-1 currently infects approximately 20 million individuals worldwide. It is endemic to many regions in the world including southern Japan, the Caribbean, multiple regions of sub-Saharan Africa, South America, Eastern Europe, and Oceania. The Caribbean basin and Southwestern Japan show the highest prevalence of infection (4–37%). Conversely, HTLV-2 is mainly found in native populations of South (1–58%), Central (8–10%), and North America (2–13%) as well as African pygmy tribes.

In the United States, studies done in blood donors show a seroprevalence of HTLV-1 of 0.005% and HTLV-2 of 0.014%, a decline since the early 1990s. Over 85% of the cases found in the United States are located in the West or Southwest. The virus is transmitted horizontally (sex), vertically (intrauterine, peripartum, and breast feeding), and parenterally (injection drug use and blood transfusion). Hence, a higher prevalence is seen among injection drug users.

Clinical Findings

A. Symptoms and Signs

HTLV-1 infection is associated with **HTLV-1 adult T cell lymphoma/leukemia (ATL)** and **HTLV-1 associated myelopathy/tropical spastic paraparesis (HAM/TSP)**. In contrast, HTLV-2 is significantly less pathogenic, with few reported cases of HAM/TSP as well as other neurologic manifestations. The causative association of HTLV-1 with ATL, attributed to the virally encoded oncoprotein *tax*, is well established. The lifetime risk of developing ATL among seropositive persons is estimated to be 3% in women and 7% in men, with an incubation period of at least 15 years. The mean age of diagnosis of ATL is 40–50 years in Central and South America and 60 years in Japan.

ATL clinical syndromes may be classified as chronic, acute (leukemic), smoldering, or lymphomatous. A primary cutaneous tumor is also described and shows a worse prognosis compared with the smoldering type. Clinical features of ATL include diffuse lymphadenopathy, maculopapular skin lesions that may evolve into erythroderma, organomegaly, lytic bone lesions, and hypercalcemia. Opportunistic infections, such as *Pneumocystis jirovecii* pneumonia and cryptococcal meningitis, are common.

HAM/TSP, associated with both HTLV-1 and HTLV-2, develops in 0.3–4% of seropositive individuals and is more common in women. A chronic inflammation of the spinal cord leads to progressive motor weakness and symmetric spastic paraparesis, nociceptive low back pain, and paraplegia with hyperreflexia. Bladder and sexual disorders (eg, dyspareunia), sensory disturbances, erectile dysfunction, and constipation are also common. A progressive cognitive impairment is seen with HAM/TSP in children. Both viruses can also induce motor abnormalities, such as leg weakness, impaired tandem walk, and vibration sense, without overt HTLV-associated myelopathy. Seropositivity to both viruses is also associated with increases in depression and anxiety.

An HTLV-1 provirus load in peripheral blood mononuclear cells and cerebrospinal fluid cells, and an HTLV-1 mRNA load are proposed as markers of HAM risk and progression. HTLV positivity is associated with erythrocytosis, lymphocytosis (HTLV-2) and with thrombocytosis (HTLV-1).

HTLV-1 seropositivity is associated with an increased risk of tuberculosis, *Strongyloides stercoralis* hyperinfection, crusted scabies, and infective dermatitis. Inflammatory states associated with HTLV-1 infection include arthropathy, polymyositis, uveitis, Sjögren syndrome, vasculitis, cryoglobulinemia, infiltrative pneumonitis, and ichthyosis. Bronchioloalveolar carcinoma is increased in frequency in the presence of HTLV-1.

HTLV-2 appears to cause a myelopathy that is milder and slower to progress than HAM. All-cause and cancer mortality is higher among HTLV-2 seropositive patients.

HTLV-1/HIV coinfection is associated both with higher CD4 counts and a higher risk of HAM. Coinfections are underdiagnosed.

B. Laboratory Findings

The peripheral smear can show atypical lymphoid cells with basophilic cytoplasm and convoluted nuclei (flower cells) but the diagnostic standard is evidence of clonal integration of the proviral DNA genome into tumor cell. The identification of HTLV-1 antibodies supports the diagnosis.

▶ Treatment, Prevention, & Prognosis

Management of ATL consists mainly of chemotherapy, with allogeneic stem cell transplantation and the use of monoclonal antibodies (anti-CCR4 and anti-CD25). A chemotherapy regimen in Japan using eight different agents shows a higher response rate than traditional biweekly CHOP (40% vs 25%). Therapy using interferon-alpha combined with zidovudine is effective in the smoldering type.

HAM is treated with a variety of immune-modulating agents (including corticosteroids) without consistent results. Combination therapy with antiretrovirals does not show benefit. Interferon-alpha may be of some efficacy. Small uncontrolled studies suggest plasmapheresis results in improvement in gait and sensory disturbance among some PML patients. Screening of the blood supply for HTLV-1 is required in the United States. There is significant cross-reactivity between HTLV-1 and HTLV-2 by serologic studies, but PCR can distinguish the two. Improved assays to screen organ donors for HTLV-1 and -2 infections are needed.

A 10-year follow-up study in the Gambia shows increased mortality associated with HTLV-1 or HTLV-2 seropositivity, particularly in the young.

Chang YB et al. Seroprevalence and demographic determinants of human T-lymphotropic virus type 1 and 2 infections among first-time blood donors—United States, 2000–2009. J Infect Dis. 2014 Feb;209(4):523–31. [PMID: 24068702]

Dhasmana D et al. Human T-lymphotropic virus/HIV co-infection: a clinical review. Curr Opin Infect Dis. 2014 Feb;27(1):16–28. [PMID: 24305042]

Okajima R et al. High prevalence of skin disorders among HTLV-1 infected individuals independent of clinical status. PLoS Negl Trop Dis. 2013 Nov 7;7(11):e2546. [PMID: 24244779]

OTHER SYSTEMIC VIRAL DISEASES

1. Hemorrhagic Fevers

This diverse group of illnesses results from infection with one of several single-stranded RNA viruses (members of the families Arenaviridae, Bunyaviridae, Filoviridae, and Flaviviridae). Flaviviruses, such as the pathogens causing dengue and yellow fever (both with occasional hemorrhagic complications), are discussed in separate sections.

Lassa fever (an Old World arenavirus) is rodent associated and transmission usually occurs through aerosolized particles (from rodents or infected individuals). Transmission through direct contact with infected biologic fluids or tissues is also documented and food-borne transmission, while considered, is not definitively proven. Similar modes of transmission are assumed for **Junin virus** and other members of the New World Arenaviridae (Machupo virus, Sabia virus, Guanarito virus, Whitewater Arroyo virus). Bats (fruit bats for Ebola) are the suspected reservoir for **Ebola and Marburg viruses** (Filoviridae) but their vectors are unknown. A subtype of Ebola (Bundibugyo) is reported in Uganda (earlier Ebola outbreaks occurred in Democratic Republic of Congo, Sudan, and one case in Côte d'Ivoire) and was responsible for 93 cases and 37 deaths in 2007–2008. Another widespread Ebola outbreak began in Guinea in 2014. Cases of Marburg hemorrhagic fever are reported in travelers exploring caves and mines inhabited by bats in endemic areas of sub-Saharan Africa. The bunyaviruses include the **Crimean-Congo hemorrhagic fever** (transmitted by infected animal exposure or tick bite), the **Rift Valley fever** (transmitted by exposure to infected animal products or bite of an infected mosquito or flea), and the **hantaviruses** (associated with rodent exposure and discussed separately below). The geographic distribution of Crimean-Congo hemorrhagic fever, like that of its tick vector, is widespread with cases reported in Asia, the Middle East, and Eastern Europe. In 2002, Turkey experienced the largest reported outbreak with over 2500 cases. Hospital-associated transmission of Crimean-Congo hemorrhagic fever is well documented in Iran (where at least five variants have been detected). Rift Valley fever causes outbreaks in sub-Saharan and Northern Africa, including a 2007 outbreak with 155 deaths in Kenya following heavy rainfalls and associated with three different lineages of the virus. Rift Valley cases are also confirmed outside the African continent, in Saudi Arabia, and Yemen.

A new bunyavirus, a phlebovirus, associated with fever and thrombocytopenia, was identified in 2010 in Central and Northeastern China and is named for its symptoms: the **severe fever with thrombocytopenia syndrome (SFTS)** virus. Its differential diagnosis includes anaplasmosis, hemorrhagic fever with renal syndrome, or leptospirosis. The current candidate vector is a tick of the Ixodidae family. A mortality of 12% was noted among the first 171 patients. A new pathogenic virus (**Heartland virus**) similar to the SFTS virus was isolated in Missouri in 2009 from two farmers who had with fever, diarrhea, and fatigue. Transmission occurs via the Lone Star tick (*Amblyomma americanum*). There is no evidence for the transmission of viral hemorrhagic fever through air travel.

Clinical Findings

A. Symptoms and Signs

The incubation period can be as short as 2 days for the Rift Valley fever or as long as 21 days for Lassa fever. The clinical symptoms in the early phase of a viral hemorrhagic fever are very similar, irrespective of the causative virus, and resemble a flu-like illness or gastroenteritis. Hepatitis is common.

The late phase is more specific and is characterized by organ failure, persistent leukopenia, altered mental status, and hemorrhage. Exanthemas and mucosal lesions can occur. The range of pathology described with Crimean-Congo hemorrhagic fever continues to grow and include cardiac failure, bilateral alveolar hemorrhages, and retinal hemorrhages. Rift Valley fever is reportedly associated with encephalitis and also retinitis. Adrenal dysfunction is a common sequela of this class of infections and a cause for the development of the late-stage shock associated with these infections. The case-fatality rate ranges from 5% to 30% and may be as high as 90% in Ebola fever. The convalescence period can be long and complicated. There is no evidence of chronic infection among survivors. Risk factors for complications in patients with Crimean-Congo hemorrhagic fever include advanced age, thrombocytopenia, prolonged clotting factor parameters, and hepatitis; risk factors for mortality include altered sensorium and prolonged international normalized ratio.

B. Laboratory Findings

Laboratory features usually include thrombocytopenia, leukopenia, (although with Lassa fever leukocytosis is noted), anemia, increased hematocrit, elevated liver function tests, and findings consistent with disseminated intravascular coagulation (although less prominently in Lassa fever). Urinalysis can reveal proteinuria and hematuria.

Special care should be taken for handling clinical specimens of suspected cases. Laboratory personnel should be warned about the diagnostic suspicion and the CDC must be contacted for guidance (Special Pathogens Branch, 404-639-1115). Diagnosis may be made by growing the virus from blood obtained early in the disease, antigen detection (by ELISA), nucleic acid amplification (PCR techniques), or by demonstration of a significant specific fourfold or greater rise in antibody titer. Detection of Ebola virus antigen in oral fluid samples by ELISA and RT-PCR may be possible; sample collection in this manner will be useful since certain ethnic customs prohibit blood collection. These tests are generally available only through the CDC. Crimean-Congo hemorrhagic fever is best diagnosed with an IgM serology, although IgG ELISA or immunofluorescence and quantitative reverse transcription PCR are nearly as effective.

Differential Diagnosis

The differential diagnosis for hemorrhagic fever includes meningococcemia or other septicemias, Rocky Mountain spotted fever, dengue, typhoid fever, and malaria. The likelihood of acquiring hemorrhagic fevers among travelers is low.

Treatment

Patients should be placed in private rooms with standard contact and droplet precautions. Barrier precautions to prevent contamination of skin or mucous membranes should also be adopted by the caring personnel. Airborne precautions should be considered in patients with significant pulmonary involvement or undergoing procedures that stimulate cough.

Certain arenaviruses (the Lassa pathogen, Junin virus in its viscerotropic phase, Machupo virus) and bunyaviruses (the Congo-Crimean hemorrhagic fever and Rift Valley fever pathogens) respond to oral ribavirin if it is started promptly: 30 mg/kg as loading dose, followed by 16 mg/kg every 6 hours for 4 days and then 8 mg/kg every 8 hours for 3 days. The efficacy for postexposure ribavirin in the management of Lassa fever, other arenaviruses, or hospital–associated Crimean-Congo hemorrhagic fever remains anecdotal. However, if ribavirin is used, it should be given in a high loading dose (35 mg/kg orally followed by 15 mg/kg three times daily for 10 days) and only for high-risk settings (eg, needle stick injury, mucous membrane contamination, emergency resuscitative contact, or prolonged intimate exposure during transport).

The filoviruses and the flaviviruses do not respond to ribavirin. Live attenuated vaccines are available for Junin hemorrhagic fever and the Rift Valley fever, and they are under study for the Crimean-Congo hemorrhagic fever, Ebola, and Marburg viruses. In addition, recombinant and virus-like particle vaccines are under development for most of these pathogens (including the Lassa fever virus but not the Junin hemorrhagic fever virus). Therapeutic interventions that target the hematologic system are at most only marginally effective.

When to Admit

- Persons with symptoms compatible with those of any hemorrhagic fever and who have traveled from a possible endemic area should be isolated for diagnosis and symptomatic treatment.

- Isolation is particularly important because diseases due to some of these agents, such as Ebola virus, are highly transmissible and carry a mortality rate of 50–90%.

Feldmann H et al. Ebola haemorrhagic fever. Lancet. 2011 Mar 5; 377(9768):849–62. [PMID: 21084112]

Gilsdorf A et al. Guidance for contact tracing of cases of Lassa fever, Ebola or Marburg haemorrhagic fever on an airplane: results of a European expert consultation. BMC Public Health. 2012 Nov 21;12:1014. [PMID: 23170851]

LaBeaud AD et al. Advances in Rift Valley fever research: insights for disease prevention. Curr Opin Infect Dis. 2010 Oct;23(5):403–8. [PMID: 20613512]

McMullan LK et al. A new phlebovirus associated with severe febrile illness in Missouri. N Engl J Med. 2012 Aug 30; 367(9):834–41. [PMID: 22931317]

Mertens M et al. The impact of Crimean-Congo hemorrhagic fever virus on public health. Antiviral Res. 2013 May;98(2): 248–60. [PMID: 23458713]

Nderitu L et al. Sequential Rift Valley fever outbreaks in eastern Africa caused by multiple lineages of the virus. J Infect Dis. 2011 Mar 1;203(5):655–65. [PMID: 21282193]
Russier M et al. Immune responses and Lassa virus infection. Viruses. 2012 Nov 5;4(11):2766–85. [PMID: 23202504]

2. Dengue

ESSENTIALS OF DIAGNOSIS

► Exposure 7–10 days before onset.

► Sudden onset of high fever, chills, severe myalgias and arthralgias, headache, sore throat, and depression.

► Biphasic fever curve: initial phase, 3–7 days; remission, few hours to 2 days; second phase, 1–2 days.

► Biphasic rash: evanescent, then maculopapular, scarlatiniform, morbilliform, or petechial changes from extremities to torso.

► Leukopenia and thrombocytopenia in the hemorrhagic form.

► **General Considerations**

Dengue is due to a flavivirus transmitted by the bite of the *Aedes* mosquito. It may be caused by one of four serotypes (possibly five, with a potentially new serotype from Malaysia under study) widely distributed globally between the tropics of Capricorn and Cancer. An estimated 70–500 million cases of dengue fever and several hundred thousand cases of dengue hemorrhagic fever occur each year with numbers growing in both dengue fever and dengue hemorrhagic fever as a consequence of climatic factors, travel, and urbanization. **It is thus along with malaria one of the two most common and important vector-borne diseases of humans,** with 2.5 billion people living in dengue-infected regions and regions of major intermittent outbreaks. The incubation period is 3–15 days (usually 7–10 days). When the virus is introduced into susceptible populations, usually by viremic travelers, epidemic attack rates range from 50% to 70%. Dengue is endemic in the lower Rio Grande Valley and adjacent border towns, with 40% of Brownsville, Texas residents showing serologic evidence of past infection and the virus being detected in mosquito larvae among 30% of households. The seroprevalence of Haitians by age 3 is over 53%.

Severe epidemics of dengue hemorrhagic fever (serotype 3) occurred over the past 20 years in East Africa, Sri Lanka, and Latin America. Dengue is the second most common cause of fever (after malaria) in travelers returning from developing countries. In one US series based on CDC reports, the highest proportion of laboratory-confirmed and probable cases were among travelers returning from the Dominican Republic (121 cases, 20% of total), Mexico (55 cases, 9% of total) and India (43 cases, 7% of total). The first European sustained outbreak of dengue since the 1920s occurred on the Portuguese archipelago of Madeira in 2012 with over 2000 people infected. In general, the more advanced forms of disease (hemorrhagic fever and shock) occur less often in the Americas than in Asia. Since the 1980s, locally acquired cases of dengue are reported from Guam, Puerto Rico, Samoa, the US Virgin Islands, and in the continental United States at the Texas-Mexico border, and Key West, Florida. Health care–associated transmission (needlestick, mucocutaneous exposure or transplant related) and vertical transmission occur rarely.

► **Clinical Findings**

A. Symptoms and Signs

A history of travel to a dengue-endemic area within 14 days of symptom onset is helpful in establishing a diagnosis of dengue. Dengue infection may range from asymptomatic to severe hemorrhagic fever to fatal shock (**dengue shock syndrome**). Dengue fever is usually a nonspecific, self-limited biphasic febrile illness. More than half of infected children are asymptomatic. The illness is more severe and begins more suddenly in adults. After an incubation period of 4–5 days, there is a sudden onset of high fever, chills, and "break bone" aching of the head, back, and extremities accompanied by sore throat, prostration, and malaise. There may be conjunctival redness. Initially, the skin appears flushed or blotched, but 3–4 days after the lysis of the fever, a maculopapular rash, which spares palms and soles, appears in over 50% of cases. As the rash fades, localized clusters of petechiae on the extensor surface of the limbs become apparent. Up to 25% may manifest signs of cardiac involvement. Hepatitis frequently complicates dengue fever with acute fulminant hepatitis in up to 5%.

Dengue hemorrhagic fever usually affects children living in endemic areas and is most likely to occur in secondary infections and in infections with serotype 2. A few days into the illness, signs of hemorrhage such as ecchymoses, gastrointestinal bleeding, and epistaxis appear. Symptoms found more often among the dengue hemorrhagic fever subset of patients include restlessness, epistaxis, and abdominal pain. Gastroenterologic complications, including hemorrhage, tenderness, and ascites, are more common with dengue hemorrhagic fever and often require intensive care observation.

A subset of patients (more often girls than boys) often with secondary infection, may progress to severe dengue, which is defined by the presence of serum leakage, hemorrhage, or organ involvement (typically liver, heart, CNS). Acute fever, hemorrhagic manifestations, and marked capillary leak may be prominent, with the latter manifesting as pleural effusions and ascites, and there is a tendency for shock to develop. In infants, even primary infection can lead to dengue shock syndrome. While the infection is difficult to distinguish from malaria, yellow fever, or influenza, the rash makes dengue far more likely. Continuous abdominal pain with vomiting, bleeding, a decrease in the level of consciousness, rash, conjunctival congestion, and hypothermia should raise concern about dengue shock syndrome. Acute kidney injury in dengue largely occurs with dengue shock syndrome and shows a high mortality. While acute severe hepatitis can occur with dengue, concomitant other hepatotropic agents are usually responsible.

Distinguishing between dengue and other causes of febrile illness in endemic areas is difficult. Fevers due to dengue are more often associated with neutropenia and thrombocytopenia and with myalgias, arthralgias/arthritis, and lethargy among adults.

B. Laboratory Findings

Leukopenia is characteristic, and elevated transaminases are found frequently in dengue fever. Thrombocytopenia, increased fibrinolysis, and hemoconcentration occur more often in the hemorrhagic form of the disease. Liver biochemical test abnormalities are nearly universal. Thrombocytopenia, plasma leakage, and acute hepatitis are identified as predictors of severe manifestations of dengue and higher mortality. The nonspecific nature of the illness mandates laboratory verification for diagnosis, usually with IgM and IgG ELISAs after the febrile phase. Virus may be recovered from the blood during the acute phase. PCR or detection of the specific viral protein NS1 by ELISA may be diagnostic during the first few days of infection and may be appropriate for febrile travelers. Immunohistochemistry for antigen detection in tissue samples and dried blood spots can also be used. Because the erythrocyte sedimentation rate is normal in most cases, elevation may suggest an alternative diagnosis. Chest radiographs in dengue hemorrhagic fever show infiltrates and effusions, which follow the course of laboratory abnormalities.

▶ Complications

Usual complications include pneumonia, bone marrow failure, hepatitis, iritis, retinal hemorrhages and maculopathy, orchitis, and oophoritis. Depression and chronic fatigue, occurring more often in older women, are also reported. Neurologic complications (such as encephalitis, Guillain-Barré syndrome, phrenic neuropathy, subdural hematoma, and transverse myelitis) are less common, although encephalitic complications are increasingly recognized. Aplastic anemia and hemophagocytosis syndrome are very rare complications. Dengue is rarely associated with stroke in patients with focal neurologic deficit and encephalopathy. Maternal infection poses a risk for premature birth and hemorrhage in both the mother and the infant if infection occurs near term.

Bacterial superinfection occurs more commonly with advanced age, higher fever, gastrointestinal bleeding, kidney disease, and altered consciousness.

▶ Treatment

Treatment entails the appropriate use of volume support, blood products, and pressor agents, and acetaminophen rather than nonsteroidal anti-inflammatory drugs for analgesia. Activities are gradually restored during prolonged convalescences. Endoscopic therapy is useful in evaluating and managing gastrointestinal hemorrhage, although injection therapy with sclerosing agents is not beneficial in most dengue hemorrhagic states. Platelet counts do not usefully predict clinically significant bleeding. Platelet transfusions, however, should be considered for severe thrombocytopenia (< 10,000/mcL) or when there is evidence of bleeding. Monitoring vital signs and blood volume may help in anticipating the complications of dengue hemorrhagic fever or shock syndrome.

The efficacy of corticosteroids in the management of dengue is not proven and corticosteroids do not appear to lessen the risk of progression to a shock state. There is anecdotal evidence for the efficacy of statins (which are under study) in the management of acute dengue and for the efficacy of intravenous anti-D globulin in the management of dengue hemorrhagic fever.

▶ Prognosis

Fatalities are rare but do occur (and more often among girls and the very young), especially during epidemic outbreaks, with occasional patients dying of fulminant hepatitis. Acute kidney injury in dengue shock syndrome portends an especially poor prognosis. Convalescence for most patients is slow. Factors associated with development of severe disease in Sri Lanka included elevated aspartate aminotransferase (AST), lymphopenia, and thrombocytopenia, while factors associated with mortality in Brazil included age 50 years or older, limited education, need for hospitalization, rural residency, male gender, and elevated hematocrit (but not moderate thrombocytopenia).

The 2009 classification of dengue into acute and severe has met with resistance.

▶ Prevention

Available prophylactic measures include control of mosquitoes by screening and insect repellents, particularly during early morning and late afternoon exposures. Testing of blood supplies is increasingly necessary especially in endemic areas as dengue spreads. Stochastic models using rainfall and temperature are useful in predicting geographic areas at increased risk for dengue.

A 2012 randomized, controlled trial in healthy Thai school children using a live attenuated, yellow fever backbone vaccine showed immunogenicity for all the serotypes and an overall efficacy of 30% (higher for serotypes 1, 3, and 4 and very low for serotype 2). A second live attenuated vaccine studied at the National Institutes of Health shows efficacy of at least 60%.

Anders KL et al. An evaluation of dried blood spots and oral swabs as alternative specimens for the diagnosis of dengue and screening for past dengue virus exposure. Am J Trop Med Hyg. 2012 Jul;87(1):165–70. [PMID: 22764309]

Chao DL et al. Controlling dengue with vaccines in Thailand. PLoS Negl Trop Dis. 2012;6(10):e1876. [PMID: 23145197]

Halstead SB. Dengue: the syndromic basis to pathogenesis research. Inutility of the 2009 WHO case definition. Am J Trop Med Hyg. 2013 Feb;88(2):212–5. [PMID: 23390220]

Sabchareon A et al. Protective efficacy of the recombinant, live-attenuated, CYD tetravalent dengue vaccine in Thai school-children: a randomised, controlled phase 2b trial. Lancet. 2012 Nov 3;380(9853):1559–67. [PMID: 22975340]

World Health Organization. Dengue: guidelines for diagnosis, treatment, prevention and control. New edition, 2009. http://whqlibdoc.who.int/publications/2009/9789241547871_eng.pdf

3. Hantaviruses

ESSENTIALS OF DIAGNOSIS

▶ Transmitted by rodents and cause two clinical syndromes.

▶ Hemorrhagic fever with renal syndrome (HFRS): mild to severe illness.

▶ Hantavirus pulmonary syndrome (HPS): 40% mortality rate.

▶ Ribavirin is used with some success in HFRS.

▶ General Considerations

Hantaviruses are enveloped RNA bunyaviruses naturally hosted in rodents, moles, and shrews. Currently, over 21 hantavirus strains are known to cause human disease. These differ in rodent hosts, geographic distribution, and degree of pathogenicity. Two major clinical syndromes are described: **hemorrhagic fever with renal syndrome (HFRS)** and **hantavirus pulmonary syndrome (HPS)**. Each year, over 150,000 cases of these two syndromes occur globally, with HPS being far less common. While they share many clinical features, a specific strain is not associated with a specific syndrome and overlap is seen between the syndromes. Usually seen in the southwestern United States, **Sin Nombre virus** (Muerto Canyon, Four Corners) is the most common hantavirus infection in the United States and is the main North American virus responsible for HPS. The presence of antibodies in Mexican rodents suggests HPS is probably unrecognized in Mexico. While retrospective diagnostics show that the disease occurred decades earlier in the United States, it was not until 1993 when the first outbreak was recognized. Through July 9, 2013, 624 cases were reported in 34 states, including all continental states west of the Mississippi River except Missouri and Arkansas, with over one-half the cases from the Four Corners area and another focus recognized in Yosemite National Park, California. Other strains native to North America known to cause HPS include Bayou, Black Creek Canal, New York, and Monongahela viruses. Outbreaks of HPS associated with other hantavirus types are also reported in Central and South America.

Hantaviruses are ubiquitous, with infections described in North and South America (New World hantaviruses) as well as Europe, Africa, and Asia (Old World hantaviruses). The Hantaan viruses cause severe hemorrhagic fever with renal syndrome and are found primarily in Korea, China, and eastern Russia. The Seoul viruses produce a less severe form of disease and are found primarily in Korea and China. Cases of domestically acquired Seoul hantavirus were recently described in the United States. The Puumala and Dobrava-Belgrade viruses are found in Scandinavia and

Europe and are associated with a mild form of the syndrome termed "nephropathia epidemica," which presents with fever, headache, gastrointestinal symptoms, and impaired kidney function. Between 16% and 48% of Dobrova-Belgrade virus cases, however, may require dialysis.

Aerosols of virus-contaminated rodent urine and feces are thought to be the main vehicle for transmission to humans. Person-to-person transmission is rare and confined to one hantavirus, the Andes virus. Occupation is the main risk factor for transmission of all hantavirus, with animal trappers, forestry workers, laboratory personnel, farmers, and military personnel considered to be at highest risk. Climate change appears to be impacting the incidence of hantavirus infection mainly through effects on reservoir ecology.

▶ Clinical Findings

A. Symptoms and Signs

Vascular leakage is the hallmark of the disease for both syndromes, with lungs being the main target on HPS and the kidneys on HFRS.

HPS is a more severe disease than HFRS, with a mortality rate of about 40%. The clinical course of HPS is divided into a febrile prodrome, a cardiopulmonary stage, oliguric and diuretic phase followed by convalescence. A 14- to 17-day incubation period is followed by a prodromal phase, typically lasting 3–6 days, that is associated with myalgia, malaise, gastrointestinal disturbance, headache, chills, and fever of abrupt onset. An ensuing cardiopulmonary phase is characterized by the acute onset of pulmonary edema. In this stage, cough is generally present, gastrointestinal manifestations may dominate the clinical presentations, and in severe cases, significant myocardial depression occurs. Acute kidney injury and myositis may occur. Sequelae include neuropsychological impairments in some HPS survivors.

HFRS manifests as mild, moderate, or severe illness depending on the causative strain, with a mortality rate of up to 12%. A 2- to 3-week incubation period is followed by a protracted clinical course, typically consisting of five distinct phases: febrile period, hypotension, oliguria, diuresis, and convalescence phase. Various degrees of renal involvement are usually seen, occasionally with frank hemorrhage. Pulmonary edema is not typically seen but when present usually occurs in the final stages of disease (oliguric and diuretic phase). Encephalitis and pituitary involvement are rare findings with hantavirus infection, although a few cases are reported with Puumala virus.

B. Laboratory Findings

Laboratory features include hemoconcentration and elevation in lactate dehydrogenase, serum lactate, and hepatocellular enzymes. Early thrombocytopenia and leukocytosis (as high as 90,000 cells/mcL in HPS) are seen in both HFRS and HPS. In HPS, immunoblasts (activated lymphocytes with plasmacytoid features) can be seen in blood, lungs, kidneys, bone marrow, liver, and spleen. The severity of "nephropathia epidemica" correlates with plasma interleukin-6 levels.

The viremia of human hantavirus infections is short-term, and therefore, viral RNA cannot be readily detected in the blood or urine of patients. An indirect fluorescent assay and enzyme immunoassay are available for detection of specific IgM or low-avidity IgG virus-specific antibodies. Seroconversion in the absence of pulmonary symptoms probably occurs often, is documented to be common in Panama.

A plaque reduction neutralization test is considered the gold standard serologic assay and distinguishes between the different hantavirus species, although cross reaction between Old World and New World viruses exist. This test needs to be performed in a laboratory with appropriate biosafety (level 3).

Differential Diagnosis

The differential diagnosis of the acute febrile syndrome seen with HFRS or early HPS includes scrub typhus, leptospirosis, and dengue. HPS requires differentiation from other respiratory infections caused by such pathogens as *Legionella*, *Chlamydia*, and *Mycoplasma*. Coxsackievirus infections should also be considered in the differential diagnosis.

Treatment

Treatment is mainly supportive. Cardiorespiratory support with vasopressors and sometimes extracorporeal membrane oxygenation are frequently needed in severe cases. Intravenous ribavirin is used in HFRS (Hantaan virus) with some success in decreasing the severity of the kidney injury. Its effectiveness in HPS, however, is not established. A randomized, controlled trial in Chile showed high-dose corticosteroids have no clinical benefit in the treatment of HPS and suggests there may be no benefit with HFRS as well.

Prognosis

The outcome is highly variable depending on severity of disease. In Sin Nombre virus infections, the persistence of elevated IgG titers correlates with a favorable outcome.

Prevention

Because infection is thought to occur by inhalation of rodent wastes, prevention is aimed at eradication of rodents in houses and avoidance of exposure to rodent excreta in rural settings, including forest service facilities. Potential vaccines are being studied in animals.

Hartline J et al. Hantavirus infection in North America: a clinical review. Am J Emerg Med. 2013 Jun;31(6):978–82. [PMID: 23680331]

Hooper JW et al. A novel Sin Nombre virus DNA vaccine and its inclusion in a candidate pan-hantavirus vaccine against hantavirus pulmonary syndrome (HPS) and hemorrhagic fever with renal syndrome (HFRS). Vaccine. 2013 Sep 13;31(40):4314–21. [PMID: 23892100]

Knust B et al. Twenty-year summary of surveillance for human hantavirus infections, United States. Emerg Infect Dis. 2013 Dec;19(12):1934–7. [PMID: 24274585]

Vaheri A et al. Hantavirus infections in Europe and their impact on public health. Rev Med Virol. 2013 Jan;23(1):35–49. [PMID: 22761056]

Vial PA et al; Hantavirus Study Group in Chile. High-dose intravenous methylprednisolone for hantavirus cardiopulmonary syndrome in Chile: a double-blind, randomized controlled clinical trial. Clin Infect Dis. 2013 Oct;57(7):943–51. [PMID: 23784924]

4. Yellow Fever

ESSENTIALS OF DIAGNOSIS

- ► Endemic area exposure (tropical South and Central America, Africa, but not Asia).
- ► Sudden onset of severe headache, aching in legs, and tachycardia.
- ► Brief (1 day) remission, followed by bradycardia, hypotension, jaundice, hemorrhagic tendency.
- ► Proteinuria, leukopenia, bilirubinemia, bilirubinuria.
- ► Rare and potentially fatal reactions to vaccination.

General Considerations

Yellow fever is a zoonotic flavivirus infection transmitted by *Aedes* and jungle mosquitoes. It occurs in an urban and jungle cycle in Africa and in a jungle cycle in South America (where genetic studies suggest it arose through the slave trade 300–400 years ago). Epidemics have extended far into the temperate zone during warm seasons.

Infection is transmitted by an infected mosquito bite. The incubation period in humans is 3–6 days. Adults and children are equally susceptible, though attack rates are highest among adult males because of their work habits. Between 5% and 50% of infections are asymptomatic.

Clinical Findings

A. Symptoms and Signs

1. Mild form—Symptoms are malaise, headache, fever, retroorbital pain, nausea, vomiting, and photophobia. Relative bradycardia, conjunctival injection, and facial flushing may be present.

2. Severe form—Severe illness develops in about 15%. Initial symptoms are similar to the mild form, but a brief fever remission lasting hours to a few days is followed by a "period of intoxication" manifested by fever and relative bradycardia (Faget sign), hypotension, jaundice, hemorrhage (gastrointestinal, nasal, oral), and delirium that may progress to coma.

B. Laboratory Findings

Leukopenia occurs, although it may not be present at the onset. Kidney disease with proteinuria is present, sometimes as high as 5–6 g/L, and usually disappears completely with recovery. Levels of liver enzymes and bilirubin can be remarkably abnormal with the levels of AST usually doubling those of alanine aminotransferase (ALT). Prothrombin time may be elevated as well. Serologic diagnosis is made by using capture ELISA to measure IgM during the acute and convalescent phases. Viral culture is used in epidemic settings. Rapid test involving PCR and monoclonal antibodies assays against circulating viral antigens are available through reference laboratories. The plaque reduction neutralization assay is the most frequently used. IgM antibodies are shown to persist in up to 73% of recipients 3–4 years after vaccination.

▶ Differential Diagnosis

It may be difficult to distinguish yellow fever from hepatitis, malaria, leptospirosis, louse-borne relapsing fever, dengue, and other hemorrhagic fevers on clinical evidence alone. **Albuminuria is a constant feature in yellow fever patients** and its presence helps differentiate yellow fever from other viral hepatitides. Serologic confirmation is often needed.

▶ Treatment

No specific antiviral therapy is available. Treatment is directed toward symptomatic relief and management of complications. If not in an endemic area, the patient should be isolated from mosquitoes to prevent transmission, since blood in the acute phase is potentially infectious.

▶ Prognosis

The mortality rate of the severe form is 20–50%, with death occurring most commonly between the sixth and the tenth days. In survivors, the temperature returns to normal by the seventh or eighth day. The prognosis in any individual case is guarded at the onset, since sudden changes for the worse are common. Intractable hiccups, copious black vomitus, melena, anuria, jaundice, and elevated AST are unfavorable signs. Convalescence is prolonged, including 1–2 weeks of asthenia. Infection confers lifelong immunity to those who recover.

▶ Prevention

Transmission is prevented through mosquito control. Live virus vaccine is highly effective and should be provided for immunocompetent persons over 9 months of age living in or traveling to endemic areas. In one study of US international travelers visiting a yellow fever endemic country, only 70% were adequately vaccinated. The highest rate of seroconversion occurs 21 days after administration. Boosting at 10-year intervals, as advocated in the past, is not necessary because a single dose of vaccine provides life-long immunity. Vaccine-induced reactions—including neurotropic (encephalitis-like syndrome) and viscerotropic (resembling yellow fever; with one space-time cluster of viscerotropic disease among five patients with four deaths reported from Ica, Peru in 2007) diseases—are reported particularly among patients aged 60 years or older, patients with immune dysfunction or with multiple sclerosis (whose rate of exacerbation in increased 1–5 weeks after vaccination). The very young (< 6 months) and the aged should probably not be vaccinated and those with immune dysfunction or multiple sclerosis should not be vaccinated, although HIV-infected persons with high CD4 counts safely receive the vaccine with an adverse event rate of about 3%. The safety of the vaccine in pregnant patients is probable but not verified; it is possible that minor dysmorphisms, including pigmented nevi, are increased in frequency but this may be a bias of evaluation. Pregnant women should consider deferring travel to endemic areas (see Chapter 30). Eradication is difficult because of the sylvatic cycle (mainly maintained by non-human primates). Transmission from mother to infant during breastfeeding is documented.

The vaccine is prepared in hen eggs and those with egg allergies can be successfully desensitized.

Carrington CV et al. Evolutionary and ecological factors underlying the tempo and distribution of yellow fever virus activity. Infect Genet Evol. 2013 Jan;13:198–210. [PMID: 22981999]

Heinz FX et al. Flaviviruses and flavivirus vaccines. Vaccine. 2012 Jun 19;30(29):4301–6. [PMID: 22682286]

Hodges-Vazquez M et al. The yellow fever 17D vaccine and risk of malignant melanoma in the United States military. Vaccine. 2012 Jun 22;30(30):4476–9. [PMID: 22561488]

Jentes ES et al; Global TravEpiNet Consortium. Travel characteristics and yellow fever vaccine usage among US Global TravEpiNet travelers visiting countries with risk of yellow fever virus transmission, 2009–2011. Am J Trop Med Hyg. 2013 May;88(5):954–61. [PMID: 23458961]

LaRocque RC et al. Global TravEpiNet: a national consortium of clinics providing care to international travelers—analysis of demographic characteristics, travel destinations, and pre-travel healthcare of high-risk US international travelers, 2009–2011. Clin Infect Dis. 2012 Feb 15;54(4):455–62. [PMID: 22144534]

Patel D et al. Yellow fever vaccination: is one dose always enough? Travel Med Infect Dis. 2013 Sep–Oct;11(5):266–73. [PMID: 24074827]

Rutkowski K et al. Administration of yellow fever vaccine in patients with egg allergy. Int Arch Allergy Immunol. 2013;161(3):274–8. [PMID: 23548550]

Thomas RE et al. The safety of yellow fever vaccine 17D or 17DD in children, pregnant women, HIV+ individuals, and older persons: systematic review. Am J Trop Med Hyg. 2012 Feb;86(2):359–72. [PMID: 22302874]

World Health Organization. Vaccines and vaccination against yellow fever. WHO position paper—June 2013. Wkly Epidemiol Rec. 2013 Jul 5;88(27):269–83. [PMID: 23909008]

5. Tick-Borne Encephalitis

ESSENTIALS OF DIAGNOSIS

▶ Flaviviral encephalitis found in Eastern, Central, and occasionally Northern Europe and Asia.

▶ Transmitted via ticks or ingestion of unpasteurized milk.

▶ Long-term neurologic sequelae occur in 2–25% of cases.

▶ Therapy is largely supportive.

▶ Prevention is based on avoiding tick exposure, pasteurization of milk, and vaccination.

General Considerations

Tick-borne encephalitis (TBE), a flaviviral infection caused by TBE virus, is the most common arbovirus infection transmitted by ticks in Europe. An estimated 10,000 to 12,000 cases occur each year in parts of Eurasia (from eastern France to northern Japan, from northern Siberia to Albania), with annual increases thought to be a function of increased recognition, climatic changes, and personal or social habits. TBE is endemic in Japan and parts of China as well. TBE occurs predominantly in the late spring through fall. It is usually a consequence of exposure to infected ticks, although unpasteurized milk from viremic livestock is also a recognized form of transmission. Surges in cases over the last 20 years are thought to be a consequence of agricultural policies that alter land cover, host prevalence, climatic factors, and human behavior (including pesticide usage and travel to endemic areas). In recent years, the maximum altitude for occurrence of cases has increased to 5000 feet (about 1500 meters). The incubation period is 7–14 days for tick-borne exposures but only 3–4 days for milk ingestion. The principal reservoirs for TBE virus are small rodents; humans are an accidental host. The vectors for most cases are *Ixodes ricinus* (most of Europe, including Turkey, Iran, and the Caucasus) and *Ixodes persulcatus* (in the belt from Eastern Europe to China and Japan).

Related viruses found in Eastern and mid-Western North America are the Powassan agent and the deer tick virus. Increasing prevalence of deer ticks in North America is thought to be responsible for the increased (but still small) number of North American cases of these two serologically indistinguishable viruses.

Clinical Findings

A. Symptoms and Signs

Most cases are subclinical and many resemble a flu-like syndrome. There are two variants of clinical presentation: the Western subtype occurs mainly in the fall (but as early as April) and is most severe among the elderly, and the Eastern subtype is more severe among children.

Western subtype disease is biphasic in which after 2–10 days of fever (usually with malaise, headache, and myalgias), a 1–21 day symptom-free interval leads to a second phase with resumed fevers followed by neurologic symptoms. **Eastern subtype disease** is progressive without an asymptomatic interval. The neurologic manifestations range from febrile headache (accounting for up to 50% of Eastern subtype cases) to aseptic meningitis and encephalitis with or without myelitis (preferentially of the cervical anterior horn) and spinal paralysis (usually flaccid). A myeloradiculitic form can also develop but is less common. Peripheral facial palsies, sometimes bilaterally, tend to occur infrequently, late in the course of infection, usually after encephalitis, and usually are associated with a favorable outcome within 30–90 days. Double infection with *Borrelia burgdorferi* (the agent of Lyme disease; transmitted by the same tick vector) may result in a more severe disease. Mortality in TBE is usually a consequence of brain edema or bulbar involvement.

B. Diagnosis

Leukocytosis and neutrophilia are common. Abnormal cerebrospinal fluid findings include a pleocytosis that may persist for up to 4 months. Neuroimaging shows hyperintense lesions in the thalamus, brainstem, and basal ganglia. TBE virus IgM and IgG are detected by ELISA techniques when neurologic symptoms occur. Cross-reactivity with other flaviviruses or a vaccinated state (see below) may require confirmation by detection of TBE virus–specific antibodies in cerebrospinal fluid. RT-PCR of blood (at earlier stages of the disease) or cerebrospinal fluid can sometimes, if available, assist with the diagnosis. TBE virus can be differentiated from serologically indistinguishable viruses (Powassan agent and deer tick virus) by plaque-reduction neutralization tests.

Complications

The main sequela of disease is paresis, which occurs in up to 10% of Western and up to 25% of Eastern subtype disease. Other causes of long-term morbidity include protracted cognitive dysfunction and persistent spinal nerve paralysis. The **postencephalitic syndrome**, characterized by headache, difficulties concentrating, balance disorders, dysphasia, hearing defects, and chronic fatigue, occurs with both subtypes. A progressive motor neuron disease and partial continuous epilepsy are complications seen with the Eastern subtype. Cognitive impairments may develop in children after infection.

Differential Diagnosis

The differential diagnosis includes other causes of aseptic meningitis such as enteroviral infections, herpes simplex encephalitis, and a variety of tick-borne pathogens including tularemia, the rickettsial diseases, babesiosis, Lyme disease, poliomyelitis (no longer reported from Eastern Europe), and other flaviviral infections.

Treatment

Therapy is largely supportive. Some clinicians believe corticosteroids may be useful, although no controlled clinical trials exist.

Prevention

There are two inactivated TBE virus vaccines for adults and two vaccines for children licensed in Europe. Their effectiveness is about 99% when properly administered but cannot be given concomitantly because of immune interference. The initial vaccination schedule requires 1 year with boosters every 3–5 years. There are decreased antibody titers (quantity not quality) and booster response in recipients of TBE vaccines who are over 50 years of age, indicating the need for a modified immunization strategy in older patients.

Vaccine efficacy has been most prominent in Austria where case loads are less than 16% of pre-vaccination numbers. Neuritis and neuropathies of peripheral nerves (plexus neuropathy—paresis of lower limb muscles, polyradiculopathy) are recognized complications of TBE vaccination.

Rare cases of olfactory dysfunction and myelitis are also reported. A single-dose live attenuated vaccine with a West Nile virus backbone is under development.

Other prevention recommendations include avoidance of tick exposure and pasteurization of cow and goat milk.

Centers for Disease Control and Prevention (CDC). Tick-borne encephalitis among U.S. travelers to Europe and Asia—2000–2009. MMWR Morb Mortal Wkly Rep. 2010 Mar 26;59(11): 335–8. [PMID: 20339345]

Fowler Å et al. Tick-borne encephalitis carries a high risk of incomplete recovery in children. J Pediatr. 2013 Aug;163(2): 555–60. [PMID: 23452585]

Hudopisk N et al. Tick-borne encephalitis associated with consumption of raw goat milk, Slovenia, 2012. Emerg Infect Dis. 2013 May;19(5):806–8. [PMID: 23697658]

Lotric-Furlan S et al. Peripheral facial palsy in patients with tick-borne encephalitis. Clin Microbiol Infect. 2012 Oct;18(10): 1027–32. [PMID: 22192120]

Rumyantsev AA et al. Single-dose vaccine against tick-borne encephalitis. Proc Natl Acad Sci U S A. 2013 Aug 6;110(32): 13103–8. [PMID: 23858441]

World Health Organization. Vaccines against tick-borne encephalitis: WHO position paper—recommendations. Vaccine. 2011 Nov 8;29(48):8769–70. [PMID: 21777636]

6. Colorado Tick Fever

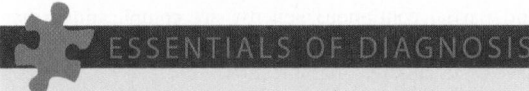

ESSENTIALS OF DIAGNOSIS

► Onset 1–19 days (average, 4 days) following tick bite.

► Fever, chills, myalgia, headache, prostration.

► Leukopenia, thrombocytopenia.

► Second attack of fever after remission lasting 2–3 days.

► General Considerations

Colorado tick fever is a reportable biphasic, febrile illness caused by a reovirus infection transmitted by *Dermacentor andersoni* tick bite. The disease is limited to the western United States and Canada and is most prevalent during the tick season (March to November). There is a discrete history of tick bite or exposure in 90% of cases. The virus infects the marrow erythrocyte precursors, leading to viremia lasting the life span of the infected red cells. Blood transfusions can be a vehicle of transmission.

► Clinical Findings

A. Symptoms and Signs

The incubation period is 3–6 days, rarely as long as 19 days. The onset is usually abrupt with fever (to 38.9–40.6°C), sometimes with chills. Severe myalgia, headache, photophobia, anorexia, nausea and vomiting, and generalized weakness are prominent. Physical findings are limited to an occasional faint rash. The acute symptoms resolve within a week. Remission is followed in 50% of cases by recurrent

fever and a full recrudescence lasting 2–4 days. In an occasional case, there may be three bouts of fever.

The differential diagnosis includes influenza, Rocky Mountain spotted fever, numerous other viral infections and, in the right setting, relapsing fevers.

B. Laboratory Findings

Leukopenia (2000–3000/mcL) with a shift to the left and atypical lymphocytes occurs, reaching a nadir 5–6 days after the onset of illness. Thrombocytopenia may occur. Viremia may be demonstrated by inoculation of blood into mice or by fluorescent antibody staining of the patient's red cells (with adsorbed virus). An RT-PCR assay may be used to detect early viremia. Detection of IgM by capture ELISA or plaque reduction neutralization is possible after 2 weeks from symptom onset and is the most frequently used diagnostic tool.

► Complications

Aseptic meningitis (particularly in children), encephalitis, and hemorrhagic fever occur rarely. Malaise may last weeks to months. Fatalities are very uncommon. Rarely, spontaneous abortion or multiple congenital anomalies may complicate Colorado tick fever infection acquired during pregnancy.

► Treatment

No specific treatment is available. Ribavirin has shown efficacy in an animal model. Antipyretics are used, although salicylates should be avoided due to potential bleeding with the thrombocytopenia seen in patients with Colorado tick fever. Tick avoidance is the best prevention.

► Prognosis

The disease is usually self-limited and benign.

► Prevention

The essence of prevention is vector (tick) control, particularly from March to November.

7. Chikungunya Fever

Chikungunya ("that which bends up" in Bantu) fever is a flaviviral infection transmitted to humans by *Aedes aegypti* and *Aedes albopictus* (the "Asian tiger mosquito") and is considered a classic "arthrogenic" virus. The virus is indigenous to tropical Africa and Asia with recent outbreaks reported from areas that adjoin the Indian Ocean, Southeast Asia and its neighboring islands (2005–2007), South India (2005) a major outbreak in Reunión Island (where women and recent immigrants from France were preferentially infected), but also from Europe (2007) including cases in Italy and France. In 2013, the first cases of locally-acquired Chikungunya Fever were found on islands in the Caribbean with a small number of travelers to that area diagnosed in Florida in 2014. The attack rates are often as high as 50%. Corneal transplants were a source of the outbreak on Reunión. Vertical transmission is documented, but teratogenicity is not established. The endemicity of

A aegypti in the Americas and the introduction of *A albopictus* into Europe and the New World raise the concerns of a global extension of the epidemic. The Rh-negative population appears to be immune. There are reports of cases of Chikungunya coinfection with yellow fever, malaria, and dengue fever.

► Clinical Findings

A. Symptoms and Signs

After an incubation period of 1–12 days (average 2–4), there is an abrupt onset of fever; headache; intestinal complaints; myalgias; and arthralgias/arthritis affecting small, large, and axial joints. The simultaneous involvement of more than 10 joints and the presence of tenosynovitis (especially in the wrist) are characteristic. The stooped posture of patients gives the disease its name. Joint symptoms persist for 4 months in 33% and linger for years in about 10%. A centrally distributed pigmented or pruritic maculopapular rash is reported in 50% of the patients, but it can be bullous with sloughing in children. Mucosal disease occurs in about 15%. Facial edema and localized petechiae are reported. Neurologic complications, including encephalitis, myelopathy, peripheral neuropathy, myeloneuropathy, and myopathy, are usually associated with a good outcome. In infants, primary manifestations of disease include fever, lethargy, acrocyanosis, and erythema evolving into vesiculobullous lesions. Hemorrhagic fever–like presentations are exceptional. Coinfection with other respiratory viruses, in particular dengue, is common. Death is rare and usually related to underlying comorbidities.

B. Laboratory Findings

Diagnosis is made epidemiologically and clinically. Mild leukopenia occurs as does thrombocytopenia, which is seldom severe. Elevated inflammatory markers do not correlate well with the severity of arthritis. Radiographs of affected joints are normal.

Serologic confirmation requires elevated IgM titers or fourfold increase in convalescent IgG levels using an ELISA. RT-PCR and culture techniques (viral isolation in insect or mammalian cell lines or by inoculation of mosquitoes or mice) are seldom available. Suspected cases in the United States should be promptly reported to public health authorities including the CDC Arboviral Diseases Branch, 970-221-6400. The differential includes other tropical febrile diseases, such as malaria, leishmaniasis, or dengue.

► Complications

A major complication of Chikungunya fever is long-term weakness, asthenia, and arthritis, noted to occur in up to 66.5% of cases at 1-year in a series from Italy but in between 4% and 25% in series from India.

► Treatment & Prevention

Treatment is largely supportive with nonsteroidal anti-inflammatory drugs. Chloroquine may be useful for managing refractory arthritis. No vaccine is available, and prevention relies on avoidance of the mosquito vectors.

Transplantation of tissue from immigrants or from travelers to known endemic areas such as Reunión should be discouraged. Prophylaxis with specific Chikungunya immunoglobulins may be useful for exposed neonates or immunosuppressed persons. Establishing the immunopathologic profile of acute versus chronic cases, new trials with immunoglobulins and vaccine development are ongoing areas of investigation.

Kucharz EJ et al. Chikungunya fever. Eur J Intern Med. 2012 Jun;23(4):325–9. [PMID: 22560378]
Moro ML et al. Long-term chikungunya infection clinical manifestations after an outbreak in Italy: a prognostic cohort study. J Infect. 2012 Aug;65(2):165–72. [PMID: 22522292]
Schilte C et al. Chikungunya virus-associated long-term arthralgia: a 36-month prospective longitudinal study. PLoS Negl Trop Dis. 2013;7(3):e2137. [PMID: 23556021]
Weaver SC et al. Chikungunya virus and prospects for a vaccine. Expert Rev Vaccines. 2012 Sep;11(9):1087–101. [PMID: 23151166]

COMMON VIRAL RESPIRATORY INFECTIONS

1. Respiratory Syncytial Virus (RSV) & Other Paramyxoviruses

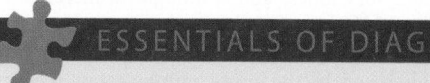
ESSENTIALS OF DIAGNOSIS

► RSV is a major cause of morbidity and mortality at the extremes of age.

► Care for patients with RSV infections is largely supportive.

► A monoclonal antibody against RSV, palivizumab, is good but expensive prophylaxis among patients with certain at-risk cardiopulmonary conditions.

► No active vaccination for RSV is available to date.

► General Considerations

Respiratory syncytial virus (RSV) is a paramyxovirus that causes annual outbreaks during the wintertime with usual onset of pulmonary symptoms between mid October and early January in the continental United States (excluding Florida). Outside the United States, RSV usually peaks during wet months in areas with high annual precipitation and during cooler months in hot and dry areas. There are two major subtypes, A and B, and it appears that the A genotype is associated with disease severity. RSV is the leading cause of hospitalization in US children, with annual hospitalization rates of 17 per 1000 children under 6 months and 3 per 1000 children under 5 years of age. Risk factors for infection in children include prematurity, low birth weight, younger age (especially younger than 6 months), bronchopulmonary dysplasia, congenital heart disease, later birth order, and day care exposure. HIV-infected children are at higher risk for hospitalization and poorer outcomes than uninfected children. RSV infection in children is associated with persistence of airway reactivity later in life.

RSV also causes upper and lower respiratory tract infection in adults with increased severity in the elderly, persons with severe combined immunodeficiency, and following lung or bone marrow transplantation (because CD8 T cells are not available for viral clearance). Recurrent infections occur throughout life. The virus enters through contact with mucosal surfaces. The average incubation period is 5 days.

In immunocompromised patients, such as bone marrow transplant recipients, serious pneumonia can occur and outbreaks with a high mortality rate (> 70%) are reported.

Other paramyxoviruses important in human disease include human metapneumovirus, parainfluenza virus, and Nipah virus.

Human metapneumovirus is less common and less pathogenic than RSV in children and is mainly a seasonal virus circulating during late winter to early spring. It is divided into subgroups A and B. Clinical presentations include mild upper respiratory tract infections to severe lower respiratory tract infections (eg, bronchiolitis, croup, and pneumonia) among slightly older children and lower respiratory tract (sometimes severe) infections among immunocompromised and elderly adults. In lung transplant recipients, human metapneumovirus is a common cause of respiratory illness and is thought to increase the risk of acute and chronic graft rejection.

Human parainfluenza viruses (HPIVs) are commonly seen in children and are the most common cause of laryngotracheitis (croup). Four different serotypes are described, and they differ in their clinical presentations as well as epidemiology. HPIV-1 and HPIV-2 are responsible for croup. HPIV-3 is associated with bronchiolitis and pneumonia. HPIV-4 is a less frequently reported pathogen. Reinfections are common throughout life. HPIVs can also cause severe disease in the elderly, immunocompromised persons, and those with chronic illnesses.

Nipah virus, is a highly virulent paramyxovirus first described in 1999. Cases are concentrated mainly in Southeast Asia (Malaysia, Singapore, Bangladesh and India). Fruit bats are identified as the natural host of the virus. Direct pig-human, cow-human, human-human, and nosocomial transmission are reported. Nipah virus causes acute encephalitis with a high fatality rate (67–92%), although respiratory symptoms are also described. Cranial nerves palsies, encephalopathy, and dystonia are among neurologic sequelae (15–32%) seen on infected individuals. Relapses occurring weeks and months after initial infection are described (3.4–7.5%).

Bocavirus infections are discussed under Erythrovirus (parvovirus) infections below.

▶ Clinical Findings

A. Symptoms and Signs

In RSV bronchiolitis, proliferation and necrosis of bronchiolar epithelium develop, producing obstruction from sloughed epithelium and increased mucus secretion. An interleukin-1 receptor polymorphism is shown to be associated with more severe bronchiolitis. Signs of infection include low-grade fever, tachypnea, and wheezes. Apnea is a common presenting symptom. Hyperinflated lungs, decreased gas exchange, and increased work of breathing are present. In children, RSV is globally the most common cause of acute lower respiratory infection and also a common cause of acute and recurrent otitis media. In patients with Down syndrome, RSV develops at a later age and is associated with more protracted hospitalizations.

B. Laboratory Findings

A rapid diagnosis of RSV infection is made by viral antigen identification of nasal washings using an ELISA or immunofluorescent assay. PCR is increasingly used in many pediatric centers. Coinfection with bacteria is relatively uncommon in industrialized countries although *Clostridium difficile*–associated diarrhea is documented to occur after RSV infections in a Canadian study. Coinfection with *Bordetella pertussis* and other viruses occurs in a subset of patients hospitalized for RSV infection. Tests for rapid detection of viral antigens with immunofluorescence or ELISA, and PCR techniques are also widely available although detection of parainfluenza by culture is also possible. RSV viral load assay values at day 3 of infection may correlate with requirement of intensive care and respiratory failure in children.

Human metapneumovirus is best diagnosed by PCR. ELISA (serum and cerebrospinal fluid) and PCR (urine, respiratory secretions but not blood) are both used for Nipah virus infection diagnosis.

▶ Treatment & Prevention

Treatment of RSV consists of supportive care, including hydration, humidification of inspired air, and ventilatory support as needed. Neither bronchodilating agents nor corticosteroids have demonstrated efficacy in bronchiolitis although individual patients with significant bronchospasm or history of asthma might respond to them.

The use of aerosolized ribavirin can be considered in high-risk patients, such as those with a history of bone marrow transplantation, and appears to lessen mortality. Pregnant women, including hospital staff, should avoid ribavirin exposure. Therapy with surfactant lacks evidence to make recommendations on its use. In the United States, RSV immunoglobulin G is no longer available and has been replaced with palivizumab, a monoclonal RSV antibody. Prophylactic administration of palivizumab (15 mg/kg intramuscularly monthly during the season of high transmission) is recommended for infants with high-risk factors, such as chronic lung disease of prematurity, bronchopulmonary dysplasia, and congenital heart disease. There are data to support the use of palivizumab in upper airway anomalies, other pulmonary diseases, and cystic fibrosis as well as in children with Down syndrome. Future studies may entail the use of small inhibitory RNA molecules and variants of palivizumab that target prefusion proteins.

No RSV vaccine is licensed to date. An encouraging phase 1 study using RSV fusion protein (F) shows that it is well tolerated and induces high levels of several antibodies associated with decreased rates of hospitalization. The use of RNA interference therapy in lung transplant patients may have some beneficial effects.

Prevention in hospitals entails rapid diagnosis, hand-washing, contact isolation, and perhaps passive immunization. The use of conjugated pneumococcal vaccination appears to decrease the incidence of concomitant pneumonia associated with viral infections in children in some countries.

Therapeutic modalities for human metapneumovirus and parainfluenza virus infections under investigation include intravenous ribavirin administration. During the initial Nipah virus outbreak, ribavirin was used empirically, although its efficacy remains questionable. Humanized monoclonal antibodies used in animal models show promising results.

Chu HY et al. Respiratory syncytial virus disease: prevention and treatment. Curr Top Microbiol Immunol. 2013;372:235–58. [PMID: 24362693]

El Saleeby CM et al. Respiratory syncytial virus load, viral dynamics, and disease severity in previously healthy naturally infected children. J Infect Dis. J Infect Dis. 2011 Oct 1;204(7):996–1002. [PMID: 21881113]

Glenn GM et al. Safety and immunogenicity of a Sf9 insect cell-derived respiratory syncytial virus fusion protein nanoparticle vaccine. Vaccine. 2013 Jan 7;31(3):524–32. [PMID: 23153449]

Haynes AK et al. Respiratory syncytial virus circulation in seven countries with Global Disease Detection Regional Centers. J Infect Dis. 2013 Dec 15;208(Suppl 3):S246–54. [PMID: 24265484]

Moyes J et al; South African Severe Acute Respiratory Illness Surveillance Group. Epidemiology of respiratory syncytial virus-associated acute lower respiratory tract infection hospitalizations among HIV-infected and HIV-uninfected South African children, 2010–2011. J Infect Dis. 2013 Dec 15;208 (Suppl 3):S217–26. [PMID: 24265481]

Sánchez-Solis M et al. Is palivizumab effective as a prophylaxis of respiratory syncytial virus infections in cystic fibrosis patients? A meta-analysis. Allergol Immunopathol (Madr). 2013 Nov 11. [Epub ahead of print] [PMID: 24231153]

Waghmare A et al. Respiratory syncytial virus lower respiratory disease in hematopoietic cell transplant recipients: viral RNA detection in blood, antiviral treatment, and clinical outcomes. Clin Infect Dis. 2013 Dec;57(12):1731–41. [PMID: 24065324]

2. Seasonal Influenza

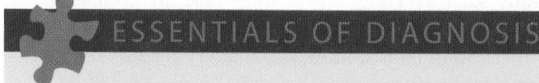

ESSENTIALS OF DIAGNOSIS

▶ Cases usually in epidemic pattern.

▶ Onset with fever, chills, malaise, cough, coryza, and myalgias.

▶ Aching, fever, and prostration out of proportion to catarrhal symptoms.

▶ Leukopenia.

▶ General Considerations

Influenza (an orthomyxovirus) is a highly contagious disease transmitted by the respiratory route in humans.

Transmission occurs primarily by droplet nuclei rather than fomites or direct contact. There are three types of influenza viruses. While type A can infect a variety of mammals (humans, swine, horses, etc) and birds, types B and C almost exclusively infect humans. Type A viruses are further divided into subtypes based on the hemagglutinin (H) and the neuraminidase (N) expressed in their surface. There are 18 subtypes of hemagglutinin and 10 subtypes of neuraminidase. Annual epidemics usually appear in the fall or winter in temperate climatic areas (although sporadic cases occur as summer outbreaks in northern areas such as Alaska or the southern hemisphere). Epidemics affect 10–20% of the global population on average each year and are typically the result of frequent minor antigenic variations of the virus, or antigenic drift, which are more common in influenza A virus. On the other hand, pandemics—associated with higher mortality—appear at longer and varying intervals (decades) as a consequence of a major genetic reassortment of the virus (antigenic shift) or the mutation of an avian virus that adapts to the human (as with the pandemic virus of 1918 with H1N1 properties).

The main circulating seasonal influenza viruses that are the target of current vaccines are a human-origin A (H3N2) subtype (H3N2 from 2011, A/Victoria/361/2011), the 2009 H1N1 strain (which replaced the seasonal H1N1 variants that circulated before 2009, A/California/7/2009) and two lineages of type B (B/Brisbane/60/2008 and B/Massachusetts/2/2012). The highly pathogenic avian (H5N1) and the H7N9 subtypes are discussed in the next section. The novel swine-origin influenza A (pandemic H1N1) virus, which emerged in Mexico in March 2009, and quickly spread through North America, is of particular concern, as with other pathogenic influenza viruses for pregnant women and immunosuppressed persons.

The outbreak of swine-origin (H1N1) influenza virus (formerly Swine-Origin Influenza Virus [S-OIV] or H1N1/A/California/04/2009, currently "A [H1N1] pdm09") emerged in Mexico City in March 2009. After initially spreading in the United States and Canada, the virus spread globally with cases reported from over 40 nations by mid-2009. The WHO declared a pandemic on June 11, 2009, which lasted until August 10, 2010. This was the first pandemic since 1968 with circulation outside the usual influenza season in the Northern Hemisphere. The **2009 pandemic H1N1** influenza virus replaced seasonal A (H1N1), previously the most common disease causing subtype was influenza A. It is estimated that this strain will continue to spread for years to come, akin to past spreading of seasonal influenza viruses. This virus originates from triple-reassortment North American swine, human and avian virus lineages and Eurasian swine virus lineages.

▶ Clinical Findings

A. Symptoms and Signs

Seasonal influenza viruses of types A and B produce clinically indistinguishable infections, whereas type C usually causes a minor illness. The incubation period is 1–4 days. In unvaccinated persons, uncomplicated influenza often begins abruptly. Symptoms include fever, chills, malaise, myalgias, substernal soreness, headache, nasal stuffiness, and occasionally nausea. Fever lasts 1–7 days (usually 3–5). Coryza, nonproductive cough, and sore throat are present. Elderly patients may present with only lassitude and confusion, often without fever or respiratory symptoms. Signs include mild pharyngeal injection, flushed face, and conjunctival redness. Moderate enlargement of the cervical lymph nodes may be observed. The presence of fever (> to 38.2°C) and cough during influenza season is highly predictive of influenza infection in those older than 4 years of age.

The pandemic 2009 strain of H1N1 showed a similarly broad range of clinical symptoms ranging from typical symptoms (fever, malaise, myalgias, cough, sore throat, rhinorrhea, shortness of breath) commonly accompanied by gastrointestinal (especially diarrhea) and respiratory (pneumonia) manifestations. The principal clinical syndrome leading to hospitalization and ICU admission is diffuse viral pneumonitis with severe hypoxemia and sometimes shock and renal failure. Neurologic complications, including seizures and encephalopathy, and cardiac dysfunction, including myocarditis and pulmonary thromboemboli, have occurred. While most patients with asthma have uncomplicated courses, asthmatic patients with pneumonia are at higher risk for ICU admission and death. Cases with pandemic H1N1 associated hemophagocytic syndrome are reported. Most patients with mild disease make full recovery, but 9–31% of hospitalized cases require ICU admission, where the mortality ranges between 14% and 46%. Adult hospitalized patients with H1N1 infection, when compared with patients with seasonal influenza, show statistically more significant complications and a higher mortality despite younger age. The disease has an incubation period of 1.5 to 7 days.

Attack rates with this pandemic strain are highest in children and young adults, particularly Hispanics, blacks, and Native Americans, with relative sparing of adults older than 60 years of age presumably due to previous exposure with related strains (conferring some degree of cross-protection). High-risk groups include patients with severe obesity, asthma, immunosuppression, or neurologic disorders, and especially pregnant and postpartum women. Infection during pregnancy increases the risk for hospitalization and may be associated with severe illness, sepsis, pneumothorax and respiratory failure, spontaneous abortion, preterm labor, and fetal distress. Overall case fatality rate is < 0.5% with 90% of deaths in those under 65 years of age and higher mortality recognized among men and patients with liver disease or a cancer diagnosis within the last year.

B. Laboratory Findings

Leukopenia is common, but leukocytosis can occur. Proteinuria may be present. The virus may be isolated from throat swabs or nasal washings by inoculation of embryonated eggs or cell cultures. Rapid immunofluorescence assays and enzyme immunoassays for detection of influenza antigens from nasal or throat swabs are becoming widely available. The sensitivity of such assays is suboptimal (at most 60–80%), especially among adults, and with very significant intertest variability, only a few can distinguish between influenza A and B. More sensitive nucleic acid (PCR) techniques are increasingly accessible. Complement-fixing and hemagglutination-inhibiting antibodies (for which fourfold or greater rises in levels are needed to establish diagnosis) appear during the second week. With the pandemic strain, elevated alkaline phosphatase, creatine kinase, creatinine, thrombocytopenia and metabolic acidosis suggest a poor prognosis. A nasopharyngeal swab, nasal aspirate, combined nasopharyngeal swab with oropharyngeal swab, or material from a bronchoalveolar lavage can be tested for any influenza strain.

Local laboratories can perform rapid influenza antigen enzyme or direct immunofluorescent assays to distinguish influenza viruses types A and B, but the results of these assays should be interpreted with caution due to a limited sensitivity (11–70%) and difficulties distinguishing seasonal influenza and the 2009 pandemic H1N1 influenza viruses. Test material can be kept at 4°C up to 4 days (not frozen) and shipped with an ice pack. The CDC or many state public health laboratories can then perform a real-time PCR or viral culture. Chest radiographic findings rarely show lobal infiltrates and pathologic findings show similar particular propensities toward diffuse alveolar damage.

▶ Differential Diagnosis

The differential diagnoses for influenza-like infections includes parainfluenza infections and RSV infections.

▶ Complications

Influenza causes necrosis of the respiratory epithelium, which predisposes to secondary bacterial infections. In turn, bacterial enzymes (eg, proteases, trypsin-like compounds, and streptokinase) activate influenza viruses. Frequent complications are acute sinusitis, otitis media, purulent bronchitis, and pneumonia. Children under 5 years of age, pregnant women, residents of nursing homes and long-term–care facilities, the elderly (aged 65 years or older), children and teens under 19 years of age who are receiving long-term aspirin therapy, and persons with underlying medical conditions (pulmonary, renal, cardiovascular, hepatic, hematologic, neurologic and neurodevelopmental conditions and immune-deficient conditions such as HIV) are at high risk for complications. Persons who are morbidly obese (body mass index > 40), American Indians, and Alaskan natives are also at high risk for complications.

Primary influenza pneumonia may occur, particularly in young children with cardiovascular disease and pregnant women, and is associated with a high mortality. Secondary bacterial pneumonia due to pneumococci, staphylococci, or *Haemophilus* spp is not uncommon. Pericarditis and myocarditis occur rarely. There is an association of acute myocardial infarction with preceding respiratory infection, including influenza; a UK study showed that influenza vaccination is associated with a lower rate of acute myocardial infarction. Rhabdomyolysis and leukocytoclastic vasculitis are rare complications of influenza.

Reye syndrome (fatty liver with encephalopathy) is a rare and severe complication of influenza (usually B type) and other viral diseases (eg, varicella), particularly in young children. It consists of rapidly progressive hepatic failure and encephalopathy, and there is a 30% mortality rate. The pathogenesis is unknown, but the syndrome is associated with aspirin use in the management of viral infections. Hypoglycemia, elevation of serum aminotransferases and blood ammonia, prolonged prothrombin time, and change in mental status all occur within 2–3 weeks after onset of the viral infection. Histologically, the periphery of liver lobules shows striking fatty infiltration and glycogen depletion. Treatment is supportive and directed toward the management of cerebral edema.

Other encephalopathic complications of influenza are uncommon and include an acute necrotizing encephalopathy associated with disseminated intravascular coagulation and cytokine storm, with worsening when treated with certain nonsteroidal anti-inflammatory drugs (diclofenac and mefenamic acid), and an acute encephalopathy associated with febrile seizures and the use of theophylline. Influenza infections are an infrequent trigger of the Guillain-Barré syndrome. A recent analysis of Medicare utilization data shows no increase in the Guillain-Barré syndrome following either seasonal or H1N1 influenza vaccination.

▶ **Treatment**

Many patients with influenza prefer to rest in bed. Analgesics and a cough mixture may be used. Treatment should be considered for all persons with acute illness, in particular those with a suggestive clinical presentation or with laboratory confirmed influenza and at high risk for developing complications (nursing home residents; patients with chronic pulmonary, cardiovascular, kidney, or liver disease; those with diabetes mellitus, active malignancy, immunosuppression, or impairment for managing respiratory secretions), or living with persons at significant risk for them. Maximum benefit is expected with the earliest initiation of therapy. Although the benefit of antiviral therapy after 48 hours of illness is reduced, it should be considered if the patient is hospitalized. There is no benefit to double-dose oseltamivir in severe influenza infections although some influenza experts continue to recommend double-dose therapy among immunocompromised patients.

The neuraminidase inhibitors, either inhaled **zanamivir,** 10 mg (2 inhalations) twice daily for 5 days, or oral **oseltamivir,** 75 mg twice daily for 5 days, are equally effective in the treatment of susceptible strains of influenza. Clinical trials show a reduction in the duration of symptoms as well as secondary complications, such as otitis, sinusitis, or pneumonia, but not in the rate of hospitalizations or mortality when using these agents. When administered early (within the first 2 days of illness), antiviral medications (neuraminidase inhibitors) are most effective. Patients with asthma who are hospitalized with pneumonia should be treated early with antivirals.

Since high levels of resistance to the adamantanes (amantadine and rimantadine) persist among 2009 influenza A (H1N1) and A (H3N2) viruses and these agents are not effective against influenza B viruses, adamantanes are generally not recommended for treatment. Resistance to neuraminidase inhibitors (oseltamivir and zanamivir) can occur with prolonged use in immunocompromised patients or in avian (H5N1)-infected patients.

Zanamivir is relatively contraindicated among persons with asthma because of the risk of bronchospasm and is not formulated for use in mechanically ventilated patients. Transient neuropsychiatric events, occasionally resulting in self-injury and death, have been reported post marketing for both neuraminidase inhibitors. Patients receiving these drugs should be closely monitored for any unusual behavior, and healthcare professionals should be notified immediately if such signs occur. Laninamivir is a long-acting inhaled neuraminidase inhibitor used for the treatment of seasonal influenza, including infection caused by oseltamivir-resistant virus. It is licensed in Japan but is awaiting FDA approval in the United States. Antibacterial antibiotics should be reserved for treatment of bacterial complications. Acetaminophen or ibuprofen rather than aspirin should be used for fever in children.

Oseltamivir-resistant virus is recognized and such virus usually remains sensitive to zanamivir, available through compassionate use programs available through GlaxoSmithKline at 877-626-8019 or 866-341-9160 or gskclinicalsupportHD@gsk.com (http://www.clinicalsupporthd.gsk.com/) (http://www.flu.nc.gov/providers/documents/IVzanamivir RequestInformation.pdf).

Person-to-person transmission with oseltamivir-resistant pandemic H1N1 is documented.

For oseltamivir-resistant 2009 H1N1 viral infection, intravenous zanamivir is preferred. While a case of multidrug-resistant pandemic H1N1 virus with resistance to oseltamivir, zanamivir, and peramivir is reported, this particular isolate is less pathogenic in animal studies than standard H1N1 strains. The use of high frequency oscillatory ventilation and extracorporeal membrane oxygenation can improve oxygenation but the impact on mortality in unknown. Corticosteroids for an associated ARDS are not useful and may increase the mortality except that the use of corticosteroids are associated with a lower rate of mechanical ventilation if used in high doses (1 mg/kg prednisone equivalence orally at the time of diagnosis) in patients with a history of hematologic stem cell transplantation.

Updated advice is available at http://www.cdc.gov/h1n1flu/recommendations.htm.

▶ **Prognosis**

The duration of the uncomplicated illness is 1–7 days, and the prognosis is excellent in healthy, nonelderly adults. Hospitalization typically occurs in those with underlying medical disease, at the extremes of age and in pregnant woman. Young adults and obese individuals were also at increased risk for hospitalization during the 2009 H1N1 pandemic. Purulent bronchitis and bronchiectasis may result in chronic pulmonary disease and fibrosis that persist throughout life. Most fatalities are due to bacterial pneumonia although exacerbations of other diseases processes, in particular cardiac diseases, occur which contributed to the overall increase in fatalities. Pneumonia resulting from influenza (in particular the H1N1 strain) has a high mortality rate among pregnant women and persons with a history of rheumatic heart disease. Mortality among adults hospitalized with influenza ranges from 4% to 8%, although higher mortality (>10–15%) may be seen during pandemics and among immunocompromised individuals.

If the fever recurs or persists for more than 4 days with productive cough and white cell count over 10,000/ mcL, secondary bacterial infection should be suspected. Pneumococcal pneumonia is the most common secondary infection, and staphylococcal pneumonia is the most serious.

▶ Prevention

Annual administration of influenza vaccine is the most effective measure for preventing influenza and its complications. Vaccines available for use in the United States are the FDA-approved trivalent inactivated influenza vaccine (TIV) and the quadrivalent live attenuated influenza vaccine (LAIV). They both contain antigens from 1 strain each of pandemic influenza A (H1N1), influenza A (H3N2), and influenza B. The 2013–2014 seasonal influenza vaccines contain A/California/7/2009 (H1N1), A/Victoria/ 361/2011 (H3N2)-like, and B/Massachusetts/2/2012-like virus antigens. The quadrivalent alternative contains an additional influenza B antigen (B/Brisbane/60/2008-like virus) and the CDC recommend that either trivalent or quadrivalent vaccine may be used. New cell-culture technologies for the manufacture of influenza vaccines that will supplement egg-based growth media are available and may contribute to improved strain selection and more robust vaccine supplies.

Chemotherapeutic regimens containing rituximab show persistent perturbations of B cell and Ig synthesis and these modifications decrease humoral responses to the influenza vaccine.

The Advisory Committee on Immunization Practices (ACIP) and the American College of Obstetricians and Gynecologists' Committee recommend annual influenza vaccination for all persons over 6 months of age. In particular, vaccination is emphasized for women who will be pregnant through the influenza season (October through May in the United States) and vaccination early in the season regardless of gestational age. No study to date has shown any major adverse consequence of inactivated influenza vaccine in pregnant women or their offspring. Fluzone High-Dose is an FDA-approved TIV containing four times more hemagglutinin than standard TIV and is recommended for persons age 65 or older. Fluzone intradermal trivalent vaccine (15 mcg hemagglutinin per strain, with current data suggesting 60 mg is the more appropriate dose) is an intradermal vaccine that is equally immunogenic and safe but more expensive than the traditional intramuscular vaccine.

The LAIV is available for use in healthy individuals between 2 and 49 years of age; it should not be given to asthmatic patients or pregnant women. For children, the LAIV shows superior efficacy compared with the TIV in most but not all studies.

Among the HIV-infected and the elderly, preliminary data suggest that a quadruple-dose influenza vaccine is associated with higher seroconversion rates.

The seasonal influenza vaccines can reduce influenza hospitalizations by an estimated 61%. All of these vaccines are contraindicated in persons with well-substantiated hypersensitivity to chicken eggs or other components of the vaccine (skin testing can be performed by an allergist), in persons with a history of vaccine-associated Guillain-Barré syndrome, or in persons with an acute febrile illness until symptomatic improvement. Concomitant warfarin or corticosteroid therapy is not a contraindication to influenza vaccination. Side effects are infrequent and include tenderness, redness, or induration at the intramuscular site of the TIV and mild upper respiratory symptoms for the LAIV.

Chemoprophylaxis is considered for individuals who are unvaccinated, for those in whom vaccination is contraindicated, and in those exposed to an infected patient within 2 weeks after vaccination with TIV. Chemoprophylaxis is not necessary and is contraindicated for those vaccinated with the LAIV, since this vaccine confers more rapid protection. Other circumstances that warrant consideration of chemoprophylaxis include outbreaks in long-term–care facilities, persons living with or in close contact with high-risk individuals, persons with immune deficiencies who might not respond to vaccination, unvaccinated staff during response to an outbreak in a closed institutional setting with residents at high risk, and first responders to epidemic situations.

Winter school breaks during periods of high influenza transmission appear to decrease rates of visits to primary care practitioners for influenza illness among children and adults.

Chemoprophylaxis against influenza A and B is accomplished with a single daily dose of the neuraminidase inhibitors oseltamivir (75 mg/d, oral) or zanamivir (10 mg/d, inhaled). These agents reduce the attack rate among unvaccinated individuals if begun within 48 hours after exposure. The CDC recommends chemoprophylaxis for up to 10 days after exposure. For outbreak control in long-term–care facilities and hospitals, a minimum of 2 weeks is recommended, including in vaccinated person, and until 1 week after identification of the last known case. Zanamivir should not be given as chemoprophylaxis to asthmatic persons, nursing home residents, or children under 5 years of age. Hand hygiene and surgical facemasks appear to prevent household transmission of influenza virus isolates when implemented within 36 hours of recognition of symptoms in an index patient. Such nonpharmaceutical interventions assist in mitigating the spread of pandemic and interpandemic influenza to nonvaccinated persons. Patients with 2009 H1N1 influenza infection should be considered potentially infectious from 1 day before to about 7 days following illness onset. Children and immunosuppressed persons exhibit prolonged viral shedding and may be infectious longer. Any hospital patient in whom the infection is suspected should be isolated in individual rooms with standard and contact precautions plus eye protection.

For pandemic H1N1 infection, the WHO guidelines recommend surgical masks for all patient care with the exception of N95 masks for aerosol generating procedures (eg, bronchoscopy, elective intubation, suctioning, administering nebulized medications). For such procedures, an airborne infection isolation room can be used, with air exhausted directly outside or recirculated after filtration by a high efficiency particulate air (HEPA) filter. Strict adherence to hand hygiene with soap and water or an alcohol-based hand sanitizer and immediate removal of gloves and other equipment after contact with respiratory secretions is essential. Precautions should be maintained until 7 days from symptom onset or until the resolution of symptoms, whichever is longer. Postexposure prophylaxis should be considered for close contacts of patients (confirmed, probable, or suspected) who are at high risk for complications of influenza (see section on seasonal influenza) as well as for healthcare personnel, public health workers, or first responders who experienced a recognized, unprotected close contact exposure to a person with novel (H1N1) influenza virus infection (confirmed, probable, or suspected) during that person's infectious period. The CDC continues to recommend considering postexposure prophylaxis with neuraminidase inhibitors to contacts of the infected person.

The MMWR and WHO website (http://www.who.int/csr/disease/swineflu/en/) provide updates about this pandemic.

▶ When to Admit

- Limited availability of supporting services.
- Pneumonia or decreased oxygen saturation.
- Changes in mental status.
- Consider with pregnancy.

Baden LR. For an influenza vaccine, are two Bs better than one? N Engl J Med. 2013 Dec 26;369(26):2547–9. [PMID: 24328439]

Centers for Disease Control and Prevention (CDC). Evaluation of 11 commercially available rapid influenza diagnostic tests—United States, 2011–2012. MMWR Morb Mortal Wkly Rep. 2012 Nov 2;61(43):873–6. [PMID: 23114254]

Centers for Disease Control and Prevention (CDC). FluView: a weekly influenza surveillance report. http://www.cdc.gov/flu/weekly

Centers for Disease Control and Prevention (CDC). Prevention and control of seasonal influenza with vaccines. Recommendations of the Advisory Committee on Immunization Practices—United States, 2013–2014. MMWR Recomm Rep. 2013 Sep 20;62(RR-07):1–43. [PMID: 24048214]

Chen LF et al. Cluster of oseltamivir-resistant 2009 pandemic influenza A (H1N1) virus infections on a hospital ward among immunocompromised patients—North Carolina, 2009. J Infect Dis. 2011 Mar 15;203(6):838–46. [PMID: 21343149]

Garza RC et al. Effect of winter school breaks on influenza-like illness, Argentina, 2005–2008. Emerg Infect Dis. 2013 Jun;19(6):938–44. [PMID: 23735682]

Hansen C et al. A large, population-based study of 2009 pandemic Influenza A virus subtype H1N1 infection diagnosis during pregnancy and outcomes for mothers and neonates. J Infect Dis. 2012 Oct;206(8):1260–8. [PMID: 22859826]

McKenna JJ et al; 2009 Pandemic Influenza A (H1N1) Virus Hospitalizations Investigation Team. Asthma in patients hospitalized with pandemic influenza A(H1N1)pdm09 virus infection—United States, 2009. BMC Infect Dis. 2013 Jan 31;13:57. [PMID: 23369034]

McKittrick N et al. Improved immunogenicity with high-dose seasonal influenza vaccine in HIV-infected persons: a single-center, parallel, randomized trial. Ann Intern Med. 2013 Jan 1;158(1):19–26. [PMID: 23277897]

South East Asia Infectious Disease Clinical Research Network. Effect of double dose oseltamivir on clinical and virological outcomes in children and adults admitted to hospital with severe influenza: double blind randomised controlled trial. BMJ. 2013 May 30;346:f3039. [PMID: 23723457]

3. Avian Influenza (H5N1 & Analogues)

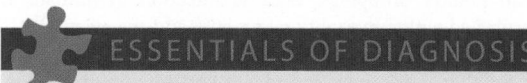

ESSENTIALS OF DIAGNOSIS

- ▶ Cases to date in humans, mostly from Southeast Asia and Egypt.
- ▶ Clinically indistinguishable from seasonal influenza.
- ▶ Epidemiologic factors assist in diagnosis.
- ▶ Rapid antigen assays confirm diagnosis but do not distinguish avian from seasonal influenza.

▶ General Considerations

The normal hosts for avian influenza viruses are aquatic waterfowl. Although avian influenza was first recognized in Italy in 1878, the current outbreak of highly pathogenic influenza A subtype (H5N1) in poultry was recognized in 1997 in Hong Kong and was followed by the first documented human cases. A massive slaughter of poultry contained the disease. Outbreaks of H5N1 influenza in poultry reemerged in 2003 and now involve more than 65 countries of East and Southeast Asia, Eurasia, Western and Eastern Europe, Northern Africa, and Haiti. The 641 confirmed human cases as of October 2013 include 380 deaths (59% of cases and 75% of deaths are reported from Egypt, Indonesia, and Vietnam) (the details are maintained and updated by the Global Outbreak Alert and Response Network, WHO:

http://www.who.int/influenza/human_animal_interface/EN_GIP_20131008CumulativeNumberH5N1cases.pdf).

Although highly contagious among birds, the transmission of this H5N1 strain from human-to-human is inefficient and not sustained although recent studies documented transmissibility of laboratory mutated virus via aerosols between ferrets. Evidence from cluster outbreaks suggests that host genetic susceptibility limits human-to-human transmission. The result is only rare cases of person-to-person infection. Occasional transmission to other mammals, including domestic cats and dogs, is also documented. Cases of influenza H7N7, transmitted from poultry to persons, especially poultry handlers and their contacts in the Netherlands occurred in 2003. More recently, two cases of conjunctivitis without fever or respiratory symptoms of H7N3 occurred this year in Mexico and one case with H7N2 occurred in New York. Cases of H7N9 are reported from China, initially in poultry, but an outbreak of 11 cases was reported in 2013 with 76.6% requiring ICU care and 27% dying. Unique characteristics were bilateral ground-glass opacities, lymphocytopenia, and thrombocytopenia. ARDS developed in patients who had underlying coexisting medical conditions. Person-to-person transmission was also documented.

Rare cases of influenza H9N2, another poultry pathogen, are reported from Bangladesh and human-to-human transmission of this pathogen is not documented.

Most human cases of H5N1 and analogous viruses occur after exposure to infected poultry or surfaces contaminated with poultry droppings. Because infection in humans is associated with a mortality rate > 50% and the avian H5N1 subtype continues to spread among birds (with many parts of Southeast Asia now considered endemic for the virus), there is worldwide concern that the virus may undergo genetic reassortment or mutation (as with the 1918 strain) and develop greater human-to-human transmissibility with the potential to produce a global pandemic.

▶ Clinical Findings

A. Symptoms and Signs

Distinguishing avian influenza from regular influenza is difficult. History of exposure to dead or ill poultry in the prior 10 days, recent travel to Southeast Asia or Egypt, or contact with known cases should be investigated. The symptoms and signs include fever and predominantly respiratory symptoms (cough and dyspnea), but a variety of other systems may be involved, producing headaches and gastrointestinal complaints in particular. Subclinical disease is relatively rare. With cytokines responsible for much of the pathology, prolonged febrile states and generalized malaise are common. Children are preferentially impacted. Respiratory failure is the usual cause of death.

B. Laboratory Findings

Current commercial rapid antigen tests are not optimally sensitive or specific for detection of H5N1 influenza but are still first-line diagnostic tests because of their widespread availability. Diagnostic yield can be improved by early collection of samples. More sensitive RT-PCR assays are available through many hospitals and state health departments. An initial negative result in the right clinical setting warrants retesting. Throat or lower respiratory swabs may provide higher yield of detection than nasal swabs. When highly pathogenic strains (eg, H5N1) are suspected, extreme care in the handling of these samples must be observed during preliminary testing. Positive samples must then be forwarded to the appropriate public health authorities for further investigations (eg, culture) in laboratories with the adequate level of biosafety (level 3).

▶ Treatment

Resistance of avian H5N1 influenza strains to amantadine and rimantadine is present in most geographic areas. The current first-line recommendation is to use the neuraminidase inhibitor oseltamivir, 75 mg orally twice daily for 5 days administered within 48 hours from onset of illness. Overall oseltamivir, by modeling, is associated with a 49% reduction in mortality from H5N1 infections. A higher dose (150 mg twice daily), longer duration (7–10 days), and possible combination therapy with amantadine or rimantadine (in countries where A [H5N1] viruses are likely to be susceptible to adamantanes) may be considered in patients with pneumonia or progressive disease. Twice daily oseltamivir is also recommended for H7N9 influenza infections. Evidence of resistance to oseltamivir is reported. Although inhaled zanamivir is proven effective in treating seasonal influenza, no data of its efficacy against H5N1 strains are available. Zanamivir is recommended, intravenously, for patients not improving with oseltamivir after 2 days of treatment.

▶ Prevention

Postexposure prophylaxis with 75 mg of oseltamivir orally once daily for 7–10 days should be given to close contacts and considered for moderate contacts of documented cases of H5N1 and H7N9 influenza infections although human-to-human transmission appears to be limited. Personnel exposed to patients should be monitored for symptoms. Careful surveillance for human cases and prudent stockpiling of medications with establishment of an infrastructure for dissemination are essential modalities of control. Nonpharmacologic means of control include masks, social distancing, quarantine, travel limitations, and infrastructure development, particularly for emergency departments.

Human vaccines against H5N1 influenza are licensed by Sanofi Pasteur (but not marketed) in the United States with the government stockpiling supplies in the event of need. Other vaccines are licensed by GlaxoSmithKline in Europe and CS Limited in Australia. It appears to be only moderately immunogenic. A vaccine candidate made with an oil-in-water emulsion-based adjuvant is highly immunogenic and well tolerated. Several other vaccine candidates are undergoing clinical trials. A major concern with H5N1 vaccinology is the evolution of the virus in vaccinated poultry, especially in the endemic nations of Egypt and Indonesia, and the need to maintain current surveillance and update vaccine development should avian influenza become more pathogenic in humans. Seasonal and H5N1 vaccines in phase 2 studies can be given either combined or in sequence safely and without affecting immunogenicity. Contrary to popular belief, persons born before 1968 are not necessarily (as had been seen in earlier studies) more likely to respond to an avian influenza A/H9N2 vaccine than those born after 1968. Prevention of exposure to avian influenza strains also includes hygienic practices during handling of poultry products, including hand washing and prevention of cross-contamination, as well as thorough cooking of poultry products (to 70°C). There is no risk of acquiring avian influenza through the consumption of cooked poultry products, although there is a risk associated with handling feathers or birds from endemic areas, and the US government bans the importation of poultry from infected areas. While no commercial H7N9 vaccines are available, two large trials are underway with vaccine and treatment evaluation units. Culling of infected H7N9 poultry is difficult because most animals are asymptomatic.

Atmar RL et al. Evaluation of age-related differences in the immunogenicity of a G9 H9N2 influenza vaccine. Vaccine. 2011 Oct 19;29(45):8066–72. [PMID: 21864622]

Centers for Disease Control and Prevention (CDC). Notes from the field: highly pathogenic avian influenza A (H7N3) virus infection in two poultry workers—Jalisco, Mexico, July 2012. MMWR Morb Mortal Wkly Rep. 2012 Sep 14;61(36):726–7. [PMID: 22971746]

Gao HN et al. Clinical findings in 111 cases of influenza A (H7N9) virus infection. N Engl J Med. 2013 Jun 13;368(24): 2277–894. [PMID: 23697469]

Herfst S et al. The future of research and publication on altered H5N1 viruses. J Infect Dis. 2012 Jun;205(11):1628–31. [PMID: 22454474]

Khurana S et al. H5N1-SeroDetect EIA and rapid test: a novel differential diagnostic assay for serodiagnosis of H5N1 infections and surveillance. J Virol. 2011 Dec;85(23):12455–63. [PMID: 21957281]

Lopez P et al. Combined, concurrent, and sequential administration of seasonal influenza and MF59-adjuvanted A/H5N1 vaccines: a phase II randomized, controlled trial of immunogenicity and safety in healthy adults. J Infect Dis. 2011 Jun 15; 203(12):1719–28. [PMID: 21606530]

Qi X et al. Probable person to person transmission of novel avian influenza A (H7N9) virus in Eastern China, 2013: epidemiological investigation. BMJ. 2013 Aug 6;347:f4752. [PMID: 23920350]

4. Severe Acute Respiratory Syndrome (SARS)

ESSENTIALS OF DIAGNOSIS

- ► Mild, moderate, or severe respiratory illness.
- ► Travel to endemic area within 10 days before symptom onset, including mainland China, Hong Kong, Singapore, Taiwan, Vietnam, and Toronto.
- ► Persistent fever; dry cough, dyspnea in most.
- ► Diagnosis confirmed by antibody testing or isolation of virus.
- ► No specific treatment; mortality as high as 14% in clinically diagnosed cases.

► General Considerations

SARS is a respiratory syndrome caused by a unique coronavirus, transmitted through direct or indirect contact of mucous membranes with infectious respiratory droplets. The virus is shed in stools but the role of fecal–oral transmission is unknown. The natural reservoir appears to be the horseshoe bat.

The earliest cases were traced to a health care worker in Guangdong Province in China in late 2002, with rapid spread thereafter throughout Asia and Canada, considered a consequence of spread through travel. The most recent cases were reported in 2004.

► Clinical Findings

A. Symptoms and Signs

SARS is an atypical pneumonia that affects persons in all age groups. Severity ranges from asymptomatic disease to severe respiratory illness. Many subclinical cases probably go undiagnosed. Seasonality, as with influenza, is not established. The incubation period is 2–7 days, and it can be spread to contacts of affected patients for 10 days. The mean time from onset of clinical symptoms to hospital admission is 3–5 days. In all clinical cases, persistent fever is present; chills or rigor (or both), cough, shortness of breath, rales, and rhonchi are the rule. Headache, myalgias, and sore throat are common with watery diarrhea occurring in a subset of patients. Elderly patients may report malaise and delirium, without the typical febrile response.

B. Laboratory Findings and Imaging

Leukopenia (particularly lymphopenia) and low-grade disseminated intravascular coagulation are common. Modest elevations of ALT and creatine kinase are frequently seen. Arterial oxygen saturation < 95% with associated nonspecific pulmonary infiltrates is evident in 80% of affected individuals. A high-resolution CT scan is abnormal in 67% of patients with initially normal chest radiographs.

Serum serologies, including enzyme immunoassays and fluorescent antibody assays, are available through public health departments at the state level, although seroconversion may not occur until 3 weeks after the onset of symptoms. The detection rates for the virus using conventional RT-PCR are generally low in the first week of illness. Urine, nasopharyngeal aspirate, and stool specimens are positive in 42%, 68%, and 97%, respectively, on day 14 of illness. Although viral isolation is possible, it is a technically laborious and time-consuming procedure.

► Complications

ARDS, with extensive bilateral consolidation, occurs in about 16% patients, and about 20–30% of patients require intubation and mechanical ventilation.

► Treatment

Severe cases require intensive supportive management. Different agents including, lopinavir/ritonavir, ribavirin, interferon, IVIG, and systemic corticosteroids were used during the 2003 epidemic, but the treatment efficacy of these agents remains inconclusive. In vitro studies with ribavirin show no activity against the virus, and a retrospective analysis of the epidemic in Toronto suggests worse outcomes in patients who received the drug. A meta-analysis studying the use of Chinese herbs failed to show any efficacy in treating SARS. Studies using monoclonal antibodies are underway based on the response of some patients to immune convalescent sera of convalescent patients.

► Prognosis

The overall mortality rate of identified cases is about 14%. Poor prognostic factors include advanced age (mortality rate > 50% in those over 65 years of age compared to < 1% for those under 2 years of age), chronic hepatitis B infection treated with lamivudine, high initial or high peak lactate dehydrogenase concentration, high neutrophil count on presentation, diabetes mellitus, acute kidney disease, and low counts of CD4 and CD8 on presentation.

► Prevention

Health care workers engaged in procedures that involve contact with respiratory droplets are at risk. Isolation of high-risk patients is essential, and simple hygienic measures may help reduce transmission.

Control measures include quarantining in the home for high-risk exposed persons and the use of facemasks for preventing hospital-acquired infections. The validity of using such masks in the community remains unsubstantiated. Continual reporting of suspected cases is crucial, as is awareness of restrictions on international travel. The most cautious modalities include monitoring for 10 days after the last potential exposure and confinement of recovering patients for a similar interval.

Balboni A et al. The SARS-like coronaviruses: the role of bats and evolutionary relationships with SARS coronavirus. New Microbiol. 2012 Jan;35(1):1–16. [PMID: 22378548]

Elshabrawy HA et al. Human monoclonal antibodies against highly conserved HR1 and HR2 domains of the SARS-CoV spike protein are more broadly neutralizing. PLoS One. 2012;7(11):e50366. [PMID: 23185609]

Liu X et al. Chinese herbs combined with Western medicine for severe acute respiratory syndrome (SARS). Cochrane Database Syst Rev. 2012 Oct 17;10:CD004882. [PMID: 23076910]

Yang L et al. Novel SARS-like beta coronaviruses in bats, China, 2011. Emerg Infect Dis. 2013 Jun;19(6):989–91. [PMID: 23739658]

5. Middle East Respiratory Syndrome–Coronavirus (MERS-CoV)

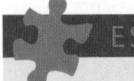

ESSENTIALS OF DIAGNOSIS

- Mild, moderate, or severe respiratory illness.
- Travel to endemic area, including Saudi Arabia, Qatar, and Jordan, within 10 days before symptom onset.
- Fever, cough, and dyspnea are most common symptoms.
- Serologic assays are not developed for diagnosis; CDC can assist with real time-PCR using serum, respiratory samples, or stool.
- No specific treatment available; mortality as high as 45%.

► General Considerations

Middle East respiratory syndrome (MERS) is a newly described syndrome that appears to be due to a coronavirus similar to that which causes SARS. All patients with MERS have had a history of residence or travel in the Middle East, in particular Saudi Arabia, or contact with such patients. The virus is probably transmitted through direct or indirect contact of mucous membranes with infectious respiratory droplets. The virus is shed in stools but the role of fecal–oral transmission is unknown. The natural reservoir is unknown.

The earliest cases were identified in 2012 in Saudi Arabia. As of November 15, 2013, 153 cases have been recognized worldwide and 64 of these have been fatal (42%). Cases in the Middle East have also occurred in Jordan, Oman, Qatar, and the United Arab Emirates, while 9 cases are currently reported from other countries, including North Africa (Tunisia, 3) and Europe (France, 2; Italy, 1; and United Kingdom, 3).

Person-to-person transmission occurs, both within families and at the hospital, although in series to date it is not common (5 cases among 217 household contacts and 2 among 200 hospital contacts). The median incubation period in hospital cases was 5.2 days but the reported range is 2–13 days.

► Clinical Findings

A. Symptoms and Signs

MERS is an acute respiratory syndrome, with the most common symptoms being fever (98%), cough (83%), and dyspnea (72%). Chills and rigors are common (87%) and gastrointestinal symptoms may occur with diarrhea the most common (26%), followed by nausea and abdominal pain. Patients often have several comorbid conditions, including diabetes mellitus (68%), hypertension (34%), or chronic heart or kidney disease. Middle-aged persons are most affected (median age of 50 years), although all ages are affected (age range of 2–94 year), and men outnumber women.

B. Laboratory Findings and Imaging

Hematologic findings in the largest series to date include thrombocytopenia (36%), lymphopenia (34%), and lymphocytosis (11%). Moderate elevations in lactate dehydrogenase (49%), AST (15%), and ALT (11%) are recognized. Chest radiograph abnormalities are nearly universal and include increased bronchovascular markings, patchy infiltrates or consolidations, interstitial changes, opacities (reticular and nodular) as well as pleural effusions and total lung opacification. The findings mimic those of many other causes of pneumonia.

A case definition is available from the CDC. Serum serologies remain a research and surveillance tool. RT-PCR is available through CDC (contact information below, on MMWR reference site) and can be performed on airway washings, serum, or stool.

► Complications

Respiratory failure is such a common complication that in a series from Saudi Arabia, 89% of patients required intensive care and mechanical ventilation and patients with MERS-CoV appear to advance faster to respiratory failure than do those with the SARS agent.

► Treatment

Respiratory support is essential. No antivirals are effective.

Prognosis

The overall mortality rate of identified cases is about 45%. Advance age is associated with a poor prognosis.

Prevention

Isolation and quarantine of cases is authorized by CDC. Strict infection control measures are essential as well as care and management of household contacts and hospital workers engaged in the care of patients. Travelers to Saudi Arabia (including the many pilgrims to the holy sites) should practice frequent hand washing and avoid contact with those who have respiratory ailments. Evaluation of patients with suspect symptoms within 14 days of return from Saudi Arabia is essential. Because health care workers engaged in procedures that involve contact with respiratory droplets are at risk, isolation of high-risk patients is essential, as are simple hygienic measures. Control measures, including quarantining in the home for high-risk exposed persons and the use of facemasks for preventing hospital-acquired infections, are prudent but not fully proven recommendations. Assisting public health authorities with case reporting and surveillance is essential. Mathematical models to date do not suggest a potential for a global pandemic.

MMWR periodically updates the infection control recommendations and the extent of the outbreak.

Assiri A et al. Epidemiological, demographic, and clinical characteristics of 47 cases of Middle East respiratory syndrome coronavirus disease from Saudi Arabia: a descriptive study. Lancet Infect Dis. 2013 Sep;13(9):752–61. [PMID: 23891402]

Assiri A et al; KSA MERS-CoV Investigation Team. Hospital outbreak of Middle East respiratory syndrome coronavirus. N Engl J Med. 2013 Aug 1;369(5):407–16. Erratum in: N Engl J Med. 2013 Aug 29;369(9):886. [PMID: 23782161]

Breban R et al. Interhuman transmissibility of Middle East respiratory syndrome coronavirus: estimation of pandemic risk. Lancet. 2013 Aug 24;382(9893):694–9. [PMID: 23831141]

Centers for Disease Control and Prevention (CDC). Updated information on the epidemiology of Middle East respiratory syndrome coronavirus (MERS-CoV) infection and guidance for the public, clinicians, and public health authorities, 2012–2013. MMWR Morb Mortal Wkly Rep. 2013 Sep 27;62(38):793–6. [PMID: 24067584]

Memish ZA et al. Family cluster of Middle East respiratory syndrome coronavirus infections. N Engl J Med. 2013 Jun 27;368(26):2487–94. Erratum in: N Engl J Med. 2013 Aug 8;369(6):587. [PMID: 23718156]

ADENOVIRUS INFECTIONS

General Considerations

About a half of the existing adenoviruses (there are over 52 serotypes described to date and divided into 7 subgroups A–G) produce a variety of clinical syndromes. Adenoviruses show a worldwide distribution and occur throughout the year. These infections are usually self-limited or clinically inapparent and most common among infants, young children, and military recruits. However, these infections may cause significant morbidity and mortality in immunocompromised persons, such as HIV-infected persons and COPD patients, as well as in patients who have undergone solid organ and hematopoietic stem cell transplantation or cardiac surgery or in those who have received cancer chemotherapy. A few cases of donor-transmitted adenoviral infection are reported in the past years. Adenoviruses, although a common cause of human disease, also receive particular recognition through their role as vectors in gene therapy.

Clinical Findings

A. Symptoms and Signs

The incubation period is 4–9 days. Clinical syndromes of adenovirus infection, often overlapping, include the following. The **common cold** (see Chapter 8) is characterized by rhinitis, pharyngitis, and mild malaise without fever. **Nonstreptococcal exudative pharyngitis** is characterized by fever lasting 2–12 days and accompanied by malaise and myalgia. Conjunctivitis is often present. **Lower respiratory tract infection** may occur, including bronchiolitis, suggested by cough and rales, or pneumonia (types 1 to 3, 4, and 7 commonly cause acute respiratory disease and atypical pneumonia) and infections are especially severe in Native American children. Adenovirus type 14 is increasingly reported as a cause of severe and sometimes fatal pneumonia in those with chronic lung disease, but it is also seen in healthy young adults and military recruit outbreaks. Viral or bacterial coinfections occur with adenovirus in 15–20% of cases. **Pharyngoconjunctival fever** is manifested by fever and malaise, conjunctivitis (often unilateral), mild pharyngitis, and cervical adenitis. **Epidemic keratoconjunctivitis** (transmissible person-to-person, most often types 8 (and showing considerable variation by season), 19, and 37) occurs in adults and is manifested by bilateral conjunctival redness, pain, tearing, and an enlarged preauricular lymph node (multiple types may be involved in a single outbreak). Keratitis may lead to subepithelial opacities (especially with the above types). **Acute hemorrhagic cystitis** is a disorder of children often associated with adenovirus type 11 and 21. **Sexually transmitted genitourinary ulcers and urethritis** may be caused by types 2, 8, and 37 in particular. Adenoviruses also cause **acute gastroenteritis** (types 40 and 41), **mesenteric adenitis**, **acute appendicitis**, and **intussusception**. Rarely, they are associated with encephalitis, acute flaccid paralysis, and pericarditis. Adenovirus is commonly identified in endomyocardial tissue of patients with **myocarditis** and dilated cardiomyopathy. Risk factors associated with severity of infection include youth, chronic underlying infections, recent transplantation, and serotypes 5 or 21.

Hepatitis (type 5 adenovirus), **pneumonia**, and **hemorrhagic cystitis** (types 11 and 34) tend to develop in infected liver, lung, or kidney transplant recipients, respectively. Syndromes that may develop in hematopoietic stem cell transplant patients include hepatitis, pneumonia, hemorrhagic cystitis, tubulointerstitial nephritis, colitis, and encephalitis.

B. Laboratory Findings and Imaging

Antigen detection assays including direct fluorescence assay or enzyme immunoassay are rapid and show sensitivity of 40–60% compared with viral culture (considered the standard). Samples with negative rapid assays require PCR assays or viral cultures for diagnosis. Quantitative real-time rapid-cycle PCR is useful in distinguishing disease from colonization, especially in hematologic cell transplant patients. Adenovirus differs from other viral and bacterial respiratory infections seen on chest CT imaging, appearing as a multifocal consolidation or ground-glass opacity without airway inflammatory findings.

▶ Treatment & Prognosis

Treatment is symptomatic. Ribavirin and cidofovir are used in immunocompromised individuals with occasional success, although cidofovir is attendant with significant renal toxicity and reduced immunosuppression is often required. Adoptive immunotherapy with transfusion of adenovirus-specific T cells is currently being investigated. IVIG is used in immunocompromised patients, but data are still limited. Typing of isolates is useful epidemiologically and in distinguishing transmission from endogenous reactivation. Complications of adenovirus pneumonia in children include bronchiolitis obliterans. Deaths are reported on occasion (eight in one season among the American military).

Vaccines are not available for general use.

Kim JK et al. Epidemiology of respiratory viral infection using multiplex rt-PCR in Cheonan, Korea (2006–2010). J Microbiol Biotechnol. 2013 Feb;23(2):267–73. [PMID: 23412071]

Lu MP et al. Clinical characteristics of adenovirus associated lower respiratory tract infection in children. World J Pediatr. 2013 Nov;9(4):346–9. [PMID: 24235068]

Miller WT Jr et al. CT of viral lower respiratory tract infections in adults: comparison among viral organisms and between viral and bacterial infections. AJR Am J Roentgenol. 2011 Nov;197(5):1088–95. [PMID: 22021500]

Potter RN et al. Adenovirus-associated deaths in US military during postvaccination period, 1999–2010. Emerg Infect Dis. 2012 Mar;18(3):507–9. [PMID: 22377242]

OTHER EXANTHEMATOUS VIRAL INFECTIONS

1. Erythrovirus (Parvovirus) Infections

Erythrovirus, formerly parvovirus B19, infects human erythroid precursor cells. It is quite widespread (by age 15 years about 50% of children have detectable IgG) and its transmission occurs through respiratory secretions and saliva, through the placenta (vertical transmission with 30–50% of pregnant women nonimmune), and through administration of blood products. The incubation period is 4–14 days. Chronic forms of the infection can occur. Bocavirus, another erythrovirus (parvovirus), is a cause of winter acute respiratory disease in children and adults.

▶ Clinical Findings

A. Symptoms and Signs

Erythrovirus (parvovirus B19) causes several syndromes and manifests differently in various populations.

1. Children—In children, an exanthematous illness ("fifth disease," erythema infectiosum) is characterized by a fiery red "slapped cheek" appearance, circumoral pallor, and a subsequent lacy, maculopapular, evanescent rash on the trunk and limbs. Malaise, headache, and pruritus (especially on the palms and soles) occur. Systemic symptoms and fever are mostly abated by the time of rash appearance. Eosinophilic cellulitis (Well syndrome) is also reported with parvovirus. Parvovirus is also one of the most common causes of myocarditis in childhood.

2. Immunocompromised patients—In immunosuppressed patients, including those with HIV infection or transplanted organs, or with hematologic conditions such as sickle cell disease, transient aplastic crisis and pure red blood cell aplasia may occur. Bone marrow aspirates reveal absence of mature erythroid precursors and characteristic giant pronormoblasts. The parvovirus B19 gene is detected in 16–19% of acute leukemic and chronic myeloid leukemia patients.

3. Adults—A limited nonerosive symmetric polyarthritis that mimics lupus erythematosus and rheumatoid arthritis, which may in some cases be a type II mixed cryoglobulinemia, can develop in middle-aged persons (especially women) but can also occur in children. Rashes, especially facial, are less common in adults.

Chloroquine and its derivatives exacerbate erythrovirus (parvovirus)-associated anemia and are linked with significantly lower hematocrit in hospital admissions in malaria endemic areas. Rare reported presentations include myocarditis with infarction, constrictive pericarditis, chronic dilated cardiomyopathy, hepatitis, pneumonitis, neutropenia, thrombocytopenia, a lupus-like syndrome, glomerulopathy, CNS vasculitis, papular-purpuric "gloves and socks" syndrome, and a chronic fatigue syndrome. A subclinical infection is documented among patients with sickle cell disease. Other CNS manifestations of erythrovirus (parvovirus) include encephalitis, meningitis, stroke (usually in sickle cell anemia patients with aplastic crises), and peripheral neuropathy (brachial plexitis and carpal tunnel syndrome) with occasional chronic residua.

The symptoms of erythrovirus (parvovirus) infection can mimic those of autoimmune states such as lupus, systemic sclerosis, antiphospholipid syndrome, or vasculitis. The molecular mimicry of erythrovirus (parvovirus) to human cytokeratin and transcription factors engaged in hematopoiesis is the basis for theories that implicate erythrovirus (parvovirus) in the pathogenesis of these autoimmune states.

In pregnancy, premature labor, hydrops fetalis, and fetal loss are reported sequelae. Pregnant women with a recent exposure or with suggestive symptoms should be tested for the disease and carefully monitored if results are positive.

B. Laboratory Findings

The diagnosis is clinical (Table 32–2) but may be confirmed by an elevated titer of IgM anti-erythrovirus (parvovirus) antibodies in serum or with PCR in serum or bone marrow. Autoimmune antibodies (antiphospholipid and antineutrophil cytoplasmic antibodies) can be present and are thought to be a consequence of molecular mimicry.

► Complications

Uncommon complications include the CNS diseases listed above, chronic hemolytic anemia, thrombotic thrombocytopenic purpuric syndrome, acute postinfectious glomerulonephritis, and hepatitis.

► Treatment

Treatment in healthy persons is symptomatic (nonsteroidal anti-inflammatory drugs are used to treat arthralgias, and transfusions are used to treat transient aplastic crises). In immunosuppressed patients including those infected with HIV, IVIG is very effective in the short-term reduction of anemia. Relapses tend to occur about 4 months after administration of IVIG. There is no reduction in encephalitic complications with IVIG. Intrauterine blood transfusion can be considered in severe fetal anemia, although such transfusions have been linked to impaired neurologic development.

► Prevention & Prognosis

Several nosocomial outbreaks are documented. In these cases, standard containment guidelines, including handwashing after patient exposure and avoiding contact with pregnant women are paramount.

The prognosis is generally excellent in immunocompetent individuals. In immunosuppressed patients, persistent anemia may require prolonged transfusion dependence. Remission of erythrovirus (parvovirus) infection in AIDS patients may occur with HAART, though the immune restoration syndrome is also reported.

Crabol Y et al; Groupe d'experts de l'Assistance Publique-Hôpitaux de Paris. Intravenous immunoglobulin therapy for pure red cell aplasia related to human parvovirus b19 infection: a retrospective study of 10 patients and review of the literature. Clin Infect Dis. 2013 Apr;56(7):968–77. [PMID: 23243178]

da Costa AC et al. Investigation of human parvovirus B19 occurrence and genetic variability in different leukaemia entities. Clin Microbiol Infect. 2013 Jan;19(1):E31–43. [PMID: 23167493]

De Jong EP et al. Intrauterine transfusion for parvovirus B19 infection: long-term neurodevelopmental outcome. Am J Obstet Gynecol. 2012 Mar;206(3):204.e1–5. [PMID: 22381602]

Lamont RF et al. Parvovirus B19 infection in human pregnancy. BJOG. 2011 Jan;118(2):175–86. [PMID: 21040396]

Molina KM et al. Parvovirus B19 myocarditis causes significant morbidity and mortality in children. Pediatr Cardiol. 2013 Feb;34(2):390–7. [PMID: 22872019]

2. Poxvirus Infections

Among the nine poxviruses causing disease in humans, the following are the most clinically important: variola/vaccinia, molluscum contagiosum, orf and paravaccinia, and monkeypox.

1. Variola/vaccinia—Smallpox (variola) was a highly contagious disease associated with high mortality and disabling sequelae. Its manifestations include severe headache, acute onset of fever, prostration and a rash characterized by the uniform progression from macules to papules to firm, deep-seated vesicles or pustules. The synchronous progression in smallpox readily differentiates lesions from those of varicella (see also Chapter 6).

Complications of smallpox include bacterial superinfections (cellulitis and pneumonia), encephalitis, and keratitis with corneal ulcerations (risk factor for blindness). **Effective vaccination led to its global elimination by 1979 and routine vaccination stopped in 1985.** Despite the recommendation of destroying remaining samples of this virus, significant concern exists for the potential misuse of these repositories in military or terrorist activities.

Smallpox should be considered, in concordance with the CDC's Smallpox Response Plan (www.bt.cdc.gov/agent/smallpox/response-plan/index.asp), in any patient with fever and a characteristic rash (see above) for which other etiologies—such as herpes infections, erythema multiforme, drug reactions (eczema herpeticum may be differentiated from suspect smallpox by appropriate serologic stains), or other infections—are unlikely. One hundred and fifteen cases of vaccine-related disease from contact with a smallpox vaccinee in the United States between 2003 and 2011 (including sexually transmission) were reported. Two cases of vaccinia infection after contact with oral rabies animal baits (which uses the vaccinia vector) are reported. Patients with suspected infection should be placed in airborne and contact isolation and the official agency contacted (CDC Emergency Preparedness and Response Branch; 770-488-7100). Original smallpox vaccine was crudely manufactured with a significant side-effect profile, including eczema vaccinatum and acute vaccinia syndrome (fatigue, headaches, myalgias, and fever). Subsequent smallpox vaccines had similar side-effect profiles, but myocarditis and pericarditis also developed in some patients. The most recent vaccine, ACAM2000 (Acambis, Inc) shows similar safety profiles and is currently used by the US military and stockpiled in the event of biologic warfare.

Contraindications to vaccination include immunosuppression, eczema or other dermatitis in the vaccinee or household contacts, allergy to any component of the vaccine, infants younger than 1 year and pregnant or breastfeeding women. According to current recommendation, it is unnecessary for anyone not handling the smallpox vaccine to be vaccinated. Israeli studies suggest about 4% of their population show contraindications to vaccination. Inoculation of the vaccine in inappropriate sites (eg, eyes) is unfortunately common. Asymptomatic vaccinia viremia can be detected up to 21 days post vaccination and no blood donation should occur during this interval. Cidofovir may be considered for treatment of poxviral conditions and intravenous human vaccinia immunoglobulin may be useful for vaccinia.

2. Molluscum contagiosum—Molluscum contagiosum may be transmitted sexually or by other close contact. It may occur also in an extensive form in children with genetic defects in dendritic and T cell migration (the DOCK8 [dedicator of cytokinesis] deficiency). The disease is manifested by pearly, raised, umbilicated skin nodules sparing the palms and soles. Keratoconjunctivitis can occur. There may be an association with atopic dermatitis or eczema. Marked and persistent lesions in AIDS patients respond readily to combination antiretroviral therapy. Treatment options include destructive therapies (curettage, cryotherapy, cantharidin, and keratolytics, among others), immunomodulators (imiquimod, cimetidine, and *Candida* antigen), and antiviral agents (topical cidofovir is effective anecdotally in refractory cases and there is some efficacy suggested for a new lipid acyclic nucleoside phosphonate called CMX001, an agent used for other viral infections, including in particular CMV). No treatment is uniformly effective and multiple courses of therapy are often needed. Cryptococcal skin lesions can mimic molluscum contagiosum.

3. Orf and paravaccinia—Orf (contagious pustular dermatitis, or ecthyma contagiosa) and paravaccinia (milker's nodules) are occupational diseases acquired by contact with sheep and cattle, respectively. Recently, household meat processing and animal slaughter have been implicated as non-traditional risk factors. A nosocomial outbreak occurred in 2012 in Turkey in a burn unit. Five cases in France were due to sheep exposures during the Muslim Feast of the Sacrifice (Eid al-Adha). Orf also occurs among children with ruminant exposures. Orf anecdotally responds to imiquimod.

4. Monkeypox—First identified in 1970, monkeypox is enzootic in the rain forests of equatorial Africa and presents in humans as a syndrome similar to smallpox. The incubation period is about 12 days, and limited person-to-person spread occurs. African mortality rates vary from 3% to 11% depending on the immune status of the patient. Secondary attack rates appear to be about 10%. The first community-acquired outbreak in the United States of monkeypox occurred in 2003 in Wisconsin and other states of the upper Midwest. Recent African outbreaks have been reported from the Sudan and the Democratic Republic of Congo. The source appeared to be imported Gambian giant rats via consequent exposure of prairie dogs. Other susceptible animals include nonhuman primates, rabbits, and rodents. Confusion with smallpox and varicella occurs; however, both lymphadenopathy (seen in up to 90% of unvaccinated persons) and a febrile prodrome are prominent features in monkeypox infection. Distinguishing characteristics of the monkeypox rash are its deep seated and well-circumscribed nature, it appears at the same stage of development (unlike varicella but like smallpox), and is centrifugal (including the palms and soles). Suspected cases should be placed on standard, contact and droplet precautions; and local and state public health officials, and the CDC should be notified for assistance with confirmation of the diagnosis (electron microscopy, viral culture, ELISA, PCR). Cidofovir is effective against monkeypox, and IVIG can be used in selected cases.

Other general precautions that should be taken are avoidance of contact with prairie dogs and Gambian giant rats (whose illness is manifested by alopecia, rash, and ocular or nasal discharge), appropriate care and isolation of those exposed within 3 prior weeks to such animals, and veterinary examination and investigation of suspect animals through health departments. Vaccinia immunization is effective against monkeypox and is recommended, if no contraindication exists (outlined above), for those involved in the investigation of the outbreak and for healthcare workers caring for those infected with monkeypox. Post exposure vaccination is also advised for documented contacts of infected persons or animals. US federal agencies currently prohibit the importation of African rodents.

Centers for Disease Control and Prevention (CDC). Human Orf virus infection from household exposures—United States, 2009–2011. MMWR Morb Mortal Wkly Rep. 2012 Apr 13;61(14):245–8. [PMID: 22495228]

Centers for Disease Control and Prevention (CDC). Secondary and tertiary transmission of vaccinia virus after sexual contact with a smallpox vaccine—San Diego, California, 2012. MMWR Morb Mortal Wkly Rep. 2013 Mar 1;62(8):145–7. [PMID: 23446513]

Centers for Disease Control and Prevention (CDC). Updated interim CDC guidance for use of smallpox vaccine, cidofovir, and vaccinia immune globulin (VIG) for prevention and treatment in the setting of an outbreak of monkeypox infections. http://www.cdc.gov/ncidod/monkeypox/treatment-guidelines.htm

Chen X et al. Molluscum contagiosum virus infection. Lancet Infect Dis. 2013 Oct;13(10):877–88. [PMID: 23972567]

Levy Y et al. Estimated size of the population at risk of severe adverse events after smallpox vaccination in Israel. Vaccine. 2012 Oct 19;30(47):6632–5. [PMID: 22963804]

Midilli K et al. Nosocomial outbreak of disseminated orf infection in a burn unit, Gaziantep, Turkey, October to December 2012. Euro Surveill. 2013 Mar 14;18(11):20425. Erratum in: Euro Surveill. 2013;18(14):20442. [PMID: 23517869]

Nougairede A et al. Sheep-to-human transmission of Orf virus during Eid al-Adha religious practices, France. Emerg Infect Dis. 2013 Jan;19(1):102–5. [PMID: 23260031]

Wertheimer ER et al. Contact transmission of vaccinia virus from smallpox vaccinees in the United States, 2003–2011. Vaccine. 2012 Feb 1;30(6):985–8. [PMID: 22192851]

VIRUSES & GASTROENTERITIS

Viruses are responsible for at least 30–40% of cases of infectious diarrhea in the United States. These agents include rotaviruses; caliciviruses, including noroviruses such as Norwalk virus; astroviruses; enteric adenoviruses; and, less often, toroviruses, coronaviruses, picornaviruses (including the Aichi virus), and pestiviruses. Rotaviruses and noroviruses are responsible for most of nonbacterial cases of gastroenteritis.

Rotavirus infections follow an endemic pattern, especially in the tropics and low-income countries, although they peak during the winter in temperate regions. The virus is transmitted by fecal-oral route and can be shed in feces for up to 3 weeks in severe infections. In outbreak settings (eg, daycare centers), the virus is ubiquitously found in the environment, and secondary attack rates are between 16% and 30% (including household contacts). Nosocomial outbreaks are reported. The disease is usually mild and self-limiting. A 2- to 3-day prodrome of fever and vomiting is followed by nonbloody diarrhea (up to 10–20 bowel movements per day) lasting for 1–4 days. The method of choice for diagnosis is PCR of the stool. It is thought that rarely systemic disease occurs and rare reported presentations include cerebellitis and pancreatitis. Treatment is largely symptomatic, with fluid and electrolyte replacement. A trial with nitazoxanide was attendant with moderate success among a small cohort of patients with gastroenteritis from Egypt with efficacy in both the rotavirus and norovirus subgroups. The enkephalinase inhibitor racecadotril (also known as acetorphan, given 1.5 mg/kg every 8 hours orally) is available in many countries (but not the United States), and in a meta-analysis appears to be clinically effective in reducing diarrheal symptoms. Local intestinal immunity gives protection against successive infection.

Two oral rotavirus vaccines are available in the United States: a live, oral, pentavalent human-bovine reassortment rotavirus vaccine (PRV, RotaTeq; to be given at 2, 4, and 6 months of age) and a live, oral attenuated monovalent human rotavirus vaccine (HRV, Rotarix; to be given at 2 and 4 months of age). The two vaccines show equal efficacy and the RotaTeq shows efficacy even with incomplete two-dose regimens. The pentavalent vaccine showed 40% efficacy in reducing the rate of new acute water diarrhea in a study among children under age 5 in Nicaragua. Contraindications include allergy to any of the vaccine ingredients, previous allergic reaction to the vaccine, and immunodeficiency. The risk of intussusception, which is far lower with this than earlier rotavirus preparations, is small (1:51,000 to 1:68,000 vaccinated infants) and is considered significantly lower than the risk associated with untreated rotavirus gastroenteritis.

The finding of small segments of a porcine circovirus in both Rotarix and RotaTeq is thought to be a contaminant derivative of the manufacturing process. These porcine circoviruses are abbreviated PCV and are not to be confused with pneumococcal conjugate vaccine. The manufacturers assure the public that both products are safe. Vaccine coverage is inadequate in the United States for rotavirus (68% in the 2012 National Immunization Study), particularly among the poor.

A new live, oral vaccine given as two doses at 2-month intervals, Rotavin-M1, was released in Vietnam in April 2012, and appears to be safe, effective, and easy to administer. A new oral vaccine in India is awaiting approval. This vaccine, RotaVac, is to be given at 6, 10, and 14 months, is safely coadministered with oral polio vaccines, and costs only a tenth of standard rotavirus vaccines. Neonatal viral strains are being used for vaccine development in Australia, the United States, and India, and alternative parenteral modes of immunization remain under study.

Noroviruses, such as Norwalk virus (one of a variety of small round viruses divided into 5 genogroups and at least 34 genotypes), are major causes of severe diarrhea in adults and are recognized as the major cause of epidemic gastroenteritis (with food handlers largely responsible and

associated foods most often leafy vegetables, fruits/nuts, and molluscs). They are responsible for a significant percentage of childhood hospitalizations for gastroenteritis in the developing world (15% in surveys from India, 31% from Peru) and about 13% of gastroenteritis-associated ambulatory visits in the United States. The efficacy of the rotavirus vaccination is increasing the percentage of gastroenteritis caused by norovirus. The noroviruses appear to evolve by antigenic drift (similar to influenza). While 90% of young adults show serologic evidence of past infection, no long-lasting protective immunity develops and reinfections are common. In the United States, noroviruses are responsible for over 90% of reported nonbacterial gastroenteritis outbreaks during cold weather intervals (hence the colloquial name "gastric flu"). Outbreak environments include long-term–care facilities (nursing homes in particular), restaurants, hospitals, schools, daycare centers, vacation destinations (including cruise ships), and military bases. Persons at particular risk are the young, the elderly, the institutionalized, and the immunosuppressed. A new strain that began in Australia (GII.4 Sydney) is responsible for increasing proportions of US cases and is transmitted most often in long-term–care facilities. Although transmission is usually fecal, oral, airborne, person-to-person, and waterborne transmission are also documented. A short incubation period (24–48 hours), a short symptomatic illness (12–60 hours, but up to 5 days in hospital-associated cases and in children under 11 years of age), a high frequency (> 50%) of vomiting, and absence of bacterial pathogens in stool samples are highly predictive of norovirus gastroenteritis. RT-PCR of stool samples is used for epidemiologic purposes. Treatment is largely symptomatic. Deaths are rare, and the more common associated diseases are aspiration pneumonia, septicemia, and necrotizing enterocolitis.

Outbreak control for both rotavirus and norovirus infections include strict adherence to general hygienic measures. Despite the promise of alcohol-based sanitizers for the control of pathogen transmission, such cleansers may be relatively ineffective against the noroviruses compared with antibacterial soap and water, reinforcing the need for new hygienic agents against this prevalent group of viruses. Cohorting of sick patients, contact precautions for symptomatic hospitalized patients, exclusion from work of symptomatic staff until symptom resolution (or 48–72 h after this for norovirus disease), and proper decontamination procedures are crucial.

The reports of efficacy with nitazoxanide or racecadotril in acute gastroenteritis suggest that new avenues of therapy may become more widely available in the future. Vaccine developments are attendant with the complications associated with the rapid evolution ("antigenic drift") of noroviruses, duration of immunity, and the probable need for annual strain selection to match circulating variants. Studies for an intranasally derived vaccine remain underway.

Atmar RL et al. Norovirus vaccine development: next steps. Expert Rev Vaccines. 2012 Sep;11(9):1023–5. [PMID: 23151158]

Becker-Dreps S et al. Community diarrhea incidence before and after rotavirus vaccine introduction in Nicaragua. Am J Trop Med Hyg. 2013 Aug;89(2):246–50. [PMID: 23817336]

Bresee JS et al; US Acute Gastroenteritis Etiology Study Team. The etiology of severe acute gastroenteritis among adults visiting emergency departments in the United States. J Infect Dis. 2012 May 1;205(9):1374–81. [PMID: 22454468]

Centers for Disease Control and Prevention (CDC). Building laboratory capacity to support the global rotavirus surveillance network. MMWR Morb Mortal Wkly Rep. 2013 May 24;62(20):409–12. [PMID: 23698607]

Cortese MM et al. Effectiveness of monovalent and pentavalent rotavirus vaccine. Pediatrics. 2013 Jul;132(1):e25–33. [PMID: 23776114]

Gastañaduy PA et al. Burden of norovirus gastroenteritis in the ambulatory setting—United States, 2001–2009. J Infect Dis. 2013 Apr;207(7):1058–65. [PMID: 23300161]

Hall AJ et al. Epidemiology of foodborne norovirus outbreaks, United States, 2001–2008. Emerg Infect Dis. 2012 Oct;18(10):1566–73. [PMID: 23017158]

Payne DC et al. Norovirus and medically attended gastroenteritis in U.S. children. N Engl J Med. 2013 Mar 21;368(12): 1121–30. [PMID: 23514289]

Soares-Weiser K et al. Vaccines for preventing rotavirus diarrhoea: vaccines in use. Cochrane Database Syst Rev. 2012 Nov 14;11:CD008521. [PMID: 23152260]

Trivedi TK et al. Hospitalizations and mortality associated with norovirus outbreaks in nursing homes, 2009–2010. JAMA. 2012 Oct 24;308(16):1668–75. [PMID: 23079758]

Vesikari T. Rotavirus vaccination: a concise review. Clin Microbiol Infect. 2012 Oct;18(Suppl 5):57–63. [PMID: 22882248]

ENTEROVIRUSES THAT PRODUCE SEVERAL SYNDROMES

The most famous enterovirus, the poliomyelitis virus, is discussed above under Vaccine Preventable Diseases. Other clinically relevant enteroviral infections are discussed in this section.

1. Coxsackievirus Infections

Coxsackievirus infections cause several clinical syndromes. As with other enteroviruses, infections are most common during the summer. Two groups, A and B, are defined either serologically or by mouse bioassay. There are more than 50 serotypes.

▶ **Clinical Findings**

A. Symptoms and Signs

The clinical syndromes associated with coxsackievirus infection are summer grippe; herpangina; epidemic pleurodynia; aseptic meningitis and other neurologic syndromes; acute nonspecific pericarditis; myocarditis; hand, foot, and mouth disease; epidemic conjunctivitis; and other syndromes.

1. Summer grippe (A and B)—A febrile illness, principally of children, summer grippe usually lasts 1–4 days. Minor symptoms of upper respiratory tract infection are often present.

2. Herpangina (A2–6, 10: B3)—There is sudden onset of fever, which may be as high as 40.6°C, sometimes with febrile convulsions. Other symptoms are headache, myalgia, and vomiting. The sore throat is characterized early by petechiae or papules on the soft palate that ulcerate in about 3 days and then heal. An outbreak in Taiwan with A2 was associated with herpangina and coincided with an enterovirus 71 (below) outbreak, characterized by hand, foot, and mouth disease. Dual A6/A10 outbreaks are reported from Europe. Treatment is symptomatic.

3. Epidemic pleurodynia (Bornholm disease) (B1–5)—Pleuritic pain is prominent. Tenderness, hyperesthesia, and muscle swelling are present over the area of diaphragmatic attachment. Other findings include headache, sore throat, malaise, nausea, and fever. Orchitis and aseptic meningitis occur in < 10% of patients. Most patients are ill for 4–6 days.

4. Aseptic meningitis (A and B) and other neurologic syndromes—Fever, headache, nausea, vomiting, stiff neck, drowsiness, and cerebrospinal fluid lymphocytosis without chemical abnormalities may occur, and pediatric clusters of group B (especially B5) meningitis are reported. Focal encephalitis and transverse myelitis are reported with coxsackievirus group A. Disseminated encephalitis occurs after group B infection, and acute flaccid paralysis is reported with both coxsackievirus group A and B. An outbreak of aseptic meningitis occurred in central China (Gansu Province) in 2008, with 85 cases reported of coxsackie A9 disease. Severe neonatal illnesses are reported with B1 infections, including encephalomyocarditis and neonatal deaths due to multiorgan failure.

5. Acute nonspecific pericarditis (B types)—Sudden onset of anterior chest pain, often worse with inspiration and in the supine position, is typical. Fever, myalgia, headache, and pericardial friction rub appear early and these symptoms are often transient. Evidence for pericardial effusion on imaging studies is often present, and the occasional patient has a paradoxical pulse. Electrocardiographic evidence of pericarditis is often present. Relapses may occur.

6. Myocarditis (B1–5)—Heart failure in the neonatal period secondary to in utero myocarditis and over 20% of adult cases of myocarditis and dilated cardiomyopathy are associated with group B (especially B3) infections.

7. Hand, foot, & mouth disease (A5, 6, 10, 12, and 16, B5)—This disease is sometimes epidemic and is characterized by stomatitis, a vesicular rash on hands and feet, nail dystrophies and onychomadesis (nail shedding). Enterovirus 71 is also a causative agent (see below).

8. Epidemic conjunctivitis—As with enterovirus 70 (see below), the A24 variant of coxsackievirus is associated with acute epidemic hemorrhagic conjunctivitis in tropical areas with outbreaks reported in the last few years in southern China, Pakistan, southern Sudan, the Comoros, Uganda, and Cuba.

9. Other syndromes associated with coxsackievirus infections—These include rhabdomyolysis, fulminant neonatal hepatitis (occurs rarely), infant sepsis (A10), glomerulopathy (group B infections), onychomadesis (B1), types 1 and 2 diabetes mellitus (mainly group B infections), and thyroid disease (group B4), although definitive causality is not established. A pathogenic role in primary Sjögren syndrome and acute myocardial infarction has also been proposed for group B coxsackievirus infections. A recent report of confirmed infective endocarditis due to coxsackievirus B2 in a patient with a prosthetic cardiac device suggests that viral etiologies of culture-negative infective endocarditis should be considered.

B. Laboratory Findings

Routine laboratory studies show no characteristic abnormalities. Neutralizing antibodies appear during convalescence. The virus may be isolated from throat washings or stools inoculated into suckling mice. Viral culture is expensive, labor demanding, and requires several days for results. A PCR test for enterovirus RNA is available and, although it cannot identify the serotype, it appears to be useful, particularly in cases of meningitis.

▶ Treatment & Prognosis

Treatment is symptomatic. With the exception of meningitis, myocarditis, pericarditis, diabetes, and rare illnesses such as pancreatitis or poliomyelitis-like states, the syndromes caused by coxsackieviruses are benign and self-limited. Two controlled trials showed a potential clinical benefit with pleconaril for patients with enteroviral meningitis although the compassionate use of this drug has stopped. There are anecdotal reports of success with IVIG in severe disease. Coxsackie A16 and enterovirus 71 (see below) in outbreaks of hand, foot, and mouth disease can be controlled with 5 minutes of exposure to 3120 ppm sodium hypochlorite.

Abzug MJ. The enteroviruses: problems in need of treatments. J Infect. 2014 Jan;68(Suppl 1):S108–14. [PMID: 24119825]

Centers for Disease Control and Prevention (CDC). Notes from the field: severe hand, foot, and mouth disease associated with coxsackievirus A6—Alabama, Connecticut, California, and Nevada, November 2011–February 2012. MMWR Morb Mortal Wkly Rep. 2012 Mar 30;61(12):213–4. [PMID: 22456122]

Gkrania-Klotsas E et al. The association between prior infection with five serotypes of Coxsackievirus B and incident type 2 diabetes mellitus in the EPIC-Norfolk study. Diabetologia. 2012 Apr;55(4):967–70. [PMID: 22231126]

Xu M et al. Enterovirus genotypes causing hand foot and mouth disease in Shanghai, China: a molecular epidemiological analysis. BMC Infect Dis. 2013 Oct 22;13:489. [PMID: 24148902]

2. Echovirus Infections

Echoviruses are enteroviruses that produce several clinical syndromes, particularly in children. Infection is most common during summer. Among reported specimens, death ensues in about 3%. Males younger than 20 years are more commonly infected than other persons.

Over 30 serotypes of echoviruses are recognized and the most common serotypes for disease are types 6, 9, 11, and 30. Most can cause aseptic meningitis, which may be associated with a rubelliform rash. Transmission is primarily fecal–oral. Handwashing is an effective control measure

in outbreaks of aseptic meningitis. Outbreaks related to fecal contamination of water sources, including drinking water and swimming and bathing pools, were reported in the past.

Besides meningitis, other conditions associated with echoviruses range from common respiratory diseases (bronchiolitis occurs often in children) and epidemic diarrhea to myocarditis, a hemorrhagic obstetric syndrome, keratoconjunctivitis, hepatitis with coagulopathy, leukocytoclastic vasculitis, and neonatal as well as adult cases of encephalitis and sepsis, interstitial pneumonitis, hemophagocytic syndromes (in children with cancer), sudden deafness, encephalitis, optic neuritis, uveitis, and septic shock. Echoviruses and enteroviruses are also a common cause of nonspecific exanthems.

As with other enterovirus infections, diagnosis is best established by correlation of clinical, epidemiologic, and laboratory evidence. Cytopathic effects are produced in tissue culture after recovery of virus from throat washings, blood, or cerebrospinal fluid. An enterovirus PCR of the cerebrospinal fluid can assist in the diagnosis and is associated with a shorter duration of hospitalization in febrile neonates. Fourfold or greater rises in antibody titer signify systemic infection.

Treatment is usually symptomatic, and the prognosis is excellent, though there are reports of mild paralysis after CNS infection. In vitro data suggest some role for amantadine or ribavirin but clinical studies supporting these findings are not available. Pleconaril is no longer available for compassionate use.

From a public health standpoint, clustered illnesses such as swimming in sewage-infested sea water in travelers suggest point-source exposure. Prevention of fecal–oral contamination and maintenance of pool hygiene through chlorination and pH control are important public health control measures.

Centers for Disease Control and Prevention (CDC). Nonpolio enterovirus and human parechovirus surveillance—United States, 2006–2008. MMWR Morb Mortal Wkly Rep. 2010 Dec 10;59(48):1577–80. [PMID: 21150865]

Maan HS et al. Genetic variants of echovirus 13, northern India, 2010. Emerg Infect Dis. 2013 Feb;19(2):293–6. [PMID: 23343581]

Wildenbeest JG et al. Pleconaril revisited: clinical course of chronic enteroviral meningoencephalitis after treatment correlates with in vitro susceptibility. Antivir Ther. 2012;17(3): 459–66. [PMID: 22293148]

3. Enteroviruses 70, 71, & Related Agents

Several distinct clinical syndromes are being described in association with enteroviruses. **Enterovirus 70 (HEV-70),** a ubiquitous agent first identified in 1969 and responsible for abrupt bilateral eye discharge and subconjunctival hemorrhage with occasional systemic symptoms, is most commonly associated with **acute hemorrhagic conjunctivitis.** Enterovirus infection of the pancreas can trigger cell-mediated autoimmune destruction of beta-cells resulting in diabetes. Enterovirus myocarditis can be a serious infection in neonates, complicated by cardiac dysfunction and arrhythmias. **Enterovirus 71 (HEV-71)** almost always occurs in the Asia-Pacific region and is associated with **hand, foot, and mouth disease** (HFMD), herpangina as well as a form of **epidemic encephalitis** associated on occasion with pulmonary edema, and **acute flaccid paralysis** often mimicking poliomyelitis. An outbreak of HFMD in Fuyang China in 2008 was caused by a recombinant virus between HEV-71 and coxsackievirus A16. In Taiwan, 29% of HEV-71 in children is asymptomatic. There is an association reported between gastrointestinal enterovirus infection and type 1 diabetes.

Human enteroviruses are neurotropic and a potential role for these viruses in amyotropic lateral sclerosis is the subject of some investigation.

Mortality is especially high in enterovirus 71-associated brainstem encephalitis, which is often complicated by pulmonary edema, particularly when it occurs in children younger than 5 years. A complication is autonomic nervous system dysregulation, which may develop prior to the pulmonary edema. Because of lower herd immunity, HFMD tends to infect the very young (under age 5) in nonendemic areas. Disease is usually more severe and sequelae more common than with other enteroviruses. Some children with enterovirus-associated cardiopulmonary failure require the usage of extracorporeal life support, which can improve the outcome. Recognized sequelae include central hypoventilation, dysphagia, and limb weakness.

Diagnosis of both entities is facilitated by the clinical and epidemiologic findings with the isolation of the suspect agent from conjunctival scraping for enterovirus 70 or vesicle swabs, body secretions, or cerebrospinal fluid for enterovirus 71. Enzyme immunoassays and complement fixation tests show good specificity but poor sensitivity (< 80%). RT-PCR may increase the detection rate in enterovirus infections and is useful in the analysis of cerebrospinal fluid samples among patients with meningitis and of blood samples among infants with a sepsis-like illness.

Treatment of both entities remains largely symptomatic. The role of immunoglobulins is under investigation. The major complication associated with enterovirus 70 is the rare development of an acute neurologic illness with motor paralysis akin to poliomyelitis. Attention-deficit with hyperactivity occurs in about 20% with confirmed infection.

Household contacts, especially children under 6 months of age, are at particular risk for enterovirus 71 acquisition. A commercial disinfectant, Virkon S, at 1–2% application, appears to reduce infectivity titers. A stage-based supportive treatment for enterovirus 71 infections, recognizing the potential for late onset CNS disease and cardiopulmonary failure is important. An E71 vaccine is in phase III clinical trials.

Enterovirus 72 (HEV-2) is another term for hepatitis A virus (see Chapter 16). Enterovirus EV-104A is related to rhinoviruses and associated with respiratory illness in reports from Italy and Switzerland.

Enterovirus 68 (HEV-68) is a unique enterovirus that shares epidemiologic characteristics with human rhinovirus and is typically associated with respiratory illness. Several clusters are reported from the Netherlands, Japan, the Philippines, the United States, and Thailand. The agent is implicated in a recent, fatal case of meningomyeloencephalitis.

Centers for Disease Control and Prevention (CDC). Clusters of acute respiratory illness associated with human enterovirus 68—Asia, Europe, and United States, 2008–2010. MMWR Morb Mortal Wkly Rep. 2011 Sep 30;60(38):1301–4. [PMID: 21956405]

Li YP et al. Immunogenicity, safety, and immune persistence of a novel inactivated human enterovirus 71 vaccine: a phase II, Randomized, double-blind, placebo-controlled Trial. J Infect Dis. 2014 Jan 1;209(1):46–55. [PMID: 23922377]

Oikarinen M et al. Type 1 diabetes is associated with enterovirus infection in gut mucosa. Diabetes. 2012 Mar;61(3):687–91. [PMID: 22315304]

4. Human Parechovirus Infection (HPeV)

HPeV is a member of the Picornaviridae family. The pathogen mainly affects small children although disease can also occur in older adults. Cases are spread worldwide. There were 16 genotypes recognized worldwide by 2013. Clinical presentation is mainly driven by gastrointestinal and respiratory illness, although otitis, neonatal sepsis, flaccid paralysis, myalgias, diffuse maculopapular and palmar-plantar rashes, aseptic meningitis, and encephalitis are described in the literature.

The added screening with a human parechovirus-specific PCR provides a significant increase in determining the viral cause of neonatal sepsis or CNS symptoms in children younger than 5 years. Human parechoviruses are one of the leading causes of viral sepsis and meningitis in young children. HPeV1 is the most prevalent genotype found among stool and nasopharyngeal samples in children (under 2 years old), whereas HPeV6 affects older individuals (> 20 years old). HPeV3 is responsible for encephalitis, neonatal sepsis, and was recently reported in association with necrotizing enterocolitis and hepatitis. It is the most prevalent picornavirus type found in cerebrospinal fluid samples of CNS-related infections in very young children. Respiratory and gastrointestinal illnesses are seen with types HPeV4–HPeV6, HPeV10, HPeV13-HPeV15. Neonatal deaths are reported with HPeV3 and HPeV6. Treatment is largely supportive and rapid identification of the viral antigen by PCR in stools, respiratory samples, and cerebrospinal fluid may decrease use of unnecessary antibiotics and shorten hospital stay, although current PCR assays are not always sufficiently sensitive to exclude parechoviruses. Reported complications of neonatal cerebral infections include learning disabilities, epilepsy, and cerebral palsy.

Alam MM et al. Human parechovirus genotypes -10, -13 and -15 in Pakistani children with acute dehydrating gastroenteritis. PLoS One. 2013 Nov 12;8(11):e78377. [PMID: 24265685]

Chen H et al. Molecular detection of human parechovirus in children with acute gastroenteritis in Guangzhou, China. Arch Virol. 2013 Nov 13. [Epub ahead of print] [PMID: 24221251]

Eis-Hübinger AM et al. Two cases of sepsis-like illness in infants caused by human parechovirus traced back to elder siblings with mild gastroenteritis and respiratory symptoms. J Clin Microbiol. 2013 Feb;51(2):715–8. [PMID: 23241372]

RICKETTSIAL DISEASES

TYPHUS GROUP

1. Epidemic Louse-Borne Typhus

ESSENTIALS OF DIAGNOSIS

▶ Prodrome of headache, then chills and fever.

▶ Severe, intractable headaches, prostration, persisting high fever.

▶ Macular rash appearing on the fourth to seventh days on the trunk and in the axillae, spreading to the rest of the body but sparing the face, palms, and soles.

▶ Diagnosis confirmed by specific antibodies using complement fixation, microagglutination, or immunofluorescence.

▶ General Considerations

Epidemic louse-borne typhus is caused by *Rickettsia prowazekii*, an obligate parasite of the body louse *Pediculus humanus corporis* (Table 32–3). Transmission is favored by crowded, unsanitary living conditions, famine, war, or any circumstances that predispose to heavy infestation with lice. After biting a person infected with *R prowazekii*, the louse becomes infected by the organism, which persists in the louse gut and is excreted in its feces. When the same louse bites an uninfected individual, the feces gain entry into the bloodstream when the person scratches the itching wound. Dry, infectious louse feces may also enter via the respiratory tract. Cases can be acquired by travel to pockets of infection (eg, central and northeastern Africa, Central and South America). Outbreaks have been reported from Peru, Burundi, and Russia. Because of aerosol transmissibility, *R prowazekii* is considered a possible bioterrorism agent. In the United States, cases occur among the homeless, refugees, and the unhygienic, most often in the winter.

R prowazekii can survive in lymphoid and adipose (in endothelial reservoirs) tissues after primary infection, and years later, produce recrudescence of disease (**Brill-Zinsser disease**) without exposure to infected lice. This phenomenon can serve as a point source for future outbreaks.

An extrahuman reservoir of *R prowazekii* in the United States is flying squirrels, *Glaucomys volans*. Transmission to humans can occur through their ectoparasites, usually causing atypical mild disease. A case of recrudescent (Brill-Zinsser) disease 11 years after disease acquired by contact with flying squirrels is reported. Foci of sylvatic typhus are found in the eastern United States and are reported to occur in Brazil, Ethiopia, and Mexico.

▶ Clinical Findings

A. Symptoms and Signs

(Table 32–2). Prodromal malaise, cough, headache, backache, arthralgia, and chest pain begin after an incubation period of 10–14 days, followed by an abrupt onset of chills, high fever, and prostration, with flu-like symptoms progressing to delirium and stupor. The headache is severe and the fever is prolonged.

Other findings consist of conjunctivitis, mild vitritis, retinal lesions, optic neuritis, and hearing loss from neuropathy of the eighth cranial nerve, flushed facies, rales at the lung bases, abdominal pain, myalgias, and often splenomegaly. A macular rash (that may become confluent) appears first in the axillae and then over the trunk, spreading to the extremities but rarely involving the face, palms, or soles. In severely ill patients, the rash becomes hemorrhagic, and hypotension becomes marked. There may be acute kidney injury, stupor, seizures, and delirium. Improvement begins 13–16 days after onset with a rapid drop of fever and typically a spontaneous recovery.

B. Laboratory Findings

The white blood cell count is variable. Thrombocytopenia, elevated liver enzymes, proteinuria and hematuria commonly occur. Serum obtained 5–12 days after onset of symptoms usually shows specific antibodies for *R prowazekii* antigens as demonstrated by complement fixation, microagglutination, or immunofluorescence. In primary rickettsial infection, early antibodies are IgM; in recrudescence (Brill-Zinsser disease), early antibodies are predominantly IgG. A PCR test exists, but its availability is limited. *R prowazekii* is differentiated into 7 genotypes.

C. Imaging

Radiographs of the chest may show patchy consolidation.

▶ Differential Diagnosis

The prodromal symptoms and the early febrile stage lack enough specificity to permit diagnosis in nonepidemic situations. The rash is sufficiently distinctive for diagnosis, but it may be absent in up to 50% of cases or may be difficult to observe in dark-skinned persons. A variety of other acute febrile diseases should be considered, including typhoid fever, meningococcemia, and measles.

▶ Complications

Pneumonia, thromboses, vasculitis with major vessel obstruction and gangrene, circulatory collapse, myocarditis, and uremia may occur.

▶ Treatment

Treatment consists of either doxycycline (100 mg orally twice daily) or chloramphenicol (50–100 mg/kg/d in four divided doses, orally or intravenously) for 4–10 days. Chloramphenicol is considered less effective than doxycycline, but it is still the drug of choice in pregnancy. In epidemic conditions, a single dose of doxycycline can be effective and is less costly.

Table 32–3. Rickettsial diseases.

Disease	Rickettsial Pathogen	Geographic Areas of Prevalence	Insect Vector	Mammalian Reservoir	Travel Association
Typhus group					
Epidemic (louse-borne) typhus	*Rickettsia prowazekii*	South America, Northeastern and Central Africa	Louse	Humans, flying squirrels	Rare
Endemic (murine) typhus	*Rickettsia typhi*	Worldwide; small foci (United States: southeastern Gulf coast)	Flea	Rodents, opossums	Often
Scrub typhus group					
Scrub typhus	*Orientia tsutsugamushi*	Southeast Asia, Japan, Australia, Western Siberia	Mite[1]	Rodents	Often
Spotted fever group					
Rocky Mountain spotted fever	*Rickettsia rickettsii*	Western Hemisphere; United States (especially mid-Atlantic coast region)	Tick[1]	Rodents, dogs, porcupines	Rare
California flea rickettsiosis	*Rickettsia felis*	Worldwide	Flea	Cats, opossums	
Mediterranean spotted fever, Boutonneuse fever, Kenya tick typhus, South African tick fever, Indian tick typhus	*Rickettsia conorii*	Africa, India, Mediterranean regions	Tick[1]	Rodents, dogs	Often
Queensland tick typhus	*Rickettsia australis*	Eastern Australia	Tick[1]	Rodents, marsupials	Rare
Siberian Asian tick typhus	*Rickettsia sibirica*	Siberia, Mongolia	Tick[1]	Rodents	Rare
African tick bite fever	*Rickettsia africae*	Rural sub-Saharan Africa, Eastern Caribbean	Tick[1]	Cattle	Often
Rickettsialpox	*Rickettsia akari*	United States, Korea, former USSR	Mite[1]	Mice	
Other					
Ehrlichiosis and anaplasmosis, human Monocytic	*Ehrlichia chaffeensis, Anaplasma equi, Ehrlichia canis*	Southeastern United States	Tick[1]	Dogs	
Granulocytic	*Anaplasma phago-cytophilum, Ehrlichia ewingii*	Northeastern United States	Tick[1]	Rodents, deer, sheep	
Q fever	*Coxiella burnetii*	Worldwide	None[2]	Cattle, sheep, goats	

[1]Also serve as arthropod reservoirs by maintaining rickettsiae through transovarian transmission.
[2]Human infection results from inhalation of dust.

▶ Prognosis

The prognosis depends greatly on the patient's age and immune status. In children under age 10 years, the disease is usually mild. The mortality rate is 10% in the second and third decades but in the past reached 60% in the sixth decade. Brill-Zinsser disease (recrudescent epidemic typhus) has a more gradual onset than primary *R prowazekii* infection, fever and rash are of shorter duration, and the disease is milder and rarely fatal.

▶ Prevention

Prevention consists of louse control with insecticides, particularly by applying chemicals to clothing or treating it with heat, and frequent bathing. The control of typhus in Finland during World War II is attributed to sauna use.

A deloused and bathed typhus patient is not infectious. The disease is not transmitted from person to person. Patients are infectious for the lice during the febrile period and perhaps 2–3 days after the fever returns to normal. Infected lice pass rickettsiae in their feces within 2–6 days after the blood meal and can be infectious earlier if crushed. Rickettsiae remain viable in a dead louse for weeks.

No vaccine is currently available for the prevention of *R prowazekii* infection.

Badiaga S et al. Human louse-transmitted infectious diseases. Clin Microbiol Infect. 2012 Apr;18(4):332–7. [PMID: 22360386]

Faucher JF et al. Brill-Zinsser disease in Moroccan man, France, 2011. Emerg Infect Dis. 2012 Jan;18(1):171–2. [PMID: 22261378]

2. Endemic Flea-Borne Typhus (Murine Typhus)

Rickettsia typhi, a ubiquitous pathogen recognized on all continents, is transmitted from rat to rat through the rat flea (Table 32–3). Serosurveys of animals show high prevalence of antibodies to *R typhi* in opossums, followed by dogs and cats. Humans usually acquire the infection in an urban or suburban setting when bitten by an infected flea, which releases infected feces while sucking blood. Rare human cases in the developed world follow travel, usually to Southeast Asia, Africa (Burundi and Ethiopia have foci of infection), or the Mediterranean area although other pockets of infection are also known to occur in the Andes. In the United States, cases are mainly reported from Texas and Southern California.

Endemic typhus resembles recrudescent epidemic typhus in that it has a gradual onset, less severe symptoms, and a shorter duration of illness than epidemic typhus (7–10 days versus 14–21 days). The presentation is nonspecific, including fever, headache, and chills. Maculopapular rash occurs in around 50% of cases; it is concentrated on the trunk and fades fairly rapidly. Liver dysfunction occurs in the majority of cases. Peripheral facial paralysis and splenic infarction are reported to occur. Severe disease with mental confusion and signs of hepatic, cardiac, renal, and pulmonary involvement may develop. Postinfectious optic neuritis is rare and may occur weeks after successful treatment. Rare complications include a respiratory distress syndrome and a hemophagocytosis syndrome. Jaundice, bradycardia, and the absence of a headache are correlated with a delayed defervescence (in both epidemic and endemic typhus).

The most common entity in the differential diagnosis is Rocky Mountain spotted fever, usually occurring after a rural exposure and with a different rash (centripetal versus centrifugal for epidemic or endemic typhus). Serologic confirmation may be necessary for differentiation, with complement-fixing or immunofluorescent antibodies detectable within 15 days after onset, with specific *R typhi* antigens. A fourfold rise in serum antibody titers between the acute and the convalescence phase is diagnostic.

Antibiotic treatment is the same as for epidemic typhus (see above). Ciprofloxacin (500–750 mg orally twice a day) and ampicillin (500 mg orally three times a day) are reportedly successful in pregnant women. Mortality is usually low with (1%) or without (4%) appropriate antibiotics. Preventive measures are directed at control of rats and ectoparasites (rat fleas) with insecticides, rat poisons, and rat-proofing of buildings.

Anyfantakis D et al. Liver function test abnormalities in murine typhus in Greece: a retrospective study of 165 cases. Infez Med. 2013 Sep;21(3):207–10. [PMID: 24008853]

Badiaga S et al. Murine typhus in the homeless. Comp Immunol Microbiol Infect Dis. 2012 Jan;35(1):39–43. [PMID: 22093517]

Raby E et al. Endemic (murine) typhus in returned travelers from Asia, a case series: clues to early diagnosis and comparison with dengue. Am J Trop Med Hyg. 2013 Apr;88(4):701–3. [PMID: 23358638]

3. Scrub Typhus (Tsutsugamushi Fever)

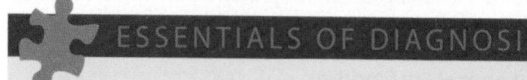

ESSENTIALS OF DIAGNOSIS

▶ Exposure to mites in endemic area of Southeast Asia, the western Pacific (including Korea), and Australia.

▶ Black eschar at site of the bite, with regional and generalized lymphadenopathy.

▶ High fever, headache, myalgia, and a short-lived macular rash.

▶ Frequent pneumonitis, encephalitis, and cardiac failure.

▶ General Considerations

Scrub typhus is caused by *Orientia tsutsugamushi*, which is principally a parasite of rodents and is transmitted by larval trombiculid mites (chiggers). The disease is endemic in Korea, China, Taiwan, Japan, Pakistan, India, Thailand, Malaysia and Queensland, Australia (Table 32–3), which form an area known as the "tsutsugamushi triangle". Transmission is often more common at higher altitudes. The mites live on vegetation but complete their maturation cycle by biting humans who come in contact with infested vegetation. Therefore, the disease is more common in rural areas within these countries. Vertical transmission occurs, and blood transfusions may transmit the pathogen as well. Rare occupational transmission via inhalation is documented among laboratory workers.

▶ Clinical Findings

A. Symptoms and Signs

After a 1- to 3-week incubation period, malaise, chills, severe headache and backache develop. At the site of the bite, a papule evolves into a flat black eschar, a finding which is usually helpful for diagnosis. The regional lymph nodes are commonly enlarged and tender, and sometimes a more generalized adenopathy occurs. Fever rises gradually during the first week of infection and the rash is usually macular and primarily on the trunk area. The rash can be fleeting or more severe, peaking at 8 days but lasting up to 21 days after onset of infection. The patient may become obtunded. Gastrointestinal symptoms including nausea, vomiting, and diarrhea occur in nearly two-thirds of patients and correspond to the presence of superficial mucosal hemorrhage, multiple erosions, or ulcers in the gastrointestinal tract. Both acalculous cholecystitis and acute abdominal attacks are reported. Transient parkinsonism, opsoclonus, or myoclonus may occur. Severe complications, such as pneumonitis, myocarditis and heart failure, encephalitis or meningitis, acute abdominal pain, peritonitis, granulomatous hepatitis, disseminated intravascular coagulation, cerebrovascular hemorrhage or infarction, ARDS, hemophagocytosis, or acute kidney disease may develop during the second or third week. An attack confers prolonged immunity against homologous strains and transient immunity against heterologous strains. Heterologous strains produce mild disease if infection occurs within a year after the first episode.

B. Laboratory Findings

Thrombocytopenia and elevation of liver enzymes, bilirubin, and creatinine are common. Serologic testing with immunofluorescence and immunoperoxidase assays or commercial dot-blot ELISA dipstick assays are convenient diagnostic aids, but a conclusive diagnosis requires documentation of a fourfold increase between acute and convalescence titers of antibodies. An indirect immunofluorescence assay is the mainstay of serologic diagnosis and titers quickly lose sensitivity so should be read as soon as possible after collection. A rapid immunochromatographic test for IgM and IgG detection is more sensitive and specific than the standard immunofluorescence assay. PCR (from the eschar or blood) may be the most sensitive diagnostic test but remains positive even after the initiation of treatment. Culture of the organism (by mouse inoculation) from blood obtained in the first few days of illness is another diagnostic modality but requires a specialized BioSafety Level 3 laboratory. Filter paper immunofluorescent assays are as sensitive and specific as paired sera and may be especially useful in field settings.

▶ Differential Diagnosis

Leptospirosis, typhoid, dengue, malaria, Q fever, hemorrhagic fevers, and other rickettsial infections should be considered. The headache may mimic trigeminal neuralgia. Scrub typhus is a recognized cause of obscure tropical fevers, especially in children.

▶ Treatment & Prognosis

Without treatment, fever subsides spontaneously after 2 weeks, but the mortality rate may be 10–30%. Empiric treatment for 3 days with doxycycline, 100 mg orally twice daily, or with minocyline, 100 mg intravenously twice daily, or for 7 days with chloramphenicol, 25 mg/kg/d orally or intravenously in four divided doses, eliminates most deaths and relapses. Chloramphenicol- and tetracycline-resistant strains have been reported from Southeast Asia, where azithromycin or roxythromycin may become the drug of choice for children, pregnant women, and patients with refractory disease. Rifampin reduces the duration of fever by 1 day when used with doxycycline.

Poor prognostic factors include requiring care in an ICU, high APACHE-II scores, age over 60 years, absence of an eschar (making the diagnosis difficult) and laboratory findings such as leukocytosis or hypoalbuminemia. HIV infection does not appear to influence the severity of scrub typhus.

▶ Prevention

Repeated application of long-acting miticides can make endemic areas safe. Insect repellents on clothing and skin as well as protective clothing are effective preventive measures. For short exposure, chemoprophylaxis with doxycycline (200 mg weekly) can prevent the disease but permits infection. No effective vaccines are available.

Chiou YH et al. Scrub typhus associated with transient parkinsonism and myoclonus. J Clin Neurosci. 2013 Jan;20(1):182–3. [PMID: 23010430]

Chung JH et al. Scrub typhus and cerebrovascular injury: a phenomenon of delayed treatment? Am J Trop Med Hyg. 2013 Jul;89(1):119–22. [PMID: 23716407]

Lee CH et al. Peritonitis in patients with scrub typhus. Am J Trop Med Hyg. 2012 Jun;86(6):1046–8. [PMID: 22665616]

Silpasakorn S et al. Development of new, broadly reactive, rapid IgG and IgM lateral flow assays for diagnosis of scrub typhus. Am J Trop Med Hyg. 2012 Jul;87(1):148–52. [PMID: 22764306]

SPOTTED FEVERS

1. Rocky Mountain Spotted Fever

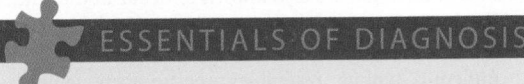

ESSENTIALS OF DIAGNOSIS

▶ Exposure to tick bite in an endemic area.

▶ An influenza-like prodrome followed by chills, fever, severe headache, and myalgias; occasionally, delirium and coma.

▶ Red macular rash appears between the second and sixth days of fever, first on the wrists and ankles and then spreading centrally; it may become petechial.

▶ Serial serologic examinations by indirect fluorescent antibody confirm the diagnosis retrospectively.

▶ General Considerations

Despite its name, most cases of Rocky Mountain spotted fever (RMSF) occur outside the Rocky Mountain area. Passive surveillance data from 2002 to 2007 reported cases from 46 states and the District of Columbia. More than half (64%) of these cases were from only five states: North Carolina, Tennessee, Oklahoma, Missouri, and Arkansas. RMSF is endemic in Central and Southern America with a small fatal familiar cluster reported from Panama (Table 32–3). Native American residents are at high risk for infection. The causative agent, *R rickettsii*, is transmitted to humans by the bite of ticks, including the Rocky Mountain wood tick, *D andersoni*, in the western United States, and the American dog tick, *Dermacentor variabilis*, in the eastern United States. Several hours of contact between the tick and the human host are required for transmission. The brown dog tick, *Rhipicephalus sanguineus*, is a vector in eastern Arizona and responsible for many Native American cases. Other hard ticks transmit the organism in the southern United States and in Central and South America and are responsible for transmitting it among rodents, dogs, porcupines, and other animals. There are 25 genotypes of *R rickettsii* in four different groups, and potential genomic-clinical correlations are underway.

In the United States, the estimated annual incidence of RMSF is increasing to as high as seven cases per million persons (primarily occurring from April through September), with a higher incidence among children and men.

Better diagnostic capacity and improved surveillance are thought responsible for the changing epidemiology.

▶ Clinical Findings

A. Symptoms and Signs

RMSF can cause severe multiorgan dysfunction and fatality rates of up to 73% if left untreated, making it the most serious rickettsial disease. Two to 14 days (mean, 7 days) after the bite of an infectious tick, symptoms begin with the abrupt onset of high fevers, chills, headache, nausea and vomiting, myalgias, restlessness, insomnia, and irritability. The characteristic rash (faint macules that progress to maculopapules and then petechiae) appears between days 2 and 6 of fever. It initially involves the wrists and ankles, spreading *centrally* to the arms, legs, and trunk over the next 2–3 days. Involvement of the palms and soles is characteristic. Facial flushing, conjunctival injection, and hard palatal lesions (Figure 32–6) may occur. In about 10% of cases, however, no rash or only a minimal rash is seen. Cough and pneumonitis may develop and delirium, lethargy, seizures, stupor, and coma may also appear in more severe cases. Splenomegaly, hepatomegaly, jaundice, myocarditis (which may mimic an acute coronary syndrome), adrenal hemorrhage, or uremia are occasionally present. ARDS and necrotizing vasculitis, when present, are of greatest concern.

B. Laboratory Findings

Thrombocytopenia, hyponatremia, elevated aminotransferases, and hyperbilirubinemia are common. Cerebrospinal fluid may show hypoglycorrhachia and mild pleocytosis. Disseminated intravascular coagulation is observed in severe cases. Diagnosis during the acute phase of the illness can be made by immunohistologic (including PCR) demonstration of *R rickettsiae* in skin biopsy specimens (or cutaneous swabs of eschars or skin lesions), but sensitivity is maximized by performing such studies as soon as skin lesions become apparent and before antibiotics commence. Isolation of the organism using the shell-vial technique is available in some laboratories but is hazardous.

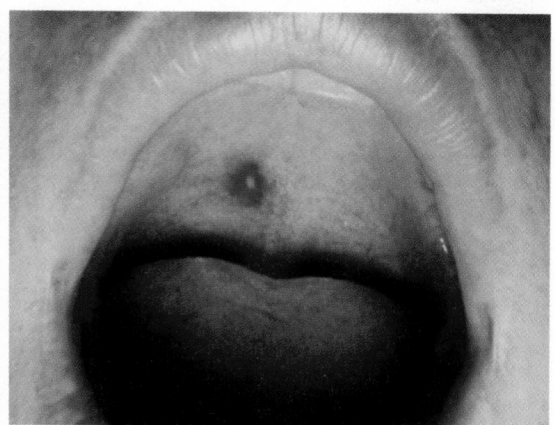

▲ **Figure 32–6.** Hard palate lesion caused by Rocky Mountain spotted fever. (Public Health Image Library, CDC.)

Serologic studies confirm the diagnosis, but most patients do not mount an antibody response until the second week of illness. The indirect fluorescent antibody test is most commonly used. No commercial PCR technique is validated for serologic use.

▶ Differential Diagnosis

The diagnosis is challenging because early symptoms resemble those of many other infections. The classic triad of fever, rash, and tick bite is rarely recognized, with up to 40% of patients not recalling a tick bite. Moreover, the rash may be confused with that of measles, typhoid, and ehrlichiosis, or—most importantly—meningococcemia. Blood cultures and examination of cerebrospinal fluid establish the latter. Some spotted fever rickettsioses may also mimic RMSF.

▶ Treatment & Prognosis

Treatment with doxycycline at similar doses and duration as for epidemic typhus (100 mg orally twice daily for 4–10 days) is recommended, including for children. Similarly, chloramphenicol (50–100 mg/kg/d in four divided doses, orally or intravenously for 4–10 days) is the preferred alternative during pregnancy. Patients usually defervesce within 48–72 hours and therapy should be maintained for at least 3 days after defervescence occurs. Mild cases in low-risk individuals may be observed without treatment.

The reported mortality rate in the United States is about 3–5%. The following features are associated with increased mortality: (1) infection in very young children, the elderly, or Native Americans; (2) the presence of atypical clinical features (absence of headache, no history of tick attachment, gastrointestinal symptoms) and underlying chronic diseases; (3), and a delay in initiation of appropriate antibiotic therapy. The usual cause of death is pneumonitis with respiratory or cardiac failure. Sequelae may include seizures, encephalopathy, peripheral neuropathy, paraparesis, bowel and bladder incontinence, cerebellar and vestibular dysfunction, hearing loss, and motor deficits.

▶ Prevention

Protective clothing, tick-repellent chemicals, and the removal of ticks at frequent intervals are helpful measures. Prophylactic therapy after a tick bite is not currently recommended.

Dahlgren FS et al. Fatal Rocky Mountain spotted fever in the United States, 1999–2007. Am J Trop Med Hyg. 2012 Apr;86(4):713–9. [PMID: 22492159]

Mosites E et al. Knowledge, attitudes, and practices regarding Rocky Mountain spotted fever among healthcare providers, Tennessee, 2009. Am J Trop Med Hyg. 2013 Jan;88(1):162–6. [PMID: 23243110]

Woods CR. Rocky Mountain spotted fever in children. Pediatr Clin North Am. 2013 Apr;60(2):455–70. [PMID: 23481111]

2. Rickettsialpox

Rickettsialpox is an acute, self-limiting, febrile illness caused by *Rickettsia akari,* a parasite of mice, transmitted by the mite *Liponyssoides sanguineus* (Table 32–3). Infections are reported globally. Seroprevalence studies done on injection drug users in inner Baltimore showed antibody positivity as high as 16%. The illness has also been found in farming communities. Crowded conditions and mouse-infested housing allow transmission of the pathogen to humans. The primary lesion is a painless red papule that vesiculates and forms a black eschar followed by an incubation period of 7–12 days. Onset of symptoms is sudden, with chills, fever, headache, photophobia, and disseminated aches and pains. Two to 4 days later, a widespread papular eruption appears. The rash becomes vesicular and forms crusts that are shed in about 10 days. Early lesions may resemble those of chickenpox (typically vesicular versus papulovesicular in rickettsialpox). Pathologic findings include dermal edema, subepidermal vesicles, and at times a lymphocytic vasculitis.

Transient leukopenia and thrombocytopenia and acute hepatitis can occur. A fourfold rise in serum antibody titers to rickettsial antigen, detected by complement fixation or indirect fluorescent assays, is diagnostic. Conjugated antirickettsial globulin can identify antigen in punch biopsies of skin lesions. PCR detection of rickettsial DNA in fresh tissue also appears of value. *R akari* can reportedly also be isolated from eschar biopsy specimens.

Treatment consists of oral doxycycline (200 mg/d) for 7 days. The disease is usually mild and self-limited without treatment, but occasionally severe symptoms may require hospitalization. Control requires the elimination of mice from human habitations and insecticide applications.

Eremeeva ME et al. Investigation of an outbreak of rickettsial febrile illness in Guatemala, 2007. Int J Infect Dis. 2013 May;17(5):e304–11. [PMID: 23266334]
Renvoisé A et al. A case of rickettsialpox in Northern Europe. Int J Infect Dis. 2012 Mar;16(3):e221–2. [PMID: 22257655]

3. Tick Typhus (Rickettsial Fever)

The term "tick typhus" denotes a variety of spotted rickettsial fevers, often named by their geographic location (eg, Mediterranean spotted fever, Queensland tick typhus, Oriental spotted fever, African tick bite fever, Siberian tick typhus, North Asian tick typhus), or by morphology (eg, boutonneuse fever). These illnesses are transmitted by tick vectors of the rickettsial organisms *R africae*, *R australis*, *R conorii*, *R japonica*, *R massiliae*, *R parkeri*, and *R sibirica* (Table 32–3). Dogs and wild animals, usually rodents and even reptiles, may serve as reservoirs. Travel is a risk factor for disease, particularly among elderly ecotourists. In a series of 280 international travelers with rickettsial disease, the most common cause was spotted fever rickettsiosis (231 cases, 82.5% of the total) followed by scrub typhus (16, 5.7%). The pathogens usually produce an eschar or black spot (tâche noire) at the site of the tick bite that may be useful in diagnosis, though spotless boutonneuse fever occurs. Symptoms include fever, headache, myalgias, and rash. Rarely, papulovesicular lesions may resemble rickettsialpox. Endothelial injury produces perivascular edema and dermal necrosis. Regional adenopathy, disseminated lesions, kidney disease, splenic rupture, and focal hepatic necrosis may occur. Neurologic manifestations, including encephalitis, internuclear ophthalmoplegia, coronary involvement, and the hemophagocytic syndrome, are rare.

The diagnosis is clinical, with serologic or PCR (culture can be used but is less sensitive than either) used for confirmation, and treatment should be started upon clinical suspicion since delayed therapy is the usual cause of increased morbidity. Oral treatment with doxycycline (200 mg/d) or chloramphenicol (50–75 mg/kg/d in four divided doses) for 7–10 days is indicated. Caution is advised with the use of ciprofloxacin because it is associated with a poor outcome and increases the severity of disease in Mediterranean spotted fever. The combination of azithromycin and rifampin is effective and safe in pregnancy. Prevention entails protective clothing, repellents, and inspection for and removal of ticks.

Formerly classified as an endemic or murine typhus, the cat-flea typhus, caused by *Rickettsia felis* is now more properly classified as a spotted fever. The causative agent has been linked to the cat flea and opossum exposure. Most cases in the United States (southern Texas and California, and possibly Hawaii) occur in the spring and summer. Treatment is the same as for other rickettsial fevers.

A rickettsial infection recognized as a cause of eschar-associated illness was recognized in northern California and is referred to as the spotted fever group rickettsia 364D.

Angelakis E et al. Comparison of real-time quantitative PCR and culture for the diagnosis of emerging Rickettsioses. PLoS Negl Trop Dis. 2012;6(3):e1540. [PMID: 22413026]
Blanton LS. Rickettsial infections in the tropics and in the traveler. Curr Opin Infect Dis. 2013 Oct;26(5):435–40. [PMID: 23842049]
Wilson PA et al. Queensland tick typhus: three cases with unusual clinical features. Intern Med J. 2013 Jul;43(7):823–5. [PMID: 23841762]

OTHER RICKETTSIAL & RICKETTSIAL-LIKE DISEASES

1. Ehrlichiosis & Anaplasmosis

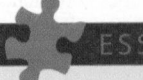
ESSENTIALS OF DIAGNOSIS

▶ Infection of monocyte or granulocyte by tick-borne gram-negative bacteria.

▶ Nine-day incubation period, with variable clinical illness, ranging from asymptomatic to persistent or life threatening.

▶ Common symptoms are malaise, nausea, fever, and headaches.

▶ US cases are largely in elderly white men in the summer.

▶ Excellent response to therapy with tetracyclines.

▶ General Considerations

Ehrlichiae and anaplasmae are small tick-borne gram-negative obligate intracellular bacteria that infect monocytes or granulocytes. Human monocytic ehrlichiosis is caused by *Ehrlichia chaffeensis* (Table 32–3). Human granulocytic anaplasmosis is caused by *Anasplasma phagocytophilium*. *Ehrlichia ewingii* (infecting primarily dogs) can rarely cause human granulocytic ehrlichiosis (also referred to as *E ewingii* ehrlichiosis) similar to human granulocytic anaplasmosis. A third *Ehrlichia* species that infects humans appears to be related to *Ehrlichia muris*. An *Ehrlichia*-like organism, *Neorickettsia sennetsu,* is the etiologic agent of sennetsu fever, which is confined to western Japan.

Human monocytic ehrlichiosis is seen primarily in the South Central states (especially Arkansas, Missouri, and Oklahoma) of the United States, although cases are also recognized in Israel, Japan, Mexico, South America, and Europe. Human granulocytic anaplasmosis is more frequent in the upper Midwestern United States; but infections in Europe and China are also well documented. Human infection with *E ewingii* is limited to Missouri, Oklahoma, and Tennessee and occurs mainly among the immunocompromised. In North America, the major vectors for these pathogens are the Lone Star tick (*Amblyomma americanus* for *E chaffeensis* and *E ewingii*), the western black-legged tick (*Ixodes pacificus*, for *E chaffeensis*), and *Ixodes scapularis* (the same vector for Lyme disease and babesiosis for *A phagocytophilium*). Reported incidences of both human monocytic and granulocytic ehrlichiosis are increasing and both are now at about 3 per million, respectively, with higher rates in the summer among whites and among men. Up to 4.9% of *Amblyomma americatus* and *D variabilis* ticks are seropositive for *Ehrlichia*.

The principal reservoirs for human monocytic ehrlichiosis and human granulocytic anaplasmosis are the white tail deer and the white footed mouse, respectively. Other mammals are implicated as well. A nosocomial outbreak was reported from China (where nine patients had exposure to body fluids and none reported tick bites). Perinatal and blood product transmission of human granulocytic anaplasmosis is also documented.

Clinical Findings

A. Symptoms and Signs

Clinical disease of human monocytic ehrlichiosis ranges from mild to life threatening. Typically, after about a 9-day incubation period and a prodrome consisting of malaise, rigors, and nausea, worsening fever and headache develop. A pleomorphic rash may occur. Presentation in immunosuppressed patients (including transplant patients) and the elderly tends to be more severe. Serious sequelae include acute respiratory failure and ARDS, encephalopathy, and acute kidney disease, which may mimic thrombotic thrombocytopenic purpura.

The symptoms of human granulocytic ehrlichiosis and *E ewingii* infection are similar to those seen with human monocytic ehrlichiosis. Rash, however, is infrequent in human granulocytic ehrlichiosis and should prompt the consideration of other infections (eg, Lyme disease). Persistent fever and malaise are reported to occur for 2 or more years.

The clinical manifestations of anaplasmosis are similar to those of ehrlichiosis. Coinfection with anaplasmosis and Lyme disease or babesiosis may occur, but the clinical manifestations (including fever and cytopenias) are greater with anaplasmosis than with Lyme disease. A newly discovered spirochete, *Borrelia miyamotoi,* may mimic anaplasmosis in its clinical manifestations.

B. Laboratory Findings

Diagnosis can be made by the history of tick exposure followed by a characteristic clinical presentation. Leukopenia, absolute lymphopenia, thrombocytopenia, and transaminitis occur often. Thrombocytopenia occurs more often than leukopenia in human granulocytic ehrlichiosis. Examination of peripheral blood with Giemsa stain may reveal characteristic intraleukocytic vacuoles (morulae). An indirect fluorescent antibody assay is available through the CDC and requires acute and convalescent sera. A PCR assay, if available, is a rapid diagnostic tool, especially for early disease.

► Treatment & Prevention

Treatment for all forms of ehrlichiosis is with doxycycline, 100 mg twice daily (orally or intravenously) for at least 10 days or until 3 days of defervescence. Rifampin is an alternative in pregnant women and children. Treatment should not be withheld while awaiting confirmatory serology when suspicion is high. Lack of clinical improvement and defervescence 48 hours after doxycycline initiation suggests an alternate diagnosis. Tick control is the essence of prevention.

Chowdri HR et al. *Borrelia miyamotoi* infection presenting as human granulocytic anaplasmosis: a case report. Ann Intern Med. 2013 Jul 2;159(1):21–7. [PMID: 23817701]

Dahlgren FS et al. Increasing incidence of *Ehrlichia chaffeensis* and *Anaplasma phagocytophilum* in the United States, 2000–2007. Am J Trop Med Hyg. 2011 Jul;85(1):124–31. [PMID: 21734137]

Fritzen CM et al. Infection prevalences of common tick-borne pathogens in adult lone star ticks (*Amblyomma americanum*) and American dog ticks (*Dermacentor variabilis*) in Kentucky. Am J Trop Med Hyg. 2011 Oct;85(4):718–23. [PMID: 21976578]

Horowitz HW et al. Lyme disease and human granulocytic anaplasmosis coinfection: impact of case definition on coinfection rates and illness severity. Clin Infect Dis. 2013 Jan;56(1):93–9. [PMID: 23042964]

Pritt BS et al. Emergence of a new pathogenic Ehrlichia species, Wisconsin and Minnesota, 2009. N Engl J Med. 2011 Aug 4;365(5):422–9. [PMID: 21812671]

2. Q Fever

ESSENTIALS OF DIAGNOSIS

► Exposure to sheep, goats, cattle, or their products; some infections are laboratory acquired.

► An acute or chronic febrile illness with severe headache, cough, prostration, and abdominal pain.

► Extensive pneumonitis, hepatitis, or encephalopathy; less often, endocarditis, vascular infections, or chronic fatigue syndrome.

► A common cause of culture-negative endocarditis.

General Considerations

Q fever (for "query" in view of its formerly unknown cause), a reportable disease in the United States, is caused by *Coxiella burnetii*, an organism previously classified as a rickettsia but now considered a proteobacteria. Unlike rickettsiae, *C burnetii* is usually transmitted to humans not by arthropods but by inhalation or ingestion. *Coxiella* infections occur globally, mostly in cattle, sheep, and goats, in which they cause mild or subclinical disease (Table 32–3). In these animals, reactivation of the infection occurs during pregnancy and causes abortions or low birth weight offspring. *Coxiella* is resistant to heat and drying and remains infective in the environment for months.

Humans become infected by inhalation of aerosolized bacteria (in dust or droplets) from feces, urine, milk (in particular raw milk), or products of conception of infected animals. Ingestion and skin penetration are other recognized routes of transmission. Outbreaks associated with other mammals such as cats and dogs are also described. A major outbreak in Netherlands that began in 2007 was thought to be due to exposure to aborting ruminants and was associated with over 3000 cases through 2010. There is a known occupational risk for animal handlers, slaughterhouse workers, veterinarians, laboratory workers, and other workers exposed to animal products. Outbreaks in military personnel returning from Iraq and Afghanistan were described. Transmission through aerosols is possible in that *Coxiella* can be pathogens of other organisms (free living amoebae), which are transmitted through air ducts.

Endocarditis, an uncommon but serious form of *Coxiella* infection, is linked to preexisting valvular conditions, immunocompromised states, urban residence, and raw milk ingestion. Horizontal spread from one human to another does not seem to occur even in the presence of florid pneumonitis, but maternal–fetal infection can occur.

Clinical Findings

A. Symptoms and Signs

Asymptomatic infection is common. For the remaining cases, a febrile illness develops after an incubation period of 2–3 weeks, usually accompanied by headache, relative bradycardia, prostration, and muscle pains. The clinical course may be acute, chronic (duration ≥ 6 months), or relapsing. Pneumonia and granulomatous hepatitis are the predominant manifestation in the acute form, whereas other less common manifestations include skin rashes (maculopapular or purpuric), fever of unknown origin, myocarditis, pericarditis, aseptic meningitis, encephalitis, hemolytic anemia, orchitis, acute kidney disease, spondylodiscitis, tenosynovitis, and regional (mediastinal) or diffuse lymphadenopathies. Cases of Q fever mimicking autoimmune and systemic inflammatory disease are reported. The most common presentation of chronic Q fever is culture-negative endocarditis, which occurs in < 1% of infected individuals. It is found mainly in the setting of preexisting valve disease. Vascular infections, particularly of the aorta (causing mycotic aneurysms), are the second most common form of Q fever and are associated with a high mortality (25%). A post-Q fever chronic fatigue syndrome (1 year after acute infection with chronic symptoms not explained by chronic Q fever) is controversial and of unknown pathophysiology although the basis may be immunogenetic.

Reactivation of Q fever in pregnant women may cause spontaneous abortions, intrauterine growth retardation, intrauterine fetal death, premature delivery, and oligamnios.

B. Laboratory Findings

Laboratory examination during the acute phase may show elevated liver function tests and occasional leukocytosis. Patients with acute Q fever usually produce antibodies to *C burnetii* phase II antigen. A fourfold rise between acute and convalescent sera by indirect immunofluorescence is diagnostic. Realtime PCR for *C burnetii* DNA is helpful only in early diagnosis of Q fever with *C burnetii* DNA becoming undetectable in serum as serologic responses develop. The positive predictive value of antibodies to phase II antigens in acute disease is at most 65%.

While chronic Q fever can be diagnosed on the basis of serologic tests done at 3- and 6-month intervals (with an IgG titer against phase I antigen of 1:1600 or greater), it is now recommended that clinical criteria be used for diagnosis of chronic disease. Diagnosis is often made at the time of valve replacement with PCR of tissue samples. *C burnetti* may also be isolated from affected valves using the shell-vial technique. The organism is highly transmissible to laboratory workers and culture techniques require a biosafety level 3 setting. In one series, at 6 years after infection, reversion to seronegativity occurred in 7 of 38 patients, and none showed the organism in peripheral blood mononuclear cells. Antiphospholipid antibodies and anti-ADAMTS 13 antibodies may be present and account for thrombotic and other clinical symptoms.

C. Imaging

Radiographs of the chest show patchy pulmonary infiltrates, often more prominent than the physical signs suggest.

Differential Diagnosis

Viral, mycoplasmal, and bacterial pneumonias, viral hepatitis, brucellosis, Legionnaire disease, Kawasaki disease, tuberculosis, psittacosis, and other animal-borne diseases must be considered. Q fever should be considered in cases of unexplained fevers with negative blood cultures in association with embolic or cardiac disease.

Treatment & Prognosis

For acute infection, treatment with doxycycline (100 mg orally twice daily) for 14 days or at least 3 full days after defervescence is recommended. Even in untreated patients, the mortality rate is usually low, except when endocarditis develops.

For chronic infection, there is no agreement on the type and duration of antimicrobial therapy. Most experts recommend a combination oral therapy with doxycycline (100 mg twice a day) plus ciprofloxacin (typically 750 mg twice a day) or rifampin (300 mg twice a day) or hydroxychloroquine (200 mg three times a day) for approximately 2 years or more for the treatment of endocarditis. A study reported in 1999 of 35 patients with Q fever endocarditis showed favorable outcomes with oral doxycycline (100 mg twice a day) plus oral hydroxychloroquine (200 mg three times a day) for 18 months for native valves and 24 months for prosthetic valves. A randomized study assessing antibiotics and cognitive therapy in chronic Q fever is underway in the Netherlands.

Serologic responses can be monitored during and after completion of therapy and treatment extended in the absence of favorable serologic response (considered a titer of 1:1600 or greater to phase I antigen). The general variability of serologic data, however, limits their usefulness and providers usually rely on clinical criteria. Patients should be monitored for at least 5 years due to risk of relapse. Heart valve replacement may be necessary in refractory disease. **Given the difficulty in treating endocarditis, transthoracic echocardiography is recommended for all patients with acute Q fever, and the same aforementioned therapy for 1 year should be offered in the presence of valvulopathy.**

Because of the obstetric complications (which appear to have a strain specificity) that occur among pregnant women in whom Q fever develops, a regimen of long-term trimethoprim-sulfamethoxazole (320/1600 mg orally for the duration of pregnancy) should be given to all infected pregnant women. However, a randomized controlled study of pregnant women in Holland did not show that serologic surveillance and treatment of seropositive women were effective in preventing obstetric complications. Other data from Denmark among pregnant women exposed in the past to *Coxiella* also suggest the risk of obstetric complications may not be high. The official recommendations nonetheless remain as stated.

Prevention

Prevention is based on detection of the infection in livestock, reduction of contact with infected and, in particular, parturient animals or contaminated dust, special care when working with animal tissues, and effective pasteurization of milk. No vaccine is approved for use in the United States, although a whole-cell Q fever vaccine, with a 5-year efficacy of > 95%, is available in Australia for persons with high-risk exposures where some seroprevalence studies show 7% seropositivity.

C burnetii is a category B bioterrorism agent. In the setting of a bioterrorist attack, postexposure prophylaxis with doxycycline (100 mg orally twice daily) for 5 days should be started 8–12 days after exposure.

Pregnant women should take trimethoprim-sulfamethoxazole (160 mg/800 mg orally twice daily) for the duration of the pregnancy.

Anderson A et al. Diagnosis and management of Q fever—United States, 2013: recommendations from CDC and the Q Fever Working Group. MMWR Recomm Rep. 2013 Mar 29;62(RR-03):1–30. Erratum in: MMWR Recomm Rep. 2013 Sep 6;62(35):730. [PMID: 23535757]

Gunn TM et al. Cardiac manifestations of Q fever infection: case series and a review of the literature. J Card Surg. 2013 May;28(3):233–7. [PMID: 23574261]
Keijmel SP et al. The Qure study: Q fever fatigue syndrome—response to treatment; a randomized placebo-controlled trial. BMC Infect Dis. 2013 Mar 27;13:157. [PMID: 23536997]
Munster JM et al. Routine screening for *Coxiella burnetii* infection during pregnancy: a clustered randomised controlled trial during an outbreak, the Netherlands, 2010. Euro Surveill. 2013 Jun 13;18(24). [PMID: 23787163]
Nielsen SY et al. No excess risk of adverse pregnancy outcomes among women with serological markers of previous infection with *Coxiella burnetii*: evidence from the Danish National Birth Cohort. BMC Infect Dis. 2013 Feb 17;13:87. [PMID: 23413787]
van der Hoek W et al. Follow-up of 686 patients with acute Q fever and detection of chronic infection. Clin Infect Dis. 2011 Jun 15;52(12):1431–6. [PMID: 21628483]

KAWASAKI DISEASE

ESSENTIALS OF DIAGNOSIS

► Fever, conjunctivitis, oral mucosal changes, rash, cervical lymphadenopathy, peripheral extremity changes.

► Elevated erythrocyte sedimentation rate and C-reactive protein levels.

General Considerations

Kawasaki disease is a worldwide multisystemic disease initially described by Tomisaku Kawasaki in 1967. It is also known as the "mucocutaneous lymph node syndrome." It occurs mainly in children between the ages of 3 months and 5 years but can occur occasionally in adults as well. Kawasaki disease occurs significantly more often in Asians or native Pacific Islanders than in whites. It is an acute, self-limiting, mucocutaneous vasculitis characterized by the infiltration of vessel walls with mononuclear cells and later by IgA secreting plasma cells that can result in the destruction of the tunica media and aneurysm formation. Several infectious agents (New Haven coronavirus, parvovirus, bocavirus, CMV, *Yersinia pseudotuberculosis*, meningococcus), bacterial superantigens, and genetic polymorphisms (confirmed in whole genome analysis) in components of the immune system (interleukin 10 and 18) are implicated in its pathogenesis. A "new" RNA virus was considered a trigger of the disease, based on the finding of intracytoplasmic inclusion bodies in ciliated bronchial epithelium of Kawasaki patients. Epidemiologic studies from Seattle show an increased risk with advanced maternal age, mother of foreign birth, maternal group B streptococcus colonization, and early infancy hospitalization. Whole genomic analysis, mostly from China, is identifying target gene products.

Clinical Findings

A clinical diagnosis of "complete" Kawasaki disease requires, in the absence of other processes, explaining the current illness of fever and four of the following criteria for at least 5 days: bilateral nonexudative conjunctivitis, mucous membrane changes of at least one type (injected pharynx, erythema, swelling and fissuring of the lips, strawberry tongue), peripheral extremity changes of at least one type (edema, desquamation, erythema of the palms and soles, induration of the hands and feet, Beau lines [transverse grooves of the nails]), a polymorphous rash, and cervical lymphadenopathy > 1.5 cm (most worrisome when retropharyngeal with edema is present). An "incomplete" form is diagnosed when only two criteria are met. The classic syndrome is often preceded by nonspecific symptoms including irritability, vomiting, anorexia, cough, and diarrhea for up to 10 days.

Major complications include arteritis and aneurysms of the coronary vessels, occurring in about 25% of untreated patients (and slightly over 10% of treated patients in a recent Danish review), on occasion causing myocardial infarction. The "incomplete" form appears more frequently to result in cardiac complications. The pathogenesis of infarction is often thrombus formation, vasospasm, stenosis, or aneurysm rupture. Coronary complications are more common among patients older than 6 years or younger than 1 year of age. Noninvasive diagnosis of coronary complications can be made with CT coronary angiography (preferred in one series to MR), magnetic resonance angiography or transthoracic echocardiography (advocated for early screening). Other factors associated with the development of coronary artery aneurysms are male sex, relentless fever (even after the administration of IVIG), high C-reactive protein, urticarial exanthems, anemia, hypoalbuminemia, hyponatremia, and thrombocytopenia. Pericardial effusions, myocarditis, and mitral regurgitation (usually mild) are also common. Coronary artery fistulas occur in up to 5% of patients and diastolic dysfunction is also reported. Arteritis of extremity vessels, peripheral gangrene, syndrome of inappropriate secretion of antidiuretic hormone (SIADH), and the hemophagocytic syndrome are also reported. Cases of pancreatitis and bile duct stenosis due to underlying vasculitis are reported. Cerebrospinal fluid pleocytosis is found in one-third of cases and encephalitis is rarely reported. Other CNS complications include seizures, oculomotor palsies, and sensorineural hearing loss which, when sought, can be found in as many as 55% of cases. Rare case reports of atypical presentations (eg, retropharyngeal abscess) are described.

Differentiation from disseminated adenovirus infection is important and can be performed with rapid adenovirus assays.

▶ **Treatment & Prevention**

Every patient with a clinical diagnosis of Kawasaki disease (complete or incomplete) should be treated. IVIG (2 g/kg over 10–12 hours) is given within the first 10 days of illness. Patients in whom persistent fever, ongoing systemic inflammation, or aneurysm formation presents later should be offered IVIG as well. Concomitant aspirin should be started at 80–100 mg/kg/d orally (divided into four doses and not exceeding 4 g/d) until the patient is

afebrile for 48 hours and then reduced to 3–5 mg/kg/d until markers of acute inflammation normalize. Aspirin therapy is continued if coronary aneurysm develops. If fevers persist beyond 36 hours after the initial IVIG infusion, a second dose of IVIG at 2 g/kg should be given if no other source of fever is found. Rare cases of aseptic meningitis are reported with IVIG, and this complication may be hard to distinguish from the occasional CNS disease associated with Kawasaki syndrome itself although the time course and the cerebrospinal fluid differential (more polymorphonuclear with IVIG, more lymphocytic with Kawasaki syndrome) may help differentiate the two. Methylprednisolone (30 mg/kg/d intravenously if possible for a maximum of 3 days) followed by tapering dose of corticosteroids in addition to IVIG administration improve coronary artery outcomes in severe Kawasaki disease. Routine childhood vaccinations should be given and live vaccines (eg, MMR) should be delayed for at least 9 months only if IVIG was administered (IVIG can block the immune response to live vaccines). If vaccine preventable disease endemicity requires urgent vaccination, it is prudent to revaccinate 11 months after the IVIG and first vaccination were given.

Further options for refractory cases include TNF blockers (infliximab or etanercept), cyclophosphamide or cyclosporine, methotrexate, and plasmapheresis, but not further pulse corticosteroid or IVIG. Abciximab therapy may be associated with coronary vessel remodeling in large coronary artery aneurysms. An echocardiogram is essential in the acute phase of illness and 6–8 weeks after onset. Anticoagulation with warfarin or low-molecular-weight heparin (the latter is preferable for children where dosage adjustments are difficult using warfarin) is indicated along with aspirin, 81 mg orally daily, in patients with aneurysms > 8 mm in diameter. If myocardial infarction occurs, therapy with thrombolytics, percutaneous coronary intervention, coronary artery bypass grafts, and even cardiac transplantation should be considered. Manifestation of coronary artery aneurysms can occur as late as in the third or fourth decade of life with a study showing a prevalence of 5% coronary sequelae from Kawasaki disease among young adults evaluated with angiography. Data are equivocal on the development of accelerated atherosclerosis among those with a history of Kawasaki disease.

While secondary prevention of complications entails the modalities described above, primary prevention is difficult in the absence of a clear explanation for the disease.

▶ **Prognosis**

Cases that develop recurrent disease tend to more often show cardiac complications. Patients with a parental history of Kawasaki disease show more recurrent disease and more cardiac complications. The long-term prognosis for adults with a history of Kawasaki disease but without coronary artery aneurysms is excellent. A heart-healthy lifestyle, however, is essential. The prognosis of patients with a history of cardiac complications requires regular follow-up with risk stratification based on published guidelines and under cardiologic supervision. Children with Kawasaki disease show an increased risk for subsequent allergic diseases.

▶ When to Refer

All cases of Kawasaki disease merit referral to specialists.

Dominguez SR et al. Advances in the treatment of Kawasaki disease. Curr Opin Pediatr. 2013 Feb;25(1):103–9. [PMID: 23283289]

Hayward K et al. Perinatal exposures and Kawasaki disease in Washington State: a population-based, case-control study. Pediatr Infect Dis J. 2012 Oct;31(10):1027–31. [PMID: 22653485]

Kobayashi T et al. Efficacy of immunoglobulin plus prednisolone for prevention of coronary artery abnormalities in severe Kawasaki disease (RAISE study): a randomised, open-label, blinded-endpoints trial. Lancet. 2012 Apr 28;379(9826): 1613–20. [PMID: 22405251]

Patel A et al. Evaluation of clinical characteristics of Kawasaki syndrome and risk factors for coronary artery abnormalities among children in Denmark. Acta Paediatr. 2013 Apr;102(4): 385–90. [PMID: 23278838]

Punnoose AR et al. JAMA patient page. Kawasaki disease. JAMA. 2012 May 9;307(18):1990. [PMID: 22570468]

Selamet Tierney ES et al. Vascular health in Kawasaki disease. J Am Coll Cardiol. 2013 Sep 17;62(12):1114–21. [PMID: 23835006]

Teraguchi M et al. Steroid pulse therapy for children with intravenous immunoglobulin therapy-resistant Kawasaki disease: a prospective study. Pediatr Cardiol. 2013 Apr;34(4):959–63. [PMID: 23184018]

Bacterial & Chlamydial Infections

Brian S. Schwartz, MD

INFECTIONS CAUSED BY GRAM-POSITIVE BACTERIA

STREPTOCOCCAL INFECTIONS

1. Pharyngitis

 ESSENTIALS OF DIAGNOSIS

▶ Abrupt onset of sore throat, fever, malaise, nausea, and headache.

▶ Throat red and edematous, with or without exudate; cervical nodes tender.

▶ Diagnosis confirmed by culture of throat.

▶ General Considerations

Group A beta-hemolytic streptococci (*Streptococcus pyogenes*) are the most common bacterial cause of pharyngitis. Transmission occurs by droplets of infected secretions. Group A streptococci producing erythrogenic toxin may cause scarlet fever in susceptible persons.

▶ Clinical Findings

A. Symptoms and Signs

"Strep throat" is characterized by a sudden onset of fever, sore throat, pain on swallowing, tender cervical adenopathy, malaise, and nausea. The pharynx, soft palate, and tonsils are red and edematous. There may be a purulent exudate. The Centor clinical criteria for the diagnosis of streptococcal pharyngitis are temperature >38°C, tender anterior cervical adenopathy, lack of a cough, and pharyngotonsillar exudate.

The rash of scarlet fever is diffusely erythematous, resembling a sunburn, with superimposed fine red papules, and is most intense in the groin and axillas. It blanches on pressure, may become petechial, and fades in 2–5 days, leaving a fine desquamation. The face is flushed, with circumoral pallor, and the tongue is coated with enlarged red papillae (strawberry tongue).

B. Laboratory Findings

Leukocytosis with neutrophil predominance is common. Throat culture onto a single blood agar plate has a sensitivity of 80–90%. Rapid diagnostic tests based on detection of streptococcal antigen are slightly less sensitive than culture. Clinical criteria, such as the Centor criteria, are useful for identifying patients in whom a rapid antigen test or throat culture is indicated. Patients who meet two or more of these criteria merit further testing. When three of the four are present, laboratory sensitivity of rapid antigen testing exceeds 90%. When only one criterion is present, streptococcal pharyngitis is unlikely. In high-prevalence settings or if clinical suspicion for streptococcal pharyngitis is high, a negative antigen test or culture should be confirmed by a follow-up culture.

▶ Complications

Suppurative complications include sinusitis, otitis media, mastoiditis, peritonsillar abscess, and suppuration of cervical lymph nodes.

Nonsuppurative complications are rheumatic fever and glomerulonephritis. Rheumatic fever may follow recurrent episodes of pharyngitis beginning 1–4 weeks after the onset of symptoms. Glomerulonephritis follows a single infection with a nephritogenic strain of streptococcus group A (eg, types 4, 12, 2, 49, and 60), more commonly on the skin than in the throat, and begins 1–3 weeks after the onset of the infection.

▶ Differential Diagnosis

Streptococcal sore throat resembles (and cannot be reliably distinguished clinically from) pharyngitis caused by viruses such as adenoviruses, Epstein-Barr virus, primary HIV, or other bacteria such as *Fusobacterium necrophorum* and *Arcanobacterium haemolyticum* (which also may cause a rash). Pharyngitis and lymphadenopathy are common findings in primary HIV infection. Generalized lymphadenopathy, splenomegaly, atypical lymphocytosis, and a positive serologic test distinguish mononucleosis from streptococcal pharyngitis. Diphtheria is characterized by a pseudomembrane; oropharyngeal candidiasis shows white patches of exudate and less erythema; and necrotizing ulcerative gingivostomatitis (Vincent fusospirochetal gingivitis or stomatitis) presents with shallow ulcers in the mouth. Retropharyngeal abscess or bacterial epiglottitis should be considered when odynophagia and difficulty in handling secretions are present and when the severity of symptoms is disproportionate to findings on examination of the pharynx. *F necrophorum* causes pharyngitis at a similar rate as group A beta-hemolytic streptococci in adolescents and young adults. *F necrophorum* pharyngitis is associated with Lemierre syndrome, suppurative thrombophlebitis of the internal jugular vein, bacteremia, and metastatic infections. Early recognition and treatment of this disease is important.

▶ Treatment

Antimicrobial therapy has a modest effect on resolution of symptoms and primarily is administered for prevention of complications. Antibiotic therapy can be safely delayed until the diagnosis is established on the basis of a positive antigen test or culture. Empiric therapy usually is not a cost-effective approach to the management of most adults with pharyngitis because the prevalence of streptococcal pharyngitis is likely to be no more than 10–20% in typical clinical settings. The positive predictive value of clinical criteria is low. Since macrolides are not reliable against *F necrophorum* infection, adolescents or young adults with pharyngitis, which is not confirmed to be due to group A beta-hemolytic streptococci, should be given penicillin or amoxicillin preferentially at the doses listed below. If the pharyngitis does not resolve quickly, symptoms worsen, or unilateral neck swelling develops, clinicians should consider suppurative complications such as peritonsillar abscess and the Lemierre syndrome.

A. Benzathine Penicillin G

Benzathine penicillin G, 1.2 million units intramuscularly as a single dose, is optimal therapy.

B. Penicillin VK

Penicillin VK, 250 mg orally four times daily or 500 mg orally twice daily for 10 days, is effective.

C. Amoxicillin

Amoxicillin, 1000 mg orally once daily or 500 mg orally twice daily for 10 days is another option.

D. Cephalosporins

Cephalexin, 500 mg orally twice daily for 10 days, cefdinir, 300 mg orally twice daily for 5–10 days or 600 mg orally once daily for 10 days, and cefpodoxime, 100 mg orally twice daily for 5–10 days, should be reserved for penicillin-allergic patients who do not have immediate-type hypersensitivity to penicillin.

E. Macrolides

Erythromycin, 500 mg orally four times a day, or azithromycin, 500 mg orally once daily for 5 days, is an alternative

for the penicillin-allergic patient. Macrolides are less effective than penicillins and are considered second-line agents. Macrolide-resistant strains almost always are susceptible to clindamycin, a suitable alternative to penicillins; a 10-day course of 300 mg orally twice daily is effective.

▶ Prevention of Recurrent Rheumatic Fever

Effectively controlling rheumatic fever depends on identification and treatment of primary streptococcal infection and secondary prevention of recurrences. Patients who have had rheumatic fever should be treated with a continuous course of antimicrobial prophylaxis for at least 5 years. Effective regimens are erythromycin, 250 mg orally twice daily, or penicillin G, 500 mg orally daily.

▶ When to Refer

Patients with peritonsillar or retropharyngeal abscess should be referred to an otolaryngologist.

▶ When to Admit

- Odynophagia resulting in dehydration.
- Suspected or known epiglottitis.

Cirilli AR. Emergency evaluation and management of the sore throat. Emerg Med Clin North Am. 2013 May;31(2):501–15. [PMID: 23601485]

Shulman ST et al. Clinical practice guideline for the diagnosis and management of group A streptococcal pharyngitis: 2012 update by the Infectious Diseases Society of America. Clin Infect Dis. 2012 Nov 15;55(10):1279–82. [PMID: 23091044]

van Driel ML et al. Different antibiotic treatments for group A streptococcal pharyngitis. Cochrane Database Syst Rev. 2013 Apr 30;4:CD004406. [PMID: 23633318]

Wessels MR. Clinical practice. Streptococcal pharyngitis. N Engl J Med. 2011 Feb 17;364(7):648–55. [PMID: 21323542]

2. Streptococcal Skin Infections

Group A beta-hemolytic streptococci are not normal skin flora. Streptococcal skin infections result from colonization of normal skin by contact with other infected individuals or by preceding streptococcal respiratory infection.

▶ Clinical Findings

A. Symptoms and Signs

Impetigo is a focal, vesicular, pustular lesion with a thick, amber-colored crust with a "stuck-on" appearance (see Chapter 6).

Erysipelas is a painful superficial cellulitis that frequently involves the face. It is well demarcated from the surrounding normal skin. It affects skin with impaired lymphatic drainage, such as edematous lower extremities or wounds.

B. Laboratory Findings

Cultures obtained from a wound or pustule are likely to grow group A streptococci. Blood cultures are occasionally positive.

▶ **Treatment**

Parenteral antibiotics are indicated for patients with facial erysipelas or evidence of systemic infection. Penicillin, 2 million units intravenously every 4 hours, is the drug of choice. However, staphylococcal infections may at times be difficult to differentiate from streptococcal infections. In practice, initial therapy for patients with risk factors for *Staphylococcus aureus* (eg, injection drug use, diabetes, wound infection) should cover this organism. Nafcillin, 1–2 g every 4–6 hours intravenously, and cefazolin, 1 g intravenously or intramuscularly every 8 hours, are reasonable choices. In the patient at risk for methicillin-resistant *S aureus* infection or with a serious penicillin allergy (ie, anaphylaxis), vancomycin, 1 g intravenously every 12 hours, or daptomycin 4 mg/kg intravenously daily, should be used (Table 33–1).

Patients who do not require parenteral therapy may be treated with amoxicillin, 875 mg twice daily for 7–10 days. A first-generation oral cephalosporin, eg, cephalexin, 500 mg four times daily, or clindamycin, 300 mg orally three times daily, is an alternative to amoxicillin. In patients with recurrent cellulitis of the leg, maintenance therapy (for at least 1 year) with penicillin, 250 mg orally twice daily, can reduce the likelihood of relapse.

Thomas KS et al; U.K. Dermatology Clinical Trials Network's PATCH I Trial Team. Penicillin to prevent recurrent leg cellulitis. N Engl J Med. 2013 May 2;368(18):1695–703. [PMID: 23635049]

3. Other Group A Streptococcal Infections

Arthritis, pneumonia, empyema, endocarditis, and necrotizing fasciitis are relatively uncommon infections that may be caused by group A streptococci. Toxic shock-like syndrome also occurs.

Arthritis generally occurs in association with cellulitis. In addition to intravenous therapy with penicillin G, 2 million units every 4 hours (or cefazolin or vancomycin in doses recommended above for penicillin-allergic patients), frequent percutaneous needle aspiration should be performed to remove joint effusions. Open surgical drainage may be necessary in many cases.

Pneumonia and **empyema** often are characterized by extensive tissue destruction and an aggressive, rapidly progressive clinical course associated with significant morbidity and mortality. High-dose penicillin and chest tube drainage are indicated for treatment of empyema. Vancomycin is an acceptable substitute in penicillin-allergic patients.

Group A streptococci can cause **endocarditis.** Endocarditis should be treated with 4 million units of penicillin G intravenously every 4 hours for 4–6 weeks. Vancomycin, 1 g intravenously every 12 hours, is recommended for persons allergic to penicillin.

Necrotizing fasciitis is a rapidly spreading infection involving the fascia of deep muscle. The clinical findings at presentation may be those of severe cellulitis, but the presence of systemic toxicity and severe pain, which may be followed by anesthesia of the involved area due to destruction of nerves as infection advances through the fascial planes, is a clue to the diagnosis. Surgical exploration is

Table 33–1. Empiric treatment of common skin and soft tissue infections (SSTI).

SSTI Type	Common Pathogens	Treatment
Purulent (abscess, furuncle, carbuncle, cellulitis with purulence)	*Staphylococcus aureus*	Incision and drainage is the primary treatment Consider the addition of antibiotics in select situations[1] **Oral antibiotic regimens** 　　Cephalexin 500 mg four times daily *or* dicloxacillin 500 mg four times daily 　　Clindamycin 300–450 mg three or four times daily[2] *or* one double-strength tablet of 　　　trimethoprim-sulfamethoxazole twice daily[2] *or* doxycycline 100 mg twice daily[2] **Intravenous antibiotic regimens**[3] 　　Cefazolin 1 g three times daily *or* nafcillin 1–2 g four to six times daily 　　Vancomycin 1 g twice daily[2] *or* daptomycin 4 mg/kg once daily[2]
Nonpurulent (cellulitis, erysipelas)	Beta-hemolytic streptococci (*S aureus* less likely)	**Oral antibiotic regimens** 　　Cephalexin 500 mg four times daily *or* dicloxacillin 500 mg four times daily 　　Clindamycin 300–450 mg three or four times daily[2] *or* amoxicillin 875 mg twice daily 　　　*plus* one double-strength tablet of trimethoprim-sulfamethoxazole twice daily[2] **Intravenous antibiotic regimens**[3] 　　Cefazolin 1 g three times daily *or* nafcillin 1–2 g four to six times daily 　　Vancomycin 1 g twice daily[2] *or* daptomycin 4 mg/kg once daily

[1]Antibiotic therapy should be given in addition to incision and drainage for purulent SSTI if the patient has any of the following: severe or extensive disease, symptoms and signs of systemic illness, purulent cellulitis/wound infection, comorbidities and extremes of age, abscess in area difficult to drain or on face/hand, associated septic phlebitis, or lack of response to incision and drainage alone.
[2]Regimens with activity against methicillin-resistant *S aureus*.
[3]Other regimens approved by the FDA for treatment of complicated skin and soft tissue infections include linezolid, 600 mg twice daily (can also be given by mouth); tigecycline, 50 mg twice daily; telavancin, at 10 mg/kg once daily; and ceftaroline, 600 mg twice daily.

mandatory when the diagnosis is suspected. Early and extensive debridement is essential for survival.

Any streptococcal infection—and necrotizing fasciitis in particular—can be associated with **streptococcal toxic shock syndrome,** typified by invasion of skin or soft tissues, acute respiratory distress syndrome, and kidney failure. The very young, the elderly, and those with underlying medical conditions are at particularly high risk for invasive disease. Bacteremia occurs in most cases. Skin rash and desquamation may not be present. Mortality rates can be up to 80%. The syndrome is due to elaboration of pyrogenic erythrotoxin (which also causes **scarlet fever),** a superantigen that stimulates massive release of inflammatory cytokines believed to mediate the shock. A beta-lactam, such as penicillin, remains the drug of choice for treatment of serious streptococcal infections, but clindamycin, which is a potent inhibitor of toxin production, should also be administered at a dose of 600 mg every 8 hours intravenously for invasive disease, especially in the presence of shock. Intravenous immune globulin has also been recommended for streptococcal toxic shock syndrome for presumed, although unproven, therapeutic benefit from specific antibody to streptococcal exotoxins in immune globulin preparations. Two dosage regimens have been used: 450 mg/kg once daily for 5 days or a single dose of 2 g/kg with a repeat dose at 48 hours if the patient remains unstable.

Outbreaks of invasive disease have been associated with colonization by invasive clones that can be transmitted to close contacts who, though asymptomatic, may be a reservoir for disease. Tracing contacts of patients with invasive disease is controversial.

Sultan HY et al. Necrotising fasciitis. BMJ. 2012 Jul 20;345:e4274. [PMID: 22822005]

4. Non-Group A Streptococcal Infections

Non-group A hemolytic streptococci (eg, groups B, C, and G) produce a spectrum of disease similar to that of group A streptococci. The treatment of infections caused by these strains is the same as for group A streptococci.

Group B streptococci are an important cause of sepsis, bacteremia, and meningitis in the neonate. Antepartum screening to identify carriers and peripartum antimicrobial prophylaxis are recommended in pregnancy. This organism, part of the normal vaginal flora, may cause septic abortion, endometritis, or peripartum infections and, less commonly, cellulitis, bacteremia, and endocarditis in adults. Treatment of infections caused by group B streptococci is with either penicillin or vancomycin in doses recommended for group A streptococci. Because of in vitro synergism, some experts recommend the addition of low-dose gentamicin, 1 mg/kg every 8 hours.

Viridans streptococci, which are nonhemolytic or alpha-hemolytic (ie, producing a green zone of hemolysis on blood agar), are part of the normal oral flora. Although these strains may produce focal pyogenic infection, they are most notable as the leading cause of native valve endocarditis (see below).

Group D streptococci include *Streptococcus bovis* and the enterococci. *S bovis* is a cause of endocarditis in association with bowel neoplasia or cirrhosis and is treated like viridans streptococci.

Desimone DC et al; Mayo Cardiovascular Infections Study Group. Incidence of infective endocarditis caused by viridans group streptococci before and after publication of the 2007 American Heart Association's endocarditis prevention guidelines. Circulation. 2012 Jul 3;126(1):60–4. [PMID: 22689929]

Deutscher M et al; Active Bacterial Core Surveillance Team. Incidence and severity of invasive *Streptococcus pneumoniae*, group A *Streptococcus*, and group B *Streptococcus* infections among pregnant and postpartum women. Clin Infect Dis. 2011 Jul 15;53(2):114–23. [PMID: 21690617]

Ohlsson A et al. Intrapartum antibiotics for known maternal Group B streptococcal colonization. Cochrane Database Syst Rev. 2013 Jan 31;1:CD007467. [PMID: 23440815]

ENTEROCOCCAL INFECTIONS

Two species, *Enterococcus faecalis* and *Enterococcus faecium*, are responsible for most human enterococcal infections. Enterococci cause wound infections, urinary tract infections, bacteremia, and endocarditis. Infections caused by penicillin-susceptible strains should be treated with penicillin 3–4 million units every 4 hours; ampicillin 3 g every 6 hours; or if the patient is penicillin-allergic, vancomycin 15 mg/kg every 12 hours intravenously. If the patient has endocarditis or meningitis, gentamicin 1 mg/kg every 8 hours intravenously should be added to the regimen in order to achieve the bactericidal activity that is required to cure these infections.

Resistance to vancomycin, penicillin, and gentamicin is common among enterococcal isolates, especially *E faecium*; it is essential to determine antimicrobial susceptibility of isolates. Infection control measures that may be indicated to limit their spread include isolation, barrier precautions, and avoidance of overuse of vancomycin and gentamicin. Consultation with an infectious diseases specialist is strongly advised when treating infections caused by resistant strains of enterococci. Quinupristin/dalfopristin and linezolid are approved by the FDA for treatment of infections caused by vancomycin-resistant strains of enterococci. Daptomycin and tigecycline are not approved by the FDA for the treatment for vancomycin-resistant strains of enterococci, although they are frequently active in vitro.

Quinupristin/dalfopristin is not active against strains of *E faecalis* and should be used only for infections caused by *E faecium*. The dose is 7.5 mg/kg intravenously every 8–12 hours. Phlebitis and irritation at the infusion site (often requiring a central line) and an arthralgia-myalgia syndrome are relatively common side effects. Linezolid, an oxazolidinone, is active against both *E faecalis* and *E faecium*. The dose is 600 mg twice daily, and both intravenous and oral preparations are available. Its two principal side effects are thrombocytopenia and bone marrow suppression; however, peripheral neuropathy, optic neuritis, and lactic acidosis have been observed with prolonged use due to mitochondrial toxicity. Emergence of resistance has occurred during therapy with both quinupristin/dalfopristin and linezolid.

Cattoir V et al. Twenty-five years of shared life with vancomycin-resistant enterococci: is it time to divorce? J Antimicrob Chemother. 2013 Apr;68(4):731–42. [PMID: 23208830]

Huskins WC et al; STAR*ICU Trial Investigators. Intervention to reduce transmission of resistant bacteria in intensive care. N Engl J Med. 2011 Apr 14;364(15):1407–18. [PMID: 21488763]

Lin E et al. Overtreatment of enterococcal bacteriuria. Arch Intern Med. 2012 Jan 9;172(1):33–8. [PMID: 22232145]

Stein GE et al. Tigecycline: an update. Diagn Microbiol Infect Dis. 2013 Apr;75(4):331–6. [PMID: 23357291]

PNEUMOCOCCAL INFECTIONS

1. Pneumococcal Pneumonia

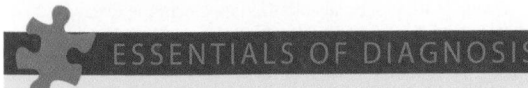

ESSENTIALS OF DIAGNOSIS

▸ Productive cough, fever, rigors, dyspnea, early pleuritic chest pain.

▸ Consolidating lobar pneumonia on chest radiograph.

▸ Gram-positive diplococci on Gram stain of sputum.

General Considerations

The pneumococcus is the most common cause of community-acquired pyogenic bacterial pneumonia. Alcoholism, asthma, HIV infection, sickle cell disease, splenectomy, and hematologic disorders are predisposing factors. The mortality rate remains high in the setting of advanced age, multilobar disease, severe hypoxemia, extrapulmonary complications, and bacteremia.

Clinical Findings

A. Symptoms and Signs

Presenting symptoms and signs include high fever, productive cough, occasionally hemoptysis, and pleuritic chest pain. Rigors occur within the first few hours of infection but are uncommon thereafter. Bronchial breath sounds are an early sign.

B. Laboratory Findings

Pneumococcal pneumonia classically is a lobar pneumonia with radiographic findings of consolidation and occasionally effusion. However, differentiating it from other pneumonias is not possible radiographically or clinically because of significant overlap in presentations. Diagnosis requires isolation of the organism in culture, although the Gram stain appearance of sputum can be suggestive. Sputum and blood cultures, positive in 60% and 25% of cases of pneumococcal pneumonia, respectively, should be obtained prior to initiation of antimicrobial therapy in patients who are admitted to the hospital. A good-quality sputum sample (< 10 epithelial cells and > 25 polymorphonuclear leukocytes per high-power field) shows gram-positive diplococci in 80–90% of cases. A rapid urinary antigen test for *Streptococcus pneumoniae,* with sensitivity of 70–80% and specificity > 95%, can assist with early diagnosis.

Complications

Parapneumonic (sympathetic) effusion is common and may cause recurrence or persistence of fever. These sterile fluid accumulations need no specific therapy. Empyema occurs in 5% or less of cases and is differentiated from sympathetic effusion by the presence of organisms on Gram-stained fluid or positive pleural fluid cultures.

Pneumococcal pericarditis is a rare complication that can cause tamponade. Pneumococcal arthritis also is uncommon. Pneumococcal endocarditis usually involves the aortic valve and often occurs in association with meningitis and pneumonia (sometimes referred to as Austrian or Osler triad). Early heart failure and multiple embolic events are typical.

Treatment

A. Specific Measures

Initial antimicrobial therapy for pneumonia is empiric (see Chapter 9 for specific recommendations) pending isolation and identification of the causative agent. Once *S pneumoniae* is identified as the infecting pathogen, any of several antimicrobial agents may be used depending on the clinical setting, community patterns of penicillin resistance, and susceptibility of the particular isolate. Uncomplicated pneumococcal pneumonia (ie, arterial $PO_2 > 60$ mm Hg, no coexisting medical problems, and single-lobe disease without signs of extrapulmonary infection) caused by penicillin-susceptible strains of pneumococcus may be treated on an outpatient basis with amoxicillin, 750 mg orally twice daily for 7–10 days. For penicillin-allergic patients, alternatives are azithromycin, one 500-mg dose orally on the first day and 250 mg for the next 4 days; clarithromycin, 500 mg orally twice daily for 10 days; doxycycline, 100 mg orally twice daily for 10 days; levofloxacin, 750 mg orally for 5 days; or moxifloxacin, 400 mg orally for 7–14 days. Patients should be monitored for clinical response (eg, less cough, defervescence within 2–3 days) because pneumococci have become increasingly resistant to penicillin and the second-line agents.

Parenteral therapy is generally recommended for the hospitalized patient at least until there has been clinical improvement. Aqueous penicillin G, 2 million units intravenously every 4 hours, or ceftriaxone, 1 g intravenously every 24 hours, is effective for strains that are not highly penicillin-resistant (ie, strains for which the minimum inhibitory concentration [MIC] of penicillin is ≤ 1 mcg/mL). For serious penicillin allergy or infection caused by a highly penicillin-resistant strain, vancomycin, 1 g intravenously every 12 hours, is effective. Alternatively, a respiratory fluoroquinolone (eg, levofloxacin, 750 mg) can be used. The total duration of therapy is not well defined but 5–7 days is appropriate for patients who have an uncomplicated infection and demonstrate a good clinical response.

B. Treatment of Complications

Pleural effusions developing after initiation of antimicrobial therapy usually are sterile, and thoracentesis need not be performed if the patient is otherwise improving. Thoracentesis is indicated for an effusion present prior to initiation of therapy and in the patient who has not responded to antibiotics after 3–4 days. Chest tube drainage may be required if pneumococci are identified by culture or Gram stain, especially if aspiration of the fluid is difficult.

Echocardiography should be done if pericardial effusion is suspected. Patients with pericardial effusion who are responding to therapy and have no signs of tamponade may be monitored and treated with indomethacin, 50 mg orally three times daily, for pain. In patients with increasing effusion, unsatisfactory clinical response, or evidence of tamponade, pericardiocentesis will determine whether the pericardial space is infected. Infected fluid must be drained either percutaneously (by tube placement or needle aspiration), by placement of a pericardial window, or by pericardiectomy. Pericardiectomy eventually may be required to prevent or treat constrictive pericarditis, a common sequela of bacterial pericarditis.

Endocarditis should be treated for 4 weeks with 3–4 million units of penicillin G every 4 hours intravenously; ceftriaxone, 2 g once daily intravenously; or vancomycin, 15 mg/kg every 12 hours intravenously. Mild heart failure from endocarditis may respond to medical therapy, but moderate to severe heart failure is an indication for prosthetic valve implantation, as are systemic emboli or large friable vegetations as determined by echocardiography.

C. Penicillin-Resistant Pneumococci

Susceptibility breakpoints defining penicillin-resistant pneumococci for isolates causing pneumonia were revised in 2008. Resistance breakpoints for parenterally administered penicillin and high-dose oral amoxicillin (2 g twice daily) are as follows: susceptible, penicillin MIC ≤ 2 mcg/mL; intermediate, MIC = 4 mcg/mL; resistant, MIC ≥ 8 mcg/mL. This change reflected results from studies demonstrating equivalent cure rates when high doses of parenteral penicillin were used for treatment of pneumococcal pneumonia due to isolates with penicillin MIC ≤ 2 mcg/mL. Note, however, that these new breakpoints do not apply to orally administered penicillin, which are the same as for use of penicillin in treatment of meningitis (see below). In cases of pneumococcal pneumonia where the isolate has a penicillin MIC > 2 mcg/mL, cephalosporin cross-resistance is common, and a non–beta-lactam antimicrobial, such as vancomycin, 1 g intravenously every 12 hours or a fluoroquinolone with enhanced gram-positive activity (eg, levofloxacin, 750 mg intravenously or orally once daily or moxifloxacin, 400 mg intravenously or orally once daily), is recommended. Penicillin-resistant strains of pneumococci may be resistant to macrolides, trimethoprim-sulfamethoxazole, and chloramphenicol, and susceptibility must be documented prior to their use. All blood and cerebrospinal fluid isolates should still be tested for resistance to penicillin. There has been no change to the penicillin susceptibility breakpoint for pneumococcal isolates causing meningitis, nor any change in treatment recommendations (see below).

▶ Prevention

See Chapter 30 for discussion of pneumococcal vaccines.

▶ When to Refer

- All patients with suspected pneumococcal endocarditis or meningitis to an infectious disease specialist.
- Extensive disease.
- Seriously ill patient with pneumonia, particularly in the setting of comorbid conditions (eg, liver disease).
- Progression of pneumonia or failure to improve on antibiotics.

▶ When to Admit

- All patients in whom pneumococcal endocarditis or meningitis is suspected or documented should be admitted for observation and empiric therapy.
- All patients with pneumococcal pneumonia that is multilobar or associated with significant hypoxemia.
- Failure of outpatient pneumonia therapy, including inability to maintain oral intake and medications.
- Exacerbations of underlying disease (eg, heart failure) by pneumonia that would benefit from hospitalization.

Blasi F et al. Understanding the burden of pneumococcal disease in adults. Clin Microbiol Infect. 2012 Oct;18(Suppl 5):7–14. [PMID: 22882668]

Carratalà J et al. Effect of a 3-step critical pathway to reduce duration of intravenous antibiotic therapy and length of stay in community-acquired pneumonia: a randomized controlled trial. Arch Intern Med. 2012 Jun 25;172(12):922–8. [PMID: 22732747]

Feldman C et al. Bacteraemic pneumococcal pneumonia: current therapeutic options. Drugs. 2011 Jan 22;71(2):131–53. [PMID: 21275443]

Moberley S et al. Vaccines for preventing pneumococcal infection in adults. Cochrane Database Syst Rev. 2013 Jan 31; 1:CD000422. [PMID: 23440780]

Moran GJ et al. Emergency management of community-acquired bacterial pneumonia: what is new since the 2007 Infectious Diseases Society of America/American Thoracic Society guidelines. Am J Emerg Med. 2013 Mar;31(3):602–12. [PMID: 23380120]

2. Pneumococcal Meningitis

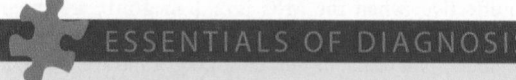

ESSENTIALS OF DIAGNOSIS

- ▶ Fever, headache, altered mental status.
- ▶ Meningismus.
- ▶ Gram-positive diplococci on Gram stain of cerebrospinal fluid.

General Considerations

S pneumoniae is the most common cause of meningitis in adults. Head trauma with cerebrospinal fluid leaks, sinusitis, and pneumonia may precede it.

Clinical Findings

A. Symptoms and Signs

The onset is rapid, with fever, headache, meningismus, and altered mentation. Pneumonia may be present. Compared with meningitis caused by the meningococcus, pneumococcal meningitis lacks a rash, and focal neurologic deficits, cranial nerve palsies, and obtundation are more prominent features.

B. Laboratory Findings

The cerebrospinal fluid typically has > 1000 white blood cells per microliter, over 60% of which are polymorphonuclear leukocytes; the glucose concentration is < 40 mg/dL (< 2.22 mmol/L), or < 50% of the simultaneous serum concentration; and the protein usually exceeds 150 mg/dL (1500 mg/L) (see Chapter 30). Not all cases of meningitis will have these typical findings, and alterations in cerebrospinal fluid cell counts and chemistries may be surprisingly minimal, overlapping with those of aseptic meningitis.

Gram stain of cerebrospinal fluid shows gram-positive cocci in 80–90% of cases, and in untreated cases, blood or cerebrospinal fluid cultures are almost always positive.

Treatment

Antibiotics should be given as soon as the diagnosis is suspected. If lumbar puncture must be delayed (eg, while awaiting results of an imaging study to exclude a mass lesion), the patient should be treated empirically for presumed meningitis with intravenous ceftriaxone, 2 g, plus vancomycin, 15 mg/kg, plus dexamethasone, 0.15 mg/kg administered concomitantly after blood cultures (positive in 50% of cases) have been obtained. Once susceptibility to penicillin has been confirmed, penicillin, 24 million units intravenously daily in six divided doses, or ceftriaxone, 2 g every 12 hours intravenously, is continued for 10–14 days in documented cases.

The best therapy for penicillin-resistant strains is not known. Penicillin-resistant strains (MIC > 0.06 mcg/mL) are often cross-resistant to the third-generation cephalosporins as well as other antibiotics. Susceptibility testing is essential to proper management of this infection. If the MIC of ceftriaxone or cefotaxime is ≤ 0.5 mcg/mL, single-drug therapy with either of these cephalosporins is likely to be effective; when the MIC is ≥ 1 mcg/mL, treatment with a combination of ceftriaxone, 2 g intravenously every 12 hours, plus vancomycin, 30 mg/kg/d intravenously in two or three divided doses, is recommended. If a patient with a penicillin-resistant organism is slow to respond clinically, repeat lumbar puncture may be indicated to assess bacteriologic response.

Dexamethasone administered with antibiotic to adults has been associated with a 60% reduction in mortality and a 50% reduction in unfavorable outcomes. It is recommended that dexamethasone, 10 mg intravenously, be given immediately prior to or concomitantly with the first dose of appropriate antibiotic and continued in those with pneumococcal disease every 6 hours thereafter for a total of 4 days. Patients with pneumococcal meningitis and AIDS who do not have access to resources may not benefit from dexamethasone. The effect of dexamethasone on outcome of meningitis caused by penicillin-resistant organisms is not known.

Borchorst S et al. The role of dexamethasone in the treatment of bacterial meningitis—a systematic review. Acta Anaesthesiol Scand. 2012 Nov;56(10):1210–21. [PMID: 22524556]

Erdem H et al. Mortality indicators in pneumococcal meningitis: therapeutic implications. Int J Infect Dis. 2014 Feb;19:13–9. [PMID: 24211227]

McIntyre PB et al. Effect of vaccines on bacterial meningitis worldwide. Lancet. 2012 Nov 10;380(9854):1703–11. [PMID: 23141619]

Thigpen MC et al; Emerging Infections Programs Network. Bacterial meningitis in the United States, 1998–2007. N Engl J Med. 2011 May 26;364(21):2016–25. [PMID: 21612470]

van de Beek D et al. Advances in treatment of bacterial meningitis. Lancet. 2012 Nov 10;380(9854):1693–702. [PMID: 23141618]

STAPHYLOCOCCUS AUREUS INFECTIONS

1. Skin & Soft Tissue Infections

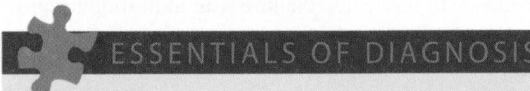

ESSENTIALS OF DIAGNOSIS

► Localized erythema with induration and purulent drainage.

► Abscess formation.

► Folliculitis commonly observed.

► Gram stain of pus with gram-positive cocci in clusters; cultures usually positive.

General Considerations

Approximately one-quarter of people are asymptomatic nasal carriers of *S aureus*, which is spread by direct contact. Carriage often precedes infection, which occurs as a consequence of disruption of the cutaneous barrier or impairment of host defenses. *S aureus* tends to cause more localized skin infections than streptococci, and abscess formation is common. The prevalence of methicillin-resistant strains in community settings is increasing, and these strains have been associated with recurrent and severe skin and soft tissue infections, including necrotizing fasciitis.

Clinical Findings

A. Symptoms and Signs

S aureus skin infections may begin around one or more hair follicles, causing folliculitis; may become localized to form

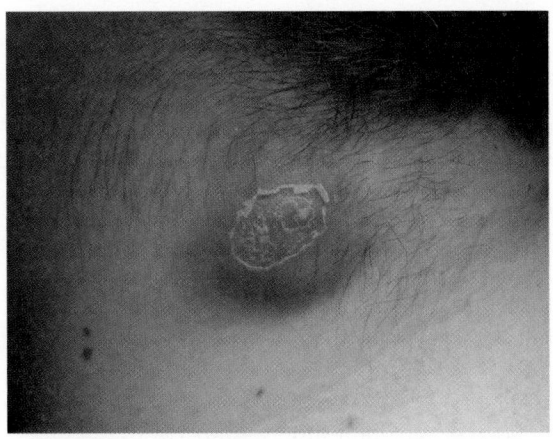

▲ **Figure 33–1.** Methicillin-resistant *Staphylococcus aureus* (MRSA) abscess of the neck. (From Edward Wright, MD; Reproduced, with permission, from Usatine RP, Smith MA, Mayeaux EJ Jr, Chumley H, Tysinger J. *The Color Atlas of Family Medicine.* McGraw-Hill, 2009.)

boils (or furuncles); or may spread to adjacent skin and deeper subcutaneous tissue (ie, a carbuncle) (Figure 33–1). Deep abscesses involving muscle or fascia may occur, often in association with a deep wound or other inoculation or injection. Necrotizing fasciitis, a rare form of *S aureus* skin and soft tissues infection, has been reported with community strains of methicillin-resistant *S aureus.*

B. Laboratory Findings

Cultures of the wound or abscess material will almost always yield the organism. In patients with systemic signs of infection, blood cultures should be obtained because of potential endocarditis, osteomyelitis, or metastatic seeding of other sites. Patients who are bacteremic should have blood cultures taken early during therapy to exclude persistent bacteremia, an indicator of severe or complicated infection.

▶ Treatment

Proper drainage of abscess fluid or other focal infections is the mainstay of therapy. Incision and drainage alone may be sufficient for cutaneous abscess. For uncomplicated skin infections, oral antimicrobial therapy is satisfactory. Before the emergence of community methicillin-resistant strains of *S aureus,* an oral penicillinase-resistant penicillin or cephalosporin, such as dicloxacillin or cephalexin, 500 mg four times a day for 7–10 days, was the drug of choice for empiric therapy. However, increasing prevalence of methicillin-resistant strains of *S aureus* among community isolates may necessitate use of other oral agents to which the isolate is susceptible in vitro, such as clindamycin, 300 mg three times daily; doxycycline or minocycline, 100 mg twice daily; or trimethoprim-sulfamethoxazole, given in two divided doses based on 5–10 mg/kg/d of the trimethoprim component. Unfortunately, the efficacy of these agents is not well defined and not evidence based. Because of the high prevalence of macrolide resistance among *S aureus*

strains, these agents should not be used unless susceptibility is documented (see Table 33–1).

For more complicated infections with extensive cutaneous or deep tissue involvement or fever, parenteral therapy is indicated initially. A penicillinase-resistant penicillin such as nafcillin or oxacillin in a dosage of 1.5 g every 6 hours intravenously or cefazolin 1 g intravenously or intramuscularly is preferred for infections caused by methicillin-susceptible isolates. In patients with a serious allergy to beta-lactam antibiotics or if the strain is methicillin-resistant, vancomycin, 1 g intravenously every 12 hours, is a drug of choice. If the local prevalence of methicillin-resistance is high (eg, 10% or more), and particularly if the patient is seriously ill, vancomycin is indicated empirically pending strain isolation and determination of susceptibility.

Linezolid is FDA-approved for treatment of skin and skin-structure infections as well as hospital-acquired pneumonia caused by methicillin-resistant strains of *S aureus* and clinically is as effective as vancomycin. The dose is 600 mg orally (bioavailability of 100%) or intravenously twice a day for 10–14 days. Its considerable cost makes it an unattractive choice for most routine outpatient infections, and its safety in treatment courses lasting longer than 2–3 weeks is not well characterized; nevertheless, it is the only proven effective oral alternative to parenteral vancomycin. Daptomycin, 4 mg/kg intravenously once daily (or every other day in the patient with creatinine clearance < 30 mL/min) for 7–14 days, is also an option for treatment of complicated skin and skin structure infections. Tigecycline (a glycylcycline class antimicrobial), telavancin (a lipoglycopeptide), and ceftaroline (a novel cephalosporin with activity against methicillin-resistant *S aureus*) are all approved by the FDA for treatment of complicated skin and skin structure infections due to methicillin-resistant strains of *S aureus.* The dosage of tigecycline is 100 mg intravenously once followed by 50 mg intravenously twice a day. The dose of telavancin is 10 mg/kg intravenously once daily for 7–14 days. The dosage of ceftaroline is 600 mg twice a day for 7–14 days.

Gaspari RJ et al. A randomized controlled trial of incision and drainage versus ultrasonographically guided needle aspiration for skin abscesses and the effect of methicillin-resistant *Staphylococcus aureus.* Ann Emerg Med. 2011 May;57(5):483–91. [PMID: 21239082]

Liu C et al. Clinical practice guidelines by the Infectious Diseases Society of America for the treatment of methicillin-resistant *Staphylococcus aureus* infections in adults and children. Clin Infect Dis. 2011 Feb 1;52(3):e18–55. [PMID: 21208910]

Pottinger PS. Methicillin-resistant *Staphylococcus aureus* infections. Med Clin North Am. 2013 Jul;97(4):601–19. [PMID: 23809716]

Skov R et al. Update on the prevention and control of community-acquired methicillin-resistant *Staphylococcus aureus* (CA-MRSA). Int J Antimicrob Agents. 2012 Mar;39(3):193–200. [PMID: 22226649]

2. Osteomyelitis

S aureus causes approximately 60% of all cases of osteomyelitis. Osteomyelitis may be caused by direct inoculation, eg, from an open fracture or as a result of surgery; by extension from a contiguous focus of infection or open wound; or by hematogenous spread. Long bones and vertebrae are the usual sites. Epidural abscess is a common complication of vertebral osteomyelitis and should be suspected if fever and severe back or neck pain are accompanied by radicular pain or symptoms or signs indicative of spinal cord compression (eg, incontinence, extremity weakness, pathologic extremity reflexes).

▶ **Clinical Findings**

A. Symptoms and Signs

The infection may be acute, with abrupt development of local symptoms and systemic toxicity, or indolent, with insidious onset of vague pain over the site of infection, progressing to local tenderness and constitutional symptoms (fever, malaise, anorexia, night sweats). Fever is absent in one-third or more of cases. Back pain is often the only symptom in vertebral osteomyelitis and may be associated with an epidural abscess and spinal cord compression. Draining sinus tracts occur in chronic infections or infections of foreign body implants.

B. Laboratory Findings

The diagnosis is established by isolation of *S aureus* from the blood, bone, or a contiguous focus of a patient with symptoms and of signs focal bone infection. Blood culture will be positive in approximately 60% of untreated cases. Bone biopsy and culture are indicated if blood cultures are sterile.

C. Imaging

Bone scan and gallium scan, each with a sensitivity of approximately 95% and a specificity of 60–70%, are useful in identifying or confirming the site of bone infection. Plain bone films early in the course of infection are often normal but will become abnormal in most cases even with effective therapy. Spinal infection (unlike malignancy) traverses the disk space to involve the contiguous vertebral body. CT is more sensitive than plain films and helps localize associated abscesses. MRI is slightly less sensitive than bone scan but has a specificity of 90%. It is indicated when epidural abscess is suspected in association with vertebral osteomyelitis.

▶ **Treatment**

Prolonged therapy is required to cure staphylococcal osteomyelitis. Durations of 4–6 weeks or longer are recommended. Although oral regimens can be effective, intravenous therapy is preferred, particularly during the acute phase of the infection for patients with systemic toxicity. Nafcillin or oxacillin, 9–12 g/d in six divided doses, is the drug of choice for infection with methicillin-sensitive isolates. Cefazolin, 2 g every 8 hours, also is effective. Patients with infections due to methicillin-resistant strains of *S aureus* or who have severe penicillin allergies should be treated with vancomycin, 30 mg/kg/d intravenously divided in two or three doses. Doses should be adjusted to achieve a vancomycin trough of 15–20 mcg/mL.

Oral step-down therapy to a rifampin combination regimen may be effective and in certain cases primary oral therapy may be effective, but consultation with an infectious diseases specialists is recommended. The role of newer agents, such as daptomycin or linezolid, remains to be defined.

Surgical treatment is often indicated under the following circumstances: (1) staphylococcal osteomyelitis with associated epidural abscess and spinal cord compression, (2) other abscesses (psoas, paraspinal), (3) extensive disease, or (4) recurrent infection following standard medical therapy.

Dhanoa A et al. Acute haematogenous community-acquired methicillin-resistant *Staphylococcus aureus* osteomyelitis in an adult: case report and review of literature. BMC Infect Dis. 2012 Oct 25;12:270. [PMID: 23098162]

Liu C et al. Clinical practice guidelines by the Infectious Diseases Society of America for the treatment of methicillin-resistant *Staphylococcus aureus* infections in adults and children. Clin Infect Dis. 2011 Feb 1;52(3):e18–55. [PMID: 21208910]

Vardakas KZ et al. Incidence, characteristics, and outcomes of patients with bone and joint infections due to community-associated methicillin-resistant *Staphylococcus aureus*: a systematic review. Eur J Clin Microbiol Infect Dis. 2013 Jun;32(6):711–21. [PMID: 23334662]

3. Staphylococcal Bacteremia

S aureus readily invades the bloodstream and infects sites distant from the primary site of infection, which may be relatively minor or even inapparent. Whenever *S aureus* is recovered from blood cultures, the possibility of endocarditis, osteomyelitis, or other metastatic deep infection must be considered. Bacteremia that persists for more than 48 to 96 hours after initiation of therapy is strongly predictive of worse outcome and complicated infection. The appropriate duration of therapy for uncomplicated bacteremia arising from a removable source (eg, intravenous device) or drainable focus (eg, skin abscess) has not been well defined, but a 10- to 14-day course of therapy appears to be the minimum. However, 5% or more of patients may relapse, usually with endocarditis or osteomyelitis, even if treated for 2 weeks.

Nafcillin or oxacillin, 2 g intravenously every 4 hours or cefazolin, 2 g every 8 hours is recommended for uncomplicated methicillin-susceptible *S aureus* bacteremia. Vancomycin, 30 mg/kg/d intravenously in two or three divided doses, as definitive therapy should be reserved for patients with serious penicillin allergy or with infections caused by methicillin-resistant strains because it is less active than beta-lactam antibiotics and treatment failures are more common than with beta-lactams. Maintaining a vancomycin trough concentration of 15–20 mcg/mL may improve outcomes and is recommended. Transesophageal echocardiography (TEE) is a sensitive and cost-effective method for excluding underlying endocarditis. It is considered for patients for whom the pretest probability of endocarditis is 5% or higher—and for all patients with unexplained *S aureus* bacteremia.

Vancomycin treatment failures are relatively common, particularly for complicated bacteremia, in foreign body infection, or when the MIC of the isolate is ≥ 2 mcg/mL.

Consultation should be sought with an infectious diseases specialist when vancomycin treatment failure is encountered. Daptomycin, 6 mg/kg intravenously once daily, is approved by the FDA for treatment of *S aureus* bacteremia and is an alternative to vancomycin, especially if a beta-lactam cannot be used or if the patient is not responding to vancomycin. Cases of vancomycin treatment failures in which the staphylococcal isolate exhibits a vancomycin MIC ≥ 4 mcg/mL should be reported to the Centers for Disease Control and Prevention (CDC) to help track this potentially serious and emerging problem of vancomycin resistance.

Empiric therapy of suspected staphylococcal infection, whether of community or hospital onset, depends on the severity of the infection and the likelihood that it is caused by methicillin-resistant strains. If the prevalence exceeds 5–10% for more seriously ill patients, initial therapy should include vancomycin, 30 mg/kg/d intravenously divided in two or three doses, until results of susceptibility tests are known. Resistance to vancomycin fortunately remains rare and should not affect the choice of empiric therapy.

Keynan Y et al. *Staphylococcus aureus* bacteremia, risk factors, complications, and management. Crit Care Clin. 2013 Jul;29(3):547–62. [PMID: 23830653]

Liu C et al. Clinical practice guidelines by the Infectious Diseases Society of America for the treatment of methicillin-resistant *Staphylococcus aureus* infections in adults and children. Clin Infect Dis. 2011 Feb 1;52(3):e18–55. [PMID: 21208910]

4. Toxic Shock Syndrome

S aureus produces toxins that cause three important entities: "scalded skin syndrome" in children, toxic shock syndrome in adults, and enterotoxin food poisoning. Toxic shock syndrome is characterized by abrupt onset of high fever, vomiting, and watery diarrhea. Sore throat, myalgias, and headache are common. Hypotension with kidney and heart failure is associated with a poor outcome. A diffuse macular erythematous rash (Figure 33–2) and nonpurulent conjunctivitis are common, and desquamation, especially

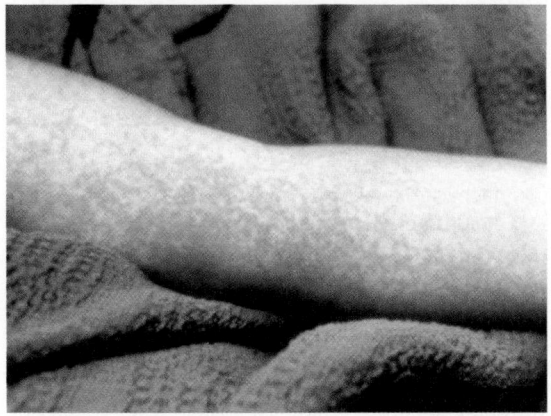

▲ **Figure 33–2.** Morbilliform rash in toxic shock syndrome caused by *Staphylococcus aureus*. (Public Health Image Library, CDC.)

of palms and soles, is typical during recovery. Fatality rates may be as high as 15%. Although originally associated with tampon use, any focus (eg, nasopharynx, bone, vagina, rectum, abscess, or wound) harboring a toxin-producing *S aureus* strain can cause toxic shock syndrome and non-menstrual cases of toxic shock syndrome are common. Classically, blood cultures are negative because symptoms are due to the effects of the toxin and not systemic infection.

Important aspects of treatment include rapid rehydration, antistaphylococcal drugs, management of kidney or heart failure, and addressing sources of toxin, eg, removal of tampon or drainage of abscess.

5. Infections Caused by Coagulase-Negative Staphylococci

Coagulase-negative staphylococci are an important cause of infections of intravascular and prosthetic devices and of wound infection following cardiothoracic surgery. These organisms infrequently cause infections such as osteomyelitis and endocarditis in the absence of a prosthesis, but rates may be increasing. Most human infections are caused by *Staphylococcus epidermidis, S haemolyticus, S hominis, S warnerii, S saprophyticus, S saccharolyticus,* and *S cohnii*. These common hospital-acquired pathogens are less virulent than *S aureus*, and infections caused by them tend to be more indolent.

Because coagulase-negative staphylococci are normal inhabitants of human skin, it is difficult to distinguish infection from contamination, the latter perhaps accounting for three-fourths of blood culture isolates. Infection is more likely if the patient has a foreign body (eg, sternal wires, prosthetic joint, prosthetic cardiac valve, pacemaker, intracranial pressure monitor, cerebrospinal fluid shunt, peritoneal dialysis catheter) or an intravascular device in place. Purulent or serosanguineous drainage, erythema, pain, or tenderness at the site of the foreign body or device suggests infection. Instability and pain are signs of prosthetic joint infection. Fever, a new murmur, instability of the prosthesis, or signs of systemic embolization are evidence of prosthetic valve endocarditis. Immunosuppression and recent antimicrobial therapy are risk factors.

Infection is also more likely if the same strain is consistently isolated from two or more blood cultures (particularly if samples were obtained at different times) and from the foreign body site. Contamination is more likely when a single blood culture is positive or if more than one strain is isolated from blood cultures. The antimicrobial susceptibility pattern and speciation are used to determine whether one or more strains have been isolated. More sophisticated typing methods, eg, pulse-field gel electrophoresis of restriction enzyme digested chromosomal DNA, may be required to identify distinct strains.

Whenever possible, the intravascular device or foreign body suspected of being infected by coagulase-negative staphylococci should be removed. However, removal and replacement of some devices (eg, prosthetic joint, prosthetic valve, cerebrospinal fluid shunt) can be a difficult or risky procedure, and it may sometimes be preferable to treat with antibiotics alone with the understanding that the probability of cure is reduced and that surgical management may eventually be necessary.

Coagulase-negative staphylococci are commonly resistant to beta-lactams and multiple other antibiotics. For patients with normal kidney function, vancomycin, 1 g intravenously every 12 hours, is the treatment of choice for suspected or confirmed infection caused by these organisms until susceptibility to penicillinase-resistant penicillins or other agents has been confirmed. Duration of therapy has not been established for relatively uncomplicated infections, such as those secondary to intravenous devices, which may be eliminated by simply removing the infected device. Infection involving bone or a prosthetic valve should be treated for 6 weeks. A combination regimen of vancomycin plus rifampin, 300 mg orally twice daily, plus gentamicin, 1 mg/kg intravenously every 8 hours, is recommended for treatment of prosthetic valve endocarditis caused by methicillin-resistant strains.

Widerström M et al. Coagulase-negative staphylococci: update on the molecular epidemiology and clinical presentation, with a focus on *Staphylococcus epidermidis* and *Staphylococcus saprophyticus*. Eur J Clin Microbiol Infect Dis. 2012 Jan;31(1):7–20. [PMID: 21533877]

CLOSTRIDIAL DISEASES

1. Clostridial Myonecrosis (Gas Gangrene)

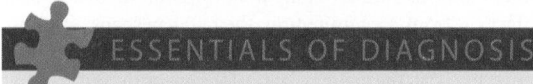

ESSENTIALS OF DIAGNOSIS

► Sudden onset of pain and edema in an area of wound contamination.

► Prostration and systemic toxicity.

► Brown to blood-tinged watery exudate, with skin discoloration of surrounding area.

► Gas in the tissue by palpation or radiograph.

► Gram-positive rods in culture or smear of exudate.

► General Considerations

Gas gangrene or clostridial myonecrosis is produced by any one of several clostridia (*Clostridium perfringens, C ramosum, C bifermentans, C histolyticum, C novyi,* etc). Trauma and injection drug use are common predisposing conditions. Toxins produced in devitalized tissues under anaerobic conditions result in shock, hemolysis, and myonecrosis.

► Clinical Findings

A. Symptoms and Signs

The onset is usually sudden, with rapidly increasing pain in the affected area, hypotension, and tachycardia. Fever is present but is not proportionate to the severity of the infection. In the last stages of the disease, severe prostration, stupor, delirium, and coma occur.

The wound becomes swollen, and the surrounding skin is pale. There is a foul-smelling brown, blood-tinged serous discharge. As the disease advances, the surrounding tissue changes from pale to dusky and finally becomes deeply discolored, with coalescent, red, fluid-filled vesicles. Gas may be palpable in the tissues.

B. Laboratory Findings

Gas gangrene is a clinical diagnosis, and empiric therapy is indicated if the diagnosis is suspected. Radiographic studies may show gas within the soft tissues, but this finding is not specific. The smear shows absence of neutrophils and the presence of gram-positive rods. Anaerobic culture confirms the diagnosis.

► Differential Diagnosis

Other bacteria can produce gas in infected tissue, eg, enteric gram-negative organisms, or anaerobes.

► Treatment

Penicillin, 2 million units every 3 hours intravenously, is effective. Clindamycin may decrease the production of bacterial toxin, and some experts recommend the addition of clindamycin, 600–900 mg every 8 hours intravenously, to penicillin. Adequate surgical debridement and exposure of infected areas are essential, with radical surgical excision often necessary. Hyperbaric oxygen therapy has been used empirically but must be used in conjunction with administration of an appropriate antibiotic and surgical debridement.

Bryant AE et al. Clostridial myonecrosis: new insights in pathogenesis and management. Curr Infect Dis Rep. 2010 Sep;12(5):383–91. [PMID: 21308521]
Stevens DL et al. Life-threatening clostridial infections. Anaerobe. 2012 Apr;18(2):254–9. [PMID: 22120198]

2. *Clostridium sordellii* Toxic Shock Syndrome

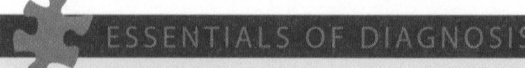

ESSENTIALS OF DIAGNOSIS

► Sudden onset after medical abortion.

► Abdominal pain.

► Absence of fever.

► Tachycardia, severe hypotension, capillary leak syndrome with edema.

► Profound leukocytosis, hemoconcentration.

► General Considerations & Clinical Findings

C sordellii is a rare cause of endometritis and toxic shock syndrome following childbirth. Fatal cases of uterine infection following medically induced abortion with mifepristone have been reported. Onset of illness was within 4–5 days of ingestion of mifepristone and the clinical course fulminant. Infection appeared to be limited to the uterus, which showed necrosis, edema, hemorrhage, and acute inflammatory changes.

Treatment

Early recognition, aggressive resuscitation from shock, immediate surgical debridement with hysterectomy, and administration of an antimicrobial that is active against *C sordellii* are essential to survival. Based on in vitro susceptibility data, any of several agents should be active, including penicillin, ampicillin, a macrolide, clindamycin, a tetracycline, or metronidazole. Whether a protein synthesis inhibitor to block further toxin production offers any advantage over a beta-lactam is unknown.

Dempsey A. Serious infection associated with induced abortion in the United States. Clin Obstet Gynecol. 2012 Dec;55(4):888–92. [PMID: 23090457]

Stevens DL et al. Life-threatening clostridial infections. Anaerobe. 2012 Apr;18(2):254–9. [PMID: 22120198]

3. Tetanus

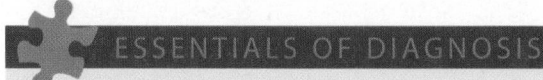

ESSENTIALS OF DIAGNOSIS

► History of wound and possible contamination.

► Jaw stiffness followed by spasms of jaw muscles (trismus).

► Stiffness of the neck and other muscles, dysphagia, irritability, hyperreflexia.

► Finally, painful convulsions precipitated by minimal stimuli.

General Considerations

Tetanus is caused by the neurotoxin tetanospasmin, elaborated by *C tetani*. Spores of this organism are ubiquitous in soil and may germinate when introduced into a wound. The vegetative bacteria produce tetanospasmin, a zinc metalloprotease that cleaves synaptobrevin, a protein essential for neurotransmitter release. Tetanospasmin interferes with neurotransmission at spinal synapses of inhibitory neurons. As a result, minor stimuli result in uncontrolled spasms, and reflexes are exaggerated. The incubation period is 5 days to 15 weeks, with the average being 8–12 days.

Most cases occur in unvaccinated individuals. Persons at risk are the elderly, migrant workers, newborns, and injection drug users. While puncture wounds are particularly prone to causing tetanus, any wound, including bites or decubiti, may become colonized and infected by *C tetani*.

Clinical Findings

A. Symptoms and Signs

The first symptom may be pain and tingling at the site of inoculation, followed by spasticity of the muscles nearby.

Stiffness of the jaw, neck stiffness, dysphagia, and irritability are other early signs. Hyperreflexia develops later, with spasms of the jaw muscles (trismus) or facial muscles and rigidity and spasm of the muscles of the abdomen, neck, and back. Painful tonic convulsions precipitated by minor stimuli are common. Spasms of the glottis and respiratory muscles may cause acute asphyxia. The patient is awake and alert throughout the illness. The sensory examination is normal. The temperature is normal or only slightly elevated.

B. Laboratory Findings

The diagnosis of tetanus is made clinically.

Differential Diagnosis

Tetanus must be differentiated from various acute central nervous system infections such as meningitis. Trismus may occasionally develop with the use of phenothiazines. Strychnine poisoning should also be considered.

Complications

Airway obstruction is common. Urinary retention and constipation may result from spasm of the sphincters. Respiratory arrest and cardiac failure are late, life-threatening events.

Prevention

Tetanus is preventable by active immunization (see Table 30–7). For primary immunization of adults, Td (tetanus and diphtheria toxoids vaccine) is administered as two doses 4–6 weeks apart, with a third dose 6–12 months later. For one of the doses, Tdap (tetanus toxoid, reduced dose diphtheria toxoid, acellular pertussis vaccine) should be substituted for Td. Booster doses are given every 10 years or at the time of major injury if it occurs more than 5 years after a dose. A single dose of Tdap is preferred to Td for wound prophylaxis if the patient has not been previously vaccinated with Tdap.

Passive immunization should be used in nonimmunized individuals and those whose immunization status is uncertain whenever a wound is contaminated or likely to have devitalized tissue. Tetanus immune globulin, 250 units, is given intramuscularly. Active immunization with tetanus toxoid is started concurrently. Table 33–2 provides a guide to prophylactic management.

Treatment

A. Specific Measures

Human tetanus immune globulin, 500 units, should be administered intramuscularly within the first 24 hours of presentation. Whether intrathecal administration has any additional benefit is controversial. An unblinded, randomized trial comparing intramuscular tetanus immune globulin to intramuscular plus intrathecal tetanus immune globulin found more rapid resolution of spasms, fewer days

Table 33–2. Guide to tetanus prophylaxis in wound management.

	Clean, Minor Wounds		All Other Wounds[1]	
History of Absorbed Tetanus Toxoid	Tdap or Td[2]	TIG[3]	Tdap or Td[2]	TIG[3]
Unknown or < 3 doses	Yes	No	Yes	Yes
3 or more doses	No[4]	No	No[5]	No

[1]Such as, but not limited to, wounds contaminated with dirt, feces, soil, saliva, etc; puncture wounds; avulsions; and wounds resulting from missiles, crushing, burns, and frostbite.
[2]Td indicates tetanus toxoid and diphtheria toxoid, adult form. Tdap indicates tetanus toxoid, reduced diphtheria toxoid, and acellular pertussis vaccine, which may be substituted as a single dose for Td. Unvaccinated individuals should receive a complete series of three doses, one of which is Tdap.
[3]Human tetanus immune globulin, 250 units intramuscularly.
[4]Yes if more than 10 years have elapsed since last dose.
[5]Yes if more than 5 years have elapsed since last dose. (More frequent boosters are not needed and can enhance side effects.) Tdap has been safely administered within 2 years of Td vaccination, although local reactions to the vaccine may be increased.

of ventilatory support, and a shorter hospital stay in the intrathecal group. However, the exact immunoglobulin preparation that was used was not specified and the total dose was 4000 units. Tetanus does not produce natural immunity, and a full course of immunization with tetanus toxoid should be administered once the patient has recovered.

B. General Measures

Minimal stimuli can provoke spasms, so the patient should be placed at bed rest and monitored under the quietest conditions possible. Sedation, paralysis with curare-like agents, and mechanical ventilation are often necessary to control tetanic spasms. Penicillin, 20 million units intravenously daily in divided doses, is given to all patients—even those with mild illness—to eradicate toxin-producing organisms.

▶ Prognosis

High mortality rates are associated with a short incubation period, early onset of convulsions, and delay in treatment. Contaminated lesions about the head and face are more dangerous than wounds on other parts of the body.

Afshar M et al. Narrative review: tetanus—a health threat after natural disasters in developing countries. Ann Intern Med. 2011 Mar 1;154(5):329–35. [PMID: 21357910]

Ataro P et al. Tetanus: a review. South Med J. 2011 Aug; 104(8):613–7. [PMID: 21886075]

Centers for Disease Control and Prevention (CDC). Updated recommendations for use of tetanus toxoid, reduced diphtheria toxoid, and acellular pertussis (Tdap) vaccine in adults aged 65 years and older—Advisory Committee on Immunization Practices (ACIP), 2012. MMWR Morb Mortal Wkly Rep. 2012 Jun 29;61(25):468–70. [PMID: 22739778]

Centers for Disease Control and Prevention (CDC). Updated recommendations for use of tetanus toxoid, reduced diphtheria toxoid, and acellular pertussis vaccine (Tdap) in pregnant women—Advisory Committee on Immunization Practices (ACIP), 2012. MMWR Morb Mortal Wkly Rep. 2013 Feb 22;62(7):131–5. [PMID: 23425962]

4. Botulism

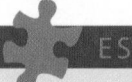

ESSENTIALS OF DIAGNOSIS

▶ History of recent ingestion of home-canned or smoked foods or of injection drug use and demonstration of toxin in serum or food.

▶ Sudden onset of diplopia, dry mouth, dysphagia, dysphonia, and muscle weakness progressing to respiratory paralysis.

▶ Pupils are fixed and dilated in most cases.

▶ General Considerations

Botulism is a paralytic disease caused by botulinum toxin, which is produced by *C botulinum*, a ubiquitous, strictly anaerobic, spore-forming bacillus found in soil. Four toxin types—A, B, E, and F—cause human disease. Botulinum toxin is a zinc metalloprotease that cleaves a specific component of the synaptic vesicle membrane docking and fusion complex at the neuromuscular junction blocking release of the neurotransmitter acetylcholine. Botulinum toxin is extremely potent and is classified by the CDC as a high-priority agent because of its potential for use as an agent of bioterrorism. Naturally occurring botulism occurs in one of three forms: food-borne botulism, infant botulism, or wound botulism. Food-borne botulism is caused by ingestion of preformed toxin present in canned, smoked, or vacuum-packed foods such as home-canned vegetables, smoked meats, and vacuum-packed fish. Commercial foods have also been associated with outbreaks of botulism. Infant botulism (associated with ingestion of honey) and wound botulism (which typically occurs in association with injection drug use) result from organisms present in the gut or wound that elaborate toxin in vivo.

Clinical Findings

A. Symptoms and Signs

Twelve to 36 hours after ingestion of the toxin, visual disturbances appear, particularly diplopia and loss of accommodation. Ptosis, cranial nerve palsies with impairment of extraocular muscles, and fixed dilated pupils are characteristic signs. The sensory examination is normal. Other symptoms are dry mouth, dysphagia, and dysphonia. Nausea and vomiting may be present, particularly with type E toxin. The sensorium remains clear and the temperature normal. Paralysis progressing to respiratory failure and death may occur unless mechanical assistance is provided.

B. Laboratory Findings

Toxin in patients' serum and in suspected foods can be demonstrated by mouse inoculation and identified with specific antiserum.

Differential Diagnosis

Because the clinical presentation of botulism is so distinctive and the differential diagnosis limited, botulism once considered is not easily confused with other diseases. Cranial nerve involvement may be seen with vertebrobasilar insufficiency, the C. Miller Fisher variant of Guillain-Barré syndrome, myasthenia gravis, or any basilar meningitis (infectious or carcinomatous). Intestinal obstruction or other types of food poisoning are considered when nausea and vomiting are present.

Treatment

If botulism is suspected, the practitioner should contact the state health authorities or the CDC for advice and help with procurement of equine serum heptavalent botulism antitoxin and for assistance in obtaining assays for toxin in serum, stool, or food. Skin testing is recommended to exclude hypersensitivity to the antitoxin preparation. Antitoxin should be administered as early as possible, ideally within 24 hours of the onset of symptoms or signs, to arrest progression of disease; its administration should not be delayed for laboratory confirmation of the diagnosis. Respiratory failure is managed with intubation and mechanical ventilation. Parenteral fluids or alimentation should be given while swallowing difficulty persists. The removal of unabsorbed toxin from the gut may be attempted. Any remnants of suspected foods should be assayed for toxin. Persons who might have eaten the suspected food must be located and observed.

Chalk C et al. Medical treatment for botulism. Cochrane Database Syst Rev. 2011 Mar 16;(3):CD008123. [PMID: 21412916]
Lavender TW et al. Acute infections in intravenous drug users. Clin Med. 2013 Oct;13(5):511–3. [PMID: 24115713]

ANTHRAX

ESSENTIALS OF DIAGNOSIS

▶ Appropriate epidemiologic setting, eg, exposure to animals or animal hides, or potential exposure from an act of bioterrorism.

▶ A painless cutaneous black eschar on exposed areas of the skin, with marked surrounding edema and vesicles.

▶ Nonspecific flu-like symptoms that rapidly progress to extreme dyspnea and shock; mediastinal widening and pleural effusions on chest radiograph.

General Considerations

The death of a Florida photo editor from inhalational anthrax acquired from a letter deliberately contaminated with spores of *Bacillus anthracis* thrust this extremely rare infection into the public awareness. Between September 18 and November 21 of 2001, there were 13 cases of cutaneous anthrax and 11 cases of inhalational anthrax associated with exposure to anthrax spores in contaminated mail.

Naturally occurring anthrax is a disease of sheep, cattle, horses, goats, and swine. *B anthracis* is a gram-positive spore-forming aerobic rod. Spores—not vegetative bacteria—are the infectious form of the organism. These are transmitted to humans from contact with contaminated animals, animal products, or animal hides, or from soil by inoculation of broken skin or mucous membranes; by inhalation of aerosolized spores; or, rarely, by ingestion resulting in cutaneous, inhalational, or gastrointestinal forms of anthrax, respectively. Spores germinate into vegetative bacteria that multiply locally in cutaneous and gastrointestinal anthrax but may also disseminate to cause systemic infection. Inhaled spores are ingested by pulmonary macrophages and carried via lymphatics to regional lymph nodes, where they germinate. The bacteria rapidly multiply within the lymphatics, causing a hemorrhagic lymphadenitis. Invasion of the bloodstream leads to overwhelming sepsis, killing the host.

Clinical Findings

A. Symptoms and Signs

1. Cutaneous anthrax—This occurs within 2 weeks after exposure to spores; there is no latency period for cutaneous disease as there is with inhalational anthrax. The initial lesion is an erythematous papule, often on an exposed area of skin that vesiculates and then ulcerates and undergoes necrosis, ultimately progressing to a purple to black eschar. The eschar typically is painless; pain indicates secondary staphylococcal or streptococcal infection. The surrounding area is edematous and vesicular but not purulent. Regional adenopathy, fever, malaise, headache, and nausea and vomiting may be present. The infection is self-limited in most cases, but hematogenous spread with sepsis or meningitis may occur.

2. Inhalational anthrax—Illness occurs in two stages, beginning on average 10 days after exposure, but may have a latent onset 6 weeks after exposure. Nonspecific viral-like symptoms such as fever, malaise, headache, dyspnea, cough, and congestion of the nose, throat, and larynx are characteristic of the initial stage. Anterior chest pain is an early symptom of mediastinitis. Within hours to a few days, progression to the fulminant stage of infection occurs in which symptoms or signs of overwhelming sepsis predominate. Delirium, obtundation, or findings of meningeal irritation suggest an accompanying hemorrhagic meningitis.

3. Gastrointestinal anthrax—Fever, diffuse abdominal pain, rebound abdominal tenderness, vomiting, constipation, and diarrhea occur 2–5 days after ingestion of meat contaminated with anthrax spores. The primary lesion is ulcerative, producing emesis that may be blood-tinged or coffee-grounds and stool that may be blood-tinged or melenic. Bowel perforation can occur. The oropharyngeal form of the disease is characterized by local lymphadenopathy, cervical edema, dysphagia, and upper respiratory tract obstruction.

B. Laboratory Findings

Laboratory findings are nonspecific. The white blood cell count initially may be normal or modestly elevated, with polymorphonuclear predominance and an increase in early forms. Pleural fluid from patients with inhalational anthrax is typically hemorrhagic with few white cells. Cerebrospinal fluid from meningitis cases is also hemorrhagic. Gram stain of pleural fluid, cerebrospinal fluid, unspun blood, blood culture, or fluid from a cutaneous lesion may show the characteristic boxcar-shaped encapsulated rods in chains.

The diagnosis is established by isolation of the organism from culture of the skin lesion (or fluid expressed from it), blood, or pleural fluid—or cerebrospinal fluid in cases of meningitis. In the absence of prior antimicrobial therapy, cultures are invariably positive. Cultures obtained after initiation of antimicrobial therapy may be negative. If anthrax is suspected on clinical or epidemiologic grounds, immunohistochemical tests (eg, to detect capsular antigen), polymerase chain reaction assays, and serologic tests (useful for documenting past cutaneous infection) are available through the CDC and should be used to establish the diagnosis. Any suspected case of anthrax should be immediately reported to the CDC so that a complete investigation can be conducted.

C. Imaging

The chest radiograph is the most sensitive test for inhalational disease, being abnormal (though the findings can be subtle) initially in every case of bioterrorism-associated disease. Mediastinal widening due to hemorrhagic lymphadenitis, a hallmark feature of the disease, was present in 70% of the bioterrorism-related cases. Pleural effusions were present initially or occurred over the course of illness in all cases, and approximately three-fourths had pulmonary infiltrates or signs of consolidation.

▶ Differential Diagnosis

Cutaneous anthrax, despite its characteristic appearance, can be confused with a variety of other also uncommon or rare conditions such as ecthyma gangrenosum, rat-bite fever, ulceroglandular tularemia, plague, glanders, rickettsialpox, orf (parapoxvirus infection), or cutaneous mycobacterial infection. Inhalational anthrax must be differentiated from mediastinitis due to other bacterial causes, fibrous mediastinitis due to histoplasmosis, coccidioidomycosis, atypical or viral pneumonia, silicosis, sarcoidosis, and other causes of mediastinal widening (eg, superior vena cava syndrome or aortic aneurysm or dissection). Gastrointestinal anthrax shares clinical features with a variety of common intra-abdominal disorders, including bowel obstruction, perforated viscus, peritonitis, gastroenteritis, and peptic ulcer disease.

▶ Treatment

Strains of *B anthracis* (including the strain isolated in the bioterrorism cases) are susceptible in vitro to penicillin, amoxicillin, chloramphenicol, clindamycin, imipenem, doxycycline, ciprofloxacin (as well as other fluoroquinolones), macrolides, rifampin, and vancomycin. *B anthracis* may express beta-lactamases that confer resistance to cephalosporins and penicillins. For this reason, penicillin or amoxicillin is no longer recommended for use as a single agent in treatment of disseminated disease. Based on results of animal experiments and because of concern for engineered drug resistance in strains of *B anthracis* used in bioterrorism, ciprofloxacin is considered the drug of choice (Table 33–3) for treatment and for prophylaxis following exposure to anthrax spores. Other fluoroquinolones with activity against gram-positive bacteria (eg, levofloxacin, moxifloxacin) are likely to be just as effective as ciprofloxacin. Doxycycline is an alternative first-line agent.

Table 33–3. Antimicrobial agents for treatment of anthrax or for prophylaxis against anthrax.

First-line agents and recommended doses
Ciprofloxacin, 500 mg twice daily orally or 400 mg every 12 hours intravenously
Doxycycline, 100 mg every 12 hours orally or intravenously
Second-line agents and recommended doses
Amoxicillin, 500 mg three times daily orally
Penicillin G, 2–4 million units every 4 hours intravenously
Alternative agents with in vitro activity and suggested doses
Rifampin, 10 mg/kg/d orally or intravenously
Clindamycin, 450–600 mg every 8 hours orally or intravenously
Clarithromycin, 500 mg orally twice daily
Erythromycin, 500 mg every 6 hours intravenously
Vancomycin, 1 g every 12 hours intravenously
Imipenem, 500 mg every 6 hours intravenously

Combination therapy with at least one additional agent is recommended for inhalational or disseminated disease and in cutaneous infection involving the face, head, and neck or associated with extensive local edema or systemic signs of infection, eg, fever, tachycardia and elevated white blood cell count. Single-drug therapy is recommended for prophylaxis following exposure to spores.

The required duration of therapy is poorly defined. In naturally occurring disease, treatment for 7–10 days for cutaneous disease and for at least 2 weeks following clinical response for disseminated, inhalational, or gastrointestinal infection have been standard recommendations. Because of concern about relapse from latent spores acquired by inhalation of aerosol in bioterrorism-associated cases, the initial recommendation was treatment for 60 days.

▶ Prevention

In 2001, the CDC offered one of two options for postal workers receiving prophylaxis for exposure to contaminated mail: (1) antibiotics for 100 days (fearing that even with 60 days of treatment late relapses might occur) or (2) vaccination with an investigative agent (three doses administered over a 1-month period) in conjunction with 40 days of antibiotic administration to cover the time required for a protective antibody response to develop. Insufficient information exists to favor one recommendation over the other.

There is also an FDA-approved vaccine for persons at high risk for exposure to anthrax spores. The vaccine is cell-free antigen prepared from an attenuated strain of B anthracis. Multiple injections over 18 months and an annual booster dose are required to achieve and maintain protection. Existing supplies have been reserved for vaccination of military personnel.

▶ Prognosis

The prognosis in cutaneous infection is excellent. Death is unlikely if the infection has remained localized, and lesions heal without complications in most cases. The reported mortality rate for gastrointestinal and inhalational infections is up to 85%. The experience with bioterrorism-associated inhalational cases in which six of eleven victims survived suggests a somewhat better outcome with modern supportive care and antibiotics provided that treatment is initiated before the patient has progressed to the fulminant stage of disease. No cases of anthrax have occurred among the several thousand individuals receiving antimicrobial prophylaxis following exposure to spores.

Artenstein AW et al. Novel approaches to the treatment of systemic anthrax. Clin Infect Dis. 2012 Apr;54(8):1148–61. [PMID: 22438345]

Meaney-Delman D et al. Prophylaxis and treatment of anthrax in pregnant women. Obstet Gynecol. 2013 Oct;122(4):885–900. [PMID: 24084549]

Sweeney DA et al. Anthrax infection. Am J Respir Crit Care Med. 2011 Dec 15;184(12):1333–41. [PMID: 21852539]

DIPHTHERIA

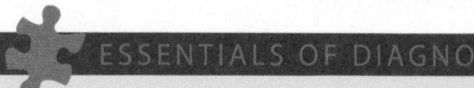

ESSENTIALS OF DIAGNOSIS

▶ Tenacious gray membrane at portal of entry in pharynx.

▶ Sore throat, nasal discharge, hoarseness, malaise, fever.

▶ Myocarditis, neuropathy.

▶ Culture confirms the diagnosis.

▶ General Considerations

Diphtheria is an acute infection caused by *Corynebacterium diphtheriae* that usually attacks the respiratory tract but may involve any mucous membrane or skin wound. The organism is spread chiefly by respiratory secretions. Exotoxin produced by the organism is responsible for myocarditis and neuropathy.

▶ Clinical Findings

A. Symptoms and Signs

Nasal, laryngeal, pharyngeal, and cutaneous forms of diphtheria occur. Nasal infection produces few symptoms other than a nasal discharge. Laryngeal infection may lead to upper airway and bronchial obstruction. In pharyngeal diphtheria, the most common form, a tenacious gray membrane covers the tonsils and pharynx. Mild sore throat, fever, and malaise are followed by toxemia and prostration.

Myocarditis and neuropathy are the most common and most serious complications. Myocarditis causes cardiac arrhythmias, heart block, and heart failure. The neuropathy usually involves the cranial nerves first, producing diplopia, slurred speech, and difficulty in swallowing.

B. Laboratory Findings

The diagnosis is made clinically but can be confirmed by culture of the organism.

▶ Differential Diagnosis

Diphtheria must be differentiated from streptococcal pharyngitis, infectious mononucleosis, adenovirus or herpes simplex infection, Vincent angina, pharyngitis due to *Arcanobacterium haemolyticum*, and candidiasis. A presumptive diagnosis of diphtheria should be made on clinical grounds without waiting for laboratory verification, since emergency treatment is needed.

▶ Prevention

Active immunization with diphtheria toxoid is part of routine childhood immunization with appropriate booster injections. The immunization schedule for adults is the same as for tetanus.

Susceptible persons exposed to diphtheria should receive a booster dose of diphtheria toxoid (or a complete series if previously unimmunized), as well as a course of penicillin or erythromycin.

▶ Treatment

Antitoxin, which is prepared from horse serum, must be given in all cases when diphtheria is suspected. For mild early pharyngeal or laryngeal disease, the dose is 20,000–40,000 units; for moderate nasopharyngeal disease, 40,000–60,000 units; for severe, extensive, or late (3 days or more) disease, 80,000–100,000 units. Diphtheria equine antitoxin can be obtained from the CDC.

Removal of membrane by direct laryngoscopy or bronchoscopy may be necessary to prevent or alleviate airway obstruction.

Either penicillin, 250 mg orally four times daily, or erythromycin, 500 mg orally four times daily, for 14 days is effective therapy, although erythromycin is slightly more effective in eliminating the carrier state. Azithromycin or clarithromycin is probably as effective as erythromycin. The patient should be isolated until three consecutive cultures at the completion of therapy have documented elimination of the organism from the oropharynx. Contacts to a case should receive erythromycin, 500 mg orally four times daily for 7 days, to eradicate carriage.

Adler NR et al. Diphtheria: forgotten, but not gone. Intern Med J. 2013 Feb;43(2):206–10. [PMID: 23402486]

Centers for Disease Control and Prevention (CDC). Updated recommendations for use of tetanus toxoid, reduced diphtheria toxoid, and acellular pertussis (Tdap) vaccine in adults aged 65 years and older—Advisory Committee on Immunization Practices (ACIP), 2012. MMWR Morb Mortal Wkly Rep. 2012 Jun 29;61(25):468–70. [PMID: 22739778]

Centers for Disease Control and Prevention (CDC). Updated recommendations for use of tetanus toxoid, reduced diphtheria toxoid, and acellular pertussis vaccine (Tdap) in pregnant women—Advisory Committee on Immunization Practices (ACIP), 2012. MMWR Morb Mortal Wkly Rep. 2013 Feb 22; 62(7):131–5. [PMID: 23425962]

LISTERIOSIS

ESSENTIALS OF DIAGNOSIS

▶ Ingestion of contaminated food product leads to primary infection.

▶ Undifferentiated fever in a pregnant woman in her third trimester.

▶ Altered mental status and fever in an elderly or immunocompromised patient.

▶ Obtain blood and cerebral spinal fluid cultures.

▶ Culture confirms the diagnosis.

▶ General Considerations

Listeria monocytogenes is a facultative, motile, gram-positive rod that is capable of invading several cell types and causes intracellular infection. Most cases of infection caused by *L monocytogenes* are sporadic, but outbreaks have been traced to eating contaminated food, including unpasteurized dairy products, hot dogs, and delicatessen meats. In 2011, a multistate outbreak of *Listeria* infection was traced to contaminated cantaloupes, and in 2012, a multistate outbreak was traced to ricotta cheese. Both outbreaks were associated with significant morbidity and mortality in infected persons.

▶ Clinical Findings

Five types of infection are recognized:

(1) **Infection during pregnancy,** usually in the last trimester, is a mild febrile illness without an apparent primary focus. This relatively benign disease for the mother may resolve without specific therapy. However, approximately one in five pregnancies complicated by listeriosis result in spontaneous abortion or stillbirth and surviving infants are at high risk for clinical neonatal listeriosis.

(2) **Granulomatosis infantisepticum** is a neonatal infection acquired in utero, characterized by disseminated abscesses, granulomas, and a high mortality rate.

(3) **Bacteremia** with or without sepsis syndrome is an infection of neonates or immunocompromised adults. The presentation is of a febrile illness without a recognized source.

(4) **Meningitis** caused by *L monocytogenes* affects infants under 2 months of age as well as older adults, ranking third after meningococcus and pneumococcus as common causes of bacterial meningitis. Cerebrospinal fluid shows a *neutrophilic* pleocytosis. Adults with meningitis are often immunocompromised, and cases have been associated with HIV infection and therapy with tumor necrosis factor (TNF) inhibitors such as infliximab.

(5) Finally, **focal infections,** including adenitis, brain abscess, endocarditis, osteomyelitis, and arthritis, occur rarely.

▶ Treatment

Ampicillin, 8–12 g/d intravenously in four to six divided doses (the higher dose for meningitis) is considered the treatment of choice. Gentamicin, 5 mg/kg/d intravenously once or in divided doses is synergistic with ampicillin against *Listeria* in vitro and in animal models, and the use of combination therapy may be considered during the first few days of treatment to enhance eradication of organisms. In patients with penicillin allergies, trimethoprim-sulfamethoxazole has excellent intracellular and cerebrospinal fluid penetration and is considered an appropriate alternative. The dose is 10–20 mg/kg/d intravenously of the trimethoprim component. Mortality and morbidity rates still are high. Therapy should be administered for at least 2–3 weeks. Longer durations—between 3 and 6 weeks—have been recommended for treatment of meningitis, especially in immunocompromised persons.

Cartwright EJ et al. Listeriosis outbreaks and associated food vehicles, United States, 1998–2008. Emerg Infect Dis. 2013 Jan;19(1):1–9. [PMID: 23260661]

Goulet V et al. What is the incubation period for listeriosis? BMC Infect Dis. 2013 Jan 10;13:11. [PMID: 23305174]

McCollum JT et al. Multistate outbreak of listeriosis associated with cantaloupe. N Engl J Med. 2013 Sep 5;369(10):944–53. [PMID: 24004121]

INFECTIVE ENDOCARDITIS

ESSENTIALS OF DIAGNOSIS

▶ Fever.

▶ Preexisting organic heart lesion.

▶ Positive blood cultures.

▶ Evidence of vegetation on echocardiography.

▶ New or changing heart murmur.

▶ Evidence of systemic emboli.

▶ General Considerations

Endocarditis is a bacterial or fungal infection of the valvular or endocardial surface of the heart. The clinical presentation depends on the infecting organism and the valve or valves that are infected. More virulent organisms—*S aureus* in particular—tend to produce a more rapidly progressive and destructive infection. Endocarditis caused by more virulent organisms often presents as an acute febrile illnesses and is complicated by early embolization, acute valvular regurgitation, and myocardial abscess formation. Viridans strains of streptococci, enterococci, other bacteria, yeasts, and fungi tend to cause a more subacute picture.

Underlying valvular disease, less common than in the past, is present in about 50% of cases. Valvular disease alters blood flow and produces jet effects that disrupt the endothelial surface, providing a nidus for attachment and infection of microorganisms that enter the bloodstream. Predisposing valvular abnormalities include rheumatic involvement of any valve, bicuspid aortic valves, calcific or sclerotic aortic valves, hypertrophic subaortic stenosis, mitral valve prolapse, and a variety of congenital disorders such as ventricular septal defect, tetralogy of Fallot, coarctation of the aorta, or patent ductus arteriosus. Rheumatic disease is no longer the major predisposing factor in developed countries. Regurgitation lesions are more susceptible than stenotic ones.

The initiating event in native valve endocarditis is colonization of the valve by bacteria or yeast that gain access to the bloodstream. Transient bacteremia is common during dental, upper respiratory, urologic, and lower gastrointestinal diagnostic and surgical procedures. It is less common during upper gastrointestinal and gynecologic procedures. Intravascular devices are increasingly implicated as a portal of access of microorganisms into the bloodstream. A large proportion of cases of *S aureus* endocarditis are attributable to health care-associated bacteremia.

Native valve endocarditis is usually caused by viridans streptococci, group D streptococci, *S aureus*, enterococci, or HACEK organisms (an acronym for *Haemophilus aphrophilus* [now *Aggregatibacter aphrophilus*], *Actinobacillus actinomycetemcomitans* [now *Aggregatibacter actinomycetemcomitans*], *Cardiobacterium hominis*, *Eikenella corrodens*, and *Kingella* species). Streptococcal species formerly accounted for the majority of native valve endocarditis cases, but the proportion of cases caused by *S aureus* has been increasing, and this organism is now the leading cause. Gram-negative organisms and fungi account for a small percentage.

In injection drug users, *S aureus* accounts for over 60% of all endocarditis cases and for 80–90% of cases in which the tricuspid valve is infected. Enterococci and streptococci comprise the balance in about equal proportions. Gram-negative aerobic bacilli, fungi, and unusual organisms may cause endocarditis in injection drug users.

The microbiology of prosthetic valve endocarditis also is distinctive. Early infections (ie, those occurring within 2 months after valve implantation) are commonly caused by staphylococci—both coagulase-positive and coagulase-negative—gram-negative organisms, and fungi. In late prosthetic valve endocarditis, streptococci are commonly identified, although coagulase-negative and coagulase-positive staphylococci still cause many cases.

▶ Clinical Findings

A. Symptoms and Signs

Virtually all patients have fever at some point in the illness, although it may be very low grade (< 38°C) in elderly individuals and in patients with heart failure or kidney failure. Rarely, there may be no fever at all.

The duration of illness typically is a few days to a few weeks. Nonspecific symptoms are common. The initial symptoms and signs of endocarditis may be caused by direct arterial, valvular, or cardiac damage. Although a changing regurgitant murmur is significant diagnostically, it is the exception rather than the rule. Symptoms also may occur as a result of embolization, metastatic infection or immunologically mediated phenomena. These include cough; dyspnea; arthralgias or arthritis; diarrhea; and abdominal, back, or flank pain.

The characteristic peripheral lesions—petechiae (on the palate or conjunctiva or beneath the fingernails), subungual ("splinter") hemorrhages (Figure 33–3), Osler nodes (painful, violaceous raised lesions of the fingers, toes, or feet) (Figure 33–4), Janeway lesions (painless erythematous lesions of the palms or soles), and Roth spots (exudative lesions in the retina)—occur in about 25% of patients. Strokes and major systemic embolic events are present in about 25% of patients, and tend to occur before or within the first week of antimicrobial therapy. Hematuria and proteinuria may result from emboli or immunologically mediated glomerulonephritis, which can cause kidney dysfunction.

▶ B. Imaging

Chest radiograph may show evidence for the underlying cardiac abnormality and, in right-sided endocarditis,

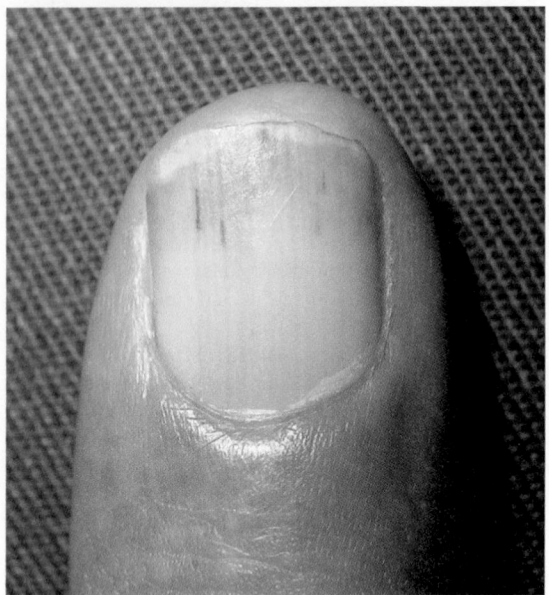

▲ **Figure 33–3.** Splinter hemorrhages appearing as red lineal streaks under the nail plate and within the nail bed, in endocarditis, psoriasis, and trauma. (Reproduced, with permission, from Richard P. Usatine, MD.)

pulmonary infiltrates. The electrocardiogram is nondiagnostic, but new conduction abnormalities suggest myocardial abscess formation. Echocardiography is useful in identifying vegetations and other characteristic features suspicious for endocarditis and may provide adjunctive information about the specific valve or valves that are infected. The sensitivity of transthoracic echocardiography is between 55% and 65%; it cannot reliably rule out endocarditis but may confirm a clinical suspicion. TEE is 90% sensitive in detecting vegetations and is particularly useful for identifying valve ring abscesses as well as prosthetic valve endocarditis.

C. Diagnostic Studies

1. Blood cultures—Blood cultures establish the diagnosis. Three sets of blood cultures at least 1 hour apart before starting antibiotics are recommended to maximize the opportunity for a microbiologic diagnosis. Approximately 5% of cases will be culture-negative, usually attributable to administration of antimicrobials prior to obtaining cultures. If antimicrobial therapy has been administered prior to obtaining cultures and the patient is clinically stable, it is reasonable to withhold further antimicrobial therapy for 2–3 days so that appropriate cultures can be obtained. Culture-negative endocarditis may also be due to organisms that require special media for growth (eg, *Legionella*, *Bartonella*, *Abiotrophia* species, formerly referred to as nutritionally deficient streptococci), organisms that do not grow on artificial media (*Tropheryma whippelii*, or pathogens of Q fever or psittacosis), or those that are slow-growing and may require prolonged incubation (eg, *Brucella*, anaerobes, HACEK organisms). *Bartonella quintana* has emerged as an important cause of culture-negative endocarditis.

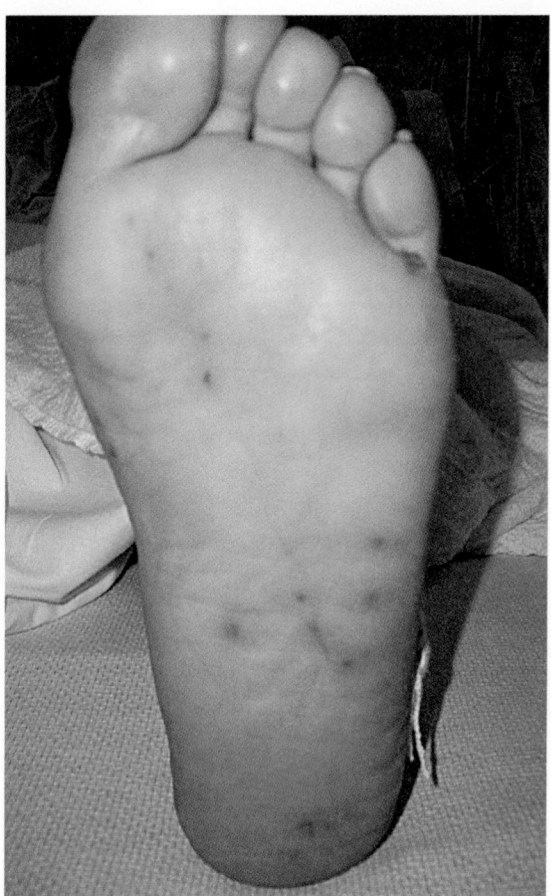

▲ **Figure 33–4.** Osler node causing pain within the pulp of the big toe and multiple painless flat Janeway lesions over the sole of the foot. (From David A. Kasper, DO, MBA; Reproduced, with permission, from Usatine RP, Smith MA, Mayeaux EJ Jr, Chumley H, Tysinger J. *The Color Atlas of Family Medicine.* McGraw-Hill, 2009.)

2. Modified Duke criteria—Clinical criteria, referred to as the Modified Duke criteria, for the diagnosis of endocarditis have been proposed. Major criteria include: (1) two positive blood cultures for a microorganism that typically causes infective endocarditis or persistent bacteremia; (2) evidence of endocardial involvement documented by echocardiography (eg, definite vegetation, myocardial abscess, or new partial dehiscence of a prosthetic valve); or (3) development of a new regurgitant murmur. Minor criteria include the presence of a predisposing condition; fever ≥ 38°C; vascular phenomena, such as cutaneous hemorrhages, aneurysm, systemic emboli, pulmonary infarction; immunologic phenomena, such as glomerulonephritis, Osler nodes, Roth spots, rheumatoid factor; and positive blood cultures not meeting the major criteria or serologic evidence of an active infection. A definite diagnosis can be made with 80% accuracy if two major criteria, one major criterion and three minor criteria, or five minor criteria are fulfilled. A possible diagnosis of endocarditis is made if one major and one minor criterion or three minor criteria are met.

If fewer criteria are found, or a sound alternative explanation for illness is identified, or the patient's febrile illness has resolved within 4 days, endocarditis is unlikely.

► **Complications**

The course of infective endocarditis is determined by the degree of damage to the heart, by the site of infection (right-sided versus left-sided, aortic versus mitral valve), by the presence of metastatic foci of infection, by the occurrence of embolization, and by immunologically mediated processes. Destruction of infected heart valves is especially common and precipitous with *S aureus* but can occur with any organism and can progress even after bacteriologic cure. The infection can also extend into the myocardium, resulting in abscesses leading to conduction disturbances, and involving the wall of the aorta, creating sinus of Valsalva aneurysms.

Peripheral embolization to the brain and myocardium may result in infarctions. Embolization to the spleen and kidneys is also common. Peripheral emboli may initiate metastatic infections or may become established in vessel walls, leading to mycotic aneurysms. Right-sided endocarditis, which usually involves the tricuspid valve, causes septic pulmonary emboli, occasionally with infarction and lung abscesses.

► **Prevention**

In 2007, the American Heart Association made major revisions to their recommendation on antibiotic prophylaxis for infective endocarditis. The committee determined that only a few cases of infective endocarditis would be prevented by antibiotic prophylaxis for dental procedures even if the prophylactic therapy were 100% effective. Therefore, they limited their recommendations for prophylaxis to a small group of patients with predisposing congenital or valvular anomalies (Table 33–4) undergoing select dental

Table 33–4. Cardiac conditions with high risk of adverse outcomes from endocarditis for which prophylaxis with dental procedures is recommended.[1,2]

Prosthetic cardiac valve
Previous infective endocarditis
Congenital heart disease (CHD)[3]
   Unrepaired cyanotic CHD, including palliative shunts and conduits
   Completely repaired congenital heart defect with prosthetic material or device, whether placed by surgery or by catheter intervention, during the first 6 months after the procedure[4]
   Repaired CHD with residual defects at the site or adjacent to the site of a prosthetic patch or prosthetic device
Cardiac transplantation recipients in whom cardiac valvulopathy develops

[1]Reproduced, with permission, from the American Heart Association. Circulation. 2007 Oct 9;116(15):1736–54.
[2]See Table 33–6 for prophylactic regimens.
[3]Except for the conditions listed above, antibiotic prophylaxis is no longer recommended for other forms of CHD.
[4]Prophylaxis is recommended because endothelialization of prosthetic material occurs within 6 months after procedure.

Table 33–5. Recommendations for administration of bacterial endocarditis prophylaxis for patients according to type of procedure.[1]

Prophylaxis Recommended	Prophylaxis Not Recommended
Dental procedures All dental procedures that involve manipulation of gingival tissue or the periapical region of the teeth or perforation of the oral mucosa **Respiratory tract procedures** Only respiratory tract procedures that involve incision of the respiratory mucosa **Procedures on infected skin, skin structure, or musculoskeletal tissue**	**Dental procedures** Routine anesthetic injections through noninfected tissue, taking dental radiographs, placement of removable prosthodontic or orthodontic appliances, adjustment of orthodontic appliances, placement of orthodontic brackets, shedding of deciduous teeth, and bleeding from trauma to the lips or oral mucosa **Gastrointestinal tract procedures** **Genitourinary tract procedures**

[1]Reproduced, with permission, from the American Heart Association. Circulation. 2007 Oct 9;116(15):1736–54.

procedures, operations involving the respiratory tract, or operations of infected skin, skin structure, or musculoskeletal tissue (Table 33–5). Current antimicrobial recommendations are given in Table 33–6.

► **Treatment**

Empiric regimens for endocarditis while culture results are pending should include agents active against staphylococci, streptococci, and enterococci. Vancomycin 1 g every 12 hours intravenously plus ceftriaxone 2 g every 24 hours provides appropriate coverage pending definitive diagnosis.

A. Viridans Streptococci

For penicillin-susceptible viridans streptococcal endocarditis (ie, MIC ≤ 0.1 mcg/mL), penicillin G, 2–3 million units intravenously every 4 hours for 4 weeks, is recommended. The duration of therapy can be shortened to 2 weeks if gentamicin, 1 mg/kg intravenously every 8 hours, is used with penicillin. Ceftriaxone, 2 g once daily intravenously or intramuscularly for 4 weeks, is also effective therapy for penicillin-susceptible strains and is a convenient regimen for home therapy. For the penicillin-allergic patient, vancomycin, 15 mg/kg intravenously every 12 hours for 4 weeks, is given. The 2-week regimen is not recommended for patients with symptoms of more than 3 months' duration or with complications such as myocardial abscess or extracardiac infection. Prosthetic valve endocarditis is treated with a 6-week course of penicillin with at least 2 weeks of gentamicin.

Viridans streptococci relatively resistant to penicillin (ie, MIC > 0.1 mcg/mL but ≤ 0.5 mcg/mL) should be

Table 33–6. American Heart Association recommendations for endocarditis prophylaxis for dental procedures for patients with cardiac conditions.[1-3]

Oral	Amoxicillin	2 g 1 hour before procedure
Penicillin allergy	Clindamycin	600 mg 1 hour before procedure
	or	
	Cephalexin	2 g 1 hour before procedure (contraindicated if there is history of a beta-lactam immediate hypersensitivity reaction)
	or	
	Azithromycin or clarithromycin	500 mg 1 hour before procedure
Parenteral	Ampicillin	2 g intramuscularly or intravenously 30 minutes before procedure
Penicillin allergy	Clindamycin	600 mg intravenously 1 hour before procedure
	or	
	Cefazolin	1 g intramuscularly or intravenously 30 minutes before procedure (contraindicated if there is history of a beta-lactam immediate hypersensitivity reaction)

[1]Data from the American Heart Association. Circulation. 2007 Oct 9;116(15):1736–54.
[2]For patients undergoing respiratory tract procedures involving incision of respiratory tract mucosa to treat an established infection or a procedure on infected skin, skin structure, or musculoskeletal tissue known or suspected to be caused by *S aureus*, the regimen should contain an anti-staphylococcal penicillin or cephalosporin. Vancomycin can be used to treat patients unable to tolerate a beta-lactam or if the infection is known or suspected to be caused by a methicillin-resistant strain of *S aureus*.
[3]See Table 33–4 for list of cardiac conditions.

treated for 4 weeks. Penicillin G, 3 million units intravenously every 4 hours, is combined with gentamicin, 1 mg/kg intravenously every 8 hours for the first 2 weeks. In the patient with IgE-mediated allergy to penicillin, vancomycin alone, 15 mg/kg intravenously every 12 hours for 4 weeks, should be administered.

Endocarditis caused by viridans streptococci with an MIC > 0.5 mcg/mL or by nutritionally deficient streptococci should be treated the same as enterococcal endocarditis (see below).

B. Other Streptococci

Endocarditis caused by *S pneumoniae*, *S pyogenes* (group A streptococcus), or groups B, C, and G streptococci is unusual. *S pneumoniae* sensitive to penicillin (MIC < 0.1 mcg/mL) can be treated with penicillin alone, 2–3 million units intravenously every 4 hours for 4–6 weeks. Vancomycin should be effective for endocarditis caused by strains resistant to penicillin. Group A streptococcal infection can be treated with penicillin, ceftriaxone, or vancomycin for 4–6 weeks. Groups B, C, and G streptococci tend to be more resistant to penicillin than group A streptococci, and some experts have recommended adding gentamicin, 1 mg/kg intravenously every 8 hours, to penicillin for the first 2 weeks of a 4- to 6-week course. Endocarditis caused by *S bovis* is associated with liver disease and gastrointestinal abnormalities, especially colon cancer. Colonoscopy should be performed to exclude the latter.

C. Enterococci

For enterococcal endocarditis, penicillin alone is inadequate; either streptomycin or gentamicin must be included in the regimen. Because aminoglycoside resistance occurs in enterococci, susceptibility should be documented. Gentamicin is the aminoglycoside of choice, because streptomycin resistance is more common and the nephrotoxicity of gentamicin is generally more easily managed than the vestibular toxicity of streptomycin. Ampicillin, 2 g intravenously every 4 hours, or penicillin G, 3–4 million units intravenously every 4 hours (or, in the penicillin-allergic patient, vancomycin, 15 mg/kg intravenously every 12 hours), plus gentamicin, 1 mg/kg intravenously every 8 hours, are recommended. The recommended duration of combination therapy is 4–6 weeks (the longer duration for patients with symptoms for more than 3 months, relapse, or prosthetic valve endocarditis), although a study from Sweden found that discontinuing the aminoglycoside before 4 weeks did not reduce efficacy. Experience is more extensive with penicillin and ampicillin than with vancomycin for treatment of enterococcal endocarditis, and penicillin and ampicillin are superior to vancomycin in vitro. Thus, whenever possible, either ampicillin or penicillin should be used. Emerging data suggest that ampicillin, 2 g intravenously every 4 hours, plus ceftriaxone, 2 g intravenously every 12 hours, for 4–6 weeks may be as effective, and less toxic, than the combination of ampicillin and an aminoglycoside.

Endocarditis caused by strains resistant to penicillin, vancomycin, or aminoglycosides is particularly difficult to treat. Such cases should be treated according to recent American Heart Association guidelines and managed in consultation with an infectious diseases specialist.

D. Staphylococci

For methicillin-susceptible *S aureus*, nafcillin or oxacillin, 1.5–2 g intravenously every 4 hours for 6 weeks, is the preferred therapy. Uncomplicated tricuspid valve endocarditis probably can be treated for 2 weeks with nafcillin or oxacillin alone. For penicillin-allergic patients, cefazolin, 2 g intravenously every 8 hours, or vancomycin, 30 mg/kg/d intravenously divided in two or three doses, may be used. For methicillin-resistant strains, vancomycin remains the preferred agent. Aminoglycoside combination regimens are probably of no benefit and in general should be avoided. The effect of rifampin with antistaphylococcal drugs is variable, and its routine use is not recommended.

Because coagulase-negative staphylococci—a common cause of prosthetic valve endocarditis—are routinely resistant to methicillin, beta-lactam antibiotics should not be used for this infection unless the isolate is demonstrated to be susceptible. A combination of vancomycin, 30 mg/kg/d intravenously divided in two or three doses for 6 weeks; rifampin, 300 mg every 8 hours for 6 weeks; and gentamicin, 1 mg/kg intravenously every 8 hours for the first 2 weeks is recommended for prosthetic valve infection. If the organism is sensitive to methicillin, either nafcillin or oxacillin or cefazolin can be used in combination with rifampin and gentamicin. Combination therapy with nafcillin or oxacillin (vancomycin for methicillin-resistant strains or patients allergic to beta-lactams), rifampin, and gentamicin is also recommended for treatment of *S aureus* prosthetic valve infection.

E. HACEK Organisms

HACEK organisms are slow-growing, fastidious gram-negative coccobacilli or bacilli (*H aphrophilus* [now *A aphrophilus*], *A actinomycetemcomitans* [now *A actinomycetemcomitans*], *C hominis, E corrodens*, and *Kingella* species) that are normal oral flora and cause < 5% of all cases of endocarditis. They may produce beta-lactamase, and thus the treatment of choice is ceftriaxone (or some other third-generation cephalosporin), 2 g intravenously once daily for 4 weeks. Prosthetic valve endocarditis should be treated for 6 weeks. In the penicillin-allergic patient, experience is limited, but trimethoprim-sulfamethoxazole, quinolones, and aztreonam have in vitro activity and should be considered; desensitization may be preferable.

F. Role of Surgery

While many cases can be successfully treated medically, operative management is frequently required. Acute heart failure unresponsive to medical therapy is an indication for valve replacement even if active infection is present, especially for aortic valve infection. Infections unresponsive to appropriate antimicrobial therapy after 7–10 days (ie, persistent fevers, positive blood cultures despite therapy) are more likely to be eradicated if the valve is replaced. Surgery is nearly always required for cure of fungal endocarditis and is more often necessary with gram-negative bacilli. It is also indicated when the infection involves the sinus of Valsalva or produces septal abscesses. Recurrent infection with the same organism prompts an operative approach, especially with infected prosthetic valves.

Continuing embolization presents a difficult problem when the infection is otherwise responding; surgery may be the proper approach. Particularly challenging is a large and fragile vegetation demonstrated by echocardiography in the absence of embolization. Most clinicians favor an operative approach, vegetectomy with valve repair if the patient is a good candidate. Embolization after bacteriologic cure does not necessarily imply recurrence of endocarditis.

G. Role of Anticoagulation

Anticoagulation is contraindicated in native valve endocarditis because of an increased risk of intracerebral hemorrhage. The role of anticoagulant therapy during active prosthetic valve endocarditis is more controversial. Reversal of anticoagulation may result in thrombosis of the mechanical prosthesis, particularly in the mitral position. On the other hand, anticoagulation during active prosthetic valve endocarditis caused by *S aureus* has been associated with fatal intracerebral hemorrhage. One approach is to discontinue anticoagulation during the septic phase of *S aureus* prosthetic valve endocarditis. In patients with *S aureus* prosthetic valve endocarditis complicated by a central nervous system embolic event, anticoagulation should be discontinued for the first 2 weeks of therapy. Indications for anticoagulation following prosthetic valve implantation for endocarditis are the same as for patients with prosthetic valves without endocarditis (eg, nonporcine mechanical valves and valves in the mitral position).

▶ Response to Therapy

If infection is caused by viridans streptococci, enterococci, or coagulase-negative staphylococci, defervescence occurs in 3–4 days on average; with *S aureus* or *Pseudomonas aeruginosa*, fever commonly persists for 9–12 days. Blood cultures should be obtained to document sterilization of the blood. Other causes of persistent fever are myocardial or metastatic abscess, sterile embolization, superimposed hospital-acquired infection, and drug reaction. Most relapses occur within 1–2 months after completion of therapy. Obtaining one or two blood cultures during this period is prudent.

▶ When to Refer

- Consider consulting an infectious diseases specialist in all cases of suspected infective endocarditis.
- Consult a cardiac surgeon in the situations mentioned in the Role of Surgery section above to prevent further embolic disease, heart failure, and other complications including death.

▶ When to Admit

Patients with infective endocarditis should be hospitalized for expedited evaluation and treatment.

Baddour LM et al. Infective endocarditis: diagnosis, antimicrobial therapy, and management of complications: a statement for healthcare professionals from the Committee on Rheumatic Fever, Endocarditis, and Kawasaki Disease, Council on Cardiovascular Disease in the Young, and the Councils on Clinical Cardiology, Stroke, and Cardiovascular Surgery and Anesthesia, American Heart Association: endorsed by the Infectious Diseases Society of America. Circulation. 2005 Jun 14;111(23):e394–434. [PMID: 15956145]

Fernández-Hidalgo N et al. Ampicillin plus ceftriaxone is as effective as ampicillin plus gentamicin for treating *Enterococcus faecalis* infective endocarditis. Clin Infect Dis. 2013 May;56(9):1261–8. [PMID: 23392394]

Hoen B et al. Clinical practice. Infective endocarditis. N Engl J Med. 2013 Apr 11;368(15):1425–33. [PMID: 23574121]

Kang DH et al. Early surgery versus conventional treatment for infective endocarditis. N Engl J Med. 2012 Jun 28;366(26):2466–73. [PMID: 22738096]

Wilson W et al. Prevention of infective endocarditis: guidelines from the American Heart Association: a guideline from the American Heart Association Rheumatic Fever, Endocarditis, and Kawasaki Disease Committee, Council on Cardiovascular Disease in the Young, and the Council on Clinical Cardiology, Council on Cardiovascular Surgery and Anesthesia, and the Quality of Care and Outcomes Research Interdisciplinary Working Group. Circulation. 2007 Oct 9;116(15):1736–54. [PMID: 17446442]

INFECTIONS CAUSED BY GRAM-NEGATIVE BACTERIA

BORDETELLA PERTUSSIS INFECTION (Whooping Cough)

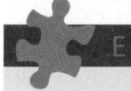

ESSENTIALS OF DIAGNOSIS

- ▶ Predominantly in infants under age 2 years. Adolescents and adults are an important reservoir of infection.

- ▶ Two-week prodromal catarrhal stage of malaise, cough, coryza, and anorexia.

- ▶ Paroxysmal cough ending in a high-pitched inspiratory "whoop."

- ▶ Absolute lymphocytosis, often striking; culture confirms diagnosis.

▶ General Considerations

Pertussis is an acute infection of the respiratory tract caused by *B pertussis* that is transmitted by respiratory droplets. The incubation period is 7–17 days. Half of all cases occur before age 2 years. Neither immunization nor disease confers lasting immunity to pertussis. Consequently, adults are an important reservoir of the disease. In 2010 and then again in 2012, large pertussis outbreaks were reported with over 40,000 cases in 2012. Following the identification of this epidemic in 2010, the CDC made significant changes to its recommendations on vaccination of adults, as detailed below.

▶ Clinical Findings

The symptoms of classic pertussis last about 6 weeks and are divided into three consecutive stages. The catarrhal stage is characterized by its insidious onset, with lacrimation, sneezing, and coryza, anorexia and malaise, and a hacking night cough that becomes diurnal. The paroxysmal stage is characterized by bursts of rapid, consecutive coughs followed by a deep, high-pitched inspiration (whoop). The convalescent stage begins 4 weeks after onset of the illness with a decrease in the frequency and severity of paroxysms of cough. The diagnosis often is not considered in adults, who may not have a typical presentation. Cough persisting more than 2 weeks is suggestive. Infection may also be asymptomatic.

The white blood cell count is usually 15,000–20,000/mcL (rarely, as high as 50,000/mcL or more), 60–80% of which are lymphocytes. The diagnosis is established by isolating the organism from nasopharyngeal culture. A special medium (eg, Bordet-Gengou agar) must be requested. Polymerase chain reaction assays for diagnosis of pertussis may be available in some clinical or health department laboratories.

▶ Prevention

Acellular pertussis vaccine is recommended for all infants, combined with diphtheria and tetanus toxoids (DTaP). Infants and susceptible adults with significant exposure should receive prophylaxis with an oral macrolide (see below). In recognition of their importance as a reservoir of disease, vaccination of adolescents and adults against pertussis is recommended (see Table 30–7 and www.cdc.gov/vaccines/schedules). The FDA licensed two tetanus toxoid, reduced diphtheria toxoid and acellular pertussis vaccine (Tdap) products (BOOSTRIX, GlaxoSmithKline and ADACEL, Sanofi Pasteur) in 2005. Adolescents aged 11–18 years (preferably between 11 and 12 years of age) who have completed the DTP or DTaP vaccination series should receive a single dose of either Tdap product instead of Td (tetanus and diphtheria toxoids vaccine) for booster immunization against tetanus, diphtheria, and pertussis. Following the 2010 pertussis outbreak, the CDC expanded its recommendations, stating that adults of all ages (including those > 64 years) should receive a single dose of Tdap. In addition, pregnant women should receive a dose of Tdap during each pregnancy regardless of prior vaccination history. The optimal timing for such Tdap administration is between 27 and 36 weeks of gestation, in order to maximize the antibody response of the pregnant woman and the passive antibody transfer to the infant. For any woman who was not previously vaccinated with Tdap and for whom the vaccine was not given during her pregnancy, Tdap should be administered immediately postpartum. The CDC eliminated the recommendation that a 2-year period window is needed between receiving the Td and Tdap vaccines based on data showing that there is not an increased risk of adverse events.

▶ Treatment

Antibiotic treatment should be initiated in all suspected cases. Treatment options include erythromycin, 500 mg four times a day orally for 7 days; azithromycin, 500 mg orally on day 1 and 250 mg for 4 more days; or clarithromycin, 500 mg orally twice daily for 7 days. Trimethoprim-sulfamethoxazole, 160 mg–800 mg orally twice a day for 7 days, also is effective. Treatment shortens the duration of carriage and may diminish the severity of coughing paroxysms. These same regimens are indicated for prophylaxis of contacts to an active case of pertussis that are exposed within 3 weeks of the onset of cough in the index case.

Centers for Disease Control and Prevention (CDC). Updated recommendations for use of tetanus toxoid, reduced diphtheria toxoid, and acellular pertussis (Tdap) vaccine in adults aged 65 years and older—Advisory Committee on Immunization Practices (ACIP), 2012. MMWR Morb Mortal Wkly Rep. 2012 Jun 29;61(25):468–70. Erratum in: MMWR Morb Mortal Wkly Rep. 2012 Jul 13;61(27):515. [PMID: 22739778]
Centers for Disease Control and Prevention (CDC). Updated recommendations for use of tetanus toxoid, reduced diphtheria toxoid, and acellular pertussis vaccine (Tdap) in pregnant women—Advisory Committee on Immunization Practices (ACIP), 2012. MMWR Morb Mortal Wkly Rep. 2013 Feb 22;62(7):131–5. [PMID: 23425962]
Spector TB et al. Pertussis. Med Clin North Am. 2013 Jul;97(4): 537–52. [PMID: 23809713]

OTHER *BORDETELLA* INFECTIONS

Bordetella bronchiseptica is a pleomorphic gram-negative coccobacillus causing kennel cough in dogs. On occasion it causes upper and lower respiratory infection in humans, principally HIV-infected patients. Infection has been associated with contact with dogs and cats, suggesting animal-to-human transmission. Treatment of *B bronchiseptica* infection is guided by results of in vitro susceptibility tests.

MENINGOCOCCAL MENINGITIS

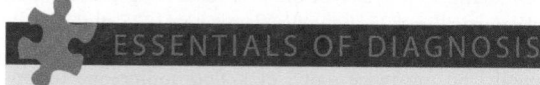

ESSENTIALS OF DIAGNOSIS

► Fever, headache, vomiting, confusion, delirium, convulsions.

► Petechial rash of skin and mucous membranes in many.

► Neck and back stiffness with positive Kernig and Brudzinski signs is characteristic.

► Purulent spinal fluid with gram-negative intracellular and extracellular diplococci.

► Culture of cerebrospinal fluid, blood, or petechial aspiration confirms the diagnosis.

General Considerations

Meningococcal meningitis is caused by *Neisseria meningitidis* of groups A, B, C, Y, and W-135, among others. Meningitis due to serogroup A is uncommon in the United States. Serogroup B generally causes sporadic cases. The frequency

of outbreaks of meningitis caused by group C *meningococcus* has increased, and this serotype is the most common cause of epidemic disease in the United States. Up to 40% of persons are nasopharyngeal carriers of meningococci, but disease develops in relatively few of these persons. Infection is transmitted by droplets. The clinical illness may take the form of meningococcemia (a fulminant form of septicemia without meningitis), meningococcemia with meningitis, or meningitis. Recurrent meningococcemia with fever, rash, and arthritis is seen rarely in patients with certain terminal complement deficiencies.

► Clinical Findings

A. Symptoms and Signs

High fever, chills, and headache; back, abdominal, and extremity pains; and nausea and vomiting are typical. Rapidly developing confusion, delirium, seizures, and coma occur in some. On examination, nuchal and back rigidity are typical. Positive Kernig and Brudzinski signs (Kernig sign is pain in the hamstrings upon extension of the knee with the hip at 90-degree flexion; Brudzinski sign is flexion of the knee in response to flexion of the neck) are specific but not sensitive findings. A petechial rash appearing in the lower extremities and at pressure points is found in most cases. Petechiae may vary in size from pinpoint lesions to large ecchymoses or even skin gangrene that may later slough if the patient survives.

B. Laboratory Findings

Lumbar puncture typically reveals a cloudy or purulent cerebrospinal fluid, with elevated pressure, increased protein, and decreased glucose content. The fluid usually contains > 1000 cells/mcL, with polymorphonuclear cells predominating and containing gram-negative intracellular diplococci. The absence of organisms in a Gram-stained smear of the cerebrospinal fluid sediment does not rule out the diagnosis. The capsular polysaccharide can be demonstrated in cerebrospinal fluid or urine by latex agglutination; this is useful in partially treated patients, though sensitivity is 60–80%. The organism is usually demonstrated by smear and culture of the cerebrospinal fluid, oropharynx, blood, or aspirated petechiae.

Disseminated intravascular coagulation is an important complication of meningococcal infection and is typically present in toxic patients with ecchymotic skin lesions.

► Differential Diagnosis

Meningococcal meningitis must be differentiated from other meningitides. In small infants and in the elderly, fever or stiff neck is often missing, and altered mental status may dominate the picture.

Rickettsial, echovirus and, rarely, other bacterial infections (eg, staphylococcal infections, scarlet fever) also cause petechial rash.

► Prevention

Two vaccines, meningococcal polysaccharide vaccine (MPSV4, indicated for vaccination of persons over age 55) and a conjugate vaccine (MCV4, indicated for persons aged 2–55 years) are effective for meningococcal groups A, C, Y, and W-135. The Advisory Committee on Immunization Practices recommends immunization with a dose of MCV4 for preadolescents ages 11–12 with a booster at age 16 (see www.cdc.gov/vaccines/schedules). For ease of program implementation, persons aged 21 years or younger should have documentation of receipt of a dose of MCV4 not more than 5 years before enrollment to college. If the primary dose was administered before the sixteenth birthday, a booster dose should be administered before enrollment. Vaccine is also recommend as a two-dose primary series administered 2 months apart for persons aged 2 through 54 years with persistent complement deficiency, persons with functional or anatomic asplenia, and for adolescents with HIV infection. All other persons at increased risk for meningococcal disease (eg, military recruits, microbiologists, or travelers to an epidemic or highly endemic country) should receive a single dose.

Eliminating nasopharyngeal carriage of meningococci is an effective prevention strategy in closed populations and to prevent secondary cases in household or otherwise close contacts. Rifampin, 600 mg orally twice a day for 2 days, ciprofloxacin, 500 mg orally once, or one intramuscular 250-mg dose of ceftriaxone is effective. A cluster of cases of fluoroquinolone-resistant meningococcal infections was recently identified in the United States. However, ciprofloxacin remains a recommended empiric agent for eradication of nasopharyngeal carriage. School and work contacts ordinarily need not be treated. Hospital contacts receive therapy only if intense exposure has occurred (eg, mouth-to-mouth resuscitation). Accidentally discovered carriers without known close contact with meningococcal disease do not require prophylactic antimicrobials.

▶ Treatment

Blood cultures must be obtained and intravenous antimicrobial therapy started immediately. This may be done prior to lumbar puncture in patients in whom the diagnosis is not straightforward and for those in whom MR or CT imaging is indicated to exclude mass lesions. Aqueous penicillin G is the antibiotic of choice (24 million units/ 24 h intravenously in divided doses every 4 hours). The prevalence of strains of N meningitidis with intermediate resistance to penicillin in vitro (MICs 0.1 to 1 mcg/mL) is increasing, particularly in Europe. At what level of resistance penicillin treatment failure can occur is not known. Penicillin-intermediate strains thus far remain fully susceptible to ceftriaxone and other third-generation cephalosporins used to treat meningitis, and these should be effective alternatives to penicillin. In penicillin-allergic patients or those in whom Haemophilus influenzae or gram-negative meningitis is a consideration, ceftriaxone, 2 g intravenously every 12 hours, should be used. Treatment should be continued in full doses by the intravenous route until the patient is afebrile for 5 days. Shorter courses—as few as 4 days if ceftriaxone is used—are also effective.

▶ When to Admit

All patients with suspected meningococcal infection including meningitis and meningococcemia should be admitted for evaluation and empiric intravenous antibiotic therapy.

Campsall PA et al. Severe meningococcal infection: a review of epidemiology, diagnosis, and management. Crit Care Clin. 2013 Jul;29(3):393–409. [PMID: 23830646]

Cohn AC et al; Centers for Disease Control and Prevention (CDC). Prevention and control of meningococcal disease: recommendations of the Advisory Committee on Immunization Practices (ACIP). MMWR Recomm Rep. 2013 Mar 22; 62(RR-2):1–28. [PMID: 23515099]

Simon MS et al. Invasive meningococcal disease in men who have sex with men. Ann Intern Med. 2013 Aug 20;159(4):300–1. [PMID: 23778867]

Zheteyeva Y et al. Safety of meningococcal polysaccharide-protein conjugate vaccine in pregnancy: a review of the Vaccine Adverse Event Reporting System. Am J Obstet Gynecol. 2013 Jun;208(6):478.e1–6. [PMID: 23453881]

INFECTIONS CAUSED BY *HAEMOPHILUS* SPECIES

H influenzae and other *Haemophilus* species may cause sinusitis, otitis, bronchitis, epiglottitis, pneumonia, cellulitis, arthritis, meningitis, and endocarditis. Nontypeable strains are responsible for most disease in adults. Alcoholism, smoking, chronic lung disease, advanced age, and HIV infection are risk factors. *Haemophilus* species colonize the upper respiratory tract in patients with chronic obstructive pulmonary disease and frequently cause purulent bronchitis.

Beta-lactamase–producing strains are less common in adults than in children. For adults with sinusitis, otitis, or respiratory tract infection, oral amoxicillin, 750 mg twice daily for 10–14 days, is adequate. For beta-lactamase–producing strains, use of the oral fixed drug combination of amoxicillin, 875 mg, with clavulanate, 125 mg, is indicated. For the penicillin-allergic patient, oral cefuroxime axetil, 250 mg twice daily; or a fluoroquinolone (ciprofloxacin, 500 mg orally twice daily; levofloxacin, 500–750 mg orally once daily; or moxifloxacin, 400 mg orally once daily) for 7 days is effective. Azithromycin, 500 mg orally once followed 250 mg daily for 4 days, is preferred over clarithromycin when a macrolide is the preferred agent. Trimethoprim-sulfamethoxazole (160/800 mg orally twice daily) can be considered, but resistance rates have been reported to be up to 25%.

In the more seriously ill patient (eg, the toxic patient with multilobar pneumonia), ceftriaxone, 1 g/d intravenously is recommended pending determination of whether the infecting strain is a beta-lactamase producer. A fluoroquinolone (see above for dosages) can be used for the penicillin-allergic patients for a 10- to 14-day course of therapy.

Epiglottitis is characterized by an abrupt onset of high fever, drooling, and inability to handle secretions. An important clue to the diagnosis is complaint of a severe sore throat despite an unimpressive examination of the pharynx. Stridor and respiratory distress result from laryngeal obstruction. The diagnosis is best made by direct visualization of the cherry-red, swollen epiglottis at laryngoscopy. Because laryngoscopy may provoke laryngospasm and obstruction, especially in children, it should be performed in an intensive care unit or similar setting, and only at a time when intubation can be performed promptly. Ceftriaxone, 1 g intravenously every 24 hours for 7–10 days, is the drug of choice. Trimethoprim-sulfamethoxazole or a fluoroquinolone (see above for dosage) may be used in the patient with serious penicillin allergy.

Meningitis, rare in adults, is a consideration in the patient who has meningitis associated with sinusitis or otitis. Initial therapy for suspected *H influenzae* meningitis should be with ceftriaxone, 4 g/d in two divided doses, until the strain is proved not to produce beta-lactamase. Meningitis is treated for 10–14 days. Dexamethasone, 0.15 mg/kg intravenously every 6 hours may reduce the incidence of long-term sequelae, principally hearing loss.

Agrawal A et al. *Haemophilus influenzae* infections in the *H influenzae* type b conjugate vaccine era. J Clin Microbiol. 2011 Nov;49(11):3728–32. [PMID: 21900515]

Okada F et al. Radiological findings in acute *Haemophilus influenzae* pulmonary infection. Br J Radiol. 2012 Feb;85(1010): 121–6. [PMID: 21224303]

INFECTIONS CAUSED BY *MORAXELLA CATARRHALIS*

M catarrhalis is a gram-negative aerobic coccus morphologically and biochemically similar to *Neisseria*. It causes sinusitis, bronchitis, and pneumonia. Bacteremia and meningitis have also been reported in immunocompromised patients. The organism frequently colonizes the respiratory tract, making differentiation of colonization from infection difficult. If *M catarrhalis* is the predominant isolate, therapy is directed against it. *M catarrhalis* typically produces beta-lactamase and therefore is usually resistant to ampicillin and amoxicillin. It is susceptible to amoxicillin-clavulanate, ampicillin-sulbactam, trimethoprim-sulfamethoxazole, ciprofloxacin, and second- and third-generation cephalosporins.

Aebi C. *Moraxella catarrhalis*—pathogen or commensal? Adv Exp Med Biol. 2011;697:107–16. [PMID: 21120723]

LEGIONNAIRES DISEASE

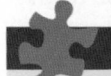

ESSENTIALS OF DIAGNOSIS

▶ Patients are often immunocompromised, smokers, or have chronic lung disease.

▶ Scant sputum production, pleuritic chest pain, toxic appearance.

▶ Chest radiograph: focal patchy infiltrates or consolidation.

▶ Gram stain of sputum: polymorphonuclear leukocytes and no organisms.

▶ General Considerations

Legionella infection ranks among the three or four most common causes of community-acquired pneumonia and is considered whenever the etiology of a pneumonia is in question. Legionnaires disease is more common in immunocompromised persons, in smokers, and in those with chronic lung disease. Outbreaks have been associated with contaminated water sources, such as showerheads and faucets in patient rooms and air conditioning cooling towers.

▶ Clinical Findings

A. Symptoms and Signs

Legionnaires disease is one of the atypical pneumonias, so called because a Gram-stained smear of sputum does not show organisms. However, many features of Legionnaires disease are more like typical pneumonia, with high fevers, a toxic patient, pleurisy, and grossly purulent sputum. Classically, this pneumonia is caused by *Legionella pneumophila*, though other species can cause identical disease.

B. Laboratory Findings

Several laboratory abnormalities can be associated with Legionnaires disease, which include hyponatremia, elevated liver enzymes, and elevated creatine kinase. Culture of *Legionella* species onto charcoal-yeast extract agar or similar enriched medium is the most sensitive method (80–90% sensitivity) for diagnosis and permits identification of infections caused by species and serotypes other than *L pneumophila* serotype 1. Dieterle silver staining of tissue, pleural fluid, or other infected material is also a reliable method for detecting *Legionella* species. Direct fluorescent antibody stains and serologic testing are less sensitive because these will detect only *L pneumophila* serotype 1. In addition, making a serologic diagnosis requires that the host respond with sufficient specific antibody production. Urinary antigen tests, which are targeted for detection of *L pneumophila* serotype 1, are also less sensitive than culture.

▶ Treatment

Azithromycin (500 mg orally once daily), clarithromycin (500 mg orally twice daily), or a fluoroquinolone (eg, levofloxacin, 750 mg orally once daily), and not erythromycin, are the drugs of choice for treatment of legionellosis because of their excellent intracellular penetration and in vitro activity, as well as desirable pharmacokinetic properties that permit oral administration and once or twice daily dosing. Duration of therapy is 10–14 days, although a 21-day course of therapy is recommended for immunocompromised patients.

Cunha BA. Legionnaires' disease: clinical differentiation from typical and other atypical pneumonias. Infect Dis Clin North Am. 2010 Mar;24(1):73–105. [PMID: 20171547]

Decker BK et al. The role of water in healthcare-associated infections. Curr Opin Infect Dis. 2013 Aug;26(4):345–51. [PMID: 23806897]

Guyard C et al. *Legionella* infections and travel associated legionellosis. Travel Med Infect Dis. 2011 Jul;9(4):176–86. [PMID: 21995862]

GRAM-NEGATIVE BACTEREMIA & SEPSIS

Gram-negative bacteremia can originate in a number of sites, the most common being the genitourinary system, hepatobiliary tract, gastrointestinal tract, and lungs. Less common sources include intravenous lines, infusion fluids, surgical wounds, drains, and pressure ulcers.

Patients with potentially fatal underlying conditions in the short term such as neutropenia or immunoparesis have a mortality rate of 40–60%; those with serious underlying diseases likely to be fatal in 5 years, such as solid tumors, cirrhosis, and aplastic anemia, die in 15–20% of cases; and individuals with no underlying diseases have a mortality rate of 5% or less.

► Clinical Findings

A. Symptoms and Signs

Most patients have fevers and chills, often with abrupt onset. However, 15% of patients are hypothermic (temperature ≤ 36.4°C) at presentation, and 5% never develop a temperature above 37.5°C. Hyperventilation with respiratory alkalosis and changes in mental status are important early manifestations. Hypotension and shock, which occur in 20–50% of patients, are unfavorable prognostic signs.

B. Laboratory Findings

Neutropenia or neutrophilia, often with increased numbers of immature forms of polymorphonuclear leukocytes, is the most common laboratory abnormality in septic patients. Thrombocytopenia occurs in 50% of patients, laboratory evidence of coagulation abnormalities in 10%, and overt disseminated intravascular coagulation in 2–3%. Both clinical manifestations and the laboratory abnormalities are nonspecific and insensitive, which accounts for the relatively low rate of blood culture positivity (approximately 20–40%). If possible, three blood cultures from separate sites should be obtained in rapid succession before starting antimicrobial therapy. The chance of recovering the organism in at least one of the three blood cultures is > 95%. The false-negative rate for a single culture of 5–10 mL of blood is 30%. This may be reduced to 5–10% (albeit with a slight false-positive rate due to isolation of contaminants) if a single volume of 30 mL is inoculated into several blood culture bottles. Because blood cultures may be falsely negative, when a patient with presumed septic shock, negative blood cultures, and inadequate explanation for the clinical course responds to antimicrobials, therapy should be continued for 10–14 days.

► Treatment

Several factors are important in the management of patients with sepsis.

A. Removal of Predisposing Factors

This usually means decreasing or stopping immunosuppressive medications and, in certain circumstances, (eg, positive blood cultures) giving granulocyte colony-stimulating factor (filgrastim; G-CSF) to the neutropenic patient.

B. Identifying the Source of Bacteremia

By simply finding the source of bacteremia and removing it (central venous catheter) or draining it (abscess), a fatal disease becomes easily treatable.

C. Supportive Measures

The use of fluids, vasopressors, and corticosteroids in septic shock are discussed in Chapter 12; management of disseminated intravascular coagulation is discussed in Chapter 13.

D. Antibiotics

Antibiotics should be given as soon as the diagnosis is suspected, since delays in therapy have been associated with increased mortality rates, particularly once hypotension develops. In general, bactericidal antibiotics should be used and given intravenously to ensure therapeutic serum levels. Penetration of antibiotics into the site of primary infection is critical for successful therapy—ie, if the infection originates in the central nervous system, antibiotics that penetrate the blood-brain barrier should be used—eg, ampicillin, chloramphenicol, or a third- or fourth-generation cephalosporin—but not first-generation cephalosporins or aminoglycosides, which penetrate poorly. Sepsis caused by gram-positive organisms cannot be differentiated on clinical grounds from that due to gram-negative bacteria. Therefore, initial therapy should include antibiotics active against both types of organisms.

The number of antibiotics necessary remains controversial and depends on the cause. Table 30–5 provides a guide for empiric therapy. Although a combination of antibiotics is often recommended for "synergism," combination therapy has not been shown to be superior to a single-drug regimen with any of several broad-spectrum antibiotics (eg, a third-generation cephalosporin, piperacillin-tazobactam, carbapenem). If multiple drugs are used initially, the regimen should be modified and coverage narrowed based on the results of culture and sensitivity testing.

Angus DC et al. Severe sepsis and septic shock. N Engl J Med. 2013 Aug 29;369(9):840–51. Erratum in: N Engl J Med. 2013 Nov 21;369(21):2069. [PMID: 23984731]

Casserly B et al. Low-dose steroids in adult septic shock: results of the Surviving Sepsis Campaign. Intensive Care Med. 2012 Dec;38(12):1946–54. [PMID: 23064466]

Patel GP et al. Systemic steroids in severe sepsis and septic shock. Am J Respir Crit Care Med. 2012 Jan 15;185(2):133–9. [PMID: 21680949]

SALMONELLOSIS

Salmonellosis includes infection by any of approximately 2000 serotypes of salmonellae. The taxonomy of *Salmonella* species has been confusing. All *Salmonella* serotypes are members of a single species, *Salmonella enterica*. Human infections are caused almost exclusively by *S enterica* subsp *enterica*, of which three serotypes—*typhi, typhimurium*, and *choleraesuis*—are predominantly isolated. Three clinical patterns of infection are recognized: (1) enteric fever, the best example of which is typhoid fever, due to serotype *typhi*; (2) acute enterocolitis, caused by serotype *typhimurium*, among others; and (3) the "septicemic" type, characterized by bacteremia and focal lesions, exemplified by infection with serotype *choleraesuis*. All types are transmitted by ingestion of the organism, usually from contaminated food or drink.

Feasey NA et al. Invasive non-typhoidal salmonella disease: an emerging and neglected tropical disease in Africa. Lancet. 2012 Jun 30;379(9835):2489–99. [PMID: 22587967]
Onwuezobe IA et al. Antimicrobials for treating symptomatic non-typhoidal *Salmonella* infection. Cochrane Database Syst Rev. 2012 Nov 14;11:CD001167. [PMID: 23152205]

1. Enteric Fever (Typhoid Fever)

ESSENTIALS OF DIAGNOSIS

- ▶ Gradual onset of malaise, headache, nausea, vomiting, abdominal pain.
- ▶ Rose spots, relative bradycardia, splenomegaly, and abdominal distention and tenderness.
- ▶ Slow (stepladder) rise of fever to maximum and then slow return to normal.
- ▶ Leukopenia; blood, stool, and urine culture positive for salmonella.

▶ General Considerations

Enteric fever is a clinical syndrome characterized by constitutional and gastrointestinal symptoms and by headache. It can be caused by any *Salmonella* species. The term "typhoid fever" applies when serotype *typhi* is the cause. Infection is transmitted by consumption of contaminated food or drink. The incubation period is 5–14 days. *Salmonella* is an intracellular pathogen. Infection begins when organisms breach the mucosal epithelium of the intestines by transcytosis, an organism-mediated transport process through the cell via an endocytic vesicle. Having crossed the epithelial barrier, organisms invade and replicate in macrophages in Peyer patches, mesenteric lymph nodes, and the spleen. Serotypes other than *typhi* usually do not cause invasive disease, presumably because they lack the necessary human-specific virulence factors. Bacteremia occurs, and the infection then localizes principally in the lymphoid tissue of the small intestine (particularly within 60 cm of the ileocecal valve). Peyer patches become inflamed and may ulcerate, with involvement greatest during the third week of disease. The organism may disseminate to the lungs, gallbladder, kidneys, or central nervous system.

▶ Clinical Findings

A. Symptoms and Signs

During the prodromal stage, there is increasing malaise, headache, cough, and sore throat, often with abdominal pain and constipation, while the fever ascends in a stepwise fashion. After about 7–10 days, it reaches a plateau and the patient is much more ill, appearing exhausted and often prostrated. There may be marked constipation, especially early, or "pea soup" diarrhea; marked abdominal distention occurs as well. If there are no complications, the patient's condition will gradually improve over 7–10 days. However, relapse may occur for up to 2 weeks after defervescence.

During the early prodrome, physical findings are few. Later, splenomegaly, abdominal distention and tenderness, relative bradycardia, and occasionally meningismus appear. The rash (rose spots) commonly appears during the second week of disease. The individual spot, found principally on the trunk, is a pink papule 2–3 mm in diameter that fades on pressure. It disappears in 3–4 days.

B. Laboratory Findings

Typhoid fever is best diagnosed by blood culture, which is positive in the first week of illness in 80% of patients who have not taken antimicrobials. The rate of positivity declines thereafter, but one-fourth or more of patients still have positive blood cultures in the third week. Cultures of bone marrow occasionally are positive when blood cultures are not. Stool culture is unreliable because it may be positive in gastroenteritis without typhoid fever. Relative bradycardia and leukopenia are typical.

▶ Differential Diagnosis

Enteric fever must be distinguished from other gastrointestinal illnesses and from other infections that have few localizing findings. Examples include tuberculosis, infective endocarditis, brucellosis, lymphoma, and Q fever. Often there is a history of recent travel to endemic areas, and viral hepatitis, malaria, or amebiasis may be in the differential as well.

▶ Complications

Complications occur in about 30% of untreated cases and account for 75% of deaths. Intestinal hemorrhage, manifested by a sudden drop in temperature and signs of shock followed by dark or fresh blood in the stool, or intestinal perforation, accompanied by abdominal pain and tenderness, is most likely to occur during the third week. Appearance of leukocytosis and tachycardia should suggest these complications. Urinary retention, pneumonia, thrombophlebitis, myocarditis, psychosis, cholecystitis, nephritis, osteomyelitis, and meningitis are less often observed.

▶ Prevention

Immunization is not always effective but should be considered for household contacts of a typhoid carrier, for travelers to endemic areas, and during epidemic outbreaks. A multiple-dose oral vaccine and a single-dose parenteral vaccine are available. Their efficacies are similar, but oral vaccine causes fewer side effects. Boosters, when indicated, should be given every 5 years and 2 years for oral and parenteral preparations, respectively.

Adequate waste disposal and protection of food and water supplies from contamination are important public health measures to prevent salmonellosis. Carriers cannot work as food handlers.

▶ Treatment

A. Specific Measures

Several antibiotics, including ampicillin, azithromycin, chloramphenicol, third-generation cephalosporins, and trimethoprim-sulfamethoxazole all are effective for treatment of enteric fever caused by drug-susceptible strains. These drugs can be given orally or intravenously depending on the patient's condition. Because many salmonella strains are resistant to ampicillin, chloramphenicol, and trimethoprim-sulfamethoxazole, a fluoroquinolone—such as ciprofloxacin 750 mg orally twice daily or levofloxacin 500 mg orally once daily, 5–7 days for uncomplicated enteric fever and 10–14 days for severe infection—is the agent of choice for treatment of salmonella infections. Ceftriaxone, 2 g intravenously for 7 days, is also effective. Although resistance to fluoroquinolones or cephalosporins occurs uncommonly, the prevalence appears to be increasing. When an infection is caused by a multidrug-resistant strain, select an antibiotic to which the isolate is susceptible in vitro. Alternatively, increasing the dose of ceftriaxone to 4 g/d and treating for 10–14 days or using azithromycin 500 mg orally for 7 days in uncomplicated cases may be effective.

B. Treatment of Carriers

Chemotherapy often is unsuccessful in eradicating the carrier state. While treatment of carriage with ampicillin, trimethoprim-sulfamethoxazole, or chloramphenicol may be successful, ciprofloxacin, 750 mg orally twice a day for 4 weeks, has proved to be highly effective. Cholecystectomy may also achieve this goal.

▶ Prognosis

The mortality rate of typhoid fever is about 2% in treated cases. Elderly or debilitated persons are likely to do poorly. With complications, the prognosis is poor. Relapses occur in up to 15% of cases. A residual carrier state frequently persists in spite of chemotherapy.

Anwar E et al. Vaccines for preventing typhoid fever. Cochrane Database Syst Rev. 2014 Jan 2;1:CD001261. [PMID: 24385413]

Butler T. Treatment of typhoid fever in the 21st century: promises and shortcomings. Clin Microbiol Infect. 2011 Jul;17(7):959–63. [PMID: 21722249]

2. *Salmonella* Gastroenteritis

By far the most common form of salmonellosis is acute enterocolitis caused by numerous *Salmonella* serotypes. The incubation period is 8–48 hours after ingestion of contaminated food or liquid.

Symptoms and signs consist of fever (often with chills), nausea and vomiting, cramping abdominal pain, and diarrhea, which may be grossly bloody, lasting 3–5 days. Differentiation must be made from viral gastroenteritis, food poisoning, shigellosis, amebic dysentery, and acute ulcerative colitis. The diagnosis is made by culturing the organism from the stool.

The disease is usually self-limited, but bacteremia with localization in joints or bones may occur, especially in patients with sickle cell disease.

In most cases, treatment of uncomplicated enterocolitis is symptomatic only. However, patients who are malnourished or severely ill, patients with sickle cell disease, and patients who are immunocompromised (including those who are HIV-positive) should be treated with ciprofloxacin, 500 mg orally twice a day; ceftriaxone, 1 g intravenously once daily; trimethoprim-sulfamethoxazole, 160 mg/80 mg orally twice a day; or azithromycin, 500 mg orally once daily for 7–14 days (14 days for immunocompromised patients).

Gaffga NH et al. Outbreak of salmonellosis linked to live poultry from a mail-order hatchery. N Engl J Med. 2012 May 31; 366(22):2065–73. [PMID: 22646629]

3. *Salmonella* Bacteremia

Salmonella infection may be manifested by prolonged or recurrent fevers accompanied by bacteremia and local infection in bone, joints, pleura, pericardium, lungs, or other sites. Mycotic abdominal aortic aneurysms may also occur. Serotypes other than typhi usually are isolated. This complication tends to occur in immunocompromised persons and is seen in HIV-infected individuals, who typically have bacteremia without an obvious source. Treatment is the same as for typhoid fever, plus drainage of any abscesses. In HIV-infected patients, relapse is common, and lifelong suppressive therapy may be needed. Ciprofloxacin, 750 mg orally twice a day, is effective both for therapy of acute infection and for suppression of recurrence. Incidence of infections caused by drug-resistant strains may be on the rise.

Abbott SL et al. Increase in extraintestinal infections caused by *Salmonella* enterica subspecies II–IV. Emerg Infect Dis. 2012 Apr;18(4):637–9. [PMID: 22469432]

Hennedige T et al. Spectrum of imaging findings in *Salmonella* infections. AJR Am J Roentgenol. 2012 Jun;198(6):W534–9. [PMID: 22623567]

Onwuezobe IA et al. Antimicrobials for treating symptomatic non-typhoidal *Salmonella* infection. Cochrane Database Syst Rev. 2012 Nov 14;11:CD001167. [PMID: 23152205]

SHIGELLOSIS

ESSENTIALS OF DIAGNOSIS

- ▸ Diarrhea, often with blood and mucus.
- ▸ Crampy abdominal pain and systemic toxicity.
- ▸ White blood cells in stools; organism isolated on stool culture.

▶ General Considerations

Shigella dysentery is a common disease, often self-limited and mild but occasionally serious. *S sonnei* is the leading cause in the United States, followed by *S flexneri*. *S dysenteriae* causes the most serious form of the illness. Shigellae are invasive organisms. The infective dose is 10^2–10^3 organisms. There has been a rise in strains resistant to multiple antibiotics.

▶ Clinical Findings

A. Symptoms and Signs

The illness usually starts abruptly, with diarrhea, lower abdominal cramps, and tenesmus. The diarrheal stool often is mixed with blood and mucus. Systemic symptoms are fever, chills, anorexia and malaise, and headache. The abdomen is tender. Sigmoidoscopic examination reveals an inflamed, engorged mucosa with punctate and sometimes large areas of ulceration.

B. Laboratory Findings

The stool shows many leukocytes and red cells. Stool culture is positive for shigellae in most cases, but blood cultures grow the organism in < 5% of cases.

▶ Differential Diagnosis

Bacillary dysentery must be distinguished from salmonella enterocolitis and from disease due to enterotoxigenic *Escherichia coli*, *Campylobacter*, and *Yersinia enterocolitica*. Amebic dysentery may be similar clinically and is diagnosed by finding amebas in the fresh stool specimen. Ulcerative colitis is also an important cause of bloody diarrhea.

▶ Complications

Temporary disaccharidase deficiency may follow the diarrhea. Reactive arthritis is an uncommon complication, usually occurring in HLA-B27 individuals infected by *Shigella*. Hemolytic-uremic syndrome occurs rarely.

▶ Treatment

Treatment of dehydration and hypotension is lifesaving in severe cases. Recommended empiric antimicrobial therapy is either a fluoroquinolone (ciprofloxacin, 750 mg orally twice daily for 7–10 days, or levofloxacin, 500 mg orally once daily for 3 days) or ceftriaxone, 1 g intravenously once daily for 5 days. If the isolate is susceptible, trimethoprim-sulfamethoxazole, 160/80 mg orally twice daily for 5 days or azithromycin, 500 mg orally once daily for 3 days, is also effective. High rates of resistance to amoxicillin make it a less effective treatment option.

DuPont HL. Approach to the patient with infectious colitis. Curr Opin Gastroenterol. 2012 Jan;28(1):39–46. [PMID: 22080825]
Pons MJ et al. Antimicrobial resistance in *Shigella* spp. causing traveller's diarrhoea (1995–2010): a retrospective analysis. Travel Med Infect Dis. 2013 Sep–Oct;11(5):315–9. [PMID: 23886737]

GASTROENTERITIS CAUSED BY *ESCHERICHIA COLI*

E coli causes gastroenteritis by a variety of mechanisms. Enterotoxigenic *E coli* (ETEC) elaborates either a heat-stable or heat-labile toxin that mediates the disease. ETEC is an important cause of traveler's diarrhea. Enteroinvasive *E coli* (EIEC) differs from other *E coli* bowel pathogens in that these strains invade cells, causing bloody diarrhea and dysentery similar to infection with *Shigella* species. EIEC is uncommon in the United States. Neither ETEC nor EIEC strains are routinely isolated and identified from stool cultures because there is no selective medium. Antimicrobial therapy against *Salmonella* and *Shigella*, such as ciprofloxacin 500 mg orally twice daily, shortens the clinical course, but the disease is self-limited.

Shiga-toxin-producing *E coli* (STEC) infection can result in asymptomatic carrier stage, nonbloody diarrhea, hemorrhagic colitis, hemolytic-uremic syndrome, or thrombotic thrombocytopenic purpura. Although *E coli* O157:H7 is responsible for most cases of STEC infection in the United States, recently in Europe, other STEC strains (such as *E coli* O104:H4) have been reported to cause severe disease. *E coli* O157:H7 has caused several outbreaks of diarrhea and hemolytic-uremic syndrome related to consumption of undercooked hamburger, unpasteurized apple juice, and spinach, while *E coli* O145 was recently linked to the consumption of contaminated lettuce. Older individuals and young children are most affected, with hemolytic-uremic syndrome being more common in the latter group. STEC identification can be difficult and the CDC recommends that all stools submitted for routine testing from patients with acute community-acquired diarrhea be simultaneously cultured for *E coli* O157:H7 and tested with an assay that detects Shiga toxins to detect non O157 STEC, such as *E coli* O145. Antimicrobial therapy does not alter the course of the disease and may increase the risk of hemolytic-uremic syndrome. Treatment is primarily supportive. Hemolytic-uremic syndrome or thrombotic thrombocytopenic purpura occurring in association with a diarrheal illness suggests the diagnosis and should prompt evaluation for STEC. Confirmed infections should be reported to public health officials.

Bettelheim KA. Non-O157 Shiga-toxin-producing *Escherichia coli*. Lancet Infect Dis. 2012 Jan;12(1):12. [PMID: 22192128]

Wu CJ et al. A new health threat in Europe: *Shiga* toxin-producing *Escherichia coli* O104:H4 infections. J Microbiol Immunol Infect. 2011 Oct;44(5):390–3. [PMID: 21862425]

CHOLERA

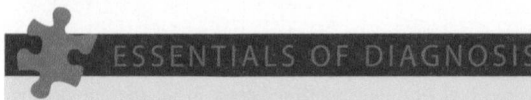

ESSENTIALS OF DIAGNOSIS

- ► History of travel in endemic area or contact with infected person.
- ► Voluminous diarrhea.
- ► Stool is liquid, gray, turbid, and without fecal odor, blood, or pus ("rice water stool").
- ► Rapid development of marked dehydration.
- ► Positive stool cultures and agglutination of vibrios with specific sera.

General Considerations

Cholera is an acute diarrheal illness caused by certain serotypes of *Vibrio cholerae*. The disease is toxin-mediated, and fever is unusual. The toxin activates adenylyl cyclase in intestinal epithelial cells of the small intestines, producing hypersecretion of water and chloride ion and a massive diarrhea of up to 15 L/d. Death results from profound hypovolemia. Cholera occurs in epidemics under conditions of crowding, war, and famine (eg, in refugee camps) and where sanitation is inadequate. Infection is acquired by ingestion of contaminated food or water. For over a century, cholera was rarely seen in the Western Hemisphere until an outbreak occurred in Peru, starting in the early 1990s and ending by 2001; the outbreak resulted in almost 400,000 cholera cases and more than 4000 deaths. Cholera again became a rare disease in the Western Hemisphere until late 2010. A massive earthquake in Haiti in January 2010 crumbled the country's already fragile infrastructure. Later that fall, a cholera outbreak erupted that has continued and resulted in thousands of deaths.

Clinical Findings

Cholera is characterized by a sudden onset of severe, frequent watery diarrhea (up to 1 L/h). The liquid stool is gray; turbid; and without fecal odor, blood, or pus ("rice water stool"). Dehydration and hypotension develop rapidly. Stool cultures are positive, and agglutination of vibrios with specific sera can be demonstrated.

Prevention

A vaccine is available that confers short-lived, limited protection and may be required for entry into or reentry after travel to some countries. It is administered in two doses 1–4 weeks apart. A booster dose every 6 months is recommended for persons remaining in areas where cholera is a hazard.

Vaccination programs are expensive and not particularly effective in managing outbreaks of cholera. When outbreaks occur, efforts should be directed toward establishing clean water and food sources and proper waste disposal.

Treatment

Treatment is by replacement of fluids. In mild or moderate illness, oral rehydration usually is adequate. A simple oral replacement fluid can be made from 1 teaspoon of table salt and 4 heaping teaspoons of sugar added to 1 L of water. Intravenous fluids are indicated for persons with signs of severe hypovolemia and those who cannot take adequate fluids orally. Lactated Ringer infusion is satisfactory.

Antimicrobial therapy will shorten the course of illness. Several antimicrobials are active against *V cholerae*, including tetracycline, ampicillin, chloramphenicol, trimethoprim-sulfamethoxazole, fluoroquinolones, and azithromycin. Multiple drug-resistant strains are increasingly encountered, so susceptibility testing, if available, is advisable. A single 1 g oral dose of azithromycin is effective for severe cholera caused by strains with reduced susceptibility to fluoroquinolones, but resistance is emerging to this drug as well.

Harris JB et al. Cholera. Lancet. 2012 Jun 30;379(9835):2466–76. [PMID: 22748592]
Schilling KA et al. Diarrheal illness among U.S. residents providing medical services in Haiti during the cholera epidemic, 2010 to 2011. J Travel Med. 2014 Jan;21(1):55–7. [PMID: 24383654]

INFECTIONS CAUSED BY OTHER *VIBRIO* SPECIES

Vibrios other than *V cholerae* that cause human disease are *Vibrio parahaemolyticus*, *V vulnificus*, and *V alginolyticus*. All are halophilic marine organisms. Infection is acquired by exposure to organisms in contaminated, undercooked, or raw crustaceans or shellfish and warm (> 20°C) ocean waters and estuaries. Infections are more common during the summer months from regions along the Atlantic coast and the Gulf of Mexico in the United States and from tropical waters around the world. Oysters are implicated in up to 90% of food-related cases. *V parahaemolyticus* causes an acute watery diarrhea with crampy abdominal pain and fever, typically occurring within 24 hours after ingestion of contaminated shellfish. The disease is self-limited, and antimicrobial therapy is usually not necessary. *V parahaemolyticus* may also cause cellulitis and sepsis, though these findings are more characteristic of *V vulnificus* infection.

V vulnificus and *V alginolyticus*—neither of which is associated with diarrheal illness—are important causes of cellulitis and primary bacteremia following ingestion of contaminated shellfish or exposure to sea water. Cellulitis with or without sepsis may be accompanied by bulla formation and necrosis with extensive soft tissue destruction, at times requiring debridement and amputation. The infection can be rapidly progressive and is particularly severe in immunocompromised individuals—especially those with cirrhosis—with death rates as high as 50%. Patients with chronic liver disease and those who are immunocompromised should be cautioned to avoid eating raw oysters.

Tetracycline at a dose of 500 mg orally four times a day for 7–10 days is the drug of choice for treatment of suspected or documented primary bacteremia or cellulitis caused by *Vibrio* species. *V vulnificus* is susceptible in vitro to penicillin, ampicillin, cephalosporins, chloramphenicol, aminoglycosides, and fluoroquinolones, and these agents may also be effective. *V parahaemolyticus* and *V alginolyticus* produce beta-lactamase and therefore are resistant to penicillin and ampicillin, but susceptibilities otherwise are similar to those listed for *V vulnificus*.

Daniels NA. *Vibrio vulnificus* oysters: pearls and perils. Clin Infect Dis. 2011 Mar 15;52(6):788–92. [PMID: 21367733]
Vugia DJ et al. Impact of 2003 state regulation on raw oyster-associated *Vibrio vulnificus* illnesses and deaths, California, USA. Emerg Infect Dis. 2013 Aug;19(8):1276–80. [PMID: 23876744]

INFECTIONS CAUSED BY *CAMPYLOBACTER* SPECIES

Campylobacter organisms are microaerophilic, motile, gram-negative rods. Two species infect humans: *Campylobacter jejuni*, an important cause of diarrheal disease, and *C fetus* subsp *fetus*, which typically causes systemic infection and not diarrhea. Dairy cattle and poultry are an important reservoir for campylobacters. Outbreaks of enteritis have been associated with consumption of raw milk. *Campylobacter* gastroenteritis is associated with fever, abdominal pain, and diarrhea characterized by loose, watery, or bloody stools. The differential diagnosis includes shigellosis, *Salmonella* gastroenteritis, and enteritis caused by *Y enterocolitica* or invasive *E coli*. The disease is self-limited, but its duration can be shortened with antimicrobial therapy. Either azithromycin, 1 g orally as a single dose, or ciprofloxacin, 500 mg orally twice daily for 3 days, is effective therapy. However, fluoroquinolone resistance among *C jejuni* isolates has been increasing, particularly in Southeast Asia, and susceptibility testing should be routinely performed.

C fetus causes systemic infections that can be fatal, including primary bacteremia, endocarditis, meningitis, and focal abscesses. It infrequently causes gastroenteritis. Patients infected with *C fetus* are often older, debilitated, or immunocompromised. Closely related species, collectively termed "campylobacter-like organisms," cause bacteremia in HIV-infected individuals. Systemic infections respond to therapy with gentamicin, chloramphenicol, ceftriaxone, or ciprofloxacin. Ceftriaxone or chloramphenicol should be used to treat infections of the central nervous system because of their ability to penetrate the blood-brain barrier.

Kollaritsch H et al. Traveler's diarrhea. Infect Dis Clin North Am. 2012 Sep;26(3):691–706. [PMID: 22963778]
Lévesque S et al. Campylobacteriosis in urban versus rural areas: a case-case study integrated with molecular typing to validate risk factors and to attribute sources of infection. PLoS One. 2013 Dec 26;8(12):e83731. [PMID: 24386265]

BRUCELLOSIS

ESSENTIALS OF DIAGNOSIS

- ► History of animal exposure, ingestion of unpasteurized milk or cheese.
- ► Insidious onset: easy fatigability, headache, arthralgia, anorexia, sweating, irritability.
- ► Intermittent and persistent fever.
- ► Cervical and axillary lymphadenopathy; hepatosplenomegaly.
- ► Lymphocytosis, positive blood culture, positive serologic test.

► General Considerations

The infection is transmitted from animals to humans. *Brucella abortus* (cattle), *B suis* (hogs), and *B melitensis* (goats) are the main agents. Transmission to humans occurs by contact with infected meat (slaughterhouse workers), placentae of infected animals (farmers, veterinarians), or ingestion of infected unpasteurized milk or cheese. The incubation period varies from a few days to several weeks. Brucellosis is a systemic infection that may become chronic. In the United States, brucellosis is very rare. Almost all US cases are imported from countries where brucellosis is endemic (eg, Mexico, Mediterranean Europe, Spain, South American countries).

► Clinical Findings

A. Symptoms and Signs

The onset may be acute, with fever, chills, and sweats, but more often is insidious with symptoms of weakness, weight loss, low-grade fevers, sweats, and exhaustion upon minimal activity. Headache, abdominal or back pain with anorexia and constipation, and arthralgias are also common. The chronic form may assume an undulant nature, with periods of normal temperature between acute attacks; symptoms may persist for years, either continuously or intermittently.

Fever, hepatosplenomegaly, and lymphadenopathy are the most common physical findings. Infection may present with or be complicated by specific organ involvement with signs of endocarditis, meningitis, epididymitis, orchitis, arthritis (especially sacroiliitis), spondylitis, or osteomyelitis.

B. Laboratory Findings

The organism can be recovered from cultures of blood, cerebrospinal fluid, urine, bone marrow, or other sites. Modern automated systems have shortened the time to detection of the organism in blood culture. Cultures are more likely to be negative in chronic cases. The diagnosis often is made by serologic testing. Rising serologic titers or an absolute agglutination titer of > 1:160 supports the diagnosis.

▶ Differential Diagnosis

Brucellosis must be differentiated from any other acute febrile disease, especially influenza, tularemia, Q fever, mononucleosis, and enteric fever. In its chronic form it resembles Hodgkin disease, tuberculosis, HIV infection, malaria, and disseminated fungal infections such as histoplasmosis and coccidioidomycosis.

▶ Complications

The most frequent complications are bone and joint lesions such as spondylitis and suppurative arthritis (usually of a single joint), endocarditis, and meningoencephalitis. Less common complications are pneumonitis with pleural effusion, hepatitis, and cholecystitis.

▶ Treatment

Single-drug regimens are not recommended because the relapse rate may be as high as 50%. Combination regimens of two or three drugs are most effective. Regimens of doxycycline (200 mg/d orally for 6 weeks) plus rifampin (600 mg/d orally for 6 weeks) or streptomycin (1 g/d intramuscularly for 2 weeks) or gentamicin (240 mg intramuscularly once daily for 7 days) have the lowest recurrence rates. Longer courses of therapy may be required to prevent relapse of meningitis, osteomyelitis, or endocarditis.

Dean AS et al. Clinical manifestations of human brucellosis: a systematic review and meta-analysis. PLoS Negl Trop Dis. 2012;6(12):e1929. [PMID: 23236528]
Solís García del Pozo J et al. Systematic review and meta-analysis of randomized clinical trials in the treatment of human brucellosis. PLoS One. 2012;7(2):e32090. [PMID: 22393379]
Yousefi-Nooraie R et al. Antibiotics for treating human brucellosis. Cochrane Database Syst Rev. 2012 Oct 17;10:CD007179. [PMID: 23076931]

TULAREMIA

ESSENTIALS OF DIAGNOSIS

- ▶ History of contact with rabbits, other rodents, and biting arthropods (eg, ticks in summer) in endemic area.
- ▶ Fever, headache, nausea, and prostration.
- ▶ Papule progressing to ulcer at site of inoculation.
- ▶ Enlarged regional lymph nodes.
- ▶ Serologic tests or culture of ulcer, lymph node aspirate, or blood confirm the diagnosis.

▶ General Considerations

Tularemia is a zoonotic infection of wild rodents and rabbits caused by *Francisella tularensis*. Humans usually acquire the infection by contact with animal tissues (eg, trapping muskrats, skinning rabbits) or from a tick or insect bite. Hamsters and prairie dogs also may carry the organism. An investigation of an outbreak of pneumonic tularemia on Martha's Vineyard in Massachusetts implicated lawn-mowing and brush-cutting as risk factors for infection, underscoring the potential for probable aerosol transmission of the organism. *F tularensis* has been classified as a high-priority agent for potential bioterrorism use because of its virulence and relative ease of dissemination. Infection in humans often produces a local lesion and widespread organ involvement but may be entirely asymptomatic. The incubation period is 2–10 days.

▶ Clinical Findings

A. Symptoms and Signs

Fever, headache, and nausea begin suddenly, and a local lesion—a papule at the site of inoculation—develops and soon ulcerates. Regional lymph nodes may become enlarged and tender and may suppurate. The local lesion may be on the skin of an extremity or in the eye. Pneumonia may develop from hematogenous spread of the organism or may be primary after inhalation of infected aerosols, which are responsible for human-to-human transmission. Following ingestion of infected meat or water, an enteric form may be manifested by gastrointestinal symptoms, stupor, and delirium. In any type of involvement, the spleen may be enlarged and tender and there may be nonspecific rashes, myalgias, and prostration.

B. Laboratory Findings

Culturing the organism from blood or infected tissue requires special media. For this reason and because cultures of *F tularensis* may be hazardous to laboratory personnel, the diagnosis is usually made serologically. A positive agglutination test (> 1:80) develops in the second week after infection and may persist for several years.

▶ Differential Diagnosis

Tularemia must be differentiated from rickettsial and meningococcal infections, cat-scratch disease, infectious mononucleosis, and various bacterial and fungal diseases.

▶ Complications

Hematogenous spread may produce meningitis, perisplenitis, pericarditis, pneumonia, and osteomyelitis.

▶ Treatment

Streptomycin is drug of choice for treatment of tularemia. The recommended dose is 7.5 mg/kg intramuscularly every 12 hours for 7–14 days. Gentamicin, which has good in vitro activity against *F tularensis*, is generally less toxic than streptomycin and probably just as effective. Doxycycline (200 mg/d orally) is also effective but has a higher relapse rate. A variety of other agents (eg, fluoroquinolones) are active in vitro but their clinical effectiveness is less well established.

Centers for Disease Control and Prevention (CDC). Tularemia—United States, 2001–2010. MMWR Morb Mortal Wkly Rep. 2013 Nov 29;62(47):963–6. [PMID: 24280916]

Weber IB et al. Clinical recognition and management of tularemia in Missouri: a retrospective records review of 121 cases. Clin Infect Dis. 2012 Nov 15;55(10):1283–90. [PMID: 22911645]

PLAGUE

ESSENTIALS OF DIAGNOSIS

- ▶ History of exposure to rodents in endemic area.
- ▶ Sudden onset of high fever, malaise, muscular pains, and prostration.
- ▶ Axillary or inguinal lymphadenitis (bubo).
- ▶ Bacteremia, pneumonitis, and meningitis may occur.
- ▶ Positive smear and culture from bubo and positive blood culture.

▶ General Considerations

Plague is an infection of wild rodents with *Yersinia pestis*, a small bipolar-staining gram-negative rod. It is endemic in California, Arizona, Nevada, and New Mexico. It is transmitted among rodents and to humans by the bites of fleas or from contact with infected animals. Following a fleabite, the organisms spread through the lymphatics to the lymph nodes, which become greatly enlarged (bubo). They may then reach the bloodstream to involve all organs. When pneumonia or meningitis develops, the outcome is often fatal. The patient with pneumonia can transmit the infection to other individuals by droplets. The incubation period is 2–10 days. Because of its extreme virulence, its potential for dissemination and person-to-person transmission, and efforts to develop the organism as an agent of biowarfare, plague bacillus is considered a high-priority agent for bioterrorism.

▶ Clinical Findings

A. Symptoms and Signs

The onset is sudden, with high fever, malaise, tachycardia, intense headache, delirium, and severe myalgias. The patient appears profoundly ill. If pneumonia develops, tachypnea, productive cough, blood-tinged sputum, and cyanosis also occur. There may be signs of meningitis. A pustule or ulcer at the site of inoculation and lymphangitis may be observed. Axillary, inguinal, or cervical lymph nodes become enlarged and tender and may suppurate and drain. With hematogenous spread, the patient may rapidly become toxic and comatose, with purpuric spots (black plague) appearing on the skin.

Primary plague pneumonia is a fulminant pneumonitis with bloody, frothy sputum and sepsis. It is usually fatal unless treatment is started within a few hours after onset.

B. Laboratory Findings

The plague bacillus may be found in smears from aspirates of buboes examined with Gram stain. Cultures from bubo aspirate or pus and blood are positive but may grow slowly. In convalescing patients, an antibody titer rise may be demonstrated by agglutination tests.

▶ Differential Diagnosis

The lymphadenitis of plague is most commonly mistaken for the lymphadenitis accompanying staphylococcal or streptococcal infections of an extremity, sexually transmitted diseases such as lymphogranuloma venereum or syphilis, and tularemia. The systemic manifestations resemble those of enteric or rickettsial fevers, malaria, or influenza. The pneumonia resembles other bacterial pneumonias, and the meningitis is similar to those caused by other bacteria.

▶ Prevention

Avoiding exposure to rodents and fleas in endemic areas is the best prevention strategy. Drug prophylaxis may provide temporary protection for persons exposed to the risk of plague infection, particularly by the respiratory route. Doxycycline, 100 mg twice daily for 7 days, is effective. No vaccine is available at this time.

▶ Treatment

Therapy should be started immediately once plague is suspected. Either streptomycin (the agent with which there is greatest experience), 1 g every 12 hours intravenously, or gentamicin, administered as a 2-mg/kg loading dose, then 1.7 mg/kg every 8 hours intravenously, is effective. Alternatively, doxycycline, 100 mg orally or intravenously, may be used. The duration of therapy is 10 days. Patients with plague pneumonia are placed in strict respiratory isolation, and prophylactic therapy is given to any person who came in contact with the patient.

Raoult D et al. Plague: history and contemporary analysis. J Infect. 2013 Jan;66(1):18–26. [PMID: 23041039]
Williamson ED et al. The natural history and incidence of *Yersinia pestis* and prospects for vaccination. J Med Microbiol. 2012 Jul;61(Pt 7):911–8. [PMID: 22442294]

GONOCOCCAL INFECTIONS

ESSENTIALS OF DIAGNOSIS

- ▶ Purulent and profuse urethral discharge, especially in men, with dysuria, yielding positive smear.
- ▶ Men: epididymitis, prostatitis, periurethral inflammation, proctitis.
- ▶ Women: cervicitis with purulent discharge, or asymptomatic, yielding positive culture; vaginitis, salpingitis, proctitis also occur.
- ▶ Fever, rash, tenosynovitis, and arthritis with disseminated disease.
- ▶ Gram-negative intracellular diplococci seen in a smear or cultured from any site, particularly the urethra, cervix, pharynx, and rectum.

General Considerations

Gonorrhea is caused by *Neisseria gonorrhoeae*, a gram-negative diplococcus typically found inside polymorphonuclear cells. It is transmitted during sexual activity and has its greatest incidence in the 15- to 29-year-old age group. The incubation period is usually 2–8 days.

Classification

A. Urethritis and Cervicitis

In men, there is initially burning on urination and a serous or milky discharge. One to 3 days later, the urethral pain is more pronounced and the discharge becomes yellow, creamy, and profuse, sometimes blood-tinged. The disorder may regress and become chronic or progress to involve the prostate, epididymis, and periurethral glands with painful inflammation. Chronic infection leads to prostatitis and urethral strictures. Rectal infection is common in homosexual men. Atypical sites of primary infection (eg, the pharynx) must always be considered. Asymptomatic infection is common and occurs in both sexes.

Gonococcal infection in women often becomes symptomatic during menses. Women may have dysuria, urinary frequency, and urgency, with a purulent urethral discharge. Vaginitis and cervicitis with inflammation of Bartholin glands are common. Infection may be asymptomatic, with only slightly increased vaginal discharge and moderate cervicitis on examination. Infection may remain as a chronic cervicitis—an important reservoir of gonococci. It can progress to involve the uterus and tubes with acute and chronic salpingitis, with scarring of tubes and sterility. In pelvic inflammatory disease, anaerobes and chlamydiae often accompany gonococci. Rectal infection may result from spread of the organism from the genital tract or from anal coitus.

Gram stain of urethral discharge in men, especially during the first week after onset, shows gram-negative diplococci in polymorphonuclear leukocytes. Gram stain is less often positive in women. Culture has been the gold standard for diagnosis, particularly when the Gram stain is negative. Nucleic acid amplification tests for *N gonorrhoeae* are FDA-approved for the testing of endocervical swabs, vaginal swabs, urethral swabs (men), and urine (from both men and women), and have excellent sensitivity and specificity, and have largely replaced culture. Identification of *N gonorrhoeae* from rectal or pharyngeal sites, blood, and in joint fluid still requires culture.

B. Disseminated Disease

Systemic complications follow the dissemination of gonococci from the primary site via the bloodstream. Two distinct clinical syndromes—either purulent arthritis or the triad of rash, tenosynovitis, and arthralgias—are commonly observed in patients with disseminated gonococcal infection, although overlap can be seen. The skin lesions can range from maculopapular to pustular or hemorrhagic, which tend to be few in number and peripherally located. The tenosynovitis is often found in the hands and wrists

and feet and ankles. These unique findings can help distinguish among other infectious syndromes. The arthritis can occur in one or more joints. Gonococci are isolated by culture from less than half of patients with gonococcal arthritis. Rarely, gonococcal endocarditis or meningitis develops.

C. Conjunctivitis

The most common form of eye involvement is direct inoculation of gonococci into the conjunctival sac. In adults, this occurs by autoinoculation of a person with genital infection. The purulent conjunctivitis may rapidly progress to panophthalmitis and loss of the eye unless treated promptly. A single 1-g dose of ceftriaxone is effective.

Differential Diagnosis

Gonococcal urethritis or cervicitis must be differentiated from nongonococcal urethritis; cervicitis or vaginitis due to *Chlamydia trachomatis*, *Gardnerella vaginalis*, *Trichomonas*, *Candida*, and many other pathogens associated with sexually transmitted diseases; and pelvic inflammatory disease, arthritis, proctitis, and skin lesions. Often, several such pathogens coexist in a patient. Reactive arthritis (urethritis, conjunctivitis, arthritis) may mimic gonorrhea or coexist with it.

Prevention

Prevention is based on education and mechanical or chemical prophylaxis. The condom, if properly used, can reduce the risk of infection. Effective drugs taken in therapeutic doses within 24 hours of exposure can abort an infection. Partner notification and referral of contacts for treatment has been the standard method used to control sexually transmitted diseases. Expedited treatment of sex partners by patient-delivered partner therapy is more effective than partner notification in reducing persistence and recurrence rates of gonorrhea and chlamydia. This strategy is being increasingly adopted as a means of disease control.

Treatment

Therapy typically is administered before antimicrobial susceptibilities are known. The choice of which regimen to use should be based on the national prevalences of antibiotic-resistant organisms. Nationwide, strains of gonococci that are resistant to penicillin, tetracycline, or ciprofloxacin have been increasingly observed. Consequently, these drugs can no longer be considered first-line therapy. All sexual partners should be treated and tested for HIV infection and syphilis, as should the patient.

A. Uncomplicated Gonorrhea

Due to increasing resistance of *N gonorrhoeae* to cephalosporins, the CDC has updated its treatment recommendation for gonorrhea. Treatment for gonorrhea should include a higher dose of intramuscular ceftriaxone in combination with a second drug (azithromycin or doxycycline) regardless of concern for possible secondary infection with chlamydia. For uncomplicated gonococcal infections of the cervix, urethra, and rectum, the recommended treatment is ceftriaxone (250 mg intramuscularly) plus either azithromycin (1000 mg orally as a single dose) or doxycycline (100 mg twice daily for 7 days). In cases where an oral cephalosporin is the only option, cefixime, 400 mg orally as a single dose, can be combined with azithromycin or doxycycline as above but a "test of cure" is recommended 1 week after treatment. Fluoroquinolones are no longer recommended for treatment due to high rates of microbial resistance. Spectinomycin, 1 g intramuscularly once, may be used for the penicillin-allergic patient but is not currently available in the United States.

Pharyngeal gonorrhea is also treated with ceftriaxone (250 mg intramuscularly) plus either azithromycin (1000 mg orally as a single dose) or doxycycline (100 mg twice daily for 7 days). All women should have a pregnancy test before a tetracycline (such as doxycycline) is prescribed.

B. Treatment of Other Infections

Disseminated gonococcal infection should be treated with ceftriaxone, 1 g intravenously daily, until 48 hours after improvement begins, at which time therapy may be switched to cefixime, 400 mg orally daily to complete at least 1 week of antimicrobial therapy. An oral fluoroquinolone (ciprofloxacin, 500 mg twice daily, or levofloxacin, 500 mg once daily) for 7 days also is effective, provided the isolate is susceptible. Endocarditis should be treated with ceftriaxone, 2 g every 24 hours intravenously, for at least 3 weeks. Postgonococcal urethritis and cervicitis, which are usually caused by chlamydia, are treated with a regimen of erythromycin, doxycycline, or azithromycin as described above.

Pelvic inflammatory disease requires cefoxitin, 2 g parenterally every 6 hours, or cefotetan, 2 g intravenously every 12 hours plus doxycycline 100 mg every 12 hours. Clindamycin, 900 mg intravenously every 8 hours, plus gentamicin, administered intravenously as a 2-mg/kg loading dose followed by 1.5 mg/kg every 8 hours, is also effective. Ceftriaxone 250 mg intramuscularly as a single dose (or cefoxitin, 2 g intramuscularly, plus probenecid, 1 g orally as a single dose) plus doxycycline, 100 mg twice a day for 14 days, with or without metronidazole, 500 mg twice daily for 14 days, is an effective outpatient regimen.

Centers for Disease Control and Prevention (CDC). Update to CDC's sexually transmitted diseases treatment guidelines, 2010: oral cephalosporins no longer a recommended treatment for gonococcal infections. MMWR Morb Mortal Wkly Rep. 2012 Aug 10;61(31):590–4. [PMID: 22874837]

Mayor MT et al. Diagnosis and management of gonococcal infections. Am Fam Physician. 2012 Nov 15;86(10):931–8. Erratum in: Am Fam Physician. 2013 Feb 1;87(3):163. [PMID: 23157146]

Torpy JM et al. JAMA patient page. Gonorrhea. JAMA. 2013 Jan 9; 309(2):196. [PMID: 23299613]

Workowski K. In the clinic. Chlamydia and gonorrhea. Ann Intern Med. 2013 Feb 5;158(3):ITC2-1. Erratum in: Ann Intern Med. 2013 Mar 19;158(6):504. [PMID: 23381058]

Workowski KA et al; Centers for Disease Control and Prevention (CDC). Sexually transmitted diseases treatment guidelines, 2010. MMWR Recomm Rep. 2010 Dec 17;59(RR-12):1–110. Erratum in: MMWR Recomm Rep. 2011 Jan 14;60(1):18. [PMID: 21160459]

CHANCROID

Chancroid is a sexually transmitted disease caused by the short gram-negative bacillus *Haemophilus ducreyi*. The incubation period is 3–5 days. At the site of inoculation, a vesicopustule develops that breaks down to form a painful, soft ulcer with a necrotic base, surrounding erythema, and undermined edges. There may be multiple lesions due to autoinoculation. The adenitis is usually unilateral and consists of tender, matted nodes of moderate size with overlying erythema. These may become fluctuant and rupture spontaneously. With lymph node involvement, fever, chills, and malaise may develop. Balanitis and phimosis are frequent complications in men. Women may have no external signs of infection. The diagnosis is established by culturing a swab of the lesion onto a special medium.

Chancroid must be differentiated from other genital ulcers. The chancre of syphilis is clean and painless, with a hard base. Mixed sexually transmitted disease is very common (including syphilis, herpes simplex, and HIV infection), as is infection of the ulcer with fusiforms, spirochetes, and other organisms.

A single dose of either azithromycin, 1 g orally, or ceftriaxone, 250 mg intramuscularly, is effective treatment. Effective multiple-dose regimens are erythromycin, 500 mg orally four times a day for 7 days, or ciprofloxacin, 500 mg orally twice a day for 3 days.

Kemp M et al. European guideline for the management of chancroid, 2011. Int J STD AIDS. 2011 May;22(5):241–4. [PMID: 21571970]

Roett MA et al. Diagnosis and management of genital ulcers. Am Fam Physician. 2012 Feb 1;85(3):254–62. [PMID: 22335265]

Workowski KA et al; Centers for Disease Control and Prevention (CDC). Sexually transmitted diseases treatment guidelines, 2010. MMWR Recomm Rep. 2010 Dec 17;59(RR-12):1–110. Erratum in: MMWR Recomm Rep. 2011 Jan 14;60(1):18. [PMID: 21160459]

GRANULOMA INGUINALE

Granuloma inguinale is a chronic, relapsing granulomatous anogenital infection due to *Calymmatobacterium (Donovania) granulomatis*. The pathognomonic cell, found in tissue scrapings or secretions, is large (25–90 mcm) and contains intracytoplasmic cysts filled with bodies (Donovan bodies) that stain deeply with Wright stain.

The incubation period is 8 days to 12 weeks. The onset is insidious. The lesions occur on the skin or mucous membranes of the genitalia or perineal area. They are relatively painless infiltrated nodules that soon slough. A shallow, sharply demarcated ulcer forms, with a beefy-red friable base of granulation tissue. The lesion spreads by contiguity. The advancing border has a characteristic rolled edge of granulation tissue. Large ulcerations may advance onto the lower abdomen and thighs. Scar formation and healing occur along one border while the opposite border advances.

Superinfection with spirochete-fusiform organisms is common. The ulcer then becomes purulent, painful, foul-smelling, and extremely difficult to treat.

Several therapies are available. Because of the indolent nature of the disease, duration of therapy is relatively long. The following recommended regimens should be given for 3 weeks or until all lesions have healed: doxycycline, 100 mg orally twice daily; or azithromycin, 1 g orally once weekly; or ciprofloxacin, 750 mg orally twice daily; or erythromycin, 500 mg orally four times a day.

Workowski KA et al; Centers for Disease Control and Prevention (CDC). Sexually transmitted diseases treatment guidelines, 2010. MMWR Recomm Rep. 2010 Dec 17;59(RR-12):1–110. Erratum in: MMWR Recomm Rep. 2011 Jan 14;60(1):18. [PMID: 21160459]

BARTONELLA SPECIES

Bartonella species are responsible for a wide variety of clinical syndromes. **Bacillary angiomatosis,** an important manifestation of bartonellosis, is discussed in Chapter 31. A variety of atypical infections, including retinitis, encephalitis, osteomyelitis, and persistent bacteremia and endocarditis have been described.

Trench fever is a self-limited, louse-borne relapsing febrile disease caused by *B quintana*. The disease has occurred epidemically in louse-infested troops and civilians during wars and endemically in residents of scattered geographic areas (eg, Central America). An urban equivalent of trench fever has been described among the homeless. Humans acquire infection when infected lice feces enter sites of skin breakdown. Onset of symptoms is abrupt and fever lasts 3–5 days, with relapses. The patient complains of weakness and severe pain behind the eyes and typically in the back and legs. Lymphadenopathy, splenomegaly, and a transient maculopapular rash may appear. Subclinical infection is frequent, and a carrier state is recognized. The differential diagnosis includes other febrile, self-limited states such as dengue, leptospirosis, malaria, relapsing fever, and typhus. Recovery occurs regularly even in the absence of treatment.

Cat-scratch disease is an acute infection of children and young adults caused by *Bartonella henselae*. It is transmitted from cats to humans as the result of a scratch or bite. Within a few days, a papule or ulcer will develop at the inoculation site in one-third of patients. One to 3 weeks later, fever, headache, and malaise occur. Regional lymph nodes become enlarged, often tender, and may suppurate. Lymphadenopathy from cat scratches resembles that due to neoplasm, tuberculosis, lymphogranuloma venereum, and bacterial lymphadenitis. The diagnosis is usually made clinically. Special cultures for bartonellae, serology, or excisional biopsy, though rarely necessary, confirm the diagnosis. The biopsy reveals necrotizing lymphadenitis and is itself not specific for cat-scratch disease. Cat-scratch disease is usually self-limited, requiring no specific therapy. Encephalitis occurs rarely.

Disseminated forms of the disease—bacillary angiomatosis, peliosis hepatis, and retinitis—occur most commonly in immunocompromised patients such as persons with late stages of HIV or solid organ transplant recipients. The lesions are vasculoproliferative and histopathologically distinct from those of cat-scratch disease. Unexplained fever in patients with late stages of HIV infection is not uncommonly due to bartonellosis. *B quintana*, the agent of trench fever, can also cause bacillary angiomatosis and persistent bacteremia or endocarditis (which will be "culture-negative" unless specifically sought), the latter two entities being associated with homelessness. Due to the fastidious nature of the organism and its special growth requirements, serologic testing (eg, demonstration of a high antibody titer in an indirect immunofluorescence assay) or nucleic acid amplification tests are often required to establish a diagnosis.

The disseminated forms of the disease (bacillary angiomatosis, peliosis hepatis, and retinitis) require a prolonged course of antibiotic therapy often in combination with a second agent. Bacteremia and endocarditis can be effectively treated with a 6-week course of doxycycline (200 mg orally or intravenously in two divided doses per day) plus either gentamicin 3 mg/kg/d intravenously or rifampin 600 mg/d orally in two divided doses. Relapse may occur.

Badiaga S et al. Human louse-transmitted infectious diseases. Clin Microbiol Infect. 2012 Apr;18(4):332–7. [PMID: 22360386]
Zangwill KM. Cat scratch disease and other *Bartonella* infections. Adv Exp Med Biol. 2013;764:159–66. [PMID: 23654065]

ANAEROBIC INFECTIONS

Anaerobic bacteria comprise the majority of normal human flora. Normal microbial flora of the mouth (anaerobic spirochetes, *Prevotella,* fusobacteria), the skin (anaerobic diphtheroids), the large bowel (bacteroides, anaerobic streptococci, clostridia), and the female genitourinary tract (bacteroides, anaerobic streptococci, fusobacteria) produce disease when displaced from their normal sites into tissues or closed body spaces.

Anaerobic infections tend to be polymicrobial and abscesses are common. Pus and infected tissue often are malodorous. Septic thrombophlebitis and metastatic infection are frequent and may require incision and drainage. Diminished blood supply that favors proliferation of anaerobes because of reduced tissue oxygenation may interfere with the delivery of antimicrobials to the site of anaerobic infection. Cultures, unless carefully collected under anaerobic conditions, may yield negative results.

Important types of infections that are most commonly caused by anaerobic organisms are listed below. Treatment of all these infections consists of surgical exploration and judicious excision in conjunction with administration of antimicrobial drugs.

1. Head & Neck Infections

Prevotella melaninogenica (formerly *Bacteroides melaninogenicus*) and anaerobic spirochetes are commonly involved in periodontal infections. These organisms, fusobacteria, and peptostreptococci may cause chronic sinusitis, peritonsillar abscess, chronic otitis media, and mastoiditis. *F necrophorum* has been recognized as a common cause of pharyngitis in adolescents and young adults. *F necrophorum* infection has been associated with septic internal jugular thrombophlebitis (Lemierre syndrome) and causes septic pulmonary embolization. Hygiene, drainage, and surgical debridement are as important in treatment as antimicrobials. Oral anaerobic organisms have been uniformly susceptible to penicillin, but there has been a recent trend of increasing penicillin resistance, usually due to beta-lactamase production. Therefore, ampicillin/sulbactam 1.5-3 g intravenously every 6 hours (if parenteral therapy is required) or amoxicillin/clavulanic acid 875/125 mg orally twice daily, or clindamycin can be used (600 mg intravenously every 8 hours or 300 mg orally every 6 hours). Antimicrobial treatment is continued for a few days after symptoms and signs of infection have resolved. Indolent, established infections (eg, mastoiditis or osteomyelitis) may require prolonged courses of therapy, eg, 4–6 weeks or longer.

Brook I. Anaerobic bacteria in upper respiratory tract and head and neck infections: microbiology and treatment. Anaerobe. 2012 Apr;18(2):214–20. [PMID: 22197951]
Brook I. Antimicrobial treatment of anaerobic infections. Expert Opin Pharmacother. 2011 Aug;12(11):1691–707. [PMID: 21506900]

2. Chest Infections

Usually in the setting of poor oral hygiene and periodontal disease, aspiration of saliva (which contains 10^8 anaerobic organisms per milliliter in addition to aerobes) may lead to necrotizing pneumonia, lung abscess, and empyema. Polymicrobial infection is the rule and anaerobes—particularly *P melaninogenica*, fusobacteria, and peptostreptococci—are common etiologic agents. Most pulmonary infections respond to antimicrobial therapy alone. Percutaneous chest tube or surgical drainage is indicated for empyema.

Penicillin-resistant *Bacteroides fragilis* and *P melaninogenica* are commonly isolated and have been associated with clinical failures. Clindamycin, 600 mg intravenously once, followed by 300 mg orally every 6–8 hours, is the treatment of choice for these infections. Metronidazole does not cover facultative streptococci, which often are present, and if used, a second agent that is active against streptococci, such as ceftriaxone 1 g intravenously or intramuscularly daily, should be added. Penicillin, 2 million units intravenously every 4 hours, followed by amoxicillin, 500 mg every 8 hours orally, is an alternative; however, increasing prevalence of beta-lactamase producing organisms is a concern. Moxifloxacin, 400 mg orally or intravenously once daily, may be used. Because these infections respond slowly, a prolonged course of therapy (eg, 4–6 weeks) is generally recommended.

Bartlett JG. Anaerobic bacterial infection of the lung. Anaerobe. 2012 Apr;18(2):235–9. [PMID: 22209937]

3. Central Nervous System

Anaerobes are a common cause of brain abscess, subdural empyema, or septic central nervous system thrombophlebitis. The organisms reach the central nervous system by direct extension from sinusitis, otitis, or mastoiditis or by hematogenous spread from chronic lung infections. Antimicrobial therapy—eg, ceftriaxone, 2 g intravenously every 12 hours, plus metronidazole, 500 mg intravenously every 8 hours—is an important adjunct to surgical drainage. Duration of therapy is 6–8 weeks but should be based on follow-up imaging. Some small multiple brain abscesses can be treated with antibiotics alone without surgical drainage.

4. Intra-abdominal Infections

In the colon there are up to 10^{11} anaerobes per gram of content—predominantly *B fragilis*, clostridia, and peptostreptococci. These organisms play a central role in most intra-abdominal abscesses following trauma to the colon, diverticulitis, appendicitis, or perirectal abscess and may also participate in hepatic abscess and cholecystitis, often in association with aerobic coliform bacteria. The bacteriology includes anaerobes as well as enteric gram-negative rods and on occasion enterococci. Therapy should be directed both against anaerobes and gram-negative aerobes. Agents that are active against *B fragilis* include metronidazole, chloramphenicol, moxifloxacin, tigecycline, ertapenem, imipenem, doripenem, ampicillin-sulbactam, ticarcillin-clavulanic acid, and piperacillin-tazobactam. Resistance to cefoxitin, cefotetan, and clindamycin is increasingly encountered. Most third-generation cephalosporins have poor efficacy.

Table 33–7 summarizes the antibiotic regimens for management of moderate to moderately severe infections (eg, patient hemodynamically stable, good surgical drainage possible or established, low APACHE score, no multiple organ failure) and severe infections (eg, major peritoneal soilage, large or multiple abscesses, patient hemodynamically unstable), particularly if drug-resistant organisms are suspected. An effective oral regimen for patients able to take it is presented also.

Brand M et al. Prophylactic antibiotics for penetrating abdominal trauma. Cochrane Database Syst Rev. 2013 Nov 18;11: CD007370. [PMID: 24249389]
Solomkin JS et al. Diagnosis and management of complicated intra-abdominal infection in adults and children: guidelines by the Surgical Infection Society and the Infectious Diseases Society of America. Clin Infect Dis. 2010 Jan 15;50(2):133–64. [PMID: 20034345]

5. Female Genital Tract & Pelvic Infections

The normal flora of the vagina and cervix includes several species of bacteroides, peptostreptococci, group B streptococci, lactobacilli, coliform bacteria, and, occasionally, spirochetes and clostridia. These organisms commonly cause genital tract infections and may disseminate from there.

Table 33–7. Treatment of anaerobic intra-abdominal infections.

Community-onset
  Oral therapy
    Moxifloxacin 400 mg every 24 hours
  Intravenous therapy
    Moderate to moderately severe infections:
      Ertapenem 1 g every 24 hours
                              or—
      Ceftriaxone 1 g every 24 hours (or ciprofloxacin 400 mg
        every 12 hours, if penicillin allergic) plus metronidazole
        500 mg every 8 hours
                              or—
      Tigecycline 100 mg once followed by 50 mg every 12 hours
                              or—
      Moxifloxacin 400 mg every 24 hours
    Severe infections:
      Imipenem, 0.5 g every 6–8 hours or meropenem 1 g every
        8 hours or doripenem 0.5 g every 8 hours or piperacillin/
        tazobactam 3.75 g every 6 hours
Health-care–associated
  Intravenous therapy
    Imipenem, 0.5 g every 6–8 hours or meropenem 1 g every
      8 hours or doripenem 0.5 g every 8 hours or piperacillin/
      tazobactam 4.5 g every 6 hours
                            or—
    Ceftazidime or cefepime 2 g every 8 hours plus metronidazole
      0.5 g every 8 hours

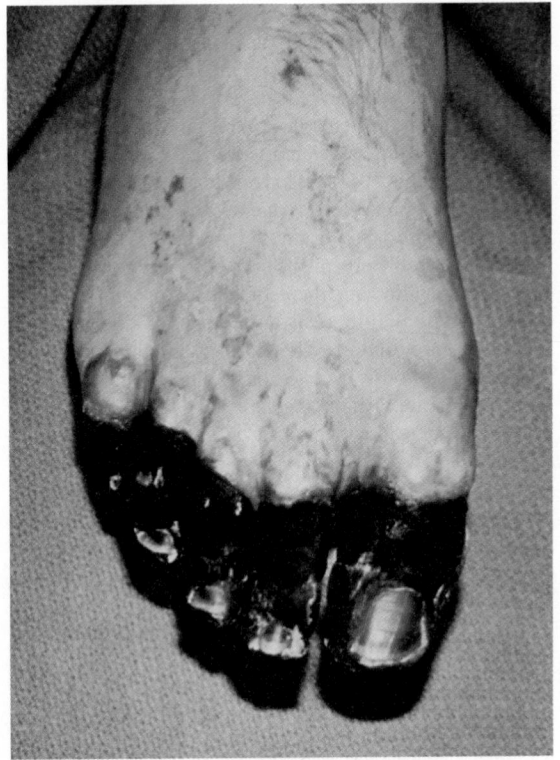

▲ **Figure 33–5.** Gangrene of the right foot causing necrosis of the toes. (From William Archibald, Public Health Image Library, CDC.)

While salpingitis is often caused by gonococci and chlamydiae, tubo-ovarian and pelvic abscesses are associated with anaerobes in most cases. Postpartum infections may be caused by aerobic streptococci or staphylococci, but anaerobes are often found, and the worst cases of postpartum or postabortion sepsis are associated with clostridia and bacteroides. These have a high mortality rate, and treatment requires both antimicrobials directed against anaerobes and coliforms (see above) and abscess drainage or early hysterectomy.

Lapinsky SE. Obstetric infections. Crit Care Clin. 2013 Jul; 29(3):509–20. [PMID: 23830651]
Sweet RL. Treatment of acute pelvic inflammatory disease. Infect Dis Obstet Gynecol. 2011;2011:561909. [PMID: 22228985]

6. Bacteremia & Endocarditis

Anaerobic bacteremia usually originates from the gastrointestinal tract, the oropharynx, decubitus ulcers, or the female genital tract. Endocarditis due to anaerobic and microaerophilic streptococci and bacteroides originates from the same sites. Most cases of anaerobic or microaerophilic streptococcal endocarditis can be effectively treated with 12–20 million units of penicillin G daily for 4–6 weeks, but optimal therapy of other types of anaerobic bacterial endocarditis must rely on laboratory guidance. Propionibacteria, clostridia, and bacteroides occasionally cause endocarditis.

7. Skin & Soft Tissue Infections

Anaerobic infections in the skin and soft tissue usually follow trauma, inadequate blood supply, or surgery and are most common in areas that are contaminated by oral or fecal flora. These infections also occur in injection drug users and persons sustaining animal to human bites. There may be progressive tissue necrosis (Figure 33–5) and a putrid odor.

Several terms, such as bacterial synergistic gangrene, synergistic necrotizing cellulitis, necrotizing fasciitis, and non-clostridial crepitant cellulitis, have been used to classify these infections. Although there are some differences in microbiology among them, their differentiation on clinical grounds alone is difficult. All are mixed infections caused by aerobic and anaerobic organisms and require aggressive surgical debridement of necrotic tissue for cure. Surgical consultation is obligatory to assist in diagnosis and treatment.

Broad-spectrum antibiotics active against both anaerobes and gram-positive and gram-negative aerobes (eg, vancomycin plus piperacillin-tazobactam) should be instituted empirically and modified by culture results (see Table 30–5). They are given for about a week after progressive tissue destruction has been controlled and the margins of the wound remain free of inflammation.

Kaafarani HM et al. Necrotizing skin and soft tissue infections. Surg Clin North Am. 2014 Feb;94(1):155–63. [PMID: 24267503]

ACTINOMYCOSIS

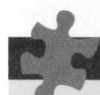

ESSENTIALS OF DIAGNOSIS

▶ History of recent dental infection or abdominal trauma.

▶ Chronic pneumonia or indolent intra-abdominal or cervicofacial abscess.

▶ Sinus tract formation.

General Considerations

Actinomyces israelii and other species of *Actinomyces* occur in the normal flora of the mouth and tonsillar crypts. They are anaerobic, gram-positive, branching filamentous bacteria (1 mcm in diameter) that may fragment into bacillary forms. When introduced into traumatized tissue and associated with other anaerobic bacteria, these actinomycetes become pathogens.

The most common site of infection is the cervicofacial area (about 60% of cases). Infection typically follows extraction of a tooth or other trauma. Lesions may develop in the gastrointestinal tract or lungs following ingestion or aspiration of the organism from its endogenous source in the mouth. Interestingly, *T whippelii*, the causative agent of Whipple disease, is an actinomycete and therefore is related to the species that cause actinomycosis.

Clinical Findings

A. Symptoms and Signs

1. Cervicofacial actinomycosis—Cervicofacial actinomycosis develops slowly. The area becomes markedly indurated, and the overlying skin becomes reddish or cyanotic. Abscesses eventually draining to the surface persist for long periods. "Sulfur granules"—masses of filamentous organisms—may be found in the pus. There is usually little pain unless there is secondary infection. Trismus indicates that the muscles of mastication are involved. Radiography may reveal bony involvement.

2. Thoracic actinomycosis—Thoracic involvement begins with fever, cough, and sputum production with night sweats and weight loss. Pleuritic pain may be present. Multiple sinuses may extend through the chest wall, to the heart, or into the abdominal cavity. Ribs may be involved. Radiography shows areas of consolidation and in many cases pleural effusion. Cervicofacial or thoracic disease may occasionally involve the central nervous system, most commonly brain abscess or meningitis.

3. Abdominal actinomycosis—Abdominal actinomycosis usually causes pain in the ileocecal region, spiking fever and chills, vomiting, and weight loss; it may be confused with Crohn disease. Irregular abdominal masses may be palpated. Pelvic inflammatory disease caused by actinomycetes has been associated with prolonged use of an intrauterine contraceptive device. Sinuses draining to the

exterior may develop. CT scanning reveals an inflammatory mass extended to involve bone.

B. Laboratory Findings

The anaerobic, gram-positive organism may be demonstrated as a granule or as scattered branching gram-positive filaments in the pus. Anaerobic culture is necessary to distinguish actinomycetes from nocardiae because specific therapy differs for the two infections.

Treatment

Penicillin G is the drug of choice. Ten to 20 million units are given via a parenteral route for 4–6 weeks, followed by oral penicillin V, 500 mg four times daily. Alternatives include ampicillin, 12 g/d intravenously for 4–6 weeks followed by oral amoxicillin 500 mg three times daily or doxycycline 100 mg twice daily intravenously or orally. Response to therapy is slow. Therapy should be continued for weeks to months after clinical manifestations have disappeared in order to ensure cure. Surgical procedures such as drainage and resection may be beneficial.

With penicillin and surgery, the prognosis is good. The difficulties of diagnosis, however, may permit extensive destruction of tissue before the diagnosis is identified and therapy is started.

Sasaki Y et al. Actinomycosis in the mandible: CT and MR findings. AJNR Am J Neuroradiol. 2014 Feb;35(2):390–4. [PMID: 23928143]

Wong VK et al. Actinomycosis. BMJ. 2011 Oct 11;343:d6099. [PMID: 21990282]

NOCARDIOSIS

Nocardia species are aerobic filamentous soil bacteria that can cause pulmonary and systemic nocardiosis. Common *Nocardia* species include members of the *Nocardia asteroides* complex and *Nocardia brasiliensis*. Bronchopulmonary abnormalities (eg, alveolar proteinosis) predispose to colonization, but infection is unusual unless the patient is also receiving systemic corticosteroids or is otherwise immunosuppressed.

Clinical Findings

Pulmonary involvement usually begins with malaise, loss of weight, fever, and night sweats. Cough and production of purulent sputum are the chief complaints. Radiography may show infiltrates accompanied by pleural effusion. The lesions may penetrate to the exterior through the chest wall, invading the ribs.

Dissemination involves any organ. Brain abscesses and subcutaneous nodules are most frequent. Even in the absence of clinical symptoms and signs of central nervous system infection, clinicians should consider brain imaging in patients with nocardiosis to rule out an occult abscess.

Nocardia species are usually found as delicate, branching, gram-positive filaments. They may be weakly acidfast, occasionally causing diagnostic confusion with tuberculosis. Identification is made by culture.

▶ Treatment

For isolated cutaneous infections, therapy is initiated with trimethoprim-sulfamethoxazole administered at a dosage of 5–10 mg/kg/d (based on trimethoprim) as an oral or intravenous formulation. Surgical procedures such as drainage and resection may be needed as adjunctive therapy. A higher dose of 15 mg/kg/d (based on trimethoprim) should be used for disseminated or pulmonary infections. Resistance to trimethoprim-sulfamethoxazole may be increasing and initiating treatment with two drugs while awaiting antibiotic susceptibilities in cases of disseminated or severe localized disease should be considered. Alternative agents or drugs that can be given in combination with trimethoprim-sulfamethoxazole include imipenem, 500 mg intravenously every 6 hours; amikacin, 7.5 mg/kg intravenously every 12 hours; or minocycline, 100–200 mg orally or intravenously twice daily. Consultation with an infectious diseases expert should be considered.

Response may be slow, and therapy should be continued for at least 6 months. The prognosis in systemic nocardiosis is poor when diagnosis and therapy are delayed.

Anagnostou T et al. Nocardiosis of the central nervous system: experience from a general hospital and review of 84 cases from the literature. Medicine (Baltimore). 2014 Jan; 93(1):19–32. [PMID: 24378740]

Lalitha P et al. Nocardia keratitis: clinical course and effect of corticosteroids. Am J Ophthalmol. 2012 Dec;154(6):934–9.e1. [PMID: 22959881]

Wilson JW. Nocardiosis: updates and clinical overview. Mayo Clin Proc. 2012 Apr;87(4):403–7. [PMID: 22469352]

▼ INFECTIONS CAUSED BY MYCOBACTERIA

NONTUBERCULOUS MYCOBACTERIAL DISEASES

About 10% of mycobacterial infections are caused by nontuberculous mycobacteria. Nontuberculous mycobacterial infections are among the most common opportunistic infections in advanced HIV disease. These organisms have distinctive laboratory characteristics, occur ubiquitously in the environment, are not communicable from person to person, and are often resistant to standard antituberculous drugs.

Nahid P et al. Update in tuberculosis and nontuberculous mycobacterial disease 2011. Am J Respir Crit Care Med. 2012 Jun 15; 185(12):1266–70. [PMID: 22707733]

1. Pulmonary Infections

Mycobacterium avium complex (MAC) causes a chronic, slowly progressive pulmonary infection resembling tuberculosis in immunocompetent patients, who typically have underlying pulmonary disease. Susceptibility testing for macrolide-resistance should be performed on clinical isolates. Treatment of nodular or bronchiectatic pulmonary disease is clarithromycin (1000 mg orally three times per week) or azithromycin (500 mg orally three times per week) plus rifampin (600 mg orally three times per week) or rifabutin (300 mg orally three times per week) plus ethambutol (25 mg/kg orally three times per week). Patients with fibrocavitary lung disease or severe nodular or bronchiectatic disease should receive three-drug therapy with clarithromycin (500–1000 mg orally daily) or azithromycin (250 orally mg daily) plus rifampin (600 mg orally daily) or rifabutin (300 mg orally daily) plus ethambutol (15 mg/kg orally daily). Therapy is continued for at least 12 months after sterilization of cultures.

M kansasii can produce clinical disease resembling tuberculosis, but the illness progresses more slowly. Most such infections occur in patients with preexisting lung disease, though 40% of patients have no known pulmonary disease. Microbiologically, *M kansasii* is similar to *M tuberculosis* and is sensitive to the same drugs except pyrazinamide, to which it is resistant. Therapy with isoniazid, ethambutol, and rifampin for 2 years (or 1 year after sputum conversion) has been successful.

Less common causes of pulmonary disease include *M xenopi*, *M szulgai*, and *M gordonae*. These organisms have variable sensitivities, and treatment is based on results of sensitivity tests. The rapid growing mycobacteria, *M abscessus*, *M chelonae*, and *M fortuitum* also can cause pneumonia in the occasional patient.

Griffith DE et al. Therapy of refractory nontuberculous mycobacterial lung disease. Curr Opin Infect Dis. 2012 Apr;25 (2):218–27. [PMID: 22327466]

2. Lymphadenitis

Most cases of lymphadenitis (scrofula) in adults are caused by *M tuberculosis* and can be a manifestation of disseminated disease. In children, the majority of cases are due to nontuberculous mycobacterial species, with MAC being the most common followed by *M scrofulaceum* in the United States and *M malmoense* and *M haemophilum* in Northern Europe. *M kansasii*, *M bovis*, *M chelonae*, and *M fortuitum* are less commonly observed. Unlike disease caused by *M tuberculosis*, which requires systemic therapy for 6 months, infection with nontuberculous mycobacteria can be successfully treated by surgical excision without antituberculous therapy.

3. Skin & Soft Tissue Infections

Skin and soft tissue infections such as abscesses, septic arthritis, and osteomyelitis can result from direct inoculation or hematogenous dissemination or may occur as a complication of surgery.

M abscessus, *M chelonae*, and *M fortuitum* are frequent causes of these types of infections. Most cases occur in the extremities and initially present as nodules. Ulceration with abscess formation often follows. The organisms are resistant to the usual antituberculosis drugs and may have susceptibility to clarithromycin, azithromycin, doxycycline, amikacin, cefoxitin, sulfonamides, imipenem, and ciprofloxacin. Given the multidrug resistant nature of these organisms, obtaining antibiotic susceptibility testing is recommended. Therapy often includes surgical debridement along with at least two active antibiotics. Antibiotic therapy is usually continued for 3 months, although this must be determined based on clinical response.

M marinum infection ("swimming pool granuloma") presents as a nodular skin lesion following exposure to nonchlorinated water. The lesions respond to therapy with clarithromycin, doxycycline, minocycline, or trimethoprim-sulfamethoxazole.

M ulcerans infection (Buruli ulcer) is seen mainly in Africa and Australia and produces a large ulcerative lesion. Therapy consists of surgical excision and skin grafting.

4. Disseminated *Mycobacterium avium* Infection

MAC causes disseminated disease in immunocompromised patients, most commonly in patients in the late stages of HIV infection, when the CD4 cell count is < 50/mcL. Persistent fever and weight loss are the most common symptoms. The organism can usually be cultured from multiple sites, including blood, liver, lymph node, or bone marrow. Blood culture is the preferred means of establishing the diagnosis and has a sensitivity of 98%.

▶ Treatment

Agents with proved activity against MAC are rifabutin, azithromycin, clarithromycin, and ethambutol. Amikacin and ciprofloxacin work in vitro, but clinical results are inconsistent. A combination of two or more active agents should be used to prevent rapid emergence of secondary resistance. Clarithromycin, 500 mg orally twice daily, plus ethambutol, 15 mg/kg/d orally as a single dose, with or without rifabutin, 300 mg/d orally, is the treatment of choice. Azithromycin, 500 mg orally once daily, may be used instead of clarithromycin. Insufficient data are available to permit specific recommendations about second-line regimens for patients intolerant of macrolides or those with macrolide-resistant organisms. MAC therapy may be discontinued in patients who have been treated with 12 months of therapy for disseminated MAC, who have no evidence of active disease, and whose CD4 counts exceed 100 cells/mcL for 6 months while receiving highly active antiretroviral therapy (HAART).

▶ Prevention

Antimicrobial prophylaxis of MAC prevents disseminated disease and prolongs survival. It is the standard of care to offer it to all HIV-infected patients with CD4 counts ≤ 50/mcL. In contrast to active infection, single-drug oral regimens of clarithromycin, 500 mg twice daily, azithromycin, 1200 mg once weekly, or rifabutin, 300 mg once daily, are appropriate. Clarithromycin or azithromycin is more effective and better tolerated than rifabutin, and therefore preferred. Primary prophylaxis for MAC infection can be stopped in patients who have responded to antiretroviral combination therapy with elevation of CD4 counts > 100 cells/mcL for 3 months.

Griffith DE et al; ATS Mycobacterial Diseases Subcommittee; American Thoracic Society; Infectious Disease Society of America. An official ATS/IDSA statement: diagnosis, treatment, and prevention of nontuberculous mycobacterial diseases. Am J Respir Crit Care Med. 2007 Feb 15;175(4):367–416. [PMID: 17277290]

Kaplan JE et al. Guidelines for prevention and treatment of opportunistic infections in HIV-infected adults and adolescents: recommendations from CDC, the National Institutes of Health, and the HIV Medicine Association of the Infectious Diseases Society of America. MMWR Recomm Rep. 2009 Apr 10;58(RR-4):1–207. [PMID: 19357635]

MYCOBACTERIUM TUBERCULOSIS INFECTIONS

Tuberculosis is discussed in Chapter 9. Further information and expert consultation can be obtained from the Francis J. Curry International Tuberculosis Center at the Web site http://www.currytbcenter.ucsf.edu or, by phone, 415-502-4600, or fax, 415-502-4620.

TUBERCULOUS MENINGITIS

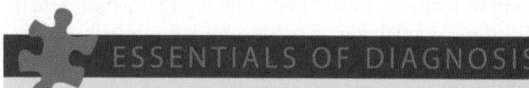

ESSENTIALS OF DIAGNOSIS

- ▶ Gradual onset of listlessness, irritability, and anorexia.
- ▶ Headache, vomiting, and seizures common.
- ▶ Cranial nerve abnormalities typical.
- ▶ Tuberculosis focus may be evident elsewhere.
- ▶ Cerebrospinal fluid shows several hundred lymphocytes, low glucose, and high protein.

▶ General Considerations

Tuberculous meningitis is caused by rupture of a meningeal tuberculoma resulting from earlier hematogenous seeding of tubercle bacilli from a pulmonary focus, or it may be a consequence of miliary spread.

▶ Clinical Findings

A. Symptoms and Signs

The onset is usually gradual, with listlessness, irritability, anorexia, and fever, followed by headache, vomiting, convulsions, and coma. In older patients, headache and behavioral changes are prominent early symptoms. Nuchal rigidity and cranial nerve palsies occur as the meningitis progresses. Evidence of active tuberculosis elsewhere or a history of prior tuberculosis is present in up to 75% of patients.

B. Laboratory Findings

The spinal fluid is frequently yellowish, with increased pressure, 100–500 cells/mcL (predominantly lymphocytes, though neutrophils may be present early during infection), increased protein, and decreased glucose. Acid-fast stains of cerebrospinal fluid usually are negative, and cultures also may be negative in 15–25% of cases. Nucleic acid amplification tests for rapid diagnosis of tuberculosis have variable sensitivity and specificity and none are FDA-approved for use in meningitis. Chest radiographs often reveal abnormalities compatible with tuberculosis but may be normal.

▶ Differential Diagnosis

Tuberculous meningitis may be confused with any other type of meningitis, but the gradual onset, the predominantly lymphocytic pleocytosis of the spinal fluid, and evidence of tuberculosis elsewhere often point to the diagnosis. The tuberculin skin test is usually (not always) positive. Fungal and other granulomatous meningitides, syphilis, and carcinomatous meningitis are in the differential diagnosis.

▶ Complications

Complications of tuberculous meningitis include seizure disorders, cranial nerve palsies, stroke, and obstructive hydrocephalus with impaired cognitive function. These result from inflammatory exudate primarily involving the basilar meninges and arteries.

▶ Treatment

Presumptive diagnosis followed by early, empiric antituberculous therapy is essential for survival and to minimize sequelae. Even if cultures are not positive, a full course of therapy is warranted if the clinical setting is suggestive of tuberculous meningitis.

Regimens that are effective for pulmonary tuberculosis are effective also for tuberculous meningitis (see Table 9–15). Rifampin, isoniazid, and pyrazinamide all penetrate into cerebrospinal fluid well. The penetration of ethambutol is more variable, but therapeutic concentrations can be achieved, and the drug has been successfully used for meningitis. Aminoglycosides penetrate less well. Regimens that do not include both isoniazid and rifampin may be effective but are less reliable and generally must be given for longer periods.

Many authorities recommend the addition of corticosteroids for patients with focal deficits or altered mental status. Dexamethasone, 0.15 mg/kg intravenously or orally four times daily for 1–2 weeks, then discontinued in a tapering regimen over 4 weeks, may be used.

Thwaites GE. Advances in the diagnosis and treatment of tuberculous meningitis. Curr Opin Neurol. 2013 Jun;26(3):295–300. [PMID: 23493162]
Thwaites GE et al. Tuberculous meningitis: more questions, still too few answers. Lancet Neurol. 2013 Oct;12(10):999–1010. [PMID: 23972913]

LEPROSY (HANSEN DISEASE)

ESSENTIALS OF DIAGNOSIS

▶ Pale, anesthetic macular—or nodular and erythematous—skin lesions.

▶ Superficial nerve thickening with associated anesthesia.

▶ History of residence in endemic area in childhood.

▶ Acid-fast bacilli in skin lesions or nasal scrapings, or characteristic histologic nerve changes.

▶ General Considerations

Leprosy (Hansen disease) is a chronic infectious disease caused by the acid-fast rod *M leprae*. The mode of transmission probably is respiratory and involves prolonged exposure in childhood. The disease is endemic in tropical and subtropical Asia, Africa, Central and South America, and the Pacific regions, and rarely seen sporadically in the southern United States.

▶ Clinical Findings

A. Symptoms and Signs

The onset is insidious. The lesions involve the cooler body tissues: skin, superficial nerves, nose, pharynx, larynx, eyes, and testicles. Skin lesions may occur as pale, anesthetic macular lesions 1–10 cm in diameter; discrete erythematous, infiltrated nodules 1–5 cm in diameter; or diffuse skin infiltration. Neurologic disturbances are caused by nerve infiltration and thickening, with resultant anesthesia, and motor abnormalities. Bilateral ulnar neuropathy is highly suggestive. In untreated cases, disfigurement due to the skin infiltration and nerve involvement may be extreme, leading to trophic ulcers, bone resorption, and loss of digits.

The disease is divided clinically and by laboratory tests into two distinct types: lepromatous and tuberculoid. The **lepromatous** type (also referred to as multibacillary leprosy) occurs in persons with defective cellular immunity. The course is progressive and malignant, with nodular skin lesions; slow, symmetric nerve involvement; abundant acid-fast bacilli in the skin lesions; and a negative lepromin skin test. In the **tuberculoid** type (paucibacillary leprosy), cellular immunity is intact and the course is more benign and less progressive, with macular skin lesions, severe asymmetric nerve involvement of sudden onset with few bacilli present in the lesions, and a positive lepromin skin test. Intermediate ("borderline") cases are frequent. Eye involvement (keratitis and iridocyclitis), nasal ulcers, epistaxis, anemia, and lymphadenopathy may occur.

B. Laboratory Findings

Laboratory confirmation of leprosy requires the demonstration of acid-fast bacilli in a skin biopsy. Biopsy of skin or of a thickened involved nerve also gives a typical histologic picture. *M leprae* does not grow in artificial media but does grow in the foot pads of armadillos.

Differential Diagnosis

The skin lesions of leprosy often resemble those of lupus erythematosus, sarcoidosis, syphilis, erythema nodosum, erythema multiforme, cutaneous tuberculosis, and vitiligo.

Complications

Kidney failure and hepatomegaly from secondary amyloidosis may occur with long-standing disease.

Treatment

Combination therapy is recommended for treatment of all types of leprosy. Single-drug treatment is accompanied by emergence of resistance, and primary resistance to dapsone also occurs. For borderline and lepromatous cases (ie, multibacillary disease), the World Health Organization recommends a triple oral drug-regimen of rifampin, 600 mg once a month; dapsone, 100 mg daily; and clofazimine, 300 mg once a month and 50 mg daily for 12 months although longer courses may be needed for patients with high burden of disease. For indeterminate and tuberculoid leprosy (paucibacillary disease), the recommendation is rifampin, 600 mg once a month, plus dapsone, 100 mg daily for 6 months.

Two reactional states—erythema nodosum leprosum and reversal reactions—may occur as a consequence of therapy. The reversal reaction, typical of borderline lepromatous leprosy, probably results from enhanced host immunity. Skin lesions and nerves become swollen and tender, but systemic manifestations are not seen. Erythema nodosum leprosum, typical of lepromatous leprosy, is a consequence of immune injury from antigen-antibody complex deposition in skin and other tissues; in addition to skin and nerve manifestations, fever and systemic involvement may be seen. Prednisone, 60 mg/d orally, or thalidomide, 300 mg/d orally (in the nonpregnant patient only), is effective for erythema nodosum leprosum. Improvement is expected within a few days after initiating prednisone, and thereafter the dose may be tapered over several weeks to avoid recurrence. Thalidomide is also tapered over several weeks to a 100-mg bedtime dose. Erythema nodosum leprosum is usually confined to the first year of therapy, and prednisone or thalidomide can be discontinued. Thalidomide is ineffective for reversal reactions, and prednisone, 60 mg/d, is indicated. Reversal reactions tend to recur, and the dose of prednisone should be slowly tapered over weeks to months. Therapy for leprosy should not be discontinued during treatment of reactional states.

Legendre DP et al. Hansen's disease (leprosy): current and future pharmacotherapy and treatment of disease-related immunologic reactions. Pharmacotherapy. 2012 Jan;32(1):27–37. [PMID: 22392826]

INFECTIONS CAUSED BY CHLAMYDIAE

Chlamydiaceae is a family of obligate intracellular parasites closely related to gram-negative bacteria. They include two important genera of human pathogens—*Chlamydia*, which includes the species of *Chlamydia trachomatis,* and *Chlamydophila,* which includes the species *Chlamydophila psittaci* (formerly known as *Chlamydia psittaci*) and *Chlamydophila pneumoniae* (formerly known as *Chlamydia pneumoniae*). The differentiation of genera is based on differences in intracellular inclusions, sulfonamide susceptibility, antigenic composition, and disease production. *C trachomatis* causes many different human infections involving the eye (trachoma, inclusion conjunctivitis), the genital tract (lymphogranuloma venereum, nongonococcal urethritis, cervicitis, salpingitis), or the respiratory tract in infants (pneumonitis). *C psittaci* causes psittacosis and *C pneumoniae* is a cause of respiratory tract infections.

CHLAMYDIA TRACHOMATIS INFECTIONS

1. Lymphogranuloma Venereum

ESSENTIALS OF DIAGNOSIS

► Evanescent primary genital lesion.
► Lymph node enlargement, softening, and suppuration, with draining sinuses.
► Proctitis and rectal stricture in women or in men who have sex with men.
► Positive complement fixation test.

General Considerations

Lymphogranuloma venereum (LGV) is an acute and chronic sexually transmitted disease caused by *C trachomatis* types L1–L3. The disease is acquired during intercourse or through contact with contaminated exudate from active lesions. The incubation period is 5–21 days. After the genital lesion disappears, the infection spreads to lymph channels and lymph nodes of the genital and rectal areas. Inapparent infections and latent disease are not uncommon.

Clinical Findings

A. Symptoms and Signs

In men, the initial vesicular or ulcerative lesion (on the external genitalia) is evanescent and often goes unnoticed. Inguinal buboes appear 1–4 weeks after exposure, are often bilateral, and have a tendency to fuse, soften, and break down to form multiple draining sinuses, with extensive scarring. In women, the genital lymph drainage is to the perirectal glands. Early anorectal manifestations are proctitis with tenesmus and bloody purulent discharge; late manifestations are chronic cicatrizing inflammation of the rectal and perirectal tissue. These changes lead to obstipation and rectal stricture and, occasionally, recto-vaginal and perianal fistulas. They are also seen in homosexual men.

B. Laboratory Findings

The complement fixation test may be positive (titers > 1:64), but cross-reaction with other chlamydiae occurs. Although a positive reaction may reflect remote infection, high titers usually indicate active disease. Nucleic acid detection tests are sensitive, but not FDA-approved for rectal specimens and cannot differentiate LGV from non-LGV strains.

▶ Differential Diagnosis

The early lesion of LGV must be differentiated from the lesions of syphilis, genital herpes, and chancroid; lymph node involvement must be distinguished from that due to tularemia, tuberculosis, plague, neoplasm, or pyogenic infection; and rectal stricture must be distinguished from that due to neoplasm and ulcerative colitis.

▶ Treatment

If diagnostic testing for LGV is not available, patients with a clinical presentation suggestive of LGV should be treated empirically. The antibiotic of choice is doxycycline (contraindicated in pregnancy), 100 mg orally twice daily for 21 days. Erythromycin, 500 mg orally four times a day for 21 days, is also effective. Azithromycin, 1 g orally once weekly for 3 weeks, may also be effective.

Roett MA et al. Diagnosis and management of genital ulcers. Am Fam Physician. 2012 Feb 1;85(3):254–62. [PMID: 22335265]
Workowski KA et al; Centers for Disease Control and Prevention (CDC). Sexually transmitted diseases treatment guidelines, 2010. MMWR Recomm Rep. 2010 Dec 17;59(RR-12):1–110. Erratum in: MMWR Recomm Rep. 2011 Jan 14;60(1):18. [PMID: 21160459]

2. Chlamydial Urethritis & Cervicitis

ESSENTIALS OF DIAGNOSIS

- ▶ *Chlamydia trachomatis* is a common cause of urethritis, cervicitis, and post-gonococcal urethritis.
- ▶ Diagnosis made by nucleic acid amplification of urine or swab specimen.

▶ General Considerations

C trachomatis immunotypes D–K are isolated in about 50% of cases of nongonococcal urethritis and cervicitis. In other cases, *Ureaplasma urealyticum* or *Mycoplasma genitalium* can be grown as a possible etiologic agent. *C trachomatis* is an important cause of postgonococcal urethritis. Coinfection with gonococci and chlamydiae is common, and post-gonococcal (ie, chlamydial) urethritis may persist after successful treatment of the gonococcal component. Occasionally, epididymitis, prostatitis, or proctitis is caused by chlamydial infection. Chlamydiae are a leading cause of infertility in females in the United States.

▶ Clinical Findings

A. Symptoms and Signs

Females infected with chlamydiae may be asymptomatic or may have symptoms and signs of cervicitis, salpingitis, or pelvic inflammatory disease. The urethral or cervical discharge due to *C trachomatis* tends to be less painful, less purulent, and watery compared with gonococcal infection.

B. Laboratory Findings

A patient with urethritis or cervicitis and absence of gram-negative diplococci on Gram stain and of *N gonorrhoeae* on culture is assumed to have chlamydial infection until proven otherwise. The diagnosis should be confirmed, whenever possible, by the FDA-approved, highly sensitive nucleic acid amplification tests for use with urine or vaginal swabs. A negative nucleic acid amplification test for chlamydia reliably excludes the diagnosis of chlamydial urethritis or cervicitis and therapy need not be administered.

C. Screening

Active screening for chlamydial infection is recommended in certain settings: pregnant women; all sexually active women 25 years of age and under; older women with risk factors for sexually transmitted diseases; and men with risk factors for sexually transmitted diseases, such as HIV-positive men or men who have sex with men.

▶ Treatment

Recommended regimens are a single oral 1-g dose of azithromycin (preferred and safe in pregnancy), 100 mg of doxycycline orally for 7 days (contraindicated in pregnancy), or 500 mg of levofloxacin once daily for 7 days (also contraindicated in pregnancy). Presumptively administered therapy still may be indicated for some patients (such as for an individual with gonococcal infection in whom no chlamydial testing was performed or a test other than a nucleic acid amplification test was used to exclude the diagnosis, or an individual for whom a test result is pending but is considered unlikely to follow-up, and for sexual contacts of documented cases). As for all patients in whom sexually transmitted diseases are diagnosed, studies for HIV and syphilis should also be performed.

Manhart LE et al. Standard treatment regimens for nongonococcal urethritis have similar but declining cure rates: a randomized controlled trial. Clin Infect Dis. 2013 Apr;56(7):934–42. [PMID: 23223595]
Mishori R et al. *Chlamydia trachomatis* infections: screening, diagnosis, and management. Am Fam Physician. 2012 Dec 15;86(12):1127–32. [PMID: 23316985]

Mylonas I. Female genital *Chlamydia trachomatis* infection: where are we heading? Arch Gynecol Obstet. 2012 May;285(5): 1271–85. [PMID: 22350326]

Seña AC et al. *Chlamydia trachomatis, Mycoplasma genitalium,* and *Trichomonas vaginalis* infections in men with nongonococcal urethritis: predictors and persistence after therapy. J Infect Dis. 2012 Aug 1;206(3):357–65. [PMID: 22615318]

Workowski KA et al; Centers for Disease Control and Prevention (CDC). Sexually transmitted diseases treatment guidelines, 2010. MMWR Recomm Rep. 2010 Dec 17;59(RR-12):1–110. Erratum in: MMWR Recomm Rep. 2011 Jan 14;60(1):18. [PMID: 21160459]

CHLAMYDOPHILA PSITTACI & PSITTACOSIS (Ornithosis)

ESSENTIALS OF DIAGNOSIS

► Fever, chills, and cough; headache common.

► Atypical pneumonia with slightly delayed appearance of signs of pneumonitis.

► Contact with infected bird (psittacine, pigeons, many others) 7–15 days previously.

► Isolation of chlamydiae or rising titer of complement-fixing antibodies.

General Considerations

Psittacosis is acquired from contact with birds (parrots, parakeets, pigeons, chickens, ducks, and many others), which may or may not be ill. The history may be difficult to obtain if the patient acquired infection from an illegally imported bird.

Clinical Findings

The onset is usually rapid, with fever, chills, myalgia, dry cough, and headache. Signs include temperature-pulse dissociation, dullness to percussion, and rales. Pulmonary findings may be absent early. Dyspnea and cyanosis may occur later. Endocarditis, which is culture-negative, may occur. The radiographic findings in typical psittacosis are those of atypical pneumonia, which tends to be interstitial and diffuse in appearance, though consolidation can occur. Psittacosis is indistinguishable from other bacterial or viral pneumonias by radiography.

The organism is rarely isolated from cultures. The diagnosis is usually made serologically; antibodies appear during the second week and can be demonstrated by complement fixation or immunofluorescence. Antibody response may be suppressed by early chemotherapy.

Differential Diagnosis

The illness is indistinguishable from viral, mycoplasmal, or other atypical pneumonias except for the history of contact with birds. Psittacosis is in the differential diagnosis of culture-negative endocarditis.

Treatment

Treatment consists of giving tetracycline, 0.5 g orally every 6 hours or 0.5 g intravenously every 12 hours, for 14–21 days. Erythromycin, 500 mg orally every 6 hours, may be effective as well.

McGuigan CC et al. Psittacosis outbreak in Tayside, Scotland, December 2011 to February 2012. Euro Surveill. 2012 May 31; 17(22):pii: 20186. [PMID: 22687915]

CHLAMYDOPHILA PNEUMONIAE INFECTION

C pneumoniae causes pneumonia and bronchitis. The clinical presentation of pneumonia is that of an atypical pneumonia. The organism accounts for approximately 10% of community-acquired pneumonias, ranking second to mycoplasma as an agent of atypical pneumonia. A putative role in coronary artery disease has not held up to close scientific scrutiny.

Like *C psittaci*, strains of *C pneumoniae* are resistant to sulfonamides. Erythromycin or tetracycline, 500 mg orally four times a day for 10–14 days, appears to be effective therapy. Fluoroquinolones, such as levofloxacin (500 mg once daily for 7–14 days) or moxifloxacin (400 mg once daily for 7–14 days), are active in vitro against *C pneumoniae* and probably are effective. It is unclear if empiric coverage for atypical pathogens in hospitalized patients with community-acquired pneumonia provides a survival benefit or improves clinical outcome.

Roulis E et al. *Chlamydia pneumoniae:* modern insights into an ancient pathogen. Trends Microbiol. 2013 Mar;21(3):120–8. [PMID: 23218799]

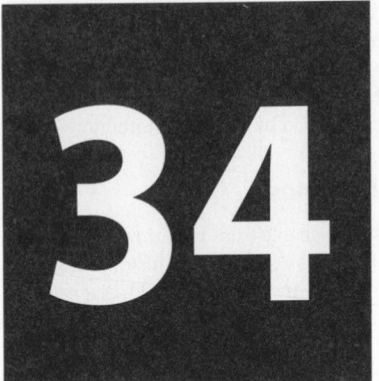

Spirochetal Infections

Susan S. Philip, MD, MPH

NATURAL HISTORY & PRINCIPLES OF DIAGNOSIS & TREATMENT

Syphilis is a complex infectious disease caused by *Treponema pallidum*, a spirochete capable of infecting almost any organ or tissue in the body and causing protean clinical manifestations (Table 34–1). Transmission occurs most frequently during sexual contact (including oral sex); sites of inoculation are usually genital but may be extragenital. The risk of acquiring syphilis after unprotected sex with an individual with infectious syphilis is approximately 30–50%. Rarely, it can also be transmitted through nonsexual contact, blood transfusion, or via the placenta from mother to fetus (congenital syphilis).

The natural history of acquired syphilis is generally divided into two major clinical stages: **early (infectious) syphilis** and **late syphilis**. The two stages are separated by a symptom-free latent phase during the first part of which (early latency) infectious lesions can recur. Infectious syphilis includes the primary lesions (chancre and regional lymphadenopathy), the secondary lesions (commonly involving skin and mucous membranes, occasionally bone, central nervous system, or liver), relapsing lesions during early latency, and congenital lesions. The hallmark of these lesions is an abundance of spirochetes; tissue reaction is usually minimal. Late syphilis consists of so-called benign (gummatous) lesions involving skin, bones, and viscera; cardiovascular disease (principally aortitis); and a variety of central nervous system and ocular syndromes. These forms of syphilis are not contagious. The lesions contain few demonstrable spirochetes, but tissue reactivity (vasculitis, necrosis) is severe and suggestive of hypersensitivity phenomena.

Public health efforts to control syphilis focus on the diagnosis and treatment of early (infectious) cases and their partners.

Most cases of syphilis in the United States continue to occur in men who have sex with men (MSM). However, despite the increase in primary and secondary syphilis in MSM in certain urban areas, such as San Francisco, a concomitant increase in the incidence of HIV has not been observed.

COURSE & PROGNOSIS

The lesions associated with primary and secondary syphilis are self-limiting, even without treatment, and resolve with few or no residua. Late syphilis may be highly destructive and permanently disabling and may lead to death. Many experts now believe that while infection is almost never completely eradicated in the absence of treatment, most infections remain latent without sequelae, and only a small number of latent infections progress to further disease.

CLINICAL STAGES OF SYPHILIS

1. Primary Syphilis

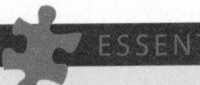 ESSENTIALS OF DIAGNOSIS

- ▶ History of sexual contact (may be unreliable).
- ▶ Painless ulcer on genitalia, perianal area, rectum, pharynx, tongue, lip, or elsewhere.
- ▶ Nontender enlargement of regional lymph nodes.
- ▶ Fluid expressed from lesion contains *T pallidum* by immunofluorescence or darkfield microscopy.
- ▶ Serologic nontreponemal and treponemal tests.

▶ Clinical Findings

A. Symptoms and Signs

This is the stage of invasion and may pass unrecognized. The typical lesion is the chancre at the site or sites of inoculation, most frequently located on the penis (Figure 34–1), labia, cervix, or anorectal region. Anorectal lesions are especially common among MSM. Chancres also occur occasionally in the oropharynx (lip, tongue, or tonsil) and rarely on the breast or finger or elsewhere. An initial small erosion appears 10–90 days (average, 3–4 weeks) after inoculation then rapidly develops into a painless superficial ulcer with a clean base and firm, indurated margins. This is associated with enlargement of regional lymph

Table 34–1. Stages of syphilis and common clinical manifestations.

Primary syphilis
   Chancre: painless ulcer with clean base and firm indurated borders
   Regional lymphadenopathy
Secondary syphilis
   Skin and mucous membranes
      Rash: diffuse (may include palms and soles), macular, papular, pustular, and combinations
      Condylomata lata
      Mucous patches: painless, silvery ulcerations of mucous membrane with surrounding erythema
   Generalized lymphadenopathy
   Constitutional symptoms
      Fever, usually low-grade
      Malaise
      Anorexia
      Arthralgias and myalgias
   Central nervous system
      Asymptomatic
      Symptomatic
         Headache
         Meningitis
         Cranial neuropathies (II–VIII)
   Ocular
      Iritis
      Iridocyclitis
   Other
      Renal: glomerulonephritis, nephrotic syndrome
      Liver: hepatitis
      Bone and joint: arthritis, periostitis
Late syphilis
   Late benign (gummatous): granulomatous lesion usually involving skin, mucous membranes and bones, but any organ can be involved
   Cardiovascular
      Aortic regurgitation
      Coronary ostial stenosis
      Aortic aneurysm
   Neurosyphilis
      Asymptomatic
      Meningovascular
         Seizures
         Hemiparesis or hemiplegia
      Tabes dorsalis
         Impaired proprioception and vibratory sensation
         Argyll Robertson pupil
         Shooting pains
         Ataxia
         Romberg sign
         Urinary and fecal incontinence
         Charcot joint
         Cranial neuropathies (II–VIII)
      General paresis
         Personality changes
         Hyperactive reflexes
         Argyll Robertson pupil
         Decreased memory
         Slurred speech
         Optic atrophy
Note: Central nervous system involvement may occur at any stage.

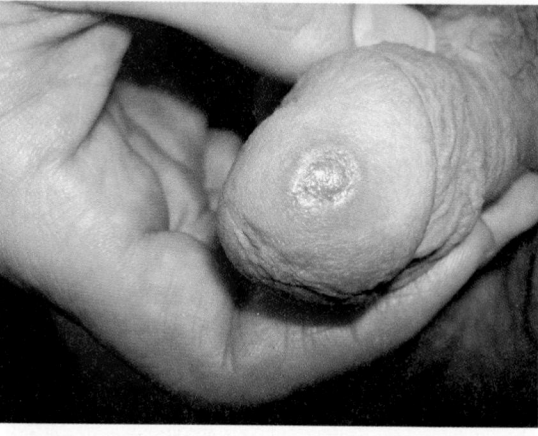

▲ **Figure 34–1.** Primary syphilis with a large chancre on the glans of the penis. (From Joseph Engelman, MD; San Francisco City Clinic.)

nodes, which are rubbery, discrete, and nontender. Bacterial infection of the chancre may occur and may lead to pain. Healing occurs without treatment, but a scar may form, especially with secondary bacterial infection. Multiple chancres may be present, particularly in HIV-positive patients. Although the "classic" ulcer of syphilis has been described as nontender, nonpurulent, and indurated, only 31% of patients have this triad.

B. Laboratory Findings

1. Microscopic examination—In early (infectious) syphilis, darkfield microscopic examination by a skilled observer of fresh exudate from lesions or material aspirated from regional lymph nodes is up to 90% sensitive for diagnosis. The darkfield examination requires expertise for proper specimen collection and identification of characteristic features of morphology and motility of pathogenic spirochetes, and repeated examinations may be necessary. Therefore, this testing is usually only available in select sexually transmitted disease clinics. Darkfield examination of oral lesions is not recommended because of the presence of nonpathogenic treponemes in the mouth. Spirochetes usually are not found in late syphilitic lesions by this technique.

An immunofluorescent staining technique for demonstrating *T pallidum* in dried smears of fluid taken from early syphilitic lesions is available through some laboratories but is not widely available.

2. Serologic tests for syphilis—(Table 34–2.) Serologic tests (the mainstay of syphilis diagnosis) fall into two general categories: (1) Nontreponemal tests detect antibodies to lipoidal antigens present in the host after modification by *T pallidum*. (2) Treponemal tests use live or killed *T pallidum* as antigen to detect antibodies specific for pathogenic treponemes.

A. NONTREPONEMAL ANTIGEN TESTS—The most commonly used nontreponemal antigen tests are the Venereal Disease Research Laboratory (VDRL) and rapid plasma

Table 34–2. Percentage of patients with positive serologic tests for syphilis.[1]

Test	Stage		
	Primary	Secondary	Tertiary
VDRL or RPR	75–85%	99–100%	40–95%
FTA-ABS, TPPA, or MHA-TP	69–100%	100%	94–98%
IgG EIA	100%	100%	NA
CIA	98	100	100

[1]Based on untreated cases.
CIA, chemiluminescence assay; EIA, enzyme immunoassay; FTA-ABS, fluorescent treponemal antibody absorption assay; MHA-TP, microhemagglutination assay for *T pallidum*; RPR, rapid plasma reagin test; TPPA, *T pallidum* particle agglutination; VDRL, Venereal Disease Research Laboratory test.

reagin (RPR) tests, which measure the ability of heated serum to flocculate a suspension of cardiolipin–cholesterol–lecithin. The flocculation tests are inexpensive, rapid, and easy to perform and have therefore been commonly used for routine screening. Quantitative expression of the reactivity of the serum, based on titration of dilutions of serum, is valuable in establishing the diagnosis and in evaluating the efficacy of treatment, since titers usually correlate with disease activity. A different, enzyme immunoassay (EIA)-based screening algorithm is discussed below.

Nontreponemal tests generally become positive 4–6 weeks after infection or 1–3 weeks after the appearance of a primary lesion; they are almost invariably positive in the secondary stage, with titers ≥ 1:16. In the late stages, titers tend to be lower (< 1:4). These serologic tests are not highly specific and must be closely correlated with other clinical and laboratory findings. The tests are positive in patients with non–sexually transmitted treponematoses (see below). More important, false-positive serologic reactions are frequently encountered in a wide variety of other conditions, including connective tissue diseases, infectious mononucleosis, malaria, febrile diseases, leprosy, injection drug use, infective endocarditis, old age, hepatitis C viral infection, and pregnancy. False-positive reactions are usually of low titer and transient and may be distinguished from true positives by performing a treponemal specific-antibody test. False-negative results can be seen when very high antibody titers are present (the prozone phenomenon). If syphilis is strongly suspected and the nontreponemal test is negative, the laboratory should be instructed to dilute the specimen to detect a positive reaction. The RPR and VDRL tests are equally reliable, but RPR titers tend to be higher than the VDRL. Thus, when these tests are used to follow disease activity, the same testing method should be used and preferably performed at the same laboratory.

Nontreponemal antibody titers are used to assess adequacy of therapy. The rate of the VDRL or RPR decline depends on various factors. In general, persons with repeat infections, higher initial titers, more advanced stages of disease, or those who are HIV-infected at the time of treatment have a slower seroconversion rate and are more likely to remain serofast (ie, titers decline but do not become nonreactive). Data based on currently recommended treatment regimens (see below) suggest that in primary and secondary syphilis it may take 6–12 months to see a fourfold decrease in titer.

B. Treponemal antibody tests—These tests measure antibodies capable of reacting with *T pallidum* antigens. The *T pallidum* hemagglutination (TPHA) test and the *T pallidum* particle agglutination (TPPA) test are comparable in specificity and sensitivity to the fluorescent treponemal antibody absorption test (FTA-ABS). The TPPA test, because of ease of performance, has supplanted the FTA-ABS test as the means of confirming the diagnosis of syphilis following a positive nontreponemal test. Newer treponemal tests used in reverse screening algorithms include EIA and chemiluminescence assay (CIA).

In traditional screening, the treponemal tests are used to determine whether a positive nontreponemal antigen test is a false-positive result (see above) or is indicative of syphilis. Because of their great sensitivity, particularly in the late stages of the disease, these tests are also of value when there is clinical evidence of syphilis but the nontreponemal serologic test for syphilis is negative. Treponemal tests are reactive in most patients with primary syphilis and in almost all patients with secondary syphilis (Table 34–2). Although a reactive treponemal-specific serologic test remains reactive throughout a patient's life in most cases, it may (like nontreponemal antibody tests) revert to negative with adequate therapy. Final decisions about the significance of the results of serologic tests for syphilis must be based on a total clinical appraisal and may require expert consultation.

C. EIA- or CIA-based screening algorithms—Newer screening algorithms reverse the traditional test order and begin with an automated treponemal antibody test, (eg, EIA or CIA) and then follow up with a nontreponemal test (RPR or VDRL) if the treponemal test is positive. This algorithm is faster and decreases labor costs to laboratories when compared with traditional screening. Compared with traditional treponemal-specific tests, the EIAs have sensitivities of 95–100% and specificities of 99–100%.

The reverse algorithms can cause challenges in clinical management. A positive treponemal test with a negative RPR or VDRL may represent prior, treated syphilis; untreated latent syphilis; or a false-positive treponemal test. Such results should be evaluated with a second treponemal test, but interpretation of discordant results is not yet fully standardized and a clinician may benefit from an expert opinion.

D. Rapid treponemal tests—A single rapid treponemal test is approved for use in the United States, with others in development. Such rapid treponemal tests are commonly used worldwide, particularly in limited-resource settings.

3. Polymerase chain reaction—Polymerase chain reaction (PCR) has been increasingly evaluated and utilized worldwide for the diagnosis of genital ulcer disease, including syphilis, but these tests are not yet commercially available in the United States.

4. Cerebrospinal fluid examination—See Neurosyphilis section.

Differential Diagnosis

The syphilitic chancre may be confused with genital herpes, chancroid (usually painful and uncommon in the United States), lymphogranuloma venereum, or neoplasm. Any genital ulcer should be considered a possible primary syphilitic lesion. Simultaneous evaluation for herpes simplex virus types 1 and 2 using PCR or culture should also be done in these cases.

Prevention & Screening

Avoidance of sexual contact is the only completely reliable method of prevention but is an impractical public health measure. Latex or polyurethane condoms are effective but protect covered areas only. Men who have sex with men should be screened every 6–12 months, and as often as every 3 months in high-risk individuals (those who have multiple encounters with anonymous partners or who have sex in conjunction with the use of drugs). Pregnant women should be screened at the first prenatal visit and again in the third trimester if there are risk indicators, including poverty, sex work, illicit drug use, history of other sexually transmitted diseases, and residing in a community with high syphilis morbidity. Patients treated for other sexually transmitted diseases should also be tested for syphilis, and persons who have known or suspected sexual contact with patients who have syphilis should be evaluated and presumptively treated to abort development of infectious syphilis (see Treating Syphilis Contacts below).

Treatment

A. Antibiotic Therapy

Penicillin remains the preferred treatment for syphilis, since there have been no documented cases of penicillin resistant *T pallidum* (Table 34–3). In pregnant women,

Table 34–3. Recommended treatment for syphilis.[1]

Stage of Syphilis	Treatment	Alternative[2]	Comment
Early			
Primary, secondary, or early latent	Benzathine penicillin G 2.4 million units intramuscularly once	Doxycycline 100 mg orally twice daily for 14 days or Tetracycline 500 mg orally four times daily for 14 days or Ceftriaxone 1 g intramuscularly or intravenously daily for 8–10 days[3]	
Late			
Late latent or uncertain duration	Benzathine penicillin G 2.4 million units intramuscularly weekly for 3 weeks	Doxycycline 100 mg orally twice daily for 28 days or Tetracycline 500 mg orally four times a day for 28 days	No routine cerebrospinal fluid evaluation unless neurologic, otologic or ocular abnormalities
Tertiary without neurosyphilis	Benzathine penicillin G 2.4 million units intramuscularly weekly for 3 weeks	Doxycycline 100 mg orally twice daily for 28 days or Tetracycline 500 mg orally four times a day for 28 days	Cerebrospinal fluid evaluation recommended in all patients
Neurosyphilis	Aqueous penicillin G 18–24 million units intravenously daily, given every 3–4 hours or as continuous infusion for 10–14 days	Procaine penicillin, 2.4 million units intramuscularly daily with probenecid 500 mg orally four times a day for 10–14 days or Ceftriaxone 2 g intramuscularly or intravenously daily for 10–14 days	Follow treatment with benzathine penicillin G 2.4 million units intramuscularly weekly for up to 3 weeks

[1]Penicillin is the only documented effective treatment in pregnancy, so pregnant patients with true allergy should be desensitized and treated with penicillin according to stage of disease as above.
[2]Patients treated with alternative therapies require close clinical and serologic monitoring.
[3]Fewer data for ceftriaxone treatment, optimal dose or duration not known.

penicillin is the only option because it reliably treats the fetus (see below).

There are some alternatives to penicillin for nonpregnant patients, including doxycycline. There are also limited data for ceftriaxone, although optimum dose and duration are not well defined. Azithromycin has been shown to be effective but should be used with caution; it should not be used at all in MSM due to demonstrated resistance. All patients treated with a non-penicillin regimen must have close clinical and serologic follow up, as noted below.

B. Managing Jarisch–Herxheimer Reaction

The Jarisch–Herxheimer reaction, manifested by fever and aggravation of the existing clinical picture in the hours following treatment, is ascribed to the sudden massive destruction of spirochetes and is not an IgE-mediated allergic reaction. It is most common in early syphilis, particularly secondary syphilis where it can occur in 66% of cases.

The reaction may be blunted by simultaneous administration of antipyretics, although no proved method of prevention exists. In cases with increased risk of morbidity due to the Jarisch–Herxheimer reaction (including central nervous system or cardiac involvement and pregnancy), consultation with an infectious disease expert is recommended. Patients should be reminded that the reaction does not signify an allergy to penicillin.

C. Local Measures (Mucocutaneous Lesions)

Local treatment is usually not necessary. No local antiseptics or other chemicals should be applied to a suspected syphilitic lesion until specimens for microscopy have been obtained.

D. Public Health Measures

Patients with infectious syphilis must abstain from sexual activity for 7–10 days after treatment. All cases of syphilis must be reported to the appropriate local public health agency in order to identify and treat sexual contacts. In addition, all patients with syphilis should have an HIV test at the time of diagnosis. In areas of high HIV prevalence, a repeat HIV test should be performed in 3 months if the initial test result was negative.

E. Treating Syphilis Contacts

Patients who have been sexually exposed to infectious syphilis within the preceding 3 months may be infected but seronegative and thus should be treated as for early syphilis even if serologic tests are negative. Persons exposed more than 3 months previously should be treated based on serologic results; however, if the patient is unreliable for follow-up, empiric therapy is indicated.

▶ Follow-Up Care

Because treatment failures and reinfection may occur, patients treated for syphilis should be monitored clinically

and serologically every 6 months. In primary and secondary syphilis, failure of nontreponemal antibody titers to decrease fourfold by 6–12 months may identify a group at high risk for treatment failure. Optimal management of these patients is unclear, but at a minimum, close clinical and serologic follow-up is indicated. In HIV-uninfected patients, an HIV test should be repeated (all patients with syphilis should have an HIV test at the time of diagnosis); a lumbar puncture should be considered since unrecognized neurosyphilis can be a cause of treatment failure; and, if careful follow-up cannot be ensured (3-month intervals for HIV-positive individuals and 6-month intervals for HIV-negative patients), treatment should be repeated with 2.4 million units of benzathine penicillin G intramuscularly weekly for 3 weeks. If symptoms or signs persist or recur after initial therapy or there is a fourfold or greater increase in nontreponemal titers, the patient has been reinfected (more likely) or the therapy failed (if a non-penicillin regimen was used). In those individuals, an HIV test should be performed, a lumbar puncture done (unless reinfection is a certainty), and re-treatment given as indicated above.

2. Secondary Syphilis

ESSENTIALS OF DIAGNOSIS

▶ Generalized maculopapular skin rash.

▶ Mucous membrane lesions, including patches and ulcers.

▶ Weeping papules (condyloma lata) in moist skin areas.

▶ Generalized nontender lymphadenopathy.

▶ Fever may be present.

▶ Meningitis, hepatitis, osteitis, arthritis, iritis may be present.

▶ Many treponemes in moist lesions by immunofluorescence or darkfield microscopy.

▶ Serologic tests for syphilis positive.

▶ Clinical Findings

The secondary stage of syphilis usually appears a few weeks (or up to 6 months) after development of the chancre, when dissemination of *T pallidum* produces systemic signs (fever, lymphadenopathy) or infectious lesions at sites distant from the site of inoculation. The most common manifestations are skin and mucosal lesions. The skin lesions are nonpruritic, macular, papular, pustular, or follicular (or combinations of any of these types, but generally *not* vesicular) and generalized; involvement of the palms and soles (Figure 34–2) occurs in 80% of cases. Annular lesions simulating ringworm may be observed in dark-skinned individuals. Mucous membrane lesions may include mucous patches (Figure 34–3), which can be found on the lips, mouth, throat, genitalia, and anus. Specific

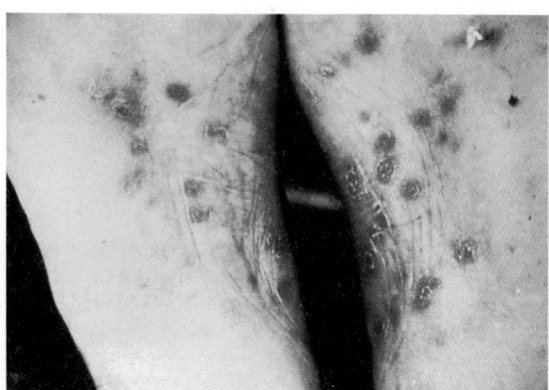

▲ **Figure 34–2.** Secondary syphilis lesions on the soles of the feet. (From Dr. Gavin Hart, Public Health Image Library, CDC.)

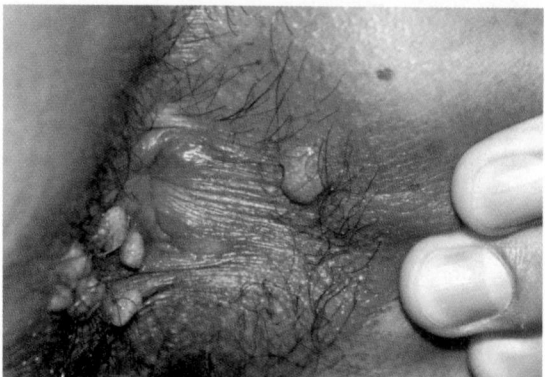

▲ **Figure 34–4.** Secondary syphilis perianal condylomata lata. (From Joseph Engelman, MD; San Francisco City Clinic.)

lesions—**condylomata lata** (Figure 34–4)—are fused, weeping papules on the moist areas of the skin and mucous membranes and are sometimes mistaken for genital warts. The mucous membrane lesions are highly infectious.

Meningeal (aseptic meningitis or acute basilar meningitis), hepatic, renal, bone, and joint invasion may occur, with resulting cranial nerve palsies, jaundice, nephrotic syndrome, and periostitis. Alopecia (moth-eaten appearance) and uveitis may also occur.

The serologic tests for syphilis are positive in almost all cases (see Primary Syphilis). The moist cutaneous and mucous membrane lesions often show *T pallidum* on darkfield microscopic examination. A transient cerebrospinal fluid (CSF) pleocytosis is seen in 40% of patients with secondary syphilis. There may be evidence of hepatitis or nephritis (immune complex type) as circulating immune complexes are deposited in blood vessel walls.

Skin lesions may be confused with the infectious exanthems, pityriasis rosea, and drug eruptions (Figure 34–5). Visceral lesions may suggest nephritis or hepatitis due to other causes.

► **Treatment**

Treatment is as for primary syphilis unless central nervous system or ocular disease is present, in which case a lumbar puncture should be performed and, if positive, treatment for neurosyphilis given (Table 34–3). See Primary Syphilis for follow-up care and treatment of contacts.

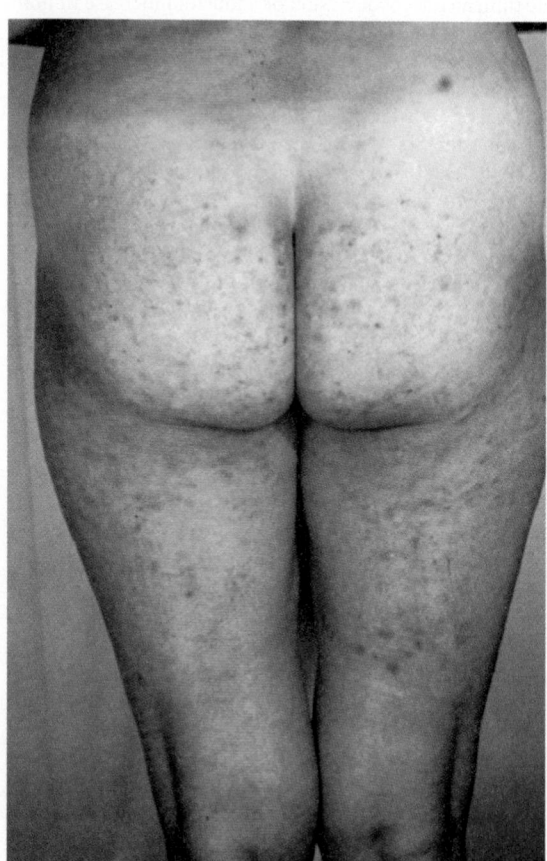

▲ **Figure 34–5.** Secondary syphilis rash of the buttocks and legs. (From J. Pledger, BSS/VD, Public Health Image Library, CDC.)

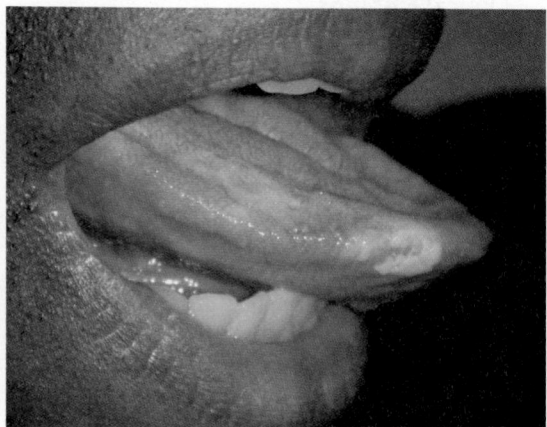

▲ **Figure 34–3.** Secondary syphilis mucous patch of the tongue. (From Kenneth Katz MD, MSc, MSCE.)

3. Latent Syphilis

ESSENTIALS OF DIAGNOSIS

▸ Early latent syphilis: infection < 1 year in duration.
▸ Late latent syphilis: infection > 1 year in duration.
▸ No physical signs.
▸ History of syphilis with inadequate treatment.
▸ Positive serologic tests for syphilis.

▸ General Considerations

Latent syphilis is the clinically quiescent phase in the absence of primary or secondary lesions. **Early latent syphilis** is defined as the first year after primary infection and may relapse to secondary syphilis if undiagnosed or inadequately treated (see above). Relapse is almost always accompanied by a rising titer in quantitative serologic tests; indeed, a rising titer may be the first or only evidence of relapse. About 90% of relapses occur during the first year after infection.

Early latent infection can be diagnosed if there was documented seroconversion or a fourfold increase in nontreponemal titers in the past 12 months; the patient can recall symptoms of primary or secondary syphilis; or the patient had a sex partner with documented primary, secondary, or early latent syphilis.

After the first year of latent syphilis, the patient is said to be in the **late latent stage** and noninfectious to sex partners. Transmission to the fetus, however, can probably occur in any phase. There are (by definition) no clinical manifestations during the latent stage, and the only significant laboratory findings are positive serologic tests. A diagnosis of late latent syphilis is justified only when the history and physical examination show no evidence of tertiary disease or neurosyphilis. The latent stage may last from months to a lifetime.

▸ Treatment

Treatment of **early latent syphilis** and follow-up is as for primary syphilis unless central nervous system disease is present (Table 34–3). Treatment of **late latent syphilis** is shown in Table 34–3. The treatment of this stage of the disease is intended to prevent late sequelae. If there is evidence of central nervous system involvement, a lumbar puncture should be performed and, if positive, the patient should receive treatment for neurosyphilis. Titers may not decline as rapidly following treatment compared to early syphilis. Nontreponemal serologic tests should be repeated at 6, 12, and 24 months. If titers increase fourfold or if initially high titers (≥ 1:32) fail to decrease fourfold by 12–24 months or if symptoms or signs consistent with syphilis develop, an HIV test should be repeated in HIV-uninfected patients, lumbar puncture should be performed, and re-treatment given according to the stage of the disease.

4. Late (Tertiary) Syphilis

ESSENTIALS OF DIAGNOSIS

▸ Infiltrative tumors of skin, bones, liver (gummas).
▸ Aortitis, aneurysms, aortic regurgitation.
▸ Central nervous system disorders, including meningovascular and degenerative changes, paresthesias, shooting pains, abnormal reflexes, dementia, or psychosis.

▸ General Considerations

This stage may occur at any time after secondary syphilis, even after years of latency, and is rarely seen in developed countries in the modern antibiotic era. Late lesions are thought to represent a delayed hypersensitivity reaction of the tissue to the organism and are usually divided into two types: (1) a localized gummatous reaction, with a relatively rapid onset and generally prompt response to therapy and (2) diffuse inflammation of a more insidious onset that characteristically involves the central nervous system and large arteries, is often fatal if untreated, and is at best arrested by treatment. Gummas may involve any area or organ of the body but most often affect the skin or long bones. Cardiovascular disease is usually manifested by aortic aneurysm, aortic regurgitation, or aortitis. Various forms of diffuse or localized central nervous system involvement may occur.

Late syphilis must be differentiated from neoplasms of the skin, liver, lung, stomach, or brain; other forms of meningitis; and primary neurologic lesions.

Although almost any tissue and organ may be involved in late syphilis, the following are the most common types of involvement: skin, mucous membranes, skeletal system, eyes, respiratory system, gastrointestinal system, cardiovascular system, and nervous system.

▸ Clinical Findings

A. Symptoms and Signs

1. Skin—Cutaneous lesions of late syphilis are of two varieties: (1) multiple nodular lesions that eventually ulcerate (lues maligna) or resolve by forming atrophic, pigmented scars and (2) solitary gummas that start as painless subcutaneous nodules, then enlarge, attach to the overlying skin, and eventually ulcerate (Figure 34–6).

2. Mucous membranes—Late lesions of the mucous membranes are nodular gummas or leukoplakia, highly destructive to the involved tissue.

3. Skeletal system—Bone lesions are destructive, causing periostitis, osteitis, and arthritis with little or no associated redness or swelling but often marked myalgia and myositis of the neighboring muscles. The pain is especially severe at night.

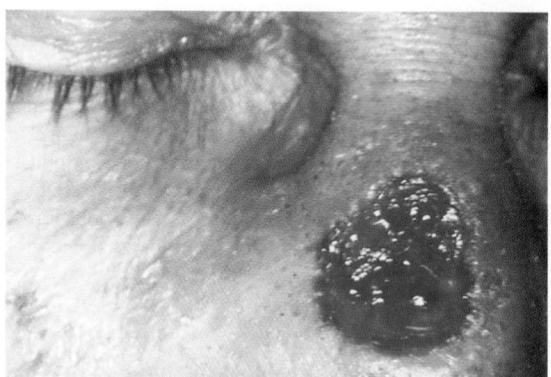

▲ Figure 34–6. Gumma of the nose due to long-standing tertiary syphilis. (From J. Pledger, Public Health Image Library, CDC.)

4. Eyes—Late ocular lesions are gummatous iritis, chorio-retinitis, optic atrophy, and cranial nerve palsies, in addition to the lesions of central nervous system syphilis.

5. Respiratory system—Respiratory involvement by late syphilis is caused by gummatous infiltrates into the larynx, trachea, and pulmonary parenchyma, producing discrete pulmonary densities. There may be hoarseness, respiratory distress, and wheezing secondary to the gummatous lesion itself or to subsequent stenosis occurring with healing.

6. Gastrointestinal system—Gummas involving the liver produce the usually benign, asymptomatic hepar lobatum. A picture resembling Laennec cirrhosis is occasionally produced by liver involvement. Gastric involvement can consist of diffuse infiltration into the stomach wall or focal lesions that endoscopically and microscopically can be confused with lymphoma or carcinoma. Epigastric pain, early satiety, regurgitation, belching, and weight loss are common symptoms.

7. Cardiovascular system—Cardiovascular lesions (10–15% of late syphilitic lesions) are often progressive, disabling, and life-threatening. Central nervous system lesions are often present concomitantly. Involvement usually starts as an arteritis in the supracardiac portion of the aorta and progresses to one or more of the following: (1) narrowing of the coronary ostia, with resulting decreased coronary circulation, angina, and acute myocardial infarction; (2) scarring of the aortic valves, producing aortic regurgitation, and eventually heart failure; and (3) weakness of the wall of the aorta, with saccular aneurysm formation (Figure 34–7) and associated pressure symptoms of dysphagia, hoarseness, brassy cough, back pain (vertebral erosion), and occasionally rupture of the aneurysm. Recurrent respiratory infections are common as a result of pressure on the trachea and bronchi.

8. Nervous system (neurosyphilis)—See following section.

▶ **Treatment**

Treatment of tertiary syphilis (excluding neurosyphilis) is the same as late latent syphilis (Table 34–3). Positive

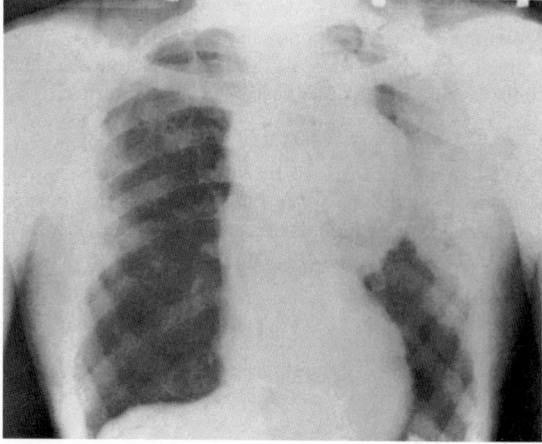

▲ Figure 34–7. Ascending saccular aneurysm of the thoracic aorta in tertiary syphilis. (Public Health Image Library, CDC.)

serologic tests do not usually become negative. Viable spirochetes are occasionally found in the eyes, in CSF, and elsewhere in patients with "adequately" treated syphilis, but claims for their capacity to cause progressive disease are speculative.

The pretreatment clinical and laboratory evaluation should include neurologic, ocular, cardiovascular, psychiatric, and CSF examinations. In the presence of definite CSF or neurologic abnormalities, one should treat for neurosyphilis.

5. Neurosyphilis

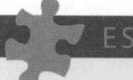

ESSENTIALS OF DIAGNOSIS

▶ Can occur at any stage of disease.

▶ Consider both clinical presentation and laboratory data.

▶ Carefully evaluate the neurologic examination in all patients and consider CSF evaluation for atypical symptoms or lack of decrease in nontreponemal serology titers.

▶ **General Considerations**

Neurosyphilis can occur at any stage of disease and can be a progressive, disabling, and life-threatening complication. CSF pleocytosis has been reported in 40% of patients with early syphilis. Asymptomatic CSF abnormalities and meningovascular syphilis occur earlier (months to years after infection, sometimes coexisting with primary and secondary syphilis) than tabes dorsalis and general paresis (2–50 years after infection).

▶ **Clinical Findings**

A. Classification

1. Asymptomatic neuroinvasion—This form is characterized by spinal fluid abnormalities (positive spinal fluid serology, increased cell count, occasionally increased protein) without symptoms or signs of neurologic involvement. There are no clear data to support that these asymptomatic CSF abnormalities have clinical significance.

2. Meningovascular syphilis—This form is characterized by meningeal involvement or changes in the vascular structures of the brain (or both), producing symptoms of acute or chronic meningitis (headache, irritability); cranial nerve palsies (basilar meningitis); unequal reflexes; irregular pupils with poor light and accommodation reflexes; and when large vessels are involved, cerebrovascular accidents. The CSF shows increased cells (100–1000/mcL), elevated protein, and may have a positive serologic test (CSF VDRL) for syphilis. The symptoms of acute meningitis are rare in late syphilis.

3. Tabes dorsalis—This form is a chronic progressive degeneration of the parenchyma of the posterior columns of the spinal cord and of the posterior sensory ganglia and nerve roots. The symptoms and signs are impairment of proprioception and vibration sense, Argyll Robertson pupils (which react poorly to light but accommodate for near focus), and muscular hypotonia and hyporeflexia. Impaired proprioception results in a wide-based gait and inability to walk in the dark. Paresthesias, analgesia, or sharp recurrent pains in the muscles of the leg ("shooting" or "lightning" pains) may occur. Crises are also common in tabes: gastric crises, consisting of sharp abdominal pains with nausea and vomiting (simulating an acute abdomen); laryngeal crises, with paroxysmal cough and dyspnea; urethral crises, with painful bladder spasms; and rectal and anal crises. Crises may begin suddenly, last for hours to days, and cease abruptly. Neurogenic bladder with overflow incontinence is also seen. Painless trophic ulcers may develop over pressure points on the feet. Joint damage may occur as a result of lack of sensory innervation (Charcot joint, Figure 34–8). The CSF may have a normal or increased cell count, elevated protein, and variable results of serologic tests.

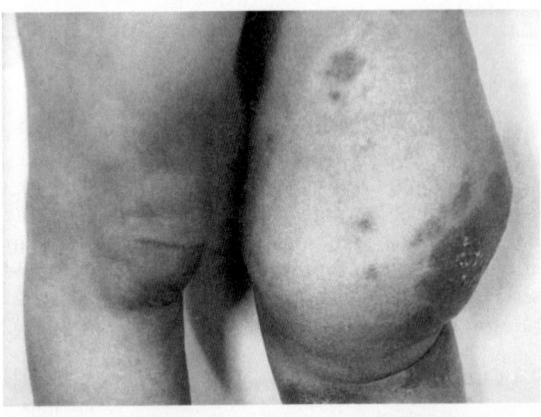

▲ **Figure 34–8.** Neuropathic arthropathy (Charcot joint) from tertiary syphilis. (From Susan Lindsley, Public Health Image Library, CDC.)

4. General paresis—This is generalized involvement of the cerebral cortex with insidious onset of symptoms. There is usually a decrease in concentrating power, memory loss, dysarthria, tremor of the fingers and lips, irritability, and mild headaches. Most striking is the change of personality; the patient may become slovenly, irresponsible, confused, and psychotic. The CSF findings resemble those of tabes dorsalis. Combinations of the various forms of neurosyphilis (especially tabes and paresis) are not uncommon.

B. Laboratory Findings

See Serologic Tests for Syphilis, above; these tests should also be performed in cases of suspected neurosyphilis.

1. Indications for a lumbar puncture—In early syphilis (primary and secondary syphilis and early latent syphilis of < 1 year duration), invasion of the central nervous system by *T pallidum* with CSF abnormalities occurs commonly, but clinical neurosyphilis rarely develops in patients who have received standard therapy. Thus, unless clinical symptoms or signs of neurosyphilis or ophthalmologic involvement (uveitis, neuroretinitis, optic neuritis, iritis) are present, a lumbar puncture in early syphilis is not routinely recommended. In latent syphilis, routine lumbar puncture is not indicated since the yield is low and findings rarely influence therapeutic decisions. CSF evaluation is recommended, however, if neurologic or ophthalmologic symptoms or signs are present, if there is evidence of treatment failure (see earlier discussion), or if there is evidence of active tertiary syphilis (eg, aortitis, iritis, optic atrophy, the presence of a gumma).

2. Spinal fluid examination—CSF findings in neurosyphilis are variable. In "classic" cases, there is an elevation of total protein, lymphocytic pleocytosis, and a positive CSF reagin test (VDRL). The serum nontreponemal titers will be reactive in most cases. In later stages of syphilis, normal CSF analysis in the presence of infection can occur, but it is unusual. False-positive reagin tests rarely occur in the CSF; a positive test confirms the presence of neurosyphilis. Because the CSF VDRL may be negative in 30–70% of cases of neurosyphilis, *a negative test does not exclude neurosyphilis*. The CSF FTA-ABS is sometimes used; it is a highly sensitive test but lacks specificity, and a high serum titer of FTA-ABS may result in a positive CSF titer in the absence of neurosyphilis.

▶ Treatment

Neurosyphilis is treated with high doses of aqueous penicillin to achieve better penetration and higher levels of drug in the CSF than is possible with benzathine penicillin G (Table 34–3). There are limited data for using ceftriaxone to treat neurosyphilis as well, but because other regimens have not been adequately studied, patients with a history of an IgE-mediated reaction to penicillin may require skin testing for allergy to penicillin and, if positive, should be desensitized. Patients treated for neurosyphilis should receive at least one dose of long-acting (benzathine) penicillin at the completion of therapy. Because of concerns about slowly dividing organisms that may persist after completing 10–14 days of therapy with short-acting aqueous penicillin G sodium or potassium, many experts recommend subsequent administration of 2.4 million units of the longer-acting benzathine penicillin G intramuscularly once weekly for up to 3 weeks as additional therapy.

All patients treated for neurosyphilis should have nontreponemal serologic tests done every 3–6 months. Guidelines established by the Centers for Disease Control and Prevention (CDC) recommend spinal fluid examinations at 6-month intervals until the CSF cell count is normal; however, there are data to suggest that in certain patients normalization of serum titers are an acceptable surrogate for CSF response. In general, CSF white blood cell count and CSF VDRL normalize more quickly (usually in 12 months) than CSF protein concentration, which can remain abnormal for extended periods. If the serum nontreponemal titers do not normalize, the CSF analysis should be repeated. A second course of penicillin therapy may be given if the CSF cell count has not decreased at 6 months or is not normal at 2 years.

6. Syphilis in HIV-Infected Patients

Syphilis is common among HIV-infected individuals. Some data suggest that syphilis coinfection is associated with an increase in HIV viral load and a decrease in CD4 count that normalizes with therapy. Researchers from a prospective cohort study of HIV-infected individuals reported that they found no association with HIV disease progression in persons with syphilis coinfection. However, for optimal patient care as well as prevention of transmission to partners, guidelines for the primary care of HIV-infected patients recommend routine syphilis screening.

Interpretation of serologic tests should be the same for HIV-positive and HIV-negative persons. All HIV-positive patients in care should be screened at least annually to identify latent disease because by establishing a serologic history, unnecessary lumbar punctures and prolonged treatment for latent syphilis of uncertain duration can be avoided. If the diagnosis of syphilis is suggested on clinical grounds but reagin tests are negative, alternative tests should be performed. These tests include darkfield examination of lesions and direct fluorescent antibody staining for *T pallidum* of lesion exudate or biopsy specimens.

HIV-positive patients with primary and secondary syphilis should have careful clinical and serologic follow-up at 3, 6, 9, 12, and 24 months. HIV-infected patients with late latent syphilis, syphilis of uncertain duration, and neurosyphilis should be treated like HIV-negative individuals, with follow-up at 6, 12, 18, and 24 months. The use of antiretroviral therapy has been associated with reduced serologic failure rates after syphilis treatment.

The diagnosis of neurosyphilis in HIV-infected patients is complicated by the fact that CSF abnormalities are frequently seen if lumbar puncture is performed. The significance of these abnormalities is unknown, and similar abnormalities are frequently seen in non–HIV-infected patients with primary or secondary syphilis. Thus, CSF testing is not recommended in those with early disease and a normal neurologic examination. In contrast, a lumbar puncture should be performed in all patients, regardless of HIV-infection status, if neurologic signs are present or if therapy has failed. Following treatment, CSF white blood cell counts normalize within 12 months regardless of HIV status, while the CSF VDRL is slower to normalize in HIV-infected individuals, especially those with CD4 counts < 200 cells/mcL. As discussed above, the same criteria for failure apply to HIV-positive and HIV-negative patients, and re-treatment regimens are the same.

Because clinical experience in treating HIV-infected patients with syphilis is based on penicillin regimens, few options exist for treating the penicillin-allergic patient. Doxycycline or tetracycline regimens can be used for primary, secondary, and early latent syphilis as well as for late latent syphilis and latent syphilis of unknown duration though with caution and close follow-up (Table 34–3). For neurosyphilis, penicillin regimens are optimal even if this requires skin testing and desensitization; limited data exist for ceftriaxone.

7. Syphilis in Pregnancy

All pregnant women should have a nontreponemal serologic test for syphilis at the time of the first prenatal visit (see Chapter 19). In women who may be at increased risk for syphilis or for populations in which there is a high prevalence of syphilis, additional nontreponemal tests should be performed during the third trimester at 28 weeks and again at delivery. The serologic status of all women who have delivered should be known before discharge from the hospital. Seropositive women should be considered infected and should be treated unless prior treatment with fall in antibody titer is medically documented.

The only acceptable treatment for syphilis in pregnancy is penicillin in dosage schedules appropriate for the stage of disease (see above). Penicillin prevents congenital syphilis in 90% of cases, even when treatment is given late in pregnancy. Tetracycline and doxycycline are contraindicated in pregnancy. Erythromycin should not be used because of failure to eradicate infection in the fetus, and insufficient data are available to justify a recommendation for ceftriaxone or azithromycin. Thus, women with a history of penicillin allergy should be skin tested and desensitized if necessary.

The infant should be evaluated immediately, as noted below, and at 6–8 weeks of age.

8. Congenital Syphilis

Congenital syphilis is a transplacentally transmitted infection that occurs in infants of untreated or inadequately treated mothers. The physical findings at birth are quite variable: The infant may have many or minimal signs or even no signs until 6–8 weeks of life (delayed form). The most common findings are on the mucous membranes and skin—maculopapular rash, condylomas, mucous membrane patches, and serous nasal discharge (snuffles). These lesions are infectious; *T pallidum* can easily be found microscopically, and the infant must be isolated. Other common findings are hepatosplenomegaly, anemia, or osteochondritis. These early active lesions subsequently heal, but if the disease is left untreated it produces the characteristic stigmas of congenital syphilis—interstitial keratitis, Hutchinson teeth, saddle nose, saber shins, deafness, and central nervous system involvement.

The presence of negative serologic tests at birth in both the mother and the infant usually means that the newborn is free of infection. However, recent infection near the time of delivery may result in negative tests because there has been insufficient time to develop a serologic response. Thus, it is necessary to maintain a high index of suspicion in infants born to high-risk mothers. All infants born to mothers with positive nontreponemal and treponemal antibody titers should have blood drawn for an RPR or VDRL test and, if positive, be referred to a pediatrician for further evaluation and therapy.

▶ **When to Refer**

- Consultation with the local public health department may help obtain all prior positive syphilis serologic results and may be helpful in complicated or atypical cases.

- Early (infectious) syphilis cases may be contacted for partner notification and treatment by local public health authorities.

▶ **When to Admit**

- Pregnant women with syphilis and true penicillin allergy should be admitted for desensitization and treatment.

- Women in late pregnancy treated for early syphilis should have close outpatient monitoring or be admitted because the Jarisch-Herxheimer reaction can induce premature labor.

- Patients with neurosyphilis usually require admission for treatment with aqueous penicillin.

Gayet-Ageron A et al. Sensitivity, specificity and likelihood ratios of PCR in the diagnosis of syphilis: a systematic review and meta-analysis. Sex Transm Infect. 2013 May;89(3):251–6. [PMID: 23024223]

Ghanem KG et al. Management of adult syphilis. Clin Infect Dis. 2011 Dec;53(Suppl 3):S110–28. [PMID: 22080265]

Seña AC et al. Novel *Treponema pallidum* serologic tests: a paradigm shift in syphilis screening for the 21st century. Clin Infect Dis. 2010 Sep 15;51(6):700–8. [PMID: 20687840]

Workowski KA et al; Centers for Disease Control and Prevention (CDC). Sexually transmitted diseases treatment guidelines, 2010. MMWR Recomm Rep. 2010 Dec 17;59(RR-12):1–110. Erratum in: MMWR Recomm Rep. 2011 Jan 14;60(1):18. [PMID: 21160459]

NON–SEXUALLY TRANSMITTED TREPONEMATOSES

A variety of treponemal diseases other than syphilis occur endemically in many tropical areas of the world. They are distinguished from disease caused by *T pallidum* by their nonsexual transmission, their relatively high incidence in certain geographic areas and among children, and their

tendency to produce less severe visceral manifestations. As in syphilis, organisms can be demonstrated in infectious lesions with darkfield microscopy or immunofluorescence but cannot be cultured in artificial media; the serologic tests for syphilis are positive; molecular methods such as PCR and genome sequencing are available but not widely used in endemic areas; the diseases have primary, secondary, and sometimes tertiary stages; and penicillin is the drug of choice. There is evidence that infection with these agents may provide partial resistance to syphilis and vice versa. Treatment with penicillin in doses appropriate to primary syphilis (eg, 2.4 million units of benzathine penicillin G intramuscularly) is generally curative in any stage of the non–sexually transmitted treponematoses. In cases of penicillin hypersensitivity, tetracycline, 500 mg orally four times a day for 10–14 days, is usually the recommended alternative. In a randomized controlled trial, oral azithromycin (30 mg/kg once) was noninferior to benzathine penicillin G for the treatment of yaws in children.

YAWS (Frambesia)

Yaws is a contagious disease largely limited to tropical regions that is caused by *T pallidum* subspecies *pertenue*. It is characterized by granulomatous lesions of the skin, mucous membranes, and bone. Yaws is rarely fatal, though if untreated it may lead to chronic disability and disfigurement. Yaws is acquired by direct nonsexual contact, usually in childhood, although it may occur at any age. The "mother yaw," a painless papule that later ulcerates, appears 3–4 weeks after exposure. There is usually associated regional lymphadenopathy. Six to 12 weeks later, secondary lesions that are raised papillomas and papules that weep highly infectious material appear and last for several months or years. Painful ulcerated lesions on the soles are called "crab yaws" because of the resulting gait. Late gummatous lesions may occur, with associated tissue destruction involving large areas of skin and subcutaneous tissues. The late effects of yaws, with bone change, shortening of digits, and contractions, may be confused with similar changes occurring in leprosy. Central nervous system, cardiac, or other visceral involvement is rare. See above for therapy. The World Health Organization has set a goal of eliminating yaws by the year 2020.

PINTA

Pinta is a non–sexually transmitted spirochetal infection caused by *T pallidum* subspecies *carateum*. It occurs endemically in rural areas of Latin America, especially in Mexico, Colombia, and Cuba, and in some areas of the Pacific. A nonulcerative, erythematous primary papule spreads slowly into a papulosquamous plaque showing a variety of color changes (slate, lilac, black). Secondary lesions resemble the primary one and appear within a year after it. These appear successively, new lesions together with older ones; are most common on the extremities; and later show atrophy and depigmentation. Some cases show pigmentary changes and atrophic patches on the soles and palms, with or without hyperkeratosis, that are indistinguishable from "crab yaws." Very rarely, central nervous system or cardiovascular disease is observed late in the course of infection. See above for therapy.

ENDEMIC SYPHILIS

Endemic syphilis is an acute or chronic infection caused by *T pallidum* subspecies *endemicum*. It has been reported in a number of countries, particularly in the eastern Mediterranean area, often with local names: bejel in Syria, Saudi Arabia, and Iraq, and dichuchwa, njovera, and siti in Africa. It also occurs in Southeast Asia. The local forms have distinctive features. Moist ulcerated lesions of the skin or oral or nasopharyngeal mucosa are the most common manifestations. Generalized lymphadenopathy and secondary and tertiary bone and skin lesions are also common. Deep leg pain points to periostitis or osteomyelitis. In the late stages of disease, destructive gummatous lesions similar to those seen in yaws can develop, resulting in loss of cartilage and saber shin deformity. Cardiovascular and central nervous system involvement are rare. See above for therapy.

Mitjà O et al. Advances in the diagnosis of endemic treponematoses: yaws, bejel, and pinta. PLoS Negl Trop Dis. 2013 Oct 24;7(10):e2283. [PMID: 24205410]

Mitjà O et al. Yaws. Lancet. 2013 Mar 2;381(9868):763–73. [PMID: 23415015]

Mitjà O et al. Single-dose azithromycin versus benzathine benzylpenicillin for treatment of yaws in children in Papua New Guinea: an open-label, non-inferiority, randomised trial. Lancet. 2012 Jan 28;379(9813):342–7. [PMID: 22240407]

SELECTED SPIROCHETAL DISEASES

RELAPSING FEVER

The infectious organisms in relapsing fever are spirochetes of the genus *Borrelia*. The infection has two forms: tick-borne and louse-borne. The main reservoir for tick-borne relapsing fever is rodents, which serve as the source of infection for ticks. Tick-borne relapsing fever may be transmitted transovarially from one generation of ticks to the next. Humans can be infected by tick bites or by rubbing crushed tick tissues or feces into the bite wound. Tick-borne relapsing fever is endemic but is not transmitted from person to person. In the United States, infected ticks are found throughout the West, especially in mountainous areas, but clinical cases are uncommon in humans.

The louse-borne form is primarily seen in the developing world, and humans are the only reservoir. Large epidemics may occur in louse-infested populations, and transmission is favored by crowding, malnutrition, and cold climate.

▶ Clinical Findings

A. Symptoms and Signs

There is an abrupt onset of fever, chills, tachycardia, nausea and vomiting, arthralgia, and severe headache. Hepatomegaly and splenomegaly may develop, as well as various types of rashes (macular, popular, petechial) that usually occur at the end of a febrile episode. Delirium occurs with high fever, and there may be various neurologic and psychic abnormalities. The attack terminates, usually abruptly, after 3–10 days. After an interval of 1–2 weeks, relapse occurs, but often it is somewhat milder. Three to ten relapses may occur before recovery in tick-borne disease, whereas louse-borne disease is associated with only one or two relapses.

B. Laboratory Findings

During episodes of fever, large spirochetes are seen in blood smears stained with Wright or Giemsa stain. The organisms can be cultured in special media but rapidly lose pathogenicity. The spirochetes can multiply in injected rats or mice and can be seen in their blood.

A variety of anti-borrelia antibodies develop during the illness; sometimes the Weil–Felix test for rickettsioses and nontreponemal serologic tests for syphilis may also be falsely positive. Infection can cause false-positive indirect fluorescent antibody and Western blot tests for *Borrelia burgdorferi*, causing some cases to be misdiagnosed as Lyme disease. PCR assays have been developed but are not widely available. CSF abnormalities occur in patients with meningeal involvement. Mild anemia and thrombocytopenia are common, but the white blood cell count tends to be normal.

▶ Differential Diagnosis

The manifestations of relapsing fever may be confused with malaria, leptospirosis, meningococcemia, yellow fever, typhus, or rat-bite fever.

▶ Prevention

Prevention of tick bites (as described for rickettsial diseases) and delousing procedures applicable to large groups can prevent illness. Arthropod vectors should be controlled if possible.

Postexposure prophylaxis with doxycycline 200 mg orally on day 1 and 100 mg daily for 4 days has been shown to prevent recurrent fever following tick bites in highly endemic areas.

▶ Treatment

A single dose of tetracycline or erythromycin, 0.5 g orally, or a single dose of procaine penicillin G, 600,000–800,000 units intramuscularly (adults) or 400,000 units intramuscularly (children), probably constitutes adequate treatment for louse-borne relapsing fevers; however, some experts advocate for longer courses of treatment to prevent persistent infection. Because of higher relapse rates, tick-borne disease is routinely treated with 0.5 g of tetracycline or erythromycin given orally four times daily for 10 days. If central nervous system invasion is suspected, penicillin G, 3 million units intravenously every 4 hours, or ceftriaxone, 1 g intravenously daily, should be given for 10–14 days. Jarisch–Herxheimer reactions occur commonly following treatment and may be life-threatening, so patients should be closely monitored (see Syphilis, above). One study in patients with louse-borne relapsing fever showed that administration of anti-TNF antibodies prior to antibiotic therapy can be effective in preventing the reaction.

► Prognosis

The overall mortality rate is usually about 5%. Fatalities are most common in old, debilitated, or very young patients. With treatment, the initial attack is shortened and relapses are largely prevented.

Balicer RD et al. Post exposure prophylaxis of tick-borne relapsing fever. Eur J Clin Microbiol Infect Dis. 2010 Mar;29(3): 253–8. [PMID: 20012878]

Cutler SJ. Relapsing fever—a forgotten disease revealed. J Appl Microbiol. 2010 Apr;108(4):1115–22. [PMID: 19886891]

Elbir H et al. Relapsing fever borreliae in Africa. Am J Trop Med Hyg. 2013 Aug;89(2):288–92. [PMID: 23926141]

RAT-BITE FEVER

Rat-bite fever is an uncommon acute infectious disease caused by the treponeme *Spirillum minus* (Asia), covered in this section, or the bacteria *Streptobacillus moniliformis* (North America). It is transmitted to humans by the bite of a rat. Inhabitants of rat-infested dwellings, owners of pet rats, and laboratory workers are at greatest risk.

► Clinical Findings

A. Symptoms and Signs

In *Spirillum* infections, the original rat bite, unless secondarily infected, heals promptly, but 1 to several weeks later the site becomes swollen, indurated, and painful; assumes a dusky purplish hue; and may ulcerate. Regional lymphangitis and lymphadenitis, fever, chills, malaise, myalgia, arthralgia, and headache are present. Splenomegaly may occur. A sparse, dusky-red maculopapular rash appears on the trunk and extremities in many cases, and there may be frank arthritis.

After a few days, both the local and systemic symptoms subside, only to reappear several days later. This relapsing pattern of fever for 3–4 days alternating with afebrile periods lasting 3–9 days may persist for weeks. The other features, however, usually recur only during the first few relapses. Endocarditis is a rare complication of infection.

B. Laboratory Findings

Leukocytosis is often present, and the nontreponemal test for syphilis is often falsely positive. The organism may be identified in darkfield examination of the ulcer exudate or aspirated lymph node material; more commonly, it is observed after inoculation of a laboratory animal with the patient's exudate or blood. It has not been cultured in artificial media.

► Differential Diagnosis

Rat-bite fever must be distinguished from the rat-bite-induced lymphadenitis and rash of streptobacillary fever. Clinically, the severe arthritis and myalgias seen in streptobacillary disease are rarely seen in disease caused by *S minus*. Reliable differentiation requires an increasing titer

of agglutinins against *S moniliformis* or isolation of the causative organism. Other diseases in the differential include tularemia, rickettsial disease, *Pasteurella multocida* infections, and relapsing fever.

► Treatment

Penicillin is given for 10–14 days. During the acute phase of illness, the intravenous route is used (1–2 million units every 4–6 hours) and once improvement has occurred, therapy is completed with oral medication, penicillin V 500 mg four times daily to complete 10–14 days of therapy. For the penicillin-allergic patient, tetracycline 500 mg orally four times daily or doxycycline 100 mg twice a day can be used.

► Prognosis

The reported mortality rate of about 10% should be markedly reduced by prompt diagnosis and antimicrobial treatment.

Khatchadourian K et al. The rise of the rats: a growing paediatric issue. Paediatr Child Health. 2010 Mar;15(3):131–4. [PMID: 21358889]

LEPTOSPIROSIS

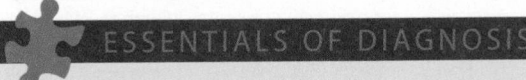

► Clinical illness can vary from asymptomatic to fatal liver and kidney disease.

► Anicteric leptospirosis is the more common and milder form of the disease.

► Icteric leptospirosis (Weil syndrome) is characterized by impaired kidney and liver function, abnormal mental status, and hemorrhagic pneumonia and has a 5–40% mortality rate.

► General Considerations

Leptospirosis is an acute and sometimes severe treponemal infection that is caused by multiple serovars of the spirochete, *Leptospira interrogans*. The disease is distributed worldwide, and it is among the most common zoonotic infections. The leptospires are often transmitted to humans by the ingestion of food and drink contaminated by the urine of an infected animal. The organism may also enter through minor skin lesions and probably via the conjunctiva. Reports of recreational cases in international travelers have been increasing, following swimming or rafting in contaminated water, and occupational cases occur among sewer workers, rice planters, abattoir workers, and farmers. Sporadic urban cases have been seen in the homeless exposed to rat urine.

► Clinical Findings

A. Symptoms and Signs

Anicteric leptospirosis, the more common and milder form of the disease, is often biphasic. After an incubation period of 2–20 days, the initial or "septicemic" phase begins with abrupt fever to 39–40°C, chills, abdominal pain, severe headache, and myalgias, especially of the calf muscles. There may be marked conjunctival suffusion. Leptospires can be isolated from blood, CSF, and tissues. Following a 1- to 3-day period of improvement in symptoms and absence of fever, the second or "immune" phase begins; however, in severe disease the phases may appear indistinct. Leptospires are absent from blood and CSF but are still present in the kidney, and specific antibodies appear. A recurrence of symptoms is seen as in the first phase of disease with the onset of meningitis. Uveitis (which can be unilateral or bilateral and usually involves the entire uveal tract), rash, and adenopathy may occur. A rare but severe manifestation is hemorrhagic pneumonia. The illness is usually self-limited, lasting 4–30 days, and complete recovery is the rule.

Icteric leptospirosis (Weil syndrome) is the most severe form of the disease, characterized by impaired kidney and liver function, abnormal mental status, hemorrhagic pneumonia, hypotension, and a 5–40% mortality rate. Symptoms and signs often are continuous and not biphasic.

Leptospirosis with jaundice must be distinguished from hepatitis, yellow fever, rickettsial disease, and relapsing fever.

B. Laboratory Findings

The leukocyte count may be normal or as high as 50,000/mcL (0.05/L), with neutrophils predominating. The urine may contain bile, protein, casts, and red cells. Oliguria is common, and in severe cases uremia may occur. Elevated bilirubin and aminotransferases are seen in 75%, and elevated creatinine (> 1.5 mg/dL) (> 132.6 mcmol/L) is seen in 50% of cases. In cases with meningeal involvement, organisms may be found in the CSF during the first 10 days of illness. Early in the disease, the organism may be identified by darkfield examination of the patient's blood (a test requiring expertise since false-positives are frequent in inexperienced hands) or by culture on a semisolid medium (eg, Fletcher EMJH). Cultures take 1–6 weeks to become positive. The organism may also be grown from the urine from the tenth day to the sixth week. Diagnosis is usually made by means of serologic tests, including the microscopic agglutination test (considered the gold standard, but not widely available), and enzyme-linked immunosorbent assay (ELISA). PCR methods (presently investigational) appear to be sensitive, specific, positive early in disease, and able to detect leptospiral DNA in blood, urine, CSF, and aqueous humor. Serum creatine kinase (CK) is usually elevated in persons with leptospirosis and normal in persons with hepatitis.

▶ Complications

Myocarditis, aseptic meningitis, acute kidney injury, and pulmonary infiltrates with hemorrhage are not common but are the usual causes of death. Iridocyclitis may occur.

▶ Prevention

The mainstay of prevention is avoidance of potentially contaminated food and water.

Prophylaxis with doxycycline has been effective in trials but is not routinely recommended. Human vaccine is used in some limited settings but is not available in the United States.

▶ Treatment

Various antimicrobial drugs, including penicillin, ceftriaxone, and tetracyclines, show antileptospiral activity; however, meta-analysis has not demonstrated a clear survival benefit for any antibiotic. Doxycycline (100 mg every 12 hours orally or intravenously), penicillin (eg, 1.5 million units every 6 hours intravenously), and ceftriaxone (1 g daily intravenously) are used in severe leptospirosis. Jarisch–Herxheimer reactions may occur (see Syphilis, above). Although therapy for mild disease is controversial, most clinicians treat with doxycycline, 100 mg orally twice daily, for 7 days, or amoxicillin 50 mg/kg, divided into three doses daily. Azithromycin is also active, but clinical experience is limited.

▶ Prognosis

Without jaundice, the disease is almost never fatal. With jaundice, the mortality rate is 5% for those under age 30 years and 40% for those over age 60 years.

▶ When to Admit

Patients with jaundice or other evidence of severe disease should be admitted for close monitoring and may require admission to an intensive care unit.

Brett-Major DM et al. Antibiotics for leptospirosis. Cochrane Database Syst Rev. 2012 Feb 15;2:CD008264. [PMID: 22336839]

Guerrier G et al. The Jarisch-Herxheimer reaction in leptospirosis: a systematic review. PLoS One. 2013;8(3):e59266. [PMID: 23555644]

Musso D et al. Laboratory diagnosis of leptospirosis: a challenge. J Microbiol Immunol Infect. 2013 Aug;46(4):245–52. [PMID: 23639380]

Schreier S et al. Leptospirosis: current situation and trends of specific laboratory tests. Expert Rev Clin Immunol. 2013 Mar;9(3):263–80. [PMID: 23445200]

LYME DISEASE (Lyme Borreliosis)

ESSENTIALS OF DIAGNOSIS

▶ Erythema migrans, a flat or slightly raised red lesion that expands with central clearing.

▶ Headache or stiff neck.

▶ Arthralgias, arthritis, and myalgias; arthritis is often chronic and recurrent.

▶ Wide geographic distribution, with most US cases in the Northeast, mid-Atlantic, upper Midwest, and Pacific coastal regions.

General Considerations

This illness, named after the town of Old Lyme, Connecticut, is the most common tick-borne disease in the United States and Europe and is caused by genospecies of the spirochete *B burgdorferi*. In the United States, the causative genospecies is *B burgdorferi senu strictu,* whereas in Europe and Asia *B garinii* and *B afzelii* predominate. Most US cases are reported from the mid-Atlantic, northeastern, and north central regions of the country. The true incidence of Lyme disease is not known for a number of reasons: (1) serologic tests are not standardized (see below); (2) clinical manifestations are nonspecific; and (3) even with reliable testing, serology is insensitive in early disease.

The tick vector of Lyme disease varies geographically and is *Ixodes scapularis* in the northeastern, north central, and mid-Atlantic regions of the United States; *Ixodes pacificus* on the West Coast; *Ixodes ricinus* in Europe; and *Ixodes persulcatus* in Asia. The disease also occurs in Australia. Mice and deer make up the major animal reservoir of *B burgdorferi*, but other rodents and birds may also be infected. Domestic animals such as dogs, cattle, and horses can also develop clinical illness, usually manifested as arthritis.

Under experimental conditions, ticks must feed for 24–36 hours or longer to transmit infections. Most cases are reported in the spring and summer months. Human epidemiologic studies have indicated that the incidence of disease is significantly higher when tick attachment is for longer than 72 hours than if it is < 72 hours, though rare cases have been documented with attachment of < 24 hours. In addition, the percentage of ticks infected varies on a regional basis. In the northeastern and midwestern regions, 15–65% of *I scapularis* ticks are infected with the spirochete; in the western United States, only 2% of *I pacificus* are infected. These are important epidemiologic features in assessing the likelihood that tick exposure will result in disease. Eliciting a history of brushing a tick off the skin (ie, the tick was not feeding) or removing a tick on the same day as exposure (ie, the tick did not feed long enough) decreases the likelihood that infection will develop.

Because the *Ixodes* tick is so small, the bite is usually painless and goes unnoticed. After feeding, the tick drops off in 2–4 days. If a tick is found, it should be removed immediately. The best way to accomplish this is to use a fine-tipped tweezers to pull firmly and repeatedly on the tick's mouth part—not the tick's body—until the tick releases its hold. Saving the tick in a bottle of alcohol for future identification may be useful, especially if symptoms develop.

Clinical Findings

Prior clinical description of Lyme disease divided the illness into three stages: stage 1, flu-like symptoms and a typical skin rash (**erythema migrans**, see Figure 6–28); stage 2, weeks to months later, facial (cranial nerve VII) palsy or meningitis; and stage 3, months to years later, arthritis. The problem with this simplified scheme is that there is a great deal of overlap, and the skin, central nervous system, and musculoskeletal system can be involved early or late. A more accurate classification divides disease into early and late manifestations and specifies whether disease is localized or disseminated.

A. Symptoms and Signs

1. Stage 1, early localized infection—Stage 1 infection is characterized by erythema migrans. About 1 week after the tick bite (range, 3–30 days; median 7–10 days), a flat or slightly raised red lesion appears at the site, which is commonly seen in areas of tight clothing such as the groin, thigh, or axilla. This lesion expands over several days. Although originally described as a lesion that progresses with central clearing ("bulls-eye" lesion), often there is a more homogeneous appearance or even central intensification. About 10–20% of patients either do not have typical skin lesions or the lesions go unnoticed. Most patients with erythema migrans will have a concomitant viral-like illness (the "summer flu") characterized by myalgias, arthralgias, headache, and fatigue. Fever may or may not be present. Even without treatment, the symptoms and signs of erythema migrans resolve in 3–4 weeks. Although the classic lesion of erythema migrans is not difficult to recognize, atypical forms can occur that may lead to misdiagnosis. Chemical reactions to tick and spider bites (these usually recede in 24–48 hours, whereas erythema migrans increases in size in this time period), drug eruptions, urticaria, and staphylococcal and streptococcal cellulitis have been mistaken for erythema migrans. Southern tick–associated rash illness (STARI) has a similar appearance, but it occurs in geographically distinct areas of the United States.

Completely asymptomatic disease, without erythema migrans or flu-like symptoms, can occur but is very uncommon in the United States.

2. Stage 2, early disseminated infection—Up to 50–60% of patients with erythema migrans are bacteremic and within days to weeks of the original infection, secondary skin lesions develop in about 50% of patients. These lesions are similar in appearance to the primary lesion but are usually smaller. Malaise, fatigue, fever, headache (sometimes severe), neck pain, and generalized achiness are common with the skin lesions. Most symptoms are transient, although fatigue may persist for months. After hematogenous spread, the organism may sequester itself in certain areas and produce focal symptoms. Some patients experience cardiac (4–10% of patients) or neurologic (10–15% of patients) manifestations. Cardiac involvement includes myopericarditis, with atrial or ventricular arrhythmias and heart block. Neurologic manifestations include both the central and peripheral nervous systems. The most common central nervous system manifestation is an aseptic meningitis with mild headache and neck stiffness. The most common peripheral manifestation is a cranial neuropathy, ie, facial palsy (usually unilateral but can be bilateral, see Figure 24–2). A sensory or motor radiculopathy and mononeuritis multiplex occur less frequently. Conjunctivitis, keratitis and, rarely, panophthalmitis can also occur. Rarely, skin involvement can be manifested as a cutaneous hypopigmented lesion called a **borrelial lymphocytoma**.

3. Stage 3, late persistent infection—Stage 3 infection occurs months to years after the initial infection and again primarily manifests itself as musculoskeletal, neurologic, and skin disease. In early reports, musculoskeletal complaints developed in up to 60% of patients, but with early recognition and treatment of disease, this has decreased to < 10%. The classic manifestation of late disease is a monarticular or oligoarticular arthritis most commonly affecting the knee or other large weight bearing joints. While these joints may be quite swollen, these patients generally report less pain compared to patients with bacterial septic arthritis. Even if untreated, the arthritis is self-limited, resolving in a few weeks to months. Multiple recurrences are common but are usually less severe than the original disease. Joint fluid reflects an inflammatory arthritis with a mean white blood cell count of 25,000/mcL (0.025/L) with a predominance of neutrophils. Chronic arthritis develops in about 10% of patients. The pathogenesis of chronic Lyme arthritis may be an immunologic phenomenon rather than persistence of infection.

Rarely, the nervous system (both central and peripheral) can be involved in late Lyme disease. In the United States, a subacute encephalopathy, characterized by memory loss, mood changes, and sleep disturbance, is seen. In Europe, a more severe encephalomyelitis caused by *B garinii* is seen and presents with cognitive dysfunction, spastic paraparesis, ataxia, and bladder dysfunction. Peripheral nervous system involvement includes intermittent paresthesias, often in a stocking glove distribution, or radicular pain.

The cutaneous manifestation of late infection, which can occur up to 10 years after infection, is **acrodermatitis chronicum atrophicans**. It has been described mainly in Europe after infection with *B afzelii*, a genospecies that commonly causes disease in Europe but not the United States. There is usually bluish-red discoloration of a distal extremity with associated swelling. These lesions become atrophic and sclerotic with time and eventually resemble localized scleroderma. Cases of diffuse fasciitis with eosinophilia, an entity that resembles scleroderma, have been rarely associated with infection with *B burgdorferi*.

B. Laboratory Findings

The diagnosis of Lyme disease is based on both clinical manifestations and laboratory findings. The National Surveillance Case Definition specifies a person with exposure to a potential tick habitat (within the 30 days just prior to developing erythema migrans) with (1) erythema migrans diagnosed by a physician or (2) at least one late manifestation of the disease and (3) laboratory confirmation as fulfilling the criteria for Lyme disease.

Nonspecific laboratory abnormalities can be seen, particularly in early disease. The most common are an elevated sedimentation rate of > 20 mm/h seen in 50% of cases, and mildly abnormal liver function tests are present in 30%. The abnormal liver function tests are transient and return to normal within a few weeks of treatment. A mild anemia, leukocytosis (11,000–18,000/mcL) (0.011–0.018/L), and microscopic hematuria have been reported in ≤10% of patients.

Laboratory confirmation requires **serologic tests** to detect specific antibodies to *B burgdorferi* in serum, preferably by ELISA and not by indirect immunofluorescence assay (IFA), which is less sensitive and specific and can cause misdiagnosis. A two-test approach is recommended for the diagnosis of active Lyme disease, with all specimens positive or equivocal by ELISA then confirmed with an Western immunoblot assay that can detect both IgM and IgG antibodies. IgM antibody appears first 2–4 weeks after onset of erythema migrans, peaks at 6–8 weeks, and then declines to low levels after 4–6 months of illness. The presence of IgM antibody in patients with prolonged symptoms persisting for several months is likely to be a false-positive result. IgG occurs later (6–8 weeks after onset of disease), peaks at 4–6 months, and may remain elevated at low levels indefinitely despite appropriate therapy and resolution of symptoms. When an Western immunoblot is done during the first 4 weeks of illness, both IgM and IgG should be tested. A positive immunoblot requires that antibodies are detected against two (for IgM) or five (for IgG) specific protein antigens from *B burgdorferi*.

If a patient with suspected early Lyme disease has negative serologic studies, acute and convalescent titers should be obtained since up to 50% of patients with early disease can be antibody negative in the first several weeks of illness. A fourfold rise in antibody titer would be diagnostic of recent infection. In patients with later stages of disease, almost all are antibody positive. False-positive reactions in the ELISA and IFA have been reported in juvenile rheumatoid arthritis, rheumatoid arthritis, systemic lupus erythematosus, infectious mononucleosis, subacute infective endocarditis, syphilis, relapsing fever, leptospirosis, enteroviral and other viral illnesses, and patients with gingival disease (presumably because of cross-reactivity with oral treponemes). False-negative serologic reactions occur early in illness, and antibiotic therapy early in disease can abort subsequent seroconversion.

The diagnosis of late **nervous system Lyme disease** is often difficult since clinical manifestations, such as subtle memory impairment, may be difficult to document. Most patients have a history of previous erythema migrans or monarticular or polyarticular arthritis, and the vast majority have antibody present in serum. When CSF is sampled from patients with encephalopathy, there may be evidence of inflammation (pleocytosis or elevated protein, or both), and localized antibody production, ie, a ratio of CSF to serum antibody of > 1.0. PCR has low sensitivity and is not recommended for routine diagnosis. Elevated CSF levels of the chemokine CXCL13 have been associated with CNS Lyme disease, but they can also occur in other infections such as neurosyphilis. Patients with late disease and peripheral neuropathy almost always have positive serum antibody tests, usually have abnormal electrophysiology tests, and may have abnormal nerve biopsies showing perivascular collections of lymphocytes; however, the CSF is usually normal and does not demonstrate local antibody production.

Caution should be exercised in interpreting serologic tests because they are not subject to national standards, and inter-laboratory variation is a major problem. In addition, some laboratories perform tests that are entirely unreliable and should never be used to support the diagnosis of Lyme disease (eg, the Lyme urinary antigen test, immunofluorescent staining for cell wall–deficient forms of *B burgdorferi*, lymphocyte transformation tests, using PCR on inappropriate specimens such as blood or urine). Finally, testing is often done in patients with nonspecific symptoms such as headache, arthralgia, myalgia, fatigue, and palpitations. Even in endemic areas, the pretest probability of having Lyme disease is low in these patients, and the probability of a false-positive test result is greater than that of a true-positive result. For these reasons, the US Centers for Disease Control and Prevention has established guidelines for laboratory evaluation of patients with suspected Lyme disease:

1. The diagnosis of early Lyme disease is clinical (ie, exposure in an endemic area, with physician-documented erythema migrans), and does *not* require laboratory confirmation. (Tests are often negative at this stage.)

2. Late disease requires objective evidence of clinical manifestations (recurrent brief attacks of monarticular or oligoarticular arthritis of the large joints; lymphocytic meningitis, cranial neuritis [facial palsy], peripheral neuropathy or, rarely, encephalomyelitis—but *not* headache, fatigue, paresthesias, or stiff neck alone; atrioventricular conduction defects with or without myocarditis) and laboratory evidence of disease (two-stage testing with ELISA or IFA followed by Western blot, as described above).

3. Patients with nonspecific symptoms without objective signs of Lyme disease should *not* have serologic testing done. It is in this setting that false-positive tests occur more commonly than true-positive tests.

4. The role of serologic testing in nervous system Lyme disease is unclear, as sensitivity and specificity of CSF serologic tests have not been determined. However, it is rare for a patient to have positive serologic tests on CSF without positive tests on serum (see below).

5. Other tests such as the T cell proliferative assay and urinary antigen detection have not yet been studied well enough to be routinely used.

Cultures for *B burgdorferi* can be performed but are not routine and are usually reserved for clinical studies.

PCR is very specific for detecting the presence of *Borrelia* DNA, but sensitivity is variable and depends on which body fluid is tested, the stage of the disease, and collection and testing technique. In general, PCR is more sensitive than culture, especially in chronic disease. Up to 85% of synovial fluid samples are positive in active arthritis. In contrast, 38% of CSF samples in acute CNS Lyme disease are PCR positive compared with only 25% in chronic CNS disease. However, whether a positive PCR indicates persistence of viable organisms that will respond to further treatment or is a marker for residual DNA (not active infection) has not been clarified. A negative PCR result does not rule out disease.

▶ **Complications**

Based on several observational studies, *B burgdorferi* infection in pregnant women has not been associated with congenital syndromes, unlike other spirochetal illnesses such as syphilis.

Some patients and advocacy groups have claimed either a post-Lyme syndrome (in the presence of positive laboratory tests and after appropriate treatment) or "chronic Lyme disease" in which tests may all be negative. Both entities include nonspecific symptoms such as fatigue, myalgias, and cognitive difficulties (see Prognosis below). Expert groups are in agreement that there are no data to support that ongoing infection is the cause of either syndrome.

▶ **Prevention**

There is no human vaccine currently available. Simple preventive measures such as avoiding tick-infested areas, covering exposed skin with long-sleeved shirts and wearing long trousers tucked into socks, wearing light-colored clothing, using repellents, and inspecting for ticks after exposure will greatly reduce the number of tick bites. Environmental controls directed at limiting ticks on residential property would be helpful, but trying to limit the deer, tick, or white-footed mouse populations over large areas is not feasible.

Prophylactic antibiotics following tick bites is recommended in certain high-risk situations if all of the following criteria are met: (1) a tick identified as an adult or nymphal *I scapularis* has been attached for at least 36 hours; (2) prophylaxis can be started within 72 hours of the time the tick was removed; (3) more than 20% of ticks in the area are known to be infected with *B burgdorferi*; and (4) there is no contraindication to the use of doxycycline (not pregnant, age > 8 years, not allergic). The drug of choice for prophylaxis is a single 200-mg dose of doxycycline. If doxycycline is contraindicated, no prophylaxis should be given and the patient should be closely monitored for early disease, since short course prophylactic therapy with other agents has not been studied, and if early disease does develop, appropriate therapy is very effective in preventing long-term sequelae. Individuals who have removed ticks (including those who have had prophylaxis) should be monitored carefully for 30 days for possible coinfections.

▶ **Coinfections**

Lyme disease, babesiosis (see Chapter 35), and human granulocytic anaplasmosis (formerly human granulocytic ehrlichiosis) (see Chapter 32) are endemic in similar areas of the country and are transmitted by the same tick, *I scapularis*. Coinfection with two or even all three of these organisms can occur, causing a clinical picture that is not "classic" for any of these diseases. The presence of erythema migrans is highly suggestive of Lyme disease, whereas flu-like symptoms without rash are more suggestive of babesiosis or anaplasmosis. The complete blood count is usually normal in Lyme disease, but in patients with Lyme disease and babesiosis, anemia and thrombocytopenia are more common. Patients with Lyme disease and anaplasmosis are more likely to have leukopenia. Coinfection should be considered and excluded in patients who have persistent high fevers 48 hours after starting appropriate therapy for Lyme disease; in patients with persistent symptoms despite resolution of rash; and in those with anemia, leukopenia, or thrombocytopenia.

Even in patients with documented Lyme disease, immunity is not complete. Reinfection, although uncommon, is predominantly seen in patients successfully treated for early disease (erythema migrans) who do not develop antibody titers. Clinical manifestations and serologic response is similar to an initial infection.

▶ Treatment

Present recommendations for therapy are outlined in Table 34–4. For erythema migrans, antibiotic therapy shortens the duration of rash and prevents late sequelae. Doxycycline is most commonly used and has the advantage of being active against *Anaplasma phagocytophilum* (formerly *Ehrlichia*). Amoxicillin is also effective and is recommended for pregnant or lactating women and for those who cannot tolerate doxycycline. Cefuroxime axetil, is as

Table 34–4. Treatment of Lyme disease.

Manifestations	Drug and Dosage
Tick bite	No treatment in most circumstances (see text); observe
Erythema migrans	Doxycycline, 100 mg orally twice daily, or amoxicillin, 500 mg orally three times daily, or cefuroxime axetil, 500 mg orally twice daily—all for 2–3 weeks
Neurologic disease	
Facial palsy (without meningitis)	Doxycycline, amoxicillin, or cefuroxime axetil as above for 2–3 weeks
Other central nervous system disease	Ceftriaxone, 2 g intravenously once daily, or penicillin G, 18–24 million units daily intravenously in six divided doses, or cefotaxime, 2 g intravenously every 8 hours—all for 2–4 weeks
Cardiac disease	
Atrioventricular block and myopericarditis[1]	An oral or parenteral (if more severe disease) regimen as described above can be used
Arthritis	
Oral dosage	Doxycycline, amoxicillin, or cefuroxime axetil as above for 28 days (see text)
Parenteral dosage	Ceftriaxone, cefotaxime, or penicillin G as above for 2–4 weeks
Acrodermatitis chronicum atrophicans	Doxycycline, amoxicillin, or cefuroxime axetil as above for 3 weeks
"Chronic Lyme disease" or "post-Lyme disease syndrome"	Symptomatic therapy; prolonged antibiotics are not recommended

[1]Symptomatic patients, those with second- or third-degree block and those with first-degree block with a PR interval ≥ 300 milliseconds should be hospitalized for observation.

effective as doxycycline, but because of its cost it should be considered an alternative choice for those who cannot tolerate doxycycline or amoxicillin or for those in whom the drugs are contraindicated. Erythromycin and azithromycin are less effective, associated with higher rates of relapse, and are not recommended as first-line therapy.

Isolated facial palsy (without meningitis or peripheral neuropathy) can be treated with doxycycline, amoxicillin, or cefuroxime axetil for 2–3 weeks. Although therapy does not affect the rate of resolution of the cranial neuropathy, it does prevent development of late manifestations of disease.

The need for a lumbar puncture in patients with seventh nerve palsy is controversial. Some clinicians perform lumbar puncture on all patients with facial palsy and others only if there are symptoms or signs of meningitis. If meningitis is present, therapy with a parenteral antibiotic is indicated. Ceftriaxone is most commonly used, but penicillin is equally efficacious. In European countries, doxycycline 400 mg/d orally for 14 days is frequently used and is comparable in efficacy to ceftriaxone.

Patients with atrioventricular block or myopericarditis (or both) can be treated with either oral or parenteral agents for 2–3 weeks. Hospitalization and observation is indicated for symptomatic patients, those with second- or third-degree block, and those with first-degree block with a PR interval ≥ 300 milliseconds. Once stabilized, hospitalized patients can be transitioned to one of the oral regimens to complete therapy.

Therapy of arthritis is difficult because some patients do not respond to any therapy, and those who do respond may do so slowly. Oral agents (doxycycline, amoxicillin, or cefuroxime axetil) are as effective as intravenous regimens (ceftriaxone, cefotaxime, or penicillin). A reasonable approach to the patient with Lyme arthritis is to start with oral therapy for 28 days, and if this fails (persistent or recurrent joint swelling), to re-treat with an oral regimen for 28 days or switch to an intravenous regimen for 2–4 weeks. If arthritis persists after re-treatment, symptomatic therapy with nonsteroidal anti-inflammatory drugs is recommended. For severe refractory pain, synovectomy may be required.

Based on the limited published data, therapy of Lyme disease in pregnancy should be the same as therapy in other patients with the exception that doxycycline should not be used.

Clinicians may encounter patients with nonspecific symptoms (such as fatigue and myalgias) and positive serologic tests for Lyme disease who request (or demand) therapy for their illness. It is important in managing these patients to remember (1) that nonspecific symptoms alone are not diagnostic; (2) that serologic tests are fraught with difficulty (as noted above), and in areas where disease prevalence is low, false-positive serologic tests are much more common than true-positive tests; and (3) that parenteral therapy with ceftriaxone for 2–4 weeks is costly and has been associated with significant adverse effects, including cholelithiasis and *Clostridium difficile* colitis. Parenteral therapy should be reserved for those most likely to benefit, ie, those with cutaneous, neurologic, cardiac, or rheumatic manifestations that are characteristic of Lyme disease.

Prognosis

Most patients respond to appropriate therapy with prompt resolution of symptoms within 4 weeks. True treatment failures are thus uncommon, and in most cases re-treatment or prolonged treatment of Lyme disease is instituted because of misdiagnosis or misinterpretation of serologic results (both IgG and IgM antibodies can persist for prolonged periods despite adequate therapy) rather than inadequate therapy or response. Prolonged courses of antibiotic therapy for nonspecific symptoms that persist after completion of appropriate assessment (and treatment, if necessary) for Lyme disease is not recommended.

The long-term outcome of adult patients with Lyme disease is generally favorable, but some patients have chronic complaints. Joint pain, memory impairment, and poor functional status secondary to pain are common subjective complaints in patients with Lyme disease, but physical examination and neurocognitive testing fail to document the presence of these symptoms as objective sequelae. Similarly, in highly endemic areas, patients with a diagnosis of Lyme disease commonly complain of pain, fatigue, and an inability to perform certain physical activities when followed for several years. However, these complaints occur just as commonly in age-matched controls without a history of Lyme disease. Attempts to document chronic cardiac disease in patients treated for Lyme disease also have been unsuccessful. The long-term outcome of treated nervous system Lyme disease is favorable, with complete recovery in 75% of patients. Of the remaining individuals, only 12% had sequelae that affected their daily activities.

When to Refer

Consultation with an infectious diseases specialist with experience in diagnosing and treating Lyme disease can be helpful in atypical or prolonged cases.

When to Admit

Admission for parenteral antibiotics is indicated for any patient with symptomatic central nervous system or cardiac disease as well as those with second- or third-degree atrioventricular block, or first-degree block with a PR interval $\geq$ 300 milliseconds.

Halperin JJ et al. Common misconceptions about Lyme disease. Am J Med. 2013 Mar;126(3):264.e1–7. [PMID: 23321431]

Stanek G et al. Lyme borreliosis. Lancet. 2012 Feb 4; 379(9814):461–73. [PMID: 21903253]

Wright WF et al. Diagnosis and management of Lyme disease. Am Fam Physician. 2012 Jun 1;85(11):1086–93. [PMID: 22962880]

Protozoal & Helminthic Infections

Philip J. Rosenthal, MD

PROTOZOAL INFECTIONS

AFRICAN TRYPANOSOMIASIS
(Sleeping Sickness)

ESSENTIALS OF DIAGNOSIS

► Exposure to tsetse flies; chancre at bite site uncommon.

► **Hemolymphatic disease:** Irregular fever, headache, joint pain, rash, edema, lymphadenopathy.

► **Meningoencephalitic disease:** Somnolence, severe headache, progressing to coma.

► Trypanosomes in blood or lymph node aspirates; positive serologic tests.

► Trypanosomes and increased white cells and protein in cerebrospinal fluid.

General Considerations

African trypanosomiasis is caused by the hemoflagellates *Trypanosoma brucei rhodesiense* and *Trypanosoma brucei gambiense*. The organisms are transmitted by bites of tsetse flies (genus *Glossina*), which inhabit shaded areas along streams and rivers. Trypanosomes ingested in a blood meal develop over 18–35 days in the fly; when the fly feeds again on a mammalian host, the infective stage is injected. Human disease occurs in rural areas of sub-Saharan Africa from south of the Sahara to about 30 degrees south latitude. *T b gambiense* causes West African trypanosomiasis, and is transmitted in the moist sub-Saharan savannas and forests of west and central Africa. *T b rhodesiense* causes East African trypanosomiasis, and is transmitted in the savannas of east and southeast Africa.

T b rhodesiense infection is primarily a zoonosis of game animals and cattle; humans are infected sporadically. Humans are the principal mammalian host for *T b gambiense*, but domestic animals can be infected. The largest number of cases is in the Democratic Republic of the Congo. The incidence of trypanosomiasis is probably decreasing, with estimates of 50,000–70,000 cases and 48,000 deaths annually, the large majority due to *T b gambiense*, leading to the loss of 1.5 million disability-adjusted life years. Infections are rare among travelers, including visitors to game parks.

► Clinical Findings

A. Symptoms and Signs

1. West African trypanosomiasis—Chancres at the site of the bite are uncommon. After an asymptomatic period that may last for months, **hemolymphatic disease** presents with fever, headache, myalgias, arthralgias, weight loss, and lymphadenopathy, with discrete, nontender, rubbery nodes, referred to as Winterbottom sign when in a posterior cervical distribution. Other common signs are mild splenomegaly, transient edema, and a pruritic erythematous rash. Febrile episodes may be broken by afebrile periods of up to several weeks. The hemolymphatic stage progresses over months to **meningoencephalitic disease**, with somnolence, irritability, personality changes, severe headache, and parkinsonian symptoms progressing to coma and death.

2. East African trypanosomiasis—Chancres at the bite site are more commonly recognized with *T b rhodesiense* infection, with a painful lesion of 3–10 cm and regional lymphadenopathy that appears about 48 hours after the tsetse fly bite and lasts 2–4 weeks. East African disease follows a much more acute course, with the onset of symptoms usually within a few days of the insect bite. The hemolymphatic stage includes intermittent fever and rash, but lymphadenopathy is less common than with West African disease. Myocarditis can cause tachycardia and death due to arrhythmias or heart failure. If untreated, East African trypanosomiasis progresses over weeks to months to meningoencephalitic disease, somnolence, coma, and death.

B. Laboratory Findings

Diagnosis can be difficult, and definitive diagnosis requires identification of trypanosomes. Microscopic examination of fluid expressed from a chancre or lymph node may show motile trypanosomes or, in fixed specimens, parasites stained with Giemsa. During the **hemolymphatic stage,** detection of parasites in Giemsa-stained blood smears is common in East African disease but difficult in West African disease. Serial specimens should be examined, since parasitemias vary greatly over time. **Meningoencephalitic (or second stage) disease** is defined by the World Health Organization (WHO) as cerebrospinal fluid (CSF) showing at least five mononuclear cells per microliter, elevated protein, or presence of trypanosomes. Concentration techniques can aid identification of parasites in blood or CSF. Serologic tests are also available. The simple card agglutination test for trypanosomes (CATT) has excellent sensitivity and specificity for West African disease and can be performed in the field; however, the diagnosis should be confirmed by identification of the parasites. Polymerase chain reaction (PCR) and related molecular diagnostic tests appear to have excellent sensitivity and specificity, but these are not yet standardized or routinely available.

▶ **Treatment**

Detection of trypanosomes is a prerequisite for treatment of African trypanosomiasis because of the significant toxicity of most available therapies. Treatment recommendations depend on the type of trypanosomiasis (Table 35–1), which is determined by geography, and stage of disease, which requires examination of CSF.

A. West African Trypanosomiasis

1. Early stage infection—Pentamidine (4 mg/kg intramuscularly or intravenously every day or every other day for 7 days) is used to treat infection that does not involve the central nervous system (CNS). The side effects of pentamidine include immediate hypotension; tachycardia; gastrointestinal symptoms during administration; sterile abscesses; and pancreatic (hypoglycemia), liver, and kidney abnormalities. An alternate drug is eflornithine (100 mg/kg/d intravenously every 6 hours for 14 days).

2. Late stage infection—Eflornithine is the drug of choice for infection that involves the CNS; the dosage is the same as that used to treat early disease. Eflornithine has less toxicity than older trypanocidal drugs, but it can cause gastrointestinal symptoms and bone marrow suppression and is limited by lack of availability and the need for infusions four times daily. Alternative therapies are melarsoprol (see below) or nifurtimox (5 mg/kg orally three times per day for 14 days), and drug combinations (eg, oral nifurtimox plus twice-daily eflornithine) may offer improved efficacy over monotherapies, with simplified regimens and decreased toxicity. Some authorities now consider nifurtimox-eflornithine combination therapy to be the standard of care for late-stage West African trypanosomiasis.

B. East African Trypanosomiasis

Pentamidine and eflornithine are not reliably effective, and early disease is treated with suramin. The dosing regimens of suramin vary (eg, 100–200 mg test dose, then 20 mg/kg [maximum 1 g] intravenously on days 1, 3, 7, 14, and 21 or weekly for 5 doses). Suramin toxicities include vomiting and, rarely, seizures and shock during infusions as well as subsequent fever, rash, headache, neuropathy, and kidney and bone marrow dysfunction.

Suramin does not enter the CNS, so East African trypanosomiasis involving the CNS is treated with melarsoprol (three series of 3.6 mg/kg/d intravenously for 3 days, with 7-day breaks between the series or a 10-day intravenous course with 0.6 mg/kg on day 1, 1.2 mg/kg on day 2, and 1.8 mg/kg on days 3–10). Melarsoprol also acts against West African disease, but eflornithine is preferred due to its lower toxicity. Immediate side effects of melarsoprol include fever and gastrointestinal symptoms. The most important side effect is a reactive encephalopathy that can progress to seizures, coma, and death. To help avoid this side effect, corticosteroids are coadministered (recommended regimens include dexamethasone 1 mg/kg/d intravenously for 2–3 days or oral prednisolone 1 mg/kg/d for 5 days, and then 0.5 mg/kg/d until treatment completion). In addition, increasing resistance to melarsoprol is a serious concern. Suramin and melarsoprol are available in the United States from the CDC Drug Service (www.cdc.gov/laboratory/drugservice).

▶ **Prevention & Control**

Individual prevention in endemic areas should include long sleeves and pants, insect repellents, and mosquito nets. Control programs focusing on vector elimination and treatment of infected persons and animals have shown good success in many areas but suffer from limited resources.

Table 35–1. Treatment of African trypanosomiasis.

Disease	Stage	Treatment	
		First Line	Alternative
West African	Early	Pentamidine	Suramin Eflornithine
	CNS involvement	Eflornithine	Melarsoprol Nifurtimox
East African	Early CNS involvement	Suramin Melarsoprol	Pentamidine

CNS, central nervous system.

Barrett MP et al. Management of trypanosomiasis and leishmaniasis. Br Med Bull. 2012;104:175–96. [PMID: 23137768]
Brun R et al. Human African trypanosomiasis. Infect Dis Clin North Am. 2012 Jun;26(2):261–73. [PMID: 22632638]
Kennedy PG. Clinical features, diagnosis, and treatment of human African trypanosomiasis (sleeping sickness). Lancet Neurol. 2013 Feb;12(2):186–94. [PMID: 23260189]

AMERICAN TRYPANOSOMIASIS
(Chagas Disease)

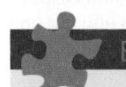

Acute stage
- ▶ Inflammatory lesion at inoculation site.
- ▶ Fever.
- ▶ Hepatosplenomegaly; lymphadenopathy.
- ▶ Myocarditis.
- ▶ Parasites in blood is diagnostic.

Chronic stage
- ▶ Heart failure, cardiac arrhythmias.
- ▶ Thromboembolism.
- ▶ Megaesophagus; megacolon.
- ▶ Serologic tests are usually diagnostic.

▶ General Considerations

Chagas disease is caused by *Trypanosoma cruzi*, a protozoan parasite found only in the Americas; it infects wild animals and to a lesser extent humans from southern South America to the southern United States. An estimated 8–10 million people are infected, mostly in rural areas. Control efforts in endemic countries have decreased disease incidence to about 40,000 new infections and 12,500 deaths per year. The disease is often acquired in childhood. In many countries in South America, Chagas disease is the most important cause of heart disease. In the United States, the vector is found, some animals are infected, and a few instances of local transmission have been reported.

T cruzi is transmitted by reduviid (triatomine) bugs infected by ingesting blood from animals or humans who have circulating trypanosomes. Multiplication occurs in the digestive tract of the bug and infective forms are eliminated in feces. Infection in humans occurs when the parasite penetrates the skin through the bite wound, mucous membranes, or the conjunctiva. Transmission can also occur by blood transfusion, organ or bone marrow transplantation, congenital transfer, or ingestion of food contaminated with vector feces. From the bloodstream, *T cruzi* invades many cell types but has a predilection for myocardium, smooth muscle, and CNS glial cells. Multiplication causes cellular destruction, inflammation, and fibrosis, with progressive disease over decades.

▶ Clinical Findings

A. Symptoms and Signs

As many as 70% of infected persons remain asymptomatic. The **acute stage** is seen principally in children and lasts 1–2 months. The earliest findings are at the site of inoculation either in the eye—Romaña sign (unilateral edema, conjunctivitis, and lymphadenopathy)—or in the skin—a chagoma (swelling with local lymphadenopathy). Subsequent findings include fever, malaise, headache, mild hepatosplenomegaly, and generalized lymphadenopathy. Acute myocarditis and meningoencephalitis are rare but can be fatal.

An asymptomatic **latent period (indeterminate phase)** may last for life, but symptomatic disease develops in 10–30% of infected individuals, commonly many years after infection.

Chronic Chagas disease generally manifests as abnormalities in cardiac and smooth muscle. Cardiac disease includes arrhythmias, heart failure, and embolic disease. Smooth muscle abnormalities lead to mega-esophagus and megacolon, with dysphagia, regurgitation, aspiration, constipation, and abdominal pain. These findings can be complicated by superinfections. In immunosuppressed persons, including AIDS patients and transplant recipients, latent Chagas disease may reactivate; findings have included brain abscesses and meningoencephalitis.

B. Diagnostic Testing

Diagnosis should be considered in persons with suggestive findings who have resided in an endemic area. The diagnosis is made by detecting parasites. With **acute infection**, evaluation of fresh blood or buffy coats may show motile trypanosomes, and fixed preparations may show Giemsa-stained parasites. Trypanosomes may be identified in lymph nodes, bone marrow, or pericardial or spinal fluid. When initial tests are unrevealing in a suspicious case, xenodiagnosis using laboratory vectors, laboratory culture, or animal inoculation may provide a diagnosis, but these methods are expensive and slow.

Chronic Chagas disease is usually diagnosed serologically. Many different serologic assays are available, but sensitivity and specificity are not ideal, so confirmatory assays are advised after an initial positive test, as is standard for blood bank testing in South America. PCR may offer an important new modality for diagnosis, but assays are not standardized, and reliability and sensitivity of assays has been disappointing.

▶ Treatment

Treatment is inadequate because the two drugs used, benznidazole and nifurtimox, often cause severe side effects, must be used for long periods, and are ineffective against chronic infection. In acute and congenital infections, the drugs can reduce the duration and severity of infection, but cure is achieved in only about 70% of patients. During the chronic phase of infection, although parasitemia may disappear in up to 70% of patients, treatment does not clearly alter the progression of the disease. Nevertheless, there is general consensus that treatment should be considered in all *T cruzi*-infected persons regardless of clinical status or time since infection. In particular, treatment is recommended for acute, congenital, and reactivated infections and for children and young adults with chronic disease. Both benznidazole and nifurtimox are available in the United States from the CDC Drug Service (www.cdc.gov/laboratory/drugservice).

Benznidazole is generally preferred due to better efficacy and safety profiles; problems with drug availability have been resolved. It is given orally at a dosage of 5 mg/kg/d in two divided doses for 60 days. Its side effects include granulocytopenia, rash, and peripheral neuropathy. Nifurtimox is given orally in daily doses of 8–10 mg/kg in four divided doses after meals for 90–120 days. Side effects include gastrointestinal (anorexia, vomiting) and neurologic (headaches, ataxia, insomnia, seizures) symptoms, which appear to be reversible and to lessen with dosage reduction. Patients with chronic Chagas disease may also benefit from antiarrhythmic therapy, standard therapy for heart failure, and conservative and surgical management of megaesophagus and megacolon.

▶ Prevention & Control

In South America, a major eradication program based on improved housing, use of residual pyrethroid insecticides and pyrethroid-impregnated bed curtains, and screening of blood donors has achieved striking reductions in new infections. In endemic areas and ideally in donors from endemic areas, blood should not be used for transfusion unless at least two serologic tests are negative.

Bern C. Antitrypanosomal therapy for chronic Chagas' disease. N Engl J Med. 2011 Jun 30;364(26):2527–34. [PMID: 21714649]
Rassi A Jr et al. American trypanosomiasis (Chagas disease). Infect Dis Clin North Am. 2012 Jun;26(2):275–91. [PMID: 22632639]
Ribeiro AL et al. Diagnosis and management of Chagas disease and cardiomyopathy. Nat Rev Cardiol. 2012 Oct;9(10):576–89. [PMID: 22847166]

LEISHMANIASIS

ESSENTIALS OF DIAGNOSIS

▶ Sand fly bite in an endemic area.

▶ **Visceral leishmaniasis:** irregular fever, progressive hepatosplenomegaly, pancytopenia, wasting.

▶ **Cutaneous leishmaniasis:** chronic, painless, moist ulcers or dry nodules.

▶ **Mucocutaneous leishmaniasis:** destructive nasopharyngeal lesions.

▶ Amastigotes in macrophages in aspirates, touch preparations, or biopsies.

▶ Positive culture, serologic tests, PCR, or skin test.

▶ General Considerations

Leishmaniasis is a zoonosis transmitted by bites of sand flies of the genus *Lutzomyia* in the Americas and *Phlebotomus* elsewhere. When sand flies feed on an infected host, the parasitized cells are ingested with the blood meal. Leishmaniasis is caused by about 20 species of *Leishmania*; taxonomy is complex. Clinical syndromes are generally dictated by the infecting species, but some species can cause more than one syndrome.

An estimated 350 million persons are at risk for leishmaniasis. The estimated annual incidence of disease is 1–1.5 million new cases of cutaneous and 500,000 cases of visceral disease, leading to an estimated 50,000–60,000 deaths. The incidence of disease is increasing in many areas.

Visceral leishmaniasis (kala azar) is caused mainly by *Leishmania donovani* in the Indian subcontinent and East Africa; *Leishmania infantum* in the Mediterranean, Middle East, China, parts of Asia, and Horn of Africa; and *Leishmania chagasi* in South and Central America. Other species may occasionally cause visceral disease. Over 90% of cases occur in five countries: India, Bangladesh, Nepal, Sudan, and Brazil. In each locale, the disease has particular clinical and epidemiologic features. The incubation period is usually 4–6 months (range: 10 days to 24 months). Without treatment, the fatality rate reaches 90%. Early diagnosis and treatment reduces mortality to 2–5%.

Old World cutaneous leishmaniasis is caused mainly by *Leishmania tropica*, *Leishmania major*, and *Leishmania aethiopica* in the Mediterranean, Middle East, Africa, Central Asia, and Indian subcontinent. **New World cutaneous leishmaniasis** is caused by *Leishmania mexicana*, *Leishmania amazonensis*, and the species listed below for mucocutaneous disease in Central and South America. **Mucocutaneous leishmaniasis** (espundia) occurs in lowland forest areas of the Americas and is caused by *Leishmania braziliensis*, *Leishmania panamensis*, and *Leishmania peruviana* .

▶ Clinical Findings

A. Symptoms and Signs

1. Visceral leishmaniasis (kala azar)—Most infections are subclinical, but a small number progress to full-blown disease. A local nonulcerating nodule at the site of the sand fly bite may precede systemic manifestations but usually is inapparent. The onset of illness may be acute, within 2 weeks of infection, or insidious. Symptoms and signs include fever, chills, sweats, weakness, anorexia, weight loss, cough, and diarrhea. The spleen progressively becomes greatly enlarged, firm, and nontender. The liver is somewhat enlarged, and generalized lymphadenopathy may occur. Hyperpigmentation of skin can be seen, leading to the name kala azar ("black fever"). Other signs include skin lesions, petechiae, gingival bleeding, jaundice, edema, and ascites. As the disease progresses, severe wasting and malnutrition are seen; death eventually occurs, often due to secondary infections, within months to a few years. Post-kala azar dermal leishmaniasis may appear after apparent cure in the Indian subcontinent and Sudan. It may simulate leprosy, with hypopigmented macules or nodules developing on preexisting lesions. Viscerotropic leishmaniasis has been reported in small numbers of American military personnel in the Middle East, with mild systemic febrile illnesses after *L tropica* infections.

2. Old World and New World cutaneous leishmaniasis—Cutaneous swellings appear 2 weeks to several months after sand fly bites and can be single or multiple. Characteristics of lesions and courses of disease vary depending on the leishmanial species and host immune response.

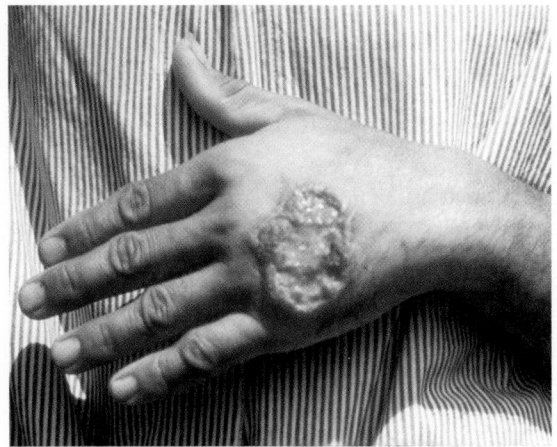

▲ **Figure 35–1.** Skin ulcer due to cutaneous leishmaniasis. (From D. S. Martin, Public Health Image Library, CDC.)

Lesions begin as small papules and develop into nonulcerated dry plaques or large encrusted ulcers with well-demarcated raised and indurated margins (Figure 35–1). Satellite lesions may be present. The lesions are painless unless secondarily infected. Local lymph nodes may be enlarged. Systemic symptoms are uncommon, but fever, constitutional symptoms, and regional lymphadenopathy may be seen. For most species, healing occurs spontaneously in months to a few years, but scarring is common.

Leishmaniasis recidivans is a relapsing form of *L tropica* infection associated with hypersensitivity, in which the primary lesion heals centrally, but spreads laterally, with extensive scarring. **Diffuse cutaneous leishmaniasis** involves spread from a central lesion to local dissemination of nodules and a protracted course. **Disseminated cutaneous leishmaniasis** involves multiple nodular or ulcerated lesions, often with mucosal involvement.

3. Mucocutaneous leishmaniasis (espundia)—In Latin America, mucosal lesions develop in a small percentage of persons infected with *L braziliensis* and some other species, usually months to years after resolution of a cutaneous lesion. Nasal congestion is followed by ulceration of the nasal mucosa and septum, progressing to involvement of the mouth, lips, palate, pharynx, and larynx. Extensive destruction can occur, and secondary bacterial infection is common.

4. Infections in patients with AIDS—Leishmaniasis is an opportunistic infection in persons with AIDS seen in southern Europe and other areas. Visceral leishmaniasis can present late in the course of HIV infection, with fever, hepatosplenomegaly, and pancytopenia. The gastrointestinal tract, respiratory tract, and skin may also be involved.

B. Laboratory Findings

Identifying amastigotes within macrophages in tissue samples provides a definitive diagnosis. In **visceral leishmaniasis,** fine-needle aspiration of the spleen for culture and tissue evaluation is generally safe, and yields a diagnosis in over 95% of cases. Bone marrow aspiration is less sensitive but safer and diagnostic in most cases, and Giemsa-stained buffy coat of peripheral blood may occasionally show organisms. Cultures with media available from the CDC will grow promastigotes within a few days to weeks. PCR can also identify the infection. Serologic tests may facilitate diagnosis, but none are sufficiently sensitive or specific to be used alone. Numerous antibody-based rapid diagnostic tests are available; these have shown good specificity but limitations in sensitivity outside of India. For **cutaneous lesions,** biopsies should be taken from the raised border of a skin lesion, with samples for histopathology, touch preparation, and culture. The histopathology shows inflammation with mononuclear cells. Macrophages filled with amastigotes may be present, especially early in infection. An intradermal leishmanin (Montenegro) skin test is positive in most individuals with cutaneous disease but negative in those with progressive visceral or diffuse cutaneous disease; this test is not approved in the United States. In **mucocutaneous leishmaniasis,** diagnosis is established by detecting amastigotes in scrapings, biopsy preparations, or aspirated tissue fluid, but organisms may be rare. Cultures from these samples may grow organisms. Serologic studies are often negative, but the leishmanin skin test is usually positive.

▶ Treatment

A. Visceral Leishmaniasis

The treatment of choice for visceral leishmaniasis is liposomal amphotericin B (approved by the FDA), which is generally effective and well tolerated but very expensive. Standard dosing is 3 mg/kg/d intravenously on days 1–5, 14, and 21. Conventional amphotericin B deoxycholate, which is much less expensive, is also highly effective but with more toxicity. It is administered as a slow intravenous infusion of 1 mg/kg/d for 15–20 days or 0.5–1 mg/kg every second day for up to 8 weeks. Infusion-related side effects with conventional or liposomal amphotericin B include gastrointestinal symptoms, fever, chills, dyspnea, hypotension, and hepatic and renal toxicity.

Pentavalent antimonials remain the most commonly used drugs to treat leishmaniasis in most areas. Response rates are good outside India, but in India, resistance is a major problem. Two preparations are available, sodium stibogluconate in the United States and many other areas and meglumine antimonate in Latin America and francophone countries; the compounds appear to have comparable activities. In the United States, sodium stibogluconate can be obtained from the CDC Drug Service (www.cdc.gov/laboratory/drugservice).

Treatment with either antimonial is given once daily at a dose of 20 mg/kg/d intravenously (preferred) or intramuscularly for 20 days for cutaneous leishmaniasis and 28 days for visceral or mucocutaneous disease. Toxicity increases over time, with development of gastrointestinal symptoms, fever, headache, myalgias, arthralgias, pancreatitis, and rash. Intramuscular injections can cause sterile abscesses. Monitoring should include serial ECGs, and changes are indications for discontinuation to avoid progression to serious arrhythmias.

Miltefosine is the first oral drug for the treatment of leishmaniasis, and it is registered in India for this indication. It has demonstrated excellent results in India, but after a decade of use, efficacy may be decreasing. It can be administered at a daily oral dose of 2.5 mg/kg in two divided doses for 28 days. A 28-day course of miltefosine (2.5 mg/kg/d) is also effective for the treatment of New World cutaneous leishmaniasis. Vomiting, diarrhea, and elevations in transaminases and kidney function studies are common, but generally short-lived, side effects.

The aminoglycoside paromomycin (11 mg/kg/d intramuscularly for 21 days) was shown to be similarly efficacious to amphotericin B for the treatment of visceral disease in India, where it is approved for this indication. It is much less expensive than liposomal amphotericin B or miltefosine. Paromomycin has shown relatively poor efficacy in Africa. The drug is well tolerated; side effects include ototoxicity and reversible elevations in liver enzymes.

The use of drug combinations to improve treatment efficacy, shorten treatment courses, and reduce the selection of resistant parasites has been actively studied. In India, compared to a standard 30-day (treatment on alternate days) course of amphotericin, noninferior efficacy and decreased adverse events were seen with a single dose of liposomal amphotericin plus a 7-day course of miltefosine, a single dose of liposomal amphotericin plus a 10-day course of paromomycin, or a 10-day course of miltefosine plus paromomycin. In East Africa, compared to a standard 30-day course of sodium stibogluconate, similar efficacy was seen with a 17-day course of sodium stibogluconate plus paromomycin.

B. Cutaneous Leishmaniasis

In the Old World, cutaneous leishmaniasis is generally self-healing over some months and does not metastasize to the mucosa, so it may be justified to withhold treatment in regions without mucocutaneous disease if lesions are small and cosmetically unimportant. Lesions on the face or hands are generally treated. New World leishmaniasis has a greater risk of progression to mucocutaneous disease, so treatment is more often warranted. Standard therapy is with pentavalent antimonials for 20 days, as described above. Other treatments include those discussed above for visceral disease, azole antifungals, and allopurinol. In studies in South America, a 28-day course of miltefosine was superior to a 20-day course of meglumine antimoniate, and oral fluconazole also showed good efficacy. In Tunisia, topical paromomycin for 20 days showed good efficacy. Topical therapy has included intralesional antimony, paromomycin ointment, cryotherapy, local heat, and surgical removal. Diffuse cutaneous leishmaniasis and related chronic skin processes generally respond poorly to therapy.

C. Mucocutaneous Leishmaniasis

Cutaneous infections from regions where parasites include those that cause mucocutaneous disease (eg, *L braziliensis* in parts of Latin America) should all be treated to help prevent disease progression. Treatment of mucocutaneous disease with antimonials is disappointing, with responses in only about 60% in Brazil. Other therapies listed above for visceral leishmaniasis may also be used, although they have not been well studied for this indication.

▶ Prevention & Control

Personal protection measures for avoidance of sand fly bites include use of insect repellants, fine-mesh insect netting, long sleeves and pants, and avoidance of warm shaded areas where flies are common. Disease control measures include destruction of animal reservoir hosts, mass treatment of humans in disease-prevalent areas, residual insecticide spraying in dwellings, limiting contact with dogs and other domesticated animals, and use of permethrin-impregnated collars for dogs.

Ben Salah A et al. Topical paromomycin with or without gentamicin for cutaneous leishmaniasis. N Engl J Med. 2013 Feb 7; 368(6):524–32. [PMID: 23388004]

Goto H et al. Cutaneous and mucocutaneous leishmaniasis. Infect Dis Clin North Am. 2012 Jun;26(2):293–307. [PMID: 22632640]

Murray HW. Leishmaniasis in the United States: treatment in 2012. Am J Trop Med Hyg. 2012 Mar;86(3):434–40. [PMID: 22403313]

Musa A et al. Sodium stibogluconate (SSG) & paromomycin combination compared to SSG for visceral leishmaniasis in East Africa: a randomised controlled trial. PLoS Negl Trop Dis. 2012;6(6):e1674. [PMID: 22724029]

Rubiano LC et al. Noninferiority of miltefosine versus meglumine antimoniate for cutaneous leishmaniasis in children. J Infect Dis. 2012 Feb 15;205(4):684–92. [PMID: 22238470]

Sundar S et al. Efficacy of miltefosine in the treatment of visceral leishmaniasis in India after a decade of use. Clin Infect Dis. 2012 Aug;55(4):543–50. [PMID: 22573856]

van Griensven J et al. Visceral leishmaniasis. Infect Dis Clin North Am. 2012 Jun;26(2):309–22. [PMID: 22632641]

MALARIA

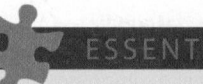

ESSENTIALS OF DIAGNOSIS

▶ Residence or exposure in a malaria-endemic area.

▶ Intermittent attacks of chills, fever, and sweating.

▶ Headache, myalgia, vomiting, splenomegaly; anemia, thrombocytopenia.

▶ Intraerythrocytic parasites identified in thick or thin blood smears.

▶ Complications of falciparum malaria: cerebral malaria, severe anemia, hypotension, noncardiogenic pulmonary edema, acute kidney injury, hypoglycemia, acidosis, and hemolysis.

▶ General Considerations

Malaria is the most important parasitic disease of humans, causing hundreds of millions of illnesses and nearly a million deaths each year. The disease is endemic in most of the tropics, including much of South and Central America, Africa, the Middle East, the Indian subcontinent, Southeast

Asia, and Oceania. Transmission, morbidity, and mortality are greatest in Africa, where most deaths from malaria are in young children. Malaria is also common in travelers from nonendemic areas to the tropics.

Four species of the genus *Plasmodium* classically cause human malaria. *Plasmodium falciparum* is responsible for nearly all severe disease. It is endemic in most malarious areas and is by far the predominant species in Africa. *Plasmodium vivax* is about as common as *P falciparum*, except in Africa. *P vivax* uncommonly causes severe disease, although this outcome may be more common than previously appreciated. *Plasmodium ovale* and *Plasmodium malariae* are much less common causes of disease, and generally do not cause severe illness. *Plasmodium knowlesi*, a parasite of macaque monkeys, is now recognized to cause occasional illnesses, including some severe disease, in humans in Southeast Asia.

Malaria is transmitted by the bite of infected female anopheline mosquitoes. During feeding, mosquitoes inject sporozoites, which circulate to the liver, and rapidly infect hepatocytes, causing asymptomatic liver infection. Merozoites are subsequently released from the liver, and they rapidly infect erythrocytes to begin the asexual erythrocytic stage of infection that is responsible for human disease. Multiple rounds of erythrocytic development, with production of merozoites that invade additional erythrocytes, lead to large numbers of circulating parasites and clinical illness. Some erythrocytic parasites also develop into sexual gametocytes, which are infectious to mosquitoes, allowing completion of the life cycle and infection of others.

Malaria may uncommonly be transmitted from mother to infant (congenital malaria), by blood transfusion, and in nonendemic areas by mosquitoes infected after biting infected immigrants or travelers. In *P vivax* and *P ovale*, parasites also form dormant liver hypnozoites, which are not killed by most drugs, allowing subsequent relapses of illness after initial elimination of erythrocytic infections. For all plasmodial species, parasites may recrudesce following initial clinical improvement after suboptimal therapy.

In highly endemic regions, where people are infected repeatedly, antimalarial immunity prevents severe disease in most older children and adults. However, young children, who are relatively nonimmune, are at high risk for severe disease from *P falciparum* infection, and this population is responsible for most deaths from malaria. Pregnant women are also at increased risk for severe falciparum malaria. In areas with lower endemicity, individuals of all ages commonly present with uncomplicated or severe malaria. Travelers, who are generally nonimmune, are at high risk for severe disease from falciparum malaria at any age.

Clinical Findings

A. Symptoms and Signs

An acute attack of malaria typically begins with a prodrome of headache and fatigue, followed by fever. A classic malarial paroxysm includes chills, high fever, and then sweats. Patients may appear to be remarkably well between febrile episodes. Fevers are usually irregular, especially early in the illness, but without therapy may become regular, with 48- (*P vivax* and *P ovale*) or 72-hour (*P malariae*) cycles, especially with non-falciparum disease. Headache, malaise, myalgias, arthralgias, cough, chest pain, abdominal pain, anorexia, nausea, vomiting, and diarrhea are common. Seizures may represent simple febrile convulsions or evidence of severe neurologic disease. Physical findings may be absent or include signs of anemia, jaundice, splenomegaly, and mild hepatomegaly. Rash and lymphadenopathy are not typical in malaria, and thus suggestive of another cause of fever.

In the developed world, it is imperative that all persons with suggestive symptoms, in particular fever, who have traveled in an endemic area be evaluated for malaria. The risk for falciparum malaria is greatest within 2 months of return from travel; other species may cause disease many months—and occasionally more than a year—after return from an endemic area.

Severe malaria is characterized by signs of severe illness, organ dysfunction, or a high parasite load (peripheral parasitemia > 5% or > 200,000 parasites/mcL). It is principally a result of *P falciparum* infection because this species uniquely infects erythrocytes of all ages and mediates the sequestration of infected erythrocytes in small blood vessels, thereby evading clearance of infected erythrocytes by the spleen.

Severe falciparum malaria can include dysfunction of any organ system, including neurologic abnormalities progressing to alterations in consciousness, repeated seizures, and coma (cerebral malaria); severe anemia; hypotension and shock; noncardiogenic pulmonary edema and the acute respiratory distress syndrome; acute kidney injury due to acute tubular necrosis or, less commonly, severe hemolysis; hypoglycemia; acidosis; hemolysis with jaundice; hepatic dysfunction; retinal hemorrhages and other fundoscopic abnormalities; bleeding abnormalities, including disseminated intravascular coagulation; and secondary bacterial infections, including pneumonia and *Salmonella* bacteremia. In the developing world, severe malaria and deaths from the disease are mostly in young children, in particular from cerebral malaria and severe anemia. Cerebral malaria is a consequence of a single severe infection while severe anemia follows multiple malarial infections, intestinal helminths, and nutritional deficiencies. In a large trial of African children, acidosis, impaired consciousness, convulsions, renal impairment, and underlying chronic illness were associated with poor outcome.

Uncommon disorders resulting from immunologic responses to chronic infection are massive splenomegaly and, with *P malariae* infection, immune complex glomerulopathy with nephrotic syndrome. HIV-infected individuals are at increased risk for malaria and for severe disease, in particular with advanced immunodeficiency.

B. Laboratory Findings

Giemsa-stained blood smears remain the mainstay of diagnosis (Figures 35–2 through 35–5), although other routine stains (eg, Wright stain) will also demonstrate parasites.

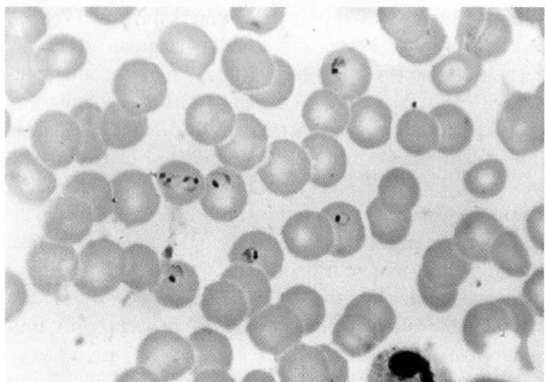

▲ **Figure 35–2.** Thin film Giemsa-stained micrograph with *Plasmodium falciparum* ring forms. (From Steven Glenn, Laboratory & Consultation Division, Public Health Image Library, CDC.)

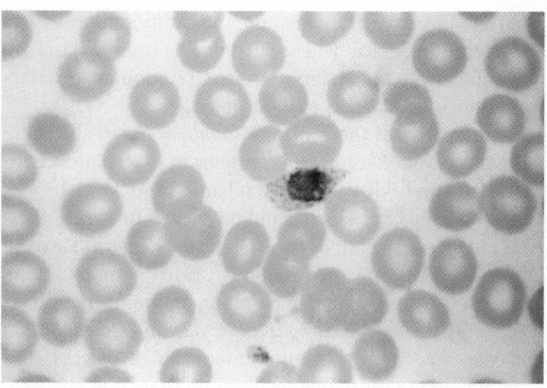

▲ **Figure 35–5.** Thin film Giemsa-stained micrograph with *Plasmodium ovale* trophozoite. (From Steven Glenn, Laboratory & Consultation Division, Public Health Image Library, CDC.)

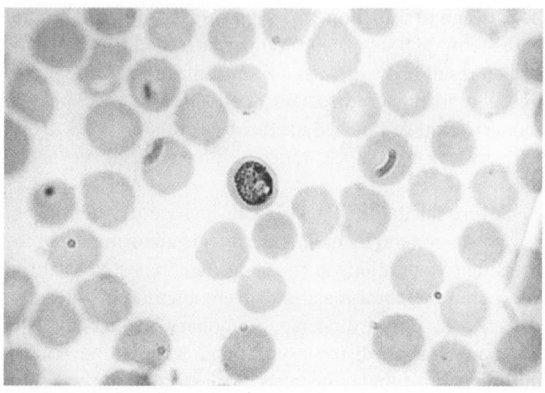

▲ **Figure 35–3.** Thin film Giemsa-stained micrograph with *Plasmodium malariae* trophozoite. (From Steven Glenn, Laboratory & Consultation Division, Public Health Image Library, CDC.)

Thick smears provide efficient evaluation of large volumes of blood, but thin smears are simpler for inexperienced personnel and better for discrimination of parasite species. Single smears are usually positive in infected individuals, although parasitemias may be very low in nonimmune individuals. If illness is suspected, repeating smears in 8- to 24-hour intervals is appropriate. The severity of malaria correlates only loosely with the quantity of infecting parasites, but high parasitemias (especially > 10–20% of erythrocytes infected or > 200,000–500,000 parasites/mcL) or the presence of malarial pigment (a breakdown product of hemoglobin) in > 5% of neutrophils are associated with a particularly poor prognosis.

A second means of diagnosis is rapid diagnostic tests to identify circulating plasmodial antigens with a simple "dipstick" format. These tests are not well standardized but are widely available. At best, they offer sensitivity and specificity near that of high-quality blood smear analysis and are simpler to perform.

Serologic tests indicate history of disease but are not useful for diagnosis of acute infection. PCR is highly sensitive but not available for routine diagnosis. In immune populations, highly sensitive tests, such as PCR, have limited value because subclinical infections, which are of uncertain significance and not routinely treated, are common.

Other diagnostic findings with uncomplicated malaria include thrombocytopenia, anemia, leukocytosis or leukopenia, liver function abnormalities, and hepatosplenomegaly. Severe malaria can present with the laboratory abnormalities expected for the advanced organ dysfunction discussed above.

▶ **Treatment**

Malaria is the most common cause of fever in much of the tropics and in travelers seeking medical attention after return from endemic areas. Fevers are often treated presumptively in endemic areas, but ideally, treatment should follow definitive diagnosis, especially in non-immune individuals.

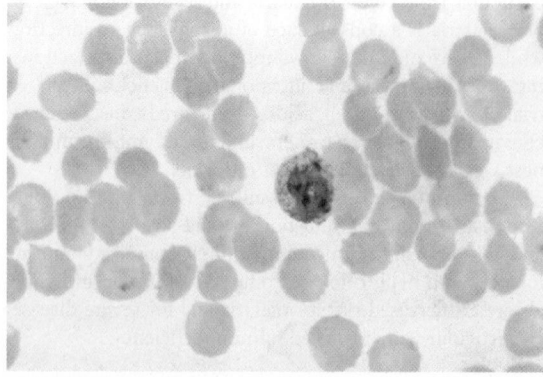

▲ **Figure 35–4.** Thin film Giemsa-stained micrograph with *Plasmodium vivax* schizont. (From Steven Glenn, Laboratory & Consultation Division, Public Health Image Library, CDC.)

Table 35–2. Major antimalarial drugs.

Drug	Class	Use
Chloroquine	4-Aminoquinoline	Treatment and chemoprophylaxis of infection with sensitive parasites
Amodiaquine[1]	4-Aminoquinoline	Treatment of *Plasmodium falciparum*, optimally in fixed combination with artesunate
Piperaquine[1]	4-Aminoquinoline	Treatment of *P falciparum* in fixed combination with dihydroartemisinin
Quinine	Quinoline methanol	Oral and intravenous[1] (for severe infections) treatment of *P falciparum*
Quinidine	Quinoline methanol	Intravenous therapy of severe infections with *P falciparum*
Mefloquine	Quinoline methanol	Chemoprophylaxis and treatment of infections with *P falciparum*
Primaquine	8-Aminoquinoline	Radical cure and terminal prophylaxis of infections with *Plasmodium vivax* and *Plasmodium ovale*; alternative for malaria chemoprophylaxis
Sulfadoxine-pyrimethamine (Fansidar)	Folate antagonist combination	Treatment of *P falciparum*, optimally in combination with artesunate; intermittent preventive therapy
Atovaquone-proguanil (Malarone)	Quinone-folate antagonist combination	Treatment and chemoprophylaxis of *P falciparum* infection
Doxycycline	Tetracycline	Treatment (with quinine) of infections with *P falciparum*; chemoprophylaxis
Halofantrine[1]	Phenanthrene methanol	Treatment of infections with some chloroquine-resistant *P falciparum*
Lumefantrine	Amyl alcohol	Treatment of *P falciparum* malaria in fixed combination with artemether (Coartem)
Artemisinins (Artesunate, artemether, dihydroartemisinin)	Sesquiterpene lactone endoperoxides	Treatment of *P falciparum* in oral combination regimens for uncomplicated disease and parenterally for severe malaria

[1]Not available in the United States.
Modified, with permission, from Katzung BG. *Basic & Clinical Pharmacology.* 11th edition. McGraw-Hill, 2009.

Symptomatic malaria is caused only by the erythrocytic stage of infection. Available antimalarial drugs (Table 35–2) act against this stage, except for primaquine, which acts principally against hepatic parasites.

A. Non-Falciparum Malaria

The first-line drug for non-falciparum malaria from most areas remains chloroquine. Due to increasing resistance of *P vivax* to chloroquine, alternative therapies are recommended when resistance is suspected, particularly for infections acquired in Indonesia, Oceania, and Peru. These infections can be treated with artemisinin-based combination therapies or other first-line regimens for *P falciparum* infections as discussed below. For *P vivax* or *P ovale*, eradication of erythrocytic parasites with chloroquine should be accompanied by treatment with primaquine (after evaluating for glucose-6-phosphate dehydrogenase [G6PD] deficiency; see below) to eradicate dormant liver stages (hypnozoites), which may lead to relapses with recurrent erythrocytic infection and malaria symptoms after weeks to months if left untreated. *P malariae* infections need only be treated with chloroquine.

B. Uncomplicated Falciparum Malaria

P falciparum is resistant to chloroquine and sulfadoxine-pyrimethamine in most areas, with the exceptions of Central America west of the Panama Canal and Hispaniola. Falciparum malaria from other areas should not be treated with these older drugs, and decisions regarding

chemoprophylaxis should follow the same geographic considerations.

Artemisinin-based combinations, all including a short-acting artemisinin and longer-acting partner drug, are now first-line therapies in nearly all endemic countries. The WHO currently recommends five artemisinin-based combinations to treat falciparum malaria (Table 35–3), but the

Table 35–3. WHO recommendations for the treatment of uncomplicated falciparum malaria.

Regimen	Notes
Artemether-lumefantrine (Coartem, Riamet)	Coformulated, first-line therapy in many countries. Approved in the United States.
Artesunate-amodiaquine (ASAQ)	Coformulated, first-line therapy in multiple African countries.
Artesunate-mefloquine	First-line therapy in parts of Southeast Asia and South America.
Artesunate-sulfadoxine-pyrimethamine	First-line in some countries, but efficacy lower than other regimens in most areas.
Dihydroartemisinin-piperaquine	Newer coformulated combination. First-line in some Southeast Asian countries.

World Health Organization: Guidelines for the Treatment of Malaria. World Health Organization. Geneva 2010. *ISBN* 978 92 4 154792 5.

Table 35–4. Treatment of malaria.

Clinical Setting	Drug Therapy[1]	Alternative Drugs
Chloroquine-sensitive *Plasmodium falciparum* and *Plasmodium malariae* infections	Chloroquine phosphate, 1 g, followed by 500 mg at 6, 24, and 48 hours –or– Chloroquine phosphate, 1 g at 0 and 24 hours, then 0.5 g at 48 hours	
Plasmodium vivax and *Plasmodium ovale* infections	Chloroquine (as above), then (if G6PD normal) primaquine, 30 mg base daily for 14 days	For infections from Indonesia, Papua New Guinea, and other areas with suspected resistance: therapies listed for uncomplicated chloroquine-resistant *P falciparum* plus primaquine
Uncomplicated infections with chloroquine-resistant *P falciparum*	Coartem (artemether 20 mg, lumefantrine 120 mg), four tablets twice daily for 3 days –or– Malarone, four tablets (total of 1 g atovaquone, 400 mg proguanil) daily for 3 days –or– Quinine sulfate, 650 mg three times daily for 3–7 days Plus one of the following (when quinine given for < 7 days) Doxycycline, 100 mg twice daily for 7 days –or– Clindamycin, 600 mg twice daily for 7 days	Mefloquine, 15 mg/kg once or 750 mg, then 500 mg in 6–8 hours –or– Dihydroartemisinin-piperaquine[2] (dihydroarte-misinin 40 mg, piperaquine 320 mg), 4 tablets daily for 3 days –or– ASAQ[2] (artesunate 100 mg, amodiaquine 270 mg), two tablets daily for 3 days
Severe or complicated infections with *P falciparum*	Artesunate 2.4 mg/kg intravenously every 12 hours for 1 day, then daily[3,6]	Quinidine gluconate,[4–6] 10 mg/kg intravenously over 1–2 hours, then 0.02 mg/kg intravenously/min –or– Quinidine gluconate,[4–6] 15 mg/kg intrave-nously over 4 hours, then 7.5 mg/kg intravenously over 4 hours every 8 hours –or– Quinine dihydrochloride,[2,4–6] 20 mg/kg intravenously over 4 hours, then 10 mg/kg intravenously every 8 hours –or– Artemether,[2,6] 3.2 mg/kg intramuscularly, then 1.6 mg/kg/d intramuscularly

[1]All dosages are oral and refer to salts unless otherwise indicated. See text for additional information on all agents, including toxicities and cautions. See Centers for Disease Control and Prevention's guidelines (phone: 877-FYI-TRIP; http://www.cdc.gov/malaria/) for additional information and pediatric dosing.
[2]Not available in the United States.
[3]Available in the United States only on an investigational basis through the CDC (phone: 770-488-7788).
[4]Cardiac monitoring should be in place during intravenous administration of quinidine or quinine.
[5]Avoid loading doses in persons who have received quinine, quinidine, or mefloquine in the prior 24 hours.
[6]With all parenteral regimens, change to an oral regimen as soon as the patient can tolerate it.
G6PD, glucose-6-phosphate dehydrogenase.

efficacy of these regimens varies. Other combination thera-pies are under development. Quinine generally remains effective for falciparum malaria, but it must be taken for an extended period to cure disease and is poorly tolerated, and should best be reserved for the treatment of severe malaria and for treatment after another regimen has failed (Table 35–4).

In developed countries, malaria is an uncommon but potentially life-threatening infection of travelers and immi-grants, many of whom are nonimmune, so they are at risk for rapid progression to severe disease. Nonimmune indi-viduals with falciparum malaria should generally be admit-ted to the hospital due to risks of rapid progression of disease. A number of options are available for the treat-ment of uncomplicated falciparum malaria in the United States (Table 35–4).

C. Severe Malaria

Severe malaria is a medical emergency. Parenteral treat-ment is indicated for severe malaria, as defined above, and with inability to take oral drugs. With appropriate prompt therapy and supportive care, rapid recoveries may be seen even in very ill individuals.

Standard therapy for severe malaria has been intrave-nous quinine in most areas and, in the United States, intravenous quinidine, which is equally effective. However, intravenous artesunate has shown superior efficacy and better tolerability than intravenous quinine for severe malaria in large randomized trials in Asian adults and African children. It is the standard of care for severe malaria, although it is not yet available in much of the developing world, where quinine remains standard therapy. In the United States, intravenous artesunate is available on an investigational basis through the CDC (for enrollment call 770-488-7788); if approved, the drug is provided emergently from CDC Quarantine Stations. The drug is administered in four doses of 2.4 mg/kg over 3 days, every 12 hours on day 1, and then daily. If artesunate cannot be obtained promptly, severe malaria should be treated with intravenous quinine or quinidine. In endemic regions, if parenteral therapy is not available, intrarectal administration of artemether or artesunate is also effective. Patients receiving intravenous quinine or quinidine should receive continuous cardiac monitoring; if QTc prolongation exceeds 25% of baseline, the infusion rate should be reduced. Blood glucose should be monitored every 4–6 hours, and 5–10% dextrose may be coadministered to decrease the likelihood of hypoglycemia.

Appropriate care of severe malaria includes maintenance of fluids and electrolytes; respiratory and hemodynamic support; and consideration of blood transfusions, anticonvulsants, antibiotics for bacterial infections, and hemofiltration or hemodialysis. With high parasitemia (> 5–10%), exchange transfusion has been used, but beneficial effects have not clearly been demonstrated, and it is generally no longer recommended.

D. Antimalarial Drugs

1. Chloroquine—Chloroquine remains the drug of choice for the treatment of sensitive *P falciparum* and other species of malaria parasites (Table 35–4). Chloroquine is active against erythrocytic parasites of all human malaria species. It does not eradicate hepatic stages, so must be used with primaquine to eradicate *P vivax* and *P ovale* infections. Chloroquine-resistant *P falciparum* is widespread in nearly all areas of the world with falciparum malaria, with the exceptions of Central America west of the Panama Canal, Mexico, and Hispaniola. Chloroquine-resistant *P vivax* has been reported from a number of areas, most notably Southeast Asia and Oceania.

Chloroquine is the drug of choice for the treatment of non-falciparum and sensitive falciparum malaria. It rapidly terminates fever (in 24–48 hours) and clears parasitemia (in 48–72 hours) caused by sensitive parasites. Chloroquine is also the preferred chemoprophylactic agent in malarious regions without resistant falciparum malaria.

Chloroquine is usually well tolerated, even with prolonged use. Pruritus is common, primarily in Africans. Nausea, vomiting, abdominal pain, headache, anorexia, malaise, blurring of vision, and urticaria are uncommon. Dosing after meals may reduce some adverse events.

2. Amodiaquine and piperaquine—Amodiaquine is a 4-aminoquinoline that is closely related to chloroquine. Amodiaquine has been widely used to treat malaria because of its low cost, limited toxicity and, in some areas, effectiveness against chloroquine-resistant strains of *P falciparum*. Use of amodiaquine decreased after recognition of rare but serious side effects, notably agranulocytosis, aplastic anemia, and hepatotoxicity. However, serious side effects are rare with short-term use, and amodiaquine is a component of a new combination therapy (artesunate-amodiaquine) recommended to treat falciparum malaria (Table 35–3). Chemoprophylaxis with amodiaquine is best avoided because of increased toxicity with long-term use.

Piperaquine is another 4-aminoquinoline that was previously heavily used in China and has been coformulated with dihydroartemisinin in an artemisinin-based therapy. Piperaquine appears to be well tolerated, to have minimal problems with resistance (despite prior reports of resistance in China), and in combination with dihydroartemisinin to offer a highly efficacious therapy for falciparum malaria.

3. Mefloquine—Mefloquine is effective against many chloroquine-resistant strains of *P falciparum* and against other malarial species. Although toxicity is a concern, mefloquine is also a recommended chemoprophylactic drug. Resistance to mefloquine has been reported sporadically from many areas, but it appears to be uncommon except in regions of Southeast Asia with high rates of multidrug resistance (especially border areas of Thailand).

For treatment of uncomplicated malaria, mefloquine can be administered as a single dose or in two doses over 1 day. It is used in combination with artesunate in Southeast Asia, where resistance to mefloquine has been seen but the combination remains effective in most areas. It should be taken with meals and swallowed with a large amount of water. Mefloquine is recommended by the CDC for chemoprophylaxis in all malarious areas except those with no chloroquine resistance (where chloroquine is preferred) and some rural areas of Southeast Asia with a high prevalence of mefloquine resistance. Eradication of *P vivax* and *P ovale* requires a course of primaquine.

Adverse effects with weekly dosing of mefloquine for chemoprophylaxis include nausea, vomiting, dizziness, sleep and behavioral disturbances, epigastric pain, diarrhea, abdominal pain, headache, rash and, uncommonly, seizures and psychosis. Concerns about neuropsychiatric toxicity, including possibly rare irreversible effects, led the FDA to add a black box warning for the drug in 2013. Mefloquine should be avoided in persons with histories of psychiatric disease or seizures.

Adverse effects are more common (up to 50% of treatments) with the higher dosages of mefloquine required for treatment. These effects may be lessened by splitting administration into two doses separated by 6–8 hours. Serious neuropsychiatric toxicities (depression, confusion, acute psychosis, or seizures) have been reported in < 1 in 1000 treatments, but some authorities believe that these are more common. Mefloquine can also alter cardiac conduction, and so it should not be coadministered with quinine, quinidine, or halofantrine, and caution is required if these drugs are used to treat malaria after mefloquine chemoprophylaxis. Mefloquine is generally considered safe in young children and pregnant women.

4. Quinine and quinidine—Quinine dihydrochloride and quinidine gluconate remain first-line therapies for falciparum malaria, especially severe disease, although toxicity concerns complicate therapy (Table 35–4). Quinine acts rapidly against the four species of human malaria parasites. Quinidine, the dextrorotatory stereoisomer of quinine, is at least as effective as quinine in the treatment of severe falciparum malaria.

Resistance of *P falciparum* to quinine is common in some areas of Southeast Asia, where the drug may fail if used alone to treat falciparum malaria. However, quinine still provides at least a partial therapeutic effect in most patients.

Quinine and quinidine are effective treatments for severe falciparum malaria, although intravenous artesunate is now the standard of care. Quinine can be administered slowly intravenously or, in a dilute solution, intramuscularly, but parenteral quinine is not available in the United States, where quinidine is used. The drugs can be administered in divided doses or by continuous intravenous infusion; treatment should begin with a loading dose to rapidly achieve effective plasma concentrations. Intravenous quinine and quinidine should be administered with cardiac monitoring because of their cardiac toxicity and the relative unpredictability of their pharmacokinetics. Therapy should be changed to an oral agent as soon as the patient has improved and can tolerate oral medications.

In areas without newer combination regimens, oral quinine sulfate is an alternative first-line therapy for uncomplicated falciparum malaria, although poor tolerance may limit compliance. Quinine is commonly used with a second drug (most often doxycycline) to shorten the duration of use (usually to 3 days) and to limit toxicity. Therapeutic dosages of quinine and quinidine commonly cause tinnitus, headache, nausea, dizziness, flushing, and visual disturbances. Hypersensitivity reactions include rash, urticaria, angioedema, and bronchospasm. Hematologic abnormalities include hemolysis (especially with G6PD deficiency), leukopenia, agranulocytosis, and thrombocytopenia. Therapeutic doses may cause hypoglycemia through stimulation of insulin release; this is a particular problem in severe infections and in pregnant patients, who have increased sensitivity to insulin. Overly rapid infusions can cause severe hypotension. ECG abnormalities (QT prolongation) are fairly common, but dangerous arrhythmias are uncommon when the drugs are administered appropriately. Blackwater fever is a rare severe illness, probably due to hypersensitivity, that includes marked hemolysis and hemoglobinuria in the setting of quinine therapy for malaria. Quinine should not be given concurrently with mefloquine and should be used with caution in a patient who has previously received mefloquine.

5. Primaquine—Primaquine phosphate, a synthetic 8-aminoquinoline, is the drug of choice for the eradication of dormant liver forms of *P vivax* and *P ovale* (Table 35–4). Primaquine is active against hepatic stages of all human malaria parasites. This action is optimal soon after therapy with chloroquine or quinine. Primaquine also acts against erythrocytic stage parasites, although this activity is too weak for the treatment of active disease, and against gametocytes.

For *P vivax* and *P ovale* infections, chloroquine or other drugs are used to eradicate erythrocytic forms, and if the G6PD level is normal, a 14-day course of primaquine (52.6 mg primaquine phosphate [30 mg base] daily) is initiated to eradicate liver hypnozoites and prevent a subsequent relapse. Some strains of *P vivax*, particularly in New Guinea and Southeast Asia, are relatively resistant to primaquine, and the drug may occasionally fail to eradicate liver forms.

Standard chemoprophylaxis does not prevent a relapse of *P vivax* or *P ovale* infections, since liver hypnozoites are not eradicated by chloroquine or other standard treatments. To diminish the likelihood of relapse, some authorities advocate the use of a treatment course of primaquine after the completion of travel to an endemic area. Primaquine can also be used for chemoprophylaxis to prevent *P falciparum* and *P vivax* infection in persons with normal levels of G6PD.

Primaquine in recommended doses is generally well tolerated. It infrequently causes nausea, epigastric pain, abdominal cramps, and headache, especially when taken on an empty stomach. Rare adverse effects include leukopenia, agranulocytosis, leukocytosis, and cardiac arrhythmias. Standard doses of primaquine may cause hemolysis or methemoglobinemia (manifested by cyanosis), especially in persons with G6PD deficiency or other hereditary metabolic defects. Patients should be tested for G6PD deficiency before primaquine is prescribed. When a patient is deficient in G6PD, treatment strategies may consist of (1) withholding therapy and treating subsequent relapses, if they occur, with chloroquine; (2) treating patients with standard dosing, paying close attention to their hematologic status; or (3) treating with weekly primaquine (45 mg base) for 8 weeks. G6PD-deficient individuals of Mediterranean and Asian ancestry are most likely to have severe deficiency, while those of African ancestry usually have a milder biochemical defect. This difference can be taken into consideration in choosing a treatment strategy. Primaquine should be discontinued if there is evidence of hemolysis or anemia and should be avoided in pregnancy.

6. Inhibitors of folate synthesis—Inhibitors of two parasite enzymes involved in folate metabolism, dihydrofolate reductase (DHFR) and dihydropteroate synthase (DHPS), are used, generally in combination regimens, for the treatment and prevention of malaria, although the drugs are rather slow acting and now limited by resistance.

Fansidar is a fixed combination of sulfadoxine (500 mg) and pyrimethamine (25 mg). The long half-lives of its components allow weekly dosing for chemoprophylaxis, but due to rare serious side effects with long-term dosing, this drug is no longer recommended for this purpose. For treatment, advantages of sulfadoxine-pyrimethamine include ease of administration (a single oral dose) and low cost. However, resistance is now a major problem. In addition, it is not reliably effective in *P vivax* infections, and its usefulness against *P ovale* and *P malariae* infections has not been adequately studied, limiting its utility outside of Africa.

Sulfadoxine-pyrimethamine is a component of two combination regimens for uncomplicated malaria recommended by the WHO (Table 35–3). Sulfadoxine-pyrimethamine plus artesunate has shown efficacy in some areas but is best replaced by more effective combination regimens in most areas. Amodiaquine plus sulfadoxine-pyrimethamine has shown quite good efficacy in Africa, despite increasing resistance to both components. It is recommended for chemoprophylaxis in areas with seasonal malaria transmission and limited drug resistance; for this purpose, the drug is administered to children monthly during the transmission season. Another antifolate combination, trimethoprim-sulfamethoxazole, is widely used to prevent coinfections in patients infected with HIV, and it offers partial protection against malaria. Malarone, a combination of proguanil with atovaquone, is discussed below.

7. Artemisinins—Artemisinin (qinghaosu) is a sesquiterpene lactone endoperoxide, the active component of an herbal medicine that has been used for various indications in China for over 2000 years. Analogs have been synthesized to increase solubility and improve antimalarial efficacy. The most important of these analogs are artesunate, artemether, and dihydroartemisinin. The WHO is encouraging availability of oral artemisinins only in coformulated combination regimens.

Artemisinins act very rapidly against all erythrocytic-stage human malaria parasites. Of concern, delayed clearance of parasites and some clinical failures have been seen after treatment with artesunate in parts of Southeast Asia, heralding the emergence of artemisinin resistance in this region.

Artemisinins are playing an increasing role in the treatment of malaria, including multidrug-resistant *P falciparum* malaria. However, due to their short plasma half-lives, recrudescence rates are unacceptably high after short-course therapy, leading to use in conjunction with another agent. Also because of their short-half lives, they are not useful in chemoprophylaxis.

Artemisinins should be used for uncomplicated malaria in combination regimens including a longer-acting partner drug, known as artemisinin-based combination therapy (ACT). The ACTs that are currently most advocated in Africa are artesunate plus amodiaquine (ASAQ) and artemether plus lumefantrine (Coartem), each of which is available as a coformulated product and is the recommended therapy for uncomplicated malaria in a number of countries. Another ACT, artesunate plus mefloquine is used mostly outside of Africa; its efficacy may be declining in parts of Asia. Dihydroartemisinin-piperaquine is a newer ACT that has shown excellent efficacy, and is now the first-line regimen in some countries in Southeast Asia.

In studies of severe malaria, intramuscular artemether was at least as effective as intramuscular quinine, and intravenous artesunate was superior to intravenous quinine in terms of efficacy and tolerability. Thus, the standard of care for severe malaria is intravenous artesunate, when it is available, although parenteral quinine and quinidine remain acceptable alternatives. Artesunate and artemether have also been effective in the treatment of severe malaria

when administered rectally, offering a valuable treatment modality when parenteral therapy is not available.

Artemisinins are very well tolerated. The most commonly reported adverse effects have been nausea, vomiting, and diarrhea, which may often be due to acute malaria, rather than drug toxicity. Neutropenia, anemia, hemolysis, and elevated levels of liver enzymes have been noted rarely. Artemisinins are teratogenic in animals, and they should be avoided in the first trimester of pregnancy for uncomplicated malaria. However, for severe malaria, for which all available treatments entail some risk, the WHO endorses the use of intravenous artesunate or quinine while additional data are gathered on artesunate safety.

8. Atovaquone plus proguanil (Malarone)—Atovaquone, a hydroxynaphthoquinone, is not effective when used alone, due to rapid development of drug resistance. However, Malarone, a fixed combination of atovaquone (250 mg) and the antifolate proguanil (100 mg), is highly effective for both the treatment and chemoprophylaxis of falciparum malaria, and it is approved for both indications in the United States (Table 35–4). It also appears to be active against other species of malaria parasites. Unlike most other antimalarials, Malarone provides activity against both erythrocytic and hepatic stage parasites.

For treatment, Malarone is given at an adult dose of four tablets daily for 3 days. For chemoprophylaxis, Malarone must be taken daily. It has an advantage over mefloquine and doxycycline in requiring shorter durations of treatment before and after the period at risk for malaria transmission, due to activity against liver-stage parasites. It should be taken with food.

Malarone is generally well tolerated. Adverse effects include abdominal pain, nausea, vomiting, diarrhea, headache, and rash, and these are more common with the higher dose required for treatment. Reversible elevations in liver enzymes have been reported. The safety of atovaquone in pregnancy is unknown.

9. Antibiotics—A number of antibacterials in addition to the folate antagonists and sulfonamides are slow-acting antimalarials. None of the antibiotics should be used as single agents for the treatment of malaria due to their slow rate of action.

Doxycycline is commonly used in the treatment of falciparum malaria in conjunction with quinidine or quinine, allowing a shorter and better-tolerated course of those drugs (Table 35–4). Doxycycline is also a standard chemoprophylactic drug, especially for use in areas of Southeast Asia with high rates of resistance to other antimalarials, including mefloquine. Doxycycline side effects include gastrointestinal symptoms, candidal vaginitis, and photosensitivity. The drug should be taken while upright with a large amount of water to avoid esophageal irritation. Clindamycin can be used in conjunction with quinine or quinidine in those for whom doxycycline is not recommended, such as children and pregnant women (Table 35–4). The most common toxicities with clindamycin are gastrointestinal. Azithromycin also has antimalarial activity and is under study for treatment and chemoprophylaxis.

10. Halofantrine and lumefantrine—Halofantrine, a phenanthrene-methanol related to quinine, is effective against erythrocytic stages of all four human malaria species. Because of toxicity concerns, it should not be taken with meals, since food enhances absorption. Halofantrine is rapidly effective against most chloroquine-resistant strains of *P falciparum*, but its use is now very limited due to risks of serious cardiac toxicity.

Lumefantrine, an aryl alcohol related to halofantrine, is available only as a fixed-dose combination with artemether (Coartem or Riamet). Oral absorption is highly variable and improved when the drug is taken with food. Use of Coartem with a fatty meal is recommended. Coartem is highly effective for the treatment of falciparum malaria, but it is fairly expensive and requires twice-daily dosing. Despite these limitations, due to its reliable efficacy against falciparum malaria, Coartem is the first-line therapy for malaria in many malarious countries. Coartem is well tolerated; side effects include headache, dizziness, loss of appetite, gastrointestinal symptoms, and palpitations. Importantly, Coartem does not generally cause QT prolongation or the serious cardiac toxicity seen with halofantrine.

▶ **Prevention**

Malaria is transmitted by night-biting anopheline mosquitoes. Bed nets, in particular nets treated with permethrin insecticides, are heavily promoted as inexpensive means of antimalarial protection, and improvement in mortality rates has been demonstrated. Extensive efforts are also underway to develop a malaria vaccine, and partial protection of African children has been demonstrated, but a vaccine offering complete protection is not anticipated in the near future. The availability of improved modalities to control mosquito vectors and treat and prevent malaria has heightened enthusiasm for malaria elimination, and there have been important gains in some areas; however, control

remains very challenging in highly endemic regions, and elimination is not expected in these areas in the foreseeable future.

When travelers from nonendemic to endemic countries are counseled on the prevention of malaria, it is imperative to emphasize measures to prevent mosquito bites (insect repellents, insecticides, and bed nets), since parasites are increasingly resistant to multiple drugs and no chemoprophylactic regimen is fully protective. Chemoprophylaxis is recommended for all travelers from nonendemic regions to endemic areas, although risks vary greatly for different locations, and some tropical areas entail no risk; specific recommendations for travel to different locales are available from the CDC (www.cdc.gov). Current recommendations from the CDC include the use of chloroquine for chemoprophylaxis in the few areas with only chloroquine-sensitive malaria parasites (principally the Caribbean and Central America west of the Panama Canal), mefloquine or Malarone for most other malarious areas, and doxycycline for areas with a high prevalence of multidrug-resistant falciparum malaria (principally parts of Southeast Asia) (Table 35–5). Recommendations should be checked regularly (Phone: 877-FYI-TRIP; Internet: http://wwwnc.cdc.gov/travel) because they may change in response to changing resistance patterns and increasing experience with new drugs. In some circumstances, it may be appropriate for travelers to not use chemoprophylaxis but to carry supplies of drugs with them in case a febrile illness develops and medical attention is unavailable. Regimens for self-treatment include ACTs, Malarone, and quinine. Most authorities do not recommend routine terminal chemoprophylaxis with primaquine to eradicate dormant hepatic stages of *P vivax* and *P ovale* after travel, but this may be appropriate in some circumstances, especially for travelers with major exposure to these parasites.

Regular chemoprophylaxis is not a standard management practice in developing world populations due to the

Table 35–5. Drugs for the prevention of malaria in travelers.[1]

Drug	Use[2]	Adult Dosage (all oral)[3]
Chloroquine	Areas without resistant *Plasmodium falciparum*	500 mg weekly
Malarone	Areas with multidrug-resistant *P falciparum*	1 tablet (250 mg atovaquone/100 mg proguanil) daily
Mefloquine	Areas with chloroquine-resistant *P falciparum*	250 mg weekly
Doxycycline	Areas with multidrug-resistant *P falciparum*	100 mg daily
Primaquine[4]	Terminal prophylaxis of *Plasmodium vivax* and *Plasmodium ovale* infections; alternative for *P falciparum* prophylaxis	30 mg base daily for 14 days after travel

[1]Recommendations may change, as resistance to all available drugs is increasing. See text for additional information on toxicities and cautions. For additional details and pediatric dosing, see Centers for Disease Control and Prevention's guidelines (phone: 800-CDC-INFO; http://wwwnc.cdc.gov/travel/). Travelers to remote areas should consider carrying effective therapy (see text) for use if a febrile illness develops, and they cannot reach medical attention quickly.
[2]Areas without known chloroquine-resistant *P falciparum* are Central America west of the Panama Canal, Haiti, Dominican Republic, Egypt, and most malarious countries of the Middle East. Malarone or mefloquine is currently recommended for other malarious areas except for border areas of Thailand, where doxycycline is recommended.
[3]For drugs other than primaquine, begin 1–2 weeks before departure (except 2 days before for doxycycline and Malarone) and continue for 4 weeks after leaving the endemic area (except 1 week for Malarone). All dosages refer to salts unless otherwise indicated.
[4]Screen for glucose-6-phosphate dehydrogenase deficiency before using primaquine.
Reproduced, with permission, from Katzung BG. *Basic & Clinical Pharmacology*. 11th edition. McGraw-Hill, 2009.

expense and potential toxicities of long-term therapy. However, intermittent preventive therapy, whereby at-risk populations (in particular pregnant women and children) receive antimalarial therapy at set intervals, is of increasing interest. This strategy may decrease the incidence of malaria while allowing antimalarial immunity to develop. During pregnancy, intermittent preventive therapy with sulfadoxine-pyrimethamine, provided once during both the second and third trimesters, has improved pregnancy outcomes. In infants, therapy with sulfadoxine-pyrimethamine following standard immunization schedules has offered benefits. With increasing resistance, it is not clear if sulfadoxine-pyrimethamine will retain prophylactic efficacy or if other drugs with shorter half-lives will be effective. In areas with seasonal malaria transmission and limited drug resistance, principally the Sahel region of West Africa, the policy is to administer amodiaquine and sulfadoxine-pyrimethamine to children monthly during the transmission season.

▶ Prognosis

When treated appropriately, uncomplicated malaria generally responds well, with resolution of fevers within 1–2 days and a mortality of about 0.1%. Severe malaria can commonly progress to death, but many children respond well to therapy. In the developed world, mortality from malaria is mostly in adults, and often follows extended illnesses and secondary complications long after eradication of the malarial infection. Pregnant women are at particular risk during their first pregnancy. Malaria in pregnancy also increases the likelihood of poor pregnancy outcomes, with increased prematurity, low birth weight, and mortality.

▶ When to Refer

Referral to an expert on infectious diseases or travel medicine is important with all cases of malaria in the United States, and in particular for falciparum malaria; referral should not delay initial diagnosis and therapy, since delays in therapy can lead to severe illness or death.

▶ When to Admit

- Admission for non-falciparum malaria is only warranted if a patient presents with specific problems that require hospital management.
- Patients with falciparum malaria are generally admitted because the disease can progress rapidly to severe illness; exceptions may be made with individuals who are from malaria-endemic areas, and thus expected to have a degree of immunity, who are without evidence of severe disease, and who are judged able to return promptly for medical attention if their disease progresses.

Baird KJ et al. Diagnosis and treatment of *Plasmodium vivax* malaria. Adv Parasitol. 2012;80:203–70. [PMID: 23199489]

Dondorp AM et al; AQUAMAT Group. Artesunate versus quinine in the treatment of severe falciparum malaria in African children (AQUAMAT): an open-label, randomised trial. Lancet. 2010 Nov 13;376(9753):1647–57. [PMID: 21062666]

Murray CJ et al. Global malaria mortality between 1980 and 2010: a systematic analysis. Lancet. 2012 Feb 4;379(9814):413–31. [PMID: 22305225]

Nadjm B et al. Malaria: an update for physicians. Infect Dis Clin North Am. 2012 Jun;26(2):243–59. [PMID: 22632637]

Olotu A et al. Four-year efficacy of RTS,S/AS01E and its interaction with malaria exposure. N Engl J Med. 2013 Mar 21;368(12):1111–20. [PMID: 23514288]

Phyo AP et al. Emergence of artemisinin-resistant malaria on the western border of Thailand: a longitudinal study. Lancet. 2012 May 26;379(9830):1960–6. [PMID: 22484134]

von Seidlein L et al. Predicting the clinical outcome of severe falciparum malaria in African children: findings from a large randomized trial. Clin Infect Dis. 2012 Apr;54(8):1080–90. [PMID: 22412067]

White NJ et al. Malaria. Lancet. 2014 Feb 22;383(9918):723–35. [PMID: 23953767]

Whitty CJ et al. Investigation and treatment of imported malaria in non-endemic countries. BMJ. 2013 May 21;346:f2900. [PMID: 23693055]

World Health Organization. *Guidelines for the treatment of malaria*, 2nd edition. Geneva, Switzerland, 2010. http://www.who.int/malaria/publications/atoz/9789241547925/en/index.html

BABESIOSIS

ESSENTIALS OF DIAGNOSIS

- ▶ History of tick bite or exposure to ticks.
- ▶ Fever, flu-like symptoms, anemia.
- ▶ Intraerythrocytic parasites on Giemsa-stained blood smears.
- ▶ Positive serologic tests.

▶ General Considerations

Babesiosis is an uncommon intraerythrocytic infection caused mainly by two *Babesia* species and transmitted by *Ixodes* ticks. In Europe, where only a few dozen cases of babesiosis have been reported, infection is caused by *Babesia divergens*, which also infects cattle. In the United States, hundreds of cases of babesiosis have been reported, and infection is caused by *Babesia microti*, which also infects wild mammals. Most babesiosis in the United States occurs in the coastal northeast, with some cases also in the upper midwest, following the geographic range of the vector *Ixodes scapularis*, and Lyme disease and anaplasmosis, which are spread by the same vector. The incidence of the disease appears to be increasing in some areas. Rare episodes of illnesses caused by *B microti*, *B divergens*, and other Babesia-like organisms have been reported from other areas. Babesiosis can also be transmitted by blood transfusion.

▶ Clinical Findings

A. Symptoms and Signs

With *B microti* infections, symptoms appear 1 to several weeks after a tick bite; parasitemia is evident after 2–4 weeks. Patients usually do not recall the tick bite. The typical flu-like illness develops gradually and is characterized by fever, fatigue, headache, arthralgia, and myalgia. Other findings may include nausea, vomiting, abdominal pain, sore throat, depression, emotional lability, anemia, thrombocytopenia, and splenomegaly. Parasitemia may continue for months to years, with or without symptoms, and the disease is usually self-limited. Severe complications are most likely to occur in older persons or in those who have had splenectomy. Serious complications include respiratory failure, hemolytic anemia, disseminated intravascular coagulation, heart failure, and acute kidney injury. In a study of hospitalized patients, the mortality rate was 6.5%. Most recognized *B divergens* infections in Europe have been in patients who have had splenectomy. These infections progress rapidly with high fever, severe hemolytic anemia, jaundice, hemoglobinuria, and acute kidney injury, with death rates over 40%.

B. Laboratory Findings

Identification of the intraerythrocytic parasite on Giemsa-stained blood smears establishes the diagnosis (Figure 35–6). These can be confused with malaria parasites, but the morphology is distinctive. Repeated smears are often necessary because well under 1% of erythrocytes may be infected, especially early in infection, although parasitemias can exceed 10%. An indirect immunofluorescent antibody test for *B microti* is available from the CDC; antibody is detectable within 2–4 weeks after the onset of symptoms and persists for months. Diagnosis can also be made by PCR or by inoculation of hamsters or gerbils.

▶ Treatment

Most patients have a mild illness and recover without therapy. Standard therapy is a 7-day course of quinine (650 mg orally three times daily) plus clindamycin (600 mg orally three times daily). An alternative is a 7-day course of atovaquone (750 mg orally every 12 hours) plus azithromycin (600 mg orally once daily). Exchange transfusion has been used successfully in severely ill asplenic patients and those with parasitemia > 10%.

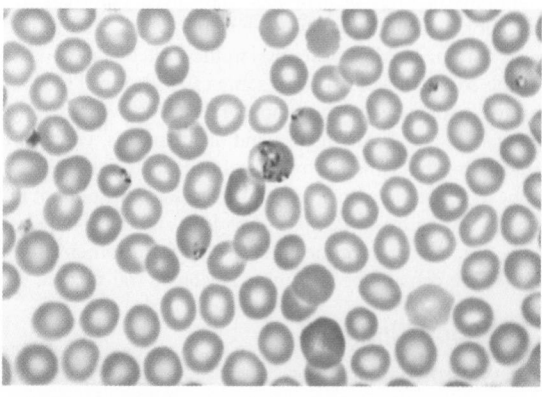

▲ **Figure 35–6.** Blood smear showing *Babesia* spp. rings with basophilic stippling. (From Dr. Mae Melvin, Public Health Image Library, CDC.)

Herwaldt BL et al. Transfusion-associated babesiosis in the United States: a description of cases. Ann Intern Med. 2011 Oct 18;155(8):509–19. [PMID: 21893613]

Vannier E et al. Human babesiosis. N Engl J Med. 2012 Jun 21;366(25):2397–407. [PMID: 22716978]

TOXOPLASMOSIS

ESSENTIALS OF DIAGNOSIS

▶ Infection confirmed by isolation of *Toxoplasma gondii* or identification of tachyzoites in tissue or body fluids.

Primary infection

▶ Fever, malaise, headache, sore throat.

▶ Lymphadenopathy.

▶ Positive IgG and IgM serologic tests.

Congenital infection

▶ Follows acute infection of seronegative mothers and leads to CNS abnormalities and retinochoroiditis.

Infection in immunocompromised persons

▶ Reactivation leads to encephalitis, retinochoroiditis, pneumonitis, myocarditis.

▶ Positive IgG but negative IgM serologic tests.

▶ General Considerations

T gondii, an obligate intracellular protozoan, is found worldwide in humans and in many species of mammals and birds. The definitive hosts are cats. Humans are infected after ingestion of cysts in raw or undercooked meat, ingestion of oocysts in food or water contaminated by cats, transplacental transmission of trophozoites or, rarely, direct inoculation of trophozoites via blood transfusion or organ transplantation. *Toxoplasma* seroprevalence varies widely. It has decreased in the United States to about 20–30%, but it is much higher in other countries in both the developed and developing worlds, where it may exceed 80%.

▶ Clinical Findings

A. Symptoms and Signs

The clinical manifestations of toxoplasmosis may be grouped into four syndromes.

1. Primary infection in the immunocompetent person— After ingestion, *T gondii* infection progresses from the gastrointestinal tract to lymphatics, and then dissemination. Most acute infections are asymptomatic. About 10–20% are symptomatic after an incubation period of 1–2 weeks. Acute infections in immunocompetent persons typically present as mild, febrile illnesses that resemble infectious mononucleosis. Nontender cervical or diffuse lymphadenopathy may persist for weeks to months. Systemic findings may include fever, malaise, headache, sore throat, rash, myalgias, hepatosplenomegaly, and atypical lymphocytosis. Rare severe manifestations are pneumonitis, meningoencephalitis, hepatitis, myocarditis, polymyositis, and retinochoroiditis. Symptoms may fluctuate, but most patients recover spontaneously within at most a few months.

2. Congenital infection—Congenital transmission occurs as a result of infection, which may be symptomatic or asymptomatic, in a nonimmune woman during pregnancy. Fetal infection follows maternal infection in 30–50% of cases, but this risk varies by trimester: 10–25% during the first, 30–50% during the second, and 60% or higher during the third trimester. In the United States, an estimated 400 to 4000 congenital infections occur yearly. While the risk of fetal infection increases, the risk of severe fetal disease decreases over the course of pregnancy. Early fetal infections commonly lead to spontaneous abortion, stillbirths, or severe neonatal disease, including neurologic manifestations. Neurologic findings can include seizures, psychomotor retardation, deafness, and hydrocephalus. Retinochoroiditis and other sight-threatening eye lesions may develop. Systemic findings include fever or hypothermia, jaundice, vomiting, diarrhea, hepatosplenomegaly, pneumonitis, myocarditis, and rash. Infections later in pregnancy less commonly lead to major fetal problems. Most infants appear normal at birth, but they may have subtle abnormalities and progress to symptoms and signs of congenital toxoplasmosis later in life. Hepatosplenomegaly and lymphadenopathy may develop in the first few months of life; CNS and eye disease often present later. The most common late presentation of congenital toxoplasmosis is retinochoroiditis.

3. Retinochoroiditis—This manifestation of congenital toxoplasmosis presents weeks to years after congenital infection, commonly in teenagers or young adults. Retinochoroiditis also is seen in persons who acquire infection early in life, and these patients more often present with unilateral disease. Uveitis is also seen. Disease presents with pain, photophobia, and visual changes, usually without systemic symptoms. Signs and symptoms eventually improve, but visual defects may persist. Rarely, progression may result in glaucoma and blindness.

4. Disease in the immunocompromised person—Reactivated toxoplasmosis occurs in patients with AIDS, cancer, or those given immunosuppressive drugs. In patients with advanced AIDS, the most common manifestation is encephalitis, with multiple necrotizing brain lesions. The encephalitis usually presents subacutely, with fever, headache, altered mental status, focal neurologic findings, and other evidence of brain lesions. Less common manifestations of toxoplasmosis in patients with AIDS are chorioretinitis and pneumonitis. Chorioretinitis presents with ocular pain and alterations in vision. Pneumonitis presents with fever, cough, and dyspnea. Toxoplasmosis can develop in seronegative recipients of solid organ or bone marrow transplants due to reactivation or, more rarely, transmission of infection. Reactivation also can occur in those with hematologic malignancies or treated with immunosuppressive drugs. With primary or reactivated disease in

those with immunodeficiency due to malignancy or immunosuppressive drugs, toxoplasmosis is similar to that in individuals with AIDS, but pneumonitis and myocarditis are more common.

B. Diagnostic Testing

1. Identification of parasites—Organisms can be seen in tissue or body fluids, although they may be difficult to identify; special staining techniques can facilitate identification. The demonstration of tachyzoites indicates acute infection; cysts may represent either acute or chronic infection. With lymphadenopathy due to toxoplasmosis, examination of lymph nodes usually does not show organisms. Parasite identification can also be made by inoculation of tissue culture or mice. PCR can be used for sensitive identification of organisms in amniotic fluid, blood, CSF, aqueous humor, and bronchoalveolar lavage fluid.

2. Serologic diagnosis—Multiple serologic methods are used, including the Sabin-Feldman dye test, enzyme-linked immunosorbent assay (ELISA), indirect fluorescent antibody test, and agglutination tests. IgG antibodies are seen within 1–2 weeks of infection, and usually persist for life. IgM antibodies peak earlier than IgG and decline more rapidly, although they may persist for years. In immunocompromised individuals in whom reactivation is suspected, a positive IgG assay indicates distant infection, and thus the potential for reactivated disease; a negative IgG argues strongly against reactivation toxoplasmosis. With reactivation in immunocompromised persons, IgM tests are generally negative.

3. During pregnancy and in newborns—Conversion from a negative to positive serologic test or rising titers are suggestive of acute infection, but tests are not routinely performed during pregnancy. When pregnant women are screened, negative IgG and IgM assays exclude active infection, but indicate the risk of infection during the pregnancy. The pattern of positive IgG with negative IgM is highly suggestive of chronic infection, with no risk of congenital disease unless the mother is severely immunocompromised. A positive IgM test is concerning for new infection because of the risk of congenital disease. Confirmatory testing should be performed before consideration of treatment or possible termination of pregnancy due to the limitations of available tests. Tests of the avidity of anti-IgG antibodies can be helpful, but a battery of tests is needed for confirmation of acute infection during pregnancy. When acute infection during pregnancy is suspected, PCR of amniotic fluid offers a sensitive assessment for congenital disease; this test should optimally be performed at 18 weeks of gestation. In newborns, positive IgM or IgA antibody tests are indicative of congenital infection, although the diagnosis is not ruled out by a negative test. Positive IgG assays may represent transfer of maternal antibodies without infection of the infant. Organisms may be identified by PCR; smears; or culture of blood, CSF, or tissue.

4. In immunocompetent individuals—Individuals with a suggestive clinical syndrome should be tested for IgG and

IgM antibodies. Seroconversion, a 16-fold rise in antibody titer, or an IgM titer > 1:64 are suggestive of acute infection, although false-positive results may occur. Acute infection can also be diagnosed by detection of tachyzoites in tissue, culture of organisms, or PCR of blood or body fluids. Histologic evaluation of lymph nodes can show characteristic morphology, with or without organisms.

5. In immunodeficient individuals—A presentation consistent with toxoplasmic encephalitis warrants imaging of the brain. CT and MRI scans typically show multiple ring-enhancing cerebral lesions, most commonly involving the corticomedullary junction and basal ganglia. MRI is the more sensitive imaging modality. In AIDS patients with a positive IgG serologic test and no recent antitoxoplasma or antiviral therapy, the predictive value of a typical imaging study is about 80%. The other common diagnosis in this setting is CNS lymphoma, which more typically causes a single brain lesion. The differential diagnosis also includes tuberculoma, bacterial brain abscess, fungal abscess, and carcinoma. Diagnosis of CNS toxoplasmosis is most typically made after a therapeutic trial, with clinical and radiologic improvement expected within 2–3 weeks. Definitive diagnosis requires brain biopsy and search for organisms and typical histology. In retinochoroiditis, funduscopic examination shows vitreous inflammatory reaction, white retinal lesions, and pigmented scars. Diagnosis of other clinical entities in immunocompromised individuals is generally based on histology.

► Treatment

A. Approach to Treatment

Therapy is generally not necessary in immunocompetent persons, since primary illness is self-limited. However, for severe, persistent, or visceral disease, treatment for 2–4 weeks may be considered. Treatment is appropriate for primary infection during pregnancy because the risk of fetal transmission or the severity of congenital disease may be reduced. For retinochoroiditis, most episodes are self-limited, and opinions vary on indications for treatment. Treatment is often advocated for episodes with decreases in visual acuity, multiple or large lesions, macular lesions, significant inflammation, or persistence for over a month. Immunocompromised patients with active infection must be treated. For those with transient immunodeficiency, therapy can be continued for 4–6 weeks after cessation of symptoms. For those with persistent immunodeficiency, such as AIDS patients, full therapy for 4–6 weeks is followed by maintenance therapy with lower doses of drugs. Immunodeficient patients who are asymptomatic but have a positive IgG serologic test should receive long-term chemoprophylaxis.

B. Medications

Drugs for toxoplasmosis are active only against tachyzoites, so they do not eradicate infection. Standard therapy is the combination of pyrimethamine (200 mg loading dose, then 50–75 mg [1 mg/kg] orally once daily) plus sulfadiazine (1–1.5 g orally four times daily), with folinic acid (10–20 mg orally once daily) to prevent bone marrow suppression. Patients should be screened for a history of sulfonamide sensitivity (skin rashes, gastrointestinal symptoms, hepatotoxicity). To prevent crystal-induced nephrotoxicity, good urinary output should be maintained. Pyrimethamine side effects include headache and gastrointestinal symptoms. Even with folinic acid therapy, bone marrow suppression may occur; platelet and white blood cell counts should be monitored at least weekly. A first-line alternative to sulfadiazine is clindamycin (600 mg orally four times daily). Other possible alternatives are trimethoprim-sulfamethoxazole or combining pyrimethamine with atovaquone, clarithromycin, azithromycin, or dapsone. Pyrimethamine is not used during the first trimester of pregnancy due to its teratogenicity. Standard therapy for the treatment of acute toxoplasmosis during pregnancy is with spiramycin (1 g orally three times daily until delivery). This therapy is used only to decrease the risk of fetal infection; it reduces the frequency of transmission to the fetus by about 60%. Spiramycin does not cross the placenta, so when fetal infection is documented or for acute infections late in pregnancy (which commonly lead to fetal transmission) treatment with combination regimens as described above is indicated.

► Prevention

Prevention of primary infection centers on avoidance of undercooked meat or contact with material contaminated by cat feces, particularly for seronegative pregnant women and immunocompromised persons. For meat, irradiation, cooking to 66°C, or freezing to –20°C kills tissue cysts. Thorough cleaning of hands and surfaces is needed after contact with raw meat or areas contaminated by cats. Oocysts passed in cat feces can remain infective for a year or more, but fresh oocysts are not infective for 48 hours. For best protection, litter boxes should be changed daily and soaked in boiling water for 5 minutes. In addition, gloves should be worn when gardening, fruits and vegetables should be thoroughly washed, and ingestion of dried meat should be avoided.

Universal screening of pregnant women for *T gondii* antibodies is conducted in some countries but not the United States. Pregnant women should ideally have their serum examined for IgG and IgM antibody, and those with negative titers should adhere to the prevention measures described above. Seronegative women who continue to have environmental exposure should undergo repeat serologic screening several times during pregnancy.

For immunocompromised individuals, chemoprophylaxis to prevent primary or reactivated infection is warranted. For transplant recipients, pyrimethamine (25 mg daily orally for 6 weeks) has been used. For advanced AIDS patients and others, chemoprophylaxis with trimethoprim-sulfamethoxazole (one double-strength tablet daily or two tablets three times weekly), used primarily for protection against *Pneumocystis,* is also effective against *T gondii.* Alternatives are pyrimethamine plus either sulfadoxine or dapsone (various regimens). In AIDS patients, chemoprophylaxis can be discontinued if antiretroviral therapy leads to immune reconstitution.

Fernàndez-Sabé N et al. Risk factors, clinical features, and outcomes of toxoplasmosis in solid-organ transplant recipients: a matched case-control study. Clin Infect Dis. 2012 Feb 1;54(3): 355–61. [PMID: 22075795]

Montoya JG et al. Management of *Toxoplasma gondii* infection during pregnancy. Clin Infect Dis. 2008 Aug 15;47(4):554–66. [PMID: 18624630]

Robert-Gangneux F et al. Epidemiology of and diagnostic strategies for toxoplasmosis. Clin Microbiol Rev. 2012 Apr;25(2): 264–96. [PMID: 22491772]

AMEBIASIS

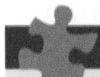 ESSENTIALS OF DIAGNOSIS

- ▶ Organisms or antigen present in stools or abscess aspirate.

- ▶ Positive serologic tests with colitis or hepatic abscess, but these may represent prior infections.

- ▶ Mild to moderate colitis with recurrent diarrhea.

- ▶ Severe colitis including bloody diarrhea, fever, and abdominal pain, with potential progression to hemorrhage or perforation.

- ▶ Hepatic abscess with fever, hepatomegaly, and abdominal pain.

▶ General Considerations

The *Entamoeba* complex contains three morphologically identical species: *Entamoeba dispar* and *Entamoeba moshkovskii*, which are avirulent, and *Entamoeba histolytica*, which may be an avirulent intestinal commensal or lead to serious disease. Disease follows penetration of the intestinal wall, resulting in diarrhea, and with severe involvement, dysentery or extraintestinal disease, most commonly liver abscess.

E histolytica infections are present worldwide but are most prevalent in subtropical and tropical areas under conditions of crowding, poor sanitation, and poor nutrition. Of the estimated 500 million persons worldwide infected with *Entamoeba,* most are infected with *E dispar* and an estimated 10% with *E histolytica*. The prevalence of *E moshkovskii* is unknown. Mortality from invasive *E histolytica* infections is estimated at 100,000 per year.

Humans are the only established *E histolytica* host. Transmission occurs through ingestion of cysts from fecally contaminated food or water, facilitated by person-to-person spread, flies and other arthropods as mechanical vectors, and use of human excrement as fertilizer. Urban outbreaks have occurred because of common-source water contamination.

▶ Clinical Findings

A. Symptoms and Signs

1. Intestinal amebiasis—In most infected persons, the organism lives as a commensal, and the carrier is without

symptoms. With symptomatic disease, diarrhea may begin within a week of infection, although an incubation period of 2–4 weeks is more common, with gradual onset of abdominal pain and diarrhea. Fever is uncommon. Periods of remission and recurrence may last days to weeks or longer. Abdominal examination may show distention, tenderness, hyperperistalsis, and hepatomegaly. Microscopic hematochezia is common. More severe presentations include colitis and dysentery, with more extensive diarrhea (10–20 stools per day) and bloody stools. With dysentery, physical findings include high fevers, prostration, vomiting, abdominal pain and tenderness, hepatic enlargement, and hypotension. Severe presentations are more common in young children, pregnant women, those who are malnourished, and those receiving corticosteroids. Thus, in endemic regions, corticosteroids should not be started for presumed inflammatory bowel disease without first ruling out amebiasis. Fulminant amebic colitis can progress to necrotizing colitis, intestinal perforation, mucosal sloughing, and severe hemorrhage, with mortality rates over 40%. More chronic complications of intestinal amebiasis include chronic diarrhea with weight loss, which may last for months to years; bowel ulcerations; and amebic appendicitis. Localized granulomatous lesions (amebomas) can present after either dysentery or chronic intestinal infection. Clinical findings include pain, obstructive symptoms, and hemorrhage and may suggest intestinal carcinoma.

2. Extraintestinal amebiasis—The most common extraintestinal manifestation is amebic liver abscess. This can occur with colitis, but more frequently presents without history of prior intestinal symptoms. Patients present with the acute or gradual onset of abdominal pain, fever, an enlarged and tender liver, anorexia, and weight loss. Diarrhea is present in a small number of patients. Physical examination may show intercostal tenderness. Abscesses are most commonly single and in the right lobe of the liver, and they are much more common in men. Without prompt treatment, amebic abscesses may rupture into the pleural, peritoneal, or pericardial space, which is often fatal. Amebic infections may rarely occur throughout the body, including the lungs, brain, and genitourinary system.

B. Laboratory Findings

Laboratory studies with intestinal amebiasis show leukocytosis and hematochezia, with fecal leukocytes not present in all cases. With extraintestinal amebiasis, leukocytosis and elevated liver function studies are seen.

C. Diagnostic Testing

Diagnosis is by finding *E histolytica* or its antigen or by serologic tests. However, each method has limitations.

1. Intestinal amebiasis—Diagnosis is most commonly made by identifying organisms in the stool. *E histolytica* and *E dispar* cannot be distinguished, but the identification of amebic trophozoites or cysts in a symptomatic patient is highly suggestive of amebiasis. Stool evaluation for organisms is not highly sensitive (~30–50% for amebic colitis), and at least three stool specimens should be evaluated after

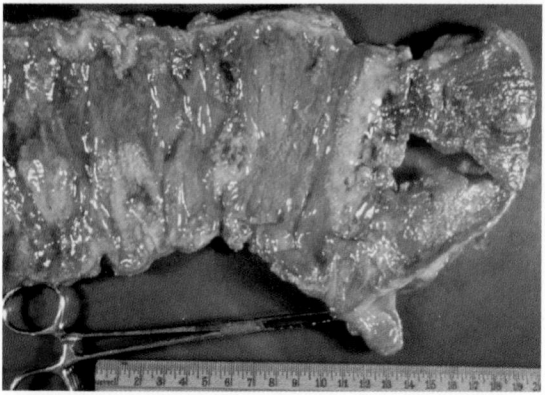

▲ **Figure 35–7.** Gross pathology showing intestinal ulcers due to amebiasis. (From Dr. Mae Melvin, Public Health Image Library, CDC.)

concentration and staining. Multiple serologic assays are available; these tests are fairly sensitive, although sensitivity is lower (~70% in colitis) early in illness, and they cannot distinguish recent and old disease, as they remain positive for years after infection. A commercially available stool antigen test (TechLab II) offers improved sensitivity (> 90% for colitis); it requires fresh or frozen (not preserved) stool specimens. PCR-based tests are available but not used routinely. Colonoscopy of uncleansed bowel typically shows no specific findings in mild intestinal disease; in severe disease, ulcers may be found with intact intervening friable mucosa, resembling inflammatory bowel disease (Figure 35–7). Examination of fresh ulcer exudate for motile trophozoites and for E histolytica antigen may yield a diagnosis.

2. Hepatic abscess—Serologic tests for anti-amebic antibodies are almost always positive, except very early in the infection. Thus, a negative test in a suspicious case should be repeated in about a week. The TechLab II antigen test can be used to test serum, with good sensitivity if used before the initiation of therapy. Examination of stools for organisms or antigen is frequently negative; the antigen test is positive in ~40% of cases. As imaging studies cannot distinguish amebic and pyogenic abscesses, when a diagnosis is not available from serologic studies, percutaneous aspiration may be indicated, ideally with an image-guided needle. Aspiration typically yields brown or yellow fluid. Detection of organisms in the aspirate is uncommon, but detection of E histolytica antigen is very sensitive and diagnostic. The key risk of aspiration is peritoneal spillage leading to peritonitis from amebas or other (pyogenic or echinococcal) organisms.

D. Imaging

Liver abscesses can be identified by ultrasonography, CT, or MRI, typically with round or oval low-density nonhomogeneous lesions, with abrupt transition from normal liver to the lesion, and hypoechoic centers. Abscesses are most commonly single, but more than one may be present. The right lobe is usually involved.

▶ Treatment

Treatment of amebiasis generally entails the use of metronidazole or tinidazole to eradicate tissue trophozoites and a luminal amebicide to eradicate intestinal cysts (Table 35–6). Asymptomatic infection with E dispar does not require therapy. This organism cannot be differentiated morphologically from E histolytica, but with negative serology E dispar colonization is likely, and treatment is not indicated. Colonization with E histolytica is generally treated with a luminal agent. Effective luminal agents are diloxanide furoate (500 mg orally three times daily with meals for 10 days), iodoquinol (diiodohydroxyquin; 650 mg orally three times daily for 21 days), and paromomycin (30 mg/kg base orally, maximum 3 g, in three divided doses after meals daily for 7 days). Side effects associated with luminal agents are flatulence with diloxanide furoate, mild diarrhea with iodoquinol, and gastrointestinal symptoms with paromomycin. Relative contraindications are thyroid disease for iodoquinol and kidney disease for iodoquinol or paromomycin.

Treatment of intestinal amebiasis requires metronidazole (750 mg orally three times daily for 10 days) or tinidazole (2 g orally once daily for 3 days for mild disease and 5 days for serious disease) plus a luminal agent (Table 35–6). Metronidazole has most commonly been used in the United States, but tinidazole offers simpler dosing and less side effects. Metronidazole often induces transient nausea, vomiting, epigastric discomfort, headache, or a metallic taste. A disulfiram-like reaction may occur if alcohol is coingested. Metronidazole should be avoided in pregnant or nursing mothers if possible. The same toxicities and concerns probably apply for tinidazole, although it appears to be better tolerated. Fluid and electrolyte replacement is also important for patients with significant diarrhea. Surgical management of acute complications of intestinal amebiasis is best avoided whenever possible. Successful therapy of severe amebic colitis may be followed by postdysenteric colitis, with continued diarrhea without persistent infection; this syndrome generally resolves in weeks to months.

Alternatives for the treatment of intestinal amebiasis are tetracycline (250–500 mg orally four times daily for 10 days) plus chloroquine (500 mg orally daily for 7 days). Emetine or dehydroemetine, which are not available in the United States, can be given subcutaneously or intramuscularly in a dose of 1–1.5 mg/kg/d; the maximum daily dose is 90 mg for dehydroemetine and 65 mg for emetine). These agents are effective but cardiotoxic with a narrow therapeutic range and should be used only until severe disease is controlled. They cause nausea, vomiting, and pain at the injection site.

Amebic liver abscess is also treated with metronidazole or tinidazole plus a luminal agent (even if intestinal infection is not documented; Table 35–6). Metronidazole can be used intravenously when necessary. With failure of initial response to metronidazole or tinidazole, chloroquine, emetine or dehydroemetine may be added. Needle aspiration may be helpful for large abscesses (over 5–10 cm), in particular if the diagnosis remains uncertain, if there is an initial lack of response, or if a patient is very ill, suggesting imminent abscess rupture. With successful therapy, abscesses disappear slowly (over months).

Table 35–6. Treatment of amebiasis.[1]

Clinical Setting	Drugs of Choice and Adult Dosage	Alternative Drugs and Adult Dosage
Asymptomatic intestinal infection	**Luminal agent:** Diloxanide furoate,[2] 500 mg orally three times daily for 10 days –or– Iodoquinol, 650 mg orally three times daily for 21 days –or– Paromomycin, 10 mg/kg orally three times daily for 7 days	
Mild to moderate intestinal infection	Metronidazole, 750 mg orally three times daily (or 500 mg intravenously every 6 hours) for 10 days –or– Tinidazole, 2 g orally daily for 3 days plus– Luminal agent (see above)	Luminal agent (see above) plus either– Tetracycline, 250 mg orally three times daily for 10 days –or– Erythromycin, 500 mg orally four times daily for 10 days
Severe intestinal infection	Metronidazole, 750 mg orally three times daily (or 500 mg intravenously every 6 hours) for 10 days –or– Tinidazole, 2 g orally daily for 3 days plus– Luminal agent (see above)	Luminal agent (see above) plus either– Tetracycline, 250 mg orally three times daily for 10 days –or– Dehydroemetine[2] or emetine,[2] 1 mg/kg subcutaneously or intramuscularly for 3–5 days
Hepatic abscess, ameboma, and other extraintestinal disease	Metronidazole, 750 mg orally three times daily (or 500 mg intravenously every 6 hours) for 10 days –or– Tinidazole, 2 g orally daily for 3 days plus– Luminal agent (see above)	Dehydroemetine[2] or emetine,[2] 1 mg/kg subcutaneously or intramuscularly for 8–10 days, followed by (liver abscess only) chloroquine, 500 mg orally twice daily for 2 days, then 500 mg daily for 21 days plus– Luminal agent (see above)

[1]See text for additional details and cautions.
[2]Not available in the United States.

▶ Prevention & Control

Prevention requires safe water supplies; sanitary disposal of human feces; adequate cooking of food; protection of food from fly contamination; handwashing; and, in endemic areas, avoidance of fruits and vegetables that cannot be cooked or peeled. Water supplies can be boiled, treated with iodine (0.5 mL tincture of iodine per liter for 20 minutes; cysts are resistant to standard concentrations of chlorine), or filtered.

Gonzales ML et al. Antiamoebic drugs for treating amoebic colitis. Cochrane Database Syst Rev. 2009 Apr 15;(2):CD006085. [PMID: 19370624]
Pritt BS et al. Amebiasis. Mayo Clin Proc. 2008 Oct;83(10): 1154–9. [PMID: 18828976]
Wright SG. Protozoan infections of the gastrointestinal tract. Infect Dis Clin North Am. 2012 Jun;26(2):323–39. [PMID: 22632642]

INFECTIONS WITH PATHOGENIC FREE-LIVING AMEBAS

ESSENTIALS OF DIAGNOSIS

▶ Acute meningoencephalitis or chronic granulomatous encephalitis after contact with warm fresh water.

▶ Keratitis, particularly in contact lens users.

The free-living amebas that cause disease in humans are of the genera *Acanthamoeba, Naegleria, Balamuthia,* and *Sappinia.* The organisms are widely distributed in soil and fresh and brackish water. *Acanthamoeba* and *Naegleria* species have been found to harbor *Legionella, Vibrio cholerae,* and other endosymbiotic bacteria and may serve as a reservoir for these organisms.

1. Primary Amebic Meningoencephalitis

Primary amebic meningoencephalitis is a fulminating, hemorrhagic, necrotizing meningoencephalitis that occurs in healthy children and young adults and is rapidly fatal. It is caused by free-living amebas, most commonly *Naegleria fowleri,* but also *Balamuthia mandrillaris* and *Acanthamoeba* species. *N fowleri* is a thermophilic organism found in fresh and polluted warm lake water, domestic water supplies, swimming pools, thermal water, and sewers. Most patients give a history of exposure to warm fresh water. The incubation period varies from 2 to 15 days. Early symptoms include headache, fever, stiff neck, and lethargy, often associated with rhinitis and pharyngitis. Vomiting, disorientation, and other signs of meningoencephalitis develop within 1 or 2 days, followed by coma and then death within 7–10 days. No distinctive clinical features distinguish the infection from acute bacterial meningoencephalitis. CSF shows hundreds to thousands of leukocytes and erythrocytes per cubic millimeter. Protein is usually elevated, and glucose is normal or moderately reduced. A fresh wet mount of the CSF may show motile trophozoites. Staining with Giemsa or Wright stain will identify the trophozoites. Species identification is based on morphology and immunologic methods. Primary amebic meningoencephalitis is nearly always fatal. Amphotericin B appears to be the drug of choice; one survivor was treated with intravenous and intrathecal amphotericin B, intravenous miconazole, and oral rifampin.

2. Granulomatous Amebic Encephalitis

Acanthamoeba species and *B mandrillaris* can cause an encephalitis that is more chronic in nature than primary amebic meningoencephalitis. One case of encephalitis caused by *Sappinia* has also been described. Neurologic disease may be preceded by skin lesions, including ulcers and nodules. After an uncertain incubation period neurologic symptoms develop slowly, with headache, meningismus, nausea, vomiting, lethargy, and low-grade fevers progressing over weeks to months to focal neurologic findings, mental status abnormalities, and eventually coma and death. CT and MRI show single or multiple nonspecific lesions. Lumbar puncture is dangerous due to increased intracranial pressure. CSF shows a lymphocytic pleocytosis with elevated protein; amebas are not typically seen. Diagnosis can be made by biopsy of skin or brain lesions. Information on the treatment of granulomatous amebic encephalitis is limited. Some patients have been successfully treated with various combinations of flucytosine, pentamidine, fluconazole or itraconazole, sulfadiazine, trimethoprim-sulfamethoxazole, and azithromycin.

3. Acanthamoeba Keratitis

Acanthamoeba keratitis is a painful, sight-threatening corneal infection. It is associated with corneal trauma, most commonly after use of contact lenses and contaminated saline solution. Symptoms include severe eye pain, photophobia, tearing, and blurred vision. The keratitis progresses slowly, with waxing and waning clinical findings over months, and can progress to blindness. Lack of response to antibacterial, antifungal, and antiviral topical treatments and potential use of contaminated contact lens solution are suggestive of the diagnosis. Ocular examination shows corneal ring infiltrates, but these can also be caused by other pathogens. The diagnosis can be made by examination or culture of corneal scrapings. Available diagnostic techniques include examination of a wet preparation for cysts and motile trophozoites, examination of stained specimens, evaluation with immunofluorescent reagents, culture of organisms, and PCR.

Acanthamoeba keratitis can be cured with local therapy. Topical propamidine isethionate (0.1%), chlorhexidine digluconate (0.02%), polyhexamethylene biguanide, neomycin-polymyxin B-gramicidin, miconazole, and combinations of these agents have been used successfully. Oral itraconazole or ketoconazole can be added for deep keratitis. Drug resistance has been reported. Use of corticosteroid therapy is controversial. In some cases, debridement and penetrating keratoplasty have been performed in addition to medical therapy. Corneal grafting can be done after the amebic infection has been eradicated.

Bravo FG et al. *Balamuthia mandrillar* is infection of the skin and central nervous system: an emerging disease of concern to many specialties in medicine. Curr Opin Infect Dis. 2011 Apr;24(2):112–7. [PMID: 21192259]

Dart JK et al. Acanthamoeba keratitis: diagnosis and treatment update, 2009. Am J Ophthalmol. 2009 Oct;148(4):487–499.e2. [PMID: 19660733]

Visvesvara GS. Amebic meningoencephalitides and keratitis: challenges in diagnosis and treatment. Curr Opin Infect Dis. 2010 Dec;23(6):590–4. [PMID: 20802332]

COCCIDIOSIS (Cryptosporidiosis, Isosporiasis, Cyclosporiasis, Sarcocystosis) & MICROSPORIDIOSIS

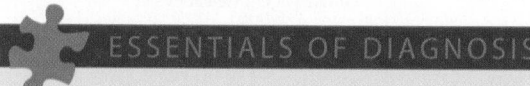
ESSENTIALS OF DIAGNOSIS

▶ Acute diarrhea, especially in children in developing countries.

▶ Outbreaks of diarrhea secondary to contaminated water or food.

▶ Prolonged diarrhea in immunocompromised persons.

▶ Diagnosis mostly by identifying organisms in specially stained stool specimens.

▶ General Considerations

The causes of coccidiosis are *Cryptosporidium* species (*C parvum, C hominis, and others)*; *Isospora belli; Cyclospora cayetanensis;* and *Sarcocystis* species. Microsporidiosis is caused by at least 14 species, most commonly *Enterocytozoon bieneusi* and *Encephalitozoon intestinalis.* These infections occur worldwide, particularly in the tropics and in regions where hygiene is poor. They are causes of endemic childhood gastroenteritis (particularly in malnourished children in developing countries); institutional and community outbreaks of diarrhea; traveler's diarrhea; and acute and chronic diarrhea in immunosuppressed patients, in particular those with AIDS. They are all notable for the potential to cause prolonged diarrhea, often lasting for a number of weeks. Clustering occurs in households, day care centers, and among sexual partners.

The infectious agents are oocysts (coccidiosis) or spores (microsporidiosis) transmitted from person to person or by contaminated drinking or swimming water or food. Ingested oocysts release sporozoites that invade and multiply in enterocytes, primarily in the small bowel. Coccidian oocysts and microsporidian cysts can remain viable in the environment for years.

I belli and *C cayetanensis* appear to infect only humans. *C cayetanensis* has caused a number of food-borne outbreaks in the United States in recent years, most commonly associated with imported fresh produce. *Sarcocystis* infects many species; humans are intermediate hosts (infected by ingestion of fecal sporocysts) for some species but definitive hosts for *Sarcocystis bovihominis* and *Sarcocystis suihominis* (infected by ingestion of tissue cysts in under-cooked beef and pork, respectively).

Cryptosporidiosis is a zoonosis (*C parvum* principally infects cattle), but most human infections are acquired from humans, in particular with *C hominus*. Cryptosporidia are highly infectious and readily transmitted in day care settings and households. They have caused large community outbreaks due to contaminated water supplies (causing ~400,000 illnesses in Milwaukee in 1993) and are the leading cause of recreational water–associated outbreaks of gastroenteritis. Of note, coccidia and microsporidians will generally be missed on routine evaluations of stool for ova and parasites, as they require special staining techniques for identification.

▶ Clinical Findings

A. Symptoms and Signs

1. Cryptosporidiosis—The incubation period appears to be 1–14 days. In developing countries, disease is primarily in children under 5 years of age, causing 5–10% of childhood diarrhea. Presenting symptoms in children include acute watery diarrhea, abdominal pain, and cramps, with rapid resolution in most patients; however, symptoms quite commonly persist for 2 weeks or more. In developed countries, most patients are adults. Diarrhea in immunocompetent individuals typically lasts from 5 to 10 days. It is usually watery, with accompanying abdominal pain and cramps, nausea, vomiting, and fever. Relapses may follow initial resolution of symptoms. Mild illness and asymptomatic infection are also common.

Cryptosporidiosis is a well-characterized cause of diarrhea in those with AIDS. It was common before the advent of highly active antiretroviral therapy, particularly with advanced immunosuppression. Clinical manifestations are variable, but patients commonly have chronic diarrhea with frequent foul smelling stools, malabsorption, and weight loss. Severe, life-threatening watery diarrhea may be seen. Cryptosporidiosis also causes extraintestinal disease with AIDS, including pulmonary infiltrates with dyspnea and biliary tract infection with sclerosing cholangitis and AIDS cholangiopathy.

2. Isosporiasis—The incubation period for *I belli* is about 1 week. In immunocompetent persons, it usually causes a self-limited watery diarrhea lasting 2–3 weeks, with abdominal cramps, anorexia, malaise, and weight loss. Fever is unusual. Chronic symptoms may persist for months. In immunocompromised patients, isosporiasis more commonly causes severe and chronic diarrhea, with complications including marked dehydration, malnutrition, and hemorrhagic colitis. Extraintestinal disease has been reported rarely.

3. Cyclosporiasis—*C cayetanensis* oocysts must undergo a period of sporulation of 7 days or more after shedding before they become infectious. Therefore, person-to-person spread is unlikely, and spread has typically been due to contaminated food (especially fresh produce) and water. The incubation period is 1–11 days. Infections can be asymptomatic. Cyclosporiasis causes an illness similar to

that described for the other pathogens described in this section, with watery diarrhea, abdominal cramps, nausea, fatigue, and anorexia. Fever is seen in 25% of cases. Symptoms typically continue for 2 weeks or longer and may persist for months. Relapses of diarrhea are common. Diarrhea may be preceded by a flu-like prodrome and followed by persistent fatigue. In immunocompromised patients, cyclosporiasis is typically more severe and prolonged, with chronic fulminant watery diarrhea and weight loss.

4. Sarcocystosis—*Sarcocystis* infection may be common in some developing countries, but it is usually asymptomatic. Infection appears to most commonly follow the ingestion of undercooked beef or pork, leading to the development of cysts in muscle, with myalgias, fever, bronchospasm, pruritic rash, lymphadenopathy, and subcutaneous nodules. Ingestion of fecal sporocysts may lead to gastrointestinal symptoms.

5. Microsporidiosis—Microsporidia are obligate intracellular protozoans that cause a wide spectrum of diseases. Many infections are of zoonotic origin, but human-to-human transmission has been documented. Infection is mainly by ingestion of spores, but also by direct inoculation of the eyes. In immunocompetent hosts, microsporidian infections most commonly present as self-limited diarrhea. Ocular infections have also been described. Disease from microsporidia is seen mainly in immunocompromised persons, particularly those with AIDS. Infections in AIDS patients are most commonly with *E bieneusi* and *E intestinalis*. They cause chronic diarrhea, with anorexia, bloating, weight loss, and wasting, especially in those with advanced immunodeficiency. Fever is usually not seen. Other illnesses in immunocompromised persons associated with microsporidians (including the genera *Enterocytozoon*, *Encephalitozoon*, *Brachiola*, *Vittaforma*, *Pleistophora*, *Trachipleistophora*, and *Microsporidium*) include biliary tract disease (AIDS cholangiopathy), genitourinary infection with cystitis, kidney disease, hepatitis, peritonitis, myositis, respiratory infections including sinusitis, central nervous system infections including granulomatous encephalitis, and disseminated infections. Ocular infections with *Encephalitozoon* species cause conjunctivitis and keratitis, presenting as redness, photophobia, and loss of visual acuity.

B. Laboratory Findings

1. Cryptosporidiosis—Typically, stool is without blood or leukocytes. Diagnosis is traditionally made by detecting the organism in stool using a modified acid-fast stain; this technique is relatively insensitive, and multiple specimens should be evaluated before ruling out the diagnosis. Of note, routine evaluation for ova and parasites typically does not include a modified acid-fast stain, so this must be specifically requested in many laboratories. Antigen detection offers improved sensitivity and specificity, both of which are well over 90% with a number of available assays, and these methods may now be considered the optimal means of diagnosis.

2. Isosporiasis—Diagnosis of isosporiasis is by examination of stool wet mounts or after modified acid-fast staining, in which the organism is clearly distinguishable from other parasites. Other stains also show the organism. Shedding of oocysts may be intermittent, so the sensitivity of stool evaluation is not high, and multiple samples should be examined. The organism may also be identified in duodenal aspirates or small bowel biopsies.

3. Cyclosporiasis—Diagnosis is made by examination of stool wet mounts or after modified acid-fast staining. Multiple specimens may need to be examined to make a diagnosis. The organism can also be identified in small bowel aspirates or biopsy specimens.

4. Sarcocystosis—Eosinophilia and elevated creatine kinase may be seen. Diagnosis is by identification of the acid-fast organisms in stool or by identification of trophozoites or bradyzoites in tissue biopsies.

5. Microsporidiosis—Diagnosis can be made by identification of organisms in specially stained stool, fluid, or tissue specimens, for example with Weber chromotrope-based stain. Electron microscopy is helpful for confirmation of the diagnosis and speciation. PCR and culture techniques are available but not used routinely.

▶ **Treatment**

Most acute infections with these pathogens in immunocompetent persons are self-limited and do not require treatment. Supportive treatment for severe or chronic diarrhea includes fluid and electrolyte replacement and, in some cases, parenteral nutrition.

1. Cryptosporidiosis—Treatment of cryptosporidiosis is challenging. No agent is clearly effective. Modest benefits have been seen in some (but not other) studies with paromomycin, a non-absorbed aminoglycoside (25–35 mg/kg orally for 14 days has been used), and nitazoxanide (500 mg–1 g orally twice daily for 3 days in nonimmunocompromised and 2–8 weeks in advanced AIDS patients), which is approved in the United States for this indication. It can cause mild gastrointestinal toxicity. Other agents that have been used with mixed success in AIDS patients with cryptosporidiosis include azithromycin, spiramycin, bovine hyperimmune colostrum, and octreotide. Reversing immunodeficiency with effective antiretroviral therapy is of greatest importance.

2. Isosporiasis—Isosporiasis is effectively treated in immunocompetent and immunosuppressed persons with trimethoprim-sulfamethoxazole (160 mg/800 mg orally two to four times daily for 10 days, with the higher dosage for patients with AIDS). An alternative therapy is pyrimethamine (75 mg orally in four divided doses) with folinic acid (10–25 mg/d orally). Maintenance therapy with low-dose trimethoprim-sulfamethoxazole (160 mg/ 800 mg daily or three times per week) or Fansidar (1 tablet weekly) prevents relapse in those with persistent immunosuppression.

3. Cyclosporiasis—Cyclosporiasis is also treated with trimethoprim-sulfamethoxazole (dosing as for isosporiasis). With AIDS, long-term maintenance therapy (160 mg/ 800 mg three times weekly) helps prevent relapse. For patients intolerant of trimethoprim-sulfamethoxazole, ciprofloxacin (500 mg orally twice daily for 7 days) showed efficacy, albeit with less ability to clear the organism than trimethoprim-sulfamethoxazole.

4. Sarcocystosis—For sarcocystosis, no specific treatment is established, but sulfadiazine cleared intestinal cysts in one study.

5. Microsporidiosis—Treatment of microsporidiosis is complex. Infections with most species, including those causing gastrointestinal and other manifestations, should be treated with albendazole (400 mg orally twice daily for 2–4 weeks), which has activity against a number of species, but relatively poor efficacy (about 50%) against *E bieneusi*, the most common microsporidial cause of diarrhea in AIDS patients. Fumagillin, which is used to treat honeybees and fish with microsporidian infections, has shown benefit in clinical trials at a dose of 20 mg three times per day for 14 days; treatment was accompanied by reversible thrombocytopenia. As with cryptosporidiosis, the best means of controlling microsporidiosis in AIDS patients is to restore immune function with effective antiretroviral therapy. Ocular microsporidiosis can be treated with fumagillin solution (3 mg/mL); this probably should be given with concurrent systemic therapy with albendazole. Adjunctive management may include corticosteroids to decrease inflammation and keratoplasty.

▶ **Prevention**

Water purification is important for control of these infections. Chlorine disinfection is not effective against cryptosporidial oocysts, so other purification measures are needed. Immunocompromised patients should boil or filter drinking water and should consider avoidance of lakes and swimming pools. Routine precautions (handwashing, gloves, disinfection) should prevent institutional patient-to-patient spread. Optimal means of preventing microsporidial infections are not well understood, but water purification and body substance precautions for immunocompromised and hospitalized individuals are likely effective.

Didier ES et al. Microsporidiosis: not just in AIDS patients. Curr Opin Infect Dis. 2011 Oct;24(5):490–5. [PMID: 21844802]

Marcos LA et al. Intestinal protozoan infections in the immuno-compromised host. Curr Opin Infect Dis. 2013 Aug;26(4):295–301. [PMID: 23806893]

O'Connor RM et al. Cryptosporidiosis in patients with HIV/AIDS. AIDS. 2011 Mar 13;25(5):549–60. [PMID: 21160413]

Shirley DA et al. Burden of disease from cryptosporidiosis. Curr Opin Infect Dis. 2012 Oct;25(5):555–63. [PMID: 22907279]

GIARDIASIS

ESSENTIALS OF DIAGNOSIS

▶ Acute diarrhea; may be profuse and watery.

▶ Chronic diarrhea with greasy, malodorous stools.

▶ Abdominal cramps, distention, flatulence, and malaise.

▶ Cysts or trophozoites in stools.

General Considerations

Giardiasis is a protozoal infection of the upper small intestine caused by the flagellate *Giardia lamblia* (also called *Giardia intestinalis* and *Giardia duodenalis*). The parasite occurs worldwide, most abundantly in areas with poor sanitation. In developing countries, young children are very commonly infected. In the United States and Europe, the infection is the most common intestinal protozoal pathogen; the US estimate is 100,000 to 2.5 million new infections leading to 5000 hospital admissions yearly. Groups at special risk include travelers to *Giardia*-endemic areas, those who swallow contaminated water during recreation or wilderness travel, men who have sex with men, and persons with impaired immunity. Outbreaks are common in households, children's day care centers, and residential facilities, and may occur as a result of contamination of water supplies.

The organism occurs in feces as a flagellated trophozoite and as a cyst. Only the cyst form is infectious by the oral route; trophozoites are destroyed by gastric acidity. Humans are a reservoir for the pathogen; dogs, cats, beavers, and other mammals have been implicated but not confirmed as reservoirs. Under suitable moist, cool conditions, cysts can survive in the environment for weeks to months. Cysts are transmitted as a result of fecal contamination of water or food, by person-to-person contact, or by anal-oral sexual contact. The infectious dose is low, requiring as few as ten cysts. After the cysts are ingested, trophozoites emerge in the duodenum and jejunum. Epithelial damage and mucosal invasion are uncommon. Hypogammaglobulinemia, low secretory IgA levels in the gut, achlorhydria, and malnutrition favor the development of infection.

Clinical Findings

A. Symptoms and Signs

It is estimated that about 50% of infected persons have no discernable infection, about 10% become asymptomatic cyst passers, and 25–50% develop an acute diarrheal syndrome. Acute diarrhea may clear spontaneously but is commonly followed by chronic diarrhea. The incubation period is usually 1–3 weeks but may be longer. The illness may begin gradually or suddenly. Cysts may not be detected in the stool at the onset of the illness. The acute phase may last days or weeks, and is usually self-limited, although cyst excretion may be prolonged. The initial illness may include profuse watery diarrhea, and hospitalization may be required due to dehydration, particularly in young children. Typical symptoms of chronic disease are abdominal cramps, bloating, flatulence, nausea, malaise, and anorexia. Fever and vomiting are uncommon. Diarrhea is usually not severe in the chronic stage of infection; stools are greasy or frothy and foul smelling, without blood, pus, or mucus. The diarrhea may be daily or recurrent; intervening periods may include constipation. Symptoms can persist for weeks to months. Weight loss is frequent. Chronic disease can include malabsorption, including fat- and protein-losing enteropathy and vitamin deficiencies.

B. Laboratory Findings

Most patients seek medical attention after having been ill for over a week, commonly with weight loss of 5 kg or more. Stool is generally without blood or leukocytes. Diagnosis is traditionally made by the identification of trophozoites or cysts in stool. A wet mount of liquid stool may identify motile trophozoites. Stained fixed specimens may show cysts or trophozoites. Sensitivity of stool analysis is not ideal, estimated at 50–80% for a single specimen and over 90% for three specimens. Sampling of duodenal contents with a string test or biopsy is no longer generally recommended, but biopsies may be helpful in very ill or immunocompromised patients. When giardiasis is suspected, antigen assays may be simpler and cheaper than repeated stool examinations, but these tests will not identify other stool pathogens. Multiple tests, which identify antigens of trophozoites or cysts, are available. They are generally quite sensitive (85–98%) and specific (90–100%).

Treatment

The treatments of choice for giardiasis are metronidazole (250 mg orally three times daily for 5–7 days) or tinidazole (2 g orally once). The drugs are not universally effective; cure rates for single courses are typically about 80–95%. Toxicities are as described for treatment of amebiasis, but the lower dosages used for giardiasis limit side effects. A meta-analysis showed albendazole (400 mg orally once daily for 5 days) to have equivalent efficacy and fewer side effects compared with metronidazole, and so it may be considered another first-line agent for giardiasis. Nitazoxanide (500 mg orally twice daily for 3 days) is generally well tolerated but may cause mild gastrointestinal side effects. Other drugs with activity against *Giardia* include furazolidone (100 mg orally four times a day for 7 days), which is about as effective as the other named drugs but causes gastrointestinal side effects, and paromomycin (500 mg orally three times a day for 7 days), which appears to have somewhat lower efficacy but unlike metronidazole, tinidazole, and furazolidone is safe in pregnancy. Symptomatic giardiasis should always be treated. Treatment of asymptomatic patients should be considered, since they can transmit the infection. With a suggestive presentation but negative diagnostic studies, an empiric course of treatment may be appropriate. Household or day care contacts with an index case should be tested and treated if infected.

Prevention

Community chlorination (0.4 mg/L) of water is relatively ineffective for inactivating cysts, so filtration is required. For wilderness or international travelers, bringing water to a boil for 1 minute or filtration with a pore size < 1 mcm are adequate. In day care centers, appropriate disposal of diapers and frequent handwashing are essential.

Granados CE et al. Drugs for treating giardiasis. Cochrane Database Syst Rev. 2012 Dec 12;12:CD007787. [PMID: 23235648]

Solaymani-Mohammadi S et al. A meta-analysis of the effectiveness of albendazole compared with metronidazole as treatments for infections with *Giardia duodenalis*. PLoS Negl Trop Dis. 2010 May 11;4(5):e682. [PMID: 20485492]

TRICHOMONIASIS

ESSENTIALS OF DIAGNOSIS

- ▶ Copious vaginal discharge in women.
- ▶ Nongonococcal urethritis in men.
- ▶ Motile trichomonads on wet mounts.

▶ General Considerations

Trichomoniasis is caused by the protozoan *Trichomonas vaginalis* and is among the most common sexually transmitted diseases, causing vaginitis in women and nongonococcal urethritis in men. It can also occasionally be acquired by other means, since it can survive in moist environments for several hours.

▶ Clinical Findings

A. Symptoms and Signs

T vaginalis is often harbored asymptomatically. For women with symptomatic disease, after an incubation period of 5 days to 4 weeks, a vaginal discharge develops, often with vulvovaginal discomfort, pruritus, dysuria, dyspareunia, or abdominal pain. Examination shows a copious discharge, which is usually not foul smelling but is often frothy and yellow or green in color. Inflammation of the vaginal walls and cervix with punctate hemorrhages are common. Most men infected with *T vaginalis* are asymptomatic, but it can be isolated from about 10% of men with nongonococcal urethritis. In men with trichomonal urethritis, the urethral discharge is generally more scanty than with other causes of urethritis.

B. Diagnostic Testing

Diagnosis is typically made by identifying the organism in vaginal or urethral secretions. Examination of wet mounts will show motile organisms. Tests for bacterial vaginosis (pH > 4.5, fishy odor after addition of potassium hydroxide) are often positive with trichomoniasis. Newer diagnostic tests include point-of-care antigen tests and nucleic acid amplification assays, both of which offer improved sensitivity compared to wet mount microscopy and excellent specificity.

▶ Treatment

The treatment of choice is tinidazole or metronidazole, each as a 2 g single oral dose. Tinidazole may be better tolerated and active against some resistant parasites. Toxicities of these drugs are discussed in the section on amebiasis. If the large single dose cannot be tolerated, an alternative metronidazole dosage is 500 mg orally twice daily for 1 week. All infected persons should be treated, even if asymptomatic, to prevent subsequent symptomatic disease and limit spread. Treatment failure suggests reinfection, but metronidazole-resistant organisms have been reported. These may be treated with tinidazole, longer courses of metronidazole, furazolidone, or other experimental therapies (see Chapter 18).

Bachmann LH et al. *Trichomonas vaginalis* genital infections: progress and challenges. Clin Infect Dis. 2011 Dec;53 (Suppl 3):S160–72. [PMID: 22080269]
Hobbs MM et al. Modern diagnosis of *Trichomonas vaginalis* infection. Sex Transm Infect. 2013 Sep;89(6):434–8. [PMID: 23633669]

HELMINTHIC INFECTIONS

TREMATODE (FLUKE) INFECTIONS

SCHISTOSOMIASIS (Bilharziasis)

ESSENTIALS OF DIAGNOSIS

- ▶ History of fresh water exposure in an endemic area.
- ▶ **Acute schistosomiasis:** fever, headache, myalgias, cough, urticaria, diarrhea, and eosinophilia.
- ▶ **Intestinal schistosomiasis:** abdominal pain, diarrhea, and hepatomegaly, progressing to anorexia, weight loss, and features of portal hypertension.
- ▶ **Urinary schistosomiasis:** hematuria and dysuria, progressing to hydroureter, hydronephrosis and urinary infections.
- ▶ Diagnosis based on characteristic eggs in feces or urine; biopsy of rectal or bladder mucosa; positive serology.

▶ General Considerations

Schistosomiasis, which affects more than 200 million persons worldwide, leads to severe consequences in 20 million persons and about 100,000 deaths annually. The disease is caused by five species of trematode blood flukes. Four species cause intestinal schistosomiasis, with infection of mesenteric venules: *Schistosoma mansoni*, which is present in Africa, the Arabian peninsula, South America, and the Caribbean; *Schistosoma japonicum*, which is endemic in China and Southeast Asia; *Schistosoma mekongi*, which is endemic near the Mekong River in Southeast Asia; and *Schistosoma intercalatum*, which occurs in parts of Africa. *Schistosoma haematobium* causes urinary schistosomiasis, with infection of venules of the urinary tract, and is endemic in Africa and the Middle East. Transmission of schistosomiasis is focal, with greatest prevalence in poor rural areas. Control efforts have diminished transmission significantly in many areas, but high level transmission remains common in sub-Saharan Africa and some other areas. Prevalence of infection and illness typically peaks at about 15–20 years of age.

Humans are infected with schistosomes after contact with fresh water containing cercariae released by infected snails. Infection is initiated by penetration of skin or mucous membranes. After penetration, schistosomulae migrate to the portal circulation, where they rapidly mature. After about 6 weeks, adult worms mate, and migrate to terminal mesenteric or bladder venules, where females deposit their eggs. Some eggs reach the lumen of the bowel or bladder and are passed with feces or urine, while others are retained in the bowel or bladder wall or transported in the circulation to other tissues, in particular the liver. Disease in endemic areas is primarily due to a host response to eggs, with granuloma formation and inflammation, eventually leading to fibrosis. Chronic infection can result in scarring of mesenteric or vesicular blood vessels, leading to portal hypertension and alterations in the urinary tract. In previously uninfected individuals, such as travelers with fresh water contact in endemic regions, acute schistosomiasis may occur, with a febrile illness 2–8 weeks after infection.

► Clinical Findings

A. Symptoms and Signs

1. Cercarial dermatitis—Following cercarial penetration, localized erythema develops in some individuals, which can progress to a pruritic maculopapular rash that persists for some days. Dermatitis can be caused by human schistosomes and, in non-tropical areas, by bird schistosomes that cannot complete their life cycle in humans (swimmer's itch).

2. Acute schistosomiasis (Katayama syndrome)—A febrile illness may develop 2–8 weeks after exposure in persons without prior infection, most commonly after heavy infection with *S mansoni* or *S japonicum*. Presenting symptoms and signs include acute onset of fever; headache; myalgias; cough; malaise; urticaria; diarrhea, which may be bloody; hepatosplenomegaly; lymphadenopathy; and pulmonary infiltrates. Localized lesions may occasionally cause severe manifestations, including CNS abnormalities and death. Acute schistosomiasis usually resolves in 2–8 weeks.

3. Chronic schistosomiasis—Many infected persons have light infections and are asymptomatic, but an estimated 50–60% have symptoms and 5–10% have advanced organ damage. Asymptomatic infected children may suffer from anemia and growth retardation. Symptomatic patients with intestinal schistosomiasis typically experience abdominal pain, fatigue, diarrhea, and hepatomegaly. Over years, anorexia, weight loss, weakness, colonic polyps, and features of portal hypertension develop. Late manifestations include hematemesis from esophageal varices, hepatic failure, and pulmonary hypertension. Urinary schistosomiasis may present within months of infection with hematuria and dysuria, most commonly in children and young adults. Fibrotic changes in the urinary tract can lead to

hydroureter, hydronephrosis, bacterial urinary infections and, ultimately, kidney disease or bladder cancer.

B. Laboratory Findings

Microscopic examination of stool or urine for eggs, evaluation of tissue, or serologic tests establish the diagnosis. Characteristic eggs can be identified on smears of stool or urine, but filtration or concentration techniques can improve yields. Quantitative tests that yield > 400 eggs per gram of feces or 10 mL of urine are indicative of heavy infections with increased risk of complications. Diagnosis can also be made by biopsy of the rectum, colon, liver, or bladder. Serologic tests include an ELISA available from the CDC that is 99% specific for all species. The test is 99% sensitive for *S mansoni*, 95% sensitive for *S haematobium*, but < 50% sensitive for *S japonicum*. Species-specific immunoblots can increase sensitivity. In acute schistosomiasis, leukocytosis and marked eosinophilia may occur; serologic tests may become positive before eggs are seen in stool or urine. After therapy, eggs may be shed in stool or urine for months, and so the identification of eggs in fluids or tissue or positive serologic tests cannot distinguish past or active disease. Tests for egg viability are available. With a diagnosis of schistosomiasis, evaluation for the extent of disease is warranted, including liver function studies and imaging of the liver with intestinal disease and ultrasound or other imaging studies of the urinary system in urinary disease.

► Treatment

Treatment is indicated for all schistosome infections. In areas where recurrent infection is common, treatment is valuable in reducing worm burdens and limiting clinical complications. The drug of choice for schistosomiasis is praziquantel. The drug is administered for 1 day at an oral dose of 40 mg/kg (in one or two doses) for *S mansoni*, *S haematobium*, and *S intercalatum* infections and a dose of 60 mg/kg (in two or three doses) for *S japonicum* and *S mekongi*. Cure rates are generally > 80% after a single treatment, and those not cured have marked reduction in the intensity of infection. Praziquantel is active against invading cercariae but not developing schistosomulae. Therefore, the drug may not prevent illness when given after exposure and, for recent infections, a repeat course after a few weeks may be appropriate. Praziquantel may be used during pregnancy. Resistance to praziquantel has been reported. Toxicities include abdominal pain, diarrhea, urticaria, headache, nausea, vomiting, and fever, and may be due both to direct effects of the drug and responses to dying worms. Alternative therapies are oxamniquine for *S mansoni* infection and metrifonate for *S haemotobium* infection. Both of these drugs currently have limited availability (they are not available in the United States), and resistance may be a problem. No second-line drug is available for *S japonicum* infections. The antimalarial drug artemether has activity against schistosomulae and adult worms and may be effective in chemoprophylaxis; however, it is expensive, and long-term use in malarious areas might select for resistant malaria parasites. With severe disease, use of corticosteroids in conjunction with praziquantel may decrease complications. Treatment should be followed by repeat examinations for eggs about every 3 months for 1 year after therapy, with re-treatment if eggs are seen.

▶ Prevention

Travelers to endemic areas should avoid fresh water exposure. Vigorous toweling after exposure may limit cercarial penetration. Chemoprophylaxis with artemether has shown efficacy but is not standard practice. Community control of schistosomiasis includes improved sanitation and water supplies, elimination of snail habitats, and intermittent treatment to limit worm burdens.

Gray DJ et al. Diagnosis and management of schistosomiasis. BMJ. 2011 May 17;342:d2651. [PMID: 21586478]

Gryseels B. Schistosomiasis. Infect Dis Clin North Am. 2012 Jun;26(2):383–97. [PMID: 22632645]

King CH et al. Utility of repeated praziquantel dosing in the treatment of schistosomiasis in high-risk communities in Africa: a systematic review. PLoS Negl Trop Dis. 2011 Sep;5 (9):e1321. [PMID: 21949893]

LIVER, LUNG, & INTESTINAL FLUKES

FASCIOLIASIS

Infection by *Fasciola hepatica,* the sheep liver fluke, results from ingestion of encysted metacercariae on watercress or other aquatic vegetables. Infection is prevalent in sheep-raising areas in many countries, especially parts of South America, the Middle East, and southern Europe. *Fasciola gigantica* has a more restricted distribution in Asia and Africa and causes similar findings. Eggs are passed from host feces into fresh water, leading to infection of snails, and then deposition of metacercariae on vegetation. In humans, metacercariae excyst, penetrate into the peritoneum, migrate through the liver, and mature in the bile ducts, where they cause local necrosis and abscess formation.

Two clinical syndromes are seen, related to acute migration of worms and chronic infection of the biliary tract. Symptoms related to migration of larvae present 6–12 weeks after ingestion. Typical findings are abdominal pain, fever, malaise, weight loss, urticaria, eosinophilia, and leukocytosis. Tender hepatomegaly and elevated liver function tests may be seen. Rarely, migration to other organs may lead to localized disease. The symptoms of worm migration subside after 2–4 months, followed by asymptomatic infection by adult worms or intermittent symptoms of biliary obstruction, with biliary colic and, at times, findings of cholangitis. Early diagnosis is difficult, as eggs are not found in the feces during the acute migratory phase of infection. Clinical suspicion should be based on clinical findings and marked eosinophilia in at risk individuals. CT and other imaging studies show hypodense migratory lesions of the liver. Definitive diagnosis is made by the identification of characteristic eggs in stool. Repeated examinations may be necessary. In chronic infection,

imaging studies show masses obstructing the extrahepatic biliary tract. Serologic assays have sensitivity and specificity > 90%, but cannot distinguish between past and current infection. Antigen tests with excellent sensitivity and specificity are available in veterinary medicine and may be appropriate for diagnosis in humans.

Fascioliasis is unusual among fluke infections, in that it does not respond well to treatment with praziquantel. The treatment of choice is triclabendazole, which is also used in veterinary medicine, but is not available in the United States. Standard dosing of 10 mg/kg orally in a single dose or two doses over 12 hours achieves a cure rate of about 80%, but repeat dosing is indicated if abnormal radiologic findings or eosinophilia do not resolve. Resistance to triclabendazole has been reported in animal but not human infections. The second-line drug for fascioliasis is bithionol (30–50 mg/kg/d orally in three divided doses on alternate days for 10–15 days); this drug is no longer available in the United States. Treatment with either drug can be accompanied by abdominal pain and other gastrointestinal symptoms. Prevention of fascioliasis involves avoidance of ingestion of raw aquatic plants.

CLONORCHIASIS & OPISTHORCHIASIS

Infection by *Clonorchis sinensis,* the Chinese liver fluke, is endemic in areas of Japan, Korea, China, Taiwan, Southeast Asia, and the far eastern part of Russia. Millions of people are affected and, in some communities, prevalence can reach over 80%. Opisthorchiasis is principally caused by *Opisthorchis felineus* (regions of the former Soviet Union) or *Opisthorchis viverrini* (Thailand, Laos, Vietnam). Clonorchiasis and opisthorchiasis are clinically indistinguishable. Parasite eggs are shed into water in human or animal feces, where they infect snails, which release cercariae, which infect fish. Human infection follows ingestion of raw, undercooked, or pickled freshwater fish containing metacercariae. These parasites excyst in the duodenum and ascend into the biliary tract, where they mature and remain for many years, shedding eggs in the bile.

Most patients harbor few parasites and are asymptomatic. An acute illness can occur 2–3 weeks after initial infection, with fever, abdominal pain, tender hepatomegaly, urticaria, and eosinophilia. The acute syndrome is difficult to diagnose, since ova may not appear in the feces until 3–4 weeks after onset of symptoms. In chronic heavy infections, findings include abdominal pain, anorexia, weight loss, and tender hepatomegaly. More serious findings can include recurrent bacterial cholangitis and sepsis, cholecystitis, liver abscess, and pancreatitis. An increased risk of cholangiocarcinoma has been documented.

Early diagnosis is presumptive, based on clinical findings and epidemiology. Subsequent diagnosis is made by finding characteristic eggs in stool or duodenal or biliary contents. Repeated concentration tests of stool may be necessary. Imaging studies show characteristic biliary tract dilatations with filling defects due to flukes. ELISA assays for clonorchiasis with sensitivities of ~90% are used in Asia.

The drug of choice is praziquantel, 25 mg/kg orally three times daily for 2 days, which provides cure rates over

95%. One day of treatment may be sufficient. Re-treatment may be required, especially in some areas with known decreased praziquantel efficacy. The second-line drug is albendazole (400 mg orally twice daily for 7 days), which appears to be somewhat less effective.

PARAGONIMIASIS

Eight species of *Paragonimus* lung flukes cause human disease. The most important is *Paragonimus westermani*. *Paragonimus* species are endemic in East Asia, Oceania, West Africa, and South America, where millions of persons are infected; rare infections have occurred in North America. Eggs are released into fresh water, where parasites infect snails, and then cercariae infect crabs and crayfish. Human infection follows consumption of raw, undercooked, or pickled freshwater shellfish. Metacercariae then excyst, penetrate into the peritoneum, and pass into the lungs, where they mature into adult worms over about 2 months.

Most persons have moderate worm burdens and are asymptomatic. In symptomatic cases, abdominal pain and diarrhea develop 2 days to 2 weeks after infection, followed by fever, cough, chest pain, urticaria, and eosinophilia. Acute symptoms may last for several weeks. Chronic infection can cause cough productive of brown sputum, hemoptysis, dyspnea, and chest pain, with progression to chronic bronchitis, bronchiectasis, bronchopneumonia, lung abscess, and pleural disease. Ectopic infections can cause disease in other organs, most commonly the CNS, where disease can present with seizures, headaches, and focal neurologic findings due to parasite meningitis and to intracerebral lesions.

The diagnosis of paragonimiasis is made by identifying characteristic eggs in sputum or stool or identifying worms in biopsied tissue. Multiple examinations and concentration techniques may be needed. Serologic tests may be helpful; an ELISA available from the CDC has sensitivity and specificity > 95%. Chest radiographs may show varied abnormalities of the lungs or pleura, including infiltrates, nodules, cavities, and fibrosis, and the findings can be confused with those of tuberculosis. With CNS disease, skull radiographs can show clusters of calcified cysts, and CT or MRI can show clusters of ring-enhancing lesions.

Treatment is with praziquantel (25 mg/kg orally three times daily for 2 days), which provides efficacy of at least 90%. Alternative therapies are bithionol and triclabendazole. As with cysticercosis, for cerebral paragonimiasis, praziquantel should generally be used with corticosteroids. Chronic infection may lead to permanent lung dysfunction and pleural disease requiring drainage procedures.

INTESTINAL FLUKES

The large intestinal fluke, *Fasciolopsis buski,* is a common parasite of pigs and humans in eastern and southern Asia. Eggs shed in stools hatch in fresh water, followed by infection of snails, and release of cercariae that encyst on aquatic plants. Humans are infected by eating uncooked plants, including water chestnuts, bamboo shoots, and watercress. Adult flukes mature in about 3 months and live in the small intestine attached to the mucosa, leading to local inflammation and ulceration. Other intestinal flukes that cause

similar syndromes include *Heterophyes* (North Africa and Turkey) and *Metagonimus* (East Asia) species; these species are transmitted by undercooked freshwater fish.

Infections with intestinal flukes are often asymptomatic, although eosinophilia may be marked. In symptomatic cases, after an incubation period of 1–2 months, manifestations include epigastric pain and diarrhea. Other gastrointestinal symptoms, ileus, edema, and ascites may be seen uncommonly. Diagnosis is based on identification of characteristic eggs or adult flukes in the stool. In contrast to other fluke infections, illness more than 6 months after travel in an endemic area is unlikely. The drug of choice is praziquantel, 25 mg/kg orally as a single dose. Alternative therapies are triclabendazole and niclosamide (for most species).

Cabada MM et al. New developments in epidemiology, diagnosis, and treatment of fascioliasis. Curr Opin Infect Dis. 2012 Oct;25(5):518–22. [PMID: 22744320]
Fürst T et al. Manifestation, diagnosis, and management of foodborne trematodiasis. BMJ. 2012 Jun 26;344:e4093. [PMID: 22736467]
Hong ST et al. *Clonorchis sinensis* and clonorchiasis, an update. Parasitol Int. 2012 Mar;61(1):17–24. [PMID: 21741496]

CESTODE INFECTIONS

NONINVASIVE CESTODE INFECTIONS

The four major tapeworms that cause noninvasive infections in humans are the beef tapeworm *Taenia saginata,* the pork tapeworm *Taenia solium,* the fish tapeworm *Diphyllobothrium latum,* each of which can reach many meters in length, and the dwarf tapeworm *Hymenolepis nana.* *Taenia* and *Hymenolepis* species are broadly distributed, especially in the tropics; *D latum* is most prevalent in temperate regions. Other tapeworms that can cause noninvasive human disease include the rodent tapeworm *Hymenolepis diminuta,* the dog tapeworm *Dipylidium caninum,* and other *Taenia* and *Diphyllobothrium* species. Invasive tapeworm infections, including *T solium* (when infective eggs, rather than cysticerci are ingested) and *Echinococcus* species, will be discussed separately.

1. Beef Tapeworm

Infection is most common in cattle breeding areas. Humans are the definitive host. Gravid segments of *T saginata* are passed in human feces to soil, where they are ingested by grazing animals, especially cattle. The eggs then hatch to release embryos that encyst in muscle as cysticerci. Humans are infected by eating raw or undercooked infected beef. Most individuals infected with *T saginata* are asymptomatic, but abdominal pain and other gastrointestinal symptoms may be present. Eosinophilia is common. The most common presenting finding is the passage of proglottids in the stool.

2. Pork Tapeworm

T solium is transmitted to pigs that ingest human feces. Humans can be either the definitive host (after consuming undercooked pork, leading to tapeworm infection) or the intermediate host (after consuming food contaminated with human feces containing *T solium* eggs, leading to cysticercosis, which is discussed under invasive tapeworm infections). As with the beef tapeworm, infection with *T solium* adult worms is generally asymptomatic, but gastrointestinal symptoms may occur. Infection is generally recognized after passage of proglottids. Autoinfection with eggs can progress to cysticercosis.

3. Fish Tapeworm

Infection with *D latum* follows ingestion of undercooked freshwater fish, most commonly in temperate regions. Eggs from human feces are taken up by crustaceans, these are eaten by fish, which are then infectious to humans. Infection with multiple worms over many years can occur. Infections are most commonly asymptomatic, but nonspecific gastrointestinal symptoms, including diarrhea, may occur. Diagnosis usually follows passage of proglottids. Prolonged heavy infection can lead to megaloblastic anemia and neuropathy from vitamin B_{12} deficiency, which is due to infection-induced dissociation of the vitamin from intrinsic factor and to utilization of the vitamin by worms.

4. Dwarf Tapeworm

H nana is the only tapeworm that can be transmitted between humans. Infections are common in warm areas, especially with poor hygiene and institutionalized populations. Infection follows ingestion of food contaminated with human feces. Eggs hatch in the intestines, where oncospheres penetrate the mucosa, encyst as cysticercoid larvae, and then rupture after about 4 days to release adult worms. Autoinfection can lead to amplification of infection. Infection with *H nana*, the related rodent tapeworm *H diminuta*, or the dog tapeworm *D caninum* can also follow accidental ingestion of infected insects. *H nana* are dwarf in size relative to other tapeworms but can reach 5 cm in length. Heavy infection is common, especially in children, and can be accompanied by abdominal discomfort, anorexia, and diarrhea.

▶ Laboratory Findings

Diagnosis is usually made based on the identification of characteristic eggs or proglottids in stool. Egg release may be irregular, so examination of multiple specimens or concentration techniques may be needed.

▶ Treatment

The treatment of choice for noninvasive tapeworm infections is praziquantel. A single dose of praziquantel (5–10 mg/kg orally) is highly effective, except for *H nana*, for which the dosage is 25 mg/kg. Treatment of *H nana* is more difficult, as the drug is not effective against maturing cysts. Therefore, a repeat treatment after 1 week and screening after therapy to document cure are appropriate with heavy infections. Therapy can be accompanied by headache, malaise, dizziness, abdominal pain, and nausea.

The alternative therapy for these infections is niclosamide. A single dose of niclosamide (2 g chewed) is effective against *D latum*, *Taenia*, and *D caninum* infections. For *H nana*, therapy is continued daily for 1 week. Niclosamide may cause nausea, malaise, and abdominal pain.

Craig P et al. Intestinal cestodes. Curr Opin Infect Dis. 2007 Oct;20(5):524–32. [PMID: 17762788]

INVASIVE CESTODE INFECTIONS

1. Cysticercosis

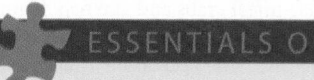

ESSENTIALS OF DIAGNOSIS

▶ Exposure to *T solium* through fecal contamination of food.

▶ Seizures, headache, and other findings of a focal CNS lesion.

▶ Brain imaging shows cysts; positive serologic tests.

▶ General Considerations

Cysticercosis is due to tissue infection with cysts of *T solium* that develop after humans ingest food contaminated with eggs from human feces, thus acting as an intermediate host for the parasite. Prevalence is high where the parasite is endemic, in particular Mexico, Central and South America, the Philippines, and Southeast Asia. An estimated 20 million persons are infected with cysticerci yearly, leading to about 400,000 persons with neurologic symptoms and 50,000 deaths. Antibody prevalence rates up to 10% are recognized in some endemic areas, and the infection is one of the most important causes of seizures in the developing world and in immigrants to the United States from endemic countries. In Latin America, it is estimated that 0.5–1.5 million people suffer from epilepsy secondary to cysticercosis.

▶ Clinical Findings

A. Symptoms and Signs

Neurocysticercosis can cause intracerebral, subarachnoid, and spinal cord lesions and intraventricular cysts. Single or multiple lesions may be present. Lesions may persist for years before symptoms develop, generally due to local inflammation or ventricular obstruction. Presenting symptoms include seizures, focal neurologic deficits, altered cognition, and psychiatric disease. Symptoms develop more quickly with intraventricular cysts, with findings of hydrocephalus and meningeal irritation, including severe headache, vomiting, papilledema, and visual loss. A particularly aggressive form of the disease, racemose cysticercosis, involves proliferation of cysts at the base of the brain, leading to alterations of consciousness and death. Spinal cord lesions can present with progressive focal findings.

Cysticercosis of other organ systems is usually clinically benign. Involvement of muscles can uncommonly cause discomfort and is identified by radiographs of muscle showing multiple calcified lesions. Subcutaneous involvement presents with multiple painless palpable skin lesions. Involvement of the eyes can present with ptosis due to extraocular muscle involvement or intraocular abnormalities.

B. Laboratory Findings

CSF examination may show lymphocytic or eosinophilic pleocytosis, decreased glucose, and elevated protein. Serology plays an important role in diagnosis. ELISAs with sensitivity and specificity over 90% are available.

C. Imaging

With neuroimaging by CT or MRI, multiple parenchymal cysts are most typically seen. Parenchymal calcification is also common. Ventricular cysts may be difficult to visualize, with MRI offering better sensitivity than CT.

▶ Treatment

The medical management of neurocysticercosis is controversial, as the benefits of cyst clearance must be weighed against potential harm of an inflammatory response to dying worms. Antihelminthic therapy hastens radiologic improvement in parenchymal cysticercosis, but some randomized trials have shown that corticosteroids alone are as effective as specific therapy plus corticosteroids for controlling seizures. Overall, most authorities recommend treatment of active lesions, in particular lesions with a high likelihood of progression, such as intraventricular cysts. At the other end of the spectrum, inactive calcified lesions probably do not benefit from therapy. When treatment is deemed appropriate, standard therapy consists of albendazole (10–15 mg/kg/d orally for 8 days) or praziquantel (50 mg/kg/d orally for 15–30 days). Albendazole is probably preferred, since it has shown better efficacy in some comparisons and since corticosteroids appear to lower circulating praziquantel levels but increase albendazole levels. Increasing the dosage of albendazole to 30 mg/kg/d orally may improve outcomes. Corticosteroids are usually administered concurrently, but dosing is not standardized. Patients should be observed for evidence of localized inflammatory responses. Anticonvulsant therapy is provided if needed, and shunting is performed if required for elevated intracranial pressure. Surgical removal of cysts may be helpful for some difficult cases of neurocysticercosis and for symptomatic non-neurologic disease.

Brunetti E et al. Cestode infestations: hydatid disease and cysticercosis. Infect Dis Clin North Am. 2012 Jun;26(2):421–35. [PMID: 22632647]
Coyle CM et al. Neurocysticercosis: neglected but not forgotten. PLoS Negl Trop Dis. 2012;6(5):e1500. [PMID: 22666505]
Nash TE et al. Diagnosis and treatment of neurocysticercosis. Nat Rev Neurol. 2011 Sep 13;7(10):584–94. [PMID: 21912406]

2. Echinococcosis

ESSENTIALS OF DIAGNOSIS

▶ History of exposure to dogs or wild canines in an endemic area.

▶ Large cystic lesions, most commonly of the liver or lung.

▶ Positive serologic tests.

▶ General Considerations

Echinococcosis occurs when humans are intermediate hosts for canine tapeworms. Infection is acquired by ingesting food contaminated with canine feces containing parasite eggs. The principal species that infect humans are *Echinococcus granulosus,* which causes cystic hydatid disease, and *Echinococcus multilocularis,* which causes alveolar hydatid disease. *E granulosus* is transmitted by domestic dogs in areas with livestock (sheep, goats, camels, and horses) as intermediate hosts, including Africa, the Middle East, southern Europe, South America, Central Asia, Australia, New Zealand, and the southwestern United States. *E multilocularis,* which much less commonly causes human disease, is transmitted by wild canines, and endemic in northern forest areas of the northern hemisphere, including central Europe, Siberia, northern Japan, northwestern Canada, and western Alaska. An increase in the fox population in Europe has been associated with an increase in human cases. The disease range has also extended southward in Central Asia and China. Other species that cause limited disease in humans are endemic in South America and China.

After humans ingest parasite eggs, the eggs hatch in the intestines to form oncospheres, which penetrate the mucosa, enter the circulation, and encyst in specific organs as hydatid cysts. *E granulosus* forms cysts most commonly in the liver (65%) and lungs (25%), but the cysts may develop in any organ, including the brain, bones, skeletal muscles, kidneys, and spleen. Cysts are most commonly single. The cysts can persist and slowly grow for many years.

▶ Clinical Findings

A. Symptoms and Signs

Infections are commonly asymptomatic and may be noted incidentally on imaging studies or present with symptoms caused by an enlarging or superinfected mass. Findings may include abdominal or chest pain, biliary obstruction, cholangitis, portal hypertension, cirrhosis, bronchial obstruction leading to segmental lung collapse, and abscesses. Cyst leakage or rupture may be accompanied by a severe allergic reaction, including fever and hypotension. Seeding of cysts after rupture may extend the infection to new areas.

E multilocularis generally causes a more aggressive disease than *E granulosus,* with initial infection of the liver, but then local and distant spread commonly suggesting a malignancy. Symptoms based on the areas of involvement gradually worsen over years, with the development of obstructive findings in the liver and elsewhere.

B. Laboratory Findings

Serologic tests, including ELISA and immunoblot, offer sensitivity and specificity over 80% for *E granulosus* liver infections, but lower sensitivity for involvement of other organs. Serologic tests may also distinguish the two major echinococcal infections.

C. Imaging

Diagnosis is usually based on imaging studies, including ultrasonography, CT, and MRI. In *E granulosus* infection, a large cyst containing daughter cysts is highly suggestive of the diagnosis. In *E multilocularis* infection, imaging shows an irregular mass, often with areas of calcification.

▶ Treatment

Treatment of cystic hydatid disease has traditionally involved cautious surgical resection of cysts, with care not to rupture cysts during removal. Injection of a cysticidal agent was used to limit spread in the case of rupture. Newer management algorithms include treatment with albendazole, often in conjunction with surgery. When used alone, as in cases where surgery is not possible, albendazole (10–15 mg/kg/d orally) has demonstrated efficacy, with courses of 3 months or longer duration, in some cases with alternating cycles of treatment and rest. Mebendazole (40–50 mg/kg/d orally) is an alternative drug, and praziquantel may also be effective. In some cases, medical therapy is begun, with surgery performed if disease persists after some months of therapy. Another approach, in particular with inoperable cysts, is percutaneous aspiration, injection, and reaspiration (PAIR). In this approach (which should not be used if cysts communicate with the biliary tract), patients receive antihelminthic therapy, and the cyst is partially aspirated. After diagnostic confirmation by examination for parasite protoscolices, a scolicidal agent (95% ethanol, hypertonic saline, or 0.5% cetrimide) is injected, and the cyst is reaspirated after about 15 minutes. PAIR includes a small risk of anaphylaxis, which has been reported in about 2% of procedures, but death due to anaphylaxis has been rare. Treatment of alveolar cyst disease is challenging, generally relying on wide surgical resection of lesions. Therapy with albendazole before or during surgery may be beneficial and may also provide improvement or even cure in inoperable cases.

Brunetti E et al. Cystic echinococcosis: chronic, complex, and still neglected. PLoS Negl Trop Dis. 2011 Jul;5(7):e1146. [PMID: 21814584]

McManus DP et al. Diagnosis, treatment, and management of echinococcosis. BMJ. 2012 Jun 11;344:e3866. [PMID: 22689886]

Nasseri-Moghaddam S et al. Percutaneous needle aspiration, injection, and re-aspiration with or without benzimidazole coverage for uncomplicated hepatic hydatid cysts. Cochrane Database Syst Rev. 2011 Jan 19;(1):CD003623. [PMID: 21249654]

INTESTINAL NEMATODE (ROUNDWORM) INFECTIONS

ASCARIASIS

ESSENTIALS OF DIAGNOSIS

▶ Transient cough, urticaria, pulmonary infiltrates, eosinophilia.

▶ Nonspecific abdominal symptoms.

▶ Eggs in stool; adult worms occasionally passed.

▶ General Considerations

Ascaris lumbricoides is the most common of the intestinal helminths, infecting about a quarter of the world's population, with estimates of over a billion infections, 12 million acute cases, and 10,000 or more deaths annually. Prevalence is high wherever there is poor hygiene and sanitation or where human feces are used as fertilizer. Heavy infections are most common in children.

Infection follows ingestion of eggs in contaminated food. Larvae hatch in the small intestine, penetrate into the bloodstream, migrate to the lungs, and then travel via airways back to the gastrointestinal tract, where they develop to adult worms, which can be up to 40 cm in length, and live for 1–2 years.

▶ Clinical Findings

Most persons with *Ascaris* infection are asymptomatic. In a small proportion of patients, symptoms develop during migration of worms through the lungs, with fever, nonproductive cough, chest pain, dyspnea, and eosinophilia, occasionally with eosinophilic pneumonia. Rarely, larvae lodge ectopically in the brain, kidney, eye, spinal cord, and other sites and may cause local symptoms.

Light intestinal infections usually produce no symptoms. With heavy infection, abdominal discomfort may be seen. Adult worms may also migrate and be coughed up, be vomited, or may emerge through the nose or anus. They may also migrate into the common bile duct, pancreatic duct, appendix, and other sites, which may lead to cholangitis, cholecystitis, pyogenic liver abscess, pancreatitis, obstructive jaundice, or appendicitis. With very heavy infestations, masses of worms may cause intestinal obstruction, volvulus, intussusception, or death. Although severe manifestations of infection are uncommon, the very high prevalence of ascariasis leads to large numbers of individuals, especially children, with important sequelae. Moderate to high worm loads in children are also associated with nutritional abnormalities due to decreased appetite and food intake, and also decreased absorption of nutrients.

The diagnosis of ascariasis is made after adult worms emerge from the mouth, nose, or anus, or by identifying characteristic eggs in the feces. Due to the very high egg burden, concentration techniques are generally not needed.

Imaging studies demonstrate worms, with filling defects in contrast studies and at times evidence of intestinal or biliary obstruction. Eosinophilia is marked during worm migration but may be absent during intestinal infection.

► Treatment

All infections should ideally be treated. Treatments of choice are albendazole (single 400 mg oral dose), mebendazole (single 500 mg oral dose or 100 mg twice daily for 3 days), or pyrantel pamoate (single 11 mg/kg oral dose, maximum 1 g). These drugs are all well tolerated but may cause mild gastrointestinal toxicity. They are considered safe for children above 1 year of age and in pregnancy, although use in the first trimester is best avoided. In endemic areas, reinfection after treatment is common. Intestinal obstruction usually responds to conservative management and antihelminthic therapy. Surgery may be required for appendicitis and other gastrointestinal complications.

TRICHURIASIS

Trichuris trichiura, the whipworm, infects about a billion persons throughout the world, particularly in humid tropical and subtropical environments. Infection is heaviest and most frequent in children. Infections are acquired by ingestion of eggs. The larvae hatch in the small intestine and mature in the large bowel to adult worms of about 4 cm in length. The worms do not migrate through tissues.

Most infected persons are asymptomatic. Heavy infections may be accompanied by abdominal cramps, tenesmus, diarrhea, distention, nausea, and vomiting. The *Trichuris* dysentery syndrome may develop, particularly in malnourished young children, with findings resembling inflammatory bowel disease including bloody diarrhea and rectal prolapse. Chronic infections in children can lead to iron deficiency anemia, growth retardation, and clubbing of the fingers.

Trichuriasis is diagnosed by identification of characteristic eggs and sometimes adult worms in stools. Concentration techniques are not needed. Eosinophilia is common. Treatment is with albendazole (400 mg/d orally) or mebendazole (200 mg/d orally), for 1–3 days for light infections or 3–7 days for heavy infections, but cure rates are lower than for ascariasis or hookworm infection. The addition of ivermectin (200 mcg/kg orally daily for 1–2 days) to these drugs improves outcomes.

HOOKWORM DISEASE

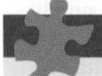

► Transient pruritic skin rash and pulmonary symptoms.

► Anorexia, diarrhea, abdominal discomfort.

► Iron deficiency anemia.

► Characteristic eggs and occult blood in the stool.

► General Considerations

Infection with the hookworms *Ancylostoma duodenale* and *Necator americanus* is very common, especially in most tropical and subtropical regions. Both worms are broadly distributed. Prevalence is estimated at about 1 billion, causing approximately 65,000 deaths each year. When eggs are deposited on warm moist soil they hatch, releasing larvae that remain infective for up to a week. With contact, the larvae penetrate skin and migrate in the bloodstream to the pulmonary capillaries. In the lungs, the larvae penetrate into alveoli and then are carried by ciliary action upward to the bronchi, trachea, and mouth. After being swallowed, they reach and attach to the mucosa of the upper small bowel, where they mature to adult worms. *Ancylostoma* infection can also be acquired by ingestion of the larvae in food or water. Hookworms attach to the intestinal mucosa and suck blood. Blood loss is proportionate to the worm burden.

► Clinical Findings

A. Symptoms and Signs

Most infected persons are asymptomatic. A pruritic maculopapular rash (ground itch) may occur at the site of larval penetration, usually in previously sensitized persons. Pulmonary symptoms may be seen during larval migration through the lungs, with dry cough, wheezing, and low-grade fever, but these symptoms are less common than with ascariasis. About 1 month after infection, as maturing worms attach to the small intestinal mucosa, gastrointestinal symptoms may develop, with epigastric pain, anorexia, and diarrhea, especially in previously unexposed individuals. Persons chronically infected with large worm burdens may have abdominal pain, anorexia, diarrhea, and findings of marked iron-deficiency anemia and protein malnutrition. Anemia can lead to pallor, weakness, dyspnea, and heart failure, and protein loss can lead to hypoalbuminemia, edema, and ascites. These findings may be accompanied by impairment in growth and cognitive development in children. Infection with the dog hookworm *Ancylostoma caninum* can uncommonly lead to abdominal pain, diarrhea, and eosinophilia, with intestinal ulcerations and regional lymphadenitis.

B. Laboratory Findings

Diagnosis is based on the demonstration of characteristic eggs in feces; concentration techniques are usually not needed. Microcytic anemia, occult blood in the stool, and hypoalbuminemia are common. Eosinophilia is common, especially during worm migration.

► Treatment

Treatment is with albendazole (single 400 mg oral dose) or mebendazole (100 mg orally twice daily for 3 days). These drugs are teratogenic, but experience suggests that they are safe in children over 1 year of age and during the second and third trimesters of pregnancy. Occasional adverse effects are diarrhea and abdominal pain. Pyrantel pamoate and levamisole are also effective. Anemia should be managed with iron replacement and, for severe symptomatic anemia, blood transfusion. Mass treatment of children with single doses of albendazole or mebendazole at regular intervals limits worm burdens and the extent of disease and is advocated by the WHO.

STRONGYLOIDIASIS

ESSENTIALS OF DIAGNOSIS

▶ Transient pruritic skin rash and pulmonary symptoms.

▶ Anorexia, diarrhea, abdominal discomfort.

▶ Hyperinfection syndrome in the immunocompromised.

▶ Larvae detected in stool.

▶ With hyperinfection, larvae detected in sputum or other fluids.

▶ Eosinophilia.

▶ General Considerations

Strongyloidiasis is caused by infection with *Strongyloides stercoralis.* Although much less prevalent than ascariasis, trichuriasis, or hookworm infections, strongyloidiasis is nonetheless a significant problem, infecting tens of millions of individuals in tropical and subtropical regions. Infection is also endemic in some temperate regions of North America, Europe, Japan, and Australia. Of particular importance is the predilection of the parasite to cause severe infections in immunocompromised individuals due to its ability to replicate in humans. A related parasite, *Strongyloides fuelleborni,* infects humans in parts of Africa and New Guinea.

Among nematodes, *S stercoralis* is uniquely capable of maintaining its full life cycle both within the human host and in soil. Infection occurs when filariform larvae in soil penetrate the skin, enter the bloodstream, and are carried to the lungs, where they escape from capillaries into alveoli, ascend the bronchial tree, and are then swallowed and carried to the duodenum and upper jejunum, where maturation to the adult stage takes place. Females live embedded in the mucosa for up to 5 years, releasing eggs that hatch in the intestines as free rhabditiform larvae that pass to the ground via the feces. In moist soil, these larvae metamorphose into infective filariform larvae. Autoinfection can occur in humans, when some rhabditiform larvae develop into filariform larvae that penetrate the intestinal mucosa or perianal skin, and enter the circulation. The most dangerous manifestation of *S stercoralis* infection is the **hyperinfection syndrome,** with dissemination of large numbers of filariform larvae to the lungs and other tissues in immunocompromised individuals. Mortality with this syndrome approaches 100% without treatment and has been about 25% with treatment. The hyperinfection syndrome is seen in patients receiving corticosteroids and other immunosuppressive medications; patients with hematologic malignancies, malnutrition, or alcoholism; or persons with AIDS. The risk seems greatest for those receiving corticosteroids.

▶ Clinical Findings

A. Symptoms and Signs

As with other intestinal nematodes, most infected persons are asymptomatic. An acute syndrome can be seen at the time of infection, with a pruritic, erythematous, maculopapular rash, usually of the feet. These symptoms may be followed by pulmonary symptoms (including dry cough, dyspnea, and wheezing) and eosinophilia after a number of days, followed by gastrointestinal symptoms after some weeks, as with hookworm infections. Chronic infection may be accompanied by epigastric pain, nausea, diarrhea, and anemia. Maculopapular or urticarial rashes of the buttocks, perineum, and thighs, due to migrating larvae, may be seen. Large worm burdens can lead to malabsorption or intestinal obstruction. Eosinophilia is common but may fluctuate.

With **hyperinfection** large numbers of larvae can migrate to many tissues, including the lungs, CNS, kidneys, and liver. Gastrointestinal symptoms can include abdominal pain, nausea, vomiting, diarrhea, and more severe findings related to intestinal obstruction, perforation, or hemorrhage. Bacterial sepsis, probably secondary to intestinal ulcerations, is a common presenting finding. Pulmonary findings include pneumonitis, cough, hemoptysis, and respiratory failure. Sputum may contain adult worms, larvae, and eggs. CNS disease includes meningitis and brain abscesses; the CSF may contain larvae. Various presentations can progress to shock and death.

B. Laboratory Findings

The diagnosis of strongyloidiasis can be difficult, as eggs are seldom found in feces. Diagnosis is usually based on the identification of rhabditiform larvae in the stool or duodenal contents. These larvae must be distinguished from hookworm larvae, which may hatch after stool collection. Repeated examinations of stool or examination of duodenal fluid may be required for diagnosis because the sensitivity of individual tests is only about 30%. Hyperinfection is diagnosed by the identification of large numbers of larvae in stool, sputum, or other body fluids. An ELISA from the CDC offers about 90% sensitivity and specificity, but cross-reactions with other helminths may occur. Eosinophilia and mild anemia are common, but eosinophilia may be absent with hyperinfection. Hyperinfection may include extensive pulmonary infiltrates, hypoproteinemia, and abnormal liver function studies.

C. Screening

It is important to be aware of the possibility of strongyloidiasis in persons with even a distant history of residence in an endemic area, since the infection can be latent for decades. Screening of at-risk individuals for infection is appropriate before institution of immunosuppressive therapy. Screening can consist of serologic tests, with stool examinations in those with positive serologic tests, but consideration of presumptive treatment even if the stool evaluations are negative (see below).

Treatment

Full eradication of *S stercoralis* is more important than with other intestinal helminths due to the ability of the parasite to replicate in humans. The treatment of choice for routine infection is ivermectin (200 mcg orally daily for 1–2 days). This treatment has replaced thiabendazole (25 mg/kg orally twice daily for 3 days), which is relatively poorly tolerated, and albendazole (400 mg orally twice daily for 3 days), which is less effective. For hyperinfection, ivermectin should be administered daily until the clinical syndrome has resolved and larvae have not been identified for at least 2 weeks. Follow-up examinations for larvae in stool or sputum are necessary, with repeat dosing if the infection persists. With continued immunosuppression, eradication may be difficult, and regular repeated doses of antihelminthic therapy (eg, monthly ivermectin) may be required.

ENTEROBIASIS

ESSENTIALS OF DIAGNOSIS

- ▶ Nocturnal perianal pruritus.
- ▶ Identification of eggs or adult worms on perianal skin or in stool.

General Considerations

Enterobius vermicularis, the pinworm, is a common cause of intestinal infections worldwide, with maximal prevalence in school-age children. Enterobiasis is transmitted person-to-person via ingestion of eggs after contact with the hands or perianal region of an infected individual, food or fomites that have been contaminated by an infected individual, or infected bedding or clothing. Auto-infection also occurs. Eggs hatch in the duodenum and larvae migrate to the cecum. Females mature in about a month, and remain viable for about another month. During this time they migrate through the anus to deposit large numbers of eggs on the perianal skin. Due to the relatively short lifespan of these helminths, continuous reinfection, as in institutional settings, is required, for long-standing infection.

Clinical Findings

A. Symptoms and Signs

Most individuals with pinworm infection are asymptomatic. The most common symptom is perianal pruritus, particularly at night, due to the presence of the female worms or deposited eggs. Insomnia, restlessness, and enuresis are common in children. Perianal scratching may result in excoriation and impetigo. Many mild gastrointestinal symptoms have also been attributed to enterobiasis, but associations are not proven. Serious sequelae are uncommon. Rarely, worm migration results in inflammation or granulomatous reactions of the gastrointestinal or

genitourinary tracts. Colonic ulceration and eosinophilic colitis have been reported.

B. Laboratory Findings

Pinworm eggs are usually not found in stool. Diagnosis is made by finding adult worms or eggs on the perianal skin. A common test is to apply clear cellophane tape to the perianal skin, ideally in the early morning, followed by microscopic examination for eggs. The sensitivity of the tape test is reported to be about 50% for a single test and 90% for three tests. Nocturnal examination of the perianal area or gross examination of stools may reveal adult worms, which are about 1 cm in length. Eosinophilia is rare.

Treatment

Treatment is with single oral doses of albendazole (400 mg), mebendazole (100 mg) or pyrantel pamoate (11 mg/kg, to a maximum of 1 g). The dose is repeated in 2 weeks due to frequent reinfection. Other infected family members should be treated concurrently, and treatment of all close contacts may be appropriate when rates of reinfection are high in family, school, or institutional settings. Standard handwashing and hygiene practices are helpful in limiting spread. Perianal scratching should be discouraged. Washing of clothes and bedding should kill pinworm eggs.

Greaves D et al. Strongyloides stercoralis infection. BMJ. 2013 Jul 30;347:f4610. [PMID: 23900531]
Jia TW et al. Soil-transmitted helminth reinfection after drug treatment: a systematic review and meta-analysis. PLoS Negl Trop Dis. 2012;6(5):e1621. [PMID: 22590656]
Knopp S et al. Nematode infections: soil-transmitted helminths and trichinella. Infect Dis Clin North Am. 2012 Jun;26(2):341–58. [PMID: 22632643]
Mejia R et al. Screening, prevention, and treatment for hyperinfection syndrome and disseminated infections caused by *Strongyloides stercoralis.* Curr Opin Infect Dis. 2012 Aug;25(4):458–63. [PMID: 22691685]
Steinmann P et al. Efficacy of single-dose and triple-dose albendazole and mebendazole against soil-transmitted helminths and *Taenia* spp.: a randomized controlled trial. PLoS One. 2011;6(9):e25003. [PMID: 21980373]
Vercruysse J et al. Assessment of the anthelmintic efficacy of albendazole in school children in seven countries where soil-transmitted helminths are endemic. PLoS Negl Trop Dis. 2011 Mar 29;5(3):e948. [PMID: 21468309]

INVASIVE NEMATODE (ROUNDWORM) INFECTIONS

DRACUNCULIASIS

ESSENTIALS OF DIAGNOSIS

- ▶ Tender cutaneous ulcer and worm protruding from the skin of an individual who has ingested untreated water in rural Africa.

General Considerations

Dracunculiasis is caused by the nematode *Dracunculus medinensis*, or Guinea worm. It causes chronic cutaneous ulcers with protruding worms in rural Africa. It occurs only in humans and is a major cause of disability, although recent control efforts have been remarkably successful, with decreased annual incidence from about 3.5 million cases in the late 1980s to 542 reported cases in 2012. Dracunculiasis has been eradicated from Asia, but remains endemic in a four countries in Africa, with > 90% of cases in South Sudan and 10 or fewer cases reported in 2012 from Mali, Chad, and Ethiopia. The disease occurs almost exclusively in isolated rural areas.

Infection occurs after swallowing water containing the infected intermediate host, the crustacean *Cyclops* (known as copepods or water fleas). In the stomach, larvae escape from the copepods and migrate through the intestinal mucosa to the retroperitoneum, where mating occurs. Females then migrate to subcutaneous tissue, usually of the legs, over about a year. A subcutaneous ulcer then forms. Upon contact with water, the parasite discharges large numbers of larvae, which are ingested by copepods. Adult worms, which can be up to a meter in length, are gradually extruded. Worm death and disintegration in tissue may provoke a severe inflammatory reaction.

Clinical Findings

Patients are usually asymptomatic until the time of worm extrusion. At that time a painful papule develops, with erythema, pruritus, and burning, usually on the lower leg. Multiple lesions may be present. At this time, some patients may also develop a short-lived systemic reaction, which may include fever, urticaria, nausea, vomiting, diarrhea, and dyspnea. The skin lesion vesiculates over a few days, followed by ulceration. The ulcer is tender, often with a visible worm. The worm is then extruded or absorbed over a few weeks, followed by ulcer healing. Secondary infections, including infectious arthritis and tetanus, are common. The disease causes significant disability; lesions commonly prevent walking for a month or more.

Diagnosis follows identification of a typical skin ulcer with a protruding worm. When the worm is not visible, larvae may be identified on smears or seen after immersion in cold water. Eosinophilia is usually present.

Treatment

No drug cures the infection, but metronidazole and mebendazole are sometimes used to limit inflammation and facilitate worm removal. Wet compresses may relieve discomfort. Occlusive dressings improve hygiene and limit shedding of infectious larvae. Worms are typically removed by sequentially rolling them out over a small stick. When available, simple surgical procedures can be used to remove worms. Corticosteroid ointments may hasten healing. Topical antibiotics may limit bacterial superinfection.

Prevention

Dracunculiasis has proven to be easier to control than most parasitic infections. The disease is prevented by avoidance of contaminated drinking water. This can be accomplished by boiling, chlorination, or filtration through finely woven cloth. A WHO dracunculiasis eradication program, initiated in 1986, has been highly successful.

Centers for Disease Control and Prevention (CDC). Progress toward global eradication of dracunculiasis, January 2012–June 2013. MMWR Morb Mortal Wkly Rep. 2013 Oct 25;62(42):829–33. [PMID: 24153313]

TRICHINOSIS

ESSENTIALS OF DIAGNOSIS

▶ Ingestion of inadequately cooked pork or game.

▶ Transient intestinal symptoms followed by fever, myalgias, and periorbital edema.

▶ Eosinophilia and elevated serum muscle enzymes.

General Considerations

Trichinosis (or trichinellosis) is caused worldwide by *Trichinella spiralis* and related *Trichinella* species. The disease is spread by ingestion of undercooked meat, most commonly pork in areas where pigs feed on garbage. When infected raw meat is ingested, *Trichinella* larvae are freed from cyst walls by gastric acid and pass into the small intestine. The larvae then invade intestinal epithelial cells, develop into adults, and the adults release infective larvae. These parasites travel to skeletal muscle via the bloodstream. They invade muscle cells, enlarge, and form cysts. These larvae may be viable for years. Pigs and other animals become infected by eating infected uncooked food scraps or other animals, such as rats.

The worldwide incidence of trichinosis has decreased, but human infections continue to occur sporadically or in outbreaks, with estimates of ~10,000 cases annually. In addition to undercooked pork, infections have been transmitted by ingestion of game and other animals, including bear and walrus in North America and wild boar and horse in Europe. In the United States, about 20 infections are reported annually, mostly from ingesting wild game.

Clinical Findings

A. Symptoms and Signs

Most infections are asymptomatic. In symptomatic cases, gastrointestinal symptoms, including diarrhea, vomiting, and abdominal pain, develop within the week after ingestion of contaminated meat. These symptoms usually last for less than a week but can occasionally persist for much longer. During the following week, symptoms and signs related to migrating larvae are seen. These findings include, most notably, fever, myalgias, periorbital edema, and eosinophilia. Additional findings may include headache, cough, dyspnea, hoarseness, dysphagia, macular or petechial rash, and subconjunctival and retinal hemorrhages. Systemic symptoms usually peak within 2–3 weeks, and commonly persist for about 2 months. In severe cases, generally with large parasite burdens, muscle involvement can be pronounced, with severe muscle pain, edema, and weakness, especially in the head and neck. Muscle pain may persist for months. Uncommon severe findings include myocarditis, pneumonitis, and meningoencephalitis, sometimes leading to death.

B. Laboratory Findings

The clinical diagnosis is supported by findings of elevated serum muscle enzymes (creatine kinase, lactate dehydrogenase, aspartate aminotransferase). A commercial ELISA assay is available in the United States. Serologic tests become positive 2 or more weeks after infection, but cross-reactivity can be seen with other parasites. Rising antibody titers are highly suggestive of the diagnosis. Muscle biopsy can usually be avoided, but if the diagnosis is uncertain, biopsy of a tender, swollen muscle may identify *Trichinella* larvae. For maximal yield, biopsy material should be examined histologically, and a portion enzymatically digested to release larvae, but evaluation before 3 weeks after infection may not show muscle larvae. Serum and muscle biopsy analysis are available from the CDC.

► Treatment

No effective specific therapy for full-blown trichinosis has been identified. However, if infection is suspected early in the course of illness, treatment with mebendazole (2.5 mg/kg orally twice daily) or albendazole (5–7.5 mg/kg orally twice daily) will kill intestinal worms and may limit progression to tissue invasion. Supportive therapy for systemic disease consists of analgesics, antipyretics, bed rest and, in severe illness, corticosteroids. Infection is prevented by cooking to a temperature of at least 71°C for at least 1 minute. Irradiation of meat is also effective in eliminating *Trichinella* larvae, but freezing is not reliable.

Gottstein B et al. Epidemiology, diagnosis, treatment, and control of trichinellosis. Clin Microbiol Rev. 2009 Jan;22(1):127–45. [PMID: 19136437]

ANGIOSTRONGYLIASIS

Nematodes of rats of the genus *Angiostrongylus* cause two distinct syndromes in humans. *Angiostrongylus cantonensis*, the rat lungworm, causes eosinophilic meningoencephalitis, primarily in Southeast Asia and some Pacific islands. *Angiostrongylus costaricensis* causes gastrointestinal inflammation. In both diseases, human infection follows ingestion of larvae within slugs or snails (and also crabs or prawns for *A cantonensis*) or on material contaminated by these organisms. Since the parasites are not in their natural hosts, they cannot complete their life cycles, but they can cause disease after migrating to the brain or gastrointestinal tract.

► Clinical Findings

A. *A cantonensis* Infection

The disease is caused primarily by worm larvae migrating through the CNS and an inflammatory response to dying worms. After an incubation period of 1 day to 2 weeks, presenting symptoms and signs include headache, stiff neck, nausea, vomiting, cranial nerve abnormalities, and paresthesias. Most cases resolve spontaneously after 2–8 weeks, but serious sequelae and death have been reported. The diagnosis is strongly suggested by the finding of eosinophilic CSF pleocytosis (over 10% eosinophils) in a patient with a history of travel to an endemic area. Peripheral eosinophilia may not be present. *A cantonensis* larvae have rarely been recovered from the CSF and the eyes.

B. *A costaricensis* Infection

Parasites penetrate ileocecal vasculature and develop into adults, which lay eggs, but do not complete their life cycle. Disease is due to an inflammatory response to dying worms in the intestinal tract, with an eosinophilic granulomatous response, at times including vasculitis and ischemic necrosis. Common findings are abdominal pain, vomiting, and fever. Pain is most commonly localized to the right lower quadrant, and a mass may be appreciated, all mimicking appendicitis. Symptoms may recur over months. Uncommon findings are intestinal perforation or obstruction, or disease due to migration of worms to other sites. Many cases are managed surgically, usually for suspected appendicitis. Biopsy of inflamed intestinal tissue may show worms localized to mesenteric arteries and eosinophilic granulomas.

► Treatment

Antihelminthic therapy may be harmful for *A cantonensis* infection, since responses to dying worms may worsen with therapy. If antihelminthic treatment is to be used, albendazole is probably the best choice. Corticosteroids have been used in severe cases, and these are probably appropriate if antihelminthics are provided. It is not known if antihelminthic therapy is helpful for *A costaricensis* infection.

Ramirez-Avila L et al. Eosinophilic meningitis due to *Angiostrongylus* and *Gnathostoma* species. Clin Infect Dis. 2009 Feb 1;48(3):322–7. [PMID: 19123863]
Wang QP et al. Human angiostrongyliasis. Lancet Infect Dis. 2008 Oct;8(10):621–30. [PMID: 18922484]

TOXOCARIASIS

► General Considerations

The dog roundworm *Toxocara canis*, the cat roundworm *Toxocara cati*, and less commonly other helminths may cause visceral larva migrans. *T canis* is highly prevalent in dogs. Humans are infected after ingestion of eggs in material contaminated by dog or other feces. Infection is spread principally by puppies and lactating females, and the eggs must be on the ground for several weeks before they are infectious. After ingestion by humans, larvae migrate to various tissues but cannot complete their life cycle.

► Clinical Findings

Visceral larva migrans is seen principally in young children. Most infections are asymptomatic. The most commonly involved organs are the liver and lungs. Presentations include cough, fever, wheezing, hepatomegaly, splenomegaly, lymphadenopathy, pulmonary infiltrates, and eosinophilia. Involvement of the CNS can occur rarely, leading to eosinophilic meningitis and other abnormalities. Ocular larva migrans is a distinct syndrome, usually in children older than is typical for visceral larva migrans. Children present with visual deficits, pain, and a retinal mass, which can be confused with retinoblastoma. *Baylisascaris procyonis,* a roundworm of raccoons, can rarely cause visceral larva migrans in humans, typically with similar, but more severe manifestations than *T canis.*

The diagnosis of visceral larva migrans is suggested by the finding of eosinophilia in a child with hepatomegaly or other signs of the disease, especially with a history of exposure to puppies. The diagnosis is confirmed by the identification of larvae in a biopsy of infected tissue, usually performed when other diseases are suspected. Serologic tests may be helpful; an available ELISA was estimated to have 78% sensitivity and 92% specificity. Most patients recover without specific therapy, although symptoms may persist for months.

► Treatment

Treatment with antihelminthics or corticosteroids may be considered in severe cases. No drugs have been proven to be effective, but albendazole (400 mg orally twice daily for 5 days), mebendazole, thiabendazole, diethylcarbamazine, and ivermectin have been used, and albendazole has been recommended as the treatment of choice.

CUTANEOUS LARVA MIGRANS (Creeping Eruption)

Cutaneous larva migrans is caused principally by larvae of the dog and cat hookworms, *Ancylostoma braziliense* and *A caninum.* Other animal hookworms, gnathostomiasis, and strongyloidiasis may also cause this syndrome. Infections are common in warm areas, including the southeastern United States. They are most common in children. The disease is caused by the migration of worms through skin; the non-human parasites cannot complete their life cycles, so only cause cutaneous disease.

► Clinical Findings

Intensely pruritic erythematous papules develop, usually on the feet or hands, followed within a few days by serpiginous tracks marking the course of the parasite, which may travel several millimeters per day (Figure 35–8). Several tracks may be present. The process may continue for weeks, with lesions becoming vesiculated, encrusted, or

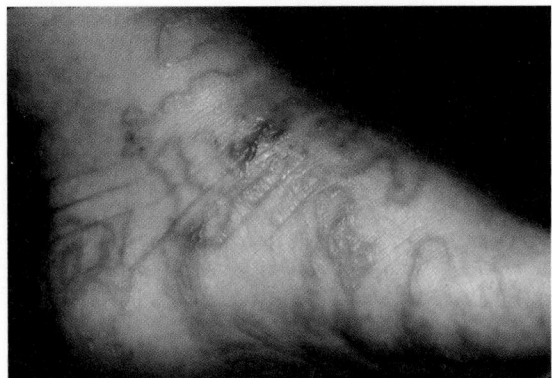

▲ **Figure 35–8.** Cutaneous larva migrans on the foot. (Reproduced, with permission, from Richard P. Usatine, MD.)

secondarily infected. Systemic symptoms or eosinophilia are uncommon.

The diagnosis is based on the characteristic appearance of the lesions. Biopsy is usually not indicated.

► Treatment

Without treatment, the larvae eventually die and are absorbed. Mild cases do not require treatment. Thiabendazole (10% aqueous suspension) can be applied topically three times daily for 5 or more days. Systemic therapy with albendazole (400 mg orally once or twice daily for 3–5 days) or ivermectin (200 mcg/kg orally single dose) is highly effective.

Heukelbach J et al. Epidemiological and clinical characteristics of hookworm-related cutaneous larva migrans. Lancet Infect Dis. 2008 May;8(5):302–9. [PMID: 18471775]

ANISAKIASIS

Anisakiasis is caused by infection with larvae of parasites of saltwater fish and squid. Multiple species of the family *Anisakidae* may occasionally infect humans. Definitive hosts for these parasites are marine mammals. Eggs are passed in the feces and ingested by crustaceans, which are then eaten by fish and squid. When ingested by humans in undercooked seafood, larvae penetrate the stomach or intestinal wall but cannot complete their life cycle. The disease is most common in Japan.

► Clinical Findings

Clinical manifestations of anisakiasis follow burrowing of worms into the stomach or intestinal wall, leading to localized ulceration, edema, and eosinophilic granuloma formation. Symptoms usually occur within 2 days of parasite ingestion and include severe epigastric or abdominal pain, nausea, and vomiting. Intestinal involvement can mimic appendicitis. Allergic symptoms, including urticaria, angioedema, and anaphylaxis, have also been attributed to acute infection. Acute symptoms generally resolve within 2 weeks, but chronic symptoms may also be seen, suggesting inflammatory bowel disease, diverticulitis, or carcinoma.

Rarely, worms may migrate to other sites or be coughed up. Eosinophilia is usually not seen.

The diagnosis is suggested in those with acute abdominal symptoms after ingestion of raw fish. Radiographic studies may identify stomach or intestinal lesions, and endoscopy may allow visualization and removal of the worm. When surgery is performed due to consideration of other diagnoses, eosinophilic inflammatory lesions and the invading worms are found.

▶ **Treatment**

Specific therapy is not indicated, but endoscopic worm removal hastens recovery. The parasites are killed by cooking or deep freezing fish.

Hochberg NS et al. Anisakidosis: perils of the deep. Clin Infect Dis. 2010 Oct 1;51(7):806–12. [PMID: 20804423]

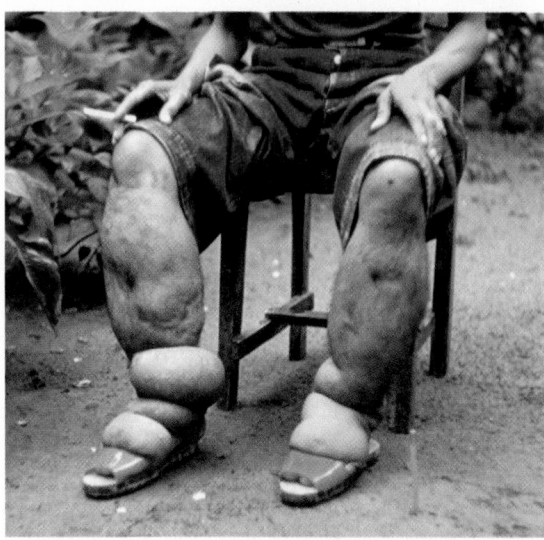

▲ **Figure 35–9.** Elephantiasis of legs due to filariasis. (Public Health Image Library, CDC.)

FILARIASIS

LYMPHATIC FILARIASIS

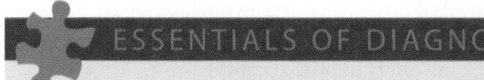

ESSENTIALS OF DIAGNOSIS

▶ Episodic attacks of lymphangitis, lymphadenitis, and fever.

▶ Chronic progressive swelling of extremities and genitals; hydrocele; chyluria; lymphedema.

▶ Microfilariae in blood, chyluria, or hydrocele fluid; positive serologic tests.

▶ **General Considerations**

Lymphatic filariasis is caused by three filarial nematodes: *Wuchereria bancrofti, Brugia malayi,* and *Brugia timori,* and is among the most important parasitic diseases of man. Approximately 120 million people are infected with these organisms in tropical and subtropical countries, about a third of these suffer clinical consequences of the infections, and many are seriously disfigured. *W bancrofti* causes about 90% of episodes of lymphatic filariasis. It is transmitted by *Culex, Aedes,* and *Anopheles* mosquitoes and is widely distributed in the tropics and subtropics, including sub-Saharan Africa, Southeast Asia, the western Pacific, India, South America, and the Caribbean. *B malayi* is transmitted by *Mansonia* and *Anopheles* mosquitoes and is endemic in parts of China, India, Southeast Asia, and the Pacific. *B timori* is found only in islands of southeastern Indonesia. *Mansonella* are filarial worms transmitted by midges and other insects in Africa and South America.

Humans are infected by the bites of infected mosquitoes. Larvae then move to the lymphatics and lymph nodes, where they mature over months to thread-like adult worms, and then can persist for many years. The adult worms produce large numbers of microfilariae, which are released into the circulation, and infective to mosquitoes,

particularly at night (except for the South Pacific, where microfilaremia peaks during daylight hours).

▶ **Clinical Findings**

A. Symptoms and Signs

Many infections remain asymptomatic despite circulating microfilariae. Clinical consequences of filarial infection are principally due to inflammatory responses to developing, mature, and dying worms. The initial manifestation of infection is often acute lymphangitis, with fever, painful lymph nodes, edema, and inflammation spreading peripherally from involved lymph nodes (in contrast to bacterial lymphangitis, which spreads centrally). Lymphangitis and lymphadenitis of the upper and lower extremities is common (Figure 35–9); genital involvement, including epididymitis and orchitis, with scrotal pain and tenderness, occurs principally only with *W bancrofti* infection. Acute attacks of lymphangitis last for a few days to a week and may recur a few times per year. Filarial fevers may also occur without lymphatic inflammation.

The most common chronic manifestation of lymphatic filariasis is swelling of the extremities or genitals due to chronic lymphatic inflammation and obstruction. Extremities become increasingly swollen, with a progression over time from pitting edema, to nonpitting edema, to sclerotic changes of the skin that are referred to as elephantiasis. Genital involvement, particularly with *W bancrofti,* occurs more commonly in men, progressing from painful epididymitis to hydroceles that are usually painless but can become very large, with inguinal lymphadenopathy, thickening of the spermatic cord, scrotal lymphedema, thickening and fissuring of the scrotal skin, and occasionally chyluria. Lymphedema of the female genitalia and breasts may also occur.

Tropical pulmonary eosinophilia is a distinct syndrome principally affecting young adult males with either

W bancrofti or *B malayi* infection but typically without microfilaremia. This syndrome is characterized by asthma-like symptoms, with cough, wheezing, dyspnea, and low-grade fevers, usually at night. Without treatment, tropical pulmonary eosinophilia can progress to interstitial fibrosis and chronic restrictive lung disease. *Mansonella* can inhabit serous cavities, the retroperitoneum, the eye, or the skin, and cause abnormalities related to inflammation at these sites.

B. Laboratory Findings

The diagnosis of lymphatic filariasis is strongly suggested by characteristic findings of lymphangitis or lymphatic obstruction in persons with risk factors for the disease. The diagnosis is confirmed by finding microfilariae, usually in blood, but microfilariae may be absent, especially early in the disease progression (first 2–3 years) or with chronic obstructive disease. To increase yields, blood samples are obtained at about midnight in most areas, but during day-light hours in the South Pacific. Smears are evaluated by wet mount to identify motile parasites and by Giemsa staining; these examinations can be delayed until the following morning, with storage of samples at room temperature. Of note, the periodicity of microfilaremia is variable, and daytime samples may yield positive results. Microfilariae may also be identified in hydrocele fluid or chylous urine. Eosinophilia is usually absent, except during acute inflammatory syndromes. Serologic tests may be helpful but cannot distinguish past and active infections. Rapid antigen tests with sensitivity and specificity over 90% are available. These can be considered the diagnostic tests of choice and are increasingly used to guide control programs. Adult worms may also be found in lymph node biopsy specimens (although biopsy is not usually clinically indicated) or by ultrasound of a scrotal hydrocele or lymphedematous breast. When microfilaremia is lacking, especially if sophisticated techniques are not available, diagnoses may need to be made on clinical grounds alone.

▶ Treatment & Control

A. Drug Treatment

Diethylcarbamazine is the drug of choice, but it cannot cure infections due to its limited action against adult worms. Asymptomatic infection and acute lymphangitis are treated with this drug (2 mg/kg orally three times daily) for 10–14 days, leading to a marked decrease in microfilaremia. Therapy may be accompanied by allergic symptoms, including fever, headache, malaise, hypotension, and bronchospasm, probably due to release of antigens from dying worms. For this reason, treatment courses may begin with a lower dosage, with escalation over the first 4 days of treatment. Single annual doses of diethylcarbamazine (6 mg/kg orally), alone or with ivermectin (400 mcg/kg orally) or albendazole (400 mg orally) may be as effective as longer courses of diethylcarbamazine. When onchocerciasis or loiasis is suspected, it may be appropriate to withhold diethylcarbamazine to avoid severe reactions to dying microfilariae; rather, ivermectin plus albendazole may be given, although these drugs are less active than diethylcarbamazine against adult worms. Appropriate management of advanced obstructive disease is uncertain. Drainage of hydroceles provides symptomatic relief, although they will recur. Therapy with diethylcarbamazine cannot reverse chronic lymphatic changes but is typically provided to lower worm burdens. An interesting approach under study is to treat with doxycycline (100–200 mg/d orally for 4–6 weeks), which kills obligate intracellular *Wolbachia* bacteria, leading to death of adult filarial worms. Doxycycline was also effective at controlling *Mansonella perstans* infection, which does not respond well to standard antifilarial drugs. Secondary bacterial infections must be treated. Surgical correction may be helpful in some cases.

B. Disease Control

Avoidance of mosquitoes is a key measure; preventive measures include the use of screens, bed nets (ideally treated with insecticide), and insect repellents. Community-based treatment with single annual doses of effective drugs offers a highly effective means of control. The current WHO strategy for control includes mass treatment of at risk communities with single annual doses of diethylcarbamazine plus albendazole or, for areas with onchocerciasis, albendazole plus ivermectin; in some circumstances, more frequent dosing offers improved control.

Hoerauf A et al. Filariasis in Africa—treatment challenges and prospects. Clin Microbiol Infect. 2011 Jul;17(7):977–85. [PMID: 21722251]

Taylor MJ et al. Lymphatic filariasis and onchocerciasis. Lancet. 2010 Oct 2;376(9747):1175–85. [PMID: 20739055]

Tisch DJ et al. Reduction in acute filariasis morbidity during a mass drug administration trial to eliminate lymphatic filariasis in Papua New Guinea. PLoS Negl Trop Dis. 2011 Jul;5(7):e1241. [PMID: 21765964]

ONCHOCERCIASIS

▶ ESSENTIALS OF DIAGNOSIS

▶ Severe pruritus; skin excoriations, thickening, and depigmentation; and subcutaneous nodules.

▶ Conjunctivitis progressing to blindness.

▶ Microfilariae in skin snips and on slit-lamp examination; adult worms in subcutaneous nodules.

▶ General Considerations

Onchocerciasis, or river blindness is caused by *Onchocerca volvulus*. An estimated 37 million persons are infected, of whom 3–4 million have skin disease, 500,000 have severe visual impairment, and 300,000 are blinded. Over 99% of infections are in sub-Saharan Africa, especially the West African savanna, with about half of cases in Nigeria and Congo. In some hyperendemic African villages, close to 100% of individuals are infected, and 10% or more of the population is blind. The disease is also prevalent in the southwestern Arabian peninsula and Latin America, including southern Mexico, Guatemala, Venezuela, Colombia, Ecuador, and northwestern Brazil. Onchocerciasis is transmitted by simulium flies (blackflies). These insects breed in fast-flowing streams and bite during the day.

After the bite of an infected blackfly, larvae are deposited in the skin, where adults develop over 6–12 months. Adult worms live in subcutaneous connective tissue or muscle nodules for a decade or more. Microfilariae are released from the nodules and migrate through subcutaneous and ocular tissues. Disease is due to responses to worms and to intracellular *Wolbachia* bacteria.

Clinical Findings

A. Symptoms and Signs

After an incubation period of up to 1–3 years, the disease typically produces an erythematous, papular, pruritic rash, which may progress to chronic skin thickening and depigmentation. Itching may be severe and unresponsive to medications, such that more disability-adjusted life years are lost to onchocercal skin problems than to blindness. Numerous firm, nontender, movable subcutaneous nodules of about 0.5–3 cm, which contain adult worms, may be present. Due to differences in vector habits, these nodules are more commonly on the lower body in Africa but on the head and upper body in Latin America. Inguinal and femoral lymphadenopathy is common, at times resulting in a "hanging groin," with lymph nodes hanging within a sling of atrophic skin. Patients may also have systemic symptoms, with weight loss and musculoskeletal pain.

The most serious manifestations of onchocerciasis involve the eyes. Microfilariae migrating through the eyes elicit host responses that lead to pathology. Findings include punctate keratitis and corneal opacities, progressing to sclerosing keratitis and blindness. Iridocyclitis, glaucoma, choroiditis, and optic atrophy may also lead to vision loss. The likelihood of blindness after infection varies greatly based on geography, with the risk greatest in savanna regions of West Africa.

B. Diagnostic Testing

The diagnosis is made by identifying microfilariae in skin snips, by visualizing microfilariae in the cornea or anterior chamber by slit-lamp examination, by identification of adult worms in a biopsy or aspirate of a nodule or, uncommonly, by identification of microfilariae in urine. Skin snips from the iliac crest (Africa) or scapula (Americas) are allowed to stand in saline for 2–4 hours or longer, and then examined microscopically for microfilariae. Deep punch biopsies are not needed, and if suspicion persists after a skin snip is negative, the procedure should be repeated. Ultrasound may identify characteristic findings suggestive of adult worms in skin nodules. When the diagnosis remains difficult, the Mazzotti test can be used; exacerbation of skin rash and pruritus after a 50-mg dose of diethylcarbamazine is highly suggestive of the diagnosis. This test should only be used after other tests are negative, since treatment can elicit severe skin and eye reactions in heavily

infected individuals. A related and safer test using topical diethylcarbamazine is also available. Eosinophilia is a common, but inconsistent finding. Antigen and antibody detection tests are under study.

Treatment & Control

The treatment of choice is ivermectin, which has replaced diethylcarbamazine due to a much lower risk of severe reactions to therapy. Ivermectin kills microfilariae, but not adult worms, so disease control requires repeat administrations. Treatment is with a single oral dose of 150 mcg/mL, but schedules for re-treatment have not been standardized. One regimen is to treat every 3 months for 1 year, followed by treatment every 6–12 months for the suspected lifespan of adult worms (about 15 years). Treatment results in marked reduction in numbers of microfilariae in the skin and eyes, although its impact on the progression of visual loss remains uncertain. Toxicities of ivermectin are generally mild; fever, pruritus, urticaria, myalgias, edema, hypotension, and tender lymphadenopathy may be seen, presumably due to reactions to dying worms. Ivermectin should be used with caution in patients also at risk for loiasis, since it can elicit severe reactions including encephalopathy. As with other filarial infections, doxycycline acts against *O volvulus* by killing intracellular *Wolbachia* bacteria. A course of 100 mg/d for 6 weeks kills the bacteria and prevents parasite embryogenesis for at least 18 months. Doxycycline shows promise as a first-line agent to treat onchocerciasis because of its improved activity against adult worms compared to other agents and limited toxicity due to the slow action of the drug.

Protection against onchocerciasis includes avoidance of biting flies. Major efforts are underway to control insect vectors in Africa. In addition, mass distribution of ivermectin for intermittent administration at the community level is ongoing, and the prevalence of severe skin and eye disease is decreasing.

Knopp S et al. Nematode infections: filariases. Infect Dis Clin North Am. 2012 Jun;26(2):359–81. [PMID: 22632644]

LOIASIS

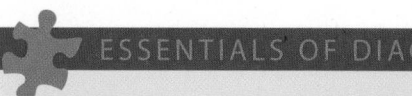

ESSENTIALS OF DIAGNOSIS

▸ Subcutaneous swellings; adult worms migrating across the eye.

▸ Encephalitis, which may be brought on by treatment.

▸ Microfilariae in the blood.

General Considerations

Loiasis is a chronic filarial disease caused by infection with *Loa loa*. The infection occurs in humans and monkeys in rainforest areas of West and central Africa. An estimated 3–13 million persons are infected. The disease is transmitted by chrysops flies, which bite during the day. Over 6–12 months after infection, larvae develop into adult worms, which migrate through subcutaneous tissues, including the subconjunctiva (leading to the term "eye worm"). Adults can live for up to 17 years.

► Clinical Findings

A. Symptoms and Signs

Many infected persons are asymptomatic, although they may have high levels of microfilaremia and eosinophilia. Transient subcutaneous swellings (Calabar swellings) develop in symptomatic persons. The swellings are nonerythematous, up to 20 cm in diameter, and may be preceded by local pain or pruritus. They usually resolve after 2–4 days but occasionally persist for several weeks. Calabar swellings are commonly seen around joints and may recur at the same or different sites. Visitors from nonendemic areas are more likely to have allergic-type reactions, including pruritus, urticaria, and angioedema. Adult worms may be seen to migrate across the eye, with either no symptoms or conjunctivitis, with pain and edema. The most serious complication of loiasis is encephalitis, which is most common in those with high level microfilaremia and microfilariae in the CSF. Symptoms may range from headache and insomnia to coma and death. Encephalitis may be brought on by treatment with diethylcarbamazine or ivermectin. Other complications of loiasis include kidney disease, with hematuria and proteinuria; endomyocardial fibrosis; and peripheral neuropathy.

B. Laboratory Findings

The diagnosis is established by identifying microfilariae in blood. Blood is evaluated as for lymphatic filariasis, but for loiasis blood should be obtained during the day. The failure to find microfilariae does not rule out the diagnosis. Identification of a migrating eye worm is also diagnostic. Serologic tests may be helpful in persons from nonendemic areas who may be acutely ill without detectable microfilaremia, but such tests have limited utility for residents of endemic areas because most of them will have positive test results. PCR methods are available to rule out loiasis before administration of ivermectin for the control of other filarial infections.

► Treatment

The treatment of choice is diethylcarbamazine, which eliminates microfilariae and has some activity against adult worms. Treatment is with 8–10 mg/kg/d orally for 21 days; repeat courses may be needed. Mild side effects are common, including fever, pruritus, arthralgias, nausea, diarrhea, and Calabar swellings. These symptoms may be lessened by antihistamines or corticosteroids. Patients with large worm burdens are at greater risk for serious complications of therapy, including kidney injury, shock, encephalitis, coma, and death. Treatment with ivermectin, which is highly active against microfilariae, but not adult worms, entails a higher risk of severe reactions. To attempt to avoid these sequelae, pretreatment with corticosteroids and antihistamines, and escalating dosage of diethylcarbamazine have been used, but this strategy does not prevent encephalitis. The circulating parasite load that indicates particular risk for severe complications with therapy has been estimated at 2500/mL. Strategies to treat patients with high parasite loads include (1) no treatment; (2) apheresis, if available, to remove microfilariae prior to therapy with diethylcarbamazine; or (3) therapy with albendazole, which appears to be well tolerated due to its slow antiparasitic effects, prior to therapy with diethylcarbamazine or ivermectin. Doxycycline is not effective for loiasis.

Fink DL et al. Rapid molecular assays for specific detection and quantitation of *Loa loa* microfilaremia. PLoS Negl Trop Dis. 2011 Aug;5(8):e1299. [PMID: 21912716]

Padgett JJ et al. Loiasis: African eye worm. Trans R Soc Trop Med Hyg. 2008 Oct;102(10):983–9. [PMID: 18466939]

Mycotic Infections

Samuel A. Shelburne, MD, PhD

Richard J. Hamill, MD

Fungal infections have assumed an increasingly important role as use of broad-spectrum antimicrobial agents has increased and the number of immunodeficient patients has grown. Some pathogens (eg, *Cryptococcus, Candida, Pneumocystis, Fusarium*) rarely cause serious disease in normal hosts. Other endemic fungi (eg, *Histoplasma, Coccidioides, Paracoccidioides*) commonly cause disease in normal hosts but tend to be more aggressive in immuno-compromised ones. Superficial mycoses are discussed in Chapter 6.

CANDIDIASIS

ESSENTIALS OF DIAGNOSIS

- ▶ Common normal flora but opportunistic pathogen.
- ▶ Gastrointestinal mucosal disease, particularly esophagitis, most common.
- ▶ Fungemia, arising from an intravenous catheter or the gastrointestinal tract occurs in patients who have sustained cutaneous or mucosal injury, undergone instrumentation, are receiving total parenteral nutrition, have kidney disease, or have received broad-spectrum antibiotics.

▶ General Considerations

Candida albicans can be cultured from the mouth, vagina, and feces of most people. Cutaneous and oral lesions are discussed in Chapters 6 and 8, respectively. The risk factors for invasive candidiasis include prolonged neutropenia, recent abdominal surgery, broad-spectrum antibiotic therapy, kidney disease, and the presence of intravascular catheters (especially when providing total parenteral nutrition). Cellular immunodeficiency predisposes to mucocutaneous disease. When no other underlying cause is found, persistent oral or vaginal candidiasis should arouse a suspicion of HIV infection.

▶ Clinical Findings

A. Mucosal Candidiasis

Esophageal involvement is the most frequent type of significant mucosal disease. Presenting symptoms include substernal odynophagia, gastroesophageal reflux, or nausea without substernal pain. Oral candidiasis, though often associated, is not invariably present. Diagnosis is best confirmed by endoscopy with biopsy and culture.

Vulvovaginal candidiasis occurs in an estimated 75% of women during their lifetime. Risk factors include pregnancy, uncontrolled diabetes mellitus, broad-spectrum antimicrobial treatment, corticosteroid use, and HIV infection. Symptoms include acute vulvar pruritus, burning vaginal discharge, and dyspareunia.

B. Candidal Funguria

Most cases of candidal funguria are asymptomatic and represent specimen contamination or bladder colonization. However, signs and symptoms of true *Candida* urinary tract infections are indistinguishable from bacterial urinary tract infections and can include urgency, hesitancy, fever, chills, or flank pain.

C. Disseminated Candidiasis

The clinical presentation of disseminated candidiasis varies from minimal fever to septic shock that can resemble a severe bacterial infection. Occasionally, patients with candidiasis will have skin lesions ranging from pustules to large nodules. Organs that may be involved in disseminated candidiasis include the liver, spleen, kidney, eyes, and heart. The diagnosis of disseminated *Candida* infection is problematic because *Candida* species are often isolated from mucosal sites in the absence of invasive disease while blood cultures are positive only 50% of the time in disseminated infection. The role of antigen tests, serologic tests (such as beta-D-glucan), and polymerase chain reaction (PCR) in diagnosing invasive candidiasis remains undefined.

Hepatosplenic candidiasis can occur following prolonged neutropenia in patients with underlying hematologic cancers. Typically, fever and variable abdominal pain present weeks after chemotherapy, when neutrophil counts have recovered. Blood cultures are generally negative. Hepatic enzymes reveal an alkaline phosphatase elevation that may be marked.

D. Candidal Endocarditis

Candidal endocarditis is a rare infection that is most frequently associated with exposure to a health care setting. Candidal endocarditis occurs with increased frequency on prosthetic valves in the first few months following surgery. The diagnosis is established definitively by culturing *Candida* from emboli or from vegetations at the time of valve replacement.

▶ Treatment

A. Mucosal Candidiasis

Therapy of **esophageal candidiasis** depends on the severity of disease. If patients are able to swallow and take adequate amounts of fluid orally, fluconazole, 100 mg/d (or itraconazole solution, 10 mg/mL, 200 mg/d), for 10–14 days usually suffices. In the individual who is more ill or in whom esophagitis has developed while taking fluconazole, options include oral or intravenous voriconazole, 200 mg twice daily; intravenous amphotericin B, 0.3 mg/kg/d; intravenous caspofungin, 50 mg/d; intravenous anidulafungin, 100 mg on day 1, then 50 mg/d; or intravenous micafungin, 150 mg/d. Relapse is common with all agents when there is underlying HIV infection without adequate immune reconstitution.

Various topical azole preparations (eg, clotrimazole, 100 mg vaginal tablet for 7 days, or miconazole, 200 mg vaginal suppository for 3 days) are effective against **vulvovaginal candidiasis**. One 150 mg oral dose of fluconazole has been shown to have equivalent efficacy with better patient acceptance. Disease recurrence is common but can be decreased with weekly fluconazole therapy (150 mg weekly).

B. Candidal Funguria

Candidal funguria frequently resolves with discontinuance of antibiotics or removal of bladder catheters. Clinical benefit from treatment of asymptomatic candiduria has not been demonstrated, but persistent funguria should raise the suspicion of disseminated infection. When symptomatic funguria persists, oral fluconazole, 200 mg/d for 7–14 days, can be used.

C. Disseminated Candidiasis

The decision to treat for disseminated *Candida* when organisms are isolated from urine or sputum (or both) needs to be individualized for each patient. A randomized trial of empiric fluconazole for patients at high risk for, but not proven to have, disseminated candidiasis showed no clinical benefit compared with placebo.

The 2009 guidelines for treatment of invasive candidiasis recommend fluconazole (loading dose of 800 mg [12 mg/kg] intravenously, then 400 mg [6 mg/kg] intravenously daily) for less critically ill patients who have had no recent azole exposure. For patients with moderately severe to severe illness or for patients who have had recent azole exposure, an echinocandin such as caspofungin (loading dose of 70 mg intravenously once, then 50 mg intravenously daily), micafungin (100 mg intravenously daily), anidulafungin (loading dose of 200 mg intravenously once, then 100 mg intravenously daily) is favored. Therapy for candidemia should be continued for 2 weeks after the last positive blood culture and resolution of symptoms and signs of infection. A dilated fundoscopic examination is recommended for all patients with candidemia to exclude endophthalmitis and repeat blood cultures should be drawn to demonstrate organism clearance. Once patients have become clinically stable, parenteral therapy can be discontinued and oral fluconazole, 200–800 mg orally given as one or two doses daily, is used to complete treatment for isolates known to be or likely to be susceptible to fluconazole. Removal or exchange of intravascular catheters is generally recommended for non-neutropenic patients, since this may decrease the duration of candidemia and overall mortality, which approaches 30%.

Non-*albicans* species of *Candida* account for over 50% of clinical bloodstream isolates and often have resistance patterns that are different from *C albicans*. An echinocandin is recommended for treatment of *Candida glabrata* infection with a transition to oral fluconazole or voriconazole reserved for patients whose isolates are known to be susceptible to these agents. Similarly, *Candida krusei* is generally fluconazole-resistant and so should be treated with an alternative agent, such as echinocandin or voriconazole. Fluconazole is the treatment of choice for *Candida parapsilosis* due to possible echinocandin resistance in such isolates.

Treatment for hepatosplenic candidiasis is with fluconazole, 400 mg orally daily, or a lipid formulation of amphotericin B, given until clinical and radiographic improvement occurs.

D. Candidal Endocarditis

Best results are achieved with a combination of medical and surgical therapy. Amphotericin, either in a lipid or standard formulation, has long been considered the optimal therapy for candidal endocarditis, given in a dosage of 3–5 mg/kg/d (lipid formulation) or 0.6–1 mg/kg/d (deoxycholate) intravenously, and can be given along with 5-flucytosine (25 mg/kg four times daily). Echinocandins are considered an alternative. Step-down or long-term suppressive therapy for nonsurgical candidates may be done with fluconazole at 6–12 mg/kg/d for susceptible organisms.

In high-risk patients undergoing induction chemotherapy, bone marrow transplantation, or liver transplantation, prophylaxis with antifungal agents has been shown to prevent invasive fungal infections although the effect on mortality and the preferred agent remain debated.

Ben-Ami R et al; Israeli Candidemia Study Group. Antibiotic exposure as a risk factor for fluconazole-resistant *Candida* bloodstream infection. Antimicrob Agents Chemother. 2012 May;56(5):2518–23. [PMID: 22314534]

Eschenauer GA et al. Fluconazole versus an echinocandin for *Candida glabrata* fungaemia: a retrospective cohort study. J Antimicrob Chemother. 2013 Apr;68(4):922–6. [PMID: 23212115]

Kullberg BJ et al. European expert opinion on the management of invasive candidiasis in adults. Clin Microbiol Infect. 2011 Sep;17(Suppl 5):1–12. [PMID: 21884296]

HISTOPLASMOSIS

ESSENTIALS OF DIAGNOSIS

▶ Epidemiologically linked to bird droppings and bat exposure; common along river valleys (especially the Ohio River and the Mississippi River valleys).

▶ Most patients asymptomatic; respiratory illness most common clinical problem.

▶ Widespread disease especially common in AIDS or other immunosuppressed states, with poor prognosis.

▶ Biopsy of affected organs with culture or urinary polysaccharide antigen most useful in disseminated disease.

▶ General Considerations

Histoplasmosis is caused by *Histoplasma capsulatum,* a dimorphic fungus that has been isolated from soil contaminated with bird or bat droppings in endemic areas (central and eastern United States, eastern Canada, Mexico, Central America, South America, Africa, and southeast Asia). Infection presumably takes place by inhalation of conidia. These convert into small budding cells that are engulfed by phagocytes in the lungs. The organism proliferates and undergoes lymphohematogenous spread to other organs.

▶ Clinical Findings

A. Symptoms and Signs

Most cases of histoplasmosis are asymptomatic or mild and thus go unrecognized. Past infection is recognized by pulmonary and splenic calcification noted on incidental radiographs. Symptomatic infection may present with mild influenza-like illness, often lasting 1–4 days. Moderately severe infections are frequently diagnosed as atypical pneumonia. These patients have fever, cough, and mild central chest pain lasting 5–15 days.

Clinically evident infections occur in several forms: (1) **Acute pulmonary histoplasmosis** frequently occurs in epidemics, often when soil containing infected bird or bat droppings is disturbed. Clinical manifestations can vary from a mild influenza-like illness to severe pneumonia. The illness may last from 1 week to 6 months but is almost never fatal. (2) **Progressive disseminated histoplasmosis** is commonly seen in patients with underlying HIV infection (with CD4 cell counts usually < 100 cells/mcL) or other conditions causing immunosuppression. Disseminated histoplasmosis has been reported in patients from endemic areas taking tumor necrosis factor (TNF)-blocking agents. It is characterized by fever and multiple organ system involvement. Chest radiographs may show a miliary pattern. Presentation may be fulminant, simulating septic shock, with death ensuing rapidly unless treatment is provided. Symptoms usually consist of fever, dyspnea, cough, loss of weight, and prostration. Ulcers of the mucous membranes of the oropharynx may be present. The liver and spleen are nearly always enlarged, and all the organs of the body are involved, particularly the adrenal glands, though this infrequently results in adrenal insufficiency. Gastrointestinal involvement may mimic inflammatory bowel disease. (3) **Chronic pulmonary histoplasmosis** is usually seen in older patients who usually have underlying chronic lung disease. Chest radiographs show various lesions including apical cavities, infiltrates, and nodules. (4) **Complications of pulmonary histoplasmosis** include granulomatous mediastinitis characterized by persistently enlarged mediastinal lymph nodes and fibrosing mediastinitis in which an excessive fibrotic response to *Histoplasma* infection results in compromise of the great vessels.

B. Laboratory Findings

Most patients with chronic pulmonary disease show anemia of chronic disease. Bone marrow involvement may be prominent in disseminated forms with occurrence of pancytopenia. Alkaline phosphatase and marked lactate dehydrogenase (LD) and ferritin elevations are also common as are mild elevations of serum aspartate aminotransferase, although alanine aminotransferase is often normal.

With pulmonary involvement, sputum culture is rarely positive except in chronic disease; antigen testing of bronchoalveolar lavage fluid may be helpful in acute disease. The combination of a first morning urine and serum antigen assays has an 83% sensitivity for the diagnosis of acute pulmonary histoplasmosis. Blood or bone marrow cultures from immunocompromised patients with acute disseminated disease are positive more than 80% of the time but may take several weeks for growth. The urine antigen assay has a sensitivity of > 90% for disseminated disease in immunocompromised patients and a declining titer can be used to follow response to therapy.

▶ Treatment

For progressive localized disease and for mild to moderately severe nonmeningeal disseminated disease in immunocompetent or immunocompromised patients, itraconazole, 200–400 mg/d orally divided into two doses, is the treatment of choice with an overall response rate of approximately 80%. The oral solution is better absorbed than the capsule formulation, which requires gastric acid for absorption. Duration of therapy ranges from weeks to several months depending on the severity of illness.

Intravenous amphotericin B formulations are used in patients with more severe illness such as meningitis, with guidelines favoring the use of liposomal or lipid complex amphotericin formulations at a dose of 3 mg/kg/d over amphotericin B deoxycholate. Patients with AIDS-related histoplasmosis require lifelong suppressive therapy with itraconazole, 200–400 mg/d orally, although secondary prophylaxis may be discontinued if immune reconstitution occurs in response to antiretroviral therapy. There is no clear evidence that antifungal or anti-inflammatory agents are of benefit for patients with granulomatous mediastinitis or fibrosing mediastinitis although oral itraconazole is often used. Reported outcomes in patients with fibrosing mediastinitis treated with either surgical procedures or nonsurgical intravascular interventions appear to be relatively good.

Assi M et al. Histoplasmosis after solid organ transplant. Clin Infect Dis. 2013 Dec;57(11):1542–9. [PMID: 24046304]
McKinsey DS et al. Pulmonary histoplasmosis. Semin Respir Crit Care Med. 2011 Dec;32(6):735–44. [PMID: 22167401]

COCCIDIOIDOMYCOSIS

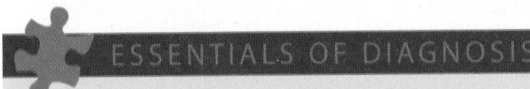

ESSENTIALS OF DIAGNOSIS

▶ Influenza-like illness with malaise, fever, backache, headache, and cough.

▶ Erythema nodosum common with acute infection.

▶ Dissemination may result in meningitis, bony lesions, or skin and soft tissue abscesses.

▶ Chest radiograph findings vary from pneumonitis to cavitation.

▶ Serologic tests useful; spherules containing endospores demonstrable in sputum or tissues.

▶ General Considerations

Coccidioidomycosis should be considered in the diagnosis of any obscure illness in a patient who has lived in or visited an endemic area. Infection results from the inhalation of arthroconidia of *Coccidioides immitis* or *C posadasii*; both organisms are molds that grow in soil in certain arid regions of the southwestern United States, in Mexico, and in Central and South America. Less than 1% of immunocompetent persons show dissemination, but among these patients, the mortality rate is high.

In HIV-infected people in endemic areas, coccidioidomycosis is a common opportunistic infection. In these patients, disease manifestations range from focal pulmonary infiltrates to widespread miliary disease with multiple organ involvement and meningitis; severity is inversely related to the extent of control of the HIV infection.

▶ Clinical Findings

A. Symptoms and Signs

Symptoms of **primary coccidioidomycosis** occur in about 40% of infections. Symptom onset (after an incubation period of 10–30 days) is usually that of a respiratory tract illness with fever and occasionally chills. Coccidioidomycosis is a common, frequently unrecognized, etiology of community-acquired pneumonia in endemic areas.

Arthralgia accompanied by periarticular swelling, often of the knees and ankles, is common. Erythema nodosum may appear 2–20 days after onset of symptoms. Persistent pulmonary lesions, varying from cavities and abscesses to parenchymal nodular densities or bronchiectasis, occur in about 5% of diagnosed cases.

Disseminated disease occurs in about 0.1% of white and 1% of nonwhite patients. Filipinos and blacks are especially susceptible, as are pregnant women of all races. Any organ may be involved. Pulmonary findings usually become more pronounced, with mediastinal lymph node enlargement, cough, and increased sputum production. Lung abscesses may rupture into the pleural space, producing an empyema. These may also extend to bones and skin, and pericardial and myocardial involvement has been occasionally observed. Fungemia may occur and is characterized clinically by a diffuse miliary pattern on chest radiograph and by early death. The course may be particularly rapid in immunosuppressed patients. Clinicians caring for immunosuppressed patients in endemic areas need to consider that patients may be latently infected.

Meningitis occurs in 30–50% of cases of dissemination. Subcutaneous abscesses and verrucous skin lesions are especially common in fulminating cases. HIV-infected persons with disseminated disease have a higher incidence of miliary infiltrates, lymphadenopathy, and meningitis, but skin lesions are uncommon.

B. Laboratory Findings

In **primary coccidioidomycosis**, there may be moderate leukocytosis and eosinophilia. Serologic testing is useful for both diagnosis and prognosis. The immunodiffusion tube precipitin test and enzyme-linked immunosorbent assay (ELISA) detect IgM antibodies and are both useful for diagnosis early in the disease process. Historically, a persistent rising IgG complement fixation titer ($\geq 1:16$) has been considered suggestive of disseminated disease; in addition, immunodiffusion complement fixation titers can be used to assess the adequacy of therapy. Serum complement fixation titer may be low when there is meningitis but no other disseminated disease. In patients with HIV-related coccidioidomycosis, the false-negative rate may be as high as 30%.

Demonstrable complement-fixing antibodies in spinal fluid are diagnostic of coccidioidal meningitis. These are found in over 90% of cases. Spinal fluid findings include increased cell count with lymphocytosis and reduced glucose. Spinal fluid culture is positive in approximately 30% of meningitis cases. Spherules filled with endospores may be found in biopsy specimens of soft tissues and bone; though they are not infectious, they convert to the highly contagious arthroconidia when grown in culture media. Blood cultures are rarely positive.

C. Imaging

Radiographic findings vary, but patchy, nodular and lobar upper lobe pulmonary infiltrates are most common. Hilar lymphadenopathy may be visible and is seen in localized disease; mediastinal lymphadenopathy suggests dissemination. There may be pleural effusions and lytic lesions in bone with accompanying complicated soft-tissue collections.

▶ Treatment

General symptomatic therapy is given as needed for disease limited to the chest with no evidence of progression. For progressive pulmonary or extrapulmonary disease, amphotericin B intravenously is used although oral azoles may be used for mild cases (see Chapter 30). Duration of therapy is determined by a declining complement fixation titer and a favorable clinical response. For meningitis, treatment usually is with high-dose oral fluconazole (400–800 mg/d, or higher) although lumbar or cisternal intrathecal administration of amphotericin B daily in increasing doses up to 1–1.5 mg/d is used initially by some physicians or in cases refractory to fluconazole. Systemic therapy with amphotericin B, 0.6 mg/kg/d intravenously, is generally given concurrently with intrathecal therapy but is not sufficient alone for the treatment of meningeal disease. Once the patient is clinically stable, oral therapy with an azole, usually with fluconazole (400 mg daily) and given lifelong, is the recommended alternative to intrathecal amphotericin B therapy.

Itraconazole, 400 mg orally daily divided into two doses, or fluconazole, 200–400 mg, or higher, orally once or twice daily should be given for disease in the chest, bones, and soft tissues; however, therapy must be continued for 6 months or longer after the disease is inactive to prevent relapse. Response to therapy should be monitored by following the clinical response and progressive decrease in serum complement fixation titers.

Surgical drainage is necessary for management of soft tissue abscesses, necrotic bone and complicated pulmonary disease (eg, rupture of coccidioidal cavity).

▶ Prognosis

The prognosis for patients with limited disease is good, but persistent pulmonary cavities may cause complications such as hemoptysis or rupture producing pyopneumothorax. Serial complement fixation titers should be performed after therapy for patients with coccidioidomycosis; rising titers warrant reinstitution of therapy because relapse is likely. Late central nervous system complications of adequately treated meningitis include cerebral vasculitis with stroke and hydrocephalitis that may require shunting. Disseminated and meningeal forms still have mortality rates exceeding 50% in the absence of therapy.

Nguyen C et al. Recent advances in our understanding of the environmental, epidemiological, immunological, and clinical dimensions of coccidioidomycosis. Clin Microbiol Rev. 2013 Jul;26(3):505–25. [PMID: 23824371]

Thompson GR 3rd. Pulmonary coccidioidomycosis. Semin Respir Crit Care Med. 2011 Dec;32(6):754–63. [PMID: 22167403]

PNEUMOCYSTOSIS
(*Pneumocystis jirovecii* Pneumonia)

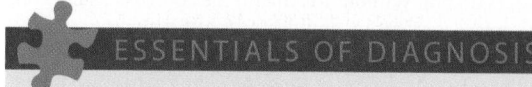

ESSENTIALS OF DIAGNOSIS

- ▶ Fever, dyspnea, nonproductive cough.
- ▶ Bilateral diffuse interstitial disease without hilar adenopathy by chest radiograph.
- ▶ Bibasilar crackles on auscultation in many cases; others have no findings.
- ▶ Reduced partial pressure of oxygen.
- ▶ *P jirovecii* in sputum, bronchoalveolar lavage fluid, or lung tissue.

▶ General Considerations

Pneumocystis jirovecii, the *Pneumocystis* species that affects humans, is distributed worldwide. Although symptomatic *P jirovecii* disease is rare in the general population, serologic evidence indicates that asymptomatic infections have occurred in most persons by a young age. The mode of transmission in primary infection is unknown, but the evidence suggests airborne transmission. Following asymptomatic primary infection, latent and presumably inactive organisms are sparsely distributed in the alveoli. De novo infection and reactivation of latent disease likely contribute to the mechanism of acute disease in older children and adults.

The overt infection is an acute interstitial plasma cell pneumonia that occurs with high frequency among two groups: (1) as epidemics of primary infections among premature or debilitated or marasmic infants on hospital wards in underdeveloped parts of the world, and (2) as sporadic cases among older children and adults who have an abnormal or altered cellular immunity. Cases occur commonly in patients with cancer or severe malnutrition and debility, in patients treated with immunosuppressive or cytotoxic drugs or irradiation for the management of organ transplants and cancer and, most frequently, in patients with AIDS (see Chapter 31).

Pneumocystis pneumonia occurs in up to 80% of AIDS patients not receiving prophylaxis and is a major cause of death. Its incidence increases in direct proportion to the fall in CD4 cells, with most cases occurring at CD4 cell counts < 200/mcL. In non-AIDS patients receiving immunosuppressive therapy, symptoms frequently begin after corticosteroids have been tapered or discontinued.

Clinical Findings

A. Symptoms and Signs

Findings are usually limited to the pulmonary parenchyma; extrapulmonary disease is reported rarely. In the sporadic form of the disease associated with deficient cell-mediated immunity, the onset is typically abrupt, with fever, tachypnea, shortness of breath, and usually nonproductive cough. Pulmonary physical findings may be slight and disproportionate to the degree of illness and the radiologic findings; many patients have bibasilar crackles, but others do not. Without treatment, the course is usually one of rapid deterioration and death. Adult patients may present with spontaneous pneumothorax, usually in patients with previous episodes or those receiving aerosolized pentamidine prophylaxis. Patients with AIDS will usually have other evidence of HIV-associated disease, including fever, fatigue, and weight loss, for weeks or months preceding the illness.

B. Laboratory Findings

Chest radiographs most often show diffuse "interstitial" infiltration, which may be heterogeneous, miliary, or patchy early in infection. There may also be diffuse or focal consolidation, cystic changes, nodules, or cavitation within nodules. Pleural effusions are not seen. About 5–10% of patients with *Pneumocystis* pneumonia have normal chest films. High-resolution chest CT scans may be quite suggestive of *P jirovecii* pneumonia, helping distinguish it from other causes of pneumonia.

Arterial blood gas determinations usually show hypoxemia with hypocapnia but may be normal; however, rapid desaturation occurs if patients exercise before samples are drawn. Serologic tests are not helpful in diagnosis, but several studies have suggested that elevated (1→3)-beta-D-glucan levels have reasonably good sensitivity and specificity for the diagnosis of *Pneumocystis* pneumonia. Specific diagnosis depends on morphologic demonstration of the organisms in clinical specimens using specific stains. The organism cannot be cultured. Adequate specimens can sometimes be obtained with induced sputum by having patients inhale an aerosol of hypertonic saline (3%) produced by an ultrasonic nebulizer. Specimens are then stained with Giemsa stain or methenamine silver, either of which allows detection of cysts. The use of monoclonal antibody with immunofluorescence has increased the sensitivity of diagnosis. Alternative techniques for obtaining specimens include bronchoalveolar lavage (sensitivity 86–97%) followed by transbronchial lung biopsy (85–97%), if necessary. Open lung biopsy and needle lung biopsy are infrequently done but may need to be performed to diagnose a granulomatous form of *Pneumocystis* pneumonia. PCR of bronchoalveolar lavage is overly sensitive in that the test is often positive in colonized, noninfected persons but quantitative values may help with identifying infected patients.

Treatment

See Table 31–5. It is appropriate to start empiric therapy for *P jirovecii* pneumonia if the disease is suspected clinically;

however, in both AIDS patients and non-AIDS patients with mild to moderately severe disease, continued treatment should be based on a proved diagnosis because of clinical overlap with other infections, the toxicity of therapy, and the possible coexistence of other infectious organisms. Oral trimethoprim-sulfamethoxazole (TMP-SMZ) is the preferred agent because of its low cost and excellent bioavailability in both AIDS patients and non-AIDS patients with mild to moderately severe disease. Patients suffering from nausea and vomiting or intractable diarrhea should be given intravenous TMP-SMZ until they can tolerate the oral formulation. The impact of resistance of *Pneumocystis* to TMP-SMZ is unclear, although increasing rates of mutations in the *DHPS* and *DHFR* genes that mediate TMP-SMZ resistance have been reported. The best-studied second-line option is a combination of primaquine and clindamycin, although dapsone/trimethoprim, pentamidine, and atovaquone have also been used. Therapy should be continued with the selected drug for at least 5–10 days before considering changing agents, as fever, tachypnea, and pulmonary infiltrates persist for 4–6 days after starting treatment. Some patients have a transient worsening of their disease during the first 3–5 days, which may be related to an inflammatory response secondary to the presence of dead or dying organisms. Early addition of corticosteroids may attenuate this response (see below). Some clinicians prefer to treat episodes of AIDS-associated *Pneumocystis* pneumonia for 21 days rather than the usual 14 days recommended for non-AIDS cases.

A. Trimethoprim-Sulfamethoxazole

The dosage of TMP/SMZ is 15–20 mg/kg/d (based on trimethoprim component) given orally or intravenously daily in three or four divided doses for 14–21 days. Patients with AIDS have a high frequency of hypersensitivity reactions (approaching 50%), which may include fever, rashes (sometimes severe), malaise, neutropenia, hepatitis, nephritis, thrombocytopenia, hyperkalemia, and hyperbilirubinemia.

B. Primaquine/Clindamycin

Although there are strong data indicating that trimethoprim-sulfamethoxazole is optimal first-line therapy for *Pneumocystis* pneumonia, the data on alternative agents are less clear. A meta-analysis suggested that primaquine, 15–30 mg/d, plus clindamycin, 600 mg three times daily, is the best second-line therapy with superior results when compared with pentamidine. Primaquine may cause hemolytic anemia in patients with glucose-6-phosphate dehydrogenase (G6PD)-deficiency.

C. Pentamidine Isethionate

The use of pentamidine has decreased as alternative agents have been studied. This drug is administered intravenously (preferred) or intramuscularly as a single dose of 3–4 mg (salt)/kg/d for 14–21 days. Pentamidine causes side effects in nearly 50% of patients. Hypoglycemia (often clinically inapparent), hyperglycemia, hyponatremia, and delayed nephrotoxicity with azotemia may occur.

D. Atovaquone

Atovaquone is approved by the US Food and Drug Administration (FDA) for patients with mild to moderate disease who cannot tolerate TMP-SMZ or pentamidine, but failure is reported in 15–30% of cases. Mild side effects are common, but no serious reactions have been reported. The dosage is 750 mg three times daily for 21 days. Atovaquone should be administered with a fatty meal.

E. Other Drugs

Trimethoprim, 15 mg/kg/d in three divided doses daily, plus dapsone, 100 mg/d, is an alternative oral regimen for mild to moderate disease or for continuation of therapy after intravenous therapy is no longer needed.

F. Prednisone

Based on studies done in patients with AIDS, prednisone is given for moderate to severe pneumonia (when Pao_2 on admission is < 70 mm Hg or oxygen saturation is < 90%) in conjunction with antimicrobials. The dosage of prednisone is 40 mg twice daily orally for 5 days, then 40 mg daily for 5 days, and then 20 mg daily until therapy is completed. The role of prednisone in non-AIDS patients is unclear, especially in patients in whom symptoms developed following tapering doses of corticosteroids.

► Prevention

Primary prophylaxis for *Pneumocystis* pneumonia in HIV-infected patients should be given to persons with CD4 counts < 200 cells/mcL, a CD4 percentage below 14%, or weight loss or oral candidiasis (see Table 31–4). Primary prophylaxis is often used in patients with hematologic malignancy and transplant recipients, although the clinical characteristics of persons with these conditions who would benefit from *Pneumocystis* prophylaxis have not been clearly defined. Patients with a history of *Pneumocystis* pneumonia should receive secondary prophylaxis until they have had a durable virologic response to antiretroviral therapy for at least 3–6 months and maintain a CD4 count of > 200 cells/mcL.

► Prognosis

In the absence of early and adequate treatment, the fatality rate for the endemic infantile form of *Pneumocystis* pneumonia is 20–50%; for the sporadic form in immunodeficient persons, the fatality rate is nearly 100%. Early treatment reduces the mortality rate to about 3% in the former and 10–20% in AIDS patients. The mortality rate in other immunodeficient patients is still 30–50%, probably because of failure to make a timely diagnosis. In immunodeficient patients who do not receive prophylaxis, recurrences are common (30% in AIDS).

Sassi M et al. Outbreaks of *Pneumocystis* pneumonia in 2 renal transplant centers linked to a single strain of *Pneumocystis*: implications for transmission and virulence. Clin Infect Dis. 2012 May;54(10):1437–44. [PMID: 22431811]

Tanaka M et al. *Pneumocystis jirovecii* pneumonia associated with etanercept treatment in patients with rheumatoid arthritis: a retrospective review of 15 cases and analysis of risk factors. Mod Rheumatol. 2012 Nov;22(6):849–58. [PMID: 22354637]

CRYPTOCOCCOSIS

ESSENTIALS OF DIAGNOSIS

► Most common cause of fungal meningitis.

► Predisposing factors: Hematologic cancer chemotherapy, Hodgkin lymphoma, corticosteroid therapy, transplant recipients, TNF inhibitor therapy, HIV infection.

► Symptoms of headache, abnormal mental status; meningismus seen occasionally, though rarely in HIV-infected patients.

► Demonstration of capsular polysaccharide antigen in cerebrospinal fluid is diagnostic.

► General Considerations

Cryptococcosis is mainly caused by *Cryptococcus neoformans*, an encapsulated budding yeast that has been found worldwide in soil and on dried pigeon dung. *C gattii* is a closely related species that also causes disease in humans although *C gattii* may affect more immunocompetent persons. It is a major cause of cryptococcosis in the Pacific Northwestern region of the United States and may result in more severe disease than *C neoformans*.

Infections are acquired by inhalation. In the lung, the infection may remain localized, heal, or disseminate. Clinically apparent cryptococcal pneumonia rarely develops in immunocompetent persons. Progressive lung disease and dissemination most often occur in the setting of cellular immunodeficiency, including underlying hematologic cancer under treatment, Hodgkin lymphoma, long-term corticosteroid therapy, solid-organ transplant, TNF-inhibitor therapy, or HIV infection.

► Clinical Findings

A. Symptoms and Signs

Pulmonary disease ranges from simple nodules to widespread infiltrates leading to respiratory failure. Disseminated disease may involve any organ, but central nervous system disease predominates. Headache is usually the first symptom of meningitis. Confusion and other mental status changes as well as cranial nerve abnormalities, nausea, and vomiting may be seen as the disease progresses. Nuchal rigidity and meningeal signs occur about 50% of the time but are uncommon in HIV-infected patients. Communicating hydrocephalus may complicate the course. *C gattii* infection frequently presents with respiratory symptoms along with neurologic signs caused by space-occupying lesions. Primary *C neoformans* infection of the skin may mimic bacterial cellulitis, especially in immunocompromised persons. Clinical worsening associated with improved immunologic status has been reported in HIV-positive and transplant patients with cryptococcosis; this entity has been labeled the immune reconstitution inflammatory syndrome (IRIS).

B. Laboratory Findings

Respiratory tract disease is diagnosed by culture of respiratory secretions or pleural fluid. For suspected meningeal disease, lumbar puncture is the preferred diagnostic procedure. Spinal fluid findings include increased opening pressure, variable pleocytosis, increased protein, and decreased glucose, though as many as 50% of AIDS patients have no pleocytosis. Gram stain of the cerebrospinal fluid usually reveals budding, encapsulated fungal cells. Cryptococcal capsular antigen in cerebrospinal fluid and culture together establish the diagnosis over 90% of the time. Patients with AIDS often have the antigen in both cerebrospinal fluid and serum, and extrameningeal disease (lungs, blood, urinary tract) is common. In patients with AIDS, the serum cryptococcal antigen is also a sensitive screening test for meningitis, being positive in over 95% of cases. MRI is more sensitive than CT in finding central nervous system abnormalities such as cryptococcomas. Antigen testing by a new lateral flow assay appears to have improved sensitivity and specificity over the conventional latex agglutination test.

▶ Treatment

Because of decreased efficacy, initial therapy with an azole alone is not recommended for treatment of acute cryptococcal meningitis. Consequently, amphotericin B, 0.7–1 mg/kg/d intravenously is used for 14 days, followed by an additional 8 weeks of fluconazole, 400 mg/d orally. This regimen has been quite effective, achieving clinical responses and cerebrospinal fluid sterilization in about 70% of patients. Lipid amphotericin B preparations (eg, liposomal amphotericin B, 3–4 mg/kg/d) have equivalent efficacy to conventional amphotericin B with reduced nephrotoxicity. The addition of flucytosine has been associated with improved survival, but toxicity is common. Flucytosine is administered orally at a dose of 100 mg/kg/d divided into four equal doses and given every 6 hours. Hematologic parameters should be closely monitored during flucytosine therapy, and it is important to adjust the dose for any decreases in renal function. Fluconazole (800–1200 mg orally daily) may be given with amphotericin B when flucytosine is not available or patients cannot tolerate it. Frequent, repeated lumbar punctures or ventricular shunting should be performed to relieve high cerebrospinal fluid pressures or if hydrocephalus is a complication. Failure to adequately relieve raised intracranial pressure is a major cause of morbidity and mortality. The end points for amphotericin B therapy and for switching to oral fluconazole are a favorable clinical response (decrease in temperature; improvement in headache, nausea, vomiting, and mini-mental status scores), improvement in cerebrospinal fluid biochemical parameters and, most importantly, conversion of cerebrospinal fluid culture to negative.

A similar approach is reasonable for patients with cryptococcal meningitis in the absence of AIDS, though the mortality rate is considerably higher. Therapy is generally continued until cerebrospinal fluid cultures become negative. Maintenance antifungal therapy is important after treatment of an acute episode in HIV-related cases, since otherwise the rate of relapse is > 50%. Fluconazole, 200 mg/d orally, is the maintenance therapy of choice, decreasing the relapse rate approximately tenfold compared with placebo and threefold compared with weekly amphotericin B in patients whose cerebrospinal fluid has been sterilized by the induction therapy. After successful therapy of cryptococcal meningitis, it is possible to discontinue secondary prophylaxis with fluconazole in individuals with AIDS who have had a satisfactory response to antiretroviral therapy (eg, CD4 cell count > 100–200 cells/mcL for at least 6 months). Among practitioners treating patients without AIDS, there has been a trend in recent years to prescribe a course (eg, 6–12 months) of fluconazole as maintenance therapy following successful treatment of the acute illness; recently published guidelines suggest this as an option.

▶ Prognosis

Factors that indicate a poor prognosis include the activity of the predisposing conditions, older age, organ failure, lack of spinal fluid pleocytosis, high initial antigen titer in either serum or cerebrospinal fluid, decreased mental status, increased intracranial pressure, and the presence of disease outside the nervous system.

Antinori S. New insights into HIV/AIDS-Associated cryptococcosis. ISRN AIDS. 2013 Feb 25;2013:471363. [PMID: 24052889]

Loyse A et al. Comparisons of the early fungicidal activity of high-dose fluconazole, voriconazole and flucytosine as second line drugs given in combination with amphotericin B for the treatment of HIV-associated cryptococcal meningitis. Clin Infect Dis. 2012 Jan;54(1):121–8. [PMID: 22052885]

McMullan BJ et al. *Cryptococcus gattii* infections: contemporary aspects of epidemiology, clinical manifestations and management of infection. Future Microbiol. 2013 Dec;8:1613–31. [PMID: 24266360]

ASPERGILLOSIS

ESSENTIALS OF DIAGNOSIS

▶ Most common cause of non-candidal invasive fungal infection in stem cell or organ transplant recipients and in patients with hematologic malignancies.

▶ Predisposing factors: leukemia, bone marrow or organ transplant, late HIV infection.

▶ Pulmonary, sinus, and CNS are most common disease sites.

▶ Detection of galactomannan by ELISA or PCR in serum or other body fluid samples is useful for early diagnosis and treatment.

General Considerations

Aspergillus fumigatus is the usual cause of aspergillosis, though many species of *Aspergillus* may cause a wide spectrum of disease. The lungs, sinuses, and brain are the organs most often involved. Clinical illness results either from an aberrant immunologic response or tissue invasion.

Clinical Findings

A. Allergic Bronchopulmonary Aspergillosis

This form of aspergillosis occurs in patients with preexisting asthma who develop worsening bronchospasm and fleeting pulmonary infiltrates accompanied by eosinophilia, high levels of IgE, and IgG *Aspergillus* precipitins in the blood. It also may complicate cystic fibrosis.

B. Invasive Aspergillosis

Invasive manifestations may be seen in immunocompetent or only mildly immunocompromised adults. These include chronic **sinusitis**, colonization of preexisting pulmonary cavities (**aspergilloma**), and chronic necrotizing pulmonary aspergillosis.

1. Sinusitis—Sinus involvement is usually diagnosed histologically after patients with chronic sinus disease undergo surgery.

2. Aspergillomas—Aspergillomas of the lung occur when preexisting lung cavities become secondarily colonized with *Aspergillus* species. These may be found by incidental radiographic studies but may also present with significant hemoptysis.

3. Chronic necrotizing aspergillosis—This invasive manifestation is a relatively rare disease seen in patients with some degree of immunocompromise and presents with a protracted course compared with the more common acute invasive form of the disease. Fibrosis and cavity formation may be prominent.

4. Life-threatening invasive aspergillosis—Severe invasive aspergillosis most commonly occurs in profoundly immunodeficient patients, particularly in patients who have undergone hematopoietic stem cell transplants; in those with prolonged, severe neutropenia; and in patients with chronic granulomatous disease. Specific risk factors in patients who have undergone a hematopoietic stem cell transplant include cytopenias, corticosteroid use, iron overload, cytomegalovirus disease, and graft-versus-host disease. Pulmonary disease is most common, with patchy infiltration leading to a severe necrotizing pneumonia. Invasive sinus disease also occurs. At any time, there may be hematogenous dissemination to the central nervous system, skin, and other organs. Early diagnosis and reversal of any correctable immunosuppression are essential. Blood cultures have very low yield. Detection of galactomannan by ELISA or PCR, or both, has been used for the early diagnosis of invasive disease, though multiple determinations should be done. Galactomannan levels and PCR can be tested in serum or in bronchoalveolar lavage fluid, which may be more sensitive compared to serum.

Higher galactomannan levels are correlated with increased mortality, and failure of galactomannan levels to fall in response to therapy portends a worse outcome. False-positive galactomannan tests have been reported in patients receiving beta-lactam antibiotics. Isolation of *Aspergillus* from pulmonary secretions does not necessarily imply invasive disease, although its positive predictive value increases with more advanced immunosuppression. Therefore, a definitive diagnosis requires demonstration of *Aspergillus* in tissue or culture from a sterile site. CT scan of the chest may show characteristics quite suggestive of invasive aspergillosis (eg, "halo sign").

Prevention

The high mortality rate and difficulty in diagnosis of invasive aspergillosis often leads clinicians to institute prophylactic therapy for patients with profound immunosuppression. The best-studied agents include itraconazole, voriconazole, and posaconazole, although patient and agent selection criteria remain undefined. Widespread use of broad-spectrum azoles raises concern for development of invasive disease by highly resistant fungi.

Treatment

A. Allergic Bronchopulmonary Aspergillosis

For acute exacerbations, oral prednisone is begun at a dose of 1 mg/kg/d and then tapered slowly over several months. Itraconazole at a dose of 200 mg daily for 16 weeks appears to improve pulmonary function and decrease corticosteroid requirements in these patients, although voriconazole may become the preferred oral agent.

B. Invasive Aspergillosis

1. Sinusitis—These patients may require protracted courses of antifungals (itraconazole, 200 mg twice daily, for weeks to months) in addition to the surgical debridement.

2. Aspergilloma—The most effective therapy for symptomatic aspergilloma remains surgical resection.

3. Chronic necrotizing aspergillosis—Guidelines suggest some benefits from prolonged oral voriconazole (200 mg twice daily) or itraconazole (200 mg twice daily) therapy.

4. Life-threatening invasive aspergillosis—When severe invasive aspergillosis is considered clinically likely or is demonstrable by laboratory testing, rapid institution of voriconazole (6 mg/kg intravenously twice on day 1 and then 4 mg/kg every 12 hours thereafter) is considered optimal therapy. Alternatives include a lipid formulation of amphotericin B (3–5 mg/kg/d), caspofungin 70 mg intravenously on day 1 and then 50 mg/d thereafter), and posaconazole oral tablets (300 mg twice daily on day 1 and then 300 mg daily thereafter). Oral dosing of voriconazole at 4 mg/kg twice daily can be used for less serious infections or as a step-down strategy after intravenous therapy. Therapeutic drug monitoring should be considered for both voriconazole and posaconazole given variations in metabolism and absorption.

In critically ill patients who are not responding to conventional antifungal treatment, there may be a role for the addition of caspofungin to liposomal amphotericin B or voriconazole therapy, although randomized trials are lacking. Surgical debridement is generally done for sinusitis, and there is increasing data regarding resection of focal pulmonary lesions, especially for treatment of life-threatening hemoptysis. The mortality rate of pulmonary or disseminated disease in the immunocompromised patient remains well above 50%, particularly in patients with refractory neutropenia.

Morrissey CO et al; Australasian Leukaemia Lymphoma Group and the Australia and New Zealand Mycology Interest Group. Galactomannan and PCR versus culture and histology for directing use of antifungal treatment for invasive aspergillosis in high-risk haematology patients: a randomised controlled trial. Lancet Infect Dis. 2013 Jun;13(6):519–28. [PMID: 23639612]

Park WB et al. The effect of therapeutic drug monitoring on safety and efficacy of voriconazole in invasive fungal infections: a randomized controlled trial. Clin Infect Dis. 2012 Oct;55(8):1080–7. [PMID: 22761409]

Schwarzinger M et al; PREVERT Investigators. Performance of serum biomarkers for the early detection of invasive aspergillosis in febrile, neutropenic patients: a multi-state model. PLoS One. 2013 Jun 14;8(6):e65776. [PMID: 2379904]

MUCORMYCOSIS

ESSENTIALS OF DIAGNOSIS

▶ Most common cause of non-*Aspergillus* invasive mold infection.

▶ Predisposing factors: poorly controlled diabetes, leukemia, bone marrow or organ transplant, trauma with wound contamination by soil.

▶ Pulmonary, rhinocerebral, and skin are most common disease sites.

▶ Rapidly fatal without multidisciplinary interventions.

▶ General Considerations

The term "mucormycosis" is applied to opportunistic infections caused by members of the genera *Rhizopus, Mucor, Lichtheimia* (formerly *Absidia*), and *Cunninghamella*. Predisposing conditions include hematologic malignancy, stem cell transplantation, solid organ transplantation, diabetic ketoacidosis, chronic kidney disease, desferoxamine therapy, and treatment with corticosteroids or cytotoxic drugs.

▶ Clinical Findings

Invasive disease of the sinuses, orbits, and the lungs may occur. Necrosis is common due to hyphal tissue invasion that may manifest as ulceration of the hard palate or nasal palate or hemoptysis. Widely disseminated disease is seen in patients who have received cytotoxic chemotherapy.

No serologic or laboratory findings assist with diagnosis, and blood cultures are unhelpful. A reverse halo sign may be seen on chest CT. Biopsy of involved tissue remains the cornerstone of diagnosis, although cultures are frequently negative. The organisms appear in tissues as broad, branching nonseptate hyphae.

▶ Treatment

Optimal therapy of mucormycosis involves reversal of predisposing conditions (if possible), surgical debridement, and prompt antifungal therapy. A prolonged course of a lipid preparation of intravenous amphotericin B (5 mg/kg) should be started early. Based on in vitro susceptibility, posaconazole tablets 300 mg/d orally is generally used after disease has been stabilized. Combination therapy with amphotericin and posaconazole is not proven but is commonly used because of the poor response to monotherapy. Other azoles are not effective. There are limited data suggesting beneficial synergistic activity when amphotericin and caspofungin are used in combination for mucormycosis. Despite favorable animal studies, a pilot study in humans incorporating adjunctive iron chelation therapy with deferasirox demonstrated a higher mortality rate than antifungal therapy alone. Control of diabetes and other underlying conditions, along with extensive repeated surgical removal of necrotic, nonperfused tissue, is essential. Even when these measures are introduced in a timely fashion, the prognosis remains guarded. The historical 4-week mortality rate is 40%, although better response rates have been noted since 2000.

Katragkou A et al. Why is mucormycosis more difficult to cure than more common mycoses? Clin Microbiol Infect. 2013 Nov 27. [Epub ahead of print] [PMID: 24279587]

Neblett Fanfair R et al. Necrotizing cutaneous mucormycosis after a tornado in Joplin, Missouri, in 2011. N Engl J Med. 2012 Dec 6;367(23):2214–25. [PMID: 23215557]

Pagano L et al. Combined antifungal approach for the treatment of invasive mucormycosis in patients with hematologic diseases: a report from the SEIFEM and FUNGISCOPE registries. Haematologica. 2013 Oct;98(10):e127–30. [PMID: 23716556]

BLASTOMYCOSIS

Blastomycosis occurs most often in men infected during occupational or recreational activities out of doors and in a geographically limited area of the south central and midwestern United States and Canada. Disease usually occurs in immunocompetent individuals.

Chronic pulmonary infection is most common and may be asymptomatic. When dissemination takes place, lesions are most frequently seen in the skin, bones, and urogenital system.

Cough, moderate fever, dyspnea, and chest pain are common. These may resolve or progress, with purulent sputum production, pleurisy, fever, chills, loss of weight, and prostration. Radiologic studies, either chest radiographs or CT scans, usually reveal airspace consolidation or masses.

Raised, verrucous cutaneous lesions are commonly present in disseminated blastomycosis. Bones—often the ribs and vertebrae—are frequently involved. Epididymitis, prostatitis, and other involvement of the male urogenital system may occur. Although they do not appear to be at greater risk for acquisition of disease, infection in HIV-infected persons may progress rapidly, with dissemination common.

Laboratory findings usually include leukocytosis and anemia, though these are not specific. The organism is found in clinical specimens, such as expectorated sputum or tissue biopsies, as a thick-walled cell 5–20 mcm in diameter that may have a single broad-based bud. It grows readily on culture. Serologic tests are not well standardized. A urinary antigen test is available, but it has considerable cross reactivity with *Histoplasma*. A serum enzyme immunoassay based on the surface protein BAD-1 appears sensitive and specific.

Itraconazole, 200–400 mg/d orally for at least 2–3 months, is the therapy of choice for nonmeningeal disease, with a response rate of over 80%. Amphotericin B, 0.7–1.0 mg/kg/d intravenously (or lipid formulation amphotericin B), is given for severe disease, treatment failures, or central nervous system involvement.

Clinical follow-up for relapse should be made regularly for several years so that therapy may be resumed or another drug instituted.

Bush JW et al. Outcomes of persons with blastomycosis involving the central nervous system. Diagn Microbiol Infect Dis. 2013 Jun;76(2):175–81. [PMID: 23566338]
López-Martínez R et al. Blastomycosis. Clin Dermatol. 2012 Nov–Dec;30(6):565–72. [PMID: 23068144]

PARACOCCIDIOIDOMYCOSIS (South American Blastomycosis)

Paracoccidioides brasiliensis infections have been found only in patients who have resided in South or Central America or Mexico. Long asymptomatic periods enable patients to travel far from the endemic areas before developing clinical problems. Weight loss, pulmonary complaints, or mucosal ulcerations are the most common symptoms. Cutaneous papules may ulcerate and enlarge both peripherally and deeper into the subcutaneous tissue. Differential diagnosis includes mucocutaneous leishmaniasis and syphilis. Extensive coalescent ulcerations may eventually result in destruction of the epiglottis, vocal cords, and uvula. Extension to the lips and face may occur. Lymph node enlargement may follow mucocutaneous lesions, eventually ulcerating and forming draining sinuses; in some patients, it is the presenting symptom. Hepatosplenomegaly may be present as well. HIV-infected patients with paracoccidioidomycosis are more likely to have extrapulmonary dissemination and a more rapid clinical disease course.

Laboratory findings are nonspecific. Serology by immunodiffusion is positive in > 80% of cases. Complement fixation titers correlate with progressive disease and fall with effective therapy. The fungus is found in clinical specimens

as a spherical cell that may have many buds arising from it. If direct examination of secretions does not reveal the organism, biopsy with Gomori staining may be helpful.

Itraconazole, 100 mg twice daily orally, is the treatment of choice and generally results in a clinical response within 1 month and effective control after 2–6 months. Trimethoprim-sulfamethoxazole (480/1200 mg) twice daily orally is equally effective and less costly but associated with more adverse effects. Amphotericin B intravenously is the drug of choice for severe and life-threatening infection.

Marques SA. Paracoccidioidomycosis: epidemiological, clinical, diagnostic and treatment up-dating. An Bras Dermatol. 2013 Sep–Oct;88(5):700-11. [PMID: 24173174]

SPOROTRICHOSIS

Sporotrichosis is a chronic fungal infection caused by *Sporothrix schenckii*. It is worldwide in distribution; most patients have had contact with soil, sphagnum moss, or decaying wood. Infection takes place when the organism is inoculated into the skin—usually on the hand, arm, or foot, especially during gardening.

The most common form of sporotrichosis begins with a hard, nontender subcutaneous nodule. This later becomes adherent to the overlying skin and ulcerates. Within a few days to weeks, lymphocutaneous spread along the lymphatics draining this area occurs, which may result in ulceration. Cavitary pulmonary disease occurs in individuals with underlying chronic lung disease.

Disseminated sporotrichosis is rare in immunocompetent persons but may present with widespread cutaneous, lung, bone, joint, and central nervous system involvement in immunocompromised patients, especially those with AIDS and alcohol abuse.

Cultures are needed to establish diagnosis. Antibody tests may be useful for diagnosis of disseminated disease, especially meningitis.

Itraconazole, 200–400 mg orally daily for several months, is the treatment of choice for localized disease and some milder cases of disseminated disease. Terbinafine, 500 mg orally twice daily, also appears to have good efficacy in lymphocutaneous disease. Amphotericin B intravenously, 1–2 g, or a lipid amphotericin B preparation, 3–5 mg/kg/d are used for severe systemic infection. Surgery may be indicated for complicated pulmonary cavitary disease, and joint involvement may require arthrodesis.

The prognosis is good for lymphocutaneous sporotrichosis; pulmonary, joint, and disseminated disease respond less favorably.

Aung AK et al. Pulmonary sporotrichosis: case series and systematic analysis of literature on clinico-radiological patterns and management outcomes. Med Mycol. 2013 Jul;51(5): 534–44. [PMID: 23286352]
de Lima Barros MB et al. *Sporothrix schenckii* and sporotrichosis. Clin Microbiol Rev. 2011 Oct;24(4):633–54. [PMID: 21976602]

PENICILLIUM MARNEFFEI INFECTIONS

Penicillium marneffei, which is endemic in southeast Asia, is a dimorphic fungus that causes systemic infection predominately in immunocompromised hosts. There have been reports of travelers with advanced AIDS returning from southeast Asia with disseminated infection. Clinical manifestations include fever, generalized umbilicated papular rash, lymphadenopathy, cough, and diarrhea. Central nervous system infection has been reported. Diagnosis is made by identification of the organism on smears or histopathologic specimens or by culture, where the fungus produces a characteristic red pigment. The best sites for isolation of the fungus include the skin, blood, bone marrow, respiratory tract, and lymph nodes. Antigen and antibody tests have been developed in endemic regions. Patients with mild to moderate infection can be treated with itraconazole, 400 mg divided into two doses daily by mouth for 8 weeks. Amphotericin B, 0.5–0.7 mg/kg/d intravenously, is the drug of choice for severe disease and should be continued until patients have had a satisfactory clinical response, at which time they can be switched to itraconazole. Because the relapse rate after successful treatment is 30%, maintenance therapy with itraconazole, 200–400 mg daily orally, is indicated indefinitely, or until immune reconstitution occurs.

Hu Y et al. *Penicillium marneffei* infection: an emerging disease in mainland China. Mycopathologia. 2013 Feb;175(1–2): 57–67. [PMID: 22983901]

CHROMOBLASTOMYCOSIS (Chromomycosis)

Chromoblastomycosis is a chronic, principally tropical cutaneous infection usually affecting young men who are agricultural workers and caused by several species of closely related black molds; *Cladophialophora carrionii* and *Fonsecaea pedrosoi* are the most common etiologic agents.

Lesions usually follow puncture wounds and are slowly progressive, occurring most frequently on a lower extremity. The lesion begins as a papule or ulcer. Over months to years, papules enlarge to become vegetating, papillomatous, verrucous elevated nodules. Satellite lesions may appear along the lymphatics. There may be secondary bacterial infection. Elephantiasis may result.

The fungus is seen as brown, thick-walled, spherical, sometimes septate cells in potassium hydroxide preparations of pus or skin scrapings (so-called Medlar bodies), which are quite sensitive for diagnosis.

Itraconazole, 200–400 mg/d orally for 6–18 months, achieves a response rate of 65%. Terbinafine at 500–1000 mg/d orally may have similar efficacy to itraconazole and may be useful in combination, especially in difficult to treat cases. Photodynamic therapy combined with antifungal drugs have been successfully used.

Queiroz-Telles F et al. Challenges in the therapy of chromoblastomycosis. Mycopathologia. 2013 Jun;175(5–6):477–88. [PMID: 23636730]

MYCETOMA (Eumycetoma & Actinomycetoma)

Mycetoma is a chronic local, slowly progressive destructive infection that usually involves the foot; it begins in subcutaneous tissues, frequently after localized trauma, and then spreads to contiguous structures. Eumycetoma (also known as maduromycosis) is the term used to describe mycetoma caused by the true fungi and by phylogenetically diverse organisms. Actinomycotic mycetoma is caused by *Actinomadura*, *Streptomyces*, and *Nocardia* species. The disease begins as a papule, nodule, or abscess that over months to years progresses slowly to form multiple abscesses and sinus tracts ramifying deep into the tissue. Secondary bacterial infection may result in large open ulcers. Radiographs may show destructive changes in the underlying bone. Larger hyphae are seen with fungal mycetoma; the causative species can often be identified by the color of the characteristic grains within the infected tissues.

The prognosis for eumycetoma is poor, though surgical debridement along with prolonged itraconazole therapy or combination therapy including itraconazole and terbinafine may result in a response rate of 70%. The various etiologic agents may respond differently to antifungal agents, so culture results are invaluable. Amputation is necessary in far advanced cases.

Estrada R et al. Eumycetoma. Clin Dermatol. 2012 Jul;30(4): 389–96. [PMID: 22682186]

OTHER OPPORTUNISTIC MOLD INFECTIONS

Fungi previously considered to be harmless colonizers, including *Pseudallescheria boydii (Scedosporium apiospermum)*, *Scedosporium prolificans*, *Fusarium*, *Paecilomyces*, *Trichoderma longibrachiatum*, and *Trichosporon*, are emerging as significant pathogens in immunocompromised patients. This occurs most often in patients being treated for hematopoietic malignancies and in those receiving broad-spectrum antifungal prophylaxis. Infection may be localized in the skin, lungs, or sinuses, or widespread disease may appear with lesions in multiple organs. Fusariosis should be suspected in severely immunosuppressed persons in whom multiple, painful skin lesions develop; blood cultures are often positive. Sinus infection may cause bony erosion. Infection in subcutaneous tissues following traumatic implantation may develop as a well-circumscribed cyst or as an ulcer.

Nonpigmented septate hyphae are seen in tissue and are indistinguishable from those of *Aspergillus* when infections are due to *S apiospermum* or species of *Fusarium*, *Paecilomyces*, *Penicillium*, or other hyaline molds. Spores or mycetoma-like granules are rarely present in tissue.

The differentiation of *S apiospermum* and *Aspergillus* is particularly important, since the former is uniformly resistant to amphotericin B but may be sensitive to azole antifungals (eg, voriconazole). Infection by any of a number of black molds is designated as phaeohyphomycosis. These black molds (eg, *Exophiala, Bipolaris, Cladophialophora, Curvularia, Alternaria*) are common in the environment, especially on decaying vegetation. Environmental molds are commonly implicated in asthma and other allergic disease but invasive disease due to these agents is rarely encountered except in persons with profound immunosuppression. Although the popular press has implicated some environmental molds, such as *Stachybotrys chartarum*, as causative agents of some toxin-induced disorders, specific toxicity from inhaled mold substances has not been scientifically established. In tissues of patients with phaeohyphomycosis, the mold is seen as black or faintly brown hyphae, yeast cells, or both. Culture on appropriate medium is needed to identify the agent. Histologic demonstration of these organisms is definitive evidence of invasive infection; positive cultures must be interpreted cautiously and not assumed to be contaminants in immunocompromised hosts. Some isolates are sensitive to antifungal agents.

A multistate outbreak of fungal infections was reported in 2012 among patients who had received contaminated preservative-free methylprednisolone acetate corticosteroid injections provided by one compounding pharmacy. Four clinical syndromes were recognized: (1) meningitis; (2) basilar stroke; (3) spinal epidural abscess/osteomyelitis; and (4) peripheral joint infections or septic arthritis.

Over 751 cases have been reported by the end of 2013 and 64 patients have died; sporadic cases continue to be reported. Most of the infections were due to the dematiaceous fungus, *Exserohilum rostratum*, a normally rare cause of human disease. Diagnosis depended on a strong index of suspicion. Routine cultures of affected tissues or fluids were performed, although the diagnosis was often made by PCR on specimens sent to the Centers for Disease Control and Prevention. Management included provision of a combination of liposomal amphotericin B, 5–6 mg/kg/d intravenously along with high-dose voriconazole, 6 mg/kg every 12 hours intravenously or orally, for severely ill patients. Less ill patients were treated with voriconazole, 6 mg/kg every 12 hours for a prolonged period of time.

Chiller TM et al; Multistate Fungal Infection Clinical Investigation Team. Clinical findings for fungal infections caused by methylprednisolone injections. N Engl J Med. 2013 Oct 24; 369(17):1610–9. [PMID: 24152260]
Pappas PG. Lessons learned in the multistate fungal infection outbreak in the United States. Curr Opin Infect Dis. 2013 Dec;26(6):545–50. [PMID: 24152763]
Shoham S. Emerging fungal infections in solid organ transplant recipients. Infect Dis Clin North Am. 2013 Jun;27(2):305–16. [PMID: 23714342]

ANTIFUNGAL THERAPY

Table 36–1 summarizes the major properties of currently available antifungal agents. Two different lipid-based amphotericin B formulations are used to treat systemic

Table 36–1. Agents for systemic mycoses.

Drug	Dosing	Renal Clearance?	CSF Penetration?	Toxicities	Spectrum of Activity
Amphotericin B	0.3–1.5 mg/kg/d intravenously	No	Poor	Rigors, fever, azotemia, hypokalemia, hypomagnesemia, renal tubular acidosis, anemia	All major pathogens except *Scedosporium*
Amphotericin B lipid complex	5 mg/kg/d intravenously	No	Poor	Fever, rigors, nausea, hypotension, anemia, azotemia, tachypnea	Same as amphotericin B, above
Amphotericin B, liposomal	3–6 mg/kg/d intravenously	No	Poor	Fever, rigors, nausea, hypotension, azotemia, anemia, tachypnea, chest tightness	Same as amphotericin B, above
Anidulafungin	100 mg intravenous loading dose, followed by 50 mg/d intravenously in one dose	< 1%	Poor	Diarrhea, hepatic enzyme elevations, histamine-mediated reactions	Mucosal and invasive candidiasis
Caspofungin acetate	70 mg intravenous loading dose, followed by 50 mg/d intravenously in one dose	< 50%[1]	Poor	Transient neutropenia; hepatic enzyme elevations when used with cyclosporine	Aspergillosis, mucosal and invasive candidiasis, empiric antifungal therapy in febrile neutropenia

(continued)

Table 36–1. Agents for systemic mycoses. (continued)

Drug	Dosing	Renal Clearance?	CSF Penetration?	Toxicities	Spectrum of Activity
Fluconazole	100–800 mg/d in one or two doses intravenously or orally	Yes	Yes	Nausea, rash, alopecia, headache, hepatic enzyme elevations	Mucosal candidiasis (including urinary tract), cryptococcosis, histoplasmosis, coccidioidomycosis
Flucytosine (5-FC)	100–150 mg/kg/d orally in four divided doses	Yes	Yes	Leukopenia,[2] rash, diarrhea, hepatitis, nausea, vomiting	Cryptococcosis,[3] candidiasis,[3] chromomycosis
Isavuconazole (investigational)	200 mg/d orally or intravenously once daily	No	Low in CSF, high in brain	Nausea, diarrhea, upper abdominal pain, dizziness	Broad range of activity including the *Mucorales*
Itraconazole	100–400 mg/d orally in one or two doses with a meal or carbonated beverage	No	Variable	Nausea, hypokalemia, edema, hypertension, peripheral neuropathy	Histoplasmosis, coccidioidomycosis, blastomycosis, paracoccidioidomycosis, mucosal candidiasis (except urinary), sporotrichosis, aspergillosis, chromomycosis
Ketoconazole	200–800 mg/d orally in one or two doses with a meal or carbonated beverage	No	Poor	Anorexia, nausea, suppression of testosterone and cortisol, rash, headache, hepatic enzyme elevations, hepatic failure	Nonmeningeal histoplasmosis and coccidioidomycosis, blastomycosis, paracoccidioidomycosis, mucosal candidiasis (except urinary)
Micafungin sodium	150 mg intravenously in one dose (treatment) 50 mg (prophylaxis)	No	Poor	Rash, rigors, headache, phlebitis	Mucosal and invasive candidiasis, prophylaxis in hematopoietic stem cell transplantation
Posaconazole	400–800 mg/d orally in one or two doses[5] (oral suspension) or 300 mg orally once daily (tablets)	No	Yes	Nausea, vomiting, abdominal pain, diarrhea, and headache	Broad range of activity including the *Mucorales*
Terbinafine	250 mg/d orally in one dose	Yes	Poor	Nausea, abdominal pain, taste disturbance, rash, diarrhea, and hepatic enzyme elevations	Dermatophytes, sporotrichosis
Voriconazole	200–400 mg/d orally in two doses or 12 mg/kg intravenously as loading dose for 2 days followed by 6 mg/kg/d intravenously in two doses[5]	Yes	Yes	Transient visual disturbances, rash, photosensitivity, fluoride excess with periostitis, peripheral neuropathy, hepatic enzyme elevations[4]	All major pathogens except the *Mucorales* and sporotrichosis

[1]No dosage adjustment required for chronic kidney disease; dosage adjustment necessary with moderate to severe hepatic dysfunction.
[2]Use should be monitored with blood levels to prevent this or the dose adjusted according to creatinine clearance.
[3]In combination with amphotericin B.
[4]Administration with drugs that are metabolized by the cytochrome P450 system is contraindicated or requires careful monitoring.
[5]Some authorities advocate therapeutic drug monitoring in patients who are not responding to therapy.

invasive fungal infections. Their principal advantage appears to be substantially reduced nephrotoxicity, allowing administration of much higher doses. Three agents of the echinocandin class, caspofungin acetate, anidulafungin, and micafungin sodium, are currently approved.

The echinocandins have relatively few adverse effects and are useful for the treatment of invasive *Candida* infections. Caspofungin acetate is also approved for use in refractory cases of invasive aspergillosis. Voriconazole has excellent activity against a broad range of fungal pathogens and has been FDA approved for use in invasive *Aspergillus* cases, *Fusarium* and *Scedosporium* infections, *Candida* esophagitis, deep *Candida* infections, and candidemia. Posaconazole has good activity against a broad range of filamentous fungi, including the *Mucorales*. Some experts now recommend therapeutic drug monitoring in individuals with severe invasive fungal infections receiving these newer azoles because of unreliable serum levels due to either metabolic alterations as a result of genetic polymorphisms (voriconazole) or erratic absorption (posaconazole). A new delayed-release tablet preparation of posaconazole provides more reliable pharmacokinetics. Isavuconazole is an investigational azole that has recently been granted orphan drug status for the treatment of aspergillosis and mucormycosis.

Falci DR et al. Profile of isavuconazole and its potential in the treatment of severe invasive fungal infections. Infect Drug Resist. 2013 Oct 22;6:163–74. [PMID: 24187505]

Paiva JA et al. New antifungal antibiotics. Curr Opin Infect Dis. 2013 Apr;26(2):168–74. [PMID: 23411420]

37

Disorders Related to Environmental Emergencies

Jacqueline A. Nemer, MD, FACEP

ACCIDENTAL SYSTEMIC HYPOTHERMIA

ESSENTIALS OF DIAGNOSIS

► Reduction of core body temperature (CBT) below 35°C.

► Accurate CBT measurement must be obtained by an intravascular, esophageal, rectal, or bladder probe that measures as low as 25°C; oral, axillary, and otic temperatures are inaccurate.

► The CBT must be over 32°C before terminating resuscitation efforts.

► Refreezing must be avoided to reduce further damage.

General Considerations

Systemic hypothermia is defined as CBT < 35°C. This may be primary (from exposure to prolonged ambient extremely low temperature) or secondary (due to thermoregulatory dysfunction); both may be present at the same time. Heat loss occurs more rapidly with high wind velocity ("wind-chill factor"), water exposure (including wet clothing), or direct contact with a cold surface.

The human body generates internal heat through muscle activity (ie, shivering or increased physical exertion) and preserves heat loss via peripheral vasoconstriction. In prolonged or repetitive cold exposure, hypothermia ensues if these thermoregulatory responses become impaired. Hypothermia should be considered in any patient with prolonged exposure to ambient or cold environment, trauma, inadequate clothing, or altered mental status.

Iatrogenic accidental hypothermia may occur in the hospital setting due to rapid infusion of intravenous fluids, prolonged exposure during resuscitation or surgical procedures, or administration of large amounts of refrigerated stored blood products (without rewarming).

Clinical Findings

Symptoms and signs of hypothermia are typically nonspecific and markedly variable based on the patient's underlying health and circumstances of hypothermia. When CBT is 32–35°C, symptoms include tachypnea, tachycardia, hypertension, shivering, impaired coordination, poor judgment, and apathy. When CBT is 28–32°C, the body slows down. Shivering stops; bradycardia, dilated pupils, slowed reflexes, cold diuresis, and confusion and lethargy ensue. The electrocardiogram (ECG) may reveal a J wave or Osborn wave (positive deflection in the terminal portion of the QRS complex, most notable in leads II, V_5, and V_6) (Figure 37–1). In extreme hypothermia (ie, CBT < 28°C), the skin may appear blue or puffy; coma, apnea, loss of reflexes, asystole, or ventricular fibrillation may lead the clinician to assume that patient is dead. Prolonged hypothermia may lead to dysrhythmias and conduction abnormalities, acidemia, hyperkalemia, rhabdomyolysis, pulmonary edema, kidney disease, pneumonia, pancreatitis, hypoglycemia or hyperglycemia, and coagulopathy.

Treatment

Resuscitation begins with rapid assessment and support of airway, breathing and circulation, initiation of rewarming, and prevention of further heat loss. *Rewarming is the initial, imperative treatment.* All cold, wet clothing must be removed and replaced with warm, dry clothing. To accurately measure hypothermia, an intravascular, esophageal, rectal or bladder probe that measures temperatures as low as 25°C is required; oral, axillary, and otic temperatures are inaccurate and unreliable. The patient should be evaluated for associated conditions (ie, hypoglycemia, trauma, infection, overdose and peripheral cold injury). Rewarming methods are determined by the degree of hypothermia and the resources available.

During rewarming, continuous monitoring of temperature, other vital signs, cardiac rhythm, and blood glucose must be done. Complications of rewarming occur as colder peripheral blood returns to central circulation. This may

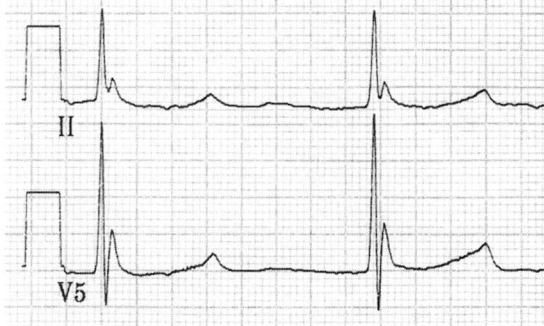

Figure 37–1. Electrocardiogram shows leads II and V5 in a patient whose body temperature is 24°C. Note the bradycardia and Osborn waves. These findings become more prominent as the body temperature lowers, and gradually resolve with rewarming. Osborn waves have an extra positive deflection in the terminal portion of the QRS complex and are best seen in the inferior and lateral precordial leads (most notably in leads II, V_5, and V_6).

result in core temperature afterdrop, rewarming lactic acidosis, rewarming shock from peripheral vasodilation and hypovolemia, ventricular fibrillation, and other cardiac arrhythmias. Extreme caution must be taken when handling the hypothermic patient to avoid triggering arrhythmias. Assessment includes acid-base status (lactate and blood gases); volume status (cold diuresis); electrolyte abnormalities (particularly potassium and glucose); metabolic acidosis; coagulopathy; rhabdomyolysis; and dysfunction of the pancreas, liver, kidneys. An ECG and a chest radiograph should be obtained. False laboratory values will occur if the blood sample is warmed to 37°C for the testing. Patient should be assessed for infection; however, antibiotics are not routinely given unless a source is identified.

A. Passive and Active External Rewarming Methods

Passive external rewarming involves removing cold wet clothing, then drying and covering the patient with blankets to prevent further heat loss. The patient will rewarm due to the body's internal heat production through shivering and increased metabolism. **Active external rewarming** is highly effective and safe for mild hypothermia. This is a noninvasive method of applying external heat to the patient's skin. Examples include warm bedding, heated blankets, heat packs, and immersion into a 40°C bath.

Afterdrop, which is the continued falling of body temperature during rewarming, can be lessened by active external rewarming of the trunk but not the extremities and by avoiding any muscle movement by the patient. Patients with mild hypothermia (CBT > 33°C) and previous good health usually respond well to passive and active external warming.

B. Active Internal (Core) Rewarming Methods

Active internal core rewarming methods are required for patients with CBT < 33°C. Patients with milder degrees of hypothermia may also benefit from these methods. Warm humidified oxygen (43–46°C) is an easy, safe, and highly effective method. Warmed intravenous saline infusions (43°C) should be used instead of lactated Ringer solution. Volume resuscitation is needed to prevent shock as vasodilation occurs during rewarming. Other rewarming methods are based on the availability of equipment and skilled personnel (ie, warm solution lavage, esophageal rewarming tubes, endovascular warming devices, and hemodialysis).

When CBT is < 30°C, initial treatment includes active rewarming, cardiopulmonary resuscitation (CPR), one shock attempt for dysrhythmia, and withholding of intravenous medications. Once the CBT reaches 30°C, cardiac medications can be given but at intervals longer than standard intervals because metabolism is slowed and there is a risk of toxic accumulation as circulation is restored. Defibrillation may be performed as needed. Resuscitative efforts should be continued until the CBT increases to at least 32°C.

Prognosis

Prognosis is directly related to the patient's underlying health and comorbidities, circumstances surrounding the hypothermia, and degree of metabolic acidosis. Prognosis is poor with low pH (≤ 6.6), elevated potassium (≥ 4.0 mEq/L or ≥ 4.0 mmol/L), serious underlying condition, or treatment delay. If treated early, most otherwise healthy patients may survive moderate or severe hypothermia.

When to Admit

Hypothermia patients must undergo close monitoring for potential complications. This is typically done during an inpatient admission or prolonged emergency department observation depending on the comorbidities and home care situation.

HYPOTHERMIA OF THE EXTREMITIES

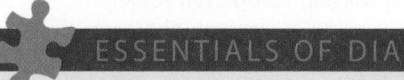

ESSENTIALS OF DIAGNOSIS

► Extremities suffering cold-induced injuries should not be exercised, rubbed, or massaged during rewarming.

► Rewarming of extremities affected by cold-induced injuries must be performed as soon as possible after there is no risk of refreezing.

Clinical Findings

Cold-induced injuries to the extremities range from mild to severe. Cold exposure of the extremities produces immediate localized vasoconstriction followed by generalized vasoconstriction. When the skin temperature falls to 25°C, tissue demand for oxygen is greater than what is supplied by the slowed circulation: the area becomes cyanotic. At 15°C, tissue damage occurs due to marked reduction in tissue metabolism and oxyhemoglobin dissociation. This results in a deceptive pink, well-oxygenated appearance to the skin. Freezing (frostbite) may occur when the skin temperature drops below –4°C to –10°C or at higher temperatures in the presence of wind, water, immobility, malnutrition, or vascular disease.

▶ Prevention

"Keep warm, keep dry, and keep moving." Individuals should wear warm, dry clothing, preferably several layers, with a windproof outer garment. Arms, legs, fingers, and toes should be exercised to maintain circulation. Wet clothing, socks, and shoes should be replaced with dry ones. Extra socks, mittens, and insoles should always be carried in a pack during travel in cold or icy areas. Caution must be taken to avoid cramped positions; constrictive clothing; prolonged dependency of the feet; use of tobacco, alcohol, and sedative medications; and exposure to wet muddy ground and windy conditions.

FROSTNIP & CHILBLAIN (Erythema Pernio)

Frostnip is a mild temporary form of cold-induced injury. The involved area has local paresthesias that completely resolve with passive external rewarming. Rewarming can be done by placing cold fingers in the armpits and, in the case of the toes or heels, by removing footwear, drying feet, rewarming, and covering with adequate dry socks or other protective footwear.

Chilblains or **erythema pernio** are inflammatory skin changes caused by exposure to cold without actual freezing of the tissues. These skin lesions may be red or purple papular lesions, which are painful or pruritic, with burning or paresthesias. They may be associated with edema or blistering and aggravated by warmth. With continued exposure, ulcerative or hemorrhagic lesions may appear and progress to scarring, fibrosis, and atrophy.

Treatment consists of elevating and passively externally rewarming the affected part. Caution must be taken to avoid rubbing or massaging injured tissues and to avoid applying ice or heat. The area must be protected from trauma, secondary infection, and further cold exposure.

IMMERSION FOOT OR TRENCH FOOT

Immersion foot (or hand) is caused by prolonged immersion in or cold water or mud, usually < 10°C. **Prehyperemic stage** is marked by early symptoms of cold and anesthesia of the affected area. **Hyperemic stage** follows with hot sensation, intense burning, and shooting pains. **Posthyperemic stage** occurs with ongoing cold exposure; the affected part becomes pale or cyanotic with diminished pulsations due to vasospasm. This may result in blistering, swelling, redness, ecchymoses, hemorrhage, necrosis,

peripheral nerve injury, or gangrene and secondary complications such as lymphangitis, cellulitis, and thrombophlebitis.

Treatment is best instituted before or during the hyperemic stage. Treatment consists of air drying, protecting the extremities from trauma and secondary infection, and gradual rewarming by exposure to air at room temperature (not ice or heat). Caution must be taken to avoid massaging or moistening the skin and to avoid further cold injury and water immersion. Affected parts are elevated to aid in removal of edema fluid. Pressure sites (ie, heels) are protected with cushions. Bed rest is required until all ulcers have healed. Prevention involves properly fitting footwear, improved foot hygiene, and sock changes to keep feet clean and dry.

FROSTBITE

Frostbite is injury from tissue freezing and formation of ice crystals in the tissue. Most tissue destruction follows the reperfusion of the frozen tissues, with damaged endothelial cells and progressive microvascular thrombosis resulting in further tissue damage. In mild cases, only the skin and subcutaneous tissues are involved; the symptoms are numbness, prickling, itching, and pallor. With increasing severity, deep frostbite involves deeper structures. The skin appears white or yellow, loses its elasticity, and becomes immobile. Edema, hemorrhagic blisters, necrosis, and gangrene may appear. This may cause paresthesias and stiffness.

▶ Treatment

A. Immediate Treatment

Evaluate and treat the patient for associated systemic hypothermia, concurrent conditions, and injury. Avoid secondary exposure to cold. Early use of systemic analgesics is recommended for nonfrozen injuries. Fluids and electrolytes should be monitored.

1. Rewarming—Rapid rewarming at temperatures slightly above body heat may significantly decrease tissue necrosis and reverse the tissue crystallization. If there is any possibility of refreezing, the frostbitten part should not be thawed. Refreezing results in increased tissue necrosis. Rewarming is best accomplished by warm bath immersion. The frozen extremity is immersed for several minutes in a moving water bath heated to 40–42°C until the distal tip of the part being thawed flushes. Dry heat (ie, stove or open fire) is not recommended because it is more difficult to regulate, and increases likelihood of accidental burns. Thawing may cause tenderness and burning pain. Once the frozen part has thawed and returned to normal temperature (usually in about 30 minutes), discontinue external heat. *In the early stage, rewarming by exercise, rubbing, or friction is contraindicated.* The patient must be kept at bed rest with the affected parts elevated and uncovered at room temperature. Casts, occlusive dressings, or bandages are not applied. Blisters should be left intact unless signs of infection supervene.

2. Anti-infective measures and wound care—Frostbite increases susceptibility to tetanus and infection. Tetanus prophylaxis must be considered. Infection risk may be reduced by aseptic wound care and protection of skin blebs from physical contact. Wounds should be kept open and allowed to dry before applying dressings. Nonadherent sterile gauze and fluffy dressing should be loosely applied to wounds and cushions used for all areas of pressure. Antibiotics should not be administered empirically. Systemic antibiotics are reserved for deep infections not responding to local wound care.

B. Medical and Surgical Treatment Options

With the availability of telemedicine, specialists are able to provide advice on early field treatment of cold-injured patients in remote areas, thereby improving outcome. Eschar formation without evidence of infection may be conservatively treated. The underlying skin may heal spontaneously with the eschar acting as a biologic dressing. Intra-arterial thrombolytic administration within 24 hours of exposure has resulted in improved tissue perfusion and has reduced amputation.

C. Follow-Up Care

Patient education must include ongoing care of the cold injury and prevention of future hypothermia and cold injury. Gentle, progressive physical therapy to promote circulation should be instituted as tolerated.

▶ Prognosis

Recovery from frostbite depends on the underlying comorbidities, the extent of initial tissue damage, the rewarming reperfusion injury, and the late sequelae. The involved extremity may be at increased susceptibility for discomfort and injury upon reexposure to cold. Neuropathic sequelae such as pain, numbness, tingling, hyperhidrosis, and cold sensitivity of the extremities, and nerve conduction abnormalities may persist for many years after the cold injury.

▶ When to Admit

- Management of tissue damage, comorbidities, associated injuries.
- Psychosocial factors (cognitive impairment, inadequate living situation) that could compromise patient safety or recovery.

Grieve AW et al. A clinical review of the management of frostbite. J R Army Med Corps. 2011 Mar;157(1):73–8. [PMID: 21465915]

Lantry J et al. Pathophysiology, management and complications of hypothermia. Br J Hosp Med (Lond). 2012 Jan;73(1):31–7. [PMID: 22241407]

McIntosh SE et al. Wilderness Medical Society practice guidelines for the prevention and treatment of frostbite. Wilderness Environ Med. 2011 Jun;22(2):156–66. [PMID: 21664561]

McMahon JA et al. Cold weather issues in sideline and event management. Curr Sports Med Rep. 2012 May;11(3):135–41. [PMID: 22580491]

DISORDERS DUE TO HEAT

ESSENTIALS OF DIAGNOSIS

▶ Spectrum of preventable heat-related illnesses: heat cramps, heat exhaustion, heat syncope, and heat stroke.

▶ **Heat stroke:** hyperthermia with cerebral dysfunction in a patient with heat exposure.

▶ **Best outcome:** early recognition, initiation of rapid cooling, and avoidance of shivering during cooling.

▶ **Best choice of cooling method:** whichever can be instituted the fastest with the least compromise the patient. Delays in cooling result in higher morbidity and mortality in heat stroke victims.

▶ General Considerations

Hyperthermia results from the body's inability to maintain normal internal temperature through heat loss. The body's heat source is a result of internal metabolic function and environmental conditions (temperature, humidity). Heat loss occurs through sweating and peripheral vasodilation.

There is a spectrum of preventable heat-related illnesses related to environmental exposure, ranging from mild forms, such as heat cramps and heat exhaustion, to severe forms, such as heat syncope and heat stroke. Risk factors include duration of exertion, hot environment, physical inactivity, and insufficient acclimatization, skin disorders or other medical conditions that inhibit sweat production or evaporation, obesity, dehydration, prolonged seizures, hypotension, reduced cutaneous blood flow, reduced cardiac output, the use of drugs that increase metabolism or muscle activity or impair sweating, and withdrawal syndromes. Nonexertional heat-related illness can also occur in a hot relaxing environment (ie, hot bath, steam room, sunbathing or sauna).

Heat cramping results from dilutional hyponatremia as sweat losses are replaced with water alone. **Heat exhaustion** results from prolonged strenuous activity with inadequate water or salt intake in a hot environment. It is characterized by dehydration, sodium depletion, or isotonic fluid loss with accompanying cardiovascular changes.

Heat syncope or sudden collapse may result in unconsciousness from volume depletion and cutaneous vasodilation with consequent systemic and cerebral hypotension. Exercise-associated postural hypotension is usually the cause of this: it may occur during or immediately following exercise. **Heat stroke,** the hallmark of which is cerebral dysfunction with CBT over 40°C, presents in one of two forms: classic and exertional. Classic heat stroke occurs in patients with impaired thermoregulatory mechanisms; exertional heat stroke occurs in healthy persons undergoing strenuous exertion in a hot or humid environment. Persons at greatest risk are those who are at the extremes of age, chronically debilitated, and taking medications that interfere with heat-dissipating mechanisms (ie, anticholinergics, antihistamines, phenothiazines).

▶ Clinical Findings

Heat cramps are slow, painful skeletal muscle contractions ("cramps") and severe muscle spasms lasting 1–3 minutes, usually of the muscles most heavily used. The examination findings typically include stable vital signs; normal or slightly increased CBT; moist and cool skin; and tender, hard, lumpy muscles that may be twitching. The patient is alert, with stable vital signs, and may be agitated and complaining of focal pain. There is almost always a history of vigorous activity just preceding the onset of symptoms. Laboratory evaluation may reveal no abnormalities or show low serum sodium, hemoconcentration, and elevated urea and creatinine.

The diagnosis of **heat exhaustion** is based on symptoms and clinical findings of a CBT over 37.8°C, increased pulse, and moist skin. Symptoms are similar to those associated with heat syncope and heat cramps. Additional symptoms include nausea, vomiting, malaise, myalgias, hyperventilation, thirst, and weakness. Central nervous system symptoms include headache, dizziness, fatigue, anxiety, paresthesias, hysteria, impaired judgment, and occasionally psychosis. Hyperventilation secondary to heat exhaustion can cause respiratory alkalosis; lactic acidosis may also occur due to poor tissue perfusion. Heat exhaustion may progress to heat stroke if sweating ceases and mental status declines.

With **heat syncope**, there is usually a history of prolonged vigorous physical activity or prolonged standing in a hot humid environment. The skin is cool and moist, the pulse is weak, and the systolic blood pressure is low.

Heat stroke is a life-threatening emergency, *the hallmarks of which are cerebral dysfunction with CBT over 40°C.* Presenting symptoms include all findings seen in heat exhaustion with additional symptoms of dizziness, weakness, emotional lability, confusion, delirium, blurred vision, convulsions, collapse, and unconsciousness. Physical examination findings include hot skin, initially covered with perspiration, then later it dries; strong pulse initially; widened pulse pressure; blood pressure is slightly elevated at first, but hypotension develops later; tachycardia; and hyperventilation (with subsequent respiratory alkalosis). Exertional heat stroke may present with sudden collapse and loss of consciousness followed by irrational behavior. Sweating may not be present. Increased mortality rates are associated with a high Simplified Acute Physiology Score II (http://clincalc.com/IcuMortality/SAPSII.aspx), high body temperature, prolonged prothrombin time, use of vasoactive drugs within the first day in the intensive care unit (ICU), and an ICU without air conditioning. Laboratory evaluation may reveal dehydration; leukocytosis; elevated blood urea nitrogen (BUN); hyperuricemia; hemoconcentration; acid-base abnormalities (lactic acidosis, respiratory alkalosis); decreased serum glucose, sodium, calcium, and phosphorus; thrombocytopenia, fibrinolysis, and coagulopathy; elevated creatine kinase; elevated aminotransferase levels and liver dysfunction; and elevated cardiac markers. Urine is concentrated, with proteinuria, hematuria, tubular casts, and myoglobinuria. Potassium may be high or low. ECG findings may include ST–T changes consistent with myocardial ischemia. Pco_2 may be < 20 mm Hg.

▶ Treatment

A. Heat Cramps

The patient should be moved to a cool environment and given oral saline solution (4 tsp of salt per gallon of water) to replace both salt and water. *Oral salt tablets are not recommended.* The patient may have to rest for 1–3 days with continued dietary supplementation before returning to work or resuming strenuous activity in the heat.

B. Heat Exhaustion

Treatment consists of moving patient to a shaded, cool environment, providing adequate fluid and electrolyte replacement, and active cooling (ie, fans, cool packs) if necessary. Physiologic saline or isotonic glucose solution should be administered intravenously when oral administration is not appropriate. At least 24 hours of rest and rehydration are recommended.

C. Heat Syncope

Treatment consists of rest and recumbency in a cool place, and fluid and electrolyte replacement by mouth (or intravenously if necessary).

D. Heat Stroke

Treatment is aimed at rapidly reducing the CBT (within 1 hour) while supporting circulatory and organ system function to prevent irreversible tissue damage and death. Clinicians must assess for possibility of concurrent conditions (infection; trauma; and drug effects, including adverse side effects, withdrawal, or overdose). Monitoring includes vital signs, temperature, and cardiac rhythm. The patient should also be observed for the following: potential complications of metabolic abnormalities, cardiac arrhythmias, coagulopathy, acute respiratory distress syndrome (ARDS), hypoglycemia, seizures, organ dysfunction, and infection. Circulatory failure in heat-related illness is mostly due to shock from relative or absolute hypovolemia. Intravascular volume status should be assessed and managed early to reduce the risk of hypovolemic shock. Hypovolemic and cardiogenic shock must be carefully distinguished and managed. Central venous monitoring is useful to guide volume status. Oral or intravenous fluid administration must be provided to ensure adequate urinary output. Fluid output should be monitored through the use of an indwelling urinary catheter. Hypokalemia frequently accompanies heat stroke but may not appear until rehydration. Maintenance of extracellular hydration and electrolyte balance should reduce the risk of acute kidney injury due to rhabdomyolysis.

Cooling methods are evaporative and conductive-based. Systemic review of the research found that there are comparable effects of these cooling methods whether used singly or in combination. No single cooling method is found to be superior. Choice of cooling method depends on which can be instituted the fastest with the least compromise to the overall care of the patient.

Evaporative cooling is a noninvasive, effective, quick and easy way to reduce temperature. Large fans circulate the room air while the entire undressed body is sprayed with lukewarm water (20°C). Inhalation of cool air or oxygen is also effective.

Conductive-based cooling involves cool fluid infusion, lavage, ice packs, and immersion into ice water or cool water. Cold water immersion includes cool baths, localized ice or ice slush application (groin, axillas, neck), and cool gastric and bladder lavage, and infusion of cool intravenous fluids. Intravascular heat exchange catheter systems as well as hemodialysis using cold dialysate (30–35°C) have been successful in reducing CBT. Research suggests that brain cooling may lessen cerebrovascular injury from heat stroke.

Shivering must be avoided because it inhibits the effectiveness of cooling by increasing internal heat production. Medications that can be used to suppress shivering include magnesium, quick-acting opioid analgesics, benzodiazepines, and quick-acting anesthetic agents. Skin massage is recommended to prevent cutaneous vasoconstriction. *Antipyretics (aspirin, acetaminophen) have no effect on environmentally induced hyperthermia and are contraindicated.* Treatment should be continued until the CBT drops to 39°C.

Prognosis

Multiorgan dysfunction is the usual cause of heat stroke–related death, and it can be predicted by elevated creatine kinase, metabolic acidosis, coagulopathy and elevated liver enzymes. Multiorgan dysfunction, rhabdomyolysis, ARDS, and inflammation may continue after temperature is normalized. Following heat stroke, immediate reexposure should be avoided.

Prevention

Public education is necessary to improve prevention and early recognition of heat-related disorders. Individuals should take steps to reduce personal risk factors and to acclimatize to the hot environment. Acclimatization is achieved by scheduled regulated exposure to hot environments and by gradually increasing the duration of exposure and the workload until the body adjusts. Proper acclimatization must be achieved before heavy physical exertion is performed in hot environments. All children's athletic programs must set heat-acclimatization guidelines. Parents, coaches, athletic trainers, and athletes must be educated about heat-related illness, specifically about prevention, risks, signs and symptoms, and treatment.

Medical evaluation and monitoring should be used to identify the individuals and the weather conditions that increase risk of heat-related disorders. Athletic events should be organized with attention to thermoregulation: the wet bulb globe temperature (WBGT) index should be monitored. Competition is not recommended when the WBGT exceeds 26–28 °C. Guidance regarding heat hazard is found in the National Weather Service's Heat Index, which rates weather conditions based on humidity and temperature measurements (http://www.nws.noaa.gov/os/heat/index.shtml).

Those who are physically active in a hot environment should increase fluid consumption before, during, and after physical activities. Fluid consumption should include balanced electrolyte fluids and water. Water consumption alone may lead to electrolyte imbalance, particularly hyponatremia. *It is not recommended to have salt tablets available for use without medical supervision because of the risk of hypertonic hypernatremia.* Close monitoring of fluid and electrolyte intake and early intervention are recommended in situations necessitating exertion or activity in hot environments. Exertional heat-related disorders are common in unconditioned participants in strenuous activities in hot humid conditions. Classic (nonexertional) heat-related disorders occur when extreme environmental conditions (heat, humidity) affect patients who are not physically active, in the extremes of ages, or with chronic medical or psychiatric illnesses.

When to Admit

All patients with suspected heat stroke must be admitted to the hospital for close monitoring.

Becker JA et al. Heat-related illness. Am Fam Physician. 2011 Jun 1;83(11):1325–30. [PMID: 21661715]

Calvello EJ et al. Management of the hyperthermic patient. Br J Hosp Med (Lond). 2011 Oct;72(10):571–5. [PMID: 22041727]

Casa DJ et al. Exertional heat stroke: new concepts regarding cause and care. Curr Sports Med Rep. 2012 May;11(3): 115–23. [PMID: 22580488]

Marom T et al. Acute care for exercise-induced hyperthermia to avoid adverse outcome from exertional heat stroke. J Sport Rehab. 2011 May;20(2):219–27. [PMID: 21576713]

THERMAL BURNS

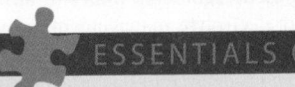
ESSENTIALS OF DIAGNOSIS

► Estimates of the burn location, size and depth greatly determine treatment plan.

► The first 48 hours of burn care offers the greatest impact on morbidity and mortality of a burn victim.

The first 48 hours after the burn injury offer the greatest opportunity to impact the survival of the patient. Early surgical intervention, wound care, enteral feeding, glucose control and metabolic management, infection control, and prevention of hypothermia and compartment syndrome have contributed to significantly lower mortality rates and shorter hospitalizations.

General Considerations

A. Classification

Burns are classified by extent, depth, patient age, and associated illness or injury. Accurate estimation of burn size and depth is important since this figure will quantify the parameters of resuscitation.

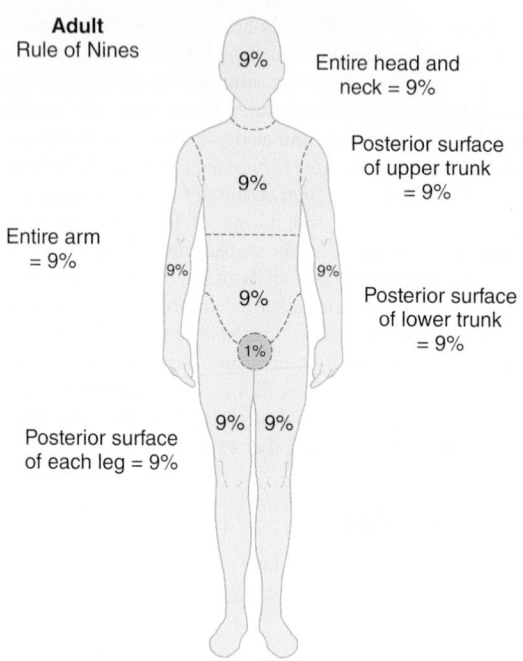

Adult
Rule of Nines

Entire head and neck = 9%

9%

Posterior surface of upper trunk = 9%

9%

Entire arm = 9%

9%

9%

9%

Posterior surface of lower trunk = 9%

1%

9% 9%

Posterior surface of each leg = 9%

▲ **Figure 37–2.** Estimation of body surface area in burns.

1. Extent—In adults, the "rule of nines" (Figure 37–2) is useful for rapidly assessing the extent of a burn. It is important to view the entire patient to make an accurate assessment of skin findings on initially and on subsequent examinations. One rule of thumb is that the palm of an open hand constitutes 1% total body surface area in adults. Only second- and third-degree burns are included in calculating the total burn surface area, since first-degree burns usually do not represent significant injury in terms of prognosis or fluid and electrolyte management. However, first- or second-degree burns may convert to deeper burns, especially if treatment is delayed or bacterial colonization or superinfection occurs.

2. Depth—Judgment of depth of injury is difficult. The **first-degree burn** may be red or gray but will demonstrate excellent capillary refill. First-degree burns are not blistered initially. If the wound is blistered, this represents a partial-thickness injury to the dermis, which is referred to as a **second-degree burn**. As the degree of burn is progressively deeper, there is a progressive loss of adnexal structures, referred to as a **third-degree burn**. Hairs can be easily extracted or are absent, sweat glands become less visible, and the skin appears smoother.

Deep second- and third-degree burns are treated in a similar fashion. Neither will heal appropriately without early debridement and grafting; the resultant skin is thin and scarred.

B. Survival after Burn Injury

The **Prognostic Burn Index** is the sum of the patient's age and percentage of full thickness or deep partial thickness burn. An additional 20% mortality is added if inhalation injury is present. The Prognostic Burn Index is most useful

at the extremes of age. Transfer to a burn unit is indicated for large burn size, circumferential burn, or burn involving a joint or high-risk body part, and patients with comorbidities. Mortality rates have been significantly reduced due to treatment advances including improvements in wound care, treatment of infection, early burn excision, skin substitute usage, and early nutritional support through parenteral or enteral feeding. Telemedicine consultation with a burn center is an alternative, cost-effective way to access burn specialists when there are barriers that prevent transfer (distance, bed unavailability, travel risks, etc).

C. Associated Injuries or Illnesses

Smoke inhalation, associated trauma, and electrical injuries are commonly associated with burns. Smoke inhalation (see Chapter 9) must be suspected when a burn victim is found in an enclosed space, or in close proximity to the fire. Electrical injury (see following section of this chapter) may cause deep tissue burns without significant superficial skin findings. Severe burns from any source may cause gastrointestinal complications including pancreatitis and stress ulcers.

D. Systemic Reactions to Burn Injury

The actual burn injury is only the incipient event leading to cascade of deleterious local tissue and systemic inflammatory reactions causing multisystem organ failure in the severely burned patient. When burns greater than approximately 20% of total body surface area are present, systemic metabolic alterations occur and require intensive support. The inflammatory cascade can result in shock.

► Treatment

Telemedicine evaluation of acute burns offers accurate, cost-effective access to a burn specialist during the crucial 48 hours after the burn injury.

A. Initial Resuscitation

1. Primary survey—The clinician must proceed with a full trauma assessment, starting with "ABCDE" (airway, breathing, circulation, disability, exposure). **Airway** assessment and management is the first priority. A patient with an inhalation injury needs to be intubated early to maintain airway patency even though he or she may appear to be breathing normally. To assess and support **breathing** and **circulation**, the clinician should administer supplemental oxygen and obtain vascular access for fluid resuscitation simultaneously with initial resuscitation. **Disability** assessment is next followed by complete patient **exposure** and thorough examination to assess the extent of burn and associated injuries. Serial assessments of airway and breathing are necessary since endotracheal intubation or tracheotomy may be needed for major burn victims, particularly those with possible inhalation injury. Generalized edema develops during fluid resuscitation, including edema of the soft tissues of the upper airway and perhaps the lungs as well. Chest radiographs are typically normal initially but may develop an ARDS picture in 24–48 hours with severe inhalation injury. The use of corticosteroids or routine use of antibiotic therapy is not indicated.

A. Airway control—Early intubation is recommended before airway edema occurs in cases of smoke inhalation or direct thermal injury to the upper airway (look for singed eyebrows or facial hair, carbonaceous sputum).

B. Vascular access—Large bore peripheral venous catheter access should be established. Intraosseous access can be obtained if venous access is unsuccessful or contraindicated. *Venous access catheters placed in the emergency department should be changed within 24 hours because of the high risk of nonsterile placement.* An arterial line is useful for monitoring mean arterial pressure and for drawing serial blood gases and other laboratory tests in critically ill patients.

C. Fluid resuscitation—Generalized capillary leak results from burn injury over more than 20% of total body surface area. This often necessitates replacement with large volumes of crystalloid. There are many guidelines for fluid resuscitation. These guidelines may be inadequate, since crystalloid solutions alone may be insufficient to restore cardiac preload during the period of burn shock. Deep electrical burns and inhalation injury increase the fluid requirement.

Adequacy of resuscitation is determined by clinical parameters, including urinary output and specific gravity, blood pressure, pulse, temperature, and central venous pressure. Overly aggressive crystalloid administration must be avoided in patients with pulmonary injury or cardiac dysfunction, since significant pulmonary edema can develop in patients with normal pulmonary capillary wedge and central venous pressures. A Foley catheter is essential for monitoring urinary output. Diuretics have no role in this phase of patient management unless fluid overload has occurred.

The need for fluid replacement of more than 150% of calculated values indicates possible unrecognized injury, possible comorbidities, and a worse prognosis.

B. Management

1. Chemoprophylaxis—

A. Tetanus immunization—For all burns deeper than superficial thickness, tetanus immunization must be updated. Tetanus toxoid-containing vaccine should be given intramuscularly to all patients with wounds regardless of how recently the patient received tetanus immunization. In addition, if a patient has not completed the recommended three doses of primary immunization or this is unknown, then tetanus immunoglobulin should also be administered intramuscularly in a different site than the tetanus toxoid. (See Chapter 33.)

B. Antibiotics—All nonsuperficial depth wounds should be covered with topical antibiotics. Prophylaxis with systemic antibiotics is not indicated.

2. Surgical management—

A. Abdominal compartment syndrome—Abdominal compartment syndrome is emerging as a potentially lethal condition in severely burned patients, even if abdominal

decompression is performed. Markedly increased intra-abdominal pressures can cause pulmonary damage and multisystem organ failure. Only 40% of patients with this complication survive. Bladder pressures over 30 mm Hg establish the diagnosis in at-risk patients. Surgical abdominal decompression may be indicated to improve ventilation and oxygen delivery, but even after this surgery, survival remains low.

B. Escharotomy—As edema fluid accumulates, ischemia may develop under any constricting eschar of an extremity, neck, chest, or trunk if the full-thickness burn is circumferential. Escharotomy incisions through the anesthetic eschar can save life and limb and can be performed in the emergency department or operating room.

C. Fasciotomy—Similar to escharotomy, fasciotomy is indicated to prevent further soft tissue, vascular, and nerve damage when soft tissue edema produces high pressures in the deep tissue compartments in the arms and legs since these compartments are divided by unyielding fascia.

D. Debridement, dressings, and topical and systemic antibiotic therapy—Minor burn wounds should be debrided at the bedside to determine the depth of the burn and then thoroughly cleansed. Thereafter, the wound should be debrided daily and dressed with a topical antibiotic and a wound dressing. Patient compliance and adequate pain treatment is essential for successful outpatient treatment. The wound should be reevaluated by the treating clinician within 24–72 hours to evaluate for signs of infection.

The goal of burn wound management is to protect the wound from desiccation and avoid further injury or infection. Regular and thorough cleansing of burned areas is a critically important intervention in burn units. Minor burn wounds (first- and superficial second-degree types, partial thickness) will spontaneously reepithelialize in 7–10 days. Topical wound agents should be applied. Topical antibiotic wound agents are painless, easy to apply, and effective against most skin pathogens.

For severely burned patients, early excision and grafting of burned areas may be performed as soon as 24 hours after burn injury or when the patient can hemodynamically tolerate the excision and grafting procedure. Meticulous prevention of infections, seromas, hypergranulation tissue formation, and malnutrition all decrease the time to complete wound healing in skin-grafted patients. Skin autograft is the most definitive treatment. Prevention of autograft infection is paramount since autograft loss is most commonly due to autograft infection.

Systemic infection remains a leading cause of morbidity among patients with major burn injuries, with nearly all severely burned patients having one or more septicemic episodes during the hospital course. Healthcare-associated infections are increasingly common. Routine use of blood culture in the severely burned population is indicated to elucidate systemic blood infections that do not manifest these clinical predictors of sepsis.

E. Wound management—The goal of therapy after fluid resuscitation is rapid and stable closure of the wound.

Wounds that do not heal spontaneously in 7–10 days (ie, deep second-degree or third-degree burns) are best treated by a specialist.

Wound infection is the top cause of skin graft rejection and failure.

C. Patient Support

Burn patients require extensive supportive care, both physiologically and psychologically. It is important to maintain normal CBT and avoid hypothermia (by maintaining environmental temperature at or above 30°C) in patients with burns over more than 20% of total body surface area. Respiratory injury, sepsis, multiorgan failure, and venous thromboembolism are common. Burn patients are at risk for developing ARDS or respiratory failure unresponsive to maximal ventilatory support.

Burn patients require careful assessment and provision of optimal nutritional needs since their metabolism is higher and they require more energy, nutrients, and antioxidants for wound healing. Enteral feedings may be started once the ileus of the resuscitation period has resolved, usually the day after the injury. There is often a markedly increased metabolic rate after burn injury, due in large part to whole body synthesis and increased fatty acid substrate cycles. If the patient does not tolerate low-residue tube feedings, total parenteral nutrition should be started without delay through a central venous catheter. Contrary to conventional teachings, data indicate that most patients can be fed adequately with energy equal to 100% to 120% of estimated basal energy expenditure (BEE). A useful guide is to provide 25 kcal/kg body weight plus 40 kcal per percent of burn surface area. Early aggressive nutrition (by parenteral or enteral routes) reduces infections, recovery time, noninfectious complications, length of hospital stay, long-term sequelae, and mortality. Occasionally, ARDS or respiratory failure unresponsive to maximal ventilatory support may develop in burn patients. Anticatabolic treatments such as beta-blockade, growth hormone, insulin, oxandrolone, and synthetic testosterone have been advocated. Melatonin, which appears to possess multifaceted antioxidant properties, may reduce proinflammatory cytokines and have beneficial chronobiotic effects in severely burned patients.

Prevention of long-term scars remains a formidable problem in seriously burned patients. The usual regimen consists of corticosteroid injections, silicone gel or patches, compression, and scar revision. Long-term sequelae can be reduced by the following strategies: (1) burn specialist consultation either directly or via telemedicine, (2) prevention of infection, (3) early nutrition, (4) early aggressive rehabilitation, (5) compressive garments, and (6) early and continual psychological support.

▶ Prognosis

Prognosis depends on the extent and location of the burn tissue damage, associated injuries, comorbidities, and complications. Hyperglycemia from poor glucose control is a predictor of worse outcomes. Psychiatric support may be necessary following burn injury.

▶ When to Admit

- Significant burns (based on location and extent).
- Patients with significant comorbidities and suboptimal home situations.

Cancio LC et al. Evolving changes in the management of burns and environmental injuries. Surg Clin North Am. 2012 Aug;92(4):959–86. [PMID: 22850157]

Wasiak J et al. Dressings for superficial and partial thickness burns. Cochrane Database Syst Rev. 2013 Mar 28;3:CD002106. [PMID: 23543513]

Zanni GR. Thermal burns and scalds: clinical complications in the elderly. Consult Pharm. 2012 Jan;27(1):16–22. [PMID: 22231994]

ELECTRICAL INJURY

ESSENTIALS OF DIAGNOSIS

▶ Extent of injury is determined by the type, amount, duration, and pathway of electrical current.

▶ Resuscitation must be attempted before assuming the electrical injury victim is dead; clinical findings are unreliable.

▶ Skin findings may be misleading and are not indicative of the degree of deeper tissue injury.

▶ General Considerations

Electricity-induced injuries are common and most are preventable. These inquiries occur by exposure to electrical current of low voltage, high voltage, or lightning. Electrical current type is either alternating current (AC) or direct current (DC). Electricity causes acute damage by direct tissue damage, muscle tetany, direct thermal injury and coagulation necrosis, and associated trauma.

Alternating current (AC) is bidirectional electrical flow that reverses direction in a sine wave pattern. This may cause muscle tetany, which prolongs the duration and amount of current exposure. AC current can be low voltage or high voltage. **Low voltage** (< 1000 V) is typically household AC current that ranges in severity from minor injury to significant damage and death. **High voltage** (> 1000 V) is most often related to occupational exposure and is associated with deep tissue damage and higher morbidity and mortality. **Direct current (DC)** is unidirectional electrical flow (eg, that associated with lightning, batteries, and automotive electrical systems). It is more likely to cause a single intense muscle contraction and asystole. **Lightning** differs from other high-voltage electrical shock in that lightning is massive DC current of millions of volts lasting a very brief duration (a small fraction of a second).

The extent of damage depends on the following factors: voltage (high or low, whether greater or lesser than 1000 volts), current type, tissue resistance, moisture, pathway; duration of exposure; associated trauma and comorbidities.

Current is the most important determinant of tissue damage. Current passes through the tissues of least resistance, and this energy produces heat causing direct thermal injury. Tissue resistance varies throughout the body. Nerve cells are the most vulnerable, and bone is the most resistant to electrical current. Skin resistance depends on thickness and condition of the skin. The entrance and exit points are the most damaged. Current passing through skeletal muscle can cause muscle necrosis and contractions severe enough to result in bone fracture.

▶ Clinical Findings

Electrical burns are of three distinct types: flash (arcing) burns, flame (clothing) burns, and the direct heating effect of tissues by the electrical current. The latter lesions are usually sharply demarcated, round or oval, painless yellow-brown areas (Joule burn) with inflammatory reaction.

Skin damage does not correlate with the degree of injury. Significant subcutaneous damage can be accompanied by little skin injury, particularly with larger skin surface area electrical contact. Symptoms and signs may range from tingling, superficial skin burns, and myalgias to coma, paralysis, massive tissue damage, or death. Not all electrical injuries cause skin damage; only very minor skin damage may be present with massive internal injuries. The presence of entrance and exit burns signifies an increased risk of deep tissue damage.

Resuscitation must be initiated on all victims of electrical injury since clinical findings are deceptive and unreliable. A victim of electrical current injury may appear dead due to dysrhythmia, respiratory arrest, or autonomic dysfunction resulting in pupils that are fixed, dilated, or asymmetric.

▶ Complications

Complications include dysrhythmias, altered mental status, seizures, paralysis, headache, pneumothorax, vascular injury, tissue edema and necrosis, compartment syndrome, associated traumatic injuries, rhabdomyolysis, acute kidney injury, hypovolemia from third spacing, infections, and acute or delayed cataract formation.

▶ Treatment

A. Emergency Measures

The patient must be assessed and treated as a trauma victim since associated traumatic injuries are common. The victim must be safely separated from the electrical current prior to initiation of CPR or other treatment. The rescuer must be protected. Separate the victim using nonconductive implements, such as dry clothing. Resuscitation must then be initiated since clinical findings of death are unreliable.

B. Hospital Measures

The initial assessment involves airway, breathing, and circulation followed by a full trauma protocol. Fluid resuscitation is important to maintain adequate urinary output (0.5 mL/kg/h if no myoglobinuria is present, 1.0 mL/kg/h if myoglobinuria is present). Initial evaluation includes cardiac monitoring and ECG, complete blood count, electrolytes, renal function tests, liver biochemical tests, urinalysis, urine myoglobin, serum creatine kinase, and cardiac enzymes. ECG does not show typical patterns of ischemia since the electrical damage is epicardial. Victims must be evaluated for hidden injury (eg, ophthalmic, otologic, muscular, compartment syndromes), organ injury (myocardium, liver, kidney, pancreas), blunt trauma, dehydration, skin burns, hypertension, posttraumatic stress, acid-base disturbances, and neurologic damage.

Electrical burn injury remains the most underrecognized and devastating burn injury, sometimes leading to amputations (often because of unrecognized compartment syndromes) and acute kidney injury, resulting in part from rhabdomyolysis (see Chapter 22).

Superficial skin may appear deceivingly benign, leading to a delayed or completely overlooked diagnosis of deep tissue injury. When electrical injury occurs, extensive deep tissue necrosis should be suspected. Deep tissue necrosis leads to profound tissue swelling and this in turn results in the high risk of a compartment syndrome. Early debridement of devitalized tissues and tetanus prophylaxis may reduce the risks of infection. In pregnant patients exposed to electrical injury, the fetus may sustain intrauterine growth retardation, fetal distress, and fetal demise. Fetal monitoring is recommended.

Pain management is important before, during, and after initial treatment and rehabilitation. Multimodal approach to pain is the most effective. Interventions include medications (opioids, acetaminophen, nonsteroidal anti-inflammatory drugs), heat therapy, massage, and cognitive-behavioral therapy.

▶ Prognosis

Prognosis depends on the degree and location of electrical injury, initial tissue damage, associated injuries, comorbidities, and complications. Complications may occur in almost any part of the body but most commonly include sepsis; gangrene requiring limb amputation; or neurologic, cardiac, cognitive, or psychiatric dysfunction. Psychiatric support may be necessary following electrical injury.

▶ When to Refer

Surgical specialists may be needed to perform fasciotomy for compartment syndrome or devitalized tissue debridement or microvascular reconstruction.

▶ When to Admit

Indications for hospitalization include high voltage exposure; dysrhythmia or ECG changes; large burn; neurologic, pulmonary, or cardiac symptoms; suspicion of significant deep tissue or organ damage; transthoracic current pathway; history of cardiac disease or other significant comorbidities or injuries; and need for surgery.

Schneider JC et al. Neurologic and musculoskeletal complications of burn injuries. Phys Med Rehabil Clin N Am. 2011 May;22(2):261–75. [PMID: 21624720]

RADIATION EXPOSURE

ESSENTIALS OF DIAGNOSIS

► Damage from radiation is determined by the source, type, quantity, duration, bodily location, and susceptibility and accumulation of exposures of the person.

► Radiation exposure from medical diagnostic imaging has dramatically risen over the past few decades.

► All patients should keep records of their medical imaging radiation exposures, and copies of the medical images and interpretations.

Exposure to radiation may occur from environmental, occupational, medical care, accidental, or intentional (ie, terrorism) exposure. With advancements in nuclear technology in the fields of medicine, energy, and industry, there is a growing risk of radiation exposure to patients, occupational workers, and the public. The extent of damage due to radiation exposure depends on the type, quantity, and duration of radiation exposure; the organs exposed; the degree of disruption to DNA; metabolic and cellular function; and the age, underlying condition, susceptibility, and accumulative exposures of the victim.

Professionals who work with radiation or its victims must have a basic understanding of radiation physics in order to identify risk, manage exposure, and minimize preventable spread of exposure. Radiation is energy waves or particles that travel through space. These energetic waves or particles radiate (move outward in all directions) from the source. Radiation occurs from both nonionizing and ionizing radiation sources. **Nonionizing radiation** is low energy, resulting in injuries related to local thermal damage (ie, microwave, ultraviolet, visible light and radiowave). **Ionizing radiation** is high energy, causing bodily damage in several ways (ie, cellular disruption, DNA damage, and mutations). Ionizing radiation is either electromagnetic (ie, x-rays and gamma rays) or particulate (ie, alpha or beta particles, neutrons, and protons). Exposure may be external, internal, or both.

► Clinical Findings

Radiation exposure results in acute and delayed effects. Acute effects involve damage of the rapidly dividing cells (ie, the mucosa, skin, and bone marrow). This may be manifested as mucositis, nausea, vomiting, gastrointestinal edema and ulcers, skin burns, and bone marrow suppression over hours to days after exposure. Delayed effects include malignancy, reproduction abnormalities, liver, kidney, and central nervous system and immune system dysfunction.

Clinicians must be educated to recognize and treat acute radiation sickness also referred to as **acute radiation syndrome.** Acute radiation syndrome is due to an exposure to high doses of ionizing radiation over a brief time course. The symptom onset is within hours to days depending on the dose. Symptoms include anorexia, nausea, vomiting, weakness, exhaustion, lassitude and, in some cases, prostration; these symptoms may occur singly or in combination. Dehydration, anemia, and infection may follow. The Centers for Disease Control and Prevention offers web-based information for clinicians regarding acute radiation syndrome (http://emergency.cdc.gov/radiation/ars-physicianfactsheet.asp).

In **acute radiation exposure**, medical care includes close monitoring of the gastrointestinal, cutaneous, hematologic, and cerebrovascular symptoms and signs from initial exposure and over time.

► Therapeutic Radiation Exposure

Radiation therapy has been a successful component to treating many malignancies. This growing population of cancer survivors treated with radiation therapy is an important resource to review and quantify associations between radiation therapy and risk of long-term adverse health and quality of life outcomes. These radiation-treated cancer survivors have a higher risk of development of a second malignancy; obesity; and pulmonary, cardiac and thyroid dysfunction as well as an increased overall risk for chronic health conditions and mortality. Ongoing study of childhood cancer survivors is needed to establish long-term risks and to evaluate the impact of newer techniques such as conformal radiation therapy or proton-beam therapy.

► Medical Imaging Radiation Exposure

Medical imaging with ionizing radiation exposure (eg, computed tomography [CT] and nuclear medicine studies) has dramatically increased over the past two decades. In addition, researchers have found that the radiation dose for the same study varies significantly among different machines and different clinicians, within and across institutions, with radiation doses varying by as much as a factor of 10. This finding highlights the urgent safety need for standardization and regulation of radiation dosing for medical diagnostics.

Clinicians and patients must be aware of the dangers of radiation when deciding on an imaging test. The risks and benefits must be carefully weighed. All patients should keep records of their cumulative medical imaging radiation exposures, as well as copies of the medical images and their interpretations. The American College of Radiology website offers additional safety information (http://www.radiologyinfo.org/en/safety/).

► Occupational & Environmental Radiation Exposure

Prevention of occupational radiation exposure involves adequate training of all persons handling radiation as well as creating safety policies and procedures. This will reduce occupational risk of radiation exposure and improve the emergency response to accidental exposure. Prehospital and hospital disaster plans are required for optimal management of radiation exposure. The Radiation Assistance Center (1-865-576-1005) provides 24-hour access to expert information. The Centers for Disease Control and Prevention "Radiation Emergency" website (http://emergency.cdc.gov/ radiation) is a useful resource for professionals.

Treatment

Treatment is focused on decontamination, symptomatic relief, supportive care, and psychosocial support. Specific treatments focus on the dose, route, and effects of exposure.

Prognosis

Prognosis is determined by the radiation dose, duration, and frequency as well as by the underlying condition of the victim. Death is usually due to hematopoietic failure, gastrointestinal mucosal damage, central nervous system damage, widespread vascular injury, or secondary infection.

Carcinogenesis is related to the total dose, duration, accumulation of exposure, and to the susceptibility of the victim. The younger the victim's age at the time of exposure, the greater the risk of acute and long-term damage from radiation. Radiation-related cancer risks persist throughout the exposed person's lifespan. X-rays are classified as carcinogens since exposure causes leukemia and cancers of the thyroid, breast, and lung.

With the increased use of ionizing radiation for medical diagnostics and treatments, there is a growing concern for the iatrogenic increase in radiation-induced cancer risks, especially in children. There are age-related sensitivities to radiation; prenatal and younger age victims are more susceptible to carcinogenesis.

When to Admit

Most patients with significant ionizing radiation exposure require admission for close monitoring and supportive treatment.

Christodouleas JP et al. Short-term and long-term health risks of nuclear-power-plant accidents. N Engl J Med. 2011 Jun 16; 364(24):2334–41. [PMID: 21506737]

Dainiak N et al. First global consensus for evidence-based management of the hematopoietic syndrome resulting from exposure to ionizing radiation. Disaster Med Public Health Prep. 2011 Oct;5(3):202–12. [PMID: 21987000]

Dainiak N et al. Literature review and global consensus on management of acute radiation syndrome affecting nonhematopoietic organ systems. Disaster Med Public Health Prep. 2011 Oct;5(3):183–201. [PMID: 21986999]

Pearce MS et al. Radiation exposure from CT scans in childhood and subsequent risk of leukaemia and brain tumours: a retrospective cohort study. Lancet. 2012 Aug 4;380(9840):499–505. [PMID: 22681860]

NEAR DROWNING

ESSENTIALS OF DIAGNOSIS

▶ The first requirement of rescue is immediate basic life support *and* CPR.

▶ Patient must also be assessed for hypothermia, hypoglycemia, concurrent injuries, and medical conditions.

▶ Clinical manifestations are hypoxemia, pulmonary edema, and hypoventilation.

General Considerations

Near drowning describes a submersion event leading to injury. Submersion injury may result in aspiration, laryngospasm, hypoxemia, and acidemia. **Drowning** describes submersion resulting in death. "Wet" drowning is due to aspiration of fluid or foreign material. "Dry" drowning is due to laryngospasm or airway obstruction. The primary effect is hypoxemia due to perfusion of poorly ventilated alveoli, intrapulmonary shunting, and decreased compliance. A patient may be deceptively asymptomatic during the initial recovery period only to deteriorate or die as a result of acute respiratory failure within the following 12–24 hours.

Clinical Findings

A. Symptoms and Signs

The patient's appearance may vary from asymptomatic, to abnormal vital signs, anxiety, dyspnea, cough, wheezing, trismus, cyanosis, chest pain, dysrhythmia, hypotension, vomiting, diarrhea, headache, altered level of consciousness, neurologic deficit, and apnea. Hypothermia is highly likely with cold water or prolonged submersion.

B. Laboratory Findings

Arterial blood gas results are helpful in determining the degree of injury since initial clinical findings may appear benign. Pao_2 is usually decreased; $Paco_2$ may be increased or decreased; pH is decreased. Bedside blood sugar must be checked rapidly. Other testing is based on clinical scenario. Metabolic acidosis is common.

Prevention

Prevention is multi-faceted. Physical barriers (ie, fences) should be placed around pools and other accessible bodies of water. Safety flotation devices and rescue supplies must be immediately available. Use of alcohol or sedative drugs must be avoided during swimming, boating, or other water-based activities. There must be close supervision of those who cannot swim, and personal flotation devices must be worn when boating or water skiing. Swimming lessons, water and boat safety, and basic life support (BLS) education is necessary for anyone involved in water-based activities.

Preventive measures should be taken to reduce morbidity and mortality from drowning. Conditions that increase risk of submersion injury include the following: (1) use of alcohol or other drugs, (2) extreme fatigue from inadequate water safety skills, (3) poor physical health, (4) hyperventilation, (5) sudden acute illness (eg, hypoglycemia, seizure, dysrhythmia, myocardial infarction, asthma flare), (6) acute trauma (particularly brain or spinal cord injury, or both), (7) venomous stings or bites, (8) decompression sickness, (9) dangerous water conditions (temperature and turbulence), and (10) carbon monoxide exposure from boat motors.

▶ Treatment

A. First Aid

1. *The first requirement of rescue is immediate BLS treatment and CPR.* CPR is provided if pulse and respirations are absent. At the scene, immediate measures to combat hypoxemia are critical to improve outcome. BLS care includes sustained ventilation, oxygenation, and circulatory support.

2. Patient must be assessed for hypothermia, hypoglycemia, concurrent medical conditions and associated trauma, especially brain and cervical spine injury.

3. Rescuer should not attempt to drain water from the victim's lungs. The Heimlich maneuver (subdiaphragmatic pressure) should be used only if foreign material airway obstruction is suspected.

4. Resuscitation and BLS efforts must be continued until core temperature reaches 32°C even for seemingly "hopeless" patients. Complete recovery has been reported after prolonged resuscitation of hypothermic patients.

B. Subsequent Management

1. Ensure optimal ventilation and oxygenation—The onset of hypoxemia exists even in the alert, conscious patient who appears to be breathing normally. Oxygen should be administered immediately at the highest available concentration. Oxygen saturation should be maintained at 90% or higher. Endotracheal intubation and mechanical ventilation are necessary for patients unable to maintain an open airway, adequate oxygenation, or ventilation. Continuous positive airway pressure (CPAP) is an effective noninvasive way of reversing hypoxia and hypercarbia in patients with spontaneous respirations and a patent airway. Positive end-expiratory pressure (PEEP) is also effective for treating respiratory insufficiency.

Serial physical examinations and chest radiographs should be carried out to detect possible pneumonitis, atelectasis, and pulmonary edema. Bronchodilators may be used to treat wheezing. Nasogastric suctioning can decompress the stomach. Antibiotics are reserved for clinical evidence of infection and should not be given prophylactically.

2. Cardiovascular support—Intravascular volume status must be monitored to determine whether vascular fluid replacement and vasopressors or diuretics are needed.

3. Correction of blood pH and electrolyte abnormalities—Metabolic acidosis is present in 70% of near-drowning victims, but it is usually corrected through adequate ventilation and oxygenation. Glycemic control improves outcome.

4. Cerebral and spinal cord injury—Central nervous system damage may progress despite apparently adequate treatment of hypoxia and shock.

5. Hypothermia—CBT should be measured and managed as appropriate (see Systemic Hypothermia, above).

▶ Course & Prognosis

Respiratory damage is often severe in the minutes to hours following a near drowning. With respiratory supportive treatment, improvements typically occur quickly over the first few days following the near drowning. Long-term complications of near drowning may include neurologic impairment, seizure disorder, and pulmonary or cardiac damage. There is a direct correlation between prognosis and the patient's age, submersion time, rapid prehospital resuscitation and rapid transport to a medical facility, clinical status at time of arrival to hospital, Glasgow Coma Scale score, pupillary reactivity, and overall health assessment (APACHE II score).

▶ When to Admit

Most patients with significant near drowning or concurrent medical or traumatic conditions require inpatient monitoring following near drowning. This includes continuous monitoring of cardiorespiratory, neurologic, renal and metabolic function. Pulmonary edema may not appear for 24 hours.

Centers for Disease Control and Prevention (CDC). Drowning—United States, 2005–2009. MMWR Morb Mortal Wkly Rep. 2012 May 18;61(19):344–7. [PMID: 22592273]

ENVIRONMENTAL DISORDERS RELATED TO ALTITUDE

DYSBARISM & DECOMPRESSION SICKNESS

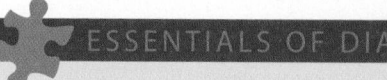

ESSENTIALS OF DIAGNOSIS

▶ Symptoms temporally related to recent altitude or pressure changes (ie, scuba diving).

▶ Early recognition and prompt treatment of decompression sickness are extremely important.

▶ Patient must also be assessed for hypothermia, hypoglycemia, concurrent injuries, and medical conditions.

▶ Consultation with diving medicine or hyperbaric oxygen specialist is indicated.

General Considerations

Dysbarism and decompression sickness are physiologic problems that result from altitude changes and the environmental pressure effects on gases in the body during underwater descent and ascent, particularly when scuba diving is followed closely by air travel or hiking to high altitudes.

Physics laws describe the mechanisms involved in dysbarism and decompression sickness. As a diver descends, the gases in the body compress; gases dissolve in blood and tissues. During the ascent, gases in the body expand. **Dysbarism** results from gas compression or expansion in parts of the body that are noncompressible or have limited compliance. Lung barotrauma results in pneumomediastinum, pneumothorax, and rupture of the pulmonary vein causing arterial gas embolism. Overpressurization of the bowels may occur, especially if there is underlying pathology. This can result in gastric rupture, bowel obstruction or perforation, or pneumoperitoneum. Less serious conditions can also occur such as mask squeeze, ear squeeze, sinus squeeze, headache, tooth squeeze.

Decompression sickness occurs when the ascent is too rapid and gas bubbles form and cause damage depending on their location (eg, coronary, pulmonary, spinal or cerebral blood vessels, joints, soft tissue). Decompression sickness symptoms depends on the size and number and location of gas bubbles released (notably nitrogen). Risk of decompression sickness depends on the dive details (depth, duration, number of dives, and interval surface time between dives, water conditions) as well as the diver's age, weight, physical condition, physical exertion, the rate of ascent, and the length of time between the low altitude (scuba dive) and high altitude (air travel or ground ascent). Predisposing factors for decompression sickness include obesity, injury, hypoxia, lung or cardiac disease, right to left cardiac shunt, diver's overall health, dehydration, alcohol and medication effects, and panic attacks. Decompression sickness also occurs in those who take hot showers after cold dives. Conservative recommendation is to avoid high altitudes (air travel or ground ascent) for at least 24 hours after surfacing from the dive.

Clinical Findings

The range of clinical manifestations varies depending on the location of the gas bubble formation or the compressibility of gases in the body. Symptom onset may be immediate, within minutes or hours (in the majority), or present up to 36 hours later. Decompression sickness symptoms include pain in the joints ("the bends"); skin pruritus or burning (skin bends); rashes; spinal cord or cerebral symptoms ("dissociation" symptoms that do not follow typical distribution patterns); labyrinthine decompression sickness ("the staggers," central vertigo); pulmonary decompression sickness ("the chokes," inspiratory pain, cough, and respiratory distress); arterial gas embolism (cerebral, pulmonary); barotrauma of the lungs, ear and sinus; dysbaric osteonecrosis; and coma.

The clinician must assess for associated conditions of hypothermia, hypoglycemia, near drowning, trauma, envenomations, or concurrent medical conditions.

Treatment

Early recognition and prompt treatment are extremely important. Decompression sickness must be considered if symptoms are temporally related to recent diving or altitude or pressure changes within the past 48 hours. Immediate consultation with a diving medicine or hyperbaric oxygen specialist is indicated even if mild symptoms resolved, since relapses with worse outcomes have occurred. Continuous administration of 100% oxygen is indicated and beneficial for all patients. Aspirin may be given for pain. Opioids should be used very cautiously, since these may obscure the response to recompression.

When to Admit

Rapid transportation to a hyperbaric treatment facility for recompression is imperative for decompression sickness. If air transportation is chosen, the aircraft must maintain pressurization near sea level to avoid worsening decompression sickness. The Divers Alert Network is an excellent worldwide resource for emergency advice 24 hours daily for the management of diving-related conditions (www.diversalertnetwork.org). For diving emergencies, contact local emergency responder first, then the Divers Alert Network.

Bennett MH et al. Recompression and adjunctive therapy for decompression illness. Cochrane Database Syst Rev. 2012 May 16;5:CD005277. [PMID: 22592704]

Vann RD et al. Decompression illness. Lancet. 2011 Jan 8; 377(9760):153–64. [PMID: 21215883]

Weaver LK. Hyperbaric oxygen in the critically ill. Crit Care Med. 2011 Jul;39(7):1784–91. [PMID: 21460713]

Webb JT et al. Fifty years of decompression sickness research at Brooks AFB, TX: 1960–2010. Aviat Space Environ Med. 2011 May;82(5 Suppl):A1–25. [PMID: 21614886]

HIGH-ALTITUDE ILLNESS

ESSENTIALS OF DIAGNOSIS

- ▶ The severity of the high-altitude illness correlates with the rate and height of ascent, and the individual's susceptibility.
- ▶ Prompt recognition and medical attention of early symptoms of high-altitude illness should prevent progression.
- ▶ Immediate descent is the definitive treatment for high-altitude cerebral edema and high-altitude pulmonary edema.

General Considerations

As altitude increases, hypobaric hypoxia results due to a decrease in both barometric pressure and oxygen partial pressure. High-altitude medical problems are due to hypobaric hypoxia at high altitudes (usually > 2000 meters or 6560 feet). Acclimatization occurs as a physiologic response to the rise in altitude and increasing hypobaric hypoxia. Physiologic changes include increases in alveolar ventilation and oxygen extraction by the tissues and increased hemoglobin level and oxygen binding.

High-altitude illness results when the hypoxic stress is greater than the individual's ability to acclimatize. Risk factors for high-altitude illness include increased physical activity with insufficient acclimatization, inadequate education and preparation, and individual susceptibility, and previous high-altitude illness. The key determinants of high-altitude illness risk and severity include both individual susceptibility factors and altitudinal factors (rapid rate and height of ascent and total change in altitude). Presentations may be acute, subacute, or chronic disturbances that result from hypobaric hypoxia.

Individual susceptibility factors include underlying conditions such as cardiac and pulmonary dysfunction, patent foramen ovale, blood disorders (ie, sickle cell disease), pregnancy, neurologic condition, recent surgery, and many other chronic medical conditions. Those with symptomatic cardiac or pulmonary disease should avoid high altitudes.

High-altitude illness comprises a spectrum of conditions based on end-organ effects, mostly cerebral and pulmonary. This is a result of fluid shifts from intravascular to extravascular spaces, especially in the brain and lungs. Manifestations of altitude illness include acute and long-term disorders. Acute high-altitude disorders are high-altitude neurologic conditions (acute mountain sickness and high-altitude cerebral edema) and high-altitude pulmonary edema. Long-term exposure to high altitude over months or years with inadequate acclimatization can result in subacute mountain sickness and chronic mountain sickness (Monge disease).

1. High-Altitude–Associated Neurologic Conditions (Acute Mountain Sickness & High-Altitude Cerebral Edema)

There is a spectrum of neurologic conditions caused by high altitude, ranging from acute mountain sickness to a more serious form, high altitude cerebral edema.

Acute mountain sickness includes both neurologic and pulmonary symptoms, such as headache (most severe and persistent symptom), lassitude, drowsiness, dizziness, chilliness, nausea and vomiting, facial pallor, dyspnea, and cyanosis. Later symptoms include facial flushing, irritability, difficulty concentrating, vertigo, tinnitus, visual and auditory disturbances, anorexia, insomnia, increased dyspnea and weakness on exertion, increased headaches (due to cerebral edema), palpitations, tachycardia, Cheyne-Stokes breathing, and weight loss. More severe manifestations include cerebral and pulmonary edema (high-altitude cerebral edema and high-altitude pulmonary edema; see below).

High-altitude cerebral edema appears to be an extension of the central nervous system symptoms of acute mountain sickness and results from cerebral vasogenic edema and cerebral cellular hypoxia. It usually occurs at elevations above 2500 meters (8250 feet) and is more common in unacclimatized individuals. Hallmarks are altered consciousness and ataxic gait. Severe headaches, confusion, truncal ataxia, urinary retention or incontinence, focal deficits, papilledema, nausea, vomiting, and seizures may also occur. Symptoms may progress to obtundation and coma.

► Treatment

Initial treatment involves oxygen administration by mask. Voluntary periodic hyperventilation will often relieve acute symptoms. Definitive treatment is immediate descent. Descent should be at least 610 meters (2000 feet) and should continue until symptoms improve. Descent is essential if the symptoms are persistent, severe, or worsening or if high-altitude pulmonary edema or high-altitude cerebral edema are present. If immediate descent is not possible, portable hyperbaric chambers can provide symptomatic relief.

Acetazolamide (125–250 mg orally every 8–12 hours, conflicting data as to the optimal dose) remains the most effective medication for treatment of acute mountain sickness and for more severe forms of altitude-related conditions. Adverse reactions include peripheral paresthesias, altered taste of carbonated beverages, polyuria, nausea, drowsiness, erectile dysfunction, and myopia. This is a sulfonamide drug and should be used with caution or avoided in persons with past reactions to this class of drug.

Dexamethasone (dose varies depending on the activity level of the individual, ranging from 2 to 4 mg orally every 6 hours) is effective for treatment of acute mountain sickness and acute cerebral edema; this medication should not be used for prophylaxis and should not be continued beyond 7 days. These medications can be continued for as long as symptoms persist and may be used together in severe cases. In most individuals, symptoms clear within 24–48 hours.

2. Acute High-Altitude Pulmonary Edema

High-altitude pulmonary edema is a serious complication of hypoxia induced pulmonary hypertension. It is the leading cause of death from high altitude illness. The hallmark is markedly elevated pulmonary artery pressure followed by pulmonary edema. It usually occurs at levels above 3000 meters (9840 feet). High altitude increases pulmonary arterial pressure and decreases the oxygen uptake and saturation and alters oxygen kinetics. Early symptoms may appear within 6–36 hours after arrival at a high-altitude area. These include incessant dry cough, shortness of breath disproportionate to exertion, headache, decreased exercise performance, fatigue, dyspnea at rest, and chest tightness. Recognition of the early symptoms may enable the patient to descend before incapacitating pulmonary edema develops. Strenuous exertion should be avoided. An early descent of even 500 or 1000 meters may result in improvement of symptoms. Later, wheezing, orthopnea, and hemoptysis may occur as pulmonary edema worsens.

Physical findings include tachycardia, mild fever, tachypnea, cyanosis, prolonged respiration, and rales and rhonchi. The clinical picture may resemble severe pneumonia.

The patient may become confused or comatose. Diagnosis is usually clinical; ancillary tests are nonspecific or unavailable on site. Prompt recognition and medical attention of early symptoms prevent progression.

Treatment

Treatment must often be initiated under field conditions. The patient must rest in the semi-Fowler position (head raised), and 100% oxygen must be administered. *Immediate descent (at least 610 meters [2000 feet]) is essential.* Recompression in a portable hyperbaric bag will temporarily reduce symptoms if rapid or immediate descent is not possible. To conserve oxygen, lower flow rates (2–4 L/min) may be used until the victim recovers or is evacuated to a lower altitude and Sao$_2$ ≥90%. Treatment for ARDS (see Chapter 9) may be is required for some patients. Calcium channel blockers and selective phosphodiesterase type 5 (PDE5) inhibitors are effective for symptomatic relief: nifedipine (30 mg slow-release tablets every 12 hours), tadalafil (10 mg by mouth every 12 hours), and sildenafil (50 mg by mouth every 8 hours) are commonly recommended alternatives.

There is an international effort to advance the understanding of high-altitude pulmonary edema through the International HAPE Database; susceptible individuals should register with this databank (http://www.altitude.org/hape.php).

3. Subacute Mountain Sickness

This occurs most frequently in unacclimatized individuals and at high altitudes (above 4500 meters) for a prolonged period of time. The hypobaric hypoxia results in pulmonary hypertension. Symptoms of dyspnea and cough are probably due to hypoxic pulmonary hypertension and secondary heart failure. Dehydration, skin dryness, and pruritus also can occur. The hematocrit may be elevated, and there may be ECG and chest radiographic evidence of right ventricular hypertrophy. Treatment consists of rest, oxygen administration, diuretics, and return to lower altitudes.

4. Chronic Mountain Sickness (Monge Disease)

This uncommon condition is seen in residents of high-altitude communities who have lost their acclimatization to such a hypobaric hypoxic environment. It is difficult to differentiate from chronic pulmonary disease.

Prevention of High-Altitude Disorders

Pre-trip preventive measures include participant education, medical prescreening, pre-trip planning, optimal physical conditioning before travel, and adequate rest and sleep the day before travel. Preventive efforts during ascent include reduced food intake; avoidance of alcohol, tobacco, and unnecessary physical activity during travel; slow ascent to allow acclimatization (300 meters per day); and a period of rest and inactivity for 1–2 days after arrival at high altitudes. Mountaineering parties at altitudes of ≥3000 meters or higher should carry a supply of oxygen and medical equipment sufficient for several days. Prophylactic medications may be prescribed if no contraindications exist. Prophylactic low-dose acetazolamide (250–500 mg every 12 hours orally or 500 mg extended-release once to twice daily orally) has been shown to reduce the incidence and severity of acute mountain sickness when started 3 days prior to ascent and continued for 48–72 hours at high altitude. Dexamethasone (4 mg every 12 hours orally beginning on the day of ascent, continuing for 3 days at the higher altitude, and then tapering over 5 days) is an alternative prophylactic medication. Research also suggests potential benefit from prophylaxis with sumatriptan, nifedipine, dexamethasone, tadalafil, sildenafil, and salmeterol (125 mcg by inhaler every 12 hours beginning 24 hours prior to ascent).

When to Admit

- All patients with high-altitude pulmonary edema or high-altitude cerebral edema must be hospitalized for further observation.
- Hospitalization must also be considered for any patient who remains symptomatic after treatment and descent. Pulmonary symptoms and hypoxia may be worsened by pulmonary embolism, bacterial pneumonia, or bronchitis.

Hall DP et al. High altitude pulmonary oedema. J R Army Med Corps. 2011 Mar;157(1):68–72. [PMID: 21465914]

Seupaul RA et al. Pharmacologic prophylaxis for acute mountain sickness: a systematic shortcut review. Ann Emerg Med. 2012 Apr;59(4):307–17. [PMID: 22153998]

SAFETY OF AIR TRAVEL & SELECTION OF PATIENTS FOR AIR TRAVEL

The medical safety of air travel depends on the nature and severity of the traveler's preflight condition and factors such as travel duration, frequency and use of inflight exercise, cabin pressurization, availability of medical supplies, and presence of health care professionals on board. Inflight medical emergencies are increasing because there are an increasing number of travelers with preexisting medical conditions. Air travel passengers are susceptible to a wide range of flight-related problems: pulmonary (eg, hypoxia, gas expansion), vascular (venous thromboembolism, VTE), infectious, cardiovascular, gastrointestinal, ocular, immunologic, syncope, neuropsychiatric, metabolic, trauma, and substance-related. These air-travel risks are higher for those air travelers with preexisting medical conditions: cardiovascular disease, thromboembolic disease, asthma, chronic obstructive pulmonary disease, epilepsy, stroke, recent surgery or trauma, diabetes mellitus, infectious disease, mental illness, and substance dependence. Occupational and frequent flyers are at risk for these as well as accumulative radiation exposure, cabin air quality, circadian disturbance, and pressurization problems.

Hypobaric hypoxia is the underlying etiology of most serious medical emergencies in flight. Requirements for commercial aircraft are to maintain cabin pressurized to the equivalent of 8000 feet or less. Despite commercial aircraft pressurization requirements, there is significant hypoxemia, dyspnea, gas expansion, and stress in travelers. Patients with underlying respiratory or cardiac conditions are at highest risk for problems stemming from hypobaric hypoxia.

Research also demonstrates an association between VTE and air travel. Air travel has a threefold higher risk of VTE, especially severe pulmonary embolism. The VTE risk increases proportionally with the flight duration. Higher risk of VTE is seen in travelers with thrombophilia, varicose veins, hormonal therapy, obesity, and pregnancy.

Air travel is not advised for anyone who is incapacitated, or who has an active pneumothorax, class III and IV pulmonary hypertension, acute worsening of an underlying lung disease, or any unstable conditions. The Air Transport Association of America defines an **incapacitated passenger** as "one who is suffering from a physical or mental disability and who, because of such disability or the effect of the flight on the disability, is incapable of self-care; would endanger the health or safety of such person or other passengers or airline employees; or would cause discomfort or annoyance of other passengers." **Unstable conditions** include poorly controlled hypertension, dysrhythmias, angina, valvular disease, heart failure, or acute psychiatric condition; severe anemia or symptomatic sickle cell disease; recent myocardial infarction; cerebrovascular accident; poorly controlled seizure disorder; deep venous thrombosis; postsurgery, especially heart surgery (unless approved by surgeon); and any active communicable disease (influenza, tuberculosis, measles, chickenpox, zoster, or other communicable virulent infections). Risk of transmission increases when there is close contact to infected passengers.

Pregnancy and Infancy

Pregnancy is a hypercoagulable state with fivefold to tenfold increase in VTE risk. Air travel increases this risk of VTE. Pregnant women may be permitted to fly during the first 8 months of pregnancy unless there is a history of pregnancy complications or premature birth. Infants younger than 1 week old should not be flown at high altitudes or for long distances. There is a higher risk of transmission of infection in-flight for pregnant women and infants due to their weaker immune response. Estimates of air travel radiation exposure are available through the Federal Aviation Administration and vary based on frequency and duration of flights.

▶ Prevention

Air travel complications may be reduced by the following preventive measures: passenger education, passenger pre-screening, and in-flight positioning and activity. Pre-screening is especially important for those who have had recent surgery or an emergency condition, and those with chronic serious medical conditions. Travelers with underlying pulmonary disease (ie, chronic obstructive pulmonary disease or pulmonary hypertension) must have preflight medical assessment to determine whether supplemental oxygen is required. Oxygen is required if the arterial oxygen tension is < 70 mm Hg or pulse oximetry < 92%. Other useful tests to determine whether oxygen is needed include the hypoxia altitude simulation test and the 6-minute walk test. Travelers can reduce VTE risk by avoiding constrictive clothing, wearing support hose, changing position frequently, avoiding leg crossing, engaging in frequent in-flight leg exercises, and walking. Low-molecular-weight heparin may be prescribed in travelers at high risk for VTE.

Bartholomew JR et al. Air travel and venous thromboembolism: minimizing the risk. Cleve Clin J Med. 2011 Feb;78(2): 111–20. [PMID: 21285343]

Edvardsen A et al. Air travel and chronic obstructive pulmonary disease: a new algorithm for pre-flight evaluation. Thorax. 2012 Nov;67(11):964–9. [PMID: 22767877]

Roubinian N et al. Effects of commercial air travel on patients with pulmonary hypertension. Chest. 2012 Oct;142(4):885–92. [PMID: 22490871]

Sugerman HJ et al. JAMA patient page. Air travel-related deep vein thrombosis and pulmonary embolism. JAMA. 2012 Dec 19;308(23):2531. [PMID: 23288474]

Withers A et al. Air travel and the risks of hypoxia in children. Paediatr Respir Rev. 2011 Dec;12(4):271–6. [PMID: 22018043]

Poisoning

Kent R. Olson, MD

INITIAL EVALUATION: POISONING OR OVERDOSE

Patients with drug overdoses or poisoning may initially have no symptoms or they may have varying degrees of overt intoxication. The asymptomatic patient may have been exposed to or may have ingested a lethal dose but not yet exhibit any manifestations of toxicity. It is important to: (1) quickly assess the potential danger, (2) consider gut decontamination to prevent absorption, (3) treat complications if they occur, and (4) observe the asymptomatic patient for an appropriate interval.

▶ Assess the Danger

If the drug or poison is known, its danger can be assessed by consulting a text or computerized information resource or by calling a regional poison control center. (In the United States, dialing 1-800-222-1222 will direct the call to the regional poison control center.) Assessment will usually take into account the dose ingested; the time since ingestion; the presence of any symptoms or clinical signs; preexisting cardiac, respiratory, kidney, or liver disease; and, occasionally, specific serum drug or toxin levels. Be aware that the history given by the patient or family may be incomplete or unreliable.

▶ Observation of the Patient

Asymptomatic or mildly symptomatic patients should be observed for at least 4–6 hours. Longer observation is indicated if the ingested substance is a sustained-release preparation or is known to slow gastrointestinal motility (opioids, anticholinergics, salicylate) or may cause a delayed onset of symptoms (such as acetaminophen, colchicine, or hepatotoxic mushrooms). After that time, the patient may be discharged if no symptoms have developed. Before discharge, psychiatric evaluation should be performed to assess suicide risk. Intentional ingestions in adolescents should raise the possibility of unwanted pregnancy or sexual abuse.

THE SYMPTOMATIC PATIENT

In symptomatic patients, treatment of life-threatening complications takes precedence over in-depth diagnostic evaluation. Patients with mild symptoms may deteriorate rapidly, which is why all potentially significant exposures should be observed in an acute care facility. The following complications may occur, depending on the type of poisoning.

COMA

▶ Assessment & Complications

Coma is commonly associated with ingestion of large doses of antihistamines (eg, diphenhydramine), benzodiazepines and other sedative-hypnotic drugs, ethanol, opioids, antipsychotic drugs, or antidepressants. The most common cause of death in comatose patients is respiratory failure, which may occur abruptly. Pulmonary aspiration of gastric contents may also occur, especially in victims who are deeply obtunded or convulsing. Hypoxia and hypoventilation may cause or aggravate hypotension, arrhythmias, and seizures. Thus, protection of the airway and assisted ventilation are the most important treatment measures for any poisoned patient.

▶ Treatment

A. Emergency Management

The initial emergency management of coma can be remembered by the mnemonic *ABCD*, for *A*irway, *B*reathing, *C*irculation, and *D*rugs (dextrose, thiamine, and naloxone or flumazenil), respectively.

1. Airway—Establish a patent airway by positioning, suction, or insertion of an artificial nasal or oropharyngeal airway. If the patient is deeply comatose or if airway reflexes are depressed, perform endotracheal intubation. These airway interventions may not be necessary if the patient is intoxicated by an opioid or a benzodiazepine and responds to intravenous naloxone or flumazenil (see below).

2. Breathing—Clinically assess the quality and depth of respiration, and provide assistance if necessary with a bag-valve-mask device or mechanical ventilator. Administer supplemental oxygen, if needed. The arterial or venous blood CO_2 tension is useful in determining the adequacy of ventilation. The arterial blood Po_2 determination may reveal hypoxemia, which may be caused by respiratory depression, bronchospasm, pulmonary aspiration, or non-cardiogenic pulmonary edema. Pulse oximetry provides an assessment of oxygenation but is not reliable in patients with methemoglobinemia or carbon monoxide poisoning, unless a pulse oximetry device capable of detecting these forms of hemoglobin is used.

3. Circulation—Measure the pulse and blood pressure and estimate tissue perfusion (eg, by measurement of urinary output, skin signs, arterial blood pH). Place the patient on continuous ECG monitoring. Insert an intravenous line, and draw blood for glucose, electrolytes, serum creatinine and liver tests, and possible quantitative toxicologic testing.

4. Drugs

A. Dextrose and thiamine—Unless promptly treated, severe hypoglycemia can cause irreversible brain damage. Therefore, in all obtunded, comatose or convulsing patients, give 50% dextrose, 50–100 mL by intravenous bolus, unless a rapid bedside blood sugar test rules out hypoglycemia. In alcoholic or very malnourished patients who may have marginal thiamine stores, give thiamine, 100 mg intramuscularly or in the intravenous fluids.

B. Opioid antagonists—Naloxone, 0.4–2 mg intravenously, may reverse opioid-induced respiratory depression and coma. It is often given empirically to any comatose patient with depressed respirations. If opioid overdose is strongly suspected, give additional doses of naloxone (up to 5–10 mg may be required to reverse the effects of potent opioids). **Note:** Naloxone has a shorter duration of action (2–3 hours) than most common opioids; repeated doses may be required, and continuous observation for at least 3–4 hours after the last dose is mandatory. Nalmefene, a newer opioid antagonist, has a duration of effect longer than that of naloxone but still shorter than that of the opioid methadone.

C. Flumazenil—Flumazenil, 0.2–0.5 mg intravenously, repeated as needed up to a maximum of 3 mg, may reverse benzodiazepine-induced coma. **Caution:** Flumazenil should **not** be given if the patient has coingested a potential convulsant drug, is a user of high-dose benzodiazepines, or has a seizure disorder because its use in these circumstances may precipitate seizures. *In most circumstances, use of flumazenil is not advised as the potential risks outweigh its benefits.* **Note:** Flumazenil has a short duration of effect (2–3 hours), and resedation requiring additional doses may occur.

HYPOTHERMIA

▶ Assessment & Complications

Hypothermia commonly accompanies coma due to opioids, ethanol, hypoglycemic agents, phenothiazines, barbiturates, benzodiazepines, and other sedative-hypnotics and central nervous system depressants. Hypothermic patients may have a barely perceptible pulse and blood pressure. Hypothermia may cause or aggravate hypotension, which will not reverse until the temperature is normalized.

▶ Treatment

Treatment of hypothermia is discussed in Chapter 37. Gradual rewarming is preferred unless the patient is in cardiac arrest.

HYPOTENSION

▶ Assessment & Complications

Hypotension may be due to poisoning by many different drugs and poisons, including antihypertensive drugs, beta-blockers, calcium channel blockers, disulfiram (ethanol interaction), iron, trazodone, quetiapine, and other antipsychotic agents and antidepressants. Poisons causing hypotension include cyanide, carbon monoxide, hydrogen sulfide, aluminum or zinc phosphide, arsenic, and certain mushrooms.

Hypotension in the poisoned or drug-overdosed patient may be caused by venous or arteriolar vasodilation, hypovolemia, depressed cardiac contractility, or a combination of these effects.

▶ Treatment

Most hypotensive patients respond to empiric treatment with repeated 200 mL intravenous boluses of 0.9% saline or other isotonic crystalloid up to a total of 1–2 L; much larger amounts may be needed if the victim is profoundly volume depleted (eg, as with *Amanita phalloides* mushroom poisoning). Monitoring the central venous pressure (CVP) can help determine whether further fluid therapy is needed. If fluid therapy is not successful, give dopamine or norepinephrine by intravenous infusion. Consider bedside cardiac ultrasound or pulmonary artery catheterization (or both) if hypotension persists.

Hypotension caused by certain toxins may respond to specific treatment. For hypotension caused by overdoses of tricyclic antidepressants or other sodium channel blockers, administer sodium bicarbonate, 50–100 mEq by intravenous bolus injection. Norepinephrine 4–8 mcg/min by intravenous infusion is more effective than dopamine in some patients with overdoses of tricyclic antidepressants or of drugs with predominantly vasodilating effects. For beta-blocker overdose, glucagon (5–10 mg intravenously) may be of value. For calcium channel blocker overdose, administer calcium chloride, 1–2 g intravenously (repeated doses may be necessary; doses of 5–10 g and more have been given in some cases). High-dose insulin (0.5–1 units/kg/h intravenously) euglycemic therapy may also be used (see the sections on Beta-Adrenergic Blockers and Calcium Channel Blockers, below). Intralipid 20% lipid emulsion has been reported to improve hemodynamics in human case reports or animal studies of intoxication by highly lipid-soluble drugs such as bupivacaine, bupropion, clomipramine, and verapamil.

Engebretsen KM et al. High-dose insulin therapy in beta-blocker and calcium channel-blocker poisoning. Clin Toxicol (Phila). 2011 Apr;49(4):277–83. [PMID: 21563902]

Waring WS. Intravenous lipid administration for drug-induced toxicity: a critical review of the existing data. Expert Rev Clin Pharmacol. 2012 Jul;5(4):437–44. [PMID: 22943123]

HYPERTENSION

▶ Assessment & Complications

Hypertension may be due to poisoning with amphetamines, anticholinergics, cocaine, performance-enhancing products (containing caffeine, phenylephrine, ephedrine, or yohimbine), monoamine oxidase (MAO) inhibitors, and other drugs.

Severe hypertension (eg, diastolic blood pressure > 105–110 mm Hg in a person who does not have chronic hypertension) can result in acute intracranial hemorrhage, myocardial infarction, or aortic dissection.

▶ Treatment

Treat hypertension if the patient is symptomatic or if the diastolic pressure is > 105–110 mm Hg—especially if there is no prior history of hypertension.

Hypertensive patients who are agitated or anxious may benefit from a sedative such as lorazepam, 2–3 mg intravenously. For persistent hypertension, administer phentolamine, 2–5 mg intravenously, or nitroprusside sodium, 0.25–8 mcg/kg/min intravenously. If excessive tachycardia is present, add propranolol, 1–5 mg intravenously, or esmolol, 25–100 mcg/kg/min intravenously, or labetalol 0.2–0.3 mg/kg intravenously. **Caution:** Do not give beta-blockers alone, since doing so may paradoxically worsen hypertension as a result of unopposed alpha-adrenergic stimulation.

Grossman E et al. Drug-induced hypertension: an unappreciated cause of secondary hypertension. Am J Med. 2012 Jan;125(1): 14–22. [PMID: 22195528]

Perruchoud C et al. Severe hypertension following accidental clonidine overdose during the refilling of an implanted intrathecal drug delivery system. Neuromodulation. 2012 Jan–Feb;15(1):31–4. [PMID: 21943355]

ARRHYTHMIAS

▶ Assessment & Complications

Arrhythmias may occur with a variety of drugs or toxins (Table 38–1). They may also occur as a result of hypoxia, metabolic acidosis, or electrolyte imbalance (eg, hyperkalemia, hypokalemia, hypomagnesemia or hypocalcemia), or following exposure to chlorinated solvents or chloral hydrate overdose. Atypical ventricular tachycardia (torsades de pointes) is often associated with drugs that prolong the QT interval.

▶ Treatment

Arrhythmias may be caused by hypoxia or electrolyte imbalance, and these conditions should be sought and treated.

Table 38–1. Common toxins or drugs causing arrhythmias.[1]

Arrhythmia	Common Causes
Sinus bradycardia	Beta-blockers, calcium channel blockers, clonidine, digitalis glycosides, organophosphates
Atrioventricular block	Beta-blockers, calcium channel blockers, class Ia antiarrhythmics (including quinidine), carbamazepine, clonidine, digitalis glycosides, lithium
Sinus tachycardia	Beta-agonists (eg, albuterol), amphetamines, anticholinergics, antihistamines, caffeine, cocaine, pseudoephedrine, tricyclic and other antidepressants
Wide QRS complex	Class Ia and class Ic antiarrhythmics, phenothiazines (eg, thioridazine), potassium (hyperkalemia), propranolol, tricyclic antidepressants, bupropion, lamotrigine, diphenhydramine (severe overdose)
QT interval prolongation and torsades de pointes	Arsenic, class Ia and class III antiarrhythmics, citalopram, droperidol, lithium, methadone, pentamidine, sertraline, sotalol, thioridazine, and many other drugs[2]
Ventricular premature beats and ventricular tachycardia	Amphetamines, cocaine, ephedrine, caffeine, chlorinated or fluorinated hydrocarbons, digoxin, aconite (found in some Chinese herbal preparations), fluoride, theophylline. QT prolongation can lead to atypical ventricular tachycardia (torsades de pointes)

[1]Arrhythmias may also occur as a result of hypoxia, metabolic acidosis, or electrolyte imbalance (eg, hyperkalemia or hypokalemia, hypocalcemia, hypomagnesemia).
[2]http://www.azcert.org/medical-pros/drug-lists/drug-lists.cfm

If ventricular arrhythmias persist, administer lidocaine or amiodarone at usual antiarrhythmic doses. **Note:** Wide QRS complex tachycardia in the setting of tricyclic antidepressant overdose (or diphenhydramine or class Ia antiarrhythmic drugs) should be treated with sodium bicarbonate, 50–100 mEq intravenously by bolus infusion. (See discussion of tricyclic antidepressant poisoning.) **Caution:** Avoid class Ia antiarrhythmic agents (eg, procainamide, disopyramide), which may aggravate arrhythmias caused by tricyclic antidepressants. Torsades de pointes associated with prolonged QT interval may respond to intravenous magnesium (2 g intravenously over 2 minutes) or overdrive pacing. Treat digitalis-induced arrhythmias with digoxin-specific antibodies (see discussion of cardiac glycoside poisoning).

For tachyarrhythmias induced by chlorinated solvents, chloral hydrate, Freons, or sympathomimetic agents, use propranolol or esmolol (see doses given above in Hypertension section).

Behr ER et al. Drug-induced arrhythmia: pharmacogenomic prescribing? Eur Heart J. 2013 Jan;34(2):89–95. [PMID: 23091201]

SEIZURES

▶ Assessment & Complications

Seizures may be due to poisoning with many poisons and drugs, including amphetamines, antidepressants (especially tricyclic antidepressants, bupropion, and venlafaxine), antihistamines (especially diphenhydramine), antipsychotics, camphor, cocaine, isoniazid (INH), chlorinated insecticides, tramadol, and theophylline. The onset of seizures may be delayed for up to 24 hours after extended-released bupropion overdose.

Seizures may also be caused by hypoxia, hypoglycemia, hypocalcemia, hyponatremia, withdrawal from alcohol or sedative-hypnotics, head trauma, central nervous system infection, or idiopathic epilepsy.

Prolonged or repeated seizures may lead to hypoxia, metabolic acidosis, hyperthermia, and rhabdomyolysis.

▶ Treatment

Administer lorazepam, 2–3 mg, or diazepam, 5–10 mg, intravenously over 1–2 minutes, or—if intravenous access is not immediately available—midazolam, 5–10 mg intramuscularly. If convulsions continue, administer phenobarbital, 15–20 mg/kg slowly intravenously over no less than 30 minutes. (For drug-induced seizures, phenobarbital is preferred over phenytoin.) Propofol infusion has also been reported effective for some resistant drug-induced seizures.

Seizures due to a few drugs and toxins may require antidotes or other specific therapies (as listed in Table 38–2).

Bekjarovski N et al. Seizures after use and abuse of tramadol. Prilozi. 2012 Jul;33(1):313–8. [PMID: 22983066]
Thundiyil JG et al. Risk factors for complications of drug-induced seizures. J Med Toxicol. 2011 Mar;7(1):16–23. [PMID: 20661684]

HYPERTHERMIA

▶ Assessment & Complications

Hyperthermia may be associated with poisoning by amphetamines (especially methylenedioxymethamphetamine [MDMA; "Ecstasy"]), atropine and other anticholinergic drugs, cocaine, salicylates, strychnine, tricyclic antidepressants, and various other medications. Overdoses of serotonin reuptake inhibitors (eg, fluoxetine, paroxetine, sertraline) or their use in a patient taking an MAO inhibitor may cause agitation, hyperactivity, myoclonus, and hyperthermia ("serotonin syndrome"). Antipsychotic agents can cause rigidity and hyperthermia (neuroleptic malignant syndrome [NMS]). (See section on schizophrenia and other psychotic disorders in Chapter 25.) Malignant hyperthermia is a rare disorder associated with general anesthetic agents.

Table 38–2. Seizures related to toxins or drugs requiring special consideration.[1]

Toxin or Drug	Comments
Methylenedioxymethamphetamine (MDMA; "Ecstasy")	Seizures may also be due to hyponatremia or hyperthermia.
Isoniazid	Administer pyridoxine.
Lithium	May indicate need for hemodialysis.
Organophosphates	Administer pralidoxime (2-PAM) and atropine in addition to usual anticonvulsants.
Strychnine	"Seizures" are actually spinally mediated muscle spasms and usually require neuromuscular paralysis and mechanical ventilation.
Theophylline	Seizures indicate need for hemodialysis.
Tricyclic antidepressants	Hyperthermia and cardiotoxicity are common complications of repeated seizures; paralyze early with neuromuscular blockers to reduce muscular hyperactivity.

[1]See text for dosages.

Hyperthermia is a rapidly life-threatening complication. Severe hyperthermia (temperature > 40–41°C) can rapidly cause brain damage and multiorgan failure, including rhabdomyolysis, acute kidney injury, and coagulopathy (see Chapter 37).

▶ Treatment

Treat hyperthermia aggressively by removing the patient's clothing, spraying the skin with tepid water, and fanning. If this is not rapidly effective, as shown by a normal rectal temperature within 30–60 minutes, or if there is significant muscle rigidity or hyperactivity, induce neuromuscular paralysis with a nondepolarizing neuromuscular blocker (eg, rocuronium, vecuronium). Once paralyzed, the patient must be intubated and mechanically ventilated and sedated. While the patient is paralyzed, the absence of visible muscular convulsive movements may give the false impression that brain seizure activity has ceased; bedside electroencephalography may be useful in recognizing continued nonconvulsive seizures.

Dantrolene (2–5 mg/kg intravenously) may be effective for hyperthermia associated with muscle rigidity that does not respond to neuromuscular blockade (ie, malignant hyperthermia). Bromocriptine, 2.5–7.5 mg orally daily, has been recommended for neuroleptic malignant syndrome. Cyproheptadine, 4 mg orally every hour for three or four doses, or chlorpromazine, 25 mg intravenously or 50 mg intramuscularly, has been used to treat serotonin syndrome.

Menaker J et al. Cocaine-induced agitated delirium with associated hyperthermia: a case report. J Emerg Med. 2011 Sep;41(3):e49–53. [PMID: 18823733]

Perry PJ et al. Serotonin syndrome vs neuroleptic malignant syndrome: a contrast of causes, diagnoses, and management. Ann Clin Psychiatry. 2012 May;24(2):155–62. [PMID: 22563571]

▼ ANTIDOTES & OTHER TREATMENT

ANTIDOTES

Give an antidote (if available) when there is reasonable certainty of a specific diagnosis (Table 38–3). Be aware that some antidotes themselves may have serious side effects. The indications and dosages for specific antidotes are discussed in the respective sections for specific toxins.

Marraffa JM et al. Antidotes for toxicological emergencies: a practical review. Am J Health Syst Pharm. 2012 Feb 1;69(3): 199–212. [PMID: 22261941]
Thanacoody RH et al. National audit of antidote stocking in acute hospitals in the UK. Emerg Med J. 2013 May;30(5):393–6. [PMID: 22875840]

Table 38–3. Some toxic agents for which there are specific antidotes.[1]

Toxic Agent	Specific Antidote
Acetaminophen	N-Acetylcysteine
Anticholinergics (eg, atropine)	Physostigmine
Anticholinesterases (eg, organophosphate pesticides)	Atropine and pralidoxime (2-PAM)
Benzodiazepines	Flumazenil (rarely used; see note below[2])
Carbon monoxide	Oxygen (hyperbaric oxygen of uncertain benefit)
Cyanide	Sodium nitrite, sodium thiosulfate; hydroxocobalamin
Digitalis glycosides	Digoxin-specific Fab antibodies
Heavy metals (eg, lead, mercury, iron) and arsenic	Specific chelating agents
Isoniazid	Pyridoxine (vitamin B$_6$)
Methanol, ethylene glycol	Ethanol (ethyl alcohol) or fomepizole (4-methylpyrazole)
Opioids	Naloxone, nalmefene
Snake venom	Specific antivenin
Sulfonylurea oral hypoglycemic drugs	Glucose, octreotide

[1]See text for indications and dosages.
[2]May induce seizures in patients with preexisting seizure disorder, benzodiazepine addiction, or concomitant tricyclic antidepressant or other convulsant overdose. If seizures occur, diazepam and other benzodiazepine anticonvulsants will not be effective. As with naloxone, the duration of action of flumazenil is short (2–3 hours) and resedation may occur, requiring repeated doses.

DECONTAMINATION OF THE SKIN

Corrosive agents rapidly injure the skin and eyes and must be removed immediately. In addition, many toxins are readily absorbed through the skin, and systemic absorption can be prevented only by rapid action.

Wash the affected areas with copious quantities of lukewarm water or saline. Wash carefully behind the ears, under the nails, and in skin folds. For oily substances (eg, pesticides), wash the skin at least twice with plain soap and shampoo the hair. Specific decontaminating solutions or solvents (eg, alcohol) are rarely indicated and in some cases may paradoxically enhance absorption. For exposure to chemical warfare poisons such as nerve agents or vesicants, some authorities recommend use of a dilute hypochlorite solution (household bleach diluted 1:10 with water), but not in the eyes.

DECONTAMINATION OF THE EYES

Act quickly to prevent serious damage. Flush the eyes with copious amounts of saline or water. (If available, instill local anesthetic drops in the eye before beginning irrigation.) Remove contact lenses if present. Direct the irrigating stream so that it will flow across the eyes after running off the nasal bridge. Lift the tarsal conjunctiva to look for undissolved particles and to facilitate irrigation. Continue irrigation for 15 minutes or until each eye has been irrigated with at least 1 L of solution. If the toxin is an acid or a base, check the pH of the tears after irrigation, and continue irrigation until the pH is between 6 and 8. Special amphoteric solutions (Diphoterine, Previn) have been introduced in Europe for treatment of alkali injuries to the eye.

After irrigation is complete, perform a careful examination of the eye, using fluorescein and a slit lamp or Wood lamp to identify areas of corneal injury. Patients with serious conjunctival or corneal injury should be immediately referred to an ophthalmologist.

GASTROINTESTINAL DECONTAMINATION

Removal of ingested poisons was a routine part of emergency treatment for decades. However, prospective randomized studies have failed to demonstrate improved clinical outcome after gastric emptying. For small or moderate ingestions of most substances, toxicologists generally recommend oral activated charcoal alone without prior gastric emptying; in some cases, when the interval after ingestion has been more than 1–2 hours and the ingestant is non–life-threatening, even charcoal is withheld. Exceptions are large ingestions of anticholinergic compounds and salicylates, which often delay gastric emptying, and ingestion of sustained-release or enteric-coated tablets, which may remain intact for several hours. In these cases, aggressive gut decontamination may be indicated.

Gastric emptying is not generally used for ingestion of corrosive agents or petroleum distillates, because further esophageal injury or pulmonary aspiration may result. However, in certain cases, removal of the toxin may be more important than concern over possible complications. Consult a medical toxicologist or regional poison control center (1-800-222-1222) for advice.

A. Emesis

Emesis using syrup of ipecac can partially evacuate gastric contents if given very soon after ingestion (eg, at work or at home). However, it may increase the risk of pulmonary aspiration and delay or prevent the use of oral activated charcoal. Therefore, it is no longer used in the routine management of ingestions.

B. Gastric Lavage

Gastric lavage is more effective for liquid poisons or small pill fragments than for intact tablets or pieces of mushroom. It is most useful when started within 60 minutes after ingestion. However, the lavage procedure may delay administration of activated charcoal and may stimulate vomiting and pulmonary aspiration in an obtunded patient.

1. Indications—Gastric lavage is sometimes used after very large ingestions (eg, massive aspirin overdose), for collection and examination of gastric contents for identification of the poison, and make it easier to administer charcoal and oral antidotes.

2. Contraindications—Do *not* use lavage for stuporous or comatose patients with depressed airway protective reflexes unless they are endotracheally intubated beforehand. Some authorities advise against lavage when caustic material has been ingested; others regard it as essential to remove liquid corrosives from the stomach.

3. Technique—In obtunded or comatose patients, the danger of aspiration pneumonia is reduced by performing endotracheal intubation with a cuffed tube before the procedure. Gently insert a lubricated, soft but noncollapsible stomach tube (at least 37–40 F) through the mouth or nose into the stomach. Aspirate and save the contents, and then lavage repeatedly with 50-to 100-mL aliquots of fluid until the return fluid is clear. Use lukewarm tap water or saline.

C. Activated Charcoal

Activated charcoal effectively adsorbs almost all drugs and poisons. Poorly adsorbed substances include iron, lithium, potassium, sodium, mineral acids, and alcohols.

1. Indications—Activated charcoal can be used for prompt adsorption of drugs or toxins in the stomach and intestine. Studies in volunteers show that activated charcoal given alone may be as effective as, or more effective, than ipecac-induced emesis or gastric lavage. However, evidence of benefit in clinical studies is lacking. Administration of charcoal, especially if mixed with sorbitol, can provoke vomiting, which could lead to pulmonary aspiration in an obtunded patient.

2. Contraindications—Activated charcoal should not be used for comatose or convulsing patients unless it can be given by gastric tube and the airway is first protected by a cuffed endotracheal tube. It is also contraindicated for patients with ileus or intestinal obstruction or those who have ingested corrosives for whom endoscopy is planned.

3. Technique—Administer activated charcoal, 60–100 g orally or via gastric tube, mixed in aqueous slurry. Repeated doses may be given to ensure gastrointestinal adsorption or to enhance elimination of some drugs (see below).

D. Catharsis

1. Indications—Cathartics are used by some toxicologists for stimulation of peristalsis to hasten the elimination of unabsorbed drugs and poisons and the activated charcoal slurry. There is no clinical evidence to support their use, and some agents (eg, sorbitol) can provoke vomiting, increasing the risk of pulmonary aspiration.

2. Contraindications and cautions—Do not give a cathartic to patients with suspected intestinal obstruction. Avoid sodium-based cathartics in patients with hypertension, advanced chronic kidney disease, and heart failure and avoid magnesium-based cathartics in patients with advanced chronic kidney disease. Sorbitol (an osmotic cathartic found in some prepackaged activated charcoal slurry products) can cause hypotension and dehydration due to third-spacing and also causes intestinal cramping and vomiting.

E. Whole Bowel Irrigation

Whole bowel irrigation uses large volumes of a balanced polyethylene glycol-electrolyte solution to mechanically cleanse the entire intestinal tract. Because of the composition of the irrigating solution, there is no significant gain or loss of systemic fluids or electrolytes.

1. Indications—Whole bowel irrigation is particularly effective for massive iron ingestion in which intact tablets are visible on abdominal radiographs. It has also been used for ingestions of lithium, sustained-release and enteric-coated tablets, and swallowed drug-filled packets.

2. Contraindications—Do not use in patients with suspected intestinal obstruction. Use with caution in patients who are obtunded or have depressed airway protective reflexes.

3. Technique—Administer a balanced polyethylene glycol-electrolyte solution (CoLyte, GoLYTELY) into the stomach via gastric tube at a rate of 1–2 L/h until the rectal effluent is clear. This may take several hours. It is most effective when patients are able to sit on a commode to pass the intestinal contents.

F. Increased Drug Removal

1. Urinary manipulation—Forced diuresis is hazardous; the risk of complications (pulmonary edema, electrolyte imbalance) usually outweighs its benefits. Acidic drugs (eg, salicylates, phenobarbital) are more rapidly excreted with an alkaline urine. Acidification (sometimes promoted for amphetamines, phencyclidine) is *not* very effective and is contraindicated in the presence of rhabdomyolysis or myoglobinuria.

Table 38–4. Recommended use of hemodialysis in poisoning.

Poison	Common Indications[1]
Carbamazepine	Seizures, severe cardiotoxicity; serum level > 60 mg/L
Ethylene glycol	Acidosis, serum level > 50 mg/dL
Lithium	Severe symptoms; level > 4 mEq/L more than 12 hours after last dose. Note: dialysis of uncertain value; CVVHD may be preferable; consult with medical toxicologist.
Methanol	Acidosis, serum level > 50 mg/dL
Phenobarbital	Intractable hypotension, acidosis despite maximal supportive care
Salicylate	Severe acidosis, CNS symptoms, level > 100 mg/dL (acute overdose) or > 60 mg/dL (chronic intoxication)
Theophylline	Serum level > 90–100 mg/L (acute) or seizures and serum level > 40–60 mg/L (chronic)
Valproic acid	Serum level > 900–1000 mg/L or deep coma, severe acidosis

[1]See text for further discussion of indications.
CNS, central nervous system; CVVHD, continuous venovenous hemodialysis.

2. Hemodialysis—The indications for dialysis are as follows: (1) Known or suspected potentially lethal amounts of a dialyzable drug (Table 38–4); (2) Poisoning with deep coma, apnea, severe hypotension, fluid and electrolyte or acid-base disturbance, or extreme body temperature changes that cannot be corrected by conventional measures; or (3) Poisoning in patients with severe kidney, cardiac, pulmonary, or hepatic disease who will not be able to eliminate toxin by the usual mechanisms.

Continuous renal replacement therapy (including continuous venovenous hemodiafiltration and similar techniques) is of uncertain benefit for elimination of most poisons but has the advantage of gradual removal of the toxin and correction of any accompanying acidosis, and its use has been reported in the management of lithium intoxication.

3. Repeat-dose charcoal—Repeated doses of activated charcoal, 20–30 g orally or via gastric tube every 3–4 hours, may hasten elimination of some drugs (eg, phenytoin, carbamazepine, dapsone) by absorbing drugs excreted into the gut lumen ("gut dialysis"). However, clinical studies have failed to prove better outcome using multiple-dose charcoal. Sorbitol or other cathartics should *not* be used with each dose, or resulting large stool volumes may lead to dehydration or hypernatremia.

Benson BE et al; American Academy of Clinical Toxicology; European Association of Poisons Centres and Clinical Toxicologists. Position paper update: gastric lavage for gastrointestinal decontamination. Clin Toxicol (Phila). 2013 Mar;51 (3):140–6. [PMID: 23418938]

Dohlman CH et al. Chemical burns to the eye: paradigm shifts in treatment. Cornea. 2011 Jun;30(6):613–4. [PMID: 21242777]
Ghannoum M et al. Enhanced poison elimination in critical care. Adv Chronic Kidney Dis. 2013 Jan;20(1):94–101. [PMID: 23265601]
Isbister GK et al. Indications for single-dose activated charcoal administration in acute overdose. Curr Opin Crit Care. 2011 Aug;17(4):351–7. [PMID: 21716104]

DIAGNOSIS OF POISONING

The identity of the ingested substance or substances is usually known, but occasionally a comatose patient is found with an unlabeled container or the patient is unable or unwilling to give a coherent history. By performing a directed physical examination and ordering common clinical laboratory tests, the clinician can often make a tentative diagnosis that may allow empiric interventions or may suggest specific toxicologic tests.

▶ Physical Examination

Important diagnostic variables in the physical examination include blood pressure, pulse rate, temperature, pupil size, sweating, and the presence or absence of peristaltic activity. Poisonings may present with one or more of the following common syndromes.

A. Sympathomimetic Syndrome

The blood pressure and pulse rate are elevated, though with severe hypertension reflex bradycardia may occur. The temperature is often elevated, pupils are dilated, and the skin is sweaty, though mucous membranes are dry. Patients are usually agitated, anxious, or frankly psychotic.

Examples: Amphetamines, cocaine, ephedrine, and pseudoephedrine.

B. Sympatholytic Syndrome

The blood pressure and pulse rate are decreased and body temperature is low. The pupils are small or even pinpoint. Patients are usually obtunded or comatose.

Examples: Barbiturates, benzodiazepines and other sedative hypnotics, gamma-hydroxybutyrate (GHB), clonidine and related antihypertensives, ethanol, opioids.

C. Cholinergic Syndrome

Stimulation of muscarinic receptors causes bradycardia, miosis, sweating, and hyperperistalsis as well as bronchorrhea, wheezing, excessive salivation, and urinary incontinence. Nicotinic receptor stimulation may produce initial hypertension and tachycardia as well as fasciculations and muscle weakness. Patients are usually agitated and anxious.

Examples: Carbamates, nicotine, organophosphates (including nerve agents), physostigmine.

D. Anticholinergic Syndrome

Tachycardia with mild hypertension is common, and the body temperature is often elevated. Pupils are widely dilated.

The skin is flushed, hot, and dry. Peristalsis is decreased, and urinary retention is common. Patients may have myoclonic jerking or choreoathetoid movements. Agitated delirium is frequently seen, and severe hyperthermia may occur.

Examples: Atropine, scopolamine, other naturally occurring and pharmaceutical anticholinergics, antihistamines, tricyclic antidepressants.

▶ Laboratory Tests

The following clinical laboratory tests are recommended for screening of the overdosed patient: measured serum osmolality and osmol gap, electrolytes and anion gap, glucose, creatinine, blood urea nitrogen (BUN), creatine kinase, urinalysis (eg, oxalate crystals with ethylene glycol poisoning, myoglobinuria with rhabdomyolysis), and electrocardiography. Serum acetaminophen and ethanol quantitative levels should be determined in all patients with drug overdoses.

A. Osmol Gap

The osmol gap (see Table 38–5) is increased in the presence of large quantities of low-molecular-weight substances, most commonly ethanol. Common poisons associated with increased osmol gap are acetone, ethanol, ethylene glycol, isopropyl alcohol, methanol, and propylene glycol. **Note:** Severe alcoholic ketoacidosis and diabetic ketoacidosis can also cause an elevated osmol gap resulting from the production of ketones and other low-molecular-weight substances.

B. Anion Gap

Metabolic acidosis associated with an elevated anion gap is usually due to an accumulation of lactic acid or other acids (see Chapter 21). Common causes of elevated anion gap in poisoning include carbon monoxide, cyanide, ethylene glycol, medicinal iron, INH, methanol, metformin, ibuprofen and salicylates. Massive acetaminophen overdose can cause early-onset anion gap metabolic acidosis.

Table 38–5. Use of the osmol gap in toxicology.

The osmol gap (Delta osm) is determined by subtracting the calculated serum osmolality from the measured serum osmolality.

$$\text{Calculated osmolality (osm)} = 2[Na^+(mEq/L)] + \frac{\text{Glucose (mg/dL)}}{18} + \frac{\text{BUN (mg/dL)}}{2.8}$$

Delta osm = Measured osmolality – Calculated osmolality = 0 ± 10

Serum osmolality may be increased by contributions of exogenous substances such as alcohols and other low-molecular-weight substances. Since these substances are not included in the calculated osmolality, there will be a gap proportionate to their serum concentration. Contact a medical toxicologist or poison control center for assistance in calculating and interpreting the osmol gap.

The osmol gap should also be checked; combined elevated anion and osmol gaps suggests poisoning by methanol or ethylene glycol, though this may also occur in patients with diabetic ketoacidosis and alcoholic ketoacidosis.

C. Toxicology Laboratory Testing

A comprehensive toxicology screen is of little value in the initial care of the poisoned patient because results usually do not return in time to influence clinical management. Specific quantitative levels of certain drugs may be extremely helpful (Table 38–6), however, especially if specific antidotes or interventions (eg, dialysis) would be indicated based on the results.

Table 38–6. Specific quantitative levels and potential therapeutic interventions.[1]

Drug or Toxin	Treatment
Acetaminophen	Specific antidote (*N*-acetylcysteine) based on serum level
Carbon monoxide	High carboxyhemoglobin level indicates need for 100% oxygen, consideration of hyperbaric oxygen
Carbamazepine	High level may indicate need for hemodialysis
Digoxin	On basis of serum digoxin level and severity of clinical presentation, treatment with Fab antibody fragments (eg, DigiFab) may be indicated
Ethanol	Low serum level may suggest nonalcoholic cause of coma (eg, trauma, other drugs, other alcohols). Serum ethanol may also be useful in monitoring ethanol therapy for methanol or ethylene glycol poisoning.
Iron	Level may indicate need for chelation with deferoxamine
Lithium	Serum levels can guide decision to institute hemodialysis
Methanol, ethylene glycol	Acidosis, high levels indicate need for hemodialysis, therapy with ethanol or fomepizole
Methemoglobin	Methemoglobinemia can be treated with methylene blue intravenously
Salicylates	High level may indicate need for hemodialysis, alkaline diuresis
Theophylline	Immediate hemodialysis or hemoperfusion may be indicated based on serum level
Valproic acid	Elevated levels may indicate need to consider hemodialysis or L-carnitine therapy, or both

[1]Some drugs or toxins may have profound and irreversible toxicity unless rapid and specific management is provided outside of routine supportive care. For these agents, laboratory testing may provide the serum level or other evidence required for administering a specific antidote or arranging for hemodialysis.

If a toxicology screen is required, urine is the best specimen. Many hospitals can perform a quick but limited screen for "drugs of abuse" (typically these screens include only opiates, amphetamines, and cocaine, and some add benzodiazepines, barbiturates, methadone, and tetrahydrocannabinol [marijuana]). There are numerous false-positive and false-negative results. For example, synthetic opioids, such as fentanyl, oxycodone, and methadone, are often not detected by routine opiate screening. Blood samples may be saved for possible quantitative testing, but blood is not generally used for screening purposes since it is relatively insensitive for many common drugs, including psychotropic agents, opioids, and stimulants.

► Abdominal Radiographs

A plain film of the abdomen may reveal radiopaque iron tablets, drug-filled condoms, or other toxic material. Studies suggest that few tablets are predictably visible (eg, ferrous sulfate, sodium chloride, calcium carbonate, and potassium chloride). Thus, the radiograph is useful only if abnormal.

► When to Refer

Consultation with a regional poison control center (1-800-222-1222) or a medical toxicologist is recommended when the diagnosis is uncertain; there are questions about what laboratory tests to order; when dialysis is being considered to remove the drug or poison; or when advice is needed regarding the indications, dose, and side effects of antidotes.

► When to Admit

- The patient has symptoms and signs of intoxication that are not expected to clear within a 6–8 hour observation period.
- Delayed absorption of the drug might be predicted to cause a later onset of serious symptoms (eg, after ingestion of a sustained-release product).
- Continued administration of an antidote is required (eg, N-acetylcysteine for acetaminophen overdose).
- Psychiatric or social services evaluation is needed for suicide attempt or suspected drug abuse.

Goldfrank LR (editor). *Goldfrank's Toxicologic Emergencies*, 9th ed. McGraw-Hill, 2010.
Holstege CP et al. Toxidromes. Crit Care Clin. 2012 Oct; 28(4):479–98. [PMID: 22998986]
Olson KR (editor). *Poisoning & Drug Overdose*, 6th ed. McGraw-Hill, 2011.

▼ SELECTED POISONINGS

ACETAMINOPHEN

Acetaminophen (paracetamol in the United Kingdom, Europe) is a common analgesic found in many nonprescription and prescription products. After absorption, it is metabolized mainly by glucuronidation and sulfation, with a small fraction metabolized via the P450 mixed-function oxidase system (2E1) to a highly toxic reactive intermediate. This toxic intermediate is normally detoxified by cellular glutathione. With acute acetaminophen overdose (> 150–200 mg/kg, or 8–10 g in an average adult), hepatocellular glutathione is depleted and the reactive intermediate attacks other cell proteins, causing necrosis. Patients with enhanced P450 2E1 activity, such as those who chronically abuse alcohol and patients taking INH, are at increased risk for developing hepatotoxicity. Hepatic toxicity may also occur after overuse of acetaminophen—eg, as a result of taking two or three acetaminophen-containing products concurrently or exceeding the recommended maximum dose of 4 g/d for several days.

► Clinical Findings

Shortly after ingestion, patients may have nausea or vomiting, but there are usually no other signs of toxicity until 24–48 hours after ingestion, when hepatic aminotransferase levels begin to increase. With severe poisoning, fulminant hepatic necrosis may occur, resulting in jaundice, hepatic encephalopathy, advanced chronic kidney disease, and death. Rarely, massive ingestion (eg, serum levels > 500–1000 mg/L [33–66 mmol/L]) can cause early onset of acute coma, seizures, hypotension, and metabolic acidosis unrelated to hepatic injury.

The diagnosis after acute overdose is based on measurement of the serum acetaminophen level. Plot the serum level versus the time since ingestion on the acetaminophen nomogram shown in Figure 38–1. Ingestion of sustained-release products or coingestion of an anticholinergic agent, salicylate, or opioid drug may cause delayed elevation of serum levels which can make it difficult to interpret the nomogram. The nomogram is also not useful after repeated overdose.

► Treatment

A. Emergency and Supportive Measures

Administer activated charcoal (see p. 1554) if it can be given within 1–2 hours of the ingestion. Although charcoal may interfere with absorption of the oral antidote acetylcysteine, this is not considered clinically significant.

B. Specific Treatment

Although the risk is greatest if the serum acetaminophen level is above the upper line on the nomogram (Figure 38–1), many clinicians and published guidelines prefer to use the lower line as a guide to treatment, as it provides an added safety margin. If the precise time of ingestion is unknown or if the patient is at higher risk for hepatotoxicity (eg, alcoholic, liver disease, long-term use of P450-inducing drugs), then some clinicians use a lower threshold for initiation of N-acetylcysteine (in some case reports, a level of 100 mg/L [66 mmol/L] at 4 hours was suggested in very high-risk patients).

The antidote N-acetylcysteine can be given orally or intravenously. Oral treatment begins with a loading dose of N-acetylcysteine, 140 mg/kg, followed by 70 mg/kg every

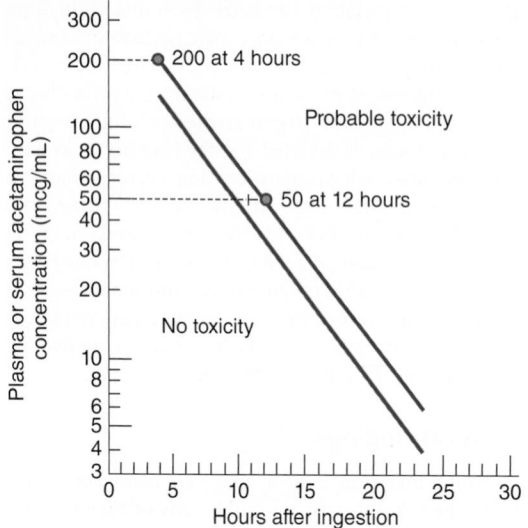

▲ **Figure 38–1.** Nomogram for prediction of acetaminophen hepatotoxicity following acute overdosage. The upper line defines serum acetaminophen concentrations associated with a risk of hepatotoxicity; the lower line defines serum levels 25% below those expected to cause hepatotoxicity. In uncomplicated cases, the upper line can be used as an indication for therapy with N-acetylcysteine. However, to provide a margin for error in the estimation of the time of ingestion and for patients at higher risk for hepatotoxicity, the lower line is usually used as a guide to treatment. (Adapted, with permission, from Rumack BH et al. Acetaminophen poisoning and toxicity. Pediatrics. 1975 Jun;55(6):871–6.)

4 hours. Dilute the solution to about 5% with water, juice, or soda. If vomiting interferes with oral N-acetylcysteine administration, consider giving the antidote intravenously (see below). The conventional oral N-acetylcysteine protocol in the United States calls for 72 hours of treatment. However, other regimens have demonstrated equivalent success with 20–48 hours of treatment.

The FDA-approved 21-hour intravenous regimen of acetylcysteine (Acetadote) calls for a loading dose of 150 mg/kg given intravenously over 60 minutes, followed by a 4-hour infusion of 50 mg/kg, and a 16-hour infusion of 100 mg/kg. (If Acetadote is not available, the conventional oral formulation may also be given intravenously using a micropore filter and a slow rate of infusion. Call a regional poison control center or medical toxicologist for assistance.)

Treatment with N-acetylcysteine is most effective if it is started within 8–10 hours after ingestion.

Hodgman MJ et al. A review of acetaminophen poisoning. Crit Care Clin. 2012 Oct;28(4):499–516. [PMID: 22998987]
Rumack BH et al. Acetaminophen and acetylcysteine dose and duration: past, present and future. Clin Toxicol (Phila). 2012 Feb;50(2):91–8. [PMID: 22320209]
Wolf MS et al. Risk of unintentional overdose with non-prescription acetaminophen products. J Gen Intern Med. 2012 Dec;27 (12):1587–93. [PMID: 22638604]

ACIDS, CORROSIVE

The strong mineral acids exert primarily a local corrosive effect on the skin and mucous membranes. Symptoms include severe pain in the throat and upper gastrointestinal tract; bloody vomitus; difficulty in swallowing, breathing, and speaking; discoloration and destruction of skin and mucous membranes in and around the mouth; and shock. Severe systemic metabolic acidosis may occur both as a result of cellular injury and from systemic absorption of the acid.

Severe deep destructive tissue damage may occur after exposure to hydrofluoric acid because of the penetrating and highly toxic fluoride ion. Systemic hypocalcemia and hyperkalemia may also occur after fluoride absorption, even following skin exposure.

Inhalation of volatile acids, fumes, or gases such as chlorine, fluorine, bromine, or iodine causes severe irritation of the throat and larynx and may cause upper airway obstruction and noncardiogenic pulmonary edema.

▶ Treatment

A. Ingestion

Dilute immediately by giving a glass (4–8 oz) of water to drink. Do *not* give bicarbonate or other neutralizing agents, and do *not* induce vomiting. Some experts recommend immediate cautious placement of a small flexible gastric tube and removal of stomach contents followed by lavage, particularly if the corrosive is a liquid or has important systemic toxicity.

In symptomatic patients, perform flexible endoscopic esophagoscopy to determine the presence and extent of injury. CT scan or plain radiographs of the chest and abdomen may also reveal the extent of injury. Perforation, peritonitis, and major bleeding are indications for surgery.

B. Skin Contact

Flood with water for 15 minutes. Use no chemical antidotes; the heat of the reaction may cause additional injury.

For hydrofluoric acid burns, soak the affected area in benzalkonium chloride solution or apply 2.5% calcium gluconate gel (prepared by adding 3.5 g calcium gluconate to 5 oz of water-soluble surgical lubricant, eg, K-Y Jelly); then arrange immediate consultation with a plastic surgeon or other specialist. Binding of the fluoride ion may be achieved by injecting 0.5 mL of 5% calcium gluconate per square centimeter under the burned area. (**Caution:** *Do not use calcium chloride.*) Use of a Bier-block technique or intra-arterial infusion of calcium is sometimes required for extensive burns or those involving the nail bed; consult with a hand surgeon or poison control center (1-800-222-1222).

C. Eye Contact

Anesthetize the conjunctiva and corneal surfaces with topical local anesthetic drops (eg, proparacaine). Flood with water for 15 minutes, holding the eyelids open. Check pH with pH 6.0–8.0 test paper, and repeat irrigation, using

0.9% saline, until pH is near 7.0. Check for corneal damage with fluorescein and slit-lamp examination; consult an ophthalmologist about further treatment.

D. Inhalation

Remove from further exposure to fumes or gas. Check skin and clothing. Treat pulmonary edema.

Singh P et al. Ocular chemical injuries and their management. Oman J Ophthalmol. 2013 May;6(2):83–86. [PMID: 24082664]

ALKALIES

The strong alkalies are common ingredients of some household cleaning compounds and may be suspected by their "soapy" texture. Those with alkalinity above pH 12.0 are particularly corrosive. Disk (or "button") batteries are also a source. Alkalies cause liquefactive necrosis, which is deeply penetrating. Symptoms include burning pain in the upper gastrointestinal tract, nausea, vomiting, and difficulty in swallowing and breathing. Examination reveals destruction and edema of the affected skin and mucous membranes and bloody vomitus and stools. Radiographs may reveal evidence of perforation or the presence of radiopaque disk batteries in the esophagus or lower gastrointestinal tract.

► Treatment

A. Ingestion

Dilute immediately with a glass of water. Do *not* induce emesis. Some gastroenterologists recommend immediate cautious placement of a small flexible gastric tube and removal of stomach contents followed by gastric lavage after ingestion of liquid caustic substances to remove residual material.

Prompt endoscopy is recommended in symptomatic patients to evaluate the extent of damage; CT scanning may also aid in assessment. If a radiograph reveals the location of ingested disk batteries in the esophagus, immediate endoscopic removal is mandatory.

The use of corticosteroids to prevent stricture formation is of no proved benefit and is definitely contraindicated if there is evidence of esophageal perforation.

B. Skin Contact

Wash with running water until the skin no longer feels soapy. Relieve pain and treat shock.

C. Eye Contact

Anesthetize the conjunctival and corneal surfaces with topical anesthetic (eg, proparacaine). Irrigate with water or saline continuously for 20–30 minutes, holding the lids open. Amphoteric solutions may be more effective than water or saline and some are available in Europe (Diphoterine, Previn). Check pH with pH test paper, and repeat irrigation for additional 30-minute periods until the pH is near 7.0. Check for corneal damage with fluorescein and slit-lamp examination; consult an ophthalmologist for further treatment.

Pavelites JJ et al. Deaths related to chemical burns. Am J Forensic Med Pathol. 2011 Dec;32(4):387–92. [PMID: 21860322]

AMPHETAMINES & COCAINE

Amphetamines and cocaine are widely abused for their euphorigenic and stimulant properties. Both drugs may be smoked, snorted, ingested, or injected. Amphetamines and cocaine produce central nervous system stimulation and a generalized increase in central and peripheral sympathetic activity. The toxic dose of each drug is highly variable and depends on the route of administration and individual tolerance. The onset of effects is most rapid after intravenous injection or smoking. Amphetamine derivatives and related drugs include methamphetamine ("crystal meth," "crank"), MDMA ("Ecstasy"), ephedrine ("herbal ecstasy"), and methcathinone ("cat" or "khat"). Methcathinone derivatives and related synthetic chemicals such as methylenedioxypyrovalerone (MDPV) have become popular drugs of abuse and are often sold as purported "bath salts." Amphetamine-like reactions have also been reported after use of synthetic cannabinoids (eg, "Spice" and "K2"). Nonprescription medications and nutritional supplements may contain stimulant or sympathomimetic drugs such as ephedrine, yohimbine, or caffeine (see also Theophylline section).

► Clinical Findings

Presenting symptoms may include anxiety, tremulousness, tachycardia, hypertension, diaphoresis, dilated pupils, agitation, muscular hyperactivity, and psychosis. Muscle hyperactivity may lead to metabolic acidosis and rhabdomyolysis. In severe intoxication, seizures and hyperthermia may occur. Sustained or severe hypertension may result in intracranial hemorrhage, aortic dissection, or myocardial infarction. Ischemic colitis has been reported. Hyponatremia has been reported after MDMA use; the mechanism is not known but may involve excessive water intake, syndrome of inappropriate antidiuretic hormone (SIADH), or both.

The diagnosis is supported by finding amphetamines or the cocaine metabolite benzoylecgonine in the urine. Note that many drugs can give a false-positive result on the immunoassay for amphetamines.

► Treatment

A. Emergency and Supportive Measures

Maintain a patent airway and assist ventilation, if necessary. Treat seizures as described at the beginning of this chapter (see p. 1552). Rapidly lower the body temperature (see hyperthermia, p. 1552) in patients who are hyperthermic (temperature > 39–40°C). Give intravenous fluids to prevent myoglobinuric renal injury in patients who have rhabdomyolysis.

B. Specific Treatment

Treat agitation, psychosis, or seizures with a benzodiazepine such as diazepam, 5–10 mg, or lorazepam, 2–3 mg intravenously. Add phenobarbital 15 mg/kg intravenously for persistent seizures. Treat hypertension with a vasodilator drug such as phentolamine (1–5 mg intravenously) or a combined alpha- and beta-adrenergic blocker such as labetalol (10–20 mg intravenously). Do *not* administer a pure beta-blocker such as propranolol alone, as this may result in paradoxic worsening of the hypertension as a result of unopposed alpha-adrenergic effects.

Treat tachycardia or tachyarrhythmias with a short-acting beta-blocker such as esmolol (25–100 mcg/kg/min by intravenous infusion). Treat hyperthermia as described above (see p. 1552). Treat hyponatremia as outlined in Chapter 21.

Gibbons S. 'Legal highs'—novel and emerging psychoactive drugs: a chemical overview for the toxicologist. Clin Toxicol (Phila). 2012 Jan;50(1):15–24. [PMID: 22248120]

Prosser JM et al. The toxicology of bath salts: a review of synthetic cathinones. J Med Toxicol. 2012 Mar;8(1):33–42. [PMID: 22108839]

ANTICOAGULANTS

Warfarin and related compounds (including ingredients of many commercial rodenticides, the so-called "superwarfarins" such as brodifacoum, difenacoum, and related compounds) inhibit the clotting mechanism by blocking hepatic synthesis of vitamin K–dependent clotting factors. After ingestion of "superwarfarins," inhibition of clotting factor synthesis may persist for several weeks or even months after a single dose. Newer oral anticoagulants include the direct thrombin inhibitors dabigatran and rivaroxaban.

Excessive anticoagulation may cause hemoptysis, gross hematuria, bloody stools, hemorrhages into organs, widespread bruising, and bleeding into joint spaces. The prothrombin time is increased within 12–24 hours (peak 36–48 hours) after overdose of warfarin or "superwarfarins" but is not as predictably abnormal after overdose of dabigatran or rivaroxiban.

▶ **Treatment**

A. Emergency and Supportive Measures

Discontinue the drug at the first sign of gross bleeding, and determine the prothrombin time (international normalized ratio, INR). If the patient has ingested an acute overdose, administer activated charcoal (see p. 1554).

B. Specific Treatment

Do *not* treat prophylactically with vitamin K—wait for evidence of anticoagulation (elevated prothrombin time). If the INR is elevated, give phytonadione (vitamin K_1), 10–25 mg orally, and increase the dose as needed to restore the prothrombin time to normal. Doses as high as 200 mg/d have been required after ingestion of "superwarfarins."

Give fresh-frozen plasma, prothrombin complex concentrate, or activated Factor VII as needed to rapidly correct the coagulation factor deficit if there is serious bleeding. If the patient is chronically anticoagulated and has strong medical indications for being maintained in that status (eg, prosthetic heart valve), give much smaller doses of vitamin K (1 mg orally) and fresh-frozen plasma (or both) to titrate to the desired prothrombin time.

If the patient has ingested brodifacoum or a related superwarfarin, prolonged observation (over weeks) and repeated administration of large doses of vitamin K may be required.

Vitamin K does not reverse the anticoagulant effects of the direct thrombin inhibitors dabigatran and rivaroxaban. The efficacy of fresh frozen plasma and clotting factor concentrates is uncertain.

Godier A et al. Evaluation of prothrombin complex concentrate and recombinant activated factor VII to reverse rivaroxaban in a rabbit model. Anesthesiology. 2012 Jan;116(1):94–102. [PMID: 22042412]

Siegal DM et al. Acute management of bleeding in patients on novel oral anticoagulants. Eur Heart J. 2013 Feb;34(7):489–498b. [PMID: 23220847]

Watson KS et al. Superwarfarin intoxication: two case reports and review of pathophysiology and patient management. J La State Med Soc. 2012 Mar–Apr;164(2):70–2. [PMID: 22685854]

ANTICONVULSANTS

Anticonvulsants (carbamazepine, phenytoin, valproic acid, and many newer agents) are widely used in the management of seizure disorders and some are also used for treatment of mood disorders or pain.

Phenytoin can be given orally or intravenously. Rapid intravenous injection of phenytoin can cause acute myocardial depression and cardiac arrest owing to the solvent propylene glycol (fosphenytoin does not contain this diluent). Chronic phenytoin intoxication can occur following only slightly increased doses because of zero-order kinetics and a small toxic-therapeutic window. Phenytoin intoxication can also occur following acute intentional or accidental overdose. The overdose syndrome is usually mild even with high serum levels. The most common manifestations are ataxia, nystagmus, and drowsiness. Choreoathetoid movements have been described.

Carbamazepine intoxication causes drowsiness, stupor and, with high levels, atrioventricular block, coma, and seizures. Dilated pupils and tachycardia are common. Toxicity may be seen with serum levels > 20 mg/L (85 mcmol/L), though severe poisoning is usually associated with concentrations > 30–40 mg/L (127–169 mcmol/L). Because of erratic and slow absorption, intoxication may progress over several hours to days.

Valproic acid intoxication produces a unique syndrome consisting of hypernatremia (from the sodium component of the salt), metabolic acidosis, hypocalcemia, elevated serum ammonia, and mild liver aminotransferase elevation. Hypoglycemia may occur as a result of hepatic metabolic dysfunction. Coma with small pupils may be seen and can mimic opioid poisoning. Encephalopathy and cerebral edema can occur.

The newer anticonvulsants **gabapentin, levetiracetam, vigabatrin,** and **zonisamide** generally cause somnolence, confusion and dizziness; **felbamate** can cause crystalluria and kidney dysfunction after overdose, and may cause idiosyncratic aplastic anemia with therapeutic use; **lamotrigine, topiramate,** and **tiagabine** have been reported to cause seizures after overdose.

▶ Treatment

A. Emergency and Supportive Measures

For recent ingestions, give activated charcoal orally or by gastric tube (see p. 1554). For large ingestions of carbamazepine or valproic acid—especially of sustained-release formulations—consider whole bowel irrigation (see p. 1554). Combined multiple-dose activated charcoal and whole-bowel irrigation may be beneficial in ensuring gut decontamination for selected large ingestions.

B. Specific Treatment

There are no specific antidotes. Naloxone was reported to have reversed valproic acid overdose in one anecdotal case. Carnitine may be useful in patients with valproic acid–induced hyperammonemia. Consider hemodialysis for massive intoxication with valproic acid or carbamazepine (eg, carbamazepine levels > 60 mg/L [254 mcmol/L] or valproic acid levels > 800 mg/L [5544 mcmol/L]).

Larkin TM et al. Overdose with levetiracetam: a case report and review of the literature. J Clin Pharm Ther. 2013 Feb;38(1):68–70. [PMID: 22725831]
Ozhasenekler A et al. Benefit of hemodialysis in carbamazepine intoxications with neurological complications. Eur Rev Med Pharmacol Sci. 2012 Mar;16(Suppl 1):43–7. [PMID: 22582484]
Pons S et al. Acute overdose of enteric-coated valproic acid and olanzapine: unusual presentation and delayed toxicity. Clin Toxicol (Phila). 2012 Apr;50(4):268. [PMID: 22385067]

ANTIPSYCHOTIC DRUGS

Promethazine, prochlorperazine, chlorpromazine, haloperidol, droperidol, risperidone, olanzapine, ziprasidone, quetiapine, and aripiprazole are used as antipsychotic agents, and sometimes as antiemetics and potentiators of analgesic and hypnotic drugs.

Phenothiazines (particularly chlorpromazine) induce drowsiness and mild orthostatic hypotension in as many as 50% of patients. Larger doses can cause obtundation, miosis, severe hypotension, tachycardia, convulsions, and coma. Abnormal cardiac conduction may occur, resulting in prolongation of QRS or QT intervals (or both) and ventricular arrhythmias. Among the newer agents, quetiapine is more likely to cause coma and hypotension.

With therapeutic or toxic doses, an acute extrapyramidal dystonic reaction may develop in some patients, with spasmodic contractions of the face and neck muscles, extensor rigidity of the back muscles, carpopedal spasm,

and motor restlessness. This reaction is more common with haloperidol and other butyrophenones and less common with newer atypical antipsychotics such as ziprasidone, olanzapine, aripiprazole, and quetiapine. Severe rigidity accompanied by hyperthermia and metabolic acidosis ("neuroleptic malignant syndrome") may occasionally occur and is life-threatening (see Chapter 25).

▶ Treatment

A. Emergency and Supportive Measures

Administer activated charcoal (see p. 1554) for large or recent ingestions. For severe hypotension, treatment with intravenous fluids and vasopressor agents may be necessary. Treat hyperthermia as outlined on p. 1552. Maintain cardiac monitoring.

B. Specific Treatment

Hypotension and cardiac arrhythmias associated with widened QRS intervals on the ECG in a patient with thioridazine poisoning may respond to intravenous sodium bicarbonate as used for tricyclic antidepressants. Prolongation of the QT interval and torsades de pointes is usually treated with intravenous magnesium or overdrive pacing.

For extrapyramidal signs, give diphenhydramine, 0.5–1 mg/kg intravenously, or benztropine mesylate, 0.01–0.02 mg/kg intramuscularly. Treatment with oral doses of these agents should be continued for 24–48 hours.

Bromocriptine (2.5–7.5 mg orally daily) may be effective for mild or moderate neuroleptic malignant syndrome. Dantrolene (2–5 mg/kg intravenously) has also been used for muscle rigidity but is not a true antidote. For severe hyperthermia, rapid neuromuscular paralysis (see p. 1552) is preferred.

Levine M et al. Overdose of atypical antipsychotics: clinical presentation, mechanisms of toxicity and management. CNS Drugs. 2012 Jul 1;26(7):601–11. Erratum in: CNS Drugs. 2012 Sep 1;26(9):812. [PMID: 22668123]
Minns AB et al. Toxicology and overdose of atypical antipsychotics. J Emerg Med. 2012 Nov;43(5):906–13. [PMID: 22555052]

ARSENIC

Arsenic is found in some pesticides and industrial chemicals and is used as a chemotherapeutic agent. A massive epidemic of chronic arsenic poisoning has occurred in Bangladesh due to naturally occurring arsenic in deep aquifers used for drinking water. Symptoms of acute poisoning usually appear within 1 hour after ingestion but may be delayed as long as 12 hours. They include abdominal pain, vomiting, watery diarrhea, and skeletal muscle cramps. Profound dehydration and shock may occur. In chronic poisoning, symptoms can be vague but often include pancytopenia, painful peripheral sensory neuropathy, and skin changes including melanosis, keratosis, and desquamating rash. Urinary arsenic levels may be falsely elevated after certain meals (eg, seafood) that contain large quantities of a nontoxic form of organic arsenic.

▶ Treatment

A. Emergency Measures

After recent ingestion (within 1–2 hours), perform gastric lavage (see p. 1554). Activated charcoal is of uncertain benefit because it binds arsenic poorly. Administer intravenous fluids to replace losses due to vomiting and diarrhea.

B. Antidote

For patients with severe acute intoxication, administer a chelating agent. The preferred drug is 2,3-dimercaptopropanesulfonic acid (DMPS, Unithiol) (3–5 mg/kg intravenously every 4 hours); although there is no FDA-approved commercial formulation of DMPS in the United States, it can be obtained from some compounding pharmacies. An alternative parenteral chelator is dimercaprol (British anti-Lewisite, BAL), which comes as a 10% solution in peanut oil, and is given 3–5 mg/kg intramuscularly every 4–6 hours for 2 days. The side effects include nausea, vomiting, headache, and hypertension. When gastrointestinal symptoms allow, switch to the oral chelator succimer (dimercaptosuccinic acid, DMSA), 10 mg/kg every 8 hours, for 1 week. Consult a medical toxicologist or regional poison control center (1-800-222-1222) for advice regarding chelation.

Hughes MF et al. Arsenic exposure and toxicology: a historical perspective. Toxicol Sci. 2011 Oct;123(2):305–32. [PMID: 21750349]
Yunus M et al. Arsenic exposure and adverse health effects: a review of recent findings from arsenic and health studies in Matlab, Bangladesh. Kaohsiung J Med Sci. 2011 Sep;27(9):371–6. [PMID: 21914523]

ATROPINE & ANTICHOLINERGICS

Atropine, scopolamine, belladonna, diphenoxylate with atropine, *Datura stramonium, Hyoscyamus niger*, some mushrooms, tricyclic antidepressants, and antihistamines are antimuscarinic agents with variable central nervous system effects. Symptoms of toxicity include dryness of the mouth, thirst, difficulty in swallowing, and blurring of vision. Physical signs include dilated pupils, flushed skin, tachycardia, fever, delirium, myoclonus, ileus, and flushed appearance. Antidepressants and antihistamines may induce convulsions.

Antihistamines are commonly available with or without prescription. Diphenhydramine commonly causes delirium, tachycardia, and seizures. Massive diphenhydramine overdose may mimic tricyclic antidepressant cardiotoxic poisoning.

▶ Treatment

A. Emergency and Supportive Measures

Administer activated charcoal (see p. 1554). External cooling and sedation, or neuromuscular paralysis in rare cases, are indicated to control high temperatures (see p. 1552).

B. Specific Treatment

For severe anticholinergic syndrome (eg, agitated delirium), give physostigmine salicylate, 0.5–1 mg slowly intravenously over 5 minutes, with ECG monitoring; repeat as needed to a total dose of no more than 2 mg. **Caution:** Bradyarrhythmias and convulsions are a hazard with physostigmine administration, and the drug should be avoided in patients with cardiotoxic effects from tricyclic antidepressants or other sodium channel blockers.

Cole JB et al. Wide complex tachycardia in a pediatric diphenhydramine overdose treated with sodium bicarbonate. Pediatr Emerg Care. 2011 Dec;27(12):1175–7. [PMID: 22158278]
Rosenbaum C et al. Timing and frequency of physostigmine redosing for antimuscarinic toxicity. J Med Toxicol. 2010 Dec;6(4):386–92. [PMID: 20405266]

BETA-ADRENERGIC BLOCKERS

There are a wide variety of beta-adrenergic blocking drugs, with varying pharmacologic and pharmacokinetic properties (see Table 11–6). The most toxic beta-blocker is propranolol, which not only blocks beta-1 and beta-2 adrenoceptors but also has direct membrane-depressant and central nervous system effects.

▶ Clinical Findings

The most common findings with mild or moderate intoxication are hypotension and bradycardia. Cardiac depression from more severe poisoning is often unresponsive to conventional therapy with beta-adrenergic stimulants such as dopamine and norepinephrine. In addition, with propranolol and other lipid-soluble drugs, seizures and coma may occur. Propranolol, oxprenolol, acebutolol, and alprenolol also have membrane-depressant effects and can cause conduction disturbance (wide QRS interval) similar to tricyclic antidepressant overdose.

The diagnosis is based on typical clinical findings. Routine toxicology screening does not usually include beta-blockers.

▶ Treatment

A. Emergency and Supportive Measures

Attempts to treat bradycardia or heart block with atropine (0.5–2 mg intravenously), isoproterenol (2–20 mcg/min by intravenous infusion, titrated to the desired heart rate), or an external transcutaneous cardiac pacemaker are often ineffective, and specific antidotal treatment may be necessary (see below).

For drugs ingested within an hour of presentation (or longer after ingestion of an extended-release formulation), administer activated charcoal (see p. 1554).

B. Specific Treatment

For persistent bradycardia and hypotension, give glucagon, 5–10 mg intravenously, followed by an infusion of 1–5 mg/h. Glucagon is an inotropic agent that acts at a different receptor site and is therefore not affected by beta-blockade. High-dose insulin (0.5-1 units/kg/h intravenously) along with glucose supplementation has been used to reverse severe cardiotoxicity. Membrane-depressant effects (wide QRS interval) may respond to boluses of sodium bicarbonate (50–100 mEq intravenously) as for tricyclic antidepressant poisoning. Intravenous lipid emulsion (Intralipid 20%, 1.5 mL/kg) has been used successfully in severe propranolol overdose.

Jovic-Stosic J et al. Severe propranolol and ethanol overdose with wide complex tachycardia treated with intravenous lipid emulsion: a case report. Clin Toxicol (Phila). 2011 Jun;49(5): 426–30. [PMID: 21740142]

CALCIUM CHANNEL BLOCKERS

In therapeutic doses, nifedipine, nicardipine, amlodipine, felodipine, isradipine, nisoldipine, and nimodipine act mainly on blood vessels, while verapamil and diltiazem act mainly on cardiac contractility and conduction. However, these selective effects can be lost after acute overdose. Patients may present with bradycardia, atrioventricular (AV) nodal block, hypotension, or a combination of these effects. Hyperglycemia is common due to blockade of insulin release. With severe poisoning, cardiac arrest may occur.

▶ Treatment

A. Emergency and Supportive Measures

For ingested drugs, administer activated charcoal (see p. 1554). In addition, whole bowel irrigation (see p. 1554) should be initiated as soon as possible if the patient has ingested a sustained-release product.

B. Specific Treatment

If bradycardia and hypotension are not reversed with atropine (0.5–2 mg intravenously), isoproterenol (2–20 mcg/ min by intravenous infusion), or a transcutaneous cardiac pacemaker, administer calcium intravenously. Start with calcium chloride 10%, 10 mL, or calcium gluconate 10%, 20 mL. Repeat the dose every 3–5 minutes. The optimum (or maximum) dose has not been established, but many toxicologists recommend raising the ionized serum calcium level to as much as twice the normal level. Calcium is most useful in reversing negative inotropic effects and is less effective for AV nodal blockade and bradycardia. High doses of insulin (0.5–1 units/kg intravenous bolus followed by 0.5–1 units/kg/h infusion) along with sufficient dextrose to maintain euglycemia have been reported to be beneficial but there are no controlled studies. Infusion of Intralipid 20% lipid emulsion has been reported to improve hemodynamics in animal models and case reports of calcium channel blocker poisoning.

Cave G et al. Intravenous lipid emulsion as antidote: a summary of published human experience. Emerg Med Australas. 2011 Apr;23(2):123–41. [PMID: 21489160]

Engebretsen KM et al. High-dose insulin therapy in beta-blocker and calcium channel-blocker poisoning. Clin Toxicol (Phila). 2011 Apr;49(4):277–83. [PMID: 21563902]

CARBON MONOXIDE

Carbon monoxide is a colorless, odorless gas produced by the combustion of carbon-containing materials. Poisoning may occur as a result of suicidal or accidental exposure to automobile exhaust, smoke inhalation in a fire, or accidental exposure to an improperly vented gas heater, generator, or other appliance. Carbon monoxide avidly binds to hemoglobin, with an affinity approximately 250 times that of oxygen. This results in reduced oxygen-carrying capacity and altered delivery of oxygen to cells (see also Smoke Inhalation in Chapter 9).

▶ Clinical Findings

At low carbon monoxide levels (carboxyhemoglobin saturation 10–20%), victims may have headache, dizziness, abdominal pain, and nausea. With higher levels, confusion, dyspnea, and syncope may occur. Hypotension, coma, and seizures are common with levels > 50–60%. Survivors of acute severe poisoning may develop permanent obvious or subtle neurologic and neuropsychiatric deficits. The fetus and newborn may be more susceptible because of high carbon monoxide affinity for fetal hemoglobin.

Carbon monoxide poisoning should be suspected in any person with severe headache or acutely altered mental status, especially during cold weather, when improperly vented heating systems may have been used. Diagnosis depends on specific measurement of the arterial or venous carboxyhemoglobin saturation, although the level may have declined if high-flow oxygen therapy has already been administered, and levels do not always correlate with clinical symptoms. Routine arterial blood gas testing and pulse oximetry are not useful because they give falsely normal PaO_2 and oxyhemoglobin saturation determinations, respectively. (A specialized pulse oximetry device, the Masimo pulse CO-oximeter, is capable of distinguishing oxyhemoglobin from carboxyhemoglobin.)

▶ Treatment

A. Emergency and Supportive Measures

Maintain a patent airway and assist ventilation, if necessary. Remove the victim from exposure. Treat patients with coma, hypotension, or seizures as described at the beginning of this chapter.

B. Specific Treatment

The half-life of the carboxyhemoglobin (CoHb) complex is about 4–5 hours in room air but is reduced dramatically by high concentrations of oxygen. Administer 100% oxygen by tight-fitting high-flow reservoir face mask or endotracheal tube. Hyperbaric oxygen (HBO) can provide 100% oxygen under higher than atmospheric pressures, further shortening the half-life; it may also reduce the incidence of subtle neuropsychiatric sequelae. Randomized controlled studies disagree about the benefit of HBO, but commonly recommended indications for HBO in patients with carbon monoxide poisoning include a history of loss of consciousness, CoHb > 25%, metabolic acidosis, age over 50 years, and cerebellar findings on neurologic examination.

Buckley NA et al. Hyperbaric oxygen for carbon monoxide poisoning. Cochrane Database Syst Rev. 2011 Apr 13;(4): CD002041. [PMID: 21491385]

Guzman JA. Carbon monoxide poisoning. Crit Care Clin. 2012 Oct;28(4):537–48. [PMID: 22998990]

CLONIDINE & OTHER SYMPATHOLYTIC ANTIHYPERTENSIVES

Overdosage with these agents (clonidine, guanabenz, guanfacine, methyldopa) causes bradycardia, hypotension, miosis, respiratory depression, and coma. (Transient hypertension occasionally occurs after acute overdosage, a result of peripheral alpha-adrenergic effects in high doses.) Symptoms are usually resolved in < 24 hours, and deaths are rare. Similar symptoms may occur after ingestion of topical nasal decongestants chemically similar to clonidine (oxymetazoline, tetrahydrozoline, naphazoline). Brimonidine and apraclonidine are used as ophthalmic preparations for glaucoma. Tizanidine is a centrally acting muscle relaxant structurally related to clonidine; it produces similar toxicity in overdose.

▶ Treatment

A. Emergency and Supportive Measures

Give activated charcoal (see p. 1554). Maintain the airway and support respiration if necessary. Symptomatic treatment is usually sufficient even in massive overdose. Maintain blood pressure with intravenous fluids. Dopamine can also be used. Atropine is usually effective for bradycardia.

B. Specific Treatment

There is no specific antidote. Although tolazoline has been recommended for clonidine overdose, its effects are unpredictable and it should not be used. Naloxone has been reported to be successful in a few anecdotal and poorly substantiated cases.

Perruchoud C et al. Severe hypertension following accidental clonidine overdose during the refilling of an implanted intrathecal drug delivery system. Neuromodulation. 2012 Jan–Feb;15(1):31–4. [PMID: 21943355]

COCAINE

See Amphetamines & Cocaine.

CYANIDE

Cyanide is a highly toxic chemical used widely in research and commercial laboratories and many industries. Its gaseous form, hydrogen cyanide, is an important component of smoke in fires. Cyanide-generating glycosides are also found in the pits of apricots and other related plants. Cyanide is generated by the breakdown of nitroprusside, and poisoning can result from rapid high-dose infusions. Cyanide is also formed by metabolism of acetonitrile, a solvent found in some over-the-counter fingernail glue removers. Cyanide is rapidly absorbed by inhalation, skin absorption, or ingestion. It disrupts cellular function by inhibiting cytochrome oxidase and preventing cellular oxygen utilization.

▶ Clinical Findings

The onset of toxicity is nearly instantaneous after inhalation of hydrogen cyanide gas but may be delayed for minutes to hours after ingestion of cyanide salts or cyanogenic plants or chemicals. Effects include headache, dizziness, nausea, abdominal pain, and anxiety, followed by confusion, syncope, shock, seizures, coma, and death. The odor of "bitter almonds" may be detected on the victim's breath or in vomitus, though this is not a reliable finding. The venous oxygen saturation may be elevated (> 90%) in severe poisonings because tissues have failed to take up arterial oxygen.

▶ Treatment

A. Emergency and Supportive Measures

Remove the victim from exposure, taking care to avoid exposure to rescuers. For suspected cyanide poisoning due to nitroprusside infusion, stop or slow the rate of infusion. (Metabolic acidosis and other signs of cyanide poisoning usually clear rapidly.)

For cyanide ingestion, administer activated charcoal (see p. 1554). Although charcoal has a low affinity for cyanide, the usual doses of 60–100 g are adequate to bind typically ingested lethal doses (100–200 mg).

B. Specific Treatment

In the United States, there are two available cyanide antidote regimens. The conventional cyanide antidote package (Taylor Pharmaceuticals) contains nitrites (to induce methemoglobinemia, which binds free cyanide) and thiosulfate (to promote conversion of cyanide to the less toxic thiocyanate). Administer amyl nitrite by crushing an ampule under the victim's nose or at the end of the endotracheal tube, and administer 3% sodium nitrite solution, 10 mL intravenously. **Caution:** Nitrites may induce hypotension and dangerous levels of methemoglobin. Also administer 25% sodium thiosulfate solution, 50 mL intravenously (12.5 g).

The other approved cyanide treatment in the United States is hydroxocobalamin (Cyanokit, EMD Pharmaceuticals), a newer and potentially safer antidote. The adult dose of hydroxocobalamin is 5 g intravenously (children's dose is, 70 mg/kg).

Anseeuw K et al. Cyanide poisoning by fire smoke inhalation: a European expert consensus. Eur J Emerg Med. 2013 Feb;20 (1):2–9. [PMID: 22828651]

Lawson-Smith P et al. Cyanide intoxication as part of smoke inhalation—a review on diagnosis and treatment from the emergency perspective. Scand J Trauma Resusc Emerg Med. 2011 Mar 3;19:14. [PMID: 21371322]

Thompson JP et al. Hydroxocobalamin in cyanide poisoning. Clin Toxicol (Phila). 2012 Dec;50(10):875–85. [PMID: 23163594]

DIETARY SUPPLEMENTS & HERBAL PRODUCTS

Unlike prescription and over-the-counter pharmaceuticals, dietary supplements do not require FDA approval, do not undergo the same premarketing evaluation of safety and efficacy as drugs, and purveyors may or may not adhere to good manufacturing practices and quality control standards. Supplements may cause illness as a result of intrinsic toxicity, misidentification or mislabeling, drug-herb reactions, or adulteration with pharmaceuticals. If you suspect a dietary supplement or herbal product may be the cause of an otherwise unexplained illness, contact the FDA (1-888-463-6332) or the regional poison control center (1-800-222-1222), or consult one of the following online databases: http://www.naturaldatabase.therapeuticresearch.com and, http://www.fda.gov/food/dietarysupplements/default.htm.

Table 38–7 lists selected examples of clinical toxicity from some of these products.

Pendleton M et al. Potential toxicity of caffeine when used as a dietary supplement for weight loss. J Diet Suppl. 2012 Dec;9 (4):293–8. [PMID: 23157583]

Posadzki P et al. Contamination and adulteration of herbal medicinal products (HMPs): an overview of systematic reviews. Eur J Clin Pharmacol. 2013 Mar;69(3):295–307. [PMID: 22843016]

Teschke R et al. Herbal hepatotoxicity: a critical review. Br J Clin Pharmacol. 2013 Mar;75(3):630–6. [PMID: 22831551]

DIGITALIS & OTHER CARDIAC GLYCOSIDES

Cardiac glycosides paralyze the Na^+-K^+-ATPase pump and have potent vagotonic effects. Intracellular effects include enhancement of calcium-dependent contractility and shortening of the action potential duration. A number of plants (eg, oleander, foxglove, lily-of-the-valley) contain cardiac glycosides. Bufotenin, a cardiotoxic steroid found in certain toad secretions and used as an herbal medicine and a purported aphrodisiac, has pharmacologic properties similar to cardiac glycosides.

▶ Clinical Findings

Intoxication may result from acute single exposure or chronic accidental overmedication. After acute overdosage, nausea and vomiting, bradycardia, hyperkalemia, and AV block frequently occur. Patients in whom toxicity develops gradually during long-term therapy may be hypokalemic and hypomagnesemic owing to concurrent diuretic treatment and more commonly present with ventricular arrhythmias (eg, ectopy, bidirectional ventricular tachycardia, or ventricular fibrillation). Digoxin levels may be only slightly elevated in patients with intoxication from cardiac glycosides other than digoxin because of limited cross-reactivity of immunologic tests.

▶ Treatment

A. Emergency and Supportive Measures

After acute ingestion, administer activated charcoal (see p. 1554). Monitor potassium levels and cardiac rhythm closely. Treat bradycardia initially with atropine (0.5–2 mg intravenously) or a transcutaneous external cardiac pacemaker.

Table 38–7. Examples of potential toxicity associated with some dietary supplements and herbal medicines.

Product	Common Use	Possible Toxicity
Azarcon (Greta)	Mexican folk remedy for abdominal pain, colic	Contains lead (see p. 1554)
Comfrey	Gastric upset, diarrhea	Contains pyrrolizidine alkaloids, can cause hepatic veno-occlusive disease
Creatine	Athletic performance enhancement	Nausea, diarrhea, abdominal cramps; elevated serum creatinine
Ginkgo	Memory improvement, tinnitus	Antiplatelet effects, hemorrhage; abdominal pain, diarrhea
Ginseng	Immune system; stress	Decreased glucose; increased cortisol
Guarana	Athletic performance enhancement, appetite suppression	Contains caffeine: can cause tremor, tachycardia, vomiting
Kava	Anxiety, insomnia	Drowsiness, hepatitis, skin rash
Ma huang	Stimulant; athletic performance enhancement	Contains ephedrine: anxiety, insomnia, hypertension, tachycardia, seizures
Spirulina	Body building	Niacin-like flushing reaction
Yohimbine	Sexual enhancement	Hallucinations, hypertension, tachycardia
Zinc	Cold/flu symptoms	Nausea, oral irritation, anosmia

Adapted, with permission, from Table II-30 by Haller C in "Herbal and Alternative Products," In: Olson KR (ed.) *Poisoning & Drug Overdose*, 5th edition, McGraw Hill, 2007.

B. Specific Treatment

For patients with significant intoxication, administer digoxin-specific antibodies (digoxin immune Fab [ovine]; Digibind or DigiFab). Estimation of the Digibind dose is based on the body burden of digoxin calculated from the ingested dose or the steady-state serum digoxin concentration, as described below. More effective binding of digoxin may be achieved if the dose is given partly as a bolus and the remainder as an infusion over a few hours.

1. From the ingested dose—Number of vials = approximately 1.5–2 × ingested dose (mg).

2. From the serum concentration—Number of vials = serum digoxin (ng/mL) × body weight (kg) × 10^{-2}. **Note:** This is based on the equilibrium digoxin level; after acute overdose, serum levels may be falsely high for several hours before tissue distribution is complete, and overestimation of the Digibind or DigiFab dose is likely.

3. Empiric dosing—Empiric titration of Digibind or Digi-Fab may be used if the patient's condition is relatively stable and an underlying condition (eg, atrial fibrillation) favors retaining a residual level of digitalis activity. Start with one or two vials and reassess the patient's clinical condition after 20–30 minutes. For cardiac glycosides other than digoxin or digitoxin, there is no formula for estimation of vials needed and treatment is entirely based on response to empiric dosing.

Note: After administration of digoxin-specific Fab antibody fragments, serum digoxin levels may be falsely elevated depending on the assay technique.

Kanji S et al. Cardiac glycoside toxicity: more than 200 years and counting. Crit Care Clin. 2012 Oct;28(4):527–35. [PMID: 22998989]

Manini AF et al. Prognostic utility of serum potassium in chronic digoxin toxicity: a case-control study. Am J Cardiovasc Drugs. 2011 Jun 1;11(3):173–8. [PMID: 21619380]

Yang EH et al. Digitalis toxicity: a fading but crucial complication to recognize. Am J Med. 2012 Apr;125(4):337–43. [PMID: 22444097]

ETHANOL, BENZODIAZEPINES, & OTHER SEDATIVE-HYPNOTIC AGENTS

The group of agents known as sedative-hypnotic drugs includes a variety of products used for the treatment of anxiety, depression, insomnia, and epilepsy. Besides common benzodiazepines, such as lorazepam, alprazolam, clonazepam, diazepam, oxazepam, chlordiazepoxide, and triazolam, this group includes the newer benzodiazepine-like hypnotics zolpidem and zaleplon, and the muscle relaxant carisoprodol. Ethanol and other selected agents are also popular recreational drugs. All of these drugs depress the central nervous system reticular activating system, cerebral cortex, and cerebellum.

▶ Clinical Findings

Mild intoxication produces euphoria, slurred speech, and ataxia. Ethanol intoxication may produce hypoglycemia, even at relatively low concentrations, in children and in fasting adults. With more severe intoxication, stupor, coma, and respiratory arrest may occur. Carisoprodol (Soma) commonly causes muscle jerking or myoclonus. Death or serious morbidity is usually the result of pulmonary aspiration of gastric contents. Bradycardia, hypotension, and hypothermia are common. Patients with massive intoxication may appear to be dead, with no reflex responses and even absent electroencephalographic activity. Diagnosis and assessment of severity of intoxication are usually based on clinical findings. Ethanol serum levels > 300 mg/dL (0.3 g/dL; 65 mmol/L) can produce coma in persons who are not chronically abusing the drug, but regular users may remain awake at much higher levels.

▶ Treatment

A. Emergency and Supportive Measures

Administer activated charcoal if the patient has ingested a massive dose and the airway is protected (see p. 1554). Repeat-dose charcoal may enhance elimination of phenobarbital, but it has not been proved to improve clinical outcome. Hemodialysis may be necessary for patients with severe phenobarbital intoxication.

B. Specific Treatment

Flumazenil is a benzodiazepine receptor-specific antagonist; it has no effect on ethanol, barbiturates, or other sedative-hypnotic agents. If used, flumazenil is given slowly intravenously, 0.2 mg over 30–60 seconds, and repeated in 0.2–0.5 mg increments as needed up to a total dose of 3–5 mg. **Caution:** Flumazenil may induce seizures in patients with preexisting seizure disorder, benzodiazepine addiction, or concomitant tricyclic antidepressant or other convulsant overdose. If seizures occur, diazepam and other benzodiazepine anticonvulsants will not be effective. As with naloxone, the duration of action of flumazenil is short (2–3 hours) and resedation may occur, requiring repeated doses.

Kuzniar TJ et al. Coma with absent brainstem reflexes resulting from zolpidem overdose. Am J Ther. 2010 Sep–Oct;17(5): e172–4. [PMID: 20862780]

Lakhal K et al. Protracted deep coma after bromazepam poisoning. Int J Clin Pharmacol Ther. 2010 Jan;48(1):79–83. [PMID: 20040343]

GAMMA-HYDROXYBUTYRATE (GHB)

GHB has become a popular drug of abuse. It originated as a short-acting general anesthetic and is occasionally used in the treatment of narcolepsy. It gained popularity among bodybuilders for its alleged growth hormone stimulation and found its way into social settings, where it is consumed as a liquid. It has been used to facilitate sexual assault ("date-rape" drug). Symptoms after ingestion include drowsiness and lethargy followed by coma with respiratory depression. Muscle twitching and seizures are sometimes observed. Recovery is usually rapid, with patients awakening within a few hours. Other related chemicals with similar effects include butanediol and gamma-butyrolactone (GBL). A prolonged withdrawal syndrome has been described in some heavy users.

▶ Treatment

Monitor the airway and assist breathing if needed. There is no specific treatment. Most patients recover rapidly with supportive care. GHB withdrawal syndrome may require very large doses of benzodiazepines.

Schep LJ et al. The clinical toxicology of gamma-hydroxybutyrate, gamma-butyrolactone and 1,4-butanediol. Clin Toxicol (Phila). 2012 Jul;50(6):458–70. [PMID: 22746383]

HYPOGLYCEMIC DRUGS

Medications used for diabetes mellitus include insulin, sulfonylureas and other insulin secretagogues, alpha-glucosidase inhibitors (acarbose, miglitol), biguanides (metformin), thiazolidinediones (pioglitazone, rosiglitazone), and newer peptide analogs (pramlintide, exenatide) or enhancers (sitagliptin) (see Chapter 27). Of these, insulin and the insulin secretagogues are the most likely to cause hypoglycemia. Metformin can cause lactic acidosis, especially in patients with renal insufficiency or after intentional drug overdose. Table 27–7 lists the duration of hypoglycemic effect of oral hypoglycemic agents and Figure 27–3 the extent and duration of various types of insulins.

▶ Clinical Findings

Hypoglycemia may occur quickly after injection of short-acting insulins or may be delayed and prolonged, especially if a large amount has been injected into a single area, creating a "depot" effect (Figure 27–3). Hypoglycemia after sulfonylurea ingestion is usually apparent within a few hours but may be delayed several hours, especially if food or glucose-containing fluids have been given (see Table 27–8).

▶ Treatment

Give sugar and carbohydrate-containing food or liquids by mouth, or intravenous dextrose if the patient is unable to swallow safely. For severe hypoglycemia, start with D50W, 50 mL intravenously (25 g dextrose); repeat, if needed. Follow up with dextrose-containing intravenous fluids (D5W or D10W) to maintain a blood glucose > 70–80 mg/dL.

For hypoglycemia caused by sulfonylureas and related insulin secretagogues, consider use of octreotide, a synthetic somatostatin analog that blocks pancreatic insulin release. A dose of 50–100 mcg octreotide subcutaneously every 6–12 hours can reduce the need for exogenous dextrose and prevent rebound hypoglycemia from excessive dextrose dosing.

Admit all patients with symptomatic hypoglycemia after sulfonylurea overdose. Observe asymptomatic overdose patients for at least 12 hours.

Furukawa S et al. Suicide attempt by an overdose of sitagliptin, an oral hypoglycemic agent: a case report and a review of the literature. Endocr J. 2012;59(4):329–33. [PMID: 22277726]
Glatstein M et al. Octreotide for the treatment of sulfonylurea poisoning. Clin Toxicol (Phila). 2012 Nov;50(9):795–804. [PMID: 23046209]

IRON

Iron is widely used therapeutically for the treatment of anemia and as a daily supplement in multiple vitamin preparations. Most children's preparations contain about 12–15 mg of elemental iron (as sulfate, gluconate, or fumarate salt) per dose, compared with 60–90 mg in most adult-strength preparations. Iron is corrosive to the gastrointestinal tract and, once absorbed, has depressant effects on the myocardium and on peripheral vascular resistance. Intracellular toxic effects of iron include disruption of Krebs cycle enzymes.

▶ Clinical Findings

Ingestion of < 30 mg/kg of elemental iron usually produces only mild gastrointestinal upset. Ingestion of > 40–60 mg/kg may cause vomiting (sometimes with hematemesis), diarrhea, hypotension, and acidosis. Death may occur as a result of profound hypotension due to massive fluid losses and bleeding, metabolic acidosis, peritonitis from intestinal perforation, or sepsis. Fulminant hepatic failure may occur. Survivors of the acute ingestion may suffer permanent gastrointestinal scarring.

Serum iron levels > 350–500 mcg/dL are considered potentially toxic, and levels > 1000 mcg/dL are usually associated with severe poisoning. A plain abdominal radiograph may reveal radiopaque tablets.

▶ Treatment

A. Emergency and Supportive Measures

Treat hypotension aggressively with intravenous crystalloid solutions (0.9% saline or lactated Ringer solution). Fluid losses may be massive owing to vomiting and diarrhea as well as third-spacing into injured intestine.

Perform whole bowel irrigation to remove unabsorbed pills from the intestinal tract (see p. 1554). Activated charcoal is not effective but may be appropriate if other ingestants are suspected.

B. Specific Treatment

Deferoxamine is a selective iron chelator. It is not useful as an oral binding agent. For patients with established manifestations of toxicity—and particularly those with markedly elevated serum iron levels (eg, > 800–1000 mcg/dL)— administer 10–15 mg/kg/h by constant intravenous infusion; higher doses (up to 40–50 mg/kg/h) have been used in massive poisonings. Hypotension may occur. The presence of an iron-deferoxamine complex in the urine may give it a "vin rosé" appearance. Deferoxamine is safe for use in pregnant women with acute iron overdose. **Caution:** Prolonged infusion of deferoxamine (> 36–48 hours) has been associated with development of acute respiratory distress syndrome (ARDS)—the mechanism is not known.

Audimoolam VK et al. Iron and acetaminophen a fatal combination? Transpl Int. 2011 Oct;24(10):e85–8. [PMID: 21883506]

Chang TP et al. Iron poisoning: a literature-based review of epidemiology, diagnosis, and management. Pediatr Emerg Care. 2011 Oct;27(10):978–85. [PMID: 21975503]

ISONIAZID

INH is an antibacterial drug used mainly in the treatment and prevention of tuberculosis. It may cause hepatitis with long-term use, especially in alcoholic patients and elderly persons. It produces acute toxic effects by competing with pyridoxal 5-phosphate, resulting in lowered brain gamma-aminobutyric acid (GABA) levels. Acute ingestion of as little as 1.5–2 g of INH can cause toxicity, and severe poisoning is likely to occur after ingestion of more than 80–100 mg/kg.

► Clinical Findings

Confusion, slurred speech, and seizures may occur abruptly after acute overdose. Severe lactic acidosis—out of proportion to the severity of seizures—is probably due to inhibited metabolism of lactate. Peripheral neuropathy and acute hepatitis may occur with long-term use.

Diagnosis is based on a history of ingestion and the presence of severe acidosis associated with seizures. INH is not usually included in routine toxicologic screening, and serum levels are not readily available.

► Treatment

A. Emergency and Supportive Measures

Seizures may require higher than usual doses of benzodiazepines (eg, lorazepam, 3–5 mg intravenously) or administration of pyridoxine as an antidote (see below).

Administer activated charcoal (see p. 1554) after large recent ingestion, but with caution because of the risk of abrupt onset of seizures.

B. Specific Treatment

Pyridoxine (vitamin B_6) is a specific antagonist of the acute toxic effects of INH and is usually successful in controlling convulsions that do not respond to benzodiazepines. Give 5 g intravenously over 1–2 minutes or, if the amount ingested is known, give a gram-for-gram equivalent amount of pyridoxine. Patients taking INH are usually given 25–50 mg of pyridoxine orally daily to help prevent neuropathy.

Eyüboğlu T et al. Rhabdomyolysis due to isoniazid poisoning resulting from the use of intramuscular pyridoxine. Turk J Pediatr. 2013 May–Jun;55(3):328–30. [PMID: 24217082]

Minns AB et al. Isoniazid-induced status epilepticus in a pediatric patient after inadequate pyridoxine therapy. Pediatr Emerg Care. 2010 May;26(5):380–1. [PMID: 20453796]

LEAD

Lead is used in a variety of industrial and commercial products, such as storage batteries, solders, paints, pottery, plumbing, and gasoline and is found in some traditional Hispanic and Ayurvedic ethnic medicines. Lead toxicity usually results from chronic repeated exposure and is rare after a single ingestion. Lead produces a variety of adverse effects on cellular function and primarily affects the nervous system, gastrointestinal tract, and hematopoietic system.

► Clinical Findings

Lead poisoning often goes undiagnosed initially because presenting symptoms and signs are nonspecific and exposure is not suspected. Common symptoms include colicky abdominal pain, constipation, headache, and irritability. Severe poisoning may cause coma and convulsions. Chronic intoxication can cause learning disorders (in children) and motor neuropathy (eg, wrist drop). Lead-containing bullet fragments in or near joint spaces can result in chronic lead toxicity.

Diagnosis is based on measurement of the blood lead level. Whole blood lead levels < 10 mcg/dL are usually considered nontoxic, although that limit has been lowered to 5 mcg/dL in children. Levels between 10 and 25 mcg/dL have been associated with impaired neurobehavioral development in children. Levels of 25–50 mcg/dL may be associated with headache, irritability, and subclinical neuropathy. Levels of 50–70 mcg/dL are associated with moderate toxicity, and levels > 70–100 mcg/dL are often associated with severe poisoning. Other laboratory findings of lead poisoning include microcytic anemia with basophilic stippling and elevated free erythrocyte protoporphyrin.

► Treatment

A. Emergency and Supportive Measures

For patients with encephalopathy, maintain a patent airway and treat coma and convulsions as described at the beginning of this chapter.

For recent acute ingestion, if a large lead-containing object (eg, fishing weight) is still visible in the stomach on abdominal radiograph, whole bowel irrigation (see p. 1554), endoscopy, or even surgical removal may be necessary to prevent subacute lead poisoning. (The acidic gastric contents may corrode the metal surface, enhancing lead absorption. Once the object passes into the small intestine, the risk of toxicity declines.)

Conduct an investigation into the source of the lead exposure.

Workers with a single lead level > 60 mcg/dL (or three successive monthly levels > 50 mcg/dL) or construction workers with any single blood lead level > 50 mcg/dL must by federal law be removed from the site of exposure. Contact the regional office of the United States Occupational Safety and Health Administration (OSHA) for more information. Several states mandate reporting of cases of confirmed lead poisoning.

B. Specific Treatment

The indications for chelation depend on the blood lead level and the patient's clinical state. A medical toxicologist or regional poison control center (1-800-222-1222) should be consulted for advice about selection and use of these antidotes.

Note: It is impermissible under the law to treat asymptomatic workers with elevated blood lead levels in order to keep their levels < 50 mcg/dL rather than remove them from the exposure.

1. Severe toxicity—Patients with severe intoxication (encephalopathy or levels > 70–100 mcg/dL) should receive edetate calcium disodium (ethylenediaminetetraacetic acid, EDTA), 1500 mg/m²/kg/d (approximately 50 mg/kg/d) in four to six divided doses or as a continuous intravenous infusion. Most clinicians also add dimercaprol (BAL), 4–5 mg/kg intramuscularly every 4 hours for 5 days, for patients with encephalopathy.

2. Less severe toxicity—Patients with less severe symptoms and asymptomatic patients with blood lead levels between 55 and 69 mcg/dL may be treated with edetate calcium disodium alone in dosages as above. An oral chelator, succimer (DMSA), is available for use in patients with mild to moderate intoxication. The usual dose is 10 mg/kg orally every 8 hours for 5 days, then every 12 hours for 2 weeks.

Centers for Disease Control and Prevention (CDC). Lead poisoning in pregnant women who used Ayurvedic medications from India—New York City, 2011–2012. MMWR Morb Mortal Wkly Rep. 2012 Aug 24;61(33):641–6. [PMID: 22914225]

Rehani B et al. Lead poisoning from a gunshot wound. South Med J. 2011 Jan;104(1):57–8. [PMID: 21079537]

Thihalolipavan S et al. Examining pica in NYC pregnant women with elevated blood lead levels. Matern Child Health J. 2013 Jan;17(1):49–55. [PMID: 22302239]

LITHIUM

Lithium is widely used for the treatment of bipolar depression and other psychiatric disorders. The only normal route of lithium elimination is via the kidney, so patients with chronic kidney disease are at risk for accumulation of lithium resulting in gradual onset (chronic) toxicity. Intoxication resulting from chronic accidental overmedication or renal impairment is more common and usually more severe than that seen after acute oral overdose.

▶ Clinical Findings

Mild to moderate toxicity causes lethargy, confusion, tremor, ataxia, and slurred speech. This may progress to myoclonic jerking, delirium, coma, and convulsions. Recovery may be slow and incomplete following severe intoxication. Laboratory studies in patients with chronic intoxication often reveal an elevated serum creatinine and an elevated BUN/creatinine ratio due to underlying volume contraction. The white blood cell count is often elevated. ECG findings include T-wave flattening or inversion, and sometimes bradycardia or sinus node arrest.

Nephrogenic diabetes insipidus can occur with overdose or with therapeutic doses. Lithium levels may be difficult to interpret. Lithium has a low toxic:therapeutic ratio and chronic intoxication can be seen with levels only slightly above the therapeutic range (0.8–1.2 mEq/L). In contrast, patients with acute ingestion may have transiently very high levels (up to 10 mEq/L reported) without any symptoms before the lithium fully distributes into tissues. **Note:** Falsely high lithium levels (as high as 6–8 mEq/L) can be measured if a green-top blood specimen tube (containing lithium heparin) is used instead of a red- or marbled-top tube.

▶ Treatment

After acute oral overdose, consider gastric lavage (see p. 1554) or whole bowel irrigation (see p. 1554) to prevent systemic absorption (lithium is not adsorbed by activated charcoal). In all patients, evaluate renal function and volume status, and give intravenous saline-containing fluids as needed. Monitor serum lithium levels, and seek assistance with their interpretation and the need for dialysis from a medical toxicologist or regional poison control center (1-800-222-1222). Consider hemodialysis if the patient is markedly symptomatic or if the serum level exceeds 10 mEq/L after an acute overdose. Continuous renal replacement hemofiltration may be an effective alternative to hemodialysis.

Chen WY et al. Reversible oro-lingual dyskinesia related to lithium intoxication. Acta Neurol Taiwan. 2013 Mar;22(1):32–5. [PMID: 23479244]

McKnight RF et al. Lithium toxicity profile: a systematic review and meta-analysis. Lancet. 2012 Feb 25;379(9817):721–8. [PMID: 22265699]

LSD & OTHER HALLUCINOGENS

A variety of substances—ranging from naturally occurring plants and mushrooms to synthetic substances such as phencyclidine (PCP), toluene and other solvents, dextromethorphan, and lysergic acid diethylamide (LSD)—are abused for their hallucinogenic properties. The mechanism of toxicity and the clinical effects vary for each substance.

Many hallucinogenic plants and mushrooms produce anticholinergic delirium, characterized by flushed skin, dry mucous membranes, dilated pupils, tachycardia, and urinary retention. Other plants and mushrooms may contain hallucinogenic indoles such as mescaline and LSD, which typically cause marked visual hallucinations and perceptual distortion, widely dilated pupils, and mild tachycardia. PCP, a dissociative anesthetic agent similar to ketamine, can produce fluctuating delirium and coma, often associated with vertical and horizontal nystagmus. Toluene and other hydrocarbon solvents (butane, trichloroethylene, "chemo," etc) cause euphoria and delirium and may sensitize the myocardium to the effects of catecholamines, leading to fatal dysrhythmias. Newer drugs used for their psychostimulant effects include synthetic cannabinoid receptor agonists (street names include "spice" and "K2"), *Salvia divinorum*, and mephedrone and related cathinone derivatives. See www.erowid.org for very thorough descriptions of a variety of hallucinogenic substances.

▶ Treatment

A. Emergency and Supportive Measures

Maintain a patent airway and assist respirations if necessary. Treat coma, hyperthermia, hypertension, and seizures as outlined at the beginning of this chapter. For recent large ingestions, consider giving activated charcoal orally or by gastric tube (see p. 1554).

B. Specific Treatment

Patients with anticholinergic delirium may benefit from a dose of physostigmine, 0.5–1 mg intravenously, not to exceed 1 mg/min. Dysphoria, agitation, and psychosis associated with LSD or mescaline intoxication may respond to benzodiazepines (eg, lorazepam, 1–2 mg orally or intravenously) or haloperidol (2–5 mg intramuscularly or intravenously) or another antipsychotic drug (eg, olanzapine or ziprasidone). Monitor patients who have sniffed solvents for cardiac dysrhythmias (most commonly premature ventricular contractions, ventricular tachycardia, ventricular fibrillation); treatment with beta-blockers such as propranolol (1–5 mg intravenously) or esmolol (250–500 mcg/kg intravenously, then 50 mcg/kg/min by infusion) may be more effective than lidocaine or amiodarone.

Cámara-Lemarroy CR et al. Clinical presentation and management in acute toluene intoxication: a case series. Inhal Toxicol. 2012 Jun;24(7):434–8. [PMID: 22642292]

Gunderson EW et al. "Spice" and "K2" herbal highs: a case series and systematic review of the clinical effects and biopsychosocial implications of synthetic cannabinoid use in humans. Am J Addict. 2012 Jul–Aug;21(4):320–6. [PMID: 22691010]

Harris CR et al. Synthetic cannabinoid intoxication: a case series and review. J Emerg Med. 2013 Feb;44(2):360–6. [PMID: 22989695]

MERCURY

Acute mercury poisoning usually occurs by ingestion of inorganic mercuric salts or inhalation of metallic mercury vapor. Ingestion of the mercuric salts causes a burning sensation in the throat, discoloration and edema of oral mucous membranes, abdominal pain, vomiting, bloody diarrhea, and shock. Direct nephrotoxicity causes acute kidney injury. Inhalation of high concentrations of metallic mercury vapor may cause acute fulminant chemical pneumonia. Chronic mercury poisoning causes weakness, ataxia, intention tremors, irritability, and depression. Exposure to alkyl (organic) mercury derivatives from highly contaminated fish or fungicides used on seeds has caused ataxia, tremors, convulsions, and catastrophic birth defects. Nearly all fish have some traces of mercury contamination; the US Environmental Protection Agency (EPA) advises consumers to avoid swordfish, shark, king mackerel, and tilefish because they contain higher levels. Fish that are generally low in mercury content include shrimp, canned light tuna (not albacore "white" tuna), salmon, pollock, and catfish. Dental fillings composed of mercury amalgam pose a very small risk of chronic mercury poisoning and their removal is rarely justified.

▶ Treatment

A. Acute Poisoning

There is no effective specific treatment for mercury vapor pneumonitis. Remove ingested mercuric salts by lavage, and administer activated charcoal (see p. 1554). For acute ingestion of mercuric salts, give dimercaprol (BAL) at once, as for arsenic poisoning. Unless the patient has severe gastroenteritis, consider succimer (DMSA), 10 mg/kg orally every 8 hours for 5 days and then every 12 hours for 2 weeks. Unithiol (DMPS) is a chelator that can be given orally or parenterally, but is not commonly available in the United States; it can be obtained from some compounding pharmacies. Maintain urinary output. Treat oliguria and anuria if they occur.

B. Chronic Poisoning

Remove from exposure. Neurologic toxicity is not considered reversible with chelation, although some authors recommend a trial of succimer or unithiol (contact a regional poison center or medical toxicologist for advice).

Mercer JJ et al. Acrodynia and hypertension in a young girl secondary to elemental mercury toxicity acquired in the home. Pediatr Dermatol. 2012 Mar–Apr;29(2):199–201. [PMID: 22409470]

Oz SG et al. Mercury vapor inhalation and poisoning of a family. Inhal Toxicol. 2012 Aug;24(10):652–8. [PMID: 22906171]

METHANOL & ETHYLENE GLYCOL

Methanol (wood alcohol) is commonly found in a variety of products, including solvents, duplicating fluids, record cleaning solutions, and paint removers. It is sometimes ingested intentionally by alcoholic patients as a substitute for ethanol and may also be found as a contaminant in bootleg whiskey. Ethylene glycol is the major constituent in most antifreeze compounds. The toxicity of both agents is caused by metabolism to highly toxic organic acids—methanol to formic acid; ethylene glycol to glycolic and oxalic acids. Diethylene glycol is a nephrotoxic solvent that has been improperly substituted for glycerine in various liquid medications (cough syrup, teething medicine, acetaminophen) causing numerous deaths in Haiti, Panama, and Nigeria.

▶ Clinical Findings

Shortly after ingestion of methanol or ethylene glycol, patients usually appear "drunk." The serum osmolality (measured with the freezing point device) is usually increased, but acidosis is often absent early. After several hours, metabolism to toxic organic acids leads to a severe anion gap metabolic acidosis, tachypnea, confusion, convulsions, and coma. Methanol intoxication frequently causes visual disturbances, while ethylene glycol often produces oxalate crystalluria and acute kidney injury.

Treatment

A. Emergency and Supportive Measures

For patients presenting within 30–60 minutes after ingestion, empty the stomach by aspiration through a nasogastric tube (see p. 1554). Charcoal is not very effective but should be administered if other poisons or drugs have also been ingested.

B. Specific Treatment

Patients with significant toxicity (manifested by severe metabolic acidosis, altered mental status, and markedly elevated osmol gap) should undergo hemodialysis as soon as possible to remove the parent compound and the toxic metabolites. Treatment with folic acid, thiamine, and pyridoxine may enhance the breakdown of toxic metabolites.

Ethanol blocks metabolism of the parent compounds by competing for the enzyme alcohol dehydrogenase. Fomepizole (4-methylpyrazole; Antizol) blocks alcohol dehydrogenase and is much easier to use than ethanol. If started before onset of acidosis, fomepizole may be used as the sole treatment for ethylene glycol ingestion in some cases. A regional poison control center (1-800-222-1222) should be contacted for indications and dosing.

Buller GK et al. When is it appropriate to treat ethylene glycol intoxication with fomepizole alone without hemodialysis? Semin Dial. 2011 Jul–Aug;24(4):441–2. [PMID: 21801226]

Coulter CV et al. Methanol and ethylene glycol acute poisonings—predictors of mortality. Clin Toxicol (Phila). 2011 Dec;49 (10):900–6. [PMID: 22091788]

Kruse JA. Methanol and ethylene glycol intoxication. Crit Care Clin. 2012 Oct;28(4):661–711. [PMID: 22998995]

METHEMOGLOBINEMIA-INDUCING AGENTS

A large number of chemical agents are capable of oxidizing ferrous hemoglobin to its ferric state (methemoglobin), a form that cannot carry oxygen. Drugs and chemicals known to cause methemoglobinemia include benzocaine (a local anesthetic found in some topical anesthetic sprays and a variety of nonprescription products), aniline, propanil (an herbicide), nitrites, nitrogen oxide gases, nitrobenzene, dapsone, phenazopyridine (Pyridium), and many others. Dapsone has a long elimination half-life and may produce prolonged or recurrent methemoglobinemia.

▶ Clinical Findings

Methemoglobinemia reduces oxygen-carrying capacity and may cause dizziness, nausea, headache, dyspnea, confusion, seizures, and coma. The severity of symptoms depends on the percentage of hemoglobin oxidized to methemoglobin; severe poisoning is usually present when methemoglobin fractions are > 40–50%. Even at low levels (15–20%), victims appear cyanotic because of the "chocolate brown" color of methemoglobin, but they have normal PO_2 results on arterial blood gas determinations. Conventional pulse oximetry gives inaccurate oxygen saturation measurements; the reading is often between 85% and 90%. (A newer pulse oximetry device

[Masimo Pulse CO-oximeter] is capable of estimating the methemoglobin level.) Severe metabolic acidosis may be present. Hemolysis may occur, especially in patients susceptible to oxidant stress (ie, those with glucose-6-phosphate dehydrogenase deficiency).

▶ Treatment

A. Emergency and Supportive Measures

Administer high-flow oxygen. If the causative agent was recently ingested, administer activated charcoal (see p. 1554). Repeat-dose activated charcoal may enhance dapsone elimination (see p. 1554).

B. Specific Treatment

Methylene blue enhances the conversion of methemoglobin to hemoglobin by increasing the activity of the enzyme methemoglobin reductase. For symptomatic patients, administer 1–2 mg/kg (0.1–0.2 mL/kg of 1% solution) intravenously. The dose may be repeated once in 15–20 minutes if necessary. Patients with hereditary methemoglobin reductase deficiency or glucose-6-phosphate dehydrogenase deficiency may not respond to methylene blue treatment. In severe cases where methylene blue is not available or is not effective, exchange blood transfusion may be necessary.

Barclay J et al. Dapsone-induced methemoglobinemia: a primer for clinicians. Ann Pharmacother. 2011 Sep;45(9):1103–15. [PMID: 21852596]

Gupta A et al. A fatal case of severe methaemoglobinemia due to nitrobenzene poisoning. Emerg Med J. 2012 Jan;29(1):70–1. [PMID: 22186264]

Shahani L et al. Acquired methaemoglobinaemia related to phenazopyridine ingestion. BMJ Case Rep. 2012 Sep 17;2012. [PMID: 22987905]

MONOAMINE OXIDASE INHIBITORS

Overdoses of MAO inhibitors (isocarboxazid, phenelzine, selegiline, moclobemide) cause ataxia, excitement, hypertension, and tachycardia, followed several hours later by hypotension, convulsions, and hyperthermia.

Ingestion of tyramine-containing foods may cause a severe hypertensive reaction in patients taking MAO inhibitors. Foods containing tyramine include aged cheese and red wines. Hypertensive reactions may also occur with any sympathomimetic drug. Severe or fatal hyperthermia (serotonin syndrome) may occur if patients receiving MAO inhibitors are given meperidine, fluoxetine, paroxetine, fluvoxamine, venlafaxine, tryptophan, dextromethorphan, tramadol, or other serotonin-enhancing drugs. This reaction can also occur with the newer selective MAO inhibitor moclobemide, and the antibiotic linezolid, which has MAO-inhibiting properties. The serotonin syndrome has also been reported in patients taking selective serotonin reuptake inhibitors (SSRIs) in large doses or in combination with other SSRIs, even in the absence of an MAO inhibitor or meperidine. It is characterized by fever, agitation, delirium, diaphoresis, hyperreflexia, and clonus (spontaneous, inducible, or ocular). Hyperthermia can be life-threatening.

▶ Treatment

Administer activated charcoal (see p. 1554). Treat severe hypertension with nitroprusside, phentolamine, or other rapid-acting vasodilators (see p. 1552). Treat hypotension with fluids and positioning, but avoid use of pressor agents if possible. Observe patients for at least 24 hours, since hyperthermic reactions may be delayed. Treat hyperthermia with aggressive cooling; neuromuscular paralysis may be required (see p. 1552 and Chapter 37). Cyproheptadine, 4 mg orally (or by gastric tube) every hour for three or four doses, or chlorpromazine, 25 mg intravenously, has been reported to be effective against serotonin syndrome.

Flockhart DA. Dietary restrictions and drug interactions with monoamine oxidase inhibitors: an update. J Clin Psychiatry. 2012;73(Suppl 1):17–24. [PMID: 22951238]

Iqbal MM et al. Overview of serotonin syndrome. Ann Clin Psychiatry. 2012 Nov;24(4):310–8. [PMID: 23145389]

Wu ML et al. Fatal serotonin toxicity caused by moclobemide and fluoxetine overdose. Chang Gung Med J. 2011 Nov–Dec; 34(6):644–9. [PMID: 22196068]

MUSHROOMS

There are thousands of mushroom species that cause a variety of toxic effects. The most dangerous species of mushrooms are *Amanita phalloides* and related species, which contain potent cytotoxins (amatoxins). Ingestion of even a portion of one amatoxin-containing mushroom may be sufficient to cause death.

The characteristic pathologic finding in fatalities from amatoxin-containing mushroom poisoning is acute massive necrosis of the liver.

▶ Clinical Findings

A. Symptoms and Signs

Amatoxin-containing mushrooms typically cause a delayed onset (8–12 hours after ingestion) of severe abdominal cramps, vomiting and profuse diarrhea, followed by hepatic necrosis, hepatic encephalopathy, and frequently acute kidney injury in 1–2 days. Cooking the mushrooms does not prevent poisoning.

Monomethylhydrazine poisoning (*Gyromitra* and *Helvella* species) is more common following ingestion of uncooked mushrooms, as the toxin is water-soluble. Vomiting, diarrhea, hepatic necrosis, convulsions, coma, and hemolysis may occur after a latent period of 8–12 hours.

The clinical effects of these and other mushrooms are described in Table 38–8.

▶ Treatment

A. Emergency Measures

After the onset of symptoms, efforts to remove the toxic agent are probably useless, especially in cases of amatoxin or gyromitrin poisoning, where there is usually a delay of 12 hours or more before symptoms occur and patients seek medical attention. However, induction of vomiting or administration of activated charcoal is recommended for any recent ingestion of an unidentified or potentially toxic mushroom (see p. 1554).

B. Specific Treatment

A variety of purported antidotes (eg, thioctic acid, penicillin, corticosteroids) have been suggested for amatoxin-type

Table 38–8. Poisonous mushrooms.

Toxin	Genus	Symptoms and Signs	Onset	Treatment
Amanitin	*Amanita (A ocreata, A phalloides, A verna, A virosa,)*	Severe gastroenteritis followed by delayed hepatic failure and acute kidney injury after 48–72 hours	6–24 hours	Supportive. Correct dehydration. Give repeated doses of activated charcoal orally. Consider intravenous silibinin (Legalon-SIL) (see text).
Muscarine	*Inocybe, Clitocybe*	Muscarinic (salivation, miosis, bradycardia, diarrhea)	30–60 minutes	Supportive. Give atropine, 0.5–2 mg intravenously, for severe cholinergic symptoms and signs.
Ibotenic acid, muscimol	*Amanita muscaria* ("fly agaric")	Anticholinergic (mydriasis,tachycardia, hyperpyrexia, delirium)	30–60 minutes	Supportive. Give physostigmine, 0.5–2 mg intravenously, for severe anticholinergic symptoms and signs.
Coprine	*Coprinus*	Disulfiram-like effect occurs with ingestion of ethanol	30–60 minutes	Supportive. Abstain from ethanol for 3–4 days.
Monomethyl-hydrazine	*Gyromitra*	Gastroenteritis; occasionally seizures, hemolysis, hepatic failure, and acute kidney injury	6–12 hours	Supportive. Correct dehydration. Pyridoxine, 2.5 mg/kg intravenously, may be helpful for seizures.
Orellanine	*Cortinarius*	Nausea, vomiting; acute kidney injury after 1–3 weeks	2–14 days	Supportive.
Psilocybin	*Psilocybe*	Hallucinations	15–30 minutes	Supportive.
Gastrointestinal irritants	Many species	Nausea and vomiting, diarrhea	1/2–2 hours	Supportive. Correct dehydration.

mushroom poisoning, but controlled studies are lacking and experimental data in animals are equivocal. Aggressive fluid replacement for diarrhea and intensive supportive care for hepatic failure are the mainstays of treatment. Sily-marin (silibinin), a derivative of milk thistle, is commonly used in Europe but is currently only commercially available in the United States as a nutritional supplement given orally. The European intravenous product (Legalon-SIL) can be obtained in the United States under an emergency IND provided by the FDA. Contact the regional poison control center (1-800-222-1222) for more information.

Interruption of enterohepatic circulation of the ama-toxin by the administration of activated charcoal or by cannulation and drainage of the bile duct may be of value in removing some of the toxin, based on animal studies and isolated case reports, but proof of efficacy and safety is lacking.

Liver transplant may be the only hope for survival in gravely ill patients—contact a liver transplant center early.

Santi L et al. Acute liver failure caused by *Amanita phalloides* poisoning. Int J Hepatol. 2012;2012:487–90. [PMID: 22811920]

Trabulus S et al. Clinical features and outcome of patients with amatoxin-containing mushroom poisoning. Clin Toxicol (Phila). 2011 Apr;49(4):303–10. [PMID: 21563906]

Ward J et al. Amatoxin poisoning: case reports and review of current therapies. J Emerg Med. 2013 Jan;44(1):116–21. [PMID: 22555054]

OPIATES & OPIOIDS

Prescription and illicit opiates and opioids (morphine, heroin, codeine, oxycodone, fentanyl, hydromorphone, etc) are popular drugs of misuse and abuse and the cause of frequent hospitalizations for overdose. These drugs have widely varying potencies and durations of action; for example, some of the illicit fentanyl derivatives are up to 2000 times more potent than morphine. All of these agents decrease central nervous system activity and sympathetic outflow by acting on opiate receptors in the brain. Trama-dol is an analgesic that is unrelated chemically to the opi-oids but acts on opioid receptors. Buprenorphine is a partial agonist-antagonist opioid used for the outpatient treatment of opioid addiction.

▶ Clinical Findings

Mild intoxication is characterized by euphoria, drowsiness, and constricted pupils. More severe intoxication may cause hypotension, bradycardia, hypothermia, coma, and respi-ratory arrest. Pulmonary edema may occur. Death is usu-ally due to apnea or pulmonary aspiration of gastric contents. Methadone has been associated with QT interval prolongation and torsades de pointes. Tramadol, dextro-methorphan, and meperidine also occasionally cause sei-zures. With meperidine, the metabolite normeperidine is probably the cause of seizures and is most likely to accu-mulate with repeated dosing in patients with chronic kid-ney disease. While the duration of effect for heroin is usually 3–5 hours, methadone intoxication may last for

48–72 hours or longer. Propoxyphene may cause seizures and prolongs the QRS interval; it has now been removed from the US market by the FDA. Many opioids, including fentanyl, tramadol, oxycodone, and methadone, are not detected on routine urine toxicology "opiate" screening. Wound botulism has been associated with skin-popping, especially involving "black tar" heroin. Buprenorphine added to an opioid regimen may produce acute narcotic withdrawal symptoms.

▶ Treatment

A. Emergency and Supportive Measures

Protect the airway and assist ventilation. Administer acti-vated charcoal (see p. 1554) for recent large ingestions.

B. Specific Treatment

Naloxone is a specific opioid antagonist that can rapidly reverse signs of narcotic intoxication. Although it is struc-turally related to the opioids, it has no agonist effects of its own. Administer 0.2–2 mg intravenously, and repeat as needed to awaken the patient and maintain airway protec-tive reflexes and spontaneous breathing. Very large doses (10–20 mg) may be required for patients intoxicated by some opioids (eg, codeine, fentanyl derivatives). **Caution:** The duration of effect of naloxone is only about 2–3 hours; repeated doses may be necessary for patients intoxicated by long-acting drugs such as methadone. Continuous obser-vation for at least 3 hours after the last naloxone dose is mandatory.

Alford DP et al. JAMA patient page. Misuse of opioid medica-tion. JAMA. 2013 May 15;309(19):2055. [PMID: 23677318]

Beletsky L et al. Prevention of fatal opioid overdose. JAMA. 2012 Nov 14;308(18):1863–4. [PMID: 23150005]

Bohnert AS et al. Association between opioid prescribing pat-terns and opioid overdose-related deaths. JAMA. 2011 Apr 6;305(13):1315–21. [PMID: 21467284]

Bowman S et al. Reducing the health consequences of opioid addiction in primary care. Am J Med. 2013 Jul;126(7):565–71. [PMID: 23664112]

Centers for Disease Control and Prevention (CDC). Vital signs: risk for overdose from methadone used for pain relief— United States, 1999–2010. MMWR Morb Mortal Wkly Rep. 2012 Jul 6;61(26):493–7. [PMID: 22763888]

PESTICIDES: CHOLINESTERASE INHIBITORS

Organophosphorus and carbamate insecticides (organo-phosphates: parathion, malathion, etc; carbamates: carba-ryl, aldicarb, etc) are widely used in commercial agriculture and home gardening and have largely replaced older, more environmentally persistent organochlorine compounds such as DDT and chlordane. The organophosphates and carbamates—also called anticholinesterases because they inhibit the enzyme acetylcholinesterase—cause an increase in acetylcholine activity at nicotinic and muscarinic recep-tors and in the central nervous system. There are a variety of chemical agents in this group, with widely varying potencies. Most of them are poorly water-soluble, are often formulated with an aromatic hydrocarbon solvent such as xylene, and are well absorbed through intact skin. Most chemical warfare "nerve agents" (such as GA [tabun], GB [sarin], GD [soman] and VX) are organophosphates.

► Clinical Findings

Inhibition of cholinesterase results in abdominal cramps, diarrhea, vomiting, excessive salivation, sweating, lacrimation, miosis (constricted pupils), wheezing and bronchorrhea, seizures, and skeletal muscle weakness. Initial tachycardia is usually followed by bradycardia. Profound skeletal muscle weakness, aggravated by excessive bronchial secretions and wheezing, may result in respiratory arrest and death. Symptoms and signs of poisoning may persist or recur over several days, especially with highly lipid-soluble agents such as fenthion or dimethoate.

The diagnosis should be suspected in patients who present with miosis, sweating, and hyperperistalsis. Serum and red blood cell cholinesterase activity is usually depressed at least 50% below baseline in those victims who have severe intoxication.

► Treatment

A. Emergency and Supportive Measures

If the agent was recently ingested, consider gut decontamination by aspiration of the liquid using a nasogastric tube followed by administration of activated charcoal (see p. 1554). If the agent is on the victim's skin or hair, wash repeatedly with soap or shampoo and water. Providers should take care to avoid skin exposure by wearing gloves and waterproof aprons. Dilute hypochlorite solution (eg, household bleach diluted 1:10) is reported to help break down organophosphate pesticides and nerve agents on equipment or clothing.

B. Specific Treatment

Atropine reverses excessive muscarinic stimulation and is effective for treatment of salivation, bronchial hypersecretion, wheezing, abdominal cramping, and sweating. However, it does not interact with nicotinic receptors at autonomic ganglia and at the neuromuscular junction and has no direct effect on muscle weakness. Administer 2 mg intravenously, and if there is no response after 5 minutes, give repeated boluses in rapidly escalating doses (eg, doubling the dose each time) as needed to dry bronchial secretions and decrease wheezing; as much as several hundred milligrams of atropine has been given to treat severe poisoning.

Pralidoxime (2-PAM, Protopam) is a specific antidote that reverses organophosphate binding to the cholinesterase enzyme; therefore, it should be effective at the neuromuscular junction as well as other nicotinic and muscarinic sites. It is most likely to be clinically effective if started very soon after poisoning, to prevent permanent binding of the organophosphate to cholinesterase. However, clinical studies have yielded conflicting results regarding the effectiveness of pralidoxime in reducing mortality. Administer 1–2 g intravenously as a loading dose, and begin a continuous infusion (200–500 mg/h, titrated to clinical response).

Continue to give pralidoxime as long as there is any evidence of acetylcholine excess. Pralidoxime is of questionable benefit for carbamate poisoning, because carbamates have only a transitory effect on the cholinesterase enzyme. Other, unproven therapies for organophosphate poisoning include magnesium, sodium bicarbonate, clonidine, and extracorporeal removal.

Blain PG. Organophosphorus poisoning (acute). Clin Evid (Online). 2011 May 17;2011. pii2102. [PMID: 21575287]

Buckley NA et al. Oximes for acute organophosphate pesticide poisoning. Cochrane Database Syst Rev. 2011 Feb 16;(2): CD005085. [PMID: 21328273]

Nurulain SM. Different approaches to acute organophosphorus poison treatment. J Pak Med Assoc. 2012 Jul;62(7):712–7. [PMID: 23866522]

Thiermann H et al. Atropine maintenance dosage in patients with severe organophosphate pesticide poisoning. Toxicol Lett. 2011 Sep 25;206(1):77–83. [PMID: 21771644]

PETROLEUM DISTILLATES & SOLVENTS

Petroleum distillate toxicity may occur from inhalation of the vapor or as a result of pulmonary aspiration of the liquid during or after ingestion. Acute manifestations of aspiration pneumonitis are vomiting, coughing, and bronchopneumonia. Some hydrocarbons—ie, those with aromatic or halogenated subunits—can also cause severe systemic poisoning after oral ingestion. Hydrocarbons can also cause systemic intoxication by inhalation. Vertigo, muscular incoordination, irregular pulse, myoclonus, and seizures occur with serious poisoning and may be due to hypoxemia or the systemic effects of the agents. Chlorinated and fluorinated hydrocarbons (trichloroethylene, Freons, etc) and many other hydrocarbons can cause ventricular arrhythmias due to increased sensitivity of the myocardium to the effects of endogenous catecholamines.

► Treatment

Remove the patient to fresh air. For simple aliphatic hydrocarbon ingestion, gastric emptying and activated charcoal are not recommended, but these procedures may be indicated if the preparation contains toxic solutes (eg, an insecticide) or is an aromatic or halogenated product. Observe the victim for 6–8 hours for signs of aspiration pneumonitis (cough, localized crackles or rhonchi, tachypnea, and infiltrates on chest radiograph). Corticosteroids are not recommended. If fever occurs, give a specific antibiotic only after identification of bacterial pathogens by laboratory studies. Because of the risk of arrhythmias, use bronchodilators with caution in patients with chlorinated or fluorinated solvent intoxication. If tachyarrhythmias occur, use esmolol intravenously 25–100 mcg/kg/min.

Argo A et al. A fatal case of a paint thinner ingestion: comparison between toxicological and histological findings. Am J Forensic Med Pathol. 2010 June;31(2):186–91. [PMID: 20010286]

Phatak DR et al. Huffing air conditioner fluid: a cool way to die? Am J Forensic Med Pathol. 2012 Mar;33(1):64–7. [PMID: 22442834]

QUINIDINE & RELATED ANTIARRHYTHMICS

Quinidine, procainamide, and disopyramide are class Ia antiarrhythmic agents, and flecainide and propafenone are class Ic agents. These drugs have membrane-depressant effects on the sodium-dependent channel responsible for cardiac cell depolarization. Manifestations of cardiotoxicity include arrhythmias, syncope, hypotension, and widening of the QRS complex on the ECG (> 100–120 ms). With type Ia drugs, a lengthened QT interval and atypical or polymorphous ventricular tachycardia (torsades de pointes) may occur. The antimalarials chloroquine and hydroxychloroquine, and the tricyclic antidepressants, have similar cardiotoxic effects in overdose.

▶ Treatment

A. Emergency and Supportive Measures

Administer activated charcoal (see p. 1554); consider gastric lavage (see p. 1554) after large recent overdose. Assist ventilation if needed. Perform continuous cardiac monitoring.

B. Specific Treatment

Treat cardiotoxicity (hypotension, QRS interval widening) with intravenous boluses of sodium bicarbonate, 50–100 mEq. Torsades de pointes may be treated with intravenous magnesium or overdrive pacing.

Camm J. Antiarrhythmic drugs for the maintenance of sinus rhythm: risks and benefits. Int J Cardiol. 2012 Mar 22; 155(3):362–71. [PMID: 21708411]

Phipps C et al. Fatal chloroquine poisoning: a rare cause of sudden cardiac arrest. Ann Acad Med Singapore. 2011 Jun;40(6):296–7. [PMID: 21779619]

SALICYLATES

Salicylates (aspirin, methyl salicylate, bismuth subsalicylate, etc) are found in a variety of over-the-counter and prescription medications. Salicylates uncouple cellular oxidative phosphorylation, resulting in anaerobic metabolism and excessive production of lactic acid and heat, and they also interfere with several Krebs cycle enzymes. A single ingestion of more than 200 mg/kg of salicylate is likely to produce significant acute intoxication. Poisoning may also occur as a result of chronic excessive dosing over several days. Although the half-life of salicylate is 2–3 hours after small doses, it may increase to 20 hours or more in patients with intoxication.

▶ Clinical Findings

Acute ingestion often causes nausea and vomiting, occasionally with gastritis. Moderate intoxication is characterized by hyperpnea (deep and rapid breathing), tachycardia, tinnitus, and elevated anion gap metabolic acidosis. Serious intoxication may result in agitation, confusion, coma, seizures, cardiovascular collapse, pulmonary edema, hyperthermia, and death. The prothrombin time is often elevated owing to salicylate-induced hypoprothrombinemia. Central nervous system intracellular glucose depletion can occur despite normal measured serum glucose levels.

Diagnosis of salicylate poisoning is suspected in any patient with metabolic acidosis and is confirmed by measuring the serum salicylate level. Patients with levels >100 mg/dL (1000 mg/L or 7.2 mcmol/L) after an acute overdose are more likely to have severe poisoning. On the other hand, patients with subacute or chronic intoxication may suffer severe symptoms with levels of only 60–70 mg/dL (4.3–5 mcmol/L). The arterial blood gas typically reveals a respiratory alkalosis with an underlying metabolic acidosis.

▶ Treatment

A. Emergency and Supportive Measures

Administer activated charcoal orally (see p. 1554). Gastric lavage followed by administration of extra doses of activated charcoal may be needed in patients who ingest more than 10 g of aspirin (see p. 1554). The desired ratio of charcoal to aspirin is about 10:1 by weight; while this cannot always be given as a single dose, it may be administered over the first 24 hours in divided doses every 2–4 hours along with whole bowel irrigation (see p. 1554). Give glucose-containing fluids to reduce the risk of cerebral hypoglycemia. Treat metabolic acidosis with intravenous sodium bicarbonate. This is critical because acidosis (especially acidemia, pH < 7.40) promotes greater entry of salicylate into cells, worsening toxicity. **Warning:** Sudden and severe deterioration can occur after rapid sequence intubation and controlled ventilation if the pH is allowed to fall during the apneic period.

B. Specific Treatment

Alkalinization of the urine enhances renal salicylate excretion by trapping the salicylate anion in the urine. Add 100 mEq (two ampules) of sodium bicarbonate to 1 L of 5% dextrose in 0.2% saline, and infuse this solution intravenously at a rate of about 150–200 mL/h. Unless the patient is oliguric or hyperkalemic, add 20–30 mEq of potassium chloride to each liter of intravenous fluid. Patients who are volume-depleted often fail to produce an alkaline urine (paradoxical aciduria) unless potassium is given.

Hemodialysis may be lifesaving and is indicated for patients with severe metabolic acidosis, markedly altered mental status, or significantly elevated salicylate levels (eg, > 100–120 mg/dL [1000–1200 mg/L or 7.2–8.6 mcmol/L] after acute overdose or > 60–70 mg/dL [600–700 mg/L or 4.3–5 mcmol/L] with subacute or chronic intoxication).

Glisson JK et al. Current management of salicylate-induced pulmonary edema. South Med J. 2011 Mar;104(3):225–32. [PMID: 21297545]

Minns AB et al. Death due to acute salicylate intoxication despite dialysis. J Emerg Med. 2011 May;40(5):515–7. [PMID: 20347249]

SEAFOOD POISONINGS

A variety of intoxications may occur after eating certain types of fish or other seafood. These include scombroid, ciguatera, paralytic shellfish, and puffer fish poisoning.

Table 38–9. Common seafood poisonings.

Type of Poisoning	Mechanism	Clinical Presentation
Ciguatera	Reef fish ingest toxic dinoflagellates, whose toxins accumulate in fish meat. Commonly implicated fish in the United States are barracuda, jack, snapper, and grouper.	1–6 hours after ingestion, victims develop abdominal pain, vomiting, and diarrhea accompanied by a variety of neurologic symptoms, including paresthesias, reversal of hot and cold sensation, vertigo, headache, and intense itching. Autonomic disturbances, including hypotension and bradycardia, may occur.
Scombroid	Improper preservation of large fish results in bacterial degradation of histidine to histamine. Commonly implicated fish include tuna, mahimahi, bonita, mackerel, and kingfish.	Allergic-like (anaphylactoid) symptoms are due to histamine, usually begin within 15–90 minutes, and include skin flushing, itching, urticaria, angioedema, bronchospasm, and hypotension as well as abdominal pain, vomiting, and diarrhea.
Paralytic shellfish poisoning	Dinoflagellates produce saxitoxin, which is concentrated by filter-feeding mussels and clams. Saxitoxin blocks sodium conductance and neuronal transmission in skeletal muscles.	Onset is usually within 30–60 minutes. Initial symptoms include perioral and intraoral paresthesias. Other symptoms include nausea and vomiting, headache, dizziness, dysphagia, dysarthria, ataxia, and rapidly progressive muscle weakness that may result in respiratory arrest.
Puffer fish poisoning	Tetrodotoxin is concentrated in liver, gonads, intestine, and skin. Toxic effects are similar to those of saxitoxin. Tetrodotoxin is also found in some North American newts and Central American frogs.	Onset is usually within 30–40 minutes but may be as short as 10 minutes. Initial perioral paresthesias are followed by headache, diaphoresis, nausea, vomiting, ataxia, and rapidly progressive muscle weakness that may result in respiratory arrest.

The mechanisms of toxicity and clinical presentations are described in Table 38–9. In the majority of cases, the seafood has a normal appearance and taste (scombroid may have a peppery taste).

▶ **Treatment**

A. Emergency and Supportive Measures

Caution: Abrupt respiratory arrest may occur in patients with acute paralytic shellfish and puffer fish poisoning. Observe patients for at least 4–6 hours. Replace fluid and electrolyte losses from gastroenteritis with intravenous saline or other crystalloid solution.

For recent ingestions, it may be possible to adsorb residual toxin in the gut with activated charcoal, 50–60 g orally (see p. 1554).

B. Specific Treatment

There is no specific antidote for paralytic shellfish or puffer fish poisoning.

1. Ciguatera—There are anecdotal reports of successful treatment of acute neurologic symptoms with mannitol, 1 g/kg intravenously, but this approach is not widely accepted.

2. Scombroid—Antihistamines such as diphenhydramine, 25–50 mg intravenously, and the H_2-blocker cimetidine, 300 mg intravenously, are usually effective. For severe reactions, give also epinephrine, 0.3–0.5 mL of a 1:1000 solution subcutaneously.

Goodman DM et al. JAMA patient page. Ciguatera fish poisoning. JAMA. 2013 Jun 26;309(24):2608. [PMID: 23800938]

Hungerford JM. Scombroid poisoning: a review. Toxicon. 2010 Aug 15;56(2):231–43. [PMID: 20152850]
Schlaich C et al. Outbreak of ciguatera fish poisoning on a cargo ship in the port of hamburg. J Travel Med. 2012 Jul;19 (4):238–42. [PMID: 22776385]

SNAKE BITES

The venom of poisonous snakes and lizards may be predominantly neurotoxic (coral snake) or predominantly cytolytic (rattlesnakes, other pit vipers). Neurotoxins cause respiratory paralysis; cytolytic venoms cause tissue destruction by digestion and hemorrhage due to hemolysis and destruction of the endothelial lining of the blood vessels. The manifestations of rattlesnake envenomation are mostly local pain, redness, swelling, and extravasation of blood. Perioral tingling, metallic taste, nausea and vomiting, hypotension, and coagulopathy may also occur. Thrombocytopenia can persist for several days after a rattlesnake bite. Neurotoxic envenomation may cause ptosis, dysphagia, diplopia, and respiratory arrest.

▶ **Treatment**

A. Emergency Measures

Immobilize the patient and the bitten part in a neutral position. Avoid manipulation of the bitten area. Transport the patient to a medical facility for definitive treatment. Do *not* give alcoholic beverages or stimulants; do *not* apply ice; do *not* apply a tourniquet. The potential trauma to underlying tissues resulting from incision and suction performed by unskilled people is probably not justified in view of the small amount of venom that can be recovered.

B. Specific Antidote and General Measures

1. Pit viper (eg, rattlesnake) envenomation—For local signs such as swelling, pain, and ecchymosis but no systemic symptoms, give 4–6 vials of crotalid antivenin (CroFab) by slow intravenous drip in 250–500 mL saline. Repeated doses of 2 vials every 6 hours for up to 18 hours has been recommended. For more serious envenomation with marked local effects and systemic toxicity (eg, hypotension, coagulopathy), higher doses and additional vials may be required. Monitor vital signs and the blood coagulation profile. Type and cross-match blood. The adequacy of venom neutralization is indicated by improvement in symptoms and signs, and the rate that swelling slows. Prophylactic antibiotics are not indicated after a rattlesnake bite.

2. Elapid (coral snake) envenomation—Give 1–2 vials of specific antivenom as soon as possible. To locate antisera for exotic snakes, call a regional poison control center (1-800-222-1222).

Lavonas EJ et al; Rocky Mountain Poison and Drug Center, Denver Health and Hospital Authority. Unified treatment algorithm for the management of crotaline snakebite in the United States: results of an evidence-informed consensus workshop. BMC Emerg Med. 2011 Feb 3;11:2. [PMID: 21291549]

Punguyire D et al. Bedside whole-blood clotting times: validity after snakebites. J Emerg Med. 2013 Mar;44(3):663–7. [PMID: 23047197]

Spano S et al. Snakebite Survivors Club: retrospective review of rattlesnake bites in Central California. Toxicon. 2013 Jul;69:38–41. [PMID: 23200707]

SPIDER BITES & SCORPION STINGS

The toxin of most species of spiders in the United States causes only local pain, redness, and swelling. That of the more venomous black widow spiders (*Latrodectus mactans*) causes generalized muscular pains, muscle spasms, and rigidity. The brown recluse spider (*Loxosceles reclusa*) causes progressive local necrosis as well as hemolytic reactions (rare).

Stings by most scorpions in the United States cause only local pain. Stings by the more toxic *Centruroides* species (found in the southwestern United States) may cause muscle cramps, twitching and jerking, and occasionally hypertension, convulsions, and pulmonary edema. Stings by scorpions from other parts of the world are not discussed here.

► Treatment

A. Black Widow Spider Bites

Pain may be relieved with parenteral opioids or muscle relaxants (eg, methocarbamol, 15 mg/kg). Calcium gluconate 10%, 0.1–0.2 mL/kg intravenously, may transiently relieve muscle rigidity, though its effectiveness is unproven. *Latrodectus* antivenom is very effective, but because of concerns about acute hypersensitivity reactions (horse serum-derived), it is often reserved for very young or elderly patients or those who do not respond promptly to the above measures. Horse serum sensitivity testing is required. (Instruction and testing materials are included in the antivenin kit.)

B. Brown Recluse Spider Bites

Because bites occasionally progress to extensive local necrosis, some authorities recommend early excision of the bite site, whereas others use oral corticosteroids. Anecdotal reports have claimed success with dapsone and colchicine. All of these treatments remain of unproved value.

C. Scorpion Stings

No specific treatment other than analgesics is required for envenomations by most scorpions found in the United States. An FDA-approved specific antivenom is now available for *Centruroides* stings.

Isbister GK et al. Spider bite. Lancet. 2011 Dec 10;378 (9808):2039–47. [PMID: 21762981]

Khattabi A et al; Scorpion Consensus Expert Group. Classification of clinical consequences of scorpion stings: consensus development. Trans R Soc Trop Med Hyg. 2011 Jul;105(7):364–9. [PMID: 21601228]

Monte AA. Black widow spider (*Latrodectus mactans*) antivenom in clinical practice. Curr Pharm Biotechnol. 2012 Aug;13(10):1935–9. [PMID: 22352727]

THEOPHYLLINE & CAFFEINE

Theophylline may cause intoxication after an acute single overdose, or intoxication may occur as a result of chronic accidental repeated overmedication or reduced elimination resulting from hepatic dysfunction or interacting drug (eg, cimetidine, erythromycin). The usual serum half-life of theophylline is 4–6 hours, but this may increase to more than 20 hours after overdose. Caffeine in herbal or dietary supplement products can produce similar toxicity.

► Clinical Findings

Mild intoxication causes nausea, vomiting, tachycardia, and tremulousness. Severe intoxication is characterized by ventricular and supraventricular tachyarrhythmias, hypotension, and seizures. Status epilepticus is common and often intractable to the usual anticonvulsants. After acute overdose (but not chronic intoxication), hypokalemia, hyperglycemia, and metabolic acidosis are common. Seizures and other manifestations of toxicity may be delayed for several hours after acute ingestion, especially if a sustained-release preparation such as Theo-Dur was taken.

Diagnosis is based on measurement of the serum theophylline concentration. Seizures and hypotension are likely to develop in acute overdose patients with serum levels > 100 mg/L (555 mcmol/L). Serious toxicity may develop at lower levels (ie, 40–60 mg/L [222–333 mcmol/L]) in patients with chronic intoxication.

▶ Treatment

A. Emergency and Supportive Measures

After acute ingestion, administer activated charcoal (see p. 1514). Repeated doses of activated charcoal may enhance theophylline elimination by "gut dialysis." Addition of whole bowel irrigation should be considered for large ingestions involving sustained-release preparations (see p. 1514).

Hemodialysis is effective in removing theophylline and is indicated for patients with status epilepticus or markedly elevated serum theophylline levels (eg, > 100 mg/L [555 mcmol/L] after acute overdose or > 60 mg/L [333 mcmol/L] with chronic intoxication).

B. Specific Treatment

Treat seizures with benzodiazepines (lorazepam, 2–3 mg intravenously, or diazepam, 5–10 mg intravenously) or phenobarbital (10–15 mg/kg intravenously). Phenytoin is not effective. Hypotension and tachycardia—which are mediated through excessive beta-adrenergic stimulation—may respond to beta-blocker therapy even in low doses. Administer esmolol, 25–50 mcg/kg/min by intravenous infusion, or propranolol, 0.5–1 mg intravenously.

Kneser J et al. Successful treatment of life threatening theophylline intoxication in a pregnant patient by hemodialysis. Clin Nephrol. 2013 Jul;80(1):72–4. [PMID: 22541679]

Trabulo D et al. Caffeinated energy drink intoxication. Emerg Med J. 2011 Aug;28(8):712–4. [PMID: 21788240]

Vaglio JC et al. Arrhythmogenic Munchausen syndrome culminating in caffeine-induced ventricular tachycardia. J Electrocardiol. 2011 Mar–Apr;44(2):229–31. [PMID: 20888004]

Wolk BJ et al. Toxicity of energy drinks. Curr Opin Pediatr. 2012 Apr;24(2):243–51. [PMID: 22426157]

TRICYCLIC & OTHER ANTIDEPRESSANTS

Tricyclic and related cyclic antidepressants are among the most dangerous drugs involved in suicidal overdose. These drugs have anticholinergic and cardiac depressant properties ("quinidine-like" sodium channel blockade). Tricyclic antidepressants produce more marked membrane-depressant cardiotoxic effects than the phenothiazines.

Newer antidepressants such as trazodone, fluoxetine, citalopram, paroxetine, sertraline, bupropion, venlafaxine, and fluvoxamine are not chemically related to the tricyclic antidepressant agents and do not generally produce quinidine-like cardiotoxic effects. However, they may cause seizures in overdoses and they may cause serotonin syndrome (see Monoamine Oxidase Inhibitors section).

▶ Clinical Findings

Signs of severe intoxication may occur abruptly and without warning within 30–60 minutes after acute tricyclic overdose. Anticholinergic effects include dilated pupils, tachycardia, dry mouth, flushed skin, muscle twitching, and decreased peristalsis. Quinidine-like cardiotoxic effects include QRS interval widening (> 0.12 s; Figure 38–2), ventricular arrhythmias, AV block, and hypotension. Rightward-axis deviation of the terminal 40 ms of the QRS has

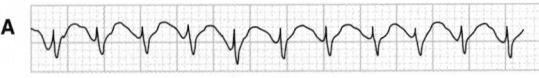

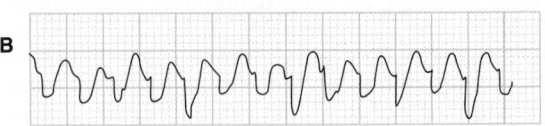

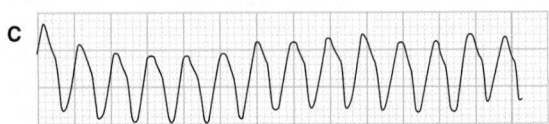

▲ **Figure 38–2.** Cardiac arrhythmias resulting from tricyclic antidepressant overdose. **A:** Delayed intraventricular conduction results in prolonged QRS interval (0.18 s). **B** and **C:** Supraventricular tachycardia with progressive widening of QRS complexes mimics ventricular tachycardia. (Reproduced, with permission, from Benowitz NL, Goldschlager N. Cardiac disturbances in the toxicologic patient. In: Haddad LM, Winchester JF [editors], *Clinical Management of Poisoning and Drug Overdose,* 3rd edition. Saunders/Elsevier, 1998.)

also been described. Prolongation of the QT interval and torsades de pointes have been reported with several of the newer antidepressants. Seizures and coma are common with severe intoxication. Life-threatening hyperthermia may result from status epilepticus and anticholinergic-induced impairment of sweating. Among newer agents, bupropion and venlafaxine have been associated with a greater risk of seizures.

The diagnosis should be suspected in any overdose patient with anticholinergic side effects, especially if there is widening of the QRS interval or seizures. For intoxication by most tricyclic antidepressants, the QRS interval correlates with the severity of intoxication more reliably than the serum drug level.

Serotonin syndrome should be suspected if agitation, delirium, diaphoresis, tremor, hyperreflexia, clonus (spontaneous, inducible, or ocular), and fever develop in a patient taking serotonin reuptake inhibitors.

▶ Treatment

A. Emergency and Supportive Measures

Observe patients for at least 6 hours, and admit all patients with evidence of anticholinergic effects (eg, delirium, dilated pupils, tachycardia) or signs of cardiotoxicity (see above). Administer activated charcoal (see p. 1554) and consider gastric lavage (see p. 1554) after recent large ingestions. All of these drugs are highly tissue-bound and are not effectively removed by hemodialysis procedures.

B. Specific Treatment

Cardiotoxic sodium channel-depressant effects of tricyclic antidepressants may respond to boluses of sodium bicarbonate (50–100 mEq intravenously). Sodium bicarbonate provides a large sodium load that alleviates depression of the sodium-dependent channel. Reversal of acidosis may also have beneficial effects at this site. Maintain the pH between 7.45 and 7.50. Alkalinization does not promote excretion of tricyclic antidepressants. Prolongation of the QT interval or torsades de pointes is usually treated with intravenous magnesium or overdrive pacing. Severe cardiotoxicity in patients with overdoses of lipid-soluble drugs (eg, amitriptyline, bupropion) has responded to intravenous lipid emulsion (Intralipid), 1.5 mL/kg repeated one or two times if needed. Plasma exchange using albumin has been reported successful in a few cases.

Mild serotonin syndrome may be treated with benzodiazepines and withdrawal of the antidepressant. Moderate cases may respond to cyproheptadine (4 mg orally or via gastric tube hourly for three or four doses) or chlorpromazine (25 mg intravenously). Severe hyperthermia should be treated with neuromuscular paralysis and endotracheal intubation in addition to external cooling measures.

Body R et al. Guidelines in Emergency Medicine Network (GEMNet): guideline for the management of tricyclic antidepressant overdose. Emerg Med J. 2011 Apr;28(4):347–68. [PMID: 21436332]

Kiberd MB et al. Lipid therapy for the treatment of a refractory amitriptyline overdose. CJEM. 2012 May;14(3):193–7. [PMID: 22575302]

Sari I et al. Therapeutic plasma exchange in amitriptyline intoxication: case report and review of the literature. Transfus Apher Sci. 2011 Oct;45(2):183–5. [PMID: 21872530]

Smith JC et al. Prolonged toxicity after amitriptyline overdose in a patient deficient in CYP2D6 activity. J Med Toxicol. 2011 Sep;7(3):220–3. [PMID: 21614669]

39

Cancer

Patricia A. Cornett, MD

Tiffany O. Dea, PharmD

The major features of this chapter are the clinical aspects of cancer, including etiology and prevention; staging; diagnosis and treatment of common cancers; and recognition and management of complications from cancer. Additional information may be obtained from the National Cancer Institute (NCI) website at http://www.cancer.gov/cancer-topics, the American Society of Clinical Oncology website at www.asco.org, and the National Comprehensive Cancer Network (NCCN) website at www.nccn.org. The NCCN website provides detailed, evidence-based recommendations for management of specific cancers as well as guidelines for cancer screening and supportive care.

▶ Etiology

Cancer is the second most common cause of death in the United States. In 2013, an estimated 1,660,290 cases of cancer were diagnosed, and 580,350 persons died as a result of cancer. Based on current statistics, one in three Americans will be diagnosed with cancer in their lifetime. Table 39–1 lists the 10 leading cancer types in men and women by site.

However, the death rates from cancer in both men and women are decreasing. In 2012, the American Cancer Society, NCI, and the Centers for Disease Control and Prevention reported that between 2004 and 2008 the cancer death rates for men declined by more than 1.8% per year and by 1.6% per year for women. Importantly, these declines in death rates have been seen in the four most common cancer types (lung, colon-rectum, breast, and prostate).

Reductions in cancer mortality reflect a successful implementation of a broad strategy of prevention, detection, and treatment.

▶ Modifiable Risk Factors

Tobacco is the most common preventable cause of cancer death; it is estimated that at least 30% of all cancer deaths in the United States are directly linked to tobacco. In 2013, a total of 174,100 cancer deaths in the United States could be directly attributed to tobacco abuse. Clear evidence links at least 15 cancers to tobacco use. The most dramatic link is with lung cancer, the most common non-dermatologic malignancy; 80% of lung cancer cases occur in smokers.

Any strategy for cancer control must include the goal of markedly reducing, if not eliminating, tobacco use.

Strategies for tobacco control should involve a focus on the individual as well as society as a whole. Tobacco cessation directed toward the individual should start with the clinician providing counseling. Simple, concise advice from a clinician can yield cessation rates of 10–20%. Additive strategies include more intensive counseling; nicotine replacement therapy with patches, gum, or lozenges; and prescription medication with bupropion or varenicline (see Chapter 1). Perhaps a more intriguing phenomenon, with potential for significant impact on cessation rates, is the influence of social contact behavior on an individual smoker's abstinence decision. For instance, analysis of the Framingham Heart Study demonstrated that smoking cessation by a spouse resulted in a 67% decrease in the subject's likelihood of continuing to smoke, and smoking cessation by a friend resulted in a 36% decrease in the subject's likelihood of smoking.

On a societal level, many initiatives have been put into place to actively discourage tobacco use. State or local laws regulating tobacco use in restaurants, the workplace, and other public places have resulted in declines in tobacco use. Countermarketing with aggressive anti-tobacco advertisements has also contributed to tobacco cessation and abstinence. The key recipients of these messages are children; 80% of smokers will start by age 18. Preventing the start of addiction in this vulnerable population should be a top priority (see Chapter 1).

There are encouraging signs of success with tobacco control. The prevalence of smoking for US adults based on the 2013 National Health Interview Survey is 18.0%, which is a remarkable reduction from the 1955 peak of 57% for males and the 1965 peak of 34% for females though it still falls short of the Healthy People 2020 goal of < 12%.

For those Americans who do not use tobacco, the most modifiable risk factors would be nutrition and physical activity. Epidemiologic studies suggest that fruit- and vegetable-rich diets lower risks of several gastrointestinal malignancies, including esophageal, stomach, and colon cancers. Excessive consumption of alcohol is linked to increased risks of head and neck cancers as well as cancers of the esophagus and liver. Lastly, being overweight is linked to several malignancies, including breast and uterine

Table 39–1. Estimated 10 most common cancer cases in the United States in males and females (all races).

Rank	Males Total Cases = 854,790 (percent)	Females Total Cases = 805,500 (percent)
1	Prostate (28)	Breast (29)
2	Lung and bronchus (14)	Lung and bronchus (14)
3	Colon and rectum (9)	Colon and rectum (9)
4	Urinary bladder (6)	Uterine corpus (6)
5	Melanoma (5)	Thyroid (6)
6	Lymphoma (5)	Lymphoma (5)
7	Kidney and renal pelvis (5)	Melanoma (4)
8	Oral cavity and pharynx (3)	Kidney and renal pelvis (3)
9	Leukemia (3)	Pancreas (3)
10	Pancreas (3)	Ovary (3)
	Other sites (19)	Other sites (18)

Data from the American Cancer Society, 2013.

cancers in women and colorectal, esophageal, and kidney cancers in both men and women. More importantly, weight reduction can decrease the risks of these cancers.

Another modifiable risk factor is radiation from radiographic studies. A 2009 study reported that the use of computed tomography (CT) in diagnostic algorithms exposes individuals to significant radiation doses that may increase the lifetime risk of developing cancer. Both standardization of CT radiation doses and limiting testing have been important steps in minimizing this risk. Both the American Society of Hematology and the American Society of Clinical Oncology now have guidelines for limiting radiograph testing in cancer patients.

Healthy People 2020 Tobacco Use Objectives: Reduce Tobacco Use by Adults http://www.healthypeople.gov/2020/topicsobjectives2020/objectiveslist.aspx?topicId=41

Siegel R et al. Cancer treatment and survivorship statistics. 2012. CA Cancer J Clin. 2012 Jul–Aug;62(4):220–41. [PMID: 22700443]

Smith-Bindman R et al. Radiation dose associated with common computed tomography examinations and the associated lifetime attributable risk of cancer. Arch Intern Med. 2009 Dec 14;169(22):2078–86. [PMID: 20008690]

▶ **Staging**

The most commonly used staging system at the time of diagnosis is the TNM (Tumor, Nodes, Metastasis) system (see www.cancerstaging.org). Rules for staging for individual cancers are established and published by the American Joint Committee on Cancer (AJCC). The elements used for staging are tumor location, size and level of tumor invasion (T), absence or presence and extent of nodal metastases (N), and presence or absence of systemic metastases (M). Once the TNM designations have been determined, an overall stage is assigned, stage I, II, III, or IV.

Clinical staging utilizes physical examination, laboratory and imaging tests as well as results from biopsies; pathologic staging relies on the results from surgery. In some instances, other classifications may be used for certain cancers such as the Ann Arbor staging system for lymphomas.

Other characteristics of cancers, not reflected in the TNM stage, may be used as another indicator of prognosis and guidelines for treatment. Pathologic features seen on routine histologic examination for some cancers are very important; examples include the Gleason score for prostate cancer and the grade of sarcomas. Cancer specimens may also be sent for targeted molecular diagnostic testing. Examples include testing for *HER2* in breast and gastric cancers, *K-ras* and *BRAF* mutations in colorectal cancers, *BRAF* mutations in melanoma, and epidermal growth factor receptor (EGFR) and *K-ras* mutations in lung cancer. As pathways for oncogenesis and relationships of mutations to treatment and prognosis continue to be delineated, analysis for detection of chromosomal alterations and oncogene products will be increasingly incorporated into routine practice.

THE PARANEOPLASTIC SYNDROMES

The clinical manifestations of cancer are usually due to pressure effects of local tumor growth, infiltration or metastatic deposition of tumor cells in a variety of organs in the body, or certain systemic symptoms. General problems observed in many patients with advanced or widespread metastatic cancer include anorexia, malaise, weight loss, and sometimes fever. These characteristics must be considered when evaluating a patient with an undiagnosed illness. Except in the case of functioning tumors such as those of the endocrine glands, systemic symptoms of cancer usually are not specific, often consisting of weakness, anorexia, and weight loss. The term "paraneoplastic" refers to features of disease considered to be due to the remote effects of a cancer. These features cannot be attributed either to a cancer's direct invasive or metastatic properties. Instead, symptoms are due to aberrant tumor production of hormones, peptides, or cytokines or to the body's immune attack on normal tissues due to shared antigens with tumor tissues. In the paraneoplastic syndromes, clinical findings may resemble those of primary endocrine, dermatologic, rheumatologic, hematologic, or neuromuscular disorders. In paraneoplastic syndromes associated with ectopic hormone production, tumor tissue itself secretes the hormone that produces the syndrome. Ectopic hormones secreted by neoplasms are often pro-hormones of higher molecular weight than those secreted by the more differentiated normal endocrine cell. Such ectopic hormone production by cancer cells is believed to result from activation of genes in the malignant cells that are suppressed in the normal tissue equivalent and in most somatic cells. Autocrine growth factors secreted by neoplastic cells may also result in paraneoplastic syndromes. Small cell lung cancer is the one type of cancer most likely to be associated with paraneoplastic syndromes.

The paraneoplastic syndromes are clinically important for the following reasons:

(1) They sometimes accompany relatively limited neoplastic growth and may provide the clinician with an early

clue to the presence of certain types of cancer, prompting the clinician to obtain screening tests for cancers known to be associated with those findings.

(2) The metabolic or toxic effects of the syndrome may constitute a more urgent hazard to the patient's life than the underlying cancer (eg, hypercalcemia, hyponatremia).

(3) Effective treatment of the tumor should be accompanied by resolution of the paraneoplastic syndrome and, conversely, recurrence of the cancer may be heralded by return of the systemic symptoms. In some instances, rapid response to cytotoxic chemotherapy may briefly increase the severity of the paraneoplastic syndrome in association with tumor lysis (eg, hyponatremia with inappropriate antidiuretic hormone excretion). In some instances the identical symptom complex (eg, hypercalcemia) may be induced by entirely different mechanisms. A single syndrome such as hypercalcemia may be due to any one of a variety of humoral factors, such as secretion of parathyroid hormone precursors or homologs (parathyroid hormone–related protein or PTHrP) or 1,25 dihydroxyvitamin D. Effective antitumor treatment usually results in return of serum calcium to normal.

Common paraneoplastic syndromes and endocrine secretions associated with functional cancers are summarized in Table 39–2.

Antoine JC et al. Paraneoplastic disorders of the peripheral nervous system. Presse Med. 2013 Jun;42(6 pt 2):e235–44. [PMID: 23608019]

Azar L et al. Paraneoplastic rheumatologic syndromes. Curr Opin Rheumatol. 2013 Jan;25(1):44–9. [PMID: 23026875]

Giometto B et al. Treatment for paraneoplastic neuropathies. Cochrane Database Syst Rev. 2012 Dec 12;12:CD007625. [PMID: 23235647]

Pelosof LC et al. Paraneoplastic syndromes: an approach to diagnosis and treatment. Mayo Clin Proc. 2010 Sep;85(9):838–54. Erratum in: Mayo Clin Proc. 2011 Apr;86(4):364. Dosage error in article text. [PMID: 20810794]

TYPES OF CANCER

LUNG CANCER

Sunny Wang, MD

BRONCHOGENIC CARCINOMA

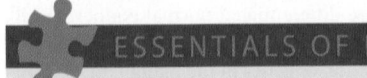

ESSENTIALS OF DIAGNOSIS

▸ New cough, or change in chronic cough.

▸ Dyspnea, hemoptysis, anorexia, weight loss.

▸ Enlarging nodule or mass; persistent opacity, atelectasis, or pleural effusion on chest radiograph or CT scan.

▸ Cytologic or histologic findings of lung cancer in sputum, pleural fluid, or biopsy specimen.

► General Considerations

Lung cancer is the leading cause of cancer deaths in both men and women. The American Cancer Society estimates 228,190 new diagnoses and 159,480 deaths from lung cancer in the United States in 2013, accounting for approximately 14% of new cancer diagnoses and 27% of all cancer deaths. More Americans die of lung cancer than of colorectal, breast, and prostate cancers combined.

Cigarette smoking causes 85–90% of cases of lung cancer. The causal connection between cigarettes and lung cancer is established not only epidemiologically but also through identification of carcinogens in tobacco smoke and analysis of the effect of these carcinogens on specific oncogenes expressed in lung cancer.

Other environmental risk factors for the development of lung cancer include exposure to environmental tobacco smoke, radon gas, asbestos (60- to 100-fold increased risk in smokers with asbestos exposure), metals (arsenic, chromium, nickel, iron oxide), and industrial carcinogens (bischloromethyl ether). A familial predisposition to lung cancer is recognized. Certain diseases are associated with an increased risk of lung cancer, including pulmonary fibrosis, chronic obstructive pulmonary disease, and sarcoidosis. Second primary lung cancers are more frequent in patients who survive their initial lung cancer.

The median age at diagnosis of lung cancer in the United States is 70; it is unusual under the age of 40. The combined relative 5-year survival rate for all stages of lung cancer is currently 16%.

Five histologic categories of bronchogenic carcinoma account for more than 90% of cases of primary lung cancer. **Squamous cell carcinoma** (20% of cases) arises from the bronchial epithelium, typically as a centrally located, intraluminal sessile or polypoid mass. Squamous cell cancers are more likely to present with hemoptysis and more frequently diagnosed by sputum cytology. They spread locally and may be associated with hilar adenopathy and mediastinal widening on chest radiography. **Adenocarcinoma** (35–40% of cases) arises from mucus glands or, in the case of **bronchioloalveolar cell carcinoma** (2% of cases), from any epithelial cell within or distal to the terminal bronchioles. Adenocarcinomas usually present as peripheral nodules or masses. Bronchioloalveolar cell carcinoma, now known as **adenocarcinoma in situ**, spreads along preexisting alveolar structures (lepidic growth) without evidence of invasion. **Large cell carcinoma** (3–5% of cases) is a heterogeneous group of relatively undifferentiated cancers that share large cells and do not fit into other categories. Large cell carcinomas typically have rapid doubling times and an aggressive clinical course. They present as central or peripheral masses. Cancers that are not better differentiated on pathologic review other than "carcinoma unspecified" make up about 20–25% of cases. **Small cell carcinoma** (10–15% of cases) is a tumor of bronchial origin that typically begins centrally, infiltrating submucosally to cause narrowing or obstruction of the bronchus without a discrete luminal mass.

For purposes of staging and treatment, bronchogenic carcinoma is divided into small cell lung cancer (SCLC) and the other four types, conveniently labeled non–small

Table 39–2. Paraneoplastic syndromes associated with cancer.

Hormone Excess or Syndrome	Non–Small Cell Lung Cancer	Small Cell Lung Cancer	Breast Cancer	Renal Cell Carcinoma	Adrenal Cancer	Hepatocellular Carcinoma	Gastrointestinal Cancers	Multiple Myeloma	Lymphoma	Thymoma	Prostatic Cancer	Ovarian Cancer	Chorio-carcinoma	Germ Cell Cancers
Endocrine														
Hypercalcemia	++		++	++	++			++	+		++			
Cushing syndrome	+	++		+	++					++	+			
SIADH	++	++			++									
Hypoglycemia				+	+	++	+							
Gonadotropin secretion	+	++		+	+	+	+						++	++
Hyperthyroidism			+										++	+
Hematologic														
Erythrocytosis				++	+	++								
Pure red cell aplasia									+	++				
Coagulopathy			++				++				++	+		
Thrombophlebitis			+				++				++	+		
Neurologic														
Lambert-Eaton myasthenic syndromes	+	++	+				+		+	+		+		
Subacute cerebellar syndrome		++	+				+		+			+		
Sensory motor peripheral neuropathy		++												
Stiff man syndrome			+											
Dermatologic														
Dermatomyositis	++	++	+				+		++			+		
Acanthosis nigricans	+		+				++				+			
Fever				++		++			++					
Hypertrophic osteoarthropathy	++									+				

+, reported associated; ++, strong association.
SIADH, syndrome of inappropriate antidiuretic hormone.

cell lung cancer (NSCLC). This practical classification reflects different natural histories and different treatment. SCLC is prone to early hematogenous spread. It is rarely amenable to surgical resection and has a very aggressive course with a median survival (untreated) of 6–18 weeks. The four histologic categories comprising NSCLC spread more slowly. They may be cured in the early stages following resection, and for advanced disease, chemotherapy is tailored to specific histologies and molecular mutations found within NSCLC.

► Clinical Findings

Lung cancer is symptomatic at diagnosis in 75–90% of patients. The clinical presentation depends on the type and location of the primary tumor, the extent of local spread, and the presence of distant metastases and any paraneoplastic syndromes.

A. Symptoms and Signs

Anorexia, weight loss, or asthenia occurs in 55–90% of patients presenting with a new diagnosis of lung cancer. Up to 60% of patients have a new cough or a change in a chronic cough; 6–31% have hemoptysis; and 25–40% complain of pain, either nonspecific chest pain or pain from bony metastases to the vertebrae, ribs, or pelvis. Local spread may cause endobronchial obstruction with atelectasis and postobstructive pneumonia, pleural effusion (12–33%), change in voice (compromise of the recurrent laryngeal nerve), superior vena cava syndrome (obstruction of the superior vena cava with supraclavicular venous engorgement), and Horner syndrome (ipsilateral ptosis, miosis, and anhidrosis from involvement of the inferior cervical ganglion and the paravertebral sympathetic chain). Distant metastases to the liver are associated with asthenia and weight loss. Brain metastases (10% in NSCLC, more common in adenocarcinoma, and 20–30% in SCLC) may present with headache, nausea, vomiting, seizures, dizziness, or altered mental status.

Paraneoplastic syndromes are incompletely understood patterns of organ dysfunction related to immune-mediated or secretory effects of neoplasms. These syndromes occur in 10–20% of lung cancer patients. They may precede, accompany, or follow the diagnosis of lung cancer and do not necessarily indicate metastatic disease. In patients with small cell carcinoma, the syndrome of inappropriate antidiuretic hormone (SIADH) can develop in 10–15%; in those with squamous cell carcinoma, hypercalcemia can develop in 10% (Table 39–2). Digital clubbing is seen in up to 20% of patients at diagnosis (see Figure 6–41). Other common paraneoplastic syndromes include increased ACTH production, anemia, hypercoagulability, peripheral neuropathy, and the Lambert-Eaton myasthenic syndrome. Their recognition is important because treatment of the primary tumor may improve or resolve symptoms even when the cancer is not curable.

B. Laboratory Findings

The diagnosis of lung cancer rests on examination of a tissue or cytology specimen. **Sputum cytology** is highly specific but insensitive; the yield is highest when there are lesions in the central airways. **Thoracentesis** (sensitivity 50–65%) can be used to establish a diagnosis of lung cancer in patients with malignant pleural effusions. If cytologic examination of an adequate sample (50–100 mL) of pleural fluid is nondiagnostic, the procedure should be repeated; approximately 30% of second samples are positive when the first sample is negative. If results remain negative, **thoracoscopy** is preferred to blind pleural biopsy. Fine-needle aspiration (FNA) of palpable supraclavicular or cervical lymph nodes is frequently diagnostic. Serum tumor markers are neither sensitive nor specific enough to aid in diagnosis.

Fiberoptic bronchoscopy allows visualization of the major airways, cytology brushing of visible lesions or lavage of lung segments with cytologic evaluation of specimens, direct biopsy of endobronchial abnormalities, blind transbronchial biopsy of the pulmonary parenchyma or peripheral nodules, and FNA biopsy of mediastinal lymph nodes. Diagnostic yield varies widely (10–90%) depending on the size of the lesion and its location. The use of fluorescence bronchoscopy improves the ability to identify early endobronchial lesions, while endobronchial and transesophageal endoscopic ultrasound enhance the direction and yield of FNA of mediastinal nodes. Transthoracic needle aspiration (TTNA) has a sensitivity between 50% and 97%. Mediastinoscopy, video-assisted thoracoscopic surgery (VATS), and thoracotomy are necessary in cases where less invasive techniques fail to yield a diagnosis.

C. Imaging

Nearly all patients with lung cancer have abnormal findings on chest radiography or CT scan. These findings are rarely specific for a particular diagnosis. Interpretation of characteristic findings in isolated nodules is described in Chapter 9.

D. Special Examinations

1. Staging—Accurate staging is crucial (1) to provide the clinician with information to guide treatment, (2) to provide the patient with accurate information regarding prognosis, and (3) to standardize entry criteria for clinical trials to allow interpretation of results.

There are two essential principles of staging **NSCLC**. First, the more extensive the disease, the worse the prognosis; second, surgical resection offers the best chance for cure. Staging of NSCLC uses two integrated systems. The **TNM international staging system** attempts a physical description of the neoplasm: T describes the size and location of the primary tumor; N describes the presence and location of nodal metastases; and M refers to the presence or absence of distant metastases. These TNM stages are grouped into prognostic categories (stages I–IV) using the results of clinical trials. This classification is used to guide therapy. Many patients with stage I and stage II disease are cured through surgery. Patients with stage IIIB and stage IV disease do not benefit from surgery (Table 39–3). Patients with stage IIIA disease have locally invasive disease that may benefit from surgery in certain circumstances as part of multimodality therapy.

Table 39–3. Five-year survival rates for non-small cell lung cancer, based on TNM staging.

Stage	TNM subset	5-Year Survival for Clinical TNM	5-Year Survival for Pathologic TNM
0	Carcinoma in situ		
IA	T1a/T1b, N0M0	50–80%	73%
IB	T2aN0M0	47%	58%
IIA	T1a/T1b, N1M0 T2aN1M0 T2bN0M0	36%	46%
IIB	T2bN1M0 T3N0M0	26%	36%
IIIA	T1/T2, N2M0 T3, N1/N2, M0 T4, N0/N1, M0	19%	24%
IIIB	T4N2M0 Any T, N3, M0	7%	9%
IV	Any T, Any N, M1a/M1b	2%	13%

Data from multiple sources. Modified and reproduced, with permission, from Tsim S et al. Staging of non-small-cell lung cancer (NSCLC): a review. Respir Med. 2010 Dec;104(12):1767–74. and Goldstraw P et al. The IASLC Lung Cancer Staging Project: proposals for the revision of the TNM stage groupings in the forthcoming (seventh) edition of the TNM Classification of malignant tumours. J Thorac Oncol. 2007 Aug;2(8):706–14.

SCLC is traditionally divided into two categories: **limited disease** (30%), when the tumor is limited to the unilateral hemithorax (including contralateral mediastinal nodes); or **extensive disease** (70%), when the tumor extends beyond the hemithorax (including pleural effusion).

For both SCLC and NSCLC, staging begins with a thorough history and physical examination. A complete examination is essential to exclude obvious metastatic disease to lymph nodes, skin, and bone. A detailed history is essential because the patient's performance status is a powerful predictor of disease course. All patients should have measurement of a complete blood count (CBC), serum electrolytes, calcium, creatinine, liver tests, lactate dehydrogenase, albumin, and a chest radiograph. Further evaluation will follow the results of these tests.

NSCLC patients being considered for surgery require meticulous evaluation to identify those with resectable disease. CT imaging is the most important modality for staging candidates for resection. A chest CT scan precisely defines the size of parenchymal lesions and identifies atelectatic lung or pleural effusions. However, CT imaging is less accurate at determining invasion of the chest wall (sensitivity 62%) or mediastinum (sensitivity 60–75%). The sensitivity and specificity of CT imaging for identifying lung cancer metastatic to the mediastinal lymph nodes are 57% (49–66%) and 82% (77–86%), respectively. Therefore, chest CT imaging does not provide definitive information on staging. CT imaging does help in making the decision about whether to proceed to resection of the primary tumor and sample the mediastinum at thoracotomy (common if there are no lymph nodes > 1 cm) or to use TTNA, mediastinoscopy, endobronchial ultrasound, endoscopic ultrasound with transesophageal needle aspiration, or limited thoracotomy to biopsy suspected metastatic disease (common where there are lymph nodes > 1–2 cm).

Positron emission tomography (PET) using 2-[^{18}F] fluoro-2-deoxyglucose (FDG) is an important modality for identifying metastatic foci in the mediastinum or distant sites. The sensitivity and specificity of PET for detecting mediastinal spread of primary lung cancer depend on the size of mediastinal nodes or masses. When only normal-sized (< 1 cm) mediastinal lymph nodes are present, the sensitivity and specificity of PET for tumor involvement of nodes are 74% and 96%, respectively. When CT shows enlarged (> 1 cm) lymph nodes, the sensitivity and specificity are 95% and 76%, respectively.

The combination of PET and CT imaging have improved preoperative staging compared with CT or PET alone. Many lung cancer specialists find whole body fusion PET-CT imaging most useful to confirm lack of metastatic disease in NSCLC patients who are candidates for surgical resection. Disadvantages of PET imaging include limited resolution below 1 cm; the expense of FDG; limited availability; and false-positive scans due to sarcoidosis, tuberculosis, or fungal infections. PET-CT scans are also inadequate for evaluating brain metastases due to the high FDG uptake there. Obtaining an MRI of the brain is important to rule out brain metastases in patients with at least stage II disease.

2. Preoperative assessment—See Chapter 3.

3. Pulmonary function testing—Many patients with NSCLC have moderate to severe chronic lung disease that increases the risk of perioperative complications as well as long-term pulmonary insufficiency following lung resection. All patients considered for surgery require spirometry. In the absence of other comorbidities, patients with good lung function (preoperative $FEV_1 \geq 2$ L) are at low risk for complications from lobectomy or pneumonectomy. If the FEV_1 is < 2 L, then an estimated postoperative FEV_1 should be calculated. The postresection FEV_1 may be estimated from considering preoperative spirometry and the amount of lung to be resected; in severe obstructive disease, a quantitative lung perfusion scan may improve the estimate. A predicted post-lung resection FEV_1 > 800 mL (or > 40% of predicted FEV_1) is associated with a low incidence of perioperative complications. High-risk patients include those with a predicted postoperative FEV_1 < 700 mL (or < 40% of predicted FEV_1). In these patients and in those with borderline spirometry, cardiopulmonary exercise testing may be helpful. A maximal oxygen uptake ($\dot{V}o_2$) of > 15 mL/kg/min identifies patients with an acceptable incidence of complications and mortality. Patients with a $\dot{V}o_2$ of < 10 mL/kg/min have a very high mortality rate at thoracotomy.

4. Screening—Screening with low-dose helical CT scans has been shown to improve mortality rates for lung cancer. The National Lung Screening Trial, a multicenter randomized US trial involving over 53,000 current and former heavy smokers, showed that screening annually with low-dose helical CT for 3 years yielded a 20% relative reduction in lung cancer mortality and 6.7% reduction in all-cause mortality compared to chest radiographs. Given these findings, US professional organizations, including the US Preventive Services Task Force, have recommended screening with low-dose helical CT for lung cancer. Initial analyses indicate that lung cancer screening based on NLST may be cost-effective, but these results have yet to be published. The results of ongoing European trials on lung cancer screening, in particular the NELSON trial in the Netherlands, are awaited. The implications of widespread screening of smokers raise issues of false positives (96% in this study), surgical and medical complications from additional testing, risks of cumulative exposure to radiation, and risks of increasing patient anxiety and stress on an already limited pool of resources. Improved risk stratification to target a higher risk population for low-dose CT screening may help alleviate these costs and concerns. Smoking cessation policies and efforts should be integrated with any screening program.

▶ Treatment

A. Non–Small Cell Lung Carcinoma

Cure of NSCLC is unlikely without resection. Therefore, the initial approach to the patient is determined by answering two questions: (1) Is complete surgical resection technically feasible? (2) If yes, is the patient able to tolerate the surgery with acceptable morbidity and mortality? Clinical features that preclude complete resection include extrathoracic metastases or a malignant pleural effusion; or tumor involving the heart, pericardium, great vessels, esophagus, recurrent laryngeal or phrenic nerves, trachea, main carina, or contralateral mediastinal lymph nodes. Accordingly, stage I and stage II patients are treated with surgical resection where possible. Stage II, and possibly a subset of stage IB, are additionally recommended to receive adjuvant chemotherapy. Stage IIIA patients have poor outcomes when treated with resection alone. They should be referred to multimodality protocols, including chemotherapy or radiotherapy, or both. Stage IIIB patients treated with concurrent chemotherapy and radiation therapy have improved survival. Stage IV patients are treated with chemotherapy or symptom-based palliative therapy, or both (see below).

Surgical approach affects outcome. In 1994, the North American Lung Cancer Study Group conducted a prospective trial of stage IA patients randomized to lobectomy versus limited resection. They reported a threefold increased rate of local recurrence in the limited resection group ($P = 0.008$) and a trend toward an increase in overall death rate (increase of 30%, $P = 0.08$) and increase in death rate due to cancer (increase of 50%, $P = 0.09$), compared with patients receiving lobectomy. However, for patients who cannot tolerate lobectomy or those with very small peripheral tumors < 2 cm with indolent imaging or histologic features, sublobar resection may be considered. A large randomized study is evaluating this question given improved technology in detecting smaller tumors.

VATS has become an acceptable and reasonable alternative to standard thoracotomy, if there are no anatomic or surgical contraindications, based on large case series showing equivalent long-term outcomes and less short-term morbidity. Radiation therapy following surgery is considered for margin-positive disease or pathologic mediastinal lymph node involvement.

Patients with small early-stage primary lung cancers who are not candidates for surgery because of significant comorbidity or other surgical contraindication may be candidates for stereotactic body radiotherapy. Stereotactic body radiotherapy, which is composed of multiple nonparallel radiation beams that converge, allows the delivery of a relatively large dose of radiation to a small, well-defined target. For small, early-stage cancers, 3-year primary tumor control rates with cyberknife exceed 95%, and 3-year survival is estimated at over 55%. Patients with locally advanced disease (stages IIIA and IIIB) who are not surgical candidates have improved survival when treated with concurrent chemotherapy and radiation therapy compared with no therapy, radiation alone, or even sequential chemotherapy and radiation.

Neoadjuvant chemotherapy consists of giving antineoplastic drugs in advance of surgery or radiation therapy. There is no consensus on the impact of neoadjuvant therapy on survival in stage I and stage II NSCLC. Such therapy is not recommended outside of ongoing clinical trials. Neoadjuvant therapy is more widely used in selected patients with stage IIIA or select stage IIIB disease. Some studies suggest a survival advantage. This remains an area of active research.

Adjuvant chemotherapy consists of administering antineoplastic drugs following surgery or radiation therapy. Cisplatin-containing regimens have been shown to confer an overall survival benefit in at least stage II disease and possibly a subset of stage IB disease. The Lung Adjuvant Cisplatin Evaluation Collaborative Group published a meta-analysis of the five largest cisplatin-based adjuvant trials. They reported a 5% absolute benefit in 5-year overall survival with a cisplatin-containing doublet regimen following surgery ($P = 0.005$) in patients with at least stage II disease. For patients with poor performance status (Eastern Cooperative Oncology Group Score ≥ 2), there is no evidence of survival benefit for adjuvant chemotherapy; rather, it may be detrimental.

Although not curative, chemotherapy has been shown in multiple clinical trials to provide a modest increase in overall survival and performance status in patients with stage IIIB and stage IV NSCLC compared with supportive care alone, with median survival increased from 5 months to a range of 7–11 months. Palliative chemotherapy also leads to improved quality of life and symptom control, with first-line therapy involving a platinum-based regimen. Platinum-based doublet regimens consist of cisplatin or carboplatin (agents that bind DNA to form adducts that inhibit their synthesis and function) combined with another agent, such as pemetrexed, gemcitabine, taxane, or vinorelbine. Investigators have shown that the choice of chemotherapeutic agent should be tailored to histologic subtype in NSCLC. For nonsquamous histologies, patients have modestly improved overall survival when treated with a platinum agent plus pemetrexed (an inhibitor of folate-dependent enzymes important in purine and pyrimidine synthesis). Patients with squamous cell lung carcinomas have modestly improved overall survival when a platinum agent is combined with gemcitabine (a deoxycytidine analog that inhibits DNA synthesis). For good performance status patients with nonsquamous histologies, bevacizumab (a monoclonal antibody to vascular endothelial growth factor [VEGF]) can be added to a traditional platinum doublet regimen with further modest increase in survival benefit. Finally, maintenance chemotherapy, that is, ongoing chemotherapy after an induction period of 4–6 cycles, has also been shown to improve overall survival.

With the advent of molecular profiling, targeted therapy has played a significant role in NSCLC. For the subgroup of patients with EGFR mutations, an EGFR tyrosine kinase inhibitor (erlotinib and gefitinib) rather than platinum-based chemotherapy is the first-line treatment. Response rates with EGFR inhibitors in patients with EGFR mutation are at least 60%, and median overall survival is estimated at 27–30 months. EGFR mutations are found in approximately 10–15% of the white population and 30–40% in the Asian population and are usually found among nonsmokers to light-smokers, females, and persons with nonsquamous histologies (particularly adenocarcinomas). Approximately 5% of all patients with NSCLC carry another mutation, the EML4-ALK fusion gene product. This is usually found in a comparatively younger population, with adenocarcinoma histology, and nonsmoking to light-smoking history. In a phase III trial of ALK-rearranged lung cancer patients, treatment with crizotinib (an ALK, cMET and ROS-1 tyrosine kinase inhibitor) showed a response rate of 60% compared with a rate of 20% among those treated with standard second-line cytotoxic chemotherapy. Crizotinib therapy also produced a statistically significant improvement in median progression-free survival over standard chemotherapy (7.7 vs 3 months, respectively). Finally, *K-ras* mutations are found among 25% of patients with adenocarcinomas, are associated with smoking, indicate a poor prognosis, and typically do not respond to EGFR inhibition. These three mutations (in *EGFR*, *EML4-ALK*, and *K-ras*) are mutually exclusive. Difficulties may arise when only small fine-needle aspirate biopsies are obtained; clinicians are recommended to get at least core biopsies for sufficient tissue for molecular analysis. Ongoing research seeks to define the role of these targeted agents in early stage and locally advanced lung cancers, mechanisms of resistance, and identification of new novel mutations, especially in squamous cell carcinomas where no approved targeted therapy exists.

B. Small Cell Lung Carcinoma

Response rates of SCLC to cisplatin and etoposide are excellent with 80–90% response in limited-stage disease (50–60% complete response), and 60–80% response in extensive stage disease (15–20% complete response). However, remissions tend to be short-lived with a median

Table 39–4. Median survival for small cell lung carcinoma following treatment.

Stage	Mean 2-Year Survival	Median Survival
Limited	20–40%	15–20 months
Extensive	5%	8–13 months

Data from multiple sources, including Van Meerbeeck JP et al. Small-cell lung cancer. Lancet. 2011 Nov 12;378(9804):1741–55.

duration of 6–8 months. Once the disease has recurred, median survival is 3–4 months. Overall 2-year survival is 20–40% in limited-stage disease and 5% in extensive-stage disease. (Table 39–4). Thoracic radiation therapy improves survival in patients with limited SCLC and is given concurrently with chemotherapy. Definitive thoracic radiation therapy is not considered beneficial for patients with extensive disease, and they should receive chemotherapy alone. There is a high rate of brain metastasis in patients with SCLC, even following a good response to chemotherapy, because chemotherapy does not adequately penetrate the blood-brain barrier. Prophylactic cranial irradiation has been shown to decrease the incidence of central nervous system disease and improve survival in patients with limited stage disease who respond to chemotherapy and a subset of patients with extensive stage disease who have had an excellent response to chemotherapy.

Occasionally, very early limited-stage disease (T1N0M0) may be detected on PET-CT, MRI of the brain, or mediastinoscopy. It may be also be identified after a peripheral nodule proves to be SCLC on resection. These patients are recommended to receive adjuvant chemotherapy following surgery given the high risk of micrometastases in SCLC. Five-year survival following resection of stage I SCLC can reach upwards to 50%.

C. Palliative Therapy

Photoresection with the Nd:YAG laser is sometimes performed on central tumors to relieve endobronchial obstruction, improve dyspnea, and control hemoptysis. External beam radiation therapy is also used to control dyspnea, hemoptysis, endobronchial obstruction, pain from bony metastases, obstruction from superior vena cava syndrome, and symptomatic brain metastases. Resection of a *solitary* brain metastasis improves quality of life when combined with radiation therapy, and if there is no evidence of other metastatic disease, may improve survival. Intraluminal radiation (brachytherapy) is an alternative approach to endobronchial disease. Pain syndromes are very common in advanced disease. As patients approach the end of life, meticulous efforts at pain control are essential (see Chapter 5). In addition to standard oncologic care, early consultation with—or referral to—a palliative care specialist is recommended in advanced disease to aid in symptom management and can modestly improve survival.

► **Prognosis**

The overall 5-year survival rate for lung cancer is approximately 15%. Predictors of survival include the type of tumor (SCLC versus NSCLC), molecular typing, the stage of the tumor, the patient's performance status, and weight loss in the past 6 months. Patients with EGFR mutation have better overall survival when compared with those without EGFR mutation, even when receiving similar cytotoxic chemotherapy.

Boiselle PM et al. JAMA patient page. Lung cancer screening. JAMA. 2013 May 8;309(18):1948. [PMID: 23652527]
Cufer T et al. Systemic therapy of advanced non-small cell lung cancer: major developments of the last 5-years. Eur J Cancer. 2013 Apr;49(6):1216–25. [PMID: 23265700]
Detterbeck FC et al. The stage classification of lung cancer: diagnosis and management of lung cancer, 3rd ed: American College of Chest Physicians evidence-based clinical practice guidelines. Chest. 2013 May;143(5 Suppl):e191S–210S. [PMID: 23649438]
Field JK et al. Prospects for population screening and diagnosis of lung cancer. Lancet. 2013 Aug 24;382(9893):732–41. [PMID: 23972816]
Jones CD et al. Does surgery improve prognosis in patients with small-cell lung carcinoma? Interact Cardiovasc Thorac Surg. 2013 Mar;16(3):375–80. [PMID: 23169878]
Kong FM et al; Expert Panel on Radiation Oncology-Lung. ACR Appropriateness Criteria® radiation therapy for small-cell lung cancer. Am J Clin Oncol. 2013 Apr;36(2):206–13. [PMID: 23511336]
Reck M et al. Management of non-small-cell lung cancer: recent developments. Lancet. 2013 Aug 24;382(9893):709–19. [PMID: 23972814]
Shaw AT et al. Crizotinib versus chemotherapy in advanced ALK-positive lung cancer. N Engl J Med. 2013 Jun 20;368 (25):2385–94. [PMID: 23724913]
Travis WD et al. New pathologic classification of lung cancer: relevance for clinical practice and clinical trials. J Clin Oncol. 2013 Mar 10;31(8):992–1001. [PMID: 23401443]

PULMONARY METASTASIS

Pulmonary metastasis results from the spread of an extrapulmonary malignant tumor through vascular or lymphatic channels or by direct extension. Almost any cancer can metastasize to the lung, including primary lung carcinomas. Metastases usually occur via the pulmonary artery and typically present as multiple nodules or masses on chest radiography. The radiographic differential diagnosis of multiple pulmonary nodules also includes pulmonary arteriovenous malformation, pulmonary abscesses, granulomatous infection, sarcoidosis, rheumatoid nodules, and granulomatosis with polyangiitis (formerly Wegener granulomatosis). Metastases to the lungs are found in 20–55% of patients dying of various malignancies. Most are intraparenchymal. Carcinoma of the kidney, breast, rectum, colon, and cervix and malignant melanoma are the most likely primary tumors. Head and neck cancers with extensive or lower cervical nodal involvement have a 30% risk for distant metastasis; half of these metastases present in the lungs. Pulmonary metastases are common in patients with osteosarcomas, but pulmonary metastases develop in only 20% of patients with soft tissue sarcomas.

Lymphangitic carcinomatosis denotes diffuse involvement of the pulmonary lymphatic network by primary or metastatic lung cancer, probably a result of extension of tumor from lung capillaries to the lymphatics. **Tumor embolization** from extrapulmonary cancer (renal cell carcinoma, hepatocellular carcinoma, choriocarcinoma) is an uncommon route for tumor spread to the lungs. Metastatic cancer may also present as a malignant pleural effusion.

► **Clinical Findings**

A. Symptoms and Signs

Symptoms are uncommon but include cough, hemoptysis and, in advanced cases, dyspnea and hypoxemia. Symptoms are more often referable to the site of the primary tumor.

B. Laboratory Findings

The diagnosis of metastatic cancer involving the lungs is usually established by identifying a primary tumor. Appropriate studies should be ordered if there is a suspicion of any primary cancer, such as breast, thyroid, testis, colorectal, or prostate, for which specific treatment is available. For example, an elevated prostate-specific antigen (PSA) may indicate prostate cancer, carcinoembryonic antigen (CEA) tests for colorectal cancer, and beta-human chorionic gonadotropin (beta-hCG) and alpha-fetoprotein test for germ cell tumors. Based on the clinical setting, imaging studies should be ordered (see below). If the history, physical examination, and initial studies fail to reveal the site of the primary tumor, attention is better focused on the lung, where tissue samples obtained by bronchoscopy, percutaneous needle biopsy, VATS, or thoracotomy may establish the histologic diagnosis and suggest the most likely primary cancer. Occasionally, cytologic studies of pleural fluid or pleural biopsy reveal the diagnosis.

If the initial histologic review does not reveal a primary diagnosis, immunohistochemical staining should be done on the biopsy specimen. For example, PSA and thyroglobulin staining are highly specific for prostate and thyroid cancer, respectively. Thyroid transcription factor-1 (TTF-1) and napsin-A are relatively specific for primary lung adenocarcinoma, while the former can be positive in cases of SCLC and thyroid carcinoma and the latter can be positive in papillary and clear cell renal cell carcinomas. An adenocarcinoma that demonstrates negative TTF-1 and napsin-A staining strongly suggests a nonpulmonary primary cancer. Positive estrogen receptor (ER) and progesterone receptor (PR) stains suggest primary breast cancer.

C. Imaging

Chest radiographs usually show multiple spherical densities with sharp margins. The size of metastatic lesions varies from a few millimeters (miliary densities) to large masses. The lesions are usually bilateral, pleural or subpleural in location, and more common in lower lung zones. Cavitation suggests squamous cell tumor; calcification suggests osteosarcoma. Lymphangitic spread and solitary pulmonary nodule are less common radiographic presentations of pulmonary metastasis. Mammography should be considered in women to search for possible primary breast cancer. CT imaging of the chest, abdomen, and pelvis may reveal the site of a primary tumor and will help determine feasibility of surgical resection of the metastatic lung tumors. PET-CT scan may also help in identifying the site of a primary cancer or identifying other areas of extrathoracic metastasis.

▶ Treatment

Once the diagnosis has been established, management consists of treatment of the primary neoplasm and any pulmonary complications. Surgical resection of a *solitary* pulmonary nodule is often prudent in the patient with known current or previous extrapulmonary cancer. Local resection of one or more pulmonary metastases is feasible in a few carefully selected patients with various sarcomas and carcinomas (such as testis, colon, and kidney). Surgical resection should be considered only if the primary tumor is under control, if the patient is a good surgical risk, if all of the metastatic tumor can be resected, if effective nonsurgical approaches are not available, and if there are no metastases elsewhere in the body. Relative contraindications to resection of pulmonary metastases include (1) malignant melanoma primary, (2) requirement for pneumonectomy, and (3) pleural involvement. Data from the International Registry of Lung Metastases report an overall 5-year survival rate of 36% and 10-year survival rate of 26% after complete resection of pulmonary metastases. Patients who are not surgical candidates but have solitary or limited metastatic disease to the lungs may be candidates for stereotactic radiosurgery, radioablation, or cryotherapy. For patients with unresectable progressive disease, diligent attention to palliative care is essential (see Chapter 5).

Hornbech K et al. Current status of pulmonary metastasectomy. Eur J Cardiothorac Surg. 2011 Jun;39(6):955–62. [PMID: 21115259]

Hornbech K et al. Outcome after pulmonary metastasectomy: analysis of 5 years consecutive surgical resections 2002–2006. J Thorac Oncol. 2011 Oct;6(10):1733–40. [PMID: 21869715]

Mitry E et al. Epidemiology, management and prognosis of colorectal cancer with lung metastases: a 30-year population-based study. Gut. 2010 Oct;59(10):1383–8. [PMID: 20732912]

Ordóñez NG. Napsin A expression in lung and kidney neoplasia: a review and update. Adv Anat Pathol. 2012 Jan;19(1):66–73. [PMID: 22156835]

Treasure T et al. Pulmonary metastasectomy in colorectal cancer: the PulMiCC Trial. J Thor Oncol. 2010 Jun;5(6 Suppl 2):S203–6. [PMID: 20502265]

MESOTHELIOMA

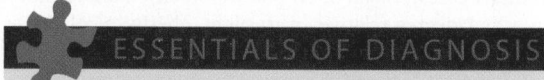

ESSENTIALS OF DIAGNOSIS

- ▶ Unilateral, nonpleuritic chest pain and dyspnea.
- ▶ Distant (> 20 years earlier) history of exposure to asbestos.
- ▶ Pleural effusion or pleural thickening or both on chest radiographs.
- ▶ Malignant cells in pleural fluid or tissue biopsy.

▶ General Considerations

Mesotheliomas are primary tumors arising from the surface lining of the pleura (80% of cases) or peritoneum (20% of cases). About three-fourths of pleural mesotheliomas are diffuse (usually malignant) tumors, and the remaining one-fourth are localized (usually benign). Men outnumber women by a 3:1 ratio. Numerous studies have confirmed the association of **malignant pleural mesothelioma** with exposure to asbestos (particularly the amphibole form). The lifetime risk to asbestos workers of developing malignant pleural mesothelioma is as high as 10%. The latent period between exposure and onset of symptoms ranges from 20 to 40 years. The clinician should inquire about asbestos exposure through mining, milling, manufacturing, shipyard work, insulation, brake linings, building construction and demolition, roofing materials, and a variety of asbestos products (pipe, textiles, paint, tile, gaskets, panels). Although cigarette smoking significantly increases the risk of bronchogenic carcinoma in asbestos workers and aggravates asbestosis, there is no association between smoking and mesothelioma.

▶ Clinical Findings

A. Symptoms and Signs

The average interval between onset of symptoms and diagnosis is 2–3 months; the median age at diagnosis is 72–74 years in Western countries. Symptoms include the insidious onset of shortness of breath, nonpleuritic chest pain, and weight loss. Physical findings include dullness to percussion, diminished breath sounds and, in some cases, digital clubbing.

B. Laboratory Findings

Pleural fluid is exudative and often hemorrhagic. Cytologic tests of pleural fluid are often negative. VATS biopsy is usually necessary to obtain an adequate specimen for histologic diagnosis. The histologic variants of malignant pleural mesothelioma are epithelial (50–60%), sarcomatoid (10%), and biphasic (30–40%). Since distinction from benign inflammatory conditions and metastatic adenocarcinoma may be difficult, immunohistochemical stains are important to confirm the diagnosis. Epithelial mesothelioma stains are positive for calretinin, keratin 5/6, WT1, and D2-40 and are negative for epithelial markers, such as p63, MOC-31, TTF-1, CD15, and Ber.EP4 (usually three needed).

C. Imaging

Radiographic abnormalities consist of nodular, irregular, unilateral pleural thickening and varying degrees of unilateral pleural effusion. Sixty percent of patients have right-sided disease, while only 5% have bilateral involvement. CT scans demonstrate the extent of pleural involvement. PET-CT is increasingly used to help differentiate benign from malignant pleural disease, improve staging accuracy, and identify candidates for aggressive surgical approaches.

Complications

Malignant pleural mesothelioma progresses rapidly as the tumor spreads along the pleural surface to involve the pericardium, mediastinum, and contralateral pleura. The tumor may eventually extend beyond the thorax to involve abdominal lymph nodes and organs. Progressive pain and dyspnea are characteristic. Local invasion of thoracic structures may cause superior vena cava syndrome, hoarseness, Horner syndrome, arrhythmias, and dysphagia.

Treatment

Chemotherapy is the mainstay of treatment, with surgery only included in multimodality treatment if there is localized disease that can be surgically resected. The optimal surgical approach is still under debate. For localized disease, surgical options include pleurectomy and decortication (surgical stripping of the pleura and pericardium from apex of the lung to diaphragm) or extrapleural pneumonectomy (a radical surgical procedure involving removal of the ipsilateral lung, parietal and visceral pleura, pericardium, and most of the hemidiaphragm). Limited nonrandomized data have shown that a trimodality approach for localized disease with extrapleural pneumonectomy, adjuvant radiation, and (neo-adjuvant or adjuvant) chemotherapy can prolong survival in highly selected patients. However, the benefit of extrapleural pneumonectomy has been brought into question with the results of the Mesothelioma and Radical Surgery (MARS) trial. This small randomized study, comparing extrapleural pneumonectomy with no extrapleural pneumonectomy after induction chemotherapy in 50 patients, showed that extrapleural pneumonectomy offers no survival benefit and may cause more harm. In advanced disease, palliative chemotherapy with cisplatin and pemetrexed can achieve response rates of 30–40%, extend median overall survival to 12 months, and improve quality of life. For patients with comorbidities, where cisplatin may not be tolerated, carboplatin can be substituted and given with pemetrexed. Other alternative chemotherapy regimens include gemcitabine, anthracyclines, or vinorelbine. Drainage of pleural effusions, pleurodesis, radiation therapy, and even surgical resection may offer palliative benefit in some patients.

Prognosis

Most patients die of respiratory failure and complications of local extension. Median survival time from diagnosis ranges from 7 months to 17 months. Five-year survival is 5–10%. Tumors that are predominantly sarcomatoid are more resistant to therapy and have a worse prognosis, with median survivals < 1 year. Poor prognostic features include poor performance status, non-epithelioid histology, male gender, nodal involvement, elevated lactate dehydrogenase, high white blood cell count, low hemoglobin, and high platelet count.

Husain AN et al. Guidelines for pathologic diagnosis of malignant mesothelioma: 2012 update of the consensus statement from the International Mesothelioma Interest Group. Arch Pathol Lab Med. 2013 May;137(5):647–67. [PMID: 22929121]

Lindenmann J et al. Multimodal therapy of malignant pleural mesothelioma: is the replacement of radical surgery imminent? Interact Cardiovasc Thorac Surg. 2013 Mar;16(3):237–43. [PMID: 23171517]

Pasello G et al. An overview of neoadjuvant chemotherapy in the multimodality treatment of malignant pleural mesothelioma. Cancer Treat Rev. 2013 Feb;39(1):10–7. [PMID: 22459200]

Pinto C et al. Second Italian Consensus Conference on Malignant Pleural Mesothelioma: state of the art and recommendations. Cancer Treat Rev. 2013 Jun;39(4):328–39. [PMID: 23244777]

Remon J et al. Malignant mesothelioma: new insights into a rare disease. Cancer Treat Rev. 2013 Oct;39(6):584–91. [PMID: 23276688]

HEPATOBILIARY CANCERS

Lawrence S. Friedman, MD

HEPATOCELLULAR CARCINOMA

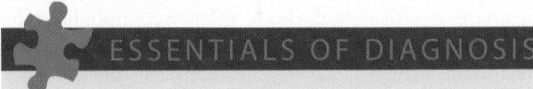

ESSENTIALS OF DIAGNOSIS

▶ In Western countries, usually a complication of cirrhosis.

▶ Characteristic CT and MRI features and elevated serum alpha-fetoprotein may obviate the need for a confirmatory biopsy.

General Considerations

Malignant neoplasms of the liver that arise from parenchymal cells are called hepatocellular carcinomas; those that originate in the ductular cells are called cholangiocarcinomas.

Hepatocellular carcinomas are associated with cirrhosis in 80% of cases. In Africa and most of Asia, hepatitis B virus (HBV) infection is a major etiologic factor, and a family history of hepatocellular carcinoma increases the risk synergistically. In the United States and other Western countries, incidence rates are rising rapidly (twofold since 1978), presumably because of the increasing prevalence of cirrhosis caused by chronic hepatitis C virus (HCV) infection and nonalcoholic fatty liver disease. In Western countries, risk factors for hepatocellular carcinoma in patients known to have cirrhosis are male gender, age > 55 years (although there has been an increase in the number of younger cases), Asian or Hispanic ethnicity, family history in a first-degree relative, overweight, obesity, alcohol use (especially in combination with obesity), diabetes mellitus, hypothyroidism (in women), a prolonged prothrombin time, a low platelet count, and an elevated serum transferrin saturation. The risk of hepatocellular carcinoma is higher in persons with a viral rather than nonviral cause of cirrhosis. Other associations include high levels of HBV replication; HBV genotype C; hepatitis D coinfection; elevated serum ALT levels in persons with chronic hepatitis B (in whom antiviral therapy to suppress HBV replication appears to reduce the risk); HCV genotype

1b; hemochromatosis (and possibly the C282Y carrier state); aflatoxin exposure (associated with mutation of the *TP53* gene); alpha-1-antiprotease (alpha-1-antitrypsin) deficiency; tyrosinemia; and radiation exposure. In patients with the metabolic syndrome, hepatocellular carcinoma may arise from a hepatocellular adenoma in the absence of cirrhosis. Evidence for an association with long-term use of oral contraceptives is inconclusive. Consumption of coffee and n-3 polyunsaturated fatty acids, the use of aspirin and, in diabetic patients, the use of statins and metformin appear to be protective, whereas use of sulfonylureas and insulin may increase the risk. The fibrolamellar variant of hepatocellular carcinoma occurs in young women and is characterized by a distinctive histologic picture, absence of risk factors, and indolent course. Vinyl chloride exposure is associated with angiosarcoma of the liver. Hepatoblastoma, the most common malignant liver tumor in infants and young children, occurs rarely in adults.

► Clinical Findings

A. Symptoms and Signs

The presence of a hepatocellular carcinoma may be unsuspected until there is deterioration in the condition of a cirrhotic patient who was formerly stable. Cachexia, weakness, and weight loss are associated symptoms. The sudden appearance of ascites, which may be bloody, suggests portal or hepatic vein thrombosis by tumor or bleeding from a necrotic tumor.

Physical examination may show tender enlargement of the liver, occasionally with a palpable mass. In Africa, the typical presentation in young patients is a rapidly expanding abdominal mass. Auscultation may reveal a bruit over the tumor or a friction rub when the tumor has extended to the surface of the liver.

B. Laboratory Findings

Laboratory tests may reveal leukocytosis, as opposed to the leukopenia that is frequently encountered in cirrhotic patients. Anemia is common, but a normal or elevated hematocrit value may be found in up to one-third of patients owing to elaboration of erythropoietin by the tumor. Sudden and sustained elevation of the serum alkaline phosphatase in a patient who was formerly stable is a common finding. HBsAg is present in a majority of cases in endemic areas, whereas in the United States anti-HCV is found in up to 40% of cases. Alpha-fetoprotein levels are elevated in up to 70% of patients with hepatocellular carcinoma in Western countries (although the sensitivity is lower in blacks and levels are not elevated in patients with fibrolamellar hepatocellular carcinoma); however, mild elevations (10–200 ng/mL [10–200 mcg/L]) are also often seen in patients with chronic hepatitis. Serum levels of des-gamma-carboxy prothrombin are elevated in up to 90% of patients with hepatocellular carcinoma, but they may also be elevated in patients with vitamin K deficiency, chronic hepatitis, and metastatic cancer. Cytologic study of ascitic fluid rarely reveals malignant cells.

C. Imaging

Multiphasic helical CT and MRI with contrast enhancement are the preferred imaging studies for determining the location and vascularity of the tumor. Lesions smaller than 1 cm may be difficult to characterize. Arterial phase enhancement of the lesion followed by delayed hypointensity ("washout") is most specific for hepatocellular carcinoma. Ultrasonography is less sensitive and operator dependent but is used to screen for hepatic nodules in high-risk patients. Contrast-enhanced ultrasonography has a sensitivity and specificity approaching those of arterial phase helical CT but, unlike CT and MRI, cannot image the entire liver during the short duration of the arterial phase and is thus associated with false-positive results. In selected cases, endoscopic ultrasonography may be useful. PET is under study.

D. Liver Biopsy and Staging

Liver biopsy is diagnostic, although seeding of the needle tract by tumor is a potential risk (1–3%). For lesions < 1 cm, ultrasonography may be repeated every 3 months followed by further investigation of enlarging lesions. For lesions ≥ 1 cm, biopsy can be deferred when characteristic arterial hypervascularity and delayed washout are demonstrated on either multiphasic helical CT or MRI with contrast enhancement (or both) or if surgical resection is planned. Staging in the TNM classification includes the following definitions: T0: no evidence of primary tumor; T1: solitary tumor without vascular invasion; T2: solitary tumor with vascular invasion or multiple tumors none more than 5 cm; T3: multiple tumors more than 5 cm (3a) or tumor involving a major branch of the portal or hepatic vein (3b); and T4: tumor(s) with direct invasion of adjacent organs other than the gallbladder or with perforation of the visceral peritoneum; N1, regional lymph node metastasis; M1, distant metastasis; F0, no to moderate hepatic fibrosis; F1, severe hepatic fibrosis to cirrhosis. The Barcelona Clinic Liver Cancer (BCLC) staging system is preferred and includes the Child-Turcotte-Pugh stage, tumor stage, and liver function and has the advantage of linking overall stage with preferred treatment modalities and with an estimation of life expectancy.

► Screening & Prevention

Surveillance for the development of hepatocellular carcinoma is recommended in patients with chronic hepatitis B (beginning as early as age 20 in Africans, age 40 in Asians or those with a family history of hepatocellular carcinoma, and age 50 in others) or cirrhosis caused by HCV, HBV, or alcohol. The standard approach is ultrasonography and alpha-fetoprotein testing every 6 months, although the value of alpha-fetoprotein screening has been questioned because of its low sensitivity. CT and MRI are considered too expensive for screening, but the sensitivity of ultrasonography for detecting early hepatocellular carcinoma is only 63%. The risk of hepatocellular carcinoma in a patient with cirrhosis is 3–5% a year, and patients with tumors detected by surveillance have a less advanced stage on average and greater likelihood that treatment will prolong survival than those not undergoing surveillance. In a population of patients with cirrhosis, over 60% of nodules < 2 cm in diameter detected on a screening ultrasonography prove to be hepatocellular carcinoma. Mass vaccination programs against HBV in developing countries are leading to reduced rates of hepatocellular carcinoma. Successful treatment of hepatitis B and of hepatitis C in patients with cirrhosis also reduces the subsequent risk of hepatocellular carcinoma.

► Treatment

Surgical resection of a solitary hepatocellular carcinoma may result in cure if liver function is preserved (Child class A or possibly B) and portal vein thrombosis is not present. Laparoscopic liver resection has been performed in selected cases. Treatment of underlying chronic viral hepatitis, adjuvant chemotherapy, and adaptive immunotherapy may lower postsurgical recurrence rates. Liver transplantation may be appropriate for small unresectable tumors in a patient with advanced cirrhosis, with reported 5-year survival rates of up to 75%. The recurrence-free survival may be better for liver transplantation than for resection in patients with well-compensated cirrhosis and small tumors (one tumor < 5 cm or three or fewer tumors each < 3 cm in diameter [Milan criteria]) and in those with expanded (University of California, San Francisco) criteria of one tumor ≥ 6.5 cm or three or fewer tumors ≥ 4.5 cm. Patients with stage 2 hepatocellular carcinoma receive an additional 22 points on their Model for End-Stage Liver Disease (MELD) score (see Chapter 16), markedly increasing their chances of undergoing transplantation. However, liver transplantation is often impractical because of the donor organ shortage, and living donor liver transplantation may be considered in these cases. Patients with larger tumors (3–5 cm), a serum alpha-fetoprotein level ≥ 455 ng/mL (455 mcg/L), or a MELD score ≥20 have poor posttransplantation survival. Chemotherapy, hormonal therapy with tamoxifen, and long-acting octreotide have not been shown to prolong life, but transarterial chemoembolization (TACE), transarterial chemoinfusion (TACI), and transarterial radioembolization (TARE) via the hepatic artery are palliative and may prolong survival in patients with a large or multifocal tumor in the absence of extrahepatic spread. TACI and TARE are suitable for patients with portal vein thrombosis. Radiofrequency ablation of, cryotherapy of, microwave ablation of, or injection of absolute ethanol into small tumors (< 2 cm) may prolong survival in patients who are not candidates for resection and have tumors that are accessible; these interventions may also provide a "bridge" to liver transplantation. Radiofrequency ablation is superior to ethanol injection for tumors > 2 cm in diameter (but no larger than 5 cm) and can be performed after TACE in select cases. Sorafenib (an oral multikinase inhibitor of Raf kinase, the VEGF receptor, and the platelet-derived growth factor receptor [and others]), prolongs median survival as well as the time to radiologic progression by 3 months in patients with advanced hepatocellular carcinoma; sorafenib is the standard of care in these patients. New chemotherapy and radiation therapy techniques (eg, radioembolization with yttrium-90 microspheres), novel biologic approaches (eg, bortezomib, a proteasome inhibitor; antiangiogenesis agents; other inhibitors of growth-factor signaling; and gene therapy), and multimodal approaches are under study. For patients whose disease progresses despite treatment or who present with advanced tumors, vascular invasion, or extrahepatic spread, meticulous efforts at palliative care are essential (see Chapter 5). Severe pain may develop in such patients due to expansion of the liver capsule by the tumor and requires concerted efforts at pain management, including the use of opioids (see Chapter 5).

► Prognosis

In the United States, overall 1- and 5-year survival rates for patients with hepatocellular carcinoma are 23% and 5%, respectively. Five-year survival rates rise to 56% for patients with localized resectable disease (T1, T2, selected T3 and T4; N0; M0) but are virtually nil for those with locally unresectable or advanced disease. In patients with HCV-related hepatocellular carcinoma, the serum alpha-fetoprotein level at the time of diagnosis of cancer has been reported to be an independent predictor of mortality. In patients who are not eligible for surgery, an elevated serum C-reactive protein level is associated with poor survival. Contrary to traditional opinion, the fibrolamellar variant does not have a better prognosis than conventional hepatocellular carcinoma without cirrhosis.

► When to Refer

All patients with hepatocellular carcinoma should be referred to a specialist.

► When to Admit

- Complications of cirrhosis.
- Severe pain.
- For surgery and other interventions.

Forner A et al. Hepatocellular carcinoma. Lancet. 2012 Mar 31;379(9822):1245–55. [PMID: 22353262]

Morgan RL et al. Eradication of hepatitis C virus infection and the development of hepatocellular carcinoma: a meta-analysis of observational studies. Ann Intern Med. 2013 Mar 5;158 (5 Pt 1):329–37. [PMID: 23460056]

Sieghart W et al. Single determination of C-reactive protein at the time of diagnosis predicts long-term outcome of patients with hepatocellular carcinoma. Hepatology. 2013 Jun;57(6): 2224–34. [PMID: 22961713]

Singh S et al. Anti-diabetic medications and the risk of hepatocellular cancer: a systematic review and meta-analysis. Am J Gastroenterol. 2013 Jun;108(6):881–91. [PMID: 23381014]

Singh S et al. Statins are associated with a reduced risk of hepatocellular cancer: a systematic review and meta-analysis. Gastroenterology. 2013 Feb;144(2):323–32. [PMID: 23063971]

CARCINOMA OF THE BILIARY TRACT

ESSENTIALS OF DIAGNOSIS

▸ Presents with obstructive jaundice, usually painless, often with dilated biliary tree.

▸ Pain is more common in gallbladder carcinoma than cholangiocarcinoma.

▸ A dilated (Courvoisier) gallbladder may be palpable.

▸ Diagnosis by cholangiography with biopsy and brushings for cytology.

▸ General Considerations

Carcinoma of the gallbladder occurs in approximately 2% of all people operated on for biliary tract disease; the incidence may be decreasing in the United States. It is notoriously insidious, and the diagnosis is often made unexpectedly at surgery. Cholelithiasis (often large, symptomatic stones) is usually present. Other risk factors are chronic infection of the gallbladder with *Salmonella typhi*, gallbladder polyps over 1 cm in diameter, mucosal calcification of the gallbladder (porcelain gallbladder), and anomalous pancreaticobiliary ductal junction. Genetic factors include *K-ras* and *TP53* mutations. Spread of the cancer—by direct extension into the liver or to the peritoneal surface—may be the initial manifestation. The TNM classification includes the following stages: Tis, carcinoma in situ; T1a, tumor invades lamina propria, and T1b, tumor invades muscle layer; T2, tumor invades perimuscular connective tissue, no extension beyond serosa (visceral peritoneum) or into liver; T3, tumor perforates the serosa or directly invades the liver or adjacent organ or structure; T4, tumor invades the main portal vein or hepatic artery or invades multiple extrahepatic organs or structures; N1, regional lymph node metastasis; and M1, distant metastasis.

Carcinoma of the bile ducts (cholangiocarcinoma) accounts for 10–25% of all hepatobiliary malignancies and 3% of all cancer deaths in the United States. It is more prevalent in persons aged 50–70, with a slight male predominance, and more common in Asia. Two-thirds arise at the confluence of the hepatic ducts (perihilar, or so-called Klatskin, tumors), and one-fourth arise in the distal extrahepatic bile duct; the remainder are intrahepatic (peripheral), the incidence of which has risen dramatically since the 1970s. Staging for extrahepatic cholangiocarcinoma is as follows: T1, tumor is confined to bile duct; T2, tumor spreads beyond the wall of the bile duct (2a) or to the adjacent liver (2b); T3, tumor spreads to unilateral branches of the portal vein or hepatic artery; T4, tumor spreads to main portal vein or its branches bilaterally, common hepatic artery, second-order biliary radicals bilaterally, or various combinations; N1, regional lymph node metastasis; M1, distant metastasis. Staging for intrahepatic cholangiocarcinoma is as follows: T1, solitary tumor without vascular invasion; T2, solitary tumor with vascular invasion or

multiple tumors ≤ 5 cm; T3, multiple tumors > 5 cm or involving major branch of portal or hepatic veins; T4, tumor invades adjacent organ (except gallbladder) or perforation of visceral peritoneum; N1, regional lymph node metastasis; and M1, distant metastasis. Other staging systems consider tumor extent and form, vascular encasement, hepatic lobe atrophy, and underlying liver disease. The frequency of carcinoma in persons with choledochal cysts has been reported to be over 14% at 20 years, and surgical excision is recommended. Most cases of cholangiocarcinoma are sporadic. There is an increased incidence of cholangiocarcinoma in patients with bile duct adenoma; biliary papillomatosis; Caroli disease; a biliary-enteric anastomosis; ulcerative colitis, especially those with primary sclerosing cholangitis; biliary cirrhosis; diabetes mellitus; hyperthyroidism; chronic pancreatitis; heavy alcohol consumption; smoking; and past exposure to thorotrast, a contrast agent. In diabetic patients, metformin use is associated with a reduced risk of intrahepatic cholangiocarcinoma. In Southeast Asia, hepatolithiasis, chronic typhoid carriage, and infection of the bile ducts with helminths (*Clonorchis sinensis, Opisthorchis viverrini*) are associated with an increased risk of cholangiocarcinoma. Hepatitis C virus (and possibly hepatitis B virus) infection, cirrhosis, HIV infection, nonalcoholic fatty liver disease, diabetes mellitus, obesity, and tobacco smoking are risk factors for intrahepatic cholangiocarcinoma. Mixed hepatocellular carcinoma-cholangiocarcinoma is a tumor that is being increasingly recognized.

▸ Clinical Findings

A. Symptoms and Signs

Progressive jaundice is the most common and usually the first sign of obstruction of the extrahepatic biliary system. Pain in the right upper abdomen with radiation into the back is usually present early in the course of gallbladder carcinoma but occurs later in the course of bile duct carcinoma. Anorexia and weight loss are common and may be associated with fever and chills due to cholangitis. Rarely, hematemesis or melena results from erosion of tumor into a blood vessel (hemobilia). Fistula formation between the biliary system and adjacent organs may also occur. The course is usually one of rapid deterioration, with death occurring within a few months.

Physical examination reveals profound jaundice. Pruritus and skin excoriations are common. A palpable gallbladder with obstructive jaundice usually is said to signify malignant disease (Courvoisier sign); however, this clinical generalization has been proved to be accurate only about 50% of the time. Hepatomegaly due to hypertrophy of the unobstructed liver lobe is usually present and is associated with liver tenderness. Ascites may occur with peritoneal implants.

B. Laboratory Findings

With biliary obstruction, laboratory examination reveals predominantly conjugated hyperbilirubinemia, with total serum bilirubin values ranging from 5 to 30 mg/dL.

There is usually concomitant elevation of the alkaline phosphatase and serum cholesterol. AST is normal or minimally elevated. The serum CA 19-9 level is elevated in up to 85% of patients and may help distinguish cholangiocarcinoma from a benign biliary stricture (in the absence of cholangitis) but is neither sensitive nor specific.

C. Imaging

Ultrasonography and contrast-enhanced, triple-phase, helical CT may show a gallbladder mass in gallbladder carcinoma and intrahepatic mass or biliary dilatation in carcinoma of the bile ducts. CT may also show involved regional lymph nodes and atrophy of a hepatic lobe because of vascular encasement with compensatory hypertrophy of the unaffected lobe. MRI with magnetic resonance cholangiopancreatography (MRCP) and gadolinium enhancement permits visualization of the entire biliary tree and detection of vascular invasion and obviates the need for angiography and, in some cases, direct cholangiography; it is the imaging procedure of choice but may understage malignant hilar strictures. The sensitivity and image quality can be increased with use of ferumoxide enhancement. The features of intrahepatic cholangiocarcinoma on MRI appear to differ from those of hepatocellular carcinoma, with contrast washout in the latter but not the former. In indeterminate cases, PET can detect cholangiocarcinomas as small as 1 cm and lymph node and distant metastases, but false-positive results occur. The most helpful diagnostic studies before surgery are either endoscopic retrograde or percutaneous transhepatic cholangiography with biopsy and cytologic specimens, although false-negative biopsy and cytology results are common. Digital image analysis and fluorescent in situ hybridization of cytologic specimens for polysomy improve sensitivity. Endoscopic ultrasonography with FNA of tumors, choledochoscopy, and intraductal ultrasonography may confirm a diagnosis of cholangiocarcinoma in a patient with bile duct stricture and an otherwise indeterminate evaluation, but FNA can result in tumor seeding and is often avoided if the tumor is potentially resectable.

▶ Treatment

In young and fit patients, curative surgery may be attempted if the tumor is well localized. The 5-year survival rate for carcinoma of the gallbladder invading the lamina propria or muscularis (stage 1, T1a or 1b, N0, M0) is as high as 85% with laparoscopic cholecystectomy but drops to 60%, even with a more extended open resection, if there is perimuscular invasion (T2). The role of radical surgery for T3 and T4 tumors is debatable. If the tumor is unresectable at laparotomy, biliary-enteric bypass (eg, Roux-en-Y hepaticojejunostomy) can be performed. Carcinoma of the bile ducts is curable by surgery in < 10% of cases. If resection margins are negative, the 5-year survival rate may be as high as 47% for intrahepatic cholangiocarcinomas, 41% for hilar cholangiocarcinoma, and 37% for distal cholangiocarcinomas, but the perioperative mortality rate may be as high as 10%. Palliation can be achieved by placement of a self-expandable metal stent via an endoscopic or percutaneous transhepatic route. Covered metal stents may be more cost-effective than uncovered metal stents because of a longer duration of patency, but they are associated with a higher rate of stent migration and cholecystitis due to occlusion of the cystic duct and are not associated with longer survival. For perihilar tumors, there is controversy as to whether unilateral or bilateral stents should be inserted. Plastic stents are less expensive but more prone to occlude than metal ones; they are suitable for patients expected to survive only a few months. Photodynamic therapy in combination with stent placement has been demonstrated to prolong survival when compared with stent placement alone in patients with nonresectable cholangiocarcinoma. Radiotherapy may relieve pain and contribute to biliary decompression. There is limited response to chemotherapy with gemcitabine alone, but the combination of cisplatin and gemcitabine prolongs survival by about 3 months in patients with locally advanced or metastatic cholangiocarcinoma. Few patients survive for more than 24 months. Although cholangiocarcinoma is generally considered to be a contraindication to liver transplantation because of rapid tumor recurrence, a 75% 5-year survival rate has been reported in patients with stage I and II perihilar cholangiocarcinoma undergoing chemoradiation and exploratory laparotomy followed by liver transplantation.

For those patients whose disease progresses despite treatment, meticulous efforts at palliative care are essential (see Chapter 5).

▶ When to Refer

All patients with carcinoma of the biliary tract should be referred to a specialist.

▶ When to Admit

- Biliary obstruction.
- Cholangitis.

Almadi MA et al. No benefit of covered vs. uncovered self-expandable metal stents in patients with malignant distal biliary obstruction: a meta-analysis. Clin Gastroenterol Hepatol. 2013 Jan;11(1):27–37. [PMID: 23103324]

American Society for Gastrointestinal Endoscopy (ASGE) Standards of Practice Committee; Anderson MA et al. The role of endoscopy in the evaluation and treatment of patients with biliary neoplasia. Gastrointest Endosc. 2013 Feb;77(2):167–74. [PMID: 23219047]

Chaiteerakij R et al. Risk factors for intrahepatic cholangiocarcinoma: association between metformin use and reduced cancer risk. Hepatology. 2013 Feb;57(2):648–55. [PMID: 23055147]

Razumilava N et al. Classification, diagnosis, and management of cholangiocarcinoma. Clin Gastroenterol Hepatol. 2013 Jan;11(1):13–21.e1. [PMID: 22982100]

Rizvi S et al. Pathogenesis, diagnosis, and management of cholangiocarcinoma. Gastroenterology. 2013 Dec;145(6):1215–29. [PMID: 24140396]

CARCINOMA OF THE PANCREAS & AMPULLA OF VATER

- ► Obstructive jaundice (may be painless).
- ► Enlarged gallbladder (may be painful).
- ► Upper abdominal pain with radiation to back, weight loss, and thrombophlebitis are usually late manifestations.

General Considerations

Carcinoma is the most common neoplasm of the pancreas. About 75% are in the head and 25% in the body and tail of the organ. Pancreatic carcinomas account for 2% of all cancers and 5% of cancer deaths. Risk factors include age, tobacco use (which is thought to cause 20–25% of cases), heavy alcohol use, obesity, chronic pancreatitis, prior abdominal radiation, family history, and possibly gastric ulcer and exposure to arsenic and cadmium. New-onset diabetes mellitus after age 45 years occasionally heralds the onset of pancreatic cancer. In diabetic patients, metformin use may reduce the risk of pancreatic cancer slightly, but insulin use and glucagon-like peptide-1-based therapy (eg, sitagliptin) may increase the risk. About 7% of patients with pancreatic cancer have a family history of pancreatic cancer in a first-degree relative, compared with 0.6% of control subjects. In 5–10% of cases, pancreatic cancer occurs as part of a hereditary syndrome, including familial breast cancer (carriers of *BRCA-2* have a 7% lifetime risk of pancreatic cancer), hereditary pancreatitis (*PSS1* mutation), familial atypical multiple mole melanoma (*p16/CDKN2A* mutation), Peutz-Jeghers syndrome (*STK11/LKB1* mutation), ataxia-telangiectasia, and Lynch syndrome (hereditary nonpolyposis colorectal cancer). Neuroendocrine tumors account for 1–2% of pancreatic neoplasms and may be functional (producing gastrin, insulin, glucagon, vasoactive intestinal peptide, somatostatin, growth hormone-releasing hormone, adrenocorticotropic hormone, and others) or nonfunctional. Cystic neoplasms account for only 1% of pancreatic cancers, but they are important because they are often mistaken for pseudocysts. A cystic neoplasm should be suspected when a cystic lesion in the pancreas is found in the absence of a history of pancreatitis. At least 15% of all pancreatic cysts are neoplasms. Whereas serous cystadenomas (which account for 32–39% of cystic pancreatic neoplasms and also occur in patients with von Hippel-Lindau disease) are benign, mucinous cystic neoplasms (defined by the presence of ovarian stroma) (10–45%), intraductal papillary mucinous neoplasms (21–33%), solid pseudopapillary tumors (< 5%), and cystic islet cell tumors (3–5%) may be malignant, although their prognoses are better than the prognosis of adenocarcinoma of the pancreas, unless the neoplasm is at least locally advanced.

Clinical Findings

A. Symptoms and Signs

Pain is present in over 70% of cases and is often vague, diffuse, and located in the epigastrium or left upper quadrant when the lesion is in the tail. Radiation of pain into the back is common and sometimes predominates. Sitting up and leaning forward may afford some relief, and this usually indicates that the lesion has spread beyond the pancreas and is inoperable. Diarrhea, perhaps due to maldigestion, is an occasional early symptom. Migratory thrombophlebitis is a rare sign. Weight loss is a common but late finding and may be associated with depression. Occasionally a patient presents with acute pancreatitis in the absence of an alternative cause. Jaundice is usually due to biliary obstruction by a cancer in the pancreatic head. A palpable gallbladder is also indicative of obstruction by neoplasm (Courvoisier sign), but there are frequent exceptions. A hard, fixed, occasionally tender mass may be present. In advanced cases, a hard periumbilical (Sister Joseph's) nodule may be palpable.

B. Laboratory Findings

There may be mild anemia. Glycosuria, hyperglycemia, and impaired glucose tolerance or true diabetes mellitus are found in 10–20% of cases. The serum amylase or lipase level is occasionally elevated. Liver biochemical tests may suggest obstructive jaundice. Steatorrhea in the absence of jaundice is uncommon. Occult blood in the stool is suggestive of carcinoma of the ampulla of Vater (the combination of biliary obstruction and bleeding may give the stools a distinctive silver appearance). CA 19-9, with a sensitivity of 70% and a specificity of 87%, has not proved sensitive enough for early detection of pancreatic cancer; increased values are also found in acute and chronic pancreatitis and cholangitis. Plasma chromogranin A levels are elevated in 88–100% of patients with pancreatic neuroendocrine tumors.

C. Imaging

Multiphase thin-cut helical CT is generally the initial diagnostic procedure and detects a mass in over 80% of cases. CT identifies metastases, delineates the extent of the tumor, and allows for percutaneous FNA for cytologic studies and tumor markers. MRI is an alternative to CT. Ultrasonography is not reliable because of interference by intestinal gas. PET is a sensitive technique for detecting pancreatic cancer and metastases, but PET-CT is not a routine staging procedure. Selective celiac and superior mesenteric arteriography may demonstrate vessel invasion by tumor, a finding that would preclude attempts at surgical resection, but it is used less commonly since the advent of multiphase helical CT. Endoscopic ultrasonography is more sensitive than CT for detecting pancreatic cancer and equivalent to CT for determining nodal involvement and resectability. A normal endoscopic ultrasonogram excludes pancreatic cancer. Endoscopic ultrasonography may also be used to guide FNA for tissue diagnosis, tumor markers, and DNA analysis. Endoscopic retrograde cholangiopancreatography

(ERCP) may clarify an ambiguous CT scan or MRI study by delineating the pancreatic duct system or confirming an ampullary or biliary neoplasm. MRCP appears to be at least as sensitive as ERCP in diagnosing pancreatic cancer. In some centers, pancreatoscopy or intraductal ultrasonography can be used to evaluate filling defects in the pancreatic duct and assess resectability of intraductal papillary mucinous tumors. With obstruction of the splenic vein, splenomegaly or gastric varices are present, the latter detected by endoscopy, endoscopic ultrasonography, or angiography.

Cystic neoplasms can be distinguished by their appearance on CT, endoscopic ultrasonography, and ERCP and features of the cyst fluid on gross and cytologic analysis. For example, serous cystadenomas may have a central scar or honeycomb appearance; mucinous cystadenomas are unilocular or multilocular and contain mucin-rich fluid with high carcinoembryonic antigen levels (> 200 ng/mL) (200 mcg/L) and *K-ras* mutations; and intraductal papillary mucinous neoplasms are associated with a dilated pancreatic duct and extrusion of gelatinous material from the ampulla.

▶ Staging

Staging of pancreatic cancer by the TNM classification includes the following definitions: Tis: carcinoma in situ; T1: tumor limited to the pancreas, 2 cm or less in greatest dimension; T2: tumor limited to the pancreas, more than 2 cm in greatest dimension; T3: tumor extends beyond the pancreas but without involvement of the celiac axis or the superior mesenteric artery; T4; tumor involves the celiac axis or the superior mesenteric artery (unresectable primary tumor); N1; regional lymph node metastasis; M1; distant metastasis.

▶ Treatment

Abdominal exploration is usually necessary when cytologic diagnosis cannot be made or if resection is to be attempted, which includes about 30% of patients with pancreatic carcinomas. In a patient with a localized mass in the head of the pancreas and without jaundice, laparoscopy may detect tiny peritoneal or liver metastases and thereby avoid resection in 4–13% of patients. Radical pancreaticoduodenal (Whipple) resection is indicated for cancers strictly limited to the head of the pancreas, periampullary area, and duodenum (T1, N0, M0). Five-year survival rates are 20–25% in this group and as high as 40% in those with negative resection margins and without lymph node involvement. Preoperative endoscopic decompression of an obstructed bile duct is often achieved with a plastic stent or short metal stent but does not reduce operative mortality and is associated with complications. The best surgical results are achieved at centers that specialize in the multidisciplinary treatment of pancreatic cancer. Adjuvant or neoadjuvant chemotherapy with gemcitabine or fluorouracil (or both), possibly combined with irradiation, is of benefit (Table 39–5). Chemoradiotherapy downstages about 30% of patients with locally advanced disease to allow resection. When resection is not feasible, endoscopic stenting of the bile duct is performed to relieve jaundice. A plastic stent is generally placed if the patient's anticipated survival is < 6 months (or surgery is planned).

A metal stent is preferred when anticipated survival is 6 months or greater. Whether covered metal stents designed to prevent tumor ingrowth offer an advantage over uncovered stents is uncertain because covered stents are associated with higher rates of migration and acute cholecystitis due to occlusion of the cystic duct. Surgical biliary bypass may be considered in patients expected to survive at least 6 months. Surgical duodenal bypass may be considered in patients in whom duodenal obstruction is expected to develop; alternatively, endoscopic placement of a self-expandable duodenal stent may be feasible. Chemoradiation may be used for palliation of unresectable cancer confined to the pancreas. Chemotherapy has been disappointing in metastatic pancreatic cancer, although improved response rates have been reported with the combination of oxaliplatin, irinotecan, fluorouracil, and leucovorin (FOLFIRINOX) and with the combination of gemcitabine and paclitaxel. The addition of erlotinib (an inhibitor of the EGFR receptor), capecitabine (an oral fluoropyrimidine), or a platinum agent may improve survival but also increases toxicity. The high rate of *K-ras* mutations in pancreatic cancer limits the benefit of erlotinib. Celiac plexus nerve block (under CT or endoscopic ultrasound guidance) or thoracoscopic splanchnicectomy may improve pain control. Photodynamic therapy is under study.

Surgical resection is the treatment of choice for neuroendocrine tumors, when feasible. Metastatic disease may be controlled with long-acting somatostatin analogs, interferon, peptide-receptor radionuclide therapy, and chemoembolization. There is a growing consensus that asymptomatic incidental pancreatic cysts ≤ 2 cm are at low risk for harboring invasive carcinoma. The cysts may be monitored by imaging tests at 6- to 12-month intervals and every 3–6 months in those > 2 cm, with surgery or possibly endoscopic ultrasound-guided cyst ablation performed if a cyst enlarges or exceeds 2.5 cm.

Surgical resection is indicated for mucinous cystic neoplasms, symptomatic serous cystadenomas, solid pseudopapillary tumors (which have a 15% risk of malignant transformation), and cystic tumors > 2 cm in diameter that remain undefined after helical CT, endoscopic ultrasonography, and diagnostic aspiration. All intraductal papillary mucinous neoplasms of the main pancreatic duct should be resected, but those of branch ducts may be monitored with serial imaging if they (1) are asymptomatic and exhibit benign features; (2) have a diameter < 3 cm (some authorities recommend a diameter ≤ 1.5 cm, but even lesions ≥ 3 cm may be monitored in elderly persons with no other worrisome cyst features); and (3) lack nonenhancing mural nodules, a thick wall, an abrupt change in the caliber of the pancreatic duct with distal pancreatic atrophy, or possibly bile duct dilatation and gallbladder adenomyomatosis. Most such lesions with benign features remain stable on follow-up, but the risk of pancreatic ductal carcinoma and of nonpancreatic cancers may also be increased in this group of patients. In the absence of locally advanced disease, survival is higher for malignant cystic neoplasms than for adenocarcinoma. Endoscopic resection or ablation, with temporary placement of a pancreatic duct stent, may be feasible for ampullary adenomas, but patients must be followed for recurrence.

Table 39–5. Treatment choices for cancers responsive to systemic agents.

Diagnosis	Current Treatment of Choice	Other Treatments
Acute lymphoblastic leukemia (ALL)	**Induction combination chemotherapy:** Vincristine, prednisone, daunorubicin, asparaginase, intrathecal methotrexate **Consolidation combination chemotherapy:** Cyclophosphamide, vincristine, doxorubicin, dexamethasone (hyper-CVAD) alternated with cytarabine, methotrexate **Maintenance chemotherapy:** Methotrexate, 6-mercaptopurine	Liposomal vincristine, imatinib mesylate (Philadelphia chromosome-positive ALL), autologous or allogeneic transplantation for high risk or at relapse
Acute myeloid leukemia (AML)	**Combination chemotherapy:** Cytarabine, daunorubicin or Cytarabine, idarubicin	Mitoxantrone, doxorubicin, cladribine, fludarabine, prednisone
Chronic myeloid leukemia (CML)	Imatinib mesylate or nilotinib or dasatinib	Dasatinib, nilotinib, bosutinib, omacetaxine mepesuccinate, allogeneic bone marrow transplantation, hydroxyurea, interferon-alpha, cytarabine
Chronic lymphocytic leukemia (CLL)	**Combination chemotherapy:** Fludarabine, cyclophosphamide, rituximab (FCR); or Fludarabine, or Bendamustine or Chlorambucil	Alemtuzumab, ofatumumab, bendamustine, pentostatin, cladribine, cyclophosphamide, vincristine, doxorubicin, prednisone
Hairy cell leukemia	Cladribine (2-chlorodeoxyadenosine)	Pentostatin, rituximab, interferon-alpha
Hodgkin lymphoma (stages III and IV)	**Combination chemotherapy:** Doxorubicin, bleomycin, vinblastine, dacarbazine (ABVD) or Doxorubicin, vinblastine, mechlorethamine, etoposide, vincristine, bleomycin, prednisone (Stanford V) or Bleomycin, etoposide, doxorubicin, cyclophosphamide, vincristine, procarbazine, prednisone (BEACOPP)	Gemcitabine, vinorelbine, ifosfamide, cyclophosphamide, procarbazine, bendamustine, brentuximab vedotin, autologous or allogeneic transplantation for relapse
Non-Hodgkin lymphoma (intermediate and high grade)	**Combination chemotherapy:** Cyclophosphamide, doxorubicin, vincristine, prednisone, rituximab (CHOP-R)	Combination chemotherapy second line: Dexamethasone, cisplatin, cytarabine (DHAP) or Etoposide, methylprednisolone, cytarabine, cisplatin (ESHAP) or Ifosfamide, carboplatin, etoposide (ICE) or Mesna, ifosfamide, mitoxantrone, etoposide (MINE); transplantation for high risk or first relapse
Non-Hodgkin lymphoma (low grade)	**Combination chemotherapy:** Fludarabine, cyclophosphamide, rituximab (FCR) or Fludarabine, rituximab (FR) or Bendamustine, rituximab or Cyclophosphamide, vincristine, doxorubicin, prednisone, rituximab (CHOP-R), or Cyclophosphamide, vincristine, prednisone, rituximab (CVP-R)	Chlorambucil, rituximab, ^{131}I tositumomab, ^{90}Y ibritumomab tiuxetan, bendamustine, autologous or allogeneic transplantation
Multiple myeloma	**Combination chemotherapy (transplant candidates):** Bortezomib, dexamethasone, thalidomide or Bortezomib, dexamethasone, lenalidomide or Dexamethasone, lenalidomide Followed by autologous or miniallogeneic stem cell transplantation **Combination chemotherapy (non-transplant candidates):** Lenalidomide, dexamethasone, or Melphalan, prednisone, bortezomib, or Melphalan, prednisone, lenalidomide, or Melphalan, prednisone, thalidomide	Cyclophosphamide, liposomal doxorubicin, carfilzomib

(continued)

Table 39–5. Treatment choices for cancers responsive to systemic agents. (continued)

Diagnosis	Current Treatment of Choice	Other Treatments
Waldenström macroglobulinemia	**Plasmapheresis alone or followed by combination chemotherapy:** Bortezomib with or without rituximab, or thalidomide with or without rituximab	Cladribine, cyclophosphamide, chlorambucil, bendamustine, alemtuzumab, autologous bone marrow transplantation
Polycythemia vera	Phlebotomy, hydroxyurea	Anagrelide, radiophosphorus ^{32}P, interferon-alpha
Non-small cell lung cancer	**Combination chemotherapy:** Cisplatin, vinorelbine or Cisplatin, etoposide or Paclitaxel, carboplatin or Cisplatin, gemcitabine (squamous histology) Cisplatin, pemetrexed (nonsquamous histology) All regimens with or without bevacizumab	Docetaxel, cetuximab, erlotinib (EGFR mutation positive), crizotinib (ALK mutation positive)
Small cell lung cancer	**Combination chemotherapy:** Cisplatin, etoposide or Carboplatin, etoposide	Irinotecan, cyclophosphamide, doxorubicin, vincristine, topotecan, gemcitabine, paclitaxel
Mesothelioma	**Combination chemotherapy:** Cisplatin, pemetrexed or Carboplatin, pemetrexed or Gemcitabine, cisplatin	Vinorelbine
Head and neck cancer	**Combination chemotherapy:** Cisplatin, fluorouracil or Paclitaxel, carboplatin or Docetaxel, cisplatin, fluorouracil or Cisplatin or cetuximab with radiation therapy	Methotrexate, cetuximab
Esophageal cancer	**Combination chemotherapy:** Cisplatin, fluorouracil or Paclitaxel, carboplatin	Irinotecan, oxaliplatin, capecitabine, epirubicin
Uterine cancer	**Hormone therapy:** Progestins, tamoxifen, aromatase inhibitors or **Combination chemotherapy:** Cisplatin, doxorubicin, or Cisplatin, doxorubicin or Carboplatin, paclitaxel	Liposomal doxorubicin
Ovarian cancer	**Combination chemotherapy:** Paclitaxel, carboplatin or Docetaxel, carboplatin or Paclitaxel, cisplatin	Gemcitabine, liposomal doxorubicin, topotecan, cyclophosphamide, etoposide, bevacizumab
Cervical cancer	**With radiation:** Cisplatin **Combination chemotherapy:** Cisplatin, paclitaxel or Cisplatin, topotecan or Carboplatin, paclitaxel or Cisplatin, gemcitabine	Docetaxel, ifosfamide, vinorelbine, irinotecan, mitomycin, fluorouracil, bevacizumab, docetaxel
Breast cancer	**Adjuvant hormone therapy:** *Premenopausal:* Tamoxifen *Postmenopausal:* Aromatase inhibitors (anastrozole, letrozol, exemestane) **Adjuvant chemotherapy (without trastuzumab):** Doxorubicin, cyclophosphamide, docetaxel or Doxorubicin, cyclophosphamide, paclitaxel or Docetaxel, cyclophosphamide or Doxorubicin, cyclophosphamide **Adjuvant chemotherapy (with trastuzumab):** Doxorubicin, cyclophosphamide, paclitaxel, trastuzumab or Docetaxel, carboplatin, trastuzumab	Megestrol, aminoglutethimide, capecitabine, mitoxantrone, cisplatin, etoposide, vinblastine, fluorouracil, ixabepilone, pertuzumab, gemcitabine
Choriocarcinoma (trophoblastic neoplasms)	**Single-agent chemotherapy:** Methotrexate or dactinomycin for low-risk disease **Combination chemotherapy:** Etoposide/methotrexate, dactinomycin, cyclophosphamide, vincristine (EMA-CO) for high-risk disease	Vinblastine, cisplatin, mercaptopurine, chlorambucil, doxorubicin
Testicular cancer	**Combination chemotherapy:** Cisplatin, etoposide or Bleomycin, etoposide, cisplatin (BEP) or Etoposide, mesna, ifosfamide, cisplatin (VIP)	Vinblastine, ifosfamide, paclitaxel, gemcitabine, oxaliplatin

(*continued*)

Table 39–5. Treatment choices for cancers responsive to systemic agents. (continued)

Diagnosis	Current Treatment of Choice	Other Treatments
Kidney (renal cell) cancer	**Single-agent chemotherapy:** Sunitinib or temsirolimus or bevacizumab or sorafenib or pazopanib or interleukin-2	Interferon-alpha, axitinib
Bladder cancer	**Combination chemotherapy:** Gemcitabine, cisplatin or Methotrexate, vinblastine, doxorubicin, cisplatin (MVAC)	Carboplatin, paclitaxel, docetaxel, fluorouracil, pemetrexed
Prostate cancer	**Hormone therapy:** Luteinizing hormone-releasing agonist (leuprolide, goserelin, triptorelin, degarelix) with or without an antiandrogen (flutamide, bicalutamide, nilutamide)	Ketoconazole, docetaxel, abiraterone, enzalutamide, mitoxantrone, cabazitaxel, sipuleucel-T, estramustine, prednisone
Brain cancer (anaplastic astrocytoma and glioblastoma multiforme)	**Single-agent chemotherapy with radiation therapy:** Temozolomide	Bevacizumab, irinotecan, procarbazine, carmustine, lomustine
Neuroblastoma	**Combination chemotherapy:** Cyclophosphamide, doxorubicin, cisplatin, etoposide	Vincristine, topotecan, irinotecan, ifosfamide, carboplatin, 13-cis-retinoic acid, ^{131}I-MIBG, autologous or allogeneic transplantation
Thyroid cancer	**Single-agent chemotherapy:** Radioiodine (^{131}I) or sorafenib, or sunitinib or pazopanib or vandetanib (medullary thyroid cancer)	Doxorubicin, dacarbazine
Adrenal cancer	**Single-agent chemotherapy:** Mitotane	Doxorubicin, etoposide, cisplatin
Stomach (gastric) cancer	**Combination chemotherapy:** Epirubicin, cisplatin, fluorouracil or Docetaxel, cisplatin, fluorouracil or Fluorouracil, leucovorin, oxaliplatin Trastuzumab added for *HER2*-overexpressing adenocarcinomas	Capecitabine, sorafenib, irinotecan
Pancreatic cancer	**Combination chemotherapy:** Gemcitabine, cisplatin; or Gemcitabine, paclitaxel; or Gemcitabine, erlotinib; or Fluorouracil, leucovorin, irinotecan, oxaliplatin (FOLFIRINOX) **Single-agent chemotherapy:** Gemcitabine	Capecitabine
Colon cancer	**Combination chemotherapy:** Fluorouracil, leucovorin, oxaliplatin (FOLFOX6) or Capecitabine, oxaliplatin (CapeOx) or Fluorouracil, leucovorin, irinotecan (FOLFIRI) each regimen with or without bevacizumab	Cetuximab, irinotecan, panitumumab, regorafenib, ziv-aflibercept
Rectal cancer	**Chemotherapy with radiation:** Fluorouracil; For adjuvant or advanced disease treatment, same regimens used with colon cancer	Cetuximab, irinotecan, panitumumab, regorafenib
Anal cancer	**Combination chemotherapy with radiation:** Fluorouracil, mitomycin	Cisplatin
Carcinoid	**Combination chemotherapy:** Streptozocin, fluorouracil or **Single-agent chemotherapy:** Bevacizumab or sorafenib or sunitinib	Doxorubicin, dacarbazine, octreotide, temozolomide
Osteogenic sarcoma	**Combination chemotherapy with two of these agents:** Doxorubicin, cisplatin, ifosfamide, high-dose methotrexate	Cyclophosphamide
Soft tissue sarcomas	**Combination chemotherapy:** Doxorubicin, dacarbazine (AD) or Doxorubicin, ifosfamide, mesna (AIM) or Mesna, doxorubicin, ifosfamide, dacarbazine (MAID) **Single-agent chemotherapy:** Imatinib or sunitinib (gastrointestinal stromal tumors)	Liposomal doxorubicin, methotrexate, gemcitabine, docetaxel, temozolomide
Melanoma	**Single-agent chemotherapy:** Ipilimumab or vemurafenib or high-dose interleukin-2	Dacarbazine, temozolomide, imatinib, paclitaxel, carboplatin
Hepatocellular cancer	**Single-agent chemotherapy:** Sorafenib	Doxorubicin
Kaposi sarcoma	**Single-agent chemotherapy:** Liposomal doxorubicin or liposomal daunorubicin	Paclitaxel, vinblastine, vincristine, etoposide, doxorubicin

Prognosis

Carcinoma of the pancreas, especially in the body or tail, has a poor prognosis; 80–85% of patients present with advanced unresectable disease, and reported 5-year survival rates range from 2% to 5%. Tumors of the ampulla have a better prognosis, with reported 5-year survival rates of 20–40% after resection; jaundice and lymph node involvement are adverse prognostic factors. In carefully selected patients, resection of cancer of the pancreatic head is feasible and results in reasonable survival. In persons with a family history of pancreatic cancer in at least two first-degree relatives, or with a genetic syndrome associated with an increased risk of pancreatic cancer, screening with endoscopic ultrasonography and helical CT or MRI/MRCP should be considered beginning at age 40–45 or 10 years before the age at which pancreatic cancer was diagnosed in a family member.

For those patients whose disease progresses despite treatment, meticulous efforts at palliative care are essential (see Chapter 5).

When to Refer

All patients with carcinoma involving the pancreas and the ampulla of Vater should be referred to a specialist.

When to Admit

Patients who require surgery and other interventions should be hospitalized.

Anand N et al. Cyst features and risk of malignancy in intraductal papillary mucinous neoplasms of the pancreas: a meta-analysis. Clin Gastroenterol Hepatol. 2013 Aug;11(8):913–21. [PMID: 23416279]

Canto MI et al. International Cancer of the Pancreas Screening (CAPS) Consortium summit on the management of patients with increased risk for familial pancreatic cancer. Gut. 2013 Mar;62(3):339–47. [PMID: 23135763]

Farrell JJ et al. Pancreatic cystic neoplasms: management and unanswered questions. Gastroenterology. 2013 Jun;144(6):1303–15. [PMID: 23622140]

Paulson AS et al. Therapeutic advances in pancreatic cancer. Gastroenterology. 2013 Jun;144(6):1316–26. [PMID: 23622141]

Singh S et al. Anti-diabetic medications and risk of pancreatic cancer in patients with diabetes mellitus: a systematic review and meta-analysis. Am J Gastroenterol. 2013 Apr;108(4):510–9. [PMID: 23399556]

ALIMENTARY TRACT CANCERS

Robin K. Kelley, MD

Kenneth McQuaid, MD

ESOPHAGEAL CANCER

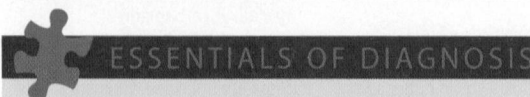

ESSENTIALS OF DIAGNOSIS

▸ Progressive solid food dysphagia.

▸ Weight loss common.

▸ Endoscopy with biopsy establishes diagnosis.

General Considerations

Esophageal cancer usually develops in persons between 50 and 70 years of age. The overall ratio of men to women is 3:1. There are two histologic types: squamous cell carcinoma and adenocarcinoma. In the United States, **squamous cell cancer** is much more common in blacks than in whites. Squamous cell cancer has a high incidence in certain regions of China and Southeast Asia. Half of all cases occur in the distal third of the esophagus. Chronic alcohol and tobacco use are strongly associated with an increased risk of squamous cell carcinoma. The risk of squamous cell cancer is also increased in patients with tylosis, achalasia, caustic-induced esophageal stricture, and other head and neck cancers. **Adenocarcinoma** is more common in whites. It is increasing dramatically in incidence and now is more common than squamous carcinoma in the United States. The majority of adenocarcinomas develop as a complication of Barrett metaplasia due to chronic gastroesophageal reflux. Thus, most adenocarcinomas arise in the distal third of the esophagus. Obesity also is strongly associated with adenocarcinoma, even after controlling for gastroesophageal reflux.

Clinical Findings

A. Symptoms and Signs

Most patients with esophageal cancer present with advanced, incurable disease. Over 90% have solid food dysphagia, which progresses over weeks to months. Odynophagia is sometimes present. Significant weight loss is common. Local tumor extension into the tracheobronchial tree may result in a tracheo-esophageal fistula, characterized by coughing on swallowing or pneumonia. Chest or back pain suggests mediastinal extension. Recurrent laryngeal involvement may produce hoarseness. Physical examination is often unrevealing. The presence of supraclavicular or cervical lymphadenopathy or of hepatomegaly implies metastatic disease.

B. Laboratory Findings

Laboratory findings are nonspecific. Anemia related to chronic disease or occult blood loss is common. Elevated aminotransferase or alkaline phosphatase concentrations suggest hepatic or bony metastases. Hypoalbuminemia may result from malnutrition.

C. Imaging

A barium esophagogram may be the first study obtained to evaluate dysphagia. The appearance of a polypoid, obstructive, or ulcerative lesion is suggestive of carcinoma and requires endoscopic evaluation. However, even lesions believed to be benign by radiography warrant endoscopic evaluation. Chest radiographs may show adenopathy, a widened mediastinum, pulmonary or bony metastases, or signs of tracheo-esophageal fistula such as pneumonia.

D. Upper Endoscopy

Endoscopy with biopsy establishes the diagnosis of esophageal carcinoma with a high degree of reliability. In some cases, significant submucosal spread of the tumor may yield nondiagnostic mucosal biopsies. Repeated biopsy may be necessary.

▶ Staging

After confirmation of the diagnosis of esophageal carcinoma, the stage of the disease should be determined since doing so influences the choice of therapy. Patients should undergo evaluation with CT of the chest and abdomen to look for evidence of pulmonary or hepatic metastases, lymphadenopathy, and local tumor extension. If there is no evidence of distant metastases or extensive local spread on CT, endoscopic ultrasonography with guided FNA biopsy of lymph nodes should be performed, which is superior to CT in demonstrating the level of local mediastinal extension and local lymph node involvement. PET with fluorodeoxyglucose or integrated PET-CT imaging is indicated to look for regional or distant spread in patients thought to have localized disease after other diagnostic studies, prior to invasive surgery. Bronchoscopy is sometimes required in esophageal cancers above the carina to exclude tracheobronchial extension. Laparoscopy to exclude occult peritoneal carcinomatosis should be considered in patients with tumors at or near the gastroesophageal junction (see Gastric Cancer).

▶ Differential Diagnosis

Esophageal carcinoma must be distinguished from other causes of progressive dysphagia, including peptic stricture, achalasia, and adenocarcinoma of the gastric cardia with esophageal involvement. Benign-appearing peptic strictures should be biopsied at presentation to exclude occult malignancy.

▶ Treatment

The approach to esophageal cancer depends on the tumor stage, patient preference and functional status, and the expertise of the surgeons, oncologists, gastroenterologists, and radiotherapists. It is helpful to classify patients into two general categories.

A. Therapy for "Curable" Disease

Superficial esophageal cancers confined to the epithelium (high-grade dysplasia or carcinoma in situ [Tis]), lamina propria (T1a), or submucosal (T1b) are increasingly recognized in endoscopic screening and surveillance programs. Esophagectomy achieves high cure rates for superficial tumors but is associated with mortality (2%) and morbidity. If performed by experienced clinicians, endoscopic mucosal resection of Tis and T1a cancers achieves equivalent long-term survival with less morbidity (see Barrett Esophagus, Chapter 15). Patients with larger tumors or deeper tumors invasive to the submucosa (T1b) have higher rates of lymph node metastasis. Frequent posttreatment endoscopic surveillance is required to ensure no residual or recurrent tumor.

1. Surgery with or without neoadjuvant chemoradiation therapy—There are multiple surgical approaches to the resection of invasive (non-superficial) but potentially "curable" esophageal cancers (stage Ib, II, or IIIA). Accepted techniques include en bloc transthoracic excision of the esophagus with extended lymph node dissection, transhiatal esophagogastrectomy (entailing laparotomy with cervical anastamosis), and minimally invasive esophagectomy techniques. Meta-analysis data suggest equivalent oncologic outcomes from minimally invasive esophagectomy and conventional open techniques. Removal of at least 15 lymph nodes is recommended for optimal surgical staging in patients who have not received neoadjuvant therapy; the optimal number of lymph nodes after neoadjuvant therapy is not known though similar lymphadenectomy is recommended by expert guidelines.

Patients with stage I tumors have high cure rates with surgery alone and do not require radiation or chemotherapy. If regional lymph node metastases have occurred (stages IIB and III), the rate of cure with surgery alone is reduced to < 20%. Meta-analysis of trials comparing neoadjuvant (preoperative) therapy followed by surgery with surgery alone suggests a 13% absolute improvement in 2-year survival with combined therapy. Preoperative (neoadjuvant) chemoradiation therapy is recommended for stage IIA, IIB, and III tumors in fit patients. The preferred neoadjuvant chemotherapy regimen used with radiation is weekly carboplatin plus paclitaxel, based on the 2012 randomized phase III CROSS trial that demonstrated improvement in median survival from 24 months with surgery alone to 49.4 months with neoadjuvant chemoradiation ($P = 0.003$). As an alternative, a combination of cisplatin plus 5-fluorouracil may be used along with radiation. Perioperative chemotherapy without radiation is also appropriate for tumors of the gastroesophageal junction based on the randomized, multicenter, phase III MAGIC trial.

2. Chemotherapy plus radiation therapy without surgery—Combined treatment with chemotherapy and radiation is superior to radiation alone and has achieved long-term survival rates in up to 25% of patients. Chemoradiation alone should be considered in patients with localized disease (stage II or IIIA) who are poor surgical candidates due to serious medical illness or poor functional status (Eastern Cooperative Oncology Group score > 2). Chemoradiation alone as definitive, nonsurgical therapy is more likely to achieve long-term disease-free survival in patients with squamous cell carcinoma than in patients with adenocarcinoma.

3. Supportive care during definitive therapy—Patients with significant tumor obstruction may require local measures such as esophageal stent placement or percutaneous feeding tube insertion to maintain adequate hydration and nutrition during neoadjuvant chemoradiation or chemotherapy. Multidisciplinary consultation is required to determine the optimal procedure. Consultation with a nutritionist also is appropriate to optimize nutrition perioperatively.

B. Therapy for Incurable Disease

More than half of patients have either locally extensive tumor spread (T4) that is unresectable or distant metastases (M1) (stage IIIB and stage IV). Surgery is not warranted in these patients. Since prolonged survival can be achieved in few patients, the primary goal is to provide relief from dysphagia and pain, optimize quality of life, and minimize treatment side effects. The optimal palliative approach depends on the presence or absence of metastatic disease, expected survival, patient preference, and institutional experience. Many patients with advanced disease may prefer concerted efforts at pain relief and care directed at symptom management (see Chapter 5).

1. Chemotherapy or chemoradiation—Combined radiation therapy and chemotherapy may achieve palliation in two-thirds of patients but is associated with significant side effects. It should be considered for patients with locally advanced tumors without distant metastases (stage IIIB) who have good functional status and no significant medical problems, in whom prolonged survival may be achieved. Improvement in dysphagia occurs within 2–4 weeks in almost 90% of patients.

Combination chemotherapy may be considered in those patients with metastatic disease who still have good functional status and expected survival of at least several months. Three-drug combinations commonly include a fluoropyrimidine (5-fluorouracil or capecitabine), a platinum drug (cisplatin or oxaliplatin), and either epirubicin or a taxane (docetaxel or paclitaxel). For patients with poor functional status, single-agent therapy with a fluoropyrimidine, a taxane, or irinotecan may be used. In patients with metastatic distal esophageal and gastroesophageal junction adenocarcinomas positive for amplification of the *HER-2* gene (approximately 15% of cases), addition of the monoclonal antibody trastuzumab (see Chapter 17) to chemotherapy is associated with prolonged survival based on the randomized, phase III ToGA trial. In a separate, randomized, phase III trial, ramucirumab, a monoclonal antibody targeting the vascular endothelial growth factor receptor-2, demonstrated a survival advantage over placebo in patients with adenocarcinoma of the gastroesophageal junction after progression on first-line therapy.

2. Local therapy for esophageal obstruction—Patients with advanced esophageal cancer often have a poor functional and nutritional status. Radiation therapy alone to the area of esophageal obstruction may afford short-term relief of pain and dysphagia and may be suitable for patients with poor functional status or underlying medical problems. This can generally be performed in a short course over a few weeks or less but may be complicated by temporary worsening of dysphagia and odynophagia. For patients with frank obstruction or near obstruction, local antitumor therapies may be preferred. Rapid palliation of dysphagia may be achieved by peroral placement of permanent expandable wire stents (alone or followed by radiation). Palliative feeding tube placement may be considered for hydration and nutrition in selected cases if the obstruction is not amenable or if it is refractory to stenting, radiation, or other local therapies. Stents are most commonly used because of their relative ease of placement. Although dysphagia and quality of life are improved, patients seldom can eat normally after stent placement. Complications occur in 20–40% and include perforation, migration, and tumor ingrowth.

Prognosis

The overall 5-year survival rate of esophageal carcinoma is < 20%. Apart from distant metastasis (M1b), the two most important predictors of poor survival are adjacent mediastinal spread (T4) and lymph node involvement. Whereas cure may be achieved in patients with regional lymph node involvement (stages IIB and III), involvement of nodes outside the chest (M1a) is indicative of metastatic disease (stage IV) that is incurable. For those patients whose disease progresses despite chemotherapy, meticulous efforts at palliative care are essential (see Chapter 5).

When to Refer

- Patients should be referred to gastroenterologist for evaluation and staging (endoscopy with biopsy, endoscopic ultrasonography) and palliative endoscopic antitumor therapy (stent).

- Patients with metastatic disease and obstructive tumors not amenable or refractory to palliative radiation or stenting may require referral to an interventional radiologist, gastroenterologist, or surgeon for feeding tube placement.

- Patients with curable and resectable disease for whom neoadjuvant therapy may be appropriate (stage IIB or IIIA) and those with locally advanced or metastatic disease should be referred to an oncologist for consideration of neoadjuvant chemotherapy or chemoradiotherapy, or for palliative chemotherapy, respectively.

When to Admit

Patients with high-grade esophageal obstruction with inability to manage oral secretions or maintain hydration should be admitted. Acute complications such as perforation, bleeding, aspiration, or fistula also may require admission.

ASGE Standards of Practice Committee. The role of endoscopy in the assessment and treatment of esophageal cancer. Gastrointest Endosc 2013 Mar;77(3):328–34. [PMID: 23410694]

Courrech Staal EF et al. Systematic review of the benefits and risks of neoadjuvant chemoradiation for oesophageal cancer. Br J Surg. 2010 Oct;97(10):1482–96. [PMID: 20645400]

Dantoc M et al. Evidence to support the use of minimally invasive esophagectomy for esophageal cancer: a meta-analysis. Arch Surg. 2012 Aug;147(8):768–76. [PMID: 22911078]

Fuchs CS et al. Ramucirumab monotherapy for previously treated advanced gastric or gastro-oesophageal junction adenocarcinoma (REGARD): an international, randomised, multicentre, placebo-controlled phase 3 trial. Lancet. 2014 Jan 4;383(9911):31–9. [PMID: 24094768]

Hanna WC et al. What is the optimal management of dysphagia in metastatic esophageal cancer? Curr Oncol. 2012 Apr;19(2):e60–6. [PMID: 22514498]

Merkow RP et al. Effect of histologic subtype on treatment and outcomes for esophageal cancer in the United States. Cancer. 2012 Jul 1;118(13):3268–76. [PMID: 22006369]

National Comprehensive Cancer Network (NCCN). NCCN Guidelines: Esophageal and Esophagogastric Junction Cancers, Version 2.2012. http://www.nccn.org/professionals/physician_gls/pdf/esophageal.pdf.

Ngamruengphong S et al. Survival of patients with superficial esophageal adenocarcinoma after endoscopic treatment vs surgery. Clin Gastroenterol Hepatol. 2013 Nov;11(11):1424–9. [PMID: 23735443]

Pennathur A et al. Oesophageal carcinoma. Lancet. 2013 Feb 2;381(9864):400–12. [PMID: 23374478]

van Hagen P et al; CROSS Group. Preoperative chemoradiotherapy for esophageal or junctional cancer. N Engl J Med. 2012 May 31;366(22):2074–84. [PMID: 22646630]

Wheeler JB et al. Epidemiology of esophageal cancer. Surg Clin North Am. 2012 Oct;92(5):1077–87. [PMID: 23026270]

GASTRIC ADENOCARCINOMA

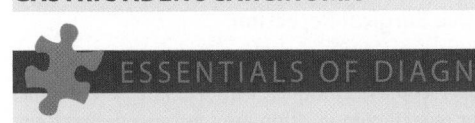

ESSENTIALS OF DIAGNOSIS

▶ Dyspeptic symptoms with weight loss in patients over age 40 years.

▶ Iron deficiency anemia: occult blood in stools.

▶ Abnormality detected on upper gastrointestinal series or endoscopy.

▶ General Considerations

Gastric adenocarcinoma remains the second most common cause of cancer death worldwide. However, its incidence has declined rapidly over the last 70 years, especially in western countries, which may be attributable to changes in diet (more fruits and vegetables), food refrigeration (allowing more fresh foods and reduced salted, smoked, and preserved foods), reduced toxic environmental exposures, and a decline in *Helicobacter pylori*. The incidence of gastric cancer remains high (70/100,000) in Japan and many developing regions, including eastern Asia, Eastern Europe, Chile, Colombia, and Central America. In the United States, there are an estimated 21,130 new cases and 10,620 deaths/year. The incidence is higher in Latinos, African Americans, and Asian Americans.

There are two main histologic variants of gastric cancer: "intestinal-type" (which resembles intestinal cancers in forming glandular structures) and "diffuse" (which is poorly differentiated, has signet-ring cells, and lacks glandular formation). The incidence of **intestinal-type gastric cancer** has declined significantly but it is still the more common type (70–80%); it occurs twice as often in men as women, primarily affects older people (mean age 63 years), and is more strongly associated with environmental factors. It is believed to arise through a gradual, multi-step progression from inflammation (most commonly due to *H pylori*), to atrophic gastritis, to intestinal metaplasia, and finally dysplasia or cancer. Chronic *H pylori* gastritis is the strong risk factor for gastric carcinoma, increasing the relative risk 3.5- to 20-fold. It is estimated that 60–90% of cases of gastric carcinomas may be attributable to *H pylori*. Other risk factors for intestinal-type gastric cancer include pernicious anemia, a history of partial gastric resection more than 15 years previously, smoking, and diets that are high in nitrates or salt and low in vitamin C.

Diffuse gastric cancer accounts for 20–30% of gastric cancer. In contrast to intestinal-type cancer, it affects men and women equally, occurs more commonly in young people, is not as strongly related to *H pylori* infection, and has a worse prognosis than intestinal-type. Most diffuse gastric cancers are attributable to acquired or hereditary mutations in the genes regulating the E-cadherin cell adhesion protein. Familial diffuse gastric cancer accounts for 1–3% of gastric cancers. The cancer may arise at a young age, is often multifocal and infiltrating with signet ring cell histology, and confers poor prognosis. Many of these families have a germline mutation of E-cadherin *CDH1*, which is inherited in an autosomal dominant pattern and carries a > 60% lifetime risk of gastric cancer. Prophylactic gastrectomy should be considered in patients known to carry this mutation.

Most gastric cancers arise in the body and antrum. These may occur in a variety of morphologic types: (1) polypoid or fungating intraluminal masses; (2) ulcerating masses; (3) diffusely spreading (linitis plastica), in which the tumor spreads through the submucosa, resulting in a rigid, atonic stomach with thickened folds (prognosis dismal); and (4) superficially spreading or "early" gastric cancer—confined to the mucosa or submucosa (with or without lymph node metastases) and associated with a favorable prognosis.

In contrast to the dramatic decline in cancers of the distal stomach, a rise in incidence of tumors of the gastric cardia has been noted. These tumors have demographic and pathologic features that resemble Barrett-associated esophageal adenocarcinomas (see Esophageal Cancer).

▶ Clinical Findings

A. Symptoms and Signs

Gastric carcinoma is generally asymptomatic until the disease is quite advanced. Symptoms are nonspecific and are determined in part by the location of the tumor. Dyspepsia, vague epigastric pain, anorexia, early satiety, and weight loss are the presenting symptoms in most patients. Patients may derive initial symptomatic relief from over-the-counter remedies, further delaying diagnosis. Ulcerating lesions can lead to acute gastrointestinal bleeding with hematemesis or melena. Pyloric obstruction results in postprandial vomiting. Lower esophageal obstruction causes progressive dysphagia. Physical examination is rarely helpful. A gastric mass is palpated in < 20% of patients. Signs of metastatic spread include a left supraclavicular lymph node (Virchow node), an umbilical nodule (Sister Mary Joseph nodule), a rigid rectal shelf (Blumer shelf), and ovarian metastases (Krukenberg tumor). Guaiac-positive stools may be detectable.

B. Laboratory Findings

Iron deficiency anemia due to chronic blood loss or anemia of chronic disease is common. Liver test abnormalities, particularly elevation of alkaline phosphatase, may be present if there is metastatic liver spread. Circulating tumor markers do not have established clinical validity in screening, diagnosis, or management of gastric cancer.

C. Endoscopy

Upper endoscopy should be obtained in all patients over age 55 years with new onset of epigastric symptoms (dyspepsia) and in anyone with dyspepsia that is persistent or fails to respond to a short trial of antisecretory therapy. Endoscopy with biopsies of suspicious lesions is highly sensitive for detecting gastric carcinoma. It can be difficult to obtain adequate biopsy specimens in linitis plastica lesions.

D. Imaging

Once a gastric cancer is diagnosed, preoperative evaluation with CT of chest and abdomen (including pelvis in females) and endoscopic ultrasonography is indicated to delineate the local extent of the primary tumor as well as to evaluate for nodal or distant metastases. Endoscopic ultrasonography is superior to CT in determining the depth of tumor penetration and is useful for evaluation of early gastric cancers that may be removed by endoscopic mucosal resection. PET or combined PET-CT imaging is recommended for detection of distant metastasis.

▶ Screening

Because of its unproven efficacy and cost-effectiveness, screening for *H pylori* infection and treating it to prevent gastric cancer is not recommended for asymptomatic adults in the general population but may be considered in patients who have immigrated from regions with a high incidence of gastric cancer or who have a family history of gastric cancer. Because of the high incidence of gastric carcinoma in Japan, screening upper endoscopy is performed there to detect early gastric carcinoma. Approximately 40% of tumors detected by screening are early, with a 5-year survival rate of almost 90%. Screening is not recommended in the United States.

▶ Staging

Staging is defined according to the TNM system, in which T1 tumors invade the lamina propria (T1a) or submucosa (T1b), T2 invade the muscularis propria, T3 penetrate the serosa, and T4 invade adjacent structures. Lymph nodes are graded as N0 if there is no involvement, and N1, N2, or N3 if there are is involvement of 1–6, 7–15, or more than 15 regional nodes. M1 signifies the presence of metastatic disease. Sampling of at least 15 lymph nodes is recommended during surgical staging (see Curative Surgical Resection below). A staging laparoscopy prior to definitive surgery to exclude peritoneal carcinomatosis should be considered in patients with stage T1b or greater disease without radiographic evidence of distant metastases. Pathologic review should include (1) grade of tumor; (2) histologic subtype; (3) depth of invasion; (4) whether lymphatic or vascular invasion is present; and (5) if there is known metastatic disease, the status of HER2 protein expression by immunohistochemistry or fluorescent in situ hybridization or both.

▶ Differential Diagnosis

Ulcerating gastric adenocarcinomas are distinguished from benign gastric ulcers by biopsies. Approximately 3% of gastric ulcers initially believed to be benign later prove to be malignant. To exclude malignancy, all gastric ulcers identified at endoscopy should be biopsied. Ulcers that are suspicious for malignancy to the endoscopist or that have atypia or dysplasia on histologic examination warrant repeat endoscopy in 2–3 months to verify healing and exclude malignancy. Nonhealing ulcers should be considered for resection. Infiltrative carcinoma with thickened gastric folds must be distinguished from lymphoma and other hypertrophic gastropathies.

▶ Treatment

A. Curative Surgical Resection

Surgical resection is the only therapy with curative potential. Laparoscopic techniques achieve similar outcomes and lower overall complication rates as open gastrectomy. After preoperative staging, about two-thirds of patients will be found to have localized disease (ie, stages I–III). In Japan and in specialized centers in the United States, endoscopic mucosal resection is performed in selected patients with small (< 1–2 cm), early (intramucosal or T1aN0) gastric cancers after careful staging with endoscopic ultrasonography. Approximately 25% of patients undergoing surgery will be found to have locally unresectable tumors or peritoneal, hepatic, or distant lymph node metastases that are incurable. The remaining patients with confirmed localized disease should undergo radical surgical resection with curative intent. For adenocarcinoma localized to the distal two-thirds of the stomach, a subtotal distal gastrectomy should be performed. For proximal gastric cancer or diffusely infiltrating disease, total gastrectomy is necessary. Vitamin B_{12} supplementation is required after gastrectomy. Current NCCN treatment guidelines recommend regional (D2) node resection with 15 or more lymph nodes sampled.

B. Perioperative Chemotherapy or Chemoradiation

The use of perioperative chemotherapy or adjuvant chemoradiation is associated with improved survival in patients with localized or locoregional gastric adenocarcinoma who undergo surgical resection. The choice of treatment depends on the location and extent of tumor, type of surgery, patient comorbidities and performance status, and institutional experience. Treatment of tumors arising in the gastroesophageal junction may be treated following algorithms for either gastric or esophageal primary tumors; multidisciplinary treatment decision-making involving the surgeon, radiation oncologist, and medical oncologist is imperative.

C. Palliative Modalities

Many patients will be found either preoperatively or at the time of surgical exploration to have advanced disease that is not amenable to "curative" surgery due to peritoneal or distant metastases or local invasion of other organs. In some of these cases, palliative resection of the tumor nonetheless may be indicated to alleviate pain, bleeding, or obstruction. For patients with unresectable disease, a surgical diversion with gastrojejunostomy may be indicated to prevent obstruction. Alternatively, unresected tumors may be treated with endoscopic laser or stent therapy, radiation therapy, or angiographic embolization to relieve bleeding or obstruction. Chemotherapy may be considered in patients with metastatic disease who still have good functional status and expected survival of at least several months. Multiple chemotherapy regimens have demonstrated activity in metastatic gastric adenocarcinoma. Two-drug combination regimens are preferred for first-line therapy, with most common regimens including a fluoropyrimidine or a taxane agent plus a platinum agent. A three-drug combination of epirubicin or docetaxel plus cisplatin and 5-fluorouracil, or a modification thereof, may be appropriate for first-line treatment in medically fit patients. A 2009 randomized, phase III study showed that addition of the biologic agent trastuzumab to standard chemotherapy prolonged survival in the subset (approximately 15%) of patients with advanced gastric adenocarcinomas harboring amplification of the EGFR-2 (HER2). Trastuzumab is not recommended for combination with anthracyclines such as epirubicin, however, due to risk for cardiotoxicity. After progression on first-line chemotherapy, treatment with irinotecan prolonged survival compared to best supportive care in a randomized, phase III trial. Ramucirumab has also demonstrated a significant survival advantage over placebo in a randomized, phase III trial in patients with advanced gastric or gastroesophageal adenocarcinoma after progression on first-line therapy.

► Prognosis

The long-term survival of gastric carcinoma is < 15%. However, 5-year survival in patients who undergo successful curative resection exceeds 45%. Survival is related to tumor stage, location, and histologic features. Stage I and stage II tumors resected for cure have a > 50% long-term survival. Patients with stage III tumors have a poor prognosis (< 20% long-term survival) and should be considered for enrollment in clinical trials. Tumors of the diffuse type have a worse prognosis than the intestinal type. Tumors of the proximal stomach (fundus and cardia) carry a far worse prognosis than distal lesions. Even with apparently localized disease, proximal tumors have a 5-year survival of < 15%. For those whose disease progresses despite therapy, meticulous efforts at palliative care are essential (see Chapter 5).

► When to Refer

- Patients with dysphagia, weight loss, protracted vomiting, iron deficiency anemia, melena, or new-onset of dyspepsia (especially if age 55 years or older or associated with other alarm symptoms) in whom gastric cancer is suspected should be referred for endoscopy.
- Patients should be referred to a surgeon for attempt at curative resection in stage I, II, or III cancer, including staging laparoscopy if indicated.
- Prior to surgery, patients should be referred to an oncologist to determine the role for neoadjuvant chemotherapy or adjuvant chemoradiation or chemotherapy.

- Patients who have undergone gastrectomy require consultation with a nutritionist due to propensity for malnutrition and complications, such as dumping syndrome and vitamin B_{12} deficiency, postoperatively.
- Patients with unresectable or metastatic disease should be referred to an oncologist for consideration of palliative chemotherapy or chemoradiation.

► When to Admit

Patients with protracted vomiting, inability to maintain hydration or nutrition, or acute bleeding.

Ajani JA et al; NCCN Gastric Cancer Panel. Gastric cancer. J Natl Compr Canc Netw. 2010 Apr;8(4):378–409. [PMID: 20410333]

Bang YJ et al; CLASSIC trial investigators. Adjuvant capecitabine and oxaliplatin for gastric cancer after D2 gastrectomy (CLASSIC): a phase 3 open-label, randomised controlled trial. Lancet. 2012 Jan 28;379(9813):315–21. [PMID: 22226517]

Bang YJ et al; ToGA Trial Investigators. Trastuzumab in combination with chemotherapy versus chemotherapy alone for treatment of HER2-positive advanced gastric or gastro-oesophageal junction cancer (ToGA): a phase 3, open-label, randomised controlled trial. Lancet. 2010 Aug 28;376(9742):687–97. [PMID: 20728210]

Fuchs CS et al. Ramucirumab monotherapy for previously treated advanced gastric or gastro-oesophageal junction adenocarcinoma (REGARD): an international, randomised, multicentre, placebo-controlled phase 3 trial. Lancet. 2014 Jan 4;383(9911):31–9. [PMID: 24094768]

Okines A et al. Gastric cancer: ESMO Clinical Practice Guidelines for diagnosis, treatment and follow-up. Ann Oncol. 2010 May;21(Suppl 5):v50–4. [PMID 20555102]

Polk DB et al. Helicobacter pylori: gastric cancer and beyond. Nat Rev Cancer. 2010 Jun;10(6):403–14. [PMID: 20495574]

Sasako M et al. Five-year outcomes of a randomized phase III trial comparing adjuvant chemotherapy with S-1 versus surgery alone in stage II or III gastric cancer. J Clin Oncol. 2011 Nov 20;29(33):4387–93. [PMID: 22010012]

Shi Y et al. The role of surgery in the treatment of gastric cancer. J Surg Oncol. 2010 Jun 15;101(8):687–92. [PMID: 20512944]

Sun J et al. Meta-analysis of randomized controlled trials on laparoscopic gastrectomy vs. open gastrectomy for distal gastric cancer. Hepatogastroenterology. 2012 Sep;59(118):1699–705. [PMID: 22626787]

Thuss-Patience PC et al. Survival advantage for irinotecan versus best supportive care as second-line chemotherapy in gastric cancer—a randomised phase III study of the Arbeitsgemeinschaft Internistische Onkologie (AIO). Eur J Cancer. 2011 Oct;47(15):2306–14. [PMID: 21742485]

GASTRIC LYMPHOMA

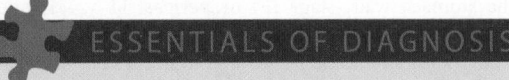

ESSENTIALS OF DIAGNOSIS

- ► Symptoms of dyspepsia, weight loss, or anemia.
- ► Variable abnormalities on upper gastrointestinal series or endoscopy including thickened folds, ulcer, mass or infiltrating lesions; diagnosis established by endoscopic biopsy.
- ► Abdominal CT and endoscopic ultrasonography required for staging.

General Considerations

Gastric lymphomas may be primary (arising from the gastric mucosa) or may represent a site of secondary involvement in patients with nodal lymphomas. Distinguishing advanced primary gastric lymphoma with adjacent nodal spread from advanced nodal lymphoma with secondary gastric spread is essential because the prognosis and treatment of primary and secondary gastric lymphomas are different. Primary lymphoma is the second most common gastric malignancy, accounting for 3% of gastric cancers. More than 95% of these are non-Hodgkin B cell lymphomas. Most primary gastric lymphomas are believed to arise from mucosa-associated lymphoid tissue (MALT).

Infection with *H pylori* is an important risk factor for the development of primary gastric lymphoma. Chronic infection with *H pylori* causes an intense lymphocytic inflammatory response that may lead to the development of lymphoid follicles. Over 90% of low-grade primary gastric MALT-type lymphomas are associated with *H pylori* infection. It is hypothesized that chronic antigenic stimulation may result in a monoclonal lymphoproliferation that may culminate in low-grade or high-grade lymphoma.

Clinical Findings & Staging

The clinical presentation and endoscopic appearance of gastric lymphoma are similar to those of adenocarcinoma. Most patients have abdominal pain, weight loss, or bleeding. Patients with diffuse large B-cell lymphoma are more likely to have systemic symptoms and advanced tumor stage. At endoscopy, lymphoma may appear as an ulcer, mass, or diffusely infiltrating lesion. The diagnosis is established with endoscopic biopsy; FNA is not adequate. Endoscopic ultrasonography is the most sensitive test for determining the level of invasion and presence of perigastric lymphadenopathy and should be performed, if available. All patients should undergo staging with CT scanning of chest, abdomen, and pelvis. For patients with diffuse large B-cell lymphomas involving the stomach, combination PET-CT imaging, bone marrow biopsy with aspirate, tumor lysis laboratory tests, and viral hepatitis and HIV serologies also may be required for staging and management (see Chapter 13).

Treatment

Treatment of primary gastric lymphomas depends on the tumor histology, grade, and stage. Marginal B-cell lymphomas of the MALT type that are low-grade and localized to the stomach wall (stage IE) or perigastric lymph nodes (stage IIE$_1$) have an excellent prognosis. Endoscopic ultrasonography should be performed to accurately determine tumor stage. Patients with primary gastric MALT-lymphoma should be tested for *H pylori* infection and treated if positive. Complete lymphoma regression after successful *H pylori* eradication occurs in approximately 75% of cases of stage IE and approximately 55% with stage II$_1$ low-grade lymphoma. Remission may take as long as a year, and relapse occurs in about 2% of cases per year. Endoscopic surveillance after *H pylori* eradication is recommended every 6 months for 2 years to look for recurrence. In patients whose tumors harbor specific gene translocations, including t(11;18) (API2-MALT1), t(1;14), or t(14;18), rates of remission after *H pylori* eradication are lower, and treatment with radiation may be required. Patients with localized marginal zone MALT-type lymphomas who either are not infected with *H pylori* or do not respond to eradication therapy may be treated with radiation therapy or rituximab, if not a candidate for radiation. Data from a 2010 study, however, suggest that many patients with minimal disease after successful *H pylori* eradication may be observed closely without further therapy. The long-term survival of low-grade MALT lymphoma for stage I is over 90% and for stage II is 35–65%. Because of a low risk of perforation with either radiation therapy or chemotherapy, surgical resection is no longer recommended. Diffuse large B-cell or other higher grade lymphomas with secondary gastrointestinal involvement usually present at an advanced stage with widely disseminated disease and are treated according to stage and subtype of lymphoma (see Chapter 13).

Alevizos L et al. Review of the molecular profile and modern prognostic markers for gastric lymphoma: how do they affect clinical practice? Can J Surg. 2012 Apr;55(2):117–24. [PMID: 22564515]

Falk S. Lymphomas of the upper GI tract: the role of radiotherapy. Clin Oncol (R Coll Radiol). 2012 Jun;24(5):352–7. [PMID: 22386892]

Gisbert JP et al. Review article: common misconceptions in the management of *Helicobacter pylori*-associated gastric MALT-lymphoma. Aliment Pharmacol Ther. 2011 Nov;34(9):1047–62. [PMID: 21919927]

Sagaert X et al. Gastric MALT lymphoma: a model of chronic inflammation-induced tumor development. Nat Rev Gastroenterol Hepatol. 2010 Jun;7(6):336–46. [PMID: 20440281]

Zullo A et al. Effects of *Helicobacter pylori* eradication on early stage gastric mucosa-associated lymphoid tissue lymphoma. Clin Gastroenterol Hepatol. 2010 Feb;8(2):105–10. [PMID: 19631287]

GASTRIC CARCINOID TUMORS

Gastric carcinoids are rare neuroendocrine tumors that make up < 1% of gastric neoplasms. They may occur sporadically or secondary to chronic hypergastrinemia that results in hyperplasia and transformation of enterochromaffin cells in the gastric fundus. The majority of carcinoids are caused by hypergastrinemia and occur in association with either pernicious anemia (75%) (type 1) or Zollinger-Ellison syndrome (5%) (type 2). Carcinoids associated with Zollinger-Ellison syndrome occur almost exclusively in patients with multiple endocrine neoplasia type 1 (MEN 1), in which chromosomal loss of 11q13 has been reported. Carcinoids caused by hypergastrinemia tend to be multicentric, < 1 cm in size, have a low potential for metastatic spread, and thus are unlikely to cause development of the carcinoid syndrome. Small lesions may be successfully treated with endoscopic resection followed by periodic endoscopic surveillance, or with observation. Antrectomy reduces serum gastrin levels and may lead to regression of small tumors. Octreotide therapy may be appropriate for patients with underlying gastrinoma and

Zollinger-Ellison syndrome. Patients with tumors > 2 cm in size should undergo endoscopic or surgical resection (see Small Intestinal Carcinoid Tumors below).

Type 3 gastric carcinoid tumors arise sporadically, independent of gastrin production, and account for up to 20% of gastric carcinoids. Most sporadic gastric carcinoids are solitary, > 2 cm in size, and have a strong propensity for hepatic or pulmonary metastases and thus the carcinoid syndrome at initial presentation. Localized sporadic carcinoids should be treated with radical gastrectomy and regional lymphadenectomy.

Hung OY et al. Hypergastrinemia, type 1 gastric carcinoid tumors: diagnosis and management. J Clin Oncol. 2011 Sep 1; 29(25):e713–5. [PMID: 21747088]

Kidd M et al. Management of gastric carcinoids (neuroendocrine neoplasms). Curr Gastroenterol Rep. 2012 Dec;14(6): 467–72. [PMID: 22976575]

Zhang L et al. Review of the pathogenesis, diagnosis, and management of type I gastric carcinoid tumor. World J Surg. 2011 Aug;35(8):1879–86. [PMID: 21559999]

GASTROINTESTINAL MESENCHYMAL TUMORS

Gastrointestinal mesenchymal tumors (which include stromal tumors, leiomyomas, and schwannomas) derive from mesenchymal stem cells and have an epithelioid or spindle cell histologic pattern, resembling smooth muscle. The most common stromal tumors are gastrointestinal stromal tumors ("GISTs"), which originate from interstitial cells of Cajal. GISTs occur throughout the gastrointestinal tract but most commonly in the stomach (60%) and small intestine (35%). Other mesenchymal tumors, such as leiomyomas, may be discovered incidentally on imaging studies or endoscopy or may cause symptoms (most commonly bleeding, pain, or obstruction). At endoscopy, they appear as a submucosal mass that may have central umbilication or ulceration. Endoscopic ultrasonography with guided FNA biopsy is the optimal study for diagnosing gastric mesenchymal tumors and distinguishing them from other submucosal lesions. Percutaneous biopsy may confer risk of bleeding or intra-abdominal seeding. CT abdomen and pelvis, MRI and PET imaging are useful in the diagnosis and staging. PET imaging also may be useful to monitor response to treatment.

While almost all GISTs have malignant potential, the risk of developing metastasis is increased with tumor size >2 cm, nongastric location, and mitotic index > 5 mitoses per high-powered field. (However, mitotic index can only be assessed after resection.) It is difficult to distinguish benign from malignant tumors before resection by endoscopic ultrasonographic appearance or FNA. In general, lesions are more likely benign if they are < 2 cm, have a smooth border, and have a homogeneous echo pattern on endoscopic ultrasonogram.

Surgery is recommended for all patients with tumors that are ≥ 2 cm or increasing in size, have an endoscopic ultrasonographic appearance suspicious for malignancy, or are symptomatic. The management of asymptomatic benign-appearing gastric lesions ≤ 2 cm in size is problematic.

Because of the low but real long-term risk of malignancy, surgical resection should be considered in younger, otherwise healthy patients; however, other patients may be followed up with serial endoscopic ultrasonographic examinations or, in selected cases, endoscopic resections. After complete surgical resection, GISTs recur within 5 years in over half of patients. Adjuvant therapy with the tyrosine kinase inhibitor imatinib delays recurrence and prolongs survival. Adjuvant imatinib is recommended for all high-risk patients for at least 1 year, though the 5-year recurrence-free survival rate is significantly better following 3 years than 1 year of such therapy (65.6% vs 47.9%). Neoadjuvant therapy with imatinib may be considered for patients with localized GIST tumors who are deemed to be at high risk for resection because of comorbidities, tumor size, or tumor location.

Untreated metastatic GIST tumors are aggressive and carry a poor prognosis. Imatinib induces disease control in up to 85% of patients with metastatic disease with a progression-free survival of 20–24 months and median overall survival of almost 5 years. Imatinib-resistant tumors may respond to high-dose imatinib or to sunitinib, another multi-targeted kinase inhibitor that is approved as second-line therapy for metastatic GIST. Patients in whom metastatic GIST develops after imatinib and sunitinib therapy may respond to the multi-targeted kinase inhibitor regorafenib. In the randomized, phase III GRID trial, patients treated with regorafenib had a significant improvement in progression-free survival compared to those receiving placebo (4.8 months vs 0.9 months).

Dematteo RP et al; American College of Surgeons Oncology Group (ACOSOG) Intergroup Adjuvant GIST Study Team. Adjuvant imatinib mesylate after resection of localised, primary gastrointestinal stromal tumor: a randomised, double-blind, placebo-controlled trial. Lancet. 2009 March 28; 373(9669):1097–104. [PMID: 19303137]

Demetri GD et al. Complete longitudinal analyses of the randomized, placebo-controlled phase III trial of sunitinib in patients with gastrointestinal stromal tumor following imatinib failure. Clin Cancer Res. 2012 Jun 1;18(11):3170–9. [PMID: 22661587]

Demetri GD et al; GRID study investigators. Efficacy and safety of regorafenib for advanced gastrointestinal stromal tumours after failure of imatinib and sunitinib (GRID): an international, multicentre, randomised, placebo-controlled, phase 3 trial. Lancet. 2013 Jan 26;381(9863):295–302. [PMID: 23177515]

Essat M et al. Imatinib as adjuvant therapy for gastrointestinal stromal tumors: a systematic review. Int J Cancer. 2011 May 1;128(9):2202–14. [PMID: 21387287]

Joensuu H et al. One vs three years of adjuvant imatinib for operable gastrointestinal stromal tumor: a randomized trial. JAMA. 2012 Mar 28;307(12):1265–72. [PMID: 22453568]

Mullady DK et al. A multidisciplinary approach to the diagnosis and treatment of gastrointestinal stromal tumor. J Clin Gastroenterol. 2013 Aug;47(7):578–85. [PMID: 23751846]

MALIGNANCIES OF THE SMALL INTESTINE

1. Small Intestinal Adenocarcinomas

These are aggressive tumors that occur most commonly in the duodenum or proximal jejunum. The incidence is rare, with approximately 6000 new diagnoses per year in the

United States. Overall, prognosis is poor, with 5-year disease-specific survival of 65% for stage I, 48% for stage II, 35% for stage III, and 4% for stage IV disease (overall, 32% of patients are stage IV at diagnosis). The ampulla of Vater is the most common site of small bowel carcinoma. The incidence of ampullary carcinoma is increased more than 200-fold in patients with familial adenomatous polyposis. Periodic endoscopic surveillance to detect early ampullary neoplasms is therefore recommended. Ampullary carcinoma may present with jaundice due to bile duct obstruction or bleeding. Surgical resection of early lesions is curative in up to 40% of patients.

2. Small Intestinal Lymphomas

Lymphomas may arise primarily in the gastrointestinal tract or involve it secondarily in patients with disseminated disease. In Western countries, primary gastrointestinal lymphomas account for 5% of lymphomas and 20% of small bowel malignancies. They occur most commonly in the small intestine. There is an increased incidence of small intestinal lymphomas in patients with AIDS, immunosuppressive therapy, and Crohn disease. The most common histologic subtype is non-Hodgkin extranodal marginal zone (MALT) B cell lymphoma. Enteropathy-associated T cell lymphomas appear to be increasing in incidence in the United States. They are associated with the diagnosis of celiac disease. Other types of intestinal lymphomas include primary intestinal follicular cell lymphoma, mantle cell lymphoma, and Burkitt lymphoma (see Chapter 13).

Presenting symptoms or signs of primary small bowel lymphoma include abdominal pain, weight loss, nausea and vomiting, distention, anemia, and occult blood in the stool. Fevers are unusual. Protein-losing enteropathy may result in hypoalbuminemia, but other signs of malabsorption are unusual. Barium radiography or CT enterography helps localize the site of the lesion. The diagnosis requires endoscopic, percutaneous, or laparoscopic biopsy. Imaging and bone marrow biopsy are required to determine stage.

Treatment depends on the tumor histologic subtype and stage of disease (see Chapter 13). Surgical resection of primary intestinal lymphoma, if feasible, may be appropriate for localized tumors. In patients with limited disease (stage IE) in whom resection is performed with negative margins, the role of adjuvant chemotherapy is unclear. Locoregional radiation should be considered if surgical margins are positive. Patients with more extensive disease generally are treated according to the tumor histology.

3. Intestinal Carcinoid Tumors

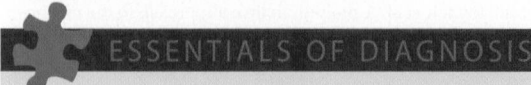

ESSENTIALS OF DIAGNOSIS

- ▶ Majority are asymptomatic and discovered incidentally at endoscopy or surgery.
- ▶ Carcinoid syndrome occurs in < 10%; hepatic metastases are generally present.
- ▶ Risk of metastasis related to tumor size and location.

▶ General Considerations

Gastrointestinal carcinoid tumors are generally slow growing neuroendocrine tumors that account for approximately one-third of tumors arising in the small bowel. Gastrointestinal carcinoid tumors most commonly occur in the small intestine (45%) but are also found in the rectum (20%), appendix (17%), and colon (11%), with the remainder occurring in the stomach (< 10%; see Gastric Carcinoid Tumors above). Carcinoid tumors may contain a variety of hormones, including serotonin, somatostatin, gastrin, and substance P, each of which may or may not be secreted.

Small intestinal carcinoids most commonly arise in the distal ileum within 60 cm of the ileocecal valve. Up to 30% are multicentric. Although many carcinoids behave in an indolent fashion, the overall 5-year survival rates for patients with locoregional and metastatic small bowel carcinoids are approximately 65% and 35%, respectively. The risk of metastatic spread increases with tumor sizes ≥ 1 cm and > 2 cm as well as with invasion beyond muscularis propria. Appendiceal carcinoids are identified in 0.3% of appendectomies, usually as an incidental finding. Almost 80% of these tumors are < 1 cm in size, and 90% are < 2 cm. However, in patients with appendiceal carcinoid tumors > 2 cm in size, approximately 90% develop nodal and distant metastases; right hemicolectomy is recommended in these cases.

Rectal carcinoids are usually detected incidentally as submucosal nodules during proctoscopic examination and often locally excised by biopsy or snare polypectomy before the histologic diagnosis is known. Endorectal ultrasound is usually recommended to assess the size, presence and depth of invasion, and presence of lymph node metastases. Rectal carcinoids < 1 cm virtually never metastasize and are treated effectively with local endoscopic or transanal excision. Larger tumors are associated with the development of metastasis in 10%. Hence, a more extensive cancer resection operation is warranted in fit patients with rectal carcinoid tumors > 1–2 cm or with high risk features (such as invasion of muscularis propria or evidence of nodal involvement), or both.

▶ Clinical Findings

A. Symptoms and Signs

Most smaller lesions (< 1–2 cm) are asymptomatic and difficult to detect by endoscopy or imaging studies. Through local extension or metastasis to mesenteric lymph nodes, carcinoids engender a fibroblastic reaction with contraction and kinking of the bowel or encasement of mesenteric vessels. Small intestinal carcinoids may present with abdominal pain, bowel obstruction, bleeding, or bowel infarction. Appendiceal and rectal carcinoids usually are small and asymptomatic but large lesions can cause bleeding, obstruction, or altered bowel habits. **Carcinoid syndrome** occurs in < 10% of patients. More than 90% of patients with carcinoid syndrome have hepatic metastases, usually from carcinoids of small bowel origin. About 10% of patients with carcinoid syndrome have primary bronchial or ovarian tumors without hepatic metastases. Carcinoid syndrome is caused by tumor secretion of hormonal mediators. The manifestations include facial flushing, edema of the head and neck (especially with bronchial carcinoid), abdominal cramps and diarrhea, bronchospasm, cardiac lesions (pulmonary or tricuspid stenosis or regurgitation in 10–30%), and telangiectases.

B. Laboratory Findings

Serum chromogranin A (CgA) is elevated in the majority of neuroendocrine tumors, although its sensitivity for small, localized carcinoid tumors is unknown. CgA is elevated in almost 90% of patients with advanced small bowel carcinoid. Urinary 5-hydroxyindoleacetic acid (5-HIAA) and platelet serotonin levels are also elevated in patients with metastatic carcinoid; however, these tests are less sensitive than CgA. There is increased urinary 5-HIAA in carcinoid syndrome; symptomatic patients usually excrete more than 25 mg of 5-HIAA per day in the urine. Ideally, all drugs should be withheld for several days prior to a 24-hour urine collection.

C. Imaging

Abdominal CT may demonstrate a mesenteric mass with tethering of the bowel, lymphadenopathy, and hepatic metastasis. Abdominal CT or enterography may reveal kinking of the bowel, but because the lesion is extraluminal, the diagnosis may be overlooked for several years. Somatostatin receptor scintigraphy, which is positive in up to 90% of patients with metastatic carcinoid, is routinely used in staging. Most patients with carcinoid syndrome have liver metastasis on abdominal imaging.

▶ Treatment & Outcomes

Small intestinal carcinoids generally are indolent tumors with slow spread. Patients with disease confined to the small intestine should be treated with surgical excision. There is no proven role for adjuvant therapy after complete resection. Five-year survival rates for patients with stage I and II disease are 96% and 87%, respectively. In patients with resectable disease who have lymph node involvement (stage III), the 5-year survival is 74%; however, by 25 years, < 25% remain disease free. Even patients with metastatic disease may have an indolent course with a 5-year survival of 43%.

In patients with advanced disease, therapy historically has been deferred until the patient is symptomatic, although one phase III, randomized, placebo-controlled trial demonstrated that early initiation of somatostatin analog therapy significantly delayed time to progression of hepatic metastases compared to placebo (14.3 vs 6 months, respectively). Conventional cytotoxic chemotherapy agents do not achieve significant responses in carcinoid tumors and have not been associated with improved outcomes. Radiolabeled somatostatin analogs are under investigation as another treatment modality for patients with somatostatin-receptor positive advanced carcinoid tumors. In patients with metastatic disease, surgery should be directed toward palliation of obstructive symptoms or bleeding.

In patients with carcinoid syndrome, the somatostatin analog octreotide, 150–250 mcg subcutaneously three times daily or administered as a long-acting intramuscular depot formulation, inhibits hormone secretion from the carcinoid tumor. This results in dramatic relief of symptoms of carcinoid syndrome, including diarrhea or flushing, in 90% of patients for a median period of 1 year. Thereafter, many patients stop responding to octreotide. In selected patients with refractory carcinoid syndrome, resection of hepatic metastases may provide dramatic improvement. Hepatic artery occlusion, liver-directed debulking procedures, and chemotherapy also may provide symptomatic improvement in some patients with hepatic metastases. Studies of peptide receptor radionuclide therapy, which consists of somatostatin analogs conjugated to a radioactive isotope such as yttrium-90 or lutetium-177, are underway in patients with metastatic small bowel neuroendocrine tumors based on preliminary evidence for antitumor activity.

4. Small Intestine Sarcoma

Most small intestine sarcomas arise from stromal tumors (GISTs) that stain positive for CD117; a minority arise from smooth muscle tumors (leiomyosarcomas) (see Gastrointestinal Mesenchymal Tumors above).

Kaposi sarcoma was at one time a common complication in AIDS, but the incidence is declining with highly active antiretroviral therapy (HAART). It can also occur in the setting of immunosuppression after organ transplant. It is caused by infection with human herpesvirus 8 (HHV8). Lesions may be present anywhere in the intestinal tract. Visceral involvement usually is associated with cutaneous disease. Most lesions are clinically silent; however, large lesions may be symptomatic. Widespread involvement may be best treated by systemic chemotherapy using single-agent therapy or combinations of pegylated-doxorubicin (Doxil), paclitaxel, vincristine, bleomycin, or etoposide. Surgery or radiation may be indicated for isolated high-risk lesions.

Bilimoria KY et al. Small bowel cancer in the United States: changes in epidemiology, treatment, and survival over the last 20 years. Ann Surg. 2009 Jan;249(1):63–71. [PMID: 19106677]

Dittmer DP et al. Treatment of Kaposi sarcoma-associated herpesvirus-associated cancers. Front Microbiol. 2012 Apr 18;3:141. [PMID: 22529843]

Holinga J et al. Metastatic risk of diminutive rectal carcinoid tumors: a need for surveillance rectal ultrasound? Gastrointest Endosc. 2012 Apr;75(4):913–16. [PMID: 22284087]

Neoptolemos JP et al; European Study Group for Pancreatic Cancer. Effect of adjuvant chemotherapy with fluorouracil plus folinic acid or gemcitabine vs observation on survival in patients with resected periampullary adenocarcinoma: the ESPAC-3 periampullary cancer randomized trial. JAMA. 2012 Jul 11;308(2):147–56. [PMID: 22782416]

Rinke A et al. Placebo-controlled, double-blind, prospective, randomized study on the effect of octreotide LAR in the control of tumor growth in patients with metastatic neuroendocrine midgut tumors: a report from the PROMID Study Group. J Clin Oncol. 2009 Oct 1;27(28):4656–63. [PMID: 19704057]

Sharaiha RZ et al. Increasing incidence of enteropathy-associated T-cell lymphoma in the United States, 1973–2008. Cancer. 2012 Aug 1;118(15):3786–92. [PMID: 22169928]

Strosberg J. Neuroendocrine tumors of the small intestine. Best Pract Res Clin Gastroenterol. 2012 Dec;26(6):755–73. [PMID: 23582917]

Toumpanakis C et al. Update on the role of somatostatin analogs for the treatment of patients with gastroenteropancreatic neuroendocrine tumors. Semin Oncol. 2013 Feb;40(1):56–68. [PMID: 23391113]

COLORECTAL CANCER

ESSENTIALS OF DIAGNOSIS

- ▶ Personal or family history of adenomatous polyps or colorectal cancer are important risk factors.
- ▶ Symptoms or signs depend on tumor location.
- ▶ Proximal colon: fecal occult blood, anemia.
- ▶ Distal colon: change in bowel habits, hematochezia.
- ▶ Diagnosis established with colonoscopy.

▶ General Considerations

Colorectal cancer is the second leading cause of death due to malignancy in the United States. Colorectal cancer will develop in approximately 6% of Americans and 40% of those will die of the disease. In 2012, there were an estimated 103,170 new cases of colon cancer and 40,290 new cases of rectal cancer in the United States, with combined estimated 51,960 deaths. The mortality has decreased by approximately 35% between 1990 and 2007, possibly due to improved screening and treatment modalities.

Colorectal cancers are almost all adenocarcinomas, which tend to form bulky exophytic masses or annular constricting lesions. The majority of colorectal cancers are thought to arise from malignant transformation of an adenomatous polyp (tubular, tubulovillous, or villous adenoma) or serrated polyp (hyperplastic polyp, traditional serrated adenoma, or sessile serrated adenoma). Polyps that are "advanced" (ie, polyps at least 1 cm in size, adenomas with villous features, or adenomas with high-grade dysplasia) are associated with a greater risk of cancer. Approximately 85% of sporadic colorectal cancers arise from adenomatous polyps and have loss of function of one or more tumor suppressor genes (eg, *p53*, *APC*, or *DCC*) due to a combination of spontaneous mutation of one allele combined with chromosomal instability and aneuploidy (abnormal DNA content) that leads to deletion and loss of heterozygosity of the other allele (eg, 5q, 17q, or 18p deletion). Activation of oncogenes such as *K-ras* and *B-raf* is present in a subset of colorectal cancers with prognostic and therapeutic implications discussed further below.

Approximately 10–20% of colorectal cancers arise from serrated polyps, most of which have hypermethylation of CpG-rich promoter regions that leads to inactivation of the DNA mismatch repair gene *MLH1*, resulting in microsatellite instability, and activation of mutations of the *BRAF* gene. Serrated colon cancers have distinct clinical and pathologic characteristics, including diploid DNA content, predominance in the proximal colon, poor differentiation, and more favorable prognosis.

Up to 5% of colorectal cancers are caused by inherited germline mutations resulting in polyposis syndromes (eg, familial adenomatous polyposis) or hereditary nonpolyposis colorectal cancer (HNPCC or Lynch syndrome). These conditions are discussed further in Chapter 15.

▶ Risk Factors

A number of factors increase the risk of developing colorectal cancer. Recognition of these has impact on screening strategies. However, 75% of all cases occur in people with no known predisposing factors.

A. Age

The incidence of colorectal cancer rises sharply after age 45 years, and 90% of cases occur in persons over the age of 50 years.

B. Family History of Neoplasia

A family history of colorectal cancer is present in approximately 20% of patients with colon cancer. Hereditary factors are believed to contribute to 20–30% of colorectal cancers; however, the genes responsible for most of these cases have not yet been identified. (See Chapter 15 for discussion of inherited polyposis syndromes.) Approximately 6% of the Ashkenazi Jewish population has a missense mutation in the *APC* gene *(APC I1307K)* that confers a modestly increased lifetime risk of developing colorectal cancer (OR 1.4–1.9) but phenotypically resembles sporadic colorectal cancer rather than familial adenomatous polyposis. Genetic screening is available, and patients harboring the mutation merit intensive screening.

A family history of colorectal cancer or adenomatous polyps is one of the most important risk factors for colorectal cancer. The risk of colon cancer is proportionate to the number and age of affected first-degree family members with colon neoplasia. People with one first-degree family member with colorectal cancer have an increased risk approximately two times that of the general population; however, the risk is almost four times if the family member's cancer was diagnosed at < 45 years of age. Patients with two first-degree relatives have a fourfold, or 25–30% lifetime, risk of developing colon cancer. First-degree relatives of patients with adenomatous polyps also have a twofold increased risk for colorectal neoplasia, especially if the polyp was large (≥ 10 mm) or detected before age 60 years.

C. Inflammatory Bowel Disease

The risk of adenocarcinoma of the colon begins to rise 8 years after disease onset in patients with ulcerative colitis and Crohn colitis. The cumulative risk approaches 5–10% after 20 years and 20% after 30 years. Chronic treatment with 5-ASA agents and folate is associated with a lower risk of cancer in patients with ulcerative colitis.

D. Dietary and Lifestyle Factors and Chemoprevention in Colorectal Cancer Risk

In epidemiologic studies, diets rich in fats and red meat are associated with an increased risk of colorectal adenomas and cancer, whereas diets high in fruits, vegetables, and fiber are associated with a decreased risk. However, prospective, randomized controlled trials failed to demonstrate a risk reduction in the recurrence of adenomatous polyps after treatment with a diet low in fat and high in fiber, fruits, and vegetables, or with fiber supplementation.

A US Preventive Services Task Force meta-analysis of cohort and case-control studies suggest that prolonged (> 6 years) regular use of aspirin (at least 325 mg twice weekly) or NSAIDs is associated with a 22–33% relative risk reduction in the incidence of colorectal cancer. Two prospective, blinded clinical trials have shown that daily low-dose aspirin (80–325 mg) reduces the number of recurrent adenomas at 1–3 years in patients with a history of colorectal adenomas or cancer; however, two large randomized controlled trials in the United States did not demonstrate a reduction in colorectal cancer incidence in patients taking low-dose aspirin over a 5–10 years. Because long-term aspirin use is associated with a low incidence of serious complications (gastrointestinal hemorrhage, stroke), the US Preventive Services Task Force concluded that it should not be prescribed as a chemopreventive agent in people without polyps or with small adenomas unless there are other medical indications. Long-term administration of low-dose aspirin may be considered in patients with a personal or family history of colorectal cancer or advanced adenomas; however, they do not obviate the need for colonoscopy screening and surveillance.

Retrospective analysis of randomized phase III trial data and a meta-analysis have shown that patients with higher levels of pre- and post-diagnosis physical activity experience reduced colorectal cancer–specific mortality and all-cause mortality. Maintaining a healthy body weight, a healthy diet, and a physically active lifestyle are recommended in colorectal cancer survivors.

E. Other Factors

The incidence of colon adenocarcinoma is higher in blacks than in whites. It is unclear whether this is due to genetic or socioeconomic factors (eg, diet or reduced access to screening). Diabetes mellitus, metabolic syndrome, obesity, and cigarette smoking are associated with a modest increase in cancer risk.

► Clinical Findings

A. Symptoms and Signs

Adenocarcinomas grow slowly and may be present for several years before symptoms appear. However, some asymptomatic tumors may be detected by the presence of fecal occult blood (see Colorectal Cancer Screening, below). Symptoms depend on the location of the carcinoma. Chronic blood loss from right-sided colonic cancers may cause iron deficiency anemia, manifested by fatigue and weakness. Obstruction, however, is uncommon because of the large diameter of the right colon and the liquid consistency of the fecal material. Lesions of the left colon often involve the bowel circumferentially. Because the left colon has a smaller diameter and the fecal matter is solid, obstructive symptoms may develop with colicky abdominal pain and a change in bowel habits. Constipation may alternate with periods of increased frequency and loose stools. The stool may be streaked with blood, though marked bleeding is unusual. With rectal cancers, patients note tenesmus, urgency, and recurrent hematochezia. Weight loss is uncommon. Physical examination is usually normal except in advanced disease. A mass may be palpable in the abdomen. The liver should be examined for hepatomegaly, suggesting metastatic spread. For cancers of the distal rectum, digital examination is necessary to determine whether there is extension into the anal sphincter or fixation, suggesting extension to the pelvic floor.

B. Laboratory Findings

A CBC is obtained to look for evidence of anemia. Elevated liver function tests, particularly the alkaline phosphatase, are suspicious for metastatic disease. Carcinoembryonic antigen (CEA) should be measured in all patients with proved colorectal cancer but is not appropriate for screening. A preoperative CEA level > 5 ng/mL is a poor prognostic indicator. After complete surgical resection, CEA levels should normalize; persistently elevated levels suggest the presence of persistent disease and warrant further evaluation.

C. Colonoscopy

Colonoscopy is the diagnostic procedure of choice in patients with a clinical history suggestive of colon cancer or in patients with an abnormality suspicious for cancer detected on radiographic imaging. Colonoscopy permits biopsy for pathologic confirmation of malignancy (Figure 39–1). In patients in whom the colonoscope is unable to reach the cecum (< 5% of cases) or when a nearly obstructing tumor precludes passage of the colonoscope, barium enema or CT colonography examination should be performed.

D. Imaging

Chest, abdominal, and pelvic CT scans are required for preoperative staging. CT scans may demonstrate distal metastases but are less accurate in the determination of the level of local tumor extension (T stage) or lymphatic spread (N stage). Intraoperative assessment of the liver by direct palpation and ultrasonography is more accurate than CT scanning for the detection of hepatic metastases. For rectal cancers (generally defined as tumors arising ≤ 12 cm proximal to the anal verge), pelvic MRI or endorectal ultrasonography is required to determine the depth of penetration of the cancer through the rectal wall (T stage) and perirectal lymph nodes, informing decisions about preoperative (neoadjuvant) chemoradiotherapy and operative management. PET is not routinely used for staging or surveillance in colorectal cancers.

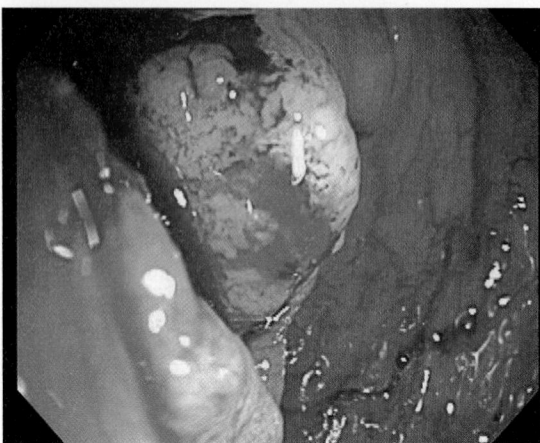

▲ **Figure 39–1.** Cecal adenocarcinoma on colonoscopy. (From Marvin Derezin, MD; Reproduced, with permission, from Usatine RP, Smith MA, Mayeaux EJ Jr, Chumley H, Tysinger J. *The Color Atlas of Family Medicine*. McGraw-Hill, 2009.)

► Staging

The TNM system is the commonly used classification to stage colorectal cancer. Staging is important not only because it correlates with the patient's long-term survival but also because it is used to determine which patients should receive adjuvant therapy.

► Differential Diagnosis

The nonspecific symptoms of colon cancer may be confused with those of irritable bowel syndrome, diverticular disease, ischemic colitis, inflammatory bowel disease, infectious colitis, and hemorrhoids. Neoplasm must be excluded in any patient over age 40 years who reports a change in bowel habits or hematochezia or who has an unexplained iron deficiency anemia or occult blood in stool samples.

► Treatment

A. Surgery

Resection of the primary colonic or rectal cancer is the treatment of choice for almost all patients who have resectable lesions and can tolerate general anesthesia. For colon cancer, multiple studies demonstrate that minimally invasive, laparoscopically assisted colectomy results in similar outcomes and rates of recurrence to open colectomy. Regional dissection of at least 12 lymph nodes should be performed to determine staging, which guides decisions about adjuvant therapy.

For rectal carcinoma, preoperative (neoadjuvant) chemoradiation with 5-fluorouracil is recommended in all node-positive tumors, and in T3 and greater tumors, due to increased risk of local recurrence (see below). After neoadjuvant therapy, the operative approach depends on the level of the tumor above the anal verge, the size and depth of

penetration, and the patient's overall condition. Clinical staging by endorectal ultrasound or MRI with endorectal coil is important in guiding the clinical approach. In carefully selected patients with small, mobile (< 4 cm), well-differentiated T1 or T2 rectal tumors that are < 8 cm from the anal verge, transanal excision may be considered. This approach avoids laparotomy and spares the rectum and anal sphincter, preserving normal bowel continence. All other patients will require either a low anterior resection with a colorectal anastomosis or an abdominoperineal resection with a colostomy, depending on how far above the anal verge the tumor is located and the extent of local tumor spread. Careful dissection of the entire mesorectum at the time of surgery reduces local recurrence to 8%. Although low anterior resections obviate a colostomy, they are associated with increased immediate postsurgical complications (eg, leak, dehiscence, stricture) and defecatory complaints (eg, increased stool frequency, and incontinence). With unresectable rectal cancer, the patient may be palliated with a diverting colostomy or placement of an expandable wire stent.

B. Systemic Chemotherapy for Colon Cancer

Chemotherapy and radiotherapy have been demonstrated to improve overall and tumor-free survival in selected patients with colorectal cancers depending on stage.

1. Stage I—Because of the excellent 5-year survival rate (90–100%), no adjuvant therapy is recommended.

2. Stage II (node-negative disease)—The 5-year survival rate is approximately 80%. A significant survival benefit from adjuvant chemotherapy has not been demonstrated in most controlled trials for stage II colon cancer (see discussion for stage III disease). However, otherwise healthy patients with stage II disease that is at higher risk for recurrence (perforation, obstruction, T4 tumors, or fewer than 12 lymph nodes sampled) may benefit from adjuvant chemotherapy.

3. Stage III (node-positive disease)—With surgical resection alone, the expected 5-year survival rate is 30–50%. Postoperative adjuvant chemotherapy significantly increases disease-free survival as well as overall survival up to 30% and is recommended for all fit patients. Large, well-designed studies of adjuvant therapy for stage III colon cancer reported a higher rate of disease-free survival at 5 years for patients treated for 6 months postoperatively with a combination of oxaliplatin, 5-fluorouracil, and leucovorin (FOLFOX) (73.3%) than with 5-fluorouracil and leucovorin (FL) alone (67.4%). The addition of oxaliplatin is associated with an increased incidence of diarrhea, myelosuppression, and peripheral sensory neuropathy, all of which generally are reversible. Based on these studies, FOLFOX currently is the preferred adjuvant therapy for most patients with stage III colon cancer (see Table 39–12). The addition of a biologic agent (bevacizumab or cetuximab) to FOLFOX does not improve outcomes in the adjuvant setting.

4. Stage IV (metastatic disease)—Approximately 20% of patients have metastatic disease at the time of initial diagnosis, and an additional 30% eventually develop metastasis. A subset of these patients has limited disease that is potentially curable with surgical resection. Resection of isolated liver or lung metastases may result in long-term (over 5 years) survival in 35–55% of cases. For those with unresectable hepatic metastases, local ablative techniques (cryosurgery, radiofrequency or microwave coagulation, embolization, hepatic intra-arterial chemotherapy) may provide long-term tumor control. The majority of patients with metastatic disease do not have resectable (curable) disease. In the absence of other treatment, the median survival is < 12 months; however, with current therapies, median survival approaches 24 months. The goals of therapy for patients with metastatic colorectal cancer are to slow tumor progression while maintaining a reasonable quality of life for as long as possible. Currently, either FOLFOX (the addition of oxaliplatin to 5-fluorouracil and folinic acid) or FOLFIRI (the addition of irinotecan to 5-fluorouracil and folinic acid) is the preferred first-line treatment regimens for fit patients. For convenience, oral capecitabine (instead of intravenous 5-fluorouracil and leucovorin) can be used in combination with oxaliplatin; however, combination with irinotecan is not recommended due to increased toxicity (diarrhea). Addition of a biologic agent to combination chemotherapy improves response rates and overall survival and is recommended in the first-line of treatment in suitable patients. Bevacizumab is a monoclonal antibody targeting VEGF. Combination therapy with bevacizumab and FOLFOX or FOLFIRI prolongs mean survival 2–5 months compared with either regimen alone (see Table 39–12). Cetuximab and panitumumab are monoclonal antibodies targeting EGFR. Activating codon 12 and 13 *K-ras* gene mutations downstream of EGFR are present in approximately 35% of patients with metastatic colorectal cancer and are a biomarker for nonresponse to cetuximab and panitumumab, for which reason the use of these agents is restricted to patients with tumors wild-type for *K-ras*. In stage IV patients with *K-ras* wild-type tumors, the addition of panitumumab or cetuximab to FOLFOX or FOLFIRI prolongs survival by approximately 4 months. Bevacizumab may cause serious side effects, including arterial thromboembolic events, bowel perforation, or serious bleeding, in up to 5% of patients. EGFR-targeted agents cause an acneiform rash in the majority of patients. Cetuximab is associated with severe infusion reactions in approximately 2–5%.

When disease progresses despite treatment either with FOLFOX or with FOLFIRI (often in conjunction with bevacizumab or an EGFR-targeted antibody), therapy is switched to the alternate regimen; patients may respond to the alternate regimen, prolonging mean survival to > 20 months. The novel anti-angiogenic agent, aflibercept, is FDA-approved for use in second-line colorectal cancer in combination with FOLFIRI. Palliative therapy with cetuximab or panitumumab can benefit patients with *K-ras* wild-type tumors whose disease has progressed after first-line and second-line chemotherapies. The multi-targeted kinase inhibitor, regorafenib, was approved by the FDA in 2012 for patients with metastatic, refractory colorectal cancer after progression on standard regimens based on results of the randomized, phase III CORRECT trial showing improved overall survival compared to placebo.

C. Neoadjuvant and Adjuvant Therapy for Rectal Cancer

Compared with colon cancer, rectal cancer has lower long-term survival rates and significantly higher rates of local tumor recurrence with surgery alone (approximately 25%) attributed in part to the difficulty of achieving adequate surgical resection margins and to lack of serosal encasement of the rectum. When initial imaging studies suggest stage I disease, surgery may be performed first (see Surgery above). For stage II and III tumors by clinical staging (including endorectal ultrasound or pelvic MRI), preoperative chemoradiation with 5-fluorouracil or capecitabine as a radiation-sensitizing agent improves disease-free survival and decreases pelvic recurrence rate (see Table 39–12). Preoperative chemoradiation has been shown to be superior to postoperative chemoradiation with lower local recurrence and toxicity rates in the randomized, phase III CAO/ARO/AIO-94 trial. Following surgical resection with total mesorectal excision (see Surgery above), adjuvant 5-fluorouracil–based therapy (generally with the FOLFOX regimen extrapolating from its benefit in patients with similarly-staged colon cancers) is recommended for a total of approximately 6 months of perioperative therapy inclusive of neoadjuvant chemoradiation.

▶ Follow-Up after Surgery

Patients who have undergone resections for cure are monitored closely to look for evidence of symptomatic or asymptomatic tumor recurrence that may be amenable to curative resection in a small number of patients. The optimal cost-effective strategy is not clear. Patients should be evaluated every 3–6 months for 5 years with history, physical examination, and laboratory surveillance, including serum CEA levels. The NCCN and ASCO guidelines recommend surveillance CT scans of chest, abdomen, and pelvis annually for up to 5 years post-resection in high-risk stage II and all stage III patients. Patients who had a complete preoperative colonoscopy should undergo another colonoscopy 1 year after surgical resection. Patients who did not undergo full colonoscopy preoperatively also should undergo colonoscopy within 3–6 months postoperatively to exclude other synchronous colorectal neoplasms. If a colonoscopy does not detect new adenomatous polyps 1 year postoperatively, surveillance colonoscopy should be performed every 3–5 years thereafter to look for metachronous polyps or cancer. Because of the high incidence of local tumor recurrence in patients with rectal cancer, proctoscopy surveillance of the low anterior resection anastomotic site may also be performed periodically. New onset of symptoms or a rising CEA warrants investigation with chest, abdominal, and pelvic CT and colonoscopy to look for a new primary tumor or recurrence, or metachronous metastatic disease that may be amenable to curative or palliative therapy. For patients with a rising CEA level with unrevealing CT imaging, a PET scan may be more sensitive for the detection of occult metastatic disease.

▶ Prognosis

The stage of disease at presentation is the most important determinant of long-term survival in colon cancer: stage I, > 90%; stage II, 70–85%; stage III with < 4 positive lymph nodes, 67%; stage III with > 4 positive lymph nodes, 33%; and stage IV, 5–7%. For each stage, rectal cancers have a worse prognosis. For those patients whose disease progresses despite therapy, meticulous efforts at palliative care are essential (see Chapter 5).

▶ Screening for Colorectal Neoplasms

Colorectal cancer is ideal for screening because it is a common disease that is fatal in almost 50% of cases yet is curable if detected at an earlier stage. Furthermore, most cases arise from benign adenomatous or serrated polyps that progress over many years to cancer, and removal of these polyps has been shown to prevent the majority of cancers. Colorectal cancer screening is endorsed by the US Preventive Services Task Force, the Agency for Health Care Policy and Research, the American Cancer Society, and every professional gastroenterology and colorectal surgery society. Although there is continued debate about the optimal cost-effective means of providing population screening, there is unanimous consent that screening of some kind should be offered to every patient over the age of 50 years. Several analyses suggest that screening is cost-effective.

It is important for primary care providers to understand the relative merits of various options and to discuss them with their patients. Due to growing awareness of the importance of screening on the part of medical professionals and the public, 65% of patients between 50 and 75 years of age have undergone screening. Discussion and encouragement by the primary care provider are the most important factors in achieving patient compliance with screening programs.

Recommendations for screening from the US Multi-Society Task Force are listed in Table 39–6. Screening is recommended for all men and women ages 50 through 75 years of age who are at average risk for cancer. Some guidelines recommend screening for African Americans beginning at age 45. The potential for harm from screening must be weighed against the likelihood of benefit, especially in elderly patients with comorbid illnesses and shorter life expectancy. Although routine screening is not recommended in adults above age 75, it may be considered on a case-by-case basis in adults age 76 through 85 years who have excellent health and functional status. Patients with first-degree relatives with colorectal neoplasms (cancer or adenomatous polyps) are at increased risk; earlier and earlier, more frequent screening may be recommended (preferably with colonoscopy) for these individuals. Recommendations for screening in families with inherited cancer syndromes or inflammatory bowel disease are provided in Chapter 15. For patients at average risk for colorectal cancer, the recommendations of the Task Force are discussed below. Screening tests may be classified into two broad categories: stool-based tests and examinations that visualize the structure of the colon by direct endoscopic inspection or radiographic imaging.

Table 39–6. Recommendations for colorectal cancer screening.[1]

Average-risk individuals ≥ 50 years old[2]
Annual fecal occult blood testing using higher sensitivity tests (Hemoccult SENSA)
Annual fecal immunochemical test (FIT)
Fecal DNA test (interval uncertain)
Flexible sigmoidoscopy every 5 years
Colonoscopy every 10 years
CT colonography every 5 years
Individuals with a family history of a first-degree member with colorectal neoplasia[3]
Single first-degree relative with colorectal cancer diagnosed at age ≥ 60 years: Begin screening at age 40. Screening guidelines same as average-risk individual; however, preferred method is colonoscopy every 10 years.
Single first-degree relative with colorectal cancer or advanced adenoma diagnosed at age < 60 years, or two first-degree relatives: Begin screening at age 40 or at age 10 years younger than age at diagnosis of the youngest affected relative, whichever is first in time. Recommended screening: colonoscopy every 5 years.

[1]For recommendations for families with inherited polyposis syndromes or hereditary nonpolyposis colon cancer, see Chapter 15.
[2]Joint Guideline from the American Cancer Society, the US Multi-Society Task Force on Colorectal Cancer, and the American College of Radiology. Gastroenterology 2008 May; 134(5):1570.
[3]American College of Gastroenterology. Guidelines for Colorectal Cancer Screening. Am J Gastroenterol. 2009 Mar;104(3):739.

A. Stool-based Tests

1. Fecal occult blood test—Most colorectal cancers and some large adenomas result in increased chronic blood loss. A variety of tests for fecal occult blood are commercially available that have varying sensitivities and specificities for colorectal neoplasia. These include guaiac-based tests (Hemoccult I and II and Hemoccult SENSA) that detect the pseudoperoxidase activity of heme or hemoglobin and fecal immunochemical tests (FITs) that detect human globin.

Guaiac-based tests have undergone the most extensive testing. For optimal detection, annual testing is required. One specimen card must be prepared from three consecutive bowel movements. To reduce the likelihood of false-positive tests, patients should abstain from aspirin (in doses > 325 mg/d), NSAIDs, red meat, poultry, fish, and vegetables with peroxide activity (turnips, horseradish) for 72 hours. Vitamin C may cause a false-negative test. Slides should be developed within 7 days after preparation. The reported sensitivities of a single guaiac-based test for detection of colorectal cancer vary widely, but are lower for Hemoccult II (35%) than Hemoccult SENSA (65%). When fecal occult blood test is administered to the general population as part of a screening program, 2–6% of tests are positive. Of those with positive tests, 5–18% have colorectal cancer that is more likely to be at an earlier stage (stage I or II). Among 46,551 participants in the Minnesota Colon Cancer Control Study, annual fecal occult blood testing showed reduced colorectal cancer mortality with relative risk 0.68 (95% CI: 0.56 to 0.82).

Several FITs are commercially available. These tests are highly specific for detecting human globin and therefore eliminate the need for pretest dietary restrictions. The optimal interval (yearly or every 2 years) and number of stool samples (one or two) required for optimal FIT testing is undetermined. In clinical trials that compare FIT with guaiac-based tests, FIT had at least comparable sensitivity to Hemoccult SENSA for detection of cancers (60–85%) with higher specificity. Because FITs are not affected by diet or medications and have superior accuracy, they are increasingly being substituted for guaiac-based tests despite a higher cost per test ($10–20). Randomized controlled trials comparing one-time colonoscopy with FIT testing for colorectal cancer screening are ongoing. Preliminary results of the ColonPrev study reported higher rates of participation in patients randomized to the FIT testing (34%) versus colonoscopy (25%). Among patients who participated in screening, the proportion with advanced neoplasia (colorectal cancer or advanced adenomas) was significantly greater in the colonoscopy group (10.3%) versus the FIT group (2.7%).

The US Multi-Society Task Force emphasizes that colon cancer prevention should be the primary goal of screening. For that reason, the lower sensitivity of fecal occult blood tests for advanced neoplasia (cancer and advanced adenomatous polyps) makes them a less attractive choice for population-based screening than endoscopic or radiographic tests. Currently, fecal occult blood tests are most suitable in settings where health care resources are limited or in patients who desire a noninvasive method of screening. The Task Force recommends that tests with higher sensitivity for colorectal cancer (Hemoccult SENSA or FIT) be used rather than less sensitive tests (Hemoccult II). Regardless of which stool-based test is used, patients should understand that annual testing is required to achieve the maximum screening benefit and that a positive test will require evaluation by colonoscopy accompanied by removal of any polyps identified. If colonoscopy reveals no colorectal neoplasm, further screening for colorectal cancer can be deferred for 10 years. In a meta-analysis of four large, prospective, longitudinal studies, annual or biennial screening with Hemoccult or Hemoccult II reduced mortality from colorectal cancer by 25% among those who were compliant with regular testing. Long-term studies with more sensitive stool tests (Hemoccult SENSA or FIT) have not been performed.

2. Multitarget DNA assay—Stool DNA tests measure a variety of mutated genes and methylated gene markers from exfoliated tumor cells. The commercially available first-generation fecal DNA panel detected only one-half of cancers; however, newer generation assays (under investigation) detect > 85% of cancers and 50% of adenomas > 1 cm. Although the Multi-Society Task Force concluded that fecal DNA is an acceptable option for colorectal cancer screening, currently available tests are not yet practical for population-based screening due to high cost and cumbersome requirements for stool collection and mailing.

B. Endoscopic Examinations of the Colon

1. Flexible sigmoidoscopy—Use of a 60-cm flexible sigmoidoscope permits visualization of the rectosigmoid and descending colon. It requires no sedation and in many centers is performed by a nurse specialist or physician's assistant. Adenomatous polyps are identified in 10–20% and colorectal cancers in 1% of patients. The risk of serious complications (perforation) associated with flexible sigmoidoscopy is < 1:10,000 patients. A 2010 randomized controlled trial in 170,000 participants in the United Kingdom comparing a one-time flexible sigmoidoscopy screening to usual care confirmed a 50% reduction in distal colorectal cancer incidence and 43% reduction in mortality after a median follow-up of 11 years. Likewise, a 2012 US study of almost 155,000 participants randomized to sigmoidoscopy screening or usual care between 1993 and 2001 reported a 50% reduction in distal colorectal cancer mortality in the sigmoidoscopy group after 11 years median follow up.

The chief disadvantage of screening with flexible sigmoidoscopy is that is does not examine the proximal colon. The prevalence of proximal versus distal neoplasia is higher in people over age 65 years of age, African Americans, and women. In men, approximately 50% of advanced neoplasms (cancer, adenomas ≥ 1 cm in size, polyps with villous histology, or high-grade dysplasia) are located in the proximal colon, compared with 60–70% in women. The finding at sigmoidoscopy of an adenomatous polyp in the distal colon increases the likelihood at least twofold that an advanced neoplasm is present in the proximal colon. Therefore, patients found on screening sigmoidoscopy to have an adenomatous polyp of any size should subsequently undergo colonoscopy to evaluate the proximal colon.

2. Colonoscopy—Colonoscopy permits examination of the entire colon. In addition to detecting early cancers, colonoscopy allows removal of adenomatous polyps by biopsy or polypectomy, which is believed to reduce the risk of subsequent cancer. Over the past decade, there has been a dramatic increase in screening colonoscopy and a similar decrease in screening sigmoidoscopy due to poor reimbursement and the perceived inferiority of sigmoidoscopy compared with colonoscopy. Almost 62% of US adults have undergone colonoscopy in the past 10 years. Colonoscopy requires aggressive bowel cleansing prior to the examination. To alleviate discomfort, intravenous sedation is used for most patients. The incidence of serious complications after colonoscopy (perforation, bleeding, cardiopulmonary events) is 0.1%. In asymptomatic individuals between 50 and 75 years of age undergoing screening colonoscopy, the prevalence of advanced neoplasia is 4–11% and of cancer is 0.1–1%.

Although colonoscopy is believed to be the most sensitive test for detecting adenomas and cancer, it is not infallible. In several studies, the rate of colorectal cancer within 3 years of a screening colonoscopy was 0.7–0.9%, ie, approximately 1 in 110 patients. This may be attributable to adenomatous and serrated polyps and early cancers that were overlooked during colonoscopy. Studies of back-to-back colonoscopies confirm that endoscopists overlook 6–12% of polyps > 1 cm and up to 25% of smaller adenomas. Polyps that are small, flat, or located behind folds are easily missed, especially if the bowel preparation is poor. Population-based case-control and cohort studies suggest that colonoscopy is associated with greater reduction in colorectal cancer incidence and mortality in the distal colon than the proximal colon. This may be attributable to incomplete examination of the proximal colon, and differences between the proximal and distal colon that include worse bowel preparation, suboptimal colonoscopic technique, and a higher prevalence of serrated polyps and flat adenomas. The latter are more common than previously recognized, are more likely to contain advanced pathology, and are more difficult to identify than raised (sessile or pedunculated) polyps. To optimize diagnostic accuracy as well as patient safety and comfort, colonoscopy should be performed after optimal bowel preparation by a well-trained endoscopist who spends sufficient time (at least 7 minutes) carefully examining the colon (especially the proximal colon) while withdrawing the endoscope.

C. Radiographic Examinations of the Colon

1. CT colonography—Using helical CT with computer-assisted image reconstruction, two- and three-dimensional views can be generated of the colon lumen that simulate the view of colonoscopy (virtual colonoscopy). CT colonography requires a similar bowel cleansing regimen as colonoscopy as well as insufflation of air into the colon through a rectal tube, which may be associated with discomfort. Nonetheless, this examination is performed rapidly and requires no sedation or intravenous contrast. It has minimal acute risk although there is controversy about potential long-term risks related to radiation exposure from CT examinations. Several large studies have compared the accuracy of virtual colonoscopy with colonoscopy for colorectal screening. Using current imaging software with multidetector helical scanners, the sensitivity is > 95% for the detection of cancer and > 84–92% for the detection of polyps ≥ 10 mm in size. The sensitivity for polyps 6–9 mm in size ranges from 57% to 84%; for polyps 5 mm or less, the sensitivity is extremely poor.

Patients undergoing screening with CT colonography should be managed appropriately. If no polyps are found, the interval for repeat screening examination is uncertain; however, 5 years may be reasonable. All patients with polyps ≥ 10 mm in size should be referred for colonoscopy with polypectomy because of the high prevalence (30%) of advanced pathology (cancer, high-grade dysplasia, or villous features) within these polyps. The optimal management of patients with polyps < 10 mm in size is controversial. The US Multi-Society Task Force currently recommends that colonoscopy with polypectomy be offered to patients with one or more 6–9 mm polyps. Patients who refuse or who have increased risk of carcinoma should undergo surveillance CT colonography in 3–5 years. At the present time, there is no consensus on the management of patients with polyps < 6 mm; however, some radiologists choose not even to report these findings.

2. Barium enema—Double-contrast barium enema was previously used as a screening technique because it was widely available, relatively inexpensive, and safe. However, compared to CT colonography, it is more time-consuming and difficult to perform, less comfortable, and less accurate. Although it continues to be included among recommended screening options, it has been supplanted by CT colonography, where available.

▶ When to Refer

- Patients with symptoms (change in bowel habits, hematochezia), signs (mass on abdominal examination or digital rectal examination [DRE]), or laboratory tests (iron deficiency anemia) suggestive of colorectal neoplasia should be referred for colonoscopy.
- Patients with suspected colorectal cancer or adenomatous polyps of any size should be referred for colonoscopy.
- Virtually all patients with proven colorectal cancer should be referred to a surgeon for resection. Patients with clinical stage T3 or node-positive rectal tumors (or both) also should be referred to an oncologist preoperatively for neoadjuvant therapy. Patients with stage III or IV colorectal tumors should be referred to an oncologist.

▶ When to Admit

- Patients with complications of colorectal cancer (obstruction, acute bleeding) requiring urgent evaluation and intervention.
- Patients with severe complications of chemotherapy.
- Patients with advanced metastatic disease requiring palliative care.

Ahlquist DA et al. Next-generation stool DNA test accurately detects colorectal cancer and large adenomas. Gastroenterology. 2012 Feb;142(2):248–56. [PMID: 22062357]

André T et al. Improved overall survival with oxaliplatin, fluorouracil, and leucovorin as adjuvant treatment in stage II or III colon cancer in the MOSAIC trial. N Engl J Med. 2009 Jul 1;27(19):3109–16. [PMID: 19451431]

Bennouna J et al; ML18147 Study Investigators. Continuation of bevacizumab after first progression in metastatic colorectal cancer (ML18147): a randomised phase 3 trial. Lancet Oncol. 2013 Jan;14(1):29–37. [PMID: 23168366]

Bokemeyer C et al. Addition of cetuximab to chemotherapy as first-line treatment for KRAS wild-type metastatic colorectal cancer: pooled analysis of the CRYSTAL and OPUS randomised clinical trials. Eur J Cancer. 2012 Jul;48(10):1466–75. [PMID: 22446022]

Brenner H et al. Protection from colorectal cancer after colonoscopy: a population-based, case-control study. Ann Intern Med. 2011 Jan 4;154(1):22–30. [PMID: 21200035]

Day LW et al. Colorectal cancer screening and surveillance in the elderly patient. Am J Gastroenterol. 2011 Jul;106(7):1197–206. [PMID: 21519362]

Douillard JY et al. Randomized, phase III trial of panitumumab with infusional fluorouracil, leucovorin, and oxaliplatin (FOLFOX4) versus FOLFOX4 alone as first-line treatment in patients with previously untreated metastatic colorectal cancer: the PRIME study. J Clin Oncol. 2010 Nov 1;28(31):4697–705. [PMID: 20921465]

Grothey A et al; CORRECT Study Group. Regorafenib monotherapy for previously treated metastatic colorectal cancer (CORRECT): an international, multicentre, randomised, placebo-controlled, phase 3 trial. Lancet. 2013 Jan 26; 381(9863):303–12. [PMID: 23177514]

Je Y et al. Association between physical activity and mortality in colorectal cancer: a meta-analysis of prospective cohort studies. Int J Cancer. 2013 Oct 15;133(8):1905–13. [PMID: 23580314]

Kahi CJ et al. Screening and surveillance for colorectal cancer: state of the art. Gastrointest Endosc. 2013 Mar;77(3):335–50. [PMID: 23410695]

Lieberman DA. Clinical Practice. Screening for colorectal cancer. N Engl J Med. 2009 Sep 17;361(12):1179–87. [PMID: 19759380]

Limketkai BN et al. The cutting edge of serrated polyps: a practical guide to approaching and managing serrated colon polyps. Gastrointest Endosc. 2013 Mar;77(3):360–75. [PMID: 23410696]

Nishihara R et al. Long-term colorectal-cancer incidence and mortality after lower endoscopy. N Engl J Med. 2013 Sep 19; 369(12):1095–105. [PMID: 24047059]

Quintero E et al; COLONPREV Study Investigators. Colonoscopy versus fecal immunochemical testing in colorectal-cancer screening. N Engl J Med. 2012 Feb 23;366(8):697–706. [PMID: 22356323]

Rex D et al. American College of Gastroenterology Guidelines for colorectal cancer screening 2009. Am J Gastroenterol. 2009 Mar;104(3):739–50. [PMID: 19240699]

Sauer R et al. Preoperative versus postoperative chemoradiotherapy for locally advanced rectal cancer: results of the German CAO/ARO/AIO-94 randomized phase III trial after a median follow-up of 11 years. J Clin Oncol. 2012 Jun 1;30(16):1926–33. [PMID: 22529255]

Schoen RE et al; PLCO Project Team. Colorectal-cancer incidence and mortality with screening flexible sigmoidoscopy. N Engl J Med. 2012 Jun 21;366(25):2345–57. [PMID: 22612596]

Shaukat A et al. Long-term mortality after screening for colorectal cancer. N Engl J Med. 2013 Sept 19;369(12):1106–14. [PMID: 24047060]

Siegel R et al. Cancer statistics, 2012. CA Cancer J Clin. 2012 Jan–Feb;62(1):10–29. [PMID: 22237781]

Van Cutsem E et al. Addition of aflibercept to fluorouracil, leucovorin, and irinotecan improves survival in a phase III randomized trial in patients with metastatic colorectal cancer previously treated with an oxaliplatin-based regimen. J Clin Oncol. 2012 Oct 1;30(28):3499–506. [PMID: 22949147]

CARCINOMA OF THE ANUS

The anal canal is lined from its proximal to distal extent by columnar, transitional and non-keratinized squamous epithelium, which merges at the anal verge with the keratinized perianal skin. Tumors arising from the mucosa of the anal canal are relatively rare, comprising only 1–2% of all cancers of the anus and large intestine. Squamous cancers make up the majority of anal cancers. Anal cancer is increased among people practicing receptive anal intercourse and those with a history of anorectal warts. In over 80% of cases, HPV may be detected, suggesting that this virus is a major causal factor. In a large controlled trial, HPV vaccination of healthy men (16- to 26-years-old) who have sex with men decreased the incidence of anal intraepithelial neoplasia by 50%. Women with anal cancer are at increased risk for cervical cancer, which may be due to a field effect of oncogenic HPV infection, and require gynecologic screening and surveillance. Anal cancer is increased

in HIV-infected individuals, possibly due to interaction with HPV. Bleeding, pain, and local tumor are the most common symptoms. The lesion is often confused with hemorrhoids or other common anal disorders. These tumors tend to become annular, invade the sphincter, and spread upward via the lymphatics into the perirectal mesenteric lymphatic nodes. CT or MRI scans of the abdomen and pelvis are required to identify regional lymphadenopathy or metastatic disease at diagnosis. PET imaging may be used in conjunction.

Treatment depends on the tumor location and histologic stage. Small (< 3 cm) superficial lesions of the perianal skin may be treated with wide local excision. Adenocarcinoma of the anal canal is treated in similar fashion to rectal cancer (see above), commonly by abdominoperineal resection with neoadjuvant chemoradiotherapy and adjuvant chemotherapy. Squamous cancer of the anal canal and large perianal tumors invading the sphincter or rectum are treated with combined-modality therapy that includes external radiation with simultaneous chemotherapy (5-fluorouracil plus mitomycin). Local control is achieved in approximately 80% of patients. Radical surgery (abdominoperineal resection) is reserved for patients who fail chemotherapy and radiation therapy. Metastatic disease is generally treated with 5-fluorouracil in combination with cisplatin. The 5-year survival rate is 60–70% for localized tumors and over 25% for metastatic (stage IV) disease.

Eng C et al. Long-term results of weekly/daily cisplatin-based chemoradiation for locally advanced squamous cell carcinoma of the anal canal. Cancer. 2013 Nov 1;119(21):3769–75. [PMID: 24037775]

Glynne-Jones R et al. Anal cancer: ESMO Clinical Practice Guidelines for diagnosis, treatment and follow-up. Ann Oncol. 2010 May;21(Suppl 5):v87–92. [PMID: 20555110]

Lim F et al. Chemotherapy/chemoradiation in anal cancer: a systematic review. Cancer Treat Rev. 2011 Nov;37(7):520–32. [PMID: 21450408]

National Cancer Institute. Anal Cancer Treatment (PDQ). http://www.cancer.gov/cancertopics/pdq/treatment/anal/HealthProfessional

Palefsky JM et al. HPV vaccine against anal HPV infection and anal intraepithelial neoplasia. N Engl J Med. 2011 Oct 27;365(17):1576–85. [PMID: 22029979]

Shia J. An update on tumors of the anal canal. Arch Pathol Lab Med. 2010 Nov;134(11):1601–11. [PMID: 21043813]

CANCERS OF THE GENITOURINARY TRACT

Maxwell V. Meng, MD, FACS

PROSTATE CANCER

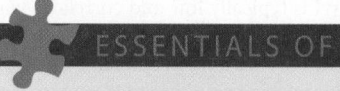

ESSENTIALS OF DIAGNOSIS

▶ Prostatic induration on DRE or elevation of PSA.

▶ Most often asymptomatic.

▶ Rarely: systemic symptoms (weight loss, bone pain).

General Considerations

Prostatic cancer is the most common noncutaneous cancer detected in American men and the second leading cause of cancer-related death. In the United States, in 2012 an estimated 238,590 new cases of prostate cancer were diagnosed, and 29,720 deaths resulted. However, the clinical incidence of the disease does not match the prevalence noted at autopsy, where more than 40% of men over 50 years of age are found to have prostatic carcinoma. Most such occult cancers are small and contained within the prostate gland; few are associated with regional or distant disease. The incidence of prostatic cancer increases with age. Whereas 30% of men aged 60–69 years will have the disease, autopsy incidence increases to 67% in men aged 80–89 years. Although the global prevalence of prostatic cancer at autopsy is relatively consistent, the clinical incidence varies considerably (high in North America and European countries, intermediate in South America, and low in the Far East), suggesting that environmental or dietary differences among populations may be important for prostatic cancer growth. A 50-year-old American man has a lifetime risk of 40% for latent cancer, 16% for developing clinically apparent cancer, and a 2.9% risk of death due to prostatic cancer. Blacks, men with a family history of prostatic cancer, and those with a history of high dietary fat intake are at increased risk for developing prostate cancer.

Clinical Findings

A. Symptoms and Signs

Prostate cancer may manifest as focal nodules or areas of induration within the prostate at the time of DRE. However, currently most prostate cancers are associated with palpably normal prostates and are detected solely on the basis of elevations in serum PSA.

Patients rarely present with signs of urinary retention or neurologic symptoms as a result of epidural metastases and cord compression. Obstructive voiding symptoms are most often due to benign prostatic hyperplasia, which occurs in the same age group. Nevertheless, large or locally extensive prostatic cancers can cause obstructive voiding symptoms while lymph node metastases can lead to lower extremity lymphedema. As the axial skeleton is the most common site of metastases, patients may present with back pain or pathologic fractures.

B. Laboratory Findings

1. Serum tumor markers—PSA is a glycoprotein produced only by cells, either benign or malignant, of the prostate gland. The serum level is typically low and correlates with the volume of both benign and malignant prostate tissue. Measurement of serum PSA is useful in detecting and staging prostate cancer, monitoring response to treatment, and detecting recurrence before it becomes clinically evident. As a screening test, PSA will be elevated in 10–15% of men. Approximately 18–30% of men with intermediate degrees of elevation (4.1–10 ng/mL [4.1–10 mcg/L]) will be found

to have prostate cancer. Between 50% and 70% of those with elevations >10 ng/mL (10 mcg/L) will have prostate cancer. Patients with intermediate levels of PSA usually have localized and therefore potentially curable cancers. It should be remembered that approximately 20% of patients who undergo radical prostatectomy for localized prostate cancer have normal levels of PSA.

In untreated patients with prostate cancer, the level of PSA correlates with the volume and stage of the disease. Whereas most organ-confined cancers are associated with PSA levels <10 ng/mL (10 mcg/L), advanced disease (seminal vesicle invasion, lymph node involvement, or occult distant metastases) is more common in patients with PSA levels in excess of 40 ng/mL (40 mcg/L). Approximately 98% of patients with metastatic prostate cancer will have elevated PSA. However, there are rare cancers that are localized despite substantial elevations in PSA. Therefore, initial treatment decisions cannot be made on the basis of PSA testing alone. A rising PSA after therapy is usually consistent with progressive disease, either locally recurrent or metastatic.

2. Miscellaneous laboratory testing—Patients in urinary retention or those with ureteral obstruction due to locoregionally advanced prostate cancers may present with elevations in blood urea nitrogen or creatinine. Patients with bony metastases may have elevations in alkaline phosphatase or hypercalcemia. Laboratory and clinical evidence of disseminated intravascular coagulation can occur in patients with advanced prostate cancers.

3. Prostate biopsy—Transrectal ultrasound-guided biopsy is the standard method for detection of prostate cancer. The use of a spring-loaded, 18-gauge biopsy needle has allowed transrectal biopsy to be performed with minimal patient discomfort and morbidity. Local anesthesia is routinely used and increases the tolerability of the procedure. The specimen preserves glandular architecture and permits accurate grading. Prostate biopsy specimens are taken from the apex, mid-portion, and base in men who have an abnormal DRE or an elevated serum PSA, or both. Extended-pattern biopsies, including a total of at least ten biopsies, are associated with improved cancer detection and risk stratification of patients with newly diagnosed disease. Patients with abnormalities of the seminal vesicles can have these structures specifically biopsied to identify local tumor invasion.

C. Imaging

Transrectal ultrasonography has primarily been used for the staging of prostate carcinomas, where tumors typically appear as hypoechoic areas. In addition, transrectal ultrasound-guided, rather than digitally-guided, biopsy of the prostate is a more accurate way to evaluate suspicious lesions. Use of imaging should be tailored to the likelihood of advanced disease in newly diagnosed cases. Asymptomatic patients with well-differentiated to moderately differentiated cancers, thought to be localized to the prostate on DRE and transurethral ultrasound and associated with modest elevations of PSA (ie, < 10 ng/mL [10 mcg/L]), need no further imaging.

MRI allows for evaluation of the prostate as well as regional lymph nodes. The positive predictive value for detection of both capsular penetration and seminal vesicle invasion is similar for transrectal ultrasound and MRI. MRI-guided biopsy may improve not only overall cancer detection but discovery of clinically relevant disease. CT plays little role because of its inability to accurately identify or stage prostate cancers, but it can be used to detect regional lymphatic metastases and intra-abdominal metastases.

Radionuclide bone scan is superior to conventional plain skeletal radiographs in detecting bony metastases. Most prostate cancer metastases are multiple and most commonly localized to the axial skeleton. Men with more advanced local lesions, symptoms of metastases (eg, bone pain), high-grade disease, or elevations in PSA > 20 ng/mL (20 mcg/L) should undergo radionuclide bone scan. Because of the high frequency of abnormal scans in patients in this age group resulting from degenerative joint disease, plain films are often necessary in evaluating patients with indeterminate findings on bone scan. Cross-sectional imaging either by CT or MRI is usually indicated only in those patients in the latter group who have negative bone scans in an attempt to detect lymph node metastases. Patients found to have enlarged pelvic lymph nodes are candidates for FNA.

Intravenous urography and cystoscopy are not routinely needed to evaluate patients with prostate cancer.

Despite application of modern, sophisticated techniques, understaging of prostate cancer occurs in at least 20% of patients.

► Screening for Prostate Cancer

Whether screening for prostate cancer results in a decrease in mortality rates due to the disease is the subject of much debate. The screening tests currently available include DRE, PSA testing, and transrectal ultrasound. Depending on the patient population being evaluated, detection rates using DRE alone vary from 1.5% to 7%. Unfortunately, most cancers detected in this manner are advanced (stage T3 or greater). Transrectal ultrasound should not be used as a first-line screening tool because of its expense, low specificity (and therefore high biopsy rate), and minimal improvement in detection rate when compared with the combined use of DRE and PSA testing.

PSA testing increases the detection rate of prostate cancers compared with DRE. Approximately 2–2.5% of men older than 50 years of age will be found to have prostate cancer using PSA testing compared with a rate of approximately 1.5% using DRE alone. PSA is not specific for cancer, and there is considerable overlap of values with men with benign prostate hyperplasia. The sensitivity, specificity, and positive predictive value of PSA and DRE are listed in Table 39–7. PSA-detected cancers are more likely to be localized compared with those detected by DRE alone. The Prostate Cancer Prevention Trial provided data demonstrating a significant risk of prostate cancer even in men with PSA < 4.0 ng/mL (4.0 mcg/L) (Table 39–8) and a web-based calculator has been developed to estimate the risk of harboring both cancer and high-grade prostate cancer (http://deb.uthscsa.edu/URORiskCalc/Pages/uroriskcalc.jsp).

To improve the performance of PSA as a screening test, several investigators have developed alternative methods for its use. These include establishment of age- and race-specific reference ranges, measurement of free serum and protein-bound levels of PSA (percent free PSA), and calculation of changes in PSA over time (PSA velocity). Generally, men with PSA free fractions exceeding 25% are unlikely to have prostate cancer, whereas those with free fractions < 10% have an approximately 50% chance of having prostate cancer. The frequency of PSA testing also remains a matter of debate. The traditional yearly screening approach may not be the most efficient; rather, earlier PSA testing at younger age may allow less frequent testing as well as provide information regarding PSA velocity. Studies from the Baltimore Longitudinal Study of Aging suggest that men with PSA above the age-based median

Table 39–7. Screening for prostatic cancer: Test performance.

Test	Sensitivity	Specificity	Positive Predictive Value
Abnormal PSA (> 4 ng/ mL or mcg/L)	0.67	0.97	0.43
Abnormal DRE	0.50	0.94	0.24
Abnormal PSA or DRE	0.84	0.92	0.28
Abnormal PSA and DRE	0.34	0.995	0.49

DRE, digital rectal examination; PSA, prostate-specific antigen.
Modified, with permission, from Kramer BS et al. Prostate cancer screening: what we know and what we need to know. Ann Intern Med. 1993 Nov 1;119(9):914–23.

Table 39–8. Risk of prostate cancer in men with PSA ≤ 4.0 ng/mL (or mcg/L).

PSA level (ng/mL [or mcg/L])	Percentage with prostate cancer	Percentage with high-grade prostate cancer
≤ 0.5	6.6	12.5
0.6–1.0	10.1	10.0
1.1–2.0	17.0	11.8
2.1–3.0	23.9	19.1
3.1–4.0	26.9	25.0

Data from Thompson IM et al. Prevalence of prostate cancer among men with a prostate-specific antigen level ≤ 4.0 ng per milliliter. N Engl J Med. 2004 May 27;350(22):2239–46.
High-grade cancer was defined as Gleason score ≥ 7.

when tested between 40 and 60 years are at significantly increased risk for subsequent cancer detection over 25 years. Therefore, men with lower PSA (0.6 ng/mL [0.6 mcg/L] ages 40–50 and 0.71 ng/mL [0.71 mcg/L] ages 50–60) may require less frequent PSA tests. In addition, men with PSA velocity greater than 0.35 ng/mL (0.35 mcg/L) per year measured 10–15 years before diagnosis had significantly worse cancer-specific survival compared with those with lower PSA velocity. The current NCCN guidelines (http://www.nccn.org/professionals/physician_gls/f_guidelines.asp) for prostate cancer early detection incorporate many of these factors (Figure 39–2).

Two large, randomized trials question the benefit of screening men for prostate cancer. In the US Prostate, Lung, Colorectal, and Ovarian (PLCO) Cancer Screening Trial, no mortality benefit was observed after combined

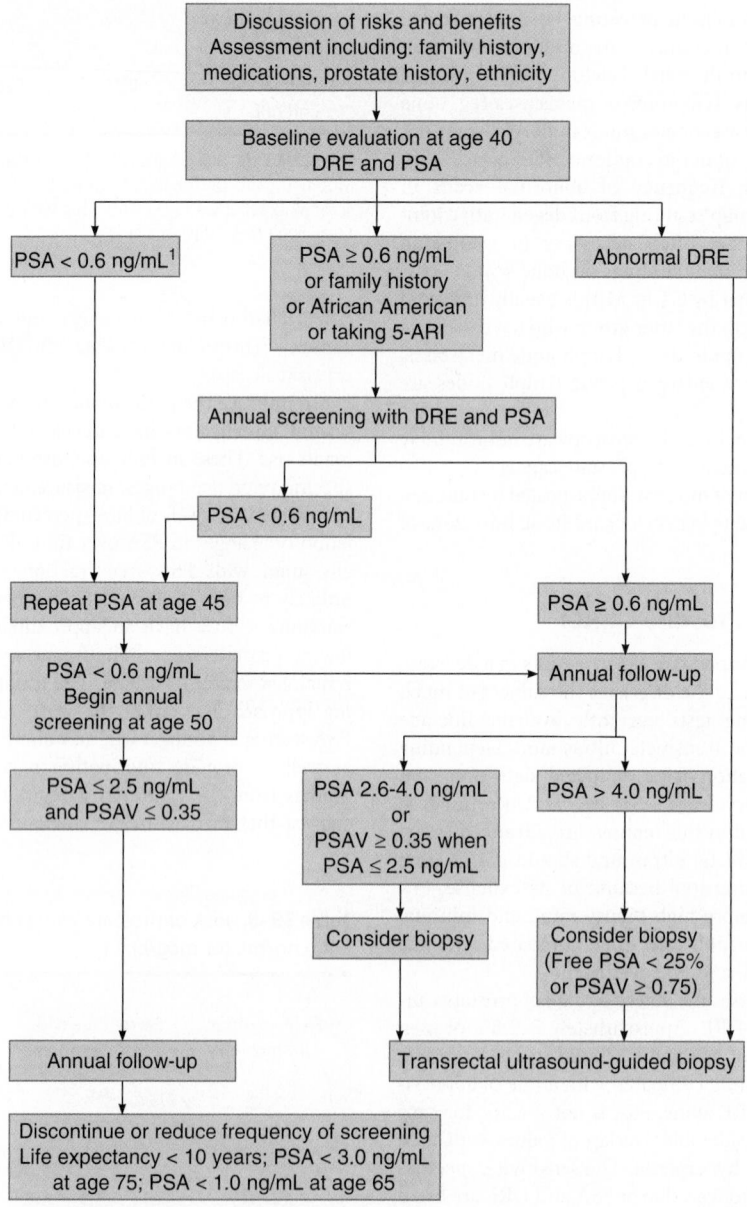

▲ **Figure 39–2.** An algorithm for prostate cancer early detection. DRE, digital rectal examination; 5-ARI, 5-alpha-reductase inhibitor; PSAV, PSA velocity (ng/mL/year) calculated on at least three consecutive values over at least an 18–24 month period. (Based on NCCN guidelines, data from the Baltimore Longitudinal Study on Aging, and Prostate Cancer Prevention Trial.)

screening with PSA testing and digital rectal examination during follow-up of 13 years. Although screening resulted in a 12% increase in prostate cancer detection, the cancer-specific mortality rate was similar in the screening and control arms (3.7 and 3.4 deaths per 10,000 person-years, respectively). Similarly, in the European Randomized Study of Screening for Prostate Cancer (ERSPC) trial, the benefit of PSA screening was minimal with a 21% relative reduction in death rate from prostate cancer at follow-up of 11 years, with an absolute reduction of 10.7 prostate cancer deaths per 10,000 men screened. A subset of these patients from Göteborg, Sweden, in an independently designed and initiated population-based screening trial, was analyzed separately. During a median follow-up of 14 years, the absolute risk reduction of death from prostate cancer in the screening group was 40% and the relative risk of prostate-cancer death in the attendees of screening was 0.44. Based on these data, the US Preventive Services Task Force recommended against PSA-based screening for prostate cancer in asymptomatic men (grade D recommendation). Criticisms of the negative PLCO study include use of a relatively high PSA threshold (4.0 ng/mL [4.0 mcg/L]), significant screening of men in the 3 years prior to enrolling in the trial (44%), and significant number of men in the control arm undergoing screening during the trial (> 50%).

Staging

The majority of prostate cancers are adenocarcinomas. Most arise in the periphery of the prostate (peripheral zone), though a small percentage arise in the central (5–10%) and transition zones (20%) of the gland. Pathologists utilize the Gleason grading system whereby a "primary" grade is applied to the architectural pattern of malignant glands occupying the largest area of the specimen and a "secondary" pattern is assigned to the next largest area of cancer. Grading is based on architectural rather than histologic criteria, and five "grades" are possible (Figure 39–3). Adding the score of the primary and secondary patterns (grades) gives a Gleason score. Grade correlates with tumor volume, pathologic stage, and prognosis (Figure 39–4).

Treatment

A. Localized Disease

The optimal treatment for patients with clinically localized prostate cancers remains controversial. Patients need to be advised of all treatment options, including active surveillance, with the specific benefits, risks, and limitations. Currently, treatment decisions are made based on tumor grade and stage as well as the age and health of the patient. Although selected patients may be candidates for surveillance based on age or health and evidence of small-volume or well-differentiated cancers, most men with an anticipated life expectancy in excess of 10 years should be considered for treatment. Newly introduced genomic tests may provide novel information to help guide treatment decisions. Both radiation therapy and radical prostatectomy result in acceptable levels of local control. A large,

prospective, randomized trial compared surveillance with radical prostatectomy in 695 men with clinically localized and well-differentiated to moderately differentiated tumors for a median of 12.8 years. Radical prostatectomy significantly reduced disease-specific mortality, overall mortality, and risks of metastasis and local progression. The relative reduction in the risk of death at 15 years was 0.62 in the prostatectomy group, with the number needed to treat to avert one death of 15; the benefit was confined to men younger than 65 years of age. This trial accrued patients in Sweden between 1989 and 1999, thus likely including patients with greater cancer burden compared with that in patients currently diagnosed using PSA screening. Nevertheless, the survival benefit in the trials was still observed in men with low-risk prostate cancer.

B. Radical Prostatectomy

During radical prostatectomy, the seminal vesicles, prostate, and ampullae of the vas deferens are removed. Refinements in technique have allowed preservation of urinary continence in most patients and erectile function in selected patients. Radical prostatectomy can be performed via open retropubic, transperineal, or laparoscopic (with or without robotic assistance) surgery. Local recurrence is uncommon after radical prostatectomy, and the incidence is related to pathologic stage. Organ-confined cancers rarely recur; however, cancers with adverse pathologic features (capsular penetration, seminal vesicle invasion) are associated with higher local (10–25%) and distant (20–50%) relapse rates.

Ideal candidates for prostatectomy include healthy patients with stages T1 and T2 prostate cancers. Patients with advanced local tumors (T4) or lymph node metastases are rarely candidates for prostatectomy alone, although surgery is sometimes used in combination with hormonal therapy and postoperative radiation therapy for select high-risk patients.

Patients with advanced pathologic stage or positive surgical margins are at an increased risk for local and distant tumor relapse. Such patients are candidates for adjuvant therapy (radiation for positive margins or androgen deprivation for lymph node metastases). Two randomized clinical trials (EORTC 22911 and SWOG 8794) have demonstrated improved progression-free and metastasis-free survival with early radiotherapy in these men, and subsequent analysis of SWOG 8794 showed improved overall survival in men receiving adjuvant radiation therapy. Evidence suggests that salvage radiotherapy after radical prostatectomy, within 2 years of PSA relapse, increases prostate cancer-specific survival in men with shorter PSA doubling time (< 6 months).

C. Radiation Therapy

Radiation can be delivered by a variety of techniques including use of external beam radiotherapy and transperineal implantation of radioisotopes. Morbidity is limited, and the survival of patients with localized cancers (T1, T2, and selected T3) approaches 65% at 10 years. As with surgery, the likelihood of local failure correlates with

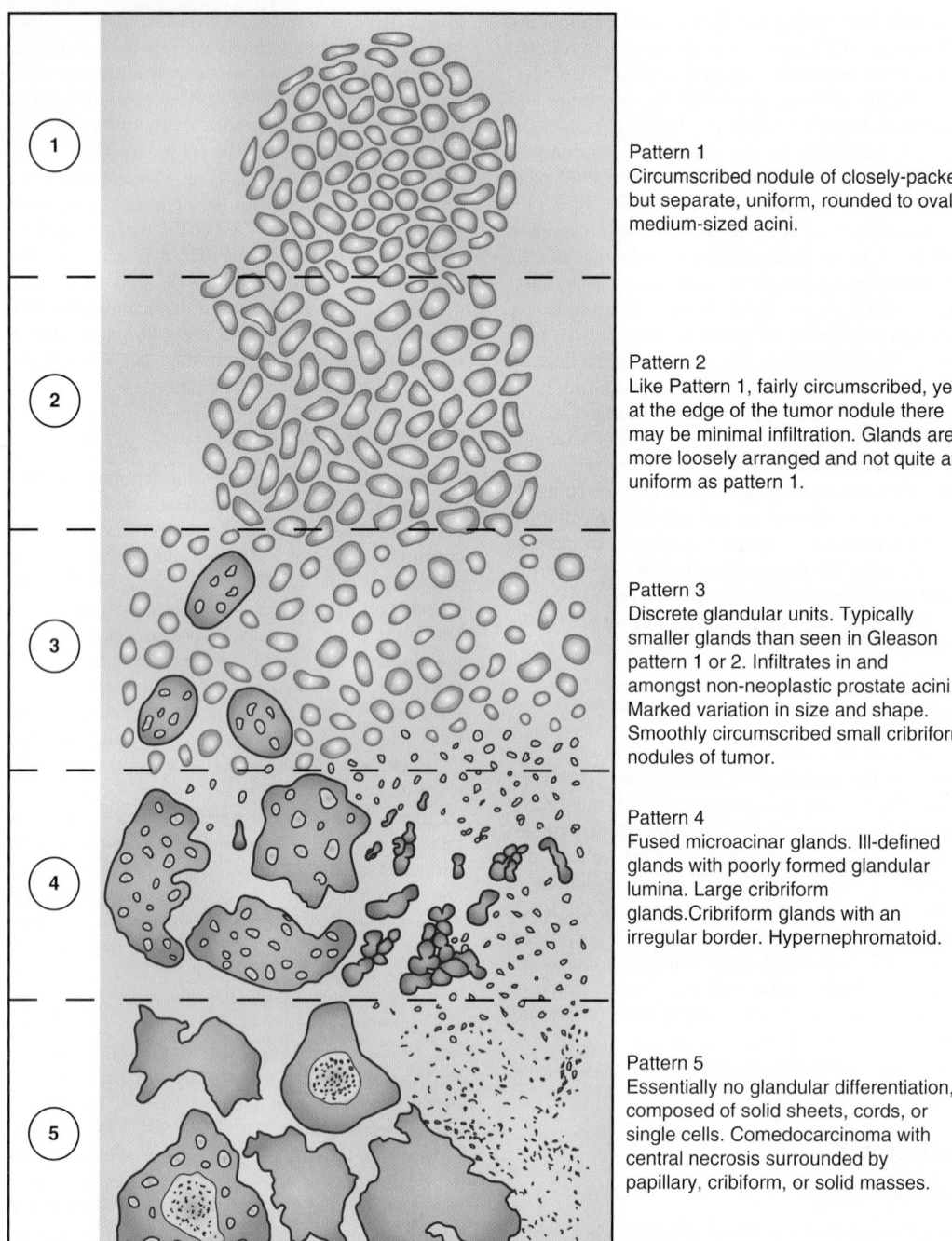

Pattern 1
Circumscribed nodule of closely-packed but separate, uniform, rounded to oval, medium-sized acini.

Pattern 2
Like Pattern 1, fairly circumscribed, yet at the edge of the tumor nodule there may be minimal infiltration. Glands are more loosely arranged and not quite as uniform as pattern 1.

Pattern 3
Discrete glandular units. Typically smaller glands than seen in Gleason pattern 1 or 2. Infiltrates in and amongst non-neoplastic prostate acini. Marked variation in size and shape. Smoothly circumscribed small cribriform nodules of tumor.

Pattern 4
Fused microacinar glands. Ill-defined glands with poorly formed glandular lumina. Large cribriform glands. Cribriform glands with an irregular border. Hypernephromatoid.

Pattern 5
Essentially no glandular differentiation, composed of solid sheets, cords, or single cells. Comedocarcinoma with central necrosis surrounded by papillary, cribriform, or solid masses.

▲ **Figure 39–3.** Patterns of prostate cancer according to the 2005 International Society of Urological Pathology modified Gleason system. (Adapted with permission from Epstein JI et al. The 2005 International Society of Urological Pathology (ISUP) Consensus Conference on Gleason Grading of Prostatic Carcinoma. Am J Surg Pathol. 2005;29(9):1228–42.)

technique and tumor characteristics. The likelihood of a positive prostate biopsy more than 18 months after radiation varies between 20% and 60%. Patients with local recurrence are at an increased risk of cancer progression and cancer death compared with those who have negative biopsies. Ambiguous target definitions, inadequate radiation doses, and understaging of the tumor may be responsible for the failure noted in some series. Newer techniques of radiation (implantation, conformal therapy using three-dimensional reconstruction of CT-based tumor volumes, heavy particle, charged particle, and heavy charged particle) may improve local control rates. Three-dimensional

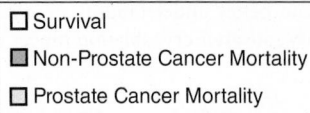

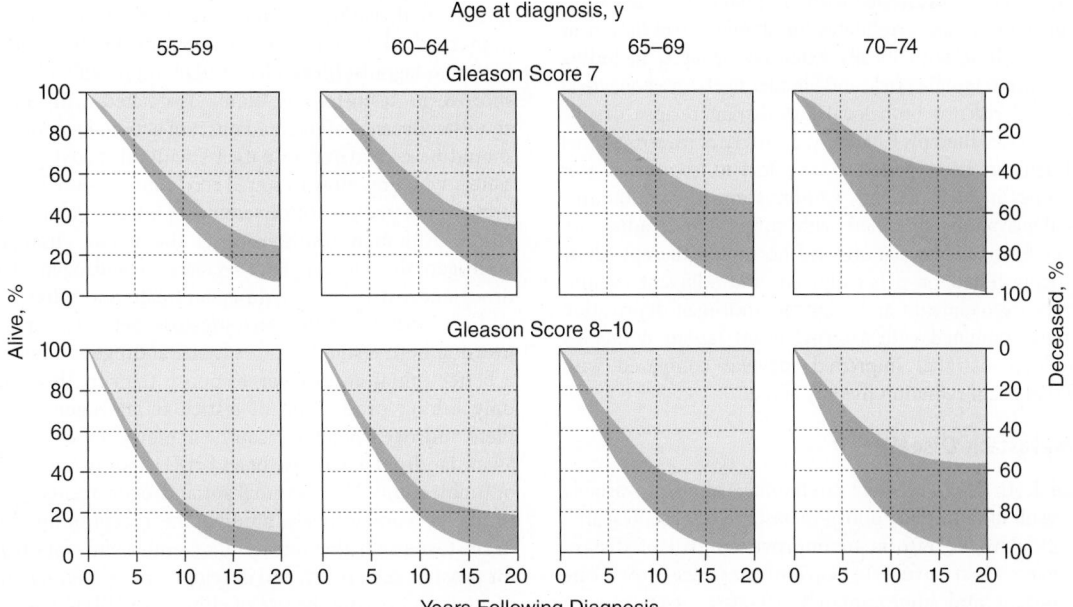

▲ **Figure 39–4.** Prostate cancer mortality as a factor of Gleason grade and age at diagnosis in men managed conservatively. (Adapted, with permission, from Albertsen PC et al. 20-year outcomes following conservative management of clinically localized prostate cancer. JAMA. 2005 May 4;293(17):2095–101.)

conformal radiation delivers a higher dose because of improved targeting and appears to be associated with greater efficacy as well as lower likelihood of adverse side effects compared with previous techniques. As a result of improvements in imaging, most notably transrectal ultrasound, there has been a resurgence of interest in brachytherapy—the implantation of permanent or temporary radioactive sources (palladium, iodine, or iridium) into the prostate. Brachytherapy can be combined with external beam radiation in patients with higher-grade or higher-volume disease or as monotherapy in those with low-grade or low-volume malignancies. The PSA may rise after brachytherapy because of prostate inflammation and necrosis. This transient elevation (PSA bounce) should not be mistaken for recurrence and may occur up to 20 months after treatment.

D. Surveillance

A beneficial impact of treating localized prostate cancer with respect to survival has not been conclusively demonstrated. Therefore, surveillance alone may be an appropriate form of management for selected patients with prostate cancer. Patients included in observational series are typically older with small volume, well-differentiated cancers. Many men with prostate cancer may be candidates for surveillance due to the significant migration to lower stage as well as lower grade, resulting from screening for prostate cancer using PSA testing. Depending on the age and health of the patient, some of these very low-volume, low-grade cancers may never become clinically relevant and can be monitored with serial PSA levels, rectal examinations, and periodic prostate biopsies to assess grade and extent of tumor. The goal of surveillance is to avoid treatment in men who never experience disease progression while recognizing and effectively treating men with evidence of progression. End points for intervention in patients on surveillance, particularly PSA changes, have not been clearly defined and surveillance regimens remain an active area of research; nonetheless, they are increasingly accepted by patients and clinicians.

E. Cryosurgery

Cryosurgery is a technique whereby liquid nitrogen is circulated through small hollow-core needles inserted into the prostate under ultrasound guidance. The freezing process results in tissue destruction. There has been a resurgence of interest in less invasive forms of therapy for localized prostate cancer as well as several modern technical innovations, including improved percutaneous techniques, expertise in transrectal ultrasound, improved cryotechnology, and better understanding of cryobiology. The positive biopsy rate after cryoablation ranges between 7% and 23%.

F. Locally and Regionally Advanced Disease

Prostate cancers associated with minimal degrees of capsular penetration are candidates for standard irradiation or surgery. Those with locally extensive cancers, including those with seminal vesicle and bladder neck invasion, are at increased risk for both local and distant relapse despite conventional therapy. Currently, a variety of investigational regimens are being tested in an effort to improve cancer outcomes in such patients. Combination therapy (androgen deprivation combined with surgery or irradiation), newer forms of irradiation, and hormonal therapy alone are being tested, as is neoadjuvant and adjuvant chemotherapy. Neoadjuvant and adjuvant androgen deprivation therapy combined with external beam radiation therapy have demonstrated improved survival compared with external beam radiation therapy alone.

G. Metastatic Disease

Since death due to prostate carcinoma is almost invariably the result of failure to control metastatic disease, research has emphasized efforts to improve control of distant disease. Most prostate carcinomas are hormone dependent and approximately 70–80% of men with metastatic prostate carcinoma will respond to various forms of androgen deprivation. Androgen deprivation may be affected at several levels along the pituitary–gonadal axis using a variety of methods or agents (Table 39–9). Use of luteinizing hormone-releasing hormone (LHRH) agonists (leuprolide, goserelin) achieves androgen deprivation without orchiectomy or administration of diethylstilbestrol and is currently the most common method of reducing testosterone levels. A single LHRH antagonist (degarelix) is FDA approved and has no short-term testosterone "flare" associated with LHRH agonists. Because of its rapid onset of action, ketoconazole should be considered in patients with advanced prostate cancer who present with spinal cord compression, bilateral ureteral obstruction, or disseminated intravascular coagulation. Although testosterone is the major circulating androgen, the adrenal gland secretes the androgens dehydroepiandrosterone, dehydroepiandrosterone sulfate, and androstenedione. Some investigators believe that suppressing both testicular and adrenal androgens allows for a better initial and longer response than methods that only inhibit production of testicular androgens. Complete androgen blockade can be achieved by combining an antiandrogen with use of an LHRH agonist/antagonist or orchiectomy. Nonsteroidal antiandrogen agents appear to act by competitively binding the receptor for dihydrotestosterone, the intracellular androgen responsible for prostate cell growth and development. A meta-analysis of trials comparing the use of either an LHRH agonist or orchiectomy alone with the use of either in combination

Table 39–9. Androgen deprivation for prostatic cancer.

Level	Agent	Dose	Sequelae
Pituitary, hypothalamus	Diethylstilbestrol	1–3 mg orally daily	Gynecomastia, hot flushes, thromboembolic disease, erectile dysfunction
	LHRH agonists Leuprolide Goserelin Triptorelin Histrelin	Monthly to annual depot injection Subcutaneous implant	Erectile dysfunction, hot flushes, gynecomastia, rarely anemia
	LHRH antagonist Degarelix	240 mg subcutaneously initial dose, then 80 mg subcutaneously monthly	Hot flushes, weight gain, erectile dysfunction, increased liver function tests
Adrenal	Ketoconazole	400 mg three times orally daily	Adrenal insufficiency, nausea, rash, ataxia
	Aminoglutethimide	250 mg four times orally daily	Adrenal insufficiency, nausea, rash, ataxia
	Corticosteroids Prednisone	20–40 mg orally daily	Gastrointestinal bleeding, fluid retention
	CYP17a1 inhibitor Abiraterone	500 mg orally daily	Weight gain, fluid retention, hypokalemia, hypertension
Testis	Orchiectomy		Gynecomastia, hot flushes, erectile dysfunction
Prostate cell	**Antiandrogens** Flutamide Bicalutamide Enzalutamide	250 mg three times orally daily 50 mg orally daily 160 mg orally daily	No erectile dysfunction when used alone; nausea, diarrhea Seizures, dizziness, asthenia

LHRH, luteinizing-hormone-releasing hormone.

with an antiandrogen agent shows little benefit of combination therapy. However, patients at risk for disease-related symptoms (bone pain, obstructive voiding symptoms) due to the initial elevation of serum testosterone that accompanies the use of an LHRH agonist should receive antiandrogens initially. Bisphosphonates can prevent osteoporosis associated with androgen deprivation, decrease bone pain from metastases, and reduce skeletal-related events. Denosumab, a RANK ligand inhibitor, is approved for the prevention of skeletal-related events in patients with bone metastases from prostate cancer and also appears to delay the development of these metastases.

Docetaxel is the first cytotoxic chemotherapy agent to improve survival in patients with hormone-refractory prostate cancer. Current research is underway combining docetaxel with androgen deprivation therapy, radiation therapy, and surgery to determine whether combinations are effective in patients with high-risk prostate cancer. Immune therapies are also under investigation and have shown promise for patients with advanced prostate cancer. Sipuleucel-T, an autologous cellular immunotherapy, is FDA approved in asymptomatic or minimally symptomatic men with metastatic hormone-refractory prostate cancer. Other agents—cabazitaxel, abiraterone, and enzalutamide—are also approved for advanced prostate cancer after clinical trials have demonstrated improvements in survival in men having received prior docetaxel. Radium-223 dichloride was approved in 2013 for the treatment of men with castration-resistant, symptomatic bone metastases, with significant improvements in both overall survival and time to skeletal-related events (eg, fractures).

Prognosis

The likelihood of success of surveillance or treatment can be predicted using risk assessment tools that usually combine stage, grade, PSA level, and number and extent of positive prostate biopsies. Several tools are available on the Internet (eg, http://mskcc.org/cancer-care/prediction-tools). One of the most widely used is the Kattan nomogram; it incorporates tumor stage, grade, and PSA level to predict the likelihood that a patient will be disease-free after radical prostatectomy or radiation therapy.

The University of California San Francisco CAPRA nomogram uses serum PSA, Gleason grade, clinical stage, percent positive biopsies, and patient age in a point system to risk stratify and predict the likelihood of PSA recurrence 3 and 5 years after radical prostatectomy (Tables 39–10 and 39–11) as well as metastasis, prostate cancer-specific, and overall survival. The CAPRA nomogram has been validated on large multicenter and international radical prostatectomy cohorts.

The patterns of prostate cancer progression have been well defined. Small and well-differentiated cancers (Gleason grades 1 and 2) are usually confined within the prostate, whereas large-volume (> 4 mL) or poorly differentiated (Gleason grades 4 and 5) cancers are more often locally extensive or metastatic to regional lymph nodes or bone. Penetration of the prostate capsule by cancer is common and occurs along perineural spaces. Seminal vesicle invasion is associated with a high likelihood of regional or distant disease, and disease recurrence. The most common sites of lymph node metastases are the obturator and internal iliac lymph node chains and of distant metastases, the axial skeleton.

When to Refer

- Refer all patients to a urologist.
- Low-risk disease may be managed by active surveillance, surgery or radiation therapy.
- High-risk disease often requires multimodal treatment strategies.

Table 39–10. The UCSF Cancer of the Prostate Risk Assessment (CAPRA).

Variable	Level	Points
PSA (ng/mL [or mcg/L])	0–6	0
	6.1–10	1
	10.1–20	2
	20.1–30	3
	> 30	4
Gleason grade	1–3/1–3	0
	1–3/4–5	1
	4–5/1–5	3
T-stage	T1 or T2	0
	T3a	1
% positive biopsies (biopsy cores positive divided by the number of biopsies obtained)	< 34%	0
	> 34%	1
Age	< 50 years	0
	> 50 years	1

Table 39–11. CAPRA: Probability of freedom from PSA recurrence after radical prostatectomy by CAPRA point total.

CAPRA Score	3-Year Recurrence Free Survival (%) (95% CI)	5-Year Recurrence Free Survival (%) (95% CI)
0–1	91 (85–95)	85 (73–92)
2	89 (83–94)	81 (69–89)
3	81 (73–87)	66 (54–76)
4	81 (69–89)	59 (40–74)
5	69 (51–82)	60 (37–77)
6	54 (27–75)	34 (12–57)
7+	24 (9–43)	8 (0–28)

PSA, prostate-specific antigen.

Andriole GL et al; PLCO Project Team. Prostate cancer screening in the randomized Prostate, Lung, Colorectal, and Ovarian Cancer Screening Trial: mortality results after 13 years of follow-up. J Natl Cancer Inst. 2012 Jan 18;104(2):125–32. [PMID: 22228146]

Bill-Axelson A et al; SPCG-4 Investigators. Radical prostatectomy versus watchful waiting in early prostate cancer. N Engl J Med. 2011 May 5;364(18):1708–17. [PMID: 21542742]

Gupta RT et al. The state of prostate MRI in 2013. Oncology (Williston Park). 2013 Apr;27(4):262–70. [PMID: 23781689]

Ha YS et al. Enzalutamide for the treatment of castration-resistant prostate cancer. Drugs Today (Barc). 2013 Jan;49(1):7–13. [PMID: 23362491]

Hoffman-Censits J et al. Chemotherapy and targeted therapies: are we making progress in castrate-resistant prostate cancer? Semin Oncol. 2013 Jun;40(3):361–74. [PMID: 23806500]

Ilic D et al. Screening for prostate cancer. Cochrane Database Syst Rev. 2013 Jan 31;1:CD004720. [PMID: 23440794]

Kollmeier MA et al. How to select the optimal therapy for early-stage prostate cancer. Crit Rev Oncol Hematol. 2012 Dec; 84(Suppl 1):e6–e15. [PMID: 23273666]

MacVicar GR et al. Emerging therapies in metastatic castration-sensitive and castration-resistant prostate cancer. Curr Opin Oncol. 2013 May;25(3):252–60. [PMID: 23511665]

Meng MV et al. Treatment of patients with high risk localized prostate cancer: results from cancer of the prostate strategic urological research endeavor (CaPSURE). J Urol. 2005 May; 173(5):1557–61. [PMID: 15821485]

Morris MJ et al. Monitoring the clinical outcomes in advanced prostate cancer: what imaging modalities and other markers are reliable? Semin Oncol. 2013 Jun;40(3):375–92. [PMID: 23806501]

Niraula S et al. Treatment of prostate cancer with intermittent versus continuous androgen deprivation: a systematic review of randomized trials. J Clin Oncol. 2013 Jun 1;31(16):2029–36. [PMID: 23630216]

Pal SK et al. Enzalutamide for the treatment of prostate cancer. Expert Opin Pharmacother. 2013 Apr;14(5):679–85. [PMID: 23441761]

Palmbos PL et al. Non-castrate metastatic prostate cancer: have the treatment options changed? Semin Oncol. 2013 Jun; 40(3):337–46. [PMID: 23806498]

Rathkopf D et al. Androgen receptor antagonists in castration-resistant prostate cancer. Cancer J. 2013 Jan–Feb;19(1):43–9. [PMID: 23337756]

Ryan CJ et al. Abiraterone acetate for the treatment of prostate cancer. Expert Opin Pharmacother. 2013 Jan;14(1):91–6. [PMID: 23199349]

Schröder FH et al; ERSPC Investigators. Prostate-cancer mortality at 11 years of follow-up. N Engl J Med. 2012 Mar 15;366(11): 981–90. Erratum in: N Engl J Med. 2012 May 31;366(22):2137. [PMID: 22417251]

Seisen T et al. Current role of image-guided robotic radiosurgery (Cyberknife®) for prostate cancer treatment. BJU Int. 2013 May;111(5):761–6. [PMID: 23368740]

Thompson IM Jr et al. Long-term survival of participants in the prostate cancer prevention trial. N Engl J Med. 2013 Aug 15;369(7):603–10. [PMID: 23944298]

Qaseem A et al. Screening for prostate cancer: a guidance statement from the Clinical Guidelines Committee of the American College of Physicians. Ann Intern Med. 2013 May 21;158 (10): 761–9. [PMID: 23567643]

Wilt TJ et al; Prostate Cancer Intervention versus Observation Trial (PIVOT) Study Group. Radical prostatectomy versus observation for localized prostate cancer. N Engl J Med. 2012 Jul 19;367(3):203–13. Erratum in: N Engl J Med. 2012 Aug 9; 367(6):582. [PMID: 22808955]

BLADDER CANCER

ESSENTIALS OF DIAGNOSIS

► Gross or microscopic hematuria.

► Irritative voiding symptoms.

► Positive urinary cytology in most patients.

► Filling defect within bladder noted on imaging.

► General Considerations

Bladder cancer is the second most common urologic cancer; it occurs more commonly in men than women (3.1:1), and the mean age at diagnosis is 73 years. Cigarette smoking and exposure to industrial dyes or solvents are risk factors for the disease and account for approximately 60% and 15% of new cases, respectively. In the United States, almost all primary bladder cancers (98%) are epithelial malignancies, usually urothelial cell carcinomas (90%). Adenocarcinomas and squamous cell cancers account for approximately 2% and 7%, respectively. The latter is often associated with schistosomiasis, vesical calculi, or prolonged catheter use.

► Clinical Findings

A. Symptoms and Signs

Hematuria—gross or microscopic, chronic or intermittent—is the presenting symptom in 85–90% of patients with bladder cancer. Irritative voiding symptoms (urinary frequency and urgency) occur in a small percentage of patients as a result of the location or size of the cancer. Most patients with bladder cancer do not have signs of the disease because of its superficial nature. Abdominal masses detected on bimanual examination may be present in patients with large-volume or deeply infiltrating cancers. Hepatomegaly or palpable lymphadenopathy may be present in patients with metastatic disease, and lymphedema of the lower extremities result from locally advanced cancers or metastases to pelvic lymph nodes.

B. Laboratory Findings

Urinalysis reveals microscopic or gross hematuria in the majority of cases. On occasion, hematuria is accompanied by pyuria. Azotemia may be present in a small number of cases associated with ureteral obstruction. Anemia may occasionally be due to chronic blood loss or to bone marrow metastases. Exfoliated cells from normal and abnormal urothelium can be readily detected in voided urine specimens. Cytology can be useful to detect the disease initially or to detect its recurrence. Cytology is sensitive in detecting cancers of higher grade and stage (80–90%) but less so in detecting superficial or well-differentiated lesions (50%). There are numerous urinary tumor markers under investigation for screening, assessing recurrence, progression, prognosis or response to therapy.

C. Imaging

Bladder cancers may be identified using ultrasound, CT, or MRI as masses within the bladder. However, the presence of cancer is confirmed by cystoscopy and biopsy, with imaging primarily used to evaluate the upper urinary tract and to stage more advanced lesions.

D. Cystourethroscopy and Biopsy

The diagnosis and staging of bladder cancers are made by cystoscopy and transurethral resection. If cystoscopy—performed usually under local anesthesia—confirms the presence of bladder cancer, the patient is scheduled for transurethral resection under general or regional anesthesia. Random bladder and, on occasion, transurethral prostate biopsies are performed to detect occult disease in the bladder or elsewhere and potentially identify patients at greater risk for tumor recurrence and progression.

▶ Pathology & Staging

Grading is based on cellular features: size, pleomorphism, mitotic rate, and hyperchromatism. Bladder cancer staging is based on the extent of bladder wall penetration and the presence of regional or distant metastases.

The natural history of bladder cancer is based on two separate but related processes: tumor recurrence within the bladder and progression to higher-stage disease. Both are correlated with tumor grade and stage.

▶ Treatment

Patients with superficial cancers (Ta, T1) are treated with complete transurethral resection and selective use of intravesical chemotherapy. The subset of patients with carcinoma in situ and those undergoing resection of large, high-grade, recurrent Ta lesions or T1 cancers are good candidates for adjuvant intravesical therapy.

Patients with invasive (T2, T3) but still localized cancers are at risk for both nodal metastases and progression and require radical cystectomy, irradiation, or the combination of chemotherapy and selective surgery or irradiation due to the much higher risk of progression compared with patients with lower-stage lesions.

For patients with muscle invasive (T2 or greater) transitional cell carcinoma, neoadjuvant systemic chemotherapy prior to radical cystectomy is superior to radical cystectomy alone. This is particularly important for higher stage or bulky tumors in order to improve their surgical resectability.

A. Intravesical Chemotherapy

Immunotherapeutic or chemotherapeutic agents delivered directly into the bladder via a urethral catheter can reduce the likelihood of recurrence in those who have undergone complete transurethral resection. Most agents are administered weekly for 6–12 weeks. Efficacy may be increased by prolonging contact time to 2 hours. The use of maintenance therapy after the initial induction regimen is beneficial. Common agents include thiotepa, mitomycin, doxorubicin, valrubicin, and BCG, the last being the most effective agent when compared with the others with respect to reducing disease progression. Side effects of intravesical chemotherapy include irritative voiding symptoms and hemorrhagic cystitis. Patients in whom symptoms or infection develop from BCG may require antituberculous therapy.

B. Surgical Treatment

Although transurethral resection is the initial form of treatment for all bladder tumors since it is diagnostic, allows for proper staging, and controls superficial cancers, muscle-infiltrating cancers require more aggressive treatment. Partial cystectomy is indicated in selected patients with solitary lesions or those with cancers in a bladder diverticulum. Radical cystectomy entails removal of the bladder, prostate, seminal vesicles, and surrounding fat and peritoneal attachments in men and the uterus, cervix, urethra, anterior vaginal vault, and usually the ovaries in women. Bilateral pelvic lymph node dissection is performed in all patients.

Urinary diversion can be performed using a conduit of small or large bowel. However, continent forms of diversion have been developed that avoid the necessity of an external appliance and can be considered in a significant number of patients.

C. Radiotherapy

External beam radiotherapy delivered in fractions over a 6- to 8-week period is generally well tolerated, but approximately 10–15% of patients will develop bladder, bowel, or rectal complications. Local recurrence is common after radiotherapy alone (30–70%) and it is therefore combined with systemic chemotherapy in an effort to reduce the need for radical cystectomy or to treat patients who are poor candidates for radical cystectomy.

D. Chemotherapy

Metastatic disease is present in 15% of patients with newly diagnosed bladder cancer, and metastases develop within 2 years in up to 40% of patients who were believed to have localized disease at the time of cystectomy or definitive radiotherapy. Cisplatin-based combination chemotherapy results in partial or complete responses in 15–45% of patients (see Table 39–5).

Combination chemotherapy has been integrated into trials of surgery and radiotherapy. It has been used to decrease recurrence rates with both modalities and to attempt bladder preservation in those treated with radiation. Chemotherapy should be considered before surgery in those with bulky lesions or those suspected of having regional disease, and evidence suggests that neoadjuvant chemotherapy may benefit all patients with muscle-invasive disease prior to planned cystectomy. Chemoradiation is best suited for those with T2 or limited T3 disease without ureteral obstruction. Alternatively, chemotherapy has been used after cystectomy in patients at high risk for recurrence, such as those who have lymph node involvement or local invasion.

▶ Prognosis

The frequency of recurrence and progression are correlated with grade. Whereas progression may be noted in few grade I cancers (19–37%), it is common with poorly differentiated lesions (33–67%). Carcinoma in situ is most often found in association with papillary bladder cancers. Its presence identifies patients at increased risk for recurrence and progression.

At initial presentation, approximately 50–80% of bladder cancers are superficial: stage Ta, Tis, or T1. When properly treated, lymph node metastases and progression are uncommon in this population and survival is excellent at 81%. Five-year survival of patients with T2 and T3 disease ranges from 50% to 75% after radical cystectomy. Long-term survival for patients with metastatic disease at presentation is rare.

▶ When to Refer

- Refer all patients to a urologist. Hematuria often deserves evaluation with both upper urinary tract imaging and cystoscopy, particularly in a high-risk group (eg, older men).
- Refer when histologic diagnosis and staging require endoscopic resection of tumor.

Burger M et al. ICUD-EAU International Consultation on Bladder Cancer 2012: non-muscle-invasive urothelial carcinoma of the bladder. Eur Urol. 2013 Jan;63(1):36–44. [PMID: 22981672]

Calabrò F et al. Metastatic bladder cancer: anything new? Curr Opin Support Palliat Care. 2012 Sep;6(3):304–9. [PMID: 22643704]

Gakis G et al. ICUD-EAU International Consultation on Bladder Cancer 2012: radical cystectomy and bladder preservation for muscle-invasive urothelial carcinoma of the bladder. Eur Urol. 2013 Jan;63(1):45–57. [PMID: 22917985]

Hautmann RE et al. ICUD-EAU International Consultation on Bladder Cancer 2012: urinary diversion. Eur Urol. 2013 Jan;63(1):67–80. [PMID: 22995974]

International Collaboration of Trialists et al. International phase III trial assessing neoadjuvant cisplatin, methotrexate, and vinblastine chemotherapy for muscle-invasive bladder cancer: long-term results of the BA06 30894 trial. J Clin Oncol. 2011 Jun 1;29(16):2171–7. [PMID: 21502557]

Kamat AM et al. ICUD-EAU International Consultation on Bladder Cancer 2012: screening, diagnosis, and molecular markers. Eur Urol. 2013 Jan;63(1):4–15. [PMID: 23083902]

Khurana KK et al. Multidisciplinary management of patients with localized bladder cancer. Surg Oncol Clin N Am. 2013 Apr;22(2):357–73. [PMID: 23453340]

Logan C et al. Intravesical therapies for bladder cancer—indications and limitations. BJU Int. 2012 Dec;110(Suppl 4):12–21. [PMID: 23194118]

Lu YY et al. Clinical value of FDG PET or PET/CT in urinary bladder cancer: a systemic review and meta-analysis. Eur J Radiol. 2012 Sep;81(9):2411–6. [PMID: 21899971]

Nargund VH et al. Management of non-muscle-invasive (superficial) bladder cancer. Semin Oncol. 2012 Oct;39(5):559–72. [PMID: 23040252]

Sandler HM et al. Current role of radiation therapy for bladder cancer. Semin Oncol. 2012 Oct;39(5):583–7. [PMID: 23040254]

Sternberg CN et al. ICUD-EAU International Consultation on Bladder Cancer 2012: chemotherapy for urothelial carcinoma-neoadjuvant and adjuvant settings. Eur Urol. 2013 Jan;63(1):58–66. [PMID: 22917984]

Volpe A et al. Advanced bladder cancer: new agents and new approaches. A review. Urol Oncol. 2013 Jan;31(1):9–16. [PMID: 20864362]

Yafi FA et al. Contemporary outcomes of 2287 patients with bladder cancer who were treated with radical cystectomy: a Canadian multicentre experience. BJU Int. 2011 Aug;108 (4):539–45. [PMID: 21166753]

CANCERS OF THE URETER & RENAL PELVIS

Cancers of the renal pelvis and ureter are rare and occur more commonly in patients with bladder cancer, with Balkan nephropathy, with Lynch syndrome, who smoke, who were exposed to Thorotrast (a contrast agent with radioactive thorium in use until the 1960s), and who have a long history of analgesic abuse. The majority are urothelial cell carcinomas. Gross or microscopic hematuria is present in most patients, and flank pain secondary to bleeding and obstruction occurs less commonly. Like primary bladder tumors, urinary cytology is often positive. The most common signs identified at the time of intravenous urography or CT include an intraluminal filling defect, unilateral nonvisualization of the collecting system, and hydronephrosis. Ureteral and renal pelvic tumors must be differentiated from calculi, blood clots, papillary necrosis, or inflammatory and infectious lesions. On occasion, upper urinary tract lesions are accessible for biopsy, fulguration, or resection using a ureteroscope. Treatment is based on the site, size, grade, depth of penetration, and number of tumors present. Most are excised with laparoscopic or open nephroureterectomy (renal pelvic and upper ureteral lesions) or segmental excision of the ureter (distal ureteral lesions). Endoscopic resection may be indicated in patients with limited renal function or focal, low-grade, cancers.

Cordier J et al. Oncologic outcomes obtained after neoadjuvant and adjuvant chemotherapy for the treatment of urothelial carcinomas of the upper urinary tract: a review. World J Urol. 2013 Feb;31(1):77–82. [PMID: 23053212]

Gayed BA et al. The role of systemic chemotherapy in management of upper tract urothelial cancer. Curr Urol Rep. 2013 Apr;14(2):94–101. [PMID: 23344684]

Rai BP et al. Surgical management for upper urinary tract transitional cell carcinoma (UUT-TCC): a systematic review. BJU Int. 2012 Nov;110(10):1426–35. [PMID: 22759317]

Ribal MJ et al. Oncologic outcomes obtained after laparoscopic, robotic and/or single port nephroureterectomy for upper urinary tract tumours. World J Urol. 2013 Feb;31(1):93–107. [PMID: 23097034]

Tyler A. Urothelial cancers: ureter, renal pelvis, and bladder. Semin Oncol Nurs. 2012 Aug;28(3):154–62. [PMID: 22846483]

RENAL CELL CARCINOMA

ESSENTIALS OF DIAGNOSIS

▶ Gross or microscopic hematuria.

▶ Flank pain or mass in some patients.

▶ Systemic symptoms such as fever, weight loss may be prominent.

▶ Solid renal mass on imaging.

▶ General Considerations

Renal cell carcinoma accounts for 2.6% of all adult cancers. In the United States, approximately 65,150 cases of renal cell carcinoma are diagnosed and 13,680 deaths result annually. Renal cell carcinoma has a peak incidence in the sixth decade of life and a male-to-female ratio of 2:1. It may be associated with a number of paraneoplastic syndromes (see below and Table 39–2).

The cause is unknown. Cigarette smoking is the only significant environmental risk factor that has been identified. Familial causes of renal cell carcinoma have been identified (von Hippel–Lindau syndrome, hereditary papillary renal cell carcinoma, hereditary leiomyoma-renal cell carcinoma, Birt-Hogg-Dubé syndrome) and there is an association with dialysis-related acquired cystic disease and specific genetic aberrations (eg, Xp11.2 translocation), but sporadic tumors are far more common.

Renal cell carcinoma originates from the proximal tubule cells. Various histologic cell types are recognized (clear cell, papillary, chromophobe, collecting duct and sarcomatoid).

▶ Clinical Findings

A. Symptoms and Signs

Historically, 60% of patients presented with gross or microscopic hematuria. Flank pain or an abdominal mass was detected in approximately 30% of cases. The triad of flank pain, hematuria, and mass was found in only 10–15% of patients, and often a sign of advanced disease. Fever occurs as a paraneoplastic symptom (see Table 39–2). Symptoms of metastatic disease (cough, bone pain) occur in 20–30% of patients at presentation. Because of the widespread use of ultrasound and CT scanning, renal tumors are frequently detected incidentally in individuals with no urologic symptoms. There has been profound stage migration toward lower stages of disease over the past 10 years, likely due to the increased use of abdominal imaging. However, population mortality rates remain stable.

B. Laboratory Findings

Hematuria is present in 60% of patients. Erythrocytosis from increased erythropoietin production occurs in 5%, though anemia is more common; hypercalcemia may be present in up to 10% of patients. **Stauffer syndrome** is a reversible syndrome of hepatic dysfunction (with elevated liver function tests) in the absence of metastatic disease.

C. Imaging

Solid renal masses are often first identified by abdominal ultrasonography or CT. CT and MRI scanning are the most valuable imaging tests for renal cell carcinoma. These scans confirm the character of the mass and further stage the lesion with respect to regional lymph nodes, renal vein, or hepatic involvement. CT and MRI also provide valuable information regarding the contralateral kidney (function, bilaterality of neoplasm). Chest radiographs exclude pulmonary metastases, and bone scans should be performed for large tumors and in patients with bone pain or elevated alkaline phosphatase levels. MRI and duplex Doppler ultrasonography are excellent methods of assessing the presence and extent of tumor thrombus within the renal vein or vena cava.

▶ Differential Diagnosis

Solid lesions of the kidney are renal cell carcinoma until proved otherwise. Other solid masses include angiomyolipomas (fat density usually visible by CT), urothelial cell cancers of the renal pelvis (more central location, involvement of the collecting system, positive urinary cytologic tests), adrenal tumors (superoanterior to the kidney) and oncocytomas (indistinguishable from renal cell carcinoma preoperatively), and renal abscesses.

▶ Treatment

Surgical extirpation is the primary treatment for localized renal cell carcinoma. Patients with a single kidney, bilateral lesions, or significant medical renal disease should be considered for partial nephrectomy. Patients with a normal contralateral kidney and good renal function but a small cancer are also candidates for partial nephrectomy, while radical nephrectomy is indicated in cases of larger tumors (> 7 cm) and those where partial nephrectomy is not technically feasible. Radiofrequency and cryosurgical ablation are being studied; they likely yield equivalent short-term oncologic outcomes with reduced morbidity.

No effective chemotherapy is available for metastatic renal cell carcinoma. Vinblastine is the single most efficacious agent, with short-term partial response rates of 15%. Bevacizumab can prolong time to progression in those with metastatic disease (see Table 39–5). Biologic response modifiers have received much attention, including interferon-alpha and interleukin-2. Partial response rates of 15–20% and 15–35%, respectively, have been reported. Responders tend to have lower tumor burdens, metastatic disease confined to the lung, and a high performance status. Patients with metastatic kidney cancer and good performance status who have resectable primary tumors should undergo cytoreductive nephrectomy. Two randomized trials have shown a survival benefit of surgery followed by the use of systemic therapy—specifically, biologic response modifiers—compared with the use of systemic therapy alone.

Several targeted drugs, specifically VEGF, Raf-kinase, and mTOR inhibitors, are effective (40% response rates) in patients with advanced kidney cancer. The drugs are oral agents, well tolerated, and particularly active for clear cell carcinoma. The appropriate timing and combination of these agents, with and without surgery and cytokine therapy, remains to be determined.

▶ Prognosis

After radical or partial nephrectomy, tumors confined to the renal capsule (T1–T2) demonstrate 5-year disease-free survivals of 90–100%. Tumors extending beyond the renal capsule (T3 or T4) and node-positive tumors have 50–60% and 0–15% 5-year disease-free survival, respectively. One subgroup of patients with nonlocalized disease has reasonable long-term survival, namely, those with solitary resectable metastases. In this setting, radical nephrectomy with resection of the metastasis results in 5-year disease-free survival rates of 15–30%.

▶ When to Refer

- Refer patients with solid renal masses or complex cysts to a urologist for further evaluation.
- Refer patients with renal cell carcinoma to a urologic surgeon for surgical excision.
- Refer patients with metastatic disease to an oncologist.

Antonelli A et al. Elective partial nephrectomy is equivalent to radical nephrectomy in patients with clinical T1 renal cell carcinoma: results of a retrospective, comparative, multi-institutional study. BJU Int. 2012 Apr;109(7):1013–8. [PMID: 21883829]

Fan X et al. Comparison of transperitoneal and retroperitoneal laparoscopic nephrectomy for renal cell carcinoma: a systematic review and meta-analysis. BJU Int. 2013 Apr;111(4):611–21. [PMID: 23106964]

Figlin R et al. Novel agents and approaches for advanced renal cell carcinoma. J Urol. 2012 Sep;188(3):707–15. [PMID: 22818130]

Larkin J et al. Second-line treatments for the management of advanced renal cell carcinoma: systematic review and meta-analysis. Expert Opin Pharmacother. 2013 Jan;14(1):27–39. [PMID: 23256638]

Linehan WM et al. Kidney cancer. Urol Oncol. 2012 Nov–Dec; 30(6):948–51. [PMID: 23218074]

Motzer RJ et al. Axitinib versus sorafenib as second-line treatment for advanced renal cell carcinoma: overall survival analysis and updated results from a randomised phase 3 trial. Lancet Oncol. 2013 May;14(6):552–62. Erratum in: Lancet Oncol. 2013 Jun;14(7):e254. [PMID: 23598172]

Motzer RJ et al. Pazopanib versus sunitinib in metastatic renal-cell carcinoma. N Engl J Med. 2013 Aug 22;369(8):722–31. [PMID: 23964934]

Pécuchet N et al. New insights into the management of renal cell cancer. Oncology. 2013;84(1):22–31. [PMID: 23076127]

Sharma V et al. Partial nephrectomy: is there still a need for open surgery? Curr Urol Rep. 2013 Feb;14(1):1–4. [PMID: 23233109]

OTHER PRIMARY TUMORS OF THE KIDNEY

Oncocytomas account for 3–5% of renal tumors, are usually benign, and are indistinguishable from renal cell carcinoma on preoperative imaging. These tumors are seen in other organs, including the adrenals, salivary glands, and thyroid and parathyroid glands.

Angiomyolipomas are rare benign tumors composed of fat, smooth muscle, and blood vessels. They are most commonly seen in patients with tuberous sclerosis (often multiple and bilateral) or in young to middle-aged women. CT scanning may identify the fat component, which is diagnostic for angiomyolipoma. Asymptomatic lesions < 5 cm in diameter usually do not require intervention; large lesions can spontaneously bleed. Acute bleeding can be treated by angiographic embolization or, in rare cases, nephrectomy. Lesions over 5 cm are often prophylactically treated with angioembolization to reduce the risk of bleeding.

SECONDARY TUMORS OF THE KIDNEY

The kidney is not an infrequent site for metastatic disease. Of the solid tumors, lung cancer is the most common (20%), followed by breast (10%), stomach (10%), and the contralateral kidney (10%). Lymphoma, both Hodgkin and non-Hodgkin, may also involve the kidney, although it tends to appear as a diffusely infiltrative process resulting in renal enlargement rather than a discrete mass.

PRIMARY TUMORS OF THE TESTIS

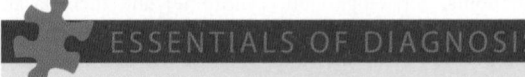

ESSENTIALS OF DIAGNOSIS

- ▶ Most common neoplasm in men aged 20–35 years.
- ▶ Patient typically discovers a painless nodule.
- ▶ Orchiectomy necessary for diagnosis.

▶ General Considerations

Malignant tumors of the testis are rare, with approximately five to six cases per 100,000 males reported in the United States each year. Ninety to 95 percent of all primary testicular tumors are germ cell tumors and can be divided into two major categories: **nonseminomas**, including embryonal cell carcinoma (20%), teratoma (5%), choriocarcinoma (< 1%), and mixed cell types (40%); and **seminomas** (35%). The remainder of primary testicular tumors are nongerminal neoplasms (Leydig cell, Sertoli cell, gonadoblastoma). The lifetime probability of developing testicular cancer is 0.3% for an American male. For the purposes of this review, only germ cell tumors will be considered.

Approximately 5% of testicular tumors develop in a patient with a history of cryptorchism, with seminoma being the most common. However, 5–10% of these tumors occur in the contralateral, normally descended testis. The relative risk of development of malignancy is highest for the intra-abdominal testis (1:20) and lower for the inguinal testis (1:80). Placement of the cryptorchid testis into the scrotum (orchidopexy) does not alter the malignant potential of the cryptorchid testis but does facilitate routine examination and tumor detection.

Testicular cancer is slightly more common on the right than the left, paralleling the increased incidence of cryptorchidism on the right side. One to 2 percent of primary testicular tumors are bilateral and up to 50% of these men have a history of unilateral or bilateral cryptorchidism. Primary bilateral testicular tumors may occur synchronously or asynchronously but tend to be of the same histology. Seminoma is the most common histologic finding in bilateral *primary* testicular tumors, while malignant lymphoma is the most common bilateral testicular tumor overall.

Clinical Findings

A. Symptoms and Signs

The most common symptom of testicular cancer is painless enlargement of the testis. Sensations of heaviness are not unusual. Patients are usually the first to recognize an abnormality, yet the typical delay in seeking medical attention ranges from 3 to 6 months. Acute testicular pain resulting from intratesticular hemorrhage occurs in approximately 10% of cases. Ten percent of patients are asymptomatic at presentation, and 10% manifest symptoms relating to metastatic disease such as back pain (retroperitoneal metastases), cough (pulmonary metastases), or lower extremity edema (vena cava obstruction).

A discrete mass or diffuse testicular enlargement is noted in most cases. Secondary hydroceles may be present in 5–10% of cases. In advanced disease, supraclavicular adenopathy may be present, and abdominal examination may reveal a mass. Gynecomastia is seen in 5% of germ cell tumors.

B. Laboratory Findings

Several serum markers are important in the diagnosis and monitoring of testicular carcinoma, including human chorionic gonadotropin (hCG), alpha-fetoprotein, and lactate dehydrogenase. Alpha-fetoprotein is never elevated with pure seminomas, and while hCG is occasionally elevated in seminomas, levels tend to be lower than those seen with nonseminomas. Lactate dehydrogenase may be elevated with either type of tumor. Liver function tests may be elevated in the presence of hepatic metastases, and anemia may be present in advanced disease.

C. Imaging

Scrotal ultrasound can readily determine whether a mass is intratesticular or extratesticular. Once the diagnosis of testicular cancer has been established by inguinal orchiectomy, clinical staging of the disease is accomplished by chest, abdominal, and pelvic CT scanning.

Staging

In a commonly used staging system for nonseminoma germ cell tumors, a stage A lesion is confined to the testis; stage B demonstrates regional lymph node involvement in the retroperitoneum; and stage C indicates distant metastasis. For seminoma, the M.D. Anderson system is commonly used. In this system, a stage I lesion is confined to

the testis, a stage II lesion has spread to the retroperitoneal lymph nodes, and a stage III lesion has supradiaphragmatic nodal or visceral involvement.

Differential Diagnosis

An incorrect diagnosis is made at the initial examination in up to 25% of patients with testicular tumors. Scrotal ultrasonography should be performed if any uncertainty exists with respect to the diagnosis. Although most intratesticular masses are malignant, a benign lesion—epidermoid cyst—may rarely be seen. Epidermoid cysts are usually very small benign nodules located just underneath the tunica albuginea; occasionally, however, they can be large.

Treatment

Inguinal exploration with early vascular control of the spermatic cord structures is the initial intervention. If cancer cannot be excluded by examination of the testis, radical orchiectomy is warranted. Scrotal approaches and open testicular biopsies should be avoided. Further therapy depends on the histology of the tumor as well as the clinical stage.

Up to 75% of clinical stage I **nonseminomas** are cured by orchiectomy alone. Selected patients who meet specific criteria may be offered surveillance after orchiectomy. These criteria are as follows: (1) tumor is confined within the tunica albuginea; (2) tumor does not demonstrate vascular invasion; (3) tumor markers normalize after orchiectomy; (4) radiographic imaging of the chest and abdomen shows no evidence of disease; and (5) the patient is reliable. Patients most likely to experience relapse on a surveillance regimen include those with predominantly embryonal cancer and those with vascular or lymphatic invasion identified in the orchiectomy specimen.

Stage I and IIa/b **seminomas** (retroperitoneal disease < 2 cm/2–5 cm in diameter) are treated by radical orchiectomy and retroperitoneal irradiation. Patients with clinical stage I disease may be candidates for surveillance or single-agent carboplatin. Seminomas of stage IIc (> 5 cm retroperitoneal involvement) and stage III receive primary chemotherapy (etoposide and cisplatin or cisplatin, etoposide, and bleomycin) (Table 39–5). Surgical resection of residual retroperitoneal masses is warranted if the mass is > 3 cm in diameter and positive on PET scan, under which circumstances 40% will harbor residual carcinoma.

Surveillance needs to be considered an active process both by the clinician and by the patient. Patients are followed every 1–2 months for the first 2 years and quarterly in the third year. Tumor markers are obtained at each visit, and chest radiographs and CT scans are obtained every 3–4 months. Follow-up continues beyond the initial 3 years; however, 80% of relapses will occur within the first 2 years. With rare exceptions, patients who relapse can be cured by chemotherapy or surgery. Alternatives to surveillance for clinical stage I nonseminoma include adjuvant chemotherapy (bleomycin, etoposide, cisplatin) (see Table 39–5) or retroperitoneal lymph node dissection.

Patients with bulky retroperitoneal disease (> 5 cm nodes) or metastatic nonseminomas are treated with primary cisplatin-based combination chemotherapy following orchiectomy (etoposide and cisplatin or cisplatin, etoposide, and bleomycin). If tumor markers normalize and a residual mass > 1 cm persists on imaging studies, the mass is resected because 15–20% of the time it will harbor viable cancer and 40% of the time it will harbor teratoma. Even if patients have a complete response to chemotherapy, some clinicians advocate retroperitoneal lymphadenectomy since 10% of patients may harbor residual carcinoma and 10% may have teratoma in the retroperitoneum. If tumor markers fail to normalize following primary chemotherapy, salvage chemotherapy is required (cisplatin, etoposide, ifosfamide).

▶ **Prognosis**

The 5-year disease-free survival rate for patients with stage A **nonseminomas** (includes all treatments) ranges from 96% to 100%. For low-volume stage B disease, 90% 5-year disease-free survival is expected. The 5-year disease-free survival rates for stage I and IIa **seminomas** (retroperitoneal disease < 2 cm in diameter) treated by radical orchiectomy and retroperitoneal irradiation are 98% and 92–94%, respectively. Ninety-five percent of patients with stage III disease attain a complete response following orchiectomy and chemotherapy. Patients with bulky retroperitoneal or disseminated disease treated with primary chemotherapy followed by surgery have a 5-year disease-free survival rate of 55–80%.

▶ **When to Refer**

Refer all patients with solid masses of the testis to a urologist.

Albers P et al; European Association of Urology. EAU guidelines on testicular cancer: 2011 update. Eur Urol. 2011 Aug; 60(2):304–19. [PMID: 21632173]

Aparicio J et al. Risk-adapted treatment in clinical stage I testicular seminoma: the third Spanish Germ Cell Cancer Study Group. J Clin Oncol. 2011 Dec 10;29(35):4677–81. [PMID: 22042940]

Ehrlich Y et al. Serum tumor markers in testicular cancer. Urol Oncol. 2013 Jan;31(1):17–23. [PMID: 20822927]

Nallu A et al. Testicular germ cell tumors: biology and clinical update. Curr Opin Oncol. 2013 May;25(3):266–72. [PMID: 23549473]

Oliver RT et al. Randomized trial of carboplatin versus radiotherapy for stage I seminoma: mature results on relapse and contralateral testis cancer rates in MRC TE19/EORTC 30982 study (ISRCTN27163214). J Clin Oncol. 2011 Mar 10;29(8): 957–62. [PMID: 21282539]

Viatori M. Testicular cancer. Semin Oncol Nurs. 2012 Aug;28(3): 180–9. [PMID: 22846486]

SECONDARY TUMORS OF THE TESTIS

Secondary tumors of the testis are rare. In men over the age of 50 years, lymphoma is the most common testis tumor, and overall it is the most common secondary neoplasm of the testis, accounting for 5% of all testicular tumors. It may be seen in three clinical settings: (1) late manifestation of widespread lymphoma, (2) the initial presentation of clinically occult disease, and (3) primary extranodal disease. Radical orchiectomy is indicated to make the diagnosis. Prognosis is related to the stage of disease.

Metastasis to the testis is rare. The most common primary site of origin is the prostate, followed by the lung, gastrointestinal tract, melanoma, and kidney.

CANCER COMPLICATIONS & EMERGENCIES

SPINAL CORD COMPRESSION

ESSENTIALS OF DIAGNOSIS

▶ Complication of metastatic solid tumor, lymphoma, or multiple myeloma.

▶ Back pain is most common presenting symptom.

▶ Prompt diagnosis is essential because once a severe neurologic deficit develops, it is often irreversible.

▶ Emergent treatment may prevent or potentially reverse paresis and urinary and bowel incontinence.

▶ **General Considerations**

Cancers that cause spinal cord compression most commonly metastasize to the vertebral bodies, resulting in physical damage to the spinal cord from edema, hemorrhage, and pressure-induced ischemia to the vasculature of the spinal cord. Persistent compression can result in irreversible changes to the myelin sheaths resulting in permanent neurologic impairment.

Prompt diagnosis and therapeutic intervention are essential, since the probability of reversing neurologic symptoms largely depends on the duration of symptoms. Patients who are treated promptly after symptoms appear may have partial or complete return of function and, depending on tumor sensitivity to specific treatment, may respond favorably to subsequent anticancer therapy.

▶ **Clinical Findings**

A. Symptoms and Signs

Back pain at the level of the tumor mass occurs in over 80% of cases and may be aggravated by lying down, weight bearing, sneezing, or coughing; it usually precedes the development of neurologic symptoms or signs. Since involvement is usually epidural, a mixture of nerve root and spinal cord symptoms often develops. Progressive weakness and sensory changes commonly occur. Bowel and bladder symptoms progressing to incontinence are late findings.

The initial findings of impending cord compression may be quite subtle, and there should be a high index of suspicion when back pain or weakness of the lower extremities develops in cancer patients.

B. Imaging

MRI is usually the initial imaging procedure of choice in a cancer patient with new-onset back pain. When there are neurologic findings suggesting spinal cord compression, an emergent MRI should be obtained; the MRI should include a survey of the entire spine in order to define all areas of tumor involvement for treatment planning purposes.

Bone radiographs, if done, may show evidence of vertebral body or pedicle destruction by the cancer. However, bone radiographs are neither sensitive nor specific and therefore are not helpful in diagnosis or treatment planning. If the back pain symptoms are nonspecific, a whole-body PET scan with ^{18}F-2-deoxyglucose may be useful as a screening procedure.

▶ Treatment

Patients found to have epidural impingement of the spinal cord should be given corticosteroids immediately. The initial dexamethasone dose is 10–100 mg intravenously followed by 4–6 mg every 6 hours intravenously or orally. Patients without a known diagnosis of cancer should have emergent surgery to relieve the impingement and obtain a pathologic specimen. Patients with a single area of compression due to solid tumors are best treated with surgical decompression followed by radiation therapy. Better outcomes (ie, improved ability to ambulate and improved bladder and bowel function) are seen in patients who undergo surgery followed by radiation therapy than in those who receive radiation therapy alone. If multiple vertebral body levels are involved with cancer, radiation therapy is the preferred treatment option. Corticosteroids are generally tapered toward the end of radiation therapy.

Kim JM et al. Clinical outcome of metastatic spinal cord compression treated with surgical excision +/– radiation versus radiation therapy alone: a systematic review of literature. Spine. 2012 Jan 1;37(1):78–84. [PMID: 21629164]

Loblaw DA et al. A 2011 updated systematic review and clinical practice guideline for the management of malignant extradural spinal cord compression. Int J Radiat Oncol Biol Phys. 2012 Oct 1;84(2):312–7. [PMID: 22420969]

McCurdy MT et al. Oncologic emergencies. Crit Care Med. 2012 Jul;40(7):2212–22. [PMID: 22584756]

MALIGNANT EFFUSIONS

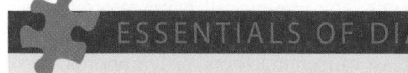

ESSENTIALS OF DIAGNOSIS

▶ Occur in pleural, pericardial, and peritoneal spaces.

▶ Caused by direct neoplastic involvement of serous surface or obstruction of lymphatic drainage.

▶ Half of undiagnosed effusions in patients not known to have cancer are malignant.

▶ General Considerations

The development of an effusion in the pleural, pericardial, or peritoneal space may be the initial finding in a patient with cancer, or an effusion may appear during the course of disease progression. Direct involvement of the serous surface with tumor is the most frequent initiating cause of the accumulation of fluid. The most common malignancies causing pleural and pericardial effusions are lung and breast cancers; the most common malignancies associated with malignant ascites are ovarian, colorectal, stomach, and pancreatic cancers.

▶ Clinical Findings

A. Symptoms and Signs

Patients with pleural and pericardial effusions complain of shortness of breath and orthopnea. Patients with ascites complain of abdominal distention and discomfort. Cardiac tamponade causing pressure equalization in the chambers impairing both filling and cardiac output can be a life-threatening event. Signs of tamponade include tachycardia, muffled heart sounds, pulsus paradoxus, and hypotension. Signs of pleural effusions include decreased breath sounds, egophony, and percussion dullness.

B. Laboratory Findings

Malignancy is confirmed as the cause of an effusion when analysis of the fluid specimen shows malignant cells in either the cytology or cell block specimen.

C. Imaging

The presence of effusions can be confirmed with radiographic studies or ultrasonography.

▶ Differential Diagnosis

The differential diagnosis of a malignant exudative pleural or pericardial effusion includes nonmalignant processes, such as infection, pulmonary embolism, heart failure, and trauma. However, malignant effusions are rarely transudative.

The differential diagnosis of malignant ascites includes similar benign processes, such as heart failure, cirrhosis, peritonitis, and pancreatic ascites.

Bloody effusions are usually due to cancer, but a bloody pleural effusion can also be due to pulmonary embolism, trauma and, occasionally, infection. Chylous pleural or ascitic fluid is generally associated with obstruction of lymphatic drainage as might occur in lymphomas.

▶ Treatment

In some cases, treatment of the underlying cancer with chemotherapy can cause regression of the effusions; however, not uncommonly, the presence of an effusion is an end-stage manifestation of the disease. In this situation, decisions regarding management are in large part dictated by the patient's symptoms and goals of care.

A. Pleural Effusion

A pleural effusion that is symptomatic may be managed initially with a **large volume thoracentesis**. With some patients, the effusion slowly reaccumulates, which allows for periodic thoracentesis when the patient becomes symptomatic. However, in many patients, the effusion reaccumulates quickly, causing rapid return of symptoms of shortness of breath. For those patients, several options exist for management. **Chest tube drainage followed by pleurodesis** is the preferred option for patients with a reasonable life expectancy. The procedure involves placement of a chest tube that is connected to closed water seal drainage. After lung expansion is confirmed on a chest radiograph, a sclerosing agent (such as talc slurry or doxycycline) is injected into the catheter. Patients should be premedicated with analgesics and placed in a variety of positions in order to distribute the drug through the pleural spaces. Previously, injection of the sclerosing agent was done only after drainage had decreased to < 100 mL/d; but it is now clear that effective sclerosis can be achieved after 24 hours of drainage regardless of the amount of the residual fluid. Pleurodesis will not be successful if the lung cannot be reexpanded; these patients may be treated with the placement of a shunt or an indwelling catheter. Placement of an indwelling catheter that can be drained by a family member or a visiting nurse may also be preferable for patients with short life expectancies or for those who do not respond to pleurodesis.

B. Pericardial Effusion

Fluid may be removed by a needle aspiration or by placement of a catheter for more thorough drainage. As with pleural effusions, most pericardial effusions will reaccumulate. Management options for recurrent, symptomatic effusions include prolonged catheter drainage for several days, sclerosis with such agents as doxycycline or bleomycin, or pericardiectomy.

C. Malignant Ascites

Patients with malignant ascites not responsive to chemotherapy are generally treated with repeated large volume paracenteses. As the frequency of drainage to maintain comfort can compromise the patient's quality of life, other alternatives include placement of a catheter or port so that the patient, family member, or visiting nurse can drain fluid as needed at home. Another option is placement of a peritoneovenous shunt; this can be considered for a select group of patients with life expectancy > 3 months and fluid that is nonviscous, nonbloody, and nonloculated.

Kastelik JA. Management of malignant pleural effusion. Lung. 2013 Apr;191(2):165–75. [PMID: 23315213]

Myers R et al. Tunneled pleural catheters: an update for 2013. Clin Chest Med. 2013 Mar;34(1):73–80. [PMID: 23411058]

Rodriguez-Panadero F et al. Management of malignant pleural effusions. Curr Opin Pulm Med. 2011 Jul;17(4):269–73. [PMID: 21519264]

White J et al. PleurX peritoneal catheter drainage system for vacuum-assisted drainage of treatment-resistant, recurrent malignant ascites: a NICE Medical Technology Guidance. Appl Health Econ Health Policy. 2012 Sep 1;10(5):299–308. [PMID: 22779402]

HYPERCALCEMIA

 ESSENTIALS OF DIAGNOSIS

▶ Usually symptomatic and severe (≥ 15 mg/dL [> 3.75 mmol/L]).

▶ Most common paraneoplastic endocrine syndrome; accounts for most inpatients with hypercalcemia.

▶ The neoplasm is clinically apparent in nearly all cases when hypercalcemia is detected.

▶ General Considerations

Hypercalcemia affects 20–30% of cancer patients at some point during their illness. The most common cancers causing hypercalcemia are myeloma, breast carcinoma, and non–small cell lung cancer. Hypercalcemia is caused by one of three mechanisms, systemic effects of tumor-released proteins, direct osteolysis of bone by tumor or vitamin D–mediated osteoabsorption.

▶ Clinical Findings

A. Symptoms and Signs

Symptoms and signs of hypercalcemia can be subtle; more severe symptoms occur with higher levels of hypercalcemia and with a rapid rate at which the calcium level rises. Early symptoms typically include anorexia, nausea, fatigue, constipation, and polyuria; later findings may include muscular weakness and hyporeflexia, confusion, psychosis, tremor, and lethargy.

B. Laboratory Findings

Symptoms and signs are caused by free calcium; as calcium is bound by protein in the serum, the measured serum calcium will underestimate the free or ionized calcium in patients with low albumin levels. In the setting of hypoalbuminemia, the corrected serum calcium should be calculated by one of several available formulas (eg, corrected calcium = measured calcium – measured albumin + 4). Alternatively, the free ionized calcium can be measured. When the corrected serum calcium rises above 12 mg/dL (3 mmol/L), sudden death due to cardiac arrhythmia or asystole may occur. The presence of hypercalcemia does not invariably indicate a dismal prognosis, especially in patients with breast cancer, myeloma, or lymphoma.

In the absence of symptoms or signs of hypercalcemia, a laboratory finding of elevated serum calcium should be retested immediately to exclude the possibility of error.

C. ECG

Electrocardiography often shows a shortening of the QT interval.

▶ Treatment

Emergency management should begin with the initiation of intravenous fluids with 0.9% saline at 100–200 mL/h to ensure rehydration with brisk urinary output of the often volume-depleted patient. If kidney function is normal or only marginally impaired, a bisphosphonate should be given. Choices include pamidronate, 60–90 mg intravenously over 2–4 hours, or zoledronic acid, 4 mg intravenously over 15 minutes. Zoledronic acid is more potent than pamidronate and has the advantage of a shorter administration time as well as a longer duration of effect, but with repeated dosing, it is more associated with the very uncommon but serious side effect of osteonecrosis of the jaw. Once hypercalcemia is controlled, treatment directed at the cancer should be initiated if possible. Commonly, though, hypercalcemia occurs in patients with cancers that are unresponsive to treatment. In the event that the hypercalcemia becomes refractory to repeated doses of bisphosphonates, other agents that can help control hypercalcemia (at least temporarily) include calcitonin, denosumab, and gallium nitrate; corticosteroids can be useful in patients with myeloma and lymphoma. Salmon calcitonin, 4–8 international units/kg given subcutaneously or intramuscularly every 12 hours, can be used in patients with severe, symptomatic hypercalcemia; its onset of action is within hours but its hypocalcemic effect wanes in 2–3 days.

Clines GA. Mechanisms and treatment of hypercalcemia of malignancy. Curr Opin Endocrinol Diabetes Obes. 2011 Dec;18(6):339–46. [PMID: 21897221]
Legrand SB. Modern management of malignant hypercalcemia. Am J Hosp Palliat Care. 2011 Nov;28(7):515–7. [PMID: 21724679]
Rosner MH et al. Onco-nephrology: the pathophysiology and treatment of malignancy-associated hypercalcemia. Clin J Am Soc Nephrol. 2012 Oct;7(10):1722–9. [PMID: 22879438]

HYPERURICEMIA & TUMOR LYSIS SYNDROME

 ESSENTIALS OF DIAGNOSIS

► Complication of treatment-associated tumor lysis of hematologic and rapidly proliferating malignancies.

► May be worsened by thiazide diuretics.

► Rapid increase in serum uric acid can cause acute urate nephropathy from uric acid crystallization.

► Reducing pre-chemotherapy serum uric acid is fundamental to preventing urate nephropathy.

General Considerations

Tumor lysis syndrome (TLS) is seen most commonly following treatment of hematologic malignancies, such as acute lymphoblastic leukemia and Burkitt lymphoma. However, TLS can develop from any tumor highly sensitive to chemotherapy. TLS is caused by the massive release of cellular material including nucleic acids, proteins, phosphorus, and potassium. If both the metabolism and excretion of these breakdown products are impaired, hyperuricemia, hyperphosphatemia, and hyperkalemia will develop abruptly. Acute kidney injury may then develop from the crystallization and deposition of uric acid and calcium phosphate within the renal tubules further exacerbating the hyperphosphatemia and hyperkalemia.

Clinical Findings

Symptoms of hyperphosphatemia include nausea and vomiting as well as seizures. Also, with high levels of phosphorus, co-precipitation with calcium can cause renal tubule blockage, further exacerbating the kidney injury. Hyperkalemia, due to release of intracellular potassium and impaired kidney excretion, can cause arrhythmias and sudden death.

Treatment

Prevention is the most important factor in the management of TLS. Published guidelines for TLS management include aggressive hydration prior to initiation of chemotherapy as well as during and after completion of the chemotherapy. Administration of fluid helps keep urine flowing and facilitates excretion of uric acid and phosphorus. For the patients with moderate risk of developing TLS, for instance, those with intermediate grade lymphomas and acute leukemias, allopurinol (which blocks the enzyme xanthine oxidase and therefore the formation of uric acid from purine breakdown) should be given before starting chemotherapy at an oral dose of 100 mg/m^2 every 8 hours (maximum 800 mg/d) with dose reductions for impaired kidney function. For patients at high risk for developing TLS, for instance, patients with high-grade lymphomas or patients with acute leukemias and markedly elevated white blood cell counts (with acute myeloid leukemia, white blood cell count > 50,000/mcL [> 50,000/10^9/L]; with acute lymphoblastic leukemia, white blood cell count > 100,000/mcL [> 100,000/10^9/L]) or in whom hyperuricemia develops despite treatment with allopurinol, rasburicase 0.1–0.2 mg/kg/d is given intravenously for 1–7 days. Rasburicase is a recombinant urate oxidase that converts uric acid into the more soluble form resulting in rapid decline in uric acid levels. Rasburicase cannot be given to patients with known glucose 6-phosphate dehydrogenase (G6PD) deficiency nor can it be given to pregnant or lactating women. One of the historic mainstays of TLS management, systemic bicarbonate infusions to alkalinize the urine, is no longer routinely recommended. Laboratory values should be monitored following initiation of chemotherapy in addition to the hyperuricemia; elevated potassium or phosphorus levels need to be promptly managed.

When to Refer

Should urinary output drop, creatinine level rise, or hyperphosphatemia persist, a nephrologist should be immediately consulted to evaluate the need for dialysis.

Howard SC et al. The tumor lysis syndrome. N Engl J Med. 2011 May 12;364(19):1844–54. [PMID: 21561350]

McBride A et al. Recognizing and managing the expanded risk of tumor lysis syndrome in hematologic and solid malignancies. J Hematol Oncol. 2012 Dec 13;5:75. [PMID: 23237230]

Wilson FP et al. Onco-nephrology: tumor lysis syndrome. Clin J Am Soc Nephrol. 2012 Oct;7(10):1730–9. [PMID: 22879434]

INFECTIONS

Chapters 30 and 31 provide more detailed discussions of infections in the immunocompromised patient.

ESSENTIALS OF DIAGNOSIS

► In patients with neutropenia, infection is a medical emergency.

► The presence of fever, although sometimes attributable to other causes, must be assumed to be due to an infection.

General Considerations

Many patients with disseminated neoplasms have increased susceptibility to infection. In some patients, this results from impaired defense mechanisms (eg, acute leukemia, Hodgkin lymphoma, multiple myeloma, chronic lymphocytic leukemia); in others, it results from the myelosuppressive and immunosuppressive effects of cancer chemotherapy or a combination of these factors. Complicating impaired defense mechanisms are the frequent presence of indwelling catheters, impaired mucosal surfaces, and colonization with more virulent hospital-acquired pathogens.

The source of a neutropenic febrile episode is determined in about 30% of cases through blood, urine, or sputum cultures. The bacterial organisms accounting for the majority of infections in cancer patients include gram-negative bacteria (*Escherichia coli, Klebsiella, Pseudomonas, Enterobacter*) and gram-positive bacteria (coagulase-negative *Staphylococcus, Staphylococcus aureus, Streptococcus pneumoniae, Corynebacterium,* and streptococci). There has been a trend over the last few decades of an increasing percentage of gram-positive organisms. The risk of bacterial infections rises when the neutrophil count is below 1000/mcL (1.0×10^9/L); the risk dramatically increases when the count falls below 100/mcL (0.1×10^9/L).

Clinical Findings

A thorough physical examination should be performed. Routine DREs are generally avoided unless symptoms suggest a rectal abscess or prostatitis. If a rectal examination is necessary, antibiotics should be administered first. Appropriate cultures (eg, blood, sputum, urine and, if indicated, cerebrospinal fluid) should always be obtained before starting therapy. Two sets of blood cultures should be drawn; if the patient has an indwelling catheter, one of the cultures should be drawn from the line. A chest radiograph should also be obtained.

► Treatment

Empiric antibiotic therapy needs to be initiated immediately in the febrile, neutropenic patient. The choice of antibiotics depends on a number of different factors including the patient's clinical status and any localizing source of infection. If the patient is clinically well, monotherapy with an intravenous beta-lactam with anti-*Pseudomonas* activity (cefepime, ceftazidime, imipenem/cilastatin, piperacillin/tazobactam) should be started (see Infections in the Immunocompromised Patient, Chapter 30). If the patient is clinically ill with hypotension or hypoxia, an aminoglycoside or fluoroquinolone should be added for "double" gram-negative bacteria coverage. If there is a strong suspicion of a gram-positive organism, such as from *S aureus* catheter infection, vancomycin can be given empirically. In some instances, patients may be treated with oral antibiotics and potentially in the outpatient setting. The Infectious Disease Society of America (IDSA) has published recommendations for antibiotic use in these low-risk patients. These patients must have an expected neutropenic timeframe of 7 days or less and not have comorbidities or signs of hemodynamic instability, gastrointestinal symptoms, altered mental status, pulmonary problems (infiltrate, hypoxia, or underlying chronic obstructive pulmonary disease), or liver or kidney disease or impairment). If a patient is to be treated as an outpatient, he or she must also have good support at home and easy access to returning to the hospital if the clinical status worsens.

Antibiotics should be continued until the neutrophil count is rising and > 500/mcL (> 0.5×10^9/L) for at least 1 day and the patient has been afebrile for 2 days. If an organism is identified through the cultures, the antibiotics should be adjusted to the antibiotic sensitivities of the isolate; treatment should be continued for the appropriate period of time and at least until the neutrophil count recovers.

For the neutropenic patient who is persistently febrile despite broad-spectrum antibiotics, an empiric antifungal drug should be added (amphotericin B, caspofungin, itraconazole, voriconazole, or liposomal amphotericin B).

Freifeld AG et al. Clinical practice guideline for the use of antimicrobial agents in neutropenic patients with cancer: 2010 Update by the Infectious Diseases Society of America. Clin Infect Dis. 2011 Feb 15;52(4):427–31. [PMID: 21205990]

PRIMARY CANCER TREATMENT

SYSTEMIC CANCER THERAPY

Detailed guidelines from the NCCN for cancer treatment can be found at www.nccn.org.

Use of cytotoxic drugs, hormones, antihormones, and biologic agents has become a highly specialized and increasingly effective means of treating cancer, with therapy administered and monitored by a medical oncologist or hematologist. Selection of specific drugs or protocols for various types of cancer is usually based on results of clinical trials. Increasingly, newer agents are being identified that target specific molecular pathways. Yet, both initial and acquired drug resistance remains a challenge. Described mechanisms of drug resistance include impaired membrane transport of drugs, enhanced drug metabolism, mutated target proteins, and blockage of apoptosis due to mutations in cellular proteins.

TOXICITY & DOSE MODIFICATION OF CHEMOTHERAPEUTIC AGENTS

Use of chemotherapy to treat cancer is generally guided by results from clinical trials in individual tumor types. The complexity of treating cancer has increased over the last decade as more drugs, including those with novel mechanisms of action, have been approved by the Food and Drug Administration and introduced into general practice. Drug side effects and toxicities must be anticipated and carefully monitored. The short- and long-term toxicities of individual drugs are listed in Tables 39–12 and 39–13. Decisions on dose modifications for toxicities should be guided by the intent of therapy. In the palliative setting where the aim of therapy is to improve symptoms and quality of life, lowering doses to minimize toxicity is commonly done. However, when the goal of treatment is cure, dosing frequency and intensity should be maintained whenever possible.

A CBC including a differential count, with absolute neutrophil count and platelet count, and liver and kidney tests should be obtained before the initiation of chemotherapy. In patients with normal CBCs as well as normal liver and kidney function, drugs are started at their full dose. When the intent of chemotherapy is cure, including treatment in the adjuvant setting, every attempt should be made to schedule chemotherapy on time and at full dose. A CBC with differential may be checked at mid cycle (to determine the nadir of the absolute neutrophil and platelet counts), and liver and kidney function tests should be obtained immediately before the next cycle of chemotherapy.

Dose reductions may be necessary for patients with impaired kidney or liver function depending on the clearance mechanism of the drug. For patients receiving chemotherapy for palliation, bone marrow toxicity can be managed with dose reductions or delaying the next treatment cycle. A schema for dose modification is shown in Table 39–14.

1. Bone Marrow Toxicity

A. Neutropenia

Granulocyte colony-stimulating factor (G-CSF), given as either daily subcutaneous injections (filgrastim, 300 mcg or 480 mcg) or as a one-time dose (pegfilgrastim, 6 mg) beginning 24 hours after cytotoxic chemotherapy is completed, has been shown to reduce the duration and severity of granulocytopenia following cytotoxic chemotherapy (Table 39–13). The American Society of Clinical Oncology and NCCN guidelines recommend primary prophylaxis with a G-CSF when there is at least a 20% risk of febrile neutropenia or when the patient's age, medical history, and disease characteristics put the patient at high risk for complications related to myelosuppression.

B. Anemia

Erythropoiesis-stimulating agents (ESAs) ameliorate the anemia and its associated symptoms that are caused by cancer chemotherapy but these drugs have untoward effects, including an increased risk of thromboembolism, and even more concerning, potentially decreased survival due to cancer-related deaths. These findings have prompted the US Food and Drug Administration and other organizations (American Society of Hematology, American Society of Clinical Oncology, and NCCN) to issue advisories and guidelines limiting their use. The NCCN recommendation that these drugs should not be used when the intent of chemotherapy is curative is based on evidence that survival may be affected by the administration of ESAs. Studies done in patients with potentially curable head and neck, breast, and cervical cancers have shown inferior outcomes when ESAs were used. It is important to point out that the target hemoglobin used in these studies was higher than is currently recommended. Nonetheless, ESAs cannot be currently recommended when the intent of therapy is cure. The alternative to managing symptomatic anemia in these patients receiving curative chemotherapy is administration of red blood cell transfusions.

ESAs can be an option in cancer patients with symptomatic anemia undergoing palliative treatment; patient preference is important in determining when to use ESAs or transfusions. When using ESAs, treatment should not be initiated until the hemoglobin is < 10 g/dL (< 100 g/L) with the medication held when the hemoglobin is > 12 g/dL (> 120 g/L). Epoetin alfa can be given subcutaneously as a weekly dose of 30,000–40,000 units with a target hemoglobin of 11–12 g/dL (110–120 g/L) (see Table 39–13). Darbepoetin alfa is given subcutaneously every 2–3 weeks at a dose of 200–300 mcg with the same target hemoglobin. Patients need to be iron replete to have maximum therapeutic effect. Uncontrolled hypertension is a contraindication to the use of ESAs; blood pressure must be controlled prior to initiation of this therapy. The FDA mandates that prescribing clinicians receive specific education on use of ESAs, and patients receiving ESAs must be provided written material describing the risks and benefits of the drug.

C. Thrombocytopenia

Drug management of chemotherapy-induced thrombocytopenia is more limited. The only available drug, oprelvekin or recombinant interleukin-11, has modest activity in improving thrombocytopenia associated with chemotherapy; however, it is rarely used due to the side effects of fluid retention, heart failure, and arrhythmias. Thrombopoietin, the protein that stimulates megakaryopoiesis in vivo, was isolated in 1994. Despite much work attempting to produce a clinically effective thrombopoietin agent for therapeutic use, no such drug is commercially available for this indication. Two drugs that activate the thrombopoietin receptor and are approved for use in idiopathic thrombocytopenia, romiplostim and eltrombopag, have not as yet been shown to be beneficial in patients receiving chemotherapy.

Table 39–12. Chemotherapeutic agents.

Chemotherapeutic Agent	Usual Adult Dosage	Adverse Effects
Alkylating Agents—Nitrogen Mustards		
Bendamustine (Treanda)	100–120 mg/m² intravenously every 3–4 weeks	Acute: hypersensitivity, nausea, vomiting Delayed: myelosuppression, rash, pyrexia, fatigue
Cyclophosphamide (Cytoxan)	500–1000 mg/m² intravenously every 3 weeks; 100 mg/m²/d orally for 14 days every 4 weeks; various doses	Acute: nausea and vomiting Delayed: myelosuppression, alopecia, hemorrhagic cystitis, cardiotoxicity (high dose)
Estramustine (Emcyt)	14 mg/kg/d orally in three or four divided doses	Acute: nausea, diarrhea Delayed: gynecomastia, edema
Ifosfamide (Ifex)	1200 mg/m² intravenously daily for 5 days every 3 weeks; various doses	Acute: nausea and vomiting Delayed: alopecia, myelosuppression, hemorrhagic cystitis, neurotoxicity
Mechlorethamine (Mustargen)	0.4 mg/kg intravenously every 3–6 weeks	Acute: nausea and vomiting Delayed: myelosuppression
Melphalan (Alkeran)	0.25 mg/kg/d or 8–10 mg/m²/d orally for 4 days every 4–6 weeks; 16 mg/m² intravenously every 2–4 weeks; various doses	Acute: nausea, vomiting, diarrhea, hypersensitivity (intravenously) Delayed: mucositis (intravenously), myelosuppression, increased risk of secondary malignancies
Alkylating Agents—Platinum Analogs		
Carboplatin (Paraplatin)	Area under the curve (AUC)-based dosing use Calvert equation [Dose (mg) = AUC × (GFR + 25)] AUC = 2–7 mg/mL/min every 2–4 weeks	Acute: nausea and vomiting Delayed: myelosuppression, electrolyte disturbances, peripheral neuropathy, nephrotoxicity, hypersensitivity
Cisplatin (Platinol)	50–100 mg/m² intravenously every 3–4 weeks; 20 mg/m²/d intravenously for 5 days every 3 weeks; various doses	Acute: nausea and vomiting Delayed: nephrotoxicity, ototoxicity, neurotoxicity, myelosuppression, electrolyte disturbances
Oxaliplatin (Eloxatin)	85–130 mg/m² intravenously every 2–3 weeks	Acute: peripheral neuropathy exacerbated by cold, nausea, vomiting, diarrhea Delayed: myelosuppression, elevated transaminases
Alkylating Agents—Triazenes		
Dacarbazine (DTIC-Dome)	375 mg/m² intravenously on day 1 and 15 every 4 weeks; 900–1000 mg/m² intravenously over 3 to 4 days; various doses	Acute: nausea, vomiting, photosensitivity Delayed: myelosuppression, anorexia, hypotension, flu-like syndrome
Procarbazine (Matulane)	60–100 mg/m² orally for 14 days every 4 weeks; various doses	Acute: nausea and vomiting Delayed: myelosuppression, disulfiram-like reaction, MAO inhibition, rash
Temozolomide (Temodar)	75 mg/m² orally daily during radiation for 42 days; 150–200 mg/m² orally for 5 days every 4 weeks	Acute: nausea, vomiting, constipation Delayed: myelosuppression, fatigue
Alkylating Agents—Miscellaneous		
Busulfan (Myleran)	1–8 mg orally daily; 0.8 mg/kg intravenously every 6 hours for 4 days	Acute: nausea and vomiting Delayed: myelosuppression, mucositis, rash, edema, electrolyte disturbances, hepatic veno-occlusive disease (high dose)
Chlorambucil (Leukeran)	0.1–0.2 mg/kg/d orally for 3–6 weeks; 0.4 mg/kg pulse every 4 weeks	Acute: nausea Delayed: myelosuppression, rash
Lomustine (CCNU)	100–130 mg/m² orally every 6 weeks	Acute: nausea and vomiting Delayed: myelosuppression
Antimetabolites—Folate Antagonists		
Methotrexate (MTX; Trexall)	**Intrathecal:** 12 mg **High dose:** 1000–12,000 mg/m² intravenously every 2–3 weeks	Acute: nausea, vomiting, mucositis Delayed: myelosuppression, nephrotoxicity, hepatotoxicity, neurotoxicity, photosensitivity, pulmonary toxicity

(continued)

Table 39–12. Chemotherapeutic agents. (continued)

Chemotherapeutic Agent	Usual Adult Dosage	Adverse Effects
Pemetrexed (Alimta)	500 mg/m^2 intravenously every 3 weeks	Acute: nausea, vomiting, diarrhea, rash Delayed: myelosuppression, fatigue, mucositis
Pralatrexate (Folotyn)	30 mg/m^2 intravenous bolus once weekly for 6 weeks in 7-week cycle	Acute: nausea, constipation Delayed: mucositis, myelosuppression, edema, fever, fatigue, cough
Antimetabolites—Purine Analogs		
Cladribine (Leustatin)	0.1 mg/kg/d subcutaneously daily for 5 days or 0.09 mg/kg/d intravenously via continuous infusion for 7 days	Acute: nausea, injection site reaction Delayed: myelosuppression, immunosuppression, fever, fatigue, rash
Clofarabine (Clolar)	52 mg/m^2 intravenously daily for 5 days every 2–6 weeks (for patients < 21 years of age)	Acute: nausea, vomiting, diarrhea Delayed: myelosuppression, hepatotoxicity, nephrotoxicity, rash, capillary leak syndrome
Fludarabine (Fludara)	25 mg/m^2 intravenously for 5 days every 4 weeks	Acute: fever, nausea, vomiting Delayed: asthenia, myelosuppression, immunosuppression, neurotoxicity, anorexia
Mercaptopurine (6-MP; Purinethol)	**Induction:** 2.5–5 mg/kg/d orally **Maintenance:** 1.5–2.5 mg/kg/d orally	Acute: nausea, vomiting, diarrhea, rash Delayed: myelosuppression, immunosuppression, hepatotoxicity, mucositis
Pentostatin (Nipent)	2–4 mg/m^2 intravenously every 2–3 weeks	Acute: nausea, vomiting, rash Delayed: myelosuppression, fever, myalgia, immunosuppression, hepatotoxicity, cough
Antimetabolites—Pyrimidine Analogs		
Azacitidine (Vidaza)	75–100 mg/m^2 subcutaneously or intravenously for 7 days every 4 weeks	Acute: injection site reaction (subcutaneously), nausea, diarrhea, fever Delayed: myelosuppression, dyspnea, arthralgia
Capecitabine (Xeloda)	1000–1250 mg/m^2 orally twice a day for 14 days every 3 weeks	Acute: nausea, vomiting, diarrhea Delayed: hand-foot syndrome, mucositis, hyperbilirubinemia, myelosuppression
Cytarabine (Ara-C, Cytosar U)	**Standard dose:** 100 mg/m^2/d intravenously via continuous infusion for 7 days **High dose:** 1000–3000 mg/m^2 intravenously every 12 hours for 2–6 days	Acute: nausea, vomiting, rash, flu-like syndrome Delayed: myelosuppression **High-dose therapy:** neurotoxicity, ocular toxicities
Decitabine (Dacogen)	15 mg/m^2 intravenously every 8 hours for 3 days every 8 weeks; 20 mg m^2 intravenously daily for 5 days	Acute: nausea, vomiting, hyperglycemia Delayed: myelosuppression, fever, fatigue, cough
Fluorouracil (Adrucil)	400 mg/m^2 intravenous bolus followed by 2400 mg/m^2 intravenously over 46 hours every 2 weeks; 1000 mg/m^2 intravenously via continuous infusion for 4–5 days every 3–4 weeks; various doses	Acute: nausea, vomiting, diarrhea Delayed: myelosuppression, hand-foot syndrome, mucositis, photosensitivity, cardiotoxicity (rare)
Gemcitabine (Gemzar)	1000–1250 mg/m^2 intravenously on days 1 and 8 every 3 weeks or days 1, 8, 15 every 4 weeks	Acute: nausea, vomiting, rash, flu-like symptoms, fever, diarrhea Delayed: myelosuppression, edema, elevated transaminases
Antimicrotubules—Vinca Alkaloids		
Vinblastine (Velban)	6 mg/m^2 intravenously on days 1 and 15 every 4 weeks; various doses	Acute: constipation Delayed: myelosuppression, alopecia, bone pain, malaise
Vincristine (Oncovin)	0.5–1.4 mg/m^2 intravenously every 3 weeks; various doses; maximum single dose usually limited to 2 mg	Acute: constipation, nausea Delayed: peripheral neuropathy, alopecia
Liposomal Vincristine (Marqibo)	2.25 mg/m^2 intravenously every 7 days	Acute: constipation, nausea Delayed: fatigue, neurotoxicity, myelosuppression

(continued)

Table 39–12. Chemotherapeutic agents. (continued)

Chemotherapeutic Agent	Usual Adult Dosage	Adverse Effects
Vinorelbine (Navelbine)	25–30 mg/m² intravenously weekly	Acute: nausea, vomiting Delayed: myelosuppression, peripheral neuropathy, constipation, alopecia, asthenia
Antimicrotubules—Taxanes		
Cabazitaxel (Jevtana)	25 mg/m² intravenously every 3 weeks	Acute: diarrhea, nausea, vomiting, hypersensitivity Delayed: myelosuppression, peripheral neuropathy, fatigue
Docetaxel (Taxotere)	60–100 mg/m² intravenously every 3 weeks	Acute: nausea, vomiting, diarrhea, hypersensitivity, rash Delayed: myelosuppression, asthenia, peripheral neuropathy, alopecia, edema, mucositis
Paclitaxel (Taxol)	135–175 mg/m² intravenously every 3 weeks; 50–80 mg/m² intravenously weekly; various doses	Acute: diarrhea, nausea, vomiting, hypersensitivity Delayed: myelosuppression, peripheral neuropathy, alopecia, mucositis, arthralgia
Paclitaxel protein-bound (Abraxane)	100–125 mg/m² on days 1, 8, 15 every 3–4 weeks; 260 mg/m² intravenously every 3 weeks	Acute: nausea, vomiting, diarrhea Delayed: myelosuppression, peripheral neuropathy, alopecia, asthenia
Antimicrotubules—Epothilone		
Ixabepilone (Ixempra)	40 mg/m² intravenously every 3 weeks	Acute: nausea, vomiting, diarrhea, hypersensitivity Delayed: peripheral neuropathy, fatigue, alopecia, myelosuppression, mucositis, arthralgia
Enzyme Inhibitors—Anthracyclines		
Daunorubicin (Cerubidine)	30–60 mg/m² intravenously for 3 days	Acute: nausea, vomiting, diarrhea, red/orange discoloration of urine, infusion-related reactions (liposomal products) Delayed: myelosuppression, mucositis, alopecia, hand-foot syndrome (liposomal doxorubicin), cardiotoxicity (dose related)
Liposomal Daunorubicin (Daunoxome)	40 mg/m² intravenously every 2 weeks	
Doxorubicin (Adriamycin)	45–75 mg/m² intravenously every 3 weeks; various doses	
Liposomal Doxorubicin (Lipodox)	20–50 mg/m² intravenously every 3–4 weeks	
Epirubicin (Ellence)	60–120 mg/m² intravenously every 3–4 weeks	
Idarubicin (Idamycin)	10–12 mg/m² intravenously for 3 days	
Enzyme Inhibitors—Topoisomerase Inhibitors		
Etoposide (Vepesid)	50–100 mg/m² intravenously for 3–5 days every 3 weeks	Acute: nausea, vomiting, diarrhea, hypersensitivity, fever, hypotension Delayed: myelosuppression, alopecia, fatigue
Etoposide phosphate (Etopophos)	35–100 mg/m² intravenously for 3–5 days every 3–4 weeks	
Irinotecan (Camptosar)	180 mg/m² intravenously every other week; various doses	Acute: diarrhea, cholinergic syndrome, nausea, vomiting Delayed: myelosuppression, alopecia, asthenia
Topotecan (Hycamtin)	1.5 mg/m² intravenously for 5 days every 3 weeks; 2.3 mg/m² orally for 5 days every 3 weeks	Acute: nausea, vomiting, diarrhea Delayed: myelosuppression, alopecia, asthenia
Immunomodulatory Therapy		
Lenalidomide (Revlimid)	5–25 mg orally once daily on days 1–21 of 28-day cycle; or continuously	Acute: diarrhea, rash Delayed: myelosuppression, fatigue, venous thromboembolism, potential for birth defects
Pomalidomide (Pomalyst)	4 mg orally once daily on days 1–21 of 28-day cycle	Acute: nausea, diarrhea, dizziness Delayed: myelosuppression, fatigue, neuropathy, upper respiratory tract infections, venous thromboembolism, potential for birth defects

(continued)

Table 39–12. Chemotherapeutic agents. (continued)

Chemotherapeutic Agent	Usual Adult Dosage	Adverse Effects
Thalidomide (Thalomid)	50–800 mg orally once daily	Acute: sedation, constipation, rash Delayed: edema, peripheral neuropathy, venous thrombo-embolism, potential for birth defects
Targeted Therapy—Monoclonal Antibodies		
Ado-trastuzumab emtansine (Kadcyla)	3.6 mg/kg intravenously every 3 weeks	Acute: infusion-related reaction, nausea Delayed: fatigue, musculoskeletal pain, thrombocytopenia, cardiotoxicity, heptatotoxicity
Alemtuzumab (Campath)	3–10 mg intravenously or subcutaneously three times weekly	Acute: infusion-related reaction, nausea, vomiting, hypotension, rash Delayed: myelosuppression, immunosuppression
Bevacizumab (Avastin)	5–15 mg/kg intravenously every 2–3 weeks	Acute: infusion-related reaction Delayed: hypertension, proteinuria, wound healing complications, gastrointestinal perforation, hemorrhage
Brentuximab vedotin (Adcetris)	1.8 mg/kg intravenously every 3 weeks	Acute: infusion-related reaction, nausea, vomiting, diarrhea Delayed: myelosuppression, peripheral neuropathy, fatigue, rash, cough
Cetuximab (Erbitux)	Loading dose 400 mg/m^2 intravenously, maintenance dose 250 mg/m^2 intravenously weekly	Acute: infusion-related reaction, nausea, diarrhea Delayed: acneiform skin rash, hypomagnesemia, asthenia, paronychial inflammation, dyspnea
Ibritumomab tiuxetan (Zevalin)	0.4 mCi/kg intravenously on day 7, 8, or 9	Acute: infusion-related reaction, nausea, diarrhea Delayed: myelosuppression, asthenia, nasopharyngitis
Ipilimumab (Yervoy)	3 mg/kg intravenously every 3 weeks for a total of four doses	Acute: infusion-related reaction Delayed: fatigue, diarrhea, colitis, pruritus, rash, hepatotoxicity, neuropathy, endocrinopathy
Obinutuzumab (Gazyva)	Cycle 1: 100 mg intravenously on day 1, 900 mg on day 2, 1000 mg on day 8 and 15 of a 28-day cycle; Cycles 2–6: 1000 mg intravenously on day 1	Acute: infusion-related reaction, tumor lysis syndrome Delayed: myelosuppression, pyrexia, cough, musculoskeletal disorder, potential hepatitis B reactivation
Ofatumumab (Arzerra)	300 mg initial dose intravenously, followed 1 week later by 2000 mg intravenously weekly for 7 doses, followed 4 weeks later by 2000 mg intravenously every 4 weeks for four doses	Acute: infusion-related reaction, diarrhea, nausea Delayed: neutropenia, infections, pyrexia, rash, fatigue, potential hepatitis B reactivation
Panitumumab (Vectibix)	6 mg/kg intravenously every 2 weeks	Acute: infusion-related reaction, nausea Delayed: acneiform skin rash, hypomagnesemia, asthenia, paronychia, fatigue, dyspnea
Pertuzumab (Perjeta)	840 mg intravenously once followed by 420 mg intravenously every 3 weeks	Acute: infusion-related reaction, diarrhea, nausea Delayed: fatigue, alopecia, neutropenia, rash, peripheral neuropathy, cardiomyopathy
Rituximab (Rituxan)	375 mg/m^2 intravenously weekly for 4 weeks, or every 3–4 weeks	Acute: infusion-related reaction, tumor lysis syndrome Delayed: lymphopenia, asthenia, rash, potential hepatitis B reactivation
Trastuzumab (Herceptin)	Initial dose 4 mg/kg intravenously then 2 mg/kg intravenously weekly; or initial dose 8 mg/kg then 6 mg/kg intravenously every 3 weeks	Acute: headache, nausea, diarrhea, infusion-related reaction Delayed: myelosuppression, pyrexia, cardiomyopathy, pulmonary toxicity (rare)
Targeted Therapy—Kinase Inhibitors		
Afatinib (Gilotrif)	40 mg orally once daily without food	Acute: diarrhea Delayed: acneiform rash, stomatitis, paronychia
Axitinib (Inlyta)	5–10 mg orally twice daily	Acute: diarrhea, nausea, vomiting Delayed: hypertension, fatigue, dysphonia, hand-foot syndrome, elevated transaminases

(Continued)

Table 39–12. Chemotherapeutic agents. (continued)

Chemotherapeutic Agent	Usual Adult Dosage	Adverse Effects
Bosutinib (Bosulif)	500–600 mg orally once daily with food	Acute: diarrhea, nausea, vomiting Delayed: myelosuppression, rash, abdominal pain, hepato-toxicity, fluid retention
Crizotinib (Xalkori)	250 mg orally twice daily	Acute: nausea, vomiting, diarrhea, constipation Delayed: vision disorder, edema, elevated transaminases, fatigue
Dabrafenib (Tafinlar)	150 mg orally twice daily without food	Acute: headache Delayed: hyperkeratosis, fever, hand-foot syndrome, hyper-glycemia, hypophosphatemia
Dasatinib (Sprycel)	100–180 mg orally once daily	Acute: diarrhea, nausea, vomiting Delayed: myelosuppression, fluid retention, fatigue, dyspnea, musculoskeletal pain, rash
Erlotinib (Tarceva)	100 or 150 mg orally once daily without food	Acute: diarrhea, nausea, vomiting Delayed: acneiform skin rash, fatigue, anorexia, dyspnea
Everolimus (Afinitor)	10 mg orally once daily	Acute: mucositis, diarrhea, nausea Delayed: myelosuppression, fatigue, edema, hypercholes-terolemia, hypertriglyceridemia, hyperglycemia
Ibrutinib (Imbruvica)	560 mg orally once daily	Acute: diarrhea, nausea Delayed: myelosuppression, fatigue, edema, rash elevated serum creatinine, hemorrhage
Imatinib (Gleevec)	100–800 mg orally once daily with food	Acute: nausea, vomiting, diarrhea Delayed: edema, muscle cramps, rash, myelosuppression, hepatotoxicity
Lapatinib (Tykerb)	1250 mg or 1500 mg orally once daily	Acute: diarrhea, nausea, vomiting Delayed: hand-foot syndrome, fatigue, hepatotoxicity (rare)
Nilotinib (Tasigna)	300 or 400 mg orally twice daily without food	Acute: nausea, vomiting, diarrhea Delayed: rash, fatigue, myelosuppression, prolonged QT interval (rare)
Pazopanib (Votrient)	800 mg orally once daily without food	Acute: diarrhea, nausea, vomiting Delayed: hypertension, hair color changes, hepatotoxicity, hemorrhage
Regorafenib (Stivarga)	160 mg orally once daily with food (low-fat breakfast)	Acute: diarrhea Delayed: asthenia, hand-foot syndrome, anorexia, hyper-tension, mucositis, myelosuppression, hepatotoxicity
Sorafenib (Nexavar)	400 mg orally twice daily without food	Acute: diarrhea and nausea Delayed: fatigue, hand-foot syndrome, rash, hypertension, hemorrhage
Sunitinib (Sutent)	50 mg orally once daily for 4 weeks followed by 2 weeks rest; 37.5 mg orally daily	Acute: diarrhea and nausea Delayed: hypertension, hand-foot syndrome, rash, yellow discoloration of skin, fatigue, hypothyroidism, mucositis, left ventricular dysfunction, bleeding, hepatotoxicity
Temsirolimus (Torisel)	25 mg intravenously weekly	Acute: hypersensitivity, rash Delayed: myelosuppression, asthenia, hyperglycemia, hyperlipidemia, elevated serum creatinine
Trametinib (Mekinist)	2 mg orally once daily without food	Acute: rash, diarrhea Delayed: elevated transaminases, lymphedema, cardiomyopathy
Vandetanib (Caprelsa)	300 mg orally once daily	Acute: diarrhea, nausea Delayed: acneiform skin rash, hypertension, prolonged QT interval

(continued)

Table 39–12. Chemotherapeutic agents. (continued)

Chemotherapeutic Agent	Usual Adult Dosage	Adverse Effects
Vemurafenib (Zelboraf)	960 mg orally twice daily	Acute: nausea, hypersensitivity (rare) Delayed: photosensitivity, rash, arthralgia, alopecia, fatigue, prolonged QT interval, cutaneous squamous cell carcinoma
Miscellaneous Agents		
Altretamine (Hexalen)	260 mg/m^2 orally in four divided doses for 14–21 days every 4 weeks	Acute: nausea, vomiting Delayed: neurotoxicity, myelosuppression
Arsenic trioxide (Trisenox)	0.15 mg/kg intravenously daily	Acute: nausea, dizziness Delayed: acute promyelocytic leukemia differentiation syndrome, prolonged QT interval
Asparaginase Erwinia chrysanthemi (Erwinaze)	25,000 international units/m^2 intramuscularly three times weekly	Acute: hypersensitivity, nausea, vomiting Delayed: coagulation abnormalities, hepatotoxicity, pancreatitis, neurotoxicity
Bleomycin (Blenoxane)	10 units/m^2 intravenously on days 1 and 15 every 28 days; 30 units intravenously on day 2, 9, and 16 every 21 days	Acute: hypersensitivity, fever Delayed: skin reaction (rash, hyperpigmentation of skin, striae), mucositis, pneumonitis
Bortezomib (Velcade)	1.3 mg/m^2 intravenous bolus or subcutaneously on days 1, 4, 8, 11 followed by a 10-day rest or weekly for 4 weeks followed by 13-day rest	Acute: nausea, vomiting, diarrhea Delayed: peripheral neuropathy, fatigue, myelosuppression
Carfilzomib (Kyprolis)	20 mg/m^2 or 27 mg/m^2 intravenously on days 1, 2, 8, 9, 15, 16 followed by a 12-day rest (28-day cycle)	Acute: nausea, dyspnea, diarrhea, infusion-related reaction Delayed: fatigue, myelosuppression, elevated serum creatinine
Dactinomycin (Cosmegen)	15 mcg/kg or 400–600 mcg/m^2 intravenously daily for 5 days	Acute: nausea, vomiting Delayed: myelosuppression, mucositis, rash, diarrhea, hepatoveno-occlusive disease (rare)
Denileukin diftitox (Ontak)	9 or 18 mcg/kg intravenously daily for 5 days every 21 days	Acute: flu-like syndrome, nausea, vomiting, hypersensitivity Delayed: diarrhea, elevated transaminases, capillary leak syndrome
Hydroxyurea (Hydrea)	20–30 mg/kg orally daily	Acute: none Delayed: myelosuppression
Mitomycin (Mutamycin)	10–20 mg/m^2 intravenously every 4–8 weeks; 20–40 mg intravesically	Acute: cystitis (intravesically), nausea, vomiting Delayed: myelosuppression, mucositis, anorexia
Mitoxantrone (Novantrone)	12–14 mg/m^2 intravenously every 3 weeks; 12 mg/m^2 intravenously for 2–3 days	Acute: nausea, vomiting, diarrhea, mucositis, blue-green discoloration of urine Delayed: myelosuppression, alopecia, cardiotoxicity
Omacetaxine mepesuccinate (Synribo)	Induction: 1.25 mg/m^2 subcutaneously twice daily for 14 days every 28 days Maintenance: 1.25 mg/m^2 subcutaneously twice daily for 7 days every 28 days	Acute: diarrhea, nausea, fatigue, injection site reaction Delayed: myelosuppression, infection
Romidepsin (Istodax)	14 mg/m^2 intravenously on days 1, 8, 15 of a 28-day cycle	Acute: nausea, vomiting Delayed: myelosuppression, fatigue, anorexia, ECG changes
Tretinoin (All-Trans-Retinoic Acid, ATRA, Vesanoid)	45 mg/m^2 orally divided twice daily for 45–90 days or 30 days past complete remission	Acute: headache, nausea Delayed: vitamin A toxicity, retinoic acid-acute promyelocytic leukemia syndrome
Vismodegib (Erivedge)	150 mg orally once daily	Acute: fatigue, nausea, diarrhea Delayed: muscle spasms, alopecia, weight loss
Ziv-aflibercept (Zaltrap)	4 mg/kg intravenously every 2 weeks	Acute: diarrhea Delayed: myelosuppression, proteinuria, elevated transaminases, stomatitis, fatigue, hypertension

(continued)

Table 39–12. Chemotherapeutic agents. (continued)

Chemotherapeutic Agent	Usual Adult Dosage	Adverse Effects
Antiandrogens		
Bicalutamide (Casodex)	50 mg orally once daily	Acute: none Delayed: hot flashes, back pain, asthenia
Enzalutamide (Xtandi)	160 mg orally once daily	Acute: asthenia, diarrhea Delayed: hot flashes, arthralgia, peripheral edema
Flutamide (Eulexin)	250 mg orally every 8 hours	Acute: diarrhea Delayed: hot flashes, hepatotoxicity
Nilutamide (Nilandron)	300 mg orally for 30 days then 150 mg orally once daily	Acute: none Delayed: visual disturbances (impaired adaptation to dark), hot flashes, disulfiram-like reaction
Selective Estrogen Receptor Modulators		
Tamoxifen (Nolvadex)	20–40 mg orally once daily	Acute: none Delayed: hot flashes, vaginal discharge, menstrual irregularities, arthralgia
Toremifene (Fareston)	60 mg orally once daily	Acute: nausea Delayed: hot flashes, vaginal discharge
Aromatase Inhibitors		
Anastrozole (Arimidex)	1 mg orally once daily	Acute: nausea Delayed: hot flashes, peripheral edema, asthenia, hypercholesterolemia, arthralgia/myalgia, osteoporosis
Exemestane (Aromasin)	25 mg orally once daily	
Letrozole (Femara)	2.5 mg orally once daily	
Pure Estrogen Receptor Antagonist		
Fulvestrant (Faslodex)	500 mg intramuscularly on days 1, 15, 29, then monthly	Acute: injection site reaction, nausea Delayed: hot flashes, bone pain, elevated transaminases
Progestins		
Megestrol acetate (Megace)	40–320 mg orally in divided doses (four times a day)	Acute: none Delayed: hot flashes, tumor flare, weight gain, edema
LHRH Analogs		
Goserelin acetate (Zoladex)	3.6 mg subcutaneously every month; 10.8 mg subcutaneously every 3 months	Acute: injection site discomfort Delayed: hot flashes, tumor flare, edema, decreased libido, erectile dysfunction, osteoporosis
Leuprolide (Lupron)	7.5 mg intramuscularly or subcutaneously every month; 22.5 mg intramuscularly or subcutaneously every 3 months; 30 mg intramuscularly or subcutaneously every 4 months; 45 mg intramuscularly or subcutaneously every 6 months	
Triptorelin pamoate (Trelstar)	3.75 mg intramuscularly every 4 weeks; 11.25 mg intramuscularly every 12 weeks; 22.5 mg every 24 weeks	
LHRH Antagonist		
Degarelix (Firmagon)	240 mg subcutaneously once then 80 mg subcutaneously every 28 days	Acute: injection site reaction Delayed: hot flashes, weight gain, elevated transaminases, QT prolongation
Adrenocorticosteroids		
Abiraterone (Zytiga)	1000 mg orally once daily	Acute: diarrhea, edema Delayed: adrenal insufficiency, hepatotoxicity, joint pain, hypokalemia
Ketoconazole	400 mg orally three times daily	Acute: nausea and vomiting Delayed: hepatotoxicity, adrenal insufficiency

(continued)

Table 39–12. Chemotherapeutic agents. (continued)

Chemotherapeutic Agent	Usual Adult Dosage	Adverse Effects
Biologic Response Modifiers		
Aldesleukin (IL-2, Proleukin)	600,000 international units/kg intravenously every 8 hours for 14 doses, repeat after 9 days rest	Acute: hypotension, nausea, vomiting, diarrhea, flu-like syndrome, capillary leak syndrome Delayed: myelosuppression, confusion, somnolence, oliguria
Interferon-alpha-2b (Intron A)	20 million international units/m² intravenously 5 days a week for 4 weeks then 10 million international units/m² subcutaneously three times a week for 48 weeks	Acute: flu-like syndrome, nausea, vomiting, diarrhea Delayed: myelosuppression, anorexia, alopecia, depression, elevated transaminases
Sipuleucel-T (Provenge)	One dose (minimum of 50 million autologous CD54+ cells) intravenously every 2 weeks for three doses	Acute: infusion-related reaction, nausea, vomiting Delayed: fatigue, back pain, arthralgia

GFR, glomerular filtration rate; LHRH, luteinizing hormone–releasing hormone; MAO, monoamine oxidase.

2. Chemotherapy-Induced Nausea & Vomiting

A number of cytotoxic anticancer drugs can induce nausea and vomiting, which can be the most anticipated and stressful side effects for patients. Chemotherapy-induced nausea and vomiting is mediated in part by the stimulation of at least two central nervous system receptors, 5-hydroxytryptamine subtype 3 ($5HT_3$) and neurokinin subtype 1 (NK_1). Chemotherapy-induced nausea and vomiting can be acute, occurring within minutes to hours of chemotherapy administration, or delayed until the second day and lasting up to 7 days. Anticipatory nausea and vomiting may even occur before the administration of chemotherapy. Chemotherapy drugs or drug regimens are classified into high, moderate, low, and minimal likelihoods of causing emesis (90%, 30–90%, 10–30%, < 10%, respectively). Highly emetogenic chemotherapy drugs include cisplatin, carmustine, cyclophosphamide at doses over 1.5 g/m², dacarbazine, mechlorethamine, and streptozocin or a combination of regularly dosed cyclophosphamide and anthracyclines. Chemotherapy drugs that are moderately emetogenic include azacitidine, bendamustine, carboplatin, cyclophosphamide, cytarabine, daunomycin, doxorubicin, epirubicin, idarubicin, ifosfamide, irinotecan, oxaliplatin, and temozolomide. Drugs with low emetic potential include bortezomib, brentuximab, docetaxel, etoposide, fluorouracil, gemcitabine, methotrexate, mitomycin, mitoxantrone, paclitaxel, pemetrexed, temsirolimus, and topotecan. Drugs with minimal risk of emesis include bevacizumab, bleomycin, cetuximab, cladribine, decitabine, fludarabine, panitumumab, rituximab, temsirolimus, trastuzumab, vinblastine, vincristine, and vinorelbine.

By understanding the physiology of chemotherapy-induced nausea and vomiting, major advances have occurred with the development of highly effective antiemetic drugs. Antagonists to the $5HT_3$-receptor include ondansetron, granisetron, dolasetron, tropisetron, and palonosetron. Ondansetron can be given either intravenously (8 mg or 0.15 mg/kg) or orally (24 mg for highly emetogenic chemotherapy, 8 mg twice daily for moderately emetogenic chemotherapy). Doses of 8 mg can be repeated parenterally or orally every 8 hours. Dosing of granisetron is 1 mg or 0.01 mg/kg intravenously or 1–2 mg orally. Dolasetron is given 1.8 mg/kg or a fixed dose of 100 mg intravenously or 100 mg can be given orally. Tropisetron is given at a dose of 5 mg either orally or intravenously. Palonosetron, a long-acting $5HT_3$ with high affinity for the $5HT_3$-receptor given at a dose of 0.25 mg intravenously, is effective for not only acute but also delayed emesis. The efficacy of the $5HT_3$-blockers is improved by adding 6–10 mg of either oral or intravenous dexamethasone.

Aprepitant and fosaprepitant are antagonists to the NK_1 receptor. Aprepitant is given as a 125-mg oral dose followed by 80 mg on the second and third day with a $5HT_3$-receptor antagonist (such as ondansetron or granisetron), the immediate and delayed protective effect for highly emetogenic chemotherapy is increased. Fosaprepitant, the intravenous formulation of aprepitant, can be given at a dose of 115 mg if followed by 2 days of aprepitant or at a dose of 150 mg if given alone.

Standard therapy for highly emetogenic chemotherapy includes a $5HT_3$-antagonist given on the first day, and both dexamethasone and a neurokinin-1 receptor antagonist given on the first day as well as the second and third days. Moderately emetogenic chemotherapy regimens are best managed with a two-drug regimen of palonosetron and dexamethasone. Palonosetron is now the preferred $5HT_3$-blocker due to its greater affinity for the $5HT_3$-receptor and its longer half-life.

Other adjunctive medications that may be helpful include lorazepam, 0.5–1.0 mg given orally every 6–8 hours, and prochlorperazine, 5–10 mg orally or intravenously every 8 hours. Lorazepam, in addition to antianxiety effects, has an antinausea effect. Prochlorperazine is generally sufficient to treat patients receiving low emetogenic chemotherapy. A suppository form of prochlorperazine, 25 mg, may be used for patients who are unable to swallow oral medications.

Table 39–13. Supportive care agents.

Agent	Indication	Usual Dose	Adverse Effects
Allopurinol (Xyloprim)	Prevent hyperuricemia from tumor lysis syndrome	600–800 mg/d orally	Acute: none Delayed: rash
Rasburicase (Elitek)	Prevent hyperuricemia from tumor lysis syndrome	3–6 mg intravenously once	Acute: hypersensitivity, nausea, vomiting, diarrhea, fever, headache Delayed: rash, peripheral edema
Mesna (Mesnex)	Prevent ifosfamide-induced hemorrhagic cystitis	20% of ifosfamide dose intravenously at 0, 4, and 8 hours; various doses	Acute: nausea, vomiting Delayed: fatigue
Leucovorin	Rescue after high-dose methotrexate; in combination with fluorouracil for colon cancer	10 mg/m^2 intravenously or orally every 6 hours; 20 mg/m^2 or 200–500 mg/m^2 intravenously before fluorouracil; various doses	Acute: nausea, vomiting, diarrhea Delayed: stomatitis, fatigue
Levoleucovorin (Fusilev)	Rescue after high-dose methotrexate; in combination with fluorouracil for colon cancer	7.5 mg intravenously every 6 hours for 10 doses; 100 mg/m^2 intravenously before fluorouracil	Acute: nausea, vomiting Delayed: stomatitis, diarrhea
Amifostine (Ethyol)	Prevent cisplatin nephropathy; prevent radiation-induced xerostomia	910 mg/m^2 intravenously before cisplatin; 200 mg/m^2 intravenously before radiation	Acute: nausea, vomiting, hypotension, infusion-related reaction Delayed: hypocalcemia
Dexrazoxane (Zinecard)	Prevent cardiomyopathy secondary to doxorubicin; anthracycline-induced injection site extravasation	10 times the doxorubicin dose intravenously before doxorubicin; 1000 mg/m^2 intravenously on days 1 and 2 then 500 mg/m^2 intravenously on day 3	Acute: nausea Delayed: myelosuppression, elevated transaminases
Palifermin (Kepivance)	Prevent mucositis following chemotherapy	60 mcg/kg/d intravenously for 3 days before and 3 days after chemotherapy	Acute: none Delayed: rash, fever, elevated serum amylase, erythema, edema
Pilocarpine (Salagen)	Radiation-induced xerostomia	5–10 mg orally three times a day	Acute: flushing, sweating, nausea, dizziness Delayed: increased urinary frequency, rhinitis
Radium Ra 223 Dichloride (Xofigo)	Symptomatic bone metastases	50 kilobecquerel/kg (1.35 microCurie/kg) intravenously every 4 weeks for 6 cycles	Acute: nausea, vomiting, diarrhea, peripheral edema Delayed: myelosuppression
Samarium-153 (Quadramet)	Symptomatic bone metastasis	1 milliCurie/kg intravenously	Acute: pain flare Delayed: myelosuppression
Strontium-89 (Metastron)	Symptomatic bone metastasis	148 megabecquerels (4 milliCuries) intravenously; or 1.5–2.2 megabecquerels/kg (40–60 microCuries/kg)	Acute: bone pain Delayed: myelosuppression
Bone-Modifying Agents			
Denosumab (Xgeva)	Osteolytic bone metastasis	120 mg subcutaneously every 4 weeks	Acute: nausea Delayed: hypocalcemia, hypophosphatemia, fatigue, osteonecrosis of the jaw
Pamidronate (Aredia)	Osteolytic bone metastasis, hypercalcemia of malignancy	90 mg intravenously every 3–4 weeks; 60–90 mg intravenously, may repeat after 7 days	Acute: nausea Delayed: dyspnea, arthralgia, bone pain, osteonecrosis of the jaw, nephrotoxicity, hypocalcemia
Zoledronic acid (Zometa)	Osteolytic bone metastasis, hypercalcemia of malignancy	4 mg intravenously every 3–4 weeks; 4 mg intravenously once, may repeat after 7 days	
Growth Factors			
Epoetin alfa (Epogen, Procrit)	Chemotherapy-induced anemia	40,000 units subcutaneously once weekly; 150 units/kg subcutaneously three times a week	Acute: injection site reaction Delayed: hypertension, thromboembolic events, increased risk of tumor progression or recurrence

(continued)

Table 39–13. Supportive care agents. (continued)

Agent	Indication	Usual Dose	Adverse Effects
Darbepoetin alfa (Aranesp)	Chemotherapy-induced anemia	2.25 mcg/kg subcutaneously weekly; 500 mcg subcutaneously every 3 weeks	
Filgrastim (Neupogen)	Febrile neutropenia prophy-laxis, mobilization of periph-eral stem cells	5–10 mcg/kg/d subcutaneously or intravenously once daily, treat past nadir	Acute: injection site reaction Delayed: bone pain
Pegfilgrastim (Neulasta)	Febrile neutropenia prophylaxis	6 mg subcutaneously once per chemotherapy cycle	Acute: injection site reaction Delayed: bone pain
Sargramostim (Leukine)	Myeloid reconstitution follow-ing bone marrow transplant, mobilization of peripheral blood stem cells	250 mcg/m² intravenously daily until the absolute neutrophil count is > 1500 cells/mcL for 3 consecutive days	Acute: fever, rash, pruritus, nausea, vomiting, diarrhea, injection site reaction, dyspnea Delayed: asthenia, bone pain, mucositis, edema, arrhythmia
Oprelvekin (Neumega)	Chemotherapy-induced thrombocytopenia	50 mcg/kg subcutaneously every day for 14–21 days or until post-nadir platelet count is > 50,000/mcL	Acute: hypersensitivity, nausea, vomiting, blurred vision, injection site reaction Delayed: edema, dyspnea, arrhythmias, febrile neutropenia, rash
Tbo-filgrastim (Neutroval)	Severe chemotherapy-induced neutropenia	5 mcg/kg subcutaneously once daily until neutrophil recovery	Acute: none Delayed: bone pain, leukocytosis

The importance of treating chemotherapy-induced nausea and vomiting expectantly and aggressively beginning with the first course of chemotherapy cannot be overemphasized. Patients being treated in the clinic setting should always be given antiemetics for home use with written instructions as well as contact numbers to call for advice.

3. Gastrointestinal Toxicity

Untoward effects of cancer chemotherapy include damage to the more rapidly growing cells of the body such as the mucosal lining from the mouth through the gastrointestinal tract. Oral symptoms range from mild mouth soreness to frank ulcerations in the mouth. Not uncommonly, mouth ulcerations will have superimposed candida or herpes simplex infections. In addition to receiving cytotoxic chemotherapy, a significant risk factor for development of oral mucositis is poor oral hygiene and existing caries or periodontal disease. Toxicity in the gastrointestinal tract

Table 39–14. A common scheme for dose modification of cancer chemotherapeutic agents.

Granulocyte Count (cells/mcL)	Platelet Count (/mcL)	Suggested Drug Dosage (% of Full Dose)
> 2000	> 100,000	100%
1000–2000	75,000–100,000	50%
< 2000	< 50,000	0%

usually manifests as diarrhea. Gastrointestinal symptoms can range from mild symptoms of loose stools to life-threatening diarrhea leading to dehydration and electrolyte imbalances. Drugs most commonly associated with causing mucositis in the mouth and the gastrointestinal tract are cytarabine, 5-fluorouracil, and methotrexate.

Patients undergoing treatment for head and neck cancer with concurrent chemotherapy and radiation therapy have a very high risk of developing severe mucositis.

Preventive strategies for managing oral mucositis includes a pretreatment dental examination, particularly for all head and neck cancer patients and any cancer patient with poor dental hygiene who will be receiving chemotherapy. For patients receiving fluorouracil, simple measures such as ice chips in the mouth for 30 minutes during infusion can reduce the incidence and severity of mucositis. Once mucositis is encountered, superimposed fungal infections should be treated with topical antifungal medications (oral nystatin mouth suspensions, or clotrimazole troches) or systemic therapy (fluconazole 100–400 mg orally daily). Suspected herpetic infections can be treated with acyclovir (up to 800 mg orally five times daily) or valacyclovir (1 g orally twice daily). Mucositis may also be managed with mouthwashes; it is also important to provide adequate pain medication.

Other strategies for prevention of oral mucositis include the use of the recombinant keratinocyte growth factor inhibitor, palifermin. Practice guidelines recommend prophylaxis with intravenous palifermin (60 mcg/kg/d) for patients receiving high-dose chemotherapy in order to reduce the incidence and duration of mucositis.

Diarrhea is most associated with fluorouracil, capecitabine, and irinotecan as well as the tyrosine kinase inhibitors (sorafenib, sunitinib, regorafenib, imatinib, dasatinib, nilotinib) and epithelial growth factor inhibitors (cetuximab, panitumumab, and erlotinib). Mild to moderate diarrhea can be managed with oral antidiarrheal medication (loperamide, 4 mg initially followed by 2 mg every 2–4 hours until bowel movements are formed). Occasionally, the diarrhea will be overwhelming causing dehydration, electrolyte imbalances, and acute kidney injury. These patients require inpatient management with aggressive intravenous hydration and replacement of electrolytes.

4. Skin Toxicity

Dermatologic complications from cancer chemotherapy can include hyperpigmentation (liposomal doxorubicin, busulfan, hydroxyurea), alopecia, photosensitivity, nail changes, acral erythema, and generalized rashes. Acral erythema, otherwise known as hand-foot syndrome and most commonly associated with administration of fluorouracil, capecitabine, and liposomal doxorubicin, manifests as painful palms or soles accompanied by erythema, progressing to blistering, desquamation, and ulceration in its worst forms. Management can include attempts at prevention with oral pyridoxine, 200 mg daily, and applying cold packs to the extremities while the chemotherapy is being administered. Agents targeting the epidermal growth factor pathway can cause an acne like rash; interestingly, the development of the rash may identify those who will respond to the drug. Inhibitors of the tyrosine kinase pathway are also associated with a high incidence of dermatologic complications, such as rash and acral erythema.

5. Miscellaneous Drug-Specific Toxicities

The toxicities of individual drugs have been summarized in Tables 39–12 and 39–13; however, several of these warrant additional mention, since they occur with frequently administered agents, and special measures are often indicated.

A. Hemorrhagic Cystitis Induced by Cyclophosphamide or Ifosfamide

Metabolic products of cyclophosphamide that retain cytotoxic activity are excreted into the urine. Some patients appear to metabolize more of the drug to these active excretory products; if their urine is concentrated, severe bladder damage may result. Patients receiving cyclophosphamide must maintain a high fluid intake prior to and following the administration of the drug and be counseled to empty their bladders frequently. Early symptoms suggesting bladder toxicity include dysuria and increased frequency or urination. Should microscopic hematuria develop, it is advisable to stop the drug temporarily or switch to a different alkylating agent, to increase fluid intake, and to administer a urinary analgesic such as phenazopyridine. With severe cystitis, large segments of bladder mucosa may be shed, resulting in prolonged gross hematuria. Such patients should be observed for signs of urinary obstruction and may require cystoscopy for removal of obstructing blood clots. The cyclophosphamide analog ifosfamide can cause severe hemorrhagic cystitis when used alone. However, when its use is followed by a series of doses of the neutralizing agent mesna, bladder toxicity can be prevented. Mesna can also be used for patients taking cyclophosphamide in whom cystitis develops.

B. Neuropathy Due to Vinca Alkaloids and Other Chemotherapy Drugs

Neuropathy is caused by a number of different chemotherapy drugs, the most common being vincristine. The peripheral neuropathy can be sensory, motor, autonomic, or a combination of these types. In its mildest form, it consists of paresthesias of the fingers and toes. Occasionally, acute jaw or throat pain can develop after vincristine therapy. This may be a form of trigeminal neuralgia. With continued vincristine therapy, the paresthesias extend to the proximal interphalangeal joints, hyporeflexia appears in the lower extremities, and significant weakness can develop. Other drugs in the vinca alkaloid class as well as the taxane drugs (paclitaxel and docetaxel) and agents to treat myeloma (thalidomide and bortezomib) cause similar toxicity. The presence of neurologic symptoms is not in itself a reason to stop therapy; the severity of the symptoms must be balanced against the goals of therapy. Usually though, the presence of moderate to severe paresthesias or the detection of motor impairment would result in the decision to discontinue the drug.

Constipation is the most common symptom of autonomic neuropathy associated with the vinca alkaloids. Patients receiving these drugs should be started on stool softeners and mild cathartics when therapy is begun; otherwise, severe impaction may result from an atonic bowel.

More serious autonomic involvement can lead to acute intestinal obstruction with signs indistinguishable from those of an acute abdomen. Bladder neuropathies are uncommon but may be severe. These two complications are absolute contraindications to continued vincristine therapy.

C. Methotrexate Toxicity

Methotrexate, a folate antagonist, is a commonly used drug and a key component of regimens to treat patients with leptomeningeal disease, acute lymphoblastic leukemia, and sarcomas. The dose used in intrathecal therapy is 12 mg. Methotrexate is almost entirely eliminated by the kidney. The methotrexate toxicity affects cells with rapid turnover, including the bone marrow and mucosa resulting in myelosuppression and mucositis. Methotrexate can also damage the liver and kidney manifesting as elevated liver enzymes and creatinine. High-dose methotrexate, usually defined as a dose of 500 mg/m^2 or more given over 4–36 hours, would be lethal without "rescue" of the normal tissues. Leucovorin, a form of folate, will reverse the toxic effects of methotrexate and is given until serum methotrexate levels are in the safe range (< 0.05 mmol/L). It is crucial that high-dose methotrexate and leucovorin are given precisely according to protocol as deviations of the timing of methotrexate delivery or delay in rescue can result in patient death. Lower doses of methotrexate can be problematic in patients with kidney disease who cannot clear the drug normally or with patients who have effusions. In the latter instance, methotrexate distributes itself in effusions and will leak out continuously, exposing normal tissue to small but cumulatively toxic amounts of the drug. If methotrexate is given to a patient who either has or develops kidney disease or to a patient with an effusion, prolonged rescue with leucovorin will be necessary.

Vigorous hydration and bicarbonate loading also appear to be important in preventing crystallization of high-dose methotrexate in the renal tubular epithelium and minimizing the possibility of nephrotoxicity. Daily monitoring of the serum creatinine is mandatory. Drugs impairing methotrexate excretion include aspirin, nonsteroidal anti-inflammatory drugs, amiodarone, omeprazole, penicillin, phenytoin, and sulfa compounds; these drugs should be stopped if possible before methotrexate administration.

D. Anthracycline Cardiotoxicity

A number of cancer chemotherapy drugs can cause cardiotoxicity. The most common class of drugs associated with cardiotoxicity is the anthracycline antibiotics, including doxorubicin, daunomycin, idarubicin, and epirubicin. They can produce acute (during administration), subacute (days to months following administration), and delayed (years following administration) cardiac toxicity. The most feared complication is the delayed development of heart failure. Risk factors for this debilitating toxicity include the anthracycline cumulative dose, age over 70, previous or concurrent irradiation of the chest, preexisting cardiac disease, and concurrent administration of chemotherapy drugs such as trastuzumab. The problem is greatest with doxorubicin because this drug is the most commonly administered anthracycline due to its major role in the treatment of lymphomas, sarcomas, breast cancer, and certain other solid tumors. Patients receiving anthracyclines should have a baseline multiple-gated radionuclide cardiac scan (MUGA) to calculate the left ventricular-ejection fraction (LVEF). If the LVEF is > 50%, anthracyclines can be administered; if the LVEF is < 30%, these drugs should not be given. For patients with intermediate cardiac function, anthracycline dosing, if necessary, should be cautiously done with LVEF monitoring between doses. Studies of left ventricular function and endomyocardial biopsies indicate that some changes in cardiac dynamics occur in most patients by the time they have received 300 mg/m^2 of doxorubicin. In general, patients should not receive a total dose of doxorubicin in excess of 450 mg/m^2; the dose should be lower if prior chest radiotherapy has been given. The appearance of a high resting pulse may herald the appearance of overt cardiac toxicity. Unfortunately, toxicity may be irreversible and frequently fatal at dosage levels above 550 mg/m^2. At lower doses (eg, 350 mg/m^2 of doxorubicin), the symptoms and signs of cardiac failure generally respond well to medical therapy as well as the discontinuation of anthracycline. Laboratory studies suggest that cardiac toxicity may be due to a mechanism involving the formation of intracellular free radicals in cardiac muscle. The iron chelator dexrazoxane has been approved for use as a cardioprotectant for patients receiving anthracyclines; however, some evidence suggests that the anthracycline anticancer effect may be compromised by the coadministration of dexrazoxane. In general, dexrazoxane should not be used when the goal of chemotherapy is for curative intent either in the settings of adjuvant or definitive treatment. Doxorubicin and daunomycin have been formulated as liposomal products; these drugs, approved for use in patients with Kaposi sarcoma and sometimes used in certain cancers as a substitute for conventional anthracyclines, appear to have minimal potential for cardiac toxicity.

E. Cisplatin Nephrotoxicity and Neurotoxicity

Cisplatin is effective in treating a wide range of malignancies, including testicular, bladder, lung, and ovarian cancers. Although nausea and vomiting are the side effects most commonly associated with cisplatin, the more serious side effects of nephrotoxicity and neurotoxicity must also be anticipated and aggressively managed. Patients must be vigorously hydrated prior, during, and after cisplatin administration. Both kidney function and electrolytes must be monitored. Low magnesium and potassium levels as well as hyponatremia can develop. The neurotoxicity is usually manifested as a peripheral neuropathy of mixed sensorimotor type and may be associated with painful paresthesias. Development of neuropathy typically occurs after cumulative doses of 300 mg/m^2. Ototoxicity is a potentially serious manifestation of neurotoxicity and can progress to deafness. Amifostine, developed initially as a radioprotective agent and given intravenously at a dose of 910 mg/m^2 over 15 minutes prior to cisplatin, is used to protect against nephrotoxicity and neuropathy. Use of amifostine does not appear to compromise the antineoplastic effect of cisplatin. The second-generation platinum analog, carboplatin, is non-nephrotoxic, although it is myelosuppressive. In the setting of preexisting kidney disease or neuropathy, carboplatin is occasionally substituted for cisplatin.

F. Bleomycin Toxicity

Bleomycin is used for the treatment of testicular cancer, Hodgkin lymphoma, and non-Hodgkin lymphoma. Bleomycin produces edema of the interphalangeal joints and hardening of the palmar and plantar skin. The more serious toxicities include an anaphylactic or serum sickness-like reaction and a serious or fatal pulmonary fibrotic reaction (seen especially in elderly patients receiving a total dose of over 300 units). If nonproductive cough, dyspnea, and pulmonary infiltrates develop, the drug is discontinued, and high-dose corticosteroids are instituted as well as empiric antibiotics pending cultures. Fever alone or with chills is an occasional complication of bleomycin treatment and is not an absolute contraindication to continued treatment. The fever may be avoided by intravenous premedication with hydrocortisone administration. Moreover, fever alone is not predictive of pulmonary toxicity. About 1% of patients (especially those with lymphoma) may have a severe or even fatal hypotensive reaction after the initial dose of bleomycin. In order to identify such patients, a test dose of 5 units of bleomycin is administered first with adequate monitoring and emergency facilities available should they be needed. Patients exhibiting a hypotensive reaction should not receive further bleomycin therapy.

PROGNOSIS

A valuable sign of clinical improvement is the general well-being of the patient. Although this finding is a combination of subjective and objective factors and may be partly a placebo effect, it nonetheless serves as a sign of clinical improvement in assessing some of the objective observations listed above. Factors included in the assessment of general well-being are improved appetite and weight gain and increased "performance status" (eg, ambulatory versus bedridden). Evaluation of factors such as activity status enables the clinician to judge whether the net effect of chemotherapy is worthwhile palliation (see Chapter 5).

Basch E et al. Antiemetics: American Society of Clinical Oncology clinical practice guideline update. 2011 Nov 1;29(31): 4189–98. [PMID: 21947834]

Sugerman DT. JAMA patient page. Chemotherapy. JAMA. 2013 Jul 10;310(2):218. [PMID: 23839767]

Clinical Genetic Disorders

Reed E. Pyeritz, MD, PhD

40

ACUTE INTERMITTENT PORPHYRIA

ESSENTIALS OF DIAGNOSIS

▶ Unexplained abdominal crisis, generally in young women.

▶ Acute peripheral or central nervous system dysfunction; recurrent psychiatric illnesses.

▶ Hyponatremia.

▶ Porphobilinogen in the urine during an attack.

General Considerations

Though there are several different types of porphyrias, the one with the most serious consequences and the one that usually presents in adulthood is acute intermittent porphyria (AIP), which is inherited as an autosomal dominant, though it remains clinically silent in most patients who carry a mutation in *HMBS*. Clinical illness usually develops in women. Symptoms begin in the teens or 20s, but onset can begin after menopause in rare cases. The disorder is caused by partial deficiency of hydroxymethylbilane synthase activity, leading to increased excretion of aminolevulinic acid and porphobilinogen in the urine. The diagnosis may be elusive if not specifically considered. The characteristic abdominal pain may be due to abnormalities in autonomic innervation in the gut. In contrast to other forms of porphyria, cutaneous photosensitivity is absent in AIP. Attacks are precipitated by numerous factors, including drugs and intercurrent infections. Harmful and relatively safe drugs for use in treatment are listed in Table 40–1. Hyponatremia may be seen, due in part to inappropriate release of antidiuretic hormone, although gastrointestinal loss of sodium in some patients may be a contributing factor.

Clinical Findings

A. Symptoms and Signs

Patients show intermittent abdominal pain of varying severity, and in some instances it may so simulate acute abdomen as to lead to exploratory laparotomy. Because the origin of the abdominal pain is neurologic, there is an absence of fever and leukocytosis. Complete recovery between attacks is usual. Any part of the nervous system may be involved, with evidence for autonomic and peripheral neuropathy. Peripheral neuropathy may be symmetric or asymmetric and mild or profound; in the latter instance, it can even lead to quadriplegia with respiratory paralysis. Other central nervous system manifestations include seizures, altered consciousness, psychosis, and abnormalities of the basal ganglia. Hyponatremia may further cause or exacerbate central nervous system manifestations.

B. Laboratory Findings

Often there is profound hyponatremia. The diagnosis can be confirmed by demonstrating an increased amount of porphobilinogen in the urine during an acute attack. Freshly voided urine is of normal color but may turn dark upon standing in light and air.

Most families have different mutations in *HMBS* causing AIP. Mutations can be detected in 90% of patients and used for presymptomatic and prenatal diagnosis.

Prevention

Avoidance of factors known to precipitate attacks of AIP—especially drugs—can reduce morbidity. Sulfonamides and barbiturates are the most common culprits; others are listed in Table 40–1 and on the Internet (www.drugs-porphyria.org). Starvation diets or prolonged fasting also cause attacks and so must be avoided. Hormonal changes during pregnancy can precipitate crises.

Treatment

Treatment with a high-carbohydrate diet diminishes the number of attacks in some patients and is a reasonable empiric gesture considering its benignity. Acute attacks may be life-threatening and require prompt diagnosis, withdrawal of the inciting agent (if possible), and treatment with analgesics and intravenous glucose in saline and hematin. A minimum of 300 g of carbohydrate per day should be provided orally or intravenously. Electrolyte balance requires close attention. Hematin therapy should be

Table 40–1. Some of the "unsafe" and "probably safe" drugs used in the treatment of acute porphyrias.

Unsafe	Probably Safe
Alcohol	Acetaminophen
Alkylating agents	Beta-adrenergic blockers
Barbiturates	Amitriptyline
Carbamazepine	Aspirin
Chloroquine	Atropine
Chlorpropamide	Chloral hydrate
Clonidine	Chlordiazepoxide
Dapsone	Corticosteroids
Ergots	Diazepam
Erythromycin	Digoxin
Estrogens, synthetic	Diphenhydramine
Food additives	Guanethidine
Glutethimide	Hyoscine
Griseofulvin	Ibuprofen
Hydralazine	Imipramine
Ketamine	Insulin
Meprobamate	Lithium
Methyldopa	Naproxen
Metoclopramide	Nitrofurantoin
Nortriptyline	Opioid analgesics
Pentazocine	Penicillamine
Phenytoin	Penicillin and derivatives
Progestins	Phenothiazines
Pyrazinamide	Procaine
Rifampin	Streptomycin
Spironolactone	Succinylcholine
Succinimides	Tetracycline
Sulfonamides	Thiouracil
Theophylline	
Tolazamide	
Tolbutamide	
Valproic acid	

undertaken with full recognition of adverse consequences, especially phlebitis and coagulopathy. The intravenous dosage is up to 4 mg/kg once or twice daily. Liver transplantation may provide an option for patients with disease poorly controlled by medical therapy.

▶ When to Refer

- For management of severe abdominal pain, seizures, or psychosis.
- For preventive management when a patient with porphyria contemplates pregnancy.
- For genetic counseling and molecular diagnosis.

▶ When to Admit

The patient should be hospitalized when he or she has an acute attack accompanied by mental status changes, seizure, or hyponatremia.

Kuo HC et al. Neurological complications of acute intermittent porphyria. Eur Neurol. 2011;66(5):247–52. [PMID: 21986212]

Stein PE et al. Acute intermittent porphyria: fatal complications of treatment. Clin Med. 2012 Jun;12(3):293–4. [PMID: 22783787]

Whatley SD et al. Role of genetic testing in the management of patients with inherited porphyria and their families. Ann Clin Biochem. 2013 May;50(Pt 3):204–16. [PMID: 23605133]

ALKAPTONURIA

 ESSENTIALS OF DIAGNOSIS

- ▶ Ochronosis (gray-black discoloration of connective tissue, including the sclerae, ears, and cartilage).
- ▶ Characteristic radiologic dense intervertebral disks in the spine.
- ▶ Arthropathy.
- ▶ Urine darkens on standing.

▶ Clinical Findings

A. Symptoms and Signs

Alkaptonuria is caused by a recessively inherited deficiency of the enzyme homogentisic acid oxidase. This acid derives from metabolism of both phenylalanine and tyrosine and is present in large amounts in the urine throughout the patient's life. A dark oxidation product accumulates slowly in cartilage and other connective tissues throughout the body, leading to degenerative joint disease of the spine and peripheral joints. Examination of patients in the third and fourth decades shows a slight darkish blue color below the skin in areas overlying cartilage, such as in the ears, a phenomenon called **ochronosis**. In some patients, a more severe hyperpigmentation can be seen in the sclera, conjunctiva, and cornea. Kidney, biliary, and salivary stones can occur. Accumulation of metabolites in heart valves can lead to aortic or mitral stenosis. A predisposition to coronary artery disease may also be present. Although the syndrome causes considerable morbidity, life expectancy is reduced only modestly. Symptoms are more often attributable to spondylitis with back pain, leading to a clinical picture difficult to distinguish from that of ankylosing spondylitis, though on radiographic assessment the sacroiliac joints are not fused in alkaptonuria. The disorder is uncommon in most populations (< 1 per 100,000) but much more common in Slovakia and the Dominican Republic.

B. Laboratory Findings

The diagnosis is established by demonstrating homogentisic acid in the urine, which turns black spontaneously on exposure to the air; this reaction is particularly noteworthy if the urine is alkaline or when alkali is added to a specimen. Molecular analysis of the homogentisic acid oxidase gene (*HGD*) is available but not necessary for diagnosis.

Prevention

Carrier screening and prenatal diagnosis are possible by testing for genetic mutations.

Treatment

Treatment of the arthritis is similar to that for other arthropathies and joint replacement can be effective. Although, in theory, rigid dietary restriction or medications might reduce accumulation of the pigment, this has not proved to be of practical benefit. Since the aortic valve becomes involved by the fifth decade, screening echocardiography of affected adults is indicated. Nitisinone, a drug that inhibits the formation of homogentisic acid, is in development.

Pettit SJ et al. Cardiovascular manifestations of alkaptonuria. J Inherit Metab Dis. 2011 Dec;34(6):1177–81. [PMID: 21506017]

DOWN SYNDROME

ESSENTIALS OF DIAGNOSIS

► Typical craniofacial features (flat occiput, epicanthal folds, large tongue).

► Intellectual disability.

► Congenital heart disease (eg, atrioventricular canal defects) in 50% of patients.

► Dementia of the Alzheimer type in early-to-mid adulthood.

► Three copies of chromosome 21 (trisomy 21) or a chromosome rearrangement that results in three copies of a region of the long arm of chromosome 21.

General Considerations

Nearly 0.5% of all human conceptions are trisomic for chromosome 21. Because of increased fetal mortality, birth incidence of Down syndrome is 1 per 700 but varies from 1 per 1000 in young mothers to more than three times as frequent in women of advanced maternal age. The presence of a fetus with Down syndrome can be detected in many pregnancies in the first or early second trimester through screening maternal serum for alpha-fetoprotein and other biomarkers ("multiple marker screening") and by detecting increased nuchal thickness and underdevelopment of the nasal bone on ultrasonography. Prenatal diagnosis with high sensitivity and specificity can be achieved by assaying fetal DNA that is circulating in maternal blood. The chance of bearing a child with Down syndrome increases exponentially with the age of the mother at conception and begins a marked rise after age 35. By age 45 years, the odds of having an affected child are as high as 1 in 40. The risk of other conditions associated with trisomy also increases, because of the predisposition of older

oocytes to nondisjunction during meiosis. There is little risk of trisomy associated with increased paternal age. However, older men do have an increased risk of fathering a child with a new autosomal dominant condition. Because there are so many distinct conditions, though, the chance of fathering an offspring with any given one is extremely small.

Clinical Findings

A. Symptoms and Signs

Down syndrome is usually diagnosed at birth on the basis of the typical craniofacial features, hypotonia, and single palmar crease. Several serious problems that may be evident at birth or may develop early in childhood include duodenal atresia, congenital heart disease (especially atrioventricular canal defects), and hematologic malignancy. The intestinal and cardiac anomalies usually respond to surgery. A transient neonatal leukemia generally responds to conservative management. The incidences of both acute lymphoblastic and myeloid leukemias are increased in childhood. Intelligence varies across a wide spectrum. Many people with Down syndrome do well in sheltered workshops and group homes, but few achieve full independence in adulthood. Other frequent complications include atlanto-axial instability, celiac disease, frequent infections due to immune deficiency, and hypothyroidism. An Alzheimer-like dementia usually becomes evident in the fourth or fifth decade. Patients with Down syndrome who survive childhood and who develop dementia have a reduced life expectancy; on average, they live to about age 55 years.

B. Laboratory Findings

Cytogenomic analysis should always be performed—even though most patients will have simple trisomy for chromosome 21—to detect unbalanced translocations; such patients may have a parent with a balanced translocation, and there will be a substantial recurrence risk of Down syndrome in future offspring of that parent and potentially that parent's relatives.

Treatment

Duodenal atresia should be treated surgically. Congenital heart disease should be treated as in any other patient. No medical treatment has been proven to affect the intellectual capacity.

When to Refer

• For comprehensive evaluation of infants to investigate congenital heart disease, hematologic malignancy, and duodenal atresia.

• For genetic counseling of the parents.

• For signs of dementia in an adult patient.

When to Admit

An affected young patient should be hospitalized when he or she has failure to thrive, regurgitation, breathlessness, or easy bruising.

Andriolo RB et al. Aerobic exercise training programmes for improving physical and psychosocial health in adults with Down syndrome. Cochrane Database Syst Rev. 2010 May 12;5: CD005176. [PMID: 20464738]

Bartesaghi R et al. Is it possible to improve neurodevelopmental abnormalities in Down syndrome? Rev Neurosci. 2011;22(4): 419–55. [PMID: 21819263]

Lott IT et al. Cognitive deficits and associated neurological complications in individuals with Down's syndrome. Lancet Neurol. 2010 Jun;9(6):623–33. [PMID: 20494326]

Ram G et al. Infections and immunodeficiency in Down syndrome. Clin Exp Immunol. 2011 Apr;164(1):9–16. [PMID: 21352207]

FRAGILE X MENTAL RETARDATION

ESSENTIALS OF DIAGNOSIS

► Expanded trinucleotide repeat (> 200) in the *FMR1* gene.

► Mental retardation and autism in males; large testes after puberty.

► Learning disabilities or mental retardation in females; premature ovarian failure.

► Late-onset tremor and ataxia in males and females with moderate trinucleotide repeat (55–200) expansion (premutation carriers).

► Clinical Findings

A. Symptoms and Signs

This X-linked condition accounts for more cases of mental retardation in males than any condition except Down syndrome; about 1 in 4000 males is affected. The central nervous system phenotype includes autism spectrum, impulsivity and aggressiveness, and repetitive behaviors. The condition also affects intellectual function in females, although less severely and about 50% less frequently than in males. Affected (heterozygous) young women show no physical signs other than early menopause, but they may have learning difficulties, anxiety, sensory issues, or frank retardation. Affected males show macro-orchidism (enlarged testes) after puberty, large ears and a prominent jaw, a high-pitched voice, autistic characteristics, and mental retardation. Some males show evidence of a mild connective tissue defect, with joint hypermobility and mitral valve prolapse.

Women who are premutation carriers (55–200 CGG repeats) are at increased risk for premature ovarian failure and mild cognitive abnormalities. Male and female premutation carriers are at risk for mood and anxiety disorders and the development of tremor and ataxia beyond middle age (fragile-X tremor-ataxia syndrome, FXTAS). Changes in the cerebellar white matter may be evident on MRI before symptoms appear. Because of the relatively high prevalence of premutation carriers in the general population (1/130–1/600), older people in whom any of these behavioral or neurologic problems develop should undergo testing of the *FMR1* locus.

B. Laboratory Findings

The first marker for this condition was a small gap, or fragile site, evident near the tip of the long arm of the X chromosome. Subsequently, the condition was found to be due to expansion of a trinucleotide repeat (CGG) near a gene called *FMR1*. All individuals have some CGG repeats in this location, but as the number increases beyond 52, the chances of further expansion during spermatogenesis or oogenesis increase.

Being born with one *FMR1* allele with 200 or more repeats results in mental retardation in most men, and in about 60% of women. The more repeats, the greater the likelihood that further expansion will occur during gametogenesis; this results in anticipation, in which the disorder can worsen from one generation to the next.

► Prevention

DNA diagnosis for the number of repeats has supplanted cytogenetic analysis for both clinical and prenatal diagnosis. This should be done on any male or female who has unexplained mental retardation. Newborn screening based on hypermethylation of the *FMR1* gene is being considered as a means of early detection and intervention.

► Treatment

Several treatments that address the imbalances in neurotransmission have been developed based on the mouse model and are in clinical trials. Valproic acid may reduce symptoms of hyperactivity and attention deficit, but standard therapies should be tried first.

► When to Refer

• For otherwise unexplained mental retardation or learning difficulties in boys and girls.

• For otherwise unexplained tremor or ataxia in middle-aged individuals.

• For premature ovarian failure.

• For genetic counseling.

Gallagher A et al. Fragile X-associated disorders: a clinical overview. J Neurol. 2012 Mar;259(3):401–13. [PMID: 21748281]

Hagerman R et al. Advances in clinical and molecular understanding of the *FMR1* premutation and fragile X-associated tremor/ataxia syndrome. Lancet Neurol. 2013 Aug;12(8): 786–98. [PMID: 23867198]

GAUCHER DISEASE

ESSENTIALS OF DIAGNOSIS

► Deficiency of beta-glucocerebrosidase.

► Anemia and thrombocytopenia; hypersplenism.

► Pathologic fractures.

Clinical Findings

A. Symptoms and Signs

Gaucher disease has an autosomal recessive pattern of inheritance. A deficiency of beta-glucocerebrosidase causes an accumulation of sphingolipid within phagocytic cells throughout the body. Anemia and thrombocytopenia are common and may be symptomatic; both are due primarily to hypersplenism, but marrow infiltration with Gaucher cells may be a contributing factor. Cortical erosions of bones, especially the vertebrae and femur, are due to local infarctions, but the mechanism is unclear. Episodes of bone pain (termed "crises") are reminiscent of those in sickle cell disease. A hip fracture in a patient with a palpable spleen— especially in a Jewish person of Eastern European origin— suggests the possibility of Gaucher disease. Peripheral neuropathy may develop in patients.

Two uncommon forms of Gaucher disease, called type II and type III, involve neurologic accumulation of sphingolipid and a variety of neurologic problems. Type II is of infantile onset and has a poor prognosis. Heterozygotes for Gaucher disease are at increased risk for developing Parkinson disease.

B. Laboratory Findings

Bone marrow aspirates reveal typical Gaucher cells, which have an eccentric nucleus and periodic acid–Schiff (PAS)-positive inclusions, along with wrinkled cytoplasm and inclusion bodies of a fibrillar type. In addition, the serum acid phosphatase is elevated. Definitive diagnosis requires the demonstration of deficient glucocerebrosidase activity in leukocytes. Hundreds of mutations have been found to cause Gaucher disease and some are highly predictive of the neuronopathic forms. Thus, mutation detection, especially in a young person, is of potential value. Only four mutations in glucocerebrosidase account for more than 90% of the disease among Ashkenazi Jews, in whom the carrier frequency is 1:15.

Prevention

Most clinical complications can be prevented by early institution of enzyme replacement therapy. Carrier screening, especially among Ashkenazi Jews, detects those couples at 25% risk of having an affected child. Prenatal diagnosis through mutation analysis is feasible. Because of an increased risk of malignancy, especially multiple myeloma and other hematologic cancers, regular screening of adults with Gaucher disease may be warranted.

Treatment

A recombinant form of the enzyme glucocerebrosidase (imiglucerase) for intravenous administration on a regular basis reduces total body stores of glycolipid and improves orthopedic and hematologic manifestations. Unfortunately, the neurologic manifestations of types II and III have not improved with enzyme replacement therapy. The major drawback is the exceptional cost of imiglucerase, which can exceed $100,000 per year for a severely affected patient. Early treatment of affected children normalizes growth and bone mineral density and improves liver and spleen size, anemia, and thrombocytopenia. In adults with thrombocytopenia due to splenic sequestration, enzyme replacement often obviates the need for splenectomy. Alternative or complementary therapies, including methods to reduce substrate and to provide a chaperone for a defective enzyme, are being developed. One approved medication, miglustat, does reduce the production of glucocerebroside in some patients, but can be poorly tolerated because of adverse effects.

Mistry PK et al. A reappraisal of Gaucher disease-diagnosis and disease management algorithms. Am J Hematol. 2011 Jan;86(1):110–5. [PMID: 21080341]

Mistry PK et al. Gaucher disease and malignancy: a model for cancer pathogenesis in an inborn error of metabolism. Crit Rev Oncog. 2013;18(3):235–46. [PMID: 23510066]

Sidransky E et al. Multicenter analysis of glucocerebrosidase mutation in Parkinson's disease. N Engl J Med. 2009 Oct 22; 361(17):1651–61. [PMID: 19846850]

Suzuki Y. Chaperone therapy update: Fabry disease, GM1-gangliosidosis and Gaucher disease. Brain Dev. 2013 Jun;35(6):515–23. [PMID: 23290321]

DISORDERS OF HOMOCYSTEINE METABOLISM

ESSENTIALS OF DIAGNOSIS

► For homocystinuria, dislocated ocular lenses.
► Elevated homocysteine in the urine or plasma.

General Considerations

Considerable evidence has accumulated to support the observation that patients with clinical and angiographic evidence of coronary artery disease tend to have higher levels of plasma homocysteine than persons without coronary artery disease. The relationship has been extended to cerebrovascular and peripheral vascular diseases. Although this effect was initially thought to be due at least in part to heterozygotes for cystathionine beta-synthase deficiency (see below), there is little supporting evidence. Rather, an important factor leading to hyperhomocysteinemia is folate deficiency. Pyridoxine (vitamin B_6) and vitamin B_{12} are also important in the metabolism of methionine, and deficiency of any of these vitamins can lead to accumulation of homocysteine. A number of genes influence utilization of these vitamins and can predispose to deficiency. For example, having one—and especially two—copies of an allele that causes thermolability of methylene tetrahydrofolate reductase predisposes people to elevated fasting homocysteine levels. Both nutritional and most genetic deficiencies of these vitamins can be corrected by dietary supplementation of folic acid and, if serum levels are low, vitamins B_6 and B_{12}. In the United States, cereal grains are fortified with folic acid. However, therapy with B vitamins and folate lowers homocysteine levels significantly but does not reduce the risk of either venous thromboembolism or complications of coronary artery disease. The role of lowering homocysteine as primary prevention for sequelae of atherosclerosis has received little direct support in clinical trials. Hyperhomocysteinemia occurs with end-stage chronic kidney disease.

Clinical Findings

A. Symptoms and Signs

Homocystinuria in its classic form is caused by cystathionine beta-synthase deficiency and exhibits an autosomal recessive pattern of inheritance. This results in extreme elevations of plasma and urinary homocystine levels, a basis for diagnosis of this disorder. Homocystinuria is similar in certain superficial aspects to Marfan syndrome, since patients may have a similar body habitus and ectopia lentis is almost always present. However, mental retardation is often present in homocystinuria, and the cardiovascular events are those of repeated venous and arterial thromboses whose precise cause remains obscure. Thus, the diagnosis should be suspected in patients in the second and third decades of life who have arterial or venous thromboses without other risk factors. Life expectancy is reduced, especially in untreated and pyridoxine-unresponsive patients; myocardial infarction, stroke, and pulmonary embolism are the most common causes of death. This condition is diagnosed by newborn screening for hypermethioninemia; however, pyridoxine-responsive infants may not be detected. In addition, homozygotes for a common mutant allele, p.I278T, show marked clinical variability, with some unaffected as adults.

B. Laboratory Findings

Although many mutations have been identified in the cystathionine beta-synthase gene (*CBS*), amino acid analysis of plasma remains the most appropriate diagnostic test. Patients should be studied after they have been off folate or pyridoxine supplementation for at least 1 week. Relatively few laboratories currently provide highly reliable assays for homocysteine. Processing of the specimen is crucial to obtain accurate results. The plasma must be separated within 30 minutes; otherwise, blood cells release the amino acid and the measurement will then be artificially elevated.

Prevention

About 50% of patients have a form of cystathionine beta-synthase deficiency that improves biochemically and clinically through pharmacologic doses of pyridoxine (50–500 mg/d) and folate (5–10 mg/d). For these patients, treatment from infancy can prevent retardation and the other clinical problems. Patients who are pyridoxine nonresponders must be treated with a dietary reduction in methionine and supplementation of cysteine, also from infancy. The vitamin betaine is also useful in reducing plasma methionine levels by facilitating a metabolic pathway that bypasses the defective enzyme.

Treatment

Patients with classic homocystinuria who have suffered venous thrombosis receive anticoagulation therapy, but there are no studies to support prophylactic use of warfarin or antiplatelet agents.

Blom HJ et al. Overview of homocysteine and folate metabolism. With special references to cardiovascular disease and neural tube defects. J Inherit Metab Dis. 2011 Feb;34(1):75–81. [PMID: 20814827]

Lee M et al. Efficacy of homocysteine-lowering therapy with folic acid in stroke prevention: a meta-analysis. Stroke. 2010 Jun;41(6):1205–12. [PMID: 20413740]

Schiff M et al. Treatment of inherited homocystinurias. Neuropediatrics. 2012 Dec;43(6):295–304. [PMID: 23124942]

Study of the Effectiveness of Additional Reductions in Cholesterol and Homocysteine (SEARCH) Collaborative Group et al. Effects of homocysteine-lowering with folic acid plus vitamin B$_{12}$ vs placebo on mortality and major morbidity in myocardial infarction survivors: a randomized trial. JAMA. 2010 Jun 23;303(24):2486–94. [PMID: 20571015]

KLINEFELTER SYNDROME

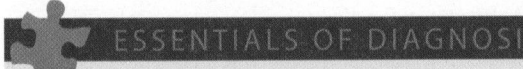
ESSENTIALS OF DIAGNOSIS

► Males with hypergonadotropic hypogonadism and small testes.

► 47,XXY karyotype.

Clinical Findings

A. Symptoms and Signs

Boys with an extra X chromosome are normal in appearance before puberty; thereafter, they have disproportionately long legs and arms, sparse body hair, a female escutcheon, gynecomastia, and small testes. Infertility is due to azoospermia; the seminiferous tubules are hyalinized. The incidence is 1 in 660 newborn males, but the diagnosis is often not made until a man is evaluated for inability to conceive. Intellectual disability is somewhat more common than in the general population. Many men with Klinefelter syndrome have language-based learning problems. However, their intelligence usually tests within the broad range of normal. As adults, detailed psychometric testing may reveal a deficiency in executive skills. The risk of osteoporosis, breast cancer and diabetes mellitus is much higher in men with Klinefelter syndrome than in 46,XY men.

B. Laboratory Findings

Low serum testosterone is common. The karyotype is typically 47,XXY, but other sex chromosome anomalies cause variations of Klinefelter syndrome.

Prevention

Screening for cancer (especially of the breast), deep venous thrombosis, and glucose intolerance are indicated.

Treatment

Treatment with testosterone after puberty is advisable but will not restore fertility. However, men with Klinefelter syndrome have had mature sperm aspirated from their testes and injected into oocytes, resulting in fertilization. After the blastocysts have been implanted into the uterus of a partner, conception has resulted. However, men with Klinefelter syndrome do have an increased risk for aneuploidy in sperm, and therefore genomic analysis of a blastocyst should be considered before implantation.

Aksglaede L et al. Testicular function and fertility in men with Klinefelter syndrome: a review. Eur J Endocrinol. 2013 Mar 15;168(4):R67-76. [PMID: 23504510]

Gravholt CH. Sex chromosome abnormalities. In: Rimoin DL et al (editors). *Emery and Rimoin's Principles and Practice of Medical Genetics*, 6th ed. Philadelphia: Churchill Livingstone, 2013.

Radicioni AF et al. Consensus statement on diagnosis and clinical management of Klinefelter syndrome. J Endocrinol Invest. 2010 Dec;33(11):839-50. [PMID: 21293172]

Sigman M. Klinefelter syndrome: how, what, and why? Fertil Steril. 2012 Aug;98(2):251-2. [PMID: 22726951]

Sokol RZ. It's not all about the testes: medical issues in Klinefelter patients. Fertil Steril. 2012 Aug;98(2):261-5. [PMID: 22704628]

MARFAN SYNDROME

ESSENTIALS OF DIAGNOSIS

- ► Disproportionately tall stature, thoracic deformity, and joint laxity or contractures.
- ► Ectopia lentis and myopia.
- ► Aortic root dilation and dissection; mitral valve prolapse.
- ► Mutation in *FBN1*, the gene encoding fibrillin-1.

General Considerations

Marfan syndrome, a systemic connective tissue disease, has an autosomal dominant pattern of inheritance. It is characterized by abnormalities of the skeletal, ocular, and cardiovascular systems; spontaneous pneumothorax; dural ectasia; and striae atrophicae. Of most concern is disease of the ascending aorta, which begins as a dilated aortic root. Histology of the aorta shows diffuse medial degeneration. Mitral valve leaflets are also abnormal and mitral prolapse and regurgitation may be present, often with elongated chordae tendineae, which on occasion may rupture.

Clinical Findings

A. Symptoms and Signs

Affected patients are typically tall, with particularly long arms, legs, and digits (arachnodactyly). However, there can be wide variability in the clinical presentation. Commonly, scoliosis and anterior chest deformity, such as pectus excavatum, are found. Ectopia lentis is present in about half of patients; severe myopia is common and retinal detachment can occur. Mitral valve prolapse is seen in about 85% of patients. Aortic root dilation is common and leads to aortic regurgitation or dissection with rupture. To diagnose Marfan syndrome, people with an affected relative need features in at least two systems. People with no family history need features in the skeletal system, two other systems, and one of the major criteria of ectopia lentis, dilation of the aortic root, or aortic dissection. Patients with homocystinuria due to cystathionine beta-synthase deficiency also have dislocated lenses, tall, disproportionate stature, and thoracic deformity. They tend to have below normal intelligence, stiff joints, and a predisposition to arterial and venous occlusive disease. Males with Klinefelter syndrome do not show the typical ocular or cardiovascular features of Marfan syndrome and are generally sporadic occurrences in the family.

B. Laboratory Findings

Mutations in the fibrillin gene (*FBN1*) on chromosome 15 cause Marfan syndrome. Nonetheless, no simple laboratory test is available to support the diagnosis in questionable cases because related conditions may also be due to defects in fibrillin. The nature of the *FBN1* mutation has little predictive value in terms of prognosis. The pathogenesis of Marfan syndrome involves aberrant regulation of transforming growth factor (TGF)-beta activity. Mutations in either of two receptors for TGF-beta (TGFBR1 and TGFBR2) can cause conditions that resemble Marfan syndrome in terms of aortic aneurysm and dissection and autosomal dominant inheritance.

Prevention

There is prenatal and presymptomatic diagnosis for patients in whom the molecular defect in *FBN1* has been found.

Treatment

Children with Marfan syndrome require regular ophthalmologic surveillance to correct visual acuity and thus prevent amblyopia, and annual orthopedic consultation for diagnosis of scoliosis at an early enough stage so that bracing might delay progression. Patients of all ages require echocardiography at least annually to monitor aortic diameter and mitral valve function. Long-term beta-adrenergic blockade, titrated to individual tolerance but enough to produce a negative inotropic effect (atenolol, 1-2 mg/kg orally daily) retards the rate of aortic dilation. A dozen clinical trials comparing the effectiveness of atenolol and losartan or other angiotensin receptor blockers, drugs that reduces activity of TGF-beta, are underway, and results from several are being reported. Restriction from vigorous physical exertion protects from aortic dissection. Prophylactic replacement of the aortic root with a composite graft when the diameter reaches 45-50 mm in an adult (normal: < 40 mm) prolongs life. A procedure to reimplant the patient's native aortic valve and replace just the aneurysmal sinuses of Valsalva and ascending aorta avoids the need for lifelong anticoagulation.

Prognosis

People with Marfan syndrome who are untreated commonly die in the fourth or fifth decade from aortic dissection or heart failure secondary to aortic regurgitation. However, because of earlier diagnosis, lifestyle modifications, beta-adrenergic blockade, and prophylactic aortic surgery, life expectancy has increased by several decades in the past 25 years.

When to Refer

- For detailed ophthalmologic examination.
- For at least annual cardiologic evaluation.
- For moderate scoliosis.
- For pregnancy in a woman with Marfan syndrome.
- For genetic counseling.

When to Admit

Any patient with Marfan syndrome in whom severe or unusual chest pain develops should be hospitalized to exclude pneumothorax and aortic dissection.

Benedetto U et al. Surgical management of aortic root disease in Marfan syndrome: a systematic review and meta-analysis. Heart. 2011 Jun;97(12):955–8. [PMID: 21228428]

David TE et al. Long-term results of aortic root repair using the reimplantation technique. J Thorac Cardiovasc Surg. 2013 Mar;145(3 Suppl):S22–5. [PMID: 23260437]

Groenink M et al. Losartan reduces aortic dilatation rate in adults with Marfan syndrome: a randomized controlled trial. Eur Heart J. 2013 Dec;34(45):3491–500. [PMID: 23999449]

Pyeritz RE. Evaluation of the adolescent or adult with some features of Marfan syndrome. Genet Med. 2012 Jan;14(1):171–7. [PMID: 22237449]

Pyeritz RE. Marfan syndrome and related disorders. In: Rimoin DL et al (editors). *Emery and Rimoin's Principles and Practice of Medical Genetics*, 6th ed. Philadelphia: Churchill Livingstone, 2013.

HEREDITARY HEMORRHAGIC TELANGIECTASIA

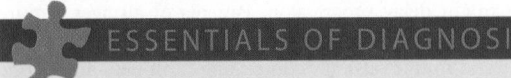

ESSENTIALS OF DIAGNOSIS

- ► Recurrent epistaxis.
- ► Mucocutaneous telangiectases.
- ► Visceral arteriovenous malformations (especially lung, liver, brain, bowel).

Clinical Findings

A. Symptoms and Signs

Hereditary hemorrhagic telangiectasia (HHT), formerly termed "Osler-Weber-Rendu syndrome," is an autosomal dominant disorder of development of the vasculature. Epistaxis may begin in childhood or later in adolescence. Punctate telangiectases of the lips, tongue, fingers, and skin generally appear in later childhood and adolescence. Arteriovenous malformations (AVMs) can occur at any age in the brain, lungs, and liver. Bleeding from the gastrointestinal tract is due to mucosal vascular malformations and usually is not a problem until mid-adult years or later. Pulmonary AVMs can cause hypoxemia (with peripheral cyanosis, dyspnea, and clubbing) and right-to-left shunting (with embolic stroke or brain abscess). The criteria for diagnosis require presence of three of the following four features: (1) recurrent epistaxis, (2) visceral AVMs, (3) mucocutaneous telangiectases, and (4) being the near relative of a clearly affected individual. Mutation analysis can be used for presymptomatic diagnosis or exclusion of the worry of HHT.

B. Laboratory Findings

MR or CT arteriography detects AVMs. Mutations in at least five genes can cause HHT. Three have been identified and molecular analysis to identify them is available; these mutations in *ENG, ALK1,* and *SMAD4* account for about 87% of families with HHT. When the familial mutation is known, molecular testing is far more cost effective than repeated screening of relatives who are at risk.

Prevention

Embolization of pulmonary AVMs with wire coils or other occlusive devices reduces the risk of stroke and brain abscess. Treatment of brain AVMs reduces the risk of hemorrhagic stroke. All patients with HHT with evidence of a pulmonary shunt should practice routine endocarditis prophylaxis (see Table 33–6). All intravenous lines (except those for transfusion of red blood cells and radiographic contrast) should have an air-filter to prevent embolization of an air bubble. Prenatal diagnosis through mutation detection is possible.

Treatment

All patients in whom the diagnosis of HHT is considered should have an MRI of the brain with contrast. A contrast echocardiogram will detect most pulmonary AVMs when "bubbles" appear on the left side of the heart after 3–6 cardiac cycles. A positive contrast echocardiogram should be followed by a high-resolution CT angiogram for localization of pulmonary AVMs. Patients who have AVMs with a feeding artery of 1–2 mm diameter or greater should undergo embolization. After successful embolization of all treatable pulmonary AVMs, the CT angiogram should be repeated in 3 years. A person with a negative contrast echocardiogram should have the test repeated every 5 years. Several recent studies suggest that treatment with anti-estrogenic agents (eg, tamoxifen), thalidomide, or anti-vascular endothelial growth factor agents (eg, bevacizumab) can reduce epistaxis and gastrointestinal bleeding and improve hepatic shunting.

Dupuis-Girod S et al. Bevacizumab in patients with hereditary hemorrhagic telangiectasia and severe hepatic vascular malformations and high cardiac output. JAMA. 2012 Mar 7; 307(9):948–55. [PMID: 22396517]

Faughnan ME et al; HHT Guidelines Working Group. International guidelines for the diagnosis and management of hereditary haemorrhagic telangiectasia. J Med Genet. 2011 Feb;48(2):73–87. [PMID: 19553198]

Guttmacher AE et al. Hereditary hemorrhagic telangiectasia. In: Rimoin DL et al (editors). *Emery and Rimoin's Principles and Practice of Medical Genetics*, 6th ed. Philadelphia: Churchill Livingstone, 2013.

Trerotola SO, Pyeritz RE. PAVM embolization: an update. AJR Am J Roentgenol. 2010 Oct;195(4):837–45. [PMID: 20858807]

Velthuis S et al. Role of transthoracic contrast echocardiography in the clinical diagnosis of hereditary hemorrhagic telangiectasia. Chest. 2013 Dec;144(6):1876–82. [PMID: 23907523]

Yaniv E et al. Anti-estrogen therapy for hereditary hemorrhagic telangiectasia—a long-term clinical trial. Rhinology. 2011 Jun;49(2):214–6. [PMID: 21743879]

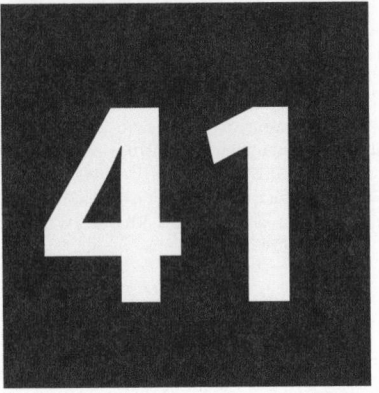

Sports Medicine & Outpatient Orthopedics

Anthony Luke, MD, MPH

C. Benjamin Ma, MD

GENERAL APPROACH TO MUSCULOSKELETAL INJURIES

 ESSENTIALS OF DIAGNOSIS

► History is most important in diagnosing musculo-skeletal problems.

► The mechanism of injury can explain the pathology and symptoms.

► Determine whether the injury is traumatic or atraumatic, acute or chronic, high or low velocity (greater velocity suggests more structural damage), or whether any movement aggravates or relieves pain associated with the injury.

► General Considerations

Musculoskeletal problems account for about 10–20% of outpatient primary care clinical visits. Orthopedic problems can be classified as traumatic (ie, injury-related) or atraumatic (ie, degenerative or overuse syndromes) as well as acute or chronic. The mechanism of injury is usually the most helpful part of the history in determining the diagnosis.

The onset of symptoms should be elicited. With acute traumatic injuries, patients typically seek medical attention within 6 weeks of onset. The patient should describe the exact location of symptoms, which helps determine anatomic structures that may be damaged. If the patient is vague, the clinician can ask the patient to point with one finger only to the point of maximal tenderness.

► Clinical Findings

A. Symptoms and Signs

The chief musculoskeletal complaints are typically pain (most common), instability or dysfunction around the joints. Since symptoms and signs are often nonspecific, recognizing the expected combination of symptoms and physical examination signs can help facilitate the

clinical diagnosis. Patients may describe symptoms of "locking" or "catching," suggesting internal derangement in joints. Symptoms of "instability" or "giving way" suggest ligamentous injury; however, these symptoms may also be due to pain causing muscular inhibition. Constitutional symptoms of fever or weight loss, swelling with no injury, or systemic illness suggest medical conditions (such as infection, cancer, or rheumatologic disease).

Initial evaluation should follow routine trauma guidelines to rule out serious joint injury. However, typical evaluations in the clinic follow the traditional components of the physical examination and should include **inspection**, **palpation**, and assessment of **range of motion** and **neurovascular status**.

Inspection includes observation of *s*welling, *e*rythema, *a*trophy, *d*eformity, and (surgical) *s*cars (mnemonic, "SEADS"). The patient should be asked to move joints of concern (for example, see Table 41–1). If motion is asymmetric, the clinician should assess the passive range of motion for any physical limitation.

There are special tests to assess each joint. Typically, **provocative tests** recreate the mechanism of injury with the goal to reproduce the patient's pain. **Stress tests** apply load to ligaments of concern. Typically, 10 to 15 pounds of force should be applied when performing stress tests. **Functional testing,** including simple tasks performed during activities of daily living, is useful to assess injury severity.

B. Imaging

Bony pathology can be assessed using standard radiographs, although there also may be characteristic soft tissue findings. However, CT scans are the most effective method for visualizing any bony pathology, including morphology of fractures. Nuclear bone scans are now less commonly used but are still valuable for identifying stress injuries, infection, malignancy, or multisite pathology. Positron emission tomography (PET) scans are useful in identifying metastatic malignant lesions. MRI provides excellent visualization of ligaments, cartilage, and soft tissues. High Field 3.0 Tesla MRI is available clinically and allows higher image resolution and decreased examination

Table 41–1. Shoulder examination.

Maneuver	Description
Inspection	Check the patient's posture and "SEADS" (*s*welling, *e*rythema, *a*trophy, *d*eformity, surgical *s*cars).
Palpation	Include important landmarks: acromioclavicular (AC) joint, long head of biceps tendon, coracoid, and greater tuberosity (supraspinatus insertion).
Range of motion testing	Check range of motion actively (patient performs) and passively (clinician performs).
Flexion 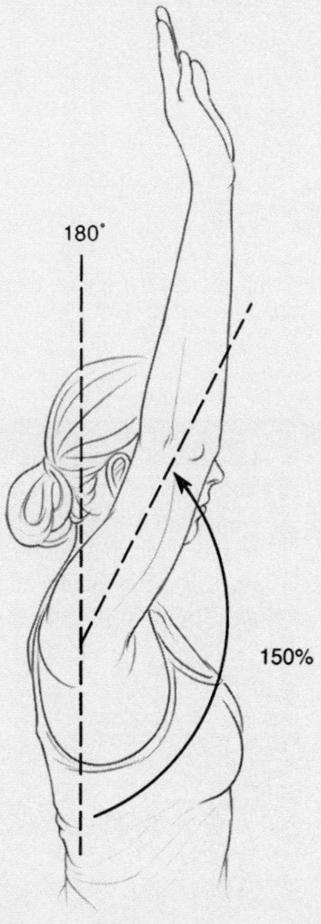	Move the arm forward as high as possible in the sagittal plane.

180°

150%

| **External rotation** 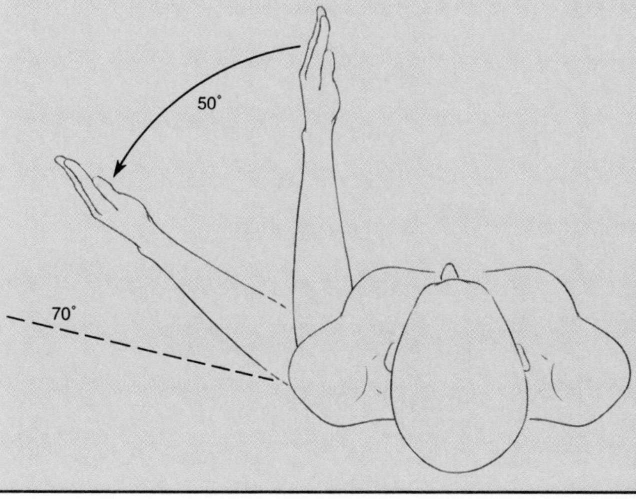 | Check with the patient's elbow touching their body so that external rotation occurs predominantly at the glenohumeral joint. |

50°

70°

(continued)

Table 41–1. Shoulder examination. (continued)

Maneuver	Description
Internal rotation T8	The patient is asked to reach the thumbs as high as possible behind the spine on each side. The clinician can record the highest spinous process that the individual can reach on each side (iliac crest = L4, inferior angle of scapula = T8).
Rotator cuff strength testing	
Supraspinatus (open can) test	Perform resisted shoulder abduction at 90 degrees with slight forward flexion to around 45 degrees to test for supraspinatus tendon strength ("open can" test), or with shoulder abduction at 30 degrees and flexion to 30 degrees ("empty can" test).
External rotation 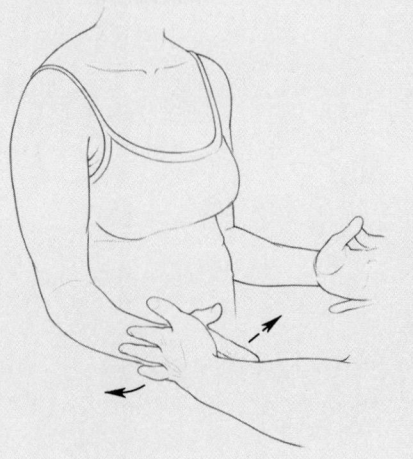	The patient resists by externally rotating the arms with elbows at his or her side.

(continued)

Table 41–1. Shoulder examination. (continued)

Maneuver	Description
Internal rotation (lift off test) 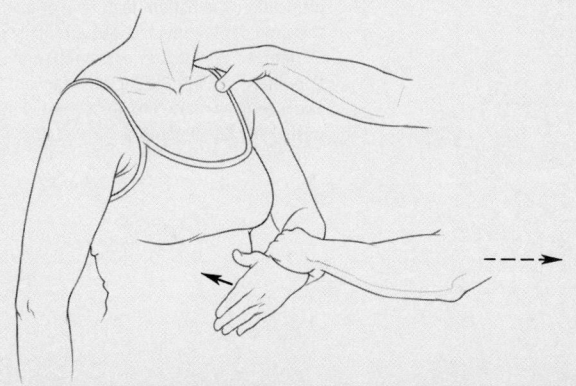	A positive "lift-off" test is the inability of the patient to hold his or her hand away from the body when reaching toward the small of the back. The clinician pushes the patient's hand toward the back while the patient resists. A positive lift-off indicates subscapularis tendon insufficiency.
Internal rotation (belly press test) 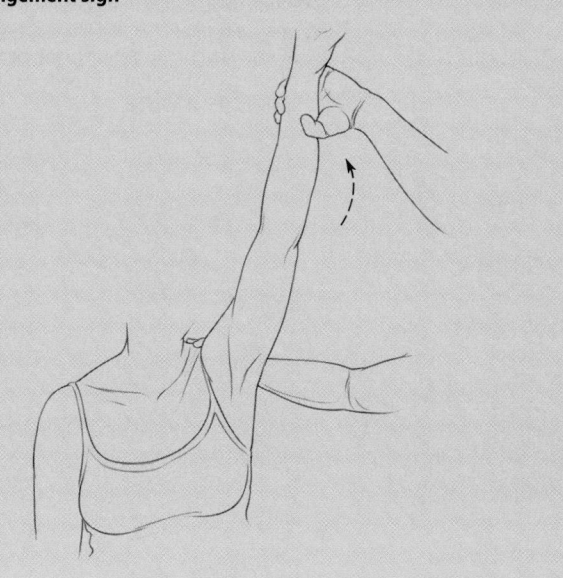	A positive "belly-press" test is the inability to hold the elbow in front of the trunk while pressing down with the hand on the belly. A positive belly press test indicates subscapularis tendon insufficiency.

Impingement tests

Neer impingement sign	Perform by having the clinician flex the shoulder maximally in an overhead position. The test is positive when pain is reproduced with full passive shoulder flexion. Sensitivity is 79%; specificity is 53%.

(continued)

Table 41–1. Shoulder examination. (continued)

Maneuver	Description
Hawkins impingement sign 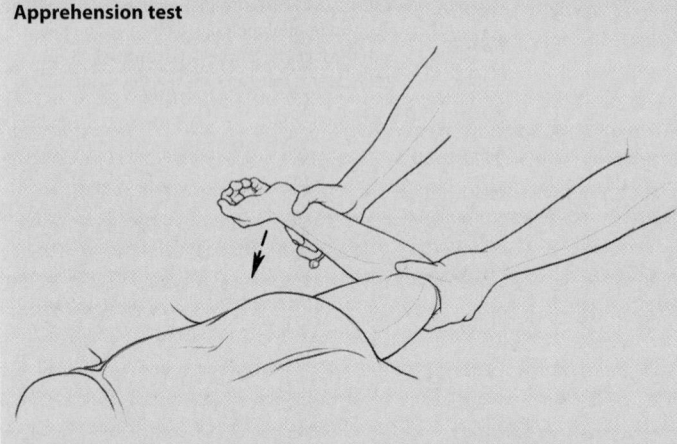	Perform with the shoulder forward flexed 90 degrees and the elbow flexed at 90 degrees. The shoulder is then maximally internally rotated to impinge the greater tuberosity on the undersurface of the acromion. The test is considered positive when the patient's pain is reproduced by this maneuver. Sensitivity is 79%; specificity is 59%.
Stability tests	
Apprehension test 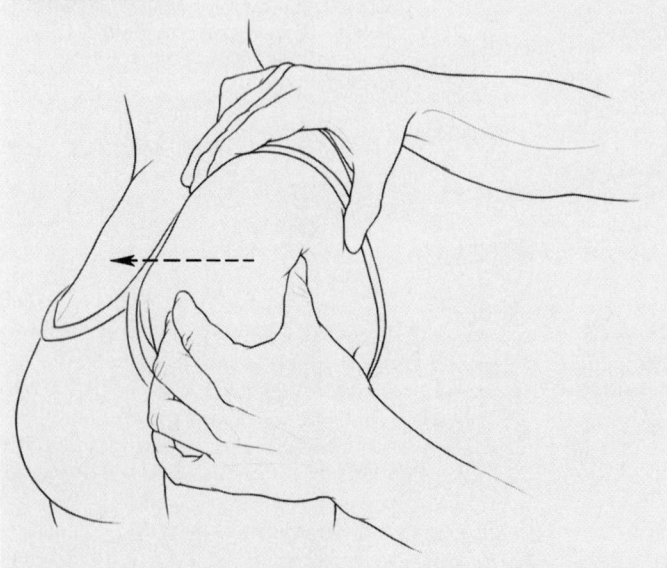	With persistent anterior instability or a recent dislocation, the patient feels pain or guards when the shoulder is abducted and externally rotated at 90 degrees. With posterior instability, the patient is apprehensive with the shoulder forward flexed and internally rotated to 90 degrees with a posteriorly directed force.
Load and shift test	Perform to determine shoulder instability by manually translating the humeral head anteriorly and posteriorly in relation to the glenoid. However, this test can be difficult to perform when the patient is not relaxed.

(continued)

Table 41–1. Shoulder examination. (continued)

Maneuver	Description
O'Brien test 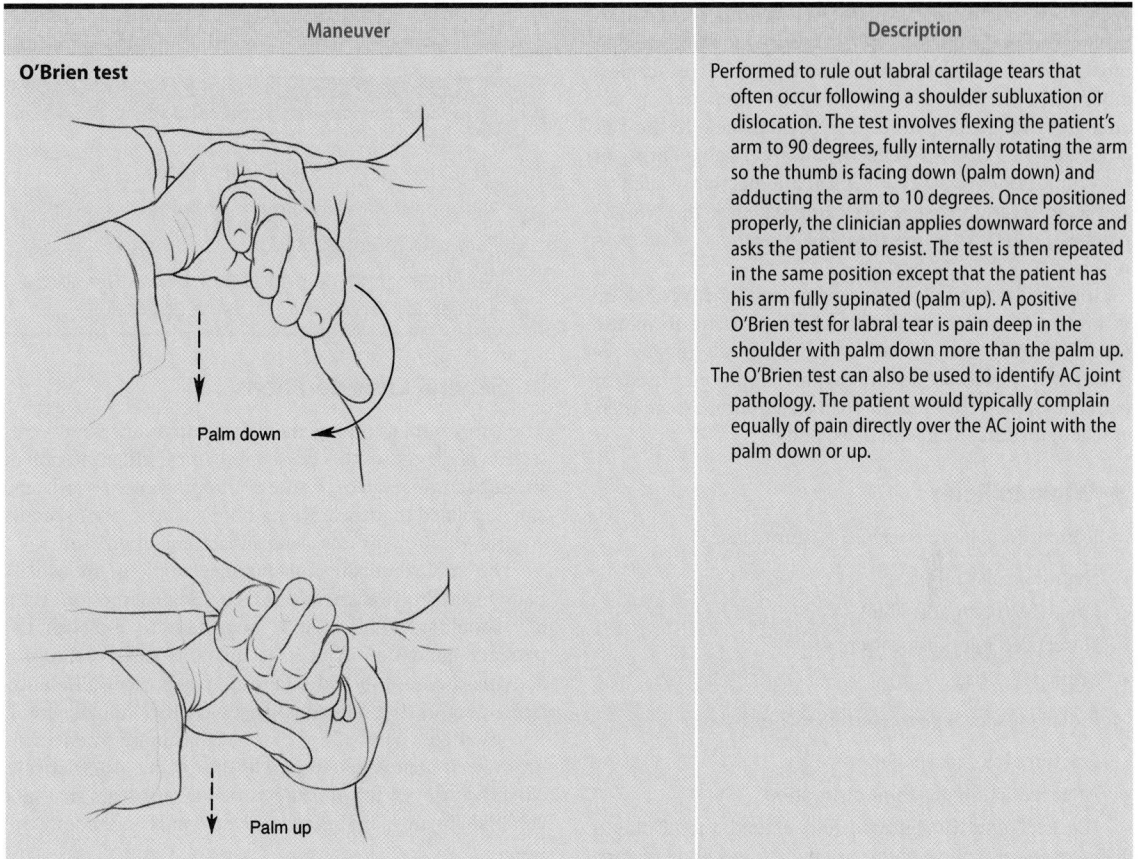 Palm down Palm up	Performed to rule out labral cartilage tears that often occur following a shoulder subluxation or dislocation. The test involves flexing the patient's arm to 90 degrees, fully internally rotating the arm so the thumb is facing down (palm down) and adducting the arm to 10 degrees. Once positioned properly, the clinician applies downward force and asks the patient to resist. The test is then repeated in the same position except that the patient has his arm fully supinated (palm up). A positive O'Brien test for labral tear is pain deep in the shoulder with palm down more than the palm up. The O'Brien test can also be used to identify AC joint pathology. The patient would typically complain equally of pain directly over the AC joint with the palm down or up.

times compared to the standard 1.5 Tesla machines. Gadolinium contrast can be injected as an MRI arthrogram to increase sensitivity of detecting certain internal derangements in joints such as labral injuries. Musculoskeletal ultrasound, where available, can be useful for identifying superficial tissue problems, including tendinopathies and synovial problems.

C. Special Tests

Arthrocentesis must be performed promptly to rule out an infection when acute knee pain with effusion and inflammation are present and the patient is unable to actively flex the joint (see Tables 20–2 and 20–3). The joint fluid should be sent for cell count, crystal analysis, and culture. Arthrocentesis and joint fluid analysis demonstrating crystals can lead to the diagnosis of gout (negatively birefringent, needle-shaped crystals) or pseudogout (positively birefringent, rectangular-shaped crystals). In large, uncomfortable knee joint effusions, removal of excessive joint fluid may improve joint range of motion (flexion) and patient comfort. To avoid infecting the joint, arthrocentesis should not be performed when there is an active cellulitis or abscess overlying the joint. It appears the risk of bleeding after arthrocentesis or joint injection is extremely low even if the patient

is taking anticoagulants. Caution should be practiced if the INR is > 3.0; however, even a supratherapeutic INR did not suggest an increased risk of hemarthrosis in one study. Markers of inflammation such as complete blood cell count, erythrocyte sedimentation rate, and C-reactive protein, and rheumatologic tests are useful in evaluating for infectious, oncologic, or rheumatologic processes. Electrodiagnostic studies such as electromyography and nerve conduction studies are useful when there are neurologic concerns; they can also help with prognostication in chronic conditions.

▶ Treatment

While most outpatient musculoskeletal problems are best treated conservatively, the first consideration is whether there is an immediate surgical need. Surgical treatment is chosen when the outcome promises better health, restoration of function, and improved quality of life. During surgery, the musculoskeletal problem is usually repaired, removed, realigned, reconstructed, or replaced (eg, joint replacement).

If surgery is not immediately indicated, conservative treatment in the outpatient setting usually includes *m*odification of activities, *i*ce, *c*ompression, and *e*levation (remembered by the mnemonic, "MICE"). Controlling pain is an early concern for most patients. Commonly prescribed medications are analgesics (nonsteroidal anti-inflammatory drugs [NSAIDs], acetaminophen, or opioids). Other medications that may also be prescribed, albeit less commonly, are muscle relaxants or co-analgesics for neuropathic pain (which include the calcium channel alpha-2-delta ligands [eg, gabapentin] or tricyclic antidepressants). Topical medications, such as capsaicin cream or patch, lidocaine patches, and NSAID patches or gels, can help provide superficial local pain relief.

Immobilization by casting, slings, and braces is helpful to protect an injured limb. Crutches are useful to reduce weight bearing. Rehabilitation and physical therapy are frequently needed. Other modalities commonly used by patients include chiropractic manipulation, massage therapy, acupuncture, heat, and osteopathy.

▶ When to Refer

Indications for *emergency* referral (immediate)

- Neurovascular injury.
- Fractures (open, unstable).
- Unreduced joint dislocation.
- Septic arthritis.

Indications for *urgent* referral (within 7 days)

- Fractures (closed, stable).
- After reduction of a joint dislocation.
- "Locked" joint (inability to fully extend a joint due to mechanical derangement, usually a loose body or torn cartilage).
- Tumor.

Indications for *early* orthopedic assessment (2–4 weeks)

- Motor weakness (neurologic).
- Constitutional symptoms (eg, weight loss, fever not due to septic arthritis).
- Multiple joint involvement.

Indications for *routine* orthopedic assessment (for further management)

- Failure of conservative treatment (persistent symptoms > 3 months).
- Persistent numbness and tingling in an extremity.

Ahmed I et al. Safety of arthrocentesis and joint injection in patients receiving anticoagulation at therapeutic levels. Am J Med. 2012 Mar;125(3):265–9. [PMID: 22340924]

Patel KV et al. Prevalence and impact of pain among older adults in the United States: findings from the 2011 National Health and Aging Trends Study. Pain. 2013 Dec;154(12):2649–57. [PMID: 24287107]

Shapiro L et al. Advances in musculoskeletal MRI: technical considerations. J Magn Reson Imaging. 2012 Oct;36(4):775–87. [PMID: 22987756]

SHOULDER

1. Subacromial Impingement Syndrome

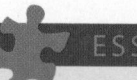
ESSENTIALS OF DIAGNOSIS

- ▶ Shoulder pain with overhead motion.
- ▶ Night pain with sleeping on shoulder.
- ▶ Pain with internal rotation.
- ▶ Numbness and pain radiation below the elbow are usually due to cervical spine disease.

▶ General Considerations

The subacromial impingement syndrome describes a collection of diagnoses that cause mechanical inflammation in the subacromial space. Causes of impingement syndrome can be related to muscle strength imbalances, poor scapula control, rotator cuff tears, and subacromial bone spurs.

The chief complaints for shoulder problems are usually pain, instability, weakness, or loss of range of motion. With any shoulder problem, it is important to establish the patient's hand dominance, occupation, and recreational activities because shoulder injuries may present differently depending on the demands placed on the shoulder joint. For example, baseball pitchers with impingement syndrome may complain of pain while throwing. Alternatively, elders with even full thickness rotator cuff tears may not complain of any pain because the demands on the joint are low.

▶ Clinical Findings

A. Symptoms and Signs

Shoulder problems classically present with one or more of the following: pain with overhead activities, nocturnal pain with sleeping on the shoulder, or pain on internal rotation (eg, putting on a jacket or bra). On inspection, there may be appreciable atrophy in the supraspinatus or infraspinatus fossa. The patient with impingement syndrome can have mild scapula winging or "dyskinesis." The patient often has a rolled-forward shoulder posture or head-forward posture. On palpation, the patient can have tenderness over the anterolateral shoulder at the edge of the greater tuberosity. The patient may lack full active range of motion (Table 41–1) but should have preserved passive range of motion. Impingement symptoms can be elicited with the Neer and Hawkins impingement signs (Table 41–1).

B. Imaging

The following four radiographic views should be ordered to evaluate subacromial impingement syndrome: the anteroposterior (AP) scapula, the AP acromioclavicular joint, the lateral scapula (scapular Y), and the axillary lateral. The AP scapula view can rule out glenohumeral joint arthritis. The AP acromioclavicular view evaluates the acromioclavicular joint for inferior spurs. The scapula

Y view evaluates the acromial shape, and the axillary lateral view visualizes the glenohumeral joint as well and for the presence of os acromiale.

MRI of the shoulder may demonstrate full or partial thickness tears or tendinosis. Ultrasound evaluation may demonstrate thickening of the rotator cuff tendons and tendinosis. Tears may also be visualized, although it is more difficult to identify partial tears from small full thickness on ultrasound than on MRI.

▶ Treatment

A. Conservative

The first-line treatment for impingement syndrome is usually a conservative approach with education, activity modification, and physical therapy exercises. Impingement syndrome can be caused by muscle weakness or tear. Rotator cuff muscle strengthening can alleviate weakness or pain, unless the tendons are seriously compromised, which may cause more symptoms. Physical therapy is directed at rotator cuff muscle strengthening, scapula stabilization, and postural exercises. There is no strong evidence supporting the effectiveness of ice and NSAIDs as a prolonged therapy. In a Cochrane review, corticosteroid injections produced slightly better relief of symptoms in the short-term when compared with placebo. Most patients respond well to conservative treatment.

B. Surgical

Procedures include arthroscopic acromioplasty with coracoacromial ligament release, bursectomy, or debridement or repair of rotator cuff tears.

▶ When to Refer

- Failure of conservative treatment over 3 months.
- Young and active patients with impingement due to full thickness rotator cuff tears.

Hegedus EJ et al. Which physical examination tests provide clinicians with the most value when examining the shoulder? Update of a systematic review with meta-analysis of individual tests. Br J Sports Med. 2012 Nov;46(14):964–78. [PMID: 22773322]

2. Rotator Cuff Tears

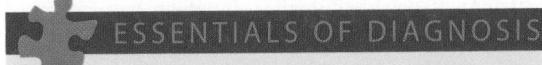

ESSENTIALS OF DIAGNOSIS

- ▶ A common cause of shoulder impingement syndrome after age 40.
- ▶ Difficulty lifting the arm with limited active range of motion.
- ▶ Weakness with resisted strength testing suggests full thickness tears.

▶ General Considerations

Rotator cuff tears can be caused by acute injuries related to falls on an outstretched arm or to pulling on the shoulder. It can also be related to chronic repetitive injuries with overhead movement and lifting. **Partial rotator cuff tears are one of the most common reasons for impingement syndrome.** Full thickness rotator cuff tears are usually more symptomatic and may require surgical treatment. The most commonly torn tendon is the supraspinatus.

▶ Clinical Findings

A. Symptoms and Signs

Most patients complain of weakness or pain with overhead movement. Night pain is also a common complaint. The clinical findings with rotator cuff tears include those of the impingement syndrome except that with full-thickness rotator cuff tears there may be more obvious weakness noted with light resistance testing of specific rotator cuff muscles. Supraspinatus tendon strength is tested with resisted shoulder abduction at 90 degrees with slight forward flexion to around 45 degrees ("open can" test) (Table 41–1). Infraspinatus/teres minor strength is tested with resisted shoulder external rotation with shoulder at 0 degrees abduction, elbow by side (Table 41–1). Subscapularis strength is tested with the "lift-off" or "belly-press" tests (Table 41–1). The affected patient usually also has positive Neer and Hawkins impingement tests.

B. Imaging

Recommended radiographs are very similar to impingement syndrome: AP scapula (glenohumeral), axillary lateral, supraspinatus outlet, and AP acromioclavicular joint views. The AP scapula view is useful in visualizing rotator cuff tears because degenerative changes can appear between the acromion and greater tuberosity of the shoulder. Axillary lateral views show superior elevation of the humeral head in relation to the center of the glenoid. Supraspinatus outlet views allow evaluation of the shape of the acromion. High-grade acromial spurs are associated with a higher incidence of rotator cuff tears. The AP acromioclavicular joint view evaluates for the presence of acromioclavicular joint arthritis, which can mimic rotator cuff tears, and for spurs that can cause rotator cuff injuries.

MRI is the best method for visualizing rotator cuff tears. The MR arthrogram can show partial or small (< 1 cm) rotator cuff tears. For patients who cannot undergo MRI testing or when postoperative artifacts limit MRI evaluations, ultrasonography can be helpful.

▶ Treatment

Partial rotator cuff tears may heal with scarring. Most partial rotator cuff tears can be treated with physical therapy and scapular and rotator cuff muscle strengthening. However, research suggests that that 40% of the partial thickness tears progress to full thickness tears in 2 years. Physical therapy can strengthen the remaining muscles to compensate for loss of strength and can have high rate of success for chronic tears. Physical therapy is also an option for older sedentary patients. On the contrary, full-thickness rotator cuff tears do not heal well and also have a tendency to increase in size with time. Fatty infiltration progresses in full thickness rotator cuff tears and it is a negative prognostic factor for successful surgical treatment. **Most young active patients with acute, full-thickness tears should be treated with operative fixation.** In particular, subscapularis tendon injuries warrant different treatment. Full-thickness subscapularis tendon tears should undergo surgical repair as they usually lead to premature osteoarthritis of the shoulder.

When to Refer

- Young and active patients with full thickness rotator cuff tears.
- Partial tears with > 50% involvement and with significant pain.
- Older and sedentary patients with full-thickness rotator cuff tears who have not responded to nonoperative treatment.
- Full thickness subscapularis tears.

Kuhn JE et al; MOON Shoulder Group. Effectiveness of physical therapy in treating atraumatic full-thickness rotator cuff tears: a multicenter prospective cohort study. J Shoulder Elbow Surg. 2013 Oct;22(10):1371–9. [PMID: 23540577]

Longo UG et al. Conservative treatment and rotator cuff tear progression. Med Sport Sci. 2012;57:90–9. [PMID: 21986048]

Pedowitz RA et al; American Academy of Orthopaedic Surgeons. Optimizing the management of rotator cuff problems. J Am Acad Orthop Surg. 2011 Jun;19(6):368–79. [PMID: 21628648]

3. Shoulder Dislocation & Instability

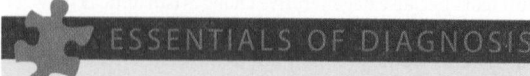

ESSENTIALS OF DIAGNOSIS

- ▶ Most dislocations (95%) are in the anterior direction.
- ▶ Pain and apprehension with an unstable shoulder that is abducted and externally rotated.
- ▶ Acute shoulder dislocations should be reduced as quickly as possible, using manual relocation techniques if necessary.

General Considerations

The shoulder is a ball and socket joint, similar to the hip. However, the bony contours of the shoulder bones are much different than the hip. Overall, the joint has much less stability than the hip, allowing greater movement and action. Stabilizing the shoulder joint relies heavily on rotator cuff muscle strength and also scapular control. If patients have poor scapular control or weak rotator cuff tendons or tears, their shoulders are more likely to have instability. Ninety-five percent of the shoulder dislocations/instability occur in the anterior direction. Dislocations

usually are caused by a fall on an outstretched and abducted arm. Patients complain of pain and feeling of instability when the arm is in the abducted and externally rotated position. Posterior dislocations are usually caused by falls from a height, epileptic seizures, or electric shocks. Traumatic shoulder dislocation can lead to instability. The rate of repeated dislocation is directly related to the patient's age: patients age 21 years or younger have a 70–90% risk of redislocation, whereas patients age 40 years or older have a much lower rate (20–30%). Ninety percent of young active individuals who had traumatic shoulder dislocation have labral injuries often described as Bankart lesions when the anterior inferior labrum is torn, which can lead to continued instability. Older patients (over age 55 years) are more likely to have rotator cuff tears or fractures following dislocation. Atraumatic shoulder dislocations are usually caused by intrinsic ligament laxity or repetitive microtrauma leading to joint instability. This is often seen in swimmers, gymnasts, and pitchers as well as other athletes involved in overhead and throwing sports.

Clinical Findings

A. Symptoms and Signs

For acute traumatic dislocations, patients usually have an obvious deformity with the humeral head dislocated anteriorly. The patient holds the shoulder and arm in an externally rotated position. The patient complains of acute pain and deformity that are improved with manual relocation of the shoulder. Reductions are usually performed in the emergency department. Even after reduction, the patient will continue to have limited range of motion and pain for 4–6 weeks, especially following a first-time shoulder dislocation.

Patients with recurrent dislocations can have less pain with subsequent dislocations. Posterior dislocations can be easily missed because the patient usually holds the shoulder and arm in an internally rotated position, which makes the shoulder deformity less obvious. Patients complain of difficulty pushing open a door.

Atraumatic shoulder instability is usually well tolerated with activities of daily living. Patients usually complain of a "sliding" sensation during exercises or strenuous activities such as throwing. Such dislocations may be less symptomatic and can often undergo spontaneous reduction of the shoulder with pain resolving within days after onset. The clinical examination for shoulder instability includes the apprehension test (Table 41–1), the load and shift test (Table 41–1) and the O'Brien test (Table 41–1). Most patients with persistent shoulder instability have preserved range of motion.

B. Imaging

Radiographs for acute dislocations should include a standard trauma series of AP and axillary lateral scapula (glenohumeral) views to determine the relationship of the humerus and the glenoid and to rule out fractures. Orthogonal views are used to identify a posterior shoulder dislocation, which can be missed easily with one AP view of the shoulder. An axillary lateral view of the shoulder can be safely performed even in the acute setting of a patient with a painful shoulder dislocation. For chronic injuries or symptomatic instability, these recommended radiographic views are helpful to identify bony injuries and Hill-Sachs lesions (indented compression fractures at the posterior-superior part of the humeral head associated with anterior shoulder dislocation). MRI is commonly used to show soft tissue injuries to the labrum and to visualize associated rotator cuff tears. MRI arthrograms better identify labral tears and ligamentous structures. Three-dimensional CT scans are being used to determine the significance of bone loss.

Treatment

For **acute dislocations,** the shoulder should be reduced as soon as possible. The Stimson procedure is the least traumatic method and is quite effective. The patient lies prone with the dislocated arm hanging off the examination table with a weight applied to the wrist to provide traction for 20–30 minutes. Afterward, gentle medial mobilization can be applied manually to assist the reduction. The shoulder can also be reduced with axial "traction" on the arm with "counter-traction" along the trunk. The patient should be sedated and relaxed. The shoulder can then be gently internally and externally rotated to guide it back into the socket.

Initial treatment of acute shoulder dislocations should include sling immobilization for 2–4 weeks along with pendulum exercises. Early physical therapy can be used to maintain range of motion and strengthening of rotator cuff muscles. Patients can also modify their activities to avoid active and risky sports. For patients with a *t*raumatic incident and *u*nilateral shoulder dislocation, a *B*ankart lesion is commonly present (remembered by the mnemonic, "TUBS") and *s*urgical treatment is often required.

The treatment of **atraumatic shoulder instability** is different than traumatic shoulder instability. Patients with chronic, recurrent shoulder dislocations should be managed with physical therapy and a regular maintenance program, consisting of scapular stabilization and postural and rotator cuff strengthening exercises. Activities may need to be modified. In patients with an *a*traumatic, *m*ultidirectional, *b*ilateral shoulder instability, *r*ehabilitation is the mainstay for treatment; *i*nferior capsular shift surgery is rarely required (remembered by the mnemonic, "AMBRI").

When to Refer

- Patients who are at risk for second dislocation, such as young patients, certain jobholders (eg, police officers, fire fighters, and rock climbers) to avoid recurrent dislocation or dislocation while at work.
- Patients who have not responded to conservative approach or who have chronic instability.

Bishop JY et al; MOON Shoulder Group. 3-D CT is the most reliable imaging modality when quantifying glenoid bone loss. Clin Orthop Relat Res. 2013 Apr;471(4):1251–6. [PMID: 22996361]

Chahal J et al. Anatomic Bankart repair compared with nonoperative treatment and/or arthroscopic lavage for first-time traumatic shoulder dislocation. Arthroscopy. 2012 Apr;28(4):565–75. [PMID: 22336435]

Rerko MA et al. Comparison of various imaging techniques to quantify glenoid bone loss in shoulder instability. J Shoulder Elbow Surg. 2013 Apr;22(4):528–34. [PMID: 22748926]

4. Adhesive Capsulitis ("Frozen Shoulder")

ESSENTIALS OF DIAGNOSIS

- ► Very painful shoulder triggered by minimal or no trauma.
- ► Pain out of proportion to clinical findings during the inflammatory phase.
- ► Stiffness during the "freezing" phase and resolution during the "thawing" phase.

General Considerations

Adhesive capsulitis ("frozen shoulder") is seen commonly in patients 40 to 65 years old. It is more commonly seen in women than men, especially in perimenopausal women or in patients with endocrine disorders, such as diabetes mellitus or thyroid disease. Adhesive capsulitis is a self-limiting but very debilitating disease.

Clinical Findings

A. Symptoms and Signs

Patients usually present with a painful shoulder that has a limited range of motion with both passive and active movements. A useful clinical sign is limitation of movement of external rotation with the elbow by the side of the trunk (Table 41–1). Strength is usually normal but it can appear diminished when the patient is in pain.

There are three phases: the inflammatory phase, the "freezing" phase, and the "thawing" phase. During the **inflammatory phase**, which usually lasts 4–6 months, patients complain of a very painful shoulder without obvious clinical findings to suggest trauma, fracture, or rotator cuff tear. During the **"freezing" phase**, which also usually lasts 4–6 months, the shoulder becomes stiffer and stiffer even though the pain is improving. The **"thawing" phase** can take up to a year as the shoulder slowly regains its motion. The total duration of an idiopathic frozen shoulder is usually about 24 months; it can be much longer for patients who have trauma or an endocrinopathy.

B. Imaging

Standard AP, axillary, and lateral glenohumeral radiographs are useful to rule out glenohumeral arthritis, which can also present with limited active and passive range of motion. However, adhesive capsulitis is usually a clinical diagnosis, and it does not need an extensive diagnostic work-up.

Treatment

Adhesive capsulitis is caused by acute inflammation of the capsule followed by scarring and remodeling. During the acute "freezing" phase, NSAIDs and physical therapy are recommended to maintain motion. There is also evidence of short-term benefit from intra-articular corticosteroid injection or oral prednisone. One study demonstrated improvement at 6 weeks but not 12 weeks following 30 mg of daily prednisone for 3 weeks. During the "freezing" phase, the shoulder is less painful but remains stiff. Anti-inflammatory medication is not as helpful during the "thawing" phase as it is during the "freezing" phase, and the shoulder symptoms usually resolve with time. Surgical treatments include manipulation under anesthesia and arthroscopic release.

When to Refer

- When the patient does not respond after more than 6 months of conservative treatment.
- When there is no progress or worsening range of motion over 3 months.

Rill BK et al. Predictors of outcome after nonoperative and operative treatment of adhesive capsulitis. Am J Sports Med. 2011 Mar;39(3):567–74. [PMID: 21160014]

Robinson CM et al. Frozen shoulder. J Bone Joint Surg Br. 2012 Jan;94(1):1–9. [PMID: 22219239]

SPINE PROBLEMS

1. Low Back Pain

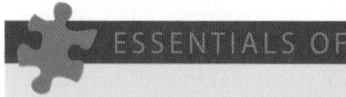

ESSENTIALS OF DIAGNOSIS

- ▶ The cause of back pain may be categorized by pain on flexion versus pain on extension.

- ▶ Nerve root impingement is suspected when pain is leg-dominant rather than back-dominant.

- ▶ Alarming signs for serious spinal disease include unexplained weight loss, failure to improve with treatment, severe pain for more than 6 weeks, and night or rest pain.

- ▶ The cauda equina syndrome often presents with bowel or bladder symptoms (or both) and is an emergency.

General Considerations

Low back pain remains the most common cause of disability for patients under the age of 45 and is the second most common cause for primary care visits. The annual prevalence of low back pain is 15–45%, and the annual cost in the United States is over $50 billion. Approximately 80% of episodes of low back pain resolve within 2 weeks and 90% resolve within 6 weeks. The exact cause of the low back pain is often difficult to diagnose; its cause is often multifactorial, although there are usually degenerative changes in the lumbar spine.

Alarming symptoms for back pain caused by cancer include unexplained weight loss, failure to improve with treatment, pain for more than 6 weeks, and pain at night or rest. History of cancer and age > 50 years are other risk factors for malignancy. Alarming symptoms for infection include fever, rest pain, recent infection (urinary tract infection, cellulitis, pneumonia), or history of immuno-compromise or injection drug use. The **cauda equina syndrome** is suggested by urinary retention or incontinence, saddle anesthesia, decreased anal sphincter tone or fecal incontinence, bilateral lower extremity weakness, and progressive neurologic deficits. Risk factors for back pain due to vertebral fracture include use of corticosteroids, age > 70 years, history of osteoporosis, recent significant trauma, or very severe focal pain. Back pain may also be the presenting symptom in other serious medical problems, including abdominal aortic aneurysm, peptic ulcer disease, kidney stones, or pancreatitis.

Clinical Findings

A. Symptoms and Signs

The physical examination is best done with the patient in the standing, sitting, supine, and then prone positions to avoid frequent repositioning of the patient. In the standing position, the patient's posture can be observed. Commonly encountered spinal asymmetries include scoliosis, thoracic kyphosis, and lumbar hyperlordosis. The active range of motion of the lumbar spine can be assessed. The common directions include flexion, rotation, and extension. The one-leg standing extension test assesses for pain as the patient stands on one leg while extending the spine. A positive test can be caused by pars interarticularis fractures (spondylolysis or spondylolisthesis) or facet joint arthritis, although sensitivity and specificity of the test is limited.

Motor strength, reflexes, and sensation can be tested in the sitting position (Table 41–2). The major muscles in the lower extremities are assessed for weakness by eliciting a resisted isometric contraction for approximately 5 seconds. It is important to compare the strength bilaterally to detect subtle muscle weakness. Similarly, sensory testing to light touch can be checked in specific dermatomes for corresponding nerve root function. Finally, the knee (femoral nerve L2–4), ankle (deep peroneal nerve L4–L5), and Babinski (sciatic nerve L5–S1) reflexes can be checked with the patient sitting.

In the supine position, the hip should be evaluated for range of motion, focusing on internal rotation. The straight leg raise test puts traction and compression forces on the lower lumbar nerve roots (Table 41–3).

Finally, in the prone position, the clinician can carefully palpate each level of the spine and sacroiliac joints for tenderness. A rectal examination is required if the cauda equina syndrome is suspected. Superficial skin tenderness to a light touch over the lumbar spine, overreaction to maneuvers in the regular back examination, low back pain on axial loading of spine in standing, inconsistency in the

Table 41–2. Neurologic testing of lumbosacral nerve disorders.

Nerve Root	Motor	Reflex	Sensory Area
L1	Hip flexion	None	Groin
L2	Hip flexion	None	Thigh
L3	Extension of knee	Knee jerk	Knee
L4	Dorsiflexion of ankle	Knee jerk	Medial calf
L5	Dorsiflexion of first toe	Babinski reflex	First dorsal web space between first and second toes
S1	Plantar flexion of foot, knee flexors or hamstrings	Ankle jerk	Lateral foot
S2	Knee flexors or hamstrings	Knee flexor	Back of the thigh
S2–S4	External anal sphincter	Anal reflex, rectal tone	Perianal area

Table 41–4. AHRQ criteria for lumbar radiographs in patients with acute low back pain.

Possible fracture
Major trauma
Minor trauma in patients > 50 years
Long-term corticosteroid use
Osteoporosis
> 70 years
Possible tumor or infection
> 50 years
< 20 years
History of cancer
Constitutional symptoms
Recent bacterial infection
Injection drug use
Immunosuppression
Supine pain
Nocturnal pain

AHRQ, Agency for Healthcare Research and Quality.
Reproduced, with permission, from Suarez-Almazor et al. Use of lumbar radiographs for the early diagnosis of low back pain. Proposed guidelines would increase utilization. JAMA. 1997 Jun; 277:1782–6.

straight leg raise test or on the neurologic examination suggest nonorthopedic causes for the pain or malingering.

B. Imaging

In the absence of alarming "red flag" symptoms suggesting infection, malignancy, or cauda equina syndrome, diagnostic imaging, including radiographs, is not typically recommended in the first 6 weeks. The Agency for Healthcare Research and Quality guidelines for obtaining lumbar radiographs are summarized in Table 41–4. Most clinicians obtain radiographs for new back pain in patients older than 50 years. If done, radiographs of the lumbar spine should include AP and lateral views. Oblique views can be useful if the neuroforamina or lesions need to be visualized. MRI is the method of choice in the evaluation of symptoms not responding to conservative treatment or in the presence of red flags of serious conditions.

C. Special Tests

Electromyography or nerve conduction studies may be useful in assessing patients with possible nerve root

Table 41–3. Spine: back examination.

Maneuver	Description
Inspection	Check the patient's posture in the standing position. Assess for hyperlordosis, kyphosis, and scoliosis.
Palpation	Include important landmarks: spinous process, facet joints, paravertebral muscles, sacroiliac joints, and sacrum.
Range of motion testing	Check range of motion actively (patient performs) and passively (clinician performs) especially with flexion and extension of the spine. Rotation and lateral bending are also helpful to assess symmetric motion or any restrictions.
Neurologic examination	Check motor strength, reflexes and dermatomal sensation in the lower extremities.
Straight leg raise test	The patient lies supine and the clinician elevates the patient's leg. A positive test for sciatica pain is classically described as "electric shock"-like pain radiating down the posterior aspect of the leg from the low back. This can occur in the setting of a disk herniation or degenerative conditions causing neural foraminal stenosis. Cross-over pain, where sciatica symptoms occur down the opposite leg during a straight leg raise, usually indicates a large disk herniation.
Indirect straight leg raise test	The patient sits on the side of the exam table with the knees bent. The clinician extends the knee fully. A positive test for sciatica pain is classically described as "electric shock"-like pain radiating down the posterior aspect of the leg from the low back. Cross-over pain, where sciatica symptoms occur down the opposite leg during a straight leg raise, usually indicates a large disk herniation.

symptoms lasting longer than 6 weeks; back pain may or may not also be present. These tests are usually not necessary if the diagnosis of radiculopathy is clear.

▶ Treatment

A. Conservative

Nonpharmacologic treatments are key in the management of low back pain. Education alone improves patient satisfaction with recovery and recurrence. Patients require information and reassurance, especially when diagnostic procedures are not necessary. Discussion must include reviewing safe and effective methods of symptom control as well as how to decrease the risk of recurrence with proper lifting techniques, abdominal wall/core strengthening, weight loss, and smoking cessation. Strengthening and stabilization effectively reduce pain and functional limitation compared with usual care.

Physical therapy exercise programs can be tailored to the patient's symptoms and pathology. Neither spinal manipulation nor traction have shown benefits for low back pain; however, the level of evidence is low quality and limited by small sample sizes. Heat and cold treatments have not shown any long-term benefits but may be used for symptomatic treatment. The efficacy of transcutaneous electrical nerve stimulation (TENS), back braces, physical agents, and acupuncture is unproven. Improvements in posture, core stability strengthening, physical conditioning, and modifications of activities to decrease physical strain are keys for ongoing management.

NSAIDs are effective in the early treatment of low back pain (see Chapter 20). There is limited evidence that muscle relaxants can provide short-term relief; since these medications have addictive potential, they should be used with care. Muscle relaxants are best used if there is true muscle spasm that is painful rather than simply a protective response. Opioids may be necessary to alleviate pain immediately. Treatment of more chronic neuropathic pain with alpha-2-delta ligands (eg, gabapentin), serotonin-norepinephrine reuptake inhibitors (eg, duloxetine) or tricyclic antidepressants (eg, nortriptyline) may be helpful. Epidural injections may provide improved pain reduction short term, although studies are limited and lack long-term follow-up.

B. Surgical

Surgical indications for back surgery include cauda equina syndrome, ongoing morbidity with no response to > 6 months of conservative treatment, cancer, infection, or severe spinal deformity. Prognosis is improved when there is an anatomic lesion that can be corrected and symptoms are neurologic. Spinal surgery has limitations. Patient selection is very important and the specific surgery recommended should have very clear indications. Patients should understand that surgery can improve their pain but is unlikely to cure it. Surgery is not generally indicated for radiographic abnormalities alone when the patient is asymptomatic. Depending on the surgery performed, possible complications include persistent pain; surgical site pain, especially if bone grafting is

needed; infection; neurologic damage; non-union; cutaneous nerve damage; implant failure; deep venous thrombosis; and death.

▶ When to Refer

- Patients with the cauda equina syndrome.
- Patients with cancer, infection, or severe spinal deformity.
- Patients who have not responded to conservative treatment.

Bicket MC et al. Epidural injections for spinal pain: a systematic review and meta-analysis evaluating the "control" injections in randomized controlled trials. Anesthesiology. 2013 Oct;119(4):907–31. [PMID: 24195874]

Goodman DM et al. JAMA patient page. Low back pain. JAMA. 2013 Apr 24;309(16):1738. [PMID: 23613079]

Lin CW et al. Cost-effectiveness of guideline-endorsed treatments for low back pain: a systematic review. Eur Spine J. 2011 Jul;20(7):1024–38. [PMID: 21229367]

Rubinstein SM et al. Spinal manipulative therapy for acute low back pain: an update of the Cochrane review. Spine (Phila Pa 1976). 2013 Feb 1;38(3):E158–77. [PMID: 23169072]

2. Spinal Stenosis

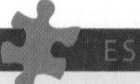

ESSENTIALS OF DIAGNOSIS

- ▶ Pain is usually worse with back extension and relieved by sitting.
- ▶ Occurs in older patients.
- ▶ May present with neurogenic claudication symptoms with walking.

▶ General Considerations

Osteoarthritis in the lumbar spine can cause narrowing of the spinal canal. A large disk herniation can also cause stenosis and compression of neural structures or the spinal artery resulting in "claudication" symptoms with ambulation. The condition usually affects patients aged 50 years or older.

▶ Clinical Findings

Patients report pain that worsens with extension. They describe reproducible single or bilateral leg symptoms that are worse after walking several minutes and that are relieved by sitting ("neurogenic claudication"). On examination, patients often exhibit limited extension of the lumbar spine, which may reproduce the symptoms radiating down the legs. A thorough neurovascular examination is recommended (Table 41–2).

▶ Treatment

Flexion-based exercises as demonstrated by a physical therapist can help relieve symptoms. Epidural or facet joint corticosteroid injections can also reduce pain symptoms. However, patients who received epidural corticosteroids had less improvement at 4 years among all patients with spinal stenosis and were associated with longer duration of surgery and longer hospital stay.

Surgical treatments for spinal stenosis include spinal decompression (widening the spinal canal or laminectomy), nerve root decompression (freeing a single nerve), and spinal fusion (joining the vertebra to eliminate motion and diminish pain from the arthritic joints). In an ongoing multicenter randomized trial, subgroups improved significantly more with surgery than with nonoperative treatment. Variables associated with greater treatment effects included lower baseline disability scores, not smoking, neuroforaminal stenosis, predominant leg pain rather than back pain, not lifting at work, and the presence of a neurologic deficit.

▶ When to Refer

- If a patient exhibits radicular or claudication symptoms > 12 weeks.
- MRI or CT confirmation of significant spinal stenosis.

Ammendolia C et al. Nonoperative treatment of lumbar spinal stenosis with neurogenic claudication: a systematic review. Spine (Phila Pa 1976). 2012 May 1;37(10):E609–16. [PMID: 22158059]

Pearson A et al. Who should have surgery for spinal stenosis? Treatment effect predictors in SPORT. Spine (Phila Pa 1976). 2012 Oct 1;37(21):1791–802. [PMID: 23018805]

Radcliff K et al. Epidural steroid injections are associated with less improvement in patients with lumbar spinal stenosis: a subgroup analysis of the spine patient outcomes research trial. Spine (Phila Pa 1976). 2013 Feb 15;38(4):279–91. [PMID: 23238485]

3. Lumbar Disk Herniation

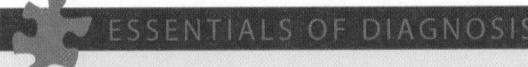

ESSENTIALS OF DIAGNOSIS

- ▶ Pain with back flexion or prolonged sitting.
- ▶ Radicular pain with compression of neural structures.
- ▶ Lower extremity numbness.
- ▶ Lower extremity weakness.

▶ General Considerations

Lumbar disk herniation is usually due to bending or heavy loading (eg, lifting) with the back in flexion, causing herniation or extrusion of disk contents (nucleus pulposus) into the spinal cord area. However, there may not be an inciting incident. Disk herniations usually occur from degenerative disk disease (dessication of the annulus fibrosis) in patients between 30- and 50-years-old. The L5–S1 disk is affected in 90% of cases. Compression of neural structures, such as the sciatic nerve, causes radicular pain. Severe compression of the spinal cord can cause the cauda equina syndrome, a surgical emergency (see above).

▶ Clinical Findings

A. Symptoms and Signs

Discogenic pain typically is localized in the low back at the level of the affected disk and is worse with activity. "Sciatica" causes electric shock-like pain radiating down the posterior aspect of the leg often to below the knee. Symptoms usually worsen with back flexion such as bending or sitting for long periods (eg, driving). A significant disk herniation can cause numbness and weakness, including weakness with plantar flexion of the foot (L5/S1) or dorsiflexion of the toes (L4/L5). The cauda equina syndrome should be ruled out if the patient complains of perianal numbness or bowel or bladder incontinence.

B. Imaging

Plain radiographs are helpful to assess spinal alignment (scoliosis, lordosis), disk space narrowing, and osteoarthritis changes. MRI is the best method to assess the level and morphology of the herniation and is recommended if surgery is planned.

▶ Treatment

For an acute exacerbation of pain symptoms, bed rest is appropriate for up to 48 hours. Otherwise, first-line treatments include modified activities; NSAIDs and other analgesics; and physical therapy, including core stabilization and McKenzie exercises. Following nonsurgical treatment for a lumbar disk for over 1 year, the incidence of low back pain recurrence is at least 40% and is predicted by longer time to initial resolution of pain. Epidural and transforaminal corticosteroid injections can be beneficial, especially in relieving acute radicular pain, although the benefit tends to last only 3 months. These injections may be effective in delaying surgery for chronic low back pain. Oral prednisone can reduce inflammation and is useful in reducing symptoms of acute sciatica; the initial dose is approximately 1 mg/kg once daily with tapering doses over 10 days. Co-analgesics for neuropathic pain, such as the calcium channel alpha-2-delta ligands (ie, gabapentin, pregabalin) or tricyclic antidepressants, may be helpful (see Chapter 5).

A large, ongoing trial has shown that patients who underwent surgery for a lumbar disk herniation achieved greater improvement than conservatively treated patients in all primary and secondary outcomes except return to work status after 4 year follow-up. So far, disk replacement surgery has not shown benefits beyond generally accepted clinically important differences in short-term pain relief, disability, and quality of life compared with spine fusion surgery.

▶ When to Refer

- Cauda equina syndrome.
- Progressive worsening of neurologic symptoms.
- Loss of motor function (sensory losses can be followed in the outpatient clinic).

Pinto RZ et al. Epidural corticosteroid injections in the management of sciatica: a systematic review and meta-analysis. Ann Intern Med. 2012 Dec 18;157(12):865–77. [PMID: 23362516]

Rihn JA et al. Duration of symptoms resulting from lumbar disc herniation: effect on treatment outcomes: analysis of the Spine Patient Outcomes Research Trial (SPORT). J Bone Joint Surg Am. 2011 Oct 19;93(20):1906–14. [PMID: 22012528]

Suri P et al. Recurrence of radicular pain or back pain after nonsurgical treatment of symptomatic lumbar disk herniation. Arch Phys Med Rehabil. 2012 Apr;93(4):690–5. [PMID: 22464091]

4. Neck Pain

ESSENTIALS OF DIAGNOSIS

▶ Most chronic neck pain is caused by degenerative joint disease and responds to conservative treatment.

▶ Cervical radiculopathy symptoms can be referred to the shoulder, arm, or upper back.

▶ Whiplash is the most common type of traumatic injury to the neck.

▶ Poor posture is often a factor for persistent neck pain.

▶ General Considerations

Most neck pain, especially in older patients, is due to mechanical degeneration involving the cervical disks, facet joints, and ligamentous structures and may occur in the setting of degenerative changes at other sites. Pain can also come from the supporting neck musculature, which often acts to protect the underlying neck structures. **Posture is a very important factor, especially in younger patients.** Many work-related neck symptoms are due to poor posture and repetitive motions over time. Acute injuries can also occur secondary to trauma. For example, whiplash occurs in 15–40% of motor vehicle accidents, with chronic pain developing in 5–7%. Neck fractures are serious traumatic injuries acutely and can lead to osteoarthritis in the long term. Ultimately, many degenerative conditions of the neck result in cervical canal stenosis or neural foraminal stenosis, sometimes affecting underlying neural structures. Cervical radiculopathy can cause neurologic symptoms in the upper extremities usually deriving from disease of the C5–C7 disks. Patients with neck pain may report associated headaches and shoulder pain. Thoracic outlet syndrome, in which there is mechanical compression of the brachial plexus and neurovascular structures with overhead positioning of the arm, should be considered in the differential diagnosis of neck pain.

Other causes of neck pain include rheumatoid arthritis, fibromyalgia, osteomyelitis, neoplasms, polymyalgia rheumatica, compression fractures, pain referred from visceral structures (eg, angina), and functional disorders. Amyotrophic lateral sclerosis, multiple sclerosis, syringomyelia, spinal cord tumors, and tropical spastic paresis from HTLV-1 infection can mimic myelopathy from cervical arthritis.

▶ Clinical Findings

A. Symptoms and Signs

Neck pain may be limited to the posterior region or, depending on the level of the symptomatic joint, may radiate segmentally to the occiput, anterior chest, shoulder girdle, arm, forearm, and hand. It may be intensified by active or passive neck motions. The general distribution of pain and paresthesias corresponds roughly to the involved dermatome in the upper extremity.

The patient's posture should be assessed, checking for shoulder rolled forward or head forward posture as well as scoliosis in the thoracolumbar spine. Patients with discogenic neck pain often complain of pain with flexion, which causes cervical disks to herniate posteriorly. Extension of the neck usually affects the neural foraminal and facet joints of the neck. Rotation and lateral flexion of the cervical spine should be measured both to the left and the right. Limitation of cervical movements is the most common objective finding.

A detailed neurovascular examination of the upper extremities should be performed, including sensory input to light touch and temperature; motor strength testing, especially the hand intrinsic muscles (thumb extension strength [C6], opponens strength (thumb to pinky) [C7], and finger abductors and adductors strength [C8–T1]); and upper extremity reflexes (biceps, triceps, brachioradialis). True cervical radiculopathy symptoms should match an expected dermatomal or myotomal distribution. The **Spurling test** involves asking the patient to rotate and extend the neck to one side (Table 41–5). The clinician can apply a gentle axial load to the neck. Reproduction of the cervical radiculopathy symptoms is a positive sign of nerve root compression. Palpation of the neck is best performed with the patient in the supine position where the clinician can palpate each level of the cervical spine with the muscles of the neck relaxed.

B. Imaging

Radiographs of the cervical spine can assist in determining the area of degenerative changes. Useful views include the AP and lateral view of the cervical spine. The odontoid view is usually added to rule out traumatic fractures and congenital abnormalities. Oblique views of the cervical spine can provide further information about arthritis changes and assess the neural foramina for narrowing. Many plain radiographs are completely normal in patients who have suffered an acute cervical strain. Loss of cervical lordosis is often seen but is nonspecific. Comparative reduction in height of the involved disk space and osteophytes are frequent findings when there are degenerative changes in the cervical spine.

CT scanning is the most useful method if bony abnormalities, such as fractures, are suspected. MRI is the best method to assess the cervical spine since the soft tissue structures (such as the disks, spinal cord, and nerve roots) can be evaluated. If the patient has signs of cervical

Table 41–5. Spine: neck examination.

Maneuver	Description
Inspection	Check the patient's posture in the standing position. Assess for cervical hyperlordosis, head forward posture, kyphosis, scoliosis, torticollis.
Palpation	Include important landmarks: spinous process, facet joints, paracervical muscles (sternocleidomastoid, scalene muscles).
Range of motion testing	Check range of motion in the cervical spine, especially with flexion and extension. Rotation and lateral bending are also helpful to assess symmetric motion or any restrictions. Pain and radicular symptoms can be exacerbated by range of motion testing.
Neurologic examination	Check motor strength, reflexes and dermatomal sensation in the upper (and lower if necessary) extremities.
Spurling test	Involves asking the patient to rotate and extend the neck to one side. The clinician can apply a gentle axial load to the neck. Reproduction of the cervical radiculopathy symptoms is a positive sign of nerve root compression.

radiculopathy with motor weakness, these more sensitive imaging modalities should be obtained urgently.

▶ **Treatment**

In the absence of trauma or evidence of infection, malignancy, neurologic findings, or systemic inflammation, the patient can be treated conservatively. A course of neck stretching, strengthening and postural exercises in physical therapy have demonstrated benefit in relieving symptoms. A soft cervical collar can be useful for short-term use (up to 1–2 weeks) in acute neck injuries. Chiropractic manual manipulation and mobilization can provide short-term benefit for mechanical neck pain. Although the rate of complications is low (5–10/million manipulations), care should be taken whenever there are neurologic symptoms present. Specific patients may respond to use of home cervical traction. NSAIDs are commonly used and opioids may be needed in cases of severe neck pain. Muscle relaxants (eg, cyclobenzaprine 5–10 mg orally three times daily) can be used short-term if there is muscle spasm or as a sedative to aid in sleeping. Acute radicular symptoms can be treated with neuropathic medications (eg, gabapentin 300–1200 mg orally three times daily), and a short course of oral prednisone (5–10 days) can be considered (starting at 1 mg/kg). Cervical foraminal or facet joint injections can also reduce symptoms. Cervical spine surgery does not have clear evidence of benefit over conservative treatment. Surgeries are successful in reducing neurologic symptoms in 80–90% of cases but are still considered as treatments of last resort.

▶ **When to Refer**

- Patients with severe symptoms with motor weakness.
- Surgical decompression surgery if the symptoms are severe and there is identifiable, correctable pathology.

Kelly JC et al. The natural history and clinical syndromes of degenerative cervical spondylosis. Adv Orthop. 2012;2012: 393642. [PMID: 22162812]
van Middelkoop M et al. Surgery versus conservative care for neck pain: a systematic review. Eur Spine J. 2013 Jan;22(1): 87–95. [PMID: 23104514]

UPPER EXTREMITY

1. Lateral & Medial Epicondylosis

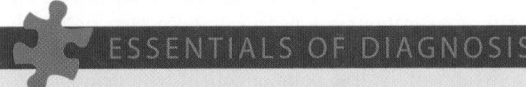

ESSENTIALS OF DIAGNOSIS

▶ Tenderness over the lateral or medial epicondyle.

▶ Diagnosis of tendinopathy is confirmed by pain with resisted strength testing and passive stretching of the affected tendon and muscle unit.

▶ Physical therapy and activity modification are more successful than anti-inflammatory treatments.

▶ **General Considerations**

Tendinopathy involving the wrist extensors, flexors, and pronators are very common complaints. The underlying mechanism is chronic repetitive overuse causing microtrauma at the tendon insertion, although acute injuries can occur as well if the tendon is strained due to excessive loading. The traditional term "epicondylitis" is a misnomer because histologically tendinosis or degeneration in the tendon is seen rather than acute inflammation. Therefore, these entities should be referred to as "tendinopathy" or "tendinosis." Lateral epicondylosis involves the wrist extensors, especially the extensor carpi radialis brevis. This is usually caused be lifting with the wrist and the elbow extended. Medial epicondylosis involves the wrist flexors and most commonly the pronator teres tendon. Ulnar neuropathy and cervical radiculopathy should be considered in the differential diagnosis.

▶ **Clinical Findings**

A. Symptoms and Signs

For lateral epicondylosis, the patient describes pain with the arm and wrist extended. For example, common complaints include pain while shaking hands, lifting objects, using a computer mouse, or hitting a backhand in tennis ("tennis elbow"). Medial epicondylosis presents with pain during motions in which the arm is repetitively pronated or the wrist is flexed. This is also known as "golfer's elbow" due to the motion of turning the hands over during the golf swing. On examination, tenderness directly over the epicondyle is present, especially over the posterior aspect where the tendon insertion occurs. The proximal tendon and musculotendinous junction can also be sore. To confirm that the pain is due to tendinopathy, pain can be reproduced over the epicondyle with resisted wrist extension and third digit extension for lateral epicondylosis and resisted wrist pronation and wrist flexion for medial epicondylosis. The pain is also often reproduced with passive stretching of the affected muscle groups, which can be performed with the arm in extension. It is useful to check the ulnar nerve (located in a groove at the posteromedial elbow) for tenderness as well as to perform a Spurling test for cervical radiculopathy.

B. Imaging

Radiographs are often normal, although a small traction spur may be present in chronic cases (enthesopathy). Diagnostic investigations are usually unnecessary, unless the patient does not improve after up to 3 months of conservative treatment. At that point, a patient who demonstrates significant disability due to the pain should be assessed with an MRI or ultrasound. Ultrasound and MRI can visualize the tendon and confirm tendinosis or tears.

▶ Treatment

Treatment is usually conservative, including patient education regarding activity modification and management of symptoms. Ice and NSAIDs can help with pain. The most important steps are to begin a good stretching program followed by strengthening exercises, particularly eccentric ones. Counterforce elbow braces might provide some symptomatic relief, although there is no published evidence to support their use. If the patient has severe or long-standing symptoms, a course of physical therapy should be performed. A randomized trial showed no differences with platelet-rich plasma, corticosteroid, or saline injections at 3 months. Corticosteroid injection had improvement at 1 month as well as evidence of decreased tendon thickness and Doppler changes. Treatments such as extracorporeal shock wave therapy and other injections have not shown clear long-term benefit. Physical therapy is still the mainstay of treatment.

▶ When to Refer

Patients not responding to 6 months of conservative treatment should be referred for surgical debridement or repair of the tendon.

Krogh TP et al. Comparative effectiveness of injection therapies in lateral epicondylitis: a systematic review and network meta-analysis of randomized controlled trials. Am J Sports Med. 2013 Jun;41(6):1435–46. [PMID: 22972856]

Krogh TP et al. Treatment of lateral epicondylitis with platelet-rich plasma, glucocorticoid, or saline: a randomized, double-blind, placebo-controlled trial. Am J Sports Med. 2013 Mar;41(3):625–35. [PMID: 23328738]

Raman J et al. Effectiveness of different methods of resistance exercises in lateral epicondylosis—a systematic review. J Hand Ther. 2012 Jan–Mar;25(1):5–25. [PMID: 22075055]

2. Carpal Tunnel Syndrome

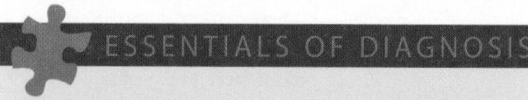
ESSENTIALS OF DIAGNOSIS

- ▶ Pain, burning, and tingling in the distribution of the median nerve.
- ▶ Initially, most bothersome during sleep.
- ▶ Late weakness or atrophy, especially of the thenar eminence.
- ▶ Can be caused by repetitive activities using the wrist.
- ▶ Commonly seen during pregnancy and in patients with diabetes mellitus or rheumatoid arthritis.

▶ General Considerations

An entrapment neuropathy, carpal tunnel syndrome is a painful disorder caused by compression of the median nerve between the carpal ligament and other structures within the carpal tunnel. The contents of the tunnel can be compressed by synovitis of the tendon sheaths or carpal joints, recent or malhealed fractures, tumors, tissue infiltration, and occasionally congenital syndromes (eg, mucopolysaccharidoses). Even though no anatomic lesion is apparent, flattening or even circumferential constriction of the median nerve may be observed during operative section of the overlying carpal ligament. The disorder may occur in fluid retention of pregnancy, in individuals with a history of repetitive use of the hands, or following injuries of the wrists. There is a familial type of carpal tunnel syndrome in which no etiologic factor can be identified. Carpal tunnel syndrome can also be a feature of many systemic diseases, such as rheumatoid arthritis and other rheumatic disorders (inflammatory tenosynovitis), myxedema, amyloidosis, sarcoidosis, leukemia, acromegaly, and hyperparathyroidism.

▶ Clinical Findings

A. Symptoms and Signs

The initial symptoms are pain, burning, and tingling in the distribution of the median nerve (the palmar surfaces of the thumb, the index and long fingers, and the radial half of the ring finger). Aching pain may radiate proximally into the forearm and occasionally proximally to the shoulder and over the neck and chest. Pain is exacerbated by manual activity, particularly by extremes of volar flexion or dorsiflexion of the wrist. It is most bothersome at night. Impairment of sensation in the median nerve distribution may or may not be demonstrable. Subtle disparity between the affected and opposite sides can be shown by testing for two-point discrimination or by requiring the patient to identify different textures of cloth by rubbing them between the tips of the thumb and the index finger. A Tinel or

Table 41–6. Wrist examination.

Maneuver	Description
Inspection	Examine for the alignment of the wrist and fingers SEADS
Palpation	Include important landmarks: scaphoid "snuff box," distal radius, scapholunate ligament, hook of hamate, ulnar joint line, distal radioulnar joint
Range of motion testing	Check range of motion actively (patient performs) and passively (clinician performs) especially with flexion and extension of the wrist. Ulnar and radial deviation and circumduction of the wrist can be screened.
Neurovascular examination	Check motor strength and dermatomal sensation in the fingers in the radial (thumb), median (3rd finger) and ulnar distribution (5th finger). Check capillary refill to digits as well as radial pulse.
Tinel sign	Tingling or shock-like pain on volar wrist percussion. The carpal compression test, in which numbness and tingling are induced by the direct application of pressure over the carpal tunnel, may be more sensitive and specific than the Tinel and Phalen tests.
Phalen sign	Pain or paresthesia in the distribution of the median nerve when the patient flexes both wrists to 90 degrees for 60 seconds.
Carpel compression test	Performed by applying direct application of pressure over the carpal tunnel.

SEADS, swelling, erythema, atrophy, deformity, and (surgical) scars.

Phalen sign may be positive. A **Tinel sign** is tingling or shock-like pain on volar wrist percussion (Table 41–6). The **Phalen sign** is pain or paresthesia in the distribution of the median nerve when the patient flexes both wrists to 90 degrees for 60 seconds (Table 41–6). The **carpal compression test,** in which numbness and tingling are induced by the direct application of pressure over the carpal tunnel, may be more sensitive and specific than the Tinel and Phalen tests (Table 41–6). Muscle weakness or atrophy, especially of the thenar eminence, can appear later than sensory disturbances as compression of the nerve worsens.

B. Imaging

Ultrasound can demonstrate flattening of the median nerve beneath the flexor retinaculum. Sensitivity of ultrasound for carpal tunnel syndrome is variable but estimated between 54% and 98%.

C. Special Tests

Electromyography and nerve conduction studies show evidence of sensory conduction delay before motor delay,

which can occur in severe cases. This syndrome should be differentiated from other cervicobrachial pain syndromes, from compression syndromes of the median nerve in the forearm or arm, and from mononeuritis multiplex. When left-sided, it may be confused with angina pectoris.

▶ Treatment

Treatment is directed toward relief of pressure on the median nerve. When a causative lesion is discovered, it should be treated appropriately. Otherwise, patients in whom carpal tunnel syndrome is suspected should modify their hand activities and have the affected wrist splinted in the neutral position for up to 3 months. A series of Cochrane reviews show limited evidence for splinting, therapeutic ultrasound, exercises, and ergonomic positioning. Oral corticosteroids or NSAIDs can also be tried. Carpal tunnel release surgery can be beneficial if the patient has a positive electrodiagnostic test, at least moderate symptoms, high clinical probability, unsuccessful nonoperative treatment, and symptoms lasting longer than 12 months. A randomized, controlled trial showed both corticosteroid injection and surgery resolved symptoms but only decompressive surgery allows resolution of neurophysiologic changes.

▶ When to Refer

- If symptoms persist > 3 months despite conservative treatment, including the use of a wrist splint.
- If thenar muscle (eg, abductor pollicis brevis) weakness or atrophy develops.

Andreu JL et al. Local injection versus surgery in carpal tunnel syndrome: neurophysiologic outcomes of a randomized clinical trial. Clin Neurophysiol. 2014 Jul;125(7):1479–84. [PMID: 24321619]

Carpal Tunnel Syndrome. In: Hegmann KT (editor). *Occupational Medicine Practice Guidelines. Evaluation and Management of Common Health Problems and Functional Recovery in Workers,* 3rd ed. Elk Grove Village (IL): American College of Occupational and Environmental Medicine (ACOEM), 2011.

3. Dupuytren Contracture

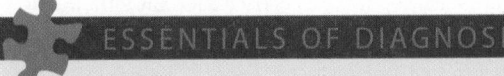

ESSENTIALS OF DIAGNOSIS

- ▶ Benign fibrosing disorder of the palmar fascia.
- ▶ Contracture of one or more fingers can lead to limited hand function.

▶ General Considerations

This relatively common disorder is characterized by hyperplasia of the palmar fascia and related structures, with nodule formation and contracture of the palmar fascia. The cause is unknown, but the condition has a genetic predisposition and occurs primarily in white men over 50 years of age, particularly in those of Celtic descent. The incidence is higher among alcoholic patients and those with chronic systemic disorders (especially cirrhosis). It is also associated with systemic fibrosing syndrome, which includes plantar fibromatosis (10% of patients), Peyronie disease (1–2%), mediastinal and retroperitoneal fibrosis, and Riedel struma. The onset may be acute, but slowly progressive chronic disease is more common.

► Clinical Findings

Dupuytren contracture manifests itself by nodular or cord-like thickening of one or both hands, with the fourth and fifth fingers most commonly affected. The patient may complain of tightness of the involved digits, with inability to satisfactorily extend the fingers, and on occasion there is tenderness. The resulting cosmetic problems may be unappealing, but in general the contracture is well tolerated since it exaggerates the normal position of function of the hand.

► Treatment

If the palmar nodule is growing rapidly, injections of triamcinolone or collagenase into the nodule may be of benefit. The injection of collagenase *Clostridium histolyticum* is a promising nonoperative treatment option that lyses collagen disrupting the contracted cords. Surgical intervention is indicated in patients with significant flexion contractures, depending on the location, but recurrence is possible. Invasive options include open fasciectomy, partial fasciectomy, or percutaneous needle aponeurotomy.

► When to Refer

Referral can be considered when one or more digits are affected by severe contractures, which interfere with everyday activities and result in functional limitations.

Baltzer H et al. Cost-effectiveness in the management of Dupuytren's contracture. A Canadian cost-utility analysis of current and future management strategies. Bone Joint J. 2013 Aug; 95-B(8):1094–100. [PMID: 23908426]

Peimer CA et al. Dupuytren contracture recurrence following treatment with collagenase clostridium histolyticum (CORD-LESS study): 3-year data. J Hand Surg Am. 2013 Jan;38(1): 12–22. [PMID: 23200951]

Worrell M. Dupuytren's disease. Orthopedics. 2012 Jan;35(1): 52–60. [PMID: 22229922]

4. Bursitis

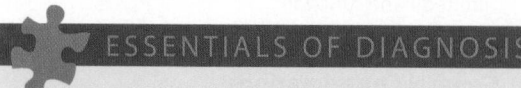

ESSENTIALS OF DIAGNOSIS

► Often occurs around bony prominences where it is important to reduce friction.

► Typically presents with local swelling that is painful acutely.

► Septic bursitis can present without fever or systemic signs.

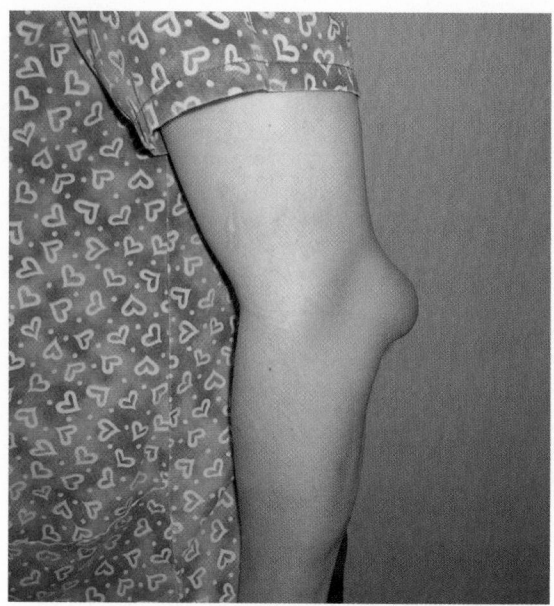

▲ **Figure 41–1.** Aseptic olecranon bursitis secondary to repetitive trauma. (Reproduced, with permission, from Richard P. Usatine, MD.)

► General Considerations

Inflammation of bursae—the synovium-like cellular membranes overlying bony prominences—may be secondary to trauma, infection, or arthritic conditions such as gout, rheumatoid arthritis, or osteoarthritis. Bursitis can result from infection. The two common sites are the olecranon (Figure 41–1) and prepatellar bursae, however, others include subdeltoid, ischial, trochanteric, and semimembranous-gastrocnemius (Baker cyst) bursae.

► Clinical Findings

A. Symptoms and Signs

Bursitis is more likely than arthritis to cause focal tenderness and swelling and less likely to affect range of motion of the adjacent joint. Olecranon bursitis, for example, causes an oval (or, if chronic, bulbous) swelling at the tip of the elbow and does not affect elbow motion, whereas an elbow joint inflammation produces more diffuse swelling and reduces range of motion. The absence of fever does not exclude infection; **one-third of those with septic olecranon bursitis are afebrile**. A bursa can also become symptomatic when it ruptures. This is particularly true for Baker cyst (see below), whose rupture can cause calf pain and swelling that mimic thrombophlebitis.

B. Imaging

Imaging is unnecessary unless there is concern for osteomyelitis, trauma or other underlying pathology. Ruptured Baker cysts are imaged easily by sonography or MRI. It may be important to exclude a deep venous thrombosis, which can be mimicked by a ruptured Baker cyst.

C. Special Tests

Acute swelling and redness at a bursal site calls for aspiration to rule out infection. A bursal fluid white blood cell count of > 1000/mcL indicates inflammation from infection, rheumatoid arthritis, or gout. In septic bursitis, the white cell count averages over 50,000/mcL. Most cases are caused by *Staphylococcus aureus;* the Gram stain is positive in two-thirds.

▶ Treatment

Bursitis caused by trauma responds to local heat, rest, NSAIDs, and local corticosteroid injections. Chronic, stable olecranon bursa swelling usually does not require aspiration. Aspiration of the olecranon bursa runs the risk of creating a chronic drainage site, which can be reduced by using a "zig-zag" approach with a small needle (25-gauge if possible) and pulling the skin over the bursa before introducing it. Applying a pressure bandage may also help prevent chronic drainage. Repetitive minor trauma to the olecranon bursa should be eliminated by avoiding resting the elbow on a hard surface or by wearing an elbow pad. Treatment of a ruptured Baker cyst includes rest, leg elevation, and injection of triamcinolone, 20–40 mg into the knee anteriorly (the knee compartment communicates with the cyst). Knowledge of trochanteric bursa anatomy is important for effective injection.

Treatment for septic bursitis involves incision and drainage and antibiotics usually delivered intravenously.

▶ When to Refer

- Surgical removal of the bursa is indicated only for cases in which repeated infections occur.
- Elective removal for persistent symptoms affecting activities of daily living can be considered.

Del Buono A et al. Diagnosis and management of olecranon bursitis. Surgeon. 2012 Oct;10(5):297–300. [PMID: 22503398]

McEvoy JR et al. Ultrasound-guided corticosteroid injections for treatment of greater trochanteric pain syndrome: greater trochanter bursa versus subgluteus medius bursa. AJR Am J Roentgenol. 2013 Aug;201(2):W313-7. [PMID: 23883246]

HIP

1. Hip Fractures

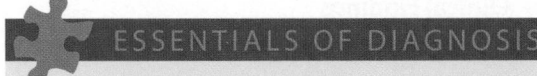

ESSENTIALS OF DIAGNOSIS

- ▶ Internal rotation of the hip is the best provocative diagnostic maneuver.
- ▶ Hip fractures should be surgically repaired as soon as possible (within 24 hours).
- ▶ Delayed treatment of hip fractures in the elderly leads to increased complications and mortality.

▶ General Considerations

Approximately 4% of the 7.9 million fractures that occur each year in the United States are hip fractures. There is a high mortality rate among elderly patients following hip fracture, with death occurring in 8–9% within 30 days and in approximately 25–30% within 1 year. Osteoporosis, female sex, height > 5-foot 8-inches, and age over 50 years are risk factors for hip fracture. Hip fractures usually occur after a fall. High velocity trauma is needed in younger patients. Stress fractures can occur in athletes or individuals with poor bone mineral density following repetitive loading activities.

▶ Clinical Findings

A. Symptoms and Signs

Patients typically report pain in the groin, though pain radiating to the lateral hip, buttock, or knee can also commonly occur. If a displaced fracture is present, the patient will not be able to bear weight and the leg may be externally rotated. Gentle logrolling of the leg with the patient supine helps rule out a fracture. Examination of the hip demonstrates pain with deep palpation in the area of the femoral triangle (similar to palpating the femoral artery). Provided the patient can tolerate it, the clinician can, with the patient supine, flex the hip to 90 degrees with the knee flexed to 90 degrees. The leg can then be internally and externally rotated to assess the range of motion on both sides. **Pain with internal rotation of the hip is the most sensitive test to identify intra-articular hip pathology.** Hip flexion, extension, abduction, and adduction strength can be tested.

Patients with hip stress fractures have less pain on physical examination than described previously but typically have pain with weight bearing. The Trendelenburg test can be performed to examine for weakness or instability of the hip abductors, primarily the gluteus medius muscle (Table 41–7). Another functional test is asking the patient to hop or jump during the examination. If the patient has a compatible clinical history of pain and is unable or unwilling to hop, then a stress fracture should be ruled out. The back should be carefully examined in patients with hip complaints, including examining for signs for sciatica.

Following displaced hip fractures, a thorough medical evaluation and treatment should be pursued to maximize the patients' ability to undergo operative intervention. Patients who are unable to get up by themselves may have been immobile for hours or even days following their falls. Thus, clinicians must exclude rhabdomyolysis, hypothermia, deep venous thrombosis, pulmonary embolism, and other conditions that can occur with prolonged immobilization. Delay of operative intervention leads to an increased risk of perioperative morbidity and mortality.

B. Imaging

Useful radiographic views of the hip include AP views of the pelvis and bilateral hips and frog-leg-lateral views of the painful hip. A CT scan or MRI may be necessary to

Table 41–7. Hip examination.

Maneuver	Description
Inspection	Examine for the alignment of the lower extremity, consider lumbar spine exam
Palpation	Include important landmarks: ASIS and AIIS (proximal quadriceps muscle insertions), greater trochanter (gluteal tendon insertions and bursa), anterior femoral triangle (hip joint and hip flexion insertion), ischial tuberosity (hamstring tendon insertion), sacroiliac joints
Range of motion testing	Check range of motion passively (clinician performs) especially internal and external rotation of the hip
Hip strength testing	Test resisted hip flexion, extension, abduction and adduction strength manually
Trendelenburg test	The patient balances first on one leg, raising the non-standing knee toward the chest. The clinician can stand behind the patient and observe for dropping of the pelvis and buttock on the non-stance side.

AIIS, anterior inferior iliac spine; ASIS, anterior superior iliac spine.

identify the hip fracture pattern or to evaluate non-displaced fractures. Hip fractures are generally described by location, including femoral neck, intertrochanteric, or subtrochanteric.

Treatment

Almost all patients with a hip fracture will require surgery and may need to be admitted to hospital for pain control while they await surgery. **Surgery is recommended within the first 24 hours** because studies have shown that delaying surgery 48 hours results in at least twice the rate of major and minor medical complications, including pneumonia, decubitus ulcers, and deep venous thrombosis.

Stress fractures in active patients require a period of protected weight-bearing and a gradual return to activities, although it may take 4–6 months before a return to normal activities. Femoral neck fractures are commonly treated with hemiarthroplasty or total hip replacement. This allows the patient to begin weight-bearing immediately postoperatively. Peritrochanteric hip fractures are treated with open reduction internal fixation, where plate and screw construct or intramedullary devices are used. The choice of implant will depend on the fracture pattern. Since fracture fixation requires the fracture to proceed to union, the patient may need to have protected weight-bearing during the early postoperative period. Dislocation, peri-prosthetic fracture, and avascular necrosis of the hip are common complications after surgery.

Patients should be mobilized as soon as possible post-operatively to avoid pulmonary complications and decubitus ulcers. Supervised physical therapy and rehabilitation is important for the patient to regain as much function as possible. Unfortunately, most patients following hip fractures will lose some degree of independence.

Prevention

Bone density screening can identify patients at risk for osteopenia or osteoporosis, and treatment can be planned accordingly. Nutrition (calcium and vitamin D intake) and bone health (bone densitometry, serum calcium and 25-OH vitamin D levels) should be reviewed with the patient (see Chapter 26). For patients with decreased mobility, systemic anticoagulation with low-molecular-weight heparin or warfarin should be considered to avoid deep venous thrombosis (see Table 14–13). Fall prevention exercise programs are available for elderly patients at risk for falls and hip fractures. Hip protectors are uncomfortable and have less use in preventing fractures.

When to Refer

All patients in whom hip fracture is suspected.

Della Rocca GJ et al. Hip fracture protocols: what have we changed? Orthop Clin North Am. 2013 Apr;44(2):163–82. [PMID: 23544822]

Moja L et al. Timing matters in hip fracture surgery: patients operated within 48 hours have better outcomes. A meta-analysis and meta-regression of over 190,000 patients. PLoS One. 2012;7(10):e46175. [PMID: 23056256]

2. Hip Osteoarthritis

ESSENTIALS OF DIAGNOSIS

► Pain deep in the groin on the affected side.
► Swelling.
► Degeneration of joint cartilage.
► Loss of active and passive range of motion in severe osteoarthritis.

General Considerations

In the United States, the prevalence of osteoarthritis will grow as the number of persons over age 65 years doubles to more than 70 million by 2030. Cartilage loss and osteoarthritis symptoms are preceded by damage to the collagen-proteoglycan matrix. The etiology of osteoarthritis is often multifactorial, including previous trauma, prior high-impact activities, genetic factors, obesity, and rheumatologic or metabolic conditions.

Clinical Findings

A. Symptoms and Signs

Osteoarthritis usually causes pain in the affected joint with loading of the joint or at the extremes of motion. Mechanical symptoms—such as swelling, grinding, catching, and locking—suggest internal derangement, which is indicated by damaged cartilage or bone fragments that affect the smooth range of motion expected at an articular joint. Pain can also produce the sensation of "buckling" or "giving way" due to muscle inhibition. As the joint degeneration becomes more advanced, the patient loses active range of motion and may lose passive range of motion as well.

Patients complain of pain deep in the groin on the affected side and have problems with weight-bearing activities such as walking, climbing stairs, and getting up from a chair. They may limp and develop a lurch during their gait, leaning toward the unaffected side as they walk to reduce pressure on the hip.

B. Imaging

Weight-bearing radiographs of the affected hip are preferred for evaluation of hip osteoarthritis. To reduce radiation exposure, obtain an AP weight-bearing radiograph of the pelvis with a lateral view of the symptomatic hip. Joint space narrowing and sclerosis suggest early osteoarthritis, while osteophytes near the femoral head or acetabulum and subchondral bone cysts are more advanced changes. After age 35, MRI of the hips already show labral changes in almost 70% of asymptomatic patients.

▶ Treatment

A. Conservative

Changes in the articular cartilage are irreversible. Therefore, a cure for the diseased joint is not possible, although symptoms or structural issues can be addressed to try to maintain activity level. Conservative treatment for patients with osteoarthritis includes activity modification, proper footwear, therapeutic exercises, weight loss, and use of assistive devices (such as a cane). In a large cohort, running significantly reduced osteoarthritis and hip replacement risk possibly since running is associated with lower BMI.

Analgesics may be effective in some cases. Corticosteroid injections can be considered for short-term relief of pain; however, hip injections are best performed under fluoroscopic, ultrasound, or CT guidance to ensure accurate injection in the joint. Use of viscosupplementation in the hip has been reported in cases with modest improvements; however, it remains an off-label use at this time.

B. Surgical

Two randomized trials demonstrate that arthroscopy does *not* improve outcomes at 1 year over placebo or routine conservative treatment of osteoarthritis. Arthroscopic surgery is indicated in patients with osteoarthritis if, rather than pain, they have mechanical symptoms and internal derangement symptoms that can be removed as the main complaint. Such surgical treatments are useful to restore range of motion by removing osteophytes, cartilage fragments, or loose bodies.

Joint replacement surgeries are effective and cost-effective for patients with significant symptoms and functional limitations, providing improvements in pain, function, and quality of life. Minimally invasive surgeries and computer-assisted navigation during operation are being investigated as methods to improve techniques (eg, accurate placement of the hardware implant) and to reduce complication rates.

Hip resurfacing surgery is a newer joint replacement technique. Rather than use a traditional artificial joint implant of the whole neck and femur, only the femoral head is removed and replaced. Concerns following resurfacing surgery include the risk of femoral neck fracture and collapse of the head. The cumulative survival rate of this implant at 10 years is estimated to be 94%. Evidence so far suggests that hip resurfacing is comparable to total hip replacement and is a viable alternative for younger patients.

Guidelines recommend prophylaxis for venous thromboembolic disease for a minimum of 14 days after arthroplasty of the hip or knee using warfarin, low-molecular-weight heparin, fondaparinux, aspirin, rivaroxaban, dabigatran, apixaban, or portable mechanical compression.

▶ When to Refer

Patients with sufficient disability, limited benefit from conservative therapy, and evidence of severe osteoarthritis can be referred for joint replacement surgery.

Lieberman JR et al. Prevention of venous thromboembolic disease after total hip and knee arthroplasty. J Bone Joint Surg Am. 2013 Oct 2;95(19):1801–11. [PMID: 24088973]

McMinn DJ et al. Mortality and implant revision rates of hip arthroplasty in patients with osteoarthritis: registry based cohort study. BMJ. 2012 Jun 14;344:e3319. [PMID: 22700782]

Register B et al. Prevalence of abnormal hip findings in asymptomatic participants: a prospective, blinded study. Am J Sports Med. 2012 Dec;40(12):2720–4. [PMID: 23104610]

KNEE

1. Knee Pain

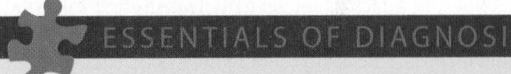

ESSENTIALS OF DIAGNOSIS

▶ Effusion can occur with intra-articular pathology, such as osteoarthritis, and meniscus and cruciate ligament tears.

▶ Acute knee swelling (due to hemarthrosis) within 2 hours may indicate ligament injuries or patellar dislocation or fracture.

▶ General Considerations

The knee is the largest joint in the body and is susceptible to injury from trauma, inflammation, infection, and degenerative changes. The knee is a hinge joint. The joint line exists between the femoral condyles and tibial plateaus. Separating and cushioning these bony surfaces is the lateral and medial meniscal cartilage, which functions as a shock absorber during weight bearing, protecting the articular cartilage. The patella is a large sesamoid bone anterior to the joint. It is embedded in the quadriceps tendon, and it articulates with the trochlear groove of the femur. Poor patellar tracking in the trochlear groove is a common source of knee pain especially when the cause is atraumatic in nature. The knee is stabilized by the collateral ligaments against varus (lateral collateral ligament) and valgus (medial collateral ligament) stresses. The tibia is limited in its anterior movement by the anterior cruciate ligament (ACL) and in its posterior movement by the posterior cruciate ligament (PCL). The bursae of the knee are located between the skin and bony prominences. They are sac-like structures with a synovial lining. They act to decrease friction of tendons and muscles as they move over adjacent bony structures. Excessive external pressure or friction can lead to swelling and pain of the bursae. The **prepatellar bursae** (located between the skin and patella), and the **pes anserine bursa** (which is medial and inferior to the patella, just below the tibial plateau) are most commonly affected. Joint fluid, when excessive due to synovitis or trauma, can track posteriorly through a potential space, resulting in a popliteal cyst (also called a **Baker cyst**). Other structures that are susceptible to overuse injury and may cause knee pain following repetitive activity include the patellofemoral joint and the iliotibial band. Osteoarthritis of the knees is common after 50 years of age and can develop due to previous trauma, aging, activities, alignment issues, and genetic predisposition.

▶ **Clinical Findings**

A. Symptoms and Signs

Evaluation of knee pain should begin with general questions regarding duration and rapidity of symptom onset and the mechanism of injury or aggravating symptoms. Overuse or degenerative problems can occur with stress or compression from sports, hobbies, or occupation. A history of trauma, previous orthopedic problems with, or surgery to, the affected knee should also be specifically queried. Symptoms of infection (fever, recent bacterial infections, risk factors for sexually transmitted infections [such as gonorrhea] or other bacterial infections [such as staphylococcal infection]) should always be elicited.

Common symptom complaints include the following:

1. Presence of grinding, clicking, or popping with bending, may be indicative of osteoarthritis or the patellofemoral syndrome.

2. "Locking" or "catching" when walking suggests an internal derangement, such as meniscal injury or a loose body in the knee.

3. Intra-articular swelling of the knee or an effusion indicates an internal derangement or a synovial pathology. Large swelling may cause a popliteal (Baker) cyst. Acute swelling within minutes to hours suggests a hemarthrosis, most likely due to an ACL injury, fracture or patellar dislocation, especially if trauma is involved.

4. Lateral "snapping" with flexion and extension of the knee may indicate inflammation of the iliotibial band.

5. Pain that is worsened with bending and walking downstairs suggests issues with the patellofemoral joint, usually degenerative such as chondromalacia of the patella or osteoarthritis.

6. Pain that occurs when rising after prolonged sitting suggests a problem with tracking of the patella.

Table 41–8. Differential diagnosis of knee pain.

Mechanical dysfunction or disruption
Internal derangement of the knee: injury to the menisci or ligaments
Degenerative changes caused by osteoarthritis
Dynamic dysfunction or misalignment of the patella
Fracture as a result of trauma
Intra-articular inflammation or increased pressure
Internal derangement of the knee: injury to the menisci or ligaments
Inflammation or infection of the knee joint
Ruptured popliteal (Baker) cyst
Peri-articular inflammation
Internal derangement of the knee: injury to the menisci or ligaments
Prepatellar or anserine bursitis
Ligamentous sprain

A careful history, coupled with a physical examination that includes observation, palpation and range of motion testing, as well as specific tests for particular anatomic structures is frequently sufficient to establish a diagnosis. When there is a knee joint effusion caused by increased fluid in the intra-articular space, physical examination will demonstrate swelling in the hollow or dimple around the patella and distention of the suprapatellar space.

Table 41–8 shows the differential diagnosis of knee pain, and Table 41–9 outlines possible diagnoses based on the location of pain.

Table 41–9. Location of common causes of knee pain.

Medial knee pain
Medial compartment osteoarthritis
Medial collateral ligament strain
Medial meniscal injury
Anserine bursitis (pain over the proximal medial tibial plateau)
Anterior knee pain
Patellofemoral syndrome (often bilateral)
Osteoarthritis
Prepatellar bursitis (associated with swelling anterior to the patella)
"Jumper's knee" (pain at the inferior pole of the patella)
Septic arthritis
Gout or other inflammatory disorder
Lateral knee pain
Lateral meniscal injury
Iliotibial band syndrome (pain superficially along the distal iliotibial band near lateral femoral condyle or lateral tibial insertion)
Lateral collateral ligament sprain (rare)
Posterior knee pain
Popliteal (Baker) cyst
Osteoarthritis
Meniscal tears
Hamstring or calf tendinopathy

B. Laboratory Findings

Laboratory testing of aspirated joint fluid, when indicated, can lead to a definitive diagnosis in most patients (see Tables 20–2 and 20–3).

C. Imaging

Knee pain is evaluated with plain (weight-bearing) radiographs and MRI most commonly, but CT and ultrasound are sometimes useful.

An acute hemarthrosis represents bloody swelling that usually occurs within the first 1–2 hours following trauma. In situations where the trauma may be activity-related and not a result of a fall or collision, the differential diagnosis most commonly includes ACL tear (responsible for almost 50% of hemarthrosis in children and > 70% in adults), fracture (patella, tibial plateau, femoral supracondylar, growth plate [physeal]), and patellar dislocation. Meniscal tears are unlikely to cause large hemarthrosis.

2. Anterior Cruciate Ligament Injury

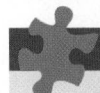

ESSENTIALS OF DIAGNOSIS

▶ An injury involving an audible pop when the knee buckles.

▶ Acute swelling immediately (or within 2 hours).

▶ Instability occurs with lateral movement activities and going down stairs.

▶ General Considerations

The anterior cruciate ligament (ACL) connects the posterior aspect of the lateral femoral condyle to the anterior aspect of the tibia. Its main function is to control anterior translation of the tibia on the femur. It also provides rotationally stability of the tibia on the femur. ACL tears are common with sporting injuries. They can result from both contact (valgus blow to the knee) and non-contact (jumping, pivoting, and deceleration) activities. The patient usually falls down following the injury, has acute swelling and difficulty with weight-bearing, and complains of instability. ACL injuries are common in skiing, soccer, football, and basketball among young adolescents and middle-age patients. Prepubertal and older patients usually sustain fractures instead of ligamentous injuries.

▶ Clinical Findings

A. Symptoms and Signs

Acute ACL injuries usually lead to acute swelling of the knee, causing difficulty with motion. After the swelling has resolved, the patient can walk with a "stiff-knee" gait or quadriceps avoidance gait because of the instability. More importantly, patients describe symptoms of instability while performing side-to-side maneuvers or descending stairs. Stability tests assess the amount of laxity of the knee while performing side-to-side maneuvers or descending stairs.

The **Lachman test** (84–87% sensitivity and 93% specificity) is performed with the patient lying supine and the knee flexed to 20–30 degrees (Table 41–10). The clinician grasps the distal femur from the lateral side and the proximal tibia with the other hand on the medial side. With the knee in neutral position, stabilize the femur, and pull the tibia anteriorly using a similar force to lifting a 10- to 15-pound weight. Excessive anterior translation of the tibia compared with the other side indicates injury to the ACL. The **anterior drawer test** (48% sensitivity and 87% specificity) is performed with the patient lying supine and the knee flexed to 90 degrees (Table 41–10). The clinician stabilizes the patient's foot by sitting on it and grasps the proximal tibia with both hands around the calf and pulls anteriorly. A positive test finds ACL laxity compared with the unaffected side. **The pivot shift** test is used to determine the amount of rotational laxity of the knee (Table 41–10). The patient is examined while lying supine with the knee in full extension. It is then slowly flexed while applying internal rotation and a valgus stress. The clinician feels for a subluxation at 20–40 degrees of knee flexion. The patient must remain very relaxed to have a positive test.

B. Imaging

Plain radiographs are usually negative in ACL tears but are useful to rule out fractures. A small avulsion injury can sometimes be seen over the lateral compartment of the knee. This is called a "Segond" fracture and is pathognomonic of an ACL injury. MRI is the best method to diagnose ACL tears. It has > 95% sensitivity and specificity for ACL tears. MRI also allows evaluation of other associated structures, such as menisci and cartilages.

▶ Treatment

Most young and active patients will require surgical reconstruction of the ACL. Common surgical techniques use the patient's own tissues, usually the patellar or hamstring tendons (autograft) or a cadaver graft (allograft) to arthroscopically reconstruct the torn ACL. Different patients groups experienced improved results with specific surgical graft choices. Recovery from surgery usually requires 6 months.

Nonoperative treatments are usually reserved for older patients or those with a very sedentary lifestyle. Physical therapy can focus on hamstring strengthening and core stability. An ACL brace can help stability. Longitudinal studies have demonstrated that nonoperative management of an ACL tear can lead to a higher incidence of meniscus tears. However, a small, randomized study demonstrated that acute ACL injuries may be treated nonoperatively initially, with similar clinical outcomes as those injuries that were operated on within 10 weeks of injury.

▶ When to Refer

• Almost all ACL tears should be referred to an orthopedic surgeon for evaluation.

• Individuals with instability in the setting of a chronic ACL tear (> 6 months) should be considered for surgical reconstruction.

Table 41–10. Knee examination.

Maneuver	Description
Inspection	Examine for the alignment of the lower extremities (varus, valgus, knee recurvatum), ankle eversion and foot pronation, gait, SEADS.
Palpation	Include important landmarks: patellofemoral joint, medial and lateral joint lines (especially posterior aspects), pes anserine bursa, distal iliotibial band and Gerdy tubercle (iliotibial band insertion).
Range of motion testing 	Check range of motion actively (patient performs) and passively (clinician performs), especially with flexion and extension of the knee normally 0–10 degrees of extension and 120–150 degrees of flexion.
Knee strength testing	Test resisted knee extension and knee flexion strength manually.
Ligament stress tests	
Lachman test 	Performed with the patient lying supine, and the knee flexed to 20–30 degrees. The examiner grasps the distal femur from the lateral side, and the proximal tibia with the other hand on the medial side. With the knee in neutral position, stabilize the femur, and pull the tibia anteriorly using a similar force to lifting a 10–15 pound weight. Excessive anterior translation of the tibia compared with the other side indicates injury to the anterior cruciate ligament.
Anterior drawer 	Performed with the patient lying supine and the knee flexed to 90 degrees. The clinician stabilizes the patient's foot by sitting on it and grasps the proximal tibia with both hands around the calf and pulls anteriorly. A positive test finds anterior cruciate ligament laxity compared with the unaffected side.

(continued)

Table 41–10. Knee examination. (continued)

Maneuver	Description
Pivot shift 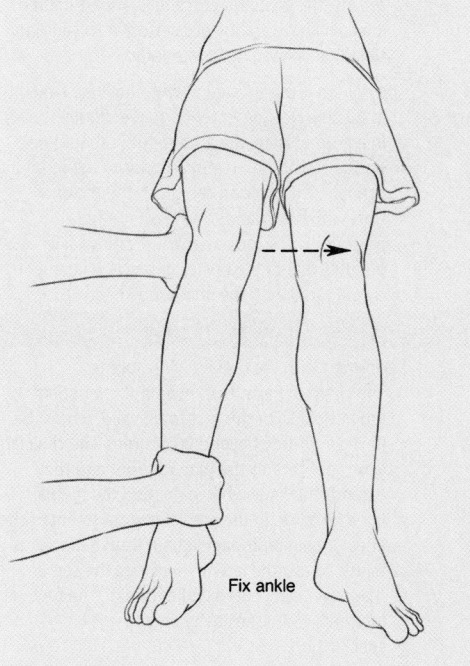	Used to determine the amount of rotational laxity of the knee. The patient is examined while lying supine with the knee in full extension. It is then slowly flexed while applying internal rotation and a valgus stress. The clinician feels for a subluxation at 20–40 degrees of knee flexion. The patient must remain very relaxed to have a positive test.
Valgus stress　　Fix ankle	Performed with the patient supine. The clinician should stand on the outside of the patient's knee. With one hand, the clinician should hold the ankle while the other hand is supporting the leg at the level of the knee joint. A valgus stress is applied at the ankle to determine pain and laxity of the medial collateral ligament. The test should be performed at both 30 degrees and at 0 degrees of knee extension.

(continued)

Table 41–10. Knee examination. (continued)

Maneuver	Description
Varus stress	The patient is again placed supine. For the right knee, the clinician should be standing on the right side of the patient. The left hand of the examiner should be holding the ankle while the right hand is supporting the lateral thigh. A varus stress is applied at the ankle to determine pain and laxity of the lateral collateral ligament. The test should be performed at both 30 degrees and at 0 degrees of knee flexion.
The sag sign	The patient is placed supine and both hips and knees are flexed up to 90 degrees. Because of gravity, the posterior cruciate ligament-injured knee will have an obvious set-off at the anterior tibia that is "sagging" posteriorly.
Posterior drawer	The patient is placed supine with the knee flexed at 90 degrees (see Anterior drawer figure above). In a normal knee, the anterior tibia should be positioned about 10 mm anterior to the femoral condyle. The clinician can grasp the proximal tibia with both hands and push the tibia posteriorly. The movement, indicating laxity and possible tear of the posterior cruciate ligament, is compared with the uninjured knee.
Meniscal signs	
McMurray test	Performed with the patient lying supine. The clinician flexes the knee until the patient reports pain. For this test to be valid, it must be flexed pain-free beyond 90 degrees. The clinician externally rotates the patient's foot and then extends the knee while palpating the medial knee for "click" in the medial compartment of the knee or pain reproducing pain from a meniscus injury. To test the lateral meniscus, the same maneuver is repeated while rotating the foot internally (53% sensitivity and 59–97% specificity).

(continued)

Table 41–10. Knee examination. (continued)

Maneuver	Description
Modified McMurray 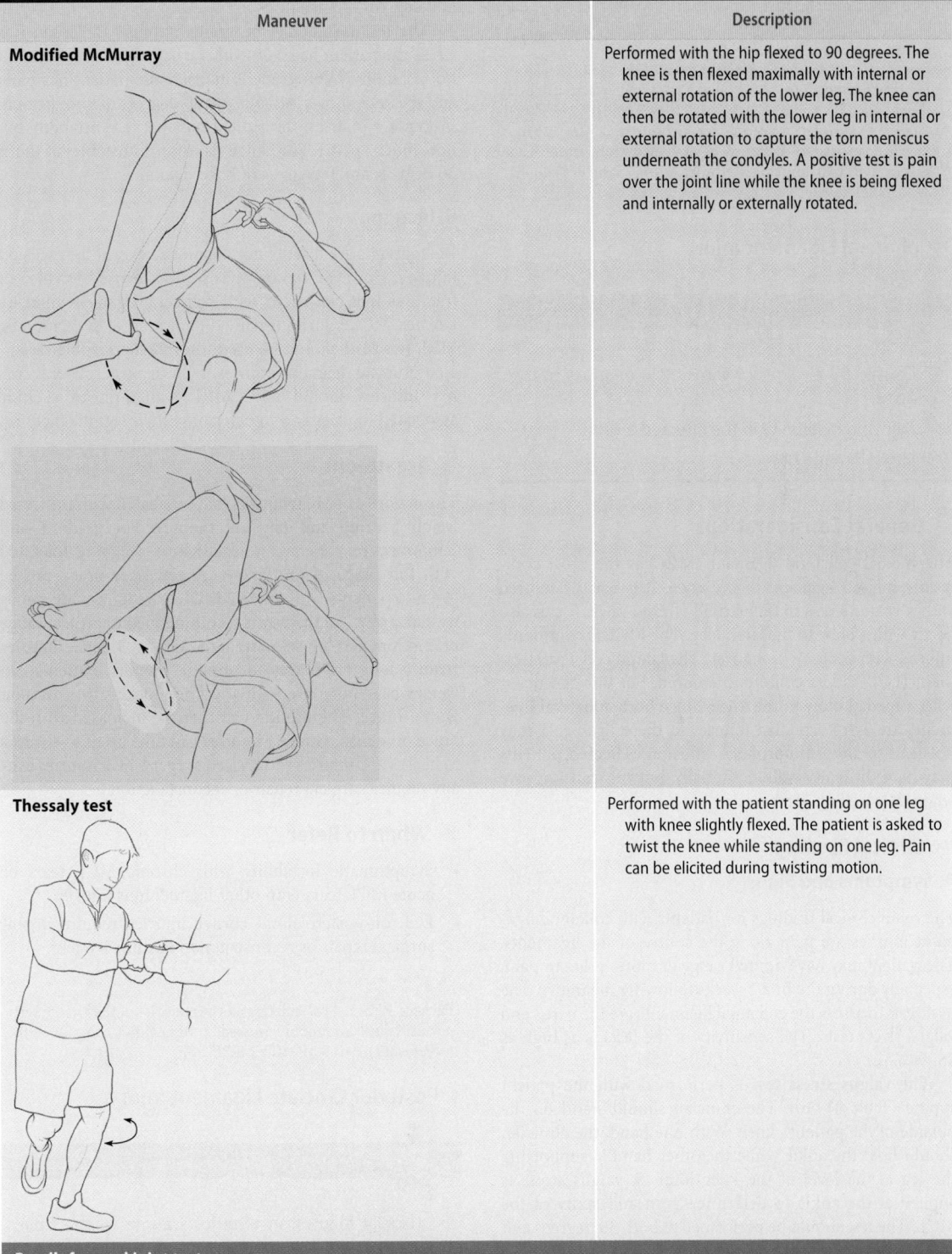	Performed with the hip flexed to 90 degrees. The knee is then flexed maximally with internal or external rotation of the lower leg. The knee can then be rotated with the lower leg in internal or external rotation to capture the torn meniscus underneath the condyles. A positive test is pain over the joint line while the knee is being flexed and internally or externally rotated.
Thessaly test	Performed with the patient standing on one leg with knee slightly flexed. The patient is asked to twist the knee while standing on one leg. Pain can be elicited during twisting motion.
Patellofemoral joint test	
Apprehension sign	Suggests instability of the patellofemoral joint and is positive when the patient becomes apprehensive when the patella is deviated laterally.

SEADS, swelling, erythema, atrophy, deformity, and (surgical) scars.

- Patients with an ACL tear and associated meniscus or articular injuries may benefit from surgery to address the other injuries.

Barrett AM et al. Anterior cruciate ligament graft failure: a comparison of graft type based on age and Tegner activity level. Am J Sports Med. 2011 Oct;39(10):2194–8. [PMID: 21784999]
Delincé P et al. Anterior cruciate ligament tears: conservative or surgical treatment? A critical review of the literature. Knee Surg Sports Traumatol Arthrosc. 2012 Jan;20(1):48–61. [PMID: 21773828]

3. Collateral Ligament Injury

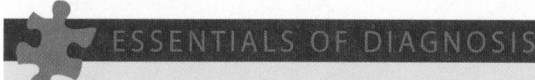
ESSENTIALS OF DIAGNOSIS

▶ Caused by a valgus or varus blow or stress to the knee.

▶ Pain and instability in the affected area.

▶ Limited range of motion.

▶ General Considerations

The medial collateral ligament (MCL) is the most commonly injured ligament in the knee. It is usually injured with a valgus stress to the partially flexed knee. It can also occur with a blow to the lateral leg. The MCL is commonly injured with acute ACL injuries. The lateral collateral ligament (LCL) is less commonly injured, but this can occur with a medial blow to the knee. Since both collateral ligaments are extra-articular, injuries to these ligaments may not lead to any intra-articular effusion. Affected patients may have difficulty walking initially, but this can improve when the swelling decreases.

▶ Clinical Findings

A. Symptoms and Signs

The main clinical findings for patients with collateral ligament injuries are pain along the course of the ligaments. The patient may have limited range of motion due to pain, especially during the first 2 weeks following the injury. The best tests to assess the collateral ligaments are the varus and valgus stress tests. The sensitivity of the tests is as high as 86–96%.

The **valgus stress test** is performed with the patient supine (Table 41–10). The clinician should stand on the outside of the patient's knee. With one hand, the clinician should hold the ankle while the other hand is supporting the leg at the level of the knee joint. A valgus stress is applied at the ankle to determine pain and laxity of the MCL. The test should be performed at both 30 degrees and at 0 degrees of knee extension.

For the **varus stress test**, the patient is again placed supine (Table 41–10). For the right knee, the clinician should be standing on the right side of the patient. The clinician's left hand should be holding the ankle while the right hand is supporting the lateral thigh. A varus stress is applied at the ankle to determine pain and laxity of the LCL. The test should be performed at both 30 degrees and at 0 degrees of knee flexion.

The test results can be graded from 1–3. Grade 1 is when the patient has pain with varus/valgus stress test but no instability. With grade 2 injuries, the patient has pain, and the knee shows instability at 30 degrees of knee flexion. In grade 3 injuries, the patient has marked instability but not much pain. The knee is often unstable at both 30 degrees and 0 degrees of knee flexion.

B. Imaging

Radiographs are usually nondiagnostic except for avulsion injuries. However, radiographs should be used to rule out fractures that can occur with collateral ligament injuries. Isolated MCL injuries usually do not require evaluation by MRI, but MRI should be used to evaluate possible associated cruciate ligament injuries. LCL or posterolateral corner injuries should have MRI evaluation to exclude associated injuries and to determine their significance.

▶ Treatment

The majority of MCL injuries can be treated with protected weight-bearing and physical therapy. For grade 1 and 2 injuries, the patient can usually bear weight as tolerated with full range of motion. A hinged knee brace can be given to patients with grade 2 MCL tears to provide stability. Early physical therapy is recommended to protect range of motion and muscle strength. Grade 3 MCL injuries require long leg braces to provide stability. Patients can weight-bear but only with the knee locked in extension with a brace. The motion can then be increased with the brace unlocked. Grade 3 injuries can take up to 6–8 weeks to heal. MCL injuries rarely need surgery. LCL injuries usually require surgical repair or reconstruction.

▶ When to Refer

- Symptomatic instability with chronic MCL tears or acute MCL tears with other ligamentous injuries.
- LCL or posterolateral corner injuries require urgent surgical repair or reconstruction (within 1 week).

Pacheco RJ et al. Posterolateral corner injuries of the knee: a serious injury commonly missed. J Bone Joint Surg Br. 2011 Feb;93(2):194–7. [PMID: 21282758]

4. Posterior Cruciate Ligament Injury

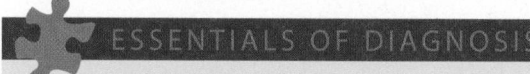
ESSENTIALS OF DIAGNOSIS

▶ Usually follows an anterior trauma to the tibia, such as a dashboard injury during a motor vehicle accident.

▶ The knee may freely dislocate and reduce.

▶ One-third of multi-ligament injuries involving the PCL have neurovascular injuries.

General Considerations

The posterior cruciate ligament (PCL) is the strongest ligament in the knee. PCL injuries usually represent significant trauma and are highly associated with multi-ligament injuries and knee dislocations. More than 70–90% of PCL injuries have associated injuries to the posterolateral corner, MCL, and ACL. Neurovascular injuries occur in up to one-third of all knee dislocations or PCL injuries. **There should be high suspicion for neurovascular injuries and a thorough neurovascular examination of the limb should be performed.**

Clinical Findings

A. Symptoms and Signs

Most patients with acute injuries have difficulty with ambulation. Patients with chronic PCL injuries can ambulate without gross instability but may complain of subjective "looseness" and often report pain and dysfunction, especially with bending. Clinical examinations of PCL injuries include the **"sag sign"** (Table 41–10). The patient is placed supine and both hips and knees are flexed up to 90 degrees. Because of gravity, the PCL-injured knee will have an obvious set-off at the anterior tibia that is "sagging" posteriorly. The PCL ligament can also be examined using the **posterior drawer test** (90% sensitivity and 99% specificity) (Table 41–10). The patient is placed supine with the knee flexed at 90 degrees. In a normal knee, the anterior tibia should be positioned about 10 mm anterior to the femoral condyle. The clinician can grasp the proximal tibia with both hands and push the tibia posteriorly. The movement, indicating laxity and possible tear of the PCL, is compared with the uninjured knee. A PCL injury is sometimes mistaken for an ACL injury during the anterior drawer test since the tibia is subluxed posteriorly in a sagged position and can be abnormally translated forward, yielding a false-positive test for an ACL injury. Pain, swelling, pallor, and numbness in the affected extremity may suggest a knee dislocation with possible injury to the popliteal artery.

B. Imaging

Radiographs are often nondiagnostic but are required to diagnose any fractures. MRI is used to diagnose PCL and other associated injuries.

Treatment

Isolated PCL injuries can be treated nonoperatively. Acute injuries are usually immobilized using a knee brace with the knee extension; the patient uses crutches for ambulation. Physical therapy can help achieve increased range of motion and improved ambulation. Many PCL injuries are associated with other injuries and may require operative reconstruction.

When to Refer

- The patient should be seen urgently within 1–2 weeks.
- If the lateral knee is also unstable with varus stress testing, the patient should be assessed for a posterolateral corner injury, which may require an urgent surgical reconstruction.
- Isolated PCL tears may require surgery if the tear is complete (grade 3) and the patient is symptomatic.

5. Meniscus Injuries

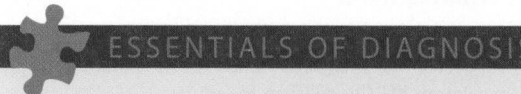

ESSENTIALS OF DIAGNOSIS

- ▶ Patient may or may not report an injury.
- ▶ Joint line pain and pain with deep squatting are the most sensitive signs.
- ▶ Difficulty with knee extension suggests an internal derangement that should be evaluated urgently with MRI.

General Considerations

The menisci act as shock absorbers within the knee. Injuries to a meniscus can lead to pain, clicking, and locking sensation. Most meniscus injuries occur with acute injuries (usually in younger patients) or repeated microtrauma, such as squatting or twisting (usually in older patients).

Clinical Findings

A. Symptoms and Signs

The patient may have an antalgic (painful) gait and difficulty with squatting. He or she may complain of catching or locking of the meniscal fragment. Physical findings can include effusion or joint line tenderness. Patients can usually point out the area of maximal tenderness along the joint line. Swelling usually occurs during the first 24 hours after the injury or later. Meniscus tears rarely lead to the immediate swelling that is commonly seen with fractures and ligament tears. Meniscus tears are commonly seen in arthritic knees. However, it is often unclear whether the pain is coming from the meniscus tear or the arthritis.

Provocative tests, including the **McMurray** test, the **modified McMurray test,** and the **Thessaly test,** can be performed to confirm the diagnosis (Table 41–10). Most symptomatic meniscus tears cause pain with deep squatting and when waddling (performing a "duck walk").

B. Imaging

Radiographs are usually normal but may show joint space narrowing, early osteoarthritis changes, or loose bodies. MRI of the knee is the best diagnostic tool for meniscal injuries (93% sensitivity and 95% specificity). High signal through the meniscus (bright on T2 images) represents a meniscal tear.

Treatment

Conservative treatment can be used for degenerative tears in older patients. The treatment is similar for patients with mild knee osteoarthritis, including analgesics and physical therapy for strengthening and core stability. Acute tears in young and active patients can be best treated arthroscopically with meniscus repair or debridement. Randomized controlled studies have demonstrated no benefit with arthroscopic meniscectomy in patients with advanced osteoarthritis.

▶ **When to Refer**

- If the patient has symptoms of internal derangement suspected as meniscus injury. The patient should receive an MRI to confirm the injury.
- If the patient cannot extend the knee due to a mechanical block, the patient should be evaluated as soon as possible. Certain shaped tears on MRI, such as bucket handle tears, are amenable to meniscal repair surgery.

McDermott I. Meniscal tears, repairs and replacement: their relevance to osteoarthritis of the knee. Br J Sports Med. 2011 Apr;45(4):292–7. [PMID: 21297172]

6. Patellofemoral Pain

ESSENTIALS OF DIAGNOSIS

- ▶ Pain experienced with bending activities (kneeling, squatting, climbing stairs).
- ▶ Lateral deviation or tilting of the patella in relation to the femoral groove.

▶ **General Considerations**

Patellofemoral pain, also known as anterior knee pain, chondromalacia, or "runner's knee," describes any pain involving the patellofemoral joint. The pain affects any or all of the anterior knee structures, including the medial and lateral aspects of the patella as well as the quadriceps and patellar tendon insertions. The patella engages the femoral trochlear groove with approximately 30 degrees of knee flexion. Forces on the patellofemoral joint increase up to three times body weight as the knee flexes to 90 degrees (eg, climbing stairs), and five times body weight when going into full knee flexion (eg, squatting). Abnormal patellar tracking during flexion can lead to abnormal articular cartilage wear and pain. When the patient has ligamentous hyperlaxity, the patella can sublux out of the groove, usually laterally. Patellofemoral pain is also associated with muscle strength and flexibility imbalances as well as altered hip and ankle biomechanics.

▶ **Clinical Findings**

A. Symptoms and Signs

Patients usually complain of pain in the anterior knee with bending movements and less commonly in full extension. Pain from this condition is localized under the kneecap but can sometimes be referred to the posterior knee or over the medial or lateral inferior patella. Symptoms may begin after a trauma or after repetitive physical activity, such as

running and jumping. When maltracking, palpable and sometimes audible crepitus can occur.

Intra-articular swelling usually does not occur unless there are articular cartilage defects or if osteoarthritis changes develop. On physical examination, it is important to palpate the articular surfaces of the patella. For example, the clinician can use one hand to move the patella laterally, and use the fingertips of the other hand to palpate the lateral undersurface of patella. Patellar mobility can be assessed by medially and laterally deviating the patella (deviation by one-quarter of the diameter of the kneecap is consider normal; greater than one-half the diameter suggests excessive mobility). The **apprehension sign** suggests instability of the patellofemoral joint and is positive when the patient becomes apprehensive when the patella is deviated laterally (Table 41–10). The **patellar grind test** is performed by grasping the knee superior to the patella and pushing it downward with the patient supine and the knee extended, pushing the patella inferiorly. The patient is asked to contract the quadriceps muscle to oppose this downward translation, with reproduction of pain or grinding being the positive sign for chondromalacia of the patella. There are two common presentations: (1) Patients whose ligaments and patella are too loose (hypermobility); (2) and patients who have soft tissues that are too tight leading to excessive pressure on the joint.

Evaluation of the quadriceps strength and hip stabilizers can be accomplished by having the patient perform a one-leg squat without support. Patients who are weak may display poor balance, with dropping of the pelvis (similar to a positive hip Trendelenburg sign) or excessive internal rotation of the knee medially. Normally, with a one-leg squat, the knee should align over the second metatarsal ray of the foot.

B. Imaging

Diagnostic imaging has limited use in younger patients and is more helpful in older patients to assess for osteoarthritis or to evaluate patients who do not respond to conservative treatment. Radiographs may show lateral deviation or tilting of the patella in relation to the femoral groove. MRI may show thinning of the articular cartilage but is not clinically necessary, except prior to surgery or to exclude other pathology.

▶ **Treatment**

A. Conservative

For symptomatic relief, use of local modalities such as ice and anti-inflammatory medications can be beneficial. If the patient has signs of patellar hypermobility, physical therapy exercises are useful to strengthen the quadriceps (especially the vastus medialis obliquus muscle) to help stabilize the patella and improve tracking. Support for the patellofemoral joint can be provided by use of a patellar stabilizer brace or special taping techniques (McConnell taping). Correcting lower extremity alignment (with appropriate footwear or over-the-counter orthotics) can help improve symptoms, especially if the patient has pronation or high arched feet. If the patient demonstrates tight peripatellar soft tissues, special focus should be put on stretching the hamstrings, iliotibial band, quadriceps, calves and hip flexors. Strengthening exercises should include the quadriceps and hip abductors.

B. Surgical

Surgery is rarely needed and is considered a last resort for patellofemoral pain. Procedures performed include lateral release or patellar realignment surgery.

▶ When to Refer

Patients with persistent symptoms.

7. Knee Osteoarthritis

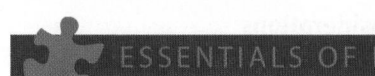

ESSENTIALS OF DIAGNOSIS

- ▶ Degeneration of joint cartilage.
- ▶ Pain with bending or twisting activities.
- ▶ Swelling.
- ▶ Loss of active and passive range of motion in severe osteoarthritis.

▶ General Considerations

In the United States, the prevalence of osteoarthritis will grow as the number of persons over age 65 years doubles to more than 70 million by 2030. The incidence of knee osteoarthritis in the United States is 240 per 100,000 person-years.

Cartilage loss and osteoarthritis symptoms are preceded by damage to the collagen-proteoglycan matrix. The etiology of osteoarthritis is often multifactorial including previous trauma, prior high-impact activities, genetic factors, obesity, and rheumatologic or metabolic conditions.

▶ Clinical Findings

A. Symptoms and Signs

Osteoarthritis usually causes pain in the affected joint with loading of the joint or at the extremes of motion. Mechanical symptoms—such as swelling, grinding, catching, and locking—suggest internal derangement, which is indicated by damaged cartilage or bone fragments that affect the smooth range of motion expected at an articular joint. Pain can also produce the sensation of "buckling" or "giving way" due to muscle inhibition. As the joint degeneration becomes more advanced, the patient loses active range of motion and may lose passive range of motion as well.

As the condition worsens, patients with knee osteoarthritis have an increasingly limited ability to walk. Symptoms include pain with bending or twisting activities, and going up and down stairs. Swelling, limping, and pain while sleeping are common complaints with osteoarthritis, especially as it progresses.

B. Imaging

The most commonly recommended radiographs include bilateral weight-bearing 45-degree bent knee posteroanterior, lateral, and patellofemoral joint views (Merchant view). Radiographic findings include diminished width of the articular cartilage causing joint space narrowing, subchondral sclerosis, presence of osteophytes, and cystic changes in the subchondral bone. MRI of the knee is most likely unnecessary unless other pathology is suspected, including ischemic osteonecrosis of the knee.

▶ Treatment

A. Conservative

Changes in the articular cartilage are irreversible. Therefore, a cure for the diseased joint is not possible, although symptoms or structural issues can be addressed to try to maintain activity level. Conservative treatment for all patients with osteoarthritis includes activity modification, therapeutic exercises, and weight loss. Lifestyle modifications also include proper footwear and avoidance of high impact activities.

Use of a cane in the hand opposite to the affected side is mechanically advantageous. Knee sleeves or braces provide some improvement in subjective pain symptoms most likely due to improvements in neuromuscular function. If patients have unicompartmental osteoarthritis in the medial or lateral compartment, joint unloader braces are available to offload the degenerative compartment. Cushioning footwear and appropriate orthotics or shoe adjustments are useful for reducing impact to the lower extremities.

The initial medication of choice for the treatment of pain in knee osteoarthritis are oral acetaminophen and topical capsaicin. If a traditional NSAID is indicated, the choice should be based on cost, side-effect profile, and adherence. The cyclooxygenase (COX)-2 inhibitor, celecoxib, is no more effective than traditional NSAIDs; it may offer short-term, but probably not long-term, advantage in preventing gastrointestinal complications. Due to its cost and potential cardiovascular risk, celecoxib should be reserved for carefully selected patients. The role of topical NSAIDs are being considered in the osteoarthritis treatment algorithm, as they do avoid many of the traditional NSAID complications. Opioids can be used appropriately in patients with severe osteoarthritis (see Chapter 5). Glucosamine and chondroitin sulfate are supplements that have been widely used and marketed for osteoarthritis. Evidence for their effectiveness in slowing or reversing cartilage loss is limited and any effect present appears to be small. Despite some initial promise, the best-controlled studies indicate these supplements are ineffective as analgesics in osteoarthritis. However, they have minimal side effects and may be appropriate if the patient experiences subjective benefit.

Knee joint corticosteroid injections are options to help reduce pain and inflammation and can provide short-term pain relief, usually lasting about 6–12 weeks. Viscosupplementation by injections of hyaluronic acid-based products improves synovial fluid viscosity by increasing the molecular weight and quantity of hyaluronic acid beyond that naturally synthesized by the synovium. Laboratory studies also demonstrate that hyaluronic acid injections decrease inflammatory cytokines and free radicals. Studies also demonstrate more prolonged effects of viscosupplementation products compared with corticosteroid injection with symptom improvement for > 6 months in some patients with mild knee osteoarthritis. One meta-analysis questions the value of viscosupplementation suggesting only a small and clinically irrelevant benefit and an increased risk of serious adverse events. However, older meta-analyses found modest improvements and did not report similar concerns regarding serious side effects.

B. Surgical

Two randomized trials demonstrate that arthroscopy does not improve outcomes at 1 year over placebo or routine conservative treatment of osteoarthritis. Arthroscopic surgery is indicated in patients with osteoarthritis if, rather than pain, they have mechanical symptoms and internal derangement symptoms. Such surgical treatments are useful to restore range of motion by removing osteophytes, cartilage fragments, or loose bodies.

Joint replacement surgeries are effective and cost-effective for patients with significant symptoms or functional limitations, providing improvements in pain, function, and quality of life. The number of total knee arthroplasty procedures jumped 162% from 1991 to 2010, along with an increase in complications and hospital readmissions. Minimally invasive surgeries and computer-assisted navigation during operation are being investigated as methods to improve techniques (eg, accurate placement of the hardware implant) and to reduce complication rates; however, major improvements have yet to be demonstrated.

Knee realignment surgery, such as high tibial osteotomy or partial knee replacement surgery, is indicated in patients younger than age 60 with unicompartmental osteoarthritis, who would benefit from delaying total knee replacement. Knee joint replacement surgery has been very successful in improving outcomes for patient with end-stage osteoarthritis. Recent long-term series describe > 95% survival rate of the implant at 15 years.

▶ When to Refer

Patients with sufficient disability, limited benefit from conservative therapy, and evidence of severe osteoarthritis can be referred for joint replacement surgery.

Cram P et al. Total knee arthroplasty volume, utilization, and outcomes among Medicare beneficiaries, 1991–2010. JAMA. 2012 Sep 26;308(12):1227–36. [PMID: 23011713]

Messier SP et al. Effects of intensive diet and exercise on knee joint loads, inflammation, and clinical outcomes among overweight and obese adults with knee osteoarthritis: the IDEA randomized clinical trial. JAMA. 2013 Sep 25;310(12): 1263–73. [PMID: 24065013]

Rutjes AW et al. Viscosupplementation for osteoarthritis of the knee: a systematic review and meta-analysis. Ann Intern Med. 2012 Aug 7;157(3):180–91. [PMID: 22868835]

ANKLE INJURIES

1. Inversion Ankle Sprains

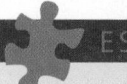

ESSENTIALS OF DIAGNOSIS

▶ Localized pain and swelling.

▶ The majority of ankle injuries involve inversion injuries affecting the lateral ligaments.

▶ Consider chronic ankle instability or associated injuries if pain persists for > 3 months following an ankle sprain.

▶ General Considerations

Ankle sprains are the most common sports injuries seen in outpatient clinics. Patients usually report "turning the ankle" during a fall or after landing on an irregular surface such as a hole or an opponent's foot. The most common mechanism of injury is an inversion and plantar flexion sprain, which injures the anterior talofibular ligament (ATF) ligament rather than the calcaneofibular ligament (CF) ligament. Other injuries that can occur with inversion ankle injuries are listed in (Table 41–11). Women appear to sustain an inversion injury more frequently than men.

▶ Clinical Findings

A. Symptoms and Signs

The usual symptoms following a sprain include localized pain and swelling over the lateral aspect of the ankle, difficulty weight bearing, and limping. The patient's ankle may feel unstable. On examination, there may be swelling or bruising over the lateral aspect of the ankle. The anterior, inferior aspect below the lateral malleolus is most often the point of maximal tenderness consistent with ATF and CF ligament injuries. The swelling may limit motion of the ankle.

Table 41–11. Injuries associated with ankle sprains.

Ligaments
Subtalar joint sprain
Sinus tarsi syndrome
Syndesmotic sprain
Deltoid sprain
Lisfranc injury
Tendons
Posterior tibial tendon strain
Peroneal tendon subluxation
Bones
Osteochondral talus injury
Lateral talar process fracture
Posterior impingement (os trigonum)
Fracture at the base of the fifth metatarsal
Jones fracture
Salter fracture (fibula)
Ankle fractures

Table 41–12. Ankle examination.

Maneuver	Description
Inspection	Examine for the alignment of the ankle. (SEADS)
Palpation	Include important landmarks: Ottawa Ankle Rules (medial and lateral malleolus, base of fifth metatarsal and navicular area), anterior tibiofibular ligament, posterior talus; tendons (Achilles, peroneals, posterior tibialis, flexor hallucis longus).
Range of motion testing	Check range of motion actively (patient performs) and passively (clinician performs), especially with flexion and extension of the spine. Rotation and lateral bending are also helpful to assess symmetric motion or any restrictions.
Ankle strength testing	Test resisted ankle dorsiflexion, plantarflexion, inversion and eversion strength manually.
Ankle anterior drawer	The clinician keeps the foot and ankle in the neutral position with the patient sitting, then uses one hand to fix the tibia and the other to hold the patient's heel and draw the ankle forward. Normally, there may be approximately 3 mm of translation until an endpoint is felt. A positive test includes increased translation of one foot compared to the other with loss of the endpoint of the anterior talofibular ligament.
Subtalar tilt test	Performed with the foot in the neutral position with the patient sitting. The clinician uses one hand to fix the tibia and the other to hold and invert the calcaneus. Normal inversion at the subtalar joint is approximately 30 degrees. A positive test consists of increased subtalar joint inversion greater than 10 degrees on the affected side with loss of endpoint for the calcaneofibular ligament.
External rotation stress test	Performed when the clinician fixes the tibia with one hand and grasps the foot in the other with the ankle in the neutral position and then dorsiflexes and externally rotates the ankle, reproducing the patient's pain.

SEADS, swelling, erythema, atrophy, deformity, and (surgical) scars.

Special stress tests for the ankle include the **anterior drawer test** (Table 41–12) and **subtalar tilt test** (Table 41–12). In order to grade the severity of ankle sprains, no laxity on stress tests is considered a grade 1 injury, laxity of the ATF ligament on anterior drawer testing but a negative tilt test is a grade 2 injury, and both positive drawer and tilt tests signify a grade 3 injury.

B. Imaging

Routine ankle radiographic views include the AP, lateral, and oblique (mortise) views. Less common views requested include the calcaneal view and subtalar view. **Ottawa Ankle Rules** are clinical prediction rules to guide the need

for radiographs and have a 97% sensitivity and 99% negative predictive value. If the patient is unable to bear weight immediately in the office setting or emergency department for four steps, then the clinician should check for (1) bony tenderness at the posterior edge of the medial or lateral malleolus and (2) bony tenderness over the navicular (medial midfoot) or at the base of the fifth metatarsal. If either malleoli demonstrates pain or deformity, then ankle radiographs should be obtained. If the foot has bony tenderness, obtain foot radiographs. An MRI is helpful when considering the associated injuries.

▶ Treatment

Immediate treatment of an ankle sprain follows the MICE mnemonic: *m*odified activities, *i*ce, *c*ompression, and *e*levation. Subsequent treatment involves protected weight bearing with crutches and use of an ankle stabilizer brace, especially for grade 2 and 3 injuries. **Early motion is essential, and patients should be encouraged to do home exercises or physical therapy.** Proprioception and balance exercises (eg, "wobble board") are useful to restore function to the ankle and prevent future ankle sprains. Regular use of an ankle support with activities can reduce the risk of lateral ankle sprains. Chronic instability can develop after acute ankle sprain in 10–20% of people and may require surgical stabilization with ligament reconstruction surgery.

▶ When to Refer

- Ankle fractures.
- Recurrent ankle sprains or signs of chronic ligamentous ankle instability.
- No response after more than 3 months of conservative treatment.
- Suspicion of associated injuries.

Doherty C et al. The incidence and prevalence of ankle sprain injury: a systematic review and meta-analysis of prospective epidemiological studies. Sports Med. 2014 Jan;44(1):123–40. [PMID: 24105612]

Kemler E et al. A systematic review on the treatment of acute ankle sprain: brace versus other functional treatment types. Sports Med. 2011 Mar 1;41(3):185–97. [PMID: 21395362]

2. Eversion ("High") Ankle Sprains

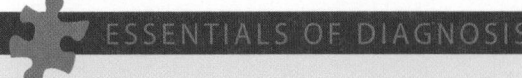
ESSENTIALS OF DIAGNOSIS

- ▶ Severe and prolonged pain.
- ▶ Limited range of motion.
- ▶ Mild swelling.
- ▶ Difficulty with weight bearing.

▶ General Considerations

A syndesmotic injury or "high ankle" sprain involves the anterior *tibio*fibular ligament in the anterolateral aspect of the ankle, superior to the anterior *talo*fibular (ATF) ligament. The injury mechanism often involves the foot being turned out or externally rotated and everted (eg, when being tackled). This injury is commonly missed or misdiagnosed as an ATF ligament sprain on initial visit.

▶ Clinical Findings

A. Symptoms and Signs

Symptoms of a high ankle sprain include severe and prolonged pain over the anterior ankle at the anterior tibiofibular ligament, worse with weight bearing. This is often more painful than the typical ankle sprain. The point of maximal tenderness involves the anterior tibiofibular ligament, which is higher than the ATF ligament. It is also important to palpate the proximal fibula to rule out any proximal syndesmotic ligament injury and associated fracture known as a "maisonneuve fracture." There is often some mild swelling in this area, and the patient may or may not have an ankle effusion. The patient usually has limited range of motion in all directions. The **external rotation stress test** reproduces the mechanism of injury (Table 41–12). (**Note:** The patient's foot should have an intact neurovascular examination before undertaking this test.)

B. Imaging

Radiographs of the ankle should include the AP, mortise, and lateral views. The mortise view may demonstrate loss of the normal overlap between the tibia and fibula, which should be at least 1–2 mm. Asymmetry in the joint space around the tibiotalar joint suggests disruption of the syndesmotic ligaments. If there is proximal tenderness in the lower leg especially around the fibula, an AP and lateral view of the tibia and fibula should be obtained to rule out a proximal fibula fracture. Radiographs during an external rotation stress test may visualize instability at the distal tibiofibular joint. MRI is the best method to visualize injury to the tibiofibular ligament and to assess status of the other ligaments and the articular cartilage.

▶ Treatment

Whereas most ankle sprains are treated with early motion and weight bearing, treatment for a high ankle sprain should be conservative with a cast or walking boot for 4–6 weeks. Thereafter, protected weight bearing with crutches is recommended until the patient can walk pain-free. Physical therapy can start early to regain range of motion and maintain strength with limited weight-bearing initially.

▶ When to Refer

If there is widening of the joint space and asymmetry at the tibiotalar joint, the patient should be referred urgently to a foot and ankle surgeon. Severe or prolonged persistent cases that do not heal may require internal fixation to avoid chronic instability at the tibiofibular joint.

Scheyerer MJ et al. Diagnostics in suspicion of ankle syndesmotic injury. Am J Orthop (Belle Mead NJ). 2011 Apr;40(4): 192–7. [PMID: 21731928]

Valkering KP et al. Isolated syndesmosis ankle injury. Orthopedics. 2012 Dec;35(12):e1705–10. [PMID: 23218625]

Women's Health Issues

Megan McNamara, MD, MSc
Judith Walsh, MD, MPH

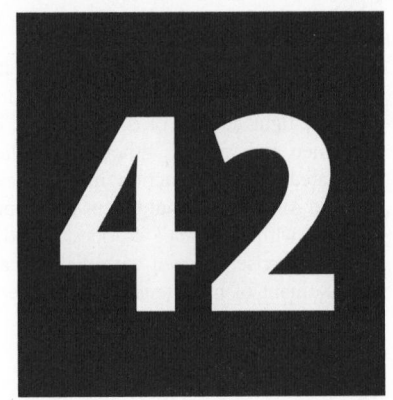

The field of women's health encompasses more than the reproductive health issues commonly addressed by obstetricians and gynecologists; it evaluates diseases and conditions only seen or experienced in women or experienced by women in ways different than men, as well as the evidence-based prevention and treatment of risk factors and diseases in women. Hence, all primary care providers, including internists and family physicians, should be well versed in women's health issues. While this chapter refers to other disease-based chapters in the textbook, it also emphasizes the understanding of issues from the particular perspective of women.

PREVENTIVE HEALTH CARE

Prevention of disease can be **primary** (preventing disease before it happens as well as identifying and modifying risk factors), **secondary** (identifying early disease), or **tertiary** (treating complications of the disease or limiting the impact of established disease). Important areas for primary prevention include encouraging women to exercise regularly to reduce the risk of coronary heart disease (CHD) and breast cancer as well as counseling women to discontinue smoking to reduce the risk of cardiac and lung diseases. Cancer screening in women focuses on secondary prevention, so that disease is detected early when prompt treatment improves outcome.

CARDIOVASCULAR DISEASE PREVENTION

Although cardiovascular disease is the leading cause of death in women, they are often more concerned about developing breast cancer (see below) than about developing heart disease. While some heart disease risk factors such as age and family history are not modifiable, as with men, other risk factors such as hypertension, hyperlipidemia, smoking, obesity, and diabetes are potentially modifiable (see also Chapter 1). The Framingham risk calculator (http://hp2010.nhlbihin.net/atpiii/calculator.asp?usertype=prof) can be used to estimate a woman's 10-year risk of CHD based on her age, smoking status, blood pressure, and cholesterol levels.

▶ Modifiable Risk Factors

A. Hypertension

Hypertension is a risk factor for CHD and stroke in both men and women (see Chapter 1). Approximately 70–80% of women over age 70 have hypertension. A woman with high blood pressure is at lower risk for CHD than a similar aged man. For many young and otherwise healthy women, medication treatment can be deferred, since their absolute risk of CHD in the next 10 years is likely to be low. When pharmacotherapy is started, the choice of medication is similar to those used in men (see Chapter 11).

B. Hyperlipidemia

Hyperlipidemia is a CHD risk factor in both men and women, but low levels of high-density lipoprotein (HDL) are more predictive of CHD risk in women. The US Preventive Services Task Force (USPSTF) recommends screening all women aged 45 and older for hyperlipidemia, whereas the National Cholesterol Education Program (NCEP) recommends screening all individuals aged 20 and over. Before screening a woman for hyperlipidemia, an important consideration is whether or not treatment recommendations will change based on the results. Since therapeutic lifestyle changes are recommended for all women, the question is at what point pharmacotherapy should be considered.

There is clear evidence that medication treatment of hyperlipidemia reduces CHD events in women who already have CHD, but when lipid-lowering medications are used in women who do not already have CHD, the evidence of benefit is less clear (see also Chapter 28). Decisions about when to initiate medication treatment should include an assessment of an individual's absolute risk of CHD in the next 10 years. Medication treatment should be targeted toward women with CHD and high-risk women who are most likely to benefit. The NCEP recommends different thresholds at which to initiate medication therapy based on individual CHD risk. For example, for a woman with known CHD, lipid-lowering medication is initiated at a low-density lipoprotein (LDL) cholesterol of > 130 mg/dL, whereas for a woman with 0–1 risk factor, medication therapy is not initiated until the LDL cholesterol measures > 190 mg/dL.

C. Diabetes

Diabetes is a CHD risk factor in both men and women. Studies have reached conflicting conclusions about the effect of tight control of diabetes on CHD outcomes in both men and women, although lipid lowering is clearly associated with a reduction in CHD events in diabetic women. All women should focus on primary prevention of diabetes with avoidance of obesity and maintenance of regular exercise. Women with diabetes also should focus on treatment of hypertension given the impact on CHD events (see Chapter 27).

D. Obesity

Obesity has been established as an independent risk factor for CHD in women. It is not known whether or not weight loss will decrease CHD risk. Since most obese women who lose weight gain it back, the overall goal should be ongoing avoidance of weight gain above normal weight (see Chapters 1 and 29).

E. Predictive Biomarkers and Clinical Tests

The use of high-sensitivity C-reactive protein (hsCRP) has increased in recent years. CRP is an inflammatory biomarker that has been shown to predict cardiovascular events. However, there is currently no evidence that screening for hsCRP improves cardiac outcomes. It has been suggested that measuring hsCRP may be useful in women for whom it would change treatment outcomes, but there is currently no evidence to support this. The USPSTF has published guidelines outlining the use of nontraditional risk factors in the evaluation of CHD. The risk factors included in the recommendation were hsCRP, ankle-brachial index, leukocyte count, fasting blood glucose, periodontal disease, carotid intima media thickness, coronary artery calcification score, electron beam CT, homocysteine, and lipoprotein (a). The USPSTF concluded that there is insufficient evidence to balance the benefits and harms of screening asymptomatic men and women with no history of CHD to predict CHD events and did not recommend routine screening.

▶ Therapeutic Options for Reducing Risk Factors

A. Aspirin

Aspirin is clearly useful for secondary prevention of CHD in women. Among women who do not have CHD, aspirin reduces the risk of stroke, whereas in men, it reduces the risk of CHD. Before starting an aspirin regimen to reduce the risk of the stroke, women should be assessed for their risk of gastrointestinal bleeding, which is the most common adverse side effect of aspirin use. The USPSTF recommends aspirin in women aged 55–79 years when the potential benefit of a reduction in ischemic strokes outweighs the potential harms of a gastrointestinal hemorrhage. For healthy or at-risk women, 81 mg/d or 100 mg every other day is the suggested dose. For high-risk women, a dose of 75–325 mg/d is recommended.

B. Exercise

Exercise has been associated with a reduction in all causes of cardiovascular mortality. Women often want to know how much exercise is necessary for health benefits. Studies have shown that walking 2.5–3 hours a week is associated with a reduction in cardiovascular disease. The Centers for Disease Control and Prevention and the American College of Sports Medicine recommend that all women accumulate at least 30 minutes a day of moderate intensity physical activity on most if not all days of the week. The Institute of Medicine recommends an hour a day for the goal of maintaining health and ideal body weight. See also Chapter 1.

Gutierrez J et al. Statin therapy in the prevention of recurrent cardiovascular events: a sex-based meta-analysis. Arch Intern Med. 2012 June 25;172(12):909–19. [PMID: 22732744]

Mosca L et al. Effectiveness-based guidelines for the prevention of cardiovascular disease in women—2011 update: a guideline from the American Heart Association. Circulation. 2011 Mar 22;123(11):1243–62. [PMID: 21325087]

U.S. Preventive Services Task Force. Screening for Lipid Disorders in Adults: U.S. Preventive Services Task Force recommendation statement. http://www.uspreventiveservicestaskforce.org/uspstf08/lipid/lipidrs.htm

CANCER PREVENTION

1. Breast Cancer

▶ Risk Factors & Risk Assessment

Breast cancer is the most commonly detected cancer in women and the second leading cause of cancer death (see also Chapter 17). Breast cancer risk is increased with age and with a family history of breast cancer. Women who drink more than two alcoholic drinks per day are at increased risk for breast cancer, and exercise is associated with a decreased risk of breast cancer. Dietary intake has not been conclusively associated with breast cancer risk. Breast density is an emerging risk factor for breast cancer; women with denser breasts as measured with mammography are at increased breast cancer risk. Although some states now mandate that women with increased breast density on mammography be notified, it is not currently known what women can do to decrease this risk.

Various models have been used to predict a woman's risk for breast cancer. The National Cancer Institute has developed the Breast Cancer Risk Assessment Tool (http://www.cancer.gov/bcrisktool/), which is based on the Gail Model, and calculates the woman's risk of developing breast cancer in the next 5 years by considering the following factors: (1) the woman's age, (2) age at which she had her first menstrual period, (3) age at delivery of first live child, (3) number of first-degree relatives with breast cancer, (4) history of any breast biopsies, and (5) history of atypical hyperplasia. The model has been validated in white women and has been evaluated in black women and found to be relatively accurate, although it may underestimate the risk in black women with a history of previous breast biopsies. It has yet to be validated in women of other ethnicities.

▶ Primary Prevention

In addition to lifestyle modifications, such as exercise and moderation of alcohol intake, chemoprevention of breast cancer is an option for some women. The selective estrogen receptor modifiers (SERMS) tamoxifen and raloxifene have both been shown to reduce invasive breast cancer in high-risk women. However, there are risks associated with SERM treatment. Tamoxifen is associated with an increased risk of endometrial cancer and deep venous thrombosis (DVT). Although raloxifene is not associated with an increased risk of endometrial cancer, the risk of DVT remains. Aromatase inhibitors, such as exemestane, show promise for breast cancer prevention but are not currently FDA approved for this indication. The USPSTF recommends that clinicians discuss chemoprevention with women at high risk for breast cancer and at low risk for the adverse effects of chemoprevention. Clinicians should inform patients of the potential benefits and harms of chemoprevention. Breast cancer risk increases with age, but the risk of adverse effects does as well. Since the clinical trials of tamoxifen and raloxifene for breast cancer prevention used a 1.66% 5-year risk, this risk level is often used as a guide for medication treatment.

▶ Breast Cancer Screening

Traditional breast cancer screening modalities include screening mammography, clinical breast examination, and breast self-examination (see also Chapter 17). Teaching women to do routine breast self-examination has not been shown to reduce breast cancer mortality. The USPSTF recommends against teaching women to do breast self-examination. The American Cancer Society states that it is acceptable not to do it, but that if women are performing breast self-examination, it is important to ensure that they are doing it correctly. The combination of breast examination done by a clinician and mammography is associated with a decrease in breast cancer mortality, but there is insufficient evidence to recommend clinical breast examination alone.

Mammography reduces breast cancer mortality in women aged 50–74 years and routine mammographic screening is recommended for women in this age group. For women aged 40–49 years, screening has been more controversial. Guidelines published by the USPSTF recommend that clinicians not routinely order mammography among 40- to 49-year-old women but rather that they individualize the decision to begin screening, since the number needed to invite to screen to prevent one breast cancer death is much higher in younger women and the number of false-positive and false-negative test results are much higher. Since women over age 75 have not been included in clinical trials and since the likelihood of comorbid diseases limiting life expectancy increases, routine screening of women in this age group is not recommended, but rather the decision making should be individualized.

Hubbard et al. Cumulative probability of false-positive recall or biopsy recommendation after 10 years of screening mammography: a cohort study. Ann Intern Med. 2011 Oct 18; 155(8):481–92. [PMID: 22007042]

Nelson HD et al. Risk factors for breast cancer for women aged 40 to 49 years: a systematic review and meta-analysis. Ann Intern Med. 2012 May 1;156(9):635–48. [PMID: 22547473]

2. Colorectal Cancer

Colorectal cancer is the third leading cause of cancer death in both men and women. In 2013 an estimated 9% of cancer deaths in women were caused by colorectal cancer. Since the risk of colorectal cancer increases with age, all women should be screened for colorectal cancer starting at the age of 50. The USPSTF recommends routine screening in men and women age 50–75, individualized decision making about screening in individuals aged 76–85, and no screening after the age of 85. Details of the screening options and suggested screening intervals are described in Chapter 1.

U.S. Preventive Services Task Force. Screening for Colorectal Cancer: U.S. Preventive Services Task Force recommendation statement. Ann Intern Med. 2008 Nov 4;149(9):627–37. [PMID: 18838716]

3. Cervical Cancer

In contrast to most other cancers for which routine screening is recommended, the incidence of cervical cancer is higher in younger women and decreases with age. The major risk factor for cervical cancer is exposure to the human papillomavirus (HPV). Primary prevention of cervical cancer includes avoidance of smoking, postponing sexual debut, and limiting the number of sexual partners. Condom use may also be protective.

▶ Primary Prevention

A quadrivalent HPV vaccine that includes capsid proteins against four HPV types (6, 11, 16, and 18) has been approved for use in girls and women aged 9–26 years to prevent disease associated with these HPV types (see also Chapter 18). A bivalent vaccine (Cervarix) is also available. The Advisory Committee on Immunization Practices (ACIP) recommends routine vaccination for girls aged 11 or 12 up to age 26, whereas the American Cancer Society recommends the vaccine for girls aged 11–18 but states that there is insufficient evidence to recommend for or against routine vaccination for women aged 19–26. Unanswered questions about the vaccine include the long-term effects and the length of protection. Receipt of vaccine should not change cervical cancer screening intervals in women.

▶ Secondary Prevention

An important focus of cervical cancer prevention is screening using the Papanicolaou smear. Cervical cancer screening is the biggest success in the history of cancer screening. Cervical cancer mortality has been reduced by about 70% with routine cervical cancer screening. One of the reasons that screening has been so successful is that there is a long preclinical phase where early changes can be detected and treated so as to avoid the development of cancer. The USP-STF updated their screening recommendations in 2012 (see Chapter 18).

U.S. Preventive Services Task Force. Screening for cervical cancer: U.S. Preventive Services Task Force recommendation statement. http://www.uspreventiveservicestaskforce.org/uspstf11/cervcancer/cervcancerrs.htm

4. Lung Cancer

Although lung cancer is not typically considered a "women's cancer," it is the leading cause of cancer mortality in both men and women. Primary prevention of lung cancer should be a high priority with encouragement of tobacco cessation among women who smoke (see Chapters 1 and 39). Consistent with a 2012 joint recommendation from the American Academy of Chest Physicians and the American Society of Clinical Oncology in December 2013, the USP-STF updated its screening recommendation based on NLST data recommending "annual screening for lung cancer with low-dose computed tomography in adults ages 55 to 80 years who have a 30 pack-year smoking history and currently smoke or have quit within the past 15 years."

Humphrey LL et al. Screening for lung cancer with low-dose computed tomography: a systematic review to update the U.S. Preventive services task force recommendation. Ann Intern Med. 2013 Sep 17;159(6):411–20. [PMID: 23897166]

National Lung Screening Trial Research Team; Aberle DR et al. Reduced lung-cancer mortality with low-dose computed tomographic screening. N Engl J Med. 2011 Aug 4;365(5):395–409. [PMID: 21714641]

5. Ovarian Cancer

Ovarian cancer is a relatively rare but dreaded cancer, with a lifetime incidence of about 1.2% in women with no family history of ovarian cancer. Because it is often detected late, treatment options may be limited.

Many of the risk factors for ovarian cancer such as age and family history are not modifiable, but there are protective factors, including having more than one full-term pregnancy, breast-feeding, and oral contraceptive use. Women at high-risk for ovarian cancer should consider the use of oral contraceptives for as long as it is feasible.

Although screening for ovarian cancer with either the serum marker CA-125 or with transvaginal ultrasound is theoretically appealing, the rarity of the disease limits their use and leads to many false-positive test results (see also Chapter 18). The USPSTF does not recommend screening for ovarian cancer.

Buys SS et al. Effect of screening on ovarian cancer mortality: the Prostate, Lung, Colorectal and Ovarian (PLCO) Cancer Screening Randomized Controlled Trial. JAMA. 2011 Jun 8; 305(22):2295–303. [PMID: 21642681]

OSTEOPOROSIS PREVENTION

Osteoporotic fractures are increasing as the population ages. Age and female sex are major risk factors for osteoporotic fractures. Hip and vertebral fractures are associated with premature mortality. Osteoporosis risk can be assessed by measuring bone mineral density (BMD). See also Chapter 26.

The World Health Organization has developed a fracture risk assessment tool (FRAX, available at http://www.shef.ac.uk/FRAX/index.jsp) that can predict a woman's 10-year risk of having any osteoporotic fracture and the 10-year risk of hip fracture. Risk factors used in the FRAX tool include age, gender, personal history of fracture, parental history of hip fracture, low body mass index, use of oral corticosteroids, secondary osteoporosis, current smoking, and alcohol intake of three or more drinks per day. It can be used with or without BMD. The FRAX tool is particularly helpful in determining which women with osteopenia are most likely to benefit from treatment. Based on the World Health Organization algorithm adopted for the United States, treatment is recommended when there is a 10-year risk of hip fracture ≥ 3% or a 10-year risk of a major osteoporotic fracture ≥ 20%.

▶ Primary Prevention

Although calcium supplementation is routinely recommended, evidence from the Women's Health Initiative showed that calcium supplementation did not reduce fracture risk in healthy postmenopausal women and other research has highlighted potential risks of calcium supplementation. Calcium appears to be necessary but not sufficient for fracture prevention. The USPSTF recommendations state that the evidence is insufficient to assess the balance of benefits and harms for the combination of vitamin D and calcium for primary prevention of fractures in men or premenopausal women. Recommended calcium intake for women younger than 50 years is 1000 mg/d and for women aged 51 and over, it is 1200 mg/d. Dietary calcium may be safer than calcium supplements, but calcium supplements can be given as either calcium citrate or calcium carbonate and should be given with vitamin D. Regular weight bearing exercise has also been associated with an increase in bone density although the effect is lost when the exercise is not continued.

Increasing evidence suggests that vitamin D supplementation is associated with a reduction in fracture risk. Vitamin D can be given as either D_2 or D_3 formulations. Recommendations are that women aged 70 and younger should consume 600 international units of vitamin D per day, whereas women aged 71 and older should consume 800 international units per day. Individuals with vitamin D deficiency (25-OH vitamin D < 20 mg/mL) may require higher doses, although most recommendations for vitamin D supplementation are based on achieving a serum 25-OH vitamin D concentration of a particular level, rather than on a clinical outcome. Whether or not women should be routinely screened for vitamin D deficiency remains an ongoing question. However, given the association of vitamin D and fractures, checking a 25-OH vitamin D level in women with osteopenia or osteoporosis is reasonable.

► Bone Mineral Density Screening

The biggest risk factor for developing osteoporosis is increasing age. Although many women expect to be screened around the time of menopause, routine BMD screening is not recommended until the age of 65. The National Osteoporosis Foundation recommends screening all women age 65 and older and screening younger postmenopausal women if there is a concern based on their risk-factor profile. The USPSTF recommends screening women aged 65 and older and only screening younger women whose fracture risk is equal to or greater than that of a 65-year-old white woman who has no additional risk factors. The Fracture Risk Assessment tool (FRAX) tool can be used to calculate 10-year risk of osteoporotic fracture. Most guidelines do not specifically address how often a woman should undergo BMD testing. However, decisions about when to rescreen should probably be based on the results of initial screening. Women with normal BMD or mild osteopenia at baseline can be screened less often than women who are near the threshold for osteoporosis.

Treatment is generally recommended in women who have a t score < –2.5, who have already had a fracture or who have a t score in the osteopenic range but are at high risk for fracture. Treatment options for osteoporosis are described in Chapter 26.

Gourlay ML et al; Study of Osteoporotic Fractures Research Group. Bone-density testing interval and transition to osteoporosis in older women. N Engl J Med. 2012 Jan 19;366(3):225–33. [PMID: 22256806]

Institute of Medicine (IOM). Dietary reference intakes for calcium and vitamin D. http://www.iom.edu/Reports/2010/Dietary-Reference-Intakes-for-Calcium-and-Vitamin-D.aspx

Li K et al. Associations of dietary calcium intake and calcium supplementation with myocardial infarction and stroke risk and overall cardiovascular mortality in the Heidelberg cohort of the European Prospective Investigation into Cancer and Nutrition study (EPIC-Heidelberg). Heart. 2012 Jun;98(12):920–5. [PMID: 22626900]

U.S. Preventive Services Task Force. Screening for osteoporosis: U.S. Preventive Services Task Force recommendation statement. Ann Intern Med. 2011 Mar 1;154(5):356–64. [PMID: 21242341]

U.S. Preventive Services Task Force. Vitamin D and calcium supplementation to prevent cancer and osteoporotic fractures. http://www.uspreventiveservicestaskforce.org/uspstf/uspsvitd.htm

World Health Organization Collaborating Centre for Metabolic Bone Diseases. Fracture Risk Assessment Tool (FRAX). http://www.shef.ac.uk/FRAX/tool.jsp

PREVENTION OF SEXUALLY TRANSMITTED INFECTIONS

Many sexually transmitted infections are asymptomatic in women and some can lead to significant consequences. Primary prevention of sexually transmitted infections includes postponing sexual debut, limiting number of sexual partners, and regular condom use.

The USPSTF and the Centers for Disease Control and Prevention recommend annual screening for *Chlamydia trachomatis* and gonorrhea in sexually active women age 25 and younger (see Chapter 30). Screening should continue in women over age 25 and in women who have high-risk sexual behaviors. The USPSTF recommends screening all women for HIV: including adolescents and women of age 15-65 years, others at high risk, as well as pregnant women. All patients who have a sexually transmitted infection or who seek testing for a sexually transmitted infection should be offered HIV testing. The CDC currently recommends screening all women born between 1945 and 1965 for hepatitis C infection.

DEPRESSION SCREENING

Since depression is approximately two times more common in women than in men, clinicians should be alert to symptoms suggesting depression in women. Symptoms include depressed mood, loss of interest in activities, sleep disturbance, change in appetite or weight, psychomotor retardation, difficulty concentrating, feelings of worthlessness, and thoughts of suicide (see also Chapter 25). Low energy or fatigue is a particularly common symptom in women.

There are several clinical surveys for depression screening. The two question screen appears to be effective. Patients are asked "Over the past 2 weeks, have you felt down, depressed or hopeless?" and "Over the past 2 weeks, have you felt little interest or pleasure in doing things?" There is no evidence to suggest that any particular screening tool is superior. A positive screening test should lead to more extensive evaluation.

The USPSTF recommends screening for depression if staff-assisted depression care supports are in place to ensure accurate diagnosis, effective treatment, and follow-up. If these supports are not in place, screening is not recommended.

U.S. Preventive Services Task Force. Screening for Depression in Adults. http://www.uspreventiveservicestaskforce.org/uspstf/uspsaddepr.htm

▼ SPECIFIC ISSUES & CONDITIONS

INTIMATE PARTNER VIOLENCE

Intimate partner violence (IPV) is a pattern of abusive behavior by a person who is in some type of intimate relationship with the victim. The abuse can be physical, sexual, or emotional and can include economic deprivation. Although anyone can be a victim of IPV, women are much more likely than men to be victims. Regardless of the type of abuse, the goal of the abuser is to gain control over the victim. IPV is common but is often not diagnosed, in part because patients try to hide the abuse.

The prevalence estimate of IPV varies depending on the setting. Rates are higher when measured in emergency departments than when measured in the general population. In a randomized controlled trial of IPV screening in emergency departments, the prevalence over 12 months ranged from 4% to 18%.

Risk factors for abuse include being young (under age 35 years); being pregnant; being single, divorced, or separated; alcohol or drug abuse in the victim or the partner; smoking; and being poor.

► Evaluation

Since patients often do not volunteer that they have been abused, clinicians must be alert to clues that suggest abuse, including an explanation of the injuries that do not fit with what is being seen; frequent visits to the emergency department; and somatic complaint such as chronic headache, abdominal pain, and fatigue. The patient may be vague about some of her symptoms and may avoid eye contact. If the abusing partner is present, he or she may answer all the questions or may decline to leave the room. **It is critical that the patient have the opportunity to speak with the clinician alone.** The patient's description of the events should be carefully detailed in case there are any subsequent legal issues.

Physical examination often reveals injuries in the central area of the body. There may be injuries on the forearms as well if the patient tried to defend herself. As with any situation of expected abuse, bruises that are in various stages of healing may be an important clue. All physical examination findings should be well documented.

In addition to the physical consequences, abuse can have psychological consequences. Posttraumatic stress disorder, depression, anxiety, and alcohol or other substance abuse can develop in victims. Somatization is also very common among victims.

Several instruments have been developed to screen for IPV. These include the HITS (Hurt, Insult, Threaten, Screamed at) tool, the Women Abuse Screening tool (WAST), the Partner Violence Screen (PVS), the Abuse Assessment Screen (AAS), and the Women's Experience with Battering (WEB) scale. A systematic review of these screening tools showed that most tools only had been evaluated in a relatively small number of studies and the sensitivities and specificities varied widely within and between the tools.

Inclusion of one question in the context of the medical history, "Have you ever been hit, kicked, punched or otherwise hurt by someone within the past year? If so, by whom?" has been shown to increase identification of IPV.

Many studies have addressed how the questions about IPV are asked. In one randomized trial, women preferred written questionnaires over face to face interviewing.

Screening for IPV (in contrast to asking questions when IPV is suspected) has been advocated by many experts, although there has been controversy about whether or not it improves outcomes. In January 2013, the USPSTF updated its previous guidelines and currently recommends that clinicians screen women of childbearing age for IPV including domestic violence, and provide or refer women who screen positive to intervention services.

► Interventions for IPV

Interventions can include encouraging the woman to leave the abusive situation, ensuring that she has a safe place to go, and counseling so that she can adequately assess her risk of danger and create a plan for safety. There is no evidence that treatment of the abuser changes abuser behavior.

► When to Refer

- Victims should be referred to social services so that they can provide information on local resources. There is a national domestic violence hotline (1-800-799-SAFE) that can provide information on local resources.
- In general, mandatory reporting of IPV or suspicion of it in adult women who are competent is not required in most states. However, mandatory reporting by clinicians is required in California, Colorado, Kentucky, Mississippi, Ohio, and Rhode Island.

Moyer VA. Screening for intimate partner violence and abuse of elderly and vulnerable adults: U.S. preventive services task force recommendation statement. Ann Intern Med. 2013 Mar 19;158(6):478–86. [PMID: 23338828]

Nelson HD et al. Screening women for intimate partner violence and elderly and vulnerable adults for abuse: systematic review to update the 2004 U.S. Preventive Services Task Force Recommendation. Evidence synthesis No. 92. AHRQ Publication No. 12-05167-EF-1. Rockville, MD: Agency for Healthcare Research and Quality; May 2012. [PMID: 22675737]

EATING DISORDERS

Eating disorders are common in women. Anorexia nervosa and bulimia nervosa are described in detail in Chapter 29. The female athlete triad, disordered eating in diabetics, and binge eating disorders are other eating disorders that should be considered in appropriate women.

1. Female Athlete Triad

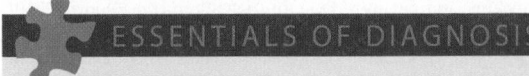

ESSENTIALS OF DIAGNOSIS

- ► Disordered eating.
- ► Menstrual disorders.
- ► Low BMD.

► General Considerations

Female athletes who participate in sports and activities valuing thinness are at increased risk for developing the female athlete triad. The definition of the triad includes disordered eating (a spectrum of abnormal patterns of eating, including bingeing; purging; food restriction; prolonged fasting; and the use of diet pills, diuretics, or laxatives), menstrual disorders, and low BMD. Half of all athletes with amenorrhea have bone density at least 1.0 standard deviation below the mean. The bone density is decreased even in those areas subjected to stress during exercise. The diagnosis is made when the individual meets the three criteria of the triad.

► Clinical Findings

A. Symptoms and Signs

Individuals with the female athlete triad display some pattern of disordered eating and have some menstrual irregularities. Many women have amenorrhea but others have irregular menses. Typically, the patient has concerns about weight and body image. A history of stress fractures should also raise the clinician's concern.

B. Laboratory Findings

Depending on the severity of the symptoms and whether or not the patient is bingeing and purging, the laboratory abnormalities can be similar to those seen in anorexia nervosa or bulimia nervosa. BMD, if measured, is decreased.

▶ Differential Diagnosis

The main differential diagnoses include anorexia nervosa, bulimia nervosa as well as endocrine disorders such as hyperthyroidism and diabetes mellitus.

▶ Treatment

Little evidence is currently available about treatment of the female athlete triad. Strategies such as counseling, cognitive behavior therapy, and possibly exercise restriction may be helpful. A multidisciplinary approach, including consultation with a nutritionist and communication with the coach and trainers, may enable common goal setting. The desire to participate in sports and the lure of a performance enhancing diet may motivate some patients to pursue treatment.

2. Disordered Eating in Diabetics

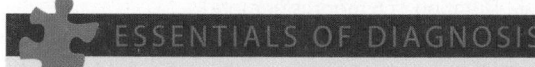

ESSENTIALS OF DIAGNOSIS

- ▶ Binge eating.
- ▶ Purging with laxatives or vomiting.
- ▶ Insulin omission.
- ▶ Taking less insulin than prescribed to lose weight.

▶ General Considerations

Eating disturbances have been estimated to be present in up to one-third of young women with diabetes. Eating disorders are more common in adolescents with diabetes than in their non-diabetic peers. Mortality is particularly high in individuals with both diabetes and eating disorders.

For diabetes, the dietary regimen emphasizes intense meal timing and consistency. In addition, the hunger associated with hypoglycemia encourages binge eating. Diabetics with disordered eating have been shown to have an increased risk of retinopathy. Given the emphasis that young women often place on body weight, maintaining optimal diabetes control is a particular challenge. The diagnosis is typically made in a diabetic who has worsening diabetic control, when other causes of worsening control have been ruled out.

▶ Clinical Findings

A. Symptoms and Signs

Diabetics may report polydipsia, polyuria, or weight loss. In addition, upon questioning, they may report disturbed eating patterns. Other symptoms associated with eating

disorders, such as disturbance of body image and menstrual irregularities, may also be present.

B. Laboratory Findings

The main laboratory finding will be a trend of increasing levels of hemoglobin A_{1C}.

▶ Differential Diagnosis

The main differential diagnosis includes looking for other causes of worsening glycemic control such as underlying infection or metabolic disease such as hyperthyroidism.

▶ Treatment

There is currently no evidence to support any particular strategies for the treatment of disordered eating in diabetic patients. Proposed strategies for at risk diabetic patients include nutritional counseling to promote healthy eating instead of dietary restraint, regular (instead of fixed) meal and snack times, less intensive insulin therapy to reduce weight gain, and family counseling to improve communication.

No studies have evaluated the optimal treatment of diabetic patients with established eating disorders. Presumably, strategies that are effective for patients without diabetes, such as cognitive behavioral therapy and medications, will be effective. In addition, diabetic management strategies that do not require the patient to constantly think about food may be beneficial.

3. Binge Eating Disorder

ESSENTIALS OF DIAGNOSIS

- ▶ Binge eating disorder consists of episodes of eating a large amount of food in a discreet period of time with a sense of lack of control.
- ▶ Binge episodes characterized by at least three of the following:
  - – Eating large amounts of food when not feeling hungry.
  - – Eating more rapidly than normal.
  - – Eating until feeling uncomfortably full.
  - – Eating alone because of embarrassment about the amount of food consumed.
  - – Feeling disgusted, depressed, or guilty after eating.
- ▶ Episodes occur at least two times a week for at least 6 months.
- ▶ No compensatory behavior (purging, fasting, or excessive exercise) after eating.

▶ General Considerations

Binge eating disorder is more common than either anorexia nervosa or bulimia nervosa, and, with the publication of the *Diagnostic and Statistical Manual of Mental Disorders,*

5th edition (DSM-V), it is recognized formally as a diagnosable eating disorder.

Binge eating disorder is much more common in women and is associated with obesity, although not all individuals with binge eating disorder are obese. Obesity-related complications are likely to occur, and the disorder may be more common in weight cycling patients.

► Clinical Findings

The patient may present with weight gain or may describe disordered eating patterns and binge eating episodes. There are no specific laboratory findings for binge eating disorder.

► Differential Diagnosis

The main differential diagnosis includes other psychiatric and eating disorders. Other diagnostic possibilities include hypothyroidism and Prader-Willi syndrome.

► Treatment

Treatment goals focus on decreasing the patient's binge eating episodes and may include weight loss and treatment of other psychiatric comorbidities. As in bulimia nervosa, cognitive behavioral therapy is the mainstay of treatment. Interpersonal therapy has also been shown to be effective. Pharmacotherapy with selective serotonin reuptake inhibitors is also helpful, but does not appear to be better than cognitive behavioral therapy.

National Institute for Health and Clinical Excellence. Eating disorders: core interventions in the treatment and management of anorexia nervosa, bulimia nervosa and related eating disorders. http://www.nice.org.uk/CG009
Young V et al. Eating problems in adolescents with Type 1 diabetes: a systematic review with meta-analysis. Diabet Med. 2013 Feb;30(2):189–98. [PMID: 22913589]

SEXUALITY & SEXUAL HEALTH

Sexual health is defined by the World Health Organization as a state of physical, emotional, mental, and social well-being in relation to sexuality. Healthy sexual functioning therefore depends on a complex interplay of physical, psychological, and societal factors. Among the more than 30,000 women who were surveyed about their sexuality in the PRESIDE study, 9–12% reported having a sexual problem that caused personal distress or interpersonal difficulties. The female sexual disorders identified in the DSM-V include female sexual interest/arousal disorder, sexual aversion disorder, female orgasmic disorder, and genito-pelvic pain/penetration disorder (these are discussed in detail in Chapters 18 and 25). Several medical conditions (depression, diabetes, urinary incontinence, and multiple sclerosis) and medications (antidepressants, hormonal therapy, antihypertensives) can contribute to the development of female sexual disorders. Clinicians should routinely assess patients' sexual health during office visits; even a brief assessment provides patients with reassurance that this is an important topic. Providers can broach the subject using a broad question, such as "What concerns or

questions do you have about your sexual functioning?" and then follow-up with more specific questions, including "Do you have difficulty with desire, arousal, or orgasm?" and "If you are not currently sexual, are there any particular problems that are contributing to your lack of sexual behavior?" Patient concerns can then be delineated more fully during the complete sexual assessment, which encompasses details about medical, surgical, and psychiatric problems, as well as medications and reproductive history. Treatment options depend on the diagnosed disorder and can include psychosexual and hormonal therapy (see Chapter 18).

Kingsberg SA et al. Female sexual disorders: assessment, diagnosis, and treatment. CNS Spectr. 2011 Feb;16(2):49–62. [PMID: 21419070]
World Health Organization. Measuring sexual health: conception and practical considerations and related indicators. World Health Organization, 2010, Geneva, Switzerland. http://www.who.int/reproductivehealth/publications/monitoring/who_rhr_10.12/en/index.html

CHRONIC PELVIC PAIN

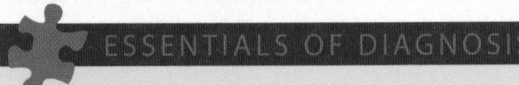
ESSENTIALS OF DIAGNOSIS

► Noncyclic pain.

► Duration of 6 months or more.

► Localized to anatomic pelvis, anterior abdominal wall at or below the umbilicus, the lumbosacral back, or buttocks.

► Associated with functional disability.

► General Considerations

Chronic pelvic pain (CPP) is defined as noncyclic pain lasting at least 6 months that localizes to the pelvic girdle region; it must be of sufficient severity to cause functional disability or necessitate medical care. CPP may result from gynecologic, urologic, gastrointestinal, musculoskeletal, or neurologic disorders. Although endometriosis is the most common gynecologic condition associated with CPP, postoperative adhesions, pelvic congestion, and chronic pelvic inflammatory disease should also be considered. Interstitial cystitis, irritable bowel syndrome, and myofascial pain syndrome arising from trigger points in the abdominal musculature or pelvic floor have all been associated with CPP. Sensation to the pelvis is supplied by nerves arising from thoracolumbar and sacral nerve roots. Thus, spinal pathology or direct injury to the pudendal nerve can produce CPP. It is important to remember that most women with CPP have multiple diagnoses contributing to their pain.

► Clinical Findings

A. Symptoms and Signs

Certain features of the history and physical examination can provide clues to the underlying diagnosis. Patients should be asked about the location, quality, and intensity of their pain as well as the relationship with the menstrual cycle, sexual activity, urination, and defecation. Dysmenorrhea and dyspareunia are often experienced by patients with endometriosis, whereas dysuria, urgency, and frequency in association with pelvic pain are characteristic of interstitial cystitis. Pain related to pelvic varices is usually postural, worsening with prolonged standing and improving with leg elevation. Patients with irritable bowel syndrome often report abdominal pain, distention, and diarrhea or constipation. Clinicians should ask patients about surgery or direct trauma involving the spine or pelvis, which may suggest musculoskeletal sources of pain. The physical examination, including the pelvic examination, is usually quite painful in the patient with CPP and should be done carefully. Palpation of the thoracic and lumbar spine, pelvic girdle, and abdomen can reveal areas of discomfort that refer to the pelvic area. A positive Carnett test (constituted by an increase in tenderness when the abdominal muscles are tensed) can be helpful for identifying abdominal wall trigger points. A single-digit internal vaginal examination should be done to localize the exact area of pain and to assess for trigger points along the pelvic floor muscles. Palpation of the pelvic viscera can help identify localized areas of tenderness in women with endometriosis or chronic pelvic inflammatory disease. The external genitalia should also be examined carefully to identify areas of vulvar discomfort because vulvodynia often coexists in patients with CPP. Notably, the absence of physical examination findings does not rule out significant pathology.

B. Laboratory Findings

Women who are at high risk for pelvic infection should be screened with cervical swabs for chlamydia and gonorrhea.

C. Diagnostic Testing and Imaging

Pelvic ultrasonography is useful for evaluating the pelvic anatomy, investigating localized areas of tenderness, and identifying pathology. Laparoscopy may be helpful for diagnosing endometriosis or pelvic adhesions, although 35% of diagnostic laparoscopies are normal in patients with CPP.

▶ Differential Diagnosis

CPP is frequently a manifestation of another disease, as noted above. When considering various diagnoses, it is important to differentiate extra-pelvic from intra-pelvic sources of pain. Musculoskeletal disorders involving the spine, hips, and sacroiliac joints may cause referred pelvic pain, whereas endometriosis, chronic pelvic inflammatory disease, and pelvic congestion are typically associated with tenderness of the pelvic viscera. Similarly, abdominal wall or hip girdle trigger points that cause CPP can be easily differentiated from trigger points in the levator ani and perineal muscles.

▶ Treatment

A. Medical Treatment

Medical treatment may focus on managing the chronic pain, the underlying condition, or both. Analgesics are commonly used, and nonsteroidal anti-inflammatory drugs (NSAIDs)

are typically helpful. However, patients and clinicians should be cautious about long-term use of these medications because long-term NSAID therapy can be associated with significant gastric toxicity. Antidepressants (eg, amitriptyline) and antiseizure medications (eg, gabapentin) (see Table 5–4), which have demonstrated efficacy in the treatment of other pain syndromes, may also be useful for CPP. Opioid therapy improves pain but not functional or psychological outcomes and should generally be avoided.

Hormonal therapies are used primarily for treating gynecologic sources of CPP. Women with endometriosis often benefit from treatment with combined oral contraceptive pills, which suppress ovulation and reduce dysmenorrhea. Gonadotropin-releasing hormone (GnRH) agonists and progestins improve pain associated with endometriosis and pelvic varices. The decrease in BMD associated with GnRH agonist treatment can be mitigated with estrogen or progesterone add-back therapy. Treatment with medroxyprogesterone improved pain scores in women with pelvic congestion, but symptoms returned with cessation of treatment.

Medical therapies directed at the treatment of nongynecologic sources of CPP, including interstitial cystitis and irritable bowel syndrome, are discussed in Chapters 15 and 23. Physical therapy and injection of identified trigger points provide significant pain relief in patients with musculoskeletal sources of pain. Psychological evaluation and treatment should also be strongly considered as many women with CPP experience anxiety and depression.

B. Surgical Treatment

Surgical treatment of CPP requires referral to a gynecologist. Condition-specific surgical treatments include ovarian or pelvic vein embolization in women with pelvic congestion syndrome or adhesiolysis in patients with pelvic adhesions. Women with endometriosis may be offered laparoscopic surgical destruction of implants or laparoscopic utero-sacral (LUNA) nerve ablation for relief of their chronic pain. Importantly, the efficacy of some of these surgical techniques is controversial. According to a recent systematic review, lysis of adhesions and LUNA were no more effective than diagnostic laparoscopy for improvement in pain scores. Women with endometriosis who have persistent disease after medical and surgical therapies may benefit from hysterectomy, although it is controversial as to whether concomitant oophorectomy improves symptoms further.

▶ When to Refer

Patients should be referred to a gynecologist for diagnostic or therapeutic surgical procedures, if the underlying diagnosis is unclear, or if the provider feels uncomfortable managing side effects associated with medical treatments (ie, GnRH agonist therapy).

Andrews J et al. Noncyclic chronic pelvic pain therapies for women: comparative effectiveness [Internet]. Rockville (MD): Agency for Healthcare Research and Quality (US); 2012 Jan. Available from http://www.ncbi.nlm.nih.gov/books/NBK84586/ [PMID: 22439157]

Engler D et al; European Association of Urology. Guidelines on chronic pelvic pain, 2012. http://www.uroweb.org/gls/pdf/24_Chronic_Pelvic_Pain_LR%20II.pdf

Shin JH et al. Management of chronic pelvic pain. Curr Pain Headache Rep. 2011 Oct;15(5):377–85. [PMID: 21556711]

Stacy J et al. Persistent pelvic pain: rising to the challenge. Aust N Z J Obstet Gynaecol. 2012 Dec;52(6):502–7. [PMID: 22998335]

MASTALGIA

ESSENTIALS OF DIAGNOSIS

► Infection, malignancy, and extramammary conditions can cause breast pain.

► Abnormal physical examination findings, such as a breast mass or skin abnormalities, should prompt radiographic imaging.

General Considerations

Breast pain, or mastalgia, is categorized as cyclical, noncyclical, or extramammary. Although minor breast discomfort is commonly associated with the normal menstrual cycle, women with cyclical mastalgia typically have moderate to severe pain that can last more than 5 days. Cyclical mastalgia can be diagnosed only in reproductive-age women who experience breast pain as a result of the hormonally-mediated proliferation in breast tissue that occurs with ovulation. In contrast, noncyclical mastalgia has no relationship to the menstrual cycle and can occur in premenopausal or postmenopausal women. Causes of noncyclical mastalgia include large breast size (with stretching of Cooper ligaments), medications, pregnancy, thrombophlebitis, or inflammatory breast cancer. Extramammary mastalgia is caused by pain that is referred from other anatomic locations, including the chest wall, heart, gallbladder, or spine. Trauma or previous surgery may also produce extramammary pain.

► Clinical Findings

A. Symptoms and Signs

Cyclical mastalgia is often described as a deep, heavy, aching pain, which is typically diffuse and bilateral and is clearly associated with the menstrual cycle. Conversely, noncyclical pain, which may be constant or intermittent, is variable in location and can involve one or both breasts. Chest wall pain, a frequent cause of extramammary mastalgia, typically causes unilateral, burning pain that may be either localized or diffuse. Malignancy-associated mastalgia is often severe, progressive, and unilateral.

Breast cancer may be associated with mastalgia, and thus a careful physical examination is essential in all women who report breast pain. Large, pendulous breasts may be observed in women who have noncyclical pain caused by stretching of Cooper ligaments. Chest wall pain is usually related to inflammation or injury to the pectoralis major muscle; it may be reproduced by palpation or by having the patient place her hand on her hip and push inward. Any palpable breast mass must be evaluated further with radiologic imaging.

B. Imaging

An ultrasound, mammogram, or both should be obtained in women who have a palpable breast mass or localized breast pain or who are at an increased risk for breast cancer. Women with diffuse breast pain who are at average risk for breast cancer and who have a normal physical examination do not require further imaging and can be reassured. However, the clinician should ensure that all patients with mastalgia are up to date on routine screening mammography, as appropriate for their age and personal risk factors.

► Differential Diagnosis

Malignancy must be ruled out in all patients with mastalgia, and this is usually accomplished through a careful history, physical examination, and diagnostic imaging in patients with clinical abnormalities, such as a palpable breast mass. Extramammary causes of breast pain include chest wall pain, spinal or gallbladder disease, and myocardial ischemia.

► Treatment

Women with cyclical mastalgia who have a normal physical examination and are up to date on routine mammographic screening should be reassured about the benign nature of their symptoms and monitored closely. Cyclical and noncyclical mastalgia often improve with use of a supportive bra. Although there is conflicting evidence regarding the benefit of vitamin E, some experts advocate its use (at a dose of 2000–3000 mg daily) for women with cyclical breast pain. Topical NSAIDs, such as diclofenac gel or patch, improve localized breast pain.

Women who experience severe and persistent cyclical mastalgia despite adherence to conservative measures may be offered hormonal treatment. Danazol, a synthetic androgen that inhibits ovulation, is the only medication that has been approved by the Food and Drug Administration (FDA) for the treatment of cyclical mastalgia. However, side effects associated with treatment are common and include weight gain, menstrual irregularities, voice deepening, and hot flashes. Tamoxifen therapy is tolerated well by most women, and many experts recommend it as first-line therapy for the treatment of cyclical mastalgia. Patients treated with tamoxifen should be counseled about the possibility of hot flashes and menstrual irregularities (experienced by up to 10% of women), as well as the risk for more serious adverse events, such as thromboembolic disease and endometrial cancer.

► Prognosis

Symptoms of cyclical and noncyclical mastalgia improve without pharmacologic treatment in most women.

► When to Refer

Patients with mastalgia and a palpable breast mass should be referred to a breast surgeon, even if the results of diagnostic imaging are normal.

Rungruang B et al. Benign breast diseases: epidemiology, evaluation, and management. Clin Obstet Gynecol. 2011 Mar; 54(1):110–24. [PMID: 21278510]

Salzman B et al. Common breast problems. Am Fam Physician. 2012 Aug 15;86(4):343–9. [PMID: 22963023]

THE PALPABLE BREAST MASS

ESSENTIALS OF DIAGNOSIS

▶ Diagnostic imaging is essential for any women with a palpable dominant breast mass, regardless of her age.

▶ Ultrasound is the initial test of choice for women under the age of 30; diagnostic mammography with or without ultrasonography is performed initially in women over the age of 30.

▶ General Considerations

Palpable breast masses may be detected by a patient during breast self-examination, or may be identified by the provider during a routine physical examination. A breast mass may be a presenting symptom of breast cancer, and thus a thorough work-up of any palpable breast mass is essential, regardless of age and personal risk factors for breast cancer (see Chapter 17). Common benign causes of palpable breast masses include fibrocystic condition, cysts, and fibroadenomas.

▶ Prognosis

In general, the benign causes of a palpable breast mass have a favorable prognosis. Many women with breast pain and palpable masses due to fibrocystic condition have spontaneous resolution or have improvement in their symptoms with menopause. Benign simple cysts that are asymptomatic may be followed clinically, and symptomatic cysts should resolve with aspiration.

Certain pathologic diagnoses increase the risk of breast cancer, including papillary lesions, radial scars, atypical ductal or lobular hyperplasia, and lobular carcinoma in situ. FNA biopsy or core-needle biopsy results that indicate one of these diagnoses necessitate referral to a breast surgeon for further evaluation and management.

▶ When to Refer

• Women with a palpable breast mass should be referred to a breast surgeon in the following situations:

– If diagnostic imaging indicates that the mass has *suspicious* features.

– If the mass persists and diagnostic imaging is *normal*.

– If the mass is categorized as *probably benign* on diagnostic imaging, but there are worrisome features on physical examination or there is a high clinical suspicion for malignancy.

– If diagnostic imaging demonstrates a complex cyst, or aspiration of a simple cyst reveals a bloody aspirate.

– If the biopsy demonstrates a lesion with an increased risk of breast cancer (papillary lesions, radial scars, atypical hyperplasia, lobular carcinoma in situ).

– If the biopsy results are discordant with the physical examination and radiographic findings.

Ferrara A. Benign breast disease. Radiol Technol. 2011 May–Jun;82(5):447M–62M. [PMID: 21572066]

Rungruang B et al. Benign breast diseases: epidemiology, evaluation, and management. Clin Obstet Gynecol. 2011 Mar; 54(1):110–24. [PMID: 21278510]

Salzman B et al. Common breast problems. Am Fam Physician. 2012 Aug 15;86(4):343–9. [PMID: 22963023]

NIPPLE DISCHARGE

Nipple discharge is a common breast complaint but is rarely indicative of malignancy. Nipple discharge that comes from multiple ducts, is bilateral, and is produced only with squeezing is considered physiologic, and no further work-up is necessary. Milky discharge that is bilateral, spontaneous, and not associated with pregnancy or breast-feeding is termed "nonlactational galactorrhea." The most common cause of nonlactational galactorrhea is an elevated prolactin level, which may be associated with pituitary or hypothalamic lesions, systemic diseases (hypothyroidism, renal disease), or medications. Women who have bloody discharge, persistent spontaneous unilateral discharge from a single duct, or discharge associated with a palpable breast mass should be referred for diagnostic mammography and ultrasonography and surgical consultation. These features are suggestive of a pathologic diagnosis, such as papilloma, duct ectasia, or malignancy. Surgical excision of the involved duct is the gold standard for diagnosis. See also Chapter 17.

Huang W et al. Evaluation and management of galactorrhea. Am Fam Physician. 2012 Jun1;85(11):1073–80. [PMID: 22962879]

Salzman B et al. Common breast problems. Am Fam Physician. 2012 Aug 15;86(4):343–9. [PMID: 22963023]

FEMALE PATTERN HAIR LOSS

Female pattern hair loss (FPHL) affects more than 20 million women in the United States. This type of alopecia is characterized by shortening of the anagen (growth) phase and follicle miniaturization. Clinically, presenting signs include diffuse thinning over the central scalp and a prominent midline part; the frontal hairline is typically spared. Although occasionally FPHL may be a sign of hyperandrogenism associated with congenital adrenal hyperplasia, androgen-secreting tumors, or polycystic ovarian syndrome, most women have normal levels of serum testosterone.

Topical minoxidil is currently the only medication that has been approved by the FDA for the treatment of FPHL. In a systematic review of several treatments for FPHL, treatment with topical minoxidil was consistently shown to result in moderate hair re-growth in affected women. When both are applied twice daily, the 2% solution of minoxidil is as effective as the 5% solution and is associated with fewer adverse events. The most common side effect of minoxidil is facial hypertrichosis, which can affect 3–5% of women, but this typically resolves after 1 year of treatment. Spironolactone and cyproterone acetate are oral antiandrogens that have been used for the treatment of FPHL, although there are limited data to support this practice. Importantly, both of these medications can cause feminization of a male fetus and should be used cautiously in reproductive-age women.

Atanaskova Mesinkovska N et al. Hair: what is new in diagnosis and management? Female pattern hair loss update: diagnosis and treatment. Dermatol Clin. 2013 Jan;31(1):119–27. [PMID: 23159181]

van Zuuren EJ et al. Evidence-based treatments for female pattern hair loss: a summary of a Cochrane systematic review. Br J Dermatol. 2012 Nov;167(5):995–1010. [PMID: 23039053]

AGE-RELATED FACIAL CHANGES

Minimally invasive aesthetic procedures are now commonly used to treat mild to moderate age-related changes in the face. These procedures are generally safe and are associated with long-lasting and natural results.

Visible signs of aging in the face result from changes in muscular tone and balance, volume loss, decreased skin elasticity, and changes in skin color and texture. Facial rejuvenation procedures can be grouped into three categories based on their mechanism of action. Neuromodulators are used to produce temporary chemodenervation of hyperactive facial muscles, thereby smoothing facial wrinkles. Soft-tissue fillers restore volume loss, and laser and light-energy based devices improve skin laxity and reflectance. Chemical peels and topical medications are considered adjunctive treatments for improving skin appearance.

For each of the three treatment categories, several options are available. The injectable neuromodulators currently approved by the FDA include various formulations of botulinum toxin A. Dermal fillers include collagen, hydroxylapatite, hyaluronic acid, and injectable poly-L-lactic acid, and differ from each other in their degree of cross-linking, gel hardness, and ability to resist dilution. Among these, hyaluronic acid fillers have become increasingly popular and have been approved by the FDA for treatment of nasolabial folds and lip augmentation; they have also been used off-label to treat wrinkles and improve facial volume. Combination therapy with botulinum toxin A and hyaluronic acid is often used in the eyebrow and eyelid regions to achieve more satisfying cosmetic results. Light-based therapy, which includes laser, radiofrequency, and infrared devices, is typically used to improve elasticity in in the upper eye area. Skin laxity may improve by as much as 30–50% with one treatment, depending on the device used.

Kontis TC et al. Contemporary review of injectable facial fillers. JAMA Facial Plast Surg. 2013 Jan;15(1):58–64. [PMID: 23183718]

Sundaram H et al. Nonsurgical rejuvenation of the upper eyelid and brow. Clin Plast Surg. 2013 Jan;40(1):55–76. [PMID: 23186756]

Wollina U et al. Minimally invasive aesthetic procedures in young adults. Clin Cosmet Investig Dermatol. 2011;4:19–26. [PMID: 21673871]

Appendix: Therapeutic Drug Monitoring & Laboratory Reference Intervals

C. Diana Nicoll, MD, PhD, MPA

Chuanyi Mark Lu, MD, PhD

Table 1. Therapeutic drug monitoring.[1]

Drug	Effective Concentrations	Half-Life (hours)	Dosage Adjustments	Comments
Amikacin	**Conventional dosing:** Peak: 20–30 mg/L; trough: < 10 mg/L **High dose once daily:** Peak: 60 mg/L; trough: < 5 mg/L	2–3; ↑ in uremia	↓ in renal dysfunction	Concomitant kanamycin or tobramycin therapy may give falsely elevated amikacin results by immunoassay.
Amitriptyline	95–250 ng/mL	9–25		Drug is highly protein-bound. Patient-specific decrease in protein binding may invalidate quoted therapeutic reference interval for effective concentration.
Carbamazepine	4–12 mg/L	10–15		Induces its own metabolism. Metabolite 10,11-epoxide exhibits 13% cross-reactivity by immunoassay. Adverse reactions: skin reactions, myelosuppression.
Cyclosporine	100–300 mcg/L (ng/mL) whole blood	6–12	↓ in renal dysfunction, liver disease	Cyclosporine is lipid-soluble (20% bound to leukocytes; 40% to erythrocytes; 40% in plasma, highly bound to lipoproteins); the binding is temperature-dependent in vitro and concentration-dependent in vivo. HPLC and LC-tandem mass spectrometry methods are highly specific for parent drug and considered as the gold standard assays. Monoclonal fluorescence polarization immunoassay (FPIA) and monoclonal chemiluminescence immunoassay also measure cyclosporine reliably; polyclonal immunoassays are less specific due to cross-reaction with drug metabolites. Anticonvulsants and rifampin increase metabolism. Erythromycin, ketoconazole, and calcium channel blockers decrease metabolism. The main adverse reaction is concentration-related nephrotoxicity.

(continued)

Table 1. Therapeutic drug monitoring.[1] (continued)

Drug	Effective Concentrations	Half-Life (hours)	Dosage Adjustments	Comments
Desipramine	100–250 ng/mL	13–23		Drug is highly protein-bound. Patient-specific decrease in protein binding may invalidate quoted therapeutic reference interval for effective concentration.
Digoxin	HF: 0.5–0.9 mcg/L Atrial fibrillation: 0.5–2 mcg/L	36–42; ↑ in uremia, HF	↓ in renal dysfunction, HF, hypothyroidism ↑ in hyperthyroidism	Bioavailability of digoxin tablets is 50–90%. Specimen must not be drawn within 4 hours of an intravenous dose or 6 hours of an oral dose. Dialysis does not remove a significant amount. Hypokalemia potentiates toxicity. Digitalis toxicity is a clinical and *not* a laboratory diagnosis. Digibind (digoxin-specific antibody) therapy of digoxin overdose can interfere with measurement of digoxin levels depending on the digoxin assay. Elimination reduced by amiodarone, quinidine, and verapamil.
Ethosuximide	40–100 mg/L	Child: 30–40 Adult: 50–60		Levels used primarily to assess clinical response and compliance. Toxicity is rare and does not correlate well with plasma concentrations.
Gentamicin	**Conventional dosing:** Peak: 4–8 mg/L; trough: < 2 mg/L **High dose once daily:** Peak: 20 mg/L; trough: undetectable	2–3; ↑ in uremia (7.3 during dialysis)	↓ in renal dysfunction	Draw peak specimen (conventional dosing) 30 minutes after end of 30- to 60-min infusion. Draw trough just before next dose. In uremic patients, some penicillins (eg, carbenicillin, ticarcillin, piperacillin) may decrease gentamicin half-life from 46 hours to 22 hours, posing a risk of reduced antibacterial efficacy. The main adverse reactions are CNS, otic, and renal toxicities.
Imipramine	180–350 ng/mL	10–16		Drug is highly protein-bound. Patient-specific decrease in protein binding may invalidate quoted therapeutic reference interval for effective concentration.
Lidocaine	1–5 mg/L	1–2; ↔ in uremia, HF; ↑ in cirrhosis	↓ in HF, liver disease	Levels increased with cimetidine therapy. CNS toxicity common in the elderly.
Lithium	0.5–1.2 mmol/L	10–35; ↑ in uremia	↓ in renal dysfunction	Thiazides and loop diuretics may increase serum lithium levels.
Methotrexate	< 1.0 mcmol/L 48 hours post high-dose therapy, or according to protocol	3–10 low dose; 8–15 high dose; ↑ in uremia	↓ in renal dysfunction	Therapeutic concentrations depend on the treatment protocol (low versus high dose) and time of specimen collection. 7-Hydroxymethotrexate cross-reacts 1.5% in immunoassay. To minimize toxicity, leucovorin should be continued if methotrexate level is > 0.1 mcmol/L at 48 hours after start of therapy. Methotrexate > 1 mcmol/L at > 48 hours requires an increase in rescue therapy. In patients with methotrexate > 1 mcmol/L and impaired renal function, glucarpidase injection can be used as the rescue.

(continued)

Table 1. Therapeutic drug monitoring.[1] (continued)

Drug	Effective Concentrations	Half-Life (hours)	Dosage Adjustments	Comments
Nortriptyline	50–140 ng/mL	18–44		Drug is highly protein-bound. Patient-specific decrease in protein binding may invalidate quoted therapeutic reference interval for effective concentration.
Phenobarbital	10–40 mg/L	Child: 37–73 Adult: 53–140; ↑ in cirrhosis	↓ in liver disease	Metabolized primarily by the hepatic microsomal enzyme system. Many drug-drug interactions.
Phenytoin	10–20 mg/L; 5–10 mg/L in uremia and severe hypoalbuminemia	Dose/concentration-dependent		Drug metabolite cross-reacts in immunoassays; the cross-reactivity may be of significance only in the presence of advanced chronic kidney disease. Metabolism is capacity-limited. Increase dose cautiously when level approaches therapeutic reference interval, since new steady-state level may be disproportionately higher. Drug is very highly protein-bound; protein binding is decreased in uremia and hypoalbuminemia. Free drug level (pharmacologically active fraction, target range 0.5–2.0 mg/L) may be indicated in certain clinical circumstances.
Sirolimus	Trough: 4–12 ng/mL when used in combination with cyclosporine A; 12–20 ng/mL if used alone	57–63	↓ in liver dysfunction and with drugs inhibiting CYP3A4 activity	Sirolimus is an immunosuppressant used in combination with cyclosporine and corticosteroids for prophylaxis of organ rejection after kidney transplantation. It has also been used in liver and heart transplantation. When used in combination with cyclosporine, careful monitoring of kidney function is required. Once the initial dose titration is complete, monitoring sirolimus trough concentrations weekly for the first month and every 2 weeks for the second month appears to be appropriate. The optimal time for specimen collection is 24 h after the previous dose or 0.5 to 1 h prior to the next dose (trough level).
Tacrolimus	Trough: 8–12 ng/mL	8.7–11.3	↓ in liver dysfunction and with drugs inhibiting CYP3A4 activity	Tacrolimus is used for prophylaxis of organ rejection in adult patients undergoing liver or kidney transplantation and in pediatric patients undergoing liver transplantation. It has also been used to prevent rejection in heart, small bowel, and allogeneic bone marrow transplant patients and to treat autoimmune diseases. Antacid or sucralfate administration should be separated from tacrolimus by at least 2 h. The optimal time for specimen collection is 12 h after the previous dose or 0.5 to 1 h prior to the next dose (trough level).

(continued)

Table 1. Therapeutic drug monitoring.[1] (continued)

Drug	Effective Concentrations	Half-Life (hours)	Dosage Adjustments	Comments
Theophylline	5–15 mg/L	4–9	↓ in HF, cirrhosis, and with cimetidine	Caffeine cross-reacts 10%. Elimination is increased 1.5–2 times in smokers. 1,3-Dimethyl uric acid metabolite increased in uremia and, because of cross-reactivity, may cause an apparent slight increase in serum theophylline.
Tobramycin	**Conventional dosing:** Peak: 5–10 mg/L; trough: < 2 mg/L **High dose once daily:** Peak: 20 mg/L; trough: undetectable	2–3; ↑ in uremia	↓ in renal dysfunction	Tobramycin, kanamycin, and amikacin may cross-react in immunoassay. Some antibiotics may decrease tobramycin half-life in uremic patients, causing reduced antibacterial efficacy.
Valproic acid (Valproate)	50–100 mg/L; 50–125 mg/L for bipolar disorder	Child: 6–8 Adult: 10–12		Significant fraction of the drug is protein-bound in vivo (concentration-dependent). Decreased binding in uremia and cirrhosis. Plasma concentrations show poor correlation with effect.
Vancomycin	Trough: 10–20 mg/L;	4–7; ↑ in uremia	↓ in renal dysfunction	Trough concentrations are recommended for monitoring vancomycin efficacy. Ototoxicity in uremic patients may lead to irreversible deafness. Monitoring serum levels to prevent ototoxicity in patients with normal renal function receiving vancomycin monotherapy is not effective since this toxicity is rarely associated with monotherapy and does not correlate with serum levels. Data do not support using peak levels to monitor nephrotoxicity. Use trough levels.

[1]Serum from a plain red-top tube is typically used for therapeutic drug monitoring except for cyclosporine, which requires whole blood sample in a lavender (EDTA) tube. In general, the specimen should be drawn just before the next dose (trough).

↑, increased; ↓, decreased; ↔, unchanged; CYP, cytochrome P450; HPLC, high performance liquid chromatography; HF, heart failure; CNS, central nervous system.

Modified, with permission, from Nicoll D et al. *Pocket Guide to Diagnostic Tests*, 6th ed. McGraw-Hill, 2012.

Table 2. Reference intervals for commonly used tests.[1,2]

		Conventional metric units × Conversion factor = SI units SI units ÷ Conversion factor = Conventional metric units			
Test	**Specimen**	**Conventional Metric Units**	**Conversion Factor**	**SI Units[2]**	**Collection[3]**
Acetaminophen	Serum	10–20 mcg/mL **Panic:** > 50 mcg/mL	6.616	66–132 mcmol/L	Serum separator tube (SST)
Acetoacetate	Serum or urine	Negative (0 mg/dL)	0.098	Negative (0 mmol/L)	SST or urine container
Activated clotting time (ACT)	Whole blood	70–180 seconds (method-specific)			Collect in a plastic syringe without anticoagulant
Adrenocorticotropic hormone (ACTH)	Plasma	9–52 pg/mL (laboratory-specific)	0.22	2–11 pmol/L	Siliconized glass or plastic lavender
Alanine aminotransferase (ALT, SGPT, GPT)	Serum or plasma	0–35 units/L (laboratory-specific)	0.02	0–0.7 mckat/L (laboratory-specific)	SST, plasma preparation tube (PPT) (green)
Albumin	Serum or plasma	3.4–4.7 g/dL	10.00	34–47 g/L	SST, PPT (green)
Aldosterone	Serum	Salt-loaded (120 mEq Na$^+$/d for 3–4 days): Supine: 3–10 ng/dL Upright: 5–30 ng/dL Salt-depleted (20 mEq Na$^+$/d for 3–4 days): Supine: 12–36 ng/dL Upright: 17–137 ng/dL	27.74	83–277 pmol/L 139–831 pmol/L 332–997 pmol/L 471–3795 pmol/L	SST
	Urine	Salt-loaded (120 mEq Na$^+$/d for 3–4 days): 1.5–12.5 mcg/24 h Salt-depleted (20 mEq Na$^+$/d for 3–4 days): 18–85 mcg/24 h	2.77	4.2–34.6 nmol/d 49.9–235.5 nmol/d	Urine bottle containing boric acid (must be refrigerated during collection)
Alkaline phosphatase	Serum or plasma	41–133 units/L (method-and age-dependent)	0.02	0.7–2.2 mckat/L (method- and age-dependent)	SST, PPT (green)
Alpha-fetoprotein (AFP)	Serum	0–15 ng/mL (age-dependent)	1.00	0–15 mcg/L (age-dependent)	SST, red
Ammonia (NH$_3$)	Plasma	18–60 mcg/dL	0.587	11–35 mcmol/L	Green (iced)
Amylase	Serum or plasma	20–110 units/L (laboratory-specific)	0.02	0.33–1.83 mckat/L (laboratory-specific)	SST, PPT (green)
Angiotensin-converting enzyme (ACE)	Serum	12–35 units/L (method-dependent)	16.67	200–583 nkat/L (method-dependent)	SST
Antithrombin (AT)	Plasma	84–123% (qualitative/activity) 80–130% (quantitative/antigen)			Blue
Alpha-1-antitrypsin, Alpha-1-antiprotease	Serum or plasma	110–270 mg/dL	0.01	1.1–2.7 g/L	SST, PPT (green)

(continued)

Table 2. Reference intervals for commonly used tests.[1,2] (continued)

		Conventional metric units × Conversion factor = SI units SI units ÷ Conversion factor = Conventional metric units			
Test	Specimen	Conventional Metric Units	Conversion Factor	SI Units[2]	Collection[3]
Aspartate aminotransferase (AST, SGOT, GOT)	Serum or plasma	0–35 units/L (laboratory-specific)	0.02	0–0.58 mckat/L (laboratory-specific)	SST, PPT (green)
Basophil count	Whole blood	$0.01–0.12 \times 10^3$/mcL	1.00	$0.01–0.12 \times 10^9$/L	Lavender
bcr/abl, t (9;22) translocation by reverse-transcriptase polymerase chain reaction (RT-PCR), qualitative	Whole blood	Negative (Positive: chronic myeloid leukemia, some acute B-lymphoblastic leukemia)			Lavender
Beta-hCG	Serum	Males and nonpregnant females: undetectable or < 5 milli-international units/mL	1.00	< 5 International Units/L	SST, red
Beta-2-microglobulin	Serum or plasma	< 0.2 mg/dL	10	< 2 mg/L	SST, PPT (green)
Bilirubin	Serum or plasma	Total: 0.1–1.2 mg/dL Direct (conjugated to glucuronide): 0.1–0.5 mg/dL Indirect (unconjugated): 0.1–0.7 mg/dL	17.10	2–21 mcmol/L < 8 mcmol/L < 12 mcmol/L	SST, PPT (green)
Blood urea nitrogen (BUN)	Serum or plasma	8–20 mg/dL	0.357	2.9–7.1 mmol/L	SST, PPT (green)
B-type natriuretic peptide (BNP)	Plasma	< 100 pg/mL	1.0	< 100 ng/L	Lavender
C-peptide	Serum or plasma	0.8–4.0 ng/mL	0.333	0.27–1.33 nmol/L	SST or green/iced (fasting)
C-reactive protein, high sensitivity (hs-CRP)	Serum or plasma	< 1.0 mg/dL	10.00	< 10 mg/L	SST, PPT (green)
C-telopeptide, beta-cross-linked (CTx)	Serum	Male: 60–850 pg/mL Female: premenopausal 60–650 pg/mL, postmenopausal 100–1000 pg/mL (age- and laboratory-specific)	1.00	Male: 60–850 ng/L Female: premenopausal 60–650 ng/L, postmenopausal 100–1000 ng/L (age- and laboratory-specific)	Red, SST
Calcitonin	Plasma or serum	Male: 0–11.5 pg/mL Female: 0–4.6 pg/mL	1.00	Male: 0–11.5 ng/L Female: 0–4.6 ng/L	Green, SST
Calcium (Ca^{2+})	Serum or plasma	8.5–10.5 mg/dL **Panic:** < 6.5 or > 13.5 mg/dL	0.25	2.1–2.6 mmol/L **Panic:** < 1.63 or > 3.37 mmol/L	SST, PPT (green)
Calcium (ionized)	Serum or whole blood	4.6–5.3 mg/dL **Panic:** < 3 or > 6.2 mg/dL	0.25	1.15–1.32 mmol/L **Panic:** < 0.75 or > 1.55 mmol/L	SST, PPT (green) (anaerobic)
Calcium (U_{Ca})	Urine	100–300 mg/24 h	0.025	2.5–7.5 mmol/24 h	Urine bottle containing hydrochloric acid
Carbon dioxide, partial pressure (Pco_2)	Whole blood	32–48 mm Hg	0.13	4.26–6.38 kPa	Heparinized syringe (iced)

(continued)

Table 2. Reference intervals for commonly used tests.[1,2] (continued)

		Conventional metric units × Conversion factor = SI units SI units ÷ Conversion factor = Conventional metric units			
Test	Specimen	Conventional Metric Units	Conversion Factor	SI Units[2]	Collection[3]
Carbon dioxide (CO_2), total (bicarbonate)	Serum or plasma	22–32 mEq/L **Panic:** < 15 or > 40 mEq/L	1.00	22–32 mmol/L **Panic:** < 15 or > 40 mmol/L	SST, PPT (green)
Carboxyhemoglobin (HbCO)	Whole blood	< 9% of total hemoglobin (Hb)	0.01	< 0.09 fraction of total hemoglobin	Heparinized syringe or Green
Carcinoembryonic antigen (CEA)	Serum	0–5 ng/mL	1.00	0–5 mcg/L	SST
Catecholamines	Urine	Norepinephrine: 15–80 mcg/24 h Epinephrine: 0–20 mcg/24 h Dopamine: 65–400 mcg/24 h	5.91 5.46 6.53	89–473 nmol/24 h 0–109 nmol/24 h 425–2610 nmol/24 h	Urine container with hydrochloride acid
CD4 T cell count	Whole blood	$0.36–1.73 \times 10^3$/mcL	1.00	$0.36–1.73 \times 10^6$/L	Lavender (order T-cell subsets and a CBC with differential)
Ceruloplasmin	Serum or plasma	20–60 mg/dL (laboratory-specific)	10.00	200–600 mg/L	SST, PPT (green)
Chloride (Cl^-)	Serum or plasma	101–112 mEq/L	1.00	101–112 mmol/L	SST, PPT (green)
Cholesterol	Serum or plasma	Desirable: < 200 mg/dL Borderline: 200–240 mg/dL High risk: > 240 mg/dL	0.0259	Desirable: < 6.0 mmol/L Borderline: 6.0–7.2 mmol/L High risk: > 7.2 mmol/L	SST, PPT (green)
Complement C3	Serum	64–166 mg/dL	10.00	640–1660 mg/L	SST
Complement C4	Serum	15–45 mg/dL	10.00	150–450 mg/L	SST
Complement CH50	Serum	(Laboratory-specific)			Red
Cortisol	Serum or plasma	8:00 AM: 5–20 mcg/dL	27.59	140–550 nmol/L	SST, PPT (green)
Cortisol (urinary free)	Urine	10–110 mcg/24 h	2.76	27.6–303.6 nmol/24 h	Urine bottle containing boric acid
Creatine kinase (CK)	Serum or plasma	32–267 units/L (method-dependent)	0.02	0.53–4.45 mckat/L (method-dependent)	SST, PPT (green)
Creatine kinase MB (CKMB)	Serum or plasma	< 16 units/L or < 4% of total CK (laboratory-specific) Mass units: 0–7 mcg/L	0.04	< 0.27 mckat/L	SST, PPT (green)
Creatinine (Cr)	Serum or plasma	0.6–1.2 mg/dL	88.4	50–100 mcmol/L	SST, PPT (green)
Creatinine clearance (Cl_{Cr})	See Collection column	Adults: 90–140 mL/min/1.73 m^2 body surface area (BSA)	0.0167	1.5–2.3 mL/s/1.73 m^2 BSA	Carefully timed 24-hour urine and simultaneous serum or plasma creatinine sample
Cryoglobulins	Serum	Negative			Red (transported at 37°C)
Cystatin C	Serum or plasma	0.5–1.3 mg/L			SST, red, PPT (green)

(continued)

Table 2. Reference intervals for commonly used tests.[1,2] (continued)

		Conventional metric units × Conversion factor = SI units SI units ÷ Conversion factor = Conventional metric units			
Test	Specimen	Conventional Metric Units	Conversion Factor	SI Units[2]	Collection[3]
D-dimer, quantitative	Plasma	< 500 ng/mL	1.00	< 500 mcg/L	Blue
Dehydroepiandrosterone sulfate (DHEA-S)	Serum or plasma	Male: 40–500 mcg/dL Female: 20–320 mcg/dL	10.00	Male: 400–5000 mcg/L Female: 200–3200 mcg/L	SST, PPT (green)
Eosinophil count	Whole blood	0.04–0.5 × 10³/mcL	1.00	0.04–0.5 × 10⁹/L	Lavender
Erythrocyte count (RBC count)	Whole blood	4.7–6.1 × 10⁶/mcL	1.00	4.7–6.1 × 10¹²/L	Lavender
Erythrocyte sedimentation rate	Whole blood	Male: < 10 mm/h Female: < 15 mm/h (laboratory-specific)		Same	Lavender (test must be run within 2 h)
Erythropoietin (EPO)	Serum	5–30 mU/mL	1.00	5–30 units/L	SST
Estradiol	Serum	Early follicular: 30–100 pg/mL Late follicular: 100–400 pg/mL Luteal: 50–150 pg/mL Postmenopausal: 2–21 pg/mL	3.671	110–367 pmol/L 367–1468 pmol/L 183–550 pmol/L 7–77 pmol/L	SST
Estrogens, total	Serum	Follicular: 60–200 pg/mL Luteal: 160–400 pg/mL Postmenopausal: < 130 pg/mL	1.00	60–200 ng/L 160–400 ng/L < 130 ng/L	SST
Ethanol	Serum or plasma	0 mg/dL Legal "driving under the influence" in many states is defined as a blood alcohol level of > 80 mg/dL (> 17 mmol/L); serum levels are 10–35% higher than whole blood alcohol levels	0.217	0 mmol/L	SST, PPT
Factor VIII assay	Plasma	50–150% of normal (varies with age)			Blue (iced)
Fecal fat	Stool	Random: < 60 droplets of fat per high-power field 72–hour: < 7 g/24 h			Qualitative: Random stool sample Quantitative: 72-hour collection following 2-day high dietary fat intake
Ferritin	Serum or plasma	Male: 16–300 ng/mL Female: 4–161 ng/mL	2.247	Male: 36–674 pmol/L Female: 9–362 pmol/L	SST, PPT (green)
Fibrinogen (functional)	Plasma	175–433 mg/dL **Panic:** < 75 mg/dL	0.0294	5.15–12.73 mcmol/L **Panic:** < 2.2 mcmol/L	Blue
Follicle-stimulating hormone (FSH)	Serum or plasma	Female: Follicular phase 4–13 mU/mL Luteal phase 2–13 mU/mL Midcycle 5–22 mU/mL Postmenopausal 30–138 mU/mL Male: 1–10 mU/mL (laboratory-specific)	1.00	Female: 4–13 units/L 2–13 units/L 5–22 units/L 30–138 units/L Male: 1–10 units/L (laboratory-specific)	SST, PPT (green)
Free erythrocyte protoporphyrin (FEP)	Whole blood	< 35 mcg/dL (method-dependent)			Lavender

(continued)

Table 2. Reference intervals for commonly used tests.[1,2] (continued)

		Conventional metric units × Conversion factor = SI units SI units ÷ Conversion factor = Conventional metric units			
Test	**Specimen**	**Conventional Metric Units**	**Conversion Factor**	**SI Units[2]**	**Collection[3]**
Fructosamine	Serum or plasma	190–270 mcmol/L	1.0	190–270 mcmol/L	SST, PPT (green)
Gamma-glutamyl trans-peptidase (GGT)	Serum or plasma	9–85 units/L (laboratory-specific)	0.02	0.15–1.42 mckat/L (laboratory-specific)	SST, PPT (green)
Gastrin	Serum	< 100 pg/mL (laboratory-specific)	1.00	< 100 ng/L (laboratory-specific)	SST
Glomerular filtration rate, estimated (eGFR)	Serum or plasma	> 60 mL/min/1.73 m² (calculated based on creatinine level)			SST, PPT (green)
Glucagon	Plasma	20–100 pg/mL	1.00	20–100 ng/L	Lavender
Glucose	Serum or plasma	60–110 mg/dL **Panic:** < 40 or > 500 mg/dL	0.0555	3.33–6.11 mmol/L **Panic:** < 2.22 or > 27.75 mmol/L	(Fasting) SST, PPT, gray
Glucose-6-phosphate dehydrogenase (G6PD) screen	Whole blood	5–14 units/g Hb	0.02	0.1–0.28 mckat/L	Lavender
Glutamine	Cerebrospinal fluid (CSF)	6–15 mg/dL **Panic:** > 40 mg/dL	68.42	411–1028 mcmol/L **Panic:** > 2737 mcmol/L	Collect CSF in a plastic tube
Glycated (glycosylated) hemoglobin (HbA₁c)	Whole blood	3.9–5.6% (method-dependent)			Lavender, pink
Growth hormone (GH)	Serum or plasma	0–5 ng/mL	1.00	0–5 mcg/L	SST, PPT (green)
Haptoglobin	Serum or plasma	46–316 mg/dL	0.01	0.5–3.2 g/L	SST, PPT (green)
HDL cholesterol	Serum or plasma	Male: 27–67 mg/dL Female: 34–88 mg/dL (HDL cholesterol > 60 mg/dL is thought to lower risk of coronary heart disease)	0.0259	0.7–1.73 mmol/L 0.88–2.28 mmol/L	SST, PPT (green)
Hematocrit (Hct)	Whole blood	Male: 39–49% Female: 35–45% (age-dependent)	0.01	Male: 0.39–0.49 Female: 0.35–0.45	Lavender, pink
Hemoglobin A₁c (See Glycated Hemoglobin)	Whole blood	3.9–5.6% (method-dependent)			
Hemoglobin A₂ (HbA₂)	Whole blood	1.5–3.5% of total hemoglobin	0.01	0.015–0.035	Lavender
Hemoglobin electrophoresis	Whole blood	HbA: > 95% HbA₂: 1.5–3.5% HbF: < 2% (age-dependent)			Lavender
Hemoglobin, total (Hb)	Whole blood	Male: 13.6–17.5 g/dL Female: 12.0–15.5 g/dL (age-dependent) **Panic:** ≤ 7 g/dL	10.00	Male: 136–175 g/L Female: 120–155 g/L (age-dependent) **Panic:** ≤ 70 g/L	Lavender
Heparin-associated antibody (heparin-induced thrombocytopenia)	Serum	Negative			SST

(continued)

Table 2. Reference intervals for commonly used tests.[1,2] (continued)

Test	Specimen	Conventional Metric Units	Conversion Factor	SI Units[2]	Collection[3]
\multicolumn{6}{c}{Conventional metric units × Conversion factor = SI units}					

<table>
<tr><td colspan="6" align="center">Conventional metric units × Conversion factor = SI units
SI units ÷ Conversion factor = Conventional metric units</td></tr>
<tr><td>Test</td><td>Specimen</td><td>Conventional Metric Units</td><td>Conversion Factor</td><td>SI Units[2]</td><td>Collection[3]</td></tr>
<tr><td>HIV antibody</td><td>Serum or plasma</td><td>EIA: Negative
Western blot: Nonreactive</td><td></td><td></td><td>SST, PPT</td></tr>
<tr><td>HIV RNA, quantitative (viral load)</td><td>Plasma</td><td>Negative (or < 75 copies/mL, assay-specific)</td><td></td><td></td><td>Lavender, PPT (white)</td></tr>
<tr><td>Homocysteine</td><td>Serum or plasma</td><td>4.5–12 mg/dL (method- and age-dependent)</td><td>7.397</td><td>33.29–88.76 mcmol/L</td><td>SST, PPT</td></tr>
<tr><td>5-Hydroxyindoleacetic acid (5-HIAA)</td><td>Urine</td><td>2–8 mg/24 h</td><td>5.23</td><td>10–40 mcmol/d</td><td>Urine bottle containing hydrochloric acid</td></tr>
<tr><td>IgG index</td><td>Serum and CSF</td><td>0.29–0.59 ratio (CSF: serum ratio)</td><td></td><td></td><td>SST (for serum) and plastic tube (for CSF)</td></tr>
<tr><td>Immunoglobulins (Ig)</td><td>Serum</td><td>IgA: 78–367 mg/dL
IgG: 583–1761 mg/dL
IgM: 52–335 mg/dL</td><td>0.01</td><td>IgA: 0.78–3.67 g/L
IgG: 5.83–17.6 g/L
IgM: 0.52–3.35 g/L</td><td>SST</td></tr>
<tr><td>Insulin, immunoreactive</td><td>Serum or plasma</td><td>6–35 mcU/mL</td><td>6.945</td><td>42–243 pmol/L</td><td>SST, PPT</td></tr>
<tr><td>Insulin-like growth factor-1</td><td>Plasma</td><td>123–463 ng/mL (age- and sex-dependent)</td><td>1.0</td><td>123–463 mcg/L</td><td>Lavender</td></tr>
<tr><td>Iron (Fe)</td><td>Serum or plasma</td><td>50–175 mcg/dL</td><td>0.179</td><td>9–31 mcmol/L</td><td>SST, PPT (green)</td></tr>
<tr><td>Iron-binding capacity, total (TIBC)</td><td>Serum or plasma</td><td>250–460 mcg/dL</td><td>0.179</td><td>45–82 mcmol/L</td><td>SST, PPT (green)</td></tr>
<tr><td>JAK2 mutations (V617F or exon 12/13 mutation), qualitative</td><td>Whole blood</td><td>Negative
(Positive: myeloproliferative neoplasms, ie, polycythemia vera, essential thrombocythemia, and primary myelofibrosis)</td><td></td><td></td><td>Lavender</td></tr>
<tr><td>Kappa and lambda free light chains, quantitative</td><td>Serum</td><td>Free kappa: 0.57–2.63 mg/dL
Free lambda: 0.33–1.94 mg/dL
Free kappa/lambda ratio: 0.26–1.65</td><td>0.01</td><td>5.7–26.3 × 10⁻³ g/L
3.3–19.4 × 10⁻³ g/L</td><td>SST, red</td></tr>
<tr><td>Ketone bodies</td><td>Serum or plasma</td><td>Qualitative: Negative
Quantitative: <10 mg/dL</td><td>10.0</td><td>< 100 mg/L</td><td>SST, PPT (green)</td></tr>
<tr><td>Lactate dehydrogenase (LDH)</td><td>Serum or plasma</td><td>88–230 units/L (laboratory-specific)</td><td>0.02</td><td>1.46–3.82 mckat/L (laboratory-specific)</td><td>SST, PPT (green)</td></tr>
<tr><td>Lactic acid (lactate)</td><td>Venous blood</td><td>0.5–2.0 mEq/L</td><td>1.00</td><td>0.5–2.0 mmol/L</td><td>Gray (iced)</td></tr>
<tr><td>LDL cholesterol (calculated or direct)</td><td>Serum or plasma</td><td>Desirable: < 130 mg/dL (< 99 mg/dL for patients with CHD);
Borderline: 130–159 mg/dL;
High risk: ≥ 160 mg/dL</td><td>0.0259</td><td>< 3.37 mmol/L (< 2.57 mmol/L);
3.38–4.13 mmol/L;
> 4.16 mmol/L</td><td>SST, PPT (green)</td></tr>
<tr><td>Lead (Pb)</td><td>Whole blood</td><td>Child: < 25 mcg/dL
Adult: < 40 mcg/dL</td><td>0.0483</td><td>Child: < 1.21 mcmol/L
Adult: < 1.93 mcmol/L</td><td>Dark blue (trace metal free)</td></tr>
<tr><td>Leukocyte (white blood cell) count, total (WBC count)</td><td>Whole blood</td><td>4.8–10.8 × 10³/mcL
Panic: < 1.5 × 10³/mcL</td><td>1.00</td><td>4.8–10.8 × 10⁹/L
Panic: < 1.5 × 10⁹/L</td><td>Lavender</td></tr>
</table>

(continued)

Table 2. Reference intervals for commonly used tests.[1,2] (continued)

Test	Specimen	Conventional Metric Units	Conversion Factor	SI Units[2]	Collection[3]
		Conventional metric units × Conversion factor = SI units SI units ÷ Conversion factor = Conventional metric units			
Lipase	Serum	0–160 units/L (laboratory-specific)	0.02	0–2.66 mckat/L (laboratory-specific)	SST
Luteinizing hormone (LH)	Serum or plasma	Female: Follicular phase 1–18 mU/mL Luteal phase 0.4–20 mU/mL Midcycle 24–105 mU/mL Postmenopausal 15–62 mU/mL Male: 1–10 mU/mL (laboratory-specific)	1.00	Female: 1–18 units/L 0.4–20 units/L 24–105 units/L 15–62 units/L Male: 1–10 units/L (laboratory-specific)	SST, PPT
Lymphocyte count	Whole blood	$0.8–3.5 \times 10^3$/mcL	1.00	$0.8–3.5 \times 10^9$/L	Lavender
Magnesium (Mg^{2+})	Serum or plasma	1.8–3.0 mg/dL **Panic:** < 0.5 or > 4.5 mg/dL	0.411	0.75–1.25 mmol/L **Panic:** < 0.2 or > 1.85 mmol/L	SST, PPT (green)
Mean corpuscular hemoglobin (MCH)	Whole blood	27–34 pg			Lavender
Mean corpuscular hemoglobin concentration (MCHC)	Whole blood	31–36 g/dL	10.00	310–360 g/L	Lavender
Mean corpuscular volume (MCV)	Whole blood	80–100 fL			Lavender
Metanephrines, free	Plasma	Normetanephrine: < 0.9 nmol/L Metanephrine: < 0.5 nmol/L			Lavender
Metanephrines	Urine	0.3–0.9 mg/24 h	5.46	1.6–4.9 mcmol/24 h	Urine bottle containing hydrochloric acid
Methemoglobin (MetHb)	Whole blood	< 1% of total hemoglobin	0.01	< 0.01 fraction of total hemoglobin	Blood gas syringe, lavender, or green
Methylmalonic acid	Serum or plasma	0–0.05 mg/L	8.475	0–0.4 mcmol/L	SST, PPT (green)
Monocyte count	Whole blood	$0.2–0.8 \times 10^3$/mcL	1.00	$0.2–0.8 \times 10^9$/L	Lavender
Neutrophil count	Whole blood	$2.2–8.6 \times 10^3$/mcL	1.00	$2.2–8.6 \times 10^9$/L	Lavender
Osmolality	Serum or plasma	275–293 mosm/kg H_2O **Panic:** < 240 or > 320 mosm/kg H_2O	1.00	275–293 mmol/kg H_2O **Panic:** < 240 or > 320 mmol/kg H_2O	SST, PPT
	Urine	Random: 100–900 mosm/kg H_2O	1.00	Random: 100–900 mmol/kg H_2O	Urine container
Osteocalcin	Serum or plasma	Child or adolescent (age 7–17 years): 25–300 ng/mL Adult: 10–15 ng/mL	1.00	Child or adolescent (age 7–17 years): 25–300 mcg/L Adult: 10–15 mcg/L	SST, PPT (green)
Oxygen, partial pressure (Po_2)	Whole blood	83–108 mm Hg	0.13	11.04–14.36 kPa	Heparinized syringe (iced)
Pancreatic elastase, fecal	Formed stool	> 200 mcg/g			Leak-proof container (freeze immediately)

(continued)

Table 2. Reference intervals for commonly used tests.[1,2] (continued)

| | | Conventional metric units × Conversion factor = SI units | | | |
| | | SI units ÷ Conversion factor = Conventional metric units | | | |
Test	Specimen	Conventional Metric Units	Conversion Factor	SI Units[2]	Collection[3]
Parathyroid hormone (PTH), intact	Serum or plasma	Intact PTH: 11–54 pg/mL (laboratory-specific)	0.11	Intact PTH: 1.2–5.7 pmol/L (laboratory-specific)	Red, SST, PPT
Partial thromboplastin time, activated (PTT)	Plasma	25–35 seconds (reference interval varies) **Panic:** ≥ 60 seconds			Blue
pH	Whole blood	Arterial: 7.35–7.45 Venous: 7.31–7.41			Heparinized syringe (iced)
Phosphorus	Serum or plasma	2.5–4.5 mg/dL **Panic:** < 1.0 mg/dL	0.323	0.8–1.45 mmol/L **Panic:** < 0.32 mmol/L	SST, PPT (green)
Plasminogen	Plasma	70–113% (activity)	1.00	70–113%	Blue
Platelet count (Plt)	Whole blood	150–450 × 10³/mcL **Panic:** < 25 × 10³/mcL	1.0	150–450 × 10⁹/L **Panic:** < 25 × 10⁹/L	Lavender
Platelet-associated IgG	Plasma or serum	Negative			Lavender, PPT, SST
Platelet function test (PFA-100 closure time) (CEPI: collagen/epineph-rine cartridge; CADP: collagen/ADP cartridge)	Whole blood	CEPI: 70–170 seconds (laboratory-specific) CADP: 50–110 seconds (laboratory-specific)	1.0	CEPI: 70–170 seconds (laboratory-specific) CADP: 50–110 seconds (laboratory-specific)	Blue
Porphobilinogen (PBG)	Urine	Negative			Protect from light
Potassium (K⁺)	Serum or plasma	3.5–5.0 mEq/L **Panic:** < 3.0 or > 6.0 mEq/L	1.00	3.5–5.0 mmol/L **Panic:** < 3.0 or > 6.0 mmol/L	SST, PPT (green)
Procalcitonin	Serum or plasma	< 0.10 ng/mL	1.00	< 0.10 mcg/L	SST, PPT (green)
Procollagen type 1 intact N-terminal propeptide (PINP)	Serum	16–105 ng/mL (age- and sex-dependent)	1.00	16–105 mcg/L (age- and sex-dependent)	SST, red
Prolactin (PRL)	Serum or plasma	< 20 ng/mL	1.00	< 20 mcg/L	SST, PPT (green)
Prostate-specific antigen (PSA)	Serum or plasma	0–4 ng/mL	1.00	0–4 mcg/L	SST, PPT
Protein C	Plasma	71–176% (functional) 60–150% (antigenic)			Blue
Protein electrophoresis	Serum	Adult: Albumin: 3.3–4.7 g/dL α₁: 0.1–0.4 g/dL α₂: 0.3–0.9 g/dL β₂: 0.7–1.5 g/dL γ: 0.5–1.4 g/dL (polyclonal)	10.00	33–47 g/L 1–4 g/L 3–9 g/L 7–15 g/L 5–14 g/L (polyclonal)	SST, red
Protein S (antigen)	Plasma	76–178%			Blue
Protein, total	Serum or plasma	6.0–8.0 g/dL	10.00	60–80 g/L	SST, PPT (green)
Prothrombin time (PT)	Plasma	11–15 seconds **Panic:** ≥ 30 seconds (laboratory-specific)			Blue

(continued)

Table 2. Reference intervals for commonly used tests.[1,2] (continued)

		Conventional metric units × Conversion factor = SI units SI units ÷ Conversion factor = Conventional metric units			
Test	Specimen	Conventional Metric Units	Conver-sion Factor	SI Units[2]	Collection[3]
Red blood cell count	Whole blood	4.7–6.1 × 10^6/mcL (male) 3.5–5.5 × 10^6/mcL (female)	1.00	4.7–6.1 × 10^{12}/L 3.5–5.5 × 10^{12}/L	Lavender
Renin activity	Plasma	High-sodium diet (75–150 mEq Na$^+$/d): Supine: 0.2–2.3 ng/mL/h Standing: 1.3–4.0 ng/mL/h Low-sodium diet (30–75 mEq Na$^+$/d): Standing: 4.0–7.7 ng/mL/h			Lavender
Reticulocyte count	Whole blood	33–137 × 10^3/mcL	1.00	33–137 × 10^9/L	Lavender
Russell viper venom clotting time (dilute) (RVVT)	Plasma	24–37 seconds			Blue
Salicylate (aspirin)	Serum	200–300 mg/L **Panic:** > 350 mg/L	0.00724	1.45–2.17 mmol/L **Panic:** > 2.53 mmol/L	Red
Sodium (Na$^+$)	Serum or plasma	135–145 mEq/L **Panic:** < 125 or > 155 mEq/L	1.00	135–145 mmol/L **Panic:** < 125 or > 155 mmol/L	SST, PPT (green)
Somatostatin	Plasma	< 25 pg/mL (laboratory-specific)	0.611	< 15.28 pmol/L (laboratory-specific)	Lavender, PPT (white)
Testosterone	Serum or plasma	Male: 175–781 ng/dL Female: 10–75 ng/dL	0.0347	Male: 6–27 nmol/L Female: 0.3–2.6 nmol/L	SST, PPT (green)
Thyroglobulin	Serum or plasma	3–42 ng/mL	1.00	3–42 mcg/L	SST, PPT (green)
Thyroid-stimulating hormone (TSH)	Serum or plasma	0.4–4 mcU/mL **Panic:** > 50 mcU/mL	1.00	0.4–4 mU/L **Panic:** > 50 mU/L	SST, PPT (green)
Thyroid-stimulating antibody, Thyroid stimulating hormone receptor antibody (TSH-R Ab [stim])	Serum	< 130% of basal activity; based on cAMP generation in thyroid cell tissue culture			
Thyroxine, free (FT$_4$)	Serum or plasma	0.7–1.86 ng/dL	12.87	9–24 pmol/L (varies with method)	SST, PPT (green)
Thyroxine (T$_4$), total	Serum or plasma	5–11 mcg/dL	12.87	64–142 nmol/L	SST, PPT (green)
Transferrin	Serum or plasma	190–375 mg/dL	0.01	1.9–3.75 g/L	SST, PPT (green)
Transferrin, carbohydrate-deficient (CDT)	Serum	< 1.3% method-dependent			SST, red
Transferrin receptor, soluble (sTfR)	Serum or plasma	2.2–5 mg/L (male) 1.9–4.4 mg/L (female) (laboratory-specific)			SST, PPT (green)
Triglycerides	Serum or plasma	< 165 mg/dL	0.0113	< 1.8 mmol/L	SST, PPT (green) (fasting)
Triiodothyronine (T$_3$), total	Serum	95–190 ng/dL	0.0154	1.5–2.9 nmol/L	Red

(continued)

Table 2. Reference intervals for commonly used tests.[1,2] (continued)

| | | Conventional metric units × Conversion factor = SI units | | | |
| | | SI units ÷ Conversion factor = Conventional metric units | | | |
Test	Specimen	Conventional Metric Units	Conversion Factor	SI Units[2]	Collection[3]
Troponin-I (cTnl)	Plasma	< 0.1 ng/mL (method-dependent)	1.0	< 0.1 mcg/L (method-dependent)	Lavender
Uric acid	Serum or plasma	Male: 2.4–7.4 mg/dL Female: 1.4–5.8 mg/dL	59.48	Male: 140–440 mcmol/L Female: 80–350 mcmol/L	SST, PPT (green)
Vanillylmandelic acid (VMA)	Urine	2–7 mg/24 h	5.05	10–35 mcmol/d	Urine bottle containing hydrochloric acid
Vitamin B_{12}	Serum or plasma	170–820 pg/mL	0.738	125–600 pmol/L	SST, PPT (green)
Vitamin D, 25-hydroxy (25[OH]D)	Serum or plasma	20–50 ng/mL	2.496	50–125 nmol/L	SST, PPT (green)
Vitamin D, 1,25-dihydroxy (1,25[OH]$_2$D)	Serum or plasma	20–76 pg/mL	2.6	48–182 pmol/L	SST, PPT (green)
von Willebrand factor (vWF)	Plasma	50–180% (activity and antigen)			Blue
White blood cell count	Whole blood	4.8–10.8 × 10^3/mcL **Panic:** < 1.5 × 10^3/mcL	1.00	4.8–10.8 × 10^9/L **Panic:** <1.5 × 10^9/L	Lavender

[1]The reference intervals given here in conventional metric units and in SI units are from several large medical centers. Always use the reference intervals provided by your clinical laboratory, since intervals may be method-dependent.

[2]References: Young DS. Implementation of SI units for clinical laboratory data. Ann Intern Med. 1987 Jan;106(1):114–29. [PMID: 3789557]; Systeme Internationale (SI) conversion factors for selected laboratory components. AMA Manual of Style. SI conversion calculator, Table 2. http://www.amamanualofstyle.com/page/si-conversion-calculator; and Stein K. Journal adopts use of conventional and SI units. J Am Diet Assoc. 2005 Aug;105(8):1186–7. [PMID: 16182628]

[3]PPT, plasma preparation tube; SST, serum separator tube.

Index

NOTE: Page numbers in **boldface** type indicate a major discussion. A *t* following a page number indicates tabular material, and *f* following page number indicates a figure. Medications are listed under their generic names. When a medication trade name is listed, the reader is referred to the generic name.